CLINICAL GYNECOLOGIC ONCOLOGY

SEVENTH EDITION

Commissioning Editor: Rebecca Gaertner
Development Editor: Deidre Simpson
Project Manager: Gemma Lawson
Design: Louis Forgione
Illustration Manager: Karen Giacomucci
Illustrator: Patty Bassman
Marketing Manager: Matt Latuchie

CLINICAL GYNECOLOGIC ONCOLOGY

SEVENTH EDITION

Philip J. DiSaia MD

The Dorothy J. Marsh Chair in Reproductive Biology Director, Division of Gynecologic Oncology Professor, Department of Obstetrics and Gynecology University of California, Irvine College of Medicine, Orange, California

William T. Creasman MD

J. Marion Sims Professor
Department of Obstetrics and Gynecology
Medical University of South Carolina
Charleston, South Carolina

MOSBY

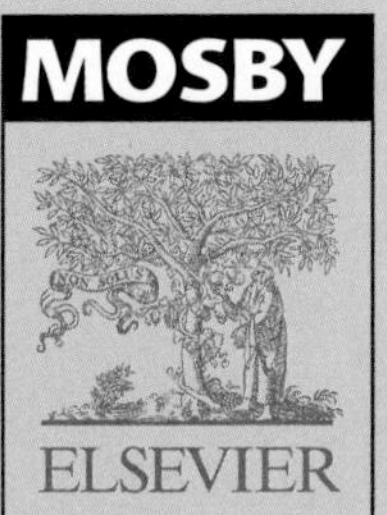

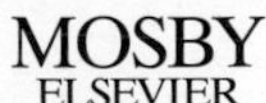

Mosby is an affiliate of Elsevier Inc.

First edition 1981
Second edition 1984
Third edition 1989
Fourth edition 1993
Fifth edition 1997
Sixth edition 2002
Seventh edition 2007

ISBN: 9780323039789

British Library Cataloguing in Publication Data
A catalogue record for this book is available from the British Library

Library of Congress Cataloging in Publication Data
A catalog record for this book is available from the Library of Congress

Notice
Medical knowledge is constantly changing. Standard safety precautions must be followed, but as new research and clinical experience broaden our knowledge, changes in treatment and drug therapy may become necessary or appropriate. Readers are advised to check the most current product information provided by the manufacturer of each drug to be administered to verify the recommended dose, the method and duration of administration, and contraindications. It is the responsibility of the practitioner, relying on experience and knowledge of the patient, to determine dosages and the best treatment for each individual patient. Neither the Publisher nor the author assume any liability for any injury and/or damage to persons or property arising from this publication.
The Publisher

Printed in China
Last digit is the print number: 9 8 7 6 5 4 3 2 1

Dedications

Cognizant of our major sources of support and comfort, we wish to dedicate this work to our loving wives Patti DiSaia and Erble Creasman and our children John DiSaia, Steven DiSaia, Dominic DiSaia, Vincent DiSaia, Vlrie Creasman-Duke, and Scott Creasman.

Also, a note of deepest gratitude to all the women, past and present, who have trusted us with their care. These women nurtured the tree of knowledge contained in this book. The roots of this tree have been founded on the courage of these women and intertwined with their lives.

Contributors

MICHAEL A. BIDUS, M.D.
Fellow, National Capital Consortium, Fellowship in Gynecologic Oncology
Walter Reed Army Medical Center, Department of Obstetrics and Gynecology
Division of Gynecologic Oncology, Washington, District of Columbia.
Germ cell, stromal, and other ovarian tumors

WENDY R. BREWSTER, M.D., Ph.D.
Associate Professor, Division of Gynecologic Oncology, UCI Medical Center, Irvine California.
Epidemiology and commonly used statistical terms, and analysis of clinical studies

CHRISTINA S. CHU, M.D.
Assistant Professor, Gynecologic Oncology, Division of Gynecologic Oncology, Hospital of the University of Pennsylvania, Philadelphia, Pennsylvania.
Basic principles of chemotherapy

DANIEL L. CLARKE-PEARSON, M.D.
Robert A Ross Professor of Obstetrics and Gynecology, University of North Carolina,
Chapel Hill, North Carolina.
Complications of disease and therapy

ROBERT L. COLEMAN, M.D.
Professor, University of Texas, MD Anderson Cancer Center, Department of Gynecologic Oncology, Houston, Texas.
Invasive cancer of the vagina and urethra

LARRY J. COPELAND, M.D.
Professor and Chair, William Greenville Pace III and Joann Norris Collins-Pace Chair, Department of Obstetrics and Gynecology, James Cancer Hospital, The Ohio State University, Columbus, Ohio.
Epithelial ovarian cancer

WILLIAM T. CREASMAN, M.D.
J Marion Sims Professor, Department of Obstetrics and Gynecology, Medical University of South Carolina, Charleston, South Carolina.

PHILIP J. DISAIA, M.D.
The Dorothy J. Marsh Chair in Reproductive Biology Director, Division of Gynecologic Oncology Professor, Department of Obstetrics and Gynecology University of California, Irvine College of Medicine,
Orange, California.

JAMES V. FIORICA, M.D.
Clinical Professor of Obstetrics & Gynecology, University of South Florida, Tampa, Florida. Director, Gynecologic Oncology, Sarasota Memorial Hospital, Sarasota, Florida.
Breast diseases

KEITH J. KAPLAN, M.D.
Assistant Professor of Pathology, Northwestern University Feinberg School of Medicine, Pathology Division, Evanston Hospital, Evanston, Illinois
Fallopian tube cancer

ROBERT S. MANNEL, M.D.
The James A Merrill Chair Professor and Chair, Department of Obstetrics and Gynecology, University of Oklahoma Health Sciences Center, Oklahoma City, Oklahoma.
Role of laparoscopic surgery in gynecologic malignancies

D. SCOTT MCMEEKIN, M.D.
Presbyterian Foundation Presidential Professor, University of Oklahoma Health Sciences Center, Oklahoma City, Oklahoma.
Sarcoma of the uterus

BRADLEY J. MONK, M.D.
Associate Professor, University of California, Irvine, Division of Gynecologic Oncology, Orange, California.
Invasive cervical cancer; Palliative care and quality of life

DAVID G. MUTCH, M.D.
Judith and Ira Gall Professor of Gynecologic Oncology, Obstetrics and Gynecology Division Chief, Washington University School of Medicine, St. Louis, Missouri.
Genes and cancer

G. SCOTT ROSE, M.D.
Director, Division of Gynecologic Oncology, Walter Reed Army Medical Center, Washington, District of Columbia.
Germ cell, stromal, and other ovarian tumors; Fallopian tube cancer

STEPHEN C. RUBIN, M.D.
Franklin Payne Professor, Chief Division of Gynecologic Oncology, Hospital of the University of Pennsylvania, Philadelphia, Pennsylvania.
Basic principles of chemotherapy

BRAIN M. SLOMOVITZ, M.D.
Assistant Professor, Department of Obstetrics and Gynecology, Weill Medical College of Cornell University, New York Presbyterian Hospital, New York, New York.
Invasive cancer of the vagina and urethra

JOHN T. SOPER, M.D.
Professor of Obstetrics & Gynecology, Division of Gynecologic Oncology, University of North Carolina School of Medicine, Chapel Hill, North Carolina.
Gestational trophoblastic neoplasia

FREDERICK B. STEHMAN, M.D.
The Clarence E. Ehrlich Professor and Chair, Department of Obstetrics and Gynecology, University Hospital, Indianapolis, Indiana.
Invasive cancer of the vulva

JAN S. SUNDE, M.D.
Fellow, National Capital Consortium, Fellowship in Gynecologic Oncology,
Walter Reed Army Medical Center, Department of Obstetrics and Gynecology
Division of Gynecologic Oncology, Washington, District of Columbia.
Fallopian tube cancer

KRISHNANSU S. TEWARI, M.D.
Associate Professor, University of California, Irvine, Division of Gynecologic Oncology, Orange, California.
Invasive cervical cancer; Cancer in pregnancy

JOAN L. WALKER, M.D.
Professor of Gynecologic Oncology, Department of Obstetrics and Gynecology, University of Oklahoma Health Sciences Center, Oklahoma City, Oklahoma.
Endometrial hyperplasia, estrogen therapy, and the prevention of endometrial cancer

LARI B. WENZEL, Ph.D.
Associate Professor, University of California, Irvine, Center for Health Policy Research, Irvine, California.
Palliative care and quality of life

CATHERYN YASHAR, M.D.
Moores Cancer Center, Radiation Oncology, La Jolla, California.
Basic principles in gynecologic radiotherapy

CHRISTOPHER M. ZAHN, M.D.
Associate Professor, Uniformed Services University of the Health Sciences, Department of Obstetrics and Gynecology, Bethesda, Maryland.
Germ cell, stromal, and other ovarian tumors

ROSEMARY E. ZUNA, M.D.
Associate Professor of Pathology, Pathology Department, University of Oklahoma Health Sciences Center, Oklahoma City, Oklahoma.
Endometrial hyperplasia, estrogen therapy, and the prevention of endometrial cancer

Preface

The first six editions of *Clinical Gynecologic Oncology* were stimulated by a recognized need for a readable text on gynecologic cancer and related subjects, addressed primarily to the community physician, resident, and other students involved with these patients. The practical aspects of the clinical presentation and management of these problems were heavily emphasized in the first six editions, and we have continued that style in this test. As in every other textbook, the authors interjected their own biases on many topics, especially in those areas where more than one approach to management has been utilized. On the other hand, most major topics are treated in depth and supplemented with ample references to current literature so that the text can provide a comprehensive resource for study by the resident, fellow, or student of gynecologic oncology and serve as a source for review material.

We continued the practice of placing an outline on the first page of each chapter as a guide to the content for that section. The reader will notice that we included topics not discussed in the former editions and expanded areas previously introduced. Some of these areas include new guidelines for managing the dying patient, current management and reporting guidelines for cervical and vulvar cancer, current management and reporting guidelines for breast cancer, expanded discussion on the basic principles of genetic alterations in cancer, techniques for laparoscopic surgery in treatment of gynecologic cancers, and new information on breast and colon cancer screening and detection. The seventh edition contains, for the first time, color photographs of key gross and microscopic specimens for the reader's review. In addition, Drs DiSaia and Creasman have included, several other authors for most of the chapters. Much more information is included to make the text as practical as possible for the practicing gynecologist. In addition, key points are highlighted for easy review.

Fortunately, many of the gynecologic malignancies have a high "cure" rate. This relatively impressive success rate with gynecologic cancers can be attributed in great part to the development of diagnostic techniques that can identify precancerous conditions, the ability to apply highly effective therapeutic modalities that are more restrictive elsewhere in the body, a better understanding of the disease spread patterns, and the development of more sophisticated and effective treatment in cancers that previously had very poor prognoses. As a result, today a patient with a gynecologic cancer my look toward more successful treatment and longer survival than at any other time. This optimism should be realistically transferred to the patient and her family. Patient denial must be tolerated until the patient decides that a frank conversation is desired. When the prognosis is discussed, some element of hope should always be introduced within the limits of reality and possibility.

The physician must be prepared to treat the malignancy in light of today's knowledge and to deal with the patient and her family in a compassionate and honest manner. The patient with gynecologic cancer needs to feel that her physician is confident and goal oriented. Although, unfortunately, gynecologic cancers will cause the demise of some individuals, it is hoped that the information collected in this book will help to increase the survical rate of these patiemts by bringing current practical knowledge to the attention of the primary care and specialized physician.

> *Our ideas are only intellectual instruments which we use to break into phenomena; we must change them when they have served their purpose, as we change a blunt lancet that we have used long enough.*
>
> Claude Bernard (1813-1878)

> *Some patients, though conscious that their condition is perilous, recover their health simply through their contentment with the goodness of their physician.*
>
> Hippocrates (440-370 BC)

Philip J. DiSaia, MD
William T. Creasman, MD

Acknowledgements

We wish to acknowledge the advice given and contributions made by several colleagues, including Robert Burger, Bradley J. Monk, David G. Mutch, Ibrahim Ramzy, Fritz Lin, Robert S. Mannel, Krishnansu Tewari, Joan Walker, Rosemary Zuna, D. Scott McMeekin, John T. Soper, Frederick B. Stehman, Robert L. Coleman, Brian M. Slomovitz, Larry J. Copeland, G. Scott Rose, Michael A. Bidus, Christopher M. Zahn, Jan S. Sunde, Keith J. Kaplan, James V. Fiorica, Daniel L. Clarke-Pearson, Christina S. Chu, Stephen C. Rubin, Lari Wenzel, wendy R. Brewster, and Catheryn Yashar. We give special thanks to Lucy Digiuseppe and, especially, Yvonne Bell for their diligent administrative support in preparing the manuscript and also to David F. Baker, MA, Carol Beckerman, Richard Crippen, Susan Stokskopf, and David Wyer for their excellent and creative contributions to many of the illustrations created for this book.

We are grateful to the sincere and diligent efforts of Rebecca Gaertner, Deirdre Simpson, Louis Forgione, and Gemma Lawson from Elsevier in bringing this book to fruition. Through their deliberate illumination and clearing of our path, this material has traversed the far distance between mere concept to a compelling reference book.

Contents

APPENDICES

1 Preinvasive Disease of the Cervix

William T. Creasman, M.D.

CERVICAL INTRAEPITHELIAL NEOPLASIA

Clinical profile

The unique accessibility of the cervix to cell and tissue study and to direct physical examination has permitted intensive investigation of the nature of malignant lesions of the cervix. Although our knowledge is incomplete, investigations have shown that most of these tumors have a gradual, rather than an explosive, onset. Their preinvasive precursors may exist in a reversible phase of surface or in situ disease for some years, although this may be changing, at least in some patients.

According to data from the Third National Cancer Survey, published by Cramer and Cutler, the mean age of patients with carcinoma in situ was 15.6 years younger than that of patients with invasive squamous cell carcinoma, exceeding the 10-year difference found by others. This difference is, at best, a rough approximation of the duration of intraepithelial carcinoma in its assumed progression to clinical invasive cancer. Data such as these serve to emphasize the essential nature of cytologic screening programs, even when performed on less than an annual basis.

Although these early phases may be asymptomatic, they can be detected by currently available methods. This concept of development of cervical malignancy has convinced many that control of this disease is well within grasp in the foreseeable future. It is possible to eradicate most deaths resulting from cervical cancer by use of the diagnostic and therapeutic techniques now available.

There is convincing evidence that cytologic screening programs are effective in reducing mortality from carcinoma of the cervix. The extent of the reduction in mortality achieved is related directly to the proportion of the population that has been screened. In fact, all studies worldwide show that screening for cancer not only decreases mortality but also probably does so by decreasing the incidence. The incidence of cervical cancer has not decreased without a screening program being implemented.

Numerous papers and lengthy discussions have focused on the optimal screening interval. Unfortunately, numerous recommendations during the last decade and a half have resulted in a confused public and dissatisfied professionals. In 1988, the American College of Obstetricians and Gynecologists (ACOG) and the American Cancer Society (ACS) agreed on the following recommendation, which has subsequently been accepted by other organizations. That recommendation was changed in 2002. ACOG guidelines are: Screening should begin about 3 years after initiation of sexual intercourse. Annual screening should begin no later than age 21 years. At age 40 and thereafter, Pap smears may be every 2–3 years after three consecutive negative test results if no history of cervical intraepithelial neoplasia (CIN) II or III, immunosuppression, human immunodeficiency virus (HIV) infection or diethylstilbestrol (DES) exposure in utero.

ACS guidelines are slightly different: Cervical cancer screening should begin about 3 years after a woman begins having vaginal intercourse but no later than 21 years of age. Screening should be done every year with conventional Pap tests or every 2 years using liquid-based Pap tests. At or after age 30, women who have had three normal test results in a row may get screened every 2–3 years. Women 70 years of age and older who have had three or more normal Pap tests and no abnormal Pap tests in the last 10 years, and women who have had a total hysterectomy, may choose to stop cervical cancer screening.

It is generally accepted by many that this recommendation advocates annual Pap smears, because most women do not satisfy the conditions for less frequent screening.

Information from many studies worldwide suggests that this recommendation is reasonable for American women. Not only has screening decreased the incidence and death rate from cervical cancer, but it has also identified many women with preinvasive neoplasia (which is the role of screening, not to diagnose cancer). As many as four million women per year will have an abnormal Pap smear in the USA. This represents 5–7% of cervical smears with 90% or more having atypical cells of undetermined significance (ASC-US) or low-grade squamous intraepithelial lesions (LSIL). In addition, women who have been screened but subsequently developed cervical cancer usually have an earlier stage of lesion. In the USA, death rates from cervical cancer have dropped from number 1 among all cancers in women to number 12. In 2005, 10,520 new cervical and 3710 cancer deaths will occur in the USA. Approximately 55,000 invasive new carcinomas in situ will be also diagnosed. Although it has not been proved in a prospective randomized study, all investigators credit screening as a major contributor to this reduction in death rate. In contrast to the industrialized world, cancer of the cervix remains the primary cancer killer in women in third world countries. Approximately 500,000 cervical cancers will be diagnosed this year worldwide, representing 12% of all cancers diagnosed in women, and almost half will die of their cancer. Because this is a poor woman's disease, not much political pressure has been brought to bear to improve the situation for this group.

Several comments are appropriate in connection with these recommendations. The high-risk woman is generally recognized to be an individual who becomes sexually active in mid adolescence and tends to have multiple sexual partners. All would agree that a woman should be screened for CIN shortly after becoming sexually active. It is believed that if an individual is virginal by the time she reaches 21 years of age, cervical cytologic testing should begin. The purpose of cytologic screening of the cervix is to identify the patient who has an intraepithelial lesion and not the patient who has invasive cancer. The latter patient will probably be symptomatic, and in many cases her diagnosis will be made because her symptoms have been investigated. The fact that a significant number of women will develop intraepithelial disease within a short time after commencement of sexual activity speaks to the propriety of these recommendations. Although invasive carcinoma of the cervix is not as common in younger women as it is in their older counterparts, an increasing number of patients with invasive cancer are in their 20s and 30s. In England and Wales in the mid-1960s, a political decision was made not to pay for Pap smears in women younger than 35 years of age unless they had three or more children. During the ensuing decade, the death rate doubled as a result of carcinoma of the cervix in women in that age group. Evidence suggests that there is an increased incidence of adenocarcinoma of the cervix, but the epidemiologic aspects of this disease have not been developed.

Subsequent data from England now suggest that there is an increasing mortality in patients aged 45 years and younger. These authors believe that current indications suggest that during the next 25 years, most of the predicted increase in incidence and mortality will occur among women younger than 50 years of age. In 1981, women younger than 50 years of age accounted for one-third of new cancer cases and one-fifth of the deaths, but by the year 2001 as many as two-thirds of new cancers and as many as one half of deaths may occur in women younger than 50 years old. Since 1986, invasive cancer incidence has increased about 3% per year in white women younger than 50 years of age, whereas the rates are still declining in African-American women. This is probably related to screening practice (as noted later).

At the same time, studies have shown that the older patient is at increased risk for cervical cancer. Mandelblatt reported that 25% of all cervical cancers and 41% of all deaths from cancer occurred in women older than 65 years of age. The prevalence of abnormal Pap smears is high in this group (16 in 1000). The chance of developing an invasive cancer is not necessarily related to prior screening habits in this age group. Another study noted that increasing age is associated with more advanced disease, yet when stage of disease was controlled, there was no effect of age on disease-free survival. Screening of the patient older than 65 years of age would benefit most, with a 63% improvement of 5-year mortality. As a result, Pap smear screening should continue for a lifetime. Data from the 1992 National Health Interview Survey indicated that one half of all women older than 60 years of age did not have a Pap smear during the last 3 years. Although screened less frequently, they have the same number of recent physician visits as do younger women. The need to educate older women and their health care providers about the importance of Pap smear screening is evident. A study from Connecticut reviewed all invasive cancers diagnosed in the state between 1985 and 1990. The purpose of the study, patterned after the investigation of puerperal deaths of the 1930s, was to assess the reason why the cancer was not detected before it became invasive. Even though cervical cytologic screening has been around for several decades, some very important facts became apparent and others need re-emphasis. More than one quarter of patients had never had a Pap smear, and almost one quarter had their last Pap smear more than 5 years before their diagnosis of cervical cancer. The average age of women who were never screened was almost 20 years older (65 vs 46 years of age) than the screened cancer patients. This suggests that many older women are not being screened for cervical cytology. Several studies have noted that many physicians may not comply with existing cancer screening guidelines. Of the previous normal Pap smears available for review after cancer diagnosis, about one-fifth were reread as abnormal. This includes those with a premalignant diagnosis. Approximately 10% of women had an incomplete evaluation after one or more abnormal smears. Adenocarcinomas were seen about twice as often in women who developed cancer within 3 years of a satisfactory negative result on a Pap smear compared with the total study group. About one quarter of women had a Pap smear within 3 years; 77% had normal reread Pap smears, which suggests that these patients may have rapidly progressive disease.

The natural history of CIN has been evaluated by reviewing the literature on the subject as well as by meta-analysis. This information may be used as a guideline in clinical management. In a review of the literature of almost 14,000 patients followed for less than 1 year up to 20 years, Östör noted that in CIN I, 60% will regress, and only 10% will progress to carcinoma in situ (CIS). In patients with CIN III, one-third will regress to normal. The initial diagnosis was by cytology, biopsy, or a combination of the two. In more than 15,000 patients, 1.7% progressed to invasive cancer with CIN I doing so in 1% compared with 12% of patients with CIN III. In a meta-analysis of almost 28,000 patients, Melnikow and colleagues found that ASCUS progressed to high-grade squamous intraepithelial lesions (HSIL) at 24 months in 7.3% and low-grade SIL in 21%. Progression to cancer was 0.25% with ASCUS, 0.15% with low-grade SIL (LSIL), and 1.44% with high-grade SIL (HSIL). Regression to normal occurred in 68% of ASCUS, 47% low-grade SIL, and 35% in high-grade SIL.

Demographic studies suggest that 9% of women older than 18 years of age have never had a Pap smear. This translates to more than one million women in the USA. Of those screened, 62% did not have a Pap smear in the past year. The group not having a Pap smear in the last year was one of older patients. More than 91% of women 65 years or older and living below the poverty level did not have a Pap smear in the last year. Approximately eleven million white women aged 65 or older in the USA did not have a Pap smear in the past year. A National Omnibus survey was conducted to ascertain women's knowledge, attitudes, and behavior toward Pap screening. Of women 18 years or older, 82% believed the Pap smear is very important. Among women who believed that the Pap smear was important, 82% stated it was to identify cancer. Among those aged 18–24, only 61% understood that the Pap smear was to detect cancer. Thirty-five percent of this same age group believed the Pap smear was important to detect vaginal infections and sexually transmitted diseases. More than one quarter of those who believed that Pap smears were important did not have a Pap test during the previous year. The older and lower-income women were less likely than others to say that Pap smears are very important, yet they had regular physical examinations. Only 51% of women stated that Pap smears identified cervical and endometrial cancers. Seven percent believed breast cancer was found on the Pap smear. Risk factors for cervical cancer were poorly understood. Approximately two-thirds of women identified a family history as a cervical cancer risk factor. One in five women could not name any risk factors for cervical cancer. Women believed that physicians did not sufficiently explain the reasons for Pap smears and the results from these tests. The need for better communication between physicians and women should be obvious. Screening patterns to some degree appear to be changing, although some habits apparently do not. The number of women who had health insurance, a higher level of education, and current employment were related to Pap smear usage. Of interest is that recently, black women have substantially increased the use of the Pap smear, with rates now exceeding those of white women. This is age-related: screening is similar for blacks and whites up to age 29; but from 30 to 49 years, blacks are significantly more compliant. Among those older than 70 years of age, compliance among white women is greater. Although screening rates appear to be higher in black women, the mortality rate is lower for white women. Age is also important in that younger women are more compliant than older women. The highest-risk group in the USA appears to be Hispanics, particularly if they speak only Spanish. Approximately 1.6 million Hispanics are not screened in the USA. This is the fastest growing segment of our population, which may explain why they are not screened. The following reasons were given for non-compliance: it was unnecessary, no problems, procrastination, physicians' non-recommendation, having a hysterectomy, and costs. One study noted that 72% of all women had a Pap smear within the last year. Yet almost 80% of women who did not have a Pap smear reported contact with medical facilities during the past 2 years, whereas more than 90% reported making contact during the last 5 years. Obviously, an educational effort should be made in this regard among health care professionals.

Another important consideration is that there is a relatively high false-negative Pap smear rate in the USA. Several studies in the USA and abroad have shown that an alarming number of patients were found to have invasive carcinoma of the cervix within a relatively short time after a reportedly normal Pap smear. A study from Seattle indicates that 27% of patients with stage I carcinoma of the cervix had a normal Pap smear within 1 year of the time of diagnosis. Berman noted that after 3 years from last screen, women who develop cervical cancer have the same incidence of advanced disease as do women who have never been screened. The false-negative rate of Pap smears is really unknown. Cervicography and colposcopic studies have suggested that the majority of women identified with CIN by these two techniques had normal Pap smears at the time of diagnosis.

Therefore, several concerns arise when determining optimal screening for cervical neoplasia. Although the transit time from CIS to invasive cancer is said to require 8, 10, or possibly 20 years, some patients make this transition in a short time. CIN does not necessarily progress in an orderly fashion to invasive cancer; an earlier CIN lesion can progress directly to invasive cancer. The inaccuracy of the Pap smear must also be considered. The purpose of screening is to identify preinvasive disease early, when the cost of treatment is considerably less than it is after the patient has developed invasive disease. Cost effectiveness is an important consideration in any screening program; however, multiple factors go into the determination of optimal screening. Essentially all investigators suggest annual screening for the high-risk patient, and it must be remembered that a substantial number of women in the

USA are at high risk. The annual Pap smear has routinely led to evaluation of the patient with regard to other malignancies and medical conditions, and this appears to be an important consideration in the health care of American women. It has been estimated that annual Pap smear testing reduces a woman's chance of dying of cervical cancer from 4 in 1000 to about 5 in 10,000—a difference of almost 90%.

Epidemiology

Numerous epidemiologic studies reported in the literature have established a positive association between cancer of the cervix and multiple, interdependent social factors. A greater incidence of cervical cancer is observed among blacks and Mexican-Americans, and this is undoubtedly related to their lower socioeconomic status. Increased occurrence of cancer of the cervix in multiparous women is probably related to other factors, such as age at first marriage and age at first pregnancy. These facts, combined with the high incidence of the disease in prostitutes, lead to a firm conclusion that first coitus at an early age and multiple sexual partners increase the probability of developing CIN. Even socioeconomic status is interrelated, because an association has long been noted between relative poverty and early marriage and youthful childbearing. The final common factors appear to be onset of regular sexual activity as a teenager and continued exposure to multiple sexual partners. Indeed, cervical cancer is rare in celibate groups such as nuns, and many have labeled cancer of the cervix a "venereal disease".

Much has been made about the sexual activity of a woman as it may affect her risk for developing CIN. Increasing data suggest that a woman may also be placed at increased risk by her sexual partner, even though she does not satisfy the requirements of early intercourse and multiple partners. The sexual history of her partner may be as important as hers. In a study by Zunzunegui, patients with cervical cancer were compared with selected controls. Both populations came from a low socioeconomic group of recent Hispanic migrants to California. All were married. Sexual histories were obtained from both sexes. Among the women the age of first coitus was earlier among the cases than among the controls (19.5 years vs 21.7 years). The average number of lifetime sexual partners did not differ between cases and controls. Interestingly, case husbands had more sexual partners than did control husbands; they had first intercourse at an earlier age and also a much greater history of venereal diseases. Visits to prostitutes were equal between the two groups, but the case husbands tended to have frequented prostitutes more often than did the husbands in the control group. Husbands in the case group smoked more than the husbands in the control group. If the number of sexual partners of the husband was greater than 20, the risk of cervical cancer increased in the wife five times more than that of a woman whose husband had fewer than 20 sexual partners. This may be related to the "infectious" agent obtained by the husband and, in turn, to the duration of exposure by the woman. (Note the following section on human papilloma virus [HPV] and the male factor.)

Even if the carcinogen is identified, its interaction with the cervix depends on the specific woman at risk. The epidemiologic data strongly suggest that the adolescent is at risk. The probable reason is that active metaplasia is occurring. Because there is active proliferation of cellular transformation from columnar to metaplastic to squamoid epithelium, the potential for interaction between the carcinogen and the cervix is increased. Once this process of metaplasia is complete, the cervix may no longer be at high risk, although CIN certainly can occur in patients who are virginal until after this process has been completed. Smoking is now considered a high-risk factor for carcinoma of the cervix, and this observation correlates with distribution of other smoking-related cancers. An increased, excess risk of preinvasive and invasive disease appears to exist among smokers, particularly among current, long-term users, high-risk intensity smokers, and users of non-filtered cigarettes. Smoking appears to be an independent risk factor, even after controlling for sexual factors. In a case-control study, the risk of HSIL increased with increasing years and pack-years of exposure. The association is for squamous cell cancers only, and no relationship with adenocarcinomas has been noted. Studies have found mutagens in cervical mucus, some of which are many times higher than those found in the blood.

One study evaluated whether smoking caused deoxyribonucleic acid (DNA) modification (addicts) in cervical epithelium. Smokers had a higher level of DNA addicts than did non-smokers. Women with abnormal Pap smears had a significantly higher number of DNA addicts than those with normal Pap smears. Women with a higher proportion of addicts may have an increased susceptibility to cervical cancer. This suggests direct biochemical evidence of smoking as a cause of cervical cancer.

It has been suggested that vitamin deficiency may have a role in certain malignancies, including cervical cancer. Butterworth evaluated 294 patients with dysplasia and 170 controls defined by cytology and colposcopy. Multiple known risk factors for cervical neoplasia were evaluated along with 12 nutritional indices on non-fasting blood specimens. Plasma nutrient levels were generally not associated with risks; however, red blood cell folate levels at or below 660 nmol/L interacted with HPV-16 infections. Chemoprevention with vitamin A may prevent some cancers. Vitamin A derivatives, particularly retinoids in vitro and in vivo, modulate the growth of normal epithelial cells, usually by inhibiting proliferation and allowing differentiation and maturation of cells to occur. Meyskens, in a randomized prospective study, treated a group of patients with CIN II and III with all-trans retinoic acid or a like placebo delivered directly to the cervix. Retinoic acid patients with CIN II had a complete histologic regression of 43% vs 27% for the placebo group ($P = 0.041$). No treatment difference was noted for the patient with CIN III. The results of this study, as well as others, suggest a chemoprevention role in the prevention of cervical neoplasia.

Human papilloma virus

Epidemiologic studies have identified the association of cervical neoplasia with sexual activity. The initial study suggests this relationship is more than 150 years old. The sexually transmitted agent that could be related to the initiation or promotion of cervical neoplasia has been sought for many years. Essentially every substance found in the genital tract has been implicated over the years. These have included sperm, smegma, spirochetes, Trichomonas, fungus, and more recently herpes simplex virus type II (HSV-2) and human papilloma virus (HPV). During the 1970s, HSV-2 was studied extensively in an attempt to develop a possible etiologic link. These endeavors mainly used case-control studies, which showed a significant higher prevalence of HSV-2 in cancer cases compared with controls. These studies encountered problems with cross-reactivity between HSV-1 and HSV-2 and standardization of assays. It could not be determined if the infection with the virus preceded the cancer. When controlled for high-risk factors, many studies found no difference among patients and controls in the prevalence of HSV-2 antibody. Most investigators today do not consider HSV-2 to be a serious candidate as an etiologic agent for cervical neoplasia, although some have postulated that it may in some way be a cofactor.

Since the mid-1970s, there has been an explosion of information concerning HPV. It was actually in the mid-1970s when zur Hausen suggested that HPV was a likely candidate as a sexually transmitted agent that may result in genital tract neoplasias. Later in that decade, Meisel published a series of articles that described a new virus-induced condylomatous lesion of the cervix. Although koilocytosis had previously been described, these workers noted the presence of intranuclear HPV in koilocytotic cells associated with CIN. In contrast to the long-identified typical cauliflower condyloma, it was noted that HPV also produced a flat, white lesion, best recognized colposcopically, that was thought to be a precursor of cervical neoplasia. The development of immunoperoxidase techniques that can identify the HPV confirmed these original observations. Subsequently, HPV has been isolated from genital lesions; with the use of hybridization techniques, the HPV DNA can be typed.

To date, about 120 different types of HPV have been isolated and characterized (Table 1–1). The identity of a new subtype has usually been based on the description of the DNA genome compared with the known HPV prototypes. A new type must share less than 50% DNA homology to any known HPV. Classification depends on the composition of DNA. About 30 HPV types primarily infect the squamous epithelium of the lower anogenital tracts of both males and females. So-called low-risk types (6, 11, 42, 43, 44) are mainly associated with benign lesions such as condyloma, which rarely progress to a malignancy. The high-risk types (16, 18, 31, 33, 35, 39, 45, 51, 52, 56, 58) are detected in intraepithelial and invasive cancers. More than 85% of all cervical cancers are said to contain high-risk HPV sequences. In benign precursor lesions, the HPV DNA is episomal (has extra chromosomal replication). In cancers, the DNA is integrated into the human genome. All HPVs contain at least seven early genes (E1-7) and two late genes (L1 and L2).

The integration usually occurs in the E1/E2 region, resulting in disrupting gene integrity and expression. These open reading frames encode DNA-binding proteins that regulate viral transcription and replication. With HPV-16 and 18, the E2 protein represses the promoter from which the E6 and E7 genes are transcribed. Because of integration, the E6 and E7 genes are expressed in HPV-positive cervical cancer. It appears that E6 and E7 are the only viral factors necessary for immortalization of human genital epithelial cells. These two oncoproteins form complexes with host regulatory proteins such as p53 and pRB (retroblastoma susceptibility gene). High-risk HPV E6, upon binding with p53, causes rapid degradation of the protein, thus preventing p53 normal function from responding to DNA damage induced by radiation or chemical mutagens. Without this binding, increased levels of p53 growth arrest of cells may occur, which allows repair of damaged DNA to take place or apoptosis (programmed cell death) to occur. E7 protein may bind to several cellular proteins, including pRB. This interaction may inactivate pRB and push the cell cycle into the S phase and induce DNA synthesis. Other regulatory genes such as c-myc may also be involved. Other factors are obviously important, because only a small percentage of women infected with high-risk HPV develop cancer. HPV-immortalized human keratinocyte cell lines will only be manifest in nude mice, for instance, after transfection with additional oncogenes such as ras. In humans, the immunologic response may contribute to this very complicated scenario.

Table 1–1 GYNECOLOGIC LESIONS ASSOCIATED WITH HUMAN PAPILLOMA VIRUS

	Common HPV types	Less common HPV types
Condyloma acuminata	6,11	2,16,30,40,41,42,44,45,54,55,61
CIN, VIN, VAIN	16,18,31	6,11,30,34,35,39,40,42–5,51,52,56–9,61,62,64,66,67,69
Cervical cancer	16,18,31,45	6,10,11,26,33,35,39,51,52,55,56,58

CIN, cervical intraepithelial neoplasia; VIN, vulvar intraepithelial neoplasia.
From Evans H, Walker PG: Infection and cervical intraepithelial neoplasia. Cont Clinical Gynecol Obstet 2:217–27, 2002.

HPVs carry their genetic information within a cellular double-stranded DNA molecule. Infections caused by these viruses are usually not systemic but result in local infections manifest as warty papillary condylomatous lesions. HPV-infected cells contain both the fully formed viral particles and their DNA. Replication of the virus occurs only in the cell nuclei, in which DNA synthesis is low. Mature HPV particles are never found in replicating basal or parabasal cells but are found in the koilocytotic cells in the superficial layer. HPV, like HSV-2, may also have a latent intranuclear form in which only fragments of the viral DNA are expressed.

Characterizations of the HPV types suggest about 40 of these can cause genital disease. These have been divided into high-risk HPV types of which 16 and 18 are the most common, probably high-risk (types 26, 53 and 66) or low-risk types with 6 and 11 being the most common. These appear to be sexually transmitted. (Fig. 1–1). Although HPV types 16 and 18 are the types most commonly isolated in cervical cancer, not all infections with type 16 and 18 progress to cancer. Reeves reported one of the largest studies of both cervical cancer and controls, and HPV-16/18 were seen in 62% of 759 cancer patients, whereas HPV-6/11 were identified in 17%. More interesting is that only 7% of 1467 randomly selected, age-matched controls were found to have HPV 6/11, whereas 32% of controls tested positive for HPV-16/18. The crude and adjusted relative risk of cervical cancer associated with HPV-16/18 or HPV-6/11 were similar. Other studies suggest that HPV-16/18 may be present in as many as 80% of the normal population. This proportion of HPV positivity in the normal population varies depending on the geographic area evaluated. Meanwell evaluated 47 cancer patients, 66% of whom had HPV-16, compared with 35% of 26

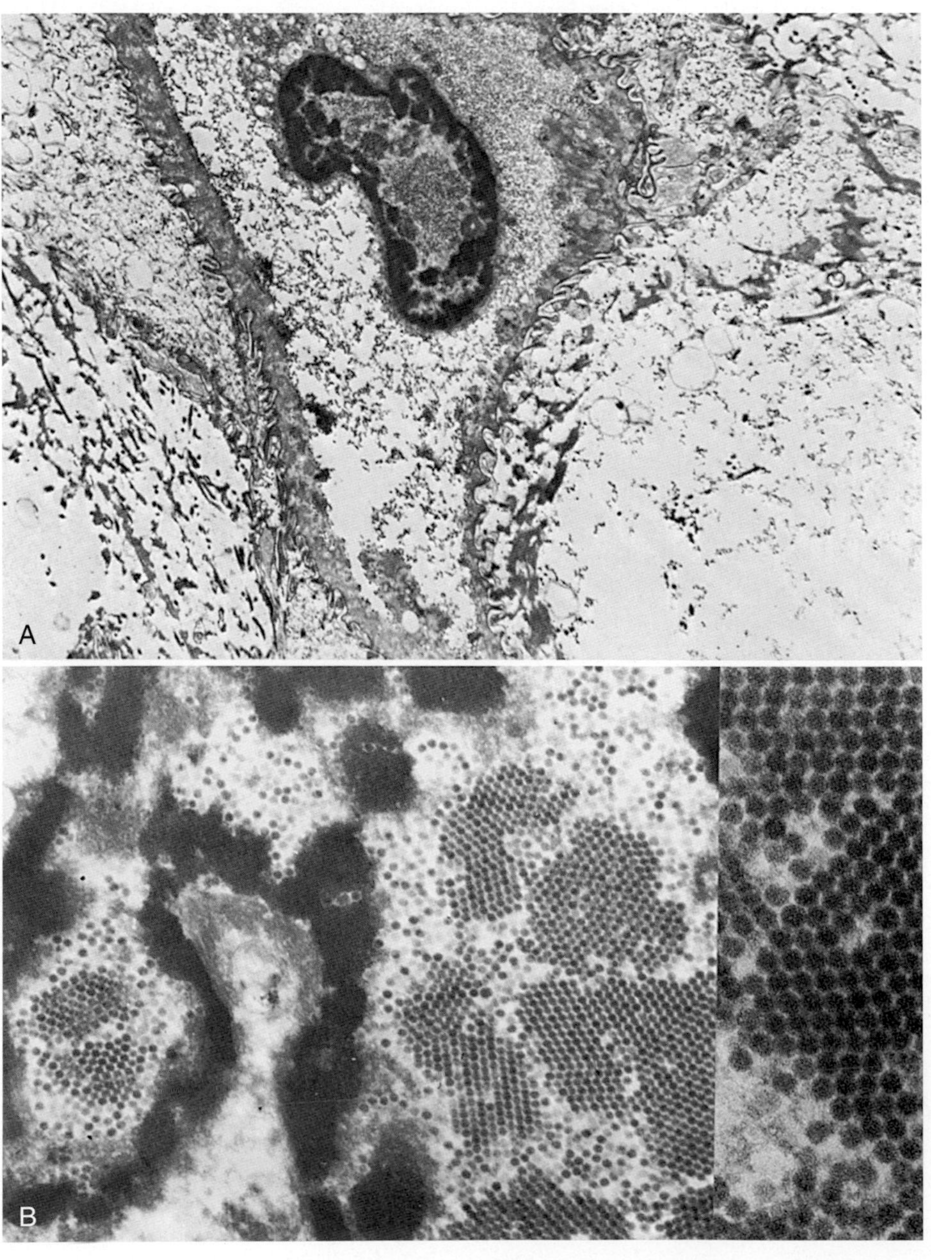

Figure 1–1 *A,* Koilocytotic cells with intranuclear virions (× 6900). *B,* Human papillomavirus particles. Note the intranuclear crystalline array ("honeycomb") arrangement of virions (× 20,500). See the insert (× 80,000). (Courtesy of Alex Ferenczy, MD, Montreal, Canada.)

controls. After controlling for age, he found no significant difference between cases and controls with regard to the frequency HPV-16 was identified.

Initially, it was suggested that in all cancers the HPV DNA was integrated, whereas in CIN lesions the HPV DNA was episomal. This suggested the role of a more virulent type of HPV (i.e., 16/18). More recently, an increased number of cancers with episomal HPV DNA have been reported. Integration has been noted in CIN lesions; therefore, it appears that integration is not a constant finding in cancers. Although integration of HPV-16 has been demonstrated, the importance of this finding in the development of cancer has not been determined.

An interesting study from Greenland and Denmark evaluated the incidence of HPV and HSV-2 in the normal population of these two countries. The cumulative incidence rate of cervical cancer in Greenland is 5.6 times higher than it is in Denmark. A total of 586 women in Greenland and 661 from Denmark were investigated. The total HPV-16/18 rate was 13% in Denmark, compared with 8.8% in Greenland; and the age-adjusted prevalence rate in Greenland was only 67% of Denmark's. HPV-6/11 prevalence was similar in the two populations (6.7% and 7.5%). The authors noted a much higher proportion of women in Greenland with HSV-2 antibodies than of those from Denmark (68.2% vs 30.9%). They also noted a higher number of sexual partners in Greenland (22% with 40 or more) compared with Denmark (0.3%). Cancer screening was similar in the two areas. Although the authors suggested that these data should be interpreted with caution and that other, similar studies need to be done, the observed HPV-16/18 infection rate in Greenland (compared with the cancer incidence in Greenland compared with Denmark) is an interesting observation.

HPV-18 may be more virulent than HPV-16 and may be a prognostic factor. Kurman and associates noted a deficit of HPV-18 in CIN compared with cancer, whereas there was no significant difference in the distribution of HPV-16 in CIN compared with cancer. These authors postulated that this deficit of HPV-18 in CIN could represent a rapid transit time through the preinvasive phase. Obviously, this is conjecture at this time. Walker noted that patients with cervical cancer and HPV-18 had a worse prognosis than did similar-staged patients with HPV-16. One other study noted that the prognosis was worse in patients with cervical cancer if no HPV subtype was identified than if any HPV type was present. Today it is generally accepted that type 18 is more frequently associated with adenocarcinoma of the cervix and type 16 with squamous cancer. There also appears to be a difference in sexual behavior and reproductive risk factors between the two histotypes. There is a positive association of high gravidity and squamous cancer and an inverse association with adenocarcinoma. Age of first intercourse and number of sexual partners is of greater risk for squamous carcinoma than adenocarcinoma. Over the last several years, many studies worldwide attempted to characterize HPV DNA with regard to specific types and correlate these findings with the cervical neoplastic process. Although the laboratory evidence of the role of HPV DNA in the carcinogenesis was being established, the epidemiologic studies were lacking. Many studies that used testing that was considered appropriate just a few years ago are today considered inadequate because of the test's insensitivity in light of current technology. For many years, the Southern blot analysis for HPV DNA was considered to be the gold standard. Because it is very laboratory and personnel intense, as well as difficult to replicate between different laboratories, other techniques were developed. The filter in situ hybridization and dot blot test were developed; the latter was used in the commercially available Vira Pap/Vira Type kits. Both techniques were insensitive. The HPV Profile kit was developed to increase the number of HPV types tested (from 7–14) but is labor intense and uses radiolabeling. This was introduced in 1993 but was replaced by hybrid capture, which is said to have greater sensitivity, requires less time and uses a chemiluminescence substrate instead of radiolabeling. The hybrid capture second generation (HC2) is Food and Drug Administration (FDA) approved for HPV testing of the cervix. Both high- and low-risk HPV types can be identified but require separate ribonucleic acid (RNA) probes. Testing for low-risk types is not usually recommended. The high-risk probe can identify 16, 18, 31, 33, 35, 39, 45, 51, 52, 56, 58, 59 and 68. A semiquantitative measure of the viral load can be obtained based on the intensity of light emitted by the sample. In many instances, more than one subtype may be present.

With our current knowledge, should HPV typing be offered or suggested as part of our routine screening or even as a triage? This question implies that we know the answer to several other questions (e.g., the incidence or prevalence in the "normal" population; what affects the positive rate; which technique is considered to be the gold standard; whether HPV DNA detection can predict future cervical neoplasia). Some investigators have stated that HPV DNA is ubiquitous and endemic. The most common method of transmittal appears to be sexual; however, nonsexual transfer is not rare. Jenison found that 28–65% of children younger than 10 years old had antibodies HPV-6, 16, or 18 fusion proteins, and 20% had (PCR) detection of HPV-6 or 16 in oral mucosa. The prevalence of HPV DNA detection appears to increase during pregnancy, and transmission from the mother to the child during delivery is accepted as a possible transfer mechanism. Although the prevalence of HPV DNA does appear to be related to sexual activity, detection of the DNA has been found in co-ed virgins. It appears that HPV DNA is detected most often in women without evidence of CIN in the 15–25 age range. The one-time prevalence of HPV DNA depends on the assay used. One study of adolescents and young women using the dot blot hybridization technique found 9–11% positive, whereas another study of similar women using PCR found HPV DNA in 33%. Studies of sexually active adolescents noted that detection of HPV DNA varied from 15–38%. The HPV detection rate was usually higher in women with more sexual partners; however, one study noted that the rate decreased significantly as the number of sexual partners increased (> 10 partners). The rate of detection did not correlate with the years of sexual activity. These usually decreased with age when other factors were controlled. Limited data are available on longitudinal studies of HPV DNA detection. de Villiers found that approximately 9% of women of all ages with normal cytology had HPV DNA present on first testing. This rate increased to 26% if repeat testing was done over a 5-year period. The actual rate is probably higher because they used a less sensitive technique (filter in situ hybridization).

Mao and associates evaluated 516 sexually active university students (18 to 24 years old). They collected genital specimens for HPV testing every 4 months for up to 4 years. During the study, over 4000 study visits were completed and at about 20% of the visits HPV positivity other than 6 and 11 was noted. Only 5% were positive for 6 and 11. Except for those with 6 and 11, all other HPV subtypes identified, the women were asymptomatic.

Ho et al followed 608 college women at 6-month intervals for 3 years. The accumulative 30- month incidence of HPV infection was 43%. The increased risk was associated with younger age, increased number of vaginal sex partners, high frequency of vaginal sex and partners with an increase of sexual partners. The median duration of new infections was 8 months. The persistence of HPV for ≥ 6 months was related to older age, type of HPV as well as multiple subtypes of HPV. The risk of an abnormal Pap smear increased with persistent HPV infection, particularly high-risk types.

Woodmar and associates recruited 2001 women, 15–19 years old, who had recently become sexually active. They took cervical smears every 6 months. In 1075 women who were cytologically normal and HPV negative at recruitment, the accumulative risk for any HPV infection was 44%. The accumulative 3-year risk of a different HPV type than present initially was 26%. 246 had abnormal smears and 28 progressed to high-grade CIN. This risk was highest in women who were positive for HPV-16 but 40% tested negative for HPV and another 33% tested positive for 1st time only at the visit as the abnormal smear. Five women who progressed to high grade CIN consistently tested negative for HPV.

Moscicki followed a small group of HPV DNA-positive women for longer than 2 years with several visits in which HPV DNA using both PCR and dot blot technique were tested. Twelve of 27 tested positive for HPV-16/18. More than half of the women had negative results spontaneously (defined as two or more negative test results) for the original HPV type detected during the first visit. The data suggested that the number of virions decreased over a relatively short period and that the infection was presumed terminated. When a new HPV type was identified, most reported acquiring a new sexual partner since the last visit. This probably reflects a new infection and not reactivation. Rosenfeld found that > 50% of young urban patients tested positive for HPV at either an initial visit or at follow-up 6–36 months later using the Southern blot test. Therefore, the prevalence and incidence of HPV DNA appear to vary greatly, depending on age, sexual activity, the number of times tested, and the laboratory technique used. More than one million people are estimated to seek medical attention each year in the USA because of virus-induced lesions. The incidence, therefore, appears to be quite high for finding HPV DNA in the female genital tract. Even with the high-risk HPV types, infections commonly cause only mild transient cytologic changes and rarely lead to significant CIN or invasive cancer. Therefore, the use of routine screening utilizing HPV DNA probes does not appear to be clinically indicated in the young patient.

HPV testing has been evaluated as an adjunct to primary cervical screening. Cuzick and associates obtained HPV testing for types 16, 18, 31, and 33 using a semiquantitative type-specific PCR test. In 1980, their study was done on evaluable women who had never been treated for CIN and who had not had an abnormal Pap smear during the previous 3 years. Cytologic abnormality or high concentrations of HPV were obtained in 11.6% (231 patients) and 81 (4%) had CIN II or III, respectively. The positive predictive value (PPV) of HSIL cytology in identifying CIN II or III was 66%. HPV testing detected 61 cases of CIN II or III (sensitivity 75% and PPV of 42%). Of the 81 cases of CIN II or III, cytology was negative in 33 and 20 had no evidence of any of the HPV types tested. Although sensitivity and PPV were noted, specificity and the negative predictive value (NPV) were not.

It has been suggested that in patients with an abnormality, HPV DNA typing may be used as a triage method to determine who may need further investigation. This is particularly true for patients with ASCUS or LSIL, because those with HSIL will most always be evaluated with a colposcopy. Goff evaluated the Vira Type kit in patients with ASCUS. Of 171 patients, 19% had detectable HPV DNA and 85% were of the high-risk HPV types. Only 6 of 28 patients with atypia and high-risk HPV types had CIN; none had CIN III. The authors thought that available HPV typing was not clinically useful in identifying patients who should have a colposcopy. Sedlacek reached similar conclusions in 334 women referred for evaluation of abnormal cytology. He could not demonstrate a relationship between the HPV type and the high-grade biopsy proven CIN using the Southern blot technique. On the other hand, using PCR with consensus primers or semiquantitative PCR suggests a significant correlation of high-risk HPV types with CIN II and III. Hatch evaluated The Hybrid Capture kit in 311 patients who were referred for evaluation of abnormal cytology. Fifty percent of LSIL, 26% of HSIL, and 44% of those with invasive cancers were HPV-DNA negative. The test missed one-third of histologic LSIL and HSIL in patients with LSIL on cytology. In the ASCUS group, the ability of the test to identify histologic HSIL noted a sensitivity of 60%, a specificity of 68%, and a PPV of 35%. With these results, most clinicians would not want to rely on this test to predict which patient may have significant cervical neoplasia, particularly invasive disease.

In a study of 1128 women referred with an abnormal Pap smear, Kaufman and associates repeated the Pap smear, obtained a sample for HPV testing (Profile kit), and did a colposcopy. They performed 1075 colposcopic-directed biopsies and endocervical curettages (ECCs). HPV DNA was identified in 488 women. Positivity of HPV increased as the severity of the referral Pap smear increased (ASCUS 25%; HSIL 44%), and this also correlated with biopsy results (HPV in CIN I 39%; CIN III 59%). The detection of high-risk HPV DNA in women with any degree of SIL on the referral Pap smear poorly predicted biopsy-proven CIN III. Sensitivity of HPV to predict CIN II and III with LSIL on a Pap smear was only 58%; specificity was 68%; and PPV was 22%. If HPV had been used as the only triage in patients with LSIL on Pap, > 40% of women with confirmed CIN II or III would not have had a colposcopy or biopsy.

In a follow-up study of these same patients with CIN II or III, the authors evaluated HPV testing using a PCR technique that is the most sensitive for the HPV tests. The PCR appeared to be more sensitive than the Profile, but the PPV was similar (21.7% and 22.8%). Approximately one quarter of the patients with negative results on biopsies were HPV-positive and almost one half of patients with CIN II or III were HPV-16-negative. When PPV and NPV were evaluated, combined triage did not improve on either HPV testing or cytology alone. Cost analysis was performed, and repeat cytology was better in identifying CIN II or III with half the cost of HPV testing. The authors thought that at present the use of these tests should be restricted to the research arena and should not be used in routine clinical practice.

In evaluation of 537 women with a referral Pap of CIN I, colposcopy and HPV typing (PCR) were done along with a repeat Pap. Based on a repeat Pap and colposcopy impression, 142 women were presumed to have CIN II or a worse lesion. In the group with CIN I, 45% tested positive for HPV and 52% tested positive in the CIN II category. In the latter group, HPV positivity among women younger than 22 years of age and with a history of current cigarette smoking in people 22 years or older were significant predictors of patients with CIN II or III. The authors believed that the age limitation would limit the usefulness of HPV screening. Most authors have noted a decrease in HPV positivity with age, even though more severe lesions appear in older patients. Manos and colleagues evaluated the use of HPV testing compared with repeat Pap smears in women with an ASCUS Pap. Of 973 patients with ASCUS and a definitive histologic diagnosis, 65 (6.7%) women had HSIL or cancer. The HPV test was positive using capture II method in 89.2%, and the repeat Pap smear was abnormal in 76.2% (not statistically significant). Triage based on HPV typing alone or on a repeat Pap smear would only refer a similar number of patients for colposcopy (39%). False-positive results for HPV testing and repeat Pap smears were similar when the histology was normal.

In a report from Italy, 221 patients with Pap smears showing minor atypia were evaluated with HPV testing, cervicography, and repeat cytology. In a multivariate analysis, only cytology and cervicography retained an association with histologic diagnosis of CIN II–III. The HPV test did not influence the decision for a biopsy nor was it associated with a histologic diagnosis. A prospective study of biopsy-proven CIN I was evaluated with regard to risk factors for progression. Of 163 women, 13 (8%) progressed to CIN III; 43% regressed; and 49% persisted. All progression occurred in women who tested positive for HPV DNA and who had an immature abnormal transformation zone on the initial evaluation. In addition, women who complained of vaginal discharge on enrollment increased the risk of progression. None of the CIN I patients with HPV DNA-positive test results progressed. Although all the patients who progressed tested HPV-positive, 89 (90%) who were HPV positive did not progress.

In a clinical opinion, Kaufman and Adams reviewed the current status of HPV testing in predicting the presence of HSIL or cancer in patients with ASCUS or LSIL cytology. Using the profile and hybrid capsule tests for HPV to identify CIN II or III, sensitivity varied from 55–93%. In the studies with the highest sensitivity, the specificity ranged from 24–67% and PPV ranged from 17–28%. To date, no data suggest that HPV testing has or will decrease morbidity and mortality from invasive cancer. Their opinion indicated that presently HPV testing has little clinical value to the practitioner. The use of HPV typing to predict progression of CIN has been suggested. In a study by Gaarenstoom, HPV 16 presence was significantly related to progression of CIN—29% vs 0% in HPV-negative lesions. All patients had colposcopically directed biopsies but were followed without being treated. PCR with a primer was used to identify HPV. In 1993, a diagnostic and therapeutic technology assessment (DATTA) was performed by the American Medical Association. Three questions were asked. Is HPV DNA testing an effective method of guiding therapy in:

1. women with atypical Pap smears;
2. LSIL, and
3. a condylomatous cervical lesion identified at colposcopy whose histologic diagnosis is indeterminate?

The scientific literature was reviewed, and a panel from the obstetric-gynecologic, pathology, oncology, infectious disease, and preventive medicine community was asked to answer the three questions. Sixty percent, 62%, and 55%, respectively, thought that HPV DNA testing was investigational with regard to the three questions posed. Only 22%, 15%, and 17% thought that HPV DNA testing may be "promising", and a similar group noted that it had "doubtful" effectiveness.

Recently cell proliferation pathways have been evaluated in regards to HPV. This has led to evaluation of genes and growth factors. Data has suggested that the progression of CIN to cancer can lead to an upregulation of epidermal growth factor receptor (EGF-R). This upregulation is common to all squamous cell cancers; however in cervical cancer, EGF-R upregulation leads to a specific up regulation of insulin-like growth factor-II (IGF-II). IGF-I but not IGF-II levels are elevated in other gyn cancers as well as breast and prostate cancers. It has been suggested that IGF-II levels could be used as a monitor for CIN as well as cervical cancers post therapy. Increased serum IGF-II levels in cervical cancer are accompanied by a significantly reduced level of serum IGF-binding protein-3 (IGF-BP3). IGF-BP3 appears to be a cell regulatory and pro-apoptotic agent and an increase in its level offers an excellent prognosis for cervical cancer regression through its downregulating effects on EGF-R, IGF-II and vascular-endothelial growth factor (VEGF). VEGF-B is known to be elevated during metastatic spread of many cancers. A reduction in IGF-BP3 levels have been observed upon treatment with VEGF in HPV-positive and negative cell lines. VEGF-C has been found to be significantly elevated in women with persistent cervical cancer or HSIL and appears to be effective in early diagnosis of metastatic cervical cancer. VEGF-C appears to be unique to cervical cancer in that it interacts with IGF-II and IGF-BP3 through EGF-R. Interestingly, VEGF-C is upregulated by nicotine in cervical cancer cell lines. This translational research may lead not only to a better understanding of cervical cancer and its precursors but may also increase our ability to predict which CIN may progress as well as monitor cervical cancer post treatment and identify persistence or recurrence at an earlier time than currently available.

It has been suggested that the sexual partners of women with CIN and HPV infection should be treated to control the infectious process among women. Campion evaluated 140 women who presented for treatment of biopsy-proven CIN. As a control group, 280 females matched for age and disease severity (two control patients for each study patient) were identified. HPV typing was performed on each control and case. The atypical T-Z was destroyed with the laser in each. Repeat HPV typing was done at 6 months. In the study group, the current sexual partners were evaluated and all HPV lesions were treated. The male partners of the control group were not treated. The primary cure rate of CIN was the same in the two groups (92% study vs 94% control group). The importance of controlling disease in the male sexual partner may be overemphasized.

It is now generally accepted that the virus itself cannot be eliminated with any known therapy. Therefore is there any benefit from knowing HPV subtypes that relates to clinical management? There probably is not. Not only is HPV commonly found in as many as 80% of normal (non-CIN) patients, but after treatment for CIN, HPV was found in 100% of 20 females with CIN who were successfully treated with laser.

Riva and associates treated 25 women with koilocytotic atypia, CIN, vaginal intraepithelial neoplasia (VAIN), or vulval intraepithelial neoplasia (VIN). All patients had laser therapy of the cervix, vagina, and vulva in continuity. Morbidity was significant. Histologic persistence of subclinical HPV infection was documented in 88% of patients after treatment. Neither treatment of male sexual consorts nor sexual abstinence significantly improved treatment outcome.

HIV and cervical neoplasia

Human immunodeficiency virus (HIV) infection is an ever-increasing disease affecting all our citizens. Initially thought to be limited to homosexual males and intravenous (IV) drug users, more and more women are being diagnosed with HIV and acquired immunodeficiency virus (AIDS). An estimated 850,000–950,000 persons in the USA are living with HIV including 180,000–220,000 who do not know they are infected. In 2003, the estimated number of AIDS was 43,171 of which 11,498 cases are in females. Eighty percent of women who contract AIDS are in the reproductive age group. Approximately 25% acquire these infections during adolescence, and over three-fourths of female cases in 2003 were contracted by heterosexual transmission. In women, early manifestations of the disease are often gynecologic, such as chronic yeast infections, pelvic inflammatory disease, genital warts, and herpes. On January 1, 1993, the Centers for Disease Control and Prevention (CDC) expanded the case definition of AIDS to include HIV-positive women with invasive cervical cancer. This inclusion remains controversial, because it apparently was based on preliminary data. These data suggested that in HIV-positive patients, there was a high incidence of CIN, Pap smears were unreliable, and other diagnostic procedures (i.e., colposcopy) should be part of routine evaluation of these patients.

It is well recognized that immunodeficiency predisposes to development of neoplasia in congenital disorders such as Wiskott–Aldrich syndrome, in which the incidence of cancer may be increased 10,000-fold. Renal transplant patients appear to be at increased risk for lower genital tract neoplasia. Cervical neoplasia has been reported to range from 5–40%, and anogenital neoplasia is reported 9 to 14 times greater in these patients compared with controls. It is not surprising, therefore, to see an increased incidence of cancers in HIV-positive patients. Kaposi sarcoma and non-Hodgkin's lymphoma are the most commonly seen cancers in patients with AIDS. Squamous cell carcinomas of the anogenital tract and oral cavity have been reported with increased frequency. Spinillo noted in 75 HIV-positive women that 22 (29%) had CIN. Sun evaluated in a cross-sectional study of 344 HIV-positive and 325 HIV-negative women. HIV-positive women were more likely to have HPV-DNA of any type, HPV-16 or 18, or more than one HPV type than HIV-negative patients. The HIV-positive patients with HPV DNA were more likely to have CIN than were HPV-infected, HIV-negative women. Essentially, all studies noted a much higher rate (up to tenfold) of CIN in HIV-positive women compared with controls. Maiman noted that 39% of HIV-positive patients but with normal cytology had CIN. He suggested in these women that Pap smears should be done every 6 months and that they should have a routine baseline colposcopy or cervicography. Subsequently, several large studies representing several hundred patients noted only a false-negative Pap smear rate of 10–19%. Wright noted that the Pap smear failed to detect abnormalities in only

Table 1–2 CDC GUIDELINES FOR THE HIV-POSITIVE PATIENT

1. All HIV-positive patients should be encouraged to have a Pap smear.
2. If the first Pap smear is negative, repeat in 6 months and then annually if normal.
3. If the first Pap smear has a severe inflammation with reactive squamous cells, repeat in 3 months.
4. For ASC-US and all SIL, perform a colposcopy.

ASC-US, atypical squamous cells of undetermined significance; CDC, Centers for Disease Control and Prevention; HIV, human immunodeficiency virus; Pap, Papanicolaou; SIL, squamous intraepithelial lesions.

0.8% of 398 HIV-positive women who actually had high-grade CIN. The CDC currently recommends that all HIV-positive women have a Pap smear (Table 1–2). If the result is normal, repeat the smear in 6 months then annually thereafter as long as the Pap smear is normal. If the first Pap has severe inflammation with reactive squamous cells, the smear should be repeated in 3 months. In patients with ASCUS or any degree of SIL, further evaluation (colposcopy) appears warranted. Not only are HIV-positive patients at greater risk for CIN, but also the severity of the disease appears to be related to T cell function. HIV-positive patients with CIN have absolute T cell counts and T4:T8 ratios of about one half of those HIV-positive patients without CIN. Wright noted in an evaluation of 398 HIV-positive and 357 HIV-negative patients that CIN was independently associated with HPV infections (odds ratio [OR] 9.8), HIV infection (OR 3.5), CD4+ T lymphocyte count < 200 (OR 2.7), and an age older than 34 years (OR 2.0). Johnson noted that one half of patients with CD4 T cell counts < 200/µL were infected with HPV-18 and that HPV-18 was detected in 19% of all HIV-positive patients.

Treatment of CIN in HIV-positive patients appears to have a high failure rate regardless of the modality used. Cryosurgery is reported to have a 48–78% failure rate, although cold knife cone has also reported a 50% failure. Loop electrosurgical excision procedure (LEEP) in one study noted a 56% failure.

Recurrence was associated with CD4 and T lymphocyte counts but not with a grade of CIN. HPV-18 may possibly account for the high failure rate. The AIDS Clinical Trial Group is currently investigating the use of topical 5-fluorouracil (5-FU) maintenance therapy as prophylaxis against recurrent CIN after initial therapy.

Data collected by the CDC for the first 6 months of 1993 noted 36,627 new patients with AIDS; 89 were signaled by the presence of cervical cancer. Palefsky noted HIV-positive women are at a higher risk of progression to invasive disease. Maiman found that women who had cervical cancer and who were HIV positive had more advanced cancer (i.e., high-grade tumors with lymph node involvement). The prognosis was poor, and most deaths were from cervical cancer and not from AIDS. Although the potential for this epidemic may be present and all should be aware of the potential, to date the death rate from cervical cancer in young patients has not increased.

Natural history

The average age of patients with carcinoma in situ reproducibly is 10–15 years less than the average age of patients with invasive cancer of the cervix. However, there are many exceptions; in the past two decades, carcinoma in situ and invasive disease have been reported in an increasing number of patients in their late teens and early 20s. Whether all invasive carcinomas begin as in situ lesions is unknown, but Peterson reported that in one-third of 127 untreated patients, invasive carcinoma developed subsequent to carcinoma in situ at the end of 9 years. Masterson found that 28% of 25 untreated patients demonstrated invasive carcinoma at the end of 5 years.

Carcinoma in situ is usually asymptomatic, and on routine examination the lesion is frequently not observed. Recognition of the lesion is assisted considerably by the use of cytologic testing and colposcopy. The mucous membrane sometimes bleeds easily on contact, and erosion or a superficial defect of the ectocervix is relatively common in patients with carcinoma in situ, but these findings are not pathognomonic. The diagnosis must always be confirmed by histologic sections of a biopsy specimen.

What happens to a patient with early CIN in regard to its natural history is important, because it relates to management. A review of the literature of the last 40 years suggests that more advanced lesions (CIN III) are more likely to persist or progress than CIN I. CIN III can regress spontaneously, but more important, it is suggested that progression to cancer occurs more than 15% of the time, whereas CIN I progresses to cancer only 1% of the time. The regression and persistence of CIN I and II appear to be similar. If the eventual outcome of a given patient with an abnormal Pap smear could be predicted, the problem of management would be greatly simplified. Certainly, not all patients with abnormal cervical cells develop cancer of the cervix or even progression of CIN. Therefore, any patient with any degree of dysplasia should be evaluated further.

Unfortunately, most of the studies performed on the natural history of this disease were carried out in the absence of the current diagnostic techniques, namely, colposcopy. Most studies used cytologic tests or biopsy as the diagnostic tools, resulting in varying progression/regression rates. Harlan reviewed many of the studies on the biologic behavior of cervical dysplasia. The occurrence of the progression of CIN lesions to either a more severe form or invasive cancer ranges from 1.4–60%. Of interest is that the two most variant studies used cytologic tests alone to follow patients. The problems of definitive diagnosis using this technique have been studied in detail, and considerable variation has been noted even in the best of hands. When biopsies are performed, particularly if the lesion is small, the natural history of the disease may be disrupted, further complicating the evaluation of this entity. Even studies on the biologic behavior of cervical carcinoma in situ are varied, with progression to invasive cancer being reported in up to 50% of cases. The differences in these findings may very well be a result of the length of follow-up once the diagnosis of carcinoma in situ was established. Some patients with CIN develop invasive cancer, whereas others, even though followed for many years, do not progress either to a more severe form of CIN or to invasive cancer.

Rapid-onset cancer in patients with normal cytology is a phenomenon that is often discussed; however, when evaluated, the cytology appears to be infrequently documented. In a study from Canada, the authors found that more than 95% of so-called rapid-onset cancers (appearing within 3 years of a "normal" Pap) were due to inadequate and false-negative smears and failure to evaluate an abnormal test. In an Italian study of 115 cervical cancer patients, 70% had never had a Pap smear; 7% were diagnosed at their first test; and 10% had false-negative cytology. The other patients had either poor compliance or inadequate evaluation.

It has become apparent from recent studies that CIN is being diagnosed at a much younger age. In our material, the median age for carcinoma in situ of the cervix has decreased from approximately 40 to 28 years of age. This may reflect only that screening of high-risk patients is done at an earlier time, resulting in a diagnosis at a younger age. Because most of these women desire children and in many cases have not started to have families, preservation of the integrity of the cervix and the uterus is important. In an analysis of approximately 800 patients with CIN at the Duke University Medical Center, 30% were 20 years of age or younger when the diagnosis was established. Nulliparity was seen in about one quarter of the population, and 60% had one child or none. More than 95% of the patients had had intercourse by the age of 20, and one half had become sexually active by 16 years of age. More than one half of these patients had three or more sexual partners. About one half of these patients had the diagnosis of CIN established within 5 years of the beginning of their sexual activity. Screening these patients at an early age, when they seek contraception or other medical attention, is important and should be done routinely. This screening probably explains why the diagnosis is being made at a much earlier age.

Certainly, it is not at all unusual to see patients in their teens or early 20s with carcinoma in situ of the cervix. Therefore, the lesion may be identified early in the spectrum of disease, and a patient may continue with CIN for a prolonged period, even after reaching the level of a CIN III lesion. Table 1–3 presents the transition time of CIN in our patients. Those patients who progress to carcinoma in situ do so within a very short time. After that level of abnormality is reached, stabilization may occur in many of the patients. To date, no method is available to predict which patient will remain within the CIN category, which will progress to a more severe form of CIN or to invasive cancer or within what time frame this transition will occur.

Table 1–3 TRANSITION TIME OF CERVICAL INTRAEPITHELIAL NEOPLASIA

Stages	Mean years
Normal to mild-to-moderate dysplasia	1.62
Normal to moderate-to-severe dysplasia	2.20
Normal to carcinoma in situ	4.51

The American Society for Colposcopy and Cervical Pathology (ASCCP) in 2001 developed consensus guidelines for management of women with CIN. As a part of that deliberation, the literature was reviewed in regards to the natural history of cervical neoplasia. The natural history of CIN I was reviewed for 4504 patients and noted spontaneous regression in 57% of patients while 11% progressed to CIN II, III or cancer. The rate of progression to cancer was 0.3%. A meta-analysis of natural history of CIN I noted similar conclusions.

Cytology

As has already been noted, genital cytology has had a major impact on the incidence of and death rate from cervical cancer. Despite general agreement about this finding, one of the problems with cervical cytology is the false-negative rate. A major concern of clinicians has been the ever changing terminology, which has resulted in a lack of meaning with regard to clinical relevance. The Pap classification has been changed so many times that the numbers have no constant meaning. Many cytologists changed to a descriptive term (dysplasia or, more recently, CIN) to indicate their diagnostic impression of the smear. In most cases, this terminology was clinically useful; however, there was an increasing tendency to use terms such as inflammatory atypia, squamous atypia but not dysplasia, which did not necessarily convey any clinical implications. In an attempt to clarify the varied terminology, the Bethesda system was developed in 1988. This new system was subsequently used in an increasing number of cytology laboratories, mainly because of federal mandates.

It became apparent within a short period of time that the Bethesda system had nomenclature and classification that was confusing with conflicting impressions to the clinician. As a result, a 2001 Bethesda system and new terminology was developed and reported in 2002. This is currently the cytology reporting system that is used in the USA today. This update has been generally accepted as an improvement and eliminated those categories that led to different interpretations. For instance, the 1991 Bethesda system had a category that had to do with specimen adequacy which was reported as "satisfactory", "less than optimal" later renamed "satisfactory but limited by…" or "unsatisfactory". The "less than" category was used mainly to note an absence of endocervical cells or squamous metaplastic cells. The 2001 Bethesda has only two categories: satisfactory for evaluation and unsatisfactory

Table 1–4 BETHESDA 2001 CLASSIFICATION
Interpretation/results
Negative for intraepithelial lesion or malignancy
Organisms may be identified
Other non-neoplastic findings may be noted
Inflammation
Radiation changes
Atrophy
Glandular cells status post hysterectomy
Atrophy
Epithelial cell abnormalities
Squamous cells
Atypical squamous cells (ASC)
Of undetermined significance (ASC-US)
Cannot exclude HSIL (ASC-H)
Low-grade squamous intraepithelial lesions (LSIL)
HPV, CIN I
High-grade squamous intraepithelial lesions (HSIL)
CIN II, CIN III
Squamous cell carcinoma
Glandular cell
Atypical glandular cells (AGC)—specify origin
Atypical glandular cells favor neoplastic—specify origin
Endocervical adenocarcinoma in situ (AIS)
Adenocarcinoma

for evaluation (specify reason). The initial general categorization listed "within normal limits" and "benign cellular changes" which were combined in 2001 as "negative for intraepithelial lesion or malignancy." These as well as other changes have improved the communication to the clinician.

One of the major changes was made in the epithelial cell abnormality designation (Table 1–4). The previous category of ASCUS represented by far the largest number of abnormal Pap smears reported each year in the US (about three million). The vast majority of these ASCUS smears on evaluation found no cervical epithelial abnormalities, although a small number did harbor CIN II, III. Cytologists were encouraged to qualify ASCUS as to whether this was a reactive process or favor SIL but these smears were mainly classified as ASCUS, not otherwise specified which was not helpful to the clinicians. The 2001 classification redefined this category and renamed it as ASC (atypical squamous cells) with the subclassification of ASC-US (of undetermined significance) and ASC-H (cannot exclude HSIL). The latter represents about 5–10% of all ASC, which can eliminate the vast majority of women with ASC undergoing unwarranted more extensive, expensive evaluation.

The low-grade SIL (HPV, CIN I) and high-grade SIL (CIN II and CIN III) classifications remain the same.

Under glandular cells, the previous AGUS (atypical glandular cells of undetermined significance) was interpreted by many clinicians as a similar process of ASCUS and managed accordingly (repeat Pap smear). The AGUS smear carried a much greater risk of having a significant number of cervical and endometrial lesions including cancer. The 2001 system has designated new categories under glandular cells: atypical glandular cells (AGC) in which the cytologist should specify origin; endocervical, endometrium, or not otherwise not specified); atypical glandular cells, favor neoplastic; endocervical adenocarcinoma in situ (AIS) and adenocarcinoma.

New diagnostic technology

Although the Pap smear has reduced dramatically the incidence in deaths from cervical cancer, false-negative smears are known to occur with various imprecise numbers being highlighted by the large financial amounts awarded in lawsuits. It is well recognized that the rate of accuracy of the Pap smear is not 100%, as in any test, although the law apparently so adjudicated it as being absolutely accurate. As a result, newer technology has been developed in an attempt to decrease the present false-negative rate. As has been previously noted, the incidence of mortality would be greatly reduced if all women were screened at regular intervals and appropriate evaluations were performed.

Fluid-based, thin layer preparations have been developed in an attempt to present to the cytologist a uniform, well-distributed layer of cells that are less likely to be distorted or obscured by blood, mucus, or inflammatory debris. The collection device, instead of being directly applied to the slide, is rinsed in a vial containing a buffered alcohol solution. The cell suspension is put through a filter system where blood and debris are removed, and a sample of cells is placed on a slide in a 20-mm diameter specimen. This preparation is much cleaner than that normally seen. This thin-prep (TP) technique has been approved by the Food and Drug Administration (FDA). Several studies have been published comparing mainly the TP with conventional Pap (CP) smears. In one of the first studies done by Wilbur and associates, a total of 3218 patients had a single cytologic sample that was split into matched pairs. A CP was made, and the other pair was prepared using the TP technique. There was exact agreement using the Bethesda terminology in 88.3% and 96% when negative/atypical vs positive findings were evaluated. The inferred false-negative rate was 15% for CP and 4% for TP (0.8% vs 3.1% respectively of total smears). No histologic correlation was reported.

The study by Lee was pivotal in obtaining FDA approval. There were 7360 women from six sites who participated in a split sample/match pair double-match study to compare TP with CP. The abstract noted that for the three screening centers, 65% more LSIL plus (LSIL, HSIL, and cancer) with the TP compared with the CP. This represented only 30% of the abnormalities. When the hospitals were evaluated, TP identified 446 abnormalities compared with 442 identified with the CP. When both screening and hospital centers were combined, there was only a 14% difference between the CP and the TP-all in the LSIL category. HSIL did not increase, and TPs missed three of four cancers noted by CP. Again, there was no path correlation.

In another study, Papillo and colleagues evaluated 16,314 TPs (subset of 80,574) compared with 18,569 CPs taken. The two groups were from different times and from different patient and physician bases. From the 16,340 TPs, 8574 TPs were chosen for the study. Using the TPs, 90.9% of the smears were normal compared with 89.4% CPs, ASCUS/atypical glandular cells of undetermined significance (AGUS) 6.5% vs 8.9% and LSIL plus 2.4% vs 1.6%, respectively. Those patients with LSIL plus on CP, 211/300 and 140/231 on the TP underwent subsequent biopsies. The authors state that a 16.3% improvement was seen with TP in patients with the histologic diagnosis of CIN and 9.3% with CIN II–III. There were 59 (28%) CPs with benign biopsies vs 27 (19%) TPs. This 8% represents a 30.7% difference. The 4.3% difference between TPs and CPs (30.7% vs 26.4%) for CIN I was noted by the authors to represent a 16.3% difference. The 50% vs 45.8% (4.2%) was said to represent a 9.3% difference for CIN II and III histologic diagnosis. The reduction of benign biopsies and the increase in confirmed CIN I–III was not statistically significant.

In a large study by Roberts and associates, 35,560 split-sample paired CP and TP slides were prepared. There was total agreement in 94.3% of the slides. Of the 1946 discordant slides, TPs showed more severe abnormalities in 1194 cases compared with CPs, and the opposite was true in 753 slides. Of these, colposcopy was recommended on the basis of the TP alone for 167 patients and CP alone for 104 patients. For those with HSIL on the TP and CP, histologic confirmation was the same with similar numbers having LSIL on the path evaluation. There were a greater number of unsatisfactory smears with CP compared with TPs (3.5%) vs 0.7%; however, a larger number of TPs had no endocervical cells (20% vs 8.3%).

In a study from Costa Rica, 8636 patients were evaluated with TP and CP along with HPV typing, cervicography, colposcopy, and biopsies as indicated. There were 323 patients identified with CIN I–III or cancer; 284 patients were identified by TP; and 222 patients were identified by CP if ASCUS was the trigger for further evaluation. If LSIL was the trigger, 257 patients and 210 patients, respectively, were identified. If only the difference of CIN I–III (on biopsy) was compared between TP and CP, 19 more lesions were identified with TP (0.22% of the total smears) using ASCUS as the trigger and only 13 (0.15%) if low-grade SIL plus cytology was the trigger for further evaluation. The false-positive result was 530 (6.9%) patients for TP and 128 (1.6%) patients for CP. The false-positive rate for TP was considerably higher than that for the true abnormalities identified. This study, which is suggestive of statistically significant better pickup with TP, must be taken with some reservation. The population screen had five times the incidence of cervical cancer than that seen in the USA and, therefore, the difference may be appreciably increased compared with the population of the USA. Also, the CPs were read in Costa Rica, whereas the TPs were evaluated in the USA. Potential bias may be considerable using different laboratories with different nuances in their interpretation. If only LSIL plus cytology was considered abnormal, 3 of 11 cancers were missed with TP compared with 2 with CP. The authors conclude by stating that TP is at least as good as CP in detecting CIN and carcinoma.

The TP has been accepted by many as the new standard method for cervical cytology. A meta-analysis of 25 studies indicated that the TP is as good or superior to the conventional Pap smear. The TP provides improved sample adequacy. There appeared to be an improved diagnosis of LSIL and HSIL but no difference in ASCUS. The US Preventive Services Task Force (USPSTF) in 2003, after a review of the literature, concluded that the evidence is insufficient to recommend for or against the routine use of new technologies to screen for cervical cancer. They found poor evidence that liquid-based, cytology computerized rescreening and algorithm-based screening are more effective than conventional Pap smears in decreasing mortality from cervical cancer. The USPSTF found few studies testing the new technologies against colposcopy or histology. Therefore, sensitivity, specificity and predictive values of the new technologies cannot be compared with tests of conventional cytology in the same population. There have been no prospective studies comparing the new technologies to conventional Pap smear screening in regards to invasive cancer, cost or cost effectiveness. They felt that the new technologies would fall within the traditional range considered to be cost effective ($50,000 per life year) only if used in screening intervals of 3 years or longer.

The USPSTF also concluded that the evidence is insufficient to recommend for or against the routine use of HPV testing as primary screening for cervical cancer.

Pathology

Cervical intraepithelial neoplasia (CIN) is the term now used to encompass all epithelial abnormalities of the cervix. The epithelial cells are malignant but confined to the epithelium. The older terminology using dysplasia and carcinoma in situ connotes a two-tier disease process that, at least in the past, has influenced therapy. That is, if only dysplasia was present, no or limited treatment was needed. If carcinoma in situ was diagnosed, in many cases a hysterectomy was recommended. This concept is inappropriate, particularly when the cervical epithelium may be no thicker than 0.25 mm. Although CIN has been arbitrarily divided into three subdivisions, it does suggest that CIN is a single neoplastic continuum. The histologic criteria for a CIN diagnosis depend on the findings of nuclear aneuploidy, abnormal mitotic figures, and a loss of normal maturation of the epithelium (Fig. 1–2). CIN is divided into grade I, II, or III, depending on the extent of cellular stratification aberration within the epithelium. In CIN I, the upper two-thirds of the epithelium, although showing some nuclear abnormalities, have undergone cytoplasmic differentiation. The cells in the lower one-third lack evidence of cytoplasmic differentiation or normal maturation (loss of polarity of the cells). Mitotic figures are few and, if present, are normal. In CIN II, the abnormal changes of CIN I involve the

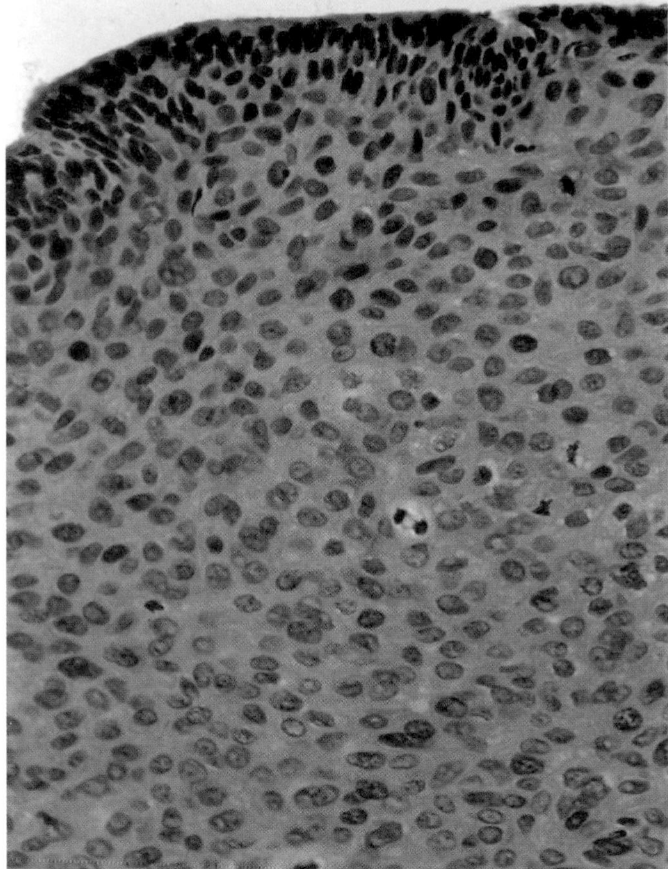

Figure 1–2 A cervical intraepithelial neoplasia lesion with multiple mitotic figures.

lower two-thirds of the epithelium. The CIN III lesions have full-thickness changes with undifferentiated non-stratified cells. Nuclear pleomorphism is common, and mitotic figures are abnormal. On the basis of nuclear DNA studies, some investigators have suggested that most lesions diagnosed as CIN I are, in fact, flat condyloma that contain human papilloma viruses 6/11 (groups). It should be remembered that HPV-16/18 are more frequently found in CIN I than other subtypes, including HPV-6/11. The impression is that these lesions, by and large, are not significant relative to this neoplastic process and have a very low risk for progressing to cancer compared with lesions containing HPV-16/18. As the epithelium becomes more involved with this intraepithelial neoplasia, there is a greater probability for HPV-16/18 identified with potential for invasion. HPV-16/18 can be present in CIN I and HPV-6/11 in higher-grade CIN.

Evaluation of an abnormal cervical cytology

As noted above, cervical cytology is a screening test. Much has been written about the reliability and the reproducibility of cervical cytology even though this has been credited with the significant decrease in cervical cancer as well as cervical cancer mortality that has occurred in the western world over the last several decades (Table 1–5). In the atypical squamous cell of undetermined significance—low-grade squamous epithelial lesion triage study (ALTS), 4948 monolayer cytological slides were obtained from patients entering into the study. This was from 3488 women who had participated in comparing alternative strategies for the initial management of women with ASC-US. There were four clinical centers that participated in this study. Cytology was interpreted in the individual institutions and then sent for central review. These specimens were independently reviewed by the pathology quality control group (QC). This review was done in a blinded fashion. Of the 1473 original interpretations of ASC-US, the QC reviewers concurred in only 43% rendering less severe readings for most of the rest. Interobserver variation also occurred in the more significant cytological interpretations as in those who had HSILs, concurrence was present in only 47.1% with 22% and 22.6% of the remainder interpreted as LSIL or ASC-US by the QC reviewers. Of further interest is the fact that histological interpretative reducibility on the biopsies was really no better than cytological reproducibilities.

Table 1–5 CAUSES OF ABNORMAL PAPANICOLAOU SMEARS
Invasive cancer
Cervical intraepithelial neoplasia
Atrophic changes
Flat condyloma
Inflammation, especially trichomoniasis and chronic cervicitis
Regeneration after injury (metaplasia)
Vaginal cancer
Vulvar cancer
Upper genital tract cancer (endometrium, fallopian tube, ovary)
Previous radiation therapy

Even with the problems of reproducibility in regards to cytology, the ALTS gave some important information as far as management of abnormalities obtained on Pap smears. As a result of these studies, a consensus conference was held in Bethesda, MD in the fall of 2001 sponsored by the American Society for Colposcopy and Cervical Pathology (ASCCP). It was felt that since about 7% of all Pap smears obtained in the USA were diagnosed with some degree of cytological abnormality with the vast majority noting only minor changes, generalized guidelines for management should be developed in order to make the most responsible use of time and resources. These guidelines may aid the clinician in the management of patients with an abnormal cytology.

Atypical squamous cells

As previously noted, the 2001 Bethesda system subdivided ASC into two categories, ASC-US and ASC-H. The patients who have ASC-US have a 5–17% chance of having CIN II or III confirmed by biopsy, whereas with ASC-H,

Table 1–6 MANAGEMENT OF WOMEN WITH ASCUS CYTOLOGY

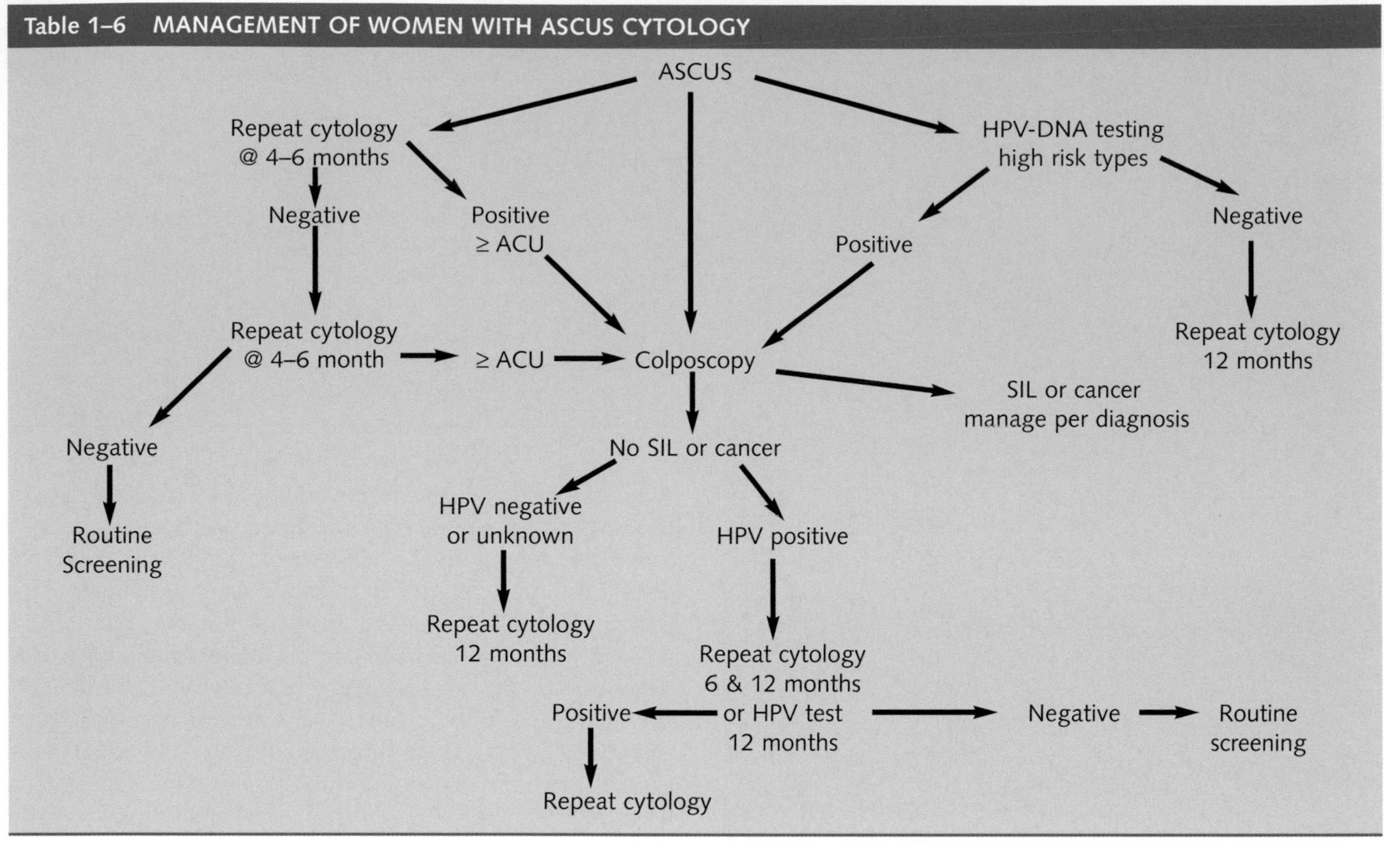

CIN II or III is identified in 24–94% of women. The risk of invasive cancer with ASC is low (approximately 0.1–0.2%).

Several approaches have been used in the management of a woman who has ASC (Table 1–6). Repeat cytology has been widely used with a sensitivity of a single test for detecting CIN II and III between 0.67 and 0.85. Colposcopy has also been used. Its advantage is that immediately the woman can be informed of the presence or absence of a significant disease. Sensitivity for distinguishing normal from abnormal tissue on the cervix by colposcopy was 0.96 and with a weighted mean specificity of 0.48. Several large studies have now been performed utilizing the DNA testing as a triage mechanism for the management of women with ASC. The sensitivity of HPV DNA testing for detection of biopsy-proven CIN II and III has been said to be 0.83–1.0. The negative predictive value for high-risk types of HPV is generally reported to be 0.98 or greater. Between 31% and 60% of all women with ASC will have high-risk types of HPV with the amount decreasing with increasing age. Recent data suggest that young women (≤ 20 years old in one study and ≤ 29 years old in another) will have a high-risk HPV type in up to 80% of individuals. This makes HPV DNA testing as part of the triage less applicable. So-called "reflex" HPV DNA testing has been used also in the triage mechanism. This utilizes liquid-based cytology employing the leftover liquid subsequent to the return of ASC cytology. With the above as a background, the following represents the 2001 consensus guidelines for cervical cytological abnormalities.

ASC-US

Acceptable methods for managing women with ASC-US may be repeat cervical cytology testing, colposcopy or DNA testing for high-risk types of HPV. When liquid-based cytology is used, then reflex testing is felt to be the preferred management of these women. Women with ASC-US who test negative for high-risk HPV DNA can then be followed up with repeat cytological testing in 12 months. For those individuals who are positive for high-risk types of HPV but do not have biopsy-confirmed CIN, it is suggested that repeat cytological testing at 6 and 12 months be carried out with referral back to colposcopy if the results of ASC-US or greater is obtained or HPV DNA testing at 12 months returns high-risk positive types.

When repeat cervical cytology testing is used, this is done at 4–6-month intervals until two consecutive "negative for intraepithelial lesions or malignancy" are obtained. Women with ASC-US or greater on repeat tests should be referred for colposcopy. If two repeat negative smears are obtained, then the woman can be returned to routine cytological screening. When immediate colposcopy is used, in those individuals not found to have CIN, they should be followed with repeat cytological testing at 12 months. It was strongly recommended that diagnostic excisional procedures such as LEEP should not be routinely used to treat women with ASC in the absence of biopsy-confirmed CIN.

There are special circumstances in women with ASC-US that should be taken into consideration.

Postmenopausal women: In women with ASC-US or

who have cytological evidence of atrophy, local intravaginal estrogen can be used for several days and then about a week after completion of therapy repeat cytology can be carried out. If the result is negative, then the test should be repeated in 4–6 months. If, in fact, the abnormality remains, then the patient should be referred for colposcopy.

Immunosuppressed women: Referral to colposcopy is recommended in all who have ASC-US. This includes women infected with HIV, irrespective of the CD4 cell count, HIV viral load, or antiretroviral therapy.

Pregnant patient: ASC-US should be managed as the non-pregnant patient.

ASC-H

Since women with ASC-H have an appreciable higher chance of having CIN II and III compared with women with ASC-US, all individuals should be referred for colposcopic evaluation. When no lesion is identified, it is suggested that a review of the cytology, colposcopy and histological results be performed. If on review a revised interpretation is submitted, then management should be follow guidelines for the revised interpretation. If cytological interpretation of ASC-H is upheld, then follow-up in 6–12 months with cytology or HPV DNA testing at 12 months is acceptable. Women who are found to have ASC or greater on repeat cervical cytology testing or who test positive for high-risk HPV DNA should be referred for colposcopy.

Low-grade squamous intraepithelial lesions (LSIL)

In most laboratories, the median rate of LSIL is 1.6%; however, this may be as high as 7–8% in laboratories serving high-risk populations. Approximately 15–30% of women with LSIL will have CIN II or III identified on subsequent cervical biopsies. In the ALT study, 83% of women referred for evaluation of LSIL cytology tested positive for high-risk HPV. With this high incidence, using HPV DNA as part of the triage in the management of LSIL is not recommended, as essentially all of these individuals would be referred for colposcopy based upon the positive HPV test. Colposcopy is the recommended management option for these women. Management then depends upon whether a lesion is identified, whether the colposcopy is satisfactory or whether the patient is pregnant. The routine use of diagnostic excisional procedures or ablative procedures is unacceptable for the initial management of these patients with LSIL in the absence of biopsy-confirmed CIN. In an individual with a satisfactory colposcopy, endocervical sampling is acceptable for the non-pregnant patient but is preferred for the non-pregnant patient in whom no lesions are identified. If after the above CIN is not confirmed, then acceptable management includes follow-up with repeat cytology at 6 and 12 months with referral for colposcopy if a result of ASC-US or greater is obtained. Follow-up with HPV DNA testing at 12 months with referral colposcopy if testing is positive for high-risk HPV is also an option.

In those patients with unsatisfactory colposcopy, endocervical sampling is preferred for the non-pregnant patient. If a biopsy fails to confirm CIN and colposcopy is unsatisfactory, accepted management can include repeat cytology at 6–12 months with referral for colposcopy if results of ASC-US or greater is obtained or with HPV DNA testing at 12-month intervals if testing is positive.

In adolescence, an acceptable option is to follow without initial colposcopy using a protocol of repeated cytological testing of 6–12 months with a threshold of ASC for referral for colposcopy. HPV DNA testing at 12 months can also be an option with colposcopy if testing is positive for high-risk HPV DNA.

If CIN is identified, then management can be performed as per the guidelines as noted later in this chapter.

High-grade squamous intraepithelial lesions (HSIL)

A cytology diagnosis of HSIL accounts for only about a half of one percent of cytological interpretations in 1996. Women with HSIL have a 70–75% chance of having biopsy confirmed CIN II and III and a 1–2% chance of having invasive cervical cancer. Traditionally in women with HSIL, colposcopy with endocervical assessment has been considered the best management. When a high-grade cervical or vaginal lesion is not identified after colposcopy, it is recommended that when possible review of cytology, colposcopy, and histological results is performed. If cytological interpretation of HSIL is upheld, a diagnostic excisional procedure is preferred by many in the non-pregnant patient. Ablation is unacceptable. In an individual with HSIL in whom colposcopy suggests a high-grade lesion, initial evaluation using a diagnostic excisional procedure is also an acceptable option. Triage using either a program of repeat cytology or HPV testing is unacceptable.

In the pregnant patient, colposcopy is preferred but carried out after the middle portion of the second trimester. Biopsy of lesions suspicious of high-grade lesions or cancer is preferred; however, endocervical curettage should not be carried out in the pregnant woman. Unless invasive cancer is identified, treatment can be postponed until postpartum. An excisional diagnostic procedure is recommended only if invasion is suspected. Reevaluation with cytology and colposcopy is recommended no sooner than 6 weeks postpartum.

In the young woman of reproductive age, when biopsy confirmed CIN II and III is not identified, observation with colposcopy and cytology at 4–6-month intervals for a year is accepted, provided that the colposcopic findings are satisfactory and the endocervical sampling is negative. If HSIL cytology persists, then further evaluation with colposcopy and excisional biopsy is indicated.

Atypical glandular cells and adenocarcinoma in situ (AGC and AIS)

As previously noted, atypical glandular cells have been redefined in the 2001 Bethesda system. If a report of AGC is obtained, then biopsy confirmed high-grade lesions or invasive cancer has been found in 9–41% with AGC not otherwise specified (NOS) compared with 27–96% with women with AGC "favored neoplasia". The cytological finding of AIS is associated with a very high risk of women having either AIS (48–69%) or invasive cervical adenocarcinoma (38%). In all women with either AGC or AIS, further evaluation is needed. Repeat cervical cytology is usually not recommended. CIN is the most common form of neoplasia identified in women with AGC and therefore inclusion of colposcopy in the initial portion of the workup of women is recommended. Endocervical sampling should also be performed at the same time. There is a higher risk of CIN II or III in ASI in premenopausal women compared with postmenopausal women. About half the women with biopsy-confirmed AIS also have a coexistent squamous abnormality.

As noted, colposcopy with endocervical sampling is recommended for all women with all subcategories of AGC. If atypical endometrial cells are also present, then an endometrial sampling should be performed. Endometrial sampling should be performed in connection with the colposcopy in all women with AGC or AIS who are 35 years of age or older. Management of a program of repeat cervical cytology is unacceptable. The role of HPV DNA testing in the management of patients with AGC or AIS is inconclusive at the present time. If invasive disease is not identified during the initial workup, it is recommended that women with AGC "favored neoplasia" or AIS undergo a diagnostic excisional procedure. A cold knife conization is preferred over a LEEP procedure. If no neoplasia is identified during the initial workup of the woman with AGC NOS, she can be followed with repeat cervical cytology at 4–6-month intervals until four consecutive negative results are obtained after which she may return to routine screening. If an abnormality is noted on repeat Pap smear, acceptable options include repeat colposcopic examinations or referral to a clinician experienced in the management of complex cytological situations.

CERVICAL GLANDULAR CELL ABNORMALITIES

Cervical glandular cell abnormalities are being identified cytologically as well as histologically in increasing numbers. In 1979, Christopherson, based on a large population-based series, estimated a 1:239 ratio of cervical adenocarcinoma in situ to squamous cell carcinoma in situ (CIS). Since then, the incidence of adenocarcinoma of the cervix has been increasing in relationship to squamous cancers. Most likely, the preinvasive glandular abnormalities are also increasing. Adenocarcinoma in situ (adenoCIS) is frequently associated with CIN. Most data would suggest that 50% or more of adenoCIS are seen with CIN. Although the entire endocervical canal may be involved, > 95% of adenoCIS occur at the squamocolumnar junction. Several studies suggest that abnormal glandular elements are associated with HPV-18. This includes adenoCIS and adenocarcinoma. Whether epidemiologic factors associated with squamous CIN are the same for adenoCIS is suggested but unknown. When cytology indicative of glandular abnormalities is present, the canal must be evaluated. A patient with AGC may want to be evaluated with repeat Pap before other procedures are done. A normal second smear may give a false-negative result. Cytology should include the canal with a brush or similar device. Even though AGC may be present, a considerable number of patients will have more significant disease on histologic evaluation. Although colposcopic findings may not be classic and subtle changes can be missed, most suggest that this is a worthwhile procedure. Colposcopic findings may include areas of whitened villi lying within immature metaplasia. The villi are thicker and blunter than normal. Long, unbranched horizontal vessels may be present. Invasive disease (either involving adenocarcinoma or squamous cells) may be suspected and confirmed with biopsies. The findings on ECC may help in the diagnosis, and this procedure is encouraged. Most investigators think that conization is the diagnostic technique of choice, unless invasion is proved earlier in the workup. Increasing data suggest that conization of the cervix may be adequate therapy for adenoCIS or less particularly if surgical margins are free. Muntz found that one-twelfth of women with uninvolved margins and seven-tenths of women with positive margins had residual disease in the hysterectomy specimen. They followed 18 women for a median interval of 3 years (1.5–5 years) who had uninvolved cone margins, and none recurred. Other data from the literature note the same findings. Hitchcock followed 21 patients with cervical glandular atypia, including adenoCIS, after conization with cytology and pelvic examinations. After 13 years, none developed abnormal cytology or invasive carcinoma, even though 13 conizations contained abnormalities that appeared to be incompletely resected. Others have, however, been more pessimistic. Poynor evaluated 28 patients with a diagnosis of adenoCIS made by conization. Only nine (43%) had a glandular lesion diagnosed on ECC before conization. Four of 10 patients with negative cone margins were found to have residual adenoCIS, either in the hysterectomy or on repeat cone specimens. Four of eight patients with positive cone margins had residual disease in the second surgical specimen (three with adenoCIS and one with invasive adenocarcinoma). Seven of 15 patients managed conservatively with close follow-up or repeat cone have had a recurrence; two patients had invasive adenocarcinoma. An increasing amount of data suggest that patients who desire future fertility may in fact be managed with cold knife conization only if surgical margins are not involved. The persistence rate is approximately 8% in these circumstances compared with a rate as high as 60% if margins are involved. In situations in which fertility is desired and positive margins are present, reconization may be considered. In patients suspected of having ACIS, the cold knife conization appears to be a better procedure than large loop excision of the transformation zone (LLETZ), because the latter tends to have a larger number with positive margins and a higher recurrence rate. In patients who are not interested in future fertility, a simple hysterectomy is suggested as definitive therapy for adenoCIS by many. Current practice mandates further evaluation of an abnormal Pap smear (dysplasia or

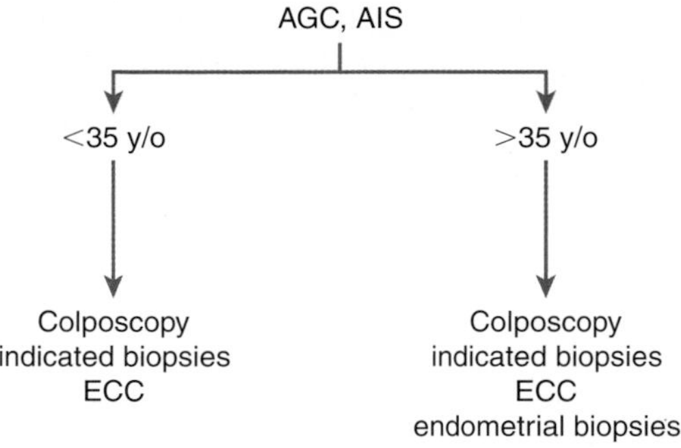

Figure 1–3 Management of Papanicolaou smears of atypical glandular cells of undetermined significance (AGC). (AIS, adenocarcinoma in situ; ECC, endocervical curettage.)

CIN), initially with colposcopy biopsies and ECC (Fig. 1–3). Further evaluation (conization) may be indicated, depending on these preliminary results.

Colposcopy

With the advent of colposcopy, a conservative schema and treatment plan for the patient with an abnormal Pap test has been generally accepted (Fig. 1–4). This schema is safe only if the steps are rigorously followed. This is particularly critical when the ECC findings are positive, even though the lesion is completely seen. In this situation, only an expert colposcopist should proceed with local treatment; otherwise, a diagnostic conization must be performed. The possibility of a coexisting unsuspected endocervical adenocarcinoma must also be considered. Omission of any of the diagnostic procedures in the evaluation may lead to the tragedy that results when invasive cancer is missed. A report by Sevin and associates of eight such cases, out of which three patients died, emphasizes the hazards of a less than optimal workup of patients before cryotherapy. Colposcopy was introduced by Hinselman in 1925 (Hamburg, Germany) as a result of his efforts to devise a practical method of more minute and comprehensive examination of the cervix. Hinselman and others during his era believed that cervical cancer began as miniature nodules on the surface epithelium and that these lesions could be detected with increased magnification and illumination. The meticulous examination of thousands of cases enabled him to clearly define the multiple physiologic and benign changes in the cervix as well as to correlate atypical changes with preinvasive and early invasive cancer. Unfortunately, Hinselman was primarily a clinician with very little pathology background, and this factor, in conjunction with the encumbrance of the tumor nodule theory, led to the development of confusing concepts and terminology associated with the use of the colposcope.

In the early 1930s, initial efforts were made to introduce colposcopy in the USA as a method of early cervical cancer detection. Because of the cumbersome terminology present at that time, the method was generally ignored; and with the introduction of reliable cytologic testing in the 1940s, North American physicians lost interest in colposcopy. The interest was renewed in the 1950s and early 1960s, but acceptance was slow because of the competitive nature of cytologic examinations, which were more economical and easier to perform and had, for the novice, a lower false-negative rate. Over the last two decades the

Figure 1–4 Evaluation and management schema for a patient with an abnormal Papanicolaou smear. (ECC, endocervical curettage.)

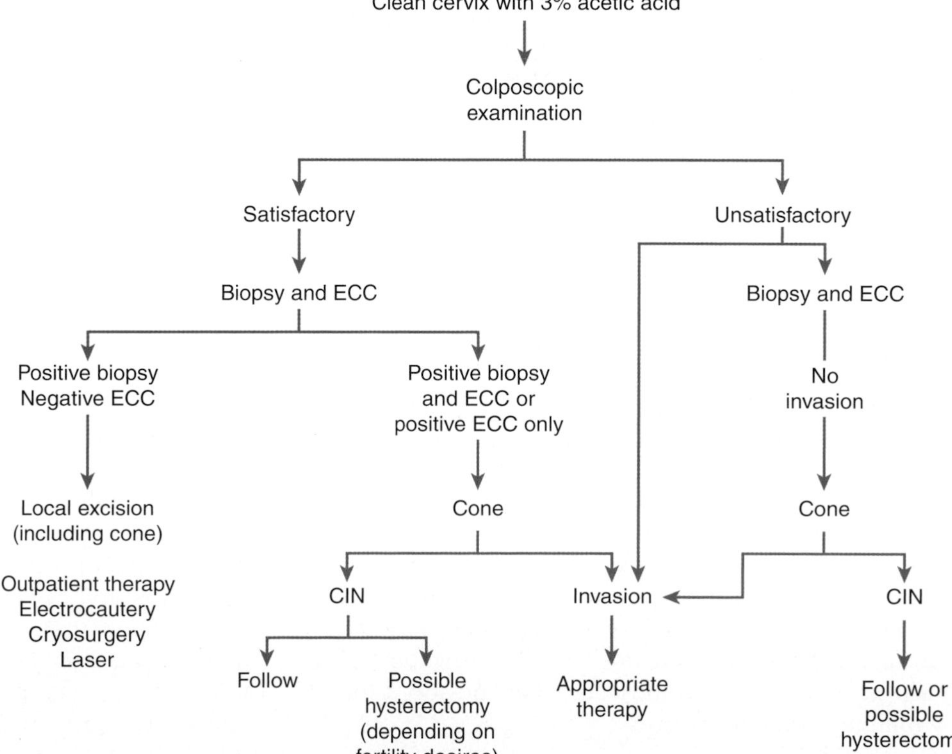

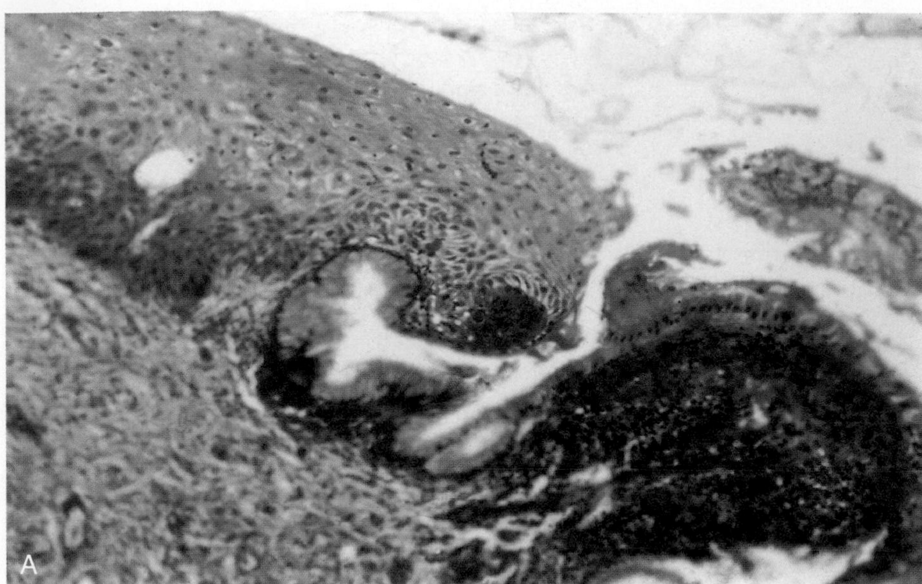

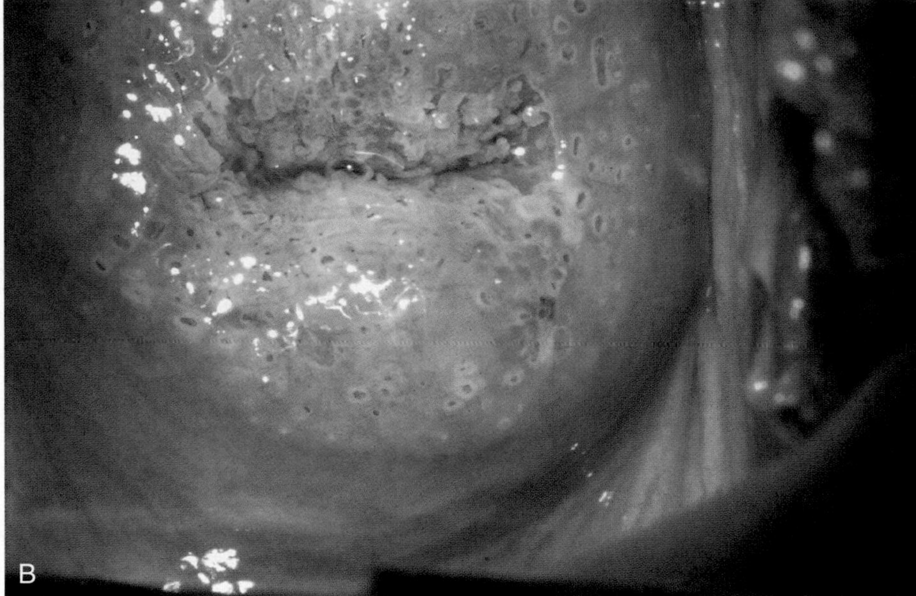

Figure 1–5 *A*, Squamocolumnar junction (transformation zone). *B*, Large transformation zone.

technique has gained long-awaited popularity and has been recognized as an adjunctive technique to cytologic testing in the investigation of genital tract epithelium. The recent popularity of colposcopy has been enhanced by the discovery of a scientific basis for most morphologic changes and the acceptance of a logical and simplified terminology for these changes.

The colposcope consists, in general, of a stereoscopic, binocular microscope with low magnification. It is provided with a center illuminating device and mounted on an adjustable stand with a transformer in the base. Several levels of magnification are available, the most useful being between 8× and 18×. A green filter is placed between the light source and the tissue to accentuate the vascular patterns and color tone differences between normal and abnormal patterns. Examination of the epithelium of the female genital tract by colposcopy takes no more than a few minutes in the usual case.

Colposcopy is based on study of the transformation zone (Fig. 1–5). The transformation zone is that area of the cervix and vagina that was initially covered by columnar epithelium and, through a process referred to as metaplasia, has undergone replacement by squamous epithelium. The wide range and variation in the colposcopic features of this tissue make up the science of colposcopy. The inheritance of variable vascular patterns, as well as the fate of residual columnar glands and clefts, determines the great variety of patterns in this zone. It had been generally taught that the cervix was normally covered by squamous epithelium and that the presence of endocervical columnar epithelium on the ectocervix portio was an abnormal finding. Studies by Coppleson and associates have established that columnar tissue can initially exist on the ectocervix in at least 70% of young women and extend into the vaginal fornix in an additional 5%. This process of transition from columnar to squamous epithelium probably occurs throughout a

Table 1–7 ABNORMAL COLPOSCOPIC FINDINGS

Atypical transformation zone
Keratosis
Aceto-white epithelium
Punctation
Mosaicism
Atypical vessels
Suspect frank invasive carcinoma
Unsatisfactory colposcopic findings

woman's lifetime. However, it has been demonstrated that this normal physiologic transformation zone is most active during three periods of a woman's life—fetal development, adolescence, and her first pregnancy. The process is enhanced by an acid pH environment and is influenced greatly by estrogen and progesterone levels.

The classification of colposcopic findings has been improved and simplified (Table 1–7), facilitating the recognition of abnormal patterns: white epithelium (Fig. 1–6), mosaic structure (Fig. 1–7), punctation (Fig. 1–8), and atypical vessels (Fig. 1–9). The term leukoplakia is generally reserved for the heavy, thick, white lesion that can frequently be seen with the naked eye. White epithelium, mosaic structure, and punctation herald atypical epithelium (CIN) and provide the target for directed biopsies. The pattern of atypical vessels is associated most often with invasive cancer, and biopsies should be performed liberally in areas with these findings. Although the abnormal colposcopic patterns reflect cytologic and histologic alterations, they are not specific enough for final diagnosis, and a biopsy is necessary. The greatest value of the colposcope is in directing the biopsy to the area that is most likely to yield the most significant histologic pattern.

When colposcopy is performed, a standard procedure is followed. First, the cervix is sampled for cytologic screening, and then it is cleansed with a 3% acetic acid solution to remove the excess mucus and cellular debris. The acetic acid also accentuates the difference between normal and abnormal colposcopic patterns. The colposcope is focused on the cervix and the transformation zone, including the squamocolumnar junction, and the area is inspected in a clockwise fashion. In most cases, the entire lesion can be outlined, and the most atypical area can be selected for biopsy. If the lesion extends up the canal beyond the vision of the colposcopist, the patient will require a diagnostic conization to define the disease. ECC is performed whether or not the lesion extends up the canal, and if invasive cancer is found at any time, plans for a cone biopsy are abandoned. This plan of investigation, which is outlined in Fig. 1–4, is based on the assumption that there are no areas of CIN higher up in the canal if indeed the upper limits of the lesion can be seen colposcopically. In other words, CIN begins in the transformation zone and extends contiguously to other areas of the cervix such that if the upper limits can be seen, one can be assured that additional disease is not present higher in the canal. The colposcope can only suggest an abnormality; final diagnosis must rest on a tissue examination by a pathologist. Selected spot biopsies in the areas showing atypical colposcopic patterns, under

Figure 1–6 White epithelium at the cervical os (a colposcopic view).

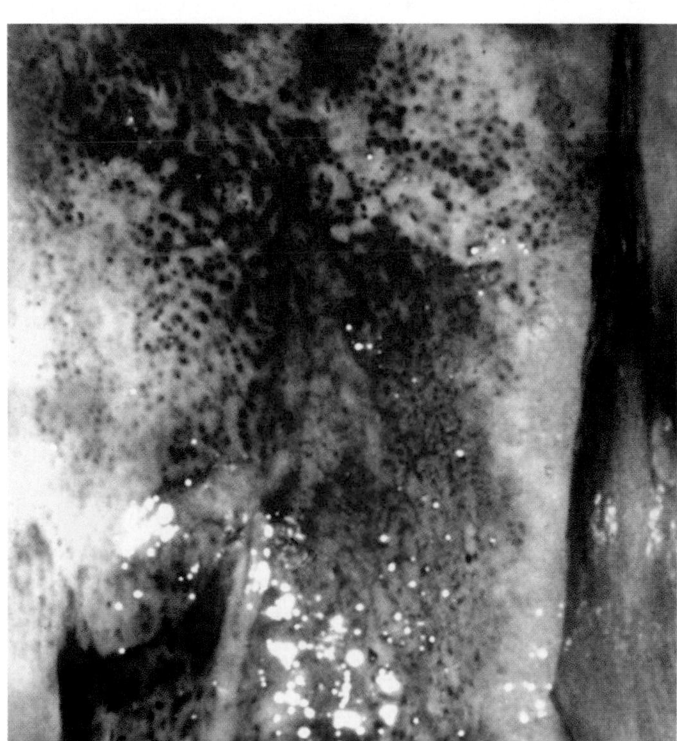

Figure 1–7 A punctation pattern is seen clearly above a mosaic structure (a colposcopic view).

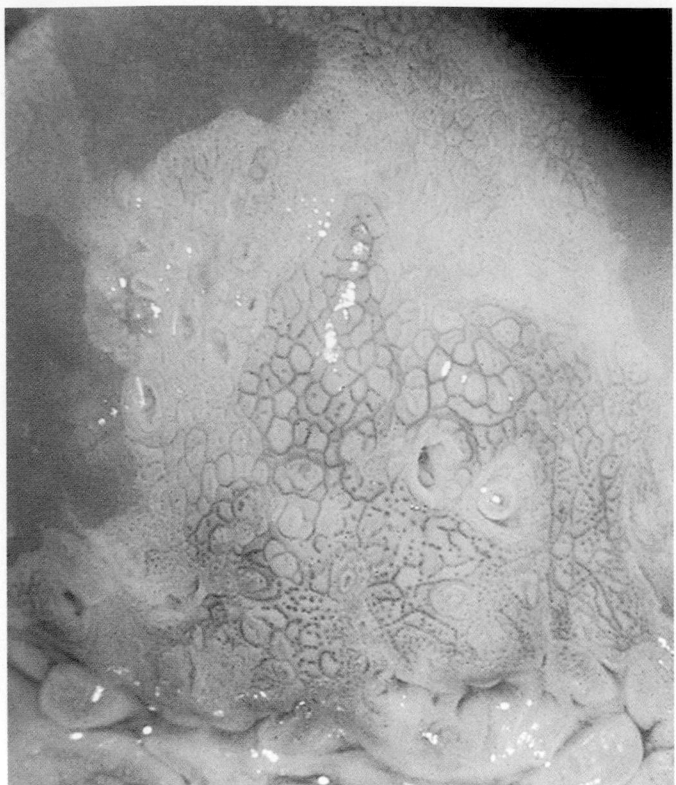

Figure 1–8 A large anterior lip lesion with white epithelium punctation and mosaic patterns.

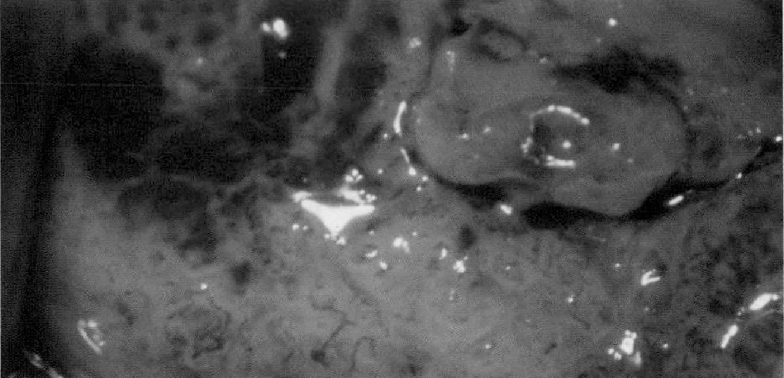

Figure 1–9 Many atypical ("corkscrew, hairpin") vessels indicative of early invasive cancer. (Courtesy of Kenneth Hatch, MD, Tucson, Arizona.)

direct colposcopic guidance and in combination with cytologic testing, give the highest possible accuracy in the diagnosis and evaluation of the cervix. Probably the greatest value of colposcopy is that in most cases a skilled colposcopist can establish and differentiate invasive cancer from CIN by direct biopsy and thus avoid the necessity of surgical conization of the cervix. This is especially valuable in the young nulliparous woman desirous of childbearing for whom cone biopsy of the cervix may result in problems of impaired fertility. The avoidance of conization is also valuable in reducing the risk to the patient from anesthesia and the additional surgical procedure with its prolonged hospitalization.

In all patients undergoing colposcopic examination, unless they are pregnant, an ECC should be performed, even if the entire lesion is seen. This gives objective proof of the absence of disease in the endocervical canal. It is believed that if the ECC had been done in several of the patients who had been reported in the literature as having invasive cancer diagnosed after outpatient therapy, the cancer would have been identified at an earlier time, and inappropriate therapy would not have been given.

ECC is performed from the internal os to the external os. The external os is the structure that is created by the opening of the bivalve speculum. A speculum as large as can be tolerated should be used to evaluate the patient with an abnormal Pap smear. During curettage, it is best to curet the entire circumference of the canal without removing the curet. This is done twice. Short, firm motions in a circumferential pattern are the most satisfactory. Patients experience some discomfort early in the procedure, but rarely does the physician have to stop because of discomfort. It is desirable to obtain endocervical stroma in the specimen if possible. On completion of the curettage, all blood, mucus, and cellular debris must be collected and placed on a 2 × 2-inch absorbent paper towel. The material is then folded into a mound and, along with the absorbent paper towel, placed into fixative. If any neoplastic tissue is found by the pathologist in the curettings, the results are considered positive. Directed punch biopsies of the cervix are done after the curettage. Using the colposcopic findings as a guide, the physician obtains punch biopsy specimens with a Kevorkian–Younge cervical biopsy instrument (or a similar tool that contains a basket in which the biopsy specimen may be collected). Biopsy specimens should be placed on a small piece of paper towel with proper orientation to minimize tangential sectioning of the specimen.

The goal of any evaluation of a patient with abnormal cervical cytologic findings is to rule out invasive cancer. Diagnostic studies may be done using outpatient facilities or may require hospitalization. No single diagnostic technique can effectively rule out invasive cancer in all patients, but with multiple diagnostic procedures the risk of missing invasive cancer is essentially eliminated. Even conization of the cervix by itself can miss an invasive cancer. Therefore, cytologic screening, colposcopy, colposcopically directed biopsies, ECC, and pelvic examination must all rule out invasive cancer. Under certain circumstances, conization is indicated, even after the full outpatient evaluation has been performed. Most important, if invasive cancer has not been ruled out by the outpatient evaluation, conization must be performed. Patients who have a positive ECC also require conization. If cytologic testing, biopsies, or colposcopic examination indicates microinvasive carcinoma of the cervix, conization must be performed to fully evaluate the extent of the invasion, which in turn determines appropriate therapy. The postmenopausal patient with abnormal cytologic findings frequently requires conization of the cervix because her lesion is usually located within the endocervical canal and cannot be adequately evaluated with outpatient techniques. The use of local estrogen for several days before colposcopy and biopsy in the postmenopausal patient will augment these diagnostic procedures tremendously.

In patients in whom conization must be done, colposcopy can aid in tailoring the conization to the individual's specific need. If the lesion extends widely onto the portio, the lateral extensions might be missed with a "standard" cone but would be included if colposcopically directed. Occasionally, the disease will extend into the vaginal fornix, and colposcopy can identify this patient so that appropriate margins may be obtained. If, however, the concern is the endocervical canal, and the portio is clean, a narrow conization can be done to remove the endocervical canal only. The use of Lugol solution as a substitute for colposcopy to determine the extent of the disease on the cervix is inappropriate and can be misleading. Both false-positive and false-negative staining with Lugol solution can occur in identifying CIN. The application of Lugol solution may be helpful to evaluate the cervix and vagina before conization. The colposcopic lesion and the non-staining area of Lugol solution should match. Failure of matching indicates that appropriate adjustments must be made at the time of conization.

This evaluation schema permits triage of patients based on the colposcopic findings (plus the results of the colposcopically directed biopsies) and ECC findings. If the results of curettage of the canal are negative and only preinvasive neoplasia is found on directed biopsy, the patient has been adequately evaluated and treatment can begin. The method of therapy chosen depends on the patient's age, desire for fertility, and reliability for follow-up, and on the histologic appearance and extent of her lesion. Cryosurgery using the double-freeze technique or destruction of the lesion with a laser beam can be performed in some patients who wish to retain their childbearing capacity but who have disease that is more extensive than can adequately be treated with a simple excisional biopsy in the office. Hysterectomy, either simple vaginal or abdominal, without preceding conization may be recommended for patients who desire sterilization. No effort is made in the performance of the hysterectomy to excise additional vaginal cuff unless there is evidence of abnormal epithelium extending to the vagina; this occurs in < 3% of patients. A final possibility for treatment is to perform a shallow conization or ring biopsy of the cervix (see Fig. 1–4).

As noted in the schema that we have presented for evaluation of the abnormal Pap smear, ECC is performed on all non-pregnant patients. Diagnostic conization must be done when ECC shows malignant cells or when colposcopic examination is unsatisfactory (the entire lesion is not seen). Because curettage is performed from the internal os to the external os, the lesion that extends only slightly into the canal is often picked up by the curet, resulting in a number of false-positive ECC results. Nonetheless, ECC should be performed on all patients unless they are pregnant; if errors are made, they should be made on the side of conization. Some physicians do not routinely perform ECC when the entire lesion is visible on the ectocervix. Although omitting this procedure may be appropriate for a few experienced colposcopists, its inclusion as a routine step will further reduce the chance of missing a lesion in the endocervix. A previously unsuspected adenocarcinoma of the endocervix is occasionally diagnosed, but even more often an early invasive squamous cell carcinoma is uncovered.

In individuals in whom ECC findings are positive and the upper limits cannot be visualized, diagnostic conization must be performed to exclude or confirm invasive cancer. Care should be taken in performing conization to include a sufficient portion of the endocervical canal to rule out occult invasive disease high in the canal.

Colposcopic evaluation of the cervix in the patient with an abnormal cervical smear has dramatically altered the management of the patient afflicted during pregnancy. The schema previously outlined is closely followed in pregnancy, when the transformation zone is everted, making visualization of the entire lesion almost a certainty. Cone biopsy is rarely indicated during pregnancy. If punch biopsy suggests microinvasion, further evaluation is needed. In many cases, a "wedge" resection of the suspicious area confirms the diagnosis of microinvasion, and conization is unnecessary. If not, then cone biopsy to allow proper management should be seriously considered. Pregnant patients with a firm diagnosis of preinvasive or microinvasive disease of the cervix should be allowed to deliver vaginally, and further therapy can be tailored to their needs after delivery. The cervix is very vascular during pregnancy, thus avoiding a cone biopsy is in the best interest of both the mother and the fetus. Small biopsies of the most colposcopically abnormal areas are recommended in an effort to minimize bleeding in the diagnostic evaluation. When a patient is in the second or third trimester and the result of the colposcopic examination is negative for any suspicion of invasion, many colposcopists will defer all biopsies to the postpartum period. Lurain and Gallup reported on 131 pregnant patients with abnormal Pap smears managed in this manner with excellent results, and no invasive cancers were missed.

Roberts and colleagues noted that only two patients had CIN III on cervical biopsies during pregnancy and also microinvasion (stage Ia1) on cold knife conization (CKC) postpartum. Whether this is progression or sampling error is unknown. Post and associates noted CIN II and III in 279 antepartum biopsies. Regression of 68% and 78% respectively among patients with CIN II and III was noted postpartum. No progression to cancer was noted. Regression rates did not depend on vaginal deliveries compared with cesarean section deliveries. Complete re-evaluation postpartum appears to be indicated so that over treatment is not done.

Treatment options

In women with CIN II or III therapy is indicated. This is applicable in those with CIN I although as noted observation is also an option. Many treatment options are available to the patient today (Table 1-8). Essentially all of these options should be considered definitive. The decision about the choice of therapy for CIN depends on many factors, including the patient's desire and the experiences of the physician involved. Probably the most compelling reasons for choosing an outpatient modality over inpatient surgery are the patient's age and desire for subsequent fertility. The recommendation that carcinoma in situ in a teenager or woman in her early 20s must be treated with a hysterectomy is outdated. Unfortunately, this type of therapy is the recommended treatment, and other alternatives, although quite effective, may not be explained to the patient. No therapy is 100% effective; the benefit:risk ratio to the patient should be explained so that she is fully informed, and a reasonable decision can be made concerning her therapy and well-being.

Observation in selected, highly individualized patients may be an option, particularly if the lesion is small and histologically of LSIL. (See the management schema in evaluation of the abnormal smear section, p 17.) There are also patients who have a small lesion that may be completely removed with the biopsy forceps. Elimination of the disease with this technique has occurred in some patients, although some investigators think that the entire transformation zone should be destroyed. Obviously, the use of observation and local excision can be made only by the experienced physician and must be highly individualized, depending on the patient's needs, desires, and ability to be followed appropriately.

Outpatient management

Electrocautery

Several modalities of treatment for the patient with CIN can be performed on an outpatient basis. If in fact these modalities are as effective as a surgical procedure accomplished in the operating room, the cost effectiveness is very important. Electrocautery has been used for many years to eradicate cervical epithelium. It was fashionable historically to destroy the "abnormal" tissue found on the cervix after delivery. Actually, this was columnar epithelium, or the transformation zone of the cervix. Some uncontrolled studies suggest that electrocautery decreased the appearance of CIN lesions in patients thus treated. Electrocautery has been shown to be effective in the treatment of CIN. The popularity of this treatment is more apparent in Europe and Australia than in the USA. In a small, controlled study, Wilbanks and associates showed that electrocautery was effective in destroying early CIN compared with tetracycline vaginal suppositories used in a control group of patients. Ortiz and colleagues treated all forms of CIN with electrocautery. In CIN I and II lesions, no failures were noted. In CIN III disease, the failure rate was approximately 13%. The failure rate in patients with carcinoma in situ did not differ whether the glands were involved or not. All the patients were treated on an outpatient basis. Chanen and Rome have used this technique extensively in Australia. Table 1–9 illustrates the excellent results that they reported. They treated more than 1700 patients, and the failure rate was only 3%. Cervical stenosis has not been a problem. Dilatation and curettage (D&C) is done at the same time that the electrocautery is performed. The patient is admitted to the hospital, and while she is under anesthesia, electrocautery is performed in the operating room to burn the tissue deep enough to destroy disease that might be present in glands. Chanen and Rome believe that this is necessary to obtain excellent results. Electrocautery, of course, is painful if the tissue is burned deeply. If a patient needs to be anesthetized to obtain these results, this negates any benefits that a

Table 1–8 TREATMENT OPTIONS FOR CERVICAL INTRAEPITHELIAL NEOPLASIA

- Observations
- Local excision
- Electrocautery
- Cryosurgery
- Laser
- Cold coagulation
- Loop electrosurgical excision procedure (LEEP)
- Conization
- Hysterectomy

Table 1–9 CONSERVATIVE TREATMENT FOR CERVICAL INTRAEPITHELIAL NEOPLASIA

Method (Based on single treatment)	Failures
Electrocoagulation[1]	47/1734 (2.7%)
Cryosurgery[2,3]	540/6143 (8.7%)
Laser[4]	119/2130 (5.6%)
Cold coagulator (CIN III)[5]	110/1628 (6.8%)
LEEP[6, 7, 8]	95/2185 (4.3%)

[1]Chanen W, Rome RM: Electrocoagulation diathermy for cervical dysplasia and carcinoma in situ: A 15-year survey. Obstet Gynecol 61:673, 1983.
[2]Richart RM, Townsend DE et al: An analysis of "long-term" follow-up results in patients with cervical intraepithelial neoplasia treated by cryosurgery. Am J Obstet Gynecol 137:823, 1980.
[3]Benedet JL, Nickerson KG, Anderson GH: Cryotherapy in the treatment or cervical intraepithelial neoplasia. Obstet Gynecol 58:72, 1981.
[4]Parashevadis E, Jandial L, Mann EMF et al: Patterns of treatment failure following laser for cervical intraepithelial neoplasia: Implications for follow-up protocol. Obstet Gynecol 78:80, 1991.
[5]Gordon HK, Duncan ID: Effective destruction of cervical intraepithelial neoplasia (CIN 3) at 100°C using the Semm cold coagulator: 14 years' experience. Br J Obstet Gynecol 98:14, 1991.
[6]Bigrigg MA, Codling BW, Pearson P et al: Colposcopic diagnosis and treatment of cervical dysplasia at a single clinic visit. Lancet 336:229, 1990.
[7]Murdoch, Murdoch JB, Grimshaw RN, Morgan PR et al: The impact of loop diathermy on management of early invasive cervical cancer. Int J Gynecol Cancer 2:129, 1992.
[8]LuesleyDM, Cullimore J, Redman CWE et al: Loop diathermy excision of the cervical transformation zone in patients with abnormal cervical smears. Br Med J 300:1090, 1990.
CIN, cervical intraepithelial neoplasia; LEEP, loop electrosurgical excision procedure.

lesser procedure than conization would obtain. The cost of hospitalization, even on an ambulatory service, would be much higher than that of outpatient treatment.

Cryosurgery

Considerable experience with cryosurgery has been obtained in the treatment of CIN. The side effects of electrocautery, mainly pain during treatment, are not present with cryosurgery and thus it is an ideal outpatient modality in terms of patient comfort.

Ample experience with cryosurgery has now been reported in the literature. In 1980, Charles and Savage reviewed the literature and reported the experience of 16 authors with approximately 3000 patients. The success rate was noted to be between 27% and 96%. Many factors accounted for the wide variation and results, including the experience of the operator, the number of patients treated, criteria established to determine a cure, as well as freezing techniques, equipment, and the refrigerant used. Subsequently, several studies have been done in the literature (see Table 1–9). Total failure for the entire group irrespective of the histologic grade was 8%. Results of cryosurgery are essentially the same as those reported for electrocautery, the advantage being that cryosurgery is essentially pain free and is effectively performed on an outpatient basis.

Ample experience has been obtained in the long-term follow-up of patients who have been treated with cryosurgery. Richart and associates noted that the recurrence rate was < 1% in almost 3000 patients with CIN who were treated with cryosurgery and followed for 5 years or more. Almost one half of the recurrences were noted within the first year after cryosurgery and to a certain extent they probably represent persistence and not a true recurrence. No cases of invasive cancer have developed in these patients. The initial failure rate can be reduced even further by a "recycling" of the patient and appropriate retreatment with cryosurgery or some other outpatient modality. Townsend states that all of the failures in the CIN I category were retreated successfully with cryosurgery, and the failure rate for the retreated patients who failed the first treatment lowered the overall failure rate to 3% for CIN II and 7% for CIN III. Although the techniques of cryosurgery are simple, several important technical points must be kept in mind to have an optimal freeze. Carbon dioxide or nitrous oxide can be used as a refrigerant for cryosurgery. The larger "D" tank is preferred over the narrow "E" tank, particularly if cryosurgery is performed on several patients over a short time interval. The pressure in the smaller tank can drop because of the cooling in the gas, even though there may be adequate volume within the tank. Pressure is very important for obtaining a satisfactory freeze. If the pressure drops below 40 kg/cm^2 during the freezing process, the treatment should be stopped; tanks should be changed; and the treatment should be started again. A thin layer of water-soluble lubricant over the tip of the probe will allow a more uniform and rapid freeze of the cervix. This allows a better heat transfer mechanism to take place between the probe and the cervix. This is particularly important in the case of a woman who may have an irregular cervix, which is common in the parous patient. The probe should cover the entire lesion, and a 4–5 mm iceball around the probe is required for an adequate freeze. This should be obtained within 1.5 to 2 minutes with most cryosurgery units today. If the 4–5 mm iceball is not obtained within this time, equipment is probably functioning incorrectly and the problem must be identified. We prefer the double-freeze technique. The cervix is allowed to thaw for 4 to 5 minutes and is then refrozen using the same technique (Table 1-10). There is usually a watery discharge for 10–14 days. The patient is instructed to refrain from intercourse and to use an external pad if necessary during the time of the watery discharge. She is then seen in 4 months for re-evaluation with a Pap smear. If the result of the Pap smear is positive, the abnormality may be a result of the healing process, and the Pap smear is then repeated in 4–6 weeks. If cytologic findings remain abnormal 6 months after cryosurgery, cryosurgery must be considered a failure; the patient should then be re-evaluated and retreated.

Attention has been drawn to the fact that several patients have been reported to have invasive carcinoma of the cervix after cryosurgery. A report from Miami details eight patients who were treated by cryosurgery for various indications and were found subsequently to have invasive cancer. Only five of the patients had abnormal cervical cytologic findings; three had colposcopic examinations; two had colposcopically directed biopsies; and only one had an ECC.

Townsend and associates reported on 66 similar patients of members of the Society of Gynecologic Oncologists. Again, an inappropriate precryosurgery evaluation was noted in most of these patients. Invasive cancer has also been reported in patients who are treated with other outpatient modalities, again emphasizing the importance of a proper evaluation before outpatient therapy.

Laser surgery

The term laser is an acronym for "light amplification by stimulated emission of radiation". The carbon dioxide laser beam is invisible and is usually guided by a second laser that emits visible light. The energy of the laser is absorbed by water with a high degree of efficiency, and the tissue is destroyed principally by vaporization. The laser is mounted on a colposcope, and the laser beam is directed

Table 1–10 CRYOSURGERY TECHNIQUE

1. N_2O or CO_2
2. KY jelly on probe
3. Double-freeze
   a. 4–5 mm iceball
   b. Thaw
   c. 4–5 mm iceball

under colposcopic control. Most instruments have a considerable power range and operate by pulse or continuous mode. The spot size may be fixed but can usually be varied. The amount of power delivered to the tissue depends on the spot size and the wattage. Because there is a high-efficiency laser beam absorption by the tissue, as well as the opportunity to precisely direct the beam, the laser is unique. It also has the ability to control the depth of destruction. Because the tissue is destroyed by vaporization, the base of destruction is clean, with little necrotic tissue and rapid healing. As experience is gained with this modality, changes in technique take place. Because the laser can precisely direct the beam, at first it was thought that only the abnormal area needed to be destroyed with the laser. This prevented the destruction of normal cervical tissue. With this technique, the failure rate was excessive, and, as a result, it was suggested that the entire transformation zone be destroyed. Masterson and colleagues noted that their change in technique from destroying the lesion to ablating the entire transformation zone did not appreciably increase their success rate. The depth of destruction appears to be important in that the failure rate was considerable when only minimal destruction (1–2 mm) was achieved. As the depth of destruction increased, the number of failures decreased. Most lasers now advocate the destruction to a depth of 5 to 7 mm. Burke, Lovell, and Antoniolo concluded that successful treatment was not related to the severity of the histologic grade or to the size of the lesion. A continuous beam gave a better result than an intermittent beam. The depth of destruction was important and must include the lamina propria. Involvement of the endocervical crypt did not preclude success (Table 1–11). Certain precautions must be taken while using the carbon dioxide laser to avoid the use of flammable agents, to protect the eyes with appropriate glasses, and to use nonreflective surfaces. As the beam is transferred, the tissue vaporizes, filling the vagina with smoke and steam, which are evacuated by a suction tube attached to the speculum. Complications with the laser include pain, which is greater than with cryosurgery but usually tolerable. Bleeding can be a problem, although spotting is more frequent than significant bleeding. Bleeding increases as the depth of tissue destruction increases, and larger vessels may be reached with the laser beam. Because 5–7 mm of tissue is destroyed, increased bleeding will probably occur more frequently.

Table 1–11 CO_2 LASER VAPORIZATION—CERVIX

Instruments	CO_2 laser, colposcope, micromanipulator
Power output	20–25 W
Power density	800–1400 W/cm^2
Spot size	1.5–2 mm diameter
Operating mode	Continuous
Depth of destruction	6–7 mm measured
Width of destruction	4–5 mm beyond the visible lesion
Bleeding control	Defocus, power density: 800 W/cm^2
Anesthesia	May need a paracervical block
Analgesia	Antiprostaglandins

Two disadvantages to the laser that have not been experienced with cryosurgery follow:

1. The process is more painful for the patient who has the procedure done in the physician's office than for the patient who has cryosurgery.
2. The destruction of all but the smallest of lesions requires much more time for both the patient and the physician.

Although the data suggest that the laser is effective in destroying CIN, it appears to be no better than other available outpatient methods, and one must question the cost effectiveness of this modality compared with cryosurgery.

In 1983, Townsend and Richart reported a study by alternating cases randomly, as much as possible, on the basis of CIN histologic grade and lesion size to compare the efficacy of cryotherapy and carbon dioxide laser therapy. In their study, 100 patients were treated with laser therapy and 100 patients were treated with cryotherapy. There were seven failures in the cryotherapy group and 11 failures in the group treated with carbon dioxide laser therapy. These authors found no significant differences in the cure rates between the two modalities. They thought that: "if the therapeutic results are equivalent, it is logical to choose the modality that provides an equivalent grade of care for the least possible cost, and, at least in an office setting, this would seem to favor cryotherapy over laser therapy."

Mitchell and associates performed a prospective randomized trial of cryosurgery, laser vaporization, and LEEP excision in 390 patients with biopsy-proven CIN. The degree of CIN, lesion size, number of quadrants involved, age, smoking history, and also HPV status were similar in all treatment groups. There was no statistical difference in complications, persistence, or recurrence between the three modalities. They noted that the risk of persistence was higher in those with large lesions. The rate of recurrence was higher among women 30 years of age or older, those with HPV-16 or 18, and those who were previously treated for CIN.

In an evaluation by Parashevadis and associates of 2130 patients treated by laser therapy, these authors noted that failures were higher in women older than 40 years of age and in those with CIN III. CIN III lesions accounted for 75% of the failures, whereas only 7% were originally CIN I. Three cases of invasive cancer were diagnosed within 2 years of laser therapy. There were 119 (5.6%) treatment failures. Of the failures, 18% had a second lesion detected colposcopically in the presence of negative cytology after laser therapy.

Cold coagulator

Gordon and Duncan have reported experience with a Semm cold coagulator in the treatment of CIN III. Over a 14-year period, 1628 women were treated, and the primary success rate was 95% at 1 year and 92% at 5 years, similar for all age groups. There were 226 pregnancies following therapy, and the rates for miscarriage, preterm, or operative delivery were not increased.

The cold coagulator essentially coagulates at a lower temperature (100°C). Therapy is performed by overlapping applications of the thermal probe so that the transformation zone and the lower endocervix are destroyed. In most cases, two to five applications were required, taking less than 2 minutes (20 seconds per application).

The exact depth of destruction is difficult to ascertain accurately. Several investigators found destruction up to 4 mm. These data suggest that this depth of destruction is adequate in patients with CIN III lesions. If this is the case, one wonders why 6–7 mm of destruction is required for adequate therapy when laser therapy is used. Even in the hands of an experienced colposcopist, subsequent carcinomas were noted in this series, as with every other treatment used in outpatient management. Microinvasion was found in two patients, and invasive cancer was found in four patients. This technique is inexpensive, quick, and essentially pain free and has very few side effects. Efficacy is excellent (see Table 1–9). One wonders why this technique has not been evaluated and used in the USA.

Loop electrosurgical excision procedure

A new approach to an old instrument has become popular. If cryosurgery was the “in” treatment of the 1970s and laser surgery was the “in” treatment of the 1980s, loop electrosurgical excision procedure (LEEP) became the instrument of the 1990s (Table 1–12). LEEP has gained a tremendous experience within a short time. After colposcopy and if the entire transformation zone is identified, it is excised with a low-voltage diathermy loop under local anesthesia. Usually less than 10 mL of local anesthesia, with epinephrine or vasopressin added to help decrease blood loss, is injected into the cervix at 12, 3, 6, and 9 o’clock. After 3–5 minutes, excision can be performed with a loop size that will excise the complete lesion.

An electrosurgical generator is used with wattage set at 25–50 W, depending on loop size (the larger the loop, the higher will be the wattage) and blended cut or coagulated. A disposable grounding plate is used, as in the operating room. The cutting loop consists of an insulated shaft with a wire loop attached. The sterilized steel wire is 0.2 mm in diameter and comes in various sizes. LEEP can be performed under colposcopy or after Lugol application (and if it matches colposcopy findings) as a guide for excision. If Lugol solution is used, saline should be applied to the cervix before LEEP, because Lugol solution tends to dehydrate the tissue. Care should be taken to avoid the vaginal walls with the loop. A smoke evacuator, used as with laser, is recommended. In some cases, the 1.5 cm loop is too small to remove the entire lesion, and an additional “pass” or two is required to remove the remaining abnormal epithelium. Depth of the excised tissue varies, but 5–8 mm is the usual depth. This allows tissue for adequate evaluation. The base of the excised tissue is then coagulated with a ball electrode, and Monsel’s paste is applied.

Table 1–12 LEEP TECHNIQUE

1. Do a colposcopy of the cervix and outline the lesion.
2. The patient is grounded with a pad return electrode.
3. Inject anesthetic solution just beneath and lateral to the lesion (at the excision site).
4. Turn on the machine and set cut/blend to 25–50 W (the larger the loop, the higher wattage is needed).
5. Set coagulation to 60 W for ball electrode use.
6. After adequate time for anesthesia to take effect, excise the lesion using the LEEP.
7. Coagulate the base of the cone, even if there is no apparent bleeding.
8. Place ferric subsulfate paste on the base.

LEEP, loop electrosurgical excision procedure.

There are several advantages to this technique. The procedure can be done on an outpatient basis. Tissue is available for study. Diagnosis and therapy are all done at one time and during the same visit. In essentially all large studies reported to date, several early invasive lesions were identified that had not been recognized on colposcopy examination. This technique tends to negate this inherent problem of destructive techniques.

Side effects are mainly secondary hemorrhage (initially reported at 10% but with experience found to be in the 1–2% range). Long-term effects such as those on pregnancy are not known; but one report noted 48 pregnancies in 1000 after LEEP. From this limited experience, it appears that pregnancies after LEEP are similar to those following laser vaporization or electrocoagulation.

Results of one large study of 1000 patients noted that 897 women were managed with only one visit. The other 103 required more than one visit, including nine women who had microinvasion or invasion. Cervical cytology at 4 months after treatment was performed in 969 women, and 41 (4.1%) were found to be abnormal. Of the nine women with invasion, only four were suspected on cervical smear and colposcopy (see Table 1–9).

LEEP appears to be the current treatment of choice even with very limited follow-up for patients with abnormal cytology. It has been estimated that many thousands of LEEPs have been performed in the USA. Several comments are probably in order. See, diagnose, and treat at one time is a philosophy that has been popularized by some, particularly our European colleagues. In some cases, LEEP has been used before colposcopy or other diagnostic procedures. As noted earlier in its guidelines for management of abnormal cervical cytology, the ASCCP-sponsored workshop stated: “Routine electroexcision of the TZ of non-staining areas as a method of evaluating a positive Pap smear diagnosed as LSIL or ASCUS is not recommended.” The indiscriminate use of LEEP should not be condoned. In essentially all studies that have addressed the subject, as many as half of LEEP specimens show no epithelial abnormalities (most studies show 15–25% with negative histology). It appears that many patients with ASCUS or LSIL on cytology are having LEEPs done that do not appear warranted. The "see and treat" fashion for patients with these degrees of abnormalities on Pap smears should not be encouraged.

Initially, it was said that LEEP caused stenosis, occurring in approximately 1% of cases. More recent data suggest that stenosis may be present four times greater than preliminary data suggested. This is still a low figure (comparable to cryosurgery and laser). Anecdotal experience has suggested that the increasing number of LEEPs being done will lead to an increase in infertility or preterm labor. Many patients with CIN are young and desire to be fertile. In the United Kingdom, where LEEP is the most frequently used therapy for CIN, 1000 patients who underwent large loop excisions of the transformation zone were evaluated for subsequent pregnancy. There were 149 women who had a singleton pregnancy progressing past 20 weeks of gestation and were matched to controls with regard to age, parity, height, father's social class, and smoking. Mean birth weights of women progressing to at least 37 weeks were equal. Following LEEP, 9.4% of deliveries were preterm (< 37 weeks) compared with 5% in the control group (not statistically significant). In a small study comparing fertility after LEEP with patients treated with a conization (79 in each group), 11 of 12 women desiring pregnancy conceived in the LEEP group compared with all 17 who desired pregnancy in the cone group.

In a retrospective study (Kennedy), 2315 women were treated with LEEP. Only 15 of the 924 new patients attending the university infertility clinic were treated with LEEP. Of the 15 patients, only 10 had good quality cervical mucus at midcycle, and three other patients had spontaneous conception.

Many physicians are reluctant to use LEEP in the young, nulliparous patient because the cervix is small and a considerable amount of the cervix can be removed very quickly with this procedure. In our practice, we have seen several young patients in whom the cervix is flush with the vagina. In this subset, fertility and preterm labor have not been evaluated to any extent.

Preliminary data on large series suggested a low persistence/recurrence rate, but follow-up time was short—only 4 months in many patients. Bigrigg has subsequently reported a longer follow-up period in 250 women out of the original 1000 treated with LEEP. During follow-up, these patients required 68 second treatments because of persistent or recurrent symptoms during their follow-up period.

Several studies have evaluated factors that predict persistence/recurrence after LEEP therapy. Baldauf and colleagues noted that on multivariate analysis, the endocervical location of the initial lesion and incomplete excision predicted treatment failure. Robinson and associates found that positive margins did not identify patients at high risk for a recurrence compared with negative margins. Nor did they find positive ECC that was worse than negative ECCs in predicting a recurrence. These authors had a high recurrence rate after LEEP (40%). Barnes and colleagues found that only positive ECC after LEEP predicted HSIL on follow-up Pap smears (16 of 219 or 7%). Margin status was not a factor. Experience after cold knife conization has shown that in many patients with positive margins, follow-up found no persistent disease. Whether this is also applicable to patients treated with LEEP will require further evaluation. It appears that routine follow-up with cytology hopefully will identify those who fail, and additional immediate therapy for positive margins can be tempered.

Thermal artifact, although reported in series to be of minimal concern, in general practice is reported to be unreadable in approximately 10% of specimens, and 20–40% have significant coagulation artifact. This is probably related to equipment power setting and technical problems such as "stalling".

Bleeding is reported to occur in approximately 5% of cases, mainly after treatment. Strict adherence to protocol reduces this problem. LEEP done when significant vaginal infection is present will increase the chance of bleeding. In almost all large series, unanticipated microinvasive cancers have been diagnosed when the histologic specimen was evaluated. This has led some authors to suggest that LEEP could be used in place of cold knife conization to evaluate patients in whom cancer has not been ruled out. Murdoch noted that 44 of 1143 LEEP specimens contained invasive cancer (18 with stage Ia, 17 with stage Ib, and 9 with stage Ib adenocarcinoma). Thirty-three (75%) of the patients had unsatisfactory or suspicious for cancer colposcopy. LEEP was compared with conization in 63 patients with a high suspicion of microinvasion. All patients had a subsequent hysterectomy. The rate of transection of disease with the LEEP was significantly higher than with conization (17% vs 0%). The high frequency of tissue fragmentation with multiple passes that were required to remove the entire lesion led to incomplete evaluation using the LEEP. Lesions high in the canal did not lend themselves to management using LEEP.

Two patients with invasion on their LEEP histology were treated with radical hysterectomies and lymphadenectomies, because the LEEP histology was inadequate to guide less radical therapy. One of the patients had no evidence of cancer in the hysterectomy specimen. These authors think that LEEP should not be used in place of conization for this purpose.

Conization of the cervix

After the extent of involvement of epithelium on the ectocervix has been clearly demarcated by colposcopy, the limits of the base of the cone biopsy on the cervix can be determined. An incision that is certain to include all the abnormal areas is made into the mucous membrane of the ectocervix. Many believe that blood loss can be reduced by injecting a dilute solution of phenylephrine (Neo-Synephrine) or pitressin into the line of incision before beginning the procedure. This incision does not need to be circular but should accommodate excision of all atypical epithelium. The depth of the incision as it tapers toward the endocervical canal should be determined by the length of the cervical canal and the suspected depth of involvement (Fig. 1–10). Often the entire limits of the lesion have been visualized, and a very shallow conization is sufficient (Fig. 1–11). Cervical conization does not need to be a fixed technical procedure for all patients, but it should always consist of adequate excision of all involved areas. Bleeding from the cone bed can usually be controlled by electrocauterization and by placing Monsel's paste on the base. The use of Sturmdorf sutures is probably unnecessary in most cases. Significant cervical stenosis, cervical incompetence, or infertility with a cervical factor are rare complications (Table 1–13) and are functions of the amount of endocervix removed. Several physicians advocate the use of the laser as a cervical tool instead of the knife in conization of the cervix (Table 1–14).

Several studies have now shown that blood loss, infection, and stenosis in laser conization are essentially equal to those occurring in cold knife conization. Some have suggested less dysmenorrhea occurs after laser conization. Complication rates, at least in one study, were equal when laser vaporization was compared with laser conization. Complications after an open cone procedure appear to be similar to those managed with a closed cone procedure (Sturmdorf or other suturing). Although it has been stated that the laser does not distort the cervical margins in regard to pathologic evaluation, one article suggests this is not the case. The authors reviewed 77 laser conizations, of which 28 (36%) showed extensive epithelial denudization, 10 (13%) contained coagulation artifact that made recognition of CIN extremely difficult or impossible, and 11 (14%) showed laser artifacts that made assessment of margins extremely difficult or impossible.

As has already been indicated, in the USA conization of the cervix is used primarily as a diagnostic tool and secondarily as therapy for patients who are young and desire further fertility. However, in other countries, conization is used as definitive therapy. Extensive experience has been obtained with this operative modality, particularly in the treatment of severe CIN.

In Europe (especially Scandinavia), conization has been used widely to treat patients with CIN, and some interesting data have been published. Bjerre and associates reported on 2099 cases of women with abnormal vaginal smears in whom conization of the cervix had been performed. The frequency of complications was considered low, and cervical carcinoma in situ was diagnosed in 1500 cases. Conization appeared to be curative in 87% of these

Table 1–13 MAJOR COMPLICATIONS OF CONIZATION

Immediate	Delayed
Hemorrhage	Bleeding (10–14 days after operation)
Uterine perforation	Cervical stenosis
Anesthetic risk	Infertility
In pregnancy	Incompetent cervix
Rupture of membranes	Increased preterm delivery (low birthweight)
Premature labor	

Table 1–14 LASER CONIZATION

Instruments	CO_2 laser, colposcope, micromanipulator
Power output	25–30 W
Power density	1400 W/cm^2
Spot size	0.5 mm
Operating mode	Continuous
Lateral margins	5 mm beyond the lesion
Endocervical margin	Surgically cut
Hemostasis	Lateral sutures, Pitressin infiltration
Anesthesia	General, local

Figure 1–10 Cone biopsy for endocervical disease. Limits of the lesion were not seen colposcopically.

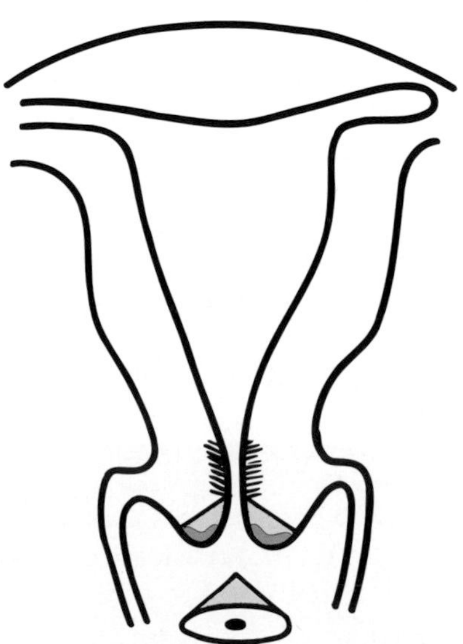

Figure 1–11 Cone biopsy for cervical intraepithelial neoplasia of the exocervix. Limits of the lesion were identified colposcopically.

1500 cases. Failure was related to whether the margins of resection were free of pathologic epithelium. If Pap smears were repeatedly negative for the first year after conization, subsequent abnormal smears were found in only 0.4% of the cases. Kolstad and Klem reported on a series of 1121 patients with carcinoma in situ who had been followed for 5–25 years. Therapeutic conization had been performed on 795 of these patients, of whom 19 (2.3%) had recurrent carcinoma in situ and 7 (0.9%) developed invasive cancer. The corresponding figures for 238 patients treated by hysterectomy were, respectively, 3 (1.2%) and 5 (2.1%). The invasive lesions noted appeared several years later, and the type of initial procedure had no significant influence. Kolstad and Klem emphasized that women who have had carcinoma in situ of the cervix will always be at some risk and, therefore, should be carefully followed for a much longer time than the conventional period of 5 years (Table 1–15).

If conization has ruled out invasive cancer, those with free surgical margins have almost a 100% disease-free follow-up. The question that is frequently asked is what should management be post cone if surgical margins, particularly the endocervical margins, have disease present? Considerable data in the literature suggest that most will have normal cytology post cone and that no further treatment is necessary. Anderson noted 58 patients with positive surgical margins, and only three (5%) had persistent disease. Lopes noted in 75 similar patients that 9 (12%) had residual disease. Grundsell found 3 of 21 patients with positive margins with residual disease. Our practice is to follow-up all post cone patients with cytology only irrespective of surgical margin status and intervene only if cytology is abnormal.

Hysterectomy

Traditionally in the USA, a vaginal hysterectomy has been the treatment of choice for patients with carcinoma in situ. This was particularly true before the establishment of reliable outpatient diagnostic techniques. Hysterectomy is an appropriate method of treatment for the CIN patient who has completed her childbearing, is interested in permanent sterilization, and has other pathology in which hysterectomy is indicated. CIN as a sole indictor for hysterectomy does not appear to be appropriate with multiple alternative therapies available today. This decision must be made jointly by the patient, her family, and the physician. For many years the removal of the upper part of the vagina has been advocated in the treatment of carcinoma in situ, yet there is no basis for this recommendation. In a study by Creasman and Rutledge, the recurrence rate for carcinoma in situ of the cervix did not depend on the amount of vagina removed with the uterus. Unless vaginal extension of disease can be identified colposcopically (this occurrence is < 5%), there is no reason for routine removal of the upper vagina. There appears to be no reason for so-called modified radical hysterectomy in the management of patients with CIN. However, even though hysterectomy is considered to be definitive therapy, patients must be followed in essentially the same manner as patients chosen for outpatient management. Although the chance of subsequent recurrence of invasive disease is small, recurrence can occur, and these patients must be followed indefinitely.

Table 1–15 CONIZATION AND HYSTERECTOMY AS TREATMENT FOR CARCINOMA IN SITU

	Persistence of CIS	Recurrence of cancer
Conization (*n* = 3103)	6.3%	0.6%
Hysterectomy (*n* = 3729)	0.9%	0.3%

From Boyes, Creasman, Kolstad, Bjerre.

Vaccines

Approximately 70–80% of all cervical cancer implicates HPV type 16 and 18. This relates not only to squamous cervical cancer, but also to adenocarcinoma. These two subtypes are also implicated in the development of high-grade cervical intraepithelial neoplasia. In a large study, almost 10% of women with HPV-16 infection and 5% of women with HPV-18 infection developed CIN-III within 36 months. The low-risk types, HPV-6 and 11, are the most common cause of genital warts and is found in over 95% of cases of condyloma acuminata. These types are also responsible for the vast majority of cases of recurrent respiratory papillomatosis (RRP). HPV currently affects about 20 million adolescents in the USA, and it is estimated that 6.2 million sexually active adults will acquire the infection each year. It is estimated that approximately 75% of sexually active men and women will acquire HPV during their lifetime.

The immunogenicity of papillomatous virus allows the possibility of developing vaccines to HPV DNA. The HPV-16 L1 virus-like particle vaccine consists of a highly purified virus-like particle of the L1 capsule of HPV-16. In a double-blind study, 23921 young women between the ages of 16 and 23 received 3 doses of the placebo or the HPV-16 virus-like particle at day 0, month 2, and month 6. Genital samples to test for HPV-16 DNA were obtained at enrollment, one month after the third vaccination and every six months thereafter. These women were followed for a median of 17.4 months after completion of the vaccination regimen. The incidence of persistent HPV-16 infection was 3.8 per 100 women years at risk in the placebo group and 0 per 100 women years in the vaccine group. All 41 cases of HPV-16 infection occurred in the placebo group, 31 were persistent HPV-16 without cervical intraepithelial neoplasia, 5 consisted of HPV-16 related CIN I and 4 consisted of CIN II. An additional 44 cases of CIN that were not associated with HPV-16 infection were detected, 22 among the placebo and 22 among the vaccine recipients.

A bivalent L1 virus-like particle vaccination with HPV type 16 and 18 has also been evaluated in a randomized controlled study. The study by Harper et al had a similar protocol as the Koutsky study as far as vaccination schedule and follow-up. Nine hundred and fifty-eight women completed the vaccination phase. These were individuals between the ages of 15 and 25 who were sexually active. According to protocol analysis, vaccine efficacy was 91.6% against incidence infection and 100% against persistent infection with HPV-16/18. It would appear that the bivalent HPV vaccine was efficacious in prevention of incidence as well as persistent cervical infections that were caused by HPV-16/18 and associated cytological abnormalities and lesions. In the placebo group, there were 27 women and 2 in the vaccine group who had HPV-16 and/or 18 associated cytological abnormalities.

A phase II study involving more than 1000 women age 16–23 randomly assigned to receive the quadrivalent vaccine or placebo on day 1, month 2 and month 6. There was an 89% and 100% efficacy in the prevention of HPV-6/11/16/18-related persistent infections and disease respectively. The quadrivalent vaccine also prevented genital warts 100% of the time. The vaccine was well tolerated and there were no significant adverse effects. Two large phase III trials of the quadrivalent vaccine (Future I and Future II) also demonstrated good results. More than 5000 women age 16–23 were evaluated in Future I, again a prospective randomized control study in much the same manner as the phase II study. Following a two-year follow-up, the vaccine appeared 100% effective in preventing all four HPV-type related CIN, genital warts, vulvovaginal neoplasia in the women who received all three vaccinations and who on day 1 were naïve to the four HPV types. The vaccine was 97% effective in the women who were naïve of all four types on day 1, but who did not receive all three injections or who had one or more of these HPV types demonstrated prior to receiving the full three courses. Future II was a similar trial involving over 12,000 women age 16–23, and again reported 100% efficacy in the prevention of HPV-16/18 related CIN-II and III, AIS and cancer through two years of follow-up. In contrast, 21 cases of CIN-II/III or AIS related to these two types developed in the group receiving the placebo.

In a recent study reported at the European Society of Paediatric Infectious Diseases, Nolan enrolled 1529 in a study of HPV-6, 11, 16, and 18 vaccines. They were divided into three groups: 510 males, 10–15 years old; 506 females, 10–15 years old; and 513 females, 16–23 years old. All received three injections of the vaccine over a 6-month period and were evaluated to determine the specific immune response. Tolerability was also assessed. Seroconversion and geometric mean titers (GMT) were determined one month after the end of the study. Seroconversion was 100% for HPV types 6, 11 and 16, and 99.9% for HPV-18 in the combined group of adolescents. For the 16–23-year-olds, again 100% seroconversion was present for HPV-6, 11 and 16 with 99.2% for HPV-18. Antibody levels (GMT) were significantly higher for all types in the adolescents compared to the 16–23 year old groups. The vaccine was generally well tolerated. Only three adolescents discontinued the vaccination due to adverse effects. Fever was more common in the adolescents compared with the 16–23 year old group; however, the febrile episodes were generally shortlived and not associated with serious clinical consequences. Currently a Phase III trial is underway with over 25,000 enrolled worldwide.

It has been estimated that if women were vaccinated against the five HPV types (16/18/31/33/45), which are mostly responsible for cervical cancer, before they become sexually active, there could be a reduction of at least 85% in the risk of cancer and a decline of 44–70% in the frequency of abnormal Pap smears attributed to HPV.

Cost-effective modeling studies have been done in regards to the potential benefit of vaccination against HPV infection. These studies concluded that if 70% of 12-year-old girls currently living in the USA were vaccinated against the high-risk HPVs, an estimated 250,000 cases of HPV infection, more than 3300 cases of cervical cancer, and more than 1300 deaths from cervical cancer would be prevented during the lifetime of these individuals. This assumes that the vaccine efficacy lasts for 10 years or longer.

The FDA has approved the quadrivalent HPV in girls and women age 9–26. There is very little data concerning efficacy in the youngest of this age spread and how long the vaccination appears effective is unknown. It is interesting to note that both girls and boys age 10–15 receiving the quadrivalent vaccine demonstrated geometric mean titers at month seven 1.67 to 2.7 times higher than those observed when the vaccine was administered to adolescents and young women aged 16–23. This does suggest, however, the high immunogenesis and the safety of the quadrivalent vaccine in young boys and girls, and has apparent stronger immune process following immunization.

Whether or not vaccinations in the future will find a place in our armamentarium, particularly in the Western world in which cytological screening is available, is unknown. It would appear that in the underdeveloped world in which cervical cancer is much more of a health care problem, vaccinations in these geographical areas might be efficacious, although logistics as well as costs certainly are formidable problems.

BIBLIOGRAPHY

EPIDEMIOLOGY AND NATURAL HISTORY

Altekruse SF, Lacey JV, Brinton LA et al: Comparison of HPV genotypes, sexual and reproductive risk factors of cervical adenocarcinoma and squamous cell carcinoma. Am J Obstet Gynecol 188: 657–663, 2003.

Amadori A, Gentiliui P, Bucchi L et al: A registry-based study of follow-up failures in the screening experience of cervical cancer patients. Int J Gynecol Cancer 8:251, 1998.

Ashley DJB: The biological status of carcinoma in situ of the uterine cervix. J Obstet Gynaecol Br Commonw 73:372, 1966.

Bauer HM, Ting Y, Greer CE et al: Genital human papilloma virus infection in female university students as determined by a PCR-based method. JAMA 265:472, 1991.

Beral V: Cancer of the cervix: A sexually transmitted infection? Lancet 1:1037, 1974.

Bower M: Women's knowledge, attitudes and behavior toward Pap screening, National Omnibus Survey Findings. The Female Patient 18:21, 1993.

Brinton LA, Fraumeni JF: Epidemiology of uterine cervical cancer. J Chron Dis 39:1051, 1986.
Butterworth CE, Hatch KD, Macaluso M et al: Folate deficiency and cervical dysplasia. JAMA 267:528, 1992.
Champion MJ et al: Increased risk of cervical neoplasia in consorts: Men with penile condyloma acuminatum. Lancet 1:943, 1985.
Champion MJ et al: Progressive potential of mild cervical atypia: Perspective cytologic, colposcopic and virological studies. Lancet 2:273, 1986.
Cohen AL, Rosenberg AJ, McCann MF: Active and passive cigarette smoke exposure and cervical neoplasia. Cancer Epidemiol Biomarkers Prev 1:349, 1992.
Coppleson M, Reid B: The etiology of squamous carcinoma of the cervix (Editorial). Obstet Gynecol 32:432, 1968.
de Villiers EM: Heterogeneity of the human papillomavirus group. J Virol 63:4898, 1989.
de Villiers EM, Wagner D, Schneider A et al: Human papilloma virus DNA in women without and with cytologic abnormalities: Results of a 5-year follow-up study. Gynecol Oncol 44:33, 1992.
Diagnostic and Therapeutic Technology Assessment (DATTA). JAMA 270:2975, 1993.
Fenoglio CM, Ferenczy A: Etiologic factors in cervical neoplasia. Semin Oncol 9:349, 1982.
Fletcher A: Screening for cancer of the cervix in elderly women. Lancet 335:97, 1990.
Fluhmann CF: Carcinoma in situ and the transitional zone of the cervix uteri. Obstet Gynecol 16:424, 1960.
Gaarenstoom KN, Melkert P, Walboomers JMM et al: Human papillomavirus DNA and genotypes: Prognostic factors for progression of CIN. Int J Gynecol Cancer 4:73, 1994.
Gagnon F: The lack of occurrence of cervical carcinoma in nuns. Proc Second Natl Cancer Conf 1:625, 1952.
Goff BA, Muntz HG, Bell DA et al: Human papillomavirus typing in patients with Pap smears showing squamous atypia. Gynecol Oncol 48:384, 1993.
Grussendorf-Conen EI, de Villiers EM, Gissmann L: Human papilloma virus genomes in penile smears of healthy men. Lancet 2:1092, 1986.
Harlan LC, Bernstein AB, Kessler LG: Cervical cancer screening: Who is not screened and why? Am J Public Health 81:885, 1991.
Hatch KD, Schneider A, Abdel-Nour MW: An evaluation of HPV testing for intermediate and high-risk types as triage before colposcopy. Am J Obstet Gynecol 172:1150–1157, 1995.
Ho GYF, Bierman R, Beardsley L et al: Natural history of cervicovaginal HPV infections in young women. NEJM 338:423–428, 1998.
Jenison SA, Yu X, Valentine JM et al: Evidence of prevalent genital-type human papillomavirus infection in adults and children. J Infect Dis 162:60, 1990.
Johnson JC, Burnett AF, Willet GD et al: High frequency of latent and clinical HPV cervical infections in immunocompromised HIV infected women. Obstet Gynecol 79:321, 1992.
Kessis TD, Siebos RJ, Nelson WG: Human papillomavirus 16 E6 expression disrupts the p-53 mediated cellular response to DNA damage. Proc Natl Acad Sci USA 90:3988, 1993.
Kjaer SK, deVilliers EM, Haugaard BJ et al: Human papillomavirus, herpes simplex virus and cervical cancer incidence in Greenland and Denmark: A population-based cross-sectional study. Int J Cancer 41:518, 1988.
Kurman RJ, Schiffman MH, Lancaster WED et al: Analysis of individual human papillomavirus types in cervical neoplasia: A possible role for type 18 in rapid progression. Am J Obstet Gynecol 159:293, 1988.
Ley C, Bauer HM, Reingold A et al: Determinants of genital human papillomavirus infection in young women. J Natl Cancer Inst 83:997, 1991.
Mao C, Hughes JP, Kiviat N et al: Clinical findings among young women with genital human HPV infections. Am J Obstet Gynecol 188:677–684, 2003.
Maiman M: Cervical neoplasia in women with HIV infection. Oncology 8:83, 1994.
Mathur SP, Mathur RS, Rust RF, Young RC: Human papilloma virus (HPV)-E6/E7 and epidermal growth factor receptor (EGF-R) protein levels in cervical cancer and cervical intraepithelial neoplasia CIN. Am J Reprod Immunol 46:280–287, 2001.
Mathur SP, Mathur RS: In vitro downregulation of growth factors by insulin-like growth factor binding protein-3 in cervical cancer. Gynecol Oncol 91:410–415, 2003.
Meanwell CA, Cox MF, Blackledge GB et al: HPV 16 DNA in normal and malignant cervical epithelium: Implications for the aetiology and behaviour of cervical neoplasia. Lancet 1:266, 1987.
Meisel A, Roy M, Fortier M et al: Condylomatous lesions of the cervix: morphologic and colposcopic diagnosis. Am J Diag Gynecol 1:109, 1979.
Melnikow J, Nuovo J, William AR et al: Natural history of cervical squamous intraepithelial lesions: A meta-analysis. Obstet Gynecol 92:727, 1998.
Meyskens FL, Surrvit E, Moon TE et al: Enhancement of regression of CIN II with topically applied all-trans-retinoic acid. J Natl Cancer Inst 86:539, 1994.
Moscicki AB, Palefsky J, Smith et al: Variability of human papillomavirus DNA testing in a longitudinal cohort of young women. Obstet Gynecol 82:578, 1993.
Munger K, Scheffra M, Huibregtse JM et al: Interaction of HPV E6 and E7 with tumor suppressor gene products. Cancer Surv 12:197, 1992.
Munoz N, Bosch X, Kaldor JM: Does human papillomavirus cause cervical cancer? The state of the epidemiological evidence. Br J Cancer 57:1, 1988.
Murphy WM, Coleman SA: The long-term course of carcinoma in situ of the uterine cervix. Cancer 38:957, 1976.
Ng A: Presidential address. Acta Cytol 22:121, 1978.
Okagaki T, Tase T, Twiggs LB et al: Histogenesis of cervical adenocarcinoma with reference to HPV 18 as a carcinogen. J Reprod Med 34:639, 1989.
Östör AG: Natural history of cervical intraepithelial neoplasia: A critical review. Int J Gynecol Pathol 12:186, 1993
Palefsky JM: Human papilloma virus-associated anogenital neoplasia and other solid tumors in HIV infected individuals. Curr Opin Oncol 3:881, 1991.
Peterson O: Spontaneous course of cervical precancerous conditions. Am J Obstet Gynecol 72:1063, 1956.
Pinion SB, Kennedy JH, Miller RW et al: Oncogene expression in cervical intraepithelial neoplasia and invasive cancer of cervix. Lancet 337:819, 1991.
Rahan T, Mann V, McLaughlin J et al: PCR-detected genital papillomavirus infection: Prevalence and association with risk factors for cervical cancer. Int J Cancer 49:856, 1991.
Ray M, Plante M: "Rapid-onset" cervical cancer due to failure in a screening program. J Lower Genital Tract Dis 1:76, 1998.
Reeves WC, Brinton LA, Garcia M et al: Human papillomavirus infection and cervical cancer in Latin America. N Engl J Med 320:1437, 1989.
Reeves WC, Rawls WE, Brinton LA: Epidemiology of genital papillomaviruses and cervical cancer. Rev Infect Dis 11:426, 1989.
Richart RM: Natural history of cervical intraepithelial neoplasia. Clin Obstet Gynecol 10:748, 1968.
Rosenfeld WD, Rose E, Vermund SH et al: Follow-up evaluation of cervicovaginal human papillomavirus in adolescents. J Pediatrics 121:307, 1992.
Sedlacek TV, Sedlacek AE, Neff DK et al: Clinical role of human papillomavirus typing. Gynecol Oncol 42:222, 1991.
Simmons AM, Phillips DH, Coleman DV: Damage to DNA in cervical epithelium related to smoking tobacco. Br Med J 306:1444, 1993.
Spinillo A, Tenti P, Zappatoe R et al: Prevalence, diagnosis, and treatment of lower genital neoplasia in women with HIV infection. Eur J Obstet Gynecol Reprod Biol 43:235, 1992.

Sun XW, Ellerbrock TV, Lungu O et al: Human papillomavirus infections in HIV seropositive women. Obstet Gynecol 85:680, 1995.

Tidy JA, Parry GCN, Ward P et al: High rate of human papillomavirus type 16 infection in cytologically normal cervices. Lancet 1:434, 1989.

Trevathan E, Loyde P, Webster LA et al: Cigarette smoking and dysplasia in carcinoma in situ of the uterine cervix. JAMA 250:499, 1983.

Walker J, Bloss JD, Liao SY et al: Human papillomavirus genotype as a prognostic indicator in carcinoma of the uterine cervix. Obstet Gynecol 74:781, 1989.

Woodman CB, Collins S, Winter H et al: Natural history of cervical human papillomavirus infection in young women: a longitudinal cohort study. Lancet 357:1831–1836, 2001.

Wright TC, Ellerbrock TV, Chiasson MA et al: CIN in women infected with HIV; prevalence, risk factors, and validity of Pap smears. Obstet Gynecol 84:591, 1994.

Zunzunegui MV, King MC, Coria CF et al: Male influence on cervical cancer risks. Am J Epidemiol 123:302, 1986.

zur Hausen H: Human papillomaviruses in the pathogenesis of anogenital cancers. Virology 184:9, 1991.

zur Hausen H, Meinhof W, Scheiber Wand Born Kamm EW: Attempts to detect virus-specific DNA in human tumors. I: Nucleic acid hybridizations with complementary RNA of human wart virus. Int J Cancer 13:650, 1974.

SCREENING AND DIAGNOSIS

Bernstein SJ, Sanchez-Ramos L, Ndubisi B: Liquid-based cervical cytologic smear study and conventional Papanicolaou smears: A meta-analysis of prospective studies comparing cytologic diagnosis and sample adequacy. Am J Obstet Gynecol 185:308–317, 2001.

Bethesda Workshop: The revised Bethesda System for reporting cervical/vaginal cytologic diagnosis: Report of the 1991 Bethesda Workshop. J Reprod Med 37:383, 1992.

Boardman LA, Stanko C, Weitzen S et al: Atypical squamous cells of undetermined significance: human papillomavirus testing in adolescents. Obstet Gynecol 105:741–746, 2005.

Calle EE, Flander D, Thun MJ: Demographic predictors of mammography and Pap smear screening in US women. Am J Public Health 83:53, 1993.

Christopherson WM, Nealon N, Gray LA: Noninvasive precursor lesions of adenocarcinoma and mixed adenosquamous carcinoma of the cervix uteri. Cancer 44(3): 975–983,1979.

Coppleson LW, Brown B: Estimation of the screening error rate from the observed detection rates in repeated cervical cytology. Am J Obstet Gynecol 119:953, 1974.

Coppleson M, Pixley E, Reid B: Colposcopy: A Scientific and Practical Approach to the Cervix in Health and Disease. Springfield, IL, Charles C Thomas, 1971.

Davis GL, Hernandez E, Davis JL et al: Atypical squamous cells in Papanicolaou smears. Obstet Gynecol 69:43, 1987.

DePetrillo AD et al: Colposcopic evaluation of the abnormal Papanicolaou test in pregnancy. Am J Obstet Gynecol 121:441, 1975.

Eddy GL, Strumpf KB, Wagtowycz MA et al: Biopsy findings in five hundred thirty-one patients with atypical glandular cells of uncertain significance as defined by the Bethesda System. Am J Obstet Gynecol 177:1188, 1997.

Ferenczy A: Screening for cervical cancer: A renewed plea for annual smears, Contemp Ob/Gyn 93, 1986.

Gad C, Koch F: The limitation of screening effect: A review of cervical disorders in previously screened women. Acta Cytol 21:719, 1978.

Gray LA, Christopherson WM: Treatment of cervical dysplasia. Gynecol Oncol 3:149, 1975.

Harlan LC, Bernstein AB, Kessler LE: Cervical cancer screening: Who is not and why? Am J Public Health 81:885, 1991.

Harper DM, Franco EL, Wheeler C et al: Efficacy of a bivalent L1 virus-like particle vaccine in prevention of infection with human papillomavirus types 16 and 18 in young women: a randomized controlled trial. Lancet 364:1757–1765, 2004.

Himmelstein LR: Evaluation of inflammatory atypia: A literature review. J Reprod Med 34:634, 1989.

Hoffman MS, Hill DA, Gordy LW et al: Comparing the yield of the standard Papanicolaou brush smears. J Reprod Med 36:267, 1991.

Janerich DT, Hadjimichael O, Schwartz PE: The screening histories of women with invasive cervical cancer, Connecticut. Am J Public Health 85:791, 1995.

Kaminski PE, Stevens CW, Wheelock JB: Squamous atypia on cytology: The influence of age. J Reprod Med 9:617, 1989.

Kaufman RH, Adams E, Icenogle J et al: Relevance of human papilloma virus screening in management of cervical intraepithelial neoplasia. Am J Obstet Gynecol 176:87, 1997.

Kim TJ, Kim HS, Park CT et al: Clinical evaluation of follow-up methods and results of atypical glandular cells of undetermined significance (AGUS) detected on cervicovaginal Pap smears. Gynecol Oncol 73:292, 1999.

Kohan S et al: Colposcopy and the management of cervical intraepithelial neoplasia. Gynecol Oncol 5:27, 1977.

Kolstad P, Klem V: Long-term follow-up of 1121 cases of carcinoma in situ. Obstet Gynecol 48:125, 1976.

Koutsky LA, Ault KA, Wheeler CM et al: A controlled trial of human papillomavirus type 16 vaccine. NEJM 347:1645–1651, 2002.

Kristensen GB, Jensen LK, Holund B: A randomized trial comparing two methods of cold knife conization with laser conization. Obstet Gynecol 76:1009, 1990.

Maier RC, Schultenover SJ: Evaluation of the atypical squamous cell Papanicolaou smear. Int J Gynecol Pathol 5:242, 1986.

Mandelblatt J, Gopaul FNP, Wistreich M: Gynecological care of elderly women. JAMA 256:367, 1986.

Manos MM, Kinney WK, Hurley LB et al: Identifying women with cervical neoplasia using human papillomavirus DNA testing for equivocal Papanicolaou result. JAMA 281:1605, 1999.

Melnikow J, Nuovo J, Willan AR et al: Natural history of cervical squamous intraepithelial lesions: a meta-analysis. Obstet Gynecol 92:727–735, 1998.

Mitchell H, Medley G: Longitudinal study of women with negative cervical smears according to endocervical status. Lancet 337:265, 1991.

NCI Workshop: The 1988 Bethesda System for reporting cervical/vaginal cytological diagnoses. JAMA 262:931, 1989.

Reiter RC: Management of initial atypical cervical cytology: A randomized prospective study. Obstet Gynecol 68:237, 1986.

Roongpisuthipone A, Grimes DA, Hodges A: Is the Papanicolaou smear useful for diagnosing sexually transmitted disease? Obstet Gynecol 69:820, 1987.

US Preventive Services Task Force (USPSTF) Screening for cervical cancer: Recommendations and rationale. www.ahrq.gov/clinic/3rduspstf/cervcan/cervcanrr.htm. Accessed July 5, 2006.

Sarode VR, Werner C, Gander R et al. Reflex human papillomavirus DNA testing on residual liquid-based (TPPT) cervical samples: focus on age-stratified clinical performance. Cancer 99:149–155, 2003.

Solomon D, Davey D, Kurman R, Moriarty A et al: The 2001 Bethesda System: terminology for reporting results of cervical cytology. JAMA 287:2114–2119, 2002.

Spitzer M, Krumholz BA, Chernys AE et al: Comparative utility of repeat Papanicolaou smears, cervicography, and colposcopy in the evaluation of atypical Papanicolaou smears. Obstet Gynecol 69:731, 1987.

Stafl A, Mattingly RF: Colposcopic diagnosis of cervical neoplasia. Obstet Gynecol 41:168, 1973.

Urcuyo R, Rome RM, Nelson J: Some observations on the value of endocervical curettage performed as an integral part of colposcopic examination of patients with abnormal cervical cytology. Obstet Gynecol 128:787, 1977.

US Preventive Services Task Force (USPSTF) Screening for cervical cancer: Recommendations and rationale. www.ahrq.gov/clinic/3rduspstf/cervcan/cervcanrr.htm. Accessed July 5, 2006.

Villa LL, Costa RL, Petta CA et al: Prophylactic quadrivalent human papillomavirus (types 6, 11, 16 and 18) L1 virus-like particle vaccine in young women: a randomised double-blind placebo-controlled multicentre phase II efficacy trial. Lancet Oncol 6: 271–278, 2005.

Walton RJ: The task force on cervical cancer screening programs (Editorial). Can Med Assoc J 114:981, 1976.

Walton RJ (Chairman): Cervical cancer screening programs: Summary of the 1982 Canadian Task Force Report. Can Med Assoc J 127:581, 1982.

Worth A: The Walton report and its subsequent impact on cervical cancer screening programs in Canada. Obstet Gynecol 63:135, 1984.

Wright TC Jr, Cox JT, Massad LS et al: 2001 consensus guidelines for the management of women with cervical intraepithelial neoplasia. Am J Obstet Gynecol 189:295–304, 2003.

Wright TC Jr, Cox JT, Massad LS et al. 2001 consensus guidelines for the management of women with cervical cytological abnormalities. JAMA 287:2120–129, 2002.

PATHOLOGY AND CYTOLOGY

ACOG Committee Opinion (206): New Pap test screening techniques. Obstet Gynecol 91:1, 1998.

Al-Nafassi AI, Calquhoun MK, Williams ARW: Accuracy of cervical smear in predicting the grade of cervical intraepithelial neoplasia. Int J Gynecol Cancer 3:89, 1993.

Brown AD, Garber AM: Cost effectiveness of 3 methods to enhance the sensitivity of Papanicolaou testing. JAMA 281:342, 1999.

Cejtin HE, Massad LS, Collins Y: Predictors of CIN in women with ASCUS and LSIL cytology (Abstract). J Lower Genital Tract 43, 1999.

Coppleson LW, Brown B: Estimation of the screening error rate from the observed detection rates in repeated cervical cytology. Am J Obstet Gynecol 119:953, 1974.

Fluhmann CF: Carcinoma in situ and the transitional zone of the cervix uteri. Obstet Gynecol 16:424, 1960.

Friedell GH, Hertig AT, Younge PA: Carcinoma in Situ of the Uterine Cervix. Springfield, IL, Charles C Thomas, 1960.

Hutchinson M, Zahniser DJ, Sherman ME et al: Utility of liquid-based cytology for cervical carcinoma screening. Cancer (Cancer Cytopathol) 87:48, 1999.

Kaufman RH, Schrieber K, Carter T: An analysis of atypical squamous (glandular) cells of undetermined significant smears by neural network-directed review. Obstet Gynecol 91:556, 1998.

Kobelin MH, Kobelin CE, Burke L et al: Incidence and predictors of cervical dysplasia in patients with minimally abnormal Papanicolaou smears. Obstet Gynecol 92:356, 1998.

Koss LG, Sherman ME, Cohen MB et al: Significant reduction in the rate of false negative cervical smears with neural network based technology: PAPNET Testing System. JAMA 281:347, 1999.

Kurman RJ, Henson DE, Herbst AL et al: Interim guidelines for management of abnormal cervical cytology. JAMA 271:1866, 1994.

Lee KR, Ashfaq R, Birdsong GG et al: Comparison of conventional Papanicolaou smears and a fluid-based thin layer system for cervical cancer screening. Obstet Gynecol 90:278, 1997.

Lonky NM, Navarre EL, Saunders S et al: Low-grade Pap smears and The Bethesda System: A prospective cytohistopathologic analysis. Obstet Gynecol 85:716, 1995.

Mitchell H, Medley G: Detection of unsuspected abnormalities by PAPNET-assisted review. Acta Cytol 42:260, 1998.

Mitchell H, Medley G: Detection of laboratory false negative smears by the PAPNET Cytologic Screening System. Acta Cytol 42:265, 1998.

O'Leary TJ, Tellado M, Buchman SB et al: PAPNET-assisted re screening of cervical smear. JAMA 279:235, 1998.

Papillo JH, Zarka MA, St Johns TL: Evaluation of the thin prep Pap test in clinical practice. Acta Cytol 90:278, 1997.

Roberts JM, Gurley AM, Thurloe JK et al: Evaluation of thin prep Pap test as an adjunct to the conventional Pap smear. MJA 167:466, 1997.

Roongpisuthipone A, Grimes DA, Hodges A: Is the Papanicolaou smear useful for diagnosing sexually transmitted disease? Obstet Gynecol 69:820, 1987.

Shingleton HM, Gore H, Austin JM Jr: Outpatient evaluation of patients with atypical Papanicolaou smears; contribution of endocervical curettage. Am J Obstet Gynecol 126:122, 1976.

Taylor RR, Guerrieri JP, Nash JD et al: Atypical cervical cytology. J Reprod Med 38:443, 1993.

Wilbur DC, Cibas ES, Merritt S et al: Thin Prep Processor clinical trials demonstrate an increase detection rate of abnormal cervical cytologic specimens. Am J Clin Pathol 101:209, 1994.

Wright TC, Sun XLO, Koulos J: Comparison of management algorithms for the evaluation of women with low-grade cytologic abnormalities. Obstet Gynecol 85:202, 1995.

MANAGEMENT

Adams E, Kaufman RH, Berkova Z et al: Is human papillomavirus testing an effective triage method for detection of high grade (grade 2 or 3) cervical intraepithelial neoplasia? Am J Obstet Gynecol 178:1235, 1998.

Anderson ES, Nielson K, Larsen G: Laser conization: Follow-up in patients with CIN in the cone margin. Gynecol Oncol 39:328, 1990.

Baggish MS: Management of cervical intraepithelial neoplasia by carbon dioxide laser. Obstet Gynecol 60:378, 1992.

Baggish MS, Barash F, Noel Y et al: Comparison of thermal injury zones in loop electrical and laser cervical excisional conization. Am J Obstet Gynecol 166:545, 1991.

Baldauf JJ, Dreyfus M, Ritter et al: Cytology and colposcopy after loop electrosurgical excision: Implications for follow-up. Obstet Gynecol 92:124, 1998.

Barnes MN, Robertson MW, Naumann RW et al: Histopathological variables predicting high-grade squamous intraepithelial lesions after large loop excision of the transformation zone. J Lower Genital Tract 2:93, 1998.

Benedet JL, Nickerson KG, Anderson GH: Cryotherapy in the treatment of cervical intraepithelial neoplasia. Obstet Gynecol 58:72, 1981.

Berget A, Andreasson B, Bock JE: Laser and cryosurgery for CIN. Acta Obstet Gynecol Scand 70:231, 1991.

Bigrigg MA, Codling BW, Pearson P et al: Colposcopic diagnosis and treatment of cervical dysplasia at a single clinic visit. Lancet 336:229, 1990.

Bigrigg MA, Codling BW, Pearson P et al: Pregnancy after cervical loop diathermy. Lancet 337:119, 1991.

Bigrigg MA, Haffenden DK, Sheehan AL et al: Efficacy and safety of large-loop excision of the TZ. Lancet 343:32, 1994.

Bjerre B et al: Conization as only treatment of carcinoma in situ of the uterine cervix. Am J Obstet Gynecol 125:143, 1976.

Bosch FX, Mano MM, Munoz N et al: Prevalence of human papillomavirus in cervical cancer: A worldwide perspective. J Natl Cancer 87:796, 1995.

Boyes DA, Worth AS, Fidler HK: The results of treatment of 4389 cases of preclinical squamous carcinoma. J Obstet Gynaecol Br Commonw 77:769, 1970.

Burke L: The use of the carbon dioxide laser in the therapy of cervical intraepithelial neoplasia. Am J Obstet Gynecol 144:337, 1982.

Burke L, Covell L, Antonioli D: Carbon dioxide laser therapy of cervical intraepithelial neoplasia: factors determining success rate. Lasers Surg Med 1(2):113–122, 1980.

Campion FM, diPaola ML, Campion MM et al: Cervical intraepithelial neoplasia—should we treat the male partner? The Colposcopist 23:5, 1991.

Chanen W, Hollyock VE: Colposcopy and the conservative management of cervical dysplasias and carcinoma in situ. Obstet Gynecol 43:527, 1974.

Chanen W, Rome RM: Electrocoagulation diathermy for cervical dysplasia and carcinoma in situ: A 15-year survey. Obstet Gynecol 61:673, 1983.

Costa S, Sideri M, Bucchi L et al: Cervicography and HPV DNA testing as triage criteria for patients with abnormal Pap smears. Gynecol Oncol 71:704, 1998.

Creasman WT, Clarke-Pearson DL, Weed JC Jr: Results of outpatient therapy of cervical intraepithelial neoplasia. Gynecol Oncol 12: S-306, 1981.

Creasman WT, Rutledge F: Carcinoma in situ of the cervix: An analysis of 861 patients. Obstet Gynecol 39:373, 1972.

Creasman WT, Weed JC Jr: Conservative management of cervical intraepithelial neoplasia. Clin Obstet Gynecol 43:281, 1980.

Creasman WT et al: Efficacy of cryosurgical treatment of severe cervical intraepithelial neoplasia. Obstet Gynecol 41:501, 1973.

Cruickshank ME, Flannelly G, Campbell DM et al: Fertility and pregnancy outcome following large loop excision of the cervical transformation zone. Br J Obstet Gynecol 102:467, 1995.

Cuzick N, Szwrewski A, Terry G et al: Human papillomavirus testing in primary cervical screening. Lancet 343:1533, 1995.

DiSaia PJ, Townsend DE, Morrow CP: The rationale for less than radical treatment for gynecologic malignancy in early reproductive years. Obstet Gynecol Surv 29:581, 1974.

Gordon HK, Duncan ID: Effective destruction of cervical intraepithelial neoplasia (CIN)3 at 100°C using the Semm cold coagulator: 14 years' experience. Br J Obstet Gynaecol 98:14, 1991.

Gray LA, Christopherson WM: Treatment of cervical dysplasia. Gynecol Oncol 3:149, 1975.

Greenberg MD, Reid R, Schiffman M et al: A prospective study of biopsy confirmed CIN I: Colposcopic, cytologic, and virological risk factors for progression. J Lower Genital Tract 2:104, 1999.

Hal R, Hammond R, Pryse-Davies J: Histologic reliability of laser cone biopsy of the cervix. Obstet Gynecol 77:905, 1991.

Harper DM, Franco EL, Wheeler C et al: Efficacy of a bivalent L1 virus-like particle vaccine in prevention of infection with human papillomavirus type 16 and 18 in young women. Lancet 364: 1757–1765, 2004.

Hitchcock A, Johnson J, McDowell K et al: A retrospective study into the occurrence of cervical glandular atypia in cone specimen from 1977–78 with clinical follow-up. Int J Gynecol Cancer 3:164, 1993.

Javaheri G, Balin M, Meltzer RM: Role of cryosurgery in the treatment of intraepithelial neoplasia of the uterine cervix. Obstet Gynecol 58:83, 1981.

Kaufman RH, Adams E: Is human papillomavirus testing a value in clinical practice? Am J Obstet Gynecol 180:1049, 1999.

Kaufman RH, Adams E, Icenogle J et al: Relevance of human papillomavirus screening in management of cervical intraepithelial neoplasia. Clin J Obstet Gynecol 176:87, 1997.

Kaufman RH, Adams E, Icenogle J, Reeves WC: Human papilloma virus testing as triage for atypical squamous cells of undetermined significance and low grade squamous intraepithelial lesions: Sensitivity, specificity and cost effectiveness. Am J Obstet Gynecol 177:930, 1997.

Kaufman RH, Irwin JF: The cryosurgical therapy of cervical intraepithelial neoplasia. Am J Obstet Gynecol 131:381, 1978.

Kennedy S, Robinson J, Hallam N: LLETZ and infertility. Br J Obstet Gynaecol 100:965, 1993.

Kolstad P, Klem V: Long-term follow-up of 1121 cases of carcinoma in situ. Obstet Gynecol 48:125, 1976.

Koutsky LA, Ault KA, Wheeler CM et al: A controlled trial of human papillomavirus type 16 vaccine. Women's Oncol Rev 3:195–197, 2003.

Lopes A, Morgan P, Murdoch J et al: The case of conservative management of "incomplete excision" of CIN after laser conization. Gynecol Oncol 49:247, 1993.

LuesleyDM, Cullimore J, Redman CWE et al: Loop diathermy excision of the cervical transformation zone in patients with abnormal cervical smears. Br Med J 300:1090, 1990.

Lurain JR, Gallup DG: Management of abnormal Papanicolaou smears in pregnancy. Obstet Gynecol 53:484, 1979.

Maiman M, Tarricone N, Viera J et al: Colposcopic evaluation of human immunity deficiency virus seropositive women. Obstet Gynecol 78:84, 1991.

Masterson BJ et al: The carbon dioxide laser in cervical intraepithelial neoplasia: A five-year experience in treating 230 patients. Am J Obstet Gynecol 139:565, 1981.

Mitchell MF, Tortolero-Luna G, Cook T et al: A randomized clinical trial of cryotherapy, laser vaporization, and loop electrosurgical excision for treatment of squamous intraepithelial lesions of the cervix. Obstet Gynecol 92:737, 1998.

Muntz HG: Can ACIS be satisfactorily managed by conization alone? Gynecol Oncol 61:303, 1996.

Muntz HG, Bell DA, Loge JM et al: Adenocarcinoma in situ of the uterine cervix. Obstet Gynecol 80:935, 1992.

Murdoch JB, Gishane RN, Monaghan JM: Loop diathermy excision of the abnormal cervical transformation zone. Int J Gynecol Cancer 1:1105, 1991.

Murdoch JB, Grimshaw RN, Morgan PR et al: The impact of loop diathermy on management of early invasive cervical cancer. Int J Gynecol Cancer 2:129, 1992.

Nichols F, Hallen MR, West J et al: LLETZ as an alternative to both local ablative and cone biopsy treatment. J Gynecol Surg 9:77, 1993.

Ortiz R, Newton M, Tsai A: Electrocautery treatment of cervical intraepithelial neoplasia. Obstet Gynecol 41:113, 1973.

Parashevadis E, Jandial L, Mann EMF et al: Patterns of treatment failure following laser for cervical intraepithelial neoplasia: Implications for follow-up protocol. Obstet Gynecol 78:80, 1991.

Popkin DR, Scali V, Ahmed MN: Cryosurgery for treatment of cervical intraepithelial neoplasia. Am J Obstet Gynecol 130:551, 1978.

Poynor EA, Barakat RR, Hoskins WJ: Management and follow-up of patients with adenocarcinoma in situ of the uterine cervix. Gynecol Oncol 57:158, 1995.

Richart RM, Townsend DE et al: An analysis of "long-term" follow-up results in patients with cervical intraepithelial neoplasia treated by cryosurgery. Am J Obstet Gynecol 137:823, 1980.

Riva JM, Sedlacek TV, Cunnane ME et al: Extended carbon dioxide laser vaporization in treatment for subclinical papillomavirus infection of the lower genital tract. Obstet Gynecol 73:25, 1989.

Roberts CH, Dinh TV, Hannigan EV et al: Management of cervical intraepithelial neoplasia during pregnancy: A simplified and cost effective approach. J Lower Genital Tract 2:67, 1998.

Robinson WR, Lund ED, Adams J: The predictive value of LEEP specimen margin status for residual/recurrent cervical intraepithelial neoplasm. Int J Gynecol Cancer 8:109, 1998.

Sevin BU et al: Invasive cancer of the cervix after cryosurgery: Pitfalls of conservative management. Obstet Gynecol 53:465, 1979.

Townsend DE: Cryosurgery for CIN. Obstet Gynecol Surv 34:838, 1979.

Townsend DE, Richart RM: Cryotherapy and carbon dioxide laser management of cervical intraepithelial neoplasia: A controlled comparison. Obstet Gynecol 61:75, 1983.

Tredway DR et al: Colposcopy and cryosurgery in cervical intraepithelial neoplasia. Am J Obstet Gynecol 114:1020, 1972.

Tseng CJ, Liang CC, Lin CI et al: A study of diagnostic failure of loop conization in microinvasive carcinoma of the cervix. Gynecol Oncol 73:91, 1999.

Turlington WT, Wright BD, Powell JL: Impact of the loop electrosurgical excision procedure on future fertility. J Reprod Med 41:815, 1996.

Urcuyo R, Rome RM, Nelson J: Some observations on the value of endocervical curettage performed as an integral part of colposcopic examination of patients with abnormal cervical cytology. Obstet Gynecol 128:787, 1977.

Vedel P, Jakobsen H, Boggsen N et al: Five-year follow-up of patients with CIN in cone margins after conization. Europ J Obstet Gynecol Reprod Biol 50:71, 1993.

Villa LL, Costa RL, Petta CA et al: Prophylactic quadrivalent human papillomavirus (types 6, 11, 16 and 18) L1 virus-like particle vaccine in young women: a randomised double-blind placebo-controlled multicentre phase II efficacy trial. Lancet Oncol 6:271–278, 2005.

Widrich T, Kennedy A, Myers TM et al: Adenocarcinoma in situ of the unterine cervix: Management and outcome. Gynecol Oncol 61:304, 1996.

Wiener JJ, Sweetnam PM, Jones JM: Long-term follow-up of women after hysterectomy with a history of preinvasive cancer of the cervix. Br J Obstet Gynecol 99:907, 1992.

Wilbanks GD, Creasman WT, Kaufman L, Parker RT: Treatment of cervical dysplasia with electrocautery and tetracycline suppositories. Am J Obstet Gynecol 117:460,1973.

Wright JC, Davies EM: The conservative management of cervical intraepithelial neoplasia: The use of cryosurgery and the carbon dioxide laser. Br J Obstet Gynaecol 88:663, 1981.

Yost NP, Santos JT, McIntire DD et al: Postpartum regression rates of antepartum cervical intraepithelial neoplasia II and III lesions. Obstet Gynecol 93:359, 1999.

VACCINES

Harper DM, Franko EL, Wheeler C et al: Efficacy of bivalent L-1 virus-like particle vaccine in prevention of infection with human papilloma type 16 and 18 in young women: A randomized controlled trial. Lancet: 364:1757–1765, 2004.

Koutsky LA, Ault KA, Wheeler CM et al: A controlled trial of a human papillomavirus type 16 vaccine. N Engl J Med 347:1645–1651, 2002.

Nolan T, Block SL, Reisinger KS et al: Comparison of the immunogenicity and tolerability of a prophylactic quadrivalent HPV 6, 11, 16, and 18 L1 virus-like particles vaccine in male and female adolescents and young women. Presented at ESPID, May 18–20, 2005, Valencia, Spain.

Sanders GD, Taira AV: Cost effectiveness of potential vaccine for human papillomavirus. Emerg Infect Dis 9:37–48, 2003.

Sattler C: Future I investigators, Efficacy of prophylactic quadrivalent human papillomavirus (HPV) (type 6, 11, 16, 18), L-1 virus-like particles (VLP), vaccine for prevention of cervical dysplasia and external genital lesions (EGL). Presented at ICAAC; December 16–19, 2005, Washington, DC.

Skjeldestad FE: Future II steering committee: Prophylactic quadrivalent human papillomavirus (HPV) (type 6, 11, 16, 18), L-1 virus-like particles, VLP vaccine (Gardasil™) reduced cervical intraepithelial neoplasia (CIN) II/III risk. Presented at IDSA October 6–9, 2005, San Francisco, California.

Taira, AV, Neukermans CP, Sanders GD: Evaluating human papillomavirus program. Emerg Infect Dis10:1915–1923, 2004.

2 Preinvasive Disease of the Vagina and Vulva and Related Disorders

William T. Creasman, M.D.

INTRAEPITHELIAL NEOPLASIA OF THE VAGINA

Clinical profile

Carcinoma in situ of the vagina has been reported sporadically in the last four decades, particularly in patients previously treated for cervical carcinoma in situ. The first report was apparently by Graham and Meigs in 1952. They reported on three patients with carcinoma of the vagina, two intraepithelial and one invasive, that were discovered 6, 7, and 10 years after total hysterectomy for carcinoma in situ of the cervix. Other reports have described multiple primary cancers of the vagina, cervix, and vulva. Several authors have commented on the "field response" of the cervix, vagina, and vulva, which suggests that the squamous epithelium of the lower genital tract may be affected in multiple sites by a similar carcinogenic trigger. Apparent extension of invasive carcinoma of the cervix to the vagina and vestibule may represent simultaneous carcinomas at sites affected by a constant carcinogenic stimulus of several end organs in the genital tract.

Carcinoma in situ of the vagina is much less common than that of the cervix or vulva. For the year 2005, the American Cancer Society estimated that 2145 cases of invasive cancer of the vagina would be diagnosed in the USA. Isolated lesions can usually be recognized colposcopically (Fig. 2–1) as white epithelium, mosaicism, and punctation, although some authors have described a "pink blush" appearance or a slightly granular texture. The diagnosis is usually confirmed by biopsy, and the limits of the lesion can be identified with the colposcope or with iodine staining (Schiller stain). Almost all lesions are asymptomatic, although a patient will occasionally have postcoital staining. An abnormal Pap smear usually initiates the diagnostic survey. Patients with abnormal squamous cytologic findings in the absence of a cervix or not explained by an adequate investigation of the cervix should be subjected to a careful examination of the vaginal epithelium. In most series, the upper third of the vagina is most frequently involved (as is the case with the invasive variety), and this in part relates to the association with the more common cervical lesions. Patients with vaginal intraepithelial neoplasia (VAIN) tend to have either an antecedent or coexistent neoplasia in the lower genital tract. This is the usual situation in at least one half to two-thirds of all patients with VAIN. In patients who have been treated for disease in the cervix or vulva, VAIN can appear many years later, necessitating long-term follow-up. First TeLinde, then Gusberg and Marshall, and later Parker and associates indicated that 2%, 1.9%, and 0.9% of patients, respectively, had vaginal recurrences after hysterectomy for a similar lesion in the cervix. On the other hand, Ferguson and Maclure reported positive cytologic findings in 151 (20.3%) of 633 previously treated patients. This large group included invasive and in situ cancers of the cervix, which were treated by irradiation or hysterectomy. Although the long-term recurrence rate for carcinoma in situ of the vagina is uncertain, it is sufficient to merit continued careful follow-up.

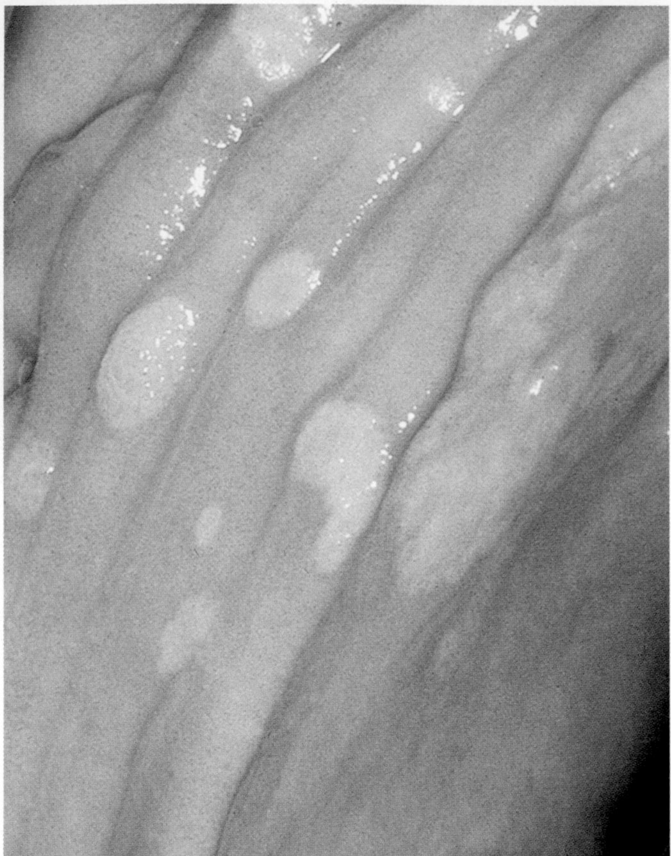

Figure 2–1 Carcinoma in situ of the vagina (colposcopic view).

Incomplete excision of sufficient vaginal cuff with hysterectomy for carcinoma in situ of the cervix with involvement of the fornices may explain an early recurrence. The finding of carcinoma in situ in the vaginal cuff area in less than 1 year after hysterectomy makes this explanation likely. It is, therefore, important to perform a preoperative evaluation of the upper vagina by Schiller tests or colposcopy at the time of hysterectomy for carcinoma in situ of the cervix. This allows the surgeon to determine accurately how much of the upper vagina has to be removed. It is also apparent that both carcinoma in situ and dysplasia may develop in the vagina as primary lesions without an association with a similar process on the cervix or vulva. Still other preinvasive lesions of the vagina may appear after irradiation therapy for invasive carcinoma of the cervix. Data from the MD Anderson Hospital suggest that these postradiation lesions are premalignant and can progress to invasive cancer if they are not treated. Without therapy, approximately 25% of the patients in this series progressed to the invasive state over varying periods of follow-up. Local therapy must be executed with care because of the previous irradiation.

Pearce and associates and Noller argued that a vaginal Pap smear after a hysterectomy for benign disease, intended to detect vaginal tumors, is not useful, even when inner-city women were studied. A prospective study has not been done and will probably never be done considering the size of the study that would be necessary. However, common series and the rarity of vaginal cancer along with reports such as that by Pearce make it difficult to justify continuing the use of routine Pap smears in patients who have had a hysterectomy for benign disease. The recently reported guidelines for cytologic screening (see Chapter 1) state that cytology is not indicated after hysterectomy for benign disease unless the woman has a history of diethylstilbestrol (DES) exposure during pregnancy or is immunosuppressed. Nonetheless, reports continue to be published of vaginal cancer developing in women who previously had hysterectomies for benign disease. This may be a matter of cost vs benefit. Interestingly, a recent survey of women who were consulted concerning the new guidelines for cytology indicated that they wanted to be followed with yearly Paps irrespective of whether they had had a hysterectomy or not.

Diagnosis

Colposcopic examination of the vagina can be difficult to perform. The largest possible speculum should be used and repositioned frequently to allow inspection of all surfaces. Colposcopic findings are similar to those described for the cervix. Our technique calls for the examination of the four walls from the apex to the introitus as separate and sequential steps. Small biopsy specimens are taken with Kevorkian–Younge alligator-jaw forceps, sometimes using a sterilized skin-hook for traction at the biopsy site. Most patients can tolerate these biopsies without local anesthesia. Lugol solution may be helpful in delineating lesions of the vagina. In the postmenopausal patient, local use of estrogen creams for several weeks helps to bring out the abnormal areas for identification by colposcopy.

In contrast to cervical intraepithelial neoplasia (CIN), VAIN tends to be multifocal; even if a lesion is identified, one must search the entire vaginal tube for coexisting multiple lesions. Although typically the lesion is more common in the upper third, disease-free skip areas may be encountered with additional VAIN in the lower vagina. In hard-to-locate lesions, selective cytologic methods, obtaining Pap smears from different locations in the vagina, can often pinpoint the area of abnormality so that attention can be paid specifically to the area of highest suspicion.

Management

Local excision of the involved area has been the mainstay of therapy. In many cases, a single isolated lesion can be removed easily in the office with biopsy forceps. If larger areas are involved, an upper colpectomy may be necessary if the lesion is to be removed by surgery. The use of a dilute solution of phenylephrine (Neo-Synephrine), which is injected submucosally at the time of surgery, will facilitate the vaginectomy greatly.

As in CIN, outpatient modalities of therapy have been investigated for VAIN. The topical application of

5-fluorouracil (5-FU) cream has been advocated by some investigators for the last three decades. Results have varied; however, studies by Petrilli and associates and Caglar, Hurtzog, and Hreshchyshyn indicate that this modality can be effective. One of the problems with 5-FU is the selection of the best mode of application, dosage, and length of treatment. Some advocate the use of a tampon or a diaphragm to keep the 5-FU cream in place. Several techniques have been suggested with equivalent results. One quarter applicator of 5% 5-FU cream is inserted high in the vagina each night after the patient is in bed. The patient can be instructed to coat the vulva and introitus with white petroleum if the cream leaks out during sleep. A small tampon or cotton ball at the introitus is also helpful to prevent leakage. The cream can be douched out with warm water the next morning. This is done every night for 5–8 days, followed by a 10-day to 2-week rest period, and then the application cycle is repeated. This usually allows an adequate treatment time without having the patient experience the tremendous local reaction that can occur with prolonged use. Treatment can be repeated if it is not successful after the first cycle. Weekly insertions of 5-FU cream, approximately 1.5 g (one third of an applicator), deep into the vagina once a week at bedtime for 10 consecutive weeks has also been shown to be efficacious. Placement of cotton balls at the introitus prevents 5-FU contamination of the perineum with resultant skin irritation. Douching the next morning, which is advocated by some, is unnecessary with the weekly instillation. We prefer the latter technique because patient compliance is high and toxicity is low.

A report by Dungar and Wilkinson noted an interesting finding in the vagina after 5-FU therapy, which we also have noted. Post treatment, a red area suggestive of a lack of squamous epithelium may be present. They found that this represented columnar epithelium consistent with a metaplastic process in which squamous epithelium is replaced with columnar epithelium. They called this finding "acquired vaginal adenosis". These changes are usually found in the upper third of the vagina but may extend into the middle third. The columnar epithelium was of a low cuboidal or mucus-secreting endocervical type. In some cases, squamous epithelium was noted overlying the glandular elements. Marked superficial chronic inflammation was also present. This has also been noted in the vagina after laser therapy.

Cryosurgery has been used in the treatment of some patients with VAIN, but it has not been found to be as successful as in the treatment of CIN. This is probably attributable to the flaccidity of the vaginal wall and the lack of good freezing contact. Also, the possibility of vesicovaginal and rectovaginal fistulas has discouraged some individuals from trying this therapy. At present, there appears to be no enthusiasm for this particular modality in the treatment of VAIN, and laser therapy is preferred. Benedet and associates evaluated 56 patients who ranged from 22–84 years of age. Over half had a prior history of CIN. Measurement of the epithelium was performed on involved as well as uninvolved tissue. The involved epithelium had a mean thickness of 0.46 mm (range of 0.1–1.4 mm). Uninvolved tissue was thinner and had a mean thickness of 0.28 mm. Of interest is that there was no statistical difference in thickness of the involved epithelium in the pre- and postmenopausal patient; however, the uninvolved epithelium was thinner in the postmenopausal patient compared with the premenopausal patient (0.25 vs 0.37 mm). Although this latter figure is statistically significant, it is certainly not clinically significant. Although Benedet did not give treatment results, the study was performed to give guidance as to the depth of vaginal destruction by the laser. Based on this study, the authors thought that destruction of 1–1.5 mm would destroy the epithelium without damaging underlying structures. Several authors have suggested that laser therapy is a very effective therapy.

Over a 6-year period, Townsend and associates treated 36 patients from two large referral hospitals with a CO_2 laser. These numbers confirm the apparent rarity of this lesion. In 92% of the patients, the lesions were completely removed by the laser without significant side effects. Almost one-fourth of the patients, however, required more than one treatment session. Pain and bleeding have been the main complications but appear to be minimal. Healing is excellent, and impaired sexual function has not been a problem. The optimal technique of laser therapy for vaginal lesions has yet to be determined. Whereas some investigators suggest removing only the identified lesions, others advocate treating the entire vaginal tube. Schellhas reported two patients treated for VAIN with the laser who subsequently developed invasive disease in the vagina. A thorough diagnostic investigation of the vagina to rule out invasive cancer can be quite difficult, but it is obviously mandatory. Multiple focal lesions, particularly post hysterectomy, with deep vaginal angles may be difficult to treat with the laser. Small skin hooks and dental mirrors have been suggested as adjuncts to successful laser therapy. Krebs treated 22 patients with topical 5-FU and 37 patients with laser therapy. The success rate was similar for the two treatments. Particularly with multifocal lesions, we prefer treatment with 5-FU.

More recently, experience with 5% imiquimod cream in the management of VAIN has been reported. In a study by Buck, 56 women with VAIN (mostly low grade) were treated with 0.25 g placed in the vagina once weekly for 3 weeks. Of 42 women available for follow-up, 36 (86%) were clear of VAIN on colposcopic evaluation one week or later after the last treatment. Five patients required two treatment cycles and one patient three treatment cycles before clearing of their lesion. Vulvar or vestibular excoriation was reported in only two individuals. No vaginal ulcerations were noted.

Some have advocated surface irradiation using an intravaginal applicator; however, our experience with this method of therapy has been discouraging, with a high recurrence rate and marked vaginal stenosis, making follow-up therapy extremely difficult. Total vaginectomy, with vaginal reconstruction using a split-thickness skin graft, should be reserved for the patient who has failed more conservative therapy. Sillman and colleagues reported on 94 patients with VAIN who were treated by various methods. The remission rate was high, but 5% of the cases progressed to invasive disease despite close follow-up.

DIETHYLSTILBESTROL-RELATED GENITAL TRACT ANOMALIES

Embryology

In any brief review of the early development of the reproductive tract, it is necessary to discuss the urinary tract, because some components of the urinary tract later become functional portions of the reproductive tract, namely the ducts. In the development of the mammalian excretory system, three successive paired kidneys are formed. The first, the pronephros, probably does not function in humans. The second kidney, the mesonephros, begins to replace the pronephros in its subdiaphragmatic location in the fourth week. It consists of tubules similar to those of its predecessor; however, instead of elaborating a duct of its own, it appropriates the pronephric duct, which thereafter is known as the mesonephric duct, or by the more familiar eponym, the wolffian duct. The definitive kidney, the metanephros, supplants it. The tubules of this final excretory organ form a little lower in the abdominal cavity than those of the kidneys that first appear in the sixth or seventh week. Its duct originates as an outpouching of the lower end of the mesonephric duct and the ureteric bud, which grows upward, eventually invaginating the metanephros and connecting with the metanephric tubules. The connection of the ureter with the mesonephric duct is interrupted at an early stage by differential growth processes that give the two ducts separate entrances to the ureterogenital sinus. A close association exists between the definitive urinary tract and those parts of the reproductive tract that are derived from the mesonephric duct. The common origin of their lining epithelium is shown in Figure 2–2.

The female reproductive tract, the paramesonephric or müllerian duct, originates during the sexually indifferent period, early in the 6th week, and is therefore present in the future male as well as the future female. In the male, it degenerates about the 10th week, at approximately the time when the mesonephric duct is degenerating in the female. The müllerian duct originates as an invagination of coelomic epithelium lateral to the upper end of the mesonephric duct. The epithelium at the base of this small pit proliferates to form a solid blind cord that grows downward toward the pelvis. This cord later becomes canalized. This mechanism, which results in a lining of coelomic epithelium, contrasts with the bulging of the gonads into the body cavity, which produces a covering of coelomic epithelium. The müllerian ducts on either side grow toward each other; they cross over the wolffian duct anteriorly to meet and fuse in the midline in the ninth week. The medial walls of the fused ducts gradually disappear and produce a single uterovaginal cavity (Fig. 2–2). The upper portions of the ducts, which do not fuse, remain as the paired uterine, or fallopian, tubes. When the lower end of the fused müllerian ducts makes contact with the urogenital sinus, the cell cords are still solid. They merge with the endodermal cells growing back from the sinus to form a temporary barrier between the uterovaginal cavity and the urogenital sinus, the müllerian tubercle. The mesonephric ducts enter the urogenital sinus immediately lateral to the tubercle. Between the openings of the mesonephric (wolffian) ducts and the müllerian tubercle, the proliferation of sinus cells occurs, producing the dorsolateral (sinovaginal) bulbs. At the same time, the simple columnar epithelium that lines the vaginal portion of the ureterovaginal canal begins to undergo transformation into stratified epithelium of polygonal cells. This transformation proceeds cranially until it reaches the columnar epithelium of the future endocervical canal. The

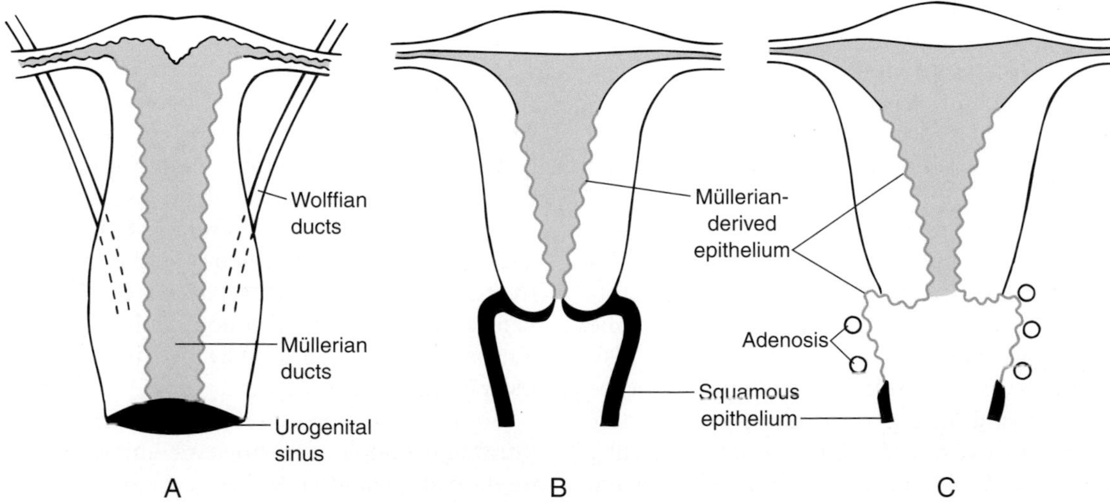

Figure 2–2 *A–C*, Schematic representations of the embryologic development of the vagina in unexposed (*A*) and diethylstilbestrol-exposed (*B* and *C*) women. (From Stillman RJ: In utero exposure to diethylstilbestrol: Adverse effects on the reproductive tract and reproductive performance in male and female offspring. Am J Obstet Gynecol 142(7):905, 1982.)

vagina, which is lined initially by simple columnar epithelium of müllerian origin, now has acquired a stratified müllerian epithelium. The base of the sinovaginal bulbs proliferates and produces a central mass with lateral wings that sweep cranially to the central mass. This entire structure, the vaginal plate, advances in a caudocranial direction, obliterating the existing vaginal lumen. By caudal cavitation of the vaginal plate, a new lumen is formed, and the stratified müllerian epithelium is replaced by a stratified squamous epithelium, which is probably of sinus origin. Local proliferation of the vaginal plate in the region of the cervicovaginal junction produces the circumferential enlargement of the vagina known as the vaginal fornices, which surround the vaginal part of the cervix. The administration of diethylstilbestrol (DES) through the 18th week of gestation can apparently result in the disruption of the transformation of columnar epithelium of müllerian origin to the stratified squamous successor. This retention of müllerian epithelium gives rise to adenosis. Adenosis may be present in any of the following forms as: a replacement, with glandular cells in place of the normal squamous lining of the vagina; glandular cells hidden beneath an intact squamous lining; or mixed with squamous metaplasia when new squamous cells attempt to replace glandular cells.

Vaginal adenosis has been observed in patients without a history of exposure to diethylstilbestrol (DES) but rarely to a clinically significant degree. Sandberg sectioned 35 vaginas obtained at autopsy, 22 of which were from postpubertal women. In nine of these vaginas (41%), Sandberg demonstrated occult glands that were consistent with adenosis. None of the 13 prepubertal specimens contained glands. However, Kurman and Scully noted six cases of vaginal adenosis among 73 prepubertal vaginal specimens that were obtained at autopsy. Robboy reported on 41 women who were born before the DES era and who had adenosis confirmed pathologically. Robboy noted that the microscopic appearances of adenosis in women born before the DES era were identical to those encountered in young women who were exposed in utero to DES. Adenosis is more common in patients whose mothers began DES treatment early in pregnancy, and its frequency is not at all increased if DES administration began after the 18th week of gestation. At least 20% of women exposed to DES show an anatomic deformity of the upper vagina and cervix. This has been variously described as a transverse vaginal and cervical ridge, cervical collar, vaginal hood, and cockscomb cervix. The transverse ridges and anatomic deformities found in one-fifth of women exposed to DES make it difficult to ascertain the boundaries of the vagina and cervix. The cervical eversion causes the cervix grossly to have a red appearance. This coloration is caused by the numerous normal-appearing blood vessels in the submucosa. By using a colposcope and applying 3% acetic acid solution, one may recognize involved areas covered with numerous papillae ("grapes") of columnar epithelium similar to those seen in the native columnar epithelium of the endocervix. The hood (Fig. 2–3) is a fold of mucous membrane surrounding the portio of the cervix; it often disappears if the portio is pulled down with a tenaculum or is displaced by the speculum. The cockscomb has an atypical peaked appearance of the anterior lip of the cervix, whereas vaginal ridges are protruding circumferential bands in the upper vagina that may hide the cervix. A pseudopolyp formation (see Fig. 2–3) has been described that occurs when the portio of the cervix is small and protrudes through a wide cervical hood.

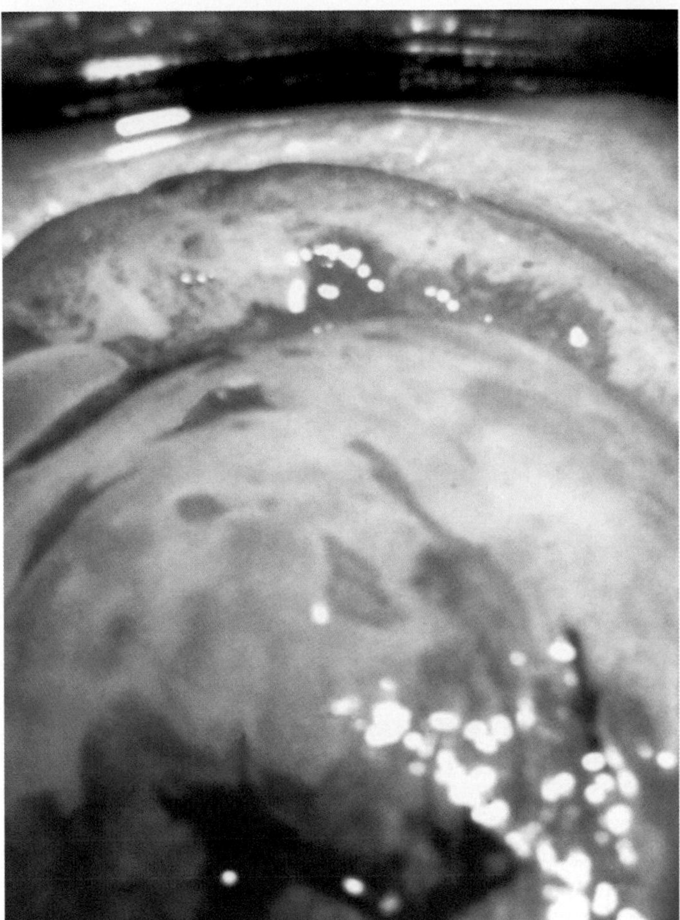

Figure 2–3 Hood surrounding the small diethylstilbestrol-exposed cervix, which is completely covered by columnar epithelium (pseudopolyp).

The striking occurrence of vaginal adenosis among young women whose mothers took no steroidal estrogens during pregnancy logically points to an occurrence during embryonic development for an explanation. The development of the müllerian system depends on and follows formation of the wolffian, or mesonephric, system. The emergence of the müllerian system as the dominant structure appears unaffected by intrauterine exposure to DES when studied in animal systems. However, it is apparent that steroidal and non-steroidal estrogens, when administered during the proper stage of vaginal embryogenesis in mice, can permanently prevent the transformation of müllerian epithelium into the adult type of vaginal epithelium, thus creating a situation like adenosis. The colposcopic and histologic features of vaginal adenosis strongly support the concept of persistent, untransformed müllerian columnar epithelia in the vagina as being the explanation of adenosis.

Table 2–1 EXAMINATION OF THE FEMALE OFFSPRING EXPOSED TO DIETHYLSTILBESTROL

1. Inspect the introitus and hymen to assess the patency of the vagina.
2. Palpate the vaginal membrane with the index finger (especially noting non-Lugol-staining areas), noting areas of induration or exophytic lesions, which should be considered for biopsy.
3. Perform a speculum examination with the largest speculum that can be comfortably inserted (virginal-type speculums are often necessary). Adenosis usually appears red and granular (strawberry surface).
4. Obtain cytologic specimens from the cervical os and the walls of the upper third of the vagina.
5. Perform a colposcopic examination or Lugol staining on the initial visit.
6. Do a biopsy of indurated or exophytic areas and colposcopically abnormal areas with a dysplastic Papanicolaou smear.
7. Perform a bimanual rectovaginal examination.

Examination and treatment of the female exposed to diethylstilbestrol

Systematic examination of the female offspring exposed to DES (Table 2–1) has disclosed that at least 60% have vaginal adenosis, that is, presence of cervical-like epithelium in the vagina; a smaller portion have minor anomalies of the cervix and vagina. Although the origin of clear cell adenocarcinoma from adenosis remains to be established, these patients warrant careful observation. Some authors have suggested that DES-exposed offspring may also have an increased risk of developing squamous neoplasia because of the large number of transformation zones inherent in this condition. Although a few cases of dysplasia and carcinoma in situ associated with adenosis have been reported, the risk of developing invasive squamous lesions remains uncertain at this time, because few DES-exposed offspring have entered the age group in which invasive squamous cell carcinoma is more prevalent.

Fowler and associates reported an increased occurrence of cervical intraepithelial neoplasia (CIN) in women with in utero exposure to DES; among 335 exposed women he found a 15% incidence of CIN. In a National Collaborative Diethylstilbestrol Adenosis Project (DESAD) report, an incidence of 15.7/1000 persons per year in the exposed group compared with 7.9/1000 persons per year of follow-up in the unexposed group was noted. In 1984, these investigators found on further evaluation of their data, that there was no increase in CIN or invasive cervical cancer in the exposed compared to the unexposed population.

All DES-exposed females should have a gynecologic examination annually beginning at age 14 or at menarche, whichever occurs first. In general, examinations of prepubertal individuals are not recommended, but they should be performed (usually under anesthesia) if any unusual symptoms, such as abnormal bleeding or discharge, develop. Mothers should be encouraged to instruct their daughters in the use of vaginal tampons during menses, because this will facilitate the physician's examination. The examination should include careful inspection of the cervix and of any suspicious area in the vagina. Careful digital palpation of the vagina must be performed. The role of colposcopy remains in the examination of suspicious areas where biopsy may be indicated. Lugol solution may be helpful in delineating abnormal areas. The purpose of regular examination is to permit detection of adenocarcinoma and squamous neoplasia during the earliest stages of development. Although many therapies have been attempted, at the present time no recommended treatment plan for vaginal adenosis exists. Some physicians have advised the use of jellies or foam to lower the vaginal pH and assist the re-epithelialization of the mucous membrane. No published studies indicate that such a practice is valid. The use of local progesterone in the vagina has been advocated by others as therapy for vaginal adenosis, but good data are similarly lacking. In most cases, the area of adenosis is physiologically transformed into squamous epithelium during varying periods of observation, and no therapy is necessary.

It is anticipated that most of the DES-associated adenocarcinomas have been identified (see Chapter 9). The past history of DES exposure is important in the follow-up of these patients, because adenocarcinoma could appear in the future. It is probably more important not to be concerned by adenosis and treat an entity that usually disappears with time. Whether these individuals will be at high risk for VAIN will be determined only in the future. Routine screening with cytology should be continued for the life of the patient.

Squamous cell cancers may arise in the metaplastic tissue that is found so extensively in females exposed to DES. Evidence for an increase in squamous cell carcinoma does not exist at present, but this possibility provides an additional reason for close follow-up of the exposed group. Colposcopic examination of these patients is hindered by the abnormal patterns (Fig. 2–4) seen with squamous metaplasia, which can be confused with neoplastic lesions, especially by the inexperienced observer. Careful histologic confirmation is essential before any treatment is undertaken. Marked mosaic (Fig. 2–5) and punctation patterns that normally herald intraepithelial neoplasia are commonly seen in the vagina of a DES-exposed female as a result of widespread metaplasia.

NON-NEOPLASTIC EPITHELIAL DISORDERS OF THE VULVA

Non-neoplastic epithelial disorders of the vulvar skin and mucosa are often seen in clinical practice and were previously categorized as vulvar dystrophies. In 1987, at a meeting of the International Society for the Study of Vulvar Disease (ISSVD), a new classification of these disorders was adopted (Table 2–2). The new classification was

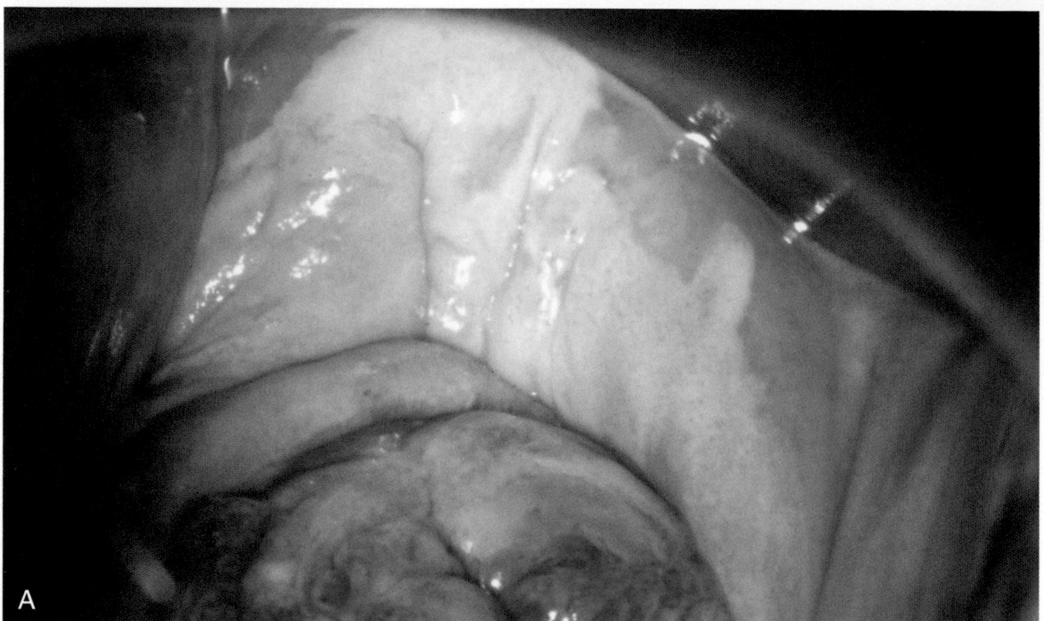

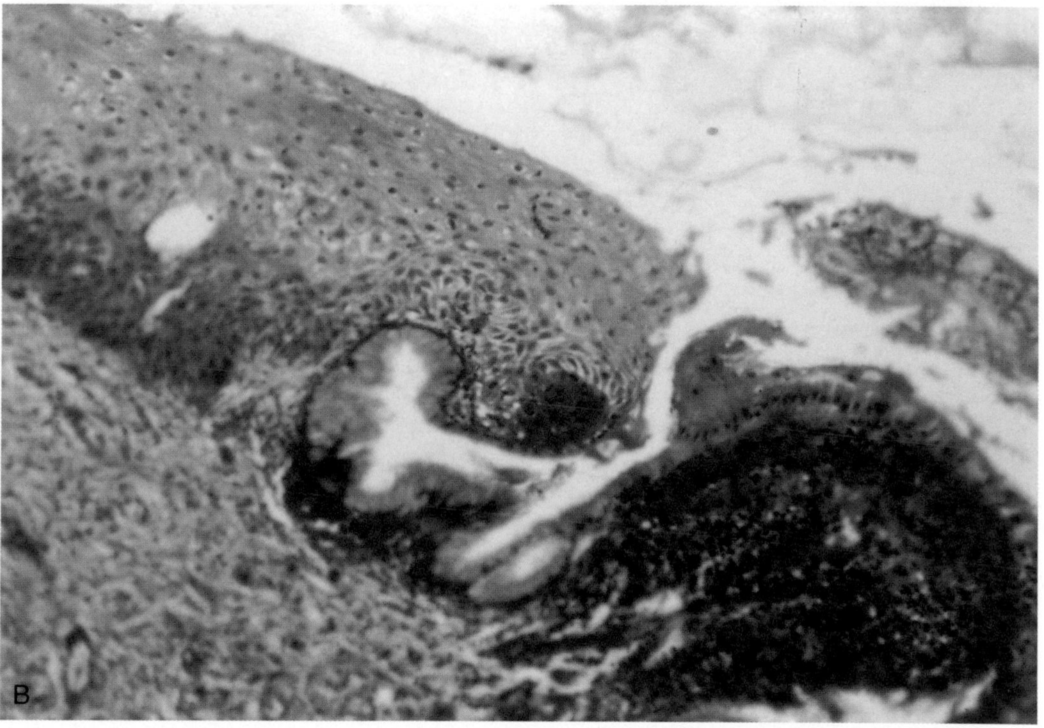

Figure 2–4 *A*, Area of white epithelium of squamous metaplasia. *B*, Histologic section of the area in *A* showing metaplasia to the left partially covering the adenosis (columnar epithelium) to the right.

developed to provide a scheme that would be accepted by gynecologists, dermatologists, and pathologists. This would encourage the standardization and comparability of vulvar pathology on an international and interdisciplinary basis.

The old terminology of "dystrophies" was replaced by "non-neoplastic epithelial disorders of skin and mucosa". The category and the specific classification system were changed involving squamous cell hyperplasia, lichen sclerosus, and other dermatoses (Table 2–3). Many previously

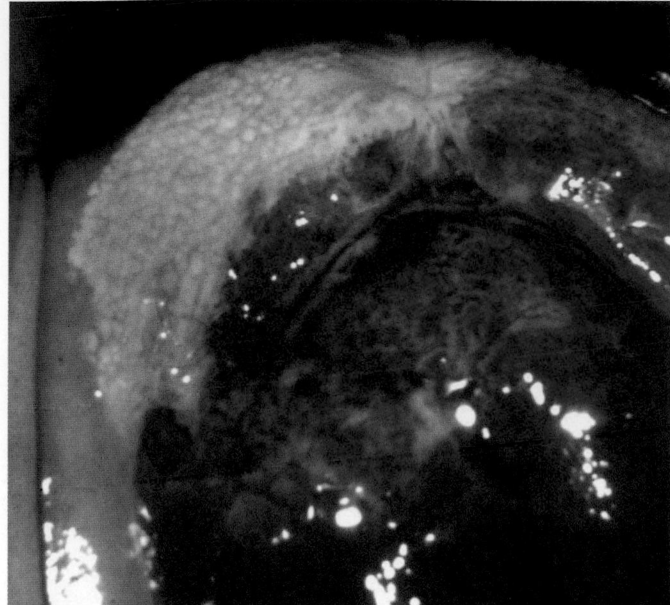

Figure 2–5 Heavy mosaic pattern (histologically proven metaplasia) in a hood surrounding the cervix of an offspring exposed to diethylstilbestrol.

used terms should be discarded (Table 2–4). It was recognized that differences in the appearance of vulvar skin were not due necessarily to separate diseases but rather, they were environmentally conditioned reactions to adverse agents. In support of this suggestion, evidence has been cited that, if the involved vulvar skin is excised and normal skin is transplanted from a site that is not usually subject to lesions characteristic of the vulvar area, the grafted epithelium may undergo the same changes that occurred in the original vulvar skin before its removal. The unique appearance of many of the dystrophies of the vulvar skin must therefore be a product of the warm moist environment of this organ.

The new classification clearly separates the non-neoplastic epithelial disorders. Lesions that demonstrate atypia do not belong within the classification of non-neoplastic epithelial disorders, because their natural history is entirely different. Unlike the prior classification, which was based purely on histopathologic features of the lesions being studied, the new classification is based on a combination of gross and histopathologic changes. Mixed disorders can occur; however, both conditions should be reported. Thus, lichen sclerosus with associated squamous cell hyperplasia (which was formerly called mixed dystrophies) should be reported as lichen sclerosus with squamous cell hyperplasia. Squamous cell hyperplasia terminology is used when the hyperplasia cannot be attributed to a more specific process. If squamous cell hyperplasia is associated with vulvar intraepithelial neoplasia (VIN), then the diagnosis should be reported as VIN.

Table 2–2 VULVAR NON-NEOPLASTIC EPITHELIAL DISORDERS

Disorder	Treatment
Lichen sclerosus	Topical high potency steroids
Squamous cell hyperplasia (formerly hyperplastic dystrophy)	Topical corticosteroids
Other dermatoses	

Table 2–3 NON-NEOPLASTIC EPITHELIAL DISORDERS OF THE VULVAR SKIN AND MUCOSA

Squamous cell hyperplasia (formerly hyperplastic dystrophy)
Lichen sclerosus
Other dermatoses

Table 2–4 DELETED TERMS

Lichen sclerosus et atrophicus
Leukoplakia
Neurodermatitis
Leukokeratosis
Bowen's disease
Carcinoma simplex
Leukoplakic vulvitis
Hyperplastic vulvitis
Kraurosis vulvae
Erythroplasia of Queyrat

Squamous cell hyperplasia

Squamous cell hyperplasia includes lesions with no known cause. Most hyperplastic lesions represent lichen simplex chronicus. The age of the patient may vary and may include both the reproductive and postmenopausal years. Pruritus is the most common symptom, and the status of the skin usually relates to the amount of scratching. Although these lesions are associated with epithelial thickening and hyperkeratosis, their appearance varies greatly. Moisture, scratching and medications may cause variations in the appearance of these lesions even in the same patient. The areas of the vulva most often involved include the labia majora, interlabial folds, outer aspects of the labia minor, and the clitoris. Changes can also extend to the lateral surfaces of the labia majora or beyond. Areas of squamous cell hyperplasia are often localized, elevated, and well delineated; however, these lesions may be extensive and sometimes poorly defined. The vulva often appears dusky-red when the degree of hyperkeratosis is slight. At other times, well-defined white patches may be seen, or a combination of red and white areas may be observed in different locations. Thickening, fissures, and excoriations require careful evaluation, because carcinoma may be exhibited by these same features.

Biopsy reveals a variable increase in the thickness of the horny layer (hyperkeratosis) and irregular thickening of the

Malpighian layer (acanthosis). This latter process produces a thickened epithelium, as well as lengthening and distortion of the rete pegs. Parakeratosis may also be present. The granular layer of the epithelium is usually prominent. An inflammatory reaction is often present within the dermis with varying numbers of lymphocytes and plasma cells.

Lichen sclerosus

Lichen sclerosus was often previously called kraurosis vulvae or atrophic leukoplakia. Lichen sclerosus represents a specific disease and can be found in non-genital sites. Children and young women may be affected, but most patients are postmenopausal. Although not seen initially, pruritus occurs with essentially all lesions, leading to scratching, which can develop into ecchymosis and ulceration. Studies have suggested that the epithelium in lichen sclerosus is metabolically active and non-atrophic. In a well-developed classic lesion, the skin of the vulva is crinkled ("cigarette paper") or appears parchment-like. The process often extends around the anal region in a figure of eight or keyhole configuration. At other times, the changes are localized, especially in the periclitoral area or the perineum. Clitoral involvement is usually associated with edema of the foreskin, which may obscure the glans clitoris. Phimosis of the clitoris is often seen late in the course of the disease. The labia minora also completely disappear as a result of atrophy. Synechiae often develop between the edges of the skin in these locations, causing pain and limited physical activity. Fissures also develop in the natural folds of the skin and especially in the posterior fourchette. The introitus may become stenosed to a point at which intercourse is impossible. In a study by Dalziel, 44 women with lichen sclerosus were evaluated for sexual dysfunction. Apareunia had been experienced by 19 women at some point. Dyspareunia and decreased frequency were noted by 80%. Orgasm was altered, and relationships were affected by half. Local steroids improved sexual function in two thirds of these patients. The microscopic features of lichen sclerosus include hyperkeratosis, epithelial thickening with flattening of the rete pegs, cytoplasmic vacuolization of the basal layer of cells, and follicular plugging. Beneath the epidermis is a zone of homogenized, pink-staining, collagenous-appearing tissue that is relatively acellular. Edema is occasionally seen in this area. Elastic fibers are absent. Immediately below this zone lies a band of inflammatory cells that is consistent with lymphocytes and some plasma cells. Lichen sclerosus is often associated with foci of both hyperplastic epithelium and thin epithelium (formerly mixed dystrophy). Squamous cell hyperplasia has been found in 27–35% of women with lichen sclerosus after microscopic study of vulvar specimens. Approximately 5% of patients with lichen sclerosus were found also to have intraepithelial neoplasia. The etiology of this condition is unknown. Wallace found that only 12 of 290 (4%) of women with lichen sclerosus, who were followed for an average of 12.5 years, developed vulvar cancer.

Other dermatoses

The term "other dermatoses" applies to the entire range of skin disorders that can affect this area of the body (Table 2–5). In reality, only a few lesions are routinely encountered in an average gynecologic practice. The new classification system gives vulvar dermatoses dermatologic names. This should help to better define the natural history, differential diagnosis, and treatment of the major skin disease. Primary lesions are the basic descriptors: *papule, plaque, nodule, tumor, vesicle, bulla, pustule, weal, telangiectasis, comedo, burrow,* or *cyst.* These generic nouns describe the skin change that results from an underlying pathologic process. When primary lesions are altered by external factors, the resultant lesion is a secondary change. Terms that describe secondary changes include *scale, crust, fissure, erosion, ulcer, excoriation, atrophy,* and *scar.* Descriptions of the skin lesions should include:

1. primary lesion form;
2. arrangement or pattern of lesions, and
3. distribution on anatomic sites.

Treatment

Before any treatment is given on a long-term basis, biopsies should be performed from representative areas to ensure the correct diagnosis. These biopsies should concentrate on sites of fissuring, ulceration, induration, and thick

Table 2–5 OTHER DERMATOSES

Disorder	Lesion	Genital	Other locations
Seborrheic dermatitis	Erythema with mild scale oval plaques	Mild scaling, also "inverse type"	Central face, neck, scalp, chest, back
Psoriasis	Annular scaly plaques that bleed easily	Red plaques with gray-white scale	Scalp, elbows, knees, sacrum
Tinea	Annular plaques with central clearing	Common	Skinfolds or single "ringworm" lesion
Lichen simplex chronicus	Lichenified plaques, some dermatitic	Scrotum or labia majora	Nape of the neck, ankle, forearm, antecubital and popliteal fossae
Lichen planus	Flat-topped lilac papules and plaques	White network, erosive vaginitis	Volar wrists, shins, buccal mucosa

plaques. Hygienic measures for keeping the vulva clean and dry should be recommended. Anxiety is frequently a factor and should be investigated. Vulvar pruritus is often seen in women with stress, and all of this promotes scratching and leads to further secondary skin changes. After lesions with malignant potential have been ruled out, local measures for control of symptoms, primarily pruritus, can be instituted. If an eczematous type of vulvitis is present as the result of infected excoriations or inappropriate medications, wet dressings with agents such as aluminum acetate (Burow's) solution applied frequently are beneficial. Lotions and creams that contain corticosteroids produce a rapid response and are more convenient to apply than are wet dressings. Squamous cell hyperplasia is best treated with local application of corticosteroids. The use of moderate and strong topical steroids two or three times daily will relieve pruritus and inflammation. Most dermatologists recommend that fluorinated steroid substances should not be used for long periods, because they may theoretically result in atrophy of treated tissues. However, in the authors' experience, prolonged use has often been necessary to keep the vulvar skin asymptomatic. A position of compromise would be to utilize fluorinated steroids until pruritus is under control and then replace the steroids with medications that contain only hydrocortisone. Friedrich has suggested a combination of Eurax (three parts) and betamethasone valerate (seven parts), because the antipruritic effect of the steroid is enhanced with the Eurax. Treatment twice daily is usually adequate, and results are expected in a few weeks. Therapy may need to be continued, particularly if a thickened hyperplastic lesion is present. If the skin returns to normal appearance, therapy can be stopped. However, experience has shown that this is infrequently the case.

Traditionally, topical testosterone has been the treatment of choice for lichen sclerosus, improving both gross and histopathologic changes. This has been replaced with the new potent steroid clobetasol propionate, which has been effective in eliminating the symptoms. A study by Bracco evaluated 79 patients using four different treatment regimens. A 3-month course of testosterone (2%), progesterone (2%), clobetasol propionate (0.05%), and a cream base preparation were used in a prospective randomized study. Patients treated with clobetasol had a better response rate with regard to relief of symptoms (75% vs 20% for testosterone and 10% for other preparations). Clobetasol therapy was the only treatment in which the gross and histologic evaluation of patients improved after treatment. The authors recommended that patients use this steroid twice daily for 1 month, then daily for 2 months. They noted that symptomatic relief is often dramatic. Recurrences after stopping the steroid occurred, but symptoms were relieved when therapy was resumed. Lorenz reported a 77% complete remission rate with clobetasol therapy. Clobetasol propionate is the treatment of choice for lichen sclerosus.

Occasionally, vulvar pruritus is so persistent that it cannot be relieved by topical measures. In such cases, intradermal injection of steroids has been reported to be effective. Others have reported subcutaneous injection of absolute alcohol to relieve symptoms. Aliquots of 0.1 mg of the alcohol are injected subcutaneously at 1 cm intervals after the vulvar tissue has been carefully mapped out, and the vulvar area is then thoroughly massaged to disperse the alcohol evenly. Vulvar burning is sometimes intense after injection of alcohol, and urinary retention occasionally occurs. Post-treatment surveillance is, therefore, appropriate. Alcohol injection has been reported to produce significant symptomatic relief of pruritus but has little effect on vulvar burning.

INTRAEPITHELIAL NEOPLASIA OF THE VULVA

Clinical profile

Vulvar intraepithelial neoplasia (VIN) had been considered to be a problem occurring in postmenopausal women in their 50s and 60s, but it can develop in women at any age. Its frequency appears to be increasing among younger women. Today, the average age for VIN is said to be about 50 years of age. A large Italian study of 370 cases had a mean age of 52.6 years: 40% had VIN I; 14% had VIN II; and 46% had VIN III. During the last two decades, the incidence of VIN has almost doubled to 2.1 per 100,000 woman-years. The incidence has almost tripled in white women younger than 35 years of age. Of interest is that during this time, the incidence of invasive vulvar cancer has not increased. The American Cancer Society estimates that in the year 2005, 3870 women will be diagnosed with invasive vulvar cancer and 870 women will die of this cancer. Neither age nor parity appears to be a risk factor in the development of intraepithelial neoplasia of the vulva. The disease is asymptomatic in > 50% of cases. In the remainder of cases, the predominant symptom is pruritus. The presence of a distinct mass, bleeding, or discharge strongly suggests invasive cancer. The most productive diagnostic technique is careful inspection of the vulva in bright light during a routine pelvic examination followed by a biopsy of suspicious lesions. A handheld lens can be very helpful, especially after application of 5% acetic acid to the skin and introitus.

Physicians should be familiar with the various premalignant conditions of the vulva. They range from dysplasia (VIN I) that is biologically and histologically similar to dysplasia of the cervix or vagina to the more aggressive carcinoma in situ (VIN III). Whether or not these lesions carry the same connotation as their counterparts in the cervix with regard to progression to invasion is unknown. Certainly, an invasive lesion can be associated with VIN, and the risk of invasive cancer has been previously reported to be as high as 30%. Kagie and associates reported on 66 women with invasive vulvar squamous cell carcinoma; 39 (62%) had synchronous VIN. In other situations, the invasive lesion may have arisen de novo.

Table 2–6 CLASSIFICATION OF VULVAR INTRAEPITHELIAL NEOPLASIA

VIN I	(mild dysplasia)	formerly mild atypia
VIN II	(moderate dysplasia)	formerly moderate atypia
VIN III	(severe dysplasia, carcinoma in situ)	formerly severe atypia

VIN, vulvar intraepithelial neoplasia.

In a study from New Zealand of 65 patients with the mean age at diagnosis was 38 years. Smokers were younger than non-smokers. Two thirds of the women also had an associated intraepithelial lesion of the lower genital tract with 43% having high-grade lesions. Three developed early vulvar invasion. In a study from Scotland, 1010 patients were seen over a 16-year period. Fifty-eight percent presented with pruritus. Over half of the women had multifocal lesions. In 39%, there were coexistent or previous genital disease and 8% had a history of invasive gyn cancer. Histologic evidence of HPV was present in 31%. There were three (3%) that progressed to invasive squamous cell carcinoma of the vulva at 6, 7 and 7 years after initial therapy. In a study from Greece, 113 women were diagnosed with VIN. The mean age was 47 years and the most common symptom was pruritus (60%). The lesion was located in the non-hairy part of the vulva in 88% of cases. Four (3.5%) subsequently developed invasive vulvar cancer. A group from the Netherlands did a systematic review of 3322 published patients. The mean age at diagnosis was 46 years although this had decreased over the last 50 years. Again over 50% of the women had symptoms usually pain and/or pruritus. Eighty-eight women were untreated or gross macroscopic VIN III was left behind and 8 (9%) progressed to invasive cancer in 12 to 96 months. Four of those had previously been treated with radiotherapy and one was immunosuppressed.

The acceptance of the new classification of VIN terminology by the ISSVD has undoubtedly clarified much of the confusion that resulted because several other terms were previously used for this disease process. This VIN-dysplasia designation replaced the previously used atypia terms. Other terms, such as *bowenoid papulosis*, *Bowen's disease*, or *erythroplasia of Queyrat*, should not be used for intraepithelial neoplasia diagnosis (Table 2–6).

Many of the squamous intraepithelial lesions of the vulva are associated with HPV, particularly types 16/18, 31, 33, 35, and 51. HPV DNA has been found in 80–90% of patients with VIN, but the incidence decreases with age. The incidence of HPV DNA in vulvar cancers also decreases with age. HPV DNA in vulvar cancers also seems to be related to the type of cancer, such as the warty or condylomatous carcinoma and basaloid types that tend to occur in the younger patient.

The ISSVD states "VIN is characterized by a loss of epithelial cell maturation with associated nuclear hyperchromatism and pleomorphism, cellular crowding, and abnormal mitosis." The thickness of the epithelial abnormality would designate further characterizations of the lesion (i.e., VIN I, VIN II, and VIN III). VIN III would suggest full-thickness changes (Fig. 2–6). The milder forms of VIN first appear clinically as pale areas that vary in density. More severe forms are seen as papules or macules, coalescent or discrete, or single or multiple. Lesions on the cutaneous surface of the vulva usually appear as lichenified or hyperkeratotic plaques, that is, white epithelium (Fig. 2–7). By contrast, lesions of mucous membranes are usually macular and pink or red. Vulvar lesions are hyperpigmented

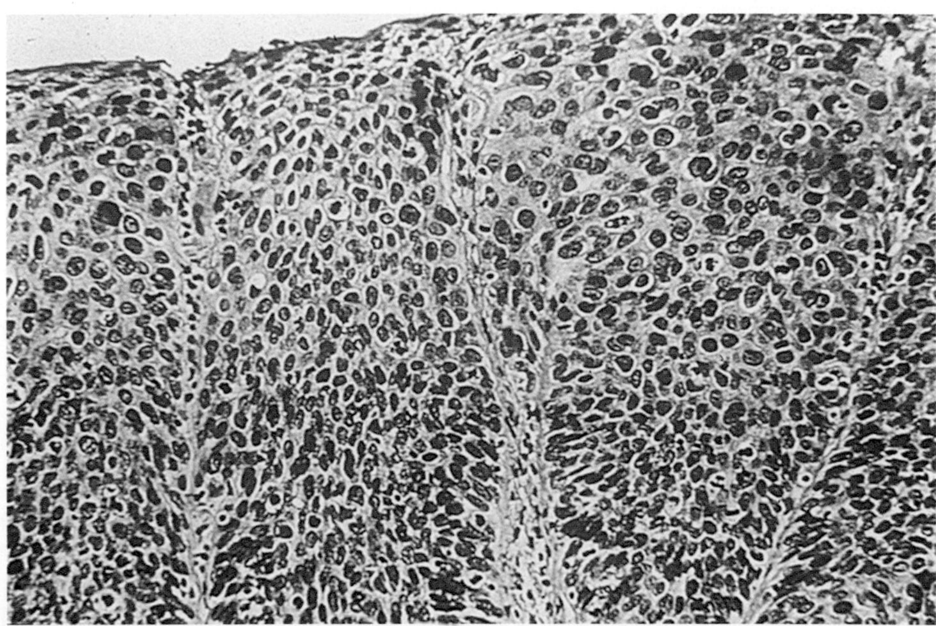

Figure 2–6 Histologic section of carcinoma in situ of the vulva.

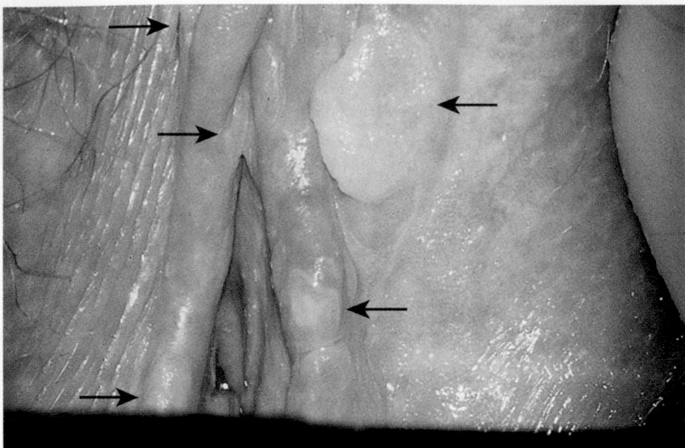

Figure 2–7 Multiple white lesions of the vulva caused by vulvar intraepithelial neoplasia.

in 10–15% of patients (Fig. 2–8). These lesions range from mahogany to dark brown, and they stand out sharply when observed solely with the naked eye.

Diagnosis

The value of careful inspection of the vulva during routine gynecologic examinations cannot be overstated; this remains the most productive diagnostic technique. The entire vulva, perineum, and perianal area must be evaluated for multifocal lesions. It is not uncommon to find intraepithelial lesions on hemorrhoid tags. The use of acetic acid is very helpful in identifying subtle lesions. In contrast to the cervix, the vulva requires application of acetic acid for 5 minutes or longer before many lesions are apparent. Placement of numerous soaked cotton balls on the vulva for the desired length of time is an effective method. After a lesion has been diagnosed, colposcopic examination of the entire vulva and perianal area should follow to rule out multicentric lesions. A handheld magnifying glass can also be used which allows greater viewing area at one time compared with the colposcope. In general, multifocal lesions are more common in premenopausal patients, whereas postmenopausal patients have a higher rate of unifocal disease.

Some investigators prefer to use toluidine blue to identify vulvar lesions. A 1% aqueous solution of the dye is applied to the external genital area. After drying for 2–3 minutes, the region is then washed with 1–2% acetic acid solution. Suspicious foci of increased nuclear activity become deeply stained (royal blue), whereas normal skin accepts little or none of the dye. Regrettably, hyperkeratotic lesions, even though neoplastic, are only lightly stained, whereas benign excoriations are often brilliant, an observation that accounts for the high false-positive and false-negative rates.

The diagnosis of VIN can be subtle. To avoid delay, the physician must exercise a high degree of suspicion. Vulvar biopsy should be used liberally. It is best accomplished under local anesthesia with a Keyes dermatologic punch (4–6 mm size). This instrument allows removal of an adequate tissue sample and orientation for future sectioning. After obtaining the biopsy specimen, we use the Keyes punch to cut out a piece of absorbable gelatin powder (e.g. Gelfoam); this is positioned in the skin defect and kept in place with a small dressing for at least 24 hours.

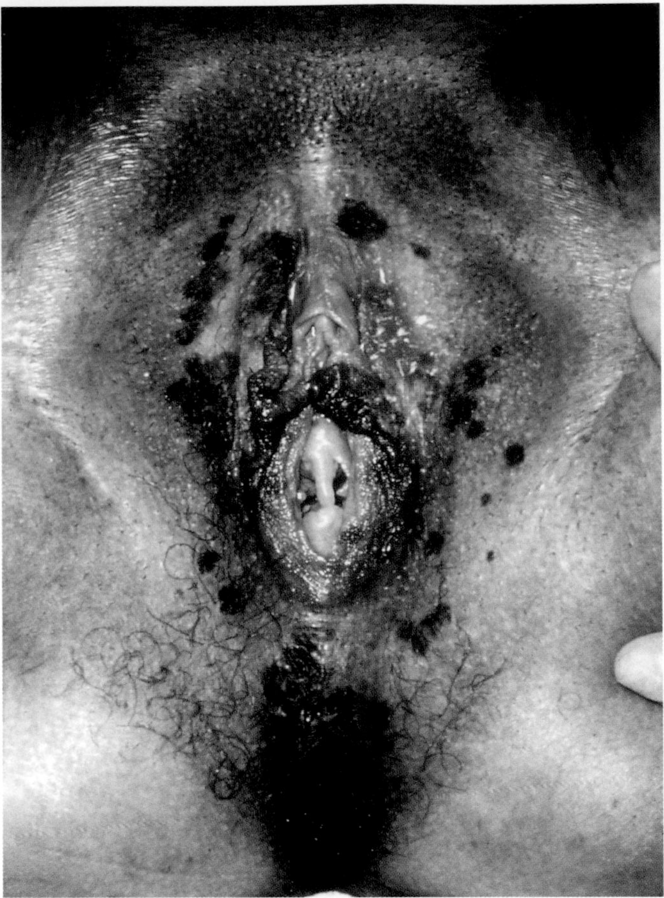

Figure 2–8 Pseudopigmented lesions of vulvar carcinoma in situ.

Adequate biopsy specimens can also be obtained with a sharp alligator-jaw instrument if one has proper traction on the skin. The problem with ordinary knife biopsies is that only superficial epithelium can be reached. If this technique is used, one must be careful to sample deeper layers.

Few reports have been made on untreated VIN (see previous section). Jones and McLean observed five of five untreated VIN lesions, which progressed to invasive cancer in 2–3 years. All had multiple focal lesions. Barbero and colleagues noted 3 of 55 patients treated with VIN whose condition progressed to carcinoma in 14 months–15 years. These three patients were 58–74 years of age. Adequate diagnosis is important. Chafe and associates noted that 19% of women who were thoroughly evaluated and thought to have only VIN had invasive cancer on the vulvectomy specimen.

Pigmented lesions

Pigmented lesions of the vulva are, for the most part, intraepithelial, with the exception of melanoma, which is discussed in Chapter 8. Pigmented lesions probably account for 10% of all vulvar disease. The most common pigmented lesion is a lentigo, which is a concentration of melanocytes in the basal layer of cells. It can have the clinical appearance of a freckle, although it is more commonly confused with a nevus. The borders are fuzzy, but it is not a raised lesion. A lentigo is benign, and the diagnosis is usually made by inspection with magnification. If there is doubt, a biopsy is performed.

VIN may appear as a pigmented lesion. Friedrich found that carcinoma in situ of the vulva was more frequent in pigmented lesions than in nevi. Characteristic raised hyperkeratotic pigmented lesions are suggestive of carcinoma in situ and should be biopsied.

A new term associated with pigmented lesions has emerged in gynecologic literature. Bowenoid papulosis is a variant of a pigmented lesion; dermatologists have noted this variant for some time. These are small pigmented papules that develop and spread rapidly. According to dermatologists, these papules often regress spontaneously. Histologically, at least on the vulva, these are squamous cell carcinomas in situ. These lesions have been reported to have an aneuploid DNA pattern. Many authorities have not found bowenoid papulosis of the vulva to spontaneously regress. Regardless of the clinical characteristics, if VIN is present histologically, the physician should treat the patient accordingly.

The management of nevi can be conservative. A nevus can often be detected only microscopically. Unfortunately, a simple nevus and an early melanoma cannot be differentiated on clinical evaluation. Excisional biopsy of these raised, smooth, pigmented areas can be done easily in the physician's office. If the nevus changes in color, size, and shape, it should be removed for diagnostic purposes. After a nevus is removed, no further therapy is needed regardless of whether it is a compound, intradermal, or junctional type.

Management

Surgical excision has been the mainstay of therapy. An important advantage is that excision allows for a complete histologic assessment; lesions with early invasion can thus be found. Most localized lesions are managed very effectively by wide local excision (a disease-free border of at least 5 mm) with end-to-end approximation of the defect. The vulvar skin and mucous membrane usually have a lot of elasticity, and cosmetic results are satisfactory after uncomplicated healing occurs. Modesitt and associates reported that recurrences were 3-fold higher when margins were positive for residual VIN II–III.

In the New Zealand study, 84% were treated with local excision and 65% had positive margins. Fifty-one percent required further therapy with histological factors being positive margins and multifocal disease. The Scotland study used wide local excision in 78% with 83% requiring treatment for recurrent disease.

In the review article, 1921 patients were surgically treated. Recurrence was noted in 19% after vulvectomy, 18% after partial vulvectomy, and 22% after local excision. Recurrences were significantly lower after free surgical margins (17%) than after positive surgical margins (47%), $P < 0.001$. Progression to invasive disease (58 patients) occurred 52% of the time after vulvectomy and 48% after local excision.

With multicentric lesions (Fig. 2–9), the involved skin can be excised and substitute a split-thickness skin graft that is taken from the buttocks or from the inner aspect of the thigh. This skinning vulvectomy and skin graft procedure was introduced by Rutledge and Sinclair in 1968 (Fig. 2–10). Its purpose was to replace the skin at risk in the vulvar site with ectopic epidermis from a donor site. We modified the procedure in that the clitoris is always preserved and any lesions on the glans are scraped off with a scalpel blade; the epithelium of the glans regenerates without loss of sensation. Some reports have questioned this approach on the basis that, at least in cases of vulvar dystrophy, the donated skin might be susceptible to a similar dystrophic process. In our experience, VIN lesions have developed outside the grafted area in preserved vulvar skin but rarely in the graft itself. This suggests that the neoplastic potential is inherent in the original vulvar skin and does not translate to skin from other parts of the body placed at the vulvar site, which may be the case in dystrophies.

The skinning vulvectomy and skin graft procedure preserves the subcutaneous tissue of the vulva and gives an optimal cosmetic and functional result. In > 100 patients treated to date, we have had no complaints of dyspareunia or diminished sexual responsiveness. In the elderly patient, simple vulvectomy may be preferred, because the skinning vulvectomy and skin graft operation requires prolonged bedrest (6–7 days) to allow the split-thickness graft to adhere to the graft bed. Thus, the potential for morbidity

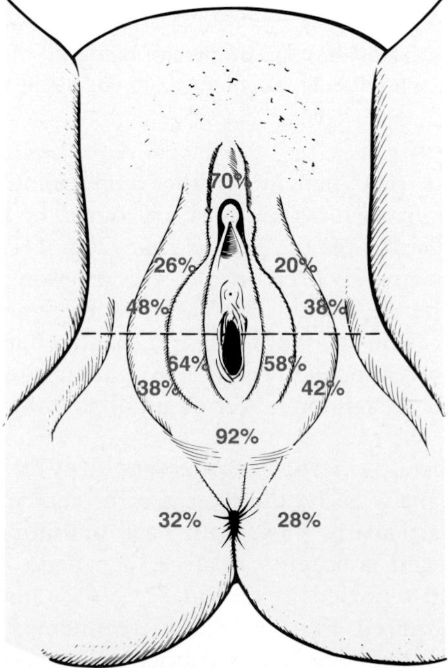

Figure 2–9 Plot of lesion locations in 36 patients treated for multifocal carcinoma in situ of the vulva.

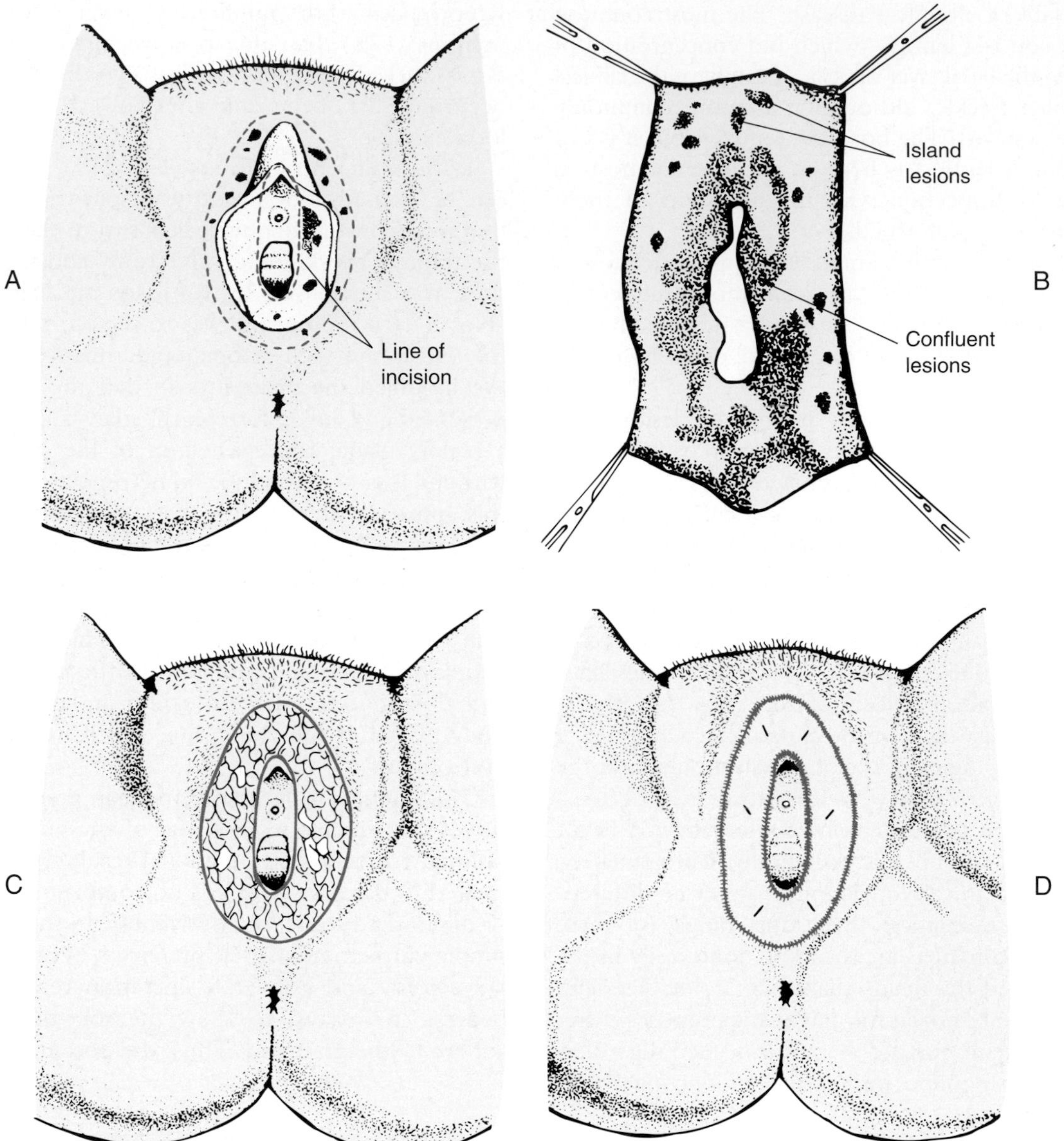

Figure 2–10 Skinning vulvectomy and skin graft. *A*, Excise all areas of involvement en bloc. *B*, Lesions may be isolated or confluent. *C*, Preserve all subcutaneous tissue as the graft bed. *D*, Suture the skin graft to the graft bed.

is increased. The patient's wishes concerning cosmetic results and sexual function must, of course, be taken into account regardless of the person's age (Fig. 2–11).

An alternative to excision of a vulvar lesion is ablative therapy. The disadvantage of ablative therapy is that a necrotic ulcer on the vulva may result and wound healing may be slow. Complete healing may take up to 3 months. The treated area is often very painful for much of that time.

Laser therapy in the management of VIN was considered by many to be the treatment of choice for many patients, particularly those who have multifocal disease. Townsend and colleagues treated 33 patients with laser therapy and reported success in 31 (94%); however, 14 patients required two or more treatments, and two patients required five laser treatments. The results published by Baggish and Dorsey were much the same, in that 32 of 35 patients were believed to have been cured from their disease; however, 26 of 35 patients required three or more treatments, and two women had six treatments. In the review article of the 253 patients treated with laser, 23% recurred. Pain, which has been severe in some patients, has been the main complication with laser therapy. Most therapists treat only a small portion of the vulva on an outpatient basis. Patients require general anesthesia if large areas of the vulva are to be treated at one time. Pain after therapy can be severe in some patients. Bleeding and infection have also been reported. The cosmetic results appear to be excellent. It appears that laser therapy can be an acceptable treatment modality; however, patients must be evaluated carefully before treatment, and invasive carcinoma must be ruled out (Table 2–7). Greater expertise with the laser is required for this therapy than is needed for cervical vaporization. The depth of destruction must be

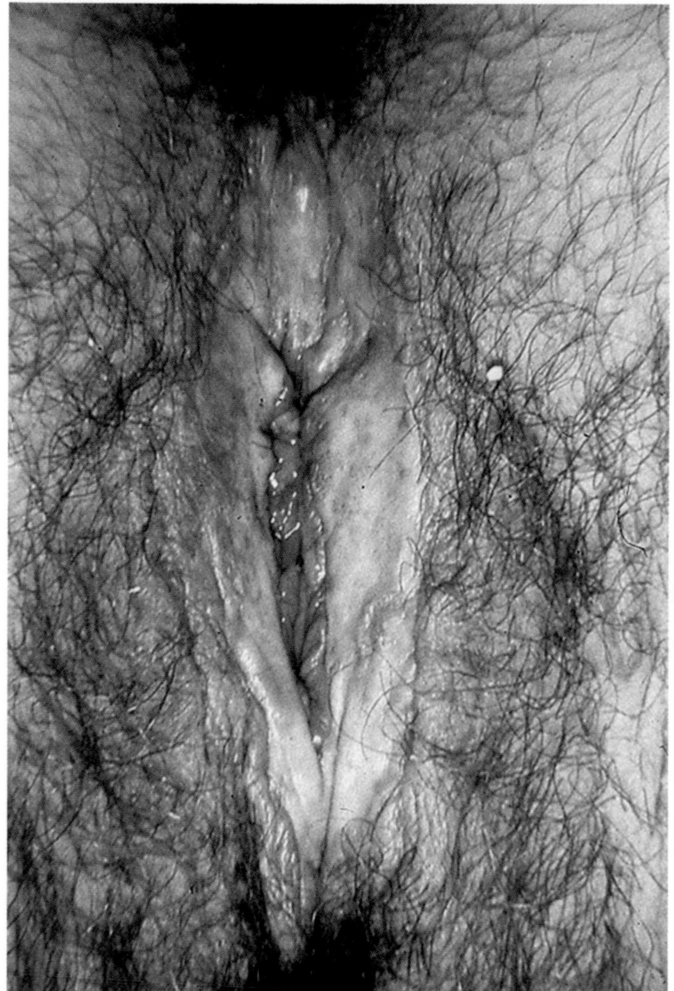

Figure 2–11 Excellent cosmetic results are present after superficial vulvectomy and skin graft for vulvar intraepithelial neoplasia (VIN).

Table 2–7 CO_2 LASER VAPORIZATION—VULVA	
Instrument	CO_2 laser, colposcopic, micromanipulator
Power density	600–1000 W/cm^2
Depth of destruction	Non-hairy areas < 1 mm
Hairy areas	> 3 mm
Lateral margins	"Brush"
Anesthesia	General, local
Analgesia	Significant post-laser pain—narcotics

controlled. Too deep a wound can result in long-term ulcers, which may take some time to heal and cause considerable discomfort. Benedet and colleagues evaluated 165 women with VIN. Of the 122 patients with VIN III, the mean thickness of the epithelium was 0.52 mm (range of 0.1–1.9 mm). In patients with hair follicles involved with VIN, the mean depth of involvement was 1.9 mm (range of 1–3.4 mm). Only 19 patients had appendiceal involvement. Age did not seem to affect the thickness of involved epithelium. Koilocytosis was present in 74% of VIN I lesions but was present in only 19% of VIN III lesions. Multifocal lesions were present in 64% of all patients. The most common sites were the labia minora, posterior fourchette, and perineum. Based on this study, the authors believe that 1 mm destruction of non-hair-bearing epithelium is adequate treatment. If skin appendages are involved, 2.5–3 mm is required (Fig. 2–12). Do not take the burn level to the subcutaneous fat. Wipe the carbon from the surgical site during the procedure and be certain that the shiny white lower dermis is preserved. Reid has defined surgical planes in the vulva as a guide to laser therapy. The first plane is the surface epithelium only, which includes the basement membrane. Opalescent cell debris is noted through the heat char. Healing is rapid with good cosmetic results. The second plane involves the dermal papillae with necrosis extending to the deep papillary area. The appearance is a homogeneous yellow color that resembles a chamois cloth. Again healing is rapid with good cosmesis. The third plane affects the upper and mid-reticular area where the pilosebaceous ducts are located. Some hypertrophy may appear in this area during the healing process. The fourth plane affects the deep reticular area, and "sand grains" can be visualized. Healing is slow and usually occurs by granulation from the sides. Skin grafting may be required. Destruction to the third plane is adequate for hair-bearing tissue; plane one to two is the depth needed for non-hair-bearing skin. Post laser therapy, the vulva is covered with topical steroids. Sitz baths and rinsing of the vulva with water after urination and defecation are important. A hair dryer is then used to dry the area. Repeat application of steroids is used after each washing and drying. A local anesthetic can be applied for mild to moderate pain control. Oral pain medication, including narcotics, may be necessary. The most severe pain is usually not evident until 3–4 days after the laser therapy. Laser therapy is particularly effective around the areas where excision can lead to external sphincter weakening.

For some time now we have used the cavitational ultrasonic surgical aspirator (CUSA) as the treatment of choice in the management of VIN, particularly multifocal lesions. The depth of destruction can be more easily controlled than with the laser. The procedure is rapid and healing is much quicker than laser therapy. Cosmesis is excellent. The CUSA easily removes the epithelium only although destruction of the underlying tissue can occur. Post therapy care is similar to that described for the laser. In a study from Wake Forest, 37 patients were treated with the CUSA. Seventy-six percent of patients had half or more of the vulva involved. A second treatment was required in three patients. Thirteen recurrences developed over a median of 16 months. Recurrence was significantly more frequent if the VIN involved the hair-bearing tissue.

Early invasive carcinoma can be very subtle. The group at the University of Florida has routinely treated carcinoma in situ of the vulva with simple vulvectomy. They noted that in 13 of 69 (19%) patients who had been evaluated with multiple biopsies, invasive cancer was noted in vulvectomy specimens. These were undetected cancers prior to

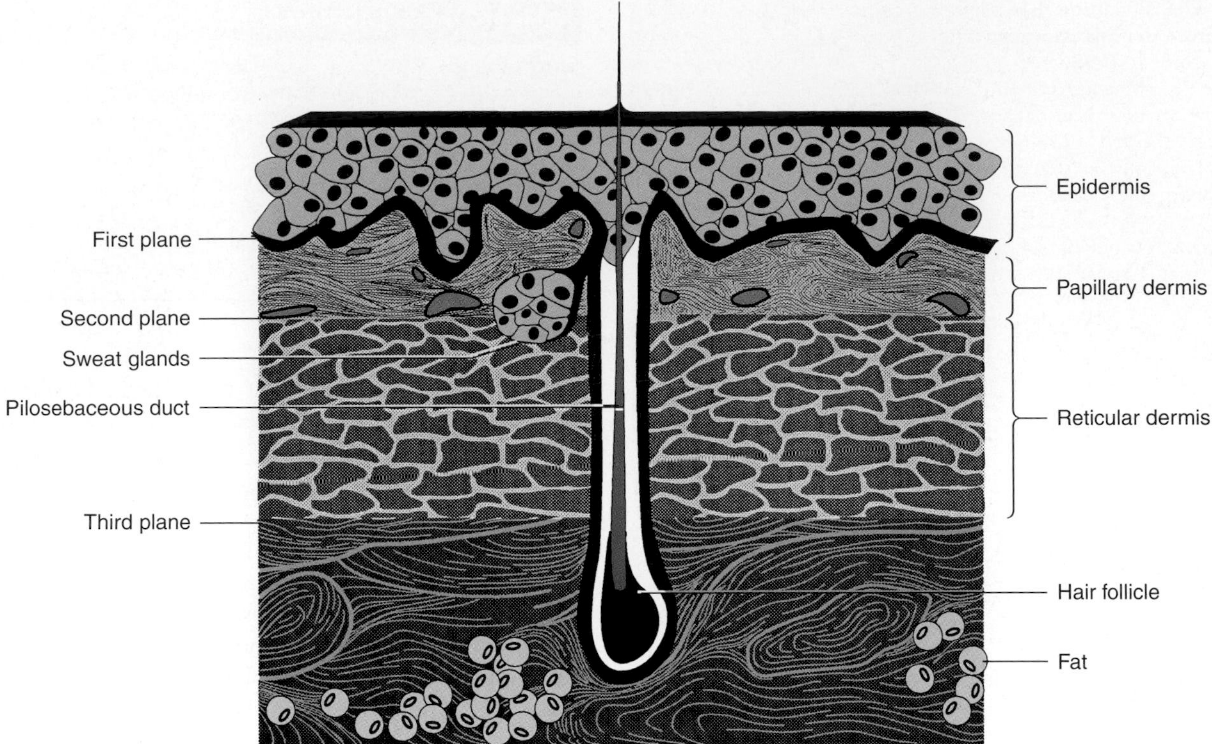

Figure 2–12 "Planes" for therapy for vulvar intraepithelial neoplasia using a laser.

vulvectomy. The temptation to preserve vulvar anatomy and prevent possible sexual dysfunction must be tempered with the necessity to rule out invasive disease. A simple vulvectomy may be the treatment of choice in such an individual and is certainly a consideration in the older patient.

Imiquimod 5% cream is an immune response modifier with indirect antiviral and antitumor properties. It has been shown to be effective and safe in the treatment of HPV-associated genital warts. Since at least some VIN lesions are HPV-related, imiquimod cream has been evaluated in a small number of patients. Todd reported 15 so treated patients and 4 had a clinical improvement and 3 had negative biopsies. Because of side effects, only two patients completed the treatment of three times per week. Christopher presented 13 patients treated, with 8 having total regression, 4 with 75% regression, and 2 had invasive cancer in the area of residual disease. Van Seters had 4 total responses and 9 partial responses in 15 patients—two did not tolerate the treatment. Marchitelli treated 8 patients with bowenoid and basaloid VIN 2/3 and had total clearance in 6 patients after 10–16 weeks of treatment. Two patients had partial response. Side effects included erythema in all patients, lesions in one and edema in one patient. During a 10–30 month followup, no relapses have occurred. The role of imiquimod cream in the treatment of VIN is encouraging but additional studies are needed before this can be accepted as desired therapy.

In summary, it is important to remember that quite often these lesions develop in young women who remain asymptomatic. Women should be taught vulvar self-examination to identify early lesions. This could lead to successful therapy that could also be less radical. Early diagnosis depends on careful vulvar examination under a bright light at regular intervals. Biopsy must be done on any suspicious lesions, and if the histologic report confirms intraepithelial neoplasia, an examination for multicentric foci should follow. The therapy of choice depends on the extent of disease; the location of the lesions; and, not least of all, on the personal desires of the patient.

BIBLIOGRAPHY

INTRAEPITHELIAL NEOPLASIA OF THE VAGINA

Benedet JL, Wilson PS, Matisic JP: Epidermal thickness measurements in VAIN. J Reprod Med 37:809, 1992.

Blumberg JM, Ober WB: Carcinoma in situ of the cervix: Recurrence in the vaginal vault. Am J Obstet Gynecol 66:421, 1952.

Buck HW and Guth KJ: Treatment of VAIN (primarily low grades) with Imiquimod 5% cream. J Lower Genital Tract Dis 7:290–293, 2003.

Caglar H, Hurtzog RW, Hreshchyshyn MM: Topical 5-FU treatment of vaginal intraepithelial neoplasia. Obstet Gynecol 58:580, 1981.

Capen CV et al: Laser therapy of vaginal intraepithelial neoplasia. Am J Obstet Gynecol 142:973, 1982.

Carter ER, Salvaggio AT, Jarkowski TL: Squamous cell carcinoma of the vagina following vaginal hysterectomy of intraepithelial carcinoma of the cervix. Am J Obstet Gynecol 82:401, 1961.

Copenhaver EH, Salzman FA, Wright KA: Carcinoma in situ of the vagina. Am J Obstet Gynecol 89:962, 1964.

Cromer JK: Invasive squamous-cell carcinoma of the vagina following surgery for carcinoma in situ of the cervix. Med Ann DC 34:115, 1965.

Diakomanolis E et al: Treatment of high grade VAIN with Imiquimod cream. N Eng J Med 347:374, 2002.

Dungar CF, Wilkinson EJ: Vaginal columnar cell metaplasia: An acquired adenosis associated with topical 5-FU therapy. J Reprod Med 40:361, 1995.

Ferguson JH, Maclure JG: Intraepithelial carcinoma, dysplasia, and exfoliation of cancer cells in the vaginal mucosa. Am J Obstet Gynecol 87:326, 1963.

Graham JB, Meigs JV: Recurrence of tumor after total hysterectomy for carcinoma in situ. Am J Obstet Gynecol 64:1159, 1952.

Gusberg SB, Marshall D: Intraepithelial carcinoma of the cervix: A clinical reappraisal. Obstet Gynecol 19:713, 1962.

Jemal A et al. Cancer statistics, 2005. CA Cancer J Clin 55:10–30, 2005.

Koss LG, Melamed MR, Daniel WW: In situ epidermoid carcinoma of the cervix and vagina following radiotherapy for cervical cancer. Cancer 14:353, 1961.

Krebs HB: Treatment of vaginal intraepithelial neoplasia with laser and topical 5FU. Obstet Gynecol 73:657, 1989.

Marcus SL: Multiple squamous cell carcinoma involving the cervix, vagina, and vulva: The theory of multicentric origin. Am J Obstet Gynecol 80:801, 1961.

McPherson HA et al: Epidermoid carcinoma of cervix, vagina, and vulva: A regional disease. Obstet Gynecol 21:145, 1963.

Moran JP, Robinson HJ: Primary carcinoma in situ of the vagina. Obstet Gynecol 20:405, 1962.

Newman W, Cromer JK: The multicentric origin of carcinoma of the female anogenital tract. Surg Gynecol Obstet 108:273, 1959.

Noller KL: Screening for vaginal cancer (Editorial). N Engl J Med 335:1599, 1996.

Ostergard DR, Morton DG: Multi-focal carcinoma of the female genitals. Am J Obstet Gynecol 99:1006, 1967.

Parker RT: Clinical problems of early cervical neoplasia. Obstet Gynecol Survey 24:684–697, 1969.

Pearce KF, Haefner HK, Sarwar SF, Nolan SF: Cytopathological findings on vaginal Papanicolaou smears after hysterectomy for benign gynecologic disease. N Engl J Med 335:1559, 1996.

Petrilli ES et al: Vaginal intraepithelial neoplasias: Biologic aspects and treatment with topical 5-fluorouracil and the carbon dioxide laser. Am J Obstet Gynecol 138:321, 1980.

Rutledge F: Cancer of the vagina. Am J Obstet Gynecol 97:635, 1967.

Samuels B, Bradburn DM, Johnson CG: Primary carcinoma in situ of the vagina. Am J Obstet Gynecol 82:393, 1961.

Schellhas HF: Personal communication, 1982.

Sillman FH, Fruchter RG, Chen YS, et al: Vaginal intraepithelial neoplasia: Risk factors for persistence, recurrence, and invasion and its management. Am J Obstet Gynecol 176:93, 1997.

Townsend DE et al: Treatment of vaginal carcinoma in situ with carbon dioxide laser. Am J Obstet Gynecol 143:565, 1982.

Woodruff JD: Treatment of recurrent carcinoma in situ in the lower genital canal. Clin Obstet Gynecol 8:757, 1965.

DIETHYLSTILBESTROL-RELATED GENITAL TRACT ANOMALIES

Fowler WC et al: Risks of cervical intraepithelial neoplasia among DES-exposed women. Obstet Gynecol 38:720, 1981.

Herbst AL, Scully RE, Robboy SJ: Problems in examination of the DES-exposed female. Obstet Gynecol 46:353, 1975.

Kurman RJ, Scully RE: The incidence and histogenesis of vaginal adenosis: An autopsy study. Hum Pathol 5:265, 1974.

Ng ABP et al: Natural history of vaginal adenosis in women exposed to diethylstilbestrol in utero. J Reprod Med 18:1, 1977.

O'Brien PC et al: Vaginal epithelial changes in young women enrolled in the National Cooperative Diethylstilbestrol Adenosis (DESAD) project. Obstet Gynecol 53:300, 1979.

Robboy SJ et al: Increased incidence of cervical and vaginal dysplasia in 3,980 diethylstilbestrol-exposed young women. JAMA 252: 2979, 1984.

Sandberg EC: The incidence and distribution of occult vaginal adenosis. Am J Obstet Gynecol 93:209, 1968.

Ulfelder H, Robboy SJ: The embryologic development of the human vagina. Am J Obstet Gynecol 126:769, 1976.

Waggoner SE, Mittendorf R, Biney N et al: Influence of in utero diethylstilbestrol exposure on the prognosis and biologic behavior of vaginal clear-cell adenocarcinoma. Gynecol Oncol 55:238, 1994.

NON-NEOPLASTIC EPITHELIAL DISORDERS OF THE VULVA

Bracco EL, Carli P, Sonni L et al: Clinical and histopathologic effects of topical treatment of vulval lichen sclerosus. J Reprod Med 38:37, 1993.

Dalziel KL: Effect of lichen sclerosus on sexual function and parturition. J Reprod Med 40:351, 1995.

Friedrich EG Jr, Julian CG, Woodruff JD: Acridine orange fluorescence in vulvar dysplasia. Am J Obstet Gynecol 90:1281, 1964.

Friedrich EG Jr: Vulvar dystrophy. Clin Obstet Gynecol 28:178, 1985.

Friedrich EG Jr, Kalra PS: Serum levels of sex hormones in vulvar lichen sclerosus, and the effect of topical testosterone. N Engl J Med 310:488, 1984.

Harrington CI, Dunsmore JR: An investigation into the incidence of auto-immune disorders in patients with lichen sclerosus et atrophicus. Br J Dermatol 104:563, 1981.

Hart WR, Norris HJ, Helwig EB: Relation of lichen sclerosus et atrophicus of vulva to the development of carcinoma. Obstet Gynecol 45:369, 1975.

International Society for the Study of Vulvovaginal Disease. J Reprod Med 43:601, 1998.

International Society for the Study of Vulvovaginal Disease(ISSVD): Classification of vulvar lesions: Report of the ISSVD Terminology Committee. Am J Obstet Gynecol 160:769, 1989.

Jeffcoat TNA: Chronic vulva dystrophies. Am J Obstet Gynecol 95:61, 1966.

Jeffcoat TNA: The dermatology of the vulva. J Obstet Gynaecol Br Comm 69:888, 1962.

Kaufman RH, Gardener HL, Brown D Jr, Beyth Y: Vulvar dystrophies: An evaluation. Am J Obstet Gynecol 120:363, 1974.

Lorenz B, Kaufman RH, Kutzner SK: Lichen sclerosus, therapy with clobetasol propionate. J Reprod Med 43:790, 1998.

Wallace HJ: Lichen sclerosus et atrophicus. Traus St. Julius Hosp. Dermatol Soc 57:9, 1971.

Woodruff JD, Borkowf HI, Holzman GB et al: Metabolic activity in normal and abnormal vulvar epithelia. Am J Obstet Gynecol 91:809, 1965.

INTRAEPITHELIAL NEOPLASIA OF THE VULVA

Abell MR, Gosling JR: Intraepithelial and infiltrative carcinoma of vulva, Bowen's type. Cancer 14:318, 1961.

Baggish MS, Dorsey HJ: CO_2 laser for treatment of vulvar carcinoma in situ. Obstet Gynecol 57:371, 1981.

Barbero M, Micheletti L, Preti M et al: Biologic behavior of vulvar intraepithelial neoplasia. J Reprod Med 38:108, 1993.

Benedet JL, Wilson PS, Matisic J: Epidermal thickness and skin appendage involvement in VIN. J Reprod Med 36:608, 1991.

Bowen JT: Precancerous dermatoses. J Cutan Dis 30:241, 1912.

Carson TE, Hoskins WJ, Wurzel JF: Topical 5-fluorouracil in the treatment of carcinoma in situ of the vulva. Obstet Gynecol 47(Suppl):59, 1976.

Chafe W, Richards A, Morgan L et al: Unrecognized invasive carcinoma in VIN. Gynecol Oncol 31:154, 1988.

Christopher J, Kaufman RH: Treatment of VIN 2/3 with imiquimod. J Reprod Med 47:395–398, 2002.

Colgan TJ: Vulvar intraepithelial neoplasia: A synopsis of recent developments. J Lower Genital Tract Dis 2:31, 1998.

Collin CG: A clinical stain for use in selecting biopsy sites in patients with vulvar diseases. Obstet Gynecol 28:158, 1966.

Costa S, Syrjanen S, Vendra C et al: Human papillomavirus infections in vulval precancerous lesions and cancer. J Reprod Med 40:291, 1995.

Crum CP et al: Vulvar intraepithelial neoplasia: Correlation of nuclear DNA content in the presence of human papilloma virus (HPV) structural antigen. Cancer 49:468, 1982.

Friedrich EG Jr: Reversible vulvar atypia. Obstet Gynecol 39:173, 1972.

Friedrich EG Jr: Vulvar carcinoma in situ in identical twins—an occupational hazard. Obstet Gynecol 39:837, 1972.

Higgins RV, Van Nagell JR, Donaldson ES et al: The efficacy of laser therapy in the treatment of cervical intraepithelial neoplasia. Gynecol Oncol 36:79, 1990.

Italian Study Group in Vulvar Disease: Clinicopathologic analysis of 370 cases of vulvar intraepithelial neoplasia. J Reprod Med 41:665, 1996.

Jones RW, McLean MR: CIS of vulva: A review of 31 treated and 5 untreated cases. Obstet Gynecol 68:499, 1986.

Jones RW, Park JS, McLean MR et al: Human papilloma virus in women with VIN III. J Reprod Med 35:1124, 1990.

Kagie MJ, Kenter GG, Hermans J et al: The relevance of various vulvar epithelial changes in the early detection of squamous cell carcinoma of the vulva. Int J Gynecol Cancer 7:50, 1997.

Krupp PJ, Bohm JW: 5-Fluorouracil topical treatment of in situ vulvar cancer. Obstet Gynecol 51:702, 1978.

Litwin MS et al: Topical chemotherapy of lentigo maligna with 5-fluorouracil cream. J Surg Oncol 35:721, 1975.

Marchitelli C, Secco G, Perrotta M et al: Treatment of bowenoid and basaloid VIN 2/3 with imiquimod 5% cream. J Reprod Med 49:876–882, 2004.

McNally OM, Mulvany NJ, Pagano R et al: VIN 3: A clinicopathologic review. In J Gynecol Can 12:490–495, 2002.

Miller BE: VIN treated with cavitational ultrasonic surgical aspiration. Gynecol Oncol 85:114–118, 2002.

Modesitt SC, Waters AB, Walton L et al: Vulvar intraepithelial neoplasia III: Occult cancer and the impact of margin status on recurrence. Obstet Gynecol 92:962, 1998.

Raaf JH et al: Treatment of Bowen's disease with topical dinitrochlorobenzene and 5-fluorouracil. Cancer 37:1633, 1976.

Reid R: Superficial laser vulvectomy. Am J Obstet Gynecol 152:504, 1985.

Report of the Committee on Terminology: New nomenclature for vulvar disease. Am J Obstet Gynecol 160:769, 1989.

Richart RM: A clinical staining test for the in vivo delineation of dysplasia and carcinoma in situ. Am J Obstet Gynecol 86:703, 1963.

Rodolakis A, Diakomanolis E, Vlachos G et al: VIN-diagnostic and therapeutic challenges. Eur J Gynaecol Oncol 24:317–322, 2003.

Rutledge F, Sinclair M: Treatment of intraepithelial carcinoma of the vulva by skin excision and graft. Am J Obstet Gynecol 102:806, 1968.

Simonsen EF: CO_2 laser used for carcinoma in situ/Bowen's disease (VIN) and lichen sclerosus in the vulvar region. Acta Obstet Gynecol Scand 68:551, 1989.

Sturgeon SS, Brinton LA, Devesa SS et al: In situ and invasive vulvar cancer incidence trends (1973 to 1987). Am J Obstet Gynecol 166:1482, 1992.

Sykes P, Smith N, McCormick P et al: High grade VIN. A retrospective analysis of patient characteristics, management, outcome and relationship to squamous cell carcinoma of the vulva 1989–1999. Aust NZ J Obstet Gynaecol 42:69–74, 2002.

Todd RW, Etherington IJ, Lineseley DM: The effects of 5% imiquimod cream on high grade VIN. Gynecol Oncol 85:67–70, 2002.

Townsend DE et al: Management of vulvar intraepithelial neoplasia by carbon dioxide laser. Obstet Gynecol 60:49, 1982.

Van Beurden M, Van Der Vange N, Ten Kate FJW et al: Restricted surgical management of vulvar intraepithelial neoplasia 3: Focus on exclusion of invasion and on relief of symptoms. Int J Gynecol Cancer 8:73, 1998.

Van Seters M, Fons G, van Beurden M: Imiquimod in the treatment of multifocal vulvar intraepithelial neoplasia 2/3. Results of a pilot study. J Reprod Med 47:501–505, 2002.

Van Seters M, van Beurden M, deCraen AJM: Is the assumed natural history of VIN IV based on enough evidence? A systematic review of 3322 published patients. Gynecol Oncol 97:645–651, 2005.

Woodruff JD et al: The contemporary challenge of carcinoma in situ of the vulva. Am J Obstet Gynecol 115:677, 1973.

3 Invasive Cervical Cancer

Bradley J. Monk, M.D. and Krishnansu S. Tewari, M.D.

GENERAL OBSERVATIONS

The uterine cervix is of major interest and importance to almost every obstetrician and gynecologist. To the gynecologic oncologist it represents a common focus for the development of malignant disease. To the obstetrician, it represents the primary barometer in the process of labor and delivery. No other organ is as accessible to the obstetrician and gynecologist in terms of both diagnosis and therapy. Its accessibility led to the great strides made possible by the Papanicolaou (Pap) smear, resulting in complete reversal of the prognosis in cancer of this organ. Easy access to the cervix also led to the skillful application of radiation techniques, which have resulted in some of the best overall cure rates for any malignancy found in humans.

The cause of cervical cancer is not completely known, but its development seems to be related to multiple insults and injuries sustained by the cervix. Squamous cell carcinoma of the cervix is almost non-existent in a celibate population: only one case has been reported in the literature. This type of cancer is more prevalent in women of lower socioeconomic groups and is correlated with first coitus at an early age and with multiple sexual partners. There is no proven correlation with the frequency of sexual intercourse. However, studies have shown that husbands of women with cervical cancer reported significantly more sexual partners than did husbands of patients in the control group. Husbands of women who had cervical cancer were also more likely to report histories of various genital conditions, including genital warts, gonorrhea, and genital herpes.

Currently, greater attention is being paid to the human papillomavirus (HPV) infection of the cervix as a link to etiology. The power, consistency, and specificity of the association between subclinical HPV infection and cervical neoplasia raise the strong possibility that this relationship is causal. The biologic plausibility of this is supported by evidence that this sexually transmitted oncogenic virus often produces persistent asymptomatic infection of metaplastic epithelium in the cervical transformation zone. The postulate that cervical neoplasia may arise by mutagenesis within papillomavirus-infected cells at the squamocolumnar junction is discussed with other corollaries in Chapter 1.

The cervix (L. *cervix,* neck) is a narrow, cylindrical segment of the uterus; it enters the vagina through the anterior vaginal wall and lies, in most cases, at right angles to it. In the average patient, the cervix measures 2–4 cm in length and is contiguous with the inferior aspect of the uterine corpus. The point of juncture of the uterus and the cervix is known as the isthmus; this area is marked by slight constriction of the lumen. Anteriorly, the cervix is separated from the bladder by fatty tissue and is connected laterally to the broad ligament and parametrium (through which it obtains its blood supply). The lower intravaginal portion of the cervix, a free segment that projects into the vault of the vagina, is covered with mucous membrane. The cervix opens into the vaginal cavity through the external os. The cervical canal extends from the anatomic external os to the internal os, where it joins the uterine cavity. The histologic internal os is where there is a transition from endocervical to endometrial glands. The intravaginal portion of the cervix (portio vaginalis, exocervix) is covered with stratified squamous epithelium that is essentially identical to the epithelium of the vagina. The endocervical mucosa is arranged in branching folds (plicae palmatae) and is lined by cylindrical epithelium. The stroma of the cervix consists of connective tissue with stratified muscle fibers and elastic tissue. The elastic tissue is found primarily around the walls of the larger blood vessels.

The stratified squamous epithelium of the portio vaginalis is composed of several layers that are conventionally described as basal, parabasal, intermediate, and superficial. The basal layer consists of a single row of cells and rests on a thin basement membrane. This is the layer in which active mitosis occurs. The parabasal and intermediate layers together constitute the prickle-cell layer, which is analogous to the same layer in the epidermis. The superficial layer varies in thickness, depending on the degree of estrogen stimulation. It consists primarily of flattened cells that show an increasing degree of cytoplasmic acidophilia toward the surface. The thickness and the glycogen content of the epithelium increase following estrogen stimulation and account for the therapeutic effect of estrogens in atrophic vaginitis. The staining of glycogen in the normal epithelium of the portio vaginalis is the basis of the Schiller test.

MICROINVASIVE CARCINOMA OF THE CERVIX

There is probably no more an area of controversy in gynecologic oncology than the diagnosis and management of microinvasive carcinoma of the cervix. The evolution and sometimes revolution concerning the diagnosis and management have occurred since Mestwerdt, in 1947, observed that invasive cervical cancer diagnosed only microscopically could be cured by non-radical surgery. During the last three decades, definitions and treatment plans have changed dramatically. It is hoped that most of these changes had occurred as new data became available and that changes were therefore logical. Much of the confusion can be related to the fact that the Federation of International Gynecologists and Obstetricians (FIGO) has changed the criteria for early stage invasive carcinoma of the cervix since 1960. These changes were made as additional information in regard to this disease process became available. Other influences, however, also contributed to the confusion. Over the years as many as 20 different definitions have been proposed and as many as 27 terms have been applied to this entity. The recommended therapy has also changed, going from radical surgery with any invasion to being more conservative with various depths of invasion.

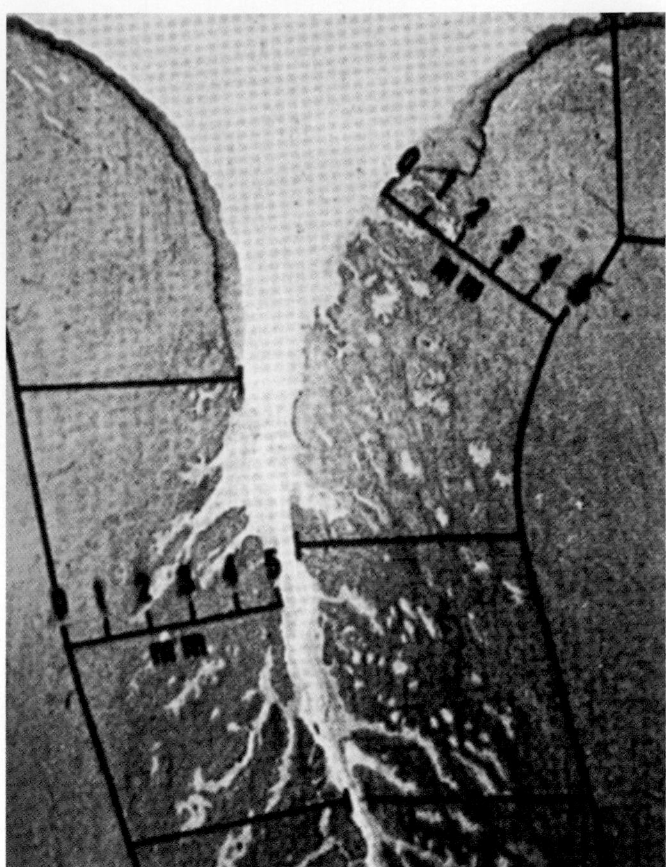

Figure 3–1 A 5 mm rule on a histologic section of a normal squamocolumnar junction. (Courtesy of Hervy Averette, MD, Miami, Florida.)

In 1971, FIGO designated stage Ia carcinoma of the cervix as those cases of preclinical carcinoma. It is obvious that preclinical invasive cancer may be only a few millimeters in depth or ≥10 mm (Fig. 3–1). In 1973, the Society of Gynecologic Oncologists (SGO) accepted the following statement concerning the definition of microinvasive carcinoma of the cervix:

1. Cases of intraepithelial carcinoma with questionable invasion should be regarded as intraepithelial carcinoma; and
2. A microinvasive lesion should be defined as one in which a neoplastic epithelium invaded the stroma in one or more places to the depth of <3 mm below the base of the epithelium (Fig. 3-2) and in which lymphatic or vascular involvement is not demonstrated.

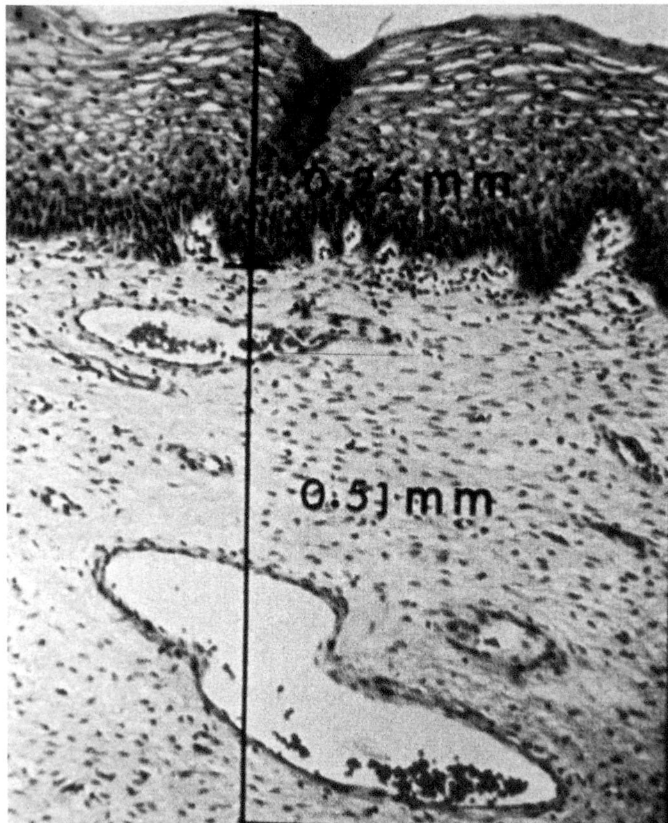

Figure 3–2 Vascular channels within 0.5 mm of the surface epithelium shown on histologic section of a normal cervix. (Courtesy of Hervy Averette, MD, Miami, Florida.)

This definition was not agreed to unanimously by the SGO; nevertheless, in the USA, it became the most quantifiable definition for this entity at that time. It was used subsequently as a guide for therapy by many physicians. FIGO has consistently stated that staging of all cancers is for comparison purposes and is not to be used as a guide for therapy. In 1979, the Japanese Society of Obstetrics and Gynecology essentially adopted the SGO definition, except that cases with confluent patterns were excluded and were considered to belong to stage Ib.

In 1985, for the first time, FIGO attempted to quantify the histologic definition of stage Ia carcinoma of the cervix. Stage Ia was defined as the earliest form of invasion in which minute foci of invasion are visible only microscopically. Stage Ia2 is a macroscopically measurable microcarcinoma that should not exceed 5 mm in depth and 7 mm in width. Vascular space involvement, either venous or lymphatic, should not alter staging. This definition has been criticized for several reasons. Although the upper limits of invasion for depth and width were stated, upper limits for measurement for stage Ia1 were not defined. It was, therefore, difficult to quantify patients in the two subgroups. Other areas of criticism were aimed at the fact that the FIGO definition could not be used as a guide for treatment, and the definition covered patients with vascular lymphatic channel involvement. These variations illustrate the problem with specific definition.

Authors have suggested various levels of invasion for this diagnosis; over the years these levels have varied from 1 to 3 to 5 and even greater depth of invasion. The width of the lesion has only recently been addressed and is included only in the FIGO definition. Some authors have even suggested that the volume of tumor should be used as a defining point. In most countries, this is impractical owing to the cost of that determination. Some authorities exclude patients with confluent growth, although this is usually ill defined. Investigators have looked at tumor grade as an independent prognostic variable, and it is generally agreed that this has no importance. As mentioned earlier, probably the most controversial aspect of the definition is whether or not patients with capillary-like space involvement (vascular lymphatic channel) should be included in the definition. FIGO does not exclude it; however, the SGO and the Japanese society do.

In 1994, FIGO, in an attempt to better qualify the definition of microinvasive carcinoma of the cervix, adopted the following definition for microinvasive carcinoma of the cervix (Table 3–1). Stage Ia1 cancers would be those with stromal invasion up to 3 mm in depth and no greater than 7 mm. Stage Ia2 would be when invasion is present at 3–5 mm in depth and no greater than 7 mm. Lymphatic vascular space involvement would not exclude a patient from this definition. The recurrence rate of patients in these two substages would probably be no more than 1–2%. Survival of stage Ia1 would approach 99%, and stage Ia2 would approach 97–98%. This new definition allows further evaluation of what might be appropriate therapy for the different substages, particularly stage Ia2 cancers.

Vascular space involvement was not excluded from the FIGO definition for several reasons. Pathologists disagree with regard to the reproducibility of this entity. At least in one study, the number of slides prepared from the cervix depended on the incidence of capillary-like space involvement. Shrinkage artifact can lead to an overdiagnosis and verification has been suggested with special staining to verify true capillary-like space involvement. In one study in which immunoperoxidase staining with Ulex Europaeus agglutinin 1 lectin (UEAI) was used, 10 of 32 cases of vascular space involvement were excluded in which involvement was initially thought to exist. In a combined study of 1004 patients at three reference centers, Burghardt et al

Table 3–1 STAGE IA CANCER OF THE CERVIX

Stage Ia: Cancer invasion identified only microscopically. All gross lesions, even with superficial invasion, are stage Ib cancers. Measured stromal invasion with maximum depth of 5 mm and no wider than 7mm*

Stage Ia1: Measured invasion of stroma up to 3 mm

Stage Ia2: Measured invasion of stroma of 3–5 mm and no wider than 7 mm

* The depth of invasion should not be >5 mm taken from the base of the epithelium, either surface or glandular, from which it originates. Vascular space involvement, either venous or lymphatic, should not alter the staging.

observed that the frequency with which angiolymphatic space involvement was detected ranged from 9% in Munich to 23% in Erlangen, and finally up to 43% in Graz.

As greater experience is obtained, the tendency has been toward conservative management involving conization of the cervix if fertility preservation is desired or simple hysterectomy for superficial invasion (0–3 mm) and even in some patients with 3–5 mm of invasion. In 1978, Lohe reported on 285 patients with early stromal invasion and 134 patients with microcarcinoma. He defined early stromal invasion as only isolated, variably shaped projections with true signs of infiltration present, whereas microcarcinomas' true confluent carcinomatosis masses were present. Tumor length and depth were 10 mm and 5 mm. He stated that the three-dimensional definition of the size of the tumor is essential to the microscopic diagnosis of early stromal invasion and of microcarcinoma. In his series, 72% with early stromal invasion and 41% with microcarcinoma were treated with conservative surgery (conization or simple hysterectomy). After long-term follow-up, no patients with early stromal invasion died. Three patients with microcarcinomas have recurred and died. In a larger collected series of 435 patients with microcarcinoma, 24 (5.5%) had a recurrence of disease. Using his criteria, Lohe predicted <1% incidence of lymph node metastasis in microcarcinoma and essentially none in early stromal invasion. Boyce and colleagues have reported a large series with both "microscopic foci" of invasion (360 cases) and "occult invasion" (390 cases). Most (283) of the patients with microscopic foci invasion were treated with simple hysterectomy and only 14 with conization. After 5–15 years of follow-up, only one patient died of the disease. Most (262) of the patients with occult invasion received irradiation therapy. Most of these lesions were greater than 5 mm in depth, and all were characterized by confluent masses of neoplastic cells. Twenty-four of the 390 patients with occult invasion died of the disease in 5 years. Benedet and colleagues reported on 180 patients with microinvasion and occult invasive squamous cell carcinoma of the cervix who were examined by colposcopy during a 10-year period. Colposcopy led to the correct management in 90% of patients with occult invasive carcinoma and in 84% of patients with microinvasive cancer. Colposcopy appeared to be less sensitive in detecting microinvasive lesions than in detecting occult carcinoma. Atypical vessels indicative of early invasive cancer are often subtle and difficult to identify. They are best visualized when the cervix has been bathed in normal saline. In many cases, acetic acid can cover atypical vessels by enhancing white epithelium that obscures the vessels. Östör in Australia has made an extensive review on this subject of the literature published since 1976. As a pathologist, he has critically reviewed many of the parameters that have historically been suggested as important prognostic factors.

0–3 mm invasion

Östör identified 3683 patients from the literature with <1 mm of invasion. Four patients had lymph node metastasis. With the incidence of lymph node metastasis in this group being essentially 0, it appears that lymphadenectomy has no place in this group of patients. There were 17 invasive recurrences and 16 cancer-related deaths. In several cases that resulted in death, patients refused further therapy or follow-up. Therefore, the death rate in this group of patients appears to be <0.1%, invasive recurrences were approximately 0.4% (Table 3–2). Östör identified 1324 patients who had invasion of 1–3 mm. Of these, 333 definitely had lymphadenectomies with seven nodal metastases. At least two of these probably had >3 mm of stromal invasion. The incidence based on these figures suggests that lymph node metastasis would be approximately 1%. There were 26 invasive recurrences and 6 deaths. Some of these patients probably had >3 mm of invasion and also included some patients with "microinvasive adenocarcinoma". In a review of reports over the last 15 years, most of which occurred within the last decade, Creasman and colleagues identified 1704 patients who had an invasion of 0–3 mm and 17 (1%) recurred. Only three (0.17%) died of their cancer. These recurrences were in patients with squamous lesions.

The management of early invasive lesions (0–3 mm of invasion, Fig. 3–3A–C) has generally been agreed on by the gynecologic oncology community. Patients with FIGO stage Ia1 and SGO criteria for microinvasion could be treated conservatively with simple hysterectomy, or if continued fertility is desired conization only, provided surgical margins are free of cancer. Most of the data in the literature concerning patients with 0–3 mm of invasion are based on conservative therapy, although some patients have had lymphadenectomies. From collected series, it would, therefore, appear that the role of vascular space involvement in this group of patients does not predict lymph node metastasis or recurrence. Although still in dis-

Table 3–2 LYMPH NODE METASTASES, RECURRENCES AND DEATHS IN STAGE IA CARCINOMA OF THE CERVIX

Invasion Depth (mm)	No. of Patients	Invasion Recurrence	Died of Cancer	No. with CLSI	No. with Positive Nodes
0–3	5007	35 (0.7%)	10 (0.2%)	182 (3.6%)	8/666 (1.2%)
3–5	674	25 (4%)	13 (2%)	124 (18.4%)	14/221 (6.3%)

CLSI, capillary-like space involvement.

Modified from Östör AG: Pandora's Box or Ariodne's Thread? Definition and prognostic significance of microinvasion into uterine cervix. Ann Pathol, 105, 1995.

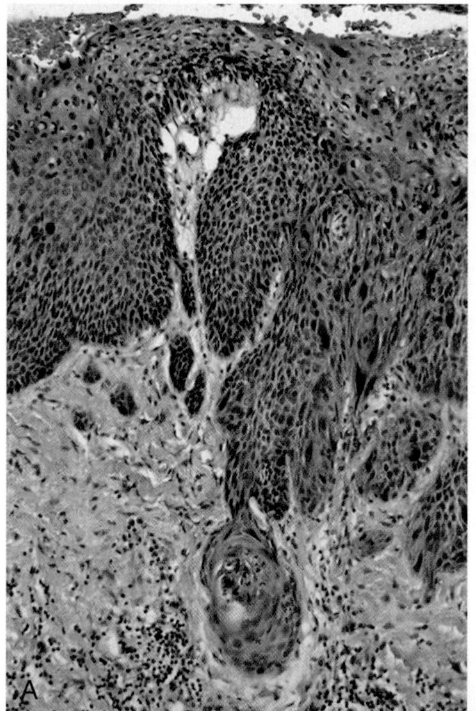

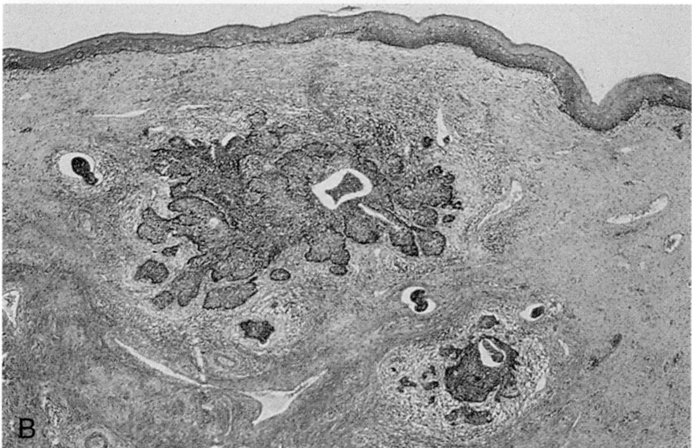

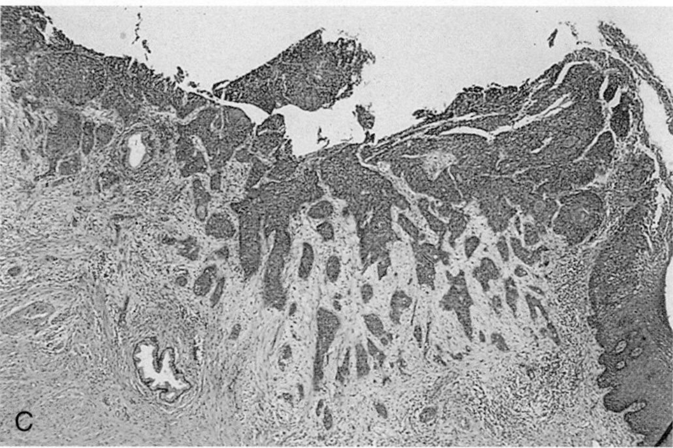

Figure 3–3 *A,* Microinvasion (stage Ia1) of squamous cell carcinoma of the cervix. Invasion of less than 1 mm, no confluency or vascular space involvement; true microinvasion. *B,* Microcarcinoma with less than 3 mm of invasion but with vascular space involvement. *C,* Microcarcinoma "spray" type with less than 1 mm of invasion.

pute, a growing number of investigators apparently do not use capillary-like space involvement as an exclusion criterion for this stage.

3–5 mm invasion

Östör identified 674 patients in this category of which 221 definitely had lymphadenectomies, 6% had nodal metastasis. If most or all of the other patients had lymphadenectomy, which is possible, and the results of all of the nodes were negative, the figure would be close to 2%. Twenty-five (4%) patients developed an invasive recurrence, and 13 (2%) died of their disease. Twenty-three percent of the patients were said to have had capillary-like space involvement. Creasman identified from the literature 264 patients with 3–5 mm invasion who had lymphadenectomy in which vascular space involvement was specifically evaluated. In patients with vascular space involvement, 2 of 83 (2.4%) and 7 of 181 (3.8%) without vascular space involvement had lymph node metastasis. In the literature, 488 patients with 3–5 mm were identified and 15 (3%) developed a recurrence with 9 (1.8%) dying of cancer deaths. The recurrence and death rates in patients with 3–5 mm approaches those with 0–3 mm invasion. Most, but not all, of patients treated for 3–5 mm invasion were managed with radical hysterectomy and pelvic lymphadenectomy. However, there are patients in this category who have been managed only with conization. In the 3–5 mm range, vascular space status does not appear to correlate with lymph node metastasis. There is limited experience with patients with these clinical lesions, but patients with limited invasion of 3–5 mm have a much greater incidence of lymph node metastasis (7%), which should be treated as a stage Ib cancer.

The data on patients with 3–5 mm invasion still remain fairly limited. With a very low incidence of lymph node metastasis (2–3%), it seems reasonable to evaluate the role of more conservative therapy in this group of patients. This may be done after consultation with the pathologist and gynecologic oncologist. If one is concerned about the 3% incidence of lymph node metastasis, these nodes can be evaluated with laparoscopy or retroperitoneal lymphadenectomy. If there is no evidence of extrauterine disease via these procedures, simple hysterectomy or even conization may be reasonable treatments. Twenty years ago, it was not unusual for investigators to suggest radical hysterectomy and pelvic lymphadenectomy for any degree of stromal invasion. With increased experience, more conservative therapy was found to be just as efficacious as radical therapy. It appears that we are now in the same arena for 3–5 mm today as we were for 0–3 mm two decades ago. Although vascular space involvement does not appear to predict lymph node metastasis with 3–5 mm invasion, anecdotal reports in the literature have suggested that recurrences are higher in patients with capillary-like space involvement but with no metastasis in the lymph nodes. It may be of significance that with progressively greater depth of stromal invasion, there is an increased risk of angiolymphatic space involvement. In point of fact, Fuller et al from the Memorial Sloan-Kettering Cancer Center detected a linear relationship between depth of cervical stromal invasion and the presence of angiolymphatic invasion. Although vascular space involvement was predictive of recurrence to the same degree it was predictive of nodal metastases, when stratified for the latter, vascular invasion lost its adverse prognostic effects. Östör noted in his review that 496 (14%) of 3597 patients who had capillary-like space involvement did not have an invasive recurrence. Morice et al retrospectively studied the clinicopathologic features of 193 patients who underwent radical surgery and lymphadenectomy for early stage cervical carcinoma, and found that both lymphovascular and nodal status were prognostic factors upon multivariate analysis. It was noteworthy that among a subgroup of 89 patients with a small tumor (<2 cm) and absence of nodal or isthmic involvement, that the overall survival was significantly correlated with the presence of lymphovascular space involvement. Recently, in an analysis of 93 patients who had undergone resection of early stage lesions, Memarzadeh et al demonstrated that the presence of lymphovascular space invasion in the parametria was an independent predictor of metastases in the pelvic ($P < 0.001$) and para-aortic ($P < 0.05$) lymphatic chains, an altogether not surprising finding. Hopefully, the role of lymphovascular space involvement will be further clarified and possibly even resolved in the future as more data are accumulated.

Conservative management for stage Ia2 carcinoma of the cervix does not seem unreasonable in light of the fact that some investigators have suggested that conservative therapy might be feasible for patients with "small stage Ib" cervical cancers. Girardi and colleagues from Graz reported on a series of 69 patients with small stage Ib carcinomas of the cervix. Treatment consisted of conization or simple hysterectomy in 27, radical hysterectomy with lymphadenectomy in 25, radical vaginal hysterectomy in 13, and conization followed by radiotherapy in 4. No patient developed a recurrence during the ensuing 2–35 years. Two of the 25 patients with lymphadenectomy had one positive lymph node each. This study comes from a group of investigators who over the years have meticulously evaluated pathologic specimens and traditionally have been surgically aggressive. Östör reviewed the literature since 1976 with regard to conization as definitive therapy for stage Ia cancers. He identified 655 patients with 0–5 mm invasion treated with conization, which resulted in 12 invasive recurrences and one death.

The Gynecologic Oncology Group (GOG) reported 50 patients with 3–5 mm invasion in the conization specimen. All underwent a radical hysterectomy and pelvic lymphadenectomy. The uterine specimen showed no evidence of residual disease. There were 23% with lymph space involvement (LSI), but none of the patients had positive nodes and there have been no recurrences. (Note that the term LSI is used interchangeably with vascular space involvement [VSI].)

In a report from Japan, 402 patients were identified with 0–5 mm invasion. These authors noted that 72 (18%), although had depth of invasion satisfying the FIGO definition, had >7 mm of horizontal spread. As the depth of invasion increased, there was a greater possibility that horizontal spread was >7 mm (6% stage Ia1 and 61% for stage Ia2). Lymph node metastasis was 1.4% for true Ia1 and 3.4% for Ia2 cancers. For those with >7 mm spread, lymph node metastasis was 7.4%. LSI was 18% in those >7 mm compared to 3.6% if <7 mm. Four patients had a recurrence, but three recurrences occurred in those with >7 mm lateral spread. Other authors have noted recurrences and deaths in patients with 0–5 mm invasion; however, when lateral spread was evaluated, it was >7 mm. Tumor volume is an important prediction for metastasis, recurrence, and cancer-related deaths. Now that there are quantifiable perimeters for stage Ia cancers, more precise data can be evaluated with regard to risk and appropriate therapy for stage Ia2 can be agreed.

CLINICAL PROFILE OF INVASIVE CANCER

A substantial and well-publicized screening program is needed to make the public and the profession more aware of *cervical* cancer as the possible cause of even minimal gynecologic symptoms. All public education should emphasize the prevention and cure of cancer, and a more optimistic attitude would help to motivate patients and physicians to seek appropriate action. The need for early diagnosis rests on the incontrovertible fact that definite cure, in actuarial terms, is readily achieved when cervical cancer is minimal—but almost impossible if the tumor is given time to grow and spread to the pelvic wall or into adjacent structures such as the bladder and rectum. The gradient of percentage curability from early invasive cancer to late, grossly invasive disease is such a steep one that even a moderate reduction in tumor size could not fail to create a substantial improvement in curability. It is true, of course, as with other cancers, that some carcinomas of the cervix grow more rapidly than others. The basis for this difference in growth rate is still beyond our knowledge, but it is not beyond our capability to prevent unnecessary growing time. Even the relatively slow-growing malignancy, if given enough time, will become incurable; and the most rapid-growing tumor, if diagnosed while of still moderate dimension, is definitely curable. The earlier that most tumors are detected and treated, the better will be the chance of cure. A Pap smear from a patient with early invasive squamous cell carcinoma illustrates a typical multinucleated "tadpole" cell (Fig. 3–4). Cytology and colposcopy are valuable tools in the eradication of cervical cancer. Every opportunity should be taken to disseminate modern concepts of cancer control to schools of nursing and other paramedical organizations, because there is still a need for more coordinated effort in these fields. The burden should not be left with the physician alone. The

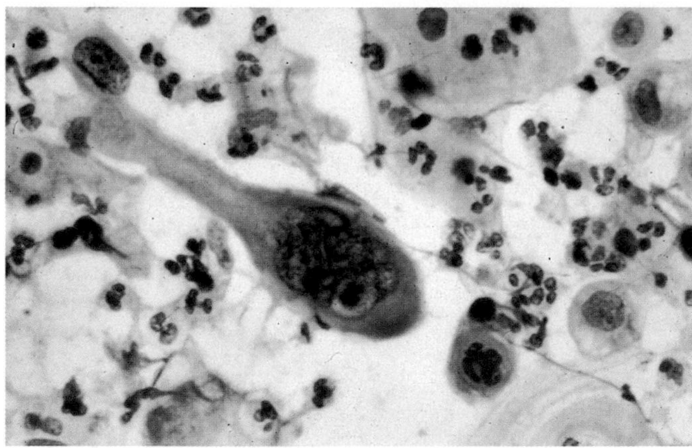

Figure 3–4 Multinucleated "tadpole" cell-early invasive squamous cell carcinoma.

frequency with which invasive cervical cancer occurs in the USA is unknown, but the best incidence data indicate a rate of approximately 8–10/100,000/yr (Fig. 3–5). The incidence and mortality rates in the US have been slowly declining (Fig 3–6). The occurrence of cervical cancer is apparently less frequent in Norway and Sweden than in the USA. However, in the underdeveloped areas of the world, the frequency of cervical cancer is more noteworthy, relative to the overall cancer problem, especially when compared with the USA (Table 3–3) and Western Europe. In many South American and Asian countries, cervical cancer accounts for the largest percentage of cancer deaths in women. One wonders whether nutritional deficiencies in these underdeveloped nations play a role in the etiology of cervical cancer. Orr reported that abnormal vitamin levels were more commonly present in patients with cervical cancer. When compared with control values, levels of

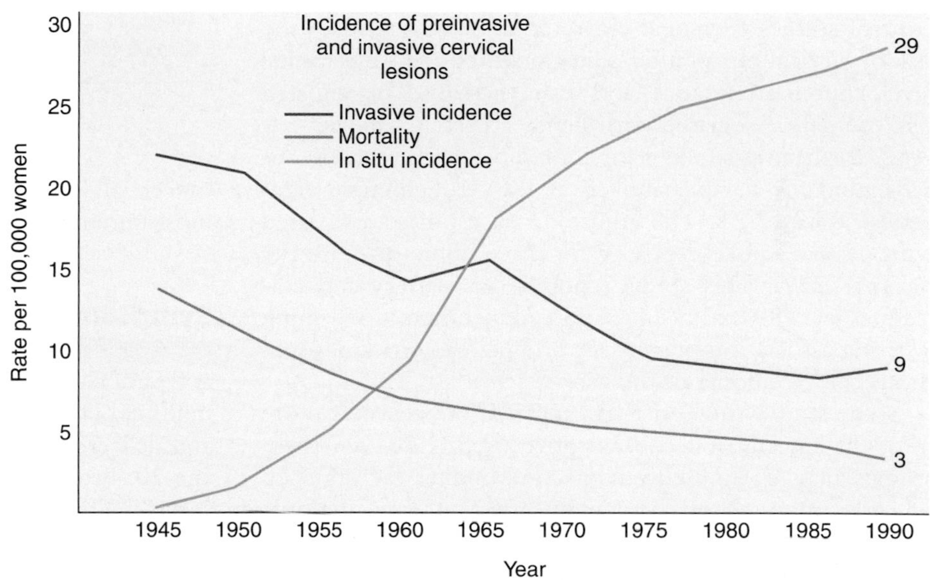

Figure 3–5 American Cancer Society data for 1991. Cervical cancer incidence and mortality.

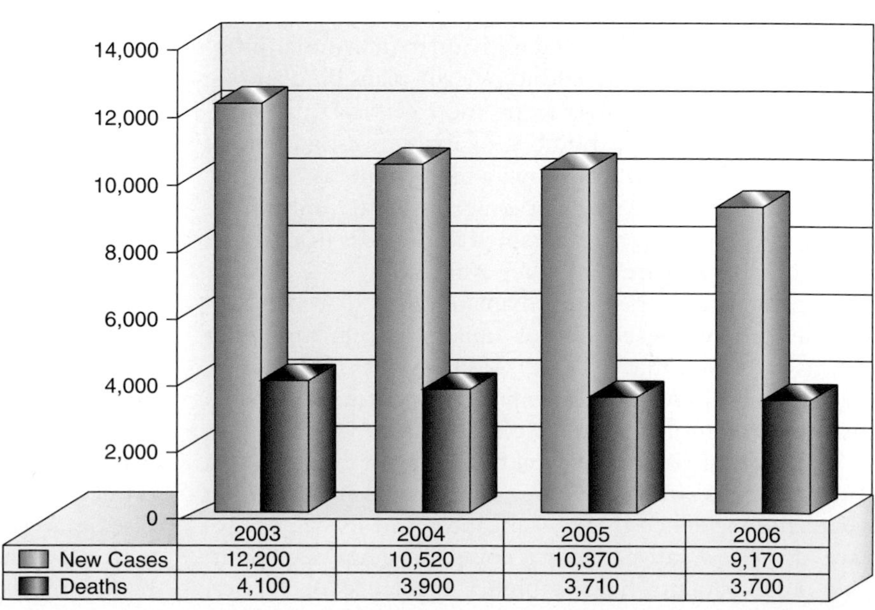

	2003	2004	2005	2006
New Cases	12,200	10,520	10,370	9,170
Deaths	4,100	3,900	3,710	3,700

Figure 3–6 Cervical Cancer in the USA: The Last Three Years. (From: Jermal et al: Cancer statistics, 2006. CA Cancer J Clin 2006;56:106–130.)

Table 3–3 AMERICAN CANCER SOCIETY ESTIMATED INCIDENCE AND DEATHS, FEMALES, 2006, USA

Type of cancer	No. of cases	No. of deaths
Breast	212,920	40,970
Colon	57,460	27,300
Corpus	41,200	7,350
Ovary	20,180	15,310
Cervix	9,710	3,700
Lung	81,770	72,130
Melanoma	27,930	2,890

From: American Cancer Society: Cancer Statistics, 2006: CA Cancer J Clin; 56:106-30.

plasma folate, beta-carotene, and vitamin C were significantly lower in patients with cervical cancer. Personal cigarette smoking and exposure to passive smoke as risk factors for cervical carcinoma have been examined in case-control studies. Personal cigarette smoking increases the risk of cervical cancer after adjustment for age, educational level, church attendance, and sexual activity. The adjusted risk estimate associated with being a current smoker was 3.42; for having smoked for 5 or more pack-years, it was 2.81; and for having smoked at least 100 lifetime cigarettes, it was 2.21. The adjusted risk estimate associated with passive smoke exposure for three hours or more per day was 2.96. This study, reported by Slattery and colleagues in 1989, has been reinforced by others, confirming a strong association of smoking and increased risk of squamous cell carcinoma of the cervix.

Some studies suggest that cancer of the cervix is more frequent among oral contraceptive users; however, these studies may be influenced by confounding factors such as early onset of sexual activity after puberty, multiple sexual partners, and previous history of sexually transmitted diseases. Ursin and colleagues reported a twofold greater risk of adenocarcinoma of the cervix, especially among those who used oral contraceptives for 12 years or more.

Because of the cervix's sensitivity to hormonal influences, it may be considered biologically plausible that oral contraceptives could induce or promote cervical carcinoma. Piver reviewed a large number of early investigations of this issue and failed to show a consistent association. Moreover, these data are based on exposure to oral contraceptive preparations that contained high doses of estrogen and progestin and are no longer available.

In most large series, approximately 85–90% of malignant lesions of the cervix are squamous cell, but other lesions are possible (Table 3–4). Most information regarding etiology and epidemiology is pertinent only to the more common squamous cell lesions.

The greatest risk for cervical cancer is not ever having a Pap test or its infrequent use. Everywhere in the world where the incidence of cervical cancer and its death rates have decreased, an active screening program is present. The older patients have a higher incidence of cervical cancer, at least in the USA, and these women have the most infrequent Pap smear screening.

Table 3–4 MALIGNANT TUMORS OF THE CERVIX

Tumors of Epithelium
Large cell nonkeratinizing
Large cell keratinizing
Small cell
Verrucous carcinoma
Common pattern
Adenoma malignum (minimal deviation adenocarcinoma)
Mucinous
Papillary
Endometrioid
Clear cell
Adenoid cystic
Stem cell carcinoma (glassy cell carcinoma)

Tumors of Mesenchymal Tissue
Leimyosarcoma
Embryonal rhabdomyosarcoma (of infants)

Tumor of the Gartner duct (true mesonephroma)

Others
Carcinoid

Symptoms

A typical patient with clinically obvious cervical cancer is a multiparous woman between 45 and 55 years who married and delivered her first child at an early age, usually before age 20. Probably the first symptom of early cancer of the cervix is a thin, watery, blood-tinged vaginal discharge that frequently goes unrecognized by the patient. The classic symptom is intermittent, painless metrorrhagia or spotting only postcoitally or after douching, although not the most common symptom. As the malignancy enlarges, the bleeding episodes become heavier and more frequent, and they last longer. The patient may also describe what seems to her to be an increase in the amount and duration of her regular menstrual flow; ultimately, the bleeding becomes continuous. In the postmenopausal woman, the bleeding is more likely to prompt early medical attention.

Late symptoms or indicators of more advanced disease include the development of pain referred to the flank, or leg, which is usually secondary to the involvement of the ureters, pelvic wall, or sciatic nerve routes. Many patients complain of dysuria, hematuria, rectal bleeding, or obstipation resulting from bladder or rectal invasion. Distant metastasis and persistent edema of one or both lower extremities as a result of lymphatic and venous blockage by extensive pelvic wall disease are late manifestations of primary disease and frequent manifestations of recurrent disease. Massive hemorrhage and development of uremia with profound inanition may also occur and occasionally be the initial presenting symptom.

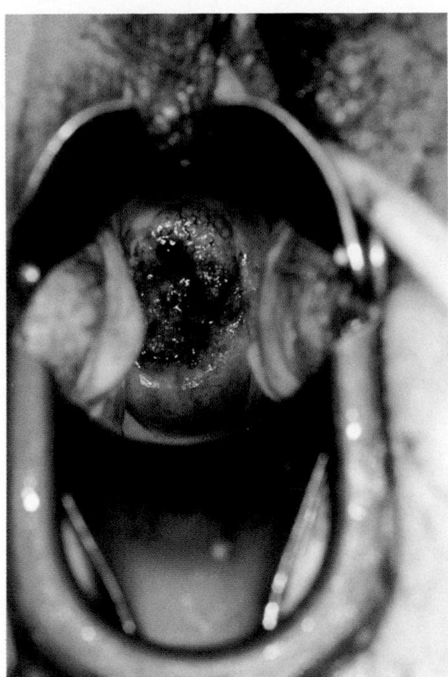

Figure 3–7 Ulcerative squamous cell carcinoma of the cervix.

Gross appearance

The gross clinical appearance of carcinoma of the cervix varies considerably and depends on the regional mode of involvement and the nature of the particular lesion's growth pattern. Three categories of gross lesions have traditionally been described. The most common is the exophytic lesion, which usually arises on the ectocervix and often grows to form a large, friable, polypoid mass that can bleed profusely. These exophytic lesions sometimes arise within the endocervical canal and distend the cervix and the endocervical canal, creating the so-called barrel-shaped lesion. A second type of cervical carcinoma is created by an infiltrating tumor that tends to show little visible ulceration or exophytic mass but is initially seen as a stone-hard cervix that regresses slowly with radiation therapy. A third category of lesion is the ulcerative tumor (Fig. 3–7) which usually erodes a portion of the cervix, often replacing the cervix and a portion of the upper vaginal vault with a large crater associated with local infection and seropurulent discharge.

Routes of spread

The main routes of spread of carcinoma of the cervix are:

1. into the vaginal mucosa, extending microscopically down beyond visible or palpable disease;
2. into the myometrium of the lower uterine segment and corpus, particularly with lesions originating in the endocervix;
3. into the paracervical lymphatics and from there to the most commonly involved lymph nodes (i.e., the obturator, hypogastric, and external iliac nodes); and
4. direct extension into adjacent structures or parametria, which may reach to the obturator fascia and the wall of the true pelvis. Extension of the disease to involve the bladder or rectum can result with or without the occurrence of a vesicovaginal or rectovaginal fistula.

The prevalence of lymph node disease correlated well with the stage of the malignancy in several anatomic studies. Lymph node involvement in stage I is between 15% and 20% and in stage II between 25% and 40%; in stage III, it is assumed that at least 50% have positive nodes. Variations are sometimes seen with different material. The best study of lymph node involvement in cervical cancer was done by Henriksen (Fig. 3–8). The nodal groups described by Henriksen follow:

Primary group

1. The parametrial nodes, which are the small lymph nodes traversing the parametria
2. The paracervical or ureteral nodes, located above the uterine artery where it crosses the ureter
3. The obturator or hypogastric nodes surrounding the obturator vessels and nerves
4. The hypogastric nodes, which course along the hypogastric vein near its junction with the external iliac vein
5. The external iliac nodes, which are a group of from six to eight nodes that tend to be uniformly larger than the nodes of the other iliac groups
6. The sacral nodes, which were originally included in the secondary group

Secondary group

1. The common iliac nodes
2. The inguinal nodes, which consist of the deep and superficial femoral lymph nodes
3. The periaortic nodes

In his autopsy studies, Henriksen plotted the percentage of nodal involvement for treated and untreated patients (Figs. 3–9 and 3–10). Distribution is, as one would expect, with a greater number of involved nodes found in the region of the cervix than in distant metastases. Although the series was an autopsy study, Henriksen found that only 27% had metastasis above the aortic chain. Cervical cancer kills by local extension with ureteral obstruction in a high percentage of patients.

In 1980, the GOG reported the results of a series of 545 patients with cancer of the cervix who were surgically staged within their institutions. This study was prompted because traditional ports of radiation therapy were destined to treatment failure when the disease extended to the periaortic nodes (Fig. 3–11). They found periaortic node involvement in 18.2% of patients with stage IIa disease and up to 33.3% in patients with stage IVa disease. Piver correlated the size of the cervical lesion with the incidence of lymph node metastasis in stage I disease (Table 3–5).

When clinical staging was compared with surgical staging, inaccuracies were found of the magnitude of a 22.9%

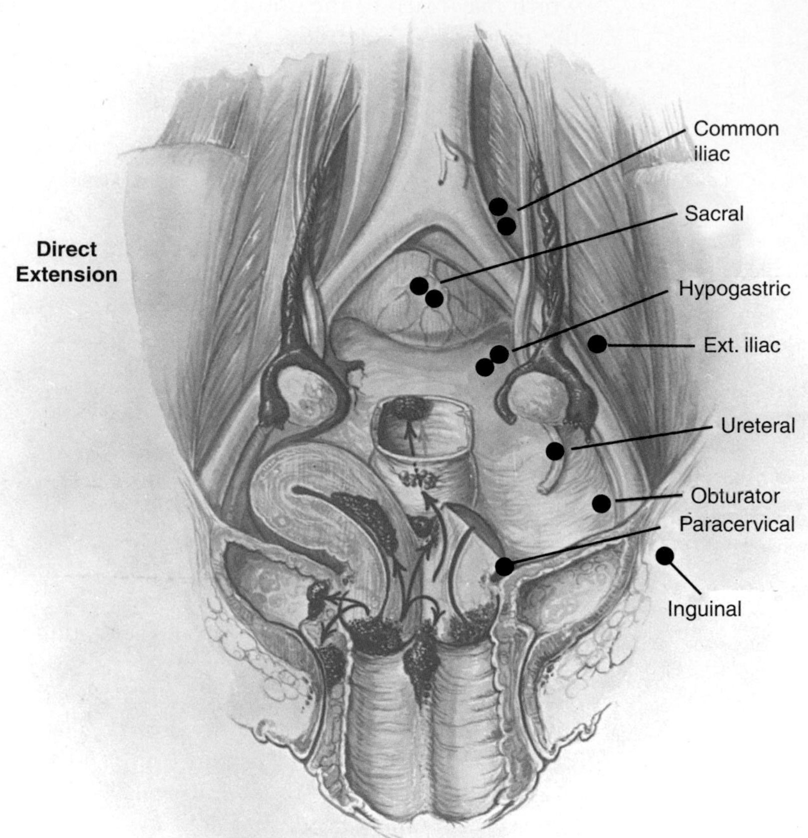

Figure 3–8 Lymph node chains draining the cervix. (From: Henriksen E: Lymphatic spread of cervix and corpus carcinoma. Am J Obstet Gynecol 58:924, 1949.)

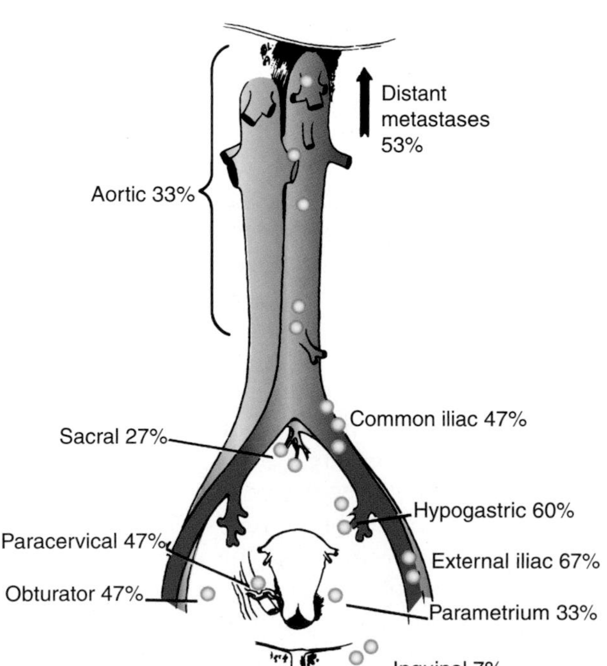

Figure 3–9 Percentage involvement of draining lymph nodes in treated patients with cervical cancer. (From: Henriksen E: Lymphatic spread of cervix and corpus carcinoma. Am J Obstet Gynecol 58:924, 1949.)

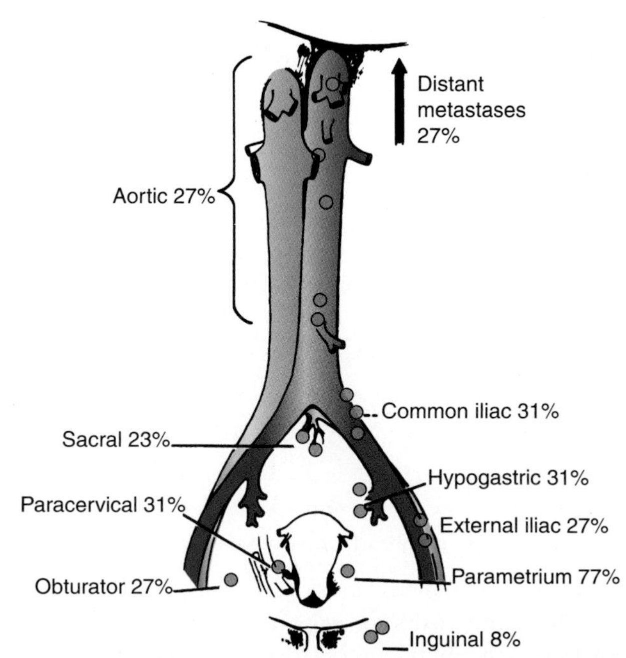

Figure 3–10 Percentage involvement of draining lymph nodes in untreated patients with cervical cancer. (From Henriksen E: Lymphatic spread of cervix and corpus carcinoma. Am J Obstet Gynecol 58:924, 1949.)

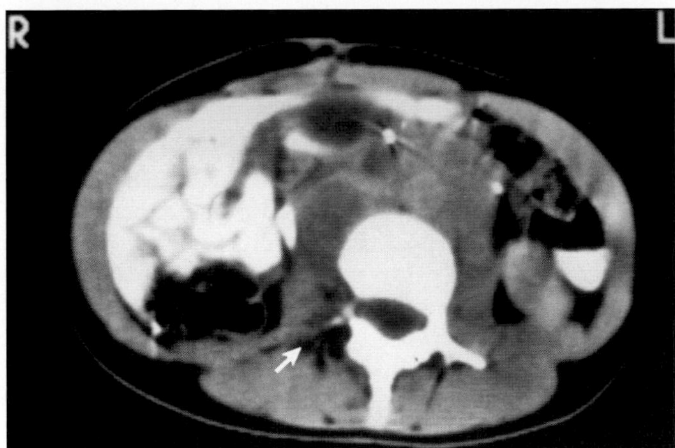

Figure 3–11 A computed tomography scan of the abdomen illustrating very enlarged peri-aortic nodes that have eroded a portion of the vertebral bone on the right.

misstaged occurrence in stage IIb disease and a 64.4% misstaged occurrence in stage IIIb disease. These data raise the question of whether knowing that disease has spread to the periaortic area enables the clinician to institute therapeutic modalities that can result in increased salvage. In other words, does the treatment of patients with spread of disease beyond the pelvis result in more cures? Berman and colleagues, reporting the GOG experience with staging laparotomy, indicated that 20% of 436 patients (stages IIb–IVa) were found to have metastatic disease to periaortic nodes. He also reported that 25% of these patients, or 5% of those surgically staged, demonstrated a 3-year, disease-free survival. Most of the patients with known periaortic node involvement received extended postoperative field irradiation.

Cumulative results from many studies utilizing lymphadenectomy in the surgical staging of cervix cancer has resulted in frequency of positive pelvic nodes as shown in Table 3–6.

Table 3–5 SIZE OF CERVICAL LESION AND LYMPH NODE METASTASIS IN STAGE IB CERVICAL CANCER

Site (cm)	No. of Patients	No. with Metastasis	(%)	
≤ 1	22	4	18.1	21.1
2–3	72	16	22.1	
4–5	45	16	35.5	35.2
≥ 6	6	3	50	
Total	145	39	26.9	

Table 3–6 PERCENTAGE INCREASE OF PELVIC AND PERIAORTIC NODE METASTASIS BY CLINICAL STAGE

Clinical Stage	Positive Pelvic Nodes	Positive Periaortic Nodes
I	15.4	6.3
II	28.6	16.5
III	47.0	8.6

GLANDULAR TUMORS OF THE CERVIX

Approximately 75–80% of cervical cancers are squamous cell, and most of the remaining 20–25% are adenocarcinomas. There appears to be an increase in the frequency of cervical adenocarcinomas, but this may be a result of the decrease in the incidence of invasive squamous cell lesions. Adenocarcinoma arises from the endocervical mucous-producing gland cells; and because of its origin within the cervix, it may be present for a considerable time before it becomes clinically evident. These lesions are characteristically bulky neoplasms that expand the cervical canal and create the so-called barrel-shaped lesions of the cervix. The spread pattern of these lesions is similar to that of squamous cell cancer, with direct extension accompanied by metastases to regional pelvic nodes as the primary routes of dissemination. Local recurrence is more common in these lesions, and this has resulted in the commonly held belief that they are more radioresistant than are their squamous counterpart. It seems more likely, however, that the bulky, expansive nature of these endocervical lesions, rather than a differential in radiosensitivity, accounts for the local recurrence.

Although debated as an entity, the term microinvasive adenocarcinoma of the cervix is appearing more frequently in the literature. Authors are reporting their experience using the 1994 FIGO definition of stage Ia cervical cancer. Kaku and associates reported 30 patients who had <5 mm invasion (21 with <3 mm), but 15 had horizontal spread >7 mm. None of the patients with <3 mm stromal invasion recurred. Östör and colleagues, in the largest and most extensive review, identified 77 women with <5 mm invasion. None of the 48 who had pelvic node dissection or the 23 in whom one or both adnexa were removed had metastasis. Twenty patients did have >7 mm horizontal spread, and LSI was present in only seven; four, however, had <3 mm invasion. None of the 24 hysterectomy specimens showed residual disease if conization margins were free. There were two recurrences, but both were in women with >7 mm horizontal spread. Schorge and associates reported 21 patients with stage Ia1 adenocarcinoma of the cervix. None of the patients had LSI. No lymph node metastasis was noted in 16 patients, and none of the 21 patients experienced a recurrence.

Two debatable issues continue with regard to adenocarcinoma of the cervix. Does this cell type carry a worse prognosis than squamous or adenosquamous cell types? For early stage disease, which therapy (radical surgery or radiation) is superior or is there a place for combined treatment? Most studies suggest no difference in survival when adenocarcinomas are compared to squamous carcinomas after correction for stage. The 1998 FIGO Annual Report, which reported >10,000 squamous carcinomas and 1138 adenocarcinomas using multivariant analysis, noted no difference in survival in stage I cancers. In a study by Chen and associates of 302 adenocarcinomas, it was noted that in early stages, multivariant analysis noted better survival in patients treated with radical surgery compared with those treated with radiation therapy.

Kjorstad and Bond investigated the metastatic potential and patterns of dissemination in 150 patients with stage Ib adenocarcinoma of the cervix treated from 1956–1977. All cases were treated with a combination of intracavitary radium followed by radical hysterectomy with pelvic lymph node dissection. The incidence of pelvic metastases and distant recurrences and the survival rates were the same as those given in previously published reports for squamous cell carcinoma treated in the same manner. In one respect, the adenocarcinomas showed a significant difference from the squamous cell cancers. The incidence of residual tumor in the hysterectomy specimens after intracavitary treatment was much higher (30% vs 11%). Kjorstad and Bond considered that this was a strong argument for surgical treatment of patients with early stages of adenocarcinoma of the cervix.

Berek and colleagues reported on 100 patients with primary adenocarcinoma of the uterine cervix. Of 48 stage I patients, 13 were treated with radical surgery, 16 with radiation alone, and 19 with combination therapy. Analysis of stage I patients by Berek and colleagues showed no significant difference in survival compared with those treated with radical surgery or combination therapy. However, both of these groups had >5-year survival ($P > 0.05$) than those treated with radiation alone. A higher tumor grade was associated with poorer survival for each stage regardless of treatment. More complications were associated with radiation therapy than with radical therapy. Radiation therapy alone did not appear to be sufficient therapy for patients with stage I or stage II disease.

Moberg and colleagues reported on 251 patients at Radiumhemmet in Stockholm with adenocarcinoma of the uterine cervix. The 5-year survival rate was compared with that in the total of cervical epithelial malignancies, and the rate was lower in the adenocarcinoma cases, with respective crude 5-year survival rates of 84%, 50%, and 9% in stages I, II, and III. Combined treatment consisting of two intracavitary radium treatments with an interval of 3 weeks followed by a radical hysterectomy with pelvic lymphadenectomy done within 3 months gave improved 5-year survival in a non-randomized series. Prempree and colleagues also suggested combined therapy for stage II lesions or for those > 4 cm.

A large series of 367 cases of adenocarcinoma of the cervix was reported by Eifel and associates. Their conclusions were that the central control of adenocarcinomas with radiation therapy is comparable to that achieved for squamous cell carcinomas of comparable bulk. They found no evidence that combined treatment (radiation therapy plus hysterectomy) improved local regional control or survival. In their study, radiation therapy alone was as effective a treatment for most patients with stage I disease. They noted, as others have, that patients with bulky stage I (>6 cm), stage II, or stage III disease, particularly with poorly differentiated lesions or evidence of nodal spread, had a very high rate of extrapelvic disease spread.

Eifel reported the results of 160 patients with adenocarcinoma of the cervix. Of those patients, 84 were treated with radiation therapy alone; 20 were treated with external and intracavitary radiation followed by hysterectomy; and 56 were treated with radical hysterectomy. Survival was strongly correlated with tumor size and grade. There was a 90% survival rate for lesions <3 cm. After 5 years, 45% of the patients treated with radical hysterectomy had a recurrence. These recurrences were strongly correlated with lymph/vascular space invasion and poorly differentiated lesions, as well as larger tumor size.

Chen and associates from Taiwan reviewed 3678 cases of cervical cancer treated between 1977 and 1994 of which 302 (8.5%) were adenocarcinoma. A higher proportion of cases with adenocarcinoma were of the lower stages and in the younger patient even within a given stage. Survival was better in all stages in patients with squamous compared with adenocarcinoma (81% vs 76% in stage I, $P = 0.0039$). When surgery was primary therapy, there was no difference in survival in stage I (83% vs 80.3% survival of squamous and adenocarcinoma, respectively). Survival with radiation therapy noted 71% vs 49%, respectively ($P = 0.0039$), in stage I. Survival decreased as age increased within a given stage.

The MD Anderson Hospital group compared 1538 patients with squamous cell carcinoma with 229 adenocarcinoma patients, all stage Ib who were treated with radiation. In patients with ≥4 cm tumors, multivariate analysis confirmed that those patients with adenocarcinoma had a significantly poorer survival than did those with squamous carcinoma (59% vs 73%). In a study by the GOG, 813 stage Ia2 and Ib cancers were evaluated. All were treated with radical hysterectomy. There were 645 squamous, 104 adenocarcinoma, and 64 adenosquamous cancers. Radiation was given postoperatively to 16% squamous, 13% adenocarcinomas, and 20% of adenosquamous patients. After adjusting for multiple risk factors, survival was worst for adenosquamous cancer compared with squamous and adenocarcinoma (71.8%, 82.1%, 88%, respectively). A similar finding was noted in a study from Taiwan in which 134 stage Ib or II cervical adenocarcinomas or adenosquamous cancers were compared with 757 similarly staged squamous carcinomas treated with radical hysterectomy. The overall survival was 72.2% for the former compared with 81.2% for the squamous cancers. The histology was an independent prognostic factor for recurrence-free survival and overall survival.

UNCOMMON AND NEUROENDOCRINE TUMORS OF THE CERVIX

Neuroendocrine small-cell cervical cancer (Fig. 3–12) is a rare malignancy, representing less than 5% of all cases of cervical cancer. These tumors provide a therapeutic challenge for the clinician, as they are characterized by frequent and early nodal and distant metastases. The pathologist's dilemma results from the large number of pathologic entities all described as "small cell cancers", including fully differentiated small cell non-keratinizing squamous cell carcinoma, reserved-cell carcinoma, and neuroendocrine (oat cell) carcinoma. Neuroendocrine carcinomas, which can be identified by characteristic light and electron microscopic criteria, are indistinguishable from oat cell cancers of the lung. In addition, they appear to have the poorest prognosis of the various small cell cancers. Therefore, it is important to distinguish this particular subtype of cancer from the rest and to consider innovative approaches to treatment. Neuroendocrine markers are commonly used to assist in classification with up to 80% of tumors staining for synaptophysin, chromogranin and/or CD56 (neural cell adhesion molecule). At least in one series, Pap smear was abnormal in only one of seven patients.

Abeler reported on 26 cases of true neuroendocrine cervical carcinoma. The 5-year survival was 14% despite aggressive therapy including surgery, radiation, and chemotherapy. Viswanathan et al observed a 66% relapse rate, with a course frequently characterized by the development of widespread hematogenous metastases. Locoregional recurrence outside irradiated fields was also frequently observed. In the group studied, the overall survival rate at 5 years was only 29%, with none of the patients who had disease more extensive than FIGO stage Ib1 or clinical evidence of lymph node metastases surviving their disease.

In our experience in the 1980s with 14 patients in stage Ib or IIa treated by radical hysterectomy with postoperative radiation therapy, all 14 have experienced recurrence, 12 before the 31st month after therapy. Innovative approaches to treating this subset of unfortunate patients are under study. Recently Chan et al updated our series and performed a multivariate analysis of different prognostic factors among 34 patients. His group documented that only those with early lesions amenable to extirpation were curable. The role of primary or postoperative radiation with or without chemotherapy is unclear and yields uniformly poor results, particularly in patients with advanced lesions.

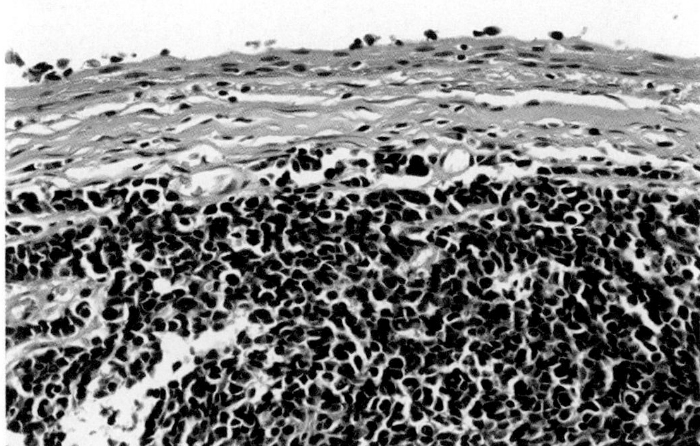

Figure 3–12 Small cell carcinoma. (Courtesy of Ibrahim Ramzy, MD, UCI, College of Medicine.)

Glassy cell carcinoma of the cervix has also been classically regarded as a poorly differentiated adenosquamous carcinoma, which is infrequently diagnosed and associated with a poor outcome regardless of the modality of therapy. Many recurrences occur in the first year after therapy, and most have occurred by 24 months. Reported survival rates are more encouraging than are those associated with neuroendocrine carcinomas; rates have been seen to be as high as 50% for stage I disease in some series. Lotocki and colleagues reported 32 cases, which accounted for 5% of all cervical carcinomas in his series. The mean age was 10 years younger than other histologic subtypes. The 5-year survival for stage Ib lesions was 45% when treated with radical hysterectomy compared with 90% for squamous cell carcinoma and 78% for adenocarcinoma.

STAGING

The staging of cancer of the cervix is a clinical appraisal, preferably confirmed with the patient under anesthesia; it cannot be changed later if findings at operation or subsequent treatment reveal further advancement of the disease.

International classification of cancer of the cervix (Fig. 3-13 A–J):

Stage 0	Carcinoma in situ, intraepithelial carcinoma
Stage I	The carcinoma is strictly confined to the cervix (extension to the corpus should be disregarded)
Stage Ia	Invasive cancer identified only microscopically; all gross lesions even with superficial invasion are stage Ib cancers. Invasion is limited to measured stromal invasion with maximum depth of 5 mm and no wider than 7 mm
Stage Ia1	Measured invasion of stroma no greater than 3 mm in depth and no wider than 7 mm
Stage Ia2	Measured invasion of stroma greater than 3 mm and no greater than 5 mm and no wider than 7 mm

The depth of invasion should not be more than 5 mm taken from the base of the epithelium, surface or glandular, from which it originates. Vascular space involvement, venous or lymphatic, should not alter the staging.

Stage Ib	Clinical lesions confined to the cervix or preclinical lesions greater than stage Ia
Stage Ib1	Clinical lesions no greater than 4 cm
Stage Ib2	Clinical lesions greater than 4 cm
Stage II	Involvement of the vagina but not the lower third, or infiltration of the parametria but not out to the sidewall
Stage IIa	Involvement of the vagina but no evidence of parametrial involvement

Stage IIb Infiltration of the parametria but not out to the sidewall

Stage III Involvement of the lower third of the vagina or extension to the pelvic sidewall; all cases with a hydronephrosis or non-functioning kidney should be included, unless they are known to be attributable to other causes

Stage IIIa Involvement of the lower third of the vagina but not out to the pelvic sidewall if the parametria are involved

Stage IIIb Extension onto the pelvic sidewall or hydronephrosis or non-functional kidney

Stage IV Extension outside the reproductive tract

Stage IVa Involvement of the mucosa of the bladder or rectum

Stage IVb Distant metastasis or disease outside the true pelvis

The clinical evaluation of patients with cervical cancer is outlined in Table 3–7. The following diagnostic aids are acceptable for determining a staging classification: physical examination, routine radiographs, colposcopy, cystoscopy, proctosigmoidoscopy, intravenous pyelogram (IVP), and barium studies of the lower colon and rectum. Other

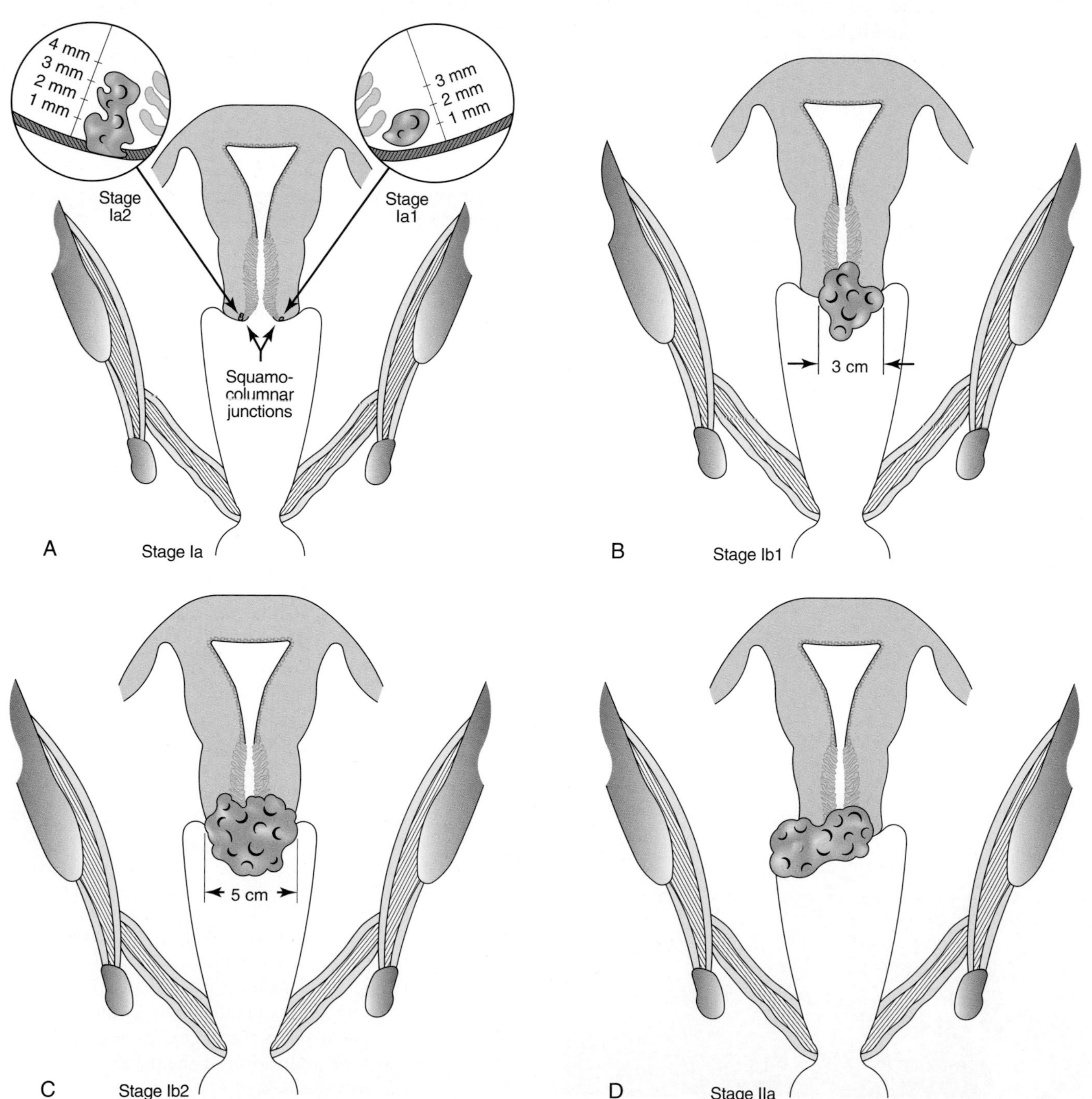

Figure 3–13 *A-J,* FIGO stagings and classification of cancer of the cervix. (From: DiSaia PJ: Staging and surgical therapy of uterine malignancies. Adv Oncol 8:15, 1992.)

Illustration continued on opposite page.

examinations, such as lymphography, computed tomography (CT) scans, magnetic resonance imaging (MRI) examinations, arteriography, venography, laparoscopy, and hysteroscopy, are not recommended for staging, because they are not uniformly available from institution to institution. It is important to emphasize that staging is a method of communicating between one institution and another. Probably more important, however, staging is a means of evaluating the treatment plans used within one institution. For these reasons, the method of staging should remain fairly constant. Staging does not define the treatment plan, and therapy can be tailored to the architecture of the malignancy in each patient.

Positron emission tomography

In 2005, the Centers for Medicare and Medicaid Services implemented coverage for 18-Fluorodeoxyglucose Positron Emission Tomography (FDG-PET) for patients with newly diagnosed and locally advanced cervical cancer undergoing pretreatment staging who have no extra-pelvic

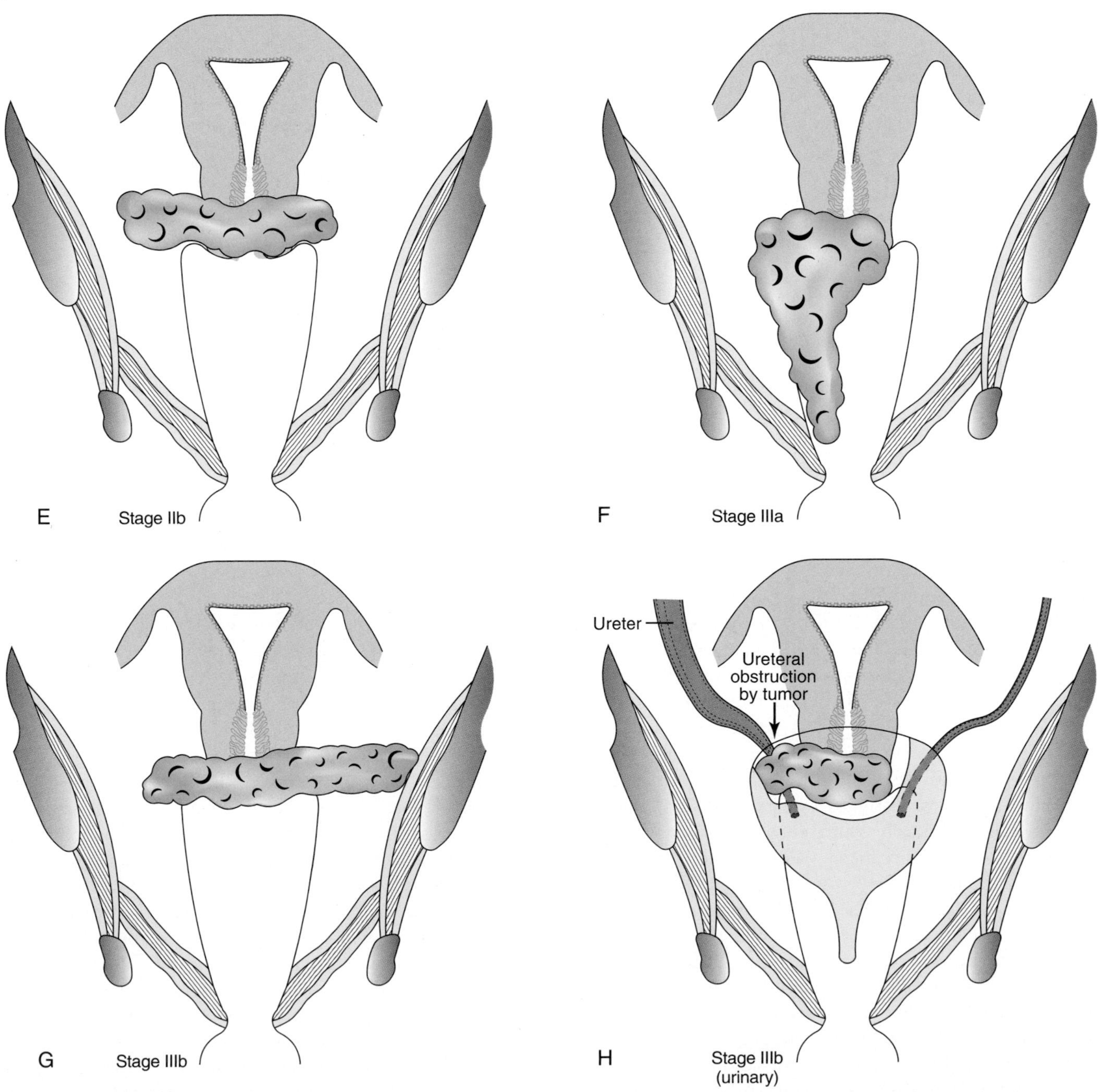

Figure 3–13, cont'd

Illustration continued on following page.

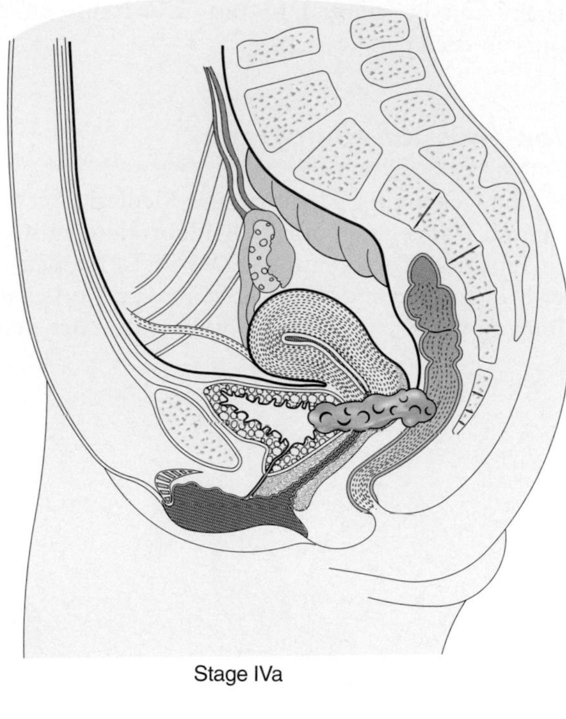

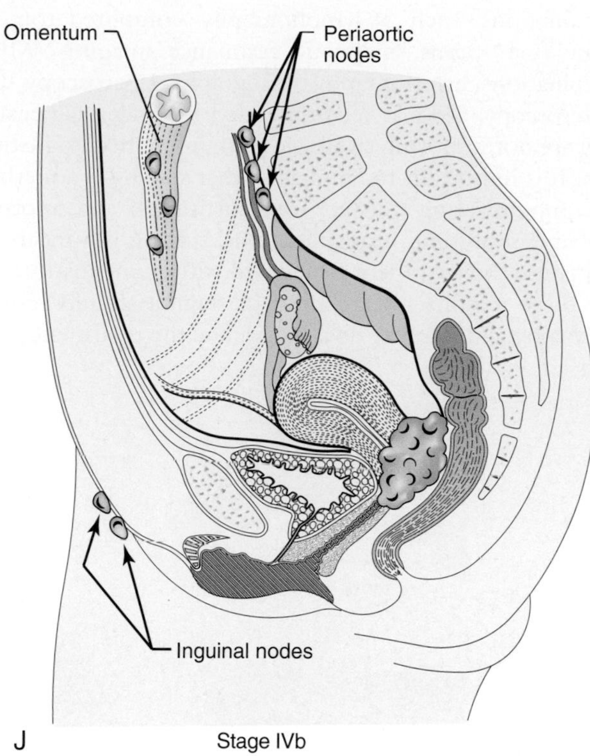

Figure 3–13, cont'd

metastases on conventional imaging studies. It should be noted that all imaging modalities are more specific than sensitive in detecting nodal metastases. The pooled sensitivity of PET in detecting pelvic nodal metastases in patients with untreated cervical cancer approaches 80% as compared with MRI (approximately 70%) or CT (approximately 48%). It is important to recognize that the available studies are limited by low numbers of patients and wide confidence intervals.

Grosu et al from Munich analyzed the results of clinical studies on the integration of PET in target volume definition for lung, head-and-neck, genitourinary, and brain tumors. FDG-PET had a significant impact on gross tumor volume and planning target volume delineation in lung cancer and was able to detect lymph node involvement and differentiate malignant tissue from atelectasis. In high-grade gliomas and meningiomas, methionine PET helped to differentiate tumor from normal tissue. Furthermore, the investigators suggest that FDG-PET seems to be particularly valuable in lymph node status definition in cervical cancer. With limited experience, several commentators have noted that FDG-PET may be superior to CT and MRI not only in the detection of lymph node metastases, but also in the detection of unknown primary cancer and in the differentiation of viable tumor tissue after treatment. The accurate delineation of gross tumor volume suggests the potential for sparing of normal tissue. The imaging of hypoxia, cell proliferation, angiogenesis, apoptosis and gene expression by new PET tracers such as choline and acetate may lead to the identification of different areas of a biologically heterogeneous tumor mass that can be individually targeted using intensity modulated radiotherapy (IMRT). In addition, a biological dose distribution can be generated permitting dose painting.

Surgical staging

Findings uncovered by fusion PET-CT or conventional MR and/or CT examinations can be used in the planning of therapy but should not influence the initial clinical staging of the lesion. Unfortunately, clinical staging is only a rough value in prognosis, because diseases of wide variability are often included under one subheading. Clinical staging is enhanced with the liberal use of rectovaginal examinations (Fig. 3–14) in that this type of pelvic examination allows more complete palpation of the parametria and cul-de-sac. The role of laparoscopic lymphadenectomy is expanding. The ability to perform pelvic and para-aortic lymphadenectomy in skilled hands allows for a more complete surgical staging of cancers of the cervix, but no conclusive data exist that indicate an advantage to this approach.

Some gynecologic oncologists believe that limited staging procedures are warranted on patients with advanced stage cervical cancer to place patients on institutional or national group protocols. The status of periaortic nodes should be known before treatment is initiated in such cases to plan appropriate modalities, such as the extent of the radiation field or concomitant chemotherapy. An extraperitoneal approach for removal of the periaortic nodes is preferred by many clinicians in an effort to reduce morbidity from the procedure. More advanced lesions have been investigated with a retroperitoneal lymphadenectomy to determine the extent of disease prior to planning radiotherapy fields (Fig. 3–15). The following figure illustrates

Table 3–7 CLINICAL EVALUATION OF PATIENTS WITH NEWLY DIAGNOSED CERVICAL CANCER

History	Review of systems	General physical examination
Risk factors (STDs, smoking, OCPs, HIV), prior abnormal Pap tests, previous dysplasia and treatment	Abnormal vaginal bleeding or discharge; pelvic pain, flank pain, sciatica, hematuria, rectal bleeding, anorexia, weight loss, bone pain	Peripheral lymphadenopathy
Evaluation	**Common procedures (FIGO)**	**Alternative procedures**
Invasive cancer	Cervical biopsy Endocervical curettage Cervical conization	Histologic diagnosis required
Tumor size; involvement of the vagina, bladder, rectum and parametria	Pelvic examination under anesthesia	MRI pelvis preferred over CT
Anemia	Complete blood count	—
Renal failure	Serum chemistries	—
Hematuria	Urinalysis	—
Bladder involvement	Cystoscopy with biopsy and urine cytology	CT, MRI pelvis
Rectal infiltration	Proctoscopy with biopsy	CT, MRI pelvis; Barium enema
Hydronephrosis	Intravenous pyelogram	Renal ultrasound; CT abdomen
Pulmonary metastases	Chest radiograph	CT chest; PET scan
Retroperitoneal lymphadenopathy	—	Lymphangiogram, CT, MRI, PET scan

STDs, sexually transmitted diseases; OCP, oral contraceptive pill; HIV, human immunodeficiency virus; MRI, magnetic resonance imaging; CT, computed tomography; PET, positron emission tomography.

one such approach (Fig. 3–16 A–J). With the increased use of PET, it is expected that the indications for surgical staging in cervical cancer will decrease.

TREATMENT

After the diagnosis of invasive cervical cancer is established, the question is how to best treat the patient. Proposed management algorithms for early stage disease, locally advanced malignancy and disseminated tumors appear in Fig. 3–17. Specific therapeutic measures are usually governed by the age and general health of the patient, by the extent of the cancer, and by the presence and nature of any complicating abnormalities. It is thus essential to carry out a complete and careful investigation of the patient (see Table 3–7) and then a joint decision regarding treatment should be made by the radiotherapist and gynecologic oncologist. The choice of treatment demands clinical

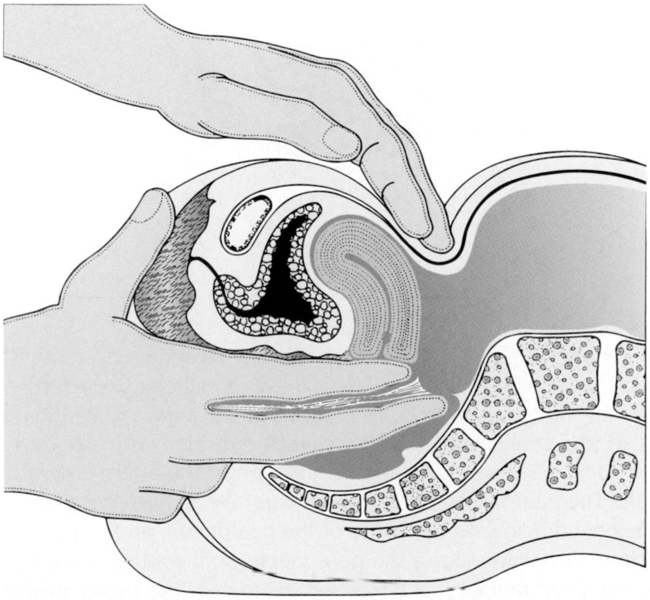

Figure 3–14 Technique of rectovaginal examination.

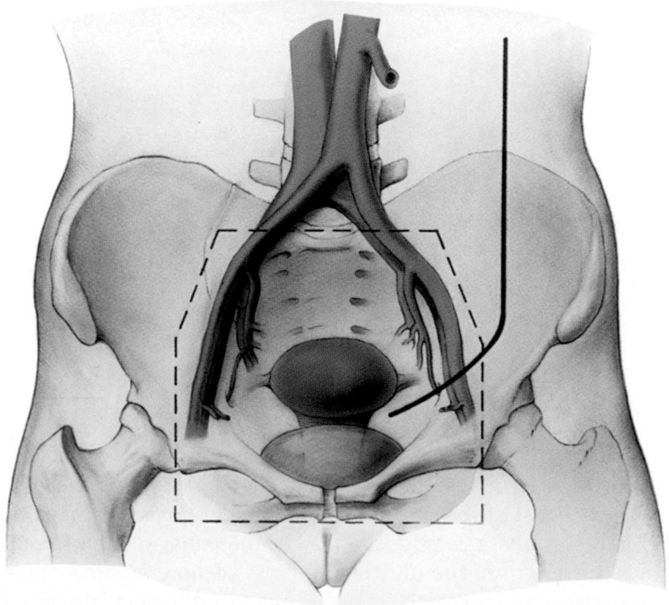

Figure 3–15 Pelvic diagram. The *dashed line* indicates the radiation field and the position of the uterus and cervix within the field. The *bold line* indicates the "J" incision path relative to the field and to the major vessels.

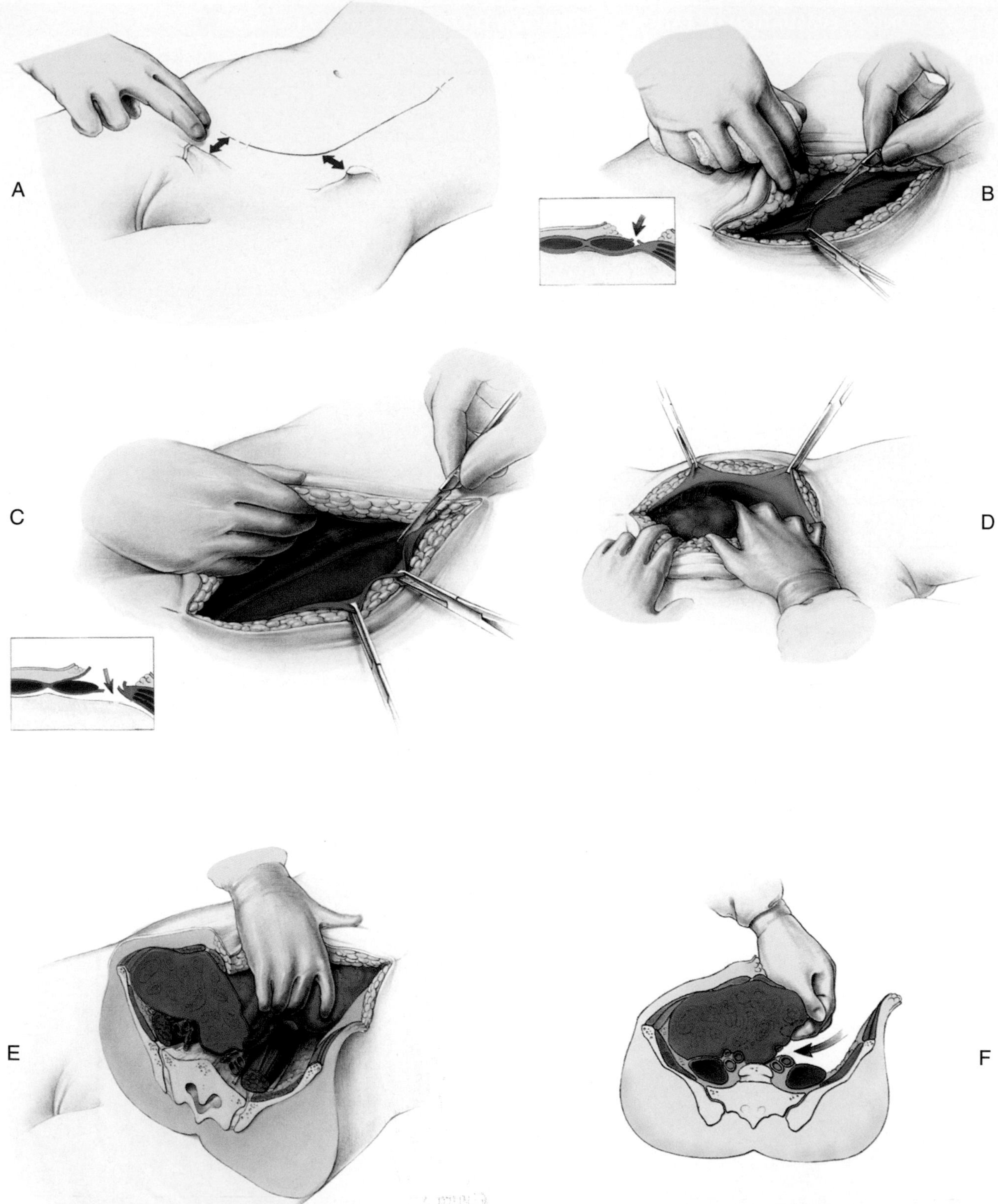

Figure 3–16 *A,* Path of incision. First measurement of 2–3 cm (two fingerwidths) above the pubic symphysis; second measurement 2–3 cm medial to the anterior superior iliac spine. A diagonal line connects these points. A *vertical line* is drawn superiorly to 3–4 cm above the level of the umbilicus. The incision begins at the lateral margin of the rectus muscle. *B,* Division of the external sheath of the rectus and a cross section. After the initial incision through the skin, the lateral margin of the sheath is divided with a bovie along the length of the muscle. On cross-section, an *arrow* points to the ideal point of separation. *C,* Division of the internal sheath of the rectus and a cross-section. The rectus muscle is mobilized medially. The internal sheath is divided carefully to preserve the underlying exposed peritoneum. *D,* Blunt dissection. Blunt dissection with a hand following the plane of the peritoneum and separating it from the transversalis fascia. *E,* Blunt dissection: perspective cross-section. Dissection along the peritoneum until contact is made with the left ureter. The ureter is preserved with the peritoneum and is mobilized medially as dissection continues. The psoas muscle and the common iliac vessels are exposed. *F,* A cross-section. Proper pathway of dissection along the peritoneum over the psoas.

Illustration continued on opposite page.

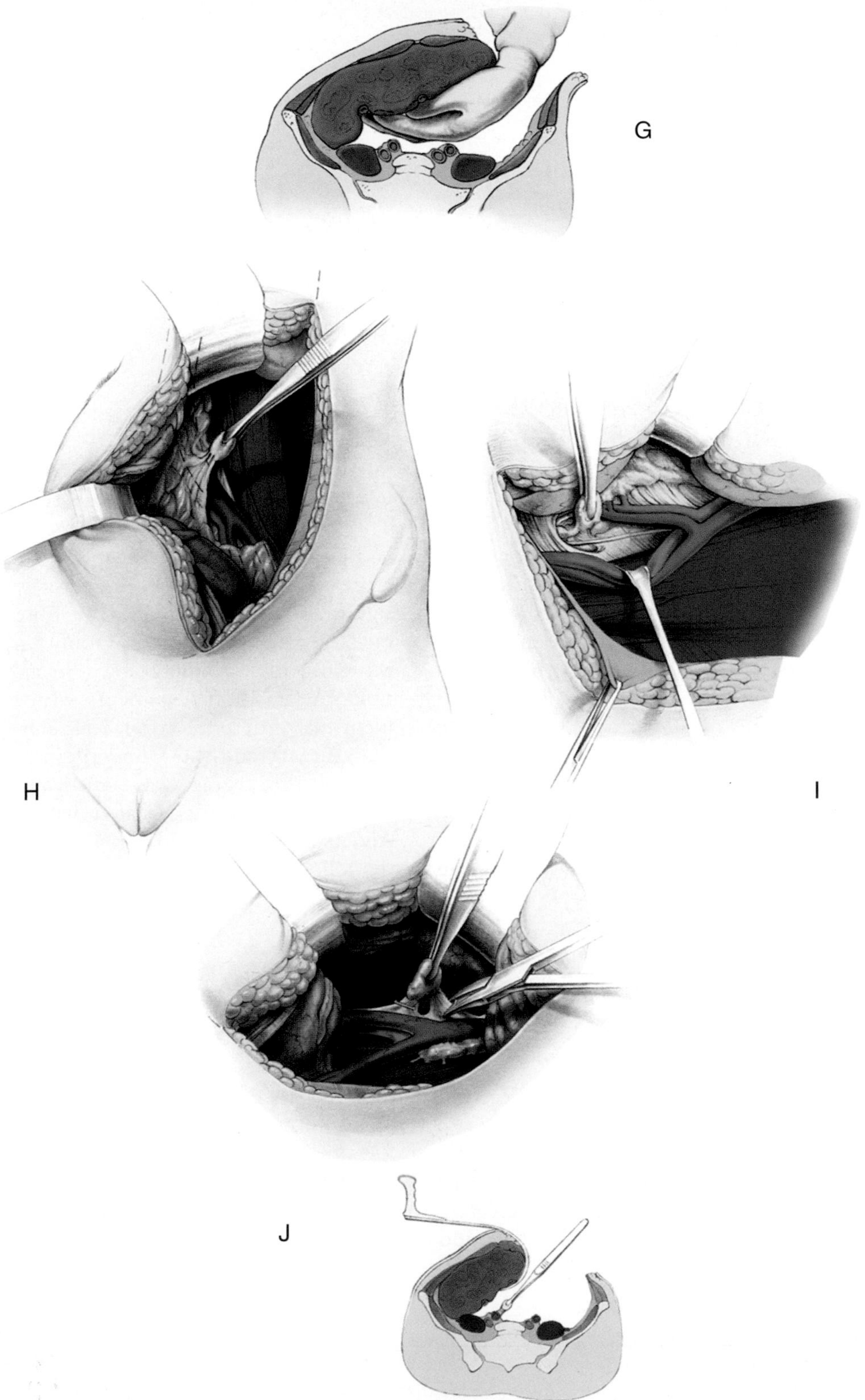

Figure 3–16, cont'd *G,* Cross-section of deep dissection. Exposure of the left and right common iliac vessels underneath the peritoneum at about the level of L5-S1. Avoid damage to the inferior mesenteric artery. *H,* Lymphadenectomy begins along the left common iliac vessels. After medial and superior retraction of the mesentery and beginning about the bifurcation of internal and external iliac vessels, lymph nodes are removed along the length of the left common iliac to the junction with the aorta. *I,* Obturator nodes. Lateral mobilization of the external iliac vessels with a vein retractor. The obturator nerve is identified, and nodes are removed. *J,* The right common iliac. The right common and para-aortic lymph nodes are clipped and removed. The diagram shows deep access to the right common iliac nodes.

Figo stage	
Ia1, 2	Cervical cone if negative surgical margins (fertility desires) or Hysterectomy, possible pelvic lymphadenectomy if nodes at risk (Ia2)
IB1, 2, IIA	Radical hysterectomy, pelvic lymphadenectomy or Chemoradiation (see table 3-14)
IIB – IVA	Chemoradiation (see table 3-14) consider GOG 219 protocol

Figure 3–17 Figure showing primary treatment of cervical cancer.

judgment, but apart from the occasional patient for whom only symptomatic treatment may be best, this choice lies between surgery and radiotherapy (almost always given with cisplatin chemotherapy). In most institutions, the initial method of treatment for locally advanced disease is chemoradiation, both intracavitary (cesium or radium) and external X-ray therapy. The controversy between surgery and radiotherapy has existed for decades and essentially surrounds the treatment of stage I and stage IIa cervical cancer (Fig. 3–17). For the most part, all stages above stage I and stage IIa are treated with combination cisplatin and radiotherapy (Fig. 3–17). The 5-year survival figures from two large series, treated with radiotherapy alone and the other with surgery, are included here. Currie reported the results of 552 radical operations for cancer of the cervix:

Preinvasive carcinoma in situ	555 cases (99.9%)
Stage I	189 cases (86.3%)
Stage IIa	103 cases (75%)
Stage IIb	78 cases (58.9%)
Other stages	41 cases (34.1%)

Some of these patients with positive nodes received postoperative radiotherapy.

In 1981 Zander and colleagues reported results of a 20-year cooperative study from Germany dealing with 1092 patients with stages Ib and II cancer of the cervix treated with radical hysterectomy of the Meigs type and bilateral pelvic lymphadenopathy. Of the 1092 patients, 50.6% had surgery only, with a 5-year survival rate of 84.5% in stage Ib and 71.1% in stage II (most were stage IIa). This correlates well with the figures reported by Currie and Falk. The rest of the patients reported by Zander received postoperative whole-pelvis irradiation therapy. No significant difference could be observed in the survival rates of patients undergoing only surgery compared with those of patients undergoing adjuvant postoperative radiation. In fact, in 199 patients with lymph node involvement, the difference in survival rates of those undergoing only surgery and those undergoing additional postoperative radiation therapy was statistically insignificant.

Of 2000 patients treated with radiotherapy at MD Anderson Hospital and Tumor Institute, Fletcher reports the following 5-year cure rates:

Stage I	91.5%
Stage IIa	83.5%
Stage IIb	66.5%
Stage IIIa	45%
Stage IIIb	36%
Stage IV	14%

Two later reports give very similar 5-year survival rates for radiotherapy alone. Perez reported 87% for stage Ib, 73% for IIa, 68% for IIb, and 44% for stage III. Montana reported 76% for IIa, 62% for IIb, and 33% for stage III.

The 1998 Annual Report of FIGO notes the following results for surgery, radiation, or combined therapy (Table 3–8).

Table 3–8 FIVE-YEAR SURVIVAL*

	Surgery only	Radiation only	Surgery + radiation
Stage Ib1	94.5% (*n* = 1125)	80.1% (*n* = 309)	83.6% (*n* = 766)
Stage Ib2	91.4% (*n* = 170)	73.7% (*n* = 225)	76.7% (*n* = 263)
Stage IIa	72.6% (*n* = 87)	64.5% (*n* = 428)	76.2% (*n* = 152)
Stage IIb	73.0% (*n* = 47)	64.2% (*n* = 1718)	64.3% (*n* = 232)

*Patients treated from 1996–1998.

Data from 2003 Annual Report of FIGO. Benedet JL, Odicino F, Maisonneuve P, et al. Carcinoma of the cervix uteri. Pecorelli S (ed). In: Int J Gynecol Obstet 2003;83(Suppl 1):41–78.

In a study from Italy, 337 patients with stage Ib–IIa were randomized to receive radiation or surgery. The median progression-free time was 87 months, and the 5-year overall PFI survival was similar between surgery and radiation (83% and 74%, respectively). Adjuvant radiotherapy was done in 62 (54%) of the surgery group with cervical diameter of (4 cm) and 46 (84%) whose diameter was > 4 cm. Survival in both 4 cm and >4 cm patients had similar survival between the two groups. As expected, severe complications were greater in the surgery and radiation group (25%) compared with radiation (18%) and surgery (10%).

In general, in early stages, comparable survival rates result from both treatment techniques. The advantage of radiotherapy is that it is applicable to almost all patients, whereas radical surgery of necessity excludes certain medically inoperable patients. The possible occurrence of immediate serious morbidity must be kept in mind when this treatment plan is selected. In many institutions, surgery for stage I and stage IIa disease is reserved for young patients in whom preservation of ovarian function is desired and improved vaginal preservation is expected. The modern operative mortality and the postoperative ureterovaginal fistula rate both have been reported to be <1%, making an objective decision for therapy even more difficult. Other reasons given for the selection of radical surgery over radiation include cervical cancer in pregnancy, concomitant inflammatory disease of the bowel, previous irradiation therapy for other disease, presence of pelvic inflammatory disease or an adnexal neoplasm along with the malignancy, as well as patient preference. Among the disadvantages of radiation therapy, one must consider the permanent injury to the tissues of the normal organ bed of the neoplasm and the possibility of second malignancies developing in this bed.

Surgical management

The use of radical hysterectomy in the USA was initiated by Joe V. Meigs at Harvard University in 1944, and shortly thereafter the radical hysterectomy with pelvic lymphadenopathy was adopted by many clinics in the USA because of dissatisfaction with the limitations of radiotherapy. Some had found that many lesions were not radiosensitive, and some patients had metastatic disease in regional lymph nodes that were alleged to be radioresistant. Radiation injuries had been reported, and one of the overriding points in favor of surgery was that gynecologists were surgeons rather than radiotherapists and thus felt more comfortable with this treatment. At the time of the popularization of this procedure, modern techniques of surgery, anesthesia, antibiotics, and electrolyte balance had emerged, reducing the enormous morbidity that once attended major operative procedures in the abdomen.

Radical hysterectomy is a procedure that must be performed by a skilled technician with sufficient experience to make the morbidity acceptable (1–5%). The procedure involves removal of the uterus, the upper 25% of the vagina, the entire uterosacral and uterovesical ligaments (Fig. 3–18), and all of the parametrium on each side, along with pelvic node dissection encompassing the four major

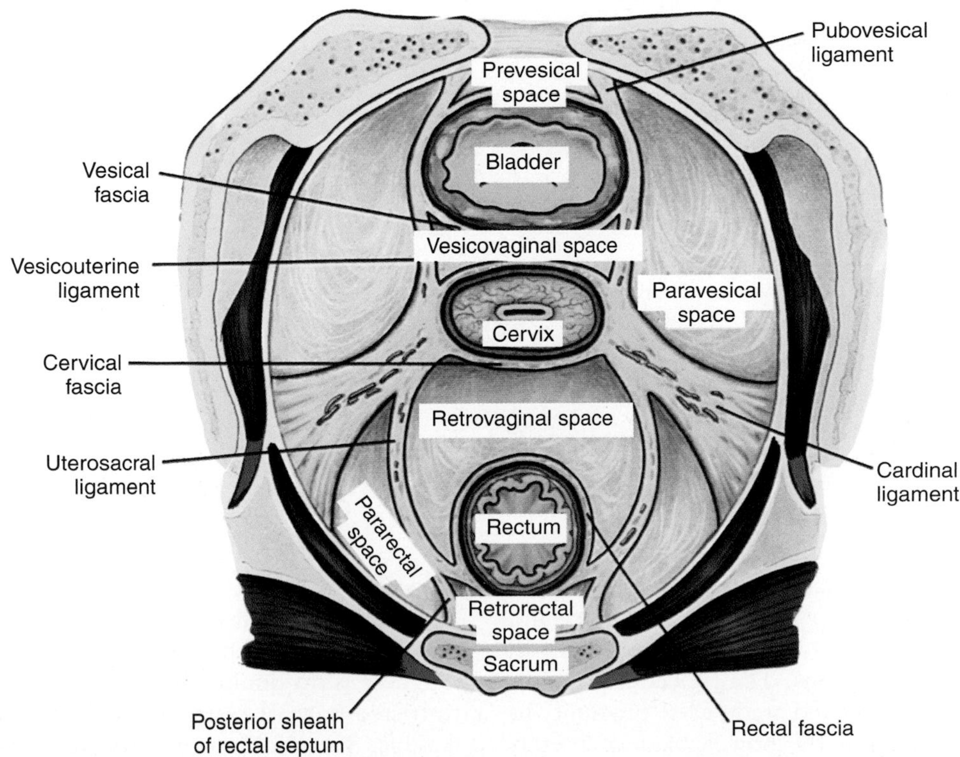

Figure 3–18 Cross-section of the pelvis at the level of the cervix.

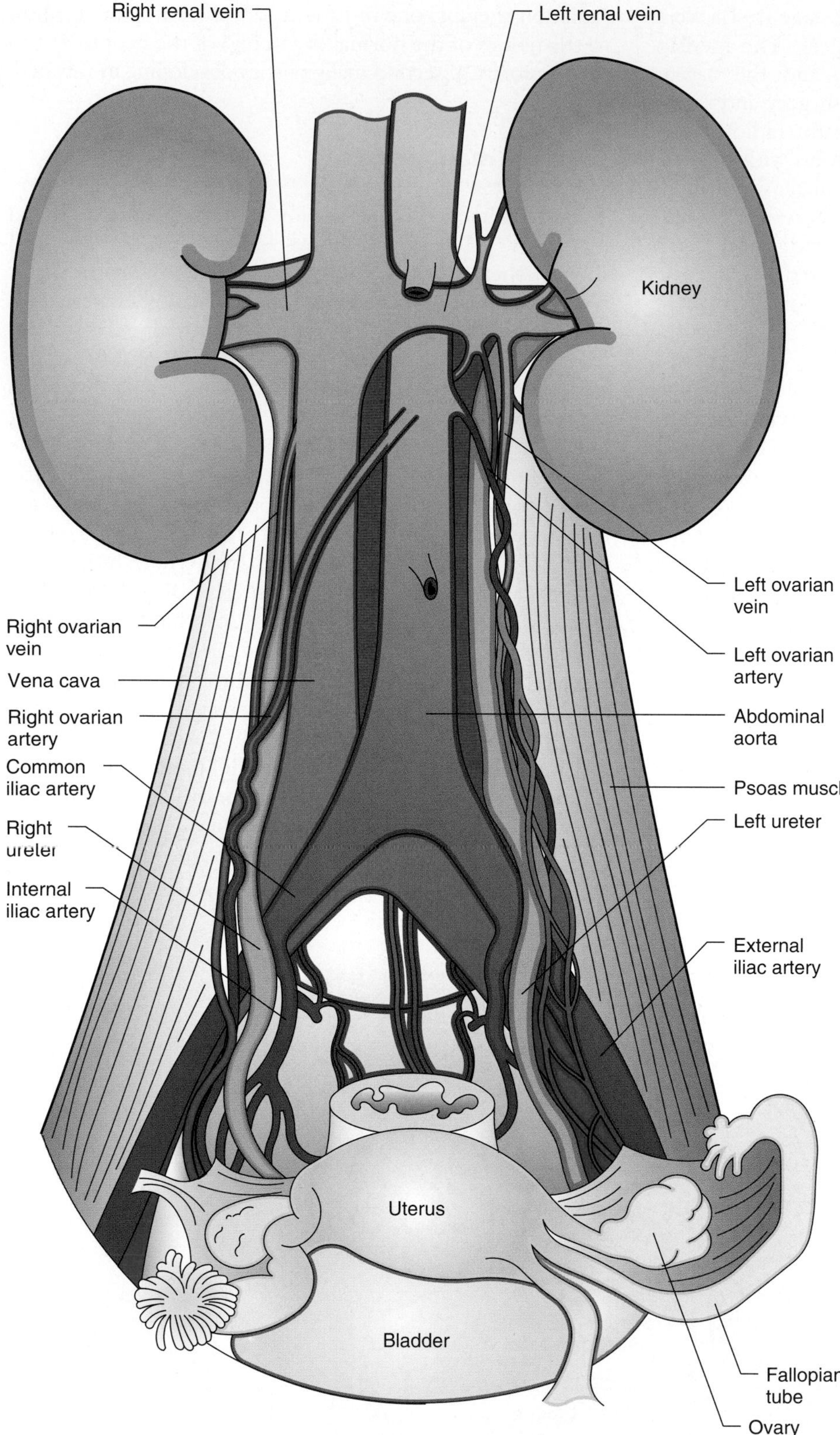

Figure 3–19 The retroperitoneal anatomy of the pelvis and lower abdomen illustrating the course of the ureters.

pelvic lymph node chains: ureteral, obturator, hypogastric, and iliac. Metastatic lesions to the ovaries are rare, and preservation of these structures is acceptable, especially in young women with small lesions. The procedure is complex, because the tissues removed are in close proximity to many vital structures such as the bowel, bladder, ureters (Figs. 3–19 and 3–20), and great vessels of the pelvis. The object of the dissection is to preserve the bladder, rectum, and ureters without injury but to remove as much of the remaining tissue of the pelvis as is feasible.

There is no doubt that in stage I, as well as the more restricted stage II cases, surgical removal of the disease is feasible. The addition of pelvic lymphadenectomy to the operative procedure caused considerable controversy in

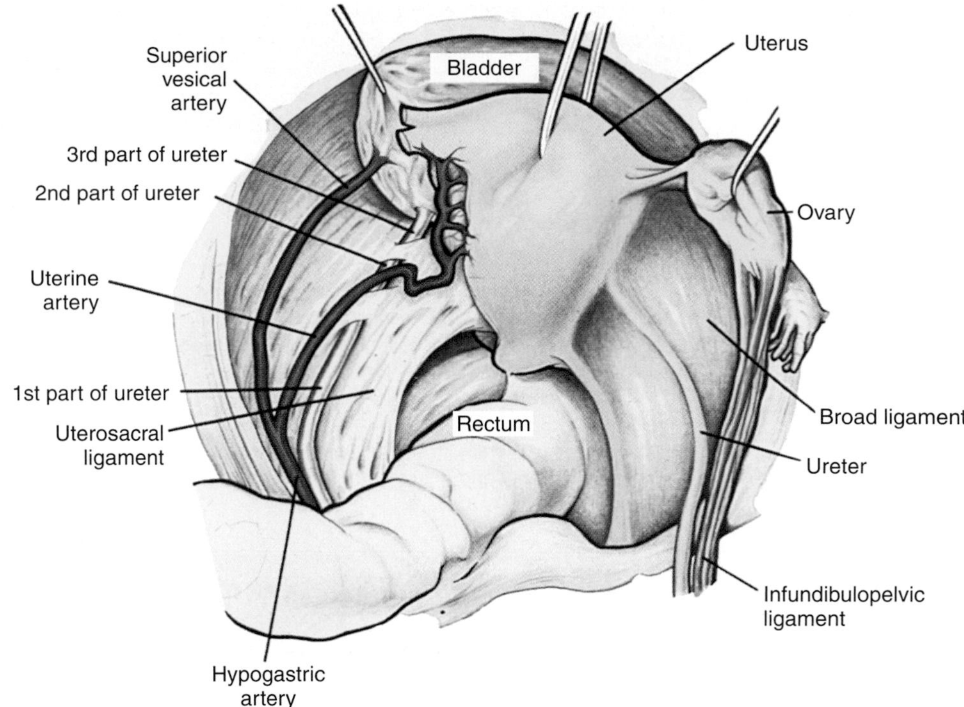

Figure 3–20 Relationship of the ureter to the uterosacral ligaments, uterine artery, infundibulopelvic ligament, and uterus.

the early part of the century. Wertheim removed nodes only if they were enlarged and then not systematically. He believed that when accessible regional nodes were involved, the inaccessible distant nodes were also involved, and removal of suspicious nodes was more for prognostic than for therapeutic value. He thought that node involvement was a measure of the lethal quality of the tumor and not merely a mechanical extension of the disease. The operative procedure popularized by Meigs included meticulous pelvic lymphadenectomy. Meigs demonstrated a 42% 5-year survival rate in another series of patients with positive nodes. Lymphadenectomy is now an established part of the operative procedure for any patient with disease greater than stage Ia1. There has been some interest in combining a radical vaginal operation with a retroperitoneal lymphadenectomy, and the results reported by Mitra, Navratil and Kastner, and McCall are surprisingly good. The survival rate in patients with negative nodes is usually in the range of 90% or more.

Tables 3–9A and 3–9B contain data sets from two randomized studies that have established the role for adjuvant therapy following radical surgery based on intermediate and high risk surgico-pathologic factors. In a GOG study (protocol 92) of 277 patients with intermediate risk factors, stage Ib cancers were randomized to radical hysterectomy with or without postoperative irradiation. Of these patients, 137 randomized to radiation therapy and 140 were not given further treatment. Based on a previous GOG study, intermediate risk was defined as greater than one third of stromal invasion, LSI, and large clinical tumor diameter. All patients had negative lymph nodes. Four combinations of the risk factors were developed. Tumor size varied from any to >4 cm. Although the two arms were equal with regard to the four combinations, in which group(s) the recurrences occurred is not stated. Using a 1-tail test, there is a greater recurrence-free survival for the combined group (84.6% compared with 72.1%). Overall survival was not significant, 11% died of cancer compared with 18% of the radical hysterectomy only group. There was a 10% non-compliance in the radiation group. These authors are able to apply this information to clinical practice because >90% of patients would be treated without benefit with regard to survival. Data were presented with an intent to treat evaluation (see Table 3–9).

Patients with positive pelvic nodes usually receive postoperative whole-pelvis irradiation and chemotherapy (Table 3–9). Peters et al randomized 268 patients with FIGO stage Ia2, Ib, and IIa carcinoma of the cervix, initially treated with radical hysterectomy and pelvic lymphadenectomy and found to have positive pelvic lymph nodes and/or positive margins and or microscopic involvement of the parametrium, to receive either pelvic radiation therapy alone or concurrent chemoirradiation. Among the 243 patients who were accessible, progression-free and overall survival were significantly improved in the patients receiving chemotherapy. The projected progression-free survival at 4 years was 63% with pelvic radiation therapy alone and 80% with concurrent chemoirradiation (hazard ratio 2.01, $P = 0.003$). The projected overall survival rate at 4 years was 71% with pelvic radiation therapy alone and 81% with concurrent chemoirradiation (hazard ratio 1.96, $P = 0.007$). The combined therapy arm had more frequent grade 3 and 4 hematologic and gastrointestinal toxicity. This landmark intergroup study of the GOG (protocol 109), the Southwest Oncology Group (protocol 8797), and the Radiation Therapy Oncology Group (protocol 91–12) was one of five randomized trials to be published between 1999 and 2000 attesting to the value of radiosensitizing chemotherapy

Table 3–9 WHEN TO USE ADJUVANT THERAPY AFTER RADICAL HYSTERECTOMY
Table 3–9A RANDOMIZED TRIAL OF ADJUVANT PELVIC RADIOTHERAPY FOR FIGO STAGE IB

GOG 92*	N	Recurrence	RR**
Adjuvant pelvic RT	137	n = 21 (15%)	0.53, P = 0.008
No further therapy	140	n = 39 (28%)	

* All patients underwent radical hysterectomy and lymphadenectomy, followed by randomization based on intermediate surgico-pathologic risk factors (i.e., depth of stromal invasion, tumor size, presence of angiolymphatic space involvement).
**Reduction in the relative risk of recurrence.
RT, radiation therapy
From Sedlis A, Bundy BN, Rotman MZ et al: A randomized trial of pelvic radiation therapy versus no further therapy in selected patients with stage IB carcinoma of the cervix after radical hysterectomy and pelvic lymphadenectomy. Gynecol Oncol 73:177, 1999.

Table 3–9 WHEN TO USE ADJUVANT THERAPY AFTER RADICAL HYSTERECTOMY
Table 3–9B RANDOMIZED TRIAL OF SYNCHRONOUS ADJUVANT RADIATION THERAPY AND CHEMOTHERAPY FOR FIGO STAGE IA2–IIA

GOG 109/SWOG 8797/RTOG 91–12*	No.	Projected PFS		Projected OS	
Adjuvant pelvic RT + CT	127	80%	HR 2.01, P = 0.003	81%	HR 1.96, P = 0.007
Adjuvant pelvic RT alone	116	63%		71%	

*All patients underwent radical hysterectomy and lymphadenectomy, followed by randomization based on high surgico-pathologic risk factors (i.e., metastatic tumor to the lymph nodes, parametria and/or vaginal margin).
From Peters WA 3rd, Liu PY, Barrett RJ 2nd et al: Concurrent chemotherapy and pelvic radiation therapy compared with pelvic radiation therapy alone as adjuvant therapy after radical surgery in high-risk early-stage cancer of the cervix. J Clin Oncol 18:1606–1613, 2000.

in the management of cervical cancer (discussed further below).

Prognostic factors have been evaluated by several authors in patients with early stage disease who have been treated surgically. In a study by Francke and associates, 105 patients with stage Ib were treated with radical hysterectomy and had negative lymph nodes. Only LSI showed significant correlation with local failure. There were 32 patients with squamous carcinoma and positive LSI, 17 received postoperative radiation with 0 of 17 recurrences, and 4 of 15 (27%) treated with surgery only developed recurrence. The overall survival at 5 years was 96% in those treated with radiation and 93.3% in those with LSI not treated with radiation. Stackler and colleagues evaluated 194 patients with stage Ib and IIa who were treated with radical hysterectomy and had negative nodes. Nuclear grade 2 or 3 (P = 0.02) and small cell squamous histology (P = 0.001) were each associated with a 4-fold increase in risk of recurrence, whereas LSI (P = 0.02), age younger than 36 years (P = 0.03), and either tumor size >28 mm (P = 0.03) or surgical clearance <5 mm (P = 0.02) were associated with a 2.5-fold increase in risk of recurrence. Survival data were not given. Delgado, in reporting a GOG study of 645 women with stage Ib squamous carcinoma, including 100 patients with positive nodes, found depth of invasion, tumor size, and LSI to be important risk factors for recurrence in multivariate analysis. The group from Boston evaluated 171 patients with lymph node-negative stage Ib and IIa cervical cancer treated primarily with surgery. One hundred and sixteen (68%) were treated with surgery only and 55 (32%) received radiation. Overall, 28 patients (16%) developed recurrent disease with no difference in the two treatment groups. After correction for other factors, patients with LSI who received radiation were less likely to develop recurrence than similar patients treated with surgery only (P = 0.04); however, overall survival was similar in the two groups. In a study from Gateshead, United Kingdom, 527 patients with stage Ib–IIb cervical cancer treated with radical hysterectomy were evaluated. There were 102 (19.3%) with lymph node metastasis. In those with lymph node metastasis, histologic differentiation (P = 0.009) and metastatic extent (P = 0.045) were the only independent prognostic factors for risk of cervical cancer deaths.

Techniques

Rutledge and colleagues devised a system of rating radicality of hysterectomy (Table 3–10) used in treating women with cervical cancer at the MD Anderson Hospital. He suggested that the term *radical hysterectomy* is not adequate to record and communicate the different amounts of therapy attempted and the subsequent risk of complications when different surgeons report their results. These authors believed that describing the technical features of five operations enabled them to evaluate more accurately

Table 3–10 RUTLEDGE'S CLASSIFICATION OF EXTENDED HYSTERECTOMY

Class	Description	Indication
I	Extrafascial hysterectomy; pubocervical ligament is incised, allowing lateral deflection of the ureter	CIN, early stromal invasion
II	Removal of the medial half of the cardinal and uterosacral ligaments; upper third of the vagina removed	Microcarcinoma postirradiation
III	Removal of the entire cardinal and uterosacral ligaments; upper third of the vagina removed	Stages Ib and IIa lesions
IV	Removal of all periureteral tissue, superior vesical artery, and three fourths of the vagina where preservation of the bladder is still possible	Anteriorly occurring central recurrences
V	Removal of portions of the distal ureter and bladder	Central recurrent cancer involving portions of the distal ureter or bladder

CIN, cervical intraepithelial neoplasia.
From Piver MS, Rutledge FN, Smith PJ: Five classes of extended hysterectomy for women with cervical cancer. Reprinted with permission from The American College of Obstetricians and Gynecologists. Obstet Gynecol 44:265,1974.

their results *and* provided a better understanding of the need to tailor each patient's treatment by using an operation that was adequate but not excessive.

The goal of the class I hysterectomy was to ensure removal of all cervical tissue. Reflection and retraction of the ureters laterally without actual dissection from the ureteral bed allows one to clamp the adjacent paracervical tissue without cutting into the side of the cervical tissue itself. Class I operations are advocated primarily for in situ and true microinvasive carcinomas of the cervix. A class I procedure is also performed after preoperative radiation in adenocarcinoma of the cervix or after preoperative radiation in the so-called barrel-shaped endocervical squamous cell carcinoma. The operation described is essentially the extrafascial hysterectomy used routinely at the MD Anderson Hospital.

Class II extended hysterectomy is described as a modified radical hysterectomy. The purpose of the class II hysterectomy is to remove more paracervical tissue (Fig. 3–21) while still preserving most of the blood supply to the distal ureters and bladder. The ureters are freed from their paracervical position but are not dissected out of the pubovesical ligament. The uterine artery is ligated just medial to the ureter as it lies in "the tunnel," ensuring preservation of the distal ureteral supply. The uterosacral ligaments are transected midway between the uterus and their sacral attachments (Fig. 3–22). The medial halves of both cardinal ligaments are removed, as well as the upper 25% of the vagina. A pelvic lymphadenectomy is usually performed with a class II hysterectomy. A class II operation is reported to be suitable for the following conditions:

1. microinvasive carcinomas in which the depth of invasion is considered greater than early stromal invasion; and
2. small postirradiation recurrences limited to the cervix.

The class III procedure is a wide radical excision of the parametrial and paravaginal tissues in addition to the removal of the pelvic lymphatic tissue. The uterine artery is ligated at its origin on the internal iliac artery. In the dissection of the ureter from the pubovesical ligament (between the lower end of the ureter and the superior vesical artery) care is taken to preserve the ligament, maintaining some additional blood supply to the distal ureter. The hazard of fistula formation is decreased by preservation

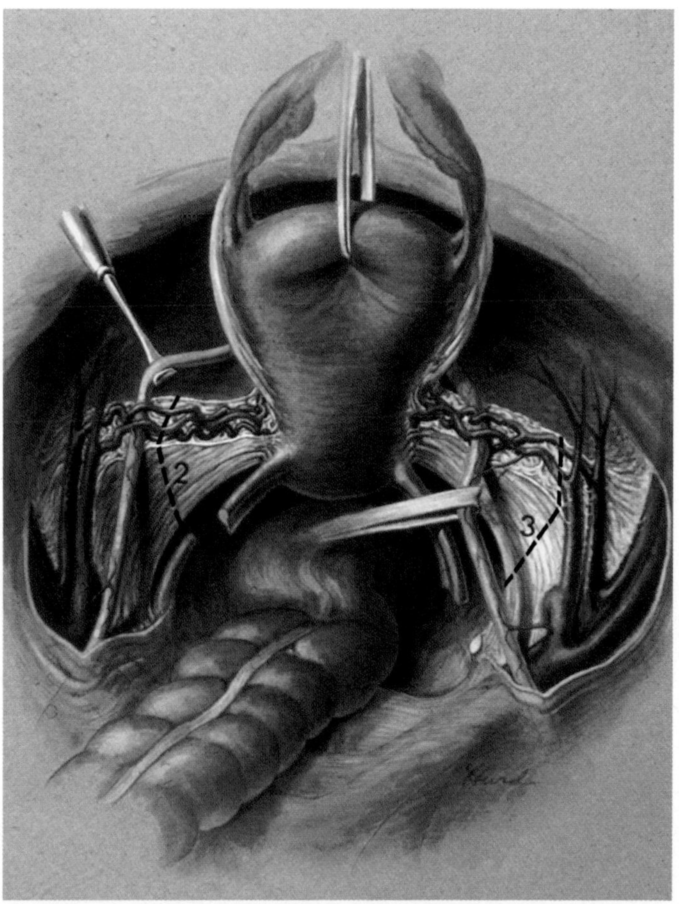

Figure 3–21 *Broken lines* identify the point of transection of the cardinal ligaments in class II and class III radical hysterectomy. (Courtesy of Gregorio Delgado, MD.)

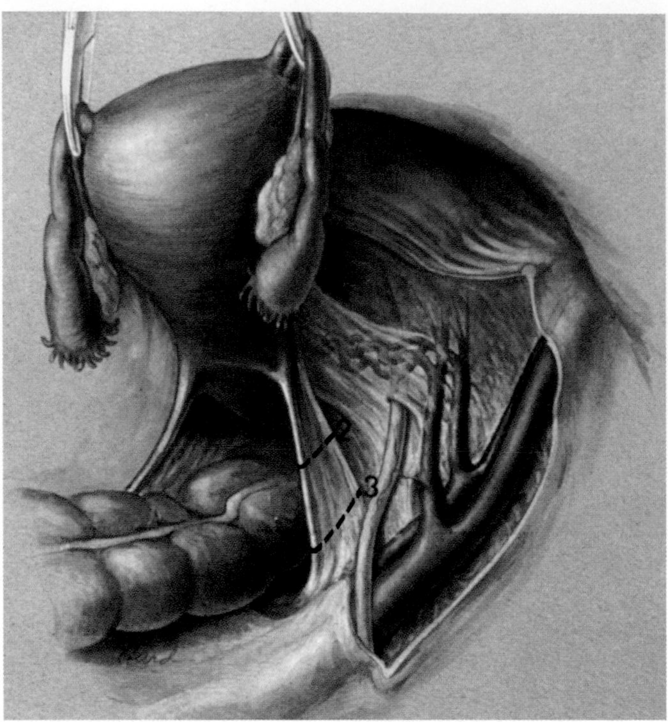

Figure 3–22 *Broken lines* identify the point of transection of the uterosacral ligaments in class II and class III radical hysterectomy. (Courtesy of Gregorio Delgado, MD.)

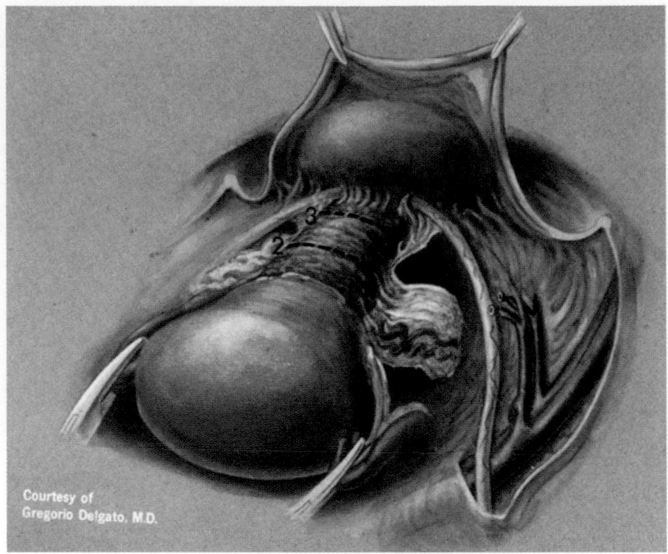

Figure 3–23 *Broken lines* illustrate the level of vaginal removal of class II and class III radical hysterectomy. (Courtesy of Gregorio Delgado, MD.)

of the superior vesical artery, along with a portion of the associated pubovesical ligament. The uterosacral ligaments are resected at the pelvic sidewall. The upper 25% of the vagina is removed (Fig. 3–23), and a pelvic lymphadenectomy is routinely performed. This operation is primarily for the patient with stage I or IIa carcinoma of the cervix with or without preservation of ovarian function.

The aim of the class IV radical hysterectomy is complete removal of all periureteral tissue, a more extensive excision of the paravaginal tissues, and, when indicated, excision of the internal iliac vessels along an involved portion of the medial pelvic wall tissue. This differs from the class III operation in three respects:

1. the ureter is completely dissected from the pubovesical ligament;
2. the superior vesical artery is sacrificed; and
3. 50% of the vagina is removed.

This procedure is used primarily for more extensive anteriorly occurring central recurrences when preservation of the bladder is seemingly still possible. Extension of the dissection laterally is needed when the disease has focally involved the medial parametrium. Sacrificing blood vessels to the bladder is unfavorable because the risk of fistula formation increases significantly. In most cases, these patients are more appropriately treated with an anterior exenteration.

The purpose of the class V hysterectomy is to remove a central recurrent cancer involving portions of the distal ureter or bladder. It differs from a class IV operation because the disease involves a portion of the distal ureter or bladder, or both, which is removed with the disease. A reimplantation of the ureter into the bladder, often as a utereroneocystostomy, is then performed. This procedure has a rare application to a small, specifically located recurrence when exenteration is considered unnecessary or has been refused by the patient.

The modified Rutledge classification of extended hysterectomies has considerable practical value. It once again underlines the necessity for the surgeon to tailor the operative procedure to the disease extent. The patient with a stage Ia2 lesion does not need an operative procedure as radical as the patient with a large IIa lesion. This is particularly pertinent in the decision between a class II and class III radical hysterectomy. In many countries the class II radical hysterectomy (called a modified radical hysterectomy) is combined with a bilateral pelvic lymphadenectomy as standard therapy for early stage cervical cancer. Indeed, the class III type of radical hysterectomy is a phenomenon of particular prevalence in the Western hemisphere and the Orient because of the dual influences of Meigs and Okabayashi. The class III or Meigs–Okabayashi procedure is a derivative of the Halstedian principle that a lesion should be removed en bloc with its draining lymphatics; thus, the class III radical hysterectomy calls for removal of all the parametria at the pelvic sidewall and transection of the uterosacral ligaments at the sacrum. Advocates of the modified radical hysterectomy or class II procedure with pelvic lymphadenectomy for stages I and IIa lesions suggest that the intervening lymphatics are not at risk in an early cancer of the cervix. Indeed, spread from the primary lesion to the draining pelvic wall nodes probably occurs as an embolic phenomenon. One virtually never finds a tumor in lymphatics except surrounding the primary lesions. However, it is prudent for the pathologist to take several sections of the most distal portion of the parametria following a class III radical hysterectomy for stage I or IIa cervical cancer in an effort to determine the presence or absence of malignant cells in lymphatics distant from the primary lesion. In the presence of a bulky central lesion, the need for an adequate surgical margin of resection often mandates a more extensive procedure than the typical class II radical hysterectomy. However, preservation of any portion of the lateral parametria appears to be associated with a greatly diminished incidence of bladder atony. Forney reported on 22 women extensively studied after undergoing radical hysterectomy; in 11 women, the cardinal ligaments had been divided completely, and in the other 11, the inferior 1–2 cm of these ligaments had been spared. Satisfactory voiding occurred significantly earlier (20 vs 51 days) in women who had had an incomplete transection. In a similar manner, preservation of a portion of the uterosacral ligaments appears to be associated with fewer complaints of postoperative obstipation. Undoubtedly, the preserved tissue contains intact nerve tracts, which avoid the extensive denervation associated with the typical class III type or radical hysterectomy.

Complications

Undoubtedly, the major complication following radical surgery for invasive cancer of the cervix is postoperative bladder dysfunction. Reports in the literature by Seski and Carenza, Nobili and Giacobini suggest that bladder dysfunction is a direct result of injury to the sensory and motor nerve supply to the detrusor muscle of the bladder. The more radical the surgery, the greater will be the extent of damage and the more likely postoperative bladder dysfunction will result. This dysfunction is usually manifested in the patient by a loss of the sense of urgency to void and an inability to empty the bladder completely without the Credé maneuver. Although most patients learn to compensate for the sensory and motor loss and return to near normal function, patients occasionally need to be taught intermittent self-catheterization, or long periods of constant bladder drainage may be necessary postoperatively. Sophisticated urodynamic studies have shown that a residual hypertonicity in the bladder detrusor muscle and urethral sphincter mechanism sometimes produces dysuria and stress incontinence. Treatment is symptomatic with near total recovery in most patients. Limitation of the extent and radicality of surgery, especially in patients with early lesions, can minimize this morbidity. Bandy and colleagues reported on the long-term effects on bladder function following radical hysterectomy (class III) with and without postoperative radiation. In his study, the necessity for bladder drainage of 30 or more days after surgery in 30% of patients was associated with significantly worse long-term residual and other bladder dysfunction. Adjunctive pelvic radiation was associated with significantly more contracted and unstable bladder. In a study reported from Greece of stage Ib cancers, 68 had a Rutledge type III and 50 a type II radical hysterectomy. Age, grade, bulky tumor, lymph node metastasis were similar in the two groups. Postoperative radiation was given to 31% of type III and 64% of type II hysterectomies. Major complications, mainly voiding problems, were significantly more common in those treated with type III hysterectomy; however, the disease-free survival was better in the class III hysterectomy (86.5% vs 76.5%, $P < 0.05$). This study would suggest type III surgery is better than type II plus radiation.

Drainage of the retroperitoneal space with continuous suction catheters can be used to help reduce the particularly troublesome complication of the lymphocyst formation. Two studies testing the hypothesis that avoiding reperitonealization of the pelvic peritoneum obviates the need for such drainage have been reported; both studies suggest that drainage is not necessary if the peritoneum is left open over the surgical site. Ligation of the lymphatics entering the obturator fossa under the external iliac vein helps reduce the flow of lymph into this area, where lymphocyst formation is prevalent. Lymphocysts, if present, rarely cause injury and are usually reabsorbed if given enough time. Choo and colleagues reported that cysts <4–5 cm usually resolve within 2 months and that only observation is necessary. Surgical intervention is necessary when there is some evidence of a significant ureteral obstruction. During laparotomy, the surgeon should unroof the lymphocyst and prevent reformation by suturing a tongue of omentum into the cavity (internal marsupialization). Percutaneous aspiration of the cyst, which is often associated with subsequent infection, should be utilized cautiously.

Pulmonary embolism is the one complication most likely to cause mortality in the period surrounding the operative therapy of cervical cancer. This must be kept in mind at all times, and particular care must be exercised during and after surgery to avoid this devastating complication. The operative period is the most dangerous period for the formation of a thrombus in the leg or pelvic veins. Care should be taken to ensure that a constriction of veins in the leg does not occur during the operative procedure, and careful dissection of the pelvic veins should lead to minimal thrombus formation in those structures. Because of the risk of pulmonary embolism and deep venous thrombosis, prophylactic heparin and/or pneumatic compression boots are strongly recommended.

Soisson and colleagues reported on 43 women undergoing radical hysterectomy for early stage cervical cancer. All patients had a body weight at least 25% greater than their ideal weight. Survival was not compromised, and the incidence of serious complications was not increased in obese patients when compared to a control group. Operative technique is more difficult; the procedure lasts longer, and surgery is associated with greater blood loss.

Preservation of ovarian function is often desirable for patients who must undergo a surgical procedure for invasive cancer of the cervix. Often, after a careful histologic examination of the operative specimen, including the pelvic lymph nodes, a postoperative recommendation for pelvic radiation is indicated. Standard pelvic placement of preserved ovaries will result in postirradiation ovarian failure;

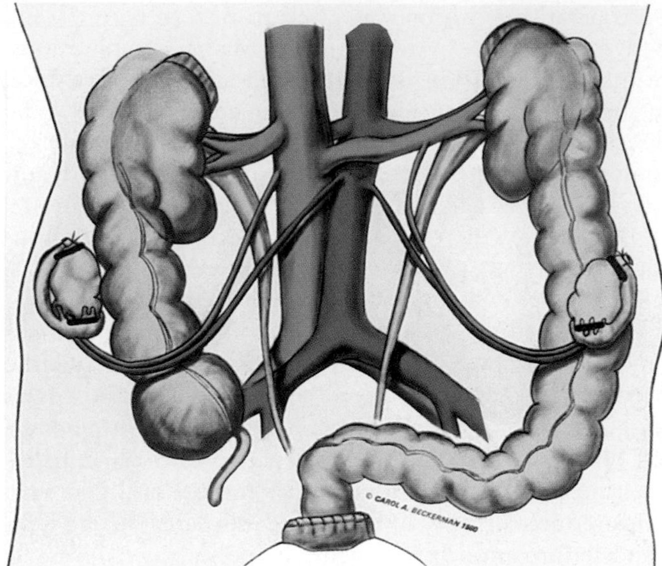

Figure 3–24 Diagram illustrating the location of transposed adnexae to a nonpelvic site where they can be spared from postoperative pelvic irradiation. (From: DiSaia PJ: Surgical aspects of cervical carcinoma. Cancer 48:548, 1981. Copyright © 1981 American Cancer Society. Reprinted by permission of Wiley-Liss, Inc., a subsidiary of John Wiley & Sons, Inc.)

therefore, a procedure for transposition of the ovaries to an extrapelvic site (Fig. 3–24) has been devised. Shielding during postoperative pelvic irradiation is possible with the ovaries so placed. The ovaries receive some radiation but not usually enough to prevent continued steroid production. A word of caution has been interjected by Mann and others regarding the rare occurrence of occult metastases to the ovary in patients with adenocarcinoma of the cervix. The two largest studies suggest that the incidence is between 0.6% and 1.3%, respectively. Most patients with metastatic disease in the ovary are postmenopausal or have had gross adnexal pathology or positive pelvic lymph nodes. These guidelines can be helpful in identifying patients for whom preservation of ovarian tissue is unwise. The incidence of occult metastasis to the ovary from squamous cell carcinoma of the cervix (stages I and IIa) is so rare that preservation of ovarian tissue does not carry the same concerns. Lateral ovarian transposition will be discussed further in the following section on fertility preservation.

Recurrent disease can be expected in 10–20% of patients treated with radical hysterectomy and bilateral lymphadenectomy. A tumor is likely to regrow from viable cancer cells left behind at the time of radical surgery. Recurrences cause rather dismal prognoses, leading to death in >85% of cases. Krebs and associates reported on 40 patients with recurrence following radical surgery for early invasive cancer of the cervix; 58% of the recurrences were found within the first 12 months after surgery and 83% within the first 2 years. The site of recurrence was found to influence diagnosis, symptoms, clinical findings, prognosis, cause of death, and therapy. The prognosis for patients with recurrent cervical cancer was poor, with only five patients (13%) surviving free of disease 5 years after recognition of the occurrence. Krebs and associates suggested radiation therapy as the treatment of choice for patients with pelvic recurrences who did not have prior radiation therapy. The survival rate in that group of patients in their study was 25%. Of their patients, 35% had recurrences outside the pelvis. The authors stressed the importance of close follow-up of patients after radical hysterectomy and bilateral node dissection. Early recognition of a recurrent lesion centrally located appears to give the best prognosis for salvage.

Table 3–11 COMPLICATIONS OF RADICAL HYSTERECTOMY WITH APPROXIMATE INCIDENCES

Complication	Incidence
Vesicovaginal fistula	1%
Ureterovaginal fistula	2%
Severe bladder atony	4%
Bowel obstruction (requiring surgery)	1%
Lymphocyst (requiring drainage)	3%
Thrombophlebitis	2%
Pulmonary embolus	1%

The major complications of radical hysterectomy are formation of ureteral fistulas and lymphocysts, pelvic infection, and hemorrhage. All these complications are preventable, and the incidence is decreasing steadily (Table 3–11). Ureteral fistulas are now infrequent (0–3%), primarily as a result of the improvement in techniques, such as avoiding excess damage to the structure itself and preserving alternate routes of blood supply. Retroperitoneal drainage of the lymphadenectomy sites by means of suction catheters or avoiding reapproximation of the pelvic peritoneum has considerably reduced the incidence of lymphocysts and pelvic infection. The use of electrocautery and hemoclips has assisted the surgeon immensely with hemostasis, and postoperative hemorrhage is rare. The broad-spectrum of antibiotics available today is invaluable in the prevention of pelvic infection, which had contributed significantly to fistula formation, adhesions, and bowel complications. Full-dose irradiation to the pelvis before radical hysterectomy will result in a significant increase in complications, particularly urinary tract fistulas and ureteral obstruction caused by fibrosis, or more frequent lymphocyst formation.

Limiting surgical morbidity in early stage disease

With highly successful surgical treatment programs in place for early stage disease, quality of life among survivors becomes important. Morbidity specifically attributable to radical surgery may result in extensive abdominal scarring as well as compromised sexual and urodynamic function. Full pelvic lymphadenectomies may predispose patients to the development of a pelvic lymphocyst, and occasionally lower extremity lymphedema. A consideration of fertility preservation will be addressed in a separate section.

Sexual function

Patients treated with full pelvic irradiation therapy (i.e., external beam and vaginal brachytherapy) will experience decreased sexual function resulting from vaginal stricture formation with obliteration and premature ovarian failure (see forthcoming discussion). Although radical hysterectomy offers an enhanced functional outcome, the procedure does not always leave sexual function undisturbed. A full disclosure of potential adverse outcomes pertaining to sexual function should be given to patients considering radical hysterectomy.

Employing a prospective, validated, self-assessment questionnaire regarding sexual function, Jensen et al prospectively evaluated 173 patients with lymph node negative early-stage cervical cancer who had undergone radical hysterectomy and pelvic lymphadenectomy. When compared with an age-matched control group from the general population in Copenhagen, patients experienced severe orgasmic problems and uncomfortable sexual intercourse due to a reduced vaginal size during the first 6 months after surgery and severe dyspareunia during the first 3 months. A persistent lack of sexual interest and lubrication were reported during the first 2 years after radical hysterectomy, while the majority of other sexual and vaginal problems disappeared over time. The authors recommend discussing these issues with patients before and after surgery.

Nerve-sparing radical hysterectomy

Lin et al evaluated the urodynamic function in 20 women with cervical cancer who underwent radical hysterectomy. Urodynamic parameters measured preoperatively and postoperatively included bladder voiding and bladder storage functions, both of which were found to be significantly impaired in all 20 cases following surgery. Surgical damage to the pelvic autonomic nerves is likely to be responsible for not only subsequent impaired bladder function, but also in defecation problems and sexual dysfunction. The development of a nerve-sparing procedure which does not compromise the radicality of the operation is highly desirable.

Trimbos et al introduced elements of the Japanese nerve-sparing technique in their Dutch population, citing that in various Japanese oncology centers it had been recognized that the anatomy of the pelvic autonomic nerve plexus permits a systematic surgical approach to preserve these structures. The investigators first identified and preserved the hypogastric nerve in a loose tissue sheath underneath the ureter and lateral to the uterosacral ligament; next, the inferior hypogastric plexus in the parametrium is lateralized and avoided during parametrial transection; finally, the most distal part of the inferior hypogastric plexus is preserved during the dissection of the posterior part of the vesicouterine ligament. Trimbos et al concluded that the procedure is feasible and safe and deserves further consideration.

An updated series was presented by Maas et al who observed that the incidence of urinary dysfunction appears to be very low after nerve-sparing. These findings have been supported by an Italian series of 23 patients reported by Raspagliesi et al, and by two recent Japanese papers for which urodynamic data was recorded for 27 patients. In the study by Sakuragi et al, none of 22 patients for whom the nerve-sparing procedure was performed had urinary dysfunction as compared to three of the five patients for whom the procedure could not be performed.

Sentinel lymph node identification

Although the risk of nodal metastases is low in women with small, early cancers (i.e., FIGO Ia2 and Ib1 lesions), the need for bilateral pelvic lymphadenectomies must still be emphasized. Controversy has centered on the existence and ability to identify sentinel lymph nodes (SLN) in cervical cancer. Two techniques for sentinel node identification are available. An injection is performed around the tumor using either a blue dye or an isotopic colloid. Ideally the two techniques are used concomitantly.

A dose of 1 mCi of technetium-99m colloidal rhenium sulphide is injected into the stroma of the cervix (half of this dose in each of the meridians) at the end of the day preceding surgery. A lymphoscintigraphy is taken just before surgery. At the beginning of surgery, a dose of 2 mL of Patent Blue Violet is injected into the stroma of the cervix after dilution in 2 mL of saline: 1 mm of the mixture in each of the four quadrants. Because the injections must be carried out in the sound tissues surrounding the tumor, only patients with FIGO stage Ia and Ib1 lesions are candidates for this investigational approach.

Dargent and Enria reported the results on 70 consecutive patients. Failure in identification of the SLN occurred in 14 of the 139 attempted dissections. One SLN was detected in 121 dissections, and two SLNs in four dissections. The investigators carried out a systematic pelvic lymphadenectomy after removal of the SN. A metastatic involvement of the SLN was put in evidence in 19 of the 129 retrieved SLNs. The other regional lymph nodes were involved in 13 cases and not involved in 6 cases. In the 110 cases where the SLN was not involved all the other regional nodes were free from metastasis.

In another study involving 23 evaluable patients from which a total of 51 SLN were detected, Martinez-Palones et al showed a 100% negative predictive value in SLN identification with technetium-99m-labeled nanocolloid combined with blue dye injection. Lin et al reported 100% SN detection rate in 30 patients with FIGO stages Ia2–IIA cervical cancer using technicium-99 intracervical injection. There were seven (23.3%) cases of microscopic lymph node metastases on pathologic analysis, all of which had sentinel node involvement. Therefore, the sensitivity of SLN identification for prediction of lymph node metastases was 100% and no false negative was found.

Silva et al reported on 56 patients with FIGO stage I (n = 53) or stage II (n = 3) cervical cancer who underwent SLN detection with preoperative lymphoscintigraphy and intraoperative lymphatic mapping with a handheld gamma probe. One or more sentinel nodes were detected in 52 of 56 eligible patients. A total of 120 SLNs were detected. Forty-four percent of SLNs were found in the external iliac area, 39% in the obturator region, 8.3% in the interiliac region, and 6.7% in the common iliac area. Unilateral SLNs were found in 31 patients (59%), and bilateral SLNs in 21 patients (41%). The negative predictive value was 92.1% and the accuracy of sentinel node in predicting lymph node status was 94.2%.

Finally, Gil-Moreno combined total laparoscopic radical hysterectomy with intraoperative SLN detection in 12 patients with FIGO Ia2 (n = 1) or Ib1 (n = 11) cervical cancer. A mean of 2.5 SLNs per patient were detected, with a mean of 2.33 SLNs per patient by gamma probe and a mean of 2 SLNs per patient after blue dye injection. No microscopic nodal metastases were found, and after a median follow-up of 20 months, all patients remain free of disease.

Dargent has demonstrated *laparoscopic identification* of the SLN using intracervical injection of Patent Blue dye. In the future we may see, combined with the radical trachelectomy (discussed below), the use of the laparoscopic SLN approach to limit the extent of the pelvic lymphadenectomy in patients with low-risk tumors. Although the approach is experimental and therefore remains unproven, it deserves further evaluation.

Vaginal radical hysterectomy

The disadvantage of the classic Shauta procedure of vaginal radical hysterectomy was the need for a second operation to remove the pelvic lymph nodes. However, in recent years it has become possible to remove these lymph nodes laparoscopically, thus decreasing the intra-abdominal scarring and enhancing postoperative convalescence. Roy et al compared the potential benefits of vaginal radical hysterectomy with radical abdominal hysterectomy for early stage cervical cancer. Fifty-two patients underwent laparoscopic lymphadenectomy followed by either a radical vaginal operation (n = 25) or a radical abdominal procedure (n = 27). The mean ages, weights, parity, histologic types, FIGO stages, and tumor volumes were comparable in both groups, as were the operating times. Perioperative morbidity included fever (vaginal group, n = 4; abdominal group, n = 9), hematoma (one in each group), wound infection/abscess (vaginal group, n = 1; abdominal group, n = 4), and two cystotomies and one vascular injury in the vaginal group. At 27 months' follow-up, one recurrence has been discovered in the abdominal group. The authors concluded that the outcomes were comparable and that the vaginal approach resulted in less febrile morbidity.

Roy's data has been supported by a United Kingdom study of 50 patients (matched successfully) who underwent laparoscopic-assisted vaginal radical hysterectomy, and a Canadian paper comparing 71 patients and 205 patients who underwent laparoscopic-assisted vaginal radical hysterectomy and radical abdominal hysterectomy, respectively. In both studies the investigators cite the major benefits of the vaginal approach being less intraoperative blood loss and shorter hospital stay.

Nam et al compared 47 cases of laparoscopic-assisted vaginal radical hysterectomy plus lymphadenectomy to 96 cases of radical abdominal hysterectomy plus lymphadenectomy. *Importantly, there was an 8.5% recurrence rate among the radical vaginal hysterectomy group as compared with 2.1% in the control group.* Because of a significantly higher recurrence-free survival in the control group, the authors have elected to limit the performance of a laparoscopic-assisted vaginal radical hysterectomy with lymphadenectomy to patients with small volume disease (tumor diameter <2 cm or volume <4.2 cm^3). The unproven benefits and potential adverse consequences of these investigational procedures cannot be overemphasized, and while some of these procedures may appear attractive to patients and family members, the oncologist must keep a critical appraisal of the available literature foremost in mind at all times.

Laparoscopic radical hysterectomy

A type III Wertheim–Meigs radical hysterectomy with bilateral pelvic and aortocaval lymphadenectomies can be accomplished via operative laparoscopy. We recommend performing the lymphadenectomy first, employing liberal use of the argon beam coagulator and countertraction using the endobabcock forceps. Serial clipping of lumbar veins permits access to the nodal tissue posterior to the inferior vena cava. Ureteral dissection with resection of the cervicovesical fascia is completed with right-angle dissectors, vascular clips and the argon beam coagulation. Application of the 2.5 mm vascular Endo-GIA stapling device employing 30 mm cartridges achieves resection of the cardinal and uterosacral ligaments at the pelvic sidewall and along the pelvic floor, respectively.

Pomel et al evaluated the outcomes of 50 patients who underwent laparoscopic radical hysterectomy over an 8-year period. The median overall operative time was 258 minutes, and there were two major urinary complications (one patient with a vesicovaginal fistula, and one with ureteral stenosis). At a median follow-up of 44 months, the overall 5-year survival rate of FIGO stage Ia2 and Ib1 patients was 96%. Spirtos et al have demonstrated that this approach is feasible and may decrease the morbidity historically associated with radical hysterectomy performed either abdominally or vaginally.

Fertility-preserving surgery for early stage tumors

For patients with microinvasive cervical carcinoma, the management depends on the depth of invasion, and select patients may undergo conservative treatment with either cervical conization (FIGO Ia1) or radical trachelectomy with lymphadenectomy (FIGO Ia1 with lymphovascular space involvement, FIGO Ia2, and FIGO Ia adenocarcinoma) (see Fig. 3–17). In addition, patients with FIGO stage Ib lesions less than 2 cm in size with limited endocervical involvement and no pathologic evidence of lymph node metastases may be candidates for radical trachelectomy. In patients who are selected for conservative therapy, there should be no clinical evidence of impaired fertility and a strong desire for future childbearing. In addition, close surveillance should be instituted with scheduled Papanicoloau testing, colposcopic evaluation, and endocervical curettage.

Cervical conization

For women with stage Ia_1 squamous cell cervical cancer, because the rates of parametrial involvement and nodal metastases are negligible, cold-knife conization alone may be suitable under certain conditions (e.g., lack of LVSI, nulliparity, desirous of childbearing etc.). Alternatively, laser CO_2 cervical conization under local anesthesia may be contemplated for microinvasive carcinoma, with a study of 62 patients by Diakomanolis et al, noting a 6.6% recurrence rate (CIN I only) over a mean follow-up period of 54 months. The use of cervical conization in the management of "microinvasive" endocervical adenocarcinoma may also be an option for select women who wish to preserve fertility. McHale et al explored the outcome on survival and fertility in women with cervical adenocarcinoma in situ and early invasive adenocarcinoma treated conservatively between 1985 and 1996. Twenty of 41 women with adenocarcinoma in situ underwent cervical conization; of five patients with positive cone margins, two recurred and one developed an invasive adenocarcinoma at 5 years of follow-up. Four of 20 women with FIGO stage Ia lesions underwent cervical conization to preserve fertility, and three subsequently delivered healthy infants. None of these women developed recurrent disease after a median follow-up of 48 months. Schorge et al prospectively employed the cervical conization technique to preserve fertility in five women with FIGO stage Ia adenocarcinoma of the uterine cervix. None of the conization specimens revealed angiolymphatic space invasion and following 6 to 20 months of follow-up, none of the patients developed recurrent disease. One must always keep in mind that the primary objective is to clear the cancer with a satisfactory margin; all concerns regarding future pregnancy are secondary.

Vaginal radical trachelectomy

Patients with stage Ia2 disease have a 6.3% risk of nodal metastases and therefore treatment must include a formal pelvic lymphadenectomy along with bilateral parametrectomy. Thus, conization is not sufficient in these cases.

In 1987, Dargent designed a fertility-preserving operation for stage Ia2 and some Ib1 lesions. A variant of the classical Shauta operation of vaginal radical hysterectomy, the vaginal radical trachelectomy (VRT) is always preceded by bilateral laparoscopic lymphadenectomies. The VRT is performed with division of the uterus underneath the isthmus, and at the completion of the procedure, the uterus is sutured to the vagina. Oncologically, the technique is satisfying as a wide margin around the lesion is obtained containing the parametria and the upper vagina, but leaving the body of the uterus in situ.

Intraoperative mandatory frozen section analysis should be performed on both the nodal tissue and the upper endocervical margins of the trachelectomy specimen. Upon a review of 61 VRT specimens, Tanguay et al recommend a complementary radical hysterectomy when the tumor extends to within 5 mm of the margin. These investigators also prefer a longitudinal rather than transverse frozen section when a macroscopic lesion is present as it permits measurement of the distance between the tumor and the endocervical margin.

Aggregate data from four centers (Dargent in France, $n = 82$; Covens et al from Toronto, $n = 58$; Roy and Plante from Quebec, $n = 44$; Shepherd et al in the United Kingdom, $n = 40$) have documented a 3.1% ($n = 7$) recurrence rate among 224 patients, three of which were at distant sites (Table 3–12). The data reflecting obstetrical outcomes are quite encouraging and have been noteworthy for 96 pregnancies, of which 51 live births have resulted (Table 3–13). Covens et al reported that all women in their series became pregnant within 12 months of attempting to conceive, giving a conception rate of 37% at one year. Importantly most women were able to become pregnant without assisted reproductive technology. There have been 12 second-trimester losses due to cervical weakness.

Bernardini et al presented the obstetric outcomes of 80 patients from the Toronto group. Thirty-nine patients attempted to conceive during a median follow-up period of 11 months, resulting in 22 pregnancies in 18 patients. Of the 22 pregnancies, 18 were viable, with 12 progressing to term and delivering by caesarean section. Preterm premature rupture of the membranes was the primary cause of preterm delivery. We currently recommend placement of

Table 3–12 RECURRENCE IN A STUDY OF 224 PATIENTS WHO UNDERWENT RADICAL VAGINAL TRACHELECTOMY WITH LAPAROSCOPIC PELVIC LYMPHADENECTOMY

Site of recurrence	No. of recurrences (%)
Parametrium	3 (1.3)
Pelvic sidewall	1 (0.4)
Distant	3 (1.3)*
Total	7 (3.1)

*Excludes two patients with small cell neuroendocrine tumors diagnosed on final pathology. Both patients died despite aggressive postoperative adjuvant chemotherapy.

Data drawn from Dargent and Mathevet, Dargent, Covens et al, Roy and Plante, and Shepherd et al.

From Stehman et al. Innovations in the treatment of invasive cervical cancer. Cancer 98(9 Suppl):2052–63, 2003.

Table 3–13 OBSTETRIC RESULTS OF A STUDY OF 224 PATIENTS WHO UNDERWENT RADICAL VAGINAL TRACHELECTOMY WITH LAPAROSCOPIC PELVIC LYMPHADENECTOMY

Event	No. of events
Pregnancy	96 (*n* = 61 women)
Live birth	51 (includes preterm birth < 34 wks, *n* = 18)
First trimester loss	22
Spontaneous abortion	16
Therapeutic abortion	5
Ectopic pregnancy	1
Second trimester loss	12
Current pregnancy	11

Data drawn from Dargent and Mathevet, Dargent, Covens et al, Roy and Plante, and Shepherd et al.
From Stehman et al. Innovations in the treatment of invasive cervical cancer. Cancer 98(9 Suppl):2052-63, 2003.

a transabdominal cerclage over the mouth of the lower uterine segment with subsequent delivery of the neonate by cesarean section.

In an updated series of 72 cases and review of the literature, the group from Quebec still maintain that the VRT is an oncologically safe procedure in well-selected patients with early stage disease. Excluding a patient with a small cell neuroendocrine tumor who rapidly recurred and died, there were two recurrences (2.8%) and one death (1.4%) at a median follow-up of 60 months. The authors suggest that lesion size beyond 2 cm appears to be associated with a higher risk of recurrence. Additionally, upon discovering a central pelvic recurrence of an endocervical adenocarcinoma 7 years after VRT, Bali et al have raised the question whether patients treated by VRT (in particular those with adenocarcinoma) should be offered hysterectomy once childbearing has been accomplished.

By allowing for the preservation of the body of the uterus and thereby the potential for reproductive function, the VRT emerges as a true breakthrough in the management of young women with early-stage cervical cancer. VRT is currently the fertility-sparing procedure with the most available data supporting its use. Although these results are encouraging, there is lack of level I evidence (i.e., randomized controlled trials) comparing safety and survival rates between conservative and radical methods. Therefore, these techniques should be used by fully trained operators, with the understanding that it is not the standard treatment for this disease at present. In our opinion, the technique can be considered in conjunction with laparoscopic transperitoneal lymphadenectomy in the patient who strongly desires future fertility and harbors a stage Ia1 lesion with LVSI, an Ia2 lesion or an Ib1 tumor < 2 cm in diameter. Additional requirements include squamous cell histology when dealing with a clinical lesion, and limited endocervical involvement as determined by colposcopy and magnetic resonance imaging.

Abdominal radical trachelectomy

Potential benefits of the abdominal approach for radical trachetectomy include wider parametrial resection, possible lower intraoperative complication rates, and techniques familiar to most gynecologic oncologists. Ungar et al performed this procedure in 30 patients, 10 with FIGO stage Ia2 tumors, 5 with stage Ib1 lesions, and 5 with stage Ib2. During a median follow-up of 47 months, no recurrences have been detected. Among five women who attempted to conceive, three women have fallen pregnant resulting in one first trimester pregnancy loss and two caesarean section deliveries at term. Although this technique has not gained wide application, the authors contend that it appears to provide equivalent oncological safety to a standard Wertheim radical hysterectomy.

The performance of a satisfactory VRT can be technically complex when dealing with the proximal endocervical margins of an adenocarcinoma. We have moved away from the vaginal approach for glandular lesions, and exclusively perform the radical trachelectomy abdominally when confronted with an early stage endocervical adenocarcinoma in patients desiring fertility preservation.

Lateral ovarian transposition

As described above, young patients with FIGO stage I–IIa cervical carcinoma who are considered to be at high risk for requiring adjuvant pelvic irradiation (with or without radiosensitizing chemotherapy) should have the ovaries transposed to the paracolic gutters at the time of radical abdominal hysterectomy. The infundibulopelvic ligament is mobilized and two large metallic clips should be placed in an 'X' formation across the mesosalpinges to assist in radiographic localization during radiation treatment planning. Patients with locally advanced carcinomas (i.e., FIGO stage Ib2–IVa) who will receive primary chemoirradiation can undergo lateral ovarian transposition via laparoscopy in anticipation of therapy.

The incidence of ovarian failure following transposition ranges from 28% to 50% when pelvic irradiation is used. There is a tendency to become postmenopausal if the scatter radiation dose at the transposed ovaries is > 300 cGy. This scatter radiation dose does not appear to depend on the distance the ovaries are placed from the linea innominata. The risk of premature ovarian failure when adjuvant radiation therapy is not required is approximately 5% in patients who have undergone lateral ovarian transposition. The risk of developing symptomatic ovarian cysts appears to be approximately 5%.

Husseinzadeh et al performed lateral ovarian transposition in 22 patients with invasive cervical cancer, 15 of whom received whole pelvic external radiation therapy. Nine patients also received one or two intracavitary insertions. Ovarian function was measured by the serum gonadotropins, follicle-stimulating hormone (FSH), and luteinizing hormone (LH). Five patients developed postmenopausal symptoms. Ovarian function was preserved in seven, all of whom received an average dose of 250 cGy to the ovaries via external radiation and intracavitary insertion(s). FSH values ranged from 3.3 to 38.8 mIU mL-1 (mean = 17.7 mIU mL-1).

Radiotherapy

Over the past century radiotherapy has emerged as a notable alternative to radical surgery, primarily because of improvements in technique. The number of radiation-resistant lesions was discovered to be small, and skilled radiologists limit radiation injury, especially with the moderate dosages used for early disease. Much evidence has been presented that proves that radiotherapy can destroy disease in lymph nodes and in the primary lesion. Over the past two decades, radical hysterectomy has been reserved in many institutions for patients who are relatively young, lean, and in otherwise good health. In other areas of the USA, radiotherapy or surgery is used alone when the alternate modality is not available. The relative safety of both treatment modalities, as well as the high curability for stages I and IIa lesions, gives physician and patient a true option for therapy.

Radiotherapy for cancer of the cervix was begun in 1903 in New York by Margaret Cleaves. In 1913, Abbe was able to report an 8-year cure. The Stockholm method was established in 1914, the Paris method in 1919, and the Manchester method in 1938. Radium was the first element used; it has always been the most important element in radiotherapy of this lesion. External irradiation was used to treat the lymphatic drainage areas in the pelvis lateral to the cervix and the paracervical tissues.

Successful radiation therapy depends on the following:

1. Greater sensitivity of the cancer cell, compared with the cells of the normal tissue bed, to ionizing radiation
2. Greater ability of normal tissue to recuperate after irradiation
3. A patient in reasonably good physical condition

The maximal effect of ionizing radiation on cancer is obtained in the presence of a good and intact circulation and adequate cellular oxygenation. Preparation of the patient for a radical course of irradiation therapy should be as careful as the preparation for radical surgery. The patient's general condition should be as well maintained as possible with a diet high in proteins, vitamins, and calories. Excessive blood loss should be controlled and hemoglobin maintained well above 10 g.

Some consideration must be given to the tolerance of normal tissues of the pelvis, which are likely to receive relatively high doses during the course of treatment of cervical malignancy. The vaginal mucosa in the area of the vault tolerates between 20,000 and 25,000 cGy. The rectovaginal septum is said to tolerate approximately 6000 cGy over 4–6 weeks without difficulty. The bladder mucosa can accept a maximal dose of 7000 cGy. The colon and rectum will tolerate approximately 5000–6000 cGy, but small bowel loops are less tolerant and are said to accept a maximal dose of between 4000 and 4200 cGy. This of course pertains to small bowel loops within the pelvis; the tolerance of the small bowel when the entire abdomen is irradiated is limited to 2500 cGy. One of the basic principles of radiotherapy is implied here: The normal tissue tolerance of any organ is inversely related to the volume of the organ receiving irradiation. External irradiation and intracavitary radium therapy must be used in various combinations (Table 3–14). Treatment plans must be tailored to each patient and her particular lesion. The size and distribution of the cancer, not the stage, should be treated. Success in curing cancer of the cervix depends on the ability of the therapy team to evaluate the lesion (as well as the geometry of the pelvis) during treatment and then make

Table 3–14 SUGGESTED THERAPY FOR CERVICAL CANCER

Stage	Whole Pelvis (cG y)	Brachytherapy (mg/hr)	Surgery
Ial true microinvasive			Extrafascial hysterectomy
Ia2	2000 (2000 parametrial)	8000 (2 applications)	Radical hysterectomy with bilateral pelvic lymphadenectmy as an option
Ib	4000	6000 (2 applications)	
IIb	4000–5000*	5000–6000 (2 applications)	Consider pelvic extenteration for tumor persistence
IIIa	5000–6000*	2000–3000 or interstitial implant	
IIIb	5000–6000*	4000 (1 application), 5000 (2 applications)†	
IVa	6000	4000 (1 application), 5000 (2 applications)‡	
IVb	500–1000 pulse 2–4 times 1 week apart	Palliative	

* Patients with larger lesions or poor vaginal geometry merit the higher dose of external radiation.

† Two applications are suggested following whole-pelvis radiation with larger lesions or when the first application has less than optimum dosimetry.

indicated changes in therapy as necessary. Intracavitary radium therapy is ideally suited to the treatment of early tumors because of the accessibility of the portio of the cervix and the cervical canal. It is possible to place radium or cesium in close proximity to the lesion and thus deliver surface doses that approximate 15,000–20,000 cGy. In addition, normal cervical and vaginal tissue has a particularly high tolerance to irradiation. One, therefore, has an ideal situation for the treatment of cancer because there are accessible lesions that lie in a bed of normal tissue (cervix and vagina) that is highly radioresistant.

Radium/cesium therapy

Radium is the isotope that has been used traditionally in the treatment of cancer of the cervix. Its greatest value is that its half-life is approximately 1620 years; therefore, it provides a very stable, durable element for therapy. In recent years, both cesium and cobalt have been used for intracavitary therapy. Cesium has a half-life of 30 years; with the current technology, cesium provides a very adequate substitute for radium. Four major technologies for the application of radium in the treatment of cervical cancer continue to be favored among gynecologists. Of these technologies, three are intracavitary techniques using specially designed applicators, and the fourth technique involves the application of radium in the form of needles directly into the tumor. The variations among the three techniques of intracavitary brachytherapy are found in the Stockholm, Paris, and Manchester schools of treatment (Fig. 3–25). The differences are mainly found in the number and length of time of applications, the size and placement of the vaginal colpostats, and radium loading. In the USA, the tendency has been to use fixed radium applicators with the intrauterine tandem and vaginal colpostats originally attached to each other. Over the last three decades, a flexible afterloading system, Fletcher-Suit, has gained increasing popularity because it provides flexibility and the safety of afterloading techniques.

The Paris method originally employed a daily insertion of 66.66 mg of radium divided equally between the uterus and the vagina. The radium remained in place for 12–14 hours, and the period of treatment varied from 5–7 days. An essential feature of the Paris method, and a part of the modification of this technique, is the vaginal colpostat, which consists of two hollow corks that serve as radium containers joined together by a steel spring that separates them into the lateral vaginal wall.

The Stockholm technique uses a tandem in the uterine cavity surrounded by a square radium plaque applied to the vaginal wall and portio vaginalis of the cervix. No radium is placed in the lower cervical canal, and vaginal sources are used to cover the cervical lesion. The uterine tandem and vaginal plaque are immobilized by packing and left in place for 12–36 hours. Two to three identical applications are made at weekly intervals.

The Manchester system is designed to yield constant isodose patterns regardless of the size of the uterus and vagina. The source placed in the neighborhood of the cervical canal is considered the unit strength. The remaining sources in the corpus and vagina are applied as multiples of this unit and are selected and arranged to produce equivalent isodose curves in each case and an optimal dose at preselected points in the pelvis. The applicator is shaped to allow an isodose curve that delivers radiation to the cervix in a uniform amount. The Fletcher-Suit system (Fig. 3–26) previously mentioned is a variation of the Manchester technique.

An effort is made in the two radium insertions to administer approximately 7000 cGy to the paracervical tissues as the total of the dose from both external and intracavitary irradiation. The isodose distribution around a Manchester system is pear-shaped (Fig. 3–27). The maximal total dose delivered by the two radium insertions is a function of the total dose to the bladder and rectum. The total dose received by the rectal mucosa from both radium applications usually ranges between 4000 and 6000 cGy. The nearest bladder mucosa may receive between 5000 and 7000 cGy. When whole-pelvis irradiation is used, the radium dose must be reduced to keep the total dose to the bladder and rectum within acceptable limits.

In conjunction with the development of a system of radium distribution, British workers have defined two anatomic areas of the parametria (see Fig. 3–27) where

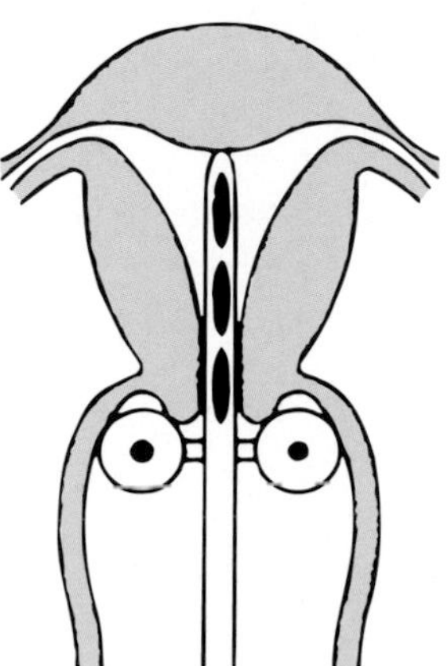

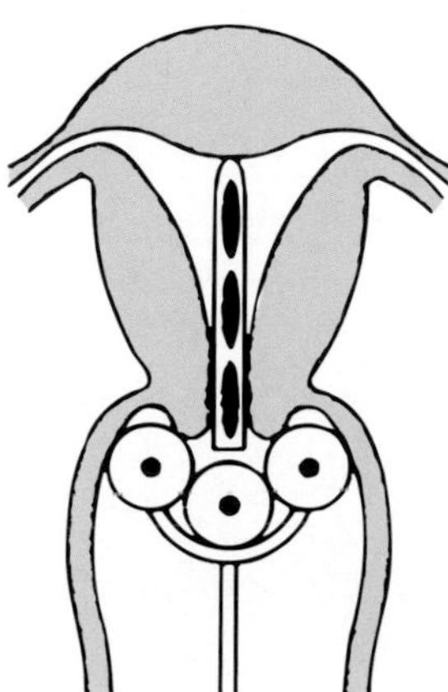

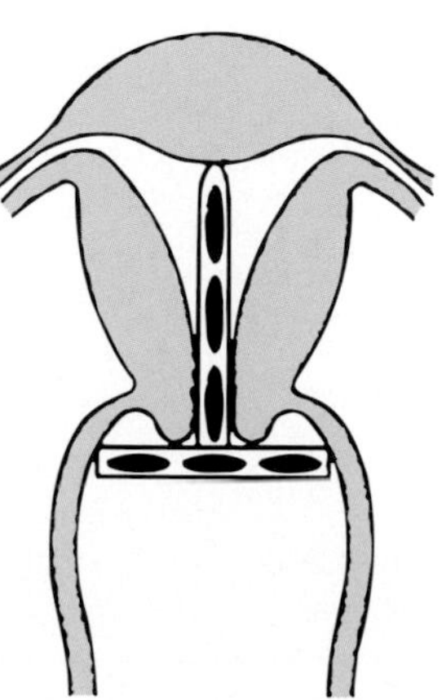

Figure 3–25 Three techniques of intracavitary brachytherapy.

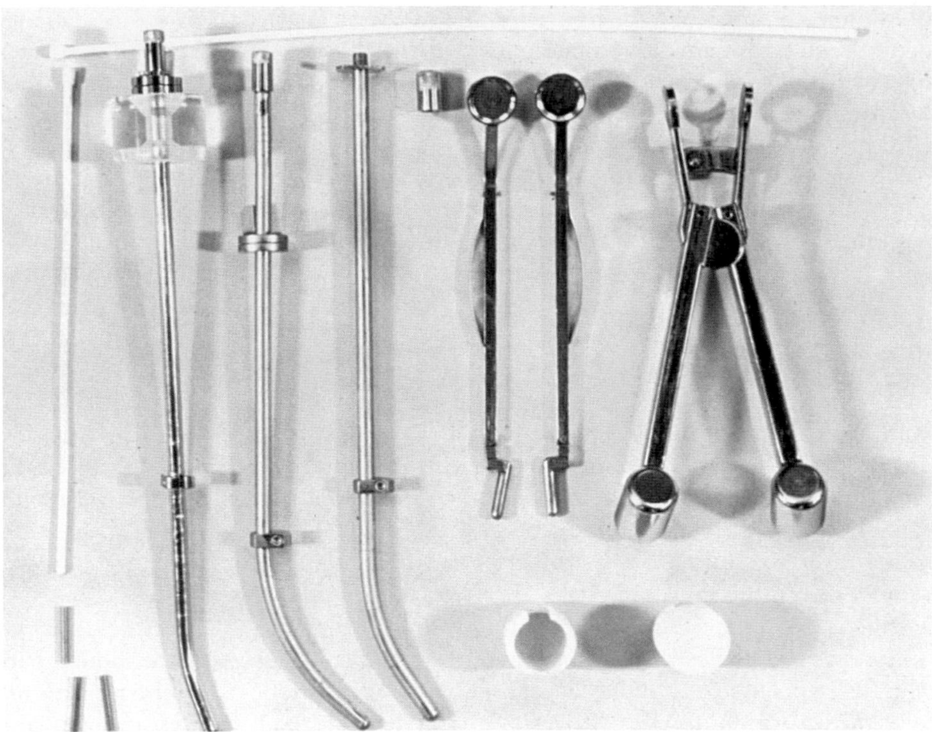

Figure 3–26 Fletcher-Suit radium applicators: Ovoids and tandem with inserts.

dose designation can be correlated with clinical effect. These are situated in the proximal parametria adjacent to the cervix at the level of the internal os and in the distal parametria in the area of the iliac lymph nodes and are designated point A and point B. The description states that point A is located 2 cm from the midline of the cervical canal and 2 cm superior to the lateral vaginal fornix. The dose at point A is representative of the dose to the paracervical triangle, which correlates well with the incidence of sequelae and with the 5-year control rate in many studies. Point B is 3 cm lateral to point A. This point, together with the tissue superior to it, is significant when considering the dose to the node-bearing tissue. It is clear from what has been said relative to points A and B that they can represent important points on a curve describing the dose gradient from the radium sources to the lateral pelvic wall. This gradient is different for the various techniques. In a comparison of the physical characteristics of radio techniques, the ratio of the dose at point A to the dose at point B should help define physical differences. In addition, determining the dose at point A relative to the calculated dose at points identified as bladder trigone and rectal mucosa provides a means of assessing the relative safety of one application over another. The concepts of points A and B have been questioned by many authors, including Fletcher and Rutledge. They remain as imaginary points but seem to provide a framework in which therapy is planned. Again, the distribution of the disease must be the primary guide in planning therapy, and the total dose to either point A or point B is relative only to their position with regard to the disease distribution.

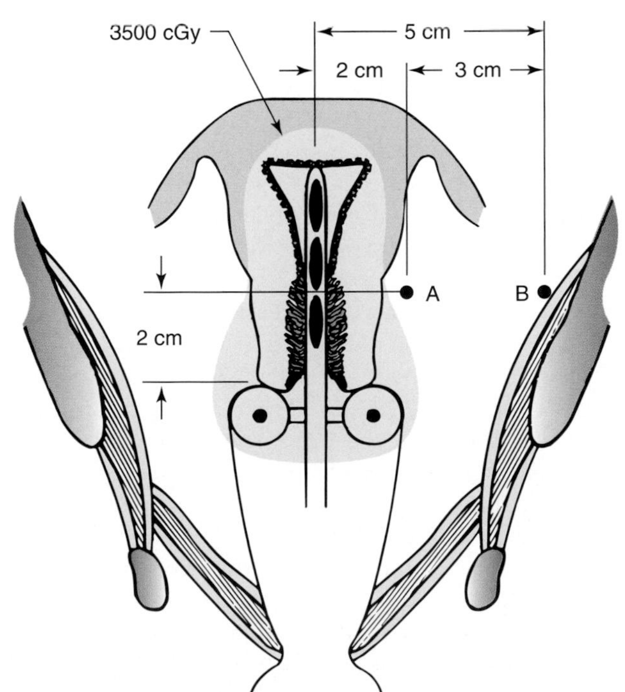

Figure 3–27 Pearshaped distribution of radiation delivered to tissues surrounding a typical radium application with the Manchester type of applicators. Points A and B are noted as reference points.

Whole-pelvis irradiation is usually administered in conjunction with brachytherapy (e.g., intracavitary radium or cesium) in a dose range of 4000–5000 cGy. Megavoltage machines such as cobalt, linear accelerators, and the betatron have the distinct advantage of giving greater homogeneity of dose to the pelvis. In addition, the hard, short rays of megavoltage pass through the skin without much absorption and cause very little injury, allowing almost unlimited amounts of radiation to be delivered to pelvic depths with little if any skin irritation. Orthovoltage, because of its relatively long wavelength and low energy, has the disadvantage that doses to the skin are particularly high and, in delivering the required amount of radiation to the pelvis, may cause temporary and permanent skin changes. Thus, for pelvis irradiation, high-energy megavoltage equipment has definite advantages over orthovoltage and even low-energy megavoltage equipment.

Interstitial therapy

In advanced carcinoma of the cervix, the associated obliteration of the fornices or contracture of the vagina may interfere with accurate placement of conventional intracavitary applicators. Poorly placed applicators fail to irradiate the lesion and the pelvis homogeneously. Syed and Feder have revived a solution to this problem by advocating transvaginal and transperineal implants. The technique employs a template to guide the insertion of a group of 18-gauge hollow steel needles into the parametria transperineally (Fig. 3–28). These hollow needles are subsequently "afterloaded" with iridium wires when the patient has returned to her hospital room. Theoretically, this technique locates a pair of paravaginal interstitial colpostats in both parametria. This approach appears promising, but long-term studies illustrating improved survival rate and reasonable morbidity are not available. Also, there is no report reflecting, prospectively, the effectiveness, in comparable groups of patients, of the interstitial technique versus the standard intracavitary approach.

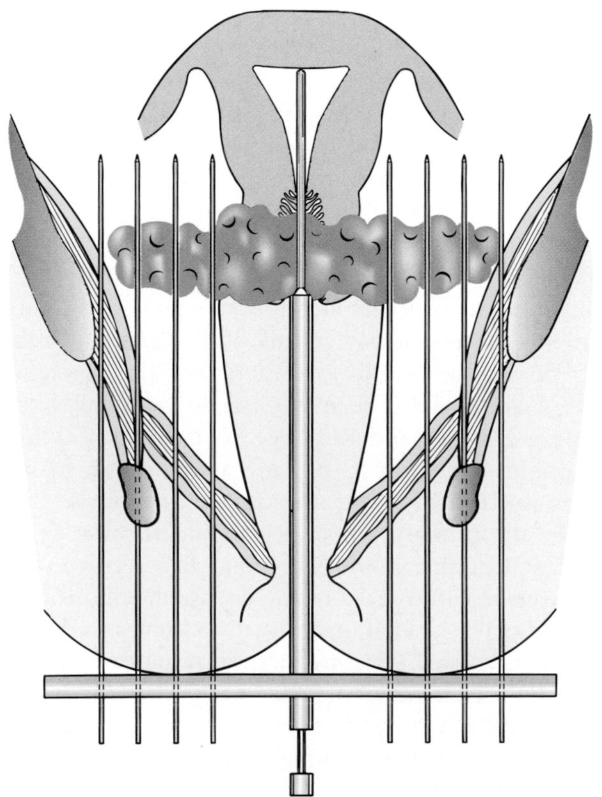

Figure 3–28 Diagram of the technique of interstitial therapy for advanced cervical cancer using a Syed–Noblett template.

Interstitial therapy may have particular value in the treatment of carcinoma of the cervical stump. Although carcinoma of the cervical stump has become a relatively rare disease, accounting for less than 1% of all gynecologic malignancies, it does create difficult problems in terms of optimal geometry for delivery of effective irradiation therapy. In some series of cervical cancer, the incidence of carcinoma of the cervical stump is approximately 10%. Prempree, Patanaphan and Scott reported excellent results with absolute survival rates of 83.3% for stage I, 75% for stage IIa, and 62.5% for stage IIb using radiation therapy with an emphasis on parametrial interstitial implants in the more advanced diseases. Similar results have been obtained by Puthawala and associates.

Extended field irradiation therapy

Over the past two decades, attempts have been made to salvage more patients with advanced cervical cancer by identifying the presence of periaortic lymph node metastases and applying extended field irradiation to the area (Fig. 3–29). The en bloc pelvic and periaortic portals extend superiorly as far as the level of the dome of the diaphragm and inferiorly to the obturator foramen. The width of the periaortic portion of the field is usually 8–10 cm, and the usual dose delivered is between 4000 and 5000 cGy in 4–6 weeks. A booster dose of 1000 cGy is often given to the pelvic field alone. Identification of periaortic lymph node involvement was initially attempted by use of lymphangiography, but this technique did not find general acceptance because of varied accuracy from institution to institution and from radiologist to radiologist. Surgical localization of periaortic involvement has been more satisfactory.

Several reports have discussed survival and complications in patients with carcinoma of the cervix and periaortic metastases who received extended field irradiation (Table 3–15). Piver and Barlow of Roswell Park Memorial Institute, Buffalo, reported on 20 women with previously untreated cervical cancer who received radical irradiation to the periaortic lymph nodes and pelvis after the diagnosis of periaortic lymph node metastases had been established by surgical staging. They noted that 90% of these patients received 6000 cGy to the periaortic nodes and pelvis in 8 weeks using a split-course technique. A later report shows that 30% died of complications of this therapy and 45% of recurrent disease. Only 25% of patients survived disease-free for 16, 18, 24, and 36 months. The criticism may be that the dose is too high, yet a lesser dose might be ineffective, and four patients did survive. It is obvious that a safe yet effective dosage level for extended field irradiation therapy has not yet been established.

Wharton and colleagues of the MD Anderson Hospital reported on 120 women treated with preirradiation celiotomy. Of these patients, 32 had severe bowel complications and 20 (16.6%) eventually died as a result of the

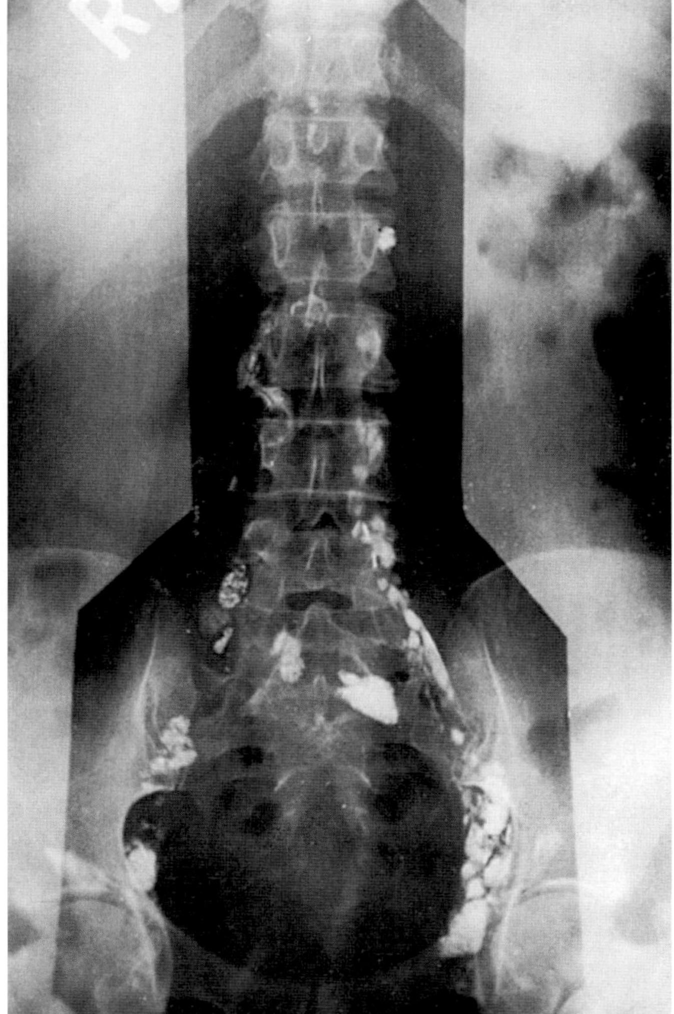

Figure 3–29 Abdominal radiograph showing portals for extended-field irradiation in cervical cancer.

surgery or of the surgery and irradiation. Four of these patients died immediately as a result of the surgical procedure. Of 64 patients with positive nodes who were irradiated, 17% lived for 13–38 months after treatment. No patient had survived for 5 years. Wharton and associates further reported that in 36 women with positive nodes it was possible to accurately determine the failure sites after completion of the full course of irradiation therapy. In 25 of these patients, distant metastases were the first evidence of treatment failure; 11 had disease or developed recurrence within the treatment fields; disease of the pelvic wall was found in only two patients.

The role of surgical staging in removal of para-aortic or pelvic nodes in cervical cancer remains controversial. The results of the aforementioned experience would question significant benefit in view of the complications and survival. Retroperitoneal lymphadenectomy, compared with the intraperitoneal approach, has decreased complications mainly due to adhesions and possible bowel complications. More recently, patients with advanced disease have had the para-aortic nodes re-evaluated so that extended fields could be added if necessary. The laparoscopic approach is

Table 3–15 LATE COMPLICATIONS OF RADIATION THERAPY WITH APPROXIMATE INCIDENCE

Sigmoiditis	3%
Rectovaginal fistula	1%
Rectal stricture	1%
Small bowel obstruction	1%
(with extended field)	20%
Vesicovaginal fistula	1%
Ureteral stricture	1%

currently being evaluated. Less invasive approaches such as lymphangiogram, CT, and MRI studies have also been evaluated. The sensitivity is less, and false-negative results may be as high as 24% in stage IIIB patients. Many gynecologic oncologists will obtain a CT scan and, if positive, will do a fine-needle aspiration. If the result is negative, then surgical removal may be done. An alternative is to radiate the para-aortic areas prophylactically. This has been done with little or no survival benefit. All the studies note that the severe complication rate essentially doubles (5–10%) when radiation was given to the para-aortic area.

Experience has shown that doses of about 4500 cGy, particularly when administered in daily fractions of 150–180 cGy, are safely tolerated by the organs in the periaortic treatment volume, and a complication rate of 5% should be expected. Extraperitoneal surgery appears to be associated with less postradiation morbidity, probably because of reduced bowel adhesions. The issues of the utility of periaortic radiation and surgical staging in the management of cervical carcinoma are closely intertwined. Although many hypotheses have been raised to support or reject the use of surgical staging, it is clear that some patients with biopsy-proven periaortic node metastases can be cured with radiotherapy employing extended fields. Approximately 20% of patients who receive extended-field radiotherapy survive cervical cancer metastatic to the periaortic lymph nodes. Rubin had a 50% survival in a group of Ib patients with documented periaortic lymph node involvement. In many reports, the true value of extended field radiation is clouded because patients with periaortic node involvement often have advanced disease in which any node or regional therapy may have little effect on long-term survival.

Radiation and chemotherapy

Five landmark papers have all reported significant improved survival for patients with cervical cancer when adjuvant chemotherapy is used in combination with radiation (Fig. 3–30 and Table 3–16). In patients with bulky (≥4 cm) stage Ib, the GOG performed a prospective randomized study of pelvic radiation with or without weekly cisplatin therapy during radiation followed by an extrafascial hysterectomy. Both progression-free survival and overall survival were significantly higher in the radiation plus cisplatin group at 4 years. Disease recurred in 37% of the radiotherapy-only group compared with 21% of patients given radiotherapy

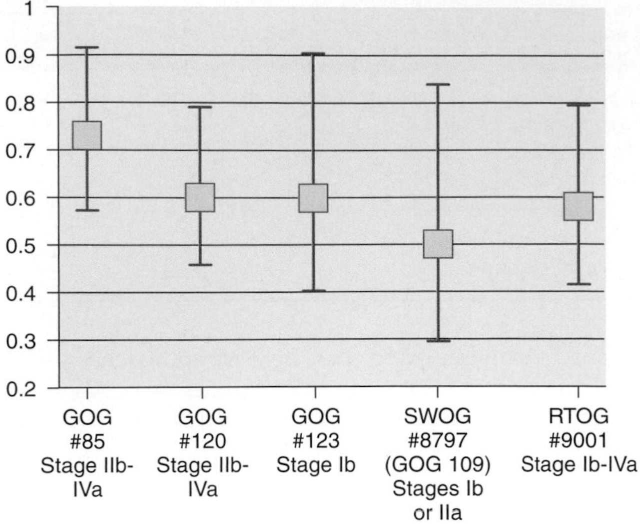

Figure 3–30 Relative risk estimate of survival from five phase III, randomized controlled clinical trials of chemoradiation in women with cervical cancer. (GOG, Gynecologic Oncology Group; RTOG, Radiation Therapy Oncology Group; SWOG, Southwestern Oncology Group.)

and cisplatin. With a median follow-up of 36 months, 83% survival was present in the combined therapy group vs 74% in the radiotherapy-alone group ($P = 0.008$).

In another GOG study, patients with stage IIb, III, or IVa cervical cancers were randomized to receive cisplatin alone; cisplatin, fluorouracil, and hydroxyurea; and hydroxyurea alone combined with radiation. All patients had negative para-aortic nodes. There were 526 women in the three-arm protocol, and both groups that received cisplatin had a higher rate of progression-free survival than the group that received hydroxyurea alone ($P < 0.001$ for both comparisons). Overall, survival was significantly better in these two groups ($P = 0.004$ and 0.002). The median follow-up time was 35 months. Survival was 66% and 67% for cisplatin groups vs 50% in the hydroxyurea group. Recurrences were less both locally and at distant site in the two cisplatin groups.

The study by the Radiation Therapy Oncology Group evaluated 386 patients with stages IIb through IVa with disease confined to pelvis (para-aortic nodes evaluated with lymphangiogram or retroperitoneal surgical exploration) or stage Ib or IIa if the tumor was > 5 cm or had biopsy-proven metastasis to pelvic lymph nodes. Details of accuracy of lymphangiogram or the number of para-aortic nodes under evaluation were not given. Patients were randomized to receive either 45 Gy to the pelvis and para-aortic nodes or 45 Gy to the pelvis alone plus two 5-day cycles of fluorouracil and cisplatin during the radiation treatment. The medical follow-up time was 43 months. Estimated accumulative survival at 5 years was 73% treated with radiation and chemotherapy compared with 58% in patients treated with radiation alone. The study is weighed toward stage I and II cancers (269 patients) compared with stage III–IVa (117 patients). When evaluating subsets of the data, the authors place IIb cancers in the same category as Ib and IIa, although their criteria for inclusion in the study are different. One wonders why IIb cancers

Table 3–16 FIVE PIVOTAL RANDOMIZED TRIALS OF CHEMORADIATION IN THE MANAGEMENT OF LOCALLY ADVANCED CERVICAL CANCER

Trial	Author	Year	FIGO stage	Arms	N	PFS at 4 yrs		OS at 4 yrs	
Intergroup	Peters et al	2000	Ia2–IIa	Adjuvant pelvic RT + cisplatin plus 5-FU	127	80%	$P = 0.003$	81%	$P = 0.007$
				Adjuvant pelvic RT alone	116	63%		71%	
						PFS at 4 yrs		OS at 4 yrs	
GOG 123	Keys et al	1999	Ib2*	Preoperative pelvic RT + cisplatin	183	80%	$P < 0.001$	86%	$P = 0.008$
				Preoperative pelvic RT	186	64%		72%	
						DFI at 5 yrs		OS at 5 yrs	
RTOG 9001	Morris et al	1999	Ib**–IVa	Pelvic RT + cisplatin plus 5-FU	193	67%	$P < 0.001$	73%	$P = 0.004$
				Pelvic RT plus para-aortic RT	193	40%		58%	
						PFS at 6 yrs		OS at 6 yrs	
GOG 85	Whitney et al	1999	IIb–IVa***	Pelvic RT + cisplatin plus 5-FU	177	60	$P = 0.033$	65	$P = 0.018$
				Pelvic RT + hydroxurea	191	48		50	
						PFS at 4 yrs		OS at 4 yrs	
GOG 120	Rose et al	1999	IIb–IVa***	Pelvic RT + cisplatin	176	60%	$P < 0.001$†	60%	$P = 0.002$ to 0.004†
				Pelvic RT + cisplatin plus 5-FU	173	60%		58%	
				Pelvic RT + Hydroxurea	177	45%		34%	

Intergroup: GOG 109/SWOG 8797/RTOG 91-12
*Negative nodes
**Ib lesions included bulky tumors as well as those with positive pelvic lymph nodes
***Negative para-aortic nodes
†Platinum-based regimens compared to hydroxurea
RT, radiation therapy; PFS, progression-free survival; OS, overall survival.

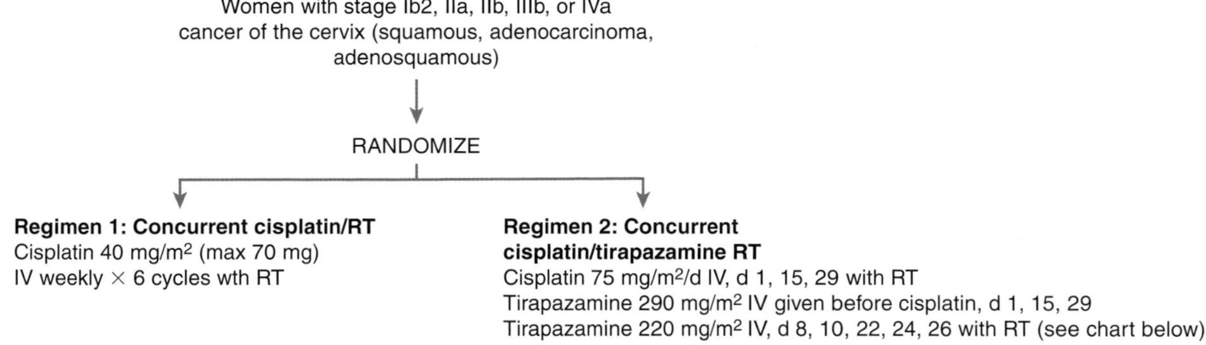

	Days				
	1	**8, 10, 12**	**15**	**22, 24, 26**	**29**
Tirapazamine	T1	T2 T2 T2	T1	T2 T2 T2	T1
Cisplatin 75 mg/m^2	X		X		X
RT	→	→	→	→	→

Figure 3–31 Schema for Gynecologic Oncology Group protocol 219.

were not included with stage III–IVa cancers. The overall survival of stage Ib–IIb cancers was 77% vs 58% ($P = 0.002$) of chemotherapy plus radiation vs radiation alone. The difference (63% vs 57% for stage III–IVa) is not statistically different ($P = 0.44$).

Two hundred and forty-one patients with stage Ia2, Ib, and IIa carcinoma of the cervix initially treated with radical hysterectomy and pelvic lymphadenectomy and who had positive pelvic nodes or positive margins or microscopic involvement of the parametrium were randomized to receive pelvic radiation with or without cisplatin and fluorouracil for 4 courses (SWOG study). Progression free survival at 4 years was 63% for radiation alone vs 81% for the combined therapy.

In another study by the GOG of stage IIb–IVa cervical cancer, 368 patients were randomized to pelvic radiation and either hydroxyurea or cisplatin and 5-fluorouracil. All had negative para-aortic nodes by surgical pathologic evaluation. At 6 years, overall survival was 59% vs 47% in the cisplatin plus 5-fluorouracil group compared with the hydroxyurea group.

Based on these studies, the National Cancer Institute issued a rare clinical announcement that strong consideration should be given to the incorporation of concurrent cisplatin-based chemotherapy with radiation therapy in women who required radiation therapy for treatment of cervical cancer. Because these studies suggest that cisplatin alone appears to be as effective as combination chemotherapy, concomitant cisplatin with radiation therapy now emerges as the treatment of choice when radiation is used in cervical cancer (Fig. 3–17).

Currently, the GOG is investigating the potential benefits of radiosensitizing chemotherapy using the combination of cisplatin (75 mg/m^2 every 14 days) and tirapazimine (TPZ) over that of weekly cisplatin (40 mg/m^2) in women with locally advanced cervical cancer receiving pelvic radiotherapy (GOG protocol 219, Fig. 3–31). TPZ is a bioreductively activated, hypoxia-selective antitumor agent of the benzotriazine series that increases cisplatin cytotoxicity both in vitro and in vivo. Two dosing schedules of TPZ are being employed: 290 mg/m^2 given on the days of cisplatin therapy, and 220 mg/m^2 given on days 8, 10, and 12 of each 14-day cycle.

Neoadjuvant chemotherapy

Although the combination of chemotherapy and radiation together is now the standard therapy for bulky (Stage Ib2) and locally advanced (Stage IIa > 4 cm, IIb–IVa) cervical carcinoma, some centers, especially those outside the USA, have explored giving chemotherapy before surgery or radiation in a neoadjuvant setting. The hypothesis is that upfront chemotherapy might reduce tumor volume and thereby increase operability or the effectiveness of radiation and thus increase cure rates. In a single institution prospective randomized study, 295 patients with stage IIb were randomized to surgery only, radiation alone, or both combined with neoadjuvant chemotherapy. At a mean of 84 months' follow-up, the survival for surgery and chemotherapy was 65%, radiation and chemotherapy 54%, 48% radiation alone, and 41% surgery alone. The best survival was in patients who received chemotherapy followed by surgery and radiation. Resectability was greater in the neoadjuvant and surgery group (80%) compared with the surgery-only group (56%), with $P < 0.0001$. Neoadjuvant chemotherapy plus surgery and radiation had a better survival rate in both tumors >5 cm and <5 cm compared with surgery and radiation.

In one of the first prospective randomized studies of neoadjuvant chemotherapy in early staged cervical cancer, Sardi and colleagues reported their final results in 205 stage Ib carcinoma of the cervix. Patients were treated with radical hysterectomy followed by 50 Gy radiotherapy to the pelvis with or without neoadjuvant chemotherapy. In patients with stage Ib1, neoadjuvant chemotherapy did not improve overall resectability or survival compared with those not receiving chemotherapy. In patients with stage Ib2, there was 83.6% (51 of 61) partial or complete response to chemotherapy. Overall survival after 9 years of follow-up was 61% for control group (no chemotherapy) and 80% for neoadjuvant group ($P < 0.01$). Resection was possible in 85% of control group and 100% in neoadjuvant group. When prognostic factors were evaluated in the operative specimen, VSI was found in 60% of control and non-responders to chemotherapy but in only 10% of the responders ($P < 0.009$). Parametrial infiltration was present in 34% of control patients, 30% non-responders, and only 2% of responders ($P < 0.0001$). Lymph node involvement was present in 41% of controls, 40% of non-responders, and 6% of responders ($P < 0.0001$). Local control was better in the neoadjuvant group compared with controls (6% vs 23% respectively, stage Ib2), although distant control was similar. Patients who responded to neoadjuvant therapy had an overall survival of 88% compared with 23% for non-responders. Interestingly, the stage Ib1, neoadjuvant groups had a 82% overall survival compared with 80% for stage Ib2. The control groups' survival was 77% and 61%, respectively. Neoadjuvant chemotherapy improved resectability and survival in the patients with stage Ib2. All patients received postoperative radiation. The impact of that therapy on patients compared with those who had surgery is unknown.

Suboptimal treatment situations

There are several situations in which patients with invasive cancer of the cervix receive suboptimal treatment:

1. cancer in a cervical stump;
2. inadequate surgery; and
3. poor vaginal geometry for radium.

Cancer that occurs in a cervical stump is fortunately a diminishing problem, because supracervical hysterectomies are performed less frequently. Carcinoma occurring in a cervical stump presents a special problem, because often an optimal dose of intracavitary radium cannot be applied because there is insufficient place to insert the central tandem, which contributes significantly to the radiation dose to the central tumor and to the pelvic sidewall. Radical surgery is also more difficult; the bladder and rectum firmly adhere to the stump and may adhere to each other. Also, the ureters are more difficult to dissect cleanly from the parametrial tissue because of fibrosis from the previous surgery. The net result is an increase in the risk of significant surgical complications involving the ureters, bladder, and rectum. In modern gynecologic surgery, supracervical hysterectomy is rarely indicated, although in recent years concerns regarding pelvic support and even sexual function have prompted some surgeons to consider the procedure.

In a report of the MD Anderson Hospital experience with 263 patients with carcinoma of the cervical stump, Miller and colleagues noted a 30% complication rate after full therapy with radiation. Urinary and bowel complications result from postsurgical adhesions, the absence of the uterus, which acts as a shield, and a tendency to emphasize external radiation therapy. We have had a similar experience, resulting in a preference for radical trachelectomy in cervical-stump patients in whom stage and medical conditions allow. The increased technical difficulty of performing such a procedure seems to be outweighed by the low complication rate and comparable survival of patients.

Inadequate surgery usually results when a simple hysterectomy is performed and frank invasive cervical cancer is subsequently discovered. This situation may occur because of poor preoperative evaluation or because the surgery was performed under emergency conditions without an adequate preoperative cervical evaluation. Such a situation may occur in a patient presenting with acute abdomen from ruptured tubo-ovarian abscesses. In any event, if an extensive cancer is found in the cervix, the prognosis is poor because optimal irradiation cannot be given with the cervix and uterus absent. An even more ominous situation occurs when a hysterectomy is performed with a "cut through" of the cancer; that is, the hysterectomy dissection passes through the cancer. The prognosis is uniformly poor in this event. In the examples just given, surgical cures are not obtained, and the probability of curative radiotherapy is greatly diminished.

In 1968, Durrance reported survival rates of 92–100% using postoperative radiation therapy in selected patients with presumed stage I or II disease after suboptimal surgery. Excellent survival rates were also reported by Andras and colleagues in 148 patients who had invasive cervical carcinoma found incidentally in the hysterectomy specimen. Of these patients, 126 were treated with postoperative radiation therapy. Patients with microscopic disease confined to the cervix had a 96% 5-year survival rate. Those with gross tumor confined to the cervix had an 84% 5-year survival. Patients with tumor cut through at the margins of surgical resection, but with no obvious residual cancer, had a 5-year survival rate of 87%. Patients with obvious residual pelvic tumor had a 47% 5-year survival rate. In 1986, Heller and colleagues reviewed the literature and reported equivalent survival rates in 35 patients who were also treated mainly with radiation.

Orr and colleagues have preferred radical parametrectomy, upper vaginectomy, and lymphadenectomy as the treatment of choice following a simple hysterectomy. We have also preferred this approach, particularly because many of these patients are young and desirous of preserving optimal sexual function. We are also concerned about postoperative small bowel adhesions and the difficulty of delivering effective irradiation to the medial parametria in the absence of a uterus. Survival rates with either approach appear to be exceptionally good; undoubtedly, this clinical situation creates a bias for smaller lesions that may be easier to eradicate.

The incidence of pelvic recurrence following irradiation alone for stages Ib, IIa, and IIb carcinomas of the cervix increases with the diameter of the tumor. Data from the MD Anderson Hospital showed an improved pelvic control rate, as well as a small increase in survival, when patients with the bulky, so-called barrel-shaped lesions were treated with preoperative irradiation followed by extrafascial hysterectomy. The subject continues to be controversial with conflicting studies in the literature. Gallion and colleagues reported on 75 patients with "bulky, barrel-shaped" stage Ib cervical cancer; 32 patients received radiation alone and 43 patients were treated with radiation followed by extrafascial hysterectomy. The incidence of pelvic recurrence was reduced from 19% to 2% and extrapelvic recurrence was reduced from 16% to 7% in patients treated by combination therapy, which produced no increase in treatment-related complications. On the other hand, Weems described 123 such patients treated from two different eras at his institution. Examination of pelvic control rates, as well as disease-free survival, showed no significant advantage in pelvic control, disease-free survival, or absolute survival for either treatment group when compared by stage and tumor size. Unfortunately, no large prospective randomized study has been done that could clarify this issue.

Adequate radiotherapy is also compromised in patients who have a vagina or cervix that cannot accommodate a complete radium application. This situation is encountered with atrophic stenotic pelvic structures. These patients are treated by inserting the tandem and ovoids in a compromised manner, such as insertion of the ovoids singly or independently of the central tandem. In any event, standard optimal doses are usually not obtained, and the possibility of sustaining a radiation injury is increased.

SURVIVAL RESULTS AND PROGNOSTIC FACTORS

Review of the annual reports on results of treatment of carcinoma of the uterus reveals a wide dispersion of 5-year recovery rates among several stages of carcinoma of the cervix. One can find data supporting any stand one wishes to take with regard to therapy. The overall survival rate in a cumulative series of 12,153 patients from 1987 to 1989 (23rd FIGO report on gynecologic cancer in 1998) was a 95% 5-year survival for both stage Ia1 and Ia2 (Fig. 3–32). Results may imply that one form of therapy has advantages over the other, but considering the rather wide dispersion that, in fact, may be unrelated to treatment, we must maintain collective openmindedness about the efficacy of individual therapeutic regimens. The best available figures for the two methods give results that are almost identical, and because the presence of other factors affect the samples being compared, large differences would be necessary to be significant. Individual physicians will probably continue to decide on the basis of personal preferences and comparison of complications and later disabilities.

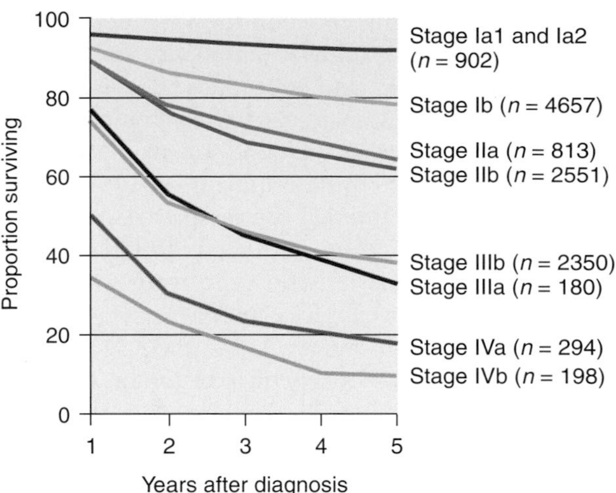

Figure 3–32 Overall survival from carcinoma of the cervix by stage, corrected for age and country. (From: Annual Report on Results of Treatment in Gynaecological Cancer, Vol 23, 1998.)

The recovery rates of patients with operative squamous cell carcinoma of the cervix depend on many factors, including the histologically documented extent of the carcinoma. Baltzer and associates studied 718 surgical specimens of patients with squamous cell carcinoma of the cervix. Lymphatic and blood vessel invasion significantly influenced survival, blood vessel invasion being much more ominous. In their study, 70% of the patients who demonstrated blood vessel invasion succumbed to the disease, whereas 31% of the patients demonstrating only lymphatic invasion succumbed to the disease process. Other studies have not found prognostic significance for vascular invasion. A definite linkage was noted between the size of the carcinomas and the frequency of metastases. Fuller and coworkers drew similar conclusions. In their study of 431 patients who underwent radical hysterectomy for stages Ib or IIa carcinoma of the cervix at Memorial Sloan–Kettering Cancer Center, they found 71 patients who had nodal spread that correlated closely with increased primary tumor size, extracervical extension of tumor, and the presence of adenocarcinoma. Although these factors were recognized as having prognostic significance, the authors were unable to demonstrate that these detrimental effects could be overcome by postoperative pelvic radiation. Patients receiving postoperative irradiation therapy seemed to have some better local control, but the problem of systemic spread of disease resulted in little overall improvement in survival. In a similar study, Abdulhayogu and associates reported on a series of patients with negative lymph nodes at the time of radical hysterectomy who subsequently developed recurrent disease. They too pointed out the histologic architecture of invasion as an important prognostic indicator. Recurrence was more likely in patients who had deep invasion of the cervical stroma, especially when it extended to the serosal surface (even when the parametria were not involved). Once again the volume of tumor correlated with the eventual prognosis for the patient. They suggested that these patients were in need of postoperative therapy, and radiation therapy for local control was recommended in the absence of any other demonstrated effective adjuvant modality for this set of circumstances. Gauthier and colleagues had similar results, and in a multifactorial analysis of clinical and pathologic factors, demonstrated that the depth of stromal invasion is the single most important determinant of survival.

The role of intraperitoneal tumor spread was evaluated by an Italian group. They evaluated 208 patients with advanced local disease who received neoadjuvant chemotherapy. There were 183 clinically responsive patients who underwent radical surgery; 7 (4%) and 13 (7%) showed macroscopic and microscopic peritoneal tumor, respectively. Multivariant analysis showed that the peritoneal tumor involvement, stage, pathologic parametrial involvement, as well as lymph node metastasis were independent factors associated with survival. About one quarter of those with pelvic lymph node metastasis had intraperitoneal involvement compared with only 6% of node-negative patients. If intraperitoneal disease was present, survival was similar, irrespective of stage (Ib–IIb compared with III–IVa).

A study from Austria evaluated 166 patients with stage Ib cancers treated with radical hysterectomy. In a multivariant analysis, microvessel density, lymph node involvement, tumor size, and postoperative radiation remained independent prognostic factors for survival. LSI failed to be a prognostic factor. Interestingly, patients with negative lymph nodes but increased microvessel density had similar survival to patients who were node positive but with low microvessel density. A study from Norway evaluated HPV DNA in 97 patients with squamous carcinoma (all stages). When corrected for stage and age, prognosis was significantly poorer for HPV-18 and -33-positive tumors; however, overall when all HPV-positive tumors were compared with HPV negative tumors, no survival difference was noted.

We have practiced a philosophy that patients with positive pelvic nodes have manifested aggressive disease, and postoperative chemoirradiation therapy should destroy microscopic residual disease in the pelvis following surgery and thus improve survival. Future prospective studies may influence this policy. To reduce possible bowel injuries as a result of postoperative radiation to the pelvis, we have also followed a practice of filling the pelvic basin with the redundant rectosigmoid (Fig. 3–33) so that small bowel loops are prevented from adhering to the operative site where they could be seriously injured by subsequent irradiation therapy. Rutledge and others have investigated the prognosis of young women with cervical cancer. In the report by Rutledge, young patients with advanced disease do poorly (stages IIb and IIIb), but those with high-volume stage Ib do better. On the other hand, Orlandi has reported on 264 patients with stages Ib and IIIa cervical squamous cancer, all of whom were treated with radical hysterectomy and pelvic lymphadenectomy. The 65 patients younger than 35 years of age had a higher incidence of lymph node metastases (46% vs 24%) and a lower 5-year survival (65% vs 76%) than the older group (199 patients). Although the conclusions are at variance, the subject matter appears to be worthy of further study.

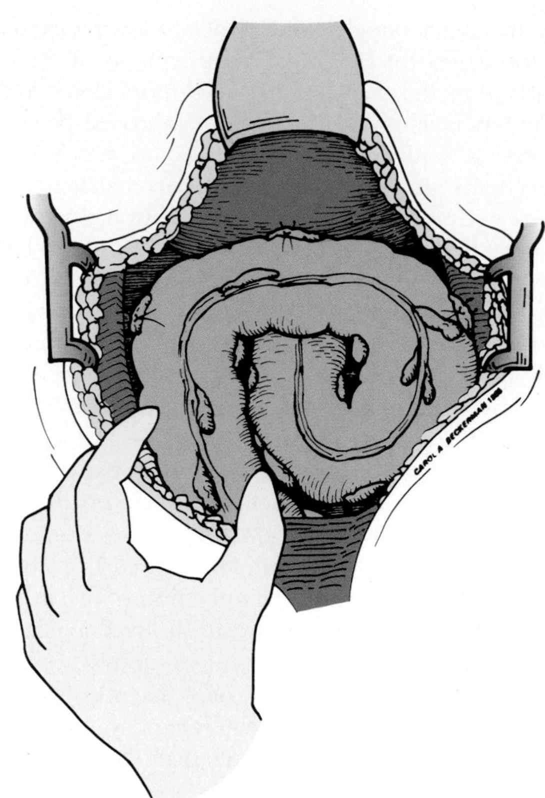

Figure 3–33 Technique of filling the pelvic basin with the redundant rectosigmoid. (From DiSaia PJ: Surgical aspects of cervical carcinoma. Cancer 48:548, 1981. Copyright © 1981 American Cancer Society. Reprinted by permission of Wiley-Liss, Inc., a subsidiary of John Wiley & Sons, Inc.)

When age was evaluated in the Annual Report, overall survival in stage I decreased with age. Stage II patients between 15 and 39 years of age had a worse survival rate compared with older patients. This was true for patients 30–49 years of age with stage IV cancers compared with patients of other ages. Mitchell and colleagues reviewed 398 patients with stages I–III cervical cancer of whom 338 patients were 35–69 years of age and 60 patients were ≥70 years old. Although elderly patients had a higher rate of comorbidity resulting in more frequent treatment breaks and less ability to receive definitive therapy with intracavity radiation, the 5-year actuarial disease-free and cause-specific survival rates were comparable between the two groups.

Sexual function after therapy for cervical cancer is a subject that is often ignored. Many patients never regain pretreatment sexual function. Andersen studied the sexual behavior, the level of sexual responsiveness, and the presence of sexual dysfunction of 41 women with uterine cancer compared with a matched group of healthy women. The two groups were similar until the onset of signs of disease, which sometimes occurred long before diagnosis, at which time the patients with cancer began experiencing significant sexual dysfunction. Sexual morbidity, therefore, begins actually in the prediagnosis period for many patients. Seibel reported on 46 patients who were interviewed >1 year after treatment for carcinoma of the cervix to establish the effects of radiation therapy and of surgical therapy on sexual feelings and performance. The irradiated patients experienced statistically significant decreases in sexual enjoyment, opportunity, and sexual dreams. The surgically treated group had no significant change in sexual function after treatment. Both groups experienced a change in self-image but did not feel that their partners or family viewed them differently. Myths about cancer and the actual effects of pelvic irradiation were found to have disrupted the sexual marital relationships of many women. Therapeutic programs with counseling and vaginal rehabilitation with the use of estrogen vaginal creams and possibly the use of dilators may be beneficial.

RECURRENT AND ADVANCED CARCINOMA OF THE CERVIX

Clinical profile

In the USA, the mortality from cervical cancer in 1945 was 15 of 100,000 female population. This had declined to approximately 4.6 of 100,000 by 1986 and 3.4 of 100,000 by 1991. It is unclear whether the mortality from cervical cancer is falling as a result of cervical cytologic screening and intervention at the in situ stage or whether cervical screening has caused an increase in the proportion of early stage cancer at diagnosis and registration. Following therapy for invasive disease, adequate follow-up is the key to early detection of a recurrence (Table 3–17). The yield of examinations such as IVP, CT scan, and chest roentgenogram in patients with initial early disease (stages I–IIa) is so low that many have discontinued their routine use. However, frequent Pap tests from the vaginal apex/cervix are recommended.

West studied the age of registration and the age of death of women with cervical cancer in South Wales. He found that the observed age at death was very close to 59 years regardless of stage and age at diagnosis. Although the 5-year survival rate of women with localized (early stage) cervical cancer was much higher than that of women with non-localized (late stage) cancer, the women with localized cancer tended to be younger than those with advanced cancer. Calculations of expected age at death of the whole population suggest that more than half the advantage in survival rate shown by women with early stage cancers is a result of the diagnosis of the former in younger women.

Christopherson and colleagues reported that the percentage of patients diagnosed as having stage I disease increased by 78% in the population studied from 1953 to 1965. The increase was most remarkable in younger women. The authors concluded that the major problem in cervical cancer control was the screening of older women. Older women had higher incidence rates; the percentage with stage I disease also decreased with each decade, reaching a low of 15% for those 70 years of age and older. These older women with cervical cancer are rarely screened and contribute heavily to the death rate. The initial advanced stage contributes heavily to the patient population with advanced recurrent cervical cancer. These patients, therefore, deserve very close post treatment observation in an effort to detect a recurrence in its earliest possible form.

It is estimated that approximately 35% of patients with invasive cervical cancer will have recurrent or persistent disease after therapy. The diagnosis of recurrent cervical cancer is often difficult to establish (Table 3–18). The optimal radiation therapy that most patients receive makes cervical cytologic findings difficult to evaluate. This is especially true immediately following completion of radiation therapy. Suit, using mammary carcinomas in C3H mice, demonstrated that persistence of histologically intact cancer cells in irradiated tissue was not indicative of the regrowth of a tumor. Radiobiologically, a viable cell is one with the capacity for sustained proliferation. A cell would be classified as non-viable if it had lost its reproductive integrity, although it could carry out diverse metabolic activities. This reproductive integrity was demonstrated by the transplantation "take" rate when histologically viable tumor cells were transplanted into a suitable recipient. It was evident from these experiments in mice that relatively normal-appearing cancer cells can persist for several months following radiation therapy but that these cells are "biologically doomed." Thus cytologic evaluation of a patient immediately after radiation therapy may erroneously lead to the supposition that persistent disease exists. In

Table 3–17 OPTIMAL INTERVAL EVALUATION OF CERVICAL CANCER FOLLOWING RADIOTHERAPY/SURGERY (ASYMPTOMATIC PATIENT*)

Year	Frequency	Examination
1	3 months	Pelvic examination, Pap smear
	6 months	Chest film, CBC,BUN, creatinine
	1 year	IVP or CT scan with contrast
2	4 months	Pelvic examination, Pap smear
	1 year	Chest films, CBC, BUN, creatinine, IVP or CT scan with contrast
3–5	6 months	Pelvic examination, Pap smear

* Symptomatic patients should have appropriate examination where indicated.
BUN, blood urea nitrogen; CBC, complete blood count; CT, tomography; IVP, intravenous pyelogram; Pap, Papanicolaou

Table 3–18 SIGNS AND SYMPTOMS OF RECURRENT CERVICAL CANCER

Weight loss (unexplained)
Leg edema (excessive and often unilateral)
Pelvic or thigh-buttock pain
Serosanguineous vaginal discharge
Progressive ureteral obstruction
Supraclavicular lymph node enlargement (usually on the left side)
Cough
Hemoptysis
Chest Pain

addition, subsequent evaluation of the irradiated cervix is also difficult because of the distortion produced in the exfoliated cells, often called *radiation effect.* Thus, histologic confirmation of recurrent cancer is essential. This can be accomplished by punch or needle biopsy of suspected areas of malignancy when they are accessible. An interval of at least 3 months should elapse following completion of radiation therapy. The clinical presentation of recurrent cervical cancer is varied and often insidious. Many patients develop a wasting syndrome with severe loss of appetite and gradual weight loss over a period of weeks to months. This is often preceded by a period of general good health following completion of radiation therapy. Because most recurrences of cancer occur within 2 years after therapy, the period of good health rarely lasts >1 year before the symptoms of cachexia become evident. Diagnostic evaluation at this time of suspected recurrence may include a chest roentgenogram and CT scan, complete blood count, blood urea nitrogen, creatinine clearance, and liver function tests.

Autopsy studies of the location of advanced recurrent and persistent disease have been reported (Figs. 3–34 and 3–35). After radical hysterectomy, about one-fourth of recurrences occur locally in the upper part of the vagina or the area previously occupied by the cervix. The location of recurrence after radiation therapy showed a 27% occurrence in the cervix, uterus, or upper vagina; 6% in the lower two-thirds of the vagina; 43% in the parametrial area, including the pelvic wall, 16% distant; and 8% unknown. Often one notes the development of ureteral obstruction in a patient who had a normal urinary tract before therapy. Although ureteral obstruction can be caused by radiation fibrosis, this is relatively rare, and 95% of the obstructions are caused by progressive tumor. Central disease may not be evident, and in the absence of other findings, a patient with ureteral obstruction and a negative evaluation for metastatic disease following therapy should undergo exploratory laparotomy and selected biopsies to confirm the diagnosis of recurrence. Patients with ureteral obstruction in the absence of recurrent malignancy should be considered for urinary diversion or internal antegrade ureteral stents.

The definition of primary healing after radiation therapy is a cervix covered with normal epithelium or an obliteration of the vaginal vault without evidence of ulceration or discharge. On rectovaginal examination, the residual induration is smooth with no nodularity. The cervix is no

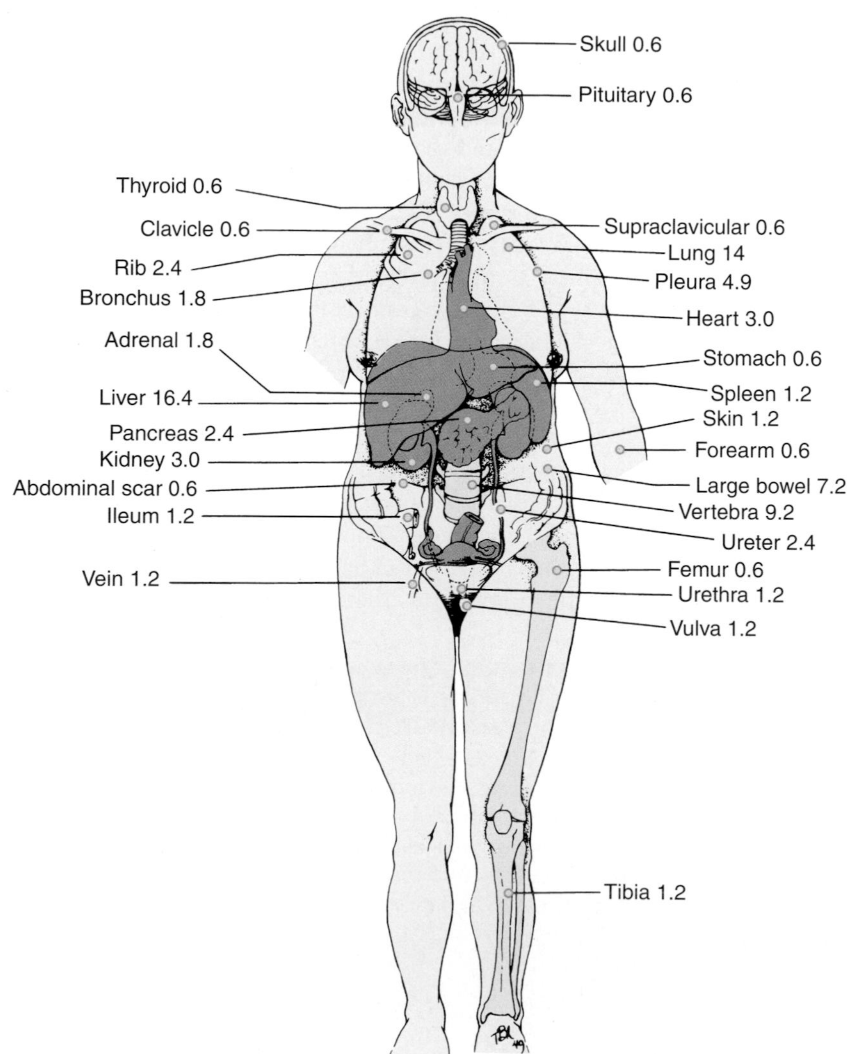

Figure 3–34 Metastatic sites of treated patients with cervical cancer and the percentage of involvement. (From Henriksen E: Lymphatic spread of cervix and corpus carcinoma. Am J Obstet Gynecol 58:924, 1949.)

>2.5 cm in width, and there is no evidence of distant metastasis. The definition of persistent disease after radiation therapy is:

1. evidence of a portion of the tumor that was clinically present before treatment, or
2. development of a new demonstrable tumor in the pelvis within the treatment period.

The definition of recurrence after radiation therapy is a regrowth of tumor in the pelvis or distally, which is noted after complete healing of the cervix and vagina.

Recurrence after surgery is defined as evidence of a tumor mass after all gross tumor was removed and the margins of the specimen were free of disease. Persistent disease after surgery is defined as persistence of gross tumor in the operative field or local recurrence of tumor within 1 year of initial surgery. A new cancer of the cervix would be a lesion that occurs locally at least 10 years after primary therapy.

The triad of weight loss accompanied by leg edema and pelvic pain is ominous. Leg edema is usually the result of progressive lymphatic obstruction, occlusion of the iliofemoral vein system, or both. The clinician should consider the possibility of thrombophlebitis, but recurrent cancer is more likely. Patients characteristically describe pain that radiates into the upper thigh either to the anterior medial aspect of the thigh or posteriorly into the buttock. Other patients describe pain in the groin or deep-seated central pelvic pain. The appearance of vaginal bleeding or watery, foul, vaginal discharge strongly suggests a central recurrence. These lesions are among the more readily detectable recurrent cervical cancers, and histologic confirmation is easily obtained.

Less than 15% of patients with recurrent cervical cancer will develop pulmonary metastasis. When this does occur, patients will complain of cough, hemoptysis, and occasionally chest pain. In many cases, there will be enlargement of supraclavicular lymph nodes, especially on the left side. Needle aspiration of enlarged lymph nodes can be accomplished easily and avoids the necessity for an open biopsy of the area.

In almost every case, the diagnosis of recurrent cervical cancer must be confirmed histologically. CT-directed needle biopsies have provided us with a tool that avoids

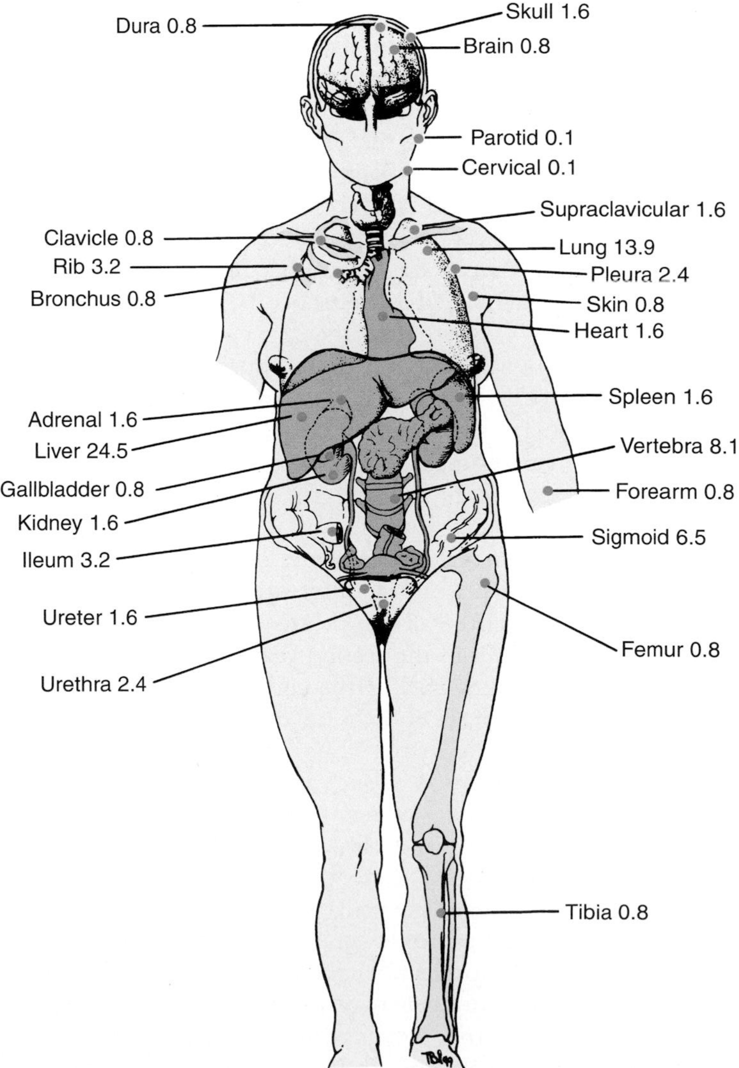

Figure 3–35 Metastatic sites of untreated patients with cervical cancer and the percentage of involvement. (From: Henriksen E: Lymphatic spread of cervix and corpus carcinoma. Am J Obstet Gynecol 58:924, 1949.)

the necessity of more elaborate operative procedures. In addition to the standard roentgenographic evaluations, such as IVP and chest roentgenogram, the clinician may find more sophisticated studies such as lymphangiography and MRI helpful in localizing deep-seated areas of recurrent cervical cancer.

Bony metastases presenting clinically are particularly rare. In a study of 644 patients with invasive cervical carcinoma, Peeples and coworkers were able to find only 29 cases of remote metastases. Of these, 15 were to the lungs, and only 12 were to the bone, which is an incidence of 1.8%. No bony metastases were found at initial staging and diagnosis. The earliest discovery of bone metastasis came 8 months after diagnosis. Therefore, a bone survey was not recommended as part of the staging examination for cervical cancer.

Blythe and associates reported on 55 patients who were treated for cervical carcinoma and who developed bony metastases. Roentgenograms were diagnostic in all except two of the patients. In 15 patients, a combination of radioactive scans and roentgenograms was used to establish the diagnosis. The most common mechanism of bony involvement from carcinoma of the cervix was extension of the neoplasia from periaortic nodes, with involvement of the adjacent vertebral bodies. The longest interval from the primary diagnosis until the discovery of bony metastases was 13 years. Sixty-nine percent of the patients were diagnosed within 30 months of initial therapy, and 96% died within 18 months. Of the 36 patients treated with radiation therapy, 4 received complete relief of symptoms, 24 gained some relief, and 8 received no relief.

Van Herik and colleagues examined the records of 2107 cases of cervical cancer for recurrence after 10 years. Sixteen (0.7%) patients had a recurrence 10–26 years after the initial therapy. Of these patients, 25% had bony metastasis or extension of the recurrence into bone. The finding of metastasis after 10 years correlates with the findings of Paunier and associates, who indicated that 92.5% of deaths resulting from carcinoma of the cervix occur in the first 5 years after diagnosis. In addition, their cumulative death rate curve was flat after 10 years.

Deaths resulting from cancer of the cervix occur most frequently in the first year of observation and decrease thereafter. About half of all the deaths occur in the first year after therapy, 25% in the second year, and 15% in the third year, for a total of 85% by the end of the third year. Because more than three-fourths of the recurrences are clinically evident in the first 2 years after initial therapy, post treatment evaluation done at frequent intervals during this critical period is mandatory. The patient should be examined every 3–4 months, and cervical cytologic testing should be done at these visits. In addition, particular attention should be paid to the parametria on rectovaginal examination to detect evidence of progressive disease. For several months after the completion of radiation therapy, the examiner may observe a progressive fibrosis in the parametria, creating the so-called horseshoe fibrosis. The amount of fibrosis may sometimes be alarming, but smoothness of the induration should be reassuring when compared with the nodular presentation of recurrent parametrial malignancy. Parametrial needle biopsies, with the patient under anesthesia, may be helpful when the palpatory findings are equivocal. Generous use of endocervical curettage at these follow-up visits is recommended, especially when central failure is suspected following radiation therapy. Every follow-up examination should include careful palpation of the abdomen for evidence of periaortic enlargement, hepatomegaly, and unexplained masses. Every follow-up examination should begin with a careful palpation of the supraclavicular areas for evidence of nodal enlargement. This frequently omitted portion of the examination will sometimes reveal the only evidence of recurrent disease.

The prognosis for the patient with recurrent or advanced cervical cancer depends on the location of the disease. Of those patients with recurrent cervical cancer, the most favorable for therapy after primary irradiation are those with a central recurrence. These patients are candidates for curative radical pelvic surgery, including pelvic exenteration. There will be further discussion of this group of patients later in this chapter. With the advent of sophisticated methods of radiation therapy, including improved methods of brachytherapy and supervoltage external irradiation therapy, patients with pure central recurrence have become a rarity.

Isolated lung metastases from pelvic malignancies have responded in very selected cases to lobectomy. Gallousis reported metastases to the lung from cervical cancer in 1.5% of 5614 cases reviewed, with solitary nodules present in 25% of the cases. A surgical attack for isolated pulmonary recurrence should be considered, especially if the latent period has been >3 years.

Other patients who deserve serious consideration are those with radiation bowel injury. Over the past decade, the limits of human tolerance to radiation therapy have been reached, with treatment techniques for advanced disease that include large extended fields to the periaortic area. Many patients with advanced stage primary lesions have been treated with large doses of pelvic radiation (6000–7000 cGy), often following intra-abdominal surgery. These techniques, as well as standard radiation therapy, can lead to a small but significant number of patients with chronic radiation injury to the large or small bowel. These patients often develop cachexia, which is indistinguishable from the clinical presentation of recurrent and progressive malignancy. These patients are often quickly and superficially diagnosed as having recurrent disease, and no further investigation is initiated. Careful investigation of these patients reveals a history of postprandial crampy abdominal pain causing anorexia and weight loss. The diagnostic evaluations discussed previously reveal no conclusive evidence of persistent malignancy. In most cases, these patients can be returned to health with appropriate bowel surgery, including internal bypass procedures. In every patient suspected of recurrent malignancy, an effort should be made to confirm this suspicion by biopsy (histologic confirmation), and patients who do not have a recurrence and who have radiation bowel injury should be identified.

Management

Prognosis

Persistent or recurrent carcinoma of the cervix is a discouraging clinical entity for the clinician, with a 1-year survival rate between 10% and 15%. Treatment failures are, as expected, much more common in patients with more advanced stages of the disease; therefore, most patients are unlikely candidates for a second curative approach with radical pelvic surgery. Cases of curative therapy applied to isolated lung metastases or lower vaginal recurrences are reported but occur rarely. Unfortunately, most recurrences are suitable for palliative management only (see Fig 3–17).

Radical hysterectomy

Radical hysterectomy has been reported as therapy for patients with a small recurrent cervical carcinoma following radiation. Coleman's series of 50 patients from the MD Anderson Hospital were treated with radical hysterectomy (type II or III). Severe postoperative complications occurred in 42% of these patients. Of these patients, 28% developed urinary tract injury. Survival was 90% at 5 years for patients with lesions <2 cm as opposed to 64% in patients with larger lesions. Excessive morbidity can be limited if an omental pedicle is placed at the operative site at the end of the procedure, bringing in a new blood supply to the operative field that has undergone previous radiation therapy.

Irradiation therapy

With recurrent disease outside the initial treatment field, irradiation is frequently successful in providing local control and symptomatic relief. External irradiation in moderate and easily delivered doses is usually effective in relieving pain from bone metastases. A dose of 3000 cGy delivered in over 2 to 3 weeks is often sufficient to relieve pain from vertebral column or long-bone metastases.

Höckel and associates reported their experience with a combined operative and radiotherapy (CORT) for recurrent tumors infiltrating the pelvic wall. Although the combination therapy is not new, these authors surgically remove the recurrence more radically than previously reported. The bony pelvis and neurovascular support of the leg is preserved. Implantation of guide tubes, which exit from the skin for brachytherapy, is done after resection of the tumor. Considerable pelvic reconstruction is usually done. Although the indications and procedure are evolving, in the first 48 patients treated, survival probabilities are 50% and 44% after 3 and 5 years, respectively.

Reirradiation of pelvic recurrences of cervical cancer occurring within the previously treated field is a subject of some controversy. The results following reirradiation of patients with recurrent cervical malignancy have varied considerably. Truelsen reported a 3-year cure rate of 1.7%. Murphy and Schmitz reported a 9% salvage rate in 1956, and Nolan and associates reported on the use of ^{60}Co teleradiation with a 25% salvage rate. At the Roswell Park Memorial Institute, Murphy adopted the policy of reirradiating patients with recurrence, delivering a full or almost full course for a second time. Among the highly selected series of 46 patients, 9–10% were living and well at the end of 5 years. Only seven patients had biopsy-proven recurrences before treatment. Others have shown that the results of reirradiation depend on many factors, including the site of recurrence, initial clinical stage, and initial dose of radiation therapy.

Careful perusal of these reports suggests that most patients who benefited from reirradiation were those who received less than optimal radiation during initial therapy. This set of circumstances has become rare in recent times, when more sophisticated radiotherapy is being delivered in many areas of the USA. Therefore, reirradiation for recurrent disease is usually not a worthwhile consideration. The potential for necrosis and fistula formation with even moderate doses of reirradiation in the pelvis by external or interstitial sources can give very unfavorable results.

Recurrence after radical hysterectomy has been treated with radiation. In a study from Holland, 271 patients were treated with radical hysterectomy and 27 recurred with 14 limited to the pelvis. Interestingly, adjuvant radiotherapy had been administered in 14 (52%) of the 27. In the four patients with isolated pelvic recurrence, only one died of disease, whereas all of the other patients with recurrences died of disease. The survivors were treated with radiation. In a study from the MD Anderson Cancer Center, 50 patients recurred after radical hysterectomy and were treated with radiation. Overall survival was 33%. In the 16 patients with central disease, 12 (69%) remained disease free. Survival of 29 patients with squamous carcinoma was 51% compared with 14% for the 14 patients with adenocarcinoma ($P = 0.05$).

Chemotherapy

The management of disseminated cervical cancer has improved with the development of modern chemotherapy. Fig. 3–17 reviews the treatment of metastatic disease.

Gynecologic Oncology Group studies

Patients with FIGO stage IVB disease and those who recur outside of the pelvis following primary therapy are destined to receive cisplatin-based palliative chemotherapy. Two recent randomized trials by the GOG (protocols 169 and 179) appear in Table 3–19. Although the combined regimen of cisplatin and paclitaxel employed in GOG 169 exhibited superior response rates (36% vs 19%), there were no singular differences demonstrated in an analysis of overall survival. There was, however, a statistically significant difference in median progression free survival (PFS) favoring the combination of paclitaxel plus cisplatin (4.8 months vs 2.8 months). Moving ahead, the GOG studied the MVAC regimen (methotrexate, vinblastine, doxorubicin, and cisplatin) and the combination

Table 3–19 GOG 169 AND 179. RECENT RANDOMIZED STUDIES BY THE GOG IN METASTATIC CERVICAL CANCER (FIGO IVB, RECURRENT)

GOG	Author	Year	Arms	N	PR%	CR%	Overall%		Median PFS		Median survival	
169	Moore et al	2004	cisplatin 50 mg/m^2 IV q 21 days	134	13	6	19	$P = 0.002$	2.8 m	$P < 0.001$	8.8 m	NS
			cisplatin 50 mg/m^2 IV q 21 days + paclitaxel 135 mg/m^2 24-hr infusion	130	21	15	36		4.8 m		9.7 m	
179	Long et al	2005	cisplatin 50 mg/m^2 IV q 21 days	145	10	13	13	$P = 0.004$	2.9 m	$P = 0.014$	6.5 m	$P = 0.017$
	Monk et al		cisplatin 50 mg/m^2 IV q 21 days + topotecan 0.75 mg/m^2 IV days 1–3	148	16	10	26		4.6 m		9.4 m	
			MVAC q 4 wks	63	9	13	22		4.4 m		9.4 m	

PR, Partial response; CR, Complete response; PFS, Progression-free survival; NS, not significant; m, months
MVAC, methotrexate, vinblastine, doxorubicin, cisplatin (note: this arm was closed due to unacceptable mortality; analysis forthcoming).
Long HJ 3rd, Monk BJ, Huang HQ, et al. Clinical results and quality of life analysis for the MVAC combination (methotrexate, vinblastine, doxorubicin, and cisplatin) in carcinoma of the uterine cervix: A Gynecologic Oncology Group study. Gynecol Oncol;100:537–543. 2006.

Table 3–20 GOG 179. IMPACT OF PRIOR RADIOSENSITIZING CISPLATIN IN GOG PROTOCOL 179

	No prior cisplatin			Pior cisplatin		
GOG Protocol 179	RR	PFS	OS	RR	PFS	OS
CDDP plus topotecan	39%	6.9 months	15.4 months	15%	3.8 months	7.9 months
CDDP	20%	3.2 months	8.8 months	8%	2.7 months	5.9 months
Hazards ratio, PFS	0.5	0.87				
Hazards ratio, OS	0.63	0.78				

CDDP, cisplatin; RR, response rate; PFS, progression-free survival (median); OS, overall survival (median).
From Long HJ 3rd, Bundy BN, Grendys EC Jr, Benda JA, McMeekin DS, Sorosky J, Miller DS, Eaton LA, Fiorica JV: Randomized phase III trial of cisplatin with or without topotecan in carcinoma of the uterine cervix: a Gynecologic Oncology Group Study. J Clin Oncol 23:4626, 2005.

of cisplatin and topotecan alongside cisplatin alone in GOG 179.

The MVAC arm was closed on July 23, 2001 by the Data Safety Monitoring Board of the GOG after four treatment-related deaths due to sepsis. The overall response rate for the three regimens ranged from 18% to 22%, although the complete response rate was higher for MVAC (13%) as compared to cisplatin (5%) and cisplatin plus topotecan (8%). Despite the early closure of the MVAC arm, the previously reported high response rate of 66% with this regimen in advanced cervical cancer was not verified. Additionally, there was no demonstrable survival advantage for those patients receiving MVAC as compared to those treated with cisplatin plus topotecan.

The comparison of cisplatin to cisplatin plus topotecan in protocol 179 has yielded the first study which has shown a statistically significant impact on the overall response rate, median PFS and median survival, with all outcome measures favoring the two-drug regimen. Because the survival curve by treatment demonstrates a separation of two months that was sustained until 18 months from study entry, the demonstrated 2.9-month improvement in median survival, although short, is taken to reflect a durable benefit of the combined regimen on long-term survival in the population studied. In addition, there was no decrease in overall quality of life among those treated with cisplatin and topotecan compared with cisplatin alone, although there was more cytopenia among those treated with the combination regimen.

It is now possible to predict failure in this population of patients. The site of recurrence appears to have prognostic significance with those that recur in a previously irradiated field having a worse prognosis. Among 110 patients with measurable disease in the pelvis in GOG protocol 149 (cisplatin plus ifosfamide with or without bleomycin), there were only 22 responders (40.2%), as compared to 69 responders among 177 patients with extrapelvic disease (78.2%; $P < 0.001$). Additionally, the time to recurrence was found to be a powerful prognostic factor in GOG 179. When analyzing the time from diagnosis to study entry for patients with recurrent disease and accounting for performance status, age and disease status at the time of study entry, it was noted that every six-month increment was associated with a 19% reduction of risk of progression, and a 21% reduction of risk of death, plateauing at 30 months.

A disparity in response rates was a phenomenon observed in GOG 179 between subjects who had been previously treated with radiosensitizing chemotherapy and those who had not (Table 3–20). Reduction in the activity of single agent cisplatin may be a consequence of the increasing use of radiosensitizing chemotherapy in primary treatment. Only 27% of patients treated on protocol 169 received prior radiosensitizing chemotherapy, as compared to 57% of patients on GOG 179, because the latter protocol was completed after concurrent chemoirradiation became standard in the upfront management of locally advanced disease. In other words, chemotherapy for patients

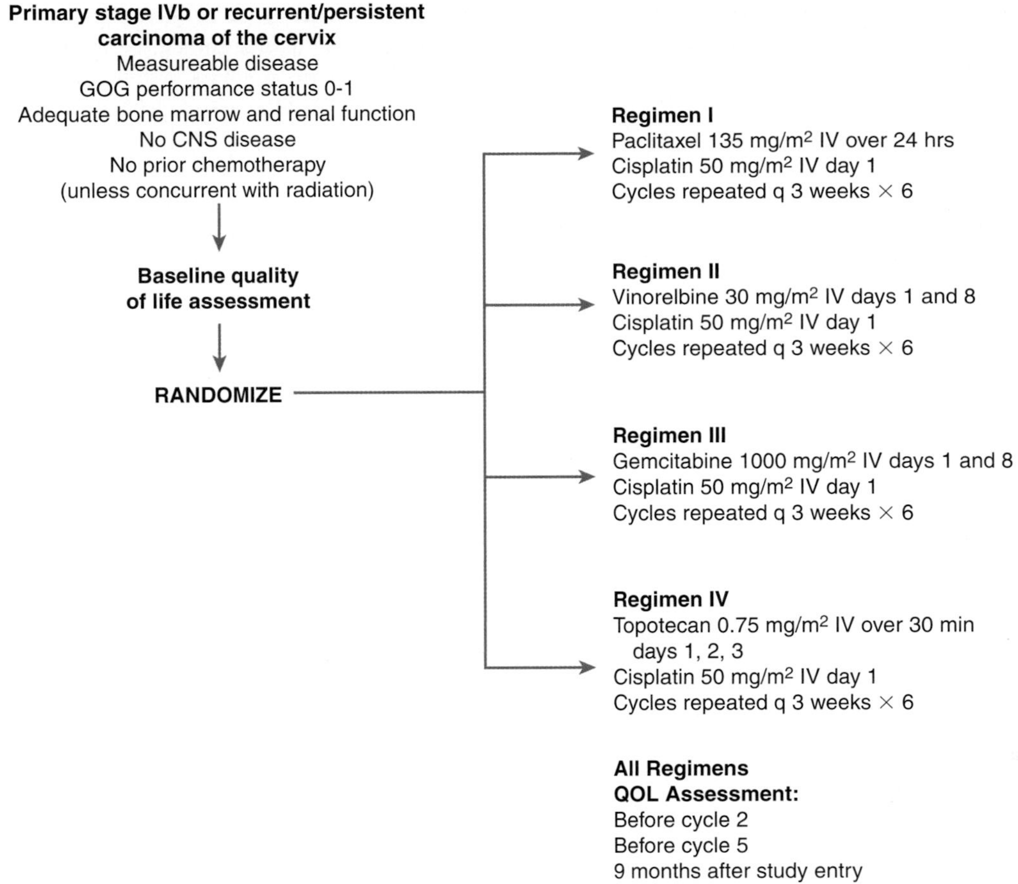

Figure 3–36 Treatment and assessment scheme for GOG 204.

on protocol 179 was for the most part "second-line" chemotherapy rather than the "first-line" chemotherapy patients on protocol 169 typically received. The implication is that if tumors have developed acquired resistance to cisplatin at the time of relapse, then the benefit observed in protocol 179 lies primarily with topotecan. Further testament to this hypothesis is the observation that in protocol 179, the response rate and PFS for the single agent cisplatin arm were lower than that observed in previous trials (GOG protocols 110, 149, and 169).

Finally, patient-reported quality of life (QOL) measures may become an important prognostic tool in advanced cervix cancer. When antineoplastic agents are combined, there is the potential for increased toxicity and QOL measures become critical endpoints. In GOG 179 after adjusting for treatment effect, age and baseline performance status, the baseline QOL scores (qualified by the Functional Assessment of Cancer Therapy-Cervix, FACT-Cx) was not found to be associated with the PFS, but was significantly associated with overall survival ($P = 0.002$).

Currently, the GOG is performing protocol 204, which constitutes the GOG's first randomized trial in advanced cervical cancer to only include cisplatin-based intravenous doublets, topotecan, paclitaxel, vinorelbine, and gemcitabine (Fig. 3–36). It is important to determine whether the activity of cisplatin plus paclitaxel in metastatic disease is sustained in the current era of concurrent chemoirradiation for locally advanced disease, and whether there is any survival advantage over the presumably more toxic regimen of cisplatin plus topotecan. The inclusion of a cisplatin-vinorelbine doublet is based on the 30% overall response rate of the combination in the phase II setting (GOG protocol 76Z), in which toxicity was only mild.

The need to study the cisplatin plus gemcitabine doublet is implicit. Through masked chain termination, which leaves a fraudulent base relatively resistant to excision repair by DNA repair enzymes, gemcitabine may overcome key mechanisms involved in the development of drug resistance. In addition, the synergy between gemcitabine and platinum observed in vitro allows for extrapolation to the clinical arena, generating an hypothesis that perhaps gemcitabine can both potentiate cisplatin cytotoxicity and reverse platinum-resistance, permitting reintroduction of platinum compounds in the salvage setting.

The inability of conventional cytotoxic agents to sustain long-term survival is likely multifactorial. Women suffering from metastatic cervical cancer typically have been previously irradiated (and therefore harbor radioresistant and chemoresistant tumor cell populations). Furthermore, such patients often have nephropathy as a consequence of a blocked kidney, limiting their ability to clear cytotoxic compounds from the bloodstream. Finally, recurrent tumors within the irradiated and therefore de-vascularized fields are difficult to bathe in chemotherapy. Clearly, this is a disease ideal for the critical study of immunotherapy, gene therapy and other novel biological stratagems.

Intra-arterial infusion for pelvic recurrence

Morrow and associates reported on a series of 20 patients from five institutions in the GOG who were treated with continuous pelvic arterial infusion of bleomycin for squamous cell carcinoma of the cervix recurrent after radiation therapy. All patients had documented unresectability and life expectancy of >8 weeks. Bleomycin was infused through a femoral arterial catheter introduced percutaneously and threaded into the lower aorta to a position between the inferior mesenteric artery and the aortic bifurcation. A few patients were treated via bilateral hypogastric artery catheters inserted at the time of exploratory laparotomy. A continuous infusion of bleomycin (20 mg/m^2/wk) for a minimum of 10 weeks or a total cumulative dose of 300 mg was given by means of low-flow portable infusion pumps. Infusion was discontinued if evidence of pulmonary toxicity appeared. Of the 20 patients studied, 10 had a moderate to severe degree of toxicity. Sixteen evaluable patients were available and no complete responses were observed. Only two partial responses were noted among 20 patients. The mean survival time was 7 months, with a range from 1–19 months. The two patients who exhibited partial tumor responses survived for 5 and 8 months, respectively. The authors concluded that continuous arterial infusion of bleomycin is not helpful in the management of squamous cell carcinoma of the cervix recurrent in the pelvis after radiation therapy.

Lifshitz and associates reported on 14 patients with a histologically confirmed recurrent pelvic malignancy who were treated with 44 courses of intra-arterial pelvic infusion of methotrexate or vincristine. Tumor regression was observed in 3 of 14 patients (21.4%). In five patients, there were major complications related to 28 intra-arterial catheter placements. The authors concluded that the value of intra-arterial infusion chemotherapy in gynecologic cancer is limited.

Intra-arterial infusion for pelvic recurrence has also been attempted with cisplatin with very discouraging results. Explanations for these failures of pelvic infusion have varied. Some believe that the malignant cells are protected in a cocoon of fibrosis, whereas others believe that those cells that have survived initial radiation therapy are resistant to chemotherapy delivered by any route. Intra-arterial infusion for large primary lesions that are considered too large for cure by radiation alone may be valuable as initial therapy, shrinking the tumor for improved presentation to the radiotherapist.

Biologic therapy on the horizon

I. Angiogenesis inhibitors

Biologic therapy in the form of angiogenesis inhibitors may be useful in retarding tumor growth and progression and even eliminating small volume residual disease. Evidence that angiogenesis plays an important role in locally advanced cervical cancer has accumulated in recent years. In one study of 111 patients, Cooper et al identified tumor angiogenesis (as reflected by the tumor microvessel density, MVD) as a significant prognostic factor within a Cox multivariate analysis, where it was associated with poor loco-regional control and overall survival. Conversely, among 166 women who underwent radical hysterectomy for stage Ib tumors, Obermair et al demonstrated enhanced 5-year survivorship when the MVD was <20 per high power field (HPF) (90% vs 63% with MVD >20 HPF). The vascular endothelial growth factor (VEGF) receptor expression has also been shown to correlate with MVD in cervical carcinomas.

Neutralizing anti-VEGF monoclonal antibodies have demonstrated therapeutic activity in a variety of preclinical solid tumor models. Bevacizumab (rhuMAb VEGF) is a recombinant humanized version of a murine anti-human VEGF monoclonal antibody, and has been advanced into clinical development by Genentech, Inc. to induce tumor growth inhibition in patients with solid tumors and for use in combination with cytotoxic chemotherapy to delay the time to progression in patients with metastatic solid tumors. In a recent study comparing carboplatin and paclitaxel with and without bevacizumab, investigators found that the addition of bevacizumab prolonged survival by 20% in patients with advanced or metastatic non-small-cell lung cancer leading to its approval by the USFDA in this disease. In another pivotal trial, 800 patients with previously untreated metastatic colorectal cancer were randomized to receive the Saltz regimen (irinotecan, 5-fluorouracil, and leucovorin, IFL) with either bevacizumab or placebo. Patients who received IFL plus bevacizumab survived a median of 20.3 months while those who received IFL plus placebo had a median survival of 15.6 months. This was the first phase III trial of an anti-angiogenesis strategy to treat human cancer. Monk is conducting a phase II evaluation of bevacizumab in cervical cancer within the GOG (protocol 227C). This immunologic molecule is being administered at a dose of 15 mg/kg intravenously on a 21-day cycle.

II. Therapeutic HPV vaccine

Therapeutic vaccines target virus-infected cells using epitopes of major histocompatibility complex (MHC)-processed peptides. Through interaction with CD8+ lymphocytes and MHC I pathways, they engage the cellular machinery resulting in production of cytotoxic T lymphocytes. The HPV oncoproteins, E6 and E7, can be targeted for the development of antigen-specific vaccination. Molecular strategies to design a therapeutic vaccine can be based on bacterial or viral vectors, peptides, proteins, DNA, and even dendritic cells. They may be useful in inducing regression and/or halting progression of preinvasive disease and/or eradicating subclinical residual neoplastic disease following therapy.

With respect to prophylactic HPV vaccines; in 2003 etc, in 2003 the WHO convened a gathering of experts from both developing and developed countries to identify the appropriate endpoint measurements for HPV vaccine efficacy. The general consensus was that it would be desirable to have a globally-agreed, measurable efficacy endpoint for considering deployment of HPV vaccines in public health settings. Because of the temporal lag between infection and the manifestation of invasive carcinoma, it was determined that a surrogate endpoint would be used to define the efficacy of HPV vaccines. Since persistent infection with the same high-risk HPV subtypes is considered a predictor for both moderate or high-grade cervical dysplasias and invasive cervical cancer, it was determined that CIN, rather than invasive cancer, would serve as the endpoint following HPV vaccine introduction.

Garcia et al from the University of Arizona conducted a randomized, multicenter, double-blind, placebo-controlled trial in 161 women with biopsy-confirmed CIN II-III. Subjects received three intramuscular doses of placebo or ZYC101a, a vaccine containing plasmid DNA-encoding fragments derived from HPV 16/18 E6 and E7 oncoproteins. The vaccine was well tolerated and had demonstrable efficacy in promoting resolution of CIN II–III in women younger than 25 years. Recently, Einstein et al presented data from their phase II trial employing the novel therapeutic vaccine, HspE7. The fusion protein consists of an M. bovis BCG heat shock protein (Hsp65) covalently linked at its C terminus to the entire sequence of HPV 16 E7. With an excellent safety profile on record, 32 HIV-negative women with CIN III were vaccinated. The investigators observed a 48% resolution of CIN III, 19% partial responses, and 33% of subjects with stable disease over a four-month follow-up period.

MANAGEMENT OF BILATERAL URETERAL OBSTRUCTION

The patient with bilateral ureteral obstruction and uremia secondary to the extension of cervical cancer presents a serious dilemma for the clinician. Management should be divided into two subsets of patients:

1. those who have received no prior radiation therapy; and
2. those who have recurrent disease after pelvic irradiation.

The patient who has bilateral ureteral obstruction from untreated cervical cancer or from recurrent pelvic disease after surgical therapy should be seriously considered for urinary diversion followed by appropriate radiation therapy. The salvage rate among this group of patients is low but realistic. Placement of antegrade ureteral stents should be attempted. When this is not possible, our preference has been to make a urinary conduit, anastomosing both ureters into an isolated loop of ileum (Bricker procedure) or creating one of a variety of continent pouches from a segment of bowel. We have also used these procedures in patients who had vesicovaginal fistulas secondary to untreated cervical malignancies. The ease with which pelvic radiation therapy can be optimally delivered is facilitated when the urinary diversion is performed before the irradiation is begun. In our experience, placement of urinary stents cystoscopically as an interim relief of the obstruction has been associated with multiple problems, leading us to favor the complete urinary diversion or antegrade ureteral stents. The traditional retrograde urinary stents are difficult to place bilaterally, and their presence in the ureter and bladder during the weeks to months of radiation therapy invariably leads to acute and chronic urinary tract infections. Interventional radiology with the use of percutaneous nephrostomy has created a reasonable option for these patients. Coddington and others have reported acceptable results after placement of internal ureteral stents via percutaneous nephrostomy. Patients require only local anesthesia for this procedure. Our experience has been favorable also, and an attempt at placement of these antegrade stents seems appropriate in patients with obstruction only and no vesicovaginal fistula before resorting to a urinary diversion.

The patient with bilateral ureteral obstruction (Fig. 3–37) following a full dose of pelvic radiation therapy is an even more complicated problem. Less than 5% of these patients will have obstruction caused by radiation fibrosis, and often this group is difficult to identify. However, simple diversion of the urinary stream in this subset of patients is lifesaving; therefore, all patients must be considered as possibly belonging to this category until recurrent malignancy is found. When the presence of recurrent disease has been unequivocally established, the decision process becomes difficult and somewhat philosophical. Numerous studies suggest that "useful life" is not achieved by urinary diversion in this subset of patients. Brin and colleagues reported on 47 cases (5 with cervical cancer) of

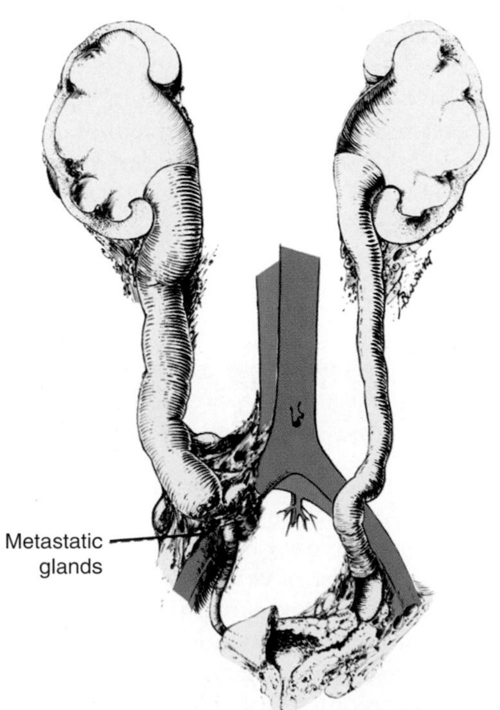

Figure 3–37 Hydroureters bilaterally secondary to a side wall recurrence on the patient's right and a parametrial recurrence on her left.

ureteral obstruction secondary to advanced pelvic malignancy. The results of this report are discouraging; the average survival time was 5.3 months, with only 50% of the patients alive at 3 months and only 22.7% alive at 6 months. After the diversion, 63.8% of the survival time was spent in the hospital. Delgato also reported on a group of patients with recurrent pelvic cancer and renal failure who underwent urinary conduit diversion. His results showed no significant increase in survival time.

It has been suggested that these patients should never undergo urinary diversion, because a more preferable method of expiration (uremia) is thus eliminated from the patient's future. It is obvious that these decisions should be made in consultation with the family and even with the patient, if possible. The decision must be heavily shared by the physician, but the attitudes of patient and family must serve as a guide. These attitudes can, in most cases, be perceived without transferring the decision-making process entirely to the family or the patient. As more sophisticated methods of chemotherapy evolve, the option for diversion may become more suitable. There are patients who need additional time to settle personal matters, and diversion with effective chemotherapy may result in a reasonable extension of life. However, in most cases, the avoidance of uremia results in an accentuation of the other clinical manifestations of recurrent pelvic cancer (i.e., severe pelvic pain, repeated infections, and hemorrhage). Pain control and progressive cachexia plague the physician and the patient. Episodes of massive pelvic hemorrhage are associated with difficult decisions for transfusion. An extension of the inpatient hospital stay is inevitable, and the financial impact that this may have on the patient and her family should also be considered.

Newer techniques, where placement of permanent ureteral stents via both the cystoscope and percutaneous insertion, have resulted in new options for this difficult clinical problem. Percutaneous placement of double J tubes with one end in the bladder and one end in the renal pelvis is now possible in many patients. As stated earlier, this is especially advantageous in patients who have bilateral ureteral obstruction before any therapy, when radiation therapy may be very useful as a palliative procedure.

PELVIC RECURRENCE AFTER SUBOPTIMAL SURGERY

A few patients who have been treated by inadequate surgery or radical hysterectomy will have isolated pelvic recurrences. These patients are candidates for radiation therapy, and this should consist of external irradiation followed by appropriate vaginal or interstitial therapy. In recent years, vaginal recurrences have been more successfully approached by use of interstitial irradiation after optimal external irradiation. The geometry of the postsurgical vagina with recurrence is such that standard vaginal applicators are often not suitable for optimal therapy. These patients are, of course, at higher risk for radiation injury because of the antecedent radical surgery. An open implant procedure, as described in Chapter 9, is often prudent.

PELVIC EXENTERATION

Extended or ultraradical surgery in the treatment of advanced and recurrent pelvic cancer is an American invention made possible by advances in the ancillary sciences that support the surgical team. The natural history of many pelvic cancers is that they may be locally advanced but still limited to the pelvis. They thus lend themselves to radical resection, unlike most other malignancies. In 1948, Brunschwig introduced the operation of pelvic exenteration for cancer of the cervix (Fig. 3–38). Since then, extensive experience with pelvic exenteration has been accumulated, and the techniques as well as patient selection have steadily improved so that now, 50 years later, this procedure has attained an important role in the treatment of gynecologic malignancies for a selected group of patients. Although pelvic exenterative surgery was subjected to severe initial criticism, it is now accepted as a respectable procedure that can offer life to selected patients when no other possibility of cure exists. The criticism of this procedure has been lessened by steadily improving mortality and morbidity and a gratifying 5-year survival record. Most important, however, patients who survive this procedure can be rehabilitated to a useful and healthful existence.

Although pelvic exenteration has been used for various pelvic malignancies, its greatest and most important role is in the treatment of advanced or recurrent carcinoma of the

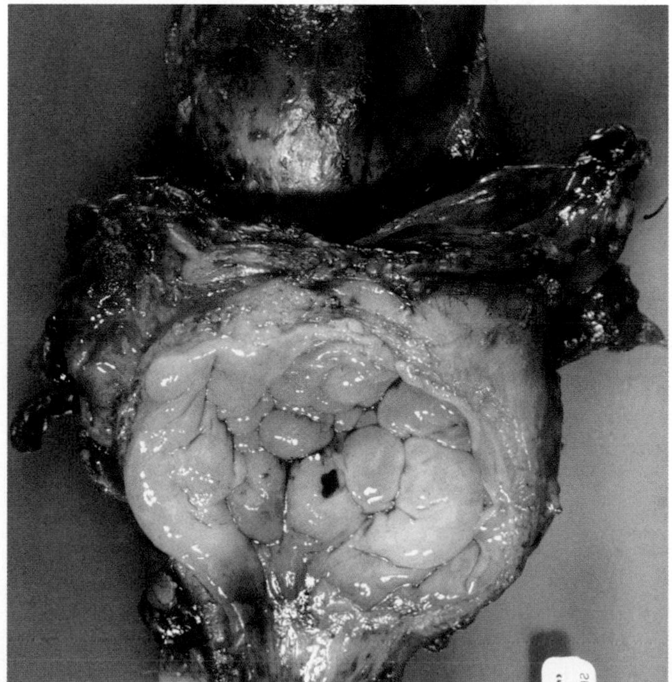

Figure 3–38 Specimen from an anterior exenteration done for recurrent cervical carcinoma; the specimen consists of the uterus, vagina, and bladder (the anterior wall has been opened to expose bullous edema of the trigone).

cervix. Total exenteration (Fig. 3–39) with removal of the pelvic viscera, including the bladder and rectosigmoid, is the procedure of choice for carcinoma of the cervix recurrent or persistent within the pelvis after irradiation. In very selected cases, the procedure may be limited to anterior exenteration (Fig. 3–40) with removal of the bladder and preservation of the rectosigmoid or posterior exenteration (Fig. 3–41) with removal of the rectosigmoid and preservation of the bladder. Cogent objections have been raised regarding these limited operations, especially in patients with carcinoma of the cervix recurrent after irradiation, because of the increased risk of an incomplete resection. In addition, those patients in whom the bladder or rectum is preserved often have multiple complications and malfunctioning of the preserved organ. Consequently, some surgeons have completely abandoned subtotal exenterations, and most oncologists use them very selectively.

One of the greatest technical advances in the evolution of pelvic exenteration is the intestinal conduit for diversion of the urinary stream. Originally, Brunschwig transplanted the ureters into the left colon just proximal to the colostomy, thus creating the so-called wet colostomy. The complication rate from this procedure, especially electrolyte imbalance and severe urinary tract infections, was unacceptable. We are indebted to Bricker for popularizing the use of an ileal segment conduit for urinary diversion. The

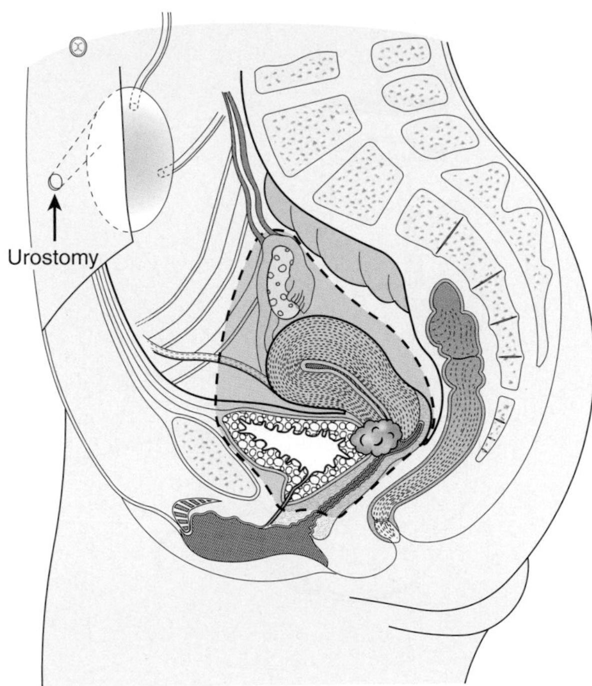

Shaded tissue within the dashed outline is permanently removed.

Figure 3–40 Anterior exenteration with removal of all pelvic viscera except the rectosigmoid. The urinary stream is diverted into an ileal or sigmoid conduit or a continent pouch. (Redrawn from DiSaia PJ, Morrow CP, Townsend DE: Cancer of the vulva. Calif Med 118:13, 1973.)

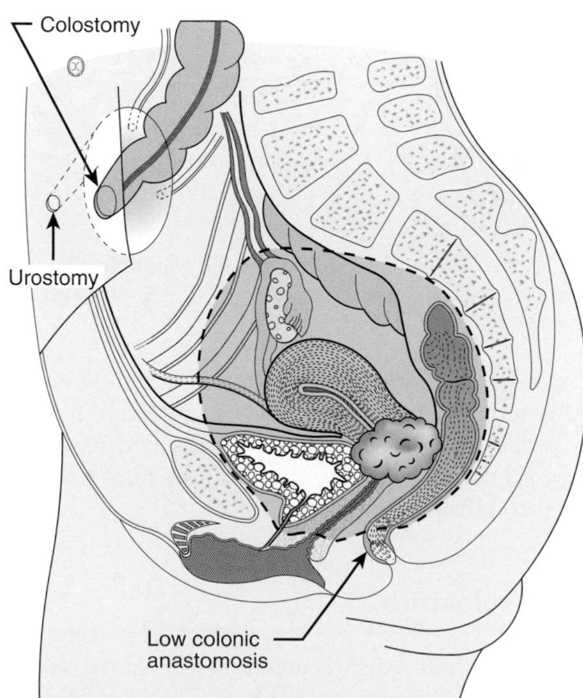

Shaded tissue within the dashed outline is permanently removed. Unshaded tissue within the dashed outline is first removed and then reconstructed.

Figure 3–39 Total exenteration with removal of all pelvic viscera. Fecal stream is diverted via a colostomy, and urinary diversion is via an ileal or sigmoid conduit or a continent pouch. (Redrawn from DiSaia PJ, Morrow CP, Townsend DE: Cancer of the vulva. Calif Med 118:13, 1973.)

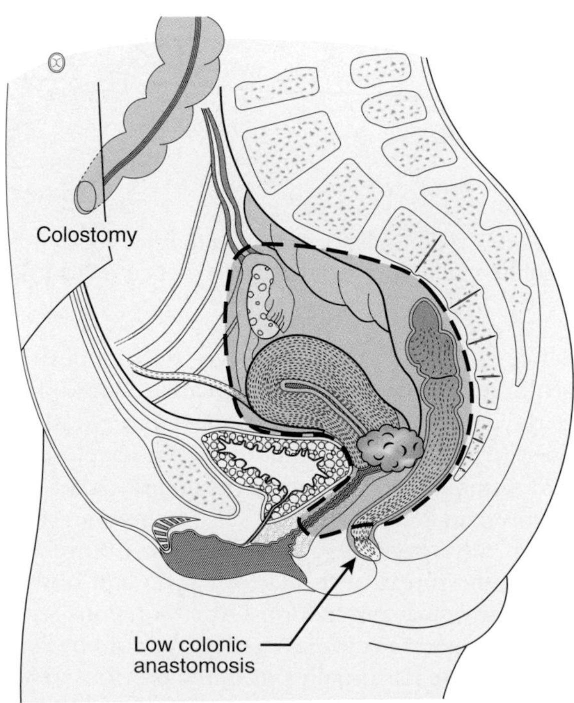

Shaded tissue within the dashed outline is permanently removed. Unshaded tissue within the dashed outline is first removed and then reconstructed.

Figure 3–41 Posterior exenteration with removal of all pelvic viscera except the bladder. The fecal stream is diverted via a colostomy. (Redrawn from DiSaia PJ, Morrow CP, Townsend DE: Cancer of the vulva. Calif Med 118:13, 1973.)

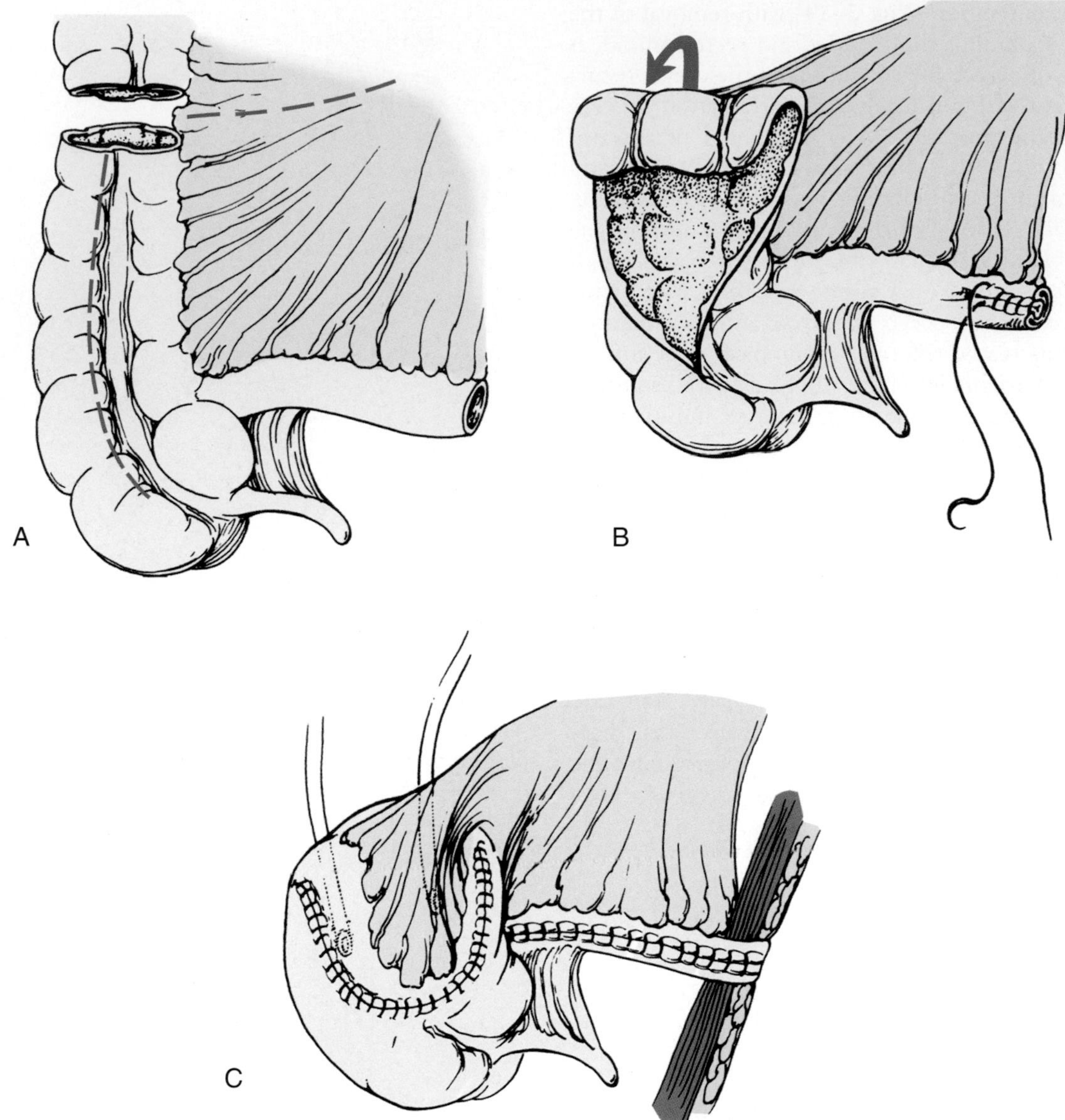

Figure 3–42 *A-C,* Construction of an Indiana pouch from the colon and the terminal ileum. (From: Amis ES, Newhouse JH, Olsson CA: Continent urinary diversions: Review of current surgical procedures and radiologic imaging. Radiology 168:395–401, 1988.)

incidence of both postoperative pyelonephritis and hypochloremic acidosis has been greatly reduced. Furthermore, the patients are dry and comfortable and, therefore, more easily rehabilitated. Some surgeons have used a segment of sigmoid colon as a urinary conduit rather than the small bowel in selected cases. This technique offers the additional advantage of avoiding a small-bowel anastomosis and the threat of fistula formation and obstruction attending any such procedure. Other surgeons have preferred the transverse colon as the segment of bowel for the conduit, because it is usually out of the previous irradiation field. This technique may avoid some of the problems that can be associated with utilizing irradiated segment of bowel for reconstructive surgery. More recent developments have resulted in several techniques for creation of a continent reservoir, again utilizing a segment of bowel (Fig. 3–42). Another significant advancement in surgical technique of these patients is the use of the intestinal stapling device. Whereas a permanent colostomy was a standard part of the exenterative procedure, today, it is rare. In many, if not most, cases, reanastomosis with the end-to-end anastomosis stapler can be performed and the fecal stream continues through the anus.

Patient selection

Only a few patients with recurrent cancer of the cervix are suitable for this operation (Table 3–21). Metastases outside the pelvis, whether manifested preoperatively or discovered at laparotomy, are an absolute contraindication to pelvic exenteration. The triad of unilateral leg edema, sciatic pain, and ureteral obstruction is pathognomonic of recurrent and unresectable disease in the pelvis. The triad must be complete, however, to be entirely reliable. Weight loss, cough, anemia, and other aberrations suggestive of

Table 3–21 MD ANDERSON HOSPITAL CENTRAL RECURRENCE RATE FOR CARCINOMA OF THE CERVIX FOLLOWING TREATMENT WITH RADIATION THERAPY

Stage I	1.5%
Stage IIb	5%
Stage IIIa	7.5%
Stage IIIb	17%

advanced disease are not sufficient justification by themselves to discontinue efforts toward surgical management. Obesity, advanced age, and systemic disease may interdict extensive surgery in direct relation to the severity of these factors. Some patients are unsuitable because of psychological reasons, and a number of women, who are otherwise candidates for pelvic exenteration, elect to accept the fate of unresected recurrence. If the time from primary treatment to recurrence is short (<2 years), this usually indicates aggressive biologic activity of the tumor and resectability is usually limited.

Although the pelvic examination plays a key role in the preoperative assessment of the patient, the examiner's impression of resectability must be tempered by the knowledge that errors are common. A small central lesion with freely mobile parametria reliably demonstrates resectability; however, immobility can be caused by radiation fibrosis or pelvic inflammatory disease (e.g., old salpingitis, inflammation from uterine perforation). Consequently, even when the disease seems inoperable on pelvic examination, if other factors are favorable, one should proceed with the investigation and exploratory laparotomy to avoid the error of a premature decision. Obviously, in many cases the finest clinical judgment must be used to avoid rejection of a potentially curable patient and also to prevent, as often as possible, subjection of an unsuitable patient to the anguish, fears, and false hopes of prolonged preparation for a fruitless operation.

Evaluation studies before surgery include chest film, CT scan of the abdomen and pelvis with intravenous contrast, creatinine clearance, liver function tests, and assessment of the patient's hemostatic mechanism. Any suspected disease outside the pelvis noted on any of the diagnostic studies should prompt an attempt at confirmation using a fine needle biopsy technique. Bone survey and liver scan are not part of the "routine" evaluation.

Preparation for pelvic exenteration is often traumatic to patients with recurrent cervical cancer, especially when the procedure is aborted. The increased use of CT-directed fine-needle aspirants has contributed greatly to lowering the fraction of patients explored who are found to be unexenterable. In a study by Miller, patients who underwent an aborted exploration were younger (median age of 49 years) than patients undergoing exenteration (median age of 54 years). On the other hand, the ratio of exenteration to aborted procedures was 1.57 among patients between the age of 30 and 39 to 3.26 in the age range 60–69. The reason for aborting the exenteration was the persistence of peritoneal tumor spread in 42% of the patients. Peritoneal cytology was predictive of peritoneal disease only in patients with adenocarcinoma. The procedure was aborted for nodal disease in 41% of patients. Parametrial fixation and other reasons for aborting the surgery made up the remaining 17%.

At laparotomy, the entire abdomen and pelvis are explored for evidence of metastatic and intraperitoneal cancer (Fig. 3–43). The liver should be carefully inspected visually and by palpation. The lymph nodes surrounding the lower aorta are the first to be sampled if the exploration of the abdomen has revealed no evidence of disease. If the lower aortic area findings are negative, a bilateral pelvic lymphadenectomy is performed. There have been almost no survivors among those patients who have undergone pelvic exenteration with multiple grossly positive pelvic wall nodes. Therefore, immediate frozen section analysis of the pelvic wall nodes is necessary to determine whether the resection should continue.

In a series of approximately 200 patients undergoing pelvic lymphadenectomy, Ketcham and associates found a positive pelvic lymph node after radiation therapy in only one 5-year survivor. In a similar series by Barber from Memorial Hospital, 148 patients with radiation failures undergoing pelvic exenteration were found to have positive nodes at the time of surgery, and only four of these patients survived for 5 years. Creasman and Rutledge suggested a slightly more optimistic view of patients with positive lymph nodes who had undergone pelvic exenteration for recurrent cervical cancer following pelvic irradiation. However, in their series most survivors with positive nodes had only microscopic disease in the nodes. Furthermore, in almost every case in the literature reported in detail of survival after exenteration for recurrent squamous cell carcinoma of the cervix in which there was a positive pelvic node, the nodal disease was not only microscopic but also unilateral.

Strenuous efforts have been made to decrease the permanent morbidity and increase patient acceptance of pelvic exenteration by tailoring the procedure to the known extent of the patient's disease. Although it is rarely justifiable to salvage the bladder because of its natural anatomic association with the cervix, the rectosigmoid may occasionally be preserved; sometimes, it is feasible to perform a lower segmental resection of the rectosigmoid and reanastomosis. A temporary diverting colostomy to protect the low anastomosis has been one practice, but with the current staple-gun anastomosis more patients can be considered for no colostomy if the surgeon feels confident of the water-tightness and viability of the reanastomosis. In most patients, the possibility of constructing a neovagina from a split-thickness skin graft or from an isolated segment of bowel at the time of initial surgery should also be considered. Others have advocated rectus abdominis or gracilis myocutaneous grafts to recreate the vaginal canal. With these modifications, exenteration for pelvic malignancy can often be performed today, leaving the patient with one stoma and a functional vagina. In the experience of the author, these neovaginas are seldom used postoperatively. This

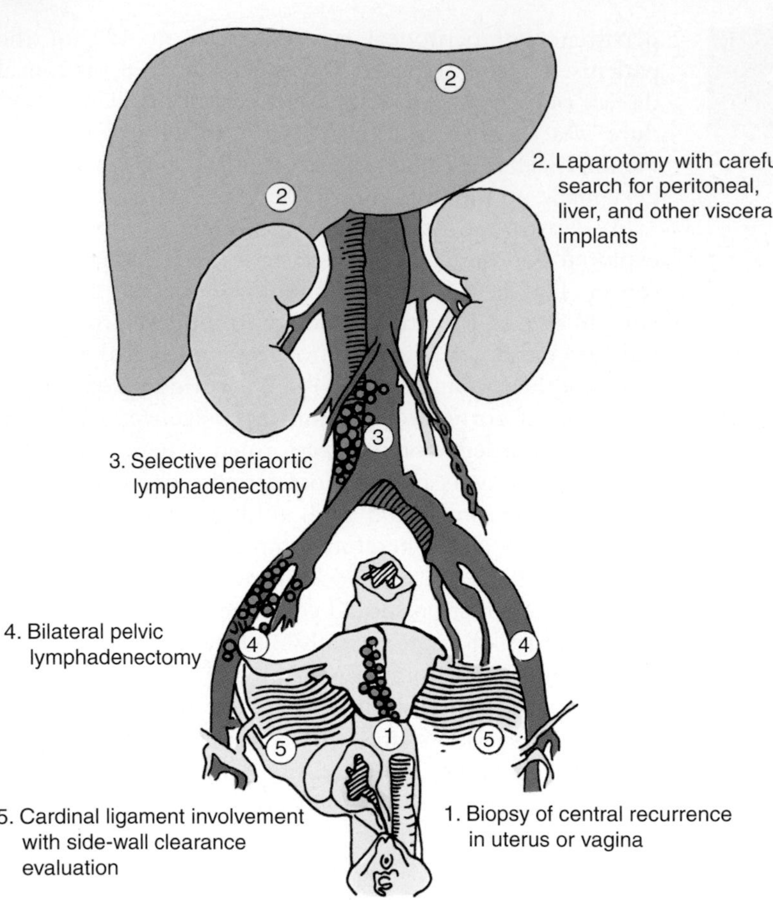

Figure 3–43 Steps in evaluation of a patient for an exenterative procedure. (Courtesy of A Robert Kagan, MD, Los Angeles, California.)

unfortunate fact has made the author prefer the more simple procedure that requires less time in what is already a very lengthy operative procedure.

Morbidity and mortality

Most of the morbidity and mortality directly related to exenteration occur within the first 18 months following the procedure. Many of the complications can be sequelae to any major surgery. These include cardiopulmonary catastrophes such as pulmonary embolism, pulmonary edema, myocardial infarction, and cerebrovascular accidents. The length of these surgical procedures and the magnitude of blood loss definitely increase the incidence of cardiovascular complications. This category of complications usually occurs within the first week after the procedure. Then there is a period when sepsis is the greatest threat to the patient's health and life. This sepsis usually originates in the pelvic cavity with occurrence of a pelvic abscess or, more commonly, diffuse pelvic cellulitis.

One of the most serious postoperative complications of exenteration is small-bowel obstruction related to the denuded pelvic floor. In the last decade, several techniques have been employed in an effort to avoid the adherence of small bowel to this large raw surface, including mobilization of omentum (Fig. 3–44) or abdominal wall peritoneum to cover the pelvic floor (Fig. 3–45). When small-bowel obstruction does occur, it is appropriately treated with conservative therapy. However, half these patients come to reoperation, and the mortality of this group is approximately 50% in some series. The risk of bowel obstruction is increased by the presence of pelvic infection. Both conditions predispose to the development of small-bowel fistulas, which always require reoperation and frequently are fatal. Lichtinger and colleagues reported 53% mortality in patients who develop a small-bowel fistula following pelvic exenteration. In general, complications are more common in patients who have recurrence after radiation therapy. Irradiated tissue is less likely to produce good wound healing, and the formation of granulation tissue is severely retarded. The tendency toward fistula formation is greatly increased. Because surgical dissection is usually more difficult in the irradiated patient, longer operating times and increased blood loss often result. Both these factors are associated with higher morbidity and mortality. Thus, the patient who has had previous radiation therapy is at much greater risk for serious complications than is the non-irradiated patient and is less capable of a competent physiologic response.

The long-term morbidity from exenteration is predominantly related to urinary diversion. Once the period of susceptibility to sepsis has passed, urinary obstruction and infection become the major non-neoplastic life-threatening complications. Recurrent cancer is forever the most likely long-term life-threatening situation after the operative

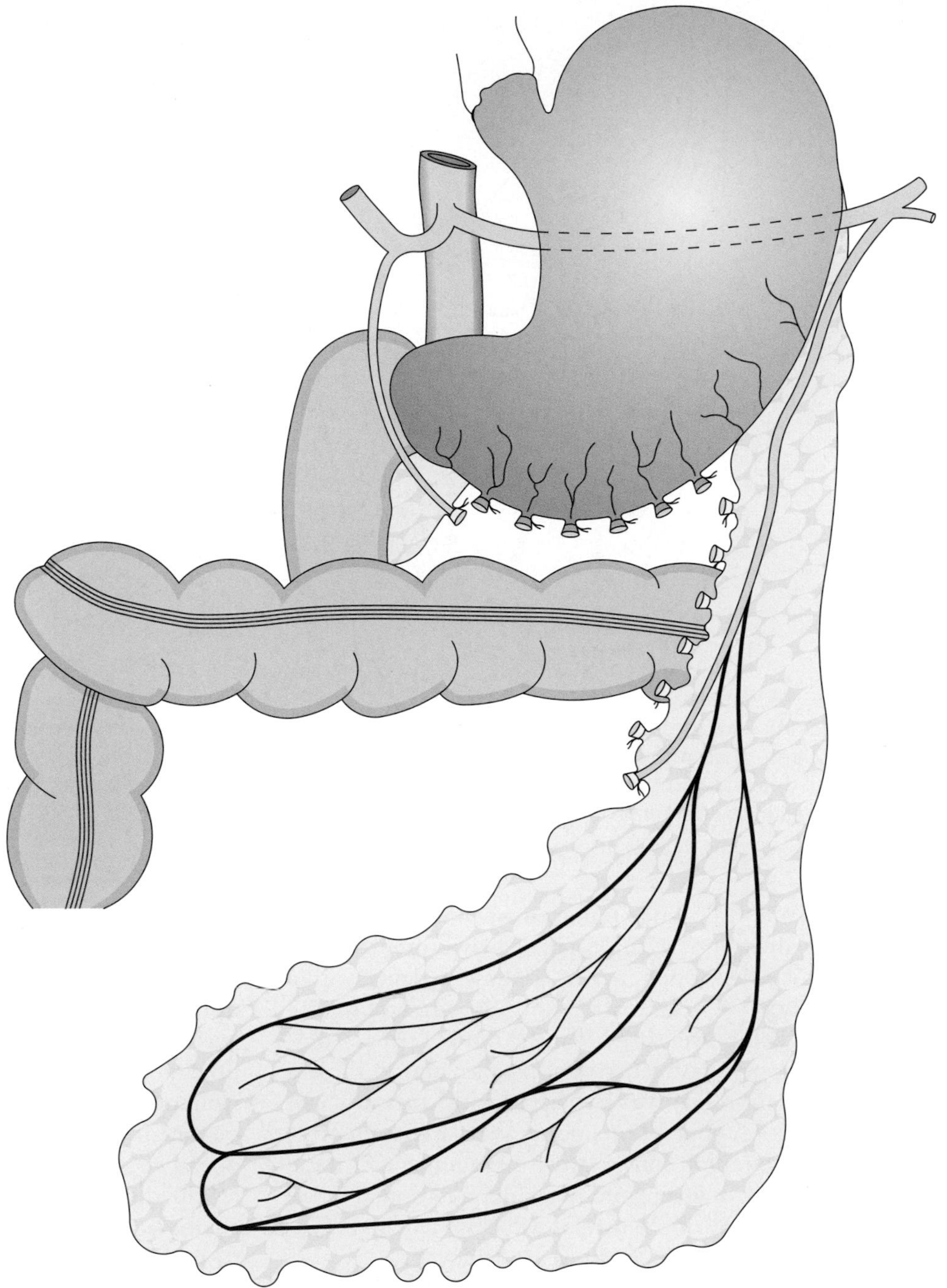

Figure 3–44 The omentum has been detached from the right transverse colon and the greater curvature of the stomach, keeping the left gastroepiploic vessels intact and creating a large "tongue of omentum" to cover the pelvic floor.

procedure, but the more preventable complications of the ileal conduit deserve primary attention. Many believe that these patients should be managed with long-term urinary antisepsis—perhaps for life. Pyelonephritis is common and should be treated promptly and vigorously. Periodic IVPs can be obtained to assess the collecting system for hydronephrosis. A mild degree of obstruction is frequently retained following construction of an ileal conduit, but progressive hydronephrosis will require correction to salvage renal function. It is tragic to lose a patient after exenteration because of resulting, but perhaps treatable, renal disease when there is no residual carcinoma.

Orr and coworkers reported on 115 urinary diversions at the time of pelvic exenteration. An ileal segment was used as a conduit in 97 patients, and a segment of transverse colon was used in 16 patients. Two patients had sigmoid colon conduits. Eighty-five patients (73.9%) had the intestinal anastomosis and conduit constructed with a gastrointestinal stapler. Fourteen patients (12.2%) required a second operation for non-cancer-related urinary complications. Complications included ureteral strictures, conduit stoma stenosis or prolapse, and renal calculi. Of these patients, 61% required rehospitalization for non-malignant indications involving the urinary tract. Late pyelonephritis was the most common reason for rehospitalization. The incidence of complications appeared to be less in patients in whom an unirradiated portion of bowel had been used for construction of the conduit.

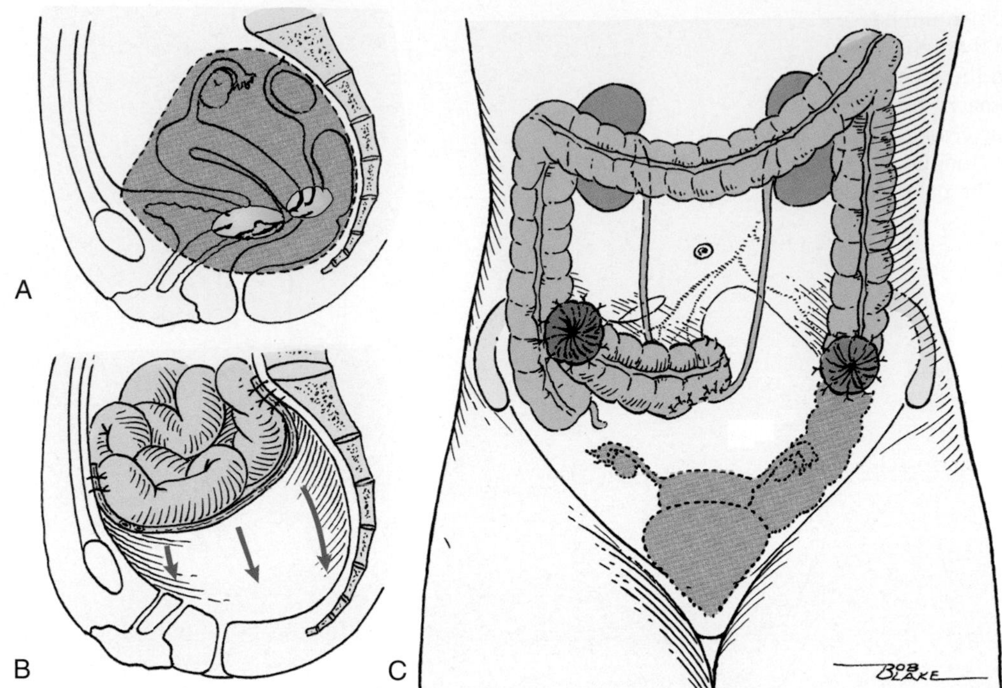

Figure 3–45 *A,* Lateral view of recurrent cancer involving the cervix and upper vagina with extension into the bladder and rectum. The *stippled area* indicates tissue to be removed by exenteration. *B,* A lateral view after pelvic viscera have been removed. The omental "carpet" is used to keep the intestines out of the pelvis during immediate postoperative period. With time, the omental "carpet" will descend into the pelvis and the "carpet" will adhere to the pelvic floor. *C,* Urinary conduit and colostomy diversion after exenteration. *Dotted areas* of the sigmoid, bladder, and internal genitalia have been removed.

Averette and colleagues reported on 88 patients who had urinary diversion at the time of pelvic exenteration. Urinary fistulas developed in 12% of these patients, with a 45% mortality on surgical correction. Also, 16% of the 92 patients who had bowel surgery at the time of pelvic exenteration developed gastrointestinal fistulas, and of these a 40% operative mortality was associated with correction. In an effort to avoid reoperation and its associated high mortality, we first attempt conservative management of these fistulas, including drainage and hyperalimentation, if sepsis is not present. Many of the fistulas will close when satisfactory patency of the bowel or ureter is achieved.

The morbidity and mortality from radical surgery can be minimized by careful selection of patients. This, however, implies a system in which some patients who may be resectable are denied an opportunity for resection in order to keep the morbidity low. This becomes a philosophical question that each physician must answer. However, the outcome of recurrent carcinoma of the cervix in a patient who is given no further treatment is clear.

Walton published a comprehensive review of the factors involved in the stress reaction of the patient after radical pelvic surgery, calling attention to the biochemical, psychological, gastrointestinal, hepatic, and cardiac effects. He concluded that with total care, the occurrence of these stress reactions will decrease but will not disappear, because the human organism reacts in such a complex manner, and derangement would occur in the weakest adaptive link to the surrounding environment.

Survival results

The 5-year cumulative survival rate after pelvic exenteration varies in the literature from 20% to 62% (Table 3–22). Symmonds et al presented a series of 198 exenterative operations performed at the Mayo Clinic for various pelvic malignant lesions. A 5-year survival rate of 33% was obtained. The investigators had noted a diminished overall operative mortality rate of 8.1%, a reduction from 13.5% (1950 through 1962) to 3% (1963 through 1971) and attributed this to better methods of urinary diversion and to better management of fluid replacement and of infectious complications. Rutledge et al evaluated the outcomes of 196 patients with recurrent carcinoma of the cervix and calculated the 5-year survival rate to be 33.8% after deaths from all causes were deducted. Finally, Sharma et al recently evaluated the outcomes of 48 exenterative procedures performed between 1980 and 1999 at the Roswell Park Cancer Institute in New York. The median survival was 35 months and the disease-free survival was 32 months. Mortality from the procedure was 4.2%. Early and later postoperative complication rates were 27% and 75%, respectively. The recurrence rate after pelvic exenteration was 60%.

Reported survival rates depend greatly on the circumstances of patient selection for exenteration. For instance, patients who undergo pelvic exenteration as a primary procedure have a 5-year survival rate 20–25% higher than a similar group of patients with recurrence following irradiation. (Pelvic exenteration may be performed as a primary

Table 3–22 PELVIC EXENTERATION

Author	Institution	No. of Patients Treated	No of Operative Deaths	No. Surviving 5 Years*
Douglas and Sweeney (1975)	New York Hospital	23	1 (4.3%)	5 (22%)
Parsons and Friedell (1964)	Harvard University	112	24 (21.4%)	24 (21.4%)
Brunschwig (1965)	Memorial Hospital	535	86 (16%)	108 (20.1%)
Bricker (1967)	Washington University	153	15 (10%)	53 (34.6%)
Krieger and Embree (1969)	Cleveland Clinics	35	4 (11%)	13 (37%)
Ketcham et al (1975)	National Cancer Institute	162	12 (7.4%)	62 (38.2%)
Symmonds et al (1975)	Mayo Clinic	198	16 (8%)	64 (32.3%)
Morley and Lindenauer (1976)	University of Michigan	34	1 (2.9%)	21 (62%)
Rutledge et al (1977)	MD Anderson Hospital	296	40 (13.5%)	99 (33.4%)
Averette et al (1984)	University of Miami			
	1966–1971	14	4 (28.5%)	5 (36%)
	1971–1976	45	15 (33.3%)	10 (22%)
	1976–1981	33	4 (12.1%)	19 (58)
		65	6 (9.2%)	15 (23%)
Lawhead (1989)	Memorial Hospital 1972–1981	65	6 (9.2%)	15 (23%)
Soper et al (1989)	Duke University	69	5 (7.2%)	28 (4.5%)
Shingleton et al (1989)	University of Alabama	143	9 (6.3%)	71 (50%)
Sharma et al (2005)	Roswell Park Cancer Institute	48	2 (4.2%)	16 (33%)
Total		1965	244 (12.4%)	663 (33.7%)

* In almost every series, the operative death rate and the 5-year survival rate improved dramatically in the later years of each series.

procedure for carcinoma of the vulva extending up the vagina and into the bladder but not out to the pelvic sidewalls.) Survival rates can be improved by excluding the elderly, the obese, the heavily irradiated, and other high-risk patients. Cumulative survival rates are always improved when no patient is exenterated who has a positive pelvic node following pelvic irradiation. In general, however, both morbidity and mortality and the 5-year survival rate have improved steadily over the last two decades. Mortality in most centers is now well below 5%, and morbidity has been similarly lowered.

The survival prognosis for many patients is related to well-defined preoperative findings. The MD Anderson Hospital series reported that 47% of the patients whose recurrences were symptomatic (pain or edema) but who were found resectable at the time of surgery survived 2 years. However, 73% of the patients who were symptom free at the time of laparotomy survived for 2 years. Of the patients who had a normal IVP at the time of laparotomy, 59% survived 2 years, whereas only 34% of the patients who had some IVP abnormality before laparotomy survived for 2 years. Forty-six percent of the patients who had recurrence within 2 years of their primary treatment survived for 2 years or more after treatment. Factors such as the status of the IVP, the presence or absence of symptoms, and the interval between primary treatment and recurrence should be considered in the preoperative assessment of the patient. One can improve the cumulative survival rate by excluding patients who have these deleterious characteristics; however, in so doing, one may be excluding some patients who are resectable and, therefore, can be cured.

Although lesions other than carcinoma of the cervix may be cured by pelvic exenteration, cervical cancer is numerically of greatest importance. This procedure offers the only possibility for cure in patients who have pelvic recurrence after receiving optimal amounts of irradiation. With improved radiotherapy techniques, the number of patients with isolated central failure is steadily diminishing, but there remain a number of patients with recurrent cancer of the cervix after radiation therapy for whom the procedure offers the only chance for life. For the mortality and morbidity to be acceptable, the surgery should be done in medical centers by experienced surgical teams who are knowledgeable in the multidisciplinary approach to cancer therapy and can tailor the management to each patient's needs. These ultraradical surgical procedures should be done only by those individuals with adequate training and background who are willing to take on the responsibility of long-term postoperative care and rehabilitation. Each patient must be assessed individually with the risks of the procedure weighed against the possible benefits. It is encouraging that technical advances continue to reduce the operative mortality and ameliorate the postoperative morbidity associated with pelvic exenteration.

Many patients can not only be cured but also rehabilitated to functional and comfortable lives; no patient should be deprived of this opportunity.

Advanced age was once considered a relative contraindication to ultraradical exenterative surgery. Matthews, however, reviewed the outcome of 63 patients, age 65 or older, who underwent pelvic exenteration between 1960 and 1991 at the University of Texas MD Anderson Cancer Center. Although 63% of the patients had pre-existing medical illnesses, tolerance of the surgery was quite good. Whereas 60% of the patients experienced one or more infectious complications, including pyelonephritis, wound infection, sepsis, and flap necrosis, accounting for the largest category of complications, 24% experienced no complications. Operative mortality was 11%; multisystem failure was the most frequent cause of death. Within a mean follow-up of 12 years after exenteration, 22 of 63 patients were alive and without clinical evidence of disease. The 5-year survival for the group was 46%. Morbidity and mortality of pelvic exenteration in elderly patients appear to be similar to those noted in previous studies of younger patients, with a similar 5-year survival rate. Therefore, age should not be considered an absolute contraindication to exenteration.

SARCOMA, LYMPHOMA, AND MELANOMA OF THE CERVIX

In the SEER report of 6549 cases of cervical carcinoma from 1973 to 1977, there were only 36 cases of cervical sarcoma, which is an incidence of 0.55%. Cervical leiomyosarcomas are rare tumors with poor prognosis regardless of the mode of therapy. Cervical stromal sarcomas arise from the basic paramesonephric stroma (mesoderm). These tumors may be homologous or combined with an epithelial element, (i.e., mixed mesodermal tumor, or carcinosarcoma). Embryonal rhabdomyosarcoma or sarcoma botryoides of the cervix usually occurs in women during their reproductive years. Although the role of adjuvant chemotherapy such as that used for children with perineal rhabdomyosarcoma has not been investigated in this group of patients, it appears to be worthy of serious consideration in patients with large lesions. Ninety-six cases of cervical sarcoma were reviewed by Rotmensch and colleagues, and no clear statement could be made regarding management, although surgery was consistently utilized for early stage lesions. Lymphangiomas and lymphosarcomas of the reticulum cell variety are also seen rarely. Identification of these lesions requires differentiation from anaplastic carcinoma, with which they can be readily confused. These lesions are usually metastatic, and further investigation of the patient reveals multiple foci.

Perren and colleagues reviewed 77 cases of the reticuloendothelial neoplasia who presented with disease apparently limited to the cervix or upper vagina. The most common clinical feature at presentation was abnormal vaginal bleeding (54%). Other presentations included vaginal mass (12%) and dyspareunia (5%). An abnormal cervical smear was noted in only two cases. The conclusion is that lymphomas of the genital tract have an unpredictable prognosis. There is no evidence that radical gynecologic surgery is advantageous, and patients are best treated as for other lymphomas with radiation therapy and combination chemotherapy.

Malignant melanoma of the uterine cervix is a rare manifestation, and neither prospective nor retrospective studies on this disease have been published. Approximately 25 published case reports have been collated in an attempt to clarify the origin, presenting symptoms, macroscopic appearance, and staging of this lesion. It is often difficult to ascertain whether the lesion is of primary or metastatic origin. A careful survey should be done of the patient's skin and mucous membranes for a possible primary site. Almost 90% of the patients are asymptomatic, and vaginal bleeding is the main complaint among 10%. Although primary cervical malignancies usually afflict women in the 40 to 50-year age range, melanoma of the cervix generally manifests in patients between 60 and 70 years of age. Most lesions present as an exophytic polypoid cervical mass with obvious coloring. Almost all patients diagnosed are stage I or II, and preferred therapy has been radical hysterectomy. The 5-year survival is very poor, not exceeding 40% of stage I and 14% of stage II.

BIBLIOGRAPHY

GENERAL OBSERVATIONS

Andersen BL, Lachenbruch PA, Andersen B et al: Sexual dysfunction and signs of gynecologic cancer. Cancer 57:1880, 1986.

Boon ME, de Graaff Guilloud JC, Kok LP et al: Efficacy of screening for cervical squamous and adenocarcinoma: The Dutch experience. Cancer 59:862, 1987.

Coppleson M, Reid B: The etiology of squamous carcinoma of the cervix (Editorial). Obstet Gynecol 32:432, 1968.

Hildesheim A, Brinton LA, Mallin K et al: Barrier and spermicidal contraceptive methods and risk of invasive cervical cancer (see comments). Epidemiology 1:266, 1990.

Pagliusi SR, Aguado MT: Efficacy and other milestones for human papillomavirus vaccine introduction. Vaccine 23:569, 2004.

Piper JM: Oral contraceptives and cervical cancer. Gynecol Oncol 22:1, 1985.

Seibel MM, Freeman MG, Graves WL: Carcinoma of the cervix and sexual function. Obstet Gynecol 55:484, 1980.

Tavassoli FA, Peter Devilee (eds): World Health Organization Classification of Tumors: Pathology and Genetics of Tumours of the Breast and Female Genital Organs. IARC Press: Lyon 2003, section 1.

Weijmar Schultz WCM, Van De Wiel HBM, Bouma J: Psychosexual functioning after treatment for cancer of the cervix: A comparative and longitudinal study. Int J Gynecol Cancer 1:37, 1991.

West RR: Cervical Cancer: Age at registration and age at death. Br J Cancer 35:236, 1977.

MICROINVASIVE CARCINOMA OF THE CERVIX

Argenta PA, Kubicek GJ, Dusenberry KE, Judson PL, Downs LS, Carson LF, Boente MP: Widespread lymph node metastases in young women with FIGO stage IA1 squamous cervical cancer. Gynecol Oncol 97:659, 2005.

Benedet JL, Anderson GH, Boyes DA: Colposcopic accuracy in the diagnosis of microinvasive and occult invasive carcinoma of the cervix. Obstet Gynecol 65:557, 1985.

Boutselis JG, Ullery JC, Charmer L: Diagnosis and management of stage Ia (microinvasive) carcinoma of the cervix. Am J Obstet Gynecol 110:984, 1971.

Boyce DA, Worth AJ: Treatment of early cervical neoplasia: Definition and management of preclinical invasive carcinoma. Gynecol Oncol 12:317, 1981.

Boyce DA, Worth AJ, Fidler HK: The results of treatment of 4389 cases of preclinical cervical squamous carcinoma. J Obstet Gynaecol Br Commonw 77:769, 1970.

Burghardt E, Girardi F, Lahousen M et al: Microinvasive carcinoma of the uterine cervix. Cancer 67:1037, 1991.

Copeland LJ, Silva EE, Gershenson DM, Morris M et al: Superficially invasive squamous cell carcinoma of the cervix. Gynecol Oncol 45:307, 1992.

Creasman WT, Fetter BF, Clarke-Pearson DL et al: Management of stage Ia carcinoma of the cervix. Am J Obstet Gynecol 153:164, 1985.

Creasman WT, Parker RT: Microinvasive carcinoma of the cervix. Clin Obstet Gynecol 16:261, 1973.

Creasman WT, Zano RJ, Major FJ et al: Early invasive carcinoma of the cervix (3–5 mm invasion): Risk factors and prognosis. Am J Obstet Gynecol 178:62, 1998.

Girardi F, Burghardt E, Pickel H: Small stage Ib cervical cancer. Gynecol Oncol 55:427, 1994.

Gurgel M, Bedone AJ, Androde L et al: Microinvasive carcinoma of the uterine cervix: Histological findings on cone specimens related to residual neoplasia on hysterectomy. Gynecol Oncol 65:437, 1997.

Halzer E: Microinvasive carcinoma of the cervix: clinical aspects, treatment, and follow-up. In Burghardt E, Halzer E (eds): Minimal Invasive Cancer. Philadelphia, WB Saunders, 1982, p 315.

Hasumi K, Sakamoto A, Sugano H: Microinvasive carcinoma of the uterine cervix. Cancer 45:928, 1980.

Hopkins MP, Morley GW: Squamous cell cancer of the cervix: Prognostic factors related to survival. Int J Gynecol Cancer 1:173, 1991.

Hopkins MP, Morley GW: Squamous cell carcinoma of the cervix: Clinical pathological features related to survival. Am J Obstet Gynecol 164:1520, 1991.

Kolstad P: Follow-up study of 232 patients with stage Ia1 and 411 patients with stage Ia2 squamous cell carcinoma of the cervix (microinvasive carcinoma). Gynecol Oncol 33:265, 1989.

Leman MH, Benson WL, Kurman RJ et al: Microinvasive carcinoma of the cervix. Obstet Gynecol 48:571, 1976.

Lohe KJ: Early squamous cell carcinoma of the uterine cervix I. Gynecol Oncol 6:10, 1978.

Lohe KJ: Early squamous cell carcinoma of the uterine cervix III. Gynecol Oncol 6:51, 1978.

Lohe KJ et al: Early squamous cell carcinoma of the uterine cervix II. Gynecol Oncol 6:31, 1979.

Maiman MA: Superficially invasive squamous cell carcinoma of the cervix. Obstet Gynecol 72 (3, pt 1):399, 1988.

Mestwerdt G. About the micro-carcinoma of the uterine cervix: colposcopy, cytology, histology and treatment. An Bras Ginecol 59:181–201, 1965.

Morice P, Piovesan P, Rey A et al: Prognostic value of lymphovascular space invasion determined with hematoxylin-eosin staining in early stage cervical carcinoma: Results of a multivariate analysis. Ann Oncol 14:1511, 2003.

Östör AG, Rome RM: Microinvasive squamous cell carcinoma of the cervix: A clinicopathologic-pathologic study of 200 cases with long-term follow-up. Int J Gynecol Cancer 4:257, 1994.

Roche WD, Norris HJ: Microinvasive carcinoma of the cervix: The significance of lymphatic invasion and confluent patterns of stromal growth. Cancer 180:180, 1985.

Sedlis A, Gall S, Tsukoda Y et al: Microinvasive carcinoma of the uterine cervix: A clinical pathologic study. Am J Obstet Gynecol 133:67, 1979.

Seski JC, Abell MR, Morley GW: Microinvasive squamous carcinoma of the cervix. Obstet Gynecol 50:410, 1977.

Sevin BU, Nadji M, Averette HE et al: Microinvasive carcinoma of the cervix. Cancer 70:2121, 1992.

Simon NL, Gore H, Shingleton HM: Study of superficially invasive carcinoma of the cervix. Obstet Gynecol 68:19, 1986.

Takeshima N, Yanoh K, Tabatat et al: Assessment of the revised International Federation of Gynecology and Obstetrics staging for early invasive squamous cervical cancer. Gynecol Oncol 74:165, 1999.

Tsukamoto N, Kaku T, Matsukuma K et al: The problem of stage Ia (FIGO 1985) carcinoma of the uterine cervix. Gynecol Oncol 34:1, 1989.

Van Nagell Jr, Greenwell N, Powell DF et al: Microinvasive carcinoma of the cervix. Am J Obstet Gynecol 145:982, 1983.

Yasgashi N, Sata S, Inque Y et al: Comparative surgical treatment in cervical cancer with 3–5 mm stromal invasion in the absence of confluent invasion and lymph-vascular pace involvement. Gynecol Oncol 54:333, 1994.

CLINICAL PROFILE OF INVASIVE CANCER

Acs J, Hildesheim A, Reeves WC et al: Regional distribution of human papillomavirus DNA and other risk factors for invasive cervical cancer in Panama. Cancer Res 49:5725, 1989.

Barron BA, Richart RM: A statistical model of the natural history of cervical carcinoma based on a prospective study of 557 cases. J Natl Cancer Inst 41:1343, 1968.

Berman ML, Keys H, Creasman W et al: Survival and patterns of recurrence in cervical cancer metastatic to periaortic lymph nodes. Gynecol Oncol 19:8, 1984.

Brinton LA: Epidemiology of cervical cancer—overview. IARC 3:1993.

Brinton LA: Oral contraceptives and cervical neoplasia. Contraception 43:58l, 1991.

Burger MP, Hollema M, Gouw AS et al: Cigarette smoking and human papillomavirus in patients with reported cervical cytological abnormality. Br Med J 306:749, 1993.

Chu J, White E: Decreasing incidence of invasive cervical cancer in young women. Am J Obstet Gynecol 157:1105, 1987.

Daling JR, Sherman KJ, Hislop TG et al: Cigarette smoking and the risk of anogenital cancer. Am J Epidemiol 135:180, 1992.

Delgado G, Bundy BN, Fowler WC Jr et al: A prospective surgical pathological study of stage I squamous carcinoma of the cervix: A Gynecologic Oncology Group study. Gynecol Oncol 35:314, 1989.

Gagnon F: The lack of occurrence of cervical carcinoma in nuns. Proc Second Natl Cancer Conf 1:625, 1952.

Henriksen E: The dispersion of cancer of the cervix. Radiology 54:812, 1950.

Henriksen E: Distribution of metastases in stage I carcinoma of the cervix. Am J Obstet Gynecol 80:919, 1960.

Henriksen E: The lymphatic spread of carcinoma of the cervix and of the body of the uterus: A study of 420 necropsies. Am J Obstet Gynecol 58:924, 1949.

Hopkins MP, Morlay GW: Squamous cell carcinoma of the cervix: Clinical pathological features related to survival. Am J Obstet Gynecol 164:1520, 1991.

Mvula M, Iwasaka T, Matsuo N et al: Detection of human papillomavirus types 16 and 18 in primary and metastatic lesions of cervical carcinomas. Gynecol Oncol 53:156, 1994.

Reeves WC, Brinton LA, Garcia M et al: Human papillomavirus infection and cervical cancer in Latin America. N Engl J Med 320:1437, 1989.

Simons AM, Philips DH, Coleman DV: Damage to DNA in cervical epithelium related to smoking tobacco. Br Med J 306:1444, 1993.

Slattery ML, Robison LM, Schuman KL et al: Cigarette smoking and exposure to passive smoke are risk factors for cervical cancer. JAMA 261:1593, 1989.

Ursin G, Peters RK, Henderson BE et al: Oral contraceptive use and adenocarcinoma of cervix. Lancet 344:1390, 1994.

GLANDULAR TUMORS OF THE CERVIX

Angel C, Dubeshter B, Lin JY: Clinical presentation and management of stage I cerical adenocarcinoma: A 25-year experience. Gynecol Oncol 44:71, 1992.

Anton-Culver H, Bloss JD, Bringman D et al: Comparison of adenocarcinoma and squamous cell carcinoma of the uterine cervix: A population based epidemiologic study. Am J Obstet Gynecol 166:1507, 1992.

Berek JS, Castaldo TW, Hacker NF et al: Adenocarcinoma of the uterine cervix. Cancer 48:2734, 1981.

Boon ME, Baak JP, Kurver PJ et al: Adenocarcinoma in situ of the cervix. Cancer 48:768, 1981.

Brand E, Berek JS, Hacker NF: Controversies in the management of cervical adenocarcinoma. Obstet Gynecol 71:261, 1988.

Chen RW, Change DY, Yen ML et al: Prognostic factors of primary adenocarcinoma of the uterine cervix. Gynecol Oncol 69:157, 1998.

Davidson SE, Symonds RP, Lamont D et al: Does adenocarcinoma of uterine cervix have a worse prognosis than squamous carcinoma when treated by radiotherapy? Gynecol Oncol 33:23, 1989.

Duk JM, Aalders JG, Fleuren GJ et al: Tumor markers CA 125, squamous cell carcinoma antigen, and carcinoembryonic antigen in patients with adenocarcinoma of the uterine cervix. Obstet Gynecol 73:661, 1989.

Eifel PJ, Burke TW, Delclos L et al: Early stage I adenocarcinoma of the uterine cervix: Treatment results in patients with tumors < 4 cm in diameter. Obstet Gynecol 41:199, 1991.

Eifel PJ, Burke TW, Morris M et al: Adenocarcinoma as an independent risk factor for disease recurrence in patients with stage IB cervical carcinoma. Gynecol Oncol 59:38, 1995.

Eifel PJ, Morris M, Oswald MJ et al: Adenocarcinoma of the uterine cervix. Cancer 65:2507, 1990.

Eifel PJ, Burke TW, Delclos L et al: Early stage I adenocarcinoma of the uterine cervix: Treatment results in patients with tumors 4 cm in diameter. Gynecol Oncol 41:199, 1991.

El-Ghobashy AA, Shaaban AM, Herod J, Herrington CS: The pathology and management of endocervical glandular neoplasia. Int J Gynecol Cancer 15:583, 2005.

Hopkins MP, Morlay GW: Comparison of adenocarcinoma and squamous cell carcinoma of the cervix. Obstet Gynecol 77:912, 1991.

Hopkins MP et al: The prognosis and treatment of stage I adenocarcinoma of the cervix. Obstet Gynecol 72:915, 1988.

Kaku T, Kamura T, Sakai K et al. Early adenocarcinoma of the uterine cervix. Gynecol Oncol 65:281–285. 1997.

Kilgore LC, Soong SJ, Gore H et al: Analysis of prognostic features in adenocarcinoma of the cervix. Gynecol Oncol 31:137, 1988.

Kjorstad KE, Bond B: Stage Ib adenocarcinoma of the cervix: Metastatic potential and patterns of dissemination. Am J Obstet Gynecol 150:297, 1984.

Kleine W, Rau K, Schwoeorer D et al: Prognosis of the adenocarcinoma of the cervix uteri: A comparative study. Gynecol Oncol 35:145, 1989.

Lai CH, Hsueh S, Hong JH et al: Are adenocarcinomas and adenosquamous carcinomas different from squamous carcinomas in stages IB and II cervical cancer patients undergoing primary surgery? Int J Gynecol Cancer 9:28, 1999.

Matthews CM, Burke TW, Tomos C et al: Stage I cervical adenocarcinoma: Prognostic evaluation of surgically treated patients. Gynecol Oncol 49:19, 1993.

McHale MT, Le TD, Burger RA, Gu M, Rutgers JL, Monk BJ: Fertility sparing treatment for in situ and early invasive adenocarcinoma of the cervix. Obstet Gynecol 98:726, 2001.

Moberg PJ, Einborn N, Silfversward C et al: Adenocarcinoma of the uterine cervix. Cancer 57:407, 1986.

Östör A, Rome R, Quinn M: Microinvasive adenocarcinoma of the cervix: A clinicopathologic study of 77 women. Obstet Gynecol 89:88, 1997.

Parazzin IF, LaVecchia C: Epidemiology of adenocarcinoma of the cervix. Gynecol Oncol 39:4, 1990.

Prempree T, Amornmarn R, Wizenberg MJ: A therapeutic approach to primary adenocarcinoma of the cervix. Cancer 56:1264, 1985.

Raju KS, Kjorstad KE, Abeler V: Prognostic factors in the treatment of stage 1b adenocarcinoma of the cervix. Int J Gynecol Cancer 1:69, 1991.

Rose PG, Reale FR: Case Report: Serous papillary carcinoma of the cervix. Gynecol Oncol 50:361, 1993.

Rutledge FN, Gutierrez AG, Fletcher GH: Management of stage I and II adenocarcinomas of the uterine cervix on intact uterus. AJR Am J Roentgenol 102:161, 1968.

Schorge JO, Lee KR, Flynn CE et al: Stage IA1 cervical adenocarcinoma: Definition and treatment. Obstet Gynecol 89:88, 1997.

Yamakawa Y, Forslund O, Teshima H et al: Human papillomavirus DNA in adenocarcinoma and adenosquamous carcinoma of the uterine cervix detected by polymerase chain reaction (PCR). Gynecol Oncol 53:190, 1994.

Young RH, Scully RE: Invasive adenocarcinoma and related tumors of the urterine cervix. Semin Diagn Pathol 7:205, 1990.

UNCOMMON AND NEUROENDOCRINE TUMORS OF THE CERVIX

Abeler VM, Holm R, Nesland JM, Kjorstad KE: Small cell carcinoma of the cervix. Cancer 73:672, 1994.

Barrett RJ, Davos I, Leuchter RS et al: Neuroendocrine features in poorly differentiated and undifferentiated carcinomas of the cervix. Cancer 60:1089, 1987.

Chan JK, Loizzi V, Burger RA, Rutgers J, Monk BJ: Prognostic factors in neuroendocrine small cell cervical carcinoma: a multivariate analysis. Cancer 97:568, 2003.

Hoskins PJ et al: Small cell carcinoma of the cervix treated with concurrent radiotherapy, cisplatin, and etoposide. Gynecol Oncol 56:218, 1995.

Lewandowski GS, Copeland LJ: Case report: A potential role for intensive chemotherapy in the treatment of small cell neuroendocrine tumors of the cervix. Gynecol Oncol 48:127, 1993.

Lotocki RJ, Krepart GV, Paraskevas M et al: Glassy cell carcinoma of the cervix: A bimodal treatment strategy. Gynecol Oncol 44:254, 1992.

Morris M, Gershenson DM, Eifel P et al: Treatment of small cell carcinoma of the cervix with cisplatin, doxorubicin, and etoposide. Gynecol Oncol 47:62, 1992.

Pazdur R, Bonomi P, Slayton R et al: Neuroendocrine carcinoma of the cervix: Implications for staging and therapy. Gynecol Oncol 12:120, 1981.

Sheets EE, Berman ML, Hrountas CK et al: Surgically treated, early-stage neuroendocrine small-cell cervical carcinoma. Obstet Gynecol 71:10, 1988.

Stoler MH, Mills SE, Gersell DJ et al: Small-cell neuroendocrine carcinoma of the cervix. Am J Surg Pathol 15:28, 1991.

Tamimi HK, Ek M, Hesla J et al: Glassy cell carcinoma of the cervix redefined. Obstet Gynecol 71:837, 1988.

Viswanathan AN, Deavers MT, Jhingran A et al. Small cell neuroendocrine carcinoma of the cervix: Outcome and patterns of recurrence. Gynecol Oncol 93:27–33, 2004.

STAGING

Belenson JL, Goldberg MI, Averette HE: Para-aortic lymphadenectomy in gynecologic cancer. Gynecol Oncol 7:188, 1979.

Brenner DE, Whitley NO, Prempree T et al: An evaluation of the computed tomographic scanner for the staging of carcinoma of the cervix. Cancer 50:2323, 1982.

Buchsbaum HJ: Extrapelvic lymph node metastases in cervical carcinoma. Am J Obstet Gynecol 133:814, 1979.

Burke TW, Heller PB, Hoskins WJ et al: Evaluation of the scalene lymph nodes in primary and recurrent cervical carcinoma. Gynecol Oncol 28:312, 1987.

Childers JM, Hatch K, Surwitt EA: The role of laparoscopic lymphadenectomy in the management of cervical carcinoma. Gynecol Oncol 47:38, 1992.

Childers JM, Hatch K, Tran AN, Surwitt EA: Laparoscopic para-aortic lymphadenectomy in gynecologic malignancies. Obstet Gynecol 82:741, 1993.

Dargent D: Laparoscopic surgery and gynecologic cancer. Curr Opin Obstet Gynecol 5:294, 1993.

Delgato G, Smith JP, Ballantyne AJ: Scalene node biopsy in carcinoma of the cervix; pelvic and para-aortic lymphadenectomy. Cancer 35:784, 1975.

Fuller AF Jr, Elliott N, Kosloff C et al: Determinants of increased risk for recurrence in patients undergoing radical hysterectomy for stage IB and IIa carcinoma of the cervix. Gynecol Oncol 33:34, 1998.

Havrilesky LJ, Kulasingam SL, Matchar DB, Myers ER: FDG-PET for management of cervical and ovarian cancer. Gynecol Oncol 97:183, 2005.

Kupets R, Covens A: Is the International Federation of Gynecology and Obstetrics staging system for cervical carcinoma able to predict survival in patients with cervical carcinoma? An assessment of clinimetric properties. Cancer 92:796, 2001.

Lagasse LD, Creasman WT, Shingleton HM et al: Results and complications of operative staging in cervical cancer: Experience of the Gynecologic Oncology Group. Gynecol Oncol 9:90, 1980.

Lanciano RM, Won M, Hanks GE: A reappraisal of the international federation of gynecology and obstetrics staging system for cervical cancer. Cancer 69:482, 1992.

Memarzadeh S, Natarajan S, Dandade DP et al: Lymphovascular and perineural invasion in the parametria: a prognostic factor for early-stage cervical cancer. Obstet Gynecol 102:612, 2003.

Nelson JH Jr, Macasaet MA, Lu T et al: The incidence and significance of para-aortic lymph node metastases in late invasive carcinoma of the cervix. Am J Obstet Gynecol 118:749, 1974.

Potish RA, Twiggs LB, Prem KA et al: The impact of extra-peritoneal surgical staging on morbidity and tumor recurrence following radiotherapy for cervical carcinoma. Am J Clin Oncol 7:245, 1984.

TREATMENT

Abbe R: The use of radium in malignant disease. Lancet 2:524, 1913.

Alberts DS, Martimbeau PW, Surwit EA et al: Mitomycin C, bleomycin, vincristine, and cis-platinum in the treatment of advanced recurrent squamous cell carcinoma of the cervix. Cancer Clin Trials 4:313, 1981.

Alberts DS, Garcia D, Mason-Liddil N: Cisplatin in advanced cancer of the cervix: An update. Semin Oncol 18:11, 1991.

Ampil F, Datta R, Datta S: Elective postoperative external radiotherapy after hysterectomy in early-stage carcinoma of the cervix: Is additional vaginal cuff irradiation necessary? Cancer 60:280, 1987.

Anderson B, LaPolla J, Turner D et al: Ovarian transposition in cervical cancer. Gynecol Oncol 49:206, 1993.

Andras EJ, Fletcher GH, Rutledge F: Radiotheraphy of carcinoma of the cervix following simple hysterectomy. Am J Obstet Gynecol 115:647, 1973.

Artman LE, Hoskins WJ, Bibro MC et al: Radical hysterectomy and pelvic lymphadenectomy for stage IB carcinoma of the cervix: 21 years' experience. Gynecol Oncol 28:8, 1987.

Bali A, Weekes A, van Trappen P et al. Central pelvic recurrence 7 years after radical vaginal trachelectomy. Gynecol Oncol 96: 854–856, 2005.

Bandy LC, Clarke-Pearson DL, Soper JT et al: Long-term effects on bladder function following radical hysterectomy with and without postoperative radiation. Gynecol Oncol 26:160, 1987.

Barnes W, Waggoner S, Delgado G et al: Manometric characterization of rectal dysfunction following radical hysterectomy. Gynecol Oncol 42:116, 1991.

Barton DPJ, Cavanagh D, Roberts WS et al: Radical hysterectomy for treatment of cervical cancer: A prospective study of two methods of closed-suction drainage. Am J Obstet Gynecol 166:533, 1992.

Bernardini M, Barrett J, Seaward G, Covens A. Pregnancy outcomes in patients after radical trachelectomy. Am J Obstet Gynecol 189:1378–1382, 2003.

Bianchi UA, Sartori E, Pecorelli S et al: Treatment of primary invasive cervical cancer; considerations on 997 consecutive cases. Eur J Gynaecol Oncol 9:47, 1988.

Bloss JD, Berman ML, Mukherejee J et al: Bulky stage IB cervical carcinoma managed by primary radical hysterectomy followed by tailored radiotherapy. Gynecol Oncol 47:21, 1992.

Bonfiglio M: The pathology of fracture of the femoral neck following irradiation. AJR Am J Roentgenol 70:449, 1953.

Bosch A, Marcial VA: Carcinoma of the uterine cervix associated with pregnancy. AJR Am J Roentgenol 96:92, 1966.

Brack CB, Everett HC, Dickson R: Irradiation therapy for carcinoma of the cervix: Its effect on urinary tract. Obstet Gynecol 7:196, 1956.

Bremer GL, van der Putten HW, Dunselman GA et al: Early stage cervical cancer: Aborted versus completed radical hysterectomy. Eur J Obstet Gynecol Reprod Biol 47:147, 1992.

Brenner DE, Gillette AW, Jones HW 3rd et al: Simultaneous radiation and chemotherapy for advanced carcinoma of the cervix. Gynecol Oncol 26:381, 1987.

Brookland RK, Rubin S, Danoff BF: Extended field irradiation in the treatment of patients with cervical carcinoma involving biopsy-proven para-aortic nodes. Radiat Oncol Biol Phys 10:1875, 1984.

Brown JV, Fu YS, Berek JS: Ovarian metastases are rare in stage I adenocarcinoma of the cervix. Obstet Gynecol 76:623, 1990.

Burghardt E, Baltzer J, Tulusan AH, Haas J: Results of surgical treatment of 1028 cervical cancers studied with volumetry. Cancer 70:648, 1992.

Carenza L, Nobili F, Giacobini S: Voiding disorders after radical hysterectomy. Gynecol Oncol 13:213, 1982.

Chambers SK et al: Sequelae of lateral ovarian transposition in unirradiated cervical cancer patients. Gynecol Oncol 39:155, 1990.

Chapman JA, Mannel RS, DiSaia PJ et al: Surgical treatment of unexpected invasive cervical cancer found at total hysterectomy. Obstet Gynecol 80:931, 1992.

Choo YC, Wong LC, Wong KP et al: The management of intractable lymphocyst following radical hysterectomy. Gynecol Oncol 24:309, 1986.

Corn BW et al: Technically accurate intracavitary insertions improve pelvic control and survival among patients with locally advanced carcinoma of the uterine cervix. Gynecol Oncol 53:294, 1994.

Covens A, Shaw P, Murphy J, et al. Is radical trachelectomy a safe alternative to radical hysterectomy for patients with stage IA–B carcinoma of the cervix? Cancer 86;2273–2279, 1999

Creasman WT, Soper JT, Clarke-Pearson D: Radical hysterectomy as therapy for early carcinoma of the cervix. Am J Obstet Gynecol 155:964, 1986.

Currie DW: Operative treatment of carcinoma of the cervix. J Obstet Gynaecol Br Commonw 78:385, 1971.

Czesnin K, Wronkowski Z: Second malignancies of the irradiated area in patients treated for uterine cervix cancer. Gynecol Oncol 6:309, 1978.

Dargent D, Enria R. Laparoscopic assessment of the sentinel lymph nodes in early cervical cancer. Technique—preliminary results and future developments. Crit Rev Oncol/Hematol 2003;48:305–310.

Delgato G, Caglar H, Walker P: Survival and complications in cervical cancer treated by pelvic and extended field radiation after para-aortic lymphadenectomy. AJR Am J Roentgenol 130:141, 1978.

Diakomanolis E, Haidopoulos D, Rodolakis A et al. Laser CO2 conization: A safe mode of treating conservatively microinvasive carcinoma of the uterine cervix. Eur J Obstet Gynecol Reprod Biol 113:229–233, 2004

DiSaia PJ, Bundy BN, Curry SL et al: Phase III study on the treatment of women with cervical cancer, stage IIb, IIIb, and IVa (confined to the pelvis and/or periaortic nodes), with radiotherapy alone versus radiotherapy plus immunotherapy with intravenous *Corynebacterium parvum:* A Gynecologic Oncology Group study. Gynecol Oncol 26:386, 1987.

DiSaia PJ: Surgical aspects of cervical carcinoma. Cancer 48:548, 1981.

DiSaia PJ: The case against the surgical concept of en bloc dissection for malignancies of the reproductive tract. Cancer 60:2025, 1987.

Dottino PR, Plaxe SC, Beddoe AM et al: Induction chemotherapy followed by radical surgery in cervical cancer. Gynecol Oncol 40:7, 1991.

Durance FY. Radiotherapy following simple hysterectomy in patients with stage I and II carcinoma of the cervix. Am J Roentgenol Radium Ther Nucl Med 102:165–169, 1968.

Einstein MH, Kadish AS, Burk RD et al: Heat shcok protein (HSP)-based immunotherapy (HspE7) for treatment of CIN III (NCI 5850, NYGOG). Gynecol Oncol 96:912a, 2005.

Falk V, Lungren N, Quarfordt L et al: Primary surgical treatment of carcinoma stage I of the uterine cervix, Acta Obstet Gynecol Scand 61:481, 1982.

Feder BH, Syed AMN, Neblett D: Treatment of extensive carcinoma of the cervix with the "transperineal parametrial butterfly." Int J Radiat Oncol Biol Phys 4:735, 1978.

Fletcher GH, Rutledge FN: Extended field technique in the management of the cancers of the uterine cervix. AJR Am J Roentgenol 114:116, 1972.

Forney JP: The effect of radical hysterectomy on bladder physiology. Am J Obstet Gynecol 138:374, 1980.

Fotiou S, Tserkezoglou A, Hatzieleftheriou G et al: Class III vs class II radical hysterectomy in stage IB cervical carcinoma: A comparison of morbidity and survival. Int J Gynecol Cancer 7:117, 1997.

Gallion HH, van Nagell JR Jr, Donaldson ES et al: Combined radiation therapy and extrafascial hysterectomy in the treatment of stage IB barrel-shaped cervical cancer. Cancer 56:262, 1985.

Garcia F, Petry KU, Muderspach L et al: ZYC101a for treatment of high-grade cervical intraepithelial neoplasia: A randomized controlled trial. Obstet Gynecol 103:317, 2004.

Giaroli A, Sananes C, Sardi JE et al: Lymph node metastases in carcinoma of the cervix uteri: Response to neoadjuvant chemotherapy and its impact on survival. Gynecol Oncol 39:34, 1990.

Gilinsky WH et al: The natural history of radiation-induced proctosigmoiditis: An analysis of 88 patients. Q J Med 205:40, 1983.

Gil-Moreno A, Diaz-Feijoo B, Roca I et al. Total laparoscopic radical hysterectomy with intraoperative sentinel node identification in patients with early invasive cervical cancer. Gynecol Oncol 2005;96:187–193.

Grosu AL, Piert M, Weber WA et al: Positron emission tomography for radiation treatment planning. Strahlenther Onkol 181:483, 2005

Hatch KD, Parham G, Shingleton HM et al: Ureteral strictures and fistulae following radical hysterectomy. Gynecol Oncol 19:17, 1984.

Heller PB, Barnhill DR, Mayer AR: Cervical carcinoma found incidentally in a uterus removed for benign indications. Obstet Gynecol 67:187, 1986.

Herzog TJ: New approaches for the management of cervical cancer. Gynecol Oncol 2003;90:S22–27.

Hopkins MP, Morley GW: Radical hysterectomy versus radiation therapy for stage IB squamous cell cancer of the cervix. Cancer 68:272, 1991.

Hreschyshn MM, Aron BS, Boronow RC et al: Hydroxyurea or placebo combined with radiation to treat stages IIIb and IV cervical cancer confined to the pelvis. Int J Radiat Oncol Biol Phys 5:317, 1979.

Hurwitz H, Fehrenbacher L, Novotny W et al: Bevacizumab plus irinotecan, fluorouracil, and leucovorin for metastatic colorectal cancer. N Engl J Med 350:2335, 2004.

Husseinzadeh N, Van Aken ML, Aron B: Ovarian transposition in young patients with invasive cervical cancer receiving radiation therapy. Int J Gynaecol Cancer 4:61, 1994.

Inoue T, Morita K: 5-year results of postoperative extended-field irradiation on 76 patients with nodal metastases from cervical carcinoma stages Ib to IIIb. Cancer 61:2009, 1988.

Ito E, SaitoT. Nerve-preserving techniques for radical hysterectomy. Eur J Surg Oncol 30:1137–1140, 2004.

Jackson KS, Das N, Naik R et al. Laparoscopically assisted radical vaginal hysterectomy vs. radical abdominal hysterectomy for cervical cancer: A matched controlled study. Gynecol Oncol 95:655–661, 2004.

Jakobsen A, Bichel P, Ahrons S et al: Is radical hysterectomy always necessary in early cervical cancer? Gynecol Oncol 39:80, 1990.

Jensen PT, Groenvold M, Klee MC et al. Early-stage cervical carcinoma, radical hysterectomy, and sexual function: A longitudinal study. Cancer 100:97–106, 2004.

Johnston CM, Dottino PR, Heller DS et al: Case report: Recurrent cervical squamous cell carcinoma in an ovary following ovarian conservation and radical hysterectomy. Gynecol Oncol 41:64, 1991.

Jolles CJ, Freedman RS, Hamberger AD et al: Complications of extended-field therapy for cervical carcinoma without prior surgery. Radiat Oncol Biol Phys 12:179, 1986.

Kagan AR, Nussbaum H, Gilbert H et al: A new staging system for irradiation injuries following treatment for cancer of the cervix uteri. Gynecol Oncol 7:166, 1979.

Keys HM, Bundy BN, Stehman FB et al: Cisplatin, radiation and adjuvant hysterectomy compared with radiation and adjuvant hysterectomy for bulky Stage IB cervical cancer. N Engl J Med 340:1154, 1999.

Khorram O, Stern JL: Case report: Bleomycin sclerotherapy of an intractable inguinal lymphocyst. Gynecol Oncol 50:244, 1993.

Kim DS, Moon H, Hwang YY et al: Preoperative adjuvant chemotherapy in the treatment of cervical cancer stage Ib, IIa, and IIb with bulky tumor. Gynecol Oncol 29:321, 1988.

Kim RY: Radiotherapeutic management in carcinoma of the uterine cervix: current status. Int J Gynecol Cancer 3:337, 1993.

Kinney WK, Alvarez RD, Reid CC et al: Value of adjuvant whole-pelvis irradiation after Wertheim hysterectomy for early-stage squamous carcinoma of the cervix with pelvic nodal metastasis: A matched-control study. Gynecol Oncol 34:258, 1989.

Kinney WK, Egorshin EV, Ballard DJ, Podratz KC: Long-term survival and sequelae after surgical management of invasive cervical carcinoma diagnosed at the time of simple hysterectomy. Gynecol Oncol 44:24, 1992.

Kirsten F, Atkinson KH, Coppleson JV et al: Combination chemotherapy followed by surgery or radiotherapy in patients with locally advanced cervical cancer. Br J Obstet Gynaecol 94:583, 1987.

Kramer C, Peschel RE, Goldberg N et al: Radiation treatment of FIGO stage IVa carcinoma of the cervix. Gynecol Oncol 32:323, 1989.

Krebs HB, Helmkamp BF, Sevin BU et al: Recurrent cancer of the cervix following hysterectomy and pelvic node dissection. Obstet Gynecol 59:422, 1982.

Landoni F, Maneo A, Colombo A et al: Randomized study of radical surgery versus radiotherapy for stage IB–IIA cervical cancer. Lancet 350:535, 1997.

Larson DM, Malone JM, Copeland LJ et al: Ureteral assessment after radical hysterectomy. Obstet Gynecol 69:612, 1987.

Larson DM, Stringer CA, Copeland LJ et al: Stage Ib cervical carcinoma treated with radical hysterectomy and pelvic lymphadenectomy: Role of adjuvant radiotherapy. Obstet Gynecol 69:378, 1987.

Lee Y, Wang KL, Lin MH et al: Radical hysterectomy with pelvic lymph node dissection for treatment of cervical cancer: A clinical review of 954 cases. Gynecol Oncol 32:135, 1989.

Lin L-Y, Wu J-H, Yang C-W et al. Impact of radical hysterectomy for cervical cancer on urodynamic findings. Int Urogynecol J 15:418–421, 2004.

Lin YS, Tzeng CC, Huang KF et al. Sentinel node detection with radiocolloid lymphatic mapping in early invasive cervical cancer. Int J Gynecol Cancer 15:273–277. 2005.

Liu W, Meigs JW: Radical hysterectomy and pelvic lymphadenectomy. Am J Obstet Gynecol 69:1, 1955.

Maas CP, Trimbos JB, DeRuiter MC et al. Nerve sparing radical hysterectomy: Latest developments and historical perspective. Crit Rev Oncol/Hematol 48:271–279, 2003.

Madhu J et al: Preliminary results of concomitant radiotherapy and chemotherapy in advanced cervical carcinoma. Gynecol Oncol 28:101, 1987.

Mann WJ, Vogel F, Pastner B et al: Management of lymphocysts after radical gynecologic surgery. Gynecol Oncol 33:248, 1989.

Mann WJ, Chumas J, Amalfitano T et al: Ovarian metastases from stage Ib adenocarcinoma of the cervix. Cancer 60:1123, 1987.

Martinez-Palones JM, Gil-Moreno A, Perez-Benavente MA et al. Intraoperative sentinel node identification in early stage cervical cancer using a combination of radiolabeled albumin injection and isosulfan blue dye injection. Gynecol Oncol 92:845–850, 2004

Maruyama Y, Donaldson E, van Nagell JR et al: Specimen findings and survival after preoperative ^{252}Cf neutron brachytherapy for stage II cervical carcinoma. Gynecol Oncol 43:252, 1991.

Massi G, Savino L, Susini T: Schauta-Amreich vaginal hysterectomy and Wertheim–Meigs abdominal hysterectomy in the treatment of cervical cancer: A retrospective analysis. Am J Obstet Gynecol 168:928, 1993.

McCall ML. A modern evaluation of the radical vaginal operation for carcinoma of the cervix. Am J Obstet Gynecol 85:295–301, 1963.

McIntyre JF, Eifel PJ, Levenback C, Oswald MJ: Ureteral stricture as a late complication of radiotherapy for stage IB carcinoma of the uterine cervix. Cancer 75:837, 1995.

Miller BE, Copeland LJ, Hamberger, AD et al: Carcinoma of the cervical stump. Gynecol Oncol 18:100, 1984.

Mitra S. Radical vaginal hysterectomy and extraperitoneal lymphadenectomy in cervical cancer. Zentralbl Gynakol 73:574–581, 1951.

Monk BJ, Cha DS, Walker JL et al: Extent of disease as an indication for pelvic radiation following radical hysterectomy and bilateral pelvic lymph node dissection in the treatment of stage IB and IIa cervical carcinoma. Gynecol Oncol 54:4, 1994.

Monk BJ, Wang J, Im S, Stock RJ, Peters WA III, Liu PY, Barrett RJ II, Berek JS, Souhami L, Grigsby PW, Gordon W Jr: Rethinking the use of radiation and chemotherapy after radical hysterectomy: a clinical-pathologic analysis of the Gynecologic Oncology Group/Southwest Oncology Group/Radiation Therapy Oncology Group trial. Gynecol Oncol 96:721, 2005

Montana GS, Fowler WC, Varia MA et al: Carcinoma of the cervix, stage III. Cancer 57:148, 1986.

Morris M, Eifel PJ, Lu J et al: Pelvic radiation with concurrent chemotherapy compared with pelvic and para-aortic radiation for high risk cervical cancer. N Engl J Med 340:1137, 1999.

Morrow CP: Is pelvic radiation beneficial in the postoperative management of stage Ib squamous cell carcinoma of the cervix with pelvic node metastasis treated by radical hysterectomy and pelvic lymphadenectomy? 10:105, 1980.

Nam JH, Kim JH, Kim DY et al. Comparative study of laparoscopico-vaginal radical hysterectomy and abdominal radical hysterectomy in patients with early cervical cancer. Gynecol Oncol 92:277–283, 2004.

Nolan JF, Anson JH, Steward M: A radium applicator for use in the treatment of cancer of the uterine cervix. AJR Am J Roentgenol 79:36, 1958.

Orr JW, Wilson K, Bodiford C: Corpus and cervix cancer: A nutritional comparison. Am J Obstet Gynecol 153:775, 1985.

Owens S et al: Ovarian management at the time of radical hysterectomy for cancer of the cervix. Gynecol Oncol 35:349, 1989.

Panici PB, Greggi S, Scambia G et al: High-dose cisplatin and bleomycin neoadjuvant chemotherapy plus radical surgery in locally advanced cervical carcinoma: A preliminary report. Gynecol Oncol 41:212, 1991.

Panici PB, Scambia G, Baiocchi G et al: Neoadjuvant chemotherapy and radical surgery in locally advanced cervical cancer: Prognostic factors for response and survival. Cancer 67:372, 1991.

Park TK, Lee SK, Kim SN et al: Combined chemotherapy and radiation for bulky stages I–II cervical cancer: Comparison of concurrent and sequential regimens. Gynecol Oncol 50:196, 1993.

Park TK, Choi DH, Kim SN et al: Role of induction chemotherapy in invasive cervical cancer. Gynecol Oncol 41:1007, 1991.

Patsner B, Sedlacek TV, Lovecchio JL: Para-aortic node sampling in small (3 cm or less) stage IB invasive cervical cancer. Gynecol Oncol 44:53, 1992.

Patsner B: Closed-suction drainage versus no drainage following radical abdominal hysterectomy with pelvic lymphadenectomy for stage IB cervical cancer. Gynecol Oncol 57:232, 1995.

Perez CA, Breaux S, Madoc-Jones H et al: Correlation between radiation dose and tumor recurrence and complications in carcinoma of the uterine cervix: stages I and IIa. Int J Radiat Oncol Biol Phys 5:373, 1979.

Perez CA, Breaux S, Askin F et al: Irradiation alone or in combination with surgery in stages Ib and IIa carcinoma of the uterine cervix: A nonrandomized comparison. Cancer 43:1062, 1979.

Petersen LK, Mamsen A, Jakobsen A: Carcinoma of the cervical stump. Gynecol Oncol 46:199, 1992.

Photopulos GJ, Vander Zuang R, Miller B et al: Vaginal radiation brachytherapy to reduce central recurrence after radical hysterectomy for cervical carcinoma. Gynecol Oncol 38:187, 1990.

Photopulos GJ, Van der Zwaag R: Class II radical hysterectomy shows less morbidity and good treatment efficacy compared to class III. Gynecol Oncol 40:21, 1991.

Piver MS, Barlow JJ: High dose irradiation to biopsy-confirmed aortic node metastases from carcinoma of the uterine cervix. Cancer 39:1243, 1977.

Piver MS, Rutledge FN, Smith PJ: Five classes of extended hysterectomy of women with cervical cancer. Obstet Gynecol 44:265, 1974.

Piver MS: Extended field irradiation in the treatment of patients with cervical carcinoma involving biopsy proven para-aortic nodes. Int J Radiat Oncol Biol Phys 10:1993, 1984.

Plante M, Renaud MC, Hoskins IA, Roy M: Vaginal radical trachelectomy: a valuable fertility-preserving option in the management of early-stage cervical cancer. A series of 50 pregnancies and review of the literature. Gynecol Oncol 98:3, 2005.

Pomel C, Atallah D, le Bouedec G et al. Laparoscopic radical hysterectomy for invasive cervical cancer: 8-year experience of a pilot study. Gynecol Oncol 91:534–539, 2003.

Potish R, Adcock L, Jones TJ Jr. et al: The morbidity and utility of periaortic radiotherapy in cervical carcinoma. Gynecol Oncol 15:1, 1983.

Puthawala A, Syed AM, Nalick R et al: Integrated external and interstitial radiation therapy for primary carcinoma of the vagina. Obstet Gynecol 62:367, 1983.

Raspagliesi F, Ditto A, Fontanelli R et al. Nerve-sparing radical hysterectomy: A surgical technique for preserving the autonomic hypogastric nerve. Gynecol Oncol 93:307–314, 2004.

Remy JC, DiMaio T, Fruchter RG et al: Adjunctive radiation after radical hysterectomy in stage Ib squamous cell carcinoma of the cervix. Gynecol Oncol 38:161, 1990.

Rettenmaier MA, Casanova DM, Micha JP et al: Radical hysterectomy and tailored postoperative radiation therapy in the management of bulky stage Ib cervical cancer. Cancer 63:2220, 1989.

Roman LD, Morris M, Mitchell MF et al: Prognostic factors for patients undergoing simple hysterectomy in the presence of invasive cancer of the cervix. Gynecol Oncol 50:179, 1993.

Rose PG, Bundy BN, Watkins ED et al: Concurrent cisplatin based radiotherapy and chemotherapy for locally advanced cervical cancer. N Engl J Med 340:1144, 1999.

Roy M, Plante M, Renaud M-C, Tetu B. Vaginal radical hysterectomy versus abdominal radical hysterectomy in the treatment of early-stage cervical cancer. Gynecol Oncol 62:336–339,1996.

Rubin SC et al: Para-aortic nodal metastases in early cervical carcinoma: Long-term survival following extended field radiotherapy. Gynecol Oncol 18:213, 1984.

Russell AH: Comtemporary radiation treatment planning for patients with cancer of the uterine cervix. Semin Oncol 21:30, 1994.

Rutledge FN, Wharton JT, Fletcher GH: Clinical studies with adjunctive surgery and irradiation therapy in the treatment of carcinoma of the cervix. Cancer 38:596, 1976.

Sakuragi N, Todo Y, Kudo M et al. A systematic nerve-sparing radical hysterectomy technique in invasive cervical cancer for preserving postsurgical bladder function. Int J Gynecol Cancer 15:389–397, 2005.

Sandler AB, Gray R, Brahmer J et al: Randomized phase II/III trial of paclitaxel (P) plus carboplatin (C) with or without bevacizumab (NSC # 704865) in patients with advanced non-squamous non-small cell lung cancer (NSCLC): An Eastern Cooperative Oncology Group (ECOG) Trial–E499. ASCO 2005 Annual Meeting, Abstract #LBA4.

Sardi JE, di Paola GR, Cachau A et al: A possible new trend in the management of the carcinoma of the cervix uteri. Gynecol Oncol 25:139, 1986.

Sardi JE, Giaroli A, Sananes C et al. Long-term follow-up of the first randomized trial using neoadjuvant chemotherapy in stage IB squamous carincoma of the cervix: The final results. Gynecol Oncol 1997;67:61-9.

Sardi JE, Sanaes CE, Giarolic AA et al: Neoadjuvant chemotherapy in cervical carcinoma stage IIB: A randomized control trial. Int J Gynecol Cancer 8:441, 1998.

Sardi JE: Neoadjuvant chemotherapy in locally advanced carcinoma of the cervix-uterus. Gynecol Oncol 38:486, 1990.

Scharge JO, Molpus KL, Koelliker D et al: Stage IB and IIa cervical cancer with negative lymph nodes: The role of adjuvant radiotherapy after radical hysterectomy. Gynecol Oncol 66:31, 1997.

Sedlis A, Bundy BN, Rotman MZ et al: A randomized trial of pelvic radiation therapy versus no further therapy in selected patients with stage IB carcinoma of the cervix after radical hysterectomy and pelvic lymphadenectomy. Gynecol Oncol 73:177, 1999.

Seibel M, Freeman MG, Graves WL: Sexual function after surgical and radiation therapy for cervical carcinoma. South Med J 75:1195, 1982.

Sekiba K: Radical hysterectomy for cancer of the uterine cervix. Semin Surg Oncol 1:95, 1985.

Silva LB, Silva-Filho AL, Traiman P et al: Sentinel node detection in cervical cancer with ^{99m}Tc-phytate. Gynecol Oncol 97:588–595, 2005.

Slater JD, Slater JM, Wahlen S: The potential for proton beam therapy in locally advanced carcinoma of the cervix. Int J Radiat Oncol Biol Phys 22:343, 1991.

Soisson AP, Soper JT, Berchuck A et al: Radical hysterectomy in obese women. Obstet Gynecol 80:940, 1992.

Soisson AP, Soper JT, Clarke-Pearson DL et al: Adjuvant radiotherapy following radical hysterectomy for patients with stage Ib and IIa cervical cancer. Gynecol Oncol 37:390, 1990.

Spirtos NM, Eisenkop SM, Schlaerth JB, Ballon SC. Laparoscopic radical hysterectomy (type III) with aortic and pelvic lymphadenectomy in patients with stage I cervical cancer: Surgical morbidity and intermediate follow-up. Am J Obstet Gynecol 87:340–348, 2002

Stallworthy J: Radical surgery following radiation treatment for cervical carcinoma. Ann R Coll Surg Engl 34:161, 1964.

Steed H, Rosen B, Murphy J et al. A comparison of laparoscopically-assisted radical vaginal hysterectomy and radical abdominal hysterectomy in the treatment of cervical cancer. Gynecol Oncol 93:588–589, 2004.

Steed H, Rosen B, Murphy J, Laframboise S, De Petrillo D, Covens A: A comparison of laparascopic-assisted radical vaginal hysterectomy and radical obdominal hysterectomy in the treatment of cervical cancer. Gynecol Oncol 93:588, 2004.

Stehman FB, Bundy BN, DiSaia PJ et al: Carcinoma of the cervix treated with radiation therapy. I: A multi-variate analysis of prognostic variables in the Gynecologic Oncology Group. Cancer 67:2776, 1991.

Stehman FB, Rose PG, Greer BE et al. Innovations in the treatment of invasive cervical cancer. Cancer 98(9 Suppl):2052–2063, 2003.

Surwit EA, Manning MR, Aristizabal SA et al: Interstitial thermoradiotherapy in recurrent gynecologic malignancies. Gynecol Oncol 15:95, 1983.

Syed AMN, Feder BH: Technique of afterloading interstitial implant. Radiol Clin 46:458, 1977.

Tabata M, Ichinoe K, Sakuragi N et al: Incidence of ovarian metastasis in patients with cancer of the uterine cervix. Gynecol Oncol 28:255, 1987.

Tanguay C, Plante M, Renaud MC et al. Vaginal radical trachelectomy in the treatment of cervical cancer: The role of frozen section. Int J Gynecol Pathol 23:170–175, 2004.

Thomas GM, Dembo AJ: Is there a role for adjuvant pelvic radiotherapy after radical hysterectomy in early stage cervical cancer? Int J Gynecol Cancer 1:1, 1991.

Trimbos JB, Maas CP, Deruiter MC et al. A nerve-sparing radical hysterectomy; Guidelines and feasibility in Western patients. Int J Gynecol Cancer 11:180–186, 2001.

Ungar L, Palfalvi L, Hogg R, et al. Abdominal radical trachelectomy: A fertility-preserving option for women with early cervical cancer. Br J Obstet Gynecol 112:366–369, 2005.

Weems DH, Mendenhall WM, Bova FJ et al: Carcinoma of the intact uterine cervix, stages Ib–IIa–b, 6 cm in diameter: Irradiation alone vs preoperative irradiation and surgery. Radiat Oncol Biol Phys 11:1911, 1985.

Wharton JT, Jones HW 3rd, Day TG Jr et al. Preirradiation celiotomy and extended field irradiation for invasive carcinoma of the cervix. Obstet Gynecol 49:333–338. 1977.

Yabuki Y, Asamoto A, Hoshiba T et al: Dissection of the cardinal ligament in radical hysterectomy for cervical cancer with emphasis on the lateral ligament. Am J Obstet Gynecol 164:7, 1991.

Yessian A, Magistris A, Burger RA, Monk BJ: Radical hysterectomy followed by tailored postoperative therapy in the treatment of stage IB2 cervical cancer: feasibility and indications for adjuvant therapy. Gynecol Oncol 94:61, 2004.

Zander J, Baltzer J, Lohe KJ et al: Carcinoma of the cervix: An attempt to individualize treatment: Results of a 20-year cooperative study. Am J Obstet Gynecol 139:752, 1981.

SURVIVAL RESULTS AND PROGNOSTIC FACTORS

Abdulhayoglu G, Rich WM, Reynolds J et al: Selective radiation therapy in stage Ib uterine cervical carcinoma following radical pelvic surgery. Gynecol Oncol 10:84, 1980.

Adcock L, Julian TM, Okagaki T et al: Carcinoma of the uterine cervix FIGO stage Ib. Gynecol Oncol 14:199, 1982.

Alvarez RD, Soong SJ, Kinney WK et al: Identification of prognostic factors and risk groups in patients found to have nodal metastasis at the time of radical hysterectomy for early-stage squamous carcinoma of the cervix. Gynecol Oncol 35:130, 1989.

Baltzer J, Lohe KJ, Kopcke W et al: Histological criteria for prognosis in patients with operative squamous cell carcinoma of the cervix. Gynecol Oncol 13:184, 1982.

Barber HRK, Brunschwig A: Gynecologic cancer complicating pregnancy. Am J Obstet Gynecol 85:156, 1963.

Berman ML, Bergen S, Salazar H: Influence of histological features and treatment on the prognosis of patients with cervical cancer metastatic to pelvic lymph nodes. Gynecol Oncol 39:127, 1990.

Burghardt E, Baltzer J, Tulusan AH, Haas J: Results of surgical treatment of 1028 cervical cancers studied with volumetry. Cancer 70:648, 1992.

Burke TW, Hoskins WJ, Heller PB et al: Prognostic factors associated with radical hysterectomy failure. Gynecol Oncol 26:153, 1987.

Chan JK, Loizzi V, Burger RA et al: Prognostic factors in neuroendocrine small cell cervical carcinoma: A multivariate analysis. Cancer 97:568, 2003.

Chen RJ, Lin YH, Chen CA et al: Influences of histologic type and age on survival rates for invasive cervical carcinoma in Taiwan. Gynecol Oncol 73:184, 1999.
Cooper RA, Wilks DP, Logue JP et al. High tumor angiogenesis is associated with poorer survival in carcinoma of the cervix treated with radiotherapy. Clin Cancer Res 4:2795–2800, 1998.
Davidson B, Goldberg I, Kopolovic J: Angiogenesis in uterine cervical intraepithelial neoplasia and squamous cell carcinoma: An immunohistochemical study. Int J Gynecol Pathol 16:335, 1997.
Dawlatly B, Laire O, Cross PA et al: Prognostic factors in surgically-treated stage IB–IIB squamous cell carcinoma of the cervix with positive lymph nodes. Int J Gynecol Cancer 8:467, 1998.
Delgado G, Bundy B, Aino R et al: Prospective surgery pathological study of disease-free interval in patients with stage IB squamous cell carcinoma cervix. Gynecol Oncol 38:352, 1990.
Delgado G: Prospective surgical pathological study of disease free interval in patients with stage Ib carcinoma of the cervix: A GOG study. Gynecol Oncol 38:352, 1990.
Dellas A, Moch H, Schultheiss E et al: Angiogenesis in cervical neoplasia; microvessel quantitation in precancerous lesions and invasive carcinomas with clinicopathlogical correlations. Gynecol Oncol 67:27, 1997.
Dobbs SP, Hewett PW, Johnson IR et al: Angiogenesis is associated with vascular endothelial growth factor expression in cervical intraepithelial neoplasia. Br J Cancer 76:1410, 1997.
Fiorica JV, Roberts WS, Greenberg H et al: Morbidity and survival patterns in patients after radical hysterectomy and postoperative adjuvant pelvic radiotherapy. Gynecol Oncol 36:343, 1990.
Francke P, Maruyama J, vanNagell J et al: Lymphovascular invasion in stage IB cervical carcinoma: Prognostic significance and role of adjuvant radiotherapy. Int J Gynecol Cancer 6:208, 1996.
Fuller AF, Elliott N, Kosloff C et al: Lymph node metastasis from carcinoma of the cervix, stages Ib and IIa: Implications for prognosis and treatment. Gynecol Oncol 13:165, 1982.
Gauthier P, Gore I, Shingleton HM et al: Identification of histopathologic risk groups in stage Ib squamous cell carcinoma of the cervix. Obstet Gynecol 66:569, 1985.
Greggi S, Benedett P, Amoroso M et al: Intraperitoneal tumor spread in locally advanced cervical carcinoma undergoing neoadjuvant chemotherapy. Int J Gynecol Cancer 8:207, 1998.
Hagmar B, Christensen JJP, Johansson B et al: Implications of human papillomavirus type for survival in cervical squamous cell carcinoma. Int J Gynecol Cancer 5:341, 1995.
Hopkins MP, Morley GW: Squamous cell cancer of the cervix: Prognostic factors related to survival. Int J Gynecol Cancer 1:173, 1991.
Hopkins MP, Morley GW: Stage IB squamous cell cancer of the cervix: Clinicopathologic feature related to survival. Am J Obstet Gynecol 164:1520, 1991.
Inoue T, Morita K: The prognostic significance of number of positive nodes in cervical carcinoma stages Ib, IIa, and IIb. Cancer 65:1923, 1990.
Kosary CL. FIGO stage, histology, histologic grade, age and race as prognostic factors in determining survival for cancers of the female gynecological system: An analysis of 1973–1987 SEER cases of cancers of the endometrium, cervix, ovary, vulva, and vagina. Semin Surg Oncol 10:31–36, 1994.
Lanciano RM, Martz K, Montant GS, Hanks GE: Influence of age, prior abdominal surgery, fraction size, and dose on complications after radiation therapy for squamous cell cancer of the uterine cervix. Cancer 69:2124, 1992.
Look KY, Brunetto VL, Clarke-Pearson DL et al: An analysis of cell type in patients with surgically staged IB carcinoma of the cervix. Gynecol Oncol 63:304, 1996.
Lovecchio JL, Averette HE, Donato D et al: 5-year survival of patients with periaortic nodal metastases in clinical stage Ib and IIa cervical carcinoma. Gynecol Oncol 34:43, 1989.
Manetta A et al: The significance of para-aortic node status in carcinoma of the cervix and endometrium. Gynecol Oncol 23:284, 1986.
Mitchell PA, Waggoner S, Rotsnensch J et al: Cervical cancer in the elderly treated with radiation therapy. Gynecol Oncol 71:291, 1998.
Montana GS, Fowler WC, Varia MA et al: Analysis of results of radiation therapy for stage II carcinoma of the cervix. Cancer 55:956, 1985.
Obermair A, Wanner C, Bilgi S et al. Tumor angiogenesis in stage IB cervical cancer: Correlation of microvessel density with survival. Am J Obstet Gynecol 178:314–319, 1998.
Orlandi C, Costa S, Terzano P et al. Presurgical assessment and therapy of microinvasive carcinoma of the cervix. Gynecol Oncol 59:255–260, 1995.
Pecorelli S (ed): FIGO Annual Report on the Results of Treatment in Gynaecological Cancer. J Epidemiol Biostat 3:5, 1998.
Perez CA, Grigsby PW, Nene SM et al: Effect of tumor size on the prognosis of carcinoma of the uterine cervix treated with irradiation alone. Cancer 69:2796, 1992.
Peterient DG, Hartenback EM, Thomas GM: Para-aortic lymph node evaluation in cervical cancer: The impact of staging upon treatment decisions and outcome. Int J Gynecol Cancer 8:353, 1998.
Prempree T, Patanaphan V, Scott R: Radiation management of carcinoma of the cervical stump. Cancer 43:1262, 1979.
Rutledge FN, Mitchell MF, Munsell M et al: Youth as a prognostic factor in carcinoma of the cervix: a matched analysis. Gynecol Oncol 44:123, 1992.
Sardi JE, di Paola GR, Giaroli A et al: Results of a phase II trial with neoadjuvant chemotherapy in carcinoma of the cervix uteri. Gynecol Oncol 31:256, 1988.
Stockler M, Russell P, McGaham S et al: Prognosis and prognostic factors in node-negative cervix cancer. Int J Gynecol Cancer 6:477, 1996.
Thomassen LV, Warshaw J, Lawhead RA, Unger ER: Invasive cervical cancer in young women. J Reprod Med 37:901, 1992.
Tinga DJ, Timmer PR, Bouma J: Prognostic significance of single vs multiple lymph node metastases in cervical carcinoma stage Ib. Gynecol Oncol 39:175, 1990.
Ulfelder H, Smith CJ, Costello JB: Invasive carcinoma of the cervix during pregnancy. Am J Obstet Gynecol 98:424, 1967.
Wang PH, Liu YC, Lai CR et al: Small cell carcinoma of the cervix: An analysis of clinical and pathological findings. Eur J Gynaecol Oncol 19:189, 1997.
Zaino RJ, Ward S, Delgado G et al: Histopathologic predictors of the behavior of surgically treated stage IB squamous cell carcinoma of the cervix: A Gynecologic Oncology Group Study. Cancer 69:1750, 1992.

RECURRENT AND ADVANCED CARCINOMA OF THE CERVIX

Alberts DS, Garcia D, Mason-Liddil N: Cisplatin in advanced cancer of the cervix: An update. Semin Oncol 18(1 suppl 3):11, 1991.
Ampil FL: Stage IVa carcinoma of the cervix. Radiat Med 8:184, 1990.
Barter JF, Soong SJ, Hatch KD et al: Diagnosis and treatment of pulmonary metastases from cervical carcinoma. Gynecol Oncol 38:347, 1990.
Bassan JS, Glaser MG: Bony metastasis in carcinoma of the uterine cervix. Clin Radiol 33:623, 1982.
Blythe JG, Cohen MH, Buchsbaum HJ, Latourette HB. Bony metastases from carcinoma of cervix. Occurrence, diagnosis, and treatment. Cancer 36:475–484, 1975.
Burke TW, Hoskins WJ, Heller PB et al: Clinical patterns of tumor recurrence after radical hysterectomy in stage Ib cervical carcinoma. Obstet Gynecol 69:382, 1987.
Christopherson WM, Lundin FE Jr, Mendez WM, Parker JE. Cervical cancer control: A study of morbidity and mortality trends over a twenty-one-year period. Cancer 38:1357–1366, 1976.
Coleman DL, Gallup DG, Wolcott HD et al: Patterns of failure of bulky-barrel carcinomas of the cervix. Am J Obstet Gynecol 166:916, 1992.

Coleman RL, Keeney ED, Freedman RS et al: Radical hysterectomy for recurrent carcinoma of the uterine cervix after radiotherapy. Gynecol Oncol 55:29, 1994.

Delgato G, Goldson AL, Ashayeri E et al: Intraoperative radiation in the treatment of advanced cervical cancer. Obstet Gynecol 63:246, 1984.

El-Minawi MF, Perez-Mesa CM: Parametrial needle biopsy follow-up of cervical cancer. Int J Obstet Gynecol 12:1, 1974.

Flint A et al: Confirmation of metastasis by fine needle aspiration biopsy in patients with gynecologic malignancies. Gynecol Oncol 14:382, 1982.

Gallousis S: Isolated lung metastases from pelvic malignancies. Gynecol Oncol 7:206, 1979.

Hartenbach EM, Saltzman AK, Carter JR et al: Nonsurgical management strategies for the function complications of ileocolonic continent urinary reservoirs. Gynecol Oncol 59:358, 1995.

Larson DM, Copeland LJ, Stringer CA et al: Recurrent cervical carcinoma after radical hysterectomy. Gynecol Oncol 30:381, 1988.

Layfield LJ, Heaps JM, Berek JS: Fine-needle aspiration cytology accuracy with palpable gynecologic neoplasms. Gynecol Oncol 40:70, 1991.

Lifshitz S, Railsback LD, Buchsbaum HJ: Intra-arterial pelvic infusion chemotherapy in advanced gynecologic cancer. Obstet Gynecol 52:476, 1978.

Lippman SM, Kavanagh JJ, Paredes-Espinoza M et al: 13-cis-retinoic acid plus interferon α-2a: Highly active systemic therapy for squamous cell carcinoma of the cervix. J Natl Cancer Inst 84:241, 1992.

Long HJ 3rd, Bundy BN, Grendys EC Jr, Benda JA, McMeekin DS, Sorosky J, Miller DS, Eaton LA, Fiorica JV: Randomized phase III trial of cisplatin with or without topotecan in carcinoma of the uterine cervix: a Gynecologic Oncology Group Study. J Clin Oncol 23:4626, 2005.

Look KY, Blessing JA, Muss HB et al: 5-Fluorouracil and low-dose leucovorin in the treatment of recurrent squamous cell carcinoma of the cervix. Am J Clin Oncol 15:497, 1992.

Monk BJ, Huang HQ, Cella D, Long HJ 3rd: Quality of life outcomes from a randomized phase III trial of cisplatin with or without topotecan in advanced carcinoma of the cervix: a Gynecologic Oncology Group Study. J Clin Oncol 23:4617, 2005.

Monk BJ, Solh S, Johnson MT, Montz FJ: Radical hysterectomy after pelvic irradiation in patients with high-risk cervical cancer or uterine sarcoma: Morbidity and outcome. Eur J Gynecol Oncol XIV:506, 1993.

Montana GS, Martz KL, Hanks GE: Patterns and sites of failure in cervix cancer treated in the USA in 1978. Int J Radiat Oncol Biol Phys 20:87, 1991.

Moore DH, Plessing JA, McQuellon RP, Thaler HT, Cella D, Brenda J, Miller DS, Olt G, King S, Boggess JF, Rocereto TF: Phase III study of cisplatin with or without paclitaxel in stave IVB, recurrent, or persistent squamous cell carcinoma of the cervix: a Gynecologic Oncology Group Study. J Clin Oncol 22:3113, 2004.

Morris M. Blessing JA, Monk BJ, McGehee R, Moore DH: Phase II study of cisplatin and vinorelbine in squamous cell carcinoma of the cervix: a Gynecologic Oncology Group Study. J Clin Oncol 22:3340, 2004.

Murphy WT, Schmitz A: The results of reirradiation of cancer of the cervix. Radiology 67:378, 1956.

Mutch DG, Bloss JD: Gemcitabine in cervical cancer. Gynecol Oncol 90:S8, 2003.

Ng HT, Kan YY, Chao HT et al: The outcome of the patients with recurrent cervical carcinoma in terms of lymph node metastasis and treatment. Gynecol Oncol 26:355, 1987.

Omura GA: Current status of chemotherapy for cancer of the cervix. Oncology 6:27, 1992.

Park RC, Thigpen JT: Chemotherapy in advanced and recurrent cervical cancer. Cancer Suppl 71:1446, 1993.

Paunier JP, Delclos L, Fletcher GH. Causes, time of death, and sites of failure in squamous-cell carcinoma of the uterine cervix on intact uterus. Radiology 88:555–562, 1967.

Peeples WJ, Inalsingh CH, Hazra TA et al: The occurrence of metastasis outside the abdomen and retroperitoneal space in invasive carcinoma of the cervix. Gynecol Oncol 4:307, 1976.

Potter ME, Alvarez RD, Gay GL et al: Optimal therapy of pelvic recurrence after radical hysterectomy for early stage cervical cancer. Gynecol Oncol 37:74, 1990.

Rettenmaier MA, Moran MF, Ramsinghani NF et al: Treatment of advanced and recurrent squamous carcinoma of the uterine cervix with constant intra-arterial infusion of cisplatin. Cancer 61:1301, 1988.

Rubin SC, Hoskins WJ, Lewis JL: Radical hysterectomy for recurrent cervical cancer following radiation therapy. Gynecol Oncol 27:316, 1987.

Russell AH, Tong DY, Figge DC et al: Adjuvant postoperative pelvic radiation for carcinoma of the uterine cervix: Pattern of cancer recurrence in patients undergoing elective radiation following radical hysterectomy and pelvic lymphadenectomy. Radiat Oncol Biol Phys 10:211, 1984.

Saphner T, Gallion HH, Van Nagell JR et al: Neurologic complications of cervical cancer: A review of 2261 cases. Cancer 64:1147, 1989.

Shield PW, Wright RG, Free K, Daunter B: The accuracy of cervicovaginal cytology in the detection of recurrent cervical carcinoma following radiotherapy. Gynecol Oncol 41:223, 1991.

Sommers GM, Grigsby PW, Perez CA et al: Outcome of recurrent cervical carcinoma following definitive irradiation. Gynecol Oncol 35:150, 1989.

Suit HD, Howes AE, Hunter N. Dependence of response of a C3H mammary carcinoma to fractionated irradiation on fractionation number and intertreatment interval. Radiat Res 72:440–454, 1977.

Sutton GP, Blessing JA, McGuire WP et al: Phase II trial of ifosfamide and mesna in patients with advanced or recurrent squamous carcinoma of the cervix who had never received chemotherapy: A Gynecologic Oncology Group Study. Am J Obstet Gynecol 168:805, 1993.

Terada K, Morley GW: Radical hysterectomy as surgical salvage therapy for gynecologic malignancy. Obstet Gynecol 70:913, 1987.

Tewari KS, Monk BJ: The evolution of systemic therapy for palliation of metastatic and relapsing cervical carcinoma. Current Oncology Reports, 2005.

Thigpen T, Shingleton H, Homesley H et al: Cis-platinum in the treatment of advanced or recurrent squamous cell carcinoma of the cervix. Cancer 48:899, 1981.

Thomas GM: Concurrent radiation and chemotherapy for carcinoma of the cervix recurrent after radical surgery. Gynecol Oncol 27: 254, 1987.

Truelsen F: Injury of bones by roentgen treatment of the uterine cervix. Acta Radiol 23:581, 1942.

Van Herik M et al: Late recurrence in carcinoma of the cervix. Am J Obstet Gynecol 108:1183, 1970.

Welander CE, Homesley HD, Barrett RJ: Combined interferon alpha and doxorubicin in the treatment of advanced cervical cancer. Am J Obstet Gynecol 165:284, 1991.

PELVIC RECURRENCE AFTER SUBOPTIMAL SURGERY

Brin EN, Schiff M Jr, Weiss RM Palliative urinary diversion for pelvic malignancy. J Urol 113:619–622, 1975.

Coddington CC, Thomas JR, Hoskins WJ. Percutaneous nephrostomy for ureteral obstruction in patients with gynecologic malignancy. Gynecol Oncol 18:339–348, 1984.

Höckel M, Baussmann E, Mitze M, Knapstein PG. Are pelvic sidewall recurrences of cervical cancer biologically different from central relapses? Cancer 74:648–655, 1994.

Feuer GA, Fruchter R, Seruri E et al: Selection for percutaneous nephrostomy in gynecologic cancer patients. Gynecol Oncol 42:60, 1991.

Ijoz T, Eifel PJ, Burke T et al: Radiation therapy of pelvic recurrence after radical hysterectomy for cervical carcinoma. Gynecol Oncol 70:241, 1998.

Orr JW, Ball GC, Soong SJ et al: Surgical treatment of women found to have invasive cervix cancer at the time of total hysterectomy. Obstet Gynecol 68:353, 1986.

Samlal RAK, Van der Velden J, Van E Erden T et al: Recurrent cervical carcinoma after radical hysterectomy: An analysis of clinical aspect and prognosis. Int J Gynecol Cancer 8:78, 1998.

PELVIC EXENTERATION

Averette HE, Lichtinger M, Sevin BU et al: Pelvic exenteration: A 15-year experience in a general metropolitan hospital. Am J Obstet Gynecol 150:179, 1984.

Barber HRK: Relative prognostic significance of preoperative and operative findings in pelvic exenteration. Surg Clin North Am 49:431, 1969.

Barber HRK, Jones W: Lymphadenectomy in pelvic exenteration for recurrent cervix cancer. JAMA 215:1949, 1971.

Behtash N, Mousavi A, Tehranian A, Khanafshar N, Hanjani P: Embryonal rhabdomyosarcoma of the uterine cervix: case report and review of the literature. Gynecol Oncol 91:452, 2003.

Berman ML, Lagasse LD, Watring WG et al: Enteroperineal fistulae following pelvic exenteration: A 10-point program of management. Gynecol Oncol 4:368, 1976.

Bricker EM: Bladder substitution after pelvic evisceration. Surg Clin North Am 30:1511, 1950.

Bricker EM, Butcher HR, McAfee A: Results of pelvic exenteration. Arch Surg 73:661, 1956.

Brunschwig A: What are the indications and results of pelvic exenteration? JAMA 194:274, 1965.

Brunschwig A, Pierce VK: Necropsy findings in patients with carcinoma of the cervix: Implications for treatment. Am J Obstet Gynecol 56:1134, 1948.

Carlson JW, Soisson AP, Fowler JM et al: Rectus abdominis myocutaneous flap for primary vaginal reconstruction. Gynecol Oncol 51:323, 1993.

Creasman WT, Rutledge F: Is positive pelvic lymphadenectomy a contraindication to radical surgery in recurrent cervical carcinoma? Gynecol Oncol 2:282, 1974.

Gruessner SE, Omwandho CO, Dreyer T, Blutters-Sawatzki R, Reiter A, Tinneburg HR, Bohle RM: Management of stage I cervical sarcoma botryoides in childhood and adolescence. Eur J Pediatr 163:452, 2004.

Hancock KC, Copeland LJ, Gershenson DM et al: Urinary conduits in gynecologic oncology. Obstet Gynecol 67:680, 1986.

Hatch KD, Shingleton HM, Potter ME et al: Low rectal resection and anastomosis at the time of pelvic exenteration. Gynecol Oncol 32:262, 1988.

Hoffman MS, Lynch CM, Gleeson NC et al: Colorectal anastomosis on a gynecologic oncology service. Gynecol Oncol 55:60, 1994.

Hökel M, Schlenger K, Hamm H et al: Five year experience with combined operative and radiotherapeutic treatment of recurrent gynecologic tumors infiltrating the pelvic wall. Cancer 77:1918, 1996.

Irvin W, Presley A, Anderson W, Taylor P, Rice L: Leiomyosarcoma of the cervix. Gynecol Oncol 91:636, 2003.

Ketcham AS, Deckers PJ, Sugarbaker EV et al: Pelvic exenteration for carcinoma of the uterine cervix: A 15-year experience. Cancer 26:513, 1970.

Lawhead RA: Pelvic exenteration for recurrent or persistent gynecologic malignancies: A 10-year review of the Memorial Sloan–Kettering Cancer Center Experience (1972–1981). Gynecol Oncol 33:279, 1989.

Lee JW, Kim YT, Min YH, Kim SH, Park KH, Lim BJ, Yang WI: Granulocytic sarcoma of the uterine cervix. Int J Gynecol Cancer 14:553, 2004.

Lichtinger M, Averette H, Girtanner R et al: Small bowel complications after supravesical urinary diversion in pelvic exenteration. Gynecol Oncol 24:137, 1986.

Magrina JF: Types of pelvic exenterations: A reappraisal. Gynecol Oncol 37:363, 1990.

Morley GW, Lindenauer SM: Pelvic exenteration therapy for gynecologic malignancies: An analysis of 70 cases. Cancer 38:581, 1976.

Morley GW, Lindenauer SM, Young D: Vaginal reconstruction following pelvic exenteration. Am J Obstet Gynecol 116:996, 1973.

Ng C, Amis S: Radiology of continent urinary diversion. Contemp Urorad 29:557, 1991.

Orr JW, Shingleton HM, Hatch KD et al: Urinary diversion in patients undergoing pelvic exenteration. Am J Obstet Gynecol 142:883, 1982.

Park TK, Choi DH, Kim SN et al: Role of induction chemotherapy in invasive cervical cancer. Gynecol Oncol 41:1007, 1991.

Penalver M, Averette H, Sevin BU et al: Gastrointestinal surgery in gynecologic oncology: Evaluation of surgical techniques. Gynecol Oncol 28:74, 1987.

Roberts WS, Cavanagh D, Bryson SC et al: Major morbidity after pelvic exenteration: A seven year experience. Obstet Gynecol 69:617, 1987.

Rutledge FN, Burns BC Jr: Pelvic exenteration. Am J Obstet Gynecol 91:692, 1965.

Rutledge FN, McGuffee VB: Pelvic exenteration: Prognostic significance of regional lymph node metastasis. Gynecol Oncol 26:374, 1987.

Rutledge FN, Smith JP, Wharton JT et al: Pelvic exenteration: Analysis of 296 patients. Am J Obstet Gynecol 129:881, 1977.

Sharma S, Odunsi K, Driscoll D, Lele S: Pelvic exenterations for gynecological malignancies: Twenty-year experience at Roswell Park Cancer Institute. Int J Gynecol Cancer 15:475, 2005.

Shingleton HM, Soong SJ, Gelder MS et al: Clinical and histopathologic factors predicting recurrence and survival after pelvic exenteration for cancer of the cervix. Obstet Gynecol 73:1027, 1989.

Snijders-Keilholz A, Ewing P, Seynaeve C, Burger CW: Primitive neuroectodermal tumor of the cervix uteri: A case report Changing concepts in therapy. Gynecol Oncol 98:516, 2005.

Soper JT, Berchuck A, Creasman WT et al: Pelvic exenteration: Factors associated with major surgical morbidity. Gynecol Oncol 35:93, 1989.

Stanhope CR, Symmonds RE, Lee RA et al: Urinary diversion with use of ileal and sigmoid conduit. Am J Obstet Gynecol 155:288, 1986.

Swan RW, Rutledge FN: Urinary conduit in pelvic cancer patients: a report of 16 years' experience. Am J Obstet Gynecol 119:6, 1974.

Symmonds RE, Pratt JH, Webb MJ: Exenteration operations: Experience with 198 patients. Am J Obstet Gynecol 121:907, 1975.

Walton LA: The stress of radical pelvic surgery: a review. Gynecol Oncol 7:25, 1979.

Wheelers CR Jr: Incidence of fecal incontinence after coloproctostomy below five centimeters in the rectum. Gynecol Oncol 27:373, 1987.

Wheelers CR Jr: Recent advances in surgical reconstrution of the gynecologic cancer patient. Curr Opin Obstet Gynecol 4:91, 1992.

NON-EPITHELIAL TUMORS OF THE CERVIX (SARCOMA, LYMPHOMA, AND MELANOMA)

Abdul-Karim RW et al: Sarcoma of the uterine cervix: Clinicopathologic findings in three cases. Gynecol Oncol 26:103, 1987.

Akine Y et al: Carcinoma of the uterine cervix treated by irradiation alone: Result of treatment at the National Cancer Center, Tokyo. Acta Oncol 29:747, 1989.

Brand E, Berek JS, Nieberg RK et al: Rhabdomyosarcoma of the uterine cervix: Sarcoma botryoides. Cancer 60:1552, 1987.

Kristiansen SB, Anderson R, Cohen DM: Case report: Primary malignant melanoma of the cervix and review of the literature. Gynecol Oncol 47:398, 1992.

Montag RW, D'Abaing G, Schlaerth JB: Embryonal rhabdomyosarcoma of the uterine corpus and cervix. Gynecol Oncol 25:171, 1986.

Mordel N, Mor-Yosef S, Ben-Baruch N et al: Malignant melanoma of the uterine cervix: Case report and review of the literature. Gynecol Oncol 32:375, 1989.

Muntz GH et al: Stage IE primary malignant lymphomas of the uterine cervix. Cancer 68:2023, 1991.

Perren T et al: Case report: Lymphomas of the cervix and upper vagina: A report of five cases and a review of the literature. Gynecol Oncol 44:87, 1992.

Rotmensch J, Rosensheim NB, Woodruff JD: Cervical sarcoma: A review. Obstet Gynecol Surg 38:456, 1983.

4 Endometrial Hyperplasia, Estrogen Therapy, and the Prevention of Endometrial Cancer

Joan L. Walker, M.D. and Rosemary E. Zuna, M.D.

INTRODUCTION

The endometrium is a very dynamic tissue in the reproductive age woman. It is continuously changing in response to hormonal, stromal, and vascular influences, with the intended goal of implanting an embryo and supporting the nutritional needs of the developing pregnancy. Estrogen stimulation is associated with the growth and proliferation of the endometrium (Fig. 4–1) while progesterone produced by the corpus luteum after ovulation inhibits proliferation and stimulates secretion in the glands and predecidual change (Fig. 4–2) in the stroma. Without conception and HCG production, the corpus luteum fails to produce progesterone and hormonal withdrawal allows menses to occur. Continuous estrogen stimulation of the endometrium bypasses the normal recycling of the endometrium. Women have transitions in their lives where the absence of ovulation predisposes them to unopposed estrogen stimulation, since no corpus luteum forms to secrete progesterone in anovulatory or menopausal women. Menarche and perimenopause are transitions of varying lengths of time, and some women (approximately 5%) have polycystic ovarian disease, which is a prolonged anovulatory condition. Obesity in the menopause also produces a state of excess estrogen production. This is due to the peripheral conversion, in the adipose tissues, of androgens secreted from the adrenal glands and ovaries into an estrogen, estrone, by the enzyme aromatase.

Unopposed estrogen stimulation will yield a continuous spectrum of change from proliferative endometrium (Fig. 4–5) through many variations of endometrial hyperplasia until a malignant neoplasm develops. Endometrial cancer (Fig. 4–8) is defined by the ability to invade local tissue and metastasize. The fact that endometrial lesions are represented by glandular and stromal variations in continuous change, explains the challenge of classifying endometrial hyperplasias into distinct categories, which are reproducible, predict neoplastic risk, as well as response to progesterone therapy. Histopathological classification of endometrial lesions provides a stratification of risk for progression to cancer by defined endometrial changes.

Understanding the pathophysiology of excess unopposed estrogen production helps the clinician better predict which women are at risk for endometrial cancer, and provides windows of opportunity for implementation of prevention strategies. These principles have also been used to treat hormonally active cancers, especially breast cancer. Tamoxifen has long been used, and now aromatase inhibitors are widely used to treat breast cancer and decrease breast cancer recurrence risk. These drugs have toxicities that the

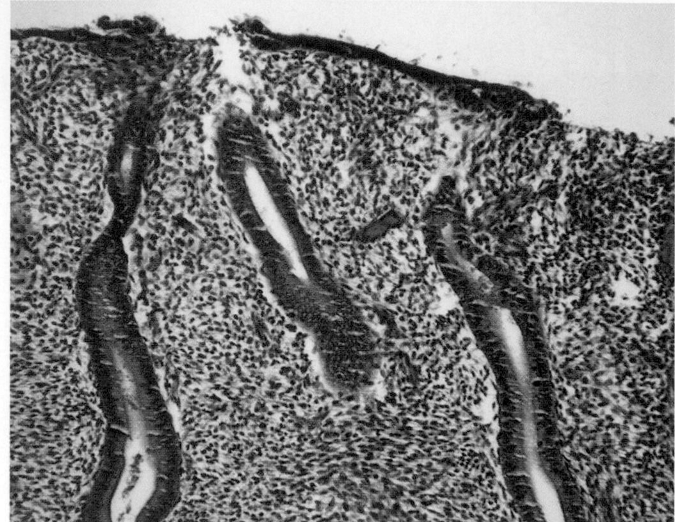

Figure 4–1 Proliferative endometrium: Simple tubular endometrial glands are set in a prominent stroma. This pattern is associated with normal estrogen stimulation in a cycling woman. (Hematoxylin and eosin, 10 × original magnification.)

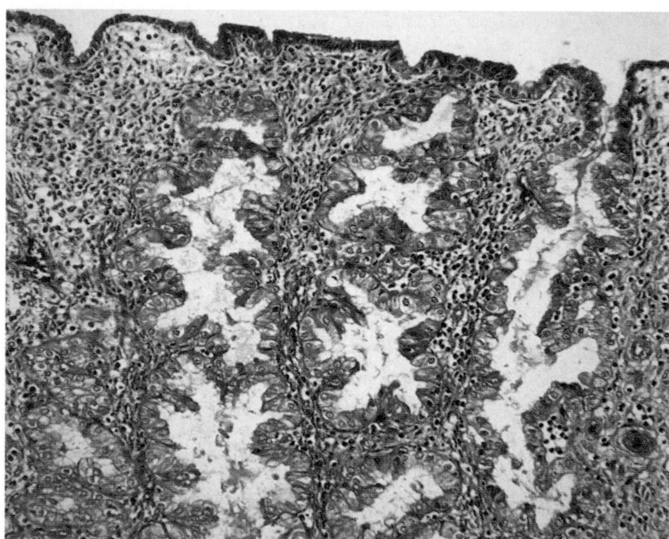

Figure 4–2 Secretory endometrium: Endometrial glands are present with a saw-tooth pattern. Each gland is an individual unit set in endometrial stroma. The epithelium has intracytoplasmic glycogen secretion that is eventually extruded into the gland lumen. (Hematoxylin and eosin, 10 × original magnification.)

obstetrician/gynecologist will be required to manage. Although Tamoxifen is an anti-estrogen in breast tissue, it paradoxically has estrogen-like properties in the endometrium and increases the risk of endometrial cancer. It is also associated with thromboembolism and stroke. While Tamoxifen provides protection against bone loss, osteoporosis and fractures, it does not appear to carry increased risk of myocardial infarction. There does appear to be an association with cataracts. Unfortunately, Tamoxifen accentuates menopausal symptoms. Aromatase inhibitors accelerate menopausal bone loss, which could lead to osteoporosis and fractures, therefore prevention of these toxicities is important when they are prescribed. Other side effects of aromatase inhibitors include hot flashes, sweats, edema, sore muscles and fatigue.

Preventative health maintenance must balance all risks and benefits, while maintaining quality of life and symptom control, and this is the central theme in this chapter. Many women want active control over these very important choices, and may value quality of life and their sexual relationship more than cancer prevention and cardiovascular risk reduction.

CLINICAL PRESENTATION OF ENDOMETRIAL HYPERPLASIA

The scientific explanation for the low incidence rates for endometrial hyperplasia is that it is a lesion that is usually unrecognized and asymptomatic until cancer develops. Until endometrial cancer screening becomes routine and cost effective, the true prevalence of the precursor lesions will remain unknown. Women with endometrial hyperplasias are identified by endometrial biopsy performed because of abnormal vaginal bleeding (menorrhagia, or postmenopausal bleeding) or because a thickened endometrial stripe is found on transvaginal ultrasound when ordered for another reason such as the identification of endometrial cells in the Pap test of a woman over the age of 40 years.

There is evidence of exogenous or endogenous unopposed estrogen stimulation of the endometrium in most women with endometrial hyperplasia. Some women have an ovarian neoplasm (the classic presentation of a granulosa cell tumor of the ovary), which produces the excess endogenous estrogen causing endometrial hyperplasia or cancer and the patient presents with vaginal bleeding. The most common causes of excess estrogen are obesity, polycystic ovarian disease, or a prolonged perimenopause with anovulatory bleeding patterns. The development of hyperplasia secondary to anovulation at menarche is very uncommon, and should be easily reversible, with normalization of cyclic menses with oral contraceptive pills. The age at presentation depends on the source of the excess estrogen. Endometrial hyperplasias and cancers that are associated with estrogen stimulation have a good prognosis. Endometrial cancers in women without evidence of excess estrogen are usually not associated with hyperplasia and can be associated with a tumor suppressor gene abnormality such as P53-associated uterine papillary serous carcinomas (Figs. 4–3 and 4–4). These are aggressive cancers, behaving similarly to ovarian cancer and have high mortality rates.

Office endometrial biopsy has replaced the dilation and curettage procedure for the diagnosis of endometrial hyperplasia or carcinoma. There is interest in the potential benefit of curettage as therapy, as well as providing more tissue for accurate histologic diagnosis. Others advocate the use of "hormonal curettage" in which medical therapy with progestogen is followed by the withdrawal bleed.

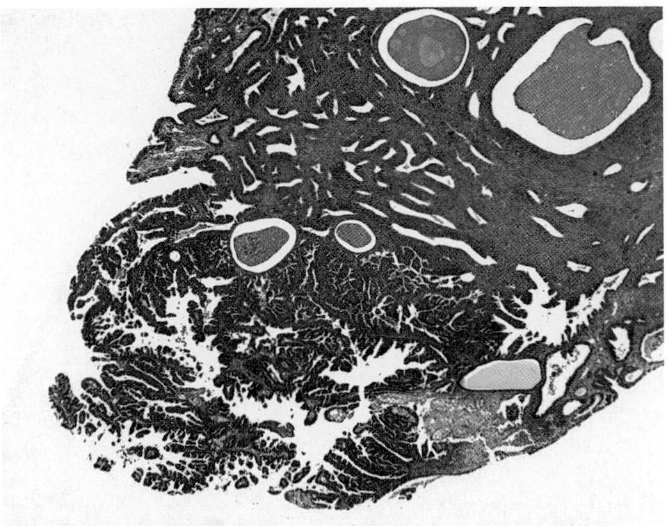

Figure 4–3 Endometrial serous carcinoma in a polyp: There is an irregular, complex pattern of papillary epithelium arising in the tip of an endometrial polyp. (Hematoxylin and eosin, 2 × original magnification.)

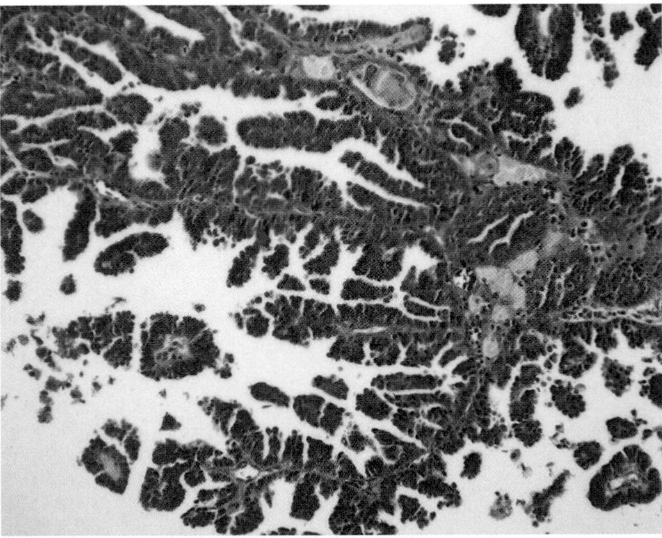

Figure 4–4 Endometrial serous carcinoma: This tumor shows a complex pattern of highly atypical cells with large irregular nuclei and prominent nucleoli. Typically, the tumor shows a papillary configuration, with abnormal epithelium covering a thin connective tissue core. (Hematoxylin and eosin, 10 × original magnification.)

This provides the same effect without the surgical cost or risk. Repeat office endometrial biopsy at three-month intervals can reassure the patient and the clinician of the therapeutic effect of the hormonal therapy. There is little to no evidence of increasing a woman's mortality risk by potentially delaying a diagnosis of cancer by three months. It is expected that an underlying cancer will be identified periodically by this technique, but no evidence that dilation and curettage reduces a women's mortality risk. This outpatient office evaluation and management has become the usual and safest way to manage these patients, until there is evidence that a hysterectomy is required. These management decisions will be discussed further in later sections of this chapter.

ENDOMETRIAL HYPERPLASIA: PATHOLOGIC DIAGNOSTIC CRITERIA

The International Society of Gynecological Pathologists (ISGYP), International Federation of Gynecology and Obstetrics (FIGO), and the World Health Organization (WHO) currently classify endometrial hyperplasia based on a 1994 classification system into four categories based on architectural structure and cytologic features. The architecture is either simple or complex and the cytologic features are described as with or without atypia (Table 4–1). This yields four separate diagnoses: simple hyperplasia without atypia (Fig. 4–5); complex hyperplasia without atypia (Fig. 4–6); simple hyperplasia with atypia (Fig. 4–7); complex hyperplasia with atypia (Fig. 4–8).

The terms adenomatous and cystic-glandular hyperplasia have been discarded, and when the abbreviation AEH is used, it refers to atypical endometrial hyperplasia, which reflects the two categories of hyperplasia with cytologic atypia (simple hyperplasia with atypia and complex hyperplasia with atypia). The presence of atypia appears to be the most important criterion for progression to adenocarcinoma, or the coexistence of endometrioid adenocarcinoma. The rates of coexisting endometrioid adenocarcinoma (new figures grade 1 and grade 3 endometrioid carcinomas) with atypical endometrial hyperplasia are reported to be as low as 13% and as high as 43%.

The pathologic diagnosis of these lesions is usually made with a small sampling of the endometrium in the office using a device called a Pipelle. This small tissue sample then has to be categorized by the pathologist. A prospective study of the reproducibility of the diagnosis of atypical endometrial hyperplasia (both simple and complex) was undertaken by the Gynecologic Oncology Group (GOG). Women with the diagnosis of atypical endometrial hyperplasia at any of 285 GOG institutions agreed to have a hysterectomy within 12 weeks to be enrolled. The study population was 302 eligible cases with a median age of 57 years and 31% were 50 years of age or younger. The endometrial biopsy specimens were re-reviewed by three gynecologic pathologists independently (study panel diagnosis) in a blinded protocol. They agreed to categorize the endometrium as normal (cycling, menstrual, or atrophic),

Table 4–1 CLASSIFICATION OF ENDOMETRIAL HYPERPLASIA
Simple hyperplasia
Complex hyperplasia (adenomatous)
Simple atypical hyperplasia
Complex atypical hyperplasia (adenomatous with atypia)

From World Health Organization
From Blaustein's Pathology of the Female Genital Tract, Fourth Edition, Robert J. Kurman Editor, Chapter 11, p 412, 1994.

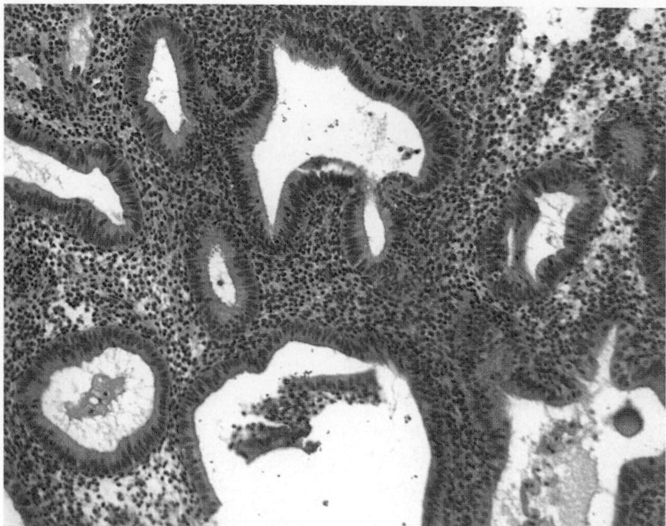

Figure 4–5 Simple hyperplasia without atypia: The endometrium shows an increase in the glandular epithelium usually due to unopposed estrogen stimulation. This results in irregular and unpredictable gland outlines that are often cystic. There is abundant stroma, so that the gland:stromal ratio is little altered from normal. (Hematoxylin and eosin, 10 × original magnification.)

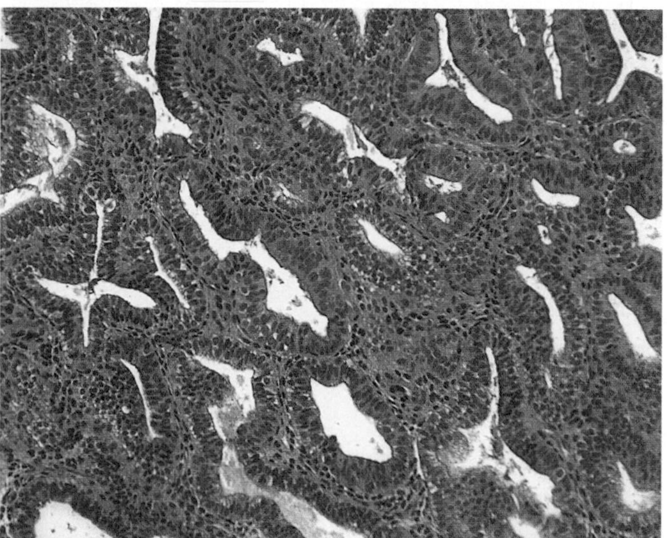

Figure 4–6 Complex hyperplasia without atypia: The gland:stromal ratio is increased with complex, closely-set, irregular gland outlines. However, there is little nuclear atypia. (Hematoxylin and eosin, 20 × original magnification.)

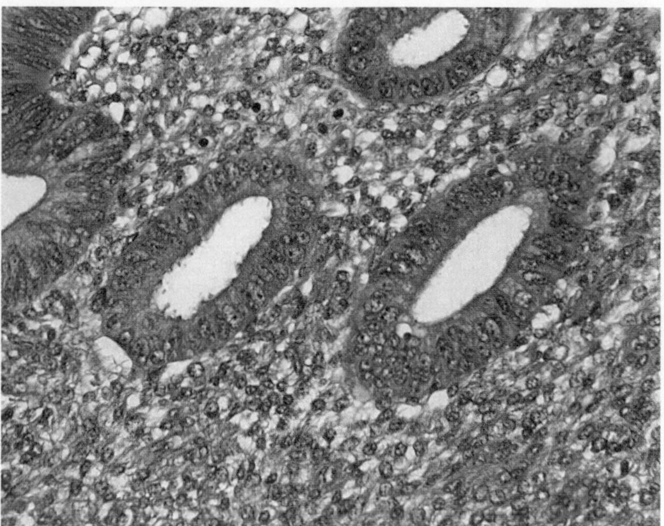

Figure 4–7 Simple hyperplasia with atypia: Uncommonly recognized form of hyperplasia in which the epithelium shows an increased gland:stromal ratio with simple glands. However, the glands are lined by epithelium with atypical nuclei. (Hematoxylin and eosin, 40 × original magnification.)

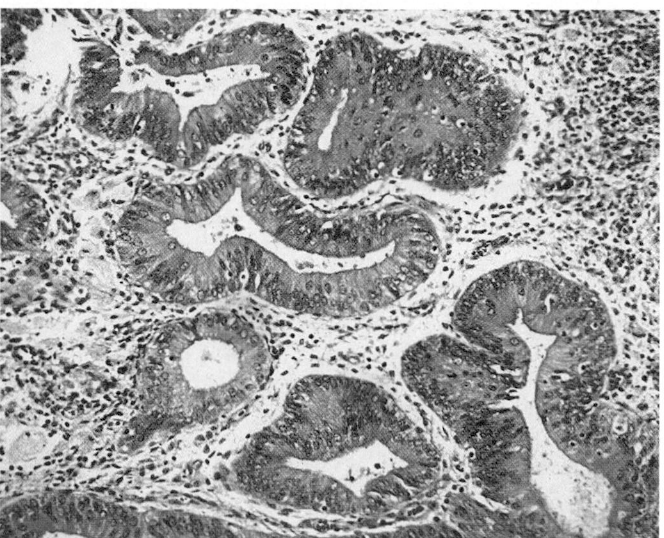

Figure 4–8 Atypical complex hyperplasia: The tissue shows a marked increase in the gland:stromal ratio with complex glandular outlines and nuclear atypia in the lining epithelium. (Hematoxylin and eosin, 20 × original magnification.)

non-atypical hyperplasia (disordered proliferative, simple or complex hyperplasia), atypical hyperplasia (Fig. 4–8) (simple or complex), adenocarcinoma (Fig. 4–9), or inadequate for evaluation. Two out of three study pathologists had to agree on one of the above five diagnoses for a study panel diagnosis to be established. Correct diagnosis was determined by consensus agreement on the hysterectomy specimen, during a panel review simultaneously with a multiheaded scope. The results found 40% of the cases had all three pathologists in agreement. The reproducibility was lowest for the diagnosis of AEH (kappa 0.28), and better for adenocarcinoma (kappa 0.51). Reproducibility was best for dilation and curettage (kappa 0.47 CI 0.41:0.53) compared to small sampling devices (kappa 0.26–0.36). Two of three study panel members agreed with the referring institution diagnosis of AEH in 38% of cases. The study panel diagnosis was less severe in 25% of cases and adenocarcinoma in 29% of cases. The most important outcome for this study was the finding that 43% of the enrolled participants were found to have adenocarcinoma in their uterus at the time of hysterectomy. The second most important finding was the rate of adenocarcinoma in each study panel majority diagnosis category: normal or non-atypical hyperplasia 14/74 (18.9%); AEH

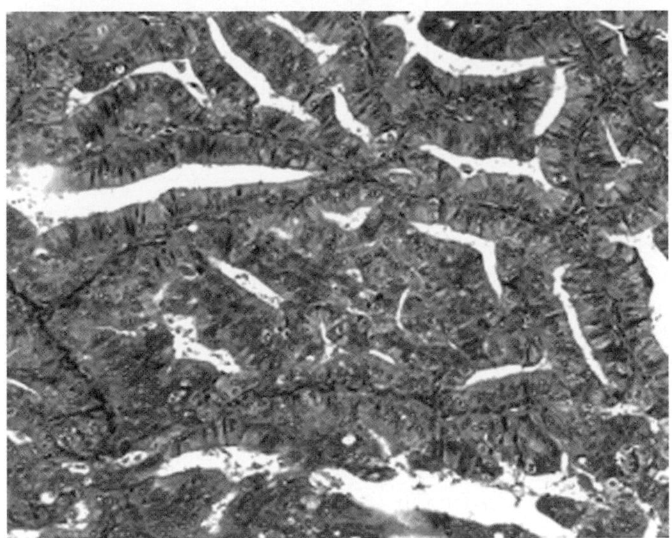

Figure 4–9 Well-differentiated (FIGO G1) endometrioid adenocarcinomas typically show a "back to back" glandular arrangement with little intervening stroma. The glands are lined by tall columnar tumor cells. (Hematoxylin and eosin, 20 × original magnification.)

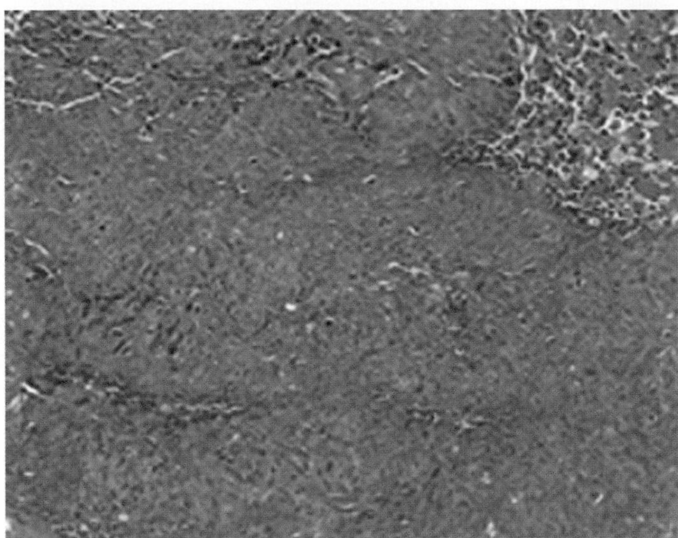

Figure 4–10 Poorly differentiated (FIGO G3) endometrioid adenocarcinomas show a loss of glandular architecture in the most of the tumor. The cells typically are round-polygonal rather than columnar in shape. Cellular necrosis (upper right) is a common feature of these lesions. (Hematoxylin and eosin, 20 × original magnification.)

45/115 (39.1%); adenocarcinoma 54/84 (64.3%). The uterine examination revealed the presence of some risk factors for metastatic disease present in 43 cases, including myometrial invasion, grade 2 or 3 lesions.

The natural history of simple hyperplasia without atypia is likely to follow a benign course. It is often seen in women near menopause when anovulatory cycles are common. The removal of the estrogenic stimulation or treatment with progestogens influences the outcome. The majority of lesions will regress (60%) without treatment, and 84% with progestin therapy. Only 3% are believed to progress to cancer. Complex hyperplasia is also expected to regress (56%) when atypia is not present. Atypical hyperplasia has a 36% progression rate, and even with progestins, 27% have been reported to progress, but it is uncertain if this is coexistent cancer that is eventually identified. Fifty five percent of atypical hyperplasia is expected to regress with progestin therapy. The best agent for progestin therapy has not yet been identified. Similarly, the pattern of administration (cyclic or continuous) and the duration of treatment remain to be established. It is assumed that unless the estrogen stimulation ceases, the progestin therapy may need to be lifelong. Alternatively, a hysterectomy is necessary to prevent the development of the most common endometrioid adenocarcinoma or Type I cancer (estrogen dependent) (Fig. 4–10). This estrogen-induced cancer is the most common histologic type and the least aggressive form of uterine malignancy and should be preventable, as well as successfully treated when detected.

Recent research involving molecular studies of endometrial lesions and objective computerized morphometrics has shown promise to increase the accuracy and reproducibility of the diagnosis of endometrial lesions. A new classification system was proposed as the 2003 WHO classification, which defines Endometrial Intraepithelial Neoplasia (EIN) as the precancerous lesion. Early evidence suggests that it may be more predictive of progression to cancer, but is not clinically used or accepted at this time.

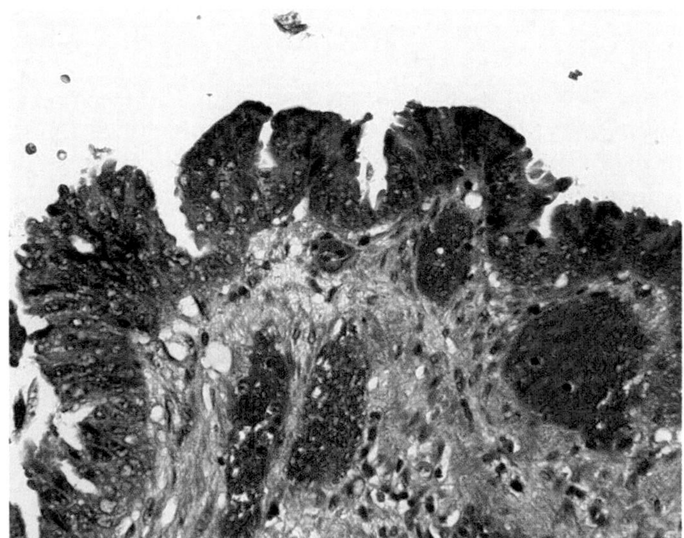

Figure 4–11 Endometrial intraepithelial carcinoma (EIC): Precursor lesion for serous carcinoma of the endometrium with markedly atypical, crowded epithelium with little architectural abnormality. This lesion is often observed on the surface of otherwise benign endometrial polyps. (Hematoxylin and eosin, 20 × original magnification.)

Endometrial carcinomas of the serous type arise in a background of atrophic endometrium. These cancers, often papillary, are not associated with excess estrogen and have been classified as Type II (estrogen-independent) endometrial cancers. Endometrial hyperplasia is not a precursor to serous carcinoma. Rather, the precursor has been identified as endometrial intraepithelial carcinoma (EIC)

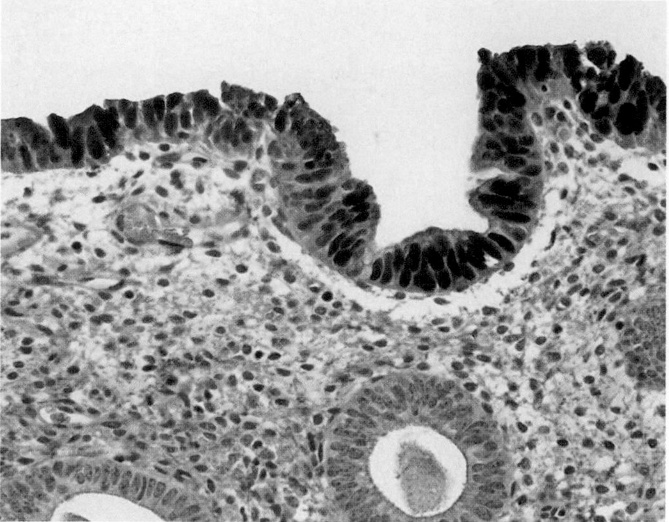

Figure 4–12 p53 immunostain of EIC: Endometrial serous carcinoma is typically accompanied by p53 mutations that allow accumulation of p53 protein in the cells that can be identified by immunostaining. Normal cells do not stain positively for p53 because the amount of normal protein is below the threshold of the staining test. (Immunoperoxidase stain for p53 with DAB chromogen, 20 × original magnification).

(Figs. 4–9 and 4–10). Serous endometrial intraepithelial carcinoma (EIC) can even be multifocal with disease found in the ovaries and omentum when no invasive component is found in the uterus. Comprehensive surgical staging is recommended, due to the difficulty in establishing the diagnosis of invasive cancer on intraoperative evaluation. Serous papillary adenocarcinoma is less likely to be identified at an early stage compared with endometrioid histologic types. Postoperative therapy can then be recommended after adequate histologic evaluation and staging. The serous lesions are often associated with abnormalities in p53 tumor suppressor gene (Fig. 4–12) that results in accumulation of p53 protein in the cell. Unlike normal cells or most endometrioid cancers, immunostaining with antibodies to p53 will be positive in the majority of serous cancers.

MANAGEMENT DECISIONS FOR ATYPICAL ENDOMETRIAL HYPERPLASIA

The patient's age, fertility plans, need for contraception, comorbidities, and personal preferences play a dramatic role in the management of these lesions. Hysterectomy is indicated when fertility is not desired and complex endometrial hyperplasia with atypia is identified. Atypical endometrial hyperplasia (AEH) is commonly found with coexisting undiagnosed cancer already present in the uterus, or progressing to endometrial cancer in untreated women. A prospective trial was conducted by the Gynecologic Oncology Group to identify the prevalence of underlying cancer and to more clearly define the diagnostic criteria for AEH compared to cancer. In this study, 306 women were enrolled who had a community-based diagnosis of AEH on endometrial biopsy, and proceeded without medical treatment to hysterectomy. Forty-three percent had invasive cancer in the uterus, some of which were high-grade lesions with deep myometrial invasion. While 63% (77/123) of the cancers identified were grade I lesions confined to the endometrium, 31% were myoinvasive, and 11% had deep myometrial invasion into the outer 50% of the myometrium. It is possible that future validation of a new EIN (endometrial intraepithelial neoplasia) scoring system, nuclear imaging technology, or a new molecular marker will allow more precise predictability for the neoplastic potential and the co-existence of cancer before hysterectomy.

The complexity of the surgical management of atypical endometrial hyperplasia is underappreciated. Intraoperative decision-making, using frozen section to determine the operative interventions, is never ideal, considering the difficulty of the diagnosis, and the variety of skill and expertise of the pathologist and gynecologists. It is to be expected that the postoperative diagnosis of cancer will be obtained in a substantial number of these cases. The recommendation is that the patient should be informed of the 20–45% risk of underlying malignancy, and hysterectomy is required for final diagnosis. She should be counseled about the desire to keep her ovaries, or have them removed, based on her age, family history, and other medical conditions or comorbidities. Vaginal hysterectomy may be all that is required, or laparoscopically assisted hysterectomy with bilateral salpingo-ophorectomy and peritoneal cytology can be considered. In the event that high-grade cancer or deep myometrial invasion is found, re-operation may be necessary for comprehensive surgical staging and removal of retained ovaries. Staging can usually be accomplished laparoscopically if a previous laparotomy was not performed. This should be necessary in approximately 10% of the cases where cancer is identified, and will depend on the entire health history of the individual. Increased cost and more errors are likely if all hyperplasia cases are subjected to laparotomy, intraoperative frozen section, and staging based on intraoperative assessment of myometrial invasion. It should be noted that pelvic radiation is no longer a substitute for accurate and thorough surgical staging in endometrial cancer, so consultation with a gynecologic oncologist is appropriate for these difficult decisions when unexpected cancer is found in the hysterectomy specimen.

Women who desire childbearing, refuse hysterectomy, or have medical conditions that make hysterectomy an undesirable first choice can be treated hormonally. Megestrol 160 mg/day, in divided doses, has been the drug of choice with acceptable results even in the face of complex endometrial hyperplasia with atypia. It is unclear whether the treatment should be continuous or cyclic, but there are theoretical advantages to the endometrial shedding provided by the progesterone withdrawal bleed. The endometrium needs to be re-evaluated histologically, by office biopsy or dilation and curettage, at 3-month intervals for at least a year. Lifelong prevention strategies must be emphasized with the patient. The pathologist finds the evaluation of the endometrial sampling more straightforward if it is not complicated by exogenous hormonal influences. For this reason, it is best to withdraw the patient from the progestogen for 7–14 days, to allow withdrawal bleeding prior to endometrial biopsies. Schedule the biopsy or dilation and curettage after the withdrawal bleeding ceases.

Ramirez reported in 2004 on successful pregnancies after treatment of grade 1 endometrial cancer with progestins. Eighty-one patients of a median age of 30 years were treated for approximately 6 months. Forty-seven were able to reverse the lesion and twenty patients were able to become pregnant. Half of the patients required assisted reproductive technologies. The ACOG Practice Bulletin on endometrial cancer includes this general guideline: Women with atypical endometrial hyperplasia (AEH) and endometrial cancer who desire to maintain their fertility may be treated with progestin therapy. Following therapy they should undergo serial complete intrauterine evaluation approximately every 3 months to document response. Hysterectomy should be reommended for women who do not desire future fertility.

Local therapy of the endometrium with a progestin-containing intrauterine device is encouraging. Wildemeersch reported on 12 women with hyperplasia from 46 to 67 years of age. Their lesions were diagnosed as simple hyperplasia without atypia in 7 and as atypical hyperplasia in 5 women. All women were without hyperplasia at 12 months. Montz et al demonstrated the successful treatment of well-differentiated endometrial adenocarcinoma with the intrauterine progestin-secreting device. Hysteroscopic removal of all hyperplastic tissue was performed and the IUD was inserted in 13 women with grade 1 endometrioid adenocarcinoma. Endometrial biopsies were performed every 3 months and six of the 12 evaluable cases were negative for carcinoma at 6 months. A total of eight women completed 12 months of therapy, six of whom were negative for carcinoma at that time. Those six women have been maintained on this therapy and undergo annual endometrial biopsies.

In conclusion, management decisions in women with atypical endometrial hyperplasia are complex, and require an understanding of the risk of invasive endometrial adenocarcinoma, the reproductive desires of the patient, her comorbidities, and risks for surgical management. Ideally, laparoscopic assisted vaginal hysterectomy with bilateral salpingo-oophorectomy can be preformed. The finding of adenocarcinoma in the uterus requires consultation with a gynecologic oncologist to determine whether observation or re-operation for surgical staging should be considered.

Table 4–2 CLASSIFICATION OF PROGESTOGENS

Progesterone (identical to endogenous progesterone)

Progestins (not identical to endogenous progesterone)

A. Structurally related to progesterone
   1. pregnane derivatives:
      a. acetylated (also called 17α–hydroxyprogesterone derivatives): medroxyprogesterone acetate, megestrol acetate, cyproterone acetate, chlormadinone acetate
      b. nonacetylated: dydrogesterone, medrogestone
   2. 19-norpregnane derivatives (also called 19-norprogesterone derivatives):
      a. acetylated: nomegestrol acetate, nestorone
      b. nonacetylated: demegestone, trimegestone, promegestone
B. Structurally related to testosterone (also called 19-nortestosterone derivatives)
   1. ethinylated:
      a. estranes: norethindrone (also called norethisterone), norethindrone acetate, norethynodrel, lynestrenol, ethynodiol diacetate
      b. 18-ethylgonanes: levonorgestrel, norgestrel, desogestrel, gestodene, norgestimate
   2. nonethinylated: dienogest, drospirenone

From Role of progestogen in hormone therapy for postmenopausal women: position statement of The North American Menopause Society, Menopause 10(2)115, 2003.

MANAGEMENT OF ENDOMETRIAL HYPERPLASIA WITHOUT ATYPIA

The diagnosis of simple or complex hyperplasia without atypia requires hormonal management and is not an indication for hysterectomy. These lesions are generally reversible with progestogen (synthetic progestin or progesterone). The classification of progestogens is seen in Table 4–2. The drugs available on the North American market are listed in Table 4–3. The initial approach is generally to treat in a cyclic fashion with the progestogen given for 14 days of the month to deliver predictable cyclic withdrawal menses. Women, including teenagers, who are premenopausal and sexually active, are usually best treated with a regimen that provides contraception such as Depo-Provera or oral contraceptives. Women who want to conceive are likely to be anovulatory and require ovulation induction agents after withdrawal bleeding is produced with a progestogen. Reassurance can be obtained from a reduction of menstrual flow and a bleeding pattern that is appropriately timed with the cyclic therapy. It is extremely important to counsel anovulatory women about the lifelong risk of endometrial cancer and methods for surveillance and prevention. Twenty-five percent of endometrial cancers occur in the premenopausal age range, and 5% are 40 years of age and younger. These cancers may be part of the polycystic ovarian syndrome or the anovulatory transition prior to menopause and are all theoretically preventable with proper counseling and active management. Premenopausal endometrial cancer patients should also be counseled

Table 4–3 PROGESTOGENS USED FOR EPT IN NORTH AMERICA

Composition	Proprietary Name	Available Dosages
Progesterone (micronized)		
Oral capsule	Prometrium	100, 200 mg
Vaginal gel	Prochieve[1] (45 mg/dose)	4% gel
Progestin		
Oral tablet		
medroxyprogesterone acetate	Provera, Gen-Medroxy[2], Alti-MPA,[2] Novo-Medrone,[2] various generics	2.5, 5.0, 10.0 mg
norethindrone (norethisterone)	Micronor, Nor-QD[1]	0.35 mg
noretindrone acetate	Aygestin,[1] Norlutate,[2] generic	5.0 mg
norgestrel	Ovrette[1]	0.075 mg
Intrauterine system		
levonorgestrel	Mirena	20 mcg/day approx release rate (52 mg/device; 5-y use)

[1]Available only in the United States.
[2]Available only in Canada.
Products not marked are available in both the United States and Canada.
From Role of progestogen in hormone therapy for postmenopausal women: position statement of The North American Menopause Society, Menopause 10(2)116, 2003.

about the possibility of Lynch syndrome. A family history should be taken and if endometrial and colon cancers are frequent in the family, the patient should be referred to genetic counseling. Colonoscopy is often recommended to endometrial cancer patients due to the association with colon cancer. There is a dramatic rise in the incidence rate of endometrial hyperplasia and endometrial cancer at 45 years of age and peaking at 65 years of age. This is likely due to the combined effects of estrone (estrogen) production in the peripheral adipose tissue particularly in obese women and to the absence of progesterone that is due to loss of ovulatory function in menopause.

PREVENTION OF ENDOMETRIAL CANCER

Endometrial stimulation by estrogens unopposed by progestins leads to endometrial hyperplastic conditions in a dose and time dependent manner. Experimental evidence has been obtained from prospective clinical trials conducted to identify the appropriate doses and schedules of hormone replacement therapies. Kurman reported a randomized trial of 1176 postmenopausal women receiving 1 mg of estradiol orally and either placebo or various doses of norethindrone acetate. Women treated with estradiol alone (247 evaluable participants) for 12 months had a 12.2% rate of simple hyperplasia without atypia, 1.6% had complex hyperplasia without atypia and 0.8% had complex atypical hyperplasia. Norethindrone acetate at all doses used in this trial, nearly eliminated that risk. The North American Menopause Society support the addition of a progestogen whenever estrogen is prescribed for menopausal symptoms in women with an intact uterus for the prevention of estrogen induced hyperplasia and adenocarcinoma. Unfortunately, the progestogen has undesirable side effects, and women have been known to discontinue this component of their prescribed hormone replacement (see Tables 4–1 and 4–2).

The prevention of endometrial cancer has been recently complicated by the publication and early closure of the estrogen plus progestin (E + P) component of the Women's Health Initiative (WHI). This randomized placebo-controlled clinical trial evaluated conjugated equine estrogens (CEE), 0.625 mg, plus medroxyprogesterone acetate (MPA), 2.5 mg orally per day (HRT). This trial enrolled 16,608 women with a range of 50–79 years of age for an average of 5.2 years, to determine the primary outcomes of coronary heart disease (CHD), invasive breast cancer and a global index (including stroke, pulmonary embolism, endometrial cancer, colorectal cancer, hip fracture and death due to other causes). In May 2002, the data safety monitoring committee recommended premature closure of the trial due to the adverse outcomes of breast cancer and, cardiovascular complications including coronary heart disease, stroke, and pulmonary embolus. Of note, overall mortality was not affected. The absolute excess risk per 10,000 person-years attributable to HRT was seven coronary heart disease events, eight strokes, eight pulmonary emboli, eight invasive breast cancers and a reduction of five hip fractures. These risks need to be reviewed with women choosing hormone replacement therapy.

The WHI trial with conjugated equine estrogen alone versus placebo had a very different outcome. There was a non-significant reduction in breast cancer risk ($P = 0.06$) and coronary heart disease risk was unaffected (HR = 0.91 [CI 0.75–1.12]), strokes were increased (HR = 1.39 [CI 1.10–1.77]) and hip fractures were reduced (HR = 0.61 [CI 0.41–0.91]). This places women with an intact uterus, and their physicians, in a difficult situation of the balancing risks. Women with a uterus can decide to accept the potential risks of the addition of a progestin, or may choose to take unopposed estrogen and follow the endometrium yearly with transvaginal ultrasound or endometrial biopsy. Unopposed estrogen use gives a woman a relative risk of endometrial cancer of 3 times the general population for less than 5 years of use, and relative risk of 10 after 10 years of use. The risk decreases, but remains elevated after discontinuing the drug. Alternatively, there are other progestins and progesterone formulations available which may carry a different, but as yet unknown risk of breast cancer. Micronized progesterone is available as oral 100 mg or 200 mg capsules (Prometrium), and has been Food and Drug Administration (FDA)-approved for use in combination with estrogen for relief of menopausal symptoms. The dose of 200 mg for 12 days per month in a cyclic fashion causes withdrawal bleeding in a predictable manner. The regimen of conjugated equine estrogen 0.625 mg daily with oral micronized progesterone at a dose of 200 mg daily for 12 days per month failed to see any increase in endometrial hyperplasia with 3 years of follow-up. There is available vaginal progesterone gel which is only FDA-approved for infertility use, but has been studied in small numbers of menopausal women. An additional provocative alternative is to use the progestin-containing intrauterine system (Mirena is FDA-approved for contraceptive use only) and unopposed estrogen, which has been studied prospectively in menopausal women. These women were only followed for one year, and they were able to convert proliferative endometrium to atrophic endometrium while using continuous estradiol 50 mcg per day via the transdermal route.

The official position statement of the North American Menopause Society is that a progestogen should be added to estrogen therapy for all postmenopausal women with an intact uterus. The type, route, or regimen can be individualized to minimize side effects, while providing adequate endometrial protection.

BENEFITS AND RISKS OF ESTROGEN REPLACEMENT THERAPY

Quality of life, vasomotor symptoms, and sexual function

The World Health Organization and the Stages of Reproductive Aging Workshop (STRAW) working group define menopause as the permanent cessation of menstrual periods that occur naturally, or is induced by surgery, chemotherapy or radiation. Menopausal transition is the time of an increase in follicle-stimulating hormone and increased variability in cycle length. Postmenopause begins at the time of the final menstrual period, but is not recognized until 12 months of amenorrhea have occurred. The NIH in the "State of the Science Conference Statement: Management of Menopause-Related Symptoms" defines menopausal symptoms as: vasomotor symptoms; vaginal dryness and painful intercourse; and sleep disturbance. Estrogen is the most consistently effective therapy for vasomotor symptoms, vaginal dryness, sleep disturbances and for improved quality of life, and a subset of women may find an improved mood with estrogen therapy. Testosterone has been demonstrated to improve libido, especially in women who have undergone oophorectomy, however, long-term risks have not been studied. Antidepressants, clonidine, gabapentin have been studied in treatment of hot flashes with some efficacy.

Symptom control is the most common reason for initiating estrogen therapy, and remains undisputed as the most appropriate indication for prescribing estrogen at the time of natural or surgical menopause. The epidemiology community recommendations are that the patient should be told that hormone replacement should be for symptom control only, prescribed at the lowest effective dose, and for the shortest duration of use possible. Women should consider tapering off after 5 years of use, to avoid the adverse events of thromboembolic disorders, breast cancer, stroke, and cardiovascular events (myocardial infarction, death). Women must be active participants in the decision-making regarding estrogen use or estrogen plus progestogen use. They must experience the symptoms, recognize the reasons they are choosing to use these agents and actively make the decision that the benefit is worth the small risk. Their own social situation or individual risk profile may influence their personal decisions.

The WHI reported the symptoms manifested by 8405 women between 8 to 12 months from the date the HRT participants were asked to discontinue conjugated equine estrogen plus medroxyprogesterone acetate. These women were mailed a survey and 21.2% had moderate to severe vasomotor symptoms, which was significantly different (CI 4.92–6.89) compared to placebo. They also reported pain and stiffness AOR 2.16, and these symptoms were reported by more than 10% of respondents. Other withdrawal effects were feeling tired, difficulty sleeping, and a feeling of bloating or gas. Depression was also significantly increased after withdrawal of hormone replacement ($P < 0.001$).

The WHI documented the beneficial effects experienced from hormone replacement therapy in women with a uterus. Relief of hot flashes (85.7%), night sweats (77.6%), vaginal or genital dryness (74.1%), joint pain or stiffness (49.1%) compared to placebo effects ranging from 57.7% to 38.4% respectively. Women taking HRT were more likely to complain of breast tenderness (9.3%) and vaginal bleeding (51%) than those on placebo 2.4% and 5% respectively.

In conclusion, the data summarized in the WHI is not generalizable to the 45–55 year old suffering from menopausal symptoms. These women must prioritize their own situation and health risks and quality of life benefits. Most will find the best symptom relief from estrogen use. Alternatives to estrogen include: progestogens, antidepressants (venlafaxine, paroxetine, fluoxetine) as well as clonidine and the anticonvulsant gabapentin. Over the counter remedies include isoflavones, black cohosh and vitamin E. None of the alternatives resolve the entire menopausal syndrome including sexual dysfunction.

Estring® (Pfizer US Pharmaceuticals) and Femring® (Warner Chilcott Laboratory) are vaginally delivered estradiol in a silicone ring. The Estring® contains 2 mg of estradiol and on average 0.02 mg per day is released over a 90 day period. Studies have demonstrated a median plasma estradiol increase from 4.5 pmol/L prior to insertion, to 12.5 pmol/L at steady state. The comparison with a 0.05 mg Estraderm patch was ten fold greater serum concentrations of estradiol. A study of endometrial thickness in 60 postmenopausal women over a 12 month period of time showed a thickness of 2.8 mm prior to Estring®, and 2.6 mm endometrial thickness after 12 months of use. This is reassuring to women unable to tolerate progestins. Another randomized controlled study demonstrated a decrease in urinary tract infections with the use of Estring®. The use of Estring® may be preferred for women wanting local therapy for vaginal dryness symptoms and inability to take progestins, or a history of breast cancer. Femring® is available when an increase in vaginal dose is desired.

Estrogen alone does not always resolve the sexual dysfunction complaints following bilateral salpingo-oophorectomy. Testosterone is currently undergoing FDA review for the use in female sexual dysfunction. Testosterone has been demonstrated in clinical trials to help with decreased sexual desire, arousal and orgasmic response. The North American Menopausal Society has developed clinical guidelines for testosterone use for women with menopausal sexual dysfunction, after thorough investigation of other psychosocial and medical reasons for these complaints.

Osteoporosis

Osteoporosis prevention strategies should begin before 40 years of age due to decline from peak bone mass. An even more dramatic loss of bone occurs at menopause with the loss of estrogen support of osteoblastic activity. Women should take active measures to protect their bones by regular weight bearing exercise, calcium supplementation (1500 mg elemental calcium for the post menopausal woman) and adequate vitamin D supplementation (800–1200 IU per day). At menopause a baseline bone density is recommended and then repeated every other year unless osteopenia or osteoporosis is detected. Most medications for treatment of osteoporosis are not yet approved for the prevention of the expected bone loss. Drugs approved for prevention include calcium carbonate (Tums), raloxifene (Evista®), Actonel® (risedronate sodium tablets), and estrogen replacement therapy. The benefit versus risk profile of a drug must be excellent for the FDA to approve it for prevention of a health problem. Randomized trial involving large numbers of healthy women must be performed over an extended period of time. Estrogen replacement therapy has been the traditional main prevention strategy to prevent this deterioration in bone strength. Unfortunately, raloxifene (Evista®) has the same thromboembolic risk of estrogen, without the benefit of menopausal symptom relief. Drugs approved for use to treat osteoporosis include raloxifene, which acts on the estrogen receptors similarly to tamoxifen. Risedronate (Actonel®), teriparatide (Forteo®) and alendronate (Fosamax®) are all tablet forms of biphosphonates, and calcitonin (Miacalcin®) is the actual bone-stimulating hormone, which can be given by injection or intranasally. Boniva® (ibandronate) is available as an intravenous form of bisphonosphonate given every three months.

Bone density readings are standardized to healthy women of similar age. Osteopenia is defined as bone loss of greater than one standard deviation from the mean and osteoporosis is bone loss greater than two standard deviations from the mean.

Osteoporosis is a disease characterized by low bone mass and microarchitectural deterioration of bone tissue, which leads to increased bone fragility and increased fracture risk. Low bone mass is related to a low peak bone mass (mainly under genetic influence) and to decrease in bone mass, which occurs after menopause and with aging. Menopause induces an accelerated bone loss within 5–8 years followed by a linear rate of bone loss.

Two anatomic areas are of interest in the bone remodeling process. The first is the axial skeleton, composed primarily of trabecular bone. The second is the appendicular skeleton, composed primarily of cortical bone. The remodeling cycle is the same in both types of bone. However, because of the greater surface area, approximately 40% of trabecular bone, as opposed to 10% of the cortical bone, is in "turnover" each year. The osteoclast is responsible for the reabsorption of old bone, which results in the formation of a resorption cavity. Osteoblasts are then attracted to the cavity where they secrete osteoid, which is primarily type I collagen. The collagen is mineralized mainly with calcium, thus producing new bone with an appropriate mechanical strength. Under normal circumstances, the amount of bone removed is replaced with fresh bone; however, this process can become uncoupled if osteoclasts remove more bone than can normally be replaced by osteoblasts, resulting in net loss of bone mass. In menopausal women, accelerated bone loss is associated with high bone turnover rate and increased osteoclast activity. Estrogen may inhibit osteoclast activity and increase proliferation of osteoblasts as well as collagen production.

The beneficial effects of estrogen in preventing or treating postmenopausal osteoporosis are becoming better recognized. At the same time, there is growing recognition that osteoporosis is a major public health problem in the USA. It is estimated that approximately eight million women in the USA have osteoporosis and another 14 million are at risk because they have low bone mass. Osteoporosis causes more than 1.5 million fractures each year, including 300,000 hip, 700,000 vertebral, and 200,000 wrist fractures. These fractures are seen mainly in women. For a 50-year-old woman, the lifetime risk of fracture of any of the three is 40%. Traditional risk factors for osteoporosis include estrogen deficiency, fair complexion, high caffeine intake, low calcium intake, small thin build, smoking, inadequate physical activities, as well as multiple disease processes and drugs. The cost of osteoporosis in the USA is estimated to be $14 billion per year, of which 70% of cases are associated with hip fractures. The risk of hip fracture is 20% by 90 years of age. Excess mortality associated with hip fracture is 12–20% during the first year after the injury. Less than one half of patients with hip fractures ever return to their prefracture activity. Many require assistance and have lost their independence and require long-term domiciliary care. Vertebral fractures may be asymptomatic in 50%, but successive fractures can lead to loss of height, kyphotic distortion of posture, and chronic back pain. Approximately 10% of patients with hip fractures die of surgical complications within 6 months of fracture. Approximately 25% of all white women older than 60 years of age have spinal compression fractures resulting from osteoporosis. The risk of hip fracture is 20% by the age of 90, and hip fractures are about 2.5 times more common in women than in men. An increased rate of loss of both cortical and cancellous bone is associated with menopause. In a follow-up study of 82 postmenopausal women 5–10 years after their first examination, Meema and coworkers concluded that:

1. as a group, menopausal women lost bone, and the beginning of this loss is less related to age than to loss of ovarian function;
2. the rate of loss was not significantly correlated with age; and
3. the bone loss was prevented by estrogen administration (i.e., 0.625 mg of conjugated estrogens).

A similar beneficial effect of estrogen administration was shown by Lindsay and colleagues (Fig. 4–13) in a short-term double-blind study of changes in metacarpal bone in oophorectomized women given an average daily dose of 25 mcg of mestranol.

Nachtigall and associates conducted a 10-year double-blind prospective study to evaluate the effects of estrogen replacement therapy (ERT). They took a sample population of 84 pairs of randomly chosen postmenopausal patients who were matched for age and diagnosis. One half of the patients received conjugated estrogens and cyclic progesterone whereas the other half received a placebo. The estrogen-treated patients whose therapy was started within 3 years of menopause showed improvement or no increase in osteoporosis. The patients in the control group demonstrated an increase in osteoporosis. A subsequent report by the same authors showed that there was no statistically significant difference in the incidence of thrombophlebitis, myocardial infarction, or uterine cancer in the two groups. Indeed, there was a lower incidence of breast cancer in the treated group. Estrogen-treated patients did show a higher incidence of cholelithiasis. The low number of cases precludes drawing any real conclusions from the data on diseases of low frequency. The study excludes a high incidence of complications from estrogens.

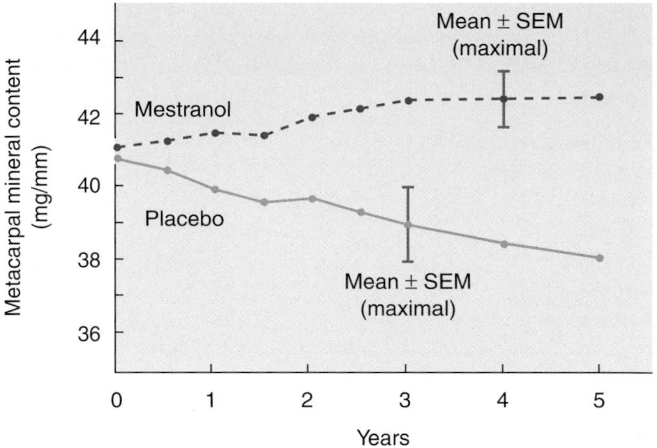

Figure 4–13 Mean metacarpal mineral content during 5-year follow-up of group observed from 3 years after bilateral oophorectomy (zero time). (From: Lindsey R. et al: Long term prevention of postmeopausal osteoporosis by oestrogen. Lancet 1:1038, 1976)

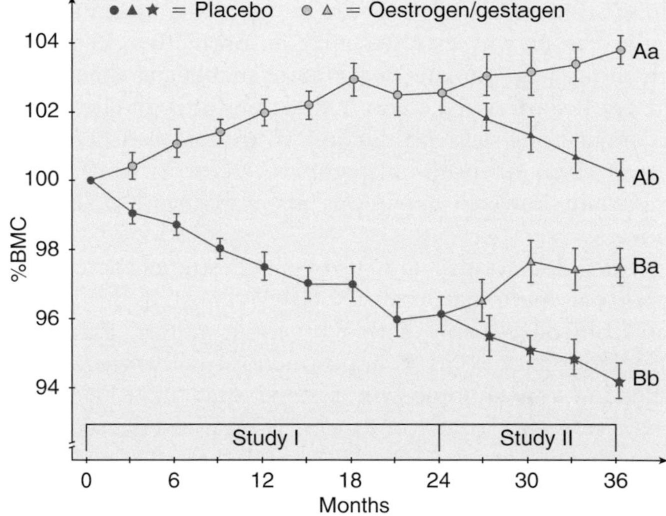

Figure 4–14 Bone mineral content as a function of time and treatment in 94 (study I) and 72 (study II) women soon after menopause. (From Christensen C et al.: Bone mass in postmenopausal women after withdrawal of oestrogen/gestagen replacement therapy. Lancet 1:459, 1981.)

In another crossover study comparing the effects of estrogen-progestin therapy with those of placebo, bone mineral content increased during the 3 years of combination hormone therapy but continued to decrease in the placebo-treated group (Fig. 4–14). When the placebo was given to some of the estrogen-progestin group, bone density decreased, whereas the placebo-treated women had an increase in bone mineral content after being given estrogen-progestin therapy. Other factors are also important in preventing osteoporosis, such as adequate dietary calcium, exercise, and vitamin D. Many case-control studies have noted considerable protection from hip fracture with HRT (Table 4–4).

Table 4–4 CASE CONTROL STUDIES OF HRT IN THE PREVENTION OF HIP FRACTURE

Authors	Relative Risk
Hutchinson et al	0.70
Weiss et al	0.43–0.77
Paganini-Hill et al	0.42
Kreiger et al	0.50
Kiel et al	0.34-0.65
Naesser et al	0.79
Kanis et al	0.55

Colorectal cancer

Colorectal cancer is the third most common cancer and the third leading cause of cancer deaths in US women. Several epidemiologic studies have noted that HRT may reduce the risk of colorectal cancers. WHI demonstrated a HR of 0.63 demonstrating slight protection from colorectal cancer in their E + P arm, but not in the estrogen alone study (HR = 1.08). There appear to be some biologic reasons why estrogen may be protective. Bile acids are thought to initiate or promote malignant changes in the epithelium of the colon. Exogenous estrogen decreases secondary bile acid production. Estrogen also decreases serum levels of insulin-like growth factor-1, which is an important mitogen apparently associated with colorectal cancer.

Both case-control and prospective studies have been reported. Kampman and associates reported the largest case-controlled study with 815 colon cancer and 1019 population base controls in postmenopausal women. After adjusting for multiple risk factors, they noted an 18% decrease in risk of colon cancer in HRT users compared with the non-users (RR = 0.82, CI 0.67–0.99). In the large study of the American Cancer Society, 897 deaths from colon cancer were identified during 7 years' follow-up of 422,373 postmenopausal women. The authors reported a 29% decrease in risk of colon cancer deaths in hormone users compared with non-users (R = 0.71, CI 0.61–0.83). In the review and meta-analysis by Grodstein and colleagues, 18 studies were evaluated. They found a 20% decrease of colon cancer in ERT users compared with the non-users (RR = 0.8, CI 0.72–0.92) and a 19% decrease in rectal cancer (RR = 0.79, CI 0.72–0.92). Ten studies provided data on timing of hormone use. Current users had an RR of 0.66 (CI 0.59–0.74) compared with that of the non-users. In the Nurses' Health Study, current users noted an RR of 0.65; in past users the RR was 0.84 (nonsignificant). Among past users, the decreased risk continued during the first 4 years after quitting ERT; however, 5 years or more after stopping ERT, the risk was similar to that of non-users (RR = 0.92, CI 0.70–1.21). Five studies evaluated the duration of current use and found similar apparent protection for all women currently on ERT, regardless of duration. Four studies evaluated ERT and colorectal adenoma. Most studies noted a significantly decreased risk of development of adenomas in women on ERT. This decrease did not appear to be caused by increased surveillance (sigmoidoscopy) in the ERT users. In several, but not all studies, there was a suggestion that colorectal cancers increased in women who were taking tamoxifen.

Cardiovascular disease

Cardiovascular morbidity (i.e. heart disease and stroke) constitutes the most frequent cause of death among women in the USA. It is estimated to account for approximately 483,800 deaths (233,900 coronary heart disease (CHD), 81,300 myocardial infarction (MI), 96,200 stroke) in the USA in 2003. The second leading cause of death in women is cancer (268,503 in 2002) followed by accidents (64,103 in 2002). Cardiovascular risk factors can be found, and potentially modulated, in women where high cholesterol levels are present. Fifty percent of women have high cholesterol levels and high blood pressure is observed in 32% of all women and 45% of black women. The prevalence of cardiovascular diseases increases dramatically with age, starting at a low level of 17.6% for women age 35–44, 36.6% for women age 45–55, 56.5% for women 55–64 years of age and 75% for women 65–74 years of age. The possible effects of estrogen and progestogen on the incidence of cardiovascular disease in women is the subject of ongoing research. Most of the cohort studies suggest that ERT effectively diminishes the risk of cardiovascular disease in women who are 50–60 years of age, but protection decreases with age (Table 4–5). Unfortunately, recent studies (WHI, HERS) reveal that initiating estrogen therapy in women with established vascular disease (mean ages of 63–67) will not prevent cardiovascular events or deaths. These studies are unable to be generalized to estrogen use in the younger perimenopausal age groups, and the cohort and epidemiologic studies reveal some benefit, but use of progestin consistently decreases benefit.

Prevention of cardiovascular disease includes smoking cessation, blood pressure control, weight control, exercise, and blood sugar and cholesterol control. Blood cholesterol level is a main risk factor for cardiovascular disease in postmenopausal women. A high positive correlation has been found between levels of low-density lipoprotein (LDL) and coronary morbidity. Conversely, the level of high-density lipoprotein (HDL) shows a high negative correlation with the probability of coronary disease and with the extent of damage to the coronary vessels. Matthews has shown the beneficial effects of ERT on LDL and HDL levels. In a prospective study, he showed clearly a corresponding rise in HDLs and a decrease in LDLs in postmenopausal patients treated with ERT. The association of increased HDL and decreased LDL levels with reduced risk of cardiovascular disease is well documented for both men and women.

Lobo reported on the impact of different dosages of MPA on metabolism and hemostasis in postmenopausal

Table 4–5 EFFECT OF ESTROGEN TREATMENT ON CARDIOVASCULAR MORBIDITY IN MENOPAUSAL WOMEN

Authors	Year	Relative risk
Bush et al	1983	0.4
Bush et al	1987	0.3
Wilson et al	1985	1.3–32*
Stampfer et al	1985	0.3
Colditz et al	1987	0.42

* Smokers

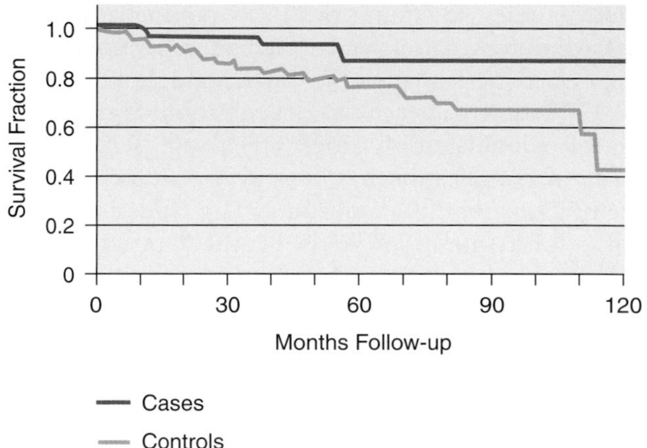

Figure 4–15 Survival in breast cancer estrogen replacement therapy users vs controls.

women treated with conjugated estrogens. In Lobo's prospective, double-blind study, 525 women were randomized to five treatment regimens at 26 sites in the USA and Europe. All participants received 0.625 mg of conjugated estrogens daily for up to 13 cycles; four groups also received MPA, either 2.5 or 5 mg/day continuously or 5 or 10 mg/day for the last 14 days of each cycle. Effects on lipid and carbohydrate metabolism and coagulation were evaluated.

All of the treatment groups experienced increases in HDL-cholesterol (HDL-C), the HDL2-C subfraction and apolipoprotein A-1 compared with baseline; however, at each time point, the increases from baseline in the conjugated estrogens-only group were significantly greater than were those for the conjugated estrogens-MPA groups. Additionally, all treatment groups had significant decreases in LDL-cholesterol (LDL-C) and apolipoprotein B. Decreases from baseline in total cholesterol (TC) levels were significantly greater than were those in the conjugated estrogens-only group. HDL3-C levels increased significantly from baseline in the conjugated estrogens-only group but not in the other treatment groups. Triglyceride levels increased significantly in all groups. The mean increase in the MPA-treated groups was less than that in the conjugated estrogens-only treatment group. Although MPA modified some of the effects of conjugated estrogens on lipid metabolism, the direction of changes in lipid parameters was unaltered.

Additional data on the conjugated estrogens regimen were reported in the results of the Postmenopausal Estrogen/Progestin Intervention (PEPI) trial. In this 3-year, randomized, double-blind, placebo-controlled trial, the investigators evaluated differences in selected heart disease risk factors among 875 postmenopausal women who received placebo, conjugated estrogens, or one of three conjugated estrogens/progestin regimens. One of the regimens utilized in this study was identical to that present in conjugated estrogens.

The investigators reported that after 3 years of therapy, women taking the conjugated estrogens regimen experienced significant increases in HDL-C levels compared with the placebo. However, the increases were significantly less than those experienced by women taking conjugated estrogens alone. Compared with the placebo, LDL-C values were significantly decreased in women taking the conjugated estrogens, with no significant difference between groups. TC levels decreased significantly among women taking the conjugated estrogens regimen compared with the placebo. Significant increases in serum triglyceride levels occurred in all treatment groups compared with the placebo group. There were no significant changes in blood pressure, fasting insulin levels, or 2-hour insulin levels among treatment groups. Treatment groups had significant increases in 2-hour glucose levels and significant decreases in fasting glucose levels compared with the placebo group. In paired comparisons, women in the placebo group had greater increases in fibrinogen than did women in the active treatment groups; no significant differences were present among active treatment groups. Among their findings, the investigators concluded that "... oral estrogen taken alone or with MPA... is associated with improved lipoprotein and lower fibrinogen levels compared with placebo and the magnitude of these differences is likely to be clinically significant."

Multiple studies have evaluated HRT and CHD. In 1998, an overview by Barrett-Connor and Grady included 25 studies. Overall, the relative risk of CHD for women who took ERT compared with those who never took ERT was 0.70 (CI 0.65–0.75). When HRT was evaluated, the relative risk was 0.66 (0.53–0.84) compared with the non-users. This analysis evaluated cohort case control and angiographic studies. The apparent benefit is limited mainly to current or recent use. These findings are consistent across diverse populations and various study designs (Fig. 4–15).

The US National Health and Nutritional Examination Survey (NHANES-1) evaluated HRT and death from all cardiovascular disease in 1944 in white women 55 years of age or older who were monitored for up to 16 years. After adjusting for risk factors of CHD, the risk of death from CHD was 0.66 (0.48–0.90) in the HRT users. The study by Ettinger and associates noted similar findings. In their patient population followed for 25 years, the death from any cause in HRT users compared with non-users was 0.54, which was mainly due to a reduction in CHD (RR 0.40) and other cardiovascular diseases (RR 0.27).

Many studies, including the PEPI randomized control trial, have noted that estrogen therapy in postmenopausal women decreased serum TC, LDL, and Lp(a) lipoproteins. HDL and triglyceride concentrations increase. The route of administration does affect the serum lipids. Transdermal application has less effect on the serum lipid concentrations than the oral route. The type of progestins can also affect the serum lipids. Synthetic progestins tend to blunt the beneficial effects on the HDL but not decrease it below the baseline. Micronized progesterone does not decrease HDL compared with estrogen alone. Estrogen tends to decrease plasma fibrinogen concentrations as do anticoagulant proteins, antithrombin III, and protein S. There also appears to be a decrease in the antifibrinolytic protein plasminogen B activator inhibitor type I with an overall increased potential for fibrinolysis. In some reports, factor VII was also lowered with estrogen. The net effect on coagulation depends on the type of estrogen, dose, and duration of treatment.

The FDA has released a statement March of 2004, recommending the use of estrogen therapy should be for the relief of moderate to severe hot flushes and when used for vulvar and vaginal atrophy, topical products should be considered first. Estrogen containing products for the treatment of osteoporosis should be used only for women where non-estrogen-containing treatments are inappropriate. They recommend the lowest dose and shortest treatment duration to achieve goals. This statement is based on the results of recent randomized trials, and warns that estrogen is not approved for prevention of heart disease or memory loss.

Two large trials (WHI and HERS) have now demonstrated that estrogen cannot protect against myocardial infarction or death in women with pre-existing heart or vascular disease. In fact, the thromboembolic properties of estrogen likely increase risk, when pre-existing vascular lesions are present, predisposing women to stroke and myocardial infarction and death. The WHI demonstrated in a trial of 16,608 women randomized to combined estrogen plus progestin (HRT) versus placebo, at a mean age of 63.6 years, an absolute excess risk per 10,000 person-years attributable to HRT was seven coronary heart disease events, eight strokes, eight pulmonary emboli, eight invasive breast cancers and a reduction of five hip fractures. The WHI trial also had women without a uterus treated with conjugated equine estrogen alone versus placebo (n = 10,739), and they had a very different outcome. There was a non-significant reduction in breast cancer risk (P = 0.06) and coronary heart disease risk was unaffected (HR = 0.91 [CI 0.75–1.12]), strokes were increased (HR = 1.39 [CI 1.10–1.77]) and hip fractures were reduced (HR = 0.61 [CI 0.41–0.91]).

HERS (Heart and Estrogen/Progestin Replacement Study) was designed to determine if hormone replacement therapy could reduce cardiovascular events in women with known coronary artery disease (CAD). A total of 2763 women with pre-existing CAD and an average age of 67 years were enrolled and randomized to conjugated estrogen 0.625 mg plus medroxyprogesterone acetate 2.5 mg daily versus placebo. After 4.1 years of follow-up there was no significant difference in the primary outcomes of CHD events, or in any secondary outcome. There was a time trend of higher risk of events in the first year of use and a decrease in events in years 3–5. HERS II was a longer-term follow-up study of the same participants, which could not substantiate any benefit of HRT with longer use. It has been speculated that the initial increase in risk of cardiovascular events with HRT might be due to prothrombotic effects of the hormonal therapy. There may be a beneficial effect on the inhibition of progression of atherosclerosis due to effects on lipoprotein cholesterol, and therefore those who were doing well on the medication, were not asked to discontinue it. The conclusion of HERS and HERS II was that postmenopausal hormone therapy should not be used to reduce risk for CHD events in women with CHD.

Manson, for the WHI investigators, published the summary of coronary heart disease outcomes. This report also emphasized the increased risk of CHD events during the first year of use, and recommend against prescribing HRT for the prevention of cardiovascular disease. The problems with these trials are that the participants were older that the usual women prescribed HRT, and were recruited due to their increased risk of CAD events. This makes the results of HERS and WHI applicable to a similar population of high risk women, and the conclusions may not be generalizable to younger women initiating HRT at the onset of menopausal symptoms. Prevention of CAD may have a different pathophysiology than the progression from CAD to death. The epidemiologic and cohort data is criticized for the likely enrollment of healthier and more active women, and may also not represent all women of a similar age.

Cardiovascular risk reduction recommendations are smoking cessation, exercise, and weight control, along with blood pressure and cholesterol management. Aspirin, recently, has been shown to lower the risk of stroke, without affecting the risk of myocardial infarction or death from cardiovascular causes in most women. This randomized trial of 39,876 healthy women 45 years of age or older, received 100 mg of aspirin or placebo on alternate days for 10 years and monitored for cardiovascular events. There was a 17% reduction of strokes for the entire study population randomized to aspirin (RR = 0.83 CI 0.69; 0.99 P = 0.04). There was benefit for prevention of myocardial infarction only in women 65 years of age and older at enrollment (RR = 0.66 CI 0.44; 0.97 P = 0.04). The conclusion of this study is that physicians should perform a careful risk assessment to determine who is likely to benefit from aspirin, versus likely to be harmed by the increase of gastrointestinal hemorrhage requiring transfusion (P = 0.05)

The current summary recommendations are that women should be prescribed estrogen or estrogen plus a progestogen (when a uterus is present), at the onset of moderate or severe menopausal symptoms. The dose should be the lowest necessary to achieve the symptom control desired, and the duration of therapy should be five years or less. Discontinuation of this medication is not without side effects, and withdrawal symptoms may be minimized by a tapering schedule over a long period of time. It is accepted, however, that once a woman is on therapy, the risk of continuing such treatment is low, risk is greatest during the first year or two after initiating treatment, especially when pre-existing vascular disease may already be present.

ESTROGEN REPLACEMENT THERAPY FOR ENDOMETRIAL AND BREAST CANCER SURVIVORS

Estrogen replacement therapy for the endometrial cancer survivor

Historically, hormone replacement therapy has been contraindicated for the patient who has been treated for cancer of the uterus. Although estrogen administration has not been shown to have adverse effects on patients who have been treated for endometrial cancer, many physicians continue to be reluctant to administer this medication to these women. No data in the literature substantiate the detrimental effects of estrogen in these patients. It is not unusual for women with endometrial cancer to have severe symptoms due to withdrawal of estrogen at the time of their diagnosis and surgical treatment.

The Gynecologic Oncology Group conducted a prospective trial to evaluate the potential risk of estrogen replacement in women after treatment of endometrial adenocarcinoma. This randomized clinical trial of estrogen replacement therapy (CEE 0.625 mg orally per day, Premarin®) compared to placebo in women treated for stage I and II endometrial cancer closed after the WHI was halted prematurely in 2002, due to decrease in accrual and lack of feasibility. 1236 eligible women were randomized and the median follow-up was 35.7 months. The median age at endometrial cancer diagnosis was 57 years (range, 26–91 years). Compliance with medication for the entire treatment period was 41%, and for those on the ERT arm, 71% knew to which arm they had been randomized. A summary of the results on the ERT arm demonstrated endometrial cancer recurrence in 14 patients (2.3%); eight patients (1.3%) developed a new malignancy, one of which was breast cancer. There were 26 deaths (4.2%) on the estrogen arm, 5 were due to endometrial cancer. An important finding is that women with stage I and II endometrial cancer are more likely to die of causes unrelated to the cancer diagnosis, therefore other health issues must take priority when planning for preventative health maintenance (Table 4–6). Women on the placebo arm of this study suffered 19 deaths (3.1% not statistically different) and four were due to endometrial cancer. Ten placebo patients developed a new malignancy (1.6%), three of which were breast cancer (0.5%).

This study was admittedly underpowered for the endpoints of new breast cancer or endometrial cancer recurrence, but at least women can be informed that the rate of recurrence of endometrial cancer was equally low on each arm of this study. This data confirms the multiple studies published by Creasman and DiSaia on the use of estrogen in women following treatment of endometrial cancer. The decision to prescribe estrogen must be individualized based on symptom control and quality of life concerns that only the patient can assess.

Many physicians do not hesitate to give ERT in patients with well-differentiated or superficially invasive cancers, because recurrences are generally very low in these patients. There is greater hesitancy to treat poorly differentiated or deeply invasive cancers with ERT. This is also true for patients with extrauterine disease. The belief is that because recurrence is more frequent, ERT may increase the risk. The data would suggest the opposite. Those patients with high-risk factors and on ERT had a lower recurrence rate than do those who are not taking ERT. Although theoretically a possible advantage, it does not appear that the addition of a progestin to estrogen is

Table 4–6 GOG RANDOMIZED TRIAL OF ESTROGEN IN ENDOMETRIAL CANCER RECURRENCE AND SURVIVAL

	Treatment group			
	Placebo*	(%)	ERT*	(%)
Alive, NED	591	(95.6)	583	(94.3)
Alive with disease recurrence	8	(1.3)	9	(1.5)
Total deaths	19	(3.1)	26	(4.2)
Endometrial cancer	4	(0.6)	5	(0.8)
MI/CHD	4	(0.6)	3	(0.5)
Pulmonary embolism	0	(0.0)	2	(0.3)
Other	6	(1.0)	9	(1.5)
Unknown	5	(0.8)	7	(1.1)

*618 evaluable patients in each treatment group
NED, no evidence of disease, MI, myocardial infarction, CHD, coronary heart disease.
From JCO 2006 Barakat et al 24(4) 587-592.

beneficial. We initially followed this routine of a combination of E + P; however, for several years now we have not done so, and we have noticed no difference in outcomes.

The optimal time to begin ERT post-treatment has not been determined. Some would suggest waiting for at least 2 years because most patients who will develop recurrences will have done so. The data currently would suggest no benefit in waiting. Within a few days of surgical treatment, many patients will develop disturbing vasomotor symptoms. These symptoms can be prolonged with subsequent adverse symptomatology, such as vaginal thinness and dryness that can lead to unpleasant intercourse. As a result, symptoms can be treated as soon as they become troublesome.

In 1993, the American College of Obstetricians and Gynecologists released the following statement: "In women with a history of endometrial cancer, estrogens could be used for the same indications as for any other woman, except that the selection of appropriate candidates should be based on prognostic indicators and the risk the patient is willing to assume."

Fear of medicolegal liability, due to the contraindication of estrogen in breast and endometrial cancer in the package insert, requires that physicians document a lengthy discussion of the risks/benefits and have the patient actively participate in the decision and understand the process of informed consent needed for this therapy.

Hormonal therapy for the breast cancer survivor

Women diagnosed with breast cancer are faced with many challenging decisions, especially if they are premenopausal. They are asked to review their family history, to determine if they may have developed breast cancer due to a genetic predisposition, (BRCA 1 or 2 gene) transmitting risk of familial breast and ovarian cancer. Genetic counseling and testing may then be recommended, in order to properly counsel the patient, and her family members, about the benefits and risks of prophylactic mastectomy and bilateral salpingo-oophorectomy. This places premenopausal breast cancer patients in the unique position of being asked to undergo surgery to remove their ovaries to prevent ovarian cancer, when they may be told they cannot take estrogen replacement for the menopausal symptoms that will occur postoperatively. Appropriate estrogen and/or testosterone replacement after premenopausal oophorectomy is not condoned in this population by oncologists. The challenges to her emotional well-being, while facing a life-threatening illness, with new menopausal symptoms, sexual dysfunction and potential problems with her marriage all at the same time, is overwhelming. The benefits to bilateral salpingo-oophorectomy in a BRCA 1 or 2 carrier is the potential reduction in risk of breast cancer recurrence, as well as the 90% risk reduction from ovarian cancer. If symptom control from the surgery were feasible, this would be a great benefit. The risk of estrogen and androgen withdrawal can be decreased libido, lubrication, hot flashes, insomnia, depression and some women conclude that the benefit is not worth the risk. For this reason the age at which prophylactic oophorectomy should be planned is not known in genetic carriers, and must be individualized. Some physicians allow patients a reversible trial period of injectable Depo-Lupron® (TAP Pharmaceuticals Inc) to simulate menopause, to help with the decision-making process.

The treatment of breast cancer may consist of tamoxifen, aromatase inhibitors, local radiation, and chemotherapy. Some would argue that the purpose of the chemotherapy is to destroy ovarian function. Oophorectomy may be able to replace the benefit of chemotherapy, but this has not yet been adequately scientifically compared. Women are also eligible for treatment with aromatase inhibitors if they are menopausal, which has demonstrated a 43% reduction in breast cancer recurrence after completion of five years of tamoxifen.

There is increasing concern for the long-term morbidity of the standard breast cancer therapies, which are poorly captured in research trials. Women report cognitive function impairment from chemotherapy, as well as fatigue, weight gain, osteoporosis, and sexual dysfunction. Further study is required to determine better supportive care: including calcium and vitamin supplementations, biphosphonates, bone density monitoring, and prevention of cognitive dysfunction, and sexual dysfunction.

The use of tamoxifen for the treatment or prevention of breast cancer has many known consequences including thromboembolic disease, strokes, and endometrial cancer. The expected annual rate of endometrial cancer in the breast cancer patient is 1 per 1000. The tamoxifen patient has an excess risk of 2 per 1000 or a total risk of 3 per 1000 per year. Studies on the appropriate monitoring of women on tamoxifen have demonstrated that transvaginal ultrasound and routine annual endometrial biopsies increase a woman's risk. The current recommendation is to "do no harm" by conducting a routine annual gynecologic examination with cervical cytology and inquire about symptoms such as bleeding or discharge.

For many years, it has been stated that ERT in patients who have had breast cancer is absolutely contraindicated; yet interestingly, no data are available to substantiate this admonition. Because the benefits of ERT are substantial and no data are available to note detrimental effect in patients with breast disease, these authors firmly believe that a reappraisal of the admonition against ERT in patients with breast cancer is needed. Historically, it has been the dictum that women who have had breast cancer should not, under any circumstances, receive ERT. When one looks in the literature for data to support that recommendation, there is a huge void. In 1989, Wile and DiSaia suggested that in the absence of prospective study of ERT in breast cancer survivors, one could analyze situations in which these patients were exposed to high levels of estrogens at a time when they may have been harboring breast cancer cells. These situations were defined as pregnancy coexistent with breast cancer, pregnancy subsequent to breast cancer, breast cancer in previous and current users of oral contraceptives, and breast cancer in women receiving ERT. After extensive evaluation of these situations, there appears to be very little, if any, relationship. Currently, approximately 185,000 cases of breast cancer occur in the USA annually. More and more of these individuals fortunately are surviving their cancer; in many, long-term survival of >90% can be expected. Because many will survive their cancer, they will experience old age. We must address the advisability of HRT in this setting.

In fact, some data suggest that ERT in the breast cancer patient is not deleterious. Historically, we must remember that before cytotoxic agents, postmenopausal women with metastatic or recurrent cancer received estrogen as a first line of therapy. We now understand that its effectiveness depended to a certain extent on the receptor status of the cancer. At least seven prospective, randomized double-blind studies have compared estrogen with tamoxifen in patients with recurrent or metastatic breast cancer. The response rate of estrogen and tamoxifen is essentially the same. In prospective randomized studies comparing estrogen and tamoxifen as adjuvant therapy, the recurrence rate was essentially the same. It would appear that we have a very short medical history memory.

At least six retrospective studies have evaluated HRT in women with breast cancer. These patients were recurrence free at the time, and they were given estrogen to combat vasomotor symptoms or to prevent the chronic illness of cardiovascular disease, osteoporosis, and colon cancer. In this selected group of >500 patients, there have been 30 (6%) recurrences and only 7 (1%) deaths. In the authors' study of 145 patients in which patients with in situ stage I–IV were treated, there have been 13 (9%) recurrences. Patients with both node-positive and node-negative disease were treated. Of the 96 node-negative patients, 11 recurred; whereas, only 1 of 34 node-positive patients to date has had a recurrence. There was 1 of 15 recurrences in individuals in whom the lymph nodes were not pathologically evaluated. It appears that evaluation of the receptor status in patients who had this performed did not have an impact one way or the other with regard to recurrences (Table 4–7).

To date, there have been three case-controlled studies and three cohort-type studies (Table 4–8) in which recurrences and deaths were similar in both the patients on ERT and the controls. A cohort study of 125 patients with breast cancer who, post cancer therapy, received HRT were compared with 362 patients with breast cancer who did not receive HRT. Patients were matched for stage, age, and year of diagnosis. All stages were included, although 78% had CIS (14%) or stage I and II cancers. There was a survival advantage for HRT users compared with non-HRT users with an odds ratio of 0.28 (CI 0.11–0.71) (see Fig. 4–13). Six endometrial cancers were subsequently diagnosed in the patients who took HRT. In 1994, ACOG, in a Committee Opinion, stated, "In conclusion, there are no data that indicate an increased risk of recurrent breast cancer in postmenopausal women receiving ERT... No woman can be guaranteed protection from recurrence... In postmenopausal women with previously treated breast cancer, consideration of ERT is an option but must be reviewed with caution." In other words, there must be informed consent. Women are interested in information from which they can make informed decisions. To not even discuss replacement therapy with these individuals is not in their best interest. In the USA today, >36,000 women who are younger than 50 years of age will develop breast cancer. Most, if not all, will go on cytotoxic chemotherapy, and a significant number will become amenorrheic even though they are younger than 35 years of age. Unfortunately, if amenorrhea occurs while on chemotherapy, permanent ovarian failure occurs in the vast

Table 4–7 HORMONE REPLACEMENT THERAPY IN WOMEN WITH BREAST CANCER

Author	Recurrence	Deaths
Stoll	0/65 (0%)	0
Powles	2/35 (8%)	0
Sellin	1/49 (2%)	0
Bluming	12/189 (6%)	1 (1%)
Brewster	13/145 (9%)	3 (2%)
Natrajan	2/50 (4%)	3 (6%)
	30/533 (6%)	7 (1%)

Table 4–8 HORMONE REPLACEMENT THERAPY FOLLOWING BREAST CANCER

	Recurrence		Deaths	
	ERT	Controls	ERT	Controls
Case Controlled				
Wile et al	1/25 (4%)	2/50 (4%)	1 (4%)	2 (4%)
DiSaia et al	6/41 (14%)	7/82 (8%)	2 (5%)	6 (7%)
Eden et al	6/90 (7%)	30/108 (17%)	0	11
Cohort				
Dew et al	?/167	/1472	2 (1%)	167 (13%)
Espie et al	5/120	/240	*	*

*No difference disease free survival.
ERT, estrogen replacement therapy.

majority. Even in the very young (<40 years of age) 86% will have ovarian failure. We, therefore, are seeing an increasing number of young women who are going through a chemotherapeutic-induced premature menopause. A significant number of these women will be cured of their breast cancer; however, because of the premature menopause, they may have significant vasomotor symptoms that are much greater than those expected with a natural menopause. Long-term benefits of replacement therapy may even be greater because of the premature menopause. These patients should be made aware of the rationale for replacement (i.e., the benefits and risks) so that intelligent decisions can be made. The breast cancer patient may be the ideal candidate for the vaginal slow release forms of estradiol rings. Estring® contains a very low dose of estradiol which can successfully treat vaginal atrophy symptoms and only increase plasma estradiol levels to one tenth the amount of a 0.05 Estraderm® patch. If menopausal symptoms remain intolerable, Femring® has a higher estradiol dose of 0.05 mg/day and may provide some relief of vasomotor symptoms as well.

BIBLIOGRAPHY

CLINICAL PRESENTATION

Chamlian DL, Taylor HB: Endometrial hyperplasia in young women. Obstet Gynecol 36:659, 1970.

Cherkis RC, Patten SF, Dickinson JC et al: Significance of atypical endometrial cells detected by cervical cytology. Obstet Gynecol 69:786, 1987.

Emge LA: Endometrial cancer and feminizing tumors of the ovary. Obstet Gynecol 1:511, 1953.

Fechner RE, Kaufman RH: Endometrial adenocarcinoma in Stein–Leventhal syndrome. Cancer 34:444, 1974.

Gallup DG, Stock RJ: Adenocarcinoma of the endometrium in women 40 years of age or younger. Obstet Gynecol 64:417, 1984.

Lyon FA, Frisch MJ: Endometrial abnormalities occurring in young women on long-term sequential oral contraception. Obstet Gynecol 47:639, 1976.

Merriam JC Jr et al: Experimental production of endometrial cancer in the rabbit. Obstet Gynecol 16:253, 1960.

Pettersson B, Bergstrom R, Johansson EDB: Serum estrogens and androgens in women with endometrial carcinoma. Gynecol Oncol 25:223, 1986.

Sirota DK, Marinoff SC: Endometrial carcinoma in Turner's syndrome following prolonged treatment with diethylstilbestrol. Mt Sinai J Med 42:586, 1975.

Weiss NS, Szekely DR, Austin DF: Increasing incidence of endometrial cancer in the USA. N Engl J Med 294:1259, 1976.

Wood GP, Boronow RC: Endometrial adenocarcinoma and the polycystic ovary syndrome. Am J Obstet Gynecol 124:140, 1976.

ENDOMETRIAL HYPERPLASIA: PATHOLOGIC DIAGNOSTIC CRITERIA

Baak JP, Mutter GL, Robboy S et al: The molecular genetics and morphometry-based endometrial intraepithelial neoplasia classification system predicts disease progression in endometrial hyperplasia more accurately than the 1994 World Health Organization classification system. Cancer 103(11):2304, 2005.

Bhagavan BS et al: Comparison of estrogen-induced hyperplasia to endometrial carcinoma. Obstet Gynecol 64:12, 1984.

Creasman WT: Estrogen replacement therapy: Is previously treated cancer a contraindication? Obstet Gynecol 77:308, 1991.

Ferenczy A, Bergeron C: Endometrial hyperplasia. In Lowe D, Fox H (eds): Advances in Gynecological Pathology. London, England, Churchill Livingstone, 1992, p 207.

Ferenczy A, Gelfand MM, Tzipris F: The cytodynamics of endometrial hyperplasia and carcinoma: A review. Ann Pathol 3:189, 1983.

Fox H, Buckley CH: The endometrial hyperplasias and their relationship to endometrial neoplasia. Histopathology 6:493, 1982.

Gusberg SB: Precursors of corpus carcinoma, estrogens, and adenomatous hyperplasia. Am J Obstet Gynecol 54:905, 1947.

Gusberg SB, Hall RE: Precursors of corpus cancer. III: The appearance of cancer of the endometrium in estrogenically-conditioned patients. Obstet Gynecol 17:397, 1961.

Gusberg SB, Kaplan AL: Precursors of corpus cancer. Am J Obstet Gynecol 87:662, 1963.

Gusberg SB, Moore DB, Martin F: Precursors of corpus cancer. II: A clinical and pathological study of adenomatous hyperplasia. Am J Obstet Gynecol 68:1472, 1954.

Hertig AT, Sommerd SC: Genesis of endometrial carcinoma: Study of prior biopsy. Cancer 2:946, 1949.

Ingram JM Jr, Novak E: Endometrial carcinoma associated with feminizing ovarian tumors. Am J Obstet Gynecol 61:774, 1951.

Jackson RL, Dockerty MB: The Stein–Leventhal syndrome analysis of 43 cases with special reference to association with endometrial carcinoma. Am J Obstet Gynecol 73:161, 1957.

Kraus FT: High-risk and premalignant lesions of the endometrium. Am J Surg Pathol 9:31, 1985.

Kurman RJ, Norris HJ: Endometrial hyperplasia and metaplasia. In Kurman RJ (ed): Blaustein's Pathology of the Female Genital Tract. New York, Springer Verlag, 1987.

Kurman RJ, Norris HJ: Evaluation of criteria for distinguishing atypical endometrial hyperplasia from well-differentiated carcinoma. Cancer 49:2547, 1982.

Kurman RJ, Kalminski PF, Norris HJ: The behavior of endometrial hyperplasia: A long term study of "untreated" hyperplasia in 170 patients. Cancer 56:403, 1985.

Maxwell GL, Risinger JI, Grumbs C, Shaw H, Bentley RC, Barrett JC, Berchuck A, Futreal PA: Mutation of the PTEN tumor suppressor gene in endometrial hyperplasias. Cancer Research, 58(12):2500, 1998.

Mutter GL, Lin M, Fitzgerald JT, Kum JB, Baak JPA, Lees JA, Weng LP, Eng C: Altered PTEN expression as a diagnostic marker for the earliest endometrial precancers. JNCI, 92(11):924, 2000.

Sherman ME, Bitterman P, Rosenshein NB et al: Uterine Serous Carcinoma: a morphologically diverse neoplasm with unifying clinicopathologic features. Am J Surg Pathol 16:600, 1992.

Silverberg SG: Hyperplasia and carcinoma of the endometrium. Semin Diagn Pathol 5:135, 1988.

Silverberg SG: Problems in the differential diagnosis of endometrial hyperplasia and carcinoma. Mod Pathol 13(3):309, 2000.

Spiegel GW. Endometrial carcinoma in situ in postmenopausal women. Am J Surg Path;19:417,1995.

Sturdee DW et al: Relations between bleeding pattern, endometrial histology, and oestrogen treatment in menopausal women. BMJ 1:1575, 1978.

Trimble CL, Kauderer J, Silverberg S, Curtin J, Lim PC, Burke JJ, Zaino R: Concurrent endometrial cancer (EC) in women with biopsy diagnosis of atypical endometrial hyperplasia (AEH): A Gynecologic Oncology Group (GOG) study. Gynecol Oncol 92(1):393 (SGO #2), 2004.

Trimble CL, Kauderer J, Zaino R, et al: Concurrent endometrial carcinoma in women with biopsy diagnosis of atypical endometrial hyperplasia: A Gynecologic Oncology Group study. Cancer, 106(4):812-819, 2006.

Welch WR, Scully RE: Precancerous lesions of the endometrium. Hum Pathol 8:503, 1977.

Winkler B, Alvarez S, Richart RM et al: Pitfalls in the diagnosis of endometrial neoplasia. Obstet Gynecol 64:185, 1984.

Wright TC Jr, Schiffman M, Solomon D, Cox JT, Garcia F, Goldie S, Hatch K, Noller KL, Roach N, Runowicz C, Saslow D: Interim Guidance for the use of human papillomavirus DNA testing as an adjunct to cervical cytology for screening. Obstet Gynecol 103:304, 2004.

Zaino, RJ: Endometrial Hyperplasia: Is it time for a Quantum Leap to a New Classification? Inter J Gynecol Path 19:314, 2000.

Zaino RJ, Kauderer J, Trimble CL, Silverberg SG, Curtin JP, Lim PC, Gallup DG: Reproducibility of the Diagnosis of Atypical Endometrial Hyperplasia (AEH): A Gynecologic Oncology Group Study. Cancer 106(4):804-811, 2006.

MANAGEMENT

Bonte J, Decoster JM, Ide P et al: Hormonoprophylaxis and hormonotherapy in the treatment of endometrial adenocarcinoma by means of medroxyprogesterone acetate. Gynecol Oncol 6:60, 1978.

Bullock JL, Massey FM, Gambrell RD Jr: Use of medroxyprogesterone acetate to prevent menopausal symptoms. Obstet Gynecol 46:165, 1975.

Chu J, Schweid AI, Weiss NS: Survival among women with endometrial cancer: A comparison of estrogen users and non-users. Am J Obstet Gynecol 143:569, 1982.

Gal D, Edman CD, Vellios F et al: Long-term effect of megestrol acetate in the treatment of endometrial hyperplasia. Am J Obstet Gynecol 146:316, 1983.

Ramirez PT, Frumovitz M, Bodurka DC et al: Hormonal therapy for the management of grade 1 endometrial adenocarcinoma: a literature review. Gynecol Oncol 95:133-138, 2004.

Rigg LA, Hermann H, Yen SS: Absorption of estrogens from vaginal creams. N Engl J Med 298:195, 1978.

Steiner GJ, Kistner RW, Craig JM: Histological effects of progestin on hyperplasia and carcinoma in situ of the endometrium—further observations. Metabolism 14:356, 1965.

Varma TR: Effect of long-term therapy with estrogen and progesterone on the endometrium of postmenopausal women. Acta Obstet Gynecol Scand 64:41, 1985.

Wilson PA, Kolstad P: Hormonal Treatment of Preinvasive and Invasive Carcinoma of the Corpus Uteri in Endometrial Cancer. London, William Heinemann Medical Books, 1973.

MANAGEMENT OF ENDOMETRIAL HYPERPLASIA WITHOUT ATYPIA

Position Statement: Role of progestogen in hormone therapy for postmenopausal women: position statement of the North American Menopause Society. Menopause 10(2)113, 2003.

PREVENTION OF ENDOMETRIAL CANCER

Grady D, Gebretsadik T, Ketlikowsli K, Ernster V, Petitti D; Hormone replacement therapy and endometrial cancer risk: a meta-analysis. Obstet Gynecol 85:304, 1995.

Kurman RJ, Felix JC, Archer DF et al: Norethindrone acetate and estradiol-induced endometrial hyperplasia. Obstet Gynecol 96: 3733, 2000.

Montz FJ, Bristow RE, Bovicelli A, et al: Intrauterine progesterone treatment of early endometrial cancer. Am J Obstet Gynecol 186: 651, 2002.

Raudaskoski T, Papanainen J, Tomas E, et al. Intrauterine 10 μg and 20 levonorgestrel systmes in postmenopausal women receiving oral oestrogen replacement therapy : clinical, endomtrial and metabolic response. Br J Obstet Gynaecol 109:136, 2002.

The Writing Group for the PEPI Trial. Effects of hormone replacement therapy on endometrial histology in postmenopausal women. The Postmenopausal Estrogen/Progestin Intervention (PEPI) Trial. JAMA 275:370, 1996.

Wildemeersch D, Dhont M: Treatment of non-atypical and atypical endometrial hyperplasia with a levonorgestrel-releasing intrauterine system. Am J Obstet Gynecol 188:1297, 2003.

Writing Group for the Women's Health Initiative Investigators; Risks and Benefits of Estrogen Plus Progestin in Healthy Postmenopausal Women: Principal Results from the Women's Health Initiative Randomized Controlled Trial; JAMA 288(3) 321, 2002.

ESTROGENS AND ENDOMETRIAL NEOPLASIA

Aitken JM, Hart DM, Anderson JB et al: Osteoporosis after oophorectomy for non-malignant disease in premenopausal women. Br Med J 2:325, 1973.

American College of Obstetricians and Gynecologists. Questions and answers on hormone therapy in response to the Women's Health Initiative Study results on estrogen and progestin hormone therapy. Available at: http://www.acog.org/from_home/publications/press_releases/nr08-30-02.cfm. Accessed March 29, 2004.

Anderson JJ, Ferguson DJP, Raab GH: Cell turnover in the "resting" human breast: Influence of parity, contraceptive pill, age and laterality. Br J Cancer 46:376, 1982.

Antunes CMF, Strolley PD, Rosenshein NB et al: Endometrial cancer and estrogen use: report of a large case-control study. N Engl J Med 300:9, 1979.

Baker DP: Estrogen replacement therapy in patients with a previous diagnosis of endometrial carcinoma. Compr Ther 16:28, 1990.

Banrabei VM, Cochrane BB, Aragaki AK, et al Menopausal symptoms and treatment-related effects of estrogen and progestin in the Women's Health Initiative. Obstet Gynecol 105:1063, 2005

Baraket JCO 24(4):587-592, 2006.

Blumel J, Castelo-Branco C, Chedraudi P et al: Patients' and clinicians' attitudes after the Women's Health Initiative study. Menopause 11:57, 2004.

Boston Collaborative Drug Surveillance Program, Boston University Medical Center: Surgical confirmed gall-bladder disease, venous thromboembolism, and breast tumors in relation to postmenopausal estrogen therapy. N Engl J Med 290:15, 1974.

Bryant GW: Administration of estrogens to patients with a previous diagnosis of endometrial adenocarcinoma (Letter). South Med J 83:725, 1990.

Chapman JA, DiSaia PJ, Osann K et al: Estrogen replacement in surgical stage I and II endometrial cancer survivors. Am J Obstet Gynecol 175:1195, 1996.

Christiansen C, Christiansen MS, Transbol I: Bone mass in postmenopausal women after withdrawal of oestrogen/progestogen replacement therapy. Lancet 1:459, 1981.

Creasman WT, Henderson D, Hinshaw W et al: Estrogen replacement therapy in the patient treated for endometrial cancer. Cancer 67:326, 1986.

Food and Drug Administration. FDA updates hormone therapy information for post menopausal women. Available at: http://www.fda.gov/bbs/topics/NEWS/2004/NEW01022.html/ Accessed July 20, 2006.

Fremont-Smith M, Meigs JV, Graham RM et al: Cancer of the endometrium and prolonged estrogen therapy. JAMA 131:805, 1946.

Gabrielsson J, Wallenback I, Birgerson L: Pharmacokinetic data on estradiol in light of the estring® concept. Acta Obstet Gynecol Scand Suppl 163; 75:26-31, 1996.

Gambrell RD Jr: Preventing endometrial cancer with progestins. Contemp Obstet Gynecol 17:133, 1981.

Gordon GE, Greenberg BG: Exogenous estrogen and endometrial cancer—an invited review. Postgrad Med 59:67, 1976.

Gray LA, Christopherson WM, Hoover RN: Estrogens and endometrial carcinoma. Obstet Gynecol 49:385, 1977.

Greene HSN: Uterine adenomata in the rabbit: Susceptibility as a function of constitutional factors. J Exp Med 73:273, 1941.

Gusberg SB, Kardon P: Proliferative endometrial response to thecal granulosa cell tumors. Am J Obstet Gynecol 3:633, 1971.

Heart Disease and Stroke Statistics—2006 Update, American Heart Association.

Henderson BE, Ross RK, Paganini-Hill A: Estrogen use and cardiovascular disease. J Reprod Med 30:814, 1985.

Hendrikson L, Stjernquist M, Boquist L, Cedergren I, Selinus I; A one-year multicenter study of efficacy and safety of a continuous, low-dose, estradiol-releasing vaginal ring (Estring®) in post-menopausal women with symptoms and signs of urogenital aging. Am J Obstet Gynecol 1996; 174:85-92.

Hoogerlan DL et al: Estrogen use:risk of endometrial carcinoma. Gynecol Oncol 64:451, 1978.

Hoover R et al: Menopausal estrogens and breast cancer. N Engl J Med 295:401, 1976.

Horowitz RI, Feinstein AR: Alternative analytic methods for case-control studies of estrogens and endometrial cancer. N Engl J Med 299:1089, 1978.

Horowitz RI, Feinstein AR: Susceptibility bias and the estrogen-endometrial cancer controversy (Abstract). Clin Res 27:222A, 1979.

Johnston Atholl, Estrogens-pharmacokinetics and pharmacodynamics with special reference to vaginal administration and the new estradiol formulation-Estring® Acta Obstet Gynecol Scand 1996; Suppl 163; 75:16-25.

Kampman E, Potter JD, Slattery ML et al: Hormone replacement therapy, reproductive history and colon cancer: A multicenter, case-control study in U.S. Cancer Causes Control 8:146, 1997.

Kay CR: Progestogens and arterial disease: Evidence from the Royal College of General Practitioners' study. Am J Obstet Gynecol 142:762, 1982.

Killacke MA, Halkes TB, Pierce VK: Endometrial endocarcinoma in breast cancer patients receiving anti-estrogens. Cancer Threat Rep 69:237, 1985.

Kistner RW: Histological effects of progestins on hyperplasia and carcinoma in situ of the endometrium. Cancer 12:1106, 1959.

Lee RB, Burke TW, Park RC: Estrogen replacement therapy following treatment for stage I endometrial carcinoma. Gynecol Oncol 36:189, 1990.

Lyon FA: The development of adenocarcinoma of the endometrium in young women receiving long-term sequential oral contraception. Am J Obstet Gynecol 123:299, 1975.

MacDonald PC, Siiteri PK: The relationship between the extraglandular production of estrone and the occurrence of endometrial neoplasia. Gynecol Oncol 2:259, 1974.

Mack TM et al: Estrogens and endometrial cancer in a retirement community. N Engl J Med 294:1262, 1976.

Mansell H, Hertig AT: Granulosa-theca cell tumor and endometrial carcinoma: A study of their relationship and survey of 80 cases. Obstet Gynecol 6:385, 1955.

Manson JE, Hsia J; Johnson KC et al: Estrogen plus Progestin and the Risk of Coronary Heart Disease; NEJM 2003; 349(6) 523–534.

Marrett LD et al: Recent trends in the incidence and mortality of cancer of the uterine corpus in Connecticut. Gynecol Oncol 6:183, 1978.

McDonald TW et al: Exogenous estrogen and endometrial carcinoma: case control and incidence study. Am J Obstet Gynecol 49:385, 1977.

Nachtigall LE et al: Estrogen replacement therapy. I: A 10-year prospective study in the relationship to osteoporosis. Obstet Gynecol 53:277, 1979.

Naessen, T, Rodriquez-Macias K; Endometrial thickness and uterine diameter not affected by ultralow doses of 17β estradiol in elderly women. Am J Obstet Gynecol 2002; 186:944-7.

NIH State-of-the-Science Panel; National Institutes of Health State-of-the-Science Conference Statement: Management of Menopause-Related Symptoms. Annals of Inter Med 142(12)1003, 2005.

Norris HJ, Taylor HB: Prognosis of granulosa-theca tumors of the ovary. Cancer 21:255, 1968.

NAMS September 8, 2005 Use of Testosterone Therapy by Post menopausal Women: Position Statement of the North American Menopausal Society. Menopause Sept/Oct 2005 The role of testosterone in postmenopausal women"

Pacheco JC, Kempers RD: Etiology of postmenopausal bleeding. Obstet Gynecol 32:40, 1968.

Ridker PM, Cook NR, Lee, IM et al. A randomized trial of low-dose aspirin in the primary prevention of cardiovascular disease in women. N Engl J Med 352(13) 1293, 2005.

Riggs BL et al: Short and long-term effects of estrogen and synthetic anabolic hormone in postmenopausal osteoporosis. J Clin Invest 51:1659, 1972.

Rosenwaks Z et al: Endometrial pathology and estrogens. Obstet Gynecol 53:403, 1979.

Scott RB, Wharton LR Jr: The effects of excessive amounts of diethylstilbestrol on experimental endometriosis in monkeys. Am J Obstet Gynecol 69:573, 1955.

Shapiro S, Kelly JP, Rosenberg L: Risk of localized and widespread endometrial cancer in relation to recent and discontinued use of conjugated estrogens. N Engl J Med 313:968, 1985.

Silverberg SQ, Makowski EL: Endometrial carcinoma in young women taking oral contraceptives. Obstet Gynecol 46:503, 1975.

Smith DC et al: Estrogens and endometrial cancer in a retirement community. N Engl J Med 293:1164, 1975.

The Women's Health Initiative Steering Committee: Effects of conjugated equine estrogen in postmenopausal women with hysterectomy. JAMA 291(14):1701, 2004.

Weiss NS, Sayretz TA: Incidence of endometrial cancer in relation to the use of oral contraceptives. N Engl J Med 302:551, 1980.

Wigle DT, Grace M, Smith ESO: Estrogen use and cancer of the uterine corpus in Alberta. Can Med Assoc J 118:1276, 1978.

Woodruff DJ, Pickar JH: Incidence of endometrial hyperplasia in postmenopausal women taking conjugated estrogens (Premarin) with medroxyprogesterones or conjugated estrogens alone. Am J Obstet Gynecol 170:1213, 1994.

Writing Group for the Women's Health Initiative Investigators: Risks and benefits if estrogen plus progestin in healthy postmenopausal women: principal results from the Women's Health Initiative randomized controlled trial. JAMA 288(3):321, 2002.

Ziel HK, Finkle WD: Increased risk of endometrial carcinoma among users of conjugated estrogens. N Engl J Med 293:1167, 1975.

ESTROGEN-PROGESTIN THERAPY

American College of Obstetricians and Gynecologists, Committee on Gynecologic Practice: Estrogen replacement therapy and endometrial cancer. ACOG Committee Opinion #80. Washington, DC, The American College of Obstetricians and Gynecologists, 1990.

Archer DF et al: Bleeding patterns in postmenopausal women taking continuous combined or sequential regimens of conjugated estrogens with medroxyprogesterone acetate. Am J Obstet Gynecol 83:686, 1994.

Armstrong BK et al: Oestrogen therapy after the menopause—boon or bane? Med J Aust 148:213, 1988.

Bain C et al: Use of postmenopausal hormones and risk of myocardial infarction. Circulation 64:42, 1981.

Jensen J, Riis BJ, Strom V et al: Continuous oestrogen-progestogen treatment and serum lipoproteins in postmenopausal women. Br J Obstet Gynaecol 94:130, 1987.

PEPI trial writing group: Effects of estrogen or estrogen/progestin regimens on heart disease risk factors in postmenopausal women. JAMA 273:199, 1995.

Prough SG, Aksel S, Wiebe RH et al: Continuous estrogen/progestin therapy in menopause. Am J Obstet Gynecol 157:1449, 1987.

Sherwin BB, Gelfand MM: A prospective one-year study of estrogen and progestin in postmenopausal women: Effects on clinical symptoms and lipoprotein lipids. Obstet Gynecol 73:759, 1989.

Weinstein L: Efficacy of a continuous estrogen-progestin regimen in the postmenopausal patient. Obstet Gynecol 69:929, 1987.

Whitehead MI et al: The effects of cyclical oestrogen and sequential oestrogen progestogen therapy on the endometrium of post-menopausal women. Acta Obstet Gynecol Scand Suppl 65:91, 1977.

Whitehead MI, Siddle N, Lane G et al: The pharmacology of progestogens. In Mishell DR (ed): Menopause: Physiology and Pharmacology. St. Louis, CV Mosby, 1987.

ESTROGENS AND BREAST CANCER

Barrett-Connor E, Grady D: Hormone replacement therapy, heart disease, and other considerations. Annu Rev Public Health 19:55, 1998.

Beatson GT: On the treatment of inoperable cases of carcinoma of the mammary glands: Suggestions for a new method of treatment with illustrative cases. Lancet 11:104, 1896.

Bergkvist L, Adami HO, Persson I et al: Prognosis after breast cancer diagnosis in women exposed to estrogen and estrogen-progestogen replacement therapy. Am J Epidemiol 130:221, 1989.

Bergkvist L, Adami HO, Persson I et al: The risk of breast cancer after estrogen and estrogen-progestin replacement. N Engl J Med 5:293, 1989.

Bonnier P et al: Clinical and biologic prognostic factors in breast cancer diagnosed during postmenopausal hormone replacement therapy. Obstet Gynecol 85:11, 1995.

Brewster WR, DiSaia PJ, McGonigle FK et al: An experience of estrogen replacement therapy in breast cancer survivors. Int J Fertil Womens Med 44:186, 1999.

Brinton LA, Hoover R, Fraumeni JF Jr: Menopausal oestrogens and breast cancer risk: An expanded case-control study. Br J Cancer 54:825, 1986.

Calle EE, Miracle-McMahill HL, Thun MJ et al: Estrogen replacement therapy and risk of fatal colon cancer in a prospective cohort of postmenopausal women. J Natl Cancer Inst 87:517, 1995.

Clinical Synthesis Panel on HRT: Hormone replacement therapy. Lancet 354:152, 1999.

Colditz GA, Walter BS, Willett C et al: Menopause and the risk of coronary heart disease in women. N Engl J Med 316:1105, 1987.

Colditz GA et al: Hormone replacement therapy and risk of breast cancer: Results from epidemiologic studies. Am J Obstet Gynecol 168:173, 1993.

Colditz GA et al: The use of estrogens and progestins and the risk of breast cancer in postmenopausal women. N Engl J Med 332: 1589, 1995.

Colditz GA et al: Type of postmenopausal hormone use and risk of breast cancer: 12-year follow-up from the Nurses' Health Study. Cancer Causes Control 3:433, 1992.

Collaborative Group on Hormonal Factors in Breast Cancer: Breast cancer and hormonal contraceptives: Collaborative reanalysis of individual data on 53,297 women with breast cancer and 100,239 women without breast cancer from 54 epidemiological studies. Lancet 347:1713, 1996.

Collaborative Group on Hormonal Factors in Breast Cancer: Breast cancer and hormone replacement therapy: Collaborative reanalysis of data from 51 epidemiologic studies of 52,705 women with breast cancer and 108,411 women without breast cancer. Lancet 350:1047, 1997.

Cooper DR, Butterfield J: Pregnancy subsequent to mastectomy for cancer of the breast. Ann Surg 171:429, 1970.

Creasman WT: Is there an association between hormone replacement therapy and breast cancer? J Women's Health Gend Based Med 7:1231, 1998.

Daly E, Vessey MP, Hawkins MM et al: Risk of venous thromboembolism in users of hormone replacement therapy. Lancet 348:977, 1996.

Dew J, Eden J, Beller E, Magarey C, Schwartz P, Crea P, Wren B. A cohort study of hormone replacement therapy given to women previously treated for breast cancer. Climacteric 1:137, 1998.

DiSaia PJ: Hormone replacement therapy in patients with breast cancer: A reappraisal. Cancer 71:1490, 1993.

DiSaia PJ et al: Hormone replace therapy in breast cancer (Letter). Lancet 232:342, 1993.

DiSaia PJ et al: Replacement therapy for breast cancer survivors: A pilot study. Cancer 476:10, 1995.

Dupont WD, Page DL: Menopausal estrogen replacement therapy and breast cancer. Arch Intern Med 151:67, 1991.

Dupont WD, Page DL: Risk factors for breast cancers in women with proliferative breast disease. N Engl J Med 312:146, 1985.

DuPont WD, Page DL, Parl FF et al: Estrogen replacement therapy in women with a history of proliferative breast disease. Cancer 85:1277, 1999.

DuPont WD, Page DL, Rogers LW et al: Influence of exogenous estrogens, proliferative breast disease and other variables on breast cancer risk. Cancer 63:948, 1989.

Eden JA: Estrogen and the breast. Med J Aust 157:125, 1992.

Espie M, Gorins A, Perret F et al: Hormone replacement therapy in patients treated for breast cancer: Analysis of a cohort of 120 patients. Proc ASCO 18:2262, 1999.

Gambrell RD Jr: Role of hormones in the etiology and prevention of endometrial and breast cancer. Acta Obstet Gynecol Scand Suppl 106:37, 1982.

Grodstein F, Martinez ME, Platz EA et al: Postmenopausal hormone use and the risk of colorectal adenoma and cancer. Ann Intern Med 128:705, 1998.

Grodstein F, Newcomb PA, Stampfer MJ: Postmenopausal hormone therapy and the risk of colorectal cancer: A review and meta-analysis. Am J Med 106:574, 1999.

Grodstein F, Stampfer M, Colditz C et al: Postmenopausal hormone therapy and mortality. N Engl J Med 336:1769, 1997.

Grodstein F, Stampfer MJ, Goldhaber SZ et al: Prospective study of exogenous hormones and risk of preliminary embolism in women. Lancet 398:983, 1996.

Grodstein F, Stampfer MJ et al: Nurses' Health Study: Postmenopausal estrogen and progestin use and risk of cardiovascular disease. N Engl J Med 335:453, 1996.

Grunfeld E, Dhesy-Thind S, Levine M: Steering Committee on Clinical Practice Guidelines for the Care and Treatment of Breast Cancer: follow-up after treatment of breast cancer. CMAJ 172;(10):1319, 2005.

Holleb AI, Farrow JH: The relation of carcinoma of the breast and pregnancy in 283 patients. Surg Gynecol Obstet 115:65, 1962.

Holli K, Isola J, Cuzick J: Low biologic aggressiveness in breast cancer in women using hormone replacement therapy. J Clin Oncol 16:1315, 1998.

Hoover R, Gray LA Sr, Cole P et al: Menopausal estrogens and breast cancer. N Engl J Med 295:401, 1976.

Hulka BS: Hormone replacement therapy and the risk of breast cancer. Cancer 40:289, 1990.

Ingle JN, Ahmann DI, Green SJ et al: Randomized clinical trial of diethylstilbestrol versus tamoxifen in postmenopausal women with advanced breast cancer. N Engl J Med 304:16, 1981.

Kaufman DW et al: Estrogen replacement therapy and the risk of breast cancer: Results from the case-control surveillance study. Am J Epidemiol 134:1375, 1991.

Korenman SG: The endocrinology of breast cancer. Cancer 46:874, 1980.

Mendelsohn ME, Karas RH: The protective effect of estrogen on the cardiovascular system. N Engl J Med 340:1801, 1999.

Mignot L, Morvan F, Berdah J et al: Pregnancy after breast cancer: Results of a case study. Presse Med 15:1961, 1986.

Nachtigall LE et al: Estrogen replacement therapy. II: A prospective study in the relationship to carcinoma and cardiovascular and metabolic problems. Obstet Gynecol 54:74, 1979.

Paganini-Hill A: Estrogen replacement therapy and stroke. Progr Cardiovas Dis 38:223, 1995.

Palmer JR et al: Breast cancer risk after estrogen replacement therapy: Results from the Toronto breast cancer study. Am J Epidemiol 134:1386, 1991.

Persson I et al: Combined oestrogen-progestogen replacement and breast cancer risk. Lancet 340:1044, 1992.

Rosner D, Lane W: Oral contraceptives use has no adverse effect on the prognosis of breast cancer. Cancer 57:591, 1986.

Sellers TA, Mink PJ, Cerban JR et al: The role of HRT in the risk for breast cancer and total mortality in women with a family history of breast cancer. Ann Intern Med 127:973, 1997.

Sillero-Arenas M et al: Menopausal hormone treatment therapy and breast cancer: A meta-analysis. Obstet Gynecol 79:286, 1992.

Stanford JL et al: Combined estrogen and progestin hormone replacement therapy in relation to risk of breast cancer in middle-aged women. JAMA 274:137, 1995.

Steinberg KK et al: A meta-analysis of the effect of estrogen replacement therapy on the risk of breast cancer. JAMA 265:1985, 1991.

Strickland DM et al: The relationship between breast cancer survival and prior postmenopausal estrogen use. Obstet Gynecol 80:400, 1992.

Sullivan JM, Vander Zwagg R, Hughes JP et al: Estrogen replacement and coronary artery disease. Arch Intern Med 150:2557, 1990.

Villarino CB, Fenster PE: Coronary heart disease. Prim Care Update Ob/Gyn 1:150, 1994.

Wile AG, DiSaia PJ: Hormones and breast cancer. Am J Surg 157:438, 1989.

Willis DB, Calle EE, Miracle-McMahill H et al: Estrogen replacement therapy and risk of fatal breast cancer in a prospective cohort of postmenopausal women in the U.S. Cancer Causes Control 7:449, 1996.

Wolf PH, Madans JH, Finucane FF et al: Reduction of cardiovascular disease-related mortality among postmenopausal women who use hormones. Am J Obstet Gynecol 164:489, 1991.

BENEFITS OF ESTROGEN REPLACEMENT THERAPY

Bain C et al: Use of postmenopausal hormones and risk of myocardial infarction. Circulation 64:42, 1981.

Barnes RB, Roy S, Lobo RA: Comparison of lipid and androgen levels after conjugated estrogens or depomedroxyprogesterone acetate treatment in postmenopausal women. Obstet Gynecol 66:216, 1985.

Bass KM: Plasma lipoproteins as predictors of cardiovascular death in women. Arch Intern Med 153:2209, 1993.

Bush TL, Barrett-Conner E, Cowan LD et al: Cardiovascular mortality and non-contraceptive use of estrogen in women: Results from the Lipid Research Clinics Program Follow-up Study. Circulation 75:1102, 1987.

Bush TL, Cowan LD, Barrett-Conner E et al: Estrogen use and all-cause mortality: Preliminary results from the Lipid Research Clinics Program Follow-up Study. JAMA 1:249, 1983.

Christiansen C, Lindsay R: Estrogens, bone loss and preservation. Osteoporosis Int 1:7, 1990.

Corson SL: Impact of estrogen replacement therapy on cardiovascular risk. J Reprod Med 34:729, 1989.

Erenus M et al: Comparison of the impact of oral vs transdermal estrogen on serum lipoproteins. Fertil Steril 61:300, 1994.

Gambrell RD Jr: The menopause: Benefits and risks of estrogen-progestogen replacement therapy. Fertil Steril 37:457, 1982.

Gambrell RD, Teran AZ: Changes in lipids and lipoproteins with long-term estrogen deficiency and hormone replacement therapy. Am J Obstet Gynecol 165:307, 1991.

Gordon GS, Picchi J, Roof BS: Antifracture efficacy of long-term estrogens for osteoporosis. Trans Assoc Am Physicians 86:326, 1973.

Gordon T et al: Menopause and coronary heart disease. Ann Intern Med 89:157, 1978.

Hammond CB et al: Effects of long-term estrogen replacement therapy. I: Metabolic effects. Am J Obstet Gynecol 133:525, 1979.

Hunt K, Vessey M, McPherson K: Mortality in a cohort of long-term users of hormone replacement therapy: An updated analysis. Br J Obstet Gynaecol 97:1080, 1990.

Knopp RH: The effect of postmenopausal estrogen therapy on the incidence of arteriosclerotic vascular disease. Obstet Gynecol 72:23S, 1988.

La Rosa JC: Estrogen: Risk vs. benefit for the prevention of coronary artery disease. Coron Artery Dis 4:588, 1993.

La Rosa JC: The varying effects of progestins on lipid levels and cardiovascular disease. Am J Obstet Gynecol 158:1621, 1988.

Lindsay R et al: Long-term prevention of post-menopausal osteoporosis by oestrogen: Evidence for an increased bone mass after delayed onset of oestrogen treatment. Lancet 1:1038, 1976.

Lobo RA: Estrogen and cardiovascular disease. N Y Acad Sci 592:286, 1990.

Lobo RA et al: Metabolic impact of adding medroxyprogesterone acetate to conjugated estrogens therapy in postmenopausal women. Obstet Gynecol 84:987, 1994.

Lufkin EG et al: Treatment of postmenopausal osteoporosis with transdermal estrogen. Ann Intern Med 117:1, 1992.

Matthews KA, Meilahn E, Kuller LH et al: Menopause and risk factors for coronary heart disease. N Engl J Med 321:641, 1989.

Meema S, Bunker ML, Meema HE: Preventive effect of estrogen on postmenopausal bone loss: A follow-up study. Arch Intern Med 135:1436, 1975.

Mendoza S et al: Postmenopausal cyclic estrogen-progestin therapy lowers lipoprotein (a). J Lab Clin Med 123:837, 1994.

Pfeffer RI, van den Noort S: Estrogen use and stroke in postmenopausal women. Am J Epidemiol 103:445, 1976.

Ross RK, Paganini-Hill A, Mack TM et al: Cardiovascular benefits of estrogen replacement therapy. Am J Obstet Gynecol 160:1301, 1989.

Ross RK et al: Menopausal oestrogen therapy and protection from death from ischemic heart disease. Lancet 1:858, 1981.

Selby PL, Peacock M: The effect of transdermal oestrogen on bone, calcium-regulating hormones and liver in postmenopausal women. Clin Endocrinol 25:543, 1986.

Stampfer MJ, Colditz GW: Estrogen replacement therapy and coronary heart disease: A quantitative assessment of the epidemiologic evidence. Prev Med 20:47, 1991.

Stampfer MJ, Colditz GA, Willett WC et al: A prospective study of postmenopausal estrogen therapy and cardiovascular diseases: A ten-year follow-up from the Nurses' Health Study, N Engl J Med 325:756, 1991.

Stampfer MJ, Colditz GW, Willett WC et al: Menopause and heart disease: A review. Ann N Y Acad Sci 592:193, 1990.

Stampfer MJ, Sacks F, Salvini S et al: A prospective study of cholesterol, apolipoproteins, and the risk of myocardial infarction. N Engl J Med 325:373, 1991.

Stampfer MJ, Willett, WC, Colditz GW et al: A prospective study of postmenopausal estrogen therapy and coronary heart disease. N Engl J Med 313:1044, 1985.

Sullivan JM, Zwaag RV, Lemp GF et al: Postmenopausal estrogen use and coronary atherosclerosis. Ann Intern Med 108:358, 1988.

Whitehead MI: Effects of hormone replacement therapy on cardiovascular disease: An interview. Am J Obstet Gynecol 69:929, 1987.

Wilson PWF, Garrison R, Castelli WP: Postmenopausal estrogen use, cigarette smoking, and cardiovascular morbidity in women over 50. N Engl J Med 313:1038, 1985.

HOW TO USE ESTROGENS

Adami HO, Bergstrom R, Holmberg L et al: The effect of female sex hormones on cancer survival. JAMA 263:2189, 1990.

Gambrell RD, Massey FM, Castaneda TA et al: Use of the progestogen challenge test to reduce the risk of endometrial cancer. Obstet Gynecol 55:732, 1980.

Henderson BE, Paganini-Hill A, Ross RK: Decreased mortality in users of estrogen replacement therapy. Arch Intern Med 151:75, 1991.

Henderson BE, Ross RK, Lobo RA et al: Reevaluating the role of progestogen therapy after the menopause. Fertil Steril 49:9S, 1988.

Mishell DR, Shoupe D, Moyer DL et al: Postmenopausal hormone replacement with a combination estrogen-progestin regimen for five days per week. J Reprod Med 36:351, 1991.

Steinberg KK, Thacker SB, Smith J et al: A meta-analysis of the effect of estrogen replacement therapy on the risk of breast cancer. JAMA 265:1985, 1991.

5 Adenocarcinoma of the Uterus

William T. Creasman, M.D.

INCIDENCE

In the USA, cancer of the uterine corpus is the most common malignant neoplasm of the female pelvis today. It is estimated by the American Cancer Society that uterine cancer will develop in approximately 40,800 women in 2005 in the USA, making it the fourth most common cancer in women. The increased incidence of carcinoma of the endometrium has been apparent only during the last three decades. In reviewing the predicted incidence for the 1970s, the American Cancer Society noted a $1\frac{1}{2}$-fold increase in the number of patients with endometrial cancer; however, there was a decline in incidence during the late 1980s. In the last several years, the incidence has remained fairly constant. During the period of increased incidence, predicted deaths from this malignant neoplasm actually decreased slightly. More recently, deaths from uterine cancer have increased. In 1990, the American Cancer Society estimated 4000 deaths from this cancer increasing to 7310 in 2005. An estimation of the most common new cancers and the percentage of female deaths for 2005 in the USA is shown in Fig. 5–1. The increased use of estrogen has been implicated in the apparent increased incidence during the 1970s and early 1980s; however, Norway and Czechoslovakia report a 50–60% increase in endometrial cancer, despite the fact that estrogens are rarely prescribed or are not generally available there. Regardless of the reason for the increased number of women with corpus cancer, this malignant neoplasm has become an important factor in the care of the female patient.

EPIDEMIOLOGY

Endometrial adenocarcinoma occurs during the reproductive and menopausal years. The median age for adenocarcinoma of the uterine corpus is 61 years; most patients are between the ages of 50 and 59 years. Approximately 5% of women will have adenocarcinoma before the age of 40 years, and 20–25% will be diagnosed before the menopause.

Increasing data note that the use of combination oral contraceptives decreases the risk for development of endometrial cancer. The Centers for Disease Control and Prevention evaluated endometrial cancer cases of all women aged 20–54 years from eight population-based cancer registries and compared them with control patients selected at random from the same centers. A comparison of the first 187 cases with 1320 control cases showed that women who used oral contraceptives at some time had a 0.5 relative risk of developing endometrial cancer compared with women who had never used oral contraceptives. This protection occurred in women who used oral contraceptives for at least 12 months, and protection continued for at least 10 years after oral contraceptive use. Protection was most notable for nulliparous women. These investigators estimate that about 2000 cases of endometrial cancer are prevented each year in the USA by past or current use of oral contraceptives. Cigarette smoking apparently decreases the risk for development of endometrial cancer. In a population-based case-control study of women aged 40–60 years, Lawrence and associates found a significant decline in relative risk of endometrial carcinoma with increased smoking ($P > 0.05$). The relative risk

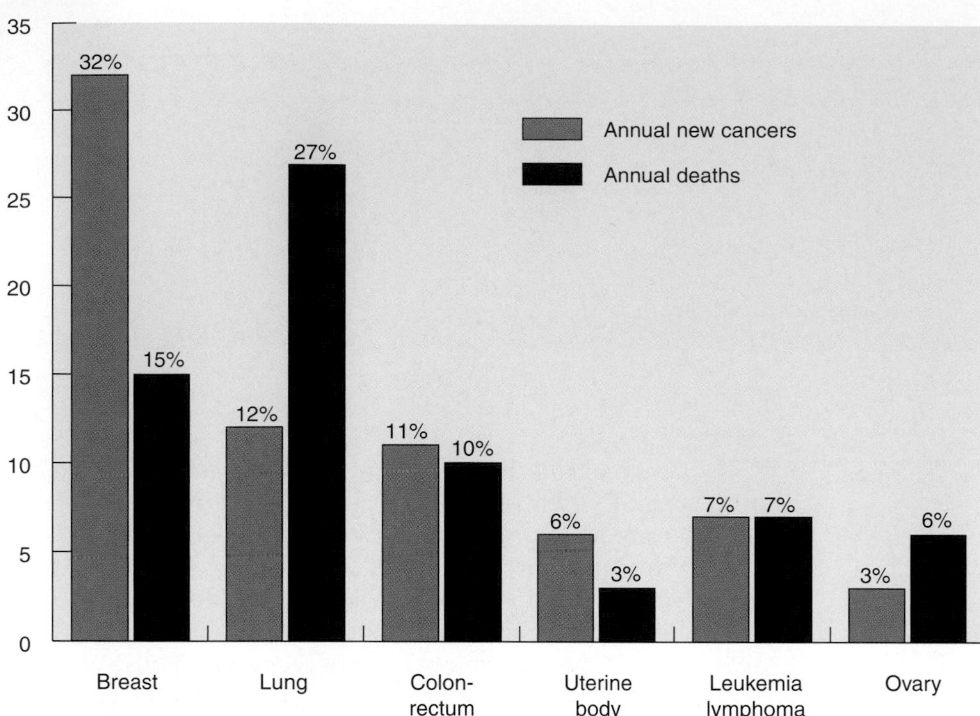

Figure 5–1 Estimated most common new cancers and female deaths (percentage) for 2005 in the USA.

decreased by about 30% when one pack of cigarettes was smoked per day and by another 30% when more than one pack was smoked per day. The effects of smoking did not appear to vary with menstrual status or exogenous estrogen. There was a 4-fold increase in smoking-related odds ratio with bodyweight; the greatest reduction in risk by smoking was in the heaviest women. On the other hand, the estimated risk increased 12-fold in overweight women who were non-smokers and whose primary source of estrogen was peripheral conversion of androgen to estrogen. Although smoking apparently reduces the risk for development of early-stage endometrial cancer, this advantage is strongly outweighed by the increased risk of lung cancer and other major health hazards associated with cigarette smoking.

Multiple risk factors for endometrial cancer have been identified, and MacMahon divides these into three categories:

- variants of normal anatomy or physiology;
- frank abnormality or disease; and
- exposure to external carcinogens.

Obesity, nulliparity, and late menopause are variants of normal anatomy or physiology classically associated with endometrial carcinoma. These three factors are evaluated in regard to the possible risk of developing endometrial cancer in Table 5–1. If a patient is nulliparous and obese and reaches menopause at age 52 years or later, she appears to have a 5-fold increase in the risk of endometrial cancer above that of the patient who does not satisfy these criteria (Table 5–2).

The type of obesity in patients with endometrial cancer has been evaluated. In a study from the University of South Florida, it was noted that women with endometrial cancer had greater waist-hip circumference ratios, abdomen-to-thigh skin ratios, and suprailiac-to-thigh skin ratios than those of matched-control women. As these ratios increased, the relative risk of endometrial cancer increased. The researchers concluded that upper-body fat localization is a significant risk factor for endometrial cancer. In a large multicenter case-control study of 403 endometrial cancer cases and 297 control cases, Swanson and associates confirmed and amplified these findings. Women whose weight exceeded 78 kg had a risk 2.3 times

Table 5–1 ENDOMETRIAL CANCER RISK FACTORS

Risk factors	Risk
Obesity	2.5–4.5×
Nulliparity	
Compared with 1 child	2×
Compared with 5 or more children	3×
Late menopause	2.4×

Table 5–2 MULTIPLE RISK FACTORS

	Risk	
Nulliparous Top 15% in weight Menopause at 52 yr	5× more than	Parous Lower two thirds in weight Menopause at <49 yr

that of women weighing less than 58 kg. For women weighing more than 96 kg, the relative risk increased to 4.3. Upper-body obesity (waist-to-height ratio) was a risk factor independent of bodyweight. Patients in the highest quartile of both weight and waist-to-thigh circumference had a risk of 5.8 times. The amount of body fat has been associated with decreased circulating levels of both progesterone and sex hormone-binding proteins. There was a strong inverse association between sitting height and risk of endometrial cancer. This may be related to serum hormone-bound globulin (SHBG), which appears to be depressed in women with endometrial cancer. The level of SHBG is progressively depressed with increasing upper-body fat localization. With lower SHBG, there is a higher endogenous production of non-protein-bound estradiol. Because endometrial cancer is related to obesity, dietary habits appear to be important. Data suggest that the levels of estriol, total estrogens, and prolactin were lower and those of SHBG were higher in postmenopausal women who were vegetarians. In a case-control study, Levi and colleagues evaluated dietary factors in 274 patients with endometrial cancer and 572 control subjects from two areas in Switzerland and northern Italy. Extensive dietary history was obtained. Their data confirmed the relationship between obesity and endometrial cancer. In relation to diet, they noted an increased association with total energy intake. After correction for total energy intake, a risk was present with the frequency of consumption of most types of meats, eggs, beans, added fats, and sugar. Conversely, significant protection was noted with an elevated intake of most vegetables, fresh fruits, wholegrain bread, and pasta. This reflected a low risk with increased intake of ascorbic acid and beta carotene. Of dietary interest is that the intake of olive oil seemed beneficial in Switzerland but resembled other added fats in the Italian women. It has been previously noted that the amount and type of dietary fat influence estrogen metabolism because estrogen reabsorption from the bowel seems to be increased by diets rich in beef or fats.

Diabetes mellitus and hypertension are frequently associated with endometrial cancer. Kaplan and Cole reported a relative risk of 2.8 associated with a history of diabetes after controlling for age, body weight, and socioeconomic status. High blood pressure is prevalent in the elderly obese patient but does not appear to be a significant factor by itself, even though 25% of endometrial cancer patients have hypertension or arteriosclerotic heart disease.

As extensively detailed in Chapter 4, the relationship of unopposed estrogen and endometrial cancer is well documented. Fortunately, the addition of a progestin appears to be protective.

Adequacy of progesterone is important in prevention of endometrial cancer. In a study from Sweden at the end of 5 years excess risk of endometrial cancer was 6.6 but with combined estrogen progestin (E + P), RR was 1.6 for 11–15 days of progestin, 2.9 for 10 days of use and 0.2 if continuous E + P was given. The Million Womens study from the United Kingdom has recently reported their findings of endometrial cancer and hormone replacement therapy (HRT). This study which first reported on HRT and breast cancer has been severely criticized mainly on methodology factors. They had an average follow-up of 3.4 years during which 1320 incident endometrial cancers were diagnosed. At time of recruitment 22% of HRT users (total number was 320,953 women) last used continuous combined therapy, 45% last used cyclic combined therapy with progestogen usually added for 10–14 days per month, 19% last used tibolone and 4% used estrogen alone. Compared with non-users, relative risk of endometrial cancer was 0.71%, CI 0.56–0.90, P = 0.005; 1.05, CI 0.91-1.22; 1.79, CI 1.43–2.25, $P < 0.001$ and 1.45, CI 1.02–2.06, p = 0.04 respectively. Interestingly, the adverse effects of tibolone and estrogen only were greatest in the non-obese woman and the beneficial effects of combined HRT were greatest in obese women. Although the risk of unopposed estrogen is present, women taking estrogen who develop endometrial cancer appear to have favorable prognostic factors. Several but not all studies suggest that risk factors such as multiparity and obesity are lower in the estrogen users. Stage of disease and histologic grade appear to be lower in estrogen users. With correction for stage and grade, estrogen users still have less myometrial invasion than non-estrogen users do. The poor prognostic subtypes, such as clear cell carcinoma and adenosquamous cancer, appear less frequently in estrogen users. As a result, survival of estrogen-related endometrial cancer is much better than that of non-estrogen cancers. In fact, some studies note just as good if not better survival in estrogen users than in women with non-estrogen, non-endometrial cancers.

Incidence and survival are higher in white women compared with black women. Reasons for these differences are unexplained. An analysis of the Gynecologic Oncology Group (GOG) database evaluated this factor in 600 white and 91 black women with clinical stage I or stage II endometrial cancer. A larger number of the African-American women were diagnosed after age 70 years, and they had a higher proportion of papillary serous and clear cell histologic types; the black women also had more advanced disease, grade, vascular space involvement, depth of invasion, and lymph node metastases than the white women did. Survival (5-year) was 77% for white women and 60% for black women. Survival difference remained even in high-risk groups such as grade 3 tumors (59% vs 37%, respectively). The unadjusted hazard rate was 2.0, which was statistically significant. With adjustment for age, cell type, and extent of disease, the relative risk dropped to 1.2. The adjusted risk rate suggests that race is not a significant factor; nevertheless, race does denote an increased risk for poor prognostic factors, which clinically may be important.

Tamoxifen is being used in an increasing amount in women with breast cancer. In addition, three studies by Fisher and coworkers, Powels and colleagues, and Veronesi and associates of the prophylactic use of tamoxifen in women without breast cancer have been reported. Several cases of endometrial cancer have been described in women receiving tamoxifen. It has not yet been determined whether this relationship placed women receiving tamoxifen at higher risk for adenocarcinoma. It is hoped that several ongoing studies will answer this question. Tamoxifen, although labeled an antiestrogen, is known to have estrogenic properties and truly is a weak estrogen. Women receiving tamoxifen also appear to have some protection from osteoporosis and against heart disease (decreased lactate dehydrogenase and cholesterol), much like women receiving estrogen replacement therapy.

During the recent past, there has been a considerable amount of lay as well as professional publicity in regard to the possible association of tamoxifen with endometrial cancer. Tamoxifen was first introduced in clinical trials in the early 1970s and approved in 1978 by the US Food and Drug Administration (FDA) for treatment of advanced breast carcinoma in the postmenopausal woman. Extensive experience with this drug has been reported. It is estimated that more than four million women in the USA have taken tamoxifen for almost eight million women-years of use. It is suggested that each year, about 80,000 women in the USA will begin taking tamoxifen because of a diagnosis of breast cancer and will probably continue it for at least 5 years. With the results of the prophylactic studies, this number is likely to increase. Tamoxifen has proved successful in efficacy, particularly in the postmenopausal patient, and is usually considered the drug of choice in this group of women. Those patients with disease spread outside of the breast also appear to benefit substantially from its use. One of its major benefits is that in women taking tamoxifen, there has been a substantial decrease in the incidence of a second cancer in the opposite breast compared with like women who were taking a placebo. In those patients in whom the drug may have been given prophylactically, recurrence has been markedly reduced compared with those not taking the drug. Initial studies suggested that the drug should be taken for 2 years, and this has been extended to 5 years. Ongoing studies are evaluating its use for up to 10 years. Therefore, there is no question that this drug, which has a relatively low toxicity rate, has proved to be extremely beneficial for women with breast cancer.

In 1985, Killackey and associates described three breast cancer patients receiving tamoxifen who subsequently developed endometrial cancer. During the last 10 years, approximately 400 endometrial cancer cases have been reported worldwide in breast cancer patients taking tamoxifen. In many instances, the literature is made up of case reports; however, several "series" have been reported. The one that has received the most notoriety is the prospective, randomized study of the National Surgical Adjuvant Breast and Bowel Project (NSABP). This study analyzed 2843 patients with node-negative estrogen receptor-positive invasive breast cancer randomly assigned to receive a placebo or 20 mg/day of tamoxifen. An additional 1220 tamoxifen-treated patients were registered and given the drug. The average time in the study was 8 years for the randomly assigned patients and 5 years for the registered patients. Of the 1419 patients randomly assigned to tamoxifen, 15 developed uterine cancer, of which two were sarcomas. One patient randomized to receive tamoxifen did not take the drug and developed endometrial cancer 78 months after randomization. In the placebo group, two developed endometrial cancer; however, both were receiving tamoxifen at the time of their uterine malignant disease. One patient had a breast recurrence and was prescribed tamoxifen, and the other was given tamoxifen after colon cancer. Two of the endometrial cancer patients had been taking tamoxifen for only 5 and 8 months before their diagnosis of uterine disease was made. There were five patients in the tamoxifen group who developed endometrial cancer after the drug had been discontinued for 7 to 73 months. In the registered patients who received tamoxifen, eight uterine tumors (seven endometrial) were subsequently diagnosed. Three of these patients had been taking tamoxifen for less than a year (2 months, 2 months, and 9 months). The authors determined the average annual hazard rate of endometrial cancer per 1000 women in their population of patients. This was 0.2 per 1000 in the placebo group and 1.6 per 1000 for the randomized tamoxifen-treated patients. In the registered patients receiving tamoxifen, the average annual hazard rate was 1.4 per 1000, similar to that of the randomized tamoxifen-treated group. The hazard rate of endometrial cancer in the placebo group was low compared with the Surveillance, Epidemiology, and End Results (SEER) data as well as with previous NSABP randomized tamoxifen-placebo studies; these data would suggest that the average annual hazard rate is 0.7 per 1000. These data, based on a limited number of patients with endometrial cancer while receiving tamoxifen, suggest that there may be a relative risk of 2.3 for development of endometrial cancer while receiving tamoxifen. This does not take into account the well-known fact that women who develop breast cancer are at an increased risk for development of endometrial cancer irrespective of subsequent treatment. The relative risk of 1.72 to more than 3 has been reported. The risks and benefits of the prevention of recurrences and new breast cancer in comparison to new endometrial cancers were evaluated in the NSABP study. The benefits suggest that 121.3 fewer breast-related events per 1000 women treated with tamoxifen were seen compared with 6.3 endometrial cancers per 1000 women. Therefore, the benefit from tamoxifen is apparent.

It was initially suggested that the rate of endometrial cancers associated with tamoxifen might be equal to that associated with unopposed estrogen replacement therapy. Because tamoxifen is a weak estrogen, similar characteristics of the endometrial cancer were also implied (i.e., well-differentiated superficially invasive cancers). Magriples and colleagues, reporting a retrospective study, identified 15 women who had breast cancer, were receiving tamoxifen, and developed uterine cancers compared with 38 other breast cancer patients who developed uterine cancer but were not receiving tamoxifen. Tamoxifen was given at 40 mg/day for 3–10 years (mean 4.2 years). These investigators noted that 67% of the tamoxifen-treated patients had high-grade tumor compared with 24% of the untreated group. Of the 15 patients, 5 died of endometrial cancer, compared with 1 in the untreated group. They suggested that tamoxifen-associated endometrial cancers carried a poor prognosis. Barakat and associates reviewed five studies, including the study by Magriples, the NSABP, their own data from Memorial Sloan-Kettering Hospital, and two studies from overseas. A total of 103 patients were evaluated in regard to histologic features, grade of tumor, International Federation of Gynecology and Obstetrics (FIGO) staging, and deaths due to uterine cancer; an increase was not found in poor prognostic histologic findings, tumor differentiation, or stage compared with what would be expected in a similar group of non-tamoxifen-treated patients with uterine cancer. Jordan, in an evaluation of the SEER data as well as of tamoxifen-associated endometrial cancer in the literature, reported similar findings.

It has been suggested by some individuals, on the basis of an extremely limited number of patients, that all women receiving tamoxifen should have the endometrium evaluated at regular intervals (i.e., yearly). The rationale for this recommendation suggests that uterine cancer is related to the tamoxifen. During the last 10 years, only 400 endometrial cancer patients have been described in the literature worldwide. During that same time, it has been estimated that there have been approximately 350,000 uterine cancers in the USA alone. With more than three million women in the USA having taken tamoxifen and only 400 women worldwide described with tamoxifen-associated endometrial cancer, cost effectiveness of yearly endometrial evaluation does not appear warranted. All women, irrespective of whether they are taking tamoxifen, should certainly have yearly gynecologic examinations. The endometrium should be evaluated if the patient is symptomatic. We do not currently recommend endometrial sampling or ultrasound evaluation of the endometrium just because an individual is taking tamoxifen. The prophylactic tamoxifen study is evaluating yearly screening, and data from that study will be most helpful in determining optimal management of these patients.

This possible concern of tamoxifen and endometrial cancer may become moot in the near future, as the aromatase inhibitors may appear to be better than tamoxifen in the prevention of recurrent or contralateral breast cancer. The role of aromatase inhibitors as prophylaxis is being investigated but data is lacking at the present time.

Recently, hereditary non-polyposis colon cancer (HNPCC) also known as Lynch II, has been identified as a risk factor for endometrial cancer. This is an autosomal-dominant inherited cancer in which a germline mutation in one of the genes in the DNA mismatch repair gene family which includes mainly MSH2, MLM1 and MSH6. Fortunately HNPCC accounts for only 1–5% of all colorectal cancers but a 39–54% lifetime risk of developing colon cancer. There is a lifetime risk of 30–61% of developing endometrial cancer. There is also an increased risk of ovarian cancers as well as other non-gyn cancers. In a study by Lu and associates, they noted that about half the time, the endometrial or ovarian cancer appeared before the colon cancer. In both instances, the age at diagnosis was in the early 40s. There was a median of 11 years between the gyn cancer and the colon cancer. In 14% of the time the gyn and colon cancer were diagnosed simultaneously. The Cancer Study Consortium suggests colonoscopy every 1–3 years beginning at age 25 in individuals with this hereditary disorder. The data suggest that if surveillance is done, survival is improved. Women should be offered surveillance with ultrasound and endometrial sampling from age 25–35, although there is no data to suggest this will improve survival if endometrial cancer is diagnosed by these means.

DIAGNOSIS

The cost of screening for adenocarcinoma and its precursors in the total population would be prohibitive. Women receiving hormone replacement therapy (estrogen and progesterone) do not need endometrial biopsy before institution of therapy or during replacement therapy unless abnormal bleeding occurs. Monthly withdrawal bleeding after progestin is not considered abnormal bleeding. On the other hand, breakthrough bleeding should be evaluated. The use of continuous estrogen alone increases the risk of adenocarcinoma. Estrogen plus progesterone appears to decrease the risk of adenocarcinoma and therefore is the preferred treatment. In asymptomatic high-risk patients, periodic screening may be advisable. All postmenopausal women with uterine bleeding must be evaluated for endometrial cancer, although only 20% of these patients will have a genital malignant neoplasm. As the patient's age increases after the menopause, there is a progressively increasing probability that her uterine bleeding is caused by endometrial cancer. Feldman and associates found that age was the greatest independent risk factor associated with endometrial cancer or complex hyperplasia. In women aged 70 years or older, the odds ratio was 9.1. If complex hyperplasia was present, the odds ratio increased to 16. When a woman was older than 70 years, her chance of having cancer when vaginal bleeding was present was about 50%. If she was also nulliparous and had diabetes, the risk was 87%. A perimenopausal patient who may have abnormal uterine bleeding indicative of endometrial cancer is frequently not evaluated because the patient or her physician interprets her new bleeding pattern as resulting from "menopause." During this time in a woman's life, the menstrual periods should become lighter and lighter and farther and farther apart. Any other bleeding pattern should be evaluated with carcinoma of the endometrium in mind.

A high index of suspicion must be maintained if the diagnosis of endometrial cancer is to be made in the young patient. Prolonged and heavy menstrual periods and intermenstrual spotting may indicate cancer, and endometrial sampling is advised. Most young patients who develop endometrial cancer are obese, in many instances massively overweight, often with anovulatory menstrual cycles. Sequential oral contraceptives, which were also incriminated in young patients with endometrial cancer, should no longer be of concern because these agents are no longer commercially available.

Historically, the fractional dilatation and curettage (D&C) has been the definitive diagnostic procedure used in ruling out endometrial cancer. In the 1920s, Kelly advocated the use of what amounts to outpatient curettage to obtain adequate endometrial tissue for diagnostic study. Today, most advocate the routine use of the endometrial biopsy as an office procedure to make a definitive diagnosis and spare the patient hospitalization and an anesthetic. Several studies have indicated that the accuracy of the endometrial biopsy in detecting endometrial cancer is approximately 90%. Hofmeister noted that 17% of the endometrial carcinomas diagnosed by routine office biopsy occurred in asymptomatic perimenopausal women. Unfortunately, in his study, in which the endometrial biopsy was used, several patients may have been missed because not all of these individuals had a subsequent D&C. Koss and associates evaluated 2586 asymptomatic women with endometrial screening and found an incidence of endometrial cancer of 1.71 per 1000 women-years. Autopsy studies identify an occult endometrial cancer in women dying of unrelated causes to be between 2.2 and 3.1 per 1000. Other procedures have been developed to be used on an outpatient basis not only for diagnosis but also for screening. Those techniques using endometrial cytology to make the diagnosis of endometrial cancer have been less successful than those in which tissue itself is evaluated.

Cytologic detection of endometrial cancer by routine cervical Papanicolaou (Pap) smear has generally been poor in comparison with the efficacy of the Pap smear in diagnosing early cervical disease. Several studies in the literature indicate that only one-third to one half of the patients with adenocarcinoma of the endometrium have abnormal Pap smears on routine cervical screening. The main reason for the poor detection with the cervical Pap smear is that cells are not removed directly from the lesion as they are on the cervix. When a cytologic preparation is obtained directly from the endometrial cavity, malignant cells are present in higher numbers than those found if routine cervical or vaginal smears are obtained. Techniques that obtain only a cytologic preparation are generally inadequate if they are used alone.

Several commercial apparatuses are available for sampling the endometrial cavity on an outpatient basis. Devices that remove tissue for histologic evaluation have generally been good if tissue is obtained from the endometrial cavity. Stovall and colleagues evaluated 40 known endometrial cancer patients with the Pipelle instrument. Ninety percent of the women were postmenopausal. Only in one patient was cancer not identified with the Pipelle. This patient had a prior D&C that revealed a grade 1 lesion. The Pipelle diagnosis was atypical adenomatous hyperplasia, and the hysterectomy specimen revealed a focus of adenocarcinoma in situ. The pathologist noted that the obtainable tissue was acceptable for analysis in 100% of patients. Discomfort was recorded as mild in 80%, and only two patients (5%) reported severe pain. Goldchmit and coworkers reported similar accuracy with the Pipelle in 176 consecutive patients undergoing D&C. In past years, we have used curets such as the Duncan and Kevorkian successfully; however, in recent years, these have been replaced by the thin disposable suction-type curets because they are as successful as the reusable instruments but appear to be less painful for the patient. In the symptomatic patient in whom inadequate tissue (or no tissue at all) is obtained for pathologic evaluation, a D&C must be considered.

The use of multiple diagnostic techniques to increase the capability of outpatient diagnosis appears to be most helpful. The use of cytologic and histologic methods will increase the detection rate of patients with endometrial cancer. If diagnosis of endometrial cancer can be made on an outpatient basis, the patient can avoid hospitalization and a minor surgical procedure. Any cytologic or histologic abnormality short of invasive cancer mandates a formal fractional curettage to rule out a small focus of invasive disease. All patients with persistent symptoms despite normal biopsy findings should submit to fractional curettage as well.

Hysterography and hysteroscopy have been suggested as adjuvants in making the diagnosis of endometrial cancer and in establishing the extent of disease. Details seen with hysterography correlate well with surgical findings. Information that can be obtained includes tumor volume, tumor origin, extent of disease within the uterine cavity, shape of the cavity, and cervical involvement. Today, hysterography is used infrequently, if at all, as a diagnostic procedure. Hysteroscopy has been used more frequently in the evaluation of patients with abnormal uterine bleeding and has the advantage of being done on an outpatient basis. Because many patients with endometrial cancer can be diagnosed with office biopsy, that is our preferred first diagnostic step. If the biopsy result is negative and further evaluation is needed, we proceed to hysteroscopy. With its use, surgeons can direct biopsies of focal lesions that might be missed by D&C. Hysteroscopy can be used to evaluate the endocervical canal.

Ultrasonography (US) has been suggested as a diagnostic tool in evaluating women with irregular bleeding, particularly the postmenopausal patient (Fig. 5–2A–C). The endometrial stripe as seen with transvaginal US appears to be indicative of endometrial thickness. Several studies suggest that if a thin endometrial stripe is present, a histologic diagnosis is not necessary, because atrophic endometrium would be present. Varner and colleagues evaluated 80 postmenopausal women; 65 were asymptomatic, of whom 38 were not receiving hormones and 27 were taking hormones. There were 60 patients with US-measured endometrial thickness of ≤4 mm, and atrophy or low estrogen stimulation was noted in all on histologic evaluation. In women with measured endometrial thickness of 5–8 mm, the type of endometrium, including cancer, could not be distinguished. Unfortunately, for evaluation, only two patients had cancer. Granberg and associates evaluated 205 women with postmenopausal bleeding, 30 postmenopausal asymptomatic women, and 30 postmenopausal patients with known endometrial cancer. In the two groups of 60 patients, the endometrial thickness was 3.2 (mean) vs 17.7, respectively. In the group of 205 women, 18 were found to have endometrial cancer. No cancers were present in the endometrium that had an endometrial thickness of ≤8 mm. There was considerable overlap of endometrial thickness by all histologic groups. The authors noted that if a cutoff of 5 mm was used, no false-negative findings were present. With this measurement, the positive predictive value was 87%, with specificity of 96% and sensitivity of 100% for identifying endometrial abnormalities. Bourne and colleagues, in evaluating 183 selected postmenopausal women of whom 34 were asymptomatic and 12 had endometrial cancer, found an overlap of endometrial thickness between women with and without cancer. Other studies have suggested similar findings. It has been suggested that if US could save a large number of endometrial biopsies, there would be a large cost savings with less discomfort to the patient. As previously noted, significant pain with the newer disposable endometrial biopsy techniques affects only a small number of patients; and a certain number of patients, because of considerable endometrial thickness, will require endometrial sampling anyway. To date, cost effectiveness has not been demonstrated. Unfortunately, endometrial cancer has been identified when the endometrial thickness is <5 mm. Although studies may evaluate several hundred patients, most do not have many cancer patients included. Wang and associates reviewed the ultrasound of 52 women who were diagnosed with papillary serous clear cell and other high-grade carcinomas. Of the 52, 34 (65%) had thickened endometrium measuring ≥5 mm, in 9 (17%) the endometrium was <5 mm and in an additional 9 women (17%) the endometrium was indistinct. In the women with non-thickened endometrium or more other ultrasound abnormalities were noted; intracavitary fluid or lesion, myometrial mass, enlarged uterus or adnexal mass. Multiple factors can affect endometrial thickness. These include estrogen, estrogen plus progestin, body mass index (BMI), diabetes, poor histotype, race, and postmenopausal status.

To date, there is no general agreement of the cutoff measurement at which endometrial sampling is not necessary. We prefer to sample the endometrium in symptomatic postmenopausal patients as the first diagnostic technique. If histologic findings are "negative" the patient is observed. A D&C is done only if the patient continues to be symptomatic after the negative biopsy result.

US has also been evaluated as a means for determining depth of myometrial invasion. Gordon and associates studied 15 known patients with endometrial cancer by US and magnetic resonance imaging (MRI). By use of criteria of ≥50% myometrial wall involvement as deep invasion and <50% as superficial invasion, US was judged to be more accurate than MRI in five; MRI was better in three, both were equally accurate in four, and neither was accurate in three. It has been suggested by some that US can accurately predict myometrial invasion in about 75% of cases. Although knowing the depth of invasion preoperatively would be important information to the clinician, the data from studies as noted before would currently appear to be too premature or too costly to use routinely. We prefer to evaluate depth of myometrial invasion intraoperatively with gross examination or frozen section.

The reliability of US in determining endometrial thickness in the postmenopausal patient does not appear to be applicable to women taking tamoxifen. In all studies, the endometrium in the tamoxifen-treated patient is considerably thicker than in the non-tamoxifen-treated patient. Histologic evaluation revealed atrophic endometrium in a large number of these tamoxifen-treated patients. Because of this discordance, Lahti and colleagues evaluated 103 asymptomatic postmenopausal patients (51 receiving tamoxifen and 52 control subjects) with US, hysteroscopy, and endometrial histologic examination. In the tamoxifen group, 84% had endometrial thickness on US of ≥5 mm vs 19% in the non-tamoxifen group (51% vs 8% >10 mm, respectively). Hysteroscopy findings noted that 28% of uterine mucosa was atrophic vs 87% in non-tamoxifen control group. Histopathologic examination noted atrophic endometrium in 60% of tamoxifen-treated patients vs 79% of control subjects. The biggest difference between the two groups was the finding of polyps in 18% of the tamoxifen group vs 0% of the control group; this appears to be a frequent finding in the tamoxifen-treated patient. So-called megapolyps measuring up to 12 cm have been described. Other uterine disease has been attributed to tamoxifen, including increased uterine volume, lower impedance to blood flow in uterine arteries, endometriosis, focal periglandular condensation of stromal cells, and epithelial metaplasia. Data now suggest that the markedly thickened endometrium (up to 40 mm) in patients receiving tamoxifen is not thickened endometrium but proximal myometrium. Goldstein suggested that US study with endometrial saline infusion may help delineate the true endometrium from the underlying myometrium. With this technique, he was able to identify large polypoid lesions and other sonolucent cystic spaces that were initially thought to represent thickened endometrium.

After a tissue diagnosis of endometrial malignant disease is established, the patient should have a thorough diagnostic evaluation before the institution of therapy. Before 1988, endometrial cancer was clinically staged. Because of the considerable discrepancy between clinical and actual stage, FIGO has now adopted a surgical-pathologic staging classification (Table 5–3; see Fig. 5–2). Approximately 75% of patients with endometrial cancer present with stage I disease (Table 5–4). Routine hematologic studies and clotting profiles are obtained for all patients. Presurgical metastatic evaluation should include a chest film and metabolic profiles, and many clinicians suggest a computed tomographic scan with contrast enhancement.

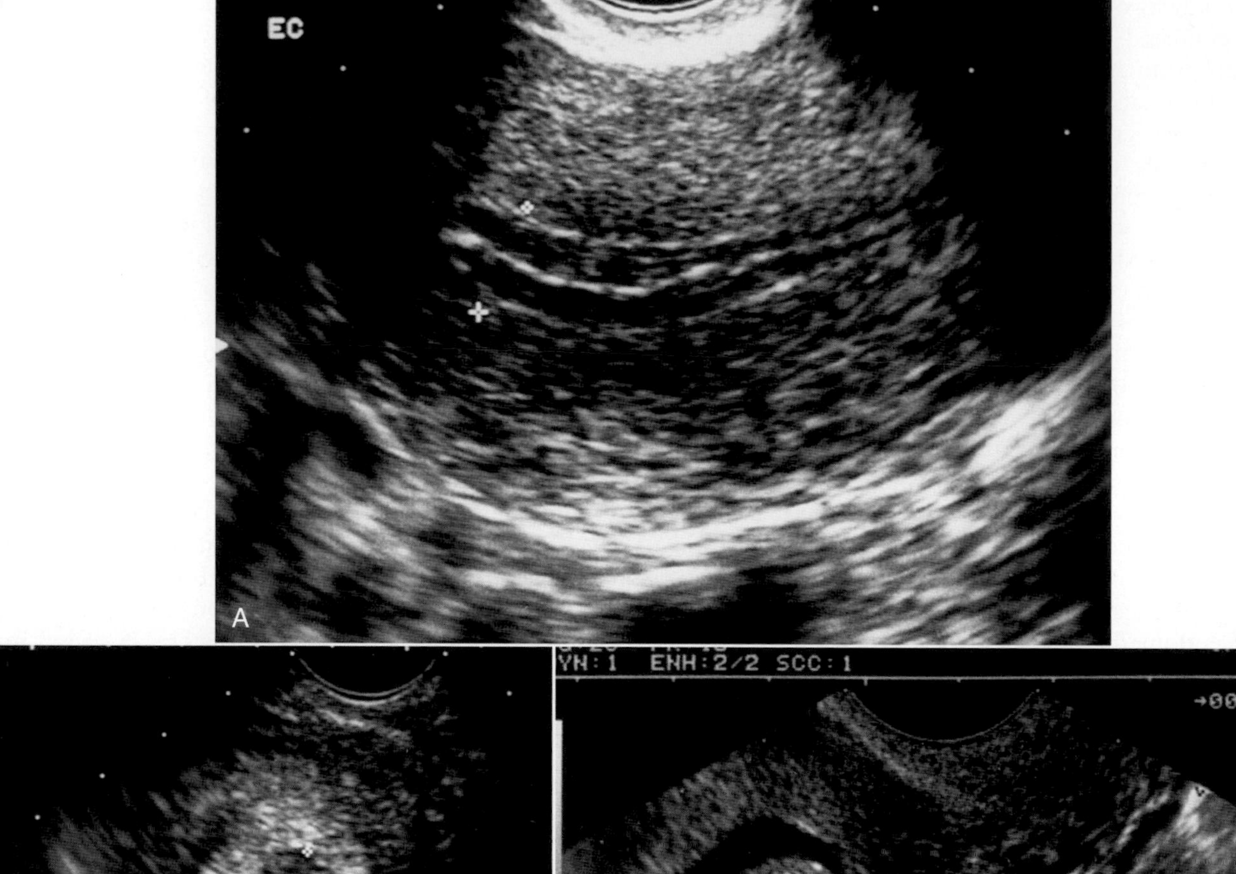

Figure 5–2 *A,* Ultrasound of the uterus showing the "triple line" indicating the thickness of the endometrium. *B,* Ultrasound of the uterus showing a "thickened endometrium" of >10 mm. *C,* Saline instillation of the endometrial cavity notes a well-defined submucous fibroid and not thickened endometrium.

Sigmoidoscopy and barium enema studies have been reserved for patients who demonstrate palpable disease outside the uterus or have recognizable symptoms of bowel disease. Brain, liver, and bone scans have been used only in patients who are thought to have extant disease.

PROGNOSTIC FACTORS

Pretreatment evaluation of patients with malignant neoplasms, coupled with clinical-pathologic experience, should allow the physician to individualize therapy for the best results. Multiple factors have been identified for endometrial carcinoma that appear to have significant predictive value for these women (Table 5–5). FIGO, in developing the classification for endometrial cancer, has taken into consideration two factors in the substage category within stage I (see Table 5–3). Essentially all reports in the literature agree that differentiation (grade) of tumor and depth of invasion are important prognostic considerations.

The patient's clinical profile as it concerns prognosis has been evaluated. Several studies indicate that the age of

Table 5–3 FIGO CLASSIFICATION OF ENDOMETRIAL CARCINOMA

Stage	
Ia G1,2,3	Tumor limited to endometrium
Ib G1,2,3	Invasion of less than half of the myometrium
Ic G1,2,3	Invasion of more than half of the myometrium
IIa G1,2,3	Endocervical glandular involvement only
IIb G1,2,3	Cervical stromal invasion
IIIa G1,2,3	Tumor invades serosa and/or adnexa and/or positive peritoneal cytology
IIIb G1,2,3	Vaginal metastases
IIIc G1,2,3	Metastases to pelvic or para-aortic lymph nodes
IVa G1,2,3	Tumor invasion of bladder or bowel mucosa
IVb	Distant metastases, including intra-abdominal or inguinal lymph node
Histopathology: Degree of differentiation	
Cases of carcinoma of the corpus should be grouped according to the degree of differentiation of the adenocarcinoma as follows:	
G1	5% or less of a non-squamous or non-morular solid growth pattern
G2	6–50% of a non-squamous or non-morular solid growth pattern
G3	More than 50% of a non-squamous or non-morular solid growth pattern

Approved by FIGO, October 1988, Rio de Janeiro.

Table 5–4 DISTRIBUTION OF ENDOMETRIAL CARCINOMA BY STAGE (SURGICAL)

Stage	Patients
I	3839 (73%)
II	574 (11%)
III	694 (13%)
IV	166 (3%)

From Pecorelli S (ed): FIGO Annual Report, years 1990–92. J Epidemiol Biostat 3:41, 1998.

Table 5–5 PROGNOSTIC FACTORS IN ENDOMETRIAL ADENOCARCINOMA

Histologic type (pathology)
Histologic differentiation
Stage of disease
Myometrial invasion
Peritoneal cytology
Lymph node metastasis
Adnexal metastasis

the patient can be directly related to prognosis in that younger women do much better than older women. This is probably because younger women tend to have more well-differentiated cancer; when corrected for grade, age does not appear to be an important prognostic factor.

Bokhman suggested that there are two pathogenic types of endometrial cancer. The first type arises in women with obesity, hyperlipidemia, and signs of hyperestrogenism, such as anovulatory uterine bleeding, infertility, late onset of menopause, and hyperplasia of the stroma of the ovaries and endometrium. The second pathogenic type of disease arises in women who have none of these disease states or in whom the disease states are not clearly defined. Bokhman's data suggest that patients with the first pathogenic type mainly have well-differentiated or moderately differentiated tumor, superficial invasion of the myometrium, high sensitivity to progestins, and favorable prognosis (85% 5-year survival in his material). The patients who fall into the second pathogenic group tend to have poorly differentiated tumors, deep myometrial invasion, high frequency of metastatic disease in the lymph nodes, decreased sensitivity to progestin, and poor prognosis (58% 5-year survival rate). Unfortunately, Bokhman does not provide a stage breakdown for the two pathogenic groups, although more than 70% of all of his patients had stage I disease. It is assumed from his description that a larger number of patients with the second pathogenic type had more advanced disease, and this may account for the poor prognosis. However, the etiologic role of hyperestrogenism suggested by this study is intriguing, particularly in view of the large number of patients with well-differentiated cancer, superficial invasion, and excellent prognosis in which exogenous estrogen association has been identified. Kauppila, Grönroos, and Nieminen, using only body weight as the determination, noted that in patients with stage I carcinoma of the endometrium, the best 5-year survival rate occurred in the heaviest patients (>75 kg), and again this seemed to be related to the fact that heavier patients had fewer anaplastic lesions than did lighter patients.

Pathology

Careful evaluation of the uterus by the pathologist is essential for proper diagnosis and treatment of corpus cancer (Fig. 5–3). Carcinoma of the endometrium may start as a focal discrete lesion, as in an endometrial polyp. It may also be diffuse in several different areas, in some situations involving the entire endometrial surface. Adenocarcinoma, the most common histologic type, is usually preceded by a predisposing lesion (atypical endometrial hyperplasia). Only those hyperplasias with cellular atypia are considered to be precursors of adenocarcinoma of the endometrium. As tumor volume increases, spread within the endometrium or myometrium occurs. As this process continues, dissemination to distant organs can take place. It is recognized that there are multiple prognostic factors in endometrial cancer (see subsequent section), including histologic type and the grade of the cancer. A clinically enlarged uterus may be caused by increasing tumor volume, but this should not be the only gauge for significant local disease.

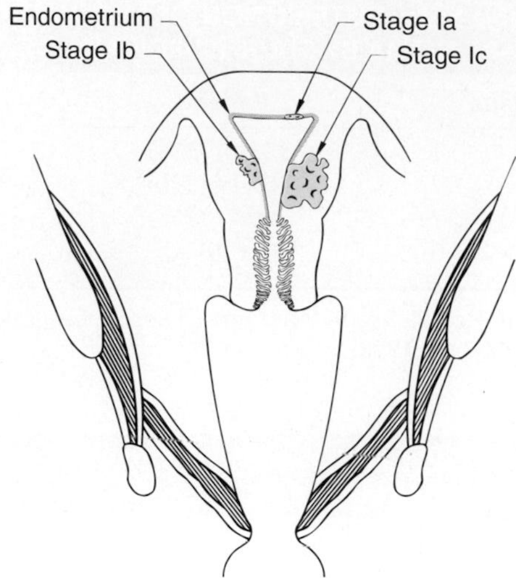

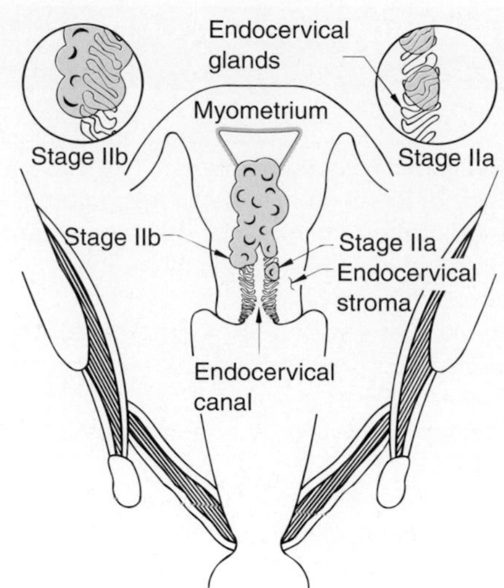

Stage Ia: Tumor limited to endometrium
Stage Ib: Invasion to less than one-half the myometrium
Stage Ic: Invasion to more than one-half the myometrium

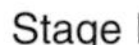

Stage I

Stage IIa: Endocervical glandular involvement only
Stage IIb: Cervical stroma invasion

Stage II

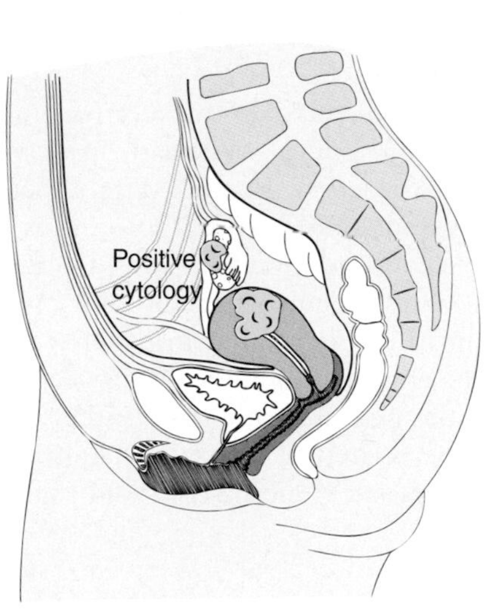

Stage IIIA

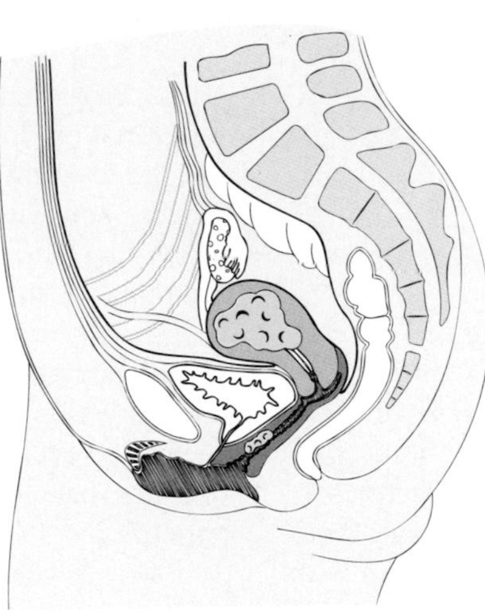

Stage IIIB

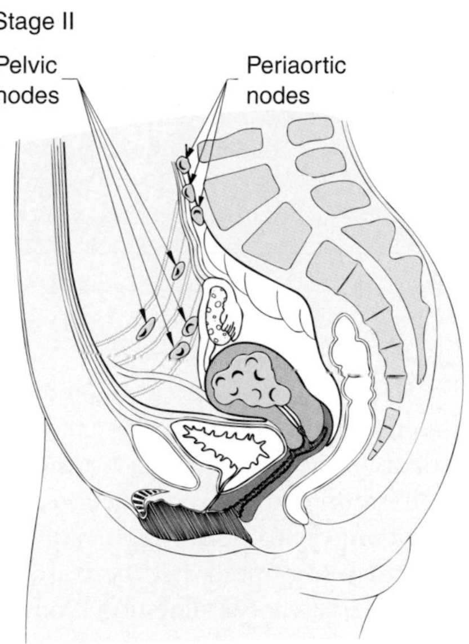

Stage IIIC

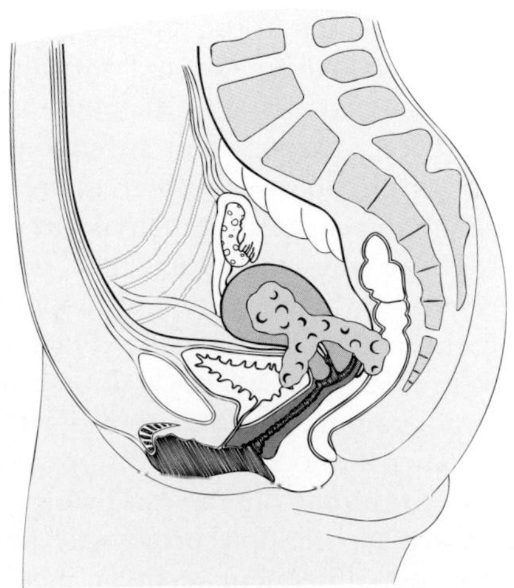

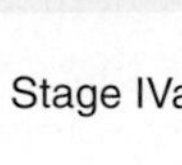

Stage IVa

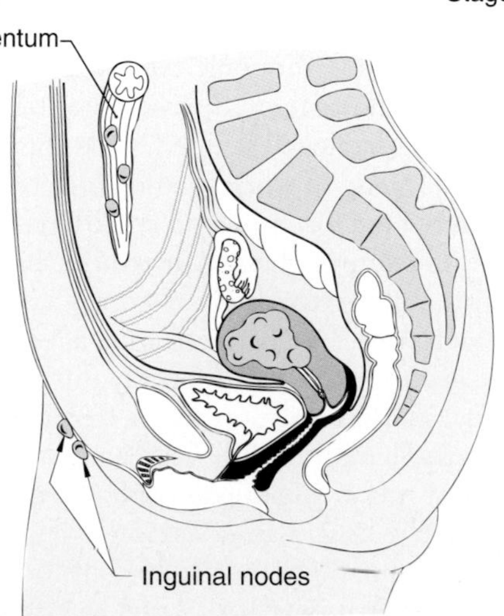

Stage IVb

FIGO staging for endometrial cancer.

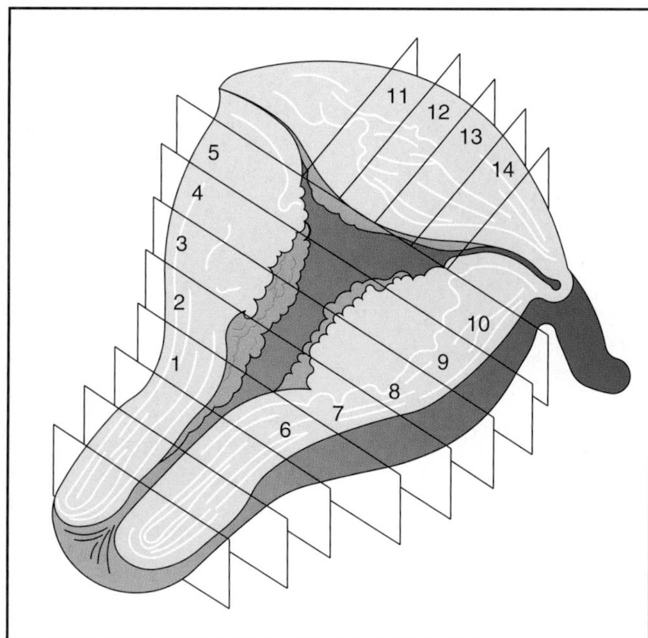

Figure 5–3 Pathologic evaluation of endometrial cancer. (Courtesy of Paul Underwood, M.D.)

Obviously, many patients can have enlarged uteri because of factors other than adenocarcinoma.

Adenocarcinoma is the most common histologic subtype that may originate in the endometrium (Table 5–6). It is characterized by the presence of glands in an abnormal relationship to each other, with the hallmark of little if any intervening stroma between the glands. There can be variations in the size of the glands, and infolding is common. The cells are usually enlarged, as are the nuclei, along with nuclear chromatin clumping and nucleolar enlargement. Mitosis may be frequent. Differentiation of adenocarcinoma (mild, moderate, and severe, or grades 1–3) is important prognostically and is incorporated into the FIGO surgical staging. Most studies suggest that approximately 60–65% of all endometrial cancers are of this subtype.

Sivridis and colleagues have suggested that there are two separate forms of endometrial carcinoma. One is associated with and is presumed to have progressed from an atypical hyperplasia of the endometrium and is thought to have a relatively good prognosis; the other develops in an atrophic or rarely cycling endometrium and is associated with a much poorer prognosis. It is believed that hyperestrogenism is the etiologic basis of those carcinomas associated with hyperplasias, but some other genetic alteration must be involved in the pathogenesis of neoplasms developing in a trophic endometrium. G1 lesions behave the same in both groups. G2 and G3 lesions are more common in the group arising from atrophic endometrium.

For almost a century, it has been recognized that a squamous component may be associated with an adenocarcinoma of the endometrium. This occurs in about 25% of patients. For many years, patients with a squamous component were further stratified according to whether the squamous component appeared benign (designated adenoacanthoma, AA) or malignant (designated adenosquamous carcinoma, AS). It was suggested that AA indicated a good prognosis, and those with AS had a poor survival. More recently, this distinction has been questioned in regard to its prognostic importance. Zaino and coworkers, in reporting data from the GOG, suggest that the notation of squamous component irrespective of differentiation does not affect survival. Patients with clinical stage I and stage II cancers were evaluated, and 456 with typical adenocarcinoma (AC) were identified as well as 175 with squamous differentiation (AC + SQ). The latter were subdivided into 99 with AA and 69 with AS. Multiple known prognostic factors were compared with differentiation of glandular and squamous component of the tumor. Age, depth of myometrial invasion, architecture, nuclear grade, and combined grade were similar for AC and AC + SQ, although patients with AA were better differentiated than those with AS and had less myometrial invasion. Both glandular and squamous differentiation correlated with frequency of pelvic and para-aortic node metastasis. Nodal metastasis, when it was stratified for grade and depth of invasion, was similar in AC and AC + SQ patients. The differentiation of squamous component is closely correlated with the differentiation of the glandular element, and the glandular element is a better predictor of outcome. It would therefore appear that the previous designation of AA and AS has no added predictive property than differentiation of glandular component and probably should be dropped as a diagnostic term. The authors suggest the term *squamous differentiation* instead, with differentiation of the glandular component noted as the important prognostic factor. Subsequently, Abeler and Kjorstad reviewed 255 cases and made the same recommendations.

Table 5–6 ENDOMETRIAL CARCINOMA SUBTYPES

Type	Number (%)
Endometrioid	6231 (84%)
Adenosquamous	317 (4.2%)
Mucinous	74 (0.9%)
Papillary serous	335 (4.5%)
Clear cell	185 (2.5%)
Squamous cell	28 (0.04%)
Other	285 (3.8%)

From Pecorelli S (ed): FIGO Annual Report, years 1996-98. Int J Gynecol Obstet 83:79-118, 203.

Increasing emphasis has been placed on the importance of the histologic subtype of papillary adenocarcinoma. This subtype represents 1–10% of all adenocarcinomas. Some authors have termed this *papillary serous adenocarcinoma* or serous papillary adenocarcinoma. Papillary carcinomas of the endometrium have been known for many years (Christopherson and associates credited Cullen with an illustration of this entity in 1900). Uterine papillary serous carcinoma (UPSC) is recognized as a distinct, highly aggressive carcinoma of the uterus. Of the two

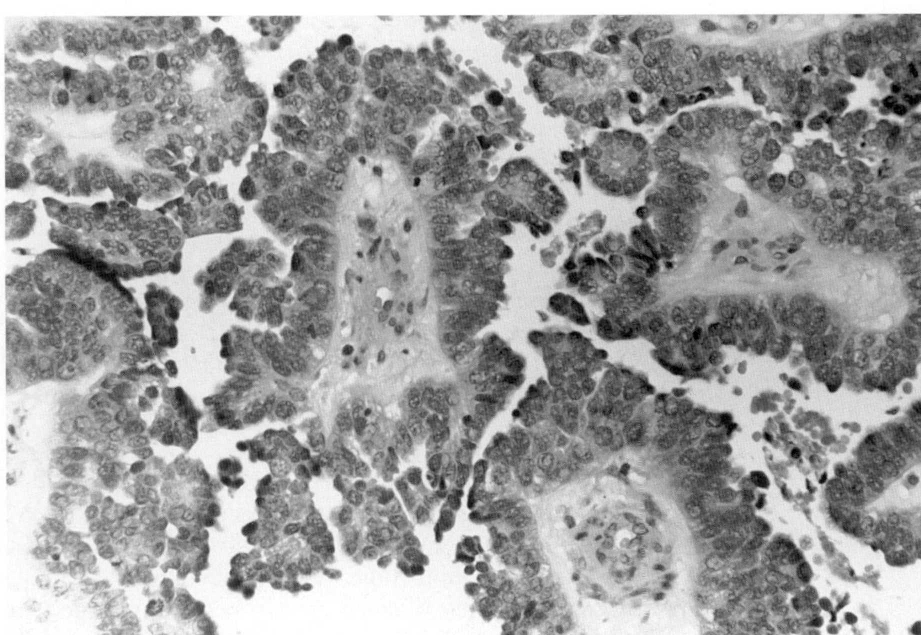

Figure 5–4 Papillary serous adenocarcinoma. Similarity to ovarian carcinoma is apparent. (Courtesy of Gregory Spiegel, MD.)

types of endometrial cancer (one type with features of hyperestrogenism, and a second type unassociated with hyperestrogenism), UPSC falls into the second. These patients tend to be elderly, not obese, and parous; they have high-grade tumor with extensive extrauterine disease and poor survival. Hendrickson, in the early 1980s, noted that in more than 250 endometrial cancers, only 10% had histologic features of UPSC, but these accounted for 50% of all treatment failures. The histopathologic appearance resembles a high-grade serous carcinoma of the ovary that has a propensity for vascular or lymphatic vascular space involvement (LVSI). Well-formed papillae are lined by neoplastic cells with grade 3 cytologic features (Fig. 5–4). Differentiation between papillary architecture and syncytial metaplasia with benign endometrial alterations must be made because the papillary architecture alone does not designate UPSC. The uterus may appear grossly normal but can have extensive myometrial invasion. Most UPSC tumors are aneuploid and have a high S-phase.

Subsequently, many small reports of this entity have appeared in the literature. One of the largest series has been reported by Goff and associates. They identified 50 patients with UPSC, 33 pure UPSC and 17 admixed with other histologic types. Indicative of poor prognostic factors, 36 (72%) had extrauterine disease. Lymph node metastasis was found in 36% with no myometrial invasion, in 50% with less than one half invasion, and in 40% with outer half invasion. Patients with LVSI had 85% incidence of extrauterine disease; however, 58% without LVSI had extrauterine disease. Grade and depth of invasion were not significant predictors of extent of disease. Of particular significance was the fact that 14 patients (28%) had disease limited to the endometrium, yet 36% had lymph node metastasis, 43% had intraperitoneal disease, and 50% had positive peritoneal cytologic findings, essentially equal to the findings in patients with outer half myometrial invasion. In this study, the only significant predictor of extrauterine disease was LVSI. Even if disease is limited to a polyp, 30–50% will have extrauterine disease. With such a poor survival, adjuvant therapy has been applied in hopes of improving survival. Radiation therapy to the pelvis has been unsuccessful because most recurrences are outside the pelvis. Interestingly, Parkash and Carcangiu described six patients treated with radiation therapy for cervical carcinoma who developed UPSC 10 years or more later (mean 16 years). This represented 7.5% of all the UPSC diagnosed at Yale during that time. Although others have also noted this relationship, prior radiation therapy does not appear to be an appreciable contributing factor. Several investigators using systemic therapy for ovarian cancer (because the two entities are histologically similar) have not noted benefits in UPSC similar to those in ovarian cancer. Levenback and colleagues from MD Anderson treated 20 patients with UPSC using cisplatin, doxorubicin, and cyclophosphamide (PAC). This included patients with measurable disease (advanced and recurrent disease) as well as adjuvant therapy. Only 2 of 11 patients with measurable disease had an objective response. Six patients had no extrauterine disease at the time of surgery and survival was better in this group, although no data were given. The 5-year survival for all patients was 23%. In contrast, Rosenberg and associates treated 10 patients with clinical stage I UPSC cancers and 21 patients assigned to clinical stage I, grade 3 with intense therapy of radical hysterectomy, bilateral pelvic lymphadenectomy, adjuvant pelvic radiation, and four courses of cisplatin and epirubicin. None of the patients with UPSC died or relapsed during a median follow-up of 32 months compared with 16 of 30 (53%) historically controlled patients who were treated less intensely ($P = 0.021$). Not all of the intensely treated patients received all planned treatment; in fact, only 53% completed the prescribed protocol. Three

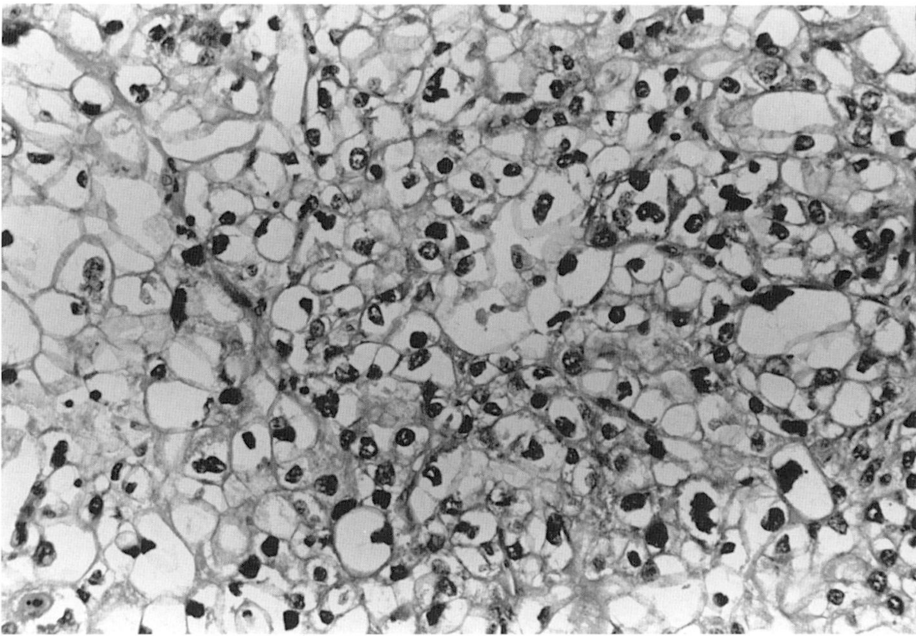

Figure 5–5 Clear cell carcinoma of the endometrium. Clear cell component is quite evident. (Courtesy of Gregory Spiegel, MD.)

patients with UPSC did not receive radiation therapy, suggesting that the chemotherapy may be the most important aspect of the adjuvant therapy. This compared with 11 of 17 (64%) historical control subjects who were treated with radiation and died of their disease. It is hoped that optimal adjuvant therapy for this aggressive subtype of endometrial cancer will be identified in the near future.

Clear cell carcinomas (Fig. 5–5) are also infrequent in number but have distinct histologic criteria. Clear cell tumors are characterized by large polyhedral epithelial cells that may be admixed with typical non-clear cell adenocarcinomas. Some authorities accept the mesonephritic-type hobnail cells as part of this pattern, whereas others believe that this histologic type should be excluded from the clear cell category. Silverberg and DeGiorgi as well as Kurman and Scully suggested a worse prognosis for clear cell adenocarcinoma than for pure adenocarcinoma. This was confirmed in studies by Christopherson and coworkers. Even in stage I disease, only 44% of patients with clear cell carcinomas survive 5 years. Neither the FIGO classification nor nuclear grade correlates with survival. Photopulos and associates, in a review of their material, noted that their patients with this entity were older and tended to have a worse prognosis. They did note that patients with stage I clear cell carcinomas had a 5-year survival similar to that of patients with stage I pure adenocarcinoma of the endometrium.

Creasman and colleagues using the FIGO Annual Report date base identified patients with UPSC and clear cell (CC) carcinoma who were surgically stage I cancers. For comparison, G3 endometrial surgically stage I cancers were reviewed. Of 3996 surgically stage I cancers, there were 148 UPSC, 59 CC (5.2% of all stage I) and 325 G3 (8.1%) cancers. These were more Ia cancers with UPSC and CC then G3. Five-year survival for UPSC and CC was 72% and 81% respectively, compared to 76% for G3 lesions. Postoperative radiation therapy improved survival somewhat (6–8%) but the difference was not significant. The role of chemotherapy was not defined in this study as few patients had this treatment.

So-called secretory adenocarcinoma (Fig. 5–6) is an uncommon type of endometrial cancer. It usually represents well-differentiated carcinoma with progestational changes. It is difficult to differentiate it from secretory endometrium. Survival is good and comparable to that associated with the pure adenocarcinoma. Although it is an interesting histologic variant, the separation of the entity as it relates to treatment and survival is probably not warranted.

Histologic differentiation

The degree of histologic differentiation of endometrial cancer has long been accepted as one of the most sensitive indicators of prognosis (Fig. 5–7). The *Annual Report on the Results of Treatment in Gynecological Cancer* has evaluated survival in regard to grade in patients with clinical stage I adenocarcinoma of the endometrium (Table 5–7). As the tumor loses its differentiation, the chance of survival decreases. In their review of 244 patients with stage I disease, Genest and colleagues noted that patients with grade 1 had a 5-year survival of 96%. This dropped to 79% and 70% for grade 2 and grade 3, respectively. In the GOG pilot study that surgically evaluated 222 clinical stage I endometrial cancers, only 42% were grade 1, and recurrences were only 4% compared with 15% and 41% in grade 2 and grade 3, respectively. Grade of tumor also correlates with other factors of prognosis. Table 5–8 shows the relationship between differentiation of the tumor and depth of myometrial invasion as reported by Creasman from the GOG study of 621 clinical stage I cancers. As the tumor

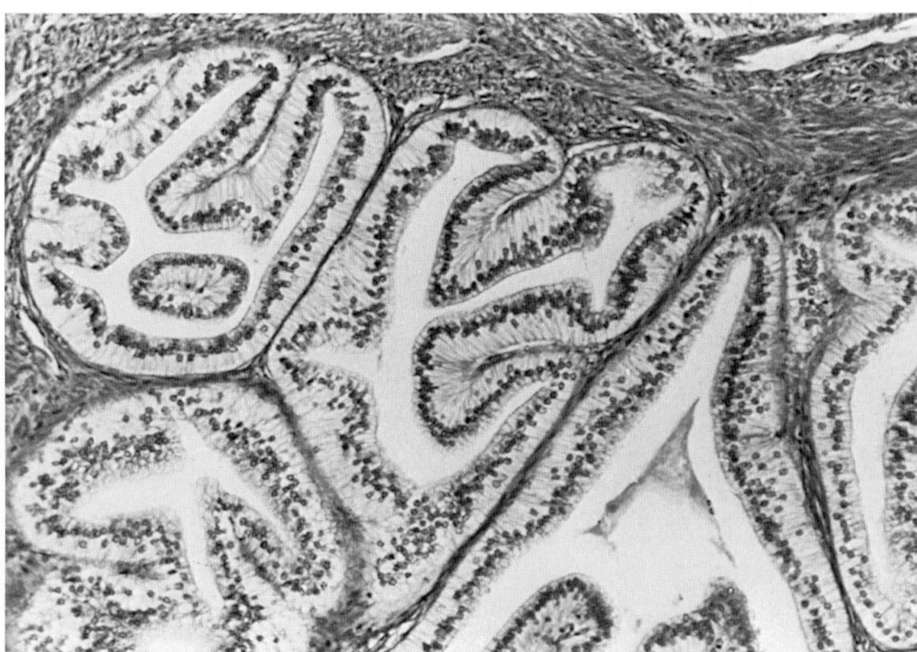

Figure 5–6 High-power view of well-differentiated secretory carcinoma invading inner one-third of the myometrium. (Courtesy of William M. Christopherson, M.D., Louisville, Kentucky.)

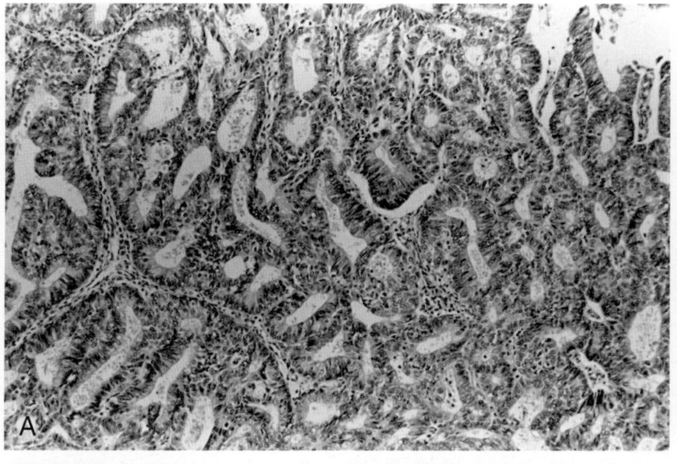

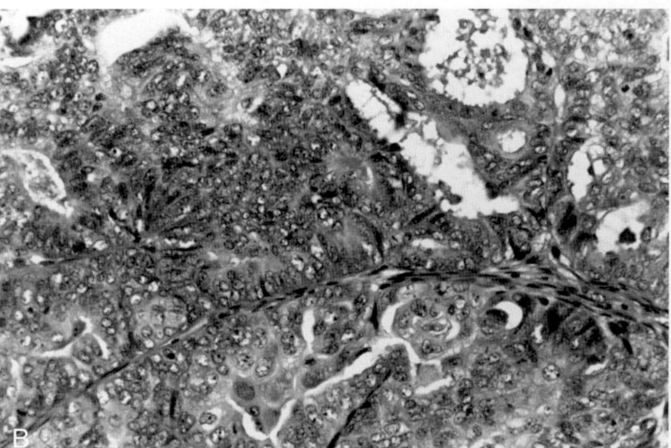

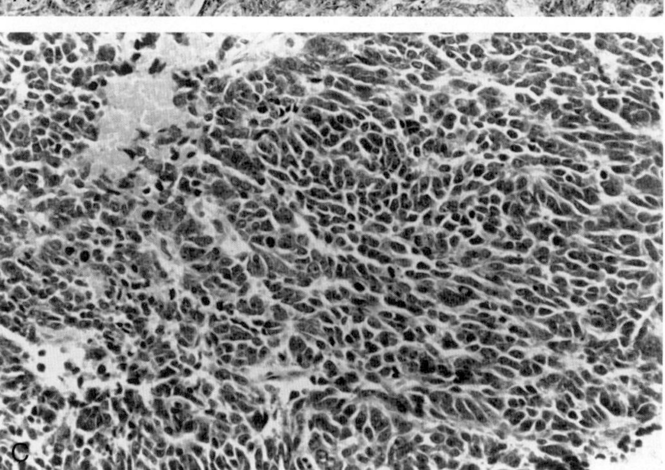

Figure 5–7 Histologic patterns of differentiation in endometrial carcinoma. *A,* Well-differentiated (G1). *B,* Moderately differentiated (G2). *C,* Poorly differentiated (G3). (Courtesy of Gregory Spiegel, M.D.)

becomes less differentiated, the chances of deep myometrial involvement increase. However, exceptions can occur: patients with a well-differentiated lesion can have deep myometrial invasion, whereas patients with a poorly differentiated malignant neoplasm might have only endometrial or superficial myometrial involvement.

Stage of disease

The pretreatment staging of patients with malignant neoplasia is designed to have prognostic value by determining the size and extent of tumor. The survival rate in regard to stage of disease has been consistent, and Table 5–9 and

Table 5–7 RELATIONSHIP BETWEEN TUMOR DIFFERENTIATION AND FIVE-YEAR SURVIVAL RATE, STAGE I (SURGICAL)

Grade	Survival (*n* = 5017)
1	91%
2	90%
3	81%

From Pecorelli S (ed), FIGO Annual Report, years 1996–98, Int J Gynecol Obstet 83:95, 2003.

Table 5–8 CORRELATION OF DIFFERENTIATION AND MYOMETRIAL INVASION IN STAGE I CANCER

	Grade		
Myometrial invasion	**1**	**2**	**3**
None	24%	11%	11%
Superficial	53%	45%	35%
Mid	12%	24%	16%
Deep	10%	20%	42%

Modified from Creasman WT, Morrow CP, Bundy L: Surgical pathological spread patterns of endometrial cancer. Cancer 60:2035, 1987.

Fig. 5–8 show the 5-year survival rate reported by FIGO. Prognosis for women with cervical involvement (stage II) is much worse than prognosis for earlier lesions. Previous endocervical curettage was used to determine whether the patient was in stage II. Many false-positives may occur through the use of this technique. The new surgical staging adopted by FIGO uses the uterine specimen as the final determination of endocervical involvement. A pretreatment endocervical curettage may guide therapy.

Table 5–9 FIVE-YEAR SURVIVAL IN ENDOMETRIAL CANCER: SURGICAL STAGE

Stage	No. of patients	Five-year survival
Ia	1063	91%
Ib	2735	90%
Ic	1219	81%
IIa	364	79%
IIb	426	71%
IIIa	484	60%
IIIb	73	30%
IIIc	293	52%
IVa	47	15%
IVb	160	17%

From Pecorelli S (ed), FIGO Annual Report, years 1996–98, Int J Gynecol Obstet 83:95, 2003.

Location of the tumor within the endometrial cavity could be significant because tumors low in the cavity can be expected to involve the cervix earlier than fundal lesions. It is shown in data from 621 patients assigned to stage I reported from the GOG that those with disease of the lower uterine segment have a higher incidence of pelvic lymph node metastases (16%) than do those with only fundal disease (8%). There is a similar pattern of occurrence of periaortic nodal metastases: a 16% incidence from disease of the lower uterine segment and a 4% incidence when only fundal disease is present.

It appears that the extent of disease within the endocervix is also of importance. Surwit and colleagues noted that the survival rate of patients with stromal invasion of the cervix was much lower at 3 years (47%) than that of patients in whom involvement was limited to the endocervical glands or in whom no stroma was present in the

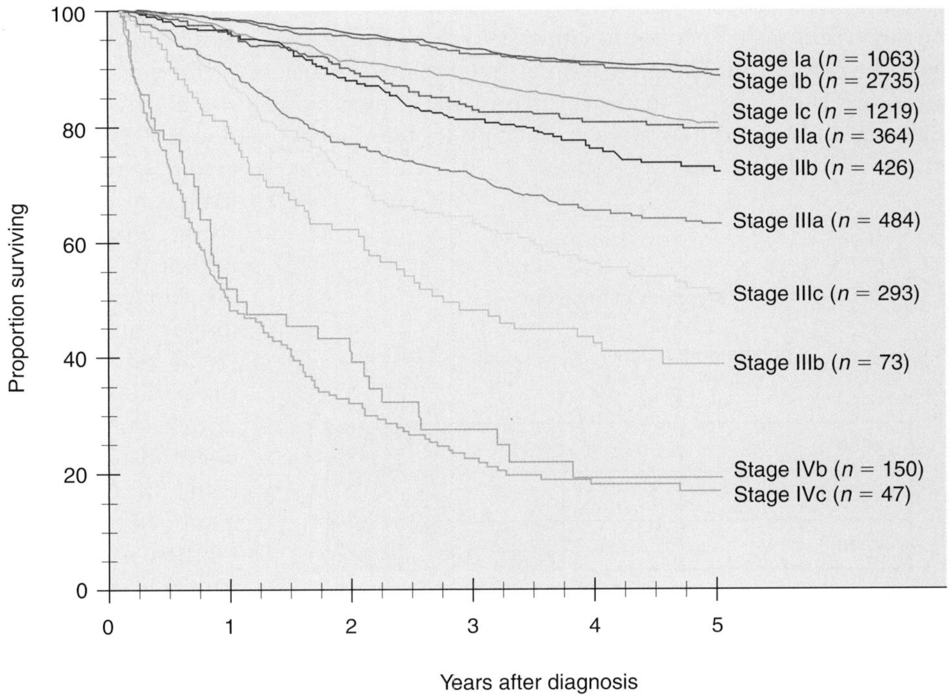

Figure 5–8 Carcinoma of the corpus uteri; patients treated in 1990–1992 (FIGO). Survival by surgical stage (*n* = 5694). (From Pecorelli S (ed), FIGO Annual Report, years 1996–1998, Int J Gynecol Obstet 83:95, 2003. © International Federation of Gynecology and Obstetrics. Reprinted with permission.)

endocervical curettage specimen (74%). The MD Anderson group, however, found no difference in survival of patients with stage II disease when gross cervical involvement was compared with occult disease. They also noted that stromal involvement made no survival difference in patients with occult disease. All these patients had preoperative radiation, and these results may not be a true representation of the disease process. In a GOG review of clinical stage II cancers that were surgically staged, more than three-fourths of patients did not have disease involving the cervix or had extant disease. Of those patients with disease limited to the endocervical glandular tissue, a smaller number had extrauterine disease (39%) compared with those with cervical stromal invasion (50%). Once corrected for true surgical stage II disease, recurrence was similar for stage IIa and stage IIb cancers.

Myometrial invasion

The degree of myometrial invasion is a consistent indicator of tumor virulence (Fig. 5–9). DiSaia and associates noted that recurrences were directly related to depth of myometrial invasion in patients with stage I cancer treated primarily with surgery (Table 5–10). The *Annual Report* of FIGO demonstrated a decrease in the survival rate as myometrial penetration increased (Table 5–11). Lutz and coworkers determined that the depth of myometrial penetration was not as important as the proximity of the invading tumor to the uterine serosa. Patients whose tumors invaded to within 5 mm of the serosa had a 65% 5-year survival rate, whereas patients whose tumors were >10 mm from the serosa had a 97% survival rate.

The depth of myometrial invasion is associated with the other prognostic factors, such as the grade of the tumor. As noted by DiSaia and associates, the survival rate of patients with poorly differentiated lesions and deep myometrial invasion is poor in contrast to that of patients who have well-differentiated lesions but no myometrial invasion. This suggests that virulence of the tumor may vary considerably, and as a result, therapy should depend on the individual prognostic factors.

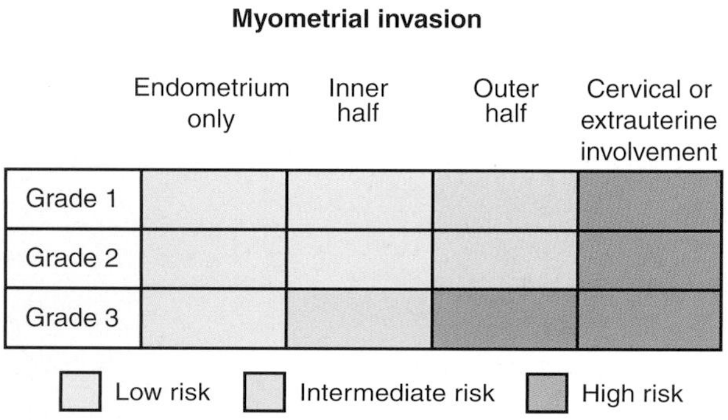

Figure 5–9 Risk assignment based on surgical staging/extent of disease in patients with endometrial cancer.

Table 5–10 RELATIONSHIP BETWEEN DEPTH OF MYOMETRIAL INVASION AND RECURRENCE IN PATIENTS WITH STAGE I ENDOMETRIAL CARCINOMA

Endometrial only	7/92 (8%)
Superficial myometrium	10/80 (13%)
Medium myometrium	2/17 (12%)
Deep myometrium	15/33 (46%)

Modified from DiSaia PJ, Creasman WT, Boronow RC, Blessing JA: Risk factors in recurrent patterns in stage I endometrial carcinoma. Am J Obstet Gynecol 151:1009, 1985.

Table 5–11 RELATIONSHIP BETWEEN DEPTH OF MYOMETRIAL INVASION AND FIVE-YEAR SURVIVAL RATE (STAGE I)

Stage	No. of patients	Five-year survival
IaG1	698	93%
IbG1	1030	88%
IcG1	442	87%
IaG2	229	91%
IbG2	1307	93%
IcG2	485	84%
IaG3	66	75%
IbG3	280	82%
IcG3	247	66%

From Pecorelli S (ed), FIGO Annual Report, years 1996–98, Int J Gynecol Obstet 83:95, 2003.

Peritoneal cytology

The cytologic evaluation of peritoneal fluids, or washings, has been recognized as an important prognostic and staging factor in pelvic malignant neoplasms. Creasman and Rutledge reported positive washings in 12% of patients with corpus cancer, although many of the patients with positive washings did have gross metastatic disease outside the uterus. When 167 patients with clinical stage I carcinoma of the endometrium treated primarily by surgery had cytologic testings of peritoneal washings, 26 (15.5%) had malignant cells identified. Recurrences developed in 10 of these 26 patients (38%), compared with 14 of 141 (9.9%) patients with negative results of cytologic testing. Of the 26 patients with positive cytologic results, 13 (50%) had disease outside the uterus at the time of operation, and 7 (54%) have died of disease. Malignant cells were found in the peritoneal washings of 13 patients, but there was no disease outside the uterus; 6 (46%) patients have died of disseminated intra-abdominal carcinomatosis. In the GOG study of 621 patients, 76 (12%) had malignant cells identified by cytologic examination of peritoneal washings. Of these patients, 25% had positive pelvic nodes, compared with 7% of patients in whom no malignant cells were found in peritoneal cytologic specimens ($P > 0.0001$). It is true that peritoneal cytology, to a certain degree, mimics other known prognostic factors; that is, if peritoneal cytologic specimens are positive, other known poor prognostic factors may also be identified.

Recurrences were evaluated according to known prognostic factors and whether malignant cells were present in peritoneal cytologic specimens. If malignant cells are not present in peritoneal cytologic specimens, the influence of known prognostic factors remains intact. However, when malignant cells are present in peritoneal fluid, this tends to neutralize the good prognostic factors, and cytologic findings become a predominantly important consideration.

A study by Yazigi and colleagues suggested that peritoneal cytology is not of prognostic significance. This study represented a population of patients of two decades earlier, in which the peritoneal cytology was not reviewed (in contrast to the pathology). In the original study, many patients were rejected because the original pathologic process could not be confirmed. Konski and associates also noted no difference in survival regardless of the cytologic findings; however, a significant number of those patients were treated with radiation therapy, which could have affected survival. More recently, Sutton, using multivariate analysis, noted that positive results of peritoneal cytology remained a significant prognostic factor. In a report from the GOG, 25 of 86 (29%) with positive cytologic findings had regional or distant recurrence, compared with 64 of 611 (10.4%) if the cytologic result was negative. In a retrospective study from the MD Anderson Hospital, 28 of 567 (5%) had positive findings of peritoneal cytologic evaluation. A positive cytologic result was associated with significantly reduced progression-free interval. In a multivariate analysis of 477 cases, cytology was significantly associated with survival and progression-free interval. Grimshaw and colleagues noted 24 of 381 patients with positive cytologic findings who had a significantly worse survival rate than those with negative cytologic results. When only patients with surgical stage I were compared, those with negative cytologic results had a better prognosis, but the difference was not statistically significant. Lo and associates described 18 patients assigned to stage I with positive cytologic findings and 127 patients with negative cytologic results. The survival was independent of results of cytologic evaluation when the tumor was confined to the uterus.

The role of peritoneal cytology and its implication in prognosis of endometrial cancer continue to be debated. Those studies that noted no or minimal effect were usually smaller in number than those that noted prognostic significance. Milosevic and colleagues reviewed 17 studies. In 3820 patients, the prevalence of positive cytologic findings was 11%. The three largest studies totaling more than 1700 patients (Haroung and associates, Turner and colleagues, Morrow and coworkers) using multivariate analysis noted that the finding of malignant cells on cytologic examination was independently significantly associated with either recurrence or reduced survival. Pooled odds ratio for the entire series was 4.7 (confidence interval 3.5–6.3) for disease recurrence. All studies note the highest correlation of malignant cytologic specimens with extrauterine disease. It does appear that with multivariate analysis, the presence of malignant cells is an important prognostic factor even when disease is limited to the uterus. Optimal therapy has not been determined to date. The use of intraperitoneal ^{32}P in patients with malignant cytologic specimens appears to be therapeutically efficacious in that patients so treated did much better than patients with positive cytologic specimens but no intraperitoneal therapy (non-randomized evaluation). Soper has reported an update of the Duke experience using ^{32}P in patients with malignant peritoneal cytologic specimens. Sixty-five patients with positive washings were treated, of whom 53 had clinical stage I disease. Disease-free survival beyond 24 months was 89% for patients in clinical stage I and 94% for patients in surgical stage I. Significant acute and chronic complications were unusual, except in combination with external irradiation. This therapy is identical to that used for ovarian cancer described in Chapter 11.

Once the peritoneal cavity is opened, an assessment of the amount of peritoneal fluid in the pelvis is made. If none is present, 100–125 mL of normal saline solution is injected into the pelvis. This can be done easily with a bulb syringe. The saline solution is admixed in the pelvis, withdrawn with the syringe, and sent for cytologic evaluation. Peritoneal cytologic evaluation is performed in all patients undergoing surgery for endometrial cancer.

Lymph node metastasis

Total abdominal hysterectomy (TAH) and bilateral salpingo-oophorectomy (BSO) have been the hallmarks of therapy for endometrial cancer. As a result, the significant incidence of lymph node metastases has been somewhat disregarded (Fig. 5–10). Although contributions to the early and recent literature indicate that a significant number of women with endometrial cancer, even stage I, will develop lymph node disease, these potential metastatic sites have not been routinely included in the treatment plan. In 1973, Morrow and coworkers reviewed the literature and noted that in a collected series of 369 patients with stage I carcinoma of the endometrium, 39 had metastasis to the pelvic lymph node area. In 1976, Creasman and associates described an additional 140 patients, 16 of whom had positive pelvic nodes. These figures have been updated as additional cases have been reported in this study (Table 5–12). In this relatively large group of patients

Table 5–12 INCIDENCE OF PELVIC NODE METASTASES

	POSITIVE NODES/PATIENTS
Stage I	81/843 (9.6%)

From Boronow RC, Morrow CP, Creasman WT et al: Surgical staging in endometrial cancer: Clinical-pathologic findings of a prospective study. Obstet Gynecol 63:825, 1984; and Creasman WT, Morrow CP, Bundy L: Surgical pathological spread patterns of endometrial cancer. Cancer 60:2035, 1987.

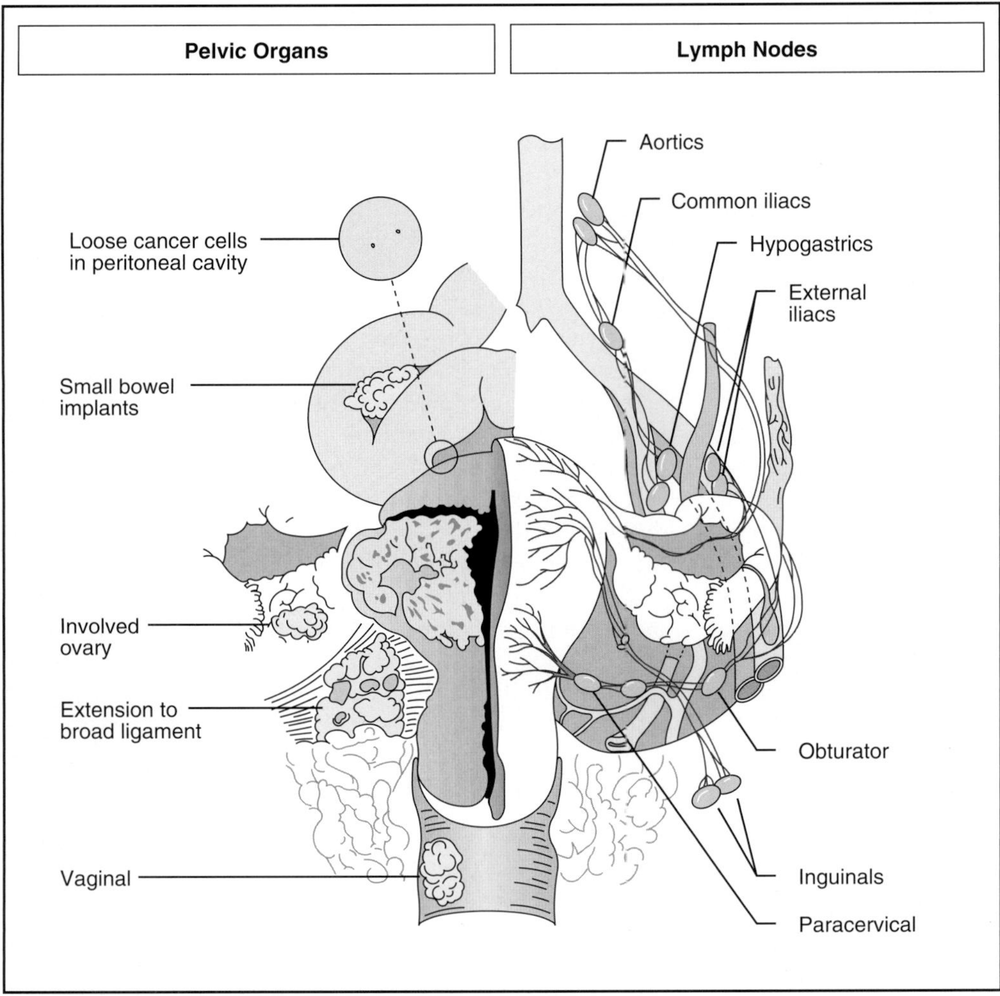

Figure 5–10 Spread pattern of endometrial cancer with particular emphasis on potential lymph node spread. Pelvic and periaortic nodes are at risk, even in stage I disease.

with clinical stage I carcinoma of the endometrium, almost 10% had metastases to the pelvic lymph node area. In the study by Morrow and coworkers, only 31% of those patients with stage I disease and positive pelvic nodes survived 5 years, and most of these had been treated with postoperative irradiation. Potish and colleagues have reported survival of patients with microscopic evidence of lymph node metastases who received irradiation therapy as part of the primary treatment. Patients with surgically confirmed lymphatic spread had a survival of 67% at 5 years. Patients with surgically confirmed periaortic spread with and without pelvic node involvement had a 5-year survival of 47% and 43%, respectively. In the study by Creasman and associates, 102 of the patients also had the periaortic fat pad removed for histologic evaluation, and it was found that 10 of these patients (9.8%) had metastasis to the periaortic area.

Boronow and colleagues, in updating the GOG pilot study, noted that of 222 patients assigned to stage I, 23 (10.4%) had pelvic node metastases. Of 156 patients in whom periaortic nodes were microscopically evaluated, 16 (10.2%) had metastases to this area. DiSaia, in reporting the long-term follow-up of these patients, noted a recurrence in 21 of 199 patients (10.5%) who had negative pelvic nodes, compared with recurrence in 13 of 23 patients (56%) whose pelvic nodes contained metastases. Recurrence with negative periaortic nodes was noted in 15 of 140 patients (11%) versus recurrence in 10 of 17 patients (59%) when periaortic nodes were positive. Creasman, in reporting the GOG data of 621 patients with stage I disease, found that 58 (9%) had positive nodes in the pelvis and 34 had positive nodes in the periaortic area. Of these patients, 11% had metastases to either pelvic nodes or periaortic nodes or to both. The occurrence of lymph node metastases in patients with stage II carcinoma of the endometrium is considerably higher than the occurrence in patients with stage I disease. Morrow and coworkers identified 85 patients in whom the pelvic lymph nodes were evaluated, and 31 (36.5%) had disease in the pelvic nodes. In the GOG study, 148 patients with clinical stage II cancers were surgically evaluated; 66 had cervical involvement. Three (17%) of the patients with only endocervical glandular involvement had pelvic node metastases compared with 35% of those with cervical stromal involvement. None of those with glandular involvement only had aortic node metastases compared with 23% of those with stromal invasion. In patients with stromal involvement, 46% had nodal metastases. The Annual Report of FIGO notes 43, 103, and 121 patients with Stage III (G1, G2, and G3 respectively. Survival (5 years) was 62%, 61% and 47% respectively.

Ben-Shachar and colleagues identified 349 patients who underwent surgical management of endometrial cancer.

Preoperatively, 52% were identified as having grade 1 disease. Surgical staging ± para-aortic lymphadenectomy was performed in 82%. In comparison of pre- and postoperative histology, 19% of patients were upgraded. Lymph node metastasis was noted in 3.9% of patients presenting with grade 1 lesions and 10.5% had extrauterine disease. High-risk features (> half myometrial invasion, grade 3 lesions, high-risk histotypes and/or cervical involvement) were found in 26% of grade 1 patients. Based on full surgical staging, 12% of patients received adjuvant therapy and 17% avoided subsequent therapy.

Since 1988 when FIGO changed endometrial staging from clinical to surgical, there have been questions raised as to whether the lymphadenectomy is only diagnostic, which is an important determinate, or could it also be therapeutic. The initial studies were conducted with selective lymphadenopathy or lymph node sampling. There is an increasing amount of data that suggests a true lymphadenectomy should be performed. Onda and colleagues carried out thorough pelvic and para-aortic lymphadenectomies on 173 patients with Stage I–III endometrial cancer. The average number of lymph nodes removed were 38 pelvic and 29 para-aortic. There were 30 patients (17%) with positive nodes; 10 to pelvis only and 2 para-aortic only and 18 with metastasis to both pelvic and para-aortic nodes. Selected patients received radiation therapy with extended fields and/or combination chemotherapy. In the 10 patients with only pelvic metastasis, 5-year survival was 100% and 75% in those with para-aortic involvement. The authors suggest that although postoperative treatment may attribute to these excellent results, systematic pelvic and para-aortic lymphadenectomy was a contributing factor. Mohan and associates evaluated 159 Stage I patients who had full pelvic lymphadenectomy followed by vaginal brachytherapy. The 15-year overall survival was 92%. Recurrence rate was 4.4%, all at distant sites. In an accompanying editorial by Podratz and associates, they identified four studies including Mohan who had performed thorough lymphadenectomies in moderate and high-risk patients who did not receive postoperative radiation therapy. There were 20 recurrences (6.6%) in 305 patients; only five recurrences were local/regional with four being in the vagina. Those four did not receive postoperative brachytherapy but were salvaged with subsequent radiation.

In a retrospective study from the Mayo clinic, 137 patients at high risk for nodal involvement who underwent para-aortic lymphadenectomy (PAL+) were compared with those who did not (PAL–). The 5-year survival was 85% for PAL+ patients compared to 77% for PAL–patients. In 51 patients with pelvic or para-aortic node metastasis, survival was 77% for PAL+ patients compared to 42% in the PAL–group. Kilgore and associates in evaluating 649 patients noted that those who underwent multiple site lymph node removal had a significantly better survival than those patients who had no lymph nodes removed (Figs. 5–13 and 5–14). Lymph node removal resulted in a better survival than those without lymph node removal plus postoperative radiation. In a small study of 41 with Stage III cancer, Bristow and coworkers noted disease-free survival was much improved if complete respected macroscopic lymphadenectomy was performed compared with patients who had gross residual disease in lymph nodes remaining after surgery (37.5 vs 8.8 months; P = 0.006).

In a study reported by Havrilesky, 91 patients were identified with Stage IIIc disease. There were 39 with microscopic involvement of the lymph nodes (LN) and 52 with grossly enlarged nodes. After surgery, 92% received some type of adjuvant therapy with 85% receiving radiation therapy. Survival (5 years) was 58% in the 39 with microscopic LN, 48% in 41 patients with grossly positive LN completely resected, and only 22% in the 11 with unresected LN. The authors felt that this data suggested a therapeutic benefit for lymphadenectomy.

Adnexal metastases

It is well recognized that endometrial cancer can and frequently does metastasize to the adnexa. Approximately 10% of patients with clinical stage I adenocarcinoma of the endometrium are found to have occult metastasis in the ovary at the time of surgery. In an analysis of 222 patients with clinical stage I carcinoma of the endometrium studied for surgical-pathologic evaluation, 16 (7%) were found to have metastasis in the adnexa. This finding correlated with many but not all of the other prognostic factors. Spread to the adnexa did not seem to be related to the size of the uterus. The grade of the disease did not appear prognostically important in regard to this in that 6% of patients with grade 1 tumors had adnexal disease compared with only 10% if poorly differentiated carcinoma was present. The depth of invasion did appear to be significant, however, in that only 4% of patients with only the endometrium involved had adnexal spread, compared with 24% who had adnexal metastases if deep muscle was involved. If tumor was limited to the fundus of the uterus, only 5% of patients had disease in the adnexa; however, if the lower uterine segment or the endocervix was involved, one-third had spread to the adnexa. Definite correlation was present in regard to adnexal metastasis and metastasis to both the pelvic and periaortic lymph node areas. When metastasis was present in the adnexa, 60% of patients had malignant cells in the peritoneal cytologic fluid, compared with only 11% if the adnexa were not involved. Recurrences appeared in only 14% of these individuals who did not have metastasis to the adnexa, compared with recurrences in 38% of patients with adnexal metastasis. In the report from the GOG, 34 of 621 patients (5%) had metastases to the adnexa. The new surgical staging classifies patients with adnexal metastases as stage IIIa.

Molecular indices

There has been an explosion of research into the molecular makeup of endometrial cancer. Cytogenetic studies have described gross chromosomal alterations including changes in the number of copies of specific chromosome. The extent of abnormalities in a given tumor is relatively low. About 80% have normal diploid DNA content. Aneuploidy in 20% is usually associated with high-grade, extrauterine disease, high-risk histotypes and poor prognosis. So-called loss of heterozygosity occurs at a relatively low frequency in comparison to other solid tumors. When chromosomal loss of heterozygosity does occur, underlying molecular genetic defects have been observed on 17p and 10q which correlates with mutational inactivation of TP53 and PTEN respectively. Individual tumors with a greater number of gains and losses are associated with a poorer prognosis and some changes seen in cancer are also present in atypical hyperplasia but not simple hyperplasia lesions.

Mutational activation or aberrant expression of some oncogenes has been described but to a lesser degree than tumor suppressor genes. RAS gene family is the most commonly identified oncogene aberration in human cancers and is present in 10–30% of endometrial cancers. This mutation appears to occur early in the neoplastic process and the incidence is the same in endometrial hyperplasia. Correlation of RAS mutation to survival has produced conflicting results. About 10–15% of endometrial cancer has overexpression of ERBB-2 (HER2/neu) protein. Overexpression appears to be confined to high-grade or advanced staged tumors.

The FMS oncogene encodes a tryosine kinase, which serves as a receptor for macrophage-colony stimulating factor (m-CSF). Expression of FMS correlates with advanced stage, high- grade, and deep myometrial invasion. Expression of C-MTC which has been observed in normal endometrium and endometriosis has a higher expression in secretory endometrium. Several studies suggest amplification is present in a fraction of endometrial cancers.

Mutation of TP53 tumor suppressor gene, the most common genetic abnormality currently recognized in human cancers, is present in 10–30% of endometrial cancers. Overexpression and/or mutation are associated with prognostic factors. In a study of over 100 endometrial hyperplasia specimens, TP53 mutation was not present. PTEN mutation analysis in endometrial cancer indicates that this gene is somatically inactivated in 30–50% of all tumors, the most frequent molecular genetic alteration defined in endometrial cancer. There does appear to be a correlation between microsatellite instability and PTEN mutation. PTEN mutation is observed in 20% of endometrial hyperplasias suggesting that this is an early event in the development of some type 1 endometrial cancers.

Inherited mutations in gene encoding DNA mismatched repair proteins, primarily MSH2 and MLM1, which are responsible for HNPCC, for which endometrial cancer is the second most common cancer in women with these mutations. Cancers in these individuals are characterized by frameshift mutations in multiple microsatellite repeat sequences throughout the genome. This instability is also seen in 20% of sporadic endometrial cancers. In these sporadic cancers, acquired mutation in mismatched repair genes is rare. Endometrial cancers that exhibit microsatellite instability tend to be type 1 which has a more favorable prognosis. This microsatellite instability is present in some cases of complex hyperplasia associated with endometrial cancer but are not seen in papillary serous cancers.

Type 1 endometrial cancers which are seen in obese and nulliparous women are well-differentiated, superficially invasive cancers with good prognosis and tend to have the following genetic features: diploid, low allelic imbalance, K-RAS, MLH1 methylation and PTEN. In contrast, type 2 with poor prognostic pathologic features have aneuploid, high allelic imbalance, K-RAS, TP53, and HER2/neu changes.

Recently, array-based technology has allowed a more comprehensive characterization of endometrial cancers. It should be noted that these new technologies are in their infancy although multiple papers using these techniques have been reported, many with DNA microassay. The effects of exogenous PTEN expression in endometrial carcinoma cell lines lacking PTEN function has been studied by Matsushima-Nishiu and associates. They observed increased expression in 99 genes and repression of 72 genes, many of which are known to be involved in cell proliferation, differentiation, and apoptosis suggesting the potential power of expression profiling identifying molecular pathways affected by critical cancer-related genes.

Proteomic profiling, which is the study of intact and fragmented proteins and their function, is being evaluated. Newer technologies allow the creating of proteomic fingerprints that reflect in serum what is happening in the end organs. The biochip is playing a major role in this evaluation. As low as a microliter of serum can be evaluated and this technology is very sensitive to low molecular weight protein regions.

The GOG is currently collecting material (tissue, serum, urine) on a large number of endometrial cancer patients to be stored in its tumor bank for in depth research using these newer technologies, which will hopefully allow us to understand the malignant process.

Other factors

Capillary-like space involvement

Hanson and colleagues described 111 patients with stage I endometrial cancer and found capillary-like space (CLS) involvement in 16. This was most frequently found in patients with poorly differentiated tumors with deep invasion. These patients had a 44% recurrence rate, compared with 2% if the CLS was not involved. This was an independently significant prognostic factor. In the GOG study of 621 patients, it was shown that 93 (15%) had CLS involvement. The incidences of pelvic and para-aortic node metastases were 27% and 19%, respectively. This compares with a 7% occurrence of pelvic node metastasis and a 3%

occurrence of para-aortic node metastasis when there is no CLS involvement.

Tumor size

Schink and coworkers evaluated tumor size in 91 patients with stage I disease. The incidence of lymph node metastases in patients with tumor size >2 cm was only 5.7%. If tumor was >2 cm in diameter, there were nodal metastases of 21% and up to 40% if the entire endometrium was involved. Patients with >2 cm lesions and less than half myometrial invasion had no nodal metastasis. Using multivariate analysis, the authors showed that tumor size was an independently significant prognostic factor. Watanabe and associates did not find cancer size was predictive of lymph node metastasis.

Hormone receptors

Using multivariate analysis to analyze hormone receptor status, Creasman and associates noted that in stage I and stage II cancers, progesterone receptor-positive status was a highly significant, independently prognostic factor in endometrial cancer. Without progesterone receptor status in the model and with the evaluation of estrogen receptor status in its stead, estrogen receptor-positive status was an independent prognostic factor but not to the degree of progesterone receptor-positive status.

Correlation of multiple prognostic factors

At the completion of the original GOG study (Creasman and associates, 1976; Boronow and colleagues, 1984; DiSaia and coworkers, 1985) of 222 patients with stage I endometrial cancer who were surgically staged, results were reported and prognostic factors correlated. A subsequent study by the entire GOG of 621 patients with stage I endometrial cancer who were treated primarily with total abdominal hysterectomy, bilateral salpingo-oophorectomy, peritoneal cytologic evaluation, and pelvic and periaortic selected lymphadenectomy has been reported. Data include size of the uterus, histologic features, grade, and depth of uterine muscle invasion, and this information is similar to that in preliminary reports as well as in others. Only 25% of these patients had poorly differentiated cancers; 22% had deep muscle invasion. Fifty eight patients (9%) had pelvic node metastases; 34 (6%) had metastases to the periaortic region. The size of the uterus, grade of tumor, and depth of muscle invasion correlated well with nodal metastasis (Tables 5–13 to 5–15). Of these patients, 35 (5%) had adnexal metastasis unappreciated before exploratory laparotomy. The chance of having disease in the adnexa increased as depth of invasion increased and when the lower uterine segment or endocervix was involved. As expected, there was a greater propensity for lymph node metastasis when disease was present in the lower uterine segment or in the cervix than when disease was limited to the fundus of the uterus. Seventy-six patients (12%) had malignant cells present on cytologic evaluation. Many of these prognostic factors interdigitated in that good prognostic factors occurred together, although it was not unusual to have several poor prognostic factors present in the same patient. When lymph node metastasis was evaluated relative to the six substages of clinical stage I disease, lymph node metastasis became more prevalent with increasing grade of tumor and increasing uterine size (Table 5–16).

Table 5–13 CLINICAL STAGE VERSUS POSITIVE PELVIC AND AORTIC NODES

Stage	Pelvic nodes	Aortic nodes
Ia (*n* = 346)	23 (7%)	11 (3%)
Ib (*n* = 275)	35 (13%)	23 (8%)

Modified from Creasman WT, Morrow CP, Bundy L: Surgical pathological spread patterns of endometrial cancer. Cancer 60:2035, 1987.

Table 5–14 GRADE VERSUS POSITIVE PELVIC AND AORTIC NODES

Grade	Pelvic nodes	Aortic nodes
G1 (*n* = 180)	5 (3%)	3 (2%)
G2 (*n* = 288)	25 (9%)	14 (5%)
G3 (*n* = 153)	28 (18%)	17 (11%)

Modified from Creasman WT, Morrow CP, Bundy L: Surgical pathological spread patterns of endometrial cancer. Cancer 60:2035, 1987.

Table 5–15 MAXIMAL INVASION AND NODE METASTASIS

Maximal invasion	Pelvic nodes	Aortic nodes
Endometrium only (*n* = 87)	1 (1%)	1 (1%)
Superficial muscle (*n* = 279)	15 (5%)	8 (3%)
Intermediate muscle (*n* = 116)	7 (6%)	1 (1%)
Deep muscle (*n* = 139)	35 (25%)	24 (17%)

Modified from Creasman WT, Morrow CP, Bundy L: Surgical pathological spread patterns of endometrial cancer. Cancer 60:2035, 1987.

Table 5–16 CLINICAL STAGE AND GRADE VERSUS PELVIC AND AORTIC NODE METASTASIS

Stage	Pelvic nodes	Aortic nodes
IaG1 (*n* = 101)	2 (2%)	0 (0%)
IaG2 (*n* = 169)	13 (8%)	6 (4%)
IaG3 (*n* = 76)	8 (11%)	5 (7%)
IbG1 (*n* = 79)	3 (4%)	3 (4%)
IbG2 (*n* = 119)	12 (10%)	8 (7%)
IbG3 (*n* = 77)	20 (26%)	12 (16%)

Modified from Creasman WT, Morrow CP, Bundy L: Surgical pathological spread patterns of endometrial cancer. Cancer 60:2035, 1987.

The patients in the GOG pilot study have been followed up for 37 to 72 months after surgery; and because most recurrences appear within the first 2 years after therapy, it can be assumed that the majority of recurrences in this group of patients have already been identified. Sixty eight patients (31%) were treated with surgery only; an additional 97 (44%) received preoperative brachytherapy, all of whom had surgery during the same hospitalization as their brachytherapy application. In at least one of the participating institutions, all patients at the beginning of the study received preoperative brachytherapy but with decreasing frequency as time elapsed; at the completion of the study, it was unusual to place brachytherapy preoperatively. Patients treated with surgery alone had a 9% recurrence; those treated with surgery plus brachytherapy had an 8% recurrence. Only 25% of the patients were thought to have disease significant enough (high risk) to require external irradiation as an individual determination. Patients treated with external irradiation had a 35% (20 of 57) recurrence. Because radiation therapy was given for patients who were thought to be at high risk, it appeared that the designation of high and low risk as determined by recurrence could be adequately determined. Only 25% of the patients in the study were determined to be at high risk, necessitating external irradiation. On the other hand, it was believed that 75% were not in need of radiation therapy, indicating a marked change in protocol as practiced by many institutions. When sites of recurrence were analyzed, only two patients (1%) had an isolated vault recurrence; one patient had been treated with surgery only, and the other had been treated with surgery plus brachytherapy. It appears from this study that the vaginal vault is not at high risk for recurrence, and the role of brachytherapy in endometrial cancer must therefore be questioned. An additional five patients had recurrence identified in the pelvis only. Of 37 recurrences, 27 (73%) were at distant sites outside the treatment field. It appears that local control with therapy was excellent, but attention must be directed in the future to control of distant metastasis.

Recurrences correlated well with other prognostic factors such as grade, depth of invasion, location of tumor within the uterus, adnexal disease, peritoneal cytologic findings, and lymph node metastasis. When recurrences were evaluated to determine whether disease was intrauterine or extrauterine (adnexal disease, positive peritoneal cytologic specimen, lymph node metastasis, or intraperitoneal disease) irrespective of other prognostic factors, only 7% of those with intrauterine disease developed recurrences, compared with 43% if extrauterine disease was present at the time of surgery.

Risk factors in 895 patients with clinical stage I and stage II disease have been reported by the GOG; 789 patients assigned to stage I and 136 patients assigned to stage II were evaluated. In some instances, not all prognostic factors were available for analysis in all patients. In multivariate analysis, those patients with disease limited to the uterus were at increased risk for recurrence if there were deep myometrial invasion, vascular space involvement, or positive washings. Figure 5–9 is the author's attempt to compartmentalize these risk factors into risk categories for predicting prognosis and guiding decisions for adjuvant therapy. The lines between categories are somewhat porous, consistent with most clinical situations.

TREATMENT

Treatment of carcinoma of the uterus, particularly stage I, has evolved considerably during the last three decades. This disease entity actually has a long history of treatment development for the last century (see previous editions for a brief treatment history). With the more general acceptance of surgical staging for this disease, preoperative irradiation has lost favor as standard therapy. Surgical staging allows a more complete identification of the true stage of disease. From surgical staging studies, it has been learned that about one-fourth of patients in clinical stage I have disease outside of the uterus and many patients in clinical stage II do not have disease involving the cervix.

More recently, a considerable amount of data has been collected to evaluate vaginal recurrence and survival rate with surgery alone or combined therapy when mainly preoperative application of brachytherapy and surgery were used. Data have also been evaluated in regard to the grade of the tumor (Table 5–17) and, in some instances, the depth of myometrial involvement (Table 5–18). In patients who had preoperative or postoperative irradiation, there

Table 5–17 SURVIVAL RATE IN STAGE I CARCINOMA OF THE ENDOMETRIUM WITH REGARD TO GRADE AND TREATMENT

	Survival	
Grade	Surgery only	Combined therapy
1	1295/1375 (94%)	2284/2389 (96%)
2	488/510 (96%)	1490/1721 (87%)
3	100/135 (74%)	398/498 (80%)

From Pettersson F (ed): Annual Report on the Results of Treatment in Gynecological Cancer, Vol 21. Stockholm, International Federation of Gynecology and Obstetrics, 1991.

Table 5–18 RECURRENCES IN STAGE I CARCINOMA OF THE ENDOMETRIUM WITH REGARD TO DEPTH OF INVASION AND TREATMENT

Recurrence	Surgery and radium	Surgery and external radiation
Endometrium only	6/88 (7%)	0/4 (0%)
Inner and mid thirds	3/68 (4%)	9/29 (31%)
Outer third	3/9 (33%)	11/24 (46%)

Modified from DiSaia PJ, Creasman WT, Boronow RC, Blessing JA: Risk factors in recurrent patterns in stage I endometrial carcinoma. Am J Obstet Gynecol 151:1009, 1985.

appeared to be a lower incidence of vaginal vault recurrences, although there does not appear to be much difference in the grade 1 and grade 2 lesions. Vaginal vault recurrence did not appear to affect survival. The survival rate of those treated by surgery only was similar to that of those treated by radiation plus surgery, particularly in the grade 1 and grade 2 lesions. Patients with poorly differentiated adenocarcinoma treated with combined therapy had a slightly better survival rate, although most studies showed no statistical difference between these patients and those treated only with surgery.

The role of preoperative irradiation in patients with endometrial carcinoma has been addressed by several authors. In a study from Germany, de Waal and Lochmuller compared patients with stage I or stage II carcinoma of the endometrium treated with preoperative intracavitary radiotherapy with those who received primary operation without radiotherapy. There was no difference in the 5-year survival rate or in the incidence of vaginal, pelvic sidewall, and distant metastases. The authors believed that preoperative radiotherapy did not appear to be of benefit in the management of patients with this malignant neoplasm. Most authorities, even those who are advocates of preoperative irradiation, agree that in stage I, grade 1 lesions, the procedure of choice is total abdominal hysterectomy and bilateral salpingo-oophorectomy alone. If extensive disease is present in the uterus or if metastasis outside the uterus is noted, appropriate irradiation, progestins, and chemotherapy are given. There is no agreement on treatment of patients with grade 2 or grade 3 disease, as noted by the various modalities advocated in the literature. Some authors prefer preoperative application of brachytherapy either by Heyman packing plus vaginal ovoid or by tandem and ovoids if the uterus is small. A total abdominal hysterectomy with bilateral salpingo-oophorectomy is done 6 weeks later. Underwood and colleagues have recommended that the hysterectomy be done immediately after the brachytherapy is removed. If deep myometrial or distant disease is present, external irradiation (4000–5000 cGy to the appropriate areas) is given. Underwood and colleagues have shown that depth of myometrial invasion is best determined by measuring the tumor-free area from serosa inward. If there is <5 mm of tumor-free area, they advocate external irradiation (4000–5000 cGy to the whole pelvis) during the postoperative period because these patients will have a high risk for recurrence. If there is >10 mm of tumor-free area, surgery alone appears adequate. Treatment of patients with 5–10 mm of tumor-free area is unresolved at present, although recurrence appears to take place more often than it does in disease with >10 mm of tumor-free area.

Bond described 1703 patients with stage Ia and stage Ib adenocarcinoma treated with or without vaginal irradiation after hysterectomy. There were fewer vaginal recurrences in those who received postoperative vaginal therapy (0% vs 3.4% in non-invasive lesions, and 4.3% vs 8.3% in invasive tumors). The vagina was the first site of recurrence in only 3.4% of cases, whereas four times as many patients developed pelvic or metastatic disease. Bond thought that postoperative vaginal irradiation was of value to a small percentage of patients but that it did not influence survival rate or the incidence of pelvic or metastatic disease in any histologic group and therefore does not recommend it as a routine measure. Chen, in a small study of 32 patients with stage I disease with deep myometrial or grade 3 lesions, noted that 18 had no extrauterine disease. None of the 18 received postoperative irradiation, and all survived for more than 5 years. Of the 15 with extrauterine disease, all received postoperative therapy, but only four survived. It is his impression that for patients with surgically determined stage I disease, even with poor prognostic factors, surgery alone may be adequate therapy.

Elliott and colleagues from Australia reported on 811 clinical stage I and 116 clinical stage II endometrial cancers treated during a 25-year interval. They have suggested that whole-vagina irradiation postoperatively decreased isolated vaginal recurrence. Forty isolated vaginal recurrences (4.3%) were detected. Unfortunately, during the years, multiple treatments were used (e.g., simple and radical hysterectomy, vault or whole-vagina irradiation, and external irradiation in various combinations). In low-risk patients (clinical stage I, grade 1 and grade 2 tumors confined to the inner third of the myometrium), vault recurrence was 2.5%, 2.5%, and 0% in patients treated with surgery alone, surgery plus vault irradiation, and surgery plus whole-vagina irradiation, respectively. The low-risk group represented 53% of all patients. In multivariate analysis, only total vaginal irradiation was independently protective. Almost 9% of patients treated with the total vaginal irradiation had complications attributable to the radiation therapy (see the section on suggested treatment).

The effectiveness of postoperative external irradiation for nodal metastases has received increased attention with the increasing popularity of surgical staging. Patients with metastases to both para-aortic and pelvic nodes have received external irradiation to the affected area. Potish and colleagues used para-aortic irradiation to treat 48 patients who had clinical or pathologic evidence of metastases to this area. In the surgically confirmed patients, the authors noted a 67% 5-year survival if pelvic nodes alone were involved, 47% if para-aortic nodes alone had metastases, and 43% if both areas were affected. Overall survival for the entire group was 52%, and 88% of the recurrences were outside of the treatment field. Morbidity appeared acceptable. Other authors, including those responsible for the follow-up of the GOG staging studies, have shown similar results. Some patients with metastases to lymph nodes have had long disease-free intervals with surgery only, but most investigators today would probably advocate postoperative radiation therapy in patients with metastases to the lymph nodes although improved survival after thorough lymphadenectomy has not been documented.

Kadar and associates retrospectively evaluated 262 surgically staged endometrial cancers. Multiple risk factors were evaluated. Tumor grade, myometrial invasion, presence of vascular invasion, cervical involvement, FIGO stage, and age of the patient were all independent prognostic factors. In patients with no risk factors or one risk factor, radiation therapy did not affect recurrence or survival. These patients had a 97% 5-year survival. Unfortunately, most patients with three or four risk factors do poorly even with radiation therapy. One wonders if adjuvant therapy has any effect on survival because only a 17% 5-year survival was appreciated, even with five of six patients receiving radiation therapy. In the risk group 2 (two risk factors), 24 of 28 received pelvic irradiation with a suggestion of improved survival although statistical significance was not reached.

To date, there have been three prospective randomized studies evaluating external radiation with or without brachytherapy in women with endometrial cancer. Onsrud, Kolstad and Normann noted no difference in survival rate between the two groups of patients. Patients who received pelvic irradiation had a 5-year survival rate of 88%, whereas those who did not receive external irradiation had a 90% survival rate. When recurrence and survival were evaluated in regard to histologic grade and myometrial involvement, no difference was noted. In patients who received external irradiation, there was less recurrence in the pelvis, but a larger number of patients had distant recurrences. Those who did not receive external irradiation had a higher number of recurrences locally in the pelvis.

In a Dutch study (PORTEC trial) Creutzberg identified 714 patients who had grade 1 lesions with ≥50% myometrial invasion, grade 2 lesions with any amount of invasion and grade 3 with <50% invasion. They were randomized postoperative to receive either external radiation or observation. These patients were not required to have been surgically staged. All histologies were eligible. In the 654 eligible for follow-up, local and regional recurrences were less frequent in the radiation therapy group (4% vs 14%) than in the observational group but 5-year survival was similar, 81% vs 85% respectively.

The GOG performed a phase III trial of surgery with or without adjunctive external pelvic radiation in intermediate risk endometrial adenocarcinomas. These included all women with any degree of myometrial invasion, any grade, and no evidence of lymph node metastasis (Stage Ib, IC, IIA occult and IIB occult). All patients were required to have surgical staging with histologic evaluation of the lymph nodes. A high intermediate risk (HIR) subgroup were defined as 1) G2-3 tumors, presence of lymphovascular invasion and outer one-third myometrial invasion; 2) age 50 or more with any two listed factors; or 3) age ≥70 with any above listed factors. All other eligible patients were considered low intermediate risk. There were 202 who received no radiation (NAT) and 190 who received pelvic radiation (RT). Median follow up was 69 months. There were 15.3% total recurrences in the NAT group compared to 6–8% in the R% (P = 0.007). Local recurrences were 8.9% vs. 1.6% respectively. The overall survival at 48 months was 86% for NAT and 92% for RT with intercurrent diseases accounting for half or more of the deaths in both groups. Deaths due to disease were 8.4% vs 7.9% in the NRT vs RT group. Grade 3 and 4 toxicity by treatment was 4.9% vs 14% in the NRT and RT groups respectively. In 12 of the 13 women who had isolated vaginal recurrences, the NAT arm were treated with radiation and 5 have died of disease.

In the group-wide GOG study, 6% of patients with clinical stage I disease were noted to have intraperitoneal disease. Chen suggests that omental biopsies as a routine procedure should be accomplished as part of the operative procedure. In 84 patients with clinical stage I cancers, 7 (8.3%) had omental metastasis and 5 were identified only microscopically. Omental metastasis was identified with other risk factors, most notably papillary serous carcinoma. Particularly in high-risk patients, omental biopsies appear to be warranted. Several studies note the role of vaginal hysterectomy in highly selected patients with endometrial cancer. These are usually obese and high-risk surgical patients. Survival rates are comparable to those of the abdominal approach. Lellé and associates identified 60 patients from two institutions during almost 30 years who were treated with vaginal hysterectomy. The 5-year survival was >90%. Two-thirds of patients had grade 1 tumors and 41% had no myometrial invasion. In fact, significant numbers of patients who were being operated on for hyperplasia or cancer were not diagnosed preoperatively. These factors are the common theme in essentially all studies in which vaginal hysterectomy was the surgical therapy.

Suggested treatment

Surgical staging has now been accepted as standard therapy in patients with endometrial cancer unless clinical conditions suggest otherwise. Of the 6260 patients with endometrial cancer reported to the last Annual Report of FIGO, 94% were surgically staged. It is appreciated that those institutions reporting to the Annual Report are academic ones and that most endometrial cancers, at least in the US, have their primary surgery not at academic hospitals. Since endometrial cancer staging has been determined by surgical staging, it has been suggested by some that these are patients who are at low risk (i.e. grade 1) for lymph node metastasis and lymphadenectomy is not worthwhile. There is increasing data that would suggest that even in grade 1, as noted on endometrial biopsy, a significant number of patients have on full surgical staging, findings that would impact on further therapy. Ben-Shacker and colleagues in evaluating 181 grade 1 endometrial cancers found 19% had grade change on hysterectomy specimen, 10.5% had extrauterine disease, 3.9% had lymph node metastasis, and 26% on final evaluation had high risk intrauterine factors. Importantly, the authors felt because of full surgical staging that 12% needed and received adjuvant therapy and 17% who may have received postoperative treatment did not, based on full surgical findings. Geisler and associates found in 349 patients that of those with grade 1 lesions, 15.9% had positive nodes and 2.6%

Table 5–19 RADIATION IN EARLY STAGE CARCINOMA OF THE ENDOMETRIUM

	Local recurrence	Survival
Aalder		
Surgery + Ra (n = 277)	6.9%[†]	91%
Surgery Ra + RT (n = 263)	1.9%[†]	89%
Creutzberg (PORTEC)		
Surgery (n = 300)	14%*	85%
Surgery + RT (n = 354)	4%*	81%
Keyes (GOG)		
Surgery (n = 202)	3.9%	86%
Surgery + RT (n = 190)	1.6%	92%

RT, radiation therapy
[†] $P < 0.01$
*$P < 0.001$

had positive para-aortic nodes only. Of all positive nodes, 31% occurred in grade 1 lesions. As a result of these as well as other studies, many feel that all endometrial cancer patients should have the benefit of full surgical staging, which includes peritoneal cytology, bilateral pelvic and para-aortic lymphadenectomy as well as total abdominal hysterectomy and bilateral salpingo-oophorectomy. Obviously, complete evaluation of the entire peritoneal cavity and its contents should be performed and any suspicious areas pathologically evaluated (Table 5–19).

Straughn and associates reported on a large number of patients who where surgically staged. Low-risk factors, stage IaG1 and 2 were present in 103 patients. None received postoperative therapy and none had recurred. Intermediate risk was defined as Stage IaG3 and all Stage Ib and Ic cancers. There were 440 patients of which 93% received no further therapy. Twenty-eight patients received postoperative therapy and one (4%) recurred compared with 5% of those not radiated. The latter patients received therapy at time of recurrence and 62% were successful. The Annual Report (2003) noted 5-year survival with surgery only of 93%, 91%, 73%, 79% and 73% respectively for stages Ia, b, c and IIa and b. This compares with 89%, 91%, 83%, 83%, and 75% respectively if surgery plus postoperative radiation is used. There is a suggestion that in Stage Ic survival is somewhat better when postoperative radiation is added than surgery alone. What factors went into decision-making re postoperative therapy is unknown. In a multi-institutional study, 220 surgically staged Ic patients were identified. High-risk histotypes were excluded. Adjuvant radiation was used in 99 (45%), 56 brachytherapy only, 19 whole-pelvis radiation, and 24 received both. Overall survival between those treated with surgery and surgery plus radiation was similar (92% vs 90%).

The role of therapy after surgery is dependent on surgical findings. As noted above, when disease is limited to the uterus, the role of postoperative radiation is questionable. All the studies suggest postoperative radiation does decrease local recurrences but not overall survival. Recurrences in the non-radiated are salvaged in about two-thirds of the time. With overall survival in some studies at 98%, it appears radiation may have very limited role as part of primary treatment (Fig. 5–11). When the cervix is involved but otherwise disease is limited to the uterus, data from the Annual Report suggests radiation does not appear to be a significant benefit.

When there is extrauterine disease (metastases to the adnexa and lymph nodes, intraperitoneally, or malignant cells in peritoneal cytologic specimens), the recurrence rate is high. Forty eight of our patients had extrauterine disease, and 21 (43%) have had recurrences, 18 at distant sites. The necessity of developing adjunctive modalities to manage these metastases is apparent. It does appear that when disease is present in the pelvic or periaortic lymph nodes, postoperative radiation therapy to these areas can be reasonably effective because 40% of patients with nodal disease were tumor free at the time of the analysis. Do all patients with metastasis to lymph nodes need radiation? There is data to suggest lymphadenectomy can be therapeutic, particularly if node disease is limited. A recent study by the GOG noted a better response when chemotherapy was used compared to radiation therapy in patients with advanced disease.

The hysterectomy should be extrafascial, and removal of the upper vagina does not appear to decrease vault recurrences (Fig. 5–12). Peritoneal cytologic specimens should be obtained immediately after opening of the peritoneal cavity. If ascites is present, appropriate samples of fluid should be sent for cytologic evaluation. When lymphadenectomy is done, the retroperitoneal spaces in the pelvis are opened in routine fashion. The vessels are outlined, and the lymph node-bearing tissue along the external iliacs from the bifurcation to the inguinal ligament is removed. The obturator fossa anterior to the obturator nerve is cleaned of lymphoid tissue. Lymph nodes along the common iliacs are also removed. No attempt to dissect lymphatic vessels behind or between the major vessels is made. The objective is to remove primarily the pelvic lymph nodes themselves. The periaortic nodes are approached by retracting the small intestine into the upper abdomen and incising the peritoneum over the upper common iliac artery and lower aorta. The main vessels are outlined, and the ureter is retracted laterally. The tissue overlying the vena cava and the aorta is removed en bloc, beginning at the bifurcation of the aorta and extending caudad. The upper limit of the dissection (unless enlarged nodes are noted above this area) is usually the second and third portion of the duodenum as it crosses the main vessels retroperitoneally. Hemostasis can usually be accomplished with hemoclips. Using this technique, one should have a total of 20–30 pelvic and periaortic lymph nodes available for histologic evaluation.

Patients with stage II carcinoma of the endometrium, because of extension of disease into the endocervix, will have a greater propensity for lymph node metastasis. Therapy should encompass likely metastatic sites and can be performed in several fashions. Primary surgery in the form of radical hysterectomy and pelvic lymphadenectomy

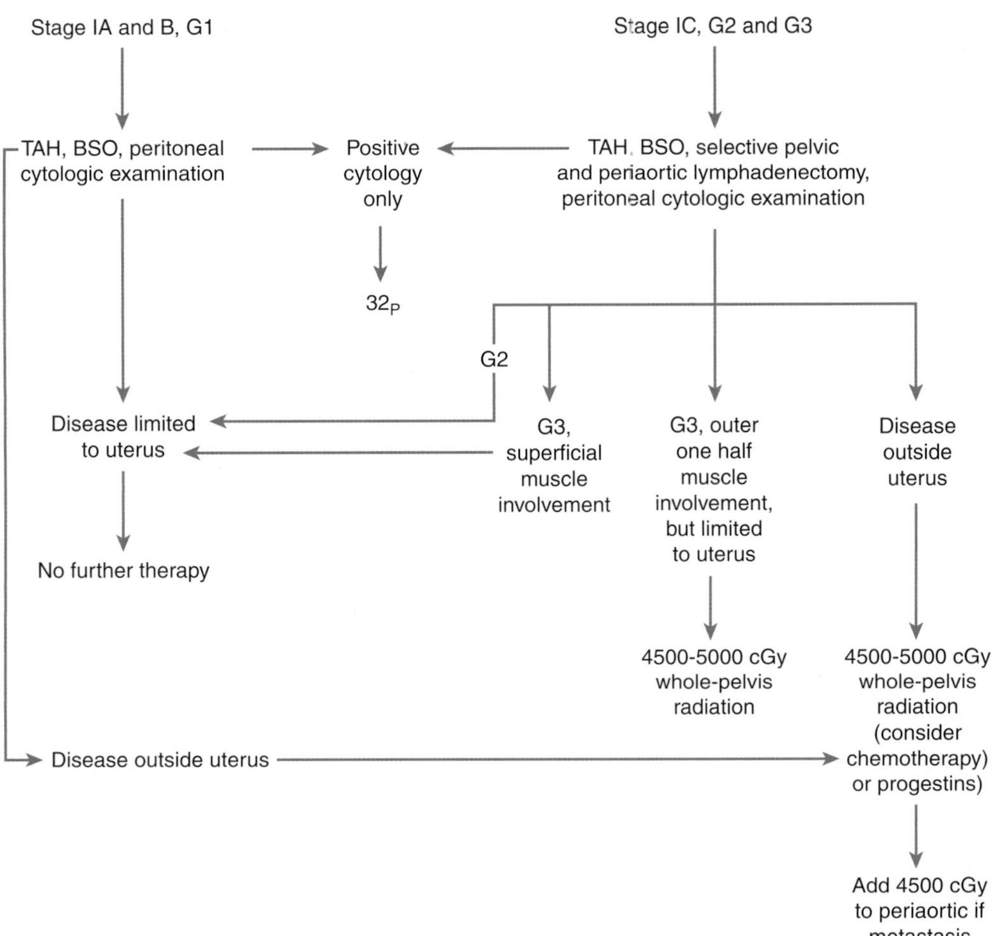

Figure 5–11 Primary surgical management of endometrial cancer. TAH, total abdominal hysterectomy; BSO, bilateral salpingo-oophorectomy.

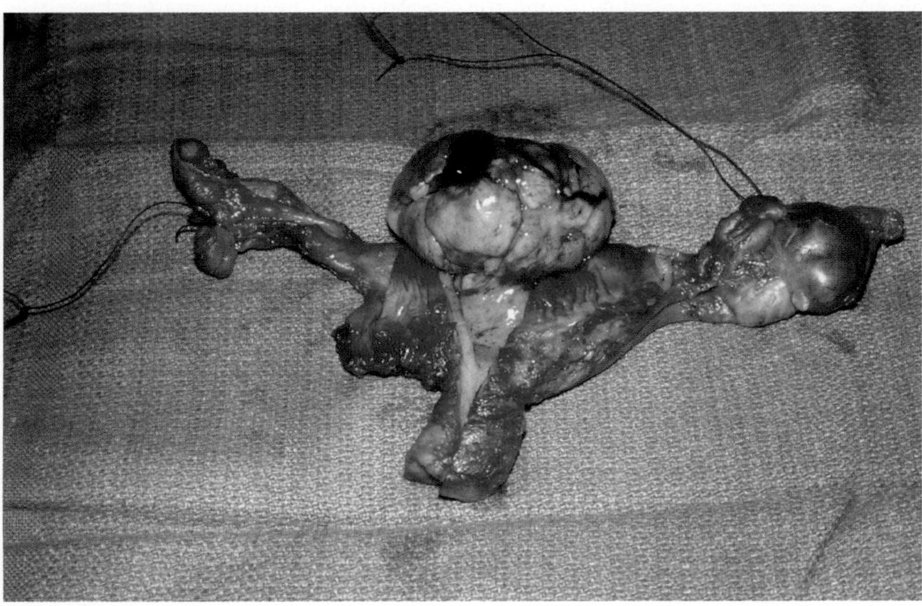

Figure 5–12 Total abdominal hysterectomy (TAH) and bilateral salpingo-oophorectomy (BSO) showing large polypoid adenocarcinoma of the endometrium with deep myometrial invasion.

has been acceptable therapy in the past, but it appears that simple hysterectomy, bilateral salpingo-oophorectomy, and pelvic and para-aortic lymphadenectomy would be adequate surgery in most cases when the amount of cervical involvement is limited. Postoperative radiation therapy can be planned, depending on surgical-pathologic findings. If disease is limited to the uterus, postoperative irradiation may not be necessary (Table 5–20).

The role of adjunctive chemotherapy in addition to surgery and radiation therapy has been addressed by the

Table 5–20 RECURRENCES IN SURGICAL STAGES I AND II IN PATIENTS TREATED WITH SURGERY ALONE OR SURGERY PLUS RADIATION (VAULT IMPLANT OR EXTERNAL)

	Surgery only	Combined therapy
Negative risk factors	13/200 (6.5%)	17/190 (8.9%)
Positive risk factors*	31/78 (39.7%)	76/118 (64.4%)

*Positive risk factors include disease outside the uterus (adnexa, lymph nodes, intraperitoneal, positive cytologic specimen), isthmus-cervix involvement, and capillary space involvement.
Based on data from Morrow CP, Bundy BN, Kurman RJ et al: Relationship between surgical pathological risk factors and outcome in clinical stage I and II carcinoma of the endometrium. Gynecol Oncol 40:55, 1991.

GOG in patients with high-risk stage I and occult stage II endometrial cancers. One hundred and eighty-one patients were treated with total abdominal hysterectomy and bilateral salpingo-oophorectomy, peritoneal cytologic evaluation, and selective pelvic and periaortic lymphadenectomy, followed by external irradiation (pelvic, with or without periaortic) and were then randomized to receive doxorubicin 60 mg/m^2 every 3 weeks for eight doses. Patients participating in the doxorubicin arm of the protocol had a higher incidence of metastases to pelvic nodes (20% vs 10%) than did those in the non-doxorubicin arm; otherwise, the risk factors were equal between the two groups. There were recurrences in 22 of 92 (23%) in the doxorubicin arm vs recurrences in 23 of 89 (26%) in the non-doxorubicin arm. Of those patients with recurrence, those who received doxorubicin had a greater chance of metastasis to the abdomen than did those not receiving it (40% vs 17%). However, distant metastases occurred more frequently without the use of doxorubicin than with it (56% vs 18%).

Patients with occult stage II disease are managed surgically, as are those with stage I, grade 2 and grade 3 disease. It is well recognized that patients with endocervical involvement have a higher risk for extrauterine disease than do those who have disease limited to the fundus. Some patients with endocervical involvement do not exhibit other poor prognostic factors. Data from the surgical-pathologic study might suggest that if only endocervical disease is found, patients do well with surgery alone. It appears, however, that once the surgery has been done, postoperative radiation therapy can be given if necessary, and studies have indicated that given in this sequence, it is just as effective as if it is given preoperatively. To proceed with surgery initially would have an added benefit of making absolutely sure that there is disease in the endocervix. It is not uncommon to designate a patient as having a stage II lesion on the basis of a fractional curettage specimen and then to find no involvement on pathologic review because tumor cells are present as "floaters." Onsrud and colleagues, from the Norwegian Radium Hospital, have addressed this problem, and they verified in a retrospective review that only 96 of 174 cases (56%) originally recorded as stage II endometrial cancer in fact were stage II. Patients who were "overdiagnosed" had a survival rate similar to that of patients with stage I disease. It is interesting that in patients who truly had stage II disease, on histologic evaluation of the uterine specimen in this prospective clinical study, survival was not improved with the use of postoperative external irradiation above that of patients who had no external irradiation. An evaluation of 140 patients with clinical stage II cancers noted that only 35 (24%) in fact had surgical stage II disease. Knowing the exact extent of disease appears to have a major impact not only on adjuvant therapy but also on survival (prognosis).

There is no question that surgical staging can more accurately identify the true extent of disease. In clinical stage I disease, about one-fourth of patients will have disease outside of the uterus; in patients thought to have stage II disease, as many as 75% will have either less than stage II or extrauterine disease. Implications in regard to therapy are great—not only in preventing unnecessary treatment but also in directing more appropriate therapy (i.e., to known nodal disease). The question of possible increased morbidity has been addressed. It is suggested that there may be a significant increased complication rate with more extensive surgical staging. Moore and associates and Larson and colleagues have addressed morbidity from lymphadenectomy and noted no increased complications compared with the patients not undergoing lymphadenectomy. Fanning and Firestein described 80 patients who were evaluated for operative time blood loss and morbidity of the lymphadenectomy. Median number of lymph nodes resected was 21 pelvic and 7 aortic. The median time of lymphadenectomy was 24 minutes, and median blood loss was 25mL. Morbidity was low and attributed primarily to the total abdominal hysterectomy and bilateral salpingo-oophorectomy.

Childers and others have advocated laparoscopic lymph node removal in conjunction with vaginal hysterectomy and bilateral salpingo-oophorectomy. In the hands of those who have acquired these surgical skills, the outcomes appear comparable and some advantages are gained, such as short hospitalization and rapid postoperative recovery. A large GOG study comparing laparoscopic approach vs laparotomy is nearing completion.

The question that has been asked since surgical staging has been proposed is whether survival may be affected. The implication of knowing the true extent of disease suggests that survival may certainly be affected in individual situations. Kilgore and colleagues in Alabama have published data suggesting that not only is lymphadenectomy therapeutic but survival appears to be improved. They evaluated 649 patients with endometrial cancers; 212 had multiple-site pelvic node sampling, 205 had limited-site pelvic node sampling, and 208 did not have nodes removed. Patients undergoing multiple-site lymphadenectomy had a significantly better survival than did those patients not undergoing lymphadenectomy ($P = 0.0002$). Low-risk patients (disease confined to the uterus) with lymphadenectomy had better survival than did those without lymphadenectomy ($P = 0.026$). High-risk patients (disease in cervix, adnexa, uterine serosa, or washings) who underwent lymphadenectomy also had a better survival than did those without lymphadenectomy ($P = 0.0006$) (Fig. 5–13). Even when subsets were evaluated, the therapeutic benefits of the lymphadenectomy were apparent. Patients in both low-risk and high-risk categories who had lymphadenectomies and no postoperative irradiation had a survival better than that of similar patients without lymphadenectomy but who received radiation therapy (Fig. 5–14). Certainly, the therapeutic benefit of the lymphadenectomy is apparent. They also noted that the extent of the lymphadenectomy was related to the number of metastatic lymph nodes identified.

Chung noted that retroperitoneal recurrence in endometrial cancer was related to status of lymphadenectomy at time of primary surgery. If nodes were positive at primary surgery, retroperitoneal recurrence was not unusual; no recurrences were noted in retroperitoneum if both pelvic and para-aortic nodes were negative at initial surgery. In multivariate analysis, only the presence of retroperitoneal nodal metastasis was significant for survival analysis.

Advanced disease presents an additional dilemma. With disease outside the uterus, therapy becomes limited with results less favorable. Behbakht and colleagues evaluated prognostic factors in 137 patients with advanced disease (stage III and stage IV). Multivariate analysis noted age, parametrial involvement, and abdominal metastasis as significant prognostic indicators. An increased frequency

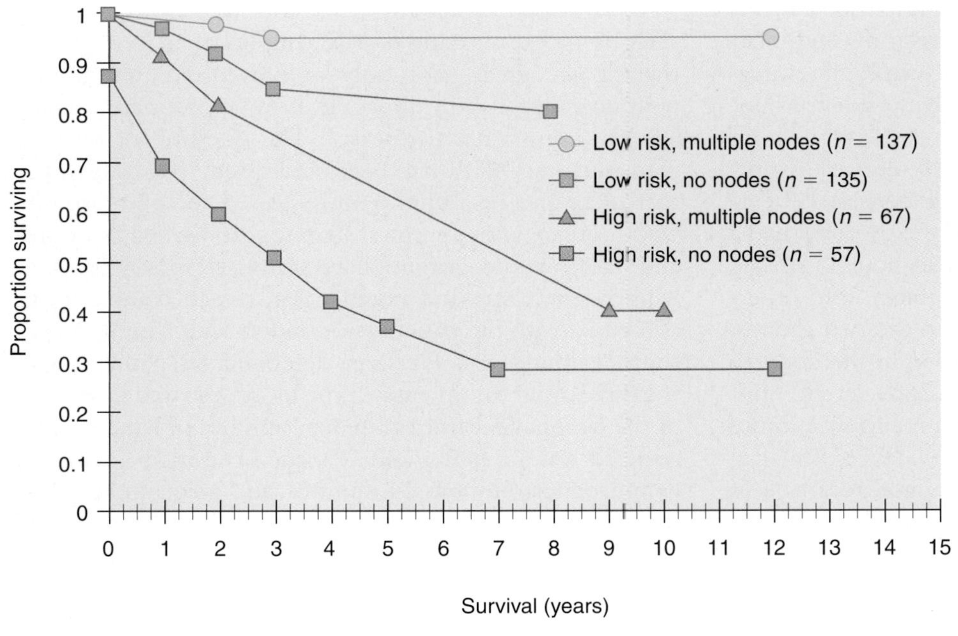

Figure 5–13 Survival by nodes sampled and risk groups: multiple-site pelvic node sampling vs no nodes. Low-risk group, $P = 0.026$; high-risk group, P = 0.0006. (From: Kilgore LC, Partridge EE, Alvarez RD et al: Adenocarcinoma of the endometrium: Survival comparison of patients with and without pelvic node sampling. Gynecol Oncol 56:29, 1995.)

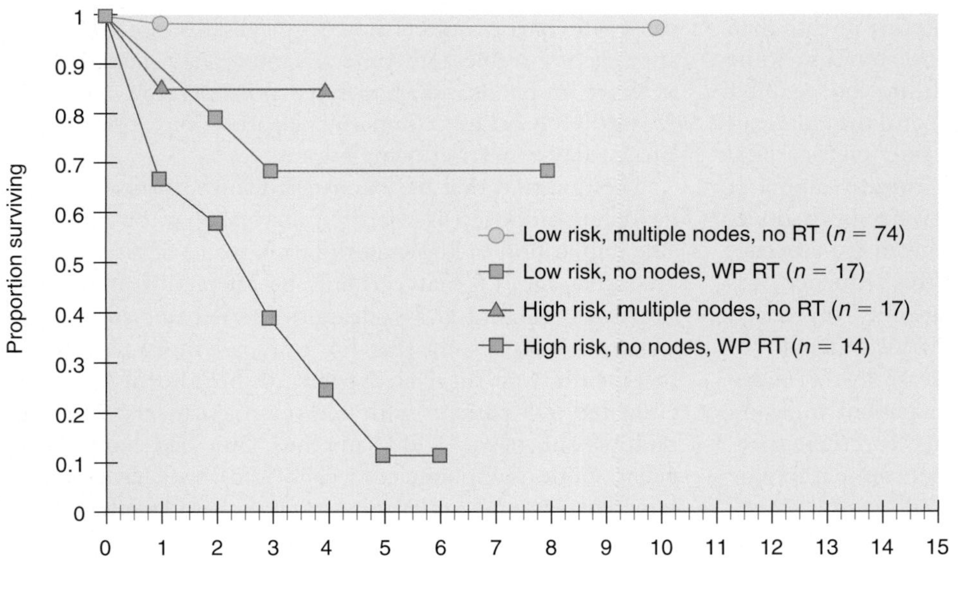

Figure 5–14 Survival comparisons of multiple-site pelvic node sampling to whole pelvic radiation therapy: Multiple nodes without RT vs no nodes plus whole pelvic RT. Low-risk, $P = 0.003$; high-risk, $P = 0.041$. (WP, whole pelvic; RT, radiation therapy.) (From: Kilgore LC, Partridge EE, Alvarez RD et al: Adenocarcinoma of the endometrium: Survival comparison of patients with and without pelvic node sampling. Gynecol Oncol 56:29, 1995.)

of advanced stage was also noted with papillary serous histology. Unfortunately, multiple therapies were used and conclusions concerning treatment cannot be made. Kadar and associates evaluated 58 patients with surgical stage III and stage IV disease. Extrapelvic peritoneal metastasis and positive peritoneal cytologic findings affected survival. If either of these factors was present, 2-year survival was only 25% compared with 83% if they were not present. Postoperative therapy varied, but it did not appear to have any effect on survival.

Several chemotherapy combinations have been used in recurrent or advanced endometrial cancer. The GOG, in a randomized trial, compared doxorubicin with or without cisplatin. The combination experienced a 66% objective response vs 35% for the single agent with a median progression-free interval of 6.2 and 3.9 months, respectively. The GOG reported a 45% response rate (22% complete response) for the combination of doxorubicin and cisplatin in advanced or recurrent endometrial cancer compared to 17% response for doxorubicin alone. The European Organization for Research and Treatment of Cancer Gynecological Cancer Cooperative Group (EORTC-GCCG) compared doxorubicin alone with doxorubicin and cisplatin. Response rate was 17% and 57% respectively. The GOG has compared doxorubicin and cisplatin to doxorubicin and paclitaxel (24 hour infusion) with filgrastim in advanced/recurrent endometrial cancer. There were 317 patients randomized to the two regimens. Response rates were similar (40% versus 43%). PFS (median 7.2 vs 6 months) and overall survival (median 12.6 vs 13.6 months) respectively. Toxicities were also similar. A phase III study by the GOG compared doxorubicin plus cisplatin with or without paclitaxel plus filgrastim in advanced endometrial cancer. There were 273 women registered and objective response (57% vs 34%, $P < 0.01$); PFS (median 8.3 vs. 5.3 months, $P < 0.01$) and overall survival (median 15.3 vs. 12.3 months, $P = 0.037$) were improved with the triple combination. Peripheral neuropathy was worse in the triple regimen.

The GOG studied patients with stage III, IV endometrial cancer with less than 2 cm residual disease (distant metastases were excluded). After surgery, they were randomized to receive doxorubicin and cisplatin every 3 weeks for 8 courses or whole abdominal radiation with 3000 cGy to the whole abdomen. A boost to the pelvic and para-aortic lymph node region (1500 cGy) could be given for positive nodes. Two years after therapy, overall survival was improved by 11% and cancer-free survival was improved by 13% with chemotherapy compared to those treated with radiation therapy. Side effects were more common in the chemotherapy treated patients.

Treatment of patients with stage III or stage IV disease must be individualized; however, in most cases, hormone treatment or chemotherapy, or both, must be used in addition to surgery and radiation therapy.

Data suggests that preoperative elevation of CA-125 dose predicts extrauterine disease. A level of > 20u/ml may be a better upper limit of normal in endometrial cancer.

The role of vaginal hysterectomy in grade 1 endometrial carcinoma has been of interest at some centers. Massi and coworkers described 180 such patients with a 90% 5-year survival rate. They proposed its use for obese and poor surgical risk patients. This seems reasonable when the surgical expertise does not exist for what can be a difficult surgical procedure and complete surgical staging is risky.

RECURRENCE

Even though the number of deaths caused by endometrial carcinoma is lower than the number associated with malignant neoplasms of the cervix and the ovary, the mortality is still significant, particularly in view of the number of patients with carcinoma of the uterus seen initially with stage I disease. Some recurrences, especially those in the vaginal vault, can be treated successfully with surgery, radiation therapy, or a combination of the two. Many patients do extremely well and are long-term survivors. Unfortunately, many of the recurrences are seen outside the confines of the upper vagina and therefore are not amenable to surgery or radiation therapy. Radiation therapy may be of limited value in other patients, particularly if it has been used as part of primary therapy. Therefore, hormone treatment or chemotherapy may be the treatment of choice in many patients with recurrent carcinoma of the endometrium.

Progestins have been evaluated as adjunctive therapy in the hope of preventing recurrences. Lewis and coworkers, in a randomized study, treated endometrial cancer patients postoperatively with medroxyprogesterone acetate (MPA) or placebo. The 4-year survival was similar in the two groups. Kauppila and associates, in describing more than 1100 patients who received adjunctive progestin therapy for 2 years after surgery and radiation therapy, found that even in stage I low-grade tumors, recurrences did appear; it was their belief that prophylactic progestins were not of benefit to these patients. In a prospective study of 363 patients with stage I disease who received adjuvant MPA for 12 months, DePalo and colleagues compared survival with that of 383 patients with stage I disease who did not receive MPA postoperatively; there was no difference in survival between the two groups. In a British study in which 429 patients with stage I or stage II cancers were randomized between postoperative MPA and observation, no difference in survival was seen after 5 years.

Progestins have been used for more than 30 years, and the objective responsiveness of recurrent carcinoma of the endometrium to these hormones has been substantiated (Fig. 5–15). Historically, approximately one-third of all patients with recurrent carcinoma of the endometrium are said to respond to the hormone, although patients with well-differentiated tumors have a response rate much higher than that of patients with moderately or poorly-differentiated lesions. The GOG described 420 patients with advanced or recurrent endometrial carcinoma treated with MPA 50 mg three times a day. Of the 219 patients with objective

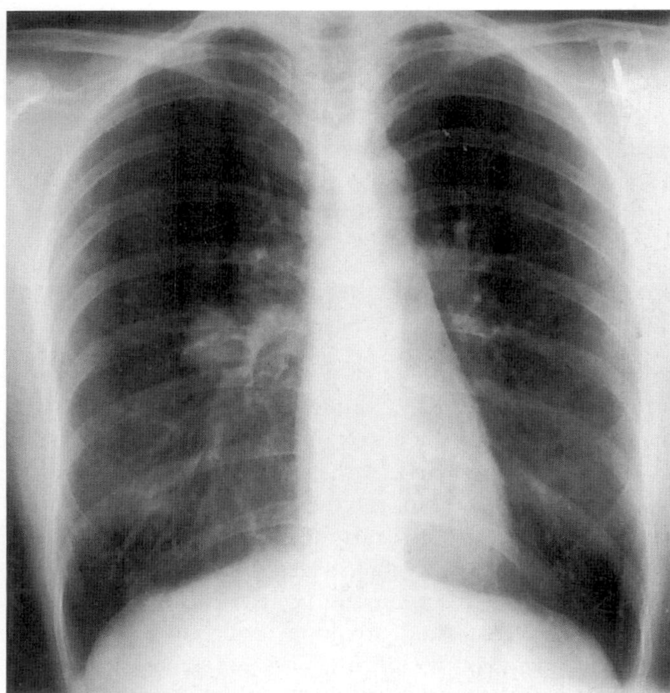

Figure 5–15 Patient with right hilar metastases that resolved completely on progestin therapy.

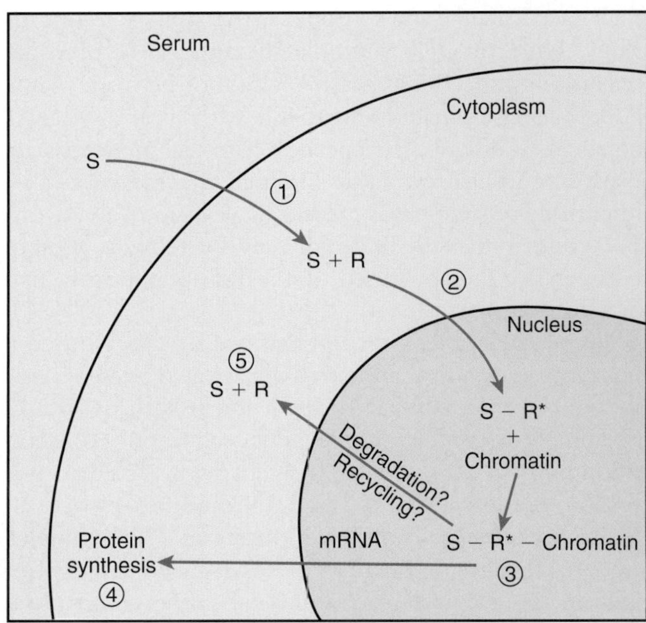

Figure 5–16 Simplified schema of steroid-receptor interactions in target tissue cell. *1,* Free steroids diffuse across the cytoplasmic membrane and are bound by specific receptors. Studies with monoclonal antibody immunohistologic techniques indicate that estrogen receptor(s) is localized within nucleus. *2,* S-R complex is translocated into the nucleus and activated (*). *3,* Activated S-R complex interacts with chromatin and initiates mRNA transcription. *4,* mRNA initiates specific protein synthesis, producing hormonal effects. *5,* S-R complex is degraded or recycled. (From: Soper JT, Christensen CW: Steroid receptors and endometrial cancer. Clin Obstet Gynecol 13:825, 1986.)

measurable disease, there were only 17 complete responders (8%) and 13 partial responders (6%). More than half of the patients remained stable and one-third progressed. Median survival was 10.5 months. Grade 1 lesions responded more frequently than poorly differentiated carcinomas did. The GOG evaluated, in randomized phase III trial, MPA at 1000 mg/day compared with 200 mg/day. In almost 300 patients, there was no difference in response rate or survival between the two groups. Lentz reported another GOG trial of high-dose megestrol acetate (800 mg/day) in patients with advanced or recurrent endometrial carcinoma. Of 58 patients, 13 (24%) responded; 6 (11%) had a partial response. Four of the responses lasted >18 months and were primarily between the grade 1 and grade 2 lesions.

More recently, considerable interest has been shown in the presence of specific estrogen and progesterone receptors in neoplastic human uterine tissue (Fig. 5–16). These receptors are definitely present and vary from tumor to tumor. It has been shown that there is a greater number of both estrogen and progesterone receptors in well-differentiated lesions than in poorly differentiated ones (Table 5–21). In a small group of patients, it was noted that about one-third of those with recurrent cancer had a positive receptor site analysis to both estrogen and progesterone. The receptor data may therefore correlate with clinical findings of responsiveness to progesterones in patients with recurrent cancer. Preliminary data suggest an excellent correlation (Table 5–22). Obviously, considerable additional data are needed to verify these findings; however, the prospects are excellent. If direct correlation can be substantiated, the receptor site analysis can guide the type of progestin therapy or chemotherapy given for recurrent endometrial cancer. If receptor site analysis is positive for both estrogen and progesterone, a patient's chances of responding to progestins are extremely good, even if she has a poorly differentiated lesion. On the other hand, if the receptor site analysis is negative, the data suggest that the patient's response to progestins may be extremely low, making it more advisable to go directly to cytotoxic agents without wasting time on progestin therapy. Kauppila noted from five studies in the literature that 89% of progesterone receptor-positive tumors were hormonally responsive, compared with only 17% of progesterone receptor-negative tumors. The GOG noted that 4 of 10 (40%) estrogen receptor-positive, progesterone receptor-positive tumors responded to progestins, compared with 5 of 41 (12%) progesterone receptor-negative tumors.

Progestin therapy may be administered in several different ways. We prefer MPA (Depo-Provera), 400 mg intramuscularly at weekly intervals. Oral MPA (Provera), in the range of 150 mg/day, and megestrol acetate (Megace), 160 mg/day, are other recommended progestins. Progestins are continued indefinitely if an objective response is obtained. If progression of disease is noted, progestins should be discontinued and chemotherapy considered.

With only modest response to progestins, other hormonal agents have been evaluated. Tamoxifen has been shown to bind estrogen receptors and thereby block access

Table 5–21 CORRELATION OF TUMOR DIFFERENTIATION WITH RECEPTOR CONTENT

Differentiation	ER and PR positive
Well	28/40 (70%)
Moderate	21/38 (55%)
Poor	11/27 (41%)

ER, estrogen receptor; PR, progesterone receptor.
From Creasman WT, Soper JT, McCarty KS Jr et al: Influence of cytoplasmic steroid receptor content on prognosis of early stage endometrial carcinoma. Am J Obstet Gynecol 151:922, 1985.

Table 5–22 RESPONSE TO PROGESTIN THERAPY IN REGARD TO RECEPTOR CONTENT

Receptor content	Progestin response
Positive	44/55 (80%)
Negative	4/76 (5%)

Based on papers by Ehrlich, Benraad, Creasman, Kauppila, Pollow, Quinn.

of the estrogen into the nucleus. It has also been suggested that tamoxifen can increase the number of progesterone receptors in vivo. Combined results of several small studies noted a response rate of 22% (complete response rate of 8%) in 257 patients. These studies suggest that grade 1 lesions are more responsive than other grades of tumors. Progestins plus tamoxifen have been evaluated in combination in recurrent carcinoma of the endometrium. Although tamoxifen is theoretically attractive (it causes an increase in progesterone receptors for better progestin effect), studies of small groups of patients have not produced favorable results. The use of tamoxifen is interesting in view of the reports of endometrial cancer in patients taking tamoxifen. This is in contrast to in vitro data suggesting that tamoxifen does not stimulate and in fact may inhibit established endometrial cell line growth.

Gonadotropin-releasing hormone (GnRH) analogues have been evaluated in the treatment of endometrial cancer in a small number of patients. These analogues suppress gonadotropins with a reduction in estrogen but not cortisol levels. Gallagher and associates treated 17 patients with recurrent endometrial cancer who had received previous progesterone therapy; 6 (35%) had a response that continued for a median of 20 months. Further study is needed, but it appears that GnRH analogues may have a direct inhibitory effect on cancer cells.

Because one-third of the patients with recurrent carcinoma of the endometrium responded to progestins and because hormone therapy is essentially non-toxic, evaluations of cytotoxic agents have not been pursued until recently. Initial data suggest that doxorubicin is an effective agent in the treatment of adenocarcinoma of the endometrium, with an approximately 35% response rate in patients not responding to progestins. In the report of the GOG experience, Thigpen and colleagues noted that 16 of 43 patients (37%) with advanced or recurrent cancer experienced an objective response with use of doxorubicin alone. Unfortunately, response lasted only 7 months. The Eastern Cooperative Oncology Group achieved only a 19% response rate in its doxorubicin trial; however, a dosage lower than the GOG dosage was used. When one evaluates the doxorubicin data, one notes that only about 10% of patients who received this drug had a complete response rate. Patients designated as giving a partial response had survival rates no greater than those of patients who had no response to this cytotoxic agent. The role of doxorubicin as a single agent may be limited in this disease.

Experience with cisplatin chemotherapy as a single agent has been reported by the MD Anderson Hospital group. Of 26 patients, 11 (42%) had objective responses (10 partial responses and one complete response). Unfortunately, the mean duration of remission was 5 months, with the complete response lasting for 8 months. The same authors had previously reported their experience with doxorubicin and cyclophosphamide: 8 of 26 patients (30%) had partial responses for a mean duration of 4 months. Experience of the GOG showed that only 1 of 23 patients treated with cisplatin responded; however, 20 of the 23 patients had previously been treated with other cytotoxic agents. Trope and coworkers noted a 36% response rate in 11 patients who were previously untreated with chemotherapy. In a subsequent study of 49 patients who had not been treated previously with a cytotoxic agent, 10 (20%) responded to cisplatin, and 2 (4%) were complete responders. Carboplatin, a cisplatin analogue, has been evaluated in 48 patients with a 30% response but only 2 (4%) complete responders.

Several other drugs have been used in phase II studies in this group of patients. These include ICRF-159 (razoxane), piperazinedione, *m*-AMSA (amsacrine), mitoxantrone (Novantrone), dianhydrogalactitol, etoposide, methotrexate, and aminothiadiazole; all showed little or no activity.

In a prospective study by the GOG, 336 patients who had advanced or recurrent adenocarcinoma were treated with doxorubicin, with or without cyclophosphamide. All these patients had failed to respond when given MPA. Only 7 (5.4%) of those treated with doxorubicin had a complete response, but 18 (12.5%) who received doxorubicin plus cyclophosphamide were complete responders. Total response was 22% for doxorubicin and 30% for doxorubicin and cyclophosphamide. The median survival was 7 months for both groups, and there was no difference in survival between the two groups. Piver and coworkers treated 50 patients with melphalan, 5-fluorouracil, and MPA, with or without tamoxifen, as first-line chemotherapy. There was a 20% complete response rate and 48% total responses. The median progression-free survival was only 5 months for the whole group, but it was 24 months for the complete responders. Several small studies have evaluated cisplatin, cyclophosphamide, and doxorubicin in phase II trials. In five studies with 127 assessable patients, responses were noted in 63 (50%), and 24 (19%) were complete

Table 5–23 RESPONSE TO CHEMOTHERAPY IN REGARD TO RECEPTOR CONTENT

	ER or PR negative	ER or PR positive
Complete or partial response (4 months)	7/10	1/5

ER, estrogen receptor; PR, progesterone receptor.
Modified from Kauppila A, Jänne O, Kujansuu E, Vihko R: Treatment of advanced endometrial adenocarcinoma with combined cytotoxic therapy. Cancer 46:2162, 1980.

responders. The GOG is currently comparing doxorubicin with cisplatin and doxorubicin.

Chemotherapy with paclitaxel has been shown to have a 14% complete response rate and a 21.4% partial response rate. In GOG studies, a complete response rate of 6.1% and a partial response rate of 18% have been achieved with ifosfamide and mesna. Tamoxifen also has some activity in recurrent endometrial cancer with response rates of up to 22% with doses of 20–40 mg/day, and patients with well-differentiated tumors are more likely to respond.

Of interest is a report by Kauppila and associates, who noted that patients with low estrogen or progesterone receptor values had a significantly greater response rate to combined cytotoxic therapy (doxorubicin, cyclophosphamide, 5-fluorouracil, and vincristine) than did patients with higher receptor values (Table 5–23). This observation must be confirmed, but the role of receptor analysis in recurrent adenocarcinoma of the endometrium may be extremely important in determining the best therapy for the individual patient.

It has been suggested by some that CA-125 can be used to monitor therapy in patients with advanced or recurrent adenocarcinoma of the endometrium, much as is done in ovarian cancer. Niloff and colleagues and others have noted that CA-125 is elevated in as many as three-fourths of these patients. Data are limited in regard to monitoring. Fanning and Piver did note in 21 women that clinical response, as well as subsequent relapse, correlated with CA-125 levels of patients with advanced or recurrent disease. Monitoring with CA-125 is helpful, primarily in patients with high risk for recurrent disease, as in patients with recurrent disease receiving therapy who have a proven elevation of their serum value.

Multiple malignant neoplasms

Simultaneous or subsequent primary cancers involving the breast, ovary, and large intestines occur more frequently in patients with endometrial cancer than might be expected. The reverse also appears true, in that women with breast or ovarian cancer have a higher than expected risk for development of subsequent primary cancers of the endometrium. As a result, the recommendation in a patient with one of these malignant neoplasms is to evaluate the other organ sites at the time of diagnosis or during follow-up visits. Appropriate screening, such as mammography, should be emphasized.

Simultaneous malignant neoplasms of the ovary and endometrium are noted in about 8% of patients with carcinoma of the uterus, and twice that rate is noted in patients with ovarian carcinoma. Ovarian involvement in cases in which endometrial cancer is present has been reported to be as high as 40% of autopsy specimens and 15% of specimens obtained at the time of hysterectomy and bilateral salpingo-oophorectomy. In approximately one-third of cases of endometrioid carcinoma of the ovary, endometrial carcinoma has also been noted. When the occurrence is simultaneous, the question arises whether these are simultaneous multiple malignant neoplasms or one is metastatic from the other. It appears that if metastasis is present, it is more common for it to go from the endometrium to the ovary than from the ovary to the endometrium. Metastasis to the ovary is suspected if the endometrial carcinoma involves significant myometrium, particularly with lymphatic or vascular channel invasion, or if the tumor is on the ovarian surface. If, on the other hand, the corpus carcinoma is small and limited to the endometrium or superficial myometrium, with associated atypical hyperplasia, and the ovarian tumor is centrally located, the tumors are probably independent of each other. Most common tumors are the endometrioid type, but they can occasionally be of different histologic types in the two organs. Most studies suggest that most of the synchronous ovarian and corpus carcinomas are independent primary tumors. The survival of patients with what is believed to be multiple primaries mimics the excellent prognosis of the individual cancer, suggesting that the two tumors are probably each stage I and not stage III. This has certainly been true when the simultaneous endometrial and ovarian carcinomas are of the endometrioid type. In one study, the survival was 100% of the 16 patients described. It appears that when such a situation is encountered (i.e., when there is no evidence of direct extension of either tumor), myometrial invasion is usually absent or superficial, there is no lymphatic or blood vessel invasion, there is atypical hyperplasia of the endometrium frequently associated with the cancer, both tumors are usually confined to the primary sites and have minimal spread, and tumor is predominantly within the ovary or the endometrium. Whether the histologic type is uniform or dissimilar, therapy should be appropriate for stage I disease, which in many instances may be treated adequately with surgery only (hysterectomy and bilateral salpingo-oophorectomy with appropriate surgical staging).

BIBLIOGRAPHY

INCIDENCE AND EPIDEMIOLOGY

Antunes CMF, Strolley PD, Rosenshein NB et al: Endometrial cancer and estrogen use (report of a large case-control study). N Engl J Med 300:9, 1979.

Barakat RR: The effects of tamoxifen on the endometrium. Oncology (Huntingt) 9:129, 1995.

Barakat RR, Eonf G, Curain JP: Tamoxifen use in breast cancer patients who subsequently develop corpus cancer is not associated with a higher incidence of adverse histological features. Gynecol Oncol 55:164, 1994.

Beresford SA, Weiss NS, Voigt LF, McKnight B: Risk of endometrial cancer in relation to use of oestrogen combined with cyclic progestogen therapy in postmenopausal women. Lancet 349:458, 1997.

Brinton LA, Berman ML, Mortel R et al: Reproductive, menstrual, and medical risk factors for endometrial cancer: Results from a case-control study. J Obstet Gynecol 167:1317, 1992.

Centers for Disease Control Cancer and Steroid Hormone Study: Oral contraceptive use and the risk of endometrial cancer. JAMA 249:1600, 1983.

Evans-Metcalf ER, Brooks SE, Reale FR, Baker SP: Profiles of women 45 years of age and younger with endometrial cancer. Obstet Gynecol 91:349, 1998.

Fisher B, Costantino JP, Wickerham DL et al: Tamoxifen for prevention of breast cancer: Report of the National Surgical Adjuvant Breast and Bowel Project P-1 study. J Natl Cancer Inst 90:1371, 1998.

Gray LA, Christopherson WM, Hoover RN: Estrogens and endometrial carcinoma. Obstet Gynecol 49:385, 1977.

Greenblatt RB, Stoddard LB: The estrogen-cancer controversy. J Am Geriatr Soc 26:1, 1978.

Gusberg SB, Kardon P: Proliferative endometrial response to thecal granulosa cell tumors. Am J Obstet Gynecol 3:633, 1971.

Hoffman K, Nekhylndov L, Deligdisch L: Endometrial carcinoma in elderly women. Gynecol Oncol 58:198, 1995.

Hoover R, Fraumeni JF, Everson R et al: Cancer of the uterine corpus after hormonal treatment for breast cancer. Lancet 1:885, 1976.

Horwitz RL, Feinstein AF: Alternative analytic methods for case-control studies of estrogens and endometrial cancer. N Engl J Med 299:1090, 1978.

Husslein H, Brietenecker G, Tatra G: Premalignant and malignant uterine changes in immunosuppressed renal transplant recipients. Acta Obstet Gynecol Scand 57:73, 1978.

Jordan VC, Assikis VJ: Endometrial carcinoma and tamoxifen: Clearing up a controversy. Clin Cancer Res 1:467, 1995.

Kaku T, Matsumura M, Sakai K et al: Endometrial carcinoma in women 65 years of age or older: A clinicopathologic study. Eur J Gynaecol 17:357, 1996.

Kaplan DS, Cole P: Epidemiology of cancer of the endometrium (in press).

Kelley HW et al: Adenocarcinoma of the endometrium in women taking sequential oral contraceptives. Obstet Gynecol 47:200, 1972.

Killackey MA, Hakes TB, Pierce VK: Endometrial adenocarcinoma in breast cancer patients receiving antiestrogens. Cancer Treat Rep 69:273, 1985.

Lawrence C et al: Smoking, body weight, and early stage endometrial cancer. Cancer 59:1665, 1987.

Levi F, Franeschi S, Negri E, LaVecchia C: Dietary factors and the risk of endometrial cancer. Cancer 71:3775, 1993.

MacMahon B: Risk factors for endometrial cancer. Gynecol Oncol 2:122, 1974.

MacMahon B: Overview of studies on endometrial cancer and other types of cancer in humans: Perspective of an epidemiologist. Semin Oncol 24:S1, 1997.

Mack TM et al: Estrogens and endometrial cancer in a retirement community. N Engl J Med 294:1262, 1976.

Mansell H, Hertig AT: Granulosa-theca cell tumor and endometrial carcinoma: A study of their relationship and survey of 80 cases. Obstet Gynecol 6:385, 1955.

McCarty KS Jr et al: Gonadal dysgenesis with adenocarcinoma of the endometrium: Electron microscopic and steroid receptor analyses with a review of the literature. Cancer 42:510, 1978.

McDonald TW, Malkasian GD, Gaffey TA: Endometrial cancer associated with feminizing ovarian tumors and polycystic ovarian disease. Obstet Gynecol 94:654, 1977.

Million Women Study Collaborators: Endometrial cancer and hormone replacement therapy in the Million Women Study. Lancet 365:1543, 2005.

Novak E, Yui E: Relationship of endometrial hyperplasia to adenocarcinoma of the endometrium. Am J Obstet Gynecol 32:674, 1936.

Nyholm NCV, Neilsen AL, Norup P: Endometrial cancer in postmenopausal women with and without previous estrogen replacement treatment: Comparison of clinical and histopathological characteristics. Gynecol Oncol 49:229, 1993.

Ostor AG et al: Endometrial carcinoma in gonadal dysgenesis with and without estrogen therapy. Gynecol Oncol 6:316, 1978.

Pacheco JC, Kempers RD: Etiology of post-menopausal bleeding. Obstet Gynecol 32:40, 1968.

Powels T, Eeles R, Ashley S et al: Interim analysis of the incidence of breast cancer in the Royal Marsden Hospital tamoxifen randomised chemoprevention trial. Lancet 352:98, 1998.

Schapira DV, Kumar NB, Lyman GH et al: Upper-body fat distribution and endometrial cancer risk. JAMA 266:1808, 1991.

Silva EG, Tornos C, Mapica A, Mitchell MF: Uterine neoplasms in patients treated with tamoxifen. J Cell Biochem Suppl 23:179, 1995.

Silverberg SG, Makowski EL: Endometrial carcinoma in young women taking oral contraceptives agents. Obstet Gynecol 46:503, 1975.

Smith DC et al: Association of exogenous estrogen and endometrial carcinoma. N Engl J Med 293:1164, 1975.

Swanson CA, Potischman N, Wilbanks GD et al: Relationship of endometrial cancer risk to past and contemporary body size and body fat distribution. Cancer Epidemiol Biomarkers Prev 2:321, 1993.

Veronesi U, Maisonneuve P, Costa A et al: Prevention of breast cancer with tamoxifen: Preliminary findings from the Italian randomised trial among hysterectomised women. Lancet 352:93, 1998.

Weiderpass E, Adami HO, Baron JA et al: Risk of Endometrial Cancer Following Estrogen Replacement With and Without Progestins, J Natl Cancer Inst 91:1131-1137, 1999

Weiss NS: Non-contraceptive estrogens and abnormalities of endometrial proliferation. Ann Intern Med 88:410, 1978.

Ziel HK, Finkle WD: Increased risk of endometrial carcinoma among users of conjugated estrogens. N Engl J Med 293:1167, 1975.

Ziel HK, Finkle WD, Greenland S: Decline in incidence of endometrial cancer following increase in prescriptions for opposed conjugated estrogens in a prepaid health plan. Gynecol Oncol 68:253, 1998.

SCREENING AND DIAGNOSIS

Abate SD, Edwards CL, Vellias F: A comparative study of the endometrial jet-washing technique and endometrial biopsy. Am J Clin Pathol 58:118, 1972.

Anderson B: Diagnosis of endometrial cancer. Clin Obstet Gynecol 13:739, 1986.

Assikis VJ, Jordan VC: A realistic assessment of the association between tamoxifen and endometrial cancer. Endocr Rel Cancer 2:1, 1995.

Berezowsky J, Chalvardjian A, Murray D: Iatrogenic endometrial mega polyps in women with breast carcinoma. Obstet Gynecol 84:727, 1994.

Bourne TH, Campbell S, Steer CV et al: Detection of endometrial cancer by transvaginal ultrasonography with color flow imaging and blood flow analysis. Gynecol Oncol 40:253, 1991.

Cacciatore B, Lehtovirta P, Wahlstrom T et al: Preoperative sonographic evaluation of endometrial cancer. Am J Obstet Gynecol 160:133, 1989.

Cohen CJ, Gusberg SB: Screening for endometrial cancer. Clin Obstet Gynecol 18:27, 1975.

Cohen I, Rosen DJD, Shapira J et al: Endometrial changes with tamoxifen: Comparison between tamoxifen-treated and non-treated asymptomatic postmenopausal breast cancer patients. Gynecol Oncol 52:185, 1994.

Creasman WT: Endometrial cancer: Incidence, prognostic factors, diagnosis, and treatment. Semin Oncol 24:S1, 1997.

Creasman WT, Weed JC Jr: Screening techniques in endometrial cancer. Cancer 38:436, 1976.

Doering DL, Barnhill DR, Weiser EB et al: Intraoperative evaluation of depth of myometrial invasion in stage I endometrial carcinoma. Obstet Gynecol 74:930, 1989.

Feldman S, Cook EF, Harlow BL, Berkowitz RS: Predicting endometrial cancer among older women who present with abnormal vaginal bleeding. Gynecol Oncol 56:376, 1995.

Fisher B, Costantino JP, Redmond CK et al: Endometrial cancer in tamoxifen treated breast cancer patients: Findings from the National Surgical Adjuvant Breast and Bowel Project (NSABP) B-14. J Natl Cancer Inst 86:527, 1994.

Giusa-Chiferi MG, Goncalves WJ, Baracat EC et al: Transvaginal ultrasound, uterine biopsy and hysteroscopy for postmenopausal bleeding. Int J Gynaecol Obstet 55:39, 1996.

Goldchmit R, Katz Z, Blickstein I et al: The accuracy of endometrial Pipelle sampling with or without sonographic measurement of endometrial thickness. Obstet Gynecol 82:727, 1993.

Goldstein SR: Unusual ultrasound appearance of the uterus in patients receiving tamoxifen. Am J Obstet Gynecol 170:447, 1994.

Gordon AN, Fleischer AC, Dudley BS et al: Preoperative assessment of myometrial invasion of endometrial adenocarcinoma by ultrasound and MRI. Gynecol Oncol 34:175, 1989.

Granberg S, Wikland M, Karlson B et al: Endometrial thickness as measured by endovaginal ultrasound for identifying endometrial abnormality. Am J Obstet Gynecol 164:47, 1991.

Gupta JK, Wilson S, Desai P, Hau C: How should we investigate women with postmenopausal bleeding? Acta Obstet Gynecol Scand 75:475, 1996.

Hofmeister FJ: Endometrial biopsy: Another look. Am J Obstet Gynecol 118:733, 1974.

Horwitz RJ, Horwitz SM, Feinstein AR et al: Necropsy diagnosis of endometrial cancer and detection bias in case/control studies, Lancet 2:66, 1981.

Ismail SM: Pathology of endometrium treated with tamoxifen. J Clin Pathol 47:827, 1994.

Kedar RP, Bourne TH, Powles TJ et al: Effects of tamoxifen on uterus and ovaries of postmenopausal women in a randomized breast cancer prevention trial. Lancet 343:1318, 1994.

Koss LG, Schreiber K, Oberlander SG et al: Detection of endometrial carcinoma in hyperplasia in asymptomatic women. Obstet Gynecol 64:1, 1984.

Lahti E, Blanco G, Kauppila A et al: Endometrial changes in postmenopausal breast cancer patients receiving tamoxifen. Obstet Gynecol 81:660, 1993.

Langer RD, Pierce JJ, O'Hanlan KA et al: Transvaginal ultrasonography compared with endometrial biopsy for the detection of endometrial disease. N Engl J Med 337:1792, 1997.

Lu KH, Dinh M, Kohlmann W et al: Gynecologic Cancer as a "Sentinel Cancer" for Women With Hereditary Nonpolyposis Colorectal Cancer Syndrome, Obstet Gynecol 105: 569, 2005.

Magriples U, Naftolin F, Schwartz PE et al: High grade endometrial carcinoma in tamoxifen treated breast cancer patients. J Clin Oncol 11:485, 1993.

Maia H Jr, Barbosa IC, Farias JP et al: Evaluation of the endometrial cavity during menopause. Int J Gynecol Obstet 52:1996.

Nasri MH, Coast CJ: Correlation of ultrasound findings and endometrial histopathology in postmenopausal women. Br J Obstet Gynaecol 96:1333, 1989.

Reich O, Winter R, Pickel H et al: Does the size of pelvic lymph nodes predict metastatic involvement in patients with endometrial cancer? Int J Gynecol Cancer 6:445, 1996.

Smith-Bindman R, Kerlikowske K, Feldstein VA et al: Endovaginal ultrasound to exclude endometrial cancer and other endometrial abnormalities. JAMA 280:1510, 1998.

Stovall TG, Photopulos GJ, Poston WM et al: Pipelle endometrial sampling in patients with known endometrial carcinoma. Obstet Gynecol 77:954, 1991.

Varner RE, Sparks JM, Cameron CD et al: Transvaginal sonography of the endometrium in postmenopausal women. Obstet Gynecol 78:195, 1991.

Vuento MH, Maatela JI, Tyrkko JE et al: A longitudinal study of screening for endometrial cancer by endometrial biopsy in diabetic females. Int J Gynecol Cancer 5:390, 1995.

Weber AM, Belinsob JL, Bradley LD, Piedmonte MR: Vaginal ultrasonography versus endometrial biopsy in women with postmenopausal bleeding. Am J Obstet Gynecol 177:924, 1997.

PROGNOSTIC FACTORS

Ambros RA, Kurman RJ: Identification of patients with stage I uterine endometrial adenocarcinoma at high risk of recurrence by DNA ploidy myometrial invasion and vascular invasion. Gynecol Oncol 45:235, 1992.

Ayhan A, Turner R, Turner ZS et al: Correlation between clinical and histopathologic risk factors; i.e., lymph node metastasis in early endometrial cancer. Int J Obstet Gynecol 4:306, 1994.

Baak JPA, Snijders WP, Van Diest PJ et al: Confirmation of the prognostic value of the ECPI-1 score in FIGO stage I endometrial cancer patients with long follow up. Int J Gynecol Cancer 5:112, 1995.

Benraad TJ et al: Do estrogen and progesterone receptors (E2R and PR) in metastasizing endometrial cancer predict the response to gestagen therapy? Acta Obstet Gynecol Scand 59:155, 1980.

Bokhman JV: Two pathogenetic types of endometrial carcinoma. Gynecol Oncol 15:10, 1983.

Boronow RC et al: Surgical staging in endometrial cancer: Clinical-pathologic findings of a prospective study. Obstet Gynecol 63: 825, 1984.

Bristow RE, Zahurak ML, Alexander CJ et al: FIGO stage IIIC endometrial carcinoma: Resection of macroscopic nodal disease and other determinants of survival. Int J Gynecol Cancer, 13:664, 2003

Britton LC, Wilson TO, Gaffey TA et al: DNA ploidy in endometrial carcinoma: Major objective prognostic factor. Mayo Clin Proc 65:643, 1990.

Connell PP, Rotmensch J, Waggoner S, Mundt AJ: Significance of adnexal involvement in endometrial carcinoma. Gynecol Oncol 74:74, 1999.

Cowles TA et al: Comparison of clinical and surgical staging in patients with endometrial cancer. Obstet Gynecol 66:413, 1985.

Creasman WT, Rutledge FN: The prognostic value of peritoneal cytology in gynecologic malignant disease. Am J Obstet Gynecol 110:773, 1971.

Creasman WT, DiSaia PJ, Blessing J: Prognostic significance of peritoneal cytology in patients with endometrial cancer and preliminary data concerning therapy with intraperitoneal radiopharmaceuticals. Am J Obstet Gynecol 141:921, 1981.

Creasman WT, McCarty KS Sr, McCarty KS Jr: Clinical correlation of estrogen, progesterone binding proteins in human endometrial adenocarcinoma. Obstet Gynecol 55:363, 1980.

Creasman WT, Morrow CP, Bundy L: Surgical pathological spread patterns of endometrial cancer. Cancer 60:2035, 1987.

Creasman WT et al: Adenocarcinoma of the endometrium: Its metastatic lymph node potential. A preliminary report. Gynecol Oncol 4:239, 1976.

Creasman WT et al: Influence of cytoplasmic steroid receptor content on prognosis of early stage endometrial carcinoma. Am J Obstet Gynecol 151:922, 1985.

Dasarahally S, Mohan MA, Samuels MA et al: Long-Term Outcomes of Therapeutic Pelvic Lymphadenectomy for Stage I Endometrial Adenocarcinoma, Gynecol Oncol 70:165-171, 1998DiSaia PJ et al: Risk factors in recurrent patterns in stage I endometrial carcinoma. Am J Obstet Gynecol 151:1009, 1985.

Ehrlich CE, Young PCM, Cleary RE: Cytoplasmic progesterone and estriol receptors in normal, hyperplastic, and carcinomatous endometria: Therapeutic implications. Am J Obstet Gynecol 141:539, 1981.

Eltabbakh GH, Moore AD: Survival of women with surgical stage II endometrial cancer. Gynecol Oncol 74:80, 1999.

Genest P et al: Prognostic factors in early carcinoma of the endometrium. Am J Clin Oncol 10:71, 1987.

Goff BA, Kato D, Schmidt RA et al: Uterine papillary serous carcinoma: Patterns of metastatic spread. Gynecol Oncol 54:264, 1994.

Grice J, Ek M, Greer B et al: Uterine papillary serous carcinoma: Evaluation of long-term survival in surgically staged patients. Gynecol Oncol 69:69, 1998.

Grimshaw RN, Tupper WC, Fraser RC et al: Prognostic value of peritoneal cytology in endometrial carcinoma. Gynecol Oncol 36:97, 1990.

Hanson NB et al: Prognostic significance of lymph-vascular space invasion in stage I endometrial cancer. Cancer 55:1753, 1985.

Haroung VR, Sutton EP, Clark SA et al: The importance of peritoneal cytology in endometrial carcinoma. Obstet Gynecol 72:394, 1988.

Havrilesky LJ, Crogum JM, Calingaert B et al: resection of lymph node metastases influences survival in Stage III endometrial cancer. Gynecol Oncol 99:689–695, 2005.

Kauppila A: Oestrogen and progestin receptors as prognostic indicators in endometrial cancer. Acta Oncol 28:561, 1989.

Kauppila A, Grönroos N, Nieminen U: Clinical outcome in endometrial cancer. Obstet Gynecol 60:473, 1982.

Kodama S, Kase H, Tanaka K, Matsui K: Multivariate analysis of prognostic factors in patients with endometrial cancer. Int J Gynecol Obstet 53:23, 1996.

Konski A, Poulter C, Keys H et al: Absence of prognostic significance, peritoneal dissemination and treatment advantage in endometrial cancer patients with positive peritoneal cytology. Int J Radiat Oncol Biol Phys 4:49, 1988.

Lefevre H: Node dissection in cancer of the endometrium. Surg Gynecol Obstet 102:649, 1956.

Levenback C, Burke TW, Silva E et al: Uterine papillary serous carcinoma treated with PAC. Gynecol Oncol 46:317, 1992.

Lo SST, Cheng DKL, Ng TY et al: The prognostic significance of positive peritoneal cytology in endometrial cancer. Int J Gynecol Cancer 6:473, 1996.

Lurian JR, Rum Sey NK, Schink JC et al: Prognostic significance of positive peritoneal cytology in clinical stage I adenocarcinoma of the endometrium. Obstet Gynecol 74:175, 1989.

Lutz MH et al: Endometrial carcinoma: A new method of classification of therapeutic and prognostic significance. Gynecol Oncol 6:83, 1978.

Mariani A, Webb MJ, Galli L, Podratz KC: Potential Therapeutic Role of Para-aortic Lymphadenectomy in Node-Positive Endometrial Cancer Gynecol Oncol 348, 2000.

Matsushima-Nishiu M. Unoki M, Ono K et al: Growth and gene expression profile analyses of endometrial cancer cells expressing exogenous PTEN. Cancer Research. 61:3741–3749, 2001.

Matthews RP, Hutchinson-Colas J, Maiman M et al: Papillary serous and clear cell type lead to poor prognosis of endometrial carcinoma in black women. Gynecol Oncol 65:265, 1997.

Milosevic MF, Dembo AD, Thomas GM: Clinical significance of malignant peritoneal cytology in stage I endometrial carcinoma. Int J Gynecol Cancer 2:225, 1992.

Morrow CP, Bundy BN, Kurman RJ et al: Relationship between surgical pathological risk factors and outcome in clinical stage I and II carcinoma of the endometrium. Gynecol Oncol 40:55, 1991.

Nolan JF, Huen A: Prognosis in endometrial cancer. Gynecol Oncol 4:384, 1976.

Nordström B, Strang P, Lindgren A et al: Endometrial carcinoma: The prognostic impact of papillary serous carcinoma (UPSC) in relation to nuclear grade, DNA ploidy and p53 expression. Anticancer Res 16:899, 1996.

Norris HJ, Taylor HG: Prognosis of granulosa thecal tumor of the ovary. Cancer 21:255, 1968.

Onda T, Yeshikawa H, Mizutani K et al: treatment of node positive endometrial cancer with complete node dissection, chemotherapy and radiation therapy. Br J Cancer 75:183, 1997

Onsrud N et al: Endometrial carcinoma with cervical involvement (stage II): Prognostic factors in value of combined radiological surgical treatment. Gynecol Oncol 13:76, 1982.

Pfisterer J, Kommoss F, Sauerbrei V et al: Prognostic value of DNA ploidy and S-phase fraction in stage I endometrial carcinoma. Gynecol Oncol 58:149, 1995.

Pisani A, Barbuto DA, Chen D et al: HER-2/neu, p53, and DNA analysis as prognosticators for survival in endometrial carcinoma. Obstet Gynecol 85:729, 1995.

Plentyl AA, Friedman EA: Lymphatic System of the Female Genitalia: The Morphologic Basis of Oncologic Diagnosis and Therapy. Philadelphia, WB Saunders, 1971.

Podratz KC, Wilson TO, Gaffey TA et al: DNA analysis facilitates the pretreatment identification of high-risk endometrial cancer patients. Am J Obstet Gynecol 168:1206, 1993.

Podratz KC, Mariani A, Webb MJ: Staging and Therapeutic Value of Lymphadenectomy in Endometrial Cancer, Gynecol Oncol 70:163-164, 1998Pollow K, Manz B, Grill JH: Estrogen progesterone receptors in endometrial carcinoma. In Jasonni VM (ed): Steroids and Endometrial Cancer. New York, Raven Press, 1989, p 101.

Potish RA et al: Para-aortic lymph node radiotherapy in the cancer of uterine corpus. Obstet Gynecol 65:251, 1985.

Quinn MA, Couchi M, Fortune V: Endometrial carcinoma: Steroid receptors and response to medroxyprogesterone acetate. Gynecol Oncol 21:314, 1985.

Rosenberg P, Boeryd B, Simonsen E: A new aggressive treatment approach to high grade endometrial cancer of possible benefit to patients with stage I uterine papillary cancer. Gynecol Oncol 48:32, 1993.

Rutledge FN, Tan S, Fletcher G: Vaginal metastases from adenocarcinoma of the corpus uteri. Am J Obstet Gynecol 75:157, 1958.

Sandstrom RE, Welch WR, Green TH Jr: Adenocarcinoma of the endometrium in pregnancy. Obstet Gynecol 53(Suppl):735, 1979.

Schink JC et al: Tumor size in endometrial cancer: A prospective factor for lymph node metastases. Obstet Gynecol 70:216, 1987.

Sherman ME, Sturgeon S, Brinton LA et al: Risk factors and hormone levels in patients with serous and endometrioid uterine carcinomas. Mod Pathol 10:963, 1997.

Soper JT et al: Intraperitoneal chromic phosphate P-32 suspension therapy in malignant peritoneal cytology and endometrial carcinoma. Am J Obstet Gynecol 153:191, 1985.

Sorbe B, Risberg B, Thonthwaite J: Nuclear morphometry and DNA flow cytometry as prognostic methods for endometrial carcinoma. Int J Gynecol Cancer 4:94, 1994.

Surwit EA et al: Stage II carcinoma of the endometrium. Int J Radiat Oncol Biol Phys 5:323, 1979.

Susini T, Rapi S, Savino L et al: Prognostic value of flow cytometric deoxyribonucleic acid in endometrial carcinoma: Comparison with other clinical-pathologic parameters. Am J Obstet Gynecol 170:527, 1994.

Sutton GP: The significance of positive peritoneal cytology in endometrial cancer. Oncology 4:21, 1990.

Takeshima N, Hirai Y, Tanaka N et al: Pelvic lymph node metastasis in endometrial cancer with no myometrial invasion. Obstet Gynecol 88:280, 1996.

Takeshima N, Hirai Y, Yano K et al: Ovarian metastasis in endometrial carcinoma. Gynecol Oncol 70:183, 1998.

Thornton JE, Ali S, O'Donovan P et al: Flow cytometric studies of ploidy and proliferative indices in the Yorkshire trial of adjuvant progestogen treatment of endometrial cancer. Br J Obstet Gynaecol 100:253, 1993.

Turner DA, Gershenson DM, Atkinson N et al: The prognostic significance of peritoneal cytology for stage I endometrial cancer. Obstet Gynecol 74:775, 1989.

Van Nostrand K, Johnson G, Monk B et al: Genetic alterations in endometrial carcinomas. Int J Gynecol Cancer 8:415, 1998.

Von Minckwitz G, Kuhn W, Kaufmann M et al: Prognostic importance of DNA ploidy and S-phase fraction in endometrial cancer. Int J Gynecol Cancer 4:250, 1994.

Yazigi R, Piver MS, Blumenson L: Malignant peritoneal cytology as prognostic indicator in stage I endometrial cancer. Obstet Gynecol 62:359, 1983.

PATHOLOGY

Abeler UA, Kjorstad KE: Endometrial adenocarcinoma with squamous cell differentiation. Cancer 69:488, 1992.

Alberhasky RC, Connely PJ, Christopherson WN: Carcinoma of the endometrium. IV: Mixed adenosquamous carcinoma. Am J Clin Pathol 77:655, 1982.

Aozasa K, Saeki K, Ohasawa M et al: Malignant lymphoma of the uterus. Cancer 72:1959, 1993.

Benedetti-Panici P, Maneschi F, Cutillo G et al: Anatomical and pathological study of retroperitoneal nodes in endometrial cancer. Int J Gynecol Cancer 8:322, 1998.

Chambers JT, Merino M, Kohorn EI et al: Uterine papillary serous carcinoma. Obstet Gynecol 69:109, 1987.

Chen JL, Trost DC, Wilkinson EJ: Endometrial papillary carcinoma: Two clinical pathological types. Int J Gynecol Pathol 4:279, 1985.

Christopherson WN, Alberhasky RC, Connely PJ: Carcinoma of the endometrium. I: A clinicopathological study of clear cell carcinoma and secretory carcinoma. Cancer 49:1511, 1982.

Christopherson WN, Alberhasky RC, Connely PJ: Carcinoma of the endometrium. II: Papillary adenocarcinoma: A clinico-pathological study of 46 patients. Am J Clin Pathol 77:534, 1982.

Connely PJ, Alberhasky RC, Christopherson WN: Carcinoma of the endometrium. III: Analysis of 865 cases of adenocarcinoma and adenocanthoma. Obstet Gynecol 59:569, 1982.

Eifel P, Hendrickson M, Ross J et al: Simultaneous presentation of carcinoma involving the ovary and uterine corpus. Cancer 50:163, 1982.

Gitsch G, Friedlander ML, Wain GV et al: Uterine papillary serous carcinoma. Cancer 75:2239, 1995.

Goff BA, Kato D, Schmidt RA et al: Uterine papillary serous carcinoma: Patterns of metastatic spread. Gynecol Oncol 54:264, 1994.

Hendrickson MR, Longacre TA, Kempson RL: Uterine papillary serous carcinoma revisited. Gynecol Oncol 54:261, 1991.

Hendrickson MR, Ross J, Eifel PJ et al: Adenocarcinoma of the endometrium: Analysis of 256 cases of carcinoma limited to the uterine corpus. Gynecol Oncol 13:373, 1982.

Jeffrey JF, Krepart GV, Lotocki RJ: Papillary serous adenocarcinomas of the endometrium. Obstet Gynecol 67:670, 1986.

Kaku T, Tsukamoto N, Hachisuga T et al: Endometrial carcinoma associated with hyperplasia. Gynecol Oncol 60:22, 1996.

Klein Z, Markovitch O, Altaras M et al: Advanced endometrial adenocarcinoma following endometrial ablation: A case report and review of the literature. Int J Gynecol Cancer 7:163, 1997.

Kurman RJ, Scully RE: Clear cell carcinoma of the endometrium: Analysis of 21 cases. Cancer 37:872, 1976.

Ng ABP, Reagan JW: Incidence and prognosis of endometrial carcinoma by histologic grade and extent. Obstet Gynecol 35:437, 1970.

Ng ABP et al: Mixed adenosquamous carcinoma of the endometrium. Am J Clin Pathol 59:765, 1973.

Parkash V, Carcangiu ML: Uterine papillary serous carcinoma after radiation therapy for carcinoma of the cervix. Cancer 69:496, 1992.

Photopulos GJ et al: Clear cell carcinoma of the endometrium. Cancer 43:1448, 1979.

Salazar OM et al: Adenosquamous carcinoma of the endometrium. Cancer 40:119, 1977.

Schwartz PE et al: Routine use of hysterography in endometrium carcinoma and postmenopausal bleeding. Obstet Gynecol 45:378, 1975.

Schwartz Z, Ohel G, Birkenfeld A et al: Second primary malignancy in endometrial carcinoma patients. Gynecol Oncol 22:40, 1985.

Sherman ME, Bur ME, Kurman RJ: P53 in endometrial cancer and its putative precursor: Evidence for diverse pathways of tumorigenesis. Hum Pathol 26:1268, 1995.

Silverberg SG, Bolin MG, DeGiorgi LS: Adenoacanthoma and mixed adenosquamous carcinoma of the endometrium. Cancer 30:1307, 1972.

Silverberg SG, DeGiorgi LS: Clear cell carcinoma of the endometrium: Clinical-pathological and ultra-structural findings. Cancer 31:1127, 1973.

Sivridis E, Fox H, Buckley CH: Endometrial carcinoma: Two or three entities? Int J Gynecol Cancer 8:183, 1998.

Umpierre SA, Burke TW, Tornos C et al: Immunocytochemical analysis of uterine papillary serous carcinomas for estrogen and progesterone receptors. Int J Gynecol Pathol 13:127, 1994.

Zaino RJ, Kurtman R, Herbald D et al: The significance of squamous differentiation. Cancer 68:2293, 1991.

Zaino RJ, Unger ER, Whitney C: Synchronous carcinomas of the uterine corpus and ovary. Gynecol Oncol 19:329, 1984.

TREATMENT AND RECURRENCE

Aapro M, Bolis G, Chevallier B et al: An EORTC-GCCG randomized phase II trial of doxorubicin versus dox-cisplatin in endometrial carcinoma. Proc Am Soc Clin Oncol 13:275, 1994.

Arneson A: Clinical results and histological changes following irradiation treatment of cancer of the corpus uteri. AJR 36:461, 1936.

Ball HG, Blessing JA, Lentz SS et al: A phase II trial of paclitaxel in patients with advanced or recurrent adenocarcinoma of the endometrium: A Gynecologic Oncology Group study. Gynecol Oncol 62:278, 1996.

Behbakht K, Jordan EL, Casey C et al: Prognostic indicators of survival in advanced endometrial cancer. Gynecol Oncol 55:363, 1994.

Ben-Shachar I, Pavelka J, Cohn DE et al: Surgical Staging for Patients Presenting With Grade 1 Endometrial Carcinoma, Obstet Gynecol 105: 487, 2005.

Bond WH: Early uterine body carcinoma: Is postoperative vaginal irradiation any value? Clin Radiol 36:619, 1985.

Bruchner HW, Deppe G: Combination chemotherapy of advanced endometrial adenocarcinoma and Adriamycin, cyclophosphamide, 5-fluorouracil, and medroxyprogesterone acetate. Obstet Gynecol 50:105, 1977.

Burke TW: Selective pelvic and para-aortic lymphadenectomy. Oper Tech Gynecol Surg 1:17, 1996.

Carcangiu ML, Chambers JT: Uterine papillary serous carcinoma. Gynecol Oncol 47:298, 1992.

Chambers JT, Chambers SK, Kohorn EI et al: Uterine papillary serous carcinoma treated with intraperitoneal cisplatin and intravenous doxorubicin and cyclophosphamide. Gynecol Oncol 60:438, 1996.

Chambers JT, Rutherford TJ, Baker L et al: Serous carcinoma of the uterus treated with cisplatin, doxorubicin and etoposide. Int J Gynecol Cancer 8:193, 1998.

Chapman JA, DiSaia PJ, Osann K et al: Estrogen replacement in surgical stage I and II endometrial cancer survivors. Am J Obstet Gynecol 175:1195, 1996.

Chen SS: Operative treatment in stage I endometrial carcinoma with deep myometrial invasion and/or grade 3 tumor surgically limited to the corpus uteri: No recurrence with only primary surgery. Cancer 63:1843, 1989.

Chi DS, Welshinger M, Venkatraman ES et al: The role of surgical cytoreduction in stage IV endometrial carcinoma. Gynecol Oncol 67:56, 1997.

Childers JM: Laparoscopic lymph node sampling. Oper Tech Gynecol Surg 1:22, 1996.

Chung C, Stryker J, Nahhas W: The role of adjuvant radiotherapy for Stage I endometrial carcinoma. Int J Radiat Oncol Biol Phys 7:1429, 1981.

Cliby WA, Clarke-Pearson DL, Dodge R et al: Acute morbidity and mortality associated with selective pelvic and para-aortic lymphadenectomy in the surgical staging of endometrial adenocarcinoma. J Gynecol Tech 1:19, 1995.

Cohen CJ et al: Multidrug treatment of advanced and recurrent endometrial carcinoma: A Gynecologic Oncology Group study. Obstet Gynecol 63:719, 1984.

Cohen CJ, Deppe G, Bruchner HW: Treatment of advanced adenocarcinoma of the endometrium with melphalan, 5-fluorouracil, and medroxyprogesterone acetate: A preliminary study. Obstet Gynecol 50:415, 1977.

Corn BW, Lanciano RM, Greven KM et al: Impact of improved irradiation technique, age and lymph node sampling on the severe complication rate of surgically staged endometrial cancer patients: A multivariate analysis. J Clin Oncol 12:510, 1994.

COSA-NZ-UK Endometrial Cancer Study Groups: Adjuvant medroxyprogesterone acetate in high risk endometrial cancer. Int J Gynecol Cancer 8:387, 1998.

COSA-NZ-UK Endometrial Cancer Study Groups: Pelvic lymphadenectomy in high-risk endometrial cancer. Int J Gynecol Cancer 6:102, 1996.

Creutzberg CL, van Putten WLJ, Koper PCM et al: Surgery and postoperative radiotherapy versus surgery alone for patients with stage-1 endometrial carcinoma: multicentre randomised trial. Lancet 355: 1404, 2000.

de Waal JC, Lochmuller H: Preoperative radium insertion in the management of carcinoma of the endometrium. Geburtshilfe Frauenheilkd 42:394, 1982.

DePalo G et al: Adjuvant treatment with medroxyprogesterone acetate in pathological stage I endometrial cancer with myometrial invasion. In Volla R, Racinet S, Vrousos A (eds): Endometrial Cancers, 5th Cancer Research Workshop, Grenoble. Basel, Karger, 1985, p 209.

Deppe G, Cohen CJ, Bruckner WH: Treatment of advanced endometrial carcinoma with cis-dichlorodiamine platinum (II) after intensive prior therapy. Gynecol Oncol 10:51, 1980.

Dotters DJ: Preoperative CA125 in endometrial cancer. Is it useful? Am J Obstet Gynecol 182:1328, 2000.

Elliott P, Green D, Coates M et al: The efficacy of postoperative vaginal irradiation in preventing vaginal recurrence in endometrial cancer. Int J Gynecol Cancer 4:84, 1994.

Fanning J, Firestein S: Prospective evaluation of the morbidity of complete lymphadenectomy in endometrial cancer. Int J Gynecol Cancer 8:270, 1998.

Fanning J, Piver MS: Serial CA125 levels during chemotherapy for metastatic or recurrent endometrial cancer. Obstet Gynecol 77: 278, 1991.

Fleming GF, Brunetto VL, Cella D et al: Phase III Trial of Doxorubicin Plus Cisplatin With or Without Paclitaxel Plus Filgrastim in Advanced Endometrial Carcinoma: A Gynecologic Oncology Group Study. J Clin Oncol 22:2159, 2004.

Fleming GF, Filiaci VL, Bentley RC et al: Phase III randomized trial of doxorubicin + cisplatin versus doxorubicin + 24-h paclitaxel + filgrastim in endometrial carcinoma: a Gynecologic Oncology Group study. Ann Oncol 15: 1173, 2004.

Gabriele A, Lissoni A, Cromio G et al: Cisplatin, doxorubicin and cyclophosphamide (PAC) followed by radiation therapy in high-risk endometrial carcinoma. Int J Gynecol Cancer 8:397, 1998.

Gallagher CJ, Oliver RTD, Oram DH et al: A new treatment for endometrial cancer with gonadotropin releasing hormonal analogue. Br J Obstet Gynaecol 98:1037, 1991.

Hyeman J: The so-called Stockholm method and the results of treatment of uterine cancer with Radium Emmet. Acta Radiol 16:129, 1935.

Kadar N, Homesley HD, Malfetano JH: Prognostic factors in surgical stage III and IV carcinoma of the endometrium. Obstet Gynecol 84:983, 1994.

Kadar N, Malfetano JH, Homesley HD: Determinants of survival of surgically staged patients with endometrial carcinoma histologically confined to the uterus. Obstet Gynecol 80:655, 1992.

Kauppila A et al: Treatment of advanced endometrial adenocarcinoma with combined cytotoxic therapy. Cancer 46:2162, 1980.

Kauppila A: Progestin therapy of endometrial, breast, and ovarian carcinoma. Acta Obstet Gynecol Scand 63:441, 1984.

Kelly H: Radium therapy and cancer of the uterus. Trans Am Gynecol Soc 41:532, 1916.

Kelly RN, Baker WH: The effect of 17-alpha-hydroxyprogesterone caproate on metastatic endometrial cancer. Conference on Experimental Clinical Cancer Chemotherapy. Bethesda, MD, National Cancer Institute, 1960, Monograph 9.

Keys HM, Roberts JA, Brunetto VL et al: A phase III trial of surgery with or without adjunctive external pelvic radiation therapy in intermediate risk endometrial adenocarcinoma: a Gynecologic Oncology Group study. Gynecol Oncol 92:744, 2004.

Kilgore LC, Partridge EE, Alvarez RD et al: Adenocarcinoma of the endometrium: Survival comparison of patients with and without pelvic node sampling. Gynecol Oncol 56:26, 1995.

Kimmig R, Strowitzki T, Muller-Hocker J et al: Conservative treatment of endometrial cancer permitting subsequent triplet pregnancy. Gynecol Oncol 58:255, 1995.

Kistner RW: The effects of progesteronal agents on hyperplasia and carcinoma in situ of the endometrium. Int J Gynaecol Obstet 8:561, 1970.

Kohorn EI: Gestagens and endometrial carcinoma. Gynecol Oncol 4:398, 1976.

Larson DM, Broste SK, Krawisz BR: Surgery without radiotherapy for primary treatment of endometrial cancer. Obstet Gynecol 91:355, 1998.

Larson DM, Johnson K, Olson FA: Pelvic and para-aortic lymphadenectomy for surgical staging of endometrial cancer: Morbidity and mortality. Obstet Gynecol 79:998, 1992.

Leijon T, Rosenberg P, Boeryd B: Total abdominal hysterectomy and bilateral salpingo-oophorectomy. A sufficient treatment for patients with low risk endometrial carcinoma. Int J Gynecol Oncol 7:376, 1997.

Lellé RJ, Morley GW, Peters WA: The role of vaginal hysterectomy in the treatment of endometrial carcinoma. Int J Gynecol Cancer 4:342, 1994.

Lentz SS, Brady MF, Major FJ et al: High-dose megestrol acetate in advanced or recurrent endometrial carcinoma: A Gynecologic Oncology Group study. J Clin Oncol 14:357, 1996.

Lentz SS: Advanced and recurrent endometrial carcinoma: Hormonal therapy. Semin Oncol 21:100, 1994.

Lewis B, Stallworthy JA, Cowdell R: Adenocarcinoma of the body of the uterus. J Obstet Gynaecol Br Commonw 77:343, 1970.

Lewis GC, Slack NH, Mortel R et al: Adjuvant progestogen therapy in primary definitive treatment of endometrial cancer. Gynecol Oncol 2:368, 1974.

Long JH, Langdon RM, Cha SS et al: Phase II trial of methotrexate, vinblastine, doxorubicin and cisplatin in advanced/recurrent endometrial carcinomas. Gynecol Oncol 58:240, 1995.

Macdonald RR, Thorogood J, Mason MK: A randomized trial of progestogens in the primary treatment of endometrial carcinoma. Br J Obstet Gynaecol 95:166, 1988.

Maggino T, Romagnolo C, Landoni F et al: An analysis of approaches to the management of endometrial cancer in North America: A CTF Study. Gynecol Oncol 68:274, 1998.

Malkasian GD et al: Progestogen treatment of recurrent endometrial carcinoma. Am J Obstet Gynecol 110:15, 1971.

Mangioni C, DePalo G, DelVecchio M: Surgical pathologic staging in apparent stage I endometrial cancer. Int J Gynecol Cancer 3:373, 1993.

Massi G, Savino L, Susini T: Vaginal hysterectomy versus abdominal hysterectomy for the treatment of stage I endometrial adenocarcinoma. Am J Obstet Gynecol 174:1320, 1996.

Mohan DS, Samuels MA, Selim MA et al: Long-term outcomes of therapeutic pelvic lymphadenectomy for stage I endometrial adenocarcinoma. Gynecol Oncol 70:165, 1998.

Monson RR, MacMahon B, Austin JH: Postoperative irradiation and carcinoma of the endometrium. Cancer 31:630, 1973.

Moore DH, Fowler WC, Walton LA et al: Morbidity of lymph node sampling in cancers of the uterine corpus and cervix. Obstet Gynecol 65:251, 1985.

Moore TO, Phillips PH, Nerenstone SR et al: Systemic treatment of advanced and recurrent endometrial carcinomas: Current status and future direction. J Clin Oncol 9:1071, 1991.

Morris M, Alvarez RD, Kinney WK, Wilson TO: Treatment of recurrent adenocarcinoma of the endometrium with pelvic exenteration. Gynecol Oncol 60:288, 1996.

Morrow CP et al: A randomized study of Adriamycin adjuvant chemotherapy for patients with high risk stage I and II (occult) endometrial carcinoma. Presented by the International Gynecologic Cancer Society, Amsterdam, October 1987.

Morrow CP, DiSaia PJ, Townsend DE: Current management of endometrial carcinoma. Obstet Gynecol 42:399, 1973.

Muss HB: Chemotherapy of metastatic endometrial cancer. Semin Oncol 21:107, 1994.

Niloff JM, Klug TL, Schaetzl E et al: Elevation of serum CA125 in carcinoma of fallopian tube, endometrium, and endocervix. Am J Obstet Gynecol 148:1057, 1984.

Onsrud M, Kolstad P, Normann T: Postoperative external pelvic irradiation in carcinoma of the corpus stage I: A controlled clinical trial. Gynecol Oncol 4:222, 1976.

Orr JW, Holloway RW, Orr PF, Halimon JL: Surgical staging of uterine cancer: An analysis of perioperative morbidity. Gynecol Oncol 42:209, 1991.

Patterson E et al: Management of stage I carcinoma of the uterus. Obstet Gynecol 59:755, 1982.

Pecorelli S (ed), FIGO Annual Report, years 1996-98, Int J Gynecol Obstet 79-118, 2003.

Piver MS et al: Melphalan, 5-FU and medroxyprogesterone acetate in metastatic endometrial carcinoma. Obstet Gynecol 67:261, 1987.

Podratz KC, Mariani A, Webb MJ: Staging and therapeutic value of lymphadenectomy in endometrial cancer (Editorial). Gynecol Oncol 70:163, 1998.

Potish RA, Twiggs LB, Adcock LL et al: Para-aortic lymph node radiotherapy in cancer of the uterine corpus. Obstet Gynecol 65:251, 1985.

Poulsen HK, Jacobsen M, Bertelsen K et al: Adjuvant radiation therapy is not necessary in the management of endometrial carcinoma stage I, low risk cases. Int J Gynecol Cancer 6:38, 1996.

Randall ME, Reisinger S: Radiation therapy and combined chemoirradiation in advanced and recurrent endometrial carcinoma. Semin Oncol 21:91, 1994.

Rose PG, Cha SD, Tak WK et al: Radiation therapy for surgically proven para-aortic node metastasis in endometrial cancer. Int J Radiat Oncol Biol Phys 24:229, 1992.

Rutledge FN: The role of radical hysterectomy in adenocarcinoma of the endometrium. Gynecol Oncol 2:331, 1974.

Selman AE, Fowler JM, Martinez-Monge R, Copeland LJ: Doxorubicin and/or cisplatin based chemotherapy for the treatment of endometrial carcinoma with retroperitoneal lymph node metastases. Int J Gynecol Cancer 8:423, 1998.

Seski JC et al: Adriamycin and cyclophosphamide chemotherapy for disseminated endometrial cancer. Obstet Gynecol 58:88, 1981.

Seski JC: Cisplatin chemotherapy for disseminated endometrial cancer. Obstet Gynecol 59:225, 1982.

Straughn JM, Jr., Huh WK, Kelly J et al: Conservative Management of Stage I Endometrial Carcinoma after Surgical Staging. Gynecol Oncol 84:194, 2002.

Straughn JM, Jr., Huh WK, Orr JW et al: Stage IC adenocarcinoma of the endometrium: survival comparisons of surgically staged patients with and without adjuvant radiation therapy. Gynecol Oncol 89: 295, 2003.

Thigpen JT et al: Phase II trial of Adriamycin in treatment of advanced or recurrent endometrial carcinoma. Cancer Treat Rep 63:21, 1979.

Thigpen JT, Blessing JA, DiSaia PJ et al: A randomized comparison of doxorubicin alone versus doxorubicin plus cyclophosphamide in the management of advanced or recurrent endometrial carcinoma: A Gynecologic Oncology Group study. J Clin Oncol 12:1408, 1994.

Thigpen JT, Blessing JA, Homesley HD et al: Phase II trial of doxorubicin with and without cisplatin in advanced or recurrent endometrial carcinoma: A Gynecologic Oncology Group (GOG) study. Proc Am Soc Clin Oncol 12:261, 1993.

Thigpen JT: Cis-platinum in the treatment of advanced or recurrent cervix and uterine cancer. In Prestayka AW, Crooke ST, Carter SK (eds): Cisplatin: Current Status and New Developments. New York, Academic Press, 1980.

Thigpen T et al: A randomized comparison of Adriamycin with or without Cytoxan in the treatment of advanced recurrent adenocarcinoma (Abstract), Vol 4. American Society of Gynecologic Oncologists, May 1985, p 115.

Thigpen T et al: Treatment of advanced early recurrent endometrial cancer with medroxyprogesterone acetate (Abstract). Society of Gynecologic Oncologists, February 1985.

Thigpen T, Blessing J, Homesley H et al: Phase III trail of doxorubicin H-cisplatin in advanced or recurrent endometrial carcinoma. Proc Am Soc Clin Oncol 12:261, 1993.

Thigpen T, Blessing J, Homesley H et al: Phase III trial of doxorubicin with and without cisplatin in advanced or recurrent endometrial carcinoma. Proc Am Soc Clin Oncol 12:26, 1993.

Trimble EL, Kosary C, Park RC: Lymph node sampling and survival in endometrial cancer. Gynecol Oncol 71:340, 1998.

Trope C et al: A phase II study of cisplatin for recurrent corpus cancer. Eur J Cancer 16:1025, 1980.

Underwood PB et al: Carcinoma of the endometrium: Radiation followed immediately by operation. Am J Obstet Gynecol 128:86, 1977.

Watanabe M, Aoki Y, Kase H et al: Low risk endometrial cancer: A study of pelvic lymph node metastasis Int J Gynecol Cancer 13:38–41, 2003.

Wharam MD, Phillips TL, Bagshawe MA: The role of radiation therapy in clinical stage I carcinoma of the endometrium. AJR Am J Roentgenol 1:1081, 1976.

Zanetta G, Gabrielle GL, Cappellini A, Manggioni C: Conservative management of endometrial carcinoma with prolonged preservation of the uterus in a young patient. Int J Gynecol Cancer 7:332, 1997.

Zanotti KM, Belinson JL, Kennedy AW et al: The use of paclitaxel and platinum-based chemotherapy in uterine papillary serous carcinoma. Gynecol Oncol 74:272, 1999.

6 Sarcoma of the Uterus

D. Scott McMeekin, M.D.

CLASSIFICATION

Sarcomas are uncommon tumors arising from mesenchymal elements, and are distinguished from carcinomas that arise from epithelial elements. Uterine sarcomas are thought to arise primarily from two tissues; endometrial stroma, and from the uterine muscle itself. When endometrial stroma undergoes malignant transformation it may be accompanied by a malignant epithelial component (carcinosarcoma, formerly referred to as malignant mixed müllerian tumor), or may be associated with a benign appearing epithelial component (adenosarcoma), or with no recognizable epithelial component (endometrial stromal sarcoma). Tumors arising from malignant transformation of uterine smooth muscle are known as uterine leiomyosarcomas. Other sarcomas, such as angiosarcoma and fibrosarcoma, arise in supporting tissues and are rare.

In 1959, Ober suggested a classification of uterine sarcomas to categorize these tumors by cell type and site of origin. Tumors were called pure sarcomas if they consisted of one cell type only, whereas those that are mixed sarcomas consisted of more than one cell type. Homologous tumors contain tissue elements entirely indigenous to the uterus, whereas heterologous tumors are defined as those that contain tissue elements that are foreign to the uterus. Several modifications of this classification have been made over time as our understanding of these tumors has evolved, such as the schema suggested by Kempson and Bari (Table 6–1). The Gynecologic Oncology Group (GOG) has developed a histologic classification that reflects current trends (Table 6–2).

The classification of tumors known as mixed müllerian sarcomas or malignant mixed müllerian tumors (MMMTs) has undergone considerable evolution. These tumors must contain both carcinoma (malignant epithelial component) and sarcoma (malignant stromal component). Kempson and Hendrickson note that the carcinoma is usually endometrioid in type, but mucinous, squamous, papillary serous, and clear cell histologies alone or in mixtures are noted. When the malignant stromal component has features that are unique to uterine tissue (stromal sarcoma, leiomyosarcoma, fibrosarcoma) the tumors are called homologous types. When the stromal component produces tissue not normally found in the uterus, such as bone, cartilage, or skeletal muscle (osteosarcoma, chondrosarcoma, rhabdomyosarcoma), the tumors are designated as heterologous. Some importance was once placed upon the presence of homologous versus heterologous elements in the stromal component of these tumors. Currently, no distinction is made in terms of behavior or prognosis based on this factor, and MMMT tumors have been reclassified by most authorities under the heading of carcinosarcoma. As our understanding of these tumors at a cellular level has increased, there is now evidence that challenges whether carcinosarcomas are actually sarcomas or if they represent an extreme manifestation of undifferentiated endometrial cancers. For example, studies comparing immunohistochemical staining or genetic mutations between epithelial and stromal components show considerable overlap suggesting a common origin of the two components. While this debate continues, research organizations such as the GOG continue to separate carcinosarcomas from endometrial cancers in clinical trials.

Table 6–1 KEMPSON AND BARI CLASSIFICATION OF UTERINE SARCOMAS

I. Non-epithelial neoplasms
  a. Pure homologous
    i. Leiomyosarcoma
    ii. Stromal sarcoma
    iii. Endolymphatic stromal myosis
    iv. Angiosarcoma
    v. Fibrosarcoma
  b. Pure heterologous
    i. Rhabdomyosarcoma
    ii. Chondrosarcoma
    iii. Osteosarcoma
    v. Liposarcoma

II. Mixed sarcomas
  a. Mixed homologous
  b. Mixed heterologous

III. Malignant mixed müllerian tumors (mixed mesodermal tumors)
  a. Homologous type
  b. Heterologous type

IV. Sarcomas, unclassified

Modified from Ober, WB, Uterine sarcomas: histogenesis and taxonomy, Ann NY Acad Sci 75,568,1959 and Kempson RL, Bari W: Uterine sarcomas: Classification, diagnosis, and prognosis. Hum Pathol 1:332, 1970.

Table 6–2 GYNECOLOGIC ONCOLOGY GROUP CLASSIFICATION OF UTERINE SARCOMA

I. Non-epithelial neoplasms
  a. Endometrial stromal tumors
    i. Stromal nodule
    ii. Low grade stromal sarcoma
    iii. High grade stromal sarcoma
  b. Smooth muscle tumor of uncertain malignant potential
  c. Leiomyosarcoma
    i. Epithelioid
    ii. Myxoid
  d. Mixed endometrial stromal and smooth muscle tumor
  e. Poorly differentiated (undifferentiated) endometrial sarcoma
  f. Other soft tissue tumors
    i. Homologous
    ii. Heterologous

II. Mixed epithelial-non-epithelial tumors
  a. Adenosarcoma
    i. Homologous
    ii. Heterologous
    iii. With high-grade stromal overgrowth (see notes)
  b. Carcinosarcoma (malignant mixed mesodermal tumor or malignant mixed müllerian tumor)
    i. Homologous
    ii. Heterologous

Incidence and epidemiology

Sarcomas arising within the uterus are relatively rare. According to the Surveillance, Epidemiology and End Results (SEER) data reported by Brooks and colleagues covering 2677 cases from 1989–1999, the age-adjusted incidence for all sarcomas (per 100,000 women age 35 and over) in US women was 2.68 for native American/Asian/Hispanic, 3.58 for white, and 7.02 for black women. By comparison, the incidence for epithelial uterine cancers, per 100,000 women, is roughly 9 for black women and 20 for white women. Uterine sarcomas represented 8% of primary uterine malignancies in the most recent analysis of the SEER database. Harlow and coworkers had previously reported from SEER databases covering 1973–1981, which suggested an annual incidence of only 1.7 cases per 100,000 women. Sarcomas have been traditionally thought to represent only 3–5% of all uterine tumors. The increasing incidence of uterine sarcomas noted in the SEER studies may reflect better diagnosis, and perhaps a true increase in an aging population. Of the sarcomas, the most common, in order of decreasing incidence, are carcinosarcoma, leiomyosarcoma, endometrial stromal sarcoma, and adenosarcoma. Of the 1452 uterine sarcomas in Harlow's study, 86% were classified as carcinosarcoma (MMMT) or leiomyosarcoma. Sherman reporting on SEER data from 1992–1998 found that 53% of all sarcomas were carcinosarcomas.

The type and frequency of uterine sarcomas is related to both age and race. As Figure 6–1 demonstrates, carcinosarcoma is unusual before 40 years of age and begins to increase steadily thereafter. Leiomyosarcoma can occur at an early age, has an incidence plateau in middle age, and declines thereafter. In a large prospective surgical-pathologic study conducted by the GOG evaluating patients with all types of sarcomas, the median age of patients with leiomyosarcoma was 55 compared to 65 for those with carcinosarcoma. Brooks suggested that white women were older at the time of diagnosis of their sarcomas compared to blacks.

Using SEER data (1992–1998), Sherman and colleagues reported on racial differences in uterine malignancies. They found that for all histopathologic categories the age-adjusted incidence of uterine cancers (per 100,000 women) was 23 for non-Hispanic white, 14 for white Hispanic, and 15 for black women. In contrast, carcinosarcomas and leiomyosarcomas are more common in black women. For carcinosarcomas, the incidence was 0.78, 0.63, and 1.82 for non-Hispanic white, white Hispanic, and black women respectively. Similarly, for leiomyosarcomas, endometrial stromal sarcomas, and adenosarcomas combined, the incidence was 1.24 for black versus 0.79 for non-Hispanic white women. Harlow found the same trend reporting on an earlier SEER data set. It has also been suggested that blacks present with Stage I disease less commonly than whites.

Given that uterine sarcomas are rare and form a heterogeneous group, little is known about other risk factors favoring development of these tumors. For carcinosarcomas, there is some evidence that exposure to radiation may increase risk. A history of pelvic irradiation is noted in 5–10% of patients with sarcoma. Sarcomas have been reported to develop from 1–37 years from radiation exposure. Meredith and colleagues reported on 1208 women with uterine malignancies and identified 30 who had a history of prior pelvic irradiation. The authors estimated that frequency of carcinosarcomas after radiation (17%) exceeded the 5% baseline rate expected. Postradiation sarcomas are predominantly carcinosarcomas.

Given the molecular evidence that carcinosarcomas are biologically related to epithelial endometrial cancers, some investigators have attempted to determine whether the two tumor types share similar risk factors. Zelmanowicz and coworkers performed a multicenter case-control study comparing risk factors associated with women diagnosed with endometrial carcinomas and those with carcinosarcomas. They found that the two tumor types share similar risk factors related to estrogen exposure (obesity, exogenous estrogen exposure, nulliparity) and suggested that the pathogenesis was similar between the two tumors. Larger studies will need to be performed to confirm these findings. Tamoxifen exposure has also been suggested to increase the risk of endometrial cancer including carcinosarcoma. For women with leiomyosarcoma, a preoperative diagnosis of uterine leiomyoma is common. However, it has not been established that leiomyosarcoma arises in benign leiomyomas; in nearly all cases the sarcoma arises independently of the benign neoplasm.

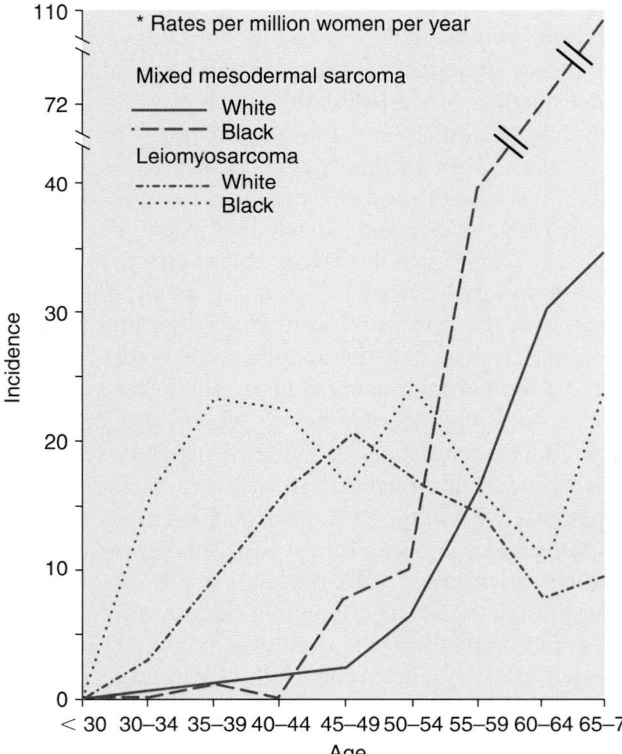

Figure 6–1 Incidence of uterine sarcoma among females by age, race, and histology: Surveillance, epidemiology, and end results (SEER) areas, 1973–1981. (From Harlow BL, Weiss NS, Lofton S: The epidemiology of sarcomas of the uterus. J Natl Cancer Inst 76:399, 1986. Reprinted with permission of Oxford University Press.)

CARCINOSARCOMA

Clinical profile

Most patients with uterine carcinosarcoma present with postmenopausal bleeding. As in other cases of postmenopausal bleeding, histologic evaluation by endometrial biopsy or curettage is mandatory, and will establish the diagnosis. Not infrequently, a large polypoid mass may extend from the endometrial cavity protruding through the cervical os which can be easily biopsied (Fig. 6–2). Carcinosarcomas have both malignant epithelial and stromal elements, but on small biopsies, the epithelial component can be the only one recognized preoperatively (Figs 6–3, 6–4). Some patients may present without bleeding, but with an enlarging pelvic mass due to tumor and hematometrium. Patients with advanced stage disease may present similarly to patients with ovarian cancer with pleural effusions, ascites, adnexal masses, and evidence of intraperitoneal disease spread.

Preoperative assessment with imaging studies is controversial. At a minimum, a chest X-ray is recommended given the potential for distant disease spread. For common endometrial cancers, routine preoperative CT scans have not shown to alter clinical management, but data are limited for patients with carcinosarcoma. Given the potential for intrauterine spread, a preoperative bowel preparation regimen is warranted. Consultation with a gynecologic oncologist should strongly be considered in cases with a preoperative diagnosis of carcinosarcoma. These tumors are aggressive and extrauterine spread is common compared to endometrial cancers.

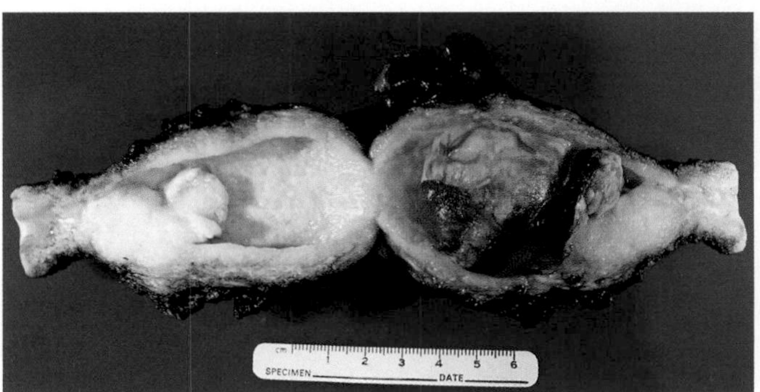

Figure 6–2 Uterine carcinosarcoma with polypoid mass filling uterine cavity, and with deep myometrial invasion. (Photo used with permission by Dr. Pablo Souza, Dept. Pathology, University of Oklahoma)

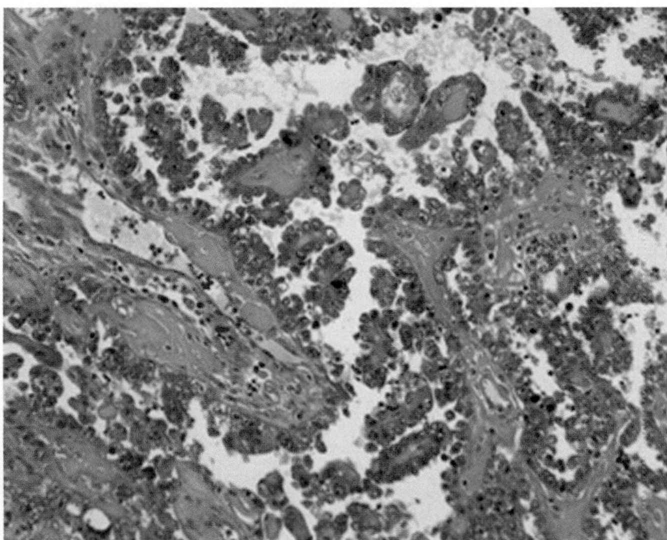

Figure 6–3 Photomicrograph of carcinosarcoma of the uterus with a high-grade epithelial component. (Photo used with permission by Dr. Pablo Souza, Dept. Pathology, University of Oklahoma)

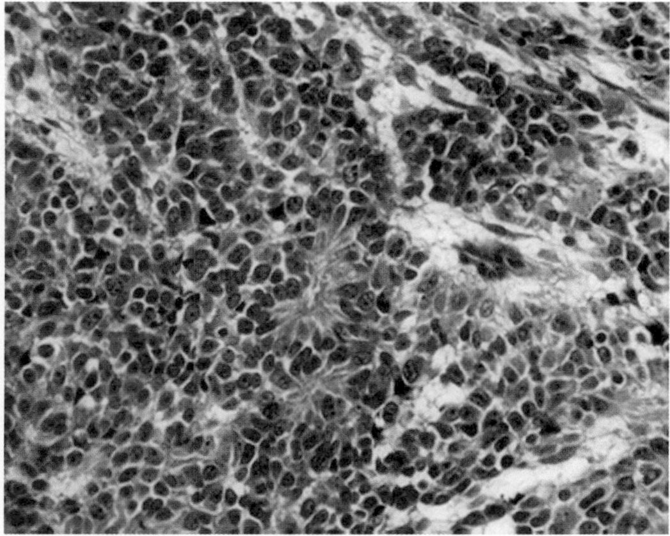

Figure 6–4 A stromal component from same tumor as Figure 6–3. (Photo used with permission by Dr. Pablo Souza, Dept. Pathology, University of Oklahoma)

Surgical management

The surgical management for patients with uterine carcinosarcoma should include collection of cytologic washings at the time of opening the abdomen, hysterectomy with bilateral salpingo-oophorectomy, and pelvic and para-aortic lymph node dissection. In cases where gross extrauterine disease is encountered, many advocate a debulking surgery akin to what is used to manage ovarian cancer. Surgical staging has been increasingly incorporated into the management of carcinosarcoma given the recognition that extrauterine disease spread is common.

In an early study by DiSaia and associates from the MD Anderson Hospital, 101 patients were evaluated, and more than 60% had disease outside the uterus at the time of diagnosis. Wolfson performed a multivariate analysis on 62 patients with uterine sarcoma, including 38 with carcinosarcoma, and found that surgical stage was the most important independent predictor for survival. The GOG conducted a large prospective study evaluating the patterns of spread in patients with uterine sarcomas, including 301 patients with clinical early staged carcinosarcoma. All patients underwent collection of pelvic washings, hysterectomy, and pelvic and para-aortic lymph node dissection. Following surgical staging, 21% were identified with positive cytologic washing, 37% had myometrial invasion into the outer half of the myometrium, 12% had adnexal metastases, and 17% had nodal involvement. Compared to a similar surgical staging study conducted by the GOG evaluating endometrial cancer patients, positive cytology was found in only 12%, deep myometrial invasion in 22%, adnexal involvement in 5%, and nodal metastases in 9% of cases (Table 6–3). For carcinosarcoma, following surgical staging 59% were Stage I, 21% Stage II, 9% were Stage III, and 11% were stage IV. In almost every case, when extrauterine metastases are encountered, only the epithelial component of the tumor is present.

Given the likelihood of spread outside of the uterus seen with carcinosarcoma, it is not unexpected that these tumors in general are thought to carry a poor prognosis. Spanos reported on 120 patients with carcinosarcoma of whom 67 recurred. Salazar reported on data from patients treated in the 1960–1970s and found only 29% of carcinosarcoma were alive at 2 years. In the GOG series, 53% of carcinosarcoma patients recurred. Even for patients with surgically staged Stage I disease, recurrences are common with about 40% of these patients recurring within 3 years of diagnosis. As in endometrial cancer, survival was related to the presence of nodal metastases, to the depth of myometrial invasion, and to whether the lower uterine segment or cervix was involved. It appears that patients with adnexal involvement also have a poor prognosis.

Even with the presumption by many that uterine carcinosarcoma represents a metaplastic high grade/undifferentiated endometrial cancer, some data indicate a different behavior between the two types. Amant and colleagues compared 104 patients with grade 3, papillary serous, or clear cell endometrial cancers to 33 with carcinosarcoma. For patients with stage I–II disease, patients with carcinosarcoma had a poorer survival and a higher incidence of pulmonary metastases. Carcinosarcoma was also an independent predictor of survival with a hazard ratio of 3.2 for recurrence compared to the other histologies. The authors suggested that carcinosarcoma should be studied separately from high-risk endometrial cancers given the difference in behavior.

The site of recurrence reflects the type of postoperative therapy used. For example, in the Spanos series, 95% of patients received adjuvant radiation therapy and 80% of all recurrences were at distant sites. The lung and abdomen accounted for 66% of all first sites of recurrence. In the larger GOG study, 40% received post-operative

Table 6–3 FREQUENCY AND DISTRIBUTION OF DISEASE SPREAD IN PATIENTS WITH UTERINE MALIGNANCIES

	Carcinosarcoma (n = 301)	Leiomyosarcoma (n = 59)	Endometrial adenocarcoma (n = 621)
Deep myometrial invasion	37%	–	22%
Positive peritoneal cytology	21%	5%	12%
Adnexal involvement	12%	3%	5%
Nodal metastases	17%	3.5%	9%

From Major FJ, Blessing JA, Silverberg SG et al: Prognostic factors in early-stage uterine sarcoma: A Gynecologic Oncology Group study. Cancer 71:1702, 1993 and Creasman WT, Morrow PC, Bundy BN et al: Surgical pathologic spread patterns of endometrial cancer: A Gynecologic Oncology Group study. Cancer 60:2035, 1987.

Table 6–4 PATTERNS OF FAILURE IN UTERINE SARCOMAS

	Carcinosarcoma (n = 301)		Leiomyosarcoma (n = 59)	
Site of 1st failure	No radiation (n = 182)	Radiation (n = 119)	No radiation (n = 46)	Radiation (n = 13)
Pelvis	24%	17%	17%	0
Extrapelvic	24%	16%	29%	8%
Lung	10%	19%	37%	54%
Other	11%	7%	4%	15%

Modified from Major FJ, Blessing JA, Silverberg SG et al: Prognostic factors in early-stage uterine sarcoma: A Gynecologic Oncology Group study. Cancer 71:1702, 1993.

pelvic radiation therapy with 17% of these patients recurring in the pelvis, 16% at an extrapelvic location, and 19% in the lung (Table 6–4). In the 60% of patients who received no radiation, 24% had a pelvic recurrence, 24% had an extrapelvic recurrence, and 10% recurred in the lung. In the GOG trial, therapy was not randomized, but was selected by the physician. Pelvic recurrences usually develop within the first 12–18 months after diagnosis and surgery.

Adjuvant therapy

To reduce the risk of recurrence, postoperative radiation therapy or chemotherapy has been used. The rarity of sarcomas has made prospective study or randomized clinical trails difficult. In older studies, all types of sarcomas were commonly grouped together so that the effect of therapy on a particular histologic type of sarcoma was largely unknown. Radiation therapy has been most commonly used in an effort to reduce pelvic failures. When radiation therapy is given, 5000–6000 cGy to the pelvis has been advocated, with some also recommending intravaginal brachytherapy to deliver a boost to the vaginal cuff or entire vagina. Preoperative radiation is infrequently used, and typically reserved to cases with bulky cervical involvement or parametrial extension.

Several retrospective series have shown improved rates of local control with the use of radiation, without necessarily improving survival compared to patients managed without radiation. Salazar and associates noted that in clinically stage I disease, there was no statistically significant difference in survival between surgery alone and surgery plus irradiation in leiomyosarcoma, carcinosarcoma, or endometrial stromal sarcoma (Table 6–5). This was true also of patients with more advanced disease. Isolated pelvic recurrence was rare showing the importance of extrapelvic sites of recurrence in this disease. In a prospective study conducted by the GOG, which included patients with Stage I–II uterine sarcomas of all types, 156 patients were randomized to postoperative treatment with doxorubicin or not. Pelvic radiation was permitted but not randomized. In this study, which included 93 patients with carcinosarcoma, 47% of patients recurred with or without the use of pelvic radiation therapy (Table 6–6). Pelvic radiation did appear to reduce local recurrences. Similarly there was not a statistically significant difference in recurrence rates, progression-free survival (PFS), or survival in patients who received doxorubicin or not.

What, then, is the possible role of radiation therapy in the management of uterine sarcomas? It appears that patients treated with radiation have a greater degree of local (pelvic) tumor control than that of patients treated with surgery only. Unfortunately, this was not reflected by an increased survival rate. In patients treated with radiation alone, the majority had recurrences, indicating that radiation therapy alone did not control these tumors. Because the main failure site is distant from the pelvis, the use of adjuvant local irradiation is ineffective in increasing the overall survival rate. This would suggest a need to identify systemic agents that could reduce distant sites of failure, or could be used in combination with radiation. Chemotherapy

Table 6–5 UTERINE SARCOMAS: SURVIVAL RATE IN TERMS OF STAGE, TREATMENT, AND PATHOLOGY

		Five-year survival rates		
	Cell Type (n)	S	S + R	R
Stage I	CS (63)	52%	48%	29%
	LMS (55)	58%	75%	33%
	ESS (24)	47%	88%	50%
Stage II–IV	CS (48)	5%	16%	0
	LMS (33)	0	13%	0
	ESS (18)	0	33%	0

Based on 142 patients with stage I disease (62% treated with S only, 30% treated with S+R, and 8% treated with R only) and 99 patients with stage II–IV disease (33% treated with S only, 46% treated with S+R, and 21% treated with R only).
S, surgery; S+R, surgery + radiation; R, radiation.
CS, carcinosarcoma; LMS, leiomyosarcoma; ESS, endometrial stromal sarcoma.
Modified from Salazar OM, Bonfiglio TA, Patten SF et al: Uterine sarcomas; natural history, treatment and prognosis. Cancer 42:1152, 1978.

Table 6–6 GYNECOLOGIC ONCOLOGY GROUP RANDOMIZED TRIAL OF DOXORUBICIN VERSUS NO FURTHER THERAPY IN COMPLETELY RESECTED STAGE I AND STAGE II UTERINE SARCOMA: RATES OF RECURRENCE

	Adjuvant doxorubicin (n = 75)		No chemotherapy (n = 53)	
CS (n = 90)	39%		51%	
LMS (n = 52)	44%		61%	
	Adjuvant doxorubicin (n = 75)		**No chemotherapy (n = 53)**	
	Radiation (n = 31)	**No Radiation (n = 44)**	**Radiation (n = 28)**	**No Radiation (n = 53)**
All sarcoma types (n = 156)	39%	43%	57%	51%
	Radiation +/– chemotherapy (n = 59)		**No radiation +/– chemotherapy (n = 97)**	
All sarcoma types (n = 156)	47%		47%	

CS, carcinosarcoma; LMS, leiomyosarcoma
Modified from Omura GA, Blessing JA, Majors F et al: A randomized clinical trial of adjuvant Adriamycin in uterine sarcoma: A Gynecologic Oncology Group study. J Clin Oncol 3:1240, 1985.

has been evaluated in an adjuvant setting, but identifying active drugs for use in upfront, adjuvant therapy has been difficult.

Wheelock reviewed a single institution's experience with 71 uterine sarcomas including 47 cases with carcinosarcoma, and found that neither radiation therapy nor chemotherapy was effective in prolonging survival. Van Rijswijk and colleagues reviewed the literature on the effects of chemotherapy on carcinosarcoma and indicated that response to doxorubicin as a single agent was low. These authors speculated on the role of cisplatin-based combinations for future development. As previously described, the GOG found no statistically significant difference in the progression-free interval or survival with the use of doxorubicin as an adjuvant therapy for treatment of uterine sarcomas. Resnik and coworkers and the group at Yale treated 42 patients with carcinosarcoma with a combination of etoposide, cisplatin, and doxorubicin. In the early-stage disease (I and II) group of 23 patients, a 2-year survival of 92% was achieved.

The GOG initially evaluated chemotherapy regimens in patient populations with advanced or recurrent disease who had all types of sarcomas. With the recognition that there are differences in prognosis and response between the histologic types, carcinosarcoma and leiomyosarcoma are now studied in separate phase II studies. To date, ifosfamide, cisplatin, and paclitaxel have shown the most promise for development for carcinosarcomas. Drawing on experience from patients with advanced and recurrent carcinosarcoma which found that the combination regimen of ifosfamide and cisplatin produced nearly a doubling in response rate and a modestly prolonged progression-free survival (PFS) compared to ifosfamide alone, the GOG initiated a randomized controlled trial comparing 3 cycles of ifosfamide and cisplatin to whole abdominal radiation therapy. This study, which recently completed planned enrollment, included 207 patients with Stages I–IV. Although data is maturing, preliminary results suggest that there may be an advantage to the chemotherapy arm. Alternatively, combining chemotherapy with radiation as a radiation sensitizer in this disease is being explored by other investigators. Although studies are ongoing, to date there is no standard proven adjuvant therapy for uterine carcinosarcoma.

Management of recurrent disease

Even in early stage disease, about half the patients with uterine sarcoma will develop a recurrence, as will approximately 90% of patients with disease extending outside of the uterus. Therapy for recurrent disease is obviously needed. Doxorubicin has been studied extensively in patients with all types of uterine sarcomas, given its importance in patients with soft tissue sarcomas. Hannigan and coworkers described 39 patients with recurrent disease treated with doxorubicin, either alone or in combination with other chemotherapeutic agents. The median survival was 7.2 months, and no patient lived >32 months after the start of chemotherapy. The response rate was only 10.3%, and there were no complete responders. The GOG performed a randomized trial comparing doxorubicin versus doxorubicin plus DTIC (dimethyl triazenoimidazole carboxamide) in 226 patients with stage III, stage IV, and recurrent sarcomas of the uterus. There were 148 patients with measurable disease; no difference in response was noted between doxorubicin and doxorubicin plus DTIC. In the non-measurable category, the PFS was similar between the two treatment arms. Response rate for leiomyosarcoma was 25% versus 15% for carcinosarcoma, and survival time of patients with leiomyosarcoma was significantly longer than that of patients with other cell types. The survival rate of the entire group was identical irrespective of the treatment given, and toxicity was appreciably increased with the addition of DTIC. This study was important as it suggested that there was a difference between sarcomas types and response to different agents.

In another GOG protocol, doxorubicin with and without cyclophosphamide was evaluated in 104 patients with stage III, stage IV, or recurrent sarcoma of the uterus. The response rate was identical for both regimens: 19% (complete and partial responses). Median survival was essentially the same: 11.6 months for doxorubicin and 10.9 months for doxorubicin and cyclophosphamide, with 80% of all patients dying by 2 years. The authors concluded that most patients in the study did not benefit from the chemotherapy used and suggested that strategies focusing on phase II trials to identify newer, more active agents rather than combinations of existing agents should be explored.

The first GOG trial to evaluate carcinosarcomas as a separate group was reported by Thigpen. This phase II study evaluated cisplatin in 28 patients with advanced or recurrent disease who had received prior chemotherapy and had measurable disease. The response rate was 18%, with two patients obtaining a complete response. A subsequent phase II study used cisplatin in a similar group of 63 patients who had not received prior chemotherapy, and noted a response rate of 19% (8% complete response).

Due to activity seen in soft tissue sarcomas, ifosfamide was selected for evaluation in uterine sarcomas. Using ifosfamide with the uroprotective agent mesna (2-mercaptoethane sodium sulfate), Sutton reported for the GOG on 28 patients with advanced or recurrent carcinosarcoma who had not received prior chemotherapy. He described a 32% response rate, including 18% of patients with a complete response. Given these promising results, interest in studying combination regimens in this disease resurfaced. The GOG evaluated ifosfamide and mesna with and without cisplatin in patients with advanced, persistent, or recurrent carcinosarcomas in a phase III study. The study evaluated 194 patients and found that response rate for ifosfamide alone was 36% compared to 54% for the combination. Patients treated with cisplatin had a modest improvement in median PFS of 2 months (6 months vs 4 months), but there was no statistically significant improvement in survival (ifosfamide, 9 months vs ifosfamide + cisplatin, 10 months, median survival). The combination regimen produced greater incidences of neutropenia, anemia, and peripheral neuropathy.

Paclitaxel has been evaluated in 44 patients with advanced or recurrent disease who all had received one prior chemotherapy regimen. Curtin for the GOG reported an 18% response rate with acceptable toxicity. A phase III trial comparing ifosphamide with and without paclitaxel has recently been conducted by the GOG. The addition of paclitaxel improved response, and progression-free and overall survival. A phase II study evaluating the combination of paclitaxel with carboplatin is ongoing. The GOG has developed a biologic queue to test novel targeted agents in patients with advanced carcinosarcoma, although the experience with these interesting agents is limited.

LEIOMYOSARCOMA

Clinical profile

As opposed to patients with carcinosarcoma who present with postmenopausal bleeding, patients with leiomyosarcoma have a median age of diagnosis of only 55 years. Many of these patients who complain of mennorhagia, are found to have a pelvic mass on examination, and will be thought to have uterine leiomyomas. Giuntoli, reporting on the Mayo Clinic experience of 208 patients with uterine leiomyosarcoma collected over a 23-year period, found that vaginal bleeding was the most common symptom (56%), followed by a palpable pelvic mass (54%), and pelvic pain (22%). A commonly described "clinical pearl" has been the relationship of a rapidly enlarging uterus to leiomyosarcoma. The data to support such an observation are mixed. Parker evaluated 1332 patients who underwent surgery for presumed leiomyoma. In the group of 371 patients who had rapid uterine growth, only one case (0.2%) of leiomyosarcoma was identified. Similarly in a subgroup of 198 patients who had carefully documented rapid uterine growth, no cases of leiomyosarcoma or carcinosarcoma were found. Leibsohn reported on 1432 patients undergoing hysterectomy for bleeding related to uterine leiomyomas and identified seven (0.49%) patients with leiomyosarcoma.

Because leiomyosarcoma arises within the uterine smooth muscle, biopsy of the malignant tissue is difficult, and many lesions are found only at final pathology. In Leibsohn's series, none of the seven patients with leiomyosarcoma was identified on preoperative biopsy, and in only three cases was there an intraoperative suspicion of sarcoma. Various authors have reported that leiomyosarcoma may be present in the submucosa of the uterus in 30–50% of patients; but even at that, biopsy diagnosis is not easily accomplished. Schwartz described the tumors to be both broad-based and pedunculated, and that in 19/20 cases the leiomyosarcoma was confined to one mass.

Several case reports have detailed the finding of leiomyosarcoma in patients who have undergone conservative management of symptomatic leiomyomas. Given the high prevalence of uterine leiomyomas in young women, fertility or uterine preserving strategies such as myomectomy, gonadotropin-releasing hormone GRNH (Lupron) treatment prior to myomectomy, and vascular embolization of leiomyomas have increasingly been used. Because of the difficulty in establishing a preoperative diagnosis of uterine leiomyosarcoma, it is not unexpected that incidental cases are occasionally encountered. These cases speak to the importance of pretreatment counseling of patients who undergo such therapies.

There is considerable discussion about the histologic criteria necessary for the diagnosis of leiomyosarcoma (Fig. 6–5). Leiomyosarcomas must be distinguished from a variety of benign smooth muscle tumors (Table 6–7). The predominant differentiating features between benign and malignant tumors include mitotic activity (as gauged by the number of mitotic figures per 10 high power fields), cellular atypia, and necrosis. Leiomyoma, cellular leiomyoma, and bizarre leiomyoma (also called atypical or symblastic leiomyoma), are considered to be benign. These entities are distinguished from leiomyosarcoma mainly by the mitotic count of the tumor. Although cellular leiomyomas and bizarre leiomyomas may appear at first sight to be malignant, they contain <5 mitoses/10 high-power fields (HPF) on histologic evaluation, and the prognosis is excellent with surgery only. Smooth muscle tumors of uncertain malignant potential (STUMP) include a group of smooth muscle tumors with 5–9 mitoses/10 HPF that can exhibit a variable behavior.

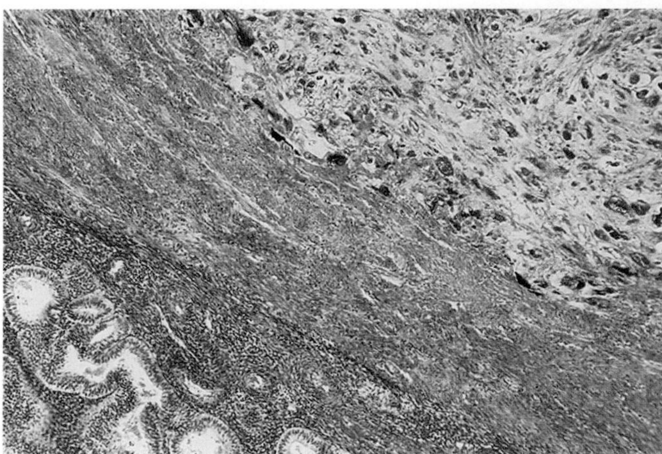

Figure 6–5 Photomicrograph of uterine leiomyosarcoma demonstrating the malignant lesion at the top right, normal endometrium at the bottom left, and normal myometrium between them.

Intravenous leiomyomatosis is a rare smooth muscle tumor characterized by nodular masses of histologically benign smooth muscle cells growing within venous channels that are lined by epithelium; arteries are not involved. Treatment involves surgical removal, and the prognosis is good. Recurrences are unusual and are usually managed successfully with further surgical excision.

Benign metastasizing leiomyoma is another rare condition in which smooth muscle tumor deposits are found in

Table 6–7 METASTATIC POTENTIAL OF SMOOTH MUSCLE TUMORS OF THE UTERUS

Mitotic figures/10 hpf	Atypia*	Diagnosis	Metastatic potential
1–4	Any degree	Leiomyoma	Very low
5–9	None	Leiomyoma with high mitotic activity	Very low
5–9	Grade 1	Smooth muscle tumor of uncertain malignant potential	Low
5–9	Grade 2 or 3	Leiomyosarcoma	Moderate
≥ 10	Grade 1	Leiomyosarcoma	High
≥ 10	Grade 2 or 3	Leiomyosarcoma	Very high

*Grade based on a scale of 3.
From O'Connor DM, Norris HJ: Mitotically active leiomyomas of the uterus. Hum Pathol 21:223, 1990.

the lung, lymph nodes, or abdomen and appear histologically like a benign leiomyoma. Most women have a history of pelvic surgery for benign leiomyomas years before these metastatic sites are recognized. Surgical excision has been the primary treatment.

Taylor and Norris believed that mitotic count was extremely important in that if <10 mitoses/10 HPF were identified, the lesion was benign regardless of the degree of cellular atypia; if >10 mitoses/10 HPF were present, the prognosis was grave. More recently, Norris stated that tumors with <5 mitoses/10 HPF can rarely metastasize. In a follow-up study from the Armed Forces Institute of Pathology, O'Connor and Norris evaluated 73 smooth muscle tumors of the uterus with 5–9 mitotic figures/10 HPF but lacking cytologic atypia. They concluded that the metastatic rate was too low to consider these as being sarcoma. Several of their patients were treated only with myomectomies with excellent results. Lissoni and colleagues have suggested extending this philosophy to additional patients.

Kempson and Bari believe that the mitotic count is important but state that prognosis is poor if >5 mitoses/10 HPF are identified. Their experience with tumors containing 5–9 mitoses/10 HPF indicates that the tumors usually behave aggressively and will metastasize. These authors believe that the degree of cellular atypia is of limited value by itself in determining the malignancy of smooth muscle tumors. In tumors with higher mitotic counts, there were usually a greater number of very atypical cells. This atypia was also seen in tumors with 5–9 mitoses/10 HPF. Tumors with <5 mitoses/10 HPF were thought to be benign regardless of the atypia of the cells. None of Kempson and Bari's patients with <5 mitoses/10 HPF had disease outside the uterus, whereas distant disease was a common finding if >5 mitoses/10 HPF were noted. The presence of coagulative necrosis, especially with diffuse significant atypia, suggests strongly that the lesion is a leiomyosarcoma regardless of the mitotic count.

On the other hand, Silverberg believes that the mitotic count alone cannot be used as a strict histologic criterion because he had patients with <10 mitoses/10 HPF who succumbed to their disease. He emphasized that the grade of the tumor, which reflects the cytologic atypia, is a better criterion than mitotic count alone. Essentially all investigators note the gravity of the situation if intravascular invasion or disease outside the uterus is found. Silverberg suggested that the single most important prognostic indicator is the menopausal status of the patient. Women who are premenopausal when the diagnosis is made tend to have a much better prognosis than that of women who are postmenopausal, even when criteria such as blood vessel invasion, growth pattern, grade, and mitotic counts are considered. Leiomyosarcomas occur in young patients and tend to be more localized when they are first diagnosed, and they probably exhibit a slower growth pattern than carcinosarcomas or endometrial stromal sarcomas do.

Surgical management

Planning the surgical management of leiomyosarcoma is difficult as many cases go unrecognized preoperatively. Patients commonly undergo myomectomy or hysterectomy for presumptive leiomyomas, which are subsequently identified as a sarcoma. In cases where a preoperative diagnosis is known, hysterectomy should be performed. Removal of the ovaries in premenopausal patients has not shown to worsen outcome in several retrospective series, and may be considered. Surgical staging with lymph node dissection is controversial, but most authorities tend to recommend biopsy of suspicious nodes only. In cases where leiomyosarcoma is recognized postoperatively, re-exploration for the purposes of completing surgical staging is not recommended. Following diagnosis, evaluation of the chest with chest x-ray or CT scan is reasonable given the propensity of spread to the lungs. Goff found that 10% of patients with leiomyosarcoma had lung metastases at presentation.

Data on patterns of spread for leiomyosarcoma are limited given the rarity of the tumor. Goff found that 16/21 patients had stage I disease at surgery, and only those patients with disseminated intra-abdominal disease had nodal involvement. Giuntoli reported that only 34/208 patients in the Mayo Clinic series had pelvic nodal dissections performed, and of the four with positive nodes, extrauterine disease was reported in three. The GOG sarcoma study on patterns of spread found that in 59 surgically-staged patients, 5% had positive extrauterine spread to peritoneal cytology, 3% had adnexal involvement, and 3.5% had nodal metastases (see Table 6–3). Following surgical staging 83% were stage I, and only 13% of patients were upstaged based on biopsies.

Leiomyosarcomas most commonly spread hematogenously. Corscaden and Singh reported the results of autopsies of 15 patients who died of leiomyosarcoma of the uterus. Of these patients, 100% had intra-abdominal visceral involvement, 80% had lung or pleural metastases, 40% had para-aortic nodal involvement, 33% had renal metastases, and 20% had liver metastases. In the GOG study the most common first site of recurrence was in the lung (41%), and only 13% had a pelvic failure (see Table 6–4).

The prognosis for leiomyosarcoma is poor, even for early stage disease. Vardi found that of the total group of 32 patients, 44% died of disease within the first 3 years after diagnosis. There was a 63.6% 5-year survival in women in whom diagnosis was made while they were premenopausal, compared with a 5.5% 5-year survival in postmenopausal women. The GOG found that only 31% of patients remained disease free at 3 years. Gadducci found that 39% of Stage I–II patients recurred with a median time to recurrence of 18 months. Berchuck reported that only 29% of patients with Stage I–II disease remained free of disease with a median follow-up of 7.5 years. Although almost all deaths and recurrences are during the 4 years after diagnosis, Gallup and coworkers reported a recurrence

25 years after initial therapy. Contrary to an older perception, these data would indicate that leiomyosarcomas have a poorer prognosis than carcinosarcomas.

Predictors of outcome have been assessed by several groups. The GOG found that patients with greater numbers of mitoses were associated with increased risk of recurrence such that 79% of patients with >20 mitoses/HPF recurred compared to 61% with 10–20 mitoses/HPF. Patients who present with extrauterine disease also have a very poor prognosis. Berchuck found no survivors beyond two years in this group of patients. Gadducci assessed 126 patients collected from a multi-institutional study and identified stage, mitotic count, and age as independent prognostic factors predicting recurrence. Giuntoli found that high grade, advanced stage, and having had ovaries removed at surgery were independent predictors of poorer survival.

Adjuvant therapy

For patients with leiomyosarcoma, no adjuvant therapy has been shown to be effective in prolonging survival. As with other high-risk uterine cancers, leiomyosarcomas have been managed postoperatively by radiation therapy or chemotherapy. Berchuck found that among patients receiving any form of adjuvant therapy, 83% recurred compared to 68% who underwent surgery alone. Given the propensity for hematogenous spread, radiation does not adequately address the high frequency of distant sites of failure (lung, liver, abdominal cavity). Supporters of radiation note that pelvic control may be obtained which can prevent bulky pelvic recurrences improving patient comfort and quality of life. In 15 Stage I–II patients treated with radiation therapy, Gadducci noted that 33% recurred, but no pelvic failures were seen. The GOG reported that only 3/13 patients who received radiation remained without recurrence, but no pelvic failures were seen. Giuntoli performed a subset analysis within his large series of patients identifying 31 patients who received adjuvant radiation therapy. In a comparison to 31 well-matched patients who did not receive radiation, there was not a statistically significant difference in survival between the groups, although 5-yr survival for those receiving radiation was 60% compared to 40% without radiation therapy. Similar to what has been reported for carcinosarcomas, radiation therapy is thought to have a limited role for the adjuvant management of leiomyosarcomas with radiation reducing pelvic failures, but not necessarily improving survival.

Given the importance of distant failures in this disease, chemotherapy has been used to manage early stage leiomyosarcomas. As discussed with carcinosarcomas, early chemotherapy trial included patients with all types of uterine sarcomas. In the GOG adjuvant trial evaluating the role of doxorubicin with or without radiation, 61% of patients with leiomyosarcoma treated without doxorubicin compared to 44% who received chemotherapy recurred (see Table 6–6). This study was too small to specifically evaluate the importance that histology played in response to therapy.

Management of recurrent disease

Data from randomized phase III trials conducted by the GOG, which included advanced and recurrent uterine sarcomas of all types, helped to identify the differential sensitivity of leiomyosarcomas compared to carcinosarcomas to different agents. In the trial comparing doxorubicin with and without DTIC, leiomyosarcomas were found to have a longer survival compared to other types when treated with a doxorubicin-containing regimen. In a subsequent study using doxorubicin with or without cyclophosphamide, histologic type was not found to be a prognostic indicator. Given that 80% of all patients died of disease within 2 years, the GOG adopted a strategy of performing phase II trials with the hope of identifying active agents that could later be tested in randomized studies. The rarity of leiomyosarcomas, however have made randomized study of this tumor impossible.

To date doxorubicin and ifosfamide have demonstrated the most promising activity inpatients with recurrent disease with responses ranging from 25–33% for doxorubicin and 18% for ifosfamide when used as single agents. Sutton and the GOG published the results of a phase II study combining ifosfamide and mesna and doxorubicin showing with an overall response rate of 30%. The duration response was 4 months, and the regimen produced substantial toxicity. Paclitaxel has been studied in leiomyosarcomas, with an 8% response seen in patients who had received prior chemotherapy, and a 9% response in those who were chemo-naïve. A novel combination of gemcitabine with docetaxel has shown a 53% response rate in a small phase II trial of patients, which included 29 patients with uterine leiomyosarcoma. This regimen is currently being evaluated by the GOG in a phase II study. Targeted biologic agents are also being explored, although no agent has yet to demonstrate activity in this tumor type. Patients with late recurrences of leiomyosarcoma in the form of isolated pulmonary metastases are candidates for thoracotomy and sequential resection of the lesions. Five-year survival of 30%–50% has been reported after such therapy.

ENDOMETRIAL STROMAL SARCOMA

Clinical profile

The most common symptom of endometrial stromal sarcoma (ESS) is irregular vaginal bleeding. Asymptomatic uterine enlargement, pelvic pain, or palpable mass are also common symptoms. The tumors are generally soft, fleshy, smooth, polypoid masses that may protrude into the endometrial cavity. The multiple-polyp form of the neoplasm has also been described, as has the characteristic yellow color of many of these lesions. On occasion, the

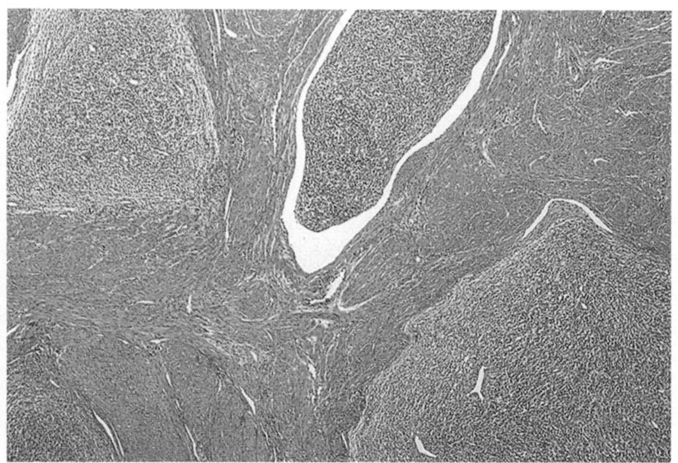

Figure 6–6 Low-power photomicrograph of a low-grade endometrial stromal sarcoma with invasion into myometrium.

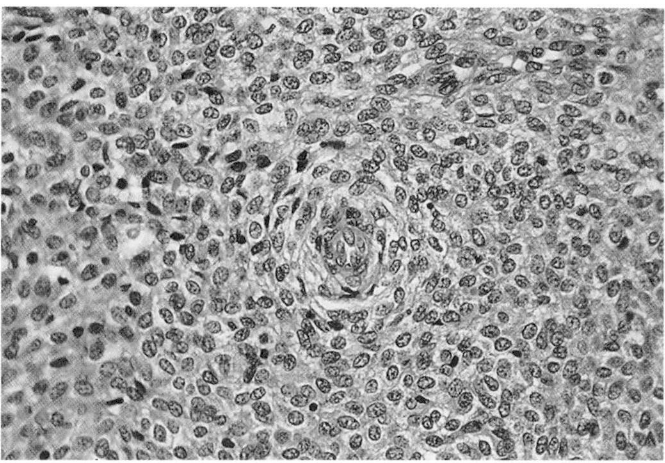

Figure 6–7 High-power view of low-grade endometrial stromal sarcoma shown in Figure 6–6.

uterine wall is diffusely enlarged by tumor without the presence of an obvious tumor mass. Preoperative diagnosis remains challenging, as endometrial biopsy may not identify the lesion in many cases.

In the past endometrial stromal tumors were largely grouped as either endolymphatic stromal myosis or endometrial stromal sarcoma. Endolymphatic stromal myosis was distinguished from stromal sarcomas by the minimal extent of tumor infiltration into the myometrium, the lack of metastases, and by an indolent clinical behavior. However, there was significant histologic overlap between the two entities, which made diagnosis difficult. Currently, endometrial stromal tumors are classified into two groups based on their metastatic potential. Stromal nodules are benign proliferations with the appearance indistinguishable from endometrial stroma of proliferative endometrium. They tend to be well-circumscribed lesions <15 cm, and do not demonstrate infiltrating margins or vascular space invasion. They behave like benign lesions without reported recurrences or metastases. Stromal sarcomas represent the second type of stromal neoplasm. Stromal sarcomas demonstrate local invasiveness or vascular and lymphatic space involvement, and infiltrate and separate the muscle fibers of the uterus. These tumors are separated into low-grade (<10 mitoses/10 HPF) and high-grade (>10 mitoses/10 HPF) stromal sarcomas, which exhibit very different behaviors.

Low-grade endometrial stromal sarcoma (LGESS), previously described as endolymphatic stromal myosis, can have an infiltrating growth pattern which on gross examination can project out in a wormlike fashion into the myometrium or into pelvic blood vessels. On microscopic examination, there is little or no cellular atypia, and there are few if any mitoses (Figs 6–6, 6–7). Although metastasis can occur, the clinical course is usually indolent, and surgery only is usually adequate treatment. Low-grade sarcomas may recur, but their clinical course is marked by late recurrences, typically greater than 5 years from diagnosis, with recurrences up to 25 years having been reported.

On the other hand, high-grade endometrial stromal sarcomas (HGESS) infiltrate the myometrium to a greater degree and have a more aggressive course, with frequent metastasis and poor prognosis. Norris and Taylor classified HGESS by the presence of ≥10 mitoses/10 HPF. From a review of 17 stromal sarcomas, Kempson and Bari noted that 10 tumors contained >20 mitoses/10 HPF, and 9/10 patients died of disease. Seven patients had tumors that contained ≤5 mitoses/10 HPF, and none have developed a recurrence. Pleomorphism was present in both groups of tumors, and thus was not a distinguishing feature. Kempson and colleagues subsequently reviewed 109 cases of endometrial stromal sarcoma and found that stage was the predominant predictor of behavior, even more so than the number of mitoses. For example, 45% of Stage I patients with rare mitosis and minimal atypia recurred. In this series, as long as the stromal cells appeared bland (similar to normal proliferative endometrial stromal cells), the 10 mitoses/10 HPF cutoff was not predictive of recurrence or survival. Patients with higher stage disease did have a greater frequency of mitoses.

Surgical management

The standard management for patients with stromal sarcoma is hysterectomy and bilateral salpingo-oophorectomy. The role of nodal dissections is unresolved, largely due to the fact there is a scarcity of data where complete surgical staging has been performed. Goff found no nodal disease, but only seven patients were evaluated. In the GOG surgical staging series, 52 stromal sarcomas were included but the frequency of nodal disease was not reported. Data suggest that bilateral salpingo-oophorectomy should be performed. Several investigators have suggested that recurrences were higher in patients who had ovaries preserved.

Patients with LGESS tend to present with disease confined to the uterus with Stage I–II disease being reported in approximately 70% of series. In contrast, patients with HGESS had Stage I–II disease in 40–50% of cases. In a retrospective review of 52 cases of LGESS by Piver and colleagues, 47% of stage I patients developed recurrence following surgery. Despite this, 5-year survival was 88% for Stage I and 100% for Stage II patients. Gadducci evaluated 66 patients with stromal sarcomas, including 26 with LGESS and 40 with HGESS. For 20 patients with Stage I–II low-grade tumors, 25% recurred (median follow-up 86 months), all in the pelvis. The median time to recurrence was 36 months, with a range of 4–108 months. For LGESS, 5-year survivals have ranged from 80–100%, despite the fact that 20–40% of patients eventually recur. Piver reported on patterns of failure in Stage I patients developed recurrences, with 12/19 recurrences being in the pelvis, 3/19 being at distant sites, and 4/19 had combined pelvic and distant failures.

The prognosis for HGESS is comparable to carcinosarcoma and leiomyosarcomas. Gadducci reported 5-year disease-free survival of only about 20% for this group of patients. The median time to recurrence is shorter than with LGESS, with a median time of 7 months. Mitotic count was an independent predictor of survival with patients with 10–20 mitoses/10 HPF having a 2-yr DFS of ~60% compared to ~10% if there were >20 mitoses/10 HPF. Other investigators have suggested 5-year survival between 20–55% for HGESS. Recurrences in the pelvis, abdomen, and lung are commonly seen, with the majority including at least some distant site of failure. A study of 24 patients with HGESS from the Mayo Clinic found that prognosis was related to the extent of disease, size of primary tumor, and grade. Mitotic count was not a prognostic factor, nor was DNA pattern.

Adjuvant therapy

As with other uterine sarcomas, adjuvant therapy has been evaluated to reduce recurrences. Gadducci had no recurrences in five low-grade patients who received adjuvant therapy versus 5/15 (33%) who did not. In the Piver study, five low-grade patients received postoperative pelvic radiation, and no recurrences were seen. Noting the sensitivity of advanced or recurrent disease to progestins, Piver suggested that adjuvant progestin therapy may be an effective strategy.

Berchuck reported recurrence rates of 57% with adjuvant chemotherapy or radiation therapy versus 56% who did not receive adjuvant therapy in 25 patients with Stage I ESS (high and low grade). Gadducci noted no benefit to adjuvant therapy in Stage I-II high-grade tumors. Given the rarity of ESS, no prospective study has been performed to identify active agents to be used in adjuvant treatment. As with other sarcoma types, radiation therapy may have a role in reducing pelvic recurrences, but with an unknown effect on survival.

Management of recurrent disease

While initial studies did allow for ESS patients, the small numbers of such patients included does not allow for interpretation of results. Low-grade endometrial sarcomas have a high frequency of progestin receptors making progestational agents reasonable. Piver found that progestins produced a 46% response rate in a small number of LGESS patients treated at recurrence. Responses lasted from 2–104. Recurrences of LGESS should be considered for local resection when they develop in the pelvis. For high-grade ESS, limited success has been reported with drugs commonly used for uterine sarcomas, including ifosfamide and doxorubicin.

OTHER SARCOMAS

Clement and Scully described 100 cases of adenosarcoma of the uterus. This is an unusual tumor with low malignant potential. Like other endometrial lesions, adenosarcoma usually presents with abnormal vaginal bleeding. On gross evaluation, the tumor is usually a polypoid mass that can fill the endometrial cavity. Involvement of the cervix and myometrium is less commonly seen. Histologic evaluation notes benign or atypical neoplastic glands with a sarcomatous stroma. In 78% of patients, the sarcomatous stroma was homologous. Stromal mitotic rate was 1–40/10 HPF. Extensive stromal fibrosis was common. Myometrial invasion was present in only 15, and it was deeply invasive in only 4. Recurrence became apparent in 23 patients and in one-third appeared 5 years after diagnosis. Recurrence was confined to the vagina, pelvis, or abdomen with two exceptions. Of those with recurrence, only 11 died with tumor. Only the presence of myometrial invasion was associated with an increased risk of recurrence. A variant of adenocarcinoma is a pattern that has been called adenosarcoma with sarcomatous overgrowth. This is characterized by overgrowth of the neoplasm by a pure sarcomatous component occupying at least 25% of the lesion. It is an ominous feature with reported recurrence rates exceeding 50% compared with the usual adenosarcoma.

Pure heterologous uterine sarcomas are rare. Of these, rhabdomyosarcoma is the most common, followed by chondrosarcoma and osteosarcoma. Rhabdomyosarcoma is derived from primitive myogenic precursors and is the most common soft tissue tumor in children and adolescents; 21% occur in genitourinary sites, and 20% of these in the uterus. Therapy has evolved from radical surgery and radiation therapy to more reliance on chemotherapy. Some authors have reported successful preservation of reproductive functions.

BIBLIOGRAPHY

CLASSIFICATION

DiSaia PJ, Pecorelli S: Gynecological sarcomas. Semin Surg Oncol 10:369, 1995.

Kempson RL, Bari W: Uterine sarcomas: Classification, diagnosis, and prognosis. Hum Pathol 1:331, 1970.

Kempson RL, Hendrickson MR. Smooth muscle, endometrial stromal, and mixed mullerian tumors of the uterus. Mod Pathol 13:328, 2000.

McCluggage WG. Uterine carcinosarcomas are metaplastic carcinomas. Int J Gynecol Cancer 12:687, 2002.

Ober WB: Uterine sarcomas: Histogenesis and taxonomy. Ann N Y Acad Sci 75:568, 1959.

Wada H, Enomoto T, Fujita M, et al: Molecular evidence that most but not all carcinosarcomas of the uterus are combination tumors. Cancer Res 57:5379, 1997.

Zhe J, Ogata S, Tamura G, et al: Carcinosarcomas (malignant mullerian mixed tumors) of the uterus and ovary: a genetic study with special reference to histogenesis. Internat J Gynecol Path 22:368, 2003.

INCIDENCE AND EPIDEMIOLOGY

Brooks SE, Zhan M, Cote T et al: Surveillance, epidemiology, and end results analysis of 2677 cases of uterine sarcoma 1989–1999. Gynecol Oncol 93:204, 2004.

Curtis RE, Freedman DM, Sherman ME et al: Risk of malignant mixed müllerian tumors after tamoxifen therapy for breast cancer. J Natl Cancer Inst 96:70, 2004.

Harlow BL, Weiss NS, Lofton S. The epidemiology of sarcomas of the uterus. J Natl Cancer Inst 76:399, 1986.

Meredith RF, Eisert DR, Kaka Z et al: An excess of uterine sarcomas after pelvic irradiation. Cancer 58:2003, 1986.

Sherman ME, Devesa SS: Analysis of racial differences in incidence, survival, and mortality for malignant tumors of the uterine corpus, Cancer 98:176, 2003.

Zelmanowicz A, Hildesheim A, Sherman ME et al: Evidence for a common etiology for endometrial carcinomas and malignant mixed müllerian tumors. Gynecol Oncol 69:253, 1998.

CARCINOSARCOMA

Amant F, Cadron I, Fuso L et al: Endometrial carcinosarcomas have a different prognosis and pattern of spread compared to high-risk epithelial endometrial cancer. Gynecol Oncol 98:274, 2005.

Arrastia CD, Fruchter RG, Clark MC et al: Uterine carcinomas: Incidence and trends in management and survival. Gynecol Oncol 65:158, 1997.

Buchsbaum HJ, Lifshitz S, Blythe JG: Prophylactic chemotherapy in stage I and II uterine sarcoma. Gynecol Oncol 8:346, 1979.

Callister M, Ramondetta LM, Jhingran A et al: Malignant mixed müllerian tumors of the uterus: analysis of patterns of failure, prognostic factors, and treatment outcome. Int J Rad Oncol Biol Phys 58:786,2004.

Chauveinc L, Deniaud E, Plancher C et al: Uterine sarcomas: The Curie Institut experience. Prognostic factors and adjuvant treatments. Gynecol Oncol 72:232, 1999.

Chi DS, Mychalczak B, Saigo PE et al: The role of whole-pelvic irradiation in the treatment of early-stage uterine carcinosarcoma. Gynecol Oncol 65:493, 1997.

Creasman WT, Morrow CP, Bundy BN et al: Surgical pathologic spread patterns of endometrial cancer: a Gynecologic Oncology Group study. Cancer 60:2035, 1987.

Connor JP, Andrews JI, Anderson B et al: Computeed tomography in endometrial cancer. Obstet Gynecol 95:692, 2000.

Curtin JP, Blessing JA, Soper JT et al: Paclitaxel in the treatment of carcinosarcoma of the uterus: A Gynecologic Oncology Group study. Gynecol Oncol 83:268, 2001

DiSaia PJ, Catro JR, Rutledge FN: Mixed mesodermal sarcoma of the uterus. AJR Am J Roentgenol 117:632, 1973.

DiSaia PJ, Morrow CP, Boronow R et al: Endometrial sarcoma; lymphatic spread pattern. Am J Obstet Gynecol 130:104, 1978.

Gerszten K, Faul C, Kounelis S et al: The impact of adjuvant radiotherapy on carcinosarcoma of the uterus. Gynecol Oncol 68:8, 1998.

Hannigan EV, Freedman RS, Rutledge FN. Adjuvant chemotherapy in early uterine sarcoma. Gynecol Oncol 15:56, 1983.

Hannigan EV, Freedman RS, Elder KW. Treatment of advanced uterine sarcoma with adriamycin. Gynecol Oncol 16:101, 1983.

Homesley H, Filiaci V, Bitterman P, Eaton L, et al. Phase III trial of ifosfamide versus ifosfamide plus paclitaxel as first-line treatment of advanced or recurrent uterine carcinosarcoma: A Gynecologic Oncology Group study. Gynecol Oncol 101 S1:S31, 2006.

Hornback NB, Omura G, Major FJ. Observations on the use of adjuvant radiation therapy in patient with stage I and II uterine sarcoma, Int J Radiation Oncol Biol Phys 12:2127, 1986.

Le T, Krepart GV, Lotocki RJ, Hewood MS: Malignant mixed mesodermal ovarian tumor treatment and prognosis: A 20 year experience. Gynecol Oncol 65:237, 1997.

Major FJ, Blessing JA, Silverberg SG et al: Prognostic factors in early stage uterine sarcoma. Int J Gynecol Pathol 11:75, 1992.

Major FJ, Blessing JA, Silverberg SG et al: Prognostic factors in early-stage uterine sarcoma: A Gynecologic Oncology Group study. Cancer 71:1702, 1993.

Marchese MJ et al: Uterine sarcomas: A clinico-pathologic study, 1965–1981. Gynecol Oncol 18:299, 1984.

Muss HB, Bundy BN, DiSaia PJ et al: Treatment of recurrent or advanced uterine sarcoma: A randomized trial of doxorubicin versus doxorubicin and cyclophosphamide. Cancer 55:1648, 1985.

Omura GA, Blessing JA, Majors F et al: A randomized clinical trial of adjuvant Adriamycin in uterine sarcoma: A Gynecologic Oncology Group study. J Clin Oncol 3:1240, 1985.

Omura GA, Major FJ, Blessing JA et al: A randomized study of adriamycin with and without demethyl triazenoimidazole carboxamide in advanced uterine sarcomas, Cancer 52:626, 1983.

Peters WA, Kumar NB, Fleming WP: Prognostic features of sarcomas and mixed tumors of the endometrium. Obstet Gynecol 63:550, 1984.

Podczaski ES, Woomert CA, Stevens CW et al: Management of malignant, mixed mesodermal tumors of the uterus. Gynecol Oncol 32:240, 1989.

Resnik E, Chambers SK, Carcangiu ML et al: A phase II study of etoposide, cisplatin and doxorubicin chemotherapy in mixed müllerian tumors of the uterus. Gynecol Oncol 56:370, 1995.

Saksela E, Lampinen V, Procopé B: Malignant mesenchymal tumors of the uterine corpus. Am J Obstet Gynecol 120:452, 1974.

Salazar OM, Bonfiglio TA, Patten SF et al: Uterine sarcomas: Natural history, treatment and prognosis. Cancer 42:1152, 1978.

Salazar OM, Bonfiglio TA, Patten SF et al: Uterine sarcomas: analysis of failures with special emphasis on the use of adjuvant radiation therapy. Cancer 42:1161, 1978.

Santos A, Tursz T, Mouridsen H et al: Doxorubicin versus CYVADIC versus doxorubicin plus ifosfamide in first line treatment of advanced soft tissue sarcoma. J Clin Oncol 13:1537, 1995.

Sartori E, Bazzurini L, Gadducci A et al: Carcinosarcoma of the uterus: A clinicopathological multicenter CTF study. Gynecol Oncol 67:70, 1997.

Spanos WJ, Peters LJ, Oswald MJ. Patterns of recurrence in malignant mixed mullerian tumor of the uterus. Cancer 57:155, 1986.

Sutton GP, Blessing JA, Rosenshein N et al: Phase II trial of ifosfamide and mesna in mixed mesodermal tumors of the uterus: a Gynecologic Oncology Group study, Am J Obstet Gynecol 12:161, 1989.

Sutton G, Brunetto VL, Kilgore L et al: A phase III trial of ifosfamide with or without cisplatin in carcinosarcoma of the uterus: A Gynecologic Oncology Group study. Gynecol Oncol 79: 147, 2000.

Thigpen JT, Blessing JA, Beecham J et al: Phase II trial of cisplatin as first line chemotherapy in patients with advanced or recurrent uterine sarcomas: a Gynecologic Oncology Group study. J Clin Oncol 9: 1962, 1991

Thigpen JT, Blessing JA, Orr JW et al: Phase II trial of cisplatin in the treatment of patients with advanced or recurrent mixed mesodermal sarcomas of the uterus: A Gynecologic Oncology Group study. Cancer Treat Rep 70:271,1986.

Van Rijswijk REN, Tognon G, Burger CW et al: The effect of chemotherapy on the different components of advanced carcinosarcomas (malignant mixed mesodermal tumors) of the female genital tract. Int J Gynecol Cancer 4:52, 1994.

Wheelock JB, Krebs HB, Schneider V et al: Uterine sarcoma: analysis of prognostic variables in 71 cases, Am J Obstet Gynecol 151:1016, 1985.

Wolfson AH, Wolfson DJ, Sittler SY et al: A multivariate analysis of clinicopathologic factors for predicting outcome in uterine sarcomas. Gynecol Oncol 52:56, 1994.

LEIOMYOSARCOMA

Amada S, Nakano H, Tsuneyoshi M. Leiomyosarcoma versus bizarre and cellular leiomyomas of the uterus: A comparative study based on the MIB-1 and proliferating cell nuclear antigen indices, p53 expression, DNA flow cytometry, and muscle specific actins. Int J Gynecol Pathol 14:134, 1995.

Bell SW, Kempson RL, Hendrickson MR: Problematic uterine smooth muscle neoplasms. A clinicopathologic study of 213 cases. Am J Surg Pathol 18:535, 1994.

Berchuck A, Rubin SC, Hoskins WJ: Treatment of uterine leiomyosarcoma. Obstet Gynecol 71:845, 1988.

Blom R, Guerrieri C, Stal O et al: Leiomyosarcoma of the uterus: A clinicopathologic, DNA flow cytometric, p53, and mdm-2 analysis of 49 cases. Gynecol Oncol 68:54, 1998.

Burns B, Curry RH, Bell ME. Morphologic features of prognostic significance in uterine smooth muscle tumors: A review of 84 cases. Am J Obstet Gynecol 135:109, 1979.

Cadducci A, Landoni F, Sartori E et al: Uterine leiomyosarcoma: Analysis of treatment failures and survival. Gynecol Oncol 62:25, 1996.

Christopherson WM, Williamson EO, Gray LA: Leiomyosarcomas of the uterus. Cancer 29:1512, 1972.

Clement PB: Intravenous leiomyomatosis of the uterus. Pathol Annu 2:153, 1988.

Corscaden JA, Singh BP: Leiomyosarcoma of the uterus. Am J Obstet Gynecol 77:286, 1959.

Currie JL, Blessing JA, Muss HB et al: Combination chemotherapy with hydroxyurea, dacarbazine (DTIC), and etoposide in the treatment of uterine leiomyosarcoma: A Gynecologic Oncology Group study. Gynecol Oncol 61:27, 1996.

D'Angelo A, Amso NM, Wood A. Uterine leiomyosarcoma discovered after uterine artery embolization. J Obstet Gynaecol 23:686, 2003.

Evans HL, Chawla SP, Simpson C et al: Smooth muscle neoplasms of the uterus other than ordinary leiomyoma: A study of 46 cases, with emphasis on diagnostic criteria and prognostic factors. Cancer 62:2239, 1988.

Gadducci A, Landone F, Sartore E et al: Uterine leiomyosarcoma: analysis of treatment failures and survival. Gynecol Oncol 62:25, 1996.

Gal AA, Brooks JJ, Pietra GG. Leiomyomatous neoplasms of the lung. Mod Pathol 2:209, 1989.

Gallup DG, Blessing JA, Anderson W et al: Evaluation of paclitaxel in previously treated leiomyosarcoma of the uterus: a gynecologic oncology group study. Gynecol Oncol 89:48, 2003.

Gallup DG, Hobbs LH, Ross WB: Recurrence of uterine leiomyosarcoma 25 years after therapy. Gynecol Oncol 13:293, 1982.

Giuntoli RL, Metzinger DS, DiMarco CS et al: Retrospective review of 208 patients with leiomyosarcoma of the uterus: prognostic indicators, surgical management, and adjuvant therapy. Gynecol Oncol 89:460, 2003.

Goff BA, Rice LW, Fleischhacker D et al: Uterine leiomyosarcoma and endometrial stromal sarcoma: Lymph node metastases and sites of recurrence. Gynecol Oncol 50:105, 1993.

Hensley ML, Maki R, Venkatranab E et al. Gemcitabine and docetaxel in patients with unresectable leiomyosarcoma: results of a phase II trial. J Clin Oncol 20:2824, 2002.

Leibsohn S, d'Ablaing G, Mishell DR et al: Leiomyosarcoma in a series of hysterectomies performed for presumed uterine leiomyomas, Am J Obstet Gynecol 76:162, 1990.

Levenback C, Rubin SC, McCormack PM et al: Resection of pulmonary metastases from uterine sarcomas. Gynecol Oncol 45:202 1992.

Lissoni A, Cormio G, Bonazzi C et al: Fertility-sparing surgery in uterine leiomyosarcoma. Gynecol Oncol 70:348, 1998.

Mayerhofer K, Obermair A, Windbichler G et al: Leiomyosarcoma of the uterus: A clinicopathologic multicenter study of 71 cases. Gynecol Oncol 74:196, 1999.

Meyer WR, Mayer AR, Diamond MP et al: Unsuspected leiomyosarcoma: treatment with a gonadotropin-releasing hormone analogue. Obstet Gynecol 75:529, 1990.

Nordal RN, Kjorstad KE, Stenweg AE, Tropé CE: Leiomyosarcoma and endometrial stromal sarcoma of the uterus. Int J Gynecol Cancer 3:110, 1993.

O'Connor DM, Norris HJ: Mitotically active leiomyomas of the uterus. Hum Pathol 21:223, 1990.

Oliva E, Young RH, Clement PB et al: Cellular benign mesenchymal tumors of the uterus. A comparative morphologic and immunohistochemical analysis of 33 highly cellular leiomyomas and six endometrial stromal nodules, two frequently confused tumors. Am J Surg Pathol 19:757, 1995.

Parker WH, Fu YS, Berek JS. Uterine sarcoma in patients operated on for presumed leiomyoma and rapidly growing leiomyoma. Obstet Gynecol 83:414, 1994.

Peters WA, Howard DR, Anderson WA, Figge DC: Uterine smooth muscle tumor of uncertain malignant potential. Obstet Gynecol 83:1015, 1994.

Rose PG, Blessing JA, Soper JT et al: Prolonged oral etoposide in recurrent or advanced leiomyosarcoma of the uterus: A Gynecologic Oncology Group study. Gynecol Oncol 70:267, 1998.

Schwartz LB, Diamond MP, Schwartz PE: Leiomyosarcomas: Clinical presentation, Am J Obstet Gynecol 180-3:168, 1993.

Silverberg SG: Leiomyosarcoma of the uterus. Obstet Gynecol 38:613, 1971.

Sutton G, Blessing JA, Ball H et al: Phase II Trial of paclitaxel in leiomyosarcoma of the uterus: a Gynecologic Oncology Group study. Gynecol Oncol 74:346, 1999.

Sutton G, Blessing JA, Malfetano JH et al: Ifosfamide and doxorubicin in the treatment of advanced leiomyosarcomas of the uterus: a Gynecologic Oncology Group study. Gynecol Oncol 62:226, 1996.

Sutton G, Blessing J, McGuire W et al: Phase II trial of ifosfamide and mesna in leiomyosarcoma of the uterus. Gynecol Oncol 36:295, 1990.

Taylor HB, Norris HJ: Mesenchymal tumors of the uterus. IV: Diagnosis and prognosis of leiomyosarcomas. Arch Pathol 82:40, 1966.

Thigpen JT, Blessing JA, Wilbanks GD: Cisplatin as second line chemotherapy in the treatment of advanced or recurrent leiomyosarcoma of the uterus. Am J Clin Oncol 9:18, 1986.

Thigpen T, Blessing JA, Yordan E et al: Phase II trial of etoposide in leiomyosarcoma of the uterus: a Gynecologic Oncology Group study. Gynecol Oncol 63:120, 1996.

Vardi JR, Tovel HM: Leiomyosarcoma of the uterus: Clinico-pathologic study, Obstet Gynecol 56:428, 1980.

ENDOMETRIAL STROMAL SARCOMA

Bohr L, Thomsen CF: Low-grade stromal sarcoma: A benign appearing malignant uterine tumour; a review of current literature. Differential diagnostic problems illustrated by four cases. Eur J Obstet Gynecol Reprod Biol 39:63, 1991.

Chang KL, Crabtree GS, Lim-Tan SK et al: Primary uterine endometrial stromal neoplasms: a clinicopathologic study of 117 cases. Am J Surg Pathol 14:415, 1990.

DiSaia PJ, Morrow CP, Boronow R et al: Endometrial sarcoma: lymphatic spread pattern. Am J Obstet Gynecol 130:104, 1978.

DeFusio PA, Gaffey TA, Malkasian GD et al: Endometrial stromal sarcomas: Review of Mayo Clinic experience, 1945–1980. Gynecol Oncol 35:8, 1989.

Evans HL: Endometrial stromal sarcoma and poorly differentiated endometrial sarcoma. Cancer 50:2170, 1982.

Gadducci A, Sartori E, Landoni F et al: Endometrial stromal sarcoma: Analysis of treatment failures and survival. Gynecol Oncol 63:247, 1996.

Lehrner LM, Miles PA, Enck RE: Complete remission of widely metastatic endometrial stromal sarcoma following combination chemotherapy. Cancer 43:1189, 1979.

Lin YC, Kudelka AP, Tresukosol D et al: Case report: Prolonged stabilization of progressive endometrial stromal sarcoma with prolonged oral etoposide therapy. Gynecol Oncol 58:262, 1995.

Lissoni A, Cormio G, Perego P et al: Conservative management of endometrial stromal sarcoma in young women. Int J Gynecol Oncol 7:364, 1997

Nordal RR, Kristensen GB, Kaeren J et al: The prognostic significance of surgery, tumor size, malignancy grade, menopausal status, and DNA ploidy in endometrial stromal sarcoma. Gynecol Oncol 62:254, 1996.

Norris HF, Taylor HB: Mesenchymal tumors of the uterus. I: A clinical and pathological study of 53 endometrial stromal tumors. Cancer 19:755, 1966.

Piver MS, Rutledge FN, Copeland L et al: Uterine endolymphatic stromal myosis: A collaborative study, Obstet Gynecol 64:173, 1984.

Scribner DR, Walker JL: Case report: Low-grade endometrial stromal sarcoma preoperative treatment with Depo-Lupron and Megace. Gynecol Oncol 71:458, 1998.

OTHER SARCOMAS

Clement PB: Müllerian adenosarcoma of the uterus with sarcomatous overgrowth: A clinicopathological analysis of 10 cases. Am J Surg Pathol 13:28, 1989.

Clement PB, Scully RE: Müllerian adenosarcoma of the uterus: A clinical pathological analysis of 100 cases with review of the literature. Hum Pathol 21:363, 1990.

Hammerman RM, Runowicz CD: Conservative management of uterine rhabdomyosarcoma. Obstet Gynecol 92:669, 1998.

Kaku T, Silverberg SG, Blessing J et al: Adenosarcoma of the uterus: a Gynecologic Oncology Group clinicopathologic study of 31 cases. Int J Gynecol Pathol 11:75, 1992.

Krivac TC, Seidman JD, McBroom JW et al: Uterine adenosarcoma with sarcomatous overgrowth versus uterine carcinosarcoma: comparison of treatment and survival. Gynecol Oncol 83:89, 2001.

Zaloudek CJ, Norris HJ: Adenofibroma and adenosarcoma of the uterus: A clinicopathologic study of 35 cases. Cancer 48:354, 1981.

7 Gestational Trophoblastic Disease

John Soper, M.D. and William T. Creasman, M.D.

Gestational trophoblastic disease comprises a spectrum of neoplastic conditions in women derived from the placenta. Complete and partial hydatidiform mole, invasive mole, gestational choriocarcinoma and placental trophoblastic tumor are histologic diagnoses, while postmolar gestational trophoblastic neoplasia (GTN) is defined by clinical and laboratory criteria. Non-invasive and invasive moles usually have a relatively self-limited course, while choriocarcinoma can have a fulminant course marked by extremely short doubling times and a propensity for widespread metastasis. The term gestational trophoblastic disease includes all of these entities, while GTN refers specifically to the forms with the potential for tissue invasion and metastasis.

Gestational trophoblastic disease has been known since antiquity. Hippocrates, writing four centuries before the birth of Christ, described hydatidiform mole as dropsy of the uterus and attributed it to unhealthy water. In the 13th century, the tombstone of Countess Henneberg noted that at 40 years of age she had delivered 365 children: half were christened John and half were christened Elizabeth; this reflected identification of individual hydropic molar villi as individual fetuses (Fig. 7–1). William Smellie, in 1700, was the first to use the terms *hydatid* and *mole*. In the early 19th century, Velpeau and Boivin recognized the hydatidiform mole as cystic dilatation of the chorionic villi. In 1895, Felix Marchand demonstrated that the hydatidiform mole, and less commonly a normal pregnancy or abortion, preceded the development of choriocarcinoma. He described proliferation of the syncytium and the cytotrophoblast of the placental villi in molar pregnancies. In the early part of the 20th century, Fels, Ehrhart, Roessler, and Zondek demonstrated that an excess of chorionic gonadotropic hormones could be identified in the urine of patients with hydatidiform moles.

Gestational trophoblastic neoplasia (GTN) is the term now commonly applied to choriocarcinoma and related malignant tumors. It appears to be appropriate, because it is indicative of the spectrum of trophoblastic diseases (e.g., postmolar GTN, invasive mole, choriocarcinoma, and placental trophoblastic tumor) that are locally proliferative, have the ability to invade normal tissue, and the potential to metastasize outside of the uterus. Before the mid-1950s the prognosis for these diseases, particularly choriocarcinoma, was dismal. Hertz, in the late 1940s, demonstrated that fetal tissues required a large amount of folic acid and could be inhibited by the antifolic compound methotrexate, but it was not until 1956 that Li and associates reported the first complete and sustained remission in a patient with metastatic choriocarcinoma by using methotrexate. Since that report, a considerable amount of knowledge and experience has been gained; GTN is recognized today as the most curable gynecologic malignancy. Several reasons are apparent for this:

1. Human chorionic gonadotropin (hCG) was identified and quantitative assays for hCG levels allowed it to become the prototype for tumor markers; the amount of hormone present in serum or urine is proportional to the number of viable tumor cells.

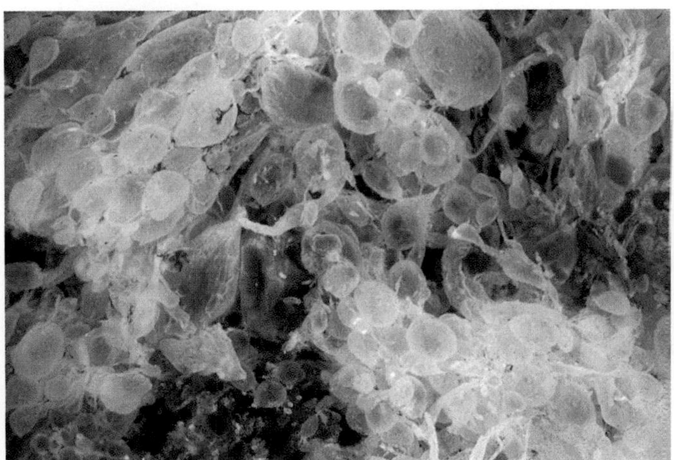

Figure 7–1 Complete hydatidiform mole, gross specimen. Note the diffuse hydropic placental villi, which make up almost the entire specimen (Courtesy of John Soper, M.D.).

2. This malignancy is extremely sensitive to various chemotherapeutic agents.
3. Identification of high-risk factors in this disease process allowed individualization of treatment.
4. The aggressive use of multiple modalities is possible, using single- and multiple-agent chemotherapy regimens, combined with radiation or surgery in selected cases.

Baergen from the University of California at San Diego noted that normal trophoblasts have an inherent propensity for invasion and metastasis, yet rarely do these processes become pathologic. For example, trophoblasts demonstrate controlled invasion at the placental site during the normal process of implantation. In addition, during pregnancy, several thousands of syncytiotrophoblasts seed the maternal circulation daily, and these are commonly identified in the pulmonary circulation. In general, GTN represents a derangement in development of the conceptus, associated with unregulated trophoblastic proliferation and invasion, with the propensity for hematogenous metastasis. The diseases are characterized by distinctive paraneoplastic disorders, which result from overexpression and secretion of gestational hormones, most notably forms of hCG. One can argue that GTD is a "sexually transmitted disease" representing the only group of female reproductive neoplasms requiring paternal genetic material (androgenetic origin). Although largely unclear, the etiology of GTD likely involves not only genetic abnormalities involved in fertilization but also abnormalities in differentiation and pronuclear cleavage, decidual implantation and myometrial invasion, and host immunologic tolerance. Several candidate tumor suppressor genes, chromosomal loci (e.g., DOC-2/hDab2, or loci chromosome 7p12–7q11,23 and 9q13,3–13,4) and oncogenes (e.g., CD9) have been implicated in the pathogenesis of GTD.

HYDATIDIFORM MOLE

Two distinct forms of molar pregnancies, complete and partial moles, are currently recognized. Previously, it was believed that hydatidiform moles with the characteristics of a fetus or fetal tissues, scattered hydropic change of the villi, and only focal trophoblastic proliferation were "incomplete" precursors to the fully developed complete moles, which present without any evidence of fetal development and generalized hydropic changes and trophoblastic proliferation. However, cytogenetic studies have conclusively demonstrated that these are completely separate, but related entities. Despite the cytogenetic, pathologic and clinical differences outlined in Table 7–1, the management of patients with complete and partial moles is similar.

Epidemiology

The incidence of molar pregnancies in the USA is approximately 1:1500 pregnancies. Race or ethnicity, age, socio-

Table 7–1 FEATURES OF PARTIAL AND COMPLETE HYDATIDIFORM MOLES

Feature	Partial mole	Complete mole
Karyotype	Most commonly 69, XXX or –,XXY	Most commonly 46, XX or –,XY
Pathology		
Fetus	Often present	Absent
Amnion, fetal RBC	Usually present	Absent
Villous edema	Variable, focal	Diffuse
Trophoblastic proliferation	Focal, slight–moderate	Diffuse, slight–severe
Clinical presentation		
Diagnosis	Missed abortion	Molar gestation
Uterine size	Small for dates	50% large for dates
Theca lutein cysts	Rare	25–30%
Medical complications	Rare	10–25%
Postmolar GTN	2.5–7.5%	6.8–20%

RBC, red blood cells; GTN, gestational trophoblastic neoplasia.

economic status, diet, and prior reproductive history all influence the risk of hydatidiform mole. The most reliable studies suggest that the incidence of hydatidiform mole is slightly less than 1 in 1000 pregnancies in most of the world, as high as 2 in 1000 in Japan, and possibly higher in Saudi Arabia. Many of the studies reporting apparent effects of race/ethnicity on the incidence of molar pregnancies may reflect reporting bias, because hospital rather than population-based populations were often used in early studies of the epidemiology of hydatidiform mole.

Extremes of reproductive age are also associated with increased risk, particularly among women older than 40 years. When analyzing the effects of maternal age on the incidence of hydatidiform mole, the Duke group studied 2202 patients with hydatidiform moles and compared them with a contemporary control group that compared all types of pregnancy events. A significant increase in the incidence of mole was seen in women 15 years old or younger and 40 years of age or older. A significantly lower incidence was seen in women aged 20–29 years. The greatest relative risks (RR) were in women 50 years of age or older (RR = 519). Mazzanti et al noted an increased risk associated with both increasing paternal age and increasing maternal age for complete moles, but did not observe similar associations between reproductive age and risk of partial mole.

Dietary factors associated with an increased risk of hydatidiform mole appear to implicate a low-protein diet and imply a link to lower socioeconomic class. Berkowitz and coworkers have suggested that a deficiency of animal fat and fat-soluble vitamin carotene is associated with increased risk of molar pregnancies. A high prevalence of vitamin A deficiency corresponds with geographic locations where there is an apparent high incidence of hydatidiform mole. Although carotene-rich vegetables are available in these countries, there is a lack of dietary fat for carotene absorption, particularly among women of lower socioeconomic status.

Previous reproductive history, in particular a history of previous complete or partial mole, increases the risk of a molar pregnancy. Women with a previous mole have more than 10 times the risk of having another mole compared with women who have never had one. This risk increases if a woman has more than one mole. Bagshawe found that the risk was 1 of 76 pregnancies for a second mole after the first mole and that this risk increased to 1 in 6.5 pregnancies among women with two prior moles. Sand reported that after two previous episodes of gestational trophoblastic disease, the risk of repeated disease is 28%. Goldstein and associates noted that 9 of 1339 patients (1 in 150) had at least two consecutive molar pregnancies. One patient had four moles. Other centers have reported incidences as high as 1 in 50 women. With recurrent molar pregnancies, there is an increased risk of malignant GTN, although patients with consecutive molar pregnancies may have subsequent normal pregnancies. Berkowitz and associates noted that four of their patients with repeated moles later had full-term pregnancies. Lurain noted that five of eight patients with consecutive moles had normal full-term pregnancies. In a case-controlled study from Baltimore, factors found to be associated with GTN included professional occupation, history of prior spontaneous abortions, and the mean number of months from last pregnancy to the index pregnancy. Contraceptive history, irradiation, ABO blood groups, and smoking factors of the male partner were not relevant.

Cytogenetics and pathology

Complete hydatidiform moles are completely derived from the paternal genome (Table 7–1). Most frequently, these have a diploid 46,XX genome with exclusively androgenetic markers on the chromosomes, implying reduplication of a haploid sperm chromosomal complement in the fertilized ovum. Approximately 5% complete moles have a 46, XY androgenetic genome, however, indicating that dispermic fertilization accounts for some complete moles. The mechanism for exclusion of the maternal polar body from the nucleus of the fertilized ovum is unknown. No 46, YY moles have been reported but aneuploid karyotypes, such as tetraploidy, have been associated with complete moles. The fetus is resorbed before development of the circulatory system in complete moles; fetal red blood cells are not observed in sections of the villi.

In contrast, partial moles are comprised of both paternal and maternal genome (Table 7–2). Usually, two paternal haploid sets of chromosomes are combined with one maternal set, resulting in complete triploidy (Fig. 7–2); 69, XXX karyotype is most common but some partial moles have a 69, XXY karyotype, implying dispermic fertilization. Sometimes other aneuploid karyotypes are observed in partial moles, but none with duplication of the y chromosome. All karyotypes reported for partial moles feature a maternal haploid set of chromosomes and multiples of the paternal chromosomal complement. Gross or histologic evidence of fetal development such as fetal red blood cells is a prominent feature of partial moles.

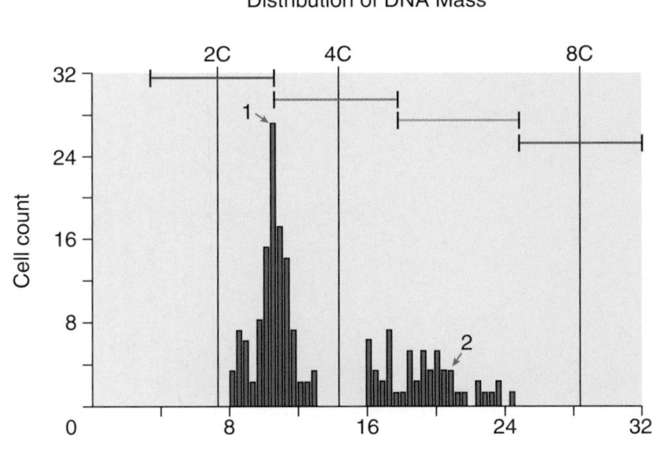

Figure 7–2 Flow cytometry of a partial mole. Note the peak at 3C, indicating triploidy (Courtesy of Dr Rex Bentley, Department of Pathology, Duke University Medical Center).

Histopathology features of partial mole can be subtle, and these are probably underdiagnosed. Focal or varying degrees of hydropic villi are observed, with scalloping of the villi and trophoblastic inclusions within villi (Fig. 7–3). Focal trophoblastic proliferation is usually subtle compared to complete moles. Fetal red blood cells are observed within vessels of the villi (Fig. 7–4) or a fetus can be grossly identified in partial moles, although the fetus is non-viable and rarely survives beyond 20 weeks' gestation. In contrast, complete moles have diffuse villous edema, often with central cisterna formation (Fig. 7–5). Trophoblastic proliferation is usually diffuse (Fig. 7–6), but may vary in extent. Histologic evidence of a fetus is lacking.

The volume and amount of trophoblastic proliferation in complete moles generally exceeds that observed in partial moles, and is reflected in the different clinical presentations (Table 7–1). Initial serum hCG levels are usually higher in patients with complete moles. Although an increasing proportion of complete moles are diagnosed as missed abortion on the basis of an early ultrasound in

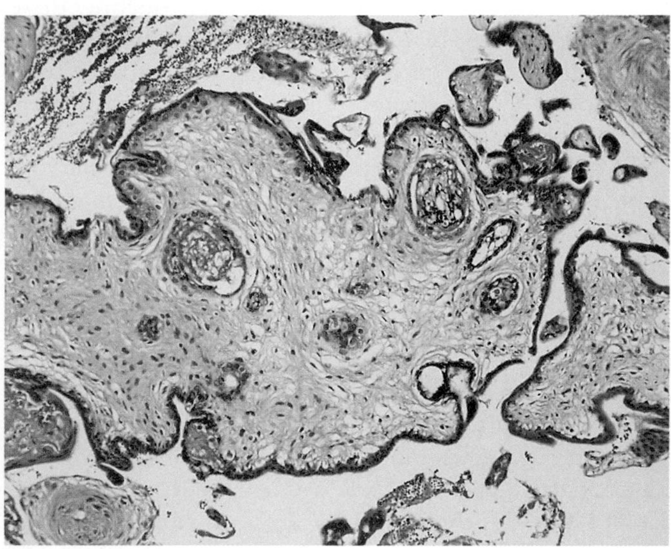

Figure 7–3 This low-power photomicrograph of a partial hydatidiform mole contains enlarged placental villi with stromal edema, scalloping at the edge of the villi, and trophoblastic inclusions within the stroma of the villi. Minimal trophoblastic proliferation is present (Courtesy of Dr Rex Bentley, Department of Pathology, Duke University Medical Center).

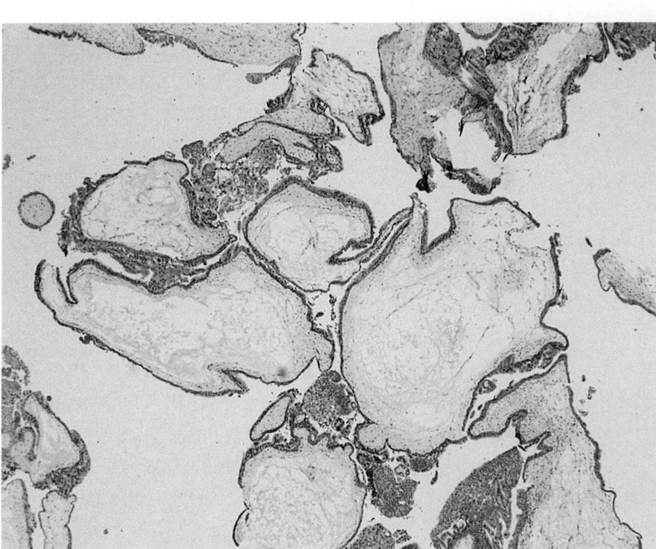

Figure 7–5 Low power photomicrograph of a complete mole illustrating diffuse hydropic change of the villi, which have marked paucity of stroma in the central zone of each villus (cisternae formation). Sheets of trophoblast cell are adjacent to the villi (Courtesy of Dr Rex Bentley, Department of Pathology, Duke University Medical Center).

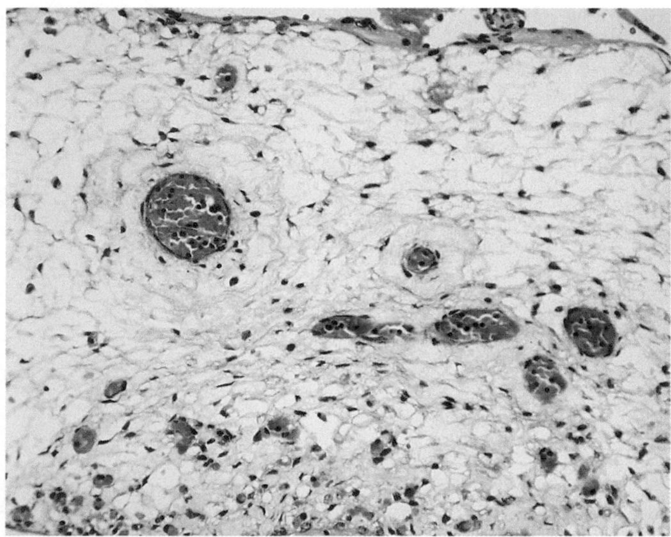

Figure 7–4 In this high-power photomicrograph of a villus from a partial mole, small vessels within the stroma are seen containing nucleated fetal red blood cells (Courtesy of Dr Rex Bentley, Department of Pathology, Duke University Medical Center).

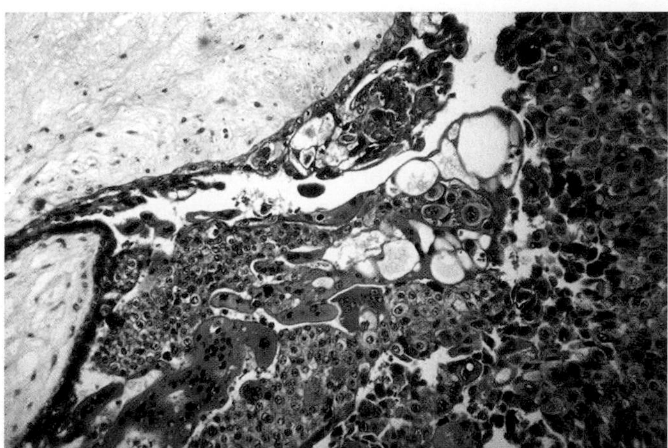

Figure 7–6 High-power photomicrograph of a complete mole. The villus (upper left) is associated with sheets of trophoblast cells, containing the multinucleated syncytiotrophoblasts and the small, polygonal cytotrophoblast cells. Production of hCG occurs mainly in the syncytiotrophoblast cells (Courtesy of Dr Rex Bentley, Department of Pathology, Duke University Medical Center).

the absence of symptoms, the majority of patients with complete moles have a clinical or sonographic diagnosis of hydatidiform mole. Uterine enlargement beyond the expected gestational age is observed in up to 50% of patients with complete moles. Medical complications of molar pregnancy, including pregnancy-induced hypertension, hyperthyroidism, anemia, and hyperemesis are more frequently seen among patients with complete moles. Approximately 15–25% of patients with complete moles will have theca-lutein cysts with ovarian enlargement >6 cm. Malignant sequelae occur in 2.5–7.5% of patients with partial moles compared to approximately 6.8–20% after evacuation of a complete hydatidiform mole (Table 7–1).

Symptoms

Essentially all patients with hydatidiform mole have delayed menses for varying periods, and most patients are considered to be pregnant. Vaginal bleeding usually occurs during the first trimester. The bleeding may vary from a dark brown spotting or discharge to significant hemorrhage in quantities sufficient to produce anemia or require a blood transfusion. In one series, bleeding was the presenting symptom in 97% of complete moles. Expulsion of recognizable molar vesicles may accompany vaginal bleeding. The majority of patients with complete moles have the diagnosis established by characteristic ultrasound findings. However, the majority of patients with partial moles and an increasing proportion of patients with complete moles are clinically diagnosed as missed abortion. This appears to be largely related to improved hCG assays and the increased use of ultrasound in early pregnancy.

Nausea and vomiting were reported in almost one-third of patients with hydatidiform mole in older studies, although Curry and coworkers, in a report on patients with hydatidiform mole, noted only 14% of 347 patients with this symptom. This symptom can be confused with hyperemesis accompanying a normal pregnancy. Pre-eclampsia in the first trimester of pregnancy has been said to be almost pathognomonic of a hydatidiform mole. This occurred in only 12% of the patients in the study by Curry and colleagues but was present in 27% of patients reported from Boston. Although proteinuria, hypertension, and hyperreflexia may be common, eclampsia appears to be rare.

Hyperthyroidism occurs rarely, but when present it can precipitate a medical emergency. Laboratory evidence of hyperthyroidism can occur in as many as 10% of patients; however, clinical manifestations occurred in less than 1% of the patients of Curry and associates, although it has been reported to be as high as 7% in other reports. Hyperthyroidism in molar pregnancy is caused by the production of thyrotrophic substances, mainly the elevated levels of normal hCG, by the molar tissue. There is correlation between hCG levels and thyroid function. With elevated levels of hCG, the hCG molecule is bound by the TSH receptor site, resulting in thyroid hyperfunction. Yoshimura and colleagues demonstrated that isoforms of hCG with higher thyrotrophic activity are more frequently produced by trophoblastic tissues in women with hydatidiform mole compared with normal pregnancies, suggesting that these isoforms of hCG may be responsible for the hyperthyroidism observed in some patients with hydatidiform moles. Clinical manifestations of hyperthyroidism disappear once the molar pregnancy is treated. Antithyroid therapy may be indicated for a short period to control hyperthyroidism during molar evacuation.

The most significant symptom of complete mole is acute respiratory distress, which may be caused by trophoblastic pulmonary embolization. Other factors, such as changes associated with toxemia, hyperthyroidism, anemia with high-output cardiac failure and other conditions, may be contributing factors. Acute respiratory distress is most often associated with a large volume of molar tissue and uterine enlargement >16 weeks gestational size.

The classic presenting symptoms of a complete mole may be changing. The New England Trophoblastic Disease Center group compared symptoms in complete moles treated at their institution from 1988–1993 to those treated in 1965–1976. Vaginal bleeding was still the most common symptom but occurred in 84% compared to 97% in the earlier interval. Excessive uterine size, pre-eclampsia, and hyperemesis were present in only 28%, 1.3%, and 8%, respectively, of patients in the most recent group, while present in 51%, 27%, and 26%, respectively, in the older group. Anemia was diagnosed in only 5% of the recent patients compared with 54% of the older group. Hyperthyroidism and respiratory distress were not diagnosed in any of the patients in the recent group, but had been diagnosed in 7% and 2% in the former group. The reason for these differences may be due to an earlier diagnosis (12 weeks versus 16 weeks) in the more recent group of patients. Earlier diagnosis may result from the use of more sensitive hCG assays and more frequent use of ultrasound in early pregnancy. The diagnosis of a mole was suspected in only 75% of the later group who had an ultrasound. It may be more difficult to make the ultrasound diagnosis of hydatidiform mole in early pregnancy, before generalized edema of the villi has occurred. Despite earlier diagnosis and lower incidence of high-risk features in the later group of patients, however, the incidence of persistent gestational trophoblastic tumor was similar between the two groups, suggesting that earlier intervention did not change the biology of complete mole.

Classically, a patient with a hydatidiform mole is said to have a uterine size excessive for gestational age, and historically this was found in approximately 50% of patients with moles; however, approximately one-third of patients have uteri smaller than expected for gestational age. In the recent Boston study, uterine size was excessive for dates in only 28%, equal to dates in 58%, and less than dates in 14% of the patients in the later group.

Theca-lutein cysts of the ovary may be large and are caused by hyperstimulation of the ovaries by excessive hCG production from the molar pregnancy. Approximately

15–25% of patients with unevacuated molar pregnancies have theca-lutein cysts >6 cm. Although theca-lutein cysts will resolve after molar evacuation, there may be considerable lag behind the decline of hCG levels. Surgical intervention is only rarely required in cases of acute torsion or bleeding from these cysts. Patients who develop theca-lutein cysts appear to have a higher incidence of malignant sequelae after molar evacuation. Furthermore, the combination of enlarged ovaries with a uterus that is large for gestational age results in an extremely high risk for malignant sequelae of trophoblastic disease. Up to 57% of patients with this combination require subsequent therapy for postmolar gestational trophoblastic neoplasia (GTN).

The symptoms outlined above are seen mainly in patients with complete moles. Patients with partial moles usually do not exhibit excessive uterine size, theca-lutein cysts, toxemia, hyperthyroidism, or respiratory problems. In most patients with a partial mole, the clinical and ultrasound diagnosis is usually missed or incomplete abortion. Because of the clinical lack of suspicion and often subtle or focal nature of the pathologic changes in the placental tissues, partial moles are frequently underdiagnosed. This emphasizes the need for a thorough histopathologic evaluation of missed or incomplete abortions.

Diagnosis

In some patients, the passage of vesicular tissue is the first evidence to suggest the presence of a hydatidiform mole (see Fig. 7–2). Several techniques are available to substantiate the diagnosis when pathologic material is not available for analysis. A quantitative pregnancy test of greater than 1,000,000 IU/L, an enlarged uterus with absent fetal heart sounds, and vaginal bleeding suggest a diagnosis of hydatidiform mole. A single hCG determination, however, is not diagnostic. A single high hCG value may be seen with a normal single or multiple pregnancy, especially if there has been bleeding or disruption of the placenta. Therefore, this should not be used as the sole determining factor in making the diagnosis of hydatidiform mole. Conversely, a "normal" hCG level for an anticipated gestational age can be seen with a mole.

Ultrasound has replaced all other radiographic means (e.g., amniography or uterine angiography) for establishing the diagnosis of hydatidiform mole. Molar tissue typically is identified as a diffuse mixed echogenic pattern replacing the placenta (Fig. 7–7), produced by villi and intrauterine blood clots, but these findings may be subtle or lacking in cases of early complete or partial mole. In most complete moles and in many partial moles, a fetus will not be identified. In rare cases, a fetus may coexist with a complete mole. The group at Yale evaluated the combined use of both ultrasound and hCG values to determine the diagnosis of hydatidiform mole. When ultrasound was used alone, 15 (42%) of 36 patients with moles did not have a definite diagnosis on first examination. When hCG value above a threshold of 82,350 mIU/ was used along with

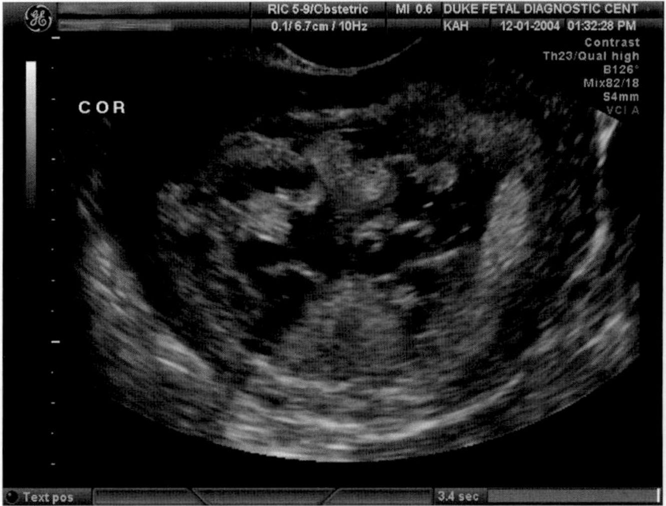

Figure 7–7 Transabdominal ultrasound of an unevacuated complete mole, illustrating the characteristic mixed echogenic pattern in the uterus (Courtesy of John Soper, M.D.).

the initial ultrasound findings, 32 patients (89%) were correctly identified as having hydatidiform moles (Fig. 7–8).

Several reports have been made of a hydatidiform mole arising in ectopic sites, such as the fallopian tube. These patients tend to present with classic symptoms and signs of ectopic non-neoplastic gestations, occasionally with hemorrhagic shock due to tubal rupture. Tubal GTN was diagnosed in 16 (0.8%) of 2100 women with GTN who were managed at the New England Trophoblastic Disease Center in the series reported by Muto. Usually tubal rupture occurs before diagnostic features suggesting molar gestation can be identified by ultrasound. Various authors have warned that the current trend of treating ectopic pregnancies with conservative surgery or single dose methotrexate necessitates close monitoring of serum hCG levels in order to avoid missing the diagnosis of ectopic GTN.

Evacuation

With increasing frequency, the diagnosis of complete or partial mole will be made only after histologic evaluation of uterine curettings after dilatation and curettage (D&C) performed for a suspected incomplete spontaneous abortion. In these cases, patients should be monitored with serial determinations of quantitative hCG values. A baseline postevacuation chest X-ray should be considered.

For patients in whom hydatidiform mole is suspected prior to evacuation, the following laboratory evaluation is recommended (Table 7–2): complete blood count with platelet determination, clotting function studies, renal and liver function studies, blood type with antibody screen, and determination of hCG level. A pre-evacuation chest X-ray should also be obtained. Medical complications of hydatidiform mole are observed in approximately 25% of patients with uterine enlargement >14–16 weeks gesta-

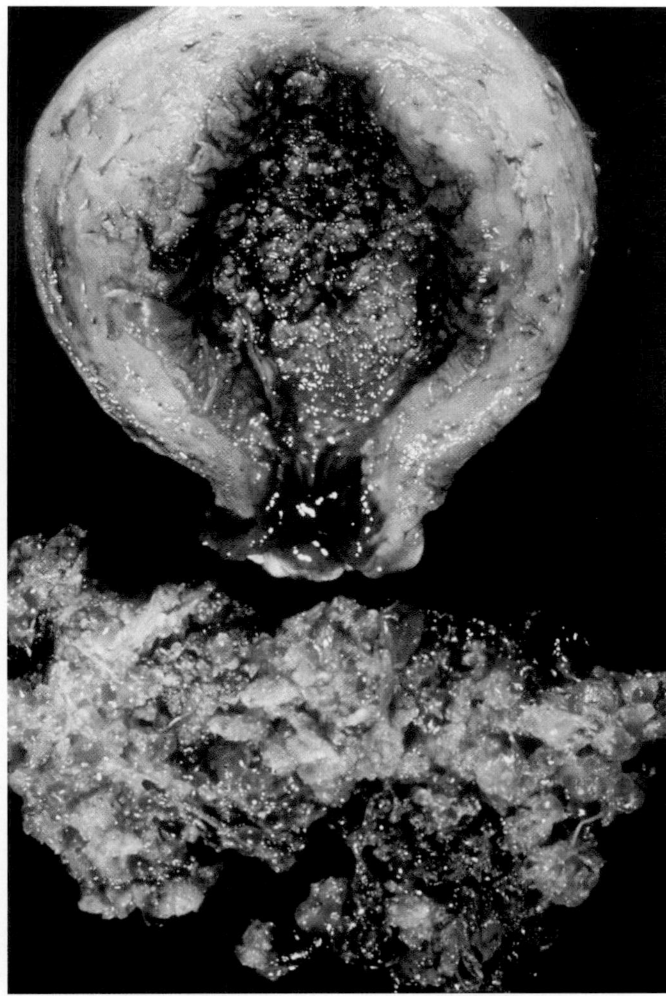

Figure 7–8 Gross specimen in a patient treated for complete hydatidiform mole with primary hysterectomy (Courtesy of John Soper, M.D.).

tional size, and seen less frequently among patients with lesser degrees of uterine enlargement. Common medical complications include anemia, hyperemesis, infection, hyperthyroidism, pregnancy-induced hypertension, and coagulopathy. The mole should be evacuated as soon as possible after stabilization of any medical complications. The choice of facilities for molar evacuation should be based on the expertise of the physician, uterine size, and ability of the facility to manage existing medical complications. In most patients, the preferred method of evacuation is suction D&C (Table 7–2).

Medical induction of labor with oxytocin or prostaglandin and hysterotomy are not recommended for evacuation because they increase blood loss and may increase the risk for malignant sequelae compared with suction D&C. The Charing Cross Group reported a significant trend toward more frequent evacuation by suction curettage compared with sharp curettage or medical induction for molar evacuation during their study interval. Postmolar GTN developed in 5.9%, 3.8%, and 9.1% of their patients evacuated with suction curettage, sharp curettage, and medical induction, respectively ($P < 0.05$, for increased postmolar GTN in the medical induction group). Furthermore, many patients require D&C to complete the evacuation of the mole after medical induction of labor.

Table 7–2 MANAGEMENT OF HYDATIDIFORM MOLE

Evacuation: suction D&C (or hysterectomy in selected patients)
Postevacuation quantitative hCG level and chest X-ray
Monitor quantitative hCG levels every 1–2 weeks until normal value or criteria for GTN
Examination every 2–4 weeks while hCG elevated
Confirm normal hCG level, then monitor hCG levels every 1–2 months for 6–12 months
Initiate chemotherapy for GTN using indications listed in Table 7–4:

1. Plateaued or rising hCG values
2. Histologic diagnosis of choriocarcinoma, invasive mole or placental site trophoblastic tumor
3. Persistent hCG >6 months after evacuation
4. Metastatic disease

D&C, dilatation and curettage; hCG, human chorionic gonadotropin; GTN, gestational trophoblastic neoplasia.

Evacuation is usually performed under general anesthesia, but local or regional anesthesia may be used for a co-operative patient with a small uterus. After serial dilatation of the cervix, uterine evacuation is accomplished with the largest cannula that can be introduced through the cervix. Intravenous oxytocin is begun after the cervix is dilated and continued for several hours postoperatively. After completion of suction D&C, gentle sharp curettage may be performed.

Hysterectomy is an alternative to suction D&C for molar evacuation in selected patients who do not wish to preserve childbearing (Fig. 7–9). Usually the adnexa may be preserved; theca-lutein cysts should be left in situ unless they are torsed or ruptured and actively bleeding. Hysterectomy reduces but does not eliminate the risk of malignant postmolar sequelae compared to evacuation by D&C. However, the risk of postmolar GTN after hysterectomy remains approximately 3–5%; therefore these patients should be monitored postoperatively with serial hCG levels.

Risk factors for postmolar gestational trophoblastic neoplasia

Many of the risk factors for development of postmolar GTN seem to indirectly reflect the amount of trophoblastic proliferation at the time of evacuation. High pre-evacuation hCG levels, uterine size larger than expected by dates, theca-lutein cysts (Fig. 7–9), and increasing maternal age increase the risk. Many of these interact: the combination of theca-lutein cysts and uterus larger than expected for dates increase the risk of postmolar GTN to 57%. Efforts

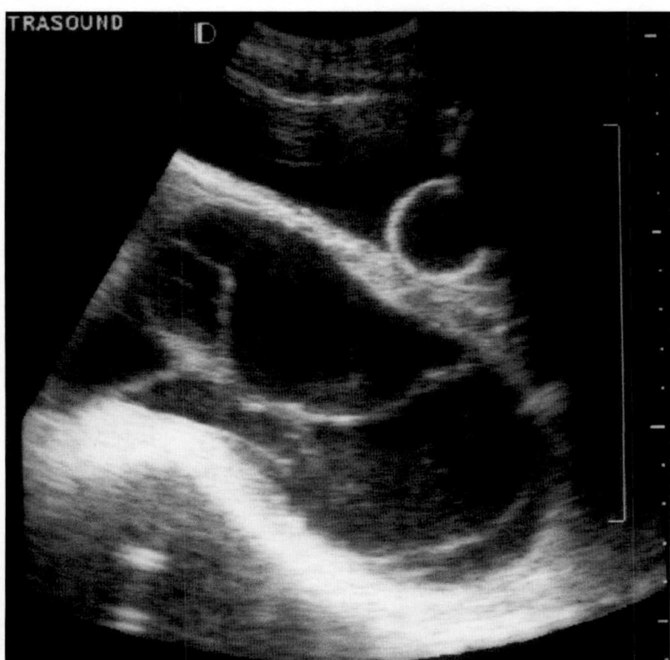

Figure 7–9 Ultrasound demonstrating a large theca-lutein ovarian cyst associated with a complete hydatidiform mole. These usually contain multiple thin septations and have an appearance similar to iatrogenic ovarian hyperstimulation during ovulation induction. Theca-lutein cysts regress spontaneously after evacuation of the molar pregnancy, but regression often lags behind hCG level decline (Courtesy of John Soper, M.D.).

to correlate outcome with the histopathologic features of uterine curettings have been inconsistent, possibly because of incomplete sampling. Multiple risk factors have been incorporated into scoring systems that might identify high-, medium-, and low-risk subsets of patients. Unfortunately, Parazzini and associates found that while 15% of their patients could be classified as high risk, these patients accounted for a minority of the cases of postmolar GTN. Of note, despite a lower incidence of clinical risk factors in the more recent cohort of patients reported by the New England Trophoblastic Disease Center, 23% of their contemporary patients required treatment for postmolar GTN, compared to 18% in the older cohort, a non-significant difference. This implies that other molecular biologic mechanisms may be responsible for the development of postmolar GTN, rather than the amount of trophoblastic proliferation at the time of evacuation. In the USA, most centers do not make treatment decisions based on risk factors; rather they rely on postmolar surveillance with serial hCG levels.

Postmolar surveillance

After molar evacuation, it is important to monitor all patients carefully in order to diagnose and treat malignant sequelae promptly. Serial quantitative serum hCG determinations should be performed using one of several commercially available assays capable of detecting beta hCG to baseline values (<5 mIU/mL). Ideally, serum hCG levels should be obtained within 48 hours of evacuation, every 1–2 weeks while elevated, and then at 1–2 month intervals for an additional 6–12 months (Table 7–2). Reliable contraception is recommended during monitoring of hCG values. Frequent pelvic examinations are performed while hCG values are elevated to monitor the involution of the uterus and to aid in the early identification of vaginal metastases. A chest X-ray is indicated if the hCG level rises. Patients with a histologic diagnosis of malignant GTN (choriocarcinoma, invasive mole, or placental site trophoblastic tumor), the development of metastatic disease, a rising hCG value, or a plateauing of the hCG values over several weeks' time are diagnosed with postmolar GTN, as discussed subsequently. Approximately 7.5–20% of patients develop postmolar GTN after evacuation of complete hydatidiform mole, while 2.5–7.5% of patients develop postmolar GTN after partial mole.

The rationale for an interval of monitoring after normalization of hCG values is to allow identification of patients who develop postmolar malignant GTN after achieving normal hCG values. Although rare instances of long latent periods between molar evacuation and postmolar GTN have been reported, the vast majority of episodes of malignant sequelae after hydatidiform moles occur within approximately 6 months of evacuation. The New England Trophoblastic Disease Center analyzed 1,029 patients followed with hCG assays after molar evacuation at their institution. Postmolar GTN developed in 153 (15%) patients. Only two women developed postmolar GTN following normalization of hCG levels; both were followed by an older assay with a sensitivity of 10 mIU/mL. None of their 82 patients who were followed with an hCG assay having a sensitivity of 5 mIU/mL developed postmolar GTN after normalizing hCG levels (95% confidence interval 0–4.5%). However, a substantial number of their patients were excluded from analysis because of incomplete follow-up, including 817 lost to follow-up after normalization of hCG and 60 patients lost to follow-up before hCG values normalized. Because this experience is relatively small, it is prudent to recommend continued surveillance after molar evacuation with hCG monitoring for several months following normalization of hCG values.

Although early pregnancies after molar evacuation are usually normal gestations, an early pregnancy obscures the value of monitoring hCG values during this interval and may result in a delayed diagnosis of postmolar malignant GTN. Oral contraceptives do not increase the incidence of postmolar GTN or alter the pattern of regression of hCG values. In a randomized study conducted by the Gynecologic Oncology Group, patients treated with oral contraceptives had half as many intercurrent pregnancies as those using barrier methods. Furthermore, the incidence of postmolar GTN was lower in patients using oral contraceptives. After completion of surveillance documenting remission for 6–12 months, pregnancy can be permitted and hCG monitoring discontinued.

Prophylactic chemotherapy after molar evacuation

Two randomized studies have evaluated prophylactic chemotherapy after molar evacuation. Kim and associates reported that a single course of methotrexate/folinic acid reduced the incidence of postmolar GTN from 47.4% to 14.3% ($P < 0.05$) in patients with high-risk moles, but the incidence was not reduced in patients with low-risk moles. Patients who had received prophylactic chemotherapy but developed postmolar trophoblastic disease required more chemotherapy than those who had not been exposed to prophylactic chemotherapy. In the second study, reported by Limpongsanurak, a single course of dactinomycin was compared to observation in patients following evacuation of high-risk moles. Postmolar GTN was 50% in the control group, compared to 13.8% in the treatment group ($P<0.05$). In both studies, there were no deaths in the treatment or control groups caused by GTN or treatment toxicity.

However, there are anecdotal cases of fatalities caused by prophylactic chemotherapy and prophylactic chemotherapy does not eliminate the need for postevacuation follow-up. Furthermore, patients are exposed to drugs most frequently used to treat postmolar GTD, which could lead to relative chemoresistance. In compliant patients the low morbidity and mortality achieved by monitoring patients with serial hCG determinations and instituting chemotherapy only in patients with postmolar GTD appears to outweigh the potential risk and small benefit of routine prophylactic chemotherapy.

Coexistent molar pregnancy with a normal fetus

Coexistence of a fetus with molar change of the placenta is relatively rare (Fig. 7–10), occurring in 1:22,000–1:100,000 pregnancies. The majority of the literature covering this relatively rare entity consists of case reports, small case series, and review of cases reported in the literature. Both complete and partial moles with a coexistent normal fetus have been reported. A variety of criteria have been used to evaluate these pregnancies. Many of the reports that antedated the histologic and cytogenetic distinction between complete and partial moles likely included twin gestations with coexistent fetus and molar gestation, in addition to singleton partial moles. While there might be an increased incidence of coexisting mole and fetus related to an increase in multifetal pregnancies caused by ovulation induction for infertility, this may only reflect reporting bias.

Most of these twin pregnancies are diagnosed antepartum by ultrasound findings of a complex, cystic placental component distinct from the fetoplacental unit. However, in a few cases the diagnosis is not suspected until examination of the placenta following delivery. Medical complications of hydatidiform mole appear to be increased, including hyperthyroidism, hemorrhage, and pregnancy-induced hypertension.

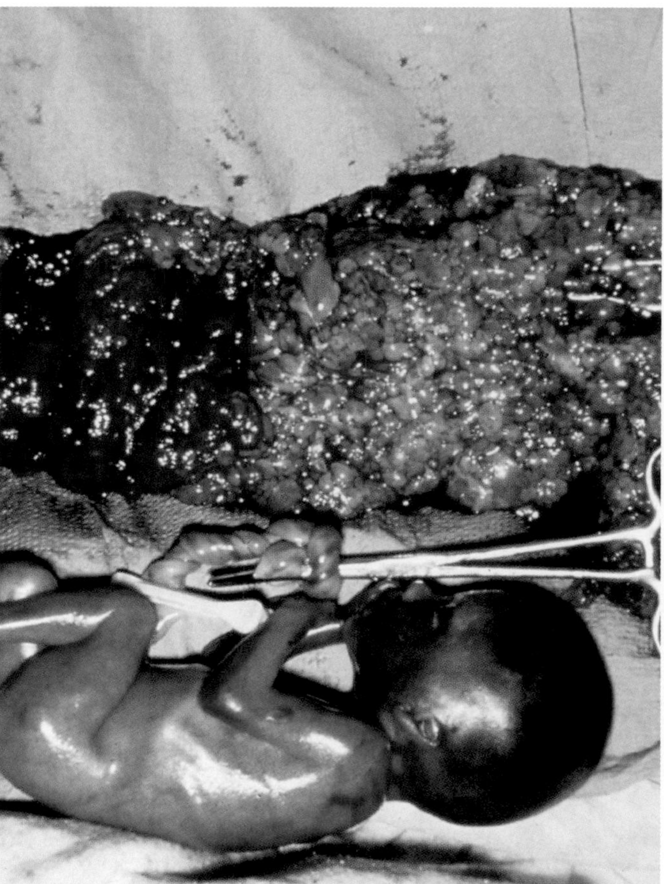

Figure 7–10 Gross photo of fetus and mole.

Compared to singleton hydatidiform moles, twin pregnancy with fetus and mole has an increased risk for postmolar GTN, with a higher proportion of patients having metastatic disease and requiring multiagent chemotherapy. Among patients with coexistent mole and fetus who continue pregnancy beyond 12 weeks, there is a subset that develops early complications leading to termination of the pregnancy before fetal viability. These patients have a markedly increased risk of postmolar GTN, compared to patients whose pregnancy continues into the third trimester. Among 72 patients collected by a national survey of physicians in Japan during 1997, 24 patients underwent first trimester evacuation with 20.8% subsequently developing postmolar GTN. In comparison, 45.2% of 31 patients who required evacuation during the second trimester and 17.6% of the 17 who delivered in the third trimester developed postmolar GTN. Nine (50%) of the 18 patients with proven androgenic mole in association with a fetus subsequently were treated for postmolar GTN, but it is not certain that this increased risk was due to selection bias. Major congenital abnormalities have not been reported in surviving infants.

For patients with coexistent hydatidiform mole and fetus suspected by ultrasound, there are no clear guidelines for management. The ultrasound should be repeated to exclude retroplacental hematoma, other placental abnormalities, or degenerating myoma, and to fully evaluate the fetoplacental unit for evidence of a partial mole or gross fetal malformations. If the diagnosis is still suspected and continuation of pregnancy is desired, fetal karyotype should be obtained, a chest X-ray performed to screen for metastases, and serial serum hCG values should be followed. Patients are at an increased risk for medical complications of pregnancy requiring evacuation, including bleeding, premature labor and pregnancy-induced hypertension. They should be counseled about these risks and the increased risk of postmolar GTN after evacuation or delivery. If fetal karyotype is normal, major fetal malformations are excluded by ultrasound, and there is no evidence of metastatic disease, it is reasonable to allow the pregnancy to continue unless pregnancy-related complications force delivery. After delivery, the placenta should be histologically evaluated and the patient followed closely with serial hCG values, similar to a singleton hydatidiform mole.

Table 7–3 DISTRIBUTION OF METASTATIC SITES FROM GTN

Metastatic site	Number	(%)	(% Metastatic)
Non-metastatic	195	(54)	
Metastatic	136	(46)	
Lung only	110		(81)
Vagina only	7		(5)
Central nervous system*	9		(7)
Gastrointestinal*	5		(4)
Liver*	2		(1.5)
Kidney*	1		(0.7)
Unknown**	4		(3)

*Concurrent lung metastases, highest risk site recorded
** Rising hCG after hysterectomy for hydatidiform mole, no identifiable metastases
Modified from Soper JT, Clarke-Pearson DL, Hammond CB: Metastatic gestational trophoblastic disease: prognostic factors in previously untreated patients. Obstet Gynecol 71: 338, 1988.

GESTATIONAL TROPHOBLASTIC NEOPLASIA

The prompt identification of malignant GTN is important because a delay in the diagnosis may increase the patient's risk and adversely affect response to treatment. All patients with malignant GTN should undergo a complete evaluation aimed at identifying metastatic sites (Table 7–3) and other clinically important prognostic factors. Several classification systems have been used to determine prognostic groups and assist in the triage of management for individual patients. The International Federation of Gynecology and Obstetrics (FIGO) revised its staging system for patients with malignant GTN in 2000 to reflect prognostic factors other than anatomic distribution of disease. These changes in FIGO staging may help facilitate classification of individual patients.

Diagnosis

Between one half to two-thirds of cases of GTN that require treatment follow evacuation of complete or partial hydatidiform moles. Because the majority of patients are treated on the basis of hCG levels rather than hysterectomy, the exact distribution of histologic lesions is not known precisely. Approximately 50–70% of patients with postmolar GTN have persistent or invasive moles, while 30–50% have postmolar gestational choriocarcinoma. Gestational choriocarcinoma (Fig. 7–11) derived from term pregnancies, spontaneous abortions and ectopic pregnancies account for the vast majority of the other cases of malignant GTN. Placental site trophoblastic tumors (PSTT) (Fig. 7–12) are rare forms of GTN that can follow any pregnancy event.

Invasive moles are characterized by presence of edematous chorionic villi with trophoblastic proliferation that invade directly into the myometrium. Metastasis of molar vesicles may occur, and usually invasive moles will undergo spontaneous resolution after many months, but they are treated with chemotherapy to prevent morbidity and mortality caused by uterine perforation, hemorrhage or infection. Gestational choriocarcinoma is a pure epithelial malignancy, comprising both neoplastic syncytiotrophoblast and cytotrophoblast elements without chorionic villi (Fig. 7–11). Gestational choriocarcinomas tend to develop early systemic metastasis and chemotherapy is clearly indicated when histologically diagnosed.

Placental site trophoblastic tumors are relatively rare. These tumors are characterized by absence of villi with proliferation of intermediate trophoblast cells (Fig 7–12). The syncytiotrophoblast population observed in choriocarcinoma is lacking in PSTT, with relatively lower levels of hCG secreted by these tumors. In general, PSTTs are not as sensitive to simple chemotherapy as other forms of malignant GTN; therefore, it is important to distinguish these tumors histologically. Surgery assumes a larger role in the management of PSTT. Fortunately, the majority of patients present with disease confined to the uterus and can be treated with hysterectomy.

Women diagnosed with GTN after evacuation of a molar pregnancy are usually identified early in the course of disease because they have been followed with serial hCG monitoring. In contrast, patients with malignant GTN following non-molar gestations often present with predominantly non-gynecologic symptoms and signs including hemoptysis or pulmonary embolism, cerebral hemorrhage, gastrointestinal or urologic hemorrhage, or widely metastatic malignancy of an unknown primary site. Most of these patients will have a history of irregular uterine bleeding, amenorrhea, or recent pregnancy event. However, the index pregnancy event may have occurred several years before presentation, or may have been a subclinical spontaneous abortion. The possibility of malignant GTN should be sus-

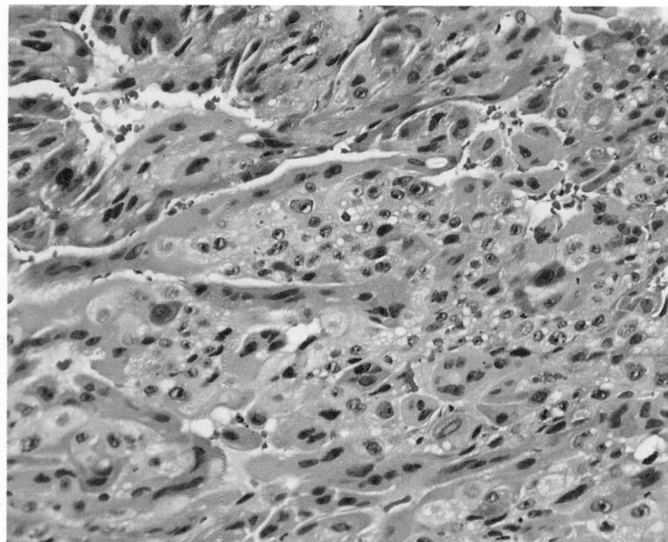

Figure 7–11 High-power photomicrograph of gestational choriocarcinoma, illustrating the dimorphic population of the polygonal cytotrophoblast and the multinucleated syncytiotrophoblast cells (Courtesy of Dr Rex Bentley, Department of Pathology, Duke University Medical Center).

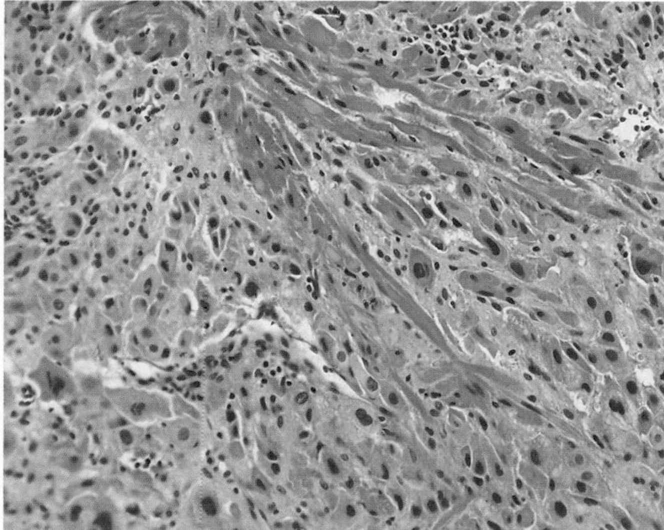

Figure 7–12 High power photomicrograph of placental site trophoblastic tumor (PSTT) treated with hysterectomy. Sheets of anaplastic polygonal cells with frequent mitoses infiltrate the smooth muscle of the uterine wall (Courtesy of Dr Rex Bentley, Department of Pathology, Duke University Medical Center).

pected in any woman of reproductive age who presents with metastatic disease from an unknown primary site or undiagnosed cerebral hemorrhage. Under these circumstances the diagnosis is facilitated by a high index of suspicion coupled with serum hCG testing and exclusion of a concurrent pregnancy, most often without the need for tissue biopsy.

Before the development of effective chemotherapy, Delfs reported that approximately 25% of patients had elevated hCG levels more than 2 months after evacuation of hydatidiform mole. Of 119 patients followed after D&C, 5 (4%) and 6 (5%) required hysterectomy for invasive mole or choriocarcinoma, respectively. Other prechemotherapy reports indicated a mortality rate of more than 20% among patients with invasive mole. Since the development of chemotherapy, between 15–36% of patients are treated after molar evacuation based on inclusive hCG level criteria for initiating chemotherapy, in an attempt to limit the morbidity and mortality caused by postmolar GTN. In contrast, Bagshawe et al used very conservative hCG criteria to initiate chemotherapy and reported treating only approximately 8% of their patients after molar evacuation.

The pattern of hCG regression after evacuation of hydatidiform mole is most often used to make a diagnosis of postmolar GTN. After evacuation, most patients will have an initial fall in hCG levels and should be followed with serial hCG values every 1–2 weeks. Almost every series has treated patients on the basis of a confirmed hCG rise. In many studies, however, chemotherapy was initiated on the basis of an hCG level plateau of relatively short (< 3 weeks) duration. Kohorn noted that 15% of his patients had hCG plateaus after molar evacuation that lasted at least two weeks, followed by spontaneous regression without intervention. Furthermore, in a chemotherapy trial of dactinomycin for patients with GTN, Schlaerth et al observed that 25% of their patients had a substantial spontaneous fall in hCG levels on the day that chemotherapy was initiated, indicating that at least some of their patients did not truly have postmolar GTN. Based on the known correlation between hCG level and tumor burden, Kohorn has suggested an approach using shorter periods of observation for patients with higher hCG level plateaus but allowing longer periods of observation for those who have hCG level plateaus at levels under 1,000 mIU/mL.

An additional criterion for initiating chemotherapy after molar evacuation in some studies has been persistence of hCG for an arbitrary length of time after molar evacuation, ranging between 6 weeks and 6 months. The initial reports of chemotherapy from the National Institutes of Health used persistence of detectable hCG for more than 60 days after molar evacuation as an indication for chemotherapy treatment. Many series have documented that persistence of hCG >60 days after evacuation increases the risk for developing postmolar GTN. However, 60–64% of patients with delayed regression of hCG beyond 60 days will ultimately undergo spontaneous hCG regression to normal values, with no deaths in those who were begun on therapy >60 days from molar evacuation. Furthermore, groups reporting from United Kingdom, where care for GTD patients is centralized, follow patients with elevated hCG levels for up to 6 months without an increase in morbidity or mortality among those treated after this prolonged follow-up.

Lurain and associates from the John I Brewer Trophoblastic Disease Center reported their experience with 738 patients with complete hydatidiform moles. In their study, 596 patients had spontaneous remission to normal of hCG values, although only 390 (65%) had done so by 60 days. An additional 206 patients reached normal values during the next 110 days. Of all of the patients, 142 (19%) were treated with chemotherapy because of rising or plateauing hCG levels. One hundred and twenty-five patients had invasive moles, and 17 had choriocarcinomas. Only 15% of the 142 treated patients, or 3% of the total, developed metastases outside of the uterus. Morrow and Kohorn treated a higher proportion of their patients (36% and 27%, respectively) using hCG criteria derived from regression curves, compared with studies in the literature that use the individual patient's hCG regression pattern. It appears that the use of the hCG regression curve may result in more patients being treated than is necessary, and it did not prevent metastatic disease in their patients. All the patients in the study by Lurain and associates, by either spontaneous or therapeutic modalities, have remained in remission.

In an effort to provide uniformity to the diagnosis of postmolar GTN, FIGO conducted workshops among members of the Society of Gynecologic Oncologists, International Society for the Study of Trophoblastic Disease, and International Gynecologic Cancer Society to formulate its current recommendations for evaluation and staging this disease. The current FIGO requirements for making a diagnosis of postmolar GTN are (Table 7–4):

1. Four values or more of plateaued hCG (+/− 10%) over at least 3 weeks: days 1, 7, 14, and 21.
2. A rise of hCG of 10% or greater for 3 values or more over at least 2 weeks: days 1, 7, and 14.
3. The histologic diagnosis of choriocarcinoma.
4. Persistence of hCG beyond 6 months after mole evacuation.

The level and duration for observation of the hCG plateau beyond 3 weeks would be determined at the discretion of the treating physician. Observation of hCG level plateau for longer than 3 weeks was permitted because this does not appear to have an adverse effect on patient survival.

The majority of centers in the USA will also treat patients if metastases are identified on examination or radiographic studies. Some pulmonary metastases result from deportation of trophoblast during molar evacuation and identification of pulmonary nodules in a post evacuation chest X-ray might not indicate true malignant behavior. Bagshawe et al, reporting the results from a centralized system for monitoring patients after evacuation of hydatidiform mole in the United Kingdom, stated that patients with pulmonary nodules were followed conservatively and treatment decisions based upon hCG regression patterns. Although the overall results from this policy were excellent, outcome for patients with pulmonary metastases was not detailed. In the USA, where care is decentralized and most patients are followed by general obstetrician-gynecologists after evacuation of hydatidiform mole, identification of metastases is included as an indication for initiation of therapy.

Table 7–4 DIAGNOSIS AND EVALUATION OF GTN

Diagnosis of GTN
After molar evacuation: 4 values or more of plateaued hCG (+/− 10%) over at least three weeks: days 1, 7, 14, and 21
After molar evacuation: a rise of hCG of 10% or greater for 3 values or more over at least 2 weeks: days 1, 7, and 14
After molar evacuation: Persistence of hCG beyond 6 months
The histologic diagnosis of choriocarcinoma, invasive mole, or PSTT
Metastatic disease without established primary site with elevated hCG; pregnancy has been excluded
Evaluation of GTN
Complete physical and pelvic examination; baseline hematologic, renal, and hepatic functions
Baseline quantitative hCG level
Chest X-ray or CT scan of chest
Brain MRI or CT scan
CT scan of abdomen and pelvis

hCG, human chorionic gonadotropin; PSTT, placental site trophoblastic tumor; CT, computed tomography; MRI, magnetic resonance imaging.

"Phantom" HCG

Rarely women present with persistently elevated hCG levels but are subsequently found to have a false positive hCG assay result, sometimes after receiving chemotherapy or surgery for presumed malignant GTN. Most patients with "phantom" hCG present with low-level hCG elevations, but occasionally values as high as 200–300 mIU/mL have been recorded. The false positive hCG values result from interference with the hCG immunometric sandwich assays caused by non-specific heterophile antibodies in the patients' sera. Many of these patients have an undefined previous pregnancy event and do not have radiographic evidence of metastatic disease. Serial hCG values usually do not substantially vary, despite often prolonged observation, and usually do not substantially change with therapeutic interventions such as surgery or chemotherapy.

"Phantom" hCG may also present after evacuation of a hydatidiform mole or following a clearly defined pregnancy event, such as an ectopic pregnancy. It should be suspected if hCG values plateau at relatively low levels and do not respond to therapeutic maneuvers such as methotrexate given for a presumed persistent mole or ectopic pregnancy. Evaluation should include evaluation of serum hCG using a variety of assay techniques at different dilutions of patient serum, combined with a urinary hCG level if the serum level is above threshold for the urinary assay. False positive hCG assays usually will not be affected by serial dilution of patient sera, and will have markedly different values using different assay techniques, with the majority of assays reflecting undetectable hCG. Heterophile antibodies are not excreted in the urine. Therefore, if they are the cause of serum hCG level elevation urinary hCG values will not be detectable. Other techniques are available to inactivate or strip the patient's serum of heterophile antibodies. It is important to exclude the possibility of "phantom" hCG before subjecting these patients to hysterectomy or chemotherapy for GTN.

Pretherapy evaluation

In contrast to epithelial endometrial cancer, GTN usually spreads by hematogenous dissemination. Invasive mole and choriocarcinoma invade locally into the myometrium, gaining access into capillaries and small veins. Venous metastasis can occur into the subvaginal venous plexus, resulting in vaginal metastases (Fig. 7–13), or into the main uterine venous system with metastases to the parametrium and lungs. While direct shunting into the systemic circulation rarely occurs, the majority of disseminated metastases develop only after pulmonary metastases have become established. From pulmonary nodules, hematogenous dissemination can occur via the systemic circulation. Brain, liver, gastrointestinal tract and kidneys are the distant organs most often affected, but metastases to virtually every organ have been reported. Although lymphatic spread can occur, it is relatively uncommon among patients with choriocarcinoma and invasive mole. The hematogenous pattern of metastatic involvement is important when considering the radiographic evaluation of patients with GTN (Table 7–3).

Pretherapy evaluation of the patient with GTN (Table 7–4) includes an assessment of history for clinical risk factors, examination, laboratory evaluation, and radiographic survey for possible sites of metastatic disease and number of lesions. Clinical risk factors important for assigning staging and treatment include duration of disease as determined by interval from antecedent pregnancy, type of antecedent pregnancy, and previous treatment. Because of different clinical characteristics, patients with histologically proven PSTT are usually classified separately from patients with gestational choriocarcinoma or postmolar GTN. The laboratory evaluation should include basic hematologic and clinical chemistry tests to determine baseline function before beginning chemotherapy, as well as a pretherapy hCG value. It should be emphasized that the hCG level obtained immediately before instituting treatment for malignant GTN is important for staging, not the hCG obtained at the time of previous molar evacuation.

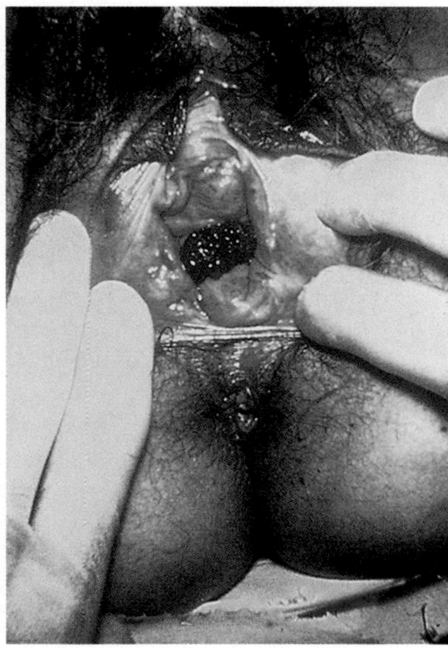

Figure 7–13 Vaginal metastasis of malignant GTN, presenting as vaginal bleeding with a discolored submucosal mass underlying the urethra. Vaginal metastases of GTN are highly vascular and should not be biopsied (Courtesy of John Soper, M.D.).

Vaginal metastases of GTN are most often diagnosed by physical examination. These lesions usually involve the submucosa of the anterior vagina and present as dark, often blue, soft nodules (Fig. 7–13). Ulceration or active bleeding may be present. Because of the highly vascular nature of these lesions, biopsy is not recommended. If vaginal metastases are the only site of metastatic disease, the majority of patients with these lesions will promptly respond to chemotherapy. A few patients will require vaginal packing or selective embolization using interventional radiology techniques to control active hemorrhage early in the course of treatment.

The recommended radiographic staging evaluation for patients with GTN includes chest X-ray or computed tomography (CT) scan, evaluation of the abdomen and pelvis with CT or magnetic resonance imaging (MRI) scan, and contrasted CT or MRI of the brain. An ultrasound of the pelvis should also be obtained to exclude the possibility of intrauterine pregnancy before instituting chemotherapy. Both ultrasound and MRI studies of the uterus can be used to identify intrauterine tumors and foci of myometrial invasion by GTN, but are not sensitive or specific enough to replace serum hCG level monitoring for establishing the diagnosis of GTN or for following patients during treatment.

Approximately 45% of patients present with metastatic disease when GTN is diagnosed. As indicated by the distribution of anatomic sites of metastatic disease encountered among patients initially treated for malignant GTN at Duke University Medical Center (Table 7–3), the lung is the most frequent site of extrauterine metastasis (Figs 7–14A and 7–14B). While the majority of patients with high-risk metastatic sites have identifiable pulmonary metastases on chest X-ray or symptoms referable to metastatic involvement, a full metastatic evaluation is recommended rather than relying upon a negative chest X-ray alone to make a determination of non-metastatic GTN. Between 29–41% of patients treated for non-metastatic GTN have pulmonary metastases identified on CT scans of the lungs that are not detected by chest X-ray. The clinical importance of occult pulmonary metastases is debated when they are the only sites of extrauterine metastases. However, many series of patients treated for high-risk metastases include patients who initially presented with normal chest X-rays. It would be a tragedy to miss the diagnosis of a high-risk metastasis in a patient on the basis of a negative chest X-ray and delay appropriate aggressive initial therapy.

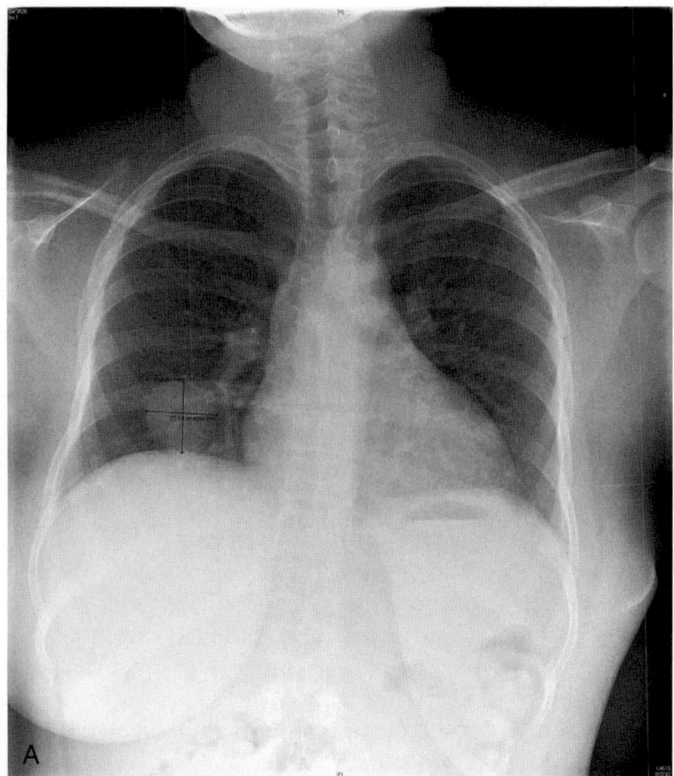

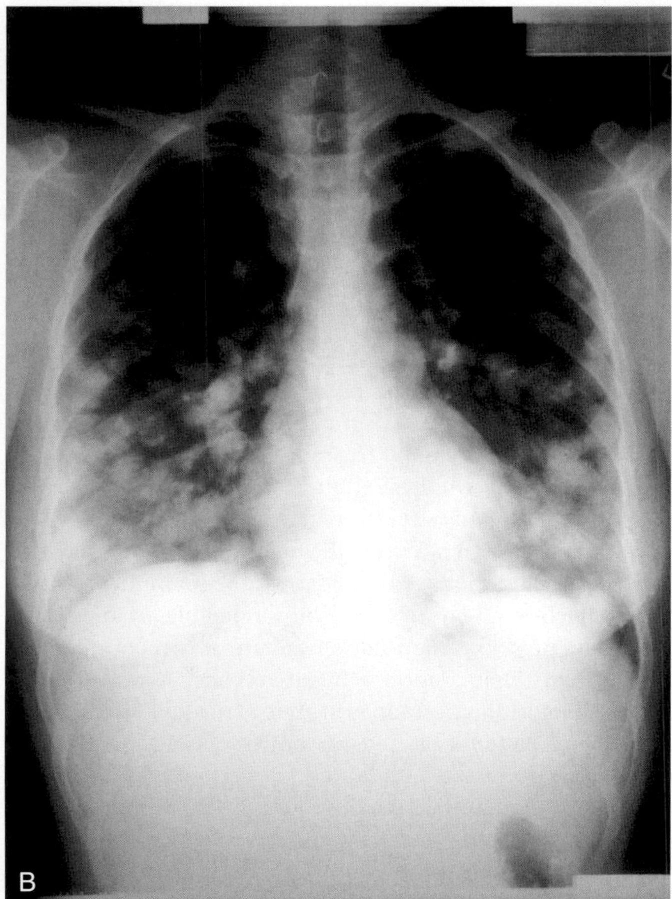

Figure 7–14 Pulmonary metastases of GTN can present as solitary (Figure 7–14A) or diffuse (Fig 7–14B) pulmonary nodules (Courtesy of John Soper, M.D.).

Although operative procedures may be integrated into the treatment of patients with malignant GTN, they are rarely indicated for establishing the diagnosis or staging. Performing a secondary D&C before beginning chemotherapy in a patient with postmolar GTN is controversial. The experience at the University of Southern California indicated that it had an effect on the need for treatment in only 20% of patients and was complicated by uterine perforation requiring hysterectomy in 8% of their patients. In contrast, Pezeshki and associates analyzed 544 women undergoing a second uterine evacuation for presumed postmolar GTN based on hCG criteria. After a second evacuation, 368 (68%) entered spontaneous remission. Ninety-six (38%) of 251 patients with a histologic diagnosis of persistent but non-invasive GTD required chemotherapy compared to 39 (38%) of 219 patients with negative histology at the second D&C. Many clinicians in the USA treat patients with postmolar GTN without performing a secondary D&C, because of the concern for preservation of fertility. Other operative procedures such as laparoscopy, thoracotomy, or craniotomy are only rarely justifiable to establish the primary diagnosis of GTN.

Classification and staging

The classification and staging of malignant GTN has evolved over the past 40 years. The Clinical Classification System based on risk factors is most frequently used in the USA (Table 7–5). In this classification system patients with non-metastatic disease are not assigned into a prognostic group because of a uniformly good outcome using simple single-agent chemotherapy. The risk factors used in this system were originally identified by retrospective analysis to predict resistance to single agent methotrexate and dactinomycin regimens among women treated for metastatic

Table 7–5 CLINICAL CLASSIFICATION SYSTEM FOR PATIENTS WITH MALIGNANT GTN

Category	Criteria
Non-metastatic GTN	No evidence of metastases; not assigned to prognostic category
Metastatic GTN	Any extrauterine metastases
Good prognosis metastatic GTN	No risk factors:
Pretherapy hCG <40,000 mIU/mL	Short duration (<4 months) Pretherapy hCG <40,000 mIU/mL No brain or liver metastases No antecedent term pregnancy No prior chemotherapy
Poor prognosis metastatic GTN	Any one risk factor: Long duration (>4 months) Pretherapy hCG >40,000 mIU/mL Brain or liver metastases Antecedent term pregnancy Prior chemotherapy

hCG, human chorionic gonadotropin; GTN, gestational trophoblastic neoplasia.

Table 7–6 WHO PROGNOSTIC INDEX SCORE COMPARED WITH CLINICAL CLASSIFICATION SYSTEM

	Who prognostic index score category			
Clinical classification	Low risk (<5)	Medium risk (5–7)	High risk (>8)	Total clinical classification
Non-metastatic GTN	99.5% (217)	100% (10)	—	99.7% (227)
Metastatic GTN				
Good prognosis	100% (86)	100% (5)		100% (91)
Poor prognosis	100% (8)	90.5% (21)	68.4% (38)	79.1% (67)
Total WHO	99.8% (311)	94.4% (36)	68.4% (38)	

WHO, World Health Organization; GTN, gestational trophoblastic neoplasia.
Data presented as life table survival percentage (number of patients).
(Modified from Soper JT, Evans AC, Conaway MR, et al: Evaluation of prognostic factors and staging in gestational trophoblastic tumor. Obstet Gynecol 84:969, 1994.)

GTN at the National Institutes of Health. Hammond et al subsequently reported essentially 100% survival among women who presented with good prognosis metastatic GTN and survival of 70% among patients with metastatic poor prognosis disease who were initially treated with multiagent chemotherapy, compared to only 14% survival for patients in this category who initially received single agent therapy. Poor tolerance of therapy was noted in the group of poor prognosis patients receiving initial single agent regimens, with toxicity causing death in half of these patients.

A more complicated classification system was adopted by the World Health Organization (WHO) in the early 1980s. This system was based on the experience of the patients treated for GTN at the Charing Cross Hospital in London between 1957 through 1973. Univariate analysis was used to retrospectively identify prognostic factors among patients treated mainly with simple chemotherapy regimens. In the original study, patient age, antecedent pregnancy, interval from antecedent pregnancy, hCG level, ABO blood type, size of the largest tumor, sites and number of metastases, and type of prior chemotherapy were each found to correlate with prognosis. The WHO prognostic index applied a weighted score to each of these factors, which were assumed to act independently. The sum of component scores was then used to determine the individual patient's risk category.

Several problems have been identified in the use of the WHO prognostic index score. One inherent problem is that multivariate analyses have not confirmed that each of the factors has an independent effect on prognosis. Paternal blood type information, identified as a risk factor by Bagshawe, is not uniformly available and has been omitted in generating WHO score values by some investigators. Others have modified the weighted scoring system using a highest risk score of 6 for each prognostic factor, while not changing the total score required to stratify patients into the graduated risk categories. In effect, this would result in a decreased number of risk factors to categorize patients into the highest risk category. Furthermore, the WHO prognostic index score provides for reassignment of a score among patients who have previously received treatment for GTN, which might obscure the prognostic effects of some of the other clinical factors on primary treatment. Finally, there has been no uniformity in use of radiographic studies to assess size of the largest tumor or assign number of metastases. Despite these limitations, various modifications of the WHO prognostic index score are useful for predicting groups of patients with malignant GTD at low and high risk for treatment failure.

In Table 7–6, the Clinical Classification System and WHO prognostic index score are compared among patients who presented for initial treatment of GTN at Duke University Medical Center. In this study, information about ABO blood type was not used to generate the WHO prognostic index score. The Clinical Classification System had a greater sensitivity for identifying patients at risk for treatment failure and death (Table 7–6). Although the WHO prognostic index score was able to provide slightly better stratification among the patients with poor prognosis metastatic disease by identifying low, intermediate and high risk populations, stratification into these three categories was considered less important than identifying patients at risk of failure for initial therapy. By multivariate analysis, both systems were roughly equivalent in efficacy for stratifying patients into risk groups.

Also in the early 1980s, FIGO proposed an anatomic staging system for malignant GTD (Table 7–7). Although this system recognized the stepwise development of metastatic disease, it did not incorporate any of the other

Table 7–7 ANATOMIC FIGO STAGING SYSTEM FOR GTN

Stage	Criteria
I	Disease confined to the uterus
II	Disease outside of uterus but is limited to the genital structures
III	Disease extends to the lungs with or without known genital tract involvement
IV	All other metastatic sites

FIGO, International Federation of Gynecology and Obstetrics; GTN, gestational trophoblastic neoplasia.
Modified from Kohorn EI: The new FIGO 2000 staging and risk factor scoring system for gestational trophoblastic disease: description and critical assessment. Int J Gynecol Cancer 11:73, 2000.

Table 7–8 THE REVISED FIGO 2000 SCORING SYSTEM FOR GTN

FIGO score	0	1	2	4
Age (years)	< 39	> 39		
Antecedent pregnancy	Hydatidiform mole	Abortion		Term pregnancy
Interval from index pregnancy (months)	< 4	4–6	6–12	> 12
Pretreatment hCG (mIU/mL)	< 1000	1000–10,000	10,000–100,000	>100,000
Largest tumor size including uterus (cm)		3–4	5	
Site of metastases		Spleen Kidney	Gastrointestinal	Brain Liver
Number of metastases identified	0	1–4	4–8	> 8
Previous failed chemotherapy			Single drug	> 2 drugs

The total score for a patient is obtained by adding the individual scores for each prognostic factor. Total score 0–6 = low risk; ≥ 7 = high risk.
From Kohorn EI: The new FIGO 2000 staging and risk factor scoring system for gestational trophoblastic disease: description and critical assessment. Int J Gynecol Cancer 11:73, 2000.

prognostic factors into the FIGO stage. While Stage I patients uniformly had low-risk disease and Stage IV patients were uniformly high risk, there could be considerable overlap of outcome within stages II and III. This failing was quickly recognized. Revision of the FIGO staging in 1992 included addition of hCG level >100,000 mIU/mL and time from antecedent pregnancy >6 months as recognized risk factors. These risk factors were used to generate substages within each anatomic stage. While this revised staging system did correlate with outcome, it resulted in a proliferation of substages with questionable importance.

In 2000, FIGO revised its staging system for GTN again. The original anatomic stages were retained but the 1992 risk factors were replaced by a risk factor score generated by a standardized modification of the WHO prognostic index score (Table 7–8). Patients with histologically diagnosed PSTT were to be reported separately, reflecting the distinct tumor biology of these lesions. Changes to the WHO classification included elimination of ABO blood group risk factors and a change in the risk score for liver metastasis from 2 to 4, reflecting high risk for patients with liver metastasis reported in many series. Chest X-ray rather than chest CT would be used to assess the number of metastatic lesions. Abdominal CT and brain MRI were recommended for the evaluation for liver and brain metastases, respectively. Finally, the three risk groups of the WHO prognostic index score were consolidated into two groups: Low Risk with a score of 6 or less and High Risk with a score of 7 or greater. Hancock et al retrospectively compared the outcomes of patients according to the risk score categories generated by modified WHO prognostic index score and the proposed FIGO score. The consolidated risk categories generated by the FIGO score correlated better with outcome than did the modified WHO prognostic index score.

Under the new FIGO system, reporting of patients will include both anatomic stage and FIGO risk score. For example: a 30-year-old patient with non-metastatic GTD diagnosed 5 months after molar evacuation with an hCG level of 8000 mIU/mL would be recorded as a FIGO Stage I: 2. Likewise, a 40-year-old with prior term pregnancy 7 months previously, hCG of 200,000 mIU/mL, brain metastases, 10 lung lesions, and uterine tumor measuring 6 centimeters would be FIGO Stage IV: 17.

It is anticipated that adoption of the newest revision of FIGO staging for GTN will allow uniformity for evaluation and reporting of outcomes. With accumulation of data through FIGO, it is hoped that multivariate analysis can confirm or refute the prognostic importance of individual factors used to generate the risk scores. While these changes are important on an international scale and the standard for reporting results of treatment, they are of lesser importance for the practicing general obstetrician-gynecologist initially encountering patients with malignant GTN. For these clinicians, the most important decisions revolve around identification of patients who should be referred out of the community to a specialist for treatment of high-risk disease. Because the clinical classification system (Table 7–5) is relatively simple, correlating well with failure of initial single agent chemotherapy, and also identifies patients who fail treatment with the greatest sensitivity, it may be the best system for use by the generalist for the purpose of appropriate triage for referral.

Treatment of non-metastatic GTN

Primary remission rates of patients treated for non-metastatic GTN are similar using a variety of chemotherapy regimens (Table 7–6). Essentially all patients with this condition can be cured, usually without the need for hysterectomy. Randomized comparisons of the regimens detailed in Table 7–9 have not been completed, and comparison of results discussed below may not be valid because of slightly different criteria used to make the diagnosis of non-metastatic GTN by different investigators.

Methotrexate 0.4 mg/kg/day given by intramuscular (IM) injection for 5 days, with cycles repeated every 12 to 14 days was the regimen originally used to treat GTN at the NIH. Hammond and colleagues reported the NIH experience treating 58 patients with non-metastatic GTN. Only four (7%) patients had disease resistant to this regimen and three of these were salvaged with single-agent dactinomycin. In Lurain's series from the Brewer

Table 7–9 CHEMOTHERAPY REGIMENS FOR NON-METASTATIC AND LOW-RISK METASTATIC GTN

Agent/Schedule	Dosage
Methotrexate (1)	
Weekly	30 mg/m^2 IM
5 day/every 2 weeks	0.4 mg/kg IM (maximum 25 mg/d total dose)
Methotrexate/folinic acid rescue	Methotrexate 1 mg/kg IM, days 1, 3, 5, 7; and
Every 2 weeks	Folinic acid 0.1 mg/kg IM, days 2, 4, 6, 8
Methotrexate infusion/folinic acid	Methotrexate 100mg/m^2 IV bolus; and
Every 2 weeks	Folinic acid 200mg/m^2 12 hr infusion 15 mg p.o. every 6 hr for four doses
Dactinomycin (2)	
5 day/every 2 weeks	9–13 mcg/kg/d IV (maximum dose 500 mcg/day)
bolus, every 2 weeks	1.25 mg/m^2 IV bolus
Etoposide (3)	200mg/m^2 /day p.o.
5 day/every 2 weeks	

(1) Dose based on ideal body weight, maximum 2 m^2; (2) Potential extravasation injury, gastrointestinal toxicity common; (3) Alopecia, small leukemogenic risk.
IM, intramuscular, IV, intravenous, p.o., oral.

Trophoblastic Disease Center, all 337 patients with non-metastatic GTN were cured. Only 10.7% of 253 patients initially treated with 5-day intramuscular (IM) methotrexate therapy required a second agent (dactinomycin), only 1.2% multiple agent chemotherapy, and in only 0.8% was a hysterectomy needed to achieve a complete remission. Factors significantly associated with the development of methotrexate resistance included pretreatment serum hCG in excess of 50,000 mIU/mL, non-molar antecedent pregnancy, and histopathologic diagnosis of choriocarcinoma. For years, 5-day IM methotrexate was the primary treatment of choice at the Southeastern Regional Center for Trophoblastic Disease, with similar results. If patients have abnormal liver function, methotrexate should not be used, because this agent is metabolized in the liver. Furthermore, significant hematologic suppression, cutaneous toxicity, mucositis, alopecia, gastrointestinal toxicity, and serositis are frequently seen in patients receiving this regimen.

Bagshawe and Wilde first reported the use of alternating daily doses of IM methotrexate (1 mg/kg) and leukovorin factor or folinic acid (0.1 mg/kg) for four doses of each agent, in an attempt to reduce the toxicity of daily methotrexate regimens. Folinic acid is a reduced form of folate that "rescues" cells from the dihydrofolate reductase block in the purine synthetic pathway produced by methotrexate. While this may be true for high doses of methotrexate, Rotmensch and associates evaluated methotrexate levels in patients after daily methotrexate therapy compared to levels in patients receiving alternating daily doses of methotrexate and folinic acid, with a higher daily dose of methotrexate given in the methotrexate/folinic acid regimen. They noted that while patients on the methotrexate/folinic acid regimen had higher peak methotrexate levels after treatment with a higher dose than those on single agent methotrexate, trough levels were both subtoxic and subtherapeutic 24 hours after methotrexate administration. This finding alone might explain therapeutic and toxicity benefit described for the low dose IM methotrexate/folinic acid regimen used for treatment in GTN.

Berkowitz and associates, at the New England Trophoblastic Center, have used methotrexate with folinic acid rescue in 185 patients with GTN. Ninety percent of 163 patients with non-metastatic disease and 68% of 22 patients with low-risk metastatic disease were placed into complete remission with methotrexate and folinic acid. Rather than recycling treatment at fixed intervals, they treated patients based on hCG level regression after chemotherapy. More than 80% were placed into remission with only one course of chemotherapy. All patients with methotrexate resistance achieved remission with other agents.

At Charing Cross Hospital in London, 347 of 348 (99.7%) low-risk patients treated with methotrexate and folinic acid survived; however, 69 (20%) had to change treatment because of drug resistance and 23 (6%) additional patients needed to change treatment because of drug-induced toxicity. An analysis of the data from the Southeastern Trophoblastic Disease Center at Duke University indicated that 8 (27.5%) of 29 patients developed resistance to methotrexate with folinic acid given at 14 day intervals, compared to 3 (7.7%) of 39 treated with standard 5-day methotrexate for non-metastatic disease. Although this difference was statistically significant, because a larger number of patients receiving standard methotrexate changed to another agent because of toxicity, a similar proportion of patients were changed to a second agent in each group. Wong and associates also compared 5-day methotrexate to methotrexate with folinic acid, resulting in comparable sustained biochemical remission rates. In their series, however, patients who received methotrexate/folinic acid achieved remission earlier but experienced a higher incidence of hepatic toxicity compared with patients receiving the 5-day regimen.

Other investigators have used higher doses of intravenous (IV) methotrexate (300–500 mg/m^2) followed by oral or intravenous folinic acid every 6 hours for 24 hours have resulted in primary remission rates of 45–86% in patients with non-metastatic and/or low-risk metastatic GTN. Overall cure rates in these series were excellent and toxicity was minimal. A major disadvantage with these regimens is the need for a prolonged (up to 12 hour) IV infusion.

Oral methotrexate is readily absorbed via the gastrointestinal tract. Barter reported a retrospective analysis of 15 patients treated solely with oral methotrexate 0.4 mg/kg for 5-day cycles that were repeated every 14 days. The primary remission rate was 87% with minimal toxicity. Concerns about patient compliance and the possibility of unpredictable absorption in individual patients have led to infrequent use for this mode of treatment in GTN.

In a prospective phase II trial, the Gynecologic Oncology Group reported an 82% primary remission rate for patients treated with weekly intramuscular methotrexate, given at a dose of 30–50 mg/m^2. Remission was achieved within a median 7 cycles of therapy. There was no apparent benefit for increasing the dose up to 50 mg/m^2. It was concluded that the weekly methotrexate regimen was most cost effective among several alternative methotrexate or dactinomycin schedules when taking efficacy, toxicity, and cost into consideration. Hoffman et al and Gleeson and associates confirmed the low toxicity and excellent overall remission rates for patients treated with this regimen. In the experience reported by Gleeson and associates, weekly methotrexate was compared with methotrexate/folinic acid, producing equivalent primary remission rates. Total doses of methotrexate required to induce remission were lower in the weekly methotrexate group. They also concluded that weekly methotrexate was minimally toxic, equally effective and their preferred regimen for non-metastatic GTN.

In contrast to IM methotrexate regimens used for treating ectopic pregnancies, chemotherapy for GTN is recycled every week until hCG values have achieved normal levels, and then an additional course is administered after the first normal hCG value has been recorded. Hematologic indices must be monitored carefully during chemotherapy, but significant hematologic toxicity is infrequent among patients treated with the weekly methotrexate regimen. Because methotrexate is excreted entirely by the kidney and can produce hepatic toxicity, patients must have normal renal and liver functions before each treatment.

Other investigators have used 5-day courses of intravenous dactinomycin 9–13 mcg/kg/day as primary therapy for non-metastatic or low-risk GTN, with equally good results. They believe that toxicity from 5-day dactinomycin is less than that from 5-day methotrexate regimens. However, alopecia, nausea, and significant myelotoxicity can result. Furthermore, dactinomycin is a vesicant; extravasation during intravenous administration can result in severe local soft tissue damage.

Treatment of non-metastatic and low-risk metastatic GTN with dactinomycin 1.25 mg/m^2 given as a single intravenous bolus dose every 2 weeks had equal remission rates in retrospective comparisons to 5-day courses of intravenous dactinomycin. The Gynecologic Oncology Group reported a phase II study of this regimen for primary treatment of GTN. Of 31 patients who were treated, 29 (94%) achieved remission after an average of 4.4 (range of 2 to 15) courses of therapy. The two patients who failed to respond to pulse therapy were subsequently cured by alternative treatment. The frequency of toxicity was quite low. The advantages of pulse dactinomycin over other dactinomycin treatment schedules include ease of administration, greater patient convenience, and improved cost effectiveness. Moreover, the single bolus administration of dactinomycin appears to reduce the risk of extravasation injuries, compared to 5-day intravenous administration.

Other investigators have alternated courses of 5-day IM methotrexate with 5-day IV dactinomycin in an attempt to limit toxicity and improve primary remission rates. Rose and Piver combined their experience using this approach in nine patients with a literature review of 40 patients treated in this manner. All patients were cured with primary therapy when the two regimens were alternated. However, given the relatively small numbers of patients and selectivity of reporting small series of patients in the literature, one cannot conclude that this strategy is superior to beginning therapy in patients with GTN using a single agent and changing to the alternative only if chemoresistance or toxicity is encountered.

5-fluorouracil (5-FU) and oral etoposide are frequently used in Asia for primary treatment of patients with non-metastatic and low-risk metastatic GTN, but are not often used in the USA. Among patients treated with a 10-day continuous intravenous infusion of 5-FU, Sung et al reported a 93% primary remission rate. Acute toxicity included diarrhea, nausea and vomiting, hepatotoxicity, and stomatitis. Likewise Wong et al reported a 98% primary remission rate among patients treated with 5-day courses of oral etoposide 100 mg/m^2, recycled at 14-day intervals. Toxicity included frequent alopecia, myelosuppression, and gastrointestinal toxicity. Furthermore, patients exposed to etoposide have a low but significant risk of developing acute myelogenous leukemia. Based on considerations of convenience, cost, and toxicity, these agents are not usually employed as first line therapy for non-metastatic GTN in the USA.

Among patients with non-metastatic GTN, early hysterectomy will shorten the duration and amount of chemotherapy required to produce remission. Therefore, each patient's desire for further childbearing should be evaluated at the onset of treatment. Hysterectomy may be performed during the first cycle of chemotherapy (Fig. 7–15). However, further chemotherapy after hysterectomy is mandatory until hCG values are normal.

Treatment for non-metastatic and low-risk metastatic GTN is outlined in Table 7–10. Most centers in the USA will begin therapy with the weekly IM methotrexate or the bolus dactinomycin regimen. Weekly hCG values should be monitored during treatment, along with hematologic and metabolic studies to monitor for toxicity. Chemotherapy

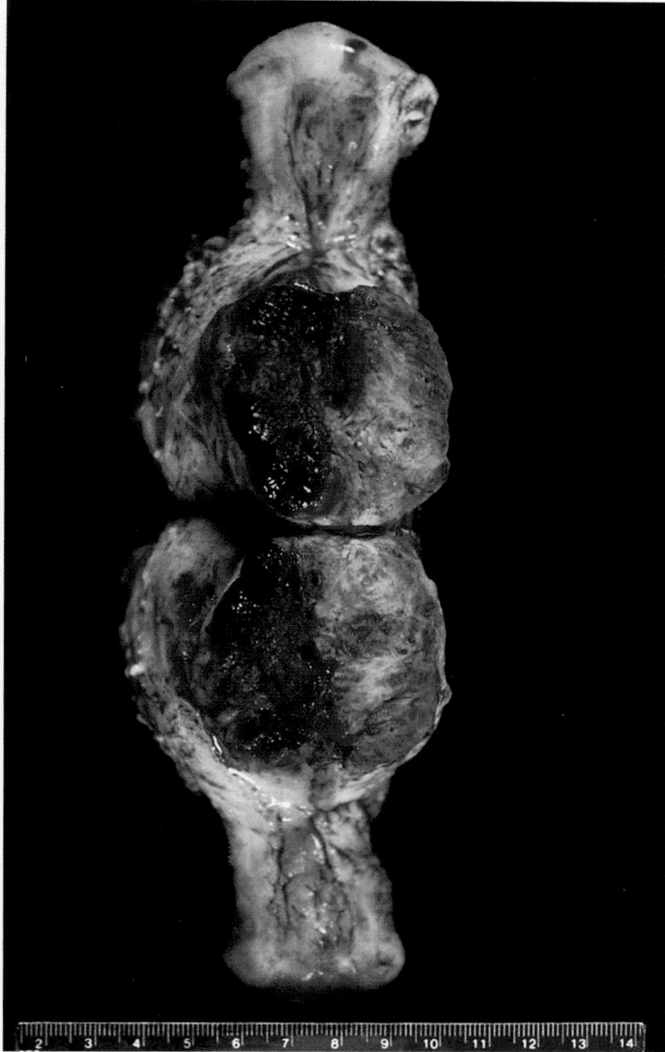

Figure 7–15 Hysterectomy specimen in a 39-year-old woman with nonmetastatic GTN who underwent surgery during her first course of methotrexate. She entered complete remission 4 weeks after initial therapy (Courtesy of John Soper, M.D.).

is repeated until hCG levels normalize and at least on cycle of chemotherapy is given as maintenance chemotherapy to prevent recurrence. Reliable contraception, preferably oral contraceptives, should be used to prevent an intercurrent pregnancy during chemotherapy or monitoring after remission is achieved.

Patients in whom the rate of fall of hCG levels has plateaued or in whom values are rising during therapy should be switched to an alternative single-agent regimen after radiographic restaging. If there is appearance of new metastases or failure of the alternative single-agent chemotherapy, the patient should be treated with multiagent regimens. Hysterectomy should be considered for the treatment of non-metastatic disease that is refractory to chemotherapy and remains confined to the uterus.

The overall cure rate for patients with non-metastatic GTN approaches 100%, and the majority of women who wish to preserve fertility can be cured without undergoing

Table 7–10 MANAGEMENT OF LOW-RISK NON-METASTATIC OR LOW-RISK METASTATIC GTN

Initiate single-agent methotrexate or dactinomycin regimen (Table 7–9)

1. Consider hysterectomy if fertility not desired

Monitor hematologic, renal, and hepatic indices before each cycle of chemotherapy
Monitor serum hCG levels weekly during therapy
Change to alternative single-agent if resistance or severe toxicity to first agent
If resistance to alternative agent:

1. Repeat metastatic evaluation
2. Consider hysterectomy if no extrauterine metastases
3. Multiagent therapy (MAC or EMA/CO, see text)

Remission: three consecutive weekly hCG values in the normal range
1–2 cycles of maintenance/consolidation chemotherapy

MAC, methotrexate, adriamycin, and cyclophosphamide; EMA/CO, etoposide, methotrexate, actinomycin D, cyclophosphamide and vincristine

hysterectomy. When chemotherapy is given for an additional 1–2 cycles after the first normal hCG value, recurrence rates are < 5%.

Low-risk metastatic GTN

Patients with metastatic GTN who lack any of the clinical high risk factors or have a total FIGO risk score of 6 or less have low-risk disease. They can be treated successfully with initial single-agent regimens similar to non-metastatic GTN (Table 7–9). Most often, this has consisted of 5-day treatment using intramuscular methotrexate or intravenous dactinomycin recycled at 14-day intervals. DuBeshter and associates used single-agent methotrexate or dactinomycin to treat 48 patients with low-risk metastatic GTN at the New England Trophoblastic Disease Center. All patients achieved sustained remission but 51% required a second drug, 14% needed combination chemotherapy and 12% required surgery to remove drug-resistant disease. Among 52 patients with low-risk metastatic GTN treated initially with the 5-day methotrexate regimen at Duke University Medical Center, 60% achieved primary remission within a median 3 cycles of methotrexate chemotherapy. Patients were treated with dactinomycin for documented methotrexate resistance or toxicity with equal frequency. All patients achieved remission with only 4% requiring multiagent regimens. Likewise, Roberts and Lurain reviewed 92 patients treated for low-risk metastatic GTN at the Brewer Trophoblastic Disease Center. Among their 70 patients who were initially treated with chemotherapy alone, 24.6% developed chemoresistant disease and 9.8% had therapy changed to an alternative single-agent regimen because of toxicity. Overall, 78% achieved remission using the primary regimen with or without hysterectomy; all eventually achieved remission and only one (1.1%) required multiagent chemotherapy.

McNeish and associates, reporting from the Charing Cross system, reviewed the results of 485 patients with low-risk GTN (prognostic index score <8, using their modification) treated with cyclical intramuscular methotrexate/folinic acid; overall survival was 100%. Two-thirds achieved remission with primary chemotherapy, while 150 patients were changed to an alternative agent because of chemoresistance. In patients with chemoresistant disease and hCG levels <100 mIU/mL, therapy was changed to single-agent dactinomycin, with 89% responding to dactinomycin and the remaining patients salvaged with multiagent regimens. If hCG levels were >100 mIU/mL, patients were treated with a multiagent regimen containing etoposide, with 98.9% responding to the first salvage regimen and all patients entering sustained remission. Based on earlier reports with excellent salvage after failure of the initial single-agent regimen using an alternative single-agent regimen regardless of hCG levels, their treatment strategy might expose patients needlessly to multiagent regimens and increase long-term risks of leukemia and early menopause.

Hysterectomy in conjunction with chemotherapy may also decrease the amount of chemotherapy required to achieve remission in these patients, but the majority of women who wish to preserve fertility can be successfully treated without hysterectomy. Similar to the treatment of women with non-metastatic GTN (Table 7–10), 1–2 cycles of maintenance chemotherapy should be given after the first normal hCG. Recurrence rates are <5% among patients successfully treated for low-risk metastatic disease.

High-risk metastatic GTN

Patients with metastatic disease and one or more of the Clinical Classification system risk factors or a FIGO risk score of >7 have high-risk disease. They will often require multiagent chemotherapy with additional surgery or radiation incorporated into treatment. It should be emphasized that patients with high-risk metastatic GTN should have their treatment directed by individuals who have experience in treating this relatively rare disease, preferably in a Trophoblastic Disease Center. Survival reported by Trophoblastic Disease Centers ranges up to 86%. In contrast to patients with non-metastatic or low-risk metastatic GTN, early hysterectomy does not appear to improve the outcome in women with high-risk metastatic disease.

Aggressive treatment with multiagent chemotherapy is an important component for management of these patients. Triple therapy (Table 7–11) with methotrexate, dactinomycin, and either chlorambucil or cyclophosphamide (MAC) was the standard regimen for many years in the USA, producing sustained remission rates of 63–73%. Studies from the Southeastern Regional and the Brewer Trophoblastic Disease Centers in the early

Table 7–11 TRIPLE AGENT (MAC) CHEMOTHERAPY FOR HIGH-RISK GTN

Day	Drug	Dose
1–5	Methotrexate	15 mg IM
	Dactinomycin	500 mcg IV
	Chlorambucil	8–10 mg p.o.
	OR	
	Cyclophosphamide	3 mg/kg IV
15–22	Begin next cycle	

IM, intramuscular, IV, intravenous, p.o., oral.

1970s documented the importance of initial combination chemotherapy for these patients; single-agent regimens followed by multiagent chemotherapy produced 14–39% remissions, while patients with high-risk GTN treated initially with MAC chemotherapy had remission rates of 65–70%. Some studies indicated that patients with extremely high WHO prognostic index scores had poor survival following MAC chemotherapy.

In the late 1970s the Charing Cross group developed a complex, alternating regimen using cyclophosphamide, hydroxyurea, dactinomycin, methotrexate/folinic acid, vincristine, and doxorubicin (CHAMOCA). Sustained remissions were reported for 56–83% of patients with high-risk GTN using modifications of this regimen, with an overall impression of reduced toxicity compared to previous experience with MAC. However, when the Gynecologic Oncology Group performed a randomized trial of MAC versus CHAMOCA, the primary remission rates were comparable at 73% and 65%, respectively. Of note, five of six patients who failed MAC were salvaged compared to only one of seven patients failing CHAMOCA. Perhaps initial exposure to marginally effective additional agents in CHAMOCA adversely affected the efficacy for savage regimens, based on multi-drug resistance, or could not be tolerated because of cumulative toxicity. Furthermore, the CHAMOCA regimen had significantly more acute life-threatening toxicity, with a 45% incidence of grade 4 toxicity compared to only 9% with MAC.

More recent regimens have incorporated etoposide into primary combination chemotherapy for GTN. Alternating weekly chemotherapy (Table 7–12) with etoposide, methotrexate/folinic acid rescue, dactinomycin/cyclophosphamide and vincristine (EMA/CO) was first developed by the Charing Cross group. Their initial report documented survival of 30 (86%) of 36 patients with high-risk GTN after primary treatment with EMA/CO. In their updated series, Bower and associates included 272 patients with high-risk GTN treated with EMA/CO. Complete remission was recorded in 213 (78%) while 33 patients who failed EMA/CO were salvaged with additional therapies, resulting in an overall 5-year survival of 86.2%. Other smaller retrospective series have reported complete response rates of 65–94% among patients with high-risk GTN treated initially with EMA/CO. As a result of these reports, EMA/CO has currently become the most widely

Table 7–12 ALTERNATING WEEKLY EMA/CO CHEMOTHERAPY FOR HIGH-RISK GTN

Day	Drug	Dose
1	Etoposide	100 mg/m^2 IV
	Methotrexate*	100 mg/m^2 IV bolus
	Methotrexate	200 mg/m^2 IV infusion over 12 hr
	Dactinomycin	350 mcg/m^2 IV
2	Etoposide	100 mg/m^2 IV
	Dactinomycin	350 mcg/m^2 IV
	Folinic acid	15 mg p.o., IM or IV every 12 hr × 4 doses, begin 24 hr after methotrexate bolus
8**	Cyclophosphamide	600 mg/m^2 IV
	Vincristine	1.0 mg/m^2 IV
15	Begin next cycle	

*Methotrexate is sometimes given as a 12 hr IV infusion at a dose of 500–1,000 mg/m^2 for treatment of brain metastases, with folinic acid rescue increased to 15 mg every 6 hours × 48 hours or 30 mg every 12 hours × 48 hours

**Some investigators give methotrexate 15 mg intrathecal injection for prophylaxis or treatment of brain metastases

IM, intramuscular, IV, intravenous, p.o., oral.

used regimen for the initial treatment of patients with high-risk GTN.

Toxicity for EMA/CO in patients receiving primary therapy usually is well tolerated; alopecia is almost universal, while stomatitis and emetogenic toxicities are frequently seen. Myelosuppression is the acute dose-limiting acute toxicity. Several investigators have used stem cell support with granulocyte colony-stimulating factor to avoid dose reductions or treatment delays during EMA/CO therapy. It is unclear whether the cyclophosphamide and vincristine are important components of the EMA/CO regimen; treatment with EMA alone has documented complete response rates of 71–78% in high-risk patients, while both cyclophosphamide and vincristine contribute to myelosuppression.

Platin-containing regimens have also been found to be active in treating GTN. Cisplatin combined with etoposide and dactinomycin (PEA) demonstrated complete responses in 57–100% of patients with high-risk GTN. A one-day course of cisplatin and etoposide (EP) were originally substituted for CO and combined with EMA to treat patients with refractory GTN. Surwit and Childers successfully treated four high-risk patients initially with EMA/EP, but concerns about acute toxicity have kept it from becoming widely accepted as primary therapy. It should be emphasized that MAC and EMA/CO are the two regimens that have been most extensively evaluated for the treatment of high-risk GTN (Table 7–13), but these have never been compared in a randomized trial. The majority of the literature for other regimens has been in the form of retrospective analyses of relatively small numbers of patients, using slightly different definitions of "high-risk" GTN. Regardless of the regimen selected, aggressive recycling of multiagent therapy is the cornerstone for management of patients with high-risk disease (Table 7–13). The need for randomized comparisons of EMA/CO or the newer combinations with MAC is obvious, but unlikely given the relative rarity of this disease.

Table 7–13 MANAGEMENT OF HIGH-RISK GTN

Evaluate for high-risk metastases: brain, liver, kidney
Stabilize medical status of patient
Multiagent therapy with EMA/CO (Table 7–12) or MAC

1. Aggressive recycling may require cytokine support

Management of brain metastases (see text):

1. Consider early neurosurgical intervention if isolated brain lesion
2. Consider stereotactic or whole brain irradiation if multiple brain lesions

Management of liver metastases (see text):

1. Consider selective angiographic embolization or irradiation

Monitor hCG weekly during therapy
At least three cycles of maintenance chemotherapy after hCG values normalize

Management of cerebral metastases is controversial. Radiation therapy has been used concurrently with chemotherapy in an attempt to limit acute hemorrhagic complications from these metastases. Brain irradiation combined with systemic chemotherapy is successful in controlling brain metastases, with cure rates up to 75% in patients who initially present with brain metastases. However, a similar primary remission rate has also been reported among patients treated with combination regimens that incorporated high-dose systemic methotrexate combined with intrathecal methotrexate infusions, without brain irradiation. The best treatment for liver or other high-risk sites of metastases has not been established. Even with intense chemotherapy, additional surgery may be necessary to control hemorrhage from metastases, remove chemoresistant disease or treat other complications in order to stabilize high-risk patients during therapy.

Treatment of patients with high-risk GTN who have developed chemoresistant disease is extremely challenging, and is largely determined by prior chemotherapy exposure and cumulative toxicity from prior treatment. Patients who have not been exposed to etoposide-containing regimens are usually treated with EMA/CO, with remission rates of 71–82% reported for this group in several studies. The Charing Cross group used EMA/EP to treat 34 high-risk patients previously exposed to EMA/CO, reporting remission rates of 95% in patients with hCG level plateau during EMA/CO compared to 75% for those with rising hCG levels. Myelosuppression is more severe in patients receiving these regimens for salvage therapy than when they are used as primary therapy.

Table 7–14 SURVEILLANCE DURING AND AFTER THERAPY OF GTN

Monitor serum quantitative hCG levels every week during chemotherapy:

1. Response: >10% decline in hCG during one cycle
2. Plateau: ±10% change in hCG during one cycle
3. Resistance: >10% rise in hCG during one cycle or plateau for two cycles of chemotherapy
   - evaluate for new metastases
   - consider alternative chemotherapy (see text)
   - consider extirpation of drug-resistant sites of disease

Remission: 3 consecutive normal weekly hCG values

1. Maintenance chemotherapy (see text)

Surveillance of remission:

1. hCG values every 2 weeks × 3 months
2. hCG values every month to complete one year of follow-up
3. hCG values every 6–12 months indefinitely; at least 3–5 years

Variations of combination regimens used in the treatment of testicular and ovarian germ cell tumors have been used as salvage therapy in patients with GTN. Etoposide-platin (+/– bleomycin +/– doxorubicin) and vinblastine-bleomycin-cisplatin have remission rates reported between 50–86% in small series of patients treated with these regimens, but with long-term survival rates of usually less than 50% and considerable myelosuppression when these combinations are used in a salvage setting. Ifosfamide-containing chemotherapy produced responses in four of five patients reported by Sutton et al, but only one patient had a sustained remission. Anecdotal case reports and small series of patients also indicate activity of paclitaxel regimens, high-dose chemotherapy with autologous bone marrow or colony-stimulating factor support, and 5-FU/dactinomycin in treating drug-resistant disease.

Chemotherapy is continued until hCG values have normalized, and this is followed by at least three courses of maintenance chemotherapy in the hope of eradicating all viable tumor (Table 7–14). Despite using sensitive hCG assays and maintenance chemotherapy, up to 13% of patients with high-risk disease will develop recurrence after achieving an initial remission.

Surgery

Brewer and associates reported that survival of patients treated with hysterectomy before effective chemotherapy was developed was only 40% for women with non-metastatic choriocarcinoma and only 19% for those with metastatic choriocarcinoma. The majority of their patients died of progressive disease within two years of surgery. The emergence of effective chemotherapy has lessened the importance of surgical procedures for managing patients with malignant GTN. However, many procedures remain useful adjuncts when integrated into the management of these patients.

Primary or delayed hysterectomy can be integrated into management to remove central disease, and surgical extirpation of metastases may cure highly selected patients with drug resistant disease. At Duke University Medical Center, extirpative procedures such as hysterectomy are usually performed during a course of chemotherapy to minimize the possibility of inducing metastases by surgical manipulation of tissues. There does not appear to be an increase in surgical morbidity using this combined modality approach. Surgical procedures are often required during therapy of patients with high-risk disease to treat complications of the disease, such as hemorrhage or abscess, and allow stabilization during chemotherapy. The use of percutaneous angiographic embolization can allow relatively non-invasive control of hemorrhagic complications of pelvic tumors or metastatic lesions. Finally, indwelling central venous catheters are useful for most patients with high-risk malignant GTN, who will often require prolonged courses of chemotherapy and intravenous support with blood products, crystalloid, antiemetics, and total parenteral nutrition during treatment.

Most patients with malignant GTN are in their peak reproductive years and do not wish sterilization. Furthermore, the majority can be cured with chemotherapy alone, especially women with non-metastatic or low-risk metastatic disease. Hysterectomy, however, continues to have a role in the management of women with malignant GTN.

Hammond et al reported an overall 100% sustained remission rate among 194 patients treated at Duke University Medical Center for non-metastatic or low risk metastatic GTN. Of these, 162 wished to retain child-bearing capacity and 89% were able to avoid hysterectomy. All 32 women treated with primary hysterectomy combined with methotrexate or dactinomycin single-agent chemotherapy regimens entered sustained remission. When compared to similar patients who had low-risk disease and were treated with chemotherapy alone, patients receiving primary hysterectomy had shorter duration of chemotherapy and lower total dosage of chemotherapy, roughly equivalent to one cycle of chemotherapy. Suzuka and associates also analyzed the total dosage of chemotherapy in women treated with etoposide for low-risk GTN. They found that the total dosage of etoposide was decreased in women with non-metastatic disease treated with adjuvant hysterectomy compared to those who were treated with chemotherapy alone, again roughly equivalent to a single cycle of chemotherapy. This effect was not observed among their patients with low-risk metastatic disease, where similar total dosages of etoposide were given to patients treated with adjuvant hysterectomy or chemotherapy alone. In other series hysterectomy was incorporated into the primary therapy of approximately 25% of patients with low-risk GTN.

Primary adjuvant hysterectomy was not effective in reducing chemotherapy requirements or improving cure rates for women with high-risk metastatic GTN in the experience reported by Hammond and colleagues. These patients usually present with disseminated disease and hysterectomy would be expected to contribute much less to reduction of tumor burden compared to patients with non-metastatic or low-risk metastatic GTN. Therefore the major role of primary hysterectomy should be as part of primary therapy of women with non-metastatic disease or with limited metastatic involvement if there is no wish to preserve fertility.

Delayed hysterectomy is often considered for patients who fail to respond to primary chemotherapy. In the Duke experience reported by Hammond et al almost all of the patients with non-metastatic or low-risk metastatic GTN who were treated with a delayed hysterectomy because of resistance to primary chemotherapy achieved remission without requiring multiagent chemotherapy. Others have reported that salvage hysterectomy is effective in producing remissions in most patients with chemoresistant non-metastatic or low-risk metastatic disease. Control of extrauterine disease is central in the success of salvage hysterectomy for these patients.

Salvage hysterectomy may be integrated into the treatment of selected patients with high-risk metastatic GTN who have a small extrauterine tumor burden, but results are not as beneficial as in patients with low-risk disease. Patients with recurrent GTN often present with limited extrauterine dissemination and may benefit from salvage hysterectomy. Among 28 women with recurrent GTN treated at Duke University Medical Center, 14 (50%) were selected to undergo salvage hysterectomy during their therapy. The majority of these patients had no radiographic evidence of extrauterine disease, and 10 (83%) have had sustained remissions. However, salvage hysterectomy performed when there is disseminated metastasis is unlikely to have a significant impact on the survival of patients with high-risk or recurrent GTN.

Placental site trophoblastic tumor (PSTT) is much more rare than invasive mole or gestational choriocarcinoma. In contrast to other forms of malignant GTN, production of hCG is relatively lower and these tumors are usually resistant to conventional methotrexate- or dactinomycin-based chemotherapy regimens. Fortunately, many patients with PSTT present with non-metastatic disease. Papadopoulos et al noted that two-thirds of their patients were cured following surgery alone if PSTT was confined to the uterus, similar to the reported experience of others in smaller series. Hysterectomy should be integrated into the primary management of PSTT unless there are widespread metastases or in the rare case of localized disease that has been removed by D&C or localized myometrial resection in a woman who strongly desires childbearing.

The majority of women undergoing hysterectomy for malignant GTN have been treated with abdominal hysterectomy, with or without preservation of the adnexa. Ovarian removal is not required, as GTN rarely metastasizes to the ovaries and these tumors are not hormonally influenced. Vaginal hysterectomy may be considered in women with non-metastatic GTN who have a small uterus and low hCG levels, but does not allow assessment of the upper abdomen for occult metastases. Laparoscopic assisted vaginal hysterectomy (LAVH) has been used in a few patients with GTN. In contrast to vaginal hysterectomy, LAVH allows surveillance of the upper abdomen combined with a shorter acute convalescence than abdominal hysterectomy.

More conservative myometrial resections combined with uterine reconstruction can be considered in highly selected patients with non-metastatic GTN who wish to avoid hysterectomy. Previous anecdotal reports of local myometrial resections of invasive moles have documented the use of resection and uterine repair for primary therapy of non-metastatic GTN and PSTT. Kanazawa et al evaluated this procedure in 22 patients with invasive moles diagnosed on the basis of abnormal hCG regression after molar evacuation. All patients had lesions localized in the myometrium and defined by pelvic angiography, ultrasound and computerized tomography techniques. Seven (32%) of their patients required chemotherapy after surgery. Pregnancies have been documented after conservative resections of invasive moles; Kanazawa et al observed that reproductive performance was similar to patients treated with chemotherapy alone. Because of the high cure rates reported following chemotherapy alone in similar patients, it is more rational to consider these as salvage procedures in women with localized chemoresistant disease. Each patient considered for this procedure should be carefully evaluated for systemic metastases and the uterine lesion localized using a combination of color-flow ultrasound, MRI, and hysteroscopy. Intraoperative frozen sections should be used to assess surgical margins. Small lesions associated with low hCG levels are more likely to be completely excised with a conservative myometrial resection than lesions >2–3 cm in diameter.

The most frequently employed surgical procedure for extirpation of extrauterine metastases of GTN is thoracotomy with pulmonary wedge resection, but there are few large series of patients reported recently, due to the relative rarity for the need to perform extirpation of metastases. Although this can safely be performed in conjunction with chemotherapy, it is not necessary to resect lung metastases in the majority of patients. Radiographic evidence of tumor regression often lags behind hCG level response to treatment and some patients will have pulmonary nodules that persist for months or years after completion of chemotherapy. In women with low-risk metastatic GTN the overall risk of recurrence is <5%. Even though women with pulmonary nodules that persist after induction of hCG level remission may be at an increased risk for recurrence, these patients can be safely followed with serial hCG levels without the need for routine surgical resection.

Many series of patients with GTN treated with thoracotomy often include patients whose disease was not suspected until after resection of a pulmonary nodule. As in the case of brain, liver, or renal metastases, any woman of reproductive age who presents with an apparent metastatic malignancy of unknown primary site should be screened for the possibility of GTN with a serum hCG level. Excisional biopsy is not indicated to histologically confirm the diagnosis of malignant GTN if the patient is not pregnant and has a high hCG value.

Resection of pulmonary nodules in highly selected patients with drug-resistant disease may successfully induce remission. Immediately before performing pulmonary resection, it is important to exclude the possibility of active disease elsewhere by performing a comprehensive metastatic survey. Patients with isolated, unilateral nodules associated with low hCG values are much more likely to benefit from thoracotomy with pulmonary resection than patients with bilateral or multiple unilateral lesions, or those with disease in other locations. Tomoda et al reported that 14 (93%) of their 15 patients with isolated nodules and low hCG values survived after pulmonary resection, compared to none of four patients with either hCG values >1,000 mIU/mL or evidence of active disease outside of the resected nodule. Others have reported that a prompt hCG level remission occurring within 1–2 weeks of surgery portends a favorable outcome. Highly selected patients will require more than one pulmonary resection during the course of treatment in order to achieve a durable remission.

Brain metastases (Fig. 7–16) occur in 8–15% of patients with metastatic GTN and are associated with a worse prognosis than vaginal or pulmonary metastases. Metastases from GTN tend to be highly vascular and have a tendency for central necrosis and hemorrhage. A significant portion of early deaths is caused by central nervous system metastases of GTN with acute neurological deterioration before effective therapy is initiated or very early in the course of treatment. The major goals of treatment include early detection of brain metastases through complete radiological metastatic survey in all patients with malignant GTN, stabilization of the patient's neurological status, and initiation of therapy. Craniotomy solely for the purpose of tissue confirmation is not justified if GTN is clinically diagnosed on the basis of metastatic disease associated with an elevated hCG level.

In series of patients with brain metastases of GTN reported from the USA, brain irradiation is usually integrated into treatment in an attempt to prevent hemorrhage and neurological deterioration. Craniotomy is usually used only to prevent deterioration. However, Rustin et al recommended an approach using early craniotomy with excision of isolated lesions combined with high-dose systemic and intrathecal chemotherapy to treat patients with brain metastases. In their experience, brain irradiation was not used routinely. Both primary radiation therapy combined with chemotherapy and the approach emphasizing early surgical intervention appear to have similar efficacy in previously untreated patients. In sharp contrast to the outlook for women with brain metastases from other solid tumors, 75–80% of women with brain metastases presenting for primary therapy and 50% of patients overall with brain metastases from malignant GTN will be cured.

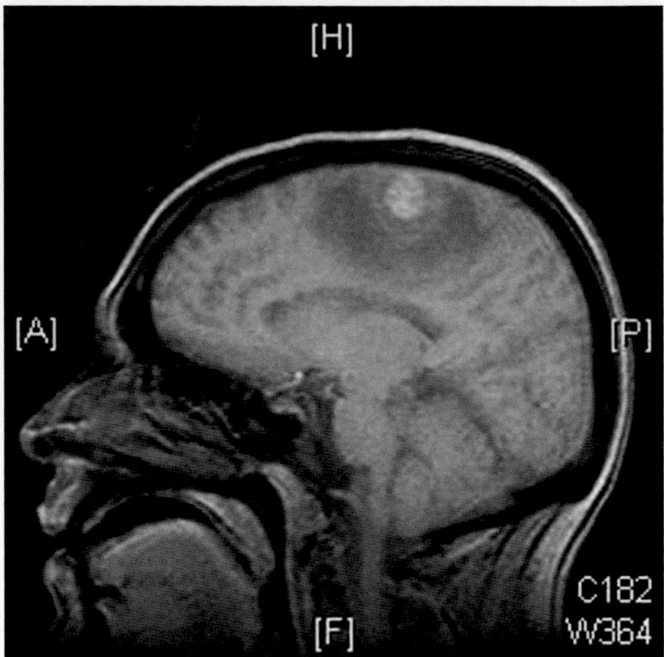

Figure 7–16 Brain MRI of a patient presenting with high-risk metastatic GTN, pulmonary metastases and seizures associated with a solitary brain metastasis. She is in remission following surgical resection of this brain lesion during her first cycle of chemotherapy followed by multiple cycles of chemotherapy with high-dose methotrexate combinations, platin-taxane, and hysterectomy (Courtesy of John Soper, M.D.).

Craniotomy for resection of drug-resistant brain lesions is only rarely performed. In these patients, it is important to exclude active disease elsewhere before attempting surgical resection. In general, craniotomy is reserved for women who require acute decompression of central nervous system hemorrhagic lesions, to allow stabilization and institution of therapy.

Surgical extirpation of metastatic disease at other sites is occasionally beneficial for primary or salvage therapy of malignant GTN. Because PSTT is more often resistant to conventional chemotherapeutic agents, multiple surgical resections of metastatic sites may be required in highly selected patients in order to produce a cure. In general, resection of distant metastases is unlikely to be successful if there is evidence of disseminated disease resistant to chemotherapy.

Vaginal metastases of malignant GTN are highly vascular, originating via metastasis through the submucosal venous plexus of the vagina. These should not be biopsied or resected unless they represent the only site of drug-resistant disease. Biopsy of a metastatic vaginal lesion often results in massive hemorrhage. Packing or angiographic localization with selective embolization are usually used in an attempt to control bleeding from vaginal metastases during initial therapy.

Renal metastases occur in 1–20% of patients treated for metastatic GTN. They are usually associated with other high-risk factors and disseminated disease. All three survivors with renal metastases treated at Duke University

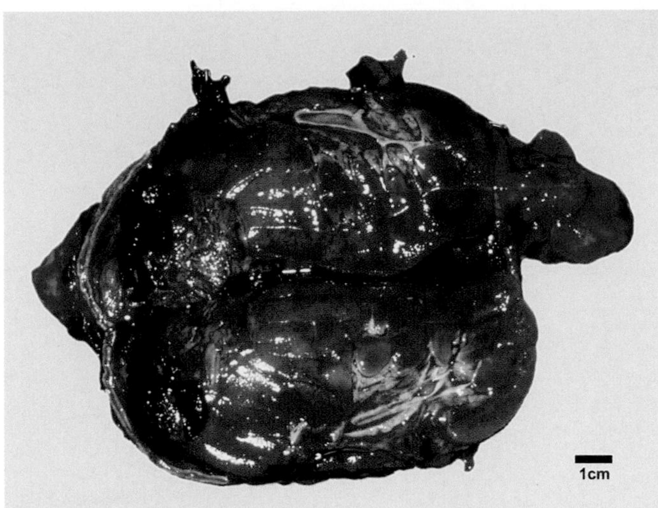

Figure 7–17 Nephrectomy specimen with a large hemorrhagic metastasis of choriocarcinoma involving the superior pole (Courtesy of John Soper, M.D.).

Medical Center underwent nephrectomy incorporated into initial therapy (Fig 7–17); however, three of the five fatalities also underwent nephrectomy. Survivors had limited metastatic involvement elsewhere when compared to patients with renal metastases who died. However, the role for this procedure appears limited, because others have reported patients with high-risk metastatic GTN involving the kidneys who entered long-term remissions after treatment with etoposide-containing chemotherapy regimens, without the need for nephrectomy.

Less than 5% of patients with metastatic GTN have initial involvement of intra-abdominal organs or the gastrointestinal tract. Most often these patients can be managed with chemotherapy alone, but occasional patients will develop bleeding that requires resection of the involved structures for stabilization during therapy. Liver metastases, while often producing catastrophic intra-abdominal hemorrhage, are less likely to be successfully controlled with surgical resection. Selective angiographic embolization techniques should be considered as an option if possible. Only rarely will resection of isolated liver metastases be feasible for treatment of drug-resistant disease because most patients will have other sites of active disease, or disseminated involvement of the liver.

Approximately 30% of patients with high-risk malignant GTN require other procedures, such as D&C or drainage of an abscess, for stabilization during therapy. Another ancillary procedure that is often employed is insertion of a multilumen Hickman catheter or subcutaneous infusion port to provide long-term venous access among patients with high-risk GTN. These patients often require prolonged courses of chemotherapy, transfusion of blood products, nutritional support, and antibiotics during the course of their treatment.

With the development of advanced interventional radiology techniques, selective angiographic localization and embolization techniques have been used to conservatively manage hemorrhage from active sites of metastatic GTN and to treat intrauterine arteriovenous malformations (AVM) that can occasionally develop after treatment of GTN. Vaginal metastases are the site of active disease most often treated with selective angiographic embolization, when simple packing or suturing techniques have failed to control hemorrhage.

Grumbine and associates managed a patient with liver metastases of GTN with the prophylactic placement of a catheter in the hepatic artery for balloon occlusion or embolization in the event of rupture, and others have successfully used selective embolization to treat hemorrhage from hepatic metastases. Lang used selective catheter placement for chemoembolization in three patients with liver metastases and two with pelvic tumors from GTN. All had chemoresistant GTN and relatively localized persistent tumors. Two of the patients with liver metastases achieved long-term remissions, with minimal hematologic toxicity recorded during treatment.

Angiographic abnormalities in the uterus caused by GTD can persist for many months after evacuation of hydatidiform mole or treatment of malignant GTN. The occurrence of intractable bleeding from intrauterine AVM after successful treatment for GTD is a relatively rare complication. Lim et al (74) reported 14 patients treated over a 20-year interval with selective angiographic embolization for this indication. Hemorrhage was initially controlled with the first procedure in 11 (78%) and 6 (45%) patients required a second embolization for treatment of recurrent bleeding, while only 2 (15%) patients required hysterectomy. Successful term pregnancies have been reported after this procedure.

Radiation therapy

With the continued evolution of chemotherapy regimens active in this disease, radiation therapy has always had a limited role in the management of patients with malignant GTD. Radiation has been employed most frequently to treat patients with brain or liver metastases, in an effort to minimize hemorrhagic complications from disease at these sites.

Brace first reported control of brain metastases using 2000 cGy whole brain irradiation for patients with GTN treated at the National Institutes of Health with single-agent regimens. He reported 5 (24%) survivors among 21 patients treated for brain metastases; three required retreatment for recurrent symptoms of intracranial disease. Whole brain irradiation has been used in the majority of series of patients with brain metastases reported from the USA. Most series report administration of between 2,000–4,000 cGy in 10–20 equal fractions that are given concurrently with combination chemotherapy, with reduced field boosts given in selected patients. Total doses correlate with control of central nervous system metastases. Schecter and colleagues reported that the 5-year actuarial local control for patients given doses <2200 cGy was only 24%, significantly worse than 91% local control among patients given 2200–600 cGy.

Survival rates of 50–75% are reported in series of patients who initially presented with brain metastases and received combined chemoradiation. Survival of these patients is influenced, in part by the extent and subsequent control of extracranial disease, in addition to the extent of central nervous system involvement. Small and colleagues reported that women who were asymptomatic at presentation had a 100% survival compared to only 38% survival in those who presented with symptoms from brain metastases, a significant difference. Evans and associates reported that patients with new brain metastases diagnosed at the time of recurrence or who developed brain metastases during chemotherapy had survivals of only 38% and 0%, respectively. These groups had significantly worse survival than the 75% survival of their patients who presented with brain metastases for primary therapy.

Chronic central nervous system toxicity such as mental retardation has been reported among long-term survivors of leukemia and other tumors treated with a combination of whole brain irradiation and concurrent moderate dose methotrexate regimens. These reports have diminished the enthusiasm for combining whole brain radiation with regimens that incorporate infusions of 300–1000 mg/m^2 of methotrexate used to treat GTN, such as EMA/CO. Stereotactic treatment of individual brain metastases could be considered in these circumstances, but concerns persist that therapeutic levels of chemotherapy might not cross the blood–brain barrier, allowing development of occult brain metastases outside of the radiated fields. However, 6- to 12-hour infusions of methotrexate >500 mg/m^2 result in therapeutic cerebrospinal fluid levels of methotrexate, suggesting that doses of methotrexate in these ranges should be used when focal irradiation or surgical resection of individual brain metastases is performed.

An alternative approach using high-dose systemic combination chemotherapy in combination with intrathecal methotrexate yields similar results to the concurrent chemoradiation approach outlined above. The group at Charing Cross Hospital reported 80% survival for patients who received primary therapy with this approach. They did not routinely administer radiotherapy to their patients and advocated early neurosurgical intervention. Although the number of patients available for randomization between concurrent chemoradiation and combined systemic/intrathecal chemotherapy is small, the need for comparative studies is obvious.

Hepatic metastases are identified in 2–8% of patients presenting for primary therapy of malignant GTN (Fig. 7–18). Involvement of the liver constitutes a poor prognostic factor, as evidenced by survival rates of 40–50% for women with primary liver involvement and dismal survival for those who develop new liver metastases during therapy. Optimal management of hepatic metastases is unknown. These are highly vascular and tend to produce catastrophic intra-abdominal hemorrhage.

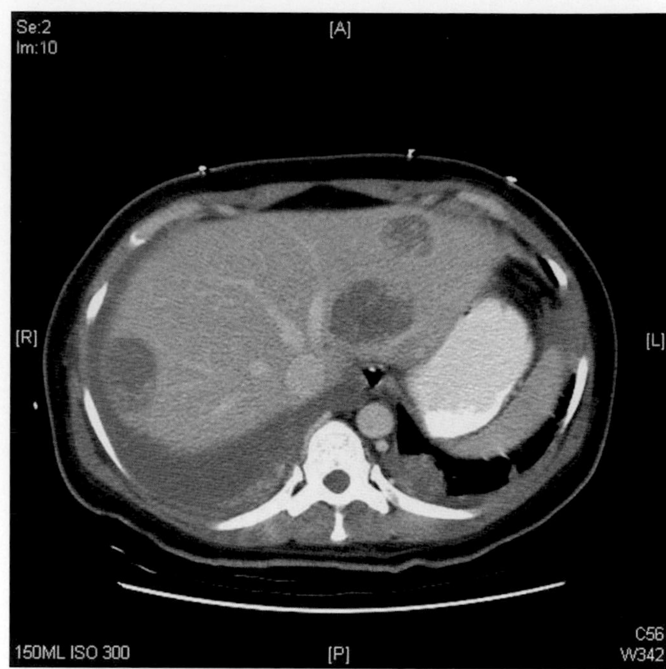

Figure 7–18 Multiple liver metastases in a woman presenting less than 4 weeks after term delivery with lung, brain, and liver metastases of GTN. Selective hepatic arterial embolization was required to control bleeding from the hepatic metastases; note fluid density around liver from intra-abdominal blood. This patient was treated aggressively with multimodality therapy and placed into remission (Courtesy of John Soper, M.D.).

In an attempt to minimize this risk, patients treated at Duke University Medical Center for liver metastases received approximately 2,000 cGy whole liver irradiation concurrently with MAC chemotherapy. Administration of chemotherapy was limited in only one of 15 patients because of hepatitis, but survival was very poor among these patients, with only two (13%) survivors overall and no survivors among patients who developed liver metastases during therapy. Bakri et al reported survival in none of their patients treated with methotrexate-dactinomycin-cyclophosphamide combined with whole liver radiation, compared with survival in five of eight patients treated with etoposide-based combination regimens. Others have reported survival of approximately 27% among patients treated with etoposide-based regimens without hepatic irradiation.

Radiation therapy is occasionally administered to other sites of disease in an attempt to treat drug-resistant foci, with anecdotal responses to multimodality therapy. However, the overall efficacy of radiation therapy to sites other than the brain is unclear. Most of the successes probably reflect the summation of an aggressive multimodality approach to individual patients with high-risk metastatic GTN.

It must be emphasized that cure rates of 75–86% for patients with high-risk metastatic GTN are reported from centers that specialize in the treatment of women with this

Table 7–15 TREATMENT RESULTS FOR GTN		
Clinical classification	**Survivors/Total**	**Life table survival**
Non-metastatic	226/227	99.7%
Metastatic		
Good prognosis	91/91	100%
Poor prognosis	54/67	79.1%
WHO classification (score)		
Low risk (< 5)	310/311	99.8%
Medium risk (5–7)	34/36	94.4%
High risk (> 7)	27/38	68.4%

Modified from Soper JT, Evans AC, Conaway MR et al: Evaluation of prognostic factors and staging in gestational trophoblastic tumor. Obstet Gynecol 84: 969, 1994

relatively rare malignancy. Patients with high-risk disease present multiple challenges for management. They often require a highly individualized approach to address the extent of their disease and treatment toxicity. All women with high-risk disease should be treated by physicians experienced in the management of patients with GTN who can coordinate all aspects of therapy. The overall treatment results for patients with malignant GTN at Duke University Medical Center through 1992 are displayed in Table 7–15.

Placental site trophoblastic tumor

This rare tumor has the potential to metastasize and cause death. Approximately 100 cases have been reported in the literature. It may be found after abortion, mole, or normal pregnancy. Bleeding, the most common symptom, can appear shortly after termination of pregnancy or years later. Bleeding is often accompanied by uterine enlargement and the diagnosis of pregnancy is often entertained. The result of a pregnancy test may be positive, but these tumors characteristically produce lower levels of hCG than other forms of GTD. Gross uterine findings may vary from a diffuse nodular enlargement of the myometrium, which is usually well circumscribed, to a large polypoid projection into the uterine cavity with involvement of the myometrium. Invasion may extend to the serosa or even with extension to the adnexae. Microscopically, it is difficult to differentiate from benign trophoblastic infiltration. It is characterized by mononuclear infiltration of the uterus and its blood vessels with occasional multinucleated giant cells. The predominant cell is an intermediate trophoblast with large polyhedral cells and pleomorphic nuclei. Occasionally, syncytial trophoblast giant cells are present. Mitotic counts have not been a reliable prognostic factor. Placental site trophoblastic tumors must be distinguished from choriocarcinoma and can occasionally be interpreted as sarcomas. Histochemical stains for human placental lactogen are usually diffusely positive but only focally positive for hCG. The serum hCG, although elevated enough to give a positive pregnancy test result, is often low, even with metastasis; therefore, it is a poor predictor of prognosis. Most of these tumors behave in a locally aggressive fashion, although they may act metastasize with at least 20 deaths reported, indicating approximately a 15–20% mortality rate. Metastases have been reported at various sites. Some patients may be cured with a D&C only, but a hysterectomy is considered optimal therapy and is usually adequate in most situations. Swisher and Drescher reported a complete response to EMA-CO in a patient with metastasis to lung and vagina. In their review, two of seven patients treated with EMA-CO had a complete response. In a review by Chang and associates of 88 patients with placental site tumor, 58 of 62 patients with FIGO stage I and II survived and were treated mainly with a hysterectomy with or without chemotherapy. Apparently, 9 of 10 patients survived after a D&C alone. Only 7 of 21 patients with stage III or IV disease survived. All received chemotherapy, and only six received a hysterectomy. Leiserowitz and Webb reported a patient whose tumor was localized with ultrasonography and magnetic resonance imaging and treated with local excision and uterine reconstruction. Surgical-free margins were present, and the patient has had three subsequent pregnancies including two spontaneous abortions and one term delivery.

OTHER CONSIDERATIONS

Future childbearing

After effective treatment for non-malignant GTN, molar pregnancies occur in only about 1–2% of subsequent pregnancies, and many patients have subsequently had normal gestations without difficulty (Table 7–16). Because of the increased risk for the development of a mole in subsequent pregnancies, it is reasonable to evaluate these pregnancies with first-trimester ultrasonography. A particular dilemma has been noted in women undergoing ovulation induction after previous molar gestations. In such cases, patients have occasionally developed repeated hydatidiform moles or malignant GTN subsequent to the implementation of assisted reproductive technologies. In one such patient, in vitro fertilization (IVF) of oocytes retrieved showed a significantly high incidence of abnormal fertilization resulting in the development of triploid embryos. The authors suggested the possible association of an oocyte defect predisposing to abnormal fertilization resulting in the high incidence of triploid embryos. Investigators have proposed the use of intracytoplasmic sperm injection (ICSI) with preimplantation genetic diagnosis or donor oocyte IVF as therapeutic alternatives in these cases.

It appears that the pregnancy outcomes in women with history of molar gestations are no different from the outcomes in women who have no such history with respect to term live births, first- and second-trimester abortions,

Table 7–16 FERTILITY AFTER TREATMENT FOR GTN

Desired fertility	109/122 (89%) patients	
Reproductive outcome		
Infertility	62/109 (57%) patients	
Pregnancies	47/109 (43%) patients	57 pregnancies
Normal infants		45*/57 (79%)
Spontaneous abortion		7/57 (12%)
Therapeutic abortion		3/57 (5%)
Mole		2/57 (4%)

*2 sets of twins

Modified from Hammond CB, Weed JC Jr, Currie JL: The role of operation in the current therapy of gestational trophoblastic disease. Am J Obstet Gynecol 136:844, 1980.

anomalies, stillbirths, prematurity, and primary cesarean section rate (Table 7–16). For individuals with prior molar gestations, subsequent pregnancy outcome appears similar irrespective of whether the mole is complete or partial.

Treatment of malignant GTN with chemotherapy is compatible with the preservation of fertility and is not associated with an increased risk of congenital malformations. Ayhan and colleagues from Turkey reported on 49 women who had received chemotherapy for GTN and subsequently became pregnant a total of 65 times with 42 (64.7%) term births and 3 (4.6%) molar pregnancies. No congenital malformations or obstetric complications were observed. Of the 63 patients in the Southeastern Trophoblastic Center study of poor prognosis metastatic GTN, only 19 were able to preserve their reproductive capacity. Only four of these patients have had subsequent pregnancies that resulted in one spontaneous abortion and four normal deliveries.

In the Charing Cross experience of women treated with EMA-CO, 56% of women who were in remission for at least 2 years and had fertility-conserving therapy achieved pregnancy after completing EMA-CO. At the time of their report there were 112 live births including three babies with congenital abnormalities. Woolas and colleagues updated the outcome data of post-treatment reproductive intent and outcome from 1121 GTN survivors. Of 728 women who had tried to become pregnant, 607 reported at least one live birth, 73 conceived but had not registered a live birth, and 48 did not conceive. No differences were apparent among the 392 women who received methotrexate as single-agent chemotherapy and the 336 treated with multiple-agent chemotherapy. Women who had registered a live birth were significantly younger. They concluded that standard chemotherapy protocols in the treatment of malignant GTN have minimal impact on the subsequent ability to reproduce.

Coexistence of normal pregnancy and gestational trophoblastic neoplasia

Rare cases of metastatic GTN coexisting with normal gestations have been reported; some have been treated successfully with delivery and subsequent chemotherapy. In one case, a patient with a normal intrauterine pregnancy of 27 weeks had a coexisting pulmonary metastatic choriocarcinoma. Treatment with single-agent methotrexate during pregnancy resulted in favorable outcomes for both the mother and the child.

Transplacental fetal metastases

Rare cases (only 15 to 20 cases have been reported, only 5 since 1990) of maternal GTN metastatic to the fetus have been described. The diagnosis of widely metastatic disease in the delivered neonate may occur in the absence of metastatic GTN in the mother (found only in retrospective examination of the term placenta) or precede diagnosis of metastatic GTN in the mother.

Survivorship issues after successful treatment of gestational trophoblastic neoplasia

Survivors of non-malignant and malignant GTN may be at risk for unique physical and psychosocial problems. This generally relates to the increased risk for the development of secondary malignancies after treatment with agents such as etoposide and to issues related to reproductive capacity.

Rustin conducted a population-based study in the United Kingdom analyzing the incidence of secondary malignancies after successful treatment of malignant GTN. Using a sophisticated epidemiologic design, an overall 50% excess of risk (RR = 1.5; 95% confidence interval [CI], 1.1–2.1; $P < 0.011$) was observed. The risk was significantly increased for myeloid leukemia (RR = 16.6; 95% CI, 5.4–38.9), colon (RR = 4.6; 95% CI, 1.5–10.7) and breast cancer when the survival exceeded 25 years (RR = 5.8; 95% CI, 1.2–16.9). The risk was not significantly increased among the 554 women who received single-agent therapy (RR = 1.3; 95% CI, 0.6–2.1). Leukemias only developed in patients who received etoposide plus other cytotoxic drugs. Wenzel and colleagues reported on 76 women with GTN from the New England Trophoblastic Disease Center in regard to chronic psychosocial effects. Across all levels of disease, they found that patients with GTN experience clinically significant levels of anxiety, anger, fatigue, confusion, and sexual problems and are significantly impacted by pregnancy concerns for protracted periods.

BIBLIOGRAPHY

EPIDEMIOLOGY AND RISK FACTORS

Aziz MF, Kampono N, Moegni EN: Epidemiology of gestational trophoblastic disease at the Doctor Cipto Mangunkusumo Hospital, Jakarta, Indonesia. Adv Exp Med Biol 176:165, 1984.

Bae SN, Kim SJ: Telomerase activity in complete hydatidiform mole. Am J Obstet Gynecol 180:328, 1999.

Baergen RN: Gestational choriocarcinoma. Gen Diagn Pathol 143:127, 1997.

Bagshawe KD: Choriocarcinoma: The Clinical Biology of the Trophoblast and its Tumours. London, Arnold, 1969.

Bagshawe KD: Risks and prognostic factors in trophoblastic neoplasia. Cancer 38:1373, 1976.

Bandy LC, Clarke-Pearson LD, Hammond CB: Malignant potential of gestational trophoblastic disease at the extreme age of reproductive life. Obstet Gynecol 64:395, 1984.

Berkowitz RS, Goldstein DP: Gestational trophoblastic disease. Cancer 76:2079, 1995.

Berkowitz RS, Goldstein DP, Bernstein MR: Choriocarcinoma following term pregnancy. Gynecol Oncol 17:32, 1984.

Brewer JI, Halpern B, Torok EE: Gestational trophoblastic disease: Selected clinical aspects and chorionic gonadotropin test methods. In Hickey RG (ed): Current Problems in Cancer. Chicago, Year Book Medical, 1979.

DiCintio E, Parazzini F, Rosa C et al: The epidemiology of gestational trophoblastic disease. Gen Diagn Pathol 143:103, 1997.

DuBeshter B: High risk factors in metastatic GTD. J Reprod Med 36:9013, 1991.

Fisher RA, Newlands ES: Gestational trophoblastic disease. Molecular and genetic studies. J Reprod Med 43:87, 1998.

Fulop V, Colitti CV, Genest D et al: DOC-2/hDab2: A candidate tumor suppressor gene involved in the development of gestational trophoblastic diseases. Oncogene 17:419, 1998.

Hertig AT, Sheldon WH: Hydatidiform mole-a pathological clinical correlation of 200 cases. Am J Obstet Gynecol 53:1, 1947.

Hirano T, Higuchi T, Katsuragawa H et al: CD9 is involved in invasion of human trophoblast-like choriocarcinoma cell line, BeWo cells. Mol Hum Reprod 5:168, 1999.

Ho Yuen B, Burch P: Relationship of oral contraceptives and the intrauterine contraceptive devices to the regression of concentrations of the beta-subunit of human chorionic gonadotropins and invasive complications after molar pregnancy. Am J Obstet Gynecol 145:214, 1983.

Ho Yuen B, Cannon W: Molar pregnancy in British Columbia: Estimated incidence and post evacuation regression pattern of the beta-subunit of human chorionic gonadotropins. Am J Obstet Gynecol 139:316, 1981.

Jones WB: Trophoblastic tumors-prognostic factors. Cancer 48:602, 1981.

Lage JM, Sheikh SS: Genetic aspects of gestational trophoblastic diseases: A general overview with emphasis on new approaches in determining genetic composition. Gen Diagn Pathol 143:109, 1997.

Matsuda T, Sasaki M, Kato H et al: Human chromosome 7 carries a putative tumor suppressor gene(s) involved in choriocarcinoma. Oncogene 15:2773, 1997.

Moglabey YB, Kircheisen R, Seoud M et al: Genetic mapping of a maternal locus responsible for familial hydatidiform moles. Hum Mol Genet 8:667, 1999.

Morrow CP et al: The influence of oral contraceptives on the postmolar human chorionic gonadotropin regression curve. Am J Obstet Gynecol 151:906, 1985.

Newlands ES, Paradinas FJ, Fisher RA: Recent advances in gestational trophoblastic disease. Hematol Oncol Clin North Am 13:225, 1999.

Nisula BC, Taliadours GS: Thyroid function in gestational trophoblastic neoplasia: Evidence that the thyrotrophic activity of chorionic gonadotropin mediates the thyrotoxicosis of choriocarcinoma. Am J Obstet Gynecol 138:77, 1980.

Ostor A: God's first cancer and man's first cure: Milestones in gestational trophoblastic disease. Anat Pathol 1:165, 1996.

Palmer JR, Driscoll SG, Rosenberg L et al: Oral contraceptive use and risk of gestational trophoblastic tumors. J Natl Cancer Inst 91:635, 1999.

Sand PK, Hurain JR, Brewer JI: Repeat gestational trophoblastic disease. Obstet Gynecol 63:140, 1984.

Smith HO: Gestational trophoblastic disease epidemiology and trends. Clin Obstet Gynecol 46:541, 2003.

Soper JT, Evans AC, Conaway MR et al: Evaluation of prognostic factors and staging in gestational trophoblastic tumor. Obstet Gynecol 84:969, 1994.

Stone N et al: Relationship of oral contraception to development of trophoblastic tumor after evacuation of a hydatidiform mole. Br J Obstet Gynaecol 83:913, 1976.

Tham KF, Ratnam SS: The classification of gestational trophoblastic disease: A critical review. Int J Gynaecol Obstet 60 (Suppl 1):S39, 1998.

World Health Organization Scientific Group: Gestational trophoblastic disease. WHO Tech Rep Ser 692:1, 1983.

MOLES

Bagshawe KD, Lawler SD, Paradmas FJ et al: Gestational trophoblastic tumours following initial diagnosis of partial hydatidiform mole. Lancet 335:1074, 1990.

Berkowitz RS, Bernstein MR, Harlow BL et al: Case-control study of risk factors for partial molar pregnancy. Am J Obstet Gynecol 173:788, 1995.

Berkowitz RS, Cramer DW, Bernstein MR: Risk factors for complete molar pregnancy from a case control study. Am J Obstet Gynecol 152:1016, 1985.

Berkowitz RS, Goldstein DP, Bernstein MR: Evolving concepts of molar pregnancy. J Reprod Med 36:40, 1991.

Berkowitz RS, Goldstein DP, Bernstein MR: Natural history of partial molar pregnancy. Obstet Gynecol 66:677, 1983.

Berkowitz RS, Goldstein DP, Bernstein MR: Reproductive experiences after complete and partial molar pregnancy and gestational trophoblastic tumors. J Reprod Med 36:3, 1991.

Berkowitz RS et al: Oral contraceptives and postmolar trophoblastic disease. Obstet Gynecol 58:474, 1981.

Bilgin T, Esmer A, Kèucèkerdoægan IB: Recurrent molar pregnancy. Int J Gynaecol Obstet 57:185, 1997.

Curry SL, Schlaerth JB, Kohorn EI et al: Hormonal contraception and trophoblastic sequelae after hydatidiform mole. Am J Obstet Gynecol 160:805, 1989.

Curry SL et al: Hydatidiform mole: Diagnosis, management, and long-term follow-up of 347 patients. Obstet Gynecol 45:1, 1975.

Davidson SA, Gottesfeld J, LaRosa FG: Molar pregnancy in a 60 year old woman. Int J Gynaecol Obstet 56:53, 1997.

Freedman RS, Tortolero-Luna G, Pandey DK et al: Gestational trophoblastic disease. Obstet Gynecol Clin North Am 23:545, 1996.

Goldstein DP, Berkowitz RS: Current management of complete and partial molar pregnancy. J Reprod Med 39:139, 1994.

Montes M, Roberts D, Berkowitz RS, Genest DR: Prevalence and significance of implantation site trophoblastic atypia in hydatidiform moles and spontaneous abortions. Am J Clin Pathol 150:411, 1996.

Mosher R, Goldstein DP, Berkowitz R et al: Complete hydatidiform mole. Comparison of clinicopathologic features, current and past. J Reprod Med 43:21, 1998.

Mungan T, Kuscu E, Dabakoæglu T et al: Hydatidiform mole: Clinical analysis of 310 patients. Int J Gynaecol Obstet 52:233, 1996.

Palmer JR: Advances in the epidemiology of gestational trophoblastic disease. J Reprod Med 39:155, 1994.

Pezeshki H, Hancock BW, Silcocks P et al: The role of repeat uterine evacuation in the management of persistent gestational trophoblastic disease. Gynecol Oncol 95:423–9, 2004.

Rice LW, Berkowitz RS, Lage JM et al: Persistent gestational trophoblastic tumor after partial hydatidiform mole. Gynecol Oncol 36:358, 1990.

Soto-Wright V, Bernstein M, Goldstein DP et al: The changing clinical presentation of complete molar pregnancy. Obstet Gynecol 86:775, 1995.

Soper JT, Mutch DG, Schink JC: Diagnosis and treatment of gestational trophoblastic disease: ACOG Practice Bulletin No. 53. Gynecol Oncol 93:575, 2004

Szulman AE, Surti U: The clinical pathologic profile of the partial hydatidiform mole. Obstet Gynecol 59:597, 1982.

Szulman AE, Surti U: The syndrome of hydatidiform mole. I: Cytogenetics and morphologic correlation. Am J Obstet Gynecol 131:665, 1978.

Szulman AE, Surti U: The syndrome of hydatidiform mole. II: Morphologic evaluation of the complete and partial mole. Am J Obstet Gynecol 132:20, 1978.

Tidy JA, Gillespie AM, Bright N et al: Gestational trophoblastic disease: a study of the mode of evacuation and the subsequent need for treatment with chemotherapy. Gynecol Oncol 78:309, 2000.

Vassilakos P, Riotton G, Kajii T: Hydatidiform mole: Two entities—a morphologic and cytogenetic study with some clinical considerations. Am J Obstet Gynecol 127:167, 1997.

van Trommel NE, Massuger LF, Verheijen RH, Sweep FC, Thomas CM: The curative effect of a second curettage in persistent trophoblastic disease: a retrospective cohort survey. Gynecol Oncol 99:6–13, 2005.

Wolfberg AJ, Feltmate C, Goldstein DP et al: Low risk of relapse after achieving undetectable hCG levels in women with complete molar pregnancy. Obstet Gynecol 104:551, 2004.

PROPHYLACTIC CHEMOTHERAPY

Goldstein DP: Five years' experience with the prevention of trophoblastic tumors by the prophylactic use of chemotherapy in patients with molar pregnancy. Clin Obstet Gynecol 13:945, 1970.

Limpongsanurak S: Prophylactic actinomycin D for high-risk complete hydatidiform mole. J Reprod Med 46:110, 2001

Kim DS et al: Effects of prophylactic chemotherapy for persistent trophoblastic disease in patients with complete hydatidiform mole. Obstet Gynecol 67:690, 1986.

DIAGNOSIS

Bagshawe KD, Lawler SD, Paradmas FJ et al: Gestational trophoblastic tumours following initial diagnosis of partial hydatidiform mole. Lancet 335:1074, 1990.

Berkowitz RS, Goldstein DP, Bernstein MR: Evolving concepts of molar pregnancy. J Reprod Med 36:40, 1991.

Cole LA: Phantom hCG and phantom choriocarcinoma. Gynecol Oncol 71:325, 1998.

Coukos G, Makrigiannakis A, Chung J et al: Complete hydatidiform mole: A disease with a changing profile. J Reprod Med 44:698, 1999.

Curry SL, Schlaerth JB, Kohorn EI et al: Hormonal contraception and trophoblastic sequelae after hydatidiform mole. Am J Obstet Gynecol 160:805, 1989.

Dobson LS, Gillespie AM, Coleman RE, Hancock BW: The presentation and management of post-partum choriocarcinoma. Br J Cancer 79:1531, 1999.

Goldstein DP, Zanten-Przybysz IV, Bernstein MR, Berkowitz RS: Reviewed FIGO staging system for gestational trophoblastic tumors: Recommendations regarding therapy. J Reprod Med 43:37, 1998.

Hancock BW, Welch EM, Gillespie AM et al: A retrospective comparison of current and proposed staging and scoring systems for persistent gestational trophoblastic disease. Int J Gynecol Cancer 10:318, 2000.

Horn LC, Bilek K: Clinicopathologic analysis of gestational trophoblastic disease? Report of 158 cases. Gen Diagn Pathol 143:173, 1997.

Horn LC, Bilek K: Histologic classification and staging of gestational trophoblastic disease. Gen Diagn Pathol 143:87, 1997.

Hunter V, Christensen RE, Olt G et al: Efficacy of the metastatic screening in the staging of gestational trophoblastic disease. Cancer 65:1647, 1990.

Kidd D, Plant GT, Scaravilli F et al: Metastatic choriocarcinoma presenting as multiple intracerebral haemorrhages: The role of imaging in the elucidation of the pathology. J Neurol Neurosurg Psychiatry 65:939, 1998.

Kohorn EI: Evaluation of the criteria used to make the diagnosis of nonmetastatic gestational trophoblastic neoplasia. Am J Obstet Gynecol 48:139, 1993.

Kohorn EI, McCarthy SM, Taylor KJ: Nonmetastatic gestational trophoblastic neoplasia: Role of ultrasonography and magnetic resonance imaging. J Reprod Med 43:14, 1998.

Kohorn EI: The new FIGO 2000 staging and risk factor scoring system for gestational trophoblastic disease: description and critical assessment. Int J Gynecol Cancer 11:73, 2000.

Lage JM, Wolf NG: Gestational trophoblastic disease: New approaches to diagnosis. Clin Lab Med 15:631, 1995.

Lele SM, Crowder SE, Grafe MR: Asymptomatic intraplacental choriocarcinoma diagnosed on routine placental examination. J Perinatol 19:244, 1999.

Massenkeil G, Crombach G, Dominik S et al: Metastatic choriocarcinoma in a postmenopausal woman. Gynecol Oncol 61:432, 1996.

Rice LW, Berkowitz RS, Lage JM et al: Persistent gestational trophoblastic tumor after partial hydatidiform mole. Gynecol Oncol 36:358, 1990.

Rodabaugh KJ, Bernstein MR, Goldstein DP, Berkowitz RS: Natural history of postterm choriocarcinoma. J Reprod Med 43:75, 1998.

Romero R et al: New criteria for diagnosis of gestational trophoblastic disease. Obstet Gynecol 66:553, 1985.

Rotmensch S, Cole LA: False diagnosis and needless therapy of presumed malignant disease in women with false-positive human chorionic gonadotropin concentrations. Lancet 355:712, 2000

Soper JT, Clarke-Pearson DL, Hammond CB: Metastatic gestational trophoblastic disease: prognostic factors in previously untreated patients. Obstet Gynecol 71:338, 1988

Soper JT, Evans AC, Conaway MR et al: Evaluation of prognostic factors and staging in gestational trophoblastic tumor. Obstet Gynecol 84:969, 1994.

Soper JT: Staging and evaluation of gestational trophoblastic disease. Clin Obstet Gynecol 46:570, 2003.

Soper JT, Mutch DG, Schink JC: Diagnosis and treatment of gestational trophoblastic disease: ACOG Practice Bulletin No. 53. Gynecol Oncol 93: 575, 2004.

TREATMENT

Ayhan A, Ergeneli MH, Yuce K et al: Pregnancy after chemotherapy for gestational trophoblastic disease. J Reprod Med 35:522, 1990.

Azab MB, Pejovic M, Theorose C et al: Prognostic factors in gestational trophoblastic tumors: A multivariant analysis. Cancer 62:585, 1988.

Azab TC, Droz JP, Assouline A et al: Treatment of high risk gestational trophoblastic disease with chemotherapy combination containing cisplatin and etoposide. Cancer 64:1824, 1989.

Bagshawe KD: Treatment of high risk choriocarcinoma. J Reprod Med 29:813, 1984.

Bagshawe KD: Treatment of trophoblastic tumors. Ann Acad Med 5:273, 1976.

Bagshawe KD, Dent J, Newlands ES et al: The role of low dose methotrexate and folic acid in gestational trophoblastic tumors (GII). Br J Obstet Gynecol 96:795, 1989.

Bagshawe KD, Wilde CE: Infusion therapy for pelvic trophoblastic tumors. J Obstet Gynaecol Br Commonw 71:565, 1964.

Bakri YN, Subhi J, Amer M et al: Liver metastasis of gestational trophoblastic tumor. Gynecol Oncol 48:110, 1993.

Barter JF, Soong SJ, Hatch KD et al: Treatment of nonmetastatic gestational trophoblastic disease with oral methotrexate. Am J Obstet Gynecol 157:1166, 1987.

Berkowitz RS, Goldstein DP: Recent advances in gestational trophoblastic disease. Curr Opin Obstet Gynecol 10:61, 1998.

Berkowitz RS, Goldstein DP, Bernstein MR: Methotrexate infusion and folinic acid in the primary therapy of non-metastatic gestational trophoblastic tumors. Gynecol Oncol 36:56, 1990.

Berkowitz RS, Goldstein DP, Bernstein MR: Methotrexate with Citrovorum factor rescue as primary therapy for gestational trophoblastic disease. Cancer 50:2024, 1982.

Berkowitz RS, Goldstein DP, Bernstein MR: Ten-year experience with methotrexate and folinic acid as primary treatment for gestational trophoblastic disease. Gynecol Oncol 23:111, 1986.

Bolis G, Bonazzi C, Landoni F et al: EMA-CO regime in high risk GTT. Gynecol Oncol 31:439, 1988.

Bower M, Newlands ES, Holden L et al: EMA-CO for high-risk gestational trophoblastic tumors: Results from a cohort of 272 patients [published erratum appears in J Clin Oncol 1997 15:3168]. J Clin Oncol 15:2636, 1997.

Brace KC: The role of irradiation in the treatment of metastatic trophoblastic disease. Radiology 91:539, 1968.

Brewer JI, Smith RT, Pratt GB: Choriocarcinoma: absolute survival rates of 122 patients treated by hysterectomy. Am J Obstet Gynecol 85:841, 1963.

Crawford RA, Newlands E, Rustin GJ et al: Gestational trophoblastic disease with liver metastases: the Charing Cross experience. Br J Obstet Gynaecol 104:105, 1997.

Curry S, Blessing J, DiSaia P et al: A prospective randomized comparison of MAC versus modified Bagshawe regimen in poor prognosis gestational trophoblastic disease. Obstet Gynecol 73:357, 1989.

DuBeshter B, Berkowitz RS, Goldstein DP: Metastatic gestational trophoblastic disease: experience at the New England Trophoblastic Disease Center, 1965–1985. Obstet Gynecol 69:390, 1987.

DuBeshter B, Berkowitz RS, Goldstein DP et al: Management of low risk metastatic gestational trophoblastic tumors. J Reprod Med 36:36, 1991.

Evans AJ, Soper JT, Clarke-Pearson DL et al: Gestational trophoblastic disease metastatic to the central nervous system. Gynecol Oncol 59:226, 1995.

Feldman S, Goldstein DP, Berkowitz RS: Low-risk metastatic gestational trophoblastic tumors. Semin Oncol 22:166, 1995.

Finkler NJ, Berkowitz RS, Driscoll SC et al: Clinical experience with placental site trophoblastic tumors at the New England Trophoblastic Disease Center. Obstet Gynecol 71:854, 1988.

Gillespie AM, Siddiqui N, Coleman RE, Hancock BW: Gestational trophoblastic disease: Does central nervous system chemoprophylaxis have a role? Br J Cancer 79:1270, 1999.

Goldstein DP et al: Methotrexate with Citrovorum factor rescue for gestational trophoblastic neoplasms. Obstet Gynecol 53:93, 1978.

Hammond CB, Lewis JL Jr: Gestational trophoblastic neoplasms. In Schirra J (ed): Davis' Gynecology and Obstetrics, Vol 1. New York, Harper & Row, 1977.

Hammond CB, Parker RT: Diagnosis and treatment of trophoblastic disease. Obstet Gynecol 35:132, 1970.

Hammond CB, Weed JC Jr, Currie JL: The role of operation in the current therapy of gestational trophoblastic disease. Am J Obstet Gynecol 135:844, 1980.

Hammond CB et al: Treatment of metastatic trophoblastic disease: Good and poor prognosis. Am J Obstet Gynecol 115:4, 1973.

Hartenbach EM, Saltzman AK, Carter JR, Twiggs LB: A novel strategy using G-CSF to support EMA-CO for high-risk gestational trophoblastic disease. Gynecol Oncol 56:105, 1995.

Herrington S: Enhancing cure and palliation: radiation therapy in the treatment of metastatic gestational trophoblastic neoplasia. Semin Oncol 22:185, 1995.

Hertz R, Lewis JL Jr, Lipsett MB: Five years' experience with chemotherapy of metastatic choriocarcinoma and related trophoblastic tumors in women. Am J Obstet Gynecol 82:631, 1961.

Hoffman MS, Fiorica JV, Gleeson NC et al: A single institution experience with weekly IM methotrexate for nonmetastatic gestational trophoblastic disease. Gynecol Oncol 60:292, 1996.

Homesley HD: Development of single-agent chemotherapy regimens for gestational trophoblastic disease. J Reprod Med 39:185, 1994.

Homesley HD: Single-agent therapy for nonmetastatic and low-risk gestational trophoblastic disease. J Reprod Med 43:69, 1998.

Homesley HD, Blessing JA, Rettenmaier M et al: Weekly intramuscular methotrexate for nonmetastatic gestational trophoblastic disease. Obstet Gynecol 72:413, 1988.

Homesley HD, Blessing JA, Schlaerth J et al: Rapid escalation of weekly IM MTX for NMGTD. Gynecol Oncol 39:305, 1990.

Jones WB, Cardinale C, Lewis JJ: Management of high-risk gestational trophoblastic disease: The Memorial Hospital experience. Int J Gynecol Cancer 7:27, 1997.

Jones WB, Schneider J, Shapiro F, Lewis JJ: Treatment of resistant gestational choriocarcinoma with taxol: A report of two cases. Gynecol Oncol 61:126, 1996.

Jones WB, Wolchok J, Lewis JJ: The role of surgery in the management of gestational trophoblastic disease. Cancer 6:261, 1996.

Kanazawa K, Sasagawa M, Suzuki T, Takeuchi S: Clinical evaluation of focal excision of myometrial lesion for treatment of invasive hydatidiform mole. Acta Obstet Gynecol Scand 67: 487, 1988.

Kim SJ, Bae SN, Kim JH et al: Risk factors for the prediction of treatment failure in gestational trophoblastic tumors treated with EMA-CO regimen. Gynecol Oncol 71:247, 1998.

Kurman RJ, Scully RE, Norris HJ: Trophoblastic pseudotumor of the uterus: An exaggerated form of "syncytial endometritis" simulating a malignant tumor. Cancer 38:1214, 1976.

Lang EK: Reduced systemic toxicity from superselective chemoembolization compared with systemic chemotherapy in patients with high-risk metastatic gestational trophoblastic disease. Cardiovasc Intervent Radiol 20:280, 1997.

Lehman E, Gershenson DM, Burke TW et al: Salvage surgery for chemoresistant gestational trophoblastic disease. J Clin Oncol 12:2737, 1994.

Leiserowitz GS, Webb MJ: Treatment of placental site trophoblast tumor with hysterotomy and uterine reconstruction. Obstet Gynecol 88:696, 1996

Li M, Hertz R, Spencer DB: Effects of methotrexate therapy upon choriocarcinoma and chorioadenoma. Proc Soc Exp Biol Med 93:361, 1956.

Lim AK, Agarwal R, Seckl MJ et al: Embolization of bleeding residual uterine vascular malformations in patients treated with gestational trophoblastic tumor. Radiol 222:640, 2002

Lurain JR: High risk metastatic gestational trophoblastic tumors. J Reprod Med 39:217, 1994.

Lurain JR: Management of high-risk gestational trophoblastic disease. J Reprod Med 43:44, 1998.

Lurain JR, Brewer JI: Treatment of high risk gestational trophoblastic disease with MAC chemotherapy. Obstet Gynecol 65:830, 1985.

Lurain JR, Elfstrand EP: Single-agent methotrexate chemotherapy for the treatment of nonmetastatic gestational trophoblastic tumors. Am J Obstet Gynecol 72:574, 1995.

Lurain JR et al: Fatal gestational trophoblastic disease, an analysis of treatment failures. Am J Obstet Gynecol 144:391, 1982.

Lurain JR et al: Gestational trophoblastic disease: treatment results at the Brewer Trophoblastic Disease Center. Obstet Gynecol 60:354, 1982.

Maroulis GB et al: Arteriography and infusional chemotherapy in localized trophoblastic disease. Obstet Gynecol 45:397, 1975.

McDonald TW, Ruffolo EH: Modern management of gestational trophoblastic disease. Obstet Gynecol 38:167, 1983.

McNeish IA, Strickland S, Holden L et al: Low-risk persistent gestational trophoblastic disease: outcome after initial treatment with low-dose methotrexate and folinic acid from 1992 to 2000. J Clin Oncol 20:1838, 2002.

Mena AM, Alastuey I: Whole brain radiotherapy for metastatic gestational trophoblastic disease [Letter; comment]. Gynecol Oncol 72:265, 1999.

Mutch DG, Soper JT, Baker et al: Role of computed axial tomography of the chest in staging patients with non-metastatic gestational trophoblastic disease. Obstet Gynecol 68:348, 1986.

Mutch DG, Soper JT, Babcock CJ et al: Recurrent gestational trophoblastic disease: Experience of the Southeastern Regional Trophoblastic Disease Center. Cancer 66:978, 1990.

Newlands ES, Bagshawe KD, Begent RHJ et al: Development in chemotherapy for medium and high risk patients with GTT. Br J Obstet Gynaecol 93:63, 1986.

Newlands ES, Bagshawe KD, Begent RHJ et al: Results with the EMA-CO regime in high risk gestation trophoblastic tumors. Br J Obstet Gynecol 98:550, 1991.

Newlands ES, Bower M, Holden L et al: The management of high-risk gestational trophoblastic tumours (GTT). Int J Gynaecol Obstet 60 (Suppl 1):S65, 1998.

Papadopoulos AJ, Foskett M, Seckel MJ et al: Twenty-five years' clinical experience with placental site trophoblastic tumors. J Reprod Med 47: 460, 2002.

Roberts JP, Lurain JR: Treatment of low-risk metastatic gestational trophoblastic tumors with single-agent chemotherapy. Am J Obstet Gynecol 174:1917, 1996.

Rose PG, Piver MS: Alternating methotrexate and dactinomycin in nonmetastatic gestational trophoblastic disease. J Surg Oncol 41:148, 1989.

Ross GT et al: Sequential use of methotrexate and actinomycin D in the treatment of metastatic choriocarcinoma and related trophoblastic diseases in women. Am J Obstet Gynecol 93:223, 1965.

Rotmensch J, Rosenschein N, Donehower R et al: Plasma methotrexate levels in patients with gestational trophoblastic regimens. Am J Obstet Gynecol 148:730, 1984.

Rustin GJ, Newlands ES, Begent RH et al: Weekly alternating etoposide, methotrexate, and actinomycin/vincristine and cyclophosphamide chemotherapy for the treatment of CNS metastases of choriocarcinoma. J Clin Oncol 7:900, 1989.

Schechter NR, Mychalczak B, Jones W, Spriggs D: Prognosis of patients treated with whole-brain radiation therapy for metastatic gestational trophoblastic disease. Gynecol Oncol 68:183, 1998.

Schink JC, Singh DK, Radmaker AW et al: EMA-CO for the treatment of metastatic, high risk gestational trophoblastic disease. Obstet Gynecol 80:817, 1992.

Schlaerth JB, Morrow DP, Rodriguez M: Diagnostic and therapeutic curettage in gestational trophoblastic disease. Am J Obstet Gynecol 162:1465, 1990.

Scully RE, Young RH: Trophoblastic pseudotumor: A reappraisal. Am J Surg Pathol 5:75, 1981.

Seckl MJ, Newlands ES: Treatment of gestational trophoblastic disease. Gen Diagn Pathol 143:159, 1997.

Small WJ, Lurain JR, Shetty RM et al: Gestational trophoblastic disease metastatic to the brain. Radiology 200:277, 1996.

Smith EB et al: Treatment of non-metastatic gestational trophoblastic disease: Results of methotrexate alone versus methotrexate-folinic acid. Am J Obstet Gynecol 144:88, 1982.

Soper JT, Mutch DG, Chin N et al: Renal metastases of gestational trophoblastic disease: a report of eight cases. Obstet Gynecol 72:796, 1988.

Soper JT: Surgical therapy for gestational trophoblastic disease. J Reprod Med 39:168, 1994.

Soper JT, Clarke-Pearson DL, Berchuck A et al: 5-day methotrexate for women with metastatic gestational trophoblastic disease. Gynecol Oncol 54:76, 1994.

Soper JT, Evans AC, Clarke-Pearson DL et al: Alternating weekly chemotherapy with etoposide-methotrexate-dactinomycin/cyclophosphamide-vincristine for high-risk gestational trophoblastic disease. Obstet Gynecol 83:113, 1994.

Soper JT, Evans AC, Rodriguez G et al: Etoposide-platin combination therapy for chemorefractory gestational trophoblastic disease. Gynecol Oncol 56:421, 1995.

Soper JT: Identification and management of high-risk gestational trophoblastic disease. Semin Oncol 22:172, 1995.

Soper JT: Role of surgery and radiation therapy in gestational trophoblastic disease. Best Prac Res Clin Obstet Gynaecol 17: 943–57, 2003.

Soper JT, Mutch DG, Schink JC: Diagnosis and treatment of gestational trophoblastic disease: ACOG Practice Bulletin No. 53. Gynecol Oncol 93:575, 2004.

Sung AC, Wu FC, Wang YB: Reevaluation of 5-FU as a single agent for gestational malignant trophoblastic disease. Adv Exp Med Biol 176:355, 1984.

Surwit EA, Childers JM: High risk metastatic GTD. J Reprod Med 39:45, 1991.

Suzuka K, Matsui H, Iitsuka Y et al: Adjuvant hysterectomy in low-risk gestational trophoblastic disease. Obstet Gynecol 97: 431, 2001.

Tidy JA, Rustin GJ, Newlands ES et al: Presentation and management of choriocarcinoma after nonmolar pregnancy. Br J Obstet Gynaecol 102:715, 1995.

Tomoda Y, Arii Y, Kaseki S et al: Surgical indications for resection in pulmonary metastasis of choriocarcinoma. Cancer 46:2723, 1980.

Twiggs LB, Hatch K, Petrilli ES: A chemotherapeutic trial of actinomycin-D with pulse fashion scheduling in the treatment of nonmetastatic trophoblastic disease (Abstracts). Gynecol Oncol 23:244, 1986.

Vaitukaitis JB, Braunstein GD, Ross GT: A radioimmunoassay which specifically measures human chorionic gonadotrophin in the presence of human luteinizing hormone. Am J Obstet Gynecol 113:751, 1972.

Weed JC Jr et al: Chemotherapy with the modified Bagshawe protocol for poor prognosis metastatic trophoblastic disease. Obstet Gynecol 59:377, 1982.

Wong LC, Choo YC, Ma HK: Methotrexate with Citrovorum rescue in gestational trophoblastic disease. Am J Obstet Gynecol 152:59, 1985.

Wong LC, Choo YC, Ma HK: Primary oral etoposide therapy in gestational trophoblastic disease: An update. Cancer 58:14, 1998.

POST-TREATMENT PREGNANCY

Goldstein DP, Berkowitz RS, Bernstein MR: Reproduction performance after molar pregnancy in gestational trophoblastic tumors. Clin Obstet Gynecol 27:221, 1984.

Kohorn EI: How soon is it safe to undertake pregnancy after trophoblastic tumor? Gynecol Oncol 73:343, 1999.

Miller JM Jr, Surwit EA, Hammond CB: Choriocarcinoma following term pregnancy. Obstet Gynecol 53:207, 1979.

Rustin GJ et al: Pregnancy after cytotoxic chemotherapy for gestational trophoblastic tumours. BMJ Clin Res 288:103, 1984.

Tuncer ZS, Bernstein MR, Goldstein DP et al: Outcome of pregnancies occurring within 1 year of hydatidiform mole. Obstet Gynecol 94:588, 1999.

Zalel Y, Dgani R: Gestational trophoblastic disease following the evacuation of partial hydatidiform mole: A review of 66 cases. Eur J Obstet Gynecol Reprod Biol 71:67, 1997.

PLACENTAL SITE TUMORS

Bettencourt E, Pinto E, Araâul E et al: Placental site trophoblastic tumour: the value of transvaginal colour and pulsed Doppler sonography (TV-CDS) in its diagnosis: Case report. Eur J Gynaecol Oncol 18:461, 1997.

Bower M, Pardinas FJ, Fisher RA et al: Placental site trophoblastic tumor: Molecular analysis and clinical experience. Clin Cancer Res 2:897, 1996.

Chang YL, Chang TC, Hseuh S et al: Prognostic factors and treatment for placental site trophoblastic tumor: report of 3 cases and analysis of 88 cases. Gynecol Oncol 73:216, 1999.

Finkler NJ, Berkowitz RS, Driscoll S et al: Clinical experience with placental site trophoblastic tumors at the New England Trophoblastic Disease Center. Obstet Gynecol 71:854, 1988.

Janni W, Hantschmann P, Rehbock J et al: Successful treatment of malignant placental site trophoblastic tumor with combined cytostatic-surgical approach: Case report and review of literature. Gynecol Oncol 75:164, 1999.

Kurman RJ (ed): Blaustein's Pathology of the Female Genital Tract. New York, Springer-Verlag, 1994, pp 1074–1078.

Kurman RJ, Scully RE, Norris HJ: Trophoblastic pseudotumor of the uterus. Cancer 38:1214, 1988.

Leiserowitz GS, Webb MJ: Treatment of placental site trophoblastic tumor with hysterotomy and uterine reconstruction. Obstet Gynecol 88:696, 1996.

Randall TC, Coukos G, Wheeler JE, Rubin SC: Prolonged remission of recurrent metastatic placental site trophoblastic tumor after chemotherapy. Gynecol Oncol 76:115, 2000.

Schneider D, Halperin R, Segal M, Bukovsky I: Placental site trophoblastic tumor following metastatic gestational trophoblastic neoplasia. Gynecol Oncol 63:267, 1996.

Silve EG, Tornos C, Lage J et al: Multiple nodules of intermediate trophoblast following hydatidiform moles. Int J Gynecol Pathol 12:324, 1993.

Swisher E, Drescher CW: Metastatic placental site trophoblastic tumor: Long-term remission in a patient treated with EMA-CO chemotherapy. Gynecol Oncol 68:62, 1998.

Twiggs LB, Hartenbach E, Saltzman AK, King LA: Metastatic placental site trophoblastic tumor. Int J Gynaecol Obstet 60 (Suppl 1):S51, 1998.

OTHER CONSIDERATIONS

Abbi M, Kriplani A, Uppal R, Takkar D: Term twin pregnancy with hydatidiform mole and normal fetus. Arch Gynecol Obstet 262:189, 1999.

Anderson CK, Deiter RW, Motz MJ, Goldstein JA: Complete hydatidiform mole with a coexistent healthy, viable fetus near term: A case report. J Reprod Med 41:55, 1996.

Basbuæg M, Aygen E, Tayyar M et al: Recurrent molar pregnancy after ovulation induction and repeated ovulation induction. A case report. J Reprod Med 42:600, 1997.

Berkowitz RS, Im SS, Bernstein MR, Goldstein DP: Gestational trophoblastic disease: Subsequent pregnancy outcome, including repeat molar pregnancy. J Reprod Med 43:81, 1998.

Bristow RE, Shumway JB, Khouzami AN, Witter FR: Complete hydatidiform mole and surviving coexistent twin. Obstet Gynecol Surv 51:705, 1996.

Chandra SA, Gilbert EF, Viseskul C et al: Neonatal intracranial choriocarcinoma. Arch Pathol Lab Med 114:1079, 1990.

Chane FP: Molar pregnancy and living normal fetus coexisting until term: prenatal biochemical and sonographic diagnosis. Hum Reprod 12:853, 1997.

Chao AS, Tsai TC, Soong YK: Clinical management of a quadruplet pregnancy combining a triplet pregnancy with a classical hydatidiform mole: Case report and review of literature. Prenat Diagn 19:1073, 1999.

Fishman DA, Padilla LA, Keh P et al: Management of twin pregnancies consisting of a complete hydatidiform mole and normal fetus. Obstet Gynecol 91:546, 1998.

Higashino M, Harada N, Hataya I et al: Trizygotic pregnancy consisting of two fetuses and a complete hydatidiform mole with dispermic androgenesis. Am J Med Genet 82:67, 1999.

Kim JH, Park DC, Bae SN et al: Subsequent reproductive experience after treatment for gestational trophoblastic disease. Gynecol Oncol 71:108, 1998.

Loret DM, Goldfarb JM: Reproductive performance of patients after gestational trophoblastic disease. Semin Oncol 22:193, 1995.

Marinoff DN, Spitzberg, EH, Cheuh JT et al: Delayed-interval delivery in a quadruplet pregnancy after intrauterine death of a partial molar pregnancy and preterm delivery: A case report. J Reprod Med 43:1051, 1998.

Montes DO, Macara L, Shaker A: Twin pregnancy with a complete hydatidiform mole and coexisting fetus following in-vitro fertilization: case report. Hum Reprod 14:2905, 1999.

Nabers J, Splinter TA, Wallenburg HC et al: Choriocarcinoma with lung metastases during pregnancy with successful delivery and outcome after chemotherapy. Thorax 45:416, 1990.

Nugent CE, Punch MR, Barr MJ et al: Persistence of partial molar placenta and severe preeclampsia after selective termination in a twin pregnancy. Obstet Gynecol 87:829, 1996.

Pal L, Toth TL, Leykin L, Isaacson KB: High incidence of triploidy in in-vitro fertilized oocytes from a patient with a previous history of recurrent gestational trophoblastic disease. Hum Reprod 11:1529, 1996.

Rustin GJ, Newlands ES, Lutz JM et al: Combination but not single-agent methotrexate for gestational trophoblastic tumors increases the incidence of second tumors. J Clin Oncol 14: 2769–73, 1996.

Steigrad SJ, Cheung AP, Osborn RA: Choriocarcinoma co-existent with an intact pregnancy: Case report and review of the literature. J Obstet Gynaecol Res 25:197, 1999.

Woolas RP, Bower M, Newlands ES et al: Influence of chemotherapy for gestational trophoblastic disease on subsequent pregnancy outcome. Br J Obstet Gynaecol 105:1032, 1998.

8 Invasive Cancer of the Vulva

Frederick B. Stehman, M.D.

In the 1998 International Federation of Gynecology and Obstetrics (FIGO) Annual Report, cancer of the vulva accounted for 5% of all female genital malignant neoplasms. During recent years, it appears that this incidence has been increasing. Green reported that in his experience, carcinoma of the vulva accounted for 5% of all gynecologic malignant neoplasms from 1927 through 1961, but in the next 12 years, it increased to 8%. He believed that this increase in incidence was a result of the continued rise in the average age of the female population in later years, causing an increase in the number at risk for development of the disease. Vulvar cancer, with the exception of the rare sarcomas, appears most frequently in women between 65 and 75 years old (Fig. 8–1); in some series, almost half are 70 years of age or older. On the other hand, vulvar cancers can also appear in young patients; Rutledge and colleagues at the MD Anderson Hospital and Tumor Institute noted that about 15% of all vulvar cancers occur in women younger than 40 years. Many of these younger patients have early stromal invasion associated with diffuse intraepithelial neoplasia of the vulvar skin.

Choo found 17 patients younger than 35 years with invasive carcinoma of the vulva. Of these, eight had microinvasion. Many of the associated features seen in patients with vulvar cancer, such as diabetes, obesity, hypertension, and arteriosclerosis, may just reflect the increased incidence of these diseases as one gets older. Al-Ghamdi evaluated 21 patients younger than 40 years with invasive vulvar cancer and found that most, but not all, had associated human papillomavirus. Outcomes in this population were excellent, but the incidence in the younger population appears to be increasing, and this increase cannot be accounted for by immunocompromised patients alone.

During the years, the possible association of vulvar carcinoma and venereal or granulomatous lesions of the vulva has been noted. The incidence tends to be greater in the older literature and much less in more recent reports, probably reflecting to a certain degree a lower incidence of syphilis. The association of condyloma acuminatum with vulvar carcinoma is well known, but no cause and effect relationship has been confirmed as yet. The human papillomavirus (HPV) is suspected in the etiology of squamous neoplasia of the vulva, as it is in similar lesions of the cervix.

INVASIVE SQUAMOUS CELL CARCINOMA

Histology

The overwhelming majority of all vulvar cancer is squamous in origin. The vulva is covered with skin, and any malignant change that appears elsewhere on the skin can occur in this region. Table 8–1 depicts the incidence of vulvar neoplasia from several collected studies in the literature. Our discussion focuses mainly on squamous cell carcinoma because of its preponderance, but as a generalization, the other lesions can be treated similarly, except as noted.

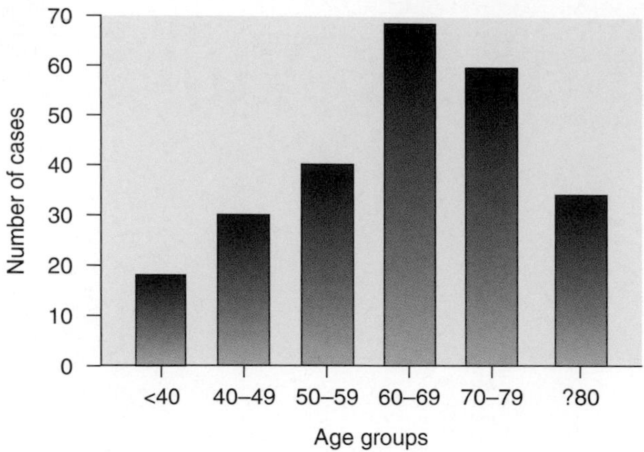

Figure 8–1 Carcinoma of the vulva: Patients treated in 1990–1992. (From the Annual Report of Gynecological Cancer. FIGO, Vol 23, 1998.)

Table 8–1 INCIDENCE OF VULVAR NEOPLASMS BY HISTOLOGIC TYPE*

Tumor type	%	
Epidermoid	86.2	
Melanoma	4.8	
Sarcoma	2.2	
Basal cell	1.4	
Bartholin gland		
Squamous	0.4	
Adenocarcinoma	0.6	1.2
Adenocarcinoma	0.6	
Undifferentiated	3.9	

*Based on 1378 reported cases.
Modified from Plentl AA, Friedman EA: Lymphatic System of the Female Genitalia. Philadelphia, WB Saunders, 1971.

Clinical profile

The development of squamous cell carcinoma of the vulva may be similar to the process that occurs on the cervix. However, no race or culture is spared, and gravidity and parity are not involved in the pathogenesis of this neoplasm. Actually, vulvar cancer is common in the poor and elderly in most parts of the world, and this has led to the hypothesis that inadequate personal hygiene and medical care are often contributing factors in this disease. In truth, the cause of cancer of the vulva is unknown—few data support the concept that these neoplasms often develop from vulvar dystrophies (Fig. 8–2). In many cases, the initial lesion appears to arise from an area of intraepithelial neoplasia that subsequently develops into a small nodule that may break down and ulcerate (Fig. 8–3). On other occasions, small, warty or cauliflower-like growths evolve, and these may be confused with condyloma acuminatum. Long-term pruritus or a lump or mass on the vulva is present in >50% of patients with invasive vulvar cancer (Table 8–2). In most reported series of carcinoma of the vulva, there is delay in treatment of the patient who has symptoms for 2–16 months before medical attention is sought, or medical treatment of vulvar lesions continues for up to 12 months or longer without biopsy for definitive diagnosis or referral.

Fortunately, vulvar cancer is commonly indolent, extends slowly, and metastasizes fairly late. Hence, we have a good opportunity for preventing the serious advanced stages of this disease through education of patients and physicians. Lawhead has proposed a technique for routine vulvar self-examination and urges that this practice be incorporated into every woman's preventive health care regimen. Biopsy must be done of all suspicious lesions of the vulva, including lumps, ulcers, and pigmented areas, even in the patient not complaining of burning or itching (Table 8–3). Our group has looked at the clinical and histologic features of vulvar carcinomas analyzed for HPV status. Of 21 invasive carcinomas of the vulva analyzed, 10 were found to contain HPV-16 DNA. Others have confirmed this observation, suggesting that HPV DNA asso-

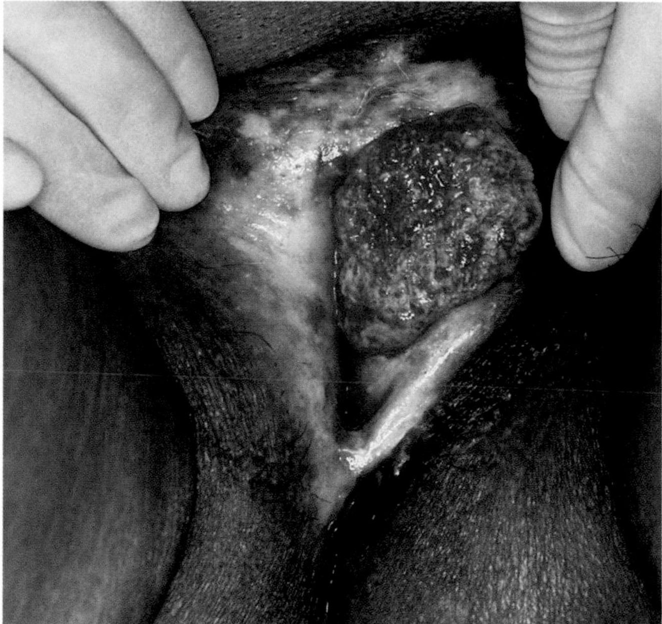

Figure 8–2 Squamous cell carcinoma arising in a bed of lichen sclerosis.

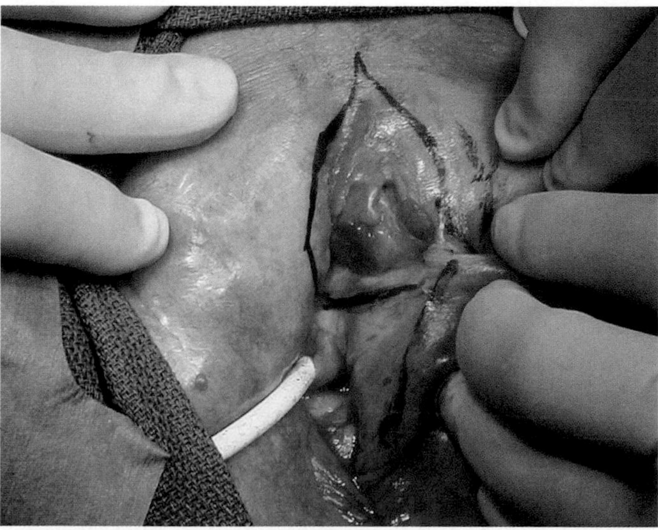

Figure 8–3 Small, well-localized lesion of the vulva.

Table 8–2 SIGNS AND SYMPTOMS OF VULVAR CANCER

Signs and symptoms	%
Pruritus	45.0
Mass	45.0
Pain	23.0
Bleeding	14.0
Ulceration	14.0
Dysuria	10.0
Discharge	8.0
Groin mass	2.5

Table 8–3 INDICATIONS FOR EXCISIONAL BIOPSY OF VULVA NEVI

Change in surface area of nevus
Change in elevation of a lesion: raised, thickened, or nodular
Change in color: especially brown to black
Change in surface: smooth to scaly or ulcerated
Change in sensation: itching or tingling

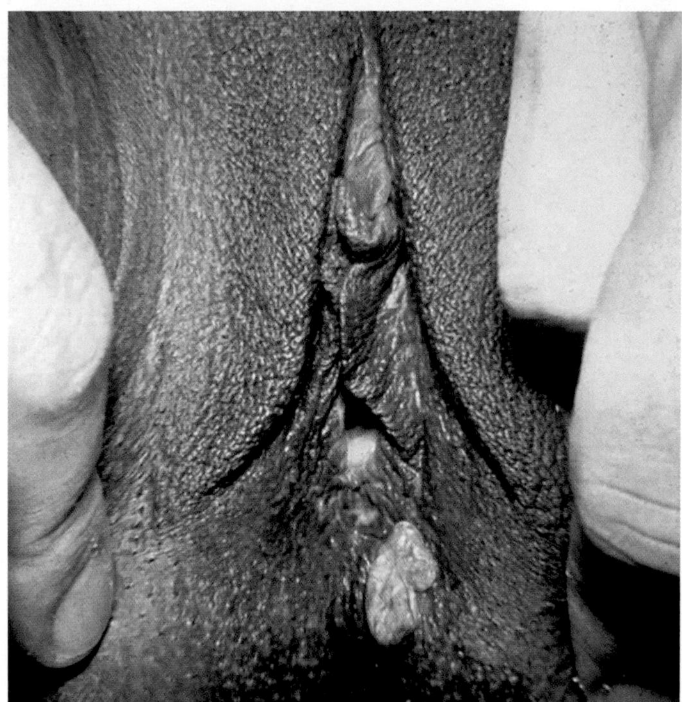

Figure 8–4 Verrucous carcinoma of the vulva.

ciations with malignant changes of the vulva are similar to those observed elsewhere in the genital tract. The correlation is not as strong as in vulvar intraepithelial neoplasia. Andersen and colleagues, among others, noted a variable detection rate of HPV nucleic acids in vulvar cancer. Only 13% of the invasive lesions contained HPV on analysis by in situ hybridization.

A rare variant of epidermoid carcinoma with distinct clinical and pathologic features is known as verrucous carcinoma (Fig. 8–4). The lesion, which may involve the cervix and vagina as well as the vulva, presents as a warty, fungating, ulcerated mass with a bulky, elevated appearance reminiscent of a benign HPV lesion. Identification of this variant is important because the biologic behavior of the disease greatly influences therapy.

Distinction from ordinary condylomata is aided by the absence of fibrovascular cores within the proliferating papillary masses of tumor. Surgical excision is the foundation of therapy; lymphadenectomy is of questionable value except when nodes are obviously involved. Historically, it was felt that radiotherapy is contraindicated because of its ineffectiveness, and reports indicate that it can be an instigator of more aggressive behavior by this tumor.

Location and spread pattern

Primary disease can appear anywhere on the vulva. Approximately 70% arises primarily on the labia. Disease more commonly occurs on the labia majora; however, it may appear on the labia minora, clitoris, and perineum. The disease is usually localized and well demarcated; although it can occasionally be so extensive that the primary location cannot be determined (Fig. 8–5). Multifocal growth pattern in invasive squamous cell carcinoma of the vulva is uncommon, except for the so-called kissing lesions that can occur as isolated lesions, usually on the upper labia.

Fundamental to the understanding of therapy for invasive cancer of the vulva is thorough knowledge of the lymphatic drainage of this organ. In general, the four histologic types of invasive cancer behave similarly and use primarily the lymphatic route for initial metastases (Fig. 8–6).

Lymphatic drainage of the external genitalia begins with minute papillae, and these are connected in turn to a multilayered meshwork of fine vessels. These fine vessels extend over the entire labium minus, the prepuce of the clitoris, the fourchette, and the vaginal mucosa up to the level of the hymenal ring (Fig. 8–7). Drainage of these lymphatics extends toward the anterior portion of the labium minus, where they emerge into three or four collecting trunks whose course is toward the mons veneris, bypassing the clitoris. Vessels from the prepuce anastomose with these lymphatics. Similarly, vessels from the labium majus proceed anteriorly to the upper part of the vulva and mons veneris, there joining the vessels of the prepuce and labium minus. These lymphatic vessels abruptly change direction, turning laterally, and terminate in ipsilateral or contralateral femoral nodes. Drainage is usually limited initially to the medial upper quadrant of the femoral node group. The nodes are medial to the great saphenous vein above the cribriform fascia and in turn may drain secondarily to the deep femoral group. The next echelon of nodes is the pelvic/iliac nodes.

The superficial inguinal lymph glands, located immediately beneath the integument and Camper fascia, are large and 8–10 in number. Most authors agree that the

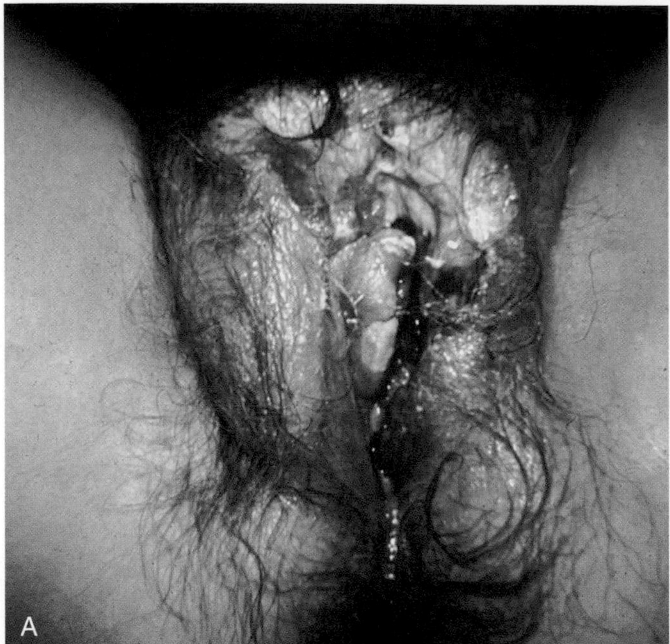

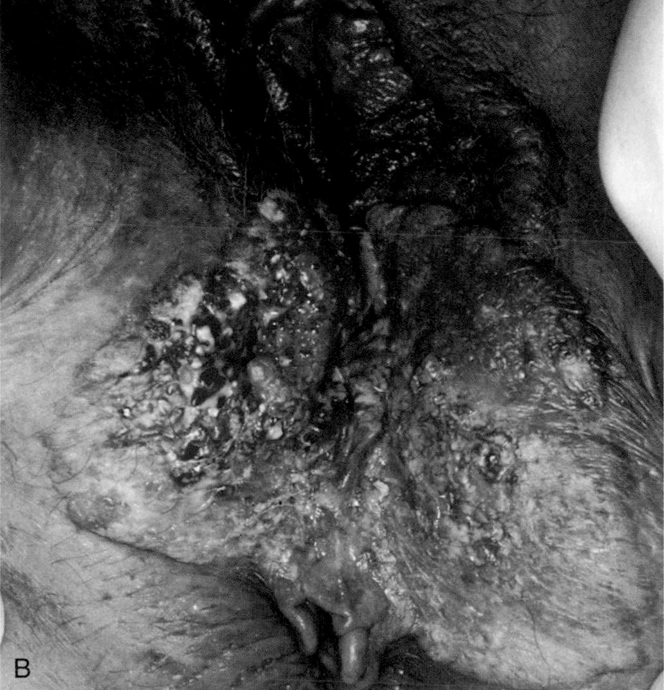

Figure 8–5 *A,* Large ulcerating squamous cell malignancy of the vulva with destruction of the clitoris and the urethra. *B,* Large exophytic squamous cell carcinoma of the vulva.

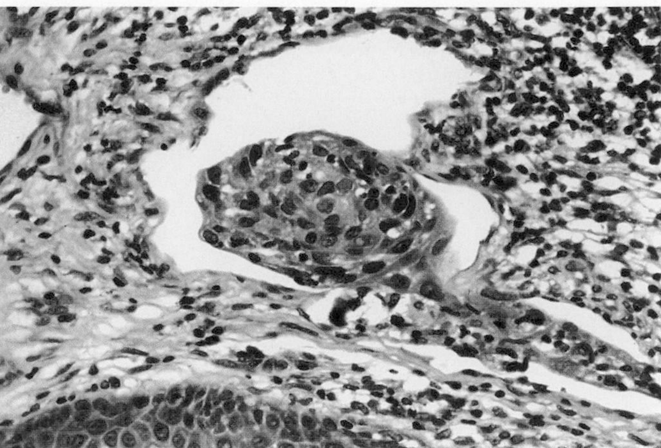

Figure 8–6 Photomicrograph of a tumor nodule invading a vulvar lymphatic.

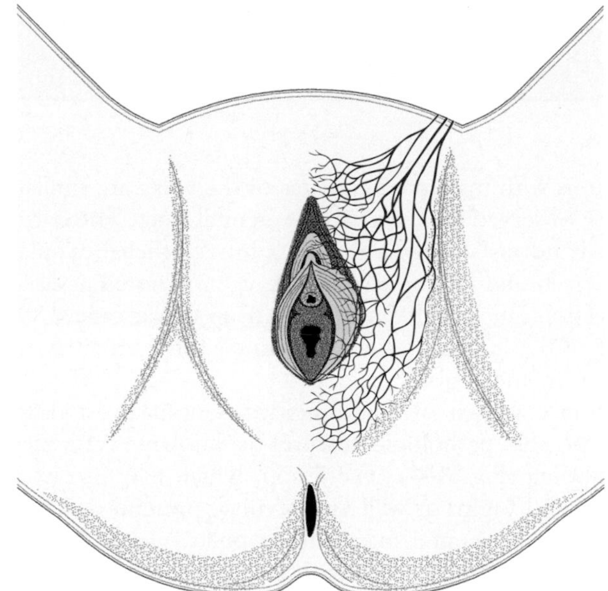

Figure 8–7 Lymphatic drainage of the external genitalia.

superficial inguinal lymph glands are the primary node group for the vulva and can serve as the sentinel lymph nodes of the vulva (Fig. 8–8). The deep femoral nodes, which are by classic teaching located beneath the cribriform fascia, are the secondary node recipients and are involved before drainage into the deep pelvic nodes occurs. The Cloquet node, the last node of the deep femoral group, is located just beneath the Poupart ligament. The multilayered meshwork of lymphatics on the vulva itself is always limited to an area medial to the genitocrural fold (Fig. 8–9). Lymphatic drainage of the vulva is a progressive systematic mechanism, and therapy can be planned according to where in the lymphatic chain tumor is present.

Borgno and colleagues examined 100 inguinal lymphadenectomy specimens at autopsy and demonstrated that the deep femoral nodes are always situated within the openings in the fascia at the fossa ovalis, and no lymph nodes are distal to the lower margin of the fossa ovalis, under the fascia cribrosa. The implication is that a carefully performed deep femoral lymphadenectomy does not require removal of the fascia lata (cribriform fascia) because no lymph nodes were found between the femoral vein and artery lateral to the artery and distal to the lower margin of the fossa ovalis beneath the cribriform fascia. They also found that the node of Cloquet or Rosenmüller, which is the uppermost node among the deep femoral lymph nodes, was absent in 54% of the specimens dissected. Their observations have been confirmed by our experience. During surgery, when traction is persistently applied to the lympho-

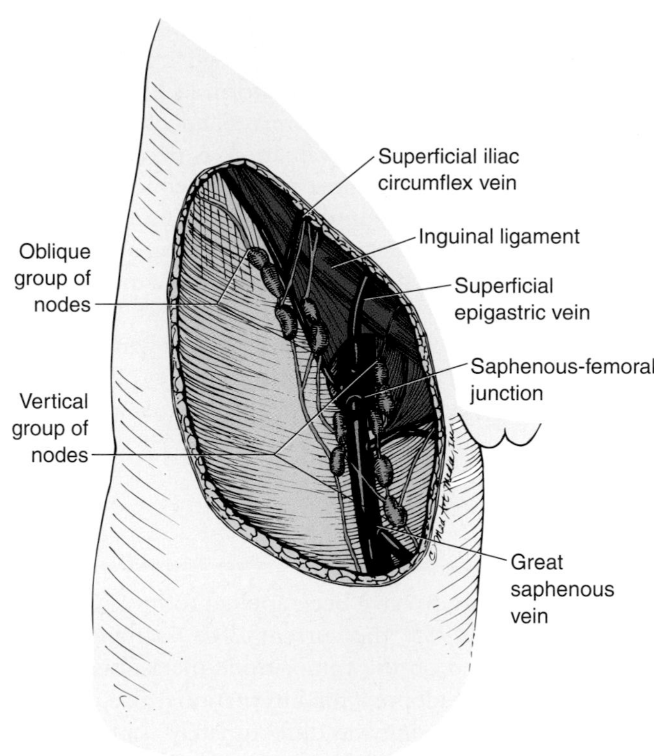

Figure 8–8 The superficial inguinal lymph nodes can be divided into the horizontal group and the perpendicular group.

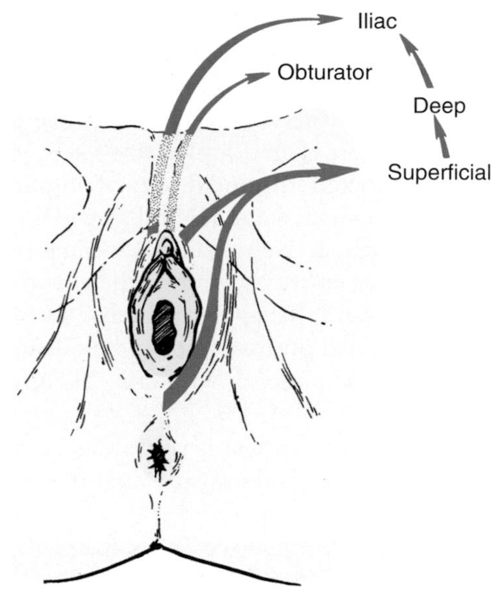

Figure 8–9 Lymphatic spread of a vulvar malignancy. See the text for details.

vascular fat tissue above the cribriform fascia, all inguinal nodes can be removed. No nodal tissue was found in our patients when the cribriform fascia and the fat beneath were submitted separately for pathologic review. Hudson et al confirmed this finding in cadaver dissection and Micheletti and co-workers found supporting evidence with careful embryologic study.

Although lymphatics from the clitoris directly to the deep pelvic lymph nodes are described, their clinical significance appears to be minimal. It is unusual to find a case in which metastasis is present in the pelvic lymph nodes without metastatic disease in the inguinal lymph nodes, even when the clitoris is involved. Curry and associates noted clitoral involvement in 58 patients of 191 studied; none had positive deep pelvic nodes without involvement of inguinal nodes also. Similar results were observed in a study of 38 patients with carcinomas of the clitoris by Ericksson and coworkers, who found also that the deep inguinal or femoral nodes were never positive in the absence of positive superficial inguinal nodes.

The incidence of positive inguinal and pelvic nodes varies considerably, as noted in Table 8–4. Unfortunately, most of these studies were unstaged, although, in general, the larger the tumor, the greater the propensity for

Table 8–4 INCIDENCE OF POSITIVE NODES

Series	No. of cases	Positive groin or pelvic nodes (%)	Positive pelvic nodes (%)
Taussig (1938)	65	46.2	7.7
Cherry and Glucksman (1955)	95	44.2	—
Green et al (1978)	142	38.0	—
Stening and Elliot (1959)	50	40.0	12.0
Way (1960)	143	42.0	16.1
Macafee (1962)	82	40.2	—
Collins et al (1963)	71	31.0	8.5
Rutledge, Smith, and Franklin (1970)	101	47.6	11.1
Faukbeudal (1973)	55	22.0	—
Morley (1976)	374	37.0	—
Krupp and Bahm (1978)	195	21.0	4.6
Curry, Wharton, and Rutledge (1980)	191	30.0	4.7
Simonsen (1984)	122	50.0	10.0
Sutton et al (1991)	150	24.0	—
Homesley (1994)	277	29.2	—
Creasman et al (1997)	1553	31.0	—

inguinal and pelvic node metastases (Table 8–5). Morley noted a 20.7% incidence of lymph node involvement if there was a T1 lesion (<2 cm in diameter). In T2 lesions (>2 cm but limited to the vulva), the incidence of lymph node involvement more than doubled to 44.8%. Malfetano and colleagues reported the incidence of inguinal node metastases in patients with stage III and stage IV lesions to be 53% and 90%, respectively. Clinical evaluation of the groin is somewhat more accurate than tumor size. Homesley (1993) found that approximately 24% of patients with N0/N1 groins had positive nodes when dissected and approximately 75% of patients with N2/N3 groins had positive nodes.

An exception to vulvar cancer is verrucous carcinoma of the vulva. This is a special and unusual variant of squamous cell carcinoma that is locally invasive but non-metastasizing. A condyloma may initially be diagnosed on microscopic examination. There is usually a uniform lack of malignant features histologically. Adequate material, including underlined stroma for pathologic evaluation, is necessary to differentiate verrucous carcinoma from the condyloma. The tumor may invade deeply into the underlying tissue, often requiring extensive surgery, and has a propensity to recur locally. Woodruff noted a lack of lymph node metastases in 27 patients (from the literature and his patients) who were treated with radical vulvectomy and inguinal lymphadenectomy. As a result, he advocated a more conservative approach, with wide excision and tumor-free margins as the therapeutic aim.

Table 8–5 GROIN NODE METASTASIS FOR EACH TUMOR DIAMETER

Tumor diameter (cm)	No.	Positive groin nodes (%)
< 1.0	61	18.0
1.1–2.0	129	19.4
2.1–3.0	175	31.4
3.1–4.0	81	54.3
4.1–5.0	48	39.6
> 5.0	85	51.8
Total	579	34.2

From Homesley HD et al: Prognostic factors for groin node metastasis in squamous cell carcinoma of the vulva (a Gynecologic Oncology Group study). Gynecol Oncol 49:279, 1993.

Staging

Many staging systems have been applied to invasive cancer of the vulva. In 1988, the current FIGO staging system (Table 8–6), based on the tumor-node-metastasis (TNM) classification, was adopted for international use. The old system of clinical staging was unfortunately contingent on the ability of the clinician to assess node involvement by palpation. The new staging system is based on surgical findings. There appears to be a large discrepancy between clinical and surgical-pathologic evaluation of lymph node status. This has been documented in a study by Iversen with 258 patients seen at the Norwegian Radium Hospital. Overdiagnosis (lymph node involvement suspected clinically

Table 8–6 FIGO STAGING OF INVASIVE CANCER OF THE VULVA

Stage 0			
Tis			Carcinoma in situ, intraepithelial carcinoma
Stage I			
T1	N0	M0	Tumor confined to the vulva and/or perineum—2 cm or less in greatest dimension (no nodal metastasis)
Stage Ia			Lesions 2 cm or less in size confined to the vulva or perineum and with stromal invasion no greater than 1.0 mm* (no nodal metastasis)
Stage b			Lesions 2 cm or less in size confined to the vulva or perineum and with stromal invasion greater than 1.0 mm (no nodal metastasis)
Stage II			
T2	N0	M0	Tumor confined to the vulva and/or perineum—more than 2 cm in greatest dimension (no nodal metastasis)
Stage III			Tumor any size with
T3	N0	M0	**1.** Adjacent spread to the lower urethra and/or the vagina, or the anus, and/or
T3	N1	M0	**2.** Unilateral regional lymph node metastasis
T1	N1	M0	
T2	N1	M0	
Stage IVa			
T1	N2	M0	Tumor invades any of the following: upper urethra, bladder, mucosa, rectal mucosa, pelvic bone, and/or bilateral regional node metastasis
T2	N2	M0	
T3	N2	M0	
T4	Any N	M0	
Stage IVb			
Any T	Any N	M1	Any distant metastasis including pelvic lymph nodes

*The depth of invasion is defined as the measurement of the tumor from the epithelial-stromal junction of the adjacent most superficial dermal papilla to the deepest point of invasion.

but negative pathologically) was seen in 40 of 258 patients (15%). Of the 100 patients with metastasis to the inguinal lymph nodes, lymph node involvement was not suspected clinically in 36 patients. Patients with "micrometastasis" (lymph node involvement not suspected clinically but positive microscopically) had a significantly better survival rate than did those with gross metastasis. As a result of these repeated findings, it was suggested that staging be based on surgical-pathologic evaluation instead of clinical evaluation alone. FIGO agreed, and a new staging has been in place since 1988. In 1995, FIGO instituted a subclassification of stage I (see Table 8–6). The reader must remain aware that many reports in the literature used the old staging system, in which data were compiled on cases treated before 1988, and must consider this when analyzing these publications.

Donaldson and coworkers thoroughly evaluated the prognostic parameters in 66 patients with squamous cell carcinomas of the vulva. The size of the lesion dictated the incidence of lymph node metastasis (19% metastasis if the lesion was <3 cm, and 72% metastasis if the lesion was >3 cm). Likewise, grade of tumor correlated with node metastasis (one-third of well-differentiated tumors had metastasis, compared with 75% of the poorly differentiated lesions). Of 38 patients, 11 (29%) had node involvement if invasion of the primary lesion was ≤5 mm, compared with 17 of 28 (61%) if invasion was >5 mm. If tumor did not involve lymphatic or vascular spaces, only 2 of 33 (6%) had positive nodes, whereas 26 of 33 patients (79%) with lymphatic or vascular space involvement had metastasis to the regional lymph nodes. None of 25 patients with lesions invading <5 mm and without lymphatic or vascular space involvement had lymph node metastasis. Iversen and colleagues, describing 117 patients with stage I cancer, noted the same prognostic factors, confirming earlier reports. Of the 690 patients with lesions ≤2 cm, 123 (18%) had node involvement compared with 359 of 863 (42%) with vulvar lesions >2 cm. Grade also related to node metastasis; 77% of grade 1 lesions had negative nodes and 4% had four or more positive nodes, whereas only 40% of grade 4 lesions had negative nodes and 30% had four or more positive nodes. From these data and from other reports by Boyce, Andreasson, and Shimm and coworkers, it appears that conservative therapy may be applied on an individual basis with minimal risk to patients.

There has been interest in using isosulfan blue dye or lymphoscintigraphy to identify and biopsy a sentinel node in the groin. Levenbach and colleagues, at the M.D. Anderson Hospital, studied 52 patients between 1993 and 1999 and found no false negatives. DeCicco used radiolabeled technetium for 37 patients and 55 groins, and was able to identify a sentinel node in all patients. De Hullu and his group (JCO 2000) advocate the use of both techniques in combination. When a sentinel node or nodes are identified, this node is removed and submitted for frozen section. If the frozen section is positive, then a complete node dissection is performed. If the frozen section is negative, then there is a low likelihood that other nodes in that groin would be positive. If this technique can be proven to be highly effective, it would offer the opportunity to reduce the morbidity of the groin dissection.

There are still unanswered questions about the technique. As Levenbach has pointed out, there is a steep learning curve, both for the operating surgeon and the institution. After the first two years at their institution, the rate of not finding a sentinel node was reduced from 16% to 7% of all patients; from 36% to 15% of all groins. Obviously, if a sentinel node cannot be identified, then an entire groin node dissection needs to be performed. Levenbach suggested that it takes 20–30 cases to achieve competence. Results to date suggest a low rate of false negativity. There are anecdotal case reports of groin recurrence after negative sentinel node procedure, however. Louis-Sylvestre notes that if a positive sentinel node is found on one side then a complete groin dissection should be done bilaterally. Also, nodes that are totally replaced by tumor may be bypassed. Step sectioning of lymph nodes may increase the yield (Puig-Tintore). This is problematic with frozen sections. The largest North American experience to date with the longest follow-up was published by Frumovitz and colleagues at the MD Anderson Hospital. Fifty-two patients underwent the procedure between 1993 and 1999, and 14 suffered a recurrence. Eight of the recurrences (15.4%) were on the vulva, three (5.8%) in the groin, and three (5.8%) distant. The pattern of recurrence is similar to that seen with standard approaches, though the rate of relapse in the groin appears somewhat high.

It will take a number of patients and longer follow-up to know if the sentinel node procedure should become the standard of care. Since 75% of patients will have negative nodes, information is only gleaned from one-fourth of the patients who are studied. We must keep in mind that the rate of groin relapse in a node-negative groin (the gold standard) is 0.3% based on the GOG experience (Homesley). De Hullu notes that this is an accurate technique with a high negative predictive value, but not yet ready for general adoption. With experience and careful patient selection, he recommends that patients with T_1/T_2 primary tumors and N_0/N_1 groins who have negative computed tomography (CT) or magnetic resonance imaging (MRI) evaluation, are potential candidates.

Management

After Way reported an improved survival rate in carcinoma of the vulva by use of the en bloc dissection of radical vulvectomy plus inguinal and pelvic lymphadenectomy, that operation became the mainstay of treatment in vulvar cancer. With this therapy, the corrected 5-year survival rate for stage I and stage II disease has been reported by many authors to be approximately 90%.

For many years, a deep pelvic lymphadenectomy was routinely performed with the radical vulvectomy and inguinal lymphadenectomy. Most surgeons now limit the initial procedure to radical vulvectomy and bilateral

Table 8–7 UNILATERAL LESIONS: PERCENTAGE OF POSITIVE GROIN NODES BY TUMOR THICKNESS

Tumor thickness (mm)	Ipsilateral positive only	Contralateral positive only	Bilateral positive	Total	*n*
≤ 2	6.8	0.0	0.0	6.8	59
3–5	20.4	1.9	2.8	25.0	108
6–10	28.8	3.8	11.3	43.8	80
≥ 11	36.7	6.7	6.7	50.0	30
Total	21.7	22.5	5.1	29.2	277

From Homesley HD et al: Prognostic factors for groin node metastasis in squamous cell carcinoma of the vulva (a Gynecologic Oncology Group study). Gynecol Oncol 49:279, 1993.

inguinal lymphadenectomy. If the presence of tumor is documented in the inguinal nodes, a pelvic lymphadenectomy is an option for therapy, on the involved side only. The deep pelvic nodes are essentially never involved with metastatic disease when the inguinal nodes are uninvolved. A study by Curry and associates at the MD Anderson Hospital showed that of 191 patients, only nine 9 (4.7%) had positive deep pelvic nodes, and all nine patients also had metastatic disease in the groin nodes. In most patients, the surgeon will elect to treat the pelvic nodes with radiation therapy.

Unilateral lesions (defined as ≥1 cm from the midline) present another possible variation for therapy. Homesley presented the Gynecologic Oncology Group (GOG) experience with such lesions (Table 8–7) and confirmed the low incidence of contralateral node involvement, making ipsilateral inguinal lymphadenectomy a rational initial approach.

The GOG did a prospective randomized study in patients with vulvar carcinoma who had positive groin nodes. As additional therapy for 114 patients with surgical findings of positive inguinal nodes, one group received radiotherapy and the other group underwent ipsilateral pelvic node dissection. In 1986, the GOG (Homesley) reported that the group receiving radiotherapy had a 68% relative 2-year survival rate, and the group undergoing pelvic node dissection had a 54% relative 2-year survival rate. The authors now recommend pelvic lymph node irradiation (Fig. 8–10) for patients with positive inguinal nodes. The National Cancer Data Base (NCDB) data noted that radiation therapy did not have an impact on patients with positive nodes. Those with one positive node had a 68% 5-year survival if no radiation was given compared with 46% if radiation was given. In those with two positive nodes, survival was 46% if no radiation was given compared with 48% if radiation was given. Radiation did not improve survival compared with surgery only for those with lesions of either ≤2 cm or >2 cm.

Combined radiation therapy and surgery, as well as radiation alone and local surgery alone, have been applied to this disease. No adequate prospective studies comparing various therapies or combinations of such are available for analysis. The older literature notes superior results with radical vulvectomy and lymphadenectomy compared with radiation therapy alone or surgery plus radiation therapy. It was also noted that patients who had vulvectomy alone did worse than patients in whom lymphadenectomy was also included.

Daly and Million advocated radical vulvectomy combined with elective node irradiation for stage I and stage II squamous cell carcinoma of the vulva. In a small number of patients, they found that this treatment combination was well tolerated with no node failures, no irradiation complications, and no delay in healing of the surgical site; the average hospitalization was 13 days. The dose to the inguinal nodes was between 5000 and 5500 cGy, and the midplane pelvic dose was between 4500 and 5000 cGy. Although this is an interesting approach, the small number of patients treated to date does not prove that elective

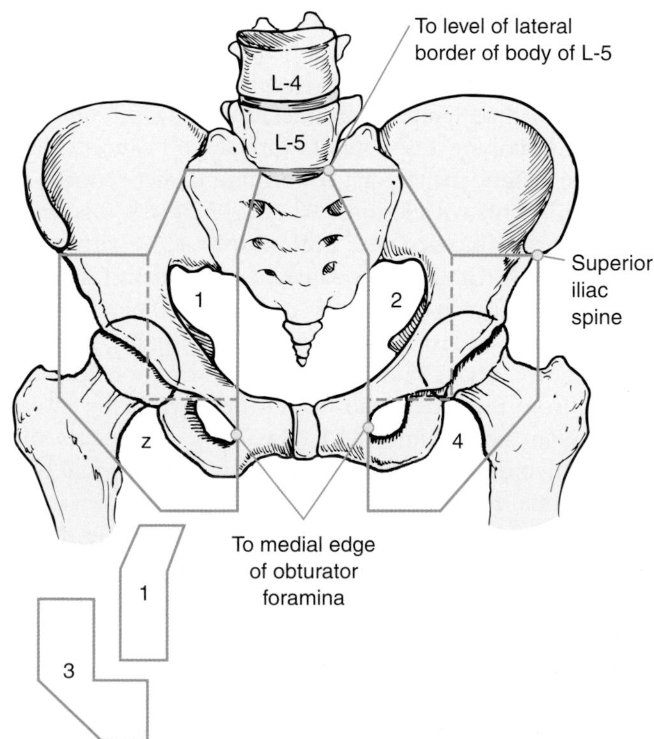

Figure 8–10 Radiation ports for inguinal and pelvic treatment. 1, 2, anteroposterior pelvic and inguinal port; 3, 4, anterior boost, or "wing." (From Prolog: Gynecologic Oncology and Surgery, 2nd ed. The American College of Obstetricians and Gynecologists, 1991, p 51.)

node irradiation will eliminate subclinical node disease from vulvar carcinoma. Because the incidence of inguinal node involvement in stage I and stage II disease is about 20–40%, it will take a reasonably large series of patients observed for a significant time to establish the validity of Daly and Million's hypothesis.

The Gynecologic Oncology Group initiated a randomized trial of groin irradiation versus groin dissection for patients with N0/N1 nodes. (Stehman, 1992). This study was closed prematurely when interim monitoring demonstrated an excess groin failure rate on the radiation arm. Though this study's radiation prescription has been criticized, a Cochrane Database Systematic Review (van der Velden, 2005) concluded that uncontrolled data do not support better groin control with radiation and that lymph node dissection continues to be the cornerstone of therapy. There may still be some role for radiation therapy, though the risk of groin failure and risk of hip fracture must be taken into account (Katz, 2003)

Boronow also emphasized the possible role of radiation therapy in vulvar vaginal cancers. His report dealt mostly with advanced disease involving vaginal mucous membrane, necessitating an exenterative procedure if a primary surgical approach was used. As an alternative, he recommends surgical extirpation of the lymph nodes with a combination of external and interstitial irradiation for control of the central lesion. In a small, highly individualized series, this approach appeared promising. Similar reports by Fairey and associates and Hacker and colleagues substantiated this initial work by Boronow. Others suggested the use of radiation therapy concomitant with chemotherapy before surgery to provide optimal reduction in the size of the central lesion. Radiotherapy has not hitherto been widely used for vulvar cancer because of the technical difficulties associated with directing the external beam to this area, and the sensitive moist vulvar skin and mucous membrane tolerate irradiation poorly. Low anterior and posterior fields must be used, resulting in intense exposure of the vulvar skin because the axis of the X-ray beam runs parallel to (and often within) the skin and mucous membrane. Vulvitis results, and interruption of therapy is often necessary because of the patient's discomfort. Similarly, radiation therapy to enlarged, obviously positive inguinal nodes becomes technically difficult, and removal of at least the enlarged nodes, with subsequent radiation therapy to the area, has been our preference. Preoperative doses of 4500–5000 cGy to either groin or vulvar areas produce a hazardous situation for any subsequent surgical approach. Russell and coworkers described 25 women with locoregionally advanced squamous cancer of the vulva. Eighteen patients were previously untreated, and all patients received external-beam radiation and synchronous radiopotentiating chemotherapy. Complete clinical response was obtained in 16 of 18 previously untreated patients and in 4 of 7 patients with recurrent disease.

Concurrent chemoradiation with cisplatin and 5-fluorouracil has been prospectively evaluated by the Gynecologic Oncology Group and found to be highly effective. Moore et al reported on 73 patients with T3/T4 tumors who would have required ultraradical surgery to clear disease. Resection was accomplished after chemoradiation in 69/71 and only three patients required urinary or fecal diversion. Montana et al reported the companion trial for patients with N3/N4 nodes. Many of these poor-prognosis patients suffered progression or intercurrent death during chemoradiation. Still, 38 of 40 who completed treatment were respectable and 15 of 37 had negative lymph nodes.

It has been suggested that in selected stage IV carcinomas of the vulva, ultraradical surgery may be applicable. Cavanagh and Shepherd, in a review of their data and the literature, identified 53 patients since 1973 who were treated with exenteration and radical vulvectomy and were eligible for a 5-year follow-up. Most of the patients were young, and 47% were alive without recurrence. In their series, Cavanagh and Shepherd found all survivors to have negative pelvic lymph nodes.

Goncalver has reported on cryovulvectomy for 107 patients with advanced and inoperable cancer. Freezing is done with continuous open spray of liquid nitrogen. Cure was obtained in 45% of patients, and local eradication was achieved in 59%. Complications occurred in 25 patients; however, a change in technique would have prevented one third of these.

Technique of radical vulvectomy

We often employ a single arching skin incision parallel to and 2 cm below the inguinal ligament. An effort should be made to spare the fat pad on the mons pubis, especially if the cancer is located posteriorly. This facilitates closure of the vulvectomy defect and provides a fat cushion over the body of the pubic bone (Fig. 8–11A). The skin incision can be tailored (Fig. 8–11B) to remove a larger amount of skin in the inguinal region if large fixed lymph nodes are found. Another possibility is to limit the skin incision to the inguinal area, especially for small posterior lesions, and thereby preserve the bridge of skin between the inguinal and vulvar incisions (three-incision technique, Fig. 8–12). All tissue is removed from the inguinal and femoral lymph node bundles and immediately sent for frozen section analysis. Closed-suction drains are then placed in the groin dissection, and the skin incision is closed by means of a running polyglycolic acid (PGA) suture. Attention is then turned to the vulvectomy itself. The line of incision extends anteriorly from the previously developed inguinal incision, laterally to the genitocrural fold, and posteriorly midway between the anus and posterior fourchette (Fig. 8–11C). A bloodless space can be dissected between vulvar fat and the subcutaneous tissue of the thigh, using a finger dissection (Fig. 8–11D). Peon clamps are then serially placed on the perivaginal fat. The tissue is transected and ligated with 0 chromic catgut at the level of the fascia of the thigh (Fig. 8–11E). The posterior dissection is performed sharply (Fig. 8–11F). Special attention is directed to the location of the anus and rectum. It is sometimes helpful for the operator to place a double-gloved finger in the rectum to ascertain its location and avoid damage during this part of the procedure. The clitoris is then isolated and its suspensory ligament clamped, divided, and suture ligated at its inferior attachment to the pubic bone. It is often helpful at this point to attempt to isolate the ischiocavernosus muscle and divide this structure as laterally as possible (Fig. 8–11G). The pudendal artery and vein are ligated bilaterally (Fig. 8–11H). At this point of the procedure, only the vagina remains attached to the vulva. A decision about the amount of vagina to be removed should be made relative to the location and size of cancer and based on knowledge of the lymphatic drainage of the vulva. For small unilateral lesions, removal of a wide margin of contralateral vagina can be avoided (Fig. 8–11I). If a unilateral lesion is present, hemivulvectomy can be done with preservation of the uninvolved side. This can be accomplished whether an en bloc dissection is performed or the separate incision technique is used (Fig. 8–12). This has been our practice now for years. Every effort should be made to avoid resection of the urethra unless it is close to the cancer. If it is indicated, the distal 1–2 cm of this organ

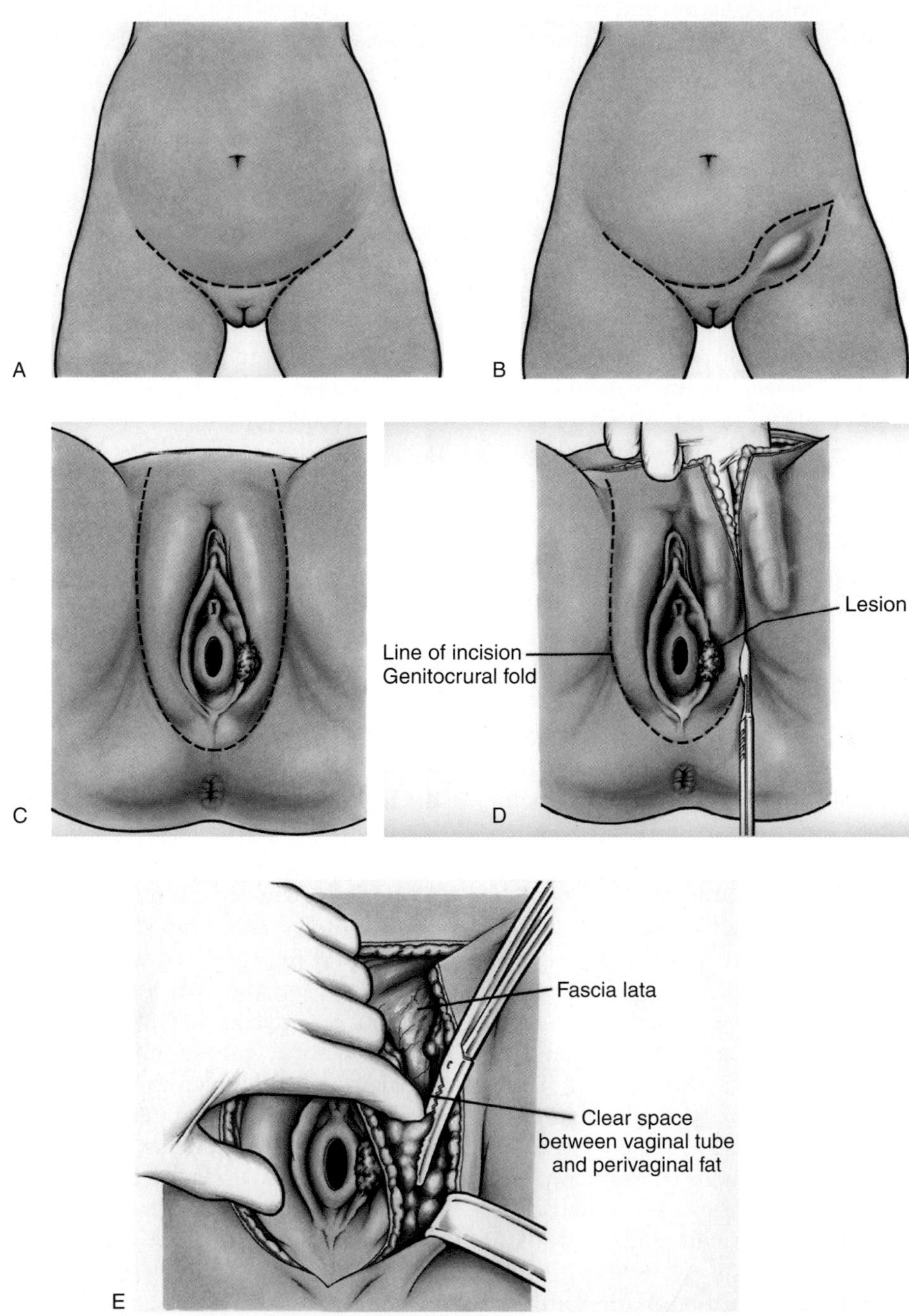

Figure 8–11 *A*, Groin incision for moderate-sized lesions. *B*, Groin incision for a patient with a matted left inguinal node. *C* and *D*, Vulvar incision along the genitocrural fold. *E*, Clamping the perivaginal tissue.

Illustration continued on opposite page.

can be removed without damage to the functional sphincter. The perineal defect is closed primarily with mattress sutures of 0 PGA laterally and posteriorly. Tension on this closure can be prevented, if necessary, by sharp and blunt mobilization of the vaginal barrel or subcutaneous tissue of the thigh. The most anterior extent of the dissection is not sutured primarily; it is allowed to granulate secondarily. This prevents distortion of the urethra and alteration of the urinary stream.

Recent studies have demonstrated that the classical radical vulvectomy can be safely modified in extent without compromising outcomes. Bell showed that a complete inguinal dissection could be achieved while leaving the fascia intact. He and his coinvestigators retrieved a mean of 10 nodes per groin without removing the cribriform fascia. Judson et al, in a randomized trial, were able to reject the hypothesis that transferring the sartorius muscle from its origin reduces morbidity. Zhang and colleagues confirmed Plaxe's observation that a complete inguinal node dissection can be performed while leaving the greater saphenous vein intact. They observed less short-term and long-term morbidity.

Patients are given a broad-spectrum cephalosporin for 1 week after surgery. Bedrest is maintained for 2–3 days. Vigorous local cleansing of the perineal and groin incisions is continued until these incisions are completely healed.

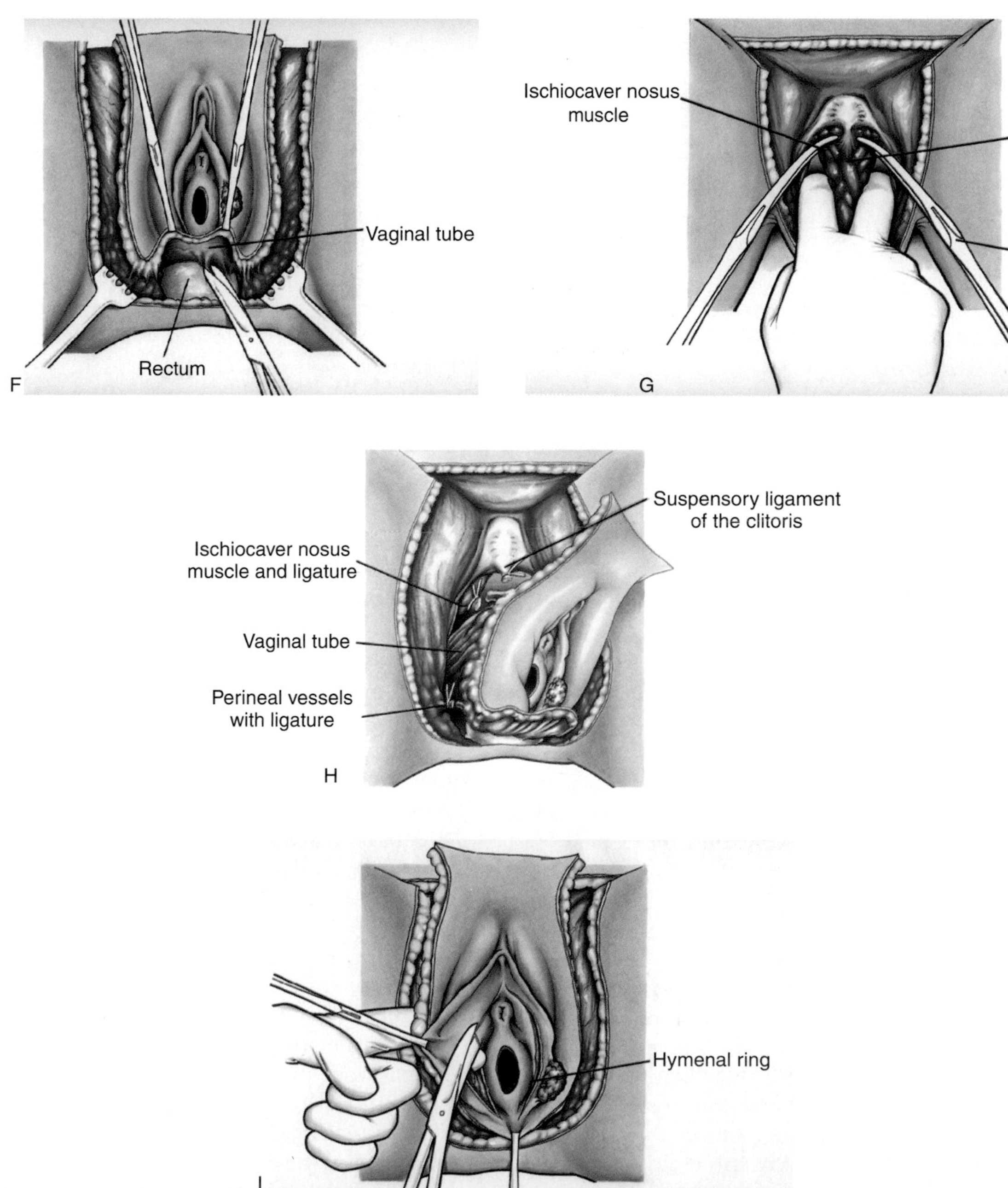

Figure 8–11, cont'd *F*, Vagina being separated from the rectum. *G*, Clamping the ischiocavernosus muscle and the crura of the clitoris. *H*, Molulized specimen is prepared for excision. *I*, Excision along the inner margin of the specimen.

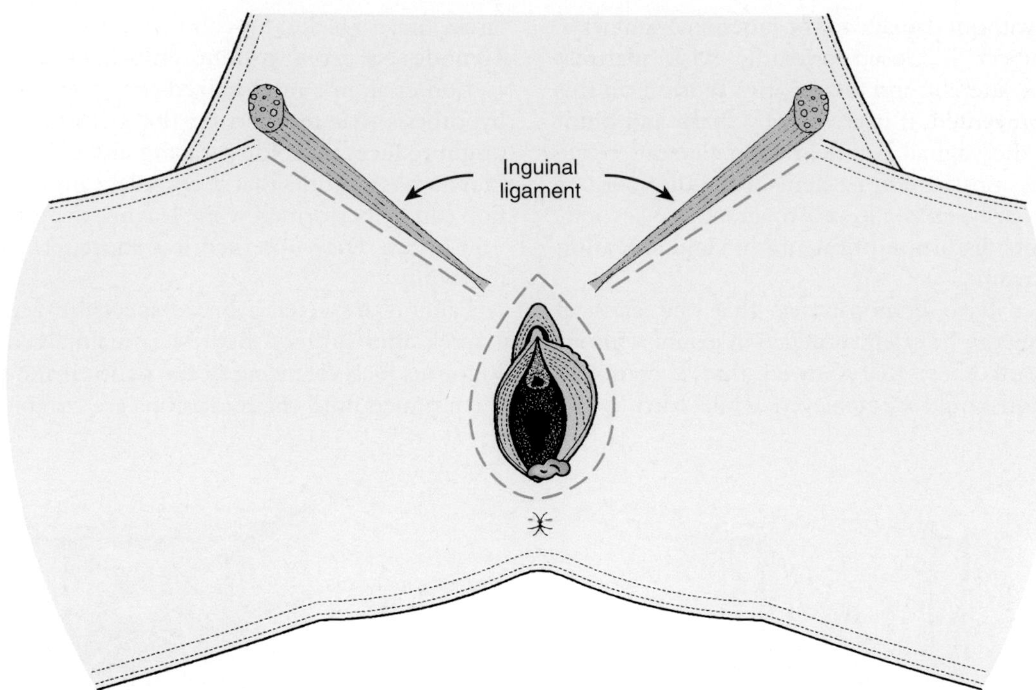

Figure 8–12 Three-incision technique for vulvar cancer.

Operative morbidity and mortality for radical vulvectomy and bilateral inguinal lymphadenectomy

In the early series of Way, operative mortality approached 20%. In the last 2 decades, this has been reduced to 1% or 2%. This procedure is frequently carried out in the 9th and 10th decades of life with surprising safety.

The complication encountered most frequently is wound breakdown, which occurs in well above 50% of patients in most series. This aspect of the morbidity is usually limited to skin loss at the margin of the groin incision. Podratz and colleagues at the Mayo Clinic noted impaired primary wound healing in 148 of 175 patients (85%) who were treated with radical vulvectomy and inguinal lymphadenectomy. Removing lesser amounts of skin and decreasing the undermining of the skin flaps have reduced the incidence of wound breakdown. Suction drainage has also added to this decreasing morbidity. Careful débridement and vigorous care to keep the wounds clean and dry almost always result in adequate healing.

Lymphedema of the lower extremities is another major problem, especially in patients who have had inguinal and deep pelvic node dissection (Fig. 8–13). In the study reported by Podratz and colleagues, varying degrees of lymphedema of the lower extremities occurred in 69% of their patients. The incidence of this debilitating long-term complication can be reduced by routine use of custom-made plastic support hose during the first postoperative year while collateral pathways of lymph drainage are being developed. Rutledge and colleagues have for many years advised that patients also receive low-dose prophylactic antibiotic therapy (similar to that used to prevent subacute bacterial endocarditis) after lymphadenectomy to prevent streptococcal lymphangitis in the lower extremities, which dramatically increases the incidence of lymphedema. Established lymphedema can be kept under control in many patients with routine use of pneumatic hose devices that have become widely available.

The development of a lymphocyst in the groin area is an infrequent occurrence, and it usually resolves spontaneously. The incidence can be reduced by careful ligation of all the lymph-bearing tissue during the groin dissection. On occasion, intermittent aseptic aspiration of the fluid facilitates resolution of these collections.

The rate of complications has been reduced in this era of modified radical operation, though it continues to be high. Three contemporary series (Rouzier, 2003; Gaarenstroom, 2003; and Gould, 2001) have shown that wound cellulitis occurs in 25–39% of patients; wound breakdown in 17–31% of patients; and lymphedema in 28–39% of patients. While these results are encouraging, it is clear that further improvements are needed.

The use of radiation therapy as a priori treatment (especially in patients with fixed inguinal nodes) can result in significant vulvar edema. This is especially true when low fields are used to include vulvar disease. Fig. 8–14 illustrates severe edema in a patient treated primarily with radiation therapy. Necrosis is seen at 5 o'clock, which is residual from the large lesion occupying that area before irradiation.

Symptoms related to stress incontinence and the development of cystocele or rectocele are sometimes reported by these patients. These conditions are secondary to the loss of the support of the lower end of the vagina and subsequent enlargement of the introitus. The findings may

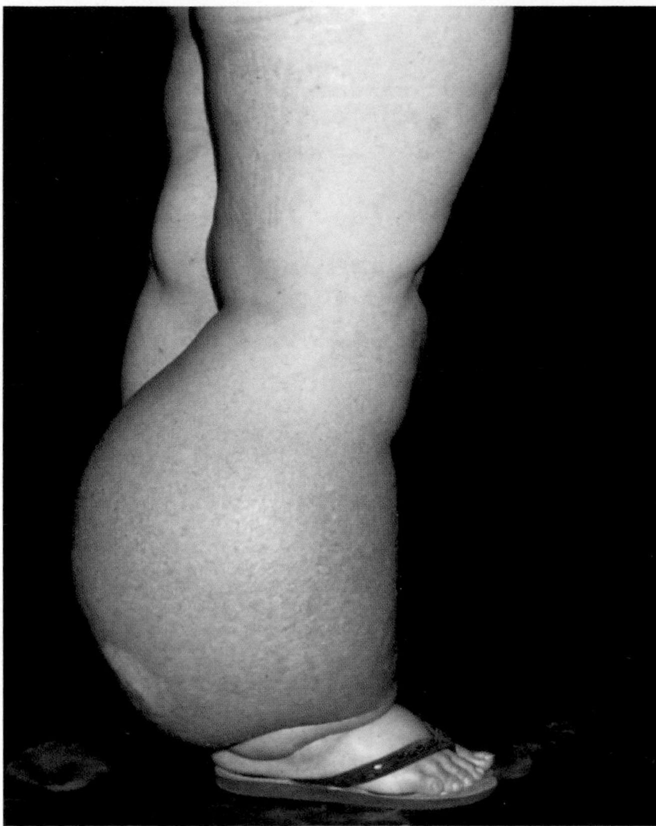

Figure 8–13 Marked lymphedema of the left leg after inguinal and pelvic lymphadenectomy.

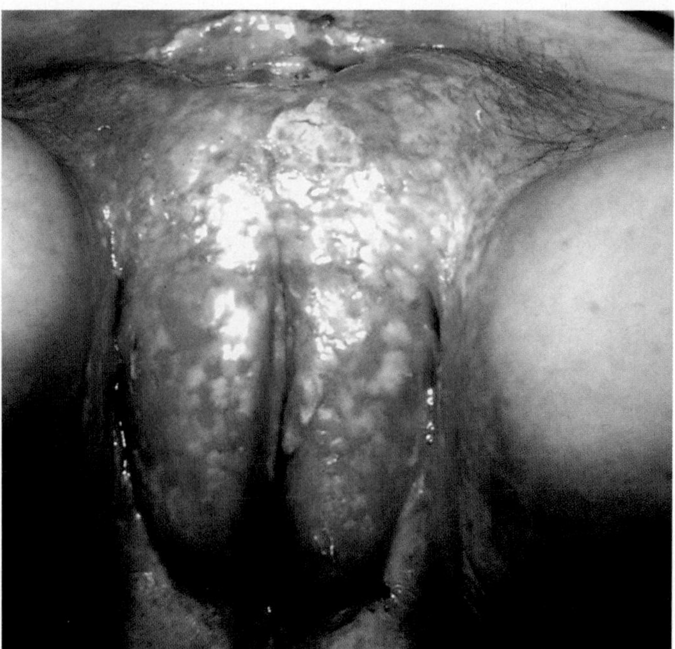

Figure 8–14 Severe edema of the vulva following radiation therapy with necrosis at the site of the primary lesion.

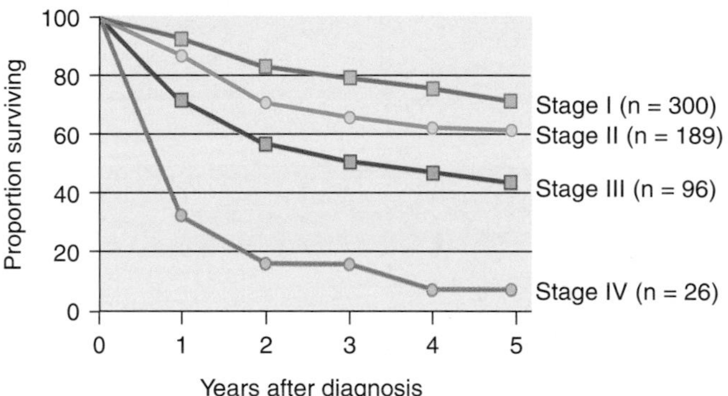

Figure 8–15 Carcinoma of the vulva: Patients treated in 1990–1992. (From the Annual Report of Gynecological Cancer. FIGO, Vol 23, 1998.)

also simply reflect the increased frequency of pelvic visceral prolapse among older women.

Removal of significant vulvar tissue, particularly the clitoris, can result in decreased sexual satisfaction. With small lesions in which the clitoris is not involved, hemivulvectomy with preservation of the clitoris can be performed. This allows sexual satisfaction to be achieved without a decrease in survival. Loss of the subcutaneous tissue prevents mobility of the external genitalia, which can also hinder sexual pleasure. Although this has been a detriment in many patients, others state that orgasm is still obtainable after vulvectomy.

Survival results

Survival in cancer of the vulva, as with all other malignant neoplasms, is directly related to the extent of disease at the time diagnosis is made and treatment is undertaken. Because this malignant neoplasm is initially diagnosed in the elderly woman, many patients succumb to intercurrent disease while they are tumor free. In stage I and stage II disease, the corrected 5-year survival rate should approach 90%. A 75% corrected 5-year survival rate for all stages of vulvar cancer is not unusual. Hacker and coworkers reported a 5-year survival rate of 98% in stage I cancer and 90% in stage II. Regardless of the stage, if negative lymph nodes were present, there was a 96% survival rate. This dropped to 66% if positive nodes were present. If only one inguinal node had metastasis, the survival rate was 94%, dropping to 80% if two positive nodes were involved. Similar results were noted from the Mayo Clinic data. If lymph nodes were negative, the 5-year survival rate was 90%. However, in that material, the survival rate dropped precipitously if even one lymph node had metastasis (57%). The NCDB reported a 5-year survival of 93% for stage I and 87% for stage II. In those patients with positive nodes, survival was 62% if the primary lesion was ≤2 cm and 43% if the primary lesion was >2 cm. Overall survival results by stage are found in Fig. 8–15.

In many series, however, if the lymph nodes are negative irrespective of stage, >90% of these patients will survive 5 years (corrected survival), whereas only 40–50% will survive if the lymph nodes are positive (Table 8–8). Curry and associates noted that in patients with three or fewer unilateral groin nodes involved with metastasis, the 5-year

Table 8–8 SURVIVAL RATES FOR CARCINOMA OF THE VULVA

Series	Status of nodes	No. of patients	Percentage surviving	
			Positive	Negative
Way (1960)	Positive	45	42	
	Negative	36		77
Macafee (1962)	Positive	33	33	
	Negative	49		70
Collins et al (1963)	Positive	19	21	
	Negative	32		69
Franklin and Rutledge (1971)	Positive	33	39	
	Negative	53		100
Morley (1976)	Positive	64	39	
	Negative	130		92
Krupp and Bahm (1978)	Positive	40	36	
	Negative	154		91
Green (1978)	Positive	46	33	
	Negative	61		87
Benedet et al (1979)	Positive	34	53	
	Negative	86		81
Boyce (1985)	Positive	30	50	
	Negative	49		82
Shimm et al (1986)	Positive	33	52	
	Negative	65		77
Cavanagh et al (1990)	Positive	77	39	
	Negative	126		85
Creasman (1997)	Positive	444	49	
	Negative	983		90

Table 8–9 SURVIVAL RATES FOR PATIENTS WITH POSITIVE PELVIC NODES

Series	Five-year survival rate (%)
Way (1957)	2/9 (22.2)
Green et al (1958)	2/16 (12.5)
Way (1960)	3/8 (37.5)
Merrill and Ross (1961)	1/3 (33.3)
Collins et al (1963)	1/6 (16.7)
Franklin and Rutledge (1971)	3/12 (25.0)
Morley (1976)	1/6 (16.7)
Curry, Wharton, and Rutledge (1980)	2/9 (22.2)
Boyce (1985)	0/6 (0)
Shimm (1986)	0/7 (0)
Total	15/82 (18.3)

survival rate was still good (17 of 25, or 68%); however, of five patients in whom more than three nodes were involved, none survived. None of the patients with three or fewer unilateral involved nodes had deep pelvic node metastases. In the large NCDB report, in those patients with negative nodes, irrespective of size or primary lesion, the 5-year survival was 90%. Survival was 55% with one positive node, 59% with two or three positive nodes, and 33% with four positive nodes. Boyce and associates and Shimm and coworkers reported similar results, with prognosis worsening not only with an increase in the number of positive nodes but to a lesser extent with bilateral inguinal node involvement. Of the patients with more than four unilateral nodes, 50% had deep pelvic node metastasis; and if bilateral groin nodes were involved, 26% had positive pelvic nodes. In patients with positive pelvic nodes, the survival rate is poor. Collected series indicate that only one-fifth of patients with deep pelvic node metastasis survived 5 years (Table 8–9).

Tolerance of the elderly patient to therapy

As stated before, many cases of squamous cell carcinoma of the vulva occur in patients who are in the 8th, 9th, and 10th decades of life. Because the average life span of women has increased, gynecologic malignant neoplasms in geriatric patients have become common. In fact, more than half of all cancers occur in elderly patients; the probability of developing cancer within a 5-year span climbs from 1 in 700 at the age of 25 years to 1 in 14 by the age of 65 years. Cancer is the second leading cause of death in persons older than 65 years. Why there is an increase in incidence of cancer in this population has not been clearly established, although a number of factors may be involved. These include the possibility of decreased immunosurveillance, the longer duration of carcinogenic exposure, and an increased susceptibility of aging cells to carcinogenesis.

In younger patients, the “clinical dictum” is to attempt to attribute all signs and symptoms of cancer to a single diagnosis. The opposite is true, however, for older patients,

Table 8–10 SITES OF RECURRENCE AFTER MODIFIED RADICAL OPERATION

Author	n	Local	Bridge	Groin	Distant
de Hullu (2002)	238	18 (8%)	1 (0.4%)	2 (0.8%)	12 (5%)
Gonzalez-Bosquet (2005)	330	64 (19%)		8 (2.4%)	37 (11%)
Maggino (2000)	502	100 (20%)		35 (6.9%)	25 (5%)
Oonk (2003)	238	49 (20%)	2 (0.8%)	6 (2.5%)	8 (3%)
Rouzier (2002)	215	26 (17%)	7 (3.3%)		

in whom the clinical features are probably caused by multiple diagnoses because of common occurrences of concomitant medical illnesses. The pervasive notion that elderly patients are less tolerant of chemotherapy, surgery, and radiation therapy is generally untrue. The majority of older people who have few concomitant medical problems can tolerate all these modalities, especially surgery, quite well. Although elderly patients should not be categorically excluded from aggressive therapy because of their age, treatment may need modification to accommodate changes that occur with age. For example, it is clear that older patients who are treated with intensive chemotherapy have a much higher initial toxicity rate because of bone marrow suppression. Therefore, doses should be initiated at a reduced level and then increased as tolerated to avoid difficulty. On the other hand, surgical therapy such as radical vulvectomy with bilateral inguinal lymphadenectomy is well tolerated by elderly patients, even those in their 90s. Undoubtedly, this is because body cavities are not violated. Much of the risk lies in the anesthesia required.

Recurrence

Recurrence may be local or distant, and >80% will occur in the first 2 years after therapy, demanding initial close follow-up. Oonk noted that 65% of recurrences were found at scheduled follow-up visits, and that half of those patients were asymptomatic. Recurrences found at scheduled follow-up tended to be smaller. Local recurrence is more common with larger tumors, and positive capillary-lymphatic space involvement. (Table 8–10). Surprisingly, more than half of the recurrences are local and near the site of the primary lesion. This is more common in patients with large primary tumors or metastatic disease in the lymph nodes revealed at initial surgery. The margin of resection has long been recognized to be a significant prognostic factor as well. Heaps et al found that if the formalin fixed margin was >8 mm (equivalent to 1 cm in fresh tissue) the risk of local recurrence was very low. This finding has been confirmed by de Hullu and Rouzier. A study from the MD Anderson Hospital suggests that local recurrences are commonly seen even when the margins are declared clear on the original operative specimen. On the other hand, the high incidence of local recurrences demands careful attention to adequate margins in the removal of the primary lesion. Some recurrences on the vulva occur at a site remote from the primary excision, often later in follow-up. Rouzier et al (2001) noted that these patients, who may have new primary lesions, had a better prognosis than those who recurred earlier and near the site of the prior excision.

Wide local excision and the triple incision technique may lead to a slightly increased risk for local recurrence (van der Velden, 2004). Care must be given to excising the entire lesion with at least a 1–2 cm margin. In many instances, local recurrences can be successfully treated by local excision or interstitial irradiation. Patients with recurrent local disease in the lymph node area or distant disease are difficult to treat, and the salvage rate is poor. Simonsen reported a 40% salvage with local recurrence and an 8% survival at 5 years with regional metastases. Both groups were treated with a combination of surgery and radiation therapy. Prempree and Amornmarn had similar results using radiation alone. Disease limited to the introitus gave the best prognosis: six of six patients survived. As expected, extensive recurrences have the poorest prognosis, especially when bone metastases occur. Patients with distant recurrences have been treated at our institution with cisplatin-based chemotherapy, and a 30% overall response rate has been achieved. Responses are more likely outside the radiation field.

EARLY VULVAR CARCINOMA

In 1974, Wharton and colleagues described an entity they called microinvasive carcinoma of the vulva. These lesions were ≤2 cm in diameter and invaded the stroma to a depth of ≤5 mm. Of 25 such patients, none had positive lymph nodes, developed recurrence, or died as a result of vulvar cancer. These results imply that microinvasive carcinoma of the vulva is a definable stage, in that this group may be treated by conservative surgery. As a result of this article, several patients with stage I lesions and limited stromal invasion were treated by radical vulvectomy only. Several of these patients subsequently developed recurrent or metastatic carcinoma and died of their disease. In 1975, Parker and coworkers at Duke University presented their evaluation of patients with early invasive epidermoid carcinoma of the vulva. They believed that the term *microinvasive* was not applicable to vulvar neoplasia. Of their patients, 60 had a stage I (T1) lesion of ≤2 cm; 58 of these patients had stromal invasion ≤5 mm in depth. Of the 58 patients, 3 (5%) had pelvic node metastases; 2 of these 3 showed invasion of vascular channels, and the third patient showed

Table 8–11 SUPERFICIALLY INVASIVE VULVAR CARCINOMA: FREQUENCY OF LYMPH NODE METASTASIS WITH LESIONS 5 mm IN DEPTH OR LESS

Author	Total cases	No. with lymphadenectomy	Node metastasis	Total with node metastasis (%)
Wharton et al	25	10	0	0.4*
Dean et al	7	1	0	0.4*
Parker et al	58	37	3	5.2*
DiPaola et al	12	11	4	33.3*
Kunschner et al	17	13	0	0.4*
Kabulski and Frankman	23	23	5	21.7*
Magrina et al	96	71	9	9.4*
DiSaia et al	19	19	1	5.3*
Barnes et al	18	7	2	11.1*
Iversen et al	70	70	5	7.1*
Donaldson et al	38	38	11	28.9*
Fu et al	13	12	2	15.4*
Buscema et al	58	40	6	10.3*
Wilkinson et al	30	27	2	6.7*
Kneale et al	92	61	6	6.5*
Hoffman et al	75	46	10	13.3*
Sedlis et al	187	187	33	18.0*
Dvoretsky et al	36	NR	6	16.7*
Rowley et al	22	22	2	9.0*
Berman et al	50	50	1	2.0*
Total	946	745	108	11.4*

*Inguinal or distant metastasis.
NR, not reported.
From Wilkinson EJ: Superficial invasive carcinoma of the vulva. Clin Obstet Gynecol 28:188, 1985.

cellular anaplasia. The Duke study concluded that if a strict histologic evaluation of the excised vulvar lesion shows invasion of ≤5 mm, an absence of vascular or lymphatic channel invasion, and no anaplasia, an operational approach less radical than radical vulvectomy, inguinal dissection, and pelvic lymphadenectomy could be used for selected patients. This would reduce the morbidity and not increase mortality.

Andreasson and coworkers constructed three different models of groups at low risk for metastasis in squamous cell carcinoma of the vulva region. They concluded that a definite, distinct profile of low-risk patients would require data from large accruals of patients and international collaboration.

There is at present no universally agreed definition for superficially invasive carcinoma of the vulva, although many authors have used the term. One of the problems of defining the lesion is determining its clinically important dimensions and how these dimensions should be measured. The measurements of the diameter of the lesion and the depth of invasion are the most commonly used. In studies that used the 5 mm depth of invasion parameter, 946 cases collected by Wilkinson with ≤5 mm depth of invasion revealed 108 patients (12.2%) with inguinal lymph node metastasis (Table 8–11). The depth of invasion by tumor acceptable as superficial invasion has been variable and is further confused by there being little agreement on how the measurement should be made. Although a 5 mm depth of invasion is accepted by many authors, others use a 3 mm depth. In patients with tumors with 3 mm depth of invasion, the frequency of lymph node metastasis is lower (Table 8–12). There remains considerable inconsistency regarding pathologists' methods of measuring depth of invasion. In most current publications, a method is described that measures from the most superficial dermal-epidermal junction of the most superficial adjacent dermal papilla. Others have used a method that measures from the surface of the lesion; although this method is simpler, it appears not to be as reflective of true invasion. The importance of vascular invasion adjacent to the vulvar carcinoma in predicting lymph node metastasis, or prognosis, remains controversial. However, data support the hypothesis that vascular space involvement by tumor at the site of the primary tumor is associated with increased frequency of lymph node metastasis.

The International Society for the Study of Vulvovaginal Disease (ISSVD) has proposed this pathologic definition of microinvasive carcinoma of the vulva: a squamous carcinoma having a diameter of ≤2 cm, as measured in the fresh state, with a depth of invasion of ≤1 mm, measured from the epithelial-stromal junction of the most superficial adjacent dermal papilla to the deepest point of invasion. Vascular space involvement by tumor excludes the lesion from this definition. These lesions probably do not need an inguinal lymphadenectomy of any type and are now classified as stage Ia. A review of the literature reveals only two cases of stage Ia with lymph node metastasis.

Table 8–12 SUPERFICIALLY INVASIVE VULVAR CARCINOMA: FREQUENCY OF LYMPH NODE METASTASIS WITH LESIONS 3 mm IN DEPTH OR LESS

Author	Total cases	No. with lymphadenectomy	Node metastasis	Total with node metastasis (%)
Jafari and Cartnick	6	6	1*	16.6
Iversen et al	48	48	2*	4.2
Chu et al	26	13	0*	0.6
Buscema et al	19	19	1*	5.3
Wilkinson et al	29	25	2*	6.8
Hoffman et al	60	NR	2*	3.3
Kneale et al	68	NR	4*	5.8
Dvoretsky et al	28	NR	2*	7.1
Rowley et al	18	18	1*	5.5
Berman et al	31	31	1*	3.2
Total	333	160	16*	4.8

*Groin recurrence.
NR, not reported.

Donaldson described a patient with 1.1 mm of stromal invasion with tumor in vascular spaces who was found to have metastatic tumor in two ipsilateral inguinal lymph nodes. There does not appear to be a definitive correlation between tumor differentiation and lymph node metastasis and survival. There may be an association between depth of tumor invasion and tumor differentiation, with deeply invasive tumors being more undifferentiated. More study of this issue is needed.

Podratz and colleagues reported a 5-year survival rate of 90% if the primary lesion was <1 cm, 89% if the lesion was 1–2 cm, and 83% if the lesion was 2–3 cm. They found that the 5- and 10-year survival rates of patients with stage I disease were independent of the extent of the surgical procedure, suggesting that more selectivity of the treatment is feasible without sacrifice of curability. There continues to be a lack of unanimity concerning the proper surgical approach to the patient with an early invasive carcinoma of the vulva. Reports illustrating metastatic disease in inguinal lymph nodes conflict with other reports that suggest radical vulvectomy only. The morbidity produced by radical vulvectomy, both to body image and with sexual function, makes this issue worthy of serious consideration. As a result, DiSaia and colleagues proposed an alternative approach to this early disease that attempts to preserve vulvar tissue without sacrificing curability when possible metastatic disease exists. This approach uses the inguinal nodes as sentinel nodes in the treatment planning when the central lesion is ≤1 cm in diameter and focal invasion is limited to ≤5 mm (see the description of metastatic lymph node spread pattern on pp 239–241).

The patient is prepared for radical vulvectomy with a bilateral inguinal lymphadenectomy if the operative findings warrant a maximal surgical effort. An 8 cm incision is made parallel to the inguinal ligament two fingerbreadths (4 cm) beneath the inguinal ligament and two fingerbreadths (4 cm) lateral to the pubic tubercle (Fig. 8–16). This allows access to the inguinal lymph nodes of both the upper oblique and inferior vertical set. The incision is carried down through the Camper fascia, and at this point skin flaps are bluntly and sharply dissected superiorly and inferiorly, allowing access to the fat pad containing the superficial nodes. The sentinel nodes are located in the fatty layer of tissue above and beneath the Camper fascia, in part anterior to the cribriform plate and also protruding from beneath the fascia lata (Fig. 8–17). The dissection should be carried superiorly to the inguinal ligament and inferiorly to a point approximately 2 cm proximal to the opening of the Hunter canal. The dissection should be carried laterally to the sartorius muscle and medially to the adductor longus muscle fascia (Fig. 8–18). Blunt dissection with the handle of the scalpel facilitates identification of

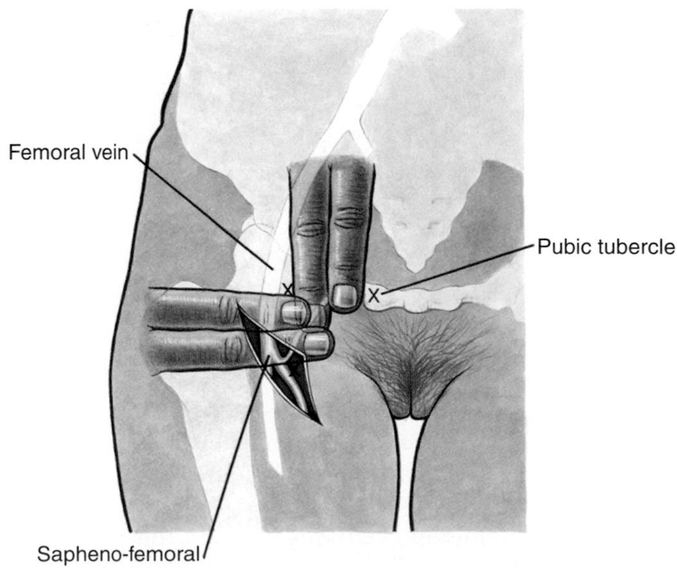

Figure 8–16 Incision can be made as noted so that superficial inguinal nodes can be removed easily. (Modified from Cabanas RM: An approach to the treatment of penile carcinoma. Cancer 39:456, 1977. Copyright © 1977 American Cancer Society. Reprinted by permission of Wiley-Liss, Inc., a subsidiary of John Wiley & Sons, Inc.)

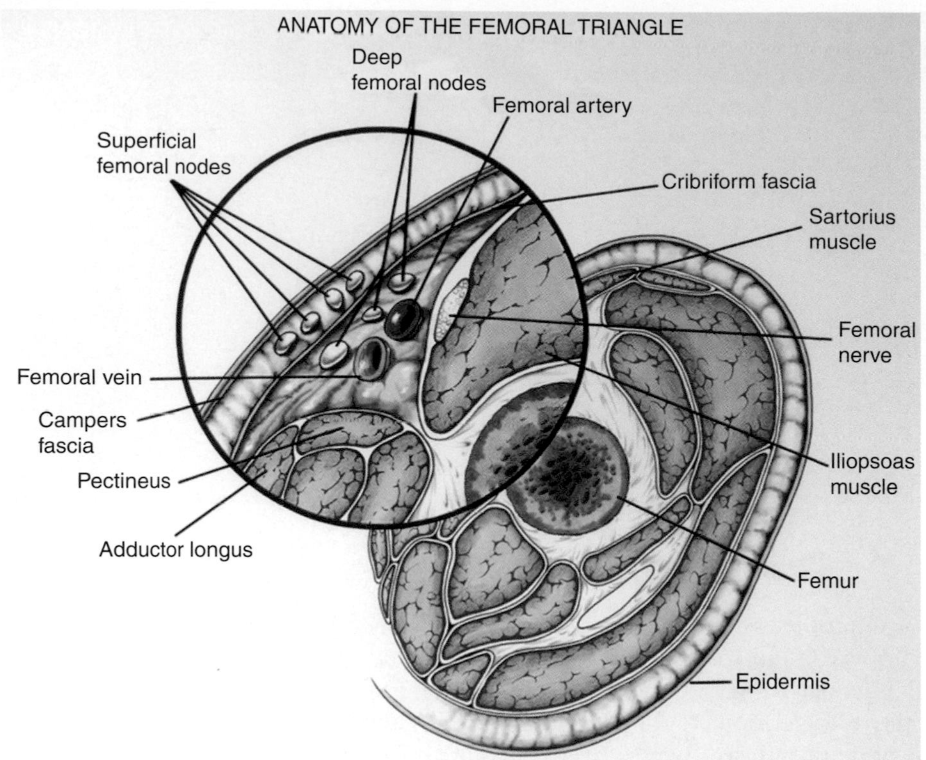

Figure 8–17 Many inguinal nodes are located between the Camper fascia and the cribriform fascia, as noted on cross-section through the femoral triangle. Additional nodes are clustered in the foramen ovalis, in the part protruding from beneath the plane of the cribriform fascia. (Modified from Cabanas RM: An approach to the treatment of penile carcinoma. Cancer 39:456, 1977. Copyright © 1977 American Cancer Society. Reprinted by permission of Wiley-Liss, Inc., a subsidiary of John Wiley & Sons, Inc.)

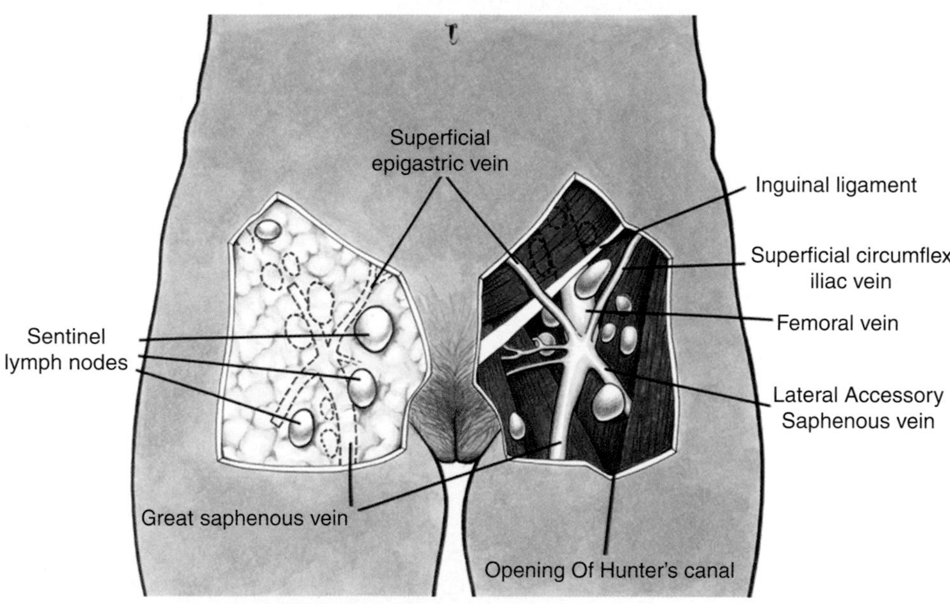

Figure 8–18 The right side demonstrates the two groups of lymph nodes making up the "sentinel" nodes. The left side notes the limits of the dissection with the cribriform fascia removed. The triangle that is dissected in a full inguinal lymphadenectomy is clearly identified on the patient's left side. The inguinal ligament forms the base of the triangle, and the opening of Hunter's canal becomes the apex. The triangle is bound laterally by the sartorius muscle and medially by the adductor muscles and fascia.

the cribriform fascia, which is most easily identified just below the inguinal ligament or in the area of the saphenous opening. The cribriform fascia unites with the fascia lata and thus is contiguous with the fascia on the surface of the adductor longus and sartorius muscles; this may facilitate its identification. The portion of the fascia covering the femoral triangle is perforated by the saphenous vein, by lymph nodes of the vertical set, and by numerous blood and lymphatic vessels, hence the name cribriform fascia. If the dissection is carried out properly, the adventitia of the femoral vessels should not be clearly seen except through the vessel openings mentioned earlier. As stated previously, Borgno and colleagues demonstrated that the deep inguinal or femoral nodes are exposed in the fossa ovalis and other openings of the cribriform fascia, allowing access to all inguinal nodes with this technique. The result is that a dissection that uses the boundaries described before and at the same time is carried out to the level of the cribriform fascia with optimal traction on the lymphovascular fat bundle of the inguinal area will produce a specimen that contains all of the inguinal and femoral nodes.

The excised nodes are immediately sent for frozen section analysis; the finding of positive nodes mandates a complete inguinal dissection. If there is no metastatic

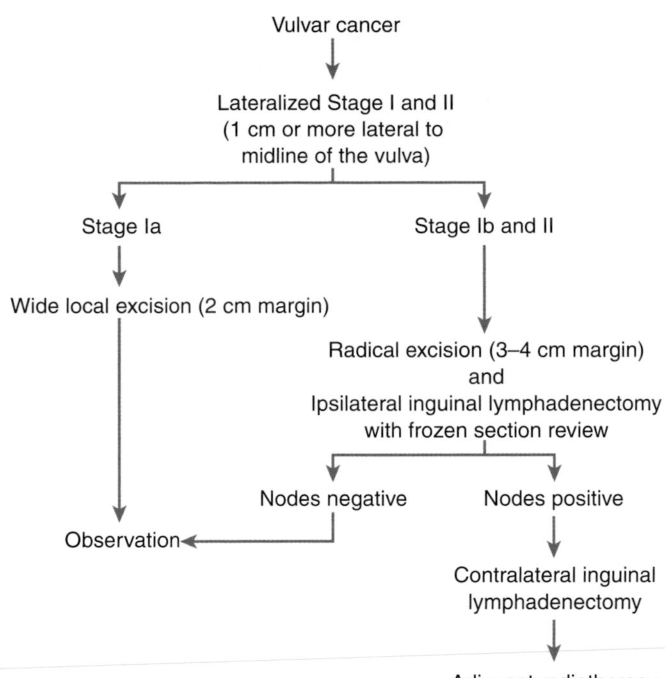

Figure 8–19 Algorithm for management of lateralized stage I or II vulvar cancer.

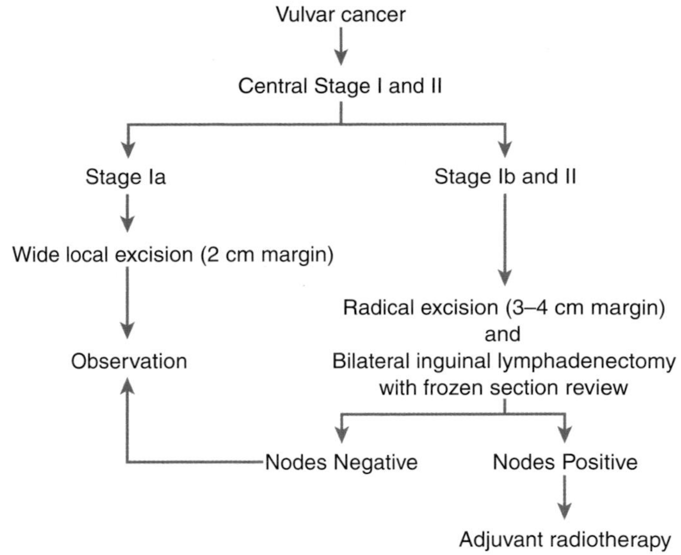

Figure 8–20 Algorithm for management of central stage I or II vulvar cancer.

disease, simple closure of the incision is done by use of a subcuticular PGA suture over two medium-sized suction drainage tubes.

A wide local excision of the vulvar skin is then performed, ensuring a margin of 2–3 cm of normal skin on all sides of the primary lesion. Adequate subcutaneous tissue should be taken down to the perineal fascia, especially beneath the primary lesion. It has been our practice to submit mucous membrane and skin margins as separate specimens.

After hemostasis is established, a decision must be made about primary closure of the defect vs intraposition of a split-thickness skin graft. When a split-thickness graft is used, the graft is usually taken from the medial aspect of the right thigh at 0.018 inch thickness. With an air-driven dermatome, this can be accomplished easily with minimal morbidity. The donor site is dressed, and an occlusive pressure dressing is applied. The skin graft is then sutured to the defect by 4–0 PGA suture and a pressure dressing applied in a manner previously described by Rutledge and Sinclair.

Berman and coworkers reported the latest series of 50 patients with use of this technique. Lesions up to 2 cm in diameter were accepted, whereas they were limited to 1 cm in the first report by DiSaia. Depth of invasion was, as in the first report, limited to 5 mm. Only 1 of 50 patients had lymph node metastases, and that patient died of her disease. Five local recurrences were noted in the other 49 patients, and these were successfully managed with re-excision of the vulvar lesion. The determination of the upper limits of size and depth of invasion acceptable for this approach is a judgment for the clinician, but we currently believe this approach should be restricted to stage I lesions with invasion of ≤5 mm.

The Mayo Clinic and Miami groups have compared radical vulvectomy and inguinal lymphadenectomy with more conservative surgical procedures. There was no difference in overall survival or development of recurrence even after adjusting for stage. Major morbidity was considerably higher in the radical group.

Stehman and colleagues reported the GOG experience with 121 patients with stage I disease and invasion <5 mm treated as described by DiSaia. There were 19 recurrences, and unlike in the reports of DiSaia and Berman, there were 5 groin only recurrences and 7 deaths. In our experience with >100 patients, there has not been any groin recurrence or death. Gordiner reported on the MD Anderson experience. They observed nine groin recurrences in 104 patients treated with superficial dissection. In these nine patients, the median number of nodes removed per groin was 7; but there were four groins with 0–2 nodes. In contrast, in Kirby's report, only an average of 2.7 nodes were retrieved per groin. The difference among all these reports is likely to be in the extent of the inguinal lymphadenectomy. Our practice is to remove all the nodes and fat in the area (shown in Fig. 8–8) down to the cribriform fascia, including nodes that are partially under the fascia appearing at the holes in that fascia. Algorithms presented in Figs. 8–19 to 8–21 are our suggestions for management.

PAGET'S DISEASE

Paget's disease of the vulva is rare. Even among vulvar neoplasias, it is an unusual finding. It occurs in women in the seventh decade of life but can be seen in young patients, just like squamous carcinoma of the vulva. Symptoms of pruritus and tenderness are most frequently seen, or a vulvar lesion is identified. These symptoms may be present for years before the patient seeks medical attention. The

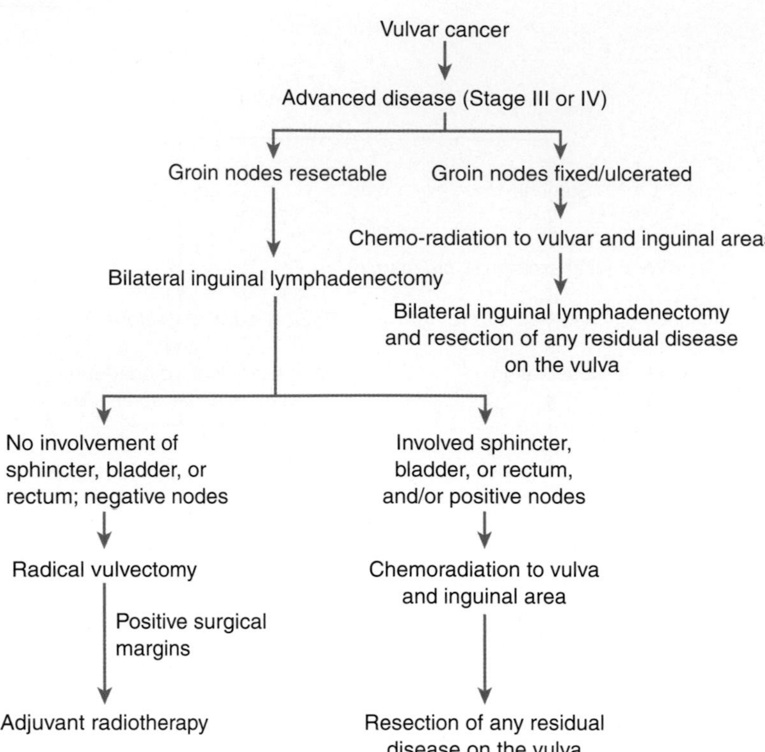

Figure 8–21 Algorithm for management of advanced (stage III or IV) vulvar cancer.

vulvar lesion may be localized to one labium or involve the entire vulvar epithelium. It is not unusual for the disease process to extend to the perirectal area, buttocks, inguinal area, or mons. Extension into the vagina has been reported.

Clinical and histologic features

On examination, the vulvar lesions are usually hyperemic, sharply demarcated, and thickened, with foci of excoriation and induration. The vulvar skin is often thick and smooth, leading to the impression of leukoplakia. It is not unusual for the hyperemic areas associated with a superficial white coating to give the impression of "cake-icing effect." This finding is classic and, if present, is almost pathognomonic for Paget's disease (Fig. 8–22). Typically, areas of leukoplakia are mixed with patches of redness where excoriation has occurred because of intense pruritus. On palpation, the vulvar changes appear to be superficial. This maneuver is extremely important, for one must rule out an underlying adenocarcinoma, which is usually evident because of thickness or a mass-like effect under the epithelial changes. It is unusual not to appreciate an underlying adenocarcinoma clinically; however, one must take adequate biopsy specimens of the lesion, relative to width as well as depth of tissue, to enable adequate histologic evaluation. Fine-needle aspiration biopsy to evaluate subcutaneous masses of the vulva, as well as other sites, should be encouraged as a rapid diagnostic technique. This procedure is associated with low morbidity and allows greater planning before major surgery is undertaken. It is our practice to perform a needle aspiration of any thickness or mass that is palpated beneath the skin involved with Paget's disease. Historically, it appears that there are two separate lesions: intraepithelial extramammary Paget's disease and pagetoid changes within the skin associated with an underlying adenocarcinoma. Today, four histologic forms of vulvar Paget's disease are recognized. Between the intraepithelial lesion in which the basement membrane is intact with Paget cells confined to the epidermis and Paget's disease with an underlying apocrine gland adenocarcinoma are two intermediate forms. Minimally invasive Paget's disease is that in which the Paget cells have broken through the basement membrane into the underlying dermis to <1 mm. Invasive vulvar Paget's disease is a lesion in which the Paget cells break through the basement membrane into the underlying dermis >1 mm. Therapy for these two lesions is considerably different, and a definitive diagnosis is therefore imperative.

A thickened, often acanthotic epidermis is the typical histologic finding. Characteristic large cells with clear granular cytoplasm are found within the epidermis (Fig. 8–23). A single layer of squamous cells often separates the Paget cells from the epidermis, but neoplastic cells may be in immediate contact with the dermis. Intraepidermal formation of glands with true lumens may also be present. The hair follicles may also be involved with Paget cells. These cells contain intracytoplasmic mucin demonstrated by Mayer's mucicarmine or alcian blue. A mixed inflammatory infiltrate of variable intensity composed usually of lymphocytes and plasma cells is present in the upper dermis. Misdiagnosis of carcinoma in situ or melanoma has been made; however, adequate tissue for evaluation and a proper clinical description tend to eliminate this confusion. Sufficient tissue for histologic evaluation will readily identify an underlying adenocarcinoma.

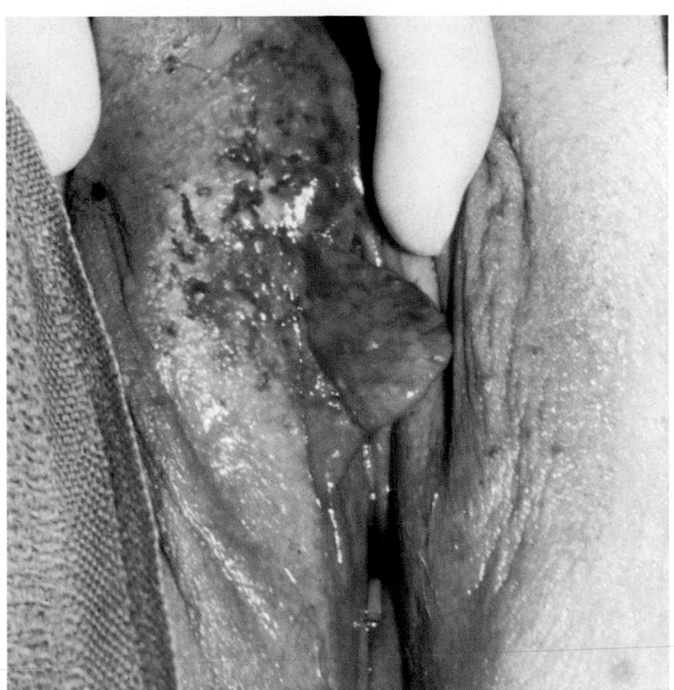

Figure 8–22 Paget's disease of the vulva involving the lower half of the left labium major and labium minor. The white medial portion is characteristic of "cake-icing effect." The red medial aspect is also commonly seen and called "violaceous coloring."

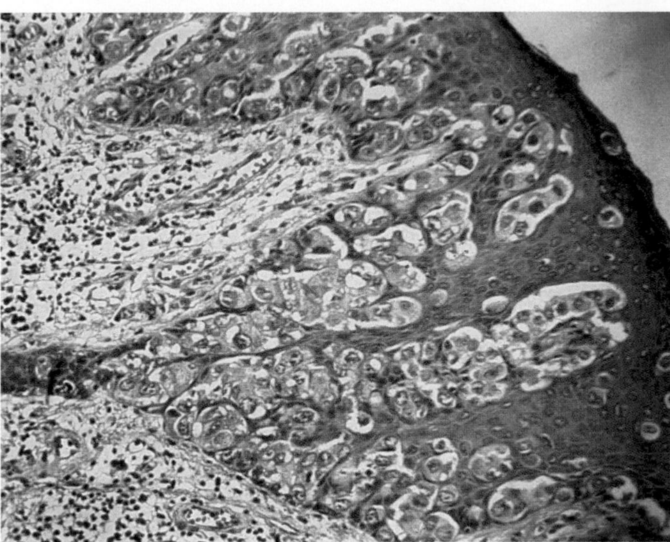

Figure 8–23 Histologic picture of Paget's disease of the vulva. Large cells with clear cytoplasm are apparent in the epidermis. Note the heavy lymphocytic infiltration in the dermis.

Clinical course and management

If only intraepithelial Paget's disease is present, the clinical course may be prolonged and indolent. In a patient with an original diagnosis of only intraepithelial Paget's disease, there can be recurrence, but it is usually seen as an intraepithelial lesion only, without an underlying adenocarcinoma. From a review of our material and the literature, we believe that when extramammary Paget's disease with an underlying adenocarcinoma is present, it is the result of simultaneous diagnoses or, more likely, a secondary infiltration of the vulvar skin by cells from a primary adenocarcinoma of underlying apocrine glands. It appears that we are dealing with two separate diseases and not a spectrum. The exclusively intraepithelial disease presentation, by far the more common one seen by the clinician, remains a local phenomenon even with recurrences. Paget's disease with an underlying adenocarcinoma can be aggressive, with metastasis to the regional lymph nodes as well as distant spread.

The literature has been confusing with regard to the association of invasive carcinoma and concomitant intraepithelial Paget's disease. Invasive underlying adenocarcinomas have been reported in up to 20% of patients with histologically confirmed pagetoid cells in the vulvar skin. Our experience suggests a much lower incidence. Similarly, older studies suggest that up to 25% of patients have a concomitant carcinoma at another site, such as the breast, colon, anus, or cervix. Here, too, our experience has not been in agreement, with only a rare patient having a simultaneous lesion. In a review of 100 cases from eight institutions, Fanning and colleagues noted 12 patients with invasive vulvar Paget's disease. A review of the literature noted an underlying adenocarcinoma in 8% and 10% with invasive Paget's disease; 20 patients had a total of 26 non-vulvar malignant neoplasms. It was thought by the authors that the non-vulvar cancers were probably related to the older age of the patients and not necessarily related to Paget's disease.

Because Paget's disease without an underlying adenocarcinoma appears to be a true intraepithelial neoplasia, it can be treated as such. Wide local excision to include the entire lesion is usually sufficient. Even with apparently wide margins, it is not unusual to find Paget's disease extending to the edge of the surgical margin. On histologic examination, one may find neoplastic cells in normal-appearing skin for a variable but often considerable distance beyond the seemingly sharp margin of the clinically evident lesion. It is difficult to avoid cutting across intraepithelial tumor, and therefore intraoperative examination of the surgical margins by cryostat frozen sectioning is imperative (Fig. 8–24). It is our custom to incise the periphery of the operative specimen and immediately send identifiable strips of surgical margin for cryostat frozen sectioning. If the presence of tumor cells is reported, additional margins can then be excised. Recurrences are common when the surgical margins contain neoplastic cells. In the Fanning study, there were 31 of 84 recurrences in those patients with intraepithelial disease. Both radical vulvectomy and hemivulvectomy as well as wide excision were used as treatment. Recurrence was similar with all three treatments. Unfortunately, surgical margins could not be determined in this retrospective review. Recurrences are also not unusual with negative margins, leading some surgeons to abandon the use of frozen

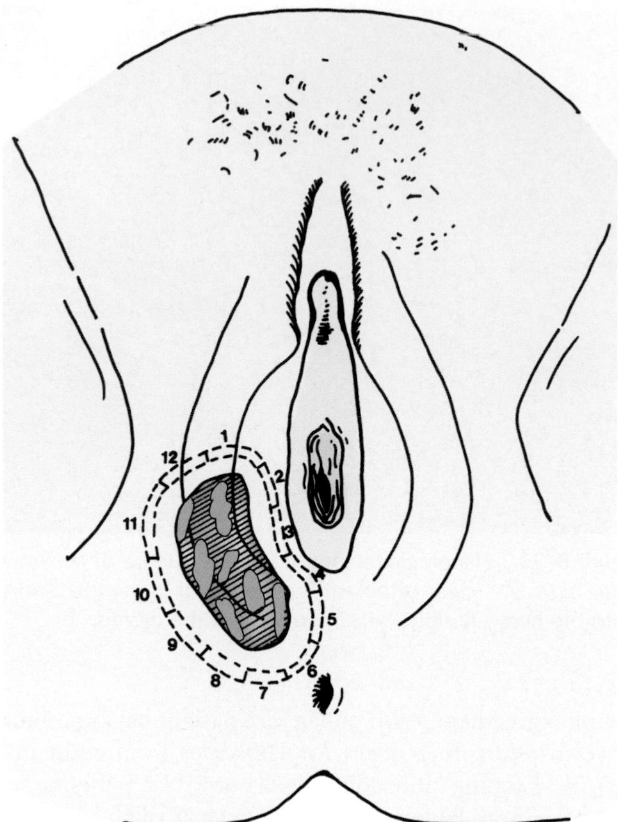

Figure 8–24 Diagram of the vulva with an area of Paget's disease involving the right labium majus. The two parallel lines lateral to the lesion represent the surgical margin sent intraoperatively for frozen section analysis. The margin is serially cut in a clockwise fashion, labeled, and analyzed. If any segment of the margin reveals Paget's disease, the resection is extended in that direction. (From Bergen S et al: Conservative management of extramammary Paget's disease of the vulva. Gynecol Oncol 33:151, 1989.)

section surgical margins. These new lesions can be handled in the same manner as the primary disease, that is, by wide local excision. Our studies show that removal of full-thickness skin plus a microscopic amount of subcutaneous fat routinely results in an operative specimen that is 6 mm thick (Fig. 8–25). Because the base of the hair follicles in vulvar skin is at a depth of 4 mm, one need not be concerned about the possibility of leaving neoplastic cells that may have involved hair shafts. Lesions can be extensive in the primary and recurrent stages, and treatment should be given accordingly. A skin graft to cover the removed tissue may be warranted and should be used freely. DiSaia described two patients who developed recurrent Paget's disease in the middle of a split-thickness skin graft. A process labeled retrodissemination was given as an explanation for this curious phenomenon whereby pagetoid cells from peripheral occult sites of persistent disease are postulated to metastasize back into a skin graft site.

Besa and coworkers reported good results when radiotherapy was used in conjunction with surgery or for patients for whom surgery was not possible. A dose of 50–55 Gy appeared to be adequate. Voigt and colleagues reported a dramatic response of extramammary Paget's carcinoma in a man with chemotherapy using carboplatin and 5-fluorouracil with folinic acid, suggesting another possible approach when surgery is not appropriate.

Patients in whom an underlying adenocarcinoma is identified in association with Paget's disease of the vulva should be treated in the same manner as patients with other invasive malignant neoplasms of the vulva. This usually includes radical vulvectomy and inguinal lymphadenectomy. If the lymph nodes have no evidence of metastatic disease, the prognosis is good; however, if metastases are present in the lymph nodes, the prognosis is guarded. Two of the four patients with an underlying adenocarcinoma had lymph node metastasis (Fanning and colleagues); one died of the disease. No statement concerning the role of radiation therapy and chemotherapy in this disease can be made because the experience has been limited and inconclusive.

MELANOMA

Melanoma of the vulva, although it is the second most common invasive cancer occurring in this area, is still rare. In a nationwide study of 198 women from Sweden, vulvar melanoma was over-represented by 2.5 times compared with cutaneous melanoma. This malignant neoplasm probably arises from a lesion containing a junctional or a compound nevus. As a result, it is suggested by some authorities that all pigmented nevi on the vulva be prophylactically excised. Table 8–13 defines the high-risk group and describes the characteristics of pigmented lesions of the vulva or any skin that determine the need for excisional biopsy.

The clinical characteristics are as elsewhere on the body; melanomas are usually pigmented and raised, and they may be ulcerated (Fig. 8–26). The median age of patients with these lesions is 65 years in a series reported by Tasseron and coworkers. In a large NCDB study of melanoma of the vulva, age ranged from 7 to 97 years with a median of 66 years; in this study, 50% were 70 years old or older, and macroscopic amelanotic tumors were present in 27% of patients. Melanomas are often misdiagnosed as undifferentiated squamous cell cancers, especially when they are histologically amelanotic. Electron microscopy can be helpful when the diagnosis continues to be in doubt. The patient may have experienced pruritus, bleeding, or enlargement of a pigmented area. Most vulvar melanomas are on the labia minora or clitoris. In the Swedish study, the clitoral area and labia majora were the most common primary sites. Of all melanomas, 46% of lesions were in glabrous (non-hairy) skin, 12% in hairy skin, and 35% in both areas. Prognosis is related to the size of the lesion and the depth of invasion. The Clark classification, commonly used for melanomas elsewhere on the skin, is of prognostic benefit for the vulva also. The Clark classification, which uses histologic levels, is outlined in Table 8–14. In 1970, Breslow recognized that survival was relative to the greatest

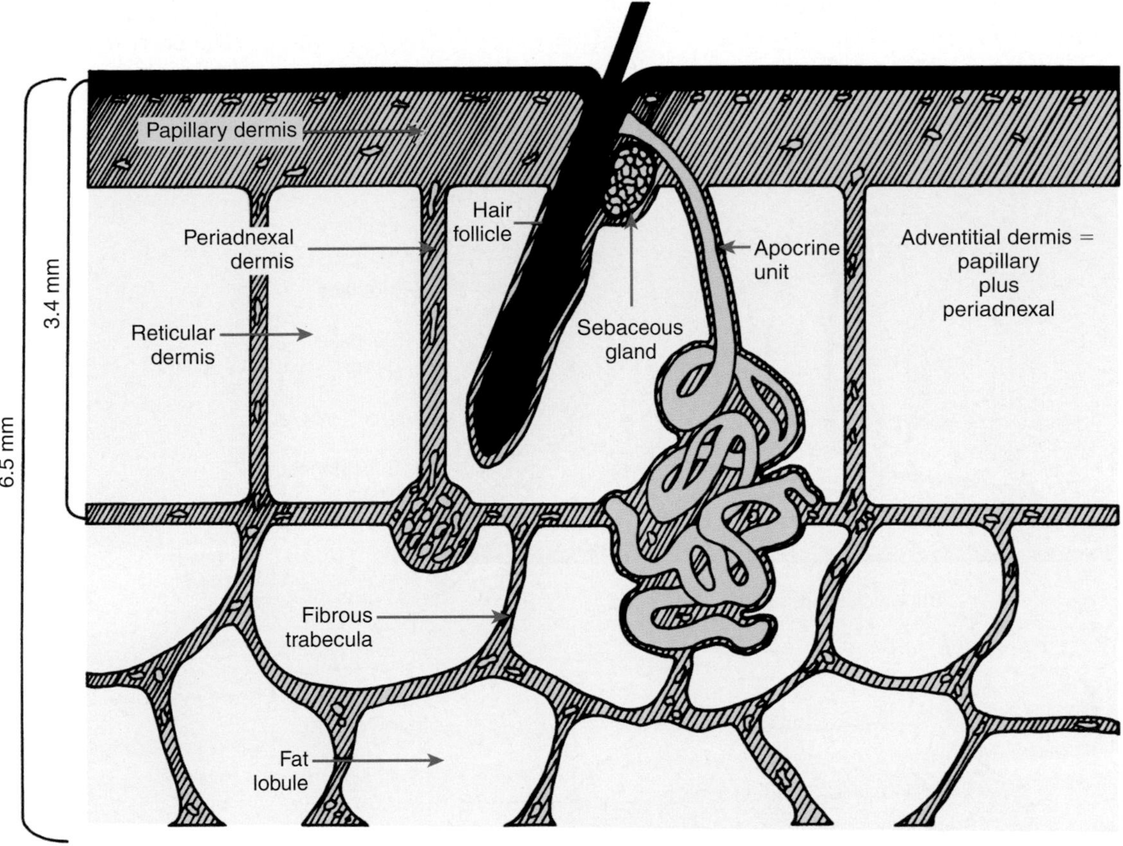

Figure 8–25 Schematic of vulvar skin anatomy showing the extension of skin appendages into the subdermal adipose tissue. (From Bergen S et al: Conservative management of extramammary Paget's disease of the vulva. Gynecol Oncol 33:151, 1989.)

Table 8–13 HIGH-RISK GROUP FOR DEVELOPMENT OF MELANOMA

Individuals at risk for development of melanoma are those who have one or more of the following:
A family history of melanoma in blood relatives
Poor or no tanning ability, often with a history of sunburn in adolescence
Unusual moles with any of the following characteristics:
Dark (blue-black) look
Speckled or splotchy color pattern
Jagged or fuzzy border
Recent change in size, shape, or color of a mole
Any mole larger than a dime

Table 8–14 CLARK'S STAGING CLASSIFICATION BY LEVELS

Level	Definition
I	In situ melanoma: all demonstrable tumor is above the basement membrane in the epidermis
II	Melanoma extends through the basement membrane into the papillary dermis
III	The tumor fills the papillary dermis and extends to the reticular dermis but does not invade it
IV	The tumor extends into the reticular dermis
V	The tumor extends into the subcutaneous fat

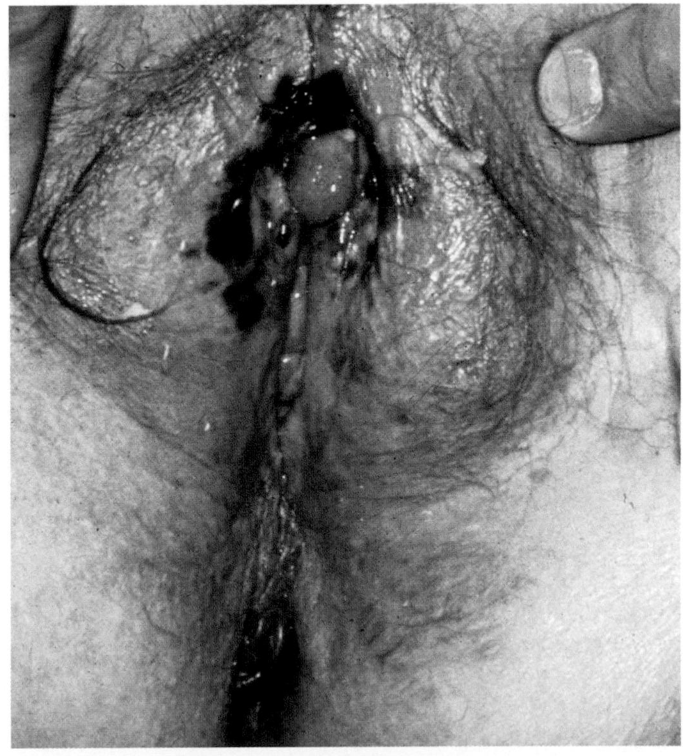

Figure 8–26 Melanoma of the vulva. A typical pigmented neoplasm is present.

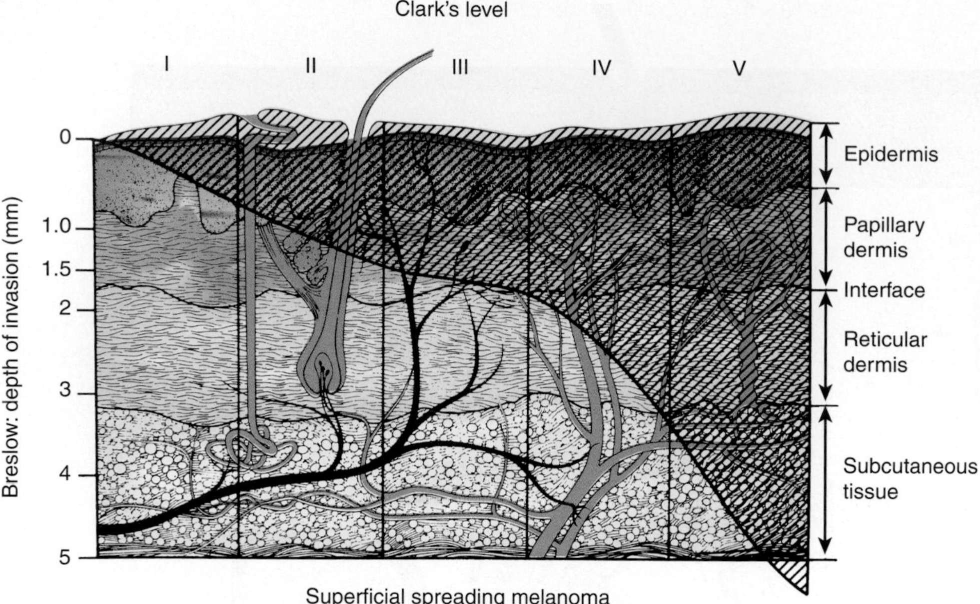

Figure 8–27 Comparison of Clark and Breslow classifications for skin melanomas.

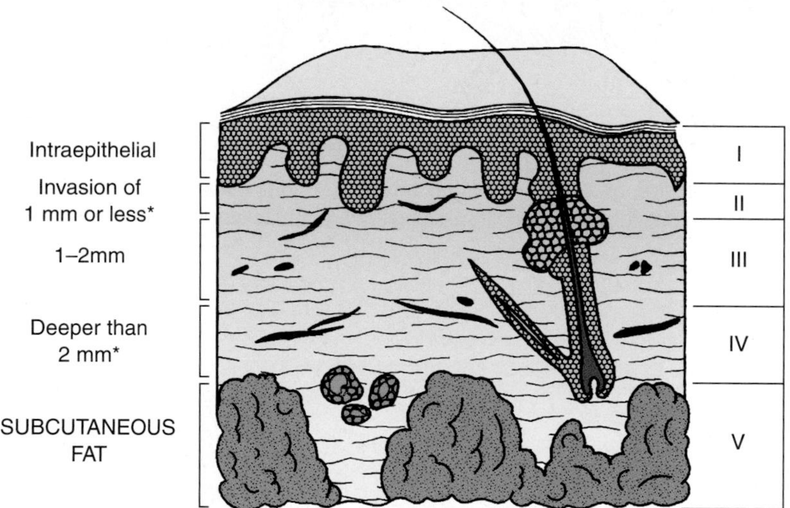

Figure 8–28 Chung system of reporting melanoma involvement.

thickness of the invasive portion of the melanoma by micrometer measure (Fig. 8–27). The Breslow technique appeals to many because of its simplicity. Evidence exists that these lesions can metastasize to deep nodes in the absence of inguinal node involvement, although this has not been our experience. In 1975, Chung and associates described a third system of reporting level of involvement of vulvar melanoma (Fig. 8–28).

Although it has been suggested that all patients with melanoma of the vulva be treated with radical vulvectomy and inguinal and pelvic lymphadenectomy, there has been a tendency of late to be more conservative. In the 596 patients described by the NCDB, surgery was used in >90% of patients with stage 0 to stage III. Local excision was used mainly in early stage (stage 0 and stage I) disease. Lymph node evaluation was performed in >50% of the patients, with greater frequency for patients with advanced disease. Radical local excision with a margin of 2 cm for thin lesions (up to 7 mm) and 3–4 cm for thicker lesions appears to be adequate for most well circumscribed lesions. Because prognosis is directly related to depth of invasion, therapy can be tailored accordingly. If the disease is intraepithelial, cure should be close to 100%. Even with level I or level II melanoma (Clark classification), a wide local excision may be adequate treatment. As the melanoma extends deeper, the chance of lymph node metastasis increases, and the prognosis decreases considerably. Podratz and colleagues reported that 10-year survival rates associated with Clark's level II, III, IV, and V tumors were 100%, 83%, 65%, and 23%, respectively. Histologic growth patterns also influence survival: 5-year survival rates for superficial spreading and nodular melanomas were 71% and 38%, respectively; 10-year survival rates were 66% and 25%, respectively. In the 323 patients described by the NCDB who had a Clark level determination, 157 had lymph nodes evaluated. Most were in level II to level V,

Table 8–15 LYMPH NODE METASTASIS AND CLARK'S LEVEL OF VULVAR MELANOMA

Clark's level	Nodes examined	Positive nodes
I (n = 38)	3 (8%)	0 (44%)
II (n = 80)	30 (60%)	3 (10%)
III (n = 70)	38 (54%)	6 (16%)
IV (n = 90)	55 (61%)	13 (23%)
V (n = 45)	31 (69%)	9 (29%)

Modified from Creasman WT, Phillips JL, Mench HR: A survey of hospital management practice for vulvar melanoma. J Am Coll Surg 188:670, 1999.

TABLE 8–16 CORRELATION OF MELANOMA THICKNESS WITH SURVIVAL OF PATIENTS

Thickness	Eight-year survival rates
< 0.85 mm	100%
0.85–1.5 mm	99%
1.5–4 mm	66%
> 4 mm	25% to 35%

From Jaramillo BA et al: Malignant melanoma of the vulva. Obstet Gynecol 66:398, 1985; and Day CL et al: The natural break points for primary tumor thickness in clinical stage I melanoma. N Engl J Med 305:1155, 1981.

and as expected, metastasis increased as level of invasion increased (Table 8–15). In the patients with negative nodes, survival of level I to level IV was 88%, 77%, 88%, and 85%, respectively. Interestingly, four of seven patients with positive nodes survived. Using the Breslow method, Jaramillo and coworkers as well as Day and coworkers reported nearly 100% survival in patients with lesions <1.5 mm in thickness, 65–70% survival in patients with lesions 1.5–4 mm, and 25–35% survival in patients with lesions > 4 mm (Table 8–16). Trimble and colleagues described 80 patients treated at Memorial Sloan–Kettering Cancer Center with a median follow-up of 193 months. By Chung level, 10-year survival for each grade was as follows:

I	100%
II	81%
III	87%
IV	11%
V	33%.

Verschraegen et al updated the experience from the M.D. Anderson hospital from 1970–1997. Thirty-two of 51 patients ultimately suffered a recurrence of their melanoma. Both Clark's and Breslow's assessments were predictive. The type of operation performed did not have an impact on recurrence. The role of lymphadenectomy in this disease is probably more prognostic than therapeutic. If disease is limited to the vulva, regardless of its extent, and the lymph nodes are negative, the survival rate is good. It is rare for a patient with positive inguinal nodes to have a long-term survival rate; most patients with positive pelvic nodes eventually succumb to the disease.

SARCOMA

Sarcoma of the vulva is rare, and the experience is limited even in large referral institutions. Symptoms and findings are the same as those noted with squamous cell carcinoma. DiSaia and colleagues, in a review of 12 patients, noted that this lesion occurred in a younger group of patients (mean age 38 years) than did other vulvar malignant neoplasms. The histologic grade of the sarcoma appears to be the most important factor in prognosis. If a patient has an undifferentiated rhabdomyosarcoma, prognosis is poor because these lesions tend to grow and metastasize rapidly. However, a well-differentiated leiomyosarcoma will grow slowly and develop late recurrences. Therapy would generally be radical vulvectomy and bilateral inguinal lymphadenectomy except in the low-grade lesions, in which node involvement is rare and wide local excision should be considered. Patients undergoing wide local excision are at risk for local recurrence and should be observed closely.

BARTHOLIN GLAND CARCINOMA

Adenocarcinoma of the Bartholin gland is a rare lesion occurring in only about 1% of all vulvar malignant neoplasms (Fig. 8–29). The peak incidence is in women in their mid-60s, although it has been reported in a teenager. Because of its location, the tumor can be of considerable size before the patient is aware of symptoms. Dyspareunia may be one of the first symptoms, although the finding of a mass or ulcerative lesion may be the first indication to the patient of her disease. An enlargement in the Bartholin gland area in a postmenopausal woman should be considered a malignant neoplasm until proven otherwise. The lesion can have a tendency to spread into the ischiorectal fossa and can have a propensity for lymphatic spread to the inguinal nodes by the common lymphatic spread pattern for vulvar cancer and for posterior spread to the pelvic nodes directly. Almost half of all carcinomas said to be of Bartholin gland origin are squamous cell carcinomas. In

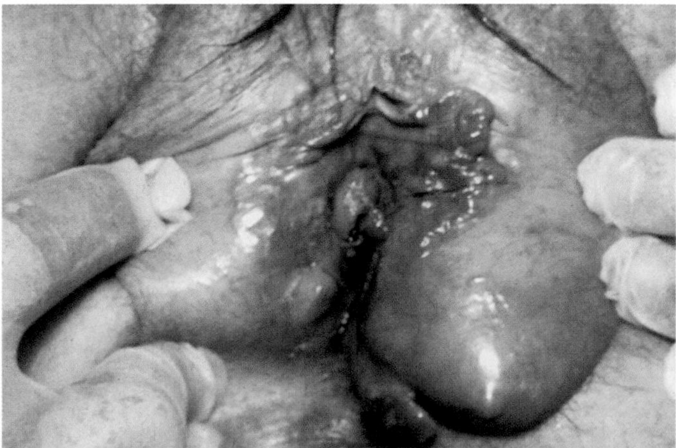

Figure 8–29 Adenocarcinoma of Bartholin's gland with local skin metastasis.

most instances, strict histologic criteria have not been followed. Every attempt should be made to differentiate between a true Bartholin gland cancer and a squamous cell carcinoma of the vulva arising in proximity to the Bartholin gland. Prognosis is good if lymph node metastasis is not present.

Therapy includes radical vulvectomy with a large, wide, extensive dissection around the gland and inguinal lymphadenectomy. To have adequate margins, there may be a need to remove a considerable amount of vagina and, on occasion, part of the rectum. It appears that pelvic lymphadenectomy is not indicated unless the inguinal nodes are involved. A more conservative approach in selected patients with early disease may be appropriate. The largest series is that reported by Copeland and associates of 36 patients whose 5-year survival was 84%. Distribution of the tumors in FIGO stages included 9 stage I, 15 stage II, 10 stage III, and 2 stage IV. Cell types were squamous, 27; adenomatous, 6; adenoid cystic, 2; and adenosquamous, 1. Of 30 patients with lymph node dissections, 14 (47%) had nodal metastasis, and 11 remain free of disease. Disease recurred in nine patients (six local recurrences, two distant, one local and distant), and four were treated successfully. Less impressive results were reported by Wheelock and coworkers in a series of 10 patients.

Adenoid cystic carcinoma of the Bartholin gland is a rare entity manifested by frequent local recurrences and slowly progressive disease, including pulmonary metastasis, sometimes many years after initial therapy. Recommended primary treatment is wide local excision, obtaining clear margins, and an ipsilateral inguinal lymphadenectomy followed by careful monitoring. Recurrences are best treated by surgery.

BASAL CELL CARCINOMA

Basal cell carcinoma is usually small, occurs on the labia majora, and may have a central ulceration (Fig. 8–30). The stromal infiltration is usually circumscribed and orderly and, as elsewhere on the body, has a slow and indolent growth rate; it rarely if ever involves the lymphatics. Metastatic basal cell carcinoma of the vulva has been reported as a rare occurrence. Of 28 patients presented by Benedet and colleagues, only 1 died of disease; 10 did have basal cell carcinomas elsewhere on the body, and 10 had 11 other malignant neoplasms diagnosed.

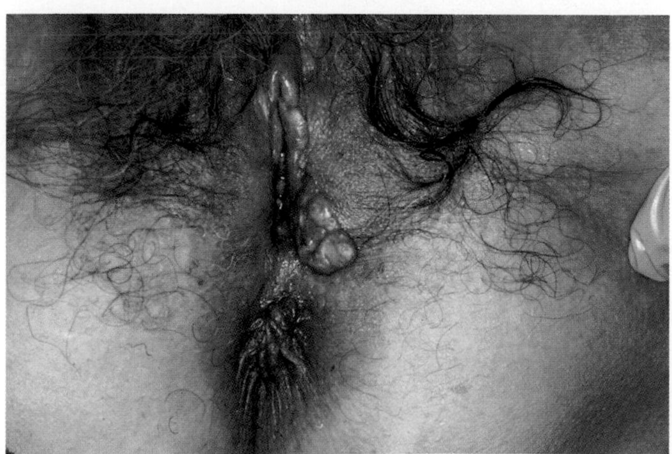

Figure 8–30 Basal cell carcinoma.

For the most part, these lesions behave like they do elsewhere on the body, with local invasion being the rule. A typical lesion has a rolled, pearly border showing fine telangiectatic vessels on the surface and a central ulceration. The patient complains that the lesion itches slightly, bleeds a little, and then seems to heal. The process repeats itself as the lesion slowly increases in size. Local excision is adequate, and primary closure is the usual rule. If a large lesion is present after local excision, a skin graft may be applied. Basal cell carcinoma must be differentiated pathologically from the so-called basosquamous cell carcinoma, which must be treated as one would treat a squamous cell carcinoma of the vulva.

BIBLIOGRAPHY

INVASIVE SQUAMOUS CELL CARCINOMA

Al-Ghamdi A, Freedman D, Miller D, Poh C, Rosin M, Zhang L, Gilks B. Vulvar squamous cell carcinoma in young women: a clinicopathologic study of 21 cases. Gynecol Oncol 84:94–101, 2002.

Andersen WA et al: Vulvar squamous cell carcinoma and papillomaviruses: Two separate entities? Am J Obstet Gynecol 165:329, 1991.

Andreasson B, Nyboe J: Value of prognostic parameters in squamous cell carcinoma of the vulva. Gynecol Oncol 22:341, 1985.

Andrews SJ et al: Therapeutic implications of lymph nodal spread in lateral T1 and T2 squamous cell carcinoma of the vulva. Gynecol Oncol 55:41, 1994.

Bell JG, Lea JS, Reid GC. Complete groin lymphadenectomy with preservation of the fascia lata in the treatment of vulvar carcinoma. Gynecol Oncol 77:314–318, 2000.

Borgno G, Micheletti L, Barbero M: Topographic distribution of groin lymph nodes: A study of 50 female cadavers. J Reprod Med 35:1127, 1990.

Boronow RC, Hickman BT, Reagan MT et al: Combined therapy as an alternative to exenteration for locally advanced vulvovaginal cancer. II: Results, complications and dosimetric and surgical considerations. Am J Clin Oncol 10:171, 1987.

Boronow RC: Therapeutic alternative to primary exenteration for advanced vulvo-vaginal cancer. Gynecol Oncol 1:233, 1973.

Boyce J et al: Prognostic factors in carcinoma of the vulva. Gynecol Oncol 20:364, 1985.

Bryson SCP, Dembo AJ, Colgan TJ et al: Invasive squamous cell carcinoma of the vulva: Defining low and high-risk groups for recurrence. Int J Gynecol Cancer 1:25, 1991.

Carson LF, Twiggs LB, Okagaki T et al: Human papillomavirus DNA in adenosquamous carcinoma and squamous cell carcinoma of the vulva. Obstet Gynecol 72:63, 1988.

Cavanagh D, Fiorica JV, Hoffman MS et al: Invasive carcinoma of the vulva: Changing trends in surgical management. Am J Obstet Gynecol 163:1007, 1990.

Cavanagh D, Shepherd JH: The place of pelvic exenteration in the primary management of advanced carcinoma of the vulva. Gynecol Oncol 13:318, 1982.

Creasman WT, Phillips JL, Mench HR: The National Cancer Data Base report on early stage invasive vulvar carcinoma. Cancer 80:505, 1997.

Crosby JH, Bryan AB, Gallup DG et al: Fine-needle aspiration of inguinal lymph nodes in gynecologic practice. Obstet Gynecol 73:281, 1989.

Curry SL, Wharton JT, Rutledge F: Positive lymph nodes in the vulvar squamous carcinoma. Gynecol Oncol 9:63, 1980.

Daly JW, Million RR: Radical vulvectomy combined with elective node irradiation for T^2N^0 squamous carcinoma of the vulva. Cancer 34:161, 1974.

de Hullu JA, Hollema H, Lolkema S, Boezen M, Boonstra H, Burger MP, Aalders JG, Mourtis MJ, van der Zee AG. Vulvar carcinoma. The price of less radical surgery. Cancer 2002, 95:2331–2338.

de Hullu JA, Hollema H, Piers DA. Verheijen RHM, van Diest PJ, Mourits MJE, Aalders JG, van der Zee AGJ. Sentinel node procedure is highly accurate in squamous cell carcinoma of the vulva. J Clin Oncol 18:2811–2816, 2000.

de Hullu JA, Oonk MHM, Ansink AC, Hollema H, Jager PL, van der Zee AGJ. Pitfalls in the sentinel lymph node procedure in vulvar cancer. Gynecol Oncol 94:10–15, 2004.

DeCicco C, Sideri M, Bartolomei M, Grana C, Cremonesi M, Fiorenza M, Maggioni A, Bocciolone L, Maggioni C, Colombo N, Paganelli G. Sentinel node biopsy in early vulvar cancer. Br J Cancer 82:295–299, 2000.

Deppe G, Cohen CJ, Bruckner HW: Chemotherapy of squamous cell carcinoma of the vulva: A review. Gynecol Oncol 7:345, 1979.

Donaldson ES et al: Prognostic parameters in invasive vulvar cancer. Gynecol Oncol 11:184, 1981.

Ericksson E, Eldh J, Peterson LE: Surgical treatment of carcinoma of the clitoris. Gynecol Oncol 17:291, 1984.

Fairey RN et al: Radiation treatment of carcinoma of the vulva, 1950 to 1980. Am J Obstet Gynecol 151:591, 1985.

Franklin EW III, Rutledge FN: Epidemiology of epidermoid carcinoma of the vulva. Obstet Gynecol 39:165, 1972.

Franklin EW III, Rutledge FN: Prognostic factors in epidermoid carcinoma of the vulva. Obstet Gynecol 37:892, 1971.

Frumovitz M, Ramirez PT, Tortolero-Luna G, Malpica A, Eifel P, Burke TW, Levenback C. Characteristics of recurrence in patients who underwent lymphatic mapping for vulvar cancer. Gynecol Oncol 92:205–210, 2004.

Gaarenstroom KN, Kenter GG, Trimbos JB, Agous I, Amant F, Peters AAW, Vergote I. Postoperative complications after vulvectomy and inguinofemoral lymphadenectomy using separate incisions. Int J Gynecol Cancer 13:522–527, 2003.

Goncalver JCA: Cryovulvectomy for advanced and inoperable cancer. J Reprod Med 43:610, 1998.

Gonzalez-Bosquet JG, Magrina JF, Gaffey TA, Hernandez JL, Webb MJ, Cliby WA, Podratz KC. Long-term survival and disease recurrence in patients with primary squamous cell carcinoma of the vulva. Gynecol Oncol 97:828–833, 2005.

Gould N, Kamelle S, Tillmans T, Scribner D, Gold M, Walker J, Mannel R. Predictors of complications after inguinal lymphadenectomy. Gynecol Oncol 82:329–332, 2001.

Green TH: Carcinoma of the vulva: A reassessment. Obstet Gynecol 52:462, 1978.

Hacker NF et al: Management of regional lymph nodes and their prognostic influence in vulvar cancer. Obstet Gynecol 61:408, 1983.

Hacker NF et al: Preoperative radiation therapy for locally advanced vulvar cancer. Cancer 54:2056, 1984.

Heaps JM, Fu YS, Montz FJ, Hacker NF, Berek JSl. Surgical-pathologic variables predictive of local recurrence in squamous cell carcinoma of the vulva. Gynecol Oncol 38:309–314,1990.

Hoffman MS, Roberts WS, La Polla JP et al: Carcinoma of the vulva involving the perianal or anal skin. Gynecol Oncol 35:215, 1989.

Hoffman MS, Roberts WS, La Polla JP et al: Recent modifications in the treatment of invasive squamous cell carcinoma of the vulva. Obstet Gynecol Surv 44:227, 1989.

Homesley HD et al: Prognostic factors for groin node metastasis in squamous cell carcinoma of the vulva (a Gynecologic Oncology Group study). Gynecol Oncol 49:279, 1993.

Homesley HD et al: Radiation therapy versus pelvic node resection for carcinoma of the vulva with positive groin nodes. Obstet Gynecol 68:733, 1986.

Homesley HD, Bundy BN, Sedlis A et al: Assessment of current International Federation of Gynecology and Obstetrics staging of vulvar carcinoma relative to prognostic factors for survival (a Gynecologic Oncology Group study). Am J Obstet Gynecol 164:997, 1991.

Homesley HD: Lymph node findings and outcome in squamous cell carcinoma of the vulva. Cancer 74:2399, 1994.

Hopkins MP, Morley GW: Pelvic exenteration for the treatment of vulvar cancer. Cancer 70:2835, 1992.

Hopkins MP, Reid GC, Morley GW: The surgical management of recurrent squamous cell carcinoma of the vulva. Obstet Gynecol 75:1001, 1990.

Hudson CN, Shulver H, Lowe DC. The surgery of inguino-femoral lymph nodes: is it adequate or excessive? Int J Gynecol Cancer 14:841–845, 2004.

Isaacs JH: Verrucous carcinoma of the female genital tract. Gynecol Oncol 4:259, 1976.

Iversen T, Aberler V, Aalders J: Individualized treatment of stage I carcinoma of the vulva. Obstet Gynecol 57:85, 1981.

Iversen T: Squamous cell carcinoma of the primary tumor and lymph node metastases. Acta Obstet Gynecol Scand 60:211, 1981.

Japaze H, Dinh TV, Woodruff JD: Verrucous carcinoma of the vulva: Study of 24 cases. Obstet Gynecol 60:462, 1982.

Judson PL, Jonson AL, Paley PJ, Bliss RL, Murray KP, Downs LS, Boente MP, Argenta PA, Carson LF. A prospective randomized study analyzing sartorius transposition following inguinal-femoral lymphadenectomy. Gynecol Oncol 95:226–230, 2004.

Katz A, Eifel PJ, Jhingran A, Levenback CF. The role of radiation therapy in preventing regional recurrences of invasive squamous cell carcinoma of the vulva. Int J Radiat Oncol Biol Phys, 57:409–418, 2003.

Kurzl R, Messerer D, Baltzer J et al: Comparative morphometric study on the depth of invasion in vulvar carcinoma. Gynecol Oncol 29:12, 1988.

Lawhead RA Jr: Vulvar self-examination. Am J Obstet Gynecol 158:4, 1988.

Levenback C, Coleman RL, Burke TW, Bodurka-Bevers D, Wolf JK, Gershenson DM. Intraoperative lymphatic mapping and sentinel node identification with blue dye in patients with vulvar cancer. Gynecol Oncol 83:276–281, 2001.

Louis-Sylvestre C, Evangelista E, Leonard F, Itti E, Meignan M, Paniel BJ. Sentinel node localzation should be interpreted with caution in midline vulvar cancer. Gynecol Oncol 97:151–154, 2005.

Maggino T, Landoni F, Sartori E, Zola P, Gadducci A, Alessi C, Solda M, Coscio S, Spinetti G, Maneo A, Ferrero A, Konishi D, Toffoli G. Patterns of recurrnence in patients with squamous cell carcinoma of the vulva. A multicenter CTF study. Cancer 89:116–122, 2000.

Magrina JF et al: Stage I squamous cell cancer of the vulva. Am J Obstet Gynecol 134:453, 1979.

Magrina JF, Gonzalez-Bosquet J, Weaver AL et al: Primary squamous cell cancer of the vulva: Radical versus modified radical vulvar surgery. Gynecol Oncol 71:116, 1998.

Malfetano J, Piver MS, Tsukada Y: Stage III and IV squamous cell carcinoma of the vulva. Gynecol Oncol 23:192, 1986.

Malmström H, Janson H, Simonsen E et al: Prognostic factors in invasive squamous cell carcinoma of the vulva treated with surgery and irradiation. Acta Oncol 29:915, 1990.

Micheletti L, Levi AC, Bogliatto F. Anatomosurgical implications derived from an embryological study of the scarpa's triangle with particular reference to groin lymphadenectomy Gynecol Oncol 70:358–364, 1998.

Montana GS, Thomas GM, Moore DH, Saxer A, Mangan CE, Lentz S, Averette HE. Preoperative chemo–radiation for carcinoma of the vulva with N2/N3 nodes: a Gynecology Oncology Group study. Int J Radiat Oncol Biol Phys 48:1007–1013, 2000.

Moore DH, Thomas GM, Montana GS, Saxer A, Gallup DG, Olt G. Preoperative chemoradiation for advanced vulvar cancer: a phase II study of the Gynecologic Oncology Group. Int J Radiat Oncol Biol Phys 42:79–85, 1998.

Morley GW: Cancer of the vulva: A review. Cancer 48:597, 1981.

Morley GW: Infiltrative carcinoma of the vulva: Results of surgical treatment. Am J Obstet Gynecol 124:874, 1976.

Morrow CP, Rutledge FN: Melanoma of the vulva. Obstet Gynecol 39:745, 1972.

Nuovo GJ et al: Correlation of histology and detection of human papillomavirus DNA in vulvar cancers. Gynecol Oncol 43:275, 1991.

Oonk MH, de Hullu JA, Hollema H, Mourtis MJ, Pras E, Wymenga AN, van der Zee AG. The value of routine follow-up in patients treated for carcinoma of the vulva. Cancer 98:2624–2629, 2003.

Piura B et al: Recurrent squamous cell carcinoma of the vulva: A study of 73 cases. Gynecol Oncol 48:189, 1993.

Planner RS, Hobbs JB: Intraepithelial and invasive neoplasia of the vulva in association with human papillomavirus infection. J Reprod Med 33:503, 1988.

Podratz KC, Symmonds RE, Taylor WF: Carcinoma of the vulva: Analysis of treatment failures. Am J Obstet Gynecol 143:340, 1982.

Prempree T, Amornmarn R: Radiation treatment of recurrent carcinoma of the vulva. Cancer 54:1943, 1984.

Puig-Tintore LM, Ordi J, Vidal-Sicart S, Lejarcegui JA, Torne A, Pahisa J, Iglesias X. Further data on the usefulness of sentinel lymph node identification and ultrastaging in vulvar squamous cell carcinoma. Gynecol Oncol 88:29–34, 2003.

Reid GC, DeLancey JO, Hopkins MP et al: Urinary incontinence following radical vulvectomy. Obstet Gynecol 75:852, 1990.

Remmenga S, Barnhill D, Nash J et al: Radical vulvectomy with partial rectal resection and temporary colostomy as primary therapy for selected patients with vulvar carcinoma. Obstet Gynecol 77:577, 1991.

Roberts WS, Hoffman MS, La Polla JP et al: Management of radionecrosis of vulva and distant vagina. Am J Obstet Gynecol 164:1235, 1991.

Rouzier R, Haddad B, Dubernard G, DuBois P, Paniel BJ. Inguinofemoral dissection for carcinoma of the vulva: effect of modifications of extent and technique on morbidity and survival. J Am Coll Surg 196:442–450, 2003

Rouzier R, Haddad B, Plantier F, DuBois P, Pelisse M, Paniel BJ. Local relapse in patients treated for squamous cell vulvar carcinoma: incidence and prognostic value. Obstet Gynecol 100:1159–1167, 2002.

Rouzier R, Morice MP, Haie-Meder C, Lhomme C, Avril MF, Duvillard P, Castaigne D. Prognostic significance of epithelial disorders adjacent to invasive vulvar carcinomas. Gynecol Oncol 81:414–419, 2001.

Rusk D, Sutton GP, Look KY: Analysis of invasive squamous cell carcinoma of the vulva and VIN for the presence of human papilloma DNA. Obstet Gynecol 77:918, 1991.

Russell AH et al: Synchronous radiation and cytotoxic chemotherapy for locally advanced or recurrent squamous cancer of the vulva. Gynecol Oncol 47:14, 1992.

Rutledge FN, Mitchell MF, Munsell MF et al: Prognostic indicators for invasive carcinoma of the vulva. Gynecol Oncol 42:239, 1991.

Shimm DS et al: Prognostic variables in the treatment of squamous cell carcinoma of the vulva. Gynecol Oncol 24:343, 1986.

Sideri M, DeCicco T, Maggioni A et al: Lymphoscintigraphy and radio guided biopsy of the sentinel node in patients with early vulvar cancer. J Reprod Med 43:613, 1998.

Siller BS et al: T2/3 vulva cancer: A case-control study of triple incision versus en bloc radical vulvectomy and inguinal lymphadenectomy. Gynecol Oncol 57:335, 1995.

Simonsen E: Invasive squamous cell carcinoma of the vulva. Ann Chir Gynaecol 73:331, 1984.

Simonsen E: Treatment of recurrent squamous cell carcinoma of the vulva. Acta Radiol Oncol 23:345, 1984.

Sutton GP et al: Trends in the operative management of invasive squamous carcinoma of the vulva at Indiana University, 1974–1988. Am J Obstet Gynecol 164:1472, 1991.

Taussig FJ: A study of the lymph glands in cancer of the cervix and cancer of the vulva. Am J Obstet Gynecol 36:1938, 1938.

Thomas GM et al: Review: Changing concepts in the management of vulvar cancer. Gynecol Oncol 42:9, 1991.

van der Velden K, Ansink A. Primary groin irradiation vs. primary groin surgery for early vulvar cancer . The Cochrane Database of Systematic Review 2005, vol 3.

van der Velden J, Schilthuis MS, Hyde SE, Ten Kate FJW, Burger MPM. Squamous cell cancer of the vulva with occult lymph nodes metastases in the groin: the impact of surgical technique on recurrence pattern and survival. Int J Gynecol Cancer 14:633–638, 2004.

Way S: The surgery of vulvar carcinoma: An appraisal. Clin Obstet Gynecol 5:623, 1978.

Zhang SH, Sood AK, Sorosky JI, Anderson B, Buller RE. Preservation of the saphenous vein during inguinal lymphadenectomy decreases morbidity in patients with carcinoma of the vulva Cancer 89:1520–1525, 2000.

EARLY VULVAR CARCINOMA

Barnes AE et al: Microinvasive carcinoma of the vulva: A clinicopathologic evaluation. Obstet Gynecol 56:234, 1980.

Berman ML, Soper JT, Creasman WT et al: Conservative surgical management of superficially invasive stage I vulvar carcinoma. Gynecol Oncol 35:352, 1989.

Burger MPM et al: The importance of the groin node status for the survival of T1 and T2 vulval carcinoma patients. Gynecol Oncol 57:327, 1995.

Burke TW, Stringer CA, Gershenson DM et al: Radical wide excision and selective inguinal node dissection for squamous cell carcinoma of the vulva. Gynecol Oncol 38:328, 1990.

Burke TW: Changing surgical approaches to vulvar cancer. Curr Opin Obstet Gynecol 4:86, 1992.

Choo YC: Invasive squamous carcinoma of the vulva in young patients. Gynecol Oncol 13:158, 1982.

Chu J et al: Stage I vulvar cancer: Criteria for microinvasion. Obstet Gynecol 59:716, 1982.

Degefu S, O'Quinn AG, Dhurandhar HN: Paget's disease of the vulva and urogenital malignancies: A case report and review of the literature. Gynecol Oncol 25:347, 1986.

DiPaola GR, Gomez-Rueda N, Arrighi L: Relevance of microinvasion in carcinoma of the vulva. Obstet Gynecol 45:647, 1975.

DiSaia PJ, Creasman WT, Rich WM: An alternate approach to early cancer of the vulva. Am J Obstet Gynecol 133:825, 1979.

Dvoretsky P et al: The pathology of superficially invasive thin vulvar squamous cell carcinoma. Int J Gynecol Pathol 3:331, 1984.

Gordinier ME, Malpica A, Burke TW, Bodurka DC, Wolf JK, Jhingran A, Ramirez PT, Levenback C. Groin recurrence in patients treated with negative nodes on superficial inguinal lymphadenectomy Gynecol Oncol 90:625–628, 2003.

Hacker NF et al: Superficially invasive vulvar cancer with nodal metastases. Gynecol Oncol 15:65, 1983.

Hoffman JS, Kumar NB, Morley GW: Microinvasive squamous carcinoma of the vulva: Search for a definition. Obstet Gynecol 61:615, 1983.

Kirby TO, Rocconi RP, Numnum TM, Kendrick JE, Wright J, Fowler, W, Mutch DG, Bhoola SM, Huh WK, Straughn JM. Outcomes of Stage I/II vulvar cancer patients after negatice superficial inguinal lymphadenectomy. Gynecol Oncol 98:309–312, 2005.

Kneale B, Elliott P, Fortune D: Microinvasive carcinoma of the vulva. Proceedings of the International Society for the Study of Vulvar Disease, 7th World Congress, Lake Buena Vista, Florida, 1983. J Reprod Med 29:454, 1984.

Nakao CY et al: "Microinvasive" epidermoid carcinoma of the vulva with an unexpected natural history. Am J Obstet Gynecol 120:1123, 1974.

Parker RT et al: Operative management of early invasive epidermoid carcinoma of the vulva. Am J Obstet Gynecol 123:349, 1975.

Plentl AA, Friedman EA: Lymphatic System of the Female Genitalia. Philadelphia, WB Saunders, 1971.

Podczaski E, Sexton M, Kaminski P et al: Recurrent carcinoma of the vulva after conservative treatment of "microinvasive" disease. Gynecol Oncol 39:65, 1990.

Rastkar G et al: Early invasive and in situ warty carcinoma of the vulva: Clinical, histologic, and electron microscopic study with particular reference to viral association. Am J Obstet Gynecol 143:814, 1982.

Rowley KC, Gallion HH, Donaldson ES et al: Prognostic factors in early vulvar cancer. Gynecol Oncol 31:43, 1988.

Sedlis A, Homesley H, Bundy BN et al: Positive groin lymph nodes in superficial squamous cell vulvar cancer: A Gynecologic Oncology Group study. Am J Obstet Gynecol 156:1159, 1987.

Stehman FB et al: Early stage I carcinoma of the vulva treated with ipsilateral superficial inguinal lymphadenectomy and modified radical hemivulvectomy: A prospective study of the Gynecologic Oncology Group. Obstet Gynecol 79:490, 1992.

Stehman FB et al: Groin dissection versus groin radiation in carcinoma of the vulva: A Gynecologic Oncology Group study. Int J Radiat Oncol Biol Phys 24:39, 1992.

Van der Velden J et al: A stage Ia vulvar carcinoma with an inguinal lymph node recurrence after local excision: A case report and literature review. Int J Gynecol Cancer 2:157, 1992.

Wharton JT, Gallager S, Rutledge FN: Microinvasive carcinoma of the vulva. Am J Obstet Gynecol 118:159, 1974.

Wilkinson EJ, Rico MJ, Pierson KK: Microinvasive carcinoma of the vulva. Int J Gynecol Pathol 1:29, 1982.

Wilkinson EJ: Superficial invasive carcinoma of the vulva. Clin Obstet Gynecol 28:188, 1985.

PAGET'S DISEASE

Baehrendtz H et al: Paget's disease of the vulva: The Radiumhemmet series 1975–1990. Int J Gynecol Cancer 4:1, 1994.

Balducci L, Athar M, Smith GF et al: Metastatic extramammary Paget's disease: Dramatic response to combined modality treatment. J Surg Oncol 38:38, 1988.

Bergen S, DiSaia PJ, Liao SY et al: Conservative management of extramammary Paget's disease of the vulva. Gynecol Oncol 33:151, 1989.

Besa P et al: Extramammary Paget's disease of the perineal skin: Role of radiotherapy. Int J Radiat Oncol Biol Phys 24:73, 1992.

Creasman WT, Gallager HS, Rutledge F: Paget's disease of the vulva. Gynecol Oncol 3:133, 1975.

Curtin JP, Rubin SC, Jones WB et al: Paget's disease of the vulva. Gynecol Oncol 39:374, 1990.

DiSaia PJ et al: A report of two cases of recurrent Paget's disease of the vulva in a split-thickness graft and its possible pathogenesis-labeled "retrodissemination." Gynecol Oncol 57:109, 1995.

Fanning J, Lambert HCL, Hale TM et al: Paget's disease of the vulva: Prevalence of associated vulvar adenocarcinoma, invasive Paget's disease, and recurrence after surgical excision. Am J Obstet Gynecol 180:24, 1999.

Fine BA et al: Case report: Minimally invasive Paget's disease of the vulva with extensive lymph node metastases. Gynecol Oncol 57:262, 1995.

Fishman DA et al: Extramammary Paget's disease of the vulva. Gynecol Oncol 56:266, 1995.

James LP: Apocrine adenocarcinoma of the vulva with associated Paget's disease. Acta Cytol 28:178, 1984.

Piura B, Rabinovich, Dgani R: Extramammary Paget's disease of the vulva. Eur J Gynaecol Oncol 20:98, 1999.

Stacy D, Burrell MO, Franklin EW: Extramammary Paget's disease of the vulva and anus: Use of intraoperative frozen-section margins. Am J Obstet Gynecol 155:519, 1986.

Taylor PT, Stenwig JT, Klausen H: Paget's disease of the vulva: A report of 18 cases. Gynecol Oncol 3:46, 1975.

Voigt H, Bassermann R, Nathrath W: Cytoreductive combination chemotherapy for regionally advanced unresectable extramammary Paget carcinoma. Cancer 70:704, 1992.

Watring WG, Roberts JA, Lagasse LD et al: Treatment of recurrent Paget's disease of the vulva with topical bleomycin. Cancer 41:10, 1978.

MELANOMA

Bailet JW, Figge DC, Tamimi HK et al: Malignant melanoma of the vulva: A case report of distal recurrence in a patient with a superficially invasive primary lesion. Obstet Gynecol 70:515, 1987.

Balch CM et al: Efficacy of 2 cm surgical margins for intermediate thickness melanomas (1 to 4 mm): Results of a multi-institutional randomized surgical trial. Ann Surg 218:262, 1993.

Blessing K, Kernohan NM, Miller ID et al: Malignant melanoma of the vulva: Clinicopathological features. Int J Gynecol Cancer 1:81, 1991.

Bradgate MG, Rollason TP, McConkey CC et al: Malignant melanoma of the vulva: A clinicopathological study of 50 women. Br J Obstet Gynaecol 97:124, 1990.

Breslow A: Thickness, cross-sectional areas and depth of invasion in the prognosis of cutaneous melanoma. Ann Surg 172:902, 1970.

Chung AF, Woodruff JM, Lewis JL: Malignant melanoma of the vulva: A report of 44 cases. Obstet Gynecol 45:638, 1975.

Clark WH Jr et al: The histogenesis and biologic behaviour of primary human malignant melanomas of the skin. Cancer Res 29:705, 1969.

Creasman WT, Phillips JL, Mench HR: A survey of hospital management practice for vulvar melanoma. J Am Coll Surg 188:670, 1999.

Day CL et al: The natural break points for primary-tumor thickness in clinical stage I melanoma. N Engl J Med 305:1155, 1981.

Jaramillo BA et al: Malignant melanoma of the vulva. Obstet Gynecol 66:398, 1985.

Look KY, Roth LM, Sutton GP: Vulvar melanoma reconsidered. Cancer 72:143, 1993.

Morris JM: A formula for selective lymphadenectomy, its application in cancer of the vulva. Obstet Gynecol 50:152, 1977.

Morrow CP, DiSaia PJ: Malignant melanoma of the female genitalia: A clinical analysis. Obstet Gynecol Surv 31:233, 1976.

Podratz KC et al: Melanoma of the vulva: An update. Gynecol Oncol 16:153, 1983.

Ragnarsson-Olding BK, Kanter-Lewensohn LR, Lagerlof B et al: Malignant melanoma of the vulva in a nationwide, 25-year study of 219 Swedish females. Cancer 86:1273, 1999.

Rose PG et al: Conservative therapy for melanoma of the vulva. Am J Obstet Gynecol 159:52, 1988.

Tasseron EWK et al: A clinicopathological study of 30 melanomas of the vulva. Gynecol Oncol 46:170, 1992.

Trimble EL, Lewis JL Jr, Williams LL et al: Management of vulvar melanoma. Gynecol Oncol 45:254, 1992.

Veronesi U, Cascinelli N: Narrow excision (1 cm margin): A safe procedure for thin cutaneous melanoma. Arch Surg 126:438, 1991.

Verschraegen CF, Benjapibal M, Supakarapongkul W, Levy LB, Ross M, Atkinson EN, Borduka-Bevers D, Kavanagh JJ, Kudelka AP, Legha SS. Vulvar melanoma at the M.D. Anderson Cancer Center; 25 years later. Int J Gynecol Cancer 11:359–364, 2001.

SARCOMA

Bakri YN et al: Case report: Vulvar sarcoma: A report of four cases. Gynecol Oncol 46:384, 1992.

DiSaia PJ, Rutledge FN, Smith JP: Sarcoma of the vulva. Obstet Gynecol 38:180, 1971.

BARTHOLIN GLAND CARCINOMA

Copeland LJ et al: Adenoid cystic carcinoma of Bartholin gland. Obstet Gynecol 67:115, 1986.

Copeland LJ et al: Bartholin gland carcinoma. Obstet Gynecol 67:794, 1986.

Flam F, Larson B: Adenoid cystic carcinoma of Bartholin's gland: A review of the literature and report of a patient with widespread metastases to the bone. Int J Gynecol Cancer 7:458, 1997.

Ghamande SA et al: Case report: Mucinous adenocarcinomas of the vulva. Gynecol Oncol 57:117, 1995.

Lelle RJ, Davis KP, Roberts JA: Adenoid cystic carcinoma of the Bartholin's gland: The University of Michigan Experience. Int J Gynecol Cancer 3:3, 1993.

Leuchter RS et al: Primary carcinoma of the Bartholin gland: A report of 14 cases and review of the literature. Obstet Gynecol 60:361, 1982.

Wheelock JB et al: Primary carcinoma of the Bartholin gland: A report of ten cases. Obstet Gynecol 63:820, 1984.

Yazigi R, Piver MS, Tsukada Y: Microinvasive carcinoma of the vulva. Obstet Gynecol 123:349, 1975.

BASAL CELL CARCINOMA

Benedet JL, Miller DM, Ehlen TG, Bertrand MA: Basal cell carcinoma of the vulva: Clinical features and treatment results in 28 patients. Obstet Gynecol 90:765, 1997.

Winkelmann SE, Llorens AS: Case report: Metastatic basal cell carcinoma of the vulva. Gynecol Oncol 38:138, 1990.

9 Invasive Cancer of the Vagina and Urethra

Brian M. Slomovitz, M.D. and Robert L. Coleman, M.D.

The vaginal tissues, in sharp contrast to the uterine cervix and other gynecologic organs, rarely undergo malignant transformation. Primary cancer of the vagina is an uncommon malignancy, accounting for only 1–3% of gynecologic malignancies (Table 9–1). The incidence of this disease is approximately 1 case in 100,000 women.

When primary cancer does occur in the vagina, it is usually in the upper third (Table 9–2), and it is usually an epithelial carcinoma. By convention, any malignant neoplasm involving both cervix and vagina that is histologically compatible with origin in either organ is classified as cervical cancer. The age incidence of this disease is between 35 and 90 years with more than 50% of the cases occurring between the seventh and ninth decades of life (Fig. 9–1).

Squamous cell carcinoma is the most frequent histologic subtype (78%). Adenocarcinoma (6%), melanoma (3%), and sarcoma (3%) have been described as primary vaginal cancers (Table 9–3). History of radiation therapy contributes to the development of vaginal sarcomas. The relationship of diethylstilbestrol (DES) intrauterine exposure to clear cell adenocarcinoma of the vagina has resulted in the reporting of significant numbers of cases of adenocarcinoma of the vagina in both exposed and unexposed individuals.

The principal focus of this chapter will address squamous cancers. Rare histologies will be discussed later in the chapter. However, the clinical evaluation and staging for vaginal tumors is the same for all types of vaginal cancers.

SQUAMOUS CELL CARCINOMA OF THE VAGINA

Epidemiology

Similar to cervix cancer, epidemiologic evidence suggests that vaginal cancer has a strong relationship with human papilloma virus (HPV) infection. HPV subtype 16 presence has been associated with the development of vaginal cancer. In addition, approximately one-third of women who develop vaginal cancer have a history of cervical dysplasia or cervix cancer more than 5 years earlier. A study from the University of South Carolina found that the median interval between cervical disease and development of vaginal cancer was 14 years. In this study, 16% of patients had a history of prior radiation. Proposed mechanisms for developing vaginal cancer with a remote history of cervix cancer include occult residual disease, radiation-induced tumorigenesis, and a new primary cancer in a high-risk individual. Regardless, a new vaginal lesion 5 years or more after treatment of cervix cancer constitutes a new primary vaginal cancer.

The natural course of vaginal intraepithelial neoplasia (VaIN) is not well understood because most patients are treated once diagnosed. Between 3% and 7% of patients with VaIN progress to invasive carcinoma despite treatment.

Chronic vaginal irritation has also been suggested to contribute to the etiology of vaginal cancer, however, the mechanism by which this promotes carcinogenesis is not well understood and has not been extensively studied.

Screening

The Papanicolaou smear is effective in detecting vaginal cancer in an asymptomatic patient. For a screening test to be effective, however, the incidence of the disease must be sufficient to justify the cost. The American Cancer Society recommends that Papanicolaou screening for cervix cancer may be discontinued at age 70 years in low-risk women. Since the incidence of vaginal cancer is so low, routine screening is not cost effective. However, women with a history of cervical dysplasia or cervical cancer are at increased risk and Pap testing should be continued.

Development of vaginal cancer is possible even in women with a history of hysterectomy for benign disease. Bell and colleagues described 87 patients with primary cancer of the vagina, 31 of whom had undergone total hysterectomy for benign disease. Benedet and colleagues found that 19 of their 97 patients (20%) with vaginal cancer had surgery for benign diseases. Peters and associates reported that 38% (25 of 68) of the patients in their series had undergone prior hysterectomies for benign disease. Guidelines aside, these observations underscore the need to individualize vaginal cancer cytological screening by careful consideration of estimated risks and benefits of such clinical activity.

Table 9–1 INCIDENCE OF VAGINAL CANCER

Series	No. of genital malignant neoplasms	Vaginal cancer (%)
Smith (1955)	8199	1.5
Ries and Ludwig (1962)	14,785	2.1
Smith (1964)	6050	1.8
Wolff and Douyon (1964)	4665	1.8
Rutledge (1967)	5715	1.2
Palumbo et al (1969)	2305	1.9
Daw (1971)	564	1.9
Gallup et al (1987)	Not given	3.1
Manetta (1988)	2149	1.3
Eddy (1991)	2929	3.1

Signs and symptoms

The signs and symptoms of invasive vaginal cancer (Fig. 9–2) are similar to those of cervical cancer. Painless vaginal discharge, often bloody, is the most frequent symptom in most series. Postcoital or postmenopausal vaginal bleeding is the initial symptom in many patients with invasive lesions, and a gross lesion is obvious on speculum examination. Urinary symptoms (pain and frequency) are more common than with cervical cancer because neoplasms lower in the vagina are close to the vesicle neck, with resulting compression of the bladder at an earlier stage of the disease. Tenesmus is commonly associated with posterior vaginal lesions. Approximately 5–10% of women have no symptoms and the disease is suspected on physical exam and confirmed by biopsy.

Diagnostic considerations

All patients who present with a vaginal cancer need to have a full workup to rule out metastatic disease. Medical history should emphasize history of cancer, radiotherapy, and surgery. Physical exam, including an adequate pelvic exam (under anesthesia if necessary), should be performed. The diagnosis is often missed on first exam, especially if the lesion is small and covered by the blades of the speculum. Definitive diagnosis is made by biopsy.

In patients with an abnormal Pap smear and no gross abnormality, careful vaginal colposcopy is necessary. In order to differentiate between an early vaginal cancer and VaIN III, it is often necessary to perform a partial upper vaginectomy because the lesion may be buried by reapproximation of the vaginal vault at the time of hysterectomy. Hoffman and associates reported on 32 patients with VaIN III who underwent an upper vaginectomy. Invasive carcinoma was found in 28% of the patients.

Metastatic carcinoma to the vagina is seen much more frequently than primary disease. Over 80% of patients with vaginal tumors have secondary lesions. In 269 patients with metastatic vaginal cancer, Mazur and colleagues found that 84% were from genital sites and the remaining 16%

Table 9–2 INVOLVEMENT OF VAGINA

Series	Upper third	Middle third	Lower third
Livingstone (1950)	34	4	42
Bivens (1953)	22	3	14
Mobius (1956)	89	0	29
Arronet, Latour, and Tremblay (1960)	14	8	3
Whelton and Kottmeier (1962)	20	13	19
Blunt (1965)	13	15	10
Daw (1971)	24	14	13
Benedet (1983)	46	3	19
Manetta et al (1990)	22	8	16
Eddy et al (1991)	33	5	8
Total	317 (56%)	73 (13%)	173 (31%)

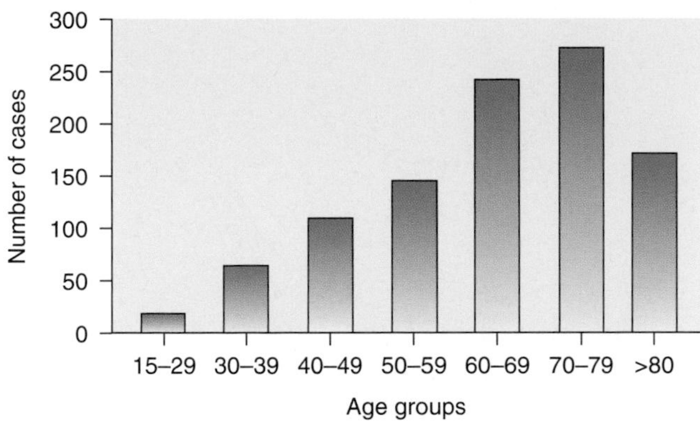

Figure 9–1 Carcinoma of the vagina. Patients treated in 1990–1992. Number of cases by age group (From the Annual Report of Gynecological Cancer. FIGO 23:105, 1998).

were most commonly metastatic from the gastrointestinal tract or breast. The cervix (32%) and endometrium (18%) are the most common primary sites of cancer. Endometrial carcinomas and choriocarcinomas often metastasize to the vagina while rectal and bladder cancers invade the vagina directly.

When the primary site of growth is in the vagina and does not involve surrounding organs (e.g., vulva or cervix), the tumor is considered a vaginal primary cancer. Special consideration needs to be made for those patients with a remote (>5 years) or questionable history of a gynecologic malignancy (especially cervix cancer) who present with a vaginal lesion. By convention, these lesions are considered primary vaginal cancers. However, patients with history of endometrial cancer and a vaginal lesion with a histologic diagnosis of adenocarcinoma consistent with recurrence are diagnosed with recurrent endometrial cancer.

Once diagnosed, patients with cancer of the vagina should be examined for evidence of local or distant spread in a manner analogous to that of cervical cancer. All patients should have at least the following diagnostic studies in addition to a thorough history and physical examination: chest x-ray, intravenous pyelography, cystoscopy, and proctosigmoidoscopy, the last two depending on the location of disease. A CT scan or MRI can replace the pyelography, cystoscopy, and proctosigmoidoscopy. If bone pain is present, further x-rays are warranted.

While staging is clinical, not surgical, an imaging evaluation should be performed to evaluate lymph node metastasis, distant metastasis, and an evaluation of the genitourinary system. Patients with vaginal cancer rarely undergo lymph node dissections. The accuracy of clinical exam for detecting lymph node involvement is probably similar to that for vulvar cancer. For patients with early-stage vulvar lesions and clinically negative lymph nodes, up to 20% will have microscopic disease in the groin nodes identified after dissection.

Table 9–3 HISTOLOGIC DISTRIBUTION OF PRIMARY VAGINAL CANCER

Cell type	%
Squamous	85
Adenocarcinoma	6
Melanoma	3
Sarcoma	3
Miscellaneous	3

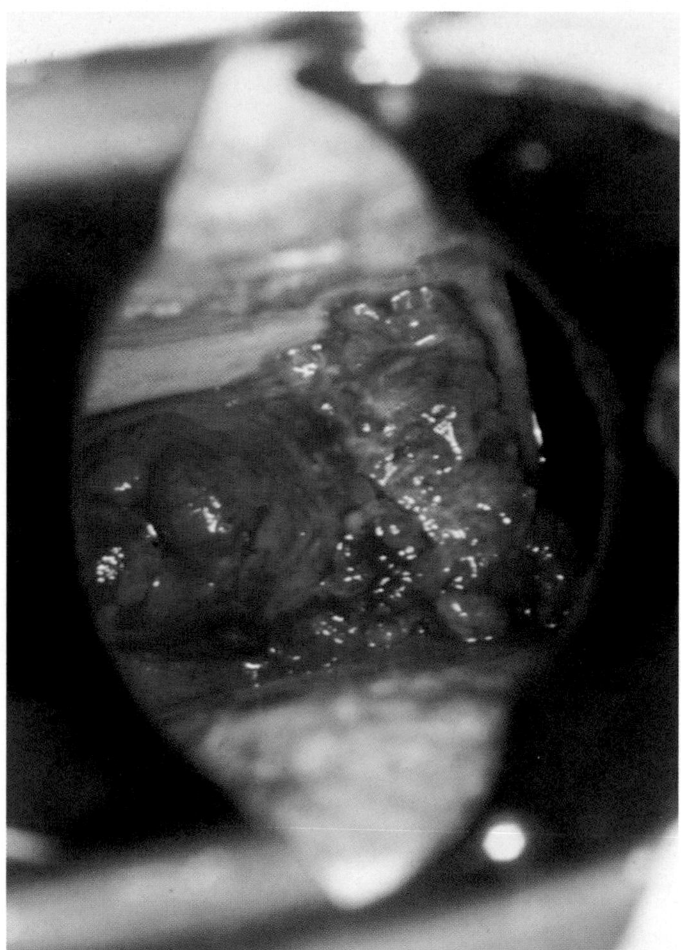

Figure 9–2 Lesion of the posterior fornix in squamous cell carcinoma.

PET/CT and vaginal cancer

CT imaging is only able to detect lymph nodes that are at least 1 cm in greatest dimension. Metabolic imaging with positron emission tomography (PET) has been shown to be more sensitive than CT and MRI, specifically for cancer of the head and neck, lung, esophagus, and cervix. In a study from Washington University, Lamoreaux and associates found that PET imaging detected primary and metastatic lesions more often than CT scans. We recommend that all patients with vaginal cancer have imaging and the PET/CT is a reasonable option for these patients.

Staging

Staging of vaginal cancer follows clinical parameters outlined by the International Federation of Gynecology and

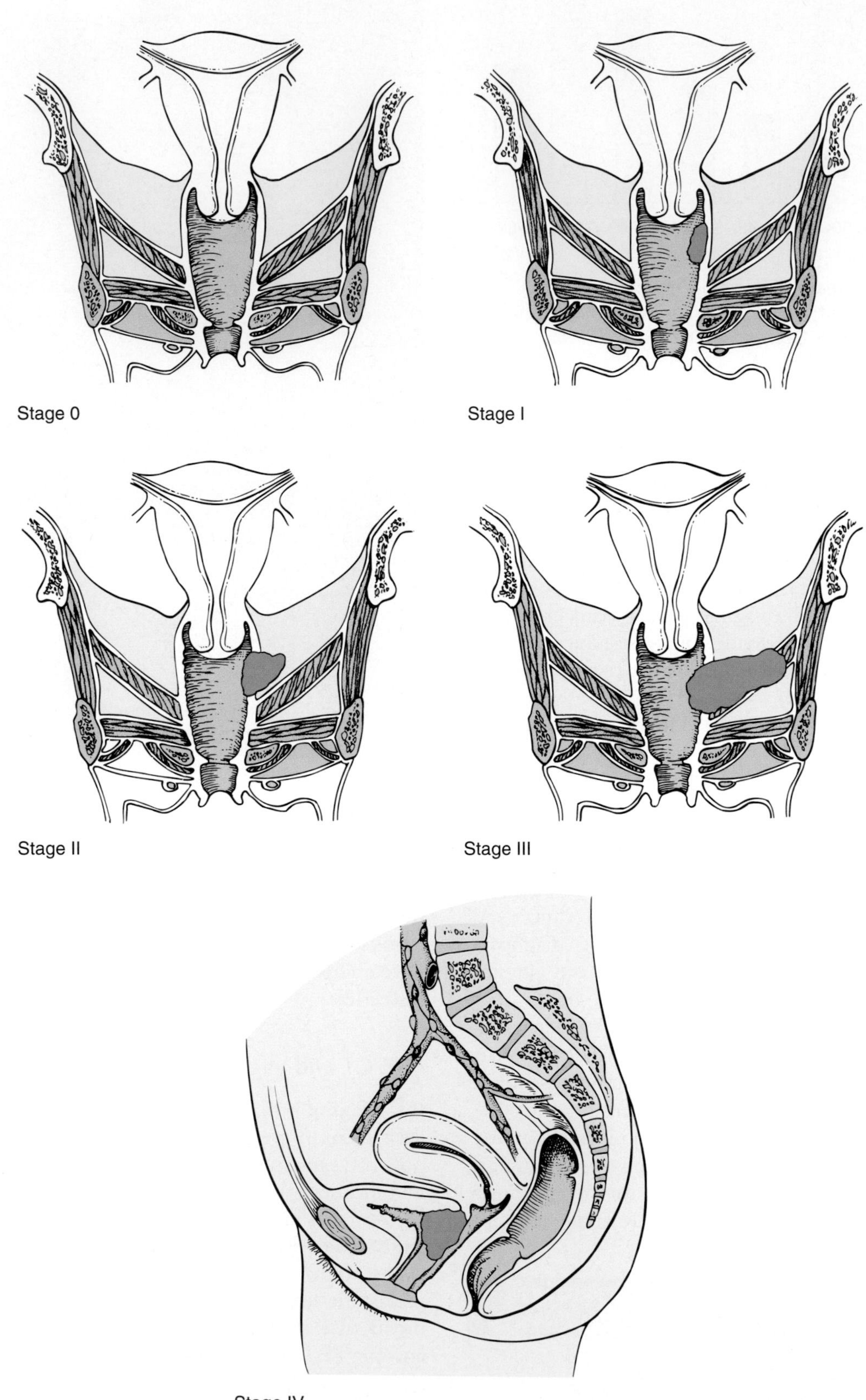

Figure 9–3 Staging diagrams for vaginal cancer.

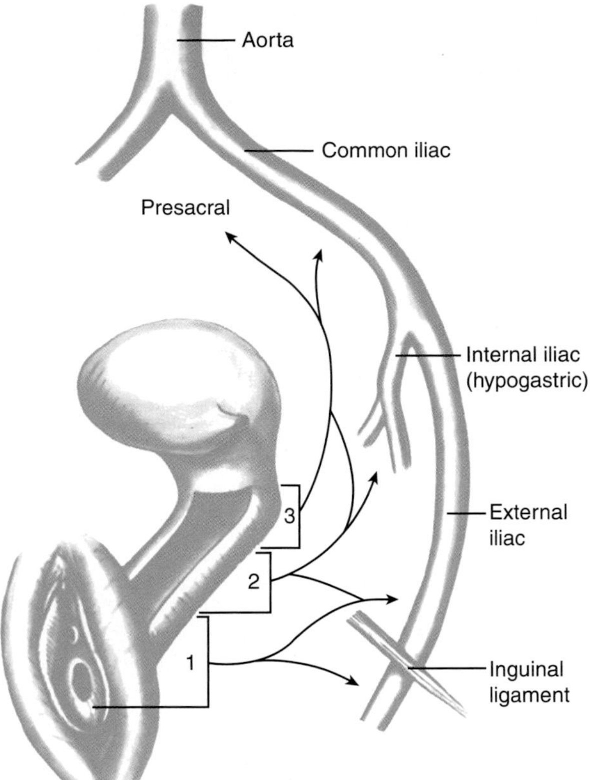

Figure 9–4 Lymphatic drainage of the vagina: (1) channels from the lower third drain into the femoral and external iliac nodes; (2) the channels from the middle third drain into the hypogastric nodes; (3) channels from the upper third drain into the common iliac, presacral, and hypogastric nodes. (Modified from Plentl AA, Friedman EA: Lymphatic System of the Female Genitalia. Philadelphia, WB Saunders, 1971.)

Obstetrics (FIGO) (Fig. 9–4); a summary of the staging classification follows:

Stage 0	Carcinoma in situ, intraepithelial carcinoma
Stage I	Carcinoma is limited to the vaginal wall
Stage II	Carcinoma has involved the subvaginal tissue but has not extended onto the pelvic wall
Stage III	Carcinoma has extended onto the pelvic wall
Stage IV	Carcinoma has extended beyond the true pelvis or has involved the mucosa of the bladder or rectum; bullous edema or tumor bulge into the bladder or rectum is not acceptable evidence of invasion of these organs
Stage IVa	Spread of the growth to adjacent organs or direct extension beyond the true pelvis
Stage IVb	Spread to distant organs

Perez and Camel have suggested modification of stage II. Stage IIa lesions would involve the submucosal area of the vagina but not extend to the parametrium. Stage IIb lesions would significantly involve the parametrium but not extend to the pelvic wall. Though useful to stratify patients with stage II disease, this staging modification has not demonstrated prognostic significance. Though FIGO does not specify the stage of patients with inguinal lymph node involvement, the American Joint Committee on Cancer (AJCC) assigns patients with T1–T3 tumors with positive inguinal lymph nodes to stage III. Involvement of the pubic symphysis places a patient in the stage III category.

Patterns of spread

Vaginal cancer metastasizes by direct extension, lymphatic dissemination and hematogenous spread. The pelvic soft tissues, pelvic bones, bladder, and rectum are commonly involved via direct extension in those patients with locally advanced disease. The lymphatic vasculature of the vagina begins as an extremely fine capillary meshwork in the mucosa and submucosa (see Fig. 9–3). In the deep layers of the submucosa and muscularis, there is a similar parallel but coarser network. Irregular anastomoses have been demonstrated between the two. Both systems drain into small trunks that coalesce at the lateral aspect of the vagina and form a number of collecting trunks. It is at this point that the efferent lymph drainage channels of the organ originate. The lymphatic trunks of the upper vagina drain into the iliac and eventually the para-aortic lymph nodes. The lower vagina is principally drained by lymphatic network that anastomose with the regional lymph nodes of the femoral triangle. All lymph nodes in the pelvis may at one time or another serve as primary sites or regional drainage nodes for vaginal lymph and its contents.

Because most patients with vaginal cancer are treated with radiation, the incidence of lymph node involvement is not well recorded. However, retrospective studies demonstrate that 30–35% of patients with vaginal cancer have lymph node metastasis. Para-aortic spread is not as common but more common in patients with concomitant pelvic node metastases.

Prognostic features

The number of patients who survive vaginal cancer has increased, which reflects our better understanding of the disease and improved radiation techniques. (Fig. 9–5, Table 9–4). Factors affecting prognosis for patients diagnosed with vaginal cancer are not well established due to the rarity of this disease. Several investigators have remarked that age at time of diagnosis is one of the most important prognostic factors. Reflecting intolerance of aggressive multimodality therapy and attendant comorbidities, age acts as a surrogate of clinical outcome. Although not well described, performance status likely reflects a factor with greater precision in determining the impact of chronological age. Tumor histology may also have prognostic relevance. It is clear that vaginal melanomas and sarcomas have the poorest prognosis when compared to squamous cell and adenocarcinomas. However, survival differences between these histologies have not been well documented.

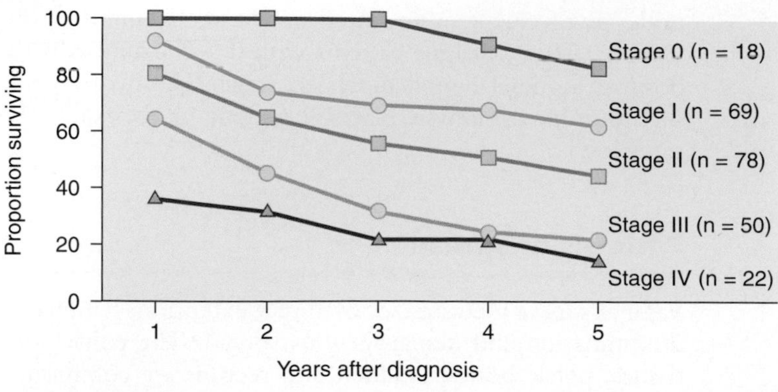

Figure 9–5 Carcinoma of the vagina. Patients treated in 1990–1992. Five-year survival rates. (From the Annual Report of Gynecological Cancer. FIGO 232:101, 1998.)

Table 9–4 VAGINAL CANCER: COMPARISON OF SURVIVAL

		Stage and survival (%)				
Authors	**No. of cases**	**I**	**II**	**III**	**IV**	**All stages**
Krepart (1979)	14*	65	60	35	39	51.8
Nori et al (1981)	36*	71	66	33	0	42.8
Perez and Camel (1982)	105*	81	42	30	9	50.8
Prempree (1982)	80*	78	57	39	0	8.8
Puthawala et al (1983)	27*	100	75	22	0	56.8
Benedet et al (1983)	75*	71	50	15	0	45.8
Reuben et al (1985)	68*	79	52	54	0	49.8
Gallup et al (1987)	28*	100	50	0	25	42.8
Eddy (1991)	84*	70	45	35	28	50.8
Stock et al (1995)	100*	67	53	0	15	46.8
Creasman et al (1998)	792*	73	58	58	58	

*5-year survival.

Stage, tumor location and tumor size also appear to impact prognosis. In a review of 843 patients with vaginal cancer, patients with stage I disease had a 64–90% 5-year survival, 31–80% for stage II, 0–79% for stage III, and 0–62% for stage IV. In this study, lesions of the distal vagina had a poorer prognosis than those originating in the proximal vagina. In a review of 104 patients, Smith (1964) found 6.8% survivors among 29 patients with cancer of the lower third of the vagina, 25% of 48 patients with tumors of the middle third, and 37% of 27 patients with lesions of the upper third. In 1958, Merrill and Bender reported a 29% survival rate in 14 patients with upper third lesions and an 11% rate in nine patients with distal third involvement. Recently, Tewari and colleagues reported that survival was better for patients less than 3 cm compared to those greater than 3 cm. Chyle and colleagues found that tumor size larger than 5 cm was associated with a higher rate of local recurrence rate when compared to smaller tumors.

Frank and colleagues at MD Anderson Cancer Center reported their 30-year experience treating patients with vaginal cancer. In this series of 193 patients, disease specific survival and pelvic disease control rates were correlated with stage (I, II, or III/IV) and tumor size (<4 cm or >4 cm).

Intuitively, lymph node status at the time of diagnosis would portend a worse prognosis, however, this has not been thoroughly evaluated. In one study by Pingley and colleagues, the 5-year survival for patients without lymph node involvement was 56% compared to 33% for those patients with lymph node involvement. Finally, as has been suggested in radiation treatment trials of patients with cervix cancer, time to treatment initiation and total treatment time affect survival. Lee and associates found that the pelvic control rate was 97% if the treatment was completed within 63 days compared to 54% if treatment lasted longer than this time.

Management

Until the 1930s, vaginal cancers were considered incurable. With advances in radiation oncology, cure rates for even advanced cancers approach those for cervix cancer. As mentioned, stage, tumor location, and size are the principle factors taken into consideration when planning treatment for patients with vaginal carcinoma. Other factors include history of surgery and/or radiation.

Stage 0 and I

Vaginal intraepithelial neoplasia (VaIN) usually occurs at the vaginal apex. It is also a multifocal disease and is common in patients with a history of cervical dysplasia.

Table 9–5 RADIOTHERAPY FOR VAGINAL CANCER

Stage	External irradiation	Vaginal therapy
0	Surgical excision preferred for localized disease	7000 cGy surface dose
I		
1–2 cm lesion		Brachytherapy irradiation, 6000–7000 cGy*
Larger lesions	4000–5000 cGy whole pelvis	Brachytherapy delivering 3000–4000 cGy
II	4000–5000 cGy whole pelvis	Same as for stage I
III	5000 cGy whole pelvis (optional 1000–2000 cGy through reduced fields)	Brachytherapy implant, 2000–3000 cGy (if tumor regression is satisfactory)
IV (pelvis only)	Same as for stage III	Same as for stage III

*Surgical excision for selected sites on 1–2 cm lesions may be used instead of brachytherapy.

Table 9–6 PRIMARY VAGINAL CARCINOMA: LOCAL CONTROL AND DISEASE-FREE SURVIVAL BY STAGE

		Five years	
FIGO stage	No.	Local control (%)	Disease-free survival
I	23	72	67
II	58	62	53
III	9	0	0
IV	10	21	15

From Stock RG et al: A 30 year experience in the management of primary carcinoma of the vagina: Analysis of prognostic factors and treatment modalities. Gynecol Oncol 56:45, 1995.

Treatment options for patients with VaIN include surgery (i.e., wide local excision or vaginectomy), 5% fluorouracil cream, local ablation (LASER, cryotherapy, electrodiathermy, etc.) and intracavitary radiation. (Table 9–5).

Creasman and associates reported the results of the National Cancer Data Base (NCDB), a large central registry of hospital data for 10 years (1984–1994). There were 4885 cases reported with 1242 in situ carcinomas (CIS) representing 26% of all vaginal lesions. CIS was almost exclusively treated with surgery; only 5% were treated with radiotherapy. Brown and colleagues reported no new cases of in situ or invasive carcinoma of the vagina developing after radiation therapy for carcinoma in situ or early invasive carcinoma. Their report discouraged overly aggressive therapy for early-stage tumors because of the good prognosis for these lesions and the adverse effects of high-dose irradiation on the pliability of the vagina and on sexual function. Lee and Symmonds reported the results in 66 patients treated previously with wide local excisions or partial vaginectomies and in seven patients with multicentric disease treated with total vaginectomies. Only one patient had recurrent carcinoma of the vagina resulting in her death. In the young, sexually active patient with diffuse involvement of the vaginal epithelium, total or subtotal vaginectomy with split-thickness skin graft reconstruction of the vagina often allows excellent long-term results. When radiation therapy is chosen, patients who have CIS and superficial stage I tumors can be treated with intracavitary insertion alone.

Surgical management is an option for lesions 0.5 cm or less in patients with invasive carcinoma. For early lesions, particularly in the upper vagina (see Fig. 9–2), surgery may be preferred in many patients. Peters and coworkers have described superficially invasive squamous cell carcinoma of the vagina as a lesion that invades <2.5 mm from the surface, is lacking involvement of lymph-vascular spaces, and is developed in a field of carcinoma in situ. Their experience with six patients suggests that local therapy was sufficient, and no attempt was made to treat pelvic nodes either surgically or with irradiation. This conservative approach might allow preservation of optimal sexual function in young patients who have these early invasive squamous and adenocarcinoma lesions.

For invasive carcinoma thicker than 0.5 cm or if the tumor is adenocarcinoma, total vaginectomy and lymphadenectomy are recommended. If the patient did not have a prior hysterectomy, a radical hysterectomy and upper vaginectomy would need to be performed. Also, pelvic external beam radiotherapy and an interstitial single-plane implant enhance the probability of tumor control.

Patients with small stage I cancers (<2 cm) who are not good surgical candidates can adequately be treated with brachytherapy alone. For large vaginal tumors, options for radiating the primary lesion are tailored by physician preference and extent of disease. Bulky stage I cancers (>2 cm) of the upper portion of the vagina in patients with intact uteri are treated with techniques similar to those used for carcinoma of the cervix. External irradiation in a dose of 4000–5000 cGy is given initially in bulky stage I and stage II cancers (Table 9–6). For young patients who require radiation therapy, pretreatment laparotomy or laparoscopy with ovarian transposition and surgical staging is a rational approach.

Stage II to IVa

For patients who have stage II–IV vaginal cancer, treatment is tailored to the extent of the disease and the radiation therapy plan should reflect consideration of the depth of invasion of the lesion. Proper planning of radiation therapy and individualization of treatment plans are essential to minimize the more serious complications of acute and long-term radiation sequelae in these organs. The difficulty in applying radiation systems to vaginal cancer led some, like Wertheim and Brunschwig, to advocate radical exenterative surgery as primary therapy. However, the complications associated with these radical procedures, especially in older patients, have become a serious limiting factor to the surgical approach.

Patients with advanced stage disease should be treated with external irradiation and brachytherapy. External irradiation to the pelvis is usually sufficient and para-aortic extension is not routinely administered. Groin radiation is often considered if the tumor involves the lower one-third of the vagina or in the presence of metastatic groin disease. Perez and associates evaluated 149 patients with vaginal carcinoma and clinically negative lymph nodes who were not treated with groin radiation. In the group of patients with tumors confined to the upper vagina, there were no recurrences, compared with an 8% recurrence rate in those patients whose tumor involved the lower third of the vagina.

If the uterus is intact and the lesion is in the upper vagina, an intrauterine tandem and ovoids would be appropriate. If the patient has had a hysterectomy, interstitial radiation alone or in combination with intracavitary therapy optimizes dose distribution.

For those patients who can be treated with brachytherapy only, a minimum of 6000–7000 cGy is delivered to the neoplasm in 5–7 days. Pelvic and groin radiation consists of a total of 45 to 50.4 Gy given in 1.8 Gy fractions daily. Use of concomitant sensitizing radiotherapy is discussed in the following section.

If there is metastatic lymph node involvement to the pelvic or groin lymph nodes, external radiation is given to a dose of 60–66 Gy. In addition, adenopathy greater than 2 cm may be best controlled with excision. The deep nodes must be included in the treatment fields because large tumors have a high incidence of regional lymphatic metastasis. After receiving 5000 cGy, the patient with a large lesion should be re-evaluated for an additional 1000–2000 cGy external radiation to reduced field. Newer treatment planning protocols utilizing intensity modulated radiation therapy (IMRT) may lead to higher tumor control with less local normal tissue effects. Long-term morbidity outcomes with this technology are awaited.

Chemotherapy

There are limited studies regarding the experience with chemotherapy for patients with vaginal cancer. In a phase II Gynecologic Oncology Group study, 26 patients with progressive or recurrent vaginal carcinoma were treated with cisplatin (50 mg/m^2 every 3 weeks). There was minimal, insignificant activity, particularly in the patients with squamous cell carcinoma. Other agents that have been used for the treatment of vaginal cancer include 5-fluorouracil, mitomycin-C, epirubicin, and the combination of two of these agents. In addition, concurrent use of cisplatin with primary radiation therapy is probably appropriate since it is beneficial in patients with cervix cancer.

Chemosensitizing radiation is standard for patients with carcinoma of the cervix. Because the natural history, the histology, and risk factors are similar for vaginal cancer, chemotherapy (cisplatin and/or 5-fluorouracil) has been recommended in patients receiving radiation for advanced stage disease. Prospective studies will likely not be performed given the rarity of this disease.

Special considerations

In vaginal cancer that develops in patients who have had a hysterectomy, the geometry is usually unfavorable for local radiation therapy. In addition, the proximity of the bladder base and urethra makes the risks of a urinary-vaginal fistula appreciable. Therapy must be individualized, and radical surgery should be reserved for failures (Fig. 9–6).

Although one is often dealing with a radiosensitive neoplasm in a relatively radioresistant bed (the vagina), serious limitations may nonetheless exist. The proximity of relatively radiosensitive normal tissues, such as the bladder and rectum, provides a challenge to the therapist, especially in the treatment of tumors in the lower third of the vagina.

The incidence of complications after radiation therapy or surgery for vaginal cancer is relatively low. Serious complications consist primarily of rectal stenosis, rectovaginal fistulas, and severe rectal bleeding often requiring diversion. As many as 35% of patients experience cystitis or proctitis during or shortly after therapy, but symptoms

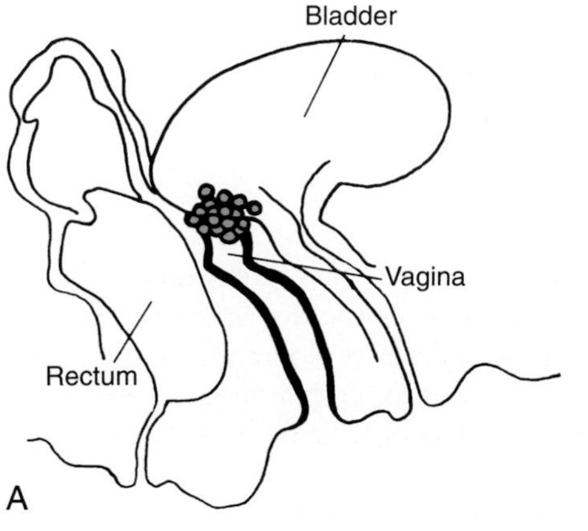

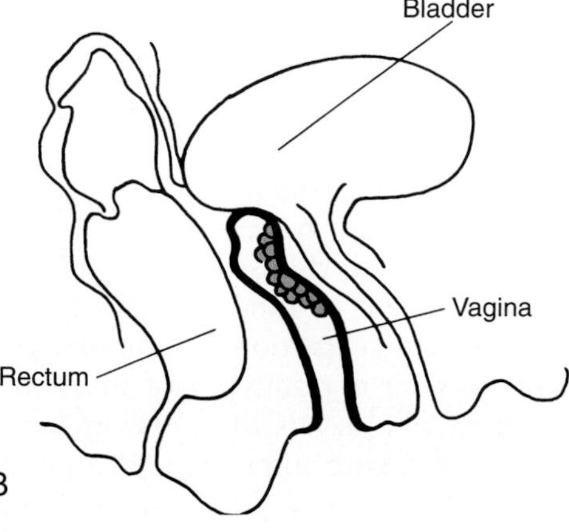

Figure 9–6 Diagrammatic representation of typical locations of vaginal cancer in a previously hysterectomized patient, illustrating the proximity of the bladder and urethra. *A,* Lesion at the vaginal apex. *B,* Lesion at the upper anterior vaginal wall. (Courtesy of A. Robert Kagan, MD, Los Angeles, California.)

usually resolve spontaneously. A few patients have extensive vaginal necrosis that usually resolves with prolonged conservative management.

Frank and associates found that the incidence of major complications associated with radiation were associated with FIGO stage. Four percent of stage I patients, 9% of stage II patients, and 21% of stage III/IVa patients suffered major complications.

Patients who are sexually active should be encouraged to continue regular intercourse. For others, vaginal dilators should be used to maintain vaginal patency during and after therapy.

Survival and recurrence

A study by Rutledge in 1967 reported 3- and 5-year survival rates of 42% and 44%, respectively, for patients treated primarily with radiotherapy. Comparable survival results at 5 years were reported by Prempree and colleagues, who used radiotherapy for stage I (83%), stage II (63%), stage III (40%), and stage IV (0%) lesions; their absolute 5-year cure rate for all stages was 55.5%.

In 1982, Perez and Camel reported their long-term follow-up of patients treated with radiation therapy for invasive carcinoma of the vagina. The actuarial disease-free 5-year survival rate for stage I (39 patients) was 90%; stage IIa (39 patients), 58%; stage IIb (21 patients), 32%; stage III (12 patients), 40%; and stage IV (8 patients), 0%. Of 39 patients with stage I carcinoma, 37 (95%) showed no evidence of vaginal or pelvic recurrence. Most of them received interstitial or intracavitary therapy or both; the addition of external-beam irradiation did not significantly increase survival or tumor control. In stage IIa (paravaginal extension), tumor was controlled in 22 of 34 patients (64.7%) with a combination of brachytherapy and external-beam irradiation; only 2 of 5 (40%) treated with brachytherapy alone exhibited tumor control in the pelvis. The incidence of complications was 9.7% for all stages.

In 1991, Eddy and coworkers published similar results for stage I and stage II lesions of the vagina treated with curative radiotherapy and reported a 5-year survival of 78% for patients assigned to stage I and 71% for patients assigned to stage II. In addition, Stock and colleagues (1995) reported local control rates of 72% for stage I and 62% for stage II disease (see Table 9–6). In the large database (NCDB) reported in 1998, the 5-year relative survival rate was 96% for stage 0, 73% for stage I, 58% for stage II, and 36% for stage III–IV. Women with stage I who were treated with surgery had a 5-year survival of 90% compared with 63% for patients treated with radiotherapy and 79% for patients treated with surgery and radiotherapy.

In the study from MD Anderson, the 5-year disease specific survival was 85% for patients with stage I disease, 78% for stage II, and 58% for stage III/IVa. In this study, external beam radiation fields and dose were determined by evaluating distribution of gross disease and possible sites of microscopic paravaginal and nodal disease.

Vaginal cancers appear to behave like cervical or vulvar cancer by first recurring locally. More than 80% of patients with recurrent disease have pelvic recurrence noted clinically, and most recurrences appear within 2 years of primary therapy. Distant sites of involvement occur later and much less frequently. Effective treatment for previously irradiated but locally recurrent or persistent vaginal cancer patients requires radical surgery (i.e., pelvic exenteration). However, for those with extrapelvic recurrence, the long-term prognosis is poor. Chyle et al reported a 12% 5-year survival rate after first recurrence. Rubin and associates reported on 33 patients with recurrent vaginal cancer. Eighteen had recurrent disease in the pelvis; 15 were extrapelvic recurrences. At the time of the report, 30 patients had died of disease. The average length of survival from recurrence was 8 months. In the past, chemotherapy for recurrent squamous cell carcinoma of the vagina has been relatively ineffective. In the only GOG study of recurrent vaginal cancer, Thigpen and coworkers described 16 patients with squamous cell carcinoma of the vagina treated in a phase II study of cisplatin 50 mg/m^2 intravenously every 3 weeks. The results were disappointing. There was only one responder, and this was a complete responder who had extrapelvic disease and who had received no prior therapy. Most of the patients with recurrence in previously irradiated fields showed no response; 5 of the remaining 15 patients had stable disease.

However, borrowing from studies in patients with cervix cancer, cisplatin is likely one of the more effective agents when it is used in a manner similar to that for recurrent cervical cancer (i.e., single agent or in combination with other active agents). Appropriate considerations would include the taxanes, camptothecin analogues, alkylating agents, vinorelbine, and gemcitabine.

RARE HISTOLOGIES

Adenocarcinoma/clear cell adenocarcinoma

Approximately 6% of vaginal cancers are adenocarcinomas. Before 1965, clear cell adenocarcinoma of the cervix in women younger than 30 years was reported only rarely, and vaginal clear cell adenocarcinoma was unknown. In April 1970, Herbst and Scully reported seven cases of primary vaginal adenocarcinoma in patients between the ages of 15 and 22 years. These seven cases exceeded the number of cases in the world literature in adolescent girls born before 1945. Because of this case clustering, an epidemiologic study of the patients and their families was initiated to identify associative factors. With the addition of another patient to the study, it was discovered that the mothers of seven of the eight patients with vaginal adenocarcinoma had been treated with DES, a non-steroidal synthetic estrogen, in the first trimester of the relevant pregnancy. Since that time, additional cases of vaginal and cervical adenocarcinoma have been reported in patients whose mothers ingested non-steroidal estrogen during pregnancy. DES and related drugs were used to support high-risk pregnancy and reduce fetal wastage in the mid-1940s and 1950s, but their use then declined. The incidence of DES-induced clear cell carcinoma peaked in the mid 1970s.

As of 1992, 594 cases of vaginal and cervical (approximately 40% involve the cervix) adenocarcinoma have been accessioned by the registry established by Herbst and colleagues. Among the cases in which a maternal history was obtainable, the proportion that was positive for medication with DES or chemically related estrogens was approximately two-thirds. Progestins had been administered in six of the cases, and a steroidal estrogen had been administered in another three cases. The risk for development of these carcinomas in the DES-exposed female patient through the age of 24 years has been estimated to be 0.14–1.4 per 1000. Ninety percent of the cases have occurred in patients 14 years of age or older. About 68% of the individuals with clear cell adenocarcinoma of the cervix and 86% of those with primary vaginal tumors had a history of hormone exposure. In addition, there was a lower risk for cancer among women whose mothers began DES after the 12th week of pregnancy. It is not known how many exposed women are in the USA, but estimates place this population at 0.5–2 million.

Patients 15 years of age and younger appeared to have more aggressive carcinomas than those of patients 19 years of age and older. Abnormal bleeding was the initial symptom in most of the patients, but 20% were asymptomatic and carcinomas were discovered on routine pelvic examinations. Cytologic testing has proved useful, but a false negative rate of up to 20% has been reported, probably because of the heavy polymorphonuclear infiltration seen with these lesions. The carcinomas may occur anywhere on the vagina or cervix, but most have been in the upper part of the vagina, particularly on the anterior wall (Fig. 9–7). Adenosis (the presence of glandular epithelium or its mucinous products in the vagina) has been found accompanying vaginal clear cell adenocarcinoma in virtually all cases. Adenosis is benign tissue, but it may be the non-neoplastic precursor of the clear cell adenocarcinoma in some cases, although direct transitions from adenosis to cancer have not been identified. The same observations apply to cervical eversion (ectropion, "congenital erosion") and clear cell adenocarcinoma of the cervix.

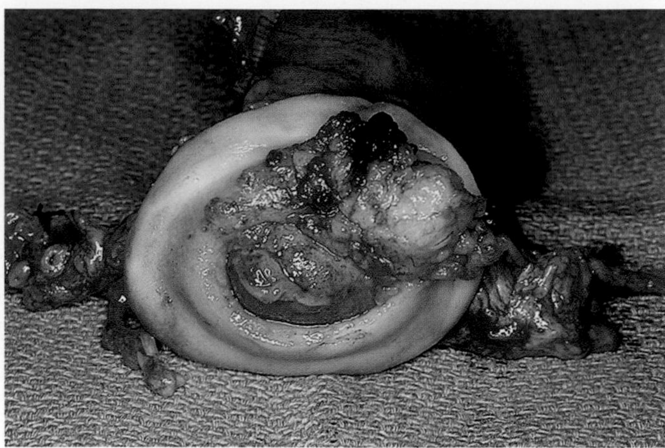

Figure 9–7 Clear cell adenocarcinoma (radical hysterectomy and upper vaginectomy specimen). Note the involvement of the cervix and the anterior wall of the upper vagina.

Both surgery and radiation have been effective in treating these tumors (Table 9–7), although follow-up for many of

Table 9–7 SUGGESTED MANAGEMENT OF CLEAR CELL ADENOCARCINOMA OF THE CERVIX AND VAGINA

Stage	Surgery	Radiation
Cervix		
Ib	Radical hysterectomy with clear vaginal margins and bilateral pelvic lymphadenectomy	5000 cGy whole pelvis in patients with positive pelvic nodes
IIa	Radical hysterectomy with bilateral pelvic lymphadenectomy and upper vaginectomy	5000 cGy whole pelvis in patients with positive pelvic nodes
IIb	Consider exenteration for radiation failures	5000 cGy whole pelvis, tandem and ovoids
IIIa and IIIb	Consider exenteration for radiation failures	6000 cGy whole pelvis, tandem and ovoids
IV	Individualize	
Vagina		
I (upper third of vagina)	Radical hysterectomy with bilateral pelvic lymphadenectomy and upper vaginectomy	5000 cGy whole pelvis in patients with positive nodes
I (lower two-thirds of vagina)	Radical hysterectomy with bilateral pelvic lymphadenectomy and total vaginectomy with vaginal reconstruction	5000 cGy whole pelvis, vaginal application or interstitial implant
II	Consider exenteration for radiation failures	5000 cGy whole pelvis, interstitial implant
III	Consider exenteration for radiation failures	6000 cGy whole pelvis, interstitial implant
IV	Individualize	

these patients is limited. Incidence of lymph node metastases is fairly high, with approximately 16% in stage I and 30% or more in stage II. The clear cell adenocarcinomas tend to remain superficial, suggesting the possibility that this disease can be treated locally, especially if the lesion is small.

The Registry for Research on Hormonal Transplacental Carcinogenesis has reported a study examining the effectiveness of various forms of therapy for early-stage vaginal clear cell adenocarcinomas. Of 219 patients with stage I vaginal clear cell adenocarcinomas, 20% received local therapy and 80% underwent conventional therapy. Actuarial survival rates at 5 and 10 years for patients managed with local therapy and conventional therapy were equivalent (92% and 88%, respectively). This study indicated that for certain early cancers, local therapy, which can conserve reproductive function, is an effective mode. Another study showed that pregnancy does not appear to affect the prognosis or behavior of clear cell adenocarcinoma. However, one instance of pelvic node metastasis has been reported in a patient with invasion of <3 mm.

If the cancer is confined to the cervix or upper vagina, or both, radical hysterectomy with upper vaginectomy and pelvic lymphadenectomy with retention of the ovaries is the recommended therapy. In young patients, avoidance of pelvic irradiation is desirable in view of the increased risks of long-term morbidity (radiation-induced carcinogenesis and progressive vasculitis) in patients surviving many decades after full-dose pelvic irradiation, and the possible decrease of optimal vaginal function.

More extensive tumors and lesions involving the lower two-thirds of the vagina are more suitable for radiation, which would include the pelvic nodes and parametrial tissues. Although some experienced surgeons have used radical hysterectomy with total vaginectomy and split-thickness skin graft vaginal reconstruction in this group of patients, it is difficult to get negative surgical margins (especially on the bladder). Herbst and coworkers reported a discouraging 37% recurrence rate among 22 patients treated by conventional irradiation, but 21 of these 22 patients had large vaginal adenocarcinomas and probably would not have been good surgical candidates for vaginectomy. Pelvic exenterations are reserved for radiation failures in patients with central persistence of the neoplasm and involvement of the lower two-thirds of the vagina.

Table 9–8 FIVE AND TEN-YEAR SURVIVAL RATES FOR 588 PATIENTS WITH CLEAR CELL ADENOCARCINOMA OF THE VAGINA AND CERVIX BY STAGE

Stage	5-year survival (%)	10-year survival (%)
I	91	85
IIa	80	67
IIb	56	47
II (vagina)	82	67
III	37	25
IV	0	0

From Herbst AL: Neoplastic diseases of the vagina. In Mishell DR Jr et al (eds): Comprehensive Gynecology, 3rd ed. St. Louis, Mosby Year Book, 1997.

Transvaginal local excision of stage I vaginal adenocarcinoma, which is associated with higher recurrence rates than transabdominal approaches, appears to be an inferior treatment. Some institutions have attempted radiation treatment with transvaginal cone or implant, especially for small vaginal tumors after local excision. The identification of the risk for pelvic lymph node spread, even in cases of small stage I tumors, led to the recommendation that retroperitoneal node dissection be carried out before the local treatment. Follow-up of many of the cases is limited. Therefore, comparing the efficacy of various modes of therapy is difficult.

Survival percentages are highly correlated with tumor stage. The following percentages were found for patients at these stages:

Stage I	91%
Stage II vaginal	82%
Stage IIa cervical	80%
Stage IIb cervical	56%
Stage III	37%.

The overall survival rate of 80% is somewhat better than the 65% crude survival rate reported for squamous cell carcinoma of the cervix and much higher than the 35–45% overall survival rate reported for squamous cell carcinoma of the vagina. The better prognosis might be the result of early detection because it is occurring mainly in young patients exposed to DES (Table 9–8).

Recurrent adenocarcinoma

A higher proportion of clear cell adenocarcinomas metastasize to the lungs and supraclavicular area when compared to squamous cancers. In the study by Herbst and colleagues, 346 patients were analyzed for frequency, site, and treatment of recurrent disease. Of the 346 patients, 20 were never free of disease after initial therapy, and 19 had died at the time of the report. Recurrence developed in 58 patients, and diagnosis was made in most of these within 3 years after primary tumor treatment: 60% had recurrence in the pelvis, almost half of these being in the vagina; 36% (21 patients) had recurrence in the lungs; and 20% (12 patients) had recurrence in the supraclavicular lymph nodes. Surgery and radiation have been effective in the control of pelvic recurrences in some cases.

The results of chemotherapy are disappointing. Objective responses (>50% reduction of tumor size for longer than 3 months) were observed in 8 of 34 cases in which chemotherapy regimens were analyzed. Two patients who received doxorubicin (Adriamycin) had objective remissions, but an alkylating agent was also given in one of these. Two patients who received combination chemotherapy (5-FU, methotrexate, vincristine, cyclophosphamide, and prednisolone; and 5-FU, dactinomycin, and cyclophosphamide) also had objective remissions. No total remissions were observed. There were no responses in nine cases in which a progestational agent alone was used.

In a 1981 report by Herbst, follow-up data of 409 patients for periods up to 15 years were published. In this study, 55 patients had an initial recurrence in the pelvis (60% of the total group with recurrence) up to 7 years after initial therapy. This emphasizes the importance of prolonged follow-up. Of the 58 patients with recurrences, 12 survived 3 years or longer after treatment of their first recurrence. A second recurrence was observed in 17 of the patients, and 12 of them died within 1 year of the diagnosis. However, three patients had survived longer than 2 years after treatment of their second recurrence.

Primary adenocarcinoma of the vagina can occur unrelated to intrauterine DES exposure. Some cases that were thought to have arisen in association with vaginal adenosis or from foci of endometriosis generally resembled endocervical or endometrial carcinomas. Because of their content of clear cells, others were considered to be of mesonephric origin. A few exceptional cases may have arisen from Gartner's duct remnants and thus may have truly been mesonephric in origin. Therapy for these adenocarcinomas is presently analogous to that for their squamous counterpart.

Vaginal metastases from adenocarcinoma of other pelvic and abdominal organs are more common than primary vaginal cancers. Lesions of cervical and endometrial origin are most common. Ovary, tube, colon, and rectum as well as renal cell neoplasms can also be present with vaginal metastasis.

Malignant melanoma

Malignant melanoma of the vagina is rare and represents <0.5% of all vaginal malignant neoplasms and 0.4–0.8% of all malignant melanomas in women. The main presenting symptoms are vaginal bleeding, vaginal discharge, and the feeling of a mass. The tumors are predominantly located in the lower third of the vagina, commonly on the anterior wall. It is primarily a disease of postmenopausal women. Lesions may be single or multiple, pigmented or nonpigmented, arising from melanocytes present in the epithelium of the vagina (Fig. 9–8).

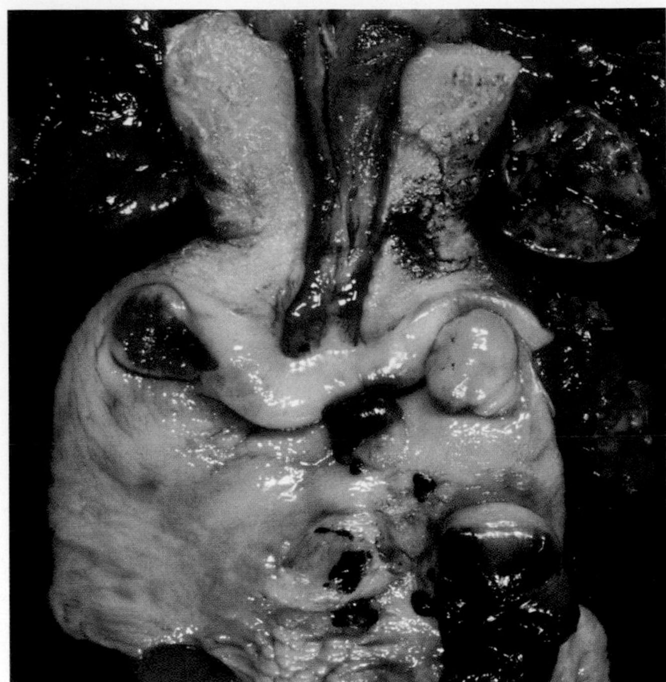

Figure 9–8 An exenteration specimen showing an open uterus, tubes, and ovaries with multifocal melanotic lesions of the vagina in a patient who underwent vaginectomy with her exenteration.

Multiple therapies have been attempted during the past several decades, and surgery remains the treatment of choice. The surgical approach must be tailored to the location of the lesions. The NCDB report noted 192 patients with vaginal melanoma; 95 (49%) were 70 years of age or older. Surgery was used as the first course of treatment in 66%, and 40% received radiotherapy. External radiation was more frequently used to treat advanced melanoma cases. Neoplasms that involve the lower third of the vagina are usually treated similarly to vulvar melanoma, with radical vulvectomy, partial vaginectomy, and inguinal and deep node dissection. Neoplasms that involve the upper two-thirds of the vagina require some form of exenteration for optimal results. Radiation therapy in general has not proved effective, and the results of chemotherapy have been equally disappointing; thus, the radical surgical approach remains the primary therapy when it is applicable.

Survival figures for this group of lesions are difficult to determine because of the infrequent occurrence of this disease. Patients with negative nodes who have disease involving the upper two-thirds of the vagina and are treated by exenteration have about a 50% probability of surviving 5 years or longer. The overall survival rate for vaginal melanoma is about 15%. Lymph node metastases portend a poorer prognosis. Many patients have advanced disease at the time of diagnosis.

Treatment must be based on the extent of the disease, location, tolerance of the patient, and depth of invasion. More and more emphasis is placed on the depth of invasion. Superficial lesions (Clark's level I and level II) can be managed with less than exenterative-type surgery, whereas more deeply invasive tumors must be managed with extended radical surgery with some expectation of a favorable outcome, as reported by Van Nostrand and associates. Survival appears to be more favorable with depths of invasion of <2 mm. In the NCDB report, the 5-year survival rate for 76 patients whose diagnosis was made between 1985 and 1989 was 14%. The number of diagnoses with Clark's level information was small (51 patients). The 3-year relative survival rate by Clark's level without regard to node status or presence of metastasis was as follows:

Level II	45%	(11 patients)
Level III	36%	(5 patients)
Level IV	27%	(4 patients)
Level V	14%	(9 patients)

No level I was reported.

The dissection of lymph nodes that are clinically negative for melanoma of the vagina, urethra, and vulva continues to be controversial. For level I and level II lesions, there appears to be little value in lymphadenectomy if nodes are clinically negative. Whether or not there is a role for selective sampling via lymphatic mapping and sentinel node localization is not known. However, in the few vulvovaginal primary lesions mapped, groin sentinel nodes have been isolated. Such dissections may provide prognostic information without extensive morbidity seen with inguinofemoral lymphadenectomy. Patients with level IV and level V lesions with positive nodes rarely survive, but local control may be achieved with lymphadenectomy. Recurrences develop primarily in the pelvis and lung. The interval to recurrence varies, but it is usually <1 year. Survival from point of recurrence averages 8 months.

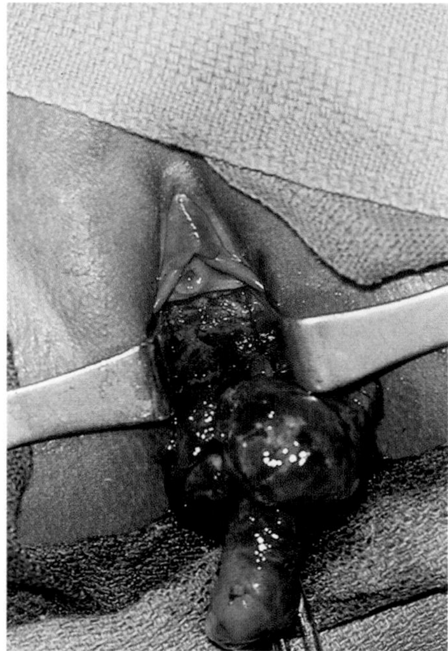

Figure 9–9 Sarcoma botryoides (rhabdomyosarcoma) in a 3-year-old child.

Sarcoma

Spindle cell sarcomas of the vagina, such as leiomyosarcoma and fibrosarcoma, occur rarely. Tavassoli and Norris reported 60 smooth muscle tumors of the vagina. Only five neoplasms recurred, and these were all >3 cm, with >5 mitotic figures per 10 high-power fields (hpf). Local excision was the treatment of choice when the tumor was well differentiated and well circumscribed and the margins were not infiltrated. In general, these lesions behave like their corresponding cell types on the vulva in that the well-differentiated lesions have a much better prognosis than the pleomorphic types, which tend to have poor prognosis regardless of therapy. The vagina, like the vulva, has a rich lymphatic and vascular network, possibly contributing to the early dissemination of these neoplasms (especially the pleomorphic types). In general, hematogenous dissemination occurs surprisingly late in the course of the disease, so that the importance of local therapy is underlined. However, after local excision of a circumscribed lesion and postoperative local radiation therapy, the value of pelvic radiation therapy is unclear. In most instances in which it has been successfully applied, the lesions were well differentiated and well circumscribed, suggesting that surgery itself was curative.

An unusual and tragic lesion that predominantly afflicts children is sarcoma botryoides (Fig. 9–9). These lesions are usually multicentric and tend to arise in the anterior wall at the apex of the vagina. There is a tendency for this tumor to originate higher in the genital tract in older patients. In all patients, the tumor may be multifocal, but this is rare and should not be taken as a basis for extensive surgery.

Whereas these lesions were formerly treated by exenterative procedures, equal success has been obtained in recent years with less radical surgery and adjuvant chemotherapy, with or without radiotherapy. There were 30 sarcomas reported in children from the NCDB; 32 patients were between the ages of 20 and 49 years, 36 patients were between 50 and 69 years, and 37 patients were 70 years or older. The diagnosis was embryonal rhabdomyosarcoma in 70% of the children (21 patients), infantile embryonal carcinoma in 20% (4 patients), and rhabdomyosarcoma in 10% (3 patients). More than three-quarters of the children received chemotherapy, including four-fifths who were treated surgically. The 12 children whose diagnosis was made between 1985 and 1989 were younger than 5 years, and their 5-year survival was 90%.

A combination of vincristine, dactinomycin, and cyclophosphamide appears to be effective in this disease and results in a marked reduction in tumor size when the drug combination is used as initial therapy, permitting more conservative surgery. Although there is continued use of external radiation therapy in many centers, its role in managing sarcoma botryoides of the female genital tract remains unclear. Small lesions appear to be adequately treated with chemotherapy and surgery. A combination of chemotherapy and radiation therapy without surgery has been reported by Flamant and colleagues to be curative of localized vaginal lesions.

The tendency for genitourinary rhabdomyosarcoma to spread to regional lymph nodes is well established. The Intergroup Rhabdomyosarcoma Study reported a 26% incidence of known lymph node metastasis. The pelvis is the most common site for primary recurrences.

Leiomyosarcoma was the most frequent type of sarcoma for adults, accounting for 50% of the cases in patients aged 20–49 years and for 35% in those aged 70 years or older. Adjuvant chemotherapy was used less with increasing age, whereas radiotherapy was used most frequently for the older patient. Survival decreased with increasing age. Relative 5-year survival was 84% for those aged 20–49 years and 48% for those 50–69 years. Those older than 70 years had a 2-year relative survival of only 30%.

Endodermal sinus tumor

This rare carcinoma occurring in the vaginas of infants is most likely of germ cell origin. Norris and coworkers use the term *mesonephroma* or *mesonephric carcinoma* because of an alternative theory of their origin. The disease usually occurs in infants younger than 2 years, and survivals have been poor, with <25% of patients alive at 2 years. Lesions most often occur on the posterior vaginal wall or fornices. Combination therapy (surgery and chemotherapy) appears appropriate. Patients who have vaginal endodermal sinus tumors are usually seen because of vaginal bleeding or discharge and have polypoid or sessile tumors. In the majority of cases, the differential diagnosis of endodermal sinus tumor is that of embryonal rhabdomyosarcoma (sarcoma botryoides). This is the most common vaginal tumor of children and almost always develops in patients younger than 5 years; the average age at the time of diagnosis is 3 years. The characteristic grapelike appearance of sarcoma botryoides differs from the usual endodermal sinus tumor. In addition, the edematous and cellular areas that are composed of immature skeletal muscle cells characteristic of embryonal rhabdomyosarcoma bear no resemblance to the histologic appearance of endodermal sinus tumor.

Young and Scully described 32 patients with endodermal sinus tumors. At the time of the report, 18 had died of their disease despite radical surgical therapy. Six patients were treated by surgery and then received vincristine, dactinomycin, and cyclophosphamide. Two of the six patients also received radiation therapy. All were alive and free of disease 2–9 years after surgery. Copeland and associates have reported similar results with the same combination. Thus, chemotherapy after conservative surgical excision can be effective in controlling this neoplasm.

Special considerations

Pride and Buchler suggested that vaginal carcinoma might occur more frequently in patients who received pelvic irradiation 10 years or longer before the appearance of the new lesion. Of patients previously treated for cervical cancer, those who had received radiation therapy (≥5 years previously) were more likely to develop vaginal cancer than were those whose cervical cancers had been treated surgically, according to Murad and colleagues. Abnormal vaginal cytologic findings are common after radiation, and many have ignored these dysplastic lesions as if they were routine results of irradiation therapy. However, a study from MD Anderson suggested that 30% of these "dysplastic" or "intraepithelial" lesions will progress to invasive cancer if they are left untreated. In this report, 28 patients with dysplasia or carcinoma in situ of the vagina after previous pelvic radiation therapy were observed for progression, and nine developed invasive carcinoma. The median length of time from diagnosis of the intraepithelial lesion to invasion was 34 months. Therefore, treatment of these intraepithelial lesions by local excision is warranted. Laser vaporization, or topical chemotherapy with 5-fluorouracil (5-FU) should be seriously considered.

URETHRAL CANCER

Primary carcinoma of the female urethra is a rare neoplasm with a relatively poor prognosis, except when disease is limited to the anterior or distal urethra. If there is any vaginal involvement, the cancer is considered a vaginal primary tumor. The incidence is 1 in 1500 female cancer admissions, which accounts for <0.1% of all female genital malignant neoplasms. Because of the rarity of the disease, only a few reports with significant numbers of treated patients have been published. The Cancer Committee of FIGO has not yet proposed a stage grouping for carcinoma of the urethra.

The majority of urethral lesions are squamous growths originating from the mucosa and, less commonly, adenocarcinomas originating from the paraurethral ducts. Sarcomas and melanomas have rarely been described. Lesions of the distal third of the urethra are elongated growths palpable through the anterior vaginal wall or exophytic neoplasms obscuring the urethral orifice. Because they can be confused with urethral carbuncle, urethral polyp, or mucosal ectropion, biopsy should be done to confirm diagnosis.

Unlike in vulvar cancer, the role of radiotherapy for this lesion is substantial. The proximal half of the urethra must be preserved to ensure urinary continence. This often leads to local failure when a surgical approach is chosen as the sole modality. Interstitial irradiation to the central lesion has thus gained wide acceptance for this site. Our recommendation has been to dissect the inguinal lymph nodes as both a diagnostic and a therapeutic procedure. Discovery of lymph node metastases should be followed by pelvic and local irradiation. Pelvic lymphadenectomy is usually omitted, even with positive inguinal nodes, because whole-pelvis irradiation should follow as soon as the groin incisions have healed. Radiation therapy alone has been less successful in controlling groin metastases, leading to the difficult problem of a fungating necrotic lesion eroding through the skin of the groin in a previously irradiated area. Local groin failure is not common after surgical resection and adjuvant radiation to the inguinal area.

Lesions of the distal urethra appear to have a better prognosis than those of the upper lumen. The poor results in carcinoma of the upper urethra appear to be caused by early lymphatic dissemination to inaccessible pelvic and periaortic nodes.

Weghaupt and colleagues described 62 women with primary carcinoma of the urethra treated with combined radiation therapy; 42 patients (67.7%) had tumors of the anterior urethra, and the posterior urethra was involved in 20 women (32.3%). In 19 patients (30.6%), the clinical diagnosis of lymph node involvement was made. Treatment was strictly individualized, but an administered tumor dose of 5500–7000 cGy was always attempted. The overall 5-year survival was 64.5%. The 5-year survival was higher for patients with anterior urethral carcinoma (71.4%) than for patients with posterior carcinoma (50%). These are the most favorable results reported in the literature and probably reflect sophisticated use of radiation therapy techniques.

BIBLIOGRAPHY

SQUAMOUS CELL CARCINOMA

Ali MM, Huang DT, Goplerud DR et al: Radiation alone for carcinoma of the vagina: Variation in response related to the location of the primary tumor. Cancer 77:1934–1939, 1996.

Al-Kurdi M, Monaghan JM. Thirty-two years experience in management of primary tumors of the vagina. BJOG 88:1145–1150, 1981.

Andersen ES: Primary carcinoma of the vagina: A study of 29 cases. Gynecol Oncol 33:317, 1989.

Ball HG, Berman ML: Management of primary vaginal carcinoma. Gynecol Oncol 14:154, 1982.

Barclay DL: Carcinoma of the vagina after hysterectomy for severe dysplasia or carcinoma in situ of the cervix. Gynecol Oncol 8:1, 1979.

Bell J et al: Vaginal cancer after hysterectomy for benign disease: Value of cytologic screening. Obstet Gynecol 64:699, 1984.

Beller V, Sideri M, Maidonneuve P, Benedet JL, Heintz APH, Ngan HYS et al. Carcinoma of the vagina: 24th annual report on the results of treatment in gynecological cancer. J Epidemiol Biostat 6:141–152, 2001.

Benedet JL et al: Primary invasive carcinoma of the vagina. Obstet Gynecol 62:715, 1983.

Benedet JL and Saunders BH. Carcinoma in situ of the vagina. Am J Obstet Gynecol 148:695–700, 1984.

Boronow RC: Therapeutic alternative to primary exenteration for advanced vulvovaginal cancer. Gynecol Oncol 1:233, 1973.

Brinton LA, Nasca PC, Mallin K et al: Case-control study of in situ and invasive carcinoma of the vagina. Gynecol Oncol 38:49, 1990.

Brown AR, Fletcher GH, Rutledge FN: Irradiation of in situ and invasive squamous cell carcinoma of the vagina. Cancer 28:1278, 1971.

Burger MPM et al: The importance of the groin node status for the survival of T1 and T2 vulval carcinoma patients. Gynecol Oncol 57:327, 1995.

Choo YC, Anderson DG. Neoplasms of the vagina following cervix carcinoma. Gynecol Oncol 14:125–132, 1982.

Chu AM, Beechinor R: Survival and recurrence in the radiation treatment of carcinoma of the vagina. Gynecol Oncol 19:298, 1984.

Chyle V, Zagars GK, Wheeler JA et al: Definitive radiotherapy for carcinoma of the vagina: Outcome and prognostic factors. Int J Radiat Oncol Biol Phys 35:891–905, 1996.

Creasman WT, Phillips J, Menck HR: The National Cancer Data Base report on cancer of the vagina. Cancer 83:1033, 1998.

Daling JR, Madeleine MM, Schwartz SM et al: A population-based study of squamous cell vaginal cancer: HPV and cofactors. Gynecol Oncol 84:263–270, 2002.

Davis KP, Stanhope CR, Garton GR et al: Invasive vaginal carcinoma: Analysis of early-stage disease. Gynecol Oncol 42:131, 1991.

DiDomenico A: Primary vaginal squamous cell carcinoma in the young patient. Gynecol Oncol 35:181, 1989.

DiSaia PJ, Syed AMN, Puthawala AA: Malignant neoplasia of the upper vagina. Endocurie Hypertherm Oncol 6:251, 1990.

Eddy GL, Marks RD Jr, Miller MC III et al: Primary invasive vaginal carcinoma. Am J Obstet Gynecol 165:292, 1991.

Eddy GL, Singh KP, Gansler TS: Superficially invasive carcinoma of the vagina following treatment for cervical cancer: A report of six cases. Gynecol Oncol 36:376, 1990.

Fine BA et al: The curative potential of radiation therapy in the treatment of primary vaginal carcinoma. Am J Clin Oncol 19:39, 1996.

Frank SJ, Jhingran A, Levenback C, Eifel PJ. Definitive radiation therapy for squamous cell carcinoma of the vagina. Int J Rad Oncol Biol Phys 62: 138–147, 2005.

Fu YS. Pathology of the uterine cervix, vagina, and vulva. 2nd edition Philadelphia: Saunders, 2002: 531.

Gallup DG et al: Invasive squamous cell carcinoma of the vagina: A 14 year study. Obstet Gynecol 69:782, 1987.

Grigsby PW, Siegel BA, Dehdashti F: Lymph node staging by positron emission tomography in patients with carcinoma of the cervix. J Clin Oncol 19:3745–3749, 2001.

Hintz BL et al: Radiation tolerance of the vaginal mucosa. Int J Radiat Oncol Biol Phys 6:711, 1980.

Hoffman MS et al: Upper vaginectomy for in situ and occult, superficially invasive carcinoma of the vagina. Am J Obstet Gynecol 166:30, 1992.

Houghton CRS, Iversen T: Squamous cell carcinoma of the vagina: A clinical study of the location of the tumor. Gynecol Oncol 13:365, 1982.

Johnston GA, Kotz J, Boutselis JG: Primary invasive carcinoma of the vagina. Surg Gynecol Obstet 156:34, 1983.

Joseph RE et al: Small cell neuroendocrine carcinoma of the vagina. Cancer 70:784, 1992.

Kanbour AI, Klionsky B, Murphy AL: Carcinoma of the vagina following cervical cancer. Cancer 34:1838, 1974.

Kirkbride P, Fyles A, Rawlings GA et al: Carcinoma of the vagina: Experience at the Princess Margaret Hospital. Gynecol Oncol 56: 435–443, 1995.

Krebs HB: Treatment of vaginal intraepithelial neoplasia with laser and topical 5-fluorouracil. Obstet and Gynecol 73:657–660, 1989.

Kucera H, Vavra N: Radiation management of primary carcinoma of the vagina: Clinical and histopathological variables associated with survival. Gynecol Oncol 40:12, 1991.

Kucera H, Langer M, Smekal G, Weghaupt K. Radiotherapy of primary carcinoma of the vagina: management and results of different therapy schemes. Gynecol Oncol 21:87–93, 1985.

Lamoreaux W, Grigsby P, Dehdashti F, Zoberi I, Powell M, Gibb R, Rader J, Mutch D, Siegel B. FDG-PET evaluation of vaginal carcinoma. International J Radiat Oncol Biol Phys 62:733–737.

Lee RA, Symmonds RE: Recurrent carcinoma in situ of the vagina in patients previously treated for in situ carcinoma of the cervix. Obstet Gynecol 48:61, 1976.

Malmström H, Enquist M: Primary invasive cancer of the vagina. Int J Gynecol Cancer 7:205, 1997.

Manetta A, Gutrecht EL, Berman ML et al: Primary invasive carcinoma of the vagina. Obstet Gynecol 76:639, 1990.

Manetta A, Pinto JL, Larson JE et al: Primary invasive carcinoma of the vagina. Obstet Gynecol 72:77, 1988.

Mazur MT, Hsueh S, Gersell DJ: Metastasis to the female genital tract: Analysis of 325 cases. Cancer 53: 1978–1984, 1984.

Merrill JA, Bender WT: Primary carcinoma of the vagina. Obstet Gynecol 11: 3–11, 1958.
Murad TM, Durant JR, Maddox WA et al: The pathologic behavior of primary vaginal carcinoma and its relationship to cervical cancer. Cancer 35:787, 1975.
Nanavati PJ et al: High-dose-rate brachytherapy in primary stage I and II vaginal cancer. Gynecol Oncol 51:67, 1993.
Nori D, Hilaris BS, Shu F: Radiation therapy of primary vaginal carcinoma. Int J Radiat Oncol Biol Phys 70:20, 1981.
Nori D et al: Radiation therapy of primary vaginal carcinoma. Int J Radiat Oncol Biol Phys 9:1471, 1983.
Perez CA, Camel HM: Long-term follow-up in radiation therapy of carcinoma of the vagina. Cancer 49:1308, 1982.
Perez CA, Arneson AN, Dehner LP, Galakatos A. Radiation therapy in carcinoma of the vagina. Obstet Gynecol 44:862–872, 1974.
Perez CA, Grigsby PW, Garipagaoglu M et al: Factors affecting long-term outcome of irradiation in carcinoma of the vagina. Int J Radiat Oncol Biol Phys 44: 37–45, 1999.
Peters WA, Kumar NB, Morley GW: Carcinoma of the vagina: Factors influencing treatment of outcome. Cancer 55:892, 1985.
Phillips B, Buchsbaum HJ, Lifshitz S: Pelvic exenteration for vulvovaginal carcinoma. Am J Obstet Gynecol 141:1038, 1981.
Pingley S, Shrivastava SK, Sarin R et al: Primary carcinoma of the vagina: Tata Memorial Hospital experience. Int J Radiat Oncol Biol Phys 46:101–108, 2000.
Piura B, Rabinvich A, Cohen Y, Glezerman M: Primary squamous cell carcinoma of the vagina: Report of four cases and review of the literature. Eur J Gynaecol Oncol 19:60–63, 1998.
Prempree T: Role of radiation therapy in the management of primary carcinoma of the vagina. Acta Radiol Oncol 21:195, 1982.
Prempree T et al: Radiation management of primary carcinoma of the vagina. Cancer 40:109, 1977.
Pride GL, Buchler DA: Carcinoma of vagina 10 or more years following pelvic irradiation therapy. Am J Obstet Gynecol 127:513, 1977.
Pride GL et al: Primary invasive squamous carcinoma of the vagina. Obstet Gynecol 53:218, 1979.
Puthawala A et al: Integrated external and interstitial radiation therapy for primary carcinoma of the vagina. Obstet Gynecol 62:367, 1983.
Reddy S, Lee MS, Graham JE, Yordan EL, Phillips R, Saxena VS et al. Radiation therapy in primary carcinoma of the vagina. Gynecol Oncol 26:19–24, 1987.
Reddy S et al: Results of radiotherapeutic management of primary carcinoma of the vagina. Int J Radiat Oncol Biol Phys 21:1041, 1991.
Rome RM, England PG. Management of vaginal intraepithelial neoplasia: a series of 132 cases with long-term follow-up. Int J Gynecol Cancer 10:382–390, 2000.
Rubin SC, Young J, Mikuta JJ: Squamous carcinoma of the vagina: Treatment, complications, and long-term follow-up. Gynecol Oncol 20:346, 1985.
Rutledge FN: Cancer of the vagina. Am J Obstet Gynecol 97:635, 1967.
Smith, FR: Clinical management of cancer of the vagina. Ann NY Acad Sci 114: 1012–1019, 1964.
Spirtos NM, Doshi BP, Kapp DS et al: Radiation therapy for primary squamous cell carcinoma of the vagina: Stanford University experience. Gynecol Oncol 35:20, 1989.
Stehman FB, Bundy BN, Thomas G et al: Groin dissection versus groin radiation in carcinoma of the vulva: A Gynecologic Oncology Group study. Int J Radiat Oncol Biol Phys 24:389–396, 1992.
Stock RG, Chen AS, Seski J: A 30-year experience in the management of primary carcinoma of the vagina: Analysis of prognostic factors and treatment modalities. Gynecol Oncol 56:45, 1995.
Sulak P, Barnhill D, Heller P, Weiser E, Hoskins W, Park P et al. Nonsquamous cancer of the vagina. Gynecol Oncol 29:309–320, 1988.
Tewari KS, Cappuccini F, Puthawala AA et al: Primary invasive carcinoma of the vagina: Treatment with interstitial brachytherapy. Cancer 91:758–770, 2001.
Thigpen JT, Blessing JA, Howresky HD et al: Phase II trial of cisplatin in advanced or recurrent cancer of the vagina. Gynecol Oncol 23:101, 1986.
Tjalma WAA, Monaghan JM, de Barros Lopes A, Naik R, Nordin AJ, Weyler JJ. The role of surgery in invasive squamous cell carcinoma of the vagina. Gynecol Oncol 81:360–365, 2001.
Urbanski K et al: Primary invasive vaginal carcinoma treated with radiotherapy: Analysis of prognostic factors. Gynecol Oncol 60:16, 1996.
Usherwood MM: Management of vaginal carcinoma after hysterectomy. Am J Obstet Gynecol 122:352, 1975.
Van Dam P, Sonnemans H, van Dam PJ, Verkinderen L, Dirix LY: Sentinel node detection in patients with vaginal carcinoma. Gynecol Oncol 92:89–92, 2004.
Woodman CB, Mould JJ, Jordan JA: Radiotherapy in the management of vaginal intraepithelial neoplasia after hysterectomy. Br J Obstet Gynaecol 95:976–979, 1988.
Wright VC, Chapman W: Intraepithelial neoplasia of the lower female genital tract: Etiology, investigation, and management. Semin Surg Oncol 8:180–190, 1992.

ADENOCARCINOMA/CLEAR CELL ADENOCARCINOMA

Bornstein J, Kaufman RH, Adam E et al: Human papillomavirus associated with vaginal intraepithelial neoplasia in women exposed to diethylstilbestrol in utero. Obstet Gynecol 70:75, 1987.
Clement PB, Benedet JL: Adenocarcinoma in situ of the vagina. Cancer 43:2479, 1979.
Demars LR et al: Case report: Primary non-clear cell adenocarcinomas of the vagina in older DES-exposed women. Gynecol Oncol 58:389, 1995.
Greenberg ER et al: Breast cancer in mothers given diethylstilbestrol in pregnancy. N Engl J Med 311:1393, 1984.
Greenwald P et al: Vaginal cancer after maternal treatment with synthetic estrogens. N Engl J Med 285:390, 1971.
Hanselaar AGJM, Van Leusen NDM, De Wilde PCM et al: Clear cell adenocarcinoma of the vagina and cervix. Cancer 67:1971, 1991.
Haskel S, Chen SS, Spiegel G: Vaginal endometrioid adenocarcinoma arising in vaginal endometriosis: A case report and literature review. Gynecol Oncol 34:232, 1989.
Herbst AL: Clear cell adenocarcinoma and the current status of DES-exposed females. Cancer 48:484, 1981.
Herbst A, Anderson D: Clear cell adenocarcinoma of the vagina and cervix secondary to intrauterine exposure to diethylstilbestrol. Semin Surg Oncol 6:343, 1990.
Herbst AL, Scully RE: Adenocarcinoma of the vagina in adolescence: A report of seven cases, including six clear cell carcinomas (so-called mesonephromas). Cancer 25:745, 1970.
Herbst AL et al: Clear cell adenocarcinoma of the genital tract in young females: Registry report. N Engl J Med 287:1259, 1972.
Herbst AL et al: Epidemiologic aspects and factors related to survival in 384 registry cases of clear cell adenocarcinoma of the vagina and cervix. Am J Obstet Gynecol 135:876, 1979.
Herbst AL et al: Risk factors of the development of diethylstilbestrol-associated clear cell adenocarcinoma. Am J Obstet Gynecol 154:814, 1986.
Hormio M, Soloheimo AM: Clear cell adenocarcinoma of the female genital tract. Acta Obstet Gynecol Scand 49:259, 1970.
Manetta A, Gutrecht EL, Berman ML et al: Primary invasive carcinoma of the vagina. Obstet Gynecol 76:639, 1990.
Rosenfeld PA, Lowe BA: Solitary metastasis of renal adenocarcinoma to the vagina: A case report. J Reprod Med 35:295, 1990.
Rutledge F: Cancer of the vagina. Am J Obstet Gynecol 97:635, 1967.
Senekjian EK, Frey KW, Anderson D et al: Local therapy in stage I clear cell adenocarcinoma of the vagina. Cancer 60:1319, 1987.
Senekjian EK, Frey K, Herbst AL: Pelvic exenteration in clear cell adenocarcinoma of the vagina and cervix. Gynecol Oncol 34:413, 1989.

Senekjian EK et al: Clear cell adenocarcinoma (CCA) of the vagina and cervix in association with pregnancy. Gynecol Oncol 24:207, 1986.

MALIGNANT MELANOMA

Borazjani G, Prem KA, Okagaki T et al: Primary malignant melanoma of the vagina: A clinicopathological analysis of 10 cases. Gynecol Oncol 37:264, 1990.

Breslow A: Thickness, cross-sectional areas, and depth of invasion in the prognosis of cutaneous melanoma. Ann Surg 172:902, 1970.

Breslow A: Tumor thickness, level of invasion, and node dissection in stage I cutaneous melanoma. Am J Surg 182:572, 1975.

Buckanan DJ, Schlaerth J, Kurosaki T: Primary vaginal melanoma. Thirteen-year disease-free survival after wide local excision and review of recent literature. Am J Obstet Gynecol 178:1177, 1998.

Clark WH Jr et al: The histogenesis and biologic behavior of primary human malignant melanomas of the skin. Cancer Res 29:705, 1969.

Geisler JP et al: Pelvic exenteration for malignant melanomas of the vagina or urethra with over 3 mm of invasion. Gynecol Oncol 59:338, 1995.

Liu L, Hou Y, Li J et al: Primary malignant melanoma of the vagina: A report of seven cases. Obstet Gynecol 70:569, 1987.

Morrow CP, DiSaia PJ: Malignant melanoma of the female genitalia: A clinical analysis. Obstet Gynecol Surv 31:233, 1976.

Reid GC, Schmidt RW, Roberts JA et al: Primary melanoma of the vagina: A clinicopathologic analysis. Obstet Gynecol 74:190, 1989.

Van Nostrand KM et al: Primary vaginal melanoma: Improved survival with radical pelvic surgery. Gynecol Oncol 55:234, 1994.

SARCOMA

Copeland LJ et al: Sarcoma botryoides of the female genital tract. Gynecol Oncol 66:262, 1985.

Curtin JP et al: Soft-tissue sarcoma of the vagina and vulva: A clinicopathologic study. Obstet Gynecol 86:269, 1995.

Flamant F et al: Embryonal rhabdomyosarcoma of the vagina in children. Eur J Cancer 15:527, 1979.

Hilgers R: Pelvic exenteration for vaginal embryonal and rhabdomyosarcoma. Gynecol Oncol 45:175, 1975.

Kaufman RH, Gardner HL: Tumors of the vulva and vagina: Benign mesodermal tumors. Clin Obstet Gynecol 8:953, 1965.

La Vecchia C, Draper J, Franceshi S: Childhood non-ovarian female genital tract cancer in Britain. Cancer 54:188, 1984.

Mahesh Kumar AP et al: Combined therapy to prevent complete pelvic exenteration for rhabdomyosarcoma of the vagina or uterus. Cancer 37:118, 1976.

Mitchell M, Talerman A, Sholl JS et al: Pseudosarcoma botryoides in pregnancy: Report of a case with ultrastructural observations. Obstet Gynecol 70:522, 1987.

Ngan HYS, Fisher C, Blake P, Shepherd JH: Vaginal sarcoma: The Royal Marsden experience. Int J Gynecol Cancer 4:337, 1994.

Norris HJ, Bagley GP, Taylor HB: Carcinoma of the infant vagina: A distinctive tumor. Arch Pathol 90:473, 1970.

O'Connell MEA et al: Intravaginal iridium-192 in the management of embryonal rhabdomyosarcoma. Clin Oncol 3:236, 1991.

Ortega JA: A therapeutic approach to childhood pelvic rhabdomyosarcoma without pelvic exenteration. J Pediatr 94:205, 1979.

Piver MS et al: Combined radical surgery, radiation therapy and chemotherapy in infants with vulvovaginal embryonal rhabdomyosarcoma. Obstet Gynecol 45:522, 1973.

Rutledge FN, Sullivan M: Sarcoma botryoides. Ann N Y Acad Sci 142:694, 1967.

Rywlin AM, Simmons RJ, Robinson MJ: Leiomyoma of vagina recurrent in pregnancy: A case with apparent hormone dependency. South Med J 62:1449, 1969.

Tavassoli FA, Norris HJ: Smooth muscle tumors of the vagina. Obstet Gynecol 53:689, 1979.

ENDODERMAL SINUS TUMOR

Aartsen EJ, Delemarre JFM, Gerretsen G: Endodermal sinus tumor of the vagina: Radiation therapy and progeny. Obstet Gynecol 81:893, 1993.

Allyn DL, Silverberg SG, Salzberg AM: Endodermal sinus tumor of the vagina. Cancer 27:1231, 1971.

Andersen WA et al: Endodermal sinus tumor of the vagina. Cancer 56:1025, 1985.

Copeland LJ et al: Endodermal sinus tumor of the vagina and cervix. Cancer 55:2558, 1985.

Young RH, Scully RE: Endodermal sinus tumor of the vagina: A report of nine cases in review of the literature. Gynecol Oncol 18:380, 1984.

URETHRAL CANCER

Bolduan JP, Farah RN: Primary urethral neoplasms: Review of 30 cases. J Urol 25:198, 1981.

Delclos L, Wharton JT, Fletcher GH et al: The role of brachytherapy in the treatment of primary carcinoma of the vagina and female urethra. In George FW (ed): Modern Interstitial and Intracavitary Radiation Management, Vol 6. New York, Masson, 1981.

Dodson MK et al: Female urethral adenocarcinoma: Evidence for more than one tissue of origin? Gynecol Oncol 59:352, 1995.

Fagan GE, Hertig AT: Carcinoma of the female urethra. Obstet Gynecol 6:1, 1955.

Geisler JP et al: Pelvic exenteration for malignant melanomas of the vagina or urethra with over 3 mm of invasion. Gynecol Oncol 59:338, 1995.

Mayer R, Fowler JE, Clayton M: Localized urethral cancer in women. Cancer 60:1548, 1987.

Meis JM, Ayala AG, Johnson DE: Adenocarcinoma of the urethra in women: A clinicopathologic study. Cancer 60:1038, 1987.

Roberts TW, Melicow MM: Pathology and natural history of urethral tumors in females: A review of 65 cases. Urology 10:583, 1977.

Taggart CG, Cortro JR, Rutledge FN: Carcinoma of the female urethra. AJR 114:145, 1972.

Weghaupt K, Gerstner GJ, Kucera H: Radiation therapy for primary carcinoma of the female urethra: A survey over 25 years. Gynecol Oncol 17:58, 1984.

10 The Adnexal Mass and Early Ovarian Cancer

Philip J. DiSaia, M.D.

ADNEXAL MASS

The adnexae consist of the fallopian tubes, broad ligament, ovaries, and structures within the broad ligament that are formed from embryologic rests. The differential diagnosis in management of the adnexal mass is complex because of the scope of the disorders that it encompasses and the numerous therapies that may be appropriate (Table 10–1). It is the risk of malignancy that propels the system as well as the fundamental concept that early diagnosis and treatment in cancer are related to lessened mortality and morbidity. An adnexal mass often involves ovarian substance because of the propensity of the ovary for neoplasia. Fewer neoplasms occur in the fallopian tube, although that structure may commonly be involved in an inflammatory process that manifests as an adnexal mass. It is estimated that 5–10% of women in the USA will undergo a surgical procedure for a suspected ovarian neoplasm during their lifetime, and 13–21% of these women will be found to have an ovarian malignant neoplasm. The overwhelming majority of adnexal masses are benign, and it is important to determine preoperatively whether a patient is at high risk for ovarian malignant disease to minimize the number of operative procedures performed for self-limited processes. To determine whether an adnexal mass requires surgery and what the appropriate preparation and intervention should be, the preoperative evaluation includes a complete history and physical examination as well as liberal use of transvaginal ultrasonography and a determination of CA-125 level. Management then depends on a combination of many predictive factors, including age and menopausal status of the patient, size of the mass, ultrasonographic features, presence or absence of symptoms, CA-125 level, and unilaterality vs bilaterality. Age is probably the most important factor for determining the potential for malignant change.

The differential diagnosis of an adnexal mass varies considerably with the age of the patient. In premenarchal girls and postmenopausal women, an adnexal mass should be considered highly abnormal and must be immediately investigated. In premenarchal patients, most neoplasms are germ cell in origin and require immediate surgical exploration (Table 10–2). Stromal, germ cell, and epithelial tumors are seen in postmenopausal women. Any enlargement of the ovary is abnormal in the group and should be considered malignant until it is proved otherwise. Many clinicians believe that any palpable ovary in a postmenopausal patient suggests malignant change and requires further study and probably laparotomy (see section on postmenopausal ovary, p 296).

In the menstruating patient (reproductive-age period), the differential diagnosis is varied; both benign and malignant tumors of multiple organs can occur. On occasion, extragenital lesions, which are often large and cystic, are found on pelvic examination; exploratory laparotomy is indicated because of the size alone. These extragenital lesions include peritoneal cysts, omental cysts, retroperitoneal

Table 10–1 DIFFERENTIAL DIAGNOSIS OF ADNEXAL MASS

Organ	Cystic	Solid
Ovary	Functional cyst Neoplastic cyst Benign Malignant Endometriosis	Neoplasm Benign Malignant
Fallopian tube	Tubo-ovarian abscess Hydrosalpinx Parovarian cyst	Tubo-ovarian abscess Ectopic pregnancy Neoplasm
Uterus	Intrauterine pregnancy in a bicornuate uterus	Pedunculated or interligamentous myoma
Bowel	Sigmoid or cecum distended with gas or feces	Diverticulitis Ileitis Appendicitis Colonic cancer
Miscellaneous	Distended bladder Pelvic kidney Urachal cyst	Abdominal wall hematoma or abscess Retroperitoneal neoplasm

Table 10–2 FREQUENCY DISTRIBUTION OF ADNEXAL MASSES IN CHILDHOOD

Mass	Age of patient at diagnosis (0–20 yr)	%
Non-neoplastic	335	64
Simple or follicular cyst	117	23
Corpus luteum cyst	143	28
Other*	75	14
Neoplastic	186	36
Benign	144	28
Malignant	42	8
Germ cell	17	3
Stromal	9	2
Epithelial	14	3
Gonadoblastoma	2	1
Total	521	

*Endometrioma, polycystic ovary syndrome, pelvic inflammatory disease, ectopic pregnancy.
Modified from Van Winter JT, Simmons PS, Podratz KC: Surgically treated adnexal masses in infancy, childhood, and adolescence. Am J Obstet Gynecol 170:1780, 1994.

lesions, and diseases of the gastrointestinal tract (cecum, appendix, sigmoid, and even small bowel, any of which can fall into the pelvis and become adherent). If one suspects gastrointestinal origin of the mass, appropriate radiographic studies usually help in the definitive diagnosis.

The adnexal mass is usually secondary to disease of one of the genital organs in the reproductive-age patient. Detection of pelvic abnormalities is more frequent in women of reproductive age because these patients have relatively frequent periodic screening for cancer detection and contraceptive counseling. Although most pelvic masses occur in this age range, fortunately the majority are histologically benign. Detection of an adnexal mass is greatly facilitated by a rectovaginal examination (see Fig. 3–14), which allows more complete access to the cul-de-sac as well as to the more superficial areas of the pelvic basin. This approach permits deeper penetration of the examining fingers. We recommend a rectovaginal examination as the primary method for examining the pelvis.

Differential diagnosis

Adnexal masses of gynecologic origin

This category includes disorders of the uterus, fallopian tubes, ovaries, and their adjacent structures. The process that creates the mass can be congenital, functional, neoplastic, or inflammatory.

Uterine masses

Pregnancy should always be kept in mind as a cause of uterine enlargement. Most physicians are familiar with the unreliability of a menstrual history, and any patient in the reproductive-age period with a pelvic mass should first have pregnancy ruled out. This can be done by any of a variety of pregnancy tests or by detection of a fetus with ultrasound examination.

Myomas of the uterus are the most common uterine neoplasms (Fig. 10-1). They are usually discrete, relatively round tumors that are firm to palpation and may be single or multiple. Myomas may be located within the myometrium (intramural), just beneath the endometrial lining (submucous), or on the surface of the uterus (serous). A myoma may frequently be found in the broad ligament attached to the lower uterine segment by a thin pedicle. This will often confuse the examiner and suggest that the mass originates

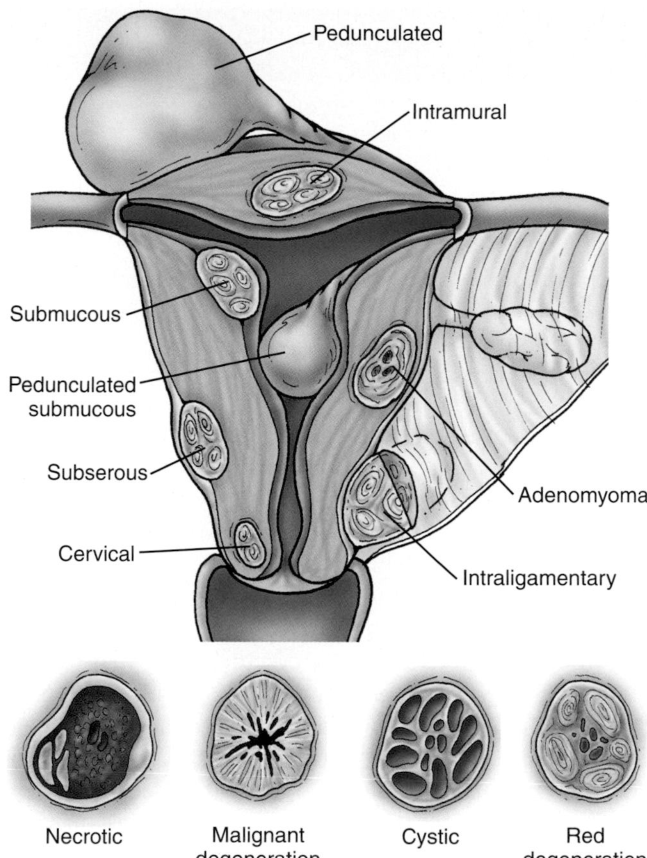

Figure 10–1 Myomas can be seen initially in multiple sizes and states of growth, disease, and degeneration. (Courtesy of Erle Henriksen, MD, Los Angeles, California.)

in the ovary or tube. In the USA, myomas are found in at least 10% of white women and 30–40% of black women older than 35 years. In the postmenopausal group, it is said that the incidence increases to 30% in white women and 50% in black women. Fortunately, these neoplasms usually shrink after menopause, especially in patients not receiving high doses of exogenous estrogen stimulation. It appears that most of these benign neoplasms are somewhat estrogen dependent. Growth is commonly seen during pregnancy, probably secondary to elevated hormone levels. Degeneration, infarction, and infection can occur in these lesions, and these complications are associated with considerable lower abdominal pain. Sarcomatous elements, associated with myomas <0.1% of the time, are most often recognized postoperatively. Symptoms of associated sarcomatous elements may include a rapidly enlarging pelvic mass, often accompanied by pain and tenderness. The mean age at diagnosis of these lesions is 50–55 years, with a range of 25–85 years.

A recent enlargement of the uterus in the postmenopausal patient is rarely caused by fibroids, particularly if the enlargement develops in a short time ("rapid" growth). The use of hormone replacement therapy in and of itself is not an explanation for such an enlargement. The most probable diagnosis is a malignant neoplasm, and physicians must prepare to do an appropriate surgical procedure even if the result of dilatation and curettage (D&C) is negative.

Other conditions that can cause enlargement of the uterus are adenomyosis and endometrial carcinoma or sarcoma. Endometrial carcinoma can enlarge the uterus to as much as four times normal size. The diagnosis of endometrial carcinoma is of course made by D&C of the endometrial cavity or other appropriate endometrial sampling.

Ovarian masses

Functional cysts. Among the most frequently found masses involving the adnexa are the non-neoplastic cysts related to the process of ovulation that are sometimes referred to as functional cysts. They are by far the most common clinically detectable enlargements of the ovary occurring during the reproductive years. They are of great significance primarily because they cannot be readily distinguished from true neoplasms on clinical grounds alone. Among the non-neoplastic cysts and hyperplasias of the ovary are functional cysts (both follicular and corpus luteum types), theca-lutein cysts, pregnancy luteoma, sclerocystic ovaries, and endometriotic cysts.

If ovulation does not occur, a clear fluid-filled follicular cyst (Fig. 10–2A,B) lined by granulosa cells may result that can reach a size as large as 10 cm in diameter. These cysts usually resolve spontaneously within a few days to 2 weeks but can persist longer. When ovulation occurs, a corpus luteum is formed that may become abnormally enlarged through internal hemorrhage or cyst formation. Such cysts are often associated with variable delays in the onset of menses and confusion regarding the possibility of an ectopic pregnancy. Pregnancy testing has greatly facilitated this differential diagnosis.

Theca-lutein cysts result from overstimulation of the ovary by human chorionic gonadotropin (hCG) and on histologic examination are characterized by extensive luteinization of the stroma surrounding the follicle. Although theca-lutein cysts do not commonly occur in a normal pregnancy, they are often associated with hydatidiform moles and choriocarcinoma. Gross examination of the ovary containing theca-lutein cysts shows a structure almost completely replaced by lobulated thin-walled cysts that vary in size and are smooth and yellow.

Corpus luteum, follicular, and theca-lutein cysts are benign and represent an exaggerated physiologic response of the ovary. In most instances, they involute over time, but they do present a problem requiring a differential diagnosis. Further discussion of the management of the suspected functional cyst is included later in this chapter. Luteomas of pregnancy are often large, solid, but not neoplastic masses originating in the ovary during pregnancy. Most cases are discovered at caesarean section in the last 2 months of pregnancy. The exact cell of origin of luteoma has not been established. It is probably a chorionic hormone-dependent non-neoplastic hyperplasia and usually regresses after delivery. Therefore, surgical excision of these lesions at the time of caesarean section is not necessary.

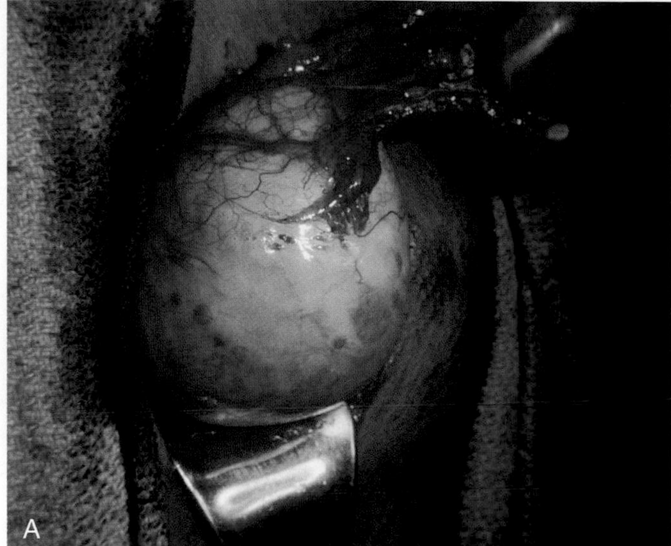

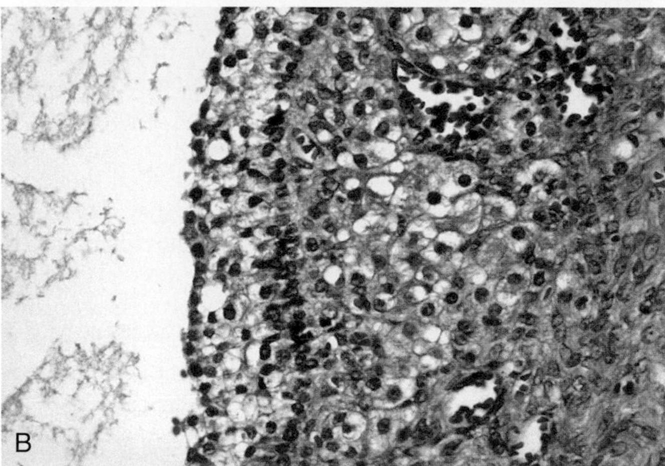

Figure 10–2 *A,* Follicular cyst (8 cm) with fimbria. *B,* Microscopic view of a follicular cyst as seen in Figure 10–2A. (Courtesy of Ibrahim Ramzy, MD, UC, Irvine, California.)

Polycystic (sclerocystic) ovaries contain multiple follicle cysts with hyperplasia and luteinization of theca interna surrounding the cysts and atretic follicles. The ovaries are two to five times normal size with a thickened capsule. The condition is found most frequently in association with the Stein–Leventhal or polycystic ovarian syndrome.

Endometriotic cysts vary in diameter from a few millimeters to 10 cm. They are usually adherent to surrounding structures. The lumen contains blood of varying color, depending on the amount and age of the hemorrhage. In most instances, it is dark brown (chocolate cyst). In at least 50% of cases, both ovaries are involved. The three cardinal features are endometrial epithelium, endometrial-type stroma, and evidence of repeated hemorrhage in the form of hemosiderin-laden macrophages in the cyst wall.

Ovarian Neoplasms. Although it is not unrealistic to consider every ovarian neoplasm or ovarian mass potentially malignant, in truth only 20% of all ovarian neoplasms are pathologically malignant. Only occasionally is it possible to differentiate benign from malignant tumors on the basis of history and physical examination findings (Table 10–3). In most instances, the diagnosis can be made only after both gross and microscopic examination of the mass. The ovary is composed of tissue derived from coelomic epithelium, germ cells, and mesenchyme, and ovarian neoplasms can be divided clinically into solid and cystic types.

Table 10–3 ADNEXAL MASS: INDICATIONS FOR SURGERY

Ovarian cystic structure >5 cm that has been observed 6–8 weeks without regression
Any solid ovarian lesion
Any ovarian lesion with papillary vegetation on the cyst wall
Any adnexal mass >10 cm in diameter
Ascites
Palpable adnexal mass in a premenarchal or postmenopausal patient
Torsion or rupture suspected

By far the most common benign cystic neoplasms of the ovary are serous and mucinous cystadenomas and cystic teratomas (dermoids). Benign cystadenomas may vary in size from 5–20 cm and are thin-walled, ovoid, and unilocular. The fluid contained within the neoplasms is usually yellow tinged and thin to viscous in quality. Benign cystic teratomas are usually no larger than 10 cm and can be identified grossly by the presence of sebaceous material, teeth or hair noted on sectioning of the neoplasm.

Malignant cystic neoplasms are usually of the serous or mucinous cystadenocarcinoma variety. In the absence of definite solid areas on imaging, these lesions may be difficult to distinguish from their benign counterparts. Papillary surface excrescences, areas of necrosis, and internal papillations are suggestive of malignancy. However, in the absence of obvious implants elsewhere in the peritoneal cavity, histologic review of the material is necessary to establish the diagnosis.

Benign solid tumors of the ovary are usually of connective tissue origin (fibromas, thecomas, or Brenner tumors). They vary in size from small nodules found on the surface of the ovary to large neoplasms weighing several thousand grams. On physical examination, these neoplasms are usually firm, slightly irregular in contour, and mobile. These neoplasms often account for the postmenopausal palpable ovary. Meigs' syndrome is an uncommon clinical entity in which a benign ovarian fibroma is seen with ascites and hydrothorax.

The malignant solid neoplasms of the ovary are most commonly adenocarcinomas arising in the ovary or metastatic from other sites. The firm masses noted on pelvic examination often appear to be associated with undifferentiated adenocarcinomas that have a poor prognosis. This clinical impression should be tempered by the knowledge that patients with inflammatory processes (e.g., chronic pelvic inflammatory disease) can demonstrate the firmest of palpable masses. In addition, elevated serum levels of several estrogens and androgens have been found in patients with solid ovarian neoplasms; fortunately, these neoplasms (arrhenoblastoma, gynandroblastoma, and hilar cell tumor) are either benign or of low malignant potential.

Most neoplasms of the ovary are asymptomatic unless they have been subject to rupture or torsion. Widespread intraperitoneal dissemination can occur in ovarian carcinoma and be totally asymptomatic until ascites causes an initial symptom of abdominal distention. On the other hand, any adnexal enlargement may cause menstrual abnormalities and a sensation of pelvic pressure from distortion of the bladder and rectum.

A true benign neoplasm of the ovary (e.g., serous and mucinous cystadenomas and benign cystic teratomas) does not resolve spontaneously. Whether these benign lesions are precursors of malignant neoplasms is as yet an unanswered question. Intraepithelial neoplasia has been reported in otherwise benign serous cystadenomas; and in early-stage invasive epithelial cancer, several authors have described the presence of transitional changes from normal epithelium to intraepithelial neoplasia to invasive cancer. Some have argued that if benign epithelial adenomas give rise to invasive cancers, it follows that surgical removal of these lesions should reduce the incidence of ovarian cancers. However, the reported increase in the incidence of surgical procedures for ovarian cysts in the past two decades has not affected the incidence of invasive ovarian cancer.

Endometriosis

Endometriosis is a condition in which implants of normal-appearing endometrial glands and stroma are found outside their normal location in the uterine cavity. The most common sites for endometriosis are the ovaries, the supporting ligaments of the uterus, and the peritoneum of the cul-de-sac and bladder. Endometriosis is most common in women 35–45 years of age and is more common in white and nulliparous women. When the ovary is involved, that structure may become enlarged and cystic as a collection of dark, chocolate-colored fluid accumulates within an ovarian cyst. These cysts rarely exceed a diameter of 12 cm, but they are often indistinguishable from ovarian neoplasms. Nodularity of the uterosacral ligaments and other structures within the cul-de-sac may be helpful in the differential diagnosis. Pelvic pain is by far the most usual symptom of endometriosis. Although physical activity and sexual intercourse usually increase the discomfort, the amount of endometriosis present does not seem to correlate with the intensity of the symptoms. For some, pain produced from small peritoneal implants appears to be incapacitating.

Tubal masses

Neoplasms arising from the fallopian tube are rare. More commonly, adnexal masses secondary to tubal disease are inflammatory or represent an ectopic pregnancy. Distinction between tubal and ovarian masses on the basis of examination alone is often difficult. In the acute phase of salpingitis, the fallopian tube is distended by grossly purulent material. This infection may be secondary to gonorrhea or other organisms, including anaerobes. As the salpingitis process progresses, the adjacent ovary may become involved, creating a so-called tubo-ovarian abscess. Although this acute process may resolve, the patient is often subject to reinfection. As a result of repeated chronic infectious processes, the tubal ostia may close or firmly adhere to the adjacent ovary, and the fallopian tube fills with a clear fluid. As the structure distends, it creates a mass that can easily be mistaken for an ovarian cyst. Although the symptoms of acute pelvic inflammatory disease are distinct (pelvic pain, fever, increased vaginal discharge, and abnormal uterine bleeding), the symptoms of chronic pelvic infection may be subtle. Even the traditional elevation of the erythrocyte sedimentation rate or leukocyte count may be absent in as many as 30% of patients with chronic pelvic inflammatory disease and adnexal masses.

A cystic mass in the adnexal region may be neither ovarian nor tubal in origin but caused instead by remnants of embryologic structures. The parovarium, located within the portion of the broad ligament containing the fallopian tube, consists of vestigial remnants of the Wolffian duct. Parovarian cysts are found as distal remnants of the Wolffian duct system. They are characteristically located between the fallopian tube and the ovary; when large, they are often found with the fallopian tube stretched over the top of the cyst. These parovarian cysts are most commonly unilocular and filled with clear yellow fluid. They often persist into the postmenopausal period and can appear as cystic structures in the adnexa on imaging studies done for other complaints.

Approximately 98% of ectopic pregnancies are tubal. Unfortunately, a pelvic mass can be found on examination in fewer than half the cases of tubal pregnancy, but urine test results for pregnancy are usually positive. Rupture usually occurs when the distended fallopian tube reaches a diameter of 4 cm. Tubal pregnancy must be distinguished from pelvic inflammatory disease, torsion of the adnexa, and bleeding corpus luteum cysts because all produce pain or abnormal bleeding.

Carcinoma of the fallopian tube is rare and accounts for <0.5% of all female genital tract malignant neoplasms. Indeed, most of these neoplasms are discovered by serendipity, a preoperative diagnosis of ovarian neoplasm being most common. On gross evaluation, the fallopian tube is usually enlarged, smooth-walled, and sausage-shaped. On occasion, patients present with the symptom of several weeks of profuse watery vaginal discharge, the so-called *hydrops tubae profluens.*

Adnexal masses of non-gynecologic origin

Bowel

By far the most common entity of the gastrointestinal tract that initially appears to be an adnexal mass is fecal material in the sigmoid colon or cecum, which may on initial pelvic examination be palpated as a soft, mobile, tubular mass. Patients should be re-examined after appropriate cleansing enemas to confirm or rule out this possibility.

Inflammatory disorders of the large and small intestine can also be detected on pelvic examination. Diarrhea, nausea

Table 10–4 DAGNOSTIC EVALUATION OF THE PATIENT WITH AN ADNEXAL MASS

Complete physical examination
Sounding of uterus (after ruling out pregnancy)
Computed tomography scan with contrast enhancement or intravenous pyelography
Colonoscopy or barium enema study, if symptomatic
Pelvic ultrasound examination (optional to rule out pregnancy)
Laparoscopy, laparotomy

Table 10–5 PELVIC FINDINGS IN BENIGN AND MALIGNANT OVARIAN TUMORS

Clinical findings	Benign	Malignant
Unilateral	+++	+++
Bilateral	+++	+++
Cystic	+++	+++
Solid	+++	+++
Mobile	+++	+++
Fixed	+++	+++
Irregular	+++	+++
Smooth	+++	+++
Ascites	+++	+++
Cul-de-sac nodules	−++	+++
Rapid growth rate	−++	+++

and vomiting, anorexia, or passage of blood or mucus per rectum should suggest these gastrointestinal tract disorders. Patients with diverticulitis, even with abscess formation, sometimes exhibit remarkably minor symptoms initially. Careful questioning to detect subtle changes in gastrointestinal symptoms is often rewarding. Periappendiceal abscesses may be formed as a result of rupture of the appendix and present as pelvic masses. Unfortunately, they vary in location, although they are generally found on the right side of the pelvis and are usually fixed, firm, and tender to palpation. Diverticulitis is a more common disorder with increasing age. Although it is usually located in the sigmoid colon, the mass may be midline or right sided. Inflammation of the ileum (regional ileitis) may occasionally present as a right-sided adnexal mass as the loops of thickened and inflamed ileum become fixed in the pelvis.

Gastrointestinal malignant disease is suggested by the presence of blood in the stool, anemia, and alterations in bowel habits. Neoplasms of the large intestine are particularly common with increasing age, and 60–70% occur on the left side within the reach of the palpating finger or flexible sigmoidoscope. On the other hand, carcinoma of the cecum often presents as a right-sided adnexal mass, and on examination, induration and irregularity may be found in the involved area. Appropriate radiographic and endoscopic studies are helpful in establishing these diagnoses (Table 10–4).

Miscellaneous

Pelvic examination should always be performed under optimal circumstances. The patient's bladder should be empty. Many patients with 10 cm midline masses thought to be ovarian neoplasms have been admitted to university hospitals. These masses disappeared with catheterization of their bladders. Whenever possible, the rectum and rectosigmoid should also be empty when a pelvic examination is done. This avoids the misdiagnosis of fecal material as an adnexal mass.

The rare pelvic kidney should always be kept in mind as a possible cause of a pelvic mass. Tragic reports of excision of such a mass in a patient with one kidney are found in the literature. Preoperative intravenous pyelography (IVP) or computed tomography (CT) with contrast enhancement in a patient with a large pelvic mass can help make this diagnosis.

Retroperitoneal disorders may also be palpated on pelvic examination. Retroperitoneal sarcomas, lymphomas, and teratomas of the sacrococcygeal areas are commonly noted on rectovaginal examination and misdiagnosed as an adnexal mass.

Management

Pelvic examination remains the most widely used method of identifying an ovarian mass in its earliest stages, although incidental discovery of a pelvic mass on CT scan, ultrasound examination, or magnetic resonance imaging (MRI) of the pelvis for other reasons is a growing method of identification. Knowledge of the size, shape, contour, and general location within the pelvis helps the physician arrive at the most likely diagnosis. Benign tumors are commonly smooth walled, cystic, mobile, unilateral, and smaller than 8 cm (7 cm is the exact diameter of a new tennis ball). Malignant tumors are usually solid or semisolid, bilateral, irregular, fixed, and associated with nodules in the cul-de-sac. Ascites is usually found with malignant neoplasms (Table 10–5). Koonings showed that the risk of malignant disease was 2.6-fold greater for women with bilateral neoplasms than for women with unilateral neoplasms. Certain studies may precede surgical exploration. Radiographic examination of the abdomen may reveal the outline of a pelvic mass, and the finding of "teeth" indicates a benign teratoma. However, not all calcifications are teeth, and psammoma bodies in serous adenocarcinoma of the ovary are other commonly found radiopaque entities also noted on radiographic examination. IVP is useful in the management of a pelvic mass because ureteral displacement and distortion of the bladder contour may be used to judge the size of the mass. Kidney position and function can also be evaluated. Ureteral obstruction or displacement should be noted before laparotomy, particularly when retroperitoneal dissection is anticipated to remove tumor bulk. Transvaginal sonography, CT scan, and MRI scans are occasionally necessary to further define the nature of the mass.

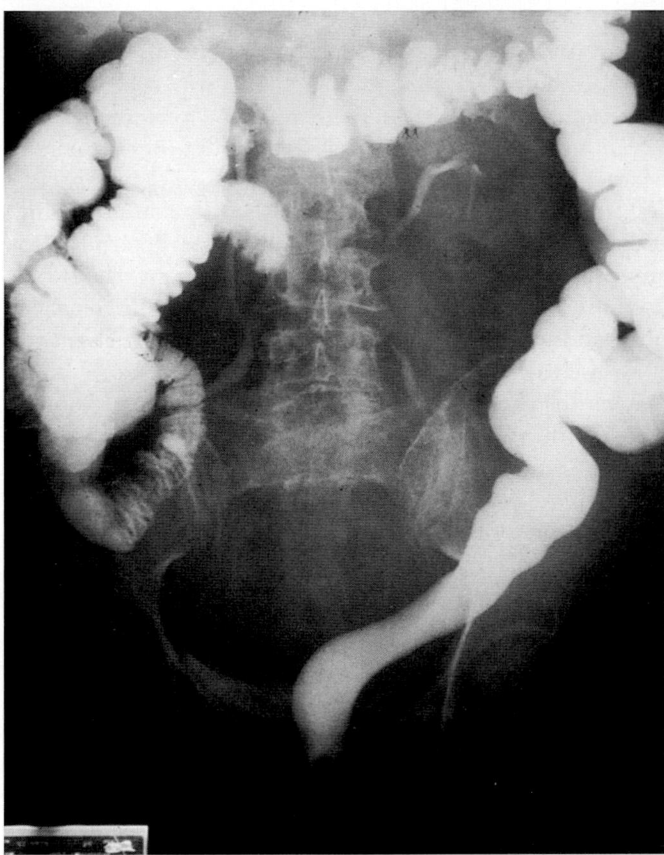

Figure 10–3 Barium enema film of a patient with a large mucinous cystadenoma of the right ovary filling the pelvis and lower abdomen.

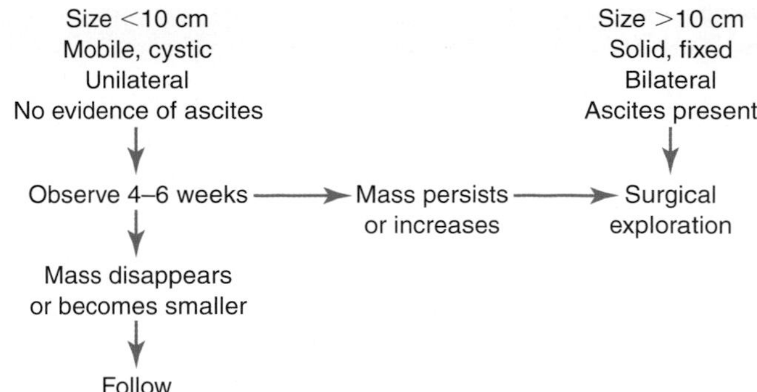

Figure 10–4 Management of a premenopausal woman with an adnexal mass.

Specific diagnostic assays (e.g., tumor markers) for ovarian cancer are also available. Some germ cell neoplasms produce hCG, lactate dehydrogenase, or α-fetoprotein, but most early-stage ovarian neoplasms are not associated with reliable tumor markers. Although serum CA-125 levels appear to be elevated in many serous cystadenocarcinomas, overall the result is positive in roughly 50% of stage I lesions.

Contrast studies of the gastrointestinal tract should be used liberally, especially when it is thought that the mass is gastrointestinal in origin (Fig. 10–3). Ultrasonography has not been as diagnostically helpful as expected, except to exclude intrauterine or extrauterine pregnancy. Although ultrasound examination can be helpful in detecting solid–fluid interfaces and distinguishing between solid and cystic masses, these determinations do not help in the eventual management of the patient and therefore seem redundant when a distinct mass has been palpated. Ultrasound examination can occasionally be helpful in confirming the suspicion of an adnexal mass in an obese or uncooperative patient. Its routine use for all adnexal masses is discouraged. Diagnostic laparoscopy may be helpful in distinguishing a uterine myoma from an ovarian neoplasm. Laparoscopy is helpful in any situation in which the source of a pelvic mass is uncertain and locating the source determines whether treatment is to be surgical or non-surgical. This is especially true in patients of reproductive age with smaller masses (≤7 cm), in whom expectant therapy should be seriously considered.

Deciding which patient needs surgical exploration can best be done by considering the characteristics of the adnexal mass. Any mass >10 cm in diameter should be surgically explored. Of ovarian cysts <5 cm in diameter, 95% are non-neoplastic. In addition, functional cysts are seldom larger than 7 cm in diameter and are usually unilateral and freely mobile. Patients usually are not taking oral contraceptive drugs. A physician can presume that during the reproductive years, an adnexal mass as described before is a functional or hyperplastic change of the ovary rather than a true neoplasm. The transitory existence of functional cysts is of prime importance in distinguishing them from true neoplasms. Tradition and clinical experience have shown that functional cysts usually persist for only a few days to a few weeks, and re-examination during a later phase of the menstrual cycle has been a reliable procedure in confirming this diagnosis. Many gynecologists prescribe oral contraceptives to accelerate the involution of the functional cyst on the presumption that these cysts are gonadotropin dependent. The unconfirmed theory is that the inhibitory effect of the contraceptive steroids on the release of pituitary gonadotropins shortens the life span of these cysts, hastening their identification as functional or non-neoplastic lesions. Failure of the enlargement to regress during one menstrual cycle (4–6 weeks) mandates operative intervention (Fig. 10–4). Spanos conducted a careful study of 286 patients who had adnexal cysts. Combination oral contraceptives were prescribed, and the women were re-examined in 6 weeks. In 72% of the women, the masses disappeared during the observation period. Of the 81 patients whose masses persisted, none was found to have a functional cyst at laparotomy. The fact that five of the removed tumors were malignant underscores the importance of avoiding unnecessary delay in the operative investigation of these patients. It has also made us slow to recommend operative laparoscopy for removal of such masses. In the premenarchal or postmenopausal period, any ovarian enlargement should result in surgical intervention.

BENIGN OVARIAN TUMORS

The differentiation between benign (Table 10–6) and malignant ovarian enlargements is often the exclusive decision of the pathologist, but a short discussion of these lesions is pertinent even in a textbook of oncology. Although functional ovarian cysts are usually asymptomatic, they can on occasion be accompanied by a minor degree of lower abdominal discomfort, pelvic pain, or dyspareunia. In addition, rupture of one of these fluid-filled structures can result in additional peritoneal irritation and possibly an accompanying hemoperitoneum; however, this is rarely serious. More intense lower abdominal discomfort results when these ovarian tumors undergo torsion or infarction. Similar to functional cysts of the ovary, benign ovarian neoplasms do not produce any symptoms that readily differentiate them from malignant tumors or from various other pelvic diseases. Although these tumors are more likely to twist, resulting in infarction, malignant neoplasms may have the same fate. Indeed, one of the most unfortunate features of benign ovarian neoplasms is that they are indistinguishable clinically from their malignant counterparts. Although it is not known whether malignant ovarian tumors arise de novo or develop from benign tumors, there is strong inferential evidence that at least some benign tumors will become malignant. All too often, the first symptom of cancer in an ovarian tumor is increasing abdominal distention, although benign ovarian neoplasms may become apparent because of increasing abdominal girth, and indeed the "giant tumors" of the ovary are often benign mucinous cystadenomas. Benign mucinous cystadenomas weighing up to 300 pounds have been reported. True functional cysts of the ovary will regress in a 4- to 6-week follow-up period of observation. All persistent adnexal enlargements must be considered malignant until proven otherwise.

Laparoscopically managed benign cysts

The operative approach for presumptively benign ovarian cysts has been the laparotomy. Advances in ultrasonography have provided an opportunity to predict benign masses preoperatively. With the use of specific ultrasound criteria, benign masses can be predicted with a high degree of certainty, especially in premenopausal women. Careful selection of patients is critical for the appropriate use of laparoscopy for removal of adnexal masses. The patient's age, the clinical examination, and the ultrasound findings provide important information that helps determine the appropriate operative approach. Laparoscopy should be used cautiously in the presence of any mass with clinical or ultrasonographic characteristics suggestive of malignancy. It is also contraindicated for management of an adnexal mass in the presence of an elevated serum CA-125 value in a postmenopausal woman.

Table 10–6 BENIGN OVARIAN TUMORS
Non-neoplastic tumors
Germinal inclusion cyst
Pregnancy luteoma
Endometrioma
Neoplastic tumors derived from coelomic epithelium
Cystic tumors
Serous cystoma
Mucinous cystoma
Mixed forms
Fibroma, adenofibroma
Brenner tumor
Tumors derived from germ cells
Dermoid (benign cystic teratoma)

Ultrasonography of the pelvis, particularly transvaginal, is a reliable and consistent method for evaluation of the size and the consistency of a pelvic mass. Masses that are cystic, unilocular, <10 cm, and unilateral and have regular borders are more likely to be benign. The presence of irregular borders, papulations, solitary thick septa, ascites, or matted bowel should raise concern about the possibility of malignancy. Using strict ultrasonographic criteria, physicians accurately predict benign masses in >95% of patients. Functional cysts, hemorrhagic cysts, dermoids, and endometriomas often have characteristic appearances on ultrasonography. Functional cysts are usually unilocular and have regular, thin borders. In premenopausal women, the majority of fairly cystic masses <7 cm resolve spontaneously within 6–8 weeks. Hemorrhagic cysts contain interior echoes that can vary in intensity from low to high levels and can be focal or diffuse. The ultrasound appearance of these cysts usually changes over time, and most regress spontaneously. Cysts that appear to be functional or hemorrhagic on ultrasonography but persist should be removed to rule out neoplasia. Dermoid cysts or mature teratomas are the most common benign neoplasms found in women under age 35 (Fig. 10–5A,B). These lesions contain mature elements derived from all three fetal layers. Dermoids have a variable appearance on ultrasonography. They may appear as a cystic mass that contains foci of echogenic material in a non-dependent distribution or a highly echogenic area suggesting bone or teeth. Endometriomas usually have regular but slightly thickened borders. They often contain low-level and diffuse internal echoes, although fresh hemorrhage may appear more highly echogenic. These masses that meet strict ultrasonic criteria for benign lesions may be considered for a laparoscopic approach. If any suspicious ultrasound findings are seen, operative laparoscopy is less appropriate, and laparotomy should be seriously considered.

CA-125, a tumor-associated antigen, has been studied to determine its value in preoperative differentiation of benign and malignant pelvic masses. In patients younger than 50 years, an elevated CA-125 level is associated with a malignant mass < 25% of the time. If the patient is older than 50 years, an elevated CA-125 level is associated with a malignant mass 80% of the time. A more detailed discussion of CA-125 is contained in Chapter 11. Of note for

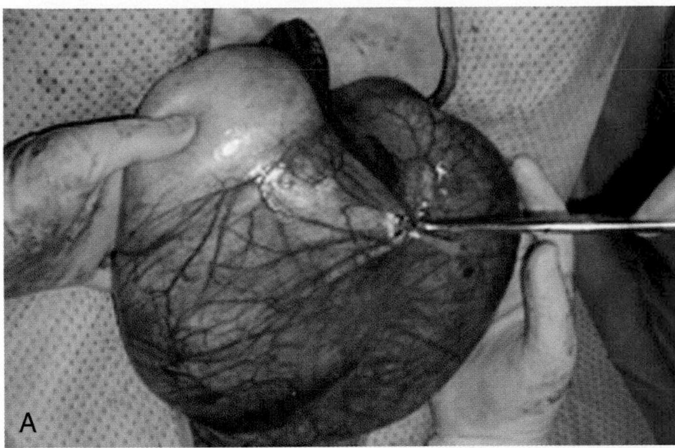

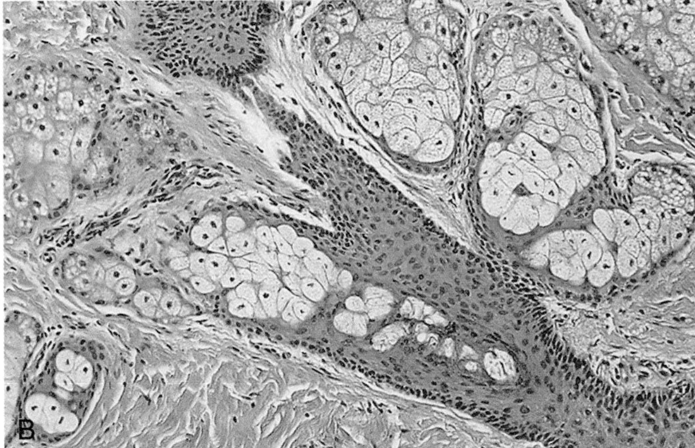

Figure 10–5 *A*, Ruptured dermoid cyst with sebaceous material seen. *B*, Photomicrograph of a mature teratoma (dermoid) of the ovary.

this discussion is that only 50% of patients with stage I epithelial cancer of the ovary have an elevated CA-125 level. The magnitude of the elevation is also of importance; CA-125 values in excess of 300 U/mL are usually associated with malignancy even in patients younger than 50 years.

All patients scheduled for operative laparoscopy with an adnexal mass should also consent to possible laparotomy; the surgeon should be prepared to proceed with staging laparotomy without delay if malignant disease is uncovered. All patients are operated on under general anesthesia in the laparoscopy stirrups. A Foley catheter is inserted into the bladder to avoid injury to that structure secondary to overdistention during prolonged cases. A 10 mm laparoscope provides a wide field of vision and excellent light. Cell washings are obtained from the pelvis and upper abdomen and saved for proper staging if a malignant neoplasm is found. Any lesions or suspicious areas are sampled and sent for frozen section analysis. If obvious carcinoma or ascites is found or the result of frozen section analysis is positive, the surgeon should proceed with immediate staging laparotomy through a midline incision. Laparoscopic fenestration of the mass and biopsy provide the most accurate method of diagnosing malignant disease by frozen section. A large window should be cut in the wall of the cyst; its size should vary with the size of the cyst, but it is usually about 2 cm smaller than the cyst to a maximum of 4–5 cm. The cavity of the cyst is carefully inspected, usually while it is being irrigated with Ringer's solution. Bleeding points from the biopsy site are controlled with hemostatic coagulation, using one of the energy sources available to the surgeon. Biopsy specimens are submitted to the laboratory for immediate tissue diagnosis. The main reasons for conversion from laparoscopy to laparotomy are:

- extensive adhesions;
- suspicion of malignancy; and
- intraoperative complications such as injury to bowel, bladder or ureter.

Nezhat and colleagues reported their experience with 1209 patients with adnexal masses who were managed laparoscopically. Of 1011 cases with surgical management, ovarian cancer was discovered intraoperatively in 4. The management of a cystic mass included aspiration of fluid, which was sent for cytologic examination, followed by opening of the cyst and inspection of the wall for any irregular thickening. Frozen section biopsy specimens were obtained if the surgeon thought any surfaces were suspicious. An ovarian cystectomy-oophorectomy was then performed, and tissue was sent for permanent histologic examination. The Nezhat study suggests that experienced surgeons using intraoperative histologic sampling may safely evaluate adnexal masses laparoscopically.

Hasson reported another series of 102 women with ovarian cysts who were managed laparoscopically. In 83 of the women, laparoscopic fenestration and biopsy were done, with or without coagulation or removal of the cyst lining. Only 1 of 56 functional, simple, or parovarian cysts recurred during the study. Two of the 18 ovarian endometriomas treated with fenestration and coagulation or removal of the lining recurred, whereas eight of nine such lesions recurred with treatment by fenestration alone. There were no surgical complications.

Canis reported his group's experience with 247 adnexal masses suspicious at ultrasound examination and managed laparoscopically. Actually, 17 patients were evaluated by laparotomy and 230 by laparoscopy. The 204 women (82.6%) who were treated by laparoscopy included 7 of 37 malignant tumors and 191 of 210 benign masses. One case of tumor dissemination did occur after a laparoscopic adenectomy and morcellation of a grade 1 immature teratoma. Some surgeons prefer to manage cystic ovarian masses with a mini laparotomy. A small incision (3–5 cm) is made over the mass and the cyst fluid is aspirated with a long needle, trocar or suction cannula after draping the field with dry laparotomy pads (see Fig. 10–20A). The collapsed mass can then be removed through the small incision (see Fig 10–20B) and submitted to pathology. Spill is minimal with this approach, but thorough irrigation of the surgical field is recommended prior to closure.

Serous cystadenoma

Serous cystadenomas are more common than the mucinous type of tumor, but as a rule, they do not attain the large size characteristic of their mucinous counterparts. On gross evaluation, the characteristic feature of the tumor is papillary projections on the surface, which at times are so numerous that a cauliflower pattern is produced. Although most of the inner wall of the cyst may be smooth (Fig. 10–6A,B), it may also contain a large number of these papillae. On microscopic examination, the epithelium is usually of the low columnar type, and cilia are present at times. Particularly characteristic of this type of cyst is the frequent finding of small cancerous granules, the so-called psammoma bodies, which are an end product of degeneration of the papillary implants. Aure and colleagues suggest that these psammoma bodies are indicative of a functional immunologic response. Associated fibrosis may lead to the so-called cystadenofibroma, which represents a similar lesion found in the breast.

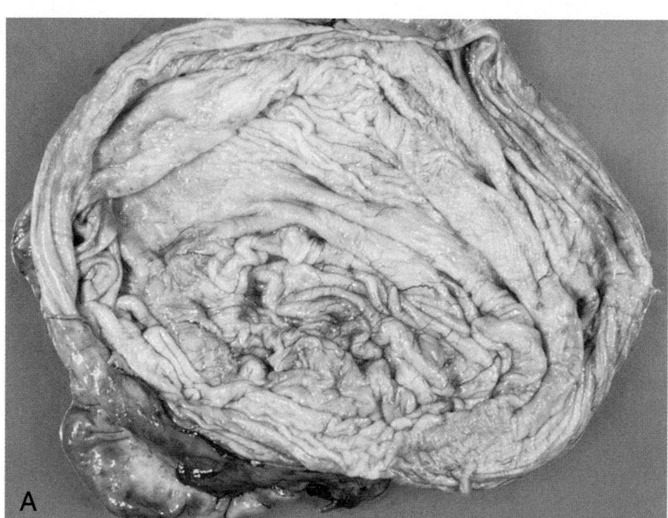

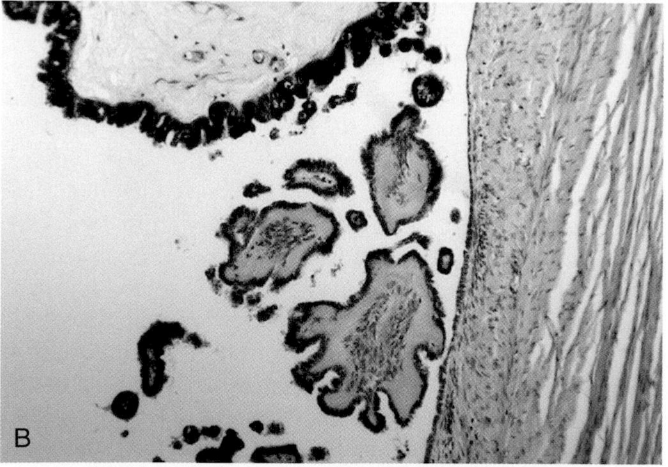

Figure 10–6 *A*, Gross photograph of an opened serous cyst adenoma that contained 500 mL of clear straw-colored fluid. Note the papillary projections on the inner surface, especially on the right. *B*, Microscopic view of a serous cystadenoma with a few papillary projections from the surface.

Mucinous cystadenoma

Mucinous cystadenomas (Fig. 10–7A,B) may become huge. Several have been reported to weigh >300 pounds. On gross evaluation, they are round or ovoid masses with smooth capsules that are usually translucent or bluish to whitish gray. The interior is divided by a number of discrete septa into loculi containing in general a clear, viscid fluid. Papillae are rarely noted. However, on microscopic examination, the lining epithelium is of a tall, pale-staining secretory type with nuclei at the basal pole; the presence of goblet cells is common. The cells will be found to be rich in mucin if suitable stains are obtained. It is believed that this type of cyst usually arises from simple metaplasia of the germinal epithelium. It may occasionally arise from a teratoma in which all the other elements have been blotted out. It rarely occurs from a Brenner tumor in which there has been mucinous transformation of the epithelium.

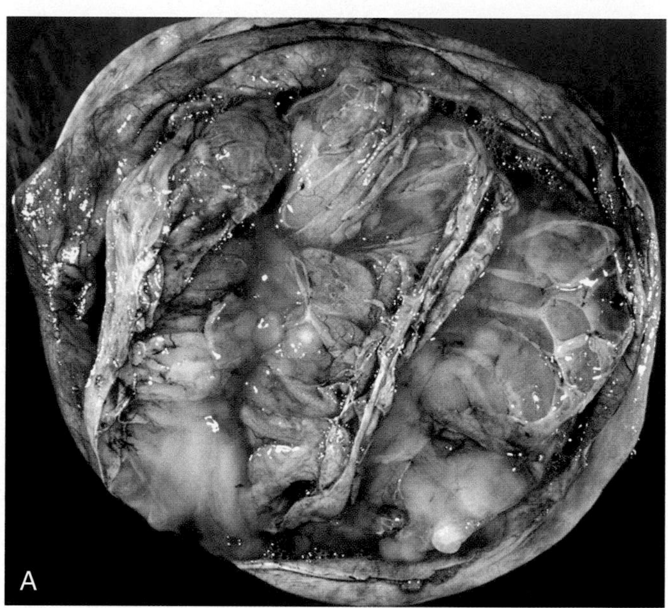

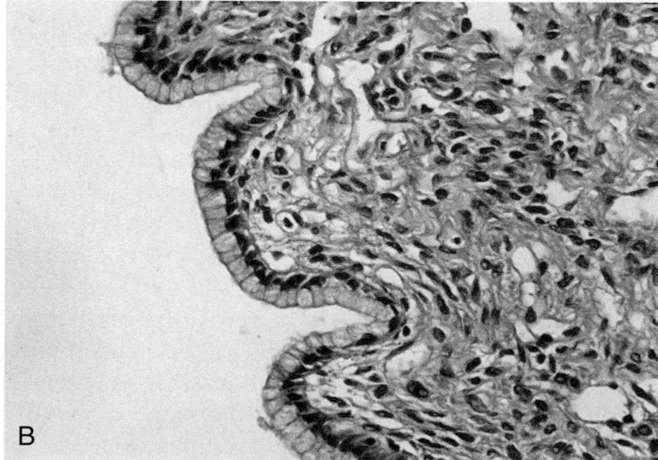

Figure 10–7A,B Mucinous cystadenoma. *A*, Gross appearance. (Courtesy of Ibrahim Ramzy, MD, UC, Irvine, California.) *B*, Histologic section showing tall epithelial lining with pale-staining nuclei at basal pole.

Bilaterality may be found in as many as 10% of patients with serous cystadenomas, in contrast with mucinous cystadenomas, for which there is essentially no significant incidence of bilaterality. This information is helpful when the surgeon needs to make a judgment about surgical inspection of the opposite ovary in a young woman desirous of further childbearing. If the other ovary is of normal size, shape, and configuration, surgical evaluation is not needed.

Pseudomyxoma peritonei

Of major concern are mucinous cysts that perforate and initiate intra-abdominal transformation of the peritoneal mesothelium to a mucin-secreting epithelium. This altered peritoneal mesothelium continues to secrete mucus, according to Woodruff and Novak, with gradual accumulation in the peritoneal cavity of huge amounts of gelatinous material, constituting the so-called pseudomyxoma peritonei (Fig. 10-8A,B). Evacuation of this material at operation is almost invariably followed by reaccumulation because of the impossibility of altering the secretion of the mucinous mesothelium.

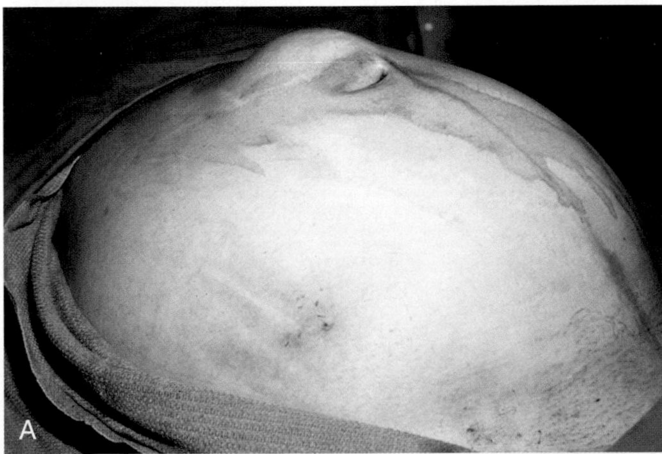

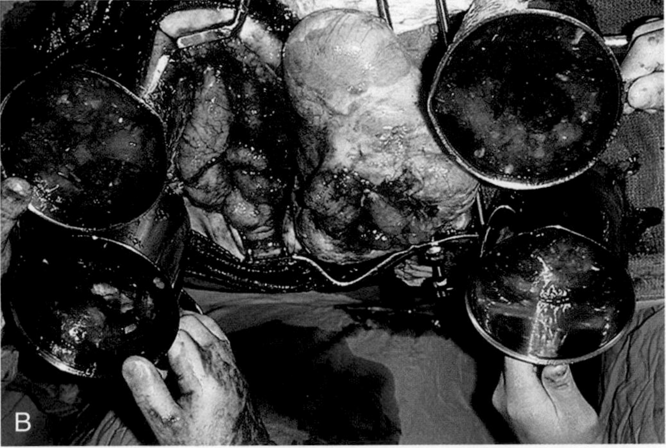

Figure 10–8 *A,* Patient with a large distended abdomen who was diagnosed as pseudomyxoma peritonei at surgery seen in Figure 10–8B (Courtesy of Hugh H. Allen, M.D., London, Ontario, Canada.) *B,* Pseudomyxomatous peritonei. Mucoid intraperitoneal material is quite evident in the operating room pitchers.

Among 13 cases of pseudomyxoma, Shanks noted that 10 cases originated in benign ovarian tumors, two cases originated in malignant ovarian tumors, and one arose from an appendiceal mucocele. Of seven survivors, two had recurrences, one after 14 years and one after 6 years.

Treatment remains primarily surgical, and because of the recurrent nature of the lesion, it may be repetitive. Intraperitoneal alkylating agents have been used with little success; however, according to Limber and associates, the use of radiation therapy, radioactive materials, and mucolytic agents has been disappointing. Long and coworkers reported a 45% 5-year and a 40% 10-year survival rate. In 1990, Mann and coworkers reported their experience with nine patients. They concluded that chemotherapy, including the use of cisplatin, was not effective, and long-term nutritional support provided a good quality of survival for select patients.

Brenner tumor

Brenner tumor (Fig. 10–9A,B), an uncommon type of ovarian neoplasm, is grossly identical to a fibroma. On microscopic examination, one finds a markedly hyperplastic fibromatous matrix interspersed with nests of epithelioid cells. The epithelioid cells under high magnification show a “coffee bean” pattern caused by the longitudinal grooving of the nuclei. The cell nests show a frequent tendency toward central cystic degeneration, producing a superficial resemblance to a follicle. Although it was originally believed that Brenner tumors arise from simple Walthard cell rests, it has been conclusively demonstrated that Brenner tumors can arise from diverse sources, including the surface epithelium, rete ovarii, and ovarian stroma itself. It was originally stressed that Brenner tumors were uniformly benign, but there have been scattered reports in the last several decades of a number of malignant Brenner tumors. Brenner tumors are generally thought to be endocrinologically inert, but several cases in recent years have been associated with postmenopausal endometrial hyperplasia, and a frequent estrogen effect has been attributed to this neoplasm. Even more recently, a characteristic Brenner tumor has been associated with virilism.

Benign lesions are managed by simple excision. Treatment of malignant Brenner tumors is unsettled, and various forms of chemotherapy have been used with little reported success.

Dermoid cyst (benign cystic teratoma)

Dermoid cysts are rarely large, are often bilateral (15–25%), and occur with disproportionate frequency in younger patients. On gross evaluation, there is a thick, opaque, whitish wall; on opening of the cyst, one frequently finds hair, bone, cartilage, and a large amount of greasy fluid, which rapidly becomes sebaceous on cooling. On microscopic examination, one may find all types of mature ectoderm, mesoderm, and such endodermal elements as gastrointestinal mucosa. Stratified squamous epithelium, hair follicles, sebaceous and sudoriferous glands, cartilage, neural and respiratory elements, and indeed all elements normally seen in fetal life may be present. When malignant degeneration occurs in these benign cystic teratomas, it is usually of a squamous type; it has been reported in 1–3% of these tumors. These neoplasms are thought to arise from early ova that have been triggered by some type of parthenogenetic process.

Management of these lesions in a patient desirous of further childbearing is cystectomy. Care must be taken to remove the entire capsule of the neoplasm to avoid recurrence. In most instances, a significant portion of normal ovary can be preserved and reconstituted. Some controversy exists relating to the necessity for creating a bivalve in the opposite ovary because of the high incidence of bilaterality with these lesions. In our experience, bilaterality is rare when the opposite ovary is normal in appearance; therefore, we do not recommend the procedure in these circumstances. Care should be taken to prevent spillage of the contents of the dermoid cyst because this material can cause a chemical peritonitis. Caspi reported 49 women with ultrasonographically diagnosed ovarian cystic teratoma <6 cm in pregnancy who were followed for change in size. A total of 68 pregnancies resulted. None of the classic complications of dermoid cysts such as torsion, dystocia, or rupture occurred. The authors concluded that such small lesions are safe to just follow especially in pregnancy.

Fibroma

The occurrence of fibromas (Fig. 10–10A, B) is not at all infrequent. Sometimes they are first noted as small nodules on the ovarian cortex. In other instances, they can be extremely large, filling the entire pelvis and lower abdomen. The tumors are characterized by their firmness and resemblance to myomas, and they are frequently misdiagnosed as such. The cut surface has a homogeneous grayish white and firm appearance, although areas of cystic degeneration

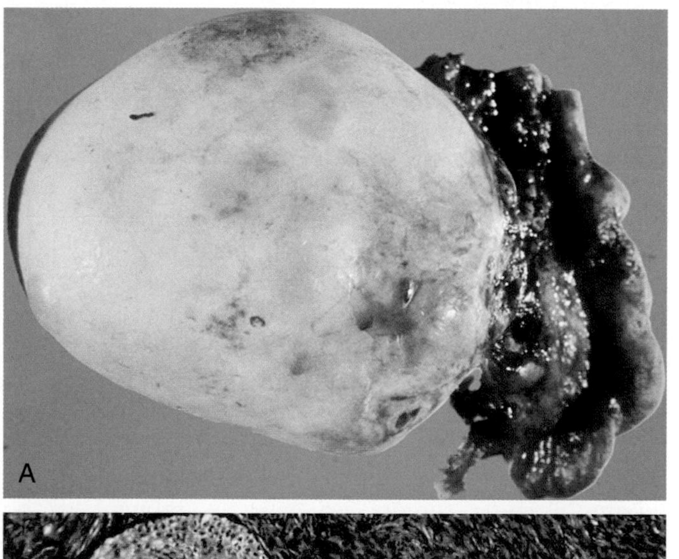

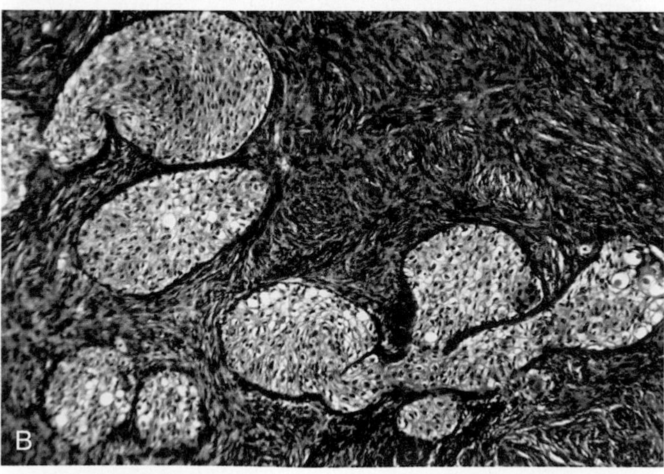

Figure 10–9A,B Brenner tumor. *A*, Gross appearance-solid, firm, white cut surface. *B*, Histologic section-hyperplastic fibromatous matrix interspersed with nests of epithelioid cells. (Courtesy of Ibrahim Ramzy, M.D., UC, Irvine, California.)

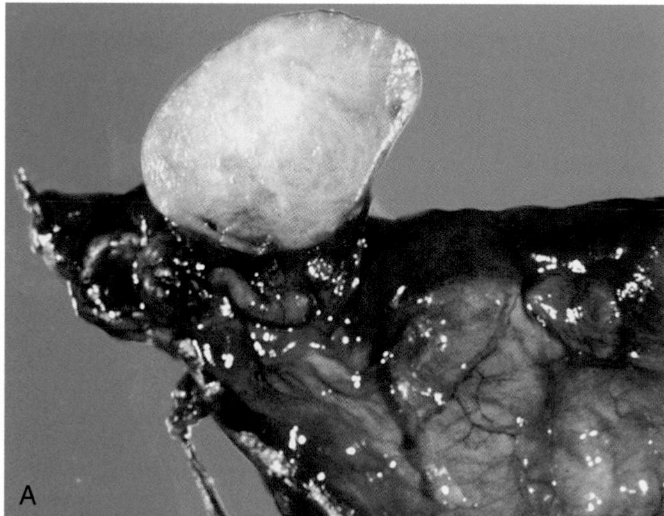

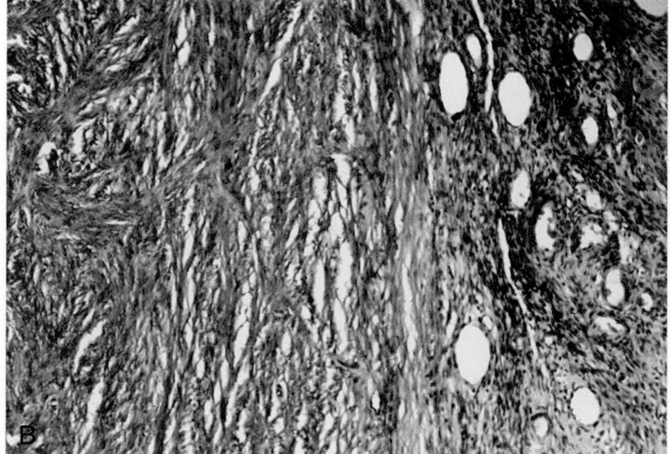

Figure 10–10A,B Ovarian fibroma. *A*, Gross appearance-solid white lesion with a firm cut surface and fallopian tube. *B*, Histologic section-whorls of fibromatous matrix. (Courtesy of Ibrahim Ramzy, M.D., UC, Irvine, California.)

are common in larger tumors. On microscopic examination, one finds stellate or spindle-shaped cells arranged in fusiform fashion. The cells are uniformly well differentiated, with nothing to suggest malignancy. Hyalinization is frequent, particularly in the larger tumors, and if fat stains are done, admixtures of theca cells may be seen. Meigs' syndrome is characterized by ascites, hydrothorax, and an ovarian tumor that was originally believed to be specifically a fibroma; however, many other types of ovarian tumors are now known to be associated with this syndrome, such as Brenner tumors and Krukenberg tumors. The cause of Meigs' syndrome is not completely understood, but it seems that the hydrothorax occurs by certain lymphatics through the diaphragm. After removal of the ovarian neoplasm, there is a prompt resolution of both abdominal and pleural fluid.

ADNEXAL MASSES IN CHILDHOOD

Figure 10–11 outlines the process of differentiating between benign and malignant masses in childhood. Whenever possible, conservative or minimally invasive surgery is preferred to preserve endocrine and reproductive functions. Dermoid cysts are among the most common ovarian masses in both pediatric and adolescent patients. These tumors are bilateral in 15–25% of cases. Two percent of dermoids (teratomas) have malignant components; these are usually found in adolescent patients but can also be found in childhood. A complete workup of a pelvic mass in this age group should include imaging and determination of serum levels of tumor markers such as CA-125, α-fetoprotein, lactate dehydrogenase, and β-hCG. The differential diagnosis should consider acute appendicitis, intussusception, gastroenteritis, chronic constipation, genitourinary problems, and pelvic infection.

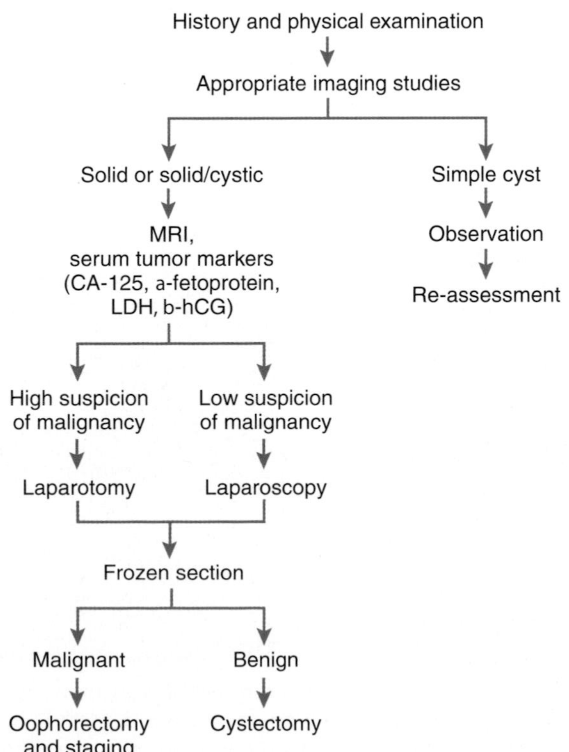

Figure 10–11 Management of an ovarian mass during childhood.

In a study by Ehren and colleagues, 63 children and adolescents with benign or malignant ovarian tumors were described. Abdominal pain was the most common complaint; 22% had torsion. The most common sign on initial examination was a palpable abdominal mass (45 of 54 patients). Benign teratoma was the final diagnosis in 41 of the patients (65%), and 29 had calcification apparent on abdominal radiography. All patients younger than 12 years with ovarian neoplasms had germ cell lesions, although an epithelial tumor has been reported in a 4-year-old patient. Two patients experienced precocious puberty, and interestingly, both had embryonal carcinoma. In this 63-patient study, appendicitis was the most usual misdiagnosis. Twenty-one percent had malignant tumors. Breen and Maxson noted that 35% of ovarian tumors in children were malignant.

Van Winter and associates reported on 521 adnexal masses in infancy, childhood, and adolescence; 92% were benign, including 335 non-neoplastic and 144 of 186 (77%) neoplastic lesions. The frequency of ovarian malignant neoplasms correlated inversely with the patient's age. Germ cell, stromal, and epithelial malignant neoplasms accounted for 40%, 21%, and 33%, respectively, of the 42 cancers. Non-conformance between preoperative and postoperative diagnoses was noted in 94 cases. The most common preoperative diagnosis necessitating reassignment was acute appendicitis. During the last decade of this study, ultrasonography and CT did not miss a single malignant neoplasm. The majority of these patients presented with a pain or a mass (Table 10–7). The histology of these lesions was presented in Table 10–2.

Table 10–7 SYMPTOMS AT INITIAL PRESENTATION OF 521 ADNEXAL MASSES IN CHILDREN

Symptom	No. of patients
Pain[1]	271
Mass[2]	151
Menstrual irregularity[3]	71
Dysmenorrhea	50
Amenorrhea, primary	12
Amenorrhea, secondary	35
Increased abdominal girth	34
Urinary complaints[4]	16
Hirsutism	13
Premature sexual development	6

[1]Mass was secondarily discovered in 150 of these patients.
[2]Without accompanying pain.
[3]Metrorrhagia, menorrhagia, oligomenorrhea.
[4]Frequency, dysuria, suprapubic pressure.
From Van Winter JT, Simmons PS, Podratz KC: Surgically treated adnexal masses in infancy, childhood, and adolescence. Am J Obstet Gynecol 170:1780, 1994.

PALPABLE OR ENLARGED POSTMENOPAUSAL OVARY

During the postmenopausal years, when the ovary becomes smaller and quiescent after cessation of menses, the presence of a palpable ovary must alert the physician to the possibility of an underlying malignant neoplasm. Physiologic enlargement and functional cysts should not be present in late postmenopausal ovaries. The postmenopausal gonad atrophies to a size of 1.5 × 1 × 0.5 cm on average (Fig. 10–12), and at that size it should not be palpable on pelvic examination. The possibility of malignant disease must therefore be carefully assessed when an ovary is palpable in a postmenopausal woman. Goswamy and colleagues studied ovaries from 2221 postmenopausal women with regard to ovarian volumes (Fig. 10–13). They noted that there were three ranges of volume and that volume appeared to be increased in obese and multiparous women.

Postmenopausal palpable ovary syndrome
The PMPO syndrome

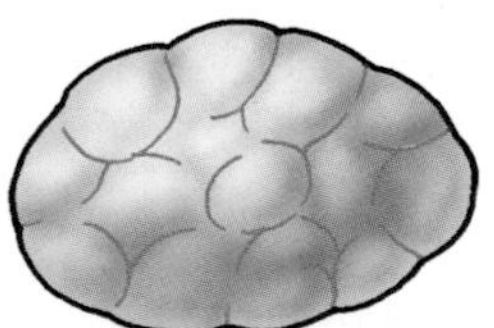
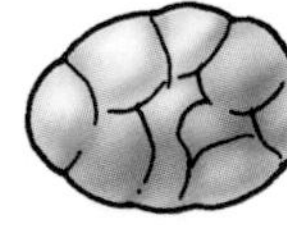
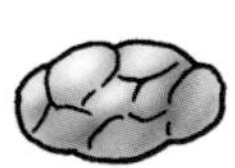

Normal ovary	Early menopause	Late menopause
Premenopause	(1–2 years)	(2–5 years)
3.5 X 2 X 1.5 cm	2 X 1.5 X 0.5 cm	1.5 X 0.75 X 0.5 cm

Figure 10–12 Comparison of the size of the ovary during progressive periods of a woman's life. (From Barber HRK, Graber EA: The PMPO syndrome [post-menopausal palpable ovary syndrome]. Obstet Gynecol Surv 28:357, 1973. Copyright 1973 The Williams & Wilkins Co, Baltimore.)

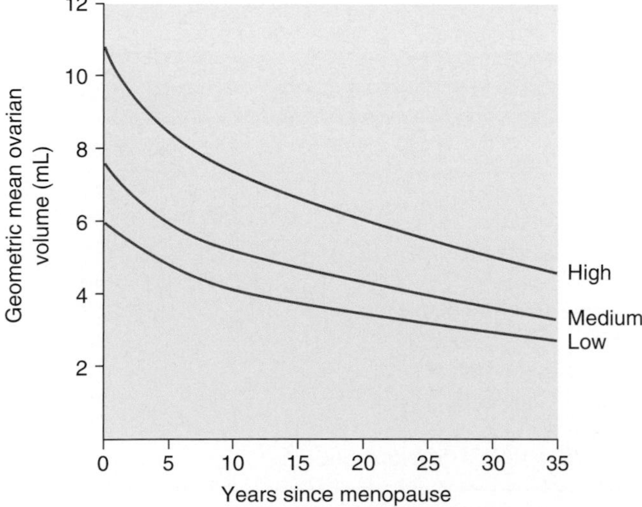

Figure 10–13 The 95th centiles for high, medium, and low expected ovarian volumes (geometric means) based on data from 2221 postmenopausal women. (From Goswamy RK et al: The size of the postmenopausal ovary. Br J Obstet Gynaecol 95(8):795, 1988. Reproduced by permission of the Royal College of Obstetrics and Gynaecologists.)

When laparoscopy or laparotomy is performed, the approach should be made with the assumption that the patient may have an early ovarian carcinoma. Cytologic washings should be obtained and careful exploration of the abdomen should be done, as in any patient being staged for ovarian cancer. A vertical abdominal incision is strongly recommended; this allows careful assessment of the subdiaphragmatic surfaces. In our experience, only 10% of patients with a palpable postmenopausal ovary who are subjected to oophorectomy are found to have a malignant ovarian neoplasm. By far the most common finding is a benign ovarian lesion such as fibroma, adenofibroma, or Brenner tumor (Fig. 10–14). This has led us to re-evaluate our former practice of recommending laparotomy in most of these patients.

Small simple cysts are not uncommon in the adnexae of postmenopausal asymptomatic women who undergo pelvic imaging. Wolf et al identified unilocular cysts in 22/149 (14.8%) of asymptomatic postmenopausal women ranging in size up to 5 cm. Conway et al performed transvaginal sonography on 1769 similar asymptomatic women and found 116 (6.6%) simple cysts up to 5 cm in diameter. Others have had a similar outcome (Table 10–8).

Goldstein described 42 postmenopausal women with simple adnexal cysts. He included only patients available for follow-up who had cysts ≤5 cm in maximal diameter that were unilocular and without ascites. Of these patients, 26 underwent prompt surgical exploration. All exhibited benign histopathologic features. In 16 patients, serial sonographic surveillance was performed every 3 to 6 months. Two of these patients had exploratory laparotomy at 6 and 9 months of observation; the first operation, for increasing size and septation, demonstrated a cystadenofibroma, and the second operation, for increasing pain, demonstrated a degenerating myoma. The remaining 14 patients were observed for 10 to 73 months without any

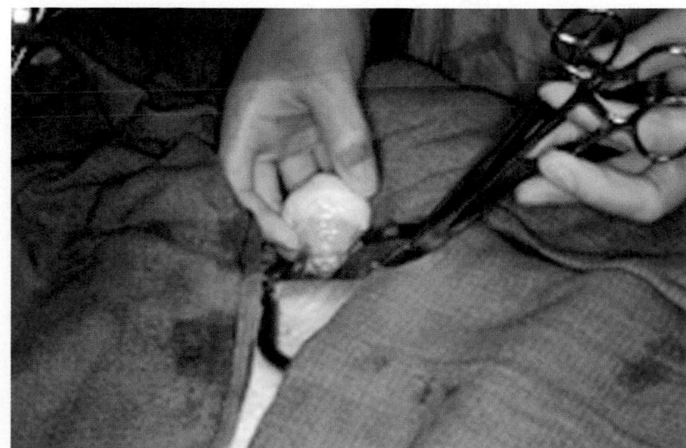

Figure 10–14 A 5 cm adenofibroma which was found in surgery in a postmenopausal woman and was detected preoperatively and diagnosed by ultrasonography as a solid mass. (Courtesy of Ibrahim Ramzy, M.D., UC, Irvine, California.)

Table 10–8 PREVALENCE OF SIMPLE OVARIAN CYSTS IN ASYMPTOMATIC POSTMENOPAUSAL WOMEN

Authors	Number of women	Number of cysts	Percentage of women with cysts
Wolf et al	149	22	14.8
Conway et al	1769	116	6.6
Andolf and Jorgensen	534	30	5.6
Aubert et al	622	36	5.7
Bailey et al	7705	256	3.3

From Oyelese Y et al: Asymptomatic postmenopausal simple ovarian cyst. Obstet Gynecol Surv 57:803, 2002. ©2002 by Lippincott Williams & Wilkins, Inc.

Table 10–9 SMALL POSTMENOPAUSAL ADNEXAL MASS STUDIES

Series	No.	Inclusion criteria	No. operative	Cancer (%)
Hall (1986)	13	Simple cyst	13	8
Goldstein (1989)	42	Unilateral cyst < 5 cm	28	0
Andolf (1989)	58	< 5 cm simple	29	0
	11	< 5 cm multicystic, echoes	10	10
	33	> 5 cm simple	27	10
	50	> 5 cm multicystic, echoes	45	30
Wolf (1991)	22	< 5 cm simple	1	0
Luxman (1991)	102	< 5 cm simple	18	10
Conway (1998)	49	< 5 cm simple	18	0

Modified from Curtin JP: Management of the adnexal mass. Gynecol Oncol 55:S42, 1994.

change in the size or character of their cysts. Goldstein concluded that small, unilocular postmenopausal cysts had a low incidence of malignant disease and that serial ultrasound follow-up, without surgical intervention, should have a major role in clinical management of such patients. Others, such as Parker and Berek, have suggested that these low-risk postmenopausal cysts be managed with operative laparoscopy.

Miller and coworkers described 20 postmenopausal patients who underwent surgical exploration for evaluation of an asymptomatic palpable ovary. Thirteen patients (65%) were found to have an ovarian neoplastic process. Three of the neoplasms were malignant or of borderline malignant potential, resulting in an overall malignancy rate of 15% for the postmenopausal palpable ovary syndrome. This is consistent with our experience and that of Flynt and Gallup, who described 11 patients, none of whom had a malignant ovarian neoplasm. The majority of neoplasms in this group of patients are benign. However, the actual number of postmenopausal women who have been observed and subsequently described in the literature is extremely small (Table 10–9). Lerner and colleagues accurately predicted a benign outcome in 247 of 248 patients studied. They used color flow Doppler analysis to improve the accuracy of ultrasonic characterization of ovarian masses. However, this technique has not been as accurate when used by others. Shalev and coworkers described 55 postmenopausal women who underwent operative laparoscopy for an adnexal cyst that was not complex and when the serum CA-125 level was normal. All of the 55 cysts were benign. During the same period, 75 women underwent exploratory laparotomy for complex cysts or an elevated serum CA-125 level. Of the 75 women, 23 had malignant lesions. Size is an important determinant of malignant potential. Cysts <5 cm in diameter are rarely malignant, whereas cysts >5 cm in diameter have a high probability of malignancy in the postmenopausal patient (Table 10–10).

Table 10–10 HISTOLOGIC FINDINGS IN POSTMENOPAUSAL WOMEN WITH PELVIC CYSTS

Author	Size (cm)	No.	Number of neoplastic (benign or malignant)
Goswamy et al	≤ 10	3	1 (33%)
Hall and McCarthy	≤ 10	10	2 (20%)
Goldstein et al	< 5	28	3 (11%)
Shalev et al	> 1	43	22 (51%)
Kroon et al	< 5	43	17 (40%)
Roman et al	5–10	5	2 (40%)
Bailey et al	≤ 10	45	36 (80%)
Total		177	83 (47%)

A diagnosis of ovarian cancer should be suspected when a postmenopausal woman presents with a pelvic mass. The presence of ascites, which can be detected clinically or by ultrasound examination, markedly increases the probability of a diagnosis of malignancy. In addition, CA-125, although non-specific in the population of premenopausal patients, is sensitive in the postmenopausal patient when it is used in combination with a clinical impression and an abnormal ultrasound finding. CT scan, which is more sensitive than ultrasonography, is often not necessary. Early surgical intervention is a key component in the treatment of these patients, and extensive diagnostic testing should be discouraged.

SCAN-DETECTED MASSES

With the increased use of CT, MRI, and ultrasonography, an increasing number of "pelvic masses" are being identified. It is not unusual today for a patient to come to the office with a scan in hand. In many instances, no mass is felt on pelvic examination. This causes a management dilemma, particularly in the postmenopausal woman. Experience has dictated that a pelvic mass in the postmenopausal woman needs surgical evaluation, but the decision to operate should be relative to identification of the mass on pelvic examination. In many cases, when surgery has been performed for scan-detected masses, no malignant neoplasms have been identified, even when the scans indicated that the masses were "solid." Hydrosalpinx and old follicular cysts have often been found. On other occasions, the mass is a fluid-filled pocket of adhesions in a patient with a history of previous pelvic surgery. Obviously, these situations must be individualized, and a false-positive rate for pelvic masses identified only by imaging must be accepted.

BORDERLINE MALIGNANT EPITHELIAL OVARIAN NEOPLASMS

In the last four decades, clear evidence has been presented that there is a group of epithelial ovarian tumors with histologic and biologic features intermediate between those of clearly benign and those of frankly malignant ovarian neoplasms. These borderline malignant neoplasms, which account for approximately 15% of all epithelial ovarian cancers, were often referred to as proliferative cystadenomas. In the younger population, these lesions tend to occur more frequently than the obviously malignant epithelial ovarian carcinomas, which are seen more frequently in older patients (Fig. 10–15). There is a 10-year survival rate of approximately 95% for stage I lesions in these borderline neoplasms. However, symptomatic recurrence and death may occur as many as 20 years after therapy in a few patients, and these neoplasms are correctly labeled as being of low malignant potential.

Borderline serous epithelial tumors (Fig. 10–16A,B) definitely occupy an intermediate position between the benign serous cystadenomas and the frankly malignant serous cystadenocarcinomas in their histologic features and prognostic aspects. On gross evaluation, the borderline serous tumors are similar to the previously described benign serous cystadenomas, which have papillary projections, but the borderline tumors possibly show an increased incidence of bilaterality. In addition, the papillary component is usually more abundant in the borderline lesions than in the perfectly benign serous cystadenoma. Survival in these lesions differs significantly from that in their obviously malignant counterpart (Fig. 10–17).

The histologic criteria characterizing the borderline tumors can be summarized as follows:

- Stratification of the epithelial lining of the papillae;
- Formation of microscopic papillary projections or tufts arising from the epithelial lining of the papillae;
- Epithelial pleomorphism;
- Atypicality;
- Mitotic activity; and
- No stromal invasion present.

According to Janovski and Paramananthon, at least two of these features must be present for the tumor to qualify as borderline. Although borderline serous epithelial tumors of the ovary (see Fig. 10–16A,B) are well established and were accepted by the International Federation of Gynecology and Obstetrics (FIGO) in 1964, they remain a controversial issue. Although there is no doubt that there exists a group of low-grade malignant tumors among the serous cystadenocarcinomas of the ovary, it is doubtful whether qualifying terms such as *borderline* are

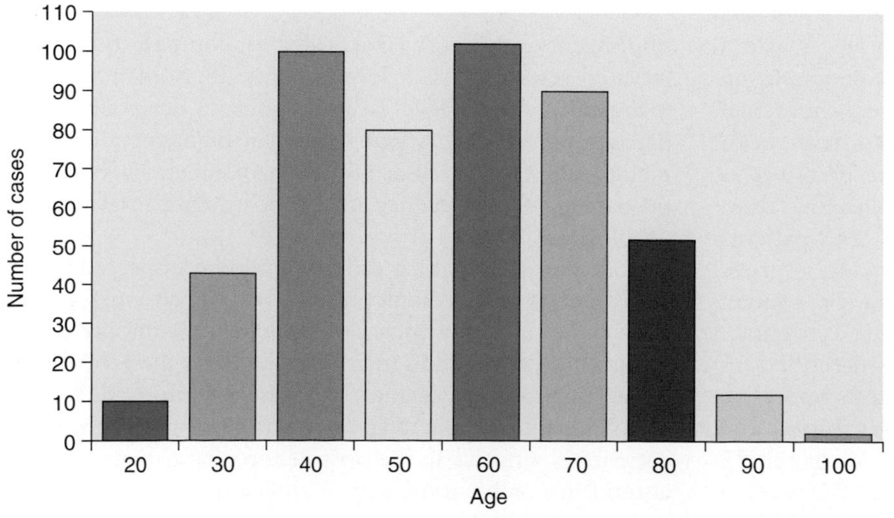

Figure 10–15 Epithelial borderline tumors of the ovary. Age distribution. (From Annual Report Gynecological Cancer. FIGO, Vol 22, 1994.)

always appropriate. Unfortunately, terms like *borderline* may create a false sense of security among some physicians. These patients should be observed as closely as any patient with ovarian cancer.

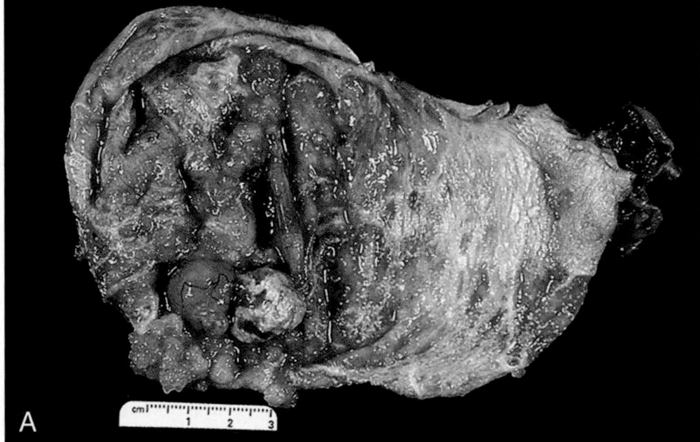

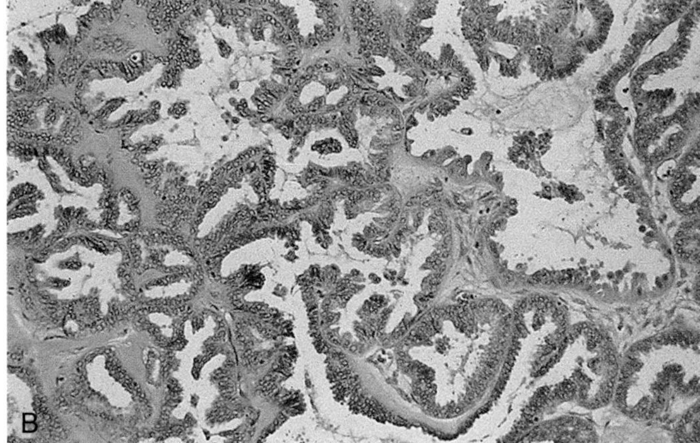

Figure 10–16A,B Borderline serous carcinoma. *A*, Gross appearance. *B*, Histologic section showing stratification of the epithelial lining in papillary projections.

In 1973, Hart and Norris reported a series of borderline mucinous tumors (Fig. 10–18A,B) confined to either ovary or both ovaries at the time of diagnosis, with a corrected 10-year actuarial survival rate of 96%. Whereas the origin of the serous tumors from germinal epithelium is generally accepted, the histogenesis of mucinous tumors is more problematic. These neoplasms do not differ significantly from their benign counterparts in gross appearance. They are multilocular, cystic, frequently voluminous masses with smooth outer surfaces. The inner lining, also similar to that of benign mucinous cystadenomas, is generally smooth, although papillary structures and solid thickening of the capsule have been observed in about 25–50% of lesions reported. On microscopic examination, in contrast to benign mucinous cystadenoma, the epithelial lining of the borderline tumor is characterized by stratification of two or three layers. In the benign tumors, the cells show no atypia or pleomorphism, but the epithelium of the borderline lesions does demonstrate atypia, with irregular, hyperchromatic nuclei and enlarged nucleoli. Mitotic figures are also seen.

For treatment of borderline lesions, the physician should strive to completely extirpate the tumor. If disease is unilateral, a salpingo-oophorectomy or a carefully performed ovarian cystectomy is appropriate, on condition that a thorough evaluation of the other ovary (biopsy if necessary), a peritoneal cytologic examination, and a partial omentectomy are done. Julian and Woodruff evaluated 65 patients who had low-grade papillary serous carcinoma of the ovary and found that 100% of the 50 patients who had unilateral adnexectomy and 90% of the 10 patients who had complete operation (total abdominal hysterectomy and bilateral salpingo-oophorectomy) were alive at 5 years. Lim-Tan and colleagues described 35 patients with ovarian serous borderline tumors treated by unilateral cystectomy or bilateral cystectomy. Tumor persisted or

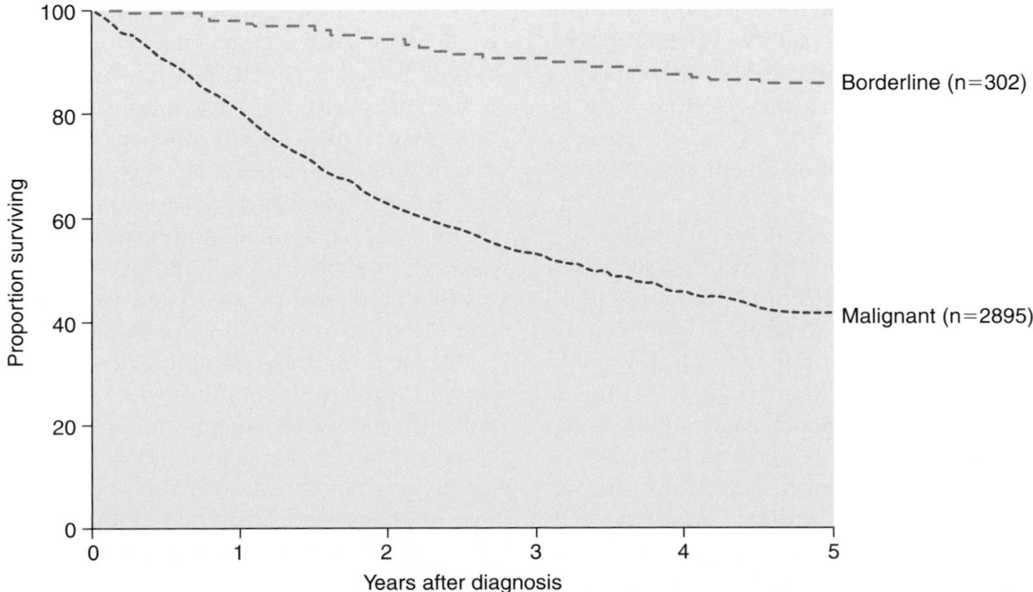

Figure 10–17 Carcinoma of the ovary: Patients treated in 1900–1992. Survival by histology (n = 3197). (From FIGO Report. J Epidemiol Biostat Vol 3, 1998. Reprinted with permission of the publisher, Taylor & Francis Ltd., http://www.tandf.co.uk/journals.)

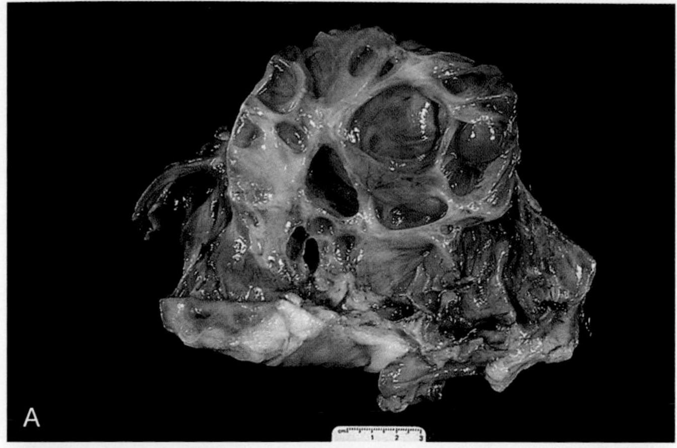

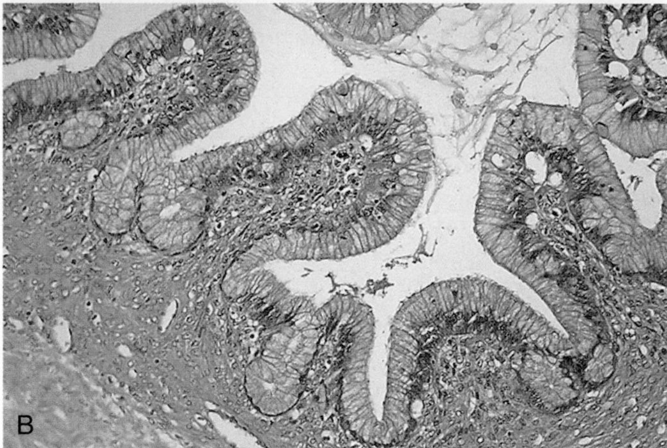

Figure 10–18 *A,* Mucinous tumor with low malignant potential. Gross appearance. *B,* Photomicrograph of mucinous tumor seen in Figure 10–18A.

recurred only in the ovary that had been subjected to cystectomy in 2 (6%) of the 33 patients, with stage I tumors in both the ipsilateral and contralateral ovary in one patient (3%) and only in the contralateral ovary in the other patient (3%). All the patients were alive without evidence of disease 3–18 years after initial operation, with the average follow-up of 7.5 years. Scattered reports of similar smaller series suggest that these lesions may be managed with ovarian cystectomy alone in patients desirous of further childbearing when acceptance of a small risk is appropriate.

If there is bilateral ovarian involvement, especially when papillary projections are found on the external surface of the tumor, or if peritoneal spread is noted, a more radical surgical approach, such as total abdominal hysterectomy with bilateral salpingo-oophorectomy and radical excision of involved pelvic peritoneum, is advocated. Peritoneal cytologic examination, partial omentectomy, and selected pelvic and periaortic lymphadenectomy should also be done in these patients with more advanced disease. Advanced (stage III) borderline lesions can occur with metastases to lymph nodes. Survival even of these advanced lesions is appreciable. Appropriate treatment of stage I borderline neoplasms of the ovary, other than surgical resection, remains uncertain. Kolstad and associates randomized patients with stage I borderline lesions into two groups, one treated by pelvic radiotherapy and the other by pelvic radiotherapy and intraperitoneal radioactive colloidal gold. The actuarial survival rates were 92.5% and 87.2%, respectively; several patients died of complications of the gold therapy. In these instances, therapy seemingly resulted in a significant lowering of survival compared with three other series. Use of intraperitoneal chromic phosphate alone, without pelvic radiotherapy, is usually associated with fewer intra-abdominal complications and may be more appropriate therapy.

Creasman described 55 patients with stage I borderline or low malignant potential lesions of the ovary. He concluded that surgical removal of the disease was as efficacious for adequate therapy as postoperative pelvic irradiation or adjunctive chemotherapy. Both Gershenson and colleagues and Bell and associates have described patients with ovarian serous borderline tumors with peritoneal implants. Gershenson had a 95% disease-free survival rate at 5 years and a 91% disease-free survival rate at 10 years. On the other hand, Bell reported that 13% of patients died of tumor and one patient was alive with widespread progressive tumor. Death due to tumor was 4% at 5 years and 23% at 10 years. Drescher and coworkers studied the significance of DNA content and nuclear morphology in these lesions. Their results suggest that measurement of DNA ploidy and nuclear morphology by image analysis can provide important prognostic information in patients with borderline ovarian tumors. Work such as this is important because some of these lesions progress in an aggressive manner, leading the clinician to consider chemotherapy. It would be comfortable to have a mechanism for distinguishing lesions that are biologically aggressive from lesions that persist in a state of equilibrium, posing no threat to the patients' health and welfare.

Some extraovarian implants are associated with irregular glandular structures in immature, desmoplastic, or inflamed stroma, and these represent a difficult diagnostic problem. Many also have a clear pattern of invasion of subjacent tissues as well as cellular features of malignancy. They thus exhibit a capacity for invasion not seen in the ovarian lesion and may represent an independent or autochthonous origin. Other bland cellular nests of cells in desmoplastic reactive granulation tissue do not invade the underlying tissue and are termed non-invasive compared with the invasive implants. Russell and Merkur have reported that invasive implants are associated with a poor clinical outcome compared with the non-invasive group.

Gershenson and colleagues described seven assessable patients with invasive implants who underwent chemotherapy and a second-look surgery. Four of the patients had a response. No clear conclusion could be drawn about which agents were most active. A total of 39 patients with invasive implants were identified at their institution, and 12 (31%) developed progressive disease or a recurrence.

Trimble and Trimble reported an excellent review of epithelial ovarian tumors of low malignant potential in 1994. For serous and mucinous tumors of low malignant potential, the mean age at diagnosis falls close to 40 years, approximately two decades earlier than the mean age at diagnosis for invasive epithelial ovarian cancer. In a meta-analysis of 12 case-control studies conducted in the USA, Harris and colleagues found a mean age of 44 years for women with tumors of low malignant potential compared with a mean age of 52.9 years for women with invasive ovarian carcinoma. The meta-analysis conducted by the Collaborative Ovarian Cancer Group found protective factors against the development of tumors of low malignant potential to be pregnancy, breastfeeding, and use of oral contraceptives. A history of infertility increased the risk of tumors of low malignant potential (odds ratio 1.9), and the use of infertility drugs further increased the risk for development of a tumor of low malignant potential above that of women with no history of infertility (odds ratio 4.0).

Kurman and Trimble reviewed survival in 22 studies of serous tumors of low malignant potential, excluding those patients with invasive peritoneal implants. For 538 patients with stage I disease, survival was 99%, with a mean follow-up of 7 years. Even in the series of 415 patients with stage II and stage III disease, survival was 92% with the mean follow-up of 7 years. In review of the causes of death in this series, three patients died of radiation-associated complications, nine died of chemotherapy-associated complications, eight died of bowel obstruction, and eight died of invasive carcinoma; 18 patients were reported as "dying of disease" without additional information. In short, more patients seemed to die with disease than of disease. In addition, more patients died of treatment-related complications than of bowel obstruction from progressive disease.

Kurman has identified an aggressive subgroup of proliferative serous lesions, which he calls micropapillary serous carcinoma. Seidman and Kurman found 11 patients with micropapillary projections, and according to Seidman and Kurman, these lesions should be classified as carcinomas, as should serous borderline tumors with invasive implants. The poor prognosis for these patients has prompted some clinicians to prescribe chemotherapy as an adjuvant to surgery.

PROPER IDENTIFICATION OF AN EARLY OVARIAN NEOPLASM

(Table 10–11)

Ultrasound has proven value in detecting ovarian cancer in asymptomatic women with advanced disease. Its utility in early stage disease is less well established. Van Nagell and coauthors reported on over 57,000 ultrasound scans performed on asymptomatic postmenopausal women and women over 25 with a family history of ovarian cancer. They identified 11 stage I ovarian, five were epithelial carcinomas, three granulosa cell tumors, and three borderline ovarian neoplasms. The sensitivity for epithelial ovarian cancer by grayscale ultrasound is very low. 3D power Doppler ultrasound may have increased clinical value and needs further study. At the same time, the combination of biologically relevant biomarkers, novel technology such as proteomics and high-resolution ultrasound may permit detection of early stage ovarian carcinoma.

Table 10–11 FIGO STAGING OF EARLY-STAGE OVARIAN CARCINOMA

FIGO stage	Description
I	Disease limited to the ovaries
Ia	Disease limited to one ovary, no ascites, no surface involvement, capsule intact
Ib	Disease limited to both ovaries, no ascites, no surface involvement, capsule intact
Ic	Either stage Ia or stage Ib with ascites containing malignant cells or positive peritoneal cytology, capsule ruptured, or surface involvement
II	Disease involving one or both ovaries with pelvic extension
IIa	Extension or metastases to the fallopian tube or uterus
IIb	Disease spread to other pelvic organs including the pelvic sidewall
IIc	Either stage IIa or stage IIb with ascites containing malignant cells or positive peritoneal cytology, capsule ruptured, or surface involvement

FIGO, International Federation of Gynecology and Obstetrics.

Table 10–12 SURVIVAL (FIVE-YEAR) IN EARLY-STAGE OVARIAN CARCINOMA

FIGO stage	No.	Five-year survival (%)
Ia	81	84
Ib	22	68
Ic	14	86
IIa	16	81
IIb	55	40
IIc	13	62

FIGO, International Federation of Gynecology and Obstetrics.

The combined 5-year survival rates quoted for stage I and stage II epithelial cancer of the ovary (Table 10–12) vary from 70–80% and from 40–70%, respectively. These survival rates are disappointing in view of the presumptive removal of all tumor at the time of surgery.

To date, several prospective studies have evaluated metastasis to the diaphragm in women with presumed stage I or stage II ovarian carcinoma (Table 10–13). In each instance, the surgeon doing the initial procedure believed that the lesion was confined to the ovary or pelvis. The incidence of such unsuspected metastases was 15.7% in the collective series (11.3% for stage I and 23.0% for stage II).

Knapp and Friedman, Delgado and coworkers, and Musumeci and associates prospectively evaluated aortic node metastasis in patients with stage I or stage II ovarian carcinoma. Collectively they found that 10.3% of patients

Table 10–13 INCIDENCE OF SUBCLINICAL METASTASES IN STAGE I AND STAGE II OVARIAN CARCINOMA

Series	Diaphragm (%)	Aortic nodes (%)	Malignant cytologic washings (%)
Knapp and Friedman	—	12.5	—
Rosenoff et al	43.7	—	—
Delgado et al	0.0	20.0	—
Spinelli et al	23.0	—	—
Musumeci et al	—	7.0	—
Keettel et al	—	—	36.0
Creasman et al	—	—	10.0
Morton, Moore, and Chang	—	—	50.0
Piver, Barlow, and Lele	3.2	0.0	25.8
Total	15.7	10.3	29.8
Stage I	11.3	10.3	32.9
Stage II	23.0	10.0	12.5

Modified from Piver MS, Barlow JJ, Lele SB: Incidence of subclinical metastases in stage I and II ovarian carcinoma. Obstet Gynecol 52:100, 1978.

assigned to stage I and 10.0% of patients assigned to stage II had aortic node disease. Knapp and Friedman found that the omentum was a site of microscopic metastasis in 4.7% of the patients with stage I and stage II ovarian epithelial cancer. Keettel and associates were among the first to report that in the absence of clinical ascites, a significant number of patients with localized ovarian cancer have free-floating intraperitoneal cancer cells, demonstrated by cytologic washings. In their report, 36% of the patients with stage I disease had malignant cells in the cytologic washings. The report and three other studies were collated by Piver and colleagues for a total of 87 women with presumed stage I or stage II ovarian carcinoma. A total of 29.8% of these patients were found to have free-floating cancer cells in the pelvis or paracolonic spaces. Therefore, many of the failures in the stage I and stage II categories were undoubtedly in patients with occult dissemination not realized at the time of the initial surgical procedure. (For recommendations on the optimal surgical procedure at initial laparotomy, see the section on diagnostic techniques and staging in Chapter 11.)

Early lesions of an epithelial nature are more common among certain histologic types (Fig. 10–19), such as mucinous, endometrial, and clear cell lesions.

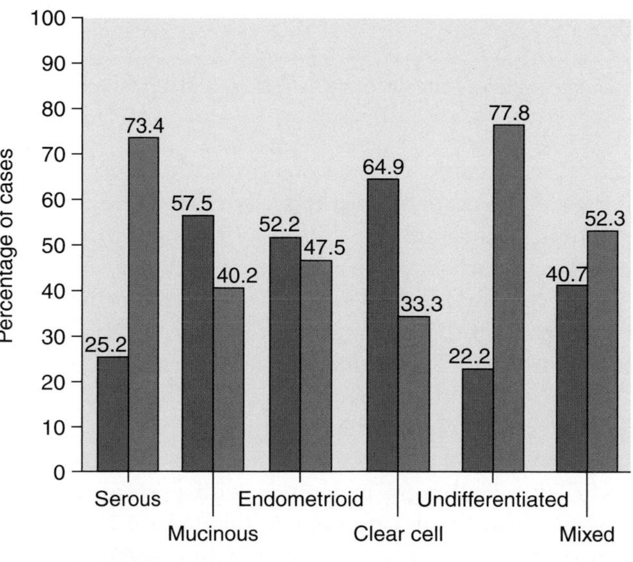

Figure 10–19 Carcinoma of the ovary. Patients treated in 1990–1992. Early versus advanced stages by histology. (From FIGO report. J Epidemiol Biostat 3:107, 1998. Reprinted with permission of the publisher, Taylor & Francis Ltd., http://www.tandf.co.uk/journals.)

MANAGEMENT OF EARLY OVARIAN CANCER IN YOUNG WOMEN

Operative treatment has traditionally been the mainstay of management in ovarian carcinoma. The technical aspects of the initial laparotomy have a greater bearing on outcome than do many subsequent therapeutic decisions. Hysterectomy with bilateral salpingo-oophorectomy continues to be the most cogent therapy for ovarian carcinoma. The opposite ovary is removed because of the frequency of bilateral synchronous tumors and the possibility of occult metastases, which in the normal-appearing opposite ovary have varied from 6–43%, depending on the report and stage of the disease. Because the uterine serosa and endometrium are often sites of occult metastasis and because the prevalence of synchronous endometrial carcinoma is relatively high, hysterectomy is also indicated. On occasion, however, unilateral oophorectomy has been done in young, childless women, and the tumors were subsequently found to be malignant. Not to proceed with further therapy is a calculated risk, the justification for which exists in statements made, summarized later, by many authoritative gynecologists.

For the young, nulliparous woman with a stage Ia tumor, the safety of more conservative operations to preserve childbearing is uncertain. Munnell reviewed 127 cases of ovarian cancer treated by operation that included bilateral salpingo-oophorectomy and 38 cases in which conservative therapy was used. Excluding the uncommon carcinomas in the series, the 5-year survival figure for the 28 patients treated conservatively and for the 105 patients treated more radically was 75%. In patients with mucinous tumors, 78% who had complete operation (23 patients) and 100% who had conservative operation (8 patients) survived 5 years. Similarly, Parker and Berek found no difference in the 5-year survival rate regardless of whether patients were treated by hysterectomy and bilateral salpingo-oophorectomy or by unilateral salpingo-oophorectomy alone. In 1990, Dembo and coworkers reported on a study of several surgical-pathologic variables using multivariate analysis to determine which tumor characteristics are important in predicting outcome. In the analysis, tumor grade, presence of dense tumor-associated adhesions, and large-volume ascites (irrespective of cytologic findings) were the only three significant independent prognostic factors. According to Dembo and coworkers, once grade, adherence, and large-volume ascites are controlled for, the traditional prognostic parameters of bilaterally positive washings, capsular invasion, tumor size, patient's age, and histologic subtype could not be shown to have any independent prognostic significance. Carey carried out the same multivariate analysis in a database from the Norwegian Radium Hospital and had similar results; tumor grade and dense tumor adhesions remained independent factors. Large-volume ascites was not in this second database.

The requirements for conservative management of stage Ia ovarian cancer are listed in Table 10–14. Unilateral salpingo-oophorectomy may be the definitive treatment of a young woman of low parity found to have a well-differentiated serous, mucinous, endometrioid, or mesonephric carcinoma of the ovary. The tumor must be unilateral, well encapsulated, free of adhesions, and not associated with ascites or evidence of extragonadal spread. Peritoneal washings for cytologic examination should be taken from the pelvis and upper abdomen, and the opposite ovary should be evaluated for disease. If the opposite ovary is of normal size, shape, and configuration, surgical evaluation is not routinely done. Munnell and others have calculated the incidence of microscopic metastases in the opposite ovary to be approximately 12%. The periaortic and pelvic wall nodes must be carefully palpated and sampled, and an adequate sample of the omentum must be taken for biopsy. In our experience, it is rare for grade 1 ovarian lesions to metastasize to pelvic or periaortic nodes. However, any grossly abnormal node tissue must be suspected of being a focus of a rare metastatic lesion. In addition, the preserved pelvic organs should be reasonably normal, because there is little to be gained by retaining the opposite ovary in a patient who is not fertile. With the finding of carcinoma in any of these areas, conservative surgery must be abandoned. After the patient has completed childbearing, some consideration should be given to the removal of the other ovary to eliminate the risk of another ovarian malignant neoplasm. Because the incidence of epithelial cancer of the ovary increases when a woman reaches the sixth decade and because a patient with a history of such a lesion harbors the unfortunate milieu that could promote another epithelial lesion, it is only logical to remove the vestigial ovarian tissue after childbearing.

The key issue in patients treated conservatively for stage Ia epithelial tumors of the ovary is the histologic type. Mucinous and endometrioid lesions fare better than serous lesions, the grade 1 and borderline lesions being the most easily treated conservatively. Serous lesions are said to be seven times more frequently bilateral than mucinous carcinomas.

Conservative therapy, designed by preservation of some ovarian tissue, appears to be safe, although no prospective trials have compared conservative surgery with bilateral salpingo-oophorectomy. Trimble and Trimble collected eight series (Table 10–15). In a study of these data, there were only 10 recurrences in 148 patients for an incidence of 6.8%. In our experience, we have observed the development of papillary serous carcinoma in a contralateral ovary 5 years after conservative therapy in the form of unilateral salpingo-oophorectomy that was performed on a 29-year-old patient.

Table 10–14 OPTIMAL REQUIREMENTS FOR CONSERVATIVE MANAGEMENT IN EPITHELIAL OVARIAN CANCER STAGE IA

- Well differentiated
- Young woman of low parity
- Otherwise normal pelvis
- Encapsulated and free of adhesions
- No invasion of capsule, lymphatics, or mesovarium
- Peritoneal washings negative
- Adequate evaluation of opposite ovary and omental biopsy result negative
- Close follow-up probable
- Excision of residual ovary after completion of childbearing

Modified from DiSaia PJ, Townsend DE, Morrow CP: The rationale for less than radical treatment for gynecologic malignancy in early reproductive years. Obstet Gynecol Surv 29:581, 1974. Copyright ©1974 by The Williams & Wilkins Co.

Table 10–15 RECURRENCE RATE IN PATIENTS WITH LOW MALIGNANT POTENTIAL LESIONS WITH CONSERVATIVE SURGERY

Author	Incidence of recurrence (%)
Casey et al	0/7 (0)
Chambers et al	2/20 (20)
Lim-Tan et al	4/35 (11)
Manchul et al	0/15 (0)
Rice et al	0/32 (0)
Sawada et al	1/5 (20)
Tazelaar et al	3/20 (15)
Tropé et al	0/14 (0)
Total	10/148 (7)

Modified from Trimble CL, Trimble EL: Management of epithelial ovarian tumors of low malignant potential. Gynecol Oncol 55:S42, 1994.

The role of adjuvant therapy, whether radiotherapy or chemotherapy, in tumors of low malignant potential has not yet been established. Several prospective, randomized studies of adjuvant therapy in patients with invasive ovarian carcinoma have included patients with tumors of low malignant potential. In one trial, conducted by the Gynecologic Oncology Group (GOG), 55 patients with stage I disease were randomized to no further therapy, pelvic radiation therapy, or oral administration of melphalan for 18 months. The investigators noted one recurrence, on the radiation therapy arm, and concluded that the total abdominal hysterectomy with bilateral salpingo-oophorectomy was adequate treatment of patients with stage I disease.

From 1983–1992, the GOG studied 414 patients with low malignant potential lesions of the ovary. The purpose of the protocol was to evaluate the biologic behavior of these tumors, the effectiveness of melphalan chemotherapy in patients with clinically detectable residual disease after surgical staging and in patients with recurrent disease, and the response rate to cisplatin in patients who failed to respond to melphalan therapy. The preliminary conclusions were that ovarian serous tumors of low malignant potential limited to the ovary rarely recur. Conservative management with unilateral salpingo-oophorectomy or ovarian cystectomy is adequate therapy for women of reproductive age. The effectiveness of melphalan and cisplatin has yet to be analyzed.

In a study from the Mayo Clinic of 33 women aged 16–29 years who had stage Ia ovarian cancer, it was shown that unilateral salpingo-oophorectomy or just resection of the ovary resulted in no recurrences in a follow-up period of 3–10 years. These results are encouraging, but they are not the final answer because many low-grade lesions are prone to late recurrence. Some centers are now studying the role of ovarian cystectomy alone for low-grade stage I epithelial neoplasms. Others have permitted stage I, grade 2 and 3 lesions, and stage Ic neoplasms to undergo ovarian tissue-sparing surgery followed by chemotherapy in an attempt to preserve fertility. These investigations await further observation and confirmation as to long-term safety. Chemotherapy administered after such ovarian tissue-sparing procedures is likely to destroy the remaining ova, especially in patients older than 30 years.

Colombo and associates reported data of 99 patients younger than 40 years with stage I ovarian cancer. Conservative surgery was performed in 56 of the patients (36 stage Ia, 1 stage Ib, and 19 stage Ic). Relapses occurred in three patients assigned to stage Ia (grades 1, 2, and 3). One recurrence was in the residual ovary and the patient was rescued by surgery; the other two patients had relapse at distant sites and died as a result of their tumors. Seventeen patients who desired to become pregnant did so, for a total of 25 conceptions. Colombo suggested a platinum-based regimen to lower the recurrence rate even further. A GOG study reported no difference in survival for patients with stage Ic or stage II or poorly differentiated stage Ia and stage Ib cancer randomized to receive either melphalan or intraperitoneal ^{32}P. The same report showed no advantage to adjuvant treatment with melphalan for patients with stage Ia or stage Ib well or moderately differentiated tumor.

Zanetta and colleagues published their results with 99 women aged 40 years or younger with stage I ovarian carcinoma. Of the 99 women, 56 underwent fertility-sparing surgery and 43 more radical surgery with a median follow-up of 7 years; they observed five recurrences (9%) of carcinoma in the women treated conservatively and five recurrences (12%) in those treated more radically. Two recurrences after conservative surgery involved the residual ovary (3.6%). These two women developed a borderline tumor in the contralateral ovary and were treated with surgery.

Only one trial testing cisplatin as adjuvant treatment of early disease has been published. In this study, 347 patients with epithelial ovarian cancer without residual tumor after primary surgery were randomized to adjuvant intraperitoneal ^{32}P therapy or six courses of cisplatin. Disease-free survival and overall survival were similar in the two arms even after adjustment for prognostic variables. Bolis and coworkers reported two multicenter clinical trials in Italy. After surgical staging and stratification by center, eligible patients were randomized according to a computer-generated list. In the first study, 92 patients with stage Ia or stage Ib grade 2 or 3 tumors were randomly assigned to receive either cisplatin for six cycles or no further treatment. With a median follow-up of 69 months, 5-year disease-free survival was 83% for the platinum group and 64% for the observation group. However, no difference in the overall survival could be detected. Indeed, the patients who had relapse in the no treatment arm appeared to be salvageable with chemotherapy begun at the time of recurrence.

The management of dysgerminoma is frequently singled out as an example for conservative surgery. Table 10–16 shows the statistics in patients treated in various manners. The exquisite radiosensitivity and chemosensitivity of dysgerminoma allows one to be somewhat liberal in its

Table 10–16 DYSGERMINOMA: STAGE I

	Cases	Treatment	Recurrence rate	Five-year survival rate
Radiumhemmet	22	UO+radiation therapy	18%	95%
AFIP	46	UO	22%	91%
AFIP	21	TAH, BSO	10%	90%

UO, unilateral oophorectomy; TAH, total abdominal hysterectomy; BSO, bilateral salpingo-oophorectomy; AFIP, Armed Forces Institute of Pathology.

management. Although the recurrence rate is approximately 20% in stage I, the overall survival rate is almost 95% because of the exceptional response to radical radiation therapy or chemotherapy. It is interesting to note that the incidence of recurrence is approximately the same despite the initial treatment. The treatment of recurrences results in an approximately 75% 5-year salvage rate. In the last decade, many centers have chosen to use multiagent chemotherapy rather than irradiation for advanced or recurrent dysgerminoma. Preferred regimens are similar to those used for other malignant germ cell tumors of the ovary (see Chapter 12).

SPILL OF TUMOR

The subject of tumor spill has been controversial in gynecologic oncology for some time. It is logical to assume that implantation and germination of cancer cells are conceivable and probable when a malignant cyst ruptures at the time of surgery. The question remains only to prove that this is so.

The early studies of Munnell did not support the theoretical possibility that rupture of a malignant ovarian tumor would enhance dissemination. He studied 99 patients with stage I or stage II ovarian cancer and had an overall 5-year survival rate of 71%. In his retrospective study, 27 of the patients had had spill at the time of surgery. Of these patients, 22 (81%) survived 5 years. Of these 27 patients, postoperative irradiation was administered to 21, and there was a 66% 5-year survival rate in this group. Six of the patients did not receive radiation therapy, and all six survived 5 years. It appears from this limited retrospective study that spill eruption does not endanger the patient's prognosis and that if spill does occur, postoperative irradiation is not necessarily indicated. Because the number of patients studied here is small, it is necessary to carefully characterize the histologic features in the six patients who did not receive radiation therapy. One might find that these were highly differentiated lesions, maybe of borderline quality. There is, in addition, an obvious bias interjected here in that the patients with more malignant lesions probably received radiation therapy. There have been few studies with enough patients to shed further light on this subject (Table 10–17). However, a report by Decker and associates of the Mayo Clinic, involving some 223 stage I cases of ovarian epithelial cancer, revealed that rupture during surgery did seem to lower the survival curve. Another study by Grogan from Harvard analyzed 124 patients with ovarian cancer. Rupture of an ovarian tumor cyst during surgery occurred in 16 of 124 patients. For our purposes, however, only nine patients should be considered, because only these patients had stage I lesions. Of these nine patients, six survived 5 years or more, one died of a massive myocardial infarction, and the other two succumbed to their malignant neoplasms. The six patients who survived had well-differentiated grade 1 histologic patterns. Both patients who died of tumor had poorly differentiated histologic pictures. They had received radiation therapy after hysterectomy and bilateral salpingo-oophorectomy, but the radiation therapy was delivered in moderate dosages of 2500–3000 cGy on a 200kV machine. This is far below optimal radiation therapy. Parker and Berek and Dembo and coworkers could find no difference in survival of patients with stage I cancers between those ovaries that ruptured at the time of surgery and those in whom rupture did not occur. Many of these retrospective studies have no information about the peritoneal cytologic status before manipulation of the neoplasm. Indeed, it is the patient with a negative peritoneal cytologic specimen who suffers spill who is of concern. Sevelda and colleagues described 60 patients with stage I disease with negative peritoneal washings at the beginning of the primary laparotomy. In 30 patients, rupture occurred; in the other 30 patients, the tumor could be removed with the capsule intact. After an average follow-up of 75 months, the probability of survival was 76% in both groups. However, all but 10 of the patients received whole-abdomen radiation postoperatively, which obscures a conclusion as to the true meaning of spill.

Table 10–17 TUMOR-FREE SURVIVAL IN STAGE I

Series	Ruptured neoplasm	Unruptured neoplasm
Purola and Nieminen (1968)	18/30 (60%)	83/100 (83%)
Williams, Symmonds, and Litwak (1973)	3/7 (43%)	57/58 (98%)
Parker, Parker, and Wilbanks (1970)	16/27 (59%)	12/20 (60%)
Dembo et al (1989)	98/119 (82%)	168/199 (84%)
Sevelda et al (1989)	23/30 (76%)	23/30 (76%)

Sainz and colleagues described 79 patients with stage I invasive epithelial ovarian cancer treated at the Massachusetts General Hospital. Of these 79 patients, 36 had stage Ia tumors; 20 had stage Ic secondary to intraoperative rupture (Ic-ruptured); and 17 had stage Ic secondary to capsule invasion, serosal disease, or positive ascites or washings. There were four recurrences and subsequent deaths among the 20 women with stage Ic-ruptured tumors (20%), compared with only one (3%) of the 36 women with stage Ia. The median follow-up time for the two groups was 97 and 78 months, respectively; overall survival was 97 and 73 months. There were two recurrences (12%) and one death (6%) among the 17 women with stage Ic disease, and no rupture. Survival experience of this last group was not significantly different from that of the stage Ic-ruptured group. Sainz de la Cuesta concluded that intraoperative rupture of malignant epithelial ovarian neoplasms may worsen the prognosis of patients with stage I ovarian epithelial cancer. In the same year (1994), Sjöval described 247 patients with stage I disease who were at risk of spill. There was no difference in survival between the patients whose tumors had intact capsules and

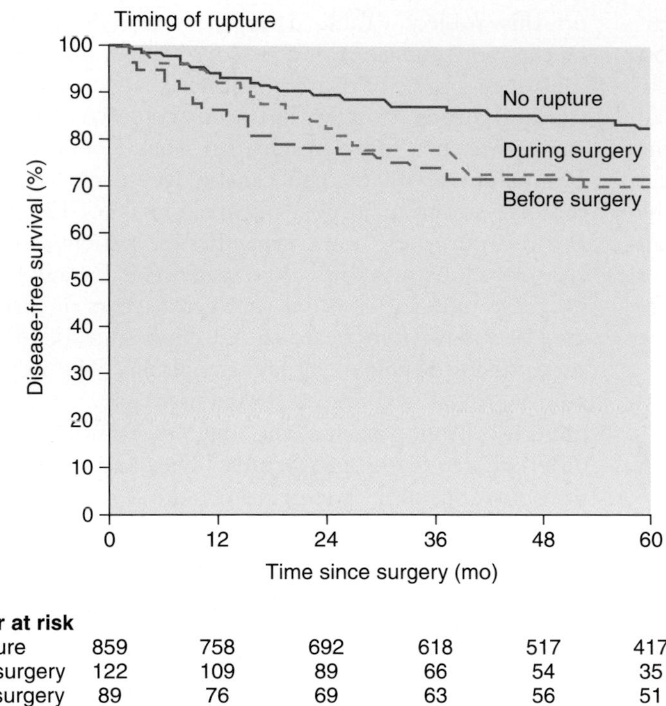

Number at risk

	0	12	24	36	48	60
No rupture	859	758	692	618	517	417
During surgery	122	109	89	66	54	35
Before surgery	89	76	69	63	56	51

Figure 10–20 Probability of survival in stage I epithelial ovarian cancer with rupture of a neoplasm during surgical removal, with and without intraperitoneal radioactive colloidal gold therapy. (From Decker DG, Webb MJ, Holbrook MA: Radiogold treatment of epithelial cancer of ovary: late results. Am J Obstet Gynecol 115:751, 1973.)

the patients in whom rupture occurred during surgery (78% and 85%, respectively). On the other hand, a significant difference in survival was found between patients in whom rupture occurred before surgery and those with intraoperative rupture (59% and 85%, respectively). The conclusion was that manipulation during surgery that results in puncture or rupture does not have a negative influence on the outcome for patients. However, rupture occurring at some interval before surgery may lead to seeding in the peritoneal cavity. Figure 10–20 illustrates the survival in stage I from FIGO data, 2001, with capsule intact vs surgical rupture vs early rupture. The issue is difficult to resolve because one is likely to treat more vigorously patients who have spill at the time of surgery, and this may equalize the survival rates in the groups of patients. In the era when whole-abdomen irradiation with pelvic boost was the only therapy that could be offered to these patients, some hesitation in instituting postoperative therapy appeared to be justified. However, we now have comparatively less morbid chemotherapeutic regimens that can be adequately used postoperatively. A reasonable and seemingly adequate recommendation in these instances is a course of chemotherapy administered in the form of a platinum-based regimen for four to six cycles and then a second-look procedure to verify the absence of disease within the pelvic and abdominal cavities. Others have recommended the use of intraperitoneal colloidal isotopes such as ^{32}P. No prospective study comparing these seemingly valid approaches has been reported. If rupture does occur, lavage of the peritoneal cavity with sterile water is recommended to cause lysis of the cells, and this may be helpful. The peritoneal surfaces absorb the water, so care should be taken to prevent delays in retrieving the fluid. Our bias is that surgical spill properly managed with adequate excision of the lesion and irrigation of the pelvis does not worsen the prognosis compared with the same patient without spill. Aspiration of a large self-contained malignant ovarian cyst by a needle attached to suction (with the area draped off with dry laparotomy pads) has been a long-time practice without apparent increased recurrences. We are convinced that this type of "controlled spill" (Fig. 10–21A,B) is safe and will not adversely affect outcome.

PROPHYLACTIC OOPHORECTOMY

The early diagnosis of ovarian carcinoma is as difficult and infrequent now as in the past. Although survival figures for this disease may be recently improving to a slight degree, the prognosis is still grave. One is therefore led to at least consider the impact of prophylactic oophorectomy for women, especially women undergoing pelvic surgery for benign disease when childbearing is completed and preservation of ovarian tissue is not essential.

At some time during their lives, 1–2% of all women develop ovarian carcinoma. The risk increases after 40 years of age, with a peak incidence between 55 and 60 years of age, closely paralleling the peak incidence of menopause in Western countries (Fig. 10–22). One is tempted to speculate that the gonadotropin changes or other factors associated with menopause might at times function as a promoting agent in the carcinogenic process. However, no scientific data are available in this regard.

The function of the ovary lies in its role of ova production for procreation and as the primary site of estrogen production. After the need for ova has passed in a woman's life, only estrogen production remains an essential func-

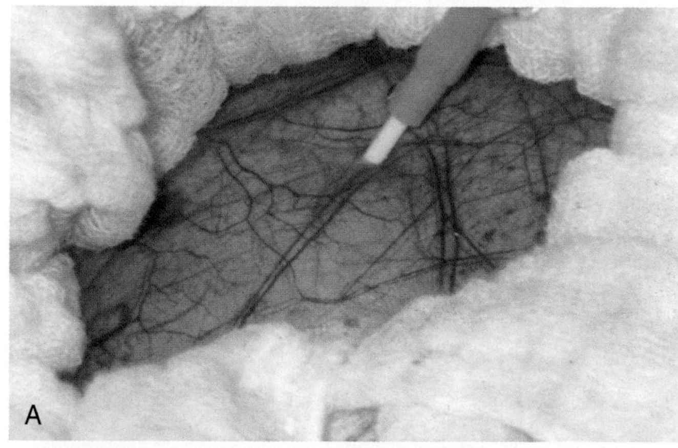

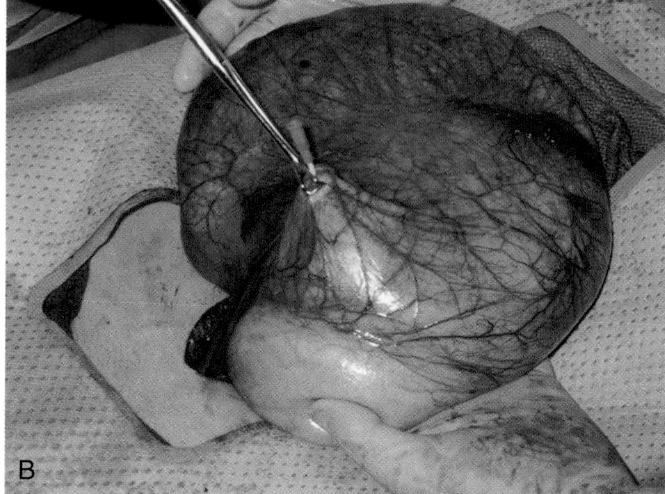

Figure 10–21A *A*, Aspiration of a large 40 cm simple cyst at laparotomy. The area around the puncture site is surrounded with dry laparotomy sponges. *B*, Collapsed cyst extracted through an 8 cm incision.

tion. The adverse effects of oophorectomy on several metabolic parameters are well known; understanding of the endocrinology, sexuality, and psychology of the postmenopausal patient (natural or surgical) has increased considerably during the past decade, and good methods of adequate substitution for the loss of ovarian function are now available.

In 1981, Grundsell and associates reported on a series of 352 women with ovarian carcinoma and studied the incidence of previous pelvic surgeries performed on these patients; 21 (6%) had undergone previous pelvic surgery, and 16 (4.6%) of these patients had surgery at some time after the age of 40 years. Others (Table 10–18) have reported similar results (Bloom, Gibbs, Grogan, Kofler, and Terz). McKenzie, Christ, and Paloucek reported that as many as 3.6% of women who have pelvic surgery with preservation of ovarian tissue will need subsequent surgery for benign lesions of the ovary, further influencing the argument for prophylactic oophorectomy.

Averette and Nguyen found that 18.2% of patients reported previous hysterectomy with ovarian conservation in a national survey of 12,316 ovarian cancer cases. Of these, hysterectomies were abdominal in 7.2%, vaginal in 4.2%, and unspecified in another 6.8%. In a subsequent analysis, Boike and associates found that 57.4% of hysterectomies were performed after the age of 40 years. Thus, a potential 1286 ovarian cancer cases could have been prevented if prophylactic oophorectomy had been practiced in women undergoing hysterectomy at the age of 40 years or later. Assuming an annual incidence of 24,000 new ovarian cases and that 5–14% of these cases had previous hysterectomies with conserved ovaries, it is estimated that at least 1000 cases could have been prevented if prophylactic oophorectomy were diligently practiced after the age of 40 years.

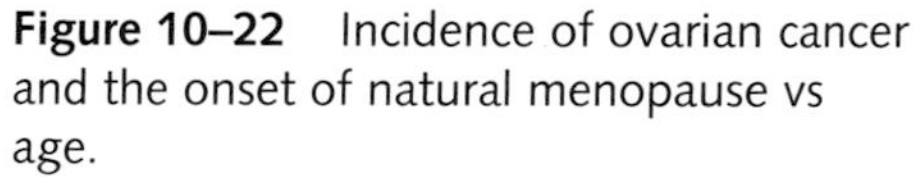

Figure 10–22 Incidence of ovarian cancer and the onset of natural menopause vs age.

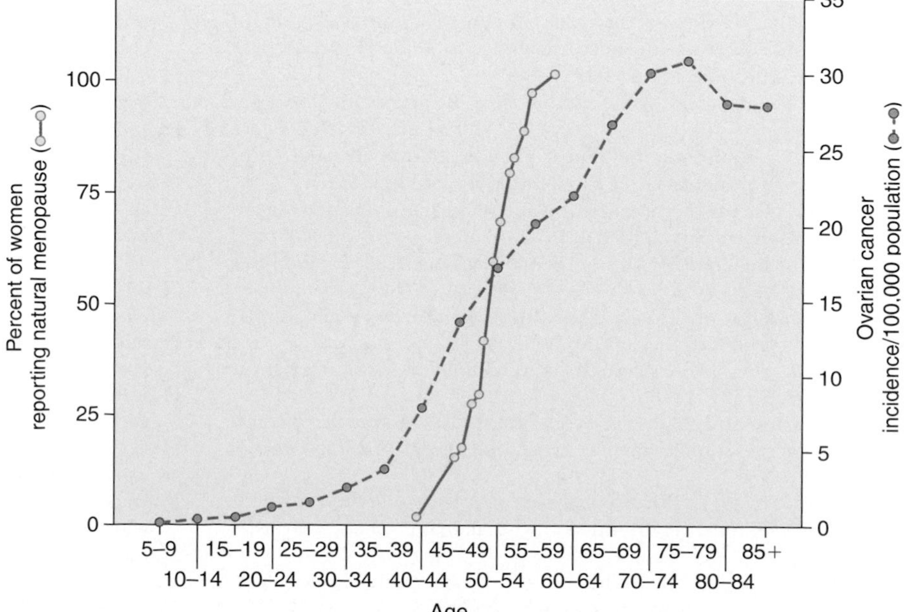

Table 10–18 OVARIAN CARCINOMA/PRESERVED OVARIES

		Previous pelvic surgery (%)	
Author	Year	All ages	> 40 yr
Bloom	1962	10.6	
Grogan	1967	8.2	
Terz	1967	8.8	3.8
Gibbs	1971	11.8	
Kofler	1972	8.1	8.1
Grundsell	1980	6.0	4.6
Averette	1994	18.2	10.1

We are obviously influenced by the frequent task of caring for patients with advanced ovarian carcinoma. The occurrence of this disease in patients who had previous pelvic surgery and in whom the ovaries could have been removed is certainly frustrating. Randall and coworkers have shown that unilateral oophorectomy does not influence the subsequent incidence of ovarian carcinoma.

All patients in whom prophylactic oophorectomy is under consideration should be thoroughly informed about the possible adverse effects as well as the advantages. The patient must make the decision without undue pressure from her physician. All thoughts of further childbearing must be settled. Open discussion should be encouraged, especially in areas of body image, libido, and other psychosexual concerns. With this as background, we believe that prophylactic oophorectomy should be offered to all perimenopausal patients (40–50 years of age) undergoing pelvic surgery.

BIBLIOGRAPHY

ADNEXAL MASS

Banks E, Beral V, Reeves G: The epidemiology of epithelial ovarian cancer: A review. Int J Gynecol Cancer 7:425, 1997.

Bergman F: Carcinoma of the ovary: A clinicopathological study of 86 autopsied cases with special reference to mode of spread. Acta Obstet Gynecol Scand 45:211, 1966.

Curtin JP: Management of the adnexal mass. Gynecol Oncol 55:S42, 1994.

Del Priore G, Robischon K, Phipps WR: Risk of ovarian cancer after treatment for infertility. N Engl J Med 332:1300, 1995.

Fathalla MF: Factors in the causation and incidence of ovarian cancer. Obstet Gynecol Surv 27:751, 1972.

Graham JB, Graham RM: Ovarian cancer and asbestosis. Environ Res 1:115, 1967.

Henderson WJ et al: Talc and carcinoma of the ovary and cervix. J Obstet Gynaecol Br Commonw 78:6, 1971.

Kurman RJ, Craig JM: Endometrioid carcinoma of the ovary. Cancer 29:1653, 1972.

Lee RA, Symmonds RE: Presacral tumors in the female: Clinical presentation, surgical management, and results. Obstet Gynecol 71:216, 1988.

Maiman M, Seltzer V, Boyce J: Laparoscopic excision of ovarian neoplasms subsequently found to be malignant. Obstet Gynecol 77:563, 1991.

McGowan L, Stein DB, Miller W: Cul-de-sac aspiration for diagnostic cytologic study. Am J Obstet Gynecol 96:413, 1966.

Menon U, Jacobs IJ: Ovarian cancer screening in the general population: current status. Int J Gynecol Cancer 11 (Suppl. 1):3, 2001.

Nezhat F et al: Four ovarian cancers diagnosed during laparoscopic management of 1011 women with adnexal masses. Am J Obstet Gynecol 167:790, 1992.

O'Hanlan KA: Case report: Resection of a 303.2-pound ovarian tumor. Gynecol Oncol 54:365, 1994.

Plaxe SC et al: Ovarian intraepithelial neoplasia demonstrated in patients with stage I ovarian carcinoma. Gynecol Oncol 38:367, 1992.

Reles AE, Gee C, Schellschmidt I et al: Prognostic significance of DNA content and S-phase fraction in epithelial ovarian carcinomas analyzed by image cytometry. Gynecol Oncol 71:3, 1998.

Shanks HGI. Pseudomyxoma peritonei. Br J Obstet Gynaecol 68:212–224, 1961.

Spiert H: The role of ionizing radiations in the causation of ovarian tumors. Cancer 5:478, 1952.

van Nagell JR Jr, Ueland FR: Ultrasound evaluation of pelvic masses: predictors of malignancy for the general gynecologist. Curr Opin Obstet Gynecol 11(1):45, 1999.

Weiner Z et al: Differentiating malignant from benign ovarian tumors with transvaginal color flow imaging. Obstet Gynecol 79:159, 1992.

Woodruff JD, Julian CG: Histologic grading and morphologic changes of significance in the treatment of semi-malignant and malignant ovarian tumors. Proc Natl Cancer Conf 6:346, 1970.

BENIGN OVARIAN TUMORS

Aure JC, Hoeg K, Kolstad P: Psammoma bodies in serous carcinoma of the ovary. Am J Obstet Gynecol 109:113, 1971.

Bourne T, Campbell S, Steer C: A possible new screening technique for ovarian cancer. Br Med J 299:1367, 1989.

Braly P: DNA content and S-phase fraction in epithelial ovarian cancer: What information do they really add? Gynecol Oncol 71:1, 1998.

Decloedt J, Berteloot P, Vergote I : The feasibility of open laparoscopy in gynecologic-oncology patients. Gynecol Oncol 66:138, 1997.

de Neef JC, Hollenbeck ZJR: The fate of ovaries preserved at the time of hysterectomy. Am J Obstet Gynecol 96:1088, 1966.

Dockerty MB, Masson JC: Ovarian fibromas: A clinical and pathologic study of 283 cases. Am J Obstet Gynecol 47:741, 1944.

Eltabbaku GH: Laparoscopic management of ovarian cysts. Contemporary OB/GYN 48(8):37, 2003.

Eltabbaku GH, Piver MS, Hempling RE et al: Analysis of failed and complicated laparoscopy on a gynecologic oncology service. Gynecol Oncol 74:477, 1999.

Finn CB et al: Can we predict a high-risk group in stage I epithelial ovarian cancer? Int J Gynecol Cancer 3:226, 1993.

Flynn MK, Niloff JLM: Outpatient minilaparotomy for ovarian cysts. J Reprod Med. 44:399, 1999.

Goede AC, Caplin ME Winslet MC: Carcinoid tumour of the appendix. British Journal of Surgery 90:1317, 2003.

Grogan RH: Reappraisal of residual ovaries. Am J Obstet Gynecol 97:124, 1967.

Harkki-Siren P, Kurki T: A nationwide analysis of laparoscopic complications. Obstet Gynecol 89:108, 1997.

Hart WR: Mucinous tumors of the ovary: a review. Int J Gynecol Pathol 24:4, 2005.

Hasson HM: Laparoscopic management of ovarian cysts. J Reprod Med 35:863, 1990.

Hasson HM, Rotman C, Rana N et al. Open laparoscopy: 29-year experience. Obstet & Gynecol 96:763, 2000.

Koonings PP et al: Bilateral ovarian neoplasms and the risk of malignancy. Am J Obstet Gynecol 162:167, 1990.

Meigs JV, Cass JW: Fibroma of the ovary with ascites and hydrothorax with a report of 7 cases. Am J Obstet Gynecol 33:249, 1937.

Ou C, Liu Y, Zabriskie V et al: Alternate method for laparoscopic management of adnexal masses greater than cm in diameter. J Laparoendosc Adv Surg Tech 11:125, 2001.

Parker WH, Childers JM, Canis M et al: Laparoscopic management of benign cystic teratomas during pregnancy. Am J Obstet Gynecol 174:1499, 1996.

Pelosi MA, Pelosi MA III: Laparoscopic removal of a 103-pound ovarian tumor. J Am Assoc Gynecol Laparosc 3:413, 1996.

Platek DN, Henderson CE, Goldberg GL: The management of a persistent adnexal mass in pregnancy. Am J Obstet Gynecol 173:1236, 1995.

Puls LE et al: Transition from benign to malignant epithelium in mucinous and serous ovarian cystadenocarcinoma. Gynecol Oncol 47:53, 1992.

Randall CL, Hall DW, Armenia CS: Pathology in the preserved ovary after unilateral oophorectomy. Am J Obstet Gynecol 84:1233, 1962.

Samanth KK, Black WC: Benign ovarian stromal tumors associated with free peritoneal fluid. Am J Obstet Gynecol 107:538, 1970.

Shozu M, Segawa T, Sumitani H et al: Leak-proof puncture of ovarian cysts: instant mounting of plastic bag using cyanoacrylate adhesive. Obstet Gynecol 97:1007, 2001.

Sigurdsson K, Alm P, Gullberg B: Prognostic factors in malignant epithelial ovarian tumors. Gynecol Oncol 15:370, 1983.

Spanos WJ: Preoperative hormonal therapy of cystic adnexal masses. Am J Obstet Gynecol 116:551, 1973.

Timmerman D, Bourne TH, Tailor A et al: A comparison of methods for preoperative discrimination between malignant and benign adnexal masses: The development of a new logistic regression model. Am J Obstet Gynecol 181:57, 1999.

Yoonessi M, Murray RA: Brenner tumors of the ovary. Obstet Gynecol 54:90, 1979.

Yuen PM, Yu KM, Yip SK et al. A randomized prospective study of laparoscopy and laparotomy in the management of benign ovarian masses. Am J Obstet Gynecol 177:109, 1997.

ADNEXAL MASSES IN CHILDHOOD

Asadourian LA, Taylor HB: Dysgerminoma: An analysis of 105 cases. Obstet Gynecol 33:370, 1969.

Blom PG, Torkildsen EM: Ovarian cystadenocarcinoma in a 4-year-old girl: Report of a case and review of the literature. Gynecol Oncol 13:242, 1982.

Breen JL, Maxson WS: Ovarian tumors in children and adolescents. Clin Obstet Gynecol 20:607, 1977.

Carlson DH, Griscom NT: Ovarian cysts in the newborn. AJR 116:664, 1972.

Deprest J et al: Case report: Ovarian borderline mucinous tumor in a premenarchal girl: Review on ovarian epithelial cancer in young girls. Gynecol Oncol 45:219, 1992.

Ehren IM, Mahour GH, Isaacs H: Benign and malignant ovarian tumors in children and adolescents. Am J Surg 147:339, 1984.

Haefner HK, Roberts JA, Schmidt RW: The university experience of clinical and pathological findings of ovarian neoplasms in children and adolescents. Adolesc Pediatr Gynecol 5:182, 1992.

Norris HG, Jensen RD: Relative frequency of ovarian neoplasms in children and adolescents. Cancer 30:713, 1972.

Plaxe SC, Braly PS, Freddo JL et al: Profiles of women age 30-39 and age less than 30 with epithelial ovarian cancer. Obstet Gynecol 81:651, 1993.

Rodriguez M, Nguyen HN, Averette HE et al: National survey of ovarian carcinoma XII. Cancer 73:1245, 1994.

Schwöbel MG, Stauffer UG: Surgical treatment of ovarian tumors in childhood. Prog Pediatr Surg 26:112, 1991.

Smith JP, Rutledge RN, Sutow WW: Malignant gynecologic tumors in children; current approaches to treatment. Am J Obstet Gynecol 116:261, 1973.

Van Winter JT, Simmons PS, Podratz KC: Surgically treated adnexal masses in infancy, childhood, and adolescence. Am J Obstet Gynecol 170:1780, 1994.

PALPABLE OR ENLARGED POSTMENOPAUSAL OVARY

Andolf E, Jorgensen C: Simple adnexal cysts diagnosed by ultrasound in postmenopausal women. J Clin Ultrasound 16:301, 1988.

Aubert JM, Rombaut C, Argacha P et al: Simple adnexal cysts in postmenopausal women: conservative management. Maturitas 30:51, 1998.

Bailey CL, Ueland FR, Land GL et al: The malignant potential of small cystic ovarian tumors in women over 50 years of age. Gynecol Oncol 69:3, 1998.

Barber HR, Graber EA: The PMPO syndrome (postmenopausal palpable ovary syndrome). Obstet Gynecol 38:921, 1971.

Conway C, Zalud I, Dilena M et al: Simple cyst in the postmenopausal patient: detection and management. J Ultrasound Med 17:369, 1998.

Creasman WT, Soper JT: The undiagnosed adnexal mass after the menopause. Clin Obstet Gynecol 29:446, 1986.

Cohen I et al: Ovarian tumors in postmenopausal breast cancer patients treated with tamoxifen. Gynecol Oncol 60:54, 1996.

Flynt JR, Gallup DG: The postmenopausal ovary syndrome: A fourteen year review. Milit Med 146:686, 1981.

Gleeson NC et al: Abdominal wall metastases from ovarian cancer after laparoscopy. Am J Obstet Gynecol 169:522, 1993.

Goldstein SR: Ultrasound for the postmenopausal patient. Female Patient 15:61, 1990.

Goldstein SR et al: The postmenopausal cystic adnexal mass: The potential role of ultrasound in conservative management. Obstet Gynecol 72:8, 1989.

Goswamy RK, Campbell S, Whitehead MI: Screening for ovarian cancer. Clin Obstet Gynecol 10:621, 1983.

Goswamy RK et al: Ovarian size in postmenopausal women. Br J Obstet Gynaecol 95:795, 1988.

Hall DA, McCarthy KA: The significance of the postmenopausal simple adnexal cyst. J Ultrasound Med 5:503, 1986.

Kroon E, Andolf E: Diagnosis and follow-up of simple ovarian cysts diagnosed by ultrasound in postmenopausal women. Obstet Gynecol 85:211, 1995.

Lerner JP et al: Transvaginal ultrasonographic characterization of ovarian masses with an improved, weighted scoring system. Am J Obstet Gynecol 170:81, 1994.

Levine D, Gosink BB, Wolf SI et al. Simple adnexal cysts; the natural history in postmenopausal women. Radiology 184:653, 1992.

Luxman D, Bergman A, Sagi J et al: The postmenopausal adnexal mass: Correlation between ultrasonic and pathologic findings. Obstet Gynecol 77:726, 1991.

Miller RC et al: The postmenopausal palpable ovary syndrome: A retrospective review with histopathologic correlates. J Reprod Med 36:568, 1991.

Parker WH, Berek JS: Management of selected cystic adnexal masses in postmenopausal women by operative laparoscopy: A pilot study. Am J Obstet Gynecol 163:1574, 1990.

Rulin MC, Preston AL: Adnexal masses in postmenopausal women. Obstet Gynecol 70:578, 1987.

Shalev E, Eliyahu S, Peleg D, Tsabari A: Laparoscopic management of adnexal cystic masses in postmenopausal women. Obstet Gynecol 83:594, 1994.

Valentin L, Akrawi D. The natural history of adnexal cysts incidentally detected at transvaginal ultrasound examination in postmenopausal women. Ultrasound Obstet Gynecol 20:174, 2002.

Vuento MH, Pirhonen JP, Makinen JI et al: Evaluation of ovarian findings in asymptomatic postmenopausal women with color Doppler ultrasound. Cancer 76:1214, 1995.

Westhoff C et al: CA 125 levels in menopausal women. Obstet Gynecol 76:428, 1990.

Wolf SI, Gosnik BB, Feldsman MR: Prevalence of simple adnexal cysts in postmenopausal women. Radiology 180:65, 1991.

SCAN-DETECTED MASSES

Andolf E, Jorgensen C: Cystic lesions in elderly women, diagnosed by ultrasound. Br J Obstet Gynaecol 96:1076, 1989.

Canis M, Pouly J, Wattiez A et al: Laparoscopic management of adnexal masses suspicious at ultrasound. Obstet Gynecol 89:679, 1997.

Granberg S, Norstrom A, Wikland M: Tumors in the lower pelvis as imaged by vaginal sonography. Gynecol Oncol 37:224, 1990.

Higgins RV, van Nagell JR, Donaldson ES: Transvaginal sonography as a screening method for ovarian cancer. Gynecol Oncol 34:402, 1989.

Kawai M et al: Transvaginal Doppler ultrasound with color flow imaging in the diagnosis of ovarian cancer. Obstet Gynecol 79:163, 1992.

Kurjak A et al: Transvaginal color Doppler assessment of pelvic circulation. Acta Obstet Gynecol Scand 68:131, 1989.

Taylor KJW, Conway DI, Hull MGR: Ultrasound and Doppler flow studies of the ovarian and uterine arteries. Br J Obstet Gynaecol 92:240, 1985.

van Nagell JR, Jr, DePriest PD, Reedy MB et al: The efficacy of transvaginal sonographic screening in asymptomatic women at risk for ovarian cancer. Gynecol Oncol 77:350, 2000.

BORDERLINE MALIGNANT EPITHELIAL OVARIAN NEOPLASMS

Barnhill DR, Kurman RJ, Brady MF et al: Preliminary analysis of the behavior of stage I ovarian serous tumors of low malignant potential: A Gynecologic Oncology Group study. J Clin Oncol 13:2752, 1995.

Bell DA, Weinstock MA, Scully RE: Peritoneal implants of ovarian serous borderline tumors: Histologic features and prognosis. Cancer 62:2212, 1988.

Burks RT, Sherman ME, Kurman RJ: Micropapillary serous carcinoma of the ovary. Am J Surg Pathol 20:1319, 1996.

Casey AC et al: Epithelial ovarian tumors of borderline malignancy: Long-term follow-up. Gynecol Oncol 50:316, 1993.

Chambers JT et al: Borderline ovarian tumors. Am J Obstet Gynecol 159:1088, 1988.

Creasman WT et al: Stage I borderline ovarian tumors. Obstet Gynecol 59:93, 1982.

Deprest J, Moerman P, Corneillie P, Ide P: Case report: Ovarian borderline mucinous tumor in a premenarchal girl: Review on ovarian epithelial cancer. Gynecol Oncol 45:219, 1992.

Drescher W et al: Prognostic significance of DNA content and nuclear morphology in borderline ovarian tumors. Gynecol Oncol 48:242, 1993.

Fort MG et al: Evidence for the efficacy of adjuvant therapy in epithelial ovarian tumors of low malignant potential. Gynecol Oncol 32:269, 1989.

Gershenson DM, Silva EG: Serous ovarian tumors of low malignant potential with peritoneal implants. Cancer 65:578, 1990.

Gershenson DM, Silva EG, Levy L et al: Ovarian serous borderline tumors with invasive peritoneal implants. Cancer 82:1096, 1998.

Harris R, Whittemore AS, Itnyre J, and the Collaborative Ovarian Cancer Group: Characteristics relating to ovarian cancer risk: Collaborative analysis of 12 US case-control studies. III: Epithelial tumors of low malignant potential in white women. Am J Epidemiol 136:1204, 1992.

Hart WR, Norris HJ: Borderline and malignant mucinous tumors of the ovary: Histologic criteria and clinical behavior. Cancer 31:1031, 1973.

Janovski NA, Paramananthon TL: Ovarian Tumors. Stuttgart, Georg Thieme Verlag, 1973.

Julian CG, Woodruff JD: The biologic behavior of the low-grade papillary serous carcinoma of the ovary. Obstet Gynecol 40:860, 1973.

Knapp RC, Friedman EA: Aortic lymph node metastases in early ovarian cancer. Am J Obstet Gynecol 119:1013, 1974.

Kurman RJ, Trimble CL: The behavior of serous tumors of low malignant potential: Are they ever malignant? Int J Gynecol Pathol 12:120, 1993.

Lim-Tan SK et al: Ovarian cystectomy for serous borderline tumors: A follow-up study of 35 cases. Obstet Gynecol 72:775, 1988.

Limber GK, King RE, Silverberg SG: Pseudomyxoma peritonei: A report of ten cases. Ann Surg 128:587, 1973.

Long RT, Spratt JS, Dowling E: Pseudomyxoma peritonei: New concepts in management with a report of 17 patients. Ann Surg 117:162, 1969.

Manchul LA et al: Borderline epithelial ovarian tumors: A review of 81 cases with an assessment of the impact of treatment. Int J Radiat Oncol Biol Phys 22:867, 1992.

Mann WG et al: The management of pseudomyxoma peritonei. Cancer 66:1636, 1990.

Parazzini F, Negri E, La Vecchia C et al: Treatment for fertility and risk of ovarian tumors of borderline malignancy. Gynecol Oncol 68:226, 1998.

Rice LW et al: Epithelial ovarian tumors of borderline malignancy. Gynecol Oncol 39:195, 1990.

Russell P, Merkur H: Proliferating ovarian "epithelial" tumours: A clinicopathological analysis of 144 cases. Aust N Z J Obstet Gynaecol 19:45, 1979.

Sawada M et al: Stage I epithelial ovarian tumors of low malignant potential. Jpn J Clin Oncol 21:30, 1991.

Seidman JD, Kurman RJ: Subclassification of serous borderline tumors of the ovary into benign and malignant types. Am J Surg Pathol 20:1331, 1996.

Shiraki M et al: Case report: Ovarian serous borderline epithelial tumors with multiple retroperitoneal nodal involvement: Metastasis or malignant transformation of epithelial glandular inclusions? Gynecol Oncol 46:255, 1992.

Silva EG et al: Symposium: Ovarian tumors of borderline malignancy. Int J Gynecol Pathol 15:281, 1996.

Silva EG et al: Tumour recurrence in stage I ovarian serous low malignant potential neoplasms (Abstract). Mod Pathol 9:987, 1996

Snider DD et al: Evaluation of surgical staging in stage I low malignant potential ovarian tumors. Gynecol Oncol 40:129, 1991.

Tazelaar HD et al: Conservative treatment of borderline ovarian tumors. Obstet Gynecol 66:417, 1985.

Trimble CL, Trimble EL: Management of epithelial ovarian tumors of low malignant potential. Gynecol Oncol 55:S52, 1994.

Tropé C, Kaern J: Management of borderline tumors of the ovary: State of the art. Semin Oncol 25:372, 1998.

Tropé C et al: Are borderline tumors of the ovary overtreated both surgically and systemically? A review of four prospective randomized trials, including 253 patients with borderline tumors. Gynecol Oncol 51:236, 1993.

Williams TJ, Dockerty MB: Status of the contralateral ovary in encapsulated low-grade malignant tumors of the ovary. Surgery 143:763, 1976.

PROPER IDENTIFICATION OF AN EARLY OVARIAN NEOPLASM

Bolis G et al: Multicenter controlled trial in patients with epithelial ovarian cancer stage I (Abstract). Proc Int Gynecol Cancer Soc 157, 1989.

Brugghe J, Baak JPA, Wiltshaw E et al: Quantitative prognostic features in FIGO I ovarian cancer patients without postoperative treatment. Gynecol Oncol 68:47, 1998.

Caspi E, Schreyer P, Bukovsky J: Ovarian lutein cysts in pregnancy. Obstet Gynecol 42:388, 1972.

Christ JE, Lotze EC: The residual ovary syndrome. Obstet Gynecol 46:551, 1975.

Colombo N et al: Controversial issues in the management of early epithelial ovarian cancer: Conservative surgery and role of adjuvant therapy. Gynecol Oncol 55:S47, 1994.

Creasman WT, Rutledge F: The prognostic value of peritoneal cytology in gynecologic malignant disease. Am J Obstet Gynecol 120:773, 1971.

Einhorn N et al: Prospective evaluation of serum CA 125 levels for early detection of ovarian cancer. Obstet Gynecol 80:14, 1992.

Eriksson L, Kjellgren O, von Schoultz B: Functional cyst or ovarian cancer: Histopathological findings during 1 year of surgery. Gynecol Obstet Invest 19:155, 1985.

Favalli G, Odicino F, Torri V et al: Early stage ovarian cancer: the Italian contribution to clinical research. An update. Int J Gynecol Cancer 11 (Suppl 1):12, 2001.

Fishman DA, Bozorgi K: The scientific basis for the early detection of early stage ovarian carcinoma. In: Fishman DA, Stack MS, eds. Ovarian Cancer. New York, NY: Kluwer Publishers; 3, 2001.

Fishman DA, Stack MS, eds: Ovarian Cancer. New York, NY: Kluwer Publishers; 2001.

Gleeson NC, Nicosia SV, Mark JE et al: Abdominal wall metastases from ovarian cancer after laparoscopy. Am J Obstet Gynecol 169:522, 1993.

Graham JB, Graham RM, Schueller EF: Preclinical detection of ovarian cancer. Cancer 17:1414, 1964.

Guerriero S, Ajossa S, Risalvato A: Diagnosis of adnexal malignancies by using color Doppler energy imaging as a secondary test in persistent masses. Obstet Gynecol 11:277, 1998.

Higgins RV, Matkins JF, Marroum MC: Comparison of fine-needle aspiration cytologic findings of ovarian cysts with ovarian histologic findings. Am J Obstet Gynecol 180:550, 1999.

Lehner R, Wenzl R, Heinzel H et al: Influence of delayed staging laparotomy after laparoscopic removal of ovarian masses later found malignant. Obstet Gynecol 92:967, 1998.

McKenzie LL: On discussion of the frequency of oophorectomy at the time of hysterectomy. Am J Obstet Gynecol 100:724, 1968.

Musumeci R et al: Lymphangiography in patients with ovarian epithelial cancer. Cancer 40:1444, 1977.

Piver MS, Barlow JJ, Lele SB: Incidence of subclinical metastases in stage I and II ovarian carcinoma. Obstet Gynecol 52:100, 1978.

Roman LD, Muderspach LI, Stein SM et al: Pelvic examination, tumor marker level, and gray-scaled and Doppler sonography in the prediction of pelvic cancer. Obstet Gynecol 89:493, 1997.

Steinberg JJ, Demopoulos RI, Bigelow B: The evaluation of the omentum in ovarian cancer. Gynecol Oncol 24:327, 1986.

Stevens EV, Liotta LA, Kohn EC: Proteomic analysis for early detection of ovarian cancer: A realistic approach? Int J Gynecol Cancer 13 (Suppl 2):133, 2003.

Trimbos JB et al: Watch and wait after careful surgical treatment and staging in well-differentiated early ovarian cancer. Cancer 67:597, 1991.

van Nagell JR, Depriest PD, Reedy MB: The efficacy of transvaginal sonographic screening in asymptomatic women at risk for ovarian cancer. Gynecol Oncol 77:350, 2000.

Vergote IB et al: Analysis of prognostic factors in stage I epithelial ovarian carcinoma: Importance of degree of differentiation and deoxyribonucleic acid ploidy in predicting relapse. Am J Obstet Gynecol 169:40, 1993.

Webb MJ et al: Factors influencing survival in stage I ovarian cancer. Am J Obstet Gynecol 116:222, 1973.

Yoshimura S, Scully RE, Taft PD, Herrington JB: Peritoneal fluid cytology in patient with ovarian cancer. Gynecol Oncol 17:161, 1984.

Young RC, Decker DG, Wharton JT et al: Staging laparotomy in early ovarian cancer. JAMA 250:3072, 1983.

MANAGEMENT OF EARLY OVARIAN CANCER IN YOUNG WOMEN

Aure JC, Hoeg K, Kolstad P: Radioactive colloidal gold in the treatment of ovarian carcinoma. Acta Radiol 10:399, 1971.

Carey M, Dembo AJ, Fyles AW, Simm J: Testing the validity of a prognostic classification in patients with surgically optimal ovarian carcinoma: a 15-year review. Int J Gynecol Cancer 3:24, 1993.

Delgado G et al: Para-aortic lymphadenectomy in gynecologic malignancies confined to the pelvis. Obstet Gynecol 50:418, 1977.

Del Priore G, Robischon K, Phipps W: Risk of ovarian cancer after treatment for infertility. N Engl J Med 332:1300, 1995.

Dembo AJ et al: Prognostic factors in patients with stage I epithelial ovarian cancer. Obstet Gynecol 75:263, 1990.

DiSaia PJ et al: Individualized treatment of ovarian cancers. Am J Obstet Gynecol 128:619, 1977.

Finn CB et al: Is stage I epithelial ovarian cancer overtreated both surgically and systemically? Results of a five-year cancer registry review. Br J Obstet Gynaecol 99:54, 1992.

Gadducci A, Sartori E, Maggino T et al: Analysis of failures in patients with stage I ovarian cancer: An Italian multicenter study. Int J Gynecol Cancer 7:445, 1997.

Helewa ME, Krepart GV, Lotocki R: Staging laparotomy in early epithelial ovarian carcinoma. Am J Obstet Gynecol 154:282, 1986.

Hester LL, White L: Radioactive colloidal chromic phosphate in the treatment of ovarian malignancies. Am J Obstet Gynecol 103: 911, 1969.

Hurwitz A, Yagel S, Zion I, et al: The management of clear pelvic cysts diagnosed by ultrasonography. Obstet Gynecol 72:320, 1988.

Kolstad P et al: Individualized treatment of ovarian cancer. Am J Obstet Gynecol 128:619, 1977.

Leblanc E, Querleu D, Narducci F et al: Laparoscopic restaging of early stage invasive adnexal tumors: a 10-year experience. Women's Oncol Rev 4:265, 2004.

Malmström H, Simonsen E, Westberg R: A phase II study of intraperitoneal carboplatin as adjuvant treatment in early-stage ovarian cancer patients. Gynecol Oncol 52:20, 1994.

Miller DM, Ehlen TG, Saleh EA: Successful term pregnancy following conservative debulking surgery for a stage IIIA serous low-malignant-potential tumor of the ovary: a case report. Gynecol Oncol 66:535, 1997.

Morris RT, Gershenson DM, Silva EG et al: Outcome and reproductive function after conservative surgery for borderline ovarian tumors. Obstet Gynecol 95:541, 2000

Munnell EW: Is conservative therapy ever justified in stage IA cancer of the ovary? Am J Obstet Gynecol 103:641, 1969.

Piver MS et al: Intraperitoneal chromic phosphate in peritoneoscopically confirmed stage I ovarian adenocarcinoma. Am J Obstet Gynecol 144:836, 1982.

Piver MS et al: Five year survival for stage Ic or stage I grade 3 epithelial ovarian cancer treated with cisplatin based chemotherapy. Gynecol Oncol 46:357, 1992.

Rossing MA et al: Ovarian tumors in a cohort of infertile women. N Engl J Med 331:771, 1994.

Rubin SC: Platinum-based chemotherapy of high-risk stage I epithelial ovarian cancer following comprehensive surgical staging. Obstet Gynecol 82:143, 1993.

Sakai K, Kamura T, Hirakawa T et al. Relationship between pelvic lymph node involvement and other disease sites in patients with ovarian cancer. Gynecol Oncol 65:164, 1997.

Spanos WJ et al: Complications in the use of intra-abdominal ^{32}P for ovarian carcinoma. Gynecol Oncol 45:243, 1992.

Walter AJ, Magrina JF: Contralateral pelvic and aortic lymph node metastasis in clinical stage 1 epithelial ovarian cancer. Gynecol Oncol 74:128, 1999.

Zanetta G, Chiari S, Rota S et al: Conservative surgery for stage I ovarian carcinoma in women of childbearing age. Br J Obstet Gynaecol 104:1030, 1997.

SPILL OF TUMOR

Decker DG, Webb MJ, Holbrook MA: Radiogold treatment of epithelial cancer of ovary: Late results. Am J Obstet Gynecol 115:751, 1973.

Grogan RH: Accidental rupture of malignant ovarian cysts during surgical removal. Obstet Gynecol 30:716, 1967.

Keettel WC, Pixley EE, Buchsbaum HJ: Experience with peritoneal cytology in the management of gynecologic malignancies. Am J Obstet Gynecol 120:174, 1974.

Purola E, Nieminen V: Does rupture of cystic carcinoma during operation influence the prognosis? Ann Chir Gynaecol Fenn 57:615, 1968.

Sainz de la Cuesta R et al: Prognostic importance of intraoperative rupture of malignant ovarian epithelial neoplasms. Obstet Gynecol 84:1, 1994.

Sevelda P, Dittrich C, Salzer H: Prognostic value of the rupture of the capsule in stage I epithelial ovarian carcinoma. Gynecol Oncol 35:321, 1989.

Sjöval K, Nilsson B, Einhorn N: Different types of rupture of the tumor capsule and the impact on survival in early ovarian carcinoma. Int J Gynecol Cancer 4:333, 1994.

PROPHYLACTIC OOPHORECTOMY

Averette HE, Nguyen HN: The role of prophylactic oophorectomy in cancer prevention. Gynecol Oncol 55:S38, 1994.

Bloom ML: Suggested prophylaxis for ovarian cancer. S Afr Med J 36:714, 1962.

Boike G et al: National survey of ovarian carcinoma. Women with prior hysterectomy: A failure of prevention? Gynecol Oncol 49:112, 1993.

Christ JE, Lotze EC: The residual ovary syndrome. Obstet Gynecol 46:551, 1975.

Gibbs EK: Suggested prophylaxis for ovarian cancer. Am J Obstet Gynecol 111:756, 1971.

Grundsell H et al: Some aspects of prophylactic oophorectomy and ovarian carcinoma. Ann Chir Gynaecol 70:36, 1981.

Kemp GM, Hsiu JG, Andrews MC: Case report: Papillary peritoneal carcinomatosis after prophylactic oophorectomy. Gynecol Oncol 47:395, 1992.

Kerlikowske K, Brown JS, Grady DG: Should women with familial ovarian cancer undergo prophylactic oophorectomy? Obstet Gynecol 80:700, 1992.

Kofler E: Uber die Häufigheit vorheriger Hysterectomien undoder unilateraler Ovarektomien. Geburtshilfe Frauenheilkd 32:873, 1972.

Paloucek FP, quoted by CL Randall. In Barber HRK and Graber EA, eds: Gynecologic Oncology, Baltimore, Williams and Wilkins, 1970, p 211.

Struwing JP, Watson P, Easton DF et al: Prophylactic oophorectomy in inherited breast/ovarian cancer families. J Natl Cancer Inst 17:33, 1995.

Terz JJ, Barber HRK, Brunchwig A: Incidence of carcinoma in the retained ovary. Am J Surg 113:511, 1967.Y

11 Epithelial Ovarian Cancer

Larry J. Copeland, M.D.

Malignant neoplasms of the ovary are the cause of more deaths than any other female genital tract cancer. About 22,220 new cases are diagnosed each year in the USA, and about 16,210 deaths occur annually as a result of this disease.

Ovarian cancer accounts for 6% of all cancers among women. In the USA, deaths from this cause occur at a rate of 1 every 44 minutes, and this disease will develop in 1 of every 68 women. The paucity of knowledge of the etiologic factors in ovarian cancer and the failure to achieve a significant reduction in mortality due to these neoplasms during the past 7 decades are areas of continuing frustration.

CLASSIFICATION

The student of ovarian pathology is often confused by the prodigious variation in histologic structure and biologic behavior. The most popular and practical scheme of classification is currently based on the histogenesis of the normal ovary, shown in Table 11–1. The early development of the ovary may be divided into four major stages. During the first stage, undifferentiated germ cells (primordial germ cells) become segregated and migrate from their sites of origin to settle in the genital ridges, which are bilateral thickenings of coelomic epithelium. The second stage occurs after arrival of the germ cells in the genital ridges and consists of proliferation of the coelomic epithelium and the underlying mesenchyme. During the third stage, the ovary becomes divided into a peripheral cortex and a central medulla. The fourth stage is characterized by the development of the cortex and the involution of the medulla. The histogenetic classification categorizes ovarian neoplasms with regard to their derivation from coelomic epithelium, germ cells, and mesenchyme.

The majority (85–90%) of malignant ovarian tumors seen in the USA are epithelial. They can be grouped into predominant histologic types as follows:

Serous cystadenocarcinoma	42%
Mucinous cystadenocarcinoma	12%
Endometrioid carcinoma	15%
Undifferentiated carcinoma	17%
Clear cell carcinoma	6%.

There seems to be limited prognostic significance to the histologic type of malignant epithelial ovarian cancer independent of clinical stage, extent of residual disease, and histologic grade. Histologic grade is an important independent prognostic factor in patients with epithelial tumors of the ovary (Fig. 11–1). Since the survival of grade 2 and 3 tumors is similar, there is some interest in simplifying the grading to low grade (grade 1) and high-grade (grade 2 and 3) tumors.

Table 11–1 HISTOGENETIC CLASSIFICATION OF OVARIAN NEOPLASMS

Neoplasms derived from coelomic epithelium
- Serous tumor
- Mucinous tumor
- Endometrioid tumor
- Mesonephroid (clear cell) tumor
- Brenner tumor
- Undifferentiated carcinoma
- Carcinosarcoma and mixed mesodermal tumor

Neoplasms derived from germ cells
- Teratoma
  - Mature teratoma
    - Solid adult teratoma
    - Dermoid cyst
    - Struma ovarii
    - Malignant neoplasms secondarily arising from mature cystic teratoma
  - Immature teratoma (partially differentiated teratoma)
- Dysgerminoma
- Embryonal carcinoma
- Endodermal sinus tumor
- Choriocarcinoma
- Gonadoblastoma

Neoplasms derived from specialized gonadal stroma
- Granulosa-theca cell tumors
  - Granulosa tumor
  - Thecoma
- Sertoli–Leydig tumors
  - Arrhenoblastoma
  - Sertoli tumor
- Gynandroblastoma
- Lipid cell tumors

Neoplasms derived from non-specific mesenchyme
- Fibroma, hemangioma, leiomyoma, lipoma
- Lymphoma
- Sarcoma

Neoplasms metastatic to the ovary
- Gastrointestinal tract (Krukenberg)
- Breast
- Endometrium
- Lymphoma

INCIDENCE, EPIDEMIOLOGY, AND ETIOLOGY

Approximately 27% of gynecologic cancers are of ovarian origin (Fig. 11–2), but 53% of all deaths from cancer of the female genital tract occur in women who have gynecologic cancer of ovarian origin. Cancer of the ovaries is the fourth most frequently occurring fatal cancer in women in the USA. It ranks high as a cause of female deaths in Canada, New Zealand, Israel, and countries of northern Europe. Ovarian cancer will develop in approximately 14 of every 1000 women in the USA older than 40 years (Table 11–2), but only 4 of the 14 will be cured. The remainder will have repeated bouts of intestinal obstruction as the tumor spreads over the surface of the bowel, develop inanition and malnutrition, and literally starve to death. In a review of mortality trends in the USA, age-adjusted (to the 2000 US standard population) ovarian cancer mortality rates from 1975–2002 show the number of deaths increased, reflecting a growing and aging population. Over the past 30 years, mortality rates have decreased for women younger than 65 years, whereas rates increased for women older than 65 years, with some plateauing over the past 10 years. This may be due to increased use of oral contraceptives in younger patients as well as a shifting of the survival curve to the right. Even when matched for stage, survival was poorer in older women. Some have suggested that this may be due to less aggressive treatment with surgery and chemotherapy in the older woman. Age-adjusted death rates were higher in whites than in blacks. Asian/Pacific Islanders, American Indian/Alaskan natives, and Hispanics have lower death rates than blacks.

Malignant neoplasms of the ovaries occur at all ages, including infancy and childhood (Fig. 11–3). Throughout childhood and adolescence, USA death rates for neoplasms of the ovary are exceeded only by those for leukemia, lymphomas, and neoplasms of the central nervous system, kidney, connective tissue, and bone. The major histologic types occur in distinctive age ranges (Table 11–3). Malignant germ cell tumors are most commonly seen in girls younger than 20 years, whereas epithelial cancers of the ovary are primarily seen in women older than 50 years. Beginning with the age group 45–49 years, which has a rate of 16.4 cases per 100,000, the incidence rates increase dramatically with age. The rate more than doubles after the age of 60 years to about 40 cases per 100,000. Highest incidence rates are found in the age group 65–85 years, in which the peak rate of 61 cases per 100,000 is found in the age group 80–84 years. The largest number of patients with ovarian cancer is found in the age group 60–64 years. More than one-third of the cases occur in patients 65 years or older. Elderly women are more likely than younger women to be in advanced stages of ovarian cancer at initial diagnosis, and the 5-year relative survival rate for elderly women is about half the rate (28.4%) observed in women younger than 65 years (56.6%). As of January 1, 2002, the prevalence of ovarian cancer in the USA was estimated to total almost 170,000 patients. This calculation was based on "First Malignant Primary Only" and so is probably an underestimate since ovarian cancer is commonly diagnosed in women with prior cancers, especially breast cancer.

Familial ovarian cancer

Familial hereditary ovarian cancer falls into three categories:

- Site-specific familial ovarian cancer;
- Breast-ovarian cancer syndrome, in which there is an increased incidence of breast and ovarian carcinomas alone or in combination; and
- Lynch syndrome type II, in which family members may develop a variety of cancers, including colorectal, endometrial, and ovarian cancer.

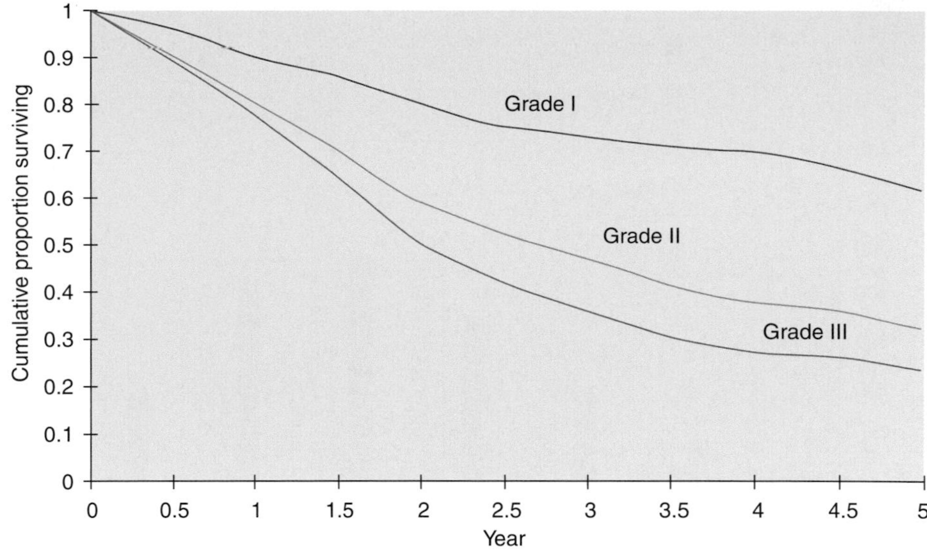

Figure 11–1 Serous cystadenocarcinoma of the ovary. Cumulative proportion surviving by degree of differentiation. (From Annual Report on the Results of Treatment in Gynecological Cancer, Vol 22. Stockholm, International Federation of Gynecology and Obstetrics, 1994.)

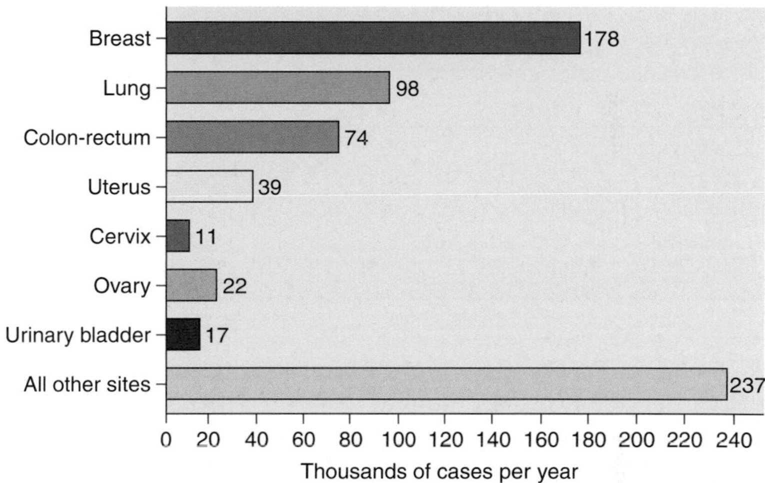

Figure 11–2 Estimated incidence of cancer of leading sites in women, USA, 2007. (From American Cancer Society. Cancer Facts and Figures 2007. Atlanta, American Cancer Society, Inc.)

Inherited genetic mutations are thought to be associated with about 10% of women who develop ovarian cancer. Thus, 90% of patients who have ovarian cancer acquired their genetic disease of cancer. Mode of inheritance observed in families is autosomal dominant (maternal or paternal transmission), and multiple family members are affected over several generations. First-degree relatives (mother or sister) are frequently involved.

True hereditary ovarian cancer as well as breast cancer is due mainly to mutation of BRCA1 and BRCA2 genes. Individuals with these mutations (BRCA1 and BRCA2) are thought to have a germline mutation (inherited mutated copy of the gene) in contrast to the more common somatic mutation (non-inherited) in most patients with ovarian cancer. BRCA1 is located on the long arm of chromosome 17q, and BRCA2 is on chromosome 13q12. Lynch II syndrome is due to inherited mutation in a family of DNA repair genes (MSH2, MLH1, PMS1, PMS2); this group accounts for only a small number of inherited ovarian cancers. Initial evaluation of these germline mutations suggested an estimated risk of ovarian cancer of 32–84% for carriers of the BRCA1 mutation if they are from a kindred with multiple cases of breast or ovarian cancer but a much lower rate for carriers of the BRCA2 mutation. With >400 mutations identified in BRCA1 and BRCA2 genes along with multiple polymorphisms, estimating risk is difficult. As more data are collected, the risk in patients with this mutation appears lower than was previously thought (65% decreasing to 20%). In most women who do develop ovarian cancer and have an ovarian familial history, the disease is sporadic in nature and not inherited. In a population-based study of 432 women with ovarian cancer, 34 (6.9%) gave a family history of the cancer, but only

Table 11–2 PROBABILITY FOR FEMALES AT BIRTH OF EVER DEVELOPING CANCER IN THE UNITED STATES

All sites	1 in 3
Breast	1 in 7
Cervix	1 in 130
Uterine corpus	1 in 38
Lung	1 in 18
Ovary	1 in 68
Colon-rectum	1 in 18

NCI. 2004. http://scrab.cancer.gov/devcan

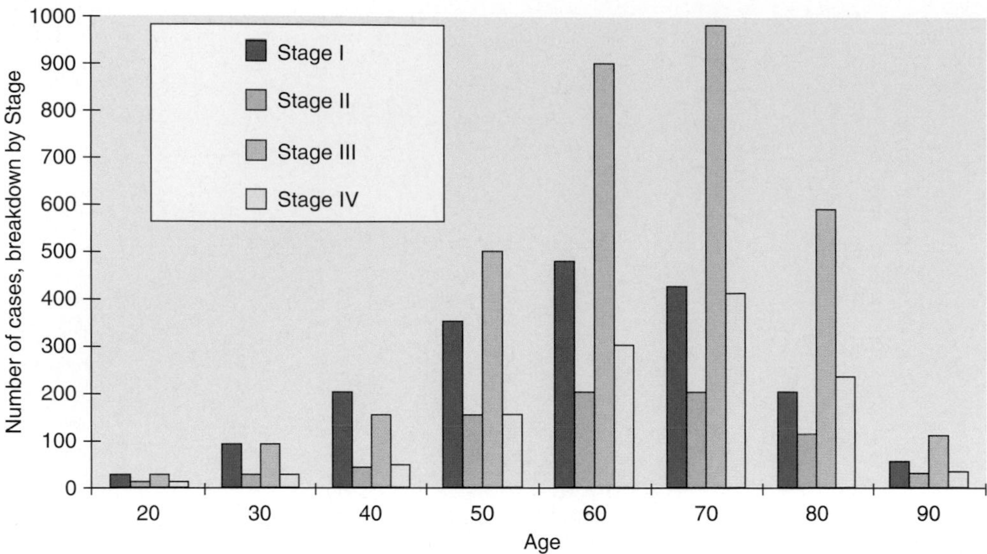

Figure 11–3 Obviously malignant ovarian epithelial tumors. Age distribution by stage. (From Annual Report on the Results of Treatment in Gynecological Cancer, Vol 22. Stockholm, International Federation of Gynecology and Obstetrics, 1994.)

Table 11–3 PRIMARY OVARIAN NEOPLASMS RELATED TO AGE

Type	< 20 yr	20–50 yr	> 50 yr
Coelomic epithelium	29%	71%	81%
Germ cell	59%	14%	6%
Specialized gonadal stroma	8%	5%	4%
Non-specific mesenchyme	4%	10%	9%

3 (0.6%) had more than one relative with the disease; the authors, after review, thought that only 1 (0.2%) may have had hereditary ovarian cancer. Houlston and colleagues evaluated 391 women who were self-referred to a screening clinic for familial ovarian cancer. Of these, 290 (74%) appeared to have no clear inheritance pattern, and there was no increased risk of cancer in the first-degree relatives. There were 82 (21%) pedigrees compatible with multisite cancer family syndrome with a relative risk of about 6, or development of ovarian cancer in 1 of 16. In the 19 families with site-specific ovarian cancer, the relative risk for first-degree relatives was 39 with a lifetime risk of 1 in 2. Kerlikowske and associates reviewed published studies of familial ovarian cancers and used ovarian cancer incidence data from the Surveillance, Epidemiology, and End Results (SEER) program to estimate lifetime probabilities of ovarian cancer in these families. They noted that the lifetime probability of ovarian cancer for a 35-year-old woman was 1.6% in an individual without a family history of ovarian cancer. It increased to 5% if she had one relative and 7% if she had two relatives with ovarian cancer. Bourne and colleagues identified 1601 high-risk patients on the basis of family history. These patients were then screened for ovarian cancers. In 1156 women who were thought to have sporadic family histories, two cancers (one low malignant potential) were identified (0.17%). Of the 288 with multiple-site designation, three cancers (two low malignant potential) were found (1.04%), and in the women with ovarian cancer, family history was identified in only 1 of 157 (0.63%). Cancers found subsequent to screening consisted of one peritoneal carcinomatosis in the sporadic group (0.08%), four (one peritoneal cancer) in the multiple-site group (1.38%), and none in the ovarian-only group. All of these studies were based on family history pedigree and preceded BRCA1 and BRCA2 testing.

Claus and associates, using a previously fit autosomal dominant genetic model to classify the breast cancer cases by carrier probability, evaluated the Cancer and Steroid Hormone Study of 4730 breast cancer patients aged 20–54 years and 4688 control subjects to estimate the proportions of breast and ovarian cases in the general population that are likely to be due to breast and ovarian cancer susceptibility genes. About 10% of patients with ovarian cancer in the general population were estimated to be carriers of a breast or ovarian cancer susceptibility gene; the proportion of ovarian cancer cases predicted to be due to the susceptibility gene ranged from 14% among patients diagnosed in their 30s to 7% among those diagnosed in their 50s. The risk for ovarian cancer in carriers to the age of 60 years and 80 years was estimated to be about 10% and 27%, respectively. Carriers were predicted to have at least a 15-fold age-specific risk of ovarian cancer compared with non-carriers. Some ethnic groups appear to be at high risk for gene mutation, and the Ashkenazi Jews have been extensively studied. In a large study by Struewing and associates, 5318 Jewish subjects had BRCA1 and BRCA2 evaluated, identifying only 120 carriers. The risk of ovarian cancer was significantly elevated in these carriers. The estimated risk was 2% by the age of 50 years and 16% by the age of 70 years compared with the non-carrier risk of 0.4% by 50 years and 1.6% by 70 years.

Frank and associates evaluated 283 women with breast cancer before 50 years of age or ovarian cancer at any age and at least one first- or second-degree relative with either diagnosis for BRCA1 followed by BRCA2 analysis. Mutations were identified in 94 women (39%) including 59 of 117 (50%) from families with ovarian cancer and 35 of 121 (29%) from families without ovarian cancer. In women with breast cancer, mutations in BRCA1 and BRCA2 were associated with a 10-fold increased risk of subsequent ovarian cancer. Mutations were noted in 24 of 38 women (63%) who had ovarian cancer. In women from breast-ovarian cancer families, 30 of the germline mutations occurred in BRCA2. Interestingly, in this study, the authors did not find Ashkenazi ancestry significantly increased in the identification of BRCA1 or BRCA2 mutation, suggesting that strong family history may be a more important factor.

In considering the woman at high risk, two questions should be addressed: Who should be tested? Are there screening or prophylactic measures that can be applied to decrease the risk? A family history of breast or ovarian cancer, particularly before the age of 50 years in a first-order relative, and Ashkenazi Jewish ancestry are risk factors for BRCA1 or BRCA2 mutation. The family history, both maternal and paternal, should be obtained (three generations is desired). Age at diagnosis should be noted. Pathology reports or death certificates verify accuracy of history; data have noted considerable error in history alone. Lifetime empirical risks developed on the basis of this information may suggest that testing for gene mutation is indicated. In general, extensive evaluation of family history and counseling should be done before genetic testing. Interpretation and plan of action that will influence medical management should be discussed in detail before genetic testing is performed. Testing of family members known to have cancer before testing of the cancer-free members is recommended. If a suspect mutation is found in the cancer member, the relatives without cancer can be tested for that specific mutation. If the cancer member does not have a mutation, other relatives probably will not benefit from testing. In one study, women sought DNA testing most commonly because of concern about the potential cancer risk to their children and secondly for their own cancer surveillance and prevention.

In a consensus statement of the Cancer Genetics Studies Consortium, annual or semiannual screening with transvaginal ultrasonography and determination of serum CA-125 levels beginning at age 25–35 years are recommended for BRCA1 mutation carriers. Both of these tests carry a relatively high false-positive and false-negative rate with low positive predictive value. Narod and associates found that oral contraceptives protected against ovarian cancer in patients with mutation in either the BRCA1 or BRCA2 gene. It has been suggested that prophylactic oophorectomy after fertility desires have been satisfied would be of benefit in protecting against ovarian cancer. The consensus statement concluded that there is insufficient evidence for or against prophylactic oophorectomy for it to be recommended as a measure to reduce ovarian cancer risk. A National Institutes of Health Consensus Conference recommended that women with two or more first-degree relatives with ovarian carcinoma be offered prophylactic oophorectomy after completion of childbearing or age 35 years. It is appreciated that carcinomatosis from a primary peritoneal cancer is not prevented with prophylactic oophorectomy; failure rates of 2–11% after prophylactic oophorectomy have been reported. Schrag and associates, in their analysis, found prophylactic oophorectomy to have small gain in life expectancy (0.3–1.7 years of life, depending on the cumulative risk of cancer). Rubin and associates identified 53 women with BRCA1 mutations. Compared with matched-control subjects, survival of patients with advanced disease was much better in women with the mutation (77 months vs 29 months; $P < 0.001$).

A recent population-based study of 232 incidents of epithelial ovarian carcinomas suggests previous studies may have underestimated the frequency of BRCA1 and BRCA2 mutations. Of 209 patients with invasive cancer, 32 patients (15%) had mutations of BRCA1 (20) or BRCA2 (12). Based on their data, Pal and colleagues suggested it may be reasonable to offer genetic counseling to any woman with an invasive, non-mucinous epithelial ovarian cancer.

As with other prevalent epithelial cancers, epidemiologic evidence strongly suggests that environmental factors are major etiologic determinants in cancer of the human ovary. The highest rates are recorded in highly industrial countries, which suggests that physical or chemical products of industry are major causes of epithelial neoplasms. A notable exception is highly industrialized Japan, where rates for malignant neoplasms of the ovary have been among the lowest recorded in the world. Interestingly, a higher rate of ovarian cancer is observed in Japanese immigrants to the USA and their offspring, eventually approaching that of Anglo-Saxon whites by the second and third generations. This suggests strongly that the causative carcinogens are probably in the immediate environment, such as food, personal customs, and other influences that change gradually during the cultural transition. To date, there are no clues as to which dietary items or other environmental contacts might be specifically carcinogenic for the ovary.

Whittemore and others have shown that the odds for invasive epithelial ovarian cancer vary with the number of term pregnancies each woman experiences. This observation coincided with the data illustrating a reduction in the disease incidence with the use of oral contraceptives (Table 11–4). The hypothesis that oral contraceptive use reduces the risk of epithelial ovarian cancer was suggested by Casagrande and associates in 1979. In 1982, Rosenberg and colleagues reported a case-control study of women younger than 60 years. Combination oral contraceptives were used by 26% of the cancer patients and 35% of the control subjects. The relative risk estimate for combination oral contraceptive use was 0.6 (Table 11–5). The reduction in risk appears to persist for as long as 10 years after use has ceased and to be greater for longer durations of use, but these results were not statistically significant. Their conclusion was that the use of combination oral contraceptives protects against epithelial ovarian cancer. The theory of "incessant ovulation" suggests that the epithelial lining of the ovary may be sensitive to the events of ovulation, which in turn can act as a promoting factor in the carcinogenic process. Gross and Schlesselman determined the

Table 11–4 ODDS RATIO FOR INVASIVE EPITHELIAL OVARIAN CANCER ACCORDING TO PARITY

			Population studies		
No. of term pregnancies	Cases	%	Controls	Percentage	Odds ratio
≥ 0	322	24	765	14	1.44
≥ 1	164	12	605	11	1.6
≥ 2	376	28	1515	27	1.53
≥ 3	265	19	1259	22	1.48
≥ 4	135	10	774	14	1.36
≥ 5	56	4	345	6	1.33
≥ 6	45	3	346	6	1.29

Adapted from Whittemore AS et al: Characteristics relating to ovarian cancer risk: Collaborative analysis of 12 US case control studies. Am J Epidemiol 136:1184, 1992.

Table 11–5 HOW ORAL CONTRACEPTIVE USE AFFECTS THE RISK OF OVARIAN CANCER

Duration of oral contraceptive use	Number of women who developed ovarian cancer	Controls	Relative risk
Never	242	1532	1.4
3–6 months	26	1280	0.6
7–11 months	14	1134	0.7
1–2 years	65	1602	0.7
3–4 years	40	1397	0.6
5–9 years	39	1594	0.4
≥ 10 years	13	1328	0.2

From the Cancer and Steroid Hormone Study of the Centers for Disease Control and the National Institute of Child Health and Human Development: The reduction in risk of ovarian cancer associated with oral contraceptive use. N Engl J Med 316:650, 1987. Reprinted, by permission, from the New England Journal of Medicine.

effect of oral contraceptive use on the cumulative incidence of epithelial ovarian cancer from ages 20–40 years, 20–50 years, and 20–55 years. The women were categorized into four groups: positive family history, negative family history, parous, and nulliparous. The Cancer and Steroid Hormone Study data were used in all four groups. The cumulative number of epithelial ovarian cancer cases estimated to occur per 100,000 oral contraceptive users compared with never-users decreased with increasing duration of use. Their results suggest that 5 years of use by nulliparous women can reduce their ovarian cancer risk to the level seen in parous women who never use oral contraceptives, and 10 years of use by women with a positive family history can reduce their risk to a level below that of women whose family history is negative and who never use oral contraceptives. On the basis of these data, the recommendation is strongly made that patients with a family history of ovarian cancer seriously consider using oral contraceptives when pregnancy is not being sought.

Studies have suggested an association between fertility drug exposure and ovarian cancer. Whittemore and associates noted that infertile women treated with infertility drugs had a 2.8 times increased risk of ovarian cancer compared with women without infertility. The risk was higher among women who did not become pregnant compared with the parous women. Specific drug exposure was not documented. The study by Franceschi and colleagues noted a non-significant decreased risk of ovarian cancer in women undergoing ovarian stimulation. Rossing and coworkers examined the risk of ovarian tumors in a cohort of 3837 women evaluated for infertility between 1974 and 1985 in Seattle, Washington. Computer linkage with a population-based tumor registry was used to identify women whose tumors were diagnosed before January 1, 1992. There were 11 invasive or borderline malignant ovarian tumors, compared with an expected number of 4.4 (odds ratio = 2.3, non-significant). Nine of the women in whom ovarian tumor developed had taken clomiphene (Clomid), and five had taken the drug during 12 or more monthly cycles. Venn and associates found no influence of ovulation induction on ovarian cancer, and Shishan in a case-control study found no increase in invasive carcinoma, although there was an increase in tumors of low malignant potential in women who used infertility drugs. There was no increase with clomiphene, but treatment with human menopausal gonadotropin was associated with increased risk, which is exactly opposite of Rossing's finding. In a large study from Denmark, Mosgaard and associates noted an increased risk of ovarian cancer in nulliparous women compared with parous women. Infertile non-treated nulliparous women had an odds ratio of 2.7 compared with non-infertile nulliparous women. The risk of ovarian carcinoma among treated nulliparous and treated parous women was less than that of non-treated nulliparous and parous infertile women. The published data suggest that there is probably little relationship of fertility drug use and ovarian cancer. Further investigations are under way to clarify this association. The concept is appealing when one considers the reduction in incidence noted with the use of oral contraceptives and parity.

Whittemore and associates, in a population-based study, noted protection against ovarian cancer with increasing parity (see Table 11–4). McGowan and colleagues, on the basis of a study of 197 women with ovarian cancer, estimated that nulligravidae were 2.45 times more likely to have malignant ovarian tumors and 2.9 times more likely to have ovarian carcinoma of low potential malignancy than were women who had been pregnant three or more times. The risk of ovarian cancer in their series was reduced to 1.27 among women who had been pregnant at least once. In Gerow's series, women with ovarian cancer demonstrated a marked decrease in the number of live births. One possible interpretation could be that the endocrinologic status of pregnancy protects against ovarian cancer and that the lack of this protection places infertile women at higher risk for ovarian cancer. A second explanation could be that infertility and ovarian cancer result from the same abnormal gonadal status. This theory would explain why infertile women are more at risk than never-married and never-pregnant women.

In the large prospective Cancer Prevention Study II, Rodriguez and coworkers evaluated the use of acetaminophen and a possible relationship to ovarian cancer mortality. Women who reported using acetaminophen daily had a death rate from ovarian cancer 45% lower than that of women reporting no use (relative risk = 0.55; confidence interval [CI] = 0.27–1.09). In a case-control study, Cramer and associates had previously reported that the odds ratio was 0.52 for development of ovarian cancer among women who used the drug at least once a week for at least 6 months; lowest risk was found in women who used the drug daily and for more than 10 years. Cramer also noted that the odds ratio of ovarian cancer was 0.75 (CI = 0.52–1.10) for aspirin and 1.03 for ibuprofen.

Parazzini and colleagues studied the influence of various menstrual factors on the risk of epithelial ovarian cancer. They reported that the risk rose with later age at menopause and with early menarche. Confirmation of this work is not yet at hand. Studies of dietary fat have been inconclusive, and other dietary factors are not at present considered well established.

Some have suggested that ovarian cancer may be initiated by a chemical carcinogen through the vagina, uterus, and fallopian tubes, and the substance promoting cancer may even be the steroid-rich antral fluid from ruptured follicles. For years, Woodruff and coworkers suggested this hypothesis of migration of chemical carcinogens from the vagina to the pelvic peritoneum. Venter demonstrated with the use of radionuclides that upward migration is possible. Certainly many different chemical substances are regularly used in the vulvovaginal areas, and some of these could be implicated in carcinogenesis. The agent most extensively studied has been talc powder. Many of the studies that noted a slight increased risk of ovarian carcinoma in association with talc did not adjust for factors (oral contraceptive use, family history) that are related to ovarian cancer. Others included low malignant potential tumors with their invasive cancers or did not correct for integrity of the female genital tract status. The relationship (if any) of talc to ovarian cancer would appear to be minimal at best.

No epidemiologic or experimental evidence exists to incriminate viruses in the development of neoplasms of the human ovary. Attempts to isolate viruses from cultures of human ovarian cancer cells have been unsuccessful to date. Because of its gonadotropic properties, mumps virus is an obvious candidate among known viruses for oncogenic activity in the ovary. Case-control studies have revealed a possible negative association with mumps parotitis, but these historical accounts were not supported by skin tests or serologic evidence of reactivity to mumps virus. Menczer and coworkers described 84 patients with ovarian cancer and 84 control subjects with non-malignant conditions matched by age and ethnic origin who were interviewed with regard to clinical mumps history, and their sera were tested for mumps complement-fixing antibodies. The patients with ovarian cancer differed from the control subjects in response to past mumps infection in two respects:

1. They appeared to be more likely to have developed subclinical mumps, as evidenced by the lower rate of clinical mumps history, despite serologic evidence of similar infection rates among those with positive and those with negative clinical mumps history; and
2. They tended to have lower persistent mumps complement-fixing antibody titers.

Menczer and coworkers interpreted these results as possibly indicating that an immunologic incompetence enables development of ovarian cancer, possibly through a direct etiologic role of mumps virus. At present, however, the evidence for mumps virus as an etiologic agent in ovarian cancer remains speculative.

Knowledge of the etiologic mechanisms involved in cancer of the ovary is limited to fragments of information. The cooperative group clinical trials programs offer an ideal population of women for case-control studies. Each patient should be questioned for a history of pre-existing gynecologic abnormalities, documented by clinical or laboratory data when possible, and for information about exposure to environmental carcinogens. There are many programs of this nature.

SIGNS, SYMPTOMS, AND ATTEMPTS AT EARLY DETECTION (SCREENING)

Although diverse ovarian tumors generally manifest in a similar manner, the diagnosis of early ovarian cancer is more a matter of chance than a triumph of the scientific method. As enlargement occurs (Fig. 11–4), there is progressive compression of the surrounding pelvic structures, producing vague abdominal discomfort, dyspepsia, urinary frequency, and "pelvic pressure" (Table 11–6). The insidious onset of ovarian cancer needs no elaboration. As the neoplasm reaches a diameter of 15 cm, it begins to rise out of the pelvis and may account for abdominal enlargement. The notion that the development of ovarian cancer is "silent" and there are no early symptoms of ovarian cancer is a focus of the patient advocacy "listen for the whisper" educational efforts. Symptoms often include vague abdominal discomfort, dyspepsia, and other mild digestive disturbances, which may be present for several months

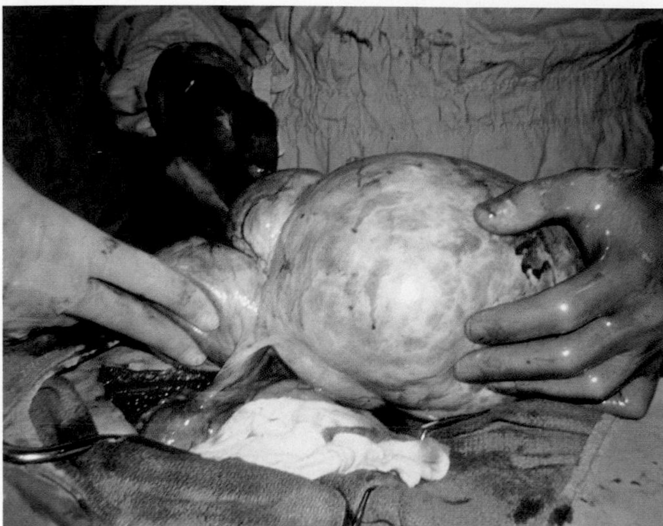

Figure 11–4 Large bilateral ovarian neoplasms: low-grade mucinous adenocarcinoma.

Table 11–6 MOST FREQUENT PRESENTING SYMPTOMS OF OVARIAN CANCER

Symptom	Relative frequency
Abdominal swelling	XXXX
Abdominal pain	XXX
Dyspepsia	XX
Urinary frequency	XX
Weight change	X

Table 11–7 SURGICAL FINDINGS

	Benign	Malignant
Surface papilla	Rare	Very common
Intracystic papilla	Uncommon	Very common
Solid areas	Rare	Very common
Bilaterality	Rare	Common
Adhesions	Uncommon	Common
Ascites (100 mL)	Rare	Common
Necrosis	Rare	Common
Peritoneal implants	Rare	Common
Capsule intact	Common	Infrequent
Totally cystic	Common	Rare

before the diagnosis. Such complaints are usually not recognized as anything more than "middle-age indigestion." A high index of suspicion is warranted in all women between the ages of 40 and 69 years who have persistent gastrointestinal symptoms that cannot be diagnosed. Unfortunately, the majority of such non-specific complaints are often functional in origin, causing the primary care physician to dismiss the possibility of ovarian cancer. Indeed, it is often only when the patient has gross enlargement of the abdomen marking the occurrence of ascites and extension of the neoplastic process to the abdominal cavity that appropriate diagnostic evaluation is undertaken.

Methods for early diagnosis have been investigated in limited studies employing cul-de-sac aspiration for peritoneal cytologic assessment and frequent pelvic examinations. All these endeavors have failed to show a significant impact on early diagnosis of this disease. These ovarian neoplasms grow quickly and painlessly. Any persistent ovarian enlargement should be an immediate indication for surgical assessment. The diagnosis rests with the pathologist. The size of the tumor does not indicate the severity of disease. Indeed, some of the largest neoplasms are benign histologically, most commonly mucinous cystadenoma. In addition, many large adnexal masses may be of non-ovarian etiology. Non-ovarian causes of apparent adnexal masses are diverticulitis, tubo-ovarian abscess, carcinoma of the cecum or sigmoid, pelvic kidney, and uterine or intraligamentous myomas. At the time of surgery, it may be difficult to discern the malignant potential of a particular ovarian neoplasm (Table 11–7). There is sufficient overlap of morphologic criteria to cause considerable confusion. The diagnosis rests with the histologic examination of the specimen, and the error rate of frozen section is about 5%.

Immunologic diagnosis of subclinical ovarian cancer by means of identification of specific tumor-associated antigens in the serum has yet to materialize. Several tumor-associated antigens, including CA-125, have been identified and purified. Recent research identifying patterns of protein fragments (proteomics) in patients with ovarian carcinoma requires validation in larger trials.

It has been suggested that every woman should have a periodic pelvic examination, pelvic ultrasound examination, and CA-125 test to make sure she does not harbor an occult ovarian cancer. Enthusiasm for early detection of ovarian cancer is laudable. However, it has been calculated that 10,000 routine pelvic examinations would be required to detect one early ovarian cancer in a population of asymptomatic patients. Jacobs and colleagues, in their large study of 22,000 women screened with CA-125 determinations, have reported a follow-up with the study population observed for a mean of 6.76 years. All women were older than 45 years and postmenopausal. There were a total of 49 index cancers (ovary and fallopian tube), of which 16 (32%) were stage I, 4 stage II, 22 stage III, and 7 stage IV at the time of diagnosis. Of the 22,000 women, 47,775 tests were obtained with 1180 tests (2.5%) and 767 women (3.5%) having a concentration of 30 U/mL. The overall specificity and positive predictive value were 96.6% and 3.1%, respectively. Sensitivity at 1 year and 7 years of follow-up was 75% and 57%, respectively. Only 49 (6.3%) of women with elevated CA-125 (16%) had cancer, or 0.0022% of women screened. The role of screening with CA-125 measurement in the general population of postmenopausal women appears non-existent. In a follow-up of 22,000 women initially undergoing a screening with CA-125 measurement, Jacobs randomized the group between yearly screening for 3 years and observation only. In the yearly screening group, six ovarian cancers were identified (468 had increased CA-125 and 781 ultrasound examinations were done, with 29 undergoing surgical evaluation—80% false-positive). During the subsequent follow-up after screening, 10 additional cancers were identified. Of the original six cancers, three were stage I and three were stage III. Eight of the subsequent cancers were stage III or stage IV. In the unscreened population, 20 cancers were subsequently diagnosed. Eight were stage III or stage IV. Although the screened cancers had a greater chance of being early stage, the total number remains low, which speaks to the prevalence rate. As already noted, the use of CA-125 measurement as a screening technique has not been rewarding, especially in premenopausal women. Many conditions of a benign nature, as well as most gastrointestinal tract malignant neoplasms, may elevate the CA-125 concentration (Table 11–8). The value of ultrasonography in screening for early ovarian carcinoma has received much attention. Herrmann analyzed data of 312 surgical patients regarding initial ultrasound readings and found a predictive value for cancer of 73%. Campbell and coworkers reported early detection of five primary ovarian cancers in approximately 5000 women screened by abdominal ultrasonography (Table 11–9). Although transvaginal ultrasonography may increase the accuracy of noting adnexal enlargements, it undoubtedly also increases costs, especially in terms of the follow-up of patients noted to have enlargement. The group from Kentucky has reported the largest number of women screened with transvaginal ultrasonography. All patients were postmenopausal unless a family history of ovarian cancer was present (24% of women). They have screened 6470 women with 14,829 scans; 90 women had persistent abnormalities on transvaginal ultrasonography and underwent surgery. Six primary ovarian cancers were found (five stage I and one stage IIIb), and only four were epithelial. Sensitivity was 0.857 and specificity was 0.987 with a positive predictive value of only 0.069 but with a negative predictive value of 0.999.

One strategy to improve the effectiveness of ovarian cancer screening would be to target populations at increased risk for the development of the disease, such as individuals with a positive family history of ovarian cancer. Bourne and colleagues reported the results of such a strategy in screening patients with transvaginal ultrasonography in combination with color flow Doppler imaging and morphologic assessment. In the screening of 1601 patients, 57% required repeated transvaginal ultrasonography to confirm the presence of a mass. Six ovarian cancers were diagnosed (two stage I, three low malignant potential tumors, and one stage III). Karlan and associates reported screening of 597 patients with a family history of cancer by CA-125 measurement, transvaginal ultrasonography, and

Table 11–8 NON-MALIGNANT CONDITIONS THAT MAY ELEVATE CA-125 CONCENTRATIONS

Gynecologic	Non-gynecologic
Acute pelvic inflammatory disease	Active hepatitis
Adenomyosis	Acute pancreatitis
Benign ovarian neoplasm	Chronic liver disease
Endometriosis	Cirrhosis
Functional ovarian cyst	Colitis
Meigs' syndrome	Congestive heart failure
Menstruation	Diabetes (poorly controlled)
Ovarian hyperstimulation	Diverticulitis
Unexplained infertility	Mesothelioma
Uterine myoma	Non-malignant ascites
	Pericarditis
	Pneumonia
	Polyarteritis nodosa
	Postoperative period
	Renal disease
	Rodent exposure (HAMA response)
	Systemic lupus erythematosus

HAMA, human anti-mouse antibody

Table 11–9 STAGE AND PREVALENCE OF SCREEN-DETECTED PRIMARY OVARIAN CANCER IN 20 PROSPECTIVE SCREENING STUDIES

	Screened	Prevalence of detected primary cancer	Screen-detected cancers per 100,000	Stage I
General population				
Ultrasound	15,834	8	51	6
Exclude LMP	6	38	4	
Multimodal[1]	27,560	14	51	7
Exclude LMP	13	47	6	
High-risk population				
Ultrasound[2]	4551	21	461	12
With family history	3146	15	477	9
Exclude LMP		8	254	2

[1]CA-125.
[2]With or without CA-125.
LMP, low malignant potential.
From Bell R et al: The performance of screening tests for ovarian cancer: Results of a systematic review. Br J Obstet Gynaecol 105:1136, 1998.

color flow Doppler imaging. Initially, 115 patients had an abnormal finding on transvaginal ultrasonography, and 68 had an abnormal CA-125 level. After repeated transvaginal ultrasonography, because of abnormal findings of color flow Doppler imaging, 19 patients underwent surgery. At the time of the report, one low malignant potential tumor had been diagnosed.

Bell and colleagues reviewed 25 studies on screening for ovarian cancer, 16 studies on women at average risk and 9 studies on women at higher risk. Many of the studies were small and imprecise on methodology; few gave follow-up details. Some studies used single screening techniques, whereas others used multimodal screening. For women at average risk, 75% of primary cancers were stage I when they were detected with ultrasonography, and 50% were stage I when they were detected by multimodal screening (see Table 11–9). In women at higher risk, 60% of tumors detected by screening were stage I; but if low malignant potential tumors were excluded, only 25% were stage I. False-negative rates were higher in the higher risk population than in the group at average risk. The false-negative data, when applied to a population with an annual incidence of 40 per 100,000, imply that 30–60 surgical procedures would be carried out for every cancer detected at annual grayscale ultrasonography (assuming 100% sensitivity), and 2.5–15 surgical procedures would be carried out for every cancer detected by multimodal screening. Even if screening detects all ovarian cancers and these are treated with 100% success, the absolute reduction in mortality would be only 1 in about 2500 screened women per year. This is much smaller than the complication rate from unnecessary diagnostic surgery or recall for further tests.

There are randomized clinical trials ongoing; however, unless results from these show differently, there are no reliable data that screening for ovarian cancer is effective in improving length and quality of life in women with ovarian cancer. Another strategy to improve sensitivity and specificity in screening for ovarian cancer involves the use of multiple serum tumor markers. Because <50% of patients with stage I ovarian cancer will have an elevated CA-125 concentration, the addition of other markers in the screening strategy could potentially improve sensitivity. While studies addressing this concept have to date not been fruitful, recent research in the area of proteomics has injected new hope into a more effective screening tool. These biomarkers may also offer useful guidelines for predicting therapeutic response and for treatment selection. The National Institutes of Health Consensus Development Conference on ovarian cancer screening in 1994 reached the following conclusions:

There is no evidence available yet that the current screening modalities of CA-125 measurement and transvaginal ultrasonography can be used effectively for widespread screening to reduce mortality from ovarian cancer or that their use will result in decreased rather than increased morbidity and mortality. Routine screening has resulted in unnecessary surgery with associated risks. Clearly, it is important to identify and validate effective screening modalities. Currently available technology for screening should be employed in the context of clinical trials to determine the efficacy of these modalities and their effect on ovarian cancer mortality. In addition, research must be continued to identify additional markers and imaging techniques that will be useful. If a woman has one first-degree relative with ovarian cancer (making her lifetime risk of developing the disease 5%) but no clinical trials are available to her, she may feel that despite the absence of prospective data, this is sufficient risk for her to be screened. This alternative and opportunity should be available to the woman and her physician.

If a woman were undergoing pelvic surgery, removal of the ovaries at that time would almost fully eliminate her risk of ovarian cancer (although there remains a minimal risk of peritoneal carcinomatosis). If the woman is premenopausal, discussion of estrogen replacement therapy is important before removal of the ovaries, because for some younger women, if estrogen replacement is not used, the risk of premature menopause and the potential for cardiovascular disease and osteoporosis may outweigh the risk of ovarian conservation and the potential for ovarian cancer.

DIAGNOSTIC TECHNIQUES AND STAGING

Routine pelvic examinations detect only 1 ovarian cancer in 10,000 asymptomatic women. However, pelvic examination remains the most practical means of detecting early disease. Pain is usually a late complication; it is seen with early disease only in association with a complication such as torsion, rupture, or, rarely, infection. The physician should have a high index of suspicion for an early ovarian neoplasm in any ovary palpated in a patient 3 years or longer after menopause. These patients should be considered for immediate laparoscopy or laparotomy when ultrasound examination findings suggest malignant change (e.g., complex mass, >5 cm, or intracystic papillations).

Routine laboratory tests are not of great value in the diagnosis of ovarian tumors. The major value of laboratory tests is in ruling out other pelvic disorders. Pelvic ultrasound examination or abdominal radiography may reveal calcifications consistent with myomas or toothlike calcifications consistent with benign teratomas. Intravenous pyelography may be helpful in ruling out disease in adjacent pelvic structures. A barium enema study is probably advisable with any pelvic mass and in a postmenopausal woman with lower intestinal symptoms. A similar comment can be made for colonoscopy and upper gastrointestinal endoscopy in patients who have lower or upper intestinal symptoms respectively. Computed tomography (CT) with contrast enhancement may be helpful in identifying the extent of clinical disease; however, a clinical pelvic mass in a postmenopausal woman needs surgical evaluation irrespective of the CT scan findings. The outcome in ovarian cancer relies so heavily on early diagnosis that procrastination with numerous diagnostic procedures is somewhat hazardous.

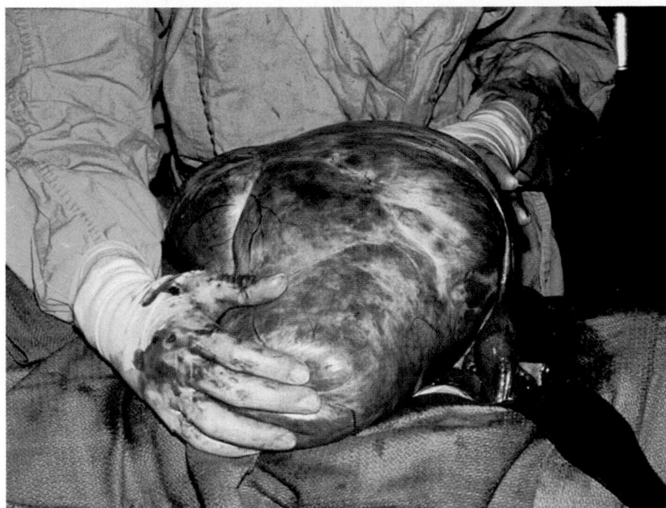

Figure 11–5 Large cystic tumors, similar to the illustration, are at risk of perforation and leakage at the time of paracentesis.

Surgical exploration is the ultimate test as to the nature of the disorder. Paracentesis for the purpose of obtaining a cell block and cytologic smear of the peritoneal fluid appears unnecessary, is occasionally dangerous, and may render a false-negative result. If one is dealing with a self-contained malignant cyst, such a procedure can result in spillage of malignant cells into the peritoneal cavity. Regardless of whether the fluid contains neoplastic cells, laparotomy is still necessary to remove the large benign neoplasm or to define the extent of the malignant process. In addition, up to 50% of ascitic fluid samples from patients with true ovarian malignant neoplasms will be negative for malignant cells on cell block analysis. Diagnostic paracentesis in a patient with ascites and a pelvic abdominal mass is therefore both unnecessary and potentially dangerous (Fig. 11–5).

The staging of ovarian cancer is surgical (Table 11–10) and based on the operative findings at the commencement of the procedure (Fig. 11–6). A longitudinal midline incision is recommended to facilitate removal of the neoplasm and to permit adequate visualization of the entire abdominal cavity, including the undersurface of the diaphragm. Ovarian cancer is classically a serosal spreading disease (Fig. 11–7), and thus all peritoneal surfaces must be carefully inspected, especially when disease is thought to be limited to the pelvis. Although lymphatic spread to retroperitoneal nodes is common in ovarian cancer, the disease most often spreads intraperitoneally; free-floating cells shed from the primary tumor are capable of implanting on any peritoneal surface. Any peritoneal fluid found when the peritoneal cavity is opened should be aspirated and submitted for cytologic examination. In the absence of peritoneal fluid, four washings should be taken by lavage of the peritoneal surfaces: the undersurface of the diaphragm as the first specimen (Fig. 11–8), lateral to the ascending and descending colon as the second and third specimens, and the pelvic peritoneal surfaces as the fourth specimen. These specimens are obtained by lavaging

Table 11–10 CARCINOMA OF THE OVARY: STAGING CLASSIFICATION USING THE FIGO NOMENCLATURE

FIGO stage	Description
I	Growth limited to the ovaries
Ia	Growth limited to one ovary; no ascites present containing malignant cells; no tumor on the external surfaces; capsule intact
Ib	Growth limited to both ovaries; no ascites present containing malignant cells; no tumor on the external surfaces; capsules intact
Ic*	Tumor stage Ia or stage Ib but with tumor on the surface of one or both ovaries; or with capsule ruptured; or with ascites present containing malignant cells or with positive peritoneal washings
II	Growth involving one or both ovaries with pelvic extension
IIa	Extension and/or metastases to the uterus and/or tubes
IIb	Extension to other pelvic tissues
IIc*	Tumor stage IIa or stage IIb but with tumor on the surface of one or both ovaries; or with capsule(s) ruptured; or with ascites present containing malignant cells or with positive peritoneal washings
III	Tumor involving one or both ovaries with peritoneal implants outside the pelvis and/or positive retroperitoneal or inguinal nodes; superficial liver metastasis equals stage III; tumor is limited to the true pelvis but with histologically verified malignant extension to small bowel or omentum
IIIa	Tumor grossly limited to the true pelvis with negative nodes with histologically confirmed microscopic seeding of abdominal peritoneal surfaces
IIIb	Tumor of one or both ovaries; histologically confirmed implants of abdominal peritoneal surfaces, none exceeding 2 cm in diameter; nodes negative
IIIc	Abdominal implants 2 cm in diameter and/or positive retroperitoneal or inguinal nodes
IV	Growth involving one or both ovaries with distant metastasis; if pleural effusion is present, there must be positive cytologic test results to allot a case to stage IV; parenchymal liver metastasis equals stage IV

*To evaluate the impact on prognosis of the different criteria for allotting cases to stage Ic or stage IIc, it would be of value to know if rupture of the capsule was (1) spontaneous or (2) caused by the surgeon and if the source of the malignant cells detected was (1) peritoneal washings or (2) ascites.

From International Federation of Gynecology and Obstetrics: Changes in definitions of clinical staging for carcinoma of the cervix and ovary. Am J Obstet Gynecol 156:263, 1987.

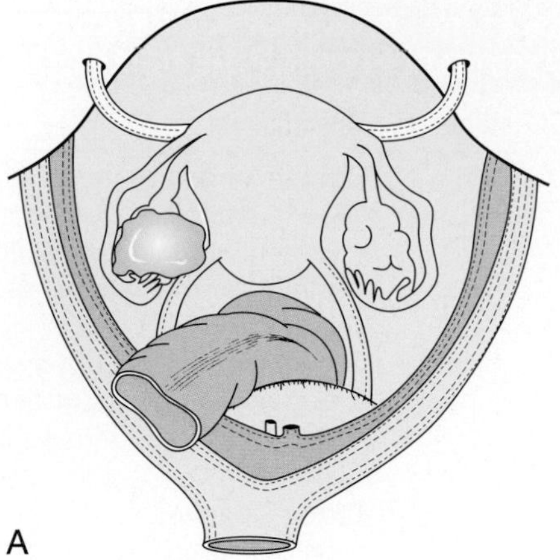

One ovary, capsule intact; no tumor on ovarian surface.

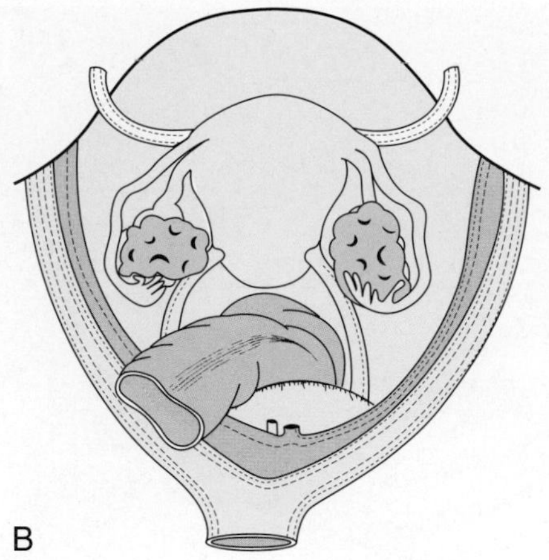

Both ovaries, capsule intact; no tumor on ovarian surface.

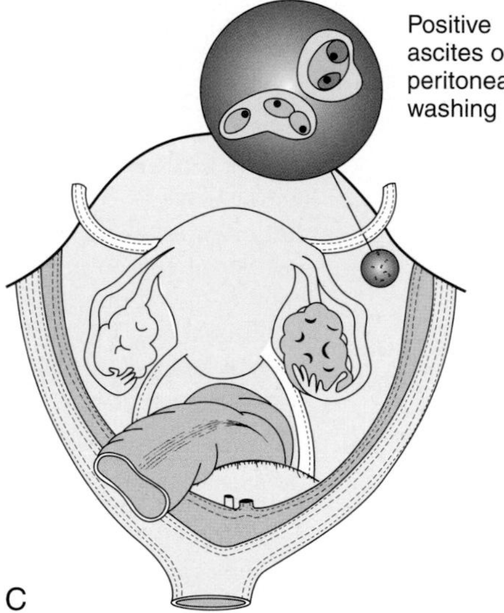

One or both ovaries with capsule ruptured or tumor on ovarian surface; malignant cells in ascites or peritoneal washings.

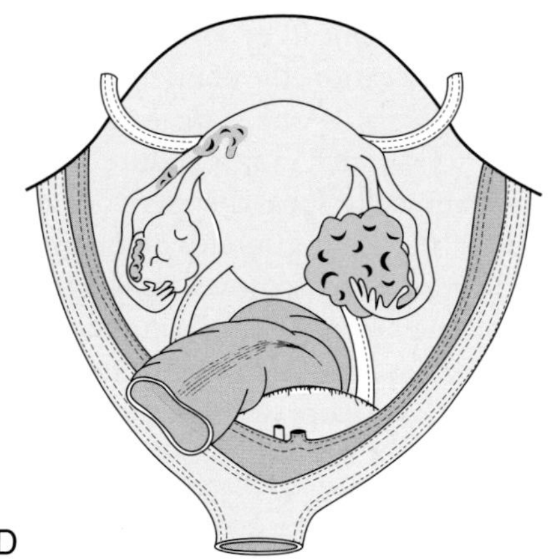

Extension and/or implants on uterus and/or tubes; adnexae.

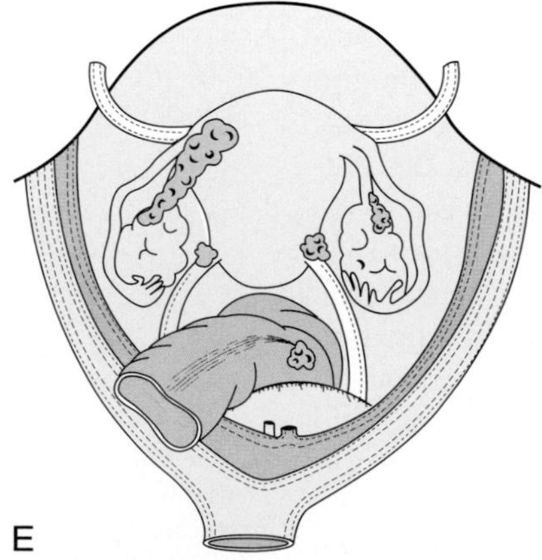

Extension and/or implants to other pelvic tissues; pelvic wall, broad ligament, adjacent peritoneum, mesovarium.

Figure 11–6 Ovarian epithelial carcinoma. *A,* Stage Ia. *B,* Stage Ib. Ovarian epithelial carcinoma. *C,* Stage Ic. *D,* Stage IIa. *E,* Stage IIb. Ovarian epithelial carcinoma.

Illustration continued on opposite page.

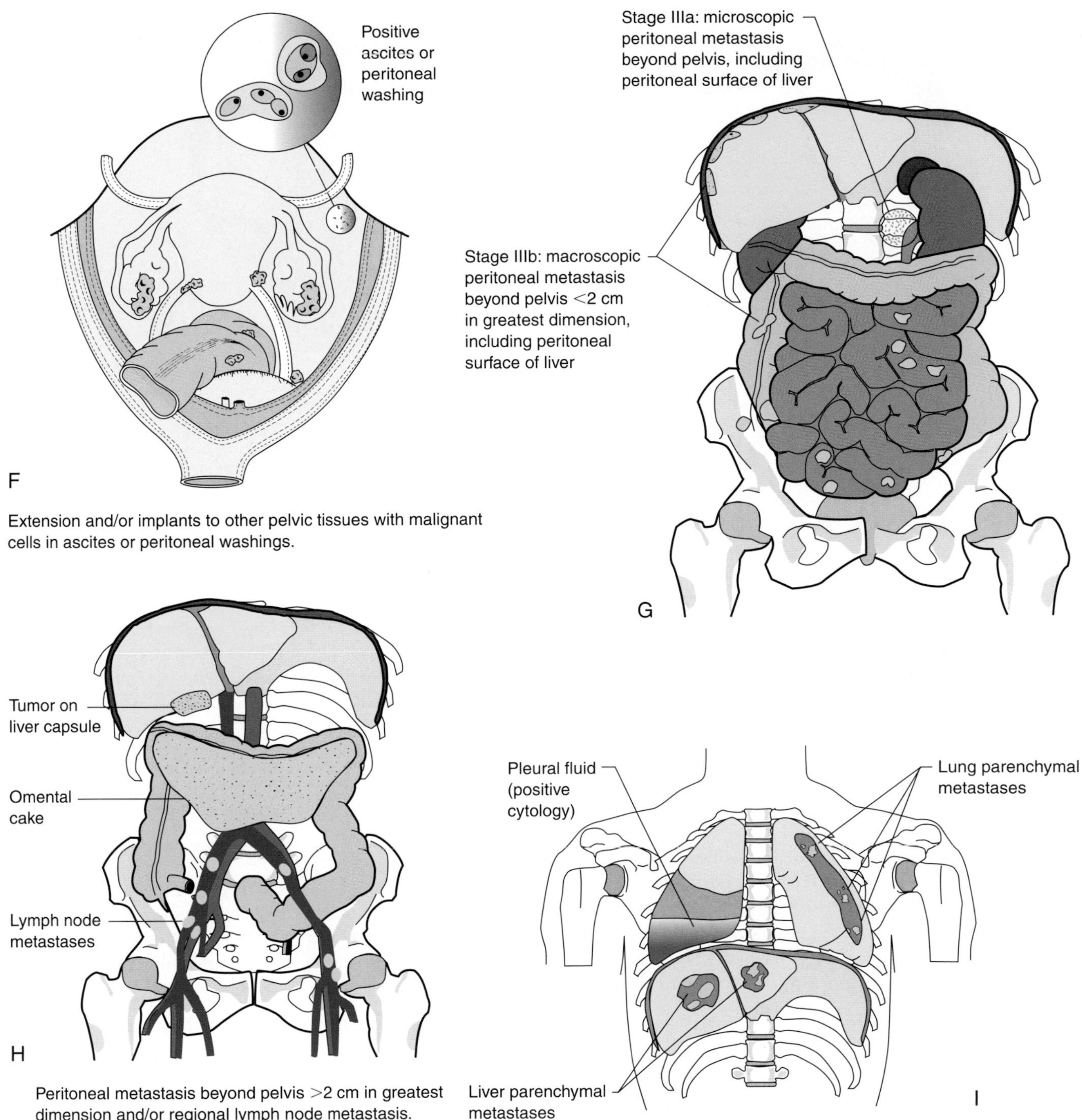

Figure 11–6 cont'd *F,* Stage IIc. *G,* Stages IIIa and IIIb. *H,* Stage IIIc. *I,* Stage IV.

these areas with 50–75 mL of saline solution and retrieving the fluid for cell block analysis. Care should be taken to visualize and palpate all peritoneal surfaces, particularly the underside of the diaphragm, the surface of the liver, the lateral abdominal gutters, and the small and large bowel mesentery. Fiberoptic light sources are particularly helpful in properly visualizing the peritoneal surfaces of the upper abdomen through a vertical lower abdominal incision. The omentum should be scrutinized and any suspicious areas removed by excision or biopsy. If the disease is apparently limited to the pelvis, it is judicious to excise the most dependent portion of the omentum or any portion of the omentum adherent to pelvic structures. Microscopic disease is often present in the omentum but not obvious grossly. It is not unusual to find only microscopic metastasis. Recommended surgical therapy is presented in sequence in Table 11–11. If the disease is limited to the pelvis, great care should be taken to avoid rupture of the neoplasm during its removal. All roughened or suspicious surfaces in the peritoneal cavity should be removed as biopsy specimens. This includes adhesions, which should be excised, not incised, because they often contain microscopic

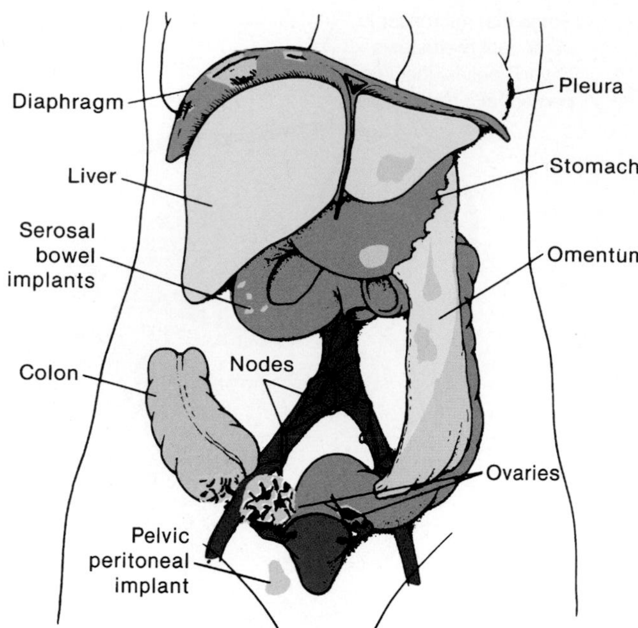

Figure 11–7 Spread pattern for epithelial cancer of the ovary. (From DiSaia PJ: Diagnosis and management of ovarian cancer. Hosp Pract [Off Ed] 22:235, 1987.)

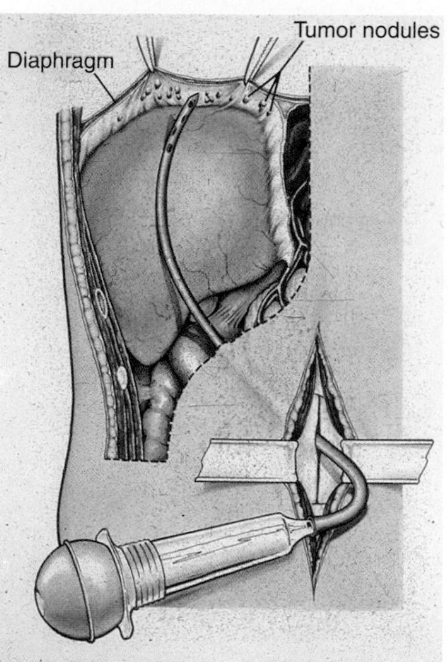

Figure 11–8 Technique of obtaining subdiaphragmatic cytologic washings at laparotomy. Saline lavage of the space between the diaphragm and the dome of the liver is easily accomplished; fluid pockets collecting in the lateral recesses are aspirated with a bulb syringe.

disease. Several studies are under way to investigate the efficacy of "blind" peritoneal biopsies and routine retroperitoneal node dissections in the proper staging of early epithelial cancer of the ovary (Table 11–12). Any abnormal-appearing surface is always regarded as suspicious, and biopsies are readily performed. Proper staging is important for treatment planning and for providing an accurate prognosis (Table 11–13).

Recent research suggests F-18-fluorodeoxyglucose position emission tomography (FDG-PET) performed sequentially may predict response to neoadjuvant chemotherapy. Avril and colleagues found the median overall survival was 38.3 months in metabolic responders (to FDG-PET) compared with 23.1 months in nonresponders, and the 2-year survival was 73% and 46% respectively.

Table 11–11 SURGICAL THERAPY IN OVARIAN CANCER

Peritoneal cytologic examination
Determination of extent of disease
- Pelvis
- Peritoneal surfaces
- Diaphragms
- Omentum
- Lymph nodes

Removal of all tumor possible (total abdominal hysterectomy and bilateral salpingo-oophorectomy) plus node sampling and omentectomy

THERAPEUTIC OPTIONS FOR PRIMARY TREATMENT

Borderline malignant epithelial neoplasms

In the last 3 decades, clear evidence has shown the existence of epithelial ovarian tumors whose histologic and biologic features are between those of clearly benign and frankly malignant ovarian neoplasms. These borderline malignant neoplasms, which account for approximately 15% of all epithelial ovarian cancers, are often referred to as proliferative cystadenomas, tumors of low malignant potential, and are more completely discussed in Chapter 10. Compared with obviously malignant epithelial neoplasms of the ovary, epithelial borderline tumors tend to afflict a younger population (see Chapter 10). A 10-year survival rate of approximately 95% has been obtained in these borderline neoplasms (see Chapter 10). However, symptomatic recurrence and death may develop as many as 20 years after therapy in a few patients. These neoplasms can correctly be labeled as being of low malignant potential. On the basis of their almost benign behavior, many gynecologists advocate conservative therapy, especially in patients who are desirous of further childbearing and have stage Ia disease (see Chapter 10).

The following can be said about ovarian tumors of low malignant potential, or so-called borderline malignant neoplasms:

- Patients have a high survival rate.
- Even lesions that behave in a malignant fashion usually have a typically indolent course.
- There is occasional spontaneous regression of peritoneal implants.
- Only a small percentage of cases are fatal.

Table 11–12 AORTIC LYMPH NODE METASTASES IN EPITHELIAL OVARIAN CANCER

	STAGE I		STAGE II		STAGE III–IV		
Series	Positive lymphangiography	Positive biopsy	Positive lymphangiography	Positive biopsy	Positive lymphangiography	Positive biopsy	Total
Hanks and Bagshaw (1969)	2/9	—	2/6	—	4/7	—	8/22
Parker et al (1974)	3/13	—	2/29	—	12/27	—	17/69
Knapp and Friedman (1974)	—	5/26	—	—	—	—	—
Delgado et al (1977)	1/5	—	1/5	—	—	3/5	2/10
Buchsbaum et al (1989)*	—	4/95	—	8/41	—	7/46	—
Burghardt (1991)	—	1/20	—	4/7	—	51/78	—
Total	10/141	12/48	61/129				

*All patients had optimal carcinoma with metastatic lesions less than 3 cm.

Table 11–13 CARCINOMA OF THE OVARY, OBVIOUSLY MALIGNANT CASES, ALL HISTOPATHOLOGIC CLASSES: FIVE-YEAR ACTUARIAL SURVIVAL BY STAGE

Stage	No.	Five-year survival (%)
Ia	342	86.9
Ib	49	71.3
Ic	352	79.2
IIa	64	66.6
IIb	92	55.1
IIc	136	57.0
IIIa	129	41.1
IIIb	137	24.9
IIIc	1193	23.4
IV	360	11.1

From Annual Report on the Results of Treatment in Gynecological Cancer, Vol 23. Stockholm, International Federation of Gynecology and Obstetrics, 1998.

- The diagnosis must be based on examination of the original ovarian tumor without considering whether it has spread.
- Extensive sectioning of the neoplasm is necessary to rule out truly invasive characteristics.
- Serous lesions appear to be more common than mucinous lesions, and mucinous lesions have a worse prognosis, possibly secondary to an unknown gastrointestinal primary site.

The majority of patients with borderline serous tumors have stage I tumors (70%–85% in most series). About 30% of patients have extraovarian tumor at the time of diagnosis, with equal numbers in stage II and stage III. Stage IV borderline tumors of low malignant potential have been described, but they are rare. Most tumor-related deaths occur in patients with stage II or stage III neoplasms, but there are several important differences from true adenocarcinoma of the ovary. More than 50% of patients with extraovarian tumors survive, even though resection is incomplete. Also, patients who ultimately die of the tumor do so many years after initial diagnosis. The protracted clinical course of these tumors makes prolonged follow-up an essential component of any scientific investigation. The long survival and the apparent cure of patients with advanced-stage proliferating serous tumors are puzzling and have led to speculation that some patients have multifocal proliferations of coelomic epithelium involving one or both ovaries and extraovarian sites, including some unusual ones, such as sites within pelvic and abdominal lymph nodes. Both clinical and pathologic evidence is available to support the hypothesis that extraovarian tumor, in at least some of these patients, represents multifocal proliferation rather than an implantation or metastasis.

Appropriate treatment of patients with serous or mucinous tumors of low malignant potential remains to be determined (see Chapter 10). The standard surgical therapy is total abdominal hysterectomy and bilateral salpingo-oophorectomy. Many believe that adjuvant therapy is unwarranted regardless of clinical stage because any extraovarian neoplasm should be viewed as multifocal and in situ, rather than metastatic. This issue obviously requires additional study that includes careful evaluation in grading of extraovarian tumor deposits, as well as ovarian neoplasms, and correlation of their appearances with outcome.

Recurrent lesions may develop after latent intervals as long as 20–50 years. After long follow-up, as many as 25% of the patients studied succumbed to their tumors. Recurrences are usually histologically similar to the primary tumors, suggesting that the cells of borderline tumors probably do not undergo progressive anaplasia

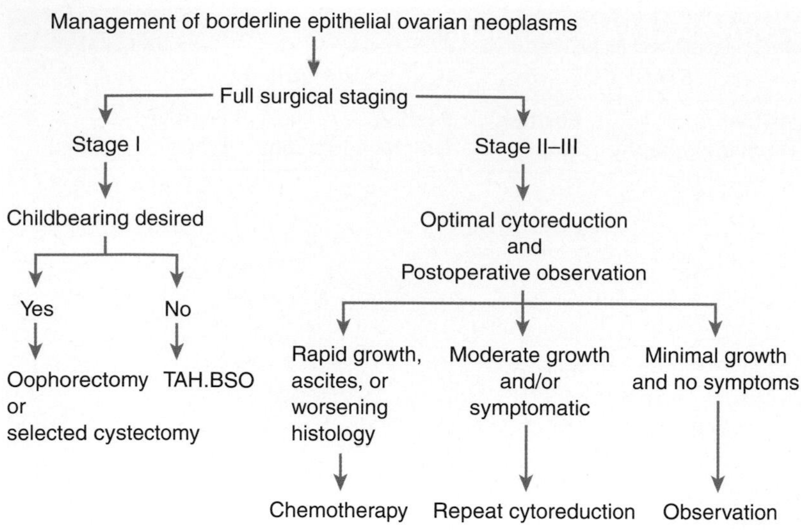

Figure 11–9 Algorithm for the management of borderline epithelial ovarian neoplasms. TAH, total abdominal hysterectomy; BSO, bilateral salpingo-oophorectomy.

with the passage of time. Lymph node metastases occasionally develop, but hematogenous metastases and extension outside the peritoneal cavity are uncommon, although subcutaneous metastases have rarely been reported.

The treatment of stage III disease remains unsettled. Many clinicians believe that neither radiation therapy nor chemotherapy is effective against these slow-dividing cell populations. No prospective or well-controlled studies of advanced disease have been conducted, although scattered reports of response to various chemotherapeutic agents have been recorded. Fort reported the experience from Memorial Sloan–Kettering Cancer Center with epithelial ovarian tumors of low malignant potential treated with chemotherapy. The study included 29 patients with stage I disease, 5 patients with stage II, 11 patients with stage III, and 1 patient with stage IV. Nineteen patients had residual disease after surgery. All 19 received adjuvant chemotherapy, radiation therapy, or a combination. Twelve patients with residual disease were found to be free of disease at second-assessment surgery after adjunctive therapy. This review indicates that adjunctive therapy can eradicate residual disease in some patients with epithelial ovarian tumors of low malignant potential. This has not been the experience of most. We have found surgical excision of disease the most effective therapy and have used repeated explorations, reserving chemotherapy for patients who develop ascites or whose tumor changes histologic features or demonstrates rapid growth (Fig. 11–9).

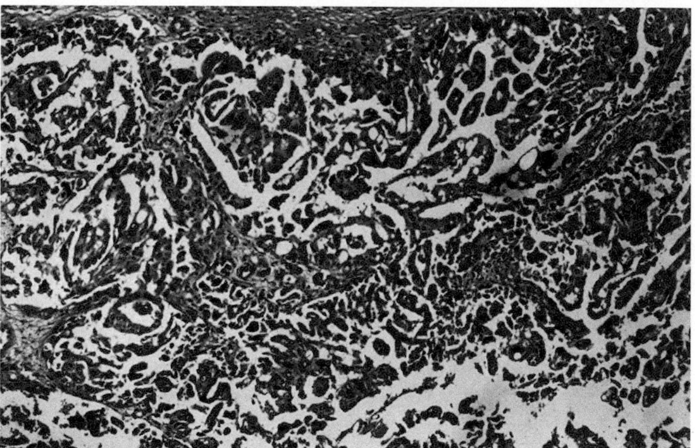

Figure 11–10 Papillary serous adenocarcinoma of ovary. Histologic appearance with prominent fibrous stalks and non-mucin-producing epithelial cells.

Treatment of malignant epithelial neoplasms

The most common epithelial cancers of the ovary are histologically categorized as serous, mucinous, endometrioid, and clear cell (mesonephroid) types (Figs 11–10 to 11–13). Although there has been some controversy in the past, it is now apparent that these different histologic varieties behave similarly, stage for stage and grade for grade. Some types, such as the mucinous and endometrioid varieties, are more commonly found in earlier stages; more well dif-

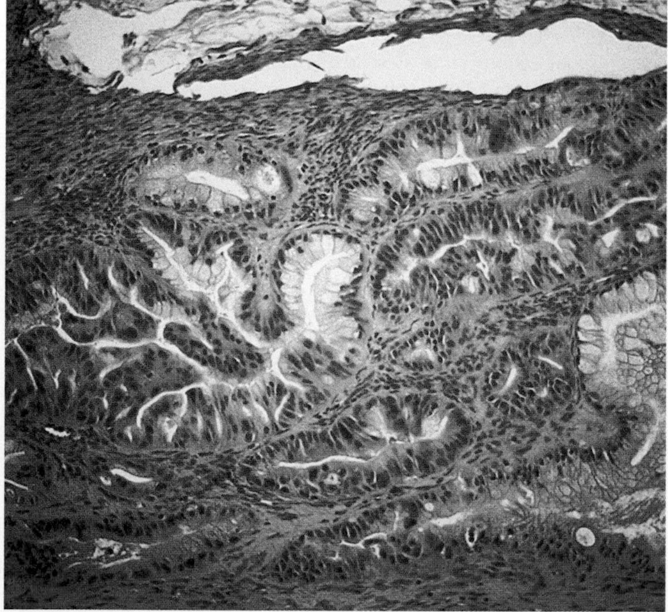

Figure 11–11 Mucinous adenocarcinoma of ovary. Microscopic appearance. Note tall, columnar, mucin-producing cells.

ferentiated lesions account for the confusion in the earlier literature. Prognosis, survival, and therapy for these various forms of epithelial cancer are hereafter considered collectively.

One theory of ovarian epithelial cancer growth suggests that the disease initially grows locally, invading the capsule and mesovarium, and then invades adjacent organs by contiguous growth and lymphatic spread. When the malignant neoplasm reaches the external surface of the capsule, cells may exfoliate into the peritoneal cavity, where they are free to circulate and later implant. Local and regional lymphatic metastasis may involve the uterus, fallopian tubes, and pelvic lymph nodes. Involvement of the periaortic lymph nodes by way of the infundibulopelvic ligament is also common.

Woodruff suggested another mechanism of disease spread that may be operational in epithelial ovarian cancer. He suggests that the entire coelomic epithelium can give rise to this lesion under the influence of carcinogenic agents that may gain access to the peritoneal cavity from the vagina through the fallopian tubes. Indeed, the lesion could then originate in a multifocal distribution, "like a measles rash," over large portions of the coelomic epithelium. This theory would explain the common observation of advanced-stage disease in a patient who was carefully examined a short time previously and was apparently free of disease with no palpable pelvic mass.

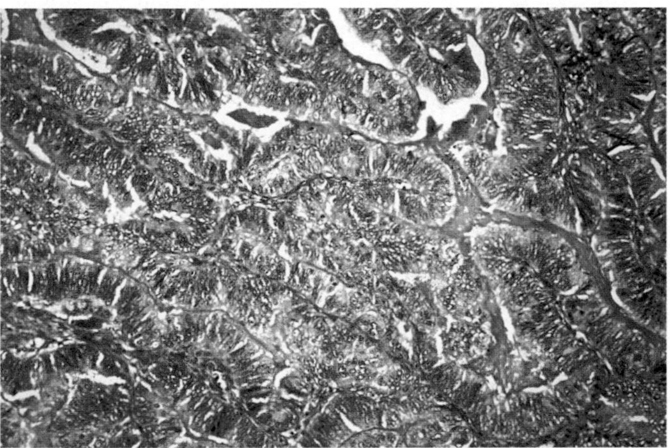

Figure 11–12 Endometrioid adenocarcinoma of ovary. Histologic appearance with columnar and pseudostratified epithelial cells showing prominent elongated hyperchromatic nuclei.

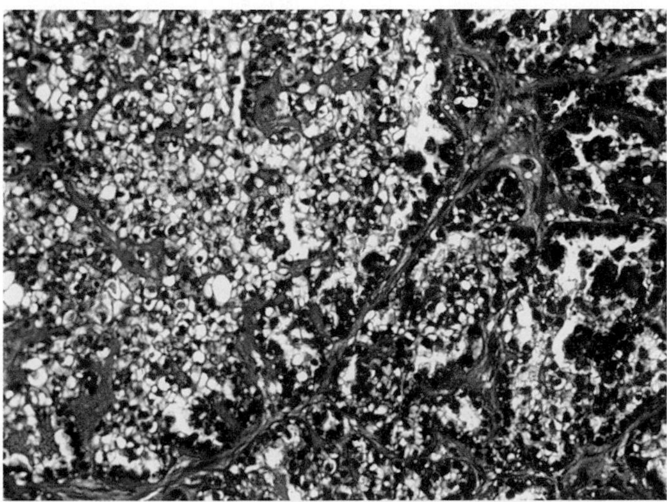

Figure 11–13 Clear cell adenocarcinoma of ovary. Microscopic view showing hobnail or peg cells.

Table 11–14 GUIDELINES FOR STAGING IN EPITHELIAL OVARIAN CANCER

Four peritoneal washings (diaphragm, right and left abdomen, pelvis)
Careful inspection and palpation of all peritoneal surfaces
Biopsy or smear from undersurface of right hemidiaphragm
Biopsy of all suspicious lesions
Infracolic omentectomy
Biopsy or resection of any adhesions
Random biopsy of normal peritoneum of bladder reflection cul-de-sac, right and left paracolic recesses, and both pelvic sidewalls (in the absence of obvious implants)
Selected lymphadenectomy of pelvic and para-aortic nodes
Total abdominal hysterectomy, bilateral salpingo-oophorectomy, and excision of masses when prudent

Probably the most important variable influencing the prognosis in each case of ovarian cancer is the stage or extent of disease. A staging system has been devised that allows a comparison of treatment results among different institutions, since treatment is usually by stage. Survival depends on the stage of the lesion, the grade of differentiation of the lesion, the gross findings at surgery (Table 11–14), the amount of residual tumor after surgery, and the additional treatment after surgery.

Stages Ia, Ib, and Ic

The best therapy for stage I lesions is undoubtedly total abdominal hysterectomy and bilateral salpingo-oophorectomy with careful surgical staging. At many institutions, omentectomy is part of staging for stage I lesions. The omentum is an organ that seems to "absorb" or attract tumor cells and may harbor microscopic disease in patients with apparent stage I lesions. The value of omentectomy in and of itself as a therapeutic modality for stage I disease has yet to be conclusively established.

Pelvic and periaortic nodes may be involved 10–20% of the time in apparent stage I disease, and lymphadenectomy is considered an important diagnostic and therapeutic procedure. Burghardt and colleagues described 23 patients with stage I epithelial cancers of the ovary, all of whom had complete pelvic lymphadenectomies; 7 patients (30%) were found to have lymph node involvement. Buchsbaum and coworkers reported a lower incidence of positive pelvic nodes from the large Gynecologic Oncology Group (GOG) study (0% for apparent stage I, 19.5% for apparent stage II, and 11.1% for apparent stage III). However, the GOG study included only patients with metastatic lesions <3 cm in diameter. Burghardt and colleagues reported on a series of patients with all sizes of lesions upon whom complete pelvic and periaortic lymphadenectomies had been done, and the involvement of pelvic nodes was much higher (15% for stage I, 57% for stage II, and 64% for stage III). Baiocchi and colleagues reviewed their experience in 242 women who had pelvic and para-aortic lymphadenectomy in whom cancer was apparently confined to the ovaries (stage I). Nodal metastasis was found in 32 patients (13.2%). Serous adenocarcinoma had the highest incidence of node metastasis (27 of 106, 25.4%). Those with grade 3 lesions had 38.5% metastasis (15 of 39) compared with 5.8% (9 of 155) with grade 1 and grade 2 disease. There were 33 women with low malignant potential tumors, and 7 (21%) had nodal metastasis. When only one to three nodes were involved, metastasis was mostly ipsilateral, but these patients could also have metastasis to the common iliac or para-aortic nodes. Para-aortic nodes were involved in the absence of pelvic metastasis. Bilateral pelvic node involvement was seen particularly if multiple nodes contained metastasis. In multivariate analysis, stage, histologic type, and grade were not predictive of survival. Lymph node status and survival noted a $P = 0.06$ (Table 11–15). Creasman and associates described four patients with ovarian cancer who, after chemotherapy or combined immunochemotherapy, were found to have retroperitoneal disease at the time of a second-look exploratory laparotomy, even though there was no evidence of intra-abdominal residual cancer. Ovarian cancer can metastasize to pelvic and periaortic lymph nodes, and therefore these areas must be evaluated for appropriate assessment of the true extent of disease in patients with ovarian cancer. Without thorough surgical staging, occult metastasis may be present and missed. This may lead to inadequate staging and subsequent inadequate therapy. Many studies have addressed this item (Table 11–16).

The use of adjuvant therapy and its role in stage I ovarian cancer continues to be investigated. In a retrospective study from England, Ahmed and associates reviewed the cases of 194 patients with stage I disease, of which 103 were thought to be "adequately" staged (low malignant potential excluded). None of the patients had postoperative therapy. Multiple factors were evaluated as to prognosis, and in multivariate analysis, only grade (grade 1 or grade 2 vs grade 3), presence of ascites, and ovarian surface tumor were significant for relapse but did not have an impact on survival. Relapse rates were 6.5%, 24.7%, and 38.1% for stage Ia, stage Ib, and stage Ic, respectively. The patients who relapsed were treated almost exclusively with carboplatin or cisplatin with 44% response rate.

Some institutions prefer chemotherapy as postoperative therapy for stage Ib and stage Ic lesions and for undifferentiated histologic types. In the more recent era, this adjuvant therapy is usually a platinum analogue alone or in combination with an alkylating agent or paclitaxel (Taxol). In the management of low-grade (grade 1) lesions, the physician must weigh the possible benefits of adjuvant chemotherapy against the risks. We have discontinued recommending chemotherapy for patients with stage Ia, Ib, grade 1 and 2 lesions, comprehensively staged. Patients with stage I, grade 3 lesions present a difficult problem. The incidence of recurrence in this group approaches 50% in some series. It is our belief that this group of patients should receive adjuvant multiple-agent chemotherapy despite the fact that no clear data show superior results compared with single-agent therapy. Philosophically, it is difficult to withhold the apparent best therapy from a group of patients who may have the best situation for a chemotherapy "cure"; in addition, this group is usually youthful and better able than older patients to tolerate vigorous adjuvant therapy.

The most appropriate adjuvant therapy for patients with stage I lesions in whom total abdominal hysterectomy and bilateral salpingo-oophorectomy have been done is a subject of considerable controversy. Some have advocated no further therapy, whereas others insist on a period of chemotherapy. Still others suggest whole-abdomen irradiation with or without chemotherapy. We favor platinum-based multiagent therapy for this group of high-risk patients.

The study by the GOG and the Ovarian Cancer Study Group has been reported in which patients with stage Ia and stage Ib grade 1 or grade 2 disease were randomized between those who received melphalan (0.2 mg/m^2/day orally for 5 days) for 12 cycles and those who received no further therapy. The 5-year survival in both arms of the

Table 11–15 LYMPH NODE METASTASIS IN STAGE I OVARIAN CANCER

Di Re	16/128
Benedetti–Panici	5/25
Wu	1/7
Burghardt	9/37
Petru	9/40
Knapp and Friedman	5/26
Tsuruchi	1/51
Chen	3/11
Lanza	3/11
Carnino	2/47
Baiocchi	32/242
	86/625 (13.7%)

Table 11–16 FREQUENCY OF SUBCLINICAL METASTASIS IN PATIENTS WITH PRESUMED EARLY-STAGE OVARIAN CANCER (BASED ON 14 STUDIES)

Localization	Frequency (%)	Range (%)
Peritoneal cytology	22	10–46
Diaphragm	9	0–44
Omentum	5	0.7
Pelvic nodes	8	0–20
Para-aortic nodes	12	0–25
Pelvic peritoneum	9	6–10
Abdominal peritoneum	8	7–9
Bowel mesentery-serosa	6	3–13

study was excellent (> 90%). Considering the toxicity, the expense, the inconvenience, and the risk of a second malignant neoplasm associated with alkylating agent therapy, defining those patients who require no additional therapy will be important should these data be confirmed. Another GOG-Ovarian Cancer Study Group trial included all patients who had stage Ic disease with no microscopic residua, patients who had stage Ia and stage Ib disease with ruptured capsule, patients who had stage Ia and stage Ib grade 3 lesions, and patients who had stage II disease when there was no evidence of macroscopic residua. These patients were randomized to receive melphalan or 15 mCi of intraperitoneal colloidal ^{32}P. Survival and disease-free survival were similar in both arms of the study (approximately 80%). The frequency of severe side effects was low in both treatment arms. However, ^{32}P was associated with fewer side effects than melphalan was, and only 25% of patients treated with ^{32}P experienced any type of toxicity. In follow-up, the GOG studied the same high risk, early stage population and compared combination chemotherapy, cyclophosphamide plus cisplatin, to intraperitoneal ^{32}P (GOG #95). The chemotherapy-treated patients' death rate was 17% lower than the radioactive colloid. While there was not a statistically significant difference in survival, the lower rate of recurrence in the chemotherapy arm and the greater complication rate in the ^{32}P arm led to the conclusion that platinum-based chemotherapy was preferred.

A study of 271 stage I ovarian cancers by the Italian Gynecologic Group was divided into two trials. Patients assigned to stage Ia and stage Ib, grade 2 or grade 3, were randomized between cisplatin (six courses) and no further therapy. Relapse rate was significantly reduced in the cisplatin arm, but survival was not statistically different between the two arms (88% cisplatin vs 82% no treatment at 76 months of median follow-up). In patients assigned to stage Ia2, stage Ib2, and stage Ic, randomization was between cisplatin and ^{32}P (intraperitoneal). Again, the relapse rate was lower in the cisplatin arm, but the overall 5-year survival was similar.

The European gynecologic groups reported a combined analysis of the ICON 1 and the ACTION trials. Over 900 patients with early-stage ovarian cancer received either platinum-based adjuvant chemotherapy or observation until chemotherapy was indicated. After a median follow-up of over four years, the overall survival at five years was 82% for patients with primary chemotherapy and 74% for the observation arms. The corresponding disease-free survivals at five years were 76% versus 65% respectively. It was concluded that the recurrence-free survival and overall survival at five years were improved by platinum-based chemotherapy. In another European Organization for Research and Treatment of Cancer (EORTC)-ACTION trial of 448 patients, they noted that the benefit of chemotherapy was limited to patients who lacked comprehensive surgical staging, again raising the necessity of adjuvant therapy in the patient with well-staged early ovarian carcinoma.

Since the treatment protocols for advanced stage disease had demonstrated improved survival by replacing cyclophosphamide with paclitaxel, the GOG then evaluated carboplatin (AUC 7.5) and paclitaxel (175mg/m^2) in high risk, early-stage disease (GOG #157). This trial compared three cycles of chemotherapy to six cycles. Over a three-year interval, 457 patients were enrolled and evaluated after a median follow-up of 6.8 years. While the recurrence rate was 24% lower with the six cycles ($P = 0.18$), the overall death rate was similar for the two arms (hazard ratio 1.02). The study concluded that the additional three cycles contributed to increased toxicity (11% grade 3 or 4 neurotoxicity versus 2% with only three cycles) without meaningfully improving outcomes.

A combined analysis of GOG #95 and #157 revealed that the stage II patients represented a disproportionate percentage of the recurrences. The GOG will now include stage II patients in their future clinical trials of patient with advanced-stage, optimally-debulked disease.

The GOG is currently evaluating the hypothesis that low-dose taxol may have anti-angiogenesis activity. GOG #175 is testing whether the addition of 24 weekly taxol treatments (60 mg/m^2) to the initial three cycles of carboplatin and paclitaxel will improve outcomes. The results of this study are pending.

In the young woman with stage Ia disease who is desirous of further childbearing, unilateral salpingo-oophorectomy may be associated with minimal increased risk of recurrence, provided a careful staging procedure is performed and due consideration is given to grade and apparent self-containment of the neoplasm.

Stages IIa, IIb, and IIc

In many institutions, the therapy of choice for stage IIa and stage IIb disease is total abdominal hysterectomy and bilateral salpingo-oophorectomy, omentectomy, and instillation of ^{32}P. Other centers prefer abdominal and pelvic irradiation as postoperative therapy. Still other institutions have had reasonable success with a combination of pelvic irradiation and systemic chemotherapy. In general, the radioisotope and irradiation treatment approaches have all but faded from frontline therapy for ovarian carcinoma. More commonly, surgery is followed with chemotherapy, usually platinum-based combination therapy. As in stage I disease, the value of omentectomy remains inconclusive. However, most authorities agree that in all stages, omentectomy serves as a valuable diagnostic tool. Careful surgical staging is essential to successful treatment planning. As previously mentioned, patients with stage II disease are managed in a similar fashion to optimally debulked stage III disease.

Stage III

In stage III, as in other stages, every effort should be made to remove the uterus with both adnexa. In addition, every effort should be made short of major bowel surgery to

Table 11–17 RELATIONSHIP OF RESIDUAL TUMOR SIZE AND MEDIAN SURVIVAL (MONTHS)

Author	No. of patients	Optimal (< 2 cm)	Suboptimal (> 2 cm)
Griffiths et al	102	28	11
Wharton et al	104	27	15
Hacker et al	47	22	6
Sutton et al	56	39	22

remove the bulk of the tumor, including the large omental cakes. Retrospective studies have strongly suggested that the survival rate in patients with stage III disease is related to the amount of residual tumor after surgery, such that patients with minimal residual tumor appear to have better prognoses with adjunctive therapy (Table 11–17). Patients with stage III disease should be treated with chemotherapy. Most centers now prefer multiple-agent platinum-based chemotherapy, usually carboplatin and paclitaxel, for this group of patients because of the excellent response rates reported in the literature (see later section on combination chemotherapy).

The duration of multiple-agent therapy is usually 6–8 cycles. If the patient survives this period and has no clinical evidence of disease, a second-look procedure was often considered in the past. This transitioned to most investigators not advocating a second-look laparotomy unless the patient is enrolled in a protocol. Subsequently, a secondary analysis on a GOG study (#158) suggested no apparent outcome advantage resulted from second-look surgery. However, second-look laparotomy is diagnostic and may offer advantages in select patients with prior inadequate surgical intervention.

Historically, reported evidence suggested that in the optimal group (patients with residua no greater than 1–2 cm in diameter at any site), the survival and response rates with chemotherapy are equivalent to those with abdominal and pelvic irradiation (Fig. 11–14). However, the long-term morbidity of radiation therapy is much greater, and this factor has considerably influenced postoperative therapy for stage III disease such that most centers prescribe multiagent chemotherapy, and radiation plays no role in primary therapy. Initial prospective studies by several groups randomized patients between those who received single-agent chemotherapy and those who received multiple-drug regimens, and most concluded (with regard to tumor response) that polychemotherapy had a significant advantage over single-agent regimens in advanced, non-optimally debulked disease. This issue is important because the morbidity of polychemotherapy is considerably greater than that of the single alkylating agent regimen.

Stage IV

The ideal management of stage IV disease is to remove as much cancer as possible and to administer chemotherapy after surgery. The overall survival is poorer for this group of patients than for those assigned to other stages, as expected (Fig. 11–15).

Maximal surgical effort

It has been axiomatic among many gynecologic oncologists that it is judicious to excise as much tumor as possible when disseminated disease is encountered at the time of primary operation for ovarian cancer. It is known that significant palliation may be achieved by reduction of a heavy tumor burden. Munnell reported a 28% 5-year survival rate among patients who had undergone a "maximal surgical effort" compared with a 9% 5-year survival rate among patients who had had partial resection and a 3% 5-year survival rate among patients who had had biopsy only. In Munnell's 14 survivors, the maximal surgical effort consisted of hysterectomy, bilateral salpingo-oophorectomy, and omentectomy.

Aure and colleagues demonstrated significant improvement in survival among patients with stage III disease only if all gross tumor had been removed (Fig. 11–16). Similar results were obtained by Griffiths and coworkers, who used a multiple linear regression equation with survival as the dependent variable to control simultaneously for the multiple therapeutic and biologic factors that contribute to the ultimate outcome in the individual patient. The most important factors proved to be histologic grade of the tumor and size of the largest residual mass after primary surgery. The operation itself contributed nothing to survival unless it effected reduction in the size of the largest residual tumor mass below the limit of 1.6 cm.

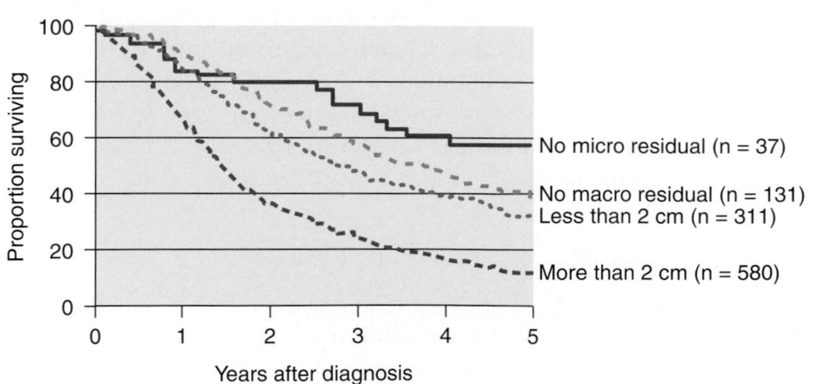

Figure 11–14 Survival in patients with stage IIIc disease by completeness of surgery (*n* = 1059). (Adapted from Annual Report on the Results of Treatment in Gynecological Cancer, Vol 23. Stockholm, International Federation of Gynecology and Obstetrics, 1998.)

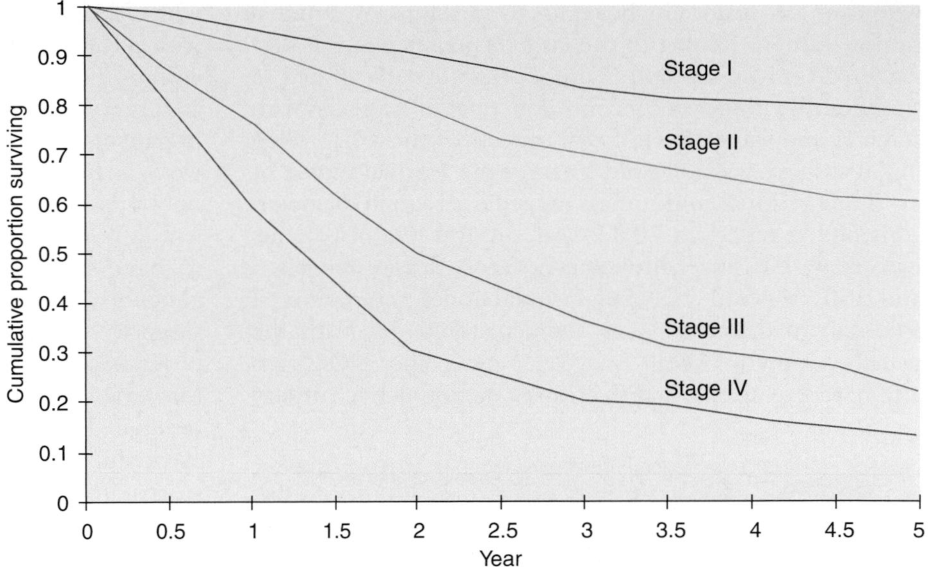

Figure 11–15 Obviously malignant cases of ovarian carcinoma. Cumulative proportion surviving by stage. (From Annual Report on the Results of Treatment in Gynecological Cancer, Vol 22. Stockholm, International Federation of Gynecology and Obstetrics, 1994.)

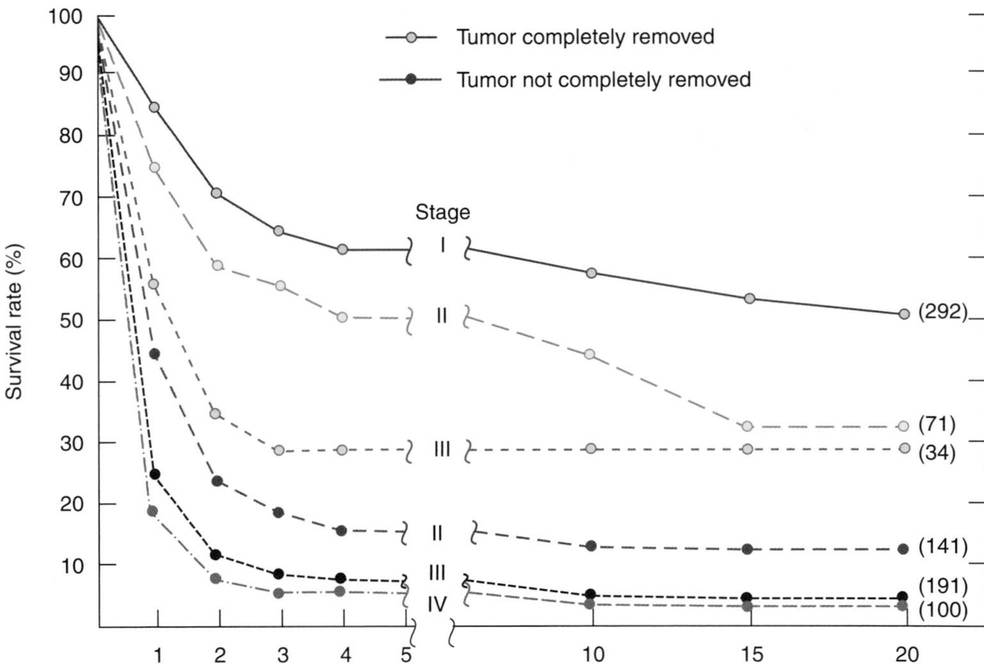

Figure 11–16 Survival rates stage for stage in patients in whom all tumor was surgically removed vs patients in whom not all tumor was completely removed. (From Aure JC, Hoeg K, Kolstad P: Clinical and histologic studies of ovarian carcinoma. Long-term follow-up of 990 cases. Obstet Gynecol 37:1, 1971.)

The so-called debulking procedure has gained considerable attention in the management of ovarian cancer. The concept is simply to diminish the residual tumor burden to a point at which adjuvant therapy will be optimally effective. All forms of adjuvant therapy are most effective when a minimal tumor burden exists. This is particularly true of ovarian carcinoma, which is one of the solid tumors more sensitive to chemotherapy. A careful and persistent surgeon can often remove large tumor masses that on first impression appear to be unresectable. Using the clear retroperitoneal spaces, one can usually identify the infundibulopelvic ligament and ureter and then isolate the vessels of the infundibulopelvic ligament and the blood supply of the ovary. Once these vessels have been ligated and transected, retrograde removal of large ovarian masses is easier and safer. The ureter, as much as possible, must be protected throughout the dissection so that the probability of traumatizing this pelvic structure is minimized. However, even in the best of hands, ureteral injuries do occur. A clear space usually exists on the transverse colon whereby large omental cakes of ovarian carcinoma can be removed after the right and left gastroepiploic vessels have been ligated (Fig. 11–17). Removal of large ovarian masses and omental involvement often reduces the tumor burden by 80–99%. The theoretical value of debulking procedures lies in the obvious reduction of cell numbers and the advantage this affords to adjuvant therapy. This is especially relevant in bulky solid tumors such as ovarian cancer, in which removal of large numbers of cells in the resting phase (G_0) may propel the residual cells into the more vulnerable proliferating pool. Several careful retrospective studies have repeatedly demonstrated improved survival rate in patients who can be surgically brought to a status of minimal tumor burden. Report of the large experience of the MD Anderson Hospital and Tumor Institute illustrated a significantly improved second-line rate in patients with stage II and stage III epithelial cancers of the ovary when initial surgery was followed by no gross residual tumor or no single residual tumor mass exceeding 1 cm in diameter. This report reflects a 70% 2-year survival rate in patients with stage III cancer in whom no gross disease remained and a 50% survival rate when residual nodules were limited to 1 cm in diameter. This compares favorably with the usually quoted overall survival rates. The GOG has attempted to better define primary cytoreductive surgery with a detailed analysis of the results of surgery in patients with advanced disease. Their initial study compared survival of the patients with stage III disease who were found at surgery to have abdominal disease of ≤1 cm with that of patients found to have disease >1 cm but whose tumors were surgically cytoreduced to ≤1 cm. If surgery was the only important factor, survival should have been equivalent in both groups. This was not the case. Patients found to have small-volume disease survived longer than did patients who had cytoreduction to small-volume disease at surgery, suggesting that the tumor biology also carries prognostic significance. In a second study, GOG investigators evaluated the effect of the diameter of the largest residual disease on survival in patients with suboptimal cytoreduction. They demonstrated that cytoreduction so that the largest residual mass was ≤2 cm resulted in a significant survival benefit, but all residual diameters >2 cm had equivalent survival (Fig. 11–18). Therefore, unless the mass can be cytoreduced to ≤2 cm, residual diameter did not influence survival. In evaluating optimal and suboptimal cytoreduction, these GOG investigators showed that three distinct groups emerged: microscopic residual, residual disease of <2 cm, and residual disease of >2 cm (Fig. 11–19). It is clear from these studies that patients with microscopic disease have a 4-year survival of about 60%, whereas patients with gross disease ≤2 cm have a 4-year survival of 35%. On the other hand, patients whose disease cannot be cytoreduced to ≤2 cm have a 4-year survival of <20%. Most striking, however, is the failure of cytoreductive surgery to have any effect on survival unless the largest diameter of residual disease is ≤2 cm.

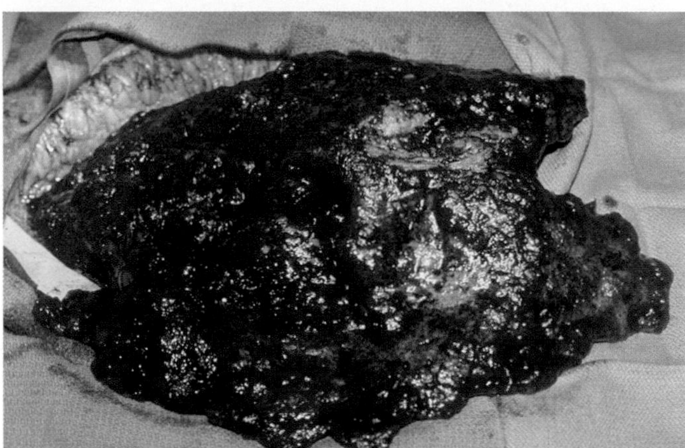

Figure 11–17 This photograph demonstrates a large omental cake of ovarian cancer exceeding 25 cm in greatest measurement.

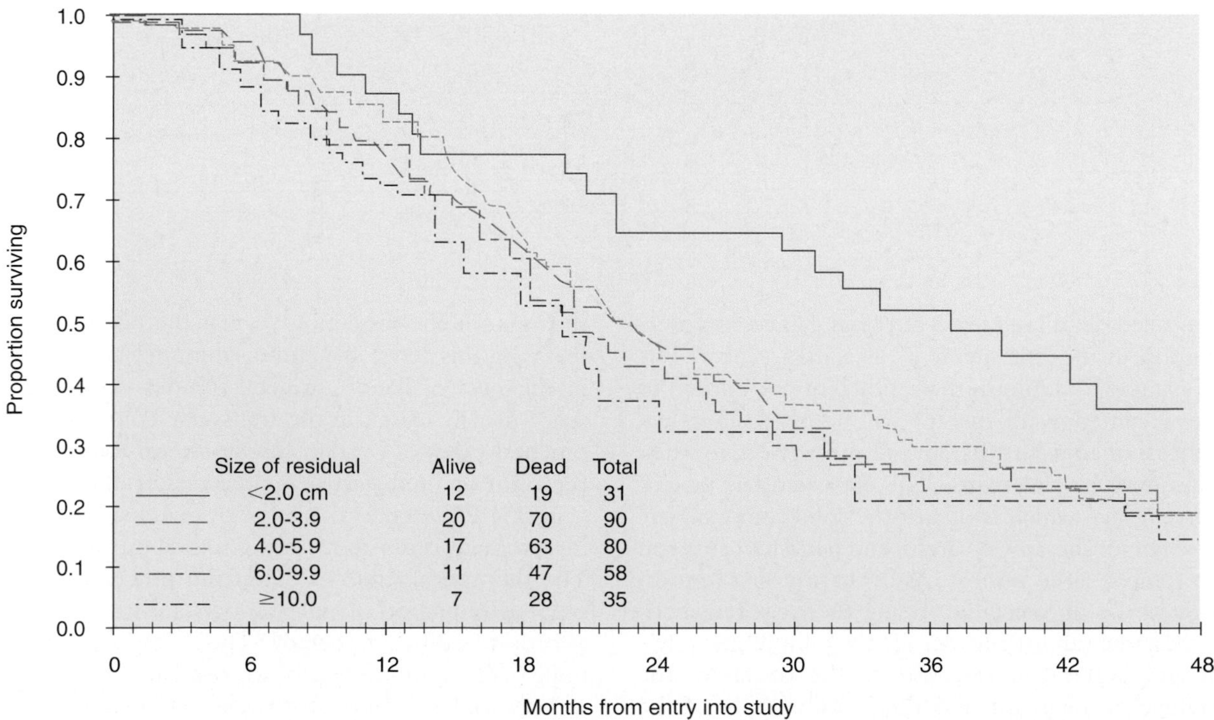

Figure 11–18 Survival by maximal diameter of residual disease. (From Hoskins WJ et al: The effect of diameter of largest residual disease on survival after primary cytoreductive surgery in patients with suboptimal residual epithelial ovarian carcinoma. Am J Obstet Gynecol 170:974, 1994.)

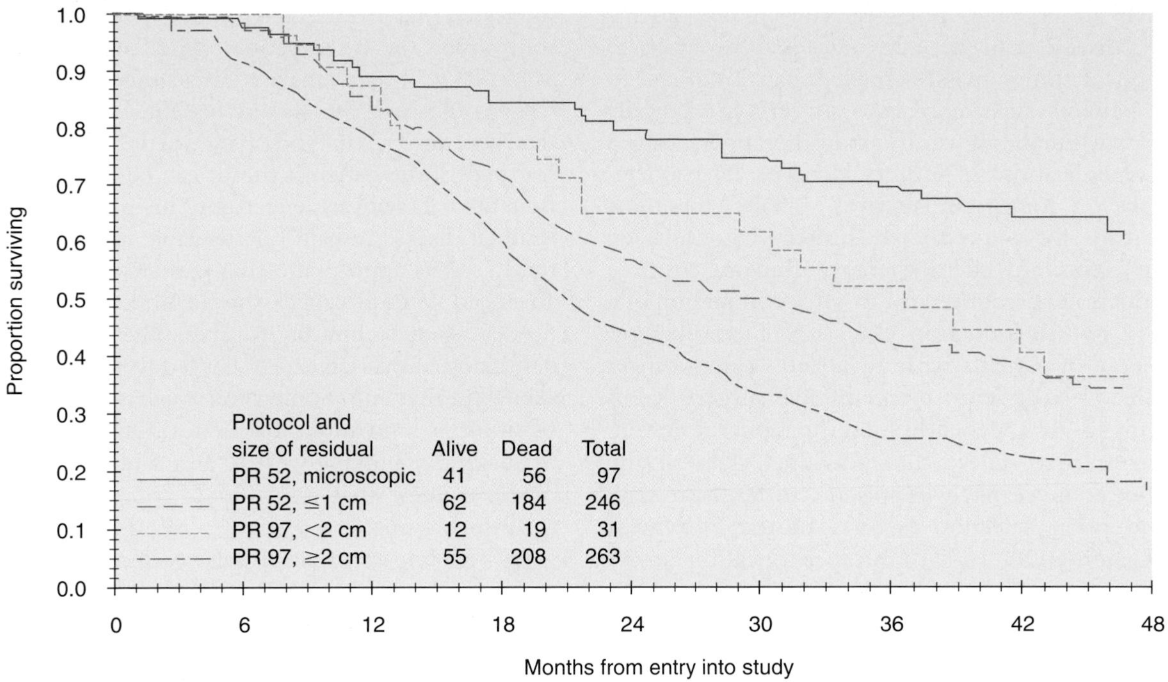

Figure 11–19 Survival by residual disease, Gynecologic Oncology Group protocols (PR) 52 and 97. (From Hoskins WJ et al: The effect of diameter of largest residual disease on survival after primary cytoreductive surgery in patients with suboptimal residual epithelial ovarian carcinoma. Am J Obstet Gynecol 170:974, 1994.)

A 2005 report analyzed the impact of cytoreductive surgery on progression-free survival. A retrospective analysis of 889 patients of the 1077 patients enrolled in the Scottish Randomised Trial in Ovarian Cancer (SCOTROC-1) was conducted. The analysis demonstrated that optimal debulking (<2 cm) was more commonly achieved in patients accrued from the USA, Europe and Australia than in patients recruited from the United Kingdom (UK) (71% vs 58%). Progression-free survival (PFS) was better in patients optimally debulked if their disease was less extensive at the onset ($P = 0.003$). Comparison of the UK and non-UK patients who had no visible residual disease demonstrated a better survival for the non-UK patients, and the authors attributed this to the fact that non-UK patients more commonly underwent primary lymphadenectomy.

The role of debulking in stage IV cancers has been questioned. Three studies have suggested that optimal debulking can be performed in many of these patients with beneficial effect. Liu and associates described 47 patients with stage IV cancers, of which 14 (30%) were optimally debulked to <2 cm residual. Median survival was 37 months in the patients in whom the cancer was optimally debulked compared with 17 months in the patients in whom the cancer was suboptimally debulked. A study from Memorial Sloan–Kettering identified 92 patients; optimal debulking was achieved in 45% with a median survival of 40 months compared with 18 months for suboptimal debulking. The MD Anderson group described 100 patients who underwent debulking. Those with optimally debulked lesions had a median survival of 25 months, whereas those with suboptimally debulked lesions survived 15 months.

The effect of maximal cytoreductive surgery can be seen in the percentage of negative second-look procedures (Table 11–18). Even though cytoreductive surgery seems to have therapeutic value, controversy continues. The primary unresolved issue is whether the poor prognosis with bulky disease is caused by the presence of increased tumor burden (in which case cytoreductive surgery is of potential benefit) or whether it is associated with differences in tumor biology or a decreased sensitivity to chemotherapeutic regimens (if these possibilities are indeed the case, cytoreductive surgery is not likely to have a major impact on survival). The implication is thus that those patients who have disease that can be cytoreduced are a select group with good prognoses on the basis of factors independent of the

Table 11–18 THE EFFECT OF CYTOREDUCTIVE SURGERY ON RESIDUAL DISEASE AS FOUND BY SECOND-ASSESSMENT SURGERY

	Negative second look (%)		
Author	**No residual**	**Optimal residual**	**Suboptimal residual**
Barnhill (1984)	67	61	14
Cain (1986)	76	50	28
Smirz (1985)	75	—	25
Webb (1982)	95	36	20
Podratz (1983)	82	44	33
Curry (1981)	79	45	22
Dauplat (1983)	100	100	40
Hoskins (1989)	75	45	25
Mean	81	52	23

cytoreductive surgery. It is not clear how many patients with bulky disease can actually successfully undergo cytoreduction of tumor masses smaller than 2 cm and in how many patients such aggressive surgery is medically contraindicated. Furthermore, if chemotherapy is delayed because of complications of surgery, this may have a deleterious effect on long-term survival. Finally, the most appropriate time for cytoreductive surgery has not been determined: before any chemotherapy, after one to three cycles of induction chemotherapy, or after completion of a full 6- to 12-month induction course of chemotherapy. The percentage of patients with advanced ovarian cancer who can effectively undergo cytoreductive surgery seems to range from 43–87%, depending on the report reviewed. This difference may reflect the individual skills of the surgeons, but it more likely represents different referral patterns and other selection factors. In the Southwest Oncology Group-GOG study of intraperitoneal therapy vs intravenous therapy in optimal stage III cancer, the median survival was 76 months, 42 months, and 32 months if microscopic only, <0.5 cm residual, and 0.5–2 cm residual was present, respectively. Eisenkop and associates described 163 consecutive patients assigned to stage IIIc and stage IV. Complete cytoreduction could be performed in 86% of patients. Overall median survival was 54 months, but it was 62 months in those whose tumor was optimally debulked.

The role of lymphadenectomy in patients with advanced disease continues to be debated. All studies show significant lymph node involvement in advanced disease (> 50%); the question is whether lymphadenectomy affects survival. Burghardt was one of the first to suggest a therapeutic benefit. His data suggested that even with positive lymph nodes, patients with advanced disease had a better survival compared with that of similar patients but without lymph nodes being evaluated. It has been suggested by some that metastases in lymph nodes do not respond to chemotherapy as well as intraperitoneal metastasis and therefore the lymph nodes should be removed. Opponents state that in patients in whom recurrence develops, it does so intraperitoneally and rarely only in the retroperitoneal space, and therefore lymph node status has little impact on the natural history of disease. Two studies from Italy, although not identical in design, came to somewhat different findings. Parazzini and associates evaluated 456 women with stage III–IV disease entered in a prospective randomized chemotherapy trial. There were 161 patients with positive nodes. They noted grade 3 tumors to have a greater number with positive nodes compared with grade 1 or grade 2 tumors. This was also true of stage IV compared with stage III cancer. They did not find a difference in survival between those with positive nodes and those with negative nodes; whether surgical removal of positive nodes affects survival is unknown. Scarabelli and colleagues evaluated lymph node status in 98 patients with stage IIIc–IV disease who had no gross residual disease after surgery compared with 44 patients who did not undergo lymphadenectomy. Survival was significantly improved if lymphadenectomy was done (Cox analysis). This study suggested that in a selected group of patients, lymphadenectomy may be therapeutic. The previously discussed SCOTROC-1 trial analysis also suggested lymphadenectomy could have therapeutic benefit. It has been our practice to do pelvic and para-aortic lymphadenectomy routinely if the patient's tumor can be optimally debulked. Benefits of lymphadenectomy in patients with bulky residual disease remain questionable in our minds. It currently seems appropriate that patients with a diagnosis of advanced ovarian cancer should undergo resection of all masses when technically feasible. The enthusiasm for the debulking of ovarian cancer has led to many techniques for achieving that end. Some clinicians have advocated the use of an ultrasound surgical aspirator. Others suggested electrosurgical debulking with an argon beam coagulator. Still others suggest that resection of the diaphragmatic peritoneum or muscle may have a role in cytoreductive surgery. The impact of all of these techniques on survival of patients is somewhat unclear. One must be cautious about techniques that are executed successfully only in the hands of the enthusiastic and await confirming reports.

There have been increasing advocates of evaluating ovarian cancer patients with laparoscopy instead of laparotomy. Technically, this can be done, although the wisdom of removing large adnexal masses through the laparoscope could be questioned. Metastases at port sites have been reported. Cancer recurrence at the site of surgical incision is well known but interestingly appears rarely even when there is considerable intra-abdominal tumor. Wang and associates reviewed the literature to determine risk factors that may contribute to early recurrence at the port site. Of the gynecologic cancers, ovarian cancer was the most common malignant neoplasm with subsequent port site metastasis. This occurred in patients with and without ascites, in patients with gross tumor within the abdominal cavity, in patients who had undergone diagnostic or palliative procedures, and in early-stage disease. Port site metastasis was also observed in patients with tumors of low malignant potential. Metastasis to the port site was more common if ascites was present and if intraperitoneal carcinomatosis was present. The earliest time from laparoscopy to port site metastasis was 8 days. Several theories about the mechanism of port site metastasis have been proposed. These include implantation of cancer cells traumatically disseminated at the time of surgical removal of the primary tumor; direct implantation by the instruments; and creation of a pressure gradient by the pneumoperitoneum, with the outflow of gas floating the tumor cells through the port sites. Although laparoscopy has been used successfully in the management of benign adnexal masses, we prefer the open laparotomy approach if ovarian cancer is expected. If unsuspected cancer is found at the time of laparoscopy, immediate laparotomy is generally performed.

As discussed later in this chapter, the role of second-look laparotomy is still controversial, although it is being used less frequently unless a patient is enrolled in a protocol. Most would agree that it has no or little impact on survival, although status of disease at a certain point in time can be ascertained. Some advocates of second-look laparotomy have suggested that secondary debulking could be beneficial and improve survival. At least five studies evaluated the role of secondary debulking in patients with known clinical disease after chemotherapy. Of a total of 193, only 11 (5.6%) had disease reduced to no residual disease and only 3 (27%) were survivors at the time of publication compared with 19% with 1–2 cm residual disease and 6% with >2 cm residual disease. There were 1207 patients (all stages) identified in 16 articles who underwent second-look laparotomy in whom no detectable clinical disease was present after chemotherapy. There were 600 patients with macroscopic disease; in 118, debulking was done to microscopic disease, and 31% survived. If debulking was to <5 mm, survival was 22%; of the 420 patients with >5 mm residual disease, only 14% survived. Of interest is that of those with debulking to microscopic disease, 31% survived compared with 47% who had microscopic disease only at the time of second-look laparotomy. Although there may be a benefit if debulking can be done to microscopic disease only, it appears from a review of the literature that this can be accomplished in <10% of patients clinically free of disease and undergoing second-look laparotomy.

The European Organization for Research and Treatment of Cancer (EORTC) group have reported their experience with interventional debulking surgery in patients with advanced ovarian carcinoma. Patients received three courses of cisplatin and cyclophosphamide and were then randomized to receive interventional debulking surgery or no surgery. All patients received six courses of chemotherapy. There were 278 patients evaluated, and median survival was 26% vs 20% (surgery vs no surgery, $P = 0.012$). Debulking surgery was an independent prognostic factor in multivariate analysis. After adjustment for all prognostic factors, surgery reduced the risk of death by 33% ($P = 0.008$).

The GOG conducted a similar study. This study, reported in 2004, enrolled 550 patients. Patients who were not optimally debulked (residual tumor >1 cm) received three cycles of paclitaxel plus cisplatin. Patients were randomized to continued chemotherapy or to a secondary surgical cytoreduction and then continued chemotherapy. Neither the PFS nor the relative risk of death were improved with the additional interval surgery. The authors speculate that the patients on the GOG study may also have undergone more aggressive surgery than the patients on the EORTC study, and this may have accounted for the difference in results. Most importantly, one could summarize these two studies by concluding that patients with advanced ovarian cancer are deserving of at least one maximal effort at cytoreduction, preferably by a gynecologic oncologist.

While a maximal primary surgical effort appears to be a cornerstone of potential long-term survival, the timing of the surgical effort remains a focus of debate. In patients with borderline performance status, based upon age, compromising medical disease, extensive effusions (especially pleural or pericardial), and in patients with extensive abdominal disease, unlikely to be effectively debulked, strong consideration should be given to initiating therapy with neoadjuvant chemotherapy. Following two to four cycles, a good clinical response to chemotherapy will often provide an opportunity for an effective surgical debulking with an acceptably low complication rate. Prior to initiating chemotherapy, it is desirable to have established a reasonable basis for a diagnosis of ovarian, tubal, or peritoneal cancer based on cytology or minimally invasive surgery. To date, neoadjuvant chemotherapy treatment (followed by surgical debulking) results have been reported in small retrospective reports of between 20 and 90 patients. These studies suggest outcomes similar to primary surgical intervention. A current clinical trial being conducted by EORTC and NCI-Canada is scheduled to complete accrual of over 700 patients in 2006. The results of this trial may provide more detailed information regarding candidate selection and outcomes for neoadjuvant chemotherapy.

Patients who undergo extensive surgery (Fig. 11–20; Fig. 11–21) are at increased risk for wound disruption; therefore, mass closure techniques for abdominal wall closure should be used (Fig. 11–22). However, in situations where edematous bowel is protruding from the abdominal cavity, an interrupted closure with delay of pulling the sutures tight may produce less fascial fracturing and less dehiscence.

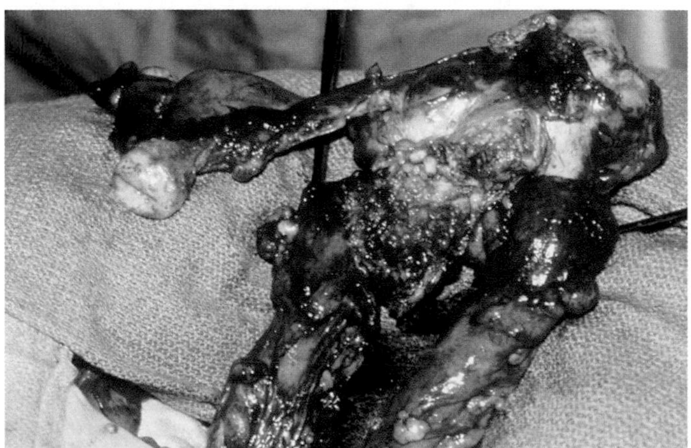

Figure 11–20 In situ surgical specimen demonstrating a large left ovarian neoplasm infiltrating a portion of sigmoid colon.

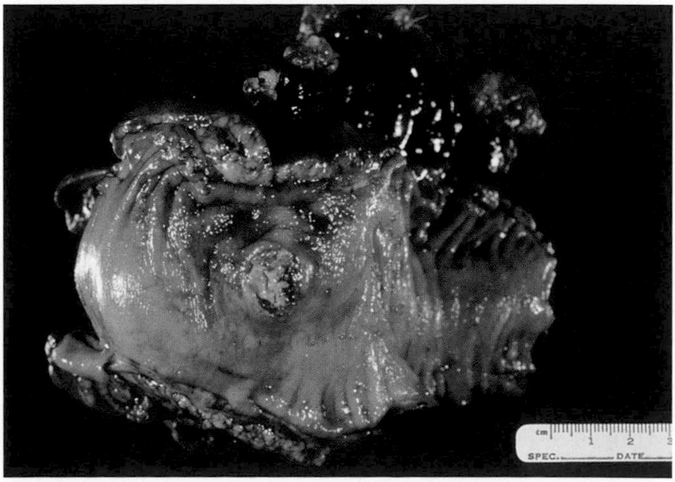

Figure 11–21 Portion of colon demonstrating transmural ovarian tumor infiltration.

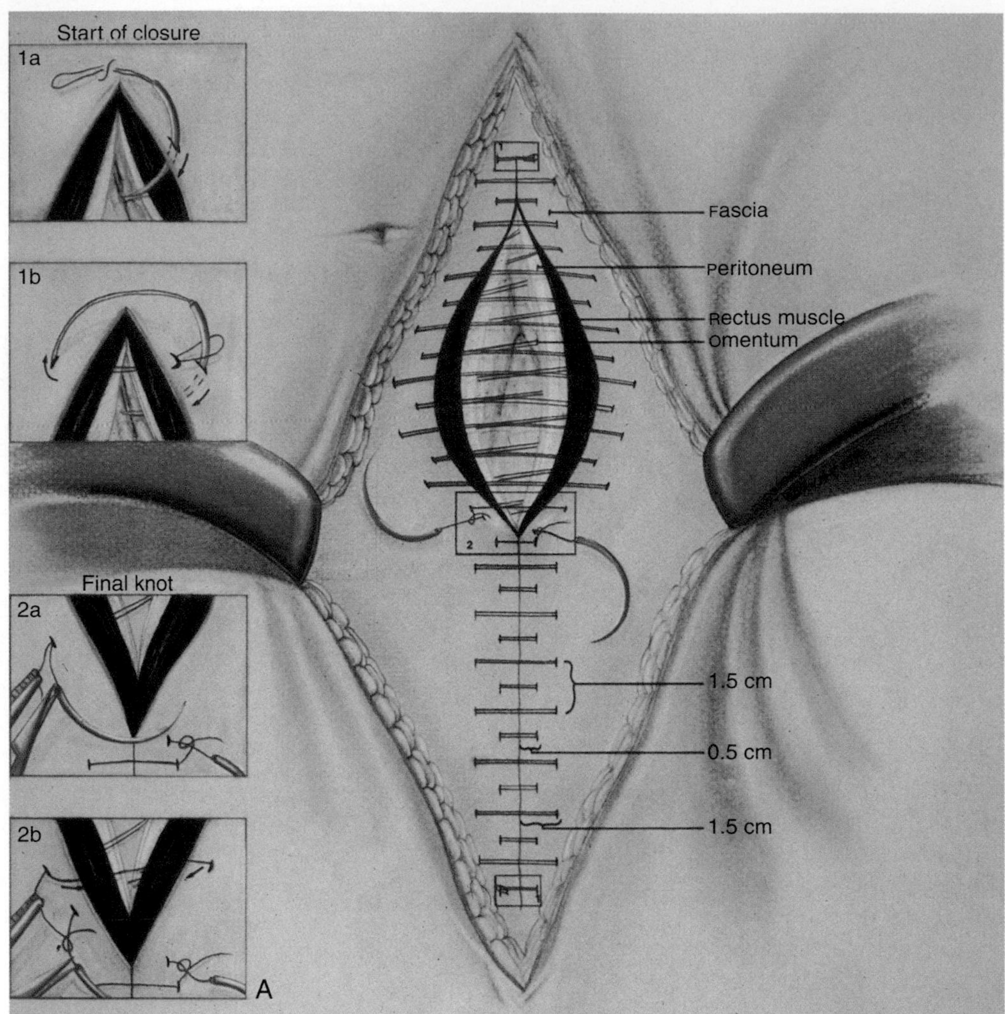

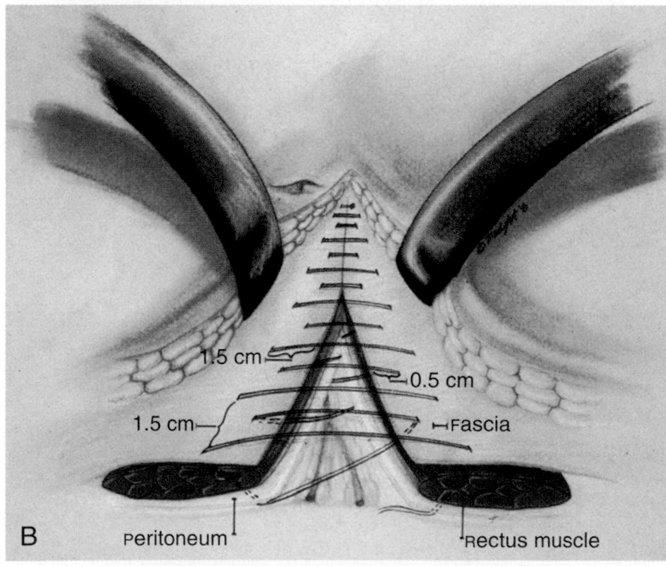

Figure 11–22 *A,* Running Smead–Jones closure techniques. After taking initial bite (*1a*), the needle, with double-stranded suture, is pulled through the open loop end (*1b*). At completion of the fascial closure, one of the two strands of the looped suture is cut from the needle (*2a*). A bilateral bite through both anterior fascial layers is taken, and the suture is tied to itself (*2b*). *B,* A mass closure technique with 0 Maxon loop suture in a running Smead–Jones technique has the value of speed and security in our experience.

Role of radiation therapy

Radiation therapy techniques include intraperitoneal instillation of radioactive chromium phosphate and external-beam radiation to the abdomen and pelvis. Patients with epithelial carcinoma of the ovary who are selected to receive postoperative irradiation should receive treatment of the entire abdomen plus additional radiation to the pelvis. This broad treatment plan is based on an analysis of postirradiation recurrences of stage I and stage II disease, which showed that most of the recurrences were outside the pelvis. There is no lid on the pelvis, and malignant cells are shed from the primary ovarian tumor and circulate throughout the entire abdominal cavity. Lymphatic dissemination is also possible.

Table 11–19 SPECIAL PROBLEMS IN OVARIAN CANCER

Limits of tumor spread often unknown
Variability of radiosensitivity
Total tumor burden usually large
Free mobility of tumor cells within the abdominal cavity
Radiation dosage restricted by neighboring organs
Infrequent detection of early disease

Table 11–20 DOSE RESTRICTIONS

Tolerance of small intestine
Limited tolerance of kidneys
Bone marrow depression
Radiation enteritis caused by large volume of intestine irradiated
Adhesive peritonitis

Two different radiation treatment techniques have been used for abdominal irradiation. Large portals may be employed, and a dose of 2500–3000 cGy can be delivered during 4–5 weeks to the entire abdomen. The kidneys and possibly the right lobe of the liver are shielded to limit the dose to 2000–2500 cGy. Nausea and vomiting may be associated with this procedure, and therapy is frequently interrupted. Historically, in some centers, abdominal irradiation was delivered by the so-called moving strip technique. Both the whole-abdomen and the moving strip techniques usually finish with a pelvic boost of approximately 2000–3000 cGy.

As a better understanding of the effects of chemotherapeutic agents in ovarian cancer has been gained, the role of radiation therapy in this disease has markedly diminished in prominence. The spread pattern of ovarian cancer and the normal tissue bed involved in the treatment of this neoplasm make effective radiation therapy difficult. Some special problems are listed in Table 11–19. When the residual disease after laparotomy is bulky, radiation therapy is particularly ineffective. The entire abdomen must be considered at risk, and therefore the volume that must be irradiated is large, resulting in multiple limitations for the radiotherapist. Dose restrictions are listed in Table 11–20.

The GOG tested the feasibility of using radiation therapy in conjunction with chemotherapy. A prospective randomized study using four arms and assessing radiation therapy alone, radiation therapy before chemotherapy (melphalan), chemotherapy alone, and chemotherapy before radiation therapy noted no significant difference in any of the four arms.

Dembo and associates reported a prospective randomized stratified trial involving 231 patients with stage I, stage II, and asymptomatic stage III ovarian carcinoma who received radiation therapy with or without chlorambucil. Chlorambucil, 6 mg daily, was given for 2 years, and patients receiving abdominal and pelvic irradiation were given 2250 cGy in 10 fractions to the pelvic portal followed immediately by 2250 cGy of cobalt given in 10 fractions to a downward moving abdominal pelvic strip. For patients with stage I or stage II disease, pelvic irradiation alone at a dose level of 4500 cGy was used. These investigators concluded that for patients who had stage Ib, stage II, or asymptomatic stage III disease, an incomplete initial pelvic operation correlated with poor survival. For patients in whom the operation was completed, abdominal and pelvic irradiation was superior to pelvic irradiation alone or pelvic irradiation followed by chlorambucil, with respect to long-term survival and control of abdominal disease. The effectiveness of abdominal and pelvic irradiation was independent of stage or histologic features. The value of abdominal and pelvic irradiation was most strikingly seen in patients with no visible residual tumor. These investigators also concluded that pelvic irradiation alone constituted inadequate and inappropriate postoperative treatment of patients with stage Ib or stage II disease. Abdominal and pelvic irradiation, which encompassed both domes of the diaphragm without liver shielding, significantly reduced tumor failure outside the pelvis and improved survival. However, adjuvant chemotherapy with daily chlorambucil after pelvic irradiation was ineffective in the management of these patients. The authors also concluded that in selecting postoperative therapy, the presence of small amounts of disease in the upper abdomen should not result in the selection of chemotherapy over radiation therapy. They seemed convinced that radiation therapy is effective, even when small amounts of disease exist in the upper abdomen. These studies by Dembo and associates reported good 5-year survival rates, such as 58% for patients with stage II and 43% for patients with stage III. In addition, Martinez and coworkers reported a 54% 5-year survival rate in 42 patients with stage II and stage III disease. Further studies to corroborate these findings are needed before renewed enthusiasm for radiotherapy in stage III and stage IV epithelial cancers of the ovary is justified.

The role of radiation therapy in localized disease also needs discussion. A prospective randomized study of stage I epithelial cancer of the ovary conducted by the GOG had the following results. Patients were randomized among three arms: no further therapy, melphalan (Alkeran), and pelvic irradiation. The patients who received melphalan did the best, with no appreciable benefit being noted from the use of pelvic irradiation. On the other hand, the role of pelvic irradiation in stage II ovarian cancer has yet to be defined. Historically, some institutions used pelvic irradiation in conjunction with systemic chemotherapy as the customary treatment of stage II disease. Retrospective studies suggest that pelvic irradiation improves survival over and above the use of surgery alone (Table 11–21). The efficacy of pelvic irradiation, compared with chemotherapy, in stage II disease has yet to be tested in a prospective randomized study. The GOG study reported by Young and coworkers compared chemotherapy with intraperitoneal colloidal ^{32}P. It is our opinion that the designation of stage II epithelial ovarian cancer mandates that the entire

Table 11–21 RADIOTHERAPY IN FIGO STAGE II DISEASE

Series	No. of patients		Five-year survival rate (%)	
	Surgery alone	Surgery and irradiation	Surgery alone	Surgery and irradiation
Van Orden et al	8	22	25.7	36.4
Barr, Cawell, and Chatfield	27	91	33.7	48.8
Kent and McKay	32	36	28.2	52.8
Munnell	16	61	0.7	40.4
Clark et al	6	51	16.7	31.4

abdomen be considered at risk. Thus, if postoperative radiation therapy is prescribed, it seems appropriate that a technique be used in which the entire abdomen and pelvis are optimally treated. There are no phase III data comparing platinum-based chemotherapy with radiation therapy in low- and intermediate-risk patients with epithelial ovarian cancer. The limitations of comparison of radiation therapy and chemotherapy results from retrospective studies are many. In many instances, the radiation therapy studies are older, and staging procedures were not done with the same accuracy. Prospective studies have failed because of low accrual. The two treatment methods are so different that investigator bias usually prevents reasonable accrual of patients. Radiation therapy techniques have advanced, lowering toxicity. This, combined with better data for selection of patients, makes an argument for another attempt at a phase III trial of this modality in ovarian carcinoma.

Radiation therapy as a second-line treatment in patients with chemotherapy-persistent or recurrent ovarian cancer has its advocates. As noted before, radiation therapy as part of the initial therapy has been abandoned in favor of chemotherapy. The impetus for renewed interest in second-line radiation therapy is that second-line chemotherapy by and large has not been successful. Cmelak and Kapp reported their experience of 41 patients who failed to respond to chemotherapy. All were treated with whole-abdomen irradiation, usually with a pelvic boost. The 5-year actuarial disease-specific survival was 40% and 50% in the platinum-refractory patients. If residual tumor was <1.5 cm, 5-year disease-free survival was 53%, but it was 0% in patients with >1.5 cm residual disease. Almost one-third of patients failed to complete the planned course of whole-abdomen irradiation because of toxicity. Three patients required surgery to correct gastrointestinal tract problems. Sedlacek and colleagues described 27 patients treated with whole-abdomen irradiation, all after platinum-based chemotherapy. All patients completed the planned course. Survival rate at 5 years was 15%. Patients with microscopic disease survived an average of 63 months, but if disease was >2 cm, average survival was 9 months. Four patients required surgery to correct gastrointestinal problems.

There may well be a role for whole-abdomen irradiation in patients after chemotherapy if residual tumor is small. Sedlacek, in a review of the literature, noted that there were 47 of 130 (36%) long-term survivors if only microscopic disease was present at the time of whole-abdomen irradiation but only 15 of 218 (6.8%) if macroscopic disease was present.

Radioisotopes

Radioisotopes have been widely used for the treatment of ovarian cancer. Both the pure beta emitter radioactive chromic phosphate (half-life of 14.2 days) and radioactive gold (10% gamma, half-life of 2.7 days) have been used. These isotopes emit radiation with an effective maximal penetration of 4–5 mm and therefore are useful only with minimal disease. Both agents are taken up by the serosal macrophages and transported to the retroperitoneal and mediastinal lymph nodes. The likelihood that the radioactive colloid will eradicate node metastases by selective lymphatic uptake is of considerable doubt because studies suggest that malignant nodes do not take up the isotope, but tumor-free nodes do. It has been estimated that 6000 cGy is delivered to the omentum and peritoneal surfaces and 7000 cGy to some retroperitoneal structures. If a free intraperitoneal distribution can be ensured, chromic phosphate with a longer half-life and no gamma irradiation is the agent of choice.

Numerous trials have been conducted comparing intraperitoneal ^{32}P with or without pelvic radiation to whole abdominal radiation or single agent chemotherapy in various clinical settings of ovarian cancer. Since intraperitoneal ^{32}P has failed to demonstrate improved outcomes, can be associated with increased complications and is "technique-intensive," it has all but evaporated from our contemporary treatment planning.

Chemotherapy

The evolution of chemotherapy for advanced ovarian cancer over the past 30 years has been significant. Ovarian cancer was one of the first solid malignant tumors demonstrating responsiveness to chemotherapy. Effectiveness of the various chemotherapy treatments has been expressed in terms of response rates (usually complete plus partial responses), negative second-look rates, and median survival. All of these outcome measures are subject to error, although the most reliable is median progression-free survival and median overall survival. However, survival outcomes are also compromised by the fact that many patients receive a number of variously active chemotherapy treatments over their treatment history.

The early agents utilized in the treatment of ovarian carcinoma (1970–1980) were predominantly the alkylating agents melphalan (also called phenylalanine mustard, Alkeran, L-PAM and L-sarcolysin), cyclophosphamide, chlorambucil and thiotepa. Response rates were usually reported in the 20–60% range, but median survival rates for patients with advanced ovarian cancer were often in the range of 10–18 months, quite inferior to most outcomes from today's clinical trials. Antimetabolites, such as 5-fluorouracil and methotrexate, were used in many of the earlier trials, especially in combination with alkylating agents. The contemporary use of these agents in epithelial ovarian cancer is rare to nonexistent.

The late 1970s and 1980s saw the introduction of combination chemotherapy regimens, Hexa CAF—hexamethylmelamine, cyclophosphamide, doxorubicin and 5-fluorouracil; and CAP—cyclophosphamide, doxorubicin and cisplatin, being two of the most common. By the early 1980s, combination therapy was the standard treatment for most patients. The 1980s also witnessed the introduction of cisplatin and later carboplatin. The introduction of the platinum compounds increased response rates to the 50–80% range and increased median survivals to the 12–30 month range in most studies. The wide range was often attributable to select patient populations with the "suboptimal" debulked patients having the 12–18 month survival and the "optimal" debulked patients having the 18–30 month survivals. The platinum compounds have remained an integral component of treatment to this day.

The 1990s saw the introduction of paclitaxel, an agent first extracted from the stripped bark of the Pacific yew tree, *taxus brevifolia*. Paclitaxel, now chemically synthesized, demonstrated a new mechanism of action by promoting microtubular assembly and stabilizing tubulin polymer formation, thus inhibiting rapidly dividing cells from completing the mitotic process. The initial single agent paclitaxel response rates in patients with refractory ovarian cancer were in the 25–35% range. Contemporary drug development is looking at various formulations of the taxane group. One study by SCOTROC (Vasey et al) demonstrated the substitution of paclitaxel with docetaxel yielded similar surgical outcomes, and the toxicity profile favored docetaxel. Other modified taxanes under investigation, such as CT-2103 (Xyotax) and Abraxane, may offer advantages of either greater activity or less toxicity.

The past five to ten years have also seen the introduction of additional active agents in ovarian cancer treatment, most noticeably topotecan, a topoisomerase I-inhibitor; a pegylated liposomal encapsulated form of doxorubicin (Doxil), and gemcitabine, a drug first tested in the pancreatic cancer setting. These three drugs were tested in the front line setting by the GOG 182/ICON-5 clinical trials, discussed later.

The current new therapeutic focus in the clinical trials is in the testing of agents targeting specific molecular targets. One such agent receiving considerable attention in current clinical trials is bevacizumab, an agent demonstrating activity in metastatic colon cancer.

Clinical trials

The relatively low rates of response to most single agents have stimulated investigators to search for combination schedules. In the "modern" era, platinum-based combinations have proven to be the most successful. Pertinent clinical trials relating to early stage disease are discussed earlier in this chapter.

A study by the GOG (GOG #47) comparing doxorubicin (Adriamycin) and cyclophosphamide (AC) with AC and cisplatin (CAP) indicated improvement with the three-drug combination. A 26% complete response was obtained with AC, and a 51% complete response was achieved with CAP. Response duration was 9 months vs 15 months, and progression-free interval was 7 months vs 13 months. Median survival was 16 months vs 19 months for CAP in all patients, but there was no statistical significance in survival between the two arms. When patients with measurable disease were evaluated separately (227 of 440 assessable patients), statistical significance for survival was present for the CAP arm. No significance in survival was noted for non-measurable residual disease. This study suggested an advantage for the platinum arm in those patients with suboptimal, measurable residual disease after debulking surgery.

Other studies at that time noted that an alkylating agent was just as effective as combinations (including platinum) containing up to four drugs. In another study by the GOG (GOG #52) of patients with stage III ovarian cancer optimally debulked to $\leq$1 cm residual disease, CAP was compared with cyclophosphamide and cisplatin. Progression-free interval and survival were not appreciably different in the two arms. Cyclophosphamide-cisplatin, therefore, became the "standard" arm for many clinical trials in the late 1980s and early 1990s.

Four trials were considered in a meta-analysis that specifically addressed the question of the role of doxorubicin in ovarian cancer. Considering only pathologic complete responses, the study shows a constant small benefit for CAP, higher for the North-West Oncology Group (GONO) and Danish Ovarian Cancer Group (DACOVA) studies. By pulling together these data in a meta-analysis, it was possible to detect a statistically significant benefit of 6% in the percentage of pathologic complete responses achieved with CAP. Moreover, this meta-analysis demonstrated a significant survival advantage of 7% at 6 years with CAP. However, because in three trials the dose intensity was greater for CAP than for cyclophosphamide-cisplatin, to what extent the benefit of CAP is from greater dose intensity or from doxorubicin itself remains unsolved. A subsequent study by the GOG (GOG #132) evaluated 614 patients with suboptimally debulked cancer who were treated in a three-arm protocol comparing cisplatin alone, paclitaxel alone, and a combination of the two drugs. Neither progression-free survival nor survival was different between the three arms. Crossover to the other drug in the single-drug arms may account for the similarity in the results. Some have interpreted the results of this study to indicate that a platinum agent should be a component of primary therapy.

The GOG (GOG #111) has randomized patients with large-volume disease to six cycles of cisplatin 75 mg/m^2 plus cyclophosphamide 750 mg/m^2 every 3 weeks or paclitaxel 135 mg/m^2 during 24 hours followed by cisplatin 75 mg/m^2 every 3 weeks. In the paclitaxel arm, administration of paclitaxel before the cisplatin was important to optimize response and minimize toxicity. A total of 386 assessable patients were entered in the study. In terms of therapeutic efficacy, the paclitaxel arm produced a significantly greater overall response rate (73% vs 60%) and clinical complete response rate, whereas the frequency of pathologic complete response was similar between the two arms. The percentage of patients achieving a state of no gross residual disease was significantly higher in the paclitaxel arm (41%) than in the control arm (25%). Progression-free survival was significantly greater in the paclitaxel arm (18 vs 13 months). The risk of progression was 32% lower among those treated with the paclitaxel regimen compared with the cyclophosphamide regimen. Survival was significantly longer in the paclitaxel arm (38 vs 24 months). The risk of death was 39% lower among those treated with the paclitaxel regimen (Fig. 11–23). A European-Canadian Intergroup trial (OV-10) had a study design similar to GOG #111, testing the replacement of cyclophosphamide with paclitaxel. This study included optimal stage III and stage IIB–C. Again, the clinical response rate was superior for the paclitaxel arm (45% vs 59%). The combination of paclitaxel and cisplatin was considered the standard for combination first-line chemotherapy for the treatment of epithelial ovarian carcinoma.

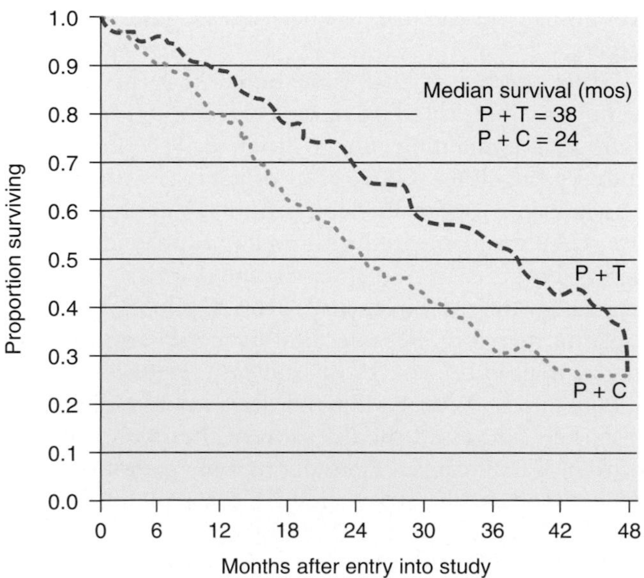

Figure 11–23 Survival by treatment group. (Modified from McGuire WP et al: Cyclophosphamide and cisplatin compared with paclitaxel and cisplatin in patients with stage III and stage IV ovarian cancer. N Engl J Med 334:1, 1996. Copyright © 1996 Massachusetts Medical society. All rights reserved. Adapted 2006 with permission.)

When combined with cisplatin, the paclitaxel requires an extended infusion interval (24 hours) to prevent unacceptable neuropathy. Accordingly, this administration was inconvenient and, since many community providers had replaced cisplatin with carboplatin, the GOG and others conducted equivalency trials to demonstrate similar efficacy of paclitaxel (175–185 mg/m^2) and carboplatin (AUC 5–7.5). The GOG conducted GOG #158 on the optimal (<1cm) patient population as a non-inferiority trial. The relative risk of progression on the paclitaxel plus carboplatin arm was 0.88 (95% CI were 0.75 to 1.03). Toxicity was greater on the paclitaxel plus cisplatin arm. A second-look laparotomy was also part of the protocol, and this will be reviewed later in the chapter.

In the International Collaborative Ovarian Neoplasm (ICON2) study, 1526 patients with ovarian cancer were randomized between carboplatin and CAP. There was no difference in survival between the two arms. Age, stage, residual disease, differentiation, and histologic features did not affect survival in either arm.

Care must always be taken in interpreting response rates as a definite indicator of trends in survival rates. Too often a chemotherapeutic regimen will produce excellent response rates but not affect the overall survival rate. Therefore, the clinician must await longer studies of cisplatin-based combination chemotherapy to accurately understand its impact on survival of patients. Omura and colleagues reported a sobering analysis of two large GOG studies of multistaging chemotherapy in epithelial ovarian cancer. In this analysis of 726 women with stage III or stage IV disease, excellent follow-up had been obtained. The authors concluded that the impact of chemotherapy to date had been modest. Less than 10% of their patients were progression free at 5 years, and late failures continued to occur, even beyond 7 years. Sutton and coworkers reported a 7% disease-free survival at 10 years. Unfortunately, the superiority of any particular combination of chemotherapeutic agents as reflected by statistically significant improvement in long-term survival remains unproved. Although carboplatin appears to be the most active agent in epithelial cancer of the ovary, there is still controversy that combining it with other agents improves outcome.

In vitro testing of chemotherapy resistance or sensitivity has been investigated for at least two decades without clarification of its role in either primary or recurrent disease. Multiple technologies are currently in use, and there is a need to identify the relative value of this testing modality.

Maintenance therapy after primary surgery and chemotherapy in patients with a complete clinical response is an area of current controversy. One clinical trial randomized this patient population to 3 versus 12 additional treatments with paclitaxel at four-week intervals. The study was closed early by the Data Safety Monitoring Board when a planned interim analysis demonstrated a progression-free interval advantage of 7 months for the extra 9 months of treatment. However, a follow-up report failed to demonstrate any survival advantage. Additional trials are in progress to clarify the potential role for maintenance therapy.

High-dose chemotherapy with autologous bone marrow support

Dose intensity refers to the amount of chemotherapy to which a cancer is exposed per unit of time; this is generally assumed to be reflected by the dose of drug in milligrams per square meter of body surface area per unit of time. The theory is well grounded in preclinical work showing that as the concentration of drug in culture medium increases, the fraction of surviving cancer cells decreases logarithmically. To determine whether dose intensity is important clinically, randomized trials are needed. The GOG did design such a trial in patients with large-volume, advanced disease. A total of 458 patients were entered into the study and were randomized to low-dose cisplatin 50 mg/m^2 plus cyclophosphamide 500 mg/m^2 every 3 weeks for eight cycles or high-dose cisplatin 100 mg/m^2 plus cyclophosphamide 1000 mg/m^2 every 3 weeks for four cycles. Each regimen delivered the same total dose of chemotherapy, but the high-dose schedule was delivered in half the time. The overall response rate of the 130 patients with measurable disease was 65% for the low-dose arm vs 59% for the high-dose arm; clinical complete response rates were 26% and 27%, respectively. These differences were not significant. There was no difference in progression-free survival in the subsets of patients with measurable or nonmeasurable disease; similarly, no difference in overall survival in either subset of patients was noted. The results of this study did not support the concept that increased dose intensity will produce greater therapeutic effect. Colombo and associates reported a randomized trial in patients with advanced disease who were given cisplatin 50 mg/m^2 per week for 9 weeks or cisplatin 75 mg/m^2 every 3 weeks for six cycles. The weekly arm delivered the same total dose of cisplatin in half the time, but each arm received the total dose of drug. Within the subsets of patients with small-volume and large-volume disease, no significant differences were observed with regard to either response rates or pathologic complete response rates. No overall differences were noted in either of these parameters or in regard to progression-free or overall survival. Whereas neither of these randomized trials of pure dose intensity showed an advantage for a higher dose intensity across a clinically relevant range of doses, other lines of evidence have been cited to support the use of higher dose schedules. In trials conducted by the National Cancer Institute of the USA, even higher dose intensities of cisplatin in conjunction with hypertonic saline to protect the kidneys have been stated to yield higher response rates than more standard doses. A closer examination of these data reported by Rothenberg and coworkers shows confusing results. In patients with large-volume disease, the National Cancer Institute results can be compared with the GOG results with cisplatin, doxorubicin, and cyclophosphamide (PAC), as reported by Omura, regimens with a 3.3-fold difference in dose intensity of cisplatin. The pathologic complete response rates for the two regimens were 12% and 11%, respectively. In patients with small-volume disease, the National Cancer Institute results can be compared with GOG results with a two-drug combination of cisplatin plus cyclophosphamide, as reported by Omura in 1989. The pathologic complete response rates in this second study for the two regimens were 38% and 30%, respectively, not significantly different. There appears to be no evidence from these data to support the importance of dose intensity of cisplatin over a 3.3-fold range of doses. At least 11 randomized trials have compared standard doses of carboplatin- or cisplatin-based chemotherapy with double doses of the same platinum analogues. Most of these trials showed no advantage in most outcome parameters. A second meta-analysis of the Levin and Hryniuk meta-analysis (in which it appeared that dose intensity had a positive impact on response rate and survival) suggested that platinum dose intensity is unimportant, although intensity of all administered drugs is important, as is tumor residual volume at initiation of therapy.

In the last decade, high-dose chemotherapy with autologous bone marrow transplantation (ABMT) has been reported for several solid tumors, and there has been a tendency for improved response rates but a relatively short period of disease-free survival in most of the reports reviewed. There have been no reports of 5-year survival studies in patients with malignant ovarian tumors treated with high-dose chemotherapy followed by ABMT. Many reports show that even in advanced cases, the most important factor for long-term survival after high-dose chemotherapy is the completeness of the primary cytoreductive surgery. Most of the reports in the literature with high-dose chemotherapy with ABMT have been phase II trials of patients who have failed to respond to first-line chemotherapy. The toxicity of high-dose chemotherapy is a serious concern, as is the additional expense. In a report from the Bone Marrow Transplant Registry, 341 patients with ovarian cancer have undergone transplantation during the last 5 years. The reported median survival was not significantly better than that with use of paclitaxel as second-line therapy. The best response and survival were in those patients who had had a complete response to pretransplantation chemotherapy. We believe that targeting of patients for high-dose therapy should be done as part of an established national protocol so that information can be obtained to increase our knowledge of this therapy, which in general does not appear promising.

Immunochemotherapy

In the last 3 decades, there has been considerable interest in combining chemotherapy with immunotherapy for better results in patients with epithelial cancer of the ovary.

Creasman and associates reported a series of patients treated with melphalan plus *Corynebacterium parvum,* a gram-positive bacterium chosen as the immunomodulating agent for this study. This agent has been shown to increase non-specific tumor resistance, to potentiate specific tumor rejections, to effect bone marrow proliferation, and to have additive antitumor effects when it is combined with alkylating agents. A prospective randomized study comparing similar treatment groups was conducted by the GOG (GOG #25). All patients had minimal residual advanced disease and participated in a randomized study comparing the effectiveness of melphalan with or without *C. parvum.* There were no significant differences between effects of the two regimens. The study did show, however, that the progression-free interval for patients with optimal disease was 16 months, compared with only 7 months in an earlier study of patients with bulky, advanced disease, and that survival was likewise strikingly better in patients with minimal residual disease (31–33 months vs 12 months). This was in part the basis for dividing these patient populations for a series of future clinical trials.

Alberts and colleagues used a combination of doxorubicin and cyclophosphamide, with or without Pasteur Institute bacille Calmette–Guérin (BCG). The median survival of patients receiving doxorubicin and cyclophosphamide plus BCG was 22.3 months versus 13.7 months for patients receiving doxorubicin and cyclophosphamide alone ($P < 0.03$). These investigators concluded that non-specific immunostimulation therapy combined with chemotherapy could improve the results in advanced epithelial carcinoma of the ovary. The GOG conducted a similar study and failed to confirm the previous report.

The potential role of biologic agents in the treatment of ovarian cancer has been investigated. Ovarian cancer is a suitable model for biologic therapies as the peritoneal cavity is capable of mounting an inflammatory response to many stimuli, and this response has been shown to induce an antitumor effect. Preliminary data of intraperitoneal administration of interleukin-2 have demonstrated that lymphokines cause the egress into the peritoneal cavity of a large number of lymphocytes, neutrophils, and macrophages as well as of the cytokines those cells produce. The peritoneal cavity is also an attractive site for the administration of antibodies as well as adoptive cellular therapies. It has been demonstrated that the intraperitoneal administration of large-molecular-weight molecules may actually lead to a deeper penetration into tumor nodules than can be achieved with small-molecular-weight chemotherapeutic agents such as doxorubicin and cisplatin. The depth of penetration into a tumor mass is a function of the rate of diffusion of the drug through the tissue and its capillary permeability. Although both factors are proportional to molecular weight, the capillary permeability is more vulnerable relative to molecular weight than is tissue diffusion. Consequently, compounds of larger molecular weight that are allowed to have a long intraperitoneal dwell time may lead to an increased depth of tissue penetration because there may be less clearance through the capillary microcirculation. It is also possible that adoptive cellular therapy may be more effective when it is administered intraperitoneally to localized tumors because monocytes or lymphocytes, when they are administered in the peritoneal cavity, may remain localized for an extended period. These experimental observations indicate that ovarian cancer is a suitable prototype tumor in which to evaluate novel immunotherapeutic and chemoimmunotherapeutic approaches. It has been reported by Berek and coworkers that recombinant interferon alfa has clinical activity in patients with small-volume residual disease. This study included only patients who had tumor masses <5 mm. Four of 11 patients evaluated by restaging laparotomy were found to be disease free after treatment with interferon alfa intraperitoneally. However, three of these patients initially had only positive cytologic findings. Nonetheless, the study demonstrates that intraperitoneal administration of a biologic agent has antitumor activity in ovarian cancer. Attempts to use biologic response modifiers in phase III trials with chemotherapy have been stalled in recent years until such time as more effective biologic response modifiers are at hand. Numerous phase II trials, using substances such as tumor necrosis factor, interleukin-2, and the like, along with other studies using combinations of cytokines have failed to demonstrate significantly improved outcomes. Combining biologic response modifiers with standard chemotherapy has proven to be more difficult than initially conceived because of overlapping toxicities. In view of this, it seems prudent to await proven efficacy before attempting to launch the phase III trials with biologic response modifiers.

Intraperitoneal (IP) chemotherapy

Ovarian cancer, while known for early extraovarian spread, is predominantly a disease limited to the peritoneal cavity for most patients. For some chemotherapeutic agents, IP administration offers pharmacokinetic advantages, including high intraperitoneal drug concentration and a longer s in the peritoneal cavity. While intraperitoneal chemotherapy proposals date back decades, it has only been over recent years that accumulative clinical trial data supports this approach.

Results from randomized trials, listed in Table 11–22, summarize the experience of clinical trials conducted since the mid-1980s. These studies, all front line therapy trials, compare intravenous (IV) chemotherapy to combined IV and IP chemotherapy. The initial IP study demonstrating that IP chemotherapy may represent an efficacy advantage was a combined SWOG/GOG trial (SWOG #8501 and GOG #104). The study compared IV cisplatin and IV cyclophosphamide to IP cisplatin and IV cyclophosphamide

Table 11–22 RANDOMIZED TRIALS COMPARING INTRAVENOUS VS INTRAPERITONEAL FIRST-LINE TREATMENT OF OVARIAN CANCER NEEDS FRAMEWORK

Study identifier/ year published	Control regimen	Experimental regimen	Target Population	No. of patients	Median duration of survival for control regimen (months)	Median duration of survival for experimental regimen (months)
SWOG/GOG-104 (Alberts et al 1996)	Cisplatin 100 mg/m^2 IV Ctx 600 mg/m^2 IV q 3 weeks × 6	Cisplatin 100 mg/m^2 IP Ctx 600 mg/m^2 IV q 3 weeks × 6	Stage III ≤2 cm residual	546	41	49
Greek (Polyzos et al 1999)	Crbpt 350 mg/m^2 IV Ctx 600 mg/m^2 IV q 3 weeks × 6	Crbpt 350 mg/m^2 IV Ctx 600 mg/m^2 IV q 3 weeks × 6	Stage III ≤ or >2 cm residual	90	52	63
GONO (Gadducci et al 2000)	Cisplatin 50 mg/m^2 IV Ctx 600 mg/m^2 IV Epidox 60 mg/m^2 IV q 4 weeks × 6	Cisplatin 50 mg/m^2 IP Ctx 600 mg/m^2 IV Epidox 60 mg/m^2 IV q 4 weeks × 6	Stage II–IV <2 cm residual	113	25	26
GOG-114/SWOG (Markman et al 2001)	Cisplatin 75 mg/m^2 IV Tax 135 mg/m^2 (24 h) IV q 3 weeks × 6	Crbpt AUC 9 IV q 28 d × 2 Cisplatin 100 mg/m^2 IP Tax 135 mg/m^2 (24 hr) IV q 3 weeks × 6	Stage III ≤1 cm residual	462	51	67
Taiwan (Yen et al 2001)	Cisplatin 50 mg/m^2 IV Ctx 500 mg/m^2 IV Epi/Adr 50 mg/m^2 IV q 3 weeks × 6	Cisplatin 100 mg/m^2 IV Ctx 500 mg/m^2 IV Epi/Adr 50 mg/m^2 IV q 3 weeks × 6	Stage III ≤1 cm residual	118	48	43
GOG-172 (Armstrong et al 2005)	Cisplatin 75 mg/m^2 IV Tax 135 mg/m^2(24 hr) IV q 3 weeks × 6 q 3 weeks × 6	Tax 135 mg/m^2(24 hr) IV Cisplatin 100 mg/m^2 IP Tax 60 mg/m^2 IV on day 8	Stage III ≤1 cm	415	49	67

in patients with less than 2 cm diameter residual disease. The IP arm produced a median survival of 49 months compared to 41 months for the IV arm, with a hazard ratio of 0.77. However, critics point out that the subsequent introduction of paclitaxel to our frontline treatment may have neutralized this apparent advantage for IP therapy. The other concern is that accrual was extended beyond the initial study design for patients with 0–0.5 cm residual disease and still this subgroup failed to demonstrate superior survival (51 months vs 46 months, HR = 0.80). One would have expected the treatment difference to be most pronounced in this patient subgroup.

Another GOG study, GOG #114, reported in 2003, compared IV cisplatin and paclitaxel (6 cycles) to high dose (AUC = 9) carboplatin IV (2 cycles) plus 6 cycles IV paclitaxel and IP cisplatin in patients with stage III disease less than or equal to 1 cm diameter residual. The median survival for the IP arm was 67 months versus 51 months for the IV arm. Obviously, this study would have had better balance and a higher degree of reliability if the patients in the IV arm had also received the extra 2 cycles of the high dose carboplatin.

The most recently reported GOG study, GOG #172, compared IV paclitaxel (135mg/m^2/24 hours), followed by either IV cisplatin (75 mg/m^2) on day 2 or by IP cisplatin (100mg/m^2) on day 2 and IP paclitaxel (60 mg/m^2) on day 8 — each arm for six cycles at 21-day intervals. The patient population was similar to GOG #114—stage III, less than 1 cm diameter residual. The median survival for the IP arm was 66.9 months compared to 49.5 months for the IV arm (hazard ratio of 0.71), results remarkably similar to the preceding study, GOG #114 (Fig. 11–24). However, this study reported significant toxicity for the IP arm, with double-digit percentage grade 3/4 toxicities. While the IP-treated patients reported a significantly worse quality of life prior to cycle four and 3–6 weeks post treatment, there was no difference in quality of life between the IP/IV arms one year post treatment, except for moderate neurotoxicity (paresthesias), which was more common in the IP arm. The GOG is currently evaluating dosing modifications to improve the tolerance to IP therapy. This study also reported catheter-related complications in 39 of 118 patients (33%). The GOG recommends use of a venous catheter with a subcutaneous access port overlying the lower ribs (Fig. 11–25). While the greatest experience with an IP platinum agent has been with cisplatin at a dose of 100 mg/m^2, substitution of carboplatin for cisplatin may limit the toxicity. Curiously, in GOG #172, only 42% of patients on the IP treatment received the complete six cycles of IP therapy, and 48% received three or four cycles of IP chemotherapy. Patients not able to receive the IP chemotherapy were switched to IV treatment, and 83% of the patients on the IP arm completed six cycles of chemotherapy (IP and/or IV). The authors postulate that the initial cycles of IP chemotherapy may render most of the benefit. The study does not provide information detailing information about IP catheter retention or management in patients converted to IV therapy. Actually,

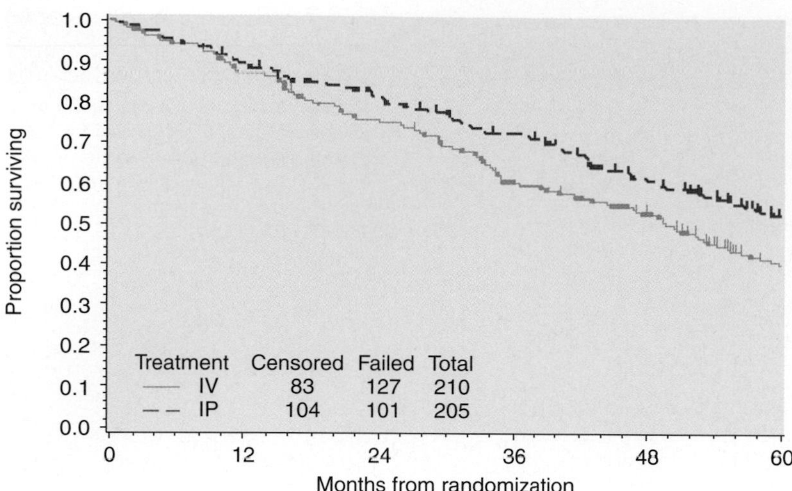

Figure 11–24 Overall survival for GOG #172–IP therapy vs IV therapy for optimally debulked advanced ovarian carcinoma.

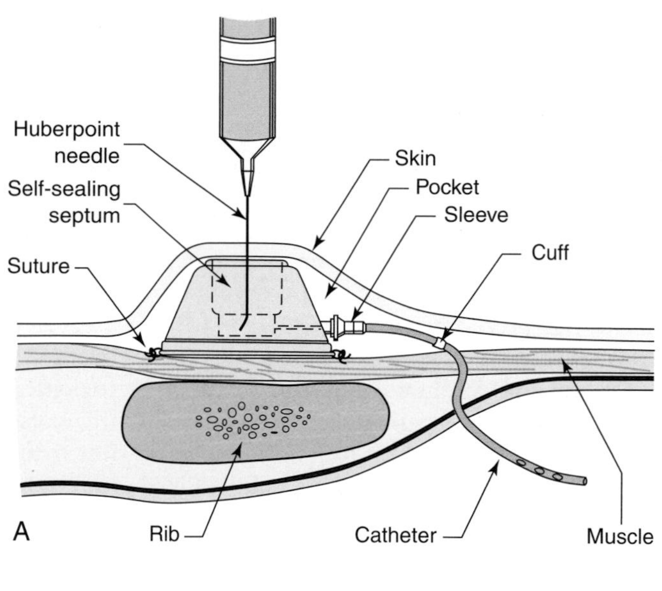

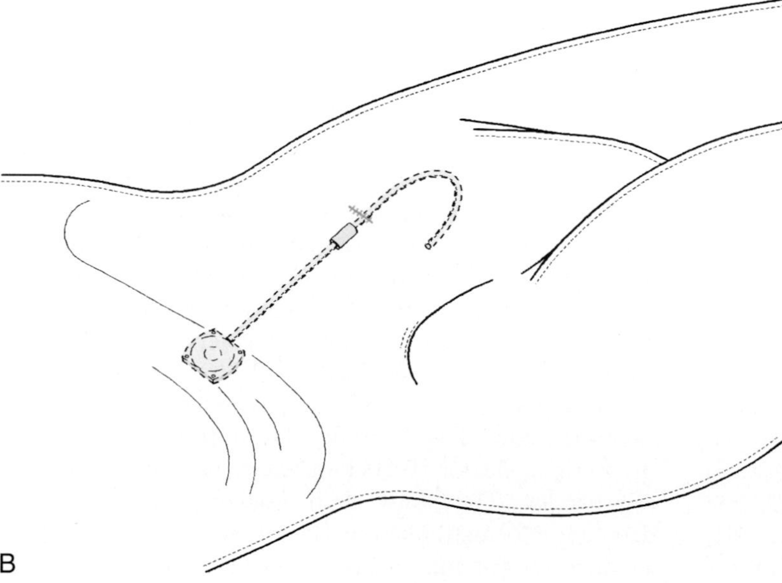

Figure 11–25 *A,* Implanted peritoneal access catheter with subcutaneous self-sealing port providing a path for intraperitoneal therapy. *B,* Intraperitoneal chemotherapy.

Figure 11–26 Treatment hazard ratios for death intraperitoneal vs. intravenous therapy. (Source: National Cancer Institute Clinical Announcement, December, 2005.)

	Rel Haz	Var (in[HR])
SWOG/GOG–104 (1996)	0.760	0.013
GONO (2000)	0.670	0.077
GOG–114/SWOG (2001)	0.810	0.012
Talwan (2001)	1.130	0.064
EORTC–55875 (2003)	0.820	0.054
GOG–172 (2005)	0.710	0.020

IP regimen better | IV regimen better

0.33 0.5 0.67 1.0 1.5 2.0 3.0

Relative hazard

χ^2 heterogeneity (5 d.f.)= 3.1, $P = 0.68$
Hazard ratio is not reported for the GONO study but it is calculated from the available data reported.
Hazard ratio is not reported for the Greek study.

none of the IP studies conducted to date has ruled out the possibility that the presence of an intraperitoneal foreign body is the inciting agent, altering host immune/cytokine response producing the more favorable outcomes. This possibility deserves further exploration (Figure 11–26).

Extraovarian peritoneal serous papillary carcinoma

Extraovarian peritoneal serous papillary carcinoma is a recognized clinical-pathologic entity in which peritoneal carcinomatosis of ovarian serous type is found in the abdomen or pelvis. Similar tumor deposits may be found on the surface of the ovary, but histologic evidence of primary or in situ ovarian carcinoma is either absent or insignificant. The tumor deposits are rarely non-invasive (borderline). This entity was first reported as "mesothelioma resembling papillary ovarian adenocarcinoma" by Swerdlow in 1959. Parmley and Woodruff, in 1974, demonstrated that pelvic peritoneum had the potential to differentiate into a müllerian type of epithelium. This entity is different from mesothelioma. The malignant neoplasm spreads inside the peritoneal cavity, invading mostly the omentum, with minimal or no involvement of the ovary. Peritoneal studding is commonly present with psammoma bodies. While usually serous, other cell types have been demonstrated. This entity has been identified in women who have had previous oophorectomies. The GOG has developed criteria for the diagnosis of extraovarian peritoneal carcinoma (Table 11–23).

Experience with extraovarian serous neoplasia of this type has been compared to clinical outcomes of homologous ovarian tumors of similar stage and grade. Fromm and colleagues reported a series of 74 patients identified as having papillary serous carcinoma of the peritoneum. The average age at diagnosis was 57 years, and the majority of the patients were white. Clinical presentation was similar to that of ovarian carcinoma. Clinical response to chemotherapy was seen in 64% of the patients; 41% had partial responses, and 23% had complete responses. Thirty-three patients came to a second-assessment surgery, and 27% were negative. Median survival for the total group was 24 months. Dalrymple reported 31 cases of extraovarian peritoneal serous papillary carcinoma. The median survival was 11.3 months for patients with this entity, compared with 13.5 months for patients with the equivalent primary ovarian neoplasms. The Roswell Park Cancer Institute described 73 patients with extraovarian peritoneal carcinoma. More than 95% were stage III–IV, ascites was present in 80%, and 95% had elevated CA-125 concentrations. Optimal debulking was performed in about two-thirds, and most received platinum-based regimens. Overall, survival was about 2 years; patients with stage III disease had a median survival of 29 months compared with only 15 months for patients with stage IV disease. In those with optimal debulking, survival was 40 months compared with 19 months if suboptimal debulking was done. In a multivariate analysis, only performance status and optimal debulking had a significant effect on overall survival. Interestingly, 10 of the patients had had previous oophorectomy. A GOG trial of cisplatin and cyclophosphamide in these patients demonstrated a response similar to that in women with papillary serous ovarian cancer.

Our experience has been that these patients generally respond to therapy in a manner similar to patients with serous papillary carcinoma of the ovary. Because many characteristics of this entity and serous ovarian cancer are similar, the GOG accepts patients with extraovarian peritoneal carcinoma into its protocols of epithelial ovarian cancer. CA-125 measurements also appear similar in both

Table 11–23 GOG CRITERIA FOR DIAGNOSIS OF EXTRAOVARIAN PERITONEAL CARCINOMA

Both ovaries must be either physiologically normal in size or enlarged by benign process.
Involvement in extraovarian sites must be greater than involvement on the surface of either ovary.
Microscopically, the ovarian involvement must be:
- Non-existent
- Confined to ovarian surface epithelium, or underlying cortical stromal involvement of no more than 5 mm

Histologic characteristics are primarily serous type, similar or identical to ovarian serous papillary adenocarcinoma.

GOG, Gynecologic Oncology Group.

groups of patients. There would appear to be an increased incidence of extraovarian peritoneal cancers in patients with a hereditary predisposition for development of ovarian cancer. In Piver's report of women at high risk for hereditary ovarian cancer, extraovarian cancer developed after prophylactic oophorectomy in almost 2%, 10 times greater than the lifetime incidence in the general population. BRCA1 mutations appear to arise in a similar number of women with extraovarian and primary ovarian cancers.

Small cell carcinoma of the ovary

Small cell carcinoma of the ovary has been identified as a specific histopathologic entity. This rare and highly aggressive malignant neoplasm primarily affects children and young women between the ages of 10 and 40 years. Few if any long-term survivors have been reported. The first 11 cases were documented by Dickersin and colleagues in 1982. Various chemotherapeutic agents have been suggested with minimal success. Senekjian and coworkers reported on a combination of vinblastine, cisplatin, cyclophosphamide, bleomycin, doxorubicin, and etoposide for this entity. One of their five patients was alive and disease free at 29 months. In general, similar chemotherapy regimens used for small cell lung carcinoma will be utilized to treat this disease. Many patients with this lesion, but not all, have an associated hypercalcemia. Neuron specific enolase may be both a histologic marker (immunohistochemistry) and a serum marker for this disease. Further study of this devastating group of tumors is necessary.

FOLLOW-UP TECHNIQUES AND TREATMENT OF RECURRENCES

Ovarian cancer is fast growing and insidious in that it is late to cause symptoms, and thus follow-up examinations are imperative to detect early recurrence. Even then, implants many centimeters in diameter can be hidden in the many crevices of the abdominal cavity and escape detection by either physical examination or imaging. There is a reasonable limit to the use of such sophisticated techniques as CT in the surveillance of a patient who has had ovarian cancer. Some have suggested that the proper assessment of the extent of disease is periodic monitoring of serum CA-125 levels and liberal use of surgical procedures (laparoscopy and laparotomy) to assay the contents of the abdominal and pelvic cavities. The role of positron emission tomography (PET) scans is evolving but appears promising in the detection of occult disease.

The optimal follow-up strategy for the asymptomatic patient who has advanced ovarian cancer after initial treatment remains undecided. Important considerations are divided between more passive and active approaches to follow-up. There is an absence of data on the benefit of second-line therapy, and these techniques are expensive, at times morbid, and certainly an inconvenience to the patient. While of possible limited therapeutic benefit, second-look laparotomy may produce information of reasonable prognostic significance, and this may aid the patient in their life planning. There is currently no evidence that intensive investigative monitoring in the symptomatic patient exerts a significant positive impact on the overall survival, symptom-free survival, or quality of life. Construction of the plan of follow-up should be individualized to each patient's needs. Trials of second-line therapy are abundant and, intuitively, early recognition of recurrent disease followed by effective second-line therapy should result in improved outcomes; whether this is valid remains to be proven.

In an era of cost containment, these considerations are even more relevant. Our practice has been to monitor these patients with physical examination and serum CA-125 measurements at regular intervals, frequently at first and decreasing as the recurrence-free interval increases. Imaging is done on an individual basis. These practices are not based on good science, and as stated before, the optimal strategy is unknown. At the 2-year anniversary, the frequency of follow-up visits is decreased to every 6 months. For patients who do not undergo reassessment laparotomy, it has been our practice to follow a similar monitoring regimen, increasing the frequency of visits to every 3 to 4 months in the first 2 years. Many patients request even more frequent examinations, in that they are greatly relieved by negative results.

Use of CA-125 levels

CA-125 is an antigenic determinant defined by Bast by a murine immunoglobulin Ig1 monoclonal antibody that was raised against an epithelial ovarian carcinoma cell line. Multiple CA-125 determinants are associated with a mucin-like glycoprotein of >200,000 daltons. Traces of the antigen are expressed in adult tissues derived from the coelomic epithelium, including mesothelial cells lining the pleura, pericardium, and peritoneum, as well as from the epithelial component of the fallopian tube, endometrium, and endocervix. CA-125 is not found in fetal or adult ovaries. Determinants are, however, expressed in >80% of non-mucinous epithelial ovarian cancers.

The radioimmune assay has been developed by Bast to detect CA-125 in serum and body fluids. The day-to-day coefficient of variability for the assay is approximately 15%. Consequently, a doubling or halving of antigen levels has been considered significant. If a cutoff of 35 U/mL is chosen for the upper limit of normal, elevated CA-125 levels should be found in 1% of apparently normal blood bank donors, 6% of patients who have benign disease, 28% of individuals who have non-gynecologic malignant neoplasms, and 82% of patients who have surgically demonstrable epithelial ovarian cancer. Niloff and coworkers reported detection of elevated CA-125 in sera from patients who have advanced fallopian tube, endometrial, and endocervical adenocarcinomas. In epithelial ovarian carcinoma, rising or falling levels of CA-125 have correlated with disease progression or regression in >90% of patients. In the report by Niloff, when CA-125 levels returned to <35 U/mL, findings of second-look surveillance procedures were in fact normal in 14 of 36 cases, but in no instance was a nodule >1 cm found. Persistently elevated CA-125 levels have been associated consistently with persistence of disease. Recurrence of disease has been heralded by elevations of CA-125 in 85% of patients whose tumors shed the antigen. Elevated CA-125 levels preceded disease recurrence by 1–14 months with a mean of 5 months in one study reported by Knapp and Friedman. Elevation of CA-125 in hepatocellular disease and in chronic peritonitis is important to note but should not compromise the utility of CA-125 as a marker for monitoring ovarian cancer.

Virtually all patients with elevated serum CA-125 levels before second-look surgery have residual ovarian cancer at laparotomy or develop disease within the next 4–6 months. Normal serum CA-125 levels before second-look surgery are of limited value. More than 50% of the patients with such findings (normal CA-125 level and normal clinical examination findings) have persistent disease. Residual disease, <2 cm in diameter, rarely elevates serum CA-125 levels. Although elevated serum CA-125 levels before second-look surgery allow the oncologist to counsel the patient with some assurance, the degree of elevation by itself does not precisely predict the amount of residual disease or the outcome. Normal levels may also accompany disease, with tumors of ≥2 cm, in one-third or more of cases. A rapid regression of the serum CA-125 level to normal limits shortly after commencement of chemotherapy is associated with a higher frequency of negative results at second-assessment surgery. Levin reported that almost all patients who subsequently come to a negative second-look laparotomy have serum CA-125 levels within normal ranges within 3 months of primary cytoreductive surgery. Buller and colleagues have shown that a favorable outcome is definitely associated with a steep regression curve of serum CA-125 levels after cytoreductive surgery and commencement of chemotherapy. These investigators demonstrated that patients in whom the CA-125 level reverts sharply to within the normal range by the third course of chemotherapy after surgery have a survival that is markedly and significantly improved over that of the patients who have an elevation of CA-125 levels before their fourth course of chemotherapy. Buller described the regression curve of the serum CA-125 level as "*s*." Indeed, he has suggested that patients with a delayed "*s*" curve (regression of the elevated value) possibly should be considered for alternative therapy rather than persisting with the same chemotherapeutic regimens. Hogberg and Kagedal demonstrated that 23 patients with a serum CA-125 half-life shorter than 16 days during induction chemotherapy had an estimated survival of 68% at 59 months after second-look operation. This compared with survival of 18% in 49 patients with a serum CA-125 half-life longer than 16 days.

All patients who have successfully completed therapy for ovarian cancer require follow-up examinations at least every 3 months. Serum CA-125 determination should be made at each visit. Patients whose clinical examination findings and tumor marker values remain normal are at a lower risk for recurrence. Those whose serum CA-125 values rise markedly have a high chance for development of clinical recurrence. Often a paracentesis will yield cytologically positive fluid, confirming the suspected diagnosis of recurrence. Patients whose serum CA-125 levels rise and then plateau and who remain clinically disease free should be observed (particularly if levels are only minimally elevated, e.g., <100 units) until recurrence is confirmed clinically or a more definitive pattern in serum CA-125 levels is apparent. Coexisting medical diseases, such as liver disease, heart disease, arthritis and others, may be the cause of a persistent abnormal plateau. The initial level of CA-125 in patients with advanced disease does not necessarily correlate with survival in women who respond to treatment. In a study by Latimer and colleagues, multivariate analysis did not show that CA-125 was a predictor of survival independent of stage. In other words, if the patient responds to treatment, survival is similar whether there is a high or low pretreatment CA-125 level.

An elevation of CA-125 in the post-treatment surveillance period is usually related to recurrence of tumor, even if clinically otherwise undetectable. Most of these patients are considered candidates for restarting chemotherapy. Unfortunately, federal regulatory authorities do not currently accept an elevated CA-125 as evidence of recurrence, complicating the interpretation of randomized clinical trials being conducted for potential drug registration purposes. However, a study by Rustin and colleagues demonstrates that "CA-125 progressions" are similar to progressions as measured by standard clinical or imaging methods.

There are other causes of elevated CA-125 concentration, particularly if it is elevated only slightly. They include both gynecologic and non-gynecologic conditions. Acute inflammatory processes involving the pelvic area as well as other regions of the body may increase CA-125. These may include acute hepatitis or pancreatitis, chronic liver disease, colitis, congestive heart failure, diverticulitis, arthritis, and pneumonia, to name a few.

Second-look operation (reassessment surgery)

The so-called second-look operation was first defined by Owen Wangenstein in the late 1940s with reference to exploratory laparotomy procedures in patients with colon cancer from whom he had previously removed all gross tumor, but in whom there was a high risk of recurrence. At varying intervals, usually 6 months initially, he would explore these patients in the hope of detecting early recurrence at a time when secondary resection still offered a chance of cure. Since then, the term *second look* has been

Table 11–24 OVARIAN CANCER: INITIAL STAGE RELATIVE TO NEGATIVE SECOND-LOOK FINDINGS

Stage	No evidence of disease (%)
I	60–79
II	45–68
III	16–48
IV	33–45

Data from collected series: Smirz, Cain, Copeland, Gershenson, and Roberts.

used to describe many procedures. With reference to ovarian cancer, it appears that a second-look (or reassessment) procedure is mainly indicated:

- for restaging in a patient who probably has localized disease but who has not had an optimal staging procedure as defined previously (see Table 11–14);
- for evaluation of the effect of chemotherapy in patients receiving both standard and investigational regimens; in this regard, some centers have instituted serial laparoscopic examinations to assess the extent of regression or progression of bulk disease several months after beginning of chemotherapy, with the option to offer therapy if a poor response is noted (less frequently necessary now when the malignant neoplasm expresses CA-125); and
- for evaluation of patients who are clinically free of disease after receiving what is considered a sufficient course of chemotherapy and are then eligible for assessment as to possible "cure" and discontinuation of therapy (Table 11–24). This last indication has been the most widely used and has resulted in small numbers of patients, even with advanced disease, who are free of detectable malignant cells at the second procedure. The most difficult second-look procedure is that in which no evidence of disease apparently exists because thorough surgery with multiple biopsies must be performed to establish lack of disease. In essence, an optimal staging procedure must be repeated.

Second-look procedures are often begun with a laparoscopic examination to rule out widespread disease. If this lesser procedure reveals diffuse miliary studding (that was not clinically detectable), a laparotomy is not necessary. It is obvious that these patients need to continue receiving therapy of some sort and are not candidates for a second attempt at surgical resection. At the time of laparotomy, a detailed exploration of the abdominal cavity must be done in a manner similar to the initial staging procedures previously described. If focal residual disease is encountered, it is surgically resected. Careful inspection of the entire abdominal cavity, including the undersurface of the diaphragm, the root of the mesentery, and all parietal and visceral peritoneal surfaces, must be tediously carried out with liberal use of biopsy for suspicious areas.

With the conscientious use of a second-look operation (Table 11–25), one can expect a relatively low subsequent recurrence rate if the results are negative. Earlier reports outlining the fate of patients with negative results of a second-look procedure after surgery and single-agent chemotherapy with alkylating agents suggested that the subsequent recurrence rate was about 10–20%. In the last 2 decades, more and more patients have been treated with platinum-based combination chemotherapy, and the fate of patients with negative results of second-look procedures has been somewhat altered. Roberts and coworkers reported a series of second-look procedures and analyzed the subsequent outcome for the patient with regard to stage. In patients with stage I and stage II disease, the negative second-look operation does not correlate with overall survival because most of these patients do not have persistent disease. The second-look laparotomy does not affect survival. In patients with advanced disease, as many as 50% with negative results of second-look operations after combination chemotherapy have experienced subsequent recurrence of their disease. This 50% figure for patients with stage III and stage IV epithelial cancers of the ovary has been confirmed by many. This discouraging statistic suggests that:

Table 11–25 STEPS TAKEN IN REASSESSMENT LAPAROTOMY

1. Midline incision
2. Cytologic washings from several areas of the abdomen and pelvis
3. Inspection of the omentum (take biopsies liberally)
4. Visualization of all peritoneal surfaces, including the undersurface of the diaphragm, serosa, and mesentery of the bowel (take biopsies of suspicious areas)
5. Submission of all excised adhesions for histologic review
6. Careful inspection of all pelvic organs and pelvic peritoneum (take biopsies liberally)
7. Retroperitoneal inspection of pelvic and periaortic nodes (take selected biopsies)

- even a thorough exploration does not reveal microscopic residuals in many patients; and
- this group of patients should be strongly considered for an adjuvant program.

The high subsequent recurrence rate after negative second-look operations after combination chemotherapy, compared with single-agent therapy, is also difficult to explain. Combination therapy appears to increase the number of patients who have regression to the point of having clinically undetectable residual disease. The fact remains: many patients are being treated almost to the point of cure, and an additional stroke of some sort is needed.

Today, the second-look laparotomy is used infrequently unless the patient is enrolled in a protocol. After several years of experience, many question its rationale. The reasons for the change in attitude are several. In patients with negative second-look laparotomy results, about half will have recurrence. The ability to optimally debulk the tumor secondarily after completion of chemotherapy was addressed earlier in this chapter and has limited success. There are no data to suggest that a second-look has an effect on survival in about 90% of patients. Unfortunately, today, if disease remains after primary therapy, second-line treatment, as far as survival is concerned, has minimal impact. In a few highly selected situations, the second-look laparotomy may be an individual benefit. The second-look laparotomy does determine, as best as is possible, the status of disease at a given point in time. It is for this reason that some investigators continue to be advocates of second-look laparotomy. Many patients want this information for purposes of life planning. Findings may guide subsequent therapy in a given patient and be beneficial. Resistant chemotherapy testing may determine which drugs appear to be ineffective and save the expense and morbidity of therapy for which the chance of benefit is low. The situation needs to be discussed in detail with the patient, and her wishes should be honored. Our experience has been that many patients want this knowledge. In this era of intraperitoneal chemotherapy and the newly introduced biologic agents, second-assessment surgery may help in selecting patients for these trials, and thus it may have some impact on survival when definitive second-line therapies have been identified. Second-look surgery may provide the managing physician with important information for selecting second-line therapy. Most patients are anxious to proceed with further therapy and insist on knowing their disease status before considering their options. For these reasons, second-assessment surgery may be helpful in a selected few. It does not appear that patients with low-risk disease (stage I and stage II) who are subjected to a full staging operation at their initial surgery will benefit from a reassessment laparotomy. In addition, there is no evidence that patients who progress during primary therapy benefit from elective repeat surgery of this nature.

Second-line therapy

Advanced epithelial ovarian cancer is a highly chemosensitive solid tumor with responses in the range of 70–80% to first-line chemotherapy, including a high proportion of complete responses. Most patients, however, eventually relapse and ultimately die of chemoresistant disease. Even with platinum-based chemotherapy, less than a quarter of the patients with an initial advanced disease diagnosis are alive at 5 years. In all forms of ovarian epithelial cancer, second-line chemotherapy has to date been disappointing. When effective drug combinations are initially used and fail, there is a very limited chance of inducing a significant response with a second or third drug or combinations. A partial response and control of malignant effusions can be achieved on occasion, but these are usually short-lived. However, most gynecologic oncologists attempt to treat these patients with use of a reasonable second-line regimen usually consisting of active chemotherapeutic agents that have not been used in the first treatment plan (Table 11–26).

Table 11–26 AGENTS USED IN EPITHELIAL OVARIAN CANCER

Active agents	Inactive agents
Alkylating agents	BCNU
Bevacizamab	Vincristine
Hexamethylmelamine	6-Mercaptopurine (6-MP)
Doxorubicin	Dactinomycin
Cisplatin	Raltitrexed (Tomudex)
Carboplatin	CI-958
5-Fluorouracil	
Methotrexate	
Etoposide (VP-16)	
Paclitaxel (Taxol)	
Vinorelbine tartrate (Navelbine)	
Gemcitabine	
Topotecan	
Liposomal doxorubicin	
Docetaxel	

BCNU, carmustine

It is hoped that as new agents evolve, more effective second and third echelon of drugs will become available. Although second-line surgery is not generally advocated, every experienced gynecologic oncologist has a group of patients who have responded well to a second surgical attack on local or regional recurrent disease that initially had not responded to chemotherapy. This is especially relevant to the patient who has what appears to be localized persistent disease at the time of second-look operation or after a prolonged disease-free interval.

Platinum sensitivity, which is defined by a sustained response to first-line platinum-based therapy, predicts the response to subsequent retreatment with a platinum-containing regimen frequently used for second-line therapy. In general, patients who progress during treatment or have stable disease in response to initial platinum-based therapy or who relapse within 6 months of this therapy are considered to have platinum-refractory disease. Patients who respond and have a progression-free interval of >6 months off treatment are defined as platinum sensitive. The response rates to second-line therapy are strikingly different in these two groups of patients. Blackledge and associates, in an analysis of 92 patients receiving five different second-line regimens, found that the interval off platinum-based therapy was a strong predictor of response. This observation held for both platinum-based and non-platinum-based second-line regimens. A response rate of <10% was observed for patients with a treatment-free interval of <6 months with the observed response rate rising as the treatment-free interval lengthened, up to 90% for those with an interval >21 months (Table 11–27).

Seltzer and coworkers reported a 72% response rate, including a 36% complete response rate, to second-line therapy with cisplatin in 11 patients who had achieved complete response to platinum-based, first-line chemotherapy. Markman and coworkers reported a 77% response rate to cisplatin in patients who had received no treatment for

Table 11–27 RESPONSE RATE VERSUS INTERVAL FROM PREVIOUS TREATMENT WITH PLATINUM-BASED REGIMEN

Interval (mo)	Total no.	Responding no.	Responding (%)
< 3	39	4	10
4–6	11	1	9
7–9	11	4	36
10–12	6	1	17
13–15	4	2	50
16–18	4	3	75
19–21	1	1	100
> 21	16	15	94

From Blackledge G et al: Response of patients in phase II studies of chemotherapy in ovarian cancer: Implications for patient treatment and the design of phase II trials. Br J Cancer 59:650, 1989.

>24 months, compared with 27% in women whose treatment-free interval remained 5–12 months. Similarly, Eisenhauer and associates reported a 43% response rate to carboplatin in patients whose treatment-free interval was >2 months compared with 10% in those whose treatment-free interval was ≤2 months. These findings make it mandatory that we define the populations of patients in clinical trials of second-line therapy. Phase II trials should include multiple adequately sized cohorts, such as patients with platinum-sensitive disease and those with platinum-refractory disease. In addition, patients should probably be stratified by the length of their treatment-free interval. In general, in phase II trials, response rates of more than 25–30% are expected for active agents being tested in the platinum sensitive population, and response rates of greater than 10–15% are considered promising in the platinum-resistant population.

Carboplatin as second-line therapy in epithelial ovarian cancer has resulted in 14–38% response rates, with one quarter to one half of the patients having complete response. Response rates increased progressively from between 6% and 13% in patients refractory to *cis*-diamminedichloroplatinum (CDDP, cisplatin) and alkylator therapy to 31% in prior CDDP responders and 45% in previously untreated patients (radiation failure). Patients whose disease progresses while they are receiving CDDP will not respond to carboplatin.

Standard dose paclitaxel has been shown to produce response rates of 22–23% in patients with platinum-resistant disease. Kohn and associates evaluated higher doses of paclitaxel, which required hematologic support, and observed a 48% response rate in platinum-refractory patients. As with other agents, these responses were generally of short duration. Nonetheless, paclitaxel should figure prominently in the consideration of second-line therapy for patients who have platinum-resistant disease. The importance of dose intensity in this setting is being explored in randomized studies throughout the world. The results will have important implications for paclitaxel dose in combination regimens, which are being evaluated both as first-line therapy and as second-line therapy.

The three chemotherapeutic agents receiving the most interest in evaluating their role in the treatment of recurrent ovarian cancer in the past 10 years have been gemcitabine, pegylated liposomal doxorubicin, and topotecan. Having demonstrated activity in the recurrent setting, these drugs have also been incorporated into frontline clinical trials.

The GOG reported a positive phase II trial with a 5-day topotecan (1.5mg/m^2) regimen (q. 21 days), demonstrating a 33% response rate and median response duration of 11.2 months. Fatigue, anemia and thrombocytopenia were the prominent toxicities. Most clinicians now use a weekly regimen of topotecan, administering 3.5–4 mg/m^2 on days 1, 8 and 15 on a 28-day cycle.

Gordon and coinvestigators reported a phase III trial in patients with refractory ovarian cancer comparing pegylated liposomal doxorubicin (Doxil), 50 mg/m^2 q. 28 d. to topotecan, 1.5 mg/m^2 per day for 5 days q. 21 days. In the platinum-refractory patient group, there was no survival difference. In the platinum-sensitive group, there was a 30% decrease in the risk of death for the pegylated liposomal doxorubicin-treated patients (median survival 108 weeks versus 70 weeks).

While gemcitabine has demonstrated modest activity as a single agent in the refractory setting, in combination with a platinum, most commonly cisplatin, the activity appears substantial. Nagourney and colleagues reported results of treatment with cisplatin (30 mg/m^2) plus gemcitabine (600–750 mg/m^2) on days 1 and 8 in a 21-day cycle. They reported 26% complete responses and 44% partial responses (70% overall response rate) with a median time to progression, for responders, of 7.9 months (range 2.1 to 13.2 months). Neutropenia, anemia, thrombocytopenia, nausea and vomiting, and peripheral neuropathy were problematic toxicities. Additional studies suggest that gemcitabine may reverse cisplatin resistance.

A current issue of debate is whether refractory ovarian cancer is better managed by sequential single agent therapy or combination chemotherapy. Two European reports suggest combination therapy is superior. One trial (ICON4/AGO-OVAR 2.2) reported over 800 patients. The patient population was "very platinum-sensitive" with over 75% of the patients having more than a 12-month platinum-free interval. After a median follow-up of 42 months, analysis showed the combination had a two-year survival of 57% versus 50% for the platinum-only treated patients, and the median survival difference was 29 months versus 24 months. This study has been the subject of some criticisms. The study was an analysis of multiple parallel trials conducted by difference groups involving five countries and 119 hospitals. The platinum agent was either cisplatin or carboplatin. The treatments were given monthly. A number of the patients had not previously received a taxane, and there was no difference in outcome if the patient previously received a taxane in their primary therapy. Thus, considering most patients receive a taxane and carboplatin for primary therapy in the USA, the application of this experience to our USA population is questioned. Other smaller studies, including a Spanish study (GEICO), also suggested the observation that combination therapy in the refractory setting may offer better outcomes. However, in general, in patients with disease-free intervals of over 12 months, the tendency is to retreat with taxane plus platinum combinations.

Another strategy is to extend the platinum-free interval by treating recurrent disease with non-platinum agents, commonly pegylated liposomal doxorubicin and topotecan. Retreatment with platinum, often in combination with gemcitabine, and retreatment with a taxane, recently in combination with a molecular targeting agent, are currently popular approaches.

Various other agents, such as hexamethylmelamine, 5-fluorouracil, etoposide, and others will rarely induce modest short duration responses.

Intraperitoneal therapy (discussed elsewhere in this chapter) has been employed with use of several antineoplastic agents as second-line therapy in ovarian cancer. Activity is essentially limited to patients with small-volume residual disease (≤ 0.5 cm in maximal diameter) when the second-line therapy program is initiated. In the absence of a randomized phase III trial, the ultimate impact of these surgically documented responses on survival is difficult to evaluate, although long-term disease-free survival (> 4 years) has been reported after intraperitoneal therapy in the rare patient with small volume refractory disease.

There is limited evidence of sustained benefit from second-line therapy in patients with ovarian cancer. Overall, only modest response rates with short durations of response have been reported. In addition, there has been a lack of consistency in these studies with regard to key definitions, such as platinum sensitivity vs platinum resistance. Future second-line trials should clearly define their patients in these two categories. It may also be necessary to discuss paclitaxel-sensitive vs paclitaxel-resistant lesions in the future. Platinum-sensitive patients are appropriate for pilot studies of platinum combinations incorporating different cytotoxic mechanisms of action and dose schedule investigations. Patients with platinum resistance are good candidates for novel investigational approaches and studies of drug resistance. Radiation to the abdomen and pelvis has been employed in select second-line situations. Whole-abdomen irradiation with a pelvic boost has been given in patients with minimal disease at second-look surgical reassessment for ovarian carcinoma. With limited follow-up, as many as 30% of such patients have remained in remission, according to some reports. However, our experience is that with longer follow-up periods, >90% of patients will have recurrence, even in this optimal group. There appears to be overlap in the resistance of cells to chemotherapy and radiotherapy. Furthermore, these patients are also at risk to develop bowel obstructions in the face of multiple prior surgeries and radiation.

Malignant effusions

The cause of malignant effusions is not known. The most common explanations are an irritant effect of the tumor on normal serous membranes, lymphatic obstruction, and venous obstruction. Graham and colleagues studied ascites circulating in patients with peritoneal carcinomatosis. They noted a large increase in the production of fluid by non-cancer-bearing peritoneal surfaces that was most marked from the omentum and small bowel surfaces. They also noted a significant elevation of portal pressure in the presence of ovarian cancer with ascites, compared with portal pressure in women without disease and in patients with ovarian cancer without ascites. Clinically troublesome ascites is rare in the absence of diffuse disease on the peritoneal surfaces underlying the right diaphragm, suggesting that large ascitic pools result from severe derangement of this absorptive surface as fluid produced in the peritoneal cavity migrates into lymphatic capillaries in its path to the thoracic duct.

Some concepts regarding the fluid kinetics of the peritoneal cavity have been relatively well substantiated. It is known that lymph vessels can carry molecules away from the tissues. The molecules can be protein, particulates, or cells. Some water also flows through the lymph vessels of tissues; it is a vehicle or solvent for the transported molecules. Removing water in bulk from tissues is a function of the blood capillaries, not of the lymphatics. Filtration and diffusion appear to be the two main processes in the exchange of substances between the blood and tissues. As blood pressure forces fluid from capillaries, the osmotic pressure of the plasma protein sucks the fluid back into the capillaries. The tissue tension tends to inhibit the exodus of fluid and to promote its re-entry into capillaries. This small amount of fluid retained in tissues exits through lymphatics.

Although diffusion accounts for the exchange of molecules across a semipermeable membrane, independent of the movement of fluid, the semipermeability restricts the process. In general, large molecules diffuse more slowly than smaller ones. This process may depend on pores in the capillaries. Large tissue molecules that cannot transgress the capillary pores can still be carried away in lymphatics. When a condition results in accumulation of large particles in the fluid outside capillaries, the osmotic pressure rises to counteract the effect of plasma proteins inside the capillaries, thus increasing filtration and hindering reabsorption. The imbalance reverses only when the tissue tension becomes high enough to counteract the filtering pressure of the capillaries. Oxygen and nutrients are diffused throughout the period of imbalance. When diffusion cannot occur, necrosis begins. In the peritoneal cavity, lymph can accumulate without diffusing and still maintain tissue viability. The constant mixing of ascitic fluid caused by the diaphragmatic contractions and intestinal peristalsis facilitates diffusion. This perhaps accounts for the continued viability of malignant cells in tissue cultures taken from ascitic fluid associated with malignant neoplasms. In neoplasia, the absorbing lymphatics may be blocked by cells or by the byproducts of cancer cells, such as large-molecular-weight mucopolysaccharides. The net effect reduces the absorption of lymph from the peritoneal cavity, resulting in accumulation of lymph fluid (ascites) in the peritoneal cavity. Normal peritoneal lymphatics can also be blocked by fluid that is too tenacious to permit absorption, predisposing to mucinous ascites of pseudomyxoma peritonei.

Malignant effusions are much more effectively managed now than they were several decades ago. Chemotherapeutic regimens control 90% of these troublesome situations. The patient who has a distended abdomen, and probable ascites, often presents for diagnosis. There is a tendency to do paracentesis for diagnostic purposes in such situations. We recommend *not* doing paracentesis in patients in whom an ovarian malignant neoplasm is highly suspected for the following reasons:

- The result of cytologic examination of fluid may be negative in the presence of malignant disease, and laparotomy is still indicated.
- Even when the result of cytologic examination of the fluid is positive, it seldom provides a definitive clue to the origin of the primary tumor, and laparotomy is indicated.
- If the patient has a large fluid-filled cyst rather than ascites, rupture of the cyst and seeding into the peritoneal cavity may occur, often long before laparotomy.
- Paracentesis may be associated with complications other than seeding, such as rupture of an intra-abdominal viscus, bleeding, infection, and depletion of electrolytes and proteins. We therefore recommend that these patients be examined short of paracentesis and that the disease be defined at laparotomy, when the situation can be controlled with more ease.

Our comments are intended to discourage paracentesis as a diagnostic tool, but in instances in which intra-abdominal pressure causes respiratory embarrassment or severe pain, the procedure should be performed as palliative therapy. Improved gastrointestinal function and relief of nausea and vomiting, as well as of constipation, may be noted after therapeutic paracentesis. Unfortunately, there are some patients whose ascites cannot be completely controlled by systemic chemotherapy, and they can often be kept comfortable by periodic paracentesis. This can be done on an outpatient basis at intervals determined by the patient's symptoms. The site of paracentesis is usually at the lateral border of the rectus muscle and at the level of the umbilicus. The site may be selected by ultrasound scanning to locate the largest pockets of fluid. The midline is avoided because tumor or adhesions are often present and complications can result. It is advisable to infiltrate the abdominal wall with a small amount of local anesthetic and then, using the same syringe and needle, to explore for a clear spot in the peritoneal cavity. A multiperforated catheter or trocar can then be inserted over the exact area of exploration. In this way, one can avoid the complication of inserting a trocar into an adherent segment of bowel. Measurements of weight and abdominal girth are recorded before and after paracentesis, and the volume of fluid is also noted. Fluid will sometimes continue to leak out of the trocar site, and attaching a urostomy bag to the area will provide some comfort for the patient. Because of this leakage from trocar sites, many physicians prefer to use a 16-gauge needle attached to the type of tubing that is used for blood donors. A needle attached to the other end of the tubing is inserted into a vacuum bottle, and the fluid is aspirated under negative pressure, eliminating the need for a large puncture site. Irradiation techniques are usually not recommended in the management of ascites.

Pleural effusion is another problem in the management of ovarian cancer. Approximately one-third of the patients with ascites will have pleural effusions. They usually respond to systemic chemotherapy. Pleural effusion in the absence of ascites usually indicates involvement of the pleura with disease. The same techniques outlined for the management of ascites can be used. Refractory reaccumulation can sometimes be managed with chest tube drainage followed by pleurodesis. Obliteration of the pleural cavity prevents the accumulation of fluid in that space. Instillation of bleomycin (60–120 mg) or talc into the pleural cavity after chest tube drainage offers the highest probability of successful palliation. A technique of pleurodesis using talc slurry reports an 81% success rate. The slurry was instilled through a chest tube at the bedside. A febrile episode frequently followed, but respiratory difficulties were rare.

Thoracentesis technique

The site of thoracentesis is selected by chest radiography, fluoroscopy, sonography, CT scan, or physical examination. When there is a large effusion of total hydrothorax, the best site of aspiration is usually the seventh or eighth interspace in the posterior axillary line. The most frequent error performed is to decide on an interspace that is too low. The physician should be aware that there is an elevation of the diaphragm and a loss of lung volume with pneumonia or trauma, and appropriately higher interspace levels should be selected. The patient is placed in a comfortable sitting position, leaning slightly forward on a padded stand or supported by an attendant. Premedication with narcotic or diazepam is often prudent. The skin of the chest wall is prepared with an antiseptic technique and then draped.

The chest wall is anesthetized with 5–10 mL of 1% lidocaine (Xylocaine), using a 22-gauge needle. Care should be taken to be sure that the skin, rib, rib periosteum, and parietal pleura are thoroughly infiltrated. Thoracentesis is virtually painless if the patient is properly anesthetized with lidocaine. A short-bevel needle (7–10 cm long, 18–30 gauge) is attached by way of a three-way stopcock to a 20–50 mL syringe. Other clinicians prefer to use a needle through which is passed a soft plastic catheter. With firm but steady pressure, the needle is passed into the pleural

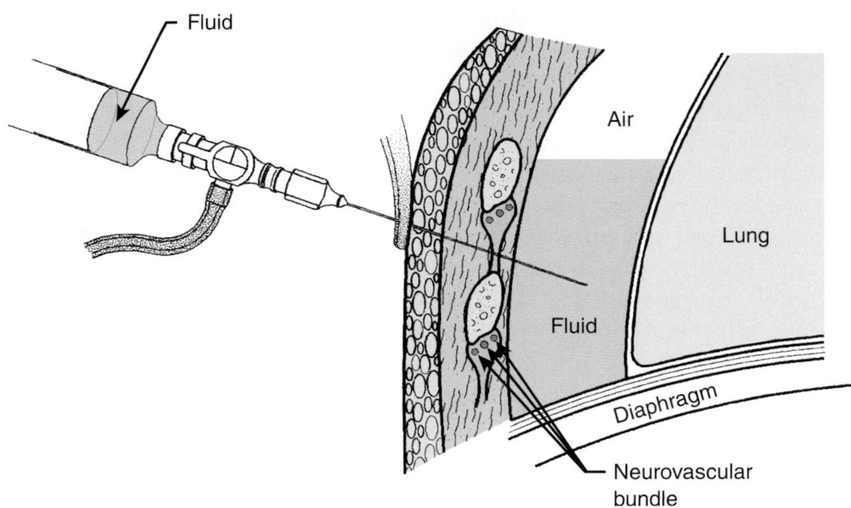

Figure 11–27 Thoracentesis.

space. In an effort to avoid injury to the intercostal nerve and vessels, the needle should be passed through the chest wall at the lower margin of the intercostal space (Fig. 11–27). A clamp may be placed on the needle to steady it on the chest wall. Care should be taken throughout the procedure to prevent air from entering the chest.

The amount of fluid removed at one setting often approaches 2000–3000 mL. If the aspiration is done slowly, the lung will accommodate to the evacuation. Where the pleural effusion has resulted from malignant implants on the pleura, the lung tissue becomes much less pliable, and a thoracostomy tube may be necessary. A small incision is made in the skin surrounding the needle entry site and a trocar is passed percutaneously into the pleural space. This technique can often be accomplished with a small tube (No. 12–14). At times, the tube must be inserted by use of a hemostat after an incision of the skin has been made with a scalpel at a previously determined site of thoracentesis. The tube, which has been clamped during insertion, should then be immediately connected to water-sealed drainage after it is secured to the chest wall with suture. These thoracostomy tubes are often left in place several days and removed 24 hours after attempts at pleurodesis. The techniques of pleurodesis are described earlier.

The surgical approach to recurrent malignant effusions has been somewhat limited. Peritoneovenous shunts for palliation of malignant ascites refractory to conventional medical management have been employed since the development of the pressure-sensitive peritoneovenous valve first reported by LeVeen and colleagues. Qazi and Savlov reported achieving palliation in 70% (28 of 40) of their patients.

For pleural effusion, decortication of the lung and pleurectomy has been used with varying results. Instillation of chemotherapeutic agents and similar caustic compounds has essentially replaced these procedures. Other agents, including hypertonic glucose and talc, have been used to create pleuritis. Again, they have variable success rates, depending on the investigator.

CURRENT AREAS OF RESEARCH

Most of the advances that have been made in the treatment of cancers of the ovary in the last 20 years have resulted from the multimodality approach proven effective in phase III trials. A combination of modalities used in a logical and flexible manner can achieve notable success on an individual basis. It is hoped that this approach, combined with improved chemotherapeutic agents, better understanding of drug resistance, and the possible addition of biologic response modifiers as a new modality, will result in improved outcome for this devastating group of malignant neoplasms (Table 11–28).

Chemotherapy has proved curative in some types of advanced cancers and is useful as an adjunct to surgery and radiotherapy in many others. That 90% of the cures with chemotherapy occur in 10% of the tumors that afflict humans is a perplexing biologic problem that appears to be related to the greater propensity of some tissue to develop specific and permanent resistance to chemotherapy of a broad nature. A discussion of tumor cell resistance is

Table 11–28 CLINICAL TRIALS: PHASES AND GOALS

Phase I
To determine the maximally tolerated dose of drug
To determine the schedule for administration
To define toxic effect to normal tissue
To generate data about the clinical pharmacology of the agent
Phase II
To identify antitumor activity in a spectrum of common metastatic tumors
To explore ability to achieve increased rates or response with changes of dose or schedule
To extend phase I data on toxicity
Phase III
To compare the investigational therapy against an established form of treatment in previously untreated patients

beyond the scope of this section. However, a few general comments can be made. The capacity to develop drug resistance is in fact an inherent and important property of malignant cell populations. It is basically not expressed by normal cell populations. It is an inherent property of malignant cells, similar to the capacity to metastasize and to invade. There appear to be two types of clinical problems. The first occurs when the malignant neoplasm is clearly sensitive at the beginning to at least some chemotherapeutic agents. There is a regression of the disease, but then the tumor recurs with treatment that was initially effective. The situation is most easily explained by the selection phenomenon, whereby killing off the population of sensitive cells leaves behind a small core of resistant cells that then proliferate. The second problem is so-called intrinsic resistance, that is, tumors appear to be resistant de novo to the application of therapy, or at least to show a high level of resistance to a broad range of chemotherapeutic agents.

Although much has been learned about ovarian cancer and treatment modalities, the surface has just been scratched. With the explosion of new techniques to explore the genetic and molecular biology of this disease, many avenues for research are opened and need exploration.

Genetic basis. The role of BRCA1 and BRCA2 has already been addressed in this chapter. Oncogenes such as K-ras are mutated in many ovarian cancers, as is the TP53 gene; erb-b2 is activated in about one-third of ovarian cancers. Technologies such as tumor loss of heterozygosity, molecular cytogenetic studies, and polymerase chain reaction-based differential expression studies have been used to identify additional genetic changes in sporadic ovarian cancers. Programmed cell senescence, probably related to reductions in telomere length, may be an important factor that may aid in our ability to increase survival.

Molecular biology. Much has been learned about the molecular biology of ovarian cancer. It is a clonal disease associated with activation of receptor tyrosine kinases, cytoplasmic kinases, and monomeric G proteins. How tumor suppressor genes may affect cell signaling is unknown at present. Invasiveness and adhesion reactions appear to be important. Paracrine interaction is obviously a factor. The role of transforming growth factor-β in progression of ovarian cancer is being studied. Epithelial-stromal interaction and activin and inhibin may be involved in the pathogenesis. The establishment of the GOG tumor and serum bank will continue to allow further investigation into these and many other aspects of molecular biology.

Experimental therapies. Gene therapy is at least theoretically attractive. If the defect is identified, the gene could be replaced. This strategy is in its infancy. Many types of gene therapy are possible: immunogene, antioncogene, and tumor suppressor gene; antigrowth factor and cytokine gene drug resistance; and genes that are associated with apoptosis. All of these may be attractive, and preliminary studies have been started. Another area receiving considerable attention is antiangiogenesis therapy.

New agents. Because chemotherapy resistance is a major problem, new agents that have non-cross-resistance properties and novel approaches to modulations or targeting are sought. Many new drugs are in the pipeline to be evaluated in phase II studies. It is to be hoped that a new platin drug is around the corner.

Quality of life. This area is receiving much deserved interest in patients with all types of cancer, including ovarian cancer. Reliable and valid tools for measuring quality of life have been developed. The GOG and others are now incorporating this item into many of their protocols. Cancer symptoms, therapy toxicity, and psychological stress need to be addressed. Pain management, sexual function, family support, and ability to deal with new genetic information are only a few items that historically have not been dealt with adequately. This area is a challenge that needs and is receiving attention.

REHABILITATION

The nature of ovarian cancer is such that the major vital organs (lungs, heart, liver, and kidneys) remain unaffected. The disease itself and its therapy appear primarily to attack the gastrointestinal tract. Indeed, the terminal event for most patients who succumb to this disease is electrolyte imbalance caused by prolonged gastrointestinal obstruction, malnutrition, and significant protein and electrolyte loss from repeated paracentesis and thoracentesis. It is necessary to support these patients with various forms of alimentation during therapy to sustain them sufficiently to tolerate the somewhat vigorous therapy often prescribed. The placement of semipermanent Silastic intravenous catheters (e.g., Hickman, Broviac, or Groshong) greatly facilitates the ability to support these patients (Fig. 11–28). Some clinicians prefer to gain intravenous access by means of a device (Port-o-cath) implanted in the subcutaneous tissue. Many centers can arrange intravenous alimentation at home for patients who are unable to take sufficient nourishment by mouth. Home pharmacy services are available in many areas, and intravenous medications, including analgesics, can be administered at home by pump infusion devices through these semipermanent intravenous catheters.

Intermittent episodes of partial small and large bowel obstruction are common, and they must be initially treated conservatively and ultimately surgically if the patient is to continue to fight. The issue of whether a patient with a high-grade small bowel obstruction from ovarian cancer carcinomatosis should undergo exploration for a possible bypass procedure to re-establish the continuity of the alimentary tract has long been debated. Management of these patients is extremely difficult because of the intactness of their vital organs and their alert mental status. Although most patients will not survive 6 months from the time of the bowel obstruction, surgical intervention should be considered because of the difficulty that all people have observing the slow process of death by starvation. Any procedure that can result in the patient's

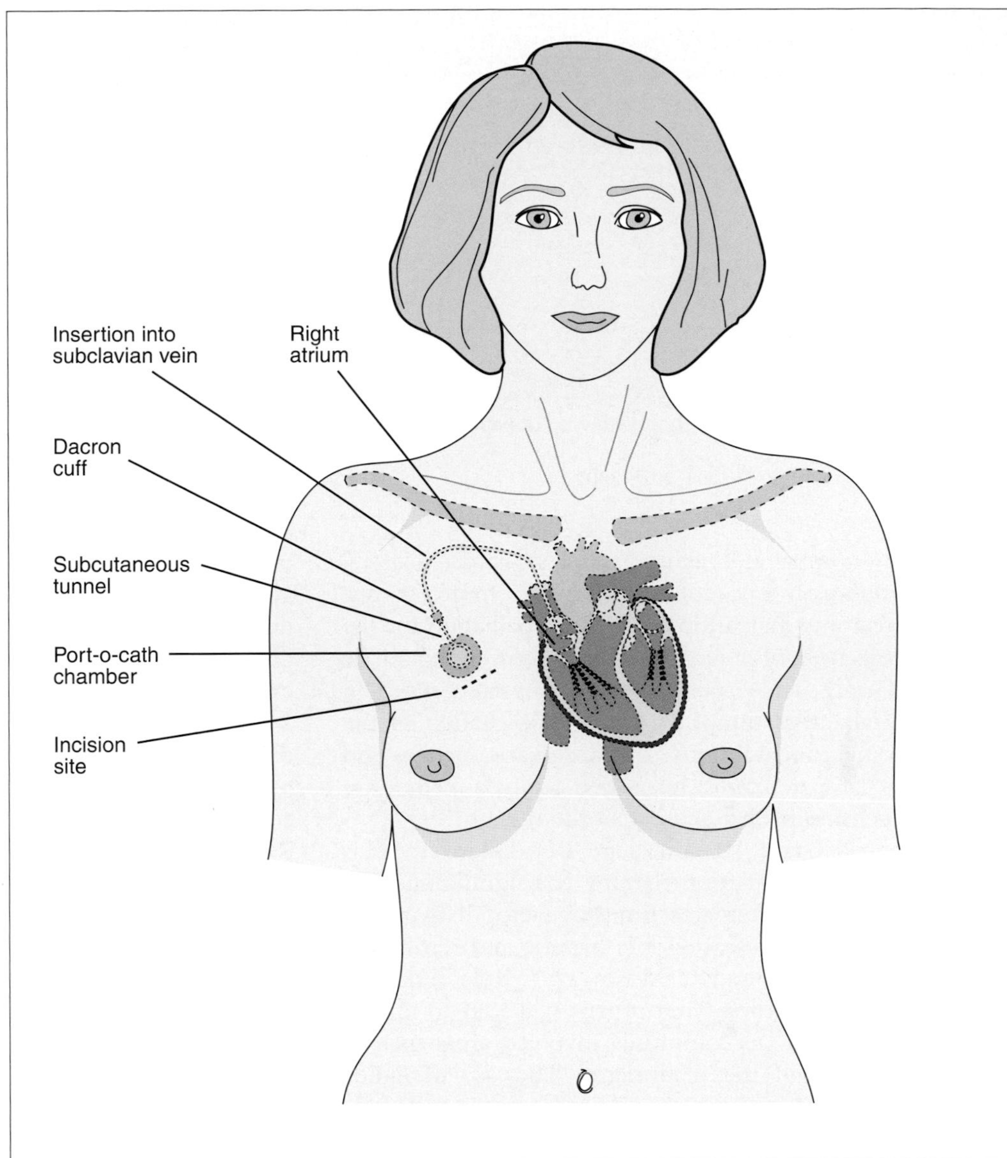

Figure 11–28 Silicone rubber catheter tunneled subcutaneously and positioned in right atrium.

returning to her home and family seems to be worthy of consideration even in these desperate cases. If nothing else, the performance of a gastrostomy to avoid uncomfortable nasogastric intubation or the persistent agony of constant vomiting is in itself humane and allows more easy return of the patient to a home setting, where the gastrostomy can be used to decompress the gastrointestinal tract as needed.

In general, the most discouraging aspect in the management of patients with ovarian cancer is the apathy of many physicians. In truth, these diseases are discouraging, but a determined attitude is medically sound and reassuring to the patient. Significant numbers of patients referred to oncologic centers as "unresectable" not only have had their tumor debulked but have responded nicely to postoperative therapy. Still other patients have survived complicated combinations of multiple surgical and adjuvant therapies. A positive approach to the disease, which restores hope in the patient with this devastating illness, is justified on that basis alone.

CONCLUSIONS ON MANAGEMENT

Although adenocarcinoma of the ovary remains one of the solid tumors most sensitive to chemotherapeutic regimens, the mortality from this disease remains high. Progress over the past 30 years has been modest and, while there has been some improvement in survival, there is significant opportunity to do better (Table 11–29). There appears, however, to be great promise with newer developments in the management of this disease. The following general principles should be kept in mind.

An optimal surgical procedure should be carried out whenever possible. This is defined as the removal of all bulk tumor with the intent to leave no gross or minimal residua (no individual mass >1–2 cm in diameter). It is not possible to advocate any one operation for all patients, and the clinician must make a judgment at the time of surgery. Unquestionably, patients with small residual tumor volumes have a better prognosis with any postoperative therapy.

Table 11–29 RELATIVE SURVIVAL PERCENTAGE* DURING THREE TIME PERIODS

	Periods, by cancer site		
Site	1974–76	1983–85	1995–2000
All sites	50	53	64
Breast	75	78	88
Colon	50	58	63
Lung & bronchus	13	14	15
Ovary	37	41	44
Prostate	67	75	99
Rectum	49	55	64

*5-year relative survival rates based on follow-up of patients through 2001.
Source: SEER Program, 1975–2001, NCI, 2004.

Even when optimal debulking is not possible, bilateral salpingo-oophorectomy, total abdominal hysterectomy, and omentectomy may afford significant palliation for the patient. Resection of a portion of the bowel should be considered only when such a resection would result in removal of all gross tumor. A careful exploration of the entire abdomen, including the diaphragmatic surfaces and retroperitoneal spaces, must be carried out by a methodical surgeon to ensure proper staging of the disease.

In advanced (stage III and stage IV) disease, there is little evidence that radiation therapy has significant value over chemotherapy. A major limiting factor with radiotherapy in advanced disease is the hepatic and renal toxicity that follows adequate doses of whole-abdomen radiation. Shielding these vital organs will lead to undertreatment, especially in commonly involved areas such as the undersurface of the diaphragm. The use of radiotherapy appears at present to be limited.

A large number of reports in the literature confirm that chemotherapy with alkylating agents can produce responses in 30–60% of patients with advanced disease. Experience with other solid tumors strongly suggests that an improved complete response rate with any particular chemotherapeutic regimen correlates well with eventual improved survival rate. Several non-alkylating agents have been identified with considerable activity in ovarian cancer, such as hexamethylmelamine, doxorubicin, cisplatin, carboplatin, and paclitaxel. Several reports have confirmed significant improvement in complete response and negative second-look laparotomy rates when a combination of drugs containing two or more of these active agents was used. It is hoped that as in other solid tumors, these reports of improved complete response rates will eventuate in later reports of improved overall survival rates.

Prognosis depends very much on stage, but other factors are also pertinent. Undifferentiated lesions have a worse prognosis regardless of stage. Patients with bulk residual disease after laparotomy are much less likely to respond to subsequent therapy.

Chemotherapy appears to be the most effective method of controlling ascites and pleural effusions. First-line chemotherapy will be effective for varying periods in 90% of patients.

Intraperitoneal chemotherapy as first-line postoperative therapy appears to be effective in patients with minimal (<1 cm) residual. Logistics of intraperitoneal therapy remain a disadvantage. There does seem to be a place for this treatment in the selected group of patients with persistent but minimal disease after the second-look laparotomy.

There appears to be a reasonable explanation of the paradox of the invariable inverse relationship between cell number and curability with drugs on the one hand and the difficulty of achieving better results in treating micrometastasis on the other. The explanation resides in the hypothesis put forth by Goldie and Coldman. They propose that as in bacteria, mutation toward resistance to drugs is an inherent property of the unstable cancer cell, and resistance occurs often by virtue of change in the cell membrane. As proposed, this tendency to mutate occurs at low cell numbers, well below the level of clinical detectability, and increases dramatically with small increases in tumor mass. Depending on the mutation rate, a tumor can go from sensitive to resistant in six doublings or a 2-log increase in cell number. The use of multiple effective drugs covers more cell lines resistant to one drug. This hypothesis is the best explanation for the effectiveness of combination chemotherapy in most human neoplasms. It is hoped this will apply also to epithelial ovarian cancer.

BIBLIOGRAPHY

INCIDENCE, EPIDEMIOLOGY, AND ETIOLOGY

Ahmed FY, Wiltshaw RP, A'Hern B et al: Natural history and prognosis of untreated stage I epithelial ovarian carcinoma. J Clin Oncol 14:2968, 1996.

Amos CI, Struewing JP: Genetic epidemiology of epithelial ovarian cancer. Cancer 71:566, 1993.

Amos CI et al: Age at onset for familial epithelial ovarian cancer. JAMA 268:1896, 1992.

Buller RE et al: Familial ovarian cancer. Gynecol Oncol 51:160, 1993.

Burke W, Daly M, Garber J et al: Recommendations for follow up care of individuals with an inherited predisposition to cancer. JAMA 277:997, 1997.

Casagrande JT et al: "Incessant ovulation" and ovarian cancer. Lancet 2:170, 1979.

Chen KTK, Schooley JL, Flam MS: Peritoneal carcinomatosis after prophylactic oophorectomy in familial ovarian cancer syndrome. Obstet Gynecol 66:935, 1985.

Claus EB, Schildkraut JM, Thompson WD et al: The genetic attributable risk of breast and ovarian cancer. Cancer 77:2318, 1996.

Franceschi S, LaVecchia C, Negri E et al: Fertility drugs and risk of epithelial ovary cancer in Italy. Hum Reprod 9:1673, 1994.

Frank TS, Manley SA, Olopade OI et al: Sequence analysis of BRCA1 and BRCA2: Correlation of mutations with family history and ovarian cancer risk. J Clin Oncol 16:2417, 1998.

Genadry R et al: Primary, papillary peritoneal neoplasia. Obstet Gynecol 58:730, 1981.

Gross TP, Schlesselman JJ: The estimated effect of oral contraceptive use on the cumulative risk of epithelial ovarian cancer. Obstet Gynecol 83:419, 1994.

Hankinson SE et al: A quantitative assessment of oral contraceptive use and risk of ovarian cancer. Obstet Gynecol 80:708, 1992.

Harlow BL et al: Perineal exposure to talc and ovarian cancer risk. Obstet Gynecol 80:19, 1992.
Heintz APM, Hacker NF, Lagasse LD: Epidemiology and etiology of ovarian cancer: A review. Obstet Gynecol 66:127, 1985.
Henderson BE, Ross RK, Pike MC: Hormonal chemoprevention of cancer in women. Science 259:633, 1993.
Jacobs I, Oram D: Prevention of ovarian cancer: A survey of the practice of prophylactic oophorectomy by fellows and members of the Royal College of Obstetricians and Gynaecologists. Br J Obstet Gynaecol 96:510, 1989.
Kerlikowske K, Brown JS, Grady DG: Should women with familial ovarian cancer undergo prophylactic oophorectomy? Obstet Gynecol 80:700, 1992.
Koch M, Gaedke H, Jenkins H: Family history of ovarian cancer patients: A case-control study. Int J Epidemiol 18:782, 1989.
Lynch HT, Severin MJ, Mooney MJ et al: Insurance adjudication favoring prophylactic surgery in hereditary breast-ovarian cancer syndrome. Gynecol Oncol 57:23, 1995.
Lynch HT, Watson P, Bewtra C et al: Hereditary ovarian cancer. Cancer 67:1460, 1991.
Lynch HT et al: Hereditary ovarian cancer: Heterogeneity in age at onset. Cancer 71:S74, 1993.
Mori M, Harabuchi I, Miyake H et al: Reproductive, genetic, and dietary risk factors for ovarian cancer. Am J Epidemiol 128:771, 1988.
Mosgaard BJ, Lidegaard O, Kjaer SK et al: Infertility, fertility, drugs, and invasive ovarian cancer: A case control study. Fertil Steril 67:1005, 1997.
Narod SA, Risch H, Moslehi R et al: Oral contraceptives and the risk of hereditary ovarian cancer. N Engl J Med 339:424, 1998.
Nguyen HN, Averette HE, Janieck M: Ovarian carcinoma. Cancer 74:545, 1994.
NIH Consensus Development Panel on Ovarian Cancer: Ovarian cancer: Screening, treatment, and follow up. JAMA 273:491, 1995.
Oriel KA, Hartenbach EM, Remington PL: Trends in U.S. ovarian cancer mortality, 1979–1995. Obstet Gynecol 93:30, 1999.
Pal T, Permuth-Wey J, Betts JA, et al: BRCA1 and BRCA2 mutations account for a large proportion of ovarian carcinoma cases. Cancer 104:2807, 2005.
Parazzini F, La Vecchia C, Negri E et al: Menstrual factor and the risk of epithelial ovarian cancer. J Clin Epidemiol 42:443, 1989.
Piver MS, Jishi MF, Tsukadu Y et al: Primary peritoneal carcinoma after prophylactic oophorectomy in women with a family history of ovarian cancer. Cancer 71:2651, 1993.
Piver MS et al: Familial ovarian cancer, a report of 558 families from the Gilda Radner familial ovarian cancer registry 1981–1991. Cancer 71:582, 1993.
Ries LAG, Eisner MP, Kosary CL, et al: SEER Cancer Statistics Review, 1975–2002, National Cancer Institute, Bethesda, MD, http://seer.cancer.gov/csr/1975_2002/, (accessed 7 August 2006) based on Nov. 2004 SEER data submission, posted to website in 2005.
Riggs JE: Rising ovarian cancer mortality in the elderly: A manifestation of differential survival. Gynecol Oncol 58:64, 1995.
Rodriguez C, Henley SJ, Calle EE et al: Paracetamol and risk of ovarian cancer mortality in a prospective study of women in the USA. Lancet 352:1354, 1998.
Rosenberg L et al: Epithelial ovarian cancer and combination oral contraceptives. JAMA 247:3210, 1982.
Rossing MA et al: Ovarian tumors in a cohort of infertile women. N Engl J Med 331:771, 1994.
Rubin SC, Benjamin I, Behbakht K et al: Clinical and pathologic features of ovarian cancer in women with germ line mutations of BRCA1. N Engl J Med 335:1413, 1996.
Schildkraut JM, Thompson WD: Familial ovarian cancer: A population-based case-control study. Am J Epidemiol 128:456, 1988.
Schrag D, Kuntz KM, Garber JE et al: Decision analysis-effects of prophylactic mastectomy and oophorectomy on life expectancy among women with BRCA1 or BRCA2 mutation. N Engl J Med 336:1465, 1997.
Stanford JL: Oral contraceptives and neoplasia of the ovary. Contraception 43:543, 1991.
Struewing JP, Hartge P, Wacholder S et al: The risk of cancer associated with specific metastasis of BRCA1 and BRCA2 among Ashkenazi Jews. N Engl J Med 336:1401, 1997.
Tobacman JK et al: Intra-abdominal carcinomatosis after prophylactic oophorectomy in ovarian cancer-prone families. Lancet 2:795, 1982.
Venn A, Watson L, Lumley J et al: Breast and ovarian cancer incidence after infertility and in vitro fertilization. Lancet 346:995, 1995.
Venter PF: Ovarian epithelial cancer and chemical carcinogenesis. Gynecol Oncol 12:281, 1981.
Whittemore AS: The risk of ovarian cancer after treatment for infertility. N Engl J Med 331:805, 1994.
Whittemore AS et al: Characteristics relating to ovarian cancer risk: Collaborative analysis of 12 US case control studies. Am J Epidemiol 136:1184, 1992.
Wong C, Hempling RE, Piver MS et al: Perineal talc exposure and subsequent epithelial ovarian cancer. Obstet Gynecol 93:372, 1999.
Yancik R, Ries LG, Yates JW: Ovarian cancer in the elderly: An analysis of Surveillance, Epidemiology, and End-results program data. Am J Obstet Gynecol 154:639, 1986.

SIGNS, SYMPTOMS, AND ATTEMPTS AT EARLY DETECTION

Alagoz T et al: What is a normal CA-125 level? Gynecol Oncol 53:93, 1994.
Bast RC et al: Coordinate elevation of serum markers in ovarian cancer but not in benign disease. Cancer 68:1758, 1991.
Bell R, Petticrew M, Sheldon T: The performance of screening tests for ovarian cancer: results of a systematic review. Br J Obstet Gynaecol 105:1136, 1998.
Bourne TH et al: Screening early familial ovarian cancer with transvaginal ultrasonography and color flow imaging. Br Med J 306:1025, 1993.
Bret PM et al: Transvaginal US-guided aspiration of ovarian cysts and solid pelvic masses. Radiology 185:377, 1992.
Burghardt E, Girardi F, LaHousen M et al: Patterns of pelvic and para-aortic lymph node involvement in ovarian cancer. Gynecol Oncol 40:103, 1991.
Carlson KJ, Skates SJ, Singer DE: Screening for ovarian cancer. Ann Intern Med 121:124, 1994.
Chung A, Birnbaum SJ: Ovarian cancer associated with pregnancy. Obstet Gynecol 41:211, 1973.
Cohen CJ, Jennings TS: Screening for ovarian cancer: The role of noninvasive imaging techniques. Am J Obstet Gynecol 170:1088, 1994.
Creasman WT, DiSaia PJ: Screening in ovarian cancer. Am J Obstet Gynecol 165:7, 1991.
Creasman WT, Abu-Ghazaleh S, Schmidt HJ: Retroperitoneal metastatic spread of ovarian cancer. Gynecol Oncol 6:447, 1978.
DePriest PD, Gallion HH, Pavlik EJ et al: Transvaginal sonography as a screening method for the detection of early ovarian cancer. Gynecol Oncol 65:408, 1997.
Droegemueller W: Screening for ovarian carcinoma: Hopeful and wishful thinking. Am J Obstet Gynecol 170:1095, 1994.
Einhorn N: Early diagnosis and screening. Ovarian Cancer 6:843, 1992.
Finkler NJ et al: Comparison of serum CA-125, clinical impression, and ultrasound in the preoperative evaluation of ovarian masses. Obstet Gynecol 72:659, 1988.
Goff BA, Mandel LS, Melancon CH et al: Frequency of symptoms of ovarian cancer in women presenting to primary care clinics. JAMA 291:2705, 2004.
Graham JB, Graham RM, Schueller EF: Pre-clinical detection of ovarian cancer. Cancer 17:1414, 1964.

Grover S et al: Screening for ovarian cancer using serum CA-125 and vaginal examination: Report on 2550 females. IGCS 5:291, 1995.

Higgins RV et al: Transvaginal sonography as a screening method for ovarian cancer. Gynecol Oncol 34:402, 1989.

Houlston R, Bourne TH, Davies A et al: Use of family history in a screening clinic for familial ovarian cancer. Gynecol Oncol 47:247, 1992.

Jacobs I et al: Prevalence screening for ovarian cancer in postmenopausal women by CA-125 measurement and ultrasonography. BMJ 306:1030, 1993.

Jacobs IJ, Skates S, Davies AP et al: Risk of diagnosis of ovarian cancer after raised serum CA125 concentration. BMJ 313:1355, 1996.

Jacobs IJ, Skates SJ, MacDonald N et al: Screening for ovarian cancer: A pilot randomized control trial. Lancet 353:1207, 1999.

Karlan BY et al: A multidisciplinary approach to early detection of ovarian cancer: Rationale, protocol design, and early results. Am J Obstet Gynecol 169:494, 1993.

Kerlikowske K, Brown JS, Grady DG: Should women with familial ovarian cancer undergo prophylactic oophorectomy? Obstet Gynecol 80:700, 1992.

Knapp RC, Friedman EA: Aortic lymph node metastases in early ovarian cancer. Am J Obstet Gynecol 119:1013, 1974.

Koch M, Gaedke H, Jenkins H: Family history of ovarian cancer patients: A case-control study. Int J Epidemiol 18:782, 1989.

Kurjak A et al: Transvaginal ultrasound, color flow, and Doppler wave form of the postmenopausal adnexal mass. Obstet Gynecol 80:917, 1992.

Layfield LJ, Heaps JM, Berek JS: Fine needle aspiration cytology accuracy with palpable gynecologic neoplasms. Gynecol Oncol 40:70, 1991.

Lifshitz S: Ascites pathophysiology and control measures. Int J Radiat Oncol Biol Phys 8:1423, 1982.

McGowan L: Ovarian cancer after hysterectomy. Obstet Gynecol 69:386, 1987.

Mills GB, Bast RC Jr., Srivastava S: Future for ovarian cancer screening: novel markers from emerging technologies of transcriptional profiling and proteomics. J Nat Cancer Inst 93:1437, 2001.

Ovarian cancer: Screening, treatment, and follow-up. NIH Consens Statement 12:1, 1994.

Posadas EM, Davidson B, Kohn EC: Proteomics and ovarian cancer: implications for diagnosis and treatment: a critical review of the recent literature. Curr Opin Oncol 16:478, 2004.

Purola E, Nieminen V: Does rupture of cystic carcinoma during operation influence the prognosis? Ann Chir Gynaecol Fenn 57:615, 1968.

Sampson JA: Endometrial carcinoma of ovary arising in endometrial tissue in that organ. Arch Surg 10:1, 1925.

Schildkraut JM, Thompson WD: Familial ovarian cancer: A population based case-control study. Am J Epidemiol 128:456, 1988.

Trimble EL et al: Diagnosing the correct ovarian cancer syndrome. Obstet Gynecol 78:1023, 1991.

Trimbos JB, Bolis B, Pecorelli S: The surgical staging of ovarian cancer: Current practice in 15 European countries. Int J Gynecol Cancer 1:89, 1991.

van Nagell JR et al: Ovarian cancer screening in asymptomatic postmenopausal women by transvaginal sonography. Cancer 68:458, 1991.

Young RC et al: Staging laparotomy in early ovarian cancer. Proc Am Assoc Cancer Res 20:399, 1979.

BORDERLINE MALIGNANT EPITHELIAL NEOPLASMS

Bell DA, Scully RE: Serous borderline tumors of the peritoneum. Am J Surg Pathol 14:230, 1990.

Bell DA, Longacre TA, Prat J et al: Serous borderline (low malignant potential, atypical proliferative) ovarian tumors: Workshop perspectives. Hum Pathol 35:934, 2004.

Berman J: Borderline Ovarian Tumor Workshop (Editorial), Bethesda, Maryland, August 27–28, 2005. Hum Path 35:907, 2004.

Carter J et al: Borderline and invasive epithelial ovarian tumors in young women. Obstet Gynecol 82:752, 1993.

Carter J et al: Pseudomyxoma peritonei: A review. Int J Gynecol Cancer 1:243, 1991.

Fort MG et al: Evidence for the efficacy of adjuvant therapy in epithelial ovarian tumors of low malignant potential. Gynecol Oncol 32:69, 1989.

Kaern J, Tropé CG, Abeler VM: A retrospective study of 370 borderline tumors of the ovary treated at the Norwegian Radium Hospital from 1970 to 1982. Cancer 71:1810, 1993.

Kurman RJ, Trimble CL: The behavior of serous tumors of low malignant potential: Are they ever malignant? Int J Gynecol Pathol 12:120, 1993.

Link CJ, Kohn E, Reed E: Review: The relationship between borderline ovarian tumors and epithelial ovarian carcinoma: Epidemiologic, pathologic, and molecular aspects. Gynecol Oncol 60:347, 1996.

Manchul LA et al: Borderline epithelial ovarian tumors: A review of 81 cases with an assessment of the impact of treatment. Int J Radiat Oncol Biol Phys 22:867, 1992.

Menzin AW et al: The accuracy of a frozen section diagnosis of borderline ovarian malignancy. Gynecol Oncol 59:183, 1995.

Nikrui N: Survey of clinical behavior of patients with borderline epithelial tumors of the ovary. Gynecol Oncol 12:107, 1981.

Ronnett BM, Kajdacsy-Balla A, Gilks CB et al: Mucinous borderline ovarian tumors: Points of general agreement and persistent controversies regarding nomenclature, diagnostic criteria, and behavior. Hum Pathol 35:949, 2004.

Seidman JD, Soslow RA, Vang R et al: Borderline ovarian tumors: Diverse contemporary viewpoints on terminology and diagnostic criteria with illustrative images. Hum Pathol 35:918, 2004.

Shanks HGI: Pseudomyxoma peritonei. J Obstet Gynaecol Br Commonw 68:212, 1961.

Sherman ME, Berman J, Birrer MJ et al: Current challenges and opportunities for research on borderline ovarian tumors. Hum Pathol 35:961, 2004.

Silverberg SG, Bell DA, Kurman RJ et al: Borderline ovarian tumors: Key points and Workshop summary. Hum Pathol 35:910, 2004.

Sutton GP et al: Stage III ovarian tumors of low malignant potential treated with cisplatin combination therapy (a Gynecologic Oncology Group study). Gynecol Oncol 41:230, 1991.

TREATMENT OF MALIGNANT EPITHELIAL NEOPLASMS

Altaras MM et al: Primary peritoneal papillary serous adenocarcinoma: Clinical and management aspects. Gynecol Oncol 40:230, 1991.

Aure JC, Hoeg K, Kolstad P: Clinical and histologic studies of ovarian carcinoma: Long-term follow-up of 990 cases. Obstet Gynecol 37:1, 1971.

Avril N, Sassen S, Schmalfeldt B et al: Prediction of response to neoadjuvant chemotherapy by sequential F-18-fluorodeoxy-glucose position emission tomography in patients with advanced-stage ovarian cancer. J Clin Oncol (In Press).

Bell JG, Young RC, Brady M et al: A randomized phase III trial of carboplatin (AUC 7.5) and paclitaxel (175mg/m^2 Q 21 days x three courses versus the same regimen x six courses) in patients with selected stage IC and II (A,B,C) and selected IA and IB ovarian cancer. Gyn Onc (In Press).

Benedry R et al: Primary, papillary peritoneal neoplasia. Obstet Gynecol 58:730, 1981.

Bertelsen K et al: A randomized study of cyclophosphamide and cisplatin with or without doxorubicin in advanced ovarian carcinoma. Gynecol Oncol 28:161, 1987.

Braly P, Doroshaw J, Hoff S: Technical aspects of intraperitoneal chemotherapy in abdominal carcinomatosis. Gynecol Oncol 25:319, 1986.

Bruckner HW et al: Improved chemotherapy for ovarian cancer with *cis*-diamminedichloroplatinum and adriamycin. Cancer 47:2288, 1981.

Bruckner HW et al: Modulation and intensification of a cyclophosphamide, hexamethylmelamine, doxorubicin, and cisplatin ovarian cancer regimen. Obstet Gynecol 73:349, 1989.

Conte PF et al: A randomized trial comparing cisplatin plus cyclophosphamide versus cisplatin, doxorubicin and cyclophosphamide in advanced ovarian cancer. J Clin Oncol 4:965, 1986.

Creasman WT et al: Chemoimmunotherapy in the management of primary stage III ovarian cancer: A Gynecologic Oncology Group study. Cancer Treat Rep 63:319, 1979.

Creasman WT et al: A randomized trial of cyclophosphamide, doxorubicin, and cisplatin with or without bacillus Calmette-Guérin in patients with suboptimal stage III and IV ovarian cancer: A Gynecologic Oncology Group study. Gynecol Oncol 39:239, 1990.

Crozier MA, Copeland LJ, Silva EG et al: Clear cell carcinoma of the ovary: A study of 59 cases. Gynecol Oncol 35:199, 1989.

Edelmann DZ et al: Carboplatin and etoposide as first line chemotherapy in advanced epithelial ovarian cancer. Int J Gynecol Oncol 5:443, 1995.

Ehrlich CE et al: Treatment of advanced epithelial ovarian cancer using cisplatin, Adriamycin, and Cytoxan-the Indiana University experience. Clin Obstet Gynecol 10:325, 1983.

Einhorn H, Williams SD: The role of *cis*-platinum in solid-tumor therapy. N Engl J Med 300:289, 1979.

Fromm G, Gershenson DM, Silva EG: Papillary serous carcinoma of the peritoneum. Obstet Gynecol 75:89, 1990.

Gaver RC et al: The disposition of carboplatin in ovarian cancer patients. Cancer Chemother Pharmacol 22:263, 1988.

Gershenson DM, Morris M, Burke TW et al: Combined cisplatin and carboplatin chemotherapy for treatment of advanced epithelial ovarian cancer. Gynecol Oncol 58:349, 1995.

Goff BA, Sainz de la Cuesta R, Muntz HG et al: Clear cell carcinoma of the ovary: A distinct histologic type with poor prognosis and resistance to platinum-based chemotherapy in stage III disease. Gynecol Oncol 60:412, 1996.

Greene MH et al: Acute non-lymphatic leukemia after therapy with alkylating agents for ovarian cancer: A study of five randomized clinical trials. N Engl J Med 307:1416, 1982.

Gruppo Interregionale Cooperativo Oncologico Ginecologia: Long-term results of a randomized trial comparing cisplatin with cisplatin and cyclophosphamide with cisplatin, cyclophosphamide and adriamycin in advanced ovarian cancer. Gynecol Oncol 45:115, 1992.

Hainsworth JD et al: The role of hexamethylmelamine in the combination chemotherapy of advanced ovarian cancer: A comparison of hexamethylmelamine, cyclophosphamide, doxorubicin, and cisplatin (H-CAP) versus cyclophosphamide, doxorubicin, and cisplatin (CAP). Am J Clin Oncol 13:410, 1990.

Hoskins WJ: The influence of cytoreductive surgery on progression-free interval and survival in epithelial ovarian cancer. Clin Obstet Gynecol 3:59, 1989.

Hreshchyshyn MM et al: The role of adjuvant therapy in stage I ovarian cancer. Am J Obstet Gynecol 138:139, 1980.

Izquierdo MA et al: Ovarian carcinoma preceded by cerebral metastasis: Review of the literature. Gynecol Oncol 45:206, 1992.

Jenison EL et al: Clear cell adenocarcinoma of the ovary: A clinical analysis and comparison with serous carcinoma. Gynecol Oncol 32:65, 1989.

Kaslow RA, Wisch N, Glass JL: Acute leukemia following cytotoxic chemotherapy. JAMA 219:75, 1972.

Kurman RJ, Craig JM: Endometrioid and clear cell carcinoma of the ovary. Cancer 29:1653, 1972.

Lele SB et al: Peritoneal papillary carcinoma. Gynecol Oncol 31:315, 1988.

Levin L, Hryniuk WM: Dose intensity analysis of chemotherapy regimens in ovarian carcinoma. J Clin Oncol 4:965, 1986.

Manetta A et al: Hexamethylmelamine as a single second-line agent in ovarian cancer. Gynecol Oncol 36:93, 1990.

Marchetti DL et al: Treatment of advanced ovarian carcinoma in the elderly. Gynecol Oncol 49:86, 1993.

McGuire WP, Hoskins WJ, Brady MF et al: Cyclophosphamide and cisplatin compared with paclitaxel and cisplatin in patients with stage III and IV ovarian cancer. N Engl J Med 334:1, 1996.

Mills SE, Andersen WA, Fechner RE, Austin MB: Serous surface papillary carcinoma: A clinicopathologic study of 10 cases and comparison with stage III–IV ovarian serous carcinoma. Am J Surg Pathol 12:827, 1988.

Munnell EW: Is conservative therapy ever justified in stage I (Ia) cancer of the ovary? Am J Obstet Gynecol 103:641, 1969.

Omura G et al: A randomized trial of cyclophosphamide and doxorubicin with or without cisplatin in advanced ovarian carcinoma. Cancer 57:1725, 1986.

Omura GA et al: Long-term follow-up and prognostic factor analysis in advanced ovarian carcinoma: The Gynecologic Oncology Group experience. J Clin Oncol 7:1138, 1991.

Omura GA et al: Randomized trial of cyclophosphamide plus cisplatin with or without doxorubicin in ovarian cancer: A Gynecologic Oncology Group study. J Clin Oncol 7:457, 1989.

Ovarian Cancer Meta-Analysis Project: Cyclophosphamide plus cisplatin versus cyclophosphamide, doxorubicin and cisplatin chemotherapy of ovarian carcinoma: A meta-analysis. J Clin Oncol 9:1668, 1991.

Ransom DT et al: Papillary serous carcinoma of the peritoneum: A review of 33 cases treated with platin-based chemotherapy. Cancer 66:1091, 1990.

Reimer RR et al: Acute leukemia after alkylating agent therapy of ovarian cancer. N Engl J Med 297:177, 1977.

Rosen GF, Lurain JR, Newton M: Hexamethylmelamine in ovarian cancer after failure of cisplatin-based multiple-agent chemotherapy. Gynecol Oncol 27:173, 1987.

Smith JP, Day TG: Review of ovarian cancer at the University of Texas Systems Cancer Center, MD Anderson Hospital and Tumor Institute. Am J Obstet Gynecol 135:984, 1979.

Sutton GP et al: Ten-year follow-up of patients receiving cisplatin, doxorubicin, and cyclophosphamide chemotherapy for advanced epithelial ovarian carcinoma. J Clin Oncol 7:223, 1989.

Tobias JS, Griffiths CT: Management of ovarian carcinoma. N Engl J Med 294:818, 1976.

Trimbos JB, Parman M, Vergote I et al: International collaborative ovarian neoplasm trial I (ICON I) and adjuvant chemotherapy in ovarian neoplasm trial (ACTION): two parallel randomized phase III trials of adjuvant chemotherapy in patients with early-stage ovarian carcinoma. J Natl Cancer Inst 95:105, 2003.

Trimbos JB, Vergote I, Bolis G et al (EORTC-ACTION collaborators): Impact of adjuvant chemotherapy and surgical staging in early-stage ovarian carcinoma: EORTC-ACTION trial. J Natl Cancer Inst 95:113, 2003.

Tropé C et al: High-dose medroxyprogesterone acetate for the treatment of advanced ovarian carcinoma. Cancer Treat Rep 66:1441, 1982.

Unzulman RF: Advanced epithelial ovarian carcinoma: Long-term survival experience at the community hospital. Am J Obstet Gynecol 166:1663, 1992.

Vogl SE et al: The CHAD and HAD regimens in advanced ovarian cancer: Combination chemotherapy including cyclophosphamide, hexamethylmelamine, Adriamycin, and *cis*-dichlorodiammineplatinum (II). Cancer Treat Rep 63:311, 1979.

Wharton JT, Edwards CL, Rutledge FN: Long-term survival after chemotherapy for advanced epithelial ovarian carcinomas. Am J Obstet Gynecol 148:997, 1984.

Young RC et al: Adjuvant therapy in stage I and stage II epithelial ovarian cancer: Results of two prospective randomized trials. N Engl J Med 322:1021, 1990.

Young RC, Walton L, Hornbeck NB, Nieberg RM: Randomized clinical trial for the treatment of women with selected stage IC and II (A,B,C) and selected stage IA and IB ovarian cancer, phage III. J Clin Oncol 2:4350, 2003.

Young RC et al: Advanced ovarian adenocarcinoma: A prospective clinical trial of melphalan (L-PAM) versus combination chemotherapy. N Engl J Med 299:1261, 1978.

MAXIMAL SURGICAL EFFORT

Baiocchi G, Raspagliese F, Grosso G et al: Early ovarian cancer. Is there a role for systematic pelvic and paraaortic lymphadenectomy? Int J Gynecol Cancer 8:103, 1998.

Barakat RR, Benjamin I: Surgery for malignant gynecologic disease. Curr Opin Obstet Gynecol 5:311, 1993.

Brand E, Pearlman N: Electrosurgical debulking of ovarian cancer: A new technique using the argon beam coagulator. Gynecol Oncol 39:115, 1990.

Bristow RE, Tomacruz RS, Armstrong DK et al: Survival effect of maximal cytoreductive surgery for advanced ovarian carcinoma during the platinum era: a meta-analysis. J Clin Oncol 20:1246, 2002.

Burghardt E et al: Pelvic lymphadenectomy in operative treatment of ovarian cancer. Am J Obstet Gynecol 155:315, 1986.

Chi DS, Franklin CC, Levine DA et al: Improved optimal cytoreduction rates for stages IIIC and IV epithelial ovarian, fallopian tube, and primary peritoneal cancer: a change in surgical approach. Gynecol Oncol 94:650, 2004.

Crawford SC, Vasey PA, Paul J et al: Does aggressive surgery only benefit patients with less advanced ovarian cancer? Results from an international comparison within the SCOTROC-1 trial. J Clin Oncol 23:8802, 2005.

Creasman WT: Second look laparotomy in ovarian cancer. Gynecol Oncol 55:S122, 1994.

Curtin JP, Malik R, Venkatraman ES et al: Stage IV ovarian cancer: Impact of surgical debulking. Gynecol Oncol 64:9, 1997.

de Gramon A: Survival after second look laparotomy in advanced ovarian endothelial cancer. Eur J Cancer Clin Oncol 25:451, 1989.

Delgado G et al: Paraaortic lymphadenectomy in gynecologic malignancies confined to the pelvis. Obstet Gynecol 50:418, 1977.

Deppe G, Malviya VK, Malone JM: Debulking surgery for ovarian cancer with the Cavitron ultrasonic surgical aspirator (CUSA): A preliminary report. Gynecol Oncol 31:223, 1988.

Eisenkop SM, Friedman RL, Wang HJ: Complete cytoreductive surgery is feasible and maximizes survival in patients with advanced ovarian cancer. Gynecol Oncol 63:103, 1998.

Goldberg GL et al: Lymph node sampling in patients with epithelial ovarian carcinoma. Gynecol Oncol 47:143, 1992.

Goodman HM et al: The role of cytoreductive surgery in the management of stage IV epithelial ovarian carcinoma. Gynecol Oncol 46:367, 1992.

Griffiths CT, Parker LM, Fuller AF: Role of cytoreductive surgical treatment in the management of advanced ovarian cancer. Cancer Treat Rep 63:235, 1979.

Guidozzi F, Ball JHS: Extensive primary cytoreductive surgery for advanced epithelial ovarian cancer. Gynecol Oncol 53:326, 1994.

Heintz APM, Hacker NF, Berek JS: Cytoreductive surgery in ovarian carcinoma: Feasibility and morbidity. Obstet Gynecol 67:783, 1986.

Hoskins WJ: The effect of diameter of largest residual disease on survival after primary cytoreductive surgery in patients with suboptimal residual epithelial ovarian carcinoma. Am J Obstet Gynecol 170:974, 1994.

Hoskins W, Rubin S, Dulaney E: The influence of secondary cytoreduction at the time of second-look laparotomy on the survival of patients with epithelial ovarian carcinoma. Gynecol Oncol 34:365, 1989.

Hoskins WJ et al: The influence of cytoreductive surgery on recurrence free interval and survival in small volume stage III epithelial ovarian cancer: A Gynecologic Oncology Group study. Gynecol Oncol 47:159, 1992.

Hunter RW, Alexander NDE, Soutter WP: Meta-analysis of surgery in advanced ovarian carcinoma: Is maximum cytoreductive surgery an independent determinant of prognosis? Am J Obstet Gynecol 166, 1992.

Jänicke F et al: Radical surgical procedure improves survival time in patients with recurrent ovarian cancer. Cancer 70:2129, 1992.

Liu PC, Benjamin I, Morgan MA et al: Effect of surgical debulking on survival in stage IV ovarian cancer. Gynecol Oncol 64:4, 1997.

Markman M et al: Characteristics of patients with small volume residual ovarian cancer unresponsive to cisplatin based IP chemotherapy: Lessons learned from a Gynecologic Oncology Group phase II trial of IP cisplatin and recombinant α-interferon. Gynecol Oncol 45:3, 1992.

Montz FJ, Schlaerth JB, Berek JS: Resection of diaphragmatic peritoneum and muscle: Role in cytoreductive surgery for advanced ovarian cancer. Gynecol Oncol 35:338, 1989.

Morris M, Gershenson DM, Wharton JT: Secondary cytoreductive surgery in epithelial ovarian cancer: Non-responders to first-line therapy. Gynecol Oncol 33:1, 1989.

Munkarah A, Levenback C, Wolf JK et al: Secondary cytoreductive surgery for localized intra-abdominal recurrences in epithelial ovarian cancer. Obstet Gynecol Surv 56:551, 2001.

Parazzini F, Valsecchi G, Bolis G et al: Pelvic and paraaortic lymph node status in advanced ovarian cancer and survival. Gynecol Oncol 74:7, 1999.

Potter ME: Secondary cytoreduction in ovarian cancer: Pro or con? Gynecol Oncol 51:131, 1993.

Rose PG, Nerenstone SR, Brady MF et al: Secondary surgical cytoreduction for advanced ovarian carcinoma. N Engl J Med 351: 2489, 2004.

Scarabelli C, Gallo A, Visentin MC et al: Systemic pelvic and paraaortic lymphadenectomy in advanced ovarian cancer patients with no residual intraperitoneal disease. Int J Gynecol Cancer 7:18, 1997.

Schueler JA, Trimbos JB, Hermans J et al: The yield of surgical staging in presumed early stage ovarian cancer: Benefits or doubts? Int J Gynecol Cancer 8:95, 1998.

Segna RA et al: Secondary cytoreduction for ovarian cancer following cisplatin therapy. J Clin Oncol 11:434, 1993.

Van der Burg MEL et al: The effect of debulking surgery after induction chemotherapy on the prognosis in advanced epithelial ovarian cancer. N Engl J Med 332:629, 1995.

Wang PH, Yuan CC, Lin G et al: Risk factors contributing to early occurrence of port site metastasis of laparoscopic surgery for malignancy. Gynecol Oncol 72:38, 1999.

Williams L: The role of secondary cytoreductive surgery in epithelial ovarian malignancies. Oncology 6:25, 1992.

ROLE OF RADIATION THERAPY AND RADIOISOTOPES

Clark DGC et al: The role of radiation therapy in the treatment of cancer of the ovary: Results of 614 patients. Prog Clin Cancer 5:227, 1973.

Cmelak AJ, Kapp DS: Long-term survival with whole abdominopelvic irradiation in platinum-refractory persistent or recurrent ovarian cancer. Gynecol Oncol 65:453, 1997.

Decker DE, Webb MJ, Holbrook MA: Radiogold treatment of epithelial cancer of ovary, late results. Am J Obstet Gynecol 115:751, 1973.

Delclos L, Fletcher GH: Postoperative irradiation for ovarian carcinoma with the cobalt-60 moving strip technique. Clin Obstet Gynecol 12:993, 1969.

Dembo AJ: Abdominopelvic radiography in ovarian cancer: A 10 year experience. Cancer 55:2285, 1985.

Dembo AJ: Epithelial ovarian cancer: The role of radiotherapy. Int J Radiat Oncol Biol Phys 22:835, 1992.

Dembo AJ et al: Prognostic factors in patients with stage I epithelial ovarian cancer. Obstet Gynecol 75:263, 1990.

Hacker NF et al: Whole abdominal radiation as second-line therapy for epithelial ovarian cancer. Obstet Gynecol 65:60, 1985.

Hoskins WJ et al: Whole abdominal and pelvic irradiation in patients with minimal disease at second-look surgical reassessment for ovarian carcinoma. Gynecol Oncol 20:271, 1985.

Martinez A, Schram MS, Howes AE, Bagshaw MA: Postoperative radiation therapy for epithelial ovarian cancer: The curative role based on a 24-year experience. J Clin Oncol 3:901, 1985.

Menczer J et al: Abdominopelvic irradiation for stage II–IV ovarian carcinoma patients with limited or no residual disease at second-look laparotomy after completion of *cis*-platinum-based combination chemotherapy. Gynecol Oncol 24:149, 1986.

Mychalczak BR, Fuks Z: The current role of radiotherapy in the management of ovarian cancer. Ovarian Cancer 6:895, 1992.

Pezner RD: Limited epithelial carcinoma of the ovary treated with curative intent by the intraperitoneal instillation of radioactive colloids. Cancer 42:2563, 1978.

Piver MS et al: Intraperitoneal chromic phosphate in peritoneoscopically confirmed stage I ovarian adenocarcinoma. Am J Obstet Gynecol 144:836, 1982.

Piver MS et al: Stage II invasive adenocarcinoma of the ovary: Results of treatment by whole abdominal radiation plus pelvic boost versus pelvic radiation plus oral melphalan chemotherapy. Gynecol Oncol 23:168, 1986.

Rosenshein N et al: The effect of volume on the distribution of substances instilled into the peritoneal cavity. Gynecol Oncol 6:106, 1978.

Sedlacek TV, Spyropoulus P, Cifaldi R et al: Whole abdomen radiation therapy as second-line-treatment for epithelial ovarian carcinoma. Cancer J Sci Am 3:358, 1997.

Sell A et al: Randomized study of whole-abdomen irradiation versus pelvic irradiation plus cyclophosphamide in treatment of early ovarian cancer. Gynecol Oncol 37:367, 1990.

Spanos WJ et al: Complications in the use of intra-abdominal ^{32}P for ovarian carcinoma. Gynecol Oncol 45:243, 1992.

Thomas GM: Radiotherapy in early ovarian cancer. Gynecol Oncol 55:S73, 1994.

Vergae IB et al: Randomized trial comparing cisplatin with radioactive phosphorus or whole abdominal irradiation as adjuvant treatment of ovarian cancer. Cancer 69:741, 1992.

CHEMOTHERAPY

Alberts D: Cisplatin versus carboplatin in advanced ovarian cancer: An economic analysis. Pharmacol Ther July, 1994.

Bertelsen K et al: A prospective randomized comparison of 6 and 12 cycles of cyclophosphamide, adriamycin, and cisplatin in advanced epithelial ovarian cancer: A Danish Ovarian Study Group trial (DACOVA). Gynecol Oncol 49:30, 1993.

Bolis G, Colombo N, Pecorelli S et al: Adjuvant treatment for early epithelial ovarian cancer: Results of two randomized trials comparing cisplatin to no further treatment or chromic phosphate. Ann Oncol 6:887, 1995.

Burger RA et al: Phase II trial of Navelbine in the treatment of women with advanced epithelial ovarian cancer. Gynecol Oncol 50:265, 1993.

Canetta R et al: Future directions for paclitaxel (Taxol) in gynecologic malignancies. Int J Gynecol Cancer 4:23, 1994.

Cavaletti G et al: Cisplatin induced peripheral neurotoxicity is dependent on total dose intensity and single dose intensity. Cancer 69:203, 1992.

Colombo N et al: Cisplatin dose intensity in advanced ovarian cancer: A randomized study of conventional dose versus dose intense cisplatin monochemotherapy. Proc ASCO 12:255, 1993.

Colombo N et al: Multimodality therapy of early-stage (FIGO I–II) ovarian cancer: Review of surgical management and postoperative adjuvant treatment. Int J Gynecol Cancer 6(Suppl 1):13, 1996.

Copeland LJ, Bookman M, Trimble E: Clinical trials of newer regimens for treatment ovarian cancer: the rationale for Gynecologic Oncology Group protocol GOG 182-ICON5. Gynecol Oncol90: S1, 2003.

Creasman WT et al: Chemoimmunotherapy in the management of primary stage III ovarian cancer: A Gynecologic Oncology Group study. Cancer Treat Rep 63:319, 1979.

duBois A, Lueck, HF, Meier V et al: Cisplatin/paclitaxel vs carboplatin/paclitaxel in ovarian cancer: update of an AGO Study Group trial. Proc ASCO 18:356a#1374.

Gershenson DM et al: The effect of prolonged cisplatin based chemotherapy on progression free survival in patients with optimal epithelial ovarian cancer; “maintenance” therapy reconsidered. Gynecol Oncol 47:7, 1992.

Gordon AN, Tonda M, Sun S et al: Long-term survival advantage for women treated with pegylated liposomal doxorubicin compared with topotecan in a phase 3 randomized study of recurrent and refractory epithelial ovarian cancer. Gynecol Oncol 95:1, 2004.

Greene MGH, Boice JD, Greer BE et al: Acute non-lymphocytic leukemia after therapy with alkylating agents for ovarian cancer. N Engl J Med 307:1416, 1982.

Hakes T et al: Randomized prospective trial of 5 versus 10 cycles of cyclophosphamide, doxorubicin, and cisplatin in advanced ovarian carcinoma. Gynecol Oncol 45:284, 1992.

ICON Collaborators: ICON2: Randomized trial of single-agent carboplatin against 3 drug combination of CAP in women with ovarian cancer. Lancet 352:1571, 1998.

Kotz KW, Schilder RJ: High dose chemotherapy and hematopoietic progenitor cell support for patients with epithelial ovarian cancer. Semin Oncol 22:250, 1995.

Loizzi V, Chan JK, Osann K et al: Survival outcomes in patients with recurrent ovarian cancer who were treated with chemoresistance assay-guided chemotherapy. Am J Obstet Gynecol 189:1301, 2003.

Markman M et al: Late effects of cisplatin-based chemotherapy on renal function in patients with ovarian cancer. Gynecol Oncol 41:217, 1991.

Markman M et al: Second-line platinum therapy in patients with ovarian cancer previously treated with cisplatin. J Clin Oncol 9:389, 1991.

Markman M et al: Control of carboplatin-induced emesis with a fixed low dose of granisetron (0.5 mg) plus dexamethasone. Gynecol Oncol 60: 435, 1996.

Markman M, Liu P, Wilczynski S et al: Phase III randomized trial of 12 months VS 3 months of paclitaxel in patients with advanced ovarian, fallopian tube or primary peritoneal cancer who attain a clinically defined complete response (CR) following platinum/paclitaxel-based chemotherapy. J Clin Oncol 21(13):2460, 2003.

Markman M, Webster K, Zanotti K et al: Phase II trial of single-agent gemcitabine in platinum-refractory ovarian cancer. Gynecol Oncol 90:593, 2003.

McGuire WP et al: Cyclophosphamide and cisplatin compared with paclitaxel and cisplatin in patients with stage III and stage IV ovarian cancer. N Engl J Med 334:1, 1996.

McGuire WP, Blessing JA, Bookman MA et al: Topotecan has substantial activity as first-line second-line therapy in platinum-sensitive epithelial ovarian carcinoma: A GOG study. J Clin Oncol 18:1062, 2000.

McMeekin DS, Tillmanns T, Chaudry T et al: Timing isn’t everything: an analysis of when to start second-line chemotherapy in ovarian cancer. Gynecol Oncol 95:157, 2004.

Morgan DP, Thigpen T: Chemotherapy in gynecologic cancer: Celomic epithelial carcinoma of the ovary. Clin Consult Obstet Gynecol 4:144, 1992.

Muggia FM, Hainsworth JD, Jeffers S et al: Phase II study of liposomal doxorubicin in refractory ovarian cancer. J Clin Oncol 15:987, 1997.

Muggia FM, Braly PS, Brady MF et al: A phase III randomized study of cisplatin versus paclitaxel versus paclitaxel and cisplatin in patients with suboptimal stage III and IV epithelial ovarian carcinoma: A GOG study. J Clin Oncol 18:106, 2000.

Murakami M et al: High dose chemotherapy with autologous bone marrow transplantation for the treatment of malignant ovarian tumors. Semin Oncol 21:29, 1994.

Nagourney RA, Brewer CA, Radecki S et al: Phase II trial of gemcitabine plus cisplatin repeating doublet therapy in previously treated, relapsed ovarian cancer patients. Gynecol Oncol 88:35, 2003.

Neijt JP, Engelholm SA, Tuxen MK et al: Exploratory phase III study of paclitaxel and cisplatin versus paclitaxel and carboplatin in advanced ovarian cancer. J Clin Oncol 18:3084, 2000.

O'Malley DM, Azodi M, Makkenchery A et al: Weekly topotecan in heavily pretreated patients with recurrent epithelial ovarian carcinoma. Gynecol Oncol 98:242, 2005.

Ozols RF, Bundy BN, Greer BE et al: Phase III trial of carboplatin and paclitaxel compared with cisplatin and paclitaxel in patients with optimally resected stage III ovarian cancer: A Gynecologic Oncology Group study (158). J Clin Oncol 21(17):3194, 2003.

Reichman B, Markman M et al: Intraperitoneal cisplatin and etoposide in the treatment of refractory/recurrent ovarian carcinoma. J Clin Oncol 7:1327, 1989.

Rose PG, Mossburger K, Fusco N et al: Gemcitabine reverses cisplatin resistance: demonstration of activity in platinum- and multidrug-resistant ovarian and peritoneal carcinoma. Gynecol Oncol 88:17, 2003.

Rothenberg M et al: Dose intensive induction therapy with cyclophosphamide, cisplatin, and consolidative abdominal radiation in the advanced stage epithelial ovarian cancer. J Clin Oncol 10:727, 1992.

Rowinsky EK, Cazenave LA, Donehower RC: Taxol: A novel investigational antimicrotubule agent. J Natl Cancer Inst 82:1247, 1990.

Santin AD et al: Development and characterization of an IL-4 secreting human ovarian carcinoma cell line. Gynecol Oncol 58:230, 1995.

Stiff P et al: A phase II trial of high dose mitoxantrone, carboplatin, and cyclophosphamide with autologous bone marrow rescue for recurrent epithelial ovarian carcinoma: Analysis of risk factors for clinical outcome. Gynecol Oncol 57:278, 1995.

Sutton G: Ifosfamide and mesna in epithelial ovarian carcinoma. Gynecol Oncol 51:104, 1993.

Swenerton KD, Peter JL: Carboplatin in the treatment of carcinoma of the ovary: The National Cancer Institute of Canada experience. Semin Oncol 19:114, 1992.

Swenerton KD et al: Cisplatin-cyclophosphamide versus carboplatin-cyclophosphamide in advanced ovarian cancer: A randomized phase III study of the National Cancer Institute of Canada Clinical Trials Group. J Clin Oncol 10:718, 1992.

Thigpen T: High dose chemotherapy with autologous bone marrow support in ovarian carcinoma: The bottom line, more or less (Editorial). Gynecol Oncol 57:275, 1995.

Van der Burg MEL et al: The role of intervention debulking surgery in advanced epithelial ovarian cancer: An EORTC Gynecological Cancer Cooperative Group study. Int J Gynecol Cancer 6(Suppl 1):30, 1996.

Vasey PA, Jayson GC, Gordon A et al: Phase III randomized trial of docetaxel-carboplatin versus paclitaxel-carboplatin as first line chemotherapy for ovarian carcinoma. J Nat'l Cancer Inst 17:1682, 2004.

Vergae IB et al: Randomized trial comparing cisplatin with radioactive phosphorus or whole abdomen irradiation as adjuvant treatment of ovarian cancer. Cancer 69:741, 1992.

Warner E: Neurotoxicity of cisplatin and Taxol. Int J Gynecol Cancer 5:161, 1995.

Wiernik PH et al: Hexamethylmelamine and low or moderate dose cisplatin with or without pyridoxine for treatment of advanced ovarian carcinoma: A study of the Eastern Cooperative Oncology Group. Cancer Invest 10:1, 1992.

INTRAPERITONEAL CHEMOTHERAPY

Alberts DS, Liu PY, Hannigan EV et al: Intraperitoneal cisplatin plus intravenous cyclophosphamide versus intravenous cisplatin plus intravenous cyclophosphamide for stage III ovarian cancer. N Engl J Med 335:1950, 1996.

Armstrong DK, Bundy B, Wenzel L et al: Randomized phase III study of intravenous (IV) paclitaxel and cisplatin versus IV paclitaxel, intraperitoneal (IP) cisplatin and IP paclitaxel in optimal stage III epithelial ovarian cancer (OC): a Gynecologic Oncology Group trial (GOG 172). Paper presented at American Society of Clinical Oncology, 2002 Annual Meeting (Abstract 803).

Armstrong DK, Bundy B, Wenzel L et al: Intraperitoneal cisplatin, and paclitaxel in ovarian cancer. N Engl J Med 354:34, 2006.

Berek JS, Hack NF, Lichtenstein A et al: Intraperitoneal recombinant a-interferon for "second-line" immunotherapy in stage III epithelial ovarian cancer: A Gynecologic Oncology Group study. Cancer Res 45:4447, 1985.

Cannistra SA: Intraperitoneal chemotherapy comes of age. N Engl J Med 354:77, 2006.

Dedrick R, Myers C, Bungay P et al: Pharmokinetic rationale for peritoneal drug administration in the treatment of ovarian cancer. Cancer Treatment Rep 62:1, 1978.

Fujiwara K, Markman M, Morgan M et al: Intraperitoneal carboplatin-based chemotherapy for epithelial ovarian cancer. Gynecol Oncol 97:10, 2005.

Gadducci A, Carnini F, Chiara S et al: Intraperitoneal versus intravenous cisplatin in combination with intravenous cyclophosphamide and epidoxorubicin in optimally cytoreduced advanced epithelial ovarian cancer: a randomized trial of the Gruppo Oncologica Nord-Ovest. Gynecol Oncol 76:157, 2000.

Howell SB, Pfeifle CL, Wung WE et al: Intraperitoneal cisplatin with systemic thiosulfate protection. Ann Intern Med 97:845, 1982.

Howell SB, Kirmani S, Lucas WE et al: kA phase II trial of intraperitoneal cisplatin and etoposide for primary treatment of ovarian epithelial cancer. J Clin Oncol 8:137, 1990.

Howell SB, Zimm S, Markman M et al: Long-term survival of advanced refractory ovarian carcinoma patients with small-volume disease treated with intraperitoneal chemotherapy. J Clin Oncol 5:1607, 1987.

Kirmani S, Braly PS, McClay EF et al: A comparison of intravenous versus intraperitoneal chemotherapy for the initial treatment of ovarian cancer. Gynecol Oncol 54:338, 1994.

Markman M et al: Responses to second line cisplatin based intraperitoneal therapy in ovarian cancer: Influence of a prior response to intravenous cisplatin. J Clin Oncol 9:1801, 1991.

Markman M et al: Impact of laparotomy finding of significant intra-abdominal adhesions on the surgically defined complete response rate to subsequent second-line intraperitoneal chemotherapy. J Cancer Res Clin Oncol 188:163, 1992.

Markman M et al: Evidence supporting the superiority of intraperitoneal cisplatin compared to intraperitoneal carboplatin for second-line therapy of small volume residual ovarian cancer. Gynecol Oncol 50:100, 1993.

Markman M et al: Rationale for the intraperitoneal administration of paclitaxel (Taxol) in the treatment of ovarian cancer. Int J Gynecol Cancer 4:19, 1994.

Markman M, Bundy BN, Alberts DS et al: Phase III trial of standard-dose intravenous cisplatin plus paclitaxel versus moderately high-dose carboplatin followed by intravenous paclitaxel and intraperitoneal cisplatin in small-volume stage III ovarian carcinoma: an intergroup study of the Gynecologic Oncology Group, Southwestern Oncology Group, and Eastern Cooperative Oncology Group. J Clin Oncol 19:1001, 2001.

Markman M, Copeland LJ, Sickel J: A phase III randomized study of intravenous cisplatin and taxol versus high dose intravenous carboplatin following by intravenous and intraperitoneal cisplatin in patients with optimal stage III epithelial ovarian carcinoma (SWOB 9227, ECOG G0114). J Clin Oncol 2(2):3814, 2003.

National Cancer Institute Clinical Announcement: Intraperitoneal chemotherapy for ovarian cancer. (In Press — January 2006).

Piccart MJ et al: Intraperitoneal chemotherapy: Technical experience at five institutions. Semin Oncol 12:90, 1985.

Piccart MJ, Floquet A, Scarfone G et al: Intraperitoneal cisplatin versus no further treatment: 8-year results of EORTC 55875, a randomized phase III study in ovarian cancer patients with a pathologically complete remission after platinum-based intravenous chemotherapy. Int J Gynecol Cancer 13(Suppl 12):196, 2003.

Polyzos A, Tasvaris N, Kosmas C et al: A comparative study of intraperitoneal carboplatin versus intravenous carboplatin with intravenous cyclophosphamide in both arms as initial chemotherapy for stage III ovarian cancer. Oncology 56:291, 1999.

Runowicz CD et al: Catheter complications associated with intraperitoneal chemotherapy. Gynecol Oncol 24:41, 1986.

Walker JL, Armstrong DA, Huang HQ et al: Intraperitoneal catheter outcomes in a phase III trial of intravenous versus intraperitoneal chemotherapy in optimal stage III ovarian or primary peritoneal cancer. A Gynecologic Oncology Group study. Gynecol Oncol 100:27, 2006.

Yen M-S, Juang C-M, Lai C-R et al: Intraperitoneal cisplatin-based chemotherapy vs. intravenous cisplatin-based chemotherapy for stage III optimally cytoreduced epithelial ovarian cancer. Int J Gynecol Obstet 72:55, 2001.

EXTRAOVARIAN PERITONEAL SEROUS PAPILLARY CARCINOMA

Bandera CA et al: BRCAl gene mutations in women with papillary serous carcinoma of the peritoneum. Obstet Gynecol 92:596, 1998.

Bloss JD, Brady M, Rocereto T et al: A phase II trial of cisplatin and cyclophosphamide in the treatment of extraovarian peritoneal serous papillary carcinoma with comparison to papillary serous ovarian carcinoma. Gynecol Oncol 68:109, 1998.

Dalrymple JC et al: Extraovarian peritoneal serous papillary carcinoma: A clinicopathologic study of 31 cases. Cancer 64:110, 1989.

Eltablakh GH, Werness BA, Piver S et al: Prognostic factors in extraovarian primary peritoneal carcinoma. Gynecol Oncol 71:230, 1998.

Fowler JM et al: Peritoneal adenocarcinoma (serous) of müllerian type: A subgroup of women presenting with peritoneal carcinomatosis. Int J Gynecol Cancer 4:43, 1994.

Killackey MA, Davis AR: Papillary serous carcinoma of the peritoneal surface: Matched-case comparison with papillary serous ovarian carcinoma. Gynecol Oncol 51:171, 1993.

Weber AM et al: Serous carcinoma of the peritoneum after oophorectomy. Obstet Gynecol 80:558, 1992.

SMALL CELL CARCINOMA OF THE OVARY

Dickersin GR, Kline IW, Scully RE: Small cell carcinoma of the ovary with hypercalcemia: A report of 11 cases. Cancer 49:188, 1982.

Patsner B, Piver MS, Lele SB et al: Small cell carcinoma of the ovary: A rapidly lethal tumor occurring in the young. Gynecol Oncol 22:233, 1985.

Pruett KM, Gordon AN, Estrada G et al: Small-cell carcinoma of the ovary: An aggressive epithelial cancer occurring in young patients. Gynecol Oncol 29:365, 1988.

Senekjian EK, Weiser PA, Talerman A, Herbst AL: Vinblastine, cisplatin, cyclophosphamide, bleomycin, doxorubicin, and etoposide in the treatment of small cell carcinoma of the ovary. Cancer 64:1183, 1989.

Taraszewski R et al: Case report: Small cell carcinoma of the ovary. Gynecol Oncol 41:149, 1991.

Ulbright TM, Roth LM, Stehman FB et al: Poorly differentiated (small cell) carcinoma of the ovary in young women: Evidence supporting a germ cell origin. Hum Pathol 18:175, 1987.

Young RH, Dickersin GR, Scully RE: Small-cell carcinoma of the ovary: An analysis of 75 cases of a distinct ovarian tumor commonly associated with hypercalcemia (Abstract). Lab Invest 56:89, 1987.

USE OF CA-125 LEVELS

Alagoz T et al: What is a normal CA-125 level? Gynecol Oncol 53:93, 1994.

Alvarez RD et al: CA-125 as a serum marker for poor prognosis in ovarian malignancies. Gynecol Oncol 26:284, 1987.

Bast RC et al: Elevation of serum CA-125 in carcinoma of the fallopian tube, endometrium, and endocervix. Am J Obstet Gynecol 148:1057, 1984.

Bast RC et al: Monitoring human ovarian carcinoma with a combination of CA-125, CA 19-9, and carcinoembryonic antigen. Am J Obstet Gynecol 149:553, 1984.

Buller RE, Vasilev S, DiSaia PJ: CA-125 kinetics: A cost-effective clinical tool to evaluate clinical trial outcomes in the 1990. Am J Obstet Gynecol 174:1241, 1996.

Gard GB, Houghton RS: An assessment of the value of serum CA-125 measurements in the management of epithelial ovarian carcinoma. Gynecol Oncol 53:283, 1994.

Hising C, Anjegard IM, Einhorn N: Clinical relevance of the CA-125 assay in monitoring of ovarian cancer patients. Am J Clin Oncol 14:111, 1991.

Hogberg T, Kagedal B: Serous half-life of the tumor marker CA-125 during induction chemotherapy as a prognostic indicator for survival in ovarian carcinoma. Acta Obstet Gynecol Scand 69:423, 1990.

Latimer JA, Beng CG, Davy MLJ: For stage III epithelial ovarian cancer, the initial level of expression of CA125 does not correlate with survival in women who respond to treatment. Int J Gynecol Cancer 6:380, 1996.

Loy TS, Quesenberry JT, Sharp SC: Distribution of CA-125 in adenocarcinomas. Am J Clin Pathol 98:175, 1992.

Maggino T et al: Prospective multicenter study on CA-125 in postmenopausal pelvic masses. Gynecol Oncol 54:117, 1994.

Markman M, Liu PY, Wilczynski S et al: Survival of ovarian cancer patients treated on SWOG 9701/GOG 178: 12 versus 3 cycles of monthly single-agent paclitaxel following attainment of a clinically-defined complete response to platinum. ASCO Proceedings 2006 (In Press).

Mogensen O, Mogensen B, Jakobsen A: Predictive value of CA-125 during early chemotherapy of advanced ovarian cancer. Gynecol Oncol 37:44, 1990.

Niloff JM et al: Predictive value of CA-125 antigen levels in second-look procedures for ovarian cancer. Am J Obstet Gynecol 151: 981, 1985.

Olt G, Berchuck A, Bast RC: The role of tumor markers in gynecologic oncology. Obstet Gynecol Surv 45:570, 1990.

Onsrud M: Tumour markers in gynaecologic oncology. Scand J Clin Lab Invest 51:60, 1991.

Podczaski E et al: Use of CA-125 to monitor patients with ovarian epithelial carcinomas. Gynecol Oncol 33:193, 1989.

Potter ME et al: Value of serum 125 CA levels: Does the result preclude second look? Gynecol Oncol 33:201, 1989.

Rustin GJS, Timmers P, Nelstrop A et al: Comparison of CA-125 and standard definitions of progression of ovarian cancer in the intergroup trial of cisplatin and paclitaxel versus cisplatin and cyclophosphamide. J Clin Oncol 24:45, 2006.

Zurawski VR Jr et al: Prospective evaluation of serum CA-125 levels in a normal population, phase I: The specifications of single and serial determinations in testing for ovarian cancer. Gynecol Oncol 36:299, 1990.

SECOND-LOOK OPERATION (REASSESSMENT SURGERY)

Childers JM, Brzechffa PR, Surwit EA: Laparoscopy using the left upper quadrant as the primary trocar site. Gynecol Oncol 50:221, 1993.

Cohen CJ, Bruckner HW, Goldberg JD et al: Improved therapy with cisplatin regimens for patients with ovarian cancer as measured by surgical end-staging—the Mount Sinai experience. Clin Obstet Gynecol 10:307, 1983.

Copeland LJ: Second-look laparotomy for ovarian carcinoma. Clin Obstet Gynecol 28:816, 1985.

Creasman WT, Gall S, Bundy BN et al: Second-look laparotomy in the patient with minimal residual stage III ovarian cancer (a Gynecologic Oncology Group study). Gynecol Oncol 35:378, 1989.

Greer BE, Bundy BN, Ozols RF et al: Implications of second-look laparotomy in the context of optimally resected stage II ovarian cancer: a non-randomized comparison using an explanatory analysis: a Gynecologic Oncology Group study. Gynecol Oncol 99:71, 2005.

Lippman SC, Alberts DS, Slymen DJ et al: Second-look laparotomy in epithelial ovarian carcinoma. Cancer 61:2571, 1988.
Miller DS et al: Critical reassessment of second look exploratory laparotomy for epithelial ovarian carcinoma. Cancer 69:502, 1992.
Peters WA et al: Intraperitoneal ^{32}P is not an effective consolidation therapy after a negative second look laparotomy for epithelial carcinoma of the ovary. Gynecol Oncol 47:146, 1992.
Podczaski ES, Stevens CW, Manetta A et al: Use of second-look laparotomy in the management of patients with ovarian epithelial malignancies. Gynecol Oncol 28:205, 1987.
Podratz KC, Schray MF, Wieand HS et al: Evaluation of treatment and survival after positive second-look laparotomy. Gynecol Oncol 31:9, 1988.
Podratz KC, Kinney WK: Second look operation in ovarian cancer. Cancer 71:1551, 1993.
Smirz LR et al: Second-look laparotomy after chemotherapy in the management of ovarian malignancy. Am J Obstet Gynecol 152:661, 1985.
Soper JT et al: Intraperitoneal chromic phosphate ^{32}P as second-line therapy for persistent carcinoma of the ovary after surgical restaging. Am J Obstet Gynecol 156:1153, 1987.
Tarraza HM et al: Consolidation intraperitoneal chemotherapy in epithelial ovarian cancer patients following negative second look laparotomy. Gynecol Oncol 50:287, 1993.
Varia M, Currie JL, Benda J: Evaluation of intraperitoneal chromic phosphate suspension therapy following negative second-look laparotomy for epithelial ovarian carcinoma (stage III), phase III. J Clin Oncol 21(15):2849, 2003.
Walton L, Ellenberg SS, Major F Jr et al: Results of second-look laparotomy in patients with early-stage ovarian carcinoma. Obstet Gynecol 80:770, 1987.

SECOND-LINE THERAPY

Abdulhay G et al: Human lymphoblastoid interferon in the treatment of advanced epithelial ovarian malignancies (a GOG study). Am J Obstet Gynecol 152:418, 1985.
Adams M: Second-line treatment for ovarian cancer. Clin Oncol 2:1, 1990.
Ben-David Y, Rossen B, Franssen E et al: Meta-analysis comparing cisplatin total dose intensity and survival. Gynecol Oncol 59:93, 1995.
Blackledge G et al: Response of patients in phase II studies of chemotherapy in ovarian cancer: Implications for patient treatment and the design of phase II trials. Br J Cancer 59:650, 1989.
Bristow RE, Giuntoli RL, Pannu HK et al: Combined PET/CT for detecting recurrent ovarian cancer limited to retroperitoneal lymph nodes. Gynecol Oncol 99:294, 2005.
Covens A et al: Phase II study of mitomycin C and 5-fluorouracil in platinum resistant ovarian cancer. Eur J Gynaecol Oncol 13:125, 1992.
Eisenhauer S et al: Carboplatin therapy for recurrent ovarian cancer: National Cancer Institute experience and review of the literature. In Bunn PA, Canetta R, Ozols RF, Rozencweig M (eds): Carboplatin (JM-8): Current Perspectives and Future Directions. Philadelphia, WB Saunders, 1990.
Fanning J, Hilgers RD, Hutson E: Carboplatin, etoposide, and ifosfamide as second line treatment for ovarian cancer. Am J Clin Oncol 17:335, 1994.
Fromm GL et al: Sequentially administered ethinyl estradiol and medroxyprogesterone acetate in the treatment of refractory epithelial ovarian carcinoma in patients with positive estrogen receptors. Cancer 68:1885, 1991.
Gonzalez-Martin AJ, Calvo E, Bover I et al: Randomized Phase II trial of carboplatin versus paclitaxel and carboplatin in platinum-sensitive recurrent advanced ovarian carcinoma: a GEICO study. Ann Oncol 16:749, 2005.
Horowitz M, Staff PJ, Verem-Stone J et al: Outcome of autotransplants for abnormal ovarian cancer. Proc Am Soc Clin Oncol 33:A1262, 1997.
Hoskins PJ, McMurtrie E, Senerton KD: A phase II trial of intravenous etoposide (VP-16-213) in epithelial ovarian cancer resistant to cisplatin or carboplatin: Clinical and serological evidence of activity. Int J Gynecol Cancer 2:35, 1992.
Hoskins WJ, Rubin SC, Dulaney E et al: Influence of secondary cytoreduction at the time of second-look laparotomy on the survival of patients with epithelial ovarian carcinoma. Gynecol Oncol 34:365, 1989.
Howell SB, Kirmani S, McClay EF et al: Intraperitoneal cisplatin-based chemotherapy for ovarian carcinoma. Semin Oncol 18(Suppl 3):5, 1991.
Kavanagh JK, Nicaise C: Carboplatin in refractory epithelial ovarian cancer. Semin Oncol 16:45, 1989.
Kohn EC et al: Dose intense Taxol: High response rate in patients with platinum resistant ovarian cancer. J Natl Cancer Inst 86:18, 1994.
Lawton F et al: A randomized trial comparing whole abdominal radiotherapy with chemotherapy following cisplatin cytoreduction in epithelial ovarian cancer: West Midlands Ovarian Cancer Group trial II. Clin Oncol 2:4, 1990.
Long HJ et al: Phase II evaluation of 5-fluorouracil and low dose leucovorin in cisplatin refractory advanced ovarian carcinoma. Gynecol Oncol 54:180, 1994.
Lucas WE, Markman M, Howell SB: Intraperitoneal chemotherapy for advanced ovarian cancer. Am J Obstet Gynecol 152:474, 1985.
Manetta A et al: Hexamethylmelamine as a single second line agent in ovarian cancer. Gynecol Oncol 36:93, 1990.
Markman M: Follow-up of the asymptomatic patient with ovarian cancer. Gynecol Oncol 55:S134, 1994.
Markman M: Second-line intraperitoneal therapy of small volume residual ovarian cancer: Impact of pretreatment finding of peritoneal carcinomatosis on the surgical complete response rate. J Cancer Res Clin Oncol 118:232, 1992.
Markman M: Second-line therapy in ovarian cancer: Is there a role for intraperitoneal drug delivery? Gynecol Oncol 51:86, 1993.
Markman M et al: Association between pretreatment CA-125 levels and surgically documented complete responses in patients with ovarian cancer treated with second-line intraperitoneal therapy. J Cancer Res Clin Oncol 118:391, 1992.
Markman M et al: Second-line platinum therapy in patients with ovarian cancer previously treated with cisplatin. J Clin Oncol 9:389, 1991.
Markman M, Markman J, Webster K et al: Duration of response to second-line, platinum-based chemotherapy for ovarian cancer: implications for patient management and clinical trial design. J Clin Oncol 22:3120, 2004.
McGuire WP et al: A unique antineoplastic agent with significant activity in advanced ovarian epithelial neoplasms. Ann Intern Med 111:273, 1989.
Menczer J: Use of the Veress needle for instillation of intraperitoneal chemotherapy. Gynecol Oncol 59:249, 1995.
Menczer J et al: Intraperitoneal chemotherapy versus no treatment in patients with ovarian carcinoma who are in complete clinical remission. Cancer 70:1956, 1992.
Miller DS, Brady FB, Barrett RJ: A phase II trial of leuprolide acetate in patients with advanced epithelial ovarian carcinoma. Am J Clin Oncol 15:125, 1992.
Moore DH et al: Hexamethylmelamine chemotherapy for persistent or recurrent epithelial ovarian cancer. Am J Obstet Gynecol 165:573, 1991.
Parmar MKB, Ledermann JA, Columbo N et al: Paclitaxel plus platinum-based chemotherapy versus conventional platinum-based chemotherapy in women with relapsed ovarian cancer. The ICON4/AGO-OVAR2.2 trial. Lancet 361:2099, 2003.
Piver MS et al: Evaluation of survival after second line intraperitoneal cisplatin based chemotherapy for advanced ovarian cancer. Cancer 73:1693, 1994.
Reed E et al: 5-Fluorouracil (5-FU) and leucovorin in platinum refractory advanced stage ovarian carcinoma. Gynecol Oncol 46:326, 1992.

Rose PG, Blessing JA, Mayer AR et al: Prolonged oral etoposide as second-line therapy for platinum-resistant and platinum-sensitive ovarian carcinoma: a GOG study. J Clin Oncol 16:405, 1998.

Rosen GF, Lurain JR, Newton M: Hexamethylmelamine in ovarian cancer after failure of cisplatin based multiple agent chemotherapy. Gynecol Oncol 27:173, 1987.

Seltzer V, Vogel S, Kaplan B: Recurrent ovarian carcinoma: Retreatment utilizing combination chemotherapy including cis-diamine dichloroplatinum in patients previously responding to this agent. Gynecol Oncol 21:167, 1985.

Shapiro JD, Millward MJ, Rischin O et al: Activity of gemcitabine in patients with advanced ovarian cancer: responses seen following platinum and paclitaxel. Gynecol Oncol 63:89, 1996.

Spencer TR et al: Intraperitoneal P-32 after negative second-look laparotomy in ovarian carcinoma. Cancer 63:2434, 1989.

Trimble EL et al: Paclitaxel for platinum refractory ovarian cancer: Results from the first 1,000 patients registered to National Cancer Institute Treatment Referral Center 9103. J Clin Oncol 11:2405, 1993.

Vergae J et al: Hexamethylmelamine as second line therapy in platin resistant ovarian cancer. Gynecol Oncol 47:282, 1992.

MALIGNANT EFFUSIONS AND SUPPORTIVE CARE

Kennedy L et al: Pleurodesis using talc slurry. Chest 106:342, 1994.

Lewin SN, Buttin BM, Powell MA et al: Resource utilization for ovarian cancer patients at the end of life: How much is too much. Gynecol Oncol 99:261, 2005.

Nagy JA et al: Pathogenesis of ascites tumor growth: Fibrinogen influx and fibrin accumulation in tissues lining the peritoneal cavity. Cancer Res 55:369, 1995.

Nagy JA et al: Pathogenesis of ascites tumor growth: Vascular permeability factor, vascular hyperpermeability, and ascites fluid accumulation. Cancer Res 55:360, 1995.

Nagy JA et al: Pathogenesis of ascites tumor growth: Angiogenesis, vascular remodeling, and stroma formation in the peritoneal lining. Cancer Res 55:376, 1995.

Ruckdeschel JD et al: Intrapleural therapy for malignant pleural effusions. Chest 100:1528, 1991.

von Gruenigen VE and Daly BJ: Treating ovarian cancer patients at the end of life: When should we stop? Gynecol Oncol 99:255, 2005.

CURRENT AREAS OF RESEARCH

Berchuck A et al: Overexpression of Her-2/neu is associated with poor survival in advanced epithelial ovarian cancer. Cancer Res 50:4087, 1990.

Berek JS et al: Intraperitoneal immunotherapy of epithelial ovarian carcinoma with *Corynebacterium parvum*. Am J Obstet Gynecol 152:1003, 1985.

Burger R, Sill MW, Monk BJ et al: Phase II trial of bevacizumab in persistent or recurrent epithelial ovarian cancer or primary peritoneal cancer: a GOG study. Proc Am Soc Clin Oncol 23:Abst 5009, 2005.

DeGregorio MW et al: Toremifene: Pharmacologic and pharmacokinetic basis of reversing multidrug resistance. Am Soc Clin Oncol 7:1359, 1989.

Enomoto T, Inoue M, Perantoni AO et al: K-ras activation in neoplasms of the human female reproductive tract. Cancer Res 50:6139, 1990.

Finlay C, Hinds P, Levine A: The p53 protooncogene can act as a suppressor of transformation. Cell 57:1083, 1989.

Foxwell BMJ et al: Identification of the multidrug resistance-related P-glycoprotein as a cyclosporine binding protein. Mol Pharmacol 36:543, 1989.

Friedlander M et al: Prediction of long-term survival by flow-cytometric analysis of cellular DNA content in patients with advanced ovarian cancer. J Clin Oncol 6:282, 1988.

Goldie JH, Coldman AJ: A mathematical model for relating the drug sensitivity to tumors of their spontaneous mutation rate. Cancer Treat Rep 63:1727, 1979.

Goldie JH, Coldman AJ: The genetic origin of drug resistance in neoplasms: Implications for systemic therapy. Cancer Res 44:3643, 1984.

Hogg R and Friedlander M: Biology of epithelial ovarian cancer: implications for screening women at high genetic risk. J Clin Oncol 22:1315, 2004.

Iverson O: Prognostic values of the flow cytometric DNA index in human ovarian carcinoma. Cancer 61:971, 1988.

Kern DH, Weisenthal LM: Highly specific prediction of antineoplastic drug resistance with an in vitro assay using suprapharmacologic drug exposures. J Natl Cancer Inst 82:582, 1990.

National Institutes of Health, Office of the Director: Ovarian cancer: Screening, treatment, and follow-up. NIH Consens Statement 12:20, 1994.

Plaxe SC et al: Ovarian intraepithelial neoplasia demonstrated in patients with stage I ovarian carcinoma. Gynecol Oncol 38:367, 1990.

Saburi Y et al: Increased expression of glutathione *S*-transferase gene in *cis*-diaminodichloroplatinum (II)-resistance variants of a Chinese hamster. Cancer Treat 49:7020, 1989.

Sharp F, Beachett AD, Berek JS et al: Conclusions and recommendations from the Helene Harris Trust Sixth Biennial International forum. Int J Gynecol Cancer 7:416, 1997.

Shilder RJ, Sill MW, Chen X et al: Phase II study of gefitinib. Clin Cancer Res 11:5539, 2005.

Slater LM et al: Cyclosporin A corrects daunorubicin resistance in Ehrlich ascites carcinoma. Br J Cancer 54:235, 1986.

Storms R, Bose H: Oncogenes, proto-oncogenes, and signal transduction: Toward a unified theory? Adv Virus Res 37:1, 1989.

Stratton JA, Braly PS, DiSaia PJ: A comparison of three assays for prediction of clinical response to chemotherapy. J Clin Lab Anal 1:67, 1987.

12 Germ Cell, Stromal, and other Ovarian Tumors

Michael A. Bidus, M.D., Christopher M. Zahn, M.D., G. Scott Rose, M.D.

GERM CELL TUMORS

Classification

This group of ovarian neoplasms consists of several histologically different tumor types and embraces all the neoplasms considered to be ultimately derived from the primitive germ cells of the embryonic gonad (Fig. 12–1). This concept of germ cell tumors as a specific group of gonadal neoplasms has evolved in the last 5 decades and become generally accepted. This acceptance is based primarily on the common histogenesis of these neoplasms, on the relatively common presence of histologically different tumor elements within the same tumor mass, on the presence of histologically similar neoplasms in extragonadal locations along the line of migration of the primitive germ cells from the wall of the yolk sac to the gonadal ridge, and on the remarkable homology between the various tumor types in men and women. In no other group of gonadal neoplasms has this homology been better illustrated. An example of this is the striking similarity between the testicular seminoma and its ovarian counterpart, the dysgerminoma. These were the first neoplasms to become accepted as originating from germ cells. A number of classifications of germ cell neoplasms of the ovary have been proposed over the past few decades. Table 12–1 shows a modification of a classification that was originally described by Teilum and is similar to that proposed by the World Health Organization, which divides the germ cell tumors into several groups and also includes neoplasms composed of germ cells and "sex" stroma derivatives.

Germ cell tumors are classified according to degree of differentiation. Two classes exist:

- undifferentiated germ cell tumors, which include dysgerminoma and gonadoblastoma; and
- differentiated tumors, which include all other germ cell tumors.

Differentiated tumors are further classified as to whether the tumor differentiates histologically into embryonic or extraembryonic structures. Extraembryonic tumors include choriocarcinoma, endodermal sinus tumor, and extraembryonal tumors. Embryonal tumors include embryonal carcinoma, polyembryoma, and teratomas that may be mature, immature, monodermal or highly specialized. Finally, it is important to recognize that germ cell tumors clinically behave in part on whether they are histologically pure, consisting of only one cell type, or mixed. Clinical behavior typically conforms to the most aggressive histologic subtype

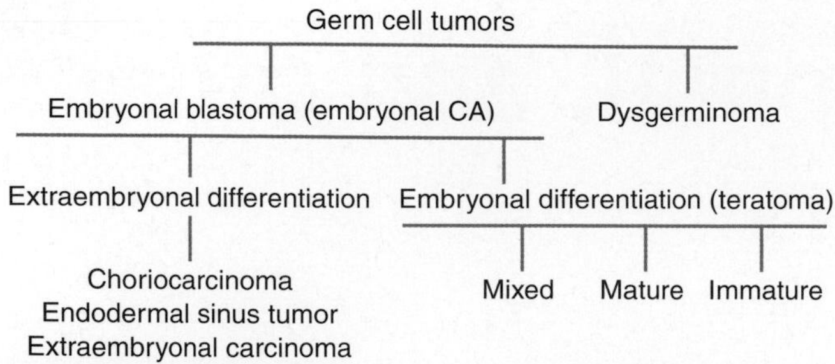

Figure 12–1 Classification schema of germ cell tumors of ovary.

Table 12–1 CLASSIFICATION OF GERM CELL NEOPLASMS OF THE OVARY

Germ cell tumors
- Dysgerminoma
- Endodermal sinus tumor
- Embryonal carcinoma
- Polyembryoma
- Choriocarcinomas
- Teratoma
  - Immature (solid, cystic, or both)
  - Mature
    - Solid
    - Cystic
      - Mature cystic teratoma (dermoid cyst)
      - Mature cystic teratoma (dermoid cyst) with malignant transformation
  - Monodermal or highly specialized
    - Struma ovarii
    - Carcinoid
    - Struma ovarii and carcinoid
    - Others
- Mixed forms (tumors composed of types A–F in any possible combination)

Tumors composed of germ cells and sex cord-stromal derivative
- Gonadoblastoma
- Mixed germ cell-sex cord-stromal tumor

Frequency ↓
- Acute abdominal pain
- Chronic abdominal pain
- Asymptomatic mass
- Abnormal vaginal bleeding
- Abdominal distention

Figure 12–2 Initial symptoms in young patients with malignant germ cell tumors.

Table 12–2 RELATIVE FREQUENCY OF OVARIAN NEOPLASMS

Type	%
Coelomic epithelium	50–70
Germ cell	15–20
Specialized gonadal stroma	5–10
Non-specific mesenchyme	5–10
Metastatic tumor	5–10

present in mixed tumors. Treatment therefore, should be predicated on this knowledge.

Clinical profile

Germ cell tumors represent a relatively small proportion (20%) of all ovarian tumors (Table 12–2) but are becoming increasingly important in the clinical practice of obstetrics and gynecology. Ninety-seven percent of these tumors are benign and only 3% are malignant. Asian and black ethnic groups are affected by malignant germ cell tumors three times as frequently as Caucasian women. Most of these neoplasms occur in young women, and extirpation of the disease involves decisions concerning childbearing and probabilities of recurrence. Recent developments in chemotherapy have dramatically changed the prognosis for many patients who develop more aggressive types of germ cell tumors. Knowledge of the classification of these lesions and how the pathologist arrives at the diagnosis, as well as the clinical significance of that diagnosis, has great practical value for the practicing obstetrician/gynecologist.

Most of these lesions are found in the second and third decades of life and are frequently diagnosed by finding a palpable abdominal mass, often associated with pain (Fig. 12–2). Except for the benign cystic teratoma, ovarian germ cell tumors are usually rapidly enlarging abdominal masses that often cause considerable abdominal pain. At times, the pain is exacerbated by rupture or torsion of the neoplasm. One of the classic initial signs of a dysgerminoma is hemoperitoneum from capsular rupture of the tumor as it rapidly enlarges, although this may occur with any germ cell tumor. Asymptomatic abdominal distension, fever, or vaginal bleeding are occasionally presenting complaints. Isosexual precocious puberty has been described, occurring in young patients whose tumors express human chorionic gonadotropin (hCG).

Because these tumors occur predominantly in the reproductive age group, it is not surprising that they are encountered commonly during pregnancy. Dysgerminomas and teratomas are the most common germ cell tumors diagnosed during pregnancy or after delivery. Surgical evaluation and treatment, including chemotherapy if necessary, can be safely performed in the second and third trimesters. Germ cell tumors are typically rapidly growing, unilateral tumors that present at an early stage (stage I). These tumors spread by direct extension, seeding of abdominal and pelvic peritoneal surfaces, and by hematogenous and lymphatic spread. Hematogenous spread to the lungs and liver parenchyma is more common in germ cell malignancies than in epithelial ovarian cancer, as is lymph node spread. Although there is not a known familial cancer syndrome for germ cell malignancies, there have been several isolated familial clusters of germ cell malignancies reported in the literature.

Many germ cell tumors produce serum markers that are specific and sensitive enough to be used clinically in following disease progression. A detailed discussion of individual tumor markers will be presented in the individual sections on specific tumor types.

Staging

Germ cell tumors should be staged surgically in the same manner as epithelial ovarian cancers, and in accordance with the International Federation of Gynecologists and Obstetrician (FIGO) guidelines. As surgical management and adjuvant therapy is predicated in part on stage of disease, accurate staging is essential. Proper staging procedures for germ cell tumors consists of a vertical midline incision, a sampling of ascitic fluid if present, cell washings, a careful exploration of the abdomen and pelvic cavity, and random staging biopsies of the omentum, paracolic gutters, pelvic sidewalls, cul de sac, vesicouterine reflection, and diaphragm. If extensive disease is present in the abdominal cavity, omentectomy and cytoreduction to optimal residual disease should be performed if possible. Pelvic and paraaortic lymph node sampling of suspicious nodes should be performed but a complete lymphadenectomy is not necessary. Bulky lymph nodes if present should be removed.

Treatment options

Surgery

The initial approach to patients with suspected germ cell tumors is surgical management for both diagnostic and therapeutic intent. The extent of primary surgery is dictated by the findings at surgery and the reproductive desires of the patient. If childbearing has been completed and future fertility is no longer a concern, then a bilateral salpingo-oophorectomy and hysterectomy are performed in addition to a full staging procedure. However, if preservation of fertility is desired, then every attempt should be made to perform a careful staging procedure followed by a unilateral salpingo-oophorectomy. The safety of such an approach has been well established in the literature. In select cases such as stage Ia dysgerminoma and stage Ia grade 1 immature teratoma, unilateral salpingo-oophorectomy is felt to be curative and is all that is required. All other cases will likely require adjuvant therapy. In all cases of apparent unilateral disease confined to the ovary, the contralateral ovary should be carefully evaluated. Although dysgerminoma is the only germ cell malignancy with a propensity for bilaterality (10–20% of cases), other histologic subtypes have occasionally involved both ovaries, so careful inspection is warranted. The contralateral ovary, if abnormal, should be biopsied or a cystectomy should be performed. If frozen section confirms a diagnosis of malignancy then the ovary should be removed. If the contralateral ovary appears normal, then it should be left alone. Some clinicians have advocated performing a wedge biopsy of a normal appearing contralateral ovary in cases of dysgerminoma to detect subclinical or microscopic disease. We recommend avoiding wedge biopsy of a normal appearing ovary because of the potential for surgical complications such as hemorrhage or adhesion formation that may impact future fertility.

The excellent response of germ cell malignancies to adjuvant chemotherapy has allowed a tailored approach to the surgical management of this disease in women desiring to preserve fertility. Although unilateral salpingo-oophorectomy should be considered the standard procedure in such cases, recently some clinicians have advocated ovarian cystectomy in select cases of immature teratoma. Beiner et al reviewed eight cases of immature teratoma (three grade 1, four grade 2, and one grade 3) treated with ovarian cystectomy. Five of the eight patients received postoperative adjuvant chemotherapy. There were no recurrences in 4.7 years of follow-up and three patients delivered a total of seven babies. The authors concluded that ovarian cystectomy with adjuvant chemotherapy appeared to be satisfactory therapy for early-stage immature teratoma if close follow-up was available, but that more studies were needed to evaluate cystectomy alone as a surgical management option. This management strategy, while exciting because of the potential for ovarian preservation, should be approached with caution, especially for other histologic germ cell subtypes which may not share the same prognosis as early stage immature teratoma.

Patients with bulk disease in the abdomen, pelvis, and retroperitoneum should be surgically cytoreduced to optimal residual disease if at all possible. Although there is not copious literature to support such a recommendation, what literature exists suggests a benefit for cytoreduction. In a Gynecologic Oncology Group (GOG) study by Slayton et al, patients with completely resected disease failed subsequent VAC (vincristine, dactinomycin, and cyclophosphamide) chemotherapy in 28% of the cases compared to 68% of cases with incomplete resection of disease. In the same study 82% of cases with bulky residual disease failed chemotherapy compared to 55% with minimal residual disease. Subsequently, the GOG published results showing that patients with clinically non-measurable disease after surgery that were treated with PVB (cisplatin, vinblastine, and bleomycin) remained progression free in 65% of cases compared to 34% of patients with measurable disease. Patients with optimal cytoreduction did better than those with unresectable bulky disease. This study helped establish the efficacy of cisplatin-based chemotherapy for germ cell tumors. Finally, Williams et al showed that patients with completely resected advanced stage (II and III) disease who were treated with cisplatin, etoposide, and bleomycin had similar tumor-free recurrence rates as those with disease limited to the ovary. These studies provide the bulk of evidence to support the thesis that cytoreduction of advanced stage disease is advantageous in germ cell cancers.

In patients with bulky metastatic disease, a normal appearing uterus and contralateral ovary may be preserved allowing for future fertility options if desired. Tangir et al reviewed 64 patients with germ cell malignancies treated with fertility preserving surgery. 10 patients were stage III (five IIIc, two IIIb, and three IIIa). Eight of the ten successfully conceived. Survival data was not included in the analysis. Zanetta et al evaluated 138 women with germ cell malignancies of all stages treated with fertility-sparing surgery, 81 of who received postoperative chemotherapy. Survival was comparable between patients treated with radical surgery and fertility-sparing surgery after a mean follow-up period of 67 months. Low et al retrospectively reviewed 74 patients with germ cell malignancies of all cell types treated with conservative surgery. Forty-seven patients were treated with adjuvant chemotherapy. Fifteen patients had stage III–IV disease. After 52 months of follow-up, patients with advanced disease had a 94% survival, comparable to historical survival rates.

The value of secondary cytoreduction procedures in patients with germ cell malignancies has not been studied. Given the sensitivity of these malignancies to combination chemotherapy regimens, it is highly likely that metastatic lesions will respond to subsequent chemotherapy, making the value of secondary cytoreduction questionable. Limited cytoreduction remains an effective management option for isolated lesions.

In summary, patients with germ cell malignancies should undergo operative evaluation, staging and management. If future fertility is not desired, surgical treatment should be identical to that for epithelial ovarian cancers. If preservation of fertility is desired, conservative management should be employed with conservation of the uterus and contralateral ovary and cytoreduction to optimal residual disease should be performed if possible. In spite of the success of surgical management, surgeons should recognize the excellent response of these tumors to chemotherapy when aggressive and potentially morbid resections of metastatic and retroperitoneal disease are considered.

Second-look laparotomy

The role of the second-look laparotomy (SLL) in epithelial carcinoma of the ovary is currently being debated. Experience with germ cell tumors of the ovary is even less well defined. Williams, when reporting the experience of the GOG, noted that in patients with complete tumor resection followed by BEP chemotherapy, 43 of 45 patients had no evidence of tumor or mature teratoma only at the time of the SLL, suggesting that there is no value of SLL in patients with completely resected disease. There were 72 patients with advanced incompletely resected tumors who received chemotherapy followed by SLL. Of 48 patients who did not have teratomatous lesions in their primary surgery, 45 had no tumor. The three patients who had persistent tumors died of their disease despite aggressive therapy. These authors think that the role of SLL is rarely, if ever, beneficial if the tumor is *almost* completely resected initially and followed by adequate chemotherapy. However, patients in this series who had incompletely resected tumors at initial surgery and had teratomatous elements present may have benefited from SLL. There were 24 patients who had teratomatous elements in the primary tumor and 16 who had progressive or bulky mature elements at SLL. Four patients had residual immature teratoma. Fourteen of the 16 with residual teratoma and 6 of the 7 with bulky disease remained tumor free after secondary cytoreduction. Therefore, the subgroup of patients that may have significant benefit from SLL are those with incompletely resected disease with teratomatous elements at primary surgery. Other authors in small series have suggested that there is a role for SLL, particularly in patients seen initially with advanced unresected disease. The use of advanced imaging technologies such as positron emission tomography (PET) and computed tomography (CT) imaging may further reduce the impact of SLL. Preliminary studies suggest positive and negative predictive values of 100% and 96% respectively for PET imaging in seminomas looking for residual disease after chemotherapy, suggesting the possibility of similar results for germ cell malignancies.

Radiation therapy

In the past, radiation therapy was traditionally employed as adjuvant therapy for patients with germ cell malignancies and dysgerminomas in particular. Historically, dysgerminomas have been extremely sensitive to radiation therapy with overall survival rates of between 70% and 100%. However, with the recent advances and success rates seen with combination chemotherapy, radiation therapy is rarely used today.

Chemotherapy

Tremendous advances have been made in the chemotherapeutic management of germ cell malignancies, such that current management strategies offer even advanced malignancies an excellent chance at long term control or cure. Historically, VAC was the first combination chemotherapy regimen widely used for treatment of these tumors. However, due to the success of cisplatin-based regimens in the treatment of testicular germ cell tumors combined with long-term survival of less than 50% in advanced stage or incompletely resected ovarian germ cell malignancies, VAC was gradually replaced by PVB. This transition resulted in an improvement in overall survival, however, failures still occurred even in patients with good prognosis at the conclusion of primary surgery.

Based on the success of etoposide therapy in testicular cancer, current combination platinum based chemotherapy for ovarian germ cell malignancies has evolved to the use of bleomycin, etoposide, and cisplatin (BEP). The GOG prospectively evaluated this regimen in women with stage I–III, completely resected, non-dysgerminoma germ cell malignancies given as three cycles of adjuvant chemotherapy.

Ninety-one of 93 patients were noted to be free of recurrence at follow-up, establishing this regimen as equivalent or superior to PVB. The toxicity profile in this series was acceptable. As a result of these findings, BEP has become the standard chemotherapeutic regimen for the adjuvant treatment of women with germ cell malignancies. Although successful, concern exists over potential long-term pulmonary toxicity of bleomycin and the risk of secondary malignancies associated with etoposide. Traditionally, cisplatin and etoposide are administered over 5 days while bleomycin is administered weekly. Recently Dimopoulos et al demonstrated safety and efficacy of outpatient BEP utilizing a lower dose of bleomycin administered over 3 days in women with early-stage, optimally debulked germ cell malignancies.

Controversy exists regarding the efficacy of high-dose cisplatin used in combination with etoposide and bleomycin (HDBEP). Several adult trials in testicular germ cell malignancies have suggested an improvement in efficacy compared to standard dose cisplatin, while other studies have not seen this association. These studies have not been replicated in adults with ovarian germ cell malignancies. Cushing et al, however, evaluated HDBEP in 74 pediatric patients with ovarian germ cell malignancies and found no difference in overall survival and increased toxicity with the HDBEP regimen. Currently, there is no established role of high-dose therapy in ovarian germ cell tumors.

Current management strategies for germ cell malignancies utilize chemotherapy in an adjuvant setting as well as to treat recurrent disease. Because approximately 20% of patients with germ cell malignancies treated with surgery alone will be expected to recur, and given the successful long term outcomes associated with BEP, all patients except those with stage Ia dysgerminoma and stage Ia grade 1 immature teratoma should be treated with adjuvant chemotherapy to reduce the risk of recurrent disease. Completely resected disease treated in this fashion can be cured nearly 100% of the time. Metastatic or incompletely resected tumors on the other hand, may fare worse but still have excellent long term survival rates and should be treated aggressively with adjuvant chemotherapy.

Recurrences in germ cell cancer

Even in cases of advanced stage disease, the majority of patients with germ cell malignancies are cured with a combination of primary surgery and adjuvant combination platinum based chemotherapy. All patients with germ cell malignancies, especially early stage disease treated with conservative therapy for curative intent, warrant close follow-up. Recurrences usually occur within two years of primary therapy. Patients with early stage dysgerminoma treated with salpingo-oophorectomy alone can be expected to recur in 15–25% of cases. For all germ cell malignancies, recurrences in many cases can be treated successfully. Recurrences after chemotherapy are defined as platinum resistant or platinum sensitive, a classification with clinical significance as platinum resistant disease is not thought to be curable. The group at the MD Anderson Hospital noted 42 primary therapy failures in 160 patients with germ cell tumors. Seventeen of these failures were treated with VAC chemotherapy. Using different chemotherapeutic regimens, 12 of 42 (29%) patients are currently disease free. Surgical debulking may have a role in the management of recurrences. In this study, 24 patients had surgery and 12 are alive, all with <2 cm of residual disease. None of the 7 patients with disease >2 cm residual survived.

Treatment toxicity

Given the favorable long-term outcomes associated with modern surgical management and combination platinum-based chemotherapy for women with germ cell malignancies, the long-term effects of treatment toxicity cannot be ignored. As many of these patients desire future fertility and undergo conservative surgery for their disease, meticulous surgical technique is essential to avoid future infertility related to surgically induced pelvic adhesive disease. Equally important is avoiding unnecessary hysterectomies and biopsies of normal-appearing contralateral ovaries. A thorough understanding of the natural history as well as management options of these tumors is essential. Women with fertility-sparing surgery can be expected to have preserved reproductive function. The long-term effect of combination chemotherapy in germ cell malignancies is less clear. Of particular concern is the risk of development of acute myelogenous leukemia (AML) associated with etoposide use. This risk appears to be dose and schedule dependent. AML has been rarely noted in patients receiving three cycles or less of etoposide, or cumulative doses of less than $2000 mg/m^2$. It is estimated that the risk of developing AML is 0.4% if these cutoff values are used. Leukemia, when it occurs, typically is seen within two to three years after treatment. Unlike in ovarian epithelial cancer where patients may not be expected to survive until the risk of developing AML is real, patients with germ cell malignancies are expected to survive well beyond the time period when AML usually occurs. In spite of this risk, an analysis of the risk:benefit ratio favors the use of etoposide in advanced germ cell malignancies, where one case of etoposide-induced AML would be expected to occur for every 20 patients cured. The long-term effects of chemotherapy on gonadal function appear to be minimal. Most younger patients can expect a return to normal ovarian function and reproductive potential. Although ovarian failure is a risk associated with chemotherapy, factors such as older age at treatment, higher drug doses and long duration of therapy appear to confer higher risk. There is a convincing body of literature to suggest that Gonadotropin-releasing hormone (GnRH)-agonists may be cytoprotective for primordial follicles when given during chemotherapy. In the setting of germ cell malignancies where younger age at diagnosis is the norm, these patients tolerate therapy quite well.

Dysgerminoma

Dysgerminoma is an uncommon tumor that accounts for 1–2% of primary ovarian neoplasms and for 3–5% of ovarian malignancies. It is the most common germ cell malignancy. Dysgerminoma may occur at any age from infancy to old age. Reported cases range between the ages of 7 months and 70 years, but most cases occur in adolescence and early adulthood (Fig. 12–3). They also present at a relatively early stage:

Stage Ia	65–75%
Stage Ib	10–15%
Stages II and III	15%
Stage IV	5%.

Dysgerminoma consists of germ cells that have not differentiated to form embryonic or extraembryonic structures (Fig. 12–4). The stroma is almost always infiltrated with lymphocytes and often contains granulomas similar to those of sarcoid. Occasionally, dysgerminoma contains isolated gonadotropin-producing syncytiotrophoblastic giant cells. An elevated serum lactate dehydrogenase or human chorionic gonadotropin (hCG) level may be present in these patients. Grossly, the tumor may be firm, fleshy, cream colored or pale tan; both its external and cut surfaces may be lobulated. A few dysgerminomas arise in sexually abnormal females, particularly those with pure (46XY) or mixed (45X,46XY) gonadal dysgenesis or testicular feminization (46XY). In such cases, the dysgerminoma often develops in a previously existing gonadoblastoma. The symptoms of dysgerminoma are not distinctive, and they are similar to those observed in patients with other solid ovarian neoplasms. The duration of symptoms is usually short; however, despite this, the tumor is often large, indicating rapid growth. The most common initial symptoms are abdominal enlargement and the presence of a mass in the lower abdomen. When the tumor is small and moves freely, its capsule is intact. Large lesions, however, may rupture or adhere to surrounding structures. Rupture can lead to peritoneal implantation, resulting in an increase in stage. In several cases, the tumor has been found incidentally at caesarean section or as a cause of dystocia. Dysgerminoma is one of the two most common malignant ovarian neoplasms observed in pregnancy, the other being serous cystadenocarcinoma of low malignant potential. The relatively common finding of dysgerminoma in pregnant patients is non-specific and relates to the age of the patient rather than to the pregnant state. Dysgerminoma may also be discovered incidentally in patients investigated for primary amenorrhea; in these cases, it is frequently associated with gonadal dysgenesis and a gonadoblastoma. Occasionally, menstrual and endocrine abnormalities may be the initial symptoms, but these symptoms tend to be more common in patients with dysgerminoma combined with other neoplastic germ cell elements—especially choriocarcinoma. Dysgerminoma is the only germ cell tumor in which the opposite ovary may be involved with the tumor process (10–20% of cases). Kurman reported a 20% incidence of disease in the serially sectioned normal appearing opposite ovary. Dysgerminomas are notable by their predilection for lymphatic spread and their acute sensitivity to irradiation and chemotherapy. Metastatic spread occurs via the lymphatic system; the lymph nodes in the vicinity of the common iliac arteries and the terminal part of the abdominal aorta are the first to be affected. Occasionally, there may be marked enlargement of these lymph nodes, with a mass evident on abdominal examination. The lesion can spread from these abdominal nodes to the mediastinal and supraclavicular nodes. Hematogenous spread to other organs occurs later. Any organ can be affected, although involvement of the liver, lungs, and bones is most common. Historically, surgery followed by radiation (in both early- and late-stage disease) has resulted in an excellent cure rate. More recently, the use of multiple-agent chemotherapy has been advocated and has produced equivalent results. In the young woman with a unilateral encapsulated dysgerminoma who is desirous of future childbearing, conservative management is indicated. In a review of the literature, more than 400 cases of dysgerminoma were reported. Seventy percent of patients were stage I at diagnosis and only 10% involved both ovaries. Because 85% of all patients with dysgerminomas are

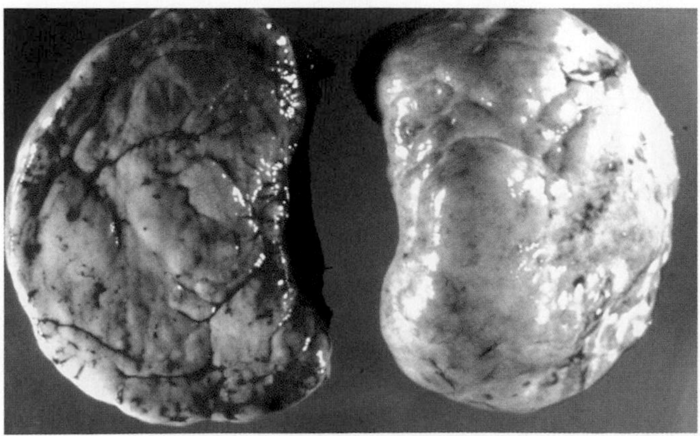

Figure 12–3 Large (25 cm) solid mass of the right ovary in a 16-year-old girl with stage Ia dysgerminoma.

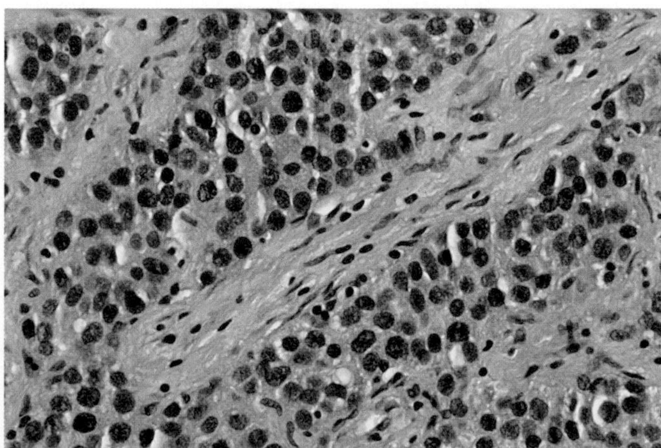

Figure 12–4 Dysgerminoma is characterized histologically by the presence of large, round, ovoid, or polygonal cells with stroma infiltrated by lymphocytes.

Table 12–3 RESULTS OF CONSERVATIVE AND NON-CONSERVATIVE SURGERY IN STAGE IA DYSGERMINOMA OF THE OVARY

	10-year survival	
	Conservative surgery	Non-conservative therapy†
Asadourian and Taylor	42/46 (91%)*	21/25 (84%)
Gordon et al	68/72 (94%)*	11/14 (79%)
Malkasian and Symmonds	23/27 (85%)*	13/14 (93%)
Total	133/145 (92%)*	45/53 (85%)

†Surgery plus radiation.
*Includes those salvaged after a recurrence (23/25–92%).

younger than 30 years, conservative therapy and preservation of fertility are major considerations. Conservative surgery without radiation in stage Ia lesions has resulted in excellent outcomes (Table 12–3). In patients in whom unilateral salpingo-oophorectomy is performed, careful inspection of the contralateral ovary and exploration to rule out disseminated disease is mandatory. Assessment of the retroperitoneal lymph nodes is an important part of the initial surgical therapy, because these neoplasms tend to spread to the lymph nodes, particularly to the high para-aortic nodes. Pelvic nodes on the same side as the primary tumor should also be evaluated through a retroperitoneal incision. Our routine is not to wedge or bivalve the opposite ovary if it has a normal size, shape, and consistency. These patients should be followed closely and have periodic examinations, because approximately 90% of recurrences appear in the first 2 years after initial therapy. Fortunately, most recurrences can be successfully eradicated by radiation therapy or chemotherapy. This knowledge permits the conservative management of patients. Recurrences can also appear in the opposite ovary, although this observation was noted after conservative surgery without careful staging surgery.

Several prognostic factors in dysgerminoma may be important, because they might influence conservative therapy in the early stage of disease. Some authors suggest that in patients with large tumors (>10 cm), there is a greater chance of a recurrence; therefore, adjuvant therapy should be given. Today, most agree that tumor size is not prognostically important and these patients do not require additional therapy. The long-term survival is almost 90% in patients who have stage I lesions. There is presently no good evidence that the behavior of an individual tumor can be assessed from its histologic appearance. Some authors consider patients older than 40 years or younger than 20 years to have a worsened prognosis, but this is not consistent in all studies. The presence of other germ cell elements definitely worsens prognosis.

Some recent series are reporting 100% survival with conservative surgery in stage Ia patients. These data strongly support an initial conservative approach with preservation of fertility. More extensive surgery and radiation therapy were not beneficial when patients had disease limited to one ovary. Schwartz reported 4 patients with metastasis to the contralateral ovary and preservation of that ovary with subsequent chemotherapy. All patients were alive and had no disease 14–56 months after diagnosis.

De Palo and associates reported on 56 patients who had pure dysgerminomas. In their study 44 patients underwent lymphangiography, and a positive study resulted in the restaging of 32% of patients. Diaphragmatic implants were not found in any patients, and positive cytologic findings were obtained in only three patients. The 5-year relapse-free survival rates were 91% in patients with stages Ia, Ib, and Ic; 74% in those with stage III retroperitoneal disease; and 24% in patients who had stage III peritoneal disease. Peritoneal involvement of any kind was associated with a poor prognosis if disease had extended to the abdominal cavity. All patients with stage III disease received postoperative radiation therapy.

Recurrences should be treated aggressively with re-exploration and tumor reduction. The removed tissue should be examined carefully for evidence of germ cell elements other than dysgerminoma. Some presumed recurrent dysgerminomas have been found to be mixed germ cell tumors and should be treated accordingly.

Although radiation therapy has been successful in treating dysgerminomas, more recently chemotherapy appears to have become the treatment of choice, as radiotherapy is associated with a high incidence of gonadal failure. The success rate of chemotherapy is as good as that of radiation, and preservation of fertility is possible in many patients, even those with bilateral ovarian disease. Weinblatt and Ortega reported on five children with extensive disease who were treated with chemotherapy as the primary therapeutic modality. Three of the five children were alive and free of disease at the time of the report, suggesting a therapeutic approach to extensive childhood dysgerminoma that spares pelvic and reproductive organs.

Chemotherapy is also being used more frequently with significant success in patients who have advanced disease. Dysgerminomas are typically very sensitive to platinum-based chemotherapy and most patients treated with combination platinum-based chemotherapy will be complete responders. Bianchi and associates reported 18 patients (6 patients with stage Ib or c and 12 patients with stage IIb, III, IV, or recurrent disease) who were treated with doxorubicin and cyclophosphamide or cisplatin, vinblastine, and bleomycin. Doxorubicin and cyclophosphamide were highly effective: 7 of 10 patients were disease-free; two of three relapsing patients were saved with cisplatin, vinblastine, and bleomycin (VBP) therapy. Of the eight patients treated with VBP, one had a recurrence in the brain and was saved with radiation therapy. Four patients who had no residual disease in the remaining ovary or in the uterus are all free of disease, and one patient has had a successful pregnancy. The optimal drug combination has not yet been determined. Because bleomycin can cause pulmonary fibrosis with resultant death, the drug is being used less frequently. Etoposide also appears to be an effective drug in the treatment of dysgerminomas. More recently, patients with advanced disease have received multiple-agent chemotherapy with results equal to or better than results for those treated with radiation. Complete responses in the 80–100% range are being reported in patients with stage II–IV disease. This is not surprising—the cure rates for stage III dysgerminomas treated with effective chemotherapy are >90%. Today, chemotherapy appears to be the treatment of choice after surgery in patients with advanced disease. The common association of dysgerminoma with gonadoblastoma, a tumor that almost always occurs in patients with dysgenetic gonads, indicates that there is a relationship between dysgerminoma and genetic and somatosexual abnormalities. Patients with these genetic abnormalities should be offered gonadectomy after puberty to prevent the development of gonadoblastoma or dysgerminoma. Phenotypically normal females suspected of having a dysgerminoma should be evaluated with a karyotype, especially if ovarian conservation is desired. Patients with pathology reports that reveal streak gonads or gonadoblastomas should also be karyotyped. If a Y chromosome is present, the retained contralateral ovary should be removed to prevent neoplasia. As stated earlier, the treatment of the usual patient with dysgerminoma should be conservative if possible. Historically, the treatment of patients with dysgerminoma associated with gonadoblastoma is radical because of the frequent occurrence of bilateral tumors and the absence of normal gonadal function. Investigation of the genotypes and karyotypes of all patients with this neoplasm is recommended by some, especially if any history of virilization or other developmental abnormalities is elicited. In vitro fertilization (IVF) can be utilized in patients without gonads. Therefore, it may be prudent to preserve the uterus in patients in whom the ovaries must be removed. In most cases, we leave the uterus. This may be particularly important in prepubertal patients, because in these patients other signs of abnormal function (e.g., primary amenorrhea, virilization, and absence of normal sexual development) are lacking.

Often lesions that consist primarily of dysgerminoma elements contain small areas of more malignant histology (e.g., embryonal carcinoma or endodermal sinus tumor). If tumor markers such as α-fetoprotein (AFP) or hCG are elevated, a strong suspicion of mixed lesions should be entertained. When the dysgerminoma is not pure and these more malignant components are present, the prognosis and therapy are determined by the more malignant germ cell elements, and the dysgerminoma component is disregarded.

Endodermal sinus tumor (yolk sac tumor)

Endodermal sinus tumors are the second most common form of malignant germ cell tumors of the ovary, accounting for 22% of germ cell lesions in one large series. The median age of the patient is 19 years. Three-fourths of the patients are initially seen with a combination of abdominal pain and abdominal or pelvic mass. Acute symptoms are typically caused by torsion of the tumor, and may lead to the diagnosis of acute appendicitis or a ruptured ectopic pregnancy. These yolk sac tumors are almost always unilateral. The tumor is usually large with most tumors measuring between 10 and 30 cm. On the cut surface, they appear gray yellow with areas of hemorrhage and cystic, gelatinous changes.

These neoplasms are highly malignant; they metastasize early and invade the surrounding structures. Intra-abdominal spread leads to extensive involvement of abdominal structures with tumor deposits. Metastases also occur via the lymphatic system. α-fetoprotein (AFP) levels are often elevated in this group of tumors. Endodermal sinus tumors are characterized by extremely rapid growth and extensive intra-abdominal spread; almost half the patients seen by a physician complain of symptoms of 1 week's duration or less.

Schiller called these neoplasms *mesonephroma*, but most pathologists now consider them to be various germ cell tumors that are unrelated to the mesonephros. The tumors were thought to originate from germ cells that differentiate into the extra embryonal yolk sac, because the tumor structure is similar to that found in the endodermal sinuses of the rat yolk sac. The tumors consist of scattered tubules or spaces lined by single layers of flattened cuboidal cells, loose reticular stroma, numerous scattered para-aminosalicylic-positive globules, and, within some spaces or clefts, a characteristic invaginated papillary structure with a central blood vessel (Schiller–Duval body) (Fig. 12–5).

Historically, the prognosis for patients with endodermal sinus tumor of the ovary has been unfavorable. Most patients have died of the disease within 12–18 months of diagnosis. Until multiple-agent chemotherapy was developed, there were only a few known 5-year survivors. Most of these patients had tumors confined to the ovary. In several cases, the tumor consisted of endodermal sinus tumors admixed with other neoplastic germ cell elements, frequently dysgerminoma. The clinical course in most patients with tumors composed of endodermal sinus tumor associated with dysgerminoma or other neoplastic germ cell elements does not differ greatly from that in patients with pure endodermal sinus tumors. Frequently, intracellular and extracellular hyaline droplets that represent deposits of AFP can be identified throughout the tumor. Mixed germ cell lesions often contain endodermal sinus tumors as one of the types present.

In the past, the treatment of patients with endodermal sinus tumor of the ovary has been frustrating. Kurman and Norris reported no long-term survivors in 17 patients with stage I tumors who were receiving adjunctive radiation or single alkylating agent, dactinomycin, or methotrexate. Gallion reviewed the literature in 1979 and found that only 27% of 96 patients with stage I endodermal sinus tumors were alive at 2 years. The tumor is not sensitive to radiation therapy, although there may be an initial response. Optimal surgical extirpation of the disease has been advocated, but this alone is unsuccessful in producing

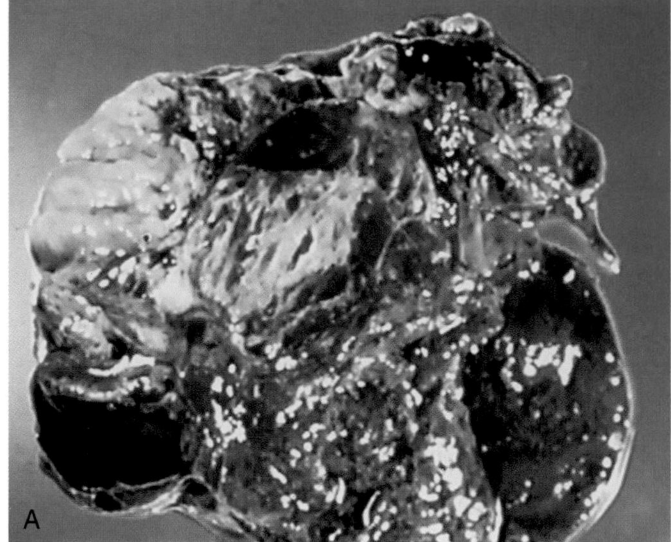
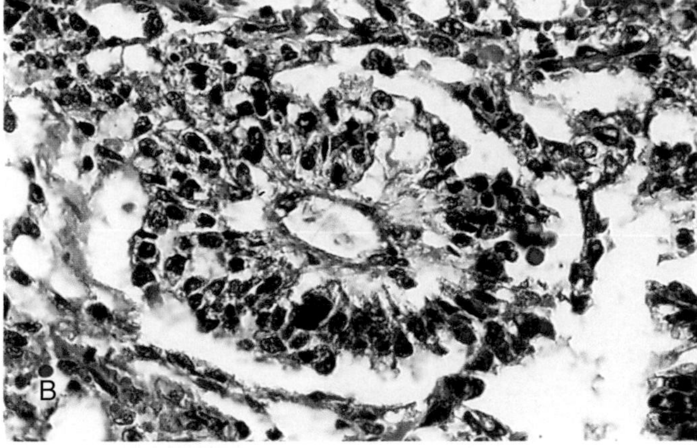

Figure 12–5 Endodermal sinus tumor. *A*, Gross appearance with areas of hemorrhage and gelatinous necrosis. *B*, Microscopic appearance with isolated papillary projections containing single blood vessels and having peripheral lining of neoplastic cells (Schiller–Duval body).

Table 12–4 VAC, VBP, AND BEP REGIMENS

Regimen	Dosage schedule
VAC	
Vincristine, 1.5 mg/m^2 (maximum dose 2.5 mg)	Weekly IV administration for 12 weeks
Dactinomycin, 0.5 mg	5-day IV course every 4 weeks
Cyclophosphamide, 5–7 mg/kg	5-day IV course every 4 weeks
VBP	
Vinblastine, 12 mg/m^2	IV every 3 weeks for 4 courses
Bleomycin, 20 U/m^2 (maximum dose 30 U/m^2)	IV weekly for 7 courses; eighth course given in week 10
Cisplatin, 20 mg/m^2	Daily × 5 every 3 weeks for 3–4 courses
BEP	
Bleomycin, 20 U/m^2 (maximum dose 30 U)	IV weekly × 9
Etoposide, 100 mg/m^2	IV days 1–5 q 3 weeks × 3
Cisplatin, 20 mg/m^2	IV days 1–5 q 3 weeks × 3

BEP, bleomycin, etoposide, cisplatin; VAC, vincristine, actinomycin D (dactinomycin), cyclophosphamide; VBP, vinblastine, bleomycin, cisplatin.

a significant number of cures. In later years, there have been optimistic reports of sustained remissions in some patients treated by surgery and multiple-agent chemotherapy. The Gynecologic Oncology Group (GOG) used VAC chemotherapy to treat 24 patients who had pure endodermal sinus tumors (EST) that were completely resected and 7 whose diseases were partially resected. Of 31 patients, 15 (48%) failed, including 11 of 24 (46%) who had complete resection. Of 15 patients with mixed germ cell tumors containing EST elements treated with VAC, 8 (53%) failed. Subsequently, the GOG treated 48 patients with stages I–III completely resected endodermal sinus tumors with VAC for six to nine courses. Thirty-five (73%) patients were free of disease with a median follow-up time of 4 years. More recently, 21 similar patients were treated with bleomycin, etoposide, and cisplatin (BEP). The first nine patients showed no evidence of disease. BEP therapy was given for three courses over 9 weeks. Gershenson and associates reported that 18 of 26 (69%) patients with pure EST were free of tumors after VAC therapy. Gallion and associates reported 17 of 25 (68%) patients with stage I disease who were alive and well 2 years or more after treatment with VAC. Sessa and associates treated 13 patients with pure EST of the ovary, 12 of whom had initial unilateral oophorectomy. All received VBP and are alive at 20 months to 6 years (Table 12–4). Three patients had a relapse but were saved. This experience is important, because nine of these patients had stage IIb or more advanced disease.

Schwartz and colleagues have used VAC for stage I disease but prefer VBP for stage II–IV patients. Of 15 patients, 12 are alive and have no evidence of disease. Their routine is to treat at least one course beyond a normal AFP titer (this has become routine in many centers). One recurrence was treated successfully with BEP. Two early VAC failures were not saved with VBP. The GOG evaluated VBP in stage III and IV and in recurrent malignant germ cell tumors, many with measurable disease after surgery. Sixteen of 29 (55%) ESTs were long-term disease-free survivors. VBP induced a substantial number of durable complete responses, even in patients with prior chemotherapy. Toxicity was significant. Although a second-look laparotomy was part of this protocol, not all patients underwent (for various reasons) second-look surgery. Smith and colleagues reported three patients whose diseases were resistant to methotrexate, actinomycin D and cyclophosphamide (MAC) and VBP and who had complete remission with regimens that contained VP-16 and cisplatin. All patients have remained free of tumor for 4 years or more. Williams noted that in disseminated germ cell tumors (primarily of the testes), BEP was more effective and had less neuromuscular toxicity than had VBP. Williams also reported the GOG experience with 93 patients who were given BEP postoperatively in an adjuvant setting for malignant germ cell cancers of the ovary. Forty-two were immature teratomas, whereas 25 were endodermal sinus tumors and 24 were mixed germ cell tumors. At the time of Williams' report, 91 of 93 had no evidence of disease (NED) after three courses of BEP with a median follow-up of 39 months. One patient developed acute myelomonocytic leukemia 22 months after diagnosis, and a second patient developed lymphoma 69 months after treatment.

Dimopoulos reported a similar result from the Hellenic Cooperative Oncology Group. Forty patients with nondysgerminomatous tumors were treated with BEP or PVB. With a median follow-up of 39 months, five patients developed progressive disease and died. Only one of the five who failed received BEP.

From Japan, Fujita reported 41 patients with endodermal sinus tumors, either pure or mixed. Although this covered a long time interval (1965–1992), 21 patients were treated surgically with unilateral oophorectomy. More aggressive surgery did not increase survival. Survival was similar whether VAC or PBV were used. All stage I patients given either VAC or PBV following surgery survived without evidence of recurrence.

From a practical point of view, serum AFP determination is considered to be a useful diagnostic tool in patients who have endodermal sinus tumors and should be considered an ideal tumor marker. It can be useful when monitoring the results of therapy and for detecting metastasis and recurrences after therapy. As noted earlier, many investigators use AFP as a guide to the number of courses needed for an individual patient. In many cases, only three or four courses have placed patients into remission with long-term survival. Conservative surgery plus chemotherapy have resulted in an appreciable number of successful pregnancies after treatment. Curtin has, nevertheless, reported two patients with normal AFPs but positive second-look laparotomies, although this finding currently must be considered the exception. Reports suggest that there may be recurrences in the retroperitoneal nodes in the absence of recognizable intraperitoneal disease.

Levels of hCG and its β subunit (β-hCG) have been found to be normal in patients with endodermal sinus tumor.

Embryonal carcinoma

Embryonal carcinoma is one of the most malignant cancers arising in the ovary (Fig. 12–6). The neoplasm closely resembles the embryonal carcinoma of the adult testes, a relatively common tumor. However, it represents only 4% of malignant ovarian germ cell tumors in the ovary, and its confusion with choriocarcinoma and endodermal sinus tumors in the past accounts for its late identification as a distinct entity. It usually manifests as an abdominal mass or pelvic mass occurring at a mean age of 15 years. More than half of the patients have hormonal abnormalities, including

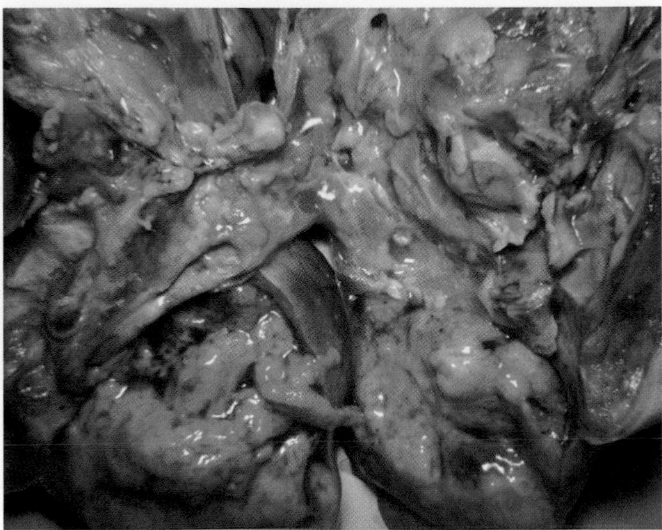

Figure 12–6 Gross photograph of embryonal carcinoma of the ovary.

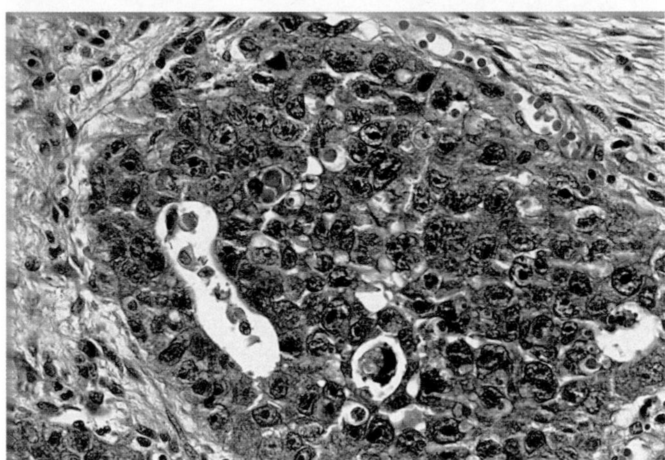

Figure 12–7 Microscopic appearance of large primitive cells with occasional papillary or gland-like formations characteristic of embryonal carcinoma.

precocious puberty, irregular uterine bleeding, amenorrhea, or hirsutism. The tumors consist of large primitive cells with occasional papillary or gland-like formations (Fig. 12–7). The cells have eosinophilic cytoplasm with distinct borders and round nuclei with prominent nucleoli. Numerous mitotic figures, many atypical, are seen; scattered throughout the tumor are multinucleated giant cells that resemble syncytial cells.

These tumors secrete hCG from syncytiotrophoblast-like cells and AFP from large primitive cells and these tumor markers can be used to monitor progress during therapy. This tumor probably arises from primordial germ cells, but it develops before there is much further differentiation toward either embryonic or extraembryonic tissue. In a review of 15 patients, Kurman and Norris reported an actuarial survival rate of 30% for the entire group; for those with stage I tumors, the survival rate was 50% (Table 12–5). This result is significantly better than survival with the endodermal sinus tumor for the same period of time

Table 12–5 COMPARISON OF EMBRYONAL CARCINOMA WITH ENDODERMAL SINUS TUMOR

	Endodermal sinus tumor (71 cases)	Embryonal carcinoma (15 cases)
Median age	19 years	15 years
Prepubertal status	23%	47%
Precocious puberty	0	43%
Positive pregnancy test	None (0/15)	All (9/9)
Vaginal bleeding	1%	33%
Amenorrhea	0	7%
Hirsutism	0	7%
Survival, stage I patients	16%	50%
Human chorionic gonadotrophin	Negative (0/15)	Positive (10/10)
α-Fetoprotein	Positive (15/15)	Positive (7/10)

From Kurman RJ, Norris HJ: Endodermal sinus tumor of the ovary: a clinical and pathological analysis of 71 cases. Cancer 38:2404, 1976.

and before the advent of vigorous multiple-agent adjuvant chemotherapy. With modern therapy, survival rates should be greatly improved. Optimal therapy, although not yet established, is probably similar to that for endodermal sinus tumor.

The VAC regimen is definitely active in this disease but does not appear to be as reliable for advanced cases as the VBP regimen. It is suggested that patients receiving VAC be watched closely for progression of disease, and the more toxic VBP regimen can be used at that point in the hope of salvage. The total number of courses of VAC therapy needed to achieve optimal numbers of disease-free patients is really not known.

The GOG has evaluated the effectiveness of the VBP regimen in stages III and IV recurrent malignant germ cell tumors of the ovary, including embryonal carcinoma. Ninety-four patients have been treated, and this therapy has produced a substantial number of durable complete responses in patients who previously received chemotherapy. The overall progression-free interval at 24 months is approximately 55%. The GOG is currently evaluating BEP in this group of patients.

Polyembryoma

Polyembryoma is a rare ovarian germ cell neoplasm that consists of numerous embryoid bodies resembling morphologically normal embryos. Similar homologous neoplasms occur more frequently in the human testes. To date, only a few ovarian polyembryomas have been reported. In most cases, the polyembryoma has been associated with other neoplastic germ cell elements, mainly the immature teratoma. Polyembryoma is a highly malignant germ cell neoplasm. It is usually associated with invasion of adjacent structures and organs and extensive metastases that are mainly confined to the abdominal cavity. The tumor is not sensitive to radiotherapy, and its response to chemotherapy is unknown.

Choriocarcinoma

Choriocarcinoma, which is a rare, highly malignant tumor that may be associated with sexual precocity, can arise in one of three ways:

1. as a primary gestational choriocarcinoma associated with ovarian pregnancy;
2. as a metastatic choriocarcinoma from a primary gestational choriocarcinoma arising in other parts of the genital tract, mainly the uterus; and
3. as a germ cell tumor differentiating in the direction of trophoblastic structures and arising admixed with other neoplastic germ cell elements.

Choriocarcinomas of the ovary may also be divided into two broad groups:

1. gestational choriocarcinoma, encompassing the first two groups mentioned above; and
2. non-gestational choriocarcinoma, a germ cell tumor that differentiates toward trophoblastic structures.

The presence of paternal DNA on analysis distinguishes gestational from non-gestational choriocarcinoma. Only non-gestational choriocarcinoma of the ovary are discussed here. In most cases, the tumor is admixed with other neoplastic germ cell elements, and their presence is diagnostic of non-gestational choriocarcinoma, except for the remote possibility of the tumor being a gestational choriocarcinoma metastatic to an ovarian germ cell tumor. The tumor, in common with other malignant germ cell neoplasms, occurs in children and young adults. Its occurrence in children has been emphasized; in some series, 50% of cases occurred in prepubescent children. This high incidence in children may result from the previous reluctance of investigators to make the diagnosis in adults.

These neoplasms secrete hCG. This is particularly noticeable in prepubescent children, who show evidence of isosexual precocious puberty with mammary development, growth of pubic and axillary hair, and uterine bleeding. Adult patients may have signs of ectopic pregnancies, because the non-gestational choriocarcinoma, like its gestational counterpart, is associated with an increased production of hCG. Estimation of urinary or plasma hCG levels is a useful diagnostic test in these cases. Historically, the prognosis of patients with choriocarcinoma of the ovary was unfavorable, but modern chemotherapy regimens appear to be effective. Creasman and associates in four cases using the MAC combination chemotherapy have achieved prolonged remissions. Some responses have been seen with combination chemotherapy using methotrexate as one of the drugs in the regimen. In most instances, the other drugs used in the combinations have been dactinomycin and an alkylating agent.

Mixed germ cell tumors

Mixed germ cell tumors contain at least two malignant germ cell elements. Dysgerminoma is the most common component (80% in Kurman and Norris' report and 69% in material from the MD Anderson Hospital). Immature teratoma and EST are also frequently identified; embryonal carcinoma and choriocarcinoma are seen only occasionally. It is not unusual to see three or four different germ cell components. In 42 patients treated at the MD Anderson Hospital, 9 patients were treated with surgery alone, and another 6 patients received radiation therapy; all developed recurrences. Of 17 patients who received VAC, 9 patients were placed into remission. Five patients received primary treatment of VBP after surgery, and 4 patients are alive and well. Of the original 42 patients, 20 patients (48%) are alive and well. Eleven patients underwent second-look laparotomies after various chemotherapeutic courses, and all had negative results. Of 14 patients who had stage I disease and were treated with combination chemotherapy after surgery, 11 (79%) survived. Creasman and colleagues treated five stage I lesions with MAC chemotherapy for three courses or fewer. Three patients also received pelvic radiation, and all five were long-term survivors. The GOG treated 10 completely resected mixed germ cell tumors with VAC, and 7 are long-term survivors. Four of five patients who had incompletely resected disease and who were treated with VAC developed recurrences. Schwartz treated eight patients with mixed tumors with VAC; seven patients are long-term survivors. Only one patient did not respond to PVB therapy. Because the most significant component of mixed tumors usually predicts results, it should determine therapy and follow-up.

Teratoma

Mature cystic teratoma

Accounting for more than 95% of all ovarian teratomas, the dermoid cyst, or mature cystic teratoma, is one of the most common ovarian neoplasms. Teratomas account for approximately 15% of all ovarian tumors. They are the most common ovarian tumors in women in the second and third decades of life. Fortunately, most benign cystic lesions contain mature tissue of ectodermal, mesodermal, or endodermal origin. The most common elements are ectodermal derivatives such as skin, hair follicles, and sebaceous or sweat glands, accounting for the characteristic histologic and gross appearance of teratomas (Fig. 12–8). These tumors are usually multicystic and contain hair intermixed with foul-smelling, sticky, keratinous and sebaceous debris.

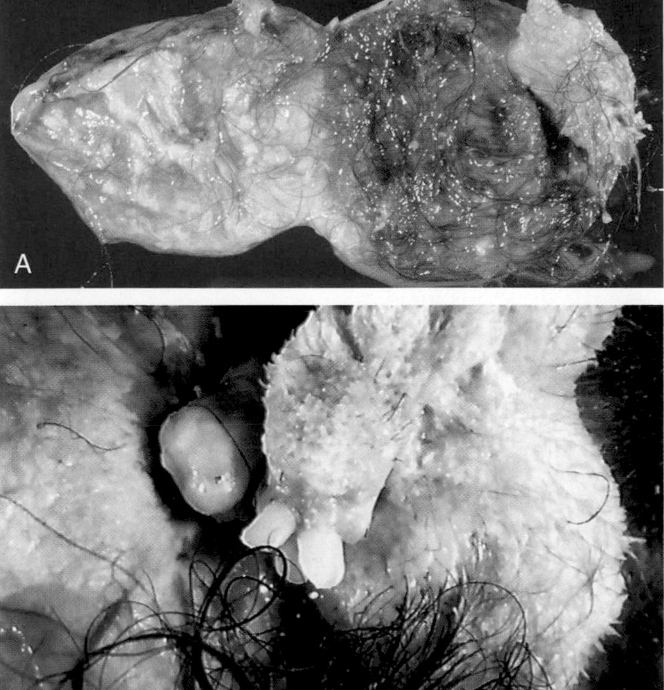

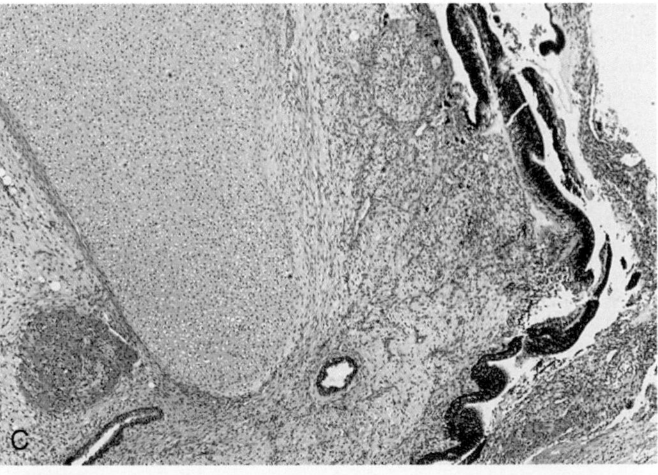

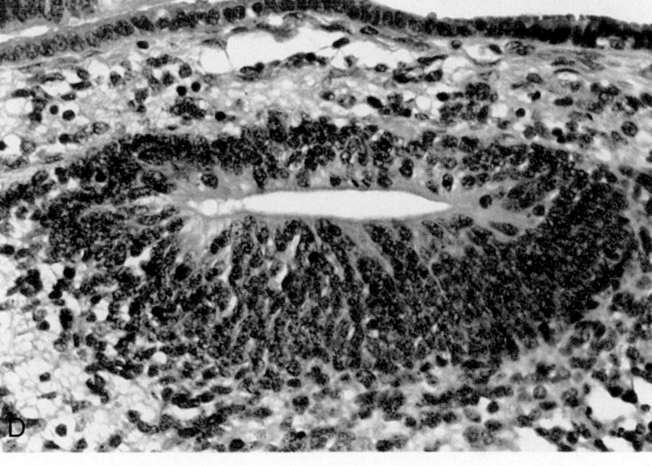

Figure 12–8 Benign cystic teratoma. *A* and *B*, Gross appearance. Benign cystic teratoma. *C*, Microscopic view of ectodermal elements (skin and skin appendages). *D*, Immature neural elements evident.

Occasionally, well-formed teeth are seen along with cartilage or bone. If the tumor consists of only ectodermal derivatives of skin and skin appendages, it is a true dermoid cyst. A mixture of other, usually mature tissues (gastrointestinal, respiratory) may be present.

The clinical manifestation of this slow-growing lesion is usually related to its size, compression, torsion, or to a chemical peritonitis secondary to intra-abdominal spill of the cholesterol-laden debris. The latter event tends to occur more commonly when the tumor is large. Torsion is the most frequent complication, observed in as many as 16% of the cases in one large series, and it tends to be more common during pregnancy and the puerperium. Mature cystic teratomas are said to comprise 22–40% of ovarian tumors in pregnancy, and 0.8–12.8% of reported cases of mature cystic teratomas have occurred in pregnancy. In general, torsion is more common in children and younger patients. Severe acute abdominal pain is usually the initial symptom, and the condition is considered to be an acute abdominal emergency. Rupture of a mature cystic teratoma is an uncommon complication, occurring in approximately 1% of cases, but it is much more common during pregnancy and may manifest during labor. The immediate result of rupture may be shock or hemorrhage, especially during pregnancy or labor, but the prognosis even in these cases is favorable. Rupture of the tumor into the peritoneal cavity may be followed by a chemical peritonitis caused by the spill of the contents of the tumor. This may result in a marked granulomatous reaction and lead to the formation of dense adhesions throughout the peritoneal cavity. Infection is an uncommon complication of mature cystic teratoma and occurs in approximately 1% of cases. The infecting organism is usually a coliform, but *Salmonella* species infection causing typhoid fever has also been reported. Removal of the neoplasm by ovarian cystectomy or, rarely, oophorectomy appears to be adequate therapy. Malignant degeneration of mature teratomas is a rare occurrence. When it occurs the most common secondary tumor is a squamous cell carcinoma. Prognosis and behavior of this secondary malignancy is similar to squamous cell cancers arising in other anatomic sites.

Mature solid teratoma

Mature solid teratoma is a rare ovarian neoplasm and a very uncommon type of ovarian teratoma. The histologic components in a mixed solid teratoma are similar to those found in an immature solid teratoma, which occurs mainly in children and young adults. The presence of immature elements immediately excludes the tumor from this group; by definition, only tumors composed entirely of mature tissues may be included. The tumor is usually unilateral and is adequately treated by unilateral oophorectomy. Although this neoplasm is considered benign, mature solid teratomas may be associated occasionally with peritoneal implants that consist entirely of mature glial tissue. Despite the extensive involvement that may be present, the prognosis is excellent.

Immature teratoma

Immature teratomas consist of tissue derived from the three germ layers—ectoderm, mesoderm, and endoderm—and, in contrast to the much more common mature teratoma, they contain immature or embryonal structures. These tumors have had a variety of names: solid teratoma, malignant teratoma, teratoblastoma, teratocarcinoma, and embryonal teratoma. These names have arisen because immature teratomas have been incorrectly considered mixed germ cell tumors or secondary malignant tumors originating in mature benign teratomas. Mature tissues are frequently present and sometimes may predominate. Immature teratoma of the ovary is an uncommon tumor, comprising less than 1% of ovarian teratomas. In contrast to the mature cystic teratoma, which is encountered most frequently during the reproductive years but occurs at all ages, the immature teratoma has a specific age incidence, occurring most commonly in the first two decades of life and almost unknown after menopause. By definition, an immature teratoma contains immature neural elements. According to Norris and associates, the quantity of immature neural tissue alone determines the grade. Neuroblastomatous elements, glial tissue, and immature cerebellar and cortical tissue may also be seen. These tumors are graded histologically on the basis of the amount and degree of cellular immaturity. The range is from grade 1 (mature teratoma containing only rare immature foci) through grade 3 (large portions of the tumor consist of embryonal tissue with atypicality and mitotic activity). Generally, older patients tend to have lower grade primary tumors compared with younger patients. When the neoplasm is solid and all elements are well differentiated histologically (solid mature teratoma), a grade 0 designation is given (Table 12–6).

Table 12–6 IMMATURE TERATOMA GRADING SYSTEM

Grade	Thurlbeck and Scully	Norris et al
0	All cells well differentiated	All tissue mature; rare mitotic activity
1	Cells well differentiated; rare small foci of embryonal tissue	Some immaturity and neuroepithelium limited to low magnification field in any slide (× 40)
2	Moderate quantities of embryonal tissue; atypia and mitosis present	Immaturity and neuroepithelium does not exceed 3 low-power microscopic fields in any one slide
3	Large quantities of embryonal tissue; atypia and mitosis present	Immaturity and neuroepithelium occupying 4 or more low magnification fields on a single slide

Table 12–7 IMMATURE (MALIGNANT) TERATOMAS

Grade	No.	Tumor deaths (%)
1	22	4 (18)
2	24	9 (37)
3	10	7 (70)

From Norris HJ, Zirkin HJ, Benson WL: Immature (malignant) teratoma of the ovary; a clinical and pathological study of 58 cases. Cancer 37:2356, 1976.

Immature teratomas are almost never bilateral, although occasionally a benign teratoma is found in the opposite ovary. These tumors may have multiple peritoneal implants at the time of initial surgery, and the prognosis is closely correlated with the histologic grade of the primary tumor and the implants. Norris and coworkers studied 58 patients with immature teratomas and reported an 82% survival rate for patients who had grade 1 primary lesions, 63% for grade 2, and 30% for grade 3 (Table 12–7). These results antedate the use of multiple-agent chemotherapy.

Multiple sections of the primary lesion and wide sampling of the peritoneal implants are necessary to properly grade the tumor. In most cases, the implants are better differentiated than the primary tumors. Both the primary lesion and the implants should be graded according to the most immature tissue present. Patients with mature glial implants have an excellent prognosis; immature implants however, do not.

To date, the histologic grade and fertility desires of the patient have been the determining factors regarding extent of surgical therapy and subsequent adjuvant therapy. Because the lesion is rarely bilateral in its ovarian involvement, the present method of therapy consists of unilateral salpingo-oophorectomy with wide sampling of peritoneal implants. Total abdominal hysterectomy with bilateral salpingo-oophorectomy does not seem to be indicated, because it does not influence the outcome for the patient. Although some authors have advocated cystectomy alone for early stage, low-grade disease, this management strategy should be approached with caution. Radiotherapy has also been shown to have little value. If the primary tumor is grade 1 and all peritoneal implants (if they exist) are grade 0, no further therapy is recommended. However, if the primary tumor is grade 2 or 3 or if implants or recurrences are grade 1, 2, or 3, triple-agent chemotherapy has been shown to be helpful. The recommendation to use adjuvant chemotherapy in high-grade stage I disease is based on studies performed before meticulous surgical staging of germ cell malignancies was routine. Cushing et al evaluated surgical therapy alone in 44 pediatric and adolescent patients under the age of 15 who had completely resected immature teratomas of all grades. Thirty-one patients had pure immature teratomas, and 13 patients had immature teratomas with microscopic endodermal sinus tumor foci. The 4-year event-free and overall survival for both groups was 97% and 100% respectively. The only endodermal sinus tumor failure was salvaged with subsequent chemotherapy. The authors concluded that surgery alone was curative for most children and adolescents with completely resected ovarian immature teratomas of any grade, and advocated avoiding adjuvant chemotherapy in this group. The VAC regimen has proved to be highly effective. DiSaia and associates have reported on several patients with disseminated disease treated with this chemotherapeutic regimen. At second-look laparotomy these patients were free of immature elements but retained peritoneal implants containing exclusively mature elements. This was labeled chemotherapeutic retroconversion of immature teratoma of the ovary, and is a similar if not identical syndrome as the "growing teratoma syndrome" described in testicular non-seminomatous germ cell tumors All these patients have had uneventful follow-ups with the mature implants apparently remaining in static states. Apparently this is a common occurrence.

Experience with the treatment of 25 patients (mean age of 19 years at diagnosis) with immature teratomas of the ovary was reported by Curry and colleagues. In their study, four patients received postoperative external radiation therapy to the pelvis or abdomen, either alone or with a single chemotherapeutic agent; two patients were treated with postoperative single-agent chemotherapy; and two patients had no treatment other than surgical removal of the tumors. All eight patients died of their disease; the longest survival time was 40 months, and six of the eight patients survived for less than 12 months after the initial treatment. Five patients received postoperative combination chemotherapy with MAC or ActFUCy. Two patients were still alive at 73 and 50 months after the initiation of chemotherapy. The combination of vincristine (1.5 mg/m^2), dactinomycin (0.5 mg), and cyclophosphamide (500 mg) (VAC) was administered to 12 patients. The drugs were administered intravenously every week for 12 consecutive weeks, and then a 5-day intravenous course was given every 4 weeks for 2 years. At the time of their report, all of the 10 patients who initially responded were surviving 16 to 28 months after the initiation of chemotherapy. Of the 12 patients, one patient died at 3 months and another patient died at 26 months.

The GOG treated 20 completely resected immature teratomas with VAC. Only one patient failed, and she was treated primarily at the time of recurrence. Of eight advanced or recurrent lesions that were incompletely resected, only four responded to VAC. The group at the MD Anderson Hospital reported that 15 of 18 patients (83%) with immature teratomas had sustained remission with primary VAC chemotherapy. VBP has been used by the GOG in patients with advanced or recurrent immature teratomas. They treated 26 patients, of whom 14 (54%) were disease-free survivors. Creasman treated six patients who had immature teratomas with MAC, and all are long-term survivors. Schwartz usually treats stage I patients with six cycles of VAC. Those with more advanced disease were given 12 cycles and a second-look operation. Of 29 patients, 24 were successfully treated. Four of the five patients with persistent lesions were successfully saved.

Today, most investigators treat stage Ia grade 1 immature teratomas with unilateral oophorectomy alone. Patients with stage Ia grade 2 or 3, as well as more advanced lesions, are treated postsurgically with VAC. Three courses appear to be as effective as longer chemotherapy regimens, particularly in patients with completely resected disease.

Bonazzi and colleagues from Italy reported their experience with 32 patients with pure immature teratomas. This represents 28% of all germ cell tumors seen by these investigators. Twenty-nine patients were stage I or II and 24 had grade 1 or 2 tumors. Twenty-two patients were treated with conservative surgery only (unilateral oophorectomy or cystectomy). Of 32 patients, 30 had fertility-sparing surgery performed. Five of six patients, who wished for subsequent pregnancies, had seven pregnancies with delivery of seven normal infants. Chemotherapy was given to patients after surgery only in the case of stage I and II grade 3 tumors or in the case of stage III tumors. Ten patients received a cisplatin-based regimen. All 32 patients were alive and disease free at a median of 47 months (11–138 months). Conservative therapy for germ cell tumors is now the norm. Even with advanced disease, unilateral oophorectomy and complete surgical staging with preservation of the uterus and other ovary may be considered. Fortunately, most germ cell tumors are early staged; these tumors are most frequently limited to one ovary. Shorter courses of chemotherapy have been shown to produce excellent results. This is important, because menstrual irregularity (even amenorrhea) during chemotherapy may be related to the duration of chemotherapy. Subsequent fertility may be affected. Fortunately, many patients with germ cell tumors have had many successful subsequent pregnancies after therapy. Although this appears to be age related in that the earlier the age at treatment the less vulnerable the patient is to menstrual irregularities and infertility, most patients with germ cell tumors are young and have apparent minimal infertility. This is in contrast to older patients (e.g., breast cancer) who are premenopausal. Most become amenorrheic during chemotherapy; very few will have resumption of their menstrual periods and, therefore, have premature ovarian failure.

Monodermal or highly specialized teratomas

Struma ovarii

Another tumor thought to represent the unilateral development of benign teratoma is struma ovarii, which consists totally or predominantly of thyroid parenchyma. This is an uncommon lesion and should not be confused with benign teratomas, which contain small foci of thyroid tissue. Between 25% and 35% of patients with strumal tumors will have clinical hyperthyroidism. The gross and microscopic appearance of these lesions is similar to that of typical thyroid tissue, although the histologic pattern may resemble that in adenomatous thyroid. These ovarian tumors may undergo malignant transformation, but they are usually benign and easily treated by simple surgical resection.

Carcinoid tumors

Primary ovarian carcinoid tumors usually arise in association with gastrointestinal or respiratory epithelium, which is present in mature cystic teratoma. They may also be observed within a solid teratoma or a mucinous tumor, or they may occur in an apparently pure form. Primary ovarian carcinoid tumors are uncommon. Approximately 50 cases have been reported. The age distribution of patients with ovarian carcinoid tumors is similar to that of patients with mature cystic teratoma, although the average age may be slightly higher in ovarian carcinoid tumors. Many patients are postmenopausal.

One-third of the reported cases have been associated with the typical carcinoid syndrome, despite the absence of metastasis. This is in contrast to intestinal carcinoid tumors, which are associated with the syndrome only when there is metastatic spread to the liver. Excision of the tumor has been associated with the rapid remission of symptoms in all of the described cases and the disappearance of 5-hydroxyindoleacetic acid from the urine. The primary ovarian carcinoids are only occasionally associated with metastasis; metastasis was observed in only 3 of 47 reported cases in one review. The prognosis after excision of the primary tumor is favorable, and in most cases a cure results.

Strumal carcinoid is an even rarer entity, which represents a close admixture of the previously discussed struma ovarii and carcinoid tumors. Strumal carcinoids may actually represent medullary carcinoma, resulting in thyroid tissue. Most cases follow a benign course.

Gonadoblastoma

Gonadoblastoma is a rare ovarian lesion that consists of germ cells that resemble those of dysgerminoma, and gonadal stroma cells that resemble those of a granulosa or Sertoli tumor. Sex chromatin studies usually show a negative nuclear pattern (45, X) or a sex chromosome mosaicism (45, X/46, XY). Patients who have a gonadoblastoma usually have primary amenorrhea, virilization, or developmental abnormalities of the genitalia. It is poorly understood as to why some patients with these lesions become virilized and others do not. Although there is a correlation between the virilization of patients with gonadoblastoma and the presence of Leydig or lutein-like cells, this relationship is not constant and some virilized patients are free of these cells. The discovery of gonadoblastoma is made in the course of investigation of these conditions. Another common initial sign is the presence of a pelvic tumor. Most patients with gonadoblastoma (80%) are phenotypic women, and the remainder are phenotypic men with cryptorchidism, hypospadias, and internal female secondary sex organs. Among the phenotypic women, 60% are virilized, and the remainder appear normal. The prognosis of patients with gonadoblastoma is excellent if the tumor and the contralateral gonad, which may be harboring a macroscopically undetectable gonadoblastoma, are excised. The association with dysgerminoma is seen in 50% of cases and with other more malignant germ cell neoplasms in an additional 10%. In view of this, the concept that these lesions represent an in situ germ cell malignancy appears valid. When gonadoblastoma is associated with or overgrown by dysgerminoma, the prognosis is still excellent. Metastases tend to occur later and more infrequently than in dysgerminoma arising de novo. Complete agreement has not been reached on whether the uterus should be excised with the gonads. In the opinion of many the uterus should be retained for psychological reasons. Exogenous estrogen therapy is given for periodic bleeding. We leave the uterus even after removing both gonads. Cyclic hormone therapy is indicated in these young women. Ovum transfer has been successful in patients who have had both ovaries removed.

TUMORS DERIVED FROM SPECIAL GONADAL STROMA

Classification, clinical profile, and staging

This category of ovarian tumors includes all those that contain granulosa cells, theca cells and luteinized derivatives, Sertoli cells, Leydig cells, and fibroblasts of gonadal stromal origin. These tumors originate from the ovarian matrix and consist of cells from the embryonic sex cord and mesenchyme. As a group, sex cord-stromal tumors (SCST) are found in all age groups with the age related incidence increasing throughout the fifth, sixth, and seventh decades. These tumors account for approximately 5% of all ovarian tumors; however, functioning neoplastic groups of this variety comprise only 2%. Approximately 90% of hormonally active ovarian tumors belong to this category and are associated with physiologic and pathologic signs of estrogen and/or androgen excess, including isosexual precocity, hirsutism, abnormal bleeding, endometrial hyperplasia or carcinoma, and breast cancer risk. Of ovarian cancers, 5–10% belong in the sex cord-stromal group; most of these (70%) are granulosa cell tumors, which are low-grade malignancies with a relapse rate of 10–33%. Because SCS tumors have a propensity for indolent growth, they tend to recur late. The average time to recurrence is between 5 and 10 years; some recur as late as 20 years after the initial diagnosis. Most authors report a 10-year survival of 90% for stage I and 0–22% for stage III. Prognostic factors shown to be responsible for survival in multivariate analysis include age less than 50, tumor size less than 10 cm, and absence of residual disease. SCST are staged surgically in accordance with FIGO guidelines and staging recommendations for ovarian epithelial tumors.

Treatment

The definitive treatment of SCST is based on findings encountered during complete surgical staging, the reproductive desires of the patient, and the histologic type of tumor. The majority of SCST are benign or low malignant potential tumors. As a result, surgical therapy is adequate in most cases. In patients who desire to retain fertility, unilateral salpingo-oophorectomy with preservation of the uterus and contralateral ovary is appropriate therapy for patients with stage Ia disease. Advanced stage disease and disease in older women should be managed with complete staging and hysterectomy with bilateral salpingo-oophorectomy. Although scientific evidence suggesting benefit is lacking, most authors recommend aggressive attempts at complete cytoreduction if possible when faced with advanced stage, metastatic, or bulky disease. Secondary cytoreduction is controversial, although there may be a survival or palliative benefit for patients with focal recurrent disease.

Two special clinical situations require additional surgical evaluation. Because estrogen-secreting ovarian tumors are associated with endometrial hyperplasia or cancer in 25–50% and 5–10% of cases respectively, surgical evaluation should include dilation and curettage of the uterine cavity, regardless of the benign or malignant nature of the ovarian primary. If malignancy in the uterus is encountered, it should be managed accordingly. Additionally, because sex cord tumors with annular tubules (SCTAT) associated with Peutz–Jeghers syndrome (discussed below) can be associated with adenoma malignum of the cervix, it is imperative that the endocervix be evaluated with an endocervical curettage. Although these ovarian tumors are benign, postoperative follow-up and surveillance of the cervix is required.

Patients with early stage disease (Ia or Ib) may be managed with surgical therapy alone and expect an excellent prognosis. However, those with stage Ic or greater disease should have strong consideration given for adjuvant therapy. Adjuvant therapy may consist of radiation or chemotherapy. The effectiveness of radiation therapy for SCST is controversial and unclear. Although experience with chemotherapy is likewise limited, active regimes are BEP or VAC. Recently, Brown et al published results demonstrating taxane activity in patients with SCST. In this study, a 42% response rate was noted in the setting of recurrent, measurable disease. Specific adjuvant therapy for individual tumor subtypes will be discussed below. In a subsequent study, Brown et al directly compared BEP to taxanes in women with SCST. In this study, there was no difference in progression free survival, overall survival, or response rates in patients with newly diagnosed tumors treated with BEP compared to taxanes. In patients with recurrent measurable disease, BEP had a higher response rate compared to the taxane regimens (71% vs 37), a finding not statistically significant. In this study, the presence of a platinum compound in the taxane regimen correlated with response, suggesting that a platinum and taxane combination is both active in SCST tumors and may have equivalent efficacy but with lower toxicity when compared to the standard BEP.

Granulosa-stromal cell tumors

Granulosa-stromal cell tumors include granulosa cell, theca cell tumors, and fibromas, and account for the majority of SCST. They occur about as frequently in women in the reproductive age group as they do in women who are postmenopausal, with a peak incidence in perimenopausal women. Only about 5% of granulosa cell tumors occur before puberty (Table 12–8). Most granulosa and theca cells produce estrogen, but a few are androgenic. The exact proportion of these neoplasms that have function is not known, because the endometrium is often not examined microscopically and appropriate preoperative laboratory tests are not done. About 80–85% of granulosa cell and theca cell neoplasms are palpable on abdominal or pelvic examination, but occasionally an unsuspected tumor is found when a hysterectomy is done on a patient who has abnormal bleeding as a result of endometrial hyperplasia or endometrial carcinoma. A study by Evans and associates from the Mayo Clinic of 76 patients who had granulosa cell tumors and in whom endometrial tissue was available shows a high incidence of endometrial stimulation (Table 12–9). In another study, one-third of patients had atypical endometrial cells.

Most patients present either with non-specific symptoms such as awareness of an abdominal mass, abdominal pain, abdominal distention, or bloating. Some patients present with an acute abdomen due to internal tumor rupture and hemorrhage with resultant hemoperitoneum. In postmenopausal women, vaginal bleeding is common due to stimulation of the endometrium. Approximately 10% of patients with this lesion will harbor an endometrial carcinoma, usually of the well-differentiated type.

Table 12–8 GRANULOSA CELL TUMOR: AGE DISTRIBUTION OF 118 CASES

Age	No.
Child	3
12–40	27
41–50	28
51–60	32
60–79	28
Total	118

Based on data from Evans AJ III et al: Clinicopathological review of 118 granulosa and 82 theca cell tumors. Obstet Gynecol 55:213, 1980.

Table 12–9 GRANULOSA CELL TUMOR (76 PATIENTS)

Endometrial histology	No.	%
Proliferative endometrium	19	25
Atrophic endometrium	5	7
Hyperplastic endometrium	42	55
Adenocarcinoma	10	13

Based on data from Evans AJ III et al: Clinicopathological review of 118 granulosa and 82 theca cell tumors. Obstet Gynecol 55:213, 1980.

Granulosa cell tumors vary greatly in gross appearance (Fig. 12–9). Sometimes they are solid tumors that are soft or firm, depending on the relative amounts of neoplastic cells and fibrothecomatous stroma that they contain. They may be yellow or gray, depending on the amount of intracellular lipid in the lesion. More commonly, the granulosa cell tumor is predominantly cystic and, on external examination, may resemble mucinous cystadenoma or cystadenocarcinoma. However, when sectioned, this cyst is generally found to be filled with serous fluid or clotted blood. About 15% of patients with cystic granulosa cell tumors are first examined for an acute abdomen associated with hemoperitoneum.

Granulosa cell tumors occur in two subtypes: adult and juvenile. Adult granulosa cell tumors account for approximately 95% of all granulosa cell tumors. They occur more commonly in the postmenopausal patient and are the most common tumor that produces estrogen. Abnormal endometria in these patients are not uncommon, such as hyperplasia or even carcinoma of the endometrium. The latter, which is usually well differentiated, has been

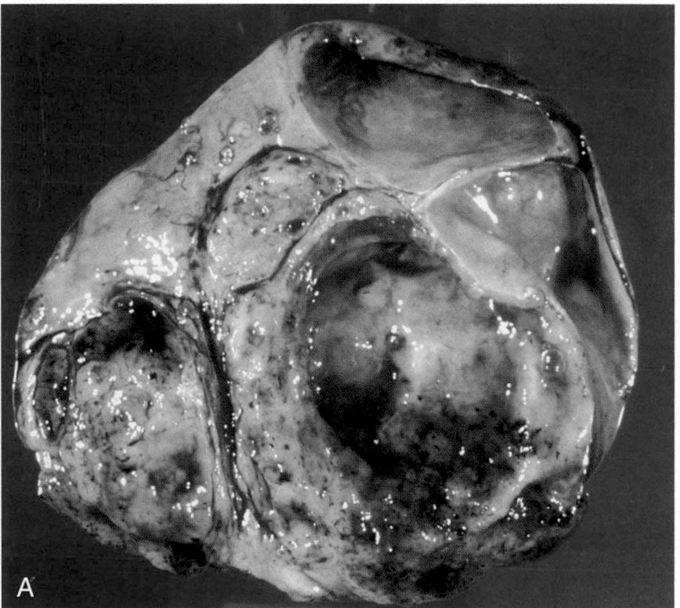

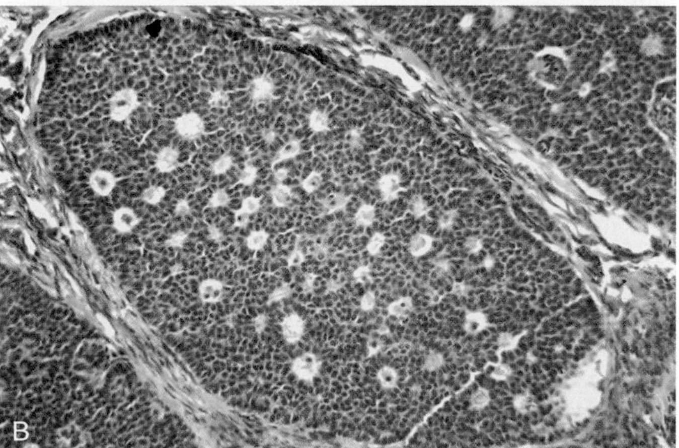

Figure 12–9 Granulosa cell tumor of the ovary. *A*, Gross appearance. *B*, Microscopic appearance with Call–Exner bodies.

reported to be as high as 25% of cases in some reports, although they probably occur in 5% or less of cases. Other estrogenic effects may also be noted (e.g., tenderness or swelling of the breast), and vaginal cytology may show an increase in maturation of the squamous cells. Rarely, androgenic effects may be present in which hirsute changes may be present, or progestational effects may be noted on histologic evaluation of the endometrium. Histologically, fibrothecomatous components are common, and the cytoplasm is usually scanty. The typical coffee-bean grooved cells are present. Cells may be arranged in clusters or rosettes surrounding a central cavity and when present, resemble primordial follicles called Call–Exner bodies and are common. Adult granulosa cell tumors are typically low-grade malignancies that demonstrate indolent growth, and present as stage I disease in over 90% of cases. Unilateral disease is most common, but bilateral disease may be found in up to 10% of cases. The most important prognostic factor is surgical stage.

In juvenile granulosa cell tumors, the great majority are found in young adults, and most occur during the first three decades of life. Most juvenile granulosa cell tumors are hormonally active, producing estradiol, progesterone, or androgens. Most of the juvenile granulosa cell tumors that occur in children result in sexual precocity with the development of breasts and pubic and axillary hair. Irregular uterine bleeding may also be present. Thyromegaly may also occur. Juvenile tumors that are hormonally active may have a more favorable prognosis than inactive tumors, presumably due to earlier presentation as a result of the signs and symptoms associated with hormonal activity. Like the adult subtype, most of these tumors are limited to one ovary. Ninety-eight percent present with stage I disease. Histologically, thecomatous components are common; cytoplasm is abundant. Mitosis may be numerous; the nuclei are dark and do not usually have the grooved coffee-bean appearance. Pleomorphism may also be present. Juvenile tumors rarely demonstrate Call–Exner bodies. Even though these tumors appear to be less well differentiated than the adult type; nevertheless, the cure rate is quite high. In contrast to adult cell types that are typically indolent and recur late, juvenile types are aggressive in advanced stage disease with recurrence and death occurring within three years after diagnosis.

On the basis of their differentiation, granulosa cell tumors should be divided into two general categories: well differentiated and moderately differentiated. The former pattern may have various presentations, including microfollicular, macrofollicular, trabecular, solid-tubular, and watered silk. Tumors in the moderately differentiated category have a diffuse pattern that has also been designated "sarcomatoid". Although many authors have made attempts, no distinct correlation between histologic structure and prognosis has yet been substantiated. It is important that undifferentiated carcinomas, adenocarcinomas, and carcinoids should not be misdiagnosed as granulosa cell tumors, which they may superficially resemble. Each of these tumors has a strikingly different prognosis. One

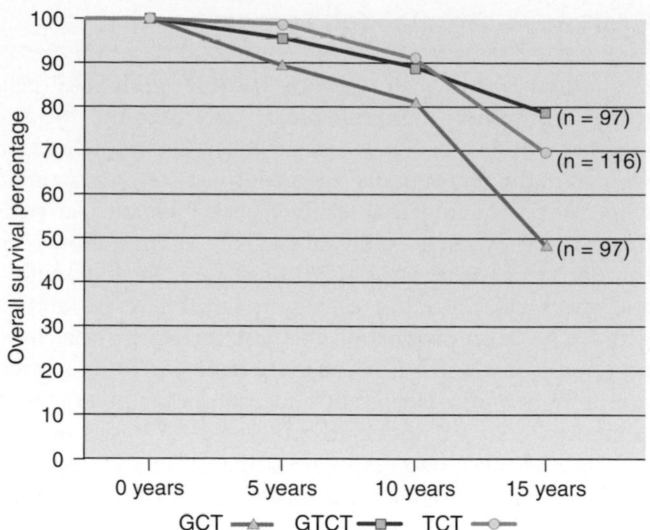

Figure 12–10 Granulosa-theca cell tumors from Emil Novak Ovarian Tumor Registry (1999). (Modified from Cronje HS, Niemand I, Bam RH, Woodruff JD: Review of the granulosa-theca cell tumors from the Emil Novak Ovarian Tumor Registry. Am J Obstet Gynecol 180(2):323, 1999.)

characteristic feature is the appearance of the nuclei. Oval or angular, grooved nuclei are typical of granulosa cell tumors (coffee-bean appearance). Call–Exner bodies also have diagnostic importance, but unfortunately they are not often sharply defined.

True granulosa tumors are low-grade malignancies, the majority of which are confined to one ovary at the time of diagnosis. Only 5–10% of the stage I cases will subsequently recur, and they often appear more than 5 years after initial therapy. The prognosis for these patients is excellent: long-term survival rates from 75–90% have been reported for all stages (Fig. 12–10). These lesions are adequately managed during the reproductive years by removing the involved ovary and ipsilateral tube. The uterus and uninvolved adnexa should be removed in the perimenopausal and postmenopausal age groups, which is the treatment for other benign or low malignant potential tumors. In a series from the Mayo Clinic, 92% of the patients had survived 5–10 years (76 patients, 82% of whom had stage I lesions). The recurrence pattern in this same series (18.6% overall recurrence rate) revealed that 23% of the recurrences were more than 13 years after initial therapy. Most of the recurrences occurred in preserved genital tract structures. These kinds of data have prompted our recommendation that the preserved internal genitalia be removed in the perimenopausal patient in whom preservation may have been appropriate during the childbearing period.

Several studies address prognostic factors in granulosa cell tumor of the ovary. The most important prognostic factor is stage. Other than stage, mitotic activity, DNA ploidy and S-phase fractions have been evaluated. In a study of 54 patients from Sweden, patients with mitotic rates of $\leq 4/10$ high-power fields (hpf) had no deaths while all patients with $\geq 10/10$ HPF died, with the longest survival being 4 years. Patients with mitotic rate of 4–10/10 HPF had a median survival of 9 years. Fortunately, most patients had mitotic counts of ≤4/10 HPF. In a small study, about two-thirds of the patients studied were found to have euploid tumors. Only one patient died of disease, whereas four of five patients with aneuploid tumors died of disease. S-phase fraction did not correlate with any clinical or histologic parameters.

Inhibin is a non-steroidal polypeptide hormone that is secreted by granulosa cells of the ovary. This hormone secretes throughout the menstrual cycle and during pregnancy but not in the postmenopausal woman. As a result, inhibin has been suggested as a tumor marker for granulosa cell tumors. In collective series, the relationship of tumor to the level of inhibin appears to be very good. However, there have been many reports denying the specificity of this substance, which may also be secreted by many other ovarian neoplasms. Nevertheless, serum inhibin levels have an important role as a marker for monitoring patients under therapy and for detection of tumor recurrence. Other tumor markers include müllerian inhibiting substance (MIS) and estradiol. Estradiol is not used clinically due to poor sensitivity, and MIS, while demonstrating excellent specificity, is only used for research purposes.

Often, recurrent tumors have been treated effectively by means of reoperation, radiation therapy, chemotherapy, or a combination thereof. Although radiation therapy has been advocated for these tumors by many authors, careful search of the literature shows little evidence relating enhanced curability to the use of radiation therapy. A prospective study has never been done to compare one form of therapy with another for patients who have advanced or recurrent disease. The question of adjuvant radiotherapy in the postmenopausal woman found to have granulosa cell tumor is often an issue.

We recommend no further therapy for patients who have stage I lesions. Adverse prognostic factors that have been reported include large tumor size, bilateral involvement, intra-abdominal rupture of the neoplasm, nuclear atypia, and a high mitotic rate. There appears to be agreement that the histologic pattern of the neoplasm has no predictive value. Stage II or III or recurrent granulosa cell tumors are probably best treated with systemic chemotherapy. Metastatic and suboptimally reduced disease should also be aggressively treated with combination chemotherapy, as response rates as high as 83% have been reported. Although the optimal chemotherapeutic regimen has not yet been determined, the following drugs have been used singly or in combination and appear to be effective: Adriamycin, bleomycin, cisplatin, and vinblastine. Colombo and associates reported 11 previously untreated women with recurrent or metastatic granulosa cell tumor of the ovary who were treated with VBP. Nine patients responded; six patients had a complete pathologic response. Patients received between two and six courses of chemotherapy. The GOG has evaluated BEP in a non-randomized study of advanced or recurrent granulosa cell tumors of the ovary. Fifty-seven evaluable patients received four cycles of BEP followed by a reassessment laparotomy. Only 38 patients agreed to a second-look laparotomy, and 14 (37%) had negative results. Obviously, BEP is an active combination in these patients with advanced disease.

The natural history of patients with recurrences is prolonged, thus making analysis of any therapy very difficult in terms of overall survival. This is especially true of therapy utilized in an adjuvant setting. Responses have been reported both with paclitaxel and gonadotropin-releasing hormone agonists.

Thecomas

Thecomas do not occur as frequently as do granulosa cell tumors, but they have similar appearances. They are solid fibromatous lesions that show varying degrees of yellow or orange coloration. Whereas granulosa cell tumors are found to be bilateral in 2–5% of patients, thecomas are almost always confined to one ovary. On microscopic examination, most tumors in the granulosa-theca cell category are found to contain both cell types. If more than a very small component of granulosa cells are present, the term *granulosa cell tumor*, rather than *granulosa-theca cell tumor*, is generally applied. The designation theca cell tumor or thecoma should be reserved for neoplasms that consist entirely of benign theca cells.

Thecomas consist of neoplastic cells of ovarian stromal origin that have accumulated moderate to large amounts of lipid. Sometimes such tumors contain clusters of lutein cells, in which case the term *luteinized thecoma* is often used. Occasionally, tumors fall into a gray zone between thecomas and fibromas. Although the latter also arise from ovarian stromal cells, they differentiate predominantly in the direction of collagen-producing fibroblasts. Tumors in the gray zone may be designated as thecoma-fibromas. They are almost always unilateral and virtually never malignant. Several tumors have been reported in the literature as malignant thecomas, but at least some of these are better interpreted as fibrosarcomas or diffuse forms of granulosa cell tumors. In cases in which preservation of fertility is important, a thecoma may be treated adequately by unilateral oophorectomy. However, total hysterectomy with bilateral salpingo-oophorectomy is recommended in most postmenopausal and perimenopausal women. As thecomas are typically one of the most hormonally active SCSTs, 15–37% and 25% of cases are associated with endometrial hyperplasia and carcinoma respectively, and endometrial sampling should be performed. Patients typically present with abnormal bleeding and an abdominal or pelvic mass.

Fibromas and sclerosing stromal cell tumors

Fibromas are the most common SCST and occur primarily in postmenopausal women, although they can occur in any age group. They are not hormonally active tumors.

Fibromas are benign tumors, however recently cellular fibromas have been described and are considered to be of low malignant potential. Fibrosarcomas by contrast are rare but considered highly aggressive tumors. Behavior of these tumors is correlated with mitotic activity and degree of anaplasia.

Fibromas may be associated with ascites or hydrothorax as a result of increased capillary permeability thought to be a result of vascular endothelial growth factor (VEGF) production. Meigs' syndrome (ovarian fibromas, ascites, and hydrothorax) is uncommon and usually resolves after surgical excision of the fibroma. Gorlin's syndrome represents an inherited predisposition to ovarian fibromas and basal cell carcinomas, and occurs rarely. Due to the benign nature of fibromas, surgical excision is all that is required.

In contrast to most SCST's, sclerosing stromal cell tumors typically present in the second and third decades of life. They may be clinically undetectable or grow to very large size. They are considered benign, occur unilaterally, and are hormonally inactive except in very rare cases.

Sertoli–Leydig cell tumors

Sertoli–Leydig cell tumors contain Sertoli cells or Leydig cells in varying proportions and degrees of differentiation. These tumors are thought to originate from the specialized gonadal stroma. The cells were able to differentiate into any of the structures derived from the embryonic gonadal mesenchyme. Because less well-differentiated neoplasms within this category may recapitulate the development of the testes, the terms *androblastoma* and *arrhenoblastoma* have been used as synonyms for Sertoli–Leydig cell tumors. However, their connotation of associated masculinization is misleading, because some of these tumors have no endocrine manifestation and others may even be accompanied by an estrogenic syndrome. Nevertheless, the World Health Organization has selected *androblastoma* as an alternate term for Sertoli–Leydig cell tumor. These neoplasms account for less than 0.5% of all ovarian tumors but are among the most fascinating from pathologic and clinical viewpoints. They are typically unilateral tumors and confined to the ovary in 97% of cases. They occur in all age groups but are most often encountered in young women (between the ages of 20 and 30), who usually become virilized (Fig. 12–11). In immunocytochemical studies, testosterone appears to be localized predominantly within the Leydig cells. Estrogen and androstenedione appear in many of the same cells. Thus, one can see the multifaceted clinical presentation of this fascinating neoplasm. Classically, there is progressive masculinization that is heralded by hirsutism, temporal balding, deepening of the voice, and enlargement of the clitoris. Other patients may manifest secondary amenorrhea, breast atrophy, and marked increase in libido.

Sertoli–Leydig cell tumors can be described in terms of differentiation and the presence or absence of heterologous elements, distinctions that have clinical relevance.

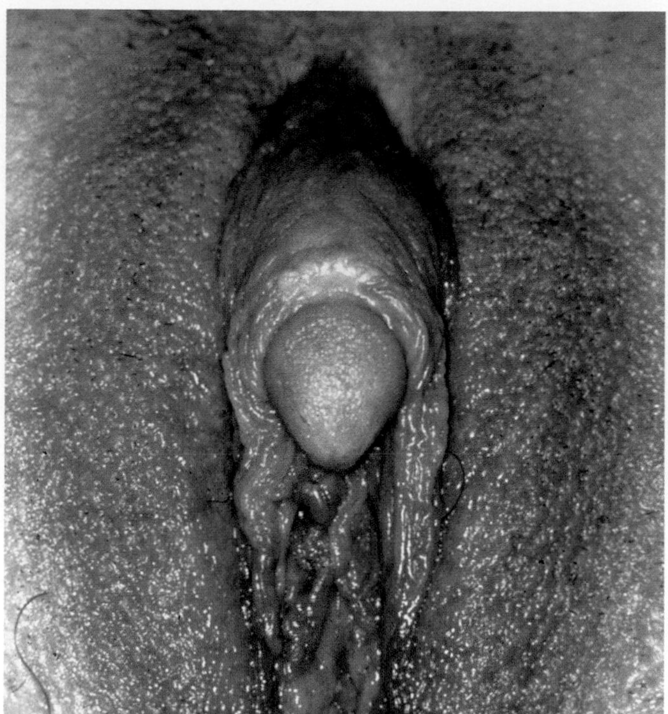

Figure 12–11 Enlarged clitoris in a patient with a Sertoli–Leydig cell tumor (arrhenoblastoma).

Sertoli–Leydig cell tumors with heterologous elements may contain various unusual cell types, but the degree of differentiation of the tumors is probably of greater importance in determining its prognosis than is its content of unexpected tissue. In the report by Young and Scully, only 29 of 220 tumors of this type have been clinically malignant. None of the 27 well-differentiated tumors and only 4 of 100 tumors of intermediate differentiation was known to be clinically malignant. Fifty-nine percent of poorly differentiated tumors, and 19 percent of heterologous tumors displayed malignant behavior. Zaloudek and Norris reported on 64 intermediately and poorly differentiated neoplasms. Only 3 of 50 patients with stage I disease developed a recurrence (Table 12–10). The 5-year survival rate in all of their patients was 92%.

The overall 5-year survival rate of patients with Sertoli–Leydig cell tumors has been reported to be slightly >70% to slightly >90%. Because these tumors occur predominantly in young women and are bilateral in less than 5% of cases, conservative removal of the tumor and adjacent fallopian tube is justifiable, if preservation of fertility is an important consideration and if there is no evidence of extension beyond the involved ovary. Removal of the tumor will halt, but not fully reverse, the masculinizing process. Like granulosa cell tumors, they are considered to have low malignant potential. There are no solid data to suggest that adjuvant therapy has any value in preventing a recurrence in patients with stage I lesions. Tumors with poor differentiation, heterologous elements, advanced stage, or recurrent lesions should be treated with adjuvant chemotherapy. Once again the VAC regimen of chemotherapy is often recommended. In the unusual patient who

Table 12–10 MANAGEMENT OF GERM CELL AND SEX CORD-STROMAL TUMORS

Neoplasms	Suggested surgery	Postoperative chemotherapy	Reassessment laparotomy
Dysgerminoma	Unilateral S&O when confined to one ovary—preserve normal-appearing ovarian tissue	BEP 3 cycles if the patient is not adequately staged or if stage II–IV staged or if stage II–IV	Not necessary unless a recurrence is suspected
Endodermal sinus	Debulk—attempt to preserve fertility	BEP 3–4 cycles Follow with AFP titers	Same as above
Embryonal carcinoma	Same as above	BEP 3–4 cycles Follow with β-hCG titers	Same as above
Malignant teratoma	Same as above	BEP or VAC 3–4 cycles	Same as above
Granulosa cell	Unilateral salpingo-oophorectomy for young patients with stage Ia disease Otherwise TAH, BSO	BEP 3–4 cycles GnRH agonists for advanced disease	Same as above
Sertoli–Leydig cell	Same as above	BEP or VAC 3–4 cycles for advanced disease	Same as above

BEP, bleomycin, etoposide, and cisplatin; S & O, salpingo-oophorectomy; VAC, vincristine, dactinomycin, and cyclophosphamide.

has an advanced or recurrent Sertoli–Leydig cell tumor, chemotherapy appears to be effective, although the experience is very limited. The combination of cisplatin and vinblastine and bleomycin therapy appears to be active in this disease. At least one case report has noted an elevated serum AFP as an early indication of a recurrence. Gershenson reported on nine patients with a poor prognosis after sex cord-stromal tumors were treated with BEP chemotherapy. The overall response rate was 83%, but the regimen lacked durability. The median survival time was 28 months, and only two of the nine patients had no evidence of disease at the time of the report.

Sex cord tumor with annular tubules

Sex cord tumor with annular tubules (SCTAT) represents a unique ovarian tumor that appears as a histologic intermediate between granulosa and Sertoli–Leydig cell tumors. This tumor typically presents in the third to fourth decade of life and is usually unilateral. Presenting complaints are usually abnormal vaginal bleeding or postmenopausal bleeding, a testament to the endocrine activity of these tumors. Both estrogen and progesterone production have been reported. SCTAT tumors are distinguished on the basis of association with Peutz–Jegher's syndrome (PJS). Tumors associated with PJS are benign but are associated with adenoma malignum of the cervix in 15% of cases. As adenoma malignum has a relatively high mortality rate, these patients deserve careful evaluation and follow-up. In contrast, SCTAT, which is not associated with PJS, has a 20% malignancy rate. There is limited experience in the literature with these tumors. Clinically, they should be managed in a similar manner to other SCSTs. Combination chemotherapy (BEP) may be helpful in patients with advanced disease. As SCTAT represents an intermediate cell type between granulosa cell and Sertoli–Leydig cell tumors, SCTAT may express inhibin, or MIS. The utility of these tumor markers in this disease is uncertain.

Gynandroblastoma

Rarely, a gonadostromal tumor contains unequivocal granulosa cell elements combined with tubules and Leydig cells that are characteristic of arrhenoblastomas. Designated as gynandroblastomas, these mixed tumors may be associated with either androgen or estrogen production, and they can be expected to behave as low-grade malignancies similar to the individual components.

Lipid cell neoplasms

Lipid cell neoplasms are a heterologous group of tumors that have in common a parenchyma composed of polygonal cells that contain lipid. They include neoplasms that have been designated as hilus cell tumors, Leydig tumors, adrenal rest tumors, stroma luteomas, or masculinovoblastomas. Leydig cell tumors are unilateral and are found commonly in the medulla or hilus regions of the ovaries. Tumors that have spread to contiguous organs or have a microscopic cellular pleomorphism with high mitotic activity should be considered malignant. Reinke crystals, which normally occur in mature Leydig cells of the testes, are often found in these neoplasms, and their presence may be interpreted as signifying a benign lesion. Regardless of the presence or absence of Reinke crystals, neoplasms that are <8 cm in diameter can be expected to act benignly.

TUMORS DERIVED FROM NON-SPECIFIC MESENCHYME

Benign and malignant tumors, including fibromas, hemangiomas, leiomyomas, soft tissue sarcomas, lymphomas, and rare neoplasms, may arise in the ovaries from non-specific supporting tissues that are common to most organs. The most common and most important tumors in this category are the fibroma and the lymphoma.

The mixed mesodermal sarcoma of the ovary (analogous to its uterine counterpart) has been more widely recognized in the last decade. This neoplasm is rare and is invariably fatal. A review by Hernandez and colleagues suggested that 50% of the patients have stage III tumors when first seen, and the patients are most commonly diagnosed in the sixth decade of life. Various forms of combination chemotherapy, including a vigorous regimen with VAC, have been advocated with varied results. Many of these lesions are carcinosarcomas, and the metastatic sites are made up predominantly of adenomatous components so that treatment with platinum and Taxol similar to high-grade epithelial ovarian carcinoma has been utilized with reasonable success. This is particularly true when the sarcomatous elements are limited to the primary lesion in the ovary.

MALIGNANT LYMPHOMA

Lymphoma is a rare tumor of the ovary and most commonly represents ovarian involvement in overt systemic disease, almost always of the non-Hodgkin's type. There has been debate as to whether lymphoma can arise de novo in the ovary; lymphoid aggregates do exist in normal ovarian tissue, which could give rise to such a lesion.

Patients with disease localized to one ovary usually do well with unilateral surgical resection followed by systemic chemotherapy. The use of chemotherapy is based on the principle that ovarian lymphoma must be considered a localized manifestation of systemic disease. The prognosis for such patients is much better than that of patients with obvious systemic disease.

METASTATIC TUMORS TO THE OVARY

Approximately 6% of ovarian cancers encountered by surgeons exploring pelvic or abdominal masses are metastases, most often either metastatic breast tumors or metastatic adenocarcinomas of large intestine origin. Metastases from carcinomas of the breast are among the more common surgical specimens of the ovary, especially if one includes those found incidentally. They are almost always incidental findings in therapeutic oophorectomy and rarely form symptomatic masses that require surgical removal. The term *Krukenberg tumor* should be reserved for metastases that contain significant numbers of signet-ring cells in a cellular stroma derived from the ovarian stroma. This restriction is important, because tumors with these microscopic characteristics also have distinctive gross pathologic and clinical features. Almost all metastasize from the stomach, but some arise in the breast, intestine, or other mucous gland-containing organs. Krukenberg tumors form a solid, often uniform mass, the sectioned surface of which typically exhibits gelatinous necrosis and hemorrhage.

Metastatic adenocarcinomas of large intestinal origin have become more common than Krukenberg tumors in the past two decades with the gradual decline in the incidence of carcinoma of the stomach. The latest reports confirm adenocarcinoma of the colon as the most frequent primary site of metastatic disease to the ovary with breast cancer in second place. These lesions are characterized microscopically by the presence of large acini similar to those of primary intestinal carcinomas. Grossly, they may form solid metastases but more often appear as large, partly cystic tumors with areas of hemorrhage and necrosis (Fig. 12–12). In such cases, they are easily confused with cystic forms of primary ovarian cancers.

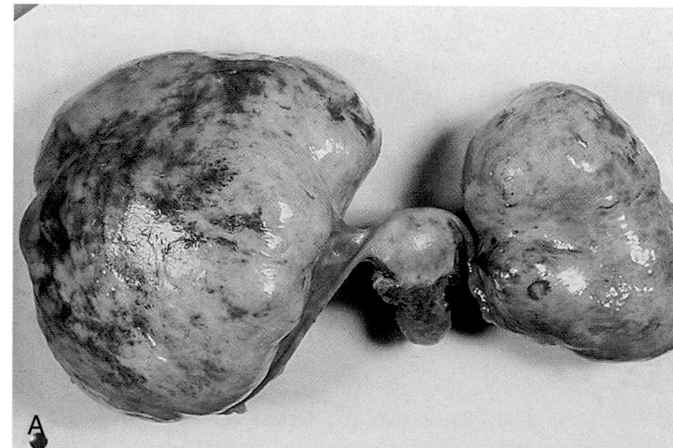

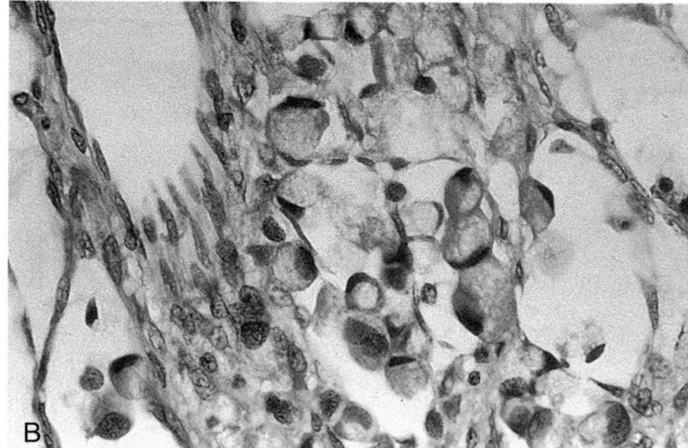

Figure 12–12 Metastatic tumor to the ovary from adenocarcinoma of the colon. *A*, Gross appearance. *B*, Histologic appearance. Note the large acini similar to those of the intestinal carcinoma.

The ovary is frequently the site of metastasis from certain primary carcinomas. Approximately 10% of ovarian tumors are not primary in origin. The most common metastasis is in the form of a carcinoma that arises in the endometrium. There is no doubt that cancer of the endometrium metastasizes to the ovaries, but it may be difficult to distinguish metastasis of an endometrial cancer from a separate ovarian tumor. This is particularly true in the case of ovarian endometrioid carcinoma, which, according to Scully, is associated with a similar tumor in the endometrium in one third of cases.

There are four possible pathways of spread to tumors to the ovary:

1. direct continuity;
2. surface papillation;
3. lymphatic metastasis; and
4. hematogenous spread.

Lymphatic metastasis is undoubtedly the most common pathway for spread to the ovary. The rich network of lymph nodes and lymphatic channels in the pelvis readily explains the metastatic pathway of tumors in the uterus and contralateral ovary. The rare finding of clusters of tumor cells limited to lymphatics in the medulla of the ovary in cases of breast carcinoma confirms that this is the pathway of spread to the ovary. As yet, no one has convincingly described the pathway of metastasis to the ovaries from cancer of the stomach. It is known that the lymphatic channels that drain the upper gastrointestinal tract ultimately link up with the lumbar chain of lymph nodes. Ovarian lymphatics drain into the lumbar nodes. This could well be the route of spread to the ovaries in these cases.

Cases of metastatic ovarian carcinoma have occurred in which a clinical presentation was consistent with hormonal activity. Both androgen and estrogen excretion have been described. Endometrial hyperplasia has been described in postmenopausal patients with metastatic ovarian carcinomas, presumably indicating estrogen activity within the metastatic lesion or its normal tissue capsule.

MALIGNANT OVARIAN TUMORS IN CHILDREN

Ovarian tumors, cysts, and torsion are more frequent indications for surgical intervention in infancy and childhood than is commonly realized. They may produce symptoms similar to appendicitis, and it is not always appreciated how often they mimic this condition. Pain is the most frequently reported symptom. The proportion of all tumors of the abdomen in this age group that are ovarian in origin has not been reported. A palpable abdominal mass is found in half of the patients with neoplasms. Approximately 10% of the patients have isosexual precocity, which includes patients who demonstrate precocious puberty and those with an early onset of sexual development. The initial signs are areolar pigmentation and breast development. Some patients have vaginal discharge or bleeding, and others have pubic hair. These changes usually completely regress after surgical extirpation of the responsible endocrine-secreting tumor. Granulosa-theca cell tumors are by far the most common ovarian neoplasms found in these patients with isosexual precocity and adnexal enlargement. Most ovarian cancers in children are of germ cell origin. Cangir and associates reported on 21 girls younger than 16 years, with a median age of 13.5. Of the 21 patients, 8 had malignant teratomas; 6 had mixed germinal tumors; 6 had endodermal sinus tumors; and 1 had a stromal cell tumor (Sertoli–Leydig type). Eight patients were at stage I; one patient was at stage II; seven patients were at stage III; and five patients were at stage IV. Ablin reported on a study of 17 children with ovarian germ cell tumors treated with multiple-agent chemotherapy. Of the 17 patients, 13 showed complete responses to therapy, suggesting that survival rates in this group of patients have improved significantly with modern chemotherapy. Lack and coworkers reported that granulosa-theca cell tumors in the premenarche patient accounted for 4% of childhood ovarian tumors at their institution from 1928–1979. The average age of diagnosis of their 10 patients was 5 years, and precocious "pseudopuberty" was the most common presentation. These 10 lesions were solitary; 5 were on the right side and 5 were on the left side, with an average diameter of 12 cm. All 10 patients survived at least 10 years, and salpingo-oophorectomy was curative despite tumor spillage in two patients.

Fortunately, the most common germ cell neoplasm is the benign teratoma. A significant number of other patients have benign functional cysts of the ovary. All patients are treated in a manner similar to that of the adolescent or the older patient in the early reproductive age period.

BIBLIOGRAPHY

GERM CELL TUMORS

Abell MR, Johnson VJ, Holtz F: Ovarian neoplasms in childhood and adolescence. I: Tumors of germ cell origin. Am J Obstet Gynecol 92:1059, 1965.

Albites V: Solid teratoma of the ovary with malignant gliomatosis peritonei. Int J Gynaecol Obstet 12:59, 1974.

Asadourian LA, Taylor HB: Dysgerminoma: An analysis of 105 cases. Obstet Gynecol 33:370, 1969.

Ashley DJB: Origin of teratomas. Cancer 32:390, 1983.

Baker BA, Frickey L, Yu IT et al: DNA content of ovarian immature teratomas and malignant germ cell tumors. Gynecol Oncol 71:14, 1998.

Beiner ME, Gotlieb WH, Korach Y et al: Cystectomy for immature teratoma of the ovary. Gynecol Oncol 93:381, 2004.

Bianchi UA, Sartori E, Favallin G: New trends in treatment of ovarian dysgerminoma. Gynecol Oncol 23:246, 1986.

Boczkowski K, Teter J, Sternadel Z: Sibship occurrence of XY gonadal dysgenesis with dysgerminoma. Am J Obstet Gynecol 113:952, 1972.

Bonazzi C, Peccatori F, Colombo N et al: Pure ovarian immature teratoma, a unique and curable disease: 10 years' experience of 32 prospectively treated patients. Obstet Gynecol 84:598, 1994.

Bower M, Eife K, Holden L et al: Chemotherapy for ovarian germ cell tumours. Eur J Cancer 32a:593, 1996.

Breen JL, Neubecker RD: Malignant teratoma of the ovary: An analysis of 17 cases. Obstet Gynecol 21:669, 1963.

Casey AC, Bhodauria S, Shapter A et al: Dysgerminoma: The role of conservative surgery. Gynecol Oncol 63:352, 1996.

Cooper MA, Einhorn LH: Maintenance chemotherapy with daily oral etoposide following salvage therapy in patients with germ cell tumors. J Clin Oncol 13:1167, 1995.

Creasman WT, Soper JT: Assessment of contemporary management of germ cell malignancies of the ovary. Am J Obstet Gynecol 153:828, 1985.

Creasman WT et al: Germ cell malignancies of the ovary. Obstet Gynecol 53:226, 1979.

Culin S, Lhomme C, Kattan J et al: Pure malignant immature teratoma of the ovary: The role of chemotherapy and second-look surgery. Int J Gynecol Oncol 5:432, 1995.

Curry SL, Smith JP, Gallagher HS: Malignant teratoma of the ovary: Prognostic factors and treatment. Am J Obstet Gynecol 131:845, 1978.

Curtin JP, Morrow CP, Ablaing GD, Schlaerth JB: Malignant germ cell tumors of the ovary: 20-year report of LAC-USC Women's Hospital. Int J Gynecol Cancer 4:29, 1994.

Curtin JP, Rubin SL, Hoskins WJ et al: Second look laparotomy in endodermal sinus tumor: A report of two patients with normal levels of alpha-fetoprotein and residual tumor at re-exploration. Obstet Gynecol 73:93, 1989.

Cushing B, Giller R, Ablin A et al: Surgical resection alone is effective treatment for ovarian immature teratoma in children and adolescents: a report of the pediatric oncology group and the children's cancer group. Am J Obstet Gynecol 181:353, 1999.

Cushing B, Giller R, Cullen JW et al: Randomized comparison of combination chemotherapy with etoposide, bleomycin, and either high-dose or standard-dose cisplatin in children and adolescents with high-risk malignant germ cell tumors: A Pediatric Intergroup Study-Pediatric Oncology Group 9049 and Children's Cancer Group 8882. J Clin Oncol 22:2691, 2004.

Dark GG, Bower M, Newlands ES et al: Surveillance policy for stage I ovarian germ cell tumours. J Clin Oncol 15:620, 1997.

De Palo G et al: Natural history of dysgerminoma. Am J Obstet Gynecol 143:799, 1982.

De Santis M, Bercherer A, Bokemyer C et al: 2-18fluoro-deoxy-D-glucose positron emission tomography is a reliable predictor for viable tumor in postchemotherapy seminoma: an update of the prospective multicentric SEMPET trial. J Clin Oncol 22(6): 1034, 2004.

Dimopoulos MA, Papadopoulou M, Andrepoulou E et al: Favorable outcome of ovarian germ cell malignancies treated with cisplatin or carboplatin-based chemotherapy: A Hellenic Cooperative Oncology Group Study. Gynecol Oncol 70:70, 1998.

Dimopoulos MA, Papadimitriou C, Hamilos G et al: Treatment of ovarian germ cell tumors with a 3-day bleomycin, etoposide, and cisplatin regimen: a prospective multicenter study. Gynecol Oncol 95:695, 2004.

DiSaia PJ et al: Chemotherapeutic retroconversion of immature teratoma of the ovary. Obstet Gynecol 49:346, 1977.

Edraki B, Schwartz PE: Fertility after conservative treatment of ovarian immature teratoma. Int J Gynecol Cancer 7:227, 1997.

Emig OR, Hertig AT, Rowe FJ: Gynandroblastoma of the ovary: Review and report of a case. Obstet Gynecol 13:135, 1959.

Favara BE, Franciosi RA: Ovarian teratoma and neuroglial implants on the peritoneum. Cancer 31:678, 1973.

Forney JP, DiSaia PJ, Morrow CP: Endodermal sinus tumor: A report of two sustained remissions treated postoperatively with a combination of actinomycin D, 5-fluorouracil and cyclophosphamide. Obstet Gynecol 45:186, 1975.

Freel JH et al: Dysgerminoma of the ovary. Cancer 43:798, 1979.

Fujita M, Inque M, Tanizawa et al: Retrospective review of 41 patients with endodermal sinus tumor of the ovary. Int J Gynecol Cancer 3:329, 1993.

Gallion HH, Van Nagell JR, Donaldson ES et al: Ovarian dysgerminoma: Report of seven cases and review of the literature. Am J Obstet Gynecol 158:591, 1988.

Gallion H, Van Nagell JR, Pall BF: Therapy of endodermal sinus tumors of the ovary. Am J Obstet Gynecol 135:447, 1979.

Gerbie MV, Brewer JI, Taminni H: Primary choriocarcinoma of the ovary. Obstet Gynecol 46:720, 1975.

Gershenson DM: Management of early ovarian cancer: Germ cell and sex-cord stromal tumors. Gynecol Oncol 55:S62, 1994.

Gershenson DM: Menstrual and reproductive function after treatment with combined chemotherapy for malignant ovarian germ cell tumors. J Clin Oncol 6:270, 1988.

Gershenson DM: Update on malignant ovarian germ cell tumors. Cancer 71:1581, 1993.

Gershenson DM, Del Junco G, Copeland LJ: Mixed germ cell tumors of the ovary. Obstet Gynecol 64:200, 1985.

Gershenson DM, Morris M, Cangir A et al: Treatment of malignant germ cell tumors of the ovary with bleomycin, etoposide, and cisplatin. J Clin Oncol 8:715, 1990.

Gershenson DM et al: Endodermal sinus tumor of the ovary. Obstet Gynecol 61:194, 1983.

Gordon A, Lipton D, Woodruff JD: Dysgerminoma: A review of 158 cases from the Emil Novak Ovarian Tumor Registry. Obstet Gynecol 58:497, 1981.

Hart WR, Burkons DM: Germ cell neoplasms arising in gonadoblastomas. Cancer 43:669, 1979.

Jacobs A et al: Treatment of recurrent and persistent germ cell tumors with cisplatin, vinblastine and bleomycin. Obstet Gynecol 59:129, 1982.

Jimerson GK, Woodruff JD: Ovarian extra-embryonal teratoma. I. Endodermal sinus tumor. Am J Obstet Gynecol 127:73, 1977.

Kammerer-Doak D, Baurick K, Black W et al: Case report: Endodermal sinus tumor and embryonal carcinoma of the ovary in a 53-year-old woman. Gynecol Oncol 63:133, 1996.

Kojs Z, Urbanski K, Mitus J et al: Pure immature teratoma of the ovary: Analysis of 22 cases. Eur J Gynecol Oncol 28:534, 1997.

Koller O, Gjonnaess H: Dysgerminoma of the ovary: A clinical report of 20 cases. Acta Obstet Gynecol Scand 43:268, 1964.

Kollmannsberger C, Hartmann JT, Kanz L et al: Therapy-related malignancies following treatment of germ cell cancer. Int J Cancer 83:860, 1999.

Kosloske AM et al: Management of immature teratoma of the ovary in children by conservative resection and chemotherapy. J Pediatr Surg 11:839, 1976.

Krepart G et al: The treatment of dysgerminoma of the ovary. Cancer 41:986, 1978.

Kurman RJ, Norris HJ: Embryonal carcinoma of the ovary—a clinicopathologic entity distinct from endodermal sinus tumor resembling embryonal carcinoma of the adult testis. Cancer 38:2420, 1976.

Kurman RJ, Norris HJ: Endodermal sinus tumor of the ovary: A clinical and pathological analysis of 71 cases. Cancer 38:2404, 1976.

Kurman RJ, Norris HJ: Malignant germ cell tumors of the ovary. Hum Pathol 8:551, 1977.

Kurman RJ, Norris HJ: Malignant mixed germ cell tumors of the ovary: A clinical and pathological analysis of 30 cases. Obstet Gynecol 48:579, 1976.

Kurman RJ, Scardino PT, Waldman TA et al: Malignant germ cell tumors of the ovary and testis: An immunologic study of 69 cases. Ann Clin Lab Sci 9:462, 1979.

La Polla JP, Bende J, Vigliotti AP et al: Dysgerminoma of the ovary. Obstet Gynecol 69:859, 1987.

Low JJ, Perrin LC, Crandon AJ et al: Conservative surgery to preserve ovarian function in patients with malignant ovarian germ cell tumors. A review of 74 cases. Cancer 89:391, 2000.

Lucraft HH: A review of 33 cases of ovarian dysgerminoma emphasizing the role of radiotherapy. Clin Radiol 30:585, 1979.

Messing MJ, Gershenson DM, Morris M et al: Primary treatment failure in patients with malignant ovarian germ cell neoplasms. Int J Gynecol Cancer 2:295, 1992.
Morris HHB, La Vecchia C, Draper GJ: Endodermal sinus tumor and embryonal carcinoma of the ovary in children. Gynecol Oncol 21:7, 1985.
Munkarah A, Gershenson DM, Leverback C et al: Salvage surgery for chemotherapy ovarian germ cell tumors. Gynecol Oncol 55:217, 1994.
Neubecker RD, Breen JL: Gynandroblastoma: A report of five cases, with a discussion of the histogenesis and classification of ovarian tumors. Am J Clin Pathol 38:60, 1982.
Newlands ES et al: Potential for cure in metastatic ovarian teratomas and dysgerminomas. Br J Obstet Gynaecol 89:555, 1982.
Norris HJ, Zirkin HJ, Benson WL: Immature (malignant) teratoma of the ovary: a clinical and pathologic study of 58 cases, Cancer 37:2359, 1976.
Parvez D et al: Long-term disease-free survival in immature teratoma of the ovary. Cancer 50:159, 1982.
Patel PS, Sharma VM, Raval GN et al: Serum lactate dehydrogenase levels in malignant germ cell tumors of the ovary. Int J Gynecol Cancer 6:328, 1996.
Peccatori F, Bonazzi C, Chiari S et al: Surgical management of malignant ovarian germ cell tumors: 10 years' experience of 129 patients. Obstet Gynecol 86:367, 1995.
Robboy SJ, Scully RE: Ovarian teratoma with glial implants on the peritoneum: an analysis of 12 cases. Hum Pathol 1:643, 1970.
Rosenshein NB et al: Pregnancy following chemotherapy for an ovarian immature embryonal teratoma. Gynecol Oncol 8:234, 1979.
Roth LM, Panganiban WG: Gonadal and extragonadal yolk sac carcinomas: A clinicopathologic study of 14 cases. Cancer 37:812, 1976.
Russell P, Pointer DM: The pathologic assessment of ovarian neoplasms. V: The germ cell tumors. Pathology 14:47, 1982.
Santesson L, Marrubini G: Clinical and pathological survey of ovarian embryonal carcinomas, including so-called "mesonephromas" (Schiller) or "mesoblastomas" (Teilum), treated at the Radiumhemmet. Acta Obstet Gynecol Scand 36:399, 1957.
Schellhas HF et al: Germ cell tumors associated with XY gonadal dysgenesis. Am J Obstet Gynecol 109:1197, 1971.
Schwartz PE, Chambers SK, Chambers JT et al: Ovarian germ cell malignancies: The Yale University experience. Gynecol Oncol 45:26, 1992.
Scully RE: Gonadoblastoma: A review of 74 cases. Cancer 25:1340, 1970.
Scully RE: Ovarian tumors: A review. Am J Pathol 87:686, 1977.
Scully RE: Special ovarian tumors and their management. Int J Radiat Oncol Biol Phys 8:1419, 1982.
Segelov E, Campbell J, Ng M et al: Cisplatin-based chemotherapy for ovarian germ cell malignancies: The Australian experience. J Clin Oncol 12:378, 1994.
Sessa C et al: Cisplatin, vinblastine, and bleomycin combination chemotherapy in endodermal sinus tumors of the ovary. Obstet Gynecol 70:220, 1987.
Shefren G, Collin J, Soriero O: Gliomatosis peritonei with malignant transformation: A case report and review of the literature. Am J Obstet Gynecol 164:1617, 1991.
Slate RE et al: Vincristine, dactinomycin and cyclophosphamide in treatment of germ cell tumors of the ovary. Cancer 56:243, 1985.
Slayton RE, Park RC, Schenberg SG et al: Vincristine, dactinomycin and cyclophosphamide in the treatment of malignant germ cell tumors of the ovary. Cancer 56:243, 1985.
Slayton RE et al: Treatment of malignant ovarian germ cell tumors; response to vincristine, dactinomycin, and cyclophosphamide (preliminary report). Cancer 42:390, 1978.
Smith EB, Clarke-Pearson DL, Creasman WT: A VP16-213- and cisplatin-containing regimen for treatment of refractory ovarian germ cell malignancies. Am J Obstet Gynecol 150:927, 1984.
Tangir J, Zelterman D, Ma W et al: Reproductive function after conservative surgery and chemotherapy for malignant germ cell tumors of the ovary. Obstet Gynecol 101:251, 2003
Teilum G: Classification of endodermal sinus tumor (mesoblastoma vitellinum) and so-called "embryonal carcinoma" of the ovary. Acta Pathol Microbiol Scand 64:407, 1965.
Tewfik HH, Tewfik FA, Latourette HB: A clinical review of seventeen patients with ovarian dysgerminoma. Int J Radiat Oncol Biol Phys 8:1705, 1982.
Thomas EM, Dembo AJ, Hacker NF et al: Current therapy for dysgerminoma of the ovary. Obstet Gynecol 70:268, 1987.
Thomas GM et al: Current therapy for dysgerminoma of the ovary. Obstet Gynecol 70:268, 1987.
Truong LD, Jurco S, McGavran MH: Gliomatosis peritonei. Am J Surg Pathol 6:443, 1982.
Ungerleider RS et al: Endodermal sinus tumor: The Stanford experience and the first reported case arising in the vulva. Cancer 41:1627, 1978.
Williams SD, Blessing JA, Liao S-Y et al: Adjuvant therapy of ovarian germ cell tumors with cisplatin, etoposide, and bleomycin: A trial of the Gynecologic Oncology Group. J Clin Oncol 12:701, 1994.
Williams SD: Current management of ovarian germ cell tumors. Oncology 8:53, 1994.
Williams SD, Birch R, Einhorn LH et al: Treatment of disseminated germ-cell tumors with cisplatin, bleomycin and either vinblastine or etoposide. N Engl J Med 316:1435, 1987.
Williams SD, Blessing JA, DiSaia PJ et al: Second look laparotomy in ovarian germ cell tumors: The Gynecologic Oncology Group Experience. Gynecol Oncol 52:287, 1994.
Williams SD, Blessing JA, Moore DM et al: Cisplatin, vinblastine and bleomycin in advanced and recurrent ovarian germ cell tumors. Ann Intern Med 111:22, 1989.
Zanetta G, Bonnazi C, Cantu M et al: Survival and reproductive function after treatment of malignant germ cell ovarian tumors. J Clin Oncol 19:1015, 2001.

TUMORS DERIVED FROM SPECIAL GONADAL STROMA

Ala-Fossi SL, Maenpaa J, Aine R et al: Prognostic significance of p53 expression in ovarian granulosa cell tumors. Gynecol Oncol 66:475, 1997.
Anderson WR, Levine AJ, MacMillan D: Granulosa-theca cell tumors: Clinical and pathologic study. Am J Obstet Gynecol 110:32, 1971.
Bremmer WJ: Inhibin: from hypothesis to clinical application. N Engl J Med 321:790, 1989.
Brewer CA, Shevlin D: Encouraging response of an advanced steroid-cell tumor to GNRH agonist therapy. Obstet Gynecol 92:661, 1998.
Brown J, Shvartsman HS, Deavers MT, Burke TW, Munsell MF, Gershenson DM: The activity of taxanes in the treatment of sex cord-stromal ovarian tumors. J Clin Oncol 22(17): 3517, 2004.
Brown J, Shvartsman HS, Deavers MT, Ramondetta LM, Burke TW, Munsell MF, Gershenson DM: The activity of taxanes compared with bleomycin, etoposide, and cisplatin in the treatment of sex cord-stromal ovarian tumors. Gynecol Oncol 97(2): 489, 2005.
Burger HG: Clinical utility of inhibin measurements. J Clin Endocrin Metab 76:1391, 1993.
Camlibel FT, Caputo TA: Chemotherapy of granulosa cell tumors. Am J Obstet Gynecol 145:763, 1983.
Chalvardjian A, Scully RE: Sclerosing stromal tumors of the ovary. Cancer 31:664, 1973.
Chan JK, Zhang M, Kaleb V, Loizzi V, Benjamin J, Vasilev S, Osann K, DiSaia PJ: Prognostic factors responsible for survival in sex cord stromal tumors of the ovary—a multivariate analysis. Gynecol Oncol 96:204–209, 2005.
Colombo N, Essa C, Landonin F et al: Cisplatin, vinblastine and bleomycin combination chemotherapy in metastatic granulosa cell tumor of the ovary. Obstet Gynecol 67:265, 1986.

Colombo N, Parma G, Franchi D: An active chemotherapy regimen for advanced ovarian sex cord-stromal tumors. Gynecol Oncol 72:129, 1999.

Cool I, O'Brien M, Charnock M et al: Inhibin as a marker for ovarian cancer. Br J Cancer 71:1046, 1995.

Cronje HS, Niemand I, Bam RH, Woodruff JD: Review of the granulosa-theca cell tumors from the Emil Novak Ovarian Tumor Registry. Am J Obstet Gynecol 180:323, 1999.

Dinnerstein AJ, O'Leary JA: Granulosa-theca cell tumors: A clinical review of 102 patients. Obstet Gynecol 31:654, 1968.

DiSaia PJ et al: A temporary response of recurrent granulosa cell tumor to Adriamycin. Obstet Gynecol 52:355, 1978.

Evans AJ III et al: Clinicopathologic review of 118 granulosa and 82 theca cell tumors. Obstet Gynecol 55:213, 1980.

Finan MA, Roberts WS, Kavanagh JJ: Ovarian Sertoli–Leydig cell tumor: success with salvage therapy. Int J Gynecol Cancer 3:189, 1993.

Gard GB, Mulvany N, Quinn MA: Alpha-fetoprotein and Sertoli–Leydig cell tumor. Int J Gynecol Cancer 8:499, 1998.

Gershenson DM: Management of early ovarian cancer: Germ cell and sex cord-stromal tumors. Gynecol Oncol 55:S62, 1994.

Gershenson DM, Copeland LJ, Kavanagh JJ et al: Treatment of metastatic stromal tumors of the ovary with cisplatin, doxorubicin, and cyclophosphamide. Obstet Gynecol 70:765, 1987.

Gershenson DM, Morris M, Burke TW et al: Treatment of poor prognosis sex cord-stromal tumors of the ovary with the combination of bleomycin, etoposide, and cisplatin. Obstet Gynecol 87(4):527, 1996.

Gillibrand PN: Granulosa-theca cell tumors of the ovary associated with pregnancy: Case report and review of the literature. Am J Obstet Gynecol 94:1108, 1966.

Gusberg SB, Kardon P: Proliferative endometrial response to theca-granulosa cell tumors. Am J Obstet Gynecol 111:633, 1971.

Healy DL, Burger HG, Mamers P et al: Elevated serum inhibin concentrations in postmenopausal women with ovarian tumors. N Engl J Med 329:1539, 1993.

Hines JF, Khalafia MA Moore JL et al: Recurrent granulosa cell tumor of the ovary 37 years after initial diagnosis: A case report and review of the literature. Gynecol Oncol 60:484, 1996.

Homesley HD, Bundy BN, Hurteau JA, Roth LM: Bleomycin, etoposide, and cisplatin combination therapy of ovarian granulosa cell tumors and other stromal malignancies: A Gynecologic Oncology Group Study. Gynecol Oncol 72:131, 1999.

Ishiko O, Yoshida H, Sumi T: Vascular endothelial growth factor levels in pleural and peritoneal fluid in Meig's syndrome. Eur J Obstet Gynecol Reprod Biol 98: 129, 2001.

Jacobs AJ, Deppe G, Cohen CJ: Combination chemotherapy of ovarian granulosa cell tumor with cisplatinum and doxorubicin. Gynecol Oncol 14:294, 1982.

Jobling T, Mamers P, Healy DL et al: A prospective study of inhibin in granulosa cell tumors of the ovary. Gynecol Oncol 55:285, 1994.

Kietlinska Z, Pietrzak K, Drabik M: The management of granulosa-cell tumors of the ovary based on long-term follow up. Eur J Gynecol Oncol 14:118, 1993.

Lack EE et al: Granulosa-theca cell tumors in premenarchal girls: a clinical and pathologic study of ten cases. Cancer 48:1846, 1981.

Malstrom H, Hogberg T, Risberg B, Simonsen E: Granulosa cell tumors of the ovary: Prognostic factors and outcome. Gynecol Oncol 52:50, 1994.

Martikainen H, Penttinen J, Huhtaniemi I, Kauppila A: Gonadotropin-releasing hormone agonist analog therapy effective in ovarian granulosa cell malignancy. Gynecol Oncol 35:406, 1989.

Maxwell GL, Soisson AP, Miles P: Failure of gonadotropin releasing hormone therapy in patients with metastatic ovarian sex cord stromal tumors. Oncology 51 (4):356, 1994.

Norris HJ, Taylor HB: Prognosis of granulosa-theca tumors of the ovary. Cancer 21:255, 1968.

Norris HJ, Taylor HB: Virilization associated with cystic granulosa tumors. Obstet Gynecol 34:629, 1969.

Novak ER, Long JH: Arrhenoblastoma of the ovary: A review of the Ovarian Tumor Registry. Am J Obstet Gynecol 92:1082, 1965.

Novak ER, Mattingly RF: Hilus cell tumor of the ovary. Obstet Gynecol 15:425, 1960.

Novak ER et al: Feminizing gonadal stromal tumors: Analysis of granulosa-theca cell tumors of the Ovarian Tumor Registry. Obstet Gynecol 38:701, 1971.

Pautier P, Lhomme C, Culine S et al: Adult granulosa cell tumor of the ovary: A retrospective study of 45 cases. Int J Gynecol Cancer 7:58, 1997.

Powell JL, Otis CN: Management of advanced juvenile granulosa cell tumor of the ovary: Case report. Gynecol Oncol 64:282, 1997.

Rey RA, Lhomme C, Marcillac I: Antimullerian hormone as a serum marker of granulosa cell tumors of the ovary: comparative study with serum alpha-inhibin and estradiol. Am J Obstet Gynecol 174:958, 1996.

Roush GR, El-Nagger AK, Abdul-Karim FW: Granulosa cell tumor of the ovary: A clinicopathologic and flow cytometric DNA analysis. Gynecol Oncol 56:430, 1995.

Segal R, DePetrillo AD, Thomas G: Clinical review of adult granulosa cell tumors of the ovary. Gynecol Oncol 56:338, 1995.

Stenwig JT, Hazekamp J, Beecham J: Granulosa cell tumors of the ovary: A clinicopathological study of 118 cases with long-term follow-up. Gynecol Oncol 7:136, 1979.

Tresukosol D, Kudelka AP, Edwards CL et al: Recurrent ovarian granulosa cell tumor: A case report of a dramatic response to Taxol. Int J Gynecol Cancer 5:156, 1995.

Young RH, Scully RE: Ovarian Sertoli-Leydig cell tumors with a retiform pattern: A problem in histopathologic diagnosis: A report of 25 cases. Am J Surg Pathol 7:755, 1983.

Young RH, Welch WR, Dickersin GR, Scully RE: Ovarian sex cord tumor with annular tubules: review of 74 cases including 27 with Peutz–Jeghers syndrome and four with adenoma malignum. Cancer 50: 1384, 1982.

Wolf JK, Mullen J, Eifel PJ et al: Radiation treatment of advanced or recurrent granulosa cell tumor of the ovary. Gynecol Oncol 73:35, 1999.

Zaloudek C, Norris HJ: Granulosa tumors of the ovary in children: A clinical and pathological study of 32 cases. Am J Surg Pathol 6:503, 1982.

Zaloudek C, Norris HJ: Sertoli–Leydig tumors of the ovary: A clinicopathologic study of 64 intermediate and poorly differentiated neoplasms. Am J Surg Pathol 8:405, 1984.

OTHER OVARIAN TUMORS

Azoury RS, Woodruff JD: Primary ovarian sarcomas: Report of 43 cases from the Emil Novak Ovarian Tumor Registry. Obstet Gynecol 37:920, 1971.

Bicher A, Levenback C, Silva EG et al: Ovarian malignant mixed müllerian tumors treated with platinum-based chemotherapy. Obstet Gynecol 85:735, 1995.

Blackwell WJ et al: Dermoid cysts of the ovary, their clinical and pathologic significance. Am J Obstet Gynecol 51:151, 1946.

Dehner LP, Norris HJ, Taylor HB: Carcinosarcomas and mixed mesodermal tumors of the ovary. Cancer 27:207, 1971.

DiSaia PJ, Pecorelli S: Gynecological sarcomas. Semin Surg Oncol 10:369, 1994.

Dunn S: Bilateral virilizing hilus (Leydig) cell tumors of the ovary. Acta Obstet Gynecol Scand 73:76, 1994.

Einhorn LH, Donohue J: Cis-diamminedichloro-platinum, vinblastine, and bleomycin combination chemotherapy in disseminated testicular cancer. Ann Intern Med 87:293, 1977.

Ferenczy A, Okagaki T, Richart RM: Para-endocrine hypercalcemia in ovarian neoplasms: Report of mesonephroma with hypercalcemia and review of literature. Cancer 27:427, 1971.

Fox H, Langley FA, Govan ADT et al: Malignant lymphoma presenting as ovarian tumor: A clinicopathologic analysis of 34 cases. Br J Obstet Gynaecol 95:386, 1998.

Fox LP, Stamm WJ: Krukenberg tumor complicating pregnancy: Report of a case with androgenic activity. Am J Obstet Gynecol 92:702, 1965.

Genadry R, Parmley T, Woodruff JD: Case report-secondary malignancies in benign cystic teratomas. Gynecol Oncol 8:246, 1979.

Hale RW: Krukenberg tumor of the ovaries: A review of 81 records. Obstet Gynecol 22:221, 1968.

Joshi VV: Primary Krukenberg tumor of ovary: A review of literature and case report. Cancer 22:1199, 1968.

Judd HL et al: Maternal virilization developing during a twin pregnancy: Demonstration of excess ovarian androgen production associated with theca-lutein cysts. N Engl J Med 288:118, 1973.

Krumerman MS, Chung A: Squamous carcinoma arising in benign cystic teratoma of the ovary. Cancer 29:1237, 1977.

Monk BJ, Nieberg R, Berek JS: Primary leiomyosarcoma of the ovary in a premenarchal female. Gynecol Oncol 48:389, 1993.

Monterroso V, Jaffe ES, Merino MJ, Medeiros LJ: Malignant lymphomas involving the ovary: A clinicopathologic analysis of 39 cases. Am J Surg Pathol 17:154, 1993.

Peterson WF et al: Benign cystic teratomas of the ovary: A clinicostatistical study of 1007 cases with a review of the literature. Am J Obstet Gynecol 70:568, 1955.

Pfeiffer P, Hardt-Madsen M, Rex S et al: Malignant mixed müllerian tumors of the ovary report of 13 cases. Acta Obstet Gynecol Scand 70:79, 1991.

Prendiville J, Murphy D, Renninson J et al: Carcinosarcoma of the ovary treated over a 10-year period at the Christie Hospital. Int J Gynecol Cancer 4:200, 1994.

Qizilbach AH et al: Functioning primary carcinoid tumor of the ovary. Am J Clin Pathol 62:629, 1974.

Robboy SJ, Scully RE, Norris HJ: Carcinoid metastatic to the ovary: A clinicopathologic analysis of 35 cases. Cancer 33:798, 1974.

Robboy SJ, Scully RE, Norris HJ: Primary trabecular carcinoid of the ovary. Obstet Gynecol 49:202, 1977.

Sood AK, Sorosky JI, Gelder MS, Buller RE: Primary ovarian sarcoma, analysis of prognostic variables and the role of surgical cytoreduction. Cancer 82:1731, 1998.

Spadoni LR et al: Virilization coexisting with Krukenberg tumor during pregnancy. Am J Obstet Gynecol 92:981, 1965.

Woodruff D, Noli Castillo RD, Novak ER: Lymphoma of the ovary: A study of 35 cases from the Ovarian Tumor Registry of the American Gynecological Society. Am J Obstet Gynecol 85:912, 1963.

Woodruff JD, Novak ER: The Krukenberg tumor: A study of 48 cases from the Ovarian Tumor Registry. Obstet Gynecol 15:351, 1960.

MALIGNANT OVARIAN TUMORS IN CHILDREN

Abell MR, Holtz F: Ovarian neoplasms in childhood and adolescence. II: Tumors of non-germ cell origin. Am J Obstet Gynecol 93:850, 1965.

Ablin AR: Malignant germ cell tumors in children. Front Radiat Ther Oncol 16:141, 1982.

Acosta A, Kaplan AL, Kaufman RH: Gynecologic cancer in children. Am J Obstet Gynecol 112:944, 1972.

Barber HRK: Ovarian cancers in childhood. Int J Radiat Oncol Biol Phys 8:1427, 1982.

Barber HRK, Graber EA: Gynecological tumors in childhood and adolescence. Obstet Gynecol Surv 28:357, 1973.

Breen JL, Bonamo JF, Maxson WS: Genital tract tumors in children. Pediatr Clin North Am 28:355, 1981.

Breen JL, Neubecker RD: Ovarian malignancy in children with special reference to the germ cell tumors. Ann N Y Acad Sci 142:208, 1962.

Cangir A, Smith J, van Eys J: Improved prognosis in children with ovarian cancers following modified VAC (vincristine, sulfate, dactinomycin, and cyclophosphamide) chemotherapy. Cancer 42:1234, 1978.

Carlson DH, Griscom NT: Ovarian cysts in the newborn. AJR Am J Roentgenol 116:664, 1972.

Groeber WR: Ovarian tumors during infancy and childhood. Am J Obstet Gynecol 86:1027, 1963.

Hernandez W et al: Mixed mesodermal sarcoma of the ovary. Obstet Gynecol 49:59, 1977.

Holtz F, Hart WR: Krukenberg tumors of the ovary: A clinicopathologic analysis of 27 cases. Cancer 50:2438, 1982.

Kempers RD et al: Struma ovarii-ascitic, hyperthyroid and asymptomatic syndromes. Ann Intern Med 72:883, 1970.

Marshall JR: Ovarian enlargement in the first year of life: Review of 45 cases. Ann Surg 161:372, 1965.

Moore JC, Schifrin BS, Erez S: Ovarian tumors in infancy, childhood and adolescence. Am J Obstet Gynecol 99:913, 1967.

Norris HJ, Jensen RD: Relative frequency of ovarian neoplasms in children and adolescents. Cancer 39:713, 1972.

Smith JP, Rutledge F, Sutow WW: Malignant gynecologic tumors in children: Current approaches to treatment. Am J Obstet Gynecol 116:261, 1973.

Weinblatt ME, Ortega JA: Treatment of children with dysgerminoma of the ovary. Cancer 49:2608, 1982.

13 Fallopian Tube Cancer

Jan S. Sunde, M.D., Keith J. Kaplan, M.D., and G. Scott Rose, M.D.

INCIDENCE AND EPIDEMIOLOGY

Adenocarcinoma of the fallopian tube is one of the rarest malignancies of the female genital tract. Its frequency in relationship to all gynecologic cancers has traditionally been considered to be 1% or less, with an average annual incidence in the USA of 3.3 per 1,000,000 women. The incidence of fallopian tube cancer (FTCA) in Finland is reported to have increased more than fourfold, from 1.2 to 5.4 per 100,000, from the 1950s to the 1990s, but a similar trend has not been reported elsewhere. Factors thought to be associated with the increase were a decrease in parity, higher socioeconomic status, and opossibly pelvic inflammatory disease, as well as improved diagnosis and increased longevity. FTCA has been associated with BRCA mutations in several recent case series, and the incidence in this subset of women is reported to be as high as 3%, an estimated 120-fold increase in risk compared with the general population.

Fallopian tube carcinoma is initially seen in many cases as an unexpected operative finding at the time of laparotomy for a pelvic mass, because of its low incidence and the difficulty in distinguishing the fallopian tube mass from ovarian or uterine pathology. Cases have been reported in patients who were undergoing prophylactic salpingo-oophorectomy for hereditary ovarian cancer syndrome, as well as tubal sterilization. Chronic tubal inflammation has been reported to be associated with fallopian tube carcinoma. The initial connection was with tuberculosis, and sporadic case reports of fallopian tube carcinoma with coexisting tubercular salpingitis continue to be published. Although histologic features of old pelvic inflammatory disease are frequently noted on gross or histologic examination of the tube, and changes consistent with chronic healed salpingitis have been found in the contralateral tube of patients with unilateral FTCA, it has not been determined whether such inflammatory changes are precursors to the development of the carcinoma. There is currently no suspected infectious agent thought to be a cocarcinogen in FTCA, as with herpes papillomavirus and cervical cancer.

Nulliparity has been reported in up to one-third of FTCA cases, and infertility has been associated in some series. Age incidence resembles the pattern seen among women who develop ovarian or endometrial malignancies, with cases occurring rarely at a young age and incidence increasing to a peak in the sixties to early seventies. Two-thirds of the patients are postmenopausal (Fig. 13–1). The similarities of age group incidence, low parity, and infertility status suggest that the etiology may be similar to that of ovarian and endometrial carcinoma. Some studies have demonstrated similar genetic abnormalities, such as c-crb, B-2, p53, and K-ras mutations. These abnormalities are also common in ovarian and endometrial carcinomas.

Molecular biology and genetics

Some studies have demonstrated a number of genetic abnormalities in FTCA that are similar to those noted in ovarian cancer, such as gene mutations, alterations in gene copy number, and loss of heterozygosity. Gene mutations include ERBB-2 (HER-2/neu), TP53 (p53), and K-RAS (K-ras) mutations. All fallopian tubal cancers showed a high frequency of copy number aberrations, with similar alterations noted by several authors, The most frequent changes detected in fallopian tube carcinoma were gains at 3q (70%) and 8q (75%), with high-level amplifications in several cases. Other common gains occurred at 1q, 5p, 7q, 12p, and 20q. The most frequent losses were found at 18q, 16q, 17p, 8p, and 5q. Similar alterations are reported in ovarian cancer, with amplifications of 8q, 1q, 20q, and

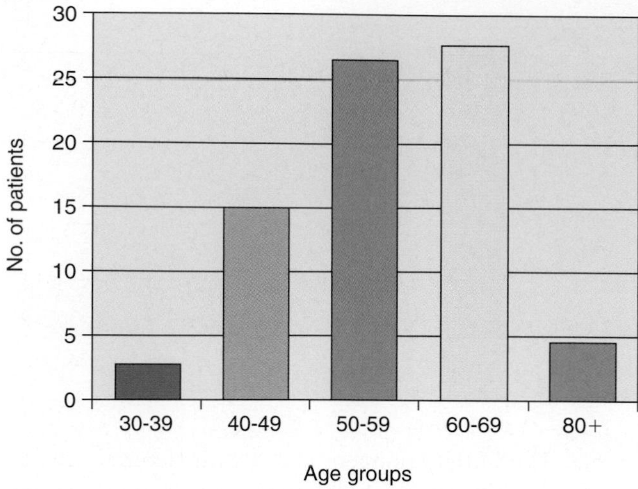

Figure 13–1 Carcinoma of the fallopian tube: patients treated in 1996–8. Distribution by age groups. (FIGO report. Int J Gynecol Obstet 83(suppl 1):119–133, 2003. © International Federation of Gynecology and Obstetrics. Reprinted with permission.)

3q, and under-representation of 18q. Loss of heterozygosity at 13q has been reported in BRCA-related fallopian tube and ovarian cancers, but the significance of this genetic alteration is unclear.

Alterations in protein levels documented by immunohistochemical staining change similarly in fallopian tube and ovarian cancer, with an increase in the proliferation-related protein MKI67 (Ki-67), and decreases in the cell cycle inhibitory proteins CDKN1A (p21) and CDKN1B (p27). Other proteins elevated in both cancer types include TP53, MYC (c-myc), ERBB-2, AKT2, WT1 (Wilms tumor 1), and PCNA. TP53 is associated with decreased survival, and is also increased in tubal dysplasia associated with FTCA. Determination of the genetic and molecular alterations of fallopian tube carcinoma, and comparison with the alterations associated with other intraperitoneal cancers, may lead to a better understanding of the relationship between these cancer types.

HEREDITARY CANCER

Fallopian tube cancer has been found with increased incidence (1.7–3%) at centers that have established screening programs for women at high risk for gynecologic malignancy, both in patients observed using a screening protocol and in patients electing prophylactic surgery (Table 13–1). The lifetime risk of FTCA in BRCA mutation carriers has been reported to be 0.6–3%. Fishman et al, in the largest series to date, reported 10 cancers in 581 BRCA mutation carriers (1.8%) undergoing prophylactic salpingo-oophorectomy, of which three were FTCAs (30%). Barakat et al reported three cancers in 180 cases (1.7%), with one of three from the fallopian tube. Meeuwissen et al found two cancers in 133 patients in their series, with one of two (50%) being a fallopian tube malignancy. Rebbeck et al, on the other hand, found six ovarian cancers in 259 patients, and no FTCA.

Several authors have recently noted a marked increase in the detection of occult gynecologic cancers, including FTCAs and carcinoma in situ (CIS), at the time of prophylactic salpingo-oophorectomy if extensive sectioning of the pathologic specimen is performed. FTCA and peritoneal papillary serous carcinoma, rather than ovarian cancer, comprise the majority of gynecologic malignancies in these high-risk women. Colgan et al found 5/60 (8%) FTCAs in their series in 2001, with 2/5 (40%) cases with disease confined to the fallopian tube; one case with disease of the fallopian tube and ovary; and one case with disease of the fallopian tube, ovary, and uterine serosa. These findings have been confirmed by others. Olivier et al reported five

Table 13–1 CANCERS DETECTED USING STANDARD PATHOLOGIC EVALUATION IN PATIENTS UNDERGOING PROPHYLACTIC BILATERAL SALPINGO-OOPHORECTOMY FOR HEREDITARY CANCER

	Reference					
	Fishman et al (2005)	Meeuwissen et al (2005)	Barakat et al for the Society of Gynecologic Oncologists (2003)	Kauff et al (2002)	Rebbeck et al (2002)	Total
Patients screened	580	133	180	98	259	1250
Cancers detected	10	2	3	3	6	24
Cancers detected (%)	1.7	1.5	1.7	3.1	—	1.9
Fallopian tube cancer	3	1	1	1	0	6
Fallopian tube cancer/all cancers (%)	30	50	33	33	—	25
Ovarian cancer	4	0	2	2	6	14
Peritoneal papillary serous carcinoma	3	0	0	0	0	3
Metastatic	0	1	3	0	0	4

Table 13–2 CANCERS DETECTED USING SERIAL SECTIONING OF THE PATHOLOGIC SPECIMENS IN PATIENTS UNDERGOING PROPHYLACTIC BILATERAL SALPINGO-OOPHORECTOMY FOR HEREDITARY CANCER

	Reference				
	Olivier et al (2004)	Leeper et al (2002)	Powell et al (2005)	Colgan et al (2001)	Total
Patients screened	58	30	67	60	215
Cancers or carcinoma in situ detected	5	5	7	5	22
Cancers detected (%)	8.6	16.7	10.4	8.3	10.2
Fallopian tube/invasive (carcinoma in situ)	2	3 (2)	4 (3)	2 (1)	11
Fallopian tube cancer/all cancers (%)	40.0	60.0	57.1	40.0	50.0
Ovarian cancer	2	1 (LMP)	3	1	7
Peritoneal papillary serous carcinoma	—	1	—	—	1
More than one site	1	—	1	2	4

cancers in 58 patients, with two (40%) cancers of the fallopian tube and one of the fallopian tube and ovary. Leeper et al reported 5/30 (17%) patients with occult malignancy at the time of risk-reducing salpingo-oophorectomy (RRSO), with 3/5 (60%) being FTCA. Powell et al found seven cancers in 67 (10%) patients, with 4/7 (57%) from the fallopian tube. Consolidating the data reported in the literature, 22 (10.2%) cancers have been detected in 215 hereditary cancer patients undergoing prophylactic RRSO, with 11 (50%) arising in the fallopian tube (Table 13–2).

Precancerous changes of the fallopian tube without the presence of cancer have also been noted with increased frequency in high-risk women. Carcangiu et al evaluated normal-appearing fallopian tubes in RRSO specimens after excluding cancers discovered at surgery to look for epithelial changes, and found that 4/22 (18%) BRCA1 patients had CIS or atypical hyperplasia, whereas 0/4 BRCA2 patients had cellular changes.

Fallopian tube cancer may be associated with BRCA mutations more frequently than ovarian cancer, with 16–43% of patients found to carry a mutation in recent series. BRCA1 appears to be associated with FTCA at a higher rate than BRCA2, although most papers linking BRCA2 with FTCA to date are case reports. The presence of a BRCA mutation also affects the histologic type of cancer that develops. In a series of 50 BRCA-associated FTCAs, Piek et al noted no non-epithelial malignancies, and 94% of the cases were papillary serous cancers compared with 62% of sporadic intraperitoneal malignancies. Improved survival of BRCA mutation carriers with FTCA, with a median survival of 148 months compared with 41 months in sporadic cases, has been reported.

Peritoneal washings and serial sectioning of pathologic specimens should be considered essential in high-risk patients, as they have improved detection of both FTCA and occult ovarian cancer. Prior to the recent association of BRCA1/2 mutations and FTCA, oophorectomy was considered by some to be adequate prophylactic surgery in high-risk patients. There has been one case report of FTCA after oophorectomy only, and the tubal epithelium is clearly at risk in these patients, so salpingectomy, along with oophorectomy, must be a part of prophylactic surgery. Hysterectomy has also been advocated to avoid the possible risk of cancer in the interstitial portion of the tube, although this remains controversial; it was recently shown by Cass et al that FTCA is a distal and mid-tube process in their series of 50 patients, and there have been no documented cases of cancer arising in the interstitial portion of the tube. Restaging, which can be done laparoscopically, is necessary if occult tumor is found at the time of RRSO, with over half the cases (5/8) of apparent early-stage FTCA upstaged in the report by Leblanc et al. Patients with FTCA or CIS appear to be at significant risk for carrying a BRCA mutation, so BRCA testing should be offered to allow appropriate counseling regarding the patient's and her family's potential increased risk of other cancers.

Patients with Peutz–Jeghers syndrome may also have a genetic predisposition to tumors of the female genital tract, including the fallopian tube. They have an increased incidence of the rare tumors, adenoma malignum, and ovarian sex cord tumor with annular tubules. There have also been reports of mucinous metaplasia and carcinosarcoma in the fallopian tubes of these patients.

CARCINOMA IN SITU

Carcinoma in situ of the fallopian tube is a diagnosis that histologically requires the epithelial cells of the endosalpingeal lining to form papillae with cytologically malignant mitotically active nuclei. CIS was present in 18% of fallopian tubes removed at RRSO in BRCA mutation carriers in one report, and can also be seen side by side with invasive adenocarcinoma (Fig. 13–2). The epithelial cells lose their polarity and grow in papillae without stromal cases. Nuclei are hyperchromatic, large, and irregular, and mitoses are numerous, but the basement membrane is intact. Atypical hyperplasia or dysplasia of the fallopian tube epithelium in high-risk women undergoing RRSO has been reported to occur in 2/22 (10%) specimens by Carcangiu et al, and in 6/12 (50%) of the tubes by Piek et al. Piek et al also reported atypical hyperplasia, considered

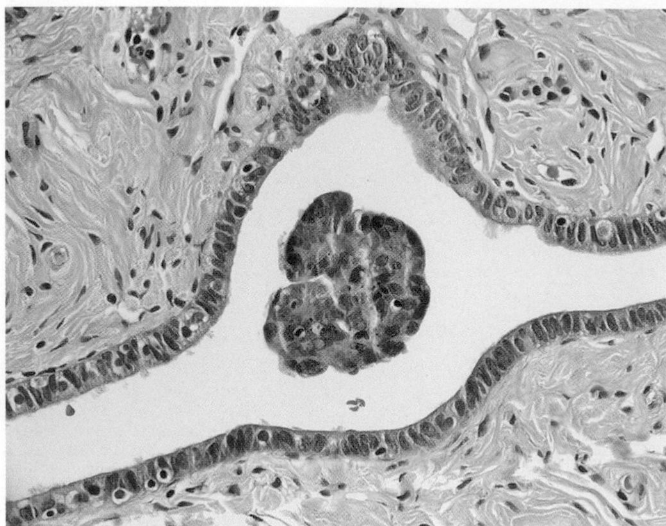

Figure 13–2 Fallopian tube carcinoma in situ seen adjacent to carcinoma in the lumen of the tube. (Courtesy of Keith Kaplan.)

to be less severe than dysplasia, in another five of the 12 patients. Of note, morphologically normal, hyperplastic, and dysplastic epithelium in the RRSO patients had molecular alterations consistent with cellular proliferation, a higher proportion of Ki-67–expressing cells, and lower fractions of cells expressing p21 and p27 when compared with control patients. Tamoxifen therapy has also been associated with diffuse bilateral atypical hyperplasia and adenocarcinoma in situ of the fallopian tube in case reports. The role of the patients' genetic predisposition vs an effect of tamoxifen therapy on the tubal epithelium remains unclear. Controversy also remains regarding the terminology of hyperplastic and dysplastic changes of the epithelium, as well as the premalignant potential of hyperplastic changes of the tubes in RRSO patients.

Mucinous metaplasia and neoplasia have been described. There are case reports of these changes noted at the time of tubal ligation, as well as in patients with Peutz–Jeghers syndrome.

Treatment of tubal CIS, if it exists alone, involves removal of the tube or tubes, with a staging procedure including careful inspection of the ovaries to rule out metastatic disease. The incidence of bilaterality of CIS is unknown and is an important consideration of this disease, which may be found incidentally in a portion of a tube removed for an ectopic pregnancy. The decision regarding therapy in this setting must consider the patient's desire for future fertility, in addition to a possible genetic predisposition for breast and gynecologic cancer. Careful surveillance for gynecologic and breast cancers, with the offer of bilateral salpingo-oophorectomy at the completion of childbearing, is probably warranted, as for women with hereditary breast cancer syndromes. When CIS is found in the portion of the tube removed at tubal ligation, the authors have routinely recommended, at a minimum, bilateral salpingo-oophorectomy, because preservation of fertility is not an issue.

INVASIVE CARCINOMA

Signs and symptoms

Most patients who have these malignancies will have symptoms such as vaginal bleeding or discharge, and/or lower abdominal pain. Less frequent symptoms include abdominal distension and urinary urgency. In many cases, these symptoms are vague and non-specific. Vaginal bleeding is the most common symptom of tubal carcinoma and is present in approximately 50% of the patients. Because this lesion occurs most frequently in the postmenopausal patient, postmenopausal bleeding is common; as a result, carcinoma of the endometrium is the first consideration in the differential diagnosis. One must seriously consider the diagnosis of fallopian tube carcinoma when the result of the dilatation and curettage is negative and symptoms persist. Vaginal bleeding is caused by blood that accumulates from the lesion in the fallopian tube, which subsequently passes into the uterine cavity and finally exits into the vagina. Pain is frequently a symptom in tubal carcinoma, is usually colicky, and often accompanies the vaginal bleeding. The pain is caused by distension of the tubal wall and stimulation of peristaltic activity. This pain, in many cases, is relieved with the passage of blood or watery discharge. Vaginal discharge, which is usually clear, occurs in approximately 25% of patients with tubal carcinoma.

The triad of pain, metrorrhagia, and leukorrhea is considered pathognomonic for tubal carcinoma, but it occurs infrequently. Pain with bloody vaginal discharge is a more common finding. Pain combined with a profuse, watery vaginal discharge, referred to as hydrops tubae profluens, is reported to be present in less than 5% of cases. If a patient is examined during the time that hydrops tubae profluens is present, a palpable pelvic mass is frequently found. The mass can decrease during the examination while the watery discharge continues. With the cessation of watery discharge and decrease in pelvic mass, the pain also decreases. Hydrops tubae profluens is caused by the effusion produced by the tumor that accumulates within the tube and causes the distension, which in turn produces the colicky pain. A pelvic mass, which is often interpreted as a pedunculated fibroid or ovarian neoplasm, is the most common physical sign. It is found in over half of patients, with an abdominal mass noted in another 25% of patients, usually adnexal in location, and in most cases it is interpreted as a pedunculated fibroid or ovarian neoplasm (Fig. 13–3). Ascites was reported to be present in 5% of patients in a meta-analysis by Nordin in 1994. Presentation with symptoms consistent with pelvic inflammatory disease should raise suspicion for FTCA in a postmenopausal patient. Presentation with metastasis to an inguinal node has been reported, as well as several cases of paraneoplastic cerebellar degeneration.

Delay of diagnosis appears to be common. In a study by Eddy and associates, symptoms had been present for as long as 48 months. One half of the patients had symp-

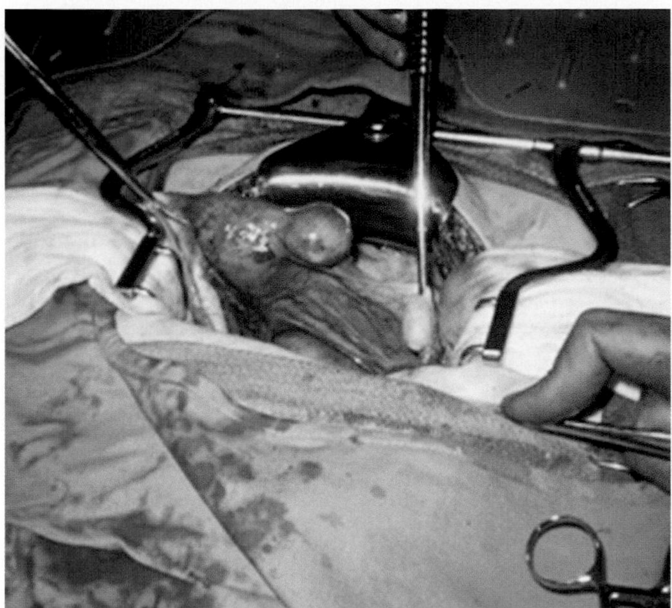

Figure 13–3 Primary tubal carcinoma. The right ovary is normal.

toms for 2 months or longer. Semrad and colleagues noted a delay from the onset of symptoms to the diagnosis of an average of 4 months in about one-half of their patients. Peters et al reported that 14% of patients were asymptomatic in their series of 115 patients.

Malignant cells are found in 11–23% of cervical cytologic preparations in patients with tubal cancer. In patients with hydrops tubae profluens, the chance of obtaining malignant cells should be relatively high. The identification of psammoma bodies in cervical cytology of postmenopausal women is often a sign of uterine or clear cell carcinoma, with serous fallopian tube or ovarian cancer occasionally being identified as the source.

Diagnosis

More than 80% of patients have either a pelvic or an abdominal mass noted before surgery. Between 10 and 25% will have abnormal cervical cytology suggestive of adenocarcinoma. Because uterine and ovarian pathology are much more common than tubal disease, it is not surprising that patients with pelvic masses are thought to have abnormalities other than tubal ones. Patients with abnormal cytology are likewise believed to have the more common diagnosis of a cervical or uterine malignancy instead of a primary tubal malignancy.

Ultrasound, both abdominal and vaginal, is reported to be very accurate in noting changes in adnexal size and its morphology. Patlas et al reported that transvaginal sonography in five of seven patients with FTCA showed normal ovaries in association with a discrete solid adnexal mass in four. In the three patients without a discrete adnexal mass, there were more extensive changes, including large, solid adnexal masses of unknown origin or gross peritoneal carcinomatosis. Presence of small cystic or solid masses shaped like a sausage, a snail, or a gourd, regardless of clinical stage, are other reported findings. Kurjak et al reported improved identification of FTCA using three-dimensional ultrasound compared with two-dimensional ultrasound. The three-dimensional ultrasound allowed precise depiction of tubal wall irregularities such as papillary protrusions and pseudosepta. Multiple sections of the tubal sausage-like structures also enabled determination of local tumor spread and capsule infiltration. Study of the vascular architecture was further enhanced using three-dimensional power Doppler imaging. Other authors have not confirmed these findings, and the role of advanced ultrasound techniques in the evaluation has not been determined.

Reports that have appeared in the literature evaluating use of ultrasound in conjunction with CA-125 testing as a method of screening for gynecologic malignancy have noted higher than expected incidence of FTCA. In the large cancer screening project of the Royal London Hospital, 22,000 patients were screened with CA-125, and if the serum CA-125 was elevated patients underwent pelvic ultrasound. Of 15 patients with pelvic malignancies identified through the elevated CA-125 screening, three (20%) had primary FTCA. The ratio of epithelial ovarian cancers to FTCAs in volunteers for ovarian cancer screening was 6:1, which is 25-fold greater than the expected ratio. Two of the patients had stage I disease, and one patient had stage II. A large screening program for high-risk women that uses both CA-125 and ultrasound every 6 months, the National Ovarian Cancer Early Detection Program, has been ongoing in the USA since 1990. Fishman et al recently reported that 12 gynecologic malignancies were discovered by screening 4426 high-risk women who elected not to have a prophylactic RRSO. Four cancers (33%) arose in the fallopian tube, four (33%) were primary peritoneal serous carcinoma, two (16%) were ovarian, and two (16%) were uterine. (Unfortunately, all the cancers detected were stage III at the time of diagnosis except for the uterine cancers, casting doubt on the value of CA-125 and transvaginal ultrasound for detecting early-stage disease.)

Both of these large screening trials found a much higher ratio of FTCA to ovarian cancer than expected based on the reported incidence of FTCA in the general population. This is in contrast to the findings of Nagall et al, who did not report an increased proportion of FTCAs in a screening program of women in the general population in Kentucky. The reason for the different ratios of FTCA to ovarian cancer in these screening trials is unclear. Whether the English study was subject to selection bias, leading to high-risk women being screened, is unknown. It may be that the diagnostic criteria for gynecologic cancers favor assessment of advanced-stage intraperitoneal cancers as ovarian in origin, and the ratio of FTCA to ovarian cancer in the general population may be higher than previously reported.

Successful use of other radiologic imaging modalities to identify FTCAs has been described in case reports. There have not been trials evaluating diagnostic imaging of FTCA prospectively, but the data on ovarian cancer are applicable to all intraperitoneal cancers, because the radiologic findings are similar. The Radiology Diagnostic Oncology Group found that magnetic resonance imaging (MRI) is superior to Doppler ultrasound and computed tomography (CT) in diagnosis of malignant ovarian masses, and that CT and MRI are preferred over ultrasound for staging. Positron emission tomography–CT with 2-fluoro-2-deoxy-D-glucose may prove to be a sensitive and accurate method for detection of metastatic disease, which may influence the clinical management of recurrent fallopian tube carcinoma.

Immunohistochemical staining for CA-125 is positive in 87% of tumors. The use of serum CA-125 levels becomes a valuable tool in monitoring these patients during and after therapy for evidence of a recurrence. It has also been evaluated in screening programs for ovarian cancer, as noted, and has been reported to be a harbinger of FTCA in this setting. Its usefulness as a screening tool remains to be determined.

Histologic diagnosis may be difficult because of the similarities of FTCA to metaplastic processes associated with inflammation of the tubal epithelium found in pelvic inflammatory disease or tuberculous salpingitis, as well as other gynecologic cancers. Another complicating factor can be multifocal neoplasia, which can occur both within the fallopian tube and in the other genital organs and the peritoneal cavity. Synchronous cancers in the fallopian tube have been reported in up to 10% of ovarian cancers. Hu has suggested diagnostic criteria for the diagnosis of tubal cancer:

- the main tumor grossly should be in the tube;
- histologically, the tubal mucosa should be involved with a papillary pattern; and
- if the tubal wall is involved to a large extent, transition from benign to malignant tubal epithelium should be identified.

When the ovaries are involved, differentiation between a primary tubal malignancy and a primary ovarian malignancy should be attempted. When ovarian cancer extends to the tube, serosal involvement is usually quite evident, and the mucosa of the endosalpinx may not be involved. In such situations, the correct diagnosis is apparent. In some cases of tubal cancer, the benign to malignant transition may not be readily apparent. It may be that these strict diagnostic criteria favor assessment of advanced-stage intraperitoneal cancers as ovarian in origin. Interestingly, in tubal carcinoma there is usually intraperitoneal involvement before the ovaries are affected. Because of the possibility of early intraperitoneal cytologic spread even with only mucosal involvement, the role of peritoneal cytology is important in this disease entity. In patients with disease limited to the tube, the exact extent should be ascertained. If an in situ lesion is present or invasion is limited to the lamina propria, the prognosis is quite good. When the muscularis is invaded or the cancer is located in the fimbria, the prognosis worsens, even with disease limited to the tube.

The late stage of the disease mimics late-staged ovarian cancer with intraperitoneal spread. It appears that FTCA, like ovarian cancer, also has a propensity for lymph node metastasis. This has been described even with apparent stage I/II disease, and with well-differentiated tumors. Klein and associates noted that the frequency of lymph node metastasis increased with intra-abdominal disease. Six of eight patients with stage III disease had lymph node metastasis. Patients frequently have para-aortic lymph node involvement only, while the majority of patients who had pelvic node metastasis had both pelvic and para-aortic involvement. Deffieux et al found that the left para-aortic chain above the level of the inferior mesenteric artery is the most frequently involved in patients with primary tubal carcinoma who have para-aortic lymph node metastasis.

Most carcinomas of the tube are cystic adenocarcinomas (Fig. 13–4), comprising 71% of cancers in one report with endometrioid, transitional cell, and mixed cell-type carcinomas each accounting for approximately 5–10% of tumors. The more indolent female adnexal tumors of probable wolffian origin tumors made up half of the endometrioid tumors at one referral center. Other rare epithelial cell types include clear cell carcinomas and adenosquamous carcinomas. Low malignant potential tumors have been reported. Sarcomas have been removed, and several case reports of other rare tumor types have been published.

Cass et al found that FTCA appears to arise primarily in the distal portion of the tube, with eight of 10 cases in the distal and mid-portion of the tube, and two cases involving the entire tube. Occult cancers were found only in the distal portion of the tube. There were no cases of only proximal involvement. Multifocal skip lesions were noted in the fallopian tubes of BRCA mutation carriers, as well as diffuse precursor lesions. Both tubes are equally affected. Bilaterality has been noted in 10–25% of patients. Tumors are usually large and noted on the pelvic examination; however, a number of cases of clinically occult cancers have been reported in patients undergoing prophylactic oophorectomy. Over-expression of p53 was found in 70% of cancers and associated dysplastic epithelium, but in only

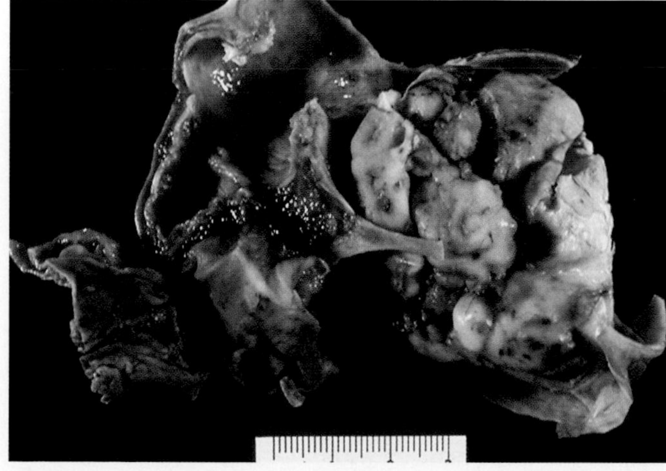

Figure 13–4 Typical cystic appearance of fallopian tube cancer. (Courtesy of Keith Kaplan.)

10% of surrounding normal epithelium in one report. The changes were present in both BRCA1 carriers and noncarriers. Meticulous histologic evaluation of the fallopian tube in apparent benign cases, including serial sectioning in high-risk patients, is obligatory.

Therapy

Because the diagnosis is rarely established preoperatively, one must be prepared to proceed with definitive therapy at the time of exploratory laparotomy for any adnexal mass or when this lesion is found coincidentally with other disease. In 1991, the International Federation of Gynecology and Obstetrics (FIGO) established a staging classification for tubal carcinoma for the first time. It follows the general outline of ovarian carcinoma that Alvarado-Cabrera et al have proposed—that depth of invasion into the lamina propria and muscularis layers of the fallopian tube and fimbrial involvement in stage I disease be incorporated into the staging classification, because these features have prognostic significance (Table 13–3).

Therapy guidelines should be essentially the same as those for ovarian carcinoma, and a total abdominal hysterectomy with bilateral salpingo-oophorectomy and surgical staging, including lymph node sampling, is optimal therapy. The safety of unilateral salpingectomy or salpingo-oophorectomy in appropriately staged young patients who desire fertility and whose disease apparently is confined to one tube has not been established. Removal of the remaining tube and ovary (or ovaries) should be performed at the completion of childbearing.

Even with apparent early disease, this malignancy can be bilateral. Peritoneal cytologic specimens should be obtained on opening the peritoneal cavity, not only from the pelvis but also from the lateral paracolonic gutters and supradiaphragmatic areas. Prognostic correlation with peritoneal cytologic findings has been noted in a report from the Mayo Clinic. Patients with negative cytologic findings had a 5-year survival of 67% compared with 20% in patients with positive cytologic findings. A partial omentectomy should be performed as well. Any disease outside the areas already extirpated should be removed if technically feasible. Debulking, as described in ovarian carcinoma, would also be applicable to this malignancy. Carcinomatous reduction to 1 cm or smaller was feasible in two-thirds of patients reported by Podratz. Optimal debulking appears to enhance survival, as in ovarian cancer. Obviously, patients with an earlier stage and complete surgical removal have a better survival than do patients with advanced disease and suboptimal removal.

Barakat and associates noted in their patients undergoing second-look laparotomy (SLL) that the absence of gross residual disease following primary surgery was the best predictor of disease-free status at SLL. These patients also had a significantly better 5-year survival rate (83%) than did those with gross residual disease (28%). Pelvic and para-aortic lymph node sampling are required for staging, even for patients with apparent early-stage disease, because of the risk of early lymphatic spread. Fallopian tube carcinoma tends to recur more often in retroperitoneal nodes and extraperitoneal sites than ovarian carcinoma. Postoperative therapy is most often needed, as in ovarian carcinoma.

Table 13–3 INTERNATIONAL FEDERATION OF GYNECOLOGY AND OBSTETRICS FALLOPIAN TUBE STAGING[a]

Stage	Definition
0	Carcinoma in situ (limited to tubal mucosa).
I[b]	Growth limited to the fallopian tubes.
Ia	Growth is limited to one tube, with extension into the submucosa or muscularis but not penetrating the serosal surface; no ascites.
Ib	Growth is limited to both tubes, with extension into the submucosa or muscularis but not penetrating the serosal surface; no ascites.
Ic	Tumor stage Ia or Ib but with tumor extension through or on to the tubal serosa; or with ascites present containing malignant cells, or with positive peritoneal washings.
II	Growth involving one or both fallopian tubes, with pelvic extension.
IIa	Extension or metastasis to the uterus or ovaries.
IIb	Extension to other pelvic tissues.
IIc	Tumor stage IIa or IIb, with ascites present containing malignant cells or with positive peritoneal washings.
III	Tumor involves one or both fallopian tubes, with peritoneal implants outside the pelvis or positive retroperitoneal or inguinal nodes. Superficial liver metastasis equals stage III. Tumor appears limited to the true pelvis but with histologically proven malignant extension to the small bowel or omentum.
IIIa	Tumor is grossly limited to the true pelvis, with negative nodes but with histologically confirmed microscopic seeding of abdominal peritoneal surfaces.
IIIb	Tumor involving one or both tubes, with histologically confirmed implants of abdominal peritoneal surfaces, none exceeding 2 cm in diameter. Lymph nodes are negative.
IIIc	Abdominal implants >2 cm in diameter or positive retroperitoneal or inguinal nodes.
IV	Growth involving one or both fallopian tubes, with distant metastases. If pleural effusion is present, there must be positive cytology to be stage IV. Parenchymal liver metastases equals stage IV.

[a]Staging for fallopian tube is by the surgical pathologic system. Operative findings designating stage are determined before tumor debulking.

[b]Alvarado-Cabrera et al have proposed that stage I disease be further subdivided based on no extension (0), extension into the lamina propria (1), and extension into the muscularis (2), with disease of the fimbria designated as a separate substage, 1(f).

(With permission of the International Federation of Gynecology and Obstetrics.)

Patients with stage Ia tumor without spread to the muscularis layer had 100% 5-year survival in the report by Alvarado-Cabrera et al and need not be treated. In contrast, patients with invasion of the muscularis layer or tumor in the fimbria, who had a 5-year survival of 71–72%, should receive additional therapy.

Fallopian tube cancers are often incorporated with ovarian cancer in chemotherapy trials, because of the small number of FTCAs and the apparent similarity of FTCA to ovarian cancer, and data regarding chemotherapy for ovarian cancer are considered applicable to FTCA. Therapy with a combination platinum/paclitaxel-based chemotherapy regimen, as in ovarian cancer, is typically used; case reports and one series reporting the outcomes of platinum/paclitaxel therapy in FTCA have also been published. Historically, the use of alkylating agent chemotherapy did not improve survival in this group of patients.

Combination chemotherapy using platinum and paclitaxel is currently the gold standard therapy for ovarian cancer. Gemignani et al have reported initial results in 24 patients (one received paclitaxel only due to hearing impairment) with this regimen in FTCA. Seven stage I and II patients had been treated, with one (14%) recurrence at a median follow-up of 42 months. In four earlier studies, adjuvant therapy in early-stage disease (I and II) had not been shown to benefit survival, although survival rates in the 50–60% range indicate that there was probably undetected disease outside the pelvis. Early experience with stage I carcinoma of the ovary showed that survival was approximately 60%. With more intense surgical staging, survival has increased to 85–90% in many series. Adjuvant therapy may have played a role in this improved survival in ovarian cancer; however, in some cases surgery only accounted for survival equal to that of those who received adjuvant therapy. Obviously, adjuvant therapy can be more optimally and judiciously utilized if the exact extent of the disease is identified surgically.

Combination platinum/paclitaxel therapy has been reported to produce complete responses and long-term survivals in advanced-stage FTCA patients. Seventeen stage III and IV patients were treated using platinum/paclitaxel therapy, with a 90% 3-year survival. (The data were not mature enough to report 5-year survival.) Five of eight patients with suboptimal cytoreduction at the time of laparotomy developed recurrence, and four were retreated with the same combination. Only two patients had died of disease at a median survival time of 51 months, so the authors were optimistic that the combination regimen would improve survival for FTCA, as it has for ovarian cancer. In an earlier report by Barakat et al, 38 patients were treated with cisplatin-based combination chemotherapy, with an overall survival of 51% at 5 years. Patients with stages II–IV who had completed resected tumors had a 5-year survival of 83%, compared with 28% if gross disease remained after surgery. It appears that cisplatin-based chemotherapy improves long-term survival in patients with advanced disease, but it may not be as effective as platinum combined with paclitaxel.

Wagenaar et al have reported the results of a phase II European Organization for Research and Treatment of Cancer trial of cyclophosphamide (C), doxorubicin (Adriamycin, A), and cisplatin (P) treating 24 patients with stage III–IV FTCA. Median overall survival at 3 and 5 years was only 25% and 19%, respectively. The group at the M.D. Anderson Hospital treated 18 patients with cisplatin, Adriamycin, and cyclophosphamide (Cytoxan) (CAP), with a mean survival rate of 44 months. No patient responded to second-line therapy.

The place of SLL has not been defined in tubal carcinoma, but it would be expected to be similar to that in ovarian cancer, where there appears to be limited benefit. Eddy and coworkers noted their experience with eight patients. Their results mimic those of ovarian cancer. The procedure may be prognostic, although two of five patients with negative SLL had a recurrence. The group at the Memorial Sloan–Kettering Cancer Center evaluated 35 patients with SLL following cytoreductive surgery and platinum-based chemotherapy. Twenty-one patients were tumor-free at the time of SLL. None of five patients with stage I or grade 1 tumors had disease at SLL. The absence of gross disease at the completion of primary surgery was the best predictor of disease-free status at SLL. Of the patients who were negative at SLL, only four (19%) had a recurrence of their tumor (mean follow-up of 50 months). Combined series in the literature also note this low recurrence rate. This, of course, is much better than in ovarian cancer. Approximately 30% of those found to have persistent disease at SLL were alive after 5 years. Whether or not an SLL has any appreciable effect on long-term survival is unknown.

Radiation therapy after surgery had been used frequently to treat FTCA prior to the advent of platinum- and taxane-based therapy, but it is not used frequently today. Much of the data regarding radiation therapy precede the era of surgical staging of apparent early-stage disease, making it difficult to draw conclusions regarding efficacy in properly staged patients. Given these constraints, Rosen et al retrospectively compared stage I and II patients who received adjuvant therapy with radiation or chemotherapy treated at multiple centers over a 25-year period ending in 1999, and found no significant difference in median survival time. They found significantly improved survival in patients undergoing surgery that included lymphadenectomy, presumably due to exclusion of advanced-stage disease in this group. They also reported that practice patterns had changed dramatically over the course of their study, with no radiation therapy for stage II patients after 1988 and for stage I patients after 1995. Baekelandt et al, in their review of 151 patients treated over many years, concluded that radiation therapy in FTCA should be abandoned due to frequent recurrences in patients receiving pelvic radiotherapy and an unacceptable complication rate in patients treated with whole abdominal radiation. Schray et al, on the other hand, reported in 1987 that eight of 10 (80%) stage I and II patients who received whole abdominal radiation (two with i.p. P-32) survived disease-free, while only four of 11 (36%) patients treated with pelvic radiation remained disease-free.

Radiation therapy appears to have fallen out of favor, and was used in only 4% of patients reported in the Surveillance, Epidemiology, and End Results (SEER) database in 2002, and in four of 105 patients in the FIGO report for 1995–8. Radiation is unlikely to be compared with combination chemotherapy in a prospective randomized trial, but preliminary data evaluating whole abdominal radiation following combination chemotherapy that indicate it may be more efficacious in preventing recurrence in ovarian cancer may be applicable in FTCA.

Prognosis

Survival with fallopian tube carcinoma has traditionally been poorer than that reported for ovarian cancer, but this has changed in two recent reports (Table 13–4). Five-year relative survival from the SEER database was reported by Kosary and Trimble as follows: stage I, 95%; stage II, 75%; stage III, 69%; and stage IV, 45%. Only 39% of patients were stage I or II, in contrast to earlier series where over half the patients were stage I or II, even though almost half of those diagnosed with stage I or II disease did not undergo surgical evaluation of lymph nodes. Most women with stage I or II disease were treated with surgery alone, while most women with stage III or IV disease were treated with surgery and chemotherapy.

Survival may improve further as a larger proportion of patients is staged and treated appropriately. Heintz et al have reported the FIGO 5-year survival data on patients treated from 1996 to 1998, with results as follows: stage I, 79%; stage II, 82%; stage III, 61%; stage IV, 29%; and an overall survival of 69%, a 24% increase from the previous 3-year reporting period. The report by Heintz et al had 57% of patients staged as stage I or II, with poorer survival when compared with the SEER data, suggesting that a greater number of patients were under-staged in their report.

Survival was better stage for stage with FTCA compared with ovarian cancer in both of these reports. Factors that contribute to the improved survival rates are improved therapeutic regimens that include chemotherapy with platinum and paclitaxel as primary therapy, upstaging of apparent stage I and II patients, and improved debulking, as well as the difficulty distinguishing the primary site of advanced-stage intraperitoneal cancer, with possible misclassification of more aggressive FTCAs. Other recent large retrospective reviews report worse survival, but these studies cover many years, with a large percentage of patients not receiving adequate staging or platinum and paclitaxel therapy.

Stage and the amount of residual disease at the time of debulking have consistently been found to be important prognostic factors, and some reports have found age, grade, lymphovascular space involvement, and a closed fimbriated end of the fallopian tube to be significant as well. Depth of invasion and involvement of the fimbria have also been reported as prognostic factors in stage I tumors, and it has been suggested that these factors be incorporated into FIGO staging by subdivision of stage I into substages based on no invasion, invasion into the lamina propria, or invasion into the muscularis layer of the tube. In patients with invasion into the tubal muscularis layer, there was a statistically significant increase in the risk of death from tumor. In these patients, the 5-year survival was only 60%, compared with 100% survival among patients who had no muscularis involvement.

SARCOMAS AND OTHER TUMORS

Sarcomas of the fallopian tube are rare. Although carcinosarcoma (mixed mesodermal or müllerian tumor) represents the largest number of sarcomas, fewer than 60 have been reported in the literature. Although 25 of the reported cases were found to contain heterologous elements, with non-müllerian tissue present this has not been shown to impact survival. Sarcomas have been reported in adolescents as well as in the elderly. Most patients present with symptoms similar to those of adenocarcinoma, are mainly in the sixth decade of life, and have low parity.

Treatment should be surgery initially, as in adenocarcinoma of the fallopian tube. Adjunctive chemotherapy with a platinum-based regimen is recommended. Sit et al reported a median survival of 19 months with paclitaxel/platinum vs 23 months with platinum/ifosfamide in carcinosarcoma of the fallopian tube. Duska et al reported combination

Table 13–4 FIVE-YEAR SURVIVAL OF FALLOPIAN TUBE CANCER PATIENTS BY STAGE DIAGNOSED AND TREATED AFTER ADOPTION OF INTERNATIONAL FEDERATION OF GYNECOLOGY AND OBSTETRICS STAGING

	Kosary and Trimble (2002)			Heintz et al (2003)		
Stage	No. of patients	% of all cases	Five-year survival (%)	No. of patients	% of cases	Five-year survival (%)
I	102	30.5	95	42	40.8	79
II	29	8.7	75	17	16.5	82
III	52	15.6	69	35	34.0	60
IV	151	45.2	45	7	6.8	29
Overall	334	—	—	103	—	69

paclitaxel/platinum therapy in 28 patients with carcinosarcoma of the ovary, with a complete response rate in 16 of 28 (55%), and a partial response rate in six patients, for a total response rate of 72%. Overall median survival was 27 months.

Prognosis in carcinosarcoma is guarded. Weber, in a review of the earlier literature, noted a survival rate of 63% at 1 year and only 47% at 2 years. Imachi noted a mean survival of all patients of only 16 months. Early-stage carcinosarcomas of the ovary have been reported to have the same prognosis as early-stage epithelial ovarian cancer when 382 cases were compared with epithelial ovarian cancer cases in the SEER database. Advanced-stage carcinosarcoma of the ovary was reported to have a 60% increased risk of death when compared with advanced-stage epithelial ovarian cancer. Presumably, carcinosarcoma of the fallopian tube has a similar prognosis, stage for stage, although there are not enough cases to make a similar evaluation of carcinosarcomas of the fallopian tube. Leiomyosarcoma of the tube has been reported but is rarer than is the carcinosarcoma. Optimal surgery combined with adjuvant therapy seems appropriate. Adjuvant therapy has yet to be defined. Pure embryonal rhabdomyosarcoma and chondrosarcoma of the tube have been reported. Trophoblastic lesions of the tube are very uncommon. Gestational trophoblastic neoplasia has been reported, including placental site nodule, placental site trophoblastic tumor, epithelioid trophoblastic tumor, and choriocarcinoma.

Metastatic tumors involving the tube are usually from the ovary or the endometrium. Low-grade stroma sarcoma may extend to involve the tube. Blood-borne metastases from breast or colon carcinoma or other extrapelvic tumors may also occur.

Other rare tumors that have been reported in the fallopian tube include neuroendocrine carcinoma, parafallopian tube transitional cell carcinoma, malignant carcinoid tumor, mixed malignant germ cell tumor, T-cell lymphoma, and marginal zone B-cell lymphoma. Benign lesions such as leiomyoma, serous cystadenofibroma, schwannoma, extraskeletal chondroma, and müllerianosis of the mesosalpinx have all been reported.

BIBLIOGRAPHY

INCIDENCE AND EPIDEMIOLOGY

Demopoulos RI, Aronov R, Mesia A: Clues to the pathogenesis of fallopian tube carcinoma: a morphological and immunohistochemical case control study. Int J Gynecol Pathol 20(2):128–132, 2001.

Gungor T, Keskin HL, Zergeroglu S et al: Tuberculous salpingitis in two of five primary fallopian tube carcinomas. J Obstet Gynaecol 23(2):193–195, 2003.

Pfeiffer P, Mogensen H, Amtrup F et al: Primary carcinoma of the fallopian tube: retrospective study of the patients reported to the Danish Cancer Registry in a five-year period. Acta Oncol 28:7, 1989.

Riska A, Leminen A, Pukkala E: Sociodemographic determinants of incidence of primary fallopian tube carcinoma, Finland 1953–97. Int J Cancer 104(5):643–645, 2003.

Starr AJ, Ruffolo EH, Shenoy BV et al: Primary carcinoma of the Fallopian tube: a surprise finding in a postpartum tubal ligation. Am J Obstet Gynecol 132(3):344–345, 1978.

Woolas R, Jacob I, Davis AP et al: What is the true incidence of primary fallopian tube carcinoma? Int J Gynecol Cancer 4:384, 1994.

MOLECULAR BIOLOGY AND GENETICS

Acs G, Pasha T, Zhang PJ: WT1 is differentially expressed in serous, endometrioid, clear cell, and mucinous carcinomas of the peritoneum, fallopian tube, ovary, and endometrium. Int J Gynecol Pathol 23(2):110–118, 2004.

Al-Hussaini M, Stockman A, Foster H et al: WT-1 assists in distinguishing ovarian from uterine serous carcinoma and in distinguishing between serous and endometrioid ovarian carcinoma. Histopathology 44(2):109–115, 2004.

Bali A, O'Brien PM, Edwards LS et al: Cyclin D1, p53, and p21Waf1/Cip1 expression is predictive of poor clinical outcome in serous epithelial ovarian cancer. Clin Cancer Res 10(15): 5168–5177, 2004.

Chung TK, Cheung TH, To KF et al: Overexpression of p53 and HER-2/neu and c-myc in primary fallopian tube carcinoma. Gynecol Obstet Invest 49(1):47–51, 2000.

Garzetti GG, Ciavattini A, Goteri G et al: Ki67 antigen immunostaining (MIB 1 monoclonal antibody) in serous ovarian tumors: index of proliferative activity with prognostic significance. Gynecol Oncol 56(2):169–174, 1995.

Ghazizadeh M, Sasaki Y, Araki T et al: Prognostic value of proliferative activity of ovarian carcinoma as revealed by PCNA and AgNOR analyses. Am J Clin Pathol 107(4):451–458, 1997.

Halon A, Rabczynski J: PCNA and laminin as prognostic factors in primary Fallopian tube carcinoma. Folia Morphol (Warsz) 62(4): 475–478, 2003.

Hashi A, Yuminamochi T, Murata S et al: Wilms tumor gene immunoreactivity in primary serous carcinomas of the fallopian tube, ovary, endometrium, and peritoneum. Int J Gynecol Pathol 22(4):374–377, 2003.

Hellstrom AC, Hue J, Silfversward C et al: DNA-ploidy and mutant p53 overexpression in primary fallopian tube cancer. Int J Gynecol Cancer 4(6):408–413, 1994.

Heselmeyer K, Hellstrom AC, Blegen H et al: Primary carcinoma of the fallopian tube: comparative genomic hybridization reveals high genetic instability and a specific, recurring pattern of chromosomal aberrations. Int J Gynecol Pathol 17(3):245–254, 1998.

Jongsma AP, Piek JM, Zweemer RP et al: Molecular evidence for putative tumour suppressor genes on chromosome 13q specific to BRCA1 related ovarian and fallopian tube cancer. Mol Pathol 55(5):305–309, 2002.

Kiechle M, Jacobsen A, Schwarz-Boeger U et al: Comparative genomic hybridization detects genetic imbalances in primary ovarian carcinomas as correlated with grade of differentiation. Cancer 91(3):534–540, 2001.

Pere H, Tapper J, Seppala M et al: Genomic alterations in fallopian tube carcinoma: comparison to serous uterine and ovarian carcinomas reveals similarity suggesting likeness in molecular pathogenesis. Cancer Res 58(19):4274–426, 1998.

Rosen AC, Ausch C, Klein M et al: p53 expression in fallopian tube carcinomas. Cancer Lett 156(1):1–7, 2000.

Snijders AM, Nowee ME, Fridlyand J et al: Genome-wide-array–based comparative genomic hybridization reveals genetic homogeneity and frequent copy number increases encompassing CCNE1 in fallopian tube carcinoma. Oncogene 22(27):4281–4286, 2003.

Taetle R, Aickin M, Yang JM et al: Chromosome abnormalities in ovarian adenocarcinoma: I. Nonrandom chromosome abnormalities from 244 cases. Genes Chromosomes Cancer 25(3): 290–300, 1999.

Zheng W, Sung CJ, Cao P et al: Early occurrence and prognostic significance of p53 alteration in primary carcinoma of the fallopian tube. Gynecol Oncol 64(1):38–48, 1997.

HEREDITARY CANCER

Agoff SN, Mendelin JE, Grieco VS et al: Unexpected gynecologic neoplasms in patients with proven or suspected BRCA-1 or -2 mutations: implications for gross examination, cytology, and clinical follow-up. Am J Surg Pathol 26(2):171–178, 2002.

Aziz S, Kuperstein G, Rosen B et al: A genetic epidemiological study of carcinoma of the fallopian tube. Gynecol Oncol 80(3): 341–345, 2001.

Barakat RR, Hensley ML, Bhaskaran D et al: Prophylactic Oophorectomy (PO) in Patients at Risk for Hereditary Ovarian Carcinoma (HOC). Chicago, Society of Gynecologic Oncologists, 2003.

Baudi F, De Paola L, Quaresima B et al: A novel Q3034R BRCA2 germline mutation identified in a fallopian tube cancer patient. Cancer Lett 191(2):211–214, 2003.

Brose MS, Rebbeck TR, Calzone KA: Cancer risk estimates for BRCA1 mutation carriers identified in a risk evaluation program. J Natl Cancer Inst 94(18):1365–1372, 2002.

Carcangiu ML, Radice P, Manoukian S et al: Atypical epithelial proliferation in fallopian tubes in prophylactic salpingo-oophorectomy specimens from BRCA1 and BRCA2 germline mutation carriers. Int J Gynecol Pathol 23(1):35–40, 2004.

Casarsa S, Puglisi F, Baudi F et al: BRCA2 germline mutations in primary cancer of the fallopian tube. Oncol Rep 12(2):313–316, 2004.

Cass I, Holschneider C, Datta N et al: BRCA-mutation Associated Fallopian Tube Carcinoma: a Distinct Clinical Phenotype? Chicago, Society of Gynecologic Oncologists, 2005.

Colgan TJ, Murphy J, Cole DE et al: Occult carcinoma in prophylactic oophorectomy specimens: prevalence and association with BRCA germline mutation status. Am J Surg Pathol 25(10): 1283–1289, 2001.

Costa J: Peutz–Jeghers syndrome: case presentation. Obstet Gynecol 50(1 suppl):15s–17s, 1977.

Demange L, Noguchi T, Sauvan R et al: A novel germline in frame deletion (4128del3) of the BRCA2 gene detected in a breast/ovarian cancer family with fallopian tube and brain tumors identified in the north of France. Hum Mutat 17(2):155, 2001.

Fishman DA, Blank SV, Singh D et al: Prophylactic Surgery for High-Risk Women. Chicago, Society of Gynecologic Oncologists, 2005.

Kauff ND, Satagopan JM, Robson ME et al: Risk-reducing salpingo-oophorectomy in women with a BRCA1 or BRCA2 mutation. N Engl J Med 346(21):1609–1615, 2002.

Lallas TA, Buekers TE, Buller RE: BRCA1 mutations in familial ovarian cancer. Mol Genet Metab 67(4):357–363, 1999.

Leeper K, Garcia R, Swisher E et al: Pathologic findings in prophylactic oophorectomy specimens in high-risk women. Gynecol Oncol 87(1):52–56, 2002.

Levine DA, Argenta PA, Yee CJ et al: Fallopian tube and primary peritoneal carcinomas associated with BRCA mutations. J Clin Oncol 21(22):4222–4227, 2003.

Lu KH, Garber JE, Cramer DW et al: Occult ovarian tumors in women with BRCA1 or BRCA2 mutations undergoing prophylactic oophorectomy. J Clin Oncol 18(14):2728–2732.

Mangili G, Taccagni G, Garavaglia E et al: An unusual admixture of neoplastic and metaplastic lesions of the female genital tract in the Peutz–Jeghers syndrome. Gynecol Oncol 92(1):337–342, 2004.

McEwen AR, McConnell DT, Kenwright DN et al: Occult cancer of the fallopian tube in a BRCA2 germline mutation carrier at prophylactic salpingo-oophorectomy. Gynecol Oncol 92(3): 992–994, 2004.

Metcalfe KA, Lynch HT, Ghadirian P et al: The risk of ovarian cancer after breast cancer in BRCA1 and BRCA2 carriers. Obstet Gynecol Surv 60(4):235–236, 2005.

Narod SA, Sun P, Ghadirian P et al: Tubal ligation and risk of ovarian cancer in carriers of BRCA1 or BRCA2 mutations: a case-control study. Lancet 357(9267):1467–1470, 2001.

Olivier RI, Lubsen-Brandsma LA, van Boven H et al: Additional salpingectomy after previous prophylactic oophorectomy in high-risk women: sense or nonsense? Gynecol Oncol 96(2):439–443, 2005.

Olivier RI, van Beurden M, Lubsen MA et al: Clinical outcome of prophylactic oophorectomy in BRCA1/BRCA2 mutation carriers and events during follow-up. Br J Cancer 90(8):1492–1497, 2004.

Paley PJ, Swisher EM, Garcia RL et al: Occult cancer of the fallopian tube in BRCA-1 germline mutation carriers at prophylactic oophorectomy: a case for recommending hysterectomy at surgical prophylaxis. Gynecol Oncol 80(2):176–180, 2001.

Peyton-Jones B, Olaitan A, Murdoch JB: Incidental diagnosis of primary fallopian tube carcinoma during prophylactic salpingo-oophorectomy in BRCA2 mutation carrier. BJOG 109(12):1413–1414, 2002.

Piek JM, Torrenga B, Hermsen B et al: Histopathological characteristics of BRCA1- and BRCA2-associated intraperitoneal cancer: a clinic-based study. Fam Cancer 2(2):73–78, 2003.

Piek JM, van Diest PJ, Zweemer RP et al: Dysplastic changes in prophylactically removed Fallopian tubes of women predisposed to developing ovarian cancer. J Pathol 195(4):451–456, 2001.

Powell CB, Kenley E, Chen LM et al: Risk-reducing salpingo-oophorectomy in BRCA mutation carriers: role of serial sectioning in the detection of occult malignancy. J Clin Oncol 23(1): 127–132, 2005.

Rebbeck TR, Lynch HT, Neuhausen SL et al: Prophylactic oophorectomy in carriers of BRCA1 or BRCA2 mutations. Prevention and Observation of Surgical End Points Study Group. N Engl J Med 346(21):1616–1622, 2002.

Rose PG, Shrigley R, Wiesner GL: Germline BRCA2 mutation in a patient with fallopian tube carcinoma: a case report. Gynecol Oncol 77(2):319–320, 2000.

Rosen B, Aziz S, Narod S et al: Hereditary and Reproductive Influences on Fallopian Tube Carcinoma. Chicago, Society of Gynecologic Oncologists, 2003.

Scheuer L, Kauff N, Robson M et al: Outcome of preventive surgery and screening for breast and ovarian cancer in BRCA mutation carriers. J Clin Oncol 20(5):1260–1268, 2002.

Schorge JO, Muto MG, Welch WR et al: Molecular evidence for multifocal papillary serous carcinoma of the peritoneum in patients with germline BRCA1 mutations. J Natl Cancer Inst 90(11):841–845, 1998.

Tong D, Stimpfl M, Reinthaller A et al: BRCA1 gene mutations in sporadic ovarian carcinomas: detection by PCR and reverse allele-specific oligonucleotide hybridization. Clin Chem 45(7):976–981, 1999.

Zweemer RP, van Diest PJ, Verheijen RH et al: Molecular evidence linking primary cancer of the fallopian tube to BRCA1 germline mutations. Gynecol Oncol 76(1):45–50, 2000.

CARCINOMA IN SITU

Carcangiu ML, Radice P, Manoukian S et al: Atypical epithelial proliferation in fallopian tubes in prophylactic salpingo-oophorectomy specimens from BRCA1 and BRCA2 germline mutation carriers. Int J Gynecol Pathol 23(1):35–40, 2004.

Keeney GL, Thrasher TV: Metaplastic papillary tumor of the fallopian tube: a case report with ultrastructure. Int J Gynecol Pathol 7(1):86–92, 1988.

Mangili G, Taccagni G, Garavaglia E et al: An unusual admixture of neoplastic and metaplastic lesions of the female genital tract in the Peutz–Jeghers syndrome. Gynecol Oncol 92(1):337–342, 2004.

Pickel H, Reich O, Tamussino K: Bilateral atypical hyperplasia of the fallopian tube associated with tamoxifen: a report of two cases. Int J Gynecol Pathol 17(3):284–285, 1998.

Piek JM, van Diest PJ, Zweemer RP et al: Dysplastic changes in prophylactically removed Fallopian tubes of women predisposed to developing ovarian cancer. J Pathol 195(4):451–456, 2001.

Robey SS, Silva EG: Epithelial hyperplasia of the fallopian tube, its association with serous borderline tumor of the ovary. Int J Gynecol Pathol 8:214, 1989.

Seidman JD: Mucinous lesions of the fallopian tube. A report of seven cases. Am J Surg Pathol 18(12):1205–1212, 1994.

Sonnendecker HE, Cooper K, Kalian KN: Primary fallopian tube adenocarcinoma in situ associated with adjuvant tamoxifen therapy for breast carcinoma. Gynecol Oncol 52(3):402–407, 1994.

Yanai-Inbar I, Siriaunkgul S, Silverberg SG: Mucosal epithelial proliferation of the fallopian tube: a particular association with ovarian serous tumor of low malignant potential? Int J Gynecol Pathol 14(2):107–113, 1995.

INVASIVE CARCINOMA

Alvarado-Cabrero I, Navani SS, Young RH et al: Tumors of the fimbriated end of the fallopian tube: a clinicopathologic analysis of 20 cases, including nine carcinomas. Int J Gynecol Pathol 16(3):189–196, 1997.

Alvarado-Cabrero I, Young RH, Vamvakas EC et al: Carcinoma of the fallopian tube: a clinicopathological study of 105 cases with observations on staging and prognostic factors. Gynecol Oncol 72(3):367–379, 1999.

Baekelandt M, Jorunn Nesbakken A, Kristensen GB et al: Carcinoma of the fallopian tube. Cancer 89(10):2076–2084, 2000.

Bannatyne P, Russell P: Early adenocarcinoma of the fallopian tubes. A case for multifocal tumorigenesis. Diagn Gynecol Obstet 3(1):49–60, 1981.

Barakat RR, Rubin SC, Saigo PE et al: Cisplatin-based combination chemotherapy in carcinoma of the fallopian tube. Gynecol Oncol 42:156, 1991.

Barakat RR, Rubin SC, Saigo PE et al: Second look laparotomy in carcinoma of the fallopian tube. Obstet Gynecol 82:748, 1993.

Deffieux X, Morice P, Thoury A et al: Anatomy of pelvic and para-aortic nodal spread in patients with primary fallopian tube carcinoma. J Am Coll Surg 200(1):45–48, 2005.

Dowdy SC, Metzinger DS, Gebhart JB et al: Salvage whole-abdominal radiation therapy after second-look laparotomy or secondary debulking surgery in patients with ovarian cancer. Gynecol Oncol 96(2):389–394, 2005.

Eddy GL et al: Fallopian tube carcinoma. Obstet Gynecol 64:546, 1984.

Euscher ED, Silva EG, Deavers MT et al: Serous carcinoma of the ovary, fallopian tube, or peritoneum presenting as lymphadenopathy. Am J Surg Pathol 28(9):1217–1223, 2004.

Fishman DA, Cohen L, Blank SV et al: The role of ultrasound evaluation in the detection of early-stage epithelial ovarian cancer. Am J Obstet Gynecol 192(4):1214–1221, 2005.

Frigerio L, Pirondini A, Pileri M et al: Primary carcinoma of the fallopian tube. Tumori 79:40, 1993.

Furneaux HM, Rosenblum MK, Dalmau J et al: Selective expression of Purkinje-cell antigens in tumor tissue from patients with paraneoplastic cerebellar degeneration. N Engl J Med 322(26): 1844–1851, 1990.

Gemignani ML, Hensley ML, Cohen R et al: Paclitaxel-based chemotherapy in carcinoma of the fallopian tube. Gynecol Oncol 80(1):16–20, 2001.

Haratz-Rubinstein N, Russell B, Gal D: Sonographic diagnosis of Fallopian tube carcinoma. Ultrasound Obstet Gynecol 24(1): 86–88, 2004.

Heintz AP, Odicino F, Maisonneuve P et al: Carcinoma of the Fallopian tube. Int J Gynaecol Obstet 83(suppl 1):119–133, 2003.

Hellström AC, Silfverswärd C, Nilsson B et al: Carcinoma of the fallopian tube: a clinical histopathologic review. Int J Cancer 4:395, 1994.

Hetzel DJ, Stanhope CR, O'Neill BP et al: Gynecologic cancer in patients with subacute cerebellar degeneration predicted by anti-Purkinje cell antibodies and limited in metastatic volume. Mayo Clin Proc 65(12):1558–1563, 1990.

Hu CY, Taylor ML, Hertig AJ: Primary carcinoma of the fallopian tube. Am J Obstet Gynecol 59:58, 1950.

Huber S, Medl M, Baumann L et al: Value of ultrasound and magnetic resonance imaging in the preoperative evaluation of suspected ovarian masses. Anticancer Res 22(4):2501–2507, 2002.

Klein M, Graf AH, Rosen A et al: Analysis of treatment failures and survival of patients with fallopian tube carcinoma: a cooperative task force study. Gynecol Oncol 84(2):351–352, 2002.

Klein M, Rosen A, Labousen M et al: Lymphogenous metastasis in the primary carcinoma of the fallopian tube. Gynecol Oncol 55:336, 1994.

Klein M, Rosen A, Lahousen M et al: The relevance of adjuvant therapy in primary carcinoma of the fallopian tube, stages I and II: irradiation vs. chemotherapy. Int J Radiat Oncol Biol Phys 48(5):1427–1431, 2000.

Klein M, Rosen AC, Lahousen M et al: Lymphadenectomy in primary carcinoma of the Fallopian tube. Cancer Lett 147(1–2): 63–66, 1999.

Kojs Z, Urbanski K, Reinfuss M et al: Whole abdominal external beam radiation in the treatment of primary carcinoma of the fallopian tube. Gynecol Oncol 65(3):473–477, 1997.

Kosary C, Trimble EL: Treatment and survival for women with Fallopian tube carcinoma: a population-based study. Gynecol Oncol 86(2):190–191, 2002.

Kupryjanczyk J, Thor AD, Beauchamp R et al: Ovarian, peritoneal, and endometrial serous carcinoma: clonal origin of multifocal disease. Mod Pathol 9(3):166–173, 1996.

Kurachi H, Maeda T, Murakami T et al: A case of fallopian tube carcinoma: successful preoperative diagnosis with MR imaging. Radiat Med 17(1):63–66, 1999.

Kurjak A, Kupesic S, Ilijas M et al: Preoperative diagnosis of primary fallopian tube carcinoma. Gynecol Oncol 68(1):29–34, 1998.

Kurjak A, Kupesic S, Jacobs I: Preoperative diagnosis of the primary fallopian tube carcinoma by three-dimensional static and power Doppler sonography. Ultrasound Obstet Gynecol 15(3):246–251, 2000.

Kurtz AB, Tsimikas JV, Tempany CM et al: Diagnosis and staging of ovarian cancer: comparative values of Doppler and conventional US, CT, and MR imaging correlated with surgery and histopathologic analysis—report of the Radiology Diagnostic Oncology Group. Radiology 212(1):19–27, 1999.

Leblanc E, Querleu D, Narducci F et al: Laparoscopic restaging of early stage invasive adnexal tumors: a 10-year experience. Gynecol Oncol 94(3):624–629, 2004.

Levite R, Fishman A, Kesler A et al: Paraneoplastic cerebellar degeneration heralding fallopian tube adenocarcinoma. Int J Gynecol Cancer 11(2):169–171, 2001.

Makhija S, Howden N, Edwards R et al: Positron emission tomography/computed tomography imaging for the detection of recurrent ovarian and fallopian tube carcinoma: a retrospective review. Gynecol Oncol 85(1):53–58, 2002.

Matsushita H, Kodama S, Aoki Y et al: Paraneoplastic cerebellar degeneration with anti-Purkinje cell antibody associated with primary tubal cancer. Gynecol Obstet Invest 45(2):140–143, 1998.

McGuire WP, Hoskins WJ, Brady MF et al: Cyclophosphamide and cisplatin compared with paclitaxel and cisplatin in patients with stage III and stage IV ovarian cancer. N Engl J Med 334(1): 1–6, 1996.

Meeuwissen PA, Seynaeve P, Brekelmans CT et al: Outcome of surveillance and prophylactic salpingo-oophorectomy in asymptomatic women at high risk for ovarian cancer. Gynecol Oncol 97(2):476–482, 2005.

Menon U, Talaat A, Rosenthal AN et al: Performance of ultrasound as a second line test to serum CA125 in ovarian cancer screening. BJOG 107(2):165–169, 2000.

Mikami M, Tei C, Kurahashi T et al: Preoperative diagnosis of fallopian tube cancer by imaging. Abdom Imaging 28(5):743–747, 2003.

Morris M, Gershenson DM, Burke TW et al: Treatment of fallopian tube carcinoma with cisplatin, doxorubicin and cyclophosphamide. Obstet Gynecol 76:1020, 1990.

Muntz HG, Rutgers JL, Tarraza HM et al: Carcinosarcomas and mixed Müllerian tumors of the fallopian tube. Gynecol Oncol 34(1):109–115, 1989.

Muntz HG, Tarraza HM, Goff BA et al: Combination chemotherapy in advanced adenocarcinoma of the fallopian tube. Gynecol Oncol 40:268, 1989.

Navani SS, Alvarado-Cabrero I, Young RH et al: Endometrioid carcinoma of the fallopian tube: a clinicopathologic analysis of 26 cases. Gynecol Oncol 63(3):371–378, 1996.

Nordin AJ: Primary carcinoma of the fallopian tube: a 20-year literature review. Obstet Gynecol Surv 49(5):349–361, 1994.

Outwater EK, Siegelman ES, Chiowanich P et al: Dilated fallopian tubes: MR imaging characteristics. Radiology 208(2):463–469, 1998.

Parkash V, Chacho MS: Psammoma bodies in cervicovaginal smears: incidence and significance. Diagn Cytopathol 26(2):81–86, 2002.

Patel PV, Cohade C, Chin BB: PET–CT localizes previously undetectable metastatic lesions in recurrent fallopian tube carcinoma. Gynecol Oncol 87(3):323–326, 2002.

Patlas M, Rosen B, Chapman W et al: Sonographic diagnosis of primary malignant tumors of the fallopian tube. Ultrasound Q 20(2):59–64, 2004.

Peters WA et al: Results of chemotherapy in advanced carcinoma of the fallopian tube. Cancer 63:836, 1989.

Peters WA, Anderson WA, Hopkins MD et al: Prognostic factors of carcinoma of the fallopian tube. Obstet Gynecol 71:757, 1988.

Pettersson F: Staging rules for gestational trophoblastic tumors and fallopian tube cancer. Acta Obstet Gynecol Scand 71(3):224–225, 1992.

Podratz KC et al: Primary carcinoma of the fallopian tube. Am J Obstet Gynecol 154:1319, 1986.

Raff JP, Anderson P, Sands C et al: Fallopian tube carcinoma presenting with a brain metastasis. Gynecol Oncol 85(2):372–375, 2002.

Romagosa C, Torne A, Iglesias X et al: Carcinoma of the fallopian tube presenting as acute pelvic inflammatory disease. Gynecol Oncol 89(1):181–184, 2003.

Rose PG, Piver MS, Tsukada Y: Fallopian tube cancer. The Roswell Park experience. Cancer 66(12):2661–2667, 1990.

Rosen AC, Ausch C, Hafner E et al: A 15-year overview of management and prognosis in primary fallopian tube carcinoma. Austrian Cooperative Study Group for Fallopian Tube Carcinoma. Eur J Cancer 34(11):1725–1729, 1998.

Rosen AC, Klein M, Hafner E et al: Management and prognosis of primary fallopian tube carcinoma. Austrian Cooperative Study Group for Fallopian Tube Carcinoma. Gynecol Obstet Invest 47(1):45–51, 1999.

Rosen AC, Reiner A, Klein M et al: Prognostic factors in primary fallopian tube carcinoma. Gynecol Oncol 53:307, 1994.

Russell P, Bannatyne PM, Solomon HJ et al: Multifocal tumorigenesis in the upper female genital tract—implications for staging and management. Int J Gynecol Pathol 4(3):192–210, 1985.

Safret A, Bosch B, Bannwart F et al: Carcinoma in situ of the fallopian tube presenting as a positive Pap smear. Acta Cytol 48(3):462–464, 2004.

Santana P, Desser TS, Teng N: Preoperative CT diagnosis of primary fallopian tube carcinoma in a patient with a history of total abdominal hysterectomy. J Comput Assist Tomogr 27(3):361–363, 2003.

Semrad N, Watring W, Fu YS et al: Fallopian tube adenocarcinoma: Common extraperitoneal recurrence. Gynecol Oncol 24:230, 1986.

Szklaruk J, Tamm EP, Choi H et al: MR imaging of common and uncommon large pelvic masses. Radiographics 23(2):403–424, 2003.

Takagi H, Matsunami K, Noda K et al: Primary fallopian tube carcinoma: a case of successful preoperative evaluation with magnetic resonance imaging. J Obstet Gynaecol 23(4):455–456, 2003.

Tamini HK, Figge DC: Adenocarcinoma of the uterine tube: potential for lymph node metastases. Am J Obstet Gynecol 141:132, 1981.

Tanaka K, Igarashi S, Yamazaki M et al: Paraneoplastic cerebellar degeneration: successful early detection and treatment of cancer through characterization of the anti-Purkinje cell antibody. Intern Med 31(12):1339–1342, 1992.

Tempany CM, Zou KH, Silverman SG et al: Staging of advanced ovarian cancer: comparison of imaging modalities—report from the Radiological Diagnostic Oncology Group. Radiology 215(3): 761–767, 2000.

Toki T, Imai T, Kobayashi H et al: Case report: adenocarcinoma of the bilateral fallopian tube occurring after tubal sterilization. Gynecol Oncol 58:400, 1995.

Tresukosol D, Kudelka AP, Edwards CL et al: Case report: primary fallopian tube adenocarcinoma: clinical complete response after salvage treatment with high-dose paclitaxel. Gynecol Oncol 58:258, 1995.

van Leeuwen BL, Pruim J, Gouw AS et al: Liver metastasis as a first sign of fallopian tube carcinoma and the role of positron emission tomography in preoperative diagnosis. Scand J Gastroenterol 37(12):1473–1474, 2002.

Wagenaar HC, Pecorelli S, Vergote I et al: Phase II study of a combination of cyclophosphamide, Adriamycin and cisplatin in advanced fallopian tube carcinoma. An EORTC Gynecological Cancer Group study. European Organization for Research and Treatment of Cancer. Eur J Gynaecol Oncol 22(3):187–193, 2001.

Winter-Roach BA, Tjalma WA, Nordin AJ et al: Inguinal lymph node metastasis: an unusual presentation of fallopian tube carcinoma. Gynecol Oncol 81(2):324–325, 2001.

Wolfson AH, Tralins KS, Greven KM et al: Adenocarcinoma of the fallopian tube: results of a multi-institutional retrospective analysis of 72 patients. Int J Radiat Oncol Biol Phys 40(1):71–76, 1998.

Woodruff JD, Solomon D, Sullivant H: Multifocal disease in the upper genital canal. Obstet Gynecol 65(5):695–698, 1985.

Yuen JH, Wong GC, Lam CH: Preoperative sonographic diagnosis of primary fallopian tube carcinoma. J Ultrasound Med 21(10): 1171–1173, 1985.

Zreik TG, Rutherford TJ: Psammoma bodies in cervicovaginal smears. Obstet Gynecol 97(5 part 1):693–695, 2001.

SARCOMAS AND OTHER TUMORS

Astall EC, Brewster JA, Lonsdale R: Malignant carcinoid tumour arising in a mature teratoma of the fallopian tube. Histopathology 36(3):282–283, 2000.

Baergen RN, Rutgers J, Young RH: Extrauterine lesions of intermediate trophoblast. Int J Gynecol Pathol 22(4):362–367, 2003.

Barnholtz-Sloan JS, Morris R, Malone JM Jr et al: Survival of women diagnosed with malignant, mixed müllerian tumors of the ovary (OMMMT). Gynecol Oncol 93(2):506–512, 2004.

Buchwalter CL, Jenison EL, Fromm M et al: Case report: pure embryonal rhabdomyosarcoma of the fallopian tube. Gynecol Oncol 67:95, 1997.

Callister M, Ramondetta LM, Jhingran A et al: Malignant mixed Müllerian tumors of the uterus: analysis of patterns of failure, prognostic factors, and treatment outcome. Int J Radiat Oncol Biol Phys 58(3):786–796, 2004.

Carlson JA, Ackerman BL, Wheeler JE: Malignant mixed müllerian tumor of the fallopian tube. Cancer 71:187, 1993.

Duran B, Guvenal T, Yildiz E et al: An unusual cause of adnexal mass: fallopian tube schwannoma. Gynecol Oncol 92(1):343–346, 2004.

Dursun P, Salman MC, Taskiran C et al: Primary neuroendocrine carcinoma of the fallopian tube: a case report. Am J Obstet Gynecol 190(2):568–571, 2004.

Duska LR, Garrett A, Eltabbakh GH et al: Paclitaxel and platinum chemotherapy for malignant mixed müllerian tumors of the ovary. Gynecol Oncol 85(3):459–463, 2002.

Gaffan J, Herbertson R, Davis P et al: Bilateral peripheral T-cell lymphoma of the fallopian tubes. Gynecol Oncol 95(3):736–738, 2004.

Han JY, Han HS, Kim YB et al: Extraskeletal chondroma of the fallopian tube. J Korean Med Sci 17(2):276–278, 2002.

Jacoby AF, Fuller AF, Thor AD et al: Primary leiomyosarcoma of the fallopian tube. Gynecol Oncol 51:404, 1993.

Kayaalp E, Heller DS, Majmudar B: Serous tumor of low malignant potential of the fallopian tube. Int J Gynecol Pathol 19(4): 398–400, 2000.

Keeney GL, Thrasher TV: Metaplastic papillary tumor of the fallopian tube: a case report with ultrastructure. Int J Gynecol Pathol 7(1): 86–92, 1988.

Kobayashi T, Suzuki K, Arai T et al: Angiomyofibroblastoma arising from the fallopian tube. Obstet Gynecol 94(5 part 2):833–834, 1999.

Li S, Zimmerman RL, LiVolsi VA: Mixed malignant germ cell tumor of the fallopian tube. Int J Gynecol Pathol 18(2):183–185, 1999.

Lim BJ, Kim JW, Yang WI et al: Malignant mixed müllerian tumor of fallopian tube with multiple distinct heterologous components. Int J Gynecol Cancer 14(4):690–693, 2004.

Misao R, Niwa K, Iwagaki S et al: Leiomyoma of the fallopian tube. Gynecol Obstet Invest 49(4):279–280, 2000.

Moore DH, Woosley JT, Reddick RL et al: Adenosquamous carcinoma of the fallopian tube. Am J Obstet Gynecol 157:903, 1987.

Noack F, Lange K, Lehmann V et al: Primary extranodal marginal zone B-cell lymphoma of the fallopian tube. Gynecol Oncol 86(3):384–386, 2002.

Paner GP, Gonzalez M, Al-Masri H et al: Parafallopian tube transitional cell carcinoma. Gynecol Oncol 86(3):379–383, 2002.

Parker A, Lee V, Dalrymple C et al: Epithelioid trophoblastic tumour: report of a case in the fallopian tube. Pathology 35(2):136–140, 2003.

Rabczynski J, Ziolkowski P: Primary endometrioid carcinoma of fallopian tube. Clinicomorphologic study. Pathol Oncol Res 5(1): 61–66, 1999.

Sills ES, Kaplan CR, Perloe M et al: Laparoscopic approach to an uncommon adnexal neoplasm associated with infertility: serous cystadenofibroma of the fallopian tube. J Am Assoc Gynecol Laparosc 10(4):545–547, 2003.

Sit AS, Price FV, Kelley JL et al: Chemotherapy for malignant mixed Müllerian tumors of the ovary. Gynecol Oncol 79(2):196–200, 2000.

Su YN, Cheng WF, Chen CA et al: Case report: pregnancy with primary tubal placental site trophoblastic tumor—a case report and literature review. Gynecol Oncol 73:322, 1999.

Vimala N, Kumar S, Dadhwal V: Primary choriocarcinoma of the Fallopian tube. Int J Gynaecol Obstet 79(1):37–38, 2002.

Weber AM, Hewett WF, Gajewski WH, Curry SL: Malignant mixed müllerian tumor of the fallopian tube. Gynecol Oncol 50:239, 1993.

Yoshioka T, Tanaka T: Mature solid teratoma of the fallopian tube: case report. Eur J Obstet Gynecol Reprod Biol 89(2):205–206, 2000.

14 Breast Diseases

James V. Fiorica, M.D.

The obstetrician-gynecologist functions as the primary care physician for many women, especially during the reproductive and perimenopausal years. Therefore the diagnosis of breast cancer in its most curable forms lies within this specialty for large numbers of women. Breast cancer will develop in one of every nine women, or about 11%. It is estimated that in 2006, about 211,000 new invasive breast cancers will have been diagnosed among women, and 58,490 in situ cases. Breast cancer incidence rates increased by about 4% every year, from 84.8 per 100,000 in 1980 to 111.9 in 1987, and from 1987 to 2002 increased in incidence by 0.3% per year. Breast cancer is the leading cause of death in women between the ages of 40 and 55. Every 2 min, a woman is diagnosed with breast cancer.

Confronted with these daunting statistics, the most direct approach in the attack against this dreaded disease is to find its cause and eradicate its inception. Unfortunately, the cause of breast cancer seems to be multifactorial, a constellation of risk factors rather than a single factor. Among many suggested causes of breast cancer are genetic predisposition, loss of the host's immunologic defense mechanism, and viruses as well as other carcinogens. Hormones, especially estrogens, were once considered to be primary carcinogenic agents, but they are now believed to be possible promoters in carcinogenesis.

While the search continues for a cause and total eradication, the most important aspect in combating the disease is diagnosis at an early stage, when the prognosis for cure with appropriate therapy is excellent. By instructing the patient in the art of monthly breast self-examination by performing careful periodic breast examinations in the office, and by judiciously using diagnostic aids, especially in patients with increased risk for the disease, the physician has a golden opportunity to detect breast cancer at an early and highly curable stage. The 5-year relative survival rate for localized breast cancer (which includes all women living at 5 years after diagnosis, whether the patient is in remission, disease-free, or under treatment) has risen to 98%, 81% for regional disease, and 26% for distant-stage disease.

ANATOMY OF THE ADULT BREAST

The location of adult breast is between the second and the sixth ribs in the vertical axis, and between the sternal edge and the mid-axillary line in the horizontal axis. The average breast is 10–12 cm in diameter, and its average thickness is 5–7 cm. Breast tissue also projects into the axilla as the axillary tail of Spence. The contour of the breast varies but is usually dome-like with a conical configuration in the nulliparous woman and a pendulous configuration in the parous woman. The breast is composed of three major structures: skin, subcutaneous tissue, and breast tissue; the breast tissue contains both parenchyma and stroma. The parenchyma is divided into 15–20 segments that converge at the nipple in a radial arrangement. The collecting ducts draining each segment are 2 mm in diameter, with subareolar lactiferous sinuses 5–8 mm in diameter; 5–10 major collecting milk ducts open at the nipple, and another 5–10 ducts at the nipple are, in reality, blind pits. Each duct drains a lobe made up of 20–40 lobules. Each lobule consists of 10–100 alveoli or tubulosaccular secretory units. The stroma and subcutaneous tissues of the breast contain fat, connective tissue, blood vessels, nerves, and lymphatics (Fig. 14–1).

The breast's skin is thin and contains hair follicles, sebaceous glands, and eccrine glands. The nipple, which is located over the fourth intercostal space in the non-

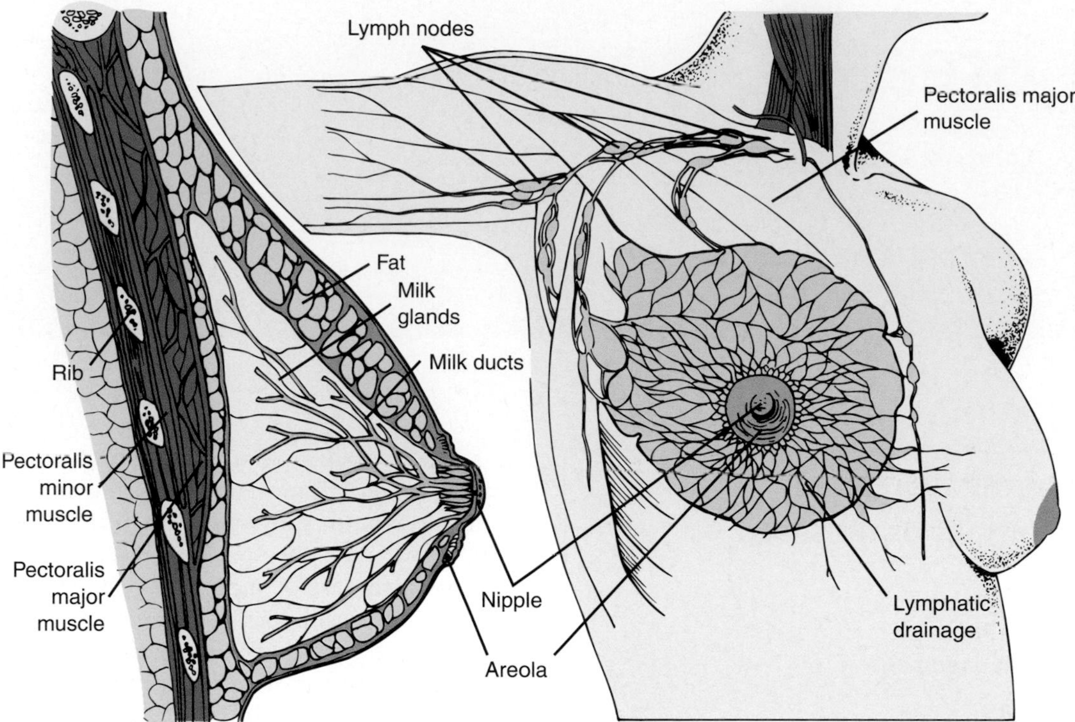

Figure 14–1 Anatomy of the female breast.

pendulous breast, contains abundant sensory nerve endings as well as sebaceous and apocrine sweat glands, but no hair follicles. The areola is circular, pigmented, and 15–60 mm in diameter. Morgagni's tubercles, located near the periphery of the areola, are elevations formed by the openings of the ducts of Montgomery's glands. Montgomery's glands are large sebaceous glands capable of secreting milk; they represent an intermediate stage between the sweat and the mammary glands. Fascial tissues envelop the breast; the superficial pectoral fascia envelops the breast and is continuous with the superficial abdominal fascia of Camper. The undersurface of the breast lies on the deep pectoral fascia, covering the pectoralis major and the anterior serratus muscles. Connecting these two fascial layers are fibrous bands (Cooper's suspensory ligaments) that are the natural means of support of the breast.

The internal mammary and the lateral thoracic arteries provide the principal blood supply to the breast. Approximately 60% of the breast, mainly the medial and central parts, is supplied by the anterior perforating branches of the internal mammary artery. About 30% of the breast, mainly the upper outer quadrant, is supplied by the lateral thoracic artery. Subepithelial or a papillary plexus of lymphatics of the breast are confluent with the subepithelial lymphatics over the surface of the body. These valveless lymphatic vessels communicate with subdermal lymphatic vessels and merge with Sappey's subareolar plexus. The subareolar plexus receives lymphatic vessels from the nipple and the areola, and communicates by way of the vertical lymphatic vessels that are equivalent to those connecting the subepithelial and subdermal plexus elsewhere in the body. Lymph flows unidirectionally from the superficial to the deep plexus, and from the subareolar plexus through the lymphatic vessels of the lactiferous duct to the perilobular and deep subcutaneous plexus. Lymph flow from the deep subcutaneous and intramammary lymphatic vessels moves centrifugally toward the axillary and internal mammary lymph nodes. It is estimated that about 3% of the lymph from the breast flows to the internal mammary chain, whereas 97% flows to the axillary nodes. Drainage of the lymph to the internal mammary chain may be observed after injection of any quadrant of the breast.

Axillary lymph nodes may be divided into the apical or subclavicular nodes, which lie medial to the pectoralis minor muscle; the axillary vein lymph nodes, which are along the axillary vein from the pectoralis minor muscle to the lateral limit of the axilla; the interpectoral nodes, which lie between the pectoralis major and minor muscles along the lateral pectoral nerve; the scapula group, which lie along the subscapular vessels; and the central nodes, which are beneath the lateral border of the pectoralis major muscle and below the pectoralis minor muscle.

Alternatively, metastatic spread, for the purposes of determining pathologic anatomy and metastatic progression, is to divide the axillary lymph nodes into arbitrary levels. Level I lymph nodes lie lateral to the lateral border of the pectoralis minor muscle, level II lymph nodes lie behind the pectoralis minor muscle, and level III lymph nodes are medial to the medial border of the pectoralis minor muscle. At the time of surgery, these levels can be determined accurately only by marking them.

BENIGN CONDITIONS OF THE BREAST

Epidemiology

The incidence of benign breast disorders cannot be accurately estimated. The subjectivity in any woman's evaluation of her breasts, as well as a variation in the physician's designation of breast disease, invalidates any clinical estimates. To gain some degree of reproducibility, most studies rely on data from women who have had biopsies for benign conditions. This approach, too, is subject to bias, because not every woman with lumpy breasts will have a biopsy, and the decision to do a biopsy is influenced by the presence of other risk factors for malignant disease.

Benign breast symptoms when clinically defined are common and have been estimated to occur in 50% of women. In a case-control study by Cole and associates in Boston from 1968 to 1969, the age-standardized incidence rates for histologically diagnosed fibrocystic disease and fibroadenoma were 89.4% and 32.8% per 100,000 women years, respectively. Cole et al found that the incidence increased in women aged 45 years or younger and then declined sharply. The results of this study are influenced by the bias inherent in using biopsies, however, and possibly underestimate the incidence in younger women. Hislop and Elwood conducted a 30-year cohort study of nurses in British Columbia and found that by the age of 50 years, the subjects' cumulative risk for benign breast disorders was 17% for those undergoing biopsy and 31% for those who had symptomatic disease. In autopsy studies, the incidence of histologic fibrocystic disease may be determined with only slightly greater accuracy. Davis summarized eight autopsy studies conducted before 1964, and found evidence of cystic disease in 58.5% of a total of 725 breasts in women who had had no symptoms of breast disease. Cystic disease was bilateral in 43% of these women. The average incidence of gross cysts was 21%, whereas the average incidence of coexisting gross and microscopic cysts and of cystic disease with epithelial hyperplasia was 58.3% and 30.6%, respectively. Kramer and Rush studied the breasts of women older than 30 years and found histologic evidence of fibrocystic disease in 67%. Thus, although the incidence of clinical features may decrease in the postmenopausal period, histologic features persist.

Physiologic changes

Breast tumors are found in most women by chance or by periodic self-examination. It is estimated that two-thirds of the tumors found by all methods during a woman's reproductive years are benign and represent cystic changes, dysplasia, fibroadenomas, and papillomas. However, 50% of the palpable masses in perimenopausal women, and the majority of lesions in postmenopausal patients, are malignant. Cystic breast changes and mammary dysplasia are common, often symptomatic, and require considerable judgment on the part of the physician in choosing the appropriate therapy. The incidence of these benign changes peaks in women 30–50 years of age and may be the result of estrogen stimulation in the absence of cyclic corpus luteum formation and the cyclic production of progesterone. Continued estrogen stimulation may be a factor in the development of the so-called macrocyst. That breast tenderness often occurs premenstrually suggests that progesterone may play a role in the development and symptoms of cystic alterations in breast tissue. However, the proportional effect of each of these hormones on the cause of benign breast conditions is unclear and needs further clarification.

A more thorough understanding of the embryologic and prepubertal development of the breast will aid in the study of benign breast lesions. The mammary glands are highly specialized skin derivatives of ectodermal origin. The epithelial ridge that will develop into breast tissue undergoes a series of proliferations to form the lactiferous ducts. Primitive breast tissue is under the gonadal control of fetal androgen production, which causes a suppression of breast growth during the period of gestation, when the tissue is under the simultaneous influence of increasing levels of growth-promoting estrogen and progesterone. After birth, breast tissue remains dormant until adolescence, when estrogen produces a proliferation of ductal epithelium, and progesterone produces rapid growth of the acini. However, breast growth and development are not totally dependent on estrogen and progesterone levels. Insulin, cortisol, thyroxine, growth hormone, and prolactin are also required for complete functional development. Minor deficiencies in any one of these hormones can be compensated for by an excess of prolactin, the interesting hormone found in mammals that suckle their young.

Increasing amounts of estrogen, progesterone, and human placental lactogen produce active growth of functional breast tissue during the course of pregnancy. Estrogen production is under the control of the fetus. Estrogen influences progesterone production, uteroplacental blood flow, mammary gland development, and fetal adrenal gland function. By the 20th week of pregnancy, most of the estrogen excreted in maternal urine comes from fetal androgens. About 90% of maternal estriol is derived from fetal precursors. Serum prolactin rises from non-pregnant levels of 10 ng/mL to term levels of 200 ng/mL. Amniotic fluid prolactin levels are more than 100 times greater than the levels in maternal or fetal blood early in pregnancy. It is not known whether the fetal pituitary gland or the trophoblast secretes the hormone into the amniotic fluid, but one hypothesis suggests that prolactin may help the embryo survive its aquatic environment much like it helps the teleost fish in its journey from salt to fresh water to spawn. Elevated levels of estradiol parallel those of prolactin, and indicate that estriol may be responsible for increases in prolactin. Although estrogen may initiate prolactin secretion, high levels block its physiologic effects. Prolactin secretion is also controlled by the prolactin-inhibiting factor. A decrease of estrogen level after delivery and suppression of the prolactin-inhibiting factor by suckling increase prolactin levels. If breast-feeding does not occur, serum prolactin levels decrease to non-pregnant levels in about 1 week.

The final episode in nature's plan to provide the newborn with milk from its mother's breast is the contraction of the duct system by the release of oxytocin from the posterior pituitary and the delivery of milk to the nipples. After 3–4 months of breast-feeding, suckling appears to be the only stimulus required for lactation.

Physical examination

A thorough breast examination remains a critical component in the early diagnosis of breast disease. Although the techniques and importance of breast examination are taught in nearly every medical school, the current trends of clinical specialization and subspecialization may cause clinicians to lose expertise in the technique or, even worse, to forget to include adequate breast examination as part of the assessment of their patients. To omit breast evaluation from routine examinations or to neglect to advise appropriate patients to undergo mammography may result in missed opportunities for early detection. This is tantamount to performing a gynecologic examination without a Papanicolaou smear, or to neglecting the examination of a stool specimen for occult blood. In diseases in which early detection is so clearly related to improved survival, the value of these relatively simple techniques cannot be overemphasized.

Examination of the patient in the sitting position

The patient should be in the sitting position during the inception of the physical breast examination. In this position, obvious asymmetry, bulging of the skin, skin or nipple retraction, and nipple ulceration should be most apparent (Fig. 14–2A). When the patient's arms are raised (see Fig. 14–2B), skin changes in the lower half of the breast, or in the inframammary fold, become accentuated. Contraction of the pectoralis major muscle, affected by the patient's pushing her hands against her hips (see Fig. 14–2C), may demonstrate an otherwise undetected skin retraction. Next, palpation of the breast with the patient still upright may allow detection of subtle lesions that would be more difficult to palpate if she were supine (see Fig. 14–2D). This is particularly true for masses high in the breast or in the axillary tail region, which are more apparent when the surrounding breast tissue is displaced inferiorly while the patient is in the sitting position. Examination of the supraclavicular areas and both sides of the neck for the purpose of detecting suspicious lymphadenopathy is also best done when the patient is in the upright position.

The axilla is examined with the patient's right arm fixed at the elbow and held there by the physician's right hand, a position that allows relaxation of the chest wall musculature (see Fig. 14–2E). Palpation with the left hand permits assessment of the lower axilla, and with extension higher toward the clavicle, the middle and upper portions of the axilla can be assessed. The left axilla is examined with the right hand, after relaxation of the patient's left arm in the physician's left hand. If lymph nodes are palpable, the clinician must assess their level and size, as well as whether they are single or multiple and mobile or fixed to underlying structures. Nodes are considered suspicious for metastases that are >1 cm in diameter, firm, irregular, and multiple or matted together. Many women, especially those subject to low-grade inflammatory processes of the hands or arms (from paper cuts, hangnails, minor abrasions, or burns) will have small, soft, mobile, and palpable axillary lymph nodes caused by lymphadenitis. These nodes are generally <1 cm in diameter and are recorded as being palpable but clinically uninvolved.

Close inspection of the skin and nipple of the breast may reveal abnormalities suggesting an underlying malignant process (Fig. 14–3). Edema of the skin of the breast (peau d'orange) is occasionally subtle but is more often extensive. This condition is frequently more prominent in the lower half of the breast than in any other region, and it is most noticeable when the patient's arms are raised. Although this edema is often attributable to lymphatic obstruction from a deep-seated carcinoma in the breast, it may also be caused by extensive axillary lymph node involvement with metastatic disease. Retraction of the skin and nipple may be accentuated by contraction of the pectoralis major muscle. Erythema of the skin of the breast is an ominous sign. Although the cause may be inflammation, such as periductal mastitis or even abscess formation, inflammatory carcinoma should be considered a possibility. Inspection of the nipple for either retraction or ulceration is important. Ulceration, which may begin as a minimal process involving a portion of the nipple, suggests Paget disease. This early form of breast carcinoma, which originates in and extends along the major ducts and expresses itself as nipple abnormality, can involve the entire nipple.

Examination of the patient lying supine

Subsequently, the patient should be asked to assume a supine position. The breast is best examined when it is positioned on top of and splayed out over the chest wall. This position is accomplished with a small pillow placed beneath the ipsilateral shoulder to elevate the breast, and with the ipsilateral arm raised above the patient's head (see Fig. 14–2F). Breast examination is most accurate when the least possible amount of breast tissue is present between the skin and the chest wall; it is least accurate when the converse is true. The examiner must assess the entire breast, extending the examination from the sternum to the mid-axillary line and superiorly from the clavicle to the lower rib cage. The examiner uses the flat of the hand or running fingers technique, remembering that the changes being sought are subtle. All quadrants are examined.

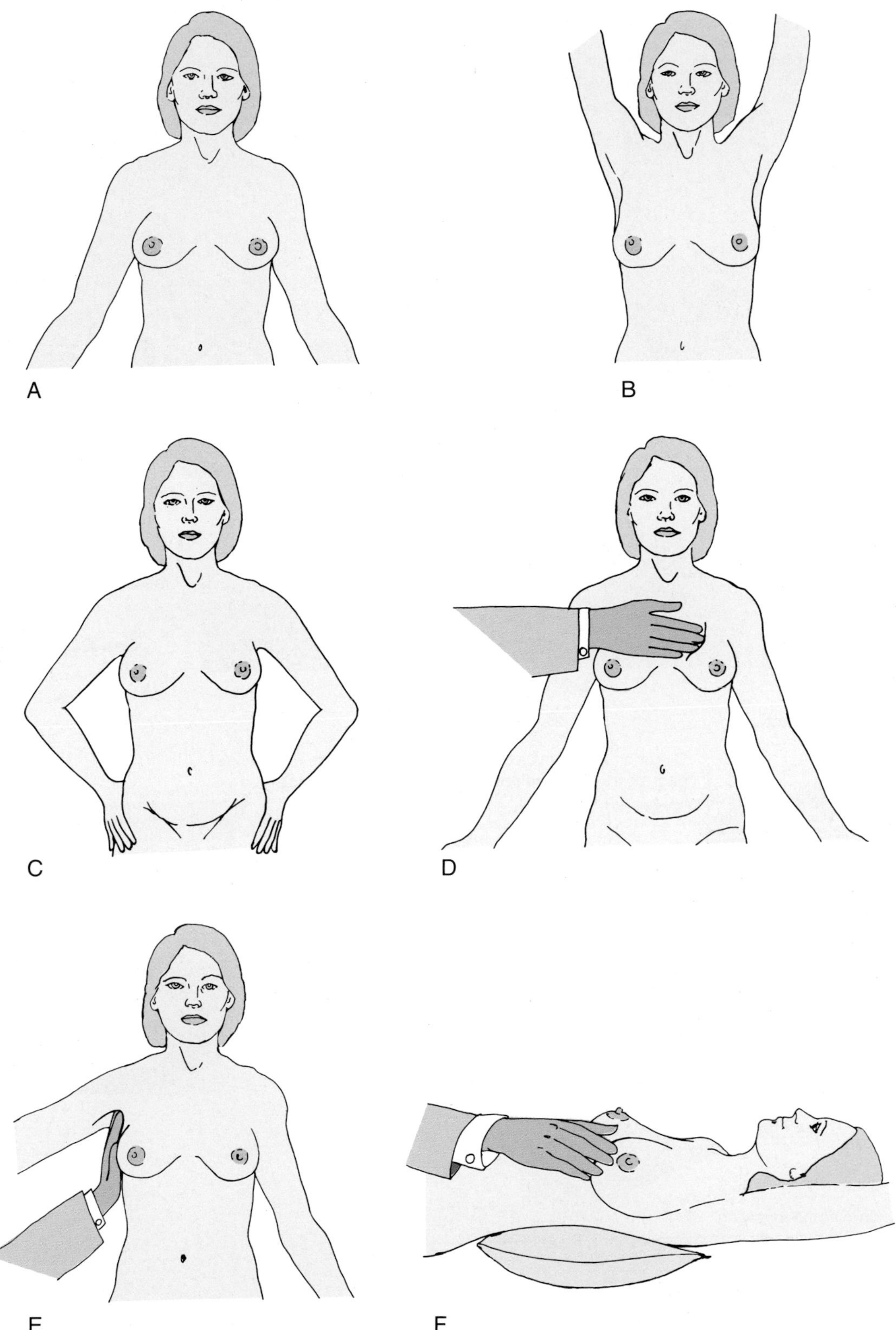

Figure 14–2 Physical examination of the breast. *A*, Upright position. *B*, Arms raised. *C*, Pushing hands against hips. *D*, Palpation in upright position. *E*, Palpation of the axilla. *F*, Palpation in supine position.

Because of the proclivity for malignant lesions to occur in the upper outer quadrant of the breast (Fig. 14–4), we make it a practice to begin in that quadrant, palpating clockwise and returning to examine the upper outer quadrant a second time. Carcinomas <1 cm in diameter are palpated in some women; in others, large lesions may be hidden. The examiner must assess the background consistency of the breast; in premenopausal patients who are examined premenstrually, clumps of engorged glandular tissue may seem impossible to assess. A repeated

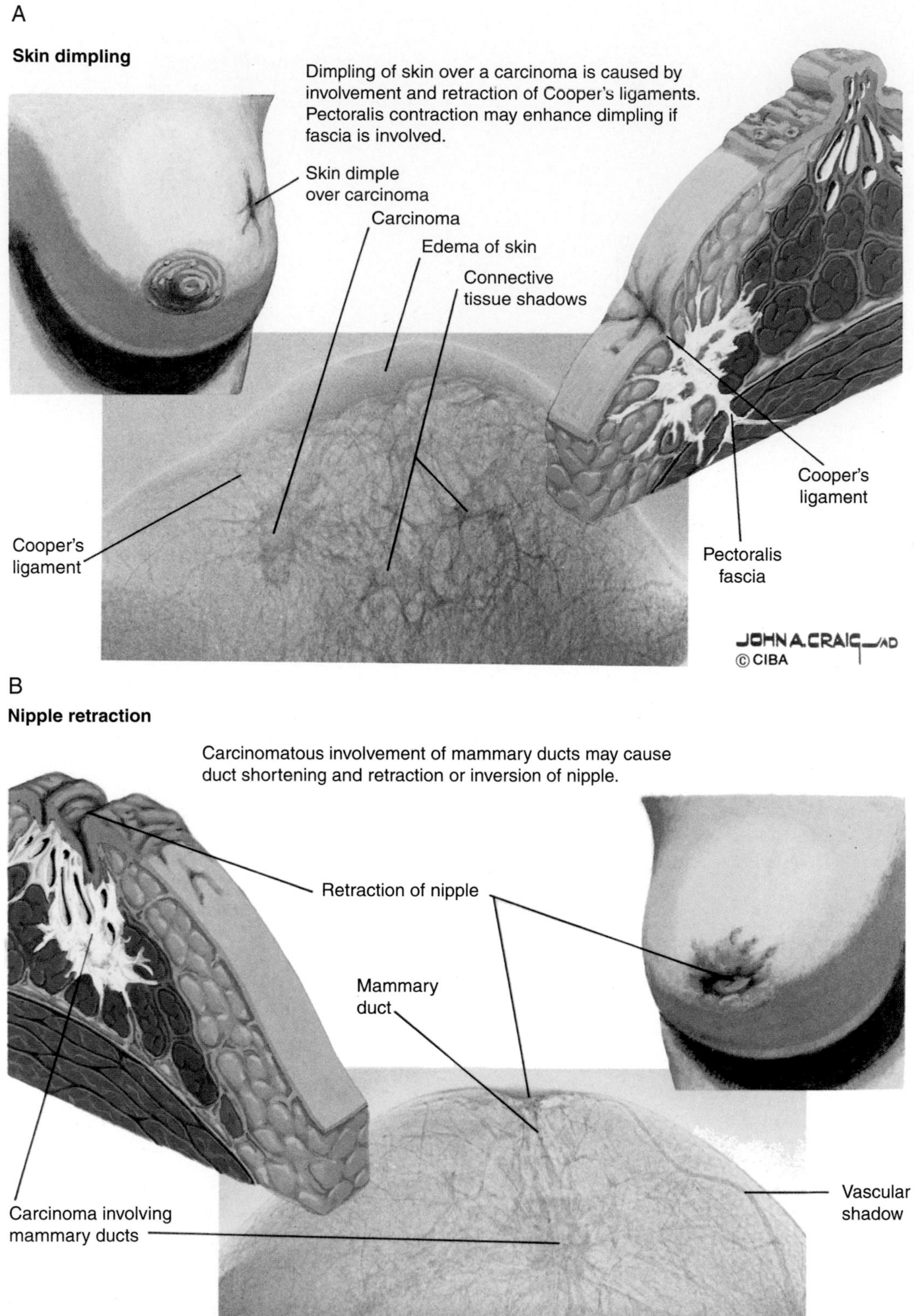

Figure 14–3 Clinical signs of cancer. *A*, Retraction of skin. *B*, Retraction of nipple. (From Townsend CM Jr: Breast lumps. Clin Symp 32:1–32, 1980. Art by John A Craig. Reprinted with permission from Elsevier Inc. All rights reserved.)

examination 1–2 weeks after a menstrual period may reveal marked improvement, with decreased glandular elements. Postmenopausal patients have a higher ratio of fat to glandular elements, making palpation and mammographic examination more accurate. No cyclic changes occur in these patients, so indiscrete thickening may be more significant in them than it is in premenopausal patients.

During the course of the examination in a supine position, the examiner searches for three-dimensional masses or significant thickenings. On palpation, firm masses or

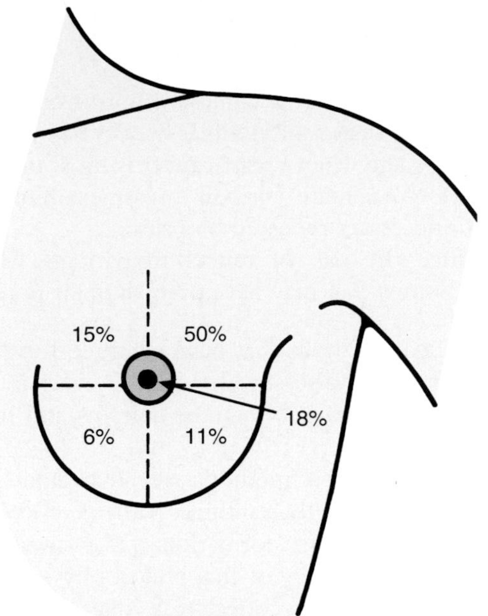

Figure 14–4 Relative location of malignant lesions of the breast.

areas that are three-dimensional, irregular, and fixed to the skin or underlying fascia are characteristic of carcinomas. Benign lesions tend to be softer and smoother, to have more regular borders, and to be freely movable. Fibroadenoma, the most common benign disease of the breast occurring in younger women, is the easiest condition to appreciate. These lesions are clearly demarcated and feel like marbles despite the dense, glandular, parenchymal tissue present in these young women.

Clinical breast examination

The question has been raised of whether a screening clinical breast examination should be done, and if so, what the best technique is. Barton and associates reviewed the literature and noted its benefits, with some caveats. One randomized trial and one case-control study compared the combination of screening clinical breast examination and mammography with no screening, and demonstrated a statistically significant decreased breast cancer mortality rate (20% and 71%, respectively) in women between the ages of 40 and 64 years. Meta-analysis of trials demonstrated that clinical breast examination or screening mammography decreased breast cancer mortality by about one-fourth in women between 40 and 69 years of age, and by 18% in women in their forties. The Canadian study of women between the ages of 50 and 59 years who were randomized between standard clinical breast examination alone and clinical breast examination with mammography annually for 5 years found that breast cancer–specific mortality rates for women in these two groups were similar at 7 years, noting the efficacy of clinical breast examination alone. The Health Insurance Plan study, which was conducted when mammography was in its infancy, concluded that most cancers were detected by clinical breast examination. Of interest, the mortality reduction after 10 years was 29%, which compared with a 30% reduction in the Swedish two-county trial that used mammography alone.

Studies certainly have noted that sensitivity of clinical breast examination and mammography seems to be improved over that of mammography alone, because clinical breast examination can identify cancers missed with mammography. Its detection rate varied between studies, and ranged from 3.4% in the Edinburgh trial to 45% in the Health Insurance Plan study. The authors, in evaluating all the data, thought that the sensitivity of clinical breast examination is approximately 54%, with a specificity of 94%.

Several factors should be taken into consideration to maximize the effectiveness of clinical breast examination. Studies have shown that the length of examination directly relates to sensitivity. It is suggested that a total of 6 min (3 min per breast) results in the best effects. Technique and the examiner's experience are obviously important. Age of the patient is a factor, in that in older women the breasts become more fatty, making lump detection easier. Size and lumpiness of the patient's breasts also affect the examiner's ability to detect cancer. These authors suggested that the MammoCare method is the best technique. This method essentially uses the pads of the index, third, and fourth fingers to make small circular motions. This palpation extends in a straight line going up and down (lawn mower technique) the breasts between the clavicle and bra line. The authors believed that a well-conducted clinical breast examination can detect at least 50% of asymptomatic cancers and may contribute to a reduction in the mortality of those patients screened.

Breast self-examination

The physician should explain the importance and technique of breast self-examination at the conclusion of the physical examination. The physician should advise the patient to perform a monthly breast self-examination at a time in her menstrual cycle when the breasts are neither engorged nor tender. A postmenopausal woman may be instructed to select her birth date each month as the time for her examination. Many physicians instruct their patients to examine themselves while bathing, because a mass is more easily felt when the hand and breasts are wet. The physician should instruct the patient then to sit before a mirror and inspect her breasts when her arms are at her sides and when her arms are raised. She should be told to look for changes in contour, dimpling, and nipple abnormality (see Fig. 14–3). Next, the patient should lie in the supine position with a small pillow under her shoulder on the side to be examined; she should then palpate the entire right breast with the flat of the fingers of the left hand and vice versa. A mass should be reported to the physician; the patient's concerns are often ill-founded, and only reassurance is required. For this reason, it is our practice to advise morning breast self-examination so that a patient need not spend a sleepless night with undue concern if she palpates a "lump."

Diagnosis and management

Fibrocystic changes (fibrocystic disease)

"Fibrocystic disease" of the breast (Fig. 14–5) includes a variety of histologic conditions. From a pathologic point of view, there is no such entity. The term encompasses a histologic spectrum of change, some normal variance, and some abnormal conditions. The breast is an inhomogeneous organ, and the non-lactating normal breast is composed primarily of adipose and fibrous tissue that is often unevenly distributed. This lack of even distribution leads to physiologic inhomogeneity, irregularity, and lumpiness. Biopsy of a lumpy area may show primarily fibrous tissue and mammary epithelium. Although normal, this finding would, in most institutions, be reported as fibrocystic disease, fibrocystic change, mammary dysplasia, chronic cystic mastitis, or any of a number of other entities.

The lesions are commonly bilateral and multiple. They are characterized by dull heavy pain, a sense of fullness, and tenderness. These symptoms increase premenstrually, as does lump size. In the case of a cyst, the patient often reports that there was a sudden appearance of a tender lump, and that she or her doctor recently examined her breast and did not notice a lump. The lumps are cystic to palpation, tender, well delineated, slightly mobile, and clear on transillumination. Aspiration (Fig. 14–6) reveals a typically turbid, non-hemorrhagic fluid that has a yellow, green, or brown tint. Deeply embedded cysts, a cluster of cysts, or dominant areas caused by sclerosing adenosis or dense fibrous dysplasia can produce a mass that clinically mimics cancer.

The three basic reasons for considering treatment of fibrocystic changes are as follow.

1. To control troublesome clinical symptoms.
2. To normalize dense and nodular breasts before a woman reaches the age when breast cancer is most prevalent in an effort to facilitate periodic breast examination and avoid unnecessary repeated biopsies.
3. To reduce the risk of cancer in patients who have benign lesions that may have premalignant potential.

A number of methods that have emerged for the treatment of fibrocystic disease can be broadly characterized into two groups: diet and vitamin therapy, and hormone manipulation.

Perhaps the simplest methods are advocated by those who maintain that dimethylxanthines (caffeine, theophylline) and nicotine stimulate the formation of fibrocystic changes in the breasts. Advocates of this philosophy suggest that patients stop consuming coffee, tea, cola, and chocolate; stop using certain respiratory drugs containing dimethylxanthines; and quit smoking.

Others have suggested that vitamin E is helpful in relieving symptoms and causing regression of fibrocystic changes of the breast. Its mechanism of action is unknown, although an alteration in serum gonadotropins and adrenal tropines has been shown to occur in patients taking high doses of vitamin E. As reported by Gonzales, a double-blind study consisted of the treatment of 20 patients and 8 control subjects with placebos for 4 weeks, followed by 600 IU of vitamin E per day for 8 weeks. Vitamin E induced a 40% complete response rate and a 46% partial

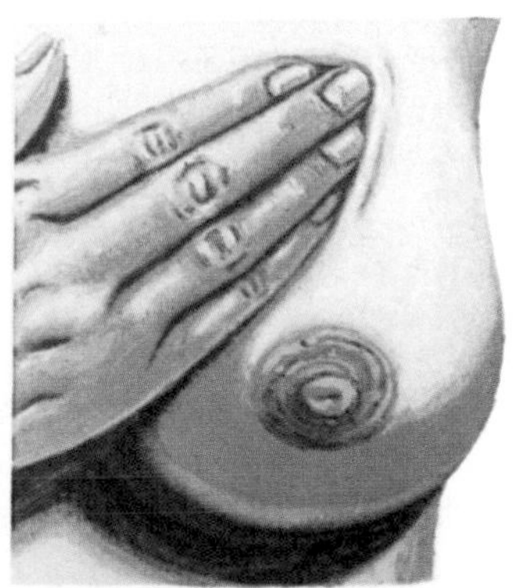

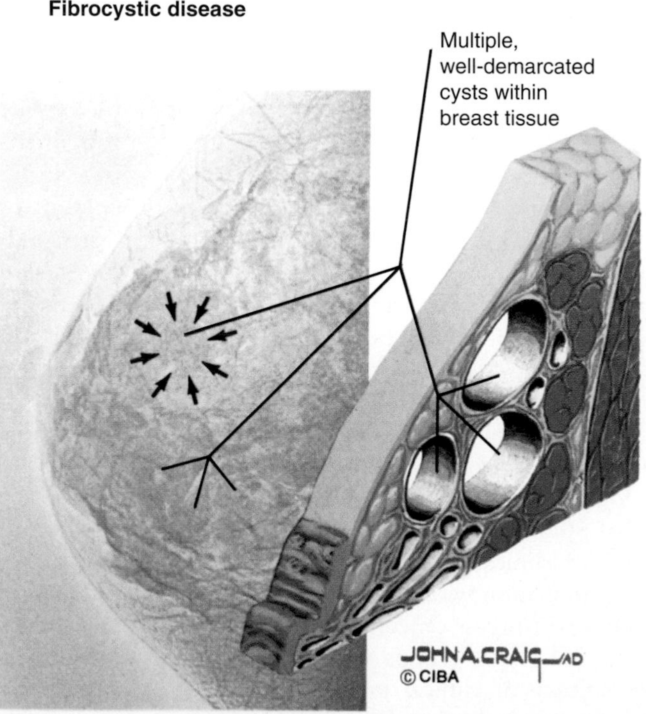

Figure 14–5 Fibrocystic disease. (From Townsend CM Jr: Breast lumps. Clin Symp 32:1–32, 1980. Art by John A Craig. Reprinted with permission from Elsevier Inc. All rights reserved.)

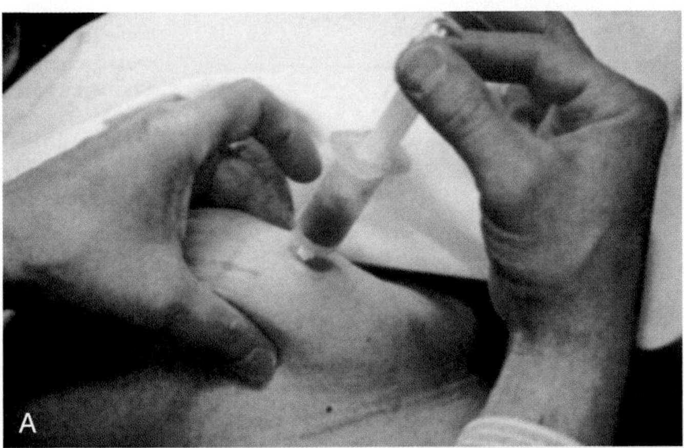

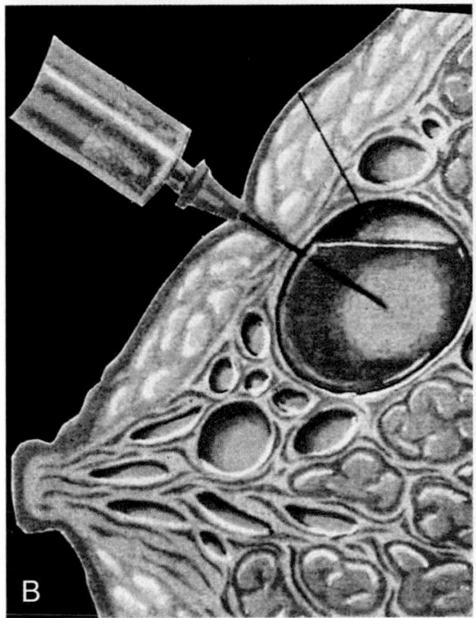

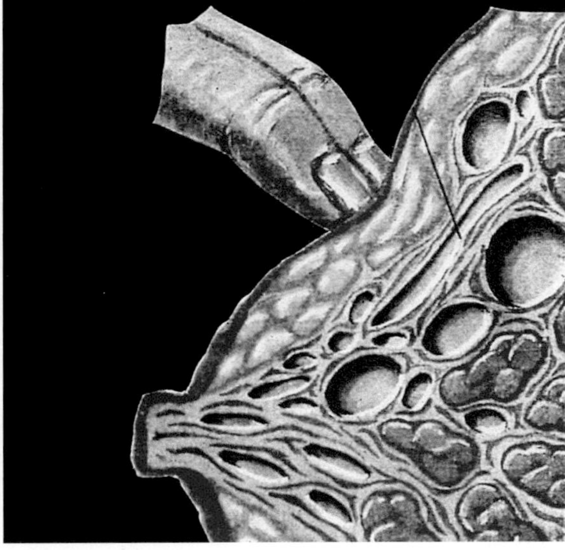

Figure 14–6 *A,* Fine-needle aspiration of a breast mass. *B,* Aspiration of a palpable mass. Hold lesion between fingers, pass needle through lesion four or five times, push air through needle on to slide, and fix slide after smearing.

response rate for a total response rate of 86%. No response was seen in the placebo group.

Danazol, an "impeded androgen" derived from 17-ethinyl testosterone, has received a great deal of attention in the treatment of endometriosis and of fibrocystic disease of the breast. As with other progestogens, the mechanism of its effect on fibrocystic disease is unclear. It has been shown to alter several parameters of endocrine function that could have bearing on the breast.

- Antigonadotropin prevents the midcycle luteinizing hormone surge.
- Antireceptor finds and translocates androgen receptors but not estrogen or progesterone receptors.
- Antiestrogen inhibits several enzymes involved in ovarian steroidogenesis.

Brookshaw described 514 patients who had benign breast disease treated with varying doses of danazol for as long as 6 months. For the best results, treatment was necessary for 4–6 months at a dose of 200–400 mg/day, with a complete response rate of 68%.

The effectiveness of tamoxifen was studied by Ricciardi and Ianniruberto with use of 10 mg/day from day 5 to day 25 of the menstrual cycle for 4 months. The response rate was 72%.

A medical treatment advocates the use of bromocriptine. Blichert-Toft and colleagues, in Copenhagen, performed a double-blind crossover study in 10 women with diffuse fibrocystic disease. By treatment with 2.5 mg/day during the first week of each menstrual cycle and 5 mg/day during the next 3 weeks, or identical placebos for 2 months, eight of the 10 women had complete relief of mastalgia and two had definite improvements, but only one had relief with the placebo.

There is considerable controversy as to whether the patient with benign cystic changes in the breast is at greater risk for the development of cancer. Some authorities believe that the risk of cancer is two to four times greater in the patient who has cystic changes. Other authorities disagree. The simplest and most common studies evaluate the coexistence of benign changes in mastectomy specimens removed because of malignant conditions. These studies show that there is no greater incidence of microscopic fibrocystic disease in cancerous breasts than in non-cancerous breasts studied at autopsy. Fibrocystic disease was found at autopsy examination in 58% of non-cancerous breasts but in only 26% of cancerous breasts. In addition, epithelial hyperplasia, often thought to be a precursor of malignant disease, was at least as common in the non-cancerous breast as in the cancerous breast (32% and

23%, respectively). Davis and coworkers concluded that the mere finding of coexistent cystic disease was not adequate evidence that cystic change had predisposed to breast carcinoma.

Two other types of epidemiologic studies have been used to assess the relationship of fibrocystic disease to cancer: a retrospective analysis of the number and histology of previous biopsy specimens in patients who subsequently had breast cancer (retrospective case-control study), and a retrospective cohort study of patients in whom biopsy specimens showed benign disease and who developed cancer later. In the retrospective case-control study, the percentage of previous biopsies in patients who had cancer was low (about 8%) compared with the percentage of previous biopsies in patients who had benign disease (about 14%). DeVitt and Chetty and associates showed that when a woman has a biopsy for benign disease, she is more likely to have a second biopsy, perhaps because of the increased surveillance or even anatomic distortion caused by the previous surgery. Evaluation of retrospective cohort studies, in which women who had benign biopsy specimens were observed to determine the subsequent incidence of cancer, poses even greater problems. There are statistical difficulties, including unspecified age distributions and periods of follow-up. In addition, only some of the investigators revealed the original histology to substantiate the diagnosis; others relied on the pathology reports as adequate evidence of fibrocystic disease. Finally, both studies used a different control to establish the expected risk of cancer.

Although the epidemiologic risk of developing cancer after biopsy has been somewhat discounted, the pathologic precursors have been clarified. Several studies have demonstrated that the most important pathologic risk factors for the subsequent development of carcinoma are the degree and nature (typical or atypical) of epithelial proliferation. The relative risks vary from study to study and depend to a great extent on the classification of various benign lesions. When biopsy results are categorized as showing non-proliferative lesions, proliferative lesions without atypia, or atypical proliferative lesions, populations with low risk for development of breast cancer may be isolated (Table 14–1). When additional factors such as family history and age are considered, subgroups that are at significantly greater risk for development of breast cancer may be identified.

In 1985, the Cancer Committee of the College of American Pathologists published a consensus statement and discouraged the use of the term *fibrocystic disease*. Their preference is *fibrocystic changes* or *fibrocystic condition*. Epithelial hyperplasias were assigned to risk categories (Table 14–2). Mild hyperplasia is defined as epithelium of more than two cells but not more than four cells deep. Moderate hyperplasia and florid hyperplasia refer to more extensive degrees of epithelial proliferation. In the absence of atypical hyperplasia, mild hyperplasia is not associated with an increased risk for invasive carcinoma. Moderate or florid hyperplasia without atypical hyperplasia is associated with slightly increased risk (one and a half to two times) for invasive carcinoma. Atypical hyperplasia refers to lesions that have some of the features of carcinomas in situ but not enough to make unequivocal diagnoses of carcinomas in situ. Although there is a moderately increased risk for invasive cancer in women who have atypical hyperplasia, the relative risk of lesser degrees of atypia (mild and moderate) has not yet been established. Carcinoma in situ is considered the end point for atypical hyperplasia. Women with carcinomas in situ established by breast biopsies who have no further treatment are at high risk for development of invasive carcinomas (8–10 times) relative to women with comparable conditions who do not have breast biopsies. Thus it seems that the use of a classification consisting of non-proliferative lesions, proliferative lesions without atypia, and atypical proliferative lesions has relevance to the malignant potential of these lesions. The following benign conditions (Table 14–3) are commonly found.

Table 14–1 PROLIFERATIVE BREAST DISEASE AND BREAST CANCER RISK

Characteristic	Relative risk (confidence interval)
Proliferative disease, no atypia	1.3 (0.69–1.9)
Complex fibroadenoma[a]	1.46 (0.53–4.0)
Atypical hyperplasia	2.53 (1.0–6.3)
Neither proliferative disease nor complex fibroadenoma	1.27 (0.89–1.8)

[a]Contains cysts, sclerosing adenosis, epithelial calcification, or papillary apocrine changes.

(After Dupont WD, Page DL, Parl FF et al: Estrogen replacement therapy in women with a history of proliferative breast disease. Cancer 85:1277–1283, 1999.)

Table 14–2 BREAST DIAGNOSIS GROUPED BY CANCER RISK

Cancer risk	Diagnosis
No increased risk	Adenosis, sclerosing or florid
	Apocrine metaplasia
	Cysts, macro or micro
	Duct ectasia
	Fibroadenoma
	Fibrosis
	Hyperplasia (mild)
	Mastitis
	Periductal mastitis
	Squamous metaplasia
Slightly increased	Hyperplasia, moderate or florid
	Papilloma, solid or papillary, with fibrovascular core
Moderately increased	Atypical hyperplasia
	Ductal
	Lobular

Fibroadenoma

A common benign lesion, the fibroadenoma (Fig. 14–7) appears predominantly in young women and occasion-

Table 14–3 BENIGN BREAST LESIONS[a]		
	Age in years (median)	Percentage
Fibrocystic changes	29–49 (30)	34
Carcinoma	40–71 (54)	27
Fibroadenoma	20–49 (30)	19
Intraductal papilloma	35–55 (40)	6
Ductal ectasia	35–55 (40)	4
Other	—	10

[a]Seventy percent of all lesions removed.

ally in adolescents. It is initially seen as a firm, painless, mobile mass and may be large, particularly in adolescents. Fibroadenomas are multiple and bilateral in about 14–25% of patients. They are the most common benign tumors of the breast. Fine-needle aspiration cytologic testing is accurate and dependable for diagnosis of fibroadenomas. Cytologic criteria for distinguishing fibroadenomas from cancers and phyllodes tumors are well established.

Management of fibroadenomas, especially in young women, has been controversial. The choice of treatment should be a shared decision between the patient and her physician. Fear of cancer and death is a paramount anxiety in women with breast tumors, but benign lesions can be monitored with regular clinical breast examinations and mammography. As with all dominant breast masses, a definitive diagnosis must be established by fine-needle aspiration cytologic testing or by histologic features on open surgical biopsy. Hindle reviewed 498 cases of biopsy-proven fibroadenomas and found no cases of coincident carcinoma within the fibroadenomas. He concluded that monitoring definitely has a role in the management of some of these lesions.

On histologic examination, fibroadenomas have both an epithelial and a stromal component. The histologic classification depends on which of these components predominates. In general, the epithelial component consists of well-defined, gland-like, and duct-like spaces lined by cuboid or columnar cells. Varying degrees of epithelial hyperplasia have been noted. The stromal component consists of connective tissue that has a variable content of collagen. Carcinoma may infrequently occur in association with fibroadenoma. The prognosis of carcinoma limited to fibroadenoma is excellent. Treatment should follow the same principle used in the management of in situ or infiltrating carcinomas that occur in breast tissue in the absence of fibroadenomas. The most common carcinoma involving fibroadenomas is lobular carcinoma in situ (LCIS), but intraductal, infiltrating ductal, and infiltrating lobular carcinoma have also been observed.

Phyllodes tumor

Phyllodes tumor is an uncommon, generally slow-growing lesion representing both epithelial and stromal proliferation. Although it can occur in women of any age, it is most common in premenopausal patients. Like fibroadenoma, it is a fibroepithelial tumor, but it is generally larger and contains a different type of connective tissue. In general, this connective tissue is hypercellular and has increased pleomorphism and mitotic activity. The cellularity of the connective tissue is the distinguishing characteristic of this tumor.

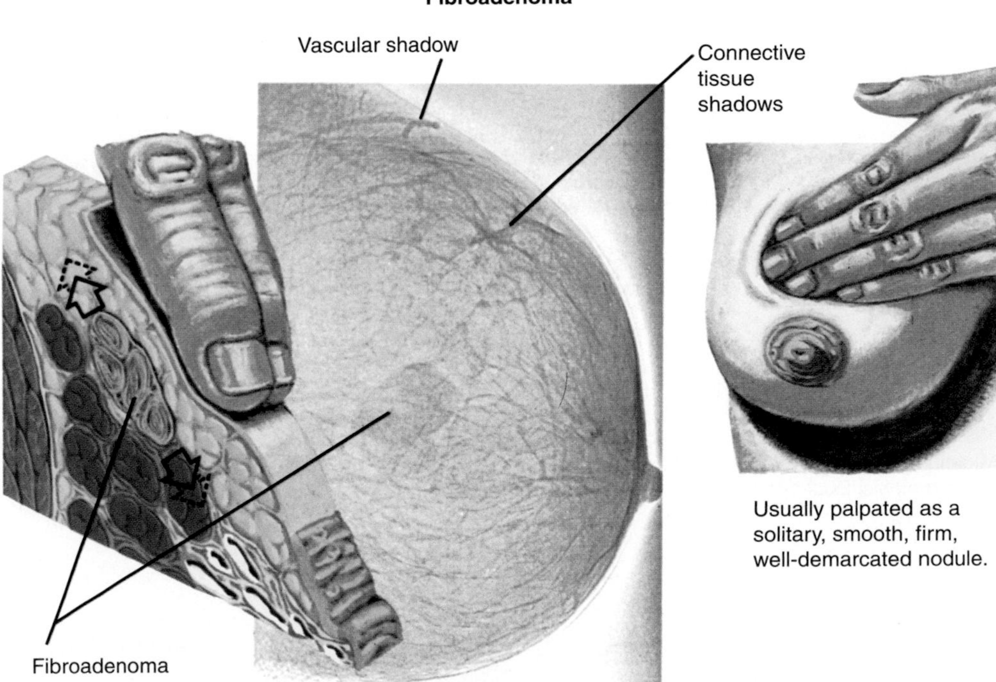

Figure 14–7 Fibroadenoma. (From Townsend CM Jr: Breast lumps. Clin Symp 32:1–32, 1980. Art by John A Craig. Reprinted with permission from Elsevier Inc. All rights reserved.)

The clinical course of a phyllodes tumor is variable and often unpredictable. Attempts to determine the degree of potential malignancy by evaluating cellularity and pleomorphism have not met with uniform success. Approximately 10% of all phyllodes tumors contain some characteristics suggestive of a frankly malignant process. Most demonstrate equivocal histopathologic characteristics or appear benign. Phyllodes tumors should be treated by total excision with a wide margin of healthy tissue. Radical mastectomy or modified radical procedures are not indicated.

Intraductal papilloma

Intraductal papilloma (Fig. 14–8) manifests as a serous, serosanguineous, or watery type of nipple discharge. In the absence of a mass, the most common cause of bloody nipple discharge is an intraductal papilloma. The discharge is usually spontaneous and from a single duct, and is commonly unilateral. Pressure on one area of the areola will result in the discharge, and that area usually contains the lesion. Intraductal papillomas are generally <1 cm in diameter, usually 3–4 mm. These lesions may occasionally be as large as 4–5 cm. On gross examination, papillomas are tan or pink viable tumors within dilated ducts or cysts. A frankly papillary configuration may or may not be apparent. The tumor is usually attached to the wall of the involved duct by a delicate stalk, but it may be sessile. To identify the papilloma, the physician should use a pair of fine scissors and carefully open the involved duct until the tumor is exposed.

On microscopic examination, these tumors are composed of multiple branching and anastomosing papillae, each with a central fibrovascular core and a covering layer of cuboid to columnar epithelial cells. There has been considerable debate in the literature about the malignant potential of solitary intraductal papillomas. Available evidence suggests that these lesions rarely undergo malignant transformation. Therefore the risk of breast carcinoma in a woman who has had an intraductal papilloma appears to be no greater than that in the general population.

Most nipple discharges are a result of benign conditions and do not require surgical intervention. The color and consistency of the discharge is important, however, and cytologic examination of the nipple discharge and, occasionally, mammography are important diagnostic aids. Even bloody nipple discharge is associated with the finding of a malignant neoplasm only 20–30% of the time. Tranquilizers, particularly the phenothiazines, may cause bilateral nipple discharge, principally because they decrease prolactin-inhibiting factor and thus elevate prolactin levels.

Ductal ectasia

Ductal ectasia (Fig. 14–9) is also commonly manifested by nipple discharge. However, this discharge is usually multicolored and sticky, bilateral, and from multiple ducts. The patient frequently experiences a burning, itching, or dull drawing type of pain around the nipple and areola, and there are palpable tortuous tubular swellings under the areola. When the condition is more advanced, a mass can develop that may resemble a locally advanced clinical stage III breast carcinoma.

The pathogenesis of this condition has not been fully established. Available evidence suggests, however, that the

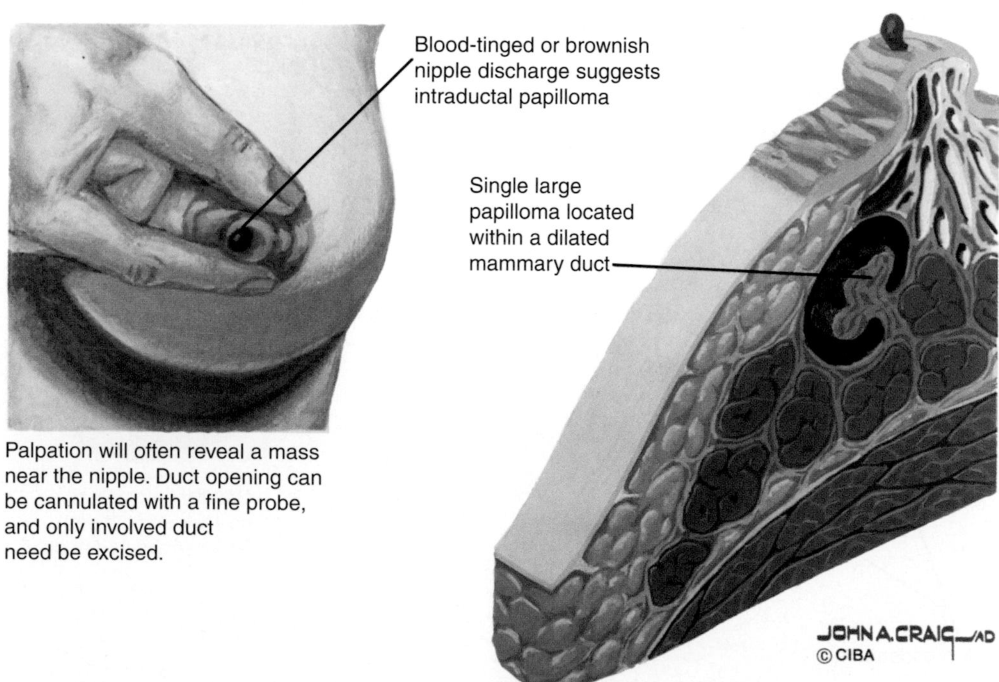

Figure 14–8 Solitary intraductal papilloma. (From Townsend CM Jr: Breast lumps. Clin Symp 32:1–32, 1980. Art by John A Craig. Reprinted with permission from Elsevier Inc. All rights reserved.)

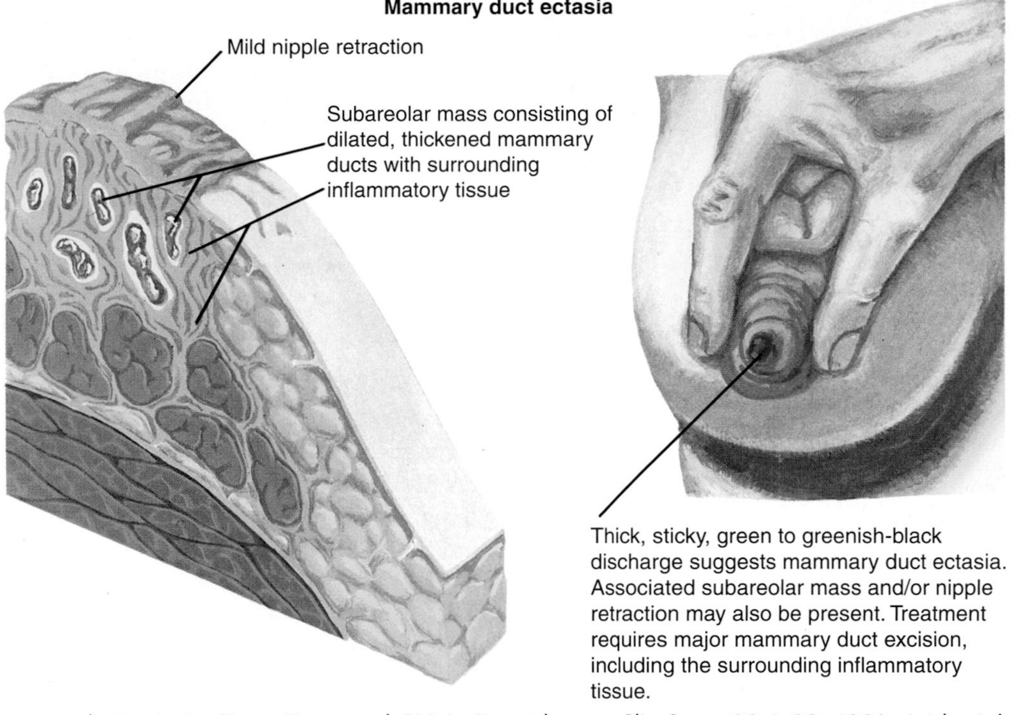

Figure 14–9 Mammary duct ectasia. (From Townsend CM Jr: Breast lumps. Clin Symp 32:1–32, 1980. Art by John A Craig. Reprinted with permission from Elsevier Inc. All rights reserved.)

primary event is periductal inflammation, and that ductal ectasia is the ultimate outcome of this disorder. The postulated sequence of events in the evolution of this disease is periductal inflammation leading to periductal fibrosis that subsequently results in ductal dilation. However, the etiology of the initial inflammatory response remains obscure. Treatment consists of local excision of the inflamed area of the breast tissue. On microscopic examination, many cases show prominence of a lipid-rich material within ducts, accompanied by periductal inflammation. Rupture or leakage of these ducts may result in release of this material into the adjacent stroma, with subsequent inflammation and fat necrosis.

Adenoma

Adenoma of the breast is a well-circumscribed tumor composed of benign epithelial elements with sparse, inconspicuous stroma, a feature that differentiates this lesion from fibroadenoma, in which the stroma is an integral part of the tumor. For practical purposes, adenomas may be divided into two major groups: tubular adenomas and lactating adenomas. Tubular adenomas in young women are well-defined, freely movable nodules that clinically resemble fibroadenomas. Lactating adenomas manifest as one or more freely movable masses during pregnancy or the postpartum period. They are grossly well circumscribed and lobulated; on cut section, they appear tan and softer than tubular adenomas. On microscopic examination, these lesions have lobulated borders and are composed of glands lined by cuboid cells with secretory activity, identical to the lactational changes normally observed in the breast tissue during pregnancy and the puerperium.

Sclerosing lesions

Sclerosing lesions have been described by a variety of names, including sclerosing papillary proliferation, nonencapsulated sclerosing lesion, indurative mastopathy, and radial scar. Their importance lies in that they may simulate carcinoma on mammographic, gross, and microscopic examinations. These lesions are typically <1 cm in diameter. On gross examination, they are irregular, gray or white, and indurated with central retraction and have an appearance identical to scirrhous carcinoma. On microscopic examination, the lesion has a stellate configuration and consists of a central, fibrotic core containing entrapped glandular elements. The surrounding breast tissue typically shows varying degrees of intraductal hyperplasia and adenosis. The significance of this lesion relative to subsequent development of carcinoma is controversial. Available evidence suggests that these lesions are part of the fibrocystic complex. It is likely that their premalignant potential is the same as that of the constituent parts. Local excision of these lesions is the treatment of choice.

Nipple discharge

Nipple discharge is usually noted to be bloody, milky, serous, or purulent. The great majority of cases of spontaneous nipple discharge are due to benign conditions. Galactorrhea presents as bilateral milky nipple discharge consisting of lipid droplets; the condition is usually idiopathic but can be found after discontinuation of oral contraceptives or as a persistent discharge after pregnancy. Plasma prolactin levels should be determined because of the possibility of a prolactin-producing pituitary adenoma.

Table 14–4 CHARACTERISTICS OF NIPPLE DISCHARGE

Color	Likely cause	Percentage caused by cancer
Milky (galactorrhea)	Pituitary adenoma, pregnancy, oral contraceptives	Rare
Green, yellow, sticky	Ductal ectasia	Rare
Clear, watery	Ductal carcinoma	30–50
Bloody, sanguineous	Fibrocystic changes, ductal papillomas	25
Pink, serosanguineous	Fibrocystic changes, ductal papillomas	10
Yellow, serous	Fibrocystic changes, ductal papillomas	5
Purulent	Bacterial infection	Rare

Bloody discharge is usually produced by a solid papilloma; green sticky discharge is characteristic of ductal ectasia (Table 14–4).

Breast mass during pregnancy and lactation

Benign lesions during pregnancy include fibroadenomas, lipomas, papillomas, fibrocystic changes, galactoceles, and inflammatory lesions.

Byrd et al, in a series of 105 biopsies with benign findings, noted that 71% of patients had conditions found in non-pregnant women, and 29% had changes particular to gestation (e.g. lobular hyperplasia, galactocele, lactational mastitis). As pregnancy progresses, the breasts become firmer, more nodular, and hypertrophic. This is of course also true of the postpartum lactation period. A subtle palpable mass may disappear as pregnancy progresses and the breast becomes more engorged. Whereas a breast mass in a menstruating woman can be re-examined just after the next menstrual period, the hormonal milieu will continue to intensify in the pregnant woman, making subsequent examinations more difficult. Fine-needle aspiration of a mass that yields fluid and causes the mass to disappear readily differentiates the fluid-filled cyst or galactocele from a solid tumor. However, cytology from fine-needle aspiration is not as accurate in the pregnant woman as in the non-pregnant woman. The hyperproliferative cellular state of the pregnant breast increases the possibility of a false-positive diagnosis. Excisional biopsy under local anesthesia may be difficult during pregnancy because of the hypervascularity and edema, but it remains the best diagnostic tool. Many clinicians attribute the advanced state and poor prognosis of breast cancer in pregnancy to delayed diagnosis. More recent theories of cancer in pregnancy have shown improved survivals undoubtedly as a result of less reluctance to perform biopsy of the breasts of pregnant women.

Breast biopsy in a pregnant or a lactating woman calls for meticulous hemostasis, because of the increased vascularity and risk of postoperative hematoma formation. The lactating breast is predisposed to postoperative infection, because milk is a good culture medium. Anesthesia by local injection may be difficult in the enlarged breast but is the method of choice. Incisional biopsy under local anesthesia is an option when excisional biopsy is a problem. Because of the significant risk of infection and milk fistula, the patient who is lactating should cease lactating before biopsy is performed.

BREAST CANCERS

Epidemiology

Over the years, multiple risk factors have been suggested for breast cancer. Many have been discarded or at the most designated a minor contributing factor. This discussion is limited to those items for which there is a consensus or recent investigations have suggested potential risk (Table 14–5). More than 75% of women with newly diagnosed breast cancer have no known risk factor. Age is considered the most important risk factor with the possible exception of gender. Breast cancer can occur in men, but 99% is found in women. Although women in their third and fourth decades of life have breast cancer, it is relatively uncommon before the menopause. The age incidence curve shows a small plateau at approximately 50 years of age, and after women undergo menopause the curve is followed by a steeper rise thereafter. The probability of development of breast cancer increases with the woman's age, with most breast cancers occurring in the postmenopausal years. Although there are some exceptions to this, such as in women in Japan, it is certainly true for the western world. The risk that a 30-year-old woman will have breast cancer is 7% that of a 60-year-old woman. By the age of 35 years, the ratio begins to change, and the risk for an individual of that age is 20% that of a 60-year-old. It is generally accepted today that a woman's risk for development of breast cancer is one in eight or nine. Although this number is frightening, women should realize that, even after the

Table 14–5 MAJOR RISK FACTORS FOR BREAST CANCER

- Age
- Family history of breast cancer
- Benign breast disease
  - Proliferative changes
  - Atypical hyperplasia
- Endogenous endocrine factors
  - Early menarche
  - Late menopause
  - Long menses duratio
  - Nulliparity
  - Late maternal age at first pregnancy
- Exogenous hormones?
  - Oral contraceptives
  - Estrogen replacement therapy

menopause, chances of developing breast cancer in a single year are low. For instance, in a 60-year-old, the risk is 1 in 420; in an 80-year-old, it is 1 in 290.

Family history of breast cancer in either the maternal or paternal line increases the risk for development of breast cancer, although this is relatively small. This relationship seems to be the greatest if there is a breast cancer history in a first-degree relative (mother, sister, or daughter) (Table 14–6). If breast cancer is present in a mother or sister, there is an approximately twofold risk. When more than two first-order relatives have breast cancer, the risk increases even more. This suggests a genetic factor; however, to date, <10% of breast cancer patients have been identified as having a genetic link (BRCA1 and BRCA2). Genetically linked breast cancers are more likely to be associated with an earlier onset of the disease and bilateral disease. In counseling patients, risk ratios are usually meaningless, and accumulated probability is a better means of relating risk. For instance, the risk of developing breast cancer for a 30-year-old woman by age 70 years if a sister has unilateral disease diagnosed before age 50 years is about 8%. If both the mother and a sister have unilateral breast disease that has developed at any age, the risk is 18%. If the normal incidence is one in eight (12.5%), the risk is increased but not markedly.

Prospective data from the Nurses' Health Study noted that the risk of breast cancer doubled among women whose mother had breast cancer diagnosed before the age of 40 years or who had a sister with breast cancer. The risk decreased with advanced maternal age; however, it remained elevated even with maternal diagnosis at age 70 years (relative risk 1.5, confidence interval [CI] 1.1–2.2). The data did show that the risk associated with a mother or sister with history of breast cancer is smaller than previously suggested. In the population of middle-aged women, the authors found that only 2.5% of breast cancer cases were attributed to a positive family history. In the large Cancer Prevention Study II by the American Cancer Society (ACS), the authors evaluated the association of fatal breast cancer and family history. They found that family history of breast cancer in a mother or sister was significantly related to fatal breast cancer risk after multivariate analysis. Association was significantly modified by age with the risk ratio of almost 5 in women younger than 40 years at enrollment compared with 1.28 in women aged 70 years or older.

Table 14–6 FIRST-DEGREE RELATIVE WITH BREAST CANCER: RELATIVE RISK FOR PATIENT

Index case	Relative risk
Premenopausal	
Unilateral	1.8
Bilateral	8.8
Postmenopausal	
Unilateral	1.2
Bilateral	4.0

Endogenous endocrine and reproductive factors have been shown to be associated with an increased risk of breast cancer. The younger a woman's age at menarche, the higher her risk for breast cancer. The relative risk for development of breast cancer in women whose menarche occurred before the age of 13 years is about twice that of women whose menarche occurred after this time. If regular ovulatory cycles began before 13 years, there may be nearly a fourfold increase in those individuals compared with those whose menarche occurred after 13 years and who have regular ovulatory cycles after an interval of about 5 years.

Early exposure to the hormone milieu is thought by some to be an important etiologic factor. In one large international case-control study, it was noted that for each 2-year delay in the onset of menstruation, breast cancer risk was reduced by about 10%. The later a woman's menopause occurs, the higher her risk for breast cancer. For every 5-year difference in age at menopause, the risk for breast cancer changes about 17%. The effect of this later age at menopause in regard to increasing breast cancer is really not seen for 10–20 years after menopause. It has been suggested that the total duration of menstruation may also be important because the risk increases in the woman who has menstruated >30 years compared with those who have had <30 years of menstruation. Among women who have undergone a natural menopause, the risk among those whose menopause occurred at age 55 years is about twice that of women whose menopause occurred before age 44 years. Those women who have undergone bilateral oophorectomy before age 50 years have a decreased risk compared with those who had a later natural or artificial menopause. However, these data are derived from observational studies, and there has not been a prospective randomized trial in which artificial menopause has been induced to specifically evaluate the risk of breast cancer development as a result of bilateral oophorectomy.

The age at first full-term pregnancy appears to be an important risk factor. If a woman whose age at first full-term birth is <19 years, there is about a 50% reduction in the risk of breast cancer compared with that of a nulliparous woman. If the first full-term pregnancy occurs at age 30–34 years, the risk of breast cancer is approximately the same as that noted in nulliparous women. Pregnancy in women after age 35 years is associated with an increased risk compared with that of a nulliparous woman. Pregnancies that are not full term do not show this protection. Some have suggested that the time interval between the onset of menarche and the first full-term pregnancy is the important factor with regard to the endocrine milieu. This importance has a possible explanation in the "estrogen open window hypothesis." There is, however, some inconsistency in reported data in regard to relationship of age at first full-term pregnancy. The association depends somewhat on control subjects used, and later studies have suggested a less strong association.

A history of benign breast disease has been suggested as a possible risk factor for development of breast cancer.

The large study of Dupont and Page evaluated benign breast biopsy specimens for subsequent risk of breast cancer. In a retrospective review of more than 3000 biopsies, reclassification was done into precise histologic category. Those individuals with non-proliferative changes (fibrocystic changes) were not at increased risk. Those individuals who had proliferative changes but without atypia had a somewhat increased risk for subsequent breast cancer; however, the highest risk was in those individuals with atypical hyperplasia. Fortunately, only 7% of the total biopsy population had atypical hyperplasia. In the 39 patients who had both atypical hyperplasia and a family history of breast cancer, the risk went up dramatically. It did appear that as the length of time increased since the breast biopsy, the risk was attenuated. In patients with either atypical hyperplasia or proliferative disease without atypia, the risk decreased by about two-thirds after one decade of follow-up.

The possible protective role of lactation and breast-feeding in the development of breast cancer is inconclusive at present. In studies from China, where breast-feeding is more common than in the USA, evidence suggests that long-term breast-feeding is protective. Studies in this country, however, have suggested only a weak protective effect and no trend of decreasing risk with increasing duration of breast-feeding. Some studies have noted a slight reduction in the risk of breast cancer among premenopausal women but not in postmenopausal women.

Early detection and diagnosis

There is general agreement that mammography screening in women aged 50–74 years has resulted in a decreased mortality from breast cancer based on multiple prospective studies (Fig. 14–10 and Table 14–7). The frequency of screening recommended differs among the various groups. The ACS recommend annual screening (Table 14–8). The American College of Obstetricians and Gynecologists (ACOG), the US Preventive Services Task Force, and the National Cancer Institute (NCI) recommend screening

Table 14–7 MAMMOGRAPHY AND REDUCED MORTALITY FROM BREAST CANCER

Study	Schedule	Percentage decrease in mortality
Health Insurance Plan	Every year for 4 years	30
Verbeek et al	Every 2 years for 4 years	33
Colette	At 1, 12, 18, and 24 months	50
Tabár et al	Every 2 years (ages 40–49 years), every 33 months (> 50 years)	31

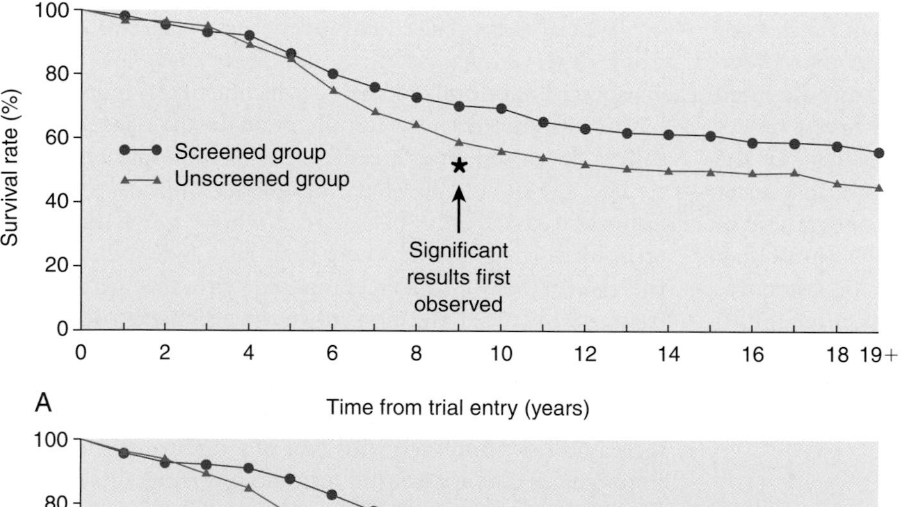

Figure 14–10 *A,* Survival rates for women in the Health Insurance Plan study aged 40–49 years at entry (all stages). *B,* Survival rates for women in the Health Insurance Plan study aged 50–64 years at entry (all stages). (After Chu KC, Smart CR, Tarone RE: Analysis of breast cancer mortality and stage distribution by age for the Health Insurance Plan clinical trial. J Natl Cancer Inst 80:1125–1132, 1988. Reprinted with permission of Oxford University Press.)

Table 14–8 RECOMMENDATIONS FOR MAMMOGRAPHIC SCREENING FOR BREAST CANCER

Age (years)	American College of Obstetricians and Gynecologists	American Cancer Society	National Cancer Institute	US Preventive Services Task Force
40–49	1–2 years	Annually	1–2 years	1–2 years
50–74	Annually	Annually	1–2 years	1–2 years

at intervals of 1–2 years. In women 40–49 years of age, there is considerable controversy in regard to the interpretation of as well as the recommendation for mammographic screening. The ACOG and the NCI recommend screening every 1–2 years. The recommendation of the ACS is annually for this age group. The ACOG recommends regular screening beginning at age 35 years for women with a family history of premenopausal breast cancer in a first-degree relative.

Clinical breast examination recommendations also varied among the organizations. The ACOG recommends clinical breast examinations during periodic evaluation, usually yearly, for women aged 18–39 years. Annual breast examinations are recommended after age 40 years by the ACOG and ACS. (For data on breast cancer frequency by age, see Fig. 14–11 and Table 14–9.)

Twelve organizations met in 1988 to develop a consensus recommendation for breast cancer screening (Fig. 14–12). They agreed to the following.

- Clinical breast examination and mammography are both essential in screening.
- Annual mammography should be performed for women aged 50 years and older.
- Mammography should be done at intervals of 1–2 years for women aged 40–49 years.

The role of breast self-examination as part of screening could not be agreed on.

In 1993, the NCI stated that it would not continue to support the recommendation of mammographic screening in women aged 40–49 years (an action not well received by many organizations and patient advocate groups) because

Table 14–9 AGE-SPECIFIC PROBABILITIES OF DEVELOPING BREAST CANCER[a]

Current age (years)	Probability of developing breast cancer in the next 10 years[b] (%)	One in:
20	0.05	1985
30	0.44	229
40	1.46	68
50	2.73	37
60	3.82	26
70	4.14	24
Lifetime risk	13.22	8

[a]Among those free of cancer at beginning of age interval. Based on cases diagnoses 2000–2. Percentages and "One in" numbers may not be numerically equivalent, due to rounding.

[b]Probability derived using National Cancer Institute DevCan software, version 6.0.

(From American Cancer Society, Surveillance Research, 2005.)

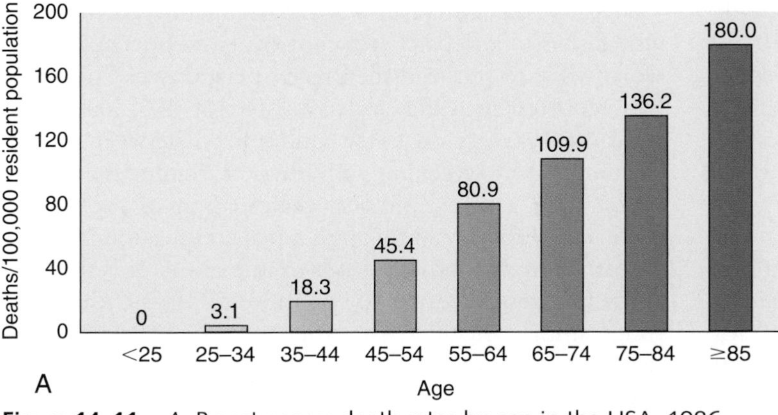

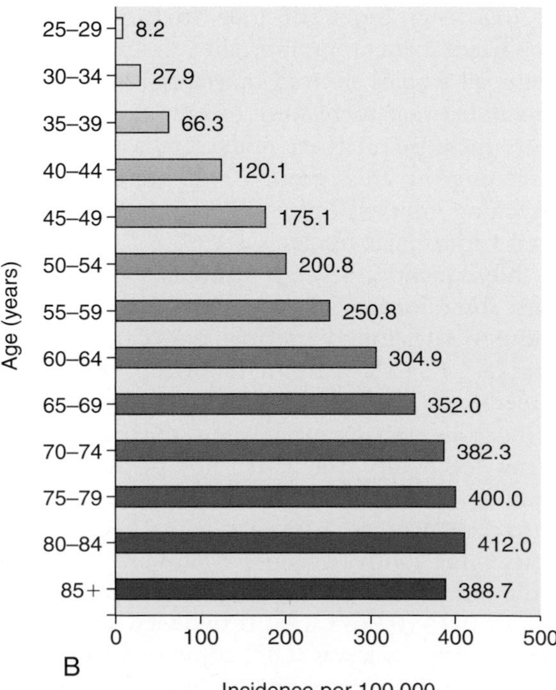

Figure 14–11 *A,* Breast cancer death rates by age in the USA, 1986. *B,* Breast cancer frequency by age. (A, source, US Department of Health and Human Services; B, based on data from Cancer Statistics Review 1973–1986. Washington, National Cancer Institute, 1989.)

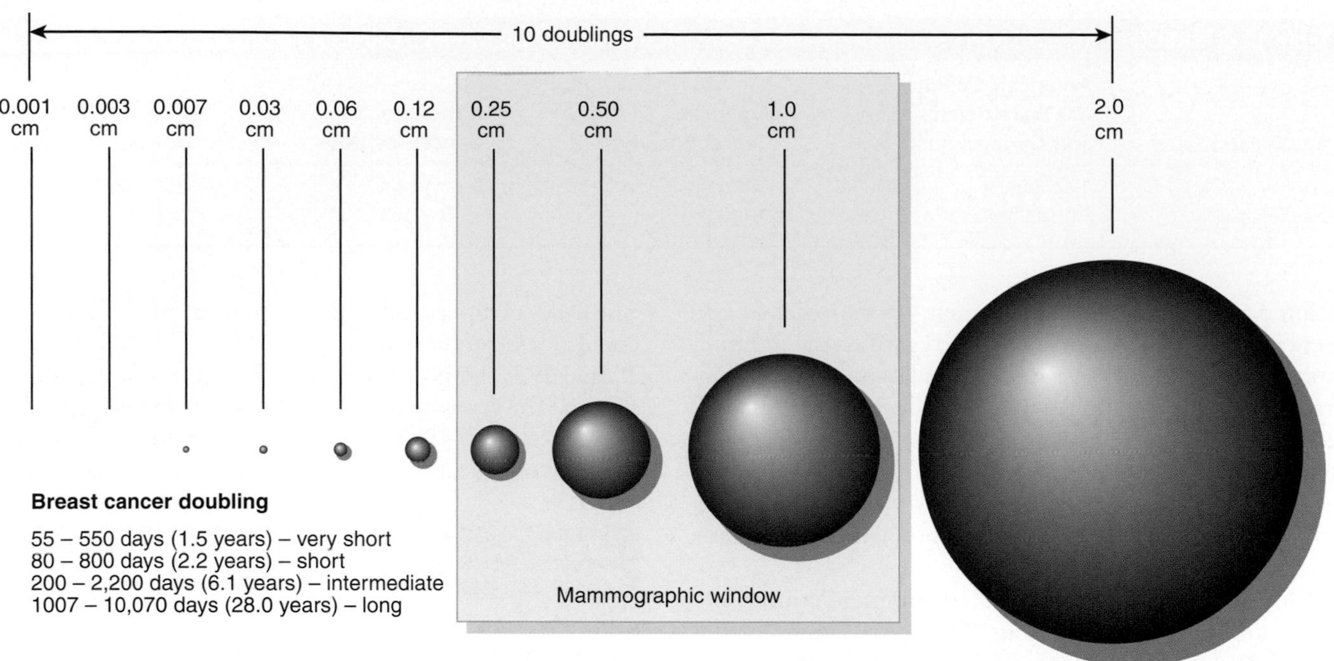

Figure 14–12 Breast cancer doubling time. (From Woodward WA, et al. Changes in the 2003 American Joint Committee on Cancer Staging for Breast Cancer Dramatically Affect Stage-specific Survival. 21(17):3244-48, 2003. © 2003 American Society for Clinical Oncology. Reprinted with permission from The American Society of Clinical Oncology.)

of lack of agreement as to the benefits of screening in this age group. This was based on Fletcher and colleagues' report of the International Workshop on Screening for Breast Cancer, published in late 1993. In eight major randomized controlled trials of breast cancer screening for women aged 40–49 years, no benefit from screening in the first 5–7 years after study entry was found. The Canadian study showed an increase in breast cancer mortality of 36% in those screened compared with the unscreened group. A meta-analysis of six trials found a relative risk of 1.08 (CI 0.85–1.39) after 7 years of follow-up. After 10–12 years of follow-up, none of four trials found a statistically significant benefit in mortality. In women aged 50–69 years, all studies showed mortality reduction. The report concluded that there were too few women older than 70 years included in these studies to assess effectiveness of screening in this group. Of interest is that various screening intervals (every 12 months to 28 months) were used with similar results.

Subsequently, several meta-analyses of these studies with some longer follow-up have been published. Smart and associates found a relative risk of 0.84 (0.69–1.02) for periods of 7–18 years of follow-up. They believed that screening of women 40–49 years of age can reduce mortality from breast cancer when it is combined with adequate follow-up (the latter not defined). Breast cancer deaths were 200 in 1,032,000 women years of follow-up in screened women, compared with 221 in 971,000 women years in the control group. Kerlikowske and colleagues also did a meta-analysis and found an overall screening relative risk of 0.93 (0.76–1.13). If two-view mammography was used, relative risk was 0.87, compared with 1.02 for those with one-view mammography. For 7–9 years of follow-up, the summary relative risk was 1.02, compared with 0.83 (CI 0.65–1.06) for those with 10–12 years of follow-up. These authors stated that there was no reduction in breast cancer mortality in women aged 40–49 years after 7–9 years of follow-up. Screening mammography may be effective in reducing breast cancer mortality in this age group, but the same benefit could probably be achieved by beginning screening at menopause or 50 years of age (two studies did not start screening until 45 years of age, and "age creep," i.e. diagnosis made after age 50 years, may account for any benefit).

Because the Canadian study has engendered considerable discussion, debate, and controversy, a brief account is worthwhile to put it in the proper perspective. This study was reported in 1992 and consisted of 40,430 women aged 40–49 years on entry randomized between annual mammography screening with physical examination of the breasts and a single physical examination of the breasts with annual follow-up through a mailed questionnaire. All women were taught breast self-examination. It is the only study that restricted the age to those of 40–49 years. The other studies included the younger patients with those who were older than 50 years. Through 7 years of follow-up, there were 331 invasive cancers in the mammographically screened patients, compared with 272 in the unscreened control subjects. There were 38 deaths from breast cancer in the screened patients, compared with 28 in the control group. The ratio of proportions of breast cancer deaths of screened compared with unscreened was 1.36 (CI 0.84–2.21). The survival rates were therefore similar. Screening with yearly mammography and physical examination of the breast detected considerably more node-negative, smaller tumors than in the usual care patients but had no impact on the rate of death from breast cancer.

Although this was the largest study to date, considerable criticism has been voiced on many accounts, such as randomization bias, mammography quality, and high prevalence rate of both groups at entry. This is the only study that has allowed outside evaluation of randomization and mammography. The authors have thought that these criticisms are unjustified, and many epistles from the two camps have appeared in the literature. Interestingly, cancer detection, survival at 7 years after diagnosis for cancers detected by mammography alone, and mortality results in the Canadian study were similar to those of other trials.

In 1997, the Canadian study was updated. During an average of 10.5 years of follow-up (range 8.75–13 years), 82 women in the screening group died of breast cancer, compared with 72 in the non-screened woman. A rate ratio of 1.14 (0.83–1.56) was present, indicating a non-significant excess of breast cancer deaths in the screened group.

In early 1997, a National Institutes of Health Consensus Development Statement on breast cancer screening for women aged 40–49 years was published. A review of the available data was performed, with updates given when they were available from previously published studies. The majority of the panel did not think that the data supported a recommendation for universal mammography screening for all women in their forties. It was noted that up to one-fourth of all invasive cancers are not detected by mammography in women 40–49 years old, compared with one-tenth of cancers in women 50–69 years old. As many as 3 of 10 women who begin annual screening at age 40 years will have an abnormal mammogram during the next decade. For women aged 40–49 years undergoing breast biopsy for an abnormal mammogram, only half as many cancers are diagnosed compared with in women aged 50–69 years. For every eight biopsies done in the younger age group, one invasive and one in situ breast cancer is found. A minority (2 of 12) report indicated that after evaluation and consideration of the evidence, women in their forties should be actively encouraged to obtain routine screening mammograms. Providing accurate information to women is essential to aid them in deciding whether to accept or reject that advice.

In the spring of 1997, the NCI accepted new guidelines from the presidentially appointed National Cancer Advisory Board, which recommended screening mammograms every 1–2 years for women aged 40–49 years if they are at average risk for breast cancer. The new guidelines also recommend screening at 1–2 years for women aged 50 years and older. Just before this new recommendation, the ACS and the American College of Radiology (ACR) recommended annual screening mammograms for women aged 40–49 years. In September 1997, the ACOG reiterated its previous recommendation in regard to breast cancer screening: mammography should be performed every 1–2 years for women 40–49 years of age, and annually thereafter.

Mammography is the most accurate technique for the detection of early-stage breast cancers. However, a false-negative rate of 5–15% has been reported for clinically palpable masses. Indications for needle aspiration of palpable masses vary depending on the clinician and the institution. We encourage liberal use of this procedure, described earlier in this chapter. Fine-needle aspiration is ideal for evaluating multiple or recurrent breast lesions—it avoids disfigurement with numerous open biopsy scars. The equipment required is available in most physicians' offices. When the diagnostic triad of physical examination, fine-needle aspiration, and mammography is employed for multiple or recurrent breast masses, open biopsy is rarely needed.

In any case, a fine-needle aspiration or open biopsy should be performed on a clinically suspicious mass whether the mammogram is suspicious or not. Some cancers, particularly the medullary type, appear well circumscribed on the mammogram and mimic cysts or fibroadenomas. It is much more common, however, for a palpable carcinoma to possess the classic characteristics of irregular or spiculated borders, with or without microcalcifications (Fig. 14–13).

The ACR Breast Imaging Reporting and Data System (BI-RADS) is the product of a collaborative effort of the ACR, the NCI, the Centers for Disease Control and Prevention, the Food and Drug Administration (FDA), the American Medical Association, the American College of Surgeons, and the College of American Pathologists. The system is a quality assurance tool designed to standardize mammographic reporting, to reduce confusion in breast imaging interpretations, and to facilitate outcome monitoring. There is no test or group of tests that can ever ensure that a woman does not have breast cancer, but

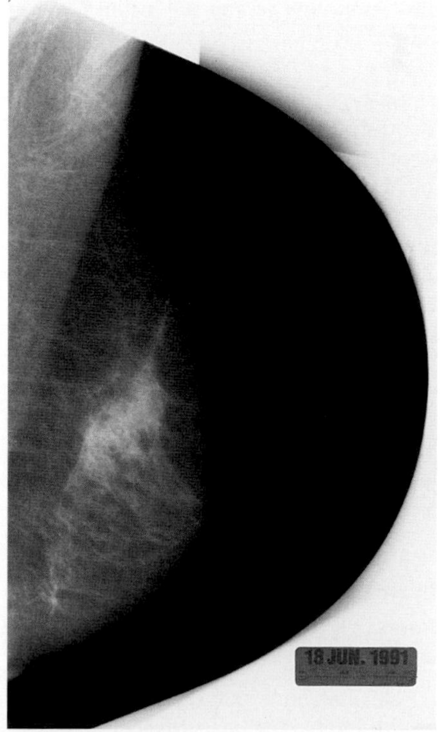

Figure 14–13 Mammogram showing an irregular configuration characteristic of malignancy.

mammography has become a useful tool for diagnosis. The excerpt from the BI-RADS guidelines lists the recommendations for a reporting system (Table 14–10). This system is clear and concise, and should be adopted by physicians treating breast disease in the interest of uniformity.

An increasing percentage of breast cancers is being suspected on mammography and needs histologic evaluation. The mammographic categories 4 and 5 require histologic study. Excisional biopsy specimens generated during breast cancer screening have many benign findings. The positive predictive value has been reported in the range of 10–40%. The study by Brown and associates of 50 community mammography facilities found an average biopsy yield of mammographic abnormalities of 21%. Because a half

Table 14–10 REPORT ORGANIZATION

The reporting system should be concise and organized using the following structure. A statement indicating that the present examination has been compared to previous mammograms should be included. If this is not included, it should be assumed that no comparison has been made.

1. Breast Composition
   A succinct description of the overall breast composition.

   This is an overall assessment of the attenuating tissues in the breast to help indicate the relative possibility that a lesion could be hidden by the normal tissues. Generally, this includes fatty, mixed or dense.

   Since mammography cannot detect all breast cancers, physical examination is always a key element of screening. It is important to alert the clinician that in the radiographically dense breast the ability of mammography to detect small cancers is reduced. Although mammography is still useful in these women, the physical examination (which is always important) is increased in importance. The available data do not support the use of mammographic patterns for determining screening frequency (i.e., risk for breast cancer).

   If an implant is present, it should be stated in the report and an implant description code added as appropriate.

   For consistency, this should be included for all patients using the following patterns:

   1. The breast is almost entirely fat.
   2. There are scattered fibroglandular densities.
   3. The breast tissue is heterogeneously dense. This may lower the sensitivity of mammography.
   4. The breast tissue is extremely dense, which could obscure a lesion on mammography.

   If an implant is present, it should be stated in the report and an implant description code added as appropriate.

2. Findings
   a. A clear description of any significant finding. (It is assumed that most significant findings are new.*)
      i. Mass:
         Size
         Lesion type and modifiers
         Associated calcifications
         Associated findings
         Location
         How changed, if previously present*
      ii. Calcifications:
         Morphology—type or shape and modifiers
         Distribution
         Associated findings
         Location
         How changed, if previously present*
      iii. Architectural Distortion:
         Associated calcifications
         Associated findings
         Location
         How changed, if previously present.*
      iv. Special Cases:
         Associated calcifications
         Associated findings
         Location
         How changed, if previously present.*
         The *clinical location* of the abnormality as extrapolated from the mammographic location (based on the face of a clock and/or quadrant).
   b. An overall (summary) impression.
      All final impressions should be complete with each lesion fully categorized and qualified. An indeterminate reading should be given only in the screening setting where additional imaging evaluation is recommended before a final opinion can be rendered.

      In the screening situation a suggestion for the next course of action should be given if the study is not conclusive (magnification, ultrasound, etc.).

      Interpretation is facilitated by recognizing that most mammograms can be categorized under a few headings. These are listed below, and suggested codes are included for computer use.

      If a suspicious abnormality is detected, the report should indicate that biopsy should be considered. This is an assessment where the radiologist has sufficient concern that biopsy is warranted unless there are other reasons why the patient and her physician might wish to defer the biopsy.

Table continued on opposite page.

Table 14–10 REPORT ORGANIZATION—CONT'D

3. Assessment Categories
   a. Assessment is Incomplete

Category 0 Need Additional Imaging Evaluation:
Finding for which additional imaging evaluation is needed. This is almost always used in a screening situation and should rarely be used after a full imaging work up. A recommendation for additional imaging evaluation includes the use of spot compression, magnification, special mammographic views, ultrasound, etc.

Whenever possible, the present mammogram should be compared to previous studies. The radiologist should use judgment in how vigorously to pursue previous studies.

   b. Assessment is Complete—**Final** Categories

Category 1 Negative:
There is nothing on which to comment. The breasts are symmetrical and no masses, architectural disturbances, or suspicious calcifications are present.

Category 2 Benign Finding:
This is also a negative mammogram, but the interpreter may wish to describe a finding. Involuting, calcified fibroadenomas, multiple secretory calcifications, fat-containing lesions such as oil cysts, lipomas, galactoceles, and mixed density hamartomas all have characteristic appearances, and may be labeled with confidence. The interpreter might wish to describe intramammary lymph nodes, implants, etc. while still concluding that there is no mammographic evidence of malignancy.

Category 3 Probably Benign Finding—Short Interval Follow-up Suggested:
A finding placed in this category should have a very high probability of being benign. It is not expected to change over the follow-up interval, but the radiologist would prefer to establish its stability. Data are becoming available that shed light on the efficacy of short interval follow-up. At the present time, most approaches are intuitive. These will likely undergo future modification as more data accrue as to the validity of an approach, the interval required, and the type of findings that should be followed.

Category 4 Suspicious Abnormality—Biopsy Should Be Considered:
These are lesions that do not have the characteristic morphologies of breast cancer but have a definite probability of being malignant. The radiologist has sufficient concern to urge a biopsy. If possible, the relevant probabilities should be cited so that the patient and her physician can make the decision on the ultimate course of action.

Category 5 Highly Suggestive of Malignancy—Appropriate Action Should Be Taken:
These lesions have a high probability of being cancer.

million to one million excisional breast biopsies are performed each year, this translates to between 300,000 and 900,000 benign breast biopsy specimens.

Fine-needle aspiration cytology, particularly in Europe, has replaced excisional biopsy for evaluation of mammographic abnormalities. This technique (Table 14–11) is not as frequently used in the USA for several reasons. Obviously, a skilled cytopathologist is required. Although reports on the sensitivity and specificity have reasonably good results, the rate of insufficient specimens ranges from 2 to 36%. Many times, a definitive diagnosis is not possible, mainly because of its inability to differentiate invasive from in situ carcinoma.

Table 14–11 TECHNIQUE OF FINE-NEEDLE ASPIRATION CYTOLOGY

Angle of needle should be at 15–20° to the skin to avoid insertion into the pleural space and development of possible pneumothorax.
Move needle back and forth in mass to obtain adequate specimen.
Keep air in barrel of syringe to allow emptying of tissue sample in the needle barrel.
Place specimen on glass slide and spread as one would do for a blood smear.
Fix immediately per cytologist's preferred method.

Stereotactically guided core needle biopsy (CNB), which uses a large-bore needle, appears to have several advantages over fine-needle aspiration cytology. The specimen can be read by a pathologist who does not have special training in cytology. Specimens are rarely insufficient, and it is easier to differentiate invasive from in situ cancers. The CNB can be performed under stereotactic mammographic or ultrasound guidance. Better results are usually obtained with a 14-gauge needle compared with small-bore needles. Studies have shown a 99% accuracy with a 14-gauge needle obtaining five specimens. Radiography should be performed routinely on women with CNB specimens of breast microcalcifications to determine whether calcifications were obtained. Certainly, false positives can occur. However, in one multi-institutional study, 5.4% who were diagnosed with benign lesions subsequently were found to have carcinoma. Up to 20% of non-palpable lesions can be missed at the time of image-directed excisional biopsy; missed lesions can be identified by radiographs taken immediately of excised specimens and be treated appropriately. Stereotactically guided CNB is less expensive than excisional biopsy, results in less morbidity, and leaves no noticeable scar. Stereotactically guided CNB can be done on most non-palpable mammographic abnormalities or on those highly suggestive, for which open biopsy would be considered. It should not be used as a substitute for poor or inadequate imaging workup.

Some patients may not be candidates for CNB. A patient may be too large to be accommodated by the system. The thickness of the breast must be adequate to accommodate to the automated biopsy device. Abnormalities just under the skin may also pose technical problems. A vague asymmetric density or diffuse group of widely separated calcifications may present difficulties. Patients who cannot remain prone or are unable to cooperate for the 20- to 40-min duration of the procedure may not be candidates.

Certain benign lesions have a relatively high incidence of coexisting carcinoma, and the CNB with its small volume of tissue may not be adequate to rule out cancer. Atypical ductal hyperplasia is the most commonly encountered of these lesions. Up to 50% of CNB diagnoses of atypical ductal hyperplasia will have carcinoma on excisional biopsy. Radial scars are reported to have a coexistent carcinoma in 20%, and therefore require a large surgical excision. The tissue obtained from a CNB may not be concordant with the imaging findings. In a study by Dershaw and associates, repeated biopsy for non-concordance found carcinoma in 47% of cases. A diagnosis of LCIS should not be accepted as consistent with imaging findings requiring biopsy. Because LCIS has no characteristic mammographic findings, a histologic diagnosis of LCIS without a second lesion should be considered non-diagnostic, and repeated biopsy may be indicated. When an open biopsy is to be performed, basic plastic surgery techniques and principles can provide a minimum of disfigurement and a nearly undetectable scar, at the same time meeting all the requirements necessary. Breast mobility allows the nipple to be rotated to any point on the breast. A periareolar incision circumscribing half the circumference of the areola will allow a linear wound 3.14 times the diameter of the areola (Fig. 14–14).

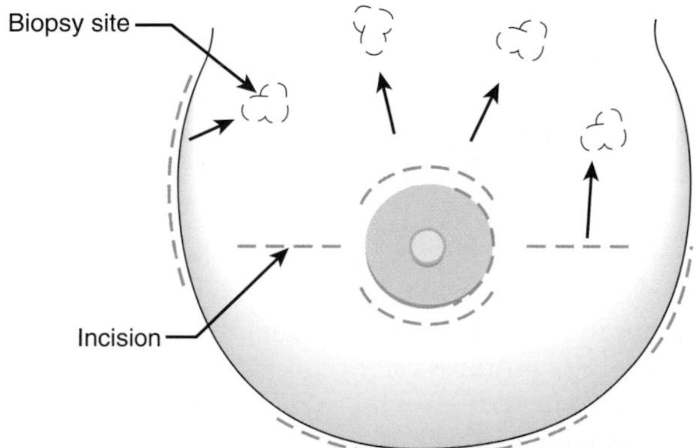

Figure 14–14 Location of incisions for breast biopsy with good cosmetic result. (From Keen G: Operative Surgery and Management. New York, Macmillan, 1987.)

Clinical staging of patients with suspected operable mammary cancer begins with measurement of the primary tumor in two or three dimensions and with a description of its location and attachments (Table 14–12). Palpation of regional lymph node areas should be thorough. Although about one-fourth of the patients with enlarged axillary nodes (clinical stage II) are without nodal metastasis, about 40% of those without palpable nodes (stage I) have nodal metastasis. The clinical staging nevertheless correlates well with the 5- to 10-year survival rate and is the basis for selection of therapy in many cases. Biopsy should be done on enlarged supraclavicular nodes before mastectomy, and other signs of local spread of tumor outside the breasts (stage III) should be sought.

The number of positive axillary nodes definitely affects survival; the 10-year disease-free survival rate is 38% for one to three positive nodes and 13% for four or more positive nodes. Size and histopathologic character of the neoplasms are correlated with curability. All patients with suspected progression of disease beyond clinical stage I, on the basis of the history and physical examination, require careful radiologic search for distant metastasis as well. The most useful tests are bone scans and x-ray films of bones with abnormal uptake on the scan, as well as films of the chest and contralateral breast.

Differences in the extent of the disease in the presence of asymptomatic but possibly detectable metastasis at the time of initial diagnosis may explain much of the variability in the results of therapy. Large clinical series indicate a frequency of clinical stage IV disease between 2 and 13% at the time of presentation. Without including the number of patients who did not have scans or x-ray examinations, Roberts and coworkers reported that 18% of new breast cancer patients with normal bone radiographs had scans with evidence of bone metastasis. Such a frequency of bone involvement in patients with clinically localized and operable breast cancer appears extensive in view of the 17% total recurrence rate at all sites observed by others in the first 18 months after surgery in patients with operable breast cancer.

With a trend toward less radical surgery and more systemic adjuvant therapy, the importance of proper staging becomes crucial. One objective of adjuvant chemotherapy is eradication of minimal "microscopic" disease. If patients with detectable primary metastatic disease contaminate the true adjuvant population, results of such therapy may be obscured. Moreover, patients with primary metastatic disease should be considered for alternative therapeutic options, such as endocrine therapy before or in combination with chemotherapy.

Chemoprevention

The search for ways to prevent breast cancer has been ongoing for many years. Tamoxifen (a triphenylethylene),

Table 14–12 AMERICAN JOINT COMMITTEE ON CANCER STAGING SYSTEMS (PATHOLOGIC)

1988		2003	
Primary tumor (T)		**Primary tumor (T)**[a]	
TX	Primary tumor cannot be assessed	TX	Primary tumor cannot be assessed
T0	No evidence of primary tumor	T0	No evidence of primary tumor
Tis	Carcinoma in situ: intraductal carcinoma, lobular carcinoma in situ, or Paget disease of the nipple with no tumor	Tis	Carcinoma in situ: intraductal carcinoma, lobular carcinoma in situ, or Paget disease of the nipple with no tumor
T1	Tumor 2 cm or less in greatest dimension[b]	T1	Tumor 2 cm or less in greatest dimension[b]
T2	Tumor more than 2 cm but not more than 5 cm in greatest dimension	T2	Tumor more than 2 cm but not more than 5 cm in greatest dimension
T3	Tumor more than 5 cm in greatest dimension	T3	Tumor more than 5 cm in greatest dimension
T4	Tumor of any size with direct extension (a) to the chest wall (b) skin, only as described below	T4	Tumor of any size with direct extension (a) to the chest wall (b) skin, only as described below
T4a	Extension to chest wall	T4a	Extension to chest wall
T4b	Edema (including peau d'orange) or ulceration of the skin of the breast or satellite skin nodules confined to the same breast	T4b	Edema (including peau d'orange) or ulceration of the skin of the breast or satellite skin nodules confined to the same breast
T4c	(a) and (b)	T4c	(a) and (b)
T4d	Inflammatory carcinoma	T4d	Inflammatory carcinoma
Regional lymph nodes (N)		**Regional lymph nodes (N)**	
NX	Regional lymph nodes cannot be assessed	NX	Regional lymph nodes cannot be assessed
N0	No regional lymph node metastasis	N0	No regional lymph node metastasis
N1	Metastasis to movable ipsilateral axillary lymph node(s)	N1	Metastasis in one to three axillary lymph nodes, and/or in internal mammary nodes with microscopic disease detected by sentinel lymph node dissection but not clinically apparent[b]
N1a	Only micrometastasis	N1mi	Micrometastasis (> 0.2 mm, ≤ 2.0 mm)
N1bi	Metastasis in one to three lymph nodes (> 0.2 cm, < 2 cm)		
N1bii	Metastasis in four or more lymph nodes (> 0.2 cm, < 2 cm)		
N1biii	Extension beyond the capsule (involved node > 0.2 cm, < 2 cm)		
N1biv	Metastasis to lymph node > 2cm		
N2	Metastasis to ipsilateral axillary lymph nodes fixed to one another or to other structures	N2	Metastasis in four to nine axillary lymph nodes, or in clinically apparent internal mammary lymph nodes in the absence of axillary lymph node metastasis
N3	Metastasis to ipsilateral internal mammary lymph node(s)	N3	Metastasis in 10 or more axillary lymph nodes, or in infraclavicular lymph nodes, or in clinically apparent ipsilateral internal mammary lymph nodes in the presence of one or more axillary lymph nodes; or in more than three axillary lymph nodes with clinically negative microscopic metastasis in internal mammary lymph nodes; or in ipsilateral supraclavicular lymph nodes

Table continued on following page.

Table 14–12 AMERICAN JOINT COMMITTEE ON CANCER STAGING SYSTEMS (PATHOLOGIC)—CONT'D

1988		2003	
Stage		**Stage**	
0	Tis, N0, M0	0	Tis, N0, M0
I	T1, N0, M0	I	T1, N0, M0
IIa	T0, N1, M0	IIa	T0, N1, M0
	T1, N1, M0		T1, N1, M0
	T2, N0, M0		T2, N0, M0
IIb	T2, N1, M0	IIb	T2, N1, M0
	T3, N0, M0		T3, N0, M0
IIIa	T0, N2, M0	IIIa	T0, N2, M0
	T1, N2, M0		T1, N2, M0
	T2, N2, M0		T2, N2, M0
	T3, N1, M0		T3, N1, M0
	T3, N2, M0		T3, N2, M0
IIIb	T4 any N, any T N3	IIIb	T4, N0, M0
			T4, N1, M0
			T4, N2, M0
		IIIc	Any T, N3
IV	Any T, any N, M1	IV	Any T, any N, M1

[a]Unchanged from 1988.
[b]Groups are further categorized in the America Joint Committee on Cancer staging guidelines.
(From http://www.jco.org and Woodward WA, Strom EA, Tucker SL et al: Changes in the 2003 American Joint Committee on Cancer staging for breast cancer dramatically affect stage-specific survival. J Clin Oncol 21:3244–3248, 2003.)

which is an antiestrogen although it is chemically related to an estrogen, was really the first selective estrogen receptor modulator. There has been more than a quarter of a century's experience with tamoxifen as an adjuvant in patients with breast cancer. The last collaborative study evaluating the efficacy of tamoxifen in patients with breast cancer concluded that tamoxifen appeared to be advantageous in all women irrespective of menopausal and lymph node status as long as the cancer was estrogen receptor–positive. The current recommendation is for 5 years of use. Because data suggested considerable protection in the development of contralateral breast cancer in women receiving tamoxifen vs those not receiving tamoxifen, a large breast cancer prevention trial (P-1) was begun in 1992 (National Surgical Adjuvant Breast Project [NSABP]/NCI). The study planned to accrue 16,000 women who were at high risk for breast cancer to participate in a prospective randomized study between a placebo and 20 mg/day tamoxifen for 5 years. Because of the high-risk status of the participants, it was thought that the accrual goal of only 13,000 women was necessary. High risk was determined by the Gail model, an algorithm for estimating breast cancer risk. This multivariate logistic regression model combines risk factors to estimate the probability of recurrence of breast cancer over time. Variables included in the model are age, number of first-degree relatives with breast cancer, nulliparity or age at first live birth, number of breast biopsies, pathologic diagnosis of atypia or hyperplasia, and age at menarche; the model then predicts the risk for breast cancer in 5 years or life expectancy. Participants eligible for this study were either 60 years of age or older, or between the ages of 35 and 59 years with a 5-year predicted risk of breast cancer of at least 1.66% or who had a history of LCIS.

A total of 368 invasive and non-invasive breast cancers occurred, of which 244 were in the placebo group and 124 in the tamoxifen group. With invasive cancer, there was a 49% reduction in the overall risk (P <0.0001), with a cumulative incidence through 69 months of 43.4 per 1000 women and 22.0 per 1000 women in each of the two groups, respectively. For the non-invasive breast cancer, reduction was 50% (P <0.002). Reduction in non-invasive cancers was related to a decrease in the incidence of both ductal carcinoma in situ (DCIS) and LCIS. Tamoxifen reduced the recurrence of estrogen receptor–positive tumors by 69%, but there was no difference in recurrence of estrogen receptor–negative tumors. There was, however, no survival difference between the two groups, with only nine deaths attributed to breast cancer, six in the placebo group and three in the tamoxifen group. There was a two and a half times greater risk for development of endometrial cancer in the tamoxifen group compared with patients receiving placebo; however, patients were not screened for endometrial cancer before going into the study. The increased risk was mainly related to those patients older than 50 years, as expected. There were 36 invasive cancers in the group receiving tamoxifen, and 15 in the placebo group. When all cancers were evaluated, the total number of cancers was equal (97) in both the placebo and the tamoxifen groups.

There appeared to be no difference in ischemic heart disease or fatal myocardial infarction in the tamoxifen group vs the control group. Vascular events including stroke, venous thrombosis, and pulmonary embolism were greater in the tamoxifen-treated patients compared with those receiving placebo (91 vs 52). There was a reduction in the risk of fracture of the hip, radius, and spine in the tamoxifen group compared with the placebo group, although not statistically significant.

Although the overall results of this study are encouraging, several questions remain. Was the beneficial effect on the breasts due to interference with initiation and promotion of tumors or hindrance of growth of occult tumors? What is the appropriate length of time for treatment with tamoxifen? The study was scheduled for 5 years in duration; however, the analysis was carried out at less than 5 years of median follow-up. What will happen after the 5 years? Will there be a rebound, with a significant number of cancers noted between 5 and 10 years? In the adjuvant studies, after 5 years of therapy, there appeared to be more recurrences in the tamoxifen group compared with the placebo group at the 5- to 10-year time.

Shortly after the NSABP study was published, two breast cancer prevention studies with tamoxifen were reported from Europe (UK and Italy). Their conclusions were different from those of the NSABP study, mainly in that there was no prevention of breast cancer in the tamoxifen group compared with the control group. In the study from the UK, there were 34 carcinomas in the tamoxifen group and 36 in the placebo group. In the Italian group, there were 19 cases of breast cancer in the tamoxifen group and 22 in the placebo group. The two studies from Europe were different from the one in the USA in that the number of patients was smaller. Although family history of breast cancer was similar in the UK and the US studies, this was not the case in the Italian study. There did seem to be a much lower risk of breast cancer in the Italian group in both the placebo and tamoxifen arms compared with in the US and UK studies, and there was a relatively high dropout rate. Breast cancer incidence in the UK study was slightly less than that in the US study as far as the placebo was concerned; however, the incidence in the tamoxifen arm was higher in the UK study compared with in the US study. The role of tamoxifen prevention, at least in the large US study, would suggest benefit. Identification of the appropriate population of patients and optimal duration of therapy may not yet be determined.

More recently, other selective estrogen receptor modulators have become available for evaluation. The Study of Tamoxifen and Raloxifene trial evaluates these drugs in the prevention of invasive breast cancer in postmenopausal women who are at high risk for this disease. This is a randomized, double-blind study of 22,000 postmenopausal women. Each participant is monitored with mammography, physical examinations, and gynecologic examinations on a regular basis for at least 7 years. This phase III trial is one of the largest trials involving breast cancer prevention, and is designed to determine the efficacy of raloxifene and tamoxifen in reducing the incidence of postmenopausal breast cancer.

Treatment

Ductal carcinoma in situ

Ductal carcinoma in situ, also known as intraductal carcinoma, is a proliferation of malignant epithelial cells within the mammary ductal system. The distribution of lesions with respect to location in the breast is similar to that seen with invasive lesions. On light microscopy, there is no evidence of invasion into the surrounding tissue. The increased use of screening mammography during the past two decades has led to a marked increase in the number of patients with a diagnosis of DCIS (Fig. 14–15), and today in many centers, one DCIS is diagnosed for every two or three mammographically detected invasive breast cancers. Today, about 85% of all DCIS is detected solely based on mammography. Age-specific time trends illustrate that the greatest rise has been in women older than 40 years who are more likely to have mammography (Fig. 14–16). In 1980, only 2% of 10,000 cancer cases were DCIS. Between 1973 and 1992, age-adjusted DCIS incidence increased almost sixfold, whereas the incidence of invasive cancer has increased only by one-third. This increase is almost entirely due to mammography screening. As a matter of fact, autopsy series suggest that latent DCIS is relatively common, ranging from 6 to 18% of women who died of causes other than breast cancer.

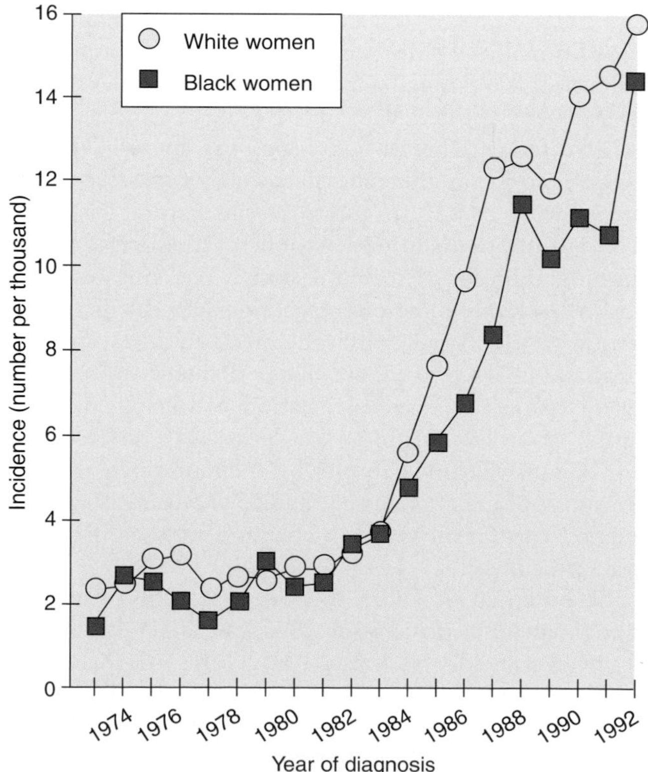

Figure 14–15 Age-adjusted incidence rates for ductal carcinoma in situ of the breast, 1973–92, for white and black women in the USA. (After National Cancer Institute Surveillance, Epidemiology, and End Results tapes.)

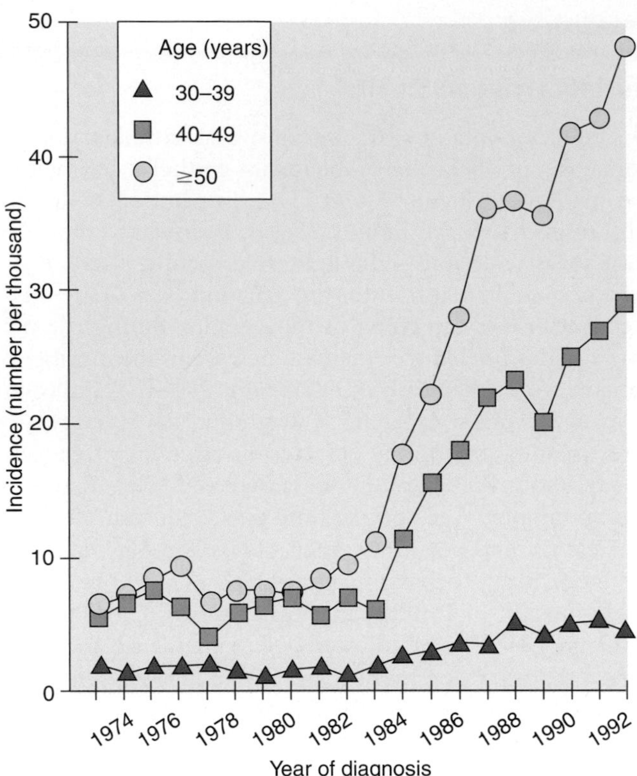

Figure 14–16 Age-specific incidence rates for ductal carcinoma in situ of the breast, 1973–92, for US women, all races combined. (After National Cancer Institute Surveillance, Epidemiology, and End Results tapes.)

Traditionally, DCIS was treated with mastectomy. However, this treatment approach has come under scrutiny because many patients with invasive breast cancer are currently treated with breast-conserving therapy, which makes it difficult to justify the generalized use of mastectomy for patients with DCIS. In addition, the natural history of DCIS is only partially understood, particularly for small mammographically detected lesions. The microcalcifications in DCIS are most often secondary to calcification of necrotic cellular debris within the involved ducts, and their extent and characteristics are better defined with magnification views of the microcalcification. Suspicious mammographic microcalcifications are generally differentiated from benign calcium deposits by their number, distribution, and appearance. Coarse granular or linear calcifications are larger clusters of varying shapes and are regarded as the most suspicious.

The potential of DCIS to progress to invasive breast cancer is an unresolved issue. Because DCIS has historically been treated with mastectomy, little information on the risk of progression to invasive disease is available. Page and coworkers' retrospective study of benign breast biopsy specimens revealed 25 patients who were subsequently identified with DCIS; seven (28%) had progressed to invasive disease during the period of observation.

Most patients with DCIS have non-palpable, mammographically detected lesions, and careful mammographic and pathologic evaluation is necessary to formulate treatment recommendations. Magnification views are obtained to clearly define the full extent of the calcification in patients who are found to have suspicious calcifications. Needle localization guides biopsy of the area. The specimen should be carefully oriented and inked for pathologic evaluation, with particular attention to the nuclear grade, the architectural subtype, the extent of disease, and the distance between DCIS and the resection margins.

Breast-conserving treatment requires removal of all microcalcification and negative microscopic margins of resection; a wide excision may be necessary to achieve this. Not every patient with DCIS who desires breast-conserving treatment will be an appropriate candidate. In general, simple mastectomy is recommended for women in whom the DCIS is too extensive to be adequately removed. Axillary resection is not routinely performed; however, a limited dissection is commonly performed in patients with extensive lesions, particularly if these are high grade. A prospective randomized study of DCIS was conducted by the NSABP (Protocol B-17), in which patients were randomized to lumpectomy alone or lumpectomy followed by breast irradiation (50 Gy). There were 818 women randomized, and surgical margins were histologically tumor-free. Mean follow-up was 90 months (67–180 months). Incidence of non-invasive ipsilateral breast tumor was reduced from 13.4 to 8.2% (P = 0.007), that of invasive from 13.4 to 3.9% (P <0.001). All women benefited from radiation therapy regardless of clinical or mammographic tumor characteristics. No difference in mortality was noted. In a subsequent report, only marked to moderate comedo necrosis was found to be a high risk predictor. Mortality due to breast carcinoma after DCIS for the entire cohort was found to be only 1.6% at 8 years. Dr. Silverstein et al published the Van Nuys experience. The results of this study demonstrated that histologic factors such as large tumor size, narrow margin width, high nuclear grade, and comedo architecture may aid in selecting which patients require the addition of radiation therapy to their treatment regimen with breast preservation.

The NSABP conducted a prospective double-blind randomized study of 1804 women with DCIS, including those with positive tumor margins (Protocol B-24). These women were randomized to lumpectomy and radiation therapy with or without tamoxifen. Median follow-up was 74 months (57–93 months). Women in the tamoxifen group had fewer breast cancer events at 5 years than did those in the placebo group (8.2 vs 13.4%, P = 0.0009). In the placebo group, 130 invasive and non-invasive breast cancer events occurred, compared with 84 in the tamoxifen group. There were 43% fewer invasive breast cancer events and 31% fewer non-invasive events in the tamoxifen group. The benefit in regard to invasive effects was present in the ipsilateral breast (P = 0.03) but not in the contralateral breast (P = 0.22). Some investigators believe that tamoxifen should be considered in all women with DCIS.

Lobular carcinoma in situ

There are important differences between intraductal carcinoma and LCIS (Table 14–13). Intraductal carcinoma has a rate of local recurrence similar to that of invasive carcinoma with breast-preserving surgery. These recurrences appear in the vicinity of the original surgery and probably represent malignant foci that persisted after the initial treatment, rather than a second primary. Approximately 50% of the recurrences will be frankly invasive ductal carcinoma; the other half will again be intraductal.

Lobular carcinoma in situ does not uniformly recur at the original excision site, and the recurrences are as likely to appear in the opposite breast as in the ipsilateral breast. The rate of recurrence of LCIS after excision alone is approximately equal to that of atypical ductal hyperplasia with a positive family history of breast cancer. Cancers that develop after excision of LCIS may be intraductal carcinoma, invasive ductal carcinoma, or lobular carcinoma. Indeed, some authorities consider LCIS a risk factor only for subsequent development of a true malignant neoplasm and not a true cancer.

In the B-17 study, women with a history of DCIS treated with lumpectomy were at greater risk for invasive breast cancer than were women in the P-1 study who had a history of LCIS or atypical hyperplasia. The annual rate of an invasive breast cancer event during the first 5 years after a diagnosis of DCIS was more than twice that after a diagnosis of LCIS, and almost three times that after a diagnosis of atypical hyperplasia. There was also a higher invasive cancer occurrence in DCIS in women who received radiation therapy than in those with LCIS or atypical hyperplasia. In the B-24 study, tamoxifen also lowered rates of invasive tumors in women with a history of LCIS and atypical hyperplasia, which are frequently estrogen receptor–positive.

Invasive disease

In recent years, a change in attitude concerning the extent of surgery for primary operable tumors has evolved. Radical mastectomy had been the standard procedure since Halsted published his first series in 1894. There was universal acceptance of his concept of wide en bloc resection of the primary tumor together with the lymphatic pathway of spread to the axillary lymph nodes. This mode of treatment was dominant for about 50 years despite undesirable cure rates. Thereafter, dissatisfaction with the standard radical mastectomy began to gain momentum, and the trend toward less radical procedures has been widespread in the past two decades.

In 1992, the American Colleges of Surgeons, Radiologists, and Pathologists, along with the ACS and the Society of Surgical Oncology, began the process of describing standard practice for breast conservation treatment. Many retrospective as well as prospective randomized trials suggested equally effective results in appropriately selected patients with early-stage breast cancer, whether they were treated with mastectomy or breast conservation surgery. The results of these deliberations were published in 1998. There have been six modern prospective randomized trials comparing mastectomy with conservative surgery plus irradiation for stage I and stage II breast cancer. Whole-breast irradiation (45–50 Gy) was used in all trials, with a boost to the primary site given in five of the six trials. Histologically negative surgical margins were required in those undergoing conservative surgery and irradiation. At a follow-up of up to 18 years, none of the trials showed significant differences in overall or disease-free survival between the two treatments (Table 14–14). In the Milan I and the NSABP B-06 study, survival was not improved in patients with positive nodes treated with mastectomy and chemotherapy. In five of the six trials, there was no significant difference in recurrence in the treated breast or chest wall after mastectomy. In the NCI study, there was a significantly higher local recurrence rate in the breast conservation group, but only gross tumor removal was required for study entry.

In a meta-analysis of nine prospective randomized trials comparing conservative surgery and irradiation with mastectomy, no survival differences were found in seven of the trials. Local recurrence was reported in 6.2% of patients treated with mastectomy and in 5.9% of those treated with breast conservation surgery. No difference was seen in the incidence of contralateral breast cancer or a second malignant neoplasm that was not breast cancer. The incidence of

Table 14–13 COMPARISON OF DUCTAL CARCINOMA IN SITU AND LOBULAR CARCINOMA IN SITU

Characteristic	Ductal carcinoma in situ	Lobular carcinoma in situ
Age	Premenopausal and postmenopausal	Predominantly premenopausal
Mammographic appearance	Microcalcification	Usually invisible
Diagnosis	Needle localization biopsy or excision of palpable lesion	Incidental finding on biopsy of benign disease
Multicentric	Infrequent	Common
Bilateral	Rare	Common
Site of recurrence	Near original site	Anywhere in either breast
Histology of recurrence	50% invasive, 50% ductal carcinoma in situ	Usually invasive ductal carcinoma
Rate of recurrence (% per year)	5	1

Table 14–14 PROSPECTIVE RANDOMIZED TRIALS COMPARING CONSERVATIVE SURGERY AND RADIATION WITH MASTECTOMY FOR EARLY-STAGE BREAST DISEASE

			Overall survival (%)	
	n	Years	Conservative surgery and radiation	Mastectomy
Milan Cancer Institute	701	18	65	65
Institut Gustave-Roussy	179	15	73	65
National Surgical Adjuvant Breast Project B-06 Project B-06	1219	12	63	59
National Cancer Institute	237	10	77	75
European Organization for Research and Treatment of Cancer	874	8	54	61
Danish Breast Cancer	904	6	79	82

(After Winchester DP, Cox JD: Standards for diagnosis and management of invasive breast carcinoma. American College of Radiology. American College of Surgeons. College of American Pathologists. Society of Surgical Oncology. CA Cancer J Clin 48:83–107, 1998.)

Table 14–15 BREAST RECURRENCE AND SURVIVAL IN TRIALS COMPARING CONSERVATIVE SURGERY ALONE WITH CONSERVATIVE SURGERY AND RADIATION

	Breast recurrence (%)		Overall survival (%)	
	Conservative surgery	Conservative surgery and radiation therapy	Conservative surgery	Conservative surgery and radiation therapy
Uppsala–Orebro	18	2	90	91
Milan	18	2	92	92
National Surgical Adjuvant Breast Project B-06	35	10	58	62
Ontario Group	40	18	72	74
Scottish Cancer	28	6	85	88
British Trial	35	13	n/a	n/a

n/a, data not available.
(After Winchester DP, Cox JD: Standards for diagnosis and management of invasive breast carcinoma. American College of Radiology. American College of Surgeons. College of American Pathologists. Society of Surgical Oncology. CA Cancer J Clin 48:83–107, 1998.)

recurrence in the treated breast ranged from 3 to 19%. Most failures in the treated breast can be salvaged with mastectomy, which can result in a 70% survival at 5 years. Mastectomy did not prevent local recurrences, which developed in 4–14% after this treatment.

There have been six randomized trials comparing conservative surgery alone with conservative surgery and irradiation. Therapy selection, extent of surgery and irradiation, and use of adjuvant systemic therapy did vary among the different trials. Despite the difference, rate of recurrence in the breast of the irradiated group noted a crude rate of reduction of 84% (range 73–97%) (Table 14–15). Subset analysis failed to consistently identify patients who would not benefit from irradiation.

For optimal breast conservation surgery to be effective, careful selection of patients and a multidisciplinary approach are necessary. Therapy selection is important and can be based on history or physical examination findings, mammographic evaluation, histologic assessment of breast resected material, and needs and expectations of the patient. Age, neither young nor old, is a contraindication to breast conservation. Skin, nipple, or breast retraction may not be a sign of locally advanced breast cancer and is not necessarily a contraindication to breast conservation.

Recent preoperative mammographic evaluation is mandatory to determine eligibility for breast conservation surgery. High-quality, certified, dedicated mammographic equipment should be used. Mammography defines the extent of disease and whether the lesion may be multicentric. Bilateral mammography should be done. An increasing number of breast conservation procedures are performed for non-palpable masses and microcalcifications. The dimensions (at least two) of the lesion should be noted. Skin of the breast over the lesion should be evaluated for possible thickness, which might suggest tumor involvement. If microcalcifications are present, determination of the extent within or outside the mass should be made. The location and distribution of microcalcifications should be described if they are the only marker of the tumor. Specialized or magnification views may be helpful.

Multiple pathologic features have been evaluated as risk factors for recurrence. Vascular or lymphatic invasion, tumor necrosis, and inflammatory infiltration have been associated with some increased risk of recurrence (10–15% at 5 years). Patients with positive nodes do not have an increased risk of breast recurrence when they are treated with conservative surgery and irradiation; however, in these patients undergoing mastectomy, the number of positive nodes correlates with chest wall recurrence. The lower recurrence rate with conservative surgery and irradiation may be due to the combined effect of chemotherapy and tamoxifen. An extensive intraductal component may be associated with a high risk of recurrence. The increased risk may be related to the presence of significant residual tumor burden after gross excision. Negative surgical margins decrease the risk of recurrence in these patients. An extensive intraductal component therefore appears to be an indicator that disease is more extensive than was clinically suggested.

Patients with positive resected margins should undergo re-excision. If resected margins remain positive on re-excision, mastectomy is the preferred treatment. Gage et al noted the 5-year actuarial breast cancer recurrence rate to be 3% for negative margins, 9% for focally positive margins, and 28% for diffusely positive margins. Recent data suggest that systemic therapy may decrease the 5-year breast cancer recurrence rate in patients with positive margins. Status of surgical margins is probably the most important aspect of pathologic evaluation of breast tumor excision specimens in patients being considered for conservative surgery.

Lobular carcinoma in situ appears to be an incidental finding (in contrast to DCIS), and is considered a marker of increased risk for subsequent breast cancer and not an indication requiring surgical re-excision because of positive margins. The increased risk applies to both breasts and appears to be lifelong.

There do appear to be absolute as well as relative contraindications to conservative surgery and radiation therapy. Pregnancy is considered an absolute contraindication to radiation therapy. Radiation therapy postpartum may be an alternative, depending on duration of pregnancy at the time of diagnosis. Women with two or more primary tumors in separate quadrants or with diffuse malignant-appearing microcalcifications are not considered candidates. The persistence of positive margins after repeated excision and previous therapeutic radiation to the breast appears to be an absolute contraindication to conservative surgery. A relative contraindication may be history of collagen-vascular disease (scleroderma or active lupus), because these patients tolerate radiation poorly. Rheumatoid arthritis does not appear to be a contraindication. Tumor size per se is not an absolute contraindication, although a large tumor in a small breast in which adequate resection may result in cosmetic disfiguration may be a relative contraindication. A family history of breast cancer does not affect survival.

The trend toward less radical surgery really began when the concept of removing the breast and axillary contents and leaving the chest wall muscles intact was first introduced. It was demonstrated that simple mastectomy followed by radiation therapy resulted in salvage rates equal to those of radical mastectomy. The trend was completed with reports advocating local excision and irradiation. The present dilemma stems from the fact that absolute data on survival in randomized controlled series are almost impossible to obtain. Many operative control studies are now in progress, but increasing restrictions of an ethical and legal nature are making it difficult to gather significant data. In most studies, survival figures are compared with those of studies based on the Halsted radical mastectomy. It is significant that all lesser procedures reveal similar end results but none surpasses those obtained with radical surgery. Accordingly, many proponents of Halsted's radical mastectomy will continue to use that operation until offered an alternative that will yield better 10-year salvage rates.

Several trials demonstrated favorable results with conservative treatment of breast cancer, but not all patients are candidates for this technique of minimal surgery and postoperative radiation therapy. Hellman described 255 patients with stage I and stage II disease who were treated in this way. The tumor was controlled locally for 97% of women with stage I disease and for 87% of women with stage II disease. The survival rate was 93% for stage I and 84% for stage II. Patients were treated with excisional biopsy to remove the tumors, followed by irradiation to the entire breast of 4500–5000 cGy in 23 treatments for 5 weeks and a booster dose to the primary tumor area of an additional 2000–2200 cGy using interstitial Ir-192. Lumpectomy (tylectomy) should be reserved for tumors <2 cm, and postoperative irradiation can be expected to achieve an 80–85% local control rate with comparable survivals.

Montague described 1073 patients with clinically favorable breast cancer who were treated at the University of Texas M.D. Anderson Hospital between 1955 and 1980. Of this group, 355 were treated with conservative surgery and radiation therapy, and 728 were treated with radical or modified radical mastectomy alone. The local regional recurrence in patients treated with conservative surgery was 4.9%; the local regional recurrence in patients who had radical or modified radical mastectomy was 5.6%. In essence, there was no significant difference in the 10-year disease-free survival rates between the two groups. Although this was a non-randomized study, there is remarkable agreement with results found in other studies.

Lichter and colleagues reported a randomized trial in 1992 from the NCI in which mastectomy was compared with breast-conserving therapy in the treatment of stage I and stage II carcinomas of the breast; 237 women were randomized between mastectomy and excisional biopsy plus irradiation. All women in both groups underwent full axillary lymph node dissection; node-positive patients in both groups received adjuvant chemotherapy with cyclophosphamide and doxorubicin every 28 days for 1 year and tamoxifen 40 mg/day for 5 years. Overall survival and disease-free survival were not significantly different in the two treatment arms. They also summarized six solid prospective randomized trials with more than 3800 patients comparing mastectomy with lumpectomy plus irradiation in the treatment of stage I and stage II breast cancer. All these studies have come to the same conclusion. It appears that the clinician can now be confident in recommending lumpectomy plus irradiation to patients, because it seems to be equivalent to mastectomy in terms of survival and optimal local-regional control.

In May 2002, the FDA approved the MammoSite Radiation Therapy Systems as a means of administering brachytherapy internally in prescribed doses over a 5-day period. During the lumpectomy, a deflated balloon is placed inside the surgical cavity. A tube connects the balloon to the outside of the breast and may be inflated with saline to fill the cavity. Radiation is delivered within the inflated balloon over 1–5 days, and the balloon is deflated then removed. The traditional length of time for radiation therapy is shortened from the traditional 6-week period to 5 days. This technology is in its infancy, and the patient inclusion criteria remain under investigation.

Surgery

Probably no area of medical therapy queries the appropriateness of the en bloc dissection for cancer more than that of surgery for breast cancer. Since the introduction of the en bloc concept by Halsted in 1894 that advocated routine removal of the pectoralis major muscle to ensure a more adequate excision of the large tumors he treated, there have been a series of modifications. The modified radical mastectomy has been popular: the entire breast, but not the pectoralis major muscle, is removed, thus avoiding the concave configuration of the anterior chest wall. Even the axillary dissection varies from complete (levels I, II, and III, with the pectoralis minor muscle) to partial (levels I and II, with sparing of the pectoralis minor muscle). Retrospective studies found that survivals were similar regardless of the extent of the operative procedure when the Halsted radical mastectomy is compared with any of the modified approaches, thus a modified approach was accepted in 1979 by the NCI Consensus Conference.

Prophylactic removal of regional axillary lymph nodes was next questioned. With the observation that clinical examination alone was not sufficiently accurate to detect small metastases, axillary node dissection quickly became routine, not only to rid the patient of clinically occult nodal metastasis but, by removal of nodes, to eliminate a secondary source of further metastases. Handley was among the first to observe that recurrence in axillary nodes after simple mastectomy was less frequent than one would expect in light of the frequency of occult metastases at this site, and suggested that some metastases were destroyed in the nodes by host defenses.

In 1971, the NSABP began a trial designed to answer the question of the value of prophylactic regional node dissection. Patients with clinically uninvolved axillary nodes (clinical stage I) were randomized for treatment among radical mastectomy, total mastectomy plus irradiation of the chest wall and regional lymphatics, and total mastectomy alone. Women who had clinically involved axillary nodes (clinical stage II) were randomized to treatment with either radical mastectomy or total mastectomy and irradiation to the chest wall and all lymph node drainage areas for the breast. If ignoring occult axillary metastases permitted continuing dissemination, the patients treated with total mastectomy alone should fare poorly; if having still-functioning nodes improves host defenses, the patients treated with total mastectomy alone should fare better than the others.

A total of 1665 patients were entered and observed for 72 months, with no difference found among the three treatment arms in stage I. Overall, patients assigned stage II survived less well, but again there was no difference between the two treatment alternatives. Only 60 (16%) of the 365 patients who did not undergo prophylactic axillary dissection developed progression in the axilla as a first sign of failure and underwent axillary dissections, predominantly in the first 30 months of follow-up but also as long as 112 months after surgery. In the group in which prophylactic axillary dissection was done, the incidence of positive nodes was 39%. More than half of the patients who should have had positive axillary nodes did not develop clinical evidence of such.

In 1985, Fisher and coworkers reported on this same group of 1665 women observed for a mean of 126 months. There were no significant differences between the two groups of patients who had clinically positive nodes treated by radical mastectomy or by total mastectomy without axillary dissection but with regional irradiation. Survival at 10 years was about 38% in both groups.

The use of the sentinel node as a means of evaluating lymph node status is quickly becoming the standard of care. Either a dye or a radioactive material is injected to identify the first (sentinel) node, and if it is negative, a full axillary node dissection can be avoided.

After the report by Moore in 1967 relating the frequency of local recurrence that followed partial mastectomy, removal of the entire breast became routine surgical practice. The problem of incomplete excision is compounded by multifocal origin; almost 50% of breast cancers have origin in more than one quadrant of the breast, and that frequency does not appear to be diminished by early detection. Later studies of less than total mastectomy have sought to determine whether irradiation of the breast can control these residua if just the primary lesion is removed. Obviously, this approach would not improve survival or preserve the function of the breast, but it may improve the cosmetic result and the patient's body image. A trial of breast preservation was conducted by the Cancer Institute of Milan in which women with tumors <2 cm in diameter and without palpable axillary nodes were randomized between radical mastectomy and a wide "quadrantectomy" of the breast with a complete axillary dissection followed by 5000 cGy of irradiation to the breast alone (an additional 1000 cGy to the tumor site). After 7 years, 701 patients could be analyzed, and there were no significant differences in local control, survival, or interval to recurrence. This study demonstrated that high-dose irradiation makes breast preservation possible for patients with small, clinically localized breast cancers. Cosmetic results were said to be satisfactory to more than 70% of the patients. Some radiation fibrosis and arm edema were reported, and the long-term carcinogenic effects on the breast from the radiation are yet to be determined.

Another study by Fisher et al and the NSABP reports the results of a randomized trial comparing total mastectomy and segmental mastectomy with or without irradiation in the treatment of breast cancer (stage I and stage II breast tumors no larger than 4 cm). In segmental resection, the surgeon removed tissue sufficient only to ensure that margins of the resected specimens were free of tumor. Women were randomly assigned to total mastectomy, segmental mastectomy alone, or segmental mastectomy followed by breast irradiation. All patients had axillary dissections, and patients with positive nodes received chemotherapy. Life table estimates based on data from 1843 women indicated that treatment by segmental mastectomy, with or without breast irradiation, resulted in disease-free, distant disease-free, and overall survivals at 5 years that were no worse than those after total breast removal. In fact, disease-free survival after segmental mastectomy plus irradiation was better than disease-free survival after total mastectomy and overall survival after total mastectomy. However, a total of 92% of women treated with radiation remained free of breast tumor at 5 years, compared with 72% of those receiving no irradiation, indicating the value of breast irradiation for reducing the incidence of tumor in the ipsilateral breast after segmental mastectomy.

The Halsted concept of tumor spread is that breast cancer starts as a local disease and spreads in an orderly, chronologic fashion from the original site to the regional lymph nodes, which serve as temporary barriers to spread, and then to distant sites such as the lung, liver, and bones. The cancer was believed to be always surgically curable if the breast, pectoral muscles, and axillary lymph nodes could be removed before the tumor had metastasized beyond that region. The findings of the NSABP and others suggest that the spread of cancer is not nearly as orderly as Halsted proposed. Cancer may metastasize to a distant site before, during, or after it spreads to the lymph nodes. The rationale for Halsted's radical surgical procedure becomes untenable if the cancer cannot be stopped at some distinct point on a supposedly orderly pathway. Breast cancer is often a systemic disease, even in its early stages.

Trials of management of primary breast cancer are long-term studies that may need at least 10 years before definitive analysis can be made. Although an early relapse rate may be helpful in an analysis, only data on long-term survival will give the final answer. Analysis of these trials must also include consideration of the heterogeneity of primary breast cancer. Subset analysis requires adequate numbers, with the various categories occurring as a result of important prognostic variables, such as size of the primary tumor, clinical and pathologic status of the axillary lymph nodes, menopausal status, and estrogen receptor content. A detailed discussion of the advantages and disadvantages of the alternatives for primary therapy in patients with potentially curable breast cancer is beyond the scope of this text. The reader is referred to the bibliography for more detailed information concerning this interesting current controversy.

Adjuvant therapy

Estrogen receptors are proteins found in hormonally dependent tissue, both malignant and non-malignant. The amount of receptor present in the breast cancer specimen is predictive of the success or failure of endocrine therapy. The identification of the estrogen receptor protein in certain human mammary cancers, and the subsequent explanation of the role of estrogen in tumor growth, clarified a clinical relationship that had been observed for a century. In 1896, Beatson produced regression of mammary cancer by oophorectomy. Huggins and Bergenstal demonstrated in 1952 that some mammary and prostatic cancers were not autonomous but were under the partial control of the endocrine system. Regressions of mammary cancers were continually obtained by removing the source of endogenous circulating hormones by oophorectomy, adrenalectomy, and hypophysectomy. Alternatively, breast cancer regressions were also achieved by administering large doses of estrogen, androgen, progesterone, and glucocorticoids.

The choice of a particular endocrine therapy has been in large part empiric, guided by certain clinical features such as menopausal status, disease-free interval, site of the dominant lesion, and response to previous therapy. As a result of basic investigations by Jensen, Smith, and DeSombre of steroid hormone metabolism, there has been development of a series of assays that can identify with considerable accuracy breast cancers that are not autonomous and that will respond to endocrine manipulation. Such a method of predicting a priori those cancers that will be responsive to changes in the endocrine milieu greatly enhances the usefulness of hormone therapy and allows recommendation of such treatments on a plausible biochemical basis.

Knowledge of the estrogen receptor content of either the primary or the recurrent mammary cancer must be viewed within the proper clinical perspective. This one determination is but a single piece in the mosaic of the subcellular biochemistry of breast cancer. To deprecate the clinical importance of this determination because some patients with significant estrogen receptor content will not respond to hormone treatment (because of eventual escape from hormone regulation or because of lack of understanding of the role of other steroid or protein hormone receptors) begs the question. Knowledge of the estrogen receptor content of either a primary or a metastatic tumor does not allow the physician to predict the hormone dependency of a tumor with enough accuracy for it to be rationally employed in the selection of appropriate palliative treatment. It does, however, allow a good assessment of the likelihood that the patient with breast cancer would benefit from endocrine therapy.

The National Comprehensive Cancer Network (NCCN) first published its comprehensive statement about the adjuvant therapy of early breast cancer in November of 2000. Since that time, refinements have occurred. The most significant change in the 2005 guidelines relating to the adjuvant therapy of breast cancer was the inclusion of HER-2 as a parameter for treatment selection, and recommendations about trastuzumab as adjuvant therapy (Table 14-19). The use of trastuzumab was suggested for patients with HER-2 3+ expression, or fluorescent in situ hybridization amplification of 2.1-fold or greater, who had tumors greater than 1 cm in size.

Ovarian ablation

Ovarian suppression is one of the oldest methods for treating premenopausal metastatic breast cancer. This can be accomplished surgically, by use of luteinizing hormone–releasing hormone analogs, or radiation. In 1996, the Collaborative Group published an overview of randomized trials concerning ovarian ablation in early breast cancer. There were 12 of 17 studies available for evaluation, all of which were begun before 1980. There were 2102 randomized women younger than 50 years and 1354 women aged 50 years and older. In women younger than 50 years, there were six fewer recurrences or deaths per 100 women allocated to ovarian ablation (45% vs 39% alive without recurrence) 15 years after randomization. Historically, ovarian ablation was used to treat premenopausal patients with metastatic or recurrent breast cancer. In this review, the benefit of ablation was most noticeable in patients with positive nodes. In patients with negative nodes, the overall survival at 10 years was not statistically significant between the two groups. There were only 473 women in the node-negative group. This group speaks to the possible role of prophylactic ovarian ablation.

The overview meta-analyses of 1995 showed a 25% reduction in relapse and 24% reduction in mortality over the control group. A prospective randomized European study by Soreide et al showed equal efficacy when ovarian ablation was compared to tamoxifen in the 320 premenopausal node-positive patients.

Tamoxifen

Many prospective double-blind randomized studies have been performed to evaluate the role of adjuvant tamoxifen among women with early breast cancer. In 1998, the Collaborative Group published an update on 55 such trials of 37,000 women. In the 18,000 women with estrogen receptor–positive tumors, the reduction in the recurrence rate at 1, 2, and 5 years of tamoxifen use was 21%, 28%, and 50%, respectively. These figures are all highly significant. Those women with estrogen receptor–positive tumors with at least 100 fmol receptor per milligram of cytosol protein had a greater reduction in recurrence than did those with positive receptors but less than 100 fmol (60% vs 43% after 5 years of tamoxifen). The reduction in mortality was also greater in those with a higher receptor level (36% vs 23%). Those patients with estrogen receptor–positive, progesterone receptor–negative tumors had results (reduction of recurrences and mortality) similar to those of patients with estrogen receptor–positive tumors (progesterone receptor status unknown). Among the 800 women with estrogen receptor–poor tumors, the reduction in recurrence was only 10%, irrespective of length of time of tamoxifen treatment. Although this reduction is statistically significant, the apparent benefit is small and the lower confidence limit is close to zero. Irrespective of the duration of tamoxifen use, the mortality reduction was only 6%. In the 2000 women with estrogen receptor–poor, progesterone receptor–poor tumors, tamoxifen had no apparent effect on recurrence or mortality rates (about 1%), but in the 602 women with estrogen receptor–poor, progesterone receptor–positive tumors, recurrence reduction was 23% and mortality reduction was 9%. There were 12,000 women with unknown estrogen receptor status. It can be estimated that about two-thirds of these women would have estrogen receptor–positive tumors if measured. The data suggest highly significant benefits among women with unknown estrogen receptor status.

In trials of 5 years of tamoxifen use, the absolute improvement in the 10-year recurrence risk was greatest for women with node-positive disease compared with those with node-negative status. The absolute improvement was 5.6% in node-negative disease compared with 10.5% in node-positive disease. In trials of 5 years, adjuvant tamoxifen reduced recurrence, and mortality appeared equally large in the absence or presence of chemotherapy.

Although the benefit of tamoxifen appears greater in the postmenopausal women, there was a 45% reduction in those younger than 50 years. This was true for those younger than 40 years (54% reduction) and in those aged 40–49 years (41%). Tamoxifen also reduced the incidence of contralateral breast cancer (47%) in those who took tamoxifen for 5 years. Risk reduction was independent of age.

The studies also evaluated possible adverse effects. There was only a slight non-significant excess of colorectal cancers in those allocated to tamoxifen. There was a significant increase in endometrial cancer (relative risk 21.58), and the relative risk was 4.2 with 5 years of use. This was based on only 32 endometrial cases among the control group. The normal incidence of endometrial cancer in the USA is 1 per 1000. The absolute excess of deaths from endometrial cancer during the decade after randomization was about 1–2 per 1000 (annual excess of about 0.2 per 1000). There was no difference in the tamoxifen group vs the control group for the aggregate of all cardiac or vascular deaths or non-breast cancer, non-endometrial cancer deaths. There was about one extra death per 5000 women years of tamoxifen attributed to pulmonary embolus.

It appears that up to 5 years of tamoxifen use reduces recurrence and mortality in women with estrogen receptor–positive tumors, irrespective of age and menopausal status and whether the lymph nodes are positive or negative, even if cytotoxic chemotherapy has been given. There is no clear evidence of benefit in women with estrogen receptor–poor tumors.

Aromatase inhibitors

Aromatase inhibitors suppress estrogen levels by inactivating aromatase, the enzyme responsible for synthesizing estrogens from androgens. In contrast to tamoxifen, these compounds lack partial agonist activity. The Anastrozole, Tamoxifen Alone or in Combination Trial compared 5 years of tamoxifen vs anastrozole vs the combination. Anastrozole was found to have a significantly better survival, prolonged time to recurrence, reduced distant metastases, and a lower incidence of contralateral breast cancer compared with tamoxifen. Letrozole, another aromatase inhibitor, was compared to tamoxifen in the multicenter Breast International Group trial of 8028 postmenopausal women with metastatic breast cancer. Letrozole reduced significantly the risk of recurrent disease when compared with tamoxifen, especially at distant sites in these postmenopausal women. Another international study of 5187 women administered letrozole after completing 5 years of tamoxifen. The results from the data indicated a nearly 50% lower recurrence rate. Therefore letrozole is now an accepted treatment choice for those postmenopausal women with hormone receptor–positive breast cancers who have utilized tamoxifen for a 5-year period. The American Society of Clinical Oncology now recommends aromatase inhibitors be used to lower the risk of recurrence in receptor-positive postmenopausal breast cancers as initial therapy or after treatment with tamoxifen. The duration of therapy has not yet been established.

There have been several studies of chemohormone therapy in patients with breast cancer. Many of these studies have included both node-negative and node-positive patients. The Eastern Cooperative Ontology Group conducted a phase III study of premenopausal women with node-positive, receptor-positive breast cancer. There were 1504 eligible patients randomized to cyclophosphamide, doxorubicin, and 5-fluorouracil (CAF); CAF plus goserelin, a luteinizing hormone–releasing hormone agonist, for 5 years; and CAF plus goserelin plus tamoxifen for 5 years. The addition of tamoxifen improved the 5-year recurrence-free interval, but the addition of goserelin did not over CAF alone. The 5-year survival was similar among the three groups (85% and 86%).

Chemotherapy (Tables 14–16 and 14–17)

The 2003 St. Gallen Consensus Panel divided the many available adjuvant chemotherapy regimens into standard efficacy and those with superior efficacy. Drugs categorized as standard efficacy included doxorubicin (Adriamycin) and cyclophosphamide (AC × 4) and cyclophosphamide, methotrexate, and 5-fluorouracil (CMF × 6). Drugs classified as superior efficacy included FA(E)C × 6, CA(E)F × 6, AE-CMF, TAC × 6, AC × 4–paclitaxel (P) × 4 or docetaxel (D) × 4, FEC × 3–D × 3.

Table 14–16 USEFUL SINGLE AGENTS IN THE TREATMENT OF BREAST CANCER

Drug	Dosage	Response rate (%)
Doxorubicin	60–75 mg/m^2 i.v. every 3 weeks	37
Cyclophosphamide	100 mg/m^2 per day p.o. 500 mg/m^2 per week i.v.	34
L-Phenylalanine mustard	6 mg/m^2 per day p.o. for 5 days every 4–6 weeks	23
5-Fluorouracil	600 mg/m^2 per week i.v.	26
Methotrexate	20 mg/m^2 i.v. or i.m. 2 times a week	34
Vincristine	1 mg/m^2 per week i.v.	21
Dibromodulcitol	180 mg/m^2 per day p.o. for 10 days every 4 weeks	27
Mitomycin C	20 mg/m^2 i.v. every 4–6 weeks	38
Paclitaxel	135–250 mg/m^2 every 3 weeks	28

Node-negative breast cancer

Clinical Practice Guidelines for the Care and Treatment of Breast Cancer (a Canadian consensus document) was published in 1998. Extensive review of the literature with a level of evidence assigned to the studies was undertaken. Although this consensus covered the entire subject of breast cancer, remarks from that report are limited to the discussion of chemotherapy.

The steering committee thought that before adjuvant systemic therapy is considered, prognosis without therapy should first be estimated. On the basis of tumor size, histologic or nuclear grade, estrogen receptor status, and lymphatic and vascular invasion, a patient's risk for recurrence could be judged to be low, intermediate, or high (Table 14–18). Premenopausal and postmenopausal patients who are at low risk for recurrence can be advised not to have adjuvant systemic therapy. In women at intermediate risk with estrogen receptor–positive tumors, tamoxifen should be the first choice of treatment. Tamoxifen should be administered daily for 5 years. Those women who are at high risk should be advised to have systemic therapy. Chemotherapy should be recommended for all women

Table 14–17 USEFUL DRUG COMBINATIONS IN THE TREATMENT OF BREAST CANCER

Abbreviation	Regimen	Dosage	Response rate (%)
CMFVP	Cyclophosphamide	80 mg/m^2 per day p.o.	62
	Methotrexate	20 mg/m^2 per week i.v.	
	5-Fluorouracil	500 mg/m^2 per week i.v.	
	Vincristine	1 mg/m^2 per week i.v.	
	Prednisone	30 mg/m^2 per day p.o. for 15 days, *then taper*	
CMF	Cyclophosphamide	100 mg/m^2 p.o. days 1 through 4	53
	Methotrexate	60 mg/m^2 i.v. days 1 and 8	
	5-Fluorouracil	600 mg/m^2 i.v. days 1 and 8	
		Repeat cycles every 4 weeks	
CMF(P)	Cyclophosphamide	100 mg/m^2 p.o. days 1 through 14	63
	Methotrexate	60 mg/m^2 i.v. days 1 and 8	
	5-Fluorouracil	600 mg/m^2 i.v. days 1 and 8	
	Prednisone	40 mg/m^2 p.o. days 1 through 14	
		Repeat cycles every 4 weeks	
CA	Cyclophosphamide	200 mg/m^2 p.o. days 3 through 6	74
	Doxorubicin	40 mg/m^2 i.v. day 1	
		Repeat cycles every 3–4 weeks	
CAF	Cyclophosphamide	100 mg/m^2 p.o. days 1 through 14	82
	Doxorubicin	30 mg/m^2 i.v. days 1 and 8	
	5-Fluorouracil	500 mg/m^2 i.v. days 1 and 8	
		Repeat cycles every 4 weeks	
DAV	Dibromodulcitol	150 mg/m^2 p.o. days 1 through 10	71
	Doxorubicin	45 mg/m^2 i.v. day 1	
	Vincristine	1.2 mg/m^2 i.v. day 1	
		Repeat cycles every 4 weeks	

Table 14–18 RISK FACTORS FOR RECURRENCE IN PATIENTS WITH NODE-NEGATIVE BREAST CANCER

Tumor size 2 cm < or >
Histologic and nuclear grade
  Grade 1: good prognosis
  Grade 2: data not conclusive as to risk
  Grade 3: poor prognosis
Hormone receptor status
  ER-positive: better survival
  Note: the use of ER and PR status is recommended
Lymphatic and vascular invasion increases recurrence
Those patients with small tumor size, low nuclear grade, and ER positivity have favorable prognostic factors

ER, estrogen receptor; PR, progesterone receptor.

with estrogen receptor–negative tumors. The two recommended regimens are:

1. six cycles of CMF, and
2. four cycles of AC (Table 14–19).

Studies comparing the two regimens have noted similar progression-free as well as overall survival. Many investigators consider AC the preferred treatment, because it requires less time for administration, fewer clinic visits are needed, and it produces similar levels of toxicity. For many women older than 70 years and at high risk, tamoxifen alone is recommended.

Node-positive breast cancer

The Canadian consensus states that chemotherapy should be offered to all premenopausal women with stage II breast cancer. Polychemotherapy is preferred to prolonged single-agent therapy. A 6-month course of CMF or a 3-month course of AC was suggested. CMF of 6 months' duration was just as effective as four courses of AC (NSABP Protocol B-15). Other studies have shown 6 months of CMF to be as effective as 12–24 months of CMF. Full standard doses should be used if possible. In the Milan study of 20 years of follow-up, only those who received 85% of the planned CMF dose benefited from adjuvant chemotherapy. Postmenopausal women with stage II, estrogen receptor–positive tumors should be offered tamoxifen.

The NCCN guidelines for chemotherapy are described in detail in the 2006 NCCN web site (http://www.NCCN.org). Paclitaxel (Taxol) has been found to be effective in the treatment of breast cancer. Paclitaxel and docetaxel (Taxotere) are now being integrated into the standard protocols for the treatment of breast cancer patients. Paclitaxel has been demonstrated to have significant antitumor activity in patients who are doxorubicin-resistant.

Table 14–19 2005 NATIONAL COMPREHENSIVE CANCER NETWORK GUIDELINES RELATING TO ADJUVANT THERAPY OF BREAST CANCER

Recommendations for ductal, not otherwise specified, lobular, mixed, medullary, and metaplastic histologies					
		ER- or PR-positive, HER-2–positive	ER- or PR-positive, HER-2–negative	ER- or PR-negative, HER-2–positive	ER- or PR-negative, HER-2–negative
NN or N1ni	T1a	No adjuvant therapy (if NN) ± E (if N1mi)			
	T1b[a]	No adjuvant therapy (if NN) ± E (if N1mi)		± C	± C
	T1b[b]	E ± C	E ± C	± C	± C
	T1c	E + C + Tr	E + C	C + Tr	C
	T2	E + C + Tr	E + C	C + Tr	C
NP	T	E + C + Tr	E + C	C + Tr	C

Recommendations for tubular and mucinous histologies			
		ER- or PR-positive	ER- or PR-negative
NN or N1mi	T1ab	No adjuvant therapy	
	T1 or T2 11–30 mm	± E ± C	± C
	T2 > 30 mm	E + C	C
NP	T	E + C	C

±, use of this therapy optional ("consider"); C, polychemotherapy; E, endocrine therapy; ER, estrogen receptor; PR, progesterone receptor; Tr, trastuzumab.

[a]Favorable: well differentiated.

[b]Unfavorable: moderately or poorly differentiated, angiolymphatic invasion, HER-2–overexpressing.

(From 2005 National Comprehensive Cancer Network guidelines relating to adjuvant therapy of breast cancer available at http://www.adjuvantonline.com/BreastHelpV8Dec05/NCCN2005.html.)

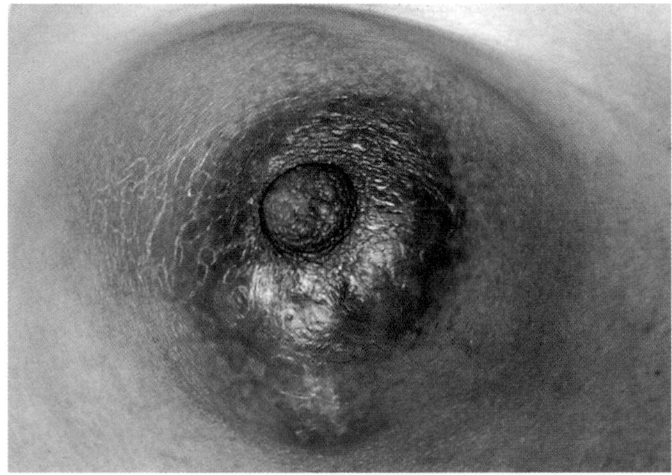

Figure 14–17 Paget disease of the breast.

In breast cancer with HER-2 over-expression, the use of trastuzumab (Herceptin), which is a recombinant DNA–derived humanized monoclonal antibody that selectively binds with high affinity to the extracellular domain of the human epidermal growth factor receptor-2 protein, has shown promise not only in recurrent disease but also in first-line combination therapy.

Paget disease of the breast

This cancer begins in the nipple area and is associated with bleeding, redness, itching, and burning (Fig. 14–17). Scaling of the nipple may be seen along with swelling of the skin surrounding the involved area of the nipple. Some consider this condition as DCIS involving the nipple, but usually associated with additional intraductal or invasive carcinoma in the underlying breast parenchyma. The extent of involvement of parenchyma determines the patient's suitability for conservative therapy. In patients with disease localized to the subareolar area, conservative surgery is appropriate, with removal of the entire nipple–areola complex and some of the underlying ductal region. The prognosis for Paget disease is related to stage and is similar to that for other breast cancer types. The need for adjuvant therapy also follows the same guidelines as ductal carcinoma.

BIBLIOGRAPHY

BENIGN CONDITIONS OF THE BREAST

American College of Obstetricians and Gynecologists: Nonmalignant conditions of the breast. ACOG Tech Bull 156:1, 1991.

American College of Obstetricians and Gynecologists: Report of Task Force on Routine Cancer Screening. ACOG Committee Opinion Number 68. Washington, ACOG, 1989.

American College of Radiology: Breast Imaging Reporting and Data System, 2nd edn. Reston, American College of Radiology, 1995.

Ariel IM: Enovid therapy for fibrocystic disease. Am J Obstet Gynecol 117:453, 1973.

Baker HW, Snedecor PA: Clinical trial of danazol for benign breast disease. Am J Surg 45:727, 1979.

Blichert-Toft M et al: Treatment of mastalgia with bromocriptine: a double-blind crossover study. Br Med J 1:237, 1979.

Byrd BF et al: Treatment of breast tumors associated with pregnancy and lactation. Ann Surg 155:940, 1962.
Chetty U et al: Benign breast disease in cancer. Br J Surg 67:789, 1979.
Cole P, Elwood JM, Kaplan SD: Incidence rates and risk factors of benign breast neoplasms. Am J Epidemiol 108:112, 1978.
Davis HH, Simons M, Davis JB: Cystic disease of the breast: relationship to carcinoma. Cancer 17:957–978, 1964.
DeVitt JE: Fibrocystic disease of the breast is not premalignant. Surg Gynecol Obstet 134:803, 1972.
Donegan WL: Pregnancy and breast cancer. Obstet Gynecol 50:244, 1977.
Gonzalez ER: Vitamin E relieves most cystic breat disease; may alter lipids, hormones. JAMA 244:1077–1078; 1980.
Hindle WH, Alonzo LJ: Conservative management of breast fibroadenomas. Am J Obstet Gynecol 164:1647, 1991.
Hislop TJ, Elwood JM: Risk factors for benign breast disease: a 30 year cohort study. Can Med Assoc J 124:283, 1981.
Kramer WM, Rush BF: Mammary duct proliferation in the elderly. Cancer 31:130, 1973.
Nezhat C et al: Danazol for benign breast disease. Am J Obstet Gynecol 137:604, 1980.
Petrek JA, Dukoff R, Rogatko A: Prognosis of pregnancy-associated breast cancer. Cancer 67:869, 1991.
Petrek JA: Surveillance and diagnosis of breast masses in pregnancy and lactation. Female Patient 18:16, 1993.
Ricciardi I, Ianniruberto A: Tamoxifen-induced regression of benign breast lesions. Obstet Gynecol 54:80, 1979.
Sitruk-Ware R, Thalabard JC, Benotmane A et al: Risk factors for breast fibroadenoma in young women. Contraception 40:251, 1989.
Wilkinson S, Anderson TJ, Rifkind E et al: Fibroadenoma of the breast: a follow-up of conservative management. Br J Surg 76:390, 1989.
Zoorob R, Anderson R, Cefalu C et al: Cancer screening guidelines. Am Family Physician 63:1–17, 2001.

EPIDEMIOLOGY

Adami HO, Krusemo UB, Bergkvist L et al: On the age-dependent associations between cancer of the breast and of the endometrium: a nationwide cohort study. Br J Cancer 47:77, 1987.
American Cancer Society: Breast Cancer Facts and Figures. Atlanta, American Cancer Society, pp 1–28.
American College of Obstetricians and Gynecologists: Carcinoma of the breast. ACOG Techn Bull 158:1, 1991.
American Joint Committee on Cancer, American Cancer Society, American College of Surgeons Commission on Cancer: American Cancer Society, 1989; 89-12M-No. 3485.01.
American Joint Committee on Cancer: Manual for Staging, 6th edn. Online. Available: http://www.jco.org/cgi/content-nw/full/21/17/3244/T1
Beral V, Hermon C, Kay C et al: Mortality associated with oral contraceptive use. Br Med J 318:96, 1999.
Calle EE, Martin LM, Thun MJ et al: Family history, age and risk of fatal breast cancer. Am J Epidemiol 138:675, 1993.
Collaborative Group: Breast cancer and hormonal contraceptives. Lancet 347:1713, 1996.
Dupont WD, Page DL, Pant FF et al: Estrogen replacement therapy in women with a history of proliferative breast disease. Cancer 85:1277, 1999.
Glass AG, Hoover RN: Rising incidence of breast cancer: relationship to stage and receptor status. J Natl Cancer Inst 82:693, 1990.
Henderson IC: Risk factors for breast cancer development. Cancer Suppl 71:2127, 1993.
Howe GR, Hirohata T, Hislop TG et al: Dietary factors and risk of breast cancer: combined analysis of 12 case-control studies. J Natl Cancer Inst 82:561, 1990.
Kritchevsky D: Nutrition and breast cancer. Cancer 66:1321, 1990.

EARLY DETECTION AND DIAGNOSIS

American College of Obstetricians and Gynecologists: ACOG, Committee Opinion Number 185. Washington, ACOG, 1997.
Anderson DE, Badzioch MD: Risk of familial breast cancer. Cancer 56:383, 1985.
Anonymous: Cancer Screening. Cancer Prevention and Early Detection Facts and Figures 2005.
Barton MB, Harris R, Fletcher SW: Does this patient have breast cancer? The screening clinical breast examination. JAMA 282:1270, 1999.
Bassett L, Winchester DP, Caplan RB et al: Stereotactic core-needle biopsy of the breast: a report of joint task force of American College of Radiology, Surgeons, and Pathologists. CA Cancer J Clin 47:171, 1997.
Boyles S: Fewer American women dying of breast cancer. WebMD. 23 Sep 2005.
Brown ML, Houn F, Sickles EA et al: Screening mammography in community practice. AJR Am J Roentgenol 165:1373, 1995.
Chu KC, Smart CR, Tarone RE: Analysis of breast cancer mortality and stage distribution by age for the Health Insurance Plan clinical trial. J Natl Cancer Inst 80:1125, 1988.
Collette HJ, Day NE, Rombach JJ et al. Evaluation of screening for breast cancer in a non-randomized study (The Dom project) by means a case-control study. Lancet 1(8388):1224–1226, 1984.
Council on Scientific Affairs: Mammographic screening in asymptomatic women ages 40 years and older. JAMA 261:2535, 1989.
Cutler SJ: Classification of extent of disease in breast cancer. Semin Oncol 1:91, 1974.
Cyrlak D, Wong CH: Mammographic changes in postmenopausal women undergoing hormonal replacement therapy. AJR Am J Roentgenol 161:1177, 1993.
Dent DM, Kirkpatrick AE, McGoogan E et al: Stereotaxic localization and aspiration cytology of impalpable breast lesions. Clin Radiol 40:380, 1989.
Dershaw DD, Morris EA, Liberman L et al: Nondiagnostic stereotactic core breast biopsy. Radiology 198:323, 1996.
Dodd GD: Quality assurance in mammography. Cancer 64:2707, 1989.
Ersek RA, Denton DR: Breast biopsy technique: a plea for cosmesis. South Med J 79:167, 1986.
Fletcher SW, Block W, Harris R et al: Report of the International Workshop on Screening for Breast Cancer. J Natl Cancer Inst 85:1644, 1993.
Gage I, Schmitt SJ, Nixon AJ et al: Pathologic margin involvement and risk of recurrence in patients treated with breast conserving therapy. Cancer 78:1921, 1996.
Hindle WH: Changing concepts in the evaluation of dominant breast masses. Female Patient 15:43, 1990.
Kerlikowske K, Grady D, Rubin SM et al: Efficacy of screening mammography. JAMA 273:149, 1995.
Leitch AM: Controversies in breast cancer screening. Cancer 76: 2064, 1995.
Lester RG: Risk versus benefit in mammography. Radiology 124:1, 1977.
Locker AP, Stickland V, Manhire AR et al: Mammography in symptomatic breast disease. Lancet 1:887, 1989.
Mettlin C: Diet and the epidemiology of human breast cancer. Cancer 53:605, 1984.
Miller AB, Baines CJ, To T et al: Canadian National Breast Screening Study: 1. Breast cancer detection and death rates among women aged 40 to 49 years. Can Med Assoc J 147:1459, 1992.
Miller AB, To T, Baines CJ et al: The Canadian National Breast Screening Study: update on breast cancer mortality. J Natl Cancer Inst Monogr 22:37, 1997.
Mitchell GW Jr, Homer MJ: Outpatient breast biopsies on a gynecologic service. Am J Obstet Gynecol 144:127, 1982.
National Breast Cancer Foundation: Early detection. Online. Available: http:www.nationalbreastcancer.org/early detection/index.html 30 Nov 2005.
National Institutes of Health: Breast cancer screening ages 40–49. NIH Consens Statement 15:1, 1997.
Nayfield SG et al: Potential role of tamoxifen in prevention of breast cancer. J Natl Cancer Inst 83:1450, 1991.

Newcomb PA, Weiss NS, Storer BE et al: Breast self-examination in relation to the occurrence of advanced breast cancer. J Natl Cancer Inst 83:260, 1991.

Nyirjesy I, Billingsley FS: Detection of breast carcinoma in gynecologic practice. Obstet Gynecol 64:747, 1984.

Parker SH, Burbank F, Jackson RJ et al: Percutaneous large core breast biopsy. Radiology 193:359, 1994.

Roberts JG, Gravelle JH, Baum M et al: Evaluation of radiolography and isotopic scintigraphy for detecting skeletal metastases in breast cancer. Lancet 1(7953):237–279, 1976.

Smart CR, Hendrick E, Rutledge JH et al: Benefits of mammography screening in women ages 40 to 49 years. Cancer 75:1619, 1995.

Smith RA, Saslow D, Sawyer KA et al: American Cancer Society Guidelines for Breast Cancer Screening: update 2003. CA Cancer J Clin 53;141–169, 2003.

Strax P: Results of mass screening for breast cancer in 50,000 examinations. Cancer 37:30, 1976.

Tabár L, Fogerberg CJ, Gad A et al: Reduction of mortality from breast cancer after mass screening with mammography. Lancet 1:829, 1985.

Vacheir H: Breast aspiration biopsy. Am J Obstet Gynecol 148:127, 1984.

Verbeek AL, Hendriks JH, Holland K et al: Mammographic screening and breast cancer mortality: age-specific effects in Nijmegen Project, 1975–82. Lancet 1(8433):865–866, 1985.

Verbeek ALM et al: Reduction of breast cancer mortality through mass screening with modern mammography: first results of Nijmegen project, 1975–1981. Lancet 1:1222, 1984.

Vogel VG, Graves DS, Vernon SW et al: Mammographic screening of women with increased risk of breast cancer. Cancer 66:1613, 1990.

Winchester DP: Evaluation and management of breast abnormalities. Cancer 66:1345, 1990.

Wolfe JN: Developments in mammography. Am J Obstet Gynecol 124:312, 1976.

TREATMENT

Adami HO, Krusemo UB, Bergkvist L et al: On the age-dependent associations between cancer of the breast and of the endometrium: a nationwide cohort study. Br J Cancer 47:77, 1987.

Barth A et al: Current management of ductal carcinoma in situ. West J Med 163:360, 1995.

Berg JW, Hutter RVP: Breast cancer. Cancer 75:257, 1995.

Blichert-Toft M, Andersen J, Dyreborg U: In situ carcinomas of the female breast. Acta Chir Scand 156:113, 1990.

Bonadonna G et al: 10-Year experience with CMF-based adjuvant chemotherapy in resectable breast cancer. Breast Cancer Res Treat 5:95, 1985.

Bonadonna G, Valagussa P: Dose response: effect of adjuvant chemotherapy in breast cancer. N Engl J Med 304:10, 1981.

Breast International Group (BIG) 1-98 Collaborative Group: A comparison of letrozole and tamoxifen in postmenopausal women with early breast cancer. N Engl J Med 353:2747–2757, 2005.

Buchanan RB, Blamey RW, Durrant KR et al: A randomized comparison of tamoxifen with surgical oophorectomy in premenopausal patients with advanced breast cancer. J Clin Oncol 4:1326, 1986.

Collaborative Group: Ovarian ablation in early breast cancer. Lancet 348:1189, 1996.

Collaborative Group: Tamoxifen for early breast cancer. Lancet 351:1451, 1998.

Davidson N, O'Neill AO, Vukov A et al: Effects of chemohormonal therapy in premenopausal, node positive, receptor positive breast cancer. ASCO Abstract 249, 1999.

Dorr FA, Friedman MA: The role of chemotherapy in the management of primary breast cancer. CA Cancer J Clin 41:231, 1991.

Early Breast Cancer Trialists' Collaborative Group: Tamoxifen for early breast cancer: an overview of the randomized trials. Lancet 351:1451, 1998.

Ernster VL et al: Incidence of and treatment for ductal carcinoma in situ of the breast. JAMA 275:913, 1996.

Fiorica JV. Lymphatic anatomy of the breast and axilla. (CH2f) In: Levenback C, van der Zee AGJ, Coleman RJ (eds): Clinical Lymphatic Mapping in Gynecologic Cancers. London: Taylor & Francis 2004; 59–65.

Fisher B et al: Five-year results of a randomized clinical trial comparing total mastectomy and segmental mastectomy with or without radiation in the treatment of breast cancer. N Engl J Med 312:665, 1985.

Fisher B et al: Ten-year results of a randomized clinical trial comparing radical mastectomy and total mastectomy with or without radiation. N Engl J Med 312:674, 1985.

Fisher B et al: Treatment of primary breast cancer with chemotherapy and tamoxifen. N Engl J Med 305:1, 1981.

Fisher B, Costantino J, Redmond C et al: Lumpectomy compared with lumpectomy and radiation therapy for the treatment of intraductal breast cancer. N Engl J Med 328:1581, 1993.

Fisher B, Costantino JP, Wickerham DL et al: Tamoxifen for prevention of breast cancer. J Natl Cancer Inst 90:1371, 1998.

Fisher B, Dignam J, Wolmark N et al: Lumpectomy and radiation therapy for the treatment of intraductal breast cancer. NSABP Project B-17. J Clin Oncol 16:441, 1998.

Fisher B, Dignam J, Wolmark N et al: Tamoxifen in treatment of intraductal breast cancer. NSABP Project B-24. Lancet 353:1993, 1999.

Fisher B, Fisher ER, Redmond C: 10-Year results from the NSABP clinical trial evaluating the use of L-phenylalanine mustard (L-PAM) in the management of primary breast cancer. J Clin Oncol 4:929, 1986.

Fisher ER, Dignam J, Tan-Chiu E et al: Pathologic findings from the NSABP eight-year update of Protocol B-17. Cancer 86:429, 1999.

Fornander T, Rutqvist LE, Cedermark B et al: Adjuvant tamoxifen in early breast cancer: occurrence of new primary cancers. Lancet 1:117, 1989.

Gelber RD, Goldhirsch A: A new end-point for the assessment of adjuvant therapy in postmenopausal women with operable breast cancer. J Clin Oncol 4:1772, 1986.

Gelber RD, Goldhirsch A: The concept of an overview of cancer clinical trials with special emphasis on early breast cancer. J Clin Oncol 4:1696, 1986.

Goldhirsch A, Glick JH, Gelber RD et al: Meeting highlights: International Expert Consensus on the Primary Therapy of Early Breast Cancer 2005. Ann Oncol 16:1569–1583, 2005.

Goss PE, Ingle JN, Martino S et al: A randomized trial of letrozole in postmenopausal women after five years of tamoxifen therapy for early-stage breast cancer. N Engl J Med 349:1793–1802, 2003.

Gusberg SB: Tamoxifen for breast cancer: associated endometrial cancer. Cancer 65:1463, 1990.

Haagensen CD: The choice of treatment for operable carcinoma of the breast. Surgery 76:685, 1974.

Halsted WS: The results of radical operations for the cure of carcinoma of the breast. Ann Surg 46:1, 1907.

Hardell L: Tamoxifen as risk factor for carcinoma of corpus uteri. Lancet 2:563, 1988.

Harris JA, Hellman S, Kinne DW. Limited surgery and radiotherapy for early breast cancer. CA Cancer J Clin 36:120–125, 1986.

Harris JR, Recht A, Connolly J et al: Conservative surgery and radiotherapy for early breast cancer. Cancer 66:1427, 1990.

Hayes DF, Henderson IC: Adjuvant therapy for node-negative breast cancer patients. Adv Oncol 6:8, 1991.

International Breast Cancer Study Group: Late effects of adjuvant oophorectomy and chemotherapy upon premenopausal breast cancer patients. Ann Oncol 1:30, 1990.

Jensen EV, Smith S, DeSombre ER. Hormone dependency in breast cancer. Journal of Steroid Biochemistry and Molecular Biology. 7:911–917, 1976.

Jones SE, Durie BGM, Salmon SE: Combination chemotherapy with Adriamycin and cyclophosphamide for advanced breast cancer. Cancer 36:90, 1975.

Kerlikowske K et al: Efficacy of screening mammography: a meta-analysis. JAMA 273:149, 1995.

Killacey MA, Hakes TB, Pierce UK: Endometrial adenocarcinoma in breast cancer patients receiving antiestrogens. Cancer Treat Rep 69:237, 1985.

Lichter AS et al: Mastectomy versus breast-conserving therapy in the treatment of stage I and II carcinoma of the breast: a randomized trial at the National Cancer Institute. J Clin Oncol 10:976, 1992.

Lippman ME: The NIH Consensus Development Conference on adjuvant chemotherapy for breast cancer: a commentary. Breast Cancer Res Treat 6:195, 1985.

Love RR, Newcomb PA, Wiebe DA: Effects of tamoxifen therapy on lipid and lipoprotein levels in postmenopausal patients with node-negative breast cancer. J Natl Cancer Inst 82:1327, 1990.

MammoSite: RTS: broadening access to breast conservation therapy. Online. Available: www.mammosite.com 1 Dec 2005.

Montague ED: Conservative surgery and radiation therapy in the treatment of operable breast cancer. Cancer 53:700, 1984.

Moore CM: On the influence of inadequate operations on the theory of cancer: Royal Medical and Chirurgical Society, London. Med Chir Trans 32:245, 1967.

National Cancer Institute: Surveillance, Epidemiology, and End Results (SEER) program public use CD-ROM (1973–1992). Bethesda, NCI, Surveillance Program, Division of Cancer Prevention and Control, Cancer Statistics Branch, 1995.

National Comprehensive Cancer Network: 2005 National Comprehensive Cancer Network, Inc. Version 2.2006. Online. Available: http:/www.NCCN.org

National Comprehensive Cancer Network: Clinical practice guidelines in oncology. V.1.2006. Breast cancer. Online. Available: http://www.nccn.org

Neville AM et al: Factors predicting treatment responsiveness and prognosis in node-negative breast cancer. J Clin Oncol 10:696, 1992.

Nielsen M et al: Breast cancer and atypia among young and middle-aged women: a study of 110 medicolegal autopsies. Br J Cancer 56:814, 1987.

Page DL et al: Continued local recurrence of carcinoma 15–25 years after a diagnosis of low grade ductal carcinoma in situ of the breast treated only with biopsy. Cancer 76:1187, 1995.

Parente JT, Amsel M, Lerner R et al: Breast cancer associated with pregnancy. Obstet Gynecol 71:861, 1988.

Piccart MJ, de Valeriola D, Dal LAgo L et al: Adjuvant chemotherapy in 2005: standards and beyond. Breast 14:439–445, 2005.

Powles T, Edes R, Ashly S et al: Interim analysis of the incidence of breast cancer in the Royal Marsden Hospital tamoxifen randomized chemoprevention trial. Lancet 362:98, 1998.

Pritchard KI: Systemic adjuvant therapy for node-negative breast cancer: proven or premature? Ann Intern Med 111:1, 1989.

Schwartz FG et al: Multicentricity of nonpalpable breast cancer. Cancer 45:2913, 1980.

Shingleton WW, McCarty KS: Breast carcinoma: an overview. Gynecol Oncol 26:271, 1987.

Silverstein MJ et al: Prognostic classification of breast ductal carcinoma-in-situ. Lancet 345:1154, 1995.

Soreide JA, Varhaug JE, Fjosne HE et al: Adjuvant endocrine treatment (goserelin vs tamoxifen) in pre-menopausal patients with operable node positive stage II breast cancer. A prospective randomized national multicenter study. Eur J Surg Oncol 28(5):505–510, 2002.

Steering Committee: Clinical practice guidelines for the care and treatment of breast cancer. A Canadian consensus document. CMAJ 158(suppl):S1, 1998.

Tancini G et al: Adjuvant CMF in breast cancer: comparative 5 year results of 12 vs. 6 cycles. Proc Am Soc Clin Oncol 1:86, 1982.

Taylor HC Jr: The coincidence of primary breast and uterine cancer. Am J Cancer 15:277,1931.

Tormey DC, Gray R, Gilchrist K et al: Adjuvant chemohormonal therapy with cyclophosphamide, methotrexate, 5-fluorouracil, and prednisone (CMFP) or CMFP plus tamoxifen compared with CMF for premenopausal breast cancer patients. Cancer 65:200, 1990.

Torres JE, Mickal A: Carcinoma of the breast in pregnancy. Clin Obstet Gynecol 18:219, 1975.

Veronesi U et al: Comparing radical mastectomy with quadrantectomy, axillary dissection, and radiotherapy in patients with small cancers of the breast. N Engl J Med 305:6, 1981.

Veronesi U, Maisonneuve P, Costa A et al: Prevention of breast cancer with tamoxifen. Lancet 362:93, 1998.

Vicini FA, Beitsch PD, Quiet CA et al: First analysis of patient demographics, technical reproducibility, cosmesis, and early toxicity: results of the American Society of Breast Surgeons MammoSite breast brachytherapy trial. Cancer 104(6);1138–1148, 2005.

Winchester DP, Strom EA: Standards for diagnosis and management of ductal carcinoma in situ of the breast. CA Cancer J Clin 48: 108, 1998.

Winer EP, Hudis C, Burstein HJ et al: American Society of Clinical Oncology technology assessment on the use of aromatase inhibitors as adjuvant therapy for postmenopausal women with hormone receptor–positive breast cancer: status report 2004. J Clin Oncol 23(3):619–629, 2005.

15 Colorectal and Bladder Cancer

Philip J. DiSaia, M.D.

COLORECTAL CANCER
Epidemiology
Screening
Polyps
Staging
Chemoprevention
Surgical therapy
Adjuvant therapy
Recurrence patterns
Therapy of recurrence

BLADDER CANCER
Pathology
Diagnosis and staging
Treatment and results

COLORECTAL CANCER

Epidemiology

Although the epidemiology of rectal cancer differs in some respects from that of colon cancer, the two share so many features that most investigators regard all large bowel cancers as a single entity. Colorectal cancer (CRC) is the western world's most common internal malignancy and one of its leading causes of cancer deaths. For the year 2005, the American Cancer Society estimated 73,470 new cases of CRC in women in the USA alone, and 35,000 women are estimated to die of this disease. In the USA, slightly more than 50% of colon cancers and slightly fewer than 45% of rectal cancers occur in women (Table 15-1). The overall incidence in the USA has remained fairly constant during the past five decades, but for unknown reasons the proportion of cases involving the rectum and the colon has changed. Approximately 70% of the incidence and 80% of deaths now involve the colon. More lesions involve the right colon (Fig. 15–1).

Colorectal cancer is the second leading cause of death of cancer in the USA. Fortunately, mortality from CRC has fallen 29% for women and 7% for men during the past 30 years. There is a trend toward earlier stage disease, even though most patients are still diagnosed with regional or distant disease. The majority of CRCs are diagnosed in patients older than 50 years of age (Fig. 15–2). A patient younger than 50 years of age is likely to belong to a high-risk group. Adenomatous polyps are the most common precursor lesion; they are estimated to occur in 93% of cases of colorectal adenocarcinoma. Adenomatous polyps occur in 30% of older individuals, however, and <10% progress to malignancy.

Because of the numbers of patients and the long periods of observation required, it has been very difficult to mount large-scale prospective studies of dietary intervention in CRC. However, observations of the epidemiologic patterns of this cancer suggest potential changes in dietary habits that may lead to a reduction in risk for populations with high incidence of disease. The observations of Burkitt and others in African populations have led many investigators to conclude that the low risk in these populations was attributable mainly to high-fiber diets, which resulted in high-bulk stools and rapid transit time. Theoretically, slow stool transit and low-bulk stools may be prone to higher concentrations of carcinogens adjacent to the bowel wall. Not all fiber may be beneficial, however, and there are no prospective intervention studies that prove the ability of fiber alone to decrease the risk of CRC. A meta-analysis of 13 case-control studies, representing nine different countries, has reported an inverse relationship between fiber-rich food and cancer of the colon and rectum, irrespective of gender or age. De Cosse et al also found that wheat bran was effective in preventing polyp recurrences in patients with a hereditary predisposition for polyps. The exact mechanism by which fiber affects the process of carcinogenesis is unknown.

Other epidemiologic studies of the low risk of colon cancer in the Far East (compared with western societies) suggest that diets that are low in unsaturated fats may be associated with a reduction in the incidence of CRC. Changes in the diet of the traditionally low-risk cultures, such as Japan, toward a diet that has a higher fat content typical of that of western countries have been associated with a rising incidence of CRC. Although the exact mechanism by which fats (and fiber) affect colon carcinogenesis is not clearly understood, these epidemiologic studies leave little doubt that there are environmental risk factors in the development of this common tumor. This conclusion is

Table 15–1 PATIENTS AT HIGH RISK FOR COLORECTAL NEOPLASMS[a]

Personal history	Family history
Breast cancer	Colorectal polyp
Endometrial cancer	Colorectal cancer
Crohn disease	
Visceral irradiation	
Ureterosigmoidostomy	
Colorectal polyp	
Previous colorectal cancer	

[a]Ulcerative colitis predisposes to malignancy but is not usually considered asymptomatic; screening is not useful in patients with familial polyposis or Gardner syndrome.
(From Gryska PV, Cohen AM: Screening asymptomatic patients at high risk for colon cancer with full colonoscopy. Dis Colon Rectum 30:18, 1987.)

supported by the alterations of risk patterns for CRC in migrating cultures that experience changing environments. For example, the migration of Japanese persons to the USA is associated with an increasing incidence of CRC in successive generations, until their risk is equivalent to that of the native-born population.

The Nurses' Health Study is a prospective cohort study of 88,751 US female nurses, aged 30–55 years, who were administered questionnaires every 2 years for 12 years regarding health habits and medical history. This study demonstrated a twofold increased risk of colon cancer among women in the highest quintile of animal fat intake compared with women in the lowest quintile. A meta-analysis of these data found that the increased risk was in fact due to red meat consumption and not fat intake. Either processed or fresh red meat, depending on the study, have been implicated in the development of cancer of the colon and rectum in three other large prospective cohort studies.

Certain micronutrients found in cruciferous vegetables (e.g. cabbage, broccoli, cauliflower, and Brussels sprouts) may reduce the risk of colon cancer. Figure 15–3 demonstrates some theories about how these agents act to interfere with initiation of malignant changes. Some of these micronutrients may directly inhibit carcinogen formation or function by binding carcinogens within the intestine; others may exert a more general systemic effect. Table 15–2 is a list of some of the foods and chemicals in foods that inhibit cancer in laboratory animals. Calcium and wheat bran have been used in various preventive trials. It has been reported that 1.5–2 g/day of calcium significantly decreases DNA-synthesizing cells of high-risk patients. Chronic wheat bran supplementation appears to decrease both rectal mucosal DNA synthesis and polyp recurrence.

The action of bile acids appears to be related to the development of colon cancer. Patients who have undergone cholecystectomy have a higher incidence of right-sided colon cancer. Cholecystectomy results in an increased concentration of secondary bile acids, particularly in the right colon. This effect of bile acids may also explain the action of dietary fiber, because the breakdown of carbohydrates (dietary fiber) by anaerobic bacteria results in the lowering of fecal pH, which inhibits conversion of the bile acids to deoxycholic acid, a potential carcinogen.

In addition to the average-risk patients (i.e. men and women age 40 and older), there are subgroups in the population at increased risk for CRC. These include:

- patients who have been cured of CRC,
- patients who have previously had adenomas,
- patients who have had universal ulcerative colitis for longer than 7 years,
- women who have had genital cancer,

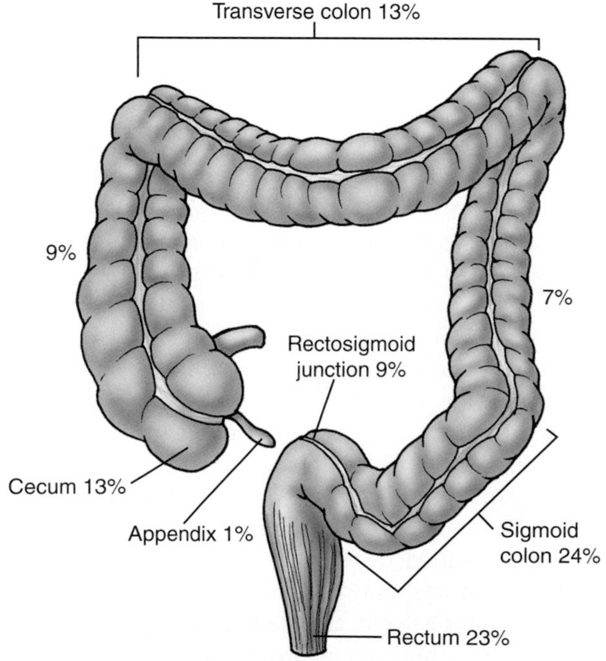

Figure 15–1 Distribution of colorectal cancer.

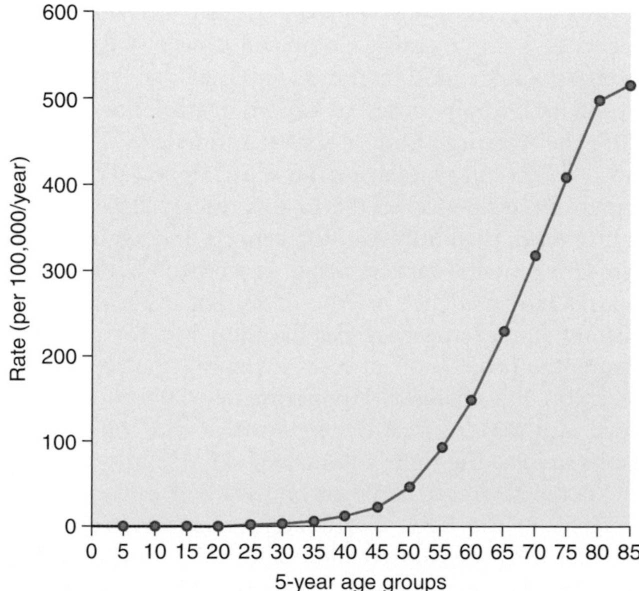

Figure 15–2 Age-specific incidence of colorectal cancer.

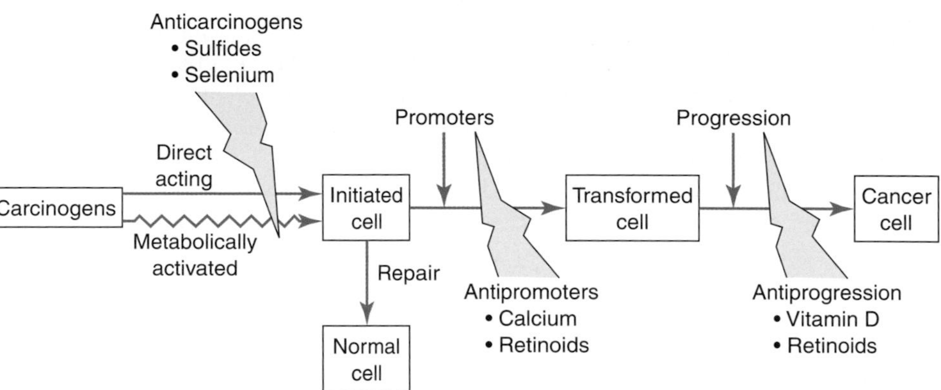

Figure 15–3 Mechanism of action of select dietary anticarcinogens and antipromoters. (From Wargovich MJ: New dietary anticarcinogens and prevention of gastrointestinal cancer. Dis Colon Rectum 31:72, 1988. Reprinted with kind permission of Springer Science and Business Media.)

Table 15–2 FOOD AND FOOD CHEMICALS THAT INHIBIT GASTROINTESTINAL CANCER IN LABORATORY ANIMALS

Food source	Chemical
Grapes, strawberries, apples	Plant phenols
Cabbage, broccoli, Brussels sprouts, cauliflower	Dithiothiones, isoflavones
Garlic, onions, leeks	Thioethers
Citrus fruits	Terpenes
Carrots, yams, watermelon	Carotenoids

- individuals who have a family history of one of the polyposis syndromes, and
- individuals who have inherited colon cancer syndromes.

Obesity, and in particular abdominal adiposity, has also been associated with an elevated risk for adenomatous polyps and colon cancer, but this has not been a universal finding.

Although much work needs to be done to clarify further these high-risk subgroups, especially those with familial factors, a much clearer picture exists today of those who are at increased risk for CRC compared with the average-risk population. Technologic advances have also occurred recently, such as new methods for fecal occult blood testing (FOBT), flexible sigmoidoscopy, colonoscopy, virtual colonoscopy, stool-based DNA testing, and refinement of the double-contrast barium enema.

A desirable goal based on these improvements is early diagnosis for improved survival. This concept is in keeping with the current emphasis on preventive measures for cancer in general and for CRC specifically. Prevention of CRC can be defined as primary or secondary. Primary prevention is the identification of factors, either genetic or environmental, responsible for CRCs, and their eradication. Secondary prevention may be defined as early detection of CRC before its more advanced, devastating, and fatal consequences, as well as detection and eradication of premalignant disease before its transformation into cancer.

The terms *hereditary*, *sporadic*, and *familial* CRC have been used by many authors. These terms are defined operationally on the basis of a family history of cancer and possibly other phenotypic information. The sporadic type occurs in the absence of a family history of CRC in a first-degree relative. The familial type occurs when at least one first-degree relative has CRC. In the case of hereditary CRC, there is a family history of CRC occurring in a pattern that indicates autosomal-dominant inheritance. Although this classification does not produce etiologically homogenous groups, it has utility in planning surveillance and management strategies. The long-term objective of study on the genetic epidemiology of CRC is primary and secondary prevention through specific management and surveillance recommendations.

In 1995, Calle and colleagues confirmed earlier studies reporting that estrogen replacement therapy decreases risk of developing colon cancer. Every use of estrogen replacement therapy was associated with significantly decreased risk of fatal colon cancer (relative risk = 0.71). The reduction in risk (relative risk = 0.55) was strongest among current users, and there was a significant trend of decreasing risk with increasing years of use among all users. These associations were not altered in multivariate analysis controlling for other risk factors.

Fernandez et al reported on a large case-control study of oral contraceptive use as well as hormone replacement therapy, and found a decreased incidence in women using either. The overall risk for women using oral contraceptives for 2 years or more was 0.52. For women using hormone replacement therapy, the odds ratio was 0.40.

Screening

The rationale for screening is based on the widely held view that most CRCs are the product of a slow and orderly progression from normal colonic mucosa to adenomatous polyp, early and surgically curable cancer, and finally advanced and incurable cancer. Screening is intended to detect and remove cancer in its earliest stages, as well as polyps thought to be precancerous (e.g. adenomatous polyps measuring more than 1 cm in diameter). However, recommendations for screening vary considerably because of the uncertainty about whether any type of screening is efficacious in reducing the morbidity or mortality of CRC.

The common clinical manifestations of CRC are bleeding and anemia, pain, and obstructive symptoms. These manifestations are most common with the advanced lesions.

Effective screening implies the examination of asymptomatic persons at high risk to detect early, highly curable lesions. Unlike the detection of many other cancers, detection of CRC at an early stage is possible with already existing resources. This includes digital examination of the rectum, examination for occult blood in the stool, and radiographic and endoscopic procedures. A large number of rectal cancers occur in the most distal 10 cm of this organ and can be easily palpated by a digital rectal examination. There are few studies that have prospectively or retrospectively evaluated the usefulness of this examination in affecting morbidity or mortality of rectal cancer. However, because of the low cost and ease with which it may be performed, this procedure is to be routinely recommended in all patients. No gynecologist should do a pelvic examination without including an examination of the rectum. Rectovaginal examination affords an excellent opportunity to accomplish an examination of the rectum and a thorough pelvic examination with more adequate evaluation of the cul-de-sac and its contents, as well as other obvious advantages.

The testing of stool for the presence of occult blood as an indicator of gastrointestinal cancer is an old concept. Seventy percent of all CRC can be detected using fecal occult blood screening; however, 30% of patients do not bleed and their cancers are not detected in this manner. In the past, patients were given no dietary restrictions and asked to bring stool samples to be tested with guaiac and hydrogen peroxide solutions. There was no quality control of the stability of the reagents used. Because of the high percentage of false-positive and false-negative results, this approach fell into disfavor. Benzidine was used in a similar matter, but it also was discarded because of an extremely high sensitivity that resulted in a high percentage of false-positive results and subsequently unnecessary diagnostic workups. Greegor reintroduced the guaiac test for occult blood in the stool: patients, while on high-fiber, meat-free diets, were asked to smear on to paper slides impregnated with guaiac two samples of stool per day for 3 days (a total of six smears). The slides were then tested with a reagent of hydrogen peroxide in denatured alcohol. CRCs were detected in several patients at an early pathologic stage.

After Greegor's reintroduction of the occult blood test in the form of an impregnated guaiac test, several studies and programs were initiated around the world using this technique in the screening of CRC. Initial observations were confirmed in other studies in the USA and in Germany. Two control trials were initiated, and these studies demonstrated the feasibility of screening patients with FOBT. The rate of positive slides reported by Winawer et al has been low (2–5%); the false positivity, low (1–2%); the predictive value for neoplasia, high (30–50%); and the Dukes staging favorable for cancers detected by screening. The false-negative rate and the long-term impact of screening on mortality have not yet been established. Patient compliance and cost effectiveness are major unresolved issues. Currently, the American Cancer Society recommends that a FOBT be done annually after the age of 50. Although hemorrhoids are common in women who have borne children, blood in the stool should never be assumed to be hemorrhoidal unless the source is visualized. Five randomized clinical trials have demonstrated a decrease in mortality between 15 and 33% by the use of serial FOBT. In one trial, patients who received FOBT in conjunction with sigmoidoscopy had a significantly higher survival probability when compared with those who received sigmoidoscopy alone (70% vs 48%, respectively).

The American Cancer Society, the American College of Obstetricians and Gynecologists, and the National Cancer Institute have similar guidelines for the screening of CRC. These guidelines are as follow.

Colorectal examination should be included as part of the periodic health examination. At age 50, FOBT should be done annually, and a sigmoidoscopy, or preferably colonoscopy, should be performed every 3–5 years. The physician should identify for special surveillance high-risk patients, including those with a strong family history of colon cancer or those with personal history of polyps, colon cancer, or inflammatory bowel disease.

Carcinoembryonic antigen (CEA) is not considered to be a screening or diagnostic test for colon cancer and is used only to monitor disease activity, especially following initial therapy. For monitoring, most investigation using serial values report that this predictor can anticipate a recurrence in about one-third of patients by approximately 3–6 months. Serial values measured at 2-month intervals the first 2 years after definitive surgery in patients with B2, C1, and C2 lesions and continuing quarterly for an additional 2 years appear useful. Endoscopic procedures have aided significantly in both colon cancer screening and therapy. In addition to assisting in the diagnosis of polyps and early cancers, the removal of polyps may be effected by the endoscopist. This may lead to a total reduction of cancer incidence. Proctosigmoidoscopy, which examines the terminal 25 cm of large bowel, has been technically the easiest for physicians to master, and it has been associated with a finding of unsuspected cancer in one of every 435 persons. However, it has been observed that <20% of physicians routinely use this procedure in their practices. Flexible sigmoidoscopes, which examine up to 60 cm of bowel, have been introduced and may improve routine endoscopic screening procedures. The results of case-control studies evaluating flexible sigmoidoscopy show a 60–80% reduction in mortality due to CRC in the distal colon and rectum.

Objections to the flexible 60-cm colonoscope for screening include cost and an examination time often exceeding 30 min. Moreover, advanced training is required to use it effectively. Subsequently, a flexible 35-cm instrument has been developed to overcome these objections: the 35-cm flexible fiberoptic proctosigmoidoscope appears to be ideally suited for office use. Its cost is relatively low, and the training required is minimal. Although examination of the entire sigmoid colon is feasible, examination to a depth of 30 cm should reveal almost 65% of bowel cancers and polyps, and pathology yield should be at least twice as great as with the rigid scope. In one investigation involving 26 women, average examination time using a 35-cm two-way tip deflection instrument was 4.3 min, and the mean insertion depth was 29 cm. The instrument's small cross-sectional diameter and ability to conform to normal bowel curvature minimized patient discomfort. The following guidelines should be observed when screening for CRC using the fiberoptic sigmoidoscope.

- Perform fiberoptic sigmoidoscopy examination every 3–5 years on women 50 years or older who have had two initial negative examination results 1 year apart.
- Identify high-risk patients (those with familial polyposis, ulcerative colitis, polyps, history of carcinoma of the colon, or family history of colon cancer; Table 15–3), begin sigmoidoscopy examinations on these patients when they are younger, and examine these patients more frequently.
- Instruct the patient to prepare herself shortly before the examination with a phosphosoda enema.
- After the rectovaginal examination, the patient should be assisted to the dorsal lithotomy position for the sigmoidoscopy examination.
- Promptly refer any abnormalities that are revealed by screening to a gastroenterologist for diagnosis.

Colonoscopy, which is the examination of the entire colon, is the only tool that combines screening capabilities with the potential for complete diagnosis and treatment. It is estimated that 80–90% of CRCs could be prevented by regular colonoscopic surveillance examinations. The examination requires a complete bowel preparation and must be done by a trained physician. Colonoscopy also carries the highest risk of available CRC screening tools, with a perforation rate that ranges from one in 500 to one in 4000 procedures.

In 2003, a new non-invasive screening test based on identifying altered DNA shed from the colon wall into the stool was made available. Multiple investigations have shown good sensitivity and high specificity for this test. To date, stool-based DNA testing combining the data from several studies illustrates a sensitivity of about 65% and a specificity of 95%.

Virtual colonoscopy is another name for computed tomography (CT) colonography, which involves the use of high-speed helical CT scanners to image the colon. Its sensitivity is the same as colonoscopy for polyps > 1 cm in size, but it shows poor sensitivity for smaller polyps. It provides three-dimensional images of the colon. A thorough bowel cleaning is required, and the value in terms of reducing mortality from CRC is under investigation. Recent data suggest that adding gastrointestinal contrast improves the accuracy.

Table 15–3 CANCER RISK FACTORS

Patient history	Family history	Associated disease
Breast cancer	Colorectal cancer	Granulomatous colitis
Colorectal adenoma	Colorectal polyp	Ulcerative colitis
Colorectal cancer	Familial polyposis	
	Gardner syndrome	
	Juvenile polyposis	

Polyps

The risk of carcinogenesis for an individual who has polyps has been debated for decades. Whether cancer arises in an observable premalignant lesion or whether it arises spontaneously in normal colonic mucosa has great implications for the prevention of colon cancer. Dukes' original analysis of 1000 cases of rectal cancer supported the concept of malignant degeneration of polyps, but the details of this event have never been fully described. Circumstantial evidence supports the concept that CRC can arise in a benign polyp. Benign adenomatous tissue is often observed to be contiguous to frank cancer, risk of cancer increases with increasing numbers and sizes of polyps, and animal–human models (familial polyposis) demonstrate that a transition does occur. Significantly, intervention studies have demonstrated that removal of benign polyps decreases the incidence of malignancies in large populations. Gilbertsen and coworkers demonstrated that, in 21,150 persons undergoing proctosigmoidoscopy with polyp removal, the subsequent development of CRC was 15% of the risk predicted for the general population.

The classifications of adenomatous polyps include tubular adenomas, villotubular or mixed adenomas, and villous adenomas. These polyps occur in all sizes and shapes, and during endoscopy they can be identified as pedunculated, sessile, or semisessile. Regardless of their gross appearance, these polyps all have cytologic characteristics of neoplasia and illustrate a serious disturbance in cell renewal where there is a loss of growth control mechanism. Mitosis is unrestricted and is observed at all levels of the adenomatous crypt. Cellular differentiation is abnormal, and differentiation into mature goblet cells is incomplete or absent. Therefore the crypts are lined with tall cells with prominent, elongated, hyperchromatic nuclei arranged in characteristic pseudostratification or picket fence pattern. The increased cellular mass produces the characteristic villous, tubular, or mixed villotubular growth pattern.

One of the most important distinctions to be made by the pathologist and the surgeon when examining adenomatous polyps is whether carcinomatous foci are confined to the area above the muscularis mucosae (in situ), or whether the lesion has traversed this boundary and invaded the submucosa and as such would be classified as invasive. Intramucosal carcinomas, that is, carcinomas that do not extend beyond the muscularis mucosae, do not metastasize (lymphatics are located in the submucosal layer). However, if left untreated these lesions progress to invasive carcinoma. Approximately two-thirds of adenomas are tubular; tubular adenomas have less premalignant

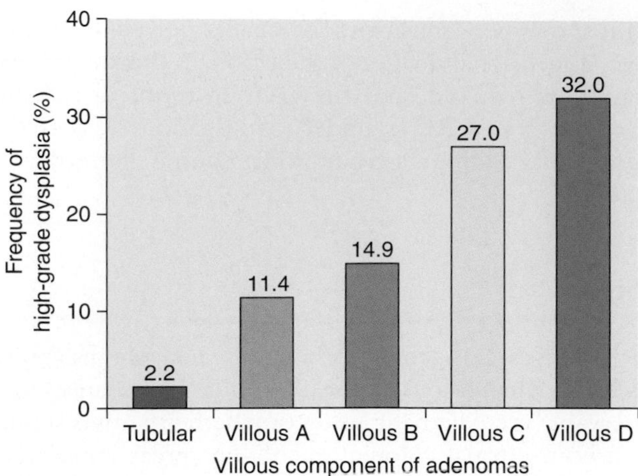

Figure 15–4 The frequency of high-grade dysplasia in adenomas according to histologic classification was determined by the National Polyp Study. (From O'Brien MJ, Winawer SJ, Zauber AG et al: The National Polyp Study: patients and polyp characteristics associated with high grade dysplasia in colorectal cancer. Gastroenterology 98[2]:371, 1990.)

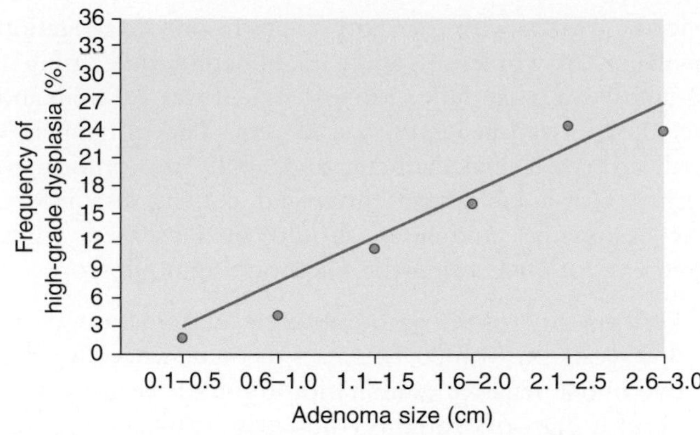

Figure 15–5 The frequency of high-grade dysplasia (severe dysplasia or carcinoma in situ) in adenomas according to size was determined from National Polyp Study data (•, observed; —, expected regression line). (From O'Brien MJ, Winawer SJ, Zauber AG et al: The National Polyp Study: patients and polyp characteristics associated with high grade dysplasia in colorectal cancer. Gastroenterology 98[2]:371, 1990.)

potential than do adenomas with villous features (Fig. 15–4). Villous features are more common with increasing size (Fig. 15–5). Approximately 5% of patients with adenomas have high-grade dysplasia, and 2–3% have invasive cancer at time of presentation. Patients presenting with an adenoma have a 40–50% likelihood of developing another adenoma in the future.

It is agreed that complete polypectomy is a definitive procedure for an in situ carcinoma in an adenomatous polyp (Fig. 15–6). However, there is controversy about treatment of an adenomatous polyp that is found to have an invasive carcinoma (penetration into the submucosa). Several investigators advocate treatment by radical surgical resection when the diagnosis of invasive malignancy has been made, whereas others advocate a more conservative approach. Other factors that should be taken into account are the type of adenomatous polyp and its size. For example, a villous adenoma is the least common of neoplastic polyps. However, it has the highest tendency toward malignant degeneration. In a collected series of cases reviewed by Coutsoftides and associates, the overall incidence of invasive malignancy was 30%. In the same reports, the incidence of positive lymph nodes ranged from 16 to 39%. In view of this finding, most surgeons advise radical surgical treatment of villous adenomas once invasive malignancy has been confirmed. Another consideration regarding the type of surgery (polypectomy vs radical surgical resection) is the degree of differentiation of the tumor in the presence of lymphatic invasion or angioinvasion.

For most patients, management of colorectal polyps should be individualized. The therapeutic decision concerning the treatment of invasive carcinomas arising in adenomatous polyps should be based on the polyp's malignant potential and its ability to metastasize. The burden of the surgeon is to confirm the presence of invasive malignancy by an excisional biopsy examination, and to weigh the risks of the presence of involved lymph nodes against the risks of radical surgery.

Hereditary non-polyposis colorectal cancer

Hereditary non-polyposis colorectal cancer (HNPCC), or Lynch syndrome, is one of the more common familial cancer syndromes, affecting one in 1000 individuals. The molecular basis for HNPCC is a defect in a DNA mismatch repair gene, usually a germline mutation in hMLH1 or hMSH2. A defective DNA mismatch repair causes microsatellite instability, and individuals with HNPCC are at increased risk for colon as well as endometrial cancers. Other malignancies of the ovary, stomach, small intestine, liver, ureter, brain, and skin may also be associated. HNPCC has been considered primarily a colon cancer–dominated syndrome, and these other cancers have been recently recognized. Two recent reports on HNPCC and cancer risk found that women with a germline mutation in hMLH1 or hMSH2 have a higher risk (40–60%) of endometrial cancer than colon cancer. The lifetime risk of ovarian cancer is lower but still between 10 and 12%. Both endometrial cancer and ovarian cancer in women with HNPCC tend to occur 15 years earlier than in their sporadic counterparts. The ovarian cancers tend to present as well-differentiated stage I lesions, as opposed to those seen with sporadic or BRCA1 or BRCA2 mutation lesions, where the majority are late stage. Colon cancers with HNPCC are also associated with an improved overall survival.

Staging

Considerable thought should be given to staging. Final staging should depend on histology, the depth of penetration, the involvement of the nodes, differentiation, muci-

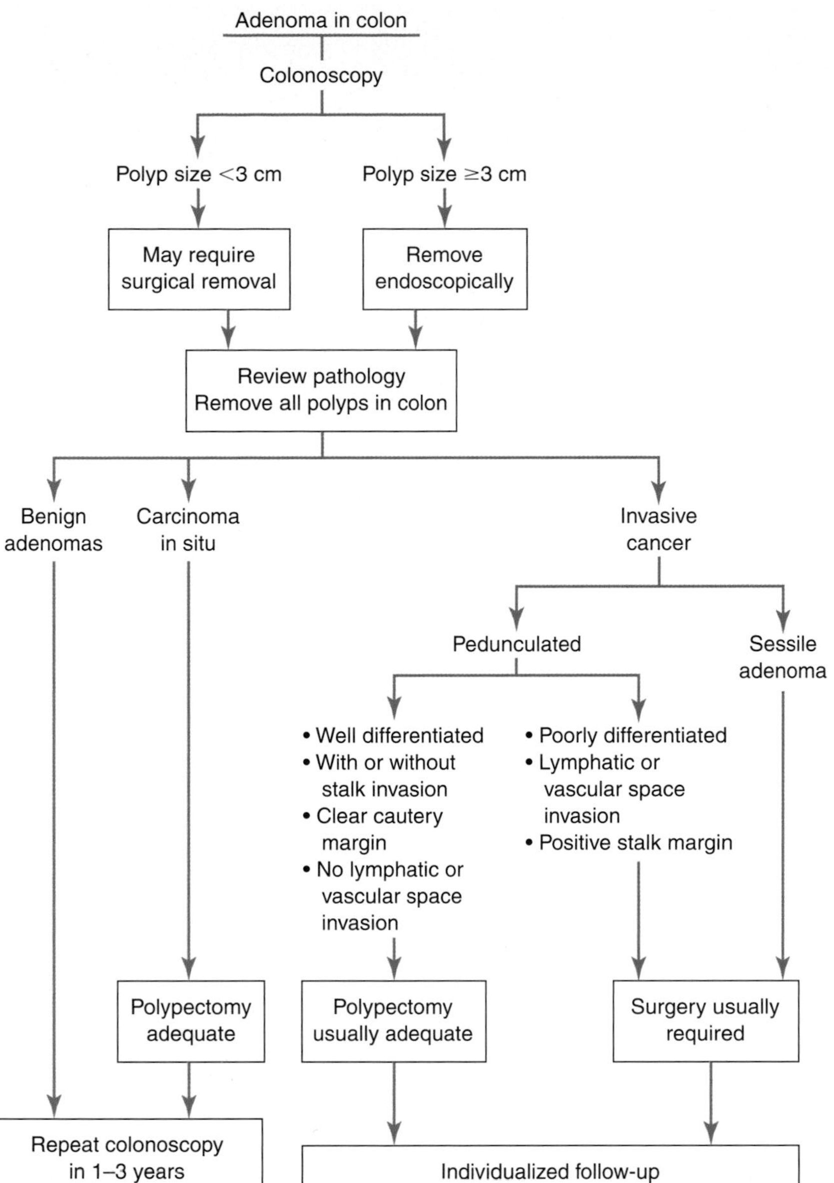

Figure 15–6 Management of adenomas. (After Hornsby-Lewis L et al: Natural history and current management of colorectal polyps. Oncology 4:142, 1990.)

nous content, signet ring appearance, pushing vs infiltrating margins, venous or perineural invasion, and lymphoplasmacytosis. Ideally, to ensure reasonably accurate staging, at least 12 lymph nodes should be found in the specimen. Various staging classifications have been proposed (Table 15–4).

Among the most commonly used staging classifications is that of Dukes and its modifications (Fig. 15–7). These modifications are based on the ability of two pathologic features of rectal cancer to predict prognosis: lymph node involvement and depth of tumor penetration. The Astler–Coller modification of this system emphasizes the depth of penetration as an independent variable in the prognosis (Table 15–5).

In addition to surgical staging, other variables have adverse effects on the prognosis of patients who have primary CRCs: ulceration of the primary tumor, fixation to adjacent organs, rectal origin, colonic perforation or obstruction, younger age, and elevated preoperative CEA. Most clinical studies indicate that the Dukes staging system, or its variations, is the single most important prognostic variable.

Chemoprevention

Several research disciplines working together in the area of chemoprevention research are contributing to the identification of effective cancer inhibitors, both synthetic and naturally occurring chemical compounds. The chemoprevention program of the National Cancer Institute is studying these basically non-toxic chemical agents that may inhibit the development of cancer in asymptomatic, mainly high-risk subjects. This program is systematically pursuing the development of effective agents through:

- information management of research leading from laboratory and epidemiology studies,

Table 15–4 STAGING FOR COLORECTAL CANCER OF THE AMERICAN JOINT COMMITTEE ON CANCER, AMERICAN CANCER SOCIETY, AND AMERICAN COLLEGE OF SURGEONS COMMISSION ON CANCER

	Definition
Primary tumor (T)	
TX	Primary tumor cannot be assessed
T0	No evidence of primary tumor
Tis	Carcinoma in situ
T1	Tumor invades submucosa
T2	Tumor invades muscularis propria
T3	Tumor invades through the muscularis propria into the subserosa, or into non-peritonealized pericolic or perirectal tissues
T4	Tumor perforates the visceral peritoneum or directly invades other organs or structures.[a]
Regional lymph nodes (N)	
NX	Regional lymph nodes cannot be assessed
N0	No regional lymph node metastasis
N1	Metastasis in one to three pericolic or perirectal lymph nodes
N2	Metastasis in four or more pericolic or perirectal lymph nodes
N3	Metastasis in any lymph node along the course of a named vascular trunk
Distant metastasis (M)	
MX	Presence of the distant metastasis cannot be assessed
M0	No distant metastasis
M1	Distant metastasis

Stage	TNM	Dukes stage[b]
0	Tis, N0, M0	—
I	T1, N0, M0	A
	T2, N0, M0	
II	T3, N0, M0	B
	T4, N0, M0	
III	Any T, N1, M0	C
	Any T, N2/3, M0	
IV	Any T, any N, M1	—

[a]Direct invasion of other organs or structures includes the invasion of other segments of the colorectum by way of the serosa (e.g. invasion of the sigmoid colon by a carcinoma of the cecum).
[b]Dukes stage B is a composite of better (T3, N0, M0) and worse (T4, N0, M0) prognostic groups, as is Dukes stage C (any T, N1, M0 and any T, N2/3, M0).

- biochemical and in vitro screening of new chemopreventive agents,
- in vivo animal model screening,
- chemopreventive agent procurement,
- toxicology testing, and
- clinical chemoprevention trials.

The National Cancer Institute is supporting several phase III colon cancer prevention trials that are designed to evaluate the effects of vitamins C and E, beta-carotene, and calcium in subjects with adenomatous polyps. In addition, smaller phase I and II trials are being conducted in high-risk subjects at various institutes to study the effectiveness of calcium citrate, calcium carbonate, wheat bran, beta-carotene, piroxicam (a prostaglandin synthesis inhibitor), difluoromethyl ornithine (DMFO), and ibuprofen.

Some of the more active compounds include non-steroidal anti-inflammatory drugs (NSAIDs), estrogen, DMFO, and micronutrients. The use of NSAIDs appears to exert an antiproliferative effect on colonic cells by inhibiting prostaglandin synthesis by reversibly binding to cyclo-oxygenase. The Nurses' Health Study determined the rate of colon cancer in women who consumed aspirin compared with women who reported no use. Regular aspirin use, at doses similar to those recommended for the prevention of cardiovascular disease, substantially reduced the risk of CRC after at least a decade of regular consumption.

Table 15–5 DUKES CLASSIFICATION: ASTLER–COLLER MODIFICATION

Stage	Extension	5-year survival (%)
A	Mucosa only	95
B	Bowel wall involvement	—
B1	Within wall	85–90
B2(m)	Microscopically through wall	60–70
B2(g)	Grossly through wall	50
B3	Adjacent structures involved	30
C	Lymph nodes positive for tumor	—
C1	Within wall	40–50
C2(m)	Microscopically through wall	40–50
C2(g)	Grossly through wall	15–25
C3	Adjacent structures involved	10–20
D	Distant metastatic disease	<5

Surgical therapy

The only curative therapy for invasive CRC is surgical resection of the primary tumor and regional mesentery lymph nodes. The extent of colorectal surgery is determined by anatomic landmarks. These include lymphatic drainage of the colon and rectum, location of the superior mesenteric artery, the middle and left colic arteries, the marginal artery, the inferior mesenteric artery, and the superior hemorrhoidal vessels. As stated by Stearns, the three essential elements of resection are:

1. wide removal of the cancer-bearing colon or rectal segments,
2. wide excision of the lymphatics draining the cancer-bearing segment of the bowel, and
3. accomplishing (1) and (2) with a minimum of cancer cell contamination and embolization.

The extent of surgery is well standardized for lesions draining into the superior mesenteric artery: a right colectomy is a well-established practice. However, as one

Classification	Dukes' A	Dukes' B	Dukes' C	Dukes' D
Development of colorectal cancer				
Cancer progression	Cancer confined to most superficial cell layer of colon or rectum (e.g. the top of the polyp)	Cancer may extend completely through wall of colon, but there is no lymph node involvement	Cancer may extend completely through wall of colon or rectum and has spread to lymph nodes	Metastatic disease the cancer has spread to distant organs such as the liver
Estimated 5-year survival rate	90%	70%	50%	5%
Percent diagnosed at stage	37%		63%	

Figure 15–7 Dukes staging of colon cancer with survival rates and distribution of cases. (From *The Female Patient,* Fidel A. Valea, author, The Critical Role of the Primary Care Physician, OB/GYN, and the Nurse Practitioner in Colorectal Cancer Screening, March 2005. Used with permission of the American Joint Committee on Cancer (AJCC), Chicago, Illinois. The original source of the material is the AJCC Cancer Staging Manual, Sixth Edition (2002) published by Springer-Verlag New York, www.springer-ny.com.)

approaches the rectosigmoid and rectum, there is controversy about treatment, and alternative procedures arise. The basic trend has been for more conservative surgery and the use of sphincter-saving approaches for lesions of the proximal two-thirds of the rectum. Another consideration for treatment of these tumors is the extension of the lymph node dissection to the retroperitoneal or pelvic nodes. Most studies of these approaches show no gain in survival but show increased morbidity and mortality. On the other hand, considerable evidence suggests that when a tumor extends to adjacent structures, particularly in rectosigmoid and rectal cancer, en bloc resection is preferable to other approaches and results in a higher level of salvage. The reason is that a significant percentage of tumors, although involving adjacent structures, do not show lymph node or distant metastases. The bladder, ureter, vagina, small bowel, abdominal wall, uterus, and ovary may all be involved contiguously with tumor and may require resection. The margin in the bowel wall itself is classically 5 cm from the gross tumor edge. This is of particular importance in rectal surgery. However, there is evidence that a 2- to 3-cm margin may be adequate in some patients. In general, the stage of CRC relates closely to the prognosis (Fig. 15–8).

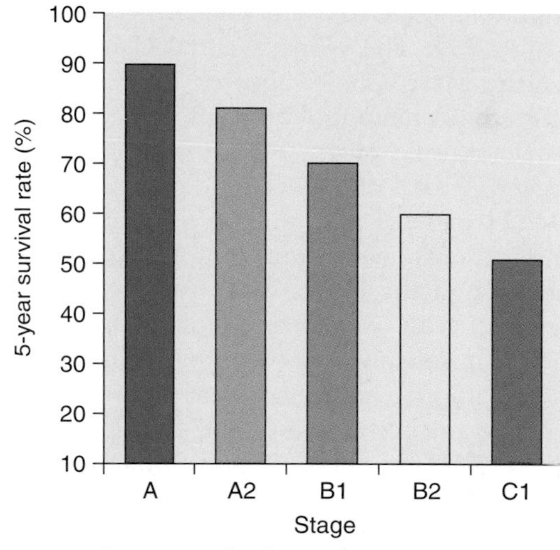

Figure 15–8 The stage of colorectal cancer relates closely to the prognosis.

Adjuvant therapy

Although CRCs are among the most highly curable neoplasms, almost half of the patients will have a relapse. The potential benefits of adjuvant therapy for CRC must therefore be seriously considered. The goals of such therapy are to prevent or delay the recurrence of the disease and to increase the percentage of patients who survive. For lesions at high risk for local recurrence, adjuvant radiation therapy has been studied. Both preoperative and postoperative radiation have been used. The goal of preoperative radiation therapy is to decrease the dissemination of cancer at surgery and to downstage the primary tumor. Postoperative radiation is used for patients at high risk for local recurrence—for example those with transmural invasion, known metastasis, and direct invasion of adjacent organs. Nonrandomized studies of postoperative therapy have suggested that such treatment has potential for decreasingly local recurrences.

Adjuvant chemotherapy programs have generally utilized 5-fluorouracil (5-FU) or 5-FU plus methyl-chloroethylcyclohexylnitrosourea (methyl-CCNU). Cooperative group studies have demonstrated a 5–10% benefit in 5-year survival for patients receiving adjuvant 5-FU. For Dukes stage C colon cancer, a significant disease-free survival benefit was noted: 40% of adjuvantly treated patients had recurrence at 5 years, compared with 52% of the control group. Several studies of large numbers of patients with Dukes stage B and C tumors suggest that adjuvant chemotherapy may delay a recurrence without necessarily prolonging survival in all treated patients. In other studies, certain subgroups of patients appear to benefit more than others, but consistent overall benefits have not been demonstrated. However, investigators have attempted to improve the therapeutic index of 5-FU by incorporating biochemical modulators or synergistically acting agents into their drug regimens. Agents such as levamisole and streptozotocin have been used in combination with 5-FU. Doses were administered to optimize objective response rates. None of the regimens demonstrated a significant statistical difference over that achieved by 5-FU alone.

The immunomodulatory agent levamisole plus 5-FU has demonstrated improved disease-free survival when compared with survival of a similar group of patients receiving no adjuvant therapy for Dukes stage C lesions. Three randomized clinical trials involving more than 400 patients have evaluated the addition of levamisole to 5-FU chemotherapy for patients with metastatic disease, with no positive results in favor of the treatment with levamisole alone. Based on this trial and the earlier positive results with levamisole, two adjuvant chemotherapy trials were reported in 1989. The North Central Cancer Treatment Group at the Mayo Clinic reported the results of a randomized study containing levamisole alone with a combination of levamisole plus 5-FU with no further therapy after surgery. A total of 101 eligible patients were chosen randomly: 21 patients had primary rectal cancer, and the remaining patients had colon cancer; 40% had tumors invading through the bowel wall that spread to regional lymph nodes. With a median follow-up in excess of 7 years, the levamisole plus 5-FU combination demonstrated a significant improvement in disease-free survival compared with no further therapy ($P = 0.02$). Overall, however, there was no improvement in survival. Subset analysis by stage demonstrated a significant decreased disease-free survival advantage for 5-FU and levamisole only in stage C patients. Subsequent studies were conducted by other cooperative groups. In 1990, the National Cancer Institute Consensus Development Conference recommended that stage II patients who were unable to participate in clinical trials should be offered adjuvant 5-FU and levamisole therapy.

The study of adjuvant therapy continues to evolve. A combination of 5-FU and leucovorin has been studied with and without a new agent, oxaliplatin, with positive early results. Capecitabine also appears to be an active agent and may be an alternative to 5-FU and leucovorin. More recently, bevacizumab, a monoclonal antibody that neutralizes vascular endothelial growth factor when combined with irinotecan, 5-FU, and leucovorin, appears to be superior to irinotecan, 5-FU, and leucovorin alone in achieving better median and progression-free survival.

Several non-randomized trials of adjuvant preoperative radiation suggested a possible survival benefit with a dose of 5000 rad. Memorial Hospital/Sloan–Kettering Cancer Center performed the first randomized prospective study, and refuted their retrospective results in that no survival advantage was seen in any subgroup. Although the rate of local recurrence was decreased by therapy, the incidence of blood-borne metastasis increased. A large-scale cooperative trial of the Veterans Administration Surgical Adjuvant Group found otherwise. Utilizing 2000–3000 rads in 2 weeks, there was a significant improvement in 5-year survival among patients undergoing abdominal peritoneal resections (from 28.4% for the control group to 40.8% in treated patients). Similar studies are under way, with conflicting preliminary results.

Combined modality for CRC has often been used in adjuvant settings. The rate of relapse for combined modality therapy appears to be significantly lower than that of surgery alone. Several randomized and non-randomized studies have been done to evaluate the impact of adjuvant therapy on both the local recurrence rate and the overall rates in patients with rectal cancer. These studies included radiotherapy administered preoperatively, postoperatively, both pre- and postoperatively, and, more recently, with concomitant chemotherapy in single and multidrug regimens. In general, these studies indicated that the incidence of local recurrence can be reduced by approximately 50% with the use of a moderate dose of radiation. However, there is no demonstrable survival benefit for this adjuvant treatment approach.

The selection of patients who are likely to benefit from adjuvant therapy of CRC is based primarily on accurate surgical staging. The application of new techniques to assess the biologic aggressiveness of a tumor may allow identification of patients who have a particularly poor prognosis. Continued progress in understanding the molecular genetics of the initiation and progression of CRC may ultimately enable the use of molecular staging to further refine our clinical prognostic ability.

Recurrence patterns

Five-year survival rates were approximately 90% for colon cancer and 80% for rectal cancer, providing that diagnosis and treatment occur before the lesions have spread beyond the bowel to regional lymph nodes or distant metastatic sites. Early detection and meticulous surgical staging are mainly responsible for this high survival rate. However, 65% of patients present with higher staged disease, leading to the lower overall 5-year survival rate of 50%.

Recurrence patterns for CRC are the result of local extension or implantation, as well as lymphatic or hematogenous dissemination. Distant failures to the lung or liver are the most dramatic, but local and regional failures also occur frequently. As an initial pattern of failure from CRC, distant metastases alone are distinctly uncommon. Autopsy studies confirm that abdominal failure is common, and almost 75% of patients will die of intra-abdominal causes. Although lung and liver metastases are also common, they account for <25% of all deaths. Patients who have isolated liver metastases form a small but highly interesting and extensively studied group of patients. Early detection of such patients by CT scan has led to a new appreciation of the long median survival rates that may be achieved in patients who have disease limited to a single or a few unilobular metastases—18–24 months in many series. A few patients treated by direct infusion of 5-FU into the portal system have had impressive remissions, although follow-up is still brief. This type of approach seems beneficial for this subgroup of patients.

The use of CEA as a tumor marker has helped in monitoring patients for recurrent cancer. Often, an elevated CEA level is the earlier sign of recurrence. Minton has reported on the use of CEA values to direct second-look surgery. The goal of such surgery was to determine whether early detection, thus early intervention, would lead to improved survival in patients who had recurrent disease. Although a 5-year survival rate of approximately 30% has been reported in such patients when they are resected with curative intent, control studies of CEA-directed second-look surgery are lacking, and further studies are indicated.

Approximately 35% of patients with colon cancer who have surgery will have disease spread to regional lymph nodes, and about 25–35% of these patients will survive 5 years. After surgical resection for colorectal carcinoma, approximately 60% of tumor recurrences are within the first 2 years, and 90% occur within 5 years of the surgical resection. Despite these recurrence rates, a potential for cure remains in a select population of patients who develop recurrent colorectal carcinomas after definitive resection. For example, the recurrence of adenocarcinoma of the colon or rectum at a site of previous anastomosis is a failure of the primary surgical treatment, which in some patients can be managed successfully by additional operative procedures. In this particular group of patients, when complete resection of the recurrent tumor can be performed, the survival rates are surprisingly high.

Close follow-up and evaluation of patients who have colorectal carcinoma must be a priority. Some guidelines for clinical application may be drawn from knowledge of the patterns of tumor spread of colorectal carcinoma. High-risk areas for recurrence can be identified, and clinical attention must be focused on these sites for early detection of recurrence and subsequent palliative or curative resection. Obviously, a complete history and a complete physical examination are important elements of this type of evaluation. The value of rectal examinations and subsequent stool guaiac testing cannot be overemphasized.

One must be aware of the conditions that can produce false readings on stool guaiac testing. The physician must ensure that the patient has not been on a diet containing rare meat, turnips, or horseradish for 48 h. No aspirin or vitamin supplements containing vitamin C in excess of 250 mg/day should be taken. A history of bleeding from the rectum or a positive stool guaiac test should be followed by rigid proctosigmoidoscopy or flexible sigmoidoscopy examination. If the result of the endoscopy is negative, the patient should undergo a double-contrast barium enema or colonoscopy. Colonoscopy also plays an important role in the patients being observed for tumor detection. Many physicians recommend a colonoscopy every 6 months for the first year or two and then annually thereafter (Table 15–6).

Table 15–6 POSTOPERATIVE FOLLOW-UP IN COLORECTAL CARCINOMA

	Timing
First year after resection of primary tumor	
Physical examination (including stool guaiac testing)	Every 3 months
Liver function tests	Every 3 months (computed tomography scan if abnormal)
Carcinoembryonic antigen	Every 3 months (begin 6 weeks after surgery)
Colonoscopy	Every 6 months
Chest roentgenogram	Every 6 months
Second year after resection of primary tumor	
Physical examination (including stool guaiac testing)	Every 6 months
Liver function tests	Every 6 months
Carcinoembryonic antigen	Every 3 months
Colonoscopy	Every 6 months
Chest roentgenogram	Every 6 months
Third year and yearly thereafter	
Physical examination and stool guaiac testing	—
Liver function tests	—
Carcinoembryonic antigen	—
Colonoscopy	—
Intravenous pyelogram (rectal carcinoma)	—
Chest roentgenogram	—

Therapy of recurrence

For purposes of therapy, patients who have recurrent colorectal carcinomas may be divided into three groups:

1. those who have local or regional recurrences,
2. those who have hepatic metastasis, and
3. those who have widely disseminated disease.

Surgery for local or regional recurrences may result in secondary cure in selected groups of patients, although controlled trials are lacking. External beam irradiation for recurrent CRC has been associated with palliation of symptoms in a reasonably large proportion of patients, but low survival rates can be expected. Detection of recurrence at the anastomotic site by barium enema remains the most favorable pattern of recurrence in terms of secondary cure.

Patients with apparently localized hepatic metastasis may survive for 2 years, even without therapy. Uncontrolled studies of surgical resection of hepatic metastases have demonstrated a 5-year survival rate of approximately 25%

in selected patients. In some series, 25% of patients who have liver metastases have resectable disease, and 25% of that group will benefit from resection. This means that 7% of patients who have hepatic metastases will benefit from surgical resection. This is a small number, and its merits have to be closely evaluated with future studies. For patients who have unresectable hepatic metastases, infusional chemotherapy has been advocated. Hepatic-directed infusional therapy via the hepatic artery circulation results in drug concentrations to the liver that are significantly higher than those achieved by systemic infusion of the same drug. Non-randomized studies suggest that the response rates are indeed higher than those seen with systemic chemotherapy.

This approach has received renewed interest because of totally implantable infusion pumps. Phase II studies with such devices indicate response rates of more than 80%, with median survival times as long as 26 months. One drug favored for such infusion therapy is floxuridine. The drug 5-FU has been the most widely tested for systemic therapy, with a 20% partial objective response rate in most studies. The optimum dose and schedule have not been determined, although numerous studies of standard bolus therapy indicate that some moderate degree of systemic toxicity is necessary to achieve objective response. Clinical trials are under way to evaluate response rates and survival with continuous infusion 5-FU therapy compared with standard bolus therapy. In addition to 5-FU, only mitomycin-C and the nitrosoureas (CCNU, BCNU, methyl-CCNU) are generally considered to have any degree of activity. The most extensively evaluated combination of 5-FU and methyl-CCNU was initially reported to have a response rate of >40%, but later trials failed to confirm this superiority to 5-FU alone.

In general, benefits from systemic chemotherapy are limited by a low partial response rate with generally low duration of response. Although some patients may achieve palliation of symptoms, prolongation of survival has to date been an illusive goal. Further investigations of new agents and promising combinations are needed.

BLADDER CANCER

More than 90% of the bladder tumors occurring in the northern hemisphere are transitional cell lesions, with adenocarcinoma, squamous carcinoma, and sarcomas making up the remainder. Tumors originating from the urothelial lining of the bladder in women have an estimated occurrence of 16,200 cases in the USA in 2005, and 4200 women are estimated to die of this disease in the year 2005. Bladder cancers are estimated to occur in men. Bladder cancer is the sixth most common form of cancer in women, and the seventh leading cause of cancer deaths in women. Hematuria, usually associated with increased frequency of urination, is the usual warning signal promoted by the American Cancer Society and others. Smoking is the greatest risk factor for bladder cancer. Smokers experience twice the risk of non-smokers, and smoking is estimated to be responsible for approximately 37% of the bladder cancer deaths among women. Overall, the incidence of bladder cancer is four times greater among men than among women, and it is higher in white people than in black people. People living in urban areas and workers exposed to dye, rubber, or leather are also at higher risk. Surgery alone or in combination with other treatments is used in more than 90% of cases.

Pathology

Over 90% of urothelial tumors are transitional (epidermoid) cell carcinoma; the remainder are squamous cell carcinoma (6–8%), adenocarcinoma, or urachal carcinoma. Most epidermoid tumors originate in the lateral and posterior bladder wall, whereas adenocarcinoma is found in the dome of the bladder and the trigone. Lesions can occur within bladder diverticula. Urachal cancer originates from the urachus, an embryonic remnant of the gut, and is similar to colonic adenocarcinoma, producing CEA.

The urinary bladder is lined with five to seven avascular layers of transitional cells attached to a lamina propria that separates mucosa from muscle. Adipose tissue surrounds the bladder, and the parietal peritoneum covers the cephalad portion of the bladder. Nerves, blood vessels, and lymphatics invade muscle and lamina propria, explaining lymphatic and hematogenous patterns of dissemination with high-grade lesions. Although 70% or more of patients are diagnosed with superficial bladder cancer, 80–90% of patients with muscle-invasive lesions already have significant invasive disease at the time of diagnosis. Patients in the latter group account for most of the bladder cancer deaths, because 50% of patients with muscle-invasive disease already have distant metastasis at diagnosis (Fig. 15–9 and Table 15–7). Improved treatment of superficial disease will have only a limited effect on the overall survival. A major reduction on mortality without highly effective treatment for the metastatic disease requires improved detection of the aggressive malignancy while it is still superficial. Metastases can involve the hypogastric lymph node chain, as well as the obturator nodes at the junction of the internal and external iliac vessels. Nodal metastases may drain from this point to the aortic bifurcation and further up the aortic chain. Common sites for metastases include, in addition to regional lymph nodes, lung, liver, and bone.

Diagnosis and staging

Cystoscopy under anesthesia with bimanual palpation and appropriate biopsies is mandatory for diagnosis. Urinary cytology is extremely useful and more often is positive after cystoscopy. Flow cytometry is being used increasingly for diagnosis and to better define the extent of tumor aneuploidy as a possible prognostic sign. Additional tests include

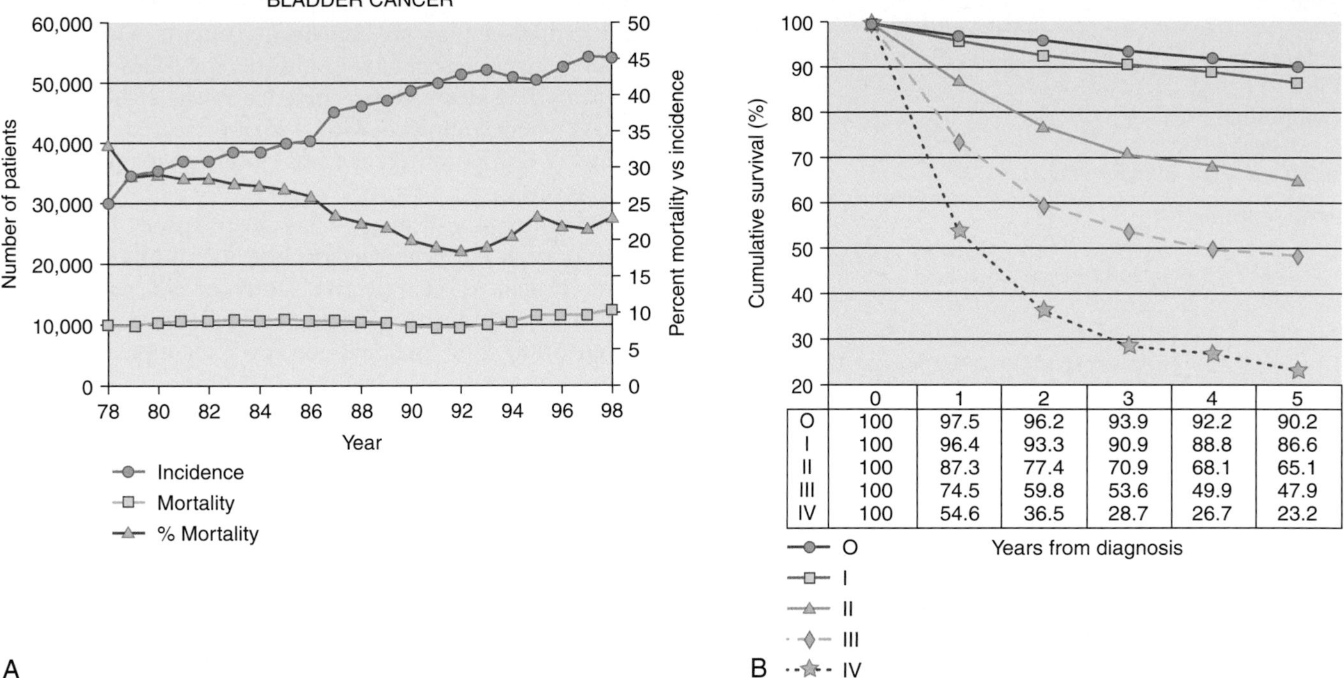

	0	1	2	3	4	5
O	100	97.5	96.2	93.9	92.2	90.2
I	100	96.4	93.3	90.9	88.8	86.6
II	100	87.3	77.4	70.9	68.1	65.1
III	100	74.5	59.8	53.6	49.9	47.9
IV	100	54.6	36.5	28.7	26.7	23.2

Figure 15–9 *A,* The overall (men and women) number of new patients with bladder cancer has increased in the USA. However, mortality has remained relatively constant despite these increased incidence numbers. *B,* Five-year cumulative relative survival rates by American Joint Committee on Cancer stage at diagnosis. (A, From Lamm DL: Bladder cancer. CA Cancer J Clin 48[5]:264, 1998.)

Table 15–7 TUMOR, NODE, METASTASIS STAGING FOR BLADDER CARCINOMA

American Joint Committee on Cancer stage	Tumor, node, metastasis staging
0	Ta-Tis, N0, M0
I	T1, N0, M0
II	T2–T3a, N0, M0
III	T3b–T4a, N0, M0
IV	T4b, any T, any N, M0/1

(From the American Joint Committee on Cancer.)

an intravenous urogram to evaluate the upper tracts, as well as the urinary bladder, and a pelvic and abdominal CT scan. The role of transvaginal and abdominal ultrasonography is still uncertain.

None of the current tumor markers (human chorionic gonadotropin, CEA, CA-125, or CA-19-9), when used alone, is elevated in more than 50% of patients, and there is no marker to detect occult disease. Whereas the Jewett–Strong–Marshall staging system has been used in the USA, the American Joint Commission on Cancer system outlined in Table 15–8 is more precise. Stage 0 indicates superficial mucosal tumors, both SIS (Tis) and exophytic papillary (Ta) lesions. Invasion into the lamina propria is stage A (T1); stage B1 (T2) denotes tumor confined to less than half of the bladder muscle, and B2 (T3a) denotes tumor involving more than half of the bladder muscle. Anaplastic tumors are deeply infiltrating in the muscle, whereas grade 1 well-differentiated lesions tend to be B1. Stage C (T3b) tumors involve perivesical fat. Stage D1 involves adjacent local extension to prostate (T4a) or lymph nodes below the sacral promontory (N1–3), and D2 (N4) denotes nodal involvement above the sacrum. Superficial tumors (Ta, Tis, T1) represent about 70% of newly diagnosed cases. Muscle infiltrating tumors (T2, T3, T4), represent about 25%, and metastatic tumors (N-positive or M-positive) represent about 5% of cases.

Treatment and results

Therapy for superficial lesions (stages 0, A, and sometimes B1) is in most cases endoscopic resection and fulguration with cystoscopy repeated every 3 months. When lesions recur frequently or are diffuse, another therapy utilized is thiotepa 60 mg/60 mL normal saline instilled intravesically for 2 h and then weekly for 6 consecutive weeks. Approximately 30–40% of patients will respond, particularly those with low-grade papillary lesions. Because this drug is absorbed after intravesical administration, severe myelosuppression can occur. Bacillus Calmette–Guérin (BCG), 120 mg/50 mL normal saline, has been found to be extremely efficacious when given weekly for 6 weeks, resulting in 80% of cases achieving complete remission after intravesical administration. Other agents utilized include mitomycin-C, 20–60 mg/20–40 mL, and doxorubicin 20–60 mg; both of these agents can cause serious bladder irritation after intravesical administration, and complete response rates are reported at only 50% compared with 80% for BCG. Radical cystectomy is utilized for

Table 15–8 BLADDER CANCER STAGING SYSTEMS

American Joint Committee on Cancer stage	Bladder cancer	Jewett–Strong–Marshall stage
Primary tumor (T)		
TX	Cannot be assessed	—
T0	No tumor clinically	—
Tis	Carcinoma in situ (flat)	0
Ta	Papillary non-invasive tumor	0
T1	No microscopic invasion beyond the lamina propria; induration on the bimanual examination; freely mobile mass that disappears after resection	A
T2	Microscopic invasion of the superficial bladder muscle; mobile induration of the bladder on bimanual examination that disappears after resection	B1
T3	Tumor invades into the muscle or perivesical fat; induration or a nodular mobile mass that persists after transurethral resection	—
T3a	Deep muscle invasion	B2
T3b	Perivesical fat invasion	C
T4	Tumor fixed or invades the neighboring structures	—
T4a	Prostate, uterus, vagina invasion	D1
T4b	Tumor fixed to the pelvic walls or invades the abdominal wall	D1
Regional lymph nodes (N)		
NX	Cannot be assessed	—
N0	No tumor	—
N1	Single homolateral regional lymph node	D1
N2	Contralateral, bilateral, multiple regional nodes	D1
N3	Fixed mass on the pelvic wall with space between the mass and the tumor	D1
N4	Tumor involves just regional lymph nodes	D2
Distant metastasis (M)		
MX	Cannot be assessed	—
M0	No known distant metastasis	—
M1	Distant metastases	D2

diffuse or recurrent superficial lesions, a procedure resulting in a 5-year survival rate of 70–90%. Clinicians vary in their judgment of precisely what existing circumstances constitute indications for radical therapy.

Preoperative radiotherapy was utilized in the 1970s, with disappointing results. A recent trial from the M.D. Anderson Hospital identified a subset for whom preoperative radiation may be beneficial. Patients with stage T3 tumors given preoperative radiotherapy followed by a cystectomy had decreased recurrence rates, 28% vs. 9% at 5 years, when compared with a group treated with cystectomy alone. No difference was observed for patients with T2 lesions.

Postoperative therapy has been used for patients with positive surgical margins, but no randomized trial has been done. A retrospective study of 92 patients from Milan reported that patients without nodal metastases given 5000 cGy after cystectomy had improved survival rates.

Five randomized trials have studied adjuvant therapy in patients with muscle invasion on pathologic review of the cystectomy specimen. Three trials with different chemotherapy requirements showed no benefit. Two other trials suggest a benefit for platinum chemotherapy over observation alone.

Standard therapy for stage B and C disease is radical cystectomy with resection of local pelvic nodes. If local organ invasion has occurred, the prostate, seminal vesicle, urethra, and part of the ureters may have to be removed. Recent modifications of urinary diversion have resulted in the contingent pouch as an option for these patients. Segmental or partial cystectomy should be used only in selected patients presenting with a single lesion outside the trigone and without areas of Tis. Most data for preoperative and postoperative radiation therapy suggest little benefit in preventing tumor dissemination. Overall 5-year survival rates for stages B and C range from 30 to 50%; in patients presenting with papillary low-grade lesions, survival is 60–75%. When surgery is medically contraindicated, supervoltage irradiation, 6000–7000 cGy in 6–8 weeks, can produce 5-year survival rates of approximately 20–30% or higher for B1-1 and C disease. A major difficulty in evaluating the efficacy of irradiation is the high clinical staging error with large bladder tumors.

For chemotherapy, active single agents are cisplatin and methotrexate, and to a lesser extent doxorubicin, vinblastine, and mitomycin-C. Single agents induce response in 15–30% of cases; few responses are complete. Cisplatin combined with paclitaxel, docetaxel, gemcitabine, or both paclitaxel and gemcitabine has been reported to have acceptable toxicity and response rates from 60 to 90%. Lymph node involvement (stage D2, N1-4) is an extremely poor prognostic sign, with 50% of the patients undergoing radical cystectomy and lymph node dissection dying in <1 year; 87% die in <2 years. The 5-year survival rate is 0–7%, and most patients are dying of disseminated disease.

Follow-up of patients after therapy consists of a chest film at 2- to 3-month intervals, urine cytology, and an intravenous urogram at 6- to 12-month intervals. Abdominal and pelvic CT scans should be performed within the first 2 months after radical cystectomy to serve as a baseline for future examination at 5- to 6-month intervals during the first 1–2 years.

BIBLIOGRAPHY

COLORECTAL CANCER

Aaltonen LA, Salovaara R, Kristo P et al: Incidence of hereditary nonpolyposis colorectal cancer and the feasibility of molecular screening for the disease. N Engl J Med 338:1481, 1998.

Aarino A, Sankila R, Pukkula E et al: Cancer risk in mutation carriers of DNA mismatch repair genes. Int J Cancer 81:214–218, 1999.

Achkar E, Carey W: Small polyps found during fiberoptic sigmoidoscopy in asymptomatic patients. Ann Intern Med 109:880, 1988.

Alexander JA, Wantanabe T, Wu T-T et al: Histopathologic identification of colon cancer with microsatellite instability. Am J Path 158:527–535, 2001.

American College of Obstetricians and Gynecologists: Committee Opinion: Routine Cancer Screening. Washington, ACOG, 1997, p 185.

American College of Obstetricians and Gynecologists: Report of task force on routine cancer screening. ACOG Committee Opinion No. 68. Washington, ACOG, 1989.

American Joint Committee on Cancer: Manual for Staging of Cancer, 3rd edn. Philadelphia, Lippincott, 1988.

André T, Boni C, Mounedji-Boudiaf L et al: Oxaliplatin, fluorouracil, and leucovorin as adjuvant treatment for colon cancer. N Engl J Med 350:2343, 2004.

Astler VB, Coller FA: The prognostic significance of direct extension of cancer of the colon and rectum. Ann Surg 139:846, 1954.

Balslev JB et al: Postoperative radiotherapy in Dukes' B and C carcinoma of the rectum and rectosigmoid: a randomized multicenter study. Cancer 58:22, 1986.

Beart RW Jr: Colon, rectum, and anus. Cancer 33:684, 1990.

Bohlman TW, Katon BM, Lipshutz GR: Fiberoptic pan sigmoidoscopy: an evaluation and comparison with rigid sigmoidoscopy. Gastroenterology 72:644, 1977.

Bostick RM, Potter JD, Kushi LH et al: Sugar, meat, and fat intake, and non-dietary risk factors for colon cancer incidence in Iowa women. Cancer Causes Control 5:38, 1994.

Brown GJE, St. John DJB, Macrae FA et al: Cancer risk in young women at risk of hereditary nonpolyposis colorectal cancer: implications for gynecologic surveillance. Gynecol Oncol 80:346, 2001.

Burke W, Petersen G, Lynch P et al: Recommendations for follow-up care of individuals with an inherited predisposition to cancer. JAMA 277:915, 1997.

Burkitt DP: Some neglected leads to cancer causation. J Natl Cancer Inst 47:913, 1971.

Buroker TR et al: A controlled evaluation of recent approaches to biochemical modulation of enhancement of 5-fluorouracil therapy in colorectal carcinoma. J Clin Oncol 3:1624, 1985.

Calle EE, Miracle-McMahill HL, Thun MJ et al: Estrogen replacement therapy and risk of fatal colon cancer in a prospective cohort of postmenopausal women. J Natl Cancer Inst 87:51, 1995.

Chau I, Norman AR, Cunningham D et al: A randomized comparison between six months of bolus fluorouracil/leucovorin and 12 weeks of protracted venous infusion fluorouracil as adjuvant treatment in colorectal cancer. Ann Oncol 16: 549, 2005.

Cole CJ, Pollack A, Zagars GK et al: Local control of muscle-invasive bladder cancer: preoperative radiotherapy and cystectomy versus cystectomy alone. Int J Radiat Oncol Biol Phys 32:331, 1995.

Coutsoftides T et al: Malignant polyps of the colon and rectum: a clinicopathologic study. Dis Colon Rectum 22:82, 1979.

Cozzarini CZ, Pelegrini D, Fallini M et al: Reappraisal of the role of adjuvant radiotherapy in muscle-invasive transitional cell carcinoma of the bladder. Int J Radiat Oncol Biol Phys 45:221, 1999.

Davis HL: Chemotherapy of large bowel cancer. Cancer 50:2638, 1982.

De Cosse JJ, Tsioulias GJ, Jacobson JS: Colorectal cancer: detection, treatment, and rehabilitation. CA Cancer J Clin 44:27, 1994.

DeVita VT, Hellman S, Rosenberg SA (eds): Cancer: Principles and Practice of Oncology, 2nd edn. Philadelphia, Lippincott, 1985.

Division of Cancer Prevention and Control, National Cancer Institute: Working Guidelines for Early Cancer Detection: Rationale and Supporting Evidence to Decrease Mortality. Bethesda, NCI, 1987, p 1.

Dukes CE, Bussey HJR: The spread of rectal cancer and its effect on prognosis. Br J Cancer 12:309, 1958.

Dwyer J: Dietary fiber and colorectal cancer risk. Nutr Rev 51:147, 1993.

Eckert R, Zeidan Z: Treatment, follow up and prevention of colorectal carcinoma: strategies and controversies in the year 2005. Schweiz Rundsch Med Prax 94:151, 2005.

Ederer F, Church TR, Mandel JS: Fecal occult blood screening in the Minnesota study: role of chance detection of lesions. J Natl Cancer Inst 89:1423, 1997.

Ehya H, O'Hara BJ: Brush cytology in the diagnosis of colonic neoplasms. Cancer 66:1563, 1990.

Enblad P, Adami HO, Glimelius B et al: The risk of subsequent primary malignant diseases after cancers of the colon and rectum. Cancer 65:2091, 1990.

Fath RB, Winawer SJ: Early diagnosis of colorectal cancer. Annu Rev Med 34:501, 1984.

Fearon ER, Cho KR, Nigro JM et al: Identification and characterization of the familial adenomatous polyposis coli gene. Cell 66:589, 1991.

Ferguson LR, Lynch JF: Towards reducing the incidence of colorectal cancer: the role of inheritance and diet. Mutagenesis 8:377, 1993.

Fernandez B, La Vecchia C, D'Avanzo B et al: Oral contraceptives, hormone replacement therapy and the risk of colorectal cancer. Br J Cancer 73:1431, 1996.

Gastrointestinal Tumor Study Group: Adjuvant therapy of colon cancer: results of a prospectively randomized trial. N Engl J Med 310:737, 1984.

Gerard A et al: Preoperative radiotherapy as adjuvant treatment in rectal cancer. Ann Surg 208:606, 1988.

Gilbertsen VA et al: The earlier detection of colorectal cancers: a preliminary report of the results of the occult blood study. Cancer 45:2899, 1980.

Gilbertsen VA, Nelms JN: The prevention of invasive cancer of the rectum. Cancer 41:1137, 1978.

Giovannucci E, Colditz GA, Stampfer MJ et al: Physical activity, obesity, and risk of colorectal adenoma in women (United States). Cancer Causes Control 7:253, 1996.

Giovannucci E, Martinez ME: Tobacco, colorectal cancer, and adenomas: a review of the evidence. J Natl Cancer Inst 88:1717, 1996.

Giovannucci E, Rimm EB, Stampfer MJ et al: Intake of fat, meat, and fiber in relation to risk of colon cancer in men. Cancer Res 54:2390, 1994.

Grabe JL, Kozarek RA, Sanowski RA: Flexible versus rigid sigmoidoscopy: a comparison using inexpensive 35 cm flexible proctosigmoidoscopy. Am J Gastroenterol 78:569, 1983.

Grage TB, Moss SE: Adjuvant chemotherapy in cancer of the colon and rectum: controlled randomized trial. Surg Clin North Am 61:1321, 1981.

Greenberg ER, Baron JA, Tosteson TD et al: A clinical trial of antioxidant vitamins to prevent colorectal adenoma. Polyp Prevention Study Group. N Engl J Med 331:141, 1994.

Greenwald P: Colon cancer overview. Cancer Suppl 70:1206, 1992.

Grem JL, Allegra CJ: Toxicity of levamisole and 5-fluorouracil in human colon carcinoma cells. J Natl Cancer Inst 81:1413, 1989.

Grodstein F, Martinez ME, Platz EA et al: Postmenopausal hormone use and risk for colorectal cancer and adenoma. Ann Intern Med 128:705, 1998.

Gryska PV, Cohen AM: Screening asymptomatic patients at high risk for colon cancer with full colonoscopy. Dis Colon Rectum 30:18, 1987.

Gunderson LL, Sosin H: Areas of failure found at reoperation (second or symptomatic look) following "curative surgery" for adenocarcinoma of the rectum. Cancer 34:1278, 1974.

Hardcastle JD, Chamberlain JO, Robinson MH et al: Randomised controlled trial of faecal occult blood screening for colorectal cancer. Lancet 348:1472, 1996.

Health and Public Policy Committee, American College of Physicians: Clinical competence in colonoscopy. Ann Intern Med 107:772, 1987.

Higgins GA et al: Preoperative radiation and surgery for cancer of the rectum, Veterans Administration Surgical Oncology Group Trial II. Cancer 58:352, 1986.

Hornsby-Lewis L, Winawer SJ: Natural history and current management of colorectal polyps. Oncology 4:139, 1990.

Howe GR, Benito E, Castelleto R et al: Dietary intake of fiber and decreased risk of cancers of the colon and rectum: evidence from the combined analysis of 13 case-controlled studies. J Natl Cancer Inst 84:1887, 1992.

Hyman J, Baron JA, Dain BJ et al: Dietary and supplemental calcium and the recurrence of colorectal adenomas. Cancer Epidemiol Biomarkers Prev 7:291, 1998.

Jacobs EJ, White E, Weiss NS: Exogenous hormones, reproductive history, and colon cancer. Cancer Causes Control 3:359, 1994.

Kearney J, Giovannucci E, Rimm EB et al: Diet, alcohol, and smoking and the occurrence of hyperplastic polyps of the colon and rectum (United States). Cancer Causes Control 6:45, 1995.

Keku TO, Millikan RC, Martin C et al: Family history of colon cancer: what does it mean and how is it useful? Am J Prev Med 24(2):170, 2003.

Kritchevsky D: Diet, nutrition, and cancer: the role of fiber. Cancer 58:1830, 1986.

Kronborg O, Fenger C, Olsen J et al: Randomised study of screening for colorectal cancer with faecal occult blood test. Lancet 348:1467, 1996.

Kuo DY, Smith HO, Runwicz CD et al: Cecal cancer in teenager presenting with a pelvic mass: a case report and review of the literature. Gynecol Oncol 55:149, 1994.

Laken SJ, Petersen GM, Gruber SB et al: Familial colorectal cancer in Ashkenazim due to a hyper mutable tract in APC. Nat Genet 79:113, 1997.

Laurie JA et al: Surgical adjuvant therapy of large-bowel carcinoma: an evaluation of levamisole and the combination of levamisole and 5-fluorouracil. J Clin Oncol 7:1447, 1989.

Letsou G, Ballantyne GH, Zdon MJ et al: Screening for colorectal neoplasms: a comparison of the fecal occult blood test and endoscopic examination. Dis Colon Rectum 30:839, 1987.

Levin B: Colorectal cancer: approach to long-term management. Adv Oncol 2:16, 1986.

Lipkin M, Newmark H: Effect of added dietary calcium on colonic epithelial cell proliferation in subjects at high risk for familial colonic cancer. N Engl J Med 313:1381, 1985.

Lush DT: Screening for colorectal cancer: use of a new protocol may reduce death rates. Postgrad Med 96:99, 1994.

Lynch HT et al: Colon cancer genetics. Cancer Suppl 70(5):1300, 1992.

Lynch HT, Smyrk TC: Identifying hereditary nonpolyposis colorectal cancer. N Engl J Med 338:1537, 1998.

Ma J, Stampfer MJ, Giovannucci E et al: Methylenetetrahydrofolate reductase polymorphism, dietary interactions, and risk of colorectal cancer. Cancer Res 57:1098, 1997.

Maclennan R, Macrae F, Bain C et al: Randomized trial of intake of fat, fiber, and beta carotene to prevent colorectal adenomas: the Australian Polyp Prevention Project. J Natl Cancer Inst 87:1760, 1995.

Mandel JS, Bond JH, Church TR et al: Reducing mortality from colorectal cancer by screening for fecal occult blood, Minnesota Colon Cancer Control Study. N Engl J Med 328:1365, 1993. Erratum N Engl J Med 1993 329(9):672.

Mansour EG et al: Combined modality therapy following resection of colorectal carcinoma in patients with non-measurable intra-abdominal metastases, an ECOG study 3282. Proc Am Soc Clin Oncol 9:107, 1990.

Metlin C et al: Management and survival of adenocarcinoma of the rectum in the United States: results of a national survey by the American College of Surgery. Oncology 39:265, 1978.

Metlin C, Cummings KM: The current status of early detection and screening of colorectal cancer. Semin Surg Oncol 2:215, 1988.

Minton JP: Colon cancer: special surgical considerations. Cancer 50:2624, 1982.

Moertel CG: Chemotherapy for colorectal cancer. N Engl J Med 330:1136, 1994.

Musinski SE: Colorectal cancer screening by obstetrician-gynecologists. Am J Obstet Gynecol 184:1054, 2001.

Ness R, Klein R, Dittus R: The cost-effectiveness of fecal DNA testing for colorectal cancer. Gastrointest Endosc 57(5):622, 2003.

Neugut AI, Pita S: Role of sigmoidoscopy in screening for colorectal cancer: a critical view. Gastroenterology 95:492, 1988.

Newcomb PA, Norfleet RG, Storer BE et al: Screening sigmoidoscopy and colorectal cancer mortality. J Natl Cancer Inst 84(20):1572, 1992.

Niederhuber JE: Colon and rectum cancer. Cancer 71:4187, 1993.

O'Brien MJ, Winawer SJ, Zauber AG et al: The national polyp study: patients and polyp characteristics associated with high-grade dysplasia in colorectal adenomas. Gastroenterology 98:371, 1990.

Page DL, Fleming ID, Fritz A et al: In Greene Fl (ed): AJCC Cancer Staging Manual, 6th edn. New York, Springer-Verlag, 2002.

Peleg II, Maibach HT, Brown SH et al: Aspirin and nonsteroidal anti-inflammatory drug use and the risk of subsequent colorectal cancer. Arch Intern Med 154:394, 1994.

Pignone M, Rich M, Teutsch SM et al: Screening for colorectal cancer in adults at average risk: a summary of the evidence for the U.S. Preventive Services Task Force. Am Intern Med 137(2):132, 2002.

Platz EA, Martinez ME, Grodstein F et al: Parity and other reproductive factors and risk of adenomatous polyps of the distal colorectum (United States). Cancer Causes Control 8:894, 1997.

Poplin EA, Benedetti JK, Estes NC et al: Phase III Southwest Oncology Group 9415/Intergroup 0153 randomized trial of fluorouracil, leucovorin, and levamisole versus fluorouracil continuous infusion and levamisole for adjuvant treatment of stage III and high-risk stage II colon cancer. J Clin Oncol 23(9):1819, 2005.

Powell SM, Zilz N, Beazer-Barclay Y et al: APC mutations occur early during colorectal tumorigenesis. Nature 359:235, 1992.

Ransohoff DF, Lang CA: Screening for colorectal cancer with the fecal occult blood test: a background paper. American College of Physicians. Ann Intern Med 126:811, 1997.

Ransohoff DF, Lang CA: Screening for colorectal cancer. N Engl J Med 325:37, 1991.

Reddy BS et al: Chemoprevention of colon carcinogenesis by concurrent administration of piroxicam, a nonsteroidal antiinflammatory drug with D, L-a-difluoromethyl ornithine, an ornithine decarboxylase inhibitor in diet. Cancer Res 50:2562, 1990.

Reddy BS, Burill C, Rigotty J: Effects of diets in omega-3 and omega-6 fatty acids on initiation and post initiation stages of colon carcinogenesis. Cancer Res 51:487, 1991.

Rosato FE, Marks SG: Changing site distribution patterns of colorectal cancer at Thomas Jefferson University Hospital. Dis Colon Rectum 24:93, 1981.

Selby JV, Friedman GD, Quesenberry CP Jr et al: A case control study of screening sigmoidoscopy and mortality from colorectal cancer. N Engl J Med 326(10):653, 1992.

Silverberg E, Lubera JA: Cancer statistics. Cancer 38:5, 1988.

Silverberg E, Lubera JA: Cancer statistics. Cancer 39:3, 1989.

Skinner DG, Daniels JR, Russell CA et al: The role of adjuvant chemotherapy following cystectomy for invasive bladder cancer: a prospective comparative trial. J Urol 145:459, 1991.

Stearns M: Benign and malignant neoplasms of the colon and rectum: diagnosis and management. Surg Clin North Am 58:695, 1978.

Stockholm Rectal Cancer Study Group: Preoperative short-term radiation therapy in operable rectal carcinoma. Cancer 66:49, 1990.

Sun W, Haller DG: Adjuvant therapy of colon cancer. Semin Oncol. 32(1):95, 2005.

Thompson WM, Trenkner SW: Staging colorectal carcinoma. Radiol Clin North Am 32:25, 1994.

Traverso G, Shuber A, Levin B et al: Detection of APC mutations in fecal DNA from patients with colorectal tumors. N Engl J Med 346(5):311, 2002.

Traverso G, Shuber A, Olsson L et al: Detection of proximal colorectal cancers through analysis of faecal DNA. Lancet 359(9304):404, 2002.

Vargus PA, Alberts DS: Primary prevention of colorectal cancer through dietary modification. Cancer Suppl 70:1229, 1992.

Verhoegen H, DeCree J, DeCock W et al: Levamisole therapy in patients with colorectal cancer. In Terry WD, Rosenberg SA (eds): Immunotherapy of Human Cancer. New York, Excerpta Medica, 1982.

Vogelstein B, Fearon ER, Hamilton SR et al: Genetic alterations during colorectal tumor development. N Engl J Med 319:525, 1988.

Voskuil DW, Kampman E, Grubben MJ et al: Meat consumption and preparation, and genetic susceptibility in relation to colorectal adenomas. Cancer Lett 114:81, 1997.

Wargovich MJ: New dietary anti carcinogens and prevention of gastrointestinal cancer. Dis Colon Rectum 31:72, 1988.

Watson P, Bützow R, Lynch HT et al: The clinical features of ovarian cancer in hereditary nonpolyposis colorectal cancer. Gynecol Oncol 82:223, 2001.

Waye JD: Techniques of polypectomy: hot biopsy forceps and snare polypectomy. Am J Gastroenterol 82:615, 1987.

Whitmore WF Jr: Bladder cancer: an overview. CA Cancer J Clin 38:213, 1988.

Wilkes GM: Therapeutic options in the management of colon cancer: 2005 update. Clin J Oncol Nurs 9(1):31, 2005.

Willett WC, Stampfer MJ, Colditz GA et al: Relation of meat, fat, and fiber intake to the risk of colon cancer in a prospective study among women. N Engl J Med 323:1664, 1990.

Willett WC: Diet, nutrition, and avoidable cancer. Environ Health Perspect 103 (suppl 8):165, 1995.

Willett WC: The search for the causes of breast and colon cancer. Nature 338:389, 1989.

Williams JT, Slack WW: A prospective study of sexual function after major colorectal surgery. Br J Surg 67:772, 1980.

Winawer S, Fletcher R, Rex D et al: Colorectal cancer screening and surveillance: clinical guidelines and rationale—update based on new evidence. Gastroenterology 124(2):544, 2003.

Winawer SJ et al: Current status of fecal occult blood testing in screening for colorectal cancer. CA Cancer J Clin 32:100, 1982.

Winawer SJ et al: Risk of colorectal cancer in the families of patients with adenomatous polyps. N Engl J Med 334:82, 1996.

Wynder EL, Bandaru SR, Weisburger JH: Environmental dietary factors in colorectal cancer: some unresolved issues. Cancer Suppl 70:1222, 1992.

Yagoda A: Chemotherapy for advanced bladder cancer. In Yagoda A (ed): Bladder Cancer: Future Directions for Treatment. New York, ParkRow, 1986, pp 87–106.

Zauber A, Winawer S: Initial management and follow-up surveillance of patients with colorectal adenomas. Gastroenterol Clin North Am 26:85, 1997.

BLADDER CANCER

Fisher HAG: Diagnosis and management of early-stage bladder cancer. Curr Concepts Oncol 4:1986.

Herr HW et al: BCG therapy alters the progression of superficial bladder cancer. J Clin Oncol 6:1450, 1988.

Herr HW, Laudone VP, Whitmore WF Jr: Review article: an overview of intravesical therapy for superficial bladder tumors. J Urol 138:363, 1987.

Herr HW: Conservative management of muscle-invading bladder cancer: prospective experience. J Urol 138:1162, 1987.

Marshall VF, McCarron JP Jr: The curability of vesical cancer: greater now or then? Cancer Res 37:2753, 1977.

Mommsen S, Aagaard J: Tobacco as a risk factor in bladder cancer. Carcinogenesis 4:335, 1983.

Murphy WM et al: Urinary cytology and bladder cancer: the cellular features of transitional cell neoplasms. Cancer 53:1555, 1984.

Prout GR Jr et al: Combined therapies in the treatment with muscle-invasive bladder carcinoma: a preliminary report of a bladder-sparing effort. J Urol 139:268, 1988.

Prout GR Jr, Griffin PP, Shipley WU: Bladder carcinoma as a systemic disease. Cancer 43:2532, 1979.

Shipley WU et al: Full-dose irradiation for patients with invasive bladder carcinoma: clinical and histological factors prognostic of improved survival. J Urol 134:679, 1985.

Shipley WU, Prout GR Jr, Kaufman DS: Bladder cancer: advances in laboratory innovations and clinical management, with emphasis on innovations allowing bladder-sparing approaches for patients with invasive tumors. Cancer 65:675, 1990.

Soloway MS: Surgery and intravesical chemotherapy in the management of superficial bladder cancer. Semin Urol 1:23, 1983.

Thompson IM: The evaluation of microscopic hematuria: a population-based study. J Urol 138:1189, 1987.

16 Cancer in Pregnancy

Krishnansu S. Tewari, M.D.

BACKGROUND AND EPIDEMIOLOGY OF CANCER IN PREGNANCY

Cancer in pregnancy appears to challenge the clinician more commonly of late. This is undoubtedly the result of the trend to defer childbearing into the fourth decade of life, when the incidence of some of the more common malignant neoplasms begins to rise (Fig. 16–1). The tragedy of the presence of a malignant neoplasm discovered during pregnancy raises many issues (Table 16–1). Fortunately, the peak incidence years for most malignant diseases do not overlap the peak reproductive years (Table 16–2). Thus, as in any unusual situation that physicians rarely encounter, clear therapeutic decisions are not readily at hand. On the other hand, a significant number of well-studied reviews can provide some guidance in this dilemma. The largest series ever reported was that of Barber and Brunschwig in 1968, which consisted of 700 cases of cancer in pregnancy. The most common malignant neoplasms in that series were breast tumors and leukemias–lymphomas as a category, melanomas, gynecologic cancer, and bone tumors, in that order. Other authors suggest that gynecologic malignant neoplasms are second only to breast carcinoma, and remind us that cancer of the colon and thyroid are also seen in pregnancy (Table 16–3).

The incidence of cancer in pregnancy is unclear but is estimated to be one in 1000. From historical case series collected at a variety of referral institutions, many commentators have concluded that cervical cancer is the most frequent malignancy to complicate pregnancy. This finding is likely to be inaccurate, as the incidence of cervical cancer in the USA and in most developed nations is steadily declining. In a 1984 population-based study, Haas reviewed the National Cancer Registry of the German Democratic Republic for the years between 1970 and 1979, and from a total of 31,353 cancer cases and 2,103,112 live births among women between the ages of 15 and 44 years, 355 pregnant women were diagnosed with a malignancy. Dinh and Warshal have emphasized that in the Haas study, the incidence of cancer in pregnancy per 1000 live births rose from 0.02 for women aged 15–19 years, to 2.3 for women aged 40–44 years. In order of decreasing frequency, cancer of the cervix, breast, ovary, lymphoma, melanoma, brain and leukemia were found to complicate pregnancy.

Data from the Surveillance, Epidemiology, and End Results program in the USA from 1992 to 1996 estimate that among women aged 15–44 years, in order of decreasing frequency, cancer of the breast, melanoma, thyroid, cervix, lymphoma, and ovary are coincident with pregnancy. The Centers for Disease Control and Prevention have highlighted pregnancy trends in the USA over the preceding 25 years. While the birth rate for women <30 years rose slowly until the early 1990s, it has steadily declined since then. In contrast, the birth rate for women aged >30 years has risen steadily over the past two decades by an average of 67%. Because of the changing attitudes regarding the role of women as part of the workforce, the delay in childbearing observed in this country will be associated with at least three considerations that are germane to the subject of this chapter.

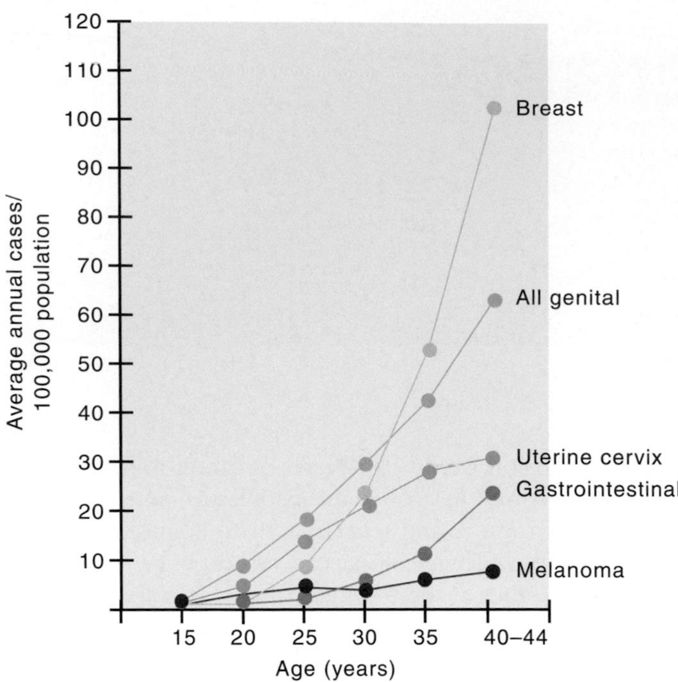

Figure 16–1 Incidence by age of more common malignancies seen in pregnancy. (Data from the American Cancer Society Facts and Figures, 1995.)

- As many malignancies manifest with advancing age, it is reasonable to expect an increase in the occurrence of some specific types of cancers during pregnancy.
- Theoretic concerns regarding possible effects of pregnancy-derived hormones among cancer survivors contemplating pregnancy will need to be addressed.
- With the popularization of investigational fertility-sparing medical and surgical therapy for nulliparous patients with seemingly early lesions who strongly desire to retain childbearing capacity, there exists an increased potential for the oncologist to encounter recurrent disease irrespective of whether pregnancy occurs.

The enormous physiologic changes of pregnancy suggest many possible influences on the malignant state. First, it has been assumed by many that malignant neoplasms arising in tissues and organs influenced by the endocrine system are possibly subject to exacerbation with pregnancy, and this has often been erroneously extrapolated to a recommendation for "therapeutic" abortion. Second, the anatomic and physiologic changes of pregnancy may obscure the subtle changes of an early neoplasm. Third, the increased vascularity and lymphatic drainage may contribute to early dissemination of the malignant process. Although all these hypotheses are interesting, the validity of each is variable, even within the same organ.

Table 16–1 CANCER IN PREGNANCY: ISSUES TO CONSIDER

Oncologic issues	Obstetric issues	Ethical, religious, medicolegal, and socioeconomic issues
Timing of surgery	Fetal effects of therapy	Pregnancy termination
Type of therapy	Antepartum fetal surveillance	Independent advocate for the fetus
Maternal effects of therapy	Corticosteroid administration	Fetal viability
Maternal surveillance	Amniocentesis	Maternal risk
Fertility-sparing therapy	Timing of delivery	Healthcare costs
	Route of delivery	Principle of beneficence
	Neonatal effects of therapy	Right to autonomy
	Long-term effects of therapy	Mother's overall prognosis[a]

[a]Important to take into account the estimated length of time the mother will realistically live to spend with the baby.

Table 16–2 CANCER AND YOUNG WOMEN

Site	Occurrence in women aged 15–44 years (%)
Cervix	35
Ovary	15
All genital	18
Lymphomas	23
Thyroid	50
Bones and joints	27
Melanoma	27
Breast	15
Leukemia	10
Soft tissues	20

Table 16–3 INCIDENCE OF THE MORE COMMON MALIGNANCIES THAT COMPLICATE PREGNANCY

Site or type	Estimated incidence per 1000 pregnancies
Cervix uteri	2.3
Non-invasive	1.3
Invasive	1.0
Breast	0.33
Melanoma	0.14
Ovary	0.10
Thyroid	Unknown
Leukemia	0.01
Lymphoma	0.01
Colorectal	0.02

(From Allen HH, Nisker JA [eds]: Cancer in Pregnancy: Therapeutic Guidelines. Mt. Kisco, Futura Publishing, 1986.)

Several additional points must be emphasized when caring for the pregnant patient with symptoms suggestive of cancer or in whom the diagnosis has been established. Although pregnancy is usually characterized by extensive medical observation, a *delay in diagnosis* can occur if attention is not paid to the subtle presentation of malignancies. Thus, although pregnancy has not been shown to increase the virulence of any tumor type, many pregnancy-associated cancers portend a poor prognosis for the mother. Although several essayists have claimed that the conduct of the pregnancy is not affected by the cohabitation of malignancy, the oncologist must recognize that some tumor types have been shown to have metastasized to the placenta and even to the fetus. In all cases of pregnancy complicated by malignancy, it is advisable to have a *multidisciplinary team of specialists* involved in the care of the patient.

When considering therapy in pregnancy, surgery is rarely contraindicated, with the optimal time being in the second trimester. Chemotherapy for the most part should have restricted use during the first trimester but can be safely administered thereafter. Certain diagnostic imaging procedures can be safely performed during pregnancy, but in most cases radiation therapy should be postponed until after delivery. Aggressive nutritional support is a mandatory requirement for the pregnant mother afflicted with cancer. In the majority of cases, with a proper coordination of effort, the pregnancy need not be terminated in order to begin treatment.

THE MORE COMMON SOLID TUMORS IN PREGNANCY

Cervical cancer

Cervical cancer complicates approximately one in 1200 pregnancies. As a consequence of widespread cytologic screening, the dramatic decrease in invasive cervical cancer observed in recent years has been paralleled by a rise in cervical intraepithelial neoplasia (CIN), especially in younger women. Because the peak incidence for both CIN and childbearing occurs during the third decade in life, abnormal Papanicolaou smears are common among gravid women, occurring at a rate of 0.5–5%. The diagnosis of cervical dysplasia in pregnancy may occur in up to 5% of some populations. For these reasons, screening for cervical neoplasia is an essential component of prenatal care. All pregnant women should have a cervical smear submitted for cytology. The ectocervix and endocervical canal should be sampled adequately. Patients noted to have a visible lesion should undergo cervical biopsy straight away, as cervical smears taken directly from tumors often contain only inflammatory cells.

In concordance with the known risk factors for invasive cervical cancer, pregnant women who develop CIN tend to marry at an earlier age, have a higher parity, and are diagnosed at an earlier age than non-pregnant women with CIN. Hacker et al compiled data from nine reports and noted that the average age of patients with carcinoma in situ (CIS) during pregnancy was 29.9 years, and the average parity was 4.0. Among non-pregnant women, the average age of CIS is 35 years. The investigators noted that the median age of patients diagnosed with invasive carcinoma of the cervix during pregnancy is 33.8 years (range 17–47 years), and the average parity is 4.5. The average parity among pregnant women with cervical cancer was 5.4 in a study reported by Creasman et al; in this group, increasing parity was not associated with a more advanced lesion, nor did it impact on prognosis.

Human papillomavirus in pregnancy

Although the human papillomavirus (HPV) is strongly associated with cervical dysplasia and carcinoma in both non-pregnant and pregnant women, a significant relationship between pregnancy and HPV prevalence has not been established. Eversion of the endocervical epithelium results in exposure to the acidity of the vaginal environment, producing a high degree of squamous metaplasia. This metaplasia is important because HPV requires active cellular machinery to reproduce and transform cells. Schneider et al examined the negative cervical smears of 92 pregnant and 96 non-pregnant, age-matched control subjects for the presence of HPV DNA by Southern blot hybridization. The investigators demonstrated both an increased prevalence of HPV (preferentially the oncolytic HPV subtype 16) and a higher replication rate of viral DNA during pregnancy. Employing the ViraPap/ViraType dot blot DNA hybridization procedure, Smith and coworkers detected an increase in HPV prevalence with advancing gestational age, suggesting that as estrogen levels rise, pregnant women may be more vulnerable to HPV infection. Using similar hybridization methods, however, Kemp et al and Chang-Claude et al were unable to demonstrate a higher prevalence of HPV infection during pregnancy.

Evaluation of the Papanicolaou smear in pregnancy

The cytopathologist frequently encounters atypical cells when reviewing the cervical smear from a pregnant patient. Cells within the endocervical canal that undergo the *Arias–Stella reaction* may contain a vacuolated clear or oxyphilic cytoplasm, intraglandular tufts, hobnail patterns, delicate filiform papillae, intranuclear pseudoinclusions, cribriform intraglandular growth, and even occasional mitotic figures. Distinguishing features of dysplastic and frankly malignant cells would include an infiltrative pattern, spectrum of cytologic atypia, a high nuclear to cytoplasmic ratio, and increased mitotic activity. Other atypical cells exfoliated by the endocervix in pregnant women include small *decidualized cells* with sharp cytoplasmic borders and hypochromatic nuclei, but unlike dysplastic cells, decidualized cells contain regular chromatin and distinct nuclei. Finally, large, multinucleated trophoblastic cells may be discharged from the uterus. At this time, it is not clear if liquid-based cytology can decrease the false-positive rate. Nevertheless, careful inspection of the cervical smear maintains its reliability as a screening test for dysplasia among pregnant patients.

The performance of colposcopy in pregnancy

Colposcopy is facilitated by the pregnancy-induced eversion of the normal cervical ectropion. However, pregnancy results in dramatic alterations in the colposcopic appearance of the cervix, the most significant changes resulting from the elevated levels of circulating estrogen, which produces a significant increase in cervical volume through hypertrophy of the fibromuscular stroma. The increased vascularity produces a bluish hue, which is then exaggerated with application of acetic acid to the metaplastic epithelium in pregnancy. Toward the end of the first trimester, eversion and metaplasia produce areas of fusion of columnar villa and distinct islands or fingers of immature metaplastic epithelium. Fine punctation and even mosaicism may accompany metaplasia, which in and of itself produces an acetowhite effect. Tenacious endocervical mucus develops, which further hinders colposcopic examination. Finally, stromal edema, enlargement of glandular structures, acute inflammatory responses, and stromal decidualization may occur in the second and third trimesters, which, while physiologic, may appear suspicious to the inexperienced colposcopist. For these reasons, colposcopy in pregnancy is difficult and should be reserved for an experienced gynecologist.

The aim of colposcopy in pregnancy is to exclude cancer, and only one directed biopsy of the site compatible with the most advanced area of dysplastic change should be performed to establish the histologic level of disease. Because of false-negative results ranging from 8 to 40%, random or non-directed biopsies should be avoided. Great care must be exercised, because the increased vascularity may lead to precipitous, heavy bleeding. A Tischler or baby Tischler biopsy forceps should be used, followed by immediate placement of a cotton-tipped applicator above the cervical epithelium. If bleeding does occur, it may be controlled with three silver nitrate sticks or with dehydrated Monsel's solution. An endocervical curettage, however, is best avoided during pregnancy.

Yoonessi et al conducted a retrospective analysis of suspected CIN associated with pregnancy, and concluded that colposcopic examination with or without directed biopsy eliminated the need for cervical conization in 104 of 107 patients. In their classic paper, Hacker et al noted that serious morbidity, such as hemorrhage, preterm labor, miscarriage, or infection, only infrequently occurs when directed biopsies are performed. For 1064 reported colposcopic examinations during pregnancy, the diagnostic accuracy was 99.5% and the complication rate was 0.6%. No case of frankly invasive carcinoma was missed, and the two cases of microinvasion missed on colposcopic biospy both had a colposcopic pattern suggestive of microinvasion, which was confirmed by subsequent conization. Thus, in experienced hands, colposcopy reduces the need for cone biopsy in pregnancy, with a false-negative rate of <0.5%.

The natural history of cervical intraepithelial neoplasia in pregnancy

It appears that in the immunocompetent host evaluated colposcopically and pathologically by experienced eyes, CIN rarely, if ever, progresses to microinvasive disease during pregnancy. In fact, there appears to be a subset of patients who will experience disease regression following delivery of the neonate. Postpartum regression rates for abnormal cervical cytology consistent with dysplasia (combining both low- and high-grade squamous intraepithelial lesions, LSILs and HSILs) have ranged from 25 to 77%. This wide range is hard to explain, with some authors postulating that regression occurs in at least one-third of patients as a consequence of resolution of pregnancy-induced changes in the maternal immunologic system. Others have advanced the theory that vaginal birth trauma may result in the complete debridement of dysplastic tissues. This phenomenon was observed by Ahdoot et al in a prospective collection of abnormal cytology during pregnancy and in the postpartum period. The investigators observed a 60% regression rate among women with HSILs delivered vaginally vs 0% in those with HSILs delivered by caesarean section (P <0.0002). A study by Siristatidis et al demonstrated a 66.6% regression rate among women with HSILs delivered vaginally vs 12.5% of those with HSILs delivered by caesarean section (P <0.002). In direct contradistinction, the cytologic study by Murta et al (LSILs in pregnancy), as well as the pregnancy-related histologic investigations by Murta et al (CIN II/III), Yost et al (CIN II/III), and Coppola et al (CIS), failed to show any statistically significant difference in postpartum regression rates for those patients who delivered vaginally vs those who labored and went on to deliver by caesarean section vs those who underwent elective caesarean delivery.

Conization and related procedures in pregnancy

The performance of a cone biopsy *during* pregnancy is a formidable undertaking, and one must weigh the risks of the procedure against the anticipated yield of microinvasive carcinoma, which would remain otherwise undetected. Maternal risk appears to be restricted to either immediate or delayed hemorrhage, occurring in up to 14% of cases and exceeding 400 mL when the procedure is performed during the third trimester. Averette et al reported the largest series of cold knife cervical conization biopsies in pregnancy, and noted that 9.4% of the study group (n = 180) required a blood transfusion. Maternal death has not been reported. Injury to the pregnancy resulting in spontaneous abortion, intrauterine infection, and preterm birth, however, place the fetus at considerable risk. Rogers and Williams presented a series of 72 pregnancy conizations and reported a perinatal complication rate of 19.4%. Across the literature, the risk of pregnancy loss when the

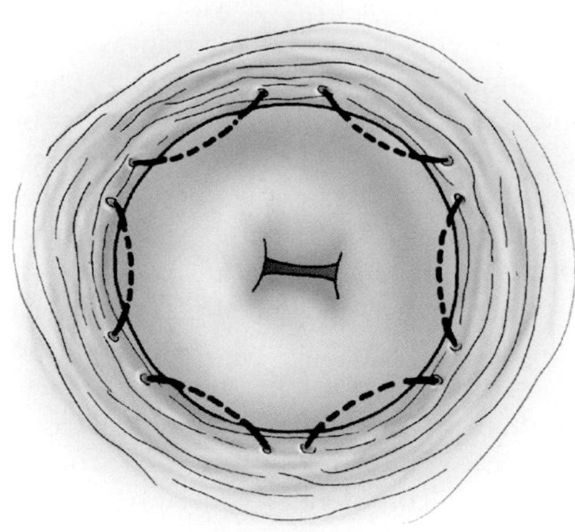

Figure 16–2 The location of six hemostatic sutures is shown. (From Creasy RK, Resnick R: Maternal–Fetal Medicine: Principles and Practice. Philadelphia, Saunders, 1987.)

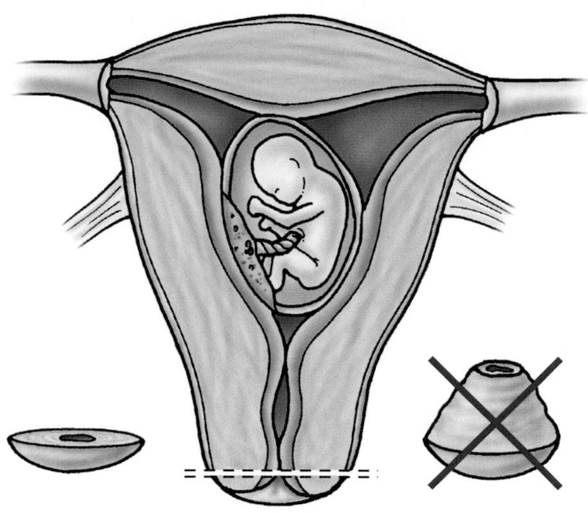

Figure 16–3 Demonstration of shallow "coin" biopsy appropriate in pregnancy. (From Creasy RK, Resnick R: Maternal–Fetal Medicine: Principles and Practice. Philadelphia, Saunders, 1987.)

procedure is performed during the first trimester ranges from 15.2 to 33%. Overall, cone biopsy in pregnancy is associated with a 3–6% risk of perinatal death as a consequence of profuse hemorrhage or from delivery of a previable or extremely premature fetus through an incompetent cervix. A further point that needs emphasizing is that 30–57% of pregnant cones will have dysplasia and/or microinvasive tumor at the endocervical or ectocervical margins. For this reason, the procedure should not be considered therapeutic in the pregnant patient.

The large-loop electrosurgical excision of the transformation zone (LLETZ) may be used in the operating room to excise a shallow cone of sufficient breadth and depth to permit treatment decisions during pregnancy. Robinson et al reported on 20 women who underwent LLETZ from 8 to 34 weeks' gestational age, and noted significant morbidity in patients treated between 27 and 34 weeks' gestational age, including two blood transfusions, three preterm births, and one unexplained intrauterine fetal demise 4 weeks post procedure. Mitsuhashi and Sekiya performed a LLETZ on nine women during the first 14 weeks of pregnancy, none of whom experienced spontaneous abortion, premature delivery, or excessive bleeding. These preliminary results would suggest that LLETZ can be performed safely during the first trimester of pregnancy, but there are insufficient data to determine whether this procedure can replace the traditional cold knife cone biopsy. LLETZ is also associated with a significant proportion of patients left with residual disease.

Hacker et al have commented that most authors reserve conization for patients in whom the transformation zone was not fully visualized, microinvasion was shown on biopsy or suspected colposcopically, or possible adenocarcinoma was found on biopsy. If colposcopy is unsatisfactory, one alternative to a full cone is a wedge resection of the cervix, removing only areas incompletely visualized colposcopically. Another option is to place six hemostatic sutures, evenly distributed around the perimetry of the cervix close to the vaginal reflection (Fig. 16–2). These sutures reduce blood flow to the cone bed, evert the squamocolumnar junction, and facilitate performance of a shallow "coin" biopsy with little interruption of the endocervical canal (Fig. 16–3).

To offset the risk of cervical incompetence, Goldberg et al performed 17 cone cerclages between 12 and 27 weeks' gestation. All procedures were performed with the patient under general anesthesia. Following injection of the entire ectocervix with vasopressin (20 units in 60 mL of normal saline), lateral hemostatic 2-0 polyglycolic acid sutures were placed at the 10 o'clock and 2 o'clock positions on the cervix, and a standard McDonald cerclage using no. 1 nylon suture material was inserted as high and as close to the internal cervical os as technically possible without reflection of the bladder. Once the cervical cone was excised, the McDonald suture was tied with the knot placed anteriorly and an iodoform vaginal pack inserted for 24 h. All 17 patients had uneventful pregnancies, delivering viable infants at or beyond 34 weeks' gestation.

Management of cervical intraepithelial neoplasia in pregnancy

An algorithm that illustrates several key points concerning the management of CIN in pregnancy is proposed in Figure 16–4. *The critical issue is to exclude the coexistence of microinvasive disease with pregnancy.* This is because everything else, the gamut between cellular atypia and CIS, can be followed expectantly during pregnancy, with treatment deferred following its conclusion. We emphasize the following steps.

- Step 1. All abnormal cervical smears in pregnancy (excluding HPV-negative atypia) should prompt an evaluation by colposcopy.
- Step 2. An experienced colposcopist must accurately assess the disease in order to determine whether a directed biopsy is indicated.

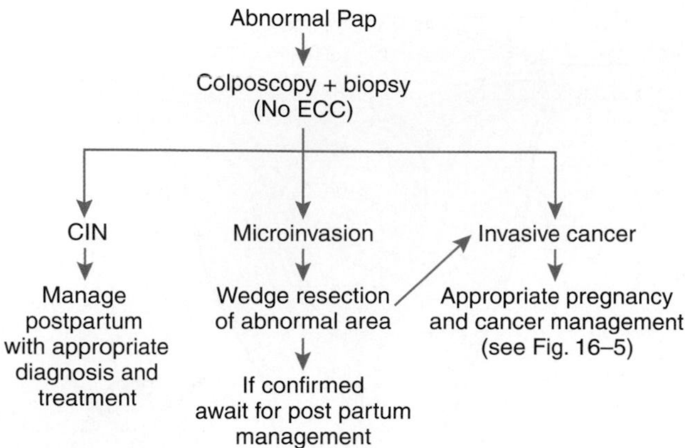

Figure 16–4 Management of abnormal cytologic findings in pregnancy. CIN, cervical intraepithelial neoplasia; ECC, endocervical curettage; Pap, Papanicolaou smear.

- Step 3. In cases involving a CIS on directed biopsy, a coordinated effort between the gynecologist and the pathologist should be undertaken to determine whether an excisional biopsy is required to exclude invasion.

Management of squamous cell abnormalities

Pregnant women with normal prenatal cytologic screening traditionally undergo repeat screening during the postpartum period. Patients with a prenatal Papanicolaou consistent with atypical squamous cells of undetermined significance (ASC-US) may undergo reflex testing for oncolytic HPV subtypes if the Hybrid Capture II test by Digene Corporation is available. Patients who test HPV-negative may be re-evaluated with cervical cytology 6–8 weeks following delivery. Pregnant women who are found to have cytology consistent with ASC-US and are high-risk HPV-positive should be referred for colposcopic evaluation. Patients with cytology consistent with atypical squamous cells favoring a high-grade lesion, LSILs, HSILs, and squamous cell carcinoma (as well as all Papanicolaou tests suggesting glandular cell abnormalities) should be referred for colposcopic evaluation. Because of the high prevalence of HPV in cytologic smears consistent with intraepithelial lesions and carcinoma, HPV testing is not indicated.

If the colposcopic impression is normal or consistent with CIN I, the Papanicolaou test with or without colposcopy can be repeated in the postpartum period provided that the original Papanicolaou test was not consistent with a high-grade lesion; if colposcopy was performed because of HSILs or squamous cell carcinoma, the colposcopic evaluation should be repeated each trimester of the pregnancy, with a directed punch biopsy taken if the impression is consistent with progressive disease (> CIN II).

Patients for whom colposcopy is consistent with CIN II or greater should undergo a single directed biopsy. If this reveals CIN III or worse, the patient should undergo repeat colposcopic evaluation each trimester, with definitive treatment reserved for after delivery, provided there is no evidence for disease progression.

Patients whose biopsies are suspicious for microinvasion should undergo one of the excisional procedures described above (i.e. conization or LLETZ with or without cerclage, coin biopsy, or wedge biopsy). If microinvasion is excluded, the patient should be observed during the pregnancy with colposcopy. If microinvasion is established either by directed punch biopsy or by excisional biopsy, recommendations specific for malignant disease must be sought (see below).

In some circumstances, the colposcopic evaluation will be unsatisfactory, in that the entire transformation zone cannot be completely evaluated. If there is no evidence of a severe lesion in the evaluable areas, and the original Papanicolaou test was not consistent with squamous cell carcinoma or adenocarcinoma in situ (AIS), close observation with repeat colposcopy during each trimester of the pregnancy may be considered. Under more dire scenarios, a coin biopsy of the cervix or a wedge biopsy of the hidden part of the transformation zone may be necessary.

Management of glandular cell abnormalities

Cervical smears containing glandular cell abnormalities may be reported as atypical cells not otherwise specified (AGC-NOS), atypical cells favor neoplasia, AIS, or even adenocarcinoma. Importantly, 40% of cervices associated with an atypical glandular cells of undetermined significance (AGUS) smear will have a significant tissue abnormality, with greater than 50% harboring a squamous intraepithelial lesion. The significance of an AGUS Papanicolaou result in the pregnant and in the postpartum woman is not yet clear. In a recent manuscript by Chhieng et al, 30 pregnant women and 5 within the immediate postpartum window were evaluated for a cytologic diagnosis of AGUS. Of 27 women for whom there was follow-up, 17 underwent colposcopic examination and biopsy. Five women (29.4%) had CIN, including three high-grade and two low-grade lesions on biopsy. Interestingly, the remaining patients (70.6%) had benign pathology, which included chronic cervicitis (n = 5), endocervical and/or endometrial polyps (n = 4), Arias–Stella reaction (n = 2), and microglandular hyperplasia (n = 1); of the 10 patients who had repeat Papanicolaou tests, only two had persistent AGUS/ASC-US. Nevertheless, the finding that up to 30% of pregnancy-associated AGUS patients had a significant preneoplastic lesion warrants careful evaluation.

The clinician's diagnostic armamentarium is limited during pregnancy. In the absence of a visible lesion or a significantly expanded cervix (i.e. the barrel-shaped cervix), all patients with AGUS smears should undergo colposcopic evaluation with directed biopsy. Patients diagnosed with a squamous lesion or AIS should be evaluated by colposcopy during subsequent trimesters. It is not known whether a patient with AIS on directed biopsy should undergo wedge resection of that area to rule out invasion in a nearby "skip" lesion. A diagnostic LLETZ and/or cold knife cervical conization during pregnancy is best reserved only for those few cases in which an AIS or squamous lesion suspicious for microinvasion is encountered on directed biopsy.

If colposcopy is unrevealing, however, the concern is raised that an endocervical lesion high in the canal or even within the endometrial compartment is being missed.

Nevertheless, an endocervical curettage, cervical dilatation with fractional uterine curettage, and/or endometrial aspiration biopsy is best deferred until the postpartum period, when even a full cervical conization can be performed if needed. Therefore, in these clinical scenarios, consultation with the cytopathologist should be arranged to determine if the original Papanicolaou slide contains troublesome features such as inflammatory cells, polyps, glandular hyperplasia, or the Arias–Stella reaction, any of which could confuse the picture, especially when dealing with an AGC-NOS Papanicolaou smear. Gravid women with a negative colposcopic survey for an AGC favor neoplasia cervical smear can be evaluated safely in pregnancy with either endovaginal ultrasonography or magnetic resonance imaging (MRI) of the pelvis to search for a lesion within the endometrium or endocervical canal. In these latter circumstances, referral to a gynecologic oncologist should be contemplated.

Intrapartum hysterectomy

Some authors have described a program in which an intrapartum hysterectomy (following either vaginal or caesarean birth) is performed for patients with CIS or AIS who have completed childbearing and/or have proven to be non-compliant. Because there is not sufficient evidence to suggest that an immunocompetent patient is at risk for rapid progression of disease during pregnancy, the need to remove the diseased segment of the cervix is not urgent. Intrapartum hysterectomies, both elective and non-elective, can be associated with significant blood loss. Furthermore, among inexperienced obstetricians, the bladder is particularly at risk for injury. One must balance the non-compliance of a given patient with the possibility that microinvasion may not have been sufficiently excluded during pregnancy, especially in cases of CIS or AIS with positive margins. The observation that postpartum regression may also occur with even CIS argues against the routine performance of an intrapartum hysterectomy for the management of CIN in pregnancy.

Invasive cervical cancer

Presenting symptoms in order of frequency among pregnant women with cervical carcinoma include abnormal vaginal bleeding (63%), vaginal discharge (13%), postcoital bleeding (4%), and pelvic pain (2%). Importantly, in the review by Hacker et al, 18% of patients were asymptomatic, as were 30% of the patients in the study by Creasman et al. When bleeding occurs, this symptom must be investigated and not automatically attributed to the pregnancy. Examination during the first trimester will not lead to abortion. Third-trimester bleeding can be adequately assessed in the operating room as a double setup procedure. Many times, visual inspection is all that is needed for diagnosis of this malignant neoplasm. The International Federation of Gynecology and Obstetrics (FIGO) staging system applies also in pregnancy. To avoid the risks of radiation exposure to a developing fetus, we recommend an ultrasound of the kidneys to evaluate for the presence of hydronephrosis, and an MRI of the pelvis when there is concern for parametrial extension of the tumor. A chest radiograph may be performed with appropriate abdominal shielding to exclude pulmonary metastases. A suggested management algorithm for the management of invasive cervical cancer in pregnancy appears in Figure 16–5.

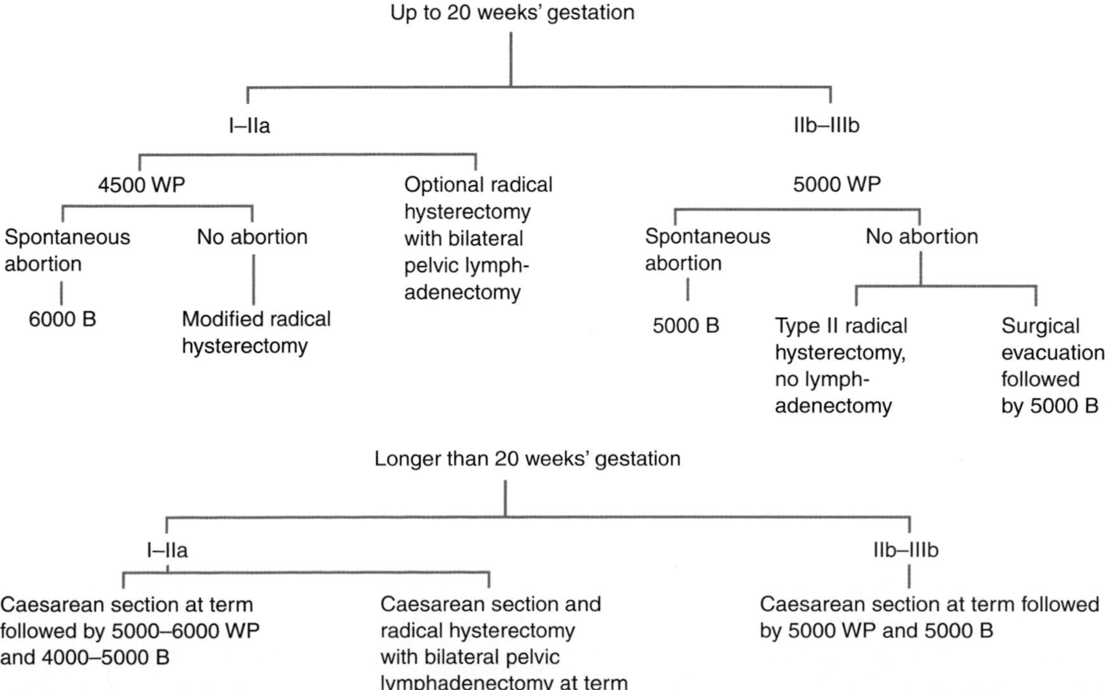

Figure 16–5 Suggested therapy for cervical cancer in pregnancy. B, brachytherapy (mg/h) vaginal radium in two applications; WP, whole-pelvis irradiation (cGy).

Microinvasive disease

The diagnosis of microinvasive carcinoma in pregnancy is typically established with colposcopic directed biopsy, and in a minority of cases in which the colposcopic biopsy cannot exclude microinvasion, a shallow coin biopsy or the cervix or wedge excision of the area under suspicion as outlined above. This is the only absolute indication for conization during pregnancy. Conization distinguishes patients who have "early stromal invasion" and who can proceed to term without appreciable risk to their survival from those with frank invasion in whom consideration must be given to early interruption of the pregnancy. We advise patients with early stromal invasion (i.e. FIGO stage Ia1) that the pregnancy may continue safely to term, provided the surgical margins are free. Caesarean section is not thought to be necessary for this group of patients, and the route of delivery should be determined by obstetric indications. Patients with FIGO stage Ia2 or occult Ib1 lesions should undergo caesarean delivery when fetal pulmonary maturation is demonstrable, followed by an immediate modified radical abdominal hysterectomy with bilateral pelvic lymphadenectomies. We advocate the deployment of a vertical uterine incision so as to leave the lower uterine segment undisturbed for subsequent detailed pathologic examination. Interestingly, the physiologic changes of pregnancy actually enhance the performance of radical surgery by providing the surgeon with multiple levels of distinct tissue planes.

Caesarean–radical hysterectomy with pelvic lymphadenectomies

In deciding on therapy for frankly invasive cervical cancer in pregnancy, the physician must consider both the stage of disease and the duration of pregnancy. The decision can often be influenced by the religious convictions of the patient and family, and the desire of the mother for the child. For FIGO stage I and FIGO stage IIa lesions, radical hysterectomy with bilateral lymphadenectomy is acceptable during any trimester (Fig. 16–6). We prefer the surgical approach because of the overall result, which includes ovarian preservation, improved sexual function, and elimination of unnecessary delays for the patient. The complication rate of radical surgery for cervical carcinoma in pregnant patients does not exceed that in non-pregnant patients when normal surgical principles are scrupulously followed.

Monk and Montz examined their institutional experience in treating invasive cervical cancer complicating intrauterine pregnancy with radical hysterectomy. They identified 13 patients treated with radical hysterectomy and bilateral pelvic lymphadenectomy with the fetus in situ, and eight others treated with caesarean delivery followed by radical hysterectomy and bilateral pelvic lymph node dissection. The mean operative time was 281 min, and the mean blood loss was 777 mL for radical hysterectomy with the fetus in situ plus lymphadenectomy, and 1750 mL when caesarean section preceded the cancer operation. The surgical morbidity was minimal for the

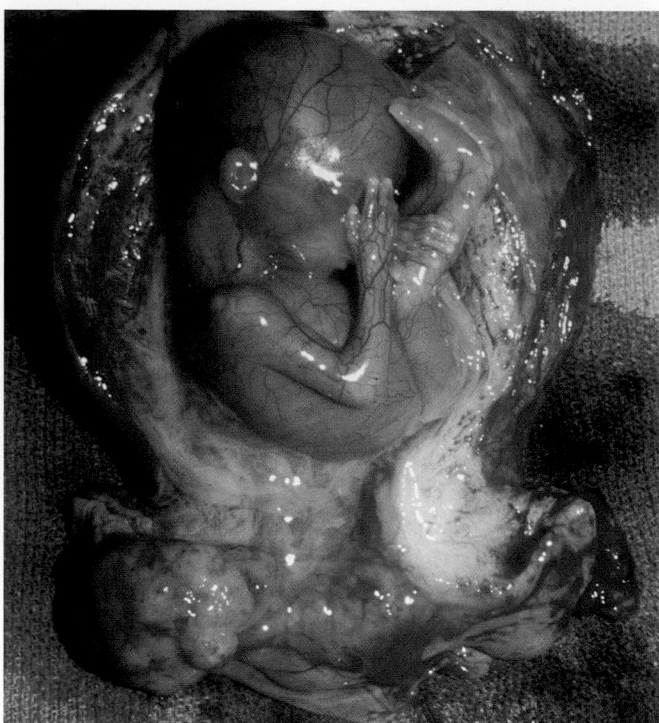

Figure 16–6 An 18-week-old fetus. Cervical cancer with a vaginal cuff and an extruding placenta are seen in a radical hysterectomy specimen from a 32-year-old patient.

whole group, and after documentation of fetal maturation, seven healthy infants were delivered. Twenty patients (95%) are alive and free of disease with a mean follow-up of 40 months. The authors concluded that radical surgery offers immediate treatment for early-stage cervical cancer during intrauterine pregnancy, with low associated morbidity, acceptable survival, and preservation of ovarian function.

Whole-pelvis radiotherapy with intracavitary brachytherapy

Radiation therapy is equally efficacious in treating patients with early-stage (i.e. FIGO stage Ib1) cervical cancer in pregnancy, and together with radiosensitizing chemotherapy is the treatment of choice in more advanced stages (FIGO stage Ib2–IVa). In the first and second trimesters when the pregnancy is to be disregarded, treatment should begin with whole-pelvis irradiation. Spontaneous abortion usually occurs during therapy, and the treatment is then completed with intracavitary radium or cesium applications. Spontaneous abortion usually occurs at about 35 days in the first trimester and at 45 days in the second trimester after onset of radiotherapy. Some second-trimester patients will go 60–70 days before abortion occurs. An alternative approach in the patient who has not aborted is to evacuate the uterus by means of a hysterotomy followed by conventional intracavitary irradiation delivered within 1–2 weeks.

If spontaneous abortion does not occur by completion of the external beam therapy, as occurs commonly after the 16th week of gestation, a modified radical hysterectomy without pelvic lymphadenectomy should be done to excise the remaining central neoplasm. This strategy delivers potentially curative doses of radiation to pelvic lymph nodes with microscopic foci of metastatic tumor followed by surgical resection of the remaining central tumor, because the gravid uterus is not suitable for intracavitary radium or cesium. Although some clinicians prefer an extrafascial hysterectomy after 5000 cGy of whole-pelvis irradiation in patients who have early lesions, we prefer the more extensive modified radical hysterectomy. This approach accomplishes adequate excision of the cervix and accompanying medial parametria and upper vagina, which includes all the tissues that would have been effectively irradiated by the pear-shaped isodose distribution of a tandem and ovoid application of radium or cesium. Those who advocate an extrafascial hysterectomy centrally often advise further vaginal vault irradiation after the surgical procedure to treat the upper vagina and medial parametria more completely.

Sood et al assessed the effects of pregnancy on tumor control, survival, and morbidity associated with radiation therapy administered to pregnant patients. They identified 26 women treated primarily with radiation therapy before the era of concurrent chemoirradiation, and matched these patients with 26 control subjects based on age, histology, stage, treatment, and year of treatment. Patients were treated with external beam radiation (mean dose 46.7 Gy) and intracavitary radiation (mean dose 56.5 Gy to point A). Three patients diagnosed during the first trimester were treated with radiation with the fetus in situ, and all had spontaneous abortions 20–24 days after the start of radiation (mean dose 34 Gy). In all these cases, radiation was interrupted for only 3 days or less. There were no statistically significant differences in recurrence rates or survival between the pregnant group and the control subjects.

Episiotomy site recurrence

Patients in whom the diagnosis of invasive cervical cancer is made in the postpartum period may have undergone vaginal delivery. This group of patients warrants immediate therapy and specialized surveillance. Recurrence of cervical cancer at the episiotomy scar is a rare event and is thought to occur through implantation at the time of vaginal delivery from an occult tumor, with subsequent early, isolated recurrence as opposed to regional spread. At least 15 cases have appeared in the literature since 1986, including one patient who relapsed along a perineal laceration scar (Table 16–4). In the majority of these patients, the primary diagnosis of cervical cancer was made during the

Table 16–4 TREATMENT MODALITIES AND SURVIVAL OF PATIENTS WITH EPISIOTOMY SITE RECURRENCE

Authors	Year	Stage	Prenatal cytology	Pathology	Time of initial diagnosis	Primary treatment	Disease-free interval	Treatment of recurrence	Status
Burgess and Waymont	1987	Ib	SCCA	SCCA	7 months pp	XRT, BT	17 months	Exenteration	n/r
Copeland et al	1987	Ib	Normal	Adenocarcinoma	3 months pp	RH	3 months	WE, XRT, BT	NED > 5 years
		Ib	Normal	Adenocarcinoma	Biopsy at delivery	RH	5 months	WE, XRT	NED 10 months
Gordon et al	1989	Ib	Normal	SCCA	Biopsy at delivery	RH	1 month	WE, XRT, BT	NED 3.5 years
van Dam et al	1992	IIIa	n/r	SCCA	6 weeks pp	Chemotherapy, XRT, BT	0 months	BT	n/r
		Ib	Normal	Adenocarcinoma	9 weeks pp	XRT, BT	3 months	WE, XRT, BT	NED > 10 years
Khalil et al	1993	IIIb	Not done	SCCA	8 weeks pp	XRT, BT	3 months	Chemotherapy, XRT	DOD 4 months
Cliby et al	1994	Ib	HSIL	SCCA	Biopsy at delivery	RH	9 weeks	Chemotherapy	DOD 6 months
		Ib	Not done	SCCA	Biopsy at 36 weeks	RH	24 months	Chemotherapy, WE, XRT	NED 1 year
		Ib	Not done	SCCA	Biopsy at delivery	RH	3 months	XRT	DOD 3.5 years
		Ib	Not done	SCCA	5 weeks pp	RH	1 month	WE, XRT	DOD 6 months
van den Broek et al	1995	Ia1	Normal	Adenocarcinoma	3 months pp	Total abdominal hysterectomy	6 weeks	WE, interstitial implants	DOD 1 year
Goldman and Goldberg	2003	Ib	Normal	SCCA	1 week pp	RH	5.5 years	WE, XRT, BT	DOD 4.5 years
Heron et al	2005	Ib	AGUS	Villoglandular	Biopsy at 31 weeks	RH, BPLND	44 months	XRT, WE	NED 10 months

AGUS, atypical glandular cells of undetermined significance; BPLND, bilateral pelvic lymphadenectomy; BT, brachytherapy; DOD, died of disease; HSIL, high-grade squamous intraepithelial lesion; n/r, not reported; no evidence of disease (NED); pp, postpartum; RH, radical hysterectomy; SCCA, squamous cell carcinoma; WE, wide excision; XRT, whole pelvic radiotherapy.

(After Goldman NA, Goldberg GL: Late recurrence of squamous cell cervical cancer in an episiotomy site after vaginal delivery. Obstet Gynecol 101:1127–1129, 2003.)

postpartum period, with recurrence at the episiotomy site typically occurring within 6 months of primary treatment.

In a matched case-control study of women with cervical cancer diagnosed during pregnancy (n = 56) or within 6 months of delivery (n = 27), Sood et al noted that among the patients diagnosed postpartum, one of seven who was delivered by caesarean section developed a local and distant recurrence, while 10 of 17 (59%) of those who delivered vaginally developed recurrences (P = 0.04). In multivariate analysis, vaginal delivery was the most significant predictor of recurrence. We recommend delivery by caesarean section when the diagnosis is known antenatally, and in those patients diagnosed in the postpartum period, vigilant examination of the episiotomy and vaginal laceration sites is warranted. Although the mode of delivery in the setting of known microinvasive disease may be based on obstetric indications, it should be pointed out that among the 14 cases of episiotomy site recurrences there was one patient who had been diagnosed with a stage Ia endocervical adenocarinoma.

Neither the time of diagnosis nor time to recurrence appears to impact survival after episiotomy site recurrence. Goldman and Goldberg noted that no patient who received chemotherapy or radiotherapy for recurrent disease without excision survived 1 year. The treatment policy should include wide local excision of the entire nodule with adjuvant external radiotherapy plus brachytherapy. Of seven patients treated by this method, 71% were without evidence of disease at longer than 1 year.

Planned delay of therapy

Historically, when invasive carcinoma was diagnosed prior to 20 weeks' gestation, recommendations included immediate treatment of the tumor, either by radical hysterectomy or radiation therapy, leaving the fetus in utero in both instances. This dogma has been challenged during the preceding decade, with multiple reports of a safe outcome for mother and child with a deliberate delay in therapy to permit gestational advancement (Table 16–5). For example, Duggan et al reported a mean diagnosis to treatment interval of 144 days (range 53–212 days) in eight patients with FIGO stage Ia or FIGO stage Ib cervical cancer who postponed therapy to optimize fetal outcome. All these women were rendered disease-free after a median follow-up of 23 months. Sorosky et al identified eight pregnant women with FIGO stage I squamous cell cervical carcinoma who declined immediate therapy in order to improve fetal outcome. They were observed

Table 16–5 DELIBERATE DELAY OF DEFINITIVE THERAPY FOR FRANKLY INVASIVE CERVICAL CARCINOMA IN PREGNANCY

Authors	Year	Stage	No.	Delay	Maternal outcome
Prem et al	1966	I	4	6 weeks	NED 5 years
		I	5	11–17 weeks	NED 3–5 years
Dudan et al	1973	Ib	2	2 and 6 months	Progression
Lee et al	1981	Ib	1	12 weeks	NED 10 years
		Ib	2	11 weeks	No progression
		II	5	1–11 weeks	No progression
Nisker and Shubat	1983	Ib	1	24 weeks	DOD
Greer et al	1989	Ib	5	6–17 weeks	NED 1–3 years (n = 4), DOD (n = 1)
Monk and Montz	1992	Ib	4	10–16 weeks	NED 3.5 years
Hopkins and Morley	1992	Ib	5	12 weeks	NED 5 years (n = 40)
Mack et al	1981	Ib	3	10–16 weeks	NED
Duggan et al	1993	Ib1	5	7–24 weeks	NED 3 years
Sivanesaratnam et al	1993	Ib	2	2 and 4 weeks	NED 5 years
Allen et al	1995	Ib	2	18–19 weeks	NED 5 years
Sorosky et al	1995	Ib1	7	7–29 weeks	NED 1.5–5.5 years
Sood et al	1996	Ib	3	3–32 weeks	NED 1–30 years
Tewari et al	1997	Ib2	1[a]	11 weeks	NED 2 years
		IIa	1[a]	18 weeks	DOD 9 months
van Vliet et al	1998	Ib	5	2–10 weeks	DOD (n = 1), NED 1.5–9 years
		IIa	1	2 weeks	NED 12 years
Marana et al	2001	IIb	1[a]	21 weeks	DOD 18 months[a]
Takushi et al	2002	Ib1	2	13 and 15 weeks	NED 8 and 9 years
		Ib2	1	6 weeks	NED 7 years
Germann et al	2005	Ib1	9	4 months	NED 5 years

DOD, died of disease; NED, no evidence of disease.

[a]Treated with neoadjuvant chemotherapy during pregnancy.

(After Tewari et al: Neoadjuvant chemotherapy in the treatment of locally advanced cervical carcinoma in pregnancy: a report of two cases and review of issues specific to the management of cervical carcinoma in pregnancy including planned delay of therapy. Cancer 82:1529–1534, 1998.)

prospectively until the late third trimester, with a mean diagnosis to treatment interval of 109 days (range 21–210 days). No clinical progression of disease was detected, and following therapy all were alive and disease-free after a mean follow-up of 37 months (range 13–68 months). Takushi et al reported a delay in treatment of 6–16 weeks for four women with FIGO stage Ia2, Ib1, or 1b2 lesions. No disease progression was documented, and following caesarean–radical hysterectomy all patients have been disease-free at a follow-up period of 70–156 months.

Although most patients with FIGO stage Ib disease have fared well with deliberate delays in therapy, four patients are noted in whom progression of disease was observed ($n = 2$) or in whom recurrence and death due to disease occurred ($n = 2$). Five patients with FIGO stage II disease who opted to delay therapy were reported by Lee et al, and although they did not progress during the pregnancy, it should be noted that their cancers were diagnosed in the third trimester and the treatment delays were relatively limited. Long-term follow-up data were not presented for this subset of patients. Thus for patients with FIGO stage Ia1–Ib1 squamous cell lesions diagnosed prior to and after 20 weeks' gestation, a limited treatment delay to await fetal maturity may be acceptable. The counseling in such situations should be analogous to obtaining an informed consent from the mother.

Neoadjuvant chemotherapy in pregnancy

Patients with advanced disease (i.e. FIGO stage Ib2 and greater) should be offered immediate therapy. A novel approach to patients with locally advanced disease who refuse interruption of pregnancy was first reported by our group in 1998. Two women with FIGO stage Ib2 and FIGO stage IIa lesions refused interruption of their pregnancies and received neoadjvuant chemotherapy consisting of vincristine (1 mg/m^2) and cisplatin (50 mg/m^2) during the early second and third trimesters. Both patients experienced significant tumor regression, rendering radical hysterectomy feasible at the time of caesarean delivery following documentation of fetal pulmonary maturation at 32 weeks' and 34 weeks' gestation. At the time of publication, one patient had remained without evidence of recurrence for over 2 years; unfortunately, the second patient experienced a lethal relapse 5 months following primary therapy. Both children have experienced normal development. Marana et al treated a pregnant woman with a FIGO stage IIb tumor with bleomycin (30 mg on day 1) and cisplatin (50 mg/m^2 on day 2 and day 3) from 17 weeks' to 38 weeks' gestation and achieved both tumor regression and a healthy infant who continued to thrive long after the mother succumbed to recurrent disease 13 months following delivery. Although such a treatment approach remains investigational, the use of neoadjuvant chemotherapy while awaiting gestational advancement may be entertained when the pregnant woman with cervical cancer, for whom a treatment delay is ill-advised, refuses interruption of therapy.

Prognosis for patients with cervical cancer in pregnancy

The overall prognosis for all stages of cervical cancer in pregnancy is similar to that in non-pregnant women (Table 16–6). The favorable overall prognosis for pregnant patients is related to a greater proportion of pregnant patients with stage I disease. In a report by Allen and Nisker of 96 cases of cervical cancer occurring in pregnancy, the disease-free survival rate for 87 patients who were available for analysis was noted to be 92.3% for FIGO stage Ia1, 68.2% for FIGO stage Ib, 54.5% for FIGO stage II, and 37.5% for FIGO stage III. The overall survival rate was 65.5%, which is slightly better than that reported by Hacker et al. They also observed an association of advanced clinical staging with diagnosis in the third trimester and postpartum. Of 49 cases of FIGO stage Ib cervical carcinoma, 64.5% were diagnosed in the third trimester and postpartum; of 22 cases of FIGO stage II cervical carcinoma, 77.3% were diagnosed in the third trimester and postpartum; and all nine cases of stage III cervical carcinoma were diagnosed in the third trimester and postpartum. Of the 32 patients who underwent pelvic

Table 16–6 FIVE-YEAR SURVIVAL RATES OF TREATED CERVICAL CANCER IN PREGNANT AND NON-PREGNANT PATIENTS

			Pregnant survival		Non-pregnant survival	
Author(s)	**Year**	**Stage**	%	*n*	%	*n*
Creasman et al	1970	I	85	24	80	371
		II	60	18	70	502
Sablinska	1977	I	72	114	76	208
		II	54	62	56	1270
Lee	1981	Ib WTH–BPLND	93	17	91	156
		Ib RT	80	4	88	32
Nisker and Shubat	1983	Ib	70	43	87	118
Sivanesaratnam et al	1993	I WTH–BPLND	78	18	92	379
Germann et al	2005	Ib1	100	14	No control group	
		Ib2	100	1		
		IIb	80	5		

BPLND, bilateral pelvic lymphadenectomy; RT, radiotherapy; WTH, Wertheim–Taussig radical abdominal hysterectomy.

lymphadenectomy, 10 were noted to have positive nodes. This increase in frequency has not been our experience.

Zemlickis et al compared 40 women who had carcinoma of the cervix in pregnancy with 89 non-pregnant women matched for age, stage, and tumor type. Long-term survival was similar between the two groups. When pregnant women were compared with a series of 1963 cervical cancers in women younger than 45 years treated during the same time, the pregnant women were three times more likely to have stage I disease and had a lower chance of having FIGO stage III–IV cancers.

In 1993, Sivanesaratnam reported surgical management of early invasive cancer of the cervix in a series of 18 patients who underwent radical hysterectomy and pelvic lymphadenectomy, with a 5-year survival of 77.7%. A comparable group of non-pregnant patients who also underwent radical surgery had a survival of 92.3%. Nisker and Shubat also reported that there was a slightly better survival in the non-pregnant group than in the pregnant group. These reports are in contrast to the previous reports by Creasman et al, Sablinska et al, and Lee et al, who found no appreciative difference in the 5-year survival rates of pregnant vs non-pregnant patients with cervical cancer.

For more advanced disease, pregnancy may have an unfavorable effect on prognosis due to problems with radiation dosimetry in pregnancy and the need to interrupt radiation therapy more frequently because of genital tract sepsis. Clinical stage remains the most important determinant of prognosis.

Ovarian cancer

Ovarian cancer is reported to occur in one per 10,000 to one per 25,000 pregnancies. Pregnancy does not alter the prognosis of most ovarian malignant neoplasms, but complications such as torsion and rupture may increase the incidence of spontaneous abortion or preterm delivery. In a survey by Kohler of the largest studies in the literature, about one in 600 pregnancies will be complicated by an adnexal mass. More contemporary accounts suggest that adnexal masses may complicate as many as one in 190 pregnancies. At least one-third of pregnant women are asymptomatic, with the adnexal mass often discovered during obstetric ultrasonography.

Most cysts in pregnant patients are follicular or corpus luteum cysts and are usually no more than 3 cm to 5 cm in diameter. Functional cysts as large as 11 cm in diameter have been reported but are rare. More than 90% of these functional cysts will disappear as pregnancy progresses and are undetectable by the 14th week of gestation. It appears that the size of the adnexal mass at the time of diagnosis is inversely related to the likelihood of spontaneous regression. Only 6% of masses less than 6 cm persisted during serial examinations, but 39% of masses greater than 6 cm persisted. The complication rate increases with increasing size of the mass. In addition, a solid or complex ultrasonographic appearance as well as the presence of bilateral

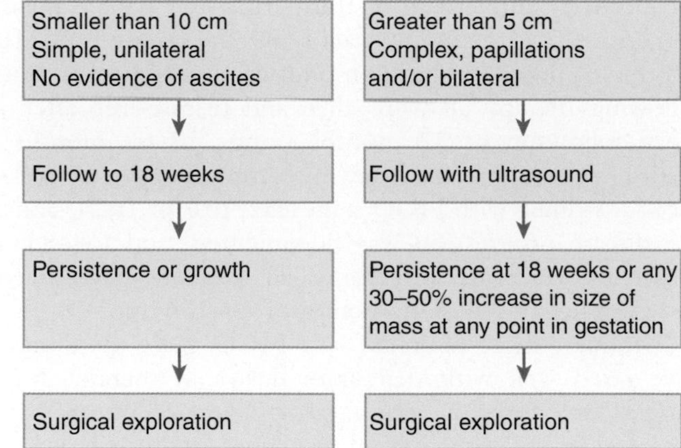

Figure 16–7 Management of an ovarian mass in pregnancy.

adnexal/ovarian abnormalities may also indications to proceed with laparotomy. Adnexal masses with blood flow characterized by a high resistive index by Doppler ultrasonography are less likely to be malignant, independent of size. MRI may be useful when ultrasonographic findings are equivocal.

The most pressing problems associated with ovarian tumors in pregnancy are the initial diagnosis and the differential diagnosis. When the tumor is palpable within the pelvis, it must be differentiated from a retroverted pregnant uterus, a pedunculated uterine fibroid, a carcinoma of the rectosigmoid, a pelvic kidney, and a congenital uterine abnormality (e.g. rudimentary uterine horn). Analysis of serum tumor markers is a complex undertaking and can be misleading because the titers for each of the markers, especially α-fetoprotein and β-human chorionic gonadotropin (hCG), and even CA-125, are routinely elevated in pregnancy for reasons unrelated to malignancy.

A proposed management algorithm for the adnexal mass in pregnancy appears in Figure 16–7. Our experience has been that patients operated on around the 18th week of gestation have negligible fetal wastage associated with the exploration. Therefore 18 weeks' gestation appears to be a judicious period for laparotomy in terms of its safety both for the fetus and for the elimination of functional ovarian cysts. If the cyst is complex and suspicious for malignancy and increases in size, the patient should undergo exploration earlier than 18 weeks. Whenever exploration is conducted, our recommendation is that the uterus not be manipulated during surgery (i.e. the so-called hands off the uterus approach) in an effort to minimize its irritability.

Torsion is common in pregnancy, with 10–15% of ovarian tumors reportedly undergo this complication. Most torsions (i.e. 60%) occur when the uterus is rising at a rapid rate (8–16 weeks) or when the uterus is involuting (in the puerperium). The usual sequence of events is sudden lower abdominal pain, nausea, vomiting, and in some cases shock-like symptoms. The abdomen is tense and tender, and there is rebound tenderness with guarding. If exploration must be undertaken during the first trimester and extraction of the ovary (or ovaries)

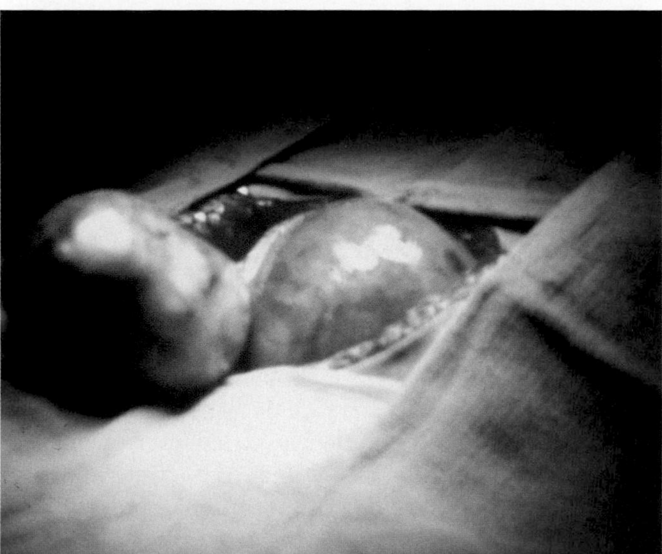

Figure 16–8 Benign cystic teratoma: Gross appearance at 18 weeks' gestation.

required, supplemental progesterone can be administered to decrease the likelihood of pregnancy loss.

In many instances, the presence of an ovarian tumor may not be suspected until delivery (Fig. 16–8). The large uterus obscures the growth of the ovarian neoplasm. The tumor may be growing in the abdomen behind the large uterus and may not fall back into the cul-de-sac until it is large. If there is a mechanical obstruction of the birth canal, exploratory laparotomy is indicated for both delivery of the baby and management of the ovarian neoplasm. Allowing labor to proceed when an ovarian neoplasm is causing obstruction of the birth canal may result in rupture of the ovarian cyst. Even if the cyst is not ruptured, the trauma of labor may cause hemorrhage into the tumor followed by necrosis and suppuration.

Ovarian masses specific to pregnancy

Two adnexal conditions may specifically be associated with pregnancy. The operating surgeon must be cognizant of their possibility so that unnecessary oophorectomies will not be performed. The luteoma of pregnancy can vary in size from microscopic to 20 cm in diameter and usually consists of multiple, well-circumscribed nodules that can be bilateral in one-third of cases. The luteoma may be associated with significant elevations in plasma testosterone and other androgens in about 25% of the cases. Maternal hirsutism or virilism may occur during the latter half of pregnancy, which may cause virilization in up to 70% of female infants born to masculinizing mothers. If the lesion is not recognized grossly, a biopsy may be taken for definitive diagnosis. Because these regress spontaneously postpartum, nothing further needs to be done. Theca-lutein cysts may occur when hCG concentrations are abnormally elevated, such as in a molar pregnancy, fetal hydrops, or multiple gestations. These are usually multiple and thin-walled. Sometimes, massive bilateral theca-lutein cysts manifest that are considerably different from the solid nodules of the luteoma of pregnancy. These also regress postpartum and should not be resected unless acute complications develop.

Histologic types of ovarian tumors

Struyk and Treffers reported on 90 pregnancies complicated by ovarian tumors. No functional cysts were noted in patients operated on after the 18th week. In eight patients, ovarian tumor enlargement was noted during a period of observation; two were malignant, one serous cystadenoma occurred, and five were teratomas. Fifty-four percent of the tumors were diagnosed in the first trimester. Severe pain occurred in 26%, torsion in 12%, obstruction of labor in 17%, and rupture in 9%. Only 37% of the patients had no complications. Fetal wastage was high, with death in utero occurring in three cases and neonatal death in seven cases.

Thornton and Wells reviewed 131 ovarian enlargements in pregnancy, 81 of which were removed (including one carcinoma and six borderline lesions). Thirty-nine were greater than 5 cm in diameter and had simple internal echo patterns and smooth walls; three of these were borderline malignant neoplasms. Hoffman reviewed 13 reports of ovarian neoplasms removed in pregnancy and found benign cystadenomas or cystic teratomas most frequently diagnosed. The Hoffman review also included a summary of 127 malignant ovarian lesions found during pregnancy (Table 16–7). Borderline and frankly malignant epithelial lesions were the most commonly encountered during pregnancy.

Borderline ovarian tumors

Adnexal masses greater than 6 cm that persist into the second trimester warrant removal at approximately 18 weeks' gestational age. Between 2 and 5% of these lesions will be malignant, with dysgerminoma being most common. Among epithelial tumors, serous carcinoma and serous tumors of low malignant potential are readily

Table 16–7 HISTOLOGY OF MALIGNANT ADNEXAL MASSES REMOVED DURING PREGNANCY

Histologic type	No. (%)
Epithelial	35 (27.6)
Borderline epithelial	26 (20.5)
Germ cell[a]	7 (5.5)
Stromal	20 (15.7)[b]
Undifferentiated	4 (3.1)
Sarcoma	2 (1.6)
Metastatic	3 (2.4)
Total	97

[a]Dysgerminoma or other.
[b]Thirteen of 64 from Novak.
(From Hoffman MS: Primary ovarian carcinoma during pregnancy, case report. Clin Consult Obstet Gynecol 7:237, 1995.)

encountered. Thirty-five cases of serous ovarian tumors of low malignant potential in conjunction with pregnancy have been reported since 1988. In the 33 cases where a FIGO stage was assigned, 30 were stage I (14 stage Ia, 1 stage Ib, 4 Stage Ic, and 11 non-substaged I). All 33 patients for whom follow-up data were available were found to be alive without disease (range 1 year to 20 years and 5 months). Recent evidence suggests that the hormonal influence of pregnancy can effect histologic changes in serous low malignant potential tumors that, if not sorted out and characterized appropriately, could be mistaken for frankly invasive carcinoma. The group at the M.D. Anderson Hospital and Tumor Institute collected 10 cases from 1944 to 1993 and conducted a slide review, noting some very peculiar histologic features distinct from those seen in non-pregnant patients, including epithelial atypia and proliferation, eosinophilic cells, mucin production, decidual changes, and frequent microinvasion. While these lesions remained within the spectrum of low malignant potential tumors, the histologic features were worrisome for a more aggressive clinical course, and yet all 10 patients remained disease-free following a variety of treatment modalities. We advise prompt recognition of these histologic findings following cystectomy and/or oophorectomy during pregnancy so as to classify them accordingly as being borderline rather than to confuse them with low-grade serous papillary carcinomas. Of additional interest is that in two cases the tumor was resected both during pregnancy and after parturition (2 months and 3 years), and there was significant regression of the epithelial proliferation, the number of eosinophilic cells, and the amount of mucin production the second time around; this regression following parturition supports a hormonal etiology of these unusual histologic features. In contrast to frankly malignant ovarian carcinomas, unilateral adnexectomy is all that is required during pregnancy for the serous low malignant potential tumor.

Frankly malignant ovarian tumors

Malignant ovarian tumors account for only 2–5% of all ovarian neoplasms found in pregnancy. The incidence for all pregnancies is one in 8000 to one in 20,000 deliveries. The diagnosis is usually fortuitous in that the patient undergoes laparotomy for an adnexal mass that is subsequently found to be malignant. In many instances, the close observation of the pregnant patient has led to the discovery of a lesion in the earlier stages. These include not only malignant germ cell tumors and sex cord–stromal cell cancers, but also some epithelial malignancies. If an ovarian malignant neoplasm is found at the time of abdominal exploration, the surgeon's first obligation is to properly stage the disease as outlined in Chapter 11. Although the gravid uterus hinders the surgeon's ability to access the retroperitoneum, every effort should be made to remove the tumor intact. The contralateral ovary should be carefully inspected and biopsied if anything suspicious is detected. In the scenario of a clinical stage I ovarian carcinoma, unilateral adnexectomy, omentectomy, unilateral pelvic and aortocaval lymph node sampling, peritoneal biopsies and four-quadrant washings can be safely carried out during pregnancy, with chemotherapy reserved for those patients who are upstaged on histopathologic analysis. The chemotherapy regimen is similar to what is used for advanced disease (e.g. a platinum compound and a taxane for the epithelial cancers); however, for patients with FIGO stage Ia–Ib, grade 1 non-clear cell tumors, no chemotherapy will be recommended.

Malignant germ cell tumors in pregnancy

Fortunately, ovarian germ cell neoplasms in pregnancy are usually benign. Dermoid cysts are by far the most common neoplastic cysts found in pregnancy; however, malignant ovarian germ cell tumors such as the dysgerminoma, embryonal carcinoma, immature teratoma, and yolk sac tumor (formerly called "endodermal sinus tumor") have also been reported. Although a considerable number of these cancers present with early-stage disease (in both pregnant and non-pregnant patients), there are several reports of advanced cancers associated with pregnancy. Combination chemotherapy during pregnancy has been given without deleterious effects on the fetus.

The management of malignant ovarian germ cell tumors is predicated on the histologic identity of the tumor (see Fig. 16–7). Patients with clinical stage Ia dysgerminoma and those with clinical stage Ia–Ib grade 1 immature teratoma require surgical staging to determine the need for adjuvant chemotherapy (Fig. 16–9). All other histologic types require adjuvant chemotherapy, and therefore unilateral adnexectomy is all that is typically accomplished at the time of laparotomy, along with removal of all gross metastatic disease. Because most malignant germ cell tumors will be unilateral (the dysgerminoma is the exception in 10% of cases), it is inappropriate to remove both ovaries. Even when the opposite side may harbor an occult dysgerminoma, it is often not necessary to remove the

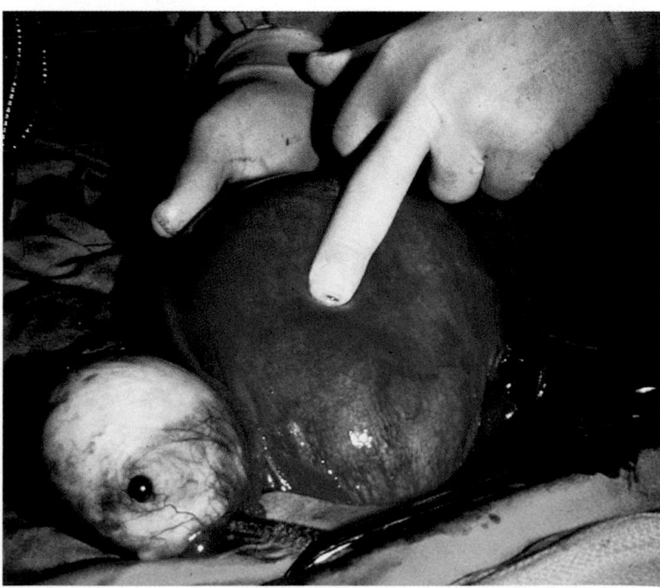

Figure 16–9 Immature teratoma in pregnancy.

entire contralateral ovary. If, however, both ovaries are grossly involved by malignancy and the pregnancy is in the second trimester and thus free from hormonal support by the corpus luteum, both ovaries should be extracted. The prognosis for this stage is not improved with more extensive surgery. Chemotherapy regimens currently used for this disease comprise bleomycin, etoposide, and cisplatin. This regimen has been used safely during pregnancy.

Combined chemotherapy has improved survival markedly for malignant germ cell ovarian tumors and can permit preservation of childbearing capacity as well as maintenance of the existing pregnancy if the disease is stage I. If the diagnosis is made during the first or second trimester, the patient must decide whether to permit the pregnancy to continue to viability before adjuvant chemotherapy is instituted. Because these tumors characteristically grow rapidly and often recur within months when therapy is withheld, delays in initiating systemic therapy can be harmful. Indeed, the high success rate obtained with adjuvant chemotherapy has been recorded with use of this modality in the immediate postoperative period. The effect of a treatment-free interval of several months before the commencement of adjuvant chemotherapy has not been tested adequately. Thus the patient with a malignant ovarian germ cell tumor discovered early in pregnancy and in need of chemotherapy is faced with a dilemma for which no data are available. Malone and colleagues described a patient with stage Ic endodermal sinus tumor diagnosed in the 25th week of gestation who received two cycles of combination chemotherapy consisting of vinblastine, bleomycin, and cisplatin and delivered a healthy boy by caesarean section at 32 weeks' gestation. She subsequently completed three more cycles of chemotherapy and remained well at the time of Malone et al's report 18 months after initial diagnosis. To our knowledge, this was the first report of a case of a patient who had endodermal sinus tumor treated with combination chemotherapy during pregnancy that apparently had a successful outcome for both mother and infant. Subsequently, we and others have had similar experiences.

Therapeutic decisions for patients who have more advanced stages of these tumors are also difficult and controversial. Many such patients can be cured with early adjuvant chemotherapy after surgery. As in earlier stages, the uterus and opposite ovary can be preserved if metastatic tumor is not found in these locations. Some clinicians preserve the uterus and opposite ovary under all conditions in the hope that postoperative chemotherapy will sterilize those organs as well. No long-term follow-up of this approach is available. Delays in withholding chemotherapy are not warranted, and uterine evacuation is often requested because of fear of potential teratogenic effects when chemotherapy is required during the first trimester. The subject of adjuvant chemotherapy in pregnancy is discussed later, but we emphasize that all chemotherapeutic agents are theoretically teratogenic. Although retrospective studies have not shown frequent congenital abnormalities in patients treated in the second and third trimesters, many newer agents have not been used frequently in pregnancy.

Dysgerminoma in pregnancy

Ovarian dysgerminomas are unique among the malignant germ cell tumors because of their overall good prognosis in FIGO stage Ia treated by surgery alone. Dysgerminoma is particularly common and accounts for 30% of ovarian malignant neoplasms in pregnancy. We believe that these tumors can be managed with a unilateral adnexectomy and continuation of the pregnancy without additional therapy in FIGO stage Ia. Optimal staging should include a pelvic and periaortic lymphadenectomy on the side of the tumor mass, because dysgerminomas metastasize primarily through the lymphatic system to the ipsilateral pelvic and periaortic lymph nodes. Because lymphangiography and computed tomography (CT) are contraindicated when the pregnancy is to be continued, patients who have not had adequate exploration at initial surgery should be considered for re-exploration before further therapy and continuation of the pregnancy are recommended. Appropriate diagnostic studies, including lymphangiography and CT scan of the abdomen and pelvis, may be performed in the postpartum period. A mass on scan or a suspicious lymph node on lymphangiography should be evaluated at re-exploration.

Emergency surgical intervention and obstetric complications are common in patients with dysgerminomas. Karlen and associates reviewed 27 cases of dysgerminoma associated with pregnancy. Torsion and incarceration were found commonly in this group of patients who had rapidly enlarging neoplasms averaging 25 cm in diameter. Obstetric complications occurred in nearly half the patients, and fetal demise occurred in one-quarter of the reviewed cases. There were recurrences in 30% of 23 stage Ia tumors treated by unilateral oophorectomy, which calls into question the philosophy of treating these patients conservatively. The extent of exploration was not known in most cases, however, and therefore accuracy of staging cannot be assessed. This information is essential for appropriate interpretation of the findings. In our experience, lesions that are confined to one ovary have a 10% recurrence rate. Although most of these lesions recur in the first 2 years after surgery, we believe that this group of patients can continue their pregnancy safely with completion of their proper evaluation in the puerperium. Because radiation therapy and chemotherapy are successful in curing greater than 75% of patients, even those with metastatic or recurrent dysgerminoma, and because there is a low incidence of recurrence in patients with FIGO stage Ia disease, we maintain a philosophy of conservatism for the treatment of these tumors.

Sex cord–stromal tumors in pregnancy

Granulosa and Sertoli–Leydig cell tumors together account for only 2–3% of all ovarian neoplasms. Although granulosa cell tumors are most commonly discovered in perimenopausal or postmenopausal women, 10–20% are encountered during the reproductive years. Sertoli–Leydig cell tumors occur in women in the reproductive age group in 74% of cases. Interestingly, sex cord–stromal tumors are rarely found in pregnancy. It is critical that these entities are distinguished from ovarian decidualization, luteoma of pregnancy, or even benign granulosa cell proliferations observed with pregnancy. Typically, the sex cord–stromal ovarian tumors behave as they do in non-pregnant women, presenting with early-stage disease and having a slow, low-grade, and indolent course. Thus, because their biologic behavior is akin to that of neoplasms of low malignant potential, it is recommended that they be managed conservatively (i.e. unilateral adnexectomy without comprehensive surgical staging) as in the young non-pregnant patient (Fig. 16–7). It is important, however, to resect all visible tumor whenever possible.

Young et al reported a series of 17 granulosa cell, 13 Sertoli–Leydig cell, and 6 unclassified sex cord–stromal tumors diagnosed during pregnancy or the puerperium. Eleven patients had abdominal pain or swelling when they were first seen by a physician, five were in shock, two had virilization, and one had vaginal bleeding. Three asymptomatic patients underwent exploration because of palpable masses, and one underwent exploration because of an adnexal mass found on ultrasound examination. In 13 patients, the tumors were discovered during caesarean sections; five patients had dystocia, and the tumors were incidental findings in eight patients. All the tumors were FIGO stage I, but 13 of the tumors had ruptured. All but one were unilateral. Hemoperitoneum was present in seven cases.

Young et al uncovered four major sources of difficulty in the interpretation of their series of 36 cases:

1. the young age of the patients,
2. an alteration in the histologic appearance of the tumors during pregnancy,
3. a decreased frequency of associated endocrine manifestations, and
4. pregnancy-induced changes in other neoplastic and non-neoplastic lesions of the ovary that cause them to simulate sex cord–stromal tumors both morphologically and in terms of endocrine function.

Indeed, the pregnancy-associated tumors commonly exhibited alterations related to the pregnant state that tended to obscure characteristics and familiar features that are apparent in tumors removed from non-pregnant patients. The most striking changes included intercellular edema and increased extent of luteinization in the granulosa cell tumors and of Leydig cell maturation in the Sertoli–Leydig cell tumors. Importantly, the edema often blurred the architectural patterns of the tumors and distorted the cytologic features of the neoplastic cells. The marked luteinization and Leydig cell maturation interfered with the recognition of these cells. The end result was that these pregnancy-associated changes made identification of the tumor type more difficult.

Granulosa cell tumors are clinically estrogenic in approximately two-thirds of cases, and Sertoli–Leydig cell tumors are virilizing in nearly 50% of cases. These hormonal manifestations often suggest the correct diagnosis to the gynecologist. However, during pregnancy the hyperestrogenic clinical manifestations do not appear, with none of the 17 tumors in the series by Young et al associated with estrogenic manifestations. It is quite probable, however, that many of these tumors were secreting estrogens in large quantities. Furthermore, only 16% ($n = 5$) of the 36 sex cord–stromal tumors were associated with clinical evidence of excess androgens (virilization in four cases, and hirsuitism in only one case). This low frequency may have been the result of the placenta's ability to aromatize androgens produced by the tumor. In fact, one of the masculinizing tumors was the largest in their series (32 cm in maximal diameter), and may have been secreting androgens in such great abundance that the aromatizing capacity of the placenta was exceeded.

Several other types of ovarian neoplasms and non-neoplastic disorders are more frequently associated with virilization during pregnancy than Sertoli–Leydig cell tumors. Tumors with functioning, proliferative ovarian stroma such as the Krukenberg and the mucinous cystic tumors may be confused morphologically with sex cord–stromal tumors. Other primary ovarian tumors that can cause virilization include luteinized thecomas, and Leydig and lipid cell tumors. Finally, as described earlier, two non-neoplastic lesions of the ovary that develop during pregnancy and can be associated with virilization include the luteoma of pregnancy and the hyperreactio luteinalis (multiple luteinized follicle cysts). All these virilizing tumors and lesions must be considered in the differential diagnosis when confronted with virilization of the pregnant mother, so as to not make an erroneous clinical diagnosis of a sex cord–stromal tumor.

With one exception, the patients in the study by Young et al were initially treated by conservative surgical procedures. Two of them received chemotherapy and two received radiation therapy postoperatively. Hysterectomies and salpingo-oophorectomies were performed as second operations in eight cases; no residual tumor was found in any of these specimens. Only one patient had a recurrence, which was treated surgically. Follow-up for the average of 4.7 years was available for 30 of the 36 patients; all of them were free of disease at their last examination. Adjuvant therapy has not been demonstrated to improve the outcome in this group of patients and is not recommended during pregnancy.

Epithelial ovarian cancer in pregnancy

Very few series of malignant ovarian carcinomas in pregnancy have been published. Reported in 2002, the most recent series contains nine ovarian cancers concurrent with pregnancy from Libya and Saudi Arabia. Among these cases were included seven epithelial cancers (four serous, two mucinous, one undifferentiated), one dysgerminoma, and one granulose cell tumor. As expected, the latter two lesions occurred in younger women, aged 18 and 21 years, respectively. All seven women with epithelial cancers were multiparous (range 3–10), which is of some interest given the epidemiologic data suggesting increasing parity to be inversely related to the risk of developing ovarian carcinoma. Four patients with FIGO stage Ia tumors, including two with epithelial lesions, underwent unilateral adnexectomy prior to 25 weeks' gestation. None of the patients with more advanced disease who went on to receive chemotherapy did so during pregnancy. The obstetric outcome was favorable for all patients except for one with a FIGO stage Ia serous cystadenocarcinoma whose infant died from complications of meconium aspiration. It is of sufficient interest that five of the epithelial tumors were early stage (three FIGO stage Ia and two FIGO stage Ic) and one was assigned FIGO stage IIa. The only death occurred in a patient with a FIGO stage III undifferentiated carcinoma. Thus, fully six of seven women with epithelial ovarian cancers were diagnosed with early or locally advanced disease only, which does not reflect what is typically observed in the general population. It is quite certain that antenatal care including serial physical examinations and ultrasonography contributed to these early pick-ups.

Once the diagnosis of ovarian carcinoma is made during pregnancy, appropriate therapy should not be withheld (Fig. 16–7). In those patients who present with metastatic disease manifest as malignant ascites and carcinomatosis, surgical exploration is warranted, with an attempt to remove as much of the tumor burden as is feasible. Depending on the degree of tumor involvement of the uterus and the mother's desire for the pregnancy, uterine preservation may be considered, and if so the "hands off" approach to the uterus, and removal of mobile intraperitoneal deposits, can be attempted. Certainly, the typical aggressive cytoreductive approach (e.g. bowel resection, splenetomy) taken in non-pregnant women with advanced-stage ovarian carcinoma can result in significant morbidity, and if the pregnancy is to be continued we advise against this approach unless the patient has presented with a bowel obstruction.

An untested option in this group of patients is measurement of the serum CA-125 and aspiration of ascites fluid under ultrasound guidance for cytologic analysis. Once malignancy is confirmed and considered likely to be of ovarian origin, systemic chemotherapy during the second and third trimesters in a "neoadjuvant" fashion can be considered, with plans for interval cytoreductive surgery following delivery. The standard regimen for metastatic epithelial ovarian cancer in non-pregnant patients includes platinum-based chemotherapy. Regimens containing cisplatin alone as well as cisplatin plus paclitaxel, and even administration of a full six cycles of carboplatin and paclitaxel (the current standard among non-pregnant women), have been used during the second and third trimesters of pregnancy. Because there does not appear to be any significant risk to the fetus when these drugs are used in the second and third trimesters, pregnant patients diagnosed during these periods should be offered the opportunity to receive platinum-based therapy without terminating their pregnancy. Postpartum, the patient may return to the operating room to undergo definitive surgical staging or comprehensive tumor debulking.

Patients remote from term (e.g. during the first trimester) with metastatic disease should be advised to undergo hysterectomy with the fetus in situ in conjunction with tumor debulking. Because the prognosis for women with advanced carcinoma is poor, patients must be counseled regarding the realities of how much time they would have with their child when making decisions regarding pregnancy termination.

Summary of the adnexal mass and ovarian cancer in pregnancy

The problem of an adnexal mass in pregnancy is simple. One must have a high index of suspicion, make the diagnosis early, and treat promptly. The difficulty arises when both patient and physician resist abdominal exploration during pregnancy because of fear of precipitating fetal wastage. However, the potential danger to the mother far exceeds the imagined danger to the child. Most of the difficulties seen with ovarian tumors are those of omission rather than of commission. The probability of ovarian cancer must be kept foremost in the minds of physicians caring for these patients. At laparotomy, most malignant ovarian tumors apparently confined to one ovary will require complete surgical staging. A technique of "hands off the uterus," whenever possible, appears to reduce postoperative uterine contractions.

Breast cancer

Pregnancy-associated breast cancer (PABC) is defined as breast cancer diagnosed during pregnancy or lactation up to 12 months postpartum. The disease is a disaster for all involved. Both patient and physician find it difficult to accept this dread disease in a healthy young pregnant woman. Because breast cancer is rare in women younger than 35 years, this problem, fortunately, is a rare complication of pregnancy, with an incidence of approximately one case for every 3000 deliveries. Conversely, of all patients with breast cancer, 1–2% are pregnant at the time of diagnosis. PABC provides a challenging scenario for the mother and oncologist. It is the second most common malignancy to complicate pregnancy but, unlike cervical cancer, it is not screened for during pregnancy, and because delays in diagnosis are common, and the diagnosis itself elusive, oftentimes patients are diagnosed with advanced tumors for which prognosis is poor. Furthermore, the management of breast cancer often involves a coordination of surgery, radiotherapy, chemotherapy, and even hormonal therapy, all of which may impact the pregnancy. Finally, there are several distinct hormonal issues related to pregnancy that may have an influence on the course of breast cancer.

Historically, PABC has been associated with a poor prognosis, with accounts from the nineteenth century describing exceedingly rapid growth and a malignant course. In 1943, Haagensen and Stout reinforced this feeling of doom when they decided that the outcome for this group of patients was so poor that they recommended surgical treatment not be offered. Contemporary opinion for the most part maintains the dismal prognosis associated with PABC. It must be acknowledged that the literature comprises mainly single-institution retrospective experiences and case reports. The only series containing greater than 100 patients are four in number (White, Bunker and Peters, Ribeiro and Palmer, Clark and Reid), none of which were published after 1978.

Although the overall survival rate for breast cancer is >60%, the overall survival rate in pregnancy is reported by some to have dropped to 15 or 20%. Pregnant patients tend to have a higher incidence of positive axillary lymph nodes. Locoregional spread of the tumor portends a poor prognosis and in all likelihood suggests that the neoplasm has metastasized at the time of the initiation of therapy. The advanced stage of the presentation of disease in the pregnant patient has been attributed to multiple factors. First, the engorged breast can successfully obscure a lesion for a much longer period. Survivals are lower for cases diagnosed late in pregnancy than for those recognized in the first trimester. Others emphasize the 30–50 multiples of increase in serum levels of estrogens and progesterone. In addition, there may be increased vascularity and lymphatic drainage from the pregnant breast, assisting the metastatic process to regional lymph nodes. If a lesion is detected early (present <3 months, smaller than 2 cm, and no positive nodes), the chance of survival (70–80%) is the same for the pregnant and the non-pregnant patient. If, on the other hand, there is involvement of the subareolar region, diffuse inflammatory carcinoma, edema or ulceration of the skin, fixation of the tumor to the breast wall, or involvement of the high axillary, supraclavicular, or internal mammary nodes, the prognosis is poor for the pregnant and the non-pregnant patient both.

Presentation

At least 10% of patients with breast cancer who are younger than 40 years will be pregnant at diagnosis. PABC typically presents as a painless mass or thickening. In some cases, there may be an associated nipple discharge, and in the lactating breast the infant may exhibit the "milk rejection sign," effectively refusing the breast that contains the cancer. The mean breast weight normally doubles in pregnancy from 200 to 400 grams, resulting in breast firmness and increased breast density. Mammographic evaluation of the pregnant breast is difficult to interpret, and the clinical examination may be deceptive. This has profound implications in terms of delays in diagnosis and treatment, which as discussed above are not uncommon in PABC. Many patients with PABC will have a delay in diagnosis ranging from 1 to 2.5 months during pregnancy, and up to 6 months during lactation. In a 1991 series from the Memorial Sloan–Kettering Cancer Center in New York, 44 of 56 patients did not have the diagnosis of cancer made until the postpartum period. Overall, in a review of the literature by Puckridge et al, a delay of 2–15 months longer from manifestation of the first symptoms to the diagnosis of cancer occurs in PABC. Given the tumor-doubling time of 130 days, a 1-month delay in primary tumor treatment increases the risk of axillary metastases by 0.9%, and a 6-month delay increases the risk by 5.1%. For this reason particularly, PABC has been considered an ominous diagnosis, but when age and stage are taken into account, there is no difference in the survival of PABC cases as compared with non-PABC cases. Pregnancy is not thought to be an independent risk factor.

Evaluation

A proposed management algorithm for PABC appears in Figure 16–10. Early diagnosis has been associated with

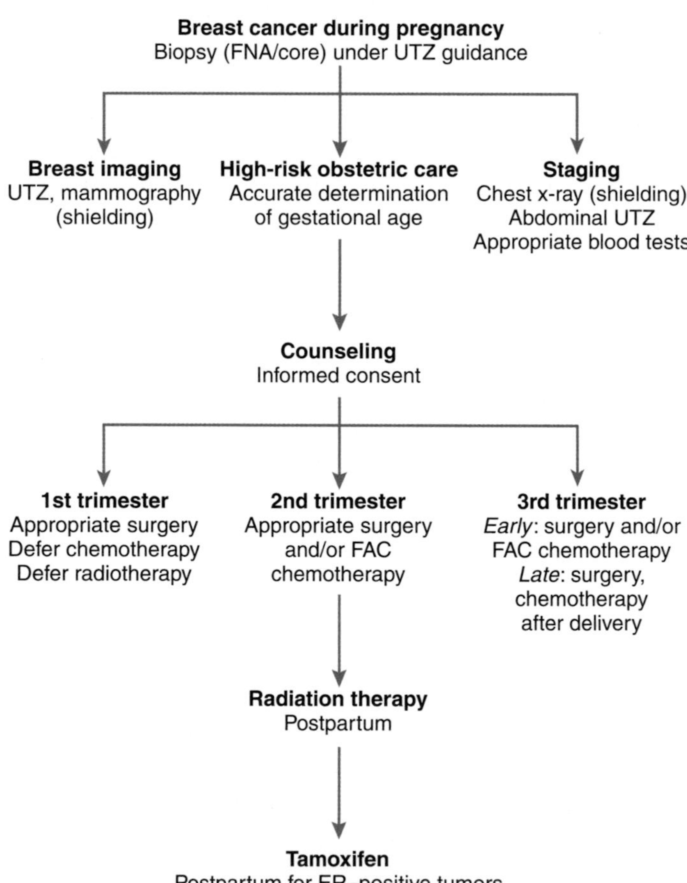

Figure 16–10 Management algorithm for pregnancy-associated breast cancer. ER, estrogen receptor; FAC, 5-fluorouracil, doxorubicin (Adriamycin), and cyclophosphamide; FNA, fine-needle aspiration; UTZ, ultrasound.

improved survivals and relies on the liberal use of imaging strategies as well as the core and fine-needle biopsy techniques for this group of patients. Mammography in conjunction with abdominal lead shielding can be safely used during pregnancy but, as discussed earlier, the engorged and lactating breast increases tissue density and may mask abnormalities. Ultrasonography yields equivalent information with no known adverse effects to the fetus. Fine-needle aspiration may be difficult to interpret cytologically secondary to cellular changes that take place during pregnancy and lactation, and is often associated with an increase in the false-negative rate. *Core biopsy remains the gold standard in making the diagnosis.* When necessary, an open biopsy under local anesthesia is also appropriate. Stopping lactation with ice packs and breast binding or bromocriptine (2.5 mg three times daily for 1 week) beforehand will reduce the risk of a milk fistula. The breasts should be emptied of milk prior to the biopsy, and a pressure dressing will decrease the risk of hematoma that may develop from the hypervascularity of the pregnant breast.

Approximately 75–90% of PABCs are ductal carcinomas, mirroring what is observed in the non-pregnant population. Historically, there was a perceived increase in inflammatory carcinoma of the breast during pregnancy; however, this has since been refuted in contemporary series, in which the incidence ranges from 1.5 to 4.2% among pregnant and non-pregnant patients. Several studies have demonstrated adverse pathologic features in PABC. Most patients with PABC have estrogen receptor (ER)–negative and progesterone receptor (PR)–negative tumors. This may be due to the production of false-negative results by the ligand-binding assay used for ER/PR when high circulating levels of estrogen and progesterone down-regulate receptors. Immunohistochemistry has not been able to detect a difference in the number of hormone receptor–positive tumors when PABC cases are compared with cases of breast cancer in non-pregnant patients of similar ages. Additionally, higher levels of c-ERBB-2 over-expression and p53 mutations have been reported in lactational carcinomas, but not in tumors diagnosed during pregnancy. Furthermore, there have been reports of increased HER-2/neu–positive tumors as compared with in non-pregnant control subjects. It is interesting that the HER-2/neu oncogene product p105 is over-expressed not only in ductal carcinomas but also in fetal epithelial cells and the placenta, and that toward the end of the third trimester of pregnancy, serum levels of p105 normally rise.

It is known from epidemiologic studies that there is an increased incidence of breast cancers in certain families; the risk increases 5–10 times if a patient's mother or sister has had the disease. Interestingly, women with a genetic predisposition to breast cancer may be over-represented among cases of PABC, with a significant family history of breast cancer being three times more common in women with PABC than among non-pregnant patients with breast cancer. Along these lines, PABC has been associated with a higher rate of BRCA2 allelic mutation compared with sporadic breast cancer. Indeed, a Swedish report of 292 women with breast cancer before the age of 40 demonstrated a greater likelihood of known BRCA1 and BRCA2 carriers to develop cancer during pregnancy.

Staging of breast cancer currently employs a complicated system jointly recommended by the International Union Against Cancer and the American Joint Committee on Cancer (see Table 14–12). The Haagensen clinical staging for breast cancer is more useful in pointing out the unfavorable prognostic indicators in this disease process. Lateral and posteroanterior chest radiographs in conjunction with lead shielding is considered safe during pregnancy, with an estimated fetal dose of only 0.6 mGy. Provided a catheter is placed to allow rapid drainage of radioactive material from the bladder, a low-dose labeled technetium-99 bone scan is also safe. The low-dose bone scan exposes the fetus to 0.0008 Gy instead of the standard 0.0019 Gy. The higher radiation exposure to the fetus excludes the use of CT in planning a metastatic workup, but MRI may be used to study the thorax and abdomen as well as to image the skeleton. MRI is preferred to ultrasonography for hepatic imaging, and is also the safest and most sensitive way to study the brain.

Surgical management

Surgery is the definitive treatment for PABC (Fig. 16–10). The extent of surgery in the treatment of breast cancer is being debated throughout the world, and that issue cannot be adequately addressed here. Lumpectomy or partial mastectomy is more commonly used, especially when the lesion is not large, although the preferred surgical treatment for stage I, stage II, and some stage III tumors involves mastectomy, thus avoiding the need for adjuvant radiotherapy in most cases (i.e. early-stage breast cancer). Because nodal metastases are commonly identified in PABC, and because nodal status dictates the choice of adjuvant chemotherapy, axillary dissection has been routinely recommended, especially in light of the potential risk to the fetus from radioisotope if sentinel node biopsy was attempted.

Recently, Keleher et al assessed the risk to the embryo/fetus associated with sentinel lymph node biopsy and lymphoscintigraphy of the breast in pregnant patients. Following peritumoral injection of 92.5 MBq (2.5 mCi) of filtered technetium-99 m sulfur colloid the day before surgery in two non-pregnant women with breast cancer, they calculated the absorbed dose to the embryo/fetus for three theoretic extreme scenarios of biodistribution and pharmacokinetics, and described the maximum absorbed dose to the fetus being 4.3 mGy calculated for the worst-case scenario. The authors concluded that breast lymphoscintigraphy during pregnancy presents a very low risk to the embryo/fetus. Further research into this area will be required to validate these findings before sentinel node identification can be safely recommended during pregnancy.

The timing of surgery for cancer diagnosed late in pregnancy is another source of debate. Some reports suggest that patients treated postpartum survive longer than those treated in the second and third trimesters. This suggests that postponement of therapy for patients near term may be of benefit. These reports fail to consider the possibility that patients selected for postponed treatment might have been those with small, more favorable cancers discovered late in pregnancy, whereas larger, aggressive, anaplastic cancers with rapid progression received immediate treatment. If such treatment bias exists, prompt treatment would not be expected to correlate with good results, and treatment after delivery would appear favorable because of a preponderance of favorable patients in that group.

Breast reconstruction

Although the performance of a transverse myocutaneous flap of the rectus abdominis muscle (TRAM flap) is a satisfying, one-step, immediate reconstruction of good aesthetic quality without need for prosthetic materials, this is not recommended in patients with PABC who undergo mastectomy. The procedure should be deferred to the postpartum period. The problem of residual functional capacities of the abdominal wall deprived of a part or of all its rectus muscle also has important implications for future pregnancies. In fact, for some authors in the past, the desire for future childbearing was a contraindication to TRAM flap breast reconstruction, because it was thought that the abdominal wall, weakened by rotation of one or both of its rectus muscles, would not be capable of withstanding the stress induced by pregnancy. To avoid the development of a hernia in the abdominal wall at the donor site, an interval of at least 12 months between breast reconstruction with a TRAM flap and pregnancy is recommended.

Adjuvant therapy

Women with early lesions may opt for a tissue-sparing procedure. In these cases, local irradiation is often required. Radiotherapy to the breast, chest wall, or axillary lymph nodes, even with shielding, results in a significant fetal dose because of scatter in excess of that which is considered safe. The doses of internal scatter of radiation have been calculated. At 12 weeks' gestation, the fetus would receive 10–15 cGy. In the third trimester, this dose can be as high as 200 cGy. This is due to the fact that although during the first trimester the fetus is in a safer position and can be better shielded, it is more sensitive to the effects of radiation. In contrast, as the fetus enlarges and is less sensitive to radiation, it moves upward out of the pelvis, where it is less readily shielded and exposed to higher levels of ionizing radiation. Local irradiation should be deferred until after delivery of the fetus (Fig. 16–10). Women treated with adjuvant radiation during the postpartum period will not be able to lactate from the irradiated breast.

Locally advanced disease is difficult to manage with the pregnancy in place. Chemotherapy or local radiotherapy, followed in 6 weeks by mastectomy, is the usual treatment plan for these lesions. For advanced disease, chemotherapy has been used after the first trimester when the mother is reluctant to terminate the pregnancy and the disease appears to be progressing at an alarming rate. The issue of whether chemotherapy should be administered to patients with node-positive breast cancer in pregnancy is complicated by reports suggesting that both single-agent and combination chemotherapy may significantly improve survival in premenopausal patients in an adjuvant setting. Follow-ups of 10 and 15 years are always necessary in breast cancer, but it would appear that the premenopausal patient is the best candidate for aggressive adjuvant chemotherapy and a resulting improved survival rate. This is especially pertinent to patients in whom positive nodes are discovered at the time of the initial procedure.

Table 16-8 contains reports of chemotherapy use during pregnancy, with favorable neonatal outcomes noted when treatment was administered only after the first trimester.

Lactation

Whether breast-feeding is safe and/or possible has also been debated. Many have postulated that breast cancer is at least in part of viral origin, and the possibility exists that the contralateral breast will be contaminated with the etiologic agent, which will be passed to the fetus. This theory has never been borne out in fact, but most surgeons recommend artificial feeding of the infant, ostensibly to avoid vascular enrichment in the opposite breast, which may also contain a neoplasm.

Reports by Higgins and Haffty and by Tralins suggest that successful lactation in the breast treated by lumpectomy and irradiation is possible. Apparently, the location of the breast incision is important. Not surprisingly, circumareolar incisions were associated with diminished ability to lactate because such incisions interrupt a large number of major milk ducts. Radial incisions in the breast interrupt fewer ducts but may be, on the other hand, cosmetically inferior. In addition, the size, shape, and orientation of the nipple are important to allow its normal mechanical function. Patients whose nipples did not extend sufficiently or were not oriented properly or were not supple found that the infant would not nurse from the treated breast. Finally, concerns have been expressed by some clinicians that attempts to breast-feed after conservative surgery may lead to a greater incidence of mastitis secondary to disruptions of the ductal system.

Hormonal considerations: pregnancy preceding breast cancer

Protective effect of human chorionic gonadotropin

The hormonal issues specific to breast cancer appear in Figure 16–11. Epidemiologic data have demonstrated a 50% reduction in the risk of breast cancer in women who

Table 16–8 CONGENITAL ANOMALIES AFTER IN UTERO EXPOSURE TO BREAST CANCER CHEMOTHERAPY

Authors	Year	*n*	Treatment	Trimester	Outcome
Tobias and Bloom	1980	1	AV, prednisone	2	No anomaly
Murray et al	1984	1	AC, radiation	1	Imperforate anus, rectovaginal fistula
Mulvihill et al	1987	1	CMF, melphalan	n/s	Spontaneous abortion
Zemlickis et al	1992	2	CMF, melphalan	1	Spontaneous abortion (both cases)
		1	CAFV, tamoxifen	1	No anomaly
		1	CAF, tamoxifen	3	No anomaly
		1	CMF	3	No anomaly
Cullins et al	1980	1	Tamoxifen	1, 2, 3	Goldenhar syndrome
Tewari et al	1997	1	Tamoxifen	1, 2	Ambiguous genitalia
Turchi and Villasis	1988	1	CAMF	1	No anomaly
Berry et al	1999	24	CAF	2, 3	No anomaly
Isaacs et al	2001	1	Tamoxifen, 0.0017 Gy RT	1, 2, 3	Preauricular skin tags
Andreadis et al	2004	1	FEC,[a] 28 Gy RT,[b] tamoxifen,[c] zolendronic acid[c]	1, 2, 3	No anomalies
Gonzalez-Angulo et al	2004	1	Neoadjuvant paclitaxel	2, 3	No anomalies

A, doxorubicin (Adriamycin); C, cyclophosphamide; E, epirubicin; F, 5-fluorouracil; M, methotrexate; n/s, not specified; RT, radiotherapy; V, vincristine.
[a]First trimester only.
[b]Second trimester.
[c]Second and third trimesters.
(After Woo et al: Breast cancer in pregnancy. A literature review. Arch Surg 138:91–98, 2003.)

complete full-term pregnancies before 20 years of age. The benefit is seen among all ethnic groups worldwide and increases with increasing parity. There is a declination in risk reduction beyond the age of 30 years. Both human and animal breast tissues and human breast cell lines contain low levels of receptors that bind hCG and its structural and functional homolog luteinizing hormone. These gonadotropins exert numerous anticancer effects in breast cancer models and cells, prompting some investigators to speculate that the elevated levels of hCG associated with full-term pregnancies may exert a protective effect against the later development of breast cancer.

Recent antecedent pregnancy

The above discussion notwithstanding, there have been concerns raised that the protective benefit of pregnancy on the risk of later breast cancer may be biphasic, with a transient increase in the risk of breast cancer shortly after pregnancy, followed by a greater long-term reduction in risk. Russo et al have postulated that this may occur via the short-term stimulation of any existing malignant clones under the influence of the hormonal milieu of pregnancy, but longer term inhibition of breast carcinogenesis is as a consequence of induction of differentiation of normal mammary stem cells in the later stages of pregnancy that otherwise have the potential for neoplastic change.

Further extrapolation leads to the possibility that a recent childbirth before the diagnosis of breast cancer may increase a woman's risk of dying from the disease. Whiteman et al observed 4299 US women enrolled between 1980 and 1982 between the ages of 20 and 54 years as incident breast cancer patients in the population-based,

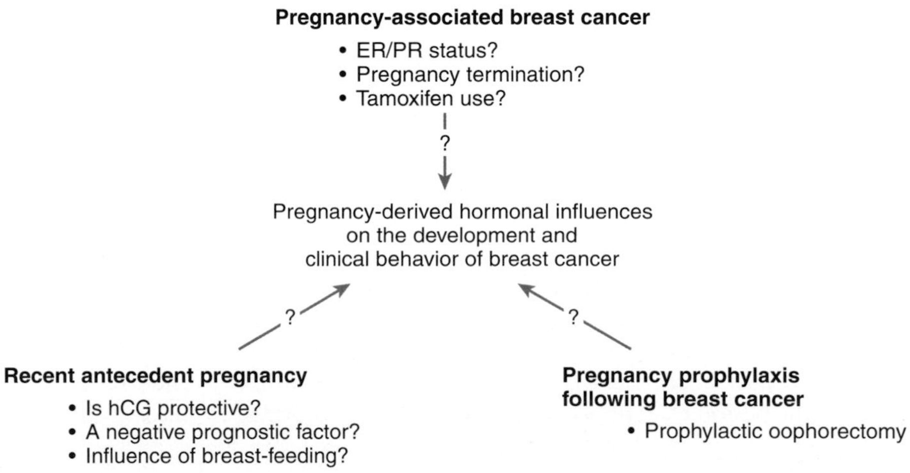

Figure 16–11 Hormonal considerations in breast cancer. ER, estrogen receptor; hCG, human chorionic gonadotropin; PR, progesterone receptor.

case-control study known as the Cancer and Steroid Hormone Study. The 15-year survival rates were 38%, 51%, and 60% among women aged 20–45 years whose last birth was 12 months or less, 13–48 months, and more than 48 months before diagnosis, respectively, compared with 65% among nulliparous women. Phillips et al prospectively studied 750 women diagnosed with breast cancer before age 45 years who were part of the population-based Australian Breast Cancer Family Study, and demonstrated that the proximity of last childbirth to subsequent breast cancer diagnosis was a predictor of mortality independent of histopathologic tumor characteristics. Specifically, compared with nulliparous women, the investigators found that women who gave birth within 2 years prior to diagnosis were more likely to have axillary node–positive (58% vs 41%, $P = 0.01$) and ER-negative (58% vs 39%, $P = 0.005$) tumors. The unadjusted hazard ratios for death were 2.3, 1.7, and 0.9 for patients who gave birth less than 2 years, 2–5 years, and 5 or more years before diagnosis, respectively.

Breast-feeding

In an effort to determine what contribution (if any) breast-feeding has on the subsequent development of breast cancer, the Collaborative Group on Hormonal Factors in Breast Cancer examined the individual data from 47 epidemiologic studies in 30 countries that included information on breast-feeding patterns. In total, 50,302 women with invasive breast cancer were compared with 96,973 control subjects. The investigators noted that women with breast cancer had fewer births than did control subjects (2.2 vs 2.6), and that fewer parous women with cancer than parous control subjects had ever breast-fed (71 vs 79%), with their average lifetime duration of breast-feeding being shorter (9.8 vs 15.6 months). The relative risk for breast cancer decreased by 4.3% for every 12 months of breast-feeding in addition to a decrease of 7.0% for each birth. Thus the longer women breast-fed, the more they were protected against breast cancer. The lack of or short lifetime duration of breast-feeding typical of women in developed countries may contribute greatly to the high incidence of breast cancer in industrialized nations.

Hormonal considerations: pregnancy coincident with breast cancer

Although there is no clear evidence that pregnancy adversely affects the course of this disease, the suspicion persists. It has been established that once the diagnosis is made, stage for stage, the pregnant patient does as well as the non-pregnant patient. However, the low incidence of stage I lesions in pregnancy strongly suggests an acceleration of the disease process in the preclinical period. As stated previously (see Ch. 14), many cell kinetic studies of breast cancer suggest that lesions are harbored within the breast for 5–8 years before becoming clinical entities. Because the period of gestation is no longer than 9 months, it is difficult to believe that the sole explanation for the high incidence of advanced disease in pregnancy is related to late diagnosis caused by the engorged breast.

The massive endogenous hormone production in pregnancy may adversely affect the course of breast cancer. Urinary excretion of all three major fractions, estrone, estradiol, and estriol, rises progressively after the eighth week of gestation, although there is a disproportionate rise in estriol production by the placenta. Serum concentrations of total estrogens rise nearly 2000-fold, from 4 μg/dL early in pregnancy to mean values of 8–22 mg/dL at term. The ability of estrogens to promote growth of breast cancer in animals and humans has been amply illustrated. Whether the stimulatory effect of increased estrogen production has an adverse effect on prognosis or whether the disproportionate rise of estriol, a relatively weak estrogen and a possible antagonist of estrone and estradiol, confers some measure of protection is unknown.

Additional hormone substances secreted in increased quantities in pregnancy that might influence neoplastic growths in the breast include the glucocorticoids and prolactin. Elevated corticosteroid levels are a regular accompaniment of pregnancy and might influence the outcome of breast cancer. Mean production of 17-hydroxycorticosteroids increases from 12 mg/24 hours to approximately 18 mg/24 hours in late pregnancy. Because glucocorticoids can reduce cellular immunity and perhaps promote the implantation and growth of malignant neoplasms, this increased production has grave clinical implications.

Similarly, elevated levels of prolactin produced by the hypophysis and of human placental lactogen by the placenta late in pregnancy and during milk production might affect breast cancer adversely. Prolactin promotes the growth of dimethyleneanthracene-induced mammary tumors in mice. Its role is not established in humans, but it is a subject of current investigation. The levels of prolactin in patients with breast cancer are not appreciably different from those in control subjects, and prolactin suppression with ergot compounds or with L-dopa has not proved to be of therapeutic value. However, the observation that women with bone pain from metastatic breast cancer sometimes obtain relief from prolactin suppression implicates prolactin as a possible promoter of breast cancer in humans.

Estrogen receptor and progesterone receptor status

A recent paper by Middleton et al detected ER positivity in seven and PR positivity in six of 25 patients with PABC whose tumors were studied by immunohistochemistry. Although most tumors associated with PABC are ER/PR-negative, a proportion will be ER-positive, thus bringing to the discussion the possibility of tamoxifen use during pregnancy (see below). There has been one report of acquired resistance to tamoxifen during the treatment of a patient with PABC, in which the investigators suggest that the changing expression of ER isoforms in pregnancy may have contributed to drug resistance.

Pregnancy termination

Historically, pregnancy was of concern to surgeons primarily because the risk of excess hemorrhage and shock with mastectomy was increased greatly in the gravid state. Billroth advocated premature induction of labor for this reason but did not find that abortion contributed to cure. More contemporary commentators have argued that the striking rise in estrogen production during pregnancy is of sufficient concern to warrant pregnancy termination, and that future pregnancy avoidance should be an important principle of continuing care. Indeed, while many clinicians think that localized breast cancer in the first trimester is a valid reason to recommend termination, reports by Peters and Rosemond illustrate that therapeutic abortion has no effect on survival, and the presence of a fetus does not compromise proper therapy in early stages. Similarly, therapy for localized disease in later pregnancy can be carried out when the diagnosis is made without pregnancy termination. Interestingly, in an updated presentation of 413 patients with PABC referred to the Princess Margaret Hospital in Canada between 1931 and 1985, Clark and Chua observed that therapeutic abortion in breast cancer with coincident, lactational, and subsequent pregnancies is associated with decreased survival. The reasons for this remain unclear. Therapeutic abortion is not currently believed to be an essential component of effective treatment of early disease, despite the theoretic advantage of removing the source of massive estrogen production.

It is critically important to emphasize that treatment of breast cancer should not be delayed provided there are no major obstetric issues. In advanced breast cancer, therapeutic abortion is usually a necessity to achieve effective palliation. In the first trimester of pregnancy, the termination can be accomplished by suction curettage of the uterus; later in pregnancy, termination is accomplished by dinoprostone (Prostin) suppositories, oxytocin (Pitocin) administration, hysterotomy, or hysterectomy. When pregnancy enters the third trimester, the decision for preterm delivery depends heavily on the patient's wishes and the urgency for palliation. A short wait until a viable fetus can be obtained might not be accompanied by significant progress of the neoplasm. Continued gestation represents no threat to the fetus, and the risk of transplacental metastases to the fetus is negligible.

Tamoxifen

Tamoxifen citrate is a non-steroidal weak estrogen that has found successful applications for each stage of breast cancer in the treatment of selected patients. Tamoxifen was originally introduced for the treatment of advanced disease in postmenopausal women; however, the drug is now also available for the palliative treatment of premenopausal women with ER-positive disease. The proven efficacy of tamoxifen and the low incidence of side effects made the drug an ideal agent to test as an adjuvant therapy for estrogen receptor-positive women with axillary lymph node–positive breast cancer. Tamoxifen is a selective ER modulator that is often prescribed for up to 5 years following completion of primary therapy.

The long-term effects of tamoxifen use and whether it may increase gynecologic cancers in daughters are unknown. In pregnant rats, tamoxifen administration has been associated with breast cancer in the female offspring. Cunha et al examined 54 genital tracts isolated from 4- to 19-week-old human female fetuses and grown for 1–2 months in untreated athymic nude mice or host mice treated by subcutaneous pellet with the antiestrogen clomiphene, tamoxifen, or the synthetic estrogen diethylstilbestrol. The investigators noted that condensation and segregation of the uterine mesenchyme was greatly impaired, and that the fallopian tube epithelium was hyperplastic and disorganized with distortion of the complex mucosal plications, in drug-treated specimens as compared with untreated age-matched control subjects.

Table 16–8 also summarizes six reports of tamoxifen use during pregnancy. In 1997, Tewari et al described the first patient to have given birth to a child with congenital anomalies following systemic tamoxifen therapy through 20 weeks of gestation. This 46 XX child had ambiguous genitalia, including labial fusion and clitoramegaly; her internal genitalia were normal by ultrasonography. Another fetus exposed to tamoxifen during all the first, second, and early part of the third trimesters was born at 26 weeks with oculoauriculovertebral dysplasia (i.e. Goldenhar syndrome). A third case appeared in 2001 and involved a fetus delivered at 31 weeks' gestation whose mother was given tamoxifen as sole systemic therapy and locoregional irradiation before pregnancy was determined. In addition to moderate hyaline membrane disease and necrotizing enterocolitis that was attributable to prematurity, the child had preauricular skin tags and an appropriate birthweight but no major malformations. At 2 years of follow-up, this last child was meeting all developmental milestones. The presentation of these three cases has prompted the creation of a tamoxifen registry. It is not clear whether women with ER-positive tumors receiving tamoxifen should temporarily discontinue the medication if and when they become pregnant.

Hormonal considerations: pregnancy following breast cancer

It has been estimated that only 7% of fertile women go on to conceive following the diagnosis and treatment of breast cancer. Nevertheless, a patient with breast cancer may have several concerns regarding future fertility, not least of which is whether she will remain fertile following treatment. In addition, the risk of recurrence conferred by subsequent pregnancy needs to be addressed, as several authors have postulated that the immunosuppressant and hormonal effects of pregnancy so close to diagnosis may have a significant deleterious effect. Finally, a patient may express fear that a child may inherit a genetic predisposition toward the later development of breast cancer.

The recommendations given to such patients should be influenced by two major considerations:

1. whether pregnancy promotes recurrence of cancer, and
2. the probability of having been cured.

Thirty percent of women under 40 years will become amenorrheic following chemotherapy for breast cancer, and 90% of women over 40 years will cease menstruating. For those who continue to ovulate and who are desirous of future childbearing, it has been common practice to recommend a waiting period of 2 years following the diagnosis of breast cancer before attempting to conceive, as most recurrences occur within the first 2 years of diagnosis. In 1985, Nugent and O'Connell described a poor prognosis for women with early subsequent pregnancy, but many investigators have since refuted this. Interestingly, women who have a subsequent pregnancy have equivalent or possibly better survival when matched for stage. Gelber et al evaluated 94 patients from the International Breast Cancer Study Group who became pregnant after the diagnosis of early-stage breast cancer, and compared them to 188 control subjects (i.e. no subsequent pregnancy) matched for nodal status, tumor size, age, and year of diagnosis. The overall 5- and 10-year survival rates from the diagnosis of early-stage breast cancer among the study group was 92% and 86%, respectively, while that of the comparison group was 85% and 74%, respectively. Some have speculated an antitumor effect of the pregnancy, but of course this could reflect the "healthy mother" bias, in that only those select women who feel healthy will go on to conceive. Although it may be presumptuous to conclude on the basis of retrospective studies that pregnancy protects against recurrence after mastectomy, it is reasonably safe to conclude that it does not promote it. In summary, therefore, it would appear that future pregnancies are safe for the mother unless she has an ER-positive tumor and has not been placed into remission. Consequently, if a pregnancy occurs there appears to be no justification for recommending its termination in patients without evidence of recurrence. The converse, that pregnancy with recurrence should be terminated in most instances and that an uneventful pregnancy in no way guarantees against a subsequent recurrence, is also true. Indeed, there are cases on record in which multiple pregnancies have eventually been followed by recurrence.

Prophylactic oophorectomy

Surgical castration for patients with early-stage breast cancer has been advocated to prevent further pregnancy, which might cause recrudescence of the disease through hormone stimulation. Oophorectomy also serves to eliminate the ovarian source of estrogen production, ideally preventing or delaying subsequent recurrence. Neither argument is substantiated by data to support a role for "prophylactic castration." In many patients, chemotherapy will cause a cessation of ovarian hormone production. Importantly, as discussed above, pregnancy after treatment for breast cancer has no influence on the disease, and a few reports even suggest that future pregnancies might be protective. The rationale for eliminating the ovarian source of estrogens in the primary treatment of early disease is based on an observation that castration in the presence of observable recurrent disease results in partial or complete temporary tumor regression in approximately one-third of cases. This argument has been refuted by two large clinical trials conducted in the USA that failed to demonstrate a significant benefit from castration and adjuvant therapy. For example, the National Surgical Adjuvant Breast Project conducted a randomized trial of prophylactic castration in premenopausal women involving 129 castrates and 70 control women. After an observation period of 10 years, there was no evidence that those who were castrated derived any benefit from the procedure.

Survival among patients with pregnancy-associated breast cancer

Most of the data-sets from the preceding few decades show that women with PABC have the same survival stage for stage as non-pregnant women with breast cancer. Women with PABC may do poorly in the aggregate because these patients tend to present with advanced disease. Table 16-9 is adapted from Keleher et al and shows selected 5-year survival data by axillary nodal status for women with PABC. Holleb and Farrow reported a series of 283 patients with carcinomas of the breast in pregnancy, including 73 who had inoperable disease and 210 who underwent surgery with or without postoperative radiation. Of those patients with inoperable disease, 93% died within 2 years of the diagnosis, including all seven of those who had interruption of pregnancy. The majority of the remaining 210 patients underwent radical mastectomy and were given postoperative radiation therapy. Of 28 patients with a diagnosis in the first trimester, seven survived for 5 years. Peters and Meakin described 70 patients with breast cancer in pregnancy, all of whom were treated with preoperative, postoperative, or palliative radiotherapy in conjunction with radical mastectomy. The overall survival rate in this series was 32.9% at 5 years and 19.5% at 10 years. Of 12 patients treated during the first and second trimesters, three survived 5 years; only one of the nine patients treated during the third trimester survived 5 years, and she had active disease at the time of the report. The remaining 49 patients who were treated postpartum had a 39% 5-year survival rate, prompting the author to suggest that a delay in the treatment of breast carcinoma until after delivery should be considered.

It is now recognized that the independent variable of youth results in an unfavorable prognosis in patients with breast cancer, presumably because of the likelihood of more aggressive tumors in these young women. Previously, only young patients had an opportunity of having breast cancer coincident with pregnancy, but as women postpone childbearing, pregnancy coincident with breast cancer will become more common. Physicians must treat patients with breast cancer in pregnancy aggressively and with curative intent.

Table 16–9 FIVE-YEAR SURVIVAL RATES BY AXILLARY NODAL STATUS IN PATIENTS WITH PREGNANCY-ASSOCIATED BREAST CANCER

Authors	Year	Institution	n	Negative lymph nodes (%)	Positive lymph nodes (%)
Haagensen et al	1943	Columbia-Presbyterian	20	0	0
Byrd et al	1962	Vanderbilt University School of Medicine	30	100	28
Bunker and Peters	1963	Princess Margaret Hospital, Toronto	50	50	30
Rosemond	1964	Not located	37	79	13
White	1954	University of Washington	40	72	6
Holleb and Farrow	1962	Memorial Sloan–Kettering	45	58	21
Applewhite et al	1973	Louisiana State University	48	56	18
Nugent and O'Connell	1985	Kaiser Permanente Los Angeles	19	100	50
King et al	1985	Mayo Clinic	63	75	33
Petrek et al	1991	Memorial Sloan–Kettering	56	82	47
Ishida et al	1992	Gunma University, Japan	172	90[a]	52[a]
Kuerer et al	1997	Mount Sinai	26	60	45
Bonnier et al[b]	1997	Multicenter French study	154	63	31

[a]Metastasis-free survival.
[b]Breast-conserving therapy used.
(After Keleher et al: Multidisciplinary management of breast cancer concurrent with pregnancy. J Am Coll Surg 194:54–64, 2001.)

EVALUATION AND THERAPEUTIC MODALITIES

Anesthesia and surgery in the pregnant patient

Anesthesia

Anesthetic considerations in the pregnant patient must take into account both the potential teratogenicity of the anesthetic agents as well as the maternal physiologic changes that result from both the pregnancy and the use of anesthetic agents. The vast majority of analgesics and anesthetics are category C drugs (see Table 16-10). When a drug has demonstrated teratogenicity in animals, it is likely to have the same effect in humans. Therefore, while category C drugs lack human studies, the existing animal studies may be useful in predicting risk to the fetus. A consensus statement published in 1998 in the pages of the *New England Journal of Medicine* did not list any anesthetic agents as definitive causes of fetal anomalies. Inhalational and local anesthetics, muscle relaxants, narcotic analgesics, and benzodiazepines are known to be safe in pregnancy.

The hyperdynamic cardiovascular system of pregnancy is characterized by an increased cardiac output and increased resting heart rate. The total blood volume is increased by 40% and that of the red blood cells by 25%, resulting in the physiologic anemia of pregnancy that decreases the hematocrit by approximately 30%. As the pregnancy progresses, a decrease in blood return to the heart from the inferior vena cava occurs via increasing intra-abdominal pressures caused by the enlarging uterus.

A 30–40% increase in the tidal volume occurs during normal pregnancy as oxygen consumption increases and the abdominal organs undergo mechanical displacement by the gravid uterus. Anesthesiologists may expect a compensatory respiratory alkalosis in pregnancy with a P_aCO_2 of 30–35 mmHg. Cricoid pressure should be applied during intubation to prevent aspiration, the risk of which is increased due to the pregnancy-associated decrease in lower esophageal sphincter pressure and delayed gastric emptying. Small-diameter endotracheal tubes are recommended to facilitate intubation later in pregnancy when airway edema is increased. Intraoperatively, the end tidal CO_2 is monitored.

Table 16–10 DRUG SAFETY CATEGORIES IN PREGNANCY

Category	Description
A	Safety established using human studies
B	Presumed safety based on animal studies
C	Uncertain safety; no human studies; animal studies show adverse effect
D	Unsafe; evidence of risk that may in certain clinical circumstances be justifiable
X	Highly unsafe

Surgery

With the improvements in neonatal care, fetal survival rates continue to increase, and although actual figures vary between different neonatal intensive care units, survival rates greater than 90% can be expected beyond 28 weeks' gestation. Table 16-11 contains neonatal intensive care unit survival statistics based on gestational age and birthweight. Patients in need of surgery during the second trimester can be permitted a short delay to attain fetal

Table 16–11 NEONATAL SURVIVAL AND MORBIDITY BY GESTATIONAL AGE AND BIRTHWEIGHT

		Mean survival rates		Moderate to severe disability (%)	
Factor		Wood et al	NICHD	Wood et al	NICHD
Gestational age (weeks)	23	11	30	56	—
	24	26	52	53	—
	25	54	76	46	—
Weight (g)	401–500	—	11	—	[a]
	501–600	—	27	—	29
	601–700	—	63	—	30
	701–800	—	74	—	28

NICHD, National Institute of Child Health and Human Development.
[a]Too few infants in study to assess.
(After Wood et al: Neurologic and developmental disability after extremely preterm birth. N Engl J Med 343:378, 2000, and Lemons et al: Very low birth weight outcomes of the National Institute of Child Health and Human Development Neonatal Research Network, January 1995 through December 1996. Pediatrics 107:1, 2000. Used with permission from Chapter 34: Preterm labor and delivery. In Creasy RK, Resnik R (eds): Maternal–Fetal Medicine: Principles and Practice, 5th edn. Pennsylvania, Saunders, 2004.)

viability in many cases. When the clinical suspicion for malignancy is high or the diagnosis established by biopsy, it is recommended that surgery not be delayed in the first or third trimesters. If an asymptomatic and clinically isolated adnexal mass is discovered during the first trimester, as discussed earlier, it is reasonable to repeat an imaging study around 17–18 weeks' gestation to determine the need for surgery.

Pregnant patients undergoing surgery during the second trimester prior to fetal viability (approximately 23–24 weeks' gestation) should have the fetal heart tones documented by Doppler pre- and postoperatively. Later in pregnancy, continuous fetal heart rate monitoring can be utilized perioperatively. Following documentation of an adequate amniotic fluid volume of approximately 10–18 mL via ultrasonography, preoperative and postoperative prophylactic indomethacin at a rectal dose of 25–50 mg can be used to minimize uterine contractions in patients undergoing surgery prior to 30 weeks' gestation. The use of indomethacin is not advisable beyond this period due to concerns of premature closure of the patent ductus arteriosus. It must be recognized that although prophylactic tocolytic agents can decrease uterine irritability, they have not been shown to decrease the incidence of preterm birth in patients undergoing surgery. The liberal use of lower extremity sequential compression devices intraoperatively and during periods of bed rest is advisable. Finally, the use of an external tocodynamometer can be used in the postoperative period to monitor uterine irritability and preterm uterine contractions.

Laparotomy

Historically, laparotomy during pregnancy was a frequent cause of fetal wastage. A 17% loss rate was reported by Brant in 1967 following appendectomy during pregnancy. In 1973, Saunders and Milton observed a 23% rate of fetal wastage after laparotomy. In modern hospitals, however, loss of the fetus as a consequence of laparotomy is uncommon. For example, Kort et al reported in 1993 that for 78 women who underwent non-obstetric operations, the perinatal mortality rate was not increased provided that fetal viability was established preoperatively. The most common indications for surgical treatment in their series were appendicitis, adnexal mass, and cholecystitis. Non-obstetric surgery was associated with an increased risk of preterm labor, and the authors identified no measurable benefit from the use of perioperative prophylactic tocolytic agents. The premature delivery rate was 21.8% after major surgery, which was twice the rate in pregnant control subjects.

With rare exceptions, when laparotomy is required to evaluate the pregnant woman for suspected or known malignancy, we utilize the midline, vertical approach. This permits excellent visualization and inspection of the entire pelvis and upper abdomen, and perhaps as importantly, facilitates the "hands off the uterus" approach we have toward surgery in the gravid patient.

Laparoscopy

Laparoscopy can be used to evaluate adnexal masses during pregnancy, and has been shown to be well tolerated by both the mother and the fetus. By the end of the second trimester, the enlarging uterus interferes with the laparoscopic view, and a celiotomy is generally required. Two million deliveries in Sweden from 1973 to 1993 were the subject of a review by Reedy et al, who evaluated 2233 laparoscopic and 2491 open laparotomy cases. The outcome measures included gestational age at delivery, birthweight, intrauterine growth restriction, congenital malformations, stillbirths, and neonatal deaths. Although both groups were at increased risk for preterm delivery and neonatal birthweights less than 2500 g, there were no statistically significant differences between the two. Highlights from the Society of American Gastrointestinal Endoscopic Surgeons recommendations for the conduct of laparoscopy in pregnancy appear in Table 16–12.

Table 16–12 RECOMMENDATIONS FOR LAPAROSCOPIC SURGERY DURING PREGNANCY

Obtain an obstetrics consult preoperatively.
When possible, delay operative intervention in elective cases until the second trimester.
Use pneumatic compression devices (pregnancy + pneumoperitoneum = hypercoagulable state).
Follow maternal and fetal physiologic status intraoperatively.
Follow maternal end tidal CO_2.
Use open technique to gain pneumoperitoneum.
Tilt table left side down to move gravid uterus off the interior vena cava.
Minimize pneumoperitoneum to 8–12 mmHg.

For seemingly isolated 6- to 10-cm adnexal masses that persist into the second trimester, we defer laparoscopic evaluation until 18 weeks' gestation, and typically use pelviscopy to determine which direction (i.e. transverse or midline-vertical) to make the laparotomy incision. For persistent masses greater than 10 cm, we recommend proceeding directly to laparotomy via a vertical incision in an effort to maximize exposure and allow surgical removal of the mass without any manipulation of the uterus.

Diagnostic and therapeutic radiation in pregnancy

The primary concern of both the oncologist and the obstetrician regarding radiation therapy during pregnancy is its possible effect on the baby. The embryo undoubtedly represents the most radiosensitive stage of human life, as many of the cells are differentiating and thus relatively more sensitive to radiation injury. In addition, the high rate of mitotic activity in the cells of the embryo contributes to its radiosensitivity, as the mitotic phase of the cell is the most radiosensitive period in the life cycle of the cell. Importantly, if the embryonic cell is genetically altered or killed during development, the fetus will be deformed or will not survive. Finally, there is the concern that irradiation of the fetal and maternal gonads may contribute to reproductive difficulties in the future, of both the mother and her offspring.

Radiobiology

For the fetus, the most sensitive period is day 18 through day 38. After day 40, primary organ systems have developed, and much larger doses of x-rays or gamma rays are necessary to produce serious abnormalities. Three periods of fetal development are highly significant from a radiologic point of view.

1. Preimplantation. In this phase, radiation produces an all or none effect, in that it either destroys the fertilized egg or does not affect it significantly.
2. Organ system formation. This is the period from day 18 through day 38, when doses of 10–40 cGy may cause visceral organ or somatic damage. Microcephaly, anencephaly, eye damage, growth retardation, spina bifida, and foot damage are reported with doses of 4 cGy or less. Cause and effect have not been proved with these lower doses.
3. Period of fetal development after day 40, when larger doses are likely to produce external malformations but organ systems, especially the nervous system, may still be undamaged.

The dose to the fetus is related to internal scatter of radiation after it enters the supradiaphragmatic tissues. Some scatter may also come from the treatment head of the machine and the collimator. Zucali et al used a tissue-equivalent phantom to measure scatter dose to the uterus. In this study, doses of 1.5% of the total dose were measured at the estimated top of the uterus, with < 1% being measurable in the true pelvis. This occurs even with abdominal shielding.

It is estimated that 1 cGy of radiation produces five mutations in every 1 million genes exposed. Fortunately, most mutants are recessive. Mutant effects are not seen in the first generation and may not be expressed for many generations until two people with the same mutation mate. Most estimates of genetic damage are empiric, but it is estimated that to double the rate of gene mutation, 25–150 cGy must be given from birth to the end of reproductive age.

Constant changes are being made in what is considered the permissible body dose of radiation. Some authorities cite 14 cGy in the first 30 years of life; others cite 10 cGy or less as the maximum. This includes medical and background sources. Radiation doses in excess of 200 cGy during the first 20 weeks of gestation will result in congenital malformations in the majority of fetuses exposed (frequently microcephaly and mental retardation). With doses above 300 cGy, there is increasing risk of abortion. If therapeutic irradiation is necessary for a pregnant patient and therapeutic abortion is refused, delay in the initiation of treatment until at least the mid-second trimester is recommended. Irradiation of even supradiaphragmatic structures during pregnancy will deliver fetal doses ranging from 1.2 to 7.1% of the total treatment dose.

Radiation-induced anomalies

There are varying sensitivities within the tissues in the human embryo. Various abnormalities have been attributed to irradiation of the embryo; microcephaly and associated conditions are most common. Other abnormalities of the central nervous system, the eye, and the skeleton have also been ascribed to irradiation. However, an accurate prediction of incidence with regard to dose has not been possible. It is widely accepted that irradiation of human beings, especially of their gonads, has certain undesirable effects. Any irradiation of gonadal tissue involves

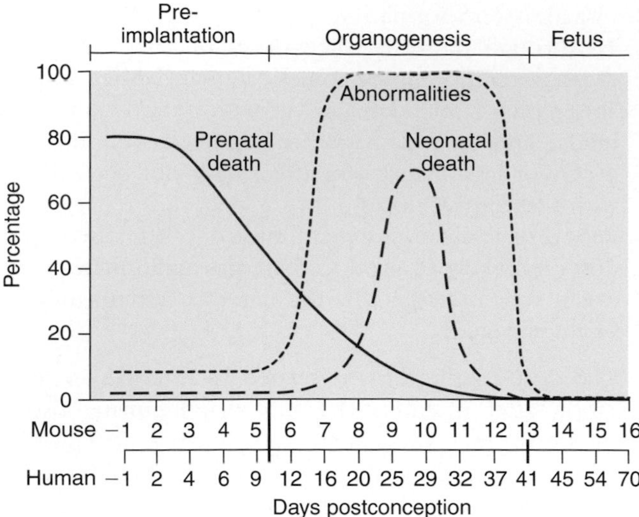

Figure 16–12 Incidence of abnormalities and of prenatal and neonatal death in mice given a dose of 200 cGy at various times post fertilization. The lower scale consists of Rugh's estimates of the equivalent stages for the human embryo. (From Hall EJ: Radiobiology for the Radiologist. New York, Harper & Row, 1973; after Russell LB et al: J Cell Comp Physiol 43[suppl 1]:103, 1954, and Rugh R: AJR Am J Roentgenol 87:559, 1962.)

possible genetic damage, because the photons can cause gene mutation or chromosome breakage with subsequent translocation, loss, deletion, and abnormal fusion of chromosome material. The effect is basically additive and cumulative; the changes are generally in direct proportion to the total dose. Unfortunately, there is no threshold for genetic damage, and even relatively small doses of irradiation can cause gene mutations, most of which can be harmful.

Doses greater than 50 cGy may produce significant mental retardation and microcephaly, even in the second trimester (Fig. 16–12). An analysis of children exposed in utero to the atomic bomb in Hiroshima and Nagasaki shows a 30 in 1600 incidence of severe mental retardation. Most of the mentally retarded children were exposed at 8–15 weeks of life; no cases were reported before the eighth week of gestation. A rough linear relationship is suggested, with a probability of mental retardation occurring at 0.4% per cGy (rad).

As noted above, the exposure dose that is associated with developmental abnormalities remains controversial. Hammer-Jacobsen suggests that 10 cGy received in the first 6 weeks of gestation should be considered a threshold for therapeutic abortion. Others disagree and suggest that the minimal level increases as the pregnancy progresses. Low-dose exposure (< 100 cGy) seems acceptable only in the third trimester. Evidence suggests that an exposure of even 3–5 cGy can result in an increase in benign or malignant tumors in the child after birth.

Most of the data to date on the effects of irradiation on the fetus are from single-dose exposure; few data are available concerning the effects of fractionated irradiation. Reported cases of fractionated irradiation during pregnancy show a low incidence of fetal anomalies.

Diagnostic radiology

The metastatic evaluation using diagnostic imaging and the treatment of malignancy by radiotherapy in the pregnant woman underscores an inherent maternal–fetal conflict, in that the mother would be the major beneficiary, whereas the fetus could be at substantial risk. Several recommendations have been widely applied in this scenario, including delaying radiation therapy for breast cancer until after delivery, avoidance of sentinel node identification procedures during pregnancy, and termination of pregnancy when doses greater than 0.05–0.1 Gy are received by the fetus. It must be recognized that these recommendations are not based on sufficient knowledge of the radiation risks to the unborn child. Although individual doses are highest in association with radiation therapy, the greatest risk to both the general population and the cancer patient comes from diagnostic procedures. Most radiologic diagnostic procedures should be avoided during the first and second trimesters of pregnancy. The exposure to the fetus and gonads will vary with the procedure performed and the precautions taken. A chest radiograph will result in an exposure of 300 mcGy per plate, whereas a barium enema study will result in a total dose to the gonads and pelvis of 6 cGy. In a pregnant patient, the barium enema study is obviously a greater threat because of the greater dose and the area irradiated.

The International Commission on Radiological Protection prepared two reports on medical irradiation in pregnant women. The biologic effects of prenatal irradiation of the embryo and fetus were derived from animal studies, data from survivors of nuclear explosions, data from children exposed in utero to diagnostic x-rays, and data on children who were exposed to radiation from the Chernobyl accident in utero. As outlined in Table 16–13, lethality, malformations, mental retardation, and cancer induction comprise the expected effects of radiation exposure of the fetus.

Ionizing radiation

In diagnostic x-ray or CT, ionizing radiation passes through the body to create an image, while ionizing radiation from radiopharmaceuticals employed in nuclear medicine procedures are retained in the tissues for a period of time and are subsequently removed by elimination from the body and by radioactive decay.

Non-ionizing radiation

Both ultrasonography imaging and MRI form images using non-ionizing radiation; however, theoretic risks to the fetus exist. Thermal effects occur in tissues with the absorption of ultrasonic energy, while cavitation (i.e. mechanical) effects may occur through motion initiated by the ultrasonic. Both thermal and cavitation effects occur only with very high-intensity ultrasonography, and no confirmed biologic effects associated with the use of diagnostic ultrasonography with standard power levels have been reported. Potential injury at the cellular level in MRI may result from exposure to high static magnetic fields. In

Table 16–13 EFFECTS AND RISKS AFTER EXPOSURE TO IONIZING RADIATION IN UTERO, AND SPONTANEOUS FREQUENCY (WITHOUT EXPOSURE)

Time after conception (weeks)	Effect(s)	Risk per 0.01 Gy	Spontaneous frequency
0–2	Prenatal death[a]	0.01–0.001	0.3–0.6
3–8	Malformation	0.005[b]	0.06
8–15	Mental retardation, IQ decrease[c]	0.004	0.005
16–25	Mental retardation, IQ decrease[d]	0.001	0.005
0–38	Leukemia, solid tumors in childhood	0.003–0.004	0.002–0.003

[a]Based on experimental data.
[b]Above threshold dose of 0.1–0.2 Gy.
[c]Reduction of 21 IQ points per 1 Gy above threshold of about 0.05 Gy; threshold dose for mental retardation about 0.06 Gy.
[d]Reduction of 13 IQ points per 0.1 Gy above threshold dose of about 0.05 Gy; threshold dose for mental retardation about 0.25 Gy.
(From Kal HB, Struikmans H: Radiotherapy during pregnancy: fact and fiction. Lancet Oncol 6:328–333, 2005.)

addition, heating can result from energy deposited by radiofrequencies used to generate the pulse sequences. The diagnostic magnets create static magnetic fields from 0.1 to 1.5T, and no adverse behavioral or physiologic effects are anticipated with fields up to 2T. Importantly, there have been no immediately observable adverse effects or delayed sequelae encountered among fetuses from an MRI examination. Table 16–14 lists the imaging modalities used to diagnose metastatic disease.

Ionic or non-ionic, iodinated intravenous contrast media used in CT appear to be safe for the fetus; however, only animal studies have been performed using iodinated contrast agents. These agents are pregnancy category B drugs. Gadolinium-based contrast medium is not advisable during pregnancy, as the gadolinium crosses the placenta, is filtered through the fetal kidneys, and is then reingested through the amniotic fluid. Gadolinium is a category C drug. The accuracy of bone scans is improved through the addition of single-photon emission computed tomography imaging. MRI is the most sensitive for studying the bone marrow, while CT is highly sensitive for cortical destruction. Positron emission tomography scanning with 2-[fluorine-18]fluoro-2-deoxy-D-glucose is being used with increasing frequency in the metastatic workup, although the potential dose to the fetus precludes its use when the pregnancy is to be preserved.

Table 16–14 IMAGING MODALITIES USED FOR TREATMENT PLANNING IN ONCOLOGY

Site of anatomic interest	Imaging modality	Type of radiation
Brain	CT scan	Ionizing
	MRI	Non-ionizing
	FDG-PET	Ionizing
Chest	Chest x-ray	Ionizing
	CT scan	Ionizing
	MRI	Non-ionizing
	FDG-PET scan	Ionizing
	Gallium scan	Ionizing
	Mammography	Ionizing
Abdomen	Ultrasound	Non-ionizing
	CT scan	Ionizing
	MRI	Non-ionizing
	FDG-PET	Ionizing
	Intravenous pyelography	Ionizing
	Upper gastrointestinal with small bowel follow-through	Ionizing
Pelvis (not bony pelvis)	Ultrasound	Non-ionizing
	CT scan	Ionizing
	MRI	Non-ionizing
	FDG-PET	Ionizing
	Barium enema	Ionizing
	Cystography	Ionizing
Skeletal	X-ray	Ionizing
	Bone scan/SPECT	Ionizing
	CT scan	Ionizing
	MRI	Non-ionizing
	FDG-PET	Ionizing
Lymph nodes	Lymphangiography	Ionizing
	CT scan	Ionizing
	MRI	Non-ionizing
	Lymphoscintigraphy	Ionizing
	Sentinel node examination	Non-ionizing and ionizing

CT, computed tomography; FDG-PET, 2-[fluorine-18]fluoro-2-deoxy-D-glucose positron emission tomography; MRI, magnetic resonance imaging; SPECT, single-photon emission computed tomography.
(After Nicklas AH, Baker ME: Imaging strategies in the pregnant cancer patient. Semin Oncol 27:623–632, 2000.)

Radionuclides

Most diagnostic nuclear medicine procedures use short-lived radionuclides (e.g. technetium-99m), resulting in a dose to the fetus generally less than 0.01Gy. Special mention should be made regarding whole-body radionuclide scanning using iodine-131 for the metastatic workup of thyroid carcinoma. It is well established that oral administration of radioactive iodine to a mother will have deleterious effects on the thyroid gland of the fetus, with placental transfer of radioactive iodine occurring as early as 8 weeks after conception. The fetal thyroid gland will concentrate iodine and synthesize thyroxine by 11–12 weeks' gestation. The radiation dose delivered by 2 μCi of iodine-131 to the fetal thyroid gland ranges from 10,000 to 40,000 cGy. Stoffer and Hamburger studied 237 cases in which radioactive iodine-131 at doses from 10 to 150 μCi was administered during pregnancy. In 55 patients, therapeutic abortion was performed on medical recommendation, and among the remaining 182 pregnancies, there were two spontaneous abortions, two stillborn infants, and two infants born with abdominal or chest anomalies. Importantly, there were six infants with hypothyroidism (3%), four of whom exhibited mental deficiencies. Pregnancy is a contraindication to the administration of iodine-131.

Radiation therapy

When the patient wishes to continue her pregnancy, delay of initiation of therapeutic radiation as long as possible without compromising cure is recommended. Fortunately, most cancers in pregnant women that require radiation therapy are remote from the pelvis. Any radiation therapy to the abdomen should be postponed until after delivery, if at all possible. Therefore, with the exception of a locally advanced cervical tumor, radiation therapy can be used during pregnancy provided that the fetal dose is precisely estimated during the radiation planning sessions. The dose to the fetus can be calculated from the internal scatter, which largely depends on the source of irradiation and on the size of the treatment fields and their proximity to the fetus. Leakage radiation from the tube head of the linear accelerator, scatter from the collimator, and blocks also contribute to the fetal dose. Leakage and scatter can be reduced by proper shielding with four to five half-value layers of lead stacked over the patient's uterus.

Kal and Struikmans have tabulated the dosimetry data and pregnancy outcomes of women who received radiation therapy during pregnancy for breast cancer (Fig. 16–13), Hodgkin disease, and brain/head and neck tumors (Table 16–15). Successful radiotherapy of breast cancers during pregnancy with fetal doses (0.039–0.18 Gy) below the deterministic threshold have resulted in the birth of healthy children. Similarly, several healthy children, some who have been observed for up to 11 years, have been delivered following radiation therapy for Hodgkin disease during pregnancy with fetal doses ranging from 0.014 to 0.136 Gy. Radiation treatment portals are now more restricted in size, and patients with stage I and II Hodgkin disease currently receive polychemotherapy followed by involved field radiotherapy, thus resulting in potentially less harm to the unborn child. Finally, the successful radiotherapeutic management of neck and cranial tumors in pregnancy suggests that high doses can be achieved with fetal exposures of less than 0.1 Gy, a dose below the deterministic threshold.

Radiation-induced carcinogenesis

The subject of the carcinogenic effects of x-ray radiation was first raised nearly half a century ago by Stewart and Webb from Oxford University in the UK. Monsoon and Macmahon summarized the bulk of the data accumulated prior to the 1980s in their monograph that focused on prenatal x-ray exposure and cancer in children. Most of the available information on radiation-induced embryonic damage during the preceding two decades is derived from animal studies, extended follow-up of individuals exposed to atomic bomb explosions in Japan, and statistical analyses.

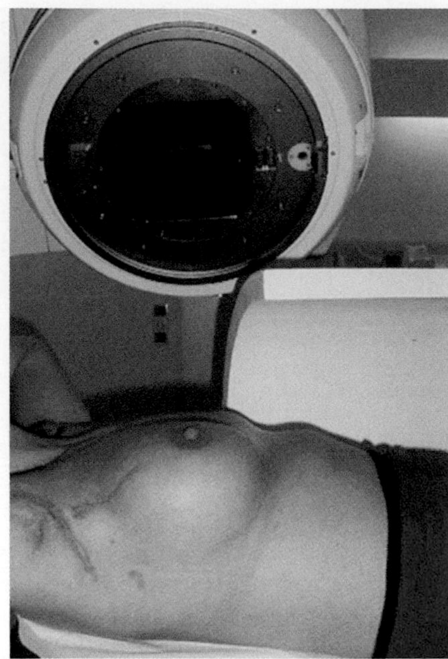

Figure 16–13 Irradiation of a pregnant woman after breast-conserving treatment. Shielding of leakage radiation is done with a mobile lead screen usually used for shielding of personnel in the brachytherapy room. (From Kal HB, Struikmans H: Radiotherapy during pregnancy: fact and fiction. Lancet Oncol 6:328–333, 2005.)

Of interest is a paper by Chen et al, who studied the records of 37 women radiated for Hodgkin disease around the time of pregnancy and of 345 women who were not pregnant. They detected a higher risk of breast cancer after irradiation around the time of pregnancy, suggesting that pregnancy represents a time of increased sensitivity of breast tissue to the carcinogenic effects of radiation.

Genetic damage and infertility

In addition, the possibility that human exposure to ionizing radiation might have a detrimental genetic consequence remains a matter of concern and uncertainty. There is concern because recessive mutations may not become apparent for several generations, and there is uncertainty because although there are no human data available, experimental animal studies have demonstrated significant radiation-induced genetic effects. There appears to be no apparent threshold dose for genetic damage, but the effect of any particular radiation dose is considerably reduced if that dose is administered during a prolonged period. Of importance also for patients planning childbearing after significant exposure of gonadal tissue to irradiation is that the genetic effect of radiation on the gonad may be minimized by delaying conception after exposure. In humans, pregnancy should be delayed 12–14 months after significant exposure.

Table 16–15 TOTAL DOSE, FETAL DOSE, AND OUTCOME OF PREGNANT PATIENTS UNDERGOING RADIOTHERAPY

Tumor type	Author(s)	Year	Maternal dose (Gy)	Fetal dose (Gy)	Trimester	*n*	Delivery
Breast[a]	van der Giessen	1997	50	0.160	3	1	Healthy boy
	Ngu et al	1992	50	0.14–0.18	3	1	—
	Antypas et al	1998	46	0.039	1	1	Healthy boy
Hodgkin disease[a]	Woo et al	1992	35–40	0.014–0.055 (6 MV) 0.100–0.136 (cobalt)	1–3	16	Healthy babies/no malignant disease
	Nuyttens et al	2002	19	0.09–0.42, head 0.114	3	1	Healthy child 8 years
	Nisce et al	1986	15–20	0.020–0.50	2–3	7	Healthy children 6–11 years
	Lishner et al	1992	15–20	0.020–0.50	2–3	16	Healthy babies
	Cygler et al	1997	35	< 0.01	2	1	Healthy child
Brain tumors, head and neck cancer[b]	Nuyttens et al	2002	64	0.027–0.086	2	1	Healthy baby
	Sharma et al	2004	45	0.020	1	1	—
	Yu et al	2003	25	0.00015–0.0031	3	1	—
	Maagne et al	2001	30	0.003	2	1	Healthy boy 3 years
	Sneed et al	1995	68	0.06	3	1	Healthy girl 2.5 years
	Sneed et ak	1995	78.2	0.030	3	1	Healthy girl 1.5 years
	Podgorsak et al	1999	66	0.033–0.086[a]	3	1	—

[a]With shielding.
[b]Without shielding.
(After Kal HB, Struikmans H: Radiotherapy during pregnancy: fact and fiction. Lancet Oncol 6:328–333, 2005.)

Chemotherapy

Because nearly all antineoplastic drugs have been shown to be teratogenic in animal studies, the available data suggest endangerment to human fetuses even for drugs for which no human data are available. Their use often evokes moral and philosophic, as well as emotional, decisions. Both mother and fetus are at risk, with abortion, intrauterine fetal demise, malformations, and growth restriction being foremost considerations. These potential dangers to the fetus must be weighed against the possible detrimental effect to the mother of withholding these agents. The long-term effect on the fetus is unknown. The problem of long-term observation has been dramatically emphasized by the occurrence of adenosis of the vagina in young women exposed to diethylstilbestrol in utero during the first trimester of pregnancy. A similar long-term effect is possible when chemotherapeutic agents are used in pregnancy.

All chemotherapeutic agents profoundly affect rapidly growing tissues, and a high rate of cell division is characteristic of the fetus. Following this reasoning, one would expect a much greater effect than is actually observed. Unquestionably, the first trimester of pregnancy is when the fetus is most vulnerable to cancer chemotherapeutic agents. The two aspects to the problem of fetal damage are:

1. death of the fetus, and
2. induction of fetal abnormalities inadequate to cause fetal death.

Most of the available data suggesting the teratogenicity and mutagenicity of chemotherapeutic agents have been derived from experiments in laboratory animals. The rat, the mouse, and the rabbit have placentas that are very similar to the human placenta, and because the teratogenic effects of a drug are species-specific, these animals provide models in which to study chemotherapy exposure in utero. These experiments indicate potential danger to the human fetus only. Teratogenic properties of chemotherapeutic agents also are predicated on the type, dose, and threshold dose of the drug. When considering an extrapolation of animal data to humans, it is important to note that the therapeutic doses used in humans are often lower than the minimum teratogenic dose studied in animal models. Thus teratogenic data are useful only if the dose resulting in injury to the model does not also cause maternal toxic effects. Another important caveat is that for many antineoplastic exposures in pregnancy that have resulted in malformations or even fetal deaths, there have typically been associated with multiagent therapy, sometimes also with concomitant radiation therapy, so that it is difficult to single out one specific agent as the cause of an adverse outcome. Importantly, in the majority of exposures, even during the first trimester, the outcome of the fetus is unremarkable. Still, unless the mother's life is in grave danger, we do not recommend chemotherapy use during the first trimester.

Teratology and embryology

Teratology is the study of the causes, mechanisms, and manifestations of abnormal fetal development. Environmental factors, such as infectious diseases, drugs, chemicals, and radiation, have been shown to cause abnormal development by inducing chromosome abnormalities, specific gene changes, vascular changes, or mechanical disruption. In many instances, the exact cause of a fetal abnormality is unknown. Although different classes of teratogens have been established, certain general principles apply to all. There are three stages of embryonic development. In the first 2 weeks of life, the blastocyst is resistant to teratogens. It is during this period that a large insult is necessary to kill the blastocyst. A surviving blastocyst will not manifest any organ's specific abnormalities as a result of that teratogen. Early embryonic cells have not differentiated sufficiently, so if one cell dies another can take over. The second stage is organogenesis, or the process of organ differentiation. The most critical period extends from the third to eighth weeks of development (fifth through tenth weeks of gestational age), when susceptibility to teratogenic agents is maximal. In the human fetus, the period of organogenesis usually ends by the 13th week of gestation. The third and final period of growth, organ development, is characterized by increase in fetal and organ size. However, brain and gonadal tissue are exceptions, because they continue to differentiate beyond the second period. Exposure to the teratogenic agent beyond the third period can affect general fetal growth but will not produce organ-specific morphologic malformations.

Figure 16–14 depicts prenatal development from implantation, through embryonic progression, and into the fetal period. Drug responses vary among individuals because of differences in absorption, protein binding, and excretion rate, as well as differences in placental transfer and fetal metabolism of the teratogen. Both polygenic and mendelian factors can be responsible for different responses to identical doses of a teratogen in two fetuses of the same species. Administration of small intermittent doses of a teratogen may enable a system to safely metabolize the teratogen and prevent malformation. The effect would be different if the total dose were administered at one time. On the other hand, small constant doses of a teratogen may interfere with cellular metabolism and cause more serious malformations than might be expected.

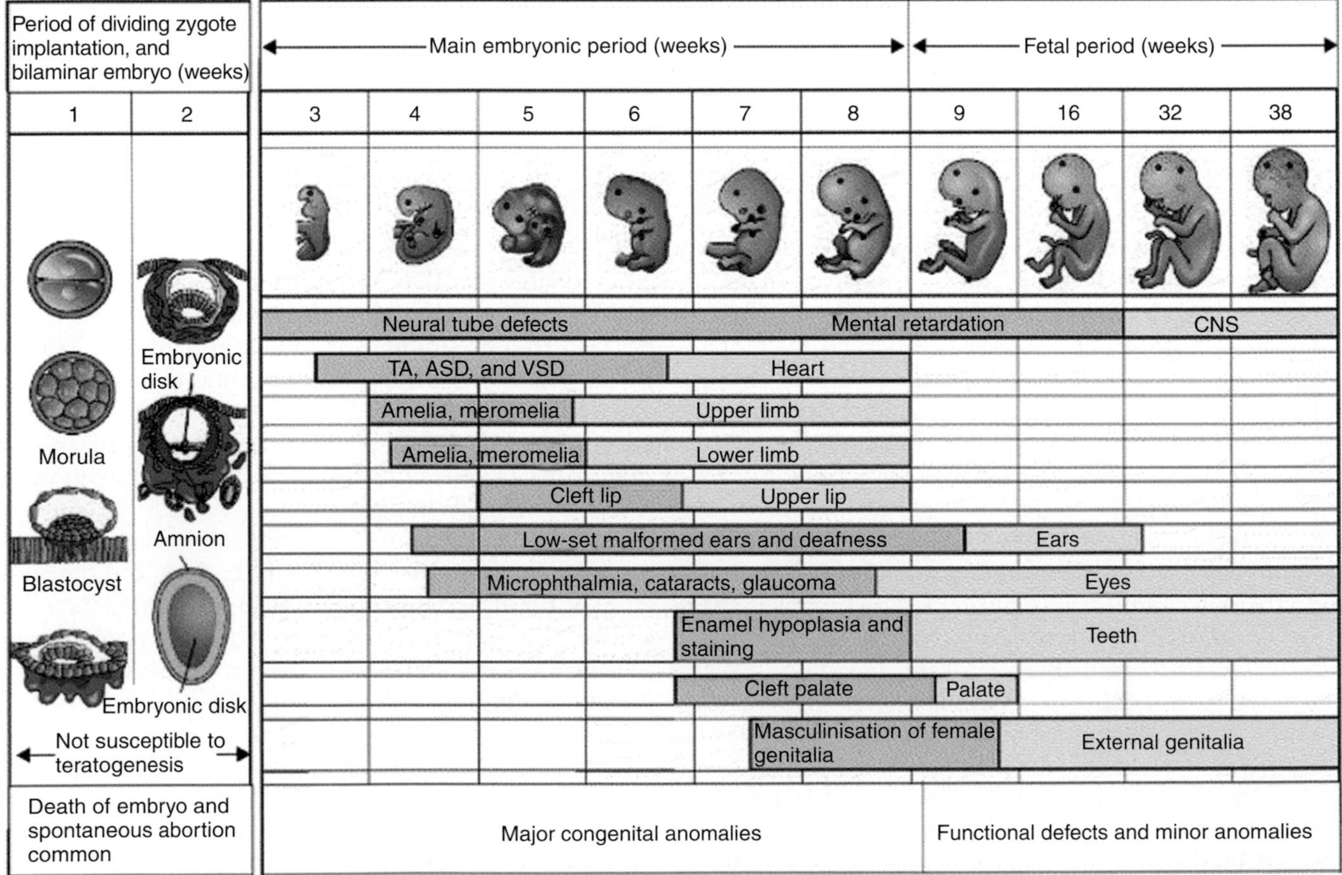

Figure 16–14 Crucial periods in prenatal development. Dots on the developing fetus show common sites of action of teratogens. Horizontal bars indicate fetal development during a highly sensitive period (purple) and a less sensitive period (green). ASD, atrial septal defect; CNS, central nervous system; TA, truncus arteriosus; VSD, ventricular septal defect. (From Moore P (ed): The Developing Human, 6th edn. Philadelphia, Saunders, 1998.)

Transplacental studies

Antineoplastic agents and/or their metabolites can be detected in placental tissue, amniotic fluid, umbilical cord blood, and breast milk. By enzyme-linked immunosorbent assay and spectrometry, Henderson et al measured cisplatin–DNA adducts in placental tissues but were unable to do so in the umbilical cord tissues or in amniotic cells. Karp et al reported high levels of doxorubicin in placental tissue; the drug was absent in umbilical cord tissue or in the blood of a healthy child born 48 h after maternal treatment. Separately, Roboz et al and Barni et al were unable to identify doxorubicin in the amniotic fluid after maternal administration. Transplacental conduct of antineoplastic drugs may occur. Although doxorubicin was not detected by liquid chromatography in the amniotic fluid, fetal brain, or fetal gastrointestinal tract 15h following its administration to the mother, d'Incalci et al found the drug in the fetal liver, kidney, and lungs after elective termination. It would have been interesting to have had data from the fetal myocardial tissue. A metabolite of doxorubicin was present in the umbilical cord, placental tissue, and neonatal spleen of a stillborn baby delivered 36h after maternal treatment. Egan et al reported a case in which milk and plasma concentrations of doxorubicin and cisplatin were measured after intravenous administration of these agents to a lactating patient who had ovarian cancer. Although the concentrations of doxorubicin in milk at times exceeded those detected in concomitant plasma samples, the total amount of drug delivered in the milk was negligible. However, the authors concluded that it is prudent to advise lactating women who are receiving these antineoplastic drugs to refrain from breast-feeding.

Classes of antineoplastic agents

Antimetabolites

Antimetabolites are small, weakly acidic molecules that are cell cycle non-specific, inhibiting cellular metabolism by acting as false substrates during RNA and DNA synthesis. Examples of these agents include methotrexate, 5-fluorouracil, aminopterin, cytarabine, thioguanine, and mercaptopurine. The *aminopterin syndrome* has been reported after in utero exposure during the first trimester, and is characterized by cranial dysostosis with delayed ossification, hypertelorism, wide nasal bridge, micrognathia, and ear anomalies. Similar malformations have been associated with methotrexate administration when doses greater than 10 mg per week are used during the first trimester. There have been 53 reported cases of exposure to 5-fluorouracil during human pregnancy; when used after the first trimester (usually in combination with other agents), the development of intrauterine growth restriction without anomalies manifested in 11% of cases ($n = 6$). There have been four reports of limb malformations following cytarabine administration during the first trimester; among 89 additional cases in which the drug was given during all trimesters (usually in combination with other agents), adverse fetal events included transient cytopenia (5%), intrauterine fetal demise (6%), intrauterine growth restriction (13%), and two neonatal deaths due to sepsis and gastroenteritis. Finally, there have been 49 women treated with mercaptopurine during pregnancy, including 29 who were exposed to the drug during the first trimester, none of whom gave birth to an anomalous neonate.

There is no doubt that the antifolics, aminopterin and methotrexate, almost invariably result in spontaneous abortion or an abnormal fetus when they are given in the first trimester of pregnancy. These drugs should not be given to the pregnant woman in the first trimester unless there is life-threatening disease that can be counteracted by the drug. If an antifolic is used and the mother does not have a spontaneous abortion, therapeutic abortion should be seriously considered. A small amount of data seem to indicate that aminopterin and methotrexate do not cause harm when they are given after the first trimester of pregnancy.

Alkylators

Alkylating agents are an integral component of many combination chemotherapy regimens and include cyclophosphamide, busulfan, ifosfamide, chlorambucil, carmustine, and dacarbazine. First-trimester use of cyclophosphamide has resulted in absent toes, eye abnormalities, low-set ears, and cleft palate. When used during the second and third trimesters, cyclophosphamide appears to be safe, although from a combined experience involving 92 cases, there have been two fetal demises, seven cases of growth restriction, and one neonatal death. A very interesting case involves the twins reported by Reynoso et al who were exposed to cyclophosphamide throughout the pregnancy: the girl had not abnormalities, but the twin boy was born with esophageal atresia right-arm deformity, abnormal inferior vena cava, and growth restriction, and went on to develop thyroid cancer at 11 years of age. There have been 19 reported cases of combined regimens containing dacarbazine in pregnancy, resulting in one case of growth restriction and possibly one minor malformation. Interestingly, although there have been eight reports of busulfan use during the first trimester without anomalies, two patients who received the drug during the second trimester delivered anomalous neonates (one case each of pyloric stenosis and unilateral renal agenesis with liver calcifications).

Anthracycline and Anti-tumor antibiotics

These high-molecular weight antibiotics interpose between DNA strands and include doxorubicin, daunorubicin, doxorubicin (Adriamycin), idarubicin, epirubicin, dactinomycin, bleomycin, and mitoxantrone. Turchi and Villasis collected 28 cases of doxorubicin and daunorubicin treatment after the first trimester. Following one elective termination, two spontaneous abortions, and two maternal deaths from malignancy with the fetus in utero, 21 pregnancies were delivered without complications. Two of three limb abnormalities seen following doxorubicin exposure during the first trimester (n = 25) may be confounded by concomitant radiation or cytarabine treatment.

It has been recognized for a number of years that children and adults receiving anthracyclines are at risk of developing dose-related cardiotoxicity due to free radical damage that results in myocardial apoptosis and hypertrophy. It is not known whether in utero exposure to these agents places the fetus at risk for this complication. Meyer-Wittkopf et al performed serial fetal echocardiograms on a pregnant patient receiving doxorubicin and on unexposed fetuses, and were unable to detect any significant differences in systolic function. Postnatal echocardiograms revealed no evidence of myocardial damage up to 2 years after birth. There have been at least two cases of transient right-sided cardiomyopathy after second-trimester exposure to anthracyclines, including one case involving idarubicin, which is more lipophilic and favors increased placental transfer. Until more information becomes available, we suggest that pregnant women requiring an anthracycline be given doxorubicin. Although the cardiac profile of fetuses exposed to anthracyclines appears to be safe in the majority of cases, because cancer treatment advances at a faster pace than the accumulation of safety data in human pregnancy, caution is always warranted before new agents are given to pregnant women.

Plant alkaloids

The vinca alkaloids are highly protein-bound and include vincristine, vinblastine, and vinorelbine. They have been regarded as less potent teratogens than the antimetabolites. One of 29 patients treated with a four-drug regimen containing vincristine during organogenesis was delivered with malformations including an atrial septal defect and no radii or fifth digits. There have been a total of 11 exposures to either vincristine or vinblastine during pregnancy, and excluding those malformations found only in first-trimester use, there have been nine cases of growth restriction, two fetal demises, and two neonatal deaths.

Taxanes

Paclitaxel and docetaxel inhibit microtubule disassembly, a process that is important for cell division as well as intracellular and intercellular functions. Because of their unique mechanism of action, many commentators have been concerned that taxanes may be detrimental to the fetus in many aspects. Animal studies have demonstrated lethality of paclitaxel to chick, rat, and rabbit embryos. Interestingly, when administered during the period of organogenesis, few malformations have been recorded. There have been only a handful of scattered reports of paclitaxel use during pregnancy in which the drug, when administered after the first trimester, has been shown to be safe for the fetus. As experience with these relatively newer chemotherapeutic agents increases, we anticipate an increase in the reporting of taxane use during pregnancy.

Platinum analogs

The precise mechanism by which the platinum agents exert their antineoplastic effect has not been fully elucidated but may be similar to that of the classic alkylators. Drugs in this group include cisplatin, carboplatin, and oxaliplatin. There have been reports of exposure to single-agent cisplatin or cisplatin-based regimens, which have resulted in sensorineural hearing loss, and cerebral atrophy due to impaired anterior cerebral circulation, respectively. In both of these cases, the babies were born before 30 weeks, and so the complications associated with extreme prematurity may be confounding the clinical picture. Nevertheless, close assessment of the fetal central nervous system may be advisable when cisplatin is used during pregnancy. Among 24 cases of cisplatin exposure, five have been complicated by growth restriction, fetal demise, hearing loss, and ventriculomegaly. The two reports that have appeared in the literature describing carboplatin use during pregnancy have been associated with unremarkable neonatal outcomes at up to 30 months of age.

Pharmacokinetics, sublethal fetal effects, and maternal risks

The increased blood volume and increased renal clearance of pregnancy should be considered when treating the mother for life-threatening disease. Together, these physiologic changes, along with the more rapid turnover of the hepatic mixed function oxidase system, may lead to a decrease in active maternal drug concentration. For example, because pregnant women receive similar weight-based dosages (adjusted with the continuing weight gain of pregnancy) as non-pregnant women, the increased drug clearance from the body may lead to a reduced area under the concentration vs time curve. In addition, changes in the gastrointestinal function may impact drug absorption of some agents. Fortunately, with the pregnancy-associated decrease in plasma albumin, the unbound active drug concentration should rise, and thus the efficacy of the drug should not be compromised when administered during pregnancy. As long as the increase in drug balances potential decrease in serum levels, toxicity should not be increased. This may indeed be the case, as Zemlickis et al have noted higher concentrations of free cisplatin in pregnant women as compared with those who were not pregnant, but all were asymptomatic. Countering this is the argument that estrogens are known to increase other plasma proteins, and thereby decrease active drug fractions. Accordingly, Cardonick and Iacobucci have reported more frequent nausea, vomiting, fatigue, alopecia, and neutropenia during postpartum chemotherapy compared with identical antenatal treatment. The volume of distribution, peak drug concentrations, and half-life of administration are likely to be changed during pregnancy, although to date we do not have pharmacokinetic data on pregnant patients receiving chemotherapy.

Concerns regarding *sublethal fetal effects* of maternally administered chemotherapy have been raised. When a multidrug regimen was used in a pregnant woman with leukemia, Morishita et al reported consistently normal fetal hematopoiesis via percutaneous umbilical cord blood sampling 2 and 5 weeks following treatment. Chemotherapy-induced neonatal alopecia is also a reasonable concern parents may have, but this condition has been reported only in three newborns, and involved administration of bleomycin, etoposide, and cisplatin, or doxorubicin, cyclophosphamide, and 5-fluorouracil. Microscopic scanning of the hair of neonates exposed to chemotherapy for maternal acute monocytic leukemia by Gokal et al did not reveal any cytotoxic damage.

Attention must also be directed to specific maternal risks associated with chemotherapy administration during pregnancy. The safe use of recombinant erythropoietin in pregnancy has been reported to offset the triple insult of pregnancy-associated dilutional anemia, iron deficiency anemia, and chemotherapy-induced marrow suppression. Along similar lines, granulocyte-colony stimulating factor has been used without adverse sequelae during human pregnancy to counter the maternal and fetal susceptibilities to infection brought about by the generalized immunosuppression of pregnancy and chemotherapy-induced neutropenia. Finally, because the pulmonary damage associated with bleomycin use is exacerbated by oxygen therapy, we do not advise the administration of oxygen during labor in women who have received bleomycin during pregnancy.

Literature review of chemotherapy use in pregnancy

Estimating the stillbirth rate

The background stillbirth rate associated with chemotherapy administration throughout pregnancy can be estimated. In 1992, Zemlickis and colleagues reported their experience with 21 pregnancies after in utero exposure to chemotherapy. Of the 13 women exposed during the first trimester, two of five whose pregnancies continued to term had major malformations in their infants, four had spontaneous abortions, and four had therapeutic abortions. Of four women with second-trimester exposure to chemotherapy, two had normal live births, one had a stillbirth, and one had a therapeutic abortion. All four pregnancies exposed to chemotherapy during the third trimester resulted in healthy live births. However, infants exposed to chemotherapy had statistically significantly lower birthweights than did matched-control infants, owing to significantly lower gestational age and substantial intrauterine growth retardation. The rate of stillbirth was one per 11; this was too small a series for comparison with matched control subjects. On the other hand, the authors analyzed 223 births in their community occurring to women who had any form of cancer in the same 30-year period, and found 10 stillbirths among the 223 deliveries, significantly more than in the general population ($P < 0.0005$); this stillbirth rate was calculated at a relative risk of 4.23 (95% confidence interval 2.0–7.8).

Combination chemotherapy

Most reports of combination chemotherapy given during pregnancy have been of patients who had leukemias and Hodgkin disease. Puzzuto and associates reported nine cases of acute leukemia treated during pregnancy with multiple chemotherapeutic agents in combination, including prednisone, cytosine arabinoside, 6-mercaptopurine, methotrexate, vincristine, and doxorubicin. Of the nine fetuses, eight were born alive and one was stillborn. No congenital anomalies were noted, although one infant had pancytopenia. Pancytopenia was confirmed in another infant whose mother was treated with combination chemotherapy for acute leukemia. Many other reports about the use of combination chemotherapy for acute leukemia during pregnancy are available. No fetal congenital anomalies have been noted with second- and third-trimester therapy, and live births have resulted.

Large series

Sokal and Lessmann collected 50 reports of pregnant women who received anticancer chemotherapy. In their series, there were eight instances of fetal abnormalities, 16 spontaneous abortions, and seven therapeutic abortions. They noted that no obvious fetal malformations were observed among these women who received chemotherapy in the second and third trimesters of pregnancy only. Although serious congenital anomalies and spontaneous abortions did occur in patients receiving chemotherapy in the first trimester of pregnancy, such complications were not inevitable.

Nicholson collected 185 cases of human pregnancies during anticancer chemotherapy. Of 110 women who received such treatment during the first trimester, the status of the fetus or infant was recorded in only 68 patients. Of these, there were 15 instances of fetal abnormalities. Ten of these women received folic acid antagonists; two had taken busulfan; and one each had received 6-mercaptopurine, chlorambucil, and cyclophosphamide. No malformations were reported in the fetuses of 75 women who received chemotherapy during the second and third trimesters of pregnancy, although the status of the fetus or the infant is recorded in only 73 instances. Gathering the remaining published data on chemotherapy during pregnancy and reviewing 39 pregnancies in which an alkylating agent was used in the first trimester, Sweet and Kinzie updated Nicholson's work. Malformations were seen in six of the 39 pregnancies, but the majority of these patients had also received radiation during pregnancy or just before conception. During the second or third trimester, 27 patients received an alkylating agent, and no congenital anomalies were noted. The authors concluded that the risk of alkylating agents given during pregnancy appears to be small, with no increased risk if they are given after the first trimester. Vinca alkaloids were given to 15 patients in the first trimester, with only one congenital malformation noted, and no abnormalities were noted in 11 pregnancies so treated after the first trimester.

In their excellent review, from 1966 to 2004, Cardonick and Iacobucci have collected a total of 376 fetuses exposed to chemotherapy in utero, most after the period of organogenesis. There have been 19 (5%) intrauterine fetal demises, and four (1%) neonatal deaths. There have been 28 cases (7%) of growth restriction, 18 (5%) premature births, and 15 (4%) babies with transient myelosuppression. Two cases of transient neonatal cardiomyopathy have occurred after exposure to idarubicin.

Occupational exposure

In a 1985 case-control study, Selevan et al examined the relation between fetal loss and occupational exposure to antineoplastic drugs in nurses in 17 Finnish hospitals. The pregnancies studied occurred in 1973 through 1980 and were identified using national sources. Each nurse with fetal loss was matched with three nurses who gave birth. A statistically significant association was observed between fetal loss and occupational exposure to antineoplastic drugs during the first trimester of pregnancy, with an odds ratio equaling 2.30 (95% confidence interval 1.20–4.39). Analyses suggested associations between fetal loss and cyclophosphamide, doxorubicin, and vincristine, although the independent effect of each individual drug could not be specifically identified, because many nurses reported handling more than one of these agents.

Recommendations on the use of chemotherapy during pregnancy

In summary, the administration of chemotherapy during the first trimester can be associated with morphologic abnormalities and fetal loss. Although first-trimester use of chemotherapy is inadvisable, if a pregnant patient has an aggressive hematologic malignancy, chemotherapy at full doses can often be safely administered, even during the first trimester, if cure of the hematologic malignancy is considered reasonable.

Chemotherapy administered in the second and third trimesters appears not to be associated with a significant risk of structural anomalies, but some reports suggest an association with preterm delivery, fetal death in utero, and intrauterine growth retardation. The background incidence of growth restriction varies according to the population, geographic location, and standard growth curves used as a reference. We must also keep in mind that the mother's underlying illness may impact perinatal complications. When more than one regimen is available and effective for a particular cancer, clearly the agents for which the most extensive investigation during pregnancy has been conducted should be selected. Some form of antepartum fetal surveillance is advisable, and close coordination with a perinatologist can determine the need and schedule for serial ultrasonography and fetal heart rate monitoring (Table 16–16). Placental pathology is mandatory in all cases following delivery or termination.

Timing of delivery

We recommend withholding chemotherapy after 35 weeks' gestation so as to avoid the maternal nadir period, as spontaneous labor may occur before the bone marrow has recovered. Chemotherapy administered to the mother within 3 weeks of delivery may not be adequately excreted by the fetus and therefore persist in the newborn.

The preterm pregnancy is also problematic. Iatrogenic preterm delivery is not advisable, and impending preterm delivery should be treated aggressively. In pregnant patients for whom preterm delivery seems inevitable, it is important to withhold chemotherapy 3 weeks prior to

Table 16–16 EXAMPLES OF TESTS USED IN THE ANTEPARTUM FETAL SURVEILLANCE OF PREGNANT PATIENTS WITH CANCER

<table>
<tr><td>Biochemical parameters</td><td colspan="2">Progesterone</td><td>E3</td><td>hCG</td><td colspan="2">Triple screen (E3, hCG, α-fetoprotein)</td><td colspan="4">Human placental lactogen</td></tr>
<tr><td>Fetal movements</td><td colspan="10">Kick counting after 25 weeks' gestation</td></tr>
<tr><td>Electronic fetal heart rate monitoring</td><td colspan="3">Non-stress test</td><td>Contraction stress test</td><td colspan="6">Sinusoidal rhythms (correlate with fetal anemia)</td></tr>
<tr><td>Ultrasonography</td><td>Accurate pregnancy dating</td><td>Confirm fetal well-being (viability)</td><td>Uterine and adnexal abnormalities</td><td>Cervical length</td><td>Serial growth assessment</td><td>Assessment of the placenta</td><td colspan="2">Assessment of fetal anomalies</td><td colspan="2">Four-dimensional imaging</td></tr>
<tr><td>Fetal echocardiography</td><td colspan="10">Evaluation for fetal cardiac defects</td></tr>
<tr><td>Color Doppler ultrasound</td><td colspan="3">Systolic:diastolic ratio in the umbilical cord artery</td><td colspan="7">Systolic:diastolic ratio in the fetal middle cerebral artery</td></tr>
<tr><td>Fetal biophysical profile</td><td colspan="3">Fetal breathing movements</td><td colspan="3">Gross body movement</td><td>Fetal tone</td><td colspan="2">Qualitative amniotic fluid volume</td><td>Reactive fetal heart rate</td></tr>
<tr><td>Chorionic villus sampling</td><td colspan="10">9 weeks</td></tr>
<tr><td>Amniocentesis</td><td colspan="4">Genetic: 16–20 weeks</td><td colspan="6">Pulmonary maturation: third trimester</td></tr>
<tr><td>Percutaneous umbilical blood sampling</td><td colspan="4">Fetal hemocrit</td><td colspan="6">Fetal infection</td></tr>
<tr><td>Fetal fibronectin</td><td colspan="10">22–34 weeks</td></tr>
<tr><td>Fetal pulse oximetry</td><td colspan="10">Acidemia with $P_aO_2 < 30\%$</td></tr>
</table>

E3, estriol; hCG, human chorionic gonadotropin.

delivery where possible. Preterm babies have limited ability to metabolize drugs, due to immaturity of the hepatic and renal systems. Neonates exposed to chemotherapy 3 weeks before delivery should be assessed for transient bone marrow suppression, and long-term neurologic and developmental follow-up is recommended.

Breast-feeding

Durodola reported one case of neonatal neutropenia occurring in a breast-fed infant whose mother was treated with cyclophosphamide during late pregnancy and early lactation. As described earlier, some drugs have been detected in the placental tissues as well as the breast milk. The ability of a drug to cross the placenta, however, has not correlated with its ability to pass into breast milk. Drug concentrations in breast milk are related to the dose and timing of therapy. Because there are no breast-feeding data available for most agents, we consider breast-feeding to be contraindicated during therapy.

Long-term neonatal follow-up

Although children and adults treated for lymphoma are at risk for secondary leukemia within 10 years, the risk of secondary malignant disease after in utero exposure to chemotherapy is unknown. No cases of secondary leukemia in exposed fetuses have been reported. As described elsewhere, only one case of malignant disease (i.e. thyroid cancer at age 11 years, and neuroblastoma at age 14 years) in an anomalous child exposed to chemotherapy in utero has been published. It must be acknowledged, however, that there is a paucity of satisfactory long-term results among children exposed to chemotherapy in utero.

In one of the few studies to address this important subject, Aviles and Neri reported the outcomes of 84 children born to mothers with hematologic malignancies who received chemotherapy during pregnancy, including 38 during the first trimester (acute leukemia, $n = 29$; Hodgkin disease, $n = 26$; malignant lymphoma, $n = 29$). These children were examined for physical health, growth, and development, and for hematologic, cytogenetic, neurologic, psychologic, and learning disorders. The occurrence of cancer or acute leukemia in these children was also considered by the investigators. In addition, some of their subjects had become parents, and their children were also considered in the analysis. In all the children studied, including the 12 second-generation children, the birthweight was normal, as was the learning and educational performance. Specifically, school performance and standardized intelligence testing did not differ significantly from unrelated matched children and unexposed siblings. No congenital, neurologic, laboratory, or psychologic abnormalities were observed. Tolerance of infections was also normal, as was secondary sexual development among the older children. With a median follow-up of 18.7 years (range 6–29 years), no cancer or acute leukemia was detected.

The lack of adequate observation of the long-term status of the fetus or infant prevents any definite conclusions as to the relative safety or danger of anticancer chemotherapy during pregnancy, even in the second and third trimesters. It is surprising how often the detailed status of the fetus is not mentioned in available reports. The infant is often described as "normal," with few if any details on the physical or laboratory profile of the baby. Long-term observation is necessary to establish normalcy, because many of the defects may not be obvious on inspection and may emerge as derangements of growth, development, function, reproduction, and heredity.

Serum tumor markers in pregnancy

Table 16–17 contains serum tumor marker ranges for pregnant and non-pregnant women. Although the serum *CA-125* has been found to fluctuate during pregnancy, comprehension of the established trends may assist in following pregnant women with a history of epithelial ovarian cancer and those being evaluated during pregnancy for a pelvic mass. Specifically, the CA-125 values are highest during the first trimester, with levels as high as 1,250 U reported. The values decrease during the late first trimester and should remain below 35 U/mL of serum until delivery, at which point the CA-125 transiently increases 1 h postpartum. It should be mentioned that Jacobs and Bast have reviewed the literature and found cases in which the maternal serum CA-125 remained within normal limits throughout uncomplicated pregnancies.

Bon et al evaluated the concentrations of maternal CA-125 and CA-15-3 (a breast cancer tumor marker) in normal and 120 pathologic pregnancies (e.g. spontaneous abortion, fetal death, growth restriction, chromosomal and structural abnormalities, and pre-eclampsia). The maternal CA-125 serum values were higher during the first and third trimesters during pregnancy, and the CA-15-3 serum levels were higher only during the third trimester. Neither antigen showed any relation with a pathologic outcome of pregnancy.

Interestingly, Kiran et al performed simultaneous measurements of CA-125, CA-15-3, CA-19-9, and *carcinoembryonic antigen* (CEA) in the maternal serum and umbilical cord blood in 53 pregnancies that were terminated by caesarean section. CA-19-9 is a pancreatic cancer tumor marker, and CEA is a marker of mucinous adenocarcinomas with levels that are normal or marginally elevated in normal pregnancy. With the exception of CEA, which was more elevated in the multigravida, all marker levels in maternal serum were significantly different to those of the umbilical cord, irrespective of fetal sex, fetal weight, and maternal parity.

Mammalian *α-fetoprotein* is classified as a member of the albuminoid gene superfamily. Molecular variants and genetic variants of α-fetoprotein differing in mRNA kilobase length have been extensively described in the biomedical literature. Following the discovery of the molten globule form in 1981, the existence of transitory, intermediate forms of α-fetoprotein was acknowledged and their physiologic significance was realized. The maternal serum α-fetoprotein is a useful marker for women harboring a malignant germ cell tumor containing an endodermal sinus

Table 16–17 SERUM TUMOR MARKERS IN NON-PREGNANT AND PREGNANT PATIENTS

Marker	Malignancy	Normal levels	Effect of pregnancy
CA-125	Serous papillary ovarian carcinoma and tumors of low malignant potential	< 35 U/mL	Elevated during the first trimester
Human chorionic gonadotropin	Gestational trophoblastic neoplasia, malignant germ cell tumors of the ovary	< 5 IU/L	Peak at 14–16 weeks: 12,000–270,000 IU/L
α-Fetoprotein	Malignant germ cell tumors of the ovary, hepatocellular carcinoma	< 15 ng/mL	Peaks at 200–300 mg/dL at 13 weeks
Lactate dehydrogenase	Dysgerminoma, tumors of the liver	45–90 U/L	Fluctuates minimally
Inhibin	Granulosa cell tumors of the ovary	33–45 pg/mL	Increased with pre-eclampsia
Testosterone	Sertoli cell tumors of the ovary	30–95 ng/dL	May rise four- to ninefold over non-pregnant levels during normal pregnancy
DHEA-S	Tumors of the adrenal gland	35–430 μg/dL	Can be increased (usually not > 700 μg/dL)
Carcinoembryonic antigen	Colorectal carcinoma, mucinous cystadenocarcinoma of the ovary, pseudomyxoma peritoneii	< 5 ng/mL	Normal or marginally elevated levels
CA-27.29	Breast cancer	≤ 38 U/mL	Not well studied
CA-15-3	Breast cancer	< 40 U/mL	Elevated during third trimester in one study
CA-19-9	Pancreatic cancer	< 40 U/mL	Not well studied
Prolactin	Pituitary tumor (prolactinoma)	< 20 ng/mL	20–400 ng/mL
Total thyroxine	Thyroid carcinoma	5–12 μg/dL	Increased due to increases in serum thyroxine-binding globulin

CA, cancer antigen; DHEA-S, dehydroepiandrosterone sulfate.

tumor or embryonal component. Initially produced by the yolk sac, and later by the fetal liver and gastrointestinal tract, α-fetoprotein is also the predominant protein synthesized during fetal development. Maternal serum α-fetoprotein levels are routinely measured between 16 and 20 weeks' gestation to screen for neural tube defects. Pregnant women with marked elevations of serum α-fetoprotein should have a germ cell cancer or liver tumor included in the differential diagnosis.

As Boulay and Podczaski point out in their excellent review on ovarian cancer complicating pregnancy, the use of α-fetoprotein levels to monitor women with a history of endodermal sinus tumor who subsequently become pregnant poses a distinct clinical dilemma. One way to distinguish between ovarian (i.e. yolk sac) α-fetoprotein and fetal (i.e. liver) α-fetoprotein is to divide the heterogeneous human α-fetoprotein into various subfractions stratified by differential reactivity with lectins, such as concanavalin A. Assay chromatography with concanavalin sepharose A will separate the α-fetoprotein into either the yolk sac or liver variant, as the yolk sac form of α-fetoprotein contains the carbonal sugar and is the type produced by the endodermal sinus tumor.

The use of the *hCG* level to monitor pregnant women in remission following treatment for gestational trophoblastic disease is also problematic. The hCG steadily increases during the first trimester of pregnancy, and may reach levels beyond 100,000 U at 10 weeks of gestation. Accordingly, women with a history of trophoblastic neoplasia must undergo transvaginal ultrasonography to document intrauterine pregnancy, and a metastatic workup should be conducted if the hCG remains markedly elevated during pregnancy or if focal symptoms manifest.

The glycolytic enzyme *lactate dehydrogenase* (LDH) is involved in the conversion of pyruvate to lactate. LDH is also a marker for gonadal and extragonadal dysgerminomas. Because the enzyme is ubiquitous, the heterogeneity afforded its multiple molecular forms permits electrophoretic separation into five isoenzymes. Isoenzyme fractions 1 and 2 are specifically elevated in women with dysgerminomas. During pregnancy and the puerperium, LDH values fluctuate very little, unless the patient is preeclamptic. In 1992, our group used the LDH level to observe two women with dysgerminoma diagnosed during pregnancy; in both cases, the LDH value was correlated to disease activity.

Inhibin is a glycoprotein hormone produced by normal ovarian granulosa cells and testicular Sertoli cells. In the ovary, it inhibits the secretion of follicle-stimulating hormone. Patients with granulosa cell tumors have elevated serum levels of inhibin, and this finding has been used to detect recurrent tumor. In pregnancy, serum levels of inhibin do not rise significantly unless the patient has preeclampsia or gestational hypertension. The use of an inhibin monoclonal antibody can preferentially mark inhibin secreted from granulosa cell tumors and Sertoli–Leydig cell tumors.

HEMATOLOGIC MALIGNANCIES IN PREGNANCY

Leukemia

Arising from bone marrow progenitor cells that have arrested along a line of differentiation, the leukemias manifest clinically when the arrested cells proliferate, overtake the bone marrow, and spill out into the peripheral blood. Without immediate therapy, patients with acute leukemia, particularly acute myelogenous leukemia (AML), survive a median of 3 months. In the USA, there are 30,000 new cases of leukemia and 20,000 deaths attributable to the disease each year. Table 16–18 summarizes a classification scheme for the leukemias, with the major subtypes being AML (comprising 46% of all leukemias), chronic lymphatic leukemia (29%), chronic myelocytic leukemia (CML, 14%), and acute lymphatic leukemia (11%). Leukemia is estimated to occur in one in 75,000 pregnancies, with AML accounting for more than 60% of reported cases, of which there are approximately 500.

The attainment of a morphologic normal bone marrow containing less than 5% blasts, the absence of any signs of extramedullary leukemia, and the return of normal neutrophil counts (>1500/μL) and platelet counts (>150,000/μL) is the treatment goal of acute leukemia. Auer rods must not appear in the peripheral blood, and anemia, if present, does not preclude complete remission, as this is often slow to recover. Bone marrow aspiration is performed weekly during the induction phase.

Because of severe myelosuppression caused by intensive chemotherapy, the achievement of complete remission is predicated on supportive care and the necessary maintenance of >500/μL circulating neutrophils and >20,000 circulating platelets, to prevent infectious and hemorrhagic deaths. Cytosine arabinoside and daunorubicin are used to induce remission in AML, with postremission therapy requiring maintenances doses of cytosine arabinoside. When the analysis of the cerebrospinal fluid establishes central nervous system involvement, intrathecal chemotherapy with or without cranial radiation is administered. Finally, the treatment and maintenance of acute lymphatic leukemia employs multiagent regimens involving vincristine and central nervous system prophylaxis.

The ability to enter into complete remission is age-dependent, with the overall rate for acute leukemia being 65%. Median survival is approximately 2 years, with 25% of patients becoming long-term, disease-free survivors. The prognosis for patients undergoing treatment of leukemia following therapy for another disease, or in the recurrent setting, is very poor. Indeed, the majority of adult patients who achieve remission subsequently experience recurrence. The long-term survival rate seen in children is not obtained in adults.

Table 16–18 CLASSIFICATION OF THE LEUKEMIAS

Acute	Chronic
Acute myelogenous leukemia	Chronic myelogenous leukemia
Acute promyelocytic leukemia	Chronic myelomonocytic leukemia
Acute myelomonocytic leukemia	Chronic lymphatic leukemia
Acute monoblastic leukemia	T cell
Acute erythroleukemia	B cell
Acute megakaryoblastic leukemia	Prolymphocytic leukemia
Acute lymphatic leukemia	Sézary syndrome
Common	Hairy cell leukemia
T cel	
B cell	
Pre-B cell	
Acute mast cell leukemia	

(From Jandi JH: Blood: Textbook of Hematology, 2nd edn. Boston, Little, Brown, 1996.)

Leukemia in pregnancy

In the pregnant patient, persistent fever, weight loss, lymphadenopathy, and/or an abnormal differential on the complete blood count should prompt an investigation and raise the clinician's suspicion for leukemia. As in the case of non-Hodgkin lymphoma (NHL) in pregnancy, patients with acute leukemia are often very ill, and the primary concern is to save the mother's life through induction chemotherapy or radiotherapy. Therefore, if the patient is remote from delivery, appropriate treatment will place the fetus at risk to exposure to chemotherapeutic agents and/or radiation therapy. Chronic myelogenous leukemia in pregnancy, on the other hand, can be managed similar to Hodgkin disease, with a justifiable delay in definitive treatment of several weeks if indicated. The outcome of pregnancy-associated acute leukemia is only worse when compared with non-pregnant cases when therapy is delayed. Regardless of gestational age, the induction of remission with combination chemotherapy is the primary objective. Seventy-five percent of pregnant women enter into complete remission following therapy for acute leukemia, owing to their favorable age. During the first and early second trimesters, termination of pregnancy should be seriously considered, especially in the acutely ill mother. When the diagnosis is made later in pregnancy, it should be recognized that there are obvious advantages of delivery before the onset of chemotherapy, and this should be encouraged if possible.

The average age of the patient with acute leukemia in pregnancy is 28 years. Premature labor is common in these women, and the average period of gestation is approximately 8 months. Postpartum hemorrhage occurs in 10–15% of cases. The fibrinogen level in patients with acute leukemia in pregnancy may be reduced from the level anticipated at that stage of gestation. Frenkel and Meyers stated that pregnancy exerts no specific effect on the course of acute leukemia except that early gestation poses an obstacle to vigorous treatment of leukemia. Other authors have observed that infants born of leukemic mothers are as well as normal control subjects. The following factors are associated with the delivery of a normal baby:

- antimetabolite drugs not administered,
- radiotherapy to the uterus not given, and
- the fetus reaches the age of viability.

Lilleyman and colleagues and Bitran and Roth have written comprehensive reports on this subject.

The decision to interrupt a pregnancy in patients discovered to have leukemia is primarily based on the desires of the patient. Prompt therapy is always advisable for the possibility of obtaining remission. However, the physician's advice to the patient should be influenced by the aggressiveness of the disease process. For instance, patients with CML are less likely to be harmed by deferring termination of pregnancy than are patients with acute myelocytic leukemia demonstrating symptoms and having a somewhat fulminating course.

Chemotherapy for acute leukemia in pregnancy

There are many reports of successful chemotherapy for patients who have acute leukemia in pregnancy, and there has been little if any significant increase in fetal wastage or congenital anomalies. In 1984, Catanzarite and Ferguson published a review of management and outcome of acute leukemia in pregnancy for the years 1972–82. The investigators collected 14 pregnancies reported in patients cured of acute lymphocytic leukemia, of which there was one early spontaneous abortion and 13 term infants. All mothers survived. They also collected 47 reports of pregnancy in association with acute leukemia. In 40 pregnancies in which acute leukemia was treated, there were five abortions, three perinatal demises, one infant "live-born in grave condition," and 31 surviving infants. Median maternal survival was at least 6 months and possibly longer than 12 months from delivery. In the remaining seven cases, the leukemia was untreated. Despite this, there were two perinatal deaths, one abortion, and four living infants.

During the years of Catanzarite's and Ferguson's study, effective combination chemotherapy was in widespread use. Previous reviews covered cases reported before the introduction of effective combination chemotherapy. There were fewer than 300 reported pregnancies, with a 36–69% perinatal mortality and a median maternal survival from diagnosis of shorter than 6 months. Advances in the fields of hematology and oncology, maternal and fetal medicine, and neonatology have resulted in marked improvements in both perinatal survival statistics and median maternal survival.

In women who refuse pregnancy termination or in whom delivery is not expected imminently, induction of remission should be attempted. When combination therapy is used during the first trimester, (and for acute leukemia in pregnancy, this is not a contraindication); the stillbirth rate is 25%—this decreases to 13% in the second and third trimesters. A combination of cytarabine, doxorubicin, and etoposide has been used with good results for both mother and fetus, and when possible we recommend this regimen. Delivery should be timed to precede the next course of chemotherapy; however, the majority of patients should be counseled to expect preterm delivery, either spontaneous or induced. It is mandatory to perform a hematologic evaluation of the newborn, as the drugs used cross the placenta and can result in pancytopenia. Although no growth or developmental abnormalities have been demonstrated, the follow-up of children exposed to in utero chemotherapy for the management of acute leukemia has been limited.

Management of chronic leukemia

Chronic myelocytic leukemia represents approximately 90% of all chronic leukemias in pregnancy. An additional 5% of the chronic leukemias in pregnancy are chronic lymphocytic leukemias. Several reports show that pregnant patients with chronic granulocytic leukemia treated during the first trimester with chemotherapy and radiation therapy to the spleen will usually deliver apparently healthy, viable babies if the uterus is protected with lead shields. Lee and coworkers reported 12 cases of leukemia associated with pregnancy. Using lead shields to protect the uterus from radiation therapy to the spleen, six of seven women with chronic leukemia who also received chemotherapy went on to delivery six apparently healthy infants. Another study that showed similar results was reported by Levin and Collea. The prognosis for these patients is poor; median survival is 45 months.

There has been some experience in treating CML during pregnancy with interferon-α. Mubarak et al reported the outcomes of three women, ages 23–32 years, with Philadelphia chromosome–positive CML who received interferon-α during the first trimester of pregnancy. No maternal complications occurred, and three normal-appearing babies were delivered, one of whom had a transient mild thrombocytopenia. Subsequently, these children were followed for 4, 12, and 30 months, and all had normal growth and development.

Hodgkin disease

The importance of staging in Hodgkin disease was recognized by Peters as early as 1950, when she devised the first clinical staging classification. Lymphangiography then

Table 16–19 CLASSIFICATION OF HODGKIN DISEASE

Subtype	Frequency (%)	Characteristics
Nodular sclerosis	40	Mediastinal and pulmonary involvement
Mixed cellularity	30	Frequently advanced at presentation
Lymphocyte predominance	15	Rare classic Reed–Sternberg cells
Lymphocyte depletion	15	Oldest median age, worst prognosis

Table 16–20 STAGING OF HODGKIN DISEASE AS PROPOSED IN THE COTSWOLDS, ENGLAND, 1990

Stage[a]	Characteristics
I	Involvement of a single lymph node or lymphoid region (e.g. spleen, thymus, Waldeyer's ring) or a single extralymphatic site (Ie)
II	Involvement of two or more lymph node regions on the same side of the diaphragm; localized contiguous involvement of only one extranodal organ or site and lymph node region(s) on the same side of the diaphragm (IIe)
III	Involvement of lymph node regions on both sides of the diaphragm, which may also include spleen (IIIs) or one extranodal localized contiguous site (IIIe), or both (IIIes)
III1	With or without involvement of splenic, hilar, celiac, or portal nodes
III2	With involvement of para-aortic, iliac, and mesenteric nodes
IV	Diffuse or disseminated involvement of one or more extranodal organs or tissues

[a]Applicable designations: a, no symptoms; b, night sweats, fever, weight loss; cs, clinical staging; e, involvement of a single extranodal site contiguous or proximal to a known nodal site; ps, pathologic staging (by laparotomy); x, bulky disease (diameter > one-third of mediastinum).

(From Peleg D, Ben-Ami M: Lymphoma and leukemia complicating pregnancy. Obstet Gynecol Clin North Am 25:365–383, 1998.)

made possible the earlier detection of retroperitoneal lymph node involvement, and it became important to distinguish two subgroups: those with widespread disease confined to lymphatic organs, and those with spread of disease beyond the lymph nodes, thymus, spleen, and Waldeyer's ring to one or more extralymphatic organs or tissues, which is now recognized as stage IV disease. The subtype classification scheme for Hodgkin lymphoma appears in Table 16–19. The staging system as proposed by the Cotswolds meeting appears in Table 16–20. Surgical staging has gained popularity in Hodgkin disease, and when evaluating young women in whom preservation of ovarian function is desired and pelvic irradiation is planned, surgical oophoropexy can be performed at the time of staging laparotomy.

The feature of the disease most helpful in selecting therapy and estimating the prognosis at the time of onset is its clinical extent. In general, the more widespread the disease, the poorer the prognosis, even if all apparent disease is confined to the lymphoid regions. The poorer prognosis of patients who have involvement of sites beyond the usual lymphoid tissues is well known. Five-year survival rates of 50% are often reported for patients who have widespread lymph node disease, and rates of 8% are reported for those who have involvement of extranodal sites such as the lung, liver, bone, and bone marrow. Survival depends more on the patient's age and stage than on the subtype. Overall, 36% survive for 20 years, and about 70% do not have a relapse after primary treatment. Those 17–34 years old have an 80% long-term survival, compared with 35% for those 60 years or older.

The treatment of Hodgkin disease has undergone radical changes in the past 40 years. Present recommendations are based on the assumptions that radiotherapy is the mainstay of treatment of early-stage disease, combination chemotherapy is the primary treatment of advanced-stage disease with parenchymal organ involvement, and a combination of the two is required for patients with bulky disease (e.g. a large mediastinal mass) or generalized abdominal lymph node involvement. Aggressive therapy has resulted in considerable improvement in overall survival rates for patients with Hodgkin disease. The most successful and widely tested combination of drugs has been developed at the National Cancer Institute (DeVita and colleagues), and consists of six 2-week cycles of therapy with nitrogen mustard, vincristine, procarbazine, and prednisone, the so-called MOPP program, although other combinations have been used successfully.

The major technical factors that determine the efficacy of radiation therapy in Hodgkin disease are the total radiation dose per field; the size, shape, and number of treatment fields; and the beam energy. Permanent eradication of any given site of involvement can be achieved consistently with doses of 3500–4500 cGy delivered at a rate of 1000 cGy/week. The desirability of irradiating apparently uninvolved lymph node regions has long been advocated by experienced radiotherapists. This approach is based on the knowledge of the clinical behavior of Hodgkin disease, the inadequacies of our diagnostic techniques to discover minute or microscopic foci of the disease, the advantage and efficacy of avoiding patchwork and overlapping fields, and the possible reseeding of previously irradiated regions from unrecognized and untreated sites. Extended field irradiation, so-called total lymphoid or total radial therapy, is technically demanding and potentially hazardous.

Hodgkin disease in pregnancy

With a peak incidence between the ages of 18 and 30 years, Hodgkin disease commonly affects young people. It is now being cured and controlled for long periods with irradiation and chemotherapy. Hodgkin disease in pregnancy occurs in approximately one in 6000 deliveries. Young women diagnosed with Hodgkin disease are usually asymptomatic. The nodular sclerosis subtype of Hodgkin disease is the most common subtype encountered in pregnancy and carries a favorable prognosis.

Most reports suggest that the onset of Hodgkin disease during pregnancy does not adversely affect survival. Chemotherapy and radiation therapy to the abdomen can usually be postponed until the pregnancy is terminated. The drugs commonly used for Hodgkin disease are contraindicated in the first trimester of pregnancy and are preferably withheld until the postpartum period. The amazing successes achieved with early stages of this disease allow much more flexibility and improved regard for the fetus. Pregnancy itself does not appear to adversely affect the course of the disease, and interruption of pregnancy during the course of the disease is not definitely indicated. The management of the pregnant patient with Hodgkin disease should be individualized and involve a multidisciplinary team of physicians and other professionals. Three of four patients diagnosed with Hodgkin disease will be cured.

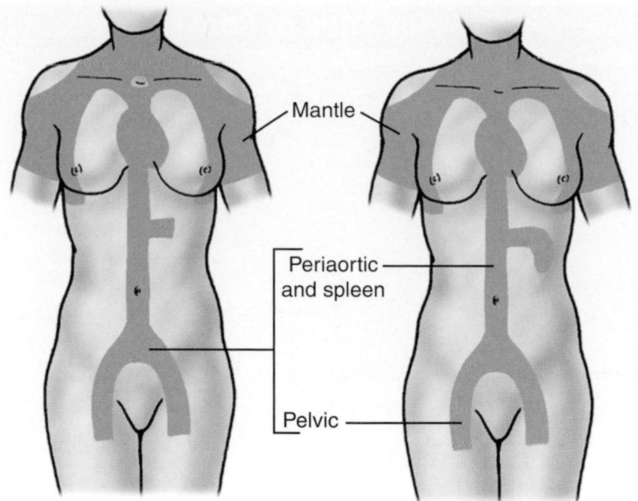

Figure 16–15 Schematic representation of "mantle" and "inverted Y" fields for total lymphoid irradiation. Left: two-field technique, with a small extension to include the splenic pedicle, used in splenectomized patients. Right: three-field technique usually used when the spleen is still present. (From Rosenberg SA, Kaplan HS: Hodgkin's disease and other malignant lymphomas. Calif Med 113:23, 1970.)

Management of Hodgkin disease in pregnancy

The complexity of the management of Hodgkin disease during pregnancy cannot be overstressed. Thorough staging of the pregnant patient is significantly compromised without termination of the pregnancy by one means or another. Surgical staging of the pregnant patient after the 18th week of pregnancy is feasible and often avoids the necessity of many of the diagnostic techniques that might be harmful to the fetus, such as lower extremity lymphangiography, intravenous pyelography, and bone and liver scans. Splenectomy is often performed at these staging procedures, and no contraindication in pregnancy is known. The purpose of staging with this disease is to achieve the best differentiation between those curable with local therapy (radiation) and those who require systemic therapy (chemotherapy or radiation) for cure. Once a criterion for systemic therapy has been uncovered, no additional diagnostic procedures are required.

Treatment is obviously easier if the pregnancy is terminated, but that may not be an option. Current data suggest that the course of Hodgkin disease does not seem to be affected by an ongoing pregnancy. Other studies have also noted a survival rate of pregnant women with Hodgkin disease comparable with that of non-pregnant patients with Hodgkin disease. Hodgkin lymphoma is not associated with an increase in miscarriage, stillbirths, or congenital anomalies unless treatment is started in the first trimester. Metastasis to the placenta has been reported, although it is rare.

Hodgkin lymphoma is a potentially curable disease, and stage I and II disease is typically treated with megavolt radiotherapy unless bulky disease is present. Given in fractions over 3.5–4.5 weeks, a dose of 3500–4500 cGy is prescribed. In early-stage disease, the lymphoid areas that need to be irradiated include the mediastinum, Waldeyer's ring and axilla (i.e. mantle field), and the para-aortic area and splenic pedicle (spade field). When necessary, total nodal irradiation includes the pelvis (inverted Y field), as illustrated in Figure 16–15.

Pregnant women with Hodgkin lymphoma present with typical manifestations, with painless enlargement of lymph nodes above the diaphragm, usually the cervical, submaxillary, or axillary nodes. In patients without obvious lymphadenopathy, a delay in diagnosis is not uncommon, as symptoms of fatigue, weight loss, chest discomfort, and anemia may be overlooked and considered "normal" during pregnancy. The role of staging laparotomy in Hodgkin disease is diminishing, and if necessary it should be delayed until after delivery, at which time bilateral oophoropexy can be performed. It has been our practice to bring the ovaries as close to the midline as possible behind the uterus, where they can be shielded underneath a protective block placed between the two arms of the Y.

Pohlman and Macklis have carefully reviewed previously published guidelines for Hodgkin disease associated with pregnancy and have proposed the following management scheme, which we have endorsed (Fig. 16–16). The earlier the pregnancy, the stronger the recommendation for pregnancy termination so that proper staging and treatment can begin. Patients diagnosed during the first trimester of pregnancy may be observed until the second trimester, when therapy can commence. Those first trimester patients with B symptoms, bulky or advanced-stage disease, or rapid progression have an indication to initiate treatment immediately and should undergo therapeutic abortion. If the mother does not wish to sacrifice the pregnancy, single-agent vinblastine, which has a 7% anomaly rate when used

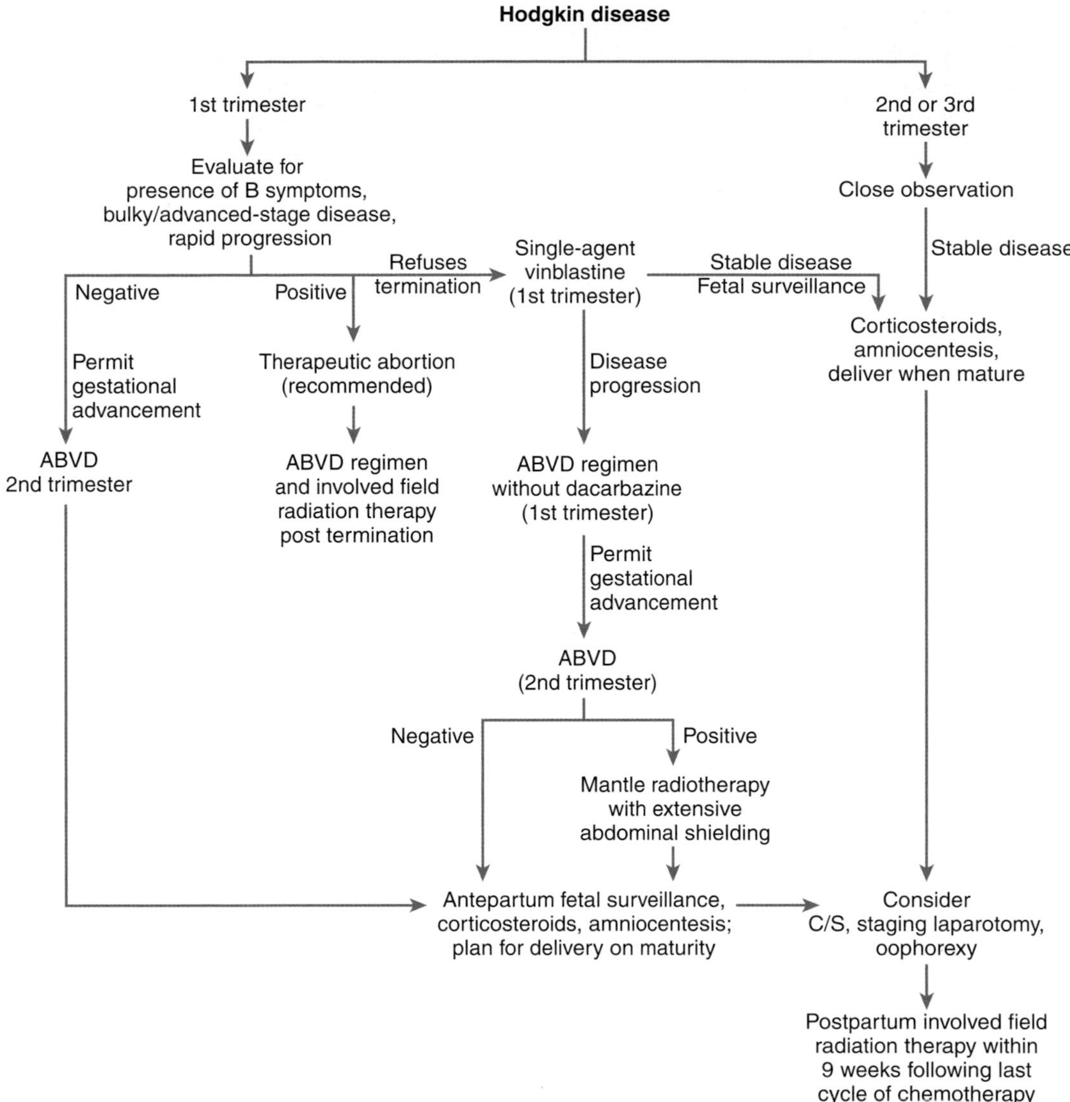

Figure 16–16 Management algorithm for Hodgkin disease in pregnancy. ABVD, doxorubicin (Adriamycin), bleomycin, vinblastine, and dacarbazine.

in the first trimester, should be administered until the second trimester or until significant disease progression. If combination chemotherapy is required, the doxorubicin (Adriamycin), bleomycin, vinblastine, and dacarbazine (ABVD) regimen without dacarbazine during the first trimester should be given, and then standard ABVD subsequently.

Patients presenting in the second or third trimester can be closely observed, and the fetus should be delivered as soon as viability and pulmonary maturation is demonstrable. Delivery should be delayed as long as possible after the last dose of chemotherapy (before the next dose) to decrease the risk of marrow suppression in the neonate. It may be worthwhile to consider a caesarean section so that surgical staging can be performed at the same time. Umbilical cord blood should be collected and stored as a possible source of human leukocyte antigen–compatible stem cells. Because the drugs used in Hodgkin disease can reach significant levels in breast milk, mothers receiving chemotherapy must avoid breast-feeding.

If treatment is necessary during the second and third trimesters of pregnancy, the standard ABVD regimen should be used. Postchemotherapy involved field radiation therapy can be postponed until after delivery but should be initiated within 9 weeks following the last cycle of chemotherapy. Mantle and spade field radiotherapy with extensive abdominal shielding is also an acceptable alternative until the third trimester, when the uterus starts to impinge on the field. The inverted Y field is not an option at any time during pregnancy.

Among those women with refractory or relapsed Hodgkin disease for whom the ABVD regimen and/or radiotherapy are not treatment options, MOPP and MOPP-like regimens have demonstrable efficacy with limited adverse effect on the fetus if administered after the first trimester.

Several older series that pre-date modern therapy suggest that Hodgkin disease has no biologic effect on pregnancy, and vice versa. More contemporary reports have substantiated these claims. Investigators from the Hospital for Sick Children and Princess Margaret Hospital in

Toronto identified 48 women with 50 pregnancies from 1958 to 1984, and matched them with three non-pregnant control subjects of similar age, stage, and year of diagnosis. Twelve women were diagnosed with Hodgkin disease before conception, 10 during pregnancy, and 27 following delivery or pregnancy termination. No statistically significant difference in stage at diagnosis, maternal outcome, or pregnancy outcome was identified between any of these subgroups and the similar control group. It should be noted that 16 patients received radiotherapy while pregnant, and five received combination chemotherapy and radiotherapy while pregnant.

In an investigation focusing on fetal effects of therapy, Ebert et al identified 24 cases in the literature between 1983 and 1995. Among 15 women who received cyclophosphamide, vincristine, procarbazine, and prednisone (COPP, $n = 1$), mechlorethamine, vincristine, procarbazine, and prednisone (MOPP, $n = 4$), doxorubicin (Adriamycin), bleomycin, vinblastine, and dacarbazine (ABVD, $n = 7$), or MOPP/ABVD ($n = 3$) beginning in the first ($n = 5$), second ($n = 8$), and third ($n = 2$) trimesters, all had healthy infants who went on to develop normally during a median follow-up of 9 years (range 0–17 years) after delivery. Of the remaining nine women, most received one of the above regimens during the first trimester and either had therapeutic abortions or experienced spontaneous abortions, delivering fetuses with multiple anomalies.

In a study from Stanford University, the outcome of 17 pregnancies associated with Hodgkin disease between 1987 and 1993 was reported. Patients received radiation therapy ($n = 6$), chemotherapy ($n = 4$), or combined modality therapy ($n = 5$), although the specific timings of therapy in relation to pregnancy were not stated. Excluding four women who had a therapeutic/spontaneous abortion, no congenital anomalies were noted at delivery, and all children were reported to be healthy at the time of last follow-up. With a median follow-up of 35 months (range 6–79 months), 15 of the 17 mothers remain in complete remission.

A final report of interest was provided by Sutcliffe, who describes three women with stage II nodular sclerosing Hodgkin disease who received ABVD chemotherapy during the second and third trimesters of pregnancy. Two of these patients also received mantle field radiation therapy following delivery. All three delivered healthy infants between 32 and 35 weeks' gestation. The chromosomal analyses of all three children were normal, and at over 1 year, 5 years, and 7 years of follow-up, all three mothers and children remain healthy.

Non-Hodgkin lymphoma

Forty-five thousand new cases of NHL are diagnosed in the USA each year. The mean age at diagnosis is 42 years. NHLs comprise a mixed family of diseases characterized by clonal neoplasms arising from one of the cellular constituents of the lymph node. Approximately 85% of NHLs are B-cell tumors, 15% are T-cell tumors, and a small percentage arise from other cells, primarily macrophages. A multitude of infectious agents (e.g. the Epstein–Barr virus, the human T-cell leukemia/lymphoma virus), non-infectious agents (e.g. radiation, radiation therapy, chemotherapy), and diseases (e.g. ataxia telangiectasia, Sjögren syndrome, systemic lupus erythematosus) are associated with NHLs. Most patients present with painless lymphadenopathy, but NHLs may arise outside the lymphoid system in any tissue accessible to lymphocytes, most commonly in the gastrointestinal tract, pharynx, central nervous system, skin, and bone. Because the disease is usually widespread when peripheral lymph nodes have become involved, staging laparotomy is not used. The prognosis of NHL has been divided into favorable, intermediate, and poor. The Working Formulation is a classification scheme for NHL that is used in determining prognosis and treatment (Table 16–21). Unfortunately, NHLs are cured in less than 25% of the general population, although women of reproductive age have a 50% cure rate.

Early-stage (I/II), low-grade NHL is treated with extended field or total lymphoid irradiation, with 5-year survival rates of 84%. Intermediate-grade tumors are managed with combination chemotherapy (prednisone, methotrexate, doxorubicin, cyclophosphamide, etoposide, cytosine arabinoside, bleomycin, vincristine, and leucovorin—ProMACE-CytaBOM) with or without radiotherapy, resulting in sustained remissions at 4 years in approximately 45% of patients.

Non-Hodgkin lymphoma in pregnancy

Most women with NHL in association with pregnancy have an aggressive histologic subtype and advanced-stage disease, possibly due to a delay in diagnosis in many cases. An unexpectedly high incidence of breast, uterine, cervical, and ovarian involvement among pregnant women has been noted when NHL is associated with pregnancy, with the predilection for these organs attributed to hormonal influences and increased blood flow to these organs. In a review of 96 women with pregnancy-associated NHL, Pohlman et al reported fully 50% of women presenting with stage IV disease. Seven percent of pregnancies ended in therapeutic abortion, and 4% of women experienced a spontaneous abortion. Eleven percent of infants were born prematurely, and 7% died. Only 31 mothers were known to have achieved a complete remission, and for 90 subjects in whom their long-term outcome was known, only 39 were alive and disease-free a median of 21 months (range 2–132 months) after delivery, 4 were alive with disease, and 47 had died a median of 6 months (range < 1 to 36 months) after delivery. Women who were diagnosed during the third trimester of pregnancy appeared to have a better outcome than those diagnosed earlier. Seventy-one of 96 children were reported alive, although the follow-up period for the majority was either under 1 month or unknown.

Aviles et al reviewed the outcome of both mother and fetus in 19 pregnancies between 1975 and 1986. All

Table 16–21 WORKING FORMULATION FOR CLASSIFICATION OF NON-HODGKIN LYMPHOMA

	Histologic type	Description	Prognosis
I	Low grade	Small lymphocytic cell Follicular (nodular) small cleaved cell Follicular mixed small cleaved cell	Favorable
II	Intermediate grade	Follicular large cell Diffuse small cleaved cell Diffuse mixed small and large cell Diffuse large cell cleaved/non-cleaved	Intermediate
III	High grade	Diffuse large cell, immunoblastic Small non-cleaved cell (Burkitt/non-Burkitt) Lymphoblastic (convoluted/non-convoluted)	Unfavorable
IV	Micellaneous	Composite Mycosis fungoides Extramedullary plasmacytoma Histiocytic Unclassified	—

(From Peleg D, Ben-Ami M: Lymphoma and leukemia complicating pregnancy. Obstet Gynecol Clin North Am 25:365–383, 1998.)

patients received doxorubicin-based combination chemotherapy during pregnancy, including eight who received chemotherapy during the first trimester. Three mothers and their fetuses died during induction, and the 16 remaining women delivered healthy infants between 35 and 39 weeks' gestation. Eight of 12 mothers remained in complete remission 4–9 years after delivery, while seven mothers died of lymphoma and one was lost to follow-up.

Overall, the prognosis for all patients with NHL is worse than the prognosis for patients with Hodgkin disease. This is explained, in part, by the dissemination of disease at presentation. For this reason, while many dispute the claims that NHL arising in pregnancy is more virulent, the management of NHL in pregnancy needs to be aggressive. A delay in treatment cannot be justified, and a woman who has not completed the first half of pregnancy should be advised to undergo therapeutic abortion unless she is willing to expose herself and her fetus to the risks of combination chemotherapy. After 24 weeks' gestation, premature delivery may be necessary, depending on the mother's medical condition.

Patients with localized disease should receive three to eight cycles of cyclophosphamide, doxorubicin, vincristine, and prednisolone (CHOP) chemotherapy and then, following delivery but within 9 weeks of the last dose of chemotherapy, involved field radiation therapy should be prescribed. Patients with advanced-stage disease should be treated with six to eight cycles of CHOP chemotherapy. Because high-dose methotrexate is an integral component of most effective regimens for Burkitt lymphoma, therapeutic abortion for women diagnosed in the first trimester is essential. Finally, for women with relapsing NHL associated with pregnancy, treatment should not be compromised as the disease is highly aggressive, and therapeutic abortion is generally advisable during the first half of pregnancy because the fetal effects of standard salvage chemotherapy regimens are unknown.

A special consideration can be made for pregnant patients with indolent or low-grade NHLs. These patients may be safely observed until delivery or significant disease progression, provided they are asymptomatic, have a relatively normal complete blood count, and show no impending organ compromise. Such a profile has not yet been reported for NHL associated with pregnancy.

Ward and Weiss reviewed the cases of 42 patients with NHL during pregnancy. Twenty-four of the cases were reported from 1976 to 1985. Three first-trimester cases resulted in two surviving infants. Twenty-one second- and third-trimester cases resulted in 15 surviving infants. Infants who were born to mothers who were untreated or treated with surgery had a 38% prenatal mortality rate, whereas 87.5% of infants of mothers treated with chemotherapy survived. Eight of the 21 second- and third-trimester patients received single-agent or combination chemotherapy. Four of these patients survived. Spitzer and coworkers reported that radiotherapy treatments given to six women in the second or third trimester of pregnancy resulted in no harm to the fetus; yet four of the mothers died of their disease. Of the four cases with a successful delivery and maternal survival, two were treated with combination chemotherapy, one with chemotherapy and radiotherapy, and one with radiotherapy alone. High-grade lymphomas have a particularly poor outcome. In the review by Ward and Weiss, none of the patients diagnosed with Burkitt lymphoma during pregnancy ($n = 18$) survived; however, only five of the patients were treated with chemotherapy. Only five cases ended with fetal survival. The most important factor influencing the well-being of the fetus is the health of the mother.

In summary then, if the hematologic malignant disease is early stage or low grade, treatment can be deferred or non-toxic therapy can be employed. However, many NHLs present with dissemination or aggressive histologic features, for which the most effective therapy is chemotherapy. The mother deserves the most effective chemotherapeutic regimen, despite its teratogenic potential.

OTHER TUMORS IN PREGNANCY

Melanoma

Melanoma accounts for one of every 50 cancer-related deaths in the USA. The incidence is rising, with approximately 10,000 cases occurring annually among women aged 20–40 years. Congenital nevi may be found within the first 6 months of life and have the highest chance of all nevi for malignant degeneration. Congenital melanocytic nevi may be found in up to 2% of newborns, and giant congenital nevi may cover large areas of the body. Nevi arising later in life are known as the common mole or acquired melanocytic nevi.

The common mole represents over 95% of nevi and may be subdivided into junctional nevi, compound nevi, and dermal nevi. The blue nevus is another type that usually appears on the dorsal aspects of the extremities and has a very low tendency to become malignant. Nevertheless, any nevi, whether congenital, acquired, or blue, that undergoes suspicious changes should be biopsied. The "ABCD" warning signs that herald changes in nevi that are associated with melanoma are *a*symmetry, irregular *b*orders, *c*olor changes, and moles that increase in *d*iameter. All melanomas masquerade as nevi before diagnosis. The average individual has 15–20 nevi, and removal of all these lesions prophylactically is hardly practical. Lesions on the feet, palms, genitals, and areas of persistent irritation from clothing are potentially dangerous nevi and should be removed during childhood.

There are five main types of melanoma, the most common of which is the superficial spreading melanoma, which accounts for 70–75% and tends toward horizontal growth prior to becoming invasive. Approximately 15% of melanomas are nodular and become invasive early. In sun-damaged areas, a lentigo maligna may develop, and in darker skinned persons the acral-lentiginous melanoma can be found on palms and soles. Finally, the least common are the amelanotic melanomas, which are difficult to diagnose.

Staging of melanoma

Reference may be made to the final version of the American Joint Committee on Cancer staging system for cutaneous melanoma that was published in 2001. Both depth of penetration of the lesion and the extent to which the lesion has involved local and regional tissues are brought into the staging system. This new system is a blend of the Clark and Breslow microstaging classifications (Table 16–22). The Clark microstaging classification provides a histologic staging scheme for classifying melanomas on the basis of level of penetration of the melanoma under the epidermis and dermis. Prognosis for the patient relates well to this microstaging system. Data indicate that a Clark level I melanoma should be viewed as an in situ lesion requiring no lymph node dissection. Clark's level II indicates superficial dermal penetration, with lymph node metastases in 1–5% of patients not justifying an elective lymph node dissection. At the other end of this pathologic spectrum are melanomas of Clark's level IV and level V, which metastasize to regional lymph nodes in approximately 40 and 70% of patients, respectively, necessitating lymphadenectomy as part of initial therapy.

Table 16–22 MICROSTAGING SYSTEMS FOR MELANOMA

Level	Clark et al	Breslow et al
I	All tumor cells above basement membrane (in situ)	<0.75-mm depth of invasion
II	Tumor extends to papillary dermis	0.76- to 1.5-mm depth of invasion
III	Tumor extends to interface between papillary and reticular dermis	1.51- to 2.25-mm depth of invasion
IV	Tumor extends between bundles of collagen of reticular dermis	2.26- to 3.0-mm depth of invasion
V	Tumor invasion of subcutaneous tissue	>3-mm depth of invasion

(From Tewari KS: Cancer of the vulva. In Manetta A (ed): Cancer Prevention and Early Diagnosis in Women. Pennsylvania, Mosby, 2004.)

An alternative classification suggested by Breslow (see Fig. 8–27) and used by some clinicians is a simple micrometer measurement of lesion thickness. Lesions greater than 4 mm have a high incidence of distant metastasis. Lesions 1.5–4 mm have a 57% incidence of regional node involvement and 15% incidence of distant metastasis. Lesions between 0.76 and 1.5 mm have a 25% incidence of regional node involvement and an 8% incidence of distant metastasis. Lesions less than or equal to 0.75 mm are usually not associated with any spread.

Melanoma in pregnancy

It is rare that pregnancy adversely affects a malignant process, but for many years melanoma was placed in this category. The average age of the patient with melanoma is 45 years, and 35% of women will be diagnosed during childbearing years. This is suggested by many case reports in which pregnancy has been incriminated in the induction or exacerbation of a melanoma. Partial or complete regressions of melanoma after delivery have been reported. In contrast, Stewart describes a case in which a tumor recurred three times; each recurrence was a few weeks after the patient delivered a child. Female patients have improved survival compared with male control subjects matched for age and tumor thickness. This suggests that some hormonally based mechanisms are operational in the biologic behavior of melanoma. Contemporary studies fail to substantiate any effect previously attributed to pregnancy.

After the second month of pregnancy, the pituitary gland increases production of melanocyte-stimulating hormone. Melanocyte-stimulating hormone activity is also increased by the pregnancy-associated increase in adrenocorticotropic hormone. This results in the increased pigmentation that is characteristic of pregnancy and often found in the nipples, vulva, linea nigra, and pre-existing nevi. In animal studies, the high circulating levels of estrogens in pregnancy have been shown to control melanocyte activity. These observations have led some to believe that pregnancy can have an inciting influence and/or a deleterious impact on the course of melanoma, and have given rise to several myths about this disease in relationship to pregnancy, including:

- pregnancy increases the risk of developing malignant melanoma,
- pregnancy worsens the prognosis,
- future pregnancies have an adverse effect both on prognosis and on recurrence,
- oral contraceptives and hormone replacement therapy are contraindicated in women with a history of melanoma due to theoretic stimulatory effects of hormones on melanocytes.

None of these claims are substantiated by the medical literature.

Historical series of melanoma in pregnancy

The original report published by Pack and Scharnagel in 1951 contained 1050 patients with melanoma. Ten of these patients were pregnant, five of whom died within 3 years of diagnosis. Later authors would cite these observations, which suggested that melanomas in pregnancy grow with unusual rapidity and metastasize widely. Subsequently, many series have challenged the findings of Pack and Scharnagel.

In 1960, George and coworkers gave a comprehensive report of 115 patients with melanoma in pregnancy compared with 330 control subjects from the same institution. In disagreement with an earlier report from their institution, they found that spread to regional nodes appeared to be more rapid in the pregnant patient, but that there was no significant difference stage for stage in the outcome for the patient. This was directly contradictory to the earlier philosophy popularized by Pack and Scharnagel that melanoma is indeed aggravated by the pregnant state.

In 1961, White and coworkers reported a study of 71 young women (aged 15–39 years), 30 of whom had melanoma during pregnancy. The 5-year survival rate in the pregnant group was 73%, and for the 41 non-pregnant patients the survival rate was 54%. They concluded that on the basis of the 5-year survival rates in pregnant and non-pregnant women with age and stage of disease taken into account, survival was equal in the two groups. No deleterious effect of pregnancy on survival of women with melanoma was demonstrated in this series.

Reintgen and colleagues described 58 women who were pregnant when the disease was diagnosed and another 43 patients who became pregnant within 5 years of diagnosis. Control groups were extracted from a total of 1424 women who were registered at the Duke University Melanoma Clinic. The mean age of patients in the series was 28 years. Both actuarial disease-free intervals and survivals were calculated for the study populations and their respective control groups. There was no statistical difference in survival between patients who had mole changes and diagnosis of melanomas during pregnancy and the control population. The results of the study also indicated no difference in survival for women who became pregnant within 5 years of diagnosis.

Despite these equivalency studies, many authorities continue to recommend survivors of melanoma to avoid pregnancy for approximately 3 years after complete surgical excision, because this is the period of highest risk of relapse. Obviously, each case must be individualized, and the recommendation should be heavily influenced by the size, depth of invasion, and any detected dissemination. The role of previous pregnancy as a protective factor in melanomas has been suggested by some but also remains controversial. Patients surviving disease-free for 5 years have a 95% chance of long-term cure. Conversely, after a woman has had a diagnosis of having a cutaneous melanoma, subsequent pregnancy has no effect on recurrence rates or survival.

Contemporary studies of melanoma in pregnancy

Contemporary studies also note no survival difference in patients with melanoma who are pregnant compared with non-pregnant patients. MacKie and associates evaluated 388 women with stage I melanoma divided into four groups: 85 treated before pregnancy, 92 treated while pregnant, 143 treated after completion of all pregnancies, and 68 treated between pregnancies. Interestingly, poor prognostic factors (e.g. tumor thickness and tumor occurring at a poor prognostic site, such as the head, neck, and trunk) occurred more frequently in the pregnant patient than in the non-pregnant patient. However, in multivariate analysis, pregnancy status was not significantly related to prognosis.

In 1998, Grin et al critically reviewed controlled clinical trials to assess the effect of pregnancy on the prognosis of melanoma and examined the available epidemiologic data to evaluate the risk of melanoma after exposure to oral contraceptives and hormone replacement therapy. The investigators concluded that pregnancy before, during, or after the diagnosis of melanoma did not influence 5-year survival rates, and exposure to oral contraceptives and hormone replacement therapy did not appear to increase the risk of melanoma.

In a recent paper retrospectively evaluating a cohort of 185 women diagnosed with melanoma during pregnancy

Table 16–23 MULTIVARIABLE COX REGRESSION ANALYSIS FOR THE 2101 WOMEN WITH MELANOMA WITH KNOWN BRESLOW THICKNESS, CLARK'S LEVEL, AND TUMOR SITE

Variable	Hazard ratio	95% confidence interval	*P*
Pregnancy at the time of diagnosis of primary melanoma[a]	1.08	0.60–1.93	0.804
Breslow thickness (per additional category)	2.16	1.80–2.58	< 0.0001
Axial site vs limb site of primary melanoma	2.51	1.78–3.56	< 0.0001
Clark's level (> 3 vs < 3)	1.39	0.92–2.14	0.12
Age (per year increase)	1.02	0.99–1.05	0.06

[a]Pregnant women at the time of diagnosis of melanoma (*n* = 185) vs non-pregnant women at the time of diagnosis of melanoma (*n* = 5348).
(From Lens MB, Rosdahl I, Ahlbom A et al: Effect of pregnancy on survival in women with cutaneous malignant melanoma. J Clin Oncol 22:4369–4375, 2004.)

and 5348 women of the same childbearing age with melanoma not associated with pregnancy, Lens et al noted no statistically significant difference in overall survival between pregnant and non-pregnant groups (Table 16–23). Women with higher Breslow tumor thickness category had a significantly higher risk of death than those with lower Breslow category. Also, women with axial tumors (head and neck, and trunk melanomas) had a poorer prognosis than those with tumors localized on the extremities. Neither pregnancy status at the time of diagnosis of melanoma nor pregnancy status after the diagnosis of melanoma was a significant predictor of survival.

The cumulative retrospective case-controlled studies have involved over 450 pregnant women with melanoma. The anatomic location of the primary tumor does not differ between pregnant and non-pregnant women, and no analysis identified any differences in survival from non-pregnant women. Multivariate analyses have been performed and have revealed that the stage of disease at diagnosis, *and not the pregnancy*, is the only consistent finding that influences prognosis. *Thus, we conclude that pregnancy does not confer a worse prognosis for this diagnosis when matched for stage of disease.*

Management of melanoma in pregnancy

It is essential that all physicians and midwives conduct a full examination of the skin of their patients. A changing skin lesion should be subjected to an excisional biopsy. Early diagnosis of stage I disease will often lead to curative therapy. Irrespective of pregnancy, treatment of melanoma is related to depth and stage. Lesions less than 1 mm in thickness usually require a wide, deep local excision with a 1-cm margin, and those between 1 and 4 mm need a 2-cm margin of excision. While a wide excision is curative for stage I lesions, the role of interferon-α for stage II and stage III disease is currently under investigation. Although the use of interferon-α in pregnancy has been reported for the management of chronic leukemia, there has been no published experience using this drug for melanoma in pregnancy.

The value of regional lymphadenectomy in clinically negative nodes has been controversial. The debate has been defused to some degree with the development of lymphatic mapping to identify the sentinel lymph node. Pathologic evaluation of the sentinel node is predictive of regional lymph node metastasis in 96–98% of cases. Thus sentinel lymph node identification and evaluation is indicated for lesions penetrating beyond 1 mm. Lloyd et al emphasizes that data regarding the effect of radioactive colloid on the fetus are insufficient to permit its use in pregnant women. The dose to the patient from lymphoscintigraphy is 0.4 mSv, with a dose to the uterus of 0.5 mGy. Most of the injected radioactivity stays at the injection site or moves to the sentinel node(s), which are resected the following day during surgery. Despite the small amounts of injected activity, the local dose rate at the injection site is high, and injection sites close to the fetus (over the lower abdomen or back) combined with next-day rather than same-day resection may result in greater doses to the fetus at any stage of the pregnancy.

It is our practice to perform a wide, deep local excision only in women under 30 weeks' gestation, and for those beyond 30 weeks' gestation we offer sentinel node identification after delivery. Because small quantities of radioactivity can be excreted into the breast milk, breastfeeding is contraindicated if sentinel node identification is performed postpartum.

Melanoma metastatic to the products of conception

The reported low incidence of metastasis of malignant neoplasms to products of conception is probably caused by several factors. One factor is the unexplained resistance of the placenta to invasion by maternal cancer, as demonstrated in many animal studies. Metastasis of maternal cancer to products of conception is rare despite the sizable number of pregnancies at risk. However, although melanoma accounts for only a small number of all cancers associated with pregnancy, almost half of all tumors metastasizing to the placenta and nearly 90% metastasizing to the fetus are melanomas.

A few cases of transplacental transmission of melanomas with subsequent death of the fetus or newborn child from disseminated melanoma have been described, but this situation is extremely rare and occurs only when the mother has widespread blood-borne metastatic disease during pregnancy. Schneiderman et al reported a case of a primary fetal melanoma fatal to a newborn. Microscopic metastases were present in the lungs and liver, and the placenta showed widespread metastases to the chorionic villi but no evidence of invasion of the intervillous spaces. The mother had no evidence of disease 1 year after delivery. To date, no instances of metastasis from fetus to mother have been documented. Moller and associates reported a case of maternal melanoma with metastasis to the placental intervillous sinuses. Tumor cells were also present in the fetal cord blood. The mother died postpartum and the infant survived. Mothers with advanced or recurrent disease should undergo ultrasound examination during pregnancy for assessment of any obvious fetal tumor masses. Attention should be directed to placental thickness as well as to the fetal liver and size of the fetal spleen. Cord blood should be examined for malignant cells, and placental tissue should be carefully inspected. A further discussion on the predilection of melanoma to metastasize to the placenta and the fetus is presented in a separate section in this chapter.

Thyroid cancer

Papillary, follicular, and anaplastic carcinomas are the most common primary thyroid malignant neoplasms, with medullary carcinoma accounting for only 5%. The disease usually manifests as a relatively asymptomatic nodular mass in the thyroid gland. The lesion is multifocal, as seen on careful sectioning in approximately 30–40% of patients, but in only 5% do these become clinically evident if thyroid tissue remains after surgery. Laboratory indices of thyroid function are contributory only if they indicate a hyperthyroid state, thus supporting the diagnosis of a toxic adenoma. Although studies show that these tumors involve regional lymphatics microscopically in 50–70% of patients, this subclinical involvement does not affect the prognosis. The growth of papillary carcinoma may depend on thyroid-stimulating hormone (TSH), and therefore thyroid hormone administration to suppress TSH is used routinely as an adjuvant in all patients. The prognosis for patients who have this cancer is favorable, especially in the younger age group. Specifically, in women younger than 49 years, a 90–95% survival at 15 years is consistently reported.

Papillary and follicular thyroid carcinomas are two to three times more common in women than in men (5.5 vs 2.4 per 100,000, respectively). This female predominance is especially notable during the reproductive years, such that the diagnosis of thyroid carcinoma in pregnancy does occur. In fact, approximately 10% of differentiated thyroid carcinomas in women of reproductive age are diagnosed during pregnancy or within the first year after delivery. The actual incidence of thyroid cancer in pregnancy has not been established.

During pregnancy, non-pathologic enlargement of the thyroid gland to twice its normal size is not uncommon. Histologic examination shows this enlargement to be caused by an apparent hyperplasia of the follicular cells and abundant colloid formation. A mild suppression of TSH and slight elevation of free thyroxine is common in early pregnancy due to the stimulation of the TSH receptor by hCG. A rise in thyroxine-binding globulin during pregnancy results in elevated levels of total thyroid hormone.

Thyroid cancer in pregnancy

Because papillary carcinomas are the most common lesions to occur in the reproductive age group, a solitary nodule in an otherwise normal gland is the most common presentation of thyroid carcinoma in pregnancy. Sam and Molitch have noted that the incidence of thyroid nodules during pregnancy may be increased, with some data suggesting a higher incidence of malignancy in these nodules. In a 1994 series of 30 pregnant women with thyroid nodules, Rosen and Walfish observed a 43% incidence of malignancy. In 1997, Doherty et al reported the incidence of malignancy to be 39% among 23 women with pregnancy-associated thyroid nodules. In contrast, the incidence of malignancy of thyroid nodules in the non-pregnant population ranges from 8 to 17%. hCG may stimulate the growth of thyroid nodules by cross-reacting with the thyrotropin-stimulating hormone receptor.

Thyroid function tests and a fine-needle aspiration should be performed in the pregnant patient with a newly discovered thyroid nodule. The latter procedure is especially important when the nodule is greater than 2 cm in size. If the results of cytologic examination are benign, a course of thyroid suppression using 0.2 mg of L-thyroxine daily is indicated for the duration of the pregnancy. Repeated cytologic evaluation may be necessary if the nodule does not diminish on suppression or if it enlarges during pregnancy, because 6% of needle aspirations give a false-negative result. The theoretic risk of two false-negative diagnoses is about 0.05%, thus providing excellent confirmation of a conservative approach if the aspirate is repeatedly negative.

If the fine-needle aspiration reveals a papillary or follicular carcinoma, we advise patients to undergo surgery in the second trimester (Fig. 16–17). If the carcinoma has been discovered in the third trimester, the workup and treatment can be delayed until after delivery. Rapidly growing tumors and medullary carcinomas should be removed on discovery, regardless of gestational age. Short treatment delays to permit gestational advancement may be acceptable for some patients with medullary carcinomas, but as soon as fetal maturity can be demonstrated labor should be induced or a caesarean section performed. Surgery is the only known effective therapy for medullary carcinomas, and results in a 50% survival at 5 years. A prophylactic lymph node dissection on the site of the lesion is indicated. Fetal loss associated with surgery has been

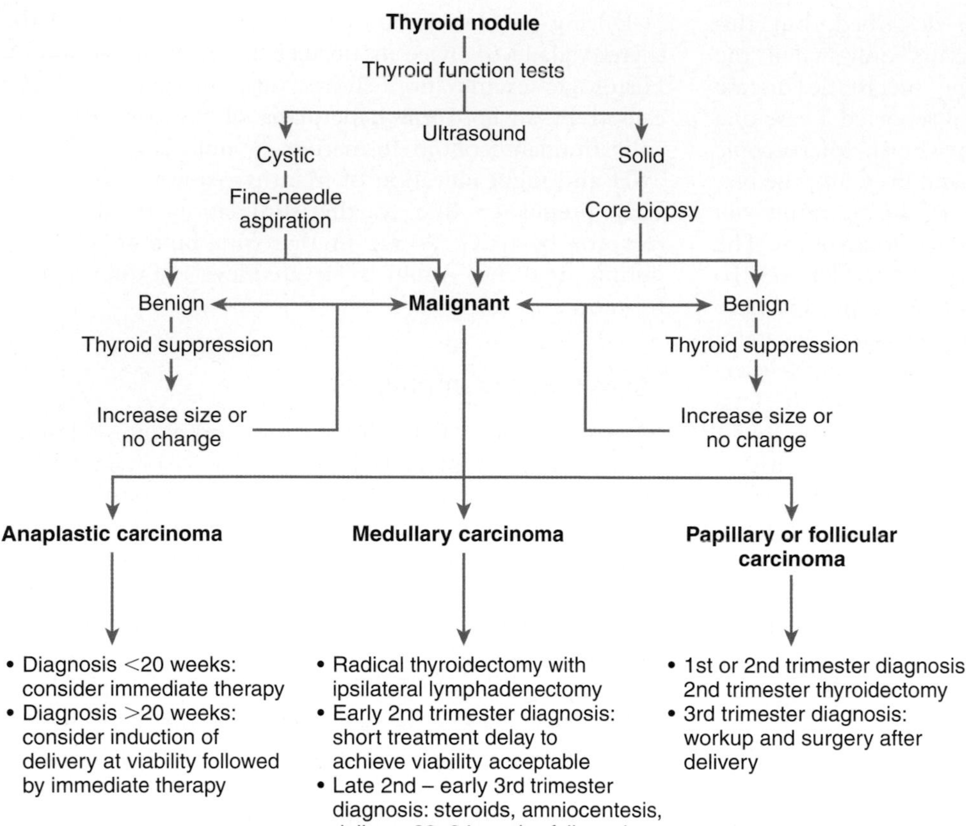

Figure 16–17 Management algorithm for the thyroid nodule and thyroid cancer in pregnancy

reported only with extensive neck exploration. Following tumor resection, suppressive doses of thyroid hormone should be administered, keeping in mind that thyroid hormone requirements may be higher in pregnancy.

Radioactive iodine is contraindicated during pregnancy and lactation. Even though trace doses are used in these uptake studies, there is still a theoretic risk of a destructive effect on the fetal thyroid and a concern for teratogenesis within the fetus. A whole-body iodine-131 can be performed 3 months after discontinuation of lactation, and if necessary, iodine-131 ablation is recommended.

The undifferentiated lesion

In the uncommon situation of an anaplastic carcinoma of the thyroid, the main concern is to keep the mother alive until the pregnancy has come to term, because these tumors are almost uniformly lethal lesions. Between 90 and 95% of patients are dead within 1 year of diagnosis. The standard treatment in these patients is radical thyroidectomy followed by radiation therapy. This obviously presents a difficult situation for the patient in the first or second trimester, and one must carefully discuss the situation with the patient and the family. Treatment of pregnant patients who have progressive, local, unresectable, or metastatic thyroid carcinoma has to be individualized and tailored to the wishes of the patient. Surgical removal of these poorly differentiated lesions will achieve the best local control. The role of radiation therapy and chemotherapy remains investigational.

Prognosis among pregnant women with thyroid cancer

Pregnancy does not negatively influence the prognosis of patients with well-differentiated thyroid carcinoma. For example, Moosa and Mazzaferri found no difference in the outcome between 61 pregnant women with thyroid cancer and a group of age-matched, non-pregnant control subjects. In addition, pregnancy has not been shown to increase the recurrence rate of women previously treated for thyroid cancer. Hill and coworkers described 70 women who conceived after the diagnosis of thyroid cancer and compared them with 109 women who remained childless. There was no difference in the overall recurrence rate. The authors concluded that subsequent pregnancy did not alter the course of the disease. Rosvoll and Winship reviewed the cases of 60 women treated for thyroid carcinoma who subsequently became pregnant, and concluded that a history of thyroid cancer is not an indication for avoidance of pregnancy or for therapeutic abortion. Friedman suggested that pregnancy was not contraindicated if the disease-free interval was at least 3–5 years. However, even in patients who had residual or recurrent disease, the prognosis did not appear to be altered by the pregnancy.

Rare gynecologic malignancies in pregnancy

Vulvar cancer

Fewer than 50 cases of invasive cancer of the vulva associated with pregnancy have been reported in the literature. Lutz et al estimated an incidence of one case per 8000 deliveries at his institution; our experience has been less frequent, at about one per 20,000 deliveries. The most common of these are invasive epidermoid carcinomas, followed by melanomas, sarcomas, and adenoid cystic adenocarcinomas. In recent years, reports of pregnancies complicated by recurrent vulvar carcinoma, metastatic vulvar melanoma, a rapidly enlarging myxoid leiomyosarcoma of the vulva, and primary choriocarcinoma of the vulva have also appeared. The majority of patients have been between 25 and 35 years of age; the youngest patient was 17 years. With the increasing frequency of the diagnosis of CIS of the vulva, the occurrence of preinvasive disease with pregnancy is common today. As is the practice with CIN, therapy for the vulvar counterpart is delayed until the postpartum period. Adequate biopsies of the most suspicious areas are essential to rule out invasive disease. The presence of intraepithelial neoplasia should not prohibit vaginal delivery but should prompt a careful colposcopic evaluation of the lower genital tract to exclude other preinvasive or invasive foci.

Historical series of vulvar cancer in pregnancy

Gitsch et al have presented a concise review of therapy and outcome for this group of patients, correctly noting that the reports have been inhomogeneous. In a review of the literature, Barclay found 31 women with vulvar cancers associated with pregnancy. The vulvar cancers were actually diagnosed and treated during pregnancy in only 12 of these women; another two were treated after termination of pregnancy. In 1974, Barclay furnished further details on nine patients, one of whom was treated with radiation therapy during pregnancy. Five patients were treated surgically before delivery, and three women underwent vulvectomy in the postpartum period. With extended follow-up, none of the patients experienced recurrent disease, although one woman developed a cervical carcinoma that was irradiated. Lutz et al reported three cases diagnosed during pregnancy but treated postpartum. Although no one survived, details concerning the stage, treatment, and survival time were not provided.

Management of vulvar cancer in pregnancy

Invasive vulvar malignant disease diagnosed during the first, second, and early third trimesters is usually treated as indicated in the non-pregnant patient some time after the 18th week of pregnancy. T1 lesions should be managed by radical wide excision with ipsilateral groin dissection if the depth of invasion is greater than 1 mm. Larger and/or more deeply invasive tumors require a radical vulvectomy and bilateral inguinofemoral lymphadenectomy. Patients with palpable inguinofemoral nodes undergoing surgery early in pregnancy present a unique challenge, as skin bridge metastases are more likely to occur in patients with bulky positive nodes. Such patients are advised to have the groin dissected using an en bloc approach because of the need to delay radiation therapy for many months. When the diagnosis is made after 36 weeks' gestation, we recommend a wide local excision with definitive surgery postponed until the postpartum period. This avoids the greatly enhanced vascularity in vulvar tissues during the later months of gestation and into the immediate postpartum period. A short delay does not appear to seriously prejudice the course of the disease.

Women treated during pregnancy may be allowed to attempt vaginal delivery provided the vulvar wounds are well healed and there are no indications for additional therapy. Patients with high risk surgicopathologic features warranting adjuvant radiation should undergo caesarean delivery as soon as fetal pulmonary maturation can be documented. Following delivery of the baby, the ovaries should be transposed to the paracolic gutters, and pelvic and/or groin irradiation can be administered postpartum.

Because this disease occurs more frequently in lower socioeconomic groups, who often do not seek prenatal care, many of these cases are diagnosed at the time of delivery or later. In this group of patients, definitive therapy should be started within 1 week after delivery during the same hospitalization. The pregnant state does not appear to significantly alter the course of the malignant process; survival of these patients stage for stage is similar to that of non-pregnant patients.

Bakour et al have carefully considered the subject of future pregnancies in this group of patients, and have found no contraindications after surveying the literature. In fact, they feel that these young patients who have undergone such extensive surgery obtain a great boost psychologically when they realize this possibility. There have been several reports of patients treated for carcinoma of the vulva with radical vulvectomy and bilateral inguinal lymphadenectomy who subsequently became pregnant and had normal deliveries. Whether the patient should deliver vaginally or by caesarean section is a decision that rests with the obstetrician, but it is heavily influenced by the state of the postsurgical vulva. In most instances, the vulva is soft and does not impede a vaginal delivery. In other instances, there may be a high degree of vaginal stenosis or other fibrosis, which makes caesarean section the more appropriate means of delivery.

Primary invasive vaginal tumors

Cancer of the vagina has been found mainly in women older than 50 years. The diagnosis of vaginal cancer during pregnancy is exceptionally uncommon, even with the clear cell adenocarcinoma of the vagina alleged to be associated with the diethylstilbestrol-exposed offspring. Although all these clear cell adenocarcinomas have occurred in women younger than 34 years, the incidence in association with pregnancy has fortunately been rare.

Senekjian et al described 24 women who were pregnant when clear cell adenocarcinoma of the vagina or cervix was diagnosed; 14 were in the first trimester, 6 in the second, and 4 in the third. Among the stage I and stage II tumors, 16 (73%) were vaginal and 6 (27%) were cervical. Thirteen long-term survivors were reported among the 16 early vaginal lesions. No significant differences were observed when the group of 24 patients with pregnancy-associated tumors and 408 never-pregnant (age-corrected) patients were compared with regard to maternal hormone history, symptoms, stage, location, predominant histologic or cell type, greatest tumor diameter, surface area, depth of invasion, grade, and number of mitoses. The overall 5- and 10-year actuarial survival rates (86% and 68%, respectively) for the group pregnant at diagnosis did not differ significantly from the rates for the never-pregnant group analyzed concomitantly ($n = 408$). Pregnancy did not seem to adversely affect the outcome of clear cell adenocarcinoma of the vagina and cervix. Jones et al have also reported a diethylstilbestrol-related clear cell carcinoma of the vagina in a patient whose tumor, observed directly over an extended period, did not appear to be influenced by elevated plasma estrogen levels during the time period when the pregnancy was carried to term.

Primary squamous cell carcinoma of the vagina discovered during pregnancy is exceedingly rare. In 1976, Collins and Barclay identified 10 patients from the literature, and while three responded well to radiation therapy, a rapidly progressive downhill course was described for four patients available for detailed analysis. In 1977, Lutz et al reported a 24-year-old patient diagnosed at 24 weeks' gestation with a stage II squamous cell carcinoma of the vagina, who despite immediate radiotherapy following preterm delivery suffered a fatal recurrence 7 months later. Three additional cases have been reported by Palumbo et al, Beck and Clayton, and Baruah and Sangupta, manifesting between 8 and 24 weeks' gestation and all resulting in maternal death within 18 months of diagnosis; in two of the cases, pregnancy termination had been performed so as to not delay radiotherapy.

Finally, Steed et al reported a 28-year-old with antepartum bleeding at 20 weeks' gestation who was found to have a 6-cm diameter anterior vaginal wall squamous cell carcinoma extending to the right lateral fornix. This patient opted to continue the pregnancy and received corticosteroids, followed by caesarean delivery at 32 weeks' gestation. Prior to delivery, gold seeds were placed transvaginally to demarcate the tumor edges. Amazingly, although the patient was debulked of multiple, enlarged, positive pelvic lymph nodes, following treatment with chemoirradiation and brachytherapy she had remained disease-free for 3 years at the time of publication. This report brings the total to 15 cases of primary invasive squamous cell carcinoma of the vulva complicating pregnancy, with an overall survivorship of 38%, similar to what is observed in non-pregnant patients.

Both cervical cancer and vaginal cancer are staged clinically, and the management principles to be discussed in detail when cervical carcinoma complicates pregnancy may be applied to vaginal tumors as well. Treatment of clear cell adenocarcinoma of the cervix and upper vagina is surgically similar to that of squamous cell cancers. Specifically, very early lesions involving the upper vagina may be treated by radical abdominal hysterectomy with pelvic lymphadenectomy, while all others are best managed radiotherapeutically. The pregnancy should be disregarded if the diagnosis is made in the first or early second trimester. Should the pregnancy be further along, the decision for appropriate time of intervention depends on the preferences of the patient and the oncologist. Patients with an early pregnancy who resist termination should be given corticosteroids and delivered as soon as fetal pulmonary maturation is demonstrable. The impact of a delay in therapy on the prognosis is impossible to predict. In instances in which there is extensive involvement of the vagina by any lesion, one should seriously consider evacuation of the uterus by a hysterotomy or caesarean section and institution of appropriate radiation therapy.

A few scattered reports of sarcoma botryoides of the cervix and vagina in pregnancy were recorded during the 1960s by Roddick and Honig, and by Schwartz et al. When these sarcomatous lesions occur in the upper half of the vagina with or without cervical involvement, the most appropriate therapy has been a radical abdominal hysterectomy, upper vaginectomy, and bilateral pelvic lymphadenectomy followed by postoperative adjuvant chemotherapy. In 2003, the first primary vaginal leiomyosarcoma diagnosed during pregnancy was reported by Behzatoglu et al in a 21-year-old woman who presented during the third trimester with a 1.5-cm firm, fleshy, pedunculated mass arising from a short stalk on the right vaginal wall. Previously, female genital tract leiomyosarcomas that have been associated with pregnancy had originated from the uterus or vulva ($n = 10$). Finally, some malignancies have been reported in pregnancy to involve the vagina secondarily by direct extension (e.g. tumors of the cervix), via lymphatic spread (e.g. endometrial carcinoma), or through hematogenous dissemination (e.g. gestational choriocarcinoma and placental site trophoblastic tumor). In fact, secondary involvement from an extravaginal site is more common than the development of a primary vaginal neoplasm, irrespective of pregnancy. While pregnancy-associated vaginal cancer is rare, the entity must remain part of the differential diagnosis of bleeding in pregnancy. Steed et al emphasize that visualization of the entire vagina and cervix is necessary during speculum examination, and the procedure should be performed in every pelvic examination and for all investigations carried out for antepartum bleeding.

Endometrial cancer

Endometrial carcinoma in conjunction with pregnancy is extremely rare. Most of the reported cases have been diagnosed at examination of uterine contents obtained by curettage for elective pregnancy termination or spontaneous abortion. Leiomyosarcoma (including a myxoid leiomyosarcoma), endometrial stromal sarcoma, and carcinosarcoma have also been reported during pregnancy. They are usually incidental findings noted in surgical specimens. The recommended therapy for endometrioid adenocarcinomas associated with pregnancy is total hysterectomy with bilateral salpingo-oophorectomy and adjuvant radiotherapy when indicated.

In 1972, Karlen and associates reviewed the literature since 1900, summarized five acceptable cases, and added a sixth. In 2004, Itoh et al collected a total of 29 patients (including one of their own), 11 of whom were older than 35 years. Twenty-one of the 29 cases had no or minimal myometrial invasion, 18 of which were histologically FIGO grade 1, and three were FIGO grade 2. This group includes a 28-year-old who received conservative treatment with high-dose medroxyprogesterone acetate following a uterine curettage that had revealed diffuse complex hyperplasia with atypia and a focus of well-differentiated adenocarcinoma showing stromal invasion. This patient subsequently conceived, and following delivery at term she underwent a total abdominal hysterectomy. Pathologic examination of the uterus revealed a persistent well-differentiated endometrioid adenocarcinoma limited to the endometrium. This case serves to illustrate a very important point. As more women opt for conservative management of invasive cancers in an effort to preserve fertility, we may anticipate a larger number of referrals than what was seen previously for patients with persistent or even recurrent malignancy during pregnancy.

All 21 patients with favorable histopathologic features were alive at the time of their report, ranging from 3 months to 10 years after treatment. Therefore most cases of endometrial carcinoma associated with pregnancy are characterized by well-differentiated tumors, an endometrioid histology with no or minimal myometrial invasion, and favorable outcome, consistent with the typical clinicopathologic features of type I endometrial carcinoma that develops in obese women. It has been hypothesized that the elevated serum progesterone level during pregnancy inhibits the growth of endometrial carcinoma cells, and this may contribute to the good outcomes observed among these 21 patients. This has prompted several authorities to argue that adenocarcinoma in pregnancy does not occur and that the reported cases were misdiagnosed Arias–Stella reactions.

However, the remaining eight of the 29 reported patients have had well-documented deep myometrial invasion or extrauterine extension. The FIGO grade distribution included grade 1 ($n = 3$), grade 2 ($n = 2$), and grade 3 ($n = 3$, including one serous papillary carcinoma), and the FIGO stage ranged from Ic to IV. Two of these eight patients died of disease, and it notable that the patient submitted by Itoh et al had deep myometrial invasion and negative expression of ER and PR. Importantly, higher grade tumors or non-endometrioid adenocarcinomas are often negative for ER/PR expression, and this group of endometrial carcinomas associated with pregnancy is characterized by high-grade histology, including non-endometrioid type, deep myometrial invasion, advanced stage, and poor outcome consistent with the type II carcinoma manifesting in non-obese patients. Thus not all endometrial carcinomas associated with pregnancy have a favorable prognosis.

Fallopian tube cancer

The fallopian tube can become secondarily involved by malignancy through direct extension of an ovarian tumor or from an endometrial carcinoma. Primary fallopian tube carcinoma was described by Starr et al as a disease of recent vintage, having been first reported in 1847 by Raymond and later, in 1861, by Rokitansky. The disease is the least common gynecologic tumor. The mean age ranges from 50 to 55 years. Thus the possibility of its presence in pregnancy is extremely remote. Cases have been reported to be associated with pregnancy; in these instances, the neoplasm is usually unilateral and most often adenocarcinoma.

The clinical presentation of carcinoma of the tube is variable and non-specific even without an associated pregnancy. The usual watery, blood-tinged vaginal discharge would be obviated in pregnancy because at 12 weeks' gestation the communication between the uterine cavity and the fallopian tube is blocked. In most instances, the diagnosis is established at laparotomy, and the treatment is total abdominal hysterectomy with bilateral salpingo-oophorectomy and postoperative radiotherapy or chemotherapy, depending on the operative findings and the residual disease after surgery. Several instances are reported in the literature of incidental findings of CIS of the tube noted in specimens submitted after postpartum tubal ligation. In these instances, a total abdominal hysterectomy with bilateral salpingo-oophorectomy has been recommended; however, simple removal of the fallopian tubes may be a reasonable alternative.

Adolph et al reported the first case of a recurrent fallopian tube carcinoma associated with pregnancy in 2001. The patient had originally underwent a limited surgical procedure to preserve fertility, followed by chemotherapy, and subsequently experienced an intraperitoneal recurrence 1 year later during her 16th week of pregnancy. Following a caesarean section at term, she underwent optimal cytoreductive surgery and was alive with stable disease 6 months following salvage chemotherapy when the paper was published. This case is included with some detail to emphasize a point made earlier, in that as fertility-preserving oncologic procedures become more widely accepted for certain early-stage malignancies, the probabilities increase for having to manage recurrent disease in pregnancy. *The criteria through which surgeons determine candidacy for fertility preservation must be carefully devised and rigorously adhered to.*

Trophoblastic tumors of the fallopian tube: "ectopic" pregnancy

Although choriocarcinoma most frequently arises in the uterus, a primary choriocarcinoma of the fallopian tube may be associated with ectopic pregnancy. In these scenarios, the biologic behavior is very aggressive, with distant metastases manifesting in 75% of cases. A review of the world literature of 93 reported cases by Ober and Maier in 1981 yielded 58 acceptable cases, to which the authors added 18 from the files of the Armed Forces Institute of Pathology. Since that time, there have been approximately 15 additional reports, bringing the total to 91 cases of primary choriocarcinoma of the fallopian tube. The mean age is 33 years, with 66% of patients presenting with acute symptoms consistent with a ruptured ectopic pregnancy. The remainder typically have presented with a gradually expanding adnexal mass clinically indistinguishable from an ovarian tumor. Endovaginal ultrasonography may offer an image compatible with an extrauterine pregnancy in the left appendages, and the quantitative serum β-hCG is elevated. Grossly, the tumor appears as a hemorrhagic friable mass, occasionally containing spongy tissue resembling the placenta. Smaller tubal choriocarcinomas are difficult to distinguish on gross inspection from the common ectopic pregnancy. Histopathologic features and the distribution of metastases are similar to gestational choriocarcinoma arising in the uterus.

The surgical approach has not been uniform, with some women undergoing unilateral salpingectomy only or unilateral adnexectomy or total abdominal hysterectomy with bilateral salpingo-oophorectomy. Most patients have gone on to receive polychemotherapy. In the review by Ober and Maier, it was noted that of 47 acceptable cases treated prior to modern chemotherapy, the mortality rate was 87% (n = 41). Of 16 cases treated with modern chemotherapy, the salvage rate was 94% (n = 15). Fewer than 10 patients have been cured by unilateral salpingectomy or unilateral salpingo-oophorectomy alone. Whenever possible, a histologic examination of the tubes should be performed in all cases of ectopic pregnancies. Serial measurements of the β-hCG is an essential component of the surveillance of all patients treated for ectopic pregnancy, and especially for those treated with methotrexate or by salpingotomy alone.

Primary choriocarcinoma of the fallopian tube coexistent with a viable intrauterine pregnancy was first reported by Lee et al in 2005, and a heterotopic pregnancy of a primary placental site trophoblastic tumor of the fallopian tube and an intrauterine pregnancy was first reported by Su et al in 1999.

Placental and fetal tumors

The placenta may be the site of origin of gestational trophoblastic neoplasia (GTN) or can be secondarily involved by other malignancies. The disease spectrum of GTN encompasses molar pregnancies (e.g. complete, partial, invasive), non-metastatic GTN, gestational choriocarcinoma (i.e. metastatic GTN), and placental site trophoblastic tumors. These entities are discussed in a separate chapter. The occurrence of gestational choriocarcinoma and placental site trophoblastic tumors in the fallopian tube has been addressed earlier in this chapter under the section concerning tumors of the fallopian tube in pregnancy. The following sections will have as their focus the occurrence of a twin pregnancy complicated by a complete mole and a normal fetus, placental and fetal metastases, and primary fetal cancers that may manifest in utero.

Complete hydatidiform mole with coexistent fetus

Ultrasonography depicting the combination of a live fetus and a molar-appearing placenta suggests three distinct possibilities:

1. a singleton pregnancy consisting of a partial mole with a live fetus,
2. a twin pregnancy comprising one placenta exhibiting a complete mole (no fetus) and the other placenta sustaining a normal twin, and
3. a twin pregnancy with a partial mole and fetus in one sac and a normal twin in the other sac.

The first possibility involves a triploid fetus that usually dies during the first trimester. The third possibility is easily eliminated by the presence of two fetuses.

The incidence of complete hydatidiform mole with coexistent fetus (CMCF) ranges from one in 10,000 to one in 100,000 pregnancies. The true incidence is difficult to establish, and the observed increased incidence of iatrogenic multiple gestations in recent years is expected to result in a higher incidence of CMCF. Vaisbuch et al have conducted a comprehensive review of the literature (Table 16–24), and after exclusion of duplicate publications they have identified 130 cases, some of which include higher order gestations (e.g. triplets and quadruplets).

Steller et al discovered eight well-documented cases of twin pregnancy with CMCF. They compared the clinical features of these eight patients with 71 women with singleton complete hydatidiform mole. Although the presenting symptoms were similar in both groups, a twin pregnancy with CMCF was diagnosed at a later gestational age (20.1 weeks vs 13 weeks), had higher pre-evacuation β-hCG levels, and had a greater propensity to develop persistent GTN (55% vs 14%).

Bristow et al reported 25 cases from the literature and one of their own, of whom 19 were evacuated before fetal viability and only seven resulted in a live-born infant. Although the previable and viable group were unremarkable with respect to mean age, gravidity, parity, uterine size, and presence of theca-lutein cysts, significant differences in gestational age at diagnosis (17.4 weeks vs 29.4 weeks) and pre-evacuation serum hCG levels (> 1,000,000 mIU/mL vs 170,000 mIU/mL) were observed. In addition, previable cases were also associated with higher frequencies of pre-eclampsia (31.6% vs 14.3%) and persistent GTN (68.4% vs 28.6%). Clinical factors that required termination of the pregnancy might have been surrogates for aggressive trophoblastic growth and therefore persistent disease and the subsequent need for adjuvant systemic therapy. Bruchim et al reported a 53.3% incidence of

Table 16–24 COMPLETE HYDATIDIFORM MOLE AND COEXISTING FETUS: SELECTED SERIES

Reference	*n*	Intended previable termination of pregnancy	Termination of pregnancy due to SAB, maternal complications, of IUFD	Live neonate	Per-eclampsia	Persistent GTN	Metastatic GTN
Bristow et al (1996)	26	19	n/a	7 (27%)	7 (27%)	15 (57%)	5/22 (lung, vagina)
Fishman et al (1998)	7	5	n/a	2 (28%)	n/a	4 (57%)	0
Matsui et al (2000)	18	5	10	3 (17%)	5 (28%)	9 (50%)	6 (lung)
Sebire et al (2002)	77	24	32	20 (26%)	n/a	15 (19%)	n/a
Vaisbuch et al (2005)	2	0	1	1	2	0	0
Marcorelles et al (2005)	4	1	1	2	1	1	0
Total 1996–2005 (5)	134	54	44/97	35 (26%)	15/46 (33%)	44 (33%)	11/49 (22%)

IUFD, intrauterine fetal death; GTN, gestational trophoblastic neoplasia; n/a, not available; SAB, spontaneous abortion.
(After Vaisbuch E et al: Twin pregnancy consisting of a complete hydatidiform mole and co-existent fetus: report of two cases and review of the literature. Gynecol Oncol 98:19–23, 2005.)

persistent GTN (including four patients with pulmonary metastasis) when they analyzed 15 cases of CMCF that had resulted in a live neonate delivered at a mean age of 34.3 weeks' gestation. Although CMCF is associated with a higher risk of persistent GTN when compared with the risk attributable to a singleton complete hydatidiform mole, the issues regarding pregnancy termination are unclear. It does not appear that advanced gestational age is an independent risk factor for developing persistent GTN in the setting of a CMCF. Once fetal anomalies and an abnormal karyotype are excluded, with some degree of caution the literature supports continuing the pregnancy provided there is no evidence of pre-eclampsia and the mother strongly wishes to do so. A declination in serum levels of hCG may also be included in the criteria through which expectant management can be offered. Patients should be informed that only 25% of such pregnancies will result in a live birth, and that there may be some serious consequences of premature delivery and prematurity.

The overall risk of developing persistent GTN is 33%, irrespective of whether the pregnancy is terminated or carried to viability and/or term. Therefore the major obstacles to continuing the pregnancy are the development of a paraneoplastic medical complication, catastrophic vaginal hemorrhage, and formation of metastatic foci antenatally. In the exceedingly rare situation in which metastatic GTN coexists with a normal gestation, intravenous systemic chemotherapy is necessary during pregnancy, unless the disease is discovered when the baby is of advanced gestational age, in which case delivery followed by immediate systemic therapy might be an option.

Placental and fetal metastases

The patient afflicted with cancer in pregnancy commonly asks whether the disease can spread to her child. Although cancer during pregnancy is not uncommon, metastases to the placental tissue or the fetus rarely occur. Most malignancies, when matched stage for stage, portend the same prognosis for the woman whether she is pregnant or not. Exceptions include hepatocellular cancer, lymphoma, thyroid, colon, and nasopharyngeal cancers. In addition to the primary cancer sites, metastatic disease to the products of conception predicts an ominous course for the mother. Metastatic lesions to the fetus or placenta remain a poorly understood subject.

The first report of metastases to the placenta and/or fetus appeared in 1866. In this case, Friedreich observed a mother with disseminated "hepatic" carcinoma that spread to and killed the fetus. There have been no other reports of "hepatic" metastases to the products of conception, and we suspect that Friedreich's patient had a melanoma, which is most likely to behave in this clinical manner. Indeed, melanoma is the most common cancer to metastasize to the placenta and fetus. Rothman and associates reported 35 cases of disseminated maternal malignant disease with either placental or fetal involvement. In only two instances was tumor demonstrated on both the maternal and fetal sides of the placenta and in the fetus. It is rare for the fetus to be involved if there is invasion only of the maternal side of the placenta. Of six cases in the literature when the villus itself was invaded, there was only one case of demonstrable fetal disease. In another report by Potter and Schoeneman, 24 cases of maternal cancer metastasizing to the fetus or placenta were reviewed. Melanoma, by far the most common tumor to spread to the fetus or placenta, was found in 11 cases. Breast cancer was found in four cases. Eight infants were found to have cancer at birth, and six of these subsequently died of their malignant neoplasms. Two infants with metastatic melanoma were noted to have complete tumor regression and ultimately survived. Seven of eight occurrences of metastasis to the fetus were found in cases of maternal melanoma, and there was one case of lymphosarcoma. Finally, Holland reported a case in which maternal, placental, and fetal disease was documented.

Table 16–25 MOST COMMON CANCERS IN PREGNANCY TO AFFECT THE PLACENTA AND/OR FETUS

Cancer type	Cases reporting placental involvement	Cases reporting only fetal metastasis	Cases reporting both placental and fetal metastasis	Total cases affecting placenta and/or fetus	Percentage of total cases
All cancers	72	10	6	88	100
Melanoma	21	3	3	27	31
Breast	15	0	0	15	17
Lung	8	1	1	10	11
Leukemia	6	3	0	9	10
Lymphoma	3	2	2	7	8

(From Alexander A et al: Metastatic melanoma in pregnancy: risk of transplacental metastases in the infant. J Clin Oncol 21:2179–2186, 2003.)

Since Friedreich's initial report, there have been fewer than 90 cases of maternal malignancy metastatic to the gestation (Table 16–25). Because of its generous blood flow, large surface area, and favorable biologic environment for growth, one would consider the placenta to be an ideal site for metastases, and therefore the relative paucity of such events remains unclear. Why have the products of conception been privileged in this way? Perhaps immunologic rejection of tumor cells, uteroplacental circulatory mechanisms, or even a protective role of the trophoblast limit the establishment of metastatic foci. Cancers that have been reported to metastasize to the intervillous space or to the placenta proper include sarcomas, carcinomas, lymphomas, leukemias, and melanomas. Importantly, 30% of the cases are melanomas, followed by breast cancer (18%) and then the hematopoietic malignancies (13%).

Nearly half of the reports contain cases of known malignancy diagnosed prior to the onset of pregnancy. Unfortunately, 93% of such women died of their disease, sometimes within hours of delivery. Gestational reactivation of malignancy has been reported in women who had been disease-free for 5 years prior to becoming pregnant. Contrasting with the unfavorable prognosis for mothers with placental metastases, the prognosis for the infant has been excellent, with 53 of the reported cases revealing no evidence of disease in the baby. In addition, since 1966 no infant has succumbed to metastatic disease, although several reports contained fetal demises as a consequence of complications of prematurity. More recently, the first case of maternal pulmonary adenocarcinoma metastatic to the fetus has been reported; the involved scalp was widely excised and skin graft coverage was applied at 3 months of life, and at the time of publication the child was 5 years old and disease-free.

Another unusual scenario is that of GTN metastatic to the fetus, with 15–20 cases reported to date. Interestingly, widely metastatic disease in the delivered neonate can occur in the absence of metastatic GTN in the mother. There are also reports of acute leukemia developing postnatally in the child of a mother with acute leukemia. In one report by Cramblett and associates, the child developed acute leukemia 9 months after delivery; in another report by Bernard, disease manifestation occurred 5 months after delivery. Transplacental transmission of maternal B-cell lymphoma was reported by Maruko et al when a 29-year-old mother developed the disease at 29 weeks and her infant developed malignant lymphoma at 8 months of life. Hypotheses relating to familial, hereditary, environmental, and viral factors can be advanced in these circumstances, but the weight of evidence suggests that acquisition of maternal malignant disease by the fetus is extremely unlikely.

Guidelines for the evaluation of children born to women with cancer are sparse in the literature. Tolar and Neglia recommend that any child born to a mother with active or suspected malignancy should initially have a thorough physical examination with a complete blood count, comprehensive metabolic panel, liver function tests, coagulation battery, serum LDH, and uric acid levels, as well as a urinalysis. In addition, the placenta should be macroscopically and microscopically examined for tumor involvement. It has been our practice to also obtain imaging studies, including an MRI of the brain and CT scans of the chest, abdomen, and pelvis, when maternal breast cancer, hematopoeitic malignancy, or melanoma is at issue or in the setting of confirmed placental metastases. Continued surveillance should be ongoing during the first year of a child's life, as some cases of maternal to fetal metastases have not presented until several months after birth. Because not all cases with documented placental involvement have corresponding fetal metastases, infants with an initially negative workup should not be prophylactically treated but should be closely observed with frequent physical examinations, laboratory tests, and imaging studies as clinically indicated.

Primary fetal tumors

Benign tumors such as *teratomas* or *lymphangiomas* may progress rapidly in utero, distorting the fetal anatomy and resulting in intrauterine fetal and obstetric complications and morbidity. In addition, several developmental tumors, including *hamartomas* and *vaginal adenosis*, are not malignant in utero, but may undergo malignant degeneration following delivery. Benign and malignant tumors present diagnostic problems and therapeutic challenges. Both typically appear as heterogeneous masses with solid and cystic components when viewed by ultrasonography. The extent and tissue characteristics of these lesions may be further evaluated by MRI, and the diagnosis can occasionally be guided by a cytologic analysis of fluid aspirated from a cystic lesion. Jauniaux et al maintain that expectant management should be the rule in the initial phase, with serial ultrasound evaluations to detect rapid enlargement, metastasis, or secondary fetal complications such as non-immune hydrops.

The *sacrococcygeal teratoma* is a tumor arising from totipotential embryonic cells of the coccyx, and has an incidence of one in 35,000–40,000 deliveries. There is a 4:1 female to male predominance, although the sex ratio in the incidence of malignant tumors is equal. With routine prenatal ultrasound, these lesions are being diagnosed increasingly when views of the spine to rule out neural tube defects are performed. The advent of antenatal ultrasound has shifted the management focus from birth to the antenatal period, where the fetal mortality rate ranges from 30 to 50%. The most common cause of perinatal loss is premature labor secondary to polyhydramnios, with one series reporting the combination of hydrops and placentomegaly as a very ominous sign with 100% mortality. On this basis, fetal surgery with tumor resection has been advocated in selected cases if the hydrops appears before 28 weeks and the tumor is deemed resectable. Because of the risk of dystocia and traumatic hemorrhage, caesarean section has been the rule for tumors greater than 5 cm. Following birth, complete excision of the tumor should not be delayed, and those who survive surgery should have a favorable prognosis. Residual tumor, however, may lead to malignant change, and although the recurrence risk is extremely low, isolated cases have been reported.

Congenital neuroblastoma is a cancer of neuronal lineage that may occur along the sites of the sympathetic ganglia from the neck to the presacral region, including the adrenal medulla. They typically contain Schwann cells, and are the most common malignant tumor of the newborn, representing 30–40% of all congenital tumors. The genetic defect is characterized by the loss of locus p36 on chromosome 1. The clinical features are a function of the size, location, and humoral activity of the neuroblastoma, with catecholamine or vasoactive intestinal polypeptide characterizing their biologic behavior. Fetal neuroblastomas are well encapsulated and may displace the kidney inferiorly and laterally, with a predilection for the right side. The presence of calcification by ultrasonography has been associated with improved survival. Importantly, neuroblastoma cells may infiltrate the placenta beyond the fetal capillaries and villous trophoblast, with metastasis to maternal tissue. Postpartum symptoms attributable to catecholamine production may be observed in the mother and include sweating, flushing, palpitations, and hypertension.

Concordance for neuroblastoma in monozygotic twins has been rarely reported, with the cause for the shared pathology unestablished. In 2001, Anderson et al described a case of infant monozygotic twins developing neuroblastomas that were morphologically, clinically, and molecularly indistinguishable, but with a delay of 6 months between times of presentation. Both tumors had metastasized and had amplification of MYCN and deletion at 1p36. The twin who developed neuroblastoma first had constitutional karyotype abnormalities in at least 5% of peripheral blood mononuclear cells. The second twin had a normal constitutional karyotype and lacked rearrangements or deletions. The authors proposed an acquired neuroblastoma predisposition specific for the first twin and in utero metastatic spread of tumor cells to the second twin (i.e. twin to twin metastasis) via the shared placental circulation.

Acute congenital leukemia is the second most common fetal cancer, occurring at an incidence of one in 4.7 million live births per year. The diagnosis requires the proliferation of blast cells together with anemia, thrombocytopenia, and leukocytosis. Important congenital infections including cytomegalovirus, rubella, and toxoplasmosis must be excluded. In utero, hepatosplenomegaly and non-immune hydrops are common at presentation.

Sporadic heritable retinoblastoma is a malignant tumor of the retina that is inherited in an autosomal dominant manner. The mutant retinoblastoma gene is mainly derived from the father and may be related to exposure of paternal germ cells to carcinogens. Primary hepatic malignant tumors of the fetus may present with an abdominal mass, and in cases of *hepatoblastoma* the serum levels of α-fetoprotein are markedly elevated and reflect the tumor burden. Finally, *rhabdomyosarcoma* is the most common soft tissue sarcoma in children, and is commonly located at the level of the head and neck. It is associated with a loss of heterozygosity of the short arm of chromosome 11. Only a few cases have been described during pregnancy, during which time the tumors manifested as rapidly growing masses of irregular contour.

BIBLIOGRAPHY

BACKGROUND AND EPIDEMIOLOGY

Barber HRK, Brunschwig A: Gynecologic cancer complicating pregnancy. Am J Obstet Gynecol 85:156, 1963.

Dinh TA, Warshal DP: The epidemiology of cancer in pregnancy. In Barnea ER, Jauniaux E, Schwartz PE (eds): Cancer and Pregnancy. London, Springer-Verlag, 2001.

Haas JF: Pregnancy in association with a newly diagnosed cancer: a population-based epidemiologic assessment. Int J Cancer 34:229–235, 1984.

Jacobs IA, Chang CK, Salti GI: Coexistence of pregnancy and cancer. Am Surgeon 70:1025–1029, 2004.

Oehler MK, Wain GV, Brand A: Gynaecological malignancies in pregnancy: a review. Aust N Z J Obstet Gynaecol 43:414–420, 2003.

Pavlidis NA: Coexistence of pregnancy and malignancy. Oncologist 7:279–287, 2002.

Ries LAG, Kosary CL, Hankey BF et al (eds): SEER Cancer Statistics Review, 1973–1996, Bethesda, National Cancer Institute, 1999.

Sivanesaratnam V: Management of the pregnant mother with malignant conditions. Curr Opin Obstet Gynecol 13:121–125, 2001.

Smith BL, Martin JA, Ventura SJ: Births and deaths. Preliminary data for July 97–June 98. National Center for Health Statistics. Vital Health Stat 22(477), 1999.
Smith LH, Dalrymple JL, Leiserowitz GS et al: Obstetrical deliveries associated with maternal malignancy in California, 1992 through 1997. Am J Obstet Gynecol 184:1504–1513, 2001.
Smith LH, Danielsen B, Allen ME et al: Cancer associated with obstetric delivery: results of linkage with the California Cancer Registry. Am J Obstet Gynecol 189:1128–1135, 2003.
Ward RM, Bristow RE: Cancer and pregnancy: recent developments. Curr Opin Obstet Gynecol 14:613–617, 2002.
Zanotti KM, Belinson JL, Kennedy AW: Treatment of gynecologic cancers in pregnancy. Semin Oncol 27:686–698, 2000.

CERVICAL CANCER IN PREGNANCY

Ahdoot D, van Nostrand KM, Nguyen NJ et al: The effect of route of delivery on regression of abnormal cervical cytologic findings in the postpartum period. Am J Obstet Gynecol 178:1116–1120, 1998.
Allen DG, Planner RS, Tang PT et al: Invasive cervical cancer in pregnancy. Aust NZ J Obstet Gynaecol 35:408–412, 1995.
Allen HH, Nisker JA, Anderson RJ: Primary surgical treatment in one hundred ninety-five cases of stage IB carcinoma of the cervix. Am J Obstet Gynecol 143:581–584, 1982.
Averette HE, Nasser N, Yankow SL et al: Cervical conization in pregnancy: analysis of 180 operations. Am J Obstet Gynecol 106:543–548, 1970.
Balderston KD, Tewari K, Gregory WT et al: Neuroendocrine small cell uterine cervix cancer in pregnancy: Long-term survival following combined therapy. Gynecol Oncol 71:128–132, 1998.
Benedet JL, Selke PA, Nickerson KG: Colposcopic evaluation of abnormal Papanicolaou smears in pregnancy. Am J Obstet Gynecol 157:932–937, 1989.
Berman ML, DiSaia PJ, Tewari KS: Cancer in pregnancy. In Creasy RK, Resnick R (eds): Maternal–Fetal Medicine: Principles and Practices, 3rd edn. Philadelphia, Saunders, 2002.
Burgess SP, Waymont B: Implantation of a cervical carcinoma in an episiotomy site. Case report. Br J Obstet Gynaecol 94:598–599, 1987.
Chang-Claude J, Schneider A, Smith E et al: Longitudinal study of the effects of pregnancy and other factors on detection of HPV. Gynecol Oncol 60:355–362, 1996.
Chhieng DC, Elqert P, Cangiarella JF et al: Significance of AGUS Pap smears in pregnant and postpartum women. Acta Cytol 45:294–299, 2001.
Cliby WA, Dodson MK, Podratz KC: Cervical cancer complicated by pregnancy: episiotomy site recurrences following vaginal delivery. Obstet Gynecol 84:179–182, 1994.
Copeland LJ, Saul PB, Sneige N: Cervical adenocarcinoma: tumor implantation in the episiotomy sites of two patients. Gynecol Oncol 28:230–235, 1987.
Coppola A, Soroksky J, Casper R et al: The clinical course of cervical carcinoma-in-situ diagnosed during pregnancy. Gynecol Oncol 67:162–165, 1997.
Creasman WT, Rutledge FN, Fletcher GH: Carcinoma of the cervix associated with pregnancy. Obstet Gynecol 36:495–501, 1970.
Daskal JL, Pitkin RM: Cone biopsy of the cervix during pregnancy. Obstet Gynecol 32:1–5, 1968.
Dudan RC, Yon JL, Ford JH et al: Carcinoma of the cervix and pregnancy. Gynecol Oncol 1:283–289, 1973.
Duggan B, Muderspach LI, Roman LD et al: Cervical cancer in pregnancy: reporting on planned delay in therapy. Obstet Gynecol 82:598–602, 1993.
Dunn TS, Ginsburg V, Wolf D: Loop-cone cerclage in pregnancy: a 5-year review. Gynecol Oncol 90:577–580, 2003.
Germann N, Haie-Meder C, Morice P et al: Management and clinical outcomes of pregnant patients with invasive cervical cancer. Ann Oncol 16:397–402, 2005.
Goldberg G, Altaras M, Block B: Cone cerclage in pregnancy. Am J Obstet Gynecol 77:315–317, 1991.
Goldman NA, Goldberg GL: Late recurrence of squamous cell cervical cancer in an episiotomy site after vaginal delivery. Obstet Gynecol 101:1127–1129, 2003.
Gordon AN, Jensen R, Jones HW III: Squamous carcinoma of the cervix complicating pregnancy: recurrence in episiotomy after vaginal delivery. Obstet Gynecol 73:850–852, 1989.
Greer BE, Easterling TR, McLennan DA et al: Fetal and maternal considerations in the management of stage IB cervical cancer during pregnancy. Gynecol Oncol 34:61–65, 1989.
Hacker NF, Berek JS, LaGasse LD et al: Carcinoma of the cervix associated with pregnancy. Obstet Gynecol 59:735–746, 1982.
Hannigan EV, Whitehouse HH, Atkinson WD et al: Cone biopsy during pregnancy. Obstet Gynecol 60:450–455, 1982.
Heron DE, Axtel A, Gerszten K et al: Villoglandular adenocarcinoma of the cervix recurrent in an episiotomy scar: a case report in a 32-year-old female. Int J Gynecol Cancer 15:366–371, 2005.
Hopkins MP, Morley GW: The prognosis and management of cervical cancer associated with pregnancy. Obstet Gynecol 80:9–13, 1992.
Jain AG, Higgins RV, Boyle MJ: Management of low-grade squamous intraepithelial lesions during pregnancy. Am J Obstet Gynecol 177:298–302, 1997.
Kaplan KJ, Dainty LA, Dolinsky B et al: Prognosis and recurrence risk for patients with cervical squamous intraepithelial lesions diagnosed during pregnancy. Cancer (Cancer Cytopathol) 102: 228–232, 2004.
Kemp EA, Hakenewerth AM, Laurent SL et al: Human papillomavirus prevalence in pregnancy. Obstet Gynecol 79:649–656, 1992.
Khalil AM, Khatib RA, Mufarrij AA et al: Squamous cell carcinoma of the cervix implanting in the episiotomy site. Gynecol Oncol 51:408–410, 1993.
Lee RB, Neglia W, Park RC: Cervical carcinoma in pregnancy. Obstet Gynecol 58:584–589, 1981.
Lurain JR, Gallup DG: Management of abnormal Papanicolaou smears in pregnancy. Obstet Gynecol 53:484–488, 1979.
Mack LA, Gottesfeld K, Johnson ML: Ultrasonic evaluation of a cervical mass in pregnancy. J Clin Ultrasound 9:49–50, 1981.
Marana HRC, de Andrade JM, da Silva Mathes AC et al: Chemotherapy in the treatment of locally advanced cervical cancer and pregnancy. Gynecol Oncol 80:272–274, 2001.
Method MW, Brost BC: Management of cervical cancer in pregnancy. Semin Surg Oncol 16:251–260, 1999.
Mitsuhashi A, Sekiya S: Loop electrosurgical excision procedure (LEEP) during first trimester of pregnancy. Int J Gynaecol Obstet 71:237–239, 2000.
Monk BJ, Montz FJ: Invasive cervical cancer complicating intrauterine pregnancy: treatment with radical hysterectomy. Obstet Gynecol 80:199–203, 1992.
Murta EF, de Andrade FC, Adad SJ et al: Low grade cervical squamous intraepithelial lesion during pregnancy: conservative antepartum management. Eur J Gynaecol Oncol 25:600–602, 2004.
Murta EF, de Souza FH, de Souza MA et al: High-grade cervical squamous intraepithelial lesion during pregnancy. Tumori 88:246–250, 2002.
Nisker JA, Shubat M: Stage IB cervical carcinoma and pregnancy: report of 49 cases. Am J Obstet Gynecol 145:203–206, 1983.
Palle C, Bangsboll S, Andreasson B: Cervical intraepithelial neoplasia in pregnancy. Acta Obstet Gynecol Scand 79:306–310, 2000.
Prem KA, Makowski EL, McKelvey JL: Carcinoma of the cervix associated with pregnancy. Am J Obstet Gynecol 95:99–108, 1966.
Robinson WR, Webb S, Tirpack J et al: Management of cervical intraepithelial neoplasia during pregnancy with LOOP excision. Gynecol Oncol 64:153–155, 1997.
Rogers RS, Williams JH: The impact of the suspicious Papanicolaou smear on pregnancy. Am J Obstet Gynecol 98:488, 1967.

Sablinska R, Tarlowska L, Stelmachow J: Invasive carcinoma of the cervix associated with pregnancy: correlation between patient age, advancement of cancer and gestation, and result of treatment. Gynecol Oncol 5:363–373, 1977.

Schneider A, Hotz M, Gissmann L: Increased prevalence of human papillomaviruses in the lower genital tract of pregnant women. Int J Cancer 40:198–201, 1987.

Siddiqui G, Kurzel RB, Lampley EC et al: Cervical dysplasia in pregnancy: progression versus regression post-partum. Int J Fertil Womens Med 46:278–280, 2001.

Siristatidis CH, Vitoratos N, Michailidis E et al: The role of the mode of delivery in the alteration of intrapartum pathological cervical cytologic findings during the postpartum period. Eur J Gynaecol Oncol 23:358–360, 2002.

Sivanesaratnam V, Jayalakshmi P, Loo C: Surgical management of early invasive cancer of the cervix associated with pregnancy. Gynecol Oncol 48:68–75, 1993.

Sood AK, Sorosky JI, Mayr N et al: Cervical cancer diagnosed shortly after pregnancy: Prognostic variables and delivery routes. Obstet Gynecol 95:832–838, 2000.

Sood AK, Sorosky JI, Mayr N et al: Radiotherapeutic management of cervical carcinoma that complicates pregnancy. Cancer 80:1073–1078, 1997.

Sood AK, Sorosky JL, Krogman S et al: Surgical management of cervical cancer complicating pregnancy: a case-control study. Gynecol Oncol 63:294–298, 1996.

Sorosky JI, Squatrito R, Ndubisi BU et al: Stage I squamous cell cervical carcinoma in pregnancy: planned delay in therapy awaiting fetal maturity. Gynecol Oncol 59:207–210, 1995.

Strinic T, Bukovic D, Karelovic D et al: The effect of delivery on regression of abnormal cervical cytologic findings. Coll Antropol 26:577–582, 2002.

Takushi M, Moromizato H, Sakumoto K et al: Management of invasive carcinoma of the uterine cervix associated with pregnancy: outcome of intentional delay of treatment. Gynecol Oncol 87: 185–189, 2002.

Tewari K, Cappuccini F, Gambino A et al: Neoadjuvant chemotherapy in the treatment of locally advanced cervical carcinoma in pregnancy: a report of two cases and review of issues specific to the management of cervical carcinoma in pregnancy including planned delay of therapy. Cancer 82:1529–1534, 1998.

van Dam PA, Irvine L, Lowe DG et al: Carcinoma in episiotomy scars. Gynecol Oncol 44:96–100, 1992.

van den Broek NR, Lopes AD, Ansink A et al: "Microinvasive" adenocarcinoma of the cervix implanting in an episiotomy scar. Gynecol Oncol 59:297–299, 1995.

van der Vange N, Weverling GJ, Ketting BW et al: The prognosis of cervical cancer associated with pregnancy: a matched cohort study. Obstet Gynecol 85:1022–1026, 1995.

van Vliet W, van Loon AJ, ten Hoor KA et al: Cervical carcinoma during pregnancy: outcome of planned delay in treatment. Eur J Obstet Gynecol Reprod Biol 79:153–157, 1998.

Woodrow N, Permezel M, Butterfield L et al: Abnormal cervical cytology in pregnancy: experience of 811 cases. Aust N Z J Obstet Gynaecol 38:161–165, 1998.

Yoonessi M, Wieckowska W, Mariniello D et al: Cervical intra-epithelial neoplasia in pregnancy. Int J Gynaecol Obstet 20:111–118, 1982.

Yost NP, Santoso JT, McIntire DD et al: Postpartum regression rates of antepartum cervical intraepithelial neoplasia II and III lesions. Obstet Gynecol 93:359–362, 1999.

OVARIAN CANCER IN PREGNANCY

Agarwal N, Parul, Kriplani A et al: Management and outcome of pregnancies complicated with adnexal masses. Arch Gynecol Obstet 267:148–152, 2003.

Ashkenazy M, Kessler I, Czernobilsky B et al: Ovarian tumors in pregnancy. Int J Gynecol Obstet 27:79–83, 1988.

Bakri YN, Given FT: Normal pregnancy and delivery following conservative surgery and chemotherapy for ovarian endodermal sinus tumor. Gynecol Oncol 19:222–225, 1984.

Bayhan G, Aban M, Yayla M et al: Cis-platinum combination chemotherapy during pregnancy for mucinous cystadenocarcinoma of the ovary. Case report. Eur J Gynaecol Oncol 20:231–232, 1999.

Baykal C, Al A, Tulunay G et al: Obstetric dilemma in an ovarian cancer patient. Acta Obstet Gynecol Scand 83:118, 2004.

Bell DA, Scully E: Ovarian serous borderline tumors with stromal microinvasion: a report of 21 cases. Hum Pathol 21:397–403, 1990.

Boulay R, Podczaski E: Ovarian cancer complicating pregnancy. Obstet Gynecol Clin North Am 25:385–399, 1998.

Buller RE, Darrow V, Manetta A et al: Conservative surgical management of dysgerminoma concomitant with pregnancy. Obstet Gynecol 79:887, 1992.

Cajigas HE, Lim-Tan SK, Scully RE: Unusual histologic changes in ovarian serous borderline tumors during pregnancy. Mod Pathol 4:55A, 1991.

Dgani R, Shoham (Schwartz) Z, Atar E et al: Ovarian carcinoma during pregnancy. A study of 23 cases in Israel between the years 1960 and 1984. Gynecol Oncol 33:326–331, 1989.

Elit L, Bocking A, Kenyon C et al: An endodermal sinus tumor diagnosed in pregnancy: case report and review of the literature. Gynecol Oncol 72:123–127, 1999.

El-Yahia AR, Rahman J, Rahman MS et al: Ovarian tumors in pregnancy. Aust N Z J Obstet Gynaecol 31:327–330, 1991.

Farahmand SM, Marchetti DL, Asirwatham JE et al: Ovarian endodermal sinus tumor associated with pregnancy: review of the literature. Gynecol Oncol 41:156–160, 2001.

Ferrandina G, Distefano M, Testa A et al: Management of an advanced ovarian cancer at 15 weeks of gestation: case report and literature review. Gynecol Oncol 97:693–696, 2005.

Gojnic M, Pervulov M, Petkovic S et al: Diagnosis of borderline ovarian cancers in pregnancy. Clin Exp Obstet Gynecol 31:45–46, 2004.

Han J-Y, Nava-Ocampo AA, Kim T-J et al: Pregnancy outcome after prenatal exposure to bleomycin, etoposide and cisplatin for malignant ovarian germ cell tumors: Report of 2 cases. Reprod Toxicol 19:557–561, 2005.

Henderson CE, Elia G, Garfinkel D et al: Platinum chemotherapy during pregnancy for serous cystadenocarcinoma of the ovary. Gynecol Oncol 49:92–94, 1993.

Horbelt D, Delmore J, Meisels R et al: Mixed germ cell malignancy of the ovary concurrent with pregnancy. Obstet Gynecol 84:662, 1984.

Huang HP, Fang CN, Kan YY: Chemotherapy for ovarian mucinous cystadenocarcinoma during pregnancy: a case report. Eur J Gynaecol Oncol 25:635–636, 2004.

Karlen JR, Akbari A, Cook WA: Dysgerminoma associated with pregnancy. Obstet Gynecol 53:330–335, 1979.

Kishimoto K, Ito K, Furukawa M et al: Immature teratoma with gliomatosis peritonei associated with pregnancy. Abdom Imaging 27:96–99, 2002.

Lee YH, Kim SG, Choi SH et al: Ovarian mature cystic teratoma containing homunculus: a case report. J Korean Med Sci 18: 905–907, 2003.

Malhotra N, Sood M: Endodermal sinus tumor in pregnancy. Gynecol Oncol 78:265–266, 2000.

Malone JM, Gershenson DM, Creasy RK et al: Endodermal sinus tumor of the ovary associated with pregnancy. Obstet Gynecol 68(3 suppl):86S–89S, 1986.

Mathevet P, Nessah K, Dargent D et al: Laparoscopic management of adnexal masses in pregnancy: a case series. Eur J Obstet Gynecol Reprod Biol 108:217–222, 2003.

Mendez LE, Mueller A, Salom E et al: Paclitaxel and carboplatin chemotherapy administered during pregnancy for advanced epithelial ovarian cancer. Obstet Gynecol 102:1200–1202, 2003.

Metz SA, Day TG, Pursell SH: Adjuvant chemotherapy in a pregnant patient with endodermal sinus tumor of the ovary. Gynecol Oncol 32:371–374, 1989.

Mikami M, Ono A, Sakaiya N et al: Case report of serous ovarian tumor of borderline malignancy (stage IC) in a pregnant woman. Eur J Obstet Gynecol Reprod Biol 98:237–239, 2001.

Mooney J, Silva E, Tornos C et al: Unusual features of serous neoplasms of low malignant potential during pregnancy. 65:30–35, 1997.

Ohara N, Teramoto K: Successful treatment of an advanced ovarian serous cystadenocarcinoma in pregnancy with cisplatin, Adriamycin and cyclophosphamide (CAP) regimen. Case report. Clin Exp Obstet Gynecol 27:123–124, 2000.

Otton G, Higgins S, Phillips KA et al: A case of early-stage epithelial ovarian cancer in pregnancy. Int J Gynecol Cancer 11:413–417, 2001.

Petrucha RA, Ruffolo E, Messina AM et al: Endodermal sinus tumor: report of a case associated with pregnancy. Obstet Gynecol 55 (3 suppl):90S–93S, 1980.

Picone O, Lhomme C, Tournaire M et al: Preservation of pregnancy in a patient with a stage IIIB ovarian epithelial carcinoma diagnosed at 22 weeks of gestation and treated with initial chemotherapy: case report and literature review. Gynecol Oncol 94:600–604, 2004.

Rahman MS, Al-Sibai MH, Rahman J et al: Ovarian carcinoma associated with pregnancy. A review of 9 cases. Acta Obstet Gynecol Scand 81:260–264, 2002.

Rajendran S, Hollingworth J, Scudamore I: Endodermal sinus tumour of the ovary in pregnancy. Eur J Gynaecol Oncol 20:272–274, 1999.

Sayedur Rahman M, Al-Sibai MH, Rahman J et al: Ovarian carcinoma associated with pregnancy. A review of 9 cases. Acta Obstet Gynecol Scand 81:260–264, 2002.

Shimizu Y, Komiyama S, Kobayashi T et al: Successful management of endodermal sinus tumor of the ovary associated with pregnancy. Gynecol Oncol 88:447–450, 2003.

Sood AK, Shahin MS, Sorosky JI: Paclitaxel and platinum chemotherapy for ovarian carcinoma during pregnancy. Gynecol Oncol 83:599–600, 2002.

Struyk AP, Treffers PE: Ovarian tumors in pregnancy. Acta Obstet Gynecol Scand 63:421–424, 1984.

Tavassoli FA: Serous tumor of low malignant potential with early stromal invasion (serous LMP with microinvasion). Mod Pathol 1:407–414, 1988.

Tewari K, Brewer C, Cappuccini F et al: Advanced stage small cell carcinoma of the ovary in pregnancy: long-term survival after surgical debulking and multiagent chemotherapy. Gynecol Oncol 66:531–534, 1997.

Thornton JG, Wells M: Ovarian cysts in pregnancy: does ultrasound make traditional management inappropriate? Obstet Gynecol 59: 717–721, 1987.

Tomlinson MW, Treadwell MC, Deppe G: Platinum based chemotherapy to treat recurrent Sertoli–Leydig cell ovarian carcinoma during pregnancy. Eur J Gynaecol Oncol 18:44–46, 1997.

Weed JC, Roh RA, Mendenhall HW: Recurrent endodermal sinus tumor during pregnancy. Obstet Gynecol 54:653–656, 1979.

Young RH, Dudley AG, Scully RE: Granulosa cell, Sertoli–Leydig cell, and unclassified sex cord–stromal tumors associated with pregnancy: a clinicopathological analysis of thirty-six cases. Gynecol Oncol 18:181–205, 1984.

BREAST CANCER IN PREGNANCY

Andreadis C, Charalampidou M, Diamantopoulos N et al: Combined chemotherapy and radiotherapy during conception and first two trimesters of gestation in a woman with metastatic breast cancer. Gynecol Oncol 95:252–255, 2004.

Applewhite RR, Smith LR, DeVicente F: Carcinoma of the breast associated with pregnancy and lactation. Am J Surg 39:101–104, 1973.

Berry D, Theriault R, Holmes F et al: Management of breast cancer during pregnancy using a standardized protocol. J Clin Oncol 17:855–861, 1999.

Bladstrom A, Anderson H, Olsson H: Worse survival in breast cancer among women with recent childbirth: results from a Swedish population-based register study. Clin Breast Cancer 4:280–285, 2003.

Blakely LJ, Buzdar AU, Lozada JA et al: Effects of pregnancy after treatment for breast carcinoma on survival and risk of recurrence. Cancer 100:465–469, 2004.

Bonnier P, Roman S, Dilhuydy JM et al: The influence of pregnancy on the outcome of breast cancer: a case-control study. Int J Cancer 72:720–727, 1997.

Bunker ML, Peters MV: Breast cancer associated with pregnancy or lactation. Am J Obstet Gynecol 85:312–321, 1963.

Byrd BF Jr, Bayer DS, Roberston JC et al: Treatment of breast tumors associated with pregnancy and lactation. Ann Surg 155: 940–947, 1962.

Clark RM, Chua T: Breast cancer and pregnancy: the ultimate challenge. Clin Oncol (R Coll Radiol) 1:11–18, 1989.

Clark RM, Reid J: Carcinoma of the breast in pregnancy and lactation. Int J Radiat Oncol Biol Phys 4:693–698, 1978.

Collaborative Group on Hormonal Factors in Breast Cancer: Breast cancer and breastfeeding: collaborative reanalysis of individual data from 47 epidemiological studies in 30 countries, including 50,302 women with breast cancer and 96,973 women without the disease. Lancet 360:187–195, 2002.

Committee on Gynecologic Practice, American College of Obstetricians and Gynecologists: ACOG committee opinion. Induced abortion and breast cancer risk. Number 285, August 2003. Int J Gynaecol Obstet 83:233–235, 2003.

Crivellari D, Lombardi D, Scuderi C et al: Breast cancer and pregnancy. Tumori 88:187–192, 2002.

Cullins SL, Pridjian G, Sutherland CM: Goldenhar's syndrome associated with tamoxifen given to the mother during gestation. Lancet 1:776, 1980.

Cunha GR, Taguchi O, Namikawa R et al: Teratogenic effects of clomiphene, tamoxifen, and diethylstilbestrol on the developing human female genital tract. Hum Pathol 18:1132–1143, 1987.

De Santis M, Lucchese A, De Carolis S et al: Metastatic breast cancer in pregnancy: first case of chemotherapy with docetaxel. Eur J Cancer Care (Engl) 9:235–237, 2000.

Falkenberry SS: Breast cancer in pregnancy. Obstet Gynecol Clin North Am 29:225–232, 2002.

Gadducci A, Cosio S, Fanucchi A et al: Chemotherapy with epirubicin and paclitaxel for breast cancer during pregnancy: case report and review of the literature. Anticancer Res 23:5225–5229, 2003.

Gelber S, Coates AS, Goldhirsch A et al: Effect of pregnancy on overall survival after the diagnosis of early stage breast cancer. J Clin Oncol 19:1671–1675, 2001.

Gemignani ML, Petrek JA: Breast cancer during pregnancy: diagnostic and therapeutic dilemmas. Adv Surg 34:273–286, 2000.

Gonzalez-Angulo AM, Walters RS, Carpenter RJ Jr et al: Paclitaxel chemotherapy in a pregnant patient with bilateral breast cancer. Clin Breast Cancer 5:317–319, 2004.

Gwyn KM, Theriault RL: Breast cancer during pregnancy. Curr Treat Options Oncol 1:239–243, 2000.

Haagensen CD, Stout AP: Carcinoma of the breast. III. Results of treatment, 1935–1942. Ann Surg 134, 1951.

Haagensen CD, Stout AP: Carcinoma of the breast: criteria for operability. Ann Surg 118:859–870, 1943.

Higgins S, Haffty BG: Pregnancy and lactation after breast-conserving therapy for early stage breast cancer. Cancer 73:2175–2180, 1994.

Holleb AI, Farrow JH: The relation of carcinoma of the breast and pregnancy in 283 patients. Surg Gynecol Obstet 115:65–71, 1962.

Ibrahim EM, Ezzat AA, Baloush A et al: Pregnancy-associated breast cancer: a case-control study in a young population with a high-fertility rate. Med Oncol 17:293–300, 2000.

Isaacs RJ, Hunter W, Clark K: Tamoxifen as systemic treatment of advanced breast cancer during pregnancy—case report and literature review. Gynecol Oncol 80:405–408, 2001.

Ishida T, Yokoe T, Kasumi F et al: Clinicopathologic characteristics and prognosis of breast cancer patients associated with pregnancy and lactation: analysis of case-control study in Japan. Jpn J Cancer Res 83:1143–1149, 1992.

Keleher AJ, Theriault RL, Gwyn KM et al: Multidisciplinary management of breast cancer concurrent with pregnancy. J Am Coll Surg 194:54–64, 2002.

King RM, Welch JS, Martin JK Jr et al: Carcinoma of the breast associated with pregnancy. Surg Gynecol Obstet 160:228–232, 1985.

Kouvaris JR, Antypas CE, Sandilos PH et al: Postoperative tailored radiotherapy for locally advanced breast carcinoma during pregnancy: a therapeutic dilemma. Am J Obstet Gynecol 183: 498–499, 2000.

Kroman N, Mouridsen HT: Prognostic influence of pregnancy before, around, and after diagnosis of breast cancer. Breast 12:516–521, 2003.

Kuerer HM, Cunningham JD, Brower ST et al: Breast carcinoma associated with pregnancy and lactation. Surg Oncol 6:93–98, 1997.

Kuerer HM, Gwyn K, Ames FC et al: Conservative surgery and chemotherapy for breast carcinoma during pregnancy. Surgery 131:108–110, 2002.

Medina D: Breast cancer: the protective effect of pregnancy. Clin Cancer Res 10:380S–384S, 2004.

Middleton LP, Amin M, Gwyn K et al: Breast carcinoma in pregnant women: assessment of clinicopathologic and immunohistochemical features. Cancer 98:1055–1060, 2003.

Moore HC, Foster RS Jr: Breast cancer and pregnancy. Semin Oncol 27:646–653, 2000.

Mueller BA, Simon MS, Deapen D et al: Childbearing and survival after breast carcinoma in young women. Cancer 98:1131–1140, 2003.

Mulvihill J, McKeen E, Rosner F et al: Pregnancy outcomes in cancer patients: experience in a large cooperative group. Cancer 60: 1143–1150, 1987.

Nugent P, O'Connell TX: Breast cancer and pregnancy. Arch Surg 120:1221–1224, 1985.

Oktay K, Sonmezer M: Ovarian tissue banking for cancer patients: fertility preservation not just ovarian cryopreservation. Hum Reprod 19:477–480, 2004.

Parodi PC, Osti M, Longhi P et al: Pregnancy and tram-flap breast reconstruction after mastectomy: case report. Scand J Plast Reconstr Surg Hand Surg 35:211–215, 2001.

Peccatori F, Martinelli G, Gentilini O et al: Chemotherapy during pregnancy: what is really safe? Lancet Oncol 5:398, 2004.

Peck JD, Hulka BS, Poole C et al: Steroid hormone levels during pregnancy and incidence of maternal breast cancer. Cancer Epidemiol Biomarkers Prev 11:361–368, 2002.

Peters MV, Meakin JW: The influence of pregnancy in carcinoma of the breast. Prog Clin Cancer 10:471–506, 1965.

Petrek J, Seltzer V: Breast cancer in pregnant and postpartum women. J Obstet Gynaecol Can 25:944–950, 2003.

Petrek JA, Dukoff R, Rogatko A: Prognosis of pregnancy associated breast cancer. Cancer 67:869–872, 1991.

Phillips KA, Milne RL, Friedlander ML et al: Prognosis of premenopausal breast cancer and childbirth prior to diagnosis. J Clin Oncol 22:699–705, 2004.

Puckridge PJ, Saunders CM, Ives AD et al: Breast cancer and pregnancy: a diagnostic and management dilemma. ANZ J Surg 73:500–503, 2003.

Rao CV: Does full-term pregnancy at a young age protect women against breast cancer through hCG? Obstet Gynecol 96:783–786, 2000.

Reed W, Hannisdal E, Skovlund E et al: Pregnancy and breast cancer: a population-based study. Virchows Arch 443:44–50, 2003.

Ribeiro GG, Palmer MK: Breast cancer associated with pregnancy: a clinician's dilemma. Br Med J 2:1524–1527, 1977.

Rosemond GP: Management of patients with carcinoma of the breast in pregnancy. Ann NY Acad Sci 114:851–856, 1964.

Rosner D, Yeh J: Breast cancer and related pregnancy: suggested management according to stages of the disease and gestational stages. J Med 33:23–62, 2002.

Rugo HS: Management of breast cancer diagnosed during pregnancy. Curr Treat Options Oncol 4:165–173, 2003.

Russo J, Moral R, Balogh GA et al: The protective role of pregnancy in breast cancer. Breast Cancer Res 7:131–142, 2006.

Schotte K, Cocquyt V, van den Broecke R et al: Breast cancer during pregnancy: cases and review of treatment and prognosis. Acta Clin Belg 55:102–109, 2000.

Tewari K, Bonebrake RG, Asrat T et al: Ambiguous genitalia in infant exposed to tamoxifen in utero. Lancet 359:183, 1997.

Tobias J, Bloom H: Doxorubicin in pregnancy. Lancet 1:776, 1980.

Tonetti DA: Prevention of breast cancer by recapitulation of pregnancy hormone levels. Breast Cancer Res 6:E8, 2004.

Tralins AH: Lactation after conservative breast surgery combined with radiation therapy. Am J Clin Oncol 18:40–43, 1995.

Turchi J, Villasis C: Anthracyclines in the treatment of malignancy in pregnancy. Cancer 61:435–440, 1988.

White TT: Carcinoma of the breast and pregnancy. Ann Surg 139:9–18, 1954.

White TT: Prognosis of breast cancer for pregnancy and nursing women: analysis of 1,413 cases. Surg Gynecol Obstet 100: 661–666, 1955.

Whiteman MK, Hillis SD, Curtis KM et al: Reproductive history and mortality after breast cancer diagnosis. Obstet Gynecol 104:146–154, 2004.

Woo JC, Yu T, Hurd TC: Breast cancer in pregnancy: a literature review. Arch Surg 138:91–98, 2003.

Zemlickis D, Lishner M, Degendorfer P et al: Fetal outcome after in utero exposure to cancer chemotherapy. Arch Intern Med 152:573–576, 1992.

Zhang J, Liu G, Wu J et al: Pregnancy-associated breast cancer: a case control and long-term follow-up study in China. J Exp Clin Cancer Res 22:23–27, 2003.

ANESTHESIA AND SURGERY

Brant HA: Acute appendicitis in pregnancy. Obstet Gynecol 29:130–138, 1967.

Koren G, Pastuszak A, Ito S: Drugs in pregnancy. N Engl J Med 338:1128–1137, 1998.

Kort B, Katz VL, Watson WJ: The effect of nonobstetric operation during pregnancy. Surg Gynecol Obstet 177:371–376, 1993.

Melnick DM, Wahl WL, Dalton VK: Management of general surgical problems in the pregnant patient. Am J Surg 187:170–180, 2004.

Reedy MB, Kallen B, Kuehl TJ: Laparoscopy during pregnancy: a study of five fetal outcome parameters with use of the Swedish Health Registry. Am J Obstet Gynecol 177:673–679, 1997.

Sam S, Molitch ME: Timing and special concerns regarding endocrine surgery during pregnancy. Endocrinol Metab Clin North Am 32:337–354, 2003.

Saunders P, Milton PJD: Laparotomy during pregnancy: an assessment of diagnostic accuracy and fetal wastage. Br Med J 3:165–167, 1973.

Society of American Gastrointestinal and Endoscopic Surgeons: SAGES publication 0023: SAGES guidelines for laparoscopic surgery during pregnancy. Online. Available: http://www.sages.org/sg_pub23 2000

DIAGNOSTIC AND THERAPEUTIC RADIATION

Antypas C, Sandilos P, Kouvaris J et al: Fetal dose evaluation during breast cancer radiotherapy. Int J Radiat Oncol Biol Phys 40: 995–999, 1998.

Chen J, Lee J, Tsodikov A et al: Does radiotherapy around the time of pregnancy for Hodgkin's disease modify the risk of breast cancer? Int J Radiat Oncol Biol Phys 58:1474–1479, 2004.

Cygler J, Ding GX, Kendal W et al: Fetal dose for a patient undergoing mantle field irradiation for Hodgkin's disease. Med Dosim 22:135–137, 1997.

Fenig E, Mishaeli M, Kalish Y et al: Pregnancy and radiation. Cancer Treat Rev 27:1–7, 2001.

Hammer-Jacobsen E: Therapeutic abortion of account of x-ray examination during pregnancy. Dan Med Bull 6:113–122, 1959.

International Commission on Radiological Protection: Pregnancy and medical radiation. Ann ICRP 30:1–43, 2000.

International Committee on Radiological Protection: Biological effects after prenatal irradiation (embryo and fetus). Ann ICRP 33:205–206, 2003.

Kal HB, Struikmans H: Radiotherapy during pregnancy: fact and fiction. Lancet Oncol 6:328–333, 2005.

Macmahon B: Prenatal x-ray exposure and childhood cancer. J Natl Cancer Inst 28:1173–1191, 1962.

Magne N, Marcie S, Pignol JP et al: Radiotherapy for a solitary brain metastasis during pregnancy: a method for reducing fetal dose. Br J Radiol 74:638–641, 2001.

Martin Rincon C, Jerez Sainz I, Modolell Farre I et al: Evaluation of the peripheral dose to uterus in breast carcinoma radiotherapy. Radiat Prot Dosim 101:469–471, 2002.

Mazonakis M, Varveris H, Damiliakis J et al: Radiation dose to conceptus resulting from tangential breast irradiation. Int J Radiat Oncol Biol Phys 55:386–391, 2003.

Ngu SL, Duval P, Collins C: Foetal radiation dose in radiotherapy for breast cancer. Australas Radiol 36:321–322, 1992.

Nicklas AH, Baker ME: Imaging strategies in the pregnant cancer patient. Semin Oncol 27:623–632, 2000.

Nuyttens JJ, Prado KL, Jenrette JM et al: Fetal dose during radiotherapy: clinical implementation and review of the literature. Cancer Radiother 6:352–357, 2002.

Podgorsak MB, Meiler RJ, Kowal H et al: Technical management of a pregnant patient undergoing radiation therapy to the head and neck. Med Dosim 24:121–128, 1999.

Sharma DS, Jalali R, Tambe CM et al: Effect of tertiary multileaf collimator (MLC) on foetal dose during three-dimensional conformal radiation therapy (3DCRT) of a brain tumour during pregnancy. Radiother Oncol 70:49–54, 2004.

Sneed PK, Albright NW, Wara WM et al: Fetal dose estimates for radiotherapy of brain tumors during pregnancy. Int J Radiat Oncol Biol Phys 32:823–830, 1995.

Stewart AM: Environmental hazards of pregnancy. J Obstet Gynaecol Br Emp 66:739–742, 1959.

Stoffer SS, Hamburger JI: Inadvertent ^{131}I therapy for hyperthyroidism in the first trimester of pregnancy. J Nucl Med 17: 146–149, 1976.

van der Giessen PH: Measurement of the peripheral dose for the tangential breast treatment technique with Co-60 gamma radiation and high energy X-rays. Radiother Oncol 42:257–264, 1997.

Woo SY, Fuller LM, Cundiff JH et al: Radiotherapy during pregnancy for clinical stages IA–IIA Hodgkin's disease. Int J Radiat Oncol Biol Phys 23:407–412, 1992.

Yu C, Jozsef G, Apuzzo ML et al: Fetal radiation doses for model C gamma knife radiosurgery. Neurosurgery 52:687–693, 2003.

Zucali R, Marchesini R, De Palo G: Abdominal dosimetry for supradiaphragmatic irradiation of Hodgkin's disease in pregnancy. Experimental data and clinical considerations. Tumori 67:203–208, 1981.

CHEMOTHERAPY

Aviles A, Diaz-Maqueo JC, Talavera A et al: Growth and development of children of mothers treated with chemotherapy during pregnancy: current status of 43 children. Am J Hematol 36:243–248, 1991.

Aviles A, Niz J: Long-term follow-up of children born to mothers with acute leukemia during pregnancy. Med Pediatr Oncol 16:3–6, 1988.

Barni S, Ardizzonia A, Zanetta G et al: Weekly doxorubicin chemotherapy for breast cancer in pregnancy: a case report. Tumori 78:349–350, 1992.

Briggs GC, Freeman RK, Yaffee SJ: A Reference Guide to Fetal and Neonatal Risk: Drugs in Pregnancy and Lactation, 5th edn. Philadelphia, Williams & Wilkins, 1998.

Cantini E, Yanes B: Acute myelogenous leukemia in pregnancy. South Med J 77:1050–1052, 1984.

Cardonick E, Iacobucci A: Use of chemotherapy during human pregnancy. Lancet Oncol 5:283–291, 2004.

d'Incalci M, Broggini M, Buscaglia M et al: Transplacental passage of doxorubicin. Lancet 75:8314–8315, 1983.

Durodola JI: Administration of cyclophosphamide during late pregnancy and early lactation: a case report. J Natl Med Assoc 71:65–66, 1979.

Earll JM, May RL: Busulfan therapy of myelocytic leukemia during pregnancy. Am J Obstet Gynecol 92:580–581, 1965.

Ebert U, Loffler H, Kirch W: Cytotoxic therapy and pregnancy. Pharmacol Ther 74:207–220, 1997.

Egan PC, Costanza ME, Dodion P et al: Doxorubicin and cisplatin excretion into human milk. Cancer Treat Rep 69:1387–1389, 1985.

Feldkamp M, Carey JC: Clinical teratology counseling and consultation case report: low dose methotrexate exposure in the early weeks of pregnancy. Teratology 47:533–539, 1993.

Giacalone PL, Laffargue F, Benos P: Chemotherapy for breast carcinoma during pregnancy: a French national survey. Cancer 89: 2266–2272, 1999.

Greenlund LJ, Letendre L, Tefferi A: Acute leukemia during pregnancy: a single institutional experience with 17 cases. Leuk Lymphoma 41:571–577, 2001.

Karp GI, von Oeyen P, Valone F et al: Doxorubicin in pregnancy: possible transplacental passage. Cancer Treat Rep 67:773–777, 1983.

Meyer-Wittkopf M, Barth H, Emons G et al: Fetal cardiac effects of doxorubicin therapy for carcinoma of the breast during pregnancy: case report and review of the literature. Ultrasound Obstet Gynecol 18:62–66, 2001.

Morishita S, Imai A, Kawabata I et al: Acute myelogenous leukemia in pregnancy: fetal blood sampling and early effects of chemotherapy. Int J Gynaecol Obstet 44:273–277, 1994.

Murray CL, Reichert JA, Anderson J et al: Multimodal cancer therapy for breast cancer in the first trimester of pregnancy: a case report. JAMA 252:2607–2608, 1984.

Nicholson HO: Cytotoxic drugs in pregnancy. Review of reported cases. J Obstet Gynaecol Br Commonw 75:307–312, 1968.

Nordlund JJ, DeVita VT, Cabbone PP: Severe vinblastine-induced leukopenia during late pregnancy with delivery of a normal infant. Ann Int Med 69:581–582, 1968.

Peres RM, Sanseverino MT, Guimaraes JL et al: Assessment of fetal risk associated with exposure to cancer chemotherapy during pregnancy: a multicenter study. Braz J Med Biol Res 34: 1551–1559, 2001.

Puzzuto J, Aviles A, Noriega L et al: Treatment of acute leukemia during pregnancy: presentation of nine cases. Cancer Treat Rep 64:679–683, 1980.

Raffles A, Williams J, Costeloe K et al: Transplacental effects of maternal cancer chemotherapy: case report. Br J Obstet Gynaecol 96:1099–1100, 1989.

Reynoso EE, Keating A, Baker MA: Acute leukemia occurring 19 years after treatment of acute lymphoblastic leukemia. Cancer 59:1963–1965, 1987.

Roboz J, Gleicher N, Wuk K et al: Does doxorubicin cross the placenta? Lancet 2:1382–1383, 1979.

Selevan SG, Lindbohm ML, Nornung RW et al: A study of occupational exposure to antineoplastic drugs and fetal loss in nurses. N Engl J Med 313:1173–1178, 1985.

Sokal JE, Lessmann EM: Effects of cancer chemotherapeutic agents on the human fetus. JAMA 172:1765–1771, 1960.

Sorosky JI, Sood AK, Buekers TE: The use of chemotherapeutic agents during pregnancy. Obstet Gynecol Clin North Am 24: 591–599, 1997.

Sweet DL Jr, Kinzie J: Consequences of radiotherapy and antineoplastic therapy for the fetus. J Reprod Med 17:241–246, 1976.

Toledo TM, Harper RC, Moser RH: Fetal effects during cyclophosphamide and irradiation therapy. Ann Int Med 74:87–91, 1971.

Turchi JJ, Villasis C: Anthracyclines in the treatment of malignancy in pregnancy. Cancer 61:435–440, 1988.

Wagner VM, Hill JS, Weaver D et al: Congenital abnormalities in baby born to cytarabine-treated mother. Lancet 2:98–99, 1980.

Warkary J, Beaudry PH, Hornstein S: Attempted abortion with aminopterin. Am J Dis Child 97:274–281, 1959.

Wiebe VJ, Sipila PEH: Pharmacology of antineoplastic agents in pregnancy. Crit Rev Oncol Hematol 16:75–112, 1994.

Zemlickis D, Klein J, Moseelhy G et al: Cisplatin protein binding in pregnancy and the neonatal period. Med Pediatr Oncol 23:476–479, 1994.

TUMOR MARKERS

Bon GG, Kenemans P, Verstraeten AA et al: Maternal serum Ca125 and Ca15-3 antigen levels in normal and pathological pregnancy. Fetal Diagn Ther 16:166–172, 2001.

Frederiksen MC, Casanova L, Schink JC: An elevated maternal serum α-fetoprotein leading to the diagnosis of an immature teratoma. Int J Gynecol Obstet 35:343, 1991.

Gon GG, Kenemans P, Verstraeten AA et al: Maternal serum Ca125 and Ca15-3 antigen levels in normal and pathologic pregnancy. Fetal Diagn Ther 16:166–172, 2001.

He S, Bremme K, Kallner A et al: Increased concentrations of lactate dehydrogenase in pregnancy with preeclampsia: a predictor of small-for-gestational age infants. Gynecol Obstet Invest 39:234, 1995.

Hohlfeld P, Dang TT, Nahoul K et al: Tumour-associated antigens in maternal and fetal blood. Prenat Diagn 14:907–912, 1994.

Jacobs I, Bast RC: The CA 125 tumor-associated antigen: a review of the literature. Hum Reprod 4:1, 1989.

Kiran G, Kiran H, Guler FI et al: Maternal serum and umbilical cord tumor marker levels at term pregnancy. Acta Obstet Gynecol Scand 84:85–89, 2005.

Kobayashi F, Sagawa N, Nakamura K et al: Mechanism and clinical significance of elevated CA 125 levels in the sera of pregnant women. Am J Obstet Gynecol 160:563, 1989.

Mizejewski GJ: Alpha-fetoprotein structure and function: relevance to isoforms, epitopes, and conformational variants. Exp Biol Med 226:377–408, 2001.

Montz FJ, Horenstein J, Platt LD et al: The diagnosis of immature teratoma by maternal serum alpha-fetoprotein screening. Obstet Gynecol 73:522, 1989.

Rishi M, Howard LN, Bratthauer GL et al: Use of monoclonal antibody against human inhibin as a marker for sex cord–stromal tumors of the ovary. Am J Surg Pathol 21:583–589, 1997.

Schwartz PE, Morris JM: Serum lactic dehydrogenase: a tumor marker for dysgerminoma. Obstet Gynecol 72:511, 1988.

Sheiko MC, Hart WR: Ovarian germinoma (dysgerminoma) with elevated serum lactic dehydrogenase: case report and review of literature. Cancer 49:994, 1982.

Silver HM, Lambert-Messerlian GM, Star JA et al: Comparison of maternal serum total activin A and inhibin A in normal , preeclamptic, and nonproteinuric gestationally hypertensive pregnancies. Am J Obstet Gynecol 180:1131–1137, 1999.

Young A, Gee H: Raised maternal serum alpha-fetoprotein levels during pregnancy following treatment of an endodermal sinus tumor: case report. BJOG 97:267, 1990.

HEMATOLOGIC MALIGNANCIES IN PREGNANCY

Aviles A, Diaz-Maqueo JC, Torras V et al: Non-Hodgkin's lymphomas and pregnancy: presentation of 16 cases. Gynecol Oncol 37:335–337, 1990.

Aviles A, Neri N: Hematological malignancies and pregnancy: a final report of 84 children who received chemotherapy in utero. Clin Lymphoma 2:173–177, 2001.

Bitran JD, Roth DG: Acute leukemia during reproductive life: its course, complications and sequelae for fertility. J Reprod Med 17:225–231, 1976.

Catanzarite VA, Ferguson JE II: Acute leukemia and pregnancy: a review of management and outcome, 1972–1982. Obstet Gynecol Surv 39(11):663–678, 1984.

DeVita VT Jr, Simon RM, Hubbard SM et al: Curability of advanced Hodgkin's disease with chemotherapy. Long-term follow-up of MOPP-treated patients at the National Cancer Institute. Ann Intern Med 92:587–595, 1980.

Frenkel EP, Meyers MC: Acute leukemia and pregnancy. Ann Intern Med 53:656–671, 1960.

Gelb AB, van de Rign M, Warnke RA et al: Pregnancy-associated lymphomas: a clinicopathologic study. Cancer 78:304–310, 1996.

Gokal R, Durrant J, Baum JD et al: Successful pregnancy in acute monocytic leukaemia. Br J Cancer 34:299–302, 1976.

Kato M, Ichimura K, Hayami Y et al: Pregnancy-associated cytotoxic lymphoma: a report of 4 cases. Int J Hematol 74:186–192, 2001.

Lilleyman JS, Hill AS, Anderton KJ: Consequences of acute myelogenous leukemia in early pregnancy. Cancer 40:1300–1303, 1977.

Lishner M, Zemlickis D, Degendorfer P et al: Maternal and foetal outcome following Hodgkin's disease in pregnancy. Br J Cancer 65:114–117, 1992.

Mubarak AAS, Kakil IR, Awidi A et al: Normal outcome of pregnancy in chronic myeloid leukemia treated with interferon-α in 1st trimester: report of 3 cases and review of the literature. Am J Hematol 69:115–118, 2002.

Nisce LZ, Tome MA, He S et al: Management of coexisting Hodgkin's disease and pregnancy. Am J Clin Oncol 9:146–151, 1986.

Peleg D, Ben-Ami M: Lymphoma and leukemia complicating pregnancy. Obstet Gynecol Clin North Am 25:365–383, 1998.

Peters MV: Summary of informal discussion on the prognostic and therapeutic implications of staging in Hodgkin's disease. Cancer Res 31:1851–1853, 1971.

Pohlman B, Lyons JA, Macklis RM: Lymphoma in pregnancy. In Trimble EL, Trimble CL (eds): Cancer Obstetrics and Gynecology. Philadelphia, Lippincott Williams & Wilkins, 1999, pp 209–238.

Pohlman B, Macklis RM: Lymphoma and pregnancy. Semin Oncol 27:657–666, 2000.

Sutcliffe SB: ABVD chemotherapy for Hodgkin's disease in pregnancy—a report of three cases and cytogenetic and clinical follow-up at 1, 5 and 7 years. Ann Oncol 7(suppl 3):113, 1996.

Terek MC, Ozkinay E, Zekioglu O et al: Acute leukemia in pregnancy with ovarian metastasis: a case report and review of the literature. Int J Gynecol Cancer 13:904–908, 2003.

Tewari K, Cappuccinni F, Rosen RB et al: Relapse of acute lymphobalstic leukemia in pregnancy: survival following chemoirradiation and autologous transfer of interleukin-2–activated stem cells. Gynecol Oncol 74:143–146, 1999.

Ward FT, Weiss RB: Lymphoma and pregnancy. Semin Oncol 16:397–409, 1989.

Wong GC: Management of haematologic malignancies in pregnancy. Ann Acad Med Singapore 31:303–310, 2002.

MELANOMA IN PREGNANCY

Borden EC: Melanoma and pregnancy. Semin Oncol 27:654–656, 2000.

George PA, Fortner JG, Pack GT: Melanoma with pregnancy. A report of 115 cases. Cancer 13:854–859, 1960.

Grin CM, Driscoll MS, Grant-Kels JM: The relationship of pregnancy, hormones and melanoma. Semin Cutan Med Surg 17:167–171, 1998.

Katz VL, Farmer RM, Dotters D: From nevus to neoplasm: myths of melanoma in pregnancy. Obstet Gynecol Surv 57:112–119, 2002.

Lens MB, Rosdahl I, Ahlbom A et al: Effect of pregnancy on survival in women with cutaneous malignant melanoma. J Clin Oncol 22:4369–4375, 2004.
Lloyd MS, Topping A, Allan R et al: Contraindications to sentinel lymph node biopsy in cutaneous malignant melanoma. Br J Plast Surg 57:725–727, 2004.
MacKie RM, Bufalino R, Morabito A et al: Lack of effect of pregnancy on outcome of melanoma. For the World Health Organisation Melanoma Programme. Lancet 337:653–657, 1991.
MacKie RM: Pregnancy and exogenous hormones in patients with cutaneous malignant melanoma. Curr Opin Oncol 11:129–131, 1999.
Moller D, Ipsen L, Asschenfeldt P: Fatal course of malignant melanoma during pregnancy with dissemination to the products of conception. Acta Obstet Gynecol Scand 65:501–502, 1986.
Pack GT, Scharnagel IM: The prognosis for malignant melanoma in the pregnant woman. Cancer 4:324–334, 1951.
Reintgen DS, McCarty KS Jr, Vollmer R et al: Malignant melanoma and pregnancy. Cancer 55:1340–1344, 1985.
Saenz-Badillos J, Brady MS: Pregnancy-associated melanoma occurring in two generations. J Surg Oncol 73:231–233, 2000.
Schneiderman H, Wu AY, Campbell WA et al: Congenital melanoma with multiple prenatal metastases. Cancer 60:1371–1377, 1987.
Smith MA, Fine JA, Barnhill RL et al: Hormonal and reproductive influences and risk of melanoma in women. Int J Epidemiol 27:751–757, 1998.
Stewart H: A case of malignant melanoma and pregnancy. Br J Med 4914:647, 1955.
White LP, Linden G, Breslow L et al: Studies on melanoma. The effect of pregnancy on survival in human melanoma. JAMA 177:235–238, 1961.

THYROID CANCER IN PREGNANCY

Doherty CM, Shindo ML, Rice DH et al: Management of thyroid nodules during pregnancy. Laryngoscopie 105:251–255, 1995.
Hod M, Sharony R, Friedman S et al: Pregnancy and thyroid carcinoma: a review of incidence, course, and prognosis. Obstet Gynecol Surv 44:774–779, 1989.
Moosa M, Mazzaferri EL: Outcome of differentiated thyroid cancer diagnosed in pregnant women. J Clin Endocrinol Metab 82:2862–2866, 1997.
Rosen IB, Walfish PG: Pregnancy as a predisposing factor in thyroid neoplasia. Arch Surg 121:1287–1290, 1986.
Rosvoll RV, Winship T: Thyroid carcinoma and pregnancy. Surg Gynecol Obstet 121:1039–1042, 1965.
Tewari K, Balderston KD, Carpenter SE et al: Papillary thyroid carcinoma manifesting as thyroid storm of pregnancy: case report. Am J Obstet Gynecol 179:818–819, 1998.
Vini L, Hyer S, Pratt B et al: Management of differentiated thyroid cancer diagnosed during pregnancy. Eur J Endocrinol 140: 404–406, 1999.

VULVAR CANCER IN PREGNANCY

Alexander A, Harris RM, Grossman D et al: Vulvar melanoma: diffuse melanosis and metastasis to the placenta. 50:293–298, 2004.
Bakour SH, Jaleel H, Weaver JB et al: Vulvar carcinoma presenting during pregnancy, associated with recurrent bone marrow hypoplasia: a case report and literature review. Gynecol Oncol 87:207–209, 2002.
Collins CG, Barclay DL: Cancer of the vulva, and cancer of the vagina in pregnancy. Clin Obstet Gynecol 30:927–942, 1963.
di Gilio AR, Cormio C, Resta L et al: Rapid growth of myxoid leiomyosarcoma of the vulva during pregnancy: a case report. Int J Gynecol Cancer 14:172–175, 2004.
Gitsch G, van Eijkeren M, Hacker NF: Surgical therapy of vulvar cancer in pregnancy. Gynecol Oncol 56:312–315, 1995.
Heller DS, Cracchiolo B, Hameed M et al: Pregnancy-associated invasive squamous cell carcinoma of the vulva in a 28-year-old, HIV-negative woman: a case report. J Reprod Med 45:659–661, 2000.
Lutz MH, Underwood PB Jr, Rozier JC et al: Genital malignancy in pregnancy. Am J Obstet Gynecol 129:536–542, 1977.
Ogunleye D, Lewin SN, Huettner P et al: Recurrent vulvar carcinoma in pregnancy. Gynecol Oncol 95:400–401, 2004.
Olayemi O, Aimakhu CO, Omigbodun AO et al: Vulval carcinoma in pregnancy. J Obstet Gyaecol 22:441–442, 2002.

PRIMARY INVASIVE VAGINAL CANCER IN PREGNANCY

Baruah N, Sangupta S: Primary carcinoma of vagina complicating pregnancy. J Indian Med Assoc 60:469–470, 1973.
Beck I, Clayton JK: Vaginal carcinoma arising in vaginal condylomata. Case report. Br J Obstet Gynaecol 91:503–505, 1984.
Behzatoglu K, Bahadir B, Inhan G et al: Primary vaginal leiomyosarcoma in pregnancy. Gynecol Oncol 91:627–629, 2003.
Davis JA, Wadehra V, McIntosh AS et al: A case of clear cell adenocarcinoma of the vagina in pregnancy. Br J Obstet Gynaecol 88:322–326, 1981.
Jones WB, Woodruff JM, Erlandson RA et al: DES-related clear cell adenocarcinoma of the vagina in pregnancy. Obstet Gynecol 57 (6 suppl):76S–80S, 1981.
Palumbo L Jr, Shingleton HM, Fishburne JI Jr et al: Primary carcinoma of the vagina. South Med J 62:1048–1053, 1969.
Roddick JW, Honig J: Sarcoma botryoides of the vagina coincident with pregnancy. Am J Obstet Gynecol 92:268–270, 1965.
Schwartz P, Klein EI, Fields C: Sarcoma botryoides in pregnancy. Am J Obstet Gynecol 85:123–124, 1963.
Senekjian EK, Hubby M, Bell DA et al: Clear cell adenocarcinoma (CCA) of the vagina and cervix in association with pregnancy. Gynecol Oncol 24:207–219, 1986.
Steed HL, Pearcey RG, Capstick V et al: Invasive squamous cell carcinoma of the vagina during pregnancy. Obstet Gynecol 100:1105–1108, 2002.

ENDOMETRIAL CANCER IN PREGNANCY

Adolph A, Le T, Khan K et al: Recurrent metastatic fallopian tube carcinoma in pregnancy. Gynecol Oncol 81:110–112, 2001.
Dekel A, van Iddekinge B, Isaacson C et al: Primary choriocarcinoma of the fallopian tube. Report of a case with survival and postoperative delivery. Review of the literature. Obstet Gynecol Surv 41:142–148, 1986.

FALLOPIAN TUBE CANCER IN PREGNANCY

Fedele M, Lanza A, Olivero F et al: Primary choriocarcinoma of the fallopian tube: report of a case. Eur J Gynaecol Oncol 6:230–232, 1985.
Galvez CR, Fernandez VC, de Los Reyes JM et al: Primary tubal choriocarcinoma. Int J Gynecol Cancer 14:1040–1044, 2004.
Ichikawa Y, Takano K, Higa S et al: Endometrial carcinoma coexisting with pregnancy, presumed to derive from adenomyosis: a case report. Int J Gynecol Cancer 11:488–490, 2001.
Itoh K, Shiozawa T, Shiohara S et al: Endometrial carcinoma in septate uterus detected 6 months after full-term delivery: case report and review of the literature. Gynecol Oncol 93:242–247, 2004.
Kagami S, Kashimura M, Toki N et al: Myxoid leiomyosarcoma of the uterus with subsequent pregnancy and delivery. Gynecol Oncol 85:538–542, 2002.
Lee SM, Kang JH, Oh SY et al: A successful treated case of primary tubal choriocarcinoma coexistent with viable intrauterine pregnancy. Gynecol Oncol 97:671–673, 2005.
Leunen K, Amant F, Debiec-Rychter M et al: Endometrial stromal sarcoma presenting as postpartum haemorrhage: report of a case with a sole t(10;17)(q22;p13) translocation. Gynecol Oncol 91:265–271, 2003.
Mitsushita J, Toki Toshihiko T, Kato K et al: Endometrial carcinoma remaining after term pregnancy following conservative treatment with medroxyprogesterone acetate. Gynecol Oncol 79:129–132, 2000.
Ober WB, Maier RC: Gestational choriocarcinoma of the fallopian tube. Diagn Gynecol Obstet 3:213–231, 1981.

Ojomo EO, Ezimokhai M, Reale FR et al: Recurrent postpartum haemorrhage caused by endometrial carcinoma co-existing with endometrioid carcinoma of the ovary in a full term pregnancy. Br J Obstet Gynaecol 100:489–491, 1993.

Schneller JA, Nicastri AD: Intrauterine pregnancy coincident with endometrial carcinoma—a case study and review of literature. Gynecol Oncol 54:87–90, 1994.

Schumann EA: Observation upon the coexistence of carcinoma fundus uteri and pregnancy. Trans A Gynecol Soc 52:245–256, 1927.

Starr AJ, Ruffolo EH, Shenoy BV et al: Primary carcinoma of the Fallopian tube: a surprise finding in a postpartum tubal ligation. Am J Obstet Gynecol 132:344–345, 1978.

Su YN, Cheng WF, Chen CA et al: Pregnancy with primary tubal placental site trophoblastic tumor: a case report and literature review. Gynecol Oncol 73:322–325, 1999.

Vaccarello L, Apte SM, Copeland LJ: Endometrial carcinoma associated with pregnancy: a report of three cases and review of the literature. Gynecol Oncol 74:118–122, 1989.

Wall JA, Lucci JA Jr: Adenocarcinoma of the corpus uteri and pelvic tuberculosis complicating pregnancy. Obstet Gynecol 2:229–235, 1953.

Wallingford AJ: Cancer of the body of the uterus complicating pregnancy. Am Gynecol 27:223–231, 1931.

Westmann A: A case of simultaneous pregnancy and cancer of the corpus uteri. Acta Obstet Gynecol Scand 14:191–194, 1934.

TWIN PREGNANCY WITH COEXISTING COMPLETE MOLE AND FETUS

Abbi M, Kriplani A, Uppal R et al: Term twin pregnancy with hydatidiform mole and normal fetus. Arch Gynecol Obstet 262:189, 1999.

Anderson CK, Deiter RW, Motz MJ et al: Complete hydatidiform mole with a coexistent healthy, viable fetus near term: a case report. J Reprod Med 41:55, 1996.

Bristow RE, Shumway JB, Khouzami AN et al: Complete hydatidiform mole and surviving coexistent twin. Obstet Gynecol Surv 51:705, 1996.

Bruchim I, Kidron D, Amiel A et al: Complete hydatidiform mole and a coexistent viable fetus: report of two cases and review of the literature. Gynecol Oncol 77:197–202, 2000.

Fishman DA, Padilla LA et al: Management of twin pregnancies consisting of a complete hydatidiform mole and normal fetus. Obstet Gynecol 91:546–550, 1998.

Hurteau JA, Roth LM, Schilder JM et al: Complete hydatidiform mole coexisting with a twin live fetus: clinical course. Gynecol Oncol 66:156–159, 1997.

Marcorelles P, Audrezet M-P, Le Bris M-J et al: Diagnosis and outcome of complete hydatidiform mole coexisting with a live twin fetus. Eur J Obstet Gynecol Reprod Biol 118:21–27, 2005.

Matsui H, Sekiya S, Hando T et al: Hydatidiform mole coexistent with a twin live fetus: a national collaborative study in Japan. Hum Reprod 15:608–611, 2000.

Sebire NJ, Foskett M, Paradinas F et al: Outcome of twin pregnancies with complete hydatidiform mole and healthy co-twin. Lancet 359:2165–2166, 2002.

Steller MA, Genest DR, Bernstein MR et al: Natural history of twin pregnancy with complete hydatidiform mole and coexisting fetus. Obstet Gynecol 83:35–42, 1994.

Vaisbuch E, Ben-Arie A, Dgani R et al: Twin pregnancy consisting of a complete hydatidiform mole and co-existent fetus: report of two cases and review of the literature. Gynecol Oncol 98:19–23, 2005.

MATERNAL MALIGNANCY METASTATIC TO THE PRODUCTS OF CONCEPTION

Ackerman J, Gilbert-Barness E: Malignancy metastatic to the products of conception: a case report with literature review. Ped Pathol Lab Med 17:577–586, 1997.

Alexander A, Samlowski WE, Grossman D et al: Metastatic melanoma in pregnancy: risk of transplacental metastases in the infant. J Clin Oncol 21:2179–2186, 2003.

Aronsson S: A case of transplacental tumor metastasis. Acta Paediatr Scand 52:123–124, 1963.

Brossard J, Abish S, Bernstein ML et al: Maternal malignancy involving the products of conception. A report of malignant melanoma and medulloblastoma. Am J Pediatr Hematol Oncol 16:380–383, 1994.

Cavell B: Transplacental metastasis of malignant melanoma. Acta Paediatr Suppl 146:37–40, 1963.

Chandra SA, Gilbert EF, Viseskul C et al: Neonatal intracranial choriocarcinoma. Arch Pathol Lab Med 114:1079, 1990.

Friedreich N: Beitrage zur pathologic des Krebses. Virchows Arch (Pathol Anat) 36:30–31, 1866.

Jackisch C, Louwen F, Schwenkhagen A et al: Lung cancer during pregnancy involving the products of conception and a review of the literature. Arch Gynecol Obstet 268:69–77, 2003.

Jauniaux E, Ogle R: Color Doppler imaging in the diagnosis and management of chorioangiomas. Ultrasound Obstet Gynecol 15:463–467, 2000.

Maruko K, Maeda T, Kamitomo M et al: Transplacental transmission of maternal B-cell lymphoma. Am J Obstet Gynecol 191:180–181, 2004.

Potter JF, Schoeneman M: Metastasis of maternal cancer to the placenta and fetus. Cancer 25:380–388, 1970.

Rothman LA, Cohen CJ, Astarloa J: Placental and fetal involvement by maternal malignancy: a report of rectal carcinoma and review of the literature. Am J Obstet Gynecol 116:1023–1034, 1973.

Tolar J, Neglia JP: Transplacental and other routes of cancer transmission between individuals. J Ped Hematol Oncol 25:430–434, 2003.

Walker JWT, Reinisch JF, Monforte HL: Maternal pulmonary adenocarcinoma metastatic to the fetus: first recorded case report and literature review. Ped Pathol Mol Med 21:57–69, 2002.

17 Complications of Disease and Therapy

Daniel L. Clarke-Pearson, M.D.

Women with gynecologic cancers frequently suffer from complications associated with their primary disease process or from the cancer-directed treatment modalities. In addition, many women are elderly and have comorbidities that further complicate therapy and impact on treatment decisions. Minimizing these problems is often accomplished by the astute clinician who is aware of potential complications and is proactive in prevention and early intervention.

Complications of disease are, in fact, commonly the primary presenting symptom (chief complaint) and subsequently the primary gynecologic cancer is discovered. Common symptoms of disease include hemorrhage (cervical and endometrial cancer), urinary tract obstruction or fistulae (cervical cancer), or intestinal obstruction (ovarian cancer). While some complications have been discussed previously in this text, it seems appropriate to devote a chapter exclusively to complications of disease and therapy. Not all possible complications can be covered, and the reader is referred to texts that expand on them. However, the most common complications and suggestions for management will be discussed.

DISEASE-ORIENTED COMPLICATIONS

Symptoms caused by cancer, such as bleeding, urinary tract obstruction, fistula, and intestinal obstruction, must be considered a complication that needs to be managed coincidentally with the cancer itself.

Hemorrhage

Bleeding from cervical or endometrial cancer is a common presenting symptom. While bleeding is rarely severe, the acute management of hemorrhage may be required before cancer therapy can be undertaken. Patients who are bleeding should be initially assessed for hemodynamic stability. On rare occasion, the bleeding is so severe that the patient may be in hypovolemic shock. Immediate management should include venous access, blood volume replacement, and supportive care. When stabilized, the patient should be examined and the source of the bleeding determined. Most commonly, massive hemorrhage is due to an exophytic cervical cancer eroding into a small cervical or vaginal artery. Prolonged slow vaginal bleeding from an endometrial cancer or sarcoma may also result in a patient presenting with profound chronic anemia. Because the bleeding has been slow over a longer period of time, the patient has often accommodated to the anemia and may be hemodynamically stable despite profound anemia. Biopsy should be obtained to document the pathology, and the patient should be examined to make a clinical estimation of the extent (stage) of disease.

Control of an actively bleeding cervical lesion is usually accomplished with a two-inch vaginal pack applied firmly to the cervix and packing the entire vagina. Monsel's solution (ferric subsulfate) may be put on the portion of the pack abutting the tumor. Soaking of the entire pack with Monsel's solution should be avoided, as it will desiccate the normal vaginal mucosa, making removal of the pack and subsequent pelvic examinations difficult. Application of acetone to the pack adjacent to the tumor has also been helpful, although acetone is often difficult to acquire in today's medical environment. An indwelling Foley catheter should be placed in the bladder, as pressure from the pack will usually obstruct the urethra. The pack should be removed slowly 24–48 h later and the patient observed. Removal of the pack under anesthesia may provide a level of safety if immediate cautery or repacking were necessary. This would also provide the opportunity to perform an examination under anesthesia and cystoscopy or proctoscopy if indicated. Suturing bleeding points in a cervical cancer is rarely successful, as the suture will tear through the tumor.

Pelvic radiation therapy for a patient with locally advanced cervical cancer who is actively bleeding should be initiated immediately. Alternatively, if the patient's cancer is an operable lesion, surgery should be performed expeditiously.

If bleeding cannot be controlled with packing, other measures must be considered. Consultation with an interventional radiologist should be obtained to consider arteriographic embolization of the hypogastric or uterine arteries. Arteriographic evaluation will usually identify the specific bleeding vessel, and selective embolization can be accomplished. Arterial access is usually obtained through the femoral artery, and the catheter is advanced to the aortic bifurcation. Using contrast injected into the artery, the arterial vascular supply of the pelvis can be investigated in order to identify the specific bleeding site. Both sides of the pelvis should be evaluated. Intravascular contrast can be nephrotoxic and therefore must be used cautiously in patients who have an element of renal failure or who are diabetic. Control of the bleeding site can be accomplished by continuous vasopressin infusion; embolization using synthetic materials (Gelfoam) or Gianturco springs, which are imbedded with Dacron; or with a balloon catheter (Fig. 17–1). Embolization is usually the procedure primarily chosen as the vasopressin infusion, and balloon catheters require that the artery remain cannulated for a longer duration.

Hypogastric (internal iliac) artery ligation is usually the procedure of last resort for bleeding from a primary gynecologic cancer, and is most commonly performed to control intraoperative hemorrhage. Details of hypogastric artery ligation will be discussed later in this chapter.

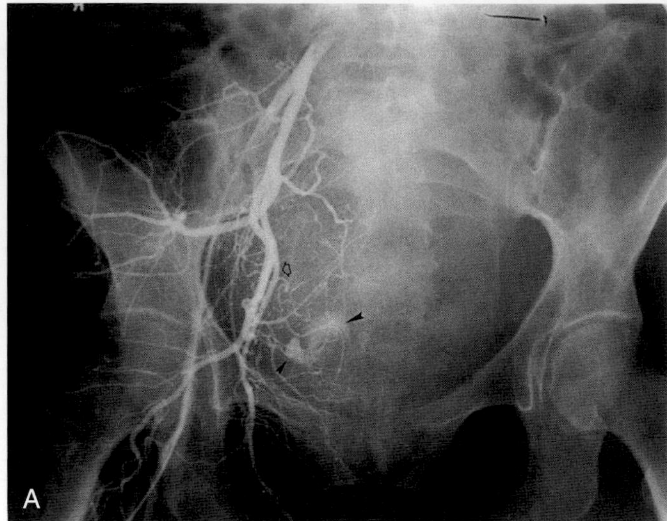

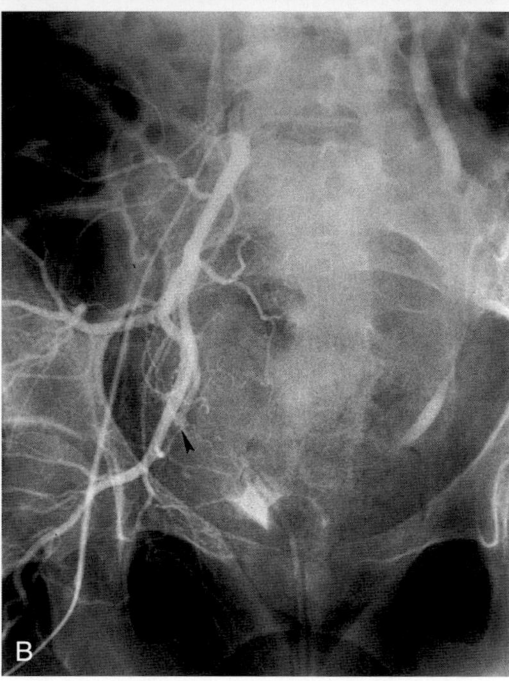

Figure 17–1 A patient who is postoperative from a vaginal hysterectomy with significant vaginal bleeding requiring multiple blood transfusions. The patient also has von Willebrand disease. *A*, Hemorrhage from the internal pudendal artery on the right. *B*, After embolization, no hemorrhage is seen from the internal pudendal artery. Dye in the pelvis is localized to the bladder, and the left ureter can be visualized. (Courtesy of Ivan Vujic, M.D., and Keeling Warburton, M.D., Medical University of South Carolina.)

Urinary tract complications

Ureteral obstruction

Ureteral obstruction may be the primary presenting symptom of a locally advanced cervical cancer and less commonly other gynecologic cancers including endometrial and ovarian cancer. The most common evidence of ureteral obstruction is an elevated serum creatinine rather than complaints of anuria. Of course, acute renal failure may arise from a number of causes that should be investigated (Table 17–1). The ureters may be obstructed due to local extension of the cancer or metastases to retroperitoneal lymph nodes, or by extrinsic compression of the ureter by large masses. Uremia secondary to bilateral ureteral obstruction is rarely encountered today but warrants immediate recognition and treatment. Given evidence of an elevated creatinine, evaluation of the ureters should avoid the use of nephrotoxic intravenous contrast dyes. Alternative methods may include a Lasix renal scan or ultrasound of the kidneys. If bilateral ureteral obstruction is diagnosed, prior to any intervention the patient should be rapidly evaluated to determine the true extent of the cancer. If the cancer appears to be locally advanced but not widely metastatic, relief of the ureteral obstruction should be attempted by cystoscopy and placement of retrograde ureteral stents. If stent placement is unsuccessful, then placement of percutaneous nephrostomy (PCN) tubes should be accomplished. Dialysis may be necessary in extreme circumstances until the obstruction can be relieved. Postobstructive diuresis and correction of electrolytes should be carefully evaluated in the several days after relief of the ureteral obstruction.

Complications of PCN placement include a high frequency of urinary tract infections and pyelonephritis (70%),

Table 17–1 MAJOR CAUSES OF ACUTE RENAL FAILURE IN GYNECOLOGY

Disorder	Example
Prerenal failure	
Hypovolemia	Skin, gastrointestinal, or renal volume loss; hemorrhage, sequestration of extracellular fluid (pancreatitis, peritonitis)
Cardiovascular failure	Impaired cardiac output (infarction, tamponade); vascular pooling (anaphylaxis, sepsis, drugs)
Postrenal failure	
Extrarenal obstruction	Urethral occlusion; bladder, pelvic, or retroperitoneal neoplasms; surgical accident; calculi
Intrarenal obstruction	Crystals (uric acid, oxalic acid, sulfonamides, methotrexate)
Bladder rupture	Trauma
Acute tubular necrosis	
Postischemic	All conditions listed above for prerenal failure
Pigment-induced	Hemolysis (transfusion reaction); rhabdomyolysis (trauma, coma, heatstroke, severe exercise, potassium or phosphate depletion)
Toxin-induced	Antibiotics; contrast material; anesthetic agents; heavy metals; organic solvents
Pregnancy-related	Septic abortion; uterine hemorrhage; eclampsia

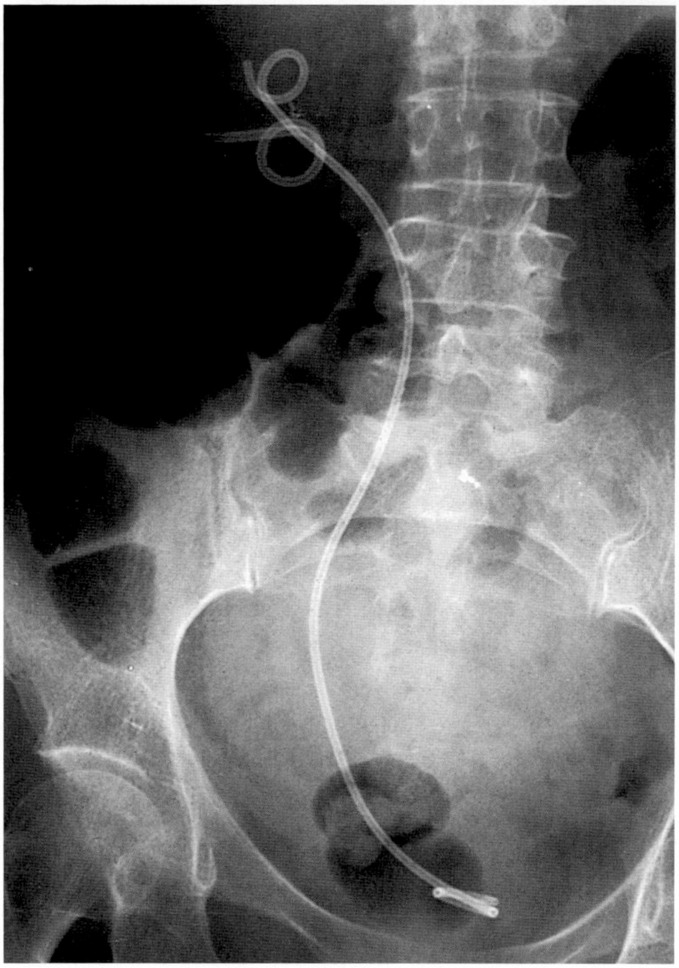

Figure 17–2 A double J stent has been inserted into the right kidney, ureter, and bladder through a percutaneous nephrostomy.

catheter occlusion (65%), and bleeding (28%). Seventy percent of the patients will have recovery of renal function after PCN placement (Dudley et al 1986).

Comment needs to be made of two sets of circumstances where the physician, patient, and family must seriously consider the possibility that relief of the obstruction may not be in the patient's best interest. These clinical situations include the following.

- The patient who presents with a widely metastatic malignancy for which there is little significant opportunity to provide effective therapy.
- The patient who has previously been treated for cervical cancer and has bilateral obstruction secondary to recurrent pelvic disease; again, a situation where there is no therapy available that would significantly prolong useful life. Careful evaluation should be made to be certain that the obstruction is not on the basis of retroperitoneal fibrosis from radiation therapy or from a lymphocyst.

Often, patients with bilateral ureteral obstruction are uremic and comatose. Decisions regarding intervention and care then fall to the next of kin, who must make the difficult decisions regarding intervention that may reverse the uremia, yet the patient will succumb from other complications of the cancer vs allowing the patient to expire peacefully in a uremic coma. Compassionate and knowledgeable consultation and advice with an experienced gynecologic oncologist is crucial in these difficult circumstances.

Unilateral ureteral obstruction at the time of initial presentation may not require stent or PCN placement if the patient's renal function is normal and therapy (e.g. pelvic radiation therapy) can be expected to control the cancer and relieve the obstruction. Placement of a PCN or stent in these circumstances must be balanced against the potential complications that might delay or interrupt therapy (Fig. 17–2).

Urinary outlet obstruction (obstruction of the urethra) by a cancer that has invaded the anterior vaginal wall (vaginal, vulvar, or cervical cancers) may usually be corrected by placement of a Foley catheter. If a Foley catheter cannot be placed, then either a suprapubic catheter or PCNs should be considered.

Urinary tract fistulas

Vesicovaginal fistula caused by a primary gynecologic cancer is relatively rare and is more commonly caused by therapy. Nonetheless, some patients will present with tumor that has eroded into the bladder, and subsequent loss of integrity between the bladder and vagina results in urinary leakage. Correction of the fistula caused by a cancer cannot be considered until the cancer has been eradicated. In the interim, while cancer therapy is initiated, the patient may be very uncomfortable from the continued loss of urine, and attempts to diminish the leakage should be undertaken. Placement of a Foley catheter will often partially divert urine from the fistula into the catheter. Modified menstrual cups or external appliances to collect urine have been used on occasion with success. Urinary diversion (ileal or transverse colon conduit) may be the only complete solution to profuse vaginal urinary leakage. Performing this major surgery should be weighed against the delay in primary cancer therapy that would be required while the patient recovers.

Gastrointestinal obstruction

Intestinal obstruction as a presenting symptom of a gynecologic cancer is most commonly caused by advanced ovarian cancer. In cases of small intestinal obstruction, initial therapy should include correction of fluid volume and electrolytes, nutritional assessment, and nasogastric tube decompression. Assessment of intestinal patency with an upper gastrointestinal series (with small bowel follow-through) or a computed tomography (CT) scan with oral contrast should be performed to develop a better understanding of the location and extent of obstruction. The colon should also be evaluated to exclude the possibility of colonic obstruction, which would need to be relieved at the same surgical procedure. In most cases, surgical exploration will be necessary in order to establish and stage the cancer diagnosis, to debulk the tumor, and to relieve the obstruction. Patients who are severely malnourished should have total parenteral nutrition (TPN) initiated perioperatively. Small bowel or colonic resection performed to relieve obstruction and to debulk primary tumor is commonly done. Linear stapling instruments have shortened operating time and create excellent anastomoses.

Short bowel syndrome may result from extensive resection of small bowel and/or colon. The syndrome is characterized by frequent diarrhea, fluid and electrolyte depletion, malabsorption, and weight loss. Depending on the extent and location of the intestinal segment(s) resected, malabsorption of the following nutrients may occur: copper, zinc, chromium, selenium, essential fatty acids, vitamins A and E, biotin, thiamine, and vitamin B_{12}. Over time, the remaining small bowel often adapts, and fluid and nutrient absorption is improved. However, in the interim, attempts to relieve short bowel syndrome should be directed at decreasing transit time by the use of an "elemental" diet and loperamide (Imodium) or diphenoxylate–atropine (Lomotil), cholestyramine (to decrease irritation of bile salts on the colonic mucosa), and somatostatin (to decrease intestinal digestive fluid production). In extreme cases, support with intravenous fluids and TPN may be necessary for several months.

On occasion, the preoperative assessment (usually with a CT scan) discovers far advanced disease that represents extensive carcinomatosis that would be unlikely to be successfully debulked. In these patients, neoadjuvant chemotherapy may be the best option rather than surgical intervention. If this therapeutic strategy is taken, gastrointestinal decompression (nasogastric tube or gastrostomy) and TPN will be required for several weeks while the neoadjuvant chemotherapy has the opportunity to result in a tumor response. Fortunately, many patients with ovarian cancer will regain intestinal function after two or three cycles of chemotherapy.

Colonic obstruction will necessitate surgical intervention in order to prevent colonic perforation, peritonitis, sepsis, and death. Given that adequate mechanical bowel preparation is impossible in the face of colonic obstruction, resection and anastomosis is out of the question and a colostomy must be formed. If the patient has an excellent response to subsequent chemotherapy, colostomy takedown in the future is reasonable to consider.

Intestinal obstruction often occurs late in the course of progressive ovarian cancer. In these situations, superb clinical judgment is required to obtain an optimal palliative outcome, for not all patients with recurrent ovarian cancer and intestinal obstruction will benefit from surgical intervention. It does seem intuitive that patients with colonic obstruction should be operated on to create a colostomy, an ileostomy, or at least a cecostomy. It is the patient with a small bowel obstruction who requires careful thought and triage. Initially, conservative management with intravenous fluid and electrolyte replacement, and nasogastric tube decompression, should be instituted. Some patients may re-establish bowel function with a few days of "bowel rest." However, if the obstruction persists, the decision to simply place a gastrostomy tube (which can often be placed percutaneously) or proceed to attempt to relieve the intestinal obstruction must be made. Of course, the patient who has a small bowel obstruction caused by adhesions should undergo surgery in all cases.

The problem in decision making comes when it is clear that the patient has recurrent ovarian cancer. Many investigators have attempted to identify factors that would predict successful outcome (often defined as surviving 30 days or being discharged from the hospital able to take oral fluids) or predict postoperative complications and death. These factors include presence of ascites, poor nutritional status, amount of prior chemotherapy regimens, availability of therapy with some potential for response, prior use of radiation therapy, length of time since prior therapy, and potential for being "platin-sensitive." If surgical intervention is deemed appropriate, surgical procedures might include bypass of involved segments of small bowel, or bowel resection with anastomosis or ileostomy. Unfortunately, in every investigator's experience there are patients who undergo laparotomy only to find such extensive carcinomatosis that they are deemed inoperable. The decision to operate, then, should be based on a clear communication between the surgeon and patient regarding expectations and definitions of "success." In our experience, which is reasonably representative of the general literature, median survival after small bowel obstruction surgery was 88 days, and only 14% of patients were alive at 12 months. In addition, 49% of patients suffered at least one significant postoperative complication, including wound infections, enterocutaneous fistula, sepsis, and recurrent obstruction.

If the decision is made not to operate, further decisions regarding management are also complex, including methods to palliate vomiting (percutaneous gastrostomy is recommended) and whether to continue intravenous fluids or even consider TPN in a hospice setting.

Gastrointestinal fistulas

Rectovaginal fistula may be discovered at the time of primary diagnosis of cervical, vaginal, or vulvar cancers. Involuntary loss of feces, flatus, and mucous discharge are the most common symptoms. If the patient has vulvar pain and excoriation, a fistula from the small intestine must be strongly suspected. In this instance, an upper gastrointestinal series (with small bowel follow-through) or a fistulogram should be performed in order to define the exact anatomic structures involved. If a rectovaginal fistula is found, diversion with a loop colostomy is suggested in order to divert the fecal stream and allow prompt treatment of the cancer (usually with radiation therapy). If vulvar cancer is so advanced as to cause a rectovaginal fistula, some surgeons would manage the cancer and the fistula in the same surgical procedure (such as a posterior pelvic exenteration and modified radical vulvectomy). Others have had excellent results treating locally advanced vulvar cancer with radiation therapy and concurrent radiosensitizing chemotherapy, thereby preserving the rectal sphincter. Colostomy diversion is still suggested for patient comfort and hygiene. If the cancer treatment is successful, attempts to close the fistula are reasonable, and if successful the colostomy may ultimately be reversed.

Enterovaginal fistulas are rare to find at initial cancer diagnosis, and more often occur as a result of complications of therapy (radiation) or at the time of cancer recurrence. The flow of intestinal contents out of the vagina is usually liquid and caustic to vulvar skin. Thorough evaluation of the upper and lower gastrointestinal tracts as well as the urinary tract is mandatory, as many of these fistula are "complex," involving more than one viscus. Surgical intervention will be necessary in most cases in order to resect the involved bowel. If resection is not possible, the fistualized bowel will need to be isolated from the intestinal stream. Because the isolated bowel will continue to create succus entericus and subsequent continued vaginal drainage, resection is advised if at all possible.

Venous thromboembolic complications

Venous thromboembolic complications may precede the diagnosis of gynecologic cancer or may be the result of cancer treatments, especially surgery and chemotherapy. Most women with gynecologic cancers have several risk factors that increase the probability of developing a venous thromboembolic event during their course of therapy.

Risk factors

The causal factors of venous thrombosis were first proposed by Virchow in 1858, and include a hypercoagulable state, venous stasis, and vessel endothelial injury. In addition to the increased risk of venous thromboembolism (VTE) due to cancer, other clinical risk factors include advanced age; major surgery; non-white race; a history of deep venous thrombosis (DVT) or pulmonary embolism; lower extremity edema or venous stasis changes; presence of varicose veins; being overweight; a history of radiation therapy; and hypercoagulable states such as factor V Leiden, pregnancy, and use of oral contraceptives, estrogens, or tamoxifen. Intraoperative factors associated with postoperative DVT included increased anesthesia time, increased blood loss, and the need for transfusion in the operating room. It is important to recognize these risk factors in order to provide the appropriate level of venous thrombosis prophylaxis. A general outline of levels of thromboembolism risk is listed in Table 17–2.

Prophylactic methods

Deep venous thrombosis and pulmonary embolism, although largely preventable, are significant complications in women with gynecologic cancers and especially those who are postoperative. The magnitude of this problem is relevant to the gynecologic oncologist, because 40% of all deaths

Table 17–2 THROMBOEMBOLISM RISK STRATIFICATION

Risk	Factors
Low	Minor surgery No other risk factors[a]
Moderate	Age >40 years and major surgery Age <40 years with other risk factors[a] and major surgery
High	Age >60 years and major surgery Cancer History of deep venous thrombosis or pulmonary embolism Thrombophilias
Highest	Age >60 and cancer or history of venous thromboembolism

[a]Risk factors: cancer; advancing age; major surgery; obesity; varicose veins; history of deep venous thrombosis or pulmonary embolism; current estrogen, tamoxifen, or oral contraceptive use; thrombophilias.

following gynecologic surgery are directly attributed to pulmonary emboli; it is the most frequent cause of postoperative death in patients with uterine or cervical carcinoma.

A number of prophylactic methods have been shown to significantly reduce the incidence of DVT in women with gynecologic cancers, and a few studies have included a large enough patient population to demonstrate a reduction in fatal pulmonary emboli. The ideal prophylactic method would be effective, free of significant side effects, well accepted by the patient and nursing staff, widely applicable to most patients, and inexpensive. Available prophylactic methods may be divided into pharmacologic agents that reduce hypercoagulable states, and mechanical methods that reduce stasis and may also enhance fibrinolysis. A key to the successful use of prophylactic methods is the understanding that women with gynecologic cancers are at very high risk, and that more intense prophylactic measures are necessary to achieve maximal success.

Low-dose heparin

The use of small doses of subcutaneously administered heparin for the prevention of DVT and pulmonary embolism is the most widely studied of all prophylactic methods. More than 25 controlled trials have demonstrated that heparin given subcutaneously 2 h preoperatively and every 8–12 h postoperatively is effective in reducing the incidence of DVT. The value of low-dose heparin (LDH) in preventing fatal pulmonary emboli was established by a randomized, controlled, multicenter international trial, which demonstrated a significant reduction in fatal postoperative pulmonary emboli in general surgery patients receiving LDH every 8 h postoperatively. Trials of LDH in gynecologic surgery patients with benign conditions have shown a significant reduction in postoperative DVT. However, in the patient with gynecologic cancer, the regimen of administering LDH 5000 U every 12 h was found to be ineffective in a randomized trial.

In a subsequent trial, two more intense heparin regimens were evaluated in high-risk gynecologic oncology patients. Heparin was given in a regimen of either 5000 U subcutaneously 2 h preoperatively and every 8 h postoperatively, or 5000 U subcutaneously every 8 h preoperatively (a minimum of three preoperative doses) and every 8 h postoperatively. Both of these prophylaxis regimens were effective in significantly reducing the incidence of postoperative DVT in patients with gynecologic cancers. We conclude that in women undergoing surgery for gynecologic malignancy, a regimen of LDH 5000 U every 8 h is necessary to provide effective prophylaxis.

Although LDH is considered to have no measurable effect on coagulation, most large series have noted an increase in the bleeding complication rate, especially a higher incidence of wound hematoma. Thrombocytopenia has been found to be associated with LDH use in 6% of patients after gynecologic surgery. If patients remain on LDH for greater than 4 days, it would be reasonable to check a platelet count to assess the possibility of the occurrence of heparin-induced thrombocytopenia.

Low molecular weight heparins

Low molecular weight heparins (LMWHs) are fragments of heparin that vary in size from 4500 to 6500 Da. When compared with unfractionated heparin, LMWHs have more anti-Xa and less antithrombin activity, leading to less effect on partial thromboplastin time (PTT), and they may also lead to fewer bleeding complications. An increased half-life of 4 h results in increased bioavailability when compared with unfractionated heparin. The increase in half-life of LMWHs also allows the convenience of once a day dosing.

Randomized controlled trials have compared LMWH to unfractionated heparin in patients undergoing gynecologic surgery. In all studies, there was a similar incidence of DVT. Bleeding complications were also similar between the unfractionated heparin and LMWH groups. A meta-analysis of general surgery and gynecologic surgery patients from 32 trials likewise indicated that daily LMWH administration is as effective as unfractionated heparin in DVT prophylaxis, without any difference in hemorrhagic complications. Again, based on randomized trials in other patients with cancer, it would appear that a more intense regimen of LMWH is necessary to obtain optimal prophylaxis. Finally, prolonged prophylaxis for 2 weeks postoperatively has resulted in improved outcomes. While this is not standard of care at the moment, consideration of providing prolonged prophylaxis should be given in extremely high-risk patients.

Mechanical methods

Stasis in the veins of the legs has been clearly demonstrated while the patient is undergoing surgery, and continues postoperatively for varying lengths of time. Stasis occurring in the capacitance veins of the calf during surgery, plus the hypercoagulable state induced by cancer and surgery, are the prime factors contributing to the development of acute postoperative DVT. Prospective studies of the natural history of postoperative venous thrombosis have shown that the calf veins are the predominant site of thrombi, and that most thrombi develop within 24 h of surgery.

Although probably of only modest benefit, reduction of stasis by short preoperative hospital stays and early postoperative ambulation should be encouraged for all patients. Elevation of the foot of the bed, raising the calf above heart level, allows gravity to drain the calf veins and should further reduce stasis.

Graduated compression stockings Controlled studies of graduated pressure stockings are limited but do suggest modest benefit when they are carefully fitted. Poorly fitted stockings may be hazardous to some patients who develop a tourniquet effect at the knee or mid-thigh. Variations in human anatomy do not allow perfect fit of all patients to available stocking sizes. The simplicity of elastic stockings and the absence of significant side effects are probably the two most important reasons that they are often included in routine postoperative care.

External pneumatic compression The largest body of literature dealing with the reduction of postoperative venous stasis deals with intermittent external compression of the leg by pneumatically inflated sleeves placed around the calf or leg during intraoperative and postoperative periods. Various pneumatic compression devices and leg sleeve designs are available, and the current literature has not demonstrated superiority of one system over another. Calf compression during and after gynecologic surgery significantly reduces the incidence of DVT on a level similar to that of LDH. In addition to increasing venous flow and pulsatile emptying of the calf veins, external pneumatic compression (EPC) also appears to augment endogenous fibrinolysis, which may result in lysis of very early thrombi before they become clinically significant.

The duration of postoperative EPC has differed in various trials. EPC may be effective when used in the operating room and for the first 24 h postoperatively in patients with benign conditions who will ambulate on the first postoperative day.

External pneumatic compression used in patients undergoing major surgery for gynecologic malignancy has been found to reduce the incidence of postoperative venous thromboembolic complications by nearly threefold. However, this was only the case if calf compression was applied intraoperatively and for the first 5 postoperative days. Patients with gynecologic malignancies may remain at risk because of stasis and hypercoagulable states for a longer period than general surgical patients, and therefore appear to benefit from longer use of EPC.

External pneumatic leg compression has no significant side effects or risks, and is considered slightly more cost effective when compared with pharmacologic methods of prophylaxis. Of course, compliance to wearing the leg compression while in bed is of utmost importance, and the patient and nursing staff should be educated to the proper regimen for maximum benefit.

We have investigated the risk factors associated with the failure of external compression to prevent DVT in a retrospective analysis of 1862 consecutive gynecologic surgery patients who received postoperative intermittent pneumatic compression at Duke University between 1992 and 1997. A history of prior DVT, diagnosis of cancer, and age >60 years were factors independently associated with the development of DVT despite EPC prophylaxis ($P < 0.05$). Patients having two or more of these factors had a 16-fold increased risk of postoperative DVT despite prophylaxis ($P < 0.05$). In these extremely high-risk patients, combined methods of prophylaxis ought to be considered.

Integrating evidence and experience

Because low-dose unfractionated heparin (LDUH), LMWH, and EPC have been shown to effectively reduce the incidence of postoperative VTE in high-risk gynecologic oncology surgery patients, the question remains, "Which is better?"

We have undertaken two randomized clinical trials in hopes of answering this critical question. In the first trial, patients were randomized to receive either LDUH (5000 U subcutaneously preoperatively and every 8 h postoperatively until hospital discharge) or EPC, which was applied to the calf prior to surgery and remained on while the patient was in bed until hospital discharge. The incidence of DVT was identical in both groups of patients, and none developed a pulmonary embolus within 30 days of follow-up. However, there were significantly more bleeding complications in the group who received LDUH. Specifically, nearly one-quarter had activated partial thromboplastin time (APTT) levels in a "therapeutic" range, and significantly more patients required blood transfusions. Following this trial, the standard of care in our institution was to use EPC because of its more favorable therapeutic ratio.

With the advent of LMWHs (which have more anti-Xa and less antithrombin activity), there was the potential that they may be associated with decreased risk of bleeding complications. We therefore undertook a second randomized trial comparing LMWH and EPC. Because higher doses of LMWH had been shown to be more effective in preventing VTE in cancer patients, we used dalteparin (Fragmin) 5000 U preoperatively and 5000 U daily postoperatively until hospital discharge. In this trial, there was a similar low frequency of DVT and no pulmonary emboli in 30 days of follow-up. In addition, we found that LMWH was not associated with increased bleeding complications or transfusion requirements. Finally, compliance and patient satisfaction with either of these prophylaxis modalities were similar. Given the results of these two randomized clinical trials, we now feel that either LMWH or EPC is our best choice for thromboembolism prophylaxis in gynecologic oncology surgery patients.

Combination prophylaxis

Combination therapy using heparin and compression stockings has been utilized in other high-risk surgical patients in an attempt to diminish both the hypercoaguability and the venous stasis that can be found in postoperative patients at high risk for thromboembolism. The prophylactic use of LDH has been compared with LDH combined with graduated compression stockings (GCS) in DVT prophylaxis among general surgery patients. Willie-Jorgensen and associates in an investigation involving 245 patients undergoing acute extensive abdominal operations, demonstrated that the rate of postoperative DVT was significantly lower among 79 patients receiving a combination regimen of GCS and LDH (i.e. 5000 U s.q. 1 h preoperatively and q 12 h postoperatively) than patients receiving only the LDH regimen ($P = 0.013$). A statistically significant improvement ($P < 0.05$) in postoperative DVT was similarly noted by the same investigators in the evaluation of 176 patients undergoing elective abdominal surgery. A meta-analysis of six studies involving 898 general surgery patients has shown that combination therapy with LDH and GCS provides significantly better DVT prophylaxis postoperatively than either single modality (odds ratio 0.40; 95% confidence interval 0.27–0.59).

Recently, a multicenter prospective randomized clinical trial demonstrated that combination prophylaxis consisting of GSC and LMWH was more effective in DVT prevention than GCS alone (relative risk 0.52; 95% confidence interval 0.17–0.95; $P = 0.04$). "Combination" prophylaxis might be considered in the highest risk gynecologic oncology patients, and is recommended by the American College of Chest Physicians Consensus Conference, although the efficacy, risks, and costs have not been fully evaluated in gynecologic oncology patients.

Management of deep venous thrombosis and pulmonary embolism

Diagnosis of deep venous thrombosis

Because pulmonary embolism is the leading cause of deaths following gynecologic surgical procedures, identification of high-risk patients and the use of prophylactic VTE regimens are an essential part of management. In addition, the early recognition of DVT and pulmonary embolism and their immediate treatment are critical. Most pulmonary emboli arise from the deep venous system of the leg, although following gynecologic surgery the pelvic veins are a known source of fatal pulmonary emboli as well.

The signs and symptoms of DVT of the lower extremities include pain, edema, erythema, and prominent vascular pattern of the superficial veins. These signs and symptoms are relatively non-specific; 50–80% of patients with these symptoms will not actually have DVT. Conversely, approximately 80% of patients with symptomatic pulmonary emboli have no signs or symptoms of thrombosis in the lower extremities. Because of the lack of specificity when signs and symptoms are recognized, additional diagnostic tests should be performed to establish the diagnosis of DVT.

Doppler ultrasound B-mode duplex Doppler imaging is currently the most common technique for the diagnosis of symptomatic venous thrombosis, especially when it arises in the proximal lower extremity. With duplex Doppler imaging, the femoral vein can be visualized and clots may be seen directly. Compression of the vein with the ultrasound probe tip allows assessment of venous collapsibility; the presence of a thrombus diminishes vein wall collapsibility. It should be recognized that Doppler imaging is less accurate when evaluating the calf and the pelvic veins.

Venogram Although venography has been the gold standard for diagnosis of DVT, other diagnostic studies are accurate when performed by a skilled technologist, and in most patients may replace the need for routine contrast venography. Venography is moderately uncomfortable, requires the injection of a contrast material that may cause allergic reaction or renal injury, and may result in phlebitis in approximately 5% of patients. However, if non-invasive imaging is normal or inconclusive and the clinician remains concerned given clinical symptoms, venography should be obtained to obtain a definitive answer.

Magnetic resonance venography Magnetic resonance venography has a sensitivity and specificity comparable with those of venography. In addition, magnetic resonance venography may detect thrombi in pelvic veins that are not imaged by venography. The primary drawback to magnetic resonance venography is the time involved in examining the lower extremity and pelvis, as well as the expense of this technology.

Treatment of deep venous thrombosis

The treatment of postoperative DVT requires the immediate institution of anticoagulant therapy. Treatment may be with either unfractionated heparin or LMWHs, followed by 6 months of oral anticoagulant therapy with warfarin. Prolonged anticoagulation (lifetime) is recommended for women who continue to have active cancer (i.e. those not in remission after treatment), as they remain at very high risk to rethrombose.

Unfractionated heparin After VTE is diagnosed, unfractionated heparin should be initiated to prevent proximal propagation of the thrombus and allow physiologic thrombolytic pathways to dissolve the clot (Table 17–3). An initial bolus of 80 U/kg is given intravenously, followed by a continuous infusion of 1000–2000 U/h (18 U/kg per h). Heparin dosage is adjusted to maintain APTT levels at a therapeutic level 1.5–2.5 times the control value. Initial APTT should be measured after 6 h of heparin administration and the dose adjusted as necessary. Patients having subtherapeutic APTT levels in the fist 24 h have a risk of recurrent thromboembolism 15 times the risk of patients

Table 17–3 ANTICOAGULATION METHOD FOR DEEP VENOUS THROMBOSIS

Obtain a pretreatment hemoglobin level, platelet count, PT, and APTT, and repeat platelet count daily until heparin is stopped.
Administer a bolus dose of heparin: 5000 U i.v.
Initiate a maintenance dose of heparin: 32,000 U i.v. per 24 h by continuous infusion, or 17,000 U s.c. to be repeated after adjustment at 12 h.
Adjust the dose of heparin at 6 h according to the nomogram; maintain APTT in the therapeutic range.
Repeat APTT every 6 h until it moves into the therapeutic range, and then daily according to the nomogram.
Start warfarin 10 mg at 24 h and 10 mg next day.
Overlap heparin and warfarin for at least 4 days.
Perform PT daily and adjust the warfarin dose to maintain the INR at 2.0–3.0.
Continue heparin for a minimum of 5 days, then stop if the INR has been in the therapeutic range for at least 2 consecutive days.
Continue warfarin for 6 months and monitor PT daily until it is in the therapeutic range, then three times during the first week, twice a week for 2 weeks or until the dose response is stable, and then every 2 weeks.

APTT, activated partial thromboplastin time; INR, international normalized ratio; PT, prothrombin time.

with appropriate levels. Patients therefore should be treated aggressively using intravenous heparin to achieve prompt anticoagulation. A weight-based nomogram has proven helpful in achieving a therapeutic APTT (Table 17–4). Oral anticoagulant (warfarin) should be started on the first day of heparin infusion. International normalized ratio (INR) should be monitored daily until a therapeutic level is achieved (INR 2.0–3.0). The change in the INR resulting from warfarin administration often precedes the anticoagulant effect by approximately 2 days, during which time low protein C levels are associated with a transient hypercoagulable state. Therefore heparin should be administered until the INR has been maintained in a therapeutic range for at least 2 days, confirming proper warfarin dose. Intravenous heparin may be discontinued in 5 days if an adequate INR level has been established.

Low molecular weight heparin Low molecular weight heparins (enoxaparin and dalteparin) have been shown to be effective in the treatment of VTE and have a cost-effective advantage over intravenous heparin in that they may be administered in the outpatient setting. The dosages used in treatment of thromboembolism are unique and weight-adjusted according to each LMWH preparation. Because LMWHs have a minimal effect on APTT, serial laboratory monitoring of PTT levels is not necessary. Similarly, monitoring of anti-Xa activity (except in difficult cases or those with renal impairment) has not been shown to be of significant benefit in a dose adjustment of LMWH. The increased bioavailability associated with LMWH allows for twice a day dosing, potentially making outpatient management an option for a subset of patients. A meta-analysis involving more than 1000 patients from 19 trials suggests that LMWH is more effective, safer, and less costly when compared with unfractionated heparin in preventing recurrent thromboembolism.

Table 17–4 HEPARIN ADMINISTRATION FOR TREATMENT OF DEEP VEIN THROMBOSIS OR PULMONARY EMBOLISM: WEIGHT-BASED NOMOGRAM

Time of administration	Dose
Initial dose	80-U/kg bolus, then 18 U/kg per h
The APTT should be measured every 6 h and the heparin dose adjusted as follows:	
APTT < 35 s (< 1.2 times control)	80-U/kg bolus, then 4 U/kg per h
APTT 35–45 s (1.2–1.5 times control)	40-U/kg bolus, then 2 U/kg per h
APTT 46–70 s (1.5–2.3 times control)	No change
APTT 71–90 s (2.3–3 times control)	Decrease infusion rate by 2 U/kg per h
APTT > 90 s (> 3 times control)	Hold infusion for 1 h, then decrease infusion rate by 3 U/kg per h

APTT, activated partial thromboplastin time.
(From Raschke RA, Reilly BM, Guidry JR et al: The weight-based heparin dosing nomogram compared with a "standard care" nomogram. Ann Intern Med 119:874–881, 1993.)

Oral anticoagulants: warfarin In most cases, the conversion from parenteral heparin or LMWH to oral warfarin may start on the initial day of therapy. Both heparin and warfarin are given, and the heparin is discontinued when the warfarin has reached a therapeutic INR of 2–3 for 2 consecutive days. Initially, the INR should be monitored frequently in order to appropriately adjust the warfarin dose. Once a stable warfarin dose is established, the INR may be checked less frequently. Patients should be cautioned to avoid the use of drugs and dietary products, which might alter the metabolism or absorption of warfarin. Warfarin may be a difficult drug to administer to some patients, especially if their nutrition is inadequate, if their oral intake is variable, or if they require prolonged use of antibiotics or other drugs that might alter the metabolism of warfarin. This is particularly common in women with advanced ovarian cancer. Given the wide variation in the INR in many of these patients, who are then predisposed to either bleeding complications or rethrombosis, we have found that it is safer to use subcutaneous LMWH (at therapeutic doses) for prolonged therapy.

Diagnosis of pulmonary embolism

Many of the signs and symptoms of pulmonary embolism are associated with other, more commonly occurring pulmonary complications following surgery. The classic findings of pleuritic chest pain, hemoptosis, shortness of breath, tachycardia, and tachypnea should alert the physician to the possibility of a pulmonary embolism. Many times, however, the signs are much more subtle and may be suggested only by a persistent tachycardia or a slight elevation in the respiratory rate. Patients suspected of pulmonary embolism should be evaluated initially by chest x-ray, electrocardiography, and arterial blood gas assessment. Any evidence of abnormality should be further evaluated by ventilation–perfusion lung scan or a spiral CT scan of the chest. Unfortunately, a high percentage of lung scans may be interpreted as "indeterminate." In this setting, careful clinical evaluation and judgment are required to decide whether pulmonary arteriography should be obtained to document or exclude the presence of a pulmonary embolism.

The treatment of pulmonary embolism is as follows.

- Immediate anticoagulant therapy, identical to that outlined for the treatment of DVT, should be initiated.
- Respiratory support, including oxygen and bronchodilators and an intensive care setting, may be necessary.
- Although massive pulmonary emboli are usually quickly fatal, pulmonary embolectomy has been performed successfully on rare occasions.
- Pulmonary artery catheterization with the administration of thrombolytic agents bears further evaluation and may be important in patients with massive pulmonary embolism.

- Vena cava interruption may be necessary in situations in which anticoagulant therapy is ineffective in the prevention of rethrombosis and repeated embolization from the lower extremities or pelvis. A vena cava umbrella or filter may be inserted percutaneously above the level of the thrombosis and caudad to the renal veins.
- In most cases, however, anticoagulant therapy is sufficient to prevent repeat thrombosis and embolism and to allow the patient's own endogenous thrombolytic mechanisms to lyse the pulmonary embolus.

Superior vena cava syndrome

Superior vena cava syndrome is caused by advanced cancers arising in or invading the mediastinum, subsequently obstructing the venous drainage of the head, neck, and upper thoracic regions. Primary tumors are most commonly the cause of this syndrome (bronchogenic carcinomas), although metastasis to the mediastinum from gynecologic cancers can also present in this manner. The vena cava has a low intravascular pressure and is easily compressed by adjacent masses. Most commonly, the symptoms caused by venous obstruction are dramatic swelling and plethora of the head, neck, upper extremities, and chest. Pleural and pericardial effusions can occur with decreased venous return to the heart and a resultant fall in cardiac output. Patients also commonly complain of a severe headache. A similar clinical syndrome is also seen associated with thrombosis of the subclavian vein and superior vena cava, which is induced by central venous catheters.

The diagnosis of the cause of superior vena cava syndrome is critical to selecting proper management. If a localized primary or metastatic neoplasm is identified, immediate radiation therapy is usually the most effective method to achieve resolution. Radiation therapy to the mediastinum in doses of 400 cGy for 3 days, and then 150–180 cGy per day for a total dose of 3000–5000 cGy, has been successful in relieving the vascular obstruction. Responses are commonly recognized in 3–4 days. Chemotherapy may also play a role, although the resolution of symptoms is usually much slower. Expandable wire stents across the constricted portion of the vena cava have also been used successfully.

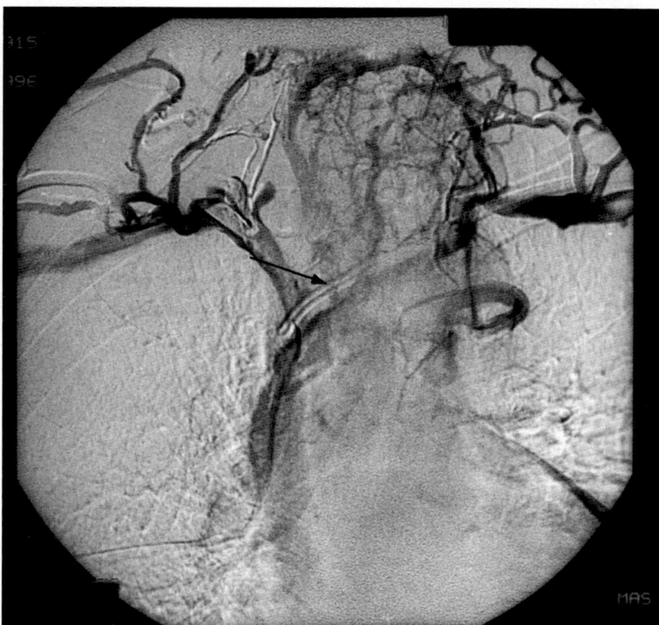

Figure 17–3 Extensive thrombosis of large vessels in the thorax. Multiple collaterals are present. The subclavian catheter is evident (arrow).

In patients where thrombosis is the etiology of venous obstruction, immediate anticoagulant therapy should be instituted (Fig. 17–3). The edema and plethora will usually diminish in 1–3 days. In many instances, the central venous catheter may be left in place and used. However, if the condition should persist or recur, the catheter should be removed.

Biliary obstruction

Obstruction of the biliary tree by gynecologic cancers is rare and is usually associated with far advanced cancers and limited life expectancy. Nonetheless, the resulting jaundice and pruritis caused by the obstruction is distressing to the patient and her family. Surgical relief of the obstruction is usually impossible due to the extent of cancer involvement in the region. However, endoscopic placement of a stent in the common duct often will resolve the symptoms and provide a better quality of life. If a stent cannot be placed due to extreme compression or other technical reasons, percutaneous placement of a drainage tube into the dilated biliary tree will also resolve symptoms.

Metastatic adenopathy high in the para-aortic chain resulting in biliary obstruction can commonly obstruct the duodenum, leading to gastric outlet obstruction. While surgical intervention (gastrojejunostomy) may correct the anatomic problem, careful consideration should be given to the patient's life expectancy. These are similar considerations to those made in women with small intestinal obstruction and recurrent ovarian cancer discussed previously. In women with just days or weeks to live, placement of a gastrostomy tube may be more prudent.

TREATMENT-RELATED COMPLICATIONS

Surgical

Intraoperative and postoperative hemorrhage

Intraoperative management of vascular complications

Surgery for gynecologic cancer often requires extensive dissection in the retroperitoneal space, which may be distorted by cancer metastatic to lymph nodes or invading other adjacent structures. It is not surprising, then, that injury to pelvic veins and arteries are common and may result in significant intraoperative blood loss and hemorrhage. Surgeons must be prepared for this eventuality and have in their armamentarium the tools and skills to bring a stop to the bleeding.

Before attempting to bring final control to a significant bleeding area, a few basic principles should be employed. First, the patient's blood volume and coagulation factors must be maintained at all times. Poor communication between the surgeon and the anesthesiologist can lead to significant hypovolemia and cardiovascular instability. Loss of coagulation factors during intraoperative hemorrhage results in continued bleeding that cannot be controlled by surgical means. The surgeon should pack the involved area to allow replacement of blood volume (packed red blood cells) and coagulation factors (fresh frozen plasma and platelets), and acquisition of appropriate assistance. When the patient is stable and the team is fully prepared, the packed area should be exposed a small area at a time in order to identify the specific bleeding site.

Before attempting to control the bleeding point, the adjacent anatomy should be identified and protected. In particular, the ureter, adjacent vessels, and viscera must be recognized in order to avoid further injury. In most cases of arterial bleeding, the artery can be isolated and controlled with sutures. Small arteries may be best controlled by vascular clips, while larger arteries may require sutures with 4-0 or 5-0 vascular suture (Prolene) (Fig. 17–4). This holds for injury to the aorta and the common and external iliac arteries. Injury to the internal iliac (hypogastric) artery may be controlled with total ligation of the artery. Patency of distal arteries should be confirmed throughout the remainder of the procedure and postoperatively. In rare instances, arterial injuries must be managed by vascular grafting.

Venous bleeding in the pelvis is probably more common given the fragility of the thin vein wall and the extensive network of pelvic venous plexus. Often, a specific bleeding point cannot be identified, but after several minutes of direct pressure on the bleeding area a clot will form over the low-pressure veins and the bleeding will resolve. If it does not, then control will have to be achieved with vascular clips, clamps, and suture ligature. Slow but persistent oozing from unidentified vessels can often be controlled by products that either serve as a matrix for clotting (Avitene, surgical Gelfoam) or that supply clotting factors which complete the clotting cascade (CoSeal, Tisseel, FloSeal). In all cases, it should be emphasized that prompt replacement of clotting factors provided by transfusion of fresh frozen plasma and platelets is critical to achieve hemostasis in the face of hemorrhage.

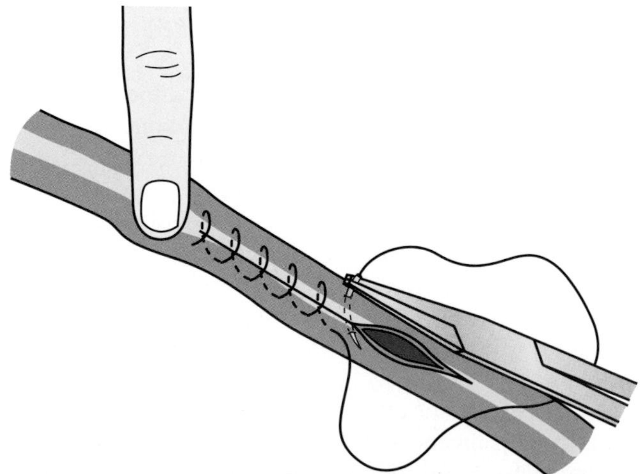

Figure 17–4 Laceration of a large pelvic wall vein. The operator's finger pressure on the vessel reduces flow to the site, while a continuous suture of fine silk or nylon is placed to close the defect.

Replacement of platelets and clotting factors in patients with massive transfusion and microvascular bleeding is dependent on clinical and surgical assessments. Guidelines have been provided by the American Society of Anesthesiologists task force regarding replacement of these products. In general, platelet transfusion is rarely indicated for counts greater than 100,000/µL and usually indicated for counts <50,000/µL (with intermediate platelet counts 50,000–100,000/µL, transfusion should be based on the risk of bleeding). Fresh frozen plasma therapy is indicated in massively transfused patients with microvascular bleeding or hemorrhage if the prothrombin or APTT values exceed 1.5 times the normal values. In cases of massive intraoperative blood loss, it may be prudent to administer fresh frozen plasma empirically (after 4 units of packed red blood cells). This strategy is aimed at preventing the patient from becoming hypocoagulable while awaiting the laboratory results (prothrombin time and PTT), which may take nearly an hour, and another hour to thaw the fresh frozen plasma before it is available to be administered. Cryoprecipitate transfusions are recommended for correction of microvascular bleeding in massively transfused patients with fibrinogen concentrations less than 80–100mg/dL.

Bleeding from the sacrum is usually not encountered except in the course of performing a total pelvic exenteration or rectosigmoid resection, or during a sacral colpopexy. If bleeding from the sacrum cannot be controlled by suture ligatures or vascular clips, placement of sterile thumbtacks pushed into the sacral bone will usually compress veins exiting the sacrum and achieve hemostasis.

Hypogastric (internal iliac) artery ligation

In situations when the usual steps to control hemorrhage have failed, hypogastric artery ligation should be performed. While the arterial blood supply to the pelvis is rich with anastomosis, ligation of the hypogastric arteries will usually decrease the arterial and venous pressure to the point where (in a patient who is not hypocoagulable) venous bleeding will slow and can either be controlled by ligature or will clot with prolonged packing.

In order to safely perform hypogastric artery ligation, the vascular anatomy must be exposed and adjacent structures, especially the ureter, must be identified. A retroperitoneal approach should be taken. The peritoneum overlying the psoas muscle (lateral to the external iliac artery) should be incised parallel to the artery. As the peritoneum is mobilized medially, the external iliac artery will first be identified. Dissection cephalad along the external iliac artery will identify the common iliac artery and the bifurcation of the internal iliac artery. Invariably, the ureter crosses the pelvic brim at the bifurcation of the common iliac artery. At this location, the ureter will be identified attached to the medial peritoneum. Further opening of the retroperitoneal space, keeping the iliac vessels lateral and the ureter medial, will open the pararectal space and further expose the internal iliac artery. Be aware that the common, external, and internal iliac veins lie just beneath their respective arteries. Without clear identification of these veins, injury can occur that will further complicate the procedure. The hypogastric artery bifurcates into an anterior and posterior branch 2–3 cm from its origin from the common iliac artery. Because most bleeding arises from the blood supply arising from the anterior division, the anterior branch should be ligated if at all possible. (Ligation of the posterior branch increases the risk of buttock pain and potential necrosis of the gluteus.) A right-angle clamp should be carefully passed from lateral to medial beneath the hypogastric artery. A heavy suture (e.g. 0-silk) should be used to ligate the artery (Fig. 17–5). There is no reason to transect the artery between two ligatures. It is usually best to perform bilateral hypogastric artery ligation, as the collateral blood supply crosses over the midline.

Finally, if all methods to control hemorrhage have been unsuccessful, the bleeding site should be packed firmly and the abdomen closed. The patient should be taken to the surgical intensive care unit and stabilized. Central monitoring and blood product replacement should be the primary focus of management. Once the patient is stabilized, attempts at angiographic embolization should be considered. Ultimately, after 24–48 h the patient should be returned to the operating room and re-explored, and the pack removed carefully. Surprisingly, many times the bleeding will have stopped due to compression of the injured veins and correction of the hypocoagulable state.

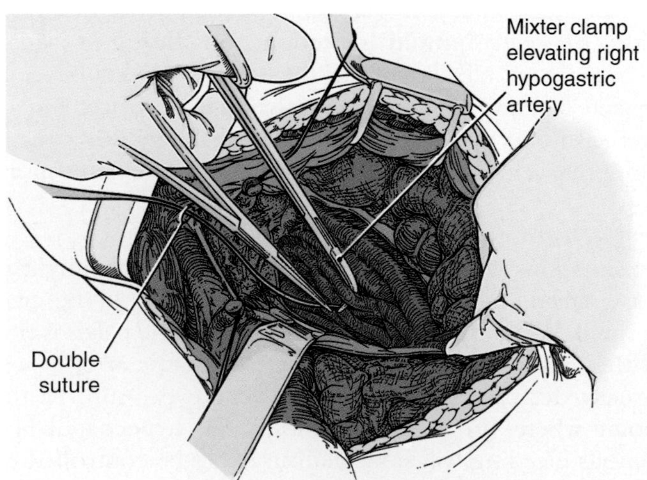

Figure 17–5 Technique for intraoperative ligation of the hypogastric artery. The ligature is placed 2–3 cm below the bifurcation so that the posterior branch will not be ligated. The clamp is passed lateral to medial to prevent trauma to the internal iliac vein. (From Nichols DH, Clarke-Pearson DL [eds]: Gynecologic, Obstetric and Related Surgery, 2nd edn. St. Louis, Mosby, 2000.)

Management of shock

During and after gynecologic surgery, blood volume deficit that results from intraoperative blood loss or postoperative hemorrhage is the most common cause of shock. This shock usually is manifested by arterial hypotension, tachycardia, a weak pulse, anxiety, skin pallor, diminished urinary output, and peripheral vasoconstriction. In addition to hemorrhage (hypovolemic shock), the differential diagnosis of shock must include many other causes, such as cardiogenic (myocardial infarction) and cardiac compressive conditions (cardiac tamponade or pneumothorax), sepsis, drug overdose, and pulmonary emboli. Appropriate studies are dictated by the patient's signs and symptoms.

Consideration should be given to obtaining arterial blood gas analysis, an electrocardiogram, a chest radiograph, blood chemistry studies, and blood cultures. The patient should be prepared for blood transfusion. The degree and duration of postoperative shock determine the need for resuscitation, central venous pressure monitoring, and Swan–Ganz pulmonary artery catheterization.

Resuscitation of a hemorrhaging patient during or after gynecologic surgery involves stabilization of the hemodynamic status and correction of the cause of the blood loss. When the hemorrhage is massive, fluid, electrolyte, and hemodynamic shifts are likewise massive. Central to stabilization efforts are the replacement and maintenance of adequate intravascular volume.

Central monitoring Invasive cardiovascular monitoring may be lifesaving for patients with massive hemorrhage or patients who are at additional risk because of pre-existing cardiopulmonary disorders. The monitoring allows the rational use of fluids and cardioactive medications while avoiding their complications.

In patients with marked hemodynamic instability, peripheral artery cannulation allows continuous monitoring of systemic arterial pressure, as well as ready access to obtain repeated analysis of arterial blood gases. The radial artery usually is chosen because of accessibility and has good collateral circulation, although the brachial and femoral arteries may be used. The complications of arterial cannulation include catheter-related septicemia (4% in one large study), local infection (as high as 18%), and arterial embolization (0.2–0.6%).

In patients without cardiopulmonary disease, monitoring of central venous pressure along with monitoring of the vital signs, urine output, and other clinical signs may be sufficient for fluid resuscitation. In addition, central venous pressure monitoring avoids several of the complications of a pulmonary artery (Swan–Ganz) catheter and may be accomplished with a simple manometer.

Table 17–5 HEMODYNAMIC CALCULATIONS[a]

Parameter	Formula	Normal range
MAP	⅓ (SBP – DBP) + DBP	0.70–105 mmHg
CO	Heart rate × stroke volume	1.4–8 L/min
Cardiac index	CO/body surface area (m^2)	2.5–4 L/min per m^2
Systemic vascular resistance	MAP – (right arterial pressure/CO)	0.10–20 U
Pulmonary vascular resistance	PAP[b] – (PCWP/CO)	1.1–3 U

CO, cardiac output; DBP, diastolic blood pressure; MAP, mean arterial pressure; PAP, mean pulmonary artery pressure; PCWP, pulmonary capillary wedge pressure; SBP, systolic blood pressure.

[a]Stroke volume can be derived from CO and heart rate. Resistance is derived from a relative change in pressure on each side of the circuit from which resistance is to be measured.

[b]PAP = [2 (pulmonary SBP) + pulmonary DBP]/3.

Central venous catheter may be introduced into the great intrathoracic veins by way of the antecubital, external or internal jugular, or subclavian veins. Cannulation of the right internal jugular vein, which provides a straight course to the right atrium, has the lowest overall complication rate. In all cases, a chest X-ray should be obtained immediately after catheter insertion to confirm proper location and to assess for possible pneumothorax.

The usefulness of the Swan–Ganz catheter in critically ill patients (even those without heart disease) who do not respond to therapy based on an initial non-invasive assessment has been well documented. Additional diagnostic information may be obtained concerning unsuspected cardiac dysfunction, pulmonary artery embolization, or sepsis. Patients without primary myocardial insult but with hypotension and evidence of inadequate perfusion of vital organs (e.g. oliguria, acidosis, mental obtundation) are better treated when data are available from central monitoring. Unnecessary fluid overload can be prevented, and the risk of congestive failure and pulmonary edema can be reduced (Table 17–5).

In patients with cardiac or pulmonary disease, cardiac output and resistance measurements allow the proper use of pressors, afterload and preload reducers, and fluids. In addition, if sepsis is part of the clinical picture, careful monitoring of pulmonary capillary wedge pressures may be necessary to prevent pulmonary edema, which is seen with even mild increases in left atrial pressures as a result of the increased permeability of the pulmonary vascular bed. This increased permeability also may be seen in patients in hypovolemic shock, again leading to pulmonary edema at relatively normal wedge pressures. Finally, invasive monitoring not only provides a direct measurement of cardiac function but also provides information within minutes about the effects of therapy.

These catheters may be placed from the antecubital fossa, although the percutaneous subclavian or internal or external jugular vein approaches are more commonly used. Complications of pulmonary artery catheters include pulmonary infarction distal to the catheter (1–2% of cases), pulmonary artery rupture (0.2% of cases), balloon rupture (3% of cases), and sepsis (2% of cases), all of which are made more likely by prolonged use of the catheter.

Intraoperative genitourinary injuries

Given the close anatomic relationships of the gynecologic organs and the urinary tract, ureteral and bladder injury are to be anticipated, even in the most skilled surgeon's hands. Of course, it is important to identify key urinary tract structures prior to embarking on a radical or extended surgery for gynecologic cancers. Retroperitoneal exploration and the opening of the lateral retroperitoneal spaces (pararectal and paravesical spaces) allows for identification of the ureter and lateral bladder. Should the medial pelvic peritoneum require resection, the ureter must be mobilized laterally (ureterolysis). This dissection of the ureter may extend throughout its entire pelvic course to the bladder, although between the uterine artery crossing the ureter and the insertion of the ureter into the bladder techniques similar to those required for a type II or III radical hysterectomy will need to be employed. Identification of the bladder is usually not a problem; however, due to anatomic distortion by advanced cancer, radiation therapy, or extensive adhesions from prior surgery, the bladder sometimes is not easily recognized. One simple method to identify the bladder is to fill it retrograde through the indwelling Foley catheter. With the bladder distended, dissection of the uterus or tumor from the bladder may be facilitated. Opening the retropubic space (space of Retzius) and the paravesical space also facilitates identification and protection of the bladder.

Injury to the bladder is usually easily corrected at the time of surgery. Incisions in the dome of the bladder should be closed in two layers with fine (3-0 or 2-0) delayed absorbable suture. Allow the bladder to heal by leaving the Foley catheter to dependent drainage for approximately 5 days. Cystotomies at the base of the bladder have a higher risk of fistula formation and ureteral occlusion. Further, they may be more difficult to recognize. Whenever there is concern about potential bladder injury, the bladder should be filled in a retrograde fashion with either sterile infant formula or indigo carmine–dyed saline. We prefer infant formula, as the formula does not stain tissues and potentially obscure the site of injury.

Once the cystotomy in the base of the bladder is identified, it is important to assess the location of the

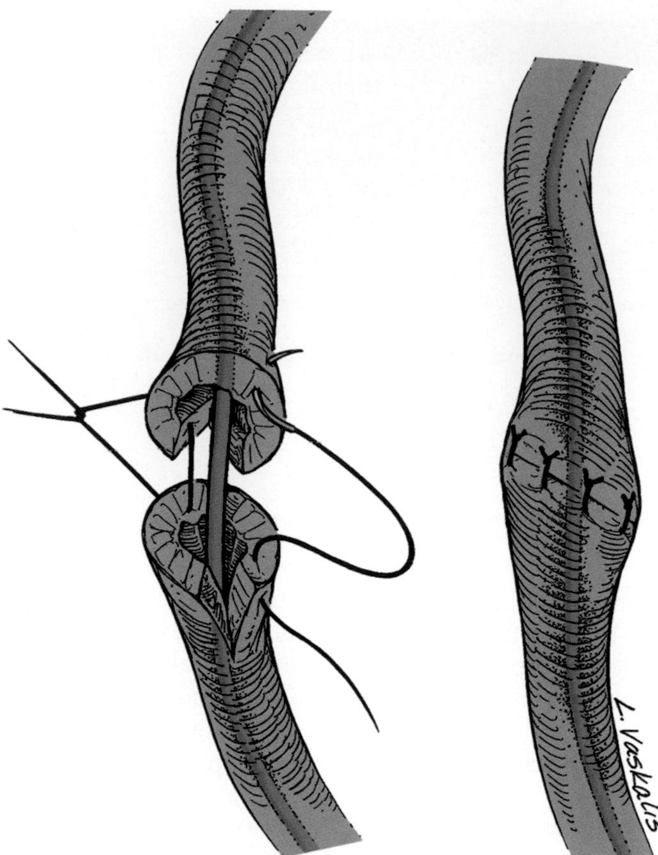

Figure 17–6 Ureteral injury at the pelvic brim repaired with an ureteroureterostomy using interrupted 4-0 delayed absorbance sutures. The ureter is spatulated to achieve a larger lumen at the anastomosis. The anastomosis is done over a ureteral stent, and the area is drained with a suction drain. (From Nichols DH, Clarke-Pearson DL [eds]: Gynecologic, Obstetric and Related Surgery, 2nd edn. St. Louis, Mosby, 2000.)

ureteral orifices. This may be accomplished by cystoscopy or by opening the dome of the bladder and directly visualizing the orifices. The administration of intravenous indigo carmine may aid in the identification of the orifices. Closure of the cystotomy should again be accomplished in two layers of delayed absorbable fine suture. If the cystotomy is near the ureteral orifice, retrograde placement of a stent may be prudent to ensure that there is no occlusion or narrowing. If the pelvis has been previously radiated, we would recommend placement of an omental J flap between the bladder and the vaginal cuff in order to bring a new, non-irradiated blood supply into this area. The Foley catheter should be left to drain for several weeks, and a cystogram should be obtained prior to the decision to remove the catheter.

Injury to the ureter as it passes through the pelvis may be managed by several methods depending on the location and extent of the injury. Ureteral injury above the pelvic brim is usually best managed by end to end anastomosis over a ureteral stent (Fig. 17–6). Injury below the pelvic brim may be best corrected by a ureteroneocystotomy with psoas hitch or a Boari flap (Fig. 17–7). In either method of repair, placement of a closed suction drain in the pelvis is advised in order to prevent a urinoma from a leak of the anastomosis.

In cases of suspected injury to the ureter, intravenous indigo carmine should be injected and the pelvis inspected for spill of dye-colored urine. If the extent of ureteral injury is a clamp crush or ligature, placement of a ureteral double-J stent left in place for 6 weeks will usually allow the injured ureter to recover and at the same time prevent ureteral stricture.

Postoperative urinary tract injury

Unless bilateral ureteral obstruction has been caused by surgery, most patients with postoperative anuria or severe oliguria will have these findings secondary to prerenal hypovolemia, which is resolved by hydration and diuresis. On the other hand, unilateral ureteral injury may not be recognized until several days postoperatively and may be manifest by flank pain, pyelonephritis, or a slight rise in serum creatinine. The volume of urinary output is rarely altered. When postoperative ureteral obstruction is suspected, evaluation may include intravenous pyelogram (IVP) or CT scan with contrast (in cases where serum creatinine is normal), or a renal ultrasound or Lasix renal scan. If ureteral obstruction is discovered, initial management should include cystoscopy with retrograde stent placement. If successful, the obstruction is likely due to tethering from nearby sutures or extrinsic compression from a mass. Leaving the stent in place for 6 weeks and then re-evaluating with follow-up IVP is recommended. If, on the other hand, a stent cannot be placed, consideration should be given to re-exploration to correct the obstruction. If reoperation is not reasonable, a PCN tube should be placed.

Radical hysterectomy for the primary treatment of cervical cancer has had urinary tract fistula considered a recognized complication. While the extensive dissection of the distal ureter and base of the bladder may lead to ischemic necrosis, in contemporary reports these fistula occur in only 1–3% of cases. The risk of fistula is increased when surgery is performed after prior pelvic radiation therapy.

Vaginal leakage of fluid during the first 10 days postoperatively is an ominous finding and requires evaluation for a urinary tract fistula. Confirming the presence of a fistula and, if present, identifying the location is the next priority. Initially, the bladder should be filled with dyed (indigo carmine) saline. A vaginal examination should reveal dye coming from the upper vagina. If there is no leakage from the bladder, then intravenous indigo carmine should be administered. Dye draining from the vagina strongly suggests a ureteral vaginal fistula. Further investigation with IVP or CT scan with intravenous contrast may further delineate the location of the fistula. Acute vesicovaginal fistula should be managed by decompression by placement of an indwelling Foley catheter to allow continuous drainage, which will often allow the fistula to close spontaneously. Similarly, if a ureterovaginal fistula is dis-

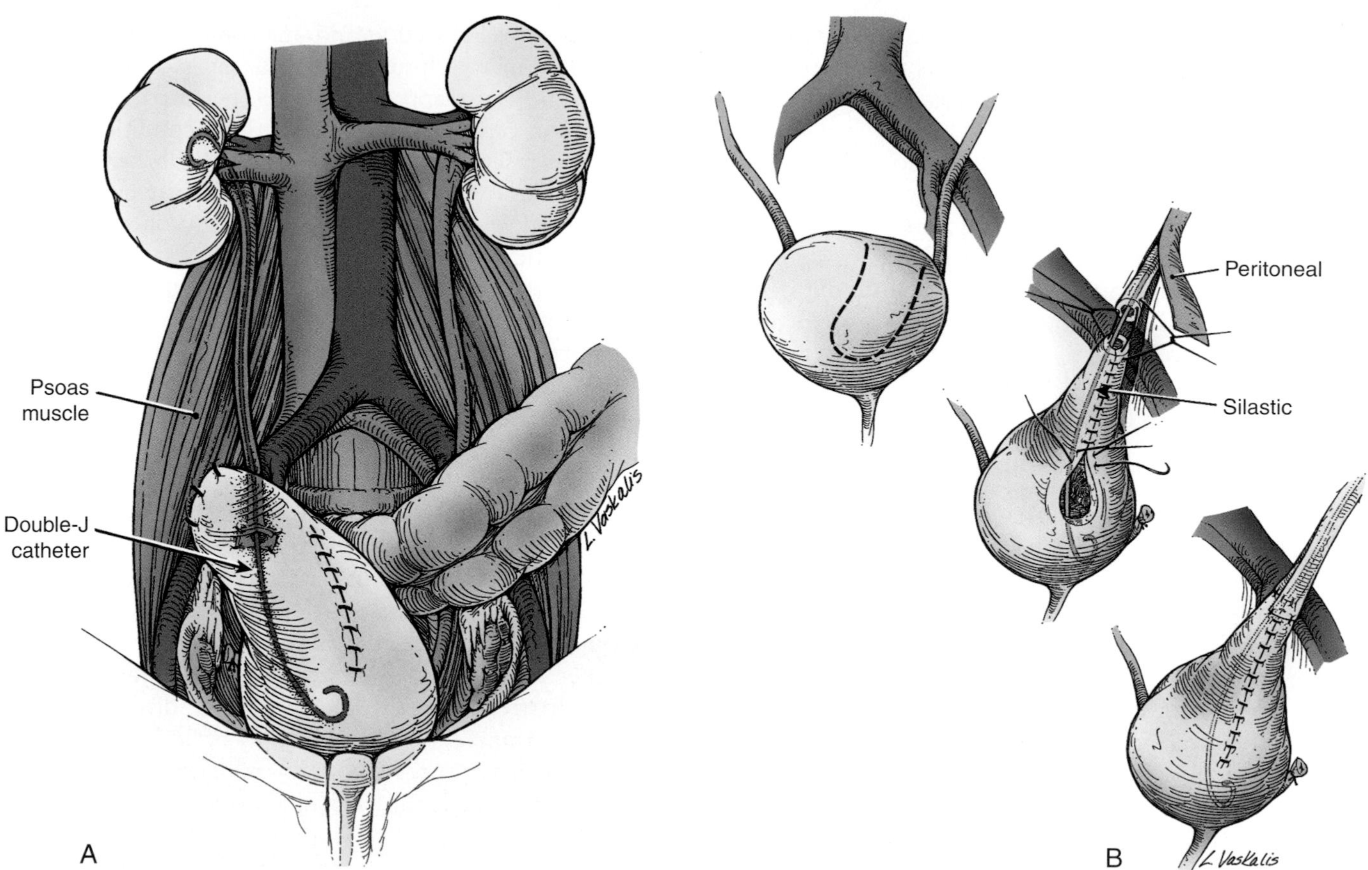

Figure 17–7 *A,* Ureteroneocystostomy with psoas hitch. Bladder is mobilized and sutured to the psoas muscle at the pelvic brim near the site of planned ureterovesical anastomosis. *B,* Boari flap. A flap from the dome of the bladder is created and "rolled" into a tube to substitute for the absent distal ureter and to reach the proximal ureter, which is reanastomosed. In either procedure, the area should be drained by closed suction. (From Nichols DH, Clarke-Pearson DL [eds]: Gynecologic, Obstetric and Related Surgery, 2nd edn. St. Louis, Mosby, 2000.)

covered a ureteral stent should be placed across the section of ureter that is fistualized. This will usually allow the ureteral injury to heal "over" the stent. Throughout attempts at conservative management, prevention of urinary tract infection is an important priority. If after 6 weeks of conservative management the vesicovaginal or ureteral fistula has not resolved, surgical correction will be required.

Bladder dysfunction after radical surgery

Voiding dysfunction following radical hysterectomy is commonly recognized and should be discussed in the preoperative informed consent. The exact frequency of occurrence depends on how the problem is diagnosed (patient report vs prospective urodynamic testing), but occurs to a greater or lesser degree in nearly all patients. It is clear that a less radical hysterectomy (type I or II) is associated with a significantly lower incidence of bladder dysfunction as compared with the traditional radical (type III) hysterectomy.

Serial cystometric studies of patients undergoing radical hysterectomy have defined the natural history of bladder function in the perioperative period. There is a nearly uniform development of detrusor hypertonia characterized by low capacity, high resting tone, and high filling pressure in the immediate postoperative phase. Bladder insensitivity to filling is also present. The patient often has difficulty initiating her stream and may have overflow incontinence when the capacity is exceeded. Hypertonia generally subsides within 3–6 months, but other abnormalities often persist for years. The duration of bladder dysfunction is also variable, with extremes recognized as full recovery of bladder function to the rare patient who will require lifetime intermittent self-catheterization to achieve adequate bladder drainage. Many patients have persistent decrease in bladder sensation or prolonged urinary hesitancy.

The pathophysiologic mechanism of voiding dysfunction after radical hysterectomy is still not clearly understood. Some investigators have proposed that incomplete innervation of the bladder produces a temporary parasympathomimetic predominance that usually resolves with nerve regeneration. The use of parasympatholytic drugs, however, has been ineffective in altering the detrusor muscle. Forney et al have suggested that disruption of the sympathetic fibers that travel through the paracervical web results in loss of inhibition for the detrusor and trigone, leaving an uncoordinated parasympathetic dominance.

This is supported by the observation that incomplete division of the cardinal ligament results in decreased post-operative detrusor hypertonia compared with complete division.

It also seems clear that over-distension of the bladder aggravates bladder dysfunction. Therefore a variety of techniques have been proposed to avoid over-distension, including short-term or long-term use of a ureteral Foley catheter, suprapubic catheter, or intermittent self-catheterization. All techniques have their proponents and varying degrees of success, but none have been proven to be superior.

Intraoperative gastrointestinal injuries

A mechanical bowel preparation should be planned for all patients undergoing major abdominal surgery. We believe that bowel preparation will reduce the risk of intestinal injury, and if injury does occur, spill of gastrointestinal contents will be minimized. Further, with the bowel empty closure is much easier and there is diminished risk of infection in the case of colonic injury. In the past, mechanical methods to prepare the bowel have included the use of cathartics such as magnesium citrate or the ingestion of 4 L of polyethelene glycol (Go-lytely). Our preference, based on a randomized clinical trial, is to use Fleets phosphosoda the day before surgery (Table 17–6).

The use of oral antibiotics (erythromycin and neomycin) has traditionally been recommended to reduce infectious complications following colonic surgery. The data on which this recommendation has been made were developed in an era prior to parenteral broad-spectrum antibiotics. Today, there is little evidence that oral antibiotic bowel preparation is necessary if the patient is to receive parenteral antibiotic prophylaxis.

Prior abdominal surgery and radiation therapy increase the probability of intraoperative injury to the small intestine. Adhesions to the anterior abdominal wall or small intestines adherent to the pelvic peritoneum increase the risk of entry into the intestines as adhesions are lysed. Interruption of the serosal and superficial muscular layers should be repaired with interrupted 2-0 or 3-0 sutures. Care should be taken to avoid narrowing of the intestinal caliber (Fig. 17–8). If the entire thickness of the intestine is entered, the segment of bowel must be assessed to decide whether primary closure should be undertaken or whether bowel resection and anastomosis should be performed. Primary closure is usually safely accomplished if the closure can reapproximate well-perfused bowel under no tension on the suture line. If these conditions cannot be met, resection and anastomosis will be necessary. Primary closure should be in two layers, the first being an interrupted layer of 2-0 or 3-0 polyglycolic acid suture incorporating the mucosa and muscularis with the knot tied into the intestinal lumen. A second imbricating layer may be of either absorbable or non-absorbable suture and incorporates the serosa and superficial muscularis (Fig. 17–9). Attention to the direction of closure of the enterotomy should ensure that the lumen is not narrowed. In most cases following closure of an enterotomy or a small bowel resection and anastomosis, a nasogastric tube is placed, although this practice is somewhat controversial.

Injury to the colon most commonly occurs in the pelvis, and the risk is increased in the face of prior pelvic surgery, cancer involving the colon, or prior radiation therapy. If colonic injury occurs, the decision must be made as to whether a primary closure is sufficiently safe or whether the fecal stream should be temporarily diverted by performing a transverse loop colostomy or ileostomy. In most cases, primary closure without diversion may be performed, especially if the patient has had a mechanical bowel preparation. The principles for closure require viable tissue and no tension on the closure. In patients who have had prior pelvic radiation, the risk of perforation of the colostomy closure is significantly increased and diversion is usually

Table 17–6 MECHANICAL BOWEL PREPARATION REGIMEN

Day before surgery:
- One bottle of phosphosoda (1.5 oz) 4 p.m.
- Four bisacodyl (Dulcolax) tablets 7 p.m.
- Oral metoclopramide (Reglan) 10 mg noon and 6 p.m.
- Clear liquids for 24 h

(From Cohen SM et al: Prospective, randomized, endoscopic-blinded trial comparing precolonoscopy bowel cleansing methods. Dis Colon Rectum 37:689, 1994.)

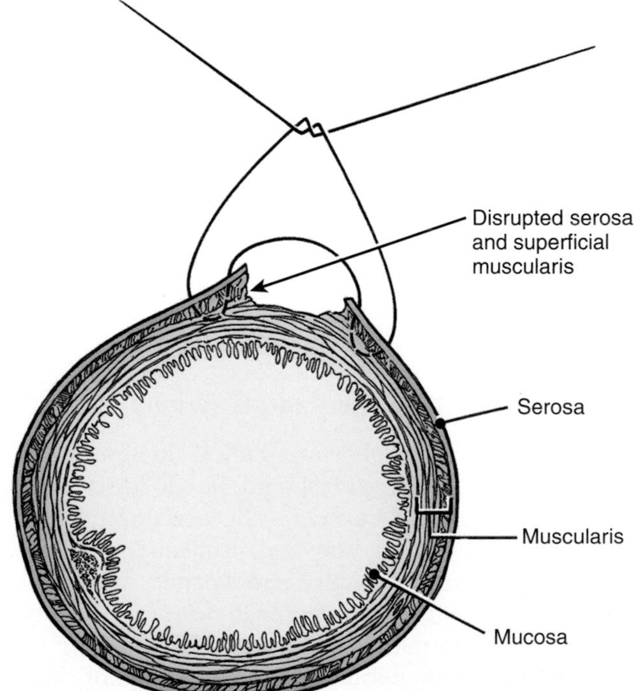

Figure 17–8 Repair of seromuscular injury of small or larger bowel. Interrupted imbricating sutures used to reap proximate the injured seromuscular layer. (From Nichols DH, Clarke-Pearson DL [eds]: Gynecologic, Obstetric and Related Surgery, 2nd edn. St. Louis, Mosby, 2000.)

advised. Following a two-layered closure of a rectosigmoid injury, we routinely perform a "bubble test" (Fig. 17–10).

Postoperative gastrointestinal complications

Ileus

Following abdominal or pelvic surgery, most patients will experience some degree of intestinal ileus. The exact mechanism by which this arrest and disorganization of gastrointestinal motility occurs is unknown, but it appears to be associated with the opening of the peritoneal cavity and is aggravated by manipulation of the intestinal tract and prolonged surgical procedures. Infection, peritonitis, and electrolyte disturbances may also result in ileus. For most patients undergoing gynecologic cancer operations, the degree of ileus is minimal and gastrointestinal function returns relatively rapidly, allowing the resumption of oral intake within a few days of surgery. Patients who have persistently diminished bowel sounds, abdominal distension, and nausea and vomiting require further evaluation and more aggressive treatment.

Ileus is usually manifest by abdominal distension and should be evaluated initially by physical examination, assessing the quality of bowel sounds and searching for tenderness or rebound on palpation. The possibility that the patient's signs and symptoms may be associated with a more serious intestinal obstruction or other intestinal complication must be considered. Pelvic examination should be performed to evaluate the possibility of a pelvic abscess or hematoma that may contribute to the ileus. Abdominal x-ray to evaluate the abdomen in the supine position as well as in the upright position usually will aid in the diagnosis of an ileus. The most common radiographic findings include dilated loops of small and large bowel, as well as air–fluid levels in the upright position. In the postoperative gynecology patient, especially in the upright position, the flat plate of the abdomen may also show evidence of free air. This is a common finding following surgery, which lasts 7–10 days in some instances and is not indicative of a perforated viscus in most patients. The remote possibility of distal colonic obstruction or pseudo-obstruction (Ogilvie syndrome) suggested by a dilated cecum should be excluded by rectal examination, proctosigmoidoscopy, or barium enema.

The initial management of a postoperative ileus is aimed at gastrointestinal tract decompression and maintenance of appropriate intravenous replacement fluids and electrolytes.

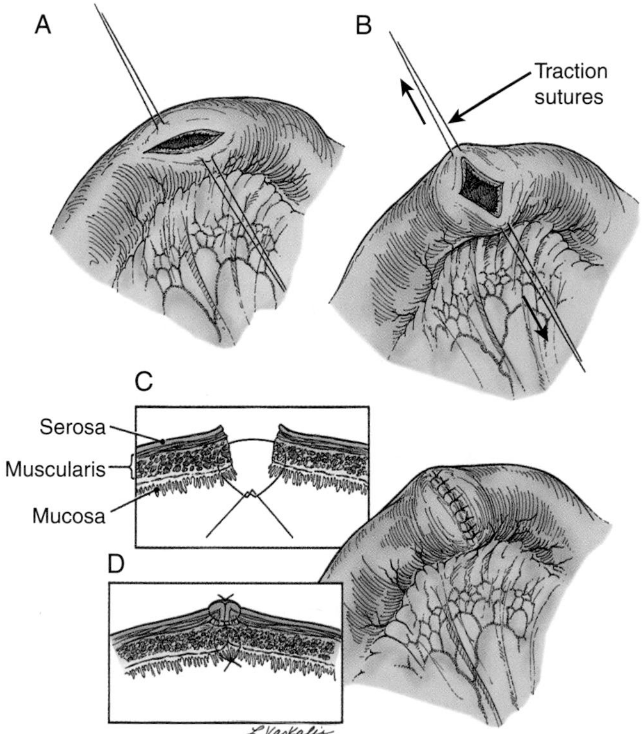

Figure 17–9 Repair of enterotomy. *A* and *B*, The repair should be performed so that the closure is perpendicular to the axis of the small bowel. *C* and *D*, Two-layer closure incorporating the mucosa and muscularis in the inner layer and the serosa and muscularis on the outer layer. (From Nichols DH, Clarke-Pearson DL [eds]: Gynecologic, Obstetric and Related Surgery, 2nd edn. St. Louis, Mosby, 2000.)

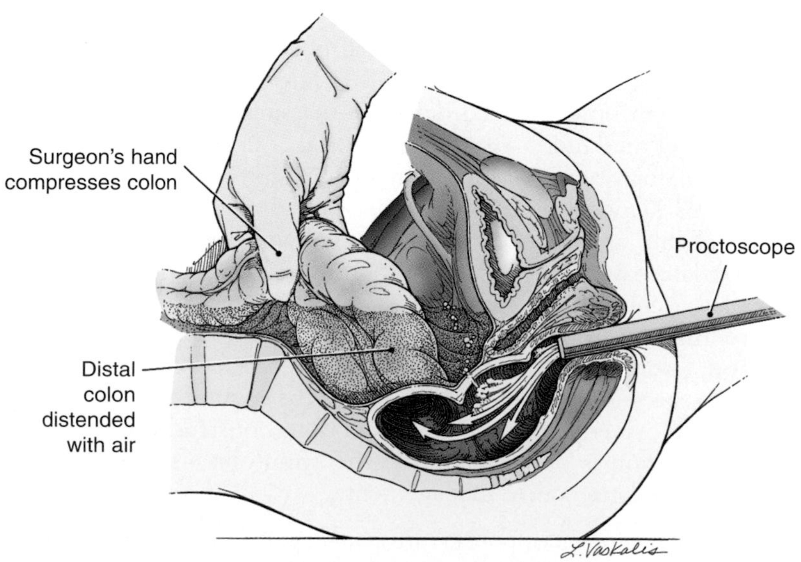

Figure 17–10 "Bubble test" to evaluate for rectosigmoid injury and to ensure a "watertight" closure of a colostomy or rectosigmoid anastomosis. The pelvis is filled with saline, and the proximal sigmoid or descending colon is occluded above the segment to be tested. Insert a proctoscope into the anus and inflate with air. Distend the occluded rectosigmoid colon with air and observe for bubbles, which would indicate a bowel defect. (From Nichols DH, Clarke-Pearson DL [eds]: Gynecologic, Obstetric and Related Surgery, 2nd edn. St. Louis, Mosby, 2000.)

- A nasogastric tube should evacuate the stomach of its fluid and gaseous contents. Prolonged nasogastric suction continues to remove swallowed air, which is the most common source of air in the small bowel.
- Fluid and electrolyte replacement must be adequate to keep the patient well perfused. Significant amounts of third-space fluid loss occur in the bowel wall, the bowel lumen, and the peritoneal cavity during the acute episode. Gastrointestinal fluid losses from the stomach may lead to a metabolic alkalosis and depletion of other electrolytes as well. Careful monitoring of serum chemistries and appropriate replacement are necessary.
- Most cases of severe ileus will begin to improve over a period of several days. In general, this is recognized by reduction in the abdominal distension, return of normal bowel sounds, and passage of flatus or stool. Follow-up abdominal x-rays should be obtained as necessary for further monitoring.
- When the gastrointestinal tract function appears to have returned to normal, the nasogastric tube may be removed and a liquid diet may be instituted.
- If a patient shows no evidence of improvement during the first 48–72 h of medical management, other causes of ileus should be sought. Such cases may include ureteral injury, peritonitis from pelvic infection, unrecognized gastrointestinal tract injury with peritoneal spill, or fluid and electrolyte abnormalities such as hypokalemia. In the evaluation of persistent ileus, the use of water-soluble upper gastrointestinal contrast studies may assist in the resolution of the ileus.

Small bowel obstruction

Obstruction of the small bowel following abdominal surgery occurs in approximately 1–2% of patients but may be more frequent after radical gynecologic oncology procedures, due to the extensive dissection and sometimes extensive manipulation of the small bowel. The most common cause of small bowel obstruction is adhesions to the operative site. If the small bowel becomes adherent in a twisted position, partial or complete obstruction may result from distension, ileus, or bowel wall edema. Less common causes of postoperative small bowel obstruction include entrapment of the small bowel into an incisional hernia and an unrecognized defect in the small bowel or large bowel mesentery. Early in its clinical course, a postoperative small bowel obstruction may exhibit signs and symptoms identical to those of ileus. Initial conservative management as outlined for the treatment of ileus is appropriate. Because of the potential for mesenteric vascular occlusion and resulting ischemia or perforation, worsening symptoms of abdominal pain, progressive distension, fever, leukocytosis, or acidosis should be evaluated carefully, because immediate surgery may be required.

In most cases of postoperative small bowel obstruction, the obstruction is only partial and the symptoms usually resolve with conservative management.

- After several days of conservative management, further investigation may be necessary. Evaluation of the gastrointestinal tract with barium enema and an upper gastrointestinal series with small bowel follow-through are appropriate. Alternatively, an abdominal and pelvic CT scan with gastrointestinal contrast may be useful in identifying the location of obstruction (and also evaluates for the presence of an abscess, a lymphocele, or a ureteral injury). In most cases, complete obstruction is not documented, although a narrowing or tethering of the segment of small bowel may indicate the site of the problem.
- Further conservative management with nasogastric decompression and intravenous fluid replacement may allow time for bowel wall edema or torsion of the mesentery to resolve.
- If resolution is prolonged and the patient's nutritional status is marginal, the use of TPN may be necessary.
- Conservative medical management of postoperative small bowel obstruction usually results in complete resolution. However, if persistent evidence of small bowel obstruction remains after full evaluation and an adequate trial of medical management, exploratory laparotomy may be necessary to surgically evaluate and manage the obstruction. In most cases, lysis of adhesions is all that is required, although a segment of small bowel that is badly damaged or extensively sclerosed from adhesions may require resection and reanastomosis.

Colonic obstruction

Postoperative colonic obstruction following gynecologic oncology surgery is exceedingly rare. Advanced ovarian carcinoma is the most common cause of colonic obstruction in postoperative gynecologic surgery patients and is caused by extrinsic impingement on the colon by the pelvic malignancy. Occult intrinsic colonic lesions (e.g. colon cancer) also may cause obstruction. When colonic obstruction is manifest by abdominal distension and abdominal radiographs reveal a dilated colon and enlarging cecum, further evaluation of the large bowel is required by barium enema or colonoscopy. Dilation of the cecum to more than 10–12 cm in diameter as viewed by abdominal x-ray requires immediate evaluation and surgical decompression by performing a colectomy or colostomy. In some circumstances, an intraluminal stent may be placed endoscopically. Surgery should be performed as soon as the obstruction is documented. Conservative management of colonic obstruction is not appropriate, because the complication of colonic perforation has an exceedingly high mortality rate.

Diarrhea

Episodes of diarrhea often occur following abdominal and pelvic surgery as the gastrointestinal tract returns to its normal function and motility. However, prolonged and multiple episodes may represent a pathologic process such as impending small bowel obstruction, colonic obstruction, or pseudomembranous colitis. Excessive amounts of diarrhea should be evaluated by abdominal x-rays and stool samples tested for the presence of ova and parasites, bacterial culture, and *Clostridium difficile* toxin. Proctoscopy and colonoscopy may also be advisable in severe cases.

Evidence of intestinal obstruction should be managed as outlined previously. Infectious causes of diarrhea should be managed with the appropriate antibiotics as well as fluid and electrolyte replacement. *Clostridium difficile*–associated pseudomembranous colitis may result from exposure to any antibiotic. Discontinuation of these antibiotics (unless they are needed for another severe infection) is advisable, along with the institution of appropriate therapy. Because of the expense of vancomycin, we usually institute therapy with oral metronidazole. Therapy should be continued until the diarrhea abates, and several weeks of oral therapy may be required in order to obtain complete resolution of the pseudomembranous colitis.

Fistula

Gastrointestinal fistulas are relatively rare following gynecologic surgery. They are most often associated with malignancy, prior radiation therapy, or surgical injury to the large or small bowel that was improperly repaired or unrecognized. Signs and symptoms of gastrointestinal fistula are often similar to those of small bowel obstruction or ileus, except that a fever is usually a more prominent component of the patient's symptoms. When fever is associated with gastrointestinal dysfunction postoperatively, evaluation should include early assessment of the gastrointestinal tract for its continuity. When fistula is suspected, the use of water-soluble gastrointestinal contrast material is advised to avoid the complication of barium peritonitis. Evaluation with abdominal pelvic CT scan may also assist in identification of a fistula and associated abscess. Recognition of an intraperitoneal gastrointestinal leak or fistula formation usually requires immediate surgery, unless the fistula has drained spontaneously through the abdominal wall or vaginal cuff.

An enterocutaneous fistula arising from the small bowel and draining spontaneously through the abdominal incision may be managed successfully with medical therapy. Therapy should include nasogastric decompression, replacement of intravenous fluids as well as TPN, and appropriate antibiotics to treat an associated mixed bacterial infection. If the infection is under control and there are no other signs of peritonitis, the surgeon may consider allowing potential resolution of the fistula over a period of up to 2 weeks. Some authors have suggested the use of somatostatin to decrease intestinal tract secretion and allow earlier healing of the fistula. In many cases, especially if the bowel was not radiated, the fistula will close spontaneously with this mode of management. If the enterocutaneous fistula does not close with conservative medical management, surgical correction with resection, bypass, or reanastomosis will be necessary.

A rectovaginal fistula that occurs following gynecologic surgery is usually the result of surgical trauma that may have been aggravated by the presence of extensive adhesions or tumor involvement of the rectosigmoid colon and cul-de-sac. Low rectal anastomoses are also at risk to break down and lead to a rectovaginal fistula. A small rectovaginal fistula may be managed with a conservative medical approach in the hope that decreasing the fecal stream will allow closure of the fistula. A small fistula that allows continence except for an occasional leak of flatus may be managed conservatively until the inflammatory process in the pelvis resolves. At that point, usually several months later, correction of the fistula is appropriate. Larger rectovaginal fistulas that have no hope of closing spontaneously are best managed by performing an initial diverting colostomy followed by repair of the fistula after inflammation has resolved. After the fistula closure is healed and deemed successful, the colostomy taken down and closed.

Lymphocysts

The occurrence of lymphocysts after pelvic and para-aortic lymphadenectomy is recognized in approximately 2% of cases. It has been suggested that prevention requires the ligation of the ascending lymphatics at the time of lymphadenectomy. Further, there is evidence that the use of LDH increases lymphatic drainage and lymphocyst formation. In years past, the parietal peritoneum was closed after lymphadenectomy and a retroperitoneal suction drain was placed in the retroperitoneal space in order to suction any lymphatic fluid. Certainly, a suction drain is reasonable and likely does prevent lymphocysts whenever the retroperitoneum is closed. Currently, most gynecologic oncologists do not close the peritoneum, allowing the lymphatic fluid to drain into the peritoneal cavity and be reabsorbed. Retrospective reports indicate that there is no increase in lymphocyst formation using this strategy. However, the problem of lymphocyst formation has not been entirely eliminated.

Lymphocysts may be recognized clinically by palpation of a mass, commonly in the iliac fossa on abdominal examination. They may also be discovered as a pelvic sidewall mass on pelvic examination. Most will be asymptomatic. However, when a lymphocyst is found, investigation should be undertaken to evaluate for ureteral or venous obstruction. If hydroureter is found, the lymphocyst should be drained. This may usually be accomplished by an interventional radiologist who can place a percutaneous drain in the lymphocyst. Suction drainage will collapse the lymphocyst and allow the cyst walls to sclerose together. If percutaneous drainage is not feasible or is unsuccessful, surgical exploration may be required to excise a wall of the lymphocyst and allow the lymphatic fluid to drain into the peritoneal cavity. Placing an omental J flap into the cavity of the lymphocyst has been suggested to provide additional routes of lymphatic drainage. When extrinsic venous compression is discovered to be associated with a lymphocyst, the patient should be evaluated for the possibility of a venous thrombosis. If a venous thrombosis is found, we would advise anticoagulation in order to stop propagation and allow stabilization of the thrombus. Thereafter, the lymphocyst should be drained. Drainage of the lymphocyst prior to anticoagulation may result in venous decompression and subsequent embolization of the thrombus. Rarely, lymphocysts will become infected and require drainage and antibiotic therapy.

Lymphocysts can also occur in the inguinal region after inguinofemoral lymphadenectomy performed as part of the staging and treatment of vulvar carcinoma. Small asymptomatic lymphocysts may be managed by observation. However, larger lymphocysts usually cause pain or lymphedema and will require drainage with placement of a closed suction drain. Repeated aspiration increases the probability of infection of the lymphocyst.

Postoperative infections

Infections are a major source of morbidity in the postoperative period. Risk factors for infectious morbidity in the gynecologic oncology patient include a lack of perioperative antibiotic prophylaxis, contamination of the surgical field from infected tissues or from spillage of large bowel contents, an immunocompromised host, diabetes, poor nutrition, chronic and debilitating severe illness, poor surgical technique, and pre-existing focal or systemic infection. Sources of postoperative infection can include the lung, urinary tract, surgical site, pelvic sidewall, vaginal cuff, abdominal wound, and sites of indwelling intravenous catheters. Early identification and treatment of any infections will result in the best outcome from these potentially serious complications.

Although infectious morbidity is an inevitable complication of surgery, the incidence of infections can be decreased by the appropriate use of simple preventive measures. In cases that involve transection of the large bowel, spillage of fecal contents also inevitably occurs. Preoperative mechanical and antibiotic bowel preparation in combination with systemic antibiotic prophylaxis will help decrease the incidence of postoperative pelvic and abdominal infections in these patients. The surgeon can further decrease the risk of postoperative infections by using meticulous surgical technique. Blood and necrotic tissue are excellent media for the growth of aerobic and anaerobic organisms. In cases in which there is higher than usual potential for serum and blood to collect in spaces that have been contaminated by bacterial spill, closed-suction drainage may reduce the risk of infection. Elective surgical procedures should be postponed in patients who have an infection preoperatively.

Historically, the standard definition of febrile morbidity for surgical patients has been the presence of a temperature higher than or equal to 38°C (100.4°F) on two occasions at least 4 h apart in the postoperative period, excluding the first 24 h. However, other sources have defined fever as two consecutive temperature elevations greater than 38.3°C (101.0°F). Febrile morbidity has been estimated to occur in as many as one-half of patients; however, it is often self-limited, resolving without therapy, and is usually non-infectious in origin. The value of 38.3°C is more useful than 38°C to distinguish patients with an infectious etiology vs an inconsequential postoperative fever.

The assessment of febrile surgical patients should include a review of the patient's history with regard to risk factors. Both the history and the physical examination should focus on the potential sites of infection. The examination should include inspection of the pharynx, a thorough pulmonary examination, percussion of the kidneys to assess for costovertebral angle tenderness, inspection and palpation of the abdominal incision, an examination of sites of intravenous catheters, and an examination of the extremities for evidence of DVT or thrombophlebitis. In gynecologic patients, an appropriate workup may also include inspection and palpation of the vaginal cuff for signs of induration, tenderness, or purulent drainage. A pelvic examination should also be performed in order to identify a mass suggesting a pelvic hematoma or abscess and to look for signs of pelvic cellulitis.

Patients with a fever in the early postoperative period should have an aggressive pulmonary toilet, including incentive spirometry. If the fever persists beyond 72 h postoperatively, additional laboratory and radiologic data may be obtained. The evaluation may include complete and differential white blood cell counts, and a urinalysis. A routine urine culture had a yield of only 9%, therefore one should not be sent unless indicated by the urinalysis results or symptoms. Routine chest x-rays have a yield of 12.5% and should be obtained in patients with and without signs and symptoms localizing to the lung. Blood cultures can also be obtained but will most likely be of little yield unless the patient has a high fever (38.9°C, 102°F). In patients with costovertebral angle tenderness, CT scan, renal ultrasound, or IVP may be indicated to rule out the presence of ureteral damage or obstruction from surgery, particularly in the absence of laboratory evidence of urinary tract infection. Patients who have persistent fevers without a clear localizing source should undergo CT scanning of the abdomen and pelvis to rule out the presence of an intra-abdominal abscess. Finally, in patients who have had gastrointestinal surgery, a barium enema or upper gastrointestinal series with small bowel follow-through may be indicated late in the course of the first postoperative week if fever persists to rule out an anastomotic leak or fistula.

Urinary tract infections

Historically, the urinary tract has been the most common site of infection in surgical patients. However, the incidence reported in the more recent gynecologic literature has been less than 4%. This decrease in urinary tract infections is most likely the result of increased perioperative use of prophylactic antibiotics.

Symptoms of a urinary tract infection may include urinary frequency, urgency, and dysuria. In patients with pyelonephritis, other symptoms include flank pain, headache, malaise, nausea, and vomiting. A urinary tract infection is diagnosed on the basis of microbiology and has been defined as the growth of 105 organisms/mL of urine cultured. Most infections are caused by coliform bacteria, with *Escherichia coli* being the most frequent pathogen. Other pathogens include *Klebsiella*, *Proteus*, and *Enterobacter* species. *Staphylococcus* organisms are the causative bacteria in fewer than 10% of cases.

Despite the high incidence of urinary tract infections in the postoperative period, few of these infections are serious. Most are confined to the lower urinary tract, and pyelonephritis is a rare complication. Catheterization of the urinary tract, either intermittently or continuously with the use of an indwelling catheter, has been implicated as a main cause of urinary tract contamination.

The treatment of urinary tract infection includes hydration and antibiotic therapy. Commonly prescribed and effective antibiotics include sulfonamide, cephalosporins, fluoroquinolones, and nitrofurantoin. The choice of antibiotic should be based on knowledge of the susceptibility of organisms cultured at a particular institution. In some institutions, for example, more than 40% of *E. coli* strains are resistant to ampicillin. For uncomplicated urinary tract infections, an antibiotic that has good activity against *E. coli* should be given in the interim while awaiting the urine culture and sensitivity data.

Patients who have a history of recurrent urinary tract infections, those with chronic indwelling catheters (Foley catheters or ureteral stents), and those who have urinary conduits should be treated with antibiotics that will be effective against the less common urinary pathogens such as *Klebsiella* and *Pseudomonas.* Chronic use of the fluoroquinolones for prophylaxis is not advised, because these agents are notorious for inducing antibiotic-resistant strains of bacteria.

Pulmonary infections

The respiratory tract is a relatively common site for complications following surgery for gynecologic cancer. Risk factors include extensive or prolonged atelectasis, pre-existent chronic obstructive pulmonary disease, severe or debilitating illness, central neurologic disease causing an inability to clear oropharyngeal secretions effectively, and nasogastric suction. In surgical patients, early ambulation and aggressive management of atelectasis are the most important preventive measures.

A significant proportion (40–50%) of hospital-acquired pneumonias are caused by gram-negative organisms. These organisms gain access to the respiratory tract from the oral pharynx. Gram-negative colonization of the oral pharynx has been shown to be increased in patients in acute care facilities and has been associated with the presence of nasogastric tubes, pre-existing respiratory disease, mechanical ventilation, tracheal intubation, and paralytic ileus, which is associated with microbial overgrowth in the stomach.

A thorough lung examination should be included in the assessment of all febrile surgical patients. In the absence of significant lung findings, a chest x-ray should nonetheless be obtained in patients at high risk for pulmonary complications. A sputum sample should also be obtained for gram stain and culture. The treatment should include postural drainage, aggressive pulmonary toilet, and antibiotics. The antibiotic chosen should be effective against both gram-positive and gram-negative organisms, and in patients who are receiving assisted ventilation the antibiotic spectrum should include drugs that are active against *Pseudomonas* organisms.

Wound infections

The results of a prospective study of more than 62,000 wounds are revealing in regard to the epidemiology of wound infections. The wound infection rate varied markedly depending on the extent of contamination of the surgical field. The wound infection rate for clean surgical cases (infection not present in the surgical field, no break in aseptic technique, no viscus entered) was lower than 2%, whereas the incidence of wound infections with dirty, infected cases was 40% or higher. Preoperative showers with hexachlorophene slightly lowered the infection rate for clean wounds, whereas preoperative shaving of the wound site with a razor increased the infection rate. A 5-min wound preparation immediately before surgery was as effective as preparation 10 min before surgery. The wound infection rate increased with the duration of the preoperative hospital stay as well as with the duration of the surgical procedure. In addition, incidental appendectomy increased the risk of wound infection in patients undergoing clean surgical procedures. The study concluded that the incidence of wound infections could be decreased by short preoperative hospital stays, hexachlorophene showers prior to surgery, minimizing shaving of the wound site, use of meticulous surgical technique, decreasing operative time as much as possible, bringing drains out through sites other than the wound, and dissemination of information to surgeons regarding their wound infection rates. A program instituting these conclusions led to a fall in the clean wound infection rate from 2.5 to 0.6% over an 8-year period. While the wound infection rate in most gynecologic services has been lower than 5%, reflective of the "clean" nature of most gynecologic operations, it is higher is the gynecologic oncology patient.

The symptoms of wound infection often occur late in the postoperative period, usually after the fourth postoperative day, and may include the presence of fever, erythema, tenderness, induration, and purulent wound drainage. Wound infections that occur on postoperative days 1 through 3 are generally caused by streptococcal and clostridial infections. The management of wound infections is mostly mechanical and involves opening the infected portion of the wound above the fascia, with cleansing and debridement of the wound edges as necessary. Wound care, consisting of debridement and dressing changes two or three times daily with mesh gauze, will promote growth of granulation tissue, with gradual filling in of the wound defect by secondary intention. The application of a Wound Vac to larger wounds speeds recovery and minimizes dressing changes. Clean, granulating wounds can often be secondarily closed with good success, shortening the time required for complete wound healing.

The technique of delayed primary wound closure can be used in contaminated surgical cases to lower the incidence of wound infection. Briefly, this technique involves leaving the wound open above the fascia at the time of the initial surgical procedure. Vertical interrupted mattress sutures though the skin and subcutaneous layers are placed 3 cm apart but are not tied. Wound care is instituted immediately after surgery and continued until the wound is noted to be granulating well. Sutures may then be tied, and the skin edges further approximated using sutures or staples. Using this technique of delayed primary wound closure, the overall wound infection rate has been shown to be decreased from 23 to 2.1% in high-risk patients.

Vaginal cuff infection following hysterectomy is characterized by erythema, induration, and tenderness at the vaginal cuff. Occasionally, a purulent discharge from the apex of the vagina may also be present. The cellulitis is often self-limited and does not require any treatment. Fever, leukocytosis, and pain localized to the pelvis may accompany severe cuff cellulitis and most often signifies extension of the cellulitis to adjacent pelvic tissues. In such cases, broad-spectrum antibiotic therapy should be instituted with coverage for gram-negative, gram-positive, and anaerobic organisms. If purulence at the vaginal cuff is excessive or if there is a fluctuant mass noted at the vaginal cuff, the vaginal cuff should be gently probed and opened with a blunt instrument. The cuff can then be left open for dependent drainage.

Intra-abdominal and pelvic abscess

The development of an abscess in the surgical field or elsewhere in the abdominal cavity is most likely to occur in contaminated cases in which the surgical site is not adequately drained, or as a secondary complication of hematomas. The causative pathogens in patients who have intra-abdominal abscess are usually polymicrobial in nature. The aerobes most commonly identified include *E. coli*, *Klebsiella*, *Streptococcus*, *Proteus*, and *Enterobacter*. Anaerobic isolates are also common, usually from the *Bacteroides* group. These pathogens are mainly from the vaginal tract but also can be derived from the gastrointestinal tract, particularly when the colon has been entered at the time of surgery.

Intra-abdominal abscess is sometimes difficult to diagnose. The evolving clinical picture is often one of persistent febrile episodes with a rising white blood cell count. Findings on abdominal examination may be equivocal. If an abscess is located deep in the pelvis, it may be palpable by pelvic or rectal examination. For abscesses above the pelvis, diagnosis will depend on radiologic confirmation.

Ultrasound can occasionally delineate fluid collections in the upper abdomen as well as in the pelvis. However, bowel gas interference makes visualization of fluid collections or abscesses in the mid-abdomen difficult to distinguish. CT scanning is therefore much more sensitive and specific for diagnosing intra-abdominal abscesses and is the radiologic procedure of choice.

Standard therapy for intra-abdominal abscess is evacuation and drainage combined with appropriate parenteral administration of antibiotics. Abscesses located low in the pelvis, particularly in the area of the vaginal cuff, can often be reached through a vaginal approach. In many patients, the ability to drain an abscess by placement of a drain percutaneously under CT guidance has obviated the need for surgical exploration. With CT guidance, a pigtail catheter is placed into an abscess cavity via percutaneous, transperineal, transrectal, or transvaginal approaches. The catheter is left in place until drainage decreases. Transperineal and transrectal drainage of deep pelvic abscesses has been successful in 90–93% of patients, obviating the need for surgical management. However, for those patients in whom radiologic drainage is not successful, surgical exploration and evacuation are indicated. The gold standard of initial antibiotic therapy has been the combination of ampicillin, gentamycin, and clindamycin. Adequate treatment can also be achieved with currently available broad-spectrum single agents (including the broad-spectrum penicillin), second- and third-generation cephalosporins, levofloxacin and metronidazole, and the sulbactam/clavulanic acid-containing preparations.

Necrotizing fasciitis

Necrotizing fasciitis is an uncommon infectious disorder; approximately 1000 cases occur annually in the USA. The disorder is characterized by a rapidly progressive bacterial infection involving the subcutaneous tissues and fascia while characteristically sparing underlying muscle. Systemic toxicity is a frequent feature of this disease, as manifest by the presence of dehydration, septic shock, disseminated intravascular coagulation, and multiorgan system failure.

The pathogenesis of necrotizing fasciitis involves a polymicrobial infection of the dermis and subcutaneous tissue. Hemolytic *Streptococcus* was initially believed to be the primary pathogen responsible for the infection in necrotizing fasciitis. However, it is now evident that numerous other organisms are present in addition to *Streptococcus*, including other gram-positive organisms, coliforms, and anaerobes. Bacterial enzymes such as hyaluronidase and lipase released in the subcutaneous space destroy the fascia and adipose tissue, and induce a liquefactive necrosis. In addition, non-inflammatory intravascular coagulation or thrombosis subsequently occurs. Intravascular coagulation results in ischemia and necrosis of the subcutaneous tissues and skin. Late in the course of the infection, destruction of the superficial nerves produces anesthesia in the involved skin. The release of bacteria and bacterial toxins into the systemic circulation can cause septic shock, acid–base disturbances, and multiorgan impairment.

The diagnostic criteria for necrotizing fasciitis include extensive necrosis of the superficial fascia and subcutaneous tissue with peripheral undermining of the normal skin, a moderate to severe systemic toxic reaction, the absence of muscle involvement, the absence of *Clostridia* in wound and blood culture, the absence of major vascular occlusion, intensive leukocytic infiltration, and necrosis of subcutaneous tissue.

Most patients with necrotizing fasciitis suffer pain, which in the early stages of the disease is often disproportionately greater than that expected from the degree of cellulitis present. Late in the course of the infection, the involved skin may actually be anesthetized secondary to necrosis of superficial nerves. Temperature abnormalities, both hyperthermia and hypothermia, are common, concomitant with the release of bacterial toxins as well as with bacterial sepsis, which is present in up to 40% of patients. The involved skin is initially tender, erythematous, and warm. Edema develops and the erythema spreads diffusely, fading into normal skin, characteristically without distinct margins or induration. Subcutaneous microvascular thrombosis induces ischemia in the skin, which becomes cyanotic and blistered. Eventually, as necrosis develops, the skin becomes gangrenous and may slough spontaneously. Most patients will have leukocytosis and acid–base abnormalities. Finally, subcutaneous gas may develop, which can be identified by palpation and by x-ray. The finding of subcutaneous gas by x-ray is often indicative of clostridial infection, although it is not a specific finding and may be caused by other organisms. These organisms include *Enterobacter*, *Pseudomonas*, anaerobic streptococci, and *Bacteroides*, which, unlike clostridial infections, spare the muscles underlying the affected area. A tissue biopsy specimen for gram stain and aerobic and anaerobic culture should be obtained from the necrotic center of the lesion in order to identify the etiologic organisms.

Predisposing risk factors for necrotizing fasciitis include diabetes mellitus, alcoholism, an immunocompromised state, hypertension, peripheral vascular disease, intravenous drug abuse, and obesity. Increased age, delay in diagnosis, inadequate debridement during initial surgery, extent of disease on initial presentation, and the presence of diabetes mellitus are all factors that have been associated with an increased likelihood of mortality from necrotizing fasciitis. Clearly, early diagnosis and aggressive management of this lethal disease have led to improved survival. In an earlier series, the mortality rate was consistently higher than 30%; in more recent series, the mortality rate has decreased to less than 10%.

Successful management of necrotizing fasciitis involves early recognition, immediate initiation of resuscitative measures (including correction of fluid, acid–base, electrolyte, and hematologic abnormalities), aggressive surgical debridement and redebridement as necessary, and broad-spectrum antibiotic therapy. Many patients will benefit from central venous monitoring, as well as from high caloric nutritional support.

During surgery, the incision should be made through the infected tissue down to the fascia. An ability to undermine the skin and subcutaneous tissues with digital palpation often will confirm the diagnosis. Multiple incisions can be made sequentially toward the periphery of the affected tissue until well-vascularized, healthy, resistant tissue is reached at all margins. The remaining affected tissue must be excised. The wound can then be packed and sequentially debrided on a daily basis as necessary until healthy tissue is displayed at all margins.

Hyperbaric oxygen therapy may be of some benefit, particularly in patients for whom culture results are positive for anaerobic organisms. Retrospective non-randomized studies have demonstrated that the addition of hyperbaric oxygen therapy to surgical debridement and antimicrobial therapy appears to significantly decrease both wound morbidity and overall mortality in patients with necrotizing fasciitis.

After the initial resuscitative efforts and surgical debridement, the primary concern is the management of the open wound. Allograft and xenograft skin can be used to cover open wounds, thus decreasing heat and evaporative water loss. Interestingly, temporary biologic closure of open wounds also seems to decrease bacterial growth. Recently, a new technology has been developed to expedite wound healing. The vacuum-assisted closure (VAC) method is a subatmospheric pressure technique that has been demonstrated in laboratory and clinical studies to significantly improve wound healing. The VAC device as a method for wound control has demonstrated significant promotion of wound healing. In situations where spontaneous closure is not likely, the VAC device may allow for the development of a suitable granulation bed and prepare the tissue for graft placement, thereby increasing the probability of graft survival. Finally, skin flaps can be mobilized to help cover open wounds once the wound infections have resolved and granulation has begun.

Obesity

Incidence and definition

Obesity is an increasing problem in America and is more frequently encountered as a risk factor for complications associated with gynecologic oncology surgery. Centers for Disease Control statistics from the year 2000 indicate that 30% of US adults greater than 20 years old are obese, an astounding 59 million adults. If these statistics are expanded to include overweight as well as obese persons, 64% of the US adult population is facing a significant medical problem.

Obesity is defined by the body mass index (BMI), which is calculated by dividing the weight in kg by the height in cm^2. Alternatively, the body weight in lbs is multiplied by 704 and then divided by the height in inches squared. Current American Gastroenterology Association guidelines use the BMI to define classes of obesity. A BMI of 25–29.9 is defined as overweight; BMI 30–34.9, class I obesity; BMI 35–39.9, class II obesity; and BMI > 40 is extreme class III obesity. In practical terms, a 5’4” American woman who is 30 lbs overweight will have a BMI > 30, classifying her in the obesity class I.

Postoperative complications and management

Obese patients are at much higher risk for postoperative complications due to the more frequent occurrence of comorbidities, including diabetes, hypertension, coronary artery disease, sleep apnea, obesity hypoventilation syndrome, and osteoarthritis of the knees and hips. These underlying alterations in physiology result in increased surgical risks and complications, including respiratory failure, cardiac failure, DVT and pulmonary embolism, aspiration, wound infection and dehiscence, postoperative asphyxia, and misdiagnosed intra-abdominal catastrophe.

Control of the airway is critical in the immediate postoperative period. Extubation may not be prudent or possible at the end of the case due to tracheal edema resulting from a difficult intubation. Alternatively, the patient may not have the physical capacity to adequately ventilate, due to suppression of the respiratory drive from anesthetics and excess chest wall weight. Many obese patients suffer from the obesity hypoventilation syndrome, which increases their baseline hypercarbia and may also delay extubation. It is often prudent to plan immediate postoperative admission to a surgical intensive care unit with mechanical ventilation and serial arterial blood sampling to aid in the proper timing for extubation.

After extubation, ventilation of the obese patient during sleep may be aided by the use of non-invasive positive pressure ventilation units, particularly if the patient has a history of sleep apnea and uses a continuous positive airway pressure (CPAP) machine at home. Respiratory therapists can be of assistance in patient instruction and management of CPAP machinery, in addition to other respiratory toilet. Monitoring with continuous pulse oximetry will assist the detection of impending respiratory failure.

There is a higher risk of aspiration in obese patients, due to increased gastric residual volumes, a higher rate of gastroesophageal reflux disease, and increased intra-abdominal pressure from mass effect. Neutralization of the stomach contents with a proton pump inhibitor can minimize the chemical burn potential of aspirated stomach contents. Gastrointestinal motility agents such as metoclopramide may decrease residual volume by increasing intestinal transit. It is also prudent to raise the head of the bed to prevent aspiration.

Prophylaxis for postoperative venous thrombosis and pulmonary embolism (as detailed above) should be ordered for obese patients, as they are at higher risk for these complications.

Venous access poses another problem. Extreme obesity obliterates anatomic landmarks and makes insertion of peripheral lines, as well as central lines, problematic. Adjunctive visualization technology such as Doppler ultrasound or fluoroscopy should increase the accuracy and safety of line placement. Arterial line placement facilitates monitoring of pressures and blood gas parameters. Ideally, central venous lines and arterial lines should be placed intraoperatively by the anesthesia team to ensure adequate access in the postoperative period. The intraoperative placement of central lines should be verified for position postoperatively by chest x-ray in the postanesthesia care unit.

Medication administration must consider the concepts of total body weight as well as ideal body weight. Certain medications are dosed on ideal body weight (corticosteroids, penicillin, cephalosporins, beta-blockers). Others are dosed on total body weight (heparin) and still others based on a calculated "dosing weight" (aminoglycosides, fluoroquinolones, vancomycin). An inpatient pharmacist should be consulted for assistance with proper dosing and monitoring of pharmacotherapy.

The elderly patient

The life expectancy of American women continues to increase. In addition, as the "baby boomer" generation ages we will see an increasingly larger population of older women who will develop gynecologic cancers. The elderly woman is at higher risk of developing gynecologic cancer, in that 65% of vulvar cancers, 43% of epithelial ovarian cancers, 45% of endometrial cancers, and 27% of cervical cancers occur in women older than 65 years of age. While many of these cancers are managed with radical surgery, careful consideration must be given in selection of surgical procedures in women who may be at high risk for surgical complications. In fact, complications of radiation therapy and chemotherapy are more likely to occur in older patients, so selection of any therapy requires consideration of patient tolerance. In past years, radical surgery was avoided in elderly women. We now know that surgery can be safely and successfully accomplished, despite a patient's age, if the patient is fully evaluated and determined to be a surgical candidate.

There is no doubt that older patients present with more advanced disease and have poorer presurgical performance status, and more intercurrent medical problems, than younger patients. Retrospective review of elderly patients with gynecologic cancers demonstrates that 90% of women over 65 years can undergo radical surgery as definitive therapy for their gynecologic cancer. When compared with women younger than 65 years, the postoperative mortality was 1.5%, and the minor complications and length of stay were similar in the two groups. In women over 65 years of age who underwent radical hysterectomy for early-stage cervical cancer, there was no perioperative mortality or ureteral fistula. Transfusion requirements and lymphedema were also similar. Febrile morbidity was less common in the older patients, although postoperative small bowel obstruction, bladder dysfunction, and pulmonary emboli were more frequently encountered in the older patients.

Perioperative management is the key to success when treating the elderly woman. Cardiac and pulmonary complications are the two most common serious problems encountered postoperatively. Careful preoperative assessment of cardiac status should include assessment for underlying coronary artery disease, valvular heart disease, and chronic congestive heart failure. There are several risk assessment algorithms that may be applied to estimate risk of major surgery. Because over 40% of elderly women have hypertension, optimal blood pressure control should be achieved preoperatively; intraoperative hypotension is one of the most common causes of myocardial ischemia and infarction. Pulmonary complications occur in nearly 40% of elderly women following major abdominal surgery. Because physiologic changes of aging diminish vital capacity, lung compliance, reduced expiratory flow rates, and increased residual volume, the elderly patient is more likely to suffer pulmonary complications following general anesthesia. These women may be at even higher risk if they have chronic obstructive pulmonary disease or asthma. Preoperative assessment may include assessment of pulmonary function by performing spirometry and obtaining an arterial blood gas measurement. Patients with underlying pulmonary disease should have their medical regimen maximized preoperatively, including the use of bronchodilators and steroids. Conduction anesthesia should be strongly considered in consultation with the anesthesiologist in order to avoid the pulmonary complications more frequently encountered with general anesthesia.

Avoiding perioperative hypothermia and hypoxemia are extremely important to avoid additional cardiac oxygen consumption. Invasive monitoring and planned intensive care unit admission should be considered in any circumstance where there is an increased risk of cardiac or pulmonary complications. Care must also be taken when ordering pharmacologic agents, as the elderly may have altered gastrointestinal absorption and decreased renal or hepatic clearance of specific drugs. Consultation with a clinical pharmacist is advised in order to establish the correct dose of drug for patients with altered renal or hepatic function.

Radiation complications in the elderly patient are also increased. The thin, hypertensive patient appears to be at greater risk for radiation therapy complications to both the gastrointestinal and genitourinary tracts. It appears that elderly women tolerate initial therapy poorly and often require delays in treatment or discontinuation of treatment due to acute toxicity such as diarrhea, dehydration, or neutropenia. Both Kennedy et al and Grant et al have described a high complication rate of radiation therapy in elderly women. This observation, then, requires carefully planned treatment decisions as to whether the patient would be best treated with surgery or radiation therapy. Neither is without risk, and it cannot be assumed that radiation therapy is necessarily less toxic.

Radiation therapy

Radiation therapy serves as a primary treatment modality for cervical and vaginal cancers (and occasionally advanced vulvar cancers), and as an adjuvant therapy for patients with high-risk endometrial cancers. Further, individualized radiation therapy may be used in nearly all gynecologic cancers to achieve palliation under specific circumstances. Morbidity resulting from properly conducted radiation therapy in patients with carcinoma of the cervix and vagina is usually minimal. However, there are unfortunate misconceptions about the magnitude of radiation morbidity in both the medical and the lay community. We believe that these misconceptions have several origins.

First, many investigators fail to distinguish that unnecessary adverse effects result from poor techniques and should not be extrapolated to the use of proper techniques. Second, there has been a failure to recognize that a great deal of radiation morbidity is usually related to compromised treatment of patients with extensive tumors in whom surgery is not applicable. Results in these patients cannot be extrapolated to the use of optimal techniques in the treatment of patients with limited malignancy. Finally, it is an often unrecognized fact that a great deal of morbidity attributed to irradiation actually results from uncontrolled tumor (i.e. rectovaginal and vesicovaginal fistulas). As in the case of surgery, the treatment-related morbidity can be minimized by good application, but it cannot be eliminated.

Because the small bowel, bladder, and rectum are adjacent to the female genital tract, most of the side effects and complications of radiation involve these adjacent organs. Radiation complications are related to the dose, field size, and type of radiation equipment used. The larger the field, the greater the risk of problems if the dose remains constant. Usually, as the fields enlarge the dose must be decreased. Conversely, as the fields become smaller a larger dose can be tolerated. The use of brachytherapy also increases the risk of local complications. Finally, the use of combined chemoradiation therapy seems to increase slightly some complications during therapy (e.g. neutropenia) but does not seem to lead to serious long-term sequelae.

The pathogenesis of radiation-induced injury may be divided into acute and delayed complications. Complications during therapy are caused by ionizing radiation injury to cells that are mitotically active, such as gastrointestinal epithelium. Damage of the mucosal cells results in mucosal thinning and denudation followed by malabsorption and fluid and electrolyte loss (due to diarrhea). The gastrointestinal mucosal stem cells generally recover totally, and the acute symptoms resolve. Late complications involve a different mechanism of tissue injury based on vascular endothelial damage. Radiation results in endarteritis and the gradual occlusion of small vessels. Subsequent tissue hypoxia leads to fibrosis of the affected tissue. These changes are progressive and may be aggravated further by other vascular compromise such as diabetes, hypertension, and aging. In severe cases, ulceration, stricture, perforation, and fistula formation may occur.

Gastrointestinal complications

Acute complications

Nearly all patients receiving external radiation to the pelvis will develop radiation proctitis or enteritis with associated diarrhea. This problem usually begins after 2 weeks of radiation therapy and is usually easily managed by dietary modification and antidiarrheal medications (diphenoxylate [Lomotil]). The diarrhea usually resolves within a week to 10 days of completing radiation. Some of the transitory symptoms are tenesmus and the passage of mucus and even blood per rectum. Diarrhea and abdominal cramping characterize small intestinal irritation. This problem is more common and more severe when a portion of the small intestine is fixed in the pelvis due to adhesions or other pathologic conditions. Anorexia may also occur during radiation therapy. If nausea and vomiting occur, the patient should be evaluated for dehydration. This is more common when concurrent chemotherapy is being given along with the radiation. Intravenous hydration and correction of electrolytes is occasionally required. If severe, radiation should be interrupted until these acute side effects are corrected. The patient should have a complete blood count weekly during radiation therapy. If the hemoglobin decreases below 10 g/dL, packed red cell transfusion is advised in order to achieve improved tumor kill. Occasionally, radiation of the pelvic bone marrow will result in neutropenia or thrombocytopenia. In severe cases, radiation will need to be temporarily interrupted. In nearly all cases, the acute side effects of radiation therapy will resolve once the radiation course is completed.

Chronic conditions

Radiation injury to the small intestine may manifest itself at any time following therapy, and may vary from diarrhea or weight loss to small bowel obstruction or fistula. A typical patient with small bowel injury will initially present with postprandial abdominal cramps and pain, anorexia, and diarrhea. About half of small bowel injuries occur within 1 year after radiation, and three-fourths occur within 2 years. These symptoms are more common in patients who have had a prior laparotomy. Initial conservative management focuses on dietary modification (avoiding green leafy vegetables, milk products, and fried foods). Antidiarrheal drugs and oral cholestyramine (which binds bile salts) are often useful in managing symptoms.

As small bowel injury progresses, fibrosis of the injured bowel wall develops, leading to stricture and partial or complete obstruction. Patients usually present with worsening abdominal pain, cramps, diarrhea, and vomiting. Sometimes, the intermittent obstruction goes unrecognized until a significant weight loss is recorded. The decision to proceed with surgical intervention in cases of intermittent obstruction is a difficult one and should be undertaken with proper preoperative preparation. Often, patients have developed a significant degree of malnutrition and should have their nutritional status corrected with preoperative TPN. Mechanical bowel preparation is mandatory although sometimes must be limited to enemas because the patient's small bowel obstruction will not allow the ingestion of oral cathartics. Dilated loops of bowel should be decompressed preoperatively with nasogastric suction. Surgical correction depends on the situation encountered at the time of surgical exploration. The obstruction is usually found to be bowel-adherent in the pelvis that has been radiated. The bowel usually is thickened, edematous, and fibrotic. Resection of the obstructed loops with reanastomosis or small bowel bypass are the two primary surgical options. In either event, it is preferable to make anastomoses to intestinal segments that have not been radiated in order to have maximum opportunity for healing. Care should be taken to have adequate perfusion and no tension on the anastomosis. Perforation or fistula, if present, must be isolated and diverted; more extensive surgery (resection and anastomosis) must be done only if it is technically feasible (Fig. 17–11).

Radiation injury to the rectum is more common after treatment for cervical cancer due to the high rectal doses from the intracavitary cesium application. Injury to the rectum may manifest itself as proctitis, stricture, or fistula. Complete colonic obstruction from radiation injury is extremely rare. The symptoms of radiation proctitis may follow an asymptomatic interval of many months to years after radiation therapy is completed. Diarrhea with or without rectal bleeding is the most common finding. Cramping abdominal pain may be associated with the diarrhea. The injury is most often located on the anterior rectal wall that received the maximal dose from the cesium brachytherapy application, and range from thickened fragile mucosa to thin atrophic mucosa or mucosal ulceration. These changes usually heal with conservative measures including low-residue diet, anticholinergic drugs, stool softeners, and steroid enemas. Hyperbaric oxygen treatments also appear to enhance healing of a rectal ulcer. If there is excessive bleeding from the rectal ulcer or proctitis, diversion of the fecal stream (colostomy) may be necessary to allow healing. Obviously, when bleeding is encountered full evaluation of the rectosigmoid colon with flexible sigmoidoscopy is mandatory to exclude recurrent cancer, rectal cancer, polyps or diverticulae, and hemorrhoids as the cause for bleeding.

Rectovaginal fistula is the most common significant radiation injury to the large bowel and is often preceded by radiation proctitis and rectal ulceration. All patients with rectovaginal fistulas should have a diverting colostomy. It is rare that diversion will result in spontaneous healing of radiated colon, and it is often necessary to decide whether repair of the fistula may be subsequently undertaken. Whenever surgical correction is considered, the use of endovascular flaps to bring a new blood supply to the radiated tissues of the rectum and vagina should be strongly considered (Fig. 17–12). Only after the fistula has completely healed and absence of obstruction of the bowel has been documented should the colostomy be reversed.

Radiation-induced strictures or obstruction of the rectosigmoid colon appear at approximately 24 months from the completion of the radiation therapy. Again, the initial step in management is a diverting colostomy. Correction will require a rectosigmoid resection with low rectal anastomosis. Harris and Wheeless reported their experience with the end to end stapler device in low colorectal anastomosis associated with rectal injury. This was accomplished in 49 patients, 17 of whom had prior radiation therapy. All five postoperative complications (two strictures, two anastomosis breakdowns, and one fecal incontinence after colostomy closure) occurred in the patients who had prior radiation.

Complex fistulas may include a variety of communications between small bowel, colon, vagina, bladder, and skin. Careful evaluation of the anatomy involved is mandatory and should include all organ systems that are possibly involved. The evaluation may include barium enema, proctosigmoidoscopy, upper gastrointestinal series with small bowel follow-through, IVP, cystogram, cystoscopy, and a "fistulogram" (injection of contrast directly into the fistula and imaging the retrograde flow of the contrast dye). These complex fistulas are often very difficult to repair, and the patients should be in optimal medical condition before surgery is performed. This usually includes antibiotics to control infection, TPN, and mechanical bowel preparation. If a fistula can be resected, it should be; however, many times the fistula must be isolated and the intestinal stream diverted around the lesion.

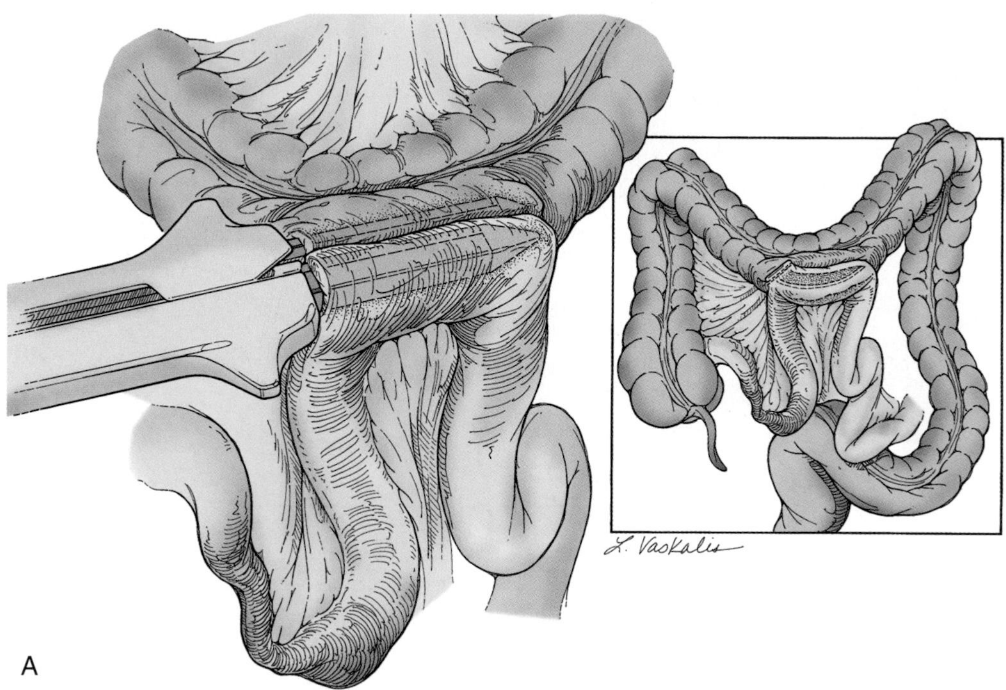

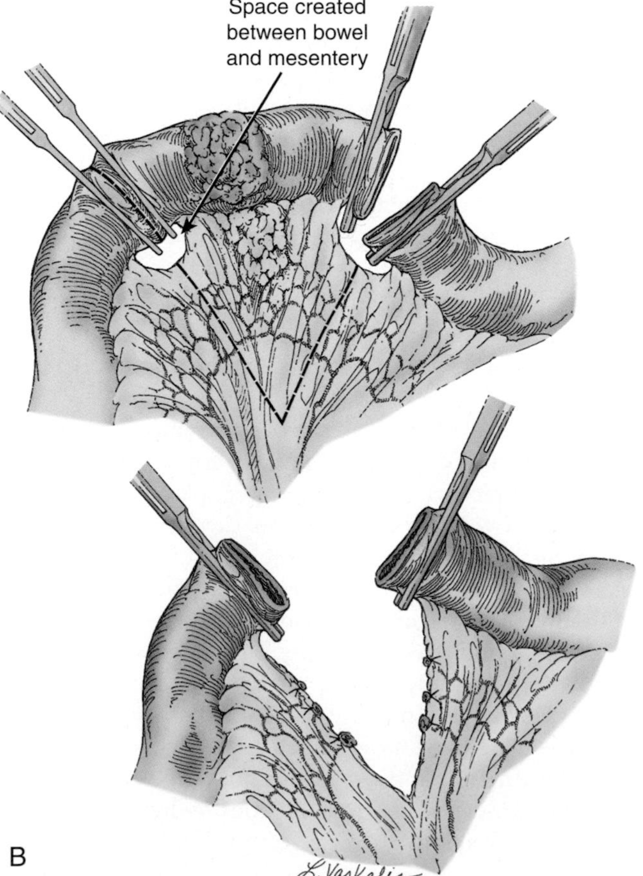

Figure 17–11 *A,* Small bowel obstruction that has been managed with a bypass ileotransverse enteroenterostomy. *B,* Resection of the involved bowel has been done with reanastomosis of the small bowel. Sufficient terminal ileum must be present for this procedure to be accomplished.

Illustration continued on following page.

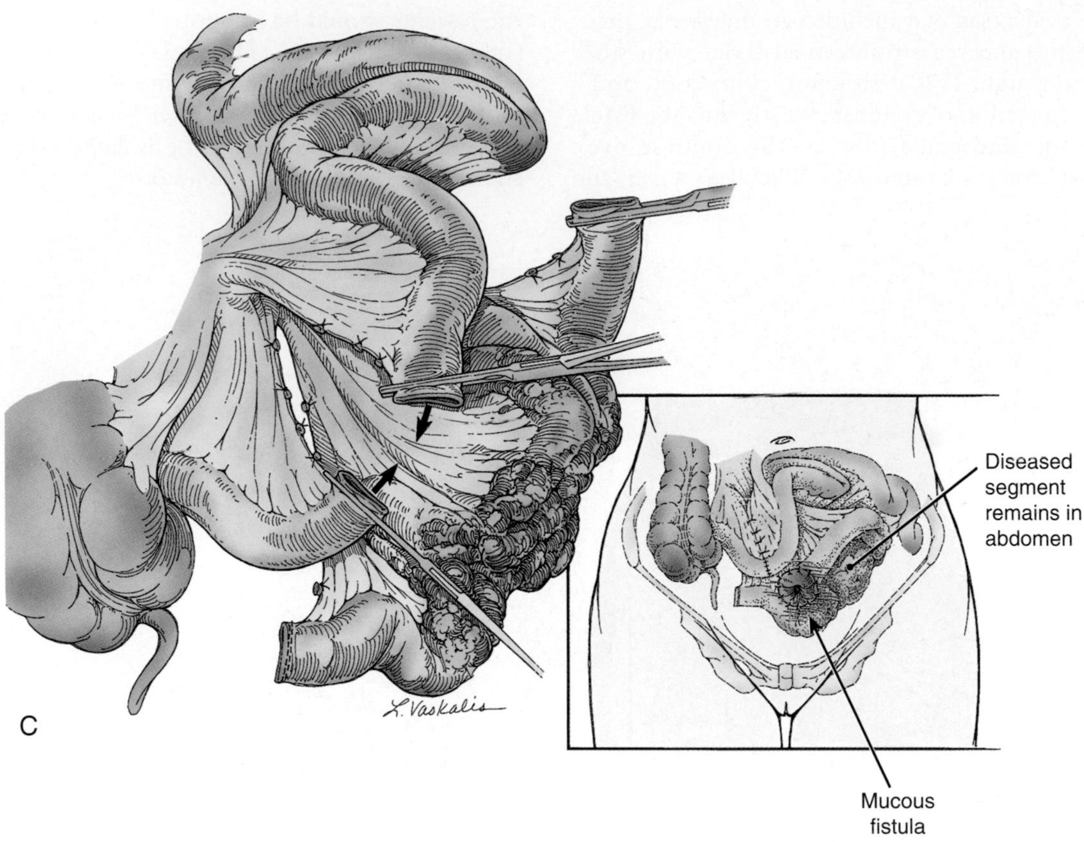

Figure 17–11, cont'd *C*, The obstructed bowel has been isolated with formation of a mucous fistula. An end to side anastomosis has also been done. (From Nichols DH, Clarke-Pearson DL [eds]: Gynecologic, Obstetric and Related Surgery, 2nd edn. St. Louis, Mosby, 2000.)

Prior pelvic radiation to the ileum (or resection or bypass surgery of the ileum) may lead to the malabsorption of vitamin B_{12} and result in a megaloblastic anemia. Because the liver usually has significant stores of B_{12}, it may be several years after radiation or surgery before the anemia is recognized. It is therefore advised that patients have annual complete blood counts indefinitely. A Shilling test can differentiate between B_{12} and folic acid deficiency. Treatment of B_{12} deficiency requires weekly B_{12} injections until the hemoglobin level returns to normal (usually 4–6 weeks), and then monthly injections to prevent recurrent anemia.

Urologic complications

Acute radiation cystitis is occasionally encountered during radiation therapy or in the period immediately after completion of therapy. Typical symptoms of cystitis are usually present, but urine cultures show no significant bacterial growth. Management includes increased oral liquid intake and urinary analgesics to relieve symptoms. The symptoms usually resolve in a short time. Chronic radiation cystitis usually presents with symptoms of urinary frequency, suprapubic pain, and hematuria. The patient should have an immediate urine culture, for a urinary tract infection further aggravates bladder mucosa damaged by radiation therapy. Gross hematuria (rather than microscopic hematuria) usually can be relieved by continuous bladder irrigation using either 0.5% or 1% acetic acid, or a 1:1000 potassium permanganate or an alum solution. Clots may need to be evacuated in the operating room to relieve bladder spasms. Cystoscopy may also be needed to identify bleeding points that may be fulgurated. An experienced urologist should be consulted, as excessive fulguration or unnecessary biopsies may lead to an iatrogenic vesicovaginal fistula. As a last resort, the bladder may be sclerosed with formaldehyde irrigation. In the most extreme cases, cystectomy and urinary diversion may be required to control bleeding.

Vesicovaginal fistulas are more common when the patient has had intensive radiation therapy, and is increased by cesium brachytherapy. Improper placement of the tandem and ovoids resulting in an excessive dose to the base of the bladder speaks to the importance of careful placement of intracavitary devices and attention to bladder doses delivered. Surgery following radiation therapy, such as a "completion" hysterectomy for bulky stage Ib2 or "barrel" lesions of the cervix, further increases the risk of vesicovaginal fistula. In many cases, upper vaginal radiation necrosis is recognized months before the occurrence of the fistula. Treatment of the necrosis may prevent the progression to a fistula. Therapy includes hydrogen peroxide douches, intravaginal estrogen, and hyperbaric oxygen therapy.

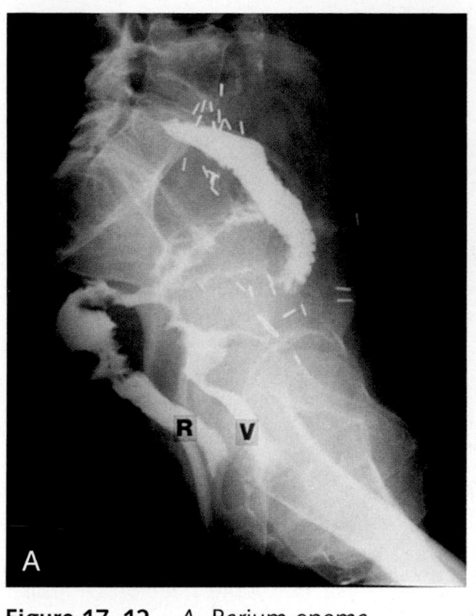

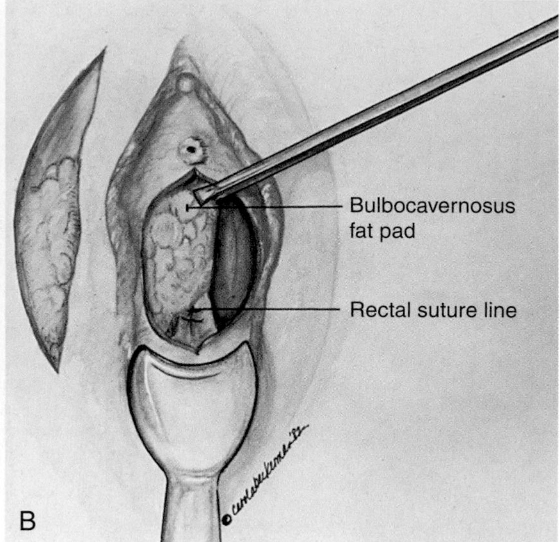

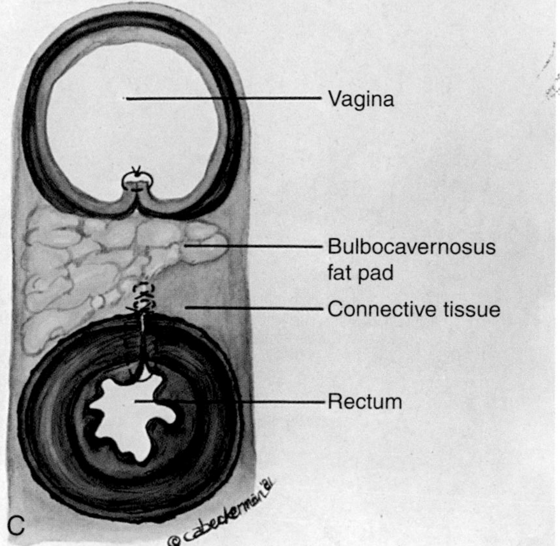

Figure 17–12 *A*, Barium enema demonstrating a rectovaginal fistula after irradiation. *B*, Repair of the rectovaginal fistula has been strengthened by interposition of the bulbocavernosus fat pad. *C*, The cross-section shows placement of the neovascular fat pad.

Evaluation of an apparent vesicovaginal fistula should include a complete evaluation of the bladder as well as the upper tracts. It is not uncommon to discover an associated ureterovaginal fistula or ureteral stricture/stenosis, which must be addressed at the time of fistula repair. Further, given the proximity of the upper vagina to the bladder and rectum, proctosigmoidoscopy is advised as the rectosigmoid colon may also communicate with the fistula.

Repair of a radiation-induced vesicovaginal fistula is difficult and less successful than fistula repair in non-irradiated areas. The primary complicating matter is diminished blood supply to the radiated tissues. Therefore techniques of repair often utilize the mobilization of a non-irradiated tissue with a good blood supply into the surgical repair. If an intra-abdominal, transvesical approach is taken to repair of a vesicovaginal fistula, the omentum and its blood supply may be mobilized and used to cover the repair of the fistula, often being interposed between the closed bladder and vagina (Fig. 17–13). Vaginal approaches to vesicovaginal fistula repair may include repair combined with colpocleisis or the use of the bulbocavernosus labial fat pad and muscle, which are mobilized and interposed between the repaired bladder and vagina (Fig. 17-14). Ureteral injury following radiation therapy may require reimplantation of the distal ureter into the bladder (ureteroneocystostomy) or permanent diversion (urinary conduit).

Chemotherapy

Chemotherapy is widely used in the initial treatment of many gynecologic malignancies. In some instances, such as gestational trophoblastic disease, ovarian germ cell malignancies, and some patients with epithelial ovarian cancer, chemotherapy can result in a cure. In many other instances, chemotherapy is palliative but can relieve symptoms and prolong meaningful life. There are numerous acute and chronic toxicities associated with chemotherapy, and the reader is referred to more comprehensive discussions in Chapter 18.

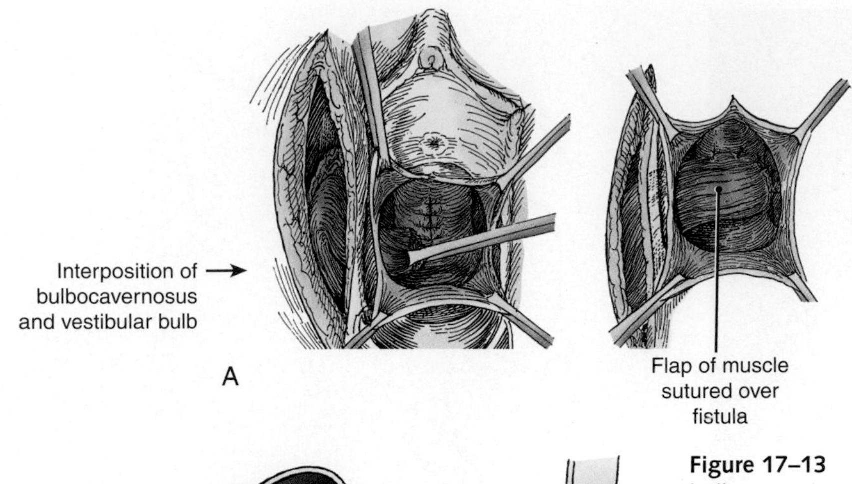

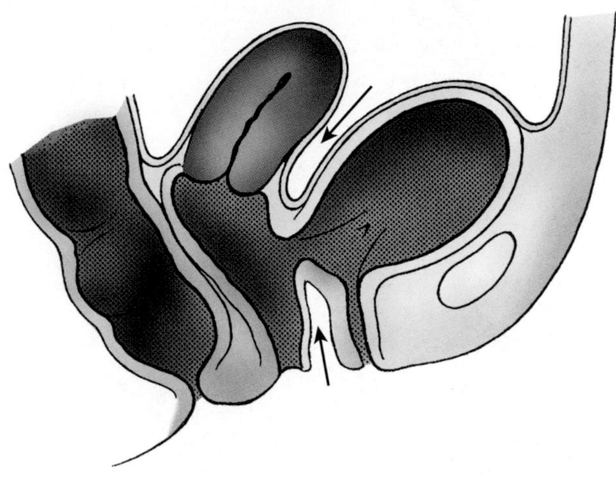

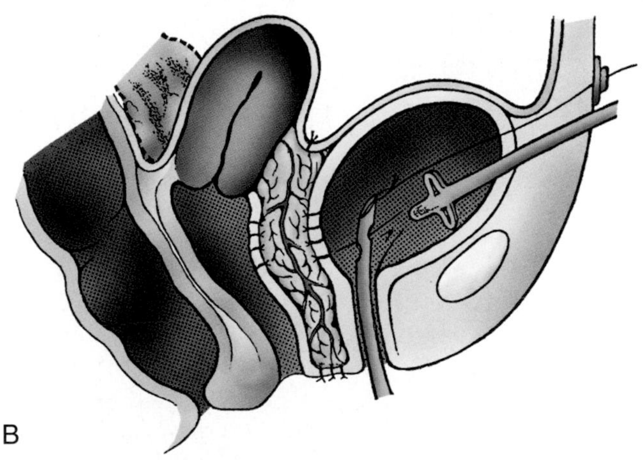

Figure 17–13 *A,* Vesicovaginal fistula repair using the bulbocavernosus fat pad as a source of neovascularization. *B,* Repair using an omental J flap for neovascularization. (From Nichols DH, Clarke-Pearson DL [eds]: Gynecologic, Obstetric and Related Surgery, 2nd edn. St. Louis, Mosby, 2000.)

Myelodysplastic syndrome and acute non-lymphocytic leukemia

This serious and usually fatal complication of chemotherapy was initially recognized in women receiving alkylating agents, and is more likely to occur after chronic administration. The risk of secondary leukemia peaks 4–5 years after completing chemotherapy. These leukemias often go through the myelodysplasia or preleukemic stage. Unfortunately, the response to leukemia therapy is poor. Modern chemotherapy for ovarian cancer, which is platin-based, has eliminated the exposure to alkylators (paclitaxel [Taxol] has been substituted for cyclophosphamide). Further, current primary therapy has reduced the number of cycles of therapy to six, avoiding chronic exposure to cytotoxic agents. The association of leukemia and the administration of cisplatin or carboplatin is uncertain. One report suggests that there is a fourfold increased risk of leukemia in women with ovarian cancer treated with platin-containing regimens. However, this conclusion is uncertain, in that most of these patients also received cyclophosphamide (Cytoxan, an alkylator) in combination with cisplatin. Etoposide (usually administered in the treatment of gestational trophoblastic disease or for ovarian germ cell

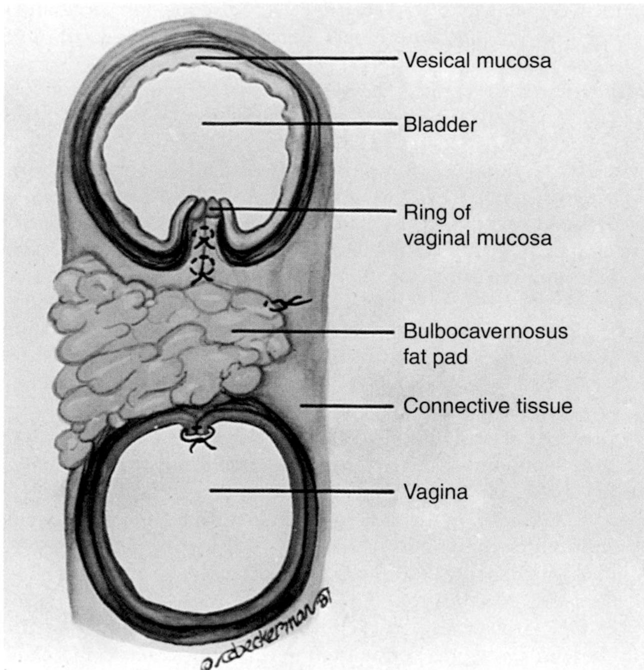

Figure 17–14 Cross-section of the vesicovaginal repair using the bulbocavernosus fat pad as a source of neovascularization.

tumors) is also associated with an increased risk of acute myeloid leukemia.

The risk seems to be associated with the total cumulative dose of drug administered over time. Therefore, especially in young women who are likely to be cured, attention should be paid to minimizing the dose and duration of etoposide therapy. Leukemia following etoposide therapy usually occurs earlier than alkylator-induced leukemias (35 months vs 4–5 years) and has a good response to chemotherapy (complete response of 50–60%). During postchemotherapy follow-up, women who have been treated with alkylating agents or etoposide should have periodic determination of complete blood counts.

Neurotoxicity

Some degree of neurotoxicity is commonly encountered with the use of cisplatin (or carboplatin) and/or paclitaxel. The most common neurologic effects of cisplatin include peripheral sensory neuropathy and ototoxicity; while paclitaxel (Taxol) commonly causes peripheral sensory toxicity. These toxicities are often the dose-limiting side effect, and are more common with cumulatively increasing doses of the drug or if the drugs are used in combination. The literature reports an incidence of neuropathy of approximately 15% if the cumulative cisplatin dose is < 300 mg/m^2, but it may be as much as 85% with doses of > 300 mg/m^2. The combination of paclitaxel and cisplatin has an even higher incidence of neuropathy and is particularly severe with the combination of cisplatin 75 mg/m^2 and paclitaxel 175 mg/m^2 (administered over 3 h). While carboplatin causes much less neurotoxicity than cisplatin, the combination of carboplatin and paclitaxel may still cause significant sensory neuropathy.

The most common neurologic side effects are due to toxicity to the peripheral sensory nerves, which results in numbness, tingling, and paresthesias of the feet and hands. Neurologic testing documents loss of ankle and knee reflexes and diminished vibratory sensation. In extreme cases, the neuropathy may progress proximally to the arms and legs, and patients may have difficulty walking and using their hands for fine motion (e.g. buttoning clothing, writing). Recovery following the onset of peripheral sensory neuropathy is common, but it may take several months to notice improvement and the improvement may never be complete. Some authors have recommended the use of vitamin B_6 (pyridoxine), amitriptyline (Elavil), and gabapentin (Neurontin) to reduce symptoms.

Cisplatin may also cause tinnitus and high-frequency hearing loss, and this is more common with high-dose regimens. In most cases, the hearing loss is not perceptible to the patient but it is readily documented with audiology testing.

Cardiac toxicity

Doxorubicin, which is commonly used to treat metastatic endometrial adenocarcinoma and leiomyosarcomas, has a potential life-threatening toxicity of causing cardiomyopathy and resultant congestive heart failure. Arrhythmias and pericarditis have also been reported. The incidence of congestive heart failure is directly related to the cumulative dose of doxorubicin, and is rarely encountered with a dose of <350 mg/m^2. Cumulative doses of >550 mg/m^2 are associated with an incidence of up to 10%. Age >70 years, hypertension, pre-existing cardiac disease, and prior mediastinal radiation may significantly increase the risk of cardiomyopathy, and a lower dose of doxorubicin should be considered in these circumstances. Prior to treatment, a cardiac ejection fraction should be evaluated (multiple-gated acquisition scan). Because a significant drop in cardiac ejection fraction precedes the onset of clinical symptoms, subsequent scans (especially as the dose exceeds 350 mg/m^2) may allow discontinuation of doxorubicin before serious myocardial damage occurs. Dexrazoxane (Zinecard) is a chemoprotective agent that reduces cardiomyopathy in women with breast cancer who are receiving a dose of doxorubicin in excess of 300 mg/m^2. Cardiotoxicity is usually irreversible, but treatment of doxorubicin-induced heart failure may reduce symptoms of congestive heart failure by improving myocardial contractility by using digitalis, diuretics, and afterload reduction. Liposomal doxorubicin is associated with minimal cardiotoxicity.

Pulmonary toxicity

Bleomycin is commonly used in a regimen of multiagent chemotherapy for the treatment of ovarian germ cell malignancies. Subacute and chronic interstitial pneumonitis is a serious, life-threatening side effect of bleomycin. This inflammatory process may progress to pulmonary fibrosis, respiratory failure, and death. Prior to the onset of fibrosis, the patient may complain of shortness of breath and cough. Risk factors for bleomycin pulmonary toxicity include age > 70 years, pre-existing chronic obstructive pulmonary disease, higher doses of bleomycin, bolus infusion, and prior chest irradiation. While toxicity has been reported at doses of < 100 mg, the incidence rises to 10% in patients receiving a dose in excess of 450 mg/m^2. In addition, general anesthesia following the use of bleomycin may be complicated by postoperative respiratory failure possibly secondary to a bleomycin-induced sensitivity of oxygen.

Pulmonary toxicity may be predicted from deteriorating pulmonary function testing, particularly the carbon monoxide diffusion capacity. When deterioration is discovered, bleomycin therapy should be discontinued. There is no specific treatment of bleomycin pulmonary toxicity. Steroid therapy may reduce inflammation and improve symptoms but will not reverse pulmonary fibrosis.

BIBLIOGRAPHY

HEMORRHAGE

American College of Obstetricians and Gynecologists: Invasive hemodynamic monitoring in obstetrics and gynecology. Technical bulletin 175. Washington, ACOG, 1992.

American Society of Anesthesiologists Task Force on Blood Component Therapy: Practice guidelines for blood component therapy. Anesthesiology 84:732–747, 1996.

D'Ambra MN, Kaplan DK: Alternatives to allogenic blood use in surgery: acute normovolemic hemodilution and preoperative autologous donation. Am J Surg 170(suppl):6A, 1995.

Development Task Force of the College of American Pathologists: Practice parameter for the use of fresh-frozen plasma, cryoprecipitate, and platelets: fresh-frozen plasma, cryoprecipitate, and platelets administration practice guidelines. JAMA 271:777, 1994.

Greenburg AG: Benefits and risks of blood transfusion in surgical patients. World J Surg 20:1189–1193, 1996.

National Institutes of Health: Summary of NIH consensus development conference on perioperative red cell transfusion. Am J Hematol 31:144–150, 1989.

Nolan TE, Gallup DG: Massive transfusion: a current review. Obstet Gynecol Surv 46:289, 1991.

GENITOURINARY TRACT

Alkhuniazi AM, Schrier RW: Management of acute renal failure: new perspectives. Am J Kidney Dis 28:315, 1996.

Boronow RC, Rutledge FN: Vesicovaginal fistula, radiation, and gynecologic cancer. Am J Obstet Gynecol 111:85, 1971.

Bricker EM: Current status of urinary diversion. Cancer 45:2986, 1980.

Carter J, Ramirez C, Waugh R et al: Percutaneous urinary diversion in gynecologic oncology. Gynecol Oncol 40:248, 1991.

Creasman WT, Weed JC Jr: Radical hysterectomy. In Schaefer G, Graber E (eds): Complications in Obstetrics and Gynecologic Surgery. New York, Harper & Row, 1981, pp 241–256.

Denton MD, Chertow GM, Brady HR: "Renal-dose" dopamine for the treatment of acute renal failure: scientific rationale, experimental studies and clinical trials. Kidney Int 50:4, 1996.

Dudley BS, Gershenson DM, Kavanagh JJ et al: Percutaneous nephrostomy catheter use in gynecologic malignancy: MD Anderson Hospital experience. Gynecol Oncol 24:273–278, 1986.

Feuer GA, Frauchter R, Souri E et al: Selection for percutaneous nephrostomy in gynecologic cancer patients. Gynecol Oncol 42:60, 1991.

Forney JP et al: Long-term effects on bladder function following radical hysterectomy with and without postoperative radiation. Gynecol Oncol 26:160, 1987.

Fyles AW, Dembo AJ, Bush RS et al: Analysis of complications in patients treated with abdomino-pelvic radiation therapy for ovarian carcinoma. Int J Radiat Oncol Biol Phys 1992; 22: 847.

Hatch KD, Parham G, Shingleton HM: Ureteral stricture and fistula following radical hysterectomy. Gynecol Oncol 19:17, 1984.

Jacobs AJ, Perez CA, Camel HM et al: Complications of patients receiving both irradiation and radical hysterectomy for carcinoma of the uterine cervix. Gynecol Oncol 22:273, 1985.

Kadar M, Saliba N, Nelson JH: The frequent causes and prevention of severe urinary dysfunction after radical hysterectomy. Br J Obstet Gynaecol 90:859, 1983.

Lee RA, Symmonds RE: Ureterovaginal fistula. Am J Obstet Gynecol 109:1032, 1971.

Liaño F, Pascual J: Epidemiology of acute renal failure: a prospective, multicenter community-based study. Kidney Int 50:811, 1996.

Mindell JA, Chertow GM: A practical approach to acute renal failure. Med Clin North Am 81:731, 1997.

Perez CA, Grigsgy BN, Lockett MA et al: Radiation therapy morbidity in carcinoma of the uterine cervix: dosimetric and clinical correlation. Ind J Radiat Oncol Biol Phys 44:855–866, 1999.

Photopulos EJ, Zwaag RV: Class II radical hysterectomy shows less morbidity and good treatment efficacy compared to class III. Gynecol Oncol 40:21, 1991.

Ralph G, Tamussino K, Lictenegger W: Urodynamics following radical abdominal hysterectomy for cervical cancer. Arch Gynecol Obstet 243:215, 1988.

Roman-Lopez JJ, Barkley DL: Bladder dysfunction following Schanta hysterectomy. Am J Obstet Gynecol 115:81, 1973.

Seski JC, Diokno AC: Bladder dysfunction after radical abdominal hysterectomy. Am J Obstet Gynecol 128:643, 1977.

Star RA: Treatment of acute renal failure. Kidney Int 54:1817, 1998.

Stern JL, Maroney TP, Lace C: Treatment of urinary conduit fistula by antegrade ureteral stent catheter. Obstet Gynecol 70:276, 1987.

Swan RW, Rutledge FN: Urinary conduit in pelvic cancer patients: a report of sixteen years' experience. Am J Obstet Gynecol 119:6, 1974.

Symmonds RE: Urological injuries: ureter. In Schaefer G, Graber E (eds): Complications in Obstetrics and Gynecologic Surgery. New York, Harper & Row, 1981.

Thadhani R, Pascual M, Bonventre JV: Acute renal failure. N Engl J Med 334:1448, 1996.

Underwood RB, Lutz MH, Smoak DL: Ureteral injury following irradiation therapy for carcinoma of the cervix. Obstet Gynecol 49:663, 1977.

GASTROINTESTINAL TRACT

Adelson MD, Kasowitz MH: Percutaneous endoscopic drainage gastrostomy in the treatment of gastrointestinal obstruction from intraperitoneal malignancy. Obstet Gynecol 81:467, 1993.

Allen-Mersch TG et al: Has the incidence of radiation-induced bowel damage following treatment of uterine carcinoma changed in the last 20 years? J Soc Med 79:387, 1986.

Barnes W, Waggoner S, Delgado G et al: Manometric characterization of rectal dysfunction following radical hysterectomy. Gynecol Oncol 42:116, 1991.

Barnhill D, Doering D, Remmenga S et al: Intestinal surgery performed on gynecologic cancer patients. Gynecol Oncol 40:38, 1991.

Beck DE, Harford FJ, DiPalma JA: Comparison of cleansing methods in preparation for colonic surgery. Dis Colon Rectum 28:491–495, 1985.

Boike GM, Sightler SE, Averett HE: Treatment of small intestinal fistulas with octreotide, a somatostatin analog. J Surg Oncol 49: 63, 1992.

Borison DI, Bloom AD, Pritchard TJ: Treatment of enterocutaneous and colocutaneous fistulas with early surgery or somatostatin analog. Dis Colon Rectum 35:635, 1992.

Bricker EM, Johnston WD: Repair of post-irradiation rectovaginal fistula and stricture. Surg Gynecol Obstet 148:499, 1979.

Bristol J, Williamson RCN: Mechanism of intestinal adaptation. Pediatr Surg Int 4:233, 1988.

Cirisano FD, Greenspoon JS, Stenson et al: The etiology and management of diarrhea in the gynecologic oncology patient. Gynecol Oncol 50:45, 1993.

Clarke JS, Condon RE, Bartlett JG et al: Preoperative oral antibiotics reduce septic complications of colon operations: results of prospective, randomized, double-blind clinical study. Ann Surg 186:251–259, 1977.

Clarke-Pearson DL, Chin NO, DeLong ER et al: Surgical management of intestinal obstruction in ovarian cancer. Gynecol Oncol 26:11, 1987.

DiCostanzo J, Cano N, Martin J et al: Treatment of external gastrointestinal fistulas by a combination of total parenteral nutrition and somatostatin. JPEN J Parenter Enteral Nutr 11:465, 1987.

Feuer DJ, Broadley KE, Shepherd JH et al: Systematic review of surgery in malignant bowel obstruction in advanced gynecological and gastrointestinal cancer. Gynecol Oncol 75:313, 1999.

Harris WJ, Wheeless CR: Use of the end-to-end anastomosis stapling device in low colorectal anastomosis associated with radical gynecologic surgery. Gynecol Oncol 23:350, 1986.

Hatch KD, Gelder MS, Soong SJ et al: Pelvic exenteration with low rectal anastomosis: survival complications and prognostic factors. Gynecol Oncol 38:462, 1990.

Iacono G, Carroccio A, Montalto G et al: Extreme short bowel syndrome: a case for reviewing the guidelines for predicting survival. J Pediatr Gastroenterol Nutr 16:216, 1993.

Jex RK, Van Heersen JA, Wolf BG et al: Gastrointestinal anastomoses: factors affecting early complications. Ann Surg 206:138, 1987.

Kagan AR, Nussbaum H, Gilbert H et al: A new staging system for irradiation injuries following treatment for cancer of the cervix uteri. Gynecol Oncol 7:166, 1979.

Kurkchubasche AG, Rowe MI, Smith SD: Adaptation in short bowel syndrome: reassessing old limits. J Pediatr Surg 28:1069, 1993.

Mangili G, Franchi M, Mariani A et al: Octreotide in the management of bowel obstruction in terminal ovarian cancer. Gynecol Oncol 61:345, 1996.

Marchant DJ: Special problems of the intestinal tract. In Schaefer G, Graber E (eds): Complications in Obstetrics and Gynecologic Surgery. New York, Harper & Row, 1981.

McIntyre PB: The short bowel. Br J Surg 72(suppl):S92, 1985.

Montz FJ, Holschneider CH, Solh S et al: Small bowel obstruction following radical hysterectomy: risk factors, incidence, and operative findings. Gynecol Oncol 53:114, 1994.

Moran BJ, Jackson AA: Function of the human colon. Br J Surg 79:1132, 1992.

Patton TJ, Mitchel MF, Atkinson EN et al: Parameters of small bowel dysfunction in cervical cancer patients undergoing radiotherapy. Int J Gynecol Cancer 3:175, 1993.

Photopulos JC et al: Intestinal anastomosis after radiation therapy by surgical stapling instruments. Obstet Gynecol 54:515, 1979.

Purdum PP, Kirby DF: Short bowel syndrome: a review of the role of nutrition support. JPEN J Parenter Enteral Nutr 15:93, 1991.

Smith JP, Golden PE, Rutledge FN: The surgical management of intestinal injuries following radiation for carcinoma of the cervix. In University of Texas MD Anderson Hospital and Tumor Institute: Cancer of the Uterus and Ovary. Chicago, Year Book Medical, 1969.

Stockbine MF, Hancock JC, Fletcher GH: Complications in 831 patients with squamous cell carcinoma of the intact cervix treated with 3000 rad or more whole pelvic irradiation. Am J Roentgenol Radium Ther Nucl Med 108:293, 1970.

Swan RW, Fowler WC, Boronow RC: Surgical management of radiation injury to the small intestine. Surg Gynecol Obstet 142: 325, 1976.

Symmonds RE: Ureteral injuries associated with gynecologic surgery: prevention and management. Clin Obstet Gynecol 19:623, 1976.

THROMBOEMBOLISM

Agnelli G, Piovella F, Buoncristiani P et al: Enoxaparin plus compression stockings alone in the prevention of venous thromboembolism after elective neurosurgery. N Engl J Surg 339:80–85, 1998.

Bergovst D, Lindgren B, Matzsch T: Comparison of the cost of preventing postoperative deep vein thrombosis with either unfractionated or low molecular weight heparin. Br J Surg 83: 1548–1552, 1996.

Borstad E, Urdal K, Handeland G et al: Comparison of low molecular weight heparin vs unfractionated heparin in gynecological surgery II: reduced dose of low molecular weight heparin. Acta Obstet Gynecol Scand 71:471–475, 1992.

Bounameaux H, de Moerloose P, Sarasin FP: Optimal duration of oral anticoagulant therapy following deep vein thrombosis of lower limbs. Blood Coagul Fibrinolysis 7:507, 1996.

Clarke-Pearson DL, DeLong ER, Synan IS et al: Variables associated with postoperative deep venous thrombosis: a prospective study of 411 gynecologic patients and the creation of a prognostic model. Obstet Gynecol 69:146, 1987.

Clarke-Pearson DL, Coleman RE, Synan IS et al: Venous thromboembolism prophylaxis in gynecologic oncology: a prospective controlled trial of low-dose heparin. Am J Obstet Gynecol 145:606, 1983.

Clarke-Pearson DL, Creasman WT: Diagnosis of deep venous thrombosis in obstetrics and gynecology by impedence phlebography. Obstet Gynecol 58:52, 1981.

Clarke-Pearson DL, Jelovsek FR, Creasman WT: Thromboembolism complicating surgery for cervical and uterine malignancy: incidence, risk factors, and prophylaxis. Obstet Gynecol 61:87, 1983.

Clarke-Pearson DL, Maxwell GL, Synan I et al: Risk factors which predispose patients to thromboembolism despite prophylaxis with external pneumatic compression. Obstet Gynecol 101:157–163, 2003.

Columbus Investigators: Low-molecular-weight heparin in the treatment of patients with venous thromboembolism. N Engl J Med 337:657, 1997.

Diugiud DL: Oral anticoagulant therapy for venous thromboembolism. N Engl J Med 336:433, 1997.

Escalante CP: Causes and management of superior vena cava syndrome. Oncology (Huntingt) 7:61, 1993.

Fishman A, Altaras M, Klein A et al: Low molecular heparin (enoxaparin) as an alternative treatment of acute deep venous thrombosis in gynecologic oncology patients. Eur J Gynaecol Oncol 17:365, 1996.

Gunnarsson PS, Sawyer WT, Montague D et al: Appropriate use of heparin. Arch Intern Med 155:526, 1995.

Hirsh J, Hoak J: Management of deep vein thrombosis and pulmonary embolism. Circulation 93:2212, 1996.

Hoffman MS, DeCesare S, Fiorica JV et al: Management of gynecologic oncology patients with a preoperative deep vein thrombosis. Gynecol Oncol 64:76, 1997.

Hommes DW, Bura A, Mazzolai L et al: Subcutaneous heparin compared with continuous intravenous heparin administration in the initial treatment of deep vein thrombosis. Ann Intern Med 116:279, 1992.

Hull RD, Delmore T, Genton E et al: Warfarin sodium versus low-dose heparin in the long-term treatment of venous thrombosis. N Engl J Med 301:855, 1979.

Hull RD, Raskob GE, Rosenbloom D et al: Treatment of proximal vein thrombosis with subcutaneous low-molecular-weight heparin vs. intravenous heparin. Arch Intern Med 157:289, 1997.

Kearon C, Hirsh J: Management of anticoagulation before and after elective surgery. N Engl J Med 336:1506, 1997.

Kuter DJ: Thrombotic complications of central venous catheters in cancer patients. Oncologist 9:207, 2004

Madura JA, Rookstool M, Wease G: The management of patients on chronic Coumadin therapy undergoing subsequent surgical procedures. Am Surg 60:542, 1994.

Maxwell GL, Myers ER, Clarke-Pearson DL: Cost-effectiveness of deep venous thrombosis prophylaxis in gynecologic oncology surgery. Obstet Gynecol 95:206–214, 2000.

Maxwell GL, Synan I, Dodge R et al: Prevention of venous thrombosis in postoperative gynecologic oncology patients: a prospective randomized trial comparing pneumatic calf compression and low molecular weight heparin (dalteparin). Obstet Gynecol 98:989–995, 2001.

Metz SA: Thromboembolism in gynecologic surgery. Female Patient 20:15, 1995.

Montgomery KD, Potter HG, Helfet DL: Magnetic resonance venography to evaluate the deep venous system of the pelvis in patients who have acetabular fracture. J Bone Joint Surg 77-A: 1639–1649, 1995.

Moser KM, Fedullo PF, LitteJohn JK et al: Frequent asymptomatic pulmonary embolism in patients with deep vein thrombosis. JAMA 271:223, 1994.

Multicenter Trial Committee: Dihydroergotamine-heparin prophylaxis of postoperative deep venous thrombosis. JAMA 251:2960, 1984.

Myhand RC, Weiss RB: Causes and management of treatment-related thrombosis. Contemp Oncol August:37, 1994.

Pearson SD, Lee TH, McCabe-Hassan S et al: A critical pathway to treat proximal lower-extremity deep vein thrombosis. Am J Med 100:283, 1996.

Pineo GF, Hull RD: Low-molecular-weight heparin: prophylaxis and treatment of venous thromboembolism. Annu Rev Med 48:79, 1997.

Prandoni P, Lensing AWA, Buller HR et al: Comparison of subcutaneous low-molecular-weight heparin with intravenous standard heparin in proximal deep-vein thrombosis. Lancet 339:441, 1992.

Prandoni P, Lensing AWA, Cogo A et al: The long-term clinical course of acute deep venous thrombosis. Ann Intern Med 125:1, 1996.

Prandoni P: Antithrombotic strategies in patients with cancer. Thromb Haemost 78:141, 1997.

Schulman S, Granqvist S, Holmstrom M et al: The duration of oral anticoagulant therapy after a second episode of venous thromboembolism. N Engl J Med 336:393, 1997.

Tapson VF, Hull RD: Management of venous thromboembolic disease: the impact of low-molecular-weight heparin. Chest 16(2):281–294, 1995.

Turkstra F, Koopman MMW, Buller HR: The treatment of deep vein thrombosis and pulmonary embolism. Thromb Haemost 78:489, 1997.

Weinmann EE, Salzman EW: Deep vein thrombosis. N Engl J Med 331:1630, 1994.

Weitz JI: Low-molecular-weight heparins. N Engl J Med 337:688, 1997.

Willie-Jorgensen P, Hauch O, Dimo B et al: Prophylaxis of deep venous thrombosis after acute abdominal operation: Surg Gynecol Obstet 172:44–48, 1991.

POSTOPERATIVE INFECTIONS

Cruse PJ, Foord R: The epidemiology of wound infection. A 10-year prospective study of 62,939 wounds. Surg Clin North Am 60:27–40, 1980.

Goldstein EJ: Possible role for the new fluoroquinolones (levofloxacin, grepafloxacin, trovafloxacin, clinafloxacin, sparfloxacin, and DU-6859a) in the treatment of anaerobic infections: review of current information on efficacy and safety. Clin Infect Dis 23(suppl 1):S25–S30, 1996.

Hemsell DL: Prophylactic antibiotics in gynecologic and obstetric surgery. Rev Infect Dis 13 (suppl 10):S821–S841, 1991.

Kingdom JC, Kitchener HC, MacLean AB: Postoperative urinary tract infection in gynecology: implications for an antibiotic prophylaxis policy. Obstet Gynecol 76:636–638, 1990.

Korhonen K, Klossner J, Hirn M et al: Management of clostridial gas gangrene and the role of hyperbaric oxygen. Ann Chir Gynaecol 88:139–142, 1999.

Lyon DS, Jones JL, Sanchez A: Postoperative febrile morbidity in the benign gynecologic patient. Identification and management. J Reprod Med 45:305–309, 2000.

Mayer HO, Petru E, Haas J et al: Perioperative antibiotic prophylaxis in patients undergoing radical surgery for gynecologic cancer: single dose versus multiple dose administration. Eur J Gynaecol Oncol 14:177–181, 1993.

Mittendorf R, Aronson MP, Berry RE et al: Avoiding serious infections associated with abdominal hysterectomy: a meta-analysis of antibiotic prophylaxis. Am J Obstet Gynecol 169:1119–1124, 1993.

Morykwas MJ, Argenta LC, Shelton-Brown EI et al: Vacuum-assisted closure: a new method for wound control and treatment: animal studies and basic foundation. Ann Plast Surg 38:553, 1997.

Nelson AL, Sinow RM, Oliak D: Transrectal ultrasonographically guided drainage of gynecologic pelvic abscesses. Am J Obstet Gynecol 182:1382–1388, 2000.

O'Grady NP, Barie PS, Bartlett J et al: Practice parameters for evaluating new fever in critically ill adult patients. Task Force of the American College of Critical Care Medicine of the Society of Critical Care Medicine in collaboration with the Infectious Disease Society of America. Crit Care Med 26:392–408, 1998.

Orr JW Jr, Sisson PF, Patsner B et al: Single-dose antibiotic prophylaxis for patients undergoing extended pelvic surgery for gynecologic malignancy. Am J Obstet Gynecol 162:718–721, 1990.

Riseman JA, Zamboni WA, Curtis A et al: Hyperbaric oxygen therapy for necrotizing fasciitis reduces mortality and the need for debridements. Surgery 108:847–850, 1990.

Sperling DC, Needleman L, Eschelman DJ et al: Deep pelvic abscesses: transperineal US-guided drainage. Radiology 208:111–115, 1998.

Sudarsky LA, Laschinger JC, Coppa GF et al: Improved results from a standardized approach in treating patients with necrotizing fasciitis. Ann Surg 206:661–665, 1989.

Umbert IJ, Winkelmann RK, Oliver GF et al: Necrotizing fasciitis: a clinical, microbiologic, and histopathologic study of 14 patients. J Am Acad Dermatol 20:774–781, 1989.

SURGICAL COMPLICATIONS

Anonymous: Perioperative total parenteral nutrition in surgical patients. The Veterans Affairs Total Parenteral Nutrition Cooperative Study Group. New Engl J Med 325:525–532, 1991.

Bandy LC, Clarke-Pearson DL, Soper JT et al: Long-term effects on bladder function following radical hysterectomy with and without postoperative irradiation. Gynecol Oncol 26:160, 1987.

Bergan JJ, Dean RH, Yao JST: Vascular injury in pelvic cancer surgery. Am J Obstet Gynecol 124:562, 1976.

Blaustein AS: Preoperative and perioperative management of cardiac patients undergoing noncardiac surgery. Cardiol Clin 13:149–161, 1995.

Connors AFJ, Speroff T, Dawson NV et al: The effectiveness of right heart catheterization in the initial care of critically ill patients. JAMA 276:889–897, 1996.

Delgado G, Smith PJ: Management of complications in gynecologic oncology. New York, John Wiley, 1982.

Ivanov R, Allen J, Calvin JE: The incidence of major morbidity in critically ill patients managed with pulmonary artery catheters: a meta-analysis. Crit Care Med 28:615–619, 2000.

Lawrence VA, Dhanda R, Hilsenbeck SG et al: Risk of pulmonary complications after elective abdominal surgery. Chest 110: 744–750, 1996.

McCraw JB, Massey FM, Shanklin KD et al: Vaginal reconstruction with gracilis myocutaneous flaps. Plast Reconstr Surg 58:176, 1976.

McDonald PT, Rich NM, Collins GJ Jr. et al: Vascular trauma secondary to diagnostic and therapeutic procedures: laparoscopy. Am J Surg 135:651, 1978.

Nelson JH: Atlas of Radical Pelvic Surgery. New York, Appleton-Century-Crofts, 1977.
O'Quinn AG, Fletcher GH, Wharton JT: Guidelines for conservative hysterectomy after irradiation. Gynecol Oncol 9:68, 1978.
Rich NM, Spencer FC: Management of Acute Injuries in Vascular Trauma. Philadelphia, Saunders, 1978.
Rosenthal DM, Colapinto R: Angiographic arterial embolization in the management of postoperative vaginal hemorrhage. Am J Obstet Gynecol 151:227, 1985.
Sandstrom R, Drott C, Hyltander A et al: The effect of postoperative intravenous feeding (TPN) on outcome following major surgery evaluated in a randomized study. Ann Surg 217:185–195, 1993.
Schwartz PE, Goldstein HM, Wallace S et al: Control of arterial hemorrhage using percutaneous arterial catheter technique in patients with gynecologic malignancies. Gynecol Oncol 3:276, 1975.
Warltier DC, Pagel PS, Kersten JR: Approaches to the prevention of perioperative myocardial ischemia. Anesthesiology 92:253–259, 2000.
Weinacker AB, Vaszar LT: Acute respiratory distress syndrome: physiology and new management strategies. Ann Rev Med 52:221–237, 2001.

LYMPHOCYSTS

American College of Obstetricians and Gynecologists: Septic shock. Technical bulletin 204. Washington, ACOG, 1995.
Bone RC, Balk RA, Cerra RF et al: Definitions for sepsis and organ failure and guidelines for the use of innovative therapies in sepsis. Chest 101:1644, 1992.
Catalona WJ, Kadmon D, Crane DB: Effect of mini-dose heparin on lymphocele formation following extraperitoneal pelvic lymphadenectomy. J Urol 123:890–895, 1979.
Dinarello CA, Gelfand JA, Wolff SM: Anticytokine strategies in the treatment of the systemic inflammatory response syndrome. JAMA 269:1829, 1993.
Fekety R, Shah AB: Diagnosis and treatment of *Clostridium difficile* colitis. JAMA 269:71, 1993.
Fisher JR, Conway MJ, Takeshita RT et al: Necrotizing fasciitis: importance of roentgenographic studies for soft-tissue gas. JAMA 241:803, 1979.
Glauser MP, Zanetta G, Baumgartner JD et al: Septic shock pathogenesis. Lancet 338:732, 1991.
Gucalp R: Management of the febrile neutropenic patient with cancer. Oncology 5:137, 1991.
Hughes WT, Armstrong D, Bodez GP et al: Guidelines for the use of antimicrobial agents in neutropenic patients with unexplained fever. J Infect Dis 161:381, 1990.
Karp JE, Merz WG, Dick JD: Management of infections in neutropenic patients: advances in therapy and prevention. Curr Opin Infect Dis 6:405, 1993.
Majeski JA, Alexander JW: Early diagnosis, nutritional support, and immediate extensive debridement improve survival in necrotizing fasciitis. Am J Surg 145:784, 1983.
Parriloo JE: Pathogenetic mechanisms of septic shock. N Engl J Med 328:1471, 1993.
Pearlman MD, Faro AE: Obstetrical septic shock: a pathophysiological basis for management. Clin Obstet Gynecol 33:485, 1990.
Piver MS, Malfetano JH, Lele SB et al: Prophylactic anticoagulation as a possible cause of inguinal lymphocyst after radical vulvectomy and inguinal lymphadenectomy. Obstet Gynecol 62:17–21, 1983.
Pizzo PA: Management of fever in patients with cancer and treatment-induced neutropenia. N Engl J Med 328:1323, 1993.
Rangel-Frausto MS, Pittet D, Costigan M et al: The natural history of systemic inflammatory response syndrome (SIRS): a prospective study. JAMA 273:117, 1995.
Roberts DB: Necrotizing fasciitis of the vulva. Am J Obstet Gynecol 157:568, 1987.

SEPSIS

Addison WA, Livengood CH III, Hill GB et al: Necrotizing fasciitis of vulvar origin in diabetic patients. Obstet Gynecol 63:157, 1987.
Soper DE: Necrotizing fasciitis and related entities. In Postosk JG III (ed): Obstetric and Gynecologic Infectious Diseases. New York, Raven Press, 1994, pp 114–1126.
Stamenkovic I, Lew PD: Early recognition of potentially fatal necrotizing fasciitis: the use of frozen-section biopsy. N Engl J Med 310:1689, 1984.
Stephenson H, Dotters DJ, Katz V et al: Necrotizing fasciitis of the vulva. Am J Obstet Gynecol 166:125, 1992.
Stevens D: Necrotizing fasciitis: don't wait to make a diagnosis. Infect Med 14:684, 1997.
Sufferdini AF: Current prospects for the treatment of clinical sepsis. Crit Care Med 22:S12, 1994.
Suzuki M, Ohwada M, Sato I: Pelvic lymphocysts following retroperitoneal lymphadenectomy: retroperitoneal partial "no closure" for ovarian and endometrial cancers. J Surg Oncol 68:149, 1998.

DRUG-RELATED LEUKEMIAS AND COMPLICATIONS

Bajorin DF, Motzer RJ, Rodriguez E et al: Acute non-lymphocytic leukemia in germ cell tumor patients treated with etoposide-containing chemotherapy. J Natl Caner Inst 85:60, 1993.
Connelly E, Markman M, Kennedy A et al: Paclitaxel delivered as a 3-hour infusion with cisplatin in patients with gynecologic cancers: unexpected incidence of neurotoxicity. Gynecol Oncol 62:166, 1996.
Gianni L, Munzone E, Capri G et al: Paclitaxel by 3-hour infusion in combination with bolus doxorubicin in women with untreated metastatic breast cancer: high antitumor efficacy and cardiac effects in a dose-finding and sequence-finding study. J Clin Oncol 13:2688, 1995.
Goldiner PL, Carlon GC, Critkovic E et al: Factors influencing postoperative morbidity and mortality in patients treated with bleomycin. Br Med J 1:1664, 1978.
Greene MH: Is cisplatin a human carcinogen? J Natl Cancer Inst 84:306, 1992.
Kaldor JM, Day NE, Petterson F et al: Leukemia following chemotherapy for ovarian cancer. N Engl J Med 322:1, 1990.
Kaye SB, Paul J, Cassidy J et al: Mature results of a randomized trial of two doses of cisplatin for the treatment of ovarian cancer. J Clin Oncol 14:2113, 1996.
Kumar L: Epipodophyllotoxins and secondary leukaemia. Lancet 342:819, 1993.
Reed E, Evans MK: Acute leukemia following cisplatin-based chemotherapy in a patient with ovarian cancer. J Natl Cancer Inst 82:431, 1990.
Schwartz RG, McKenzie WB, Alexander J et al: Congestive heart failure and left ventricular dysfunction complicating doxorubicin therapy: seven-year experience using serial radionuclide angiocardiography. Am J Med 82:1109, 1987.
Smith M, Rubinstein L, Anderson J et al: Secondary leukemia or myelodysplastic syndrome after treatment with epipodophyllotoxins. J Clin Oncol 17:569, 1999.
Stine KC, Saylors RL, Sawyer JR et al: Secondary acute myelogenous leukemia following safe exposure to etoposide. J Clin Oncol 13:2688, 1995.
Travis LB, Curtis RE, Boice JD et al: Second malignant neoplasms among long term survivors of ovarian cancer. Cancer Res 56:1564, 1996.
Travis LB, Holowaty EJ, Bergfeldt K et al: Risk of leukemia after platinum-based chemotherapy for ovarian cancer. N Engl J Med 340:351, 1999.
Verweij J, van der Burg MEL, Pinedo HM: Mitomycin C-induced hemolytic uremic syndrome: six case reports and review of the literature on renal, pulmonary and cardiac side effects of the drug. Radiother Oncol 8:33, 1987.
Von Hoff DD, Layare MW, Basa P et al: Risk factors for doxorubicin-induced congestive heart failure. Ann Intern Med 91:710, 1979.
Winick NJ, McKenna RW, Shuster JJ et al: Secondary acute myeloid leukemia in children with acute lymphoblastic leukemia treated with etoposide. J Clin Oncol 11:209, 1993.

THE ELDERLY PATIENT

Grant PT, Jeffrey JF, Frazier RC et al: Pelvic radiation therapy for gynecologic malignancy in geriatric patients. Gynecol Oncol 33:185, 1989.

Kennedy AW, Flagg JS, Webster KD: Gynecologic cancer in the very elderly. Gynecol Oncol 32:49, 1989.

Kinney WK, Egorshin EVB, Podratz KC: Wertheim hysterectomy in the geriatric population. Gynecol Oncol 31:227, 1988.

Lawton FR, Hacker N: Surgery for invasive gynecologic cancer in the elderly female population. Obstet Gynecol 76:287, 1990.

Van Le L, Fakhry S, Walton LA et al: Use of the APACHE II scoring system to determine mortality of gynecologic oncology patients in the intensive care unit. Obstet Gynecol 85:53, 1995.

INVASIVE HEMODYNAMIC MONITORING

Bandy LC, Clarke-Pearson DL, Creasman WT: Vitamin B12 deficiency following therapy in gynecologic oncology. Gynecol Oncol 17:370, 1984.

Bone RC, Balk RA, Cerra FR et al: Definitions for sepsis and organ failure and guidelines for the use of innovative therapies in sepsis. The ACCP/SCCM Consensus Conference Committee. Chest 101:1646, 1992.

Boronow RC: Management of radiation-induced vaginal fistulae. Am J Obstet Gynecol 110:1, 1971.

Ermakov S, Hoyt JW: Pulmonary artery catheterization. Crit Care Clin 8:773, 1992.

Finegan BA: The pulmonary artery catheter: when and why it should be used. Can J Anaesth 39:R71, 1992.

Heath D, Baron R: Nutrition. In Skach W, Daley CL, Forsmark CE (eds): Handbook of Medical Treatment. Greenbrae, Jones Medical Publications, 1988, pp 212–240.

Parnes HL: How to manage metabolic emergencies. Contemp Oncol September:54, 1993.

RADIATION THERAPY

Slater JM, Fletcher GH: Ureteral strictures after radiation therapy for carcinoma of the uterine cervix. Am J Roentgenol Radium Ther Nucl Med 111:269, 1971.

Smith DH, DeCosse JJ: Radiation damage to the small intestine. World J Surg 10:189, 1986.

Sola JE, Bender JS: Use of the pulmonary artery catheter to reduce operative complications. Surg Clin North Am 73:253, 1993.

Susini T, Scambia G, Margariti PA et al: Gynecologic oncology surgery in the elderly: a retrospective analysis of 213 patients. Gynecol Oncol 75:437, 1999.

Vender JS: Clinical utilization of pulmonary artery catheter monitoring. Int Anesthesiol Clin 31:57, 1993.

18 Basic Principles of Chemotherapy

Christina S. Chu, M.D., and Stephen C. Rubin, M.D.

HISTORICAL OVERVIEW

The era of modern chemotherapy began in the 1940s with the Nobel Prize–winning work of Huggins and Hodges on the antitumor effect of estrogens in prostate cancer. This observation was followed in the mid 1940s by the investigation of nitrogen mustard, a by-product of nitrogen gas used in World War I, for its effects against lymphomas and solid tumors. Between 1945 and 1965, a wide variety of chemotherapeutic agents were identified and studied, including actinomycin D, cyclophosphamide, the vinca alkaloids, 5-fluorouracil, and the progesterones. In the 1970s, cisplatin was noted to exert significant antitumor effects against ovarian and testicular cancers, and tamoxifen was found to have activity against breast cancer for both adjuvant therapy and treatment of advanced disease. In the same decade, bleomycin, etoposide, and doxorubicin came into clinical use, and derivative compounds such as carboplatin, vinorelbine, and idarubicin were developed for their ability to achieve similar antitumor effects but with less hematologic toxicity. The 1980s and 1990s have led to the widespread use of a host of new drugs, such as the taxanes (paclitaxel and docetaxel), ifosfamide, the topoisomerase inhibitors (topotecan and irinotecan), and nucleoside analogs (gemcitabine and capecitabine).

The growing number of agents in the chemotherapeutic armamentarium has been accompanied by advances in alternative dosing regimens, differing formulations using liposomal or polymer-based encapsulation, and varying schedules, sequences, and routes of administration. Fortunately, supportive therapies for gastrointestinal and hematologic toxicities have also evolved to include routine usage of 5-HT_3 receptor antagonists (such as ondansetron and granisetron) for antiemetic prophylaxis, and hematopoietic growth factors (such as epoetin) and colony-stimulating factors (such as sargramostim and filgrastim) to allow for greater chemotherapeutic dose intensity.

GENERAL PRINCIPLES

Chemotherapeutic agents are a crucial part of the physician's armamentarium in the ever-broadening fight against cancer. The physician can, with use of these drugs, ameliorate and sometimes even cure diseases that were usually fatal in the past. Until recently, in most cases chemotherapy has been reserved for relatively late stages of the disease, but its increasingly successful use, particularly in the treatment of hematologic malignancies, suggests that

Table 18–1 NATIONAL CANCER INSTITUTE RESPONSE EVALUATION CRITERIA IN SOLID TUMORS

	Evaluation
Target lesions	
Complete response	Disappearance of all target lesions
Partial response	At least a 30% decrease in the sum of the longest diameter of target lesions, taking as reference the baseline sum longest diameter
Progressive disease	At least a 20% increase in the sum of the longest diameter of target lesions, taking as reference the smallest sum longest diameter recorded since the treatment started or the appearance of one or more new lesions
Stable disease	Neither sufficient shrinkage to qualify for partial response nor sufficient increase to qualify for progressive disease, taking as reference the smallest sum longest diameter since the treatment started
Non-target lesions	
Complete response	Disappearance of all non-target lesions and normalization of tumor marker level
Incomplete response/stable disease	Persistence of one or more non-target lesion(s) or/and maintenance of tumor marker level above the normal limits
Progressive disease	Appearance of one or more new lesions and/or unequivocal progression of existing non-target lesions[a]

[a]Although a clear progression of "non target" lesions only is exceptional, in such circumstances the opinion of the treating physician should prevail and the progression status should be confirmed later on by the review panel (or study chair).

chemotherapy should be administered earlier. All physicians and surgeons must understand the nature and use of cancer chemotherapy so that they can make rational decisions about when it may be indicated. The outcome of cancer chemotherapy is not fully predictable, but the chances of remission can be improved by judicious selection of patients, careful assessment of the tumor's growth pattern, and treatment of the neoplasm with the drug or drugs most likely to be effective. The clinical response to chemotherapy may be assessed utilizing standard Response Evaluation Criteria in Solid Tumors defined by the National Cancer Institute (Table 18–1).

Unfortunately, not all patients with cancer are amenable to chemotherapy. The suitability of a patient for treatment depends on at least three critical criteria:

1. the nature of the neoplasm,
2. its extent of spread or stage, and
3. the patient's clinical condition.

Not all cancers are equally sensitive to drugs. Factors that determine a given tumor's susceptibility include how the drug is distributed to the tumor, drug transport into the cell, whether a drug-sensitive biochemical pathway is present in the tumor cell, and the relative rates of intracellular activation and inactivation of the drug. A thorough knowledge of the cell cycle and growth kinetics is fundamental to understanding of the appropriate uses of chemotherapy.

CELL CYCLE CONTROL AND GROWTH KINETICS

All living things have an inherent capacity to multiply, and they cease multiplication for various reasons. Control appears to be mediated by an unknown feedback mechanism, probably resulting from contact phenomena when cells are crowded together. Knowledge of growth patterns have aided in the derivation of chemotherapeutic principles. Strategies for therapy have evolved to take advantage of these differences in growth characteristics between normal and malignant tissues.

Normal tissues fall into three predominant categories: static, expanding, and renewing. Static populations of cells are generally well differentiated, and after a period of proliferation in fetal life rarely undergo division during adult life. Examples of static tissues include neurons and skeletal muscle. Because of the rare incidence of cell division, these cells are unlikely to be injured by chemotherapies that target rapidly dividing cells. Expanding tissue populations are also usually inactive in adult life, but unlike static populations they retain the ability to proliferate rapidly in response to stress or injury. Typical examples of expanding cells include hepatocytes and vascular endothelium. Last, the renewing cell populations are those that are constantly undergoing division, such as bone marrow and gastrointestinal epithelium. Renewing tissues are most sensitive to injury by chemotherapeutic agents (Table 18–2).

In the malignant growth, cells do not cease multiplying when they reach a critical mass. This unregulated growth appears to be due to a combination of loss of normal cell cycle controls and a failure of normal apoptotic mechanisms. Despite uncontrolled growth, malignant cell division does not appear to be more rapid than normal cell division.

In general, as tumors grow they display gompertzian growth characteristics (Fig. 18–1): as the tumor mass increases in size, the time necessary to double its size also becomes progressively longer. Thus, in the early phases of growth, tumor cells appear to grow exponentially, but as tumor mass increases there is a progressive increase in the

Table 18–2 CLASSIFICATION OF NORMAL TISSUES BY RATE OF PROLIFERATION

Renewing (rapid proliferation)	Expanding (slow proliferation)	Static (rare proliferation)
Bone marrow	Lung	Muscle
Gastrointestinal mucosa	Liver	Bone
Ovary	Kidney	Cartilage
Testis	Endocrine glands	Nerve
Hair follicles	Vascular endothelium	

doubling time, although doubling times in humans may vary greatly. For example, embryonal tumors and some lymphomas have relatively short doubling times (20–40 days), whereas adenocarcinomas and squamous cell carcinomas have relatively long doubling times (50–150 days). Three explanations have been given for this prolonged volume-doubling time:

1. an increase in cell cycle time (the time from one mitosis to the next),
2. a decrease in the growth fraction (cells participating in cell division in the tumor), and
3. an increase in cell loss from tumor cells with insufficient nutrients and vascular supply.

The gompertzian model has several important implications for cancer progression. First, metastases generally have a shorter doubling time than the primary lesion. If it is assumed that an exponential growth occurs early in the malignancy's history and that the malignancy starts from a single cell, then a 1-mm mass will have undergone approximately 20 tumor doublings. A 5-mm mass (a size that is first recognizable on an x-ray) may have undergone 27 doublings. It follows that a 1-cm mass will have undergone 30 doublings, and a clinician will be pleased to have detected such an "early" lesion. Unfortunately, this "early" lesion has already undergone 30 doublings, with significant DNA change being possible. Utilizing this rationale, clinical techniques that are currently available tend to recognize malignancies late in their growth, and metastatic disease may well have occurred long before there was obvious clinical manifestation of the primary lesion. Another implication from this kinetic information is that in late stages of tumor growth a few doublings in tumor mass make a dramatic impact on the size of the tumor and the status of the patient. Once a tumor becomes palpable (1 cm in diameter—30 doublings), only three more doublings will produce a very large tumor mass (8 cm in diameter).

The gompertzian model also has clinical implications that have guided a good deal of clinical chemotherapy research. As a mass responds to treatment (i.e. gets smaller), the doubling time has been assumed to decrease as a consequence of a greater number of cells moving into cycle. This larger percentage of metabolically active cells would therefore increase the sensitivity of the neoplastic population of cell cycle–specific agents. This has led to the sequential use of cell cycle–non-specific agents (e.g. cyclophosphamide) to bring down the mass, to be followed by cell cycle–specific agents (e.g. methotrexate). Although these sequential combinations have been theoretically attractive, none has shown clear superiority in clinical trials. Another implication of the gompertzian growth concept is that metastases can be expected to be more sensitive to chemotherapy in general, and to cell cycle–specific agents in particular, than the primary tumor from which they arise. The smaller the size of the metastatic focus, the greater is the differential sensitivity. Therefore the insensitivity of a primary tumor to a given drug regimen might not necessarily predict the response of metastasis to the same regimen.

The rationale for the use of drugs in the treatment of cancer is to achieve the selective killing of tumor cells.

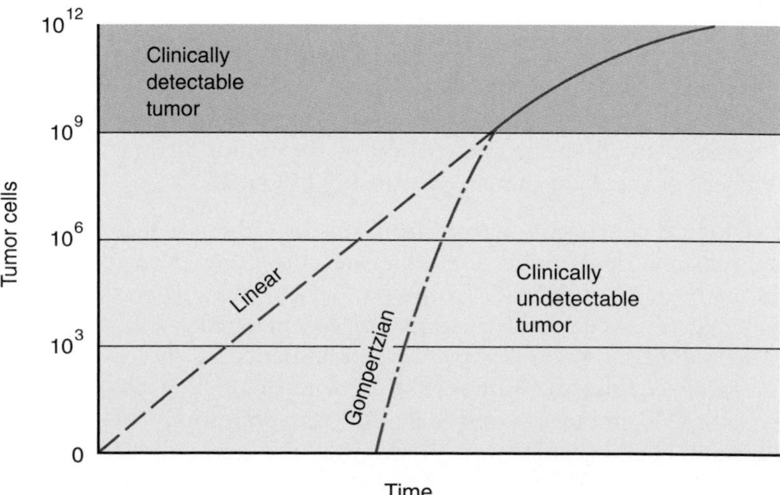

Figure 18–1 Tumor growth. As tumors grow, they display gompertzian characteristics. As tumor mass increases, doubling time becomes longer. However, a palpable tumor needs relatively few doublings to achieve a large mass.

Phase		Duration (h)
Gap 1 (G_1)	Postmitotic	4–24 (variable)
DNA synthesis (S)		10–20
Gap 2 (G_2)		2–10
Mitosis (M)		0.5–1
Gap 0 (G_0)		Resting (variable)

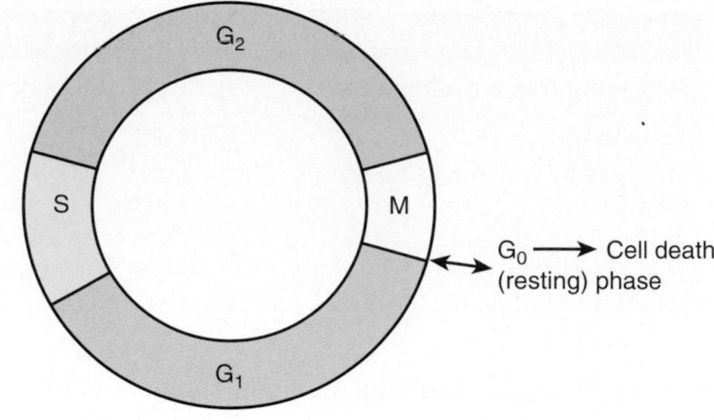

Figure 18–2 Cell generation time and sequence are similar for all mammalian cells. Tumor cells do not have faster generation times but do have more cells in the active phases of replication.

Underlying this rationale are the basic principles of the "cell kill" hypothesis first described by Skipper and associates. The following four principles were worked out in the L1210 leukemia model.

1. The survival of an animal with cancer is inversely related to the number of cancer cells.
2. A single cell is capable of multiplying and eventually killing the host.
3. For most drugs, a clear relationship exists between the dose of the drug and its ability to eradicate tumor cells.
4. A given dose of a drug kills a constant fraction of cells, not a constant number, regardless of the cell numbers present.

This fourth and most important principle implies that chemotherapeutic agents work by first-order kinetics; that is, they kill a constant fraction of cells rather than a constant number. This concept has important implications in cancer treatment. A single exposure of tumor cells to an antineoplastic drug may be capable of producing two to four logs of cell kill. With a common tumor burden of 10^{12} cells (1 kg), a single dose of chemotherapy will destroy a large number of cells but not be curative. Thus there is a need for intermittent courses of chemotherapy to achieve the magnitude of cell kill necessary to eradicate the lesion. Clinically, first-order cell kinetics dictate that to eradicate a tumor population effectively it is necessary to either:

- increase the total dose of the drug or drugs to the maximal limits tolerated by the host, or
- start treatment when the number of cells is small enough to allow the destruction of the tumor at total doses of the drug that are reasonably tolerated.

The logical conclusion derived from this hypothesis is that the maximal opportunity for achieving cure exists during the early stage of disease. In the past, chemotherapy was generally reserved for the treatment of disseminated cancer; surgery and/or radiotherapy were treatments of choice for localized disease. However, this concept of "log kill hypothesis" provides a rationale for the philosophy of adjuvant chemotherapy, which assumes the presence of undetectable cell masses of 10^1–10^4 cells after the initial surgical therapy that are capable of producing tumor relapse. This small tumor burden is particularly vulnerable to effective chemotherapy.

To better understand cell kinetics, it is imperative to visualize cell cycling. All dividing cells follow a predictable pattern for replication. The time that it takes a cell to complete one cycle of growth and division is termed its *generation time*. There are five basic phases (Fig. 18–2). The G_1 phase (G stands for gap and uncertainty as to purpose) lasts for a variable amount of time—usually between 4 and 24 h. If this phase is prolonged, the cell is usually referred to as being in the G_0, or resting, phase. The S phase is the phase of DNA synthesis and usually lasts between 10 and 20 h. The G_2 phase is a premitotic phase that lasts from 2 to 10 h, and the M phase, when actual mitosis takes place, lasts between 0.5 and 1 h. Tumors do not have faster generation times but have more cells in the active phases of replication than normal tissues. Normal tissues have a large number of cells in the G_0 phase, wherein the cell is not actively committed to division or is "out of cycle."

Some chemotherapeutic agents appear to act at several phases of the cell cycle (Fig. 18–3). Alkylating agents appear to act in all phases from G_0 to mitosis. They are called *cycle–non-specific agents.* Drugs such as hydroxyurea, doxorubicin (Adriamycin), and methotrexate appear to act primarily in the S phase. Bleomycin appears to act in the G_2 phase, and vincristine appears to act in the M phase. These drugs are called *cycle-specific agents* (Table 18–3) because they act chemotherapeutically only on cells that are in a specific phase of a cell generation cycle. Steroids, 5-fluorouracil, and cisplatin have rather uniform activity around the cell generation cycle. In theory, if certain cancer therapeutic agents attack only cells that are dividing and more tumor cells are dividing than normal tissue cells, then by properly spacing the chemotherapeutic agent and combining agents that act in different phases of the cell cycle one should be able to kill tumor cells in much greater numbers than normal cells. Kinetic studies in humans and animals suggest that tumors that have been cured by

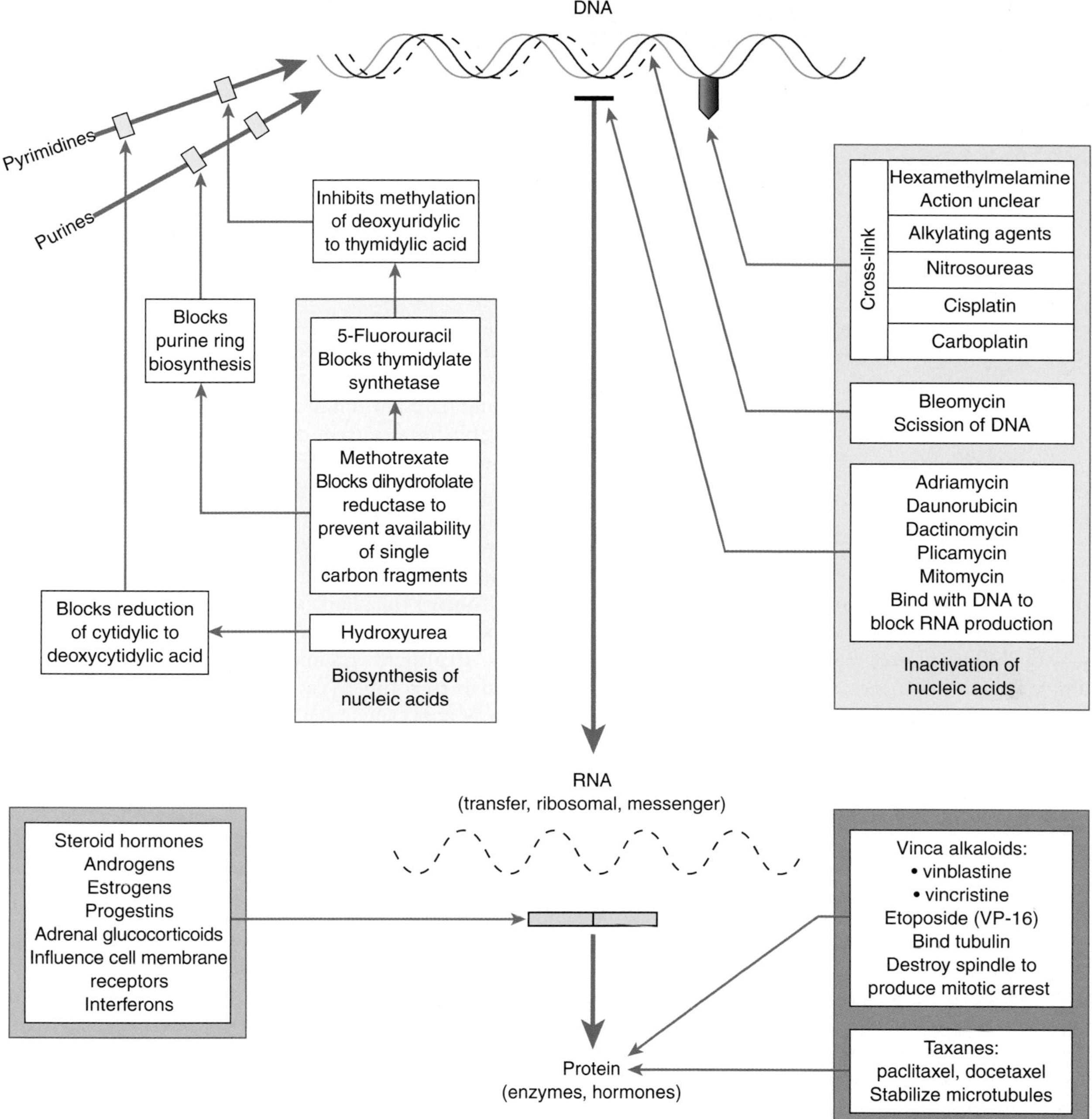

Figure 18–3 Cancer chemotherapeutic agents. (After Krakoff IH: Cancer chemotherapeutic agents. CA Cancer J Clin 37:93–105, 1987.)

chemotherapy are those with large fractions of cells in the proliferative phase (e.g. gestational choriocarcinoma and Burkitt lymphoma). The extent of the disease rather than the total mass of tumor is the most important factor when considering curative radiation or surgery, but in using chemotherapy the total mass is most important. When tumor volume is reduced, the remaining tumor cells can begin to divide actively (they are propelled from the G_0 phase into the more vulnerable cell generation cycle), thus rendering them susceptible to chemotherapy. These chemotherapeutic agents, as in radiation therapy, kill by first-order kinetics; that is, there is a reduction of the tumor population by a characteristic percentage, regardless of the actual number of tumor cells initially present (Fig. 18–4). If the tumor burden is small, fewer cycles of chemotherapy may be necessary. One milligram of tumor usually consists of 10^6 cells. One cubic centimeter of tumor usually consists of 10^9 cells. Patient death usually occurs at 10^{12} cells.

DYNAMICS OF CHEMOTHERAPY

The doubling time of a tumor depends on both generation time and cell death rate (Fig. 18–5). One cannot assume a long generation time simply because a tumor enlarges

Table 18–3 CELL CYCLE (PHASE)–SPECIFIC DRUGS

Phase dependence	Type	Drugs
S phase-dependent	Antimetabolite	Cytarabine Doxorubicin 5-Fluorouracil 6-Mercaptopurine Methotrexate Hydroxyurea Prednisone
M phase-dependent	Vinca alkaloids	Vincristine Vinblastine
	Taxanes	Paclitaxel Docetaxel
	Podophyllotoxins	Etoposide Teniposide
G_2 phase-dependent	—	Bleomycin
G_1 phase-dependent	—	Corticosteroids

slowly. Slow tumor growth can result from rapid generation time combined with a high cell death rate. For similar reasons, a small tumor discovered on radiographic or physical examination is not necessarily an early tumor; only serial studies to judge its growth rate will help establish its age. Bulky tumors (diameters >2–3 cm) enlarge more slowly than small ones because their cells, especially those of the inner core (farthest from the blood supply), have a long generation time. Competition for nutrients and other less-defined competitive pressures reduce the activity of the entire mass.

Successful chemotherapy of cancer requires a physiologic edge that can be exploited to differentially kill cancer cells but spare normal cells as much as possible. The more rapid growth rate of tumors as well as the increased synchronicity of tumor cells compared with normal tissues may be taken advantage of when designing therapeutic regimens. At any given time, comparatively large numbers of cancer cells will be in the DNA synthesis phase (S phase) of the cell cycle, the only time during which cycle-dependent agents (those inhibiting DNA synthesis) can act. Thus short-term high-dose chemotherapy with agents affecting DNA synthesis, such as methotrexate, is most effective in killing rapidly dividing tumor cells with relative sparing of normal bone marrow elements. Unfortunately, bone marrow cells, the epithelial cells that line the gastrointestinal tract, and hair follicles all have generation times comparable with those of tumors, and they are therefore vulnerable to compounds that inhibit DNA synthesis (Table 18–2). However, compared with the more synchronously growing tumor cell population, only a few of the bone marrow cells are in their S phase at any given time, and this accounts for the selective toxicity of phase-dependent compounds. A course of therapy extending over a period of several days, or even weeks, may be required to kill a slow-growing tumor in which only a few cells are in the stage of DNA synthesis at any one time.

Agents that do not depend on DNA synthesis for their effects (i.e. cycle–non–specific agents), such as alkylating agents, are most effective against bulky, slow-growing tumors. The cells remaining after treatment tend to divide more rapidly and are more susceptible to attack by cycle-specific agents. Thus there is some flexibility in the interplay of chemotherapeutic agents.

The phenomenon of increased susceptibility of tumor cells during recovery from alkylating agents is the rationale for sequentially combining cycle–non-specific and cycle-specific agents in many new regimens. If, in addition, drugs with different mechanisms of toxicity are combined, each drug can be given safely in the dose used when it is given alone. Each drug chosen for combination therapy should have antitumor activity when used alone. Whenever possible, intermittent courses of chemotherapy are used to allow restoration of normal cells if they were reduced in number by treatment. In cases in which an antidote to the chemotherapeutic agent is known, for example leucovorin (citrovorum factor, folinic acid) for methotrexate, this antidote can also be given to hasten normal cell recovery. Of course, the danger of revitalizing sublethally injured tumor cells also exists and must be evaluated with each new treatment regimen. Although careful studies are needed to compare each new combination with the single agents concerned, the trend in chemotherapy is unquestionably toward exploitation of drug combinations used simultaneously and sequentially.

PHARMACOLOGIC PRINCIPLES

Several general pharmacologic factors significantly affect the appropriate use of chemotherapeutic agents, including drug absorption, distribution, transport, metabolism, and excretion. These principles not only impinge on drug effectiveness but also dictate drug dose and schedule, as well as how drugs are selected for use in combination. The effectiveness of a given regimen depends on optimizing the *concentration x time* (also known as the area under the curve, AUC) at the site of tumor. Drug absorption influences route of administration, which in turn affects the AUC. Whether a drug is given orally, intravenously, intra-arterially, intramuscularly, or intraperitoneally is also determined by patient acceptance, feasibility, and toxicity. Drug distribution and delivery to the tumor site also affects AUC. Factors such as drug binding (to albumin or to plastic catheters), lipid solubility, and membrane transport are critical in determining effectiveness of a given agent. Certain sites in the body, such as the brain and testes, represent pharmacologic sanctuaries where drug delivery is limited. Similarly, poor tumor perfusion due to necrosis or hypoxia may also impair drug delivery and concentration. Understanding of membrane transport mechanisms is also key: certain drugs, such as 5-fluorouracil or mitomycin C, may enter cells through passive diffusion, while others, such as cisplatin and melphalan, require active transport.

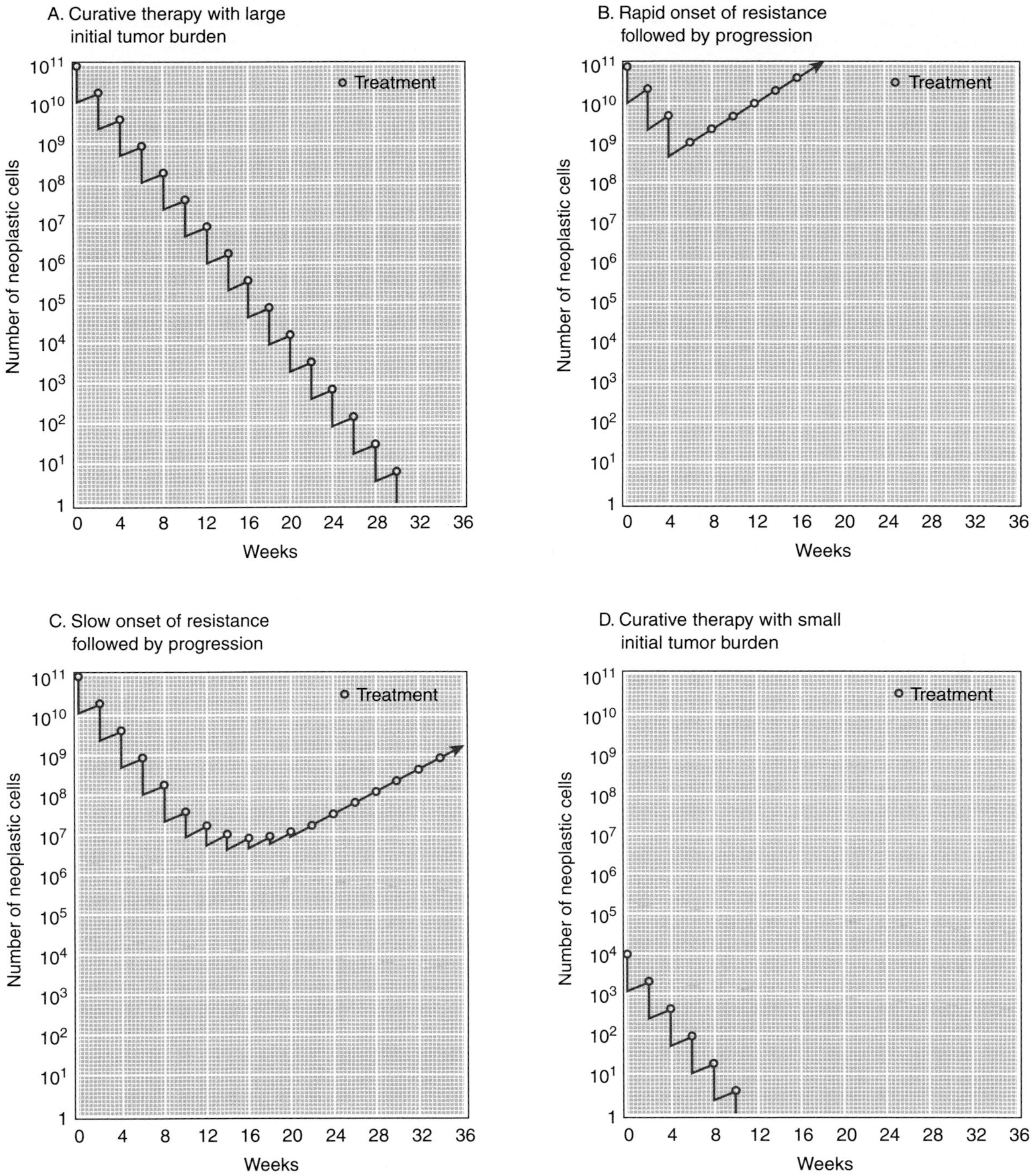

Figure 18–4 Efficacy of chemotherapy related to tumor kinetics. (After Bodye GB Sr, Frei E III, Luce JK: The systematic approach to cancer therapy. Hosp Pract 2(10):42, 1967.)

Drug metabolism is often necessary to convert an inactive prodrug into the active form. One example is cyclophosphamide, which requires cytochrome P-450 activation before antitumor effects are possible. Agents requiring hepatic metabolism to active forms are not amenable to intraperitoneal or intra-arterial administration. Conversely, metabolism and excretion of the active drug also affects AUC. The liver and the kidneys are responsible for the majority of drug elimination, although excretion in bile, stool, and respiration may also contribute in some cases. Organ dysfunction may result in increased drug toxicity and may require dose modification.

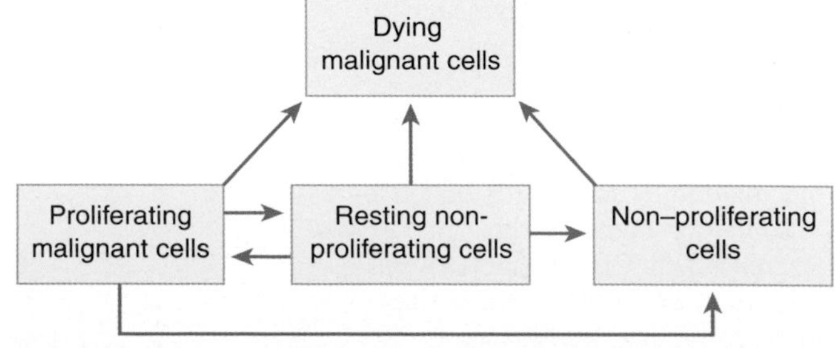

Figure 18–5 Dynamics of tumor growth, showing interrelationship of cell compartments contributing to clinical presence of tumor.

Drug interactions

Although patients undergoing chemotherapy treatment may also receive a variety of other drugs for treatment of acute side effects or chronic medical conditions, few drug interactions are clinically significant. However, a few interactions are noteworthy. In particular, doxorubicin and taxane agents are known to exert increased toxicity in the setting of impaired biliary excretion, while the platinums and methotrexate may cause increased toxicity in the setting of decreased renal function. Aspirin and sulfonamides are known to displace methotrexate from plasma proteins, and direct chemical interactions are noted between cisplatin and mannitol, and mitoxantrone and heparin.

Drug resistance

The effectiveness of any cancer treatment is limited by drug resistance, which may be intrinsic or acquired, and may develop to one drug or to multiple drugs (pleiotropic resistance). It has been suggested that spontaneous mutation is a basis for drug resistance. This spontaneous mutation occurs rapidly in malignant tumors. This concept, the Goldie–Coldman hypothesis, has been applied to the growth of malignant tumors and has important clinical implications. The theory suggests that most malignant cells begin with intrinsic sensitivity to chemotherapeutic agents but develop spontaneous resistance at variable rates. Goldie and Coldman have developed a mathematic model that relates curability to the time of recurrence of the singly or doubly resistant cells. Assuming that there is a natural mutation rate, the model predicts a variation in the size of the resistant fraction in tumors of the same size and type, which depends on that mutation rate and the point at which the mutation develops. Thus the proportion of resistant cells in any untreated tumor is likely to be small, and the initial response to treatment would not be influenced by the number of resistant cells. In clinical practice, this means that a complete remission could be obtained even if the resistant cell line were present. The failure to cure such a patient, however, would depend directly on the presence of these resistant cells. This model of spontaneous drug resistance implies that minimizing the emergence of drug-resistant clones requires that multiple effective drugs or therapies be applied as early as possible in the course of the patient's malignant disease process.

In cell lines and animal models, resistance to specific drugs likely occurs via a wide variety of mechanisms, although only a few have been confirmed to be of clinical significance in human cancers. These include increase in proficiency of DNA repair, decrease in drug uptake or increase in efflux by cells, increased levels of or alterations in target enzymes, alterations in drug activation/degradation, gene amplification, and defective drug metabolism. These mechanisms are reviewed in Table 18–4.

Multidrug resistance also occurs via various mechanisms. Some experimental evidence in murine tumors suggests that one form of multiple-drug resistance relates to the ability of drug-resistant tumor cells to limit drug accumulation of structurally unrelated agents. This cross-resistance is seen most often with natural products (e.g. doxorubicin, etoposide, paclitaxel, and vinca alkaloids); resistance to a single drug may confer a cross-resistance to structurally dissimilar drugs with different modes of action. This is the best studied mechanism for multidrug resistance and has been characterized involving the p-170 glycoprotein and its gene MDR1. Ling's coworkers initially demonstrated the appearance of a P-glycoprotein with a molecular weight of 170 kD on the cell membrane. The appearance of pleiotropic drug resistance is associated with permeability of the cell to accumulate and retain antineoplastic drugs. It has been demonstrated that this P-glycoprotein is directly related to the expression of resistance, and cells

Table 18–4 PROBABLE MECHANISMS ASSOCIATED WITH RESISTANCE TO SOME COMMONLY USED ANTICANCER DRUGS

Mechanism	Drugs
Increase in proficiency of repair of DNA	Alkylating agents, cisplatin
Decrease in cellular uptake or increase in efflux of drugs	Cisplatin, doxorubicin, etoposide, melphalan, 6-mercaptopurine, methotrexate, nitrogen mustard, vinblastine, vincristine
Increase in levels of "target" enzyme	Methotrexate
Alterations in target enzyme	5-Fluorouracil, 6-mercaptopurine, methotrexate, 6-thioguanine
Decrease in drug activation	Cytosine arabinoside, doxorubicin, 5-fluorouracil, 6-mercaptopurine, 6-thioguanine
Increase in drug degradation	Bleomycin, cytosine arabinoside, 6-mercaptopurine
Alternative biochemical pathways	Cytosine arabinoside
Inactivation of active metabolites by binding to sulfhydryl compounds	Alkylating agents, cisplatin, doxorubicin
Decreased activity of topoisomerase	Camptothecins, doxorubicin, etoposide
Alteration of tubulin-binding sites	Vincristine, paclitaxel
Increased damage tolerance	Alkylating agents, cisplatin

(After Tannock IF, Hill RT [eds]: The Basic Science of Oncology, 3rd ed., 1988. Reproduced by permission of The McGraw-Hill Companies.)

Table 18–5 EQUATIONS FOR CALCULATION OF BODY SURFACE AREA

	Equation[a]
Mostellar (m^2)	$\sqrt{\text{Weight} \times \text{height}/3600}$
DuBois and DuBois (m^2)	$(\text{Weight}^{0.425}) \times (\text{height}^{0.725}) \times 71.84$
Haycock (m^2)	$(\text{Weight}^{0.5378}) \times (\text{height}^{0.3964}) \times 0.024265$

[a]Weight in kg, height in cm.

that revert to the drug-sensitive state lose this membrane glycoprotein. DNA can be transferred from resistant cells to the sensitive cells, producing a transfer of pleiotropic resistance to unexposed cells.

Although best characterized, MDR1 is unlikely to be the most common mechanism for chemotherapy resistance among ovarian cancers, given that most do not express the MDR1 gene. Another mechanism for the multiple-drug resistance phenotype is seen among alkylating agents, cisplatin, and irradiation. Resistance in this group of agents has been linked to elevations in intracellular glutathione levels and is not associated with an overall measurable decrease in drug accumulation. Other transport proteins, including multidrug resistance–associated protein, have been identified that do not involve the p-170 glycoprotein pump. Furthermore, alterations in genes controlling apoptosis and growth arrest have also been cited. While the relative importance of these separate mechanisms in ovarian cancer remains to be established, it seems most likely that in clinical situations various combinations of mechanisms are at work.

Calculation of dosage

Dosages of chemotherapeutic agents are usually discussed in terms of mg/kg of body weight or mg/m^2 of total body surface area (Table 18–5). Dosage based on surface area is preferable to that based on weight, because surface area changes much less during the course of therapy, allowing a more consistent absolute amount of drug to be given throughout therapy. Dosages per unit are also more comparable in adults and children (Figs 18–6 and 18–7), and the variation in total dose between very obese and very thin people is minimized. Dosage in experimental animals expressed as mg/m^2 is more easily related to that in humans. In adults, mg/kg can be converted with reasonable accuracy to mg/m^2 by multiplying by 40.

Dose adjustments should be made for patients who are likely to have a compromised bone marrow reserve; that is, those older than 70 years of age, those who have received previous pelvic or abdominal irradiation, and those who have had previous chemotherapy. In these subsets of patients, the physician should consider beginning with a dose reduced by 35–50% and escalate up to a full dose with subsequent courses if initial doses are well tolerated. In a similar manner, any moderate to severe toxicity during the patient's course of therapy should direct a reduction in future doses. Many clinicians favor limiting body surface area to 2 mg/m^2 in calculation of dosage. The adverse effects criteria table used by the Gynecologic Oncology Group is included as Appendix B.

Dose adjustments are often required in patients receiving anticancer agents that are eliminated by the kidneys. These adjustments reduce the likelihood of overly

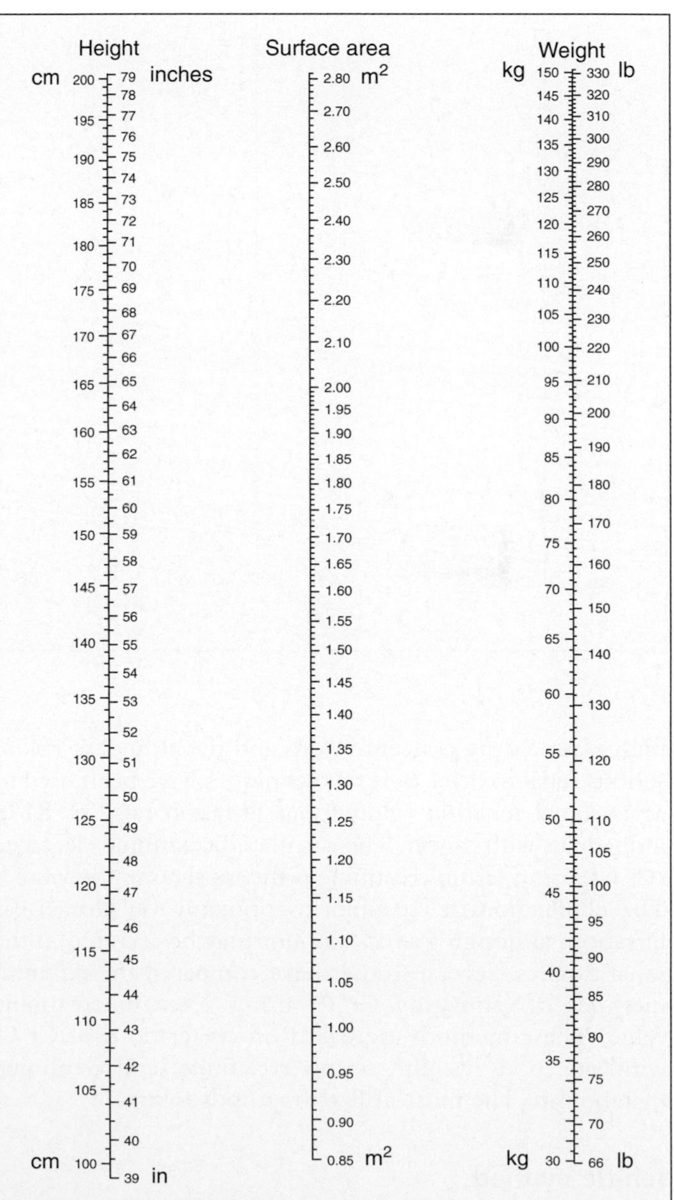

Figure 18–6 Nomogram for calculating the body surface area of adults.

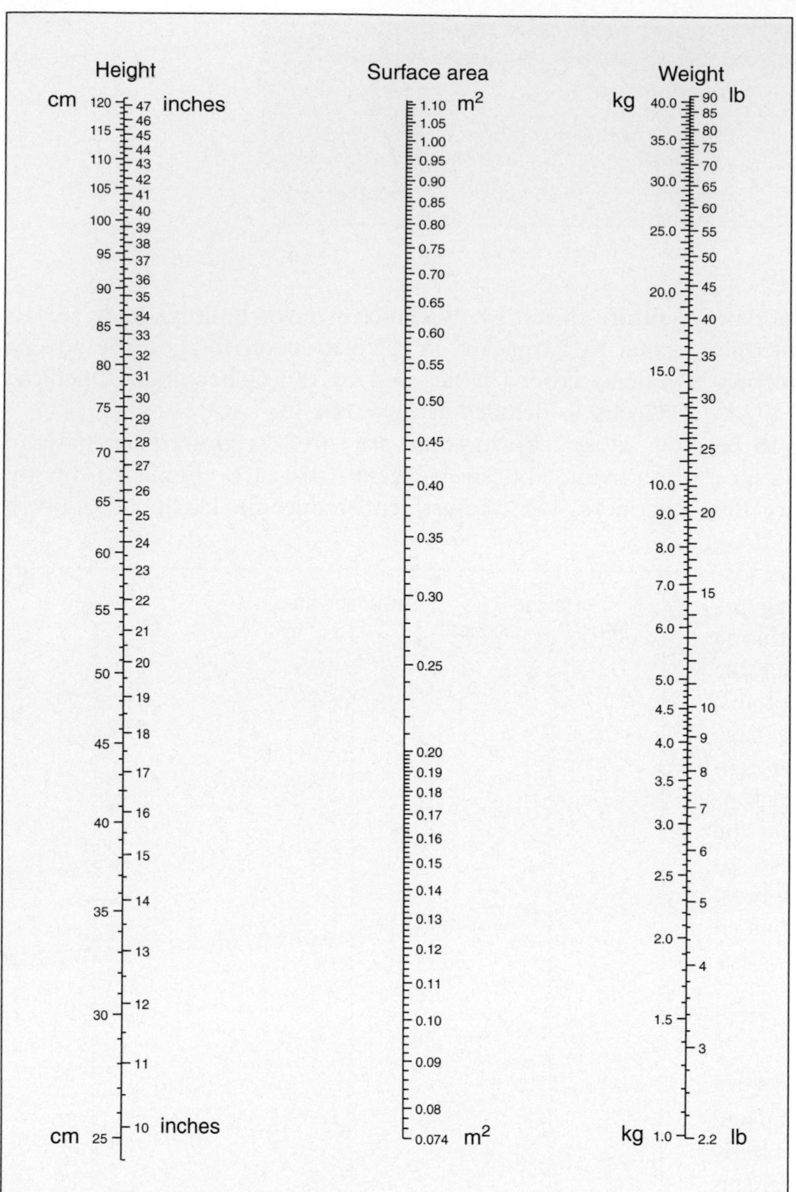

Figure 18–7 Nomogram for calculating body surface area of children.

high plasma drug concentrations and the attendant risk of serious renal toxicity. Several techniques have been used to assess renal function (glomerular filtration rate, GFR) in individuals with cancer. The calculated creatinine clearance (Cr Cl) using serum creatinine is the most commonly used. The elimination of creatinine is primarily via glomerular filtration, although a small amount may be secreted in the renal tubules. Several studies have compared the different methods of estimating Cr Cl using a serum creatinine value. These methods are based on correlations of Cr Cl with age, body weight, serum creatinine, and creatinine metabolism. The most utilized methods follow.

Jelliffe method

The Jelliffe method was used originally as a simple estimate of Cr Cl using serum creatinine, making minor adjustments in the calculation for female patients. The current Jelliffe formula takes into consideration age and renal function, and is as follows:

$$\text{Cr Cl (mL/min)} = 1.73\,[(100/\text{serum creatinine}) - 2].$$

(For female patients, use 90% of predicted Cr Cl.)

Cockroft–Gault method

This equation includes factors for lean body weight, which is especially important for obese patients, and correlation for female patients (the obtained value is multiplied by 0.85 for women). This method is similar to the Jelliffe calculation and is as follows:

$$\text{Cr Cl} = (140 - \text{age}) \times (\text{lean body weight in kg}) / (\text{serum creatinine}) \times 72.$$

Table 18–6 RECOMMENDED INDIVIDUALIZED DOSING OF CARBOPLATIN

Carboplatin dose (mg) = target AUC × (glomerular filtration rate + 25)
AUC is selected for appropriate clinical situation:
AUC 6 in untreated patients, when used in combination with taxanes
AUC 5 in previously treated patients
AUC 7 in previously untreated patients
Glomerular filtration rate is equivalent to creatinine clearance, which can be measured or can be estimated from patient's age, weight, and serum creatinine

AUC, area under the curve.

Calvert formula

The use of the Cr Cl has also been incorporated into the so-called Calvert formula. Based on good data, there is evidence showing that there is an inverse linear correlation between the GFR and the AUC of drugs such as carboplatin (Table 18–6). This finding suggests that in order to obtain the desired AUC, the dose must not only be decreased in patients with low renal function but also higher than standard doses may be required for patients with high renal clearance values. The Calvert formula is as follows:

dose (mg) = target AUC × (GFR + 25).

The original Calvert calculations were derived from GFR as measured by the chromium-51–EDTA method. Although calculated GFR is not the same as one that is measured, and Cr Cl can exceed GFR by 10–40%, the majority of physicians calculate rather than measure the GFR by using formulas such as Jelliffe or Cockcroft–Gault and then insert these numbers into the Calvert formula.

CATEGORIES OF DRUGS IN CURRENT USE (Table 18-7)

Alkylating agents

Alkylating agents prevent cell division primarily by cross-linking strands of DNA. Because of continued synthesis of other cell constituents, such as RNA and protein, growth is unbalanced and the cell dies. Activity of alkylating agents does not depend on DNA synthesis in the target cells. Cyclophosphamide, however, also inhibits DNA synthesis, which makes it distinctive among the alkylating agents in its mode and spectrum of activity. Alkylating agents now used in gynecologic oncology are:

- carboplatin,
- cisplatin,
- oxaliplatin,
- cyclophosphamide,
- chlorambucil,
- melphalan,
- triethylenethiophosphoramide,
- ifosfamide, and
- altretamine (hexmethylmelamine).

Antimetabolites

Antimetabolites act by inhibiting essential metabolic processes that are required for synthesis of purines, pyrimidines, and nucleic acids. These agents are typically S phase-specific. The currently used drugs in this category are:

- 5-fluorouracil,
- methotrexate,
- cytarabine,
- capecitabine, and
- gemcitabine.

Antitumor antibiotics

Antitumor antibiotics have generally been derived from fermentation products of various fungi, and most work via DNA intercalation. Several cytotoxic antibiotics have come into use for chemotherapy of certain neoplasms. Those used in gynecologic oncology are:

- dactinomycin (actinomycin D),
- bleomycin,
- doxorubicin and liposomal doxorubicin hydrochloride,
- mitomycin C, and
- mitoxantrone.

Agents derived from plants

Several chemotherapeutic agents have been developed from plants. The vinca alkaloids, the epipodophyllotoxins, and the taxanes act to disturb the normal assembly, disassembly, and stabilization of microtubules. The camptothecin analogs serve to inhibit topoisomerase I, thereby inducing single-stranded DNA breaks. These drugs are as follow.

- Vinca alkaloids:
  - vinblastine,
  - vincristine, and
  - vinorelbine.
- Taxanes:
  - paclitaxel and
  - docetaxel.
- Epipodophyllotoxins:
  - etoposide.
- Camptothecin analogs:
  - topotecan and
  - irinotecan.

Table 18–7 CHEMOTHERAPY AGENTS USED IN THE TREATMENT OF GYNECOLOGIC CANCER

Drug	Dosage and route of administration	Acute side effects	Toxicity	Precautions	Major indications
Alkylating agents					
Cisplatin (CDDP or Platinol)	50–100 mg/m^2 i.v. every 3 weeks; 40 mg/m^2 i.v. every week with radiation therapy; 50–100 mg/m^2 i.p. in 2 L over 30 min every 3 weeks	Nausea and vomiting, often severe	Renal damage, moderate myelosuppression, neurotoxicity; severe renal damage can be minimized by not exceeding a total dose of 500 mg/m^2 in any treatment course	Infuse at a rate not to exceed 1 mg/min and only after 10–12 h of hydration; avoid nephrotoxic antibodies; watch renal function and discontinue if blood urea nitrogen exceeds 30 or creatinine exceeds 2	Carcinoma of the ovary, endometrium, or cervix
Carboplatin (Paraplatin)	250–400 mg/m^2 i.v. bolus or by 24-h continuous infusion every 2–4 weeks (most authorities recommend dosing to area under the curve values of 5.0–8.0)	Mild nausea and vomiting	Bone marrow suppression, especially thrombocytopenia	Decreased dose in patients who have had previous chemotherapy	Carcinoma of the cervix, ovary, and endometrium
Cyclophosphamide (Cytoxan)	50–1500 mg/m^2 as a single dose i.v. or 60–120 mg/m^2 day p.o.; dose decreased if severe leukopenia develops	Nausea and vomiting	Bone marrow depression, alopecia, cystitis	Maintain adequate fluid intake to avoid cystitis	Carcinoma of the cervix, ovary, endometrium, and fallopian tube
Chlorambucil (Leukeran)	0.1–0.2 mg/kg per day p.o.; dose decreased if severe bone marrow depression develops	Nausea, vomiting (with high doses)	Bone marrow depression	None	—
Melphalan (Alkeran)	0.2 mg/kg per day p.o. for 4 days every 4–6 weeks	Nausea, vomiting (with high doses)	Bone marrow depression	None	—
Triethylenethio-phosphoramide (thiotepa)	0.2 mg/kg per day i.v. for 5 days	None	Bone marrow depression	None	—
Ifosfamide (Ifex)	7–10 g/m^2 i.v. over 3–5 days every 3–4 weeks	Nausea, vomiting	Bone marrow depression, alopecia, cystitis	Uroprotectant to prevent hemorrhagic cystitis	Carcinoma and sarcoma of ovary, cervix, and endometrium
Oxaliplatin	59–130 mg/m^2 i.v. as a 20-min or 2-h infusion every 3 weeks	Nausea, vomiting, diarrhea, mucositis	Mild to moderate myelosuppression; transaminase elevation; peripheral neuropathy	Should not be given to patient with significant renal or hepatic dysfunction	Ovarian carcinoma
Altretamine (Hexalen)	4–12 mg/kg per day p.o. in divided doses for 14–21 days, repeated every 6 weeks	Nausea and vomiting	Bone marrow depression; neurotoxicity, both central and peripheral	None	Ovarian carcinoma

Table 18–7 CHEMOTHERAPY AGENTS USED IN THE TREATMENT OF GYNECOLOGIC CANCER—cont'd

Drug	Dosage and route of administration	Acute side effects	Toxicity	Precautions	Major indications
Antimetabolites					
5-Fluorouracil (5-FU)	12 mg/kg per day i.v. for 4 days, then alternate days at 6 mg/kg for 4 days or until toxicity; repeat course monthly or give weekly i.v. dose of 12–15 mg/kg; maximal dose 1 g for either regimen; often used as one drug in combination regimens at a dose of 500 mg/m^2 i.v.	Bone marrow depression, diarrhea, stomatitis, alopecia	Occasional nausea and vomiting	Decrease dose in patients with diminished liver, renal, or bone marrow function or after adrenalectomy	Carcinoma of the ovary and endometrium
Methotrexate	Choriocarcinoma: 10–30 mg/day i.v. for 5 days Ovarian or cervical carcinoma: 200–2000 mg/m^2 i.v. with concomitant or sequential systematic antidote leucovorin ("leucovorin rescue")	None	Bone marrow depression, megaloblastic anemia, diarrhea, stomatitis, vomiting; alopecia less common; occasional hepatic fibrosis, vasculitis, pulmonary fibrosis	Adequate renal function must be present, and urine output must be maintained	Choriocarcinoma, carcinoma of the ovary and cervix
Cytarabine (Ara-C, Cytosar-U) (2′,2′-difluorodeoxy cytarabine)	200 mg/m^2 daily for 5 days by continuous infusion	Nausea and vomiting	Bone marrow depression, megaloblastosis, leukopenia, thrombocytopenia	None	Carcinoma of the ovary (intraperitoneal use)
Gemcitabine (Gemzar)	800–1000 mg/m^2 i.v. days 1, 8, 15 every 28 days; 800–1000 mg/m^2 i.v. days 1, 8 every 21 days; 900 mg/m^2 i.v. days 1, 8 every 21 days for patients with leiomyosarcoma	Mild nausea, vomiting, malaise (usually mild), transient febrile episodes, maculopapular rash	Bone marrow suppression	None	Carcinoma of the breast and ovary; leiomyosarcoma of the uterus
Capecitabine (Xeloda)	1500–2000 mg/m^2 p.o. daily in two divided doses for 2 weeks with a 1-week rest period, repeat every 3 weeks	Hand and foot syndrome (palmar–plantar erythrodysesthesia syndrome); nausea, vomiting, diarrhea; abdominal pain; constipation	Myelosuppression; hyperbilirubinemia	Should be taken in divided doses 12 h apart, administered with water 30 min after a meal	Ovarian carcinoma

Table continued on following page.

Table 18–7 CHEMOTHERAPY AGENTS USED IN THE TREATMENT OF GYNECOLOGIC CANCER—cont'd

Drug	Dosage and route of administration	Acute side effects	Toxicity	Precautions	Major indications
Antitumor antibiotics					
Dactinomycin (actinomycin D, Cosmegen)	15 μg/kg per day i.v. or 0.5 mg/day for 5 days	Pain on local infiltration with skin necrosis; nausea and vomiting in many patients 2 h after the dose; occasional cramps and diarrhea	Bone marrow depression, stomatitis, diarrhea, erythema, hyperpigmentation with occasional desquamation in areas of previous irradiation	Administer through running i.v. infusion; use with care in patients with liver disease and in the presence of inadequate marrow function; prophylactic antiemetics are helpful	Embryonal rhabdomyosarcoma, choriocarcinoma, ovarian germ cell tumors
Mitomycin C (Mutamycin)	0.05 mg/kg per day i.v. for 6 days, then alternate days until a 50-mg total dose	Nausea, vomiting, local inflammation and ulceration if extravasated	Neutropenia, thrombocytopenia, oral ulceration, nausea, vomiting, diarrhea	Administer through running i.v. infusion or inject with great care to prevent extravasation	Carcinoma of the cervix
Bleomycin	10–20 mg/m^2 i.v. or i.m. one or two times a week	Fever, chills, nausea, vomiting; local pain and phlebitis less frequent	Skin: hyperpigmentation, thickening, nail changes, ulceration, rash, peeling, alopecia Pulmonary: pneumonitis with dyspnea, rales, infiltrate can progress to fibrosis; more common in patients older than 70 years pf age and with more than a 400-mg total dose, but unpredictable	Watch for hypersensitivity in lymphoma with first one or two doses; use with extreme caution in presence of renal or pulmonary disease; start in hospital under observation; do not exceed a total dose of 400 mg	Squamous cell carcinoma of the skin, vulva, and cervix; choriocarcinoma; germ cell and sex cord–stromal tumors of the ovary
Doxorubicin (Adriamycin)	60–100 mg/m^2 i.v. every 3 weeks	Nausea, vomiting, fever, local phlebitis, necrosis if extravasated, red urine (not blood)	Bone marrow depression, alopecia, cardiac toxicity related to the cumulative dose, stomatitis; atrophy of the myocardia can occur, especially if a total dose of 450–500 mg/m^2 is exceeded	Administer through running i.v. infusion; avoid giving to patients with significant heart disease; observe for electrocardiogram abnormalities and signs of heart failure	Adenocarcinoma of the endometrium, fallopian tube, ovary, and vagina; uterine sarcoma
Mitoxantrone	—	—	—	—	—
Liposomal doxorubicin hydrochloride (Doxil)	40–50 mg/m^2 i.v. every 4 weeks	Hand and foot syndrome (palmar–plantar erythrodysesthesia syndrome); mild nausea/vomiting, mucositis, stomatitis	Mild myelosuppression; cardiomyopathy is less common compared with standard doxorubicin	Hypersensitivity reported in approximately seven patients	Ovarian carcinoma

Table 18–7 CHEMOTHERAPY AGENTS USED IN THE TREATMENT OF GYNECOLOGIC CANCER—cont'd

Drug	Dosage and route of administration	Acute side effects	Toxicity	Precautions	Major indications
Agents derived from plants					
Vinca alkaloids					
Vinblastine (Velban)	0.10–0.15 mg/kg per week i.v.	Severe, prolonged inflammation if extravasated; occasional nausea, vomiting, headache, and paresthesias	Bone marrow depression, particularly neutropenia; alopecia, muscle weakness, occasional mild peripheral neuropathy, mental depression 2–3 days after treatment, rarely stomatitis	Administer through running i.v. infusion or inject with great care to prevent extravasation; decrease dose in liver disease	Choriocarcinoma
Vincristine (Oncovin)	0.4–1.4 mg/m^2 i.v. weekly in adults; 2 mg/m^2 weekly in children	Local inflammation if extravasated	Paresthesias, weakness, loss of reflexes, constipation; abdominal, chest, and jaw pain; hoarseness, foot drop, mental depression; marrow toxicity generally mild, anemia and reticulocytopenia most prominent; alopecia	Administer through running i.v. infusion or inject with great care to prevent extravasation; decrease dose in patients with liver disease; patients with underlying neurologic problems may be more susceptible to neurotoxicity; alopecia may be prevented by use of a scalp tourniquet for 5 min during and after administration	Uterine sarcoma, germ cell tumor of the ovary
Vinorelbine (Navelbine)	30 mg/m^2 weekly i.v.	Mild nausea, 10% alopecia	Bone marrow depression, mild to moderate peripheral neuropathy	Local irritant, dose modification with hepatic dysfunction	Ovarian carcinoma
Epipodophyllotoxins					
Etoposide (VP-16)	100 mg/m^2 i.v. days 1, 3, and 5; repeat in 4 weeks	Nausea and vomiting	Leukopenia, thrombocytopenia, alopecia, headache, fever, occasional hypotension	Reduce dose by 25–50% for hematologic toxicity	Trophoblastic disease, germ cell tumors
Taxanes					
Paclitaxel (Taxol)	135–175 mg/m^2 i.v. over 3 h every 3 weeks	Allergic reaction, nausea, vomiting	Bone marrow depression, severe allergic-like reactions with facial erythema, dyspnea, tachycardia, and hypotension cardiotoxicity with bradycardia, alopecia, stomatitis, fatigue	Cardiac monitoring may be necessary	Ovarian carcinoma; endometrial cancer; cervical cancer

Table continued on following page.

Table 18–7 CHEMOTHERAPY AGENTS USED IN THE TREATMENT OF GYNECOLOGIC CANCER—cont'd					
Drug	**Dosage and route of administration**	**Acute side effects**	**Toxicity**	**Precautions**	**Major indications**
Taxanes—cont'd					
Docetaxel (Taxotere)	60–100 mg/m² i.v. over 1 h every 3 weeks	Hypersensitivity	Myelosuppression; mucositis; alopecia; fluid retention	Requires premedication with steroids	Ovarian carcinoma
Camptothecin analogs					
Topotecan	1.5 mg/m² daily for 5 days; 4 mg/m² i.v. day 1 and day 8, repeat every 21 days	Maculopapular pruritic exanthema	Bone marrow depression	Watch for neutropenic fever	Ovarian carcinoma, cervical carcinoma
Irinotecan (CPT-11)	300 mg/m² i.v. every 3 weeks; 100 mg/m² i.v. weekly for 4 weeks every 6 weeks	Nausea and vomiting, diarrhea	Myelosuppression, alopecia, rash	None	Ovarian carcinoma
Hormonal agents					
Progestational agents					
Medroxyprogesterone acetate	400–800 mg/week i.m. or p.o.	None	Occasional liver function abnormalities, occasional alopecia and hypersensitivity reactions	Use with care when liver dysfunction present	Carcinoma of the endometrium
Hydroxyprogesterone caproate	1000 mg i.m. twice weekly				
Megestrol acetate (Megace)	20–80 mg p.o. twice a day				
Antiestrogens					
Tamoxifen	10–20 mg p.o. twice daily	Nausea, usually mild	Caused by antiestrogenic action (e.g. hot flashes, pruritus vulvae, and occasionally vaginal bleeding)	None	Breast cancer, possibly useful in endometrial carcinoma (metastatic)
Miscellaneous					
Hydroxyurea (Hydrea)	80 mg/kg p.o. every 3 days or 20–30 mg/kg per day	Anorexia and nausea	Bone marrow depression, megaloblastic anemia; stomatitis, diarrhea, and alopecia less common	Decrease dose in patients with marrow and renal dysfunction	Carcinoma of the cervix (with radiotherapy)

Hormonal agents

These agents are often utilized in the treatment of endometrial, breast, and ovarian cancers and are classified in two broad categories, antiestrogens and progestational agents. Megestrol acetate may both down-regulate estrogen-responsive genes and reduce the number of available cell surface estrogen receptors. Examples of these agents are as follow.

- Antiestrogens:
  - tamoxifen.
- Progestational agents:
  - megestrol acetate,
  - medroxyprogesterone acetate, and
  - hydroxyprogesterone.

Targeted therapies

To date, traditional chemotherapy has predominantly focused on killing rapidly dividing cells. Unfortunately, normal cells may also be affected, causing significant toxicity. Targeted therapies have attempted to focus anticancer treatment on particular pathways and mechanisms that cause cancer to both increase efficacy and decrease toxicity in comparison with traditional chemotherapies. These therapies may aim to affect pathways for angiogenesis, cell cycle, and apoptosis in tumor cells. Several broad categories of targeted therapies exist. Monoclonal antibodies target receptors on the surface of tumor cells. As part of anticancer therapy, monoclonal antibodies have been used in two fashions. First, infusion of the antibody has allowed binding to target cells, which in turn triggers normal effector mechanisms of the body. Second, monoclonal antibodies have been conjugated to a strongly radioactive atom, such as iodine-131, to aid in killing the target. Other targeted therapies focus on the internal components and function of the cancer cell, using small molecules to disrupt the function of the cells, triggering apoptosis. There are several types of targeted therapy that focus on the inner parts of the cells. These therapies are currently not a replacement for traditional therapy, but may be best used in combination with chemotherapeutic agents. Some targeted therapies, along with their targets, are listed below.

- Monoclonal antibodies:
  - oregovamab (CA-125),
  - cetuximab (EGFR),
  - bevacizumab (VEGF), and
  - trastuzumab (HER-2/neu).
- Small molecules:
  - gefitinib (EGFR),
  - erlotonib (EGFR),
  - OSI-774 (EGFR-TK),
  - bortezomib (proteosome), and
  - imatinib (Bcr-Abl protein tyrosine kinase, c-kit receptor tyrosine kinase).

DRUG TOXICITY

Unfortunately, traditional chemotherapeutic agents are indiscriminate in their effects: both malignant and normal tissues are affected. Although their goal is to kill more cancerous than normal cells, many side effects, particularly those to organ systems with rapidly proliferating cell populations, are inevitable. Usually, the mechanism of toxicity is similar to the one producing the desired cytotoxic effect. Even organs with limited cell proliferation can be damaged by chemotherapeutic agents, especially if the agents are utilized at high doses. Chemotherapeutic agents must be used at doses that produce some degree of toxicity to normal tissue in order to be effective. The incidence of severe side effects of chemotherapeutic agents is greatly influenced by states such as severe disability, advancing age, poor nutrition, or direct organ involvement by primary or metastatic lesions. The physician must monitor these patients with extreme care, and appropriate dose modifications must be made (Table 18–8).

Hematologic toxicity

Hematologic toxicity is the most frequently seen side effect. Acute granulocytopenia occurs 6–12 days after the administration of most myelosuppressive chemotherapeutic agents. Recovery occurs in 10–14 days. The megakarocyte series is affected later, such that platelet suppression usually occurs 4 or 5 days after granulocytopenia and recovers several days after the white blood cell count. Mitomycin C and nitrosourea are particularly unique in their ability to produce delayed bone marrow suppression. Myelosuppression with these two drugs commonly occurs within 28–42 days, with recovery 40–60 days after treatment.

Table 18–8 DRUG DOSE MODIFICATION BASED ON COMMON HEMATOLOGIC TOXICITY

Count before next course (per mm^3)	Dose modification[a]
Leukocytes	
> 4000	100% of dose
3000–3999	100% of non-myelotoxic agents 50% of myelotoxic agents
2000–2999	100% of non-myelotoxic agents 25% of myelotoxic agents
1000–1999	25% of myelotoxic agents
≤ 999	No drug
Platelets	
> 100,000	100% of dose
50,000–100,000	100% of non-myelotoxic agents
< 50,000	No drug

[a]Based on myelosuppression.

Most clinicians consider patients with absolute granulocyte counts less than 500/mm^3 for 5 days or longer to be at a higher risk for sepsis. The practice of utilizing prophylactic broad-spectrum antibiotics in febrile granulocytopenic cancer patients has significantly decreased the incidence of life-threatening infections in this group of patients. Granulocytopenic patients should have their temperature checked every 4 h, and they should be examined frequently for evidence of infection. Thrombocytopenic patients with platelet counts less than 20,000/mm^3 are at increased risk for spontaneous hemorrhage, particularly from the gastrointestinal tract. Routine platelet transfusions for platelets under 10–20,000/mm^3 have been utilized by some clinicians. It is common to transfuse 6–10 U of random donor platelets to such patients. Others wait and watch until patients manifest some evidence of bleeding. Repeat transfusions of platelets at 2- to 3-day intervals may be necessary in patients with severe thrombocytopenia. Patients with active peptic ulcer disease and patients needing surgical procedures need to be transfused with counts lower than 50,000/mm^3.

Growth factor therapy

The application of hematopoietic factors to supportive care has been dramatic. Rapid advances in unraveling the molecular biology and biochemistry of these glycoprotein hormones that regulate hematopoiesis have led to their routine clinical use. Since their emergence in 1989, their

Table 18–9 CHARACTERISTICS OF THE HEMATOPOIETIC GROWTH FACTOR FAMILY OF CYTOKINES

Cytokine	Source	Function
Granulocyte–macrophage colony–stimulating factor (GM-CSF)	T cells, endothelial cells, stromal cells	Stimulates hematopoiesis of granulocyte and macrophage lineage; activates granulocytes and macrophages
Granulocyte colony–stimulating factor (G-CSF)	Endothelial cells, monocytes, stromal cells	Stimulates hematopoiesis of granulocyte lineage; activates granulocytes
Erythropoietin	Kidney	Stimulates erythroid growth and development
Interleukin-1	Monocytes/macrophages, B and T cells, endothelial cells	Costimulates early stages of hematopoiesis; T- and B-cell activation
Interleukin-3	T cells	Stimulates early stages of hematopoiesis
Interleukin-6	T cells, monocytes/macrophages, fibroblasts	Costimulates early stages of hematopoiesis; T- and B-cell activation

(After Kouides PA: The hematopoietic growth factors. In Haskell CM [ed]: Principles of Cancer Treatment, 4th edn. Philadelphia, Saunders, 1995.)

use has allowed amelioration of therapy-related myelosuppression, modulation of disease-related myelosuppression, and enhanced host defense to infection. This class of agents includes molecules such as granulocyte colony–stimulating factor (G-CSF) and granulocyte–macrophage colony–stimulating factor (GM-CSF). The biologic activities of these proteins are complex and multifunctional, stimulating potent changes in the growth, differentiation, distribution, and functional status of mature cells as well as their precursors (Table 18–9).

Initial studies with G-CSF and GM-CSF focused on their administration via the intravenous route. Since then, numerous studies have shown that subcutaneous administration once or twice a day is even more myelostimulatory than 2- to 4-h intravenous infusions. The recommended dose of GM-CSF is 250 μg/m^2 or 3–5 μg/kg. Interestingly, at least in some cases, a fairly low dose of GM-CSF may be more myelostimulatory than a higher dose. The enhancement of neutrophil function in terms of adherence, phagocytosis, and chemotaxis has also been noted in clinical studies, and GM-CSF may also function to activate lymphocytes. Two types of G-CSF are available: filgrastim and a long-acting pegfilgrastim. The recommended dose of filgrastim is 5 μg/kg, given subcutaneously. Treatment should begin at least 24 h after completion of chemotherapy, and should continue daily until the absolute neutrophil count exceeds 10,000/mm^3. Subsequent chemotherapy should not begin until at least 48 h have elapsed since the last dose. The recommended dose of pegfilgrastim is 6 mg. A subcutaneous injection is recommended at least 24 h after the completion of chemotherapy infusion, and should not be given within 14 days of any subsequent chemotherapy. Bone pain is the most common side effect of G-CSF. Other more rare effects include:

- a cutaneous eruption of macules and papules;
- exacerbation of underlying autoimmune disease;
- anaphylaxis, which is rare;
- mild increased risk of thrombosis; and
- a theoretic possibility of the exacerbation of the underlying malignancy.

Unquestionably, the administration of G-CSF or GM-CSF accelerates neutrophil recovery to a significant degree after standard-dose chemotherapy. G-CSF is indicated to decrease the incidence of febrile neutropenia with regimens associated with a significant incidence of neutropenia with fever.

The existence of a hormone that regulates erythropoiesis (Epo) has been proposed for 100 years. In 1985, two independent groups cloned the gene responsible for this growth factor. This gene was labeled the Epo gene. The kidney appears to be the major site of production of erythropoeitin. Apparently, the site of production in the fetus is the liver, and in the last third of the gestational period the responsibility is gradually transferred to the kidney. Erythropoietin stimulates the division and differentiation of committed erythroid progenitors in the bone marrow. Epoetin alpha is a glycoprotein manufactured by recombinant DNA technology. It is produced by mammalian cells into which the human Epo gene has been introduced. The product contains the exact amino acid sequence of natural Epo. Tissue hypoxia is the chief stimulus for the production of Epo. Relatively small blood losses (e.g. 1 U of blood) only modestly stimulate Epo production. Most patients on chemotherapy develop anemia at some point during the course of their illness. The hemoglobin concentration of these patients usually ranges from 7 to 12 g/dL, and the hematocrit is somewhere between 25 and 38%. This is sufficient to stimulate the production of Epo endogenously. However, there appears to be a large blunting of response to Epo in patients who have undergone chemotherapy.

Epoetin reduces the transfusion requirement in anemic patients and may enhance overall quality of life, and administration is indicated when hemoglobin levels have decreased below 10 mg/dL during chemotherapy treatment, or when a significant chance for blood transfusion exists. However, iron deficiency must be corrected before starting epoetin. Epoetin injected at a dose of 150 U/kg subcutaneously three times a week for 12 weeks has been used by many clinicians. The dose may be increased up to 300 U/kg. Others utilize a daily dose of 60 U/kg, progressing to a maximum dose of 90 U/kg per day. Another commonly used approach is to inject 40,000 U/week, with escalation to 60,000 U for non-responders. Darbepoetin alfa is a long-acting form that may be administered at doses of 3.0 μg/kg every 3 weeks. Adverse effects are uncommon but include worsening hypertension in patients with end-stage renal disease. Other effects include edema and diarrhea. Of more concern, recent research indicates that the erythropoietin receptor is expressed in several cancer cell lines, raising the concern of possible stimulation of tumor cell growth by these drugs. Indeed, two large randomized trials have reported significantly worse tumor control and survival rates in patients receiving epoetin. Epoetin has also been implicated in possible thromboembolic complications, possibly related to elevated hemoglobin levels.

Oprelvekin is produced in *E. coli* by recombinant DNA methods. The protein is very similar to interleukin (IL)-11, which is a thrombopoietic growth factor that directly stimulates the proliferation of hematopoietic stem cells and megakaryocyte maturation, which in turn increase platelet production. IL-11 is produced by bone marrow stromal cells and is part of the cytokine family. The usual dose is 50 μg/kg, which is given once daily subcutaneously as a single injection in either the abdomen, thigh, or hip. Treatment should begin 6–24 h after completion of chemotherapy and continued until the nadir platelet count is 50,000 cells/μL. Potential side effects include mild to moderate fluid retention, and IL-11 should be used with caution in patients with a history of atrial arrhythmia, transient mild visual blurring, and transient rashes at the injection site. Anaphylactic reactions have been reported.

Gastrointestinal toxicity

Gastrointestinal toxicity is another frequent manifestation of chemotherapeutic agents. Mucositis may be caused by direct effects on the rapidly dividing epithelial mucosa. Concomitant granulocytopenia allows the injured mucosa to become infected and serve as a portal of entry for bacteria and fungi. The onset of mucositis is frequently 3–5 days earlier than myelosuppression. The nasopharyngeal lesions are difficult to distinguish from viral lesions. Candidiasis is often seen and is difficult to distinguish from stomatitis secondary to chemotherapy; antifungal agents have been very effective in treating this condition. Necrotizing enterocolitis is another condition that is seen in patients receiving chemotherapy. Symptoms of this condition are watery or bloody diarrhea, abdominal pain, nausea, vomiting, and fever. Patients usually have abdominal tenderness and distension. They also have a history of broad-spectrum antibiotic use. Most necrotizing enterocolitis is caused by anaerobic bacteria such as *Clostridium difficile*. The treatment of choice for *C. difficile* infection is oral vancomycin, 125 mg four times daily for 10–14 days.

The most common side effect of chemotherapy is nausea and vomiting. Although the exact mechanisms are not clearly defined, most agents appear to stimulate the chemoreceptor trigger zone in the area postrema of the brain to secrete neurotransmitters such as dopamine, serotonin, and histamine. These neurotransmitters may activate the neighboring vomiting center to induce nausea and emesis. Direct stimulation of serotonin receptors in the gastrointestinal tract, direct cerebral action, and psychogenic effects may also play a role. Different patterns of emesis include acute emesis (within 24 h of chemotherapy infusion), delayed emesis (typically beginning 16–24 h after chemotherapy but persisting up to 72–96 h), and anticipatory emesis. Common antiemetic regimens are detailed in Table 18–10. Choice of agents should be governed by knowledge of the emetogenic potential of the chemotherapies administered (Table 18–11).

Highly emetogenic chemotherapies include cisplatin (>50 mg/m^2) and high-dose cyclophosphamide (>1500 mg/m^2). Cisplatin may induce both acute and delayed vomiting. A premedication regimen should consist of a combination of antiemetics given 30 min prior to chemotherapy infusion. Common regimens include use of a 5-HT$_3$ receptor antagonist with dexamethasone. Lorazepam and oral aprepitant may also be utilized. Moderately emetogenic chemotherapies include lower doses of cisplatin (<50 mg/m^2) and cyclophosphamide (750–1500 mg/m^2), as well as carboplatin, doxorubicin, methotrexate (>1000 mg/m^2), ifosfamide, and high-dose 5-fluorouracil. These agents may be premedicated with 5-HT$_3$ receptor antagonists in combination with dexamethasone. Mildly emetogenic chemotherapies include methotrexate, paclitaxel, docetaxel, liposomal doxorubicin, gemcitabine, bleomycin, and etoposide. These agents may be premedicated with single-agent antiemetics. Delayed emesis requires special consideration. Prophylaxis may include use of single-agent 5-HT$_3$ receptor antagonist therapy, or a brief pulse of dexamethasone in combination with metoclopramide, a 5-HT$_3$ receptor antagonist, or aprepitant, a substance P/NK$_1$ antagonist.

Skin reactions

Skin reactions, including alopecia and allergic hypersensitivity reactions, are also often seen with chemotherapeutic agents. Skin necrosis and sloughing at the site of intravenous extravasation is associated particularly with agents such as doxorubicin, actinomycin D, mitomycin C, vinblastine, vincristine, and nitrogen mustard. The extent of the necrosis is determined by the amount of extravasated drug. Management includes removal of the intravenous line and local infiltration of the area with corticosteroids, as well as ice pack therapy four or five times a day for 3 days. Long-term monitoring of these patients is essential. Palmar–plantar erthrodysesthesia, or hand and foot syndrome, may be a dose-limiting toxicity of liposomal doxorubicin and is characterized by painful edema and erythema. Alopecia is a common side effect of many chemotherapeutic agents. Therapies designed to reduce alopecia have not been successful. Hair growth resumes 10–20 days after treatment is completed.

Table 18–10 COMMON ANTIEMETIC REGIMENS

	Drug(s)	Dosage
Premedication		
5-HT_3 receptor antagonists	Ondansetron	8–24 mg i.v./p.o.
	Granisetron	10 μg/kg i.v.; 2 mg p.o.
	Dolasetron	1.8 mg/kg i.v.; 100 mg i.v.; 100 mg p.o.
Substance P/NK_1 receptor antagonist	Aprepitant	125 mg p.o.
Motility agent	Metoclopramide	2–3 mg/kg i.v.; 20–40 mg p.o.
Phenothiazine	Prochlorperazine	10 mg i.v./i.m./p.o.; 25 mg p.r.; 15 mg spansule
Benzodiazepine	Lorazepam	0.5–2 mg i.v./p.o./s.l.
Corticosteroid	Dexamethasone	8–20 mg i.v./p.o.
Acute-phase emesis	Dexamethasone	20 mg i.v.
	Ondansetron	8–24 mg i.v.
	Metoclopramide	3 mg/kg i.v. (repeat q 2 h p.r.n.)
	Diphenhydramine	25–50 mg i.v. (repeat q 2 h p.r.n.)
	Lorazepam	1–2 mg i.v.
Prophylaxis of delayed emesis	Dexamethasone	8 mg p.o. b.i.d. × 2 days, then 4 mg p.o. b.i.d. × 2 days
	plus metoclopramide	40 mg p.o. q.i.d. × 2–3 days[a]
	or 5-HT_3 antagonist	ondansetron 8 mg p.o. b.i.d. or t.i.d. × 2–3 days, or granisetron 1 mg p.o. b.i.d. or 2 mg p.o. q.i.d. × 2–3 days)
	5-HT_3 antagonist	p.o. × 2–3 days alone, or plus aprepitant 80 mg p.o. and dexamethasone 8 mg p.o. q.i.d. × 3 days

[a]Patients should be advised to take 50 mg of diphenhydramine p.o. at the first sign of dystonic reaction.

Hypersensitivity

Many chemotherapeutic agents may be associated with hypersensitivity reactions, although only a few agents elicit these responses in more than 5% of patients. Of the agents commonly used in gynecologic oncology, the taxanes and platinum compounds are the most likely culprits, although occasional reactions may also be seen with bleomycin, doxorubicin, etoposide, cyclophosphamide, ifosfamide, and methotrexate.

In phase I trials, the incidence of severe hypersensitivity to paclitaxel was approximately 30%; however, with adequate prophylaxis (Table 18–12) the incidence is now less than 10%. Although hypersensitivity associated with paclitaxel is often attributed to its formulation in Cremophor EL, a polyoxyethylated castor oil, docetaxel has also been associated with a similar incidence of hypersensitivity despite its formulation in Tween 80. With appropriate premedication, hypersensitivity to docetaxel has been reduced to 2–3%. The occurrence of hypersensitivity does not preclude further treatment with the drug. If additional diphenhydramine or corticosteroids do not allow the infusion to be completed after a delay, patients may undergo successful systematic desensitization.

The incidence of hypersensitivity to platinum analogs varies from 5 to 20%. Unlike reactions to taxanes, which typically occur within minutes of starting the initial dose, reactions to platinum agents typically do not manifest until several cycles have already been administered. In one series, a median of eight platinum courses were administered before hypersensitivity occurred. Routine premedication for hypersensitivity is not recommended, and patients who experience mild reactions may respond well to the addition of appropriate premedications. Patients with severe reactions may attempt systematic desensitization if indicated, although success is variable.

Hepatic toxicity

Hepatic toxicity is uncommon. Mild elevations in transaminase, alkaline phosphatase, and bilirubin are seen with many agents, but rarely is the condition severe. Psoriasis and drug-induced hepatitis can affect the amount of the chemotherapeutic agent given, as can pre-existing liver disease or exposure to other hepatic toxins.

Pulmonary toxicity

Interstitial pneumonitis with pulmonary fibrosis is seen with certain chemotherapeutic agents. The agents most likely to produce this are doxorubicin, alkylating agents, and nitrosoureas. Treatment of patients with drug-induced interstitial pneumonitis involves discontinuation of the cytotoxic agent and supportive care. Steroids may be of some benefit.

Cardiac toxicity

The risk of cardiac toxicity is seen primarily with doxorubicin. The risk increases dramatically when the cumu-

Table 18–11 EMETOGENIC POTENTIAL OF CANCER CHEMOTHERAPEUTIC AGENTS USED IN GYNECOLOGIC ONCOLOGY

Emetogenic potential (frequency, %)	Agent
< 10	Bleomycin
	Hydroxyurea
	Melphalan (p.o.)
	Methotrexate (< 50 mg/m^2)
10–30	Docetaxel
	Doxorubicin (< 20 mg/m^2)
	Etoposide
	Fluorouracil (< 1000 mg/m^2)
	Gemcitabine
	Methotrexate (50–250 mg/m^2)
	Paclitaxel
	Topotecan
30–60	Cyclophosphamide (< 750 mg/m^2)
	Dactinomycin (< 1.5 mg/m^2)
	Doxorubicin (20–60 mg/m^2)
	Ifosfamide
	Methotrexante (250–1000 mg/m^2)
60–90	Carboplatin
	Cisplatin (< 50 mg/m^2)
	Cyclophosphamide (750–1500 mg/m^2)
	Dactinomycin (> 1.5 mg/m^2)
	Doxorubicin (> 60 mg/m^2)
	Irinotecan
	Melphalan (i.v.)
	Methotrexate (> 1000 mg/m^2)
> 90	Cisplatin (> 50 mg/m^2)
	Cyclophosphamide (> 1500 mg/m^2)

(After Hesketh PJ, Kris MG, Grunberg SM et al: Proposal for classifying the acute emetogenicity of cancer chemotherapy. J Clin Oncol 15:103–109, 1997.)

lative dose exceeds 500 mg/m^2 of ideal body surface area. In recent years, this limit has rarely been exceeded, thus cardiomyopathy has diminished greatly in incidence. Acute arrhythmias may often be seen, but these disappear with a few days of supportive care. On rare occasions, cyclophosphamide has been reported to produce cardiotoxicity, particularly when it is used in massive doses. Mitomycin C has been reported to cause endocardial fibrosis and myocardial fibrosis, but again these events occur rarely.

Renal toxicity

Nephrotoxicity may be dose-limiting in up to 35% of patients receiving cisplatin. Proximal and distal tubule damage leads to electrolyte wasting, as well as increase in serum creatinine with concomitant decrease in Cr Cl. Renal toxicity may be reduced with adequate intravenous hydration and mannitol and/or furosemide-induced diuresis. Antibiotic therapy with aminoglycosides potentiates the nephrotoxicity of drugs such as cisplatin and should be avoided if possible.

Table 18–12 PROPHYLAXIS FOR TAXANE HYPERSENSITIVITY

Agent	Prophylaxis regimen
Docetaxel	Starting 1 day prior to infusion: dexamethasone 8 mg p.o. b.i.d. × 3 days
Paclitaxel	Night before and morning of infusion: dexamethasone 20 mg p.o.[a]
	30 min prior to infusion:[b] diphenhydramine 25–50 mg i.v. *plus* H_2 antagonist i.v.(cimetidine 300 mg or ranitidine 50 mg)

[a]May be repeated p.o. or i.v. 30 min prior to infusion.
[b]If the first cycle of treatment is well tolerated, subsequent cycles may be premedicated using oral doses.

Genitourinary toxicity

Metabolites of cyclophosphamide are irritants to the bladder mucosa and can cause chronic hemorrhagic cystitis. The toxic metabolite of cyclophosphamide that causes bladder toxicity is known as acrolein. Vigorous hydration and diuresis during administration of cyclophosphamide are essential. Cisplatin produces renal tubular toxicity associated with azotemia and magnesium wasting. Again, this complication can be minimized with diuresis during administration of cisplatin. Other agents known to cause genitourinary toxicity are methotrexate, nitrosoureas, and mitomycin C. Mesna or *N*-acetylcysteine has been used in recent times in conjunction with cyclophosphamide to prevent bladder toxicity. This agent acts by inactivating the toxic metabolite acrolein.

Neurologic toxicity

In general, most antineoplastic drugs are associated with mild neurologic side effects. There are some exceptions, however. Vinca alkaloids are commonly associated with peripheral motor sensory and autonomic neuropathies. Agents such as vincristine, vinblastine, paclitaxel, and vinorelbine can produce loss of deep tendon reflexes with distal paresthesias. Paclitaxel may also cause peripheral neuropathy. In most cases, these neurologic toxicities are reversible following cessation of the drug. Cisplatin produces ototoxicity and peripheral neuropathy, and occasionally retrobulbar neuritis. High doses of cisplatin, which are often used in ovarian cancer therapy, are particularly likely to produce progressive and somewhat delayed peripheral neuropathy. 5-Fluorouracil has been associated with acute cerebellar toxicity. Hexamethylmelamine is reported to produce peripheral neuropathy and encephalopathy. Ifosfamide has also been associated with encephalopathy, particularly in patients with low serum albumin.

Gonadal dysfunction

Many chemotherapeutic agents have lasting effects on testicular and ovarian functions. This is particularly true of alkylating agents, which can cause azoospermia and amenorrhea. The onset of amenorrhea and ovarian failure is accompanied by an elevation of the serum follicle stimulating hormone and a fall in serum estradiol. Indeed, these patients often end up with premature menopause. The younger the patient at the onset of therapy, the less likely it is that chemotherapy would eventuate in permanent gonadal dysfunction. In women older than 30 years of age, most chemotherapeutic regimens are associated with a high incidence of premature ovarian failure.

Supportive care

Supportive social workers, chaplains, and psychiatrists in a concentrated total care setting are of great value in enabling a patient to cope with the emotionally and financially shattering experience of having cancer. Home healthcare services have improved in most areas of the USA, so that intravenous fluids, antibiotics, intravenous alimentation, and even chemotherapy can be administered in the home if the situation allows. Although treatment of many patients must be conducted at large medical centers where new agents and multidisciplinary facilities are available, continuing collaboration between the medical center and the patient's primary physician is essential. Problems caused by the disease or its treatment often arise when the patient returns to her community. An informed local physician can rapidly evaluate these crises and take appropriate action. The performance status of the patient should be watched carefully (Table 18–13).

EVALUATION OF NEW AGENTS

The development of new, promising agents is a long, complicated, and expensive process. After identification of potential drugs in in vitro and animal models, all anticancer therapeutic agents must undergo rigorous clinical testing. Several levels of clinical trials are necessary to demonstrate that a newly developed agent should be allowed in regular medical practice. Such trials have been defined as follows.

Table 18–13 PERFORMANCE STATUS

Gynecologic Oncology Group, European Cooperative Oncology Group score	Zubrod description	Scale (%)	Karnofsky Description	Scale (%)
0	Fully active, able to carry on all predisease performance without restriction.	90–100	Normal, no complaints, no evidence of disease.	100
			Able to carry on normal activity, minor symptoms or signs of disease.	90
1	Restricted in physically strenuous activity but ambulatory and able to carry out work of a light or sedentary nature (e.g. light housework, office work).	70–80	Normal activity with effort; some signs and symptoms of disease.	80
			Cares for self, unable to perform normal activity or to do active work.	70
2	Ambulatory and capable of all self-care but unable to carry out any work activities. Up and about more than 50% of waking hours.	50–60	Requires occasional assistance but is able to care for most of own needs.	60
			Requires considerable assistance and frequent medical care.	60
3	Capable of only limited self-care, confined to bed or chair more than 50% of waking hours.	30–40	Requires special care and assistance; disabled.	40
			Severely disabled, hospitalization indicated, although death not imminent.	30
4	Completely disabled. Cannot carry on any self-care. Totally confined to bed or chair.	10–20	Very sick, hospitalization indicated.	20
			Fatal processes progressing rapidly; moribund.	10
5	Dead.	0	Dead.	0

Phase I

These initial trials are designed to test new drugs at various doses to evaluate toxicity and determine the tolerance to a particular agent. The primary end point to these trials is safety evaluation. A dose escalation design is often employed in order to define the maximum tolerated dose and to characterize the dose-limiting toxicities of the drug. Some therapeutic effects may be observed, even though the intent of these trials is not response measurement.

Phase II

Phase II studies attempt to determine the response rate of the particular agent at the dose and schedule defined by phase I trials. Secondary end points include determination of progression-free interval, determination of toxicity, and overall survival. Most phase II trials are single-arm non-randomized studies.

Phase III

Phase III trials are designed to compare a drug identified as promising in phase II trials to current standard treatment regimens. Commonly, a new drug is tested against the accepted gold standard drug therapy for a particular disease site and histology. These trials are typically large in order to provide sufficient power to detect a difference between the treatment arms. The primary end point in phase III trials is usually progression-free survival, while secondary end points usually include response rate and overall survival.

BIBLIOGRAPHY

Ball NE, Schilder RJ: Introduction and principles of chemotherapy. In Rubin SC (ed): Chemotherapy of Gynecologic Cancers, 2nd edn. Philadelphia, Lippincott Williams & Wilkins, 2004.

Bookman MA, Young RC: Principles of chemotherapy in gynecologic cancer. In Hoskins WJ, Perez CA, Young RC (eds): Principles and Practice of Gynecologic Oncology, 3rd edn. Philadelphia: Lippincott Williams & Wilkins, 2000.

Charbit A, Malaise EP, Tubiana M: Relation between the pathological nature and the growth rate of human tumors. Eur J Cancer 7:307, 1971.

DeVita VT, Hellman S, Rosenberg SA: Cancer Principles and Practice of Oncology, 4th edn. Philadelphia, Lippincott, 1993.

Dupont J, Sovak MA, Benjamin I et al: Chemotherapeutic agents used in the treatment of gynecologic malignancies. In Rubin SC (ed): Chemotherapy of Gynecologic Cancers, 2nd edn. Philadelphia: Lippincott Williams & Wilkins, 2004.

Epstein RA: Drug-induced DNA damage and tumor chemosensitivity. J Clin Oncol 8:2062, 1990.

Goldie JH, Coldman AJ: A mathematical model for relating the drug sensitivity of tumors to spontaneous mutation rate. Cancer Treat Rep 63:1727, 1979.

Goldie JH: Scientific basis for adjuvant and primary (neoadjuvant) chemotherapy. Semin Oncol 14:1, 1987.

Groopman JE, Itri LM: Chemotherapy-induced anemia in adults: incidence and treatment. J Natl Cancer Inst 91:1616–1634, 1999.

Reimer RR, Hoover R, Fraumeni JF et al: Acute leukemia after alkylating agent therapy. N Engl J Med 297:117, 1977.

Rich WM, Abdulham G, DiSaia PJ: Methylprednisolone as an antiemetic during cancer chemotherapy: a pilot study. Gynecol Oncol 9:193, 1980.

Rowinsky EK, McGuire WP, Donehower RC: The current status of Taxol. In Hoskins WJ et al (eds): Principles and Practice of Gynecologic Oncology Updates. Philadelphia, Lippincott, 1993.

Shoemaker RH et al: Potentials and drawbacks of the tumor stem cell assay. Behring Inst Mitt 74:262, 1984.

Skipper HE et al: Implications of biochemical, cytokinetic, pharmacologic, and toxicologic relationships in the design of optimal therapeutic schedules. Cancer Chemother Rep 54:431, 1950.

Skipper HE, Schabel FM Jr, Wilcox WS: Experimental evaluation of potential anticancer agents. XII: on the criteria and kinetics associated with "curability" of experimental leukemia. Cancer Chemother Rep 35:1, 1964.

Sotrel G, Jafari K, Lash AF et al: Acute leukemia in advanced ovarian carcinoma after treatment with alkylating agents. Obstet Gynecol 47:675, 1976.

Stierle A, Strobel G, Stierle D: Taxol and Taxane production by *Taxomyces andreane*: an endophytic fungus of Pacific yew. Science 260:214, 1993.

HISTORICAL OVERVIEW

Burchenal JH: The historical development of cancer chemotherapy. Semin Oncol 4:135, 1977.

Farber S, Diamond LK, Mercer RD et al: Temporary remissions in acute leukemia in children produced by folic acid antagonist, 4-aminopteroylglutamic acid (aminopterin). N Engl J Med 238: 787, 1948.

Huggins C, Hodges CV: Studies on prostatic cancer. The effect of castration, of estrogen and of androgen injection on serum phosphatases in metastatic carcinoma of the prostate. Cancer Res 1:293, 1941.

DRUG RESISTANCE

Belinsky MG, Bain LJ, Balsara BB et al: Characterization of MOAT-C and MOAT-D, new members of the MRP/cMOAT subfamily of transporter proteins. J Natl Cancer Inst 90:1735–1741, 1998.

Bell DR, Gerlach HJ, Kartner N et al: Detection of P-glycoprotein in ovarian cancer. A molecular marker associated with multidrug resistance. J Clin Oncol 3:311, 1985.

Bradley G, Juranka PF, Ling V: Mechanisms of multidrug resistance. Biochem Biophys Acta 948:87, 1988.

DeVita VT: The influence of information on drug resistance on protocol design: the Harry Kaplan Memorial Lecture given at the Fourth International Conference on malignant lymphoma, June 6–9, 1990, Lugano, Switzerland. Ann Oncol 2:93, 1991.

Endicott JA, Ling V: The biochemistry of P-glycoprotein–mediated drug resistance. Annu Rev Biochem. Berlin, Springer-Verlag, 1984.

Goldstein U et al: Expression of a multidrug resistant gene in human cancers. J Natl Cancer Inst 81:116, 1989.

Kruh GD, Chan A, Myers K et al: Expression complementary DNA library transfer establishes mrp as a multidrug resistance gene. Cancer Res 54:1649, 1994.

Ling V: Drug resistance and membrane mutase of mammalian cells. Cancer J Genet Cytol 17:503, 1975.

CALCULATION OF DOSAGE

Calvert AH, Newell DR, Gumbrell LA et al: Carboplatin dosage: prospective evaluation of a simple formula based on renal function. J Clin Oncol 7:1748, 1989.

Cockroft DW, Gault MH: Prediction of creatinine clearance from serum creatinine. Nephron 16:31, 1976.

Jelliffe RW, Jelliffe SM: A computer program for estimation of creatinine clearance from unstable serum creatinine levels, age, sex, and weight. Math Biosci 14:17, 1972.

DRUG TOXICITY

Bohlius J, Langensiepen S, Schwarzer G et al: Recombinant human erythropoietin and overall survival in cancer patients: results of a comprehensive meta-analysis. J Natl Cancer Inst 97:489–498, 2005.

Chu CS: Premedication of the chemotherapy patient. In Rubin SC (ed): Chemotherapy of Gynecologic Cancers, 2nd edn. Philadelphia: Lippincott Williams & Wilkins, 2004.

Demetri GD: Hematopoietic growth factors: current knowledge, future prospects. Curr Probl Cancer 16:179, 1992.

Henke M, Laszig R, Rube C et al: Erythropoietin to treat head and neck cancer patients with anaemia undergoing radiotherapy: randomised, double-blind, placebo-controlled trial. Lancet 362:1255–1260, 2003.

Kouides PA, Dipersio JF: The hematopoietic growth factors. In Haskell CM (ed): Principles of Cancer Treatment, 4th edn. Philadelphia, Saunders, 1995.

Leyland-Jones B, Semiglazov V, Pawlicki M et al: Maintaining normal hemoglobin levels with epoetin alfa in mainly nonanemic patients with metastatic breast cancer receiving first-line chemotherapy: a survival study. J Clin Oncol 23:5960–5972, 2005.

Lieschke GJ, Burgess AW: Granulocyte colony stimulating factor and granulocyte–macrophage colony–stimulating factor. N Engl J Med 327:28, 1992.

Lieschke GJ, Burgess AW: Granulocyte colony stimulating factor and granulocyte–macrophage colony–stimulating factor. N Engl J Med 327:99, 1992.

Miller CB, Jones RJ, Piantadosi S et al: Decreased erythropoietin response in patients with the anemia of cancer. N Engl J Med 322:1689, 1990.

Mohyeldin A, Lu H, Dalgard C et al: Erythropoietin signaling promotes invasiveness of human head and neck squamous cell carcinoma. Neoplasia 7:537–543, 2005.

Morgan MA: Use of blood products and hematologic growth factors. In Rubin SC (ed): Chemotherapy of Gynecologic Cancers, 2nd edn. Philadelphia, Lippincott Williams & Wilkins, 2004.

Neidhart JA: Hematopoietic colony–stimulating factors. Cancer 70: 913, 1992.

Piroso E, Erslev AJ, Caro J: Inappropriate increase in erythropoietin titers during chemotherapy. Am J Hematol 32:248, 1989.

Schapira L, Anbin JH, Ransil BJ et al: Serum erythropoietin levels in patients receiving intensive chemotherapy and radiotherapy. Blood 76:2354, 1990.

Tepler I, Cannistra SA, Frei E 3rd et al: Use of peripheral blood progenitor cells abrogates the myelotoxicity of repetitive outpatient high-dose carboplatin and cyclophosphamide chemotherapy. J Clin Oncol 11:1583, 1993.

Zucker S: Anemia in cancer. Cancer Invest 3:249, 1985.

19 Tumor Immunology, Host Defense Mechanisms, and Biologic Therapy

Philip J. DiSaia, M.D.

I am convinced that during development and growth, malignant cells arise frequently, but that in the majority of individuals they remain latent due to the protective action of the host. I am convinced that this natural immunity is not due to the presence of antimicrobial bodies, but is determined purely by cellular factors. These may be weakened in older age groups in which cancer is more prevalent.

Paul Ehrlich (1909)

HISTORICAL REVIEW

The word *immunity* means freedom from burden. In its original application, the burden was that of invasion by micro-organisms. In modern times, the burden is much larger and also encompasses the reaction of the body to foreign tissue, such as organ transplants, and to altered tissue, such as neoplastic growths. The 19th century saw the emergence of microbiology and immunology and witnessed the beginnings of vaccination in the prevention of disease. Edward Jenner successfully inoculated cowpox into humans and was able to offer protection against smallpox. The practices of Jenner were extended by Pasteur, who established the value of preventive inoculation against a variety of animal and human diseases. It was because of Pasteur that the skepticism about the germ theory was finally dispelled, and Koch was able to lay down the fundamental laws regarding infectious agents with the Koch postulates. The field of immunology became a firm scientific foundation around the turn of the 20th century with the recognition of immunolysis of foreign red cells by Bordet in 1898 and the description of the ABO blood groups by Landsteiner in 1904. In the early part of the 20th century, the relative importance of phagocytosis and antibody production to host defense caused a sharp division of scientific opinion. One group of scientists led by a Russian, Elie Metchnikoff, held phagocytosis to be more crucial. Paul Ehrlich and his followers attributed greater importance to antibody attack on the parasite. Ehrlich developed the theory of antigenic specificity, which depended, according to him, on chemical union between the antigen and side chains on the corresponding antibody. In 1908, the Nobel Prize was awarded to Ehrlich and Metchnikoff for their work on immunity.

Tumor immunology developed as an offshoot of transplantation immunology. The roots of transplantation immunology are found in the work of a Hungarian-born Viennese surgeon, Emerich Ullmann, who successfully transplanted a kidney into a dog. His technique was perfected by Alexis Carrel, a graduate of the University of Lyon, who was working in Chicago between 1902 and 1904. Carrel applied the principles of vascular anastomosis to transplantation of various organs. The techniques described by Carrel for developing vascular suture substances and his techniques of vascular surgery have persisted to modern times. Carrel won the Nobel Prize in medicine for his work.

In 1923 and 1924, Carol S. Williamson of the Mayo Clinic described the pathologic process of transplantation rejection, and the phenomenon of first- and second-set rejection was documented by Holman, who worked with skin allografts on a burn victim. These findings laid the foundation for the classic work of Peter Gorer, leading to the formulation of the theory of antigenic specificity of tissues from different individuals. The first clinical attempt at human kidney transplantation was at the Peter Bent Brigham Hospital in Boston by Charles A. Hufnagel, David A. Hume, and Ernest Landsteiner in 1947.

About the same time, an interesting observation made in 1945 by R. Owen, a veterinary surgeon from Wisconsin, began to be widely appreciated by the scientific community. Owen noted that in utero mixing of the circulation of monoplacental cattle led to the coexistence in the adult animal of two different blood groups, a condition called *chimerism*. In 1955, Billingham and coworkers published their landmark paper on actively acquired tolerance of foreign cells in which they showed that when fetal mice are exposed to foreign cells in utero, those mice, on attaining adult age, become tolerant to tissues from the original donor of the cells. In 1959, Macfarlane Burnet refined this concept and detailed the clonal selection theory of immunity. By 1960, teams of surgeons in the USA, France, and Britain were successfully transplanting kidneys, and their techniques have continued. Burnet and Medawar were awarded the Nobel Prize in medicine in 1960 for their monumental work. The importance of cell surface antigens in transplantation immunity became well recognized and led to advances such as those of Paul Terasaki, who developed and popularized a method for matching tissues of organ donors and recipients to prolong transplantation survival.

As transplantation immunology (Table 19–1) became more thoroughly understood, some scientists referred to the hypothesis of Paul Ehrlich, which stated that malignant neoplasms were antigenic and, as such, could be recognized by the host as foreign in much the same manner as allogeneic tissue is. Indeed, in 1908, Ehrlich indirectly suggested the theory of immunologic surveillance. Cancer-specific antigens were identified for the first time in experiments by Gross in 1943. He described the failure of mice to accept a transplant of a specific cancer after they had been immunized with material from the same cancer growing in pedigreed mice. Gross immunized mice by intradermal inoculation of tumor cells. The immunized animals rejected a subcutaneous transplant of the same tumor, but non-immunized animals did not. His work was all but ignored until 1957, when Prehn and Main reported their experiments using syngeneic methylcholanthrene-induced fibrosarcomas. They observed that mice immunized against these fibrosarcomas by inoculation of living sarcoma tissue, after surgical removal of the growing tumor, were resistant to subsequent grafts of the same tumor. In addition, immunization with normal tissue did not confer resistance to the tumor graft. The mice that had become resistant to the tumors still accepted skin grafts from the primary host of these tumors. The rejection of the tumor tissue with simultaneous acceptance of normal tissue from the same donor to the same recipient proved Ehrlich's hypothesis correct. The malignant neoplasm appeared to have acquired an antigenic moiety during the malignant transformation of the mouse tissue that allowed that malignant tissue now to be recognized as non-self, whereas corresponding normal tissue was still accepted as self.

The experiments of Prehn and Main were repeated by many others in different tumor systems, and the following conclusions have been reached. Antigenic differences exist between cancer cells and their normal counterparts, and these differences are equivalent to weak transplantation antigens. It appears that malignant tissues evoke a measurable immunologic response in most organisms in which they appear, including the human. The specificity of the cell surface tumor antigens is in doubt, and therefore they have been termed tumor-associated antigens.

In the late 1950s, the term *immunologic surveillance* was coined by Burnet, who postulated that cell-mediated immunity evolved to recognize and destroy cells that had non-self markers, such as tumor cells bearing tumor antigens. The theory of immune surveillance, then, hypothesizes that

Table 19–1 CLASSIFICATION OF IMMUNOLOGIC TERMS

Genetic relationship	Antibody	Transplant	New Term
Identical, same individual	Auto	Auto	Autologous
Identical twin (same inbred strain)	Iso	Iso	Syngeneic
Different individual, same species	Iso	Homo	Allogeneic
Different species	Hetero	Hetero	Xenogeneic

Tumor immunology is a form of transplantation immunology, and the same terminology applies.
From DiSaia PJ: Tumor immunology: General aspects. Contemp Ob Gyn 4:91, 1974, Medical Economics Co.

immune mechanisms may eliminate newly appearing tumor cells and thus serve as a surveillance system for cancer. This theory continues to be investigated from many aspects, especially with regard to the role of cell-mediated and cytokine-mediated mechanisms.

In 1959, Macfarlane Burnet conceived the clonal selection theory, which states in essence that immunocompetent cells are already endowed with the genetic ability to make a certain antibody. By combination with its specific cell through antigen-specific receptors on the surface membrane, an antigen causes that specific cell to proliferate, an activity that results in observable antibody formation. In addition, each lymphocyte carries receptor molecules of only a single specificity on its surface.

An attractive portion of the clonal selection theory is its application to specific immunologic tolerance—the failure to make an antibody to a normally antigenic material because of a previous exposure to the antigen. Burnet suggested that self-recognition occurs in neonatal life by contact of the antibody-forming cells with new antigens as the fetus first forms them. The result in utero is a functional shutdown of such a cell, so that one does not make antibodies to one's own antigens. Peter Medawar tested this hypothesis with fetal exposure to non-self antigens and measured the results. As the theory predicted, the animal, when grown to adulthood, did not respond to the antigen.

In the mid-1970s, research conducted primarily by Milstein and Köhler led to the description of immunoglobulin-sensitizing hybridomas and the discovery and development of hybridoma technology (see Fig. 19–14). Köhler and Milstein received a Nobel Prize in physiology and medicine in 1984. In 1987, the Nobel Prize in medicine and physiology was awarded to the Japanese-American Susumu Tonegawa for his important discoveries based on the analysis of immunoglobulin genes. He clearly demonstrated that more than one gene is involved in the synthesis of a single peptide or immunoglobulin.

In the last three decades, various methods to stimulate a patient's immune system non-specifically have been tried with minimal success (e.g., bacille Calmette–Guérin [BCG], *Corynebacterium parvum*). Other approaches have used monoclonal antibodies or various lymphokines and other immune system stimulatory factors (so-called biologic response modifiers).

ANATOMY OF THE IMMUNE SYSTEM

Immunogens and antigens

Acquired immune responses arise as a result of exposure to foreign stimuli. The foreign compound that evokes the response is referred to as an antigen or as an immunogen. There is a functional difference between these two terms. An *immunogen* is any substance capable of inducing an immune response. In contrast, an *antigen* is a substance capable of binding specifically to components of the immune response, such as lymphocytes or antibodies. The distinction is made between the two terms because there are many compounds incapable of inducing an immune response, yet they are capable of binding with components of the immune system that have been induced specifically against them. All immunogens are compounds such as antibiotics and many other drugs. By themselves, these compounds are not capable of inducing an immune response, but when they are coupled with much larger proteins; the resultant conjugate induces an immune response. When manipulated in this manner, the low-molecular-weight substance is referred to as a hapten. The high-molecular-weight substance to which the hapten is attached is termed the carrier. In tumor immunology, antigen is the term traditionally used, and most "foreign" substances are of high molecular weight. In general, compounds that have a molecular mass of < 1000 daltons are not immunogenic; those with a molecular mass between 1000 and 6000 daltons may or may not be immunogenic; and those with a molecular mass > 6000 daltons (e.g., human glycoproteins, lipoproteins) are usually immunogenic.

Tumor cells express most of the same cell surface antigens (e.g., transplantation or HLA antigens) that normal cells do (Fig. 19–1). In addition, many tumor cells express specific antigens not found in similar normal cells. An antigen announces its foreignness by means of intricate and characteristic shapes called epitopes or antigen determinants,

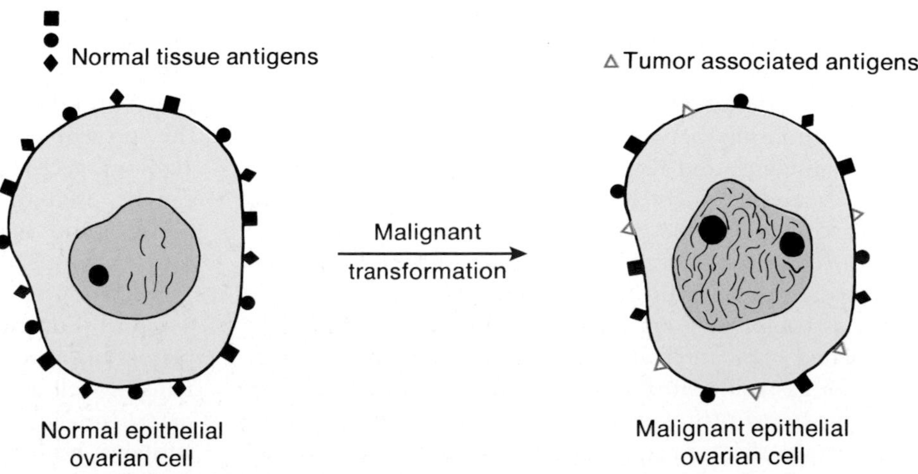

Figure 19–1 Tumor-associated antigens are additionally expressed on the tumor cell surface.

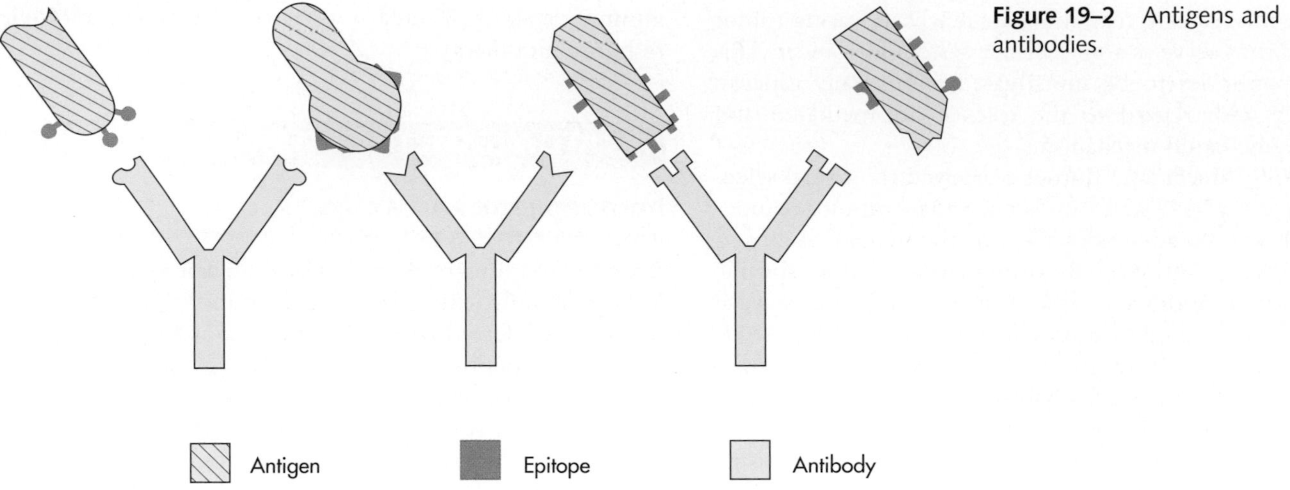

Figure 19–2 Antigens and antibodies.

which protrude from its surface. Most antigens carry several different kinds of epitopes on their surface; some may carry several hundred epitopes, and some will be more effective at stimulating an immune response (Fig. 19–2). These antigens (often rare and weak) are termed tumor-specific antigens in animal studies and tumor-associated antigens in human malignant neoplasms. Experiments to demonstrate tumor-specific antigens involve a demonstration that pretreatment with a syngeneic tumor will influence the growth of a subsequent challenge with the same tumor. In animals, this was possible after introduction of syngeneic inbred mouse strains, and Foley produced the first such evidence in 1953. This was followed by the studies of Prehn and Main (described previously). Such studies are not possible in humans; however, there are in vitro techniques for detection of tumor antigens, and these have been liberally applied to human tumors. Tumors vary widely in their immunogenicity. In general, neoplasms induced experimentally in vivo with chemical or viral agents are highly immunogenic; tumors arising spontaneously in vivo (e.g., human malignant neoplasms) are poorly immunogenic.

Oncofetal antigens have also been described; these antigens are found in fetal and malignant tissue and tend to occur more commonly than tumor-associated antigens. These normal antigens in the fetus are repressed as the process of intrauterine development proceeds toward birth and then derepressed during the malignant transformation process. Their existence supports the concept that cancer represents a dedifferentiation to a more primitive cell type. The relationship between malignant neoplasms, specific tumor antigens, and fetal antigens is not clear. The most carefully studied oncofetal antigens in gynecologic cancer are carcinoembryonic antigen (CEA) and α-fetoprotein (AFP). The most apparent importance of these antigens is not in their possible protective value but in their ability to serve as tumor markers for various cancers. CEA initially stimulated great interest as a possible accurate diagnostic assay for gastrointestinal tract malignant tumors. However, with further study, elevated levels were found in patients with benign disease (e.g., colonic polyps, severe cirrhosis, uremia, and inflammatory disease of the bowel). Indeed, CEA can be found in many non-gastrointestinal tract cancers, including several gynecologic malignant neoplasms, and its value as a clinically usable tumor marker is limited. AFP is detectable immunologically in serum from human fetuses. In the adult, it is found in patients with malignant neoplasms of endodermal origin, for example, liver tumors and gonadal tumors such as endodermal sinus tumor of the ovary. As with CEA, there does not appear to be a clear correlation between the level of AFP and the prognosis for the patient; and like CEA, AFP is not disease specific. The presence of AFP with an ovarian neoplasm strongly suggests a diagnosis of endodermal sinus tumor, and the reappearance of detectable serum levels after a period of negative titers strongly suggests recurrent disease.

With few exceptions, it has not been possible to demonstrate antigens in human neoplasms that have as high a degree of tumor specificity as that reported for most tumor-specific antigens in animals. Rather, most human tumor antigens known today are tumor-associated antigens. Some have described these as tumor-associated differentiation antigens. These tumor-associated antigens or tumor-associated differentiation antigens are sometimes referred to as fetal antigens that have relative rather than absolute specificity for cancer cells. If highly specific antigens could be found in human cancer similar to those encoded by certain tumor viruses, they would provide excellent targets for active and passive immunotherapy. However, even the weak tumor-associated antigens known today offer some promise for clinical applications in that they provide markers for diagnosis, both by histologic and cytologic techniques and through the assays of sera. They can be used to detect how cancer patients respond to therapy, and they can be used in vivo for detection of tumors by nuclear imaging.

Each human tumor may express many tumor-associated antigens. For example, melanomas, which are among the neoplasms most thoroughly studied, express different proteins as well as glycolipid antigens. There is considerable heterogenicity in the expression of many tumor-associated antigens, both between different tumors of the same type and between different cells of the same tumor. Heterogeneity is reflected even in a different expression of a tumor-associated antigen in a primary tumor and its metastases. Antigens that are expressed more in some tumor types than in others do exist, but most tumor-associated antigens are shared by neoplasms of many different types. With the development of the monoclonal technology, it is possible to identify several novel serum markers for different human tumors. One of these markers, CA-125, has been used to monitor patients who have epithelial ovarian cancer. CA-125 is recognized by the murine monoclonal G1 immunoglobulin (IgG1) OC-125. The antibody was developed with use of the technique of Köhler and Milstein. Murine myeloma cells were hybridized with spleen cells from a mouse that had been immunized with a human serous cystadenocarcinoma cell line. Stable hybrid clones were screened for reactivity against the ovarian tumor cell line used for immunization and for lack of reactivity with a B lymphocyte line established from the tumor donor by Epstein–Barr virus transformation. Clones were also screened for a lack of reactivity with allogeneic human ovary. CA-125 determinants are associated with the derivatives of the coelomic epithelium in the embryo and adult, including the pleura, pericardium, peritoneum, fallopian tube, endometrium, and endocervix. Outside of this lineage, CA-125 has also been detected in tracheobronchial epithelium and glands, amnion, amniotic fluid, milk, cervical mucus, and seminal fluid. Interestingly, CA-125 has not been found in sections of normal ovary, either in the fetus or in the adult. The antigen is present at the cell surface in >80% of non-mucinous epithelial ovarian cancers as well as in a smaller fraction of carcinomas that arise from the endometrium, fallopian tube, endocervix, pancreas, colon, breast, and lung.

An immunoradiometric assay has been developed to measure CA-125 determinants in serum or ascites fluid. In this assay, CA-125 antigen is bound to OC-125 antibody on a solid-phase immunoadsorbent. Because there are multiple CA-125 determinants on each antigen molecule or complex, ^{125}I-labeled OC-125 can be used as a probe to detect bound antigen in a double-determinant simultaneous sandwich assay. Antigen in body fluids is compared with a standard prepared from culture supernatants of an ovarian tumor cell line. Antigen activity has been expressed on an arbitrary scale from 1 to 20,000 U/mL. The daily coefficient of variation for the assay is 12–15%, and a doubling or halving of antigen levels has been considered significant.

A number of additional monoclonal antibodies that react with ovarian cancers have been generated (e.g., NB70K, CA-19-9). CA-19-9 monoclonal antibody can be coexpressed with the CA-125 determinant; CA-19-9 is found in the serum of about 25% of ovarian cancer patients. Requirements for a successful tumor marker include sensitivity, specificity, and availability of effective treatment. Sensitivity is defined as the proportion of assay positives to true positives; specificity is defined as a proportion of assay negatives to true negatives. Even when a tumor marker is highly specific and sensitive, its utility depends ultimately on its ability to influence decisions between alternative plans for management of the patient. Consequently, requirements for a useful gynecologic tumor marker must depend on the particular clinical problems for which it is applied. One of the most useful applications for a tumor marker is the detection of early disease at a time when it can be cured. In gynecologic practice, cytologic analysis has provided an appropriate screening technique for the detection of cervical carcinomas, but there has been no comparable strategy to detect neoplasms of the ovary and fallopian tube. High sensitivity is needed to detect disease at an early stage. Specificity must be sufficient to discriminate malignant disease from a broad spectrum of intercurrent benign conditions. If additional non-invasive tests could localize the site of primary tumor growth, an effective screening test might not need to distinguish different primary sites of malignant disease. If a test is sufficiently specific to identify sites of primary tumor growth, it might prove useful in evaluating patients who have malignant ascites. In this setting, tumor burden is often substantial, and high sensitivity would not be as critical as in the detection of early-stage disease.

In gynecologic practice, discrimination of benign from malignant pelvic masses would be of great value, particularly in patients who might be referred to tertiary centers for cytoreductive surgery. Because gross disease is often present, requirements for sensitivity are reduced. Specificity is still important in that the test must effectively distinguish malignant from benign conditions. Tumor markers have been used most often to monitor response to therapy in patients known to have cancer. For this application, antigen levels must parallel tumor burden. Ideally, the range of assay values should be broad relative to the precision of the assay, permitting measurement of tumor burden over several orders of magnitude. Markers with a short half-life in serum reflect decreases in tumor burden more promptly than markers with slow clearance do. For effective monitoring, the degree of specificity is somewhat less critical than that of sensitivity. The assay should not be affected by benign conditions that occur during treatment, but these conditions would include only a small subset of the broad spectrum of benign conditions that could be encountered during screening of an apparently healthy population. Assays for persistent or recurrent disease are of greatest value when there is an effective salvage therapy. If treatment with cytotoxic drugs is sufficiently morbid, however, progressive elevation of a marker might prompt discontinuation of ineffective chemotherapy in selected patients.

Humoral factors

Some immunoblasts differentiate into plasma cells, which are largely responsible for humoral immunity. Antibodies are secreted by plasma cells into the vicinity of the antigenic stimulus, and binding with the inciting antigen takes place there. A given antibody matches an antigen much like a key matches a lock. The fit varies—sometimes it is precise, at other times it is imprecise. To some degree, however, the antibody interlocks with the antigen. The basic unit of all antibodies is composed of four polypeptides, two light chains and two heavy chains linked to each other by several disulfide bridges. All immunoglobulin molecules consist of two identical heavy chains and two identical light chains. The sections that make up the tips of the Y's arms vary greatly from one antibody to another, creating a pocket uniquely shaped to lock in a specific antigen. This is called the variable region, and each arm of the Y is called the Fab fragment; the stem is termed the Fc fragment. The stem of the Y serves to link the antibody to other participants in the immune system (e.g., a T cell). This area is identical in all antibodies of the same class and is called the constant region (Fig. 19-3). The unique variable region of an antibody can itself act as an antigen. The variable region contains a number of antigen-like segments, and these are known collectively as an idiotype. Like any other antigen, an idiotype can trigger complementary antibody. This second-row antibody is known as an anti-idiotype.

There are five classes of antibodies: IgG, IgM, IgA, IgE, and IgD. The immunoglobulins of all species have been shown to consist of five different classes (isotypes) that differ in the structure of their heavy (H) chains. It is the nature of the H chain that confers on the molecule its unique biologic properties, such as its half-life in the circulation, its ability to bind to certain receptors, and its ability to activate enzymes on combination with antigen. It is estimated that a human can produce 100,000 different antibodies; specificity is a basic property of this system. An antibody directed toward a particular antigen will not confer protection against other antigens. This concept is termed the clonal selection theory, which states that each antibody-producing cell is committed to one particular antibody in production.

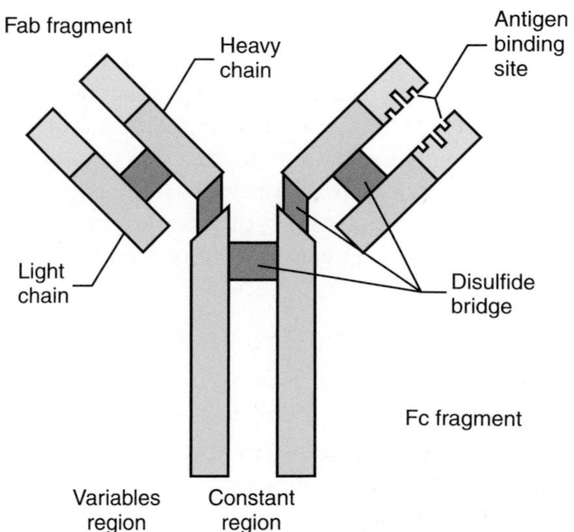

Figure 19–3 Antibody structure with antigen-binding site.

Antibodies have been demonstrated in the serum of many animals bearing a variety of experimentally induced tumors. Although these antibodies have been useful in serologic characterization and in isolation of tumor-associated antigens, the presence of a humoral response is not consistently correlated with increased tumor resistance in the host. Nonetheless, there are several ways in which tumor-specific antibodies could theoretically mediate antitumor activity. If tumor-associated antigens induce a humoral response, it is likely that the interaction of the tumor cell with some of the antibodies will activate the complement system, leading to lesions in the cell membrane and eventually lysis. Lysis by complement has been shown to be effective in vitro against certain cells in suspension; however, cell death is not usually evident in treating target cells of solid tumor tissue. Opsonization is the binding of specific antibody and complement components with particulate antigen to facilitate its phagocytosis. In vitro studies demonstrated the ability of macrophages to exert cytotoxic activity against some tumor cells by cytophagocytosis in the presence of immune serum. The relevance of this activity in vivo is difficult to assess. The ability of antibodies to bind to the surface of tumor cells in vivo may be important in antitumor activities other than those mediated by complement-dependent lysis or phagocytosis by macrophages. Antibodies bound to the membranes of malignant cells may modulate surface structures and thereby interfere with cell adhesive properties. This could have a deleterious effect on certain types of tumors because the ability to adhere to each other and to surrounding host tissue may be essential for successful establishment of the malignant clone by providing cellular organization and support. Furthermore, adherence of circulating tumor cells to the endothelium of blood vessels appears to precede metastatic spread. Antibodies specifically bound to the membranes of tumor cells may result in loss of the adhesive properties important to the establishment of bloodborne metastatic foci.

T lymphocytes (thymus-dependent)

Thymus-dependent (T) lymphocytes recognize and destroy foreign cells and regulate immune reactions. T lymphocytes carry out these functions directly by cell-to-cell contact or indirectly by using factors they produce and secrete. T cells regulate the activity of other T cells, macrophages, B cells, neutrophils, eosinophils, and basophils. T lymphocytes mature in the thymus because lymphoid cells differentiate in the thymus; they require specialized functions, and their cell membranes display distinguishing profiles or differentiation antigens. The biologic function of many of the differentiation antigens is not yet understood, but these cell surface markers are extremely useful for identifying lymphoid T cell subsets in normal and lymphoproliferative disease states. T lymphocytes, after leaving the thymus, are mainly found in the blood and thymus-dependent areas of the lymphoid tissues (e.g., spleen, lymph nodes, and

Peyer's patches). In the circulation, they make up 80–90% of the total lymphocytes. The result of antigen recognition by B and T cells is similar but also different in fundamental ways. After antigenic stimulation, both cells become activated, proliferate, and differentiate into memory cells. The end of B cell activation is simply immunoglobulin secretion, whereas T cells have major functions as a result of antigenic stimulation:

1. they produce a series of non-immunocompetent but soluble mediators called cytokines; and
2. they may kill the cell containing the antigen.

With use of the differentiation antigens, human T cells have been characterized by monoclonal antibody techniques and are divided into three functional subgroups: helper, suppressor, and cytotoxic lymphocytes. Helper T lymphocytes, which constitute about one third of the mature cell population, are programmed to produce factors that amplify the functions of other cells (B lymphocytes and other T lymphocytes). Suppressor lymphocytes also have characteristic functions and can suppress effector lymphocytes by direct interaction or by the release of soluble suppressor factors. Cytotoxic T cells also express antigens, which can be detected by monoclonal antibodies.

T lymphocytes primarily recognize cell-associated antigens. Specifically, T cells simultaneously recognize both the antigen and a portion of one of the self class I or class II major histocompatibility complex (MHC) gene products. It is not clear whether T cells have distinct receptors for this MHC and the antigenic determinant or single receptors that have both specificities combined. Activated lymphocytes can produce a variety of soluble effector substances. They participate in the complicated process called the immune response. These substances are called cytokines and include, among others, those listed in Table 19–2.

T lymphocytes are required for several types of reactions, such as regulating immunoglobulin production, mediating delayed hypersensitivity, and lysing early virus-infected cells. An important advance in understanding how T cells develop into functionally mature populations and how they mediate these functions was the demonstration that distinct stages of T cell differentiation and function correlate with the expression of specific surface molecules. These molecules are designated by the letter T followed by a number (T1–T11) and can be detected by monoclonal antibodies.

All lymphocytes are relatively indistinguishable by light microscopy, but various markers have been found that serve to identify their phenotypes. Most useful among these markers are those on the surface of the cell (Table 19–3), and although their function in many instances is unknown, their presence can be exploited for purification as well as for identification of these cells. The development of monoclonal antibodies has assisted greatly in the mapping of these cell surface molecules. Initially, these

Table 19–2 CYTOKINES

Cytokine	Biologic activity
Interferons	
IFN-α or IFN-β	Antiviral, augments NK cell activity, antiproliferative properties
IFN-γ or inhibits other cytokine activities	Activates macrophages, augments NK cell activity, augments or inhibits other cytokine activities
Interleukins	
IL-1-α or IL-1β	Activates resting T cells, induces colony-stimulating factor (CSF) production, stimulates synthesis of other cytokines
IL-2	Augments lymphocyte killer activity, induces production of other cytokines
IL-3	Stimulates early growth of monocyte, granulocyte, erythrocyte, and megakaryocyte progenitor cells
IL-4	Growth factor for activated B cells, enhances growth of most cell lines
IL-5	Induces proliferation and differentiation of eosinophil progenitors
IL-6	Induces differentiation of B cells; enhances immunoglobulin secretion by B cells
IL-7	Supports growth of pre-B cells
IL-8	Activates neutrophils; attenuates inflammatory events at blood vessel endothelium
Tumor necrosis factor, TNF-α or TNF-β	Cytotoxic for some tumor cells, activates macrophages, stimulates synthesis of other cytokines
Granulocyte colony-stimulating factor (G-CSF)	Stimulates growth of granulocyte colonies and activates mature granulocytes
Granulocyte-macrophage colony-stimulating factor (GM-CSF)	Stimulates growth of granulocyte, monocyte, and early erythrocyte progenitors; fewer megakaryocyte progenitors
Macrophage colony-stimulating factor (M-CSF)	Stimulates growth of monocyte colonies, enhances antibody-dependent monocyte-mediated cytotoxicity

Table 19–3 SURFACE ANTIGENS USEFUL FOR EXPLORING HUMAN T CELL DIFFERENTIATION AND FUNCTION

Antigens	Molecular weight	Monoclonal antibody	Comments
CD1	67,000	OKT1 Leu-1	Equivalent to murine Thy-1 antigen
CD3	20,000 23,000	OKT3 Leu-4	Associated with T cell receptor for antigen
CD4	60,000	OKT4 Leu-3	Present on helper/inducer T cells
4B4			Helper/inducer
4H4			Suppressor/inducer
CD6	44,000	OKT6 Leu-6	Equivalent to murine T1 antigens
CD8	32,000 43,000	OKT Leu-2a Leu-2b	Present on cytotoxic/suppressor cells
CD9	190,000	OKT9	Transferrin receptor, present on activated T cells
CD10	37,000	OKT10	Present on early stem cells, some B cells, activated peripheral T cells
CD11	55,000	OKT Leu	Associated with SRBC rosette receptor

monoclonal antibodies to lymphocyte markers were developed in many laboratories and given different designations. Indeed, the same antibody ended up having several designations, each applied by a laboratory involved with research using that antibody. To overcome this confusion, a uniform system of nomenclature has been adopted in which all surface markers are called CD followed by a number indicating the sequence of their acceptance. The list extends to at least CD86. The term CD (cluster determinant), describes the cluster of antigens with which antibodies react, and the number indicates its order of discovery. Thus, anti-CD4 designates antibodies that would react with a particular cell surface protein called CD4, regardless of the epitope on the CD4 they recognize. Many of these cell surface molecules have been detected by appropriate antibodies, and a list of at least 80 exists at this time. However, the functions of only a few have been adequately elaborated. With the current nomenclature, similar molecules in any species bear the same designation. The cytotoxic $CD8^+$ T cell is particularly effective against cells that have become infected by an intracellular pathogen (virus or bacterium) or that have been altered by malignancy. Cells are recognized as foreign by the peptides displayed on MHC class I molecules. The T cell binds, and this process is augmented by the binding of the CD8 surface molecule. This binding signals T cell activation, and antigen-specific directional killing may be mediated. Proliferating $CD4^+$ cells differentiate into two types of effector cells: the inflammatory T cell, which activates macrophages, and the helper T cell, which activates B cells.

B lymphocytes

The most salient characteristic of the B lymphocyte is the production of immunoglobulins on activation (Fig. 19–4). B lymphocytes are derived from the hematopoietic stem cells, and they receive their name from the discovery of their dependency on the bursa of Fabricius in birds. Studies have revealed the existence of at least seven different cell types in the B lymphocyte differentiation pathway: pro-B cells, pre-B cells, late pre-B cells, immature B cells, mature B cells, memory cells, and effector cells (plasma cells). There are also five immunoglobulin classes: IgM, IgG, IgA, IgE, and IgD. The pre-B cell is the earliest cell identifiable as belonging to the B lymphocyte lineage. Conversion of the pre-B cell to an immature B cell begins near the end of the first trimester and persists through the second trimester of pregnancy. As pregnancy progresses, the stem cell pool shifts from the liver to the bone marrow, where differentiation continues throughout life. The expression of membrane-bound immunoglobulins is the common feature of all immature B cells; this feature allows clonal selection by antigen. When stimulated by antigen, B cells undergo a series of changes in cell surface structures and in functional capabilities and differentiate into plasma cells. Plasma cells, the final stage in B cell differentiation, secrete large amounts of immunoglobulin. An individual plasma cell initially secretes antibodies of the IgM class but can switch to producing antibodies of other subclasses with the same antigen specificity.

Natural killer cells

T cell immunity and NK cell immunity represent complementary arms of the cellular immune response; they have a pivotal role in protective immunity. Natural killer (NK) cells are a subpopulation of lymphoid cells present in most normal individuals and in a variety of mammalian and avian species. They do not result from a classic cellular immune response. They are cytolytically active in a nonspecific fashion when taken from a non-immunized host. NK cells do not depend on the thymus for maturation.

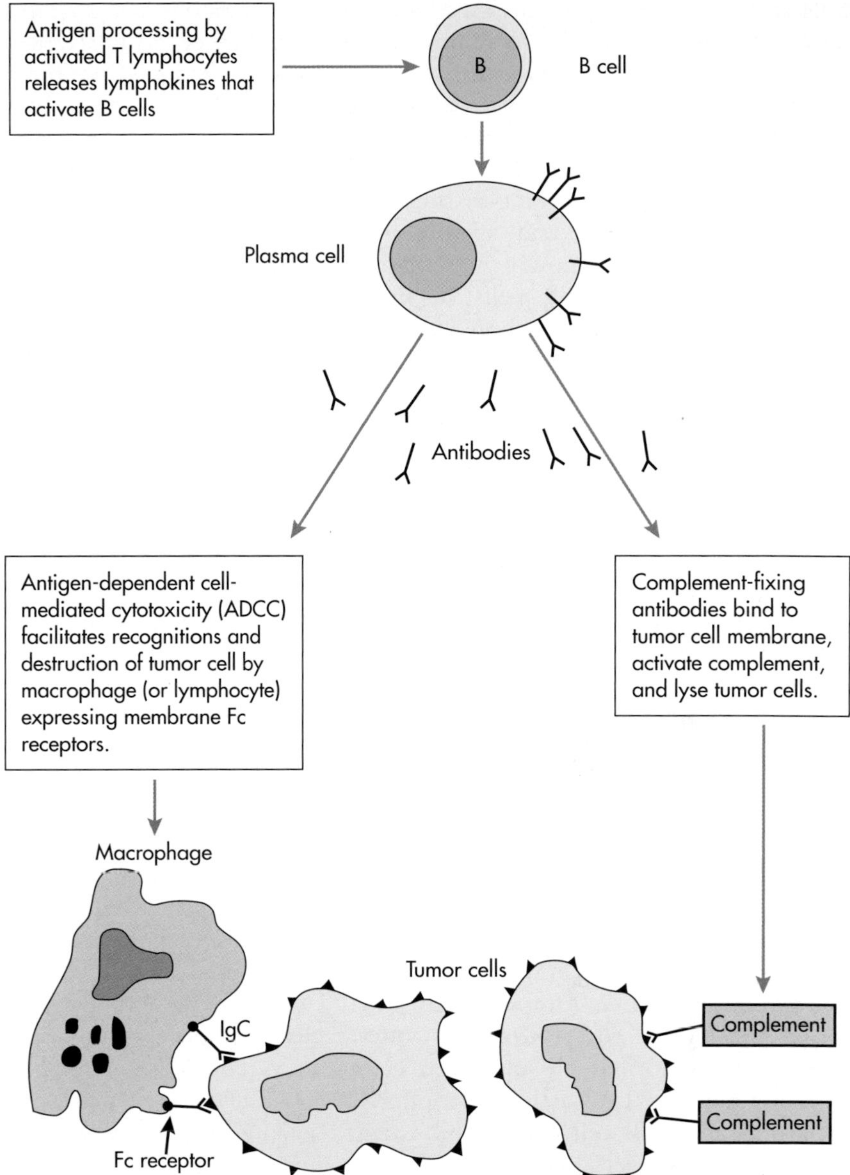

Figure 19–4 Role of the B cell in the immune response to malignant disease.

They are formed in spleen, lymph nodes, bone marrow, and peripheral blood. There is no memory response by NK cells after re-exposure of the host to a reactive target. NK cells have spontaneous cytolytic activity against a variety of tumor cells and some normal cells, and their reactivity can be rapidly augmented by interferon. They have characteristics distinct from other types of lymphoid cells and are closely associated with large granular lymphocytes, which compose about 5% of blood or splenic leukocytes. There is increasing evidence that NK cells, with the ability to mediate natural resistance against tumors in vivo, certain viruses and other microbial diseases, and bone marrow transplants, may play an important role in the immune surveillance. NK cells share several features with macrophages and polymorphonuclear leukocytes. NK cells have spontaneous activity in normal individuals, and this activity appears to be well regulated, subject to various inhibitory cells and factors. The nature of target cell recognition by NK cells seems to be intermediate between the exquisite specificity of T cells and the ill-defined or absent specificity of macrophages or polymorphonuclear leukocytes. NK cells can react against a wide variety of syngeneic, allogeneic, and xenogeneic cells. Susceptibility to cytotoxic activity is not restricted to malignant cells; fetal cells, virus-infected cells, and some subpopulations of thymus cells, bone marrow cells, and macrophages are also sensitive to lysis. It appears that NK cells can recognize at least several widely distributed antigenic specificities and that such recognition is clonally distributed. The nature of the recognition for interferon production and for cytotoxic interactions of NK cells with target cells is not clear. The mechanism of killing by NK cells is also unclear, but as with T cells, binding to target cells is first required, followed by the lytic event. The actual lysis may be mediated by neutral serine proteases, phospholipases, or both.

NK cells represent an interesting and unusual type of effector cell. Research to date has led to a good understanding of the nature and characteristics of these cells but has also raised a number of questions. For example, it would be of interest to determine more clearly the lineage of NK cells and their relation to the T cell and the myelomonocytic lineages: the nature of the recognition receptors on NK cells and of the antigens on the target cells, the detailed mechanisms for regulation of their activities, and the biochemical sequence of events that lead to their lysis of target cells. Data on the roles of NK cells in vivo suggest that these cells may be important in the first line of defense against tumor growth and against infection by some microbial agents. It is now necessary to determine more directly the role of NK cells in immunosurveillance. Ideally, one would like to show increased tumorigenesis when NK activity is selectively depressed and reduced tumor formation when such deficiencies are selectively reconstituted or normal levels of reactivity are selectively augmented. However, there are several practical problems in conducting such experiments. In addition to the long time needed for such studies and the difficulties in identifying the most relevant experimental carcinogenesis models, completely selective and sustained alterations of NK activity are not easily found or produced. If a major role for NK cells in resistance against tumor growth or other diseases can be sustained, this might lead to alternative strategies for immunoprevention or immunotherapy. Lymphokine-activated killer (LAK) cells result from culture of lymphocytes with relatively high doses of interleukin-2 (IL-2). The fundamental characteristic of LAK cells is that they selectively lyse a broad spectrum of fresh autologous, syngeneic, or allogeneic cells in an independent fashion. They are activated cells, derived largely from two sources: NK cells and T cells. The NK cells are the primary source of LAK activity generated in response to high doses of IL-2. After exposure to IL-2 for a day or more, these cells are cytotoxic for tumor cells relatively insensitive to normal NK-mediated cytotoxicity. The T cells also generate LAK activity. Peripheral blood T cells or IL-2-dependent T cell lines exhibit LAK activity after exposure to relatively high doses of IL-2. The cytotoxic mechanisms of LAK cells appear to be similar to those of NK cells and cytotoxic T lymphocytes.

Macrophage dendritic cells and antigen-presenting cells

For cells involved in the immune response to react to foreign antigens, these antigens must be presented in such a manner that the immune cells can recognize them. This requires that the foreign antigens be processed into smaller bits of information and be presented to immune cells or a part of an immune complex with cell surface MHC molecules. There are two types of MHC molecules: class I, expressed on all cells; and class II, expressed on macrophages, dendritic cells, and B cells. All three of these cell types can present antigens to CD4-bearing T cells (see Fig. 19–9).

The macrophage is emerging as a major player in the host reaction to a tumor. Recent evidence has illustrated that the macrophage can be activated by lymphocytes and exerts a killing effect on tumor cells. The mechanism of this killing is unclear, but it appears that direct contact with the target cell is necessary. The macrophage is derived from the bone marrow. Widely distributed throughout the body (blood, bone marrow, lymphoid tissue, liver, connective tissue), macrophage cells form a critical part of the immune defense system. These cells serve at least three distinct but interrelated functions in host defense (Fig. 19–5):

1. Secretion of biologically active molecules
2. Antigen clearance
3. Antigen presentation to lymphocytes (induction of the immune response)

The antigen-activated macrophage secretes a wide range of biologically active molecules that can have regulatory influences on surrounding cells in the process of tissue repair, inflammation, infection, and the immune response. Secretory products of the macrophage include enzymes, complement products, growth and differentiation factors (i.e., IL-1), cytotoxins for tumor and infectious agents, and other substances such as prostaglandins. In the immune system, prostaglandin E^2 can induce immature thymocytes, B lymphocytes, and hematopoietic cell precursors to differentiate and acquire the functional and immunologic characteristics of mature lymphocytes. Perhaps the most important role of the macrophage in the immune response is the processing and presentation of antigen to T cells to generate an immune response.

Although many in vitro studies have demonstrated the cytotoxicity of appropriately stimulated macrophages, evidence that they play a crucial role in the natural defense of the host against malignant disease has been difficult to assess directly. Nonetheless, activated macrophages isolated from donors infected with certain intracellular microorganisms or exposed to general immunopotentiating agents such as endotoxin express non-specific cytotoxicity for a wide range of tumor types but not for normal cells. Several mechanisms may be involved in generating these cytotoxic macrophages. Agents that consist of endotoxin and other stimulants may activate macrophages directly. In general, however, many agents indirectly lead to macrophage activation by functioning as specific antigen stimuli for immune lymphocytes that release a variety of lymphokines. Some of these lymphokines attract macrophages to the site of the immunologic reaction and prevent their migration away (migration inhibition factor) as well as stimulate them with macrophage-activating factor to undergo morphologic changes resulting in enhanced killing capabilities. Because the enhanced killing mediated by these mechanisms can be demonstrated against a variety of tumor target cells, the macrophage appears to be an important non-specific effector of an antigen-specific cell-mediated response.

Many consider dendritic cells the most potent antigen-presenting cells of the immune system. They are unique in their ability to stimulate naive T cells. Dendritic cells are adapted to capture proteins, to digest them by using protein enzymes, and to present the resulting peptides on their cell membranes bound to MHC antigens. Formation of this MHC-peptide complex is crucial to the activation of T cells. In addition, dendritic cells express high levels of

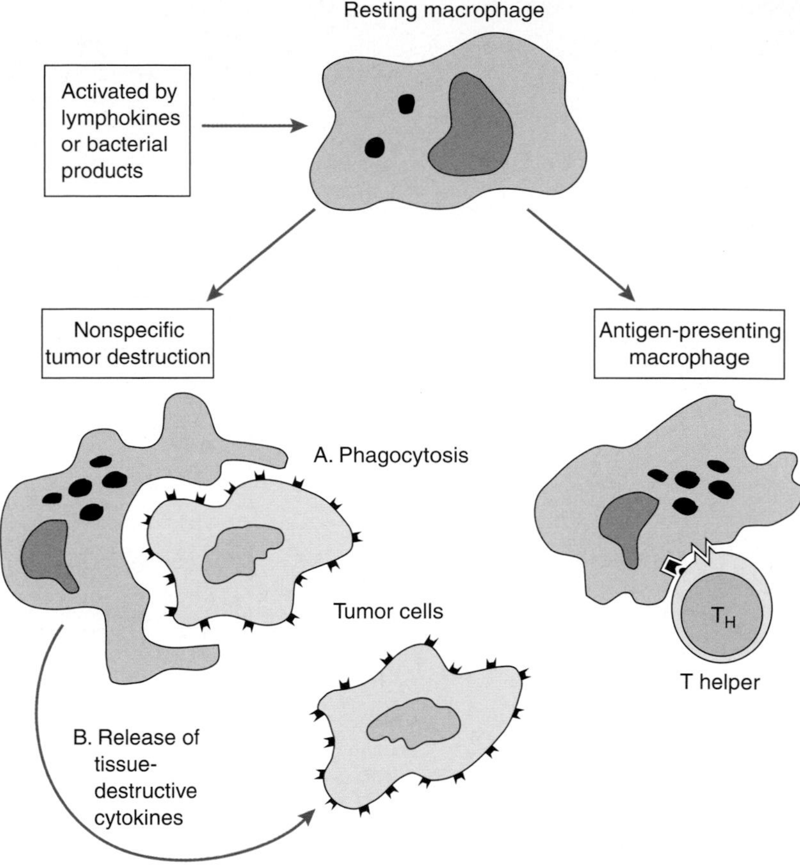

Figure 19–5 Macrophage role in the immune response to malignant disease.

the costimulatory molecules CD80 and CD86, which are required for full T cell activation. Dendritic cells are found in the peridermal layer of the skin, the respiratory and gastrointestinal tissues, and the interstitial regions of several solid organs where they function as sentinels, capturing invading substances (e.g., micro-organisms) for presentation to immune cells. Until recently, research on dendritic cells was limited because they were difficult to isolate from blood or tissues. Now dendritic cells can be isolated from peripheral blood by use of cytokines, such as granulocyte-monocyte colony-stimulating factor, IL-4, and tumor necrosis factor (TNF)-α. Dendritic cell-based cancer vaccines have been tested with some success. There is potential of autologous dendritic cells as a vehicle to deliver specific target antigens. Dendritic cell-based cancer vaccines offer the potential for an effective, non-toxic, and outpatient approach to cancer therapy. Future clinical trials will certainly incorporate dendritic cells pulsed with tumor epitopes derived from newly identified tumor-associated peptides, RNA, and lysates (Fig. 19–6). The tumor-derived compounds will be processed by dendritic cells for presentation in the context of both MHC class I and class II molecules for the priming of T cells.

Mechanisms of immunity

The immune mechanism basically consists of the initial recognition and processing of foreign matter, an afferent mechanism leading to activation of the central immune system, and an efferent mechanism leading to the elimination of the offending material. The basic study of immunology concerns the reactions of the body to certain foreign materials presented to it, both living and nonliving. The immune reaction can be defined as an interaction between the invading foreign material and the defending host tissue. The cells of the afferent arm process the antigenic information and convey it to the central immune mechanism capable of reacting specifically to this information. The cells of the central mechanism are termed immunologically competent and are of the lymphoid series. This lymphoid tissue is present in peripheral lymph nodes, bone marrow, spleen, thymus, Peyer's patches of the intestine, and thoracic duct and in the bloodstream itself. All antigens are recognized as self or non-self. It is known, however, that when recognition occurs, it is specific and precisely directed against certain molecular configurations on the antigen. In addition, antigen and immunocompetent cells apparently have physical contact to evoke a response.

Specific immune responses are mediated by two categories of effectors, with considerable interaction between the two. One category of response can be transferred from one individual to another only by transferring living immunologically competent cells or cultured products of these cells. This type of response is termed cell-mediated immunity. The second type of response can be transferred by cell-free serum and therefore is called humoral immunity (Fig. 19–7). The key to both these responses is the small lymphocyte, which until recently was relegated to a

MHC class I
MHC class I and tumor peptide
cDNA
Tumor peptides, lysates, apoptic bodies, mRNA
MHC class II
Dendritic cell
MHC class II and tumor peptide
Tumor cell

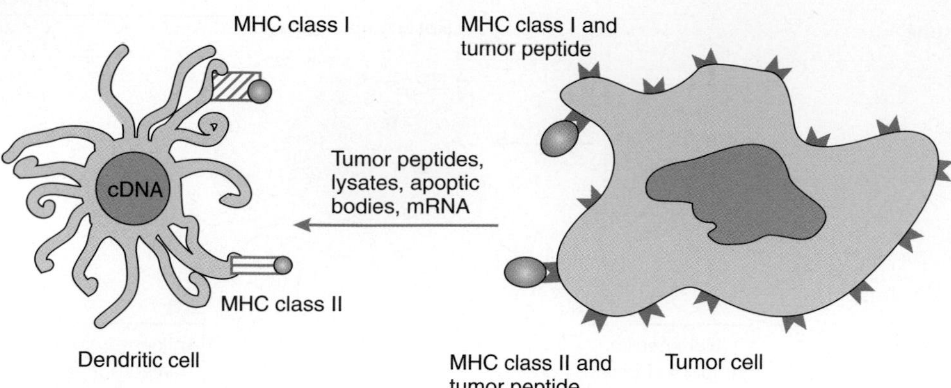

Figure 19–6 Future clinical trials with dendritic cells pulsed with tumor epitopes derived from newly identified tumor-associated peptides, RNA, lysates, and apoptotic bodies. Dendritic cells might also be genetically modified with cDNA encoding. MHC, major histocompatibility complex.

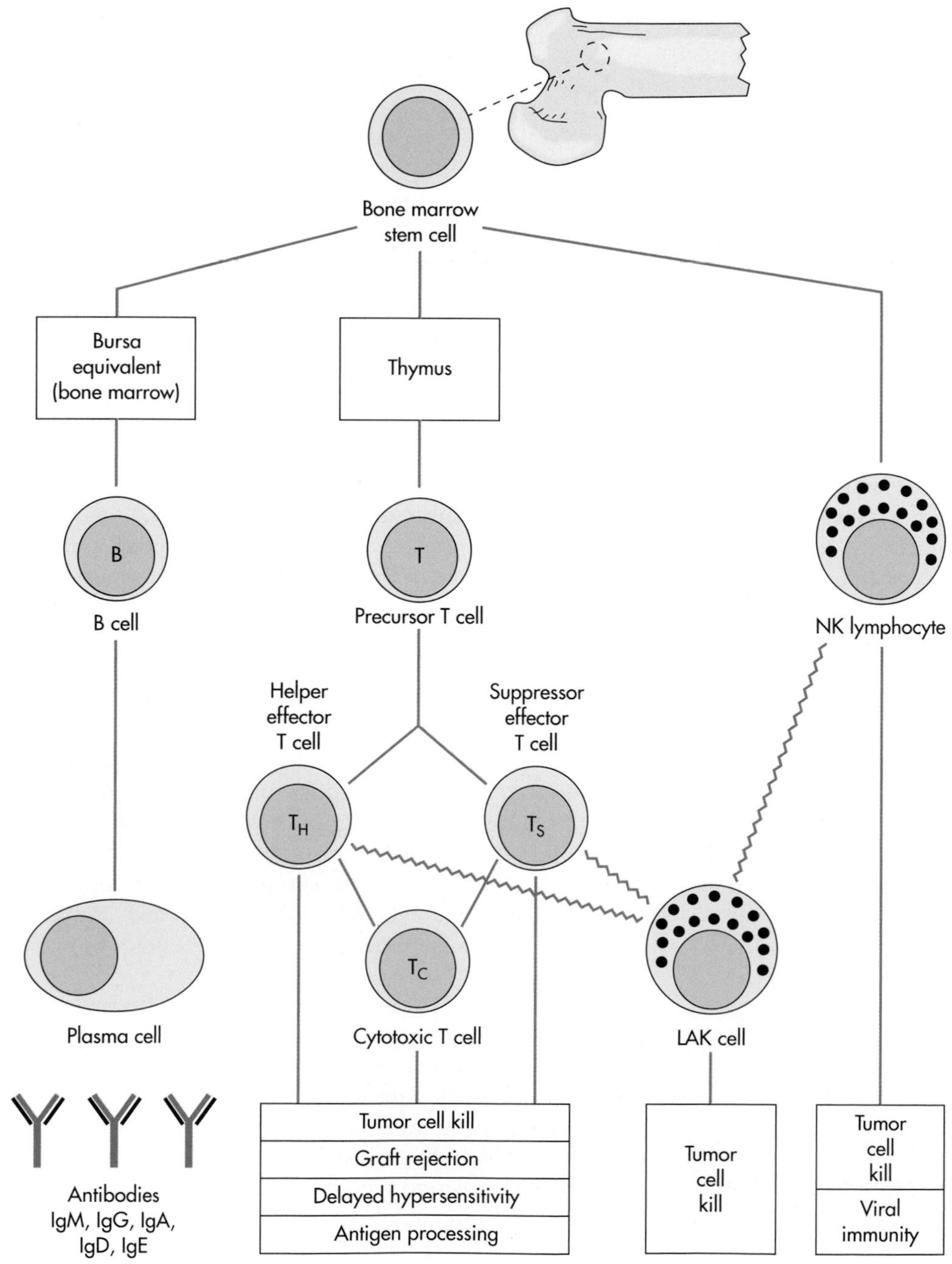

Bone marrow stem cell
Bursa equivalent (bone marrow)
Thymus
B
B cell
T
Precursor T cell
NK lymphocyte
Helper effector T cell
Suppressor effector T cell
TH
TS
TC
Plasma cell
Cytotoxic T cell
LAK cell
Antibodies IgM, IgG, IgA, IgD, IgE
Tumor cell kill
Graft rejection
Delayed hypersensitivity
Antigen processing
Tumor cell kill
Tumor cell kill
Viral immunity

Figure 19–7 Development of effector cells within the immune system. T^H, T^S, and natural killer (NK) lymphocytes require cytokine activation to differentiate into lymphokine-activated killer (LAK) cells.

position of relative obscurity in textbooks of physiology and hematology. The small lymphocyte is formed in the bone marrow from precursor stem cells and then released into the circulation, eventually coming to rest in the lymphoid organs. The small lymphocytes specialize early in their life, either by passing through the thymus gland and differentiating into cells that will participate in cell-mediated immunity (T cells) or bypassing the thymus and undergoing differentiation into cells that will mediate humoral immunity (B cells). Despite the crucial differences between these two types of cells, they are morphologically indistinguishable by light microscopy.

The interaction of antigen with antigen-specific receptors on T and B cells initiates a cascade of events that results in a proliferation and differentiation of both types of cells. The intracellular events that follow activation of the antigen-specific receptor complex are similar in both B and T cells, after receptor triggering at the cell surface. As a result of this stimulation, both B and T cells differentiate into effector cells, and a small fraction of both populations become memory cells.

Cell-mediated immunity

Cell-mediated immunity (cellular immunity, transplantation immunity, or delayed hypersensitivity) is mediated by the lymphocyte that has passed through the thymus in its development. The exact mechanism of the thymic influence is not well understood in the human organism but is suspected of being hormonal. After the lymphocyte passes through the thymus in its development, it remains under the influence of the thymus and is variously termed the thymus-dependent lymphocyte, T lymphocyte, or simply T cell (Fig. 19–8).

Many studies, both in vivo and in vitro, indicate that in addition to T cells and B cells, a central role in the inductive phase of the immune response is played by accessory cells of the monocyte-macrophage series. After the injection of antigen, macrophages, in draining lymph nodes and in the spleen, trap and concentrate the antigen. Studies in vitro have shown that the production of antibodies involves the formation of clusters of lymphocytes around central macrophages or other dendritic cells with subsequent intimate contact of these accessory cells with B and T lymphocytes. Furthermore, if accessory cells are removed from cultures of lymphocytes, the immune response is, in large part, abrogated.

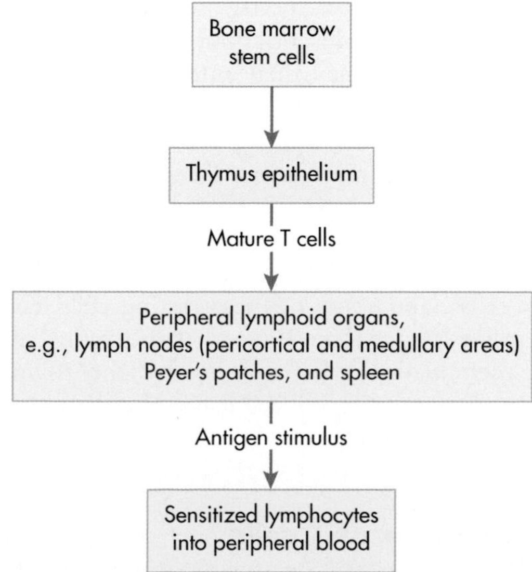

Figure 19–8 Process of T cell lymphocyte maturation.

We now have a widely accepted mechanism that follows the injection of an immunogen to elucidate the role of accessory cells in immune induction. By far the great majority of antigens involved in immune responses are proteins, and these responses depend on the presence of T cells. These antigens are therefore commonly referred to as T-dependent antigens and are to be distinguished from another major category of antigen, polysaccharides, which generally induce antibody in the absence of T cells and are thereby termed thymus-independent antigens. Unlike B cells, T cells are not activated by free antigen. The antigen involved in T cell activation must be presented by other cells, such as macrophages or even B cells. These accessory or antigen-presenting cells play a crucial role in the processing of a polypeptide. The accessory cells break the polypeptide down intracellularly into smaller peptide fragments. Some of these peptide fragments become associated with glycoprotein molecules, which are coated by genes located in the MHC. These complexes of peptides and MHC molecules are somehow transported to the surface of the cell, where they are recognized by the T cell receptor.

The key functions of the molecules encoded by the MHC and the T cell responses to such underlie the mechanism of the immunity response (Fig. 19–9). These key functions are:

1. establishing a T cell repertoire, as a consequence of the positive and negative selection events that occur when T lymphocyte precursors interact with MHC molecules expressed on the surface of accessory cells; and
2. activating mature T cells.

The activation of mature T cells is the result of the antigen-specific T cell receptor's interacting with antigen only when the polypeptide antigen is bound to the MHC molecule of an accessory cell. These polypeptide antigens are processed within an accessory cell, where smaller peptides between 10 and 20 amino acids in length are produced. When these smaller peptides become associated with MHC molecules inside the cell, the complex can then be transported to the cell surface, where it can be recognized by the T cell receptor. Each T cell bears a unique, clonally distributed receptor for antigen. As with B cells, an individual has millions of different T cells. The combination of antigen-recognizing T cell and signal transducer CD3 comprises the T cell receptor. The engagement of the T cell receptor (Ti-CD3) by the antigen-class II complex is still insufficient to activate the T cells. This may be due

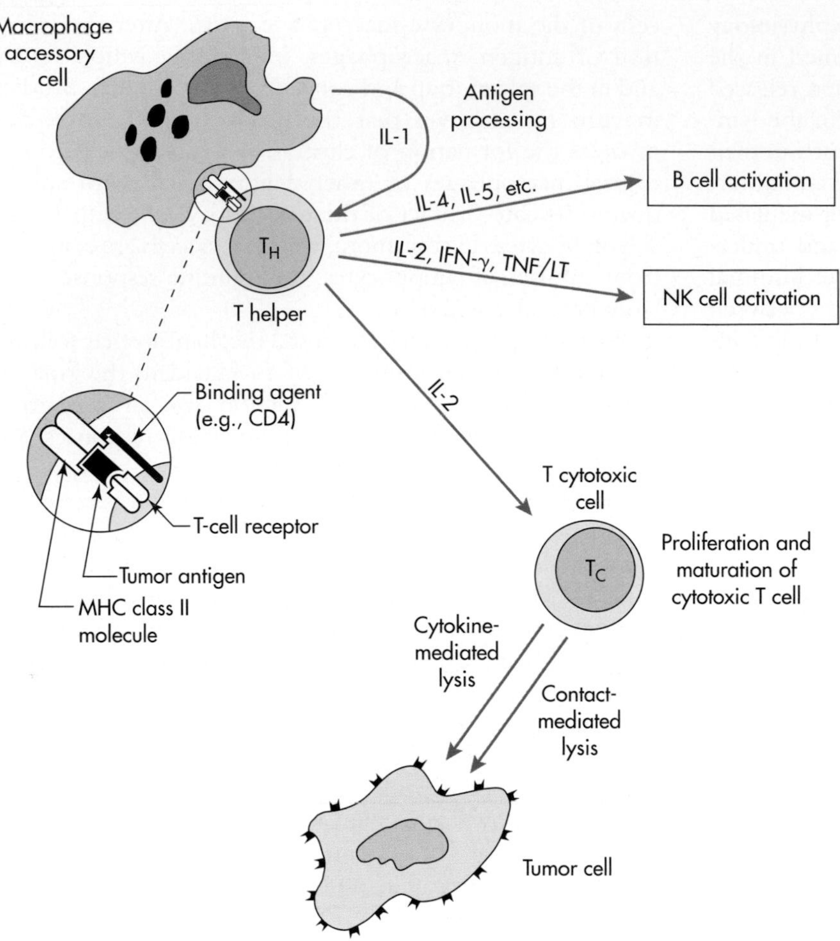

Figure 19–9 T cell activity in the immune response to malignant disease. Helper T cells (T^H MHC class II restricted) mediate effects by secretion of cytokines to activate other cells. Cytotoxic T cells (T^C MHC class I restricted) mediate effects by direct lysis of tumor cells. The complex formed by the immunogenic peptide (antigen) bound in the cleft of a class II molecule is recognized by the antigen receptor on a specific helper T cell. A binding agent such as CD4 is necessary to finally activate the T cell. NK, natural killer

to a low affinity of such reactions. This interaction of the Ti-CD3 with the peptide-MHC class II is enhanced by yet another molecule, CD4 (see Fig. 19–9), found on the surface of yet another set of T cells, the CD4 T cells. The function of the CD4 seems to be to bind to a portion of the MHC class II molecule. In summary, the sequence of events leading to the activation of CD4 T cells starts with the engagement of the Ti-CD3 receptors that recognize the specific antigen in association with the class II molecule on an accessory cell, followed by the further stabilization of this molecular interaction through CD4 class II association and through the cellular interaction of adhesion molecules. Thus, by a combination of antigen-specific and antigen-non-specific interactions, sufficient receptors are engaged with sufficient energy to start the T cell on its activation route. The way in which T cells bind antigen provides a useful mechanism for avoiding engagement of T cells by free antigen. The interaction with free antigen is a role left to antibodies.

T cell activation results in the secretion of a number of antigen-non-specific soluble factors known as lymphokines. Each lymphokine has a specific cell surface receptor, expressed on various different cell types. Soluble products released by lymphocytes, lymphokines belong to the general category of substances known as cytokines. Cytokines are soluble substances, produced by cells that have various effects on other cells (see Table 19–2). The soluble products of monocytes are known as monokines. Substances produced by one of the leukocytes, which can in turn affect other leukocytes, are known as interleukins. As a consequence of T cell activation, many different cytokines are produced. These cytokines have profound effects, not only on the proliferation and differentiation of T cells but also on the activation and growth of many different cell types.

The thymus manufactures a large number of T lymphocytes. These T cells leave the thymus to enter the bloodstream, where they represent about 80% of the peripheral blood lymphocytes. They then enter a unique pattern of recirculation, with many moving from blood to lymph node to thoracic duct; from there, they return to the blood. In the lymph node, most T cells reside in the deep cortex in areas in and between germinal centers. This pool of mature T lymphocytes is often called the recirculating pool of long-lived T lymphocytes (some undoubtedly memory cells), and some of these resting cells have been shown to live longer than 20 years without dividing. The path of recirculation does not involve the thymus; for unknown reasons, after a T cell leaves the thymus, it does not appear to return to it.

Subpopulations of T cells

There are several subpopulations of T cells, each with a different function. There is substantial evidence for separate categories of functional T lymphocytes, such as the helper cells or cytotoxic or even suppressor cells (see Fig. 19–7), but it is unclear whether these categories represent different functional states in the common differentiation pathway or have separate pathways of maturation. Normal T cells do not produce conventional immunoglobulin, as is characteristic of B cells. However, T cells do have a crucial role in the regulation of immune responses by acting as potentiators or inhibitors of the B cell transition into immunoglobulin-secreting plasma cells. The cells that potentiate this B cell transition are classified as helper cells; those that inhibit it are classified as suppressor cells. Suppressor cells have been identified in humans through a variety of circumstances. There is compelling evidence in mice and corroborating evidence in humans that help and suppression are mediated by distinct subsets of T cells, each genetically committed to mediate only one of these two functions. Other evidence suggests that immunoregulatory T cells may have an interim existence as inactive precursors, which might be referred to as pro-helper cells and pro-suppressor cells that must react with a different set of activated T cells before maturing into fully functional helper effector cells or suppressor effector cells. Physiologically, suppressor cells may terminate excessive immune responses after antigenic exposure, and they probably provide a safeguard against autoimmune reactions. It is not surprising, therefore, that recent evidence from a number of animal models of autoimmunity suggests that impaired suppressor T cell function can lead to overt autoimmune disease.

An understanding of suppressor cell function in human neoplasia may alter the perspective and direction of oncologic researchers and clinicians. There is a real possibility that chemotherapy, radiation, and surgery might, in certain cases, benefit patients with cancer by an indirect effect on suppressor cells as well as by the obvious effect on the neoplasm itself. New immunotherapeutic strategies that incorporate recent insight regarding the suppressor cell network are nullifying suppressor cell systems that oppose tumoricidal immune effector mechanisms. In addition to switching off antibody production by B cells, suppressor T cells apparently are capable of preventing lymphokine production by other T cells.

Humoral immunity

As the term suggests, humoral immunity is mediated by factors present in and transferable by serum; these include the classic antibody globulins. The cell responsible for the production of these antibodies is the second type of small lymphocyte, the B cell (Fig. 19–10). In the chicken, these lymphocytes aggregate in a small organ called the bursa of Fabricius. Removal of the bursa was noted to render the chicken unable to produce antibodies; the B cells have thus come to be known as bursa-dependent cells. In humans, there was a great deal of controversy as to the origin of these cells, but recent evidence has made it clear that these cells originate in the bone marrow and do not undergo maturation in the thymus. In humans (who have no bursa of Fabricius), no one organ appears to have control of B cell production. Rather, B cells are distributed in all areas of lymphoid tissue, including the spleen, lymph nodes, tonsils, appendix, and Peyer's patches of the small intestine. With suitable stimulation, B cells become metabolically active and begin to synthesize antibodies with great facility. The antibodies soon become detectable in the cytoplasm and are then secreted into the surrounding medium. It is at this point that the B cell has undergone transformation into a plasma cell, which is the actual antibody producer. In a typical peripheral lymph node, B cells occupy the germinal centers and T cells occupy the cortical areas; these areas are referred to, respectively, as the bursa-dependent and thymus-dependent areas of the node. Although the bone marrow appears to be the source of cells destined to make antibodies, the bone marrow itself is not the locus of large-scale antibody formation. Rather, it is the site of intense lymphocyte proliferation leading to the production of mature B lymphocytes, which quickly leave the marrow and travel to peripheral lymphoid tissues. There they may meet the appropriate antigen, become stimulated to divide and differentiate into large lymphocytes and plasma cells, and actively manufacture antibodies. Resting B lymphocytes are the typical small lymphocytes of the peripheral blood and, in fact, cannot be distinguished from resting T lymphocytes under the usual light microscope (Table 19–4). Under the scanning electron microscope, typical B cells have a hairy appearance with many small hairlike projections, whereas typical T cells are smoother (Fig. 19–11). B lymphocytes are particularly plentiful in areas where antibody production occurs, for example, in the germinal centers of the lymph nodes and in the diffuse lymphoid tissue of the gastrointestinal and respiratory tracts. They are less common in the blood, rare in the lymphatics and thoracic duct, and virtually absent from the thymus.

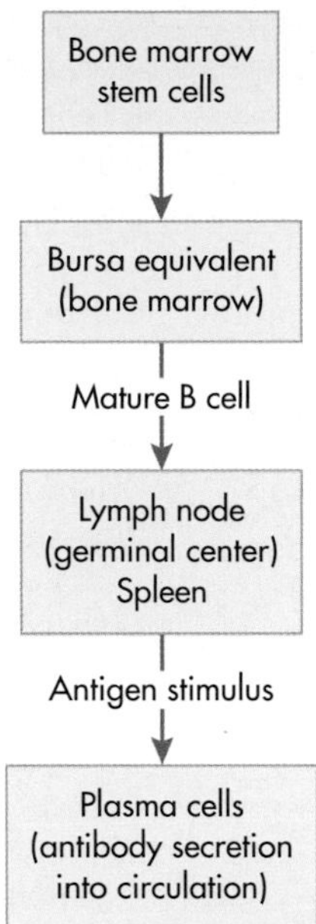

Figure 19–10 Process of B cell lymphocyte maturation.

Table 19–4 COMPARISON OF T AND B CELLS

T cells (thymus dependent)	B cells (thymus independent)
Bone marrow origin	Bone marrow origin
Mature in thymus	Mature in lymph node
Concentrated in paracortical areas of the lymph node	Concentrated in germinal centers of the lymph node
Long-lived (months to years)	Short-lived (days to weeks)
Circulate widely	Less mobile, concentrated in lymph nodes and spleen
Sensitive to phytohemagglutinin	Insensitive to phytohemagglutinin
Sensitive to pokeweed mitogen	Sensitive to pokeweed mitogen
No immunoglobulins	Synthesize immunoglobulins
Cell-mediated immunity	Humoral immunity
Delayed hypersensitivity	Antibody production
Produce lymphokines	Do not usually produce lymphokines

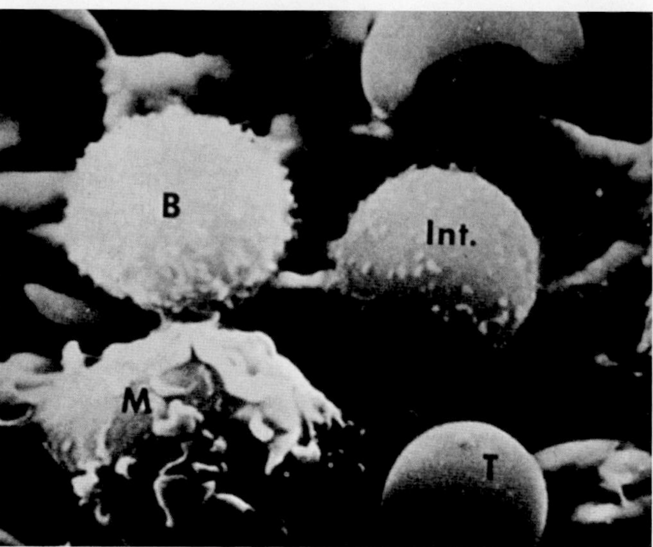

Figure 19–11 Scanning electron microscopic view of peripheral blood leukocytes. (B, B cell; M, macrophage; T, T cell; Int., intermediate form, which may be of the "double cell" variety.)

There is clear evidence that the functional separation of T cells and B cells into two systems is not as clear cut as was formerly thought. An increasing number of biologically important responses are being discovered for which interplay of two systems is essential. This has been termed T-B cooperation. The presence of healthy T cells is necessary for production by B cells of many antibodies in response to antigenic stimulation and probably for the maintenance of immunologic memory for most antigens. The precise mechanism of this T-B cooperation is unknown; it may take the form of some messenger protein or actual physical contact and cytoplasmic bridging. Under suitable circumstances, B cells are capable of secreting some of the non-immunoglobulin soluble products (lymphokines) that were formerly thought to be characteristic of T cells. The biologic role of T-B cooperation is one of the most important areas for future research. There is much controversy about the order of production of immunoglobulins by the B cell. It is currently thought that IgM is the first antibody produced, and then a switch to IgG production follows a signal possibly initiated by helper T cells. It has been theorized that IgD antedates the secretion of both IgM and IgG in embryonic life as well as in the adult. This is one of many unanswered questions. Deficiencies of either or both of the thymus-dependent and bursa-dependent systems occur in various congenital and acquired diseases. The primary immunodeficiency syndromes include chronic granulomatous disease, Chédiak–Higashi disease, Bruton's syndrome, DiGeorge's syndrome, ataxia-telangiectasia (Louis-Bar's syndrome), and Wiskott–Aldrich syndrome. The incidence of spontaneously occurring malignant disease is increased appreciably in most of these conditions.

Suppression of the immunologic responses is a natural result of certain biologic processes, such as pregnancy and aging. It also occurs in several systemic diseases, as a result of radiation or drug therapy, and after severe injuries. In most instances, cell-mediated immunity is suppressed more rapidly or profoundly than humoral immunity. With modern advances in immunologic techniques, the precise nature of the defect may be uncovered, but it is not known at present for many of these conditions. This kind of knowledge is essential if one is to treat these disorders effectively by immunologic means. Immunotherapy will be available in the near future, but its effectiveness will depend on the accurate diagnosis of the relevant immunologic defect and selective reversal. Conditions such as malnutrition, surgical trauma, burns, and accidental injuries will result in suppression of the host defense mechanism. This should be kept in mind in the design of an overall treatment plan for any patient.

Interactions that regulate immune responses

The discovery of a complex series of regulatory interactions among components of the immune system has proved to be a major advance in our understanding of the system. In the 1960s, it was demonstrated that the development of the antibody responses depended on T cell-B cell interactions, and our perspective has now widened to reveal the workings of various genes, molecules, and cells in regulation of this immune system. It is known that genes of the system produce:

1. antigen-specific receptors on lymphocyte surface membranes;
2. circulating antibodies that perform effective functions and exert feedback regulation;
3. crucial regulatory effects on various cell-cell interactions necessary for normal immunologic homeostasis; and
4. biologically active molecules capable of enhancing or suppressing T cell or B cell activity.

The cells of the system are interdependent. The development of cell-mediated or humoral immunity, therefore, is regulated by a series of essential interactions between macrophages, T cells, and B cells. Regulatory interactions between constituents of the immune system may enhance or suppress the immune responses. The qualitative or quantitative response occurring in any given time, however, reflects the net effect of the extremely dynamic interplay among the system's components.

Immunosurveillance

The mechanisms used by the host to mount a response against any antigens that are expressed by a neoplasm are called immunosurveillance. The primary function of the immune system is to recognize and degrade foreign (non-self) antigens in the body that arise de novo or are inflicted on the host. In tumor surveillance, the assumption is made that the mutant cell will express one or more antigens that can be recognized as non-self. A popular concept holds that mutant cells develop frequently in the human and are rapidly victimized by the ubiquitous and ideally competent immunologic mechanisms. Mice deprived of cell-mediated immunity and exposed to an oncogenic agent will spontaneously develop more tumors. This is regarded as evidence of an immunosurveillance mechanism. Patients with advanced disease are often more immunosuppressed than patients with early disease are. Patients taking immunosuppressive drugs after renal transplantation have an increased incidence of malignant neoplasms (100 times greater than that of matched-control subjects). Almost 50% of these tumors in immunosuppressed individuals are of mesenchymal origin, for example, reticulum cell sarcomas, but a higher incidence of epithelial neoplasia, especially cervical intraepithelial neoplasia, has also been reported. Complementary evidence for the importance of tumor surveillance comes from the relationship between congenital or acquired immunodeficiency disease and tumor development; these patients also demonstrate an incidence of malignant disease far in excess of that of matched-control subjects.

However, immune surveillance has remained a theory since first proposed in the 1950s. Some doubt is cast on the validity of the theory by the finding that the incidence of tumors in athymic mice, which have no T cell response, is not increased. Furthermore, surface antigens on tumor cells of spontaneous occurring tumors are of weak immunogenicity.

Although there are explanations of how immune surveillance may be circumvented by cancer, there is much less evidence that there is an immune mechanism for limiting tumor growth. Examples of tumor immunity have been demonstrated in experimental animals, particularly for early induced tumors and tumors induced by "strong" chemical carcinogens. However, other evidence indicates that tumors induced by "weak" carcinogens or those arising "spontaneously" are weakly antigenic or not antigenic at all. Evidence of tumor-limiting factors in humans is only circumstantial, and this is listed in Table 19-5. Although this list is impressive at first glance, the number of patients exhibiting tumor immunity is relatively low. Most untreated human tumors grow without evidence of tumor immunity. Documented spontaneous regressions are rare and occur most often in tumors of embryonal tissue such as choriocarcinomas, hypernephromas, and neuroblastomas, suggesting developmental controlling factors rather than immunity. Regression of metastases without chemotherapy or radiation is extremely rare. Reappearance of metastases after long latent periods may be explained by several factors controlling dormancy other than immunity. Although infiltration of tumors by mononuclear cells is often used to support some role of the immune response in the fate of the tumor, there is limited evidence that such infiltration actually affects the growth of the tumor. The tumors found in immunosuppressed or immunodeficient patients are frequently of lymphoid elements, suggesting an abnormality in lymphocyte-controlling mechanisms rather than specific tumor immunity. Finally, a number of immune abnormalities occur in the elderly, including loss of the thymic cortex and the appearance of a variety of autoantibodies. However, there is no directly demonstrable cause and effect relationship between an abnormality of the immune response associated with aging and the increased incidence of cancer associated with aging. In summary, the role of immunity in immunosurveillance against newly arising tumors remains controversial.

Table 19–5 CIRCUMSTANTIAL EVIDENCE FOR TUMOR-LIMITING FACTORS IN HUMANS
Spontaneous regression
Self-healing melanomas
Regression of metastases after resection of primary neoplasms
Regression of tumor after "non-cytotoxic" doses of chemotherapy
Reappearance of metastasis after long latent periods
Frequent failure of circulating tumor cells to form metastases
Infiltration of tumors by mononuclear cells
Higher incidence of tumors after clinical immunosuppression
High incidence of tumors in immune deficiency diseases
Increased incidence of malignant neoplasms with aging

Takasugi, Mickey, and Terasaki have called attention to the role of NK lymphocytes in the immunosurveillance of tumors. NK cells from several species preferentially destroy malignant target cells in vitro and appear to need no prior sensitization. Indeed, NK cells may be the effectors of tumor surveillance.

One of the major predictions of the immunosurveillance theory is that tumor development should be associated with, in fact be preceded by, depressed immunity. Several observations fit this prediction, including the fact that kidney allograft recipients who have received immunosuppressive drugs and have a high risk for development of lymphoproliferative and other tumors also have severely depressed NK cell activity. Many other observations of the animal system support the possibility that one of the requisites for tumor induction by carcinogenic agents may be interference with host defenses, including those mediated by NK cells.

Doubt is cast on the validity of the theory of immune surveillance by the finding that the incidence of tumors in athymic mice, which have no T cell-mediated response, is no higher than the incidence in their normal counterparts. However, such athymic mice have normal or in some instances increased numbers of NK cells.

Escape from surveillance (Fig. 19–12)

There are several postulated mechanisms by which mutant cells might avoid an interaction with a potentially damaging immune system.

Lowered tumor antigenicity (antigenic modulation)

Neoplasms that arise spontaneously are noted to be considerably less antigenic than those induced experimentally. Many human tumors may be weakly antigenic or nonantigenic. In addition, antigenic modulation may occur. Antigenic modulation is a loss of antigenicity or a change in the antigenic markers by which tumor cells may avoid immunologic destruction. Antigenic modulation has been demonstrated with murine leukemia cells expressing thymic lymphocyte (TL) antigens. When these tumor cells are grown in the presence of cytotoxic serum that contains anti-TL antibodies, certain cells lose their TL antigens, perhaps by shedding or internalization of membrane receptors. These variants become predominant in the culture. However, removal of the antiserum leads to the reappearance of the TL antigens. This indicates that the antigenic selection has not taken place but that specific antibodies suppress the production of the corresponding antigen.

Privileged site

Certain areas of the body (e.g., eye and nervous system) are inaccessible to effector cells of the immune system and thus may escape destruction by the immune response.

Immunoresistance

Diminished sensitivity to rejection may develop in the same way that bacteria develop resistance to antibodies after repeated exposure. The cells may develop a decrease in cell surface antigenic sites (antigenic modulation) or relevant antibody-binding sites. Another mechanism that is easy to conceive calls for antigenic molecules or receptors for cytokines on the surface of the tumor cell to be shed in large amounts into the surrounding extracellular fluid. The cell surface will then be rendered relatively immunoresistant as its locality becomes flooded with excess antigens or receptors. This may be classified then as a blocking factor. Some suggest that tumors that shed antigen rapidly are those of low immunogenicity and metastasize most rapidly.

Vascularization

Tumors probably reach 1–2 mm in diameter before vascularization takes place. Folkman and Hochberg suggested that the vessels result from ingrowth of host cells, and thus

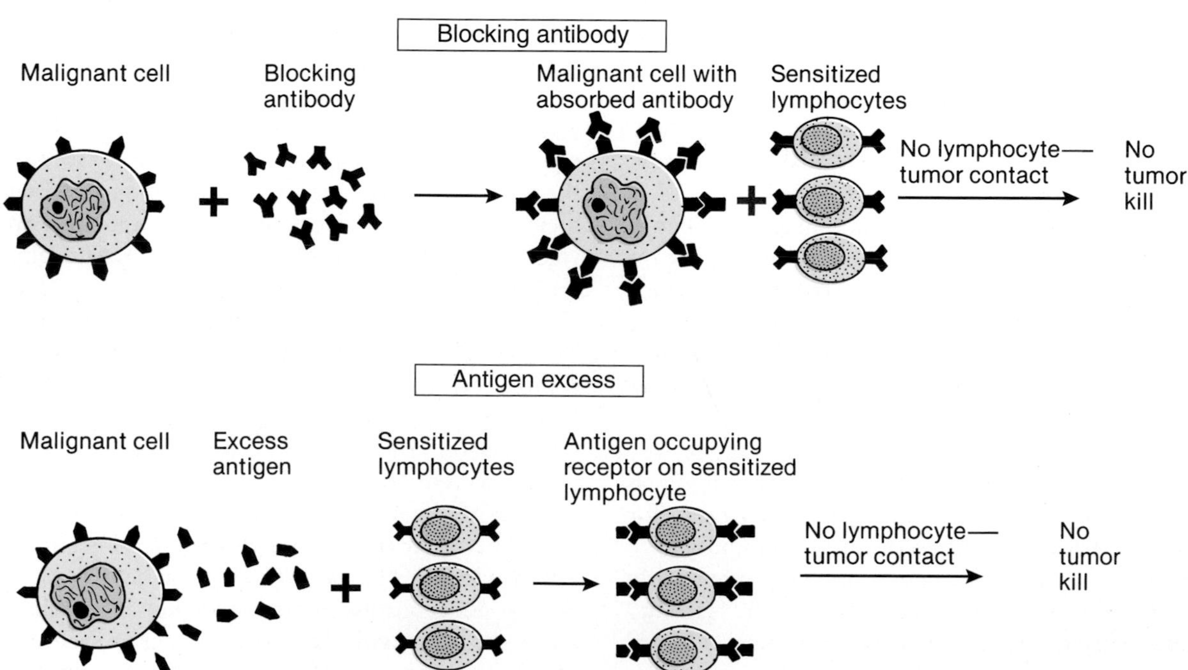

Figure 19–12 Two methods of escape from surveillance: (1) blocking antibody absorbed onto antigen sites on tumor cell surface, and (2) excess antigen flooding the tumor cell environment, preventing lymphocyte attack.

the endothelium of the tumor vessels may be recognized as self and not rejected. Therefore, some neoplasms may proliferate with their antigens locked away behind a wall of "normal" endothelial cells unpenetrated by attack lymphocytes.

Immunosuppression

It has been well established that the presence of a cancer can significantly reduce an individual's capacity to mount a response to a great variety of antigens. Immunosuppressive factors have been described in the serum of patients with cancer and confirmed in vitro. The mechanism by which these factors cause immunosuppression is not understood, but some authors have suggested that they suppress macrophage function. Some degree of immunosuppression has been found in almost all patients with cancer studied. DNCB (2,4-dinitrochlorobenzene), DNFB (2,4-dinitrofluorobenzene), and a variety of skin test antigens have been used on patients with gynecologic malignant neoplasms. An increase in tumor burden is associated with a decreased percentage of patients responding to these tests, and both are associated with poorer prognoses.

Certain types of tumors synthesize compounds, such as prostaglandins, that reduce many aspects of immune responsiveness. The role of prostaglandins in the mechanism whereby tumors escape destruction by the immune system is unclear.

Although the mechanism suggested in the preceding paragraph is non-specific suppression, antigen-specific suppressor T cells may also play an important role in the regulation of the immune response to an antigen. An increase in tumor-specific suppressor T cells has been demonstrated in many experimental systems, especially in patients with advanced malignant disease. Whether this increase can be attributed to immunologically specific suppressor mechanisms or to a more generalized suppression mediated by tumor cells is unknown.

Blocking factors

Neoplasms may escape the immune mechanism by the development of systemic factors that abrogate the usual interaction with host defense capabilities. Several serum factors have been identified in vitro: blocking antibodies, antigen-antibody complexes, and soluble antigen excess. When these blocking factors are operational, the state of the tumor-host relationship is one of tumor enhancement. The mechanisms involved may be similar to those described under immunoresistance. Excess free antibody may saturate antigenic sites on the cell surface, or conversely, excess free antigen may paralyze lymphocyte activity. In addition, studies suggest that the cellular factors of the immune system may be capable of causing tumor enhancement. In some animal and in vivo systems, small numbers of sensitized (tumor-specific) lymphocytes can enhance tumor growth, whereas larger numbers of the same cells will retard growth. This phenomenon has been referred to as immunostimulation, and if it is valid, it will help explain the emergence of neoplasms beyond the subclinical stage when tumor cell numbers are small and vulnerable. The puzzle is made more difficult because "deblocking" factors have also been described in the serum of patients with cancer undergoing remission or after surgical debulking procedures. The mechanism involved in deblocking is unknown.

IMMUNOPROPHYLAXIS

Immunoprophylaxis is the induction of resistance to a tumor before its origination and should be clearly separated from immunotherapy, which is the treatment of established neoplasms and a more difficult problem. Everyone interested in tumor immunology dreams of successes with immunoprophylaxis similar to those achieved with bacterial and viral illnesses. Immunoprophylaxis may theoretically be achieved by immunization either against the etiologic agent of the cancer, for example, an oncogenic virus, or against the tumor-specific cell surface antigens of the neoplasm. However, the oncogenic viruses of most human cancers (if they exist) have not as yet been clearly identified, and even if they exist, it is uncertain whether transmission is vertical or horizontal. The tumor-specific cell surface antigens needed for the other approach have not as yet been adequately purified. Both pathways can be made to work in animal systems but have not been truly tested in humans. Some indirect confirmation comes from studies. Rosenthal and coworkers reported a retrospective analysis of the leukemia death rate in an infant population from Chicago who received BCG vaccine compared with a similar population who had not received the vaccine. During the period 1964–1969, the death rate in the infants who were not vaccinated was six to seven times greater than the rate in the vaccinated group. At least one other study from Canada confirms the study of Rosenthal and coworkers, but others have not.

Prophylaxis against tumors by vaccination depends on immunologic reactivity between the immunogen and the tumor. Thus, at least theoretically, it should be feasible to immunize against only virally induced tumors and other tumors that exhibit immunologic reactivity. For example, positive reactivity has been demonstrated among patients who have Burkitt's lymphoma, nasopharyngeal carcinoma, melanoma, and neuroblastoma, suggesting the possibility of preparing tumor vaccines for prophylactic purposes. However, immunization would not necessarily result in protection against the tumor. It may lead to induction of immune complexes (e.g., blocking antibodies) that will enhance rather than impede tumor growth and metastasis. Such considerations must be taken into account before any trial of immunization.

Human papillomavirus (HPV) has been shown to be a primary etiologic agent of cervical cancer and cervical dysplasia. At least two prophylactic vaccines have been developed by utilizing two oncogenic proteins, E6 and E7, of the HPV virus in live vectors. Initial trials in young teenage patients have demonstrated excellent protection. An ideal prophylactic vaccine needs to possess several attributes. It must be safe, because it will be given to young, normal individuals. It should be able to be administered in settings with poor resources, be inexpensive and, hopefully, effective with a single dose. Protection should last many years and a substantial reduction in the incidence of cervix cancer should result.

Principles of immunotherapy

It is obvious that the ultimate goal of immunotherapy is the complete destruction of all neoplastic cells. Short of obtaining that, the suppression of growth of tumor cells is desired. An expression of this therapeutic effect would be the prolongation of remission and the prevention of the appearance of metastatic disease. More often than not, the immunotherapist must be satisfied with evidence that the approach has achieved at least a reduction in the mass of tumor cells. Before the institution of immunotherapy, it is crucial to reduce tumor mass to a minimum, preferably $<10^8$ cells, by whatever means at hand—radical surgical procedures, chemotherapy, or radiation therapy. It has been shown that immunotherapy can achieve little against an overwhelming tumor burden, and single-agent immunotherapy by itself appears to be relatively ineffectual. At present, it is always used with other cancericidal modalities, which are depended on to significantly reduce the tumor burden. As one would expect, immunotherapy has shown more effectiveness in neoplasms that are highly antigenic, such as Burkitt's lymphoma, malignant melanoma, and neuroblastoma.

Most clinical trials to date have used single immunoactive agents ineffectively. In fact, several elements of the immune system are probably necessary and should be orchestrated in an as yet unknown manner to achieve the desired effect. Immunotherapeutic approaches can be classified into two broad categories: active, those that attempt to induce in the host a state of immune responsiveness to the tumor; and passive, those that transfer directly to the host immunologically active substances that mediate an antitumor response themselves. There is overlap, such as monoclonal antibodies (passive) that induce a host-specific antitumor response (active). In general, however, the classification is appropriate, and both active and passive can be further subdivided into specific and non-specific. Most important, the reader should fully comprehend the embryonic nature of immunotherapy, and an attitude of cautious optimism must be maintained as this nascent area of research is brought to full term.

Table 19–6 ACTIVE IMMUNOTHERAPY

Non-specific
Biologic immunostimulants: BCG, MER, Corynebacterium parvum, OK432
Chemical immunostimulants: levamisole, cimetidine, lysosomes containing macrophage-activating substances
Chemotherapeutic agents: cyclophosphamide, doxorubicin, Vinca alkaloids, cisplatin
Cytokines: interferon, IL-2, tumor necrosis factor

Specific
Inactivated tumor vaccines (autologous, allogeneic)
Monoclonal tumor autoidiotypic antibodies
Human tumor hybrids (with xenogeneic antigen-bearing fusion partners)

Active immunotherapy (Table 19–6)

Non-specific

Central to tumor immunology and especially to active immunotherapy is the question of whether antigens recognizable by the host exist on the surface of the tumor cell. One of the theoretical concerns about active immunotherapy as a proposed modality is the apparent lack of a response in the host observed in the setting of a progressively growing tumor. Recognition of this fact has led to several approaches designed to increase the immunogenicity of these human tumors. These have included costimulation with biologic immunostimulants such as BCG, MER, *Cryptosporidium parvum*, and other products.

A substance that increases response to an antigen is an adjuvant. Adjuvants may be effective by altering the antigen itself or the immunologic reaction to the antigen. In the first instance, one can postulate a mechanism whereby the adjuvant increases the release of antigen. Non-specific immunotherapy directed toward the reaction to the antigen has focused on the cellular response. Later studies suggest, however, at least two cellular cytotoxic mechanisms. One involves thymus-processed cytotoxic cells (T cells), which recognize target antigens. The other is controlled by a thymus-independent effector cell system, which is independent of the target antigen; this system is triggered to kill by recognition of antibody bound to the target, and it refutes our previously held simplistic view that stimulation of the cellular mechanism is beneficial whereas humoral immunity is of no aid.

In the past, the most widely used non-specific immunotherapy has employed adjuvants such as BCG, *C. parvum*, levamisole, and MER. BCG is a live, attenuated strain of *Mycobacterium bovis*. *C. parvum* is a Gram-negative anaerobe given in a non-viable form. Levamisole is a synthetic anthelmintic drug that has been found to have significant effects on tumor immunity. MER is a methanol extraction of killed tuberculin bacilli (BCG).

The era of experimentation with bacterial products began in 1959, when Old and colleagues demonstrated that injection of BCG was capable of inhibiting growth of tumors in mice. BCG had been introduced into clinical medicine in 1921 with its use as a vaccine against tuberculosis. Since 1921, many effects of BCG stimulating non-specific immune responses in animals and humans have been demonstrated. Both humoral antibody synthesis and cell-mediated immunity are stimulated by BCG treatment. Mice injected with BCG show an increased resistance to infection with bacteria and are capable of clearing endotoxin and injected carbon particles much more rapidly than untreated mice are. BCG injection leads to activation of macrophages as manifested by enhanced phagocytosis, increased microbicidal activity, increased macrophage metabolism, and increased ability of macrophages to kill tumor cell monolayer cultures. The most dramatic work with BCG was that of Rapp and coworkers with transplantable hepatoma in guinea pigs. They demonstrated that injection of BCG in growing intradermal tumor nodules was capable of eliminating the local nodule and eradicating tumor cells in draining lymph nodes. The dramatic response seen with guinea pig hepatoma may be caused by cross-reactive antigens between BCG and this animal tumor. Recent evidence has shown that BCG may cross-react with antigens on human melanoma cells. In humans, BCG has been used primarily in three ways:

1. intralesional injection;
2. systemic administration, generally by scarification or intradermal injection; and
3. mixed with cells and administered as a vaccine.

Intralesional use of BCG has largely been confined to treatment of cutaneous recurrences of malignant melanoma. In one series, approximately 90% of >700 intracutaneously injected lesions in 36 patients were made to undergo complete regression by BCG injection. Subcutaneous and visceral deposits of melanoma, however, are far more resistant to BCG treatment. Uninjected nodules surrounding the injected lesion that also undergo regression are always in the drainage area of the injected nodule. It appears that direct contact between BCG and the tumor is essential for the therapeutic effect.

BCG administered intradermally by direct injection or by scarification techniques has been used in patients who have leukemia or one of a variety of solid tumors. Most of the evidence for antitumor activity of BCG used systemically is derived from experiments involving pretreatment of animals. As immunotherapy in the treatment of established experimental tumors, it is remarkably ineffective.

C. parvum, like BCG, belongs to a group of bacterial agents that have stimulatory effects on the reticuloendothelial system, increase the phagocytic capacity of macrophages, and increase the resistance of animals to both infections and subsequent implantation or induction of experimental tumors. *C. parvum* is also active by direct intralesional injection. In animal systems, *C. parvum* given intravenously can induce regression of established local and pulmonary metastasis. *C. parvum* was originally administered subcutaneously in combination with chemotherapy, and several trials now under way are using this immunopotentiator intravenously. When used intravenously, the drug produces high fever and shaking chills, and some patients have experienced thrombotic thrombocytopenic purpura. Some investigators have suggested that its action may be to cause release of TNF. Unlike BCG, *C. parvum* seems to act primarily by stimulating macrophage function; its effect on T cell immunity is less clear. Trials have been conducted in solid tumor therapy without notable success.

A second group of substances includes various synthetic compounds that are believed to be immunostimulants (e.g., levamisole, cimetidine, and others). These substances have demonstrated some effects on the immune system, including increases in delayed-type hypersensitivity response, total number of T cells, increased lymphocyte proliferation, and mitogenic response. Firm evidence that these changes in immune parameters translate to improved tumor control is not available.

Levamisole has been studied in animal systems, in which it has been shown to potentiate the antibody and delayed hypersensitivity responses to a variety of antigens. It appears that levamisole can potentiate or permit expression of established delayed-type hypersensitivity reactions in previously immunocompetent individuals. One mechanism of levamisole action may be to cause maturation of thymus-derived immature lymphocyte precursors. It has been termed an immunomodulator by some in that it seems to reconstitute immunologic competence in patients who are immunosuppressed. Administration of levamisole before or concurrently with a bacterial adjuvant may augment the activity of the bacterial adjuvant.

MER is the methanol extraction residue of BCG and was devised to overcome the problems associated with viable BCG preparations, including systemic BCG infection. This material, which is supplied as a particulate aqueous suspension, has shown both immunoprophylactic and immunotherapeutic activity comparable to that of BCG in a variety of animal models. It is administered intradermally or subcutaneously to humans. It produces severe local reactions characterized by inflammatory ulceration or sterile abscess formation. MER appears to be more immunopotentiating than BCG in humans and can restore established delayed hypersensitivity in approximately 20% of patients with widely metastatic solid tumors. A number of clinical trials with MER have been completed with little success.

A third class of drugs includes chemotherapeutic agents such as cyclophosphamide, doxorubicin, and others. These agents are presumed to work by inhibiting suppressor mechanisms.

Active non-specific immune mechanisms can also be evoked by a variety of natural and recombinant cytokines. The three major species of interferons (IFN-α, IFN-β, and IFN-γ) have in vitro and in vivo antitumor effects. IL-2 is a glycoprotein acting to cause T cell proliferation after an initial antigen recognition and presentation. Another directly cytotoxic or cytostatic cytokine is TNF.

Specific

Tumor immunotherapy has been under study with extensive clinical trials, but less has been attempted with specific immunotherapy compared with non-specific modes. Specific immunotherapy can be active, passive, or adoptive. Active specific immunotherapy calls for administration to the cancer patient of tumor cells (vaccines) or their equivalent, bearing antigens that will cross-react with the neoplasm. Tumor antigens are usually weakly antigenic, so that immunostimulants (e.g., BCG) are often administered jointly. Other ways to heighten the immunogenicity of the tumor cells have been studied, such as surface changes by enzymes, viral incorporation, physical treatments, and chemical modifications. Although this remains an exciting field for future research, trials to date in humans have been disappointing.

Several cancer vaccines are under development, and some of these have reached the point of clinical trials. Various approaches include:

1. use of synthetic peptides representing the immunoglobulin epitope of B cell malignant neoplasms;
2. fusion of cancer cells with activated B lymphocytes to increase cytotoxic T lymphocyte recognition of tumor cells; and
3. injections of gene complexes into tumor cell nuclei, which render the transformed cells capable of secreting large amounts of cytokine into the surrounding area.

Therapeutic vaccines for cervical cancer are a method of attacking already established HPV infections and HPV-related malignant lesions. E6 and E7 proteins represent good targets for developing antigen-specific immunotherapies or therapeutic vaccines for cervical cancer. Cellular immune response is the key component necessary for clearance of the HPV infection and is the main target of such a therapeutic vaccine. Whether attacking the HPV virus after the cancer is already established will result in improved outcomes is yet to be demonstrated.

Some studies suggest that antibodies to murine monoclonal antitumor antibodies (so-called anti-idiotypes) might resemble antigen and evoke a specific host antitumor response. Other modifications of the tumor cell to potentially increase antigenicity involve chemical treatment of the cell surface, including stripping off sialic acid residues. All these approaches have yet to demonstrate effectiveness in humans.

Passive adoptive immunotherapy (Table 19–7)

The use of immunologic reagents such as monoclonal antibodies or the adoptive transfer of cells to mediate direct antitumor response (without requiring a host response) has been a subject of much study. The earliest studies used heterologous sera obtained from immunized humans or animals. These did not have convincing efficacy and have largely been abandoned. The development of monoclonal antibodies allowed the evolution of potentially powerful new serologic reagents for the diagnosis and treatment of patients with cancer. The development of the lymphokine IL-2 made possible the in vitro propagation of T lymphocytes taken from the peripheral blood or directly from tumors, which allowed their use in human therapeutic protocols. The demonstration that IL-2 could also induce a subset of normal lymphoid cells to lyse tumor, a phenomenon we have called lymphokine-activated killing, has also been exploited in immunotherapy trials.

Table 19–7 PASSIVE ADOPTIVE IMMUNOTHERAPY

Non-specific
LAK cells: generated by IL-2
Activated macrophages: interferon
Cytostatic or cytotoxic cytokines: interferon and tumor necrosis factor

Specific
Heterologous antiserum from an immunized human
Monoclonal antibodies: murine or human
Radiotherapeutic: coupled to α- or β-emitting radionuclides
Chemotherapeutic: doxorubicin (Adriamycin), methotrexate, or ricin conjugates
Biologic: complement fixation or antibody-dependent and cellular cytotoxic mechanisms
T lymphocytes: autologous, allogeneic, or xenogeneic from in vitro sensitization or tumor-draining lymph nodes
Allogeneic bone marrow transplants with ablative chemotherapy or radiation therapy (graft vs tumor)

Non-specific

Non-specific immunotherapies include the use of LAK cells, activated macrophages, and directly cytotoxic or cytostatic cytokines such as interferon (IFN-α, IFN-β, and IFN-γ) and TNF.

In the mid-1980s, passive immunotherapy with sensitized cells, referred to as adoptive immunotherapy, received a resurgence of interest because of the work of Steven Rosenberg using activated lymphocytes. Leukapheresis machines were used to remove circulating lymphocytes from patients. These lymphocytes were then treated with a lymphokine called IL-2. This converted the lymphocytes into LAK cells that were capable of destroying cancer cells but not normal cells. These LAK cells were infused along with IL-2 back into the patient. The IL-2 induced the LAK cells to multiply for a short time in the body, thus enhancing their ability to destroy cancer cells. The development of the genetically engineered or recombinant form of IL-2 in 1984 made available to scientists a large amount of this substance, which was necessary for treating patients in clinical trials. Rosenberg noted that the adoptive transfer of LAK cells plus additional IL-2 administration was capable of mediating regression of established pulmonary and hepatic metastasis in a variety of human neoplasms. The dose-limiting toxicity for IL-2 was noted at 100,000 U/kg by intravenous bolus every 8 hours, and that toxicity consisted primarily of capillary permeability leak, which can lead to intravascular fluid leakage into subcutaneous tissue. In October 1987, Rosenberg described 104 patients treated in this manner. A total of seven com-

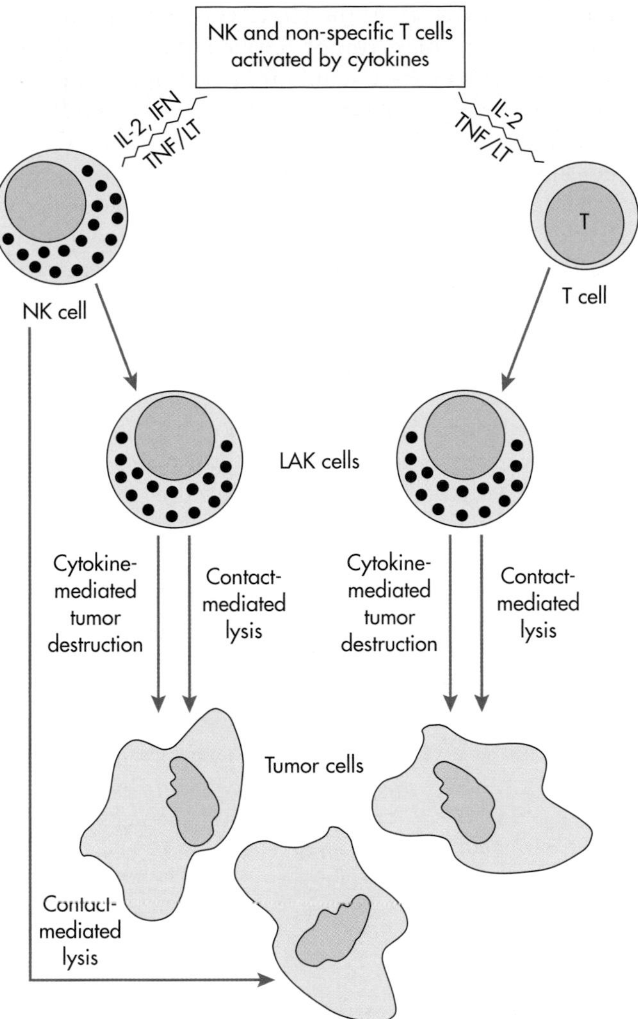

Figure 19–13 Role of the NK and LAK cells in the immune response to malignant disease. Natural killer (NK) cells are the first line of defense against growth of transformed cells. Lymphokine-activated killer (LAK) cells are IL-2 dependent and are non-genetically restricted killer cells.

plete regressions were noted in patients who had renal cell carcinoma, melanoma, colorectal cancer, or non-Hodgkin's lymphoma in an advanced state. The longest response was 36 months in a patient with widespread melanoma who received a single treatment. The mechanism by which adoptive transfer of LAK cells in conjunction with IL-2 (Fig. 19–13) is effective in humans is as yet unclear, and the role of IL-2 and the LAK cell remains to be defined. Murine studies suggest that IL-2 leads to the general proliferation of LAK cells in vivo when it is given alone and that responsiveness is in part dictated by the immunogenicity of the tumor. Refinement of the technique for improved effectiveness was pursued because of unacceptable toxicity among patient recipients.

In 1987, West and colleagues reported another series of adoptive immunotherapy involving constant infusion rather than bolus-dose recombinant IL-2 as well as LAK cells in 40 patients. There were 13 partial responses in a variety of neoplasms. The authors concluded that administration of IL-2 by constant infusion rather than by bolus dose was less toxic.

Studies of tumor-infiltrating lymphocytes (TILs) in mice suggested to Rosenberg and associates that other populations of IL-2-stimulated cytotoxic cells might provide more effective antitumor activity than LAK cells. Both human and murine tumors are known to be infiltrated by a variety of host immune cells, including significant numbers of T cells or TILs. Because tumor growth occurs despite the presence of these cells, freshly extracted TILs would not be expected to have significant antitumor activity. A method for activating and expanding these cells was required, and again IL-2 proved to be crucial. Initial experience with murine TIL therapy revealed two significant remaining limitations of adapting this therapy to protocols for patients. TILs could not be generated from nonimmunogenic tumors and were not effective against large, advanced tumor burdens in mice. Subsequent modifications of the techniques for TIL culture, as well as adjuvant therapies directed at the TIL recipient, have partially addressed these limitations. In a search for sources of lymphocytes with antitumor activity in the tumor-bearing hosts, a second site outside the tumor itself was found where T cells demonstrated this activity. Within the lymph nodes that drain the tumor site are lymphocytes with many features similar to TILs. These lymphocytes have the opportunity to be tumor sensitized, and with the proper stimulation and expansion in culture, they can be shown to have activity against established murine tumors.

The concept of generating and augmenting antitumor activity in an immune cell population, expanding these cells in vitro, and readministering them in the treatment of cancer has considerable appeal. Evidence to suggest that this can be done effectively has existed in preclinical animal systems for some time. More recently, preliminary data suggest that it can be applied successfully to the treatment of some human tumors. Models demonstrating the effectiveness of LAK cells, TILs, and tumor-draining lymph node lymphocytes have provided the technology to obtain cells for some early trials. Areas for research are related to the survival and localization of adoptively transferred cells in the tumor-bearing host and the precise mechanism and effectors of tumor regression. Ongoing investigation should be watched carefully, but the data to date suggest that this costly approach may be associated with morbidity that far outweighs the limited success.

Specific

An example of passive specific immunotherapy would be producing antisera to a patient's cancer in an animal (a great deal of absorption of foreign antigens would be necessary before use) or in another patient with cancer and then injecting the antisera into the patient. Passive transfer of antibodies has been attempted with no significant results. With further knowledge of the precarious role of antibodies, much less enthusiasm has been noted, except in the area of deblocking antibodies.

Monoclonal antibodies are produced by hybridoma techniques. This involves immunizing an animal with antigen and fusing its spleen cells with a long-lived malignant B cell line (Fig. 19–14). Subsequently, antibodies produced by the fused, normal, and malignant B cells are selected for their ability to recognize an antigen of interest. To tumor cells, this would represent a tumor differentiation antigen or a tumor-associated antigen. The advantage of this approach is that large quantities of antibodies, specific only for antigens on tumors and not antigens present on normal cells, can be produced. Similar strategies have been used in humans to produce human monoclonal antibodies from human splenocytes but with much less success.

Most currently available monoclonal antibodies come from murine sources. However, recombinant biologic techniques have also been applied to obtain monoclonal antibodies, and this technology should be helpful in promoting the development of human products. The potential use of monoclonal antibodies that recognize tumor-associated antigens is far-reaching. Whereas monoclonal antibodies directed against tumor cell surface determinants can inhibit tumor cell proliferation in culture and in animals, direct administration to patients has found limited success to date. Monoclonal antibodies could be of benefit in clearing tumor cells from the blood and in diminishing the amount of circulating tumor antigen that could have a blocking effect on subsequent immunotherapy. Monoclonal antibodies can also be attached to antitumor drugs, toxins, or radionuclides; the rationale of this approach is to target toxic substances directly to the tumor cells and spare normal cells, and it has been piloted with some success. Antibody directed against cytokines that may produce undesirable effects in certain clinical situations may provide a useful immunotherapeutic tool. For instance, passively administered antibody specific for TNF-α may be beneficial in reducing mortality associated with septic shock of infectious origin. Monoclonal antibody directed against receptor for IL-2 to T lymphocytes has been effective in preventing rejection of renal transplants.

OvaRex (MAb B43.13), an immune anti-CA-125 MAb, was radiolabeled with ^{99m}To for detection of recurrent ovarian epithelial cancer. The therapeutic potential was serendipitously discovered when a retrospective study noted that patients who received radiolabeled MAb B43.13 for immunoscintigraphy exhibited unexpected prolonged survivals. Possibly the antibody binds to circulating CA-125 antigens to form complexes that are recognized as non-self because they contain a foreign antigen.

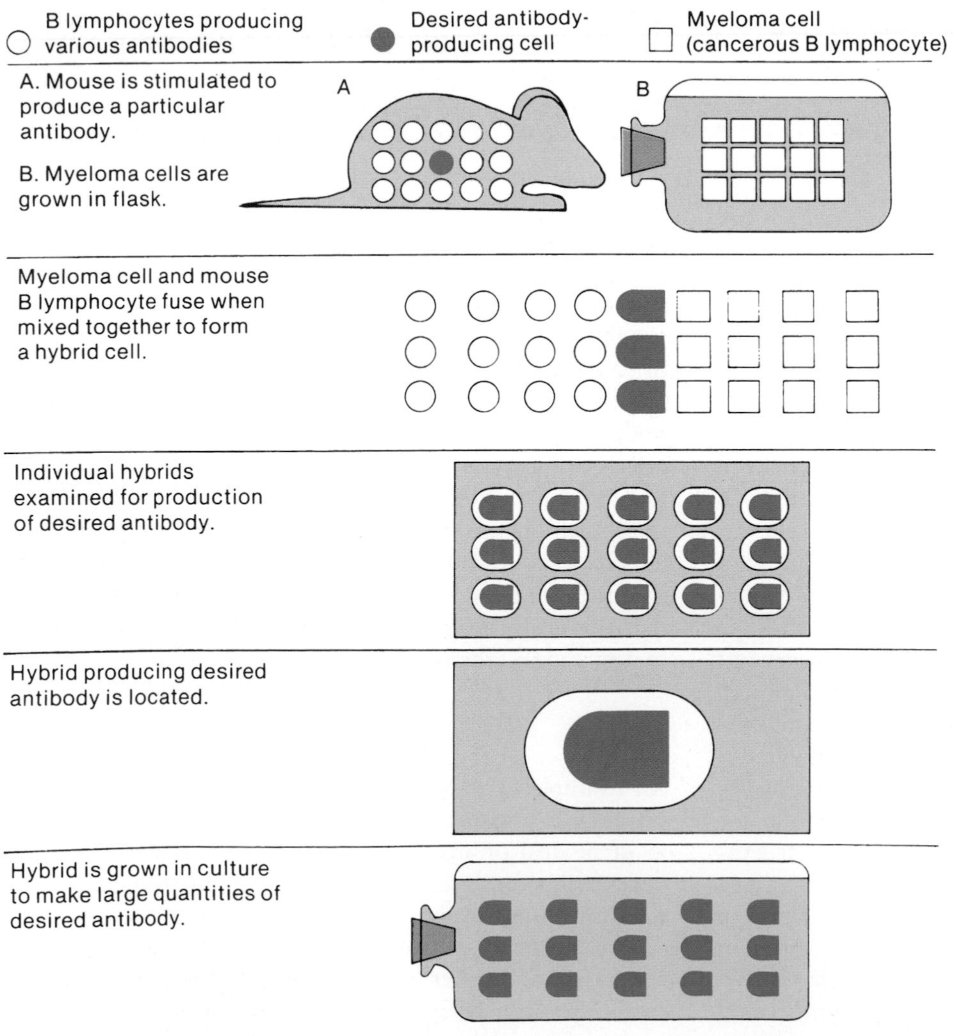

Figure 19–14 Hybridoma technique for production of monoclonal antibodies

A long-term follow-up study of 49 of the 218 patients who received injections of MAb B43.13 demonstrated notable periods of disease stabilization and showed anti-CA-125 antibody levels and some T-cell responses that correlated with the clinical impact of treatment.

One of the first randomized double-blind, placebo-controlled studies of MAb B43.13 for adjuvant consolidation in epithelial ovarian cancer was reported by Bookman. In this study, 55 patients who had no clinical evidence of disease after first-line chemotherapy, but had a CA-125 elevation, were randomized to receive MAb B43.13 or placebo. There was a trend of improved survival in the treatment group. Additional studies of OvaRex are underway and/or await analysis.

Table 19–8 TUMOR IMMUNODIAGNOSIS: DETECTION OF TUMOR CELLS AND THEIR PRODUCTS
α-Fetoprotein (e.g., liver cancer, tumor of the germ cell ovary)
Human chorionic gonadotropin (e.g., malignant trophoblastic disease)
Myeloma and Bence Jones proteins
Prostate-specific antigen
Carcinoembryonic antigen
Detection of tumor-associated antigens in other malignant neoplasms

IMMUNODIAGNOSIS

Immunodiagnosis is a field of investigative medicine largely based on the science of radioimmunoassay. Substances that are antigenic in animals or that can be bound to antigens can be measured in body fluids in low concentrations. Tumor immunodiagnosis depends on the liberation by tumors of such substances into the bloodstream or other body fluids in a form or concentration not commonly found in healthy individuals. These substances, usually called tumor markers, are sometimes referred to as antigens, although they may not necessarily produce an immune response in the tumor-bearing host. Other substances may actually play a role in immunodiagnosis, such as hormones or the pregnancy-associated proteins. Tumor-associated antigens and oncofetal antigens have been the major interest of tumor immunologists. In humans, evidence for the liberation of specific neoantigens is scanty; in ovarian cancer, early claims of the specificity of tumor extract antigenicity by Levi and by Barlow and Bhattacharya have awaited confirmation. Tumor-associated antigens have been roughly identified and characterized by Gall, Walling, and Pearl and by DiSaia. However, these antigens appear to have a unique ability to camouflage themselves among the normal proteins of the cell, defying attempts at refined isolation. Because the foundation of modern immunodiagnosis is the radioimmunoassay, one must have an absolutely pure antigen to begin the process that will lead to a clinically useful tool.

Secreted products released into the bloodstream provide the best diagnostic markers to date (Table 19–8). The most useful of these are myeloma proteins produced by plasma cell myelomas, AFP produced by hepatocellular carcinomas and teratocarcinoma containing yolk sac elements, and CEA produced by tumors of the gastrointestinal tract. Human chorionic gonadotropin is another example of an excellent tumor marker for gestational trophoblastic disease.

Monoclonal antibodies with use of the hybridoma technique (see Fig. 19–14) are being employed by investigators in many scientific disciplines and have led to a revolution in diagnostic immunology. With respect to cancer immunodiagnosis, monoclonal antibodies have aided in the recognition and identification of tumor-associated antigens (differentiation antigens and other marker molecules) with heretofore unobtainable specificity. Such antigenic determinants have been described on or in tumor cells from patients with leukemia and malignant lymphoma as well as a variety of solid tumors including melanoma and carcinomas of the lung, breast, prostate, and gastrointestinal tract. In addition to their role in detection, monoclonal agents can be used as immunoadsorbents to purify and characterize tumor-associated antigens. Although truly "tumor-specific" antigens do not appear to exist, the exquisite resolving power of monoclonal antibodies provides a means to detect antigens present on tumor cells that are not commonly found on normal adult tissue cells. These antigenic differences can conceivably be exploited in several ways relating to the diagnosis and staging of cancer and the treatment of patients. Circulating antigens secreted or shed by tumor cells can be detected by monoclonal antibodies employed as serologic reagents. Detection of circulating tumor antigen in this way would be helpful both in initial diagnosis and in serial monitoring of the results of therapy. Monoclonal antibodies to tumor and to normal tissue antigens appear valuable as immunohistologic reagents for the analysis of lymphoid infiltrates in lymph nodes, improved taxonomy of lymphomas and leukemias, and primary identification of undifferentiated carcinomas or adenocarcinomas of an unknown origin. These examples illustrate how monoclonal antibodies seem certain to lead to earlier diagnosis and more accurate classification of malignant neoplasms.

With regard to staging, monoclonal antibodies directed to tumor antigens or markers also offer a promising approach. Photoscanning after injection of radiolabeled monoclonal antibodies can be used to identify sites of tumor involvement that might otherwise go unrecognized. This reduces the likelihood of understaging disease and administering inadequate therapy. Although several problems remain, studies in animals and preliminary data in patients suggest that staging with radiolabeled monoclonal antibodies is likely to become available for clinical use in the near future.

BIOLOGIC RESPONSE MODIFIERS

Biologic response modifiers (BRMs) are the many agents and approaches to the treatment of cancer with a mechanism of action that involves modulation of the individual's own biologic responses. BRMs are molecules produced by the body to regulate cellular response. Activation of host responses, particularly the host immune response, has been the ideal of therapists for many generations, but technologic advances have improved our understanding and made manipulation of biologic responses a practical goal in therapy. Because of these advantages, biologic response-modifying therapy is now a reality, and BRMs are likely to be valuable in increasing our understanding of cancer biology and improving cancer therapeutics in this decade. Indeed, the Biological Response Modifiers Program was a comprehensive program of the Division of Cancer Treatment, National Cancer Institute, intended to investigate, develop, and bring to clinical trials potentially therapeutic agents that may alter biologic responses important in cancer growth and metastasis.

Cytokines (See Table 19–2)

The term *cytokines* defines a large group of secreted polypeptides released by living cells that act non-enzymatically to regulate cellular functions. These cellular functions include regulation of immune cell activity (interferons and interleukins), hematopoiesis (colony-stimulating factor), and regulation of proliferation and differentiation (e.g., transforming growth factor-α, epidermal growth factor). This chapter discusses only those that affect the immune system because cytokines play a crucial role in the amplification of the immune response.

Lymphokines and other cytokines have a specific ability to regulate certain components of the immune response, which may be useful in altering the growth of cancer in humans. There are early indications of a specific ability of these substances to alter immune responses in ways that may be beneficial in the host-tumor interaction. For example, it is possible that certain cytokines or lymphokines may augment the ability of T cells to respond to tumor-associated antigens, and others may induce higher responsiveness with respect to B cell activity in patients with cancer. Lymphokines also decrease suppressive functions of the immune system and may be useful in enhancing immune responses by lessening the suppressive effects of suppressive factors or suppressive cells in cancer patients. Another specific use of lymphokines may be in the pharmacologic regulation of tumors of the lymphoid system. Although many of these malignant tissues are considered to be unresponsive to normal growth-controlling mechanisms mediated by lymphokines, it is possible that the large quantities of pure lymphokines, administered pharmacologically, or certain molecular analogues of these naturally occurring lymphokines may be useful in the treatment of lymphoid malignant neoplasms. A further use of lymphokines may be the manipulation of the immune response in vitro to produce products that may subsequently be used therapeutically in vivo.

IL-1α or IL-1β activates resting T cells and makes early hematopoietic progenitors more sensitive to other factors. It also stimulates the synthesis of other cytokines, including possibly IL-2. IL-2 is also known as T cell growth factor. Pharmacologic doses of these lymphokines can conceivably be used to alter the maturation and kinetic capabilities of various T cell malignant neoplasms. Cloning of IL-1 and IL-2 has made large quantities of highly purified materials available for clinical trials. Some of these trials with LAK cells are discussed in the section on specific immunotherapy.

Interferons

The interferons are a family of glycoproteins produced by several different cell types. Type 1 interferons, IFN-α and IFN-β, which are produced, respectively, by induced leukocytes and fibroblasts, show about 30% homology of amino acids. Type 2 interferon, IFN-γ, which is produced by lymphocytes and monocytes in response to antigenic or mitogenic stimulation, differs significantly in amino acid composition. The interferons were thought at first to have only antiviral activity, but multiple other functions (previously postulated to have been related to impurities in the preparations) have been documented. Further documentation of these multiple functions as definite interferon effects is now possible because highly purified products have become available to study in clinical use. In addition to antiviral activity, the interferons have profound effects on the immune system. Relatively low doses enhance antibody formation and lymphocyte blastogenesis, whereas higher doses inhibit both of these functions. Moderate to high doses may inhibit delayed hypersensitivity while enhancing macrophage phagocytosis and cytotoxicity, sensitized lymphocyte cytotoxicity, NK activity, and surface antigenic expression. Interferons also prolong and inhibit cell division, having this effect on almost every cell system studied, whether transformed or not. Interferons also stimulate the induction of several intracellular enzyme systems, with resultant profound effects on macromolecular activities and protein synthesis.

Antitumor effects of interferon were first demonstrated in tumors considered to be induced by oncogenic viruses. Late appearance of tumors and increased animal survival have been reported with many animal tumors induced by viruses. The antitumor immune-modulating effect of interferon in vivo and the relatively low host toxicity have led to a number of clinical trials. The greatest therapeutic usefulness of interferon has been in hairy cell leukemia, a rare form of leukemia. Early trials used IFN-α purified from human leukocytes and later obtained by recombinant DNA techniques. Various recombinant forms of interferon are now in clinical trials for various malignant neoplasms.

Cytokine therapy in gynecologic tumors has been studied most extensively with IFN-8. Although the exact mode of action of IFN in patients with ovarian cancer is unknown, many mechanisms have been suggested:

1. stimulation of NK cells and macrophages;
2. through anti-angiogenic effects; and
3. inhibition of expression of oncogenes (such as HER-2/neu) and thereby improving responsiveness to cells to therapy.

In vitro studies have suggested that IFN can increase the sensitivity of tumor cells to cytotoxic drugs such as cisplatin. Several Phase II studies of IFN with cisplatin in ovarian cancer have demonstrated a trend toward improved survival, but clinical trials have not been consistently positive in ovarian cancer. A comparison of intraperitoneal (IP) carboplatin with or without IFN-8 in 111 patients with advanced ovarian cancer and minimal residual disease did not demonstrate benefit in the combination arm. Further investigations are needed.

In cervical cancer, IFN-8 alone appears to have little activity. In a multi-institutional Phase II clinical trial only a 10% response rate was achieved with INF-8 alone. The combination of IFN-8 and cisplatin plus 5-FU in patients with recurrent cervical cancer resulted in a 30% response rate. Future studies may test whether addition of IFN-8 and/or retinoic acid will provide additional benefit.

In conclusion, IP IFN appears to be well tolerated and may produce significant clinical responses in ovarian cancer patients with minimal residual disease. In advanced ovarian cancer, the combination of IFN with cytotoxic agents often adds toxicity without significant anti-tumor activity.

Interleukins

Cytokines produced by one type of leukocyte that affect other leukocytes are referred to as interleukins. The interleukins belong to a family of polypeptide growth and differentiation factors called lymphokines. These are factors, produced by lymphocytes or macrophages, that stimulate the proliferation, differentiation, and function of T lymphocytes, B lymphocytes, and certain other cells involved in the immune response (see Table 19–2). Initially discovered as soluble factors present in the growth medium of cultured lymphocytes, these substances now have several identified activities. They are usually defined by their role in stimulating an in vitro immune reaction, such as promoting the activation or proliferation of immune system cells. However, it has become clear that several of the activities previously described could be attributed to two distinct polypeptides. One of these polypeptides is IL-1, and the other is IL-2.

The term *interleukin* was chosen because it indicates the basic property of these secreted mediators to serve as intercellular signals between leukocytes. Several additional interleukins have now been identified (see Table 19–2); IL-1, IL-2, IL-3, and IL-4 have been introduced into clinical trials for various malignant diseases. IL-2 has been used in adoptive immunotherapy to stimulate clonal expansion of LAK cells and TILs. IL-3 has been used to stimulate bone marrow recovery in bone marrow or peripheral stem cell transplantation. IL-4 has been introduced as an immune system stimulator in various cancer treatment regimens. Macrophages produce IL-1 when the T cell antigen receptor interacts with antigen-MHC class II complexes on the macrophage surface. The IL-1 molecule released by the macrophage induces the T lymphocyte to express a cell surface receptor for IL-2. These events lead to the synthesis of IL-2, a growth factor produced by T cells that drives the proliferation of T cells bearing IL-2 receptors, resulting in clonal expansion of the responding T cells. In addition to the IL-2 receptor, activated T cells express other cell surface markers not found on resting T cells, including class II MHC molecules, transferrin receptors, and several antigens restricted to activated T cells. After activation, T cells of the helper-inducer subset produce a large number of mediators in addition to IL-2.

IL-2 based therapy may occasionally produce significantly long-term remissions in ovarian cancer patients. The treatment, however, can be associated with considerable toxicity. Approaches to minimize toxicity and increase efficacy are under investigation. The combination of low doses of cisplatin with IL-2 appears to be the most promising for future trials.

Tumor necrosis factor

A unique pair of cytokines produced by activated monocytes and lymphocytes are the agents referred to as TNF-α and TNF-β. These substances were originally identified by their capacity to induce hemorrhagic necrosis and regression in a mouse tumor model in vivo and by their cytotoxic-cytostatic activity against mouse L cell in vitro. There are two closely related molecules with tumor necrosis factor activity: TNF-α (a monokine) and TNF-β (a lymphotoxin), a product of activated lymphocytes. The two molecules, which are structurally related and share about 30% amino acid sequence homology, compete for the same cellular receptors. Both are now being produced by recombinant DNA technology. Only the TNF that is a monokine is currently being evaluated in the clinic. Nonetheless, it seems worthwhile to develop both species of TNF because the two molecules may have different antitumor spectra despite the fact that they share a number of functional attributes.

Because TNFs are products of normal cells, they are capable of pleiotropic biologic activities, including cytotoxic-cytostatic activity against tumor cells, immunomodulatory functions, interactions with other BRMs, and modulation of gene expression. TNFs can destroy tumor cells in vitro in the absence of cells of the immune system. Several lines of evidence suggest that TNFs may modulate cell-mediated immune defenses against tumors. TNFs can activate and enhance neutrophil and eosinophil functions and can augment expression of class I and class II histocompatibility antigens. Binding of TNF molecules to specific high-affinity receptors is an initial event in the action of TNFs, and cells that do not possess these receptors appear to be resistant to TNFs. Cytotoxic-cytostatic activity has been documented in a broad spectrum of mouse and human tumor cells in vitro. Hemorrhagic necrosis and regression have been achieved in a comparable spectrum of mouse tumors growing in syngeneic mice and in human tumors growing in the xenogeneic nude mouse model. Responsive tumor cell lines have included melanoma, colon cancer, breast cancer, cervical cancer, ovarian cancer, lung cancer, and astrocytoma. However, there is considerable heterogeneity of response within any given tumor type. Responsiveness to TNFs does not depend on tumor type or on any potentially prognostic factor.

Clinical toxicities of recombinant TNF are similar to those of recombinant interferons—primarily fever, chills, headaches, and other constitutional symptoms. A dose-dependent, reversible, local inflammatory response is not uncommon. Hypotension may occur occasionally but can be managed with intravenous hydration. Neurologic symptoms such as confusion may develop in rare cases. Myelosuppression may occur, but this is dose-dependent and reversible. These data suggest a tolerance for TNFs used in combination with myelosuppressive chemotherapy. A few patients will require transfusion for anemia, but this does not present a major clinical problem. To date, the clinical usefulness of TNF has been limited because the systemic toxicity observed after intravenous infusion limits its utility. Efforts are being made to deliver TNF directly to the tumor, which should lower toxicity.

Retinoids

Vitamin A has a number of important functions in the body. Among others, it is apparently essential for the integrity of epithelial cells. The functional and structural integrity of epithelial cells throughout the body depends on an adequate supply of vitamin A. This vitamin plays a major role in the induction of control in epithelial differentiation in mucus-secreting or keratinizing tissue. In the presence of retinol, basal epithelial cells are stimulated to produce mucus. Excessive retinol will lead to the production of a thick layer of mucin with an array of goblet cells and inhibition of keratinization. In the absence of retinol, atrophy of the epithelium is followed by a proliferation of basal cells with an increase of mucous cells. It has been established that epithelial systems need vitamin A for display of proper morphologic features and function. In vitro studies support the concept that vitamin A is directly involved in maintaining normal phenotypic expression. This concept, therefore, puts vitamin A in a special position among nutrients if one considers that most solid tumors arise from epithelial tissues.

Studies on the protective effect of vitamin A against the development of epithelial tumors have been conducted for many years. Numerous studies have been done, and in general, vitamin A either fed to the animal in its diet or applied locally appeared to have a protective and therapeutic effect on chemically produced tumors. One derivative of vitamin A, retinoic acid, has been studied most for human epithelial malignant neoplasms. Topically applied retinoic acid has been successful in certain dermatologic disorders, such as actinic keratosis, a precancerous condition, and basal cell carcinomas. Studies suggesting activity have also been done with urinary bladder papillomas and intraepithelial neoplasia of the cervix. These substances show great promise for treatment of the increasing numbers of patients who have intraepithelial neoplasia of the cervix. Vesanoid (all-*trans*-retinoic acid) is a newly approved drug that is thought to act by inducing cell differentiation and thus cell death. A related drug, 9-*cis*-retinoic acid, appears to have receptor-binding properties different from those of all-*trans*-retinoic acid and may have different biologic characteristics, which may prevent the development of resistance seen with all-*trans*-retinoic acid.

Antiangiogenesis agents

Researchers are anxiously investigating a new class of antiangiogenesis agents. Thalidomide, an old discarded drug, has been shown to prevent formation of new blood vessels in animal models. Clinical trials in humans are under way. Other antiangiogenesis agents, including angiostatin, endostatin, and matrix metalloproteinase inhibitors, are also planned for testing.

Angiogenesis is a rate-limiting step in the growth of tumors and in the development of metastases. Tumor invasion is limited by nutrient requirements; thus, vascularization is a very important step in tumor progression. A tumor mass larger than 0.125 mm^2 has outgrown the capacity to acquire nutrients by simple diffusion. Further expansion of the tumor mass requires host vessels to initiate capillary buds in the direction of the tumor.

Vascular endothelial growth factor (VEGF) has been purified from ovarian cancer xenograft ascites. VEGF induces capillary tube formation, causes increased vascular permeability and protein extravasation, stimulates endothelial cell migration and stimulates a strong endothelial-cell survival signal. Bevacizumab is a recombinant humanized version of the murine anti-human VEGF monoclonal antibody. Phase II studies have shown good tolerance as a single agent or in combination with chemotherapy. The GOG Phase II study showed considerable activity of this antibody and, therefore, a Phase III trial has been launched of standard first-line chemotherapy (carboplatin and paclitaxel [Taxol]) plus and minus bevacizumab in patients with advanced ovarian cancer.

In summary, BRM therapy and the use of various biologic products of the human genome in the clinical setting are now realities. We can expect to see the induction of partial responses and, ultimately, the induction of complete responses in patients with malignant disease that will lead to a new era in treatment. The use of these agents will become the fourth modality of cancer therapy, acting effectively and independently in patients with clinically perceptible disease but perhaps acting optimally in the minimal disease setting, especially in combination with existing treatment modalities.

ADDITIONAL IMMUNOTHERAPY TRIALS

Non-specific immunotherapy implies the stimulation of the reticuloendothelial system by injection of various substances not related to the malignant neoplasm under therapy. BCG, MER, and *C. parvum* have been used as non-specific reticuloendothelial stimulants. Various trials using non-specific immunotherapy in gynecologic malignant neoplasms have been conducted with mainly negative results. Olkowski and associates reported on the effects of combined immunotherapy with levamisole and BCG on immunocompetence of patients with squamous cell carcinoma of the cervix. Immunologic tests were performed before and immediately after a full course of radiotherapy in 25 patients with squamous cell carcinoma of the cervix, stage Ib through stage III. The patients were randomized to immunotherapy with oral levamisole and intradermal BCG or no immunotherapy. Lymphocyte responses to phytohemagglutinin and pokeweed mitogen were subnormal before radiotherapy and declined still further after radiotherapy. Both treatment groups showed a gradual recovery from immunosuppression (T and B lymphocyte counts and mitogenic responses) during follow-up, but the immunotherapy group showed a tendency (not significant in the preliminary data) toward slower recovery. Lymphocyte cytotoxicity to allogeneic tumor cells was variably affected by radiotherapy but was generally higher 8 weeks after radiotherapy than in preceding tests.

DiSaia reported the results of a Gynecologic Oncology Group (GOG) study on the treatment of women with advanced carcinoma of the uterine cervix with radiotherapy alone vs radiotherapy plus immunotherapy with intravenous *C. parvum*. At the time of analysis, 167 patients in the preliminary report and 295 patients in the final unpublished study were considered assessable. The conclusion reached was that *C. parvum* did not add any therapeutic effect as an adjuvant to radiotherapy in the study population of patients.

Alberts has an exciting report in the literature concerning non-specific immunotherapy of ovarian carcinoma. He studied the effect of adding BCG to doxorubicin (Adriamycin) and cyclophosphamide (AC) for the treatment of stage III and stage IV or recurrent epithelial ovarian carcinoma. In his study, 131 patients with no prior chemotherapy and measurable disease were randomly assigned to receive AC or AC and BCG. Doxorubicin, 40 mg/m^2 on day 1, and cyclophosphamide, 200 $mg/m^2/day$ on days 3 through 6, were given every 3 to 4 weeks for a total doxorubicin dose of 500 mg/m^2. BCG was administered by scarification to alternating upper and lower extremity sites on days 8 and 15. There was a similar distribution between the two study arms of patients with stage IV disease, bulky tumor masses, types of surgical procedures, performance status, prior radiation therapy exposure, and histologic type and grade of tumor. The complete remission and partial remission rate of 52% for patients receiving AC and BCG was significantly different ($P < 0.05$) from the 30% rate observed in the group receiving AC. The median duration of response of 13+ months for the group receiving AC plus BCG was not statistically better than the $7\frac{1}{6}$ months for the patients receiving AC. Median survival duration of the patients receiving AC plus BCG (21 months) was statistically better than that of patients receiving only AC (131/2 months) ($P < 0.005$). Therapy was well tolerated. There were no drug-related deaths and no serious systemic BCG toxicities. The addition of BCG to the standard AC treatment for far-advanced ovarian carcinoma appears to have increased response rates and overall survival duration without markedly adding to drug toxicity.

The GOG initiated another prospective randomized trial to test the efficacy of BCG by scarification in patients with advanced ovarian adenocarcinoma. Suboptimal patients with bulky residual stage III and stage IV disease were randomized between chemotherapy with cisplatin, doxorubicin, and cyclophosphamide (CAP) vs CAP plus BCG given in a manner identical to that reported by Alberts. Although the chemotherapy given in this study by the GOG is at variance with that used by Alberts, the methodology was otherwise identical. It was thought that this study would test the value of BCG in patients with advanced epithelial cancer of the ovary. In 1987, the GOG study in which BCG was used was closed, and analysis did not substantiate the efficacy of BCG as reported by Alberts.

Gall reported a prospective, randomized trial (done under the auspices of the GOG) in patients with stage III optimal epithelial carcinoma of the ovary that used melphalan vs melphalan plus *C. parvum*. There were 185 patients eligible for evaluation, 87 in the melphalan group and 98 in the melphalan plus *C. parvum* group. The comparison of the treatment regimens showed no differences regarding progression-free interval or survival. However, a 3-year survival of 50% was obtained. Both the maximal size of residual tumor and performance status were prognostically significant. In summary, this study demonstrated a lack of efficacy of the addition of *C. parvum* to melphalan for this population of patients.

Berek reported the treatment of 21 patients who had recurrent and advanced epithelial ovarian cancer with *C. parvum* administered intraperitoneally. Nineteen patients had surgically measurable disease, and two received adjuvant therapy. Surgically confirmed responses were documented in 6 of 19 patients (31.6%), which included two complete responses (10.5%) and four partial responses (21.1%). Three patients (15.8%) had stable disease, and 10 patients (52.6%) had disease progression. The mean survival of the patients who had complete response was 35.5 months; the four patients who had partial response had a median survival of 26.6 months. Of the non-responders, the mean survival was 12.6 months. Stimulation of cytotoxic lymphocytes resulted from the administration of *C. parvum*, which induced a significant increase of both intraperitoneal NK lymphocyte cytotoxicity and antibody-dependent cell-mediated cytotoxicity in six of nine patients tested. Toxicity in 86 courses of therapy included abdominal pain in 78% of cases, fever in 56%, nausea in 40%, and vomiting in 22%.

Ikic and associates studied interferon treatment of uterine cervical precancerous lesions. Human leukocyte interferon was applied topically on the uterine cervix in 10 patients with persistent cytologic findings of non-dysplastic atypia and dysplastic atypia. Patients were treated over 14–21 days with a daily dose of 1×10^6 IU. Cytologic findings after treatment were minor inflammations, that is, normalized cytologic findings (IIa according to Papanicolaou nomenclature) in all 10 patients. No relapses were found in the 6-month interval after treatment. A follow-up report in 1981 by Ikic and associates studied groups of patients with cervical intraepithelial neoplasia who were randomly selected for treatment with interferon (13 patients with cervical intraepithelial neoplasia, stages I and II) or placebo (18 patients with cervical intraepithelial neoplasia, stage I through stage III). Follow-up studies at 2 years showed significant differences between the treatment and the placebo groups with regard to cytologic findings and histologic diagnoses. In the control subjects, the pathologically changed epithelium was persistent in 7 of 18 cases, and there were 7 of 18 progressions. Among the control subjects, no regressions were observed. In the patients treated with interferon, abnormal epithelium persisted in 4 of 13 cases, progressed in 1 of 13, and regressed in 8 of 13. The results indicate that interferon has an impact on the regression of cervical intraepithelial neoplasia. Therapy with interferon may be particularly indicated in women in the reproductive age in whom fertility is to be preserved because it may obviate the need for surgery.

Einhorn and colleagues reported on a series of patients treated with interferon for advanced ovarian carcinoma. Daily intramuscular injections of 3×10^6 IU of interferon were given to five patients with advanced ovarian carcinoma, all of whom previously received other forms of treatment. Ascitic fluid production ceased in two of two patients. According to the criteria specified by Young and DeVita, a partial response was observed in one patient, and the disease was stable for more than 1 year in two other patients. Side effects of the interferon therapy were relatively mild. The introduction of interferon therapy was followed by an increase in NK cell activity of peripheral blood lymphocytes in all three patients examined. NK cell activity decreased after cessation of interferon therapy in the one patient in whom this was tested.

Abdulhay described 36 patients who had measurable epithelial ovarian cancers who failed to respond to conventional chemotherapy and were treated with lymphoblastoid interferon alone. Twenty-eight patients were assessable for response: two had complete response (7.1%), two had partial response (10.8%), 14 had stable disease (50.0%), and nine had increasing disease (32.2%). Abdulhay concluded that interferon therapy may have cytostatic and possibly cytotoxic effects. This GOG pilot study was followed by another pilot study in patients immediately after surgery who had advanced epithelial ovarian cancers who received interferon in addition to CAP chemotherapy. This study was reported by DiSaia, who noted unacceptable toxicity, especially cumulative myelotoxicity with prolonged leukopenia.

Berek described 14 patients who had persistent epithelial ovarian cancers documented at second-look laparotomy after combination chemotherapy who were treated with 146 cycles of recombinant IFN-α administered intraperitoneally. The initial dose was 5×10^6 IU, which was escalated weekly to 50×10^6 IU during 4 weeks and then continued weekly for a total of 16 weeks. Eleven patients underwent surgical re-evaluation after therapy that confirmed by pathologic examination complete responses in four patients (36%), partial response in one patient (9%), and disease progression in six patients (55%). Five of seven patients (71%) who had residual tumor <5 mm had a surgically documented response, whereas there was no response in the four patients whose tumors were ≥5 mm. Significant fever was seen in 58%, vomiting in 37%, and abdominal pain in 22%; one patient had infectious peritonitis.

On the basis of a report of Verhaegen and coworkers, who demonstrated a survival advantage in patients with colorectal carcinoma who were adjuvantly treated with levamisole, the North Central Cancer Treatment Group conducted a trial that randomly allocated 401 postoperative patients with Dukes' B or C carcinomas to:

1. observation;
2. levamisole alone; or
3. a combination of levamisole and 5-fluorouracil.

Levamisole was administered at 150 mg daily for 3 consecutive days every 2 weeks. Therapy was continued for 1 year; the median follow-up exceeded 7 years. Therapy with 5-fluorouracil and levamisole significantly reduced cancer recurrences, and an improvement in survival was observed in patients with Dukes' C colon cancer ($P = 0.03$) over that of patients receiving no additional postoperative therapy. Results in the group treated with levamisole alone suggested a reduction in recurrences ($P = 0.05$) but no influence on survival.

Many pilot studies have been initiated with use of a host of cytokines, usually as single agents alone and without chemotherapy, in an attempt at active immunotherapy. More and more is being learned about these complex and often pleiotropic molecules and the multiple populations of effector cells under their control. The future promises to allow selection of cytokines and proper orchestration of those selected to create the desired effect. The biology involved is complex and the therapeutic trials to date have been simplistic. The future promises more rational schedules, sequences, and doses of these agents, with or without chemotherapy.

Vaccine therapy

Therapeutic and prophylactic vaccine strategies that exploit the immune system on a molecular level are being developed. Vaccines are considered active immunotherapy because they elicit an immune response in the patient. Therapeutic cancer vaccines are designed to induce cellular components of the immune system to recognize and attack malignant cells. Prophylactic vaccines elicit humoral immune responses because they induce the production of antibodies capable of neutralizing an antigen (e.g., virus) before it infects the host cell. In this manner, virally induced malignant neoplasms may be prevented by inoculation with a vaccine before any exposure to a tumor virus. Therapeutic vaccines are administered to reduce or eradicate existing disease. Thus, a therapeutic tumor vaccine will target and destroy cells expressing tumor-associated antigens on their surface. As an example, in cervical cancer, these might be the viral peptides derived from human papillomavirus (HPV) E6 and E7 oncoproteins. A variety of approaches are candidates for cancer vaccines, including the adoptive transfer of antigen-presenting cells and inactivation of whole cancer cells. Antigen-presenting cells, including Langerhans cells, macrophages, B cells, and dendritic cells, can engulf exogenous proteins and present the degraded peptide antigens to T cells in an MHC-restricted manner. Given their exquisite immunostimulatory capacity, antigen-presenting cells are essential for effective immunotherapies. Peptides are attractive vaccine candidates because they can be inexpensively synthesized in large quantities and are relatively non-toxic. However, immunologically relevant target peptides must be identified for this strategy to be effective.

Dendritic cells (DC) are potent antigen-presenting cells well suited for vaccine strategies. They can be found throughout the body and are concentrated at portals of entry for infectious organisms, e.g. skin, where they are called Langerhans cells. Multiple animal studies have demonstrated cytotoxic T cell lymphocyte-mediated protective immunity and even regression of established tumors with the administration of antigen pulsed dendritic cells. Using an autologous tumor antigen-pulsed DC approach in patients with ovarian cancer ($n = 8$), Hernando harvested DCs and pulsed them with keyhole limpet hemocyanin and autologous tumor cell lysate. Significant tumor antigen specific lymphoproliferative responses were seen in two ovarian cancer patients. DC approaches are potent at inducing T cell responses, but a variety of variables require further study to enhance the approach including DC subtype, adjuvant cytokines, antigen loading method as well as route and frequency of administration.

Other immunostimulants under investigation include immune-stimulating complexes (ISCOMs), cytokines, and costimulatory molecules. An ISCOM containing a cholesterol matrix into which protein antigens can be incorporated can elicit both humoral and cell-mediated immune responses in animals. Other ISCOM adjuvants consist of cage-like microspheres made of quillaia, cholesterol, and a phospholipid. Protein or peptide antigens can be incorporated into the microspheres. The particles are taken up by the immune system and are transported to regional lymph nodes.

The potential to develop an effective prophylactic or therapeutic vaccine appears most promising for cervical cancer because of the connection between HPV infection and this malignant disease. The oncogenic potential of high-risk HPV subtypes has been linked to the E6 and E7 genes and their oncoproteins. E6 and E7 peptides appear to be expressed by tumor cells infected with this virus and can be used to generate specific cytotoxic T lymphocytes capable of tumor recognition and lysis of cervical cancer cells. In the future, the development of a therapeutic or prophylactic anti-HPV vaccine for cervical cancer may offer an attractive and cost-effective immunologic approach to reducing the worldwide morbidity from this disease. Similar comments can be made for vulvar cancer because HPV DNA has been detected in approximately 50–90% of patients with vulvar intraepithelial neoplasia and 20–60% of patients with invasive vulvar carcinoma. The HPV types most often detected are HPV-16b and HPV-18, the types that predominate in cervical cancer.

Loss of heterozygosity in the tumor suppressor genes p53 and BRCA1 on chromosomes 17p and 17q, respectively, has been detected in patients with ovarian cancer. Several other genes associated with abnormalities in the human ovary include ras, Her-2/neu, PDGF, and myc. Although this heterogeneous collection of genetic abnormalities is large, it may provide unique targets for immunotherapy. Several antibodies have been developed for ovarian cancer immunotherapy. One such approach targets the erB b2 oncoprotein. Some investigators propose to use irradiated tumor cells modified to express IL-2 or IL-4 in large amounts.

As evidence accumulates suggesting that manipulation of the immune system can induce tumor regression, many novel tumor vaccines will evolve.

Monoclonal antibody therapy

The use of monoclonal antibody and its conjugates in the treatment of cancer is in an early stage. Although it is clear that much needs to be done to clarify many of the issues surrounding the use of antibody alone or conjugates of the antibody with other toxic substances, it has been demonstrated in animal tumor models and in humans that antibody alone and antibody conjugated with drugs, toxins, and radioisotopes can have therapeutic effects. The potential for monoclonal antibodies in cancer therapeutics is enormous given the specificity that is inherent in the antibody-antigen reaction. The use of isotope-labeled antibody has enormous potential for the detection and treatment of cancer. There are still significant problems with these conjugates because of potential toxicity from the organ's non-specific accumulation of radioactivity or toxins from the conjugate or its products. In addition, any non-specific binding of the isotope-labeled conjugates will represent a significant clinical problem for the use of these conjugates in therapy. The hypothesis that lower levels of drug toxicity and greater antitumor activity may be seen by virtue of increased specificity of the drug-antibody conjugate remains to be demonstrated in humans.

Most monoclonal antibodies directed at human tumors are of murine or other rodent origin and activate human immune effector mechanisms poorly. The prospect of developing antitumor antibodies of human origin certainly will improve this situation. However, there are still few human cell lines that are as compatible as fusion partners as the murine myeloma lines, and the technique for immunizing humans to get antitumor antibodies of high affinity and IgG isotype has not yet been perfected. However, the application of recombinant DNA technology to fuse the human heavy chain constant region gene to a rearranged VDJ murine gene encoding an antitumor variable region may yield recombinant genes capable of producing high-affinity antibody with the capacity to activate the human immune response efficiently (Fig. 19–15). Thus, arming the available murine antitumor antibodies with some sort of killer molecule appears to be the most promising lead immediately available. There is considerable discussion, however, as to whether the use of conventional drugs, radionuclides, or bacterial toxins is best for this purpose. Most interest is focused on the last two.

Radionuclides have many attractive features in their use as lethal moieties on monoclonal antibodies (Fig. 19–16). They allow diagnosis through imaging that might be accomplished with conjugates of low specific activity. These results could be used in dosimetry calculations to produce a theoretical therapeutic index for the use of the conjugate at higher specific activity in the individual patient. The use of radionuclides also circumvents the problem of tumor cell antigen heterogeneity, modulation, and the need for internalization of the complex because the isotope of interest can have killing distances of many centimeters. These assumed advantages, however, by their nature decrease the specificity of the treatment, and there must be consideration as to whether, for example, a metastatic tumor in the liver with localization of the isotope-antibody complex in that organ could result in marked hepatic toxicity. In addition, there are technical limitations to the use of some of the more preferable isotopes because of incompletely defined practical and stable conjugation chemistry. The ideal isotope is of high specific activity, has a short half-life, has high energy at a short distance, is safe to work with from a radiation standpoint, possesses well-defined and stable conjugation chemistry, and is rapidly cleared from the body. At present, none of the radionuclides fulfills all of these criteria.

The use of natural toxins, for example, *Pseudomonas* exotoxin and the A chain of ricin (from the castor bean), as the cytotoxic component on a monoclonal antibody also has potential advantages (Fig. 19–17). These agents exhibit their cytotoxic effect by irreversible inhibition of protein synthesis. They catalyze the inhibition of elongation factor-2 or inhibit adenosine triphosphate ribosylation, processes essential to protein synthesis. The inhibition is so efficient that as few as one or two molecules of the toxin can kill the cell. The toxins are usually composed of two separate chains, an A chain that is the active toxic moiety, and the B chain that is responsible for binding the toxin to the cell and for getting it internalized from receptosomes to the cytoplasm. An isolated A chain is essentially nontoxic because it has no capability for entering cells. After the toxin binds its target, it is taken up by receptor-mediated endocytosis and enters the cytoplasm. Both binding and internalization into the cytoplasm must take place for toxins to exert their effects. Therefore, they are exceedingly specific. The extreme specificity of immunotoxins is a potential liability because of the tumor cell antigen heterogeneity; the use of only one monoclonal antibody would

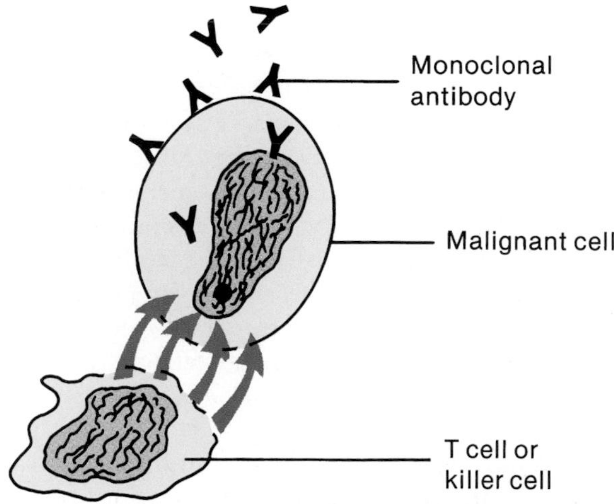

Figure 19–15 Monoclonal antibodies can be made to recognize and attach to unique proteins on the surface of cancer cells. After the cancer cell is coated with antibodies, cells of the immune system recognize and destroy the malignant cell.

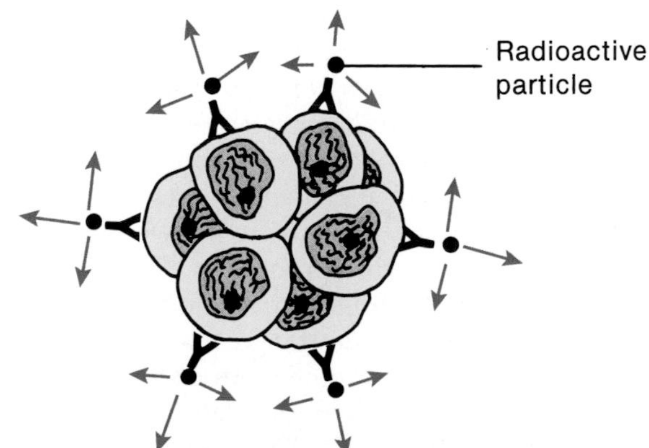

Figure 19–16 Radioactive particles can be attached to monoclonal antibodies. The antibodies carry the particles to cancer cells, where the radioactive material is then concentrated to kill the neoplastic cells.

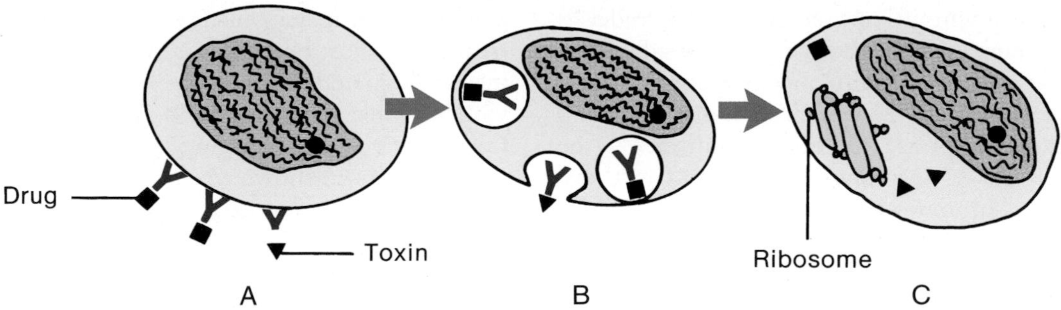

Figure 19–17 *A,* The drug-laden antibody attaches to the cancer cell's surface. *B,* The drugs or toxins-although not necessarily the antibody-are engulfed by the cell. *C,* When inside the cell, the drugs or toxins poison the cell. One toxin, for example, destroys the ribosomes, which are the cell's protein factories.

kill only those cells expressing the target antigen. A "cocktail" of toxin conjugates might circumvent this problem and yet allow retention of the killing specificity dictated by the need for internalization. Another danger relates to the fact that antigens may be shared with some normal cells so that these normal cells will also be targeted.

The need for internalization places potential constraints on some of the antibodies applicable to the production of immunotoxins. Some target antigens are shed and are poorly internalized. Therefore, in addition to the search for appropriate antitumor antibodies, antibodies must be directed against components of an actively growing cell, such as growth factor receptors and the transferrin receptor, which are potential candidates for immunotherapy. These antibodies are efficiently internalized and might quantitatively discriminate between carcinoma cells characterized by their uncontrolled growth and normal cells, which generally are dividing at a less rapid rate. Such a differential in growth rate may be particularly relevant to intraperitoneal therapy in ovarian cancer because the only rapidly dividing cells in the peritoneal cavity should be malignant ovarian cancer cells.

Few monoclonal conjugate clinical studies have been done, but preliminary results from one of these in which antiferritin antibody was linked to ^{131}I suggest some promise for the treatment of hepatocellular carcinoma. Because any monoclonal antibody conjugate is expected to be transported primarily to the liver, it is unclear what, if anything, the specific antibody contributes to the observed responses. Monoclonal antibodies directed against cell surface antigens in conjunction with immunoconjugates or complement have already proved useful in autologous bone marrow transplantation. They have been used to clear the bone marrow in vitro either of normal T cells, to decrease graft-vs-host reactions, or of malignant cells. Another useful clinical role of conjugated antibodies is to provide staging information. Such reagents have been useful in cutaneous T cell lymphoma and melanoma. The monoclonal antibody is labeled with a radioisotope such as ^{135}I or ^{131}I, the conjugate administered intravenously or intralymphatically, and the patient scanned with a gamma camera. This technique may also provide a sensitive and specific way of determining the location of metastases undetectable by other methods.

The rapid development of DNA technology has significant implication for monoclonal antibody research. For example, genetic engineering has made it possible to tailor chimeric antibodies consisting of murine light chains and human heavy chains, resulting in less immunogenicity. Recombinant technology also allows one to make novel bifunctional molecules in which one end contains the antigen-combining site and a second end binds to a drug, toxin, effector cell, or other matter. Future clinical trials may well involve the use of monoclonal antibodies or bifunctional molecules combined with other biologics such as interferon, TNF, or IL-2. The rationale for such studies stems from the preclinical data showing enhancement of the antibody-dependent cellular cytotoxicity and other immune functions generated by these cytokines. Genetically engineered monoclonal antibody constructs may eliminate several problems associated with current murine monoclonal antibodies.

Various other factors can also inhibit the efficacy of monoclonal antibody therapy: circulating tumor antigen in the serum can bind most of the antibody and prevent its effective delivery to the site of the tumor, a subset of the tumor cells may not express the tumor antigen or may express it only in low amounts, and modulation of the antigen from the cell surface will remove the antibody's target. The potential of monoclonal antibodies in cancer treatment has not yet been realized. The obvious appeal of monoclonal antibodies is their specificity and their potential for focusing immune mechanisms of the host or cytotoxic agents on the tumor cell. The initial experimental work in clinical trials defined some problems that must be resolved. These trials also provided some intriguing results that will certainly be an impetus to further work and to exploration of new approaches to the use of monoclonal antibodies in therapy. We are more optimistic for the immediate future regarding the potential use of monoclonal antibodies as a tool for imaging and diagnosis.

CONCLUSIONS

The field of tumor immunology and biologic response modifiers has grown significantly in recent years, and it is impossible to address all aspects of this highly evolving area of scientific development in one chapter. The reader is encouraged to obtain some of the references if additional information is desired. The main objective among those interested in clinical gynecologic tumor immunology and the use of biologic response modifiers continues to be determining methods of immunodiagnosis and methods of immunotherapy. Immunodiagnosis is hindered at this point by the weakness of the tumor-associated antigens in gynecologic malignant neoplasms and physicochemical and other technical problems associated with isolation of substances from the cell surface that vary only slightly from normal cellular molecules. The presence of tumor-associated antigens in gynecologic malignant neoplasms has been demonstrated by a number of indirect methods, and therefore the probability that several immunodiagnostic tools will be developed for the clinician is promising. It is hoped that the technology developed around CA-125 testing in epithelial ovarian cancer will be the first of many clinically useful immunodiagnostic methods.

The status of immunotherapy in gynecologic cancer is similar to that in other human malignant neoplasms. Immunoprophylaxis awaits identification of viral or other etiologic agents and purification of tumor-associated antigens. Both specific and non-specific immunotherapeutic trials have been performed and are currently under way in various institutions, with mixed results. These less than optimal results are understandable if one considers the following factors. Most trials have used non-specific immunotherapy, which relies on a generalized stimulation of the reticuloendothelial system with concomitant specific stimulation of clones directed toward the malignant neoplasm as a byproduct. Specific immunotherapy has not been successful because of the weak immunogenic properties of the antigens involved. In addition, most clinical trials have been conducted in patients with large tumor burdens in whom reduction of those burdens was assigned to surgery, chemotherapy, or radiotherapy. These cancericidal modalities are immunosuppressive in and of themselves and may abrogate the effectiveness of the immunopotentiator. Newer techniques, possibly using dendritic cells, may have greater promise. Tumor vaccines are another exciting area of research.

The status of most immune monitoring techniques is disappointing. Indeed, most of the immune monitoring techniques that the immunotherapist formerly relied on to demonstrate an effect from immunotherapeutic agents have been demonstrated to be unreliable or inaccurate. Thus, the immunotherapist is forced to rely on clinical response as an endpoint, and clinical response is confused by the multiplicity of other factors involved in the patient's condition, such as other tumoricidal therapies, nutrition, and genetic makeup. In many ways, the cards have been stacked against the immunotherapist, and a certain amount of patience is appropriate among clinicians as these complex issues are unraveled.

The therapeutic application of monoclonal antibodies offers perhaps the most exciting potential and the greatest challenge. Although monoclonal antibodies have already been hailed as magic bullets or guided missiles, their use in treatment is just beginning to be explored, and their ultimate role is undefined. However, early results in patients with leukemia, lymphoma, and cancer of the gastrointestinal tract have been encouraging. Monoclonal antibodies have themselves been shown to destroy tumor cells in vitro and in vivo in a nude mouse system. The mechanisms for this direct antitumor effect appear to involve antibody-dependent cellular cytotoxicity and macrophages. Other tumor cell agents, such as chemotherapy drugs, toxins, radioisotopes, and interferon, may be conjugated to carrier monoclonal antibodies for precise delivery to tumor cells.

Several obstacles must be overcome if the potential of monoclonal antibodies as a significant therapeutic modality in cancer is to be realized, including the following:

- the problem of circulating tumor antigen, which can activate the antibody and theoretically lead to immune complex disease;
- the appearance in the recipient of human antibody to mouse protein with the same consequence;
- the phenomenon of antigenic modulation (temporary disappearance of target antigen from the tumor cell surface in the presence of antibody);
- the existence of antigenic heterogeneity of tumor cells;
- the varying affinity in antitumor properties of different classes of antibodies; and
- the delineation of optimal methods of conjugating tumor cell compounds to monoclonal antibodies

Solutions to some or all of these obstacles seem likely. The development of methods to produce human hybridomas, the use of mixtures of monoclonal antibodies to enhance the affinity and specificity for tumor cells, the direct linkage of monoclonal antibodies to effector cells, and the generation of monoclonal reagents to tumor stem cell or chemoresistant cell subpopulations are examples that are currently under active investigation in many laboratories.

GLOSSARY

Accessible antigens Antigens of self that are in contact with antibody-forming tissues and to a host that is normally tolerant.

Accessory cell Cell required for, but not actually mediating, a specific immune response. Often used to describe antigen-presenting cells.

Active immunization Direct immunization of the intact individual or of immunocompetent cells derived from and returned to the individual.

Active immunotherapy May be divided into two groups: specific immunogens and non-specific adjuvants. Active specific immunotherapy is attempted by the immunization of a tumor-bearing patient with autochthonous altered (radiation, chemical) tumor cells. Non-specific immunotherapy attempts to augment antitumor immunologic activity with non-specific stimulants such as BCG or *C. Parvum.*

Adaptation A process whereby protection accorded a foreign graft from the immune reaction of the recipient renders it less vulnerable to immunologic attack by the host.

Adjuvant A substance that when mixed with an antigen enhances its antigenicity.

Adoptive immunization The transfer of immunity from one individual to another by means of specifically immune lymphoid cells or materials derived from such cells that are capable of transferring specific immunologic information to the recipient's lymphocytes.

Affinity A measure of the binding constant of a single antigen-combining site with a monovalent antigenic determinant.

AFP See α-fetoprotein.

Agglutinin Any antibody that produces aggregation or agglutination of a particular or insoluble antigen.

Allele Alternative gene acting at the same locus on the chromosome.

Allelic exclusion The ability of heterozygous lymphoid cells to produce only an allelic form of an antigen-specific receptor (immunoglobulin or T cell receptor) when they have the genetic endowment to produce both.

Allergen A substance (antigen or hapten) that incites allergy.

Allergy A state of specific increased reactivity to an antigen or hapten such as occurs in hay fever. The term is used to designate states of delayed sensitivity caused by contact allergens.

Alloantibody (isoantibody) Any antibody produced by one individual that reacts specifically with an antigen present in another individual of the same species. The term *isoantibody* is commonly used in hematology; the term *alloantibody* is used in tissue transplantation.

Alloantigen (isoantigen) Any antigen that incites the formation of antibodies in genetically dissimilar members of the same species.

Allogeneic Referring to genetically dissimilar individuals of the same species.

Allogeneic disease Any systemic illness resulting from a graft-vs-host response when the graft contains immunologically competent cells and the host is immunologically incompetent (e.g., runt disease).

Allograft (homograft) A graft derived from an allogeneic donor.

Alloimmune Specifically immune to an allogeneic antigen.

Alternative complement pathway The mechanism of complement activation that does not involve activation of the C1-C4-C2 pathway by antigen-antibody complexes and begins with the activation of C3.

Anamnestic response (recall phenomenon, memory phenomenon) An accelerated response of antibody production to an antigen that occurs in an animal that has previously responded to the antigen.

Anaphylaxis, acute Systemic shock (often fatal) that develops in a matter of minutes after subsequent exposure to a specific foreign antigen to which the host has already reacted.

Anergy Absence of a hypersensitivity reaction that would be expected in other similarly sensitized individuals.

Antibody (Ab) A substance (usually a gamma globulin) that can be incited in an animal by an antigen or by a hapten combined with a carrier and that reacts specifically with the antigen or hapten. Some antibodies can occur naturally without known antigen stimulation.

Antibody-dependent cell-mediated cytotoxicity A phenomenon in which target cells, coated with antibody, are destroyed by specialized killer cells (NK cells and macrophages), which bear receptors for the Fc portion of the coating antibody.

Antibody reaction site (antigen-binding site, antibody-combining site) The inverted surface site on antibody that reacts with the antigen determinant site on the antigen.

Antibody response The production of antibody in response to stimulation by specific antigen.

Antigen A substance that can react specifically with antibodies and under certain conditions can incite an animal to form specific antibodies. *Extrinsic:* An antigen that is not a constituent or product of the cell. *Intrinsic:* An antigen that is a constituent or product of the cell.

Antigen determinant A small, three-dimensional everted surface configuration on the antigen molecule that specifically reacts with the antibody reaction site on the antibody molecule.

Antigen-presenting cell A specialized type of cell, bearing cell antigen-presenting cell surface class II major histocompatibility complex molecules, and involved in the processing and presentation of antigen to inducer or helper T cells.

Antigen receptor The specific antigen-binding receptor on T or B lymphocytes; these receptors are transcribed and translated from rearrangements of V genes.

Antigenic modulation Loss of antigenicity or change in antigenic markers by which tumor cells may avoid immunologic identification or destruction.

Antigenic paralysis See immunologic tolerance.

Apoptosis A form of programmed cell death caused by activation of endogenous molecules leading to the fragmentation of DNA.

Arthus reaction An inflammatory reaction characterized by edema, hemorrhage, and necrosis that follows the administration of antigen to an animal that already possesses precipitating antibody to that antigen.

Atopy A hereditary predisposition of various individuals to develop immediate-type hypersensitivity on contact with certain antigens.

Auto- Self or same.

Autoantibodies Antibodies produced by an animal that react with the animal's own antigens. The stimulus is not known but could be the animal's own antigens or cross-reacting foreign antigens.

Autoantigen A self-antigen that incites the formation of autoantibodies.

Autochthonous (indigenous) Found in the same individual in which it originates, as in the case of a neoplasm; autochthonous tumor is a tumor borne by the host of origin.

Autograft A graft derived from the same individual to whom it is transplanted.

Autologous Derived from the recipient itself.

B cell or B lymphocyte A bone marrow cell. These cells mediate humoral immunity and are thymus-independent cells. In the avian species, these cells are derived from the bursa of Fabricius. In humans, they originate in the bone marrow.

Binding site A term used for the antibody-combining site and other sites of specific attachment of macromolecules to one another.

Biologic response modifier The molecule produced by the body to regulate cellular responses.

Blocking factor A humoral antibody or an antigen-antibody complex or other factor that coats antigenic sites with a protective covering so that neither complement nor killer lymphocytes can attack the cell.

Bursa of Fabricius A cloacal structure in avian species containing immature lymphoid elements (B cells) and presumed to govern the production of humoral antibodies through these B cells.

Cell-mediated cytotoxicity Killing (lysis) of a target cell by an effector lymphocyte.

Cell-mediated immunity Immune reaction mediated by T cells, in contrast to humoral immunity, which is antibody mediated. Also referred to as delayed-type hypersensitivity.

Chimera An individual composed of genetically dissimilar tissues.

Class I, class II, and class III MHC molecules Proteins encoded by genes in the major histocompatibility complex.

Clonal selection theory The prevalent concept that specificity and diversity of an immune response are the result of selection by antigen of specifically reactive clones from a large repertoire of preformed lymphocytes, each with individual specificities.

Clone A population of cells derived from a single cell by asexual division.

Colony-forming units Hematopoietic progenitors that proliferate and give rise to a colony of hematopoietic cells.

Colony-stimulating factor A polypeptide that promotes the growth of hematopoietic progenitors.

Committed cell A cell committed to the production of specific antibodies to a given antigen determinant. Committed cells include primed cells, memory cells, and antibody-producing cells.

Complement (C') A multifactorial system of one or more normal serum components characterized by their capacity to participate in certain and specific antigen-antibody reactions.

Complement activation Promotion of the killing or lytic actions of complement.

Complement cascade A precise sequence of events usually triggered by an antigen-antibody complex, in which each component of the complement system is activated in turn.

Complement fixation The fixation of C' to an antigen-antibody complex.

Conjugates Yoked or coupled substances, that is, immunoconjugates, such as monoclonal antibodies conjugated with drugs, toxins, or radioisotopes.

Cytokines Cell-derived regulatory molecules.

Cytophilic antibodies Antibodies with an affinity for cells that depend on bonding forces independent of those that bind antigen to antibody.

D cell (double cell) Lymphocytes that appear to have characteristics of both T and B cells.

Delayed hypersensitivity A specific sensitive state characterized by a delay of many hours in initiation time and course of reaction. It is transferable with cells but not with serum.

Dendritic cells White blood cells found in the spleen and other lymphoid organs. Dendritic cells typically use thread-like tentacles to enmesh antigens, which they present to T cells.

Desensitization The procedure of rendering a sensitive individual insensitive to an antigen or hapten by treatment with that specific agent.

Determinant group That part of the structure of an antigen molecule that is responsible for specific interaction with antibody molecules evoked by the same or a similar antigen.

Enhancement factor See blocking factor.

Enhancing antibodies Antibodies that enhance the survival of a graft or of a tumor.

Enzyme-linked immunosorbent assay (ELISA) The assay in which an enzyme is linked to an antibody and a colored substrate is used to measure the activity of bound enzyme and the amount of bound antibody.

Epitope An alternative term for antigenic determinant.

Exon The region of DNA coding for a protein or a segment of a protein.

Fab (fragment antigen binding) That segment of the IgG antibody molecule, derived by papain treatment and reduction, containing only one antibody reaction site. Under oxidizing conditions, Fab fragments recombine to form the divalent molecule $F(ab')^2$ devoid of the Fc segment of the original molecule.

Fc Fragment of antibody without antigen-binding sites, generated by cleavage by papain; the Fc fragment contains the C-terminal domains of the immunoglobulin heavy chains.

α-fetoprotein Synthesized in the fetus by perivascular hepatic parenchymal cells. It is found in a high percentage of patients with hepatomas and endodermal sinus tumor of the ovary or testes. It is a serum protein present in concentrations up to 400 mg/dl in early fetal life, falling to < 3 mg/dl in adults. Increased levels may be detected in the serum of adults with hepatoma (80% positive) and endodermal sinus tumor (60–80%

positive) and may be used to observe progression of the disease.

Forssman antigen An interspecies-specific antigen present in erythrocytes of many species, including some micro-organisms, that is capable of inducing the formation of lysin for sheep erythrocytes in animals devoid of such antigen.

Freund adjuvant *Complete*: Freund emulsion of mineral oil, plant waxes, and killed tubercle bacilli used to combine with antigen to stimulate antibody production. *Incomplete*: Freund mixture without tubercle bacilli.

Hapten A substance that combines specifically with antibody but does not initiate the formation of antibody unless attached to a high-molecular-weight carrier.

Helper factor Sensitized T lymphocyte subpopulations release a helper factor that enables immunocompetent B cells to respond to antigens that they otherwise are unable to recognize. The stimulated B lymphocytes differentiate into plasma cells that produce antibody. The helper factor can also stimulate the B lymphocyte to produce a variant of the B cell, termed a killer cell (K cell) that is able to attack tumor cells only after the tumor cells have been exposed to specific antibody. Complement is not required for this action. See also killer cell.

Hemagglutinin An antibody that reacts with a surface antigen determinant on red cells to cause agglutination of those red cells.

Hemolysin (amboceptor) An anti-red cell antibody that can specifically activate complement (C') to cause lysis of red cells.

Hetero- Other or different; often used to mean "of a different species".

Heterophil Pertains to antigenic specificity shared between species.

Heterophil antigens Antigens common to more than one species.

Heterozygosity The presence in a chromosome of dissimilar genes.

Histocompatibility antigens (transplantation or HLA antigens) Antigens coded for by histocompatibility genes that determine the specific compatibility of grafted tissues and organs.

HLA antigens (human leukocyte antigens) A genetic locus containing two closely linked groups of several alleles (a sublocus). They are present on the cell membranes of all nucleated cells and play a major role in determining graft take and rejection.

Homologous See allogeneic.

Homologous disease See allogeneic disease.

Horizontal transmission of viruses Transmission of viruses between individual hosts of the same generation. See also vertical transmission of viruses.

Host The organism whose body serves to sustain a graft; interchangeable with the recipient.

Humoral antibodies Antibodies present in body fluids.

Humoral immunity Pertains to the body fluids in contrast to cellular elements. It is initiated by the thymus-independent B cells. These B lymphocytes proliferate and differentiate into plasma cells that secrete immunoglobulins (IgG, IgM, IgA, IgD, and IgE).

Hybridoma A hybrid cell that results from the fusion of an antibody-creating cell with a malignant cell; the progeny secrete antibody without stimulation and proliferate continuously in vivo and in vitro.

Idiotypes The unique and characteristic parts of an antibody's variable region, which can themselves serve as antigens.

Immune The state of being secure against harmful agents (e.g., bacteria, virus, or other foreign proteins) or influences.

Immune clearance Clearance of antigen from the circulation after complexing with antibodies.

Immune response A specific response that results in immunity. The total response includes an afferent phase during which responsive cells are "primed" by antigen, a central response during which antibodies or sensitized lymphoid cells are formed, and an efferent or effector response during which immunity is effectedby antibodies or immune cells.

Immunity The state of being able to resist or overcome harmful agents or influences. *Active*: Immunity acquired as the result of experience with an organism or other foreign substance. *Passive*: Immunity resulting from acquisition of antibody or sensitized lymphoid cells.

Immunize The act or process of rendering an individual resistant or immune to a harmful agent.

Immunocompetent cell (antigen-sensitive cell) Any cell that can be stimulated by antigen to form antibodies or give rise to sensitized lymphoid cells, including inducible cells, primed cells, and memory cells.

Immunoconjugate A monoclonal antibody linked to a chemotherapy agent, radioisotope, or natural toxin to increase ability to kill target cells.

Immunogen An antigen that incites specific immunity.

Immunoglobulins Classes of globulins to which all antibodies belong.

Immunologic enhancement Enhanced survival of incompatible tissue grafts (tumor or normal tissue) caused by specific humoral or other blocking factors.

Immunologic paralysis Absence of normal specific immunologic response to an antigen, resulting from previous contact with the same antigen, administered in a quantity greatly exceeding that required to elicit an immunologic response. The normal capacity to respond to other unrelated antigens is retained.

Immunologic surveillance Effective immunologic surveillance relies on the presence of tumor-specific antigenic determinants on the surfaces of neoplastic cells, which enable these altered cells to be recognized as non-self and to be destroyed by immunologic reactions.

Immunologic tolerance (antigenic paralysis, immunologic suppression, immunologic unresponsiveness, antigen tolerance) Failure of the antibody response to a potential antigen after exposure to that antigen. Tolerance commonly results from prior exposure to antigens.

Immunoreaction Reaction between antigen and its antibody.

Immunotoxin A monoclonal antibody linked to a natural toxin.

Interferon A family of proteins released by cells in response to a virus infection. These substances represent non-specific immunity and appear to have non-specific tumoricidal characteristics.

Interleukin-1 A macrophage-derived cytokine that is necessary for the initial step in activation of specific T cells and the process of in vivo production of effector T cells.

Interleukin-2 A lymphokine with multiple in vitro and in vivo effects. It is an essential factor for the growth of T cells; it augments various T cell functions; it supports the preservation and augmentation of NK cell function; and it is critical for the generation of LAK cells.

Interleukins Polypeptides secreted by lymphocytes, monocytes, or other accessory cells that function in the regulation of the hematopoietic or immune system; these molecules have an important role in cell-to-cell communication.

Iso- Identical.

Isoantibody The term used in blood grouping studies to designate an antibody formed by one individual that reacts with antigens of another individual of the same species. See also alloantibody.

Isoantigen See alloantigen. The term *isoantigen* is commonly used in hematology.

Isogeneic See syngeneic.

Isograft See syngraft.

Isoimmune See alloimmune.

Isologous See syngeneic.

Killer cell (K cell) Sensitized T lymphocytes produce a helper factor that acts on the immunocompetent lymphoid cell to produce a population of cells, probably variants of the B cell, termed killer cells (K cells), which are able to attack tumor cells that have been exposed to a specific sensitizing antibody. Unlike in the usual humoral antibody (immunoglobulin) response, complement is not needed.

Killer T cell A T cell with a particular immune specificity and an endogenously produced receptor for antigen, capable of specifically killing its target cell after attachment to the target cell by this receptor. Also called cytotoxic T cell.

Locus The precise location of a gene on a chromosome. Different forms of the gene (alleles) are always found at the same location on the chromosome.

Lymphocyte A round cell with scanty cytoplasm and a diameter of 7-12 μm. The nucleus is round, sometimes indented, with chromatin arranged in coarse masses and without visible nucleoli. Lymphocytes may be actively mobile.

Lymphoid cell Any or all cells of the lymphocytic and plasmacytic series.

Lymphokines Substances released by sensitized lymphocytes when they come into contact with the antigen to which they are sensitized; examples include transfer factor, lymphocyte-transforming activity, migration inhibition factor, and lymphotoxin.

Macrophage Large mononuclear phagocyte. This cell may be called a histiocyte in the tissues; it is called a monocyte in the blood. An antigen must come in contact with or pass through a macrophage before it can become a processed antigen with the ability to encounter and then sensitize a small lymphocyte.

Macrophage-activating factor Sensitized T lymphocytes can release a non-specific macrophage-activating factor that creates a cytotoxic population of macrophages that appear to distinguish malignant from normal cells, killing only malignant ones.

Major histocompatibility complex (MHC) A cluster of genes encoding cell surface molecules that are polymorphic within a species and that code for antigens, which leads to rapid graft rejection between members of a single species that differ at these loci. Several classes of protein, such as MHC class I and class II proteins, are encoded in this region.

Memory cells Cells that can mount an accelerated antibody response to antigen.

MHC restriction The ability of T lymphocytes to respond only when they are presented with the appropriate antigen in association with either self MHC class I or class II molecules.

Migration inhibition factor A lymphokine produced when a sensitized lymphocyte is exposed to an antigen to which it is sensitized. Migration inhibition factor inhibits the migration of these lymphocytes.

Minor histocompatibility antigens These antigens, encoded outside the MHC, are numerous but do not generate rapid graft rejection or primary responses of T cells in vitro. They do not serve as restricting elements in cell interactions.

Mitogen A substance that induces immunocompetent lymphocytes to undergo blast transformation, mitosis, and cell division (causing mitosis or cell division).

Monoclonal antibody Antibodies with such high intrinsic specificity that only one or two antigenic determinants are recognized.

Monokines Soluble substances, secreted by monocytes, that have a variety of effects on other cells.

Mosaic An individual composed of two or more genetically dissimilar cell lines but from the same species. This can come about by somatic mutation or by grafting cells between individuals of close genetic constitution, such as dizygotic twins.

Natural antibodies Antibodies that occur naturally without deliberate antigen stimulation.

Natural killer lymphocytes (NK cells) Lymphocytes that are active in the immune surveillance of tumor. NK cells can lyse malignant target cells in vitro and appear to need no prior sensitization.

Non-specific immunization Refers to stimulation of the general immune response by the use of materials (e.g., BCG or phytohemagglutinin) that are not antigenically related to the specific tumor.

Nude mice Mice born with a congenital absence of the thymus. The blood and thymus-dependent areas of the lymph nodes and spleen are depleted of lymphocytes.

Oncogenic An agent capable of causing normal cells to acquire neoplastic characteristics. The term is often applied to viruses, such as adenoviruses.

Passive transfer of immunity The transfer of specific antibody from one individual to another.

Phytohemagglutinins Lectins extracted from the red kidney bean, *Phaseolus vulgaris* or *P. Communis*; the extract can be purified to yield a glycoprotein mitogen that stimulates lymphocyte transformation and causes agglutination of certain red cells; provides a method for calculating the pool of thymus-dependent lymphocytes (T cells).

Plasma cell End-stage differentiation of a B cell to an antibody-producing cell.

Pokeweed mitogen A mitogen extracted from the pokeweed plant; it can be purified to yield a specific glycoprotein. Pokeweed mitogen stimulates blast formation of both B and T cells.

Precipitin An antibody that reacts specifically with soluble antigen to form a precipitate.

Prophylactic immunization Represents pre-immunization of an individual against a causative agent (e.g., oncogenic virus) or tumor-specific antigen, in advance of any natural encounter with the agent or tumor.

Recombinant A gene that has been isolated and recombined with other sequences responsible for gene expression.

Runt disease A condition of dwarfing that follows the injection of mature allogeneic immunologically competent cells into immunologically immature recipients. It is characterized by failure to thrive, lymph node atrophy, hepatomegaly and splenomegaly, anemia, and diarrhea.

Sensitize The process of increasing the specific reactivity of a subject or cell to an agent. Commonly used to designate the process of increasing reactivity caused by specific antibodies or immune cells.

Shwartzman reaction A local non-immunologic inflammatory reaction with hemorrhage and necrosis produced by the injection of a bacterial endotoxin.

Suppression A mechanism for producing a specific state of immunologic unresponsiveness by the induction of suppressor T cells. This type of unresponsiveness is passively transferable by suppressor T cells or their soluble products.

Suppressor T cells Represent an important set of feedback controls, centered around sensitized T lymphocytes, through which inhibitory populations of these T cells suppress the production of sensitized lymphocytes and antibody-forming cells.

Syngeneic (isogeneic) Pertaining to genetically identical or nearly identical animals, such as identical twins or highly inbred animals.

Syngraft (isograft) A graft derived from a syngeneic donor.

T lymphocytes (T cells) Lymphocytes that have matured and differentiated under thymic influence, termed thymus-dependent lymphocytes. These cells are involved primarily in the mediation of cellular immunity as well as in tissue and organ graft rejection.

Tolerance Antigen-specific turnoff or unresponsiveness of B or T cells; usually produced as a result of contact with that antigen under non-immunizing conditions.

Topoisomerase An enzyme that controls conformational changes in DNA and aids in orderly progression of DNA replication, gene transcription, and separation of daughter chromosomes by cell division.

Transfer factor A heat-labile, dialyzable extract of human lymphocytes (a lymphokine) that is capable of conferring specific antigen reactivity to the donor.

Tumor angiogenesis factor Represents the induction of the growth of blood vessels caused by this stimulant released by tumor cells. The growth of a tumor appears to parallel the development of new blood vessels.

Tumor necrosis factor (TNF) A family of cytokines produced by activated monocytes and lymphocytes that can induce hemorrhagic necrosis and regression of tumors.

Vaccination Injection or ingestion of an immunogenic antigen for the purpose of producing active immunity.

Vaccine A suspension of dead or living micro-organisms that is injected or ingested for the purpose of producing active immunity.

Vertical transmission of viruses Transmission from one generation to another. Can include transmission from one generation to the next through milk or through the placenta.

Xenogeneic (heterologous) Pertaining to individuals of different species.

Xenograft (heterograft) A graft derived from an animal of a species different from the one receiving the graft.

BIBLIOGRAPHY

ANATOMY OF THE IMMUNE SYSTEM

Alzari PM, Lascombe MB, Poljak RJ: Three-dimensional structure of antibodies. Annu Rev Immunol 6:555, 1988.

Ashton-Rickardt PG, Tonegawa S: A differential avidity model for T cell selection. Immunol Today 15:362, 1994.

Berzofsky JA, Cease KB, Cornette JL et al: Protein antigenic structures recognized by T cells: Potential applications to vaccine design. Immunol Rev 98:9, 1987.

Billingham RE, Brent L, Medawar PB: Acquired tolerance of skin homografts. Ann N Y Acad Sci 59:409, 1955.

Broder S, Waldmann TA: The suppressor-cell network in cancer. N Engl J Med 229:1281, 1978.

Channing-Rodgers RP: Clinical laboratory methods for detection of antigens and antibodies. In Stites DP, Terr AL, Parslow TG (eds): Basic and Clinical Immunology, 8th ed. Norwalk, CT, Appleton & Lange, 1994, p 301.

Chen J, Alt FW: Gene rearrangement and B cell development. Curr Opin Immunol 5:194, 1992.

Clark EA, Ledbetter JA: How B and T cells talk to each other. Nature 367:425, 1994.
Cresswell P: Assembly, transport and function of MHC class II molecules. Annu Rev Immunol 12:259, 1994.
Currie GA: Cancer and the Immune Response. London, Edward Arnold, 1974.
DiSaia PJ: Overview of tumor immunology in gynecologic oncology. Cancer 38:566, 1976.
DiSaia PJ: Studies in cell-mediated immunity in two gynecologic malignancies. Cancer Bull 23:65, 1971.
DiSaia PJ et al: Immune competence and survival in patients with advanced cervical cancer: Peripheral lymphocyte counts. J Radiat Oncol 4:449, 1978.
Duijevestin A, Hamann A: Mechanism and regulation of lymphocyte migration. Immunol Today 10:23, 1989.
Durie FH, Foy TM, Masters SR et al: The role of CD40 in the regulation of humoral and cell mediated immunity. Immunol Today 15:406, 1994.
Engelhard VH: Structure of peptides associated with MHC class I molecules. Curr Opin Immunol 6:13, 1994.
Germain RN: MHC-dependent antigen processing and peptide presentation: Providing ligands for T lymphocyte activation. Cell 76:287, 1994.
Germain RN, Margulies DH: The biochemistry and cell biology of antigen processing and presentation. Annu Rev Immunol 11:403, 1993.
Hanna N: The role of natural killer cells in the control of tumor growth and metastasis. Biochim Biophys Acta 780:213, 1985.
Herberman RB: Animal tumor models and their relevance to tumor immunology. J Biol Response Mod 2:39, 1983.
Janeway CA Jr: How the immune system recognizes invaders. Sci Am 269:73, 1993.
Janeway CA Jr, Bottomly K: Signals and signs for lymphocyte responses. Cell 76:275, 1994.
Jefferis R: What is an idiotype? Immunol Today 14:19, 1993.
Knight SC, Stagg AJ: Antigen presenting cell types. Curr Opin Immunol 5:374, 1993.
Mackay CR, Imhof BA: Cell adhesion in the immune system. Immunol Today 14:99, 1993.
Miller JFAP: The role of the thymus in immunity—thirty years of progress. Immunologist 1:9, 1993.
Moller G: The B cell antigen receptor complex. Immunol Rev 132:5, 1993.
Moller G (ed): Lymphocyte homing. Immunol Rev 108:5, 1989.
Neefjes JJ, Momburg F: Cell biology of antigen presentation. Curr Opin Immunol 5:27, 1993.
Nossal GJV: Negative selection of lymphocytes. Cell 76:229, 1994.
Oldham RK: Natural killer cells: History and significance. J Biol Response Mod 1:217, 1982.
Paul WE, Seder RA: Lymphocyte responses and cytokines. Cell 76:241, 1994.
Rammensee H-G, Falk K, Rotzschke O: MHC molecules as peptide receptors. Curr Opin Immunol 5:35, 1993.
Rapp HJ et al: Antigenicity of new diethyl nitrosamine-induced transplantable guinea pig hepatoma. J Natl Cancer Inst 41:1, 1968.
Reth M: B cell antigen receptors. Curr Opin Immunol 6:3, 1994.
Robey E, Fowlkes BJ: Selective events in T cell development. Annu Rev Immunol 12:675, 1994.
Rothbard JB, Gefter ML: Interactions between immunogenic peptides and MHC proteins. Annu Rev Immunol 9:527, 1991.
Schatz DG, Oettinger MA, Schissel MS: V(D)J recombination: Molecular biology and regulation. Annu Rev Immunol 10:359, 1992.
Schnipper LE: Clinical implications of tumor-cell heterogeneity. N Engl J Med 314:1423, 1986.
Sherman LA, Chattopadhyay S: The molecular basis of allorecognition. Annu Rev Immunol 11:385, 1994.
Sinkovics JG, DiSaia PJ, Rutledge FN: Tumour immunology and evolution of the placenta. Lancet 2:1190, 1970.
Sjogren HO: Blocking and unblocking of cell-mediated tumour immunity. In Busch H (ed): Methods in Cancer Research. New York, Academic Press, 1973, p 92.
Stanfield RL, Fieser TM, Lerner R, Wilson IA: Crystal structures of an antibody to a peptide and its complex with peptide antigen at 2.8 A→. Science 248:712, 1990.
Takasugi M, Mickey MR, Terasaki PI: Reactivity of lymphocytes from normal persons on cultured tumor cells. Cancer Res 33:2898, 1973.
Von Boehmer H: Thymic selection: A matter of life and death. Immunol Today 13:742, 1992.
Weiss A, Littman DR: Signal transduction by lymphocyte antigen receptors. Cell 76:263, 1994.
Weissman IL: Developmental switches in the immune system. Cell 76:207, 1994.
Weissman IL, Cooper MD: How the immune system develops. Sci Am 269:64, 1993.
Welch WR, Niloff JM, Anderson D et al: Antigenic heterogeneity in human ovarian cancer. Gynecol Oncol 38:12, 1990.

IMMUNOPROPHYLAXIS

Ferris D, Koutsky L, Wehren L et al: Reduction in CIN following prophylactic HPV type 16 vaccination. Gynecol Oncol 96; 911a–912a, 2005
Goodnow CC, Adelstein S, Basten A: The need for central and peripheral tolerance in the B cell repertoire. Science 248:1373, 1990.
Harper DM, Franco EL, Wheeler C et al: Efficacy of a bivalent L1 virus-like particle vaccine in prevention of infection with human papillomavirus types 16 and 18 in young women: a randomised controlled trial. Lancet 364:1757–1765, 2004.
Hunt JS: Immunobiology of pregnancy. Curr Opin Immunol 4:591, 1992.
Nalick RH et al: Immunologic response in gynecologic malignancy as demonstrated by the delayed hypersensitivity reaction: Clinical correlations. Am J Obstet Gynecol 118:393, 1974.
Old LJ et al: Antigenic properties of chemically-induced tumors. Ann N Y Acad Sci 101:80, 1962.
Old LJ et al: The role of the reticuloendothelial system in the host reaction to neoplasia. Cancer Res 21:1281, 1961.
Romney FL et al: Retinoids and the prevention of cervical dysplasias. Am J Obstet Gynecol 1411:890, 1981.
Rosenthal SR et al: BCG vaccination and leukemia mortality. JAMA 222:1543, 1972.
Seder RA, Paul WE: Acquisition of lymphokine producing phenotype by $CD4^+$ T cell. Annu Rev Immunol 212:635, 1994.
Sprent J, Gao E, Webb SR: T cell reactivity to MHC molecules: Immunity versus tolerance. Science 248:1357, 1990.
Springer TA: Traffic signals for lymphocyte recirculation and leukocyte emigration: The multistep paradigm. Cell 76:301, 1994.
Surwit EA et al: Evaluation of topically applied *trans*-retinoic acid in the treatment of cervical intraepithelial lesions. Am J Obstet Gynecol 143:821, 1982.
Taira AV: Evaluating human papillomavirus vaccination programs. Emerg Infect Dis10:1915–1923, 2004.
Slomovitz BM, Sun CC, Frumovitz M et al: Are women ready for the cervical cancer vaccine? Gynecol Oncol 96:912a, 2005.
Padilla-Paz LA. Human papillomavirus vaccine: history, immunology, current status, and future prospects. Clin Obstet Gynecol 48:226–240, 2005.

PRINCIPLES OF IMMUNOTHERAPY

Aebersold P, Hyatt C, Johnson S et al: Lysis of autologous melanoma cells by tumor-infiltrating lymphocytes: Association with clinical response. J Natl Cancer Inst 83:932, 1991.
Alberts DS: BCG as an adjuvant to Adriamycin-Cytoxan for advanced ovarian cancer: A Southwest Oncology Group study

(Meeting Abstract). Program and abstracts of the second International Conference on the Adjuvant Therapy of Cancer, University of Arizona Cancer Center, Tucson, Arizona, March 28–31, 1979.

Arca MJ, Mulé JJ, Change AE: Genetic approaches to adoptive cellular therapy of malignancy. Semin Oncol 23:108, 1996.

Auerbach W, Auerbach R: Angiogenesis inhibition: a review. Pharmacol Ther 63:265–311, 1994.

Barnes MN, Deshane JS, Rosenfeld M et al: Gene therapy and ovarian cancer: A review. Obstet Gynecol 89:145, 1997.

Berchuck A, Lyerly HK: A phase I study of autologous human interleukin-2 (IL-2) gene modified tumor cells in patients with refractory metastatic ovarian cancer (Abstract). Human Gene Transfer Protocols. Bethesda, MD, Office of Recombinant DNA Activities, National Institutes of Health, 1995.

Berek JS, Markman M, Blessing JA et al: Intraperitoneal α-interferon alternating with cisplatin in residual ovarian carcinoma: A phase II Gynecologic Oncology Group study. Gynecol Oncol 74:48, 1999.

Berek JS, Welander C, Schink JC et al: A phase I–II trial of intraperitoneal cisplatin and alpha-interferon in patients with persistent epithelial ovarian cancer. Gynecol Oncol 40:237, 1991.

Bolle M, Niesen A, Korz W et al: Possible role of anti-CA-125 monoclonal antibody B43.13 (OvaRex) administration in long-term survival of relapsed ovarian cancer patients. Proc Am Soc Clin Oncol 19:476a, 2000.

Bookman MA, Rettenmaier M, Gordon A: Monoclonal antibody (Oregovomab) targeting of CA-125 in patients (pts) with advanced epithelial ovarian cancer (EOC) and elevated CA-125 after response to initial therapy. Clin Cancer Res 7:756s (abst 510), 2001.

Borysiewicz LK, Fiander A, Nimako M et al: A recombinant vaccinia virus encoding human papillomavirus types 16 and 18, E6 and E7 proteins as immunotherapy for cervical cancer [see comments]. Lancet 347:1523, 1996.

Bruzzone M, Rubagotti A, Gadducci A et al: Intraperitoneal carboplatin with or without interferon-alpha in advanced ovarian cancer patients with minimal residual disease at second look: a prospective randomized trial of 111 patients. GONO Gruppo Oncologic Nord Ovest. Gynecol Oncol 65:499–505, 1997.

Campo MS, Grindlay GJ, O'Neil, BW et al: Prophylactic and therapeutic vaccination against a mucosal papillomavirus. J Gen Virol 74:945, 1993.

Creasman WT et al: Chemoimmunotherapy in the management of primary stage III carcinoma of the ovary. Cancer Treat Rep 63:319, 1979.

Crowther ME, Hudson C: Experience with a pilot study of active specific intralymphatic immunotherapy. Cancer 41:2215, 1978.

Crowther ME et al: Active specific immunotherapy in ovarian cancer. Recent Results Cancer Res 68:166, 1979.

Currie GA: Eighty years of immunotherapy: A review of immunological methods used for the treatment of human cancer. Br J Cancer 26:141, 1972.

Davidson EJ, Boswell CM, Sehr P et al: Immunological and clinical responses in women with vulval intraepithelial neoplasia vaccinated with a vaccinia virus encoding human papillomavirus 16/18 oncoproteins. Cancer Res 63:6032–6041, 2003.

DiSaia PJ, Nalick RH, Townsend DE: Antibody cytotoxicity studies in ovarian and cervical malignancies. Obstet Gynecol 1:314, 1973.

DiSaia PJ et al: Preliminary report on the treatment of women with cervical cancer, stages IIB, IIIB, IVA (confined to the pelvis and/or periaortic nodes), with radiotherapy plus immunotherapy with intravenous *Corynebacterium parvum,* phase II. In Terry WD, Rosenberg SA (eds): Immunotherapy of Human Cancer. New York, Elsevier North-Holland, 1982, p 226.

Donnelly JJ, Ulmer JB, Liu MA: Immunization with polynucleotides. A novel approach to vaccination. Immunologist 2:20, 1994.

Ferrara N, Gerber HP, LeCouter J: The biology of VEGF and its receptors. Nat Med 9:669–676, 2003.

Ferrara N. Frantz G. LeCouter J et al. Differential expression of the angiogenic factor genes vascular endothelial growth factor (VEGF) and endocrine gland-derived VEGF in normal and polycystic human ovaries. Am J Pathol 162:1881–1883, 2003.

Flander AN et al: Immunocompetent for immunotherapy? A study of the immunocompetence of cervical cancer patients. Int J Gynecol Cancer 5:438, 1995.

Folkman J, Hochberg M: Self-regulation of growth in three dimensions. J Exp Med 138:745, 1973.

Foon KA, Bernard M, Oldham RK: Monoclonal antibody therapy. J Biol Response Mod 1:277, 1982.

Freedman RS et al: Novel immunologic strategies in ovarian carcinoma. Am J Obstet Gynecol 167:1470, 1992.

Gall S, Bundy B, Beecham J et al: Therapy of stage III (optimal) epithelial carcinoma of the ovary with melphalan or melphalan plus *Corynebacterium parvum* (a Gynecologic Oncology Group study). Gynecol Oncol 25:26, 1986.

Gonzales-de Leon C, Lippman SM, Kudelka AP et al. Phase II study of cisplatin, 5-fluorouracil and interferon-alpha in recurrent carcinoma of the cervix. Invest New Drugs 13:73–76, 1995.

Greten TF, Jaffee EM: Cancer vaccines. J Clin Oncol 17:1047, 1999.

Guo Y et al: Effective tumor vaccine generated by fusion of hepatoma cells with activated B cells. Science 263:518, 1994.

Hanahan D, Folkman J: Patterns and emerging mechanisms of the angiogenic switch during tumorigenesis. Cell 86:353–364, 1996.

Hawkins MJ: IL-2/LAK. In DeVita VT (ed): PPO Updates, Vol 3: Cancer, Principles and Practice of Oncology, 3rd ed. Philadelphia, JB Lippincott, 1989, p 161.

Herberman RB, Oldham RK: Cell-mediated cytotoxicity against human tumors: Lessons learned and future prospects. J Biol Response Mod 2:111, 1983.

Herberman RB, Ortaldo JR: Natural killer cells: Their role in defenses against disease. Science 214:24, 1981.

Hernando JJ, Park TW, Kubler K et al: Vaccination with autologous tumour antigen-pulsed dendritic cells in advanced gynecological malignancies: clinical and immunological evaluation of a phase I trial. Cancer Immunol Immunother 51:45–52, 2002.

Hewitt HB: Animal tumor models and their relevance to human tumor immunology. J Biol Response Mod 1:107, 1982.

HeZ, Wlazlo AP, Kowalczyk DW et al: Viral recombinant vaccines to the E6 and E7 antigens of HPV-16. Virology 270:146–161, 2000.

Hsu FJ, Kwak L, Campbell M et al: Clinical trials of idiotype specific vaccine in B cell lymphomas. Ann N Y Acad Sci 69:385, 1993.

Hwu P, Shafer GE, Treisman J et al: Lysis of ovarian cancer cells by human lymphocytes redirected with a chimeric gene composed of an antibody variable region and the Fc receptor Δ chain. J Exp Med 178:361, 1993.

Irvine KR, Restifo NP: The next wave of recombinant and synthetic anticancer vaccines. Semin Cancer Biol 6:337, 1995.

Juillard GJ, Boyer PJ, Yamashiro CH: A phase I study of active specific intralymphatic immunotherapy. Cancer 41:2215, 1978.

Kamada M, Sakamoto Y, Furumoto H et al: Treatment of malignant ascites with allogeneic and autologous lymphokine-activated killer cells. Gynecol Oncol 34:34, 1989.

Köhler G, Milstein C: Continuous cultures of fused cells secreting antibody of predefined specificity. Nature 256:495, 1975.

Langernecker BM, Maclean G: Prospects for mucin epitopes on cancer vaccines. Immunologist 1:89, 1993.

Lanzavecchia A: Identifying strategies for immune intervention. Science 260:937, 1993.

Levy R: Biological forecaster treatment: Monoclonal antibodies. Hosp Pract 20:67, 1985.

Lotze MT, Finn OJ: Recent advances in cellular immunology: Implications for immunity to cancer. Immunol Today 11:190, 1990.

Maiman M et al: Human immunodeficiency virus infection and invasive cervical carcinoma. Cancer 71:402, 1993.
Mantovani A, Bottazzi B, Colatta F et al: The origin and function of tumor associated macrophages. Immunol Today 13:265, 1992.
Meeker TC et al: A clinical trial of anti-idiotype therapy for B cell malignancy. Blood 65:1349, 1985.
Morein B: The ISCOM antigen-presenting system. Nature 332:287, 1988.
Morton DL, Goodnight JE: Clinical trials of immunotherapy. Cancer 42:2224, 1978.
Neefjes JJ, Momburg F: Cell biology of antigen presentation. Curr Opin Immunol 5:27, 1993.
Nehme A, Julia AM, Jozan S et al: Modulation of cisplatin cytotoxicity by human recombinant interferon-gamma in human ovarian cancer cell lines. Eur J Cancer 30A:520–525, 1994.
Old LJ: Immunotherapy for cancer. Sci Am 275:136, 1996.
Oldham RK, Smalley RV: Immunotherapy: The old and the new. J Biol Response Mod 2:1, 1983.
Olkowski ZL, McLaren JR, Skeen MJ: Effects of combined immunotherapy with levamisole and bacillus Calmette–Guérin on immunocompetence of patients with squamous cell carcinoma of the cervix, head and neck, and lung undergoing radiation therapy. Cancer Treat Rep 62:1651, 1978.
Onsrud M, Thorsby E: Long-term changes in natural killer activity after external pelvic radiotherapy. Int J Radiat Oncol Biol Phys 7:609, 1981.
Pardoll DM: Genetically engineered tumor vaccines. Ann NY Acad Sci 690:301, 1993.
Rabinovich NR, McInnes P, Klein DL, Hall BF: Vaccine technologies: View to the future. Science 265:1401, 1994.
Rao B et al: Intravenous *Corynebacterium parvum:* An adjunct to chemotherapy for resistant advanced ovarian cancer. Cancer 39:514, 1977.
Ressing ME, Sette A, Brandt RM et al: Human CTL epitopes encoded by human papillomavirus type 16 E6 and E7 identified through in vivo and in vitro immunogenicity studies of HLA-A*0201-binding peptides. J Immunol 154:5934, 1995.
Rosenberg SA: Adoptive immunotherapy of cancer: Accomplishments and prospects. Cancer Treat Rep 68:233, 1984.
Rosenberg SA: The development of new immunotherapies for the treatment of cancer using interleukin-2. Ann Surg 208:121, 1988.
Rosenberg SA: The immunotherapy and gene therapy of cancer. J Clin Oncol 10:180, 1992.
Rosenberg SA, Lotze MT, Yang JC et al: Experience with the use of high-dose interleukin-2 in the treatment of 652 cancer patients. Ann Surg 210:474, 1989.
Santin AD, Parham GP: Routine lymph node dissection in the treatment of early stage cancer: Are we doing the right thing? Gynecol Oncol 68:1, 1998.
Santini SM, Belardelli F: Advances in the use of dendritic cells and new adjuvants for the development of therapeutic vaccines. Stem Cells 21:495–505, 2003.
Schafer A et al: The increased frequency of cervical dysplasia-neoplasia in women infected with the human immunodeficiency virus is related to the degree of immunosuppression. Am J Obstet Gynecol 164:593, 1991.
Schiller JT, Okun MM: Papillomavirus vaccines: Current status and future prospects. Adv Dermatol 11:355, 381, 1996.
Schultes BC, Baum RP, Niesen A et al. Anti-idiotype induction therapy: anti-CA-125 antibodies (Ab3) mediated tumor killing in patients treated with Ovarex mAb B43.13 (Abl). Cancer Immunol Immunother 46:201–212, 1998.
Shu S, Plautz GE, Krauss JC, Chang AE: Tumor immunology. JAMA 278:1972, 1997.
Sotomayor EM, Borrello I, Levitsky HI: Tolerance and cancer: A critical issue in tumor immunology. Crit Rev Oncol 7:433, 1996.
Spirtos NM, Smith LH, Teng NNH: Prospective randomized trial of topical alpha-interferon (alpha-interferon gels) for the treatment of vulvar intraepithelial neoplasia III. Gynecol Oncol 37:34, 1990.
Steller MA, Schiller JT: Human papillomavirus immunology and vaccine prospects. J Natl Cancer Inst Monogr 21:145, 1996.
Stern PL: Immune control of human papillomavirus (HPV) associated anogenital disease and potential for vaccination. J Clin Virol 32(suppl 1):S72–S81, 2005.
Yancopoulos GD, Davis S, Gale NW et al. Vascular-specific growth factors and blood vessel formation. Nature 407:242–248, 2000.
Yannelli JR et al: An improved method for the generation of human lymphokine-activated killer cells. J Immunol Methods 100:137, 1987.

IMMUNODIAGNOSIS

Barlow JJ, Bhattacharya M: Tumor markers in ovarian cancer: Tumor associated antigens. Semin Oncol 11:203, 1975.
Bast RC Jr et al: A radioimmune assay using a monoclonal antibody to monitor the course of epithelial ovarian cancer. N Engl J Med 309:883, 1983.
Bast RC Jr et al: Monitoring ovarian carcinoma with a combination of CA-125, CA-19-9, and carcinoembryonic antigen. Am J Obstet Gynecol 149:553, 1984.
Berchuck A et al: Heterogeneity of antigen expression in advanced epithelial ovarian cancer. Am J Obstet Gynecol 162:883, 1990.
Cole LA et al: Urinary human chorionic gonadotropin free beta-subunit and beta-core fragment: A new marker of gynecological cancers. Cancer Res 48:1356, 1988.
Dini MM, Faiferman I: Sequential in vitro reactivity of lymphocytes from patients with cervical squamous malignancy in a cytotoxicity assay. Am J Obstet Gynecol 144:341, 1982.
DiSaia PJ, Rich WM: Value of immune monitoring in gynecologic cancer patients receiving immunotherapy. Am J Obstet Gynecol 135:907, 1979.
DiSaia PJ et al: Carcinoembryonic antigen in cancer of the female reproductive system: Serial plasma values correlated with disease state. Cancer 39:1265, 1977.
DiSaia PJ et al: Carcinoembryonic antigen in patients with gynecologic malignancies. Am J Obstet Gynecol 121:159, 1975.
Gall SA, Walling J, Pearl J: Demonstration of tumor-associated antigens in human gynecologic malignancies. Am J Obstet Gynecol 115:387, 1973.
Goldenberg DM, DeLand FH: History and status of tumor imaging with radio-labeled antibodies. J Biol Response Mod 1:121, 1982.
Kato H et al: Value of tumor-antigens (TA-4) of squamous cell carcinoma in predicting the extent of cervical cancer. Cancer 50: 1294, 1982.
Levi MM: Antigenicity of ovarian and cervical malignancy in a view toward possible immunodiagnosis. Am J Obstet Gynecol 109:689, 1971.
Molthoff CFM et al: Human ovarian cancer xenografts in nude mice: Characterization and analysis of antigen expression. Int J Cancer 43:55, 1989.
Nam JH et al: Urinary gonadotropin fragment, a new tumor marker. Gynecol Oncol 36:383, 1990.

BIOLOGIC RESPONSE MODIFIERS

Abdulhay GA et al: Human lymphoblastoid interferon in the treatment of advanced epithelial ovarian malignancies: A GOG study. Am J Obstet Gynecol 152:418, 1985.
Antman KS, Griffin JD, Elias A et al: Effect of recombinant human granulocyte-macrophage colony stimulating factor on chemotherapy-induced myelosuppression. N Engl J Med 319:1, 1988.
Balkwill F: Tumor necrosis factor: Improving on the formula. Nature 361:206, 1993.
Berchuck A, Olt GJ, Everitt L et al: The role of peptide growth factors in epithelial ovarian cancer. Obstet Gynecol 75:1, 1990.

Berek JS et al: Intraperitoneal immunotherapy of epithelial ovarian carcinoma with *Corynebacterium parvum*. Am J Obstet Gynecol 152:1003, 1985.

Berek JS et al: Intraperitoneal recombinant alpha-interferon for "salvage" immunotherapy in stage III epithelial ovarian cancer: A GOG study. Cancer Res 45:4447, 1985.

Berek JS et al: Serum interleukin-6 levels correlate with disease status in patients with epithelial ovarian cancer. Am J Obstet Gynecol 164:1038, 1991.

Bischoff J: Approaches to studying cell adhesion molecules in angiogenesis. Trends Cell Biol 5:69, 1995.

Borden EC, Sondel PM: Lymphokines and cytokines as cancer treatment: Immunotherapy realized. Cancer 65:800, 1990.

Champlin RE: Peripheral blood progenitor cells: A replacement for marrow transplantation? Semin Oncol 23:15, 1996.

Dinarello CA: Biology of interleukin 1. FASEB J 2:108, 1988.

Einhorn N et al: Human leukocyte interferon therapy for advanced ovarian carcinoma. Am J Clin Oncol 5:167, 1982.

Fidler IJ, Ellis LM: The implications of angiogenesis for the biology and therapy of cancer metastasis cells. Cell 79:185, 1994.

Folkman J: Angiogenesis in cancer, vascular, rheumatoid and other disease. Nat Med 1:27, 1995.

Folkman J, Shing Y: Angiogenesis. J Biol Chem 267:10931, 1992.

Fraser JK, Lill MCC, Figlin RA: The biology of the cytokine sequence cascade. Semin Oncol 23(Suppl 4):2, 1996.

Freedman RS, Ioannides CG: Biologic response modifiers in the treatment of gynecologic malignancies. Cancer Bull 42:98, 1990.

Freedman RS et al: Leukocyte interferon in patients with epithelial ovarian cancer. J Biol Response Mod 2:133, 1983.

Gabrilove JL, Jakubowski A, Scher H et al: Effect of granulocyte colony-stimulating factor on neutropenia and associated morbidity due to chemotherapy for transitional-cell carcinoma of the urothelium. N Engl J Med 318:1414, 1988.

Gadducci A et al: Serum levels of tumor necrosis factor (TNF), soluble receptors for TNF (55- and 75-kDa sTNFr), and soluble CD14 (sCD14) in epithelial ovarian cancer. Gynecol Oncol 58:184, 1995.

Gastl GA, Abrams JS, Nanus DM et al: Interleukin-10 production by human carcinoma cell lines and its relationship to interleukin-6 expression. Int J Cancer 55:96, 1993.

Goodman GE: The clinical evaluation of cancer chemoprevention agents: Defining and contrasting phase I, II, and III objectives. Cancer Res 52:2752, 1992.

Greenwald P, Nixon DW, Malone WF et al: Concepts in cancer chemoprevention research. Cancer 65:1483, 1990.

Grosen EA et al: Blocking factors (soluble membrane receptors) for tumor necrosis factor and lymphotoxin detected in ascites and released in short-term cultures obtained from ascites and solid tumors in women with gynecologic malignancy. Lymphokine Cytokine Res 11:347, 1992.

Grosen EA et al: Measurement of the soluble membrane receptors for tumor necrosis factor and lymphotoxin in the sera of patients with gynecologic malignancy. Gynecol Oncol 50:68, 1993.

Heo DS, Whiteside TL, Kanbour A et al: Lymphocytes infiltrating human ovarian tumors. I. Role of Leu-19 (NKH1)-positive recombinant IL-2 activated cultures of lymphocytes infiltrating human ovarian tumors. J Immunol 140:4042, 1988.

Hoover HC Jr, Surdyke MG, Dangel RB et al: Prospectively randomized trial of adjuvant active-specific immunotherapy for human colorectal cancer. Cancer 55:1236, 1985.

Horning SJ et al: Phase I study of human leukocyte interferon in patients with advanced cancer. J Biol Response Mod 2:47, 1983.

Ikic D et al: Interferon treatment of uterine cervical precancerosis. J Cancer Res Clin Oncol 101:303, 1981.

Itri LM: The interferons. Cancer 70:940, 1992.

Krusic J et al: Influence of human leukocyte interferon on squamous cell carcinoma of the uterine cervix: Clinical, histological, and histochemical observations. III. Communication. J Cancer Res Clin Oncol 101:309, 1981.

Le J, Vilcek J: Tumour necrosis factor and interleukin 1: Cytokines with multiple overlapping biological activities. Lab Invest 56:234, 1987.

Lippman SM, Benner SE, Hong WK: Cancer chemoprevention. J Clin Oncol 12:851, 1994.

Lotzova E, Savary CA, Freedman RS et al: Recombinant IL-2 activated NK cells mediate LAK activity against ovarian cancer. Int J Cancer 42:225, 1988.

Malone WF, Kelloff GJ, Boone C et al: Chemoprevention and modern cancer prevention. Prev Med 18:553, 1989.

Manetta A, Lucci J, Soopikian J et al: In vitro cytotoxicity of human recombinant tumor necrosis factor alpha in association with radiotherapy in a human ovarian carcinoma cell line. Gynecol Oncol 38:200, 1990.

Mills GB, May C, McGill M et al: A putative new growth factor in ascitic fluid from ovarian cancer patients: Identification, characterization, and mechanism of action. Cancer Res 48:1066, 1988.

Montesano R: 1992 Mack Forster Award Lecture. Review: Regulation of angiogenesis in vitro. Eur J Clin Invest 22:504, 1992.

Mutch DG, Powell CB, Kao MS et al: In vitro analysis of the anticancer potential of tumor necrosis factor in combination with cisplatin. Gynecol Oncol 34:328, 1989.

Nemunaitis J: Cytokine-mobilized peripheral blood progenitor cells. Semin Oncol 23(Suppl 4):9, 1996.

Oldham RK: Biologicals and biological response modifiers: Fourth modality of cancer treatment. Cancer Treat Rep 68:221, 1984.

Oldham RK: Biologicals and biological response modifiers: New approaches to cancer treatment. Cancer Invest 3:53, 1985.

Paul WE, Seder RA: Lymphocyte responses and cytokines. Cell 76:241, 1994.

Powrie F, Coffman RL: Cytokine regulation of T cell function: Potential for therapeutic intervention. Immunol Today 14:270, 1993.

Rosenberg SA, Packard BS, Aebersold PM et al: Use of tumor-infiltrating lymphocytes and interleukin-2 in the immunotherapy of patients with metastatic melanoma: A preliminary report. N Engl J Med 319:1676, 1988.

Rosenberg SA, Schwarz SL, Spiess PJ: Combination immunotherapy for cancer: Synergistic antitumor interactions of interleukin-2, alfa interferon, and tumor-infiltrating lymphocytes. J Natl Cancer Inst 80:1393, 1988.

Rosenberg SA, Lotze MT, Yang JC et al: Experience with the use of high dose interleukin-2 in the treatment of 652 cancer patients. Ann Surg 210:474, 1989.

Smith CA et al: The TNF receptor superfamily of cellular and viral proteins: Activation, costimulation, and death. Cell 76:959, 1994.

Tanaka T: Cancer chemoprevention. Cancer 5:11, 1992.

Topolian SL, Soloman D, Avis FP et al: Immunotherapy of patients with advanced cancer using tumor-infiltrating lymphocytes and recombinant interleukin-2: A pilot study. J Clin Oncol 6:839, 1988.

Verhaegen H, De Cree J, De Cock W et al: Levamisole therapy in patients with colorectal cancer. In Terry WD, Rosenberg SA (eds): Immunotherapy of Human Cancer. New York, Excerpta Medica, 1982, p 225.

Wadler S: The role of interferons in the treatment of solid tumors. Cancer 70:949, 1992.

Warren BS, Naylor MF, Eindberg LD: Induction and inhibition of tumor progression. Proc Soc Exp Biol Med 202:9, 1993.

Wattenberg LW: Chemoprevention of cancer. Cancer Res 45:1, 1985.

Weinstein IB: Cancer prevention: Recent progress and future opportunities. Cancer Res 51:5080s, 1991.

West WH et al: Constant-infusion recombinant interleukin-2 in adoptive immunotherapy of advanced cancers. N Engl J Med 316:898, 1987.

Young RC, DeVita VT: Cell cycle characteristics of human solid tumors in vivo. Cell Tissue Kinet 3:285, 1970.

Zimmerman RJ, Gauny S, Chan A et al: Sequence dependence of murine tumor therapy with human recombinant tumor necrosis factor and interleukin-2. J Natl Cancer Inst 981:227, 1989.

MONOCLONAL ANTIBODY THERAPY

Bast R, Klug T, St John E et al: A radioimmunoassay using a monoclonal antibody to monitor the course of epithelial ovarian cancer. N Engl J Med 309:883, 1983.

Colcher D, Esteban J, Carrasquillo JA et al: Complementation of intracavitary and intravenous administration of a monoclonal antibody (B72.3) in patients with carcinoma. Cancer Res 47:4218, 1987.

Dillman RO: Monoclonal antibodies for treating cancer. Ann Intern Med 111:592, 1989.

Epenetos AA, Spooner RA, George AJT: Application of monoclonal antibodies in clinical oncology. Immunol Today 15:559, 1994.

Fitzgerald D, Pastan I: Targeted toxin therapy for the treatment of cancer. J Natl Cancer Inst 81:1455, 1989.

Goldenberg DM: New developments in monoclonal antibodies for cancer detection and therapy. CA Cancer J Clin 44:43, 1994.

Goldenberg DM, Scholm J: The coming of age of cancer radioimmunoconjugates. Immunol Today 14:5, 1993.

Junghans RP, Waldmann TA, Landolfi NF et al: Anti-Tac-H, a humanized antibody to the interleukin 2 receptor with new features for immunotherapy in malignant and immune disorders. Cancer Res 50:1495, 1990.

Kawase I, Komuta K, Hara H et al: Combined therapy of mice bearing a lymphokine-activated killer-resistant tumor with recombinant interleukin-2 and an antitumor monoclonal antibody capable of inducing anti-dependent cellular cytotoxicity. Cancer Res 48:1173, 1988.

Köhler G, Milstein G: Continuous culture of fused cells secreting antibody of predefined specificity. Nature 256:495, 1975.

Lamki LM, Zukiwski AA, Shanken LJ et al: Radioimaging of melanoma using Tc-labeled Mab fragment reactive with a high molecular weight melanoma antigen. Cancer Res 50(Suppl):904s, 1990.

Murray JL, Unger MW: Radioimmuno-detection of cancer with monoclonal antibodies: Current status, problems, and future directions. Crit Rev Oncol Hematol 8:227, 1988.

Murray JL, Zukiwski AA, Mujoo K et al: Recombinant alpha interferon enhances tumor targeting of an anti-melanoma monoclonal antibody in vivo. J Biol Response Mod 9:556, 1990.

Oldham RK, Lewis M, Orr DW et al: Adriamycin custom-tailored immuno-conjugate in the treatment of human malignancies. Mol Biother 1:103, 1988.

Pai LH, Pastan I: Immunotoxins and recombinant toxins for cancer treatment. Important Adv Oncol 3, 1994.

Smith LH et al: Human monoclonal antibody recognizing an antigen associated with ovarian and other adenocarcinomas. Am J Obstet Gynecol 166:634, 1992.

Vitteta ES, Ghetie V: Immunotoxins in the therapy of cancer: From bench to clinic. Pharmacol Ther 63:209, 1994.

Vitteta ES, Thorpe PE, Uhr JW: Immunotoxins: Magic bullets or misguided missiles? Immunol Today 14:252, 1993.

Waldmann TA: Monoclonal antibodies in diagnosis and therapy. Science 252:1657, 1991.

20 Genes and Cancer

David G. Mutch, M.D. and Philip J. DiSaia, M.D.

INTRODUCTION

Cancer is a genetic disease that is the result of alterations in DNA; these alterations are called mutations. Mutations, if they occur in a gene or genes critical for cell growth, may allow a cell to reproduce in an uncontrolled fashion. This uncontrolled growth of a cell or tissue is known as a cancer. Cancer is seldom the result of a single mutation but usually requires several different mutations in many different genes to allow this irreversible and uncontrolled change in cell function. The concept that cancer is the result solely of genetic mutations is relatively new and comes from the last two and one half decades of cancer research. Before the 1970s, the cause of cancer was essentially a black box and its etiology largely unknown. To some extent, it is still unclear, but we no longer believe that defective immunity, viruses, or metabolic errors directly cause cancer. These factors may contribute to the development of this disease, but the basis of cancer lies in an individual organism's DNA and in that individual organism's ability to express the genetic material in a normal fashion. This is simply related to the inherited or altered DNA sequences that make up that individual's genome. Thus, cancer is a disease of abnormal DNA expression. Alterations or differences in the DNA sequences can be expressed by mutations, a change in DNA such that a protein alteration occurs, or polymorphism, a change in DNA that results in a more subtle change in gene function and protein structure. There is a fine line between a mutation and polymorphism (Figs. 20–1 and 20–2).

Heart disease is known to have an inherited component. Individuals can inherit defective genes that alter lipid metabolism, and therefore those people are at risk for development of atherosclerosis and thus have an increased risk of dying of a fatal myocardial infarction or stroke. We also know that the same individual may alter the natural history of his or her disease, to a great extent, by changing the environment. For example, an individual prone to heart disease may decrease the risk of dying by increasing the level of exercise, avoiding obesity, or eating a low-fat diet. Cancer is similar to this example of atherosclerosis in that an individual may inherit a genetic mutation or may be exposed to an environmental insult that predisposes to

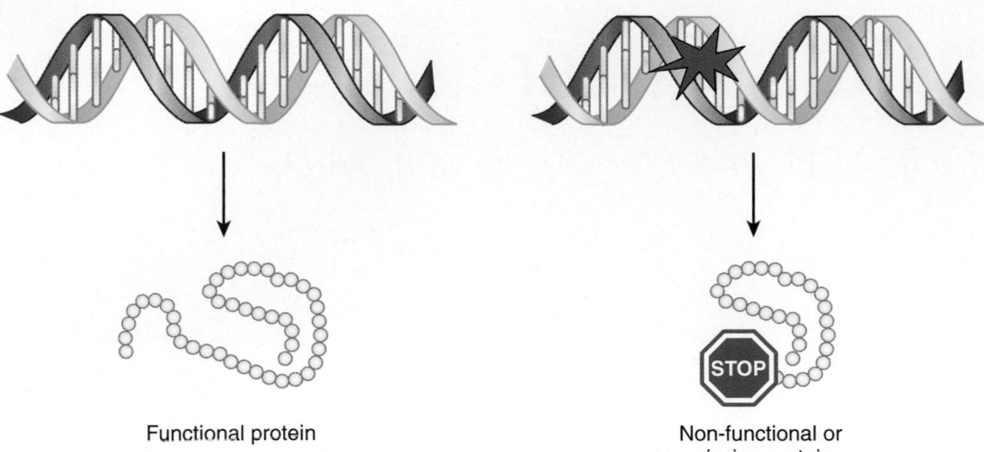

Figure 20–1 Disease-associated mutations alter protein function.

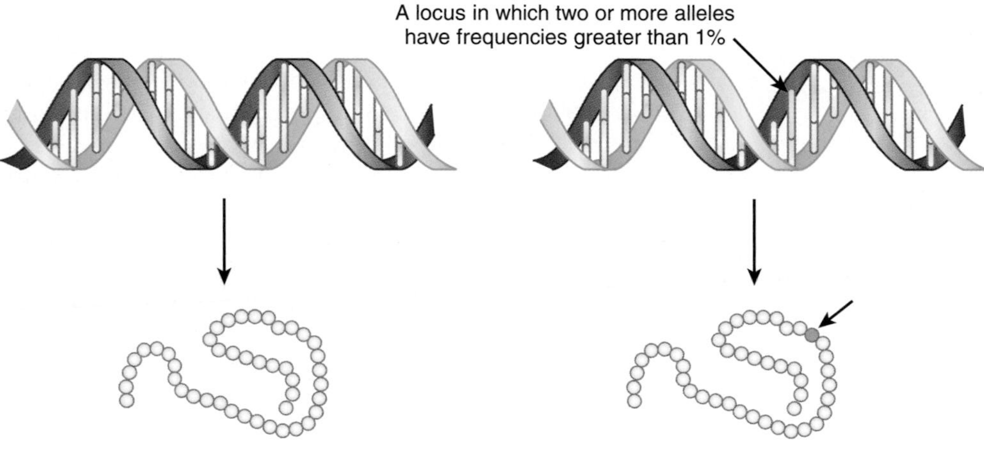

Figure 20–2 A depiction of a polymorphism.

the development of a cancer. Such insults can occur from everyday living or as the result of repetitive exposure to smoke, other substances, and other environmental factors that cause DNA damage. In addition, any process that causes cells to divide, such as ovulation, can allow an opportunity for an error in DNA replication to be made. As an example, an individual prone to the development of ovarian cancer can reduce her risk of developing this disease by taking oral contraceptives. This will inhibit ovulation and decrease the damage to the surface of the ovary that could allow a mutation to occur. Cancers, unlike many other inherited diseases, including the example of atherosclerosis that require only a single mutation, become apparent after there is an accumulation of several genetic injuries or mutations. In this respect, cancer is different than most inborn errors of metabolism because more than one genetic event is required to allow expression of the disease. One does not inherit cancers as one would inherit cystic fibrosis or sickle cell disease. One may inherit a mutation in a gene that predisposes one to the development of cancer, but most cancers are due to the accumulation of somatic mutations that result from the process of normal living. Viruses, smoking, eating charcoal-broiled steak, or simply random mistakes made during DNA replication may cause these mutations. After all, a replicating cell must copy three billion base pairs—with each division mistakes will occur.

That progression from a normal to a malignant cell is the result of the accumulation of a series of mutations has probably best been demonstrated in colon cancer by Burt Vogelstein and colleagues (Fig. 20–3). In this model, a series of mutations must occur that involve tumor suppressor genes and oncogenes; a benign tumor progresses to a malignant tumor as the necessary mutations occur during a prolonged and somewhat erratic interval.

In general, three broad classes of genes are involved in the development of cancer. These are tumor suppressor genes, oncogenes, and mismatch repair genes. Tumor suppressor genes are responsible for making a product that inhibits cell growth. These types of genes are expressed in a recessive manner, and therefore both alleles need to be lost before the phenotype becomes apparent. Oncogenes are expressed dominantly and are usually responsible for a product that promotes cell growth. If they express their protein in an uncontrolled manner, uncontrolled growth occurs. Mismatch repair genes are responsible for repairing DNA damage that results from loss of fidelity in normal DNA replication. If one of these genes does not function properly, errors in DNA can accumulate, and ultimately some of these errors will occur in genes critical for cell con-

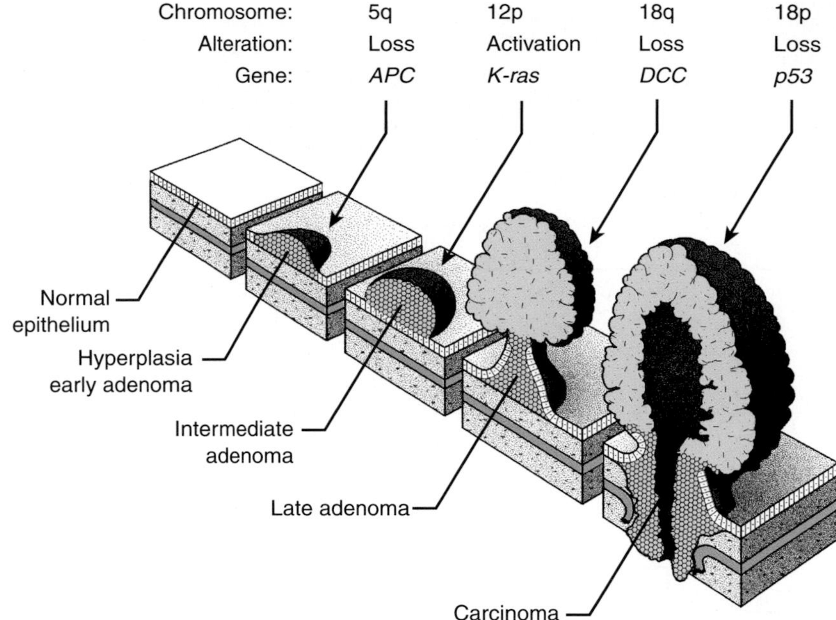

Figure 20–3 A model for colorectal tumorigenesis. This shows the molecular progression of normal colon epithelium to frank cancer.

trol, resulting in uncontrolled cell growth. The development of cancers is therefore not the result of a single error or insult but rather the accumulation of errors over time.

One thing to bear in mind is that mutations are a means of evolution. The paradox of life is that the same mutations responsible for an individual organism's death in the form of cancer or metabolic error can account for the evolution of the species as well. Mutations can be good, bad, or neutral.

GENETIC ALTERATIONS IN CANCER

Genetics is not a new field and has been a study for several centuries from Mendel in 1865 until the present. Johannsen first coined the term *gene* in 1911 as it applied to the unit of a hereditary characteristic. This was further refined to the one gene-one enzyme concept in the 1940s and put forth by Tatum and Beadle. These concepts have been clearly defined in *Drosophila* but apply equally to humans; after all, all living things are defined by their DNA. We have more DNA than other organisms and are therefore more complex, but the DNA behaves the same way in all organisms.

The one gene-one enzyme concept that developed from the ideas expressed by Tatum and Beadle can be summarized as follows:

1. All biologic processes are under genetic control.
2. These biochemical processes are expressed as a series of stepwise reactions.
3. Each biochemical reaction is ultimately under the control of different single genes.
4. Mutation of a single gene results in an alteration of the cell to carry out a single chemical reaction.

The one gene-one enzyme concept has since been refined and extended to cover proteins that are not enzymes. Now further information suggests that some genes combine with others to form unique proteins indicating that a few genes may interact to form more than one protein per gene. The human genome is estimated to contain about 3 billion base pairs and was thought to have between 50,000 and 100,000 genes. Now that the human genome has been sequenced we have discovered that there are only about 30,000 genes. These genes interact much more than we previously believed and are stored on linear strands of DNA, which are combined with certain nuclear proteins and form chromosomes. The genes are not continuous sequences of DNA but consist of coding sequences called exons interrupted by non—coding sequences called introns. Most of the DNA is not made of exons or "expressed DNA"; rather, it is composed of intronic DNA that is usually not expressed in any form and is just filler DNA. An approximation of the size of the human genome and its organization can be seen in (Fig. 20–4). The functional length of the human chromosome is expressed in centimorgans. A centimorgan (cM) is the distance over which there is a 1% chance of crossover during meiosis. Linkage studies indicate that the human genome is about 3000 cM. The average chromosome contains about 1500 genes in 130 million base pairs. Fig. 20–4 shows the estimated physical and functional size of the genome. The physical size is estimated in base pairs, whereas the functional size is estimated in centimorgans. Much of the human genome is not comprised of coded DNA and is therefore not expressed.

DNA is transcribed into RNA that is translated into protein. Therefore, the sequence of DNA base pairs ultimately determines the sequence of the functional proteins within the cell. All cellular functions are expressed in this manner (Fig. 20–5):

$$\text{DNA} \rightarrow \text{RNA} \rightarrow \text{protein}$$

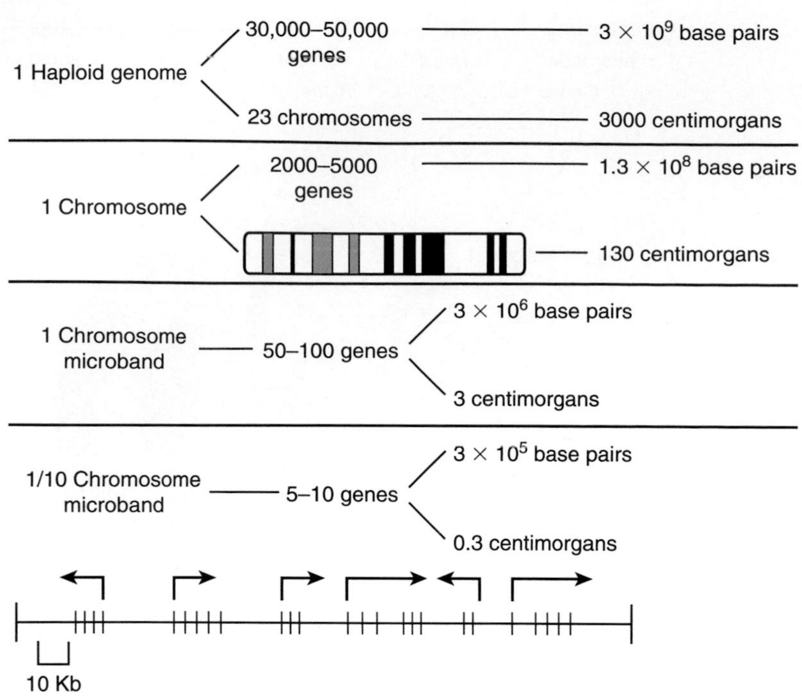

Figure 20–4 The structure of the human chromosome demonstrated in terms of functional units (centimorgans) and physical units (base pairs).

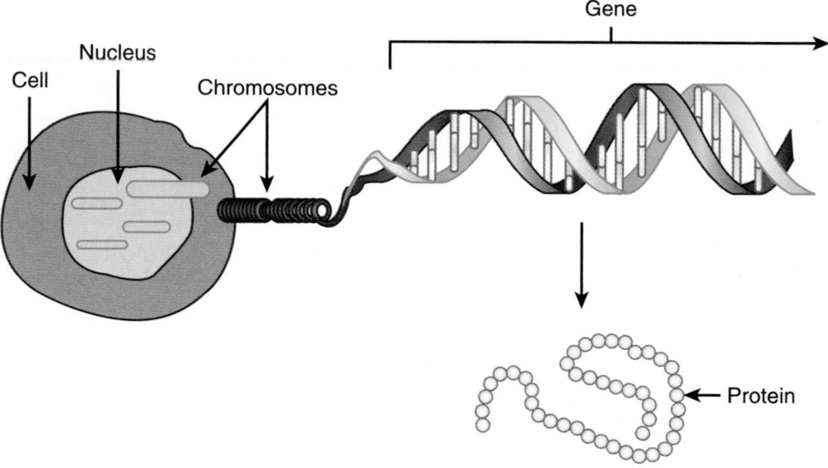

Figure 20–5 The progression of protein synthesis from DNA to RNA to protein. (From National Cancer Institute. Understanding Gene Testing. Rockville: National Cancer Institute; 1995.)

Humans and other mammals may be more complex than other organisms in that pieces of genes may combine with parts of other genes to make a totally new protein or control a separate cell function. Hence, we may essentially increase the number of genes expressed without really increasing the amount of functional DNA or the number of actual genes. Overall about 70% of the genetic material is not expressed.

MECHANISMS OF HUMAN GENE MUTATION

All cancers are due to alterations in DNA structure leading to changes in the proteins responsible for cellular function. All living organisms use the same 20 amino acids as building blocks for proteins. The translation of a nucleotide sequence from DNA to protein is dependent on a triplet code of nucleotides. Each of these triplet codes is called a codon. Some codons have very special functions. The code AUG codes for methionine and this starts the initiation of synthesis (translation) of every protein, The code UAA is a stop codon and ends translation of a protein (Fig. 20–6). Much of the data available about genetic alterations in cancers comes from studies other than of gynecologic malignant neoplasms. These studies often involve hematologic malignant neoplasms like lymphomas and leukemia because pure subsets of cells are easily obtained. More recently, we have been able to improve our study of solid carcinomas because of our ability to study pure tumor preparations and single out cells and isolate the DNA with microdissection and laser capture techniques. Using this technique and techniques like it we can dissect out a single cancer cells, replicate its DNA and evaluate the

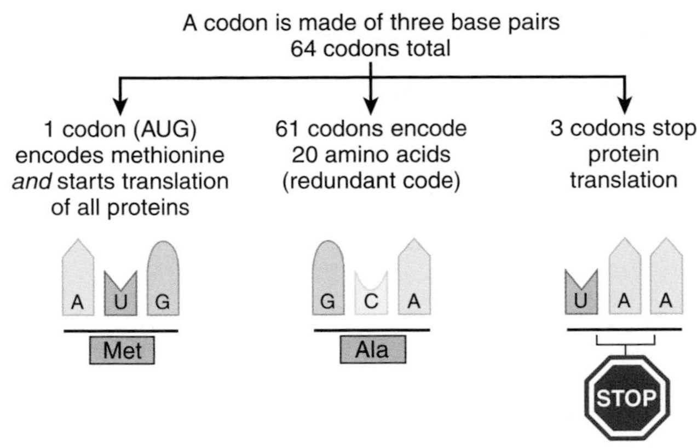

Figure 20–6 Stop codons (Reprinted with permission from ASCO Curriculum: Cancer Genetics and Cancer Predisposition Testing 2nd Edition.)

mutations that occur in this single cell or group of cells. Fig. 20–7 demonstrates the heterogeneity of cancer and why there is a need for these special techniques. Cancer is the result of clonal expansion but as the various cells replicate in and uncontrolled manner they continue to mutate. Initially, cancers usually have a single clonal origin. As the cancer progresses mutations occur and therefore some cells may become genetically different as genetic alterations often accelerate as the cancer continues to progress. Hence the term, mutator phenotype is often applied to cancers. Various types of mutations have been described. These mutations are fundamental to the understanding of cancer and of human evolution. Although many types of mutations can occur, the most common are mentioned here and are listed in Table 20–1. A listing of the specific different mutations found in cancers can be viewed on the Human Gene Mutation Database (HGMD). (*http://www.hgmd.cf.ac.uk/ac/index.php*). These mutations are periodically updated. Cartoons of common mutations can be seen in Figs. 20–8, 20–9, 20–10, 20–11, 20–12, and 20–13)

Table 20–1 CATEGORIES OF HUMAN MUTATIONS IDENTIFIED IN CANCERS

Single base pair substitutions
Types of nucleotide substitution and hypermutable nucleotides
mRNA splice junction mutations
mRNA processing and translation mutations
Regulatory mutations
Deletions
Insertions
Duplications
Inversions
Expansion or contraction of unstable repeat sequences

Single base pair substitutions and point mutations

DNA replication is the result of an accurate yet accident-prone process. The final accuracy of DNA replication depends on the fidelity of the initial process and on the ability of subsequent repair processes to correct any mistakes. Point mutations lead to single changes in the DNA sequence. These single mutations can have very different effects on the reading of a protein, as demonstrated in Figs 20–10 and 20–11. If this mutation is in a regulatory portion of a gene, loss or alteration of regulation of gene expression can occur. If the mutation is in a coding portion of the gene, an altered protein can be formed. HGMD is one of several catalogs of reported point mutations that can be obtained from the Internet.

The most common mutation as the result of substitution occurs in CpG dinucleotides (3′ cytosine-guanine 5′). Data show that these transversions account for about 30% of point mutations. Therefore, they represent the most common substitution mutation. The fidelity of this process is related to the efficiency and accuracy of the

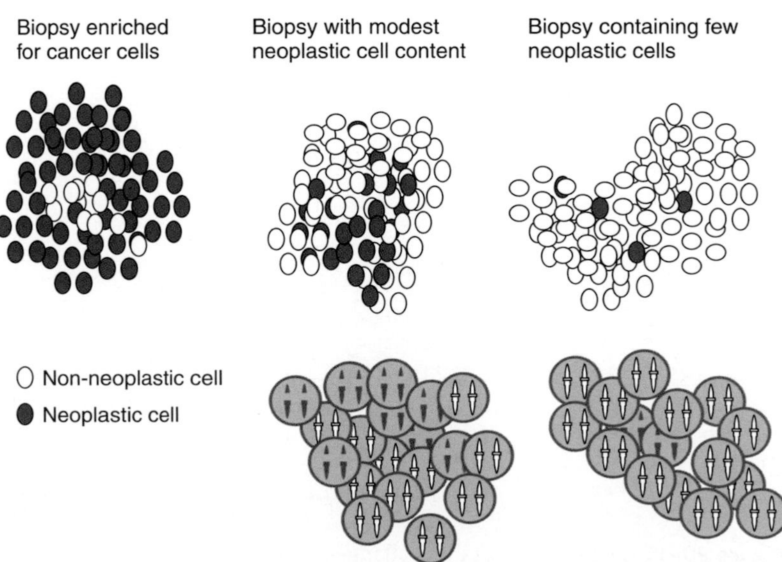

Figure 20–7 Heterogeneity within tumors often prevents accurate evaluation of tumor because of normal contamination.

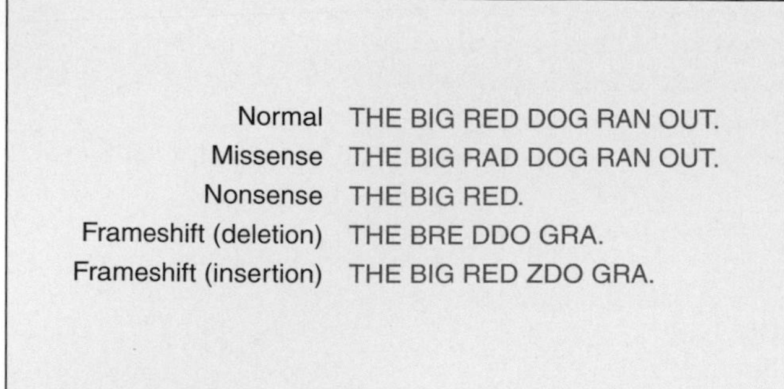

Figure 20–8 Example of how a point mutation (a change in a single base pair) can result in changing the meaning of a gene sequence using a common phrase.

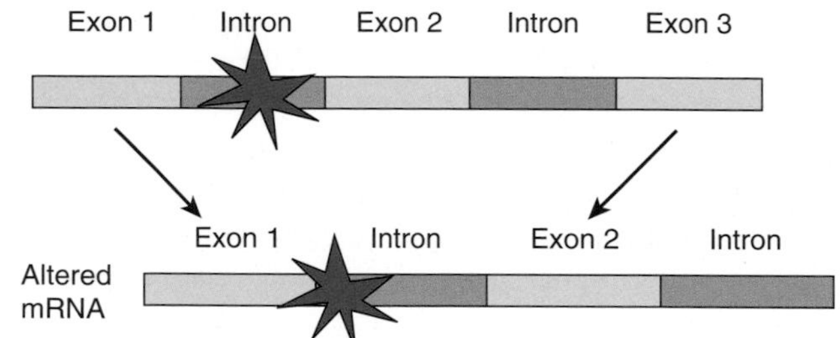

Figure 20–9 Cryptic splice site mutations. Splice site mutation, a change that results in altered RNA sequence.

DNA polymerase responsible for replication. Other types of these small nucleotide substitutions that can also occur are mRNA splice junction mutations, translational mutations, and single deletions. Alternatively, mismatches can occur by slipped mispairing, which leads to single base pair mutagenesis and deletion.

Deletion or insertion of a single nucleotide may be secondary to DNA mispairing during replication. This type of mutation often occurs in runs of identical base pairs and is the result of slippage of a single base pair (Fig. 20–14). This mechanism is similar to larger deletions caused by this same mechanism. The significance of this type of mutation to human malignant neoplasia is as yet undefined. As more information becomes available about mismatch repair, we should have a better estimate of the significance of this type of mutation to cancer formation. However, this slippage is common and similar to the errors found in individuals who have an inherited cancer syndrome, hereditary non-polyposis colon cancer (HNPCC).

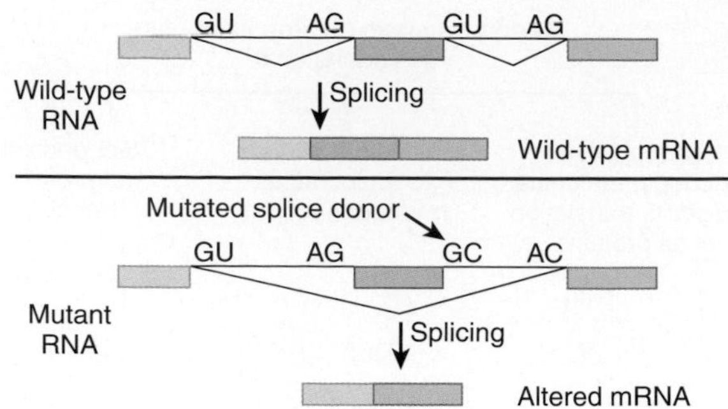

Figure 20–10 Exon skipping splice site mutations. Splice site mutation, a change that results in altered RNA sequence.

CpG dinucleotides are very susceptible to mutations. Methylation of cytosine results in a high level of mutation because of its propensity to undergo deamination. This then forms thymidine and therefore can result in a change of gene expression. The evolution of human genome seems to indicate a progressive loss of CpG islands due to this transition. The frequency of these islands is about 20–30% of the predicted frequency, probably because of the progressive loss of CpG dinucleotides. This excess of transition from cytosine to thymine (C to T) transitions was first reported by Vogel and Rohrborn in a study of the mutations responsible for variants of hemoglobin. Others now also have shown that CpG islands are associated with a high rate of transition supporting the thought that these mutations play a significant role in human disease (Fig. 20–15).

Larger deletions

Gene deletions are responsible for more than 150 inherited diseases. Deletions can range from a few base pairs to several hundred kilobases and are usually classified by size. These are also non-random in that certain sequences appear to be more prone to deletion than others are. This non-randomness is apparent when one evaluates genetic disease. Spontaneous deletions often occur in the same sequences of various genes, indicating that some sequences of DNA are more prone to deletion than others are.

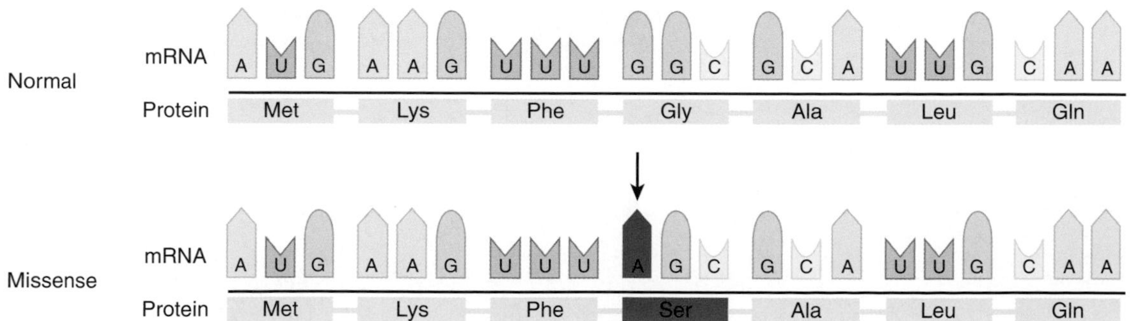

Figure 20–11 Missense mutation, changes to a codon for another amino acid (can be a harmful mutation or neutral polymorphism). (Reprinted with permission from ASCO Curriculum: Cancer Genetics and Cancer Predisposition Testing 2nd Edition.)

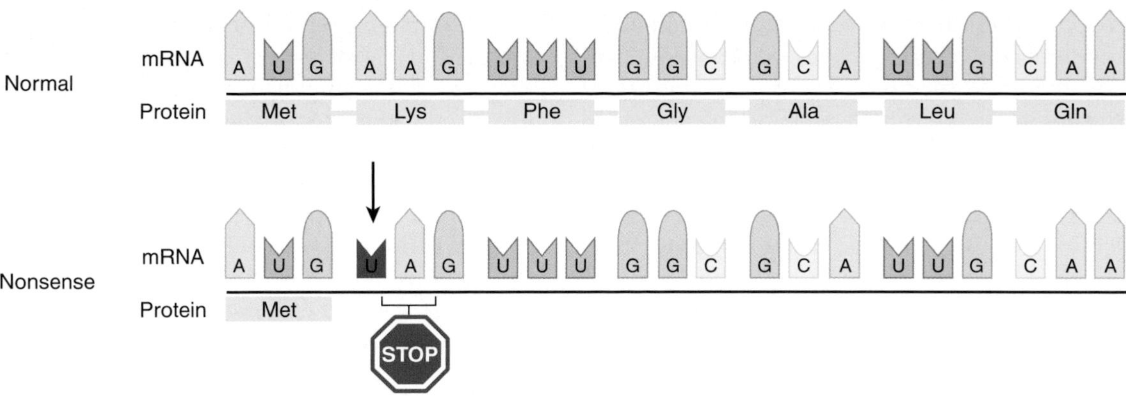

Figure 20–12 Nonsense mutation, change from an amino acid codon to a stop codon, producing a shortened protein. (Reprinted with permission from ASCO Curriculum: Cancer Genetics and Cancer Predisposition Testing 2nd Edition.)

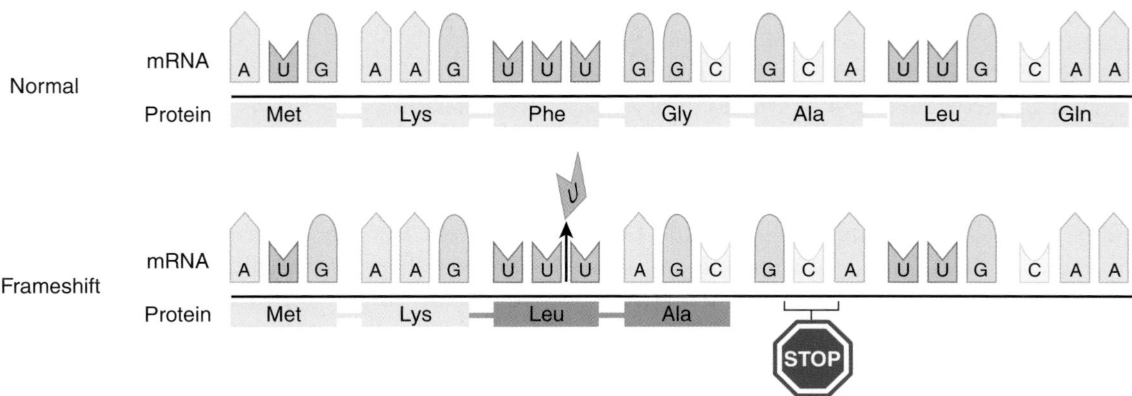

Figure 20–13 Frameshift mutation in which insertion or deletion of base pairs produces a stop codon downstream and (usually) a shortened protein. (Reprinted with permission from ASCO Curriculum: Cancer Genetics and Cancer Predisposition Testing 2nd Edition.)

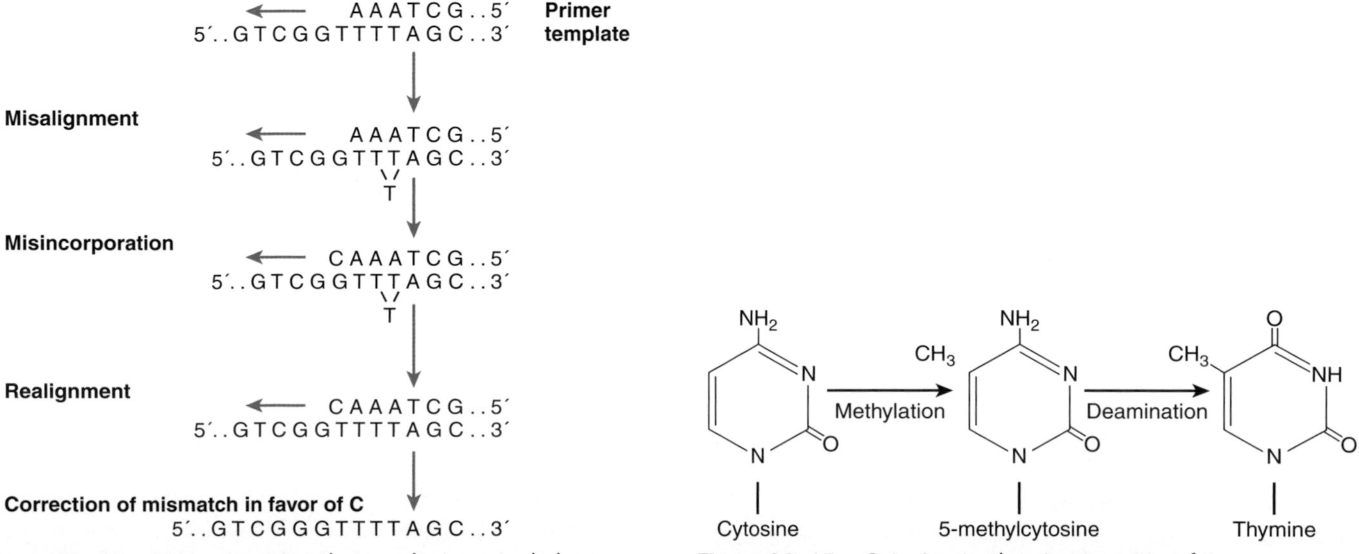

Figure 20–14 DNA mispairing that results in a single base deletion of a T. This causes a complete change of sequence. Attempt at correction adds a G or C to the sequence.

Figure 20–15 Cytosine to thymine transition from methylation. (From Korf B (ed). Human Genetics: A Problem-Based Approach, 2nd ed. Blackwell Publishers, 2000.)

Deletions occur when there is homologous but unequal recombination between gene sequences. Similar sequences in the human genome can cross over during mitosis or meiosis, resulting in a shortened portion of the gene sequence. Long areas of homology (homology boxes) are thought to be the most likely to have this type of mutation. Repetitive DNA sequences are particularly susceptible to deletions because this can allow slippage. This mechanism is called homologue or unequal recombination between repetitive sequence elements. The most common repetitive sequence is the Alu repeat (up to 10^6 Alu sequences are in the human genome). Alu repeats are characterized by an average spacing of 4 kilobases and 300-base pair length separated by a short A-rich region. The Alu element is 70–90% homologous to the consensus sequence. The 3′ ends have a polyA tail, and they contain an internal RNA polymerase III promoter. These Alu repeats are particularly prone to mutation.

There have been a total of 400 gross gene deletions recorded in the HGMD, as well as 3000 or so smaller gene deletions. Almost 2500 gene deletions of 20 base pairs or fewer have been identified. These can be the result of deletion of repeats or a part of the excision repair process. Deletion is not random; there are particular sequences that are more prone to deletion and often contain regions involving guanine repeats. The application of the techniques of molecular biology, such as gene cloning, in situ hybridization, restriction endonuclease mapping of genetic sequences, and polymerase chain reaction analysis of gene transcription, has led to the conclusion that a given chromosome abnormality may be associated with a variety of neoplasms and that a given oncogene may be activated in a variety of human cancers. The most common defects in solid tumors are deletions in specific gene sequences, observed as a loss of part of a banding region or the loss of heterozygosity of a specific genetic allele. Deletion of genetic material in a cancer cell suggests loss of function that regulates cell proliferation and differentiation. Many human solid tumors have been shown to have some type of chromosome deletion. The Tp53 tumor suppressor gene-containing region of chromosome 17p is deleted or mutated in a wide variety of human cancers. The fact that there is such commonality among cancer cell types in the loss of chromosome material suggests that these regions contain genes coding for regulating functions of a wide variety of cell types. Induction of the malignant neoplastic process must involve at least two hits when a tumor suppressor gene is involved. This implies that two mutations or deletions in each of the two alleles are necessary before the effect can be expressed. This is the two-hit theory proposed by Knudson. The possibilities for the two hits necessary to express a recessive gene can be seen in Fig. 20–16. This explained why some people could inherit a predisposition for a malignant disease and also raised the question of whether sporadic cancers could have a genetic basis. In a genetically predisposed cell, the remaining single normal allele may be sufficient to maintain normal growth and regulation; a second deletion or mutation is required to inactivate the remaining normal allele.

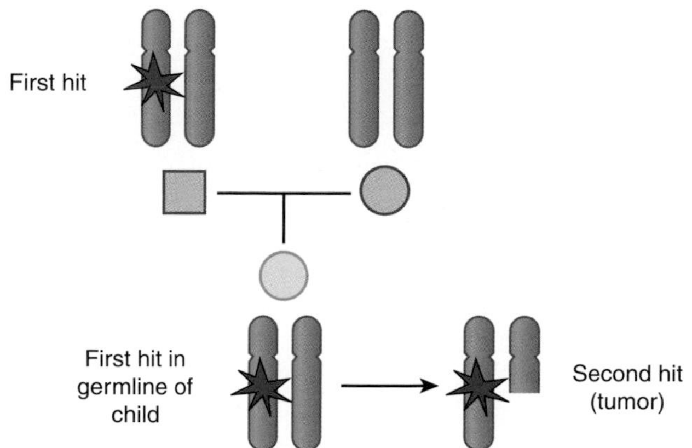

Figure 20–16 Knudsen's two-hit theory that is essential to the concept of tumor suppressor genes. (Reprinted with permission from ASCO Curriculum: Cancer Genetics and Cancer Predisposition Testing 2nd Edition.)

Insertions

Most insertions appear to be small, between one and a few base pairs. This phenomenon has been studied extensively, and these insertions often appear to be non-random in character. There are predisposing factors that lead to these insertions. These insertions can be due to slipped mispairings; they may be mediated by inverted repeat sequences or by symmetric elements. These sorts of DNA sequences are particularly prone to mutation.

Less common are large insertions. The largest insertion known is the 220-kilobase segment inserted into the DMD gene. Alu and LINE (long interspersed nucleotide elements) sequences are especially susceptible to insertion as well as deletion. Mutations are non-random, and some DNA segments are more susceptible to mutation than others are. For example, the myc gene is especially susceptible to insertions; a 50-base pair LINE element has been noted to be inserted in this gene in breast cancer cell lines. The fact that insertional mutations may not be random is underscored by the finding of Fearon who reported 10 independent examples of insertions within the same 170-bp intronic region of the DCC gene involved in the progression of colorectal cancers.

Duplications

Duplication of small parts of whole exons, or even of whole chromosomes, has played a large part in the development of cancer. This phenomenon also has a large role in the evolution of the human genome. Again, the paradox is that mutations are sometimes good and sometimes bad. Duplication of larger segments of DNA may lead to gene amplification.

Gene amplifications can occur in many ways. A gene that is usually present in a single copy in the normal cell may be duplicated or may undergo a small increase in the copy number. Another type of amplification may involve a 10-fold to 100-fold increase in copies of a genetic locus containing key regulatory genes. A third type of amplification can result in the duplication of whole chromosomes. One can envision how amplification has been important over the course of evolution. We have 23 pairs of chromosomes and all other organisms have fewer chromosomes. This is due to millions of years of evolution resulting from innumerable insertions and duplications.

Inversions

Inversions are perhaps the least common type of mutation. In this mutation, a long segment of DNA forms a loop and alters its direction; the 3′ end now becomes the 5′ end. These segments can obviously be large or quite small. The most important inversion event in human disease involves the factor VIII gene, causing severe hemophilia A. There are to date no cancers known to have resulted from a significant inversion.

Translocations

More than 100 common translocations have been observed in malignant cells. Many of these occur consistently in certain specific cancer types, which argues that they are involved in the malignant process of the cell. Some of the translocations may be secondary events in the evolution of more aggressive phenotypic changes. The inherent genetic instability of malignant cells leads to further karyotypic abnormalities as the disease progresses, reflecting additional genetic alterations that increase growth potential. Evidence that malignant transformation does not usually result from a single translocation event comes from the study of patients suffering from ataxia-telangiectasia who are at high risk for leukemia. These patients have lymphocytes with a characteristic translocation present for many years before a malignant change develops. Table 20–2 gives some examples of translocations in solid tumors.

Table 20–2 TRANSLOCATIONS IN SOLID TUMORS

Tumor	Translocation
Breast adenocarcinoma	t(1)(q21–23)
Leiomyoma (uterus)	t(12;14)(q13–15;q23–24)
Melanoma	t(1)(q11–12)
	t(1;6)(q11–12;q15–21)
	t(1;19)(q12;p13)
	t(6)(p11–q11)
	t(7)(q11)
Ovarian adenocarcinoma	t(6;14)(q21;q24)
Rhabdomyosarcoma	t(2;13)(q35–37;q14)

Modified from Solomon E, Borrow J, Goddard AD: Chromosome aberrations and cancer. Science 254:1153; 1991.

A common finding in cancers is some form of genetic instability. This is most clearly manifested in the disease called hereditary non-polyposis colon cancer (HNPCC), this is also known as Lynch II syndrome. This disease is characterized by genetic instability at microsatellite sequences and has been linked to several mismatch repair genes. Mutation rates in cells that are positive for mismatch repair defects is orders of magnitude higher than mismatch repair intact cells. Cancers in patients with this hereditary disease may serve as a model for sporadic disease as mutations that occur in the sporadic tumors are often very similar. The same genes and sequences seem to be targeted. For instance, Krawczak demonstrated that the bulk of single base substitutions in the TP53 gene in sporadic cancers strongly resemble those found in inherited cancers.

CANCER EPIGENETICS

Epigenetics refers to alternate types of gene expression that are not specifically related to differences in the genotype. This is a concept of differential expression of the genotype based on factors outside of the genome. Interestingly, these differences can be inherited and appear to be quite stable. Epigenetic changes basically refer to alterations in DNA expression not related to the actual sequence and can involve chromatin structure, histone modification, changes in transcriptional activity and most easily measured in mammals, changes in methylation of CpG loci.

Methylation is the only known covalent modification of DNA in normal mammalian cells. This change occurs at the fifth position of cytosine at 5′CG-3′ dinucleotides. About 80% of these types of dinucleotides are methylated and are probably therefore important in cell control and gene expression. Generalized hypomethylation is present in colorectal cancers and endometrial cancers early on in the development of these diseases but the exact cause and effect of this observation is unclear. Presumably, hypomethylation allows some genes to be overexpressed. Alternatively, some regions on some genes, particularly the promoter region of mismatch repair genes, can cause gene silencing (Fig. 20–17). This allows a tumor suppressor gene to be silenced, hence promoting the development of that cancer. Changes in methylation status are not clonal. Hence, some cancers can have different gene expression in the same cancer because of differential methylation. Changes in methylation status could also cause aberrant chromosome condensation during division and result in abnormal chromosome segregation. Hence, there are several ways that epigenetics could affect tumor behavior.

GENOMIC IMPRINTING AND CANCER

Genomic imprinting is a modification of DNA away from the physical gene (epigenetic modification), which alters the expression of that gene. These alterations often lead to a different expression of the gene and may be passed from

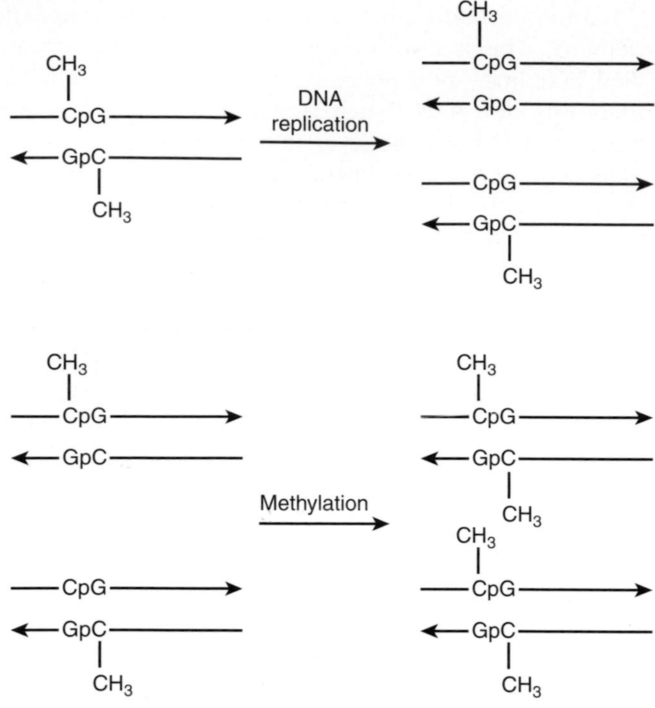

Figure 20–17 Methylation can cause gene silencing. (From Korf B (ed). Human Genetics: A Problem-Based Approach, 2nd ed. Blackwell Publishers, 2000.)

generation to generation. However, the specific expression of these modifications may change from generation to generation (Fig. 20–18). These epigenetic alterations appear to occur commonly in human malignancies and because of their unique properties may lead to novel forms of therapy.

Assumptions made in the Mendelian genetics we apply to human cancers are that the maternal and paternal allele are equivalent. We also assume that both copies of the gene are necessary for normal function. This is not true with respect to imprinting. An example of imprinting is the differences noted between the mule and the hinny. The mule is the cross between the maternal horse and paternal donkey. It is much larger than the hinny that is a cross between the maternal mule and paternal horse. Though these two have the same genomic equivalent they are distinctly different indicating differential expression of maternal and paternal genes.

Examples of genomic imprinting and cancer are the hydatidiform mole and the teratoma. The hydatidiform mole is composed of paternal chromosomes, and the teratoma is composed of only maternal chromosomes. These examples demonstrate that not only does it take 46 chromosomes to make a human being, but there must also be a balance between maternal and paternal elements.

GENETIC ALTERATIONS THAT CAUSE CANCER

Oncogenes

The past 25 years have contributed significantly to our understanding of the molecular mechanism of cancer and have identified three types of molecular aberrations that can lead to cancer: dominant transforming genes called oncogenes, recessive transforming genes called tumor suppressor genes, and genes responsible for repairing DNA errors called mismatch repair genes. Many oncogenes have been isolated as forms of proto-oncogenes acquired by RNA tumor viruses. We have known for many years that viruses can cause malignant tumors in animals. The link noted in animals spurred a great deal of research aimed at identifying the cancer-causing genes carried by the viruses and finding the human genes that were affected. These investigations surprisingly revealed that the genes implicated in malignant disease were often altered forms of viral genes. These were probably acquired when the virus

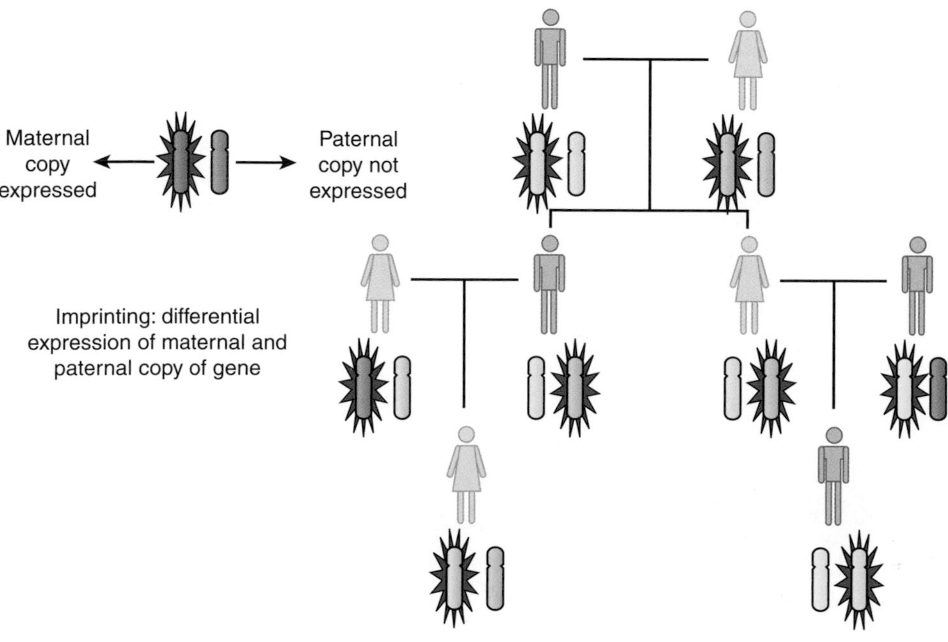

Figure 20–18 Significance and mechanism of imprinting. (From Korf B (ed). Human Genetics: A Problem-Based Approach, 2nd ed. Blackwell Publishers, 2000.)

infected the animal and then moved on to other animals. At other times, the viruses activated host genes that were normally quiescent. The normal versions of these pirated and activated genes, now termed proto-oncogenes, carried codes specifying the composition of proteins that encourage and stimulate cell replication. These growth-promoting genes come in various forms. Some specify the amino acid sequences of receptors that are found on the cell surface and bind to molecules known as growth factors. When bound by such factors, the receptor issues an intracellular signal that ultimately causes cells to replicate. Other growth-promoting genes code for proteins that lie inside the cell and govern the propagation of intracellular growth signal. A third group encodes proteins that control cell division and are under nuclear control. These oncogenes can be activated via several mechanisms. The oncogene can be amplified and many copies of the gene can become activated. Occasionally, the gene may be translocated to another chromosome where, under the influence of another promoter it promotes uncontrolled growth.

The three classes of oncogenes are controlled differently. The first is comprised of a group of peptide growth factors and their receptors. Included in this group would be the peptide growth factors and their receptors like epidermal growth factor receptor (EDGFR) or platelet-derived growth factor (PDGFR). These peptide growth factor receptors likely serve as stimulatory cofactors rather than the actual force that drives the malignant process. Targeted therapy is becoming a reality as our understanding of these cancer-promoting entities. There are unique molecules that are aimed at these gene products or proteins activated by these factors. Examples would be:

1. Herceptin (trastuzumab), a monoclonal antibody that blocks Her/2neu;
2. Gleevec (imatinib mesylate), which partially blocks the activity of c-kit, BCR-ABL, and some other tyrosine kinases;
3. Erbitux (cetuximab), a monoclonal antibody that binds epidermal growth facto receptor; and
4. Iressa (gefitinib), a small molecule that directly inhibits certain isoforms of epidermal growth factor receptor.

Another class of oncogenes comes from non-membrane traversing extranuclear growth factors. These would include G-proteins and the ras gene family. Finally, there are oncogenes of the nuclear regulatory variety such as myc. A schematic of oncogenes representing their function can be seen in Fig. 20–19.

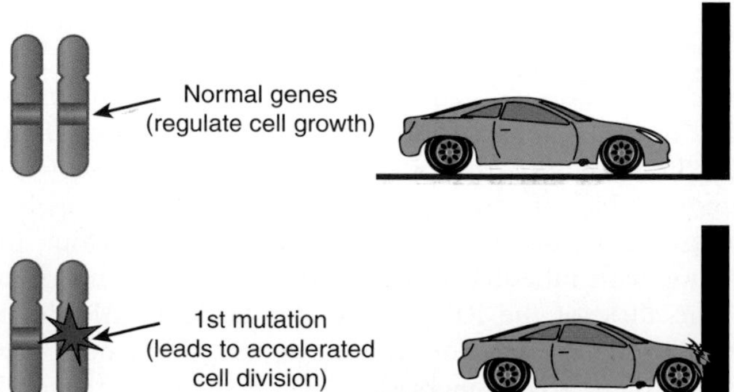

Figure 20–19 Schematic of oncogene function.

The discovery that viral genes had human counterparts introduced the intriguing possibility that human cancers, including the majority not caused by viruses, might originate from mutations that convert useful proto-oncogenes into harmful genes, that is, oncogenes. Consistent with this notion, studies indicated that alteration of just one copy, or allele, of these proto-oncogenes was enough to transform and render cancerous some types of cells growing in culture. Such dominant mutations cause cells to overproduce a normal protein or make an aberrant form that is overactive. In either case, the result is that stimulatory signals increase within the cell even when no such signals come from the outside.

It is ironic that research on animal RNA tumor viruses (retroviruses) having no ability to cause human cancer provided the first key to uncovering the identity of some oncogenes and the verification that they actually exist. These retroviruses, which infected chickens, rodents, cats, and monkeys, were extremely tumorigenic in that infected animals often showed tumors on initial exposure to the virus. One of these viruses, the Rous sarcoma virus of a chicken, was found to carry a specific gene that it used to transform infected cells to a malignant state. This type of transforming oncogene was termed a viral oncogene. A single oncogene carried onto a chicken cell by a Rous sarcoma virus was able to derail and redirect the entire metabolism of the cell, forcing it to grow in a malignant fashion.

In 1976, Varmus and Bishop found that the oncogene in the Rous sarcoma virus was not a viral gene at all; instead, it rose directly from a pre-existing cellular gene that had been captured by an ancestor of the Rous sarcoma virus. Once captured, this gene was used by the Rous sarcoma virus to transform mammalian cells. The early ancestor of the Rous sarcoma virus was capable of replicating in infected cells but was unable to transform them; it instantly gained tumorigenic potency by kidnapping this normal cellular gene, the proto-oncogene. In the end, this work by Varmus and Bishop revealed much more about the cell than it did about the Rous sarcoma virus, because it pointed to the existence of a gene residing in a normal mammalian genome that possessed potent transforming ability when appropriately activated, in this case by a retrovirus. Here was clear proof of the presence of at least one gene in the normal cellular DNA that might serve as one of the target genes activated by non-viral carcinogens of the retrovirus; such non-viral agents might also activate this proto-oncogene, converting it to a powerful oncogene. A cell carrying such a mutant gene might, in turn, respond to this damage by launching a program of deregulated growth and thus become a cancer cell.

The information uncovered concerning retroviruses and oncogenes provided little immediate comfort to investigators interested in the origins of human cancer.

Retroviruses, like Rous sarcoma virus, never infected humans and therefore could not act to mobilize human proto-oncogenes. The possible connection came from a notion that many such proto-oncogenes could be activated through an alternative route. Changes in the DNA sequence created by chemical or physical rearrangement might substitute for the virus. Mutations induced by these chemical or physical conditions in the genomes of target cells in one or another tissue might be as effective as retroviruses in activating latent carcinogenic potential in the proto-oncogenes. By the early 1980s, these suspicions were validated: mutated genes (proto-oncogenes) were found in human tumor genomes. In each case, a change in the sequence of the gene was identified as being responsible for converting a proto-oncogene into an active oncogene. For example, a ras oncogene in one human bladder carcinoma was found to have arisen through a single base change that altered the DNA sequence of a precursor proto-oncogene; myc oncogenes arose through gene amplification in various malignant neoplasms.

Next, researchers tried to ascertain how these genes succeeded in transforming cells. A simple theme emerged that makes it possible to understand and explain the mechanism of action of most if not all of the oncogenes. This comes through the understanding of how cells regulate their own growth. The growth and division of a normal cell residing in a particular tissue is controlled largely by its surroundings. A normal cell rarely if ever decides its own rate of proliferation; rather, it responds to the signals or messages from surrounding cells. These messages, which may carry growth-stimulatory or growth-inhibitory information, are conveyed by growth factors released by surrounding cells, traverse the intercellular space, and bind to the cell surfaces. These cells then respond to these growth signals by activating their synthetic machinery, copying their DNA, and dividing. A normal cell will never commit itself to such a growth program without having been simulated by these external signals. Each cell possesses complex machinery that enables it to receive these signals, process them, and launch a growth program. The machinery consists of an array of proteins that functions to acquire growth-activating signals and transmit them throughout the cell. These proteins include:

1. cell surface receptors that recognize the presence of growth factors in the extracellular space and transmit signals into the cell's interior,
2. cytoplasmic signal transducers that become activated by these receptors and then pass signals farther into the cell, and
3. nuclear transcription factors that are activated by the cytoplasmic signal transducers and in turn respond by activating entire banks of cellular genes.

These activated gene banks together orchestrate the cell's growth program; they detail events that, acting in concert, enable the cell to grow and divide. Proto-oncogenes encode many of the proteins in this complex signaling circuitry that enable a normal cell to respond to exogenous growth factors. Oncogenes participate in this signaling circuitry by selecting aberrantly functioning versions of the components of this circuitry. Oncogene proteins succeed in activating these signal circuits even in the absence of stimulation by extracellular growth factors. In doing so, they force a cell to grow even when its surroundings do not contain some of the clues that are normally required to provoke growth.

Other researchers suggest that mutations in at least two proto-oncogenes have to be present and that only certain combinations of mutations lead to malignant change. These findings suggest that individual oncogenes, although powerful controllers of cell metabolism, are not capable of causing malignant neoplasms by themselves. Thus, oncogenes cannot explain most cancers by themselves. This view was strengthened by the discovery of more than a dozen different oncogenes in human tumors (Table 20–3). However, on careful evaluation, only about 20% of tumors turned out to carry expected alterations. None of the tumors had pairs of cooperative alterations sometimes found in cultured cells. It also appeared that the inherited mutations responsible for predisposing people to cancer were not oncogenes. The concept of a recessive-type antioncogene was conceived. This type of gene is called a tumor suppressor gene. This class of gene appears to be equally important in the development of cancer.

Tumor suppressor genes

The direct identification of tumor suppressor genes has been more difficult than the identification of oncogenes. Tumor suppressor genes were first conceived of in a theoretical sense long before any were actually identified. Harris was the first to demonstrate that the malignant characteristics of a cell could be suppressed when malignant cells were fused with non-malignant cells. Furthermore, loss of portions of chromosomes can be associated with malignant transformation, and transfer of a normal chromosome can reverse these traits into the malignant cells. These data suggested a recessive type of control in normal cells. A schematic of a tumor suppressor gene can be seen in Fig. 20–20.

The first tumor suppressor gene cloned was the Rb gene; it is the defective gene in retinoblastoma. Knudson extensively studied the epidemiology of retinoblastoma. Most cases of retinoblastoma are sporadic, but there are some cases that appear to be clustered around families. He noted that cases of familial retinoblastoma were more likely to be bilateral or multifocal. On the basis of these data, he developed the two-hit hypothesis that bears his name (see Fig. 20–16). That is to say that two mutagenic events are required for retinoblastoma to develop. In patients with inherited disease, the first hit was inherited in one allele of the RB gene in the germline. Although one abnormality was not enough for development of the disease, there was an increased likelihood that the second allele would be damaged during eye development. The

Table 20–3 FUNCTIONAL CLASSIFICATION OF SELECTED ONCOGENES AND ASSOCIATED HUMAN TUMORS		
Function	**Oncogene**	**Associated tumours**
Growth factor	*hst*	Gastric cancer
	KS3	Kaposi's sarcoma
Growth factor receptor	*Neu-erB-B2*	Breast, ovary, gastric cancers
	erb-B	Breast cancer, glioblastoma
	trk	Papillary thyroid, colon cancers
Signal transducing (GTP-binding) proteins	Ha-*ras*	Bladder cancer
	Ki-*ras*	Lung, colon cancers
	N-*ras*	Leukemias
	gsp	Pituitary tumors
Protein kinases	*raf*	Gastric cancer
	met	Osteosarcoma
	abl	Leukemia/lymphoma
Nuclear transcription factor	*myc*	Lymphomas, carcinomas
	N-*myc*	Neuroblastoma
	L-*myc*	Small cell lung cancer
Membrane protein	*bcl-2*	Follicular, undifferentiated lymphoma
	mas	Breast cancer
	ret	Papillary thyroid cancer

From Mastrangelo MJ et al: Gene therapy for human cancer: An essay or clinicians. Semin Oncol 23:4, 1996.

hypothesis of two mutational events developed by Knudson applies specifically to tumor suppressor genes.

Tumor suppressor genes have proved more difficult to identify, and many techniques have been used to locate such genes within the human genome. Cytogenetic studies provide some clues to the location of tumor suppressor genes. A significant percentage of patients with retinoblastoma or some patients with Wilms' tumor have large deletions in 13q14 or 11p13, respectively. These are the regions of the respective tumor suppressor genes responsible for each malignant neoplasm. Significant loss on 5q is associated with adenomatous polyps of the colon. This can

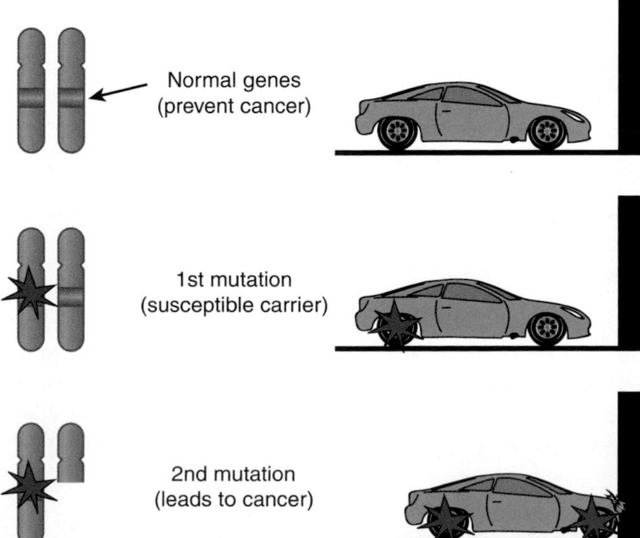

Figure 20–20 Schematic of tumor suppressor gene function. (Reprinted with permission from ASCO Curriculum: Cancer Genetics and Cancer Predisposition Testing 2nd Edition. Schematic of tumor suppressor gene function.)

be measured on a gel during electrophoresis and is called loss of heterozygosity. Although recurrent loss of a chromosome region associated with a specific malignant neoplasm is highly suggestive that this region is important in the development of the cancer, it is not sufficient to prove that there is a tumor suppressor gene in this region. Fig. 20–16 shows the possible combinations of loss that would lead to the expression of a tumor suppressor gene. Use of genome-wide linkage scans can further localize the presence of such a gene. Much smaller areas of deletion can be detected by molecular techniques such as pulsed-field electrophoresis.

When scientists were first trying to identify the regions of loss, they used DNA probes for specific regions of chromosomes. If allelic loss is noted, this is called loss of heterozygosity; and if this loss is disproportionate relative to the general population, this suggests a tumor suppressor gene in the region specific for the probe. An example of loss of heterozygosity can be seen in Fig. 20-6. Here, a region on 10q in endometrial cancers indicates the existence of a possible tumor suppressor gene. By use of various markers, a precise location of the tumor suppressor gene can be identified. A contig of the region must then be built and the region sequenced to look for specific genes. Many regions of loss have been identified by this technique. There are many more candidate regions than actual tumor suppressor genes.

The tumor suppressor gene TP53 is a gene associated with many cancers that was identified by searching for loss of heterozygosity. Several other tumor suppressor genes have been identified since. This is almost certainly only the tip of the iceberg, and many more tumor suppressor genes are likely to be discovered as investigators learn more about cancer cell genetics and as the Human Genome Project continues and reaches completion. Several generalizations

Table 20–4 COMPARISON OF ONCOGENES AND TUMOR SUPPRESSOR GENES

Characteristic	Oncogene	Tumor suppressor gene
Number of mutational events in cancer	One	Two
Role of mutation	Gain of function ("dominant")	Loss of function ("recessive")
Germline inheritance	No	Yes
Somatic mutations	Yes	Yes
Genetic alterations	Point mutations, amplifications, gene rearrangements	Point mutations, deletions
Effect on growth control	Activates cell proliferation	Negatively regulates growth-promoting genes
Result of gene transfection	Transforms cells to a partly malignant behavior	Suppresses maglinant phenotype

Table 20–5 TUMOR SUPPRESSOR GENES

Gene	Gene product	Tumor associations
RB1 (13q)*	110-kDa nuclear hypophosphorylated protein, negative cell cycle regulator	Retinoblastoma Osteosarcoma Small cell lung cancer Soft tissue sarcoma Breast cancer Bladder cancer
p53 (17p)	53-kDa sequence-specific DNA-binding protein and transcriptional activator	Li-Fraumeni syndrome Most common alteration in human cancer
DCC (18q)	1447-amino acid transmembrane protein with homology to known adhesion molecules; role in terminal cell differentiation	Colorectal cancer
APC (5q21)	2843-amino acid protein that interacts with membrane-associated cadherin-catenin complexes and with microtubules	Familial adenomatous polyposis Gardner's syndrome
MTSI (9q21)	148-amino acid protein inhibitor of cyclin-dependent kinase-4	Familial melanoma Bladder cancer
BRCAI (17q)	1863-amino acid protein with zinc finger–like domains suggesting function as a transcriptional factor	Breast cancer Ovarian cancer
BRCA2 (13q)	Possibly BRUSH I	Familial breast cancer
VHL (3p)	Protein with short homology to a glycan-anchored membrane protein of *Trypanosoma brucei*, no function assigned	Pheochromocytoma Renal cell cancer Pancreatic cancer Hemangioblastomas of CNS and retina
WT1 (11q)	50-kDa gene, related to the early growth response gene, encodes four 46- to 49-kDa proteins, which appear to function as DNA-binding transcriptional repressors	Wilms' tumor
NF1 (17q11.2)	Neurofibromin (about 2500 amino acids), probably negative regulator for p21 *ras*	von Recklinghausen's neurofibromatosis
NF2 (22q12)	Schwannomin (~600 amino acids), regulator of cellular response to external environment	Neurofibromatosis type 2

*Chromosome location.
From Mastrangelo MJ et al: Gene therapy for human cancer: An essay or clinicians. Semin Oncol 23:4, 1996.

can be made, and a comparison with the activation of oncogenes is constructive. Mutations in oncogenes are gain of function events and lead to increased cell proliferation and decreased cell differentiation. Oncogene mutations do not appear to be inherited through the germline. In contrast, tumor suppressor gene inactivations are loss of function events usually requiring a mutational event in one allele followed by a loss or inactivation of the other allele. This loss of gene function leads to loss of cellular control and unchecked growth. Tumor suppressor genes are recessive, and mutations may be inherited as a germline mutation. Somatic mutations may occur in both types of genes and accumulate throughout life. Comparison of oncogenes and tumor suppressor genes is made in Table 20–4. Common tumor suppressor genes are listed in Table 20–5.

Apoptosis

Apoptosis means programmed cell death and refers to the intentional induction of cell death. Apoptosis is important in the growth and development of an organism because as

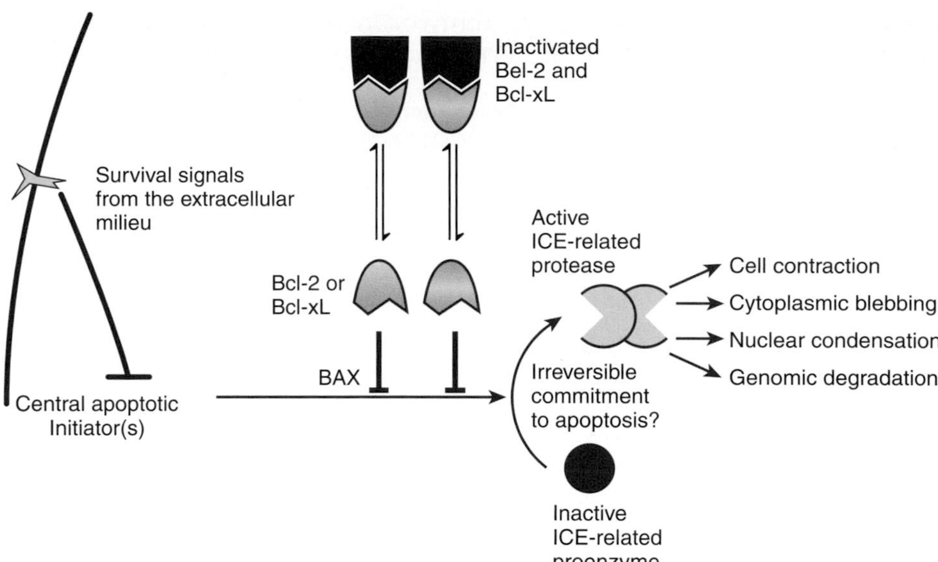

Figure 20–21 Possible pathways and possible factors controlling apoptosis. A signal from outside the cell initiates a cascade of events involving BCL2, BCL-xL, and BAX. This results in the programmed death of the cell. This pathway can be blocked at a number of points, resulting in cell immortality. (ICE, interleukin-1β-converting enzyme.) (From Rudin CM, Thompson CB: Apoptosis and disease: Regulation and clinical relevance of programmed cell death. Annu Rev Med 48:267, 1997.)

an organism matures and differentiates, cells must die to give way to more differentiated and specialized cells. If a cell does not die and becomes immortal, a cancer can result. Apoptosis was first described in the 1970s, but only recently have scientists begun to realize the importance of this phenomenon in organism development, differentiation, and cancer formation. Excitement about this process has been driven by the finding that apoptosis is controlled at the molecular level by genes associated with malignant change (i.e., oncogenes, proto-oncogenes, and tumor suppressor genes). It is also clear that many of these same controlling elements and pathways are active during development. Many believe that understanding the control of the apoptotic process is essential to understanding the control of the developing organism as well as control of senescence. Loss of these aspects of cellular control could lead to cancer.

Apoptosis is a distinct mode of cell death that is responsible for the deletion of cells in normal tissues; interestingly, it also occurs in pathologic conditions. The process of apoptosis is characterized histologically by cell contraction, blebbing of the cell membrane, and condensation of the nucleus. Apoptotic bodies are formed that contain intact organelles; these are eventually phagocytosed by surrounding cells. There is no associated inflammatory response. Cell swelling and disintegration of the cell components characterize necrotic cell death, and there is a marked inflammatory response. On a molecular level, apoptotic death causes cellular enzymes to autodigest the genome into little fragments, and this can be identified on polyacrylamide gels by multiple regular fragments seen as a DNA ladder.

Apoptosis is important in the development of the normal organism and it is important in the development and growth of cancers. It occurs spontaneously in malignant tumors, often markedly retarding their growth, and it is increased in tumors responding to radiation, chemotherapy, heat, and hormone damage. In cancer, apoptosis appears to be a mechanism for deleting cells from the population that have sustained carcinogenic DNA damage; however, when apoptosis of such cells is blocked or inhibited by mutations in genes that help control this process, such as BCL2 or Tp53, these cells are suddenly free to continue replicating and propagating their mutations. This genetic instability may be an early step in the development of cancers. Many of the current cancer treatments, such as radiotherapy and chemotherapy, kill cells by the production of DNA damage. Mutations in BCL2 and Tp53 may then influence the effectiveness of these therapies through their ability to inhibit cell death.

The primary importance of apoptosis related to cancer and cancer treatment lies in its being a regulated phenomenon subject to stimulation and inhibition. Although little is known about how to establish therapeutic agents to affect its initiation, it seems reasonable to suggest that greater understanding of the process of apoptosis might lead to the development of improved treatment possibilities. Inhibitory mechanisms such as BCL2 proto-oncogene expression may be implicated in the development of resistance to therapeutic agents and may contribute to tumor growth and perhaps to oncogenesis by allowing the inappropriate survival of cells with DNA abnormalities. It is likely that other inhibitory mechanisms will be identified, and a better understanding of the apoptotic process may lead to novel treatment regimens by allowing us to control cell death. Apoptosis is not simply a description of cell death, nor is it a spurious trend in the biology literature. It is a fundamental process and is controlled at the molecular level; as such, it can be understood and manipulated. Fig. 20–21 demonstrates how apoptosis may occur.

Mismatch repair defects

A number of mechanisms are involved in the correction of DNA changes that result from exogenous or endogenous mutagenic agents. These mechanisms include base excision repair, nucleotide excision repair, and DNA mismatch

1. 5′AGCTTGGCTGCAGGTG **CACA** GTGTCACGGTCAGGTAC3′
TCGAACCGACGTCCAC **GTGT** CACAGTGCCAGTCCATG

Replication
2. 5′AGCTTGGCTGCAGGTG **CACA** GTGTCACGGTCAGGTAC3′
GT CACAGTGCCAGTCCATG

Mismatch Repair susceptible intermediate **CA** **Slippage**
3. 5′AGCTTGGCTGCAGGTG **CA** GTGTCACGGTCAGGTAC3′
C **GT** CACAGTGCCAGTCCATG

−2Frameshift **Replication**
4. 5′AGCTTGGCTGCAGGTG **CA** GTGTCACGGTCAGGTAC3′
TCGAACCGACGTCCAC **GT** CACAGTGCCAGTCCATG

Figure 20–22 Mismatch repair occurs by slippage of CA within a CA repeat. This results in the deletion of a CA. This is the exact kind of deletion that the mismatch repair system is designed to correct. If the mismatch repair system is not working properly, errors cannot be corrected and mutations accumulate.

repair. The mismatch repair system repairs mistakes that are made in the course of normal division. These mutations often occur in regions of multiple repeats because these regions appear to be particularly prone to DNA slippage. One can intuitively see how this can happen by looking at Fig. 20–22. There are six genes that must work in concert to repair DNA damage. These genes and an example of how we think they work can be seen in Fig. 20–23.

A paradox of human tumorigenesis is that the rates of mutation in normal cells are too low to account for the transformation of benign to malignant. The instability of some colon cancers was the first strong evidence for the so-called mutator phenotype. If a cell cannot repair DNA damage that occurs during the course of normal cell division, mutations can continue to accumulate; eventually enough mutations occur in genes critical for cell control, and cancer results. This is how absence of DNA repair can lead to cancer. Many studies have shown that tumors, which have microsatellite instability, have defects in mismatch repair. Key metabolic genes usually do not have large areas of microsatellite repeats that are particularly prone to mismatch problems. The mutation rate in non-repetitive sequences is also elevated 100 to 10,000 times above that in normal cells with normal mismatch repair. Although microsatellite sequences are largely absent from functional genes, mononuclear repeats in some key genes can lead to their inactivation. Examples of such genes include TGF-BR2H (A_{10}), hMSH3 (A_8), hMSH6/GTBP (C_8), IGF2R (G_8), and BAX (G_8). Paradoxically, instability of chromosome numbers is often observed in tumors without mismatch repair defects; tumors with mismatch repair defects often have stability of chromosome number.

Germline mutations in mismatch repair genes are present in many families with hereditary cancers. These include some colon cancers (hereditary non-polyposis colorectal cancer [HNPCC]), endometrial cancers, and Lynch syndrome type II. Other cancer syndromes associated with mismatch repair are Muir–Torre and Turcot's syndromes. HNPCC accounts for about 5% of all colon cancers and is a syndrome defined by three criteria:

1. an individual must have three relatives with colon cancer, with at least two being first-degree relatives;
2. at least two successive generations must be involved; and
3. at least one of the cancers must have been diagnosed before the age of 50 years.

Seventy percent of patients with HNPCC have a germline mutation segregation around a mismatch repair gene hMLH1 (49%), hMLH2 (45%), and hPMS2 (6%). Endometrial cancers have about a 25% incidence of mismatch repair defects; approximately one-fourth of these are germline mutations, and the rest are largely the result of MLH1 inactivation due to hypermethylation of the promoter region. Mismatch repair will be increasingly investigated and more clearly defined during the next decade.

Telomerase

Normal cells divide; this process is repeated many times as an organism grows and matures. Normal cells stop dividing and terminally differentiate, but cancer cells continue to divide. Cells from younger animals divide more times than do cells from older animals. One difference between normal cells and tumor cells is at the end of their chromosomes. Telomeres, specialized structures at the ends of chromosomes, act as protective caps. In humans, telomeres are made up of 5000–15,000 base pairs of TTAGGG repeats. These terminal structures protect the chromosome ends from exonuclease digestion, prevent aberrant chromosome recombination, and form specific complexes that bind proteins.

Normal cells lose about 50–100 base pairs from the end of each chromosome every time the cell divides. When a telomere loses a critical number of base pairs, it triggers a signal for the cell to stop dividing and for senescence. Cells have developed several mechanisms to get around this terminal trigger. Some of these are uncommon, such as complex recombination and retrotransport techniques. The most common mechanism is the development of an enzyme complex called telomerase, which adds back telomere sequences lost during replication. Cells that have significant telomerase activity are immortal cells like cancer cells or germ cells.

Normal cells lack telomerase activity. Telomerase becomes reactivated in most cancer cells. It is the most prevalent cancer marker known. Therefore, telomerase may be used as a generic cancer marker and as a possible treatment.

GENE THERAPY

One approach to gene therapy for cancer involves the abrogation of oncogene activity or the restoration of

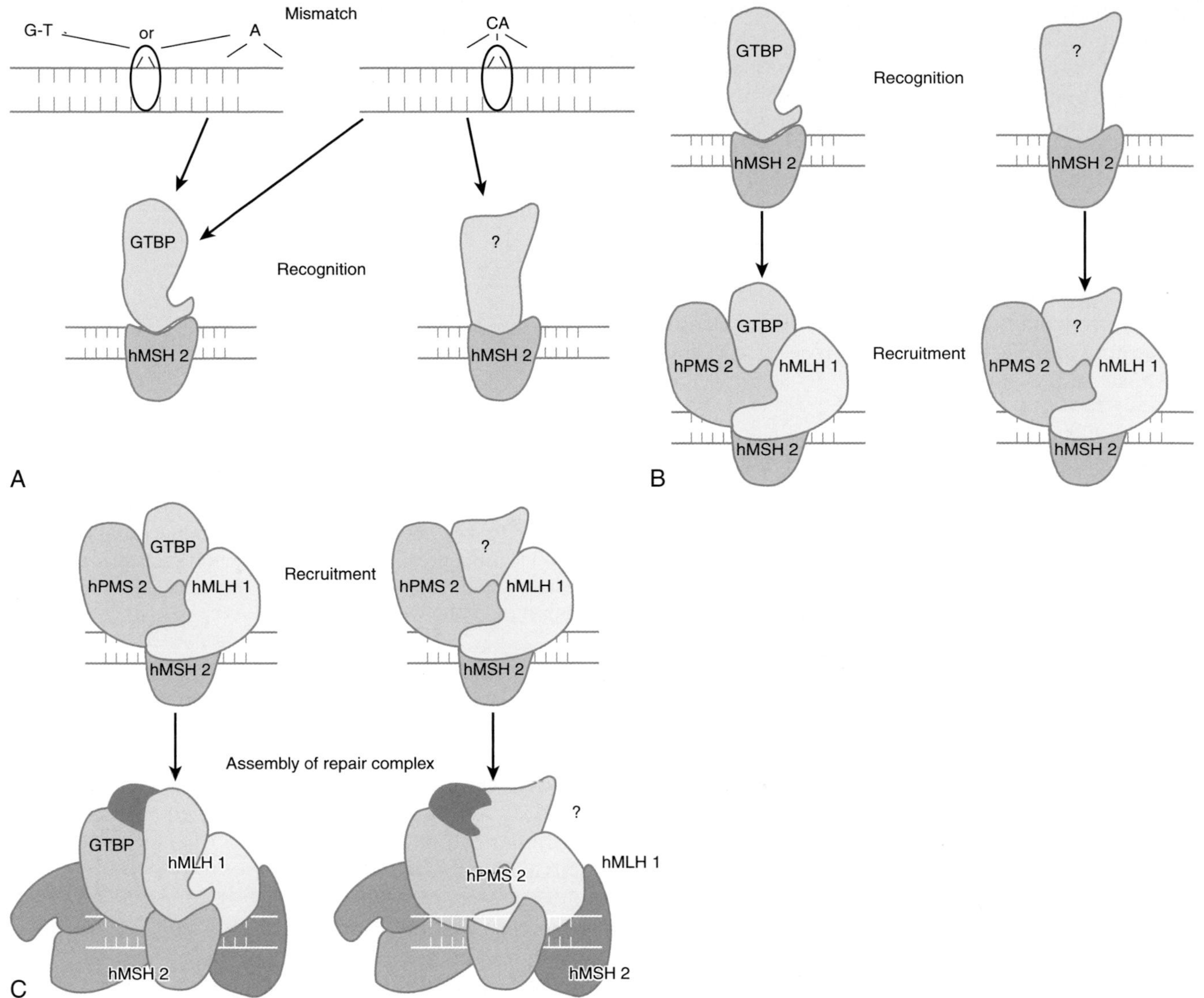

Figure 20–23 Demonstration of how mismatch repair is accomplished by the six proteins required for correction. There must be: *A*, recognition of slippage; *B*, recruitment of repair complex and finally *C*, repair (From Karran P: Microsatellite instability and DNA mismatch repair in human cancer. Semin Cancer Biol 7:15, 1996.)

tumor suppressor gene function. The defective gene could be replaced with a normal gene, a process termed homologous recombination, but progress to date has made this process too inefficient for clinical use. Available vectors can insert a gene into the genome of replicating cells on a random basis, but the faulty genes are not removed. The tumor suppressor gene Tp53 seems a likely target for gene therapy in that defects in the function of this gene are the most common alteration in human cancer. Mice genetically engineered to be without Tp53 look normal at birth; but at 6 months, all have tumors or are dead. Transfer of the wild-type Tp53 gene to deficient cells in vitro will prevent emergence of the neoplastic phenotype, even in tumor cells bearing multiple genetic abnormalities. At this point, the impact of pharmacologic doses of tumor suppressor gene protein on malignant cells is a matter of conjecture because human trials are limited.

Transforming the effects of oncogene function can take one of two approaches. One can attempt to remove the oncogene product or block its function. Alternatively, one could use exogenous or intracellularly generated antisense oligonucleotides in an attempt to block production of the oncogene by preventing the transcription of the chromosomal DNA code to RNA message. Antisense oligonucleotides can be administered systemically. Growth suppression has been achieved in vitro with exogenous antisense oligonucleotides. Several human trials are under way using exogenous antisense oligonucleotides, especially in the study of gene therapy for leukemia.

Major successes with gene therapy for cancer have been limited to in vitro systems in which tumor cells with well-defined genetic defects are easily targeted. Some success has been achieved with systemically administered antisense oligonucleotides in preclinical models. This research revolved around cytokine gene transfer to tumor cells to enhance the development of immunity. Cytokines provide stimulatory signals important for T cell activation, and enrichment of the cytokine milieu by local injection at the site of immunization can promote the acquisition of cellular immunity. By the reasoning that higher and perhaps more effective cytokine levels could be sustained at the immunization site by local production rather than by local injection, tumor cells can be genetically engineered to produce the molecule of interest when it is included in the vaccine preparation. Clinical trials are in progress in patients with squamous cell carcinoma, neuroblastoma, glioblastoma, colon cancer, small cell lung cancer, and ovarian epithelial cancer with use of this technology. Cells are engineered to produce one of several cytokines, including interleukins 2, 4, 5, and 6 as well as macrophage colony-stimulating factor, tumor necrosis factor, and the intracellular adhesion molecule.

MOLECULAR TECHNOLOGIES

Through elucidation of DNA structure by molecular techniques, we can study human genes. Molecular biology is now applied to most branches of clinical medicine. Awareness of the techniques used to assess gene function and structure is essential to understanding the basis of our current knowledge of the molecular biology of disease. DNA is a double helix composed of two coils of nucleotide chains connected by nitrogenous bases. The precise complementary nature of nitrogenous bases provides the basis for the molecular analysis of DNA structure. A gene is a strand of DNA that is transcribed into messenger RNA in the cell's nucleus. The RNA is then translated into protein on the ribosomes. The amino acid sequence is determined by groups of these base pairs of nucleotides called codons. This is referred to as the genetic code. Individual genes make up only a small percentage of the 3×10^9 base pairs of nucleotides per haploid genome in humans. The function of the remainder of the DNA is speculative, but it should be more fully understood with the completion of the Human Genome Project. Characterization of the estimated 50,000–100,000 human genes should be beneficial to the understanding and treatment of genetic disease. The majority of the mapping initiative begun in August 1989 is completed. It will be continually updated and comparison with other species should be most informative.

Restriction enzymes

Because human genomic DNA is large but specific genes are small, cutting DNA into smaller pieces greatly facilitates its study. Enzymes and bacteria make proteins called restriction enzymes or restriction endonucleases; these enzymes enable digestion of DNA into smaller pieces. These restriction enzymes are native to the organism and protect against its destruction by foreign DNA, such as viruses. The restriction enzymes recognize specific sequences and cut every time this particular array of bases is encountered. They are named for the organism in which they are identified as well as the strain. For example, EcoRI was isolated from *Escherichia coli*, strain R, and was the first such enzyme obtained from this organism. This enzyme recognizes the sequence GAATTC and cuts between the G and A (Fig. 20–24).

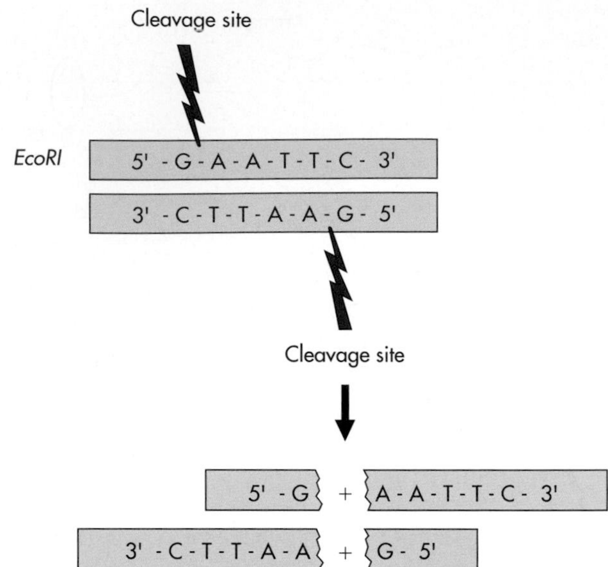

Figure 20–24 Restriction enzymes (endonucleases) recognize specific sequences and cut every time this particular array is encountered. EcoRI recognizes the sequence GAATTC, and the enzyme cuts between the G and A.

Southern blot analysis

Southern blot analysis provides a basis for studying genetic disorders at the DNA level. When a normal gene is identified, it can be used as a probe (i.e., a DNA probe to study a gene's structure in an individual's DNA). If the subject's DNA and the DNA probe are each rendered single stranded and then hybridized, complementary pairing should occur between the DNA probe and the sample DNA. If the pairing does not occur, the subject's DNA does not contain the gene structures present in the probe. For convenience, the subject's DNA is commonly placed on some type of manageable substance, usually a nylon membrane. This is the Southern blot, named for EM Southern, not for a particular geographic region. A Northern blot, which identifies a particular sequence of RNA, consists of a membrane containing immobilized RNA; a Western blot contains proteins.

A series of steps is required to create a Southern blot (Fig. 20–25). DNA is first extracted from nucleated cells (such as leukocytes, trophoblasts). The DNA is then digested with a restriction enzyme into innumerable small pieces. The gene of interest is among these many fragments, but its precise identification and size cannot be determined at this point. The DNA is loaded into an agarose gel, and electric current is applied. During this gel electrophoresis, the current causes small DNA fragments to migrate faster and farther than larger fragments. The gel is then stained

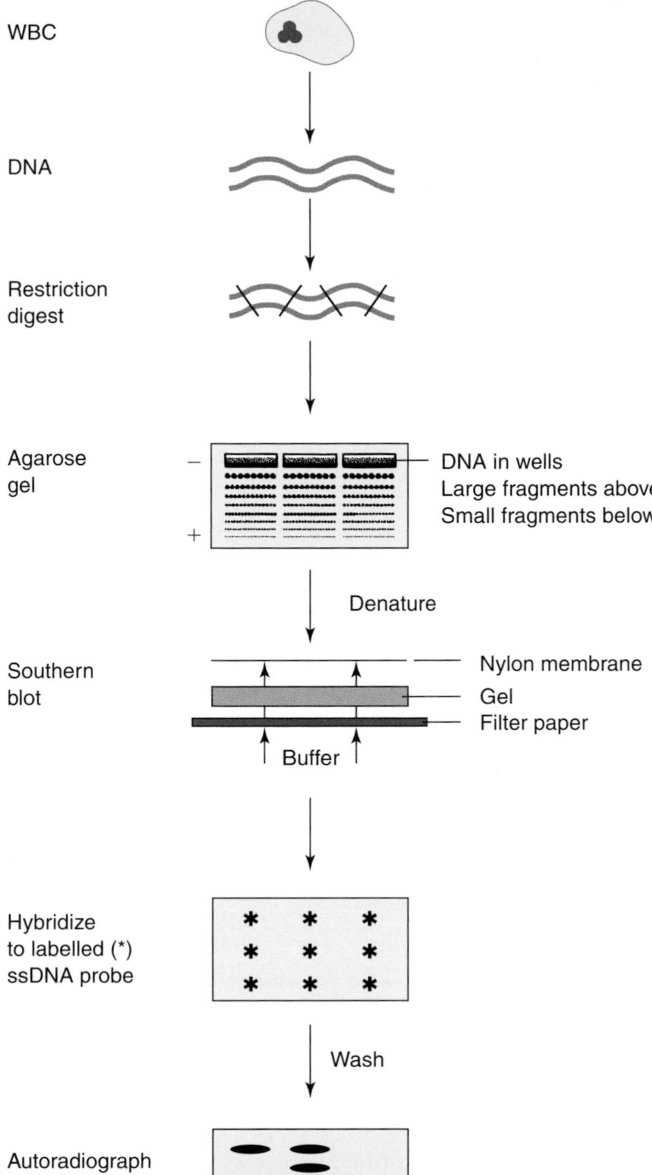

Figure 20–25 Southern blot preparation.

with ethidium bromide, which intercalates between the base pairs and allows visualization of the DNA when it is exposed to ultraviolet light. Because human genomic DNA is so large, the DNA in the lanes appears as a smear but is actually composed of many discrete fragments of varying size. Correct identification of the gene being studied is not yet possible at this point in the procedure.

The DNA contained within the agarose gel is still double stranded at this point. If the gel is exposed to alkali, the DNA will denature into single-stranded pieces. The gel now could be studied by hybridization to a single-stranded DNA probe, but because of the fragility of the gel, the DNA is usually transferred to a nylon membrane (the Southern blot). The gel is placed on a platform in a container with buffer. The nylon membrane is positioned directly above the gel, followed by paper towels on top of the membrane. The buffer passes up through the gel by capillary action, causing single-stranded DNA to migrate to the nylon membrane. The membrane is then baked in a vacuum oven to permanently fix the DNA to the nylon blot. Transfer time may be shortened by using electroblotting or vacuum blotting.

The blot, containing a number of distinct specimens from subjects and controls, can now be hybridized to a DNA probe. For example, if congenital adrenal hyperplasia due to a deletion in the 21-hydroxylase gene is suspected, the blot could be hybridized to a DNA probe for 21-hydroxylase. For hybridization, a DNA probe is labeled with some type of marker, usually a radionuclide such as ^{32}P, although non-radioactive substances such as biotin-avidin may be used. After the probe is labeled, if it is double stranded, it is denatured by boiling or by use of an alkali and placed into a bag or tube with solution and the membrane for hybridization. When hybridization is complete, the unbound, labeled DNA probe is removed by washing. Washes are performed to remove as much of the non-specific material as possible. By washing at high temperatures and low cell concentrations, only sequences that are exactly complementary remain hybridized. When washing is complete, the blot is placed in a plastic wrap inside a cassette containing film at –70°C. The film is developed, and the presence or absence of bands can be determined. If the same number and size of bands are present in the affected individuals and in the control subjects, the gene is present and no obvious large rearrangements of the gene are present. This does not preclude the possibility of the presence of smaller mutations, such as 2-base pair deletions or point mutations. Southern blot analyses are not capable of detecting changes this small unless the mutation alters a restriction enzyme's cut site.

Polymerase chain reaction

Southern blot analysis is labor intensive and generally requires 5–10 mcg of DNA for analysis. The development of polymerase chain reaction (PCR) has greatly simplified DNA analysis and shortened laboratory time. As mentioned, the target gene makes up a minority of the sequences in total chromosomal DNA. Rather than trying to identify a single gene among the many genes per haploid genome with a labeled probe such as in Southern analysis, the PCR allows the exponential amplification of the targeted gene so that its structure can be studied without the need for DNA probes. Only minute quantities of DNA (typically 0.1–1 mcg) are necessary for PCR. One important prerequisite of PCR not required for the Southern blot analysis is that the sequence of the gene, or at the borders of the region of DNA to be amplified, must be known.

The PCR procedure has three steps (Fig. 20–26). First, DNA is heated to 94–95°C to render it single stranded or denatured. Second, the temperature is lowered to 37–55°C, which results in DNA annealing. The reaction solution contains primers that are short pieces of DNA, usually about 20–30 base pairs in length. They are exactly complementary to the ends of each piece of the double-

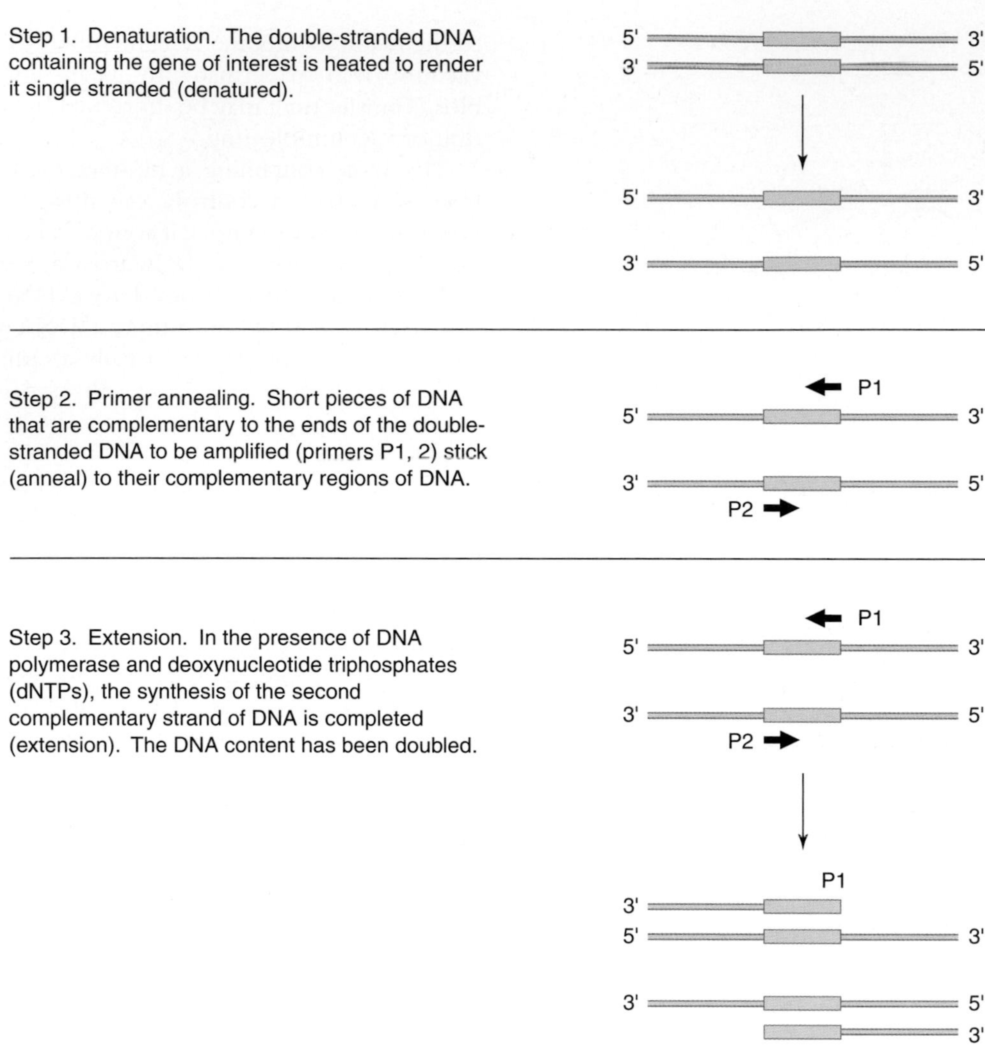

Figure 20–26 Diagram of the polymerase chain reaction. One cycle is shown. The thickened region represents the sequence to be amplified.

stranded DNA to be amplified. When the temperature is lowered, these primers will stick, or anneal, to their complementary regions of DNA. This is why the sequence part of the DNA template must be known. The primers are present in such excess that the DNA template is more likely to anneal to the primer rather than to itself. Third, the temperature is raised to about 72°C in the presence of an enzyme (a heat-stable DNA polymerase such as Taq polymerase) and the deoxynucleotide triphosphates so that the synthesis of the second complementary strand of DNA will be completed. In practice, the primers, buffer, deoxynucleotide phosphates, enzyme, and DNA are mixed together in a tube to a total volume of 25–100 ml and placed in a thermal cycler. Incubator parameters and conditions for PCR must be determined empirically for each set of primers.

After one cycle of denaturation, annealing, and primer extension, the DNA content is doubled; one piece of double-stranded DNA becomes two double-stranded pieces of DNA. Amplification increases exponentially with each cycle so that the final amount of amplified DNA is 2^n, where n equals the number of cycles. After 30 cycles, which is the typical number of cycles used, the gene of interest may be amplified from 230 to well above 1 million times. If Agarose gel electrophoresis is performed on the amplified product of PCR, the product will migrate to a specific point in the gel and appear as a distinct band. Typically, fragments several kilobases in size can be amplified, but sequences up to 10 kilobases have been successfully amplified.

Mutation detection techniques

Detection of genetic mutations is accomplished through a variety of techniques. Southern blotting, described previously, is used to detect large genomic mutations. In general, other mutation detection techniques involve the use of PCR-amplified DNA or cloned DNA. Mutations can be assessed directly through the sequencing of DNA by either a radioactive or fluorescence system. When a sequence from tumor DNA is compared with DNA from a normal tissue source or a published sequence (i.e., from an Internet database), mutations can be detected.

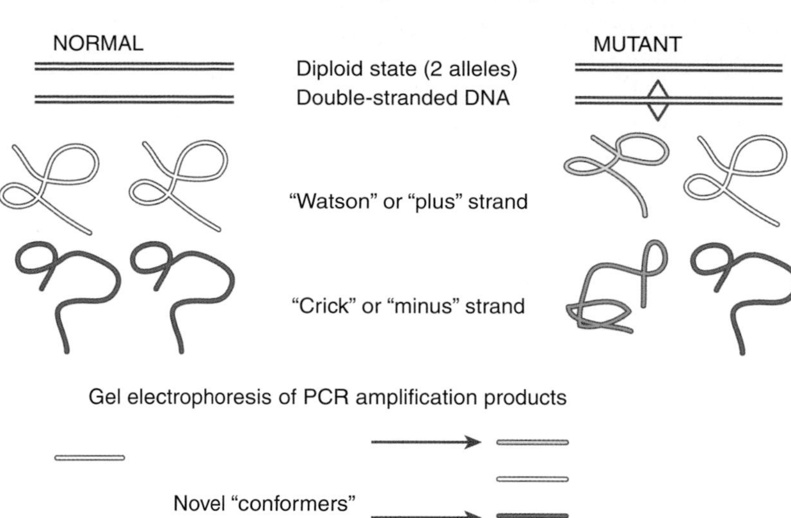

Figure 20–27 Model of the technique of single-stranded conformational variant analysis. On the left, normal alleles have the same sequence and therefore the same conformation, forming two similar bands. Alternatively, the right demonstrates a mutant allele. The dark and light segments have slightly different sequences, and these migrate at different rates through the gel. Therefore, there are four bands seen on the gel. This technique is sensitive for detecting a difference of only a few base pairs in genes.

Single-stranded conformational polymorphism analysis is a radioactive technique for mutation detection that exploits the properties of a change in shape (or conformation) of mutant DNA that can be detected by electrophoresis. Here, normal DNA and tumor DNA are PCR-amplified, denatured, and electrophoresed through gels. Mutant DNA will conform to a shape different from that of its normal counterpart and will take a different electrophoretic mobility, which is easily visualized by autoradiography. The single-stranded conformational technique is depicted in Fig. 20–27.

Denaturing high-performance liquid chromatography is a newly designed non-radioactive technique for mutation detection. Here, normal DNA and tumor DNA are amplified by PCR, mixed together, denatured to create single-stranded DNA, and slowly allowed to reanneal into double-stranded DNA. When normal DNA anneals with tumor DNA, a mismatch in the strands is created, forming a heteroduplex. This heteroduplex possesses a melting profile different from that of DNA with two normal or tumor DNA strands (homoduplexes) and is easily detected by chromatography.

Other mutation detection systems, such as denaturing gradient gel electrophoresis, allele-specific oligonucleotide analysis, and allele-specific amplification, exploit sequence differences between normal and tumor DNA in screening for mutations. Each of these mutation detection systems (except for direct sequencing) is a tool to screen for mutations and does not identify the specific sequence alteration or class of mutation responsible for the abnormal screen. There are now machines that can screen large segments of the genome and exponentially increase our ability to detect mutations, such as the microarray apparatus and transgenomic WAVE DNA Fragmentation Analysis System (Transgenomic, Santa Clara, CA).

Gene expression profiling in cancer

The ability to determine gene expression levels from thousands of genes simultaneously has recently transformed many aspects of cancer research. The ability to view gene expression on a large scale by gene expression profiling allows us to get a good view of the overall genome functioning. This technology can also be used to classify tumors by virtue of gene expression. DNA array technology uses thousands of fragments of DNA arrayed on a solid surface to probe many mRNA levels during a single experiment. Gene profiling usually begins with clustering of the genomic data as a whole in an unsupervised fashion and proceeds to more limited screening of genes known to be important in the pathologic process or supervised clustering

There are many techniques that are useful for expression profiling. Subtractive hybridization is used to produce a cDNA library that has RNA sequences present in on sample but not the other. Other techniques such as suppression subtractive hybridization and representation difference analysis are two newer techniques that allow the use of smaller samples. The subtractive techniques have been used to identify many important cancer related genes. This approach requires pair-wise analysis and a time-consuming cloning step that make it unsuitable for high throughput technology. Differential display is a newer technique that works by first producing a set of cDNA fragments that have been identically prepared from two sets of RNA samples. These are then resolved on a gel and the patterns compared. The advantage of this technique is that it can be performed in almost any lab, but the disadvantage is that to actually identify a gene it must be excised and sequenced. This requires much time, effort and specialized technology. Various DNA arrays using larger fragments of DNA can also be utilized—these are based on older technology developed by Edwin Southern.

Large-scale sequencing of cDNA libraries was first proposed as a rapid means to gain access to transcribed regions from the human genome. Transcribed sequences generated by the cDNA library sequencing effort are known as expressed sequence tags (ESTs). One of the first large scale efforts at this technology was made by a collaboration between Merck and Washington University. Counting transcripts by this method is very accurate but is expensive and laborious. Much of the EST expression data can be accessed via a variety off World Wide web sites.

Finally, serial analysis of gene expression (SAGE) was developed as an efficient means of counting large numbers of mRNA transcripts. This is largely and automated technology and relies on this efficiency to keep costs relatively low per sequence analyzed.

GENETICS OF HUMAN CANCER

Colon cancer

Colon cancer is the second leading cause of death from cancer. This figure is expected to increase as the population ages. This fact is not surprising if one considers the etiology of cancer and the histopathology of the colon. The colonic mucosa is a single layer of epithelium that turns over rapidly and is constantly exposed to carcinogenic agents. Therefore, the DNA is rapidly dividing and replicating on a regular basis. The odds are that over time, significant mistakes will be made, resulting in uncontrolled cell growth. The colon cancer model developed by Vogelstein and others illustrates some of these concepts in a clear and concise manner (see Fig. 20–3). The adenomatous polyposis coli suppressor gene (APC), when present in mutant form, appears to permit the outgrowth of early colonic polyps. In colon disease, samples are easily obtained. As a polyp becomes larger and more irregular, it becomes more readily accessible to the gastroenterologist, and serial studies can be performed. Colon cancer is also convenient to study because certain families are genetically prone to a rare disease called familial adenomatous polyposis. In affected individuals, the colon becomes carpeted with hundreds or thousands of polyps, one or more of which is likely to become malignant in midlife. It was in these patients that the defect in the APC gene was first recognized. In most human colonic tumors, the APC gene is altered by somatic mutations occurring randomly in colonic epithelial cells. In the rarer situation of familial tumors, the mutant APC gene is acquired from a parent and is thus implanted in all cells of the colon, predisposing the recipient to hundreds if not thousands of polyps. The APC somatic mutation may later activate a ras oncogene, creating a more advanced polyp that is, however, still benign. During a period of years, this polyp may sustain mutations in its DCC and p53 suppressor genes. These mutations in turn appear to lead to more autonomous uncontrolled growth of colon carcinoma cells.

Familial predisposition to colon cancer is common and can be divided into two basic groups: those with polyps and those without. Polyposis syndromes include familial adenomatous polyposis coli (FAP), Peutz–Jeghers syndrome, familial juvenile polyposis syndrome, and hyperplastic polyposis. All of these patients are at increased risk for development of colon cancer. For instance, the median age at development of cancer in a patient with familial adenomatous polyposis is about 40 years.

Non-polyposis conditions primarily include HNPCC. Patients with this inherited propensity for colon cancer also develop the disease around 40 years of age. Most patients with HNPCC have an underlying genetic defect in the mismatch repair system. This mutation most often occurs in the MLH1 gene of this system however recent data has demonstrated that MSH2 and MSH6 are also frequently involved. HNPCC is also associated with other cancers that include endometrium, ovary, breast, and neural tumors.

Colon cancers are hereditary approximately 3–5% of the time. However, patients with a family history of any colorectal cancer are at increased risk for development of this disease. Therefore, most colorectal cancers may have at least a partially inherited component. Environmental factors are also important in the development of this disease, and data suggest that a high-fiber diet will decrease the likelihood of the development of this disease. Other environmental risk factors may include diets high in fat and red meat.

Molecular changes that occur in colon cancers have been well defined by Vogelstein and colleagues. This group has nicely laid out the progression of benign epithelium to cancer. The first genes to be associated with colon cancers were ras genes originally identified in rat sarcoma viruses. They are most consistently found in intermediate non-dysplastic colon polyps. There is a distinct lack of ras mutations in early adenomas, but mutations can reliably be detected in intermediate polyps, suggesting that ras plays an early role in the development of colon cancers.

The adenomatous polyposis coli (APC) tumor suppressor gene appears to play the earliest role in development of colon cancers and was identified by simple loss of heterozygosity studies, which showed consistent loss on the long arm of chromosome 5 (5q). Another gene associated with colorectal cancers is the Tp53 tumor suppressor gene on 17p. The mutation of this gene appears to be a relatively late event in the development of colon cancer; Tp53 is an important control of cell cycle and programmed cell death (apoptosis). Loss of tumor suppressor function on chromosome 18q that includes the DCC gene is an intermediate to late event. This gene codes for a protein that is responsible for cell adhesion. DPC4, also on 18q, is involved in the signaling pathway of transforming growth factor-β.

The development of colorectal cancers requires the sequential acquisition of a series of mutations. Not every tumor requires all of the steps to progress to a cancer, but it appears that at least six or seven genetic events are required. Patients with HNPCC develop these mutations as the result of a defect in the ability of the colonic mucosa to detect and repair mismatches that occur during normal cellular division. The work of Vogelstein and colleagues demonstrates a model that may be applied to other cancers.

This work on colon cancer nicely illustrated the multistep nature of tumorigenesis and the interplay of oncogenes and tumor suppressor genes; but unfortunately it provides no clues into the later stages of tumorigenesis, including invasiveness and metastasis. Other mutant genes that yet remain to be discovered may govern these later characteristics. However, the research on colon carcinoma provides a model for researchers working on a number of other tumor types. The hope is to describe the life history of a tumor in terms of a succession of genetic lesions that are sustained in a distinct, relatively small cohort of target genes. Such genetic histories promise to provide a clear view of all the molecular changes required to transform a normal cell into a tumor cell and in turn will give us the identities of the molecular targets for future generations of diagnostic and therapeutic techniques.

Recently, microarray technologies have been used to assess genetic changes in a range of cancer types. Cancer "molecular staging" allows for the identification of genetic alterations associated with tumor progression. Knowledge of these sorts of molecular changes (either at the gene or protein level) can be used to predict disease outcome and may ultimately be used to direct therapy. Microarray approaches have and are being used in colon cancer to gain a comprehensive understanding of the genetic alterations associated with the disease. A report from Eschrich and colleagues suggests that molecular characterization of colon tumors is likely to be of clinical utility.

Breast cancer

Breast cancer is a leading cause of death among women in the USA. The most recent data suggest that one in eight women will suffer from breast cancer in her lifetime, and about one third of women with breast cancer will die of the disease. The greatest risk factor is a family history of breast cancer. Other risk factors for the development of this disease are many and varied. One hypothesis is that conclusion of breastfeeding allows terminal differentiation of breast epithelial cells; therefore, late onset of first pregnancy is a risk factor. History of repeated or high-dose radiation exposure clearly increases the risk of this disease. This is demonstrated by increased risk in atomic bomb survivors and Hodgkin's disease survivors. Other factors that may play a role in the development of this disease are alcohol consumption, high-fat diet, prolonged oral contraceptive use, and estrogen use.

The molecular biology of breast cancer is not nearly as well defined as that of colon cancer, but several significant molecular predictors of this disease are known. In 1990, linkage analysis of a small family cohort of breast cancer families identified a potential susceptibility gene on chromosome 17 near the genetic marker D17S74 on 17q21. In 1994, the gene in this region was identified and named BRCA1. BRCA1 does not appear to be a member of a known gene family.

To construct the gene from the region identified by the linkage studies, investigators used known sequences of DNA called yeast artificial chromosomes (YACs), bacterial artificial chromosomes (BACs), and cosmids (small fragments of DNA of known sequence). In this way, they were able to span the contig (the unknown area) with DNA of known sequence and determine the sequence of the gene. Once the Human Genome Project is completed, this labor intensive work will no longer be necessary because we will know the sequence of DNA in regions that we wish to study.

BRCA1 appears to be responsible for some aspect of cell cycle control. It is a nuclear phosphoprotein that is phosphorylated in S and M phases. Knockout mice with no BRCA1 genes have been constructed to study the importance of the gene. These mice are unable to live. Therefore, the gene appears to be necessary for early embryo development. How it is linked to cancer is not completely known.

A second breast susceptibility gene was identified in 1995. The initial progress toward identifying this gene was made by the linkage analysis of 22 families. This gene, named BRCA2, is located on 13q between markers 13S260 and 13S271. BRCA2 carriers have a lifetime risk for development of breast cancer of 80–90% and a risk for development of ovarian cancer. More than 100 mutations have been identified and continue to be recorded. These mutations can be found on the Breast Cancer Information Core (BIC) website at *http://research.nhgri.nih.gov/bic/*. Few mutations have been identified in sporadic breast cancers, indicating that this gene probably does not play a significant role in non-inherited breast cancer. Other inherited causes of breast cancer are Muir–Torre syndrome, ataxia-telangiectasia, Cowden disease, and Li–Fraumeni syndrome.

The study of sporadic breast cancers has yielded many other genetic mutations (Table 20–5). These include growth factors, intracellular signaling molecules, regulators of the cell cycle, and regulators of apoptosis. It is not yet clear how all of these factors act together to allow the formation of a breast cancer.

GENETIC STUDIES IN GYNECOLOGIC MALIGNANT NEOPLASMS

Ovarian cancer

Ovarian cancer is the fifth leading cause of death from cancer among women in the USA. These tumors are a heterogeneous group of cancers and are composed of a variety of histologic subtypes: serous, mucinous, endometrioid, clear cell, and other rare forms. These histologic types are similar to other tissues in the genital tract. Each histologic type presumably has different molecular mutations.

Some neoplasms with the same histologic features often have divergent clinical behavior, suggesting that the genetic alterations underlying the development and progression of these lesions may not be comparable. Studies are needed to correlate specific molecular markers with histologic subtype and clinical behavior. A few such studies have been reported. There has been controversy for decades as to whether the patterns of development in ovarian cancer support the multifocal concept. Mok and associates reported nine cases with widespread abdominal carcinomatosis in which the pattern of Tp53 gene expression was identical in cancer cells from different sites in the same patient, suggesting a unifocal origin. Tsao and coworkers used X chromosome inactivation as a molecular marker and showed similar results.

Numerous other reports have identified activation of different oncogenes in ovarian cancer. Overexpression of erb-b2 (HER-2/neu) with and without gene amplification has been reported. Using Southern blot analysis, Slamon and coworkers found erb-b2 amplification in 26% of 120 primary ovarian malignant neoplasms. Twelve percent of cases showed erb-b2 expression without evidence of gene amplification. Overexpression of erb-b2 correlates with poor clinical outcome, suggesting possible clinical use for this molecular marker in future treatment plans.

Baker and colleagues reported c-myc amplification in 29% of ovarian carcinomas. In another study, c-myc amplification was reported in 50% of ovarian carcinomas. Amplification of c-myc cannot be detected in normal ovarian tissue, benign adenomas, and tumors of low malignant potential; this observation supports the theory that different genetic alterations account for the development of benign vs malignant ovarian neoplasms. Abnormalities of other oncogenes, such as ras gene deletions, amplification, and point mutation and fos gene overexpression, have also been reported.

This carcinogenesis of ovarian cancer probably involves inactivation of tumor suppressor genes as well. Sato and colleagues reported 37 ovarian neoplasms studied with several DNA probes and found allelic losses on 6q, 13q, and 19q in serous carcinomas. They found fewer allelic losses in mucinous-type tumors. Sasano and coworkers found homogeneous deletions of the RB gene in 1 of 24 ovarian carcinomas. Mazars and associates found Tp53 gene mutations in 36% of 34 ovarian carcinomas with most mutations clustered in exons 5 and 7. Marks and colleagues examined Tp53 gene expression in >100 ovarian carcinomas and found high levels of mutant Tp53 protein in more than 50% of the tumors, whereas Tp53 was undetectable in several benign gynecologic tissue samples. Overexpression of Tp53 protein was found to correlate closely with the presence of Tp53 gene mutation in the tumors. Such studies suggest that the Tp53 gene through deletion or point mutation plays a role in the development or progression of some ovarian cancers.

Most of the preceding text applies to genetic alterations occurring in somatic cells during cancer development and progression. Primary genetic factors are thought to account for about 5% of ovarian cancer cases. A great deal of research is currently under way to identify and clone the target genes. BRCA1 is the designation given a gene located in the cells of all humans. Mutant forms of BRCA1 have been shown to be associated with disease in some families with multiple cases of ovarian cancer only. In 1995, a combined report from research centers throughout the world stated that 9(6%) of 145 families with multiple cases of ovarian and breast cancer demonstrated the presence of the BRCA1 gene.

This suggests but does not prove that an altered or mutant form (currently 50 mutants have been identified) of the normal BRCA1 gene may be passed from generation to generation in these families and that an altered BRCA1 may predispose a woman to development of breast or ovarian cancer. The data also suggest that in families in which disease is not linked to BRCA1, other genes, as yet unknown, may be responsible for ovarian cancer. In September 1994, the BRCA1 gene was isolated. This made it possible to identify specific changes in BRCA1 that are associated with disease in cancer cases of BRCA1-linked families. It also opens the possibility of identifying individuals in these families who have changes in BRCA1 but no disease. Such individuals are considered to have a high risk for development of breast or ovarian cancer. On the other hand, individuals in these families who have not inherited an altered BRCA1 gene are not known to be at high risk for development of these diseases. Thus, testing for altered BRCA1 in these families may allow better evaluation of disease risk for individual members. In 1995, a second gene associated with breast and ovarian cancer was identified, BRCA2. This gene is estimated to confer a lifetime ovarian cancer risk of 10–20%. Characterization of this gene is currently under way.

The biggest challenge of the next years is to determine what risk is known mutated genes bestow on individuals in terms of both risk and prognosis. Because experience with genetic testing for cancer is limited and it is an extremely sensitive issue, the American Society of Human Genetics has recommended that genetic testing be limited to members of families with a strong ovarian and breast cancer history and that testing be performed in conjunction with established research programs by trained professionals aware of genetic, clinical, and psychological implications of the testing and of the technical limitations of the testing methods. It is critical that individuals tested are properly counseled and that the information be used to help us understand the significance of these abnormalities.

Cervical cancer

Although the association of human papillomavirus (HPV) infection with cervical cancer suggests the virus as a causative agent, several other facts suggest that HPV infection alone is insufficient to bring about cervical carcinoma. The viral genome contains several open reading frames encoding many proteins and is stably integrated into the host DNA. Although a common point of integration has not been found, HPV sequences have been found integrated near cellular oncogenes c-myc and N-myc in at least a few cervical cancer cell lines; in most cases, integration interrupts the E1 and E2 open reading frames but leaves E6 and E7 open reading frames intact. The proteins encoded by E6 and E7 of oncogenetic HPV strains can effectively immortalize primary keratinocyctes; Barbosa and Schlegel demonstrated this in their report in 1989.

The molecular basis of differences in the oncogenic potential between various strains of HPV remains unclear. Munger and colleagues have shown some biochemical and biologic differences between E7 proteins of low-risk viruses such as HPV-6 and high-risk viruses such as HPV-16. Kastan and associates suggested that Tp53 may function as an "emergency brake" in cells that have sustained DNA damage. Cells damaged by irradiation or drugs often arrest in the G_1-S phase of the cell cycle, presumably allowing DNA repair. This cell cycle arrest is associated with transient increases in wild-type Tp53 and is not seen in cells containing mutant Tp53 genes. Kessis and associates suggested that oncogenic HPV-16 expression might also disrupt the Tp53-mediated cellular response to DNA damage. When HPV-16 E6 is transfected into cells exhibiting normal DNA damage response, Tp53 protein levels are essentially undetectable and cell cycle arrest after DNA damage is abolished. Thus, genomic instability is achieved, possibly leading to further genetic alterations and tumorigenesis.

Vulvar cancer

As in cervical cancer, a sexually transmitted agent is suspected to play a role in the pathogenesis of vulvar cancer. HPV-16 and HPV-18 have been identified in vulvar intraepithelial neoplasia and invasive squamous carcinoma. Worsham found that vulvar cancers tend to contain certain consistent chromosome abnormalities, including losses of chromosomes 3p, 8p, and 22q and gains of 3q and 11q. Losses of 10q and 18q were found only in cases that exhibited biologically aggressive behavior. As with cervical malignant neoplasms, HPV infection may play a role in the occurrence of molecular alterations that lead to tumor development and progression.

Endometrial cancer

Endometrial cancer is the most common malignant disease of the female genital tract in the USA. At least three histologic variants have been identified—endometrioid carcinomas, papillary serous cancers, and clear cell cancers. Endometrial cancers have a significant heritable component and are, for instance, the most common gynecologic cancer associated with the Lynch syndrome type II. It is estimated that as many as 6% of all endometrial cancers have a heritable component. The majority of patients with heritable endometrial cancer are from a group of women of families with HNPCC.

Endometrioid carcinomas are the most common histologic variant and account for approximately 70% of all cases of endometrial cancer. There are two histologic types of endometrioid carcinoma, termed type I and type II. Type I endometrioid carcinoma is associated with endometrial hyperplasia and is therefore known to have premalignant precursors. It is associated with obesity and estrogen use. Type II endometrioid carcinoma is associated with atrophic endometrium. Papillary serous adenocarcinoma is a particularly aggressive histologic type and often arises within endometrial hyperplasia.

The molecular events that lead to the development of endometrial cancer are poorly understood. Several studies have demonstrated loss of heterozygosity at a variety of points in endometrial cancers. This has led many investigators to search for tumor suppressor genes in these areas. Regions of loss include 3p, 10q, 17p, and 18q. Papillary serous cancers often show loss on 1p.

Several small studies have identified alterations of oncogenes, such as the ras group, K-ras, c-fms, and c-erb-1, that may play a role in the development and progression of endometrial carcinomas. Okamoto and colleagues studied 24 endometrial adenocarcinomas for allelic losses and found loss of heterozygosity in seven cases, five of which lost loci on 17p, which harbors the Tp53 gene. Risinger and coworkers reported 21 endometrial carcinomas, in which Tp53 gene point mutations were found in 3 cases (14%). Endometrial carcinoma frequently occurs in patients with HNPCC (Lynch syndrome type II), suggesting that inactivation of the same gene may participate in the development of both cancers.

Because endometrial cancers are often associated with HNPCC, and HNPCC individuals usually have a mismatch repair defect, many investigators have evaluated endometrial cancers for mismatch repair and have found that these cancers show a 20–25% chance of demonstrating microsatellite instability. However, only a small percentage of these patients demonstrate mutations in the known mismatch repair genes (MSH2, MLH1, MSH3, PMS2, PMS1). The mismatch repair phenotype appears to be conferred by methylation of the MLH1 promoter region, thus inactivating this gene. Interestingly, there are several racially based polymorphisms within the mismatch repair system. However, approximately 6% of patients with endometrial cancer have a germline mutation in one of the mismatch repair genes that may be due to a primary mutation in one of these genes. When there is a primary mutation, this may represent a germline mutation and therefore be an inherited form of endometrial cancer. Race-related polymorphisms have also been identified. Kowalski identified eight polymorphisms of MLH1 or MSH2 that were found almost exclusively in black women. This may be important in light of the known differences in survival in black women vs white women. The importance of such race-related genetic differences in cancer survival needs to be more fully investigated. These differences may be important as we identify factors that lead to stratifying patients' prognosis. One would expect tumors with a mismatch repair defect more commonly to have mutated oncogenes or tumor suppressor genes. This is often not true, again demonstrating the non-randomness of genetic mutation.

However, several tumor suppressor genes have been identified and associated with endometrial cancers. Between 5% and 50% of endometrioid endometrial cancers overexpress the p53 protein or have identifiable TP53 gene defects. This tends not to occur in endometrial hyperplasia, indicating that p53 mutations may be a late event in the genesis of endometrial cancer. The frequency of TP53 mutation is related to histologic subtype of endometrial cancer. Most uterine serous carcinomas have TP53 mutations. The rate of mutation in endometrioid cancers on the other hand is considerably lower. The histotype specificity for TP53 mutations may, in part, explain the racial predilection for black women. The expression of p53 may also be associated with a poorer prognosis. Interestingly, p53 expression appears to be inversely proportional to Bcl-2 expression; p21 and p185 have also been associated with endometrial cancer.

Several studies looking for loss of heterozygosity identified loss on chromosome 10 (Fig. 20–6). The PTEN tumor suppressor gene (phosphate and tensin homologue) has been isolated from the 10q23-10q24 region and appears to be frequently mutated in endometrial cancers. PTEN encodes a cytoplasmic protein/lipid phosphatase, the main substrate for which is phosphatidylinositol (3,4,5) triphosphate (PIP-3). Accumulation of PIP-3 at the cell membrane leads to recruitment of members of the Akt serine/threonine kinase family. The activation of Akt in turn has effects on cell survival at the levels of apoptosis and the regulation of other genes. Not only is PTEN mutated in endometrial carcinoma, it also appears to be a very early event. PTEN expression is absent in a large fraction of endometrioid carcinomas and is also missing in abnormally proliferative glands. Interestingly, PTEN defects are more common in early stage disease that more advanced endometrial carcinomas. At this time the prognostic significance of PTEN mutation and/or lack of expression in endometrial carcinoma and associations with race, stage and grade are not well understood. There appears to be a relationship between PTEN inactivation and defects in DNA mismatch repair (the MSI phenotype). Other regions of loss on 10q are not associated with the PTEN gene and may contain candidates for other tumor suppressor genes.

Oncogenes associated with endometrial cancers include the K-ras gene, which is mutated between 10% and 30% of the time. Preliminary studies suggest that this is an early event in the genesis of endometrial cancers. K-ras mutations are more common in endometrial cancers than in serous cancers. Her-2/neu is also associated with endometrial cancers. It may be overexpressed or amplified in these cancers, and its activation may portend a poorer prognosis. The molecular events associated with endometrial cancers are being intensely studied by a number of groups, and it is likely that the genesis of this cancer will be much better understood in the coming years.

Genome-wide approaches to the study of endometrial cancer genetics have just begun, as have molecular studies of mouse models for endometrial cancer. Already array-based analysis of the genetics of endometrial cancer has pointed to key molecular differences that distinguish endometrioid and the more aggressive serous histologic subtype. Furthermore, Ferguson and colleagues revealed molecular fingerprints that are predictive of outcome in a recent study. The rapid increase in understanding of what sort of molecular defects are seen in endometrial cancers is likely to lead to new approaches for the prevention, detection, and treatment of this group of malignancies.

GLOSSARY

Allele Alternative forms of the same gene. Because of the paired nature of chromosomes, every gene exists in two copies. Each is an allele.

Antioncogene See tumor suppressor gene.

c-erb-b2 proto-oncogene Also referred to as HER-2 or neu, this gene encodes a protein that is structurally similar to the receptor for epidermal growth factor. When it is amplified, the gene is of prognostic significance in breast and ovarian neoplasms.

Capping The addition of 7-methylguanosine residues to the 5′ end of most eukaryotic mRNA.

Chromosome translocation Exchange of genes or a portion of genes between different

Chromosome One mechanism for activating oncogenes.

Cloning An in vivo method to produce unlimited quantities of specific DNA fragments from as little as a single DNA molecule. Also, the process by which a DNA molecule is joined to another DNA molecule that can replicate autonomously in a specially designed host, usually a bacterium or yeast.

Codon A group of three nucleotides forming a base-coding message in the gene sequence. In ras genes, for example, the 12th, 13th, or 61st codon is often mutated, leading to oncogene activation. Complementary DNA (cDNA) DNA synthesized from mRNA template such that the DNA sequence is complementary to the mRNA.

Contig The sequence of DNA created by use of YACs, BACs, and cosmids to fill an unknown region of DNA suspected of having a candidate gene.

Cosmid Used for large-scale analysis of the human genome when large DNA fragments of known sequence are needed (40 kb).

Cytoplasmic signal transduction molecules Proteins within the cytoplasm of cells responsible for transmitting signals from one event to the next event.

DNA probe A short segment of DNA in which the base sequence is specifically complementary to a particular gene segment. The probe is used, for example, on the Southern blot assay to determine whether a certain gene is present in a tumor sample undergoing DNA analysis.

Exons The coding portion of genes.

Gel electrophoresis A molecular biology laboratory technique in which DNA, RNA, or proteins are separated according to molecular weight, charge, and spatial characteristics in an electric field applied to a gel. For example, because DNA is negatively charged, it migrates toward the positively charged electrode.

Gene amplification The presence of multiple copies of a gene within a cell that is normally present in only two copies per somatic cell. An increased number of copies of an individual gene, usually a proto-oncogene, per cell.

Gene deletion The deletion of part or all of a gene through removal of DNA sequences by any of several mechanisms.

Gene expression The active transcription of a gene into an RNA molecule followed by translation of the protein product.

Gene rearrangement The process by which part or all of a gene is moved from its normal location in the genome to another site within the genome.

Genomic imprinting An epigenetic modification of a parental allele of a gene that leads to differential expression of that allele.

Growth factor Protein that acts on cells to promote cell growth.

Growth factor receptors Proteins that interact with growth factors and transmit the growth signal to the cell.

HER-2 See c-erb-b2 proto-oncogene.

Heteronuclear RNA A form of RNA, a pre-mRNA, that exists before splicing and consists of both introns and exons.

Heterozygosity Two different forms of the same gene in a cell. An oncogene is generally heterozygous. For example, one allele may be mutated while the other copy remains normal. In addition, different forms of a gene may be normal variants. Variations in the exact base sequence within DNA are common in the genome among humans. These are called polymorphisms and are often responsible for the heterozygous state.

Informative A term used to describe the situation when the two homologous chromosomes from an individual can be distinguished from one another at a given locus; heterozygous is an alternative term.

Insertion The addition of a DNA sequence into the genome.

Introns Portions of genomic DNA that are interspersed between exons and are transcribed along with the exons into heteronuclear RNA.

Locus A general term to describe a defined chromosome region.

Loss of heterozygosity Losses of specific regions of DNA from one copy of a given chromosome that can be distinguished from the region retained on the other chromosome.

Messenger RNA (mRNA) The mature form of processed RNA used as a template for directing translation of proteins.

Myc proto-oncogenes The proto-oncogene family that includes c-myc, N-myc, L-myc, and R-myc. They encode nuclear-associated DNA-binding proteins that affect DNA replication and transcription.

Neu See c-erb-b2 proto-oncogene.

Nonsense mutation A nucleotide substitution that results in a truncated protein product by generating a stop codon specifying premature cessation of translation within an open reading frame.

Nuclear transcription factors Proteins involved in regulating the expression of genes by controlling transcription. Some factors enhance and others repress gene expression and others do both, depending on the intracellular environment.

Oncogenes Genes that regulate cell growth in a positive fashion (i.e., promote cell growth). Oncogenes include transforming genes of viruses and normal cellular genes (proto-oncogenes) that are activated by mutations to promote cell growth.

Open reading frame A sequence of DNA representing at least some of the coding portion of a gene that is transcribed and subsequently translated into a protein because it does not contain any internal translation termination codons.

Palindrome (inverted repeats) These are sequences that look the same if read forward or backward. This allows the sequence to fold back on itself, and it is particularly susceptible to mutation.

Point mutation The replacement of one nucleotide in the DNA sequence of the wild type with another nucleotide.

Polymerase chain reaction A technique by which genes or portions of genes are multiplied in vitro if the sequence of the gene is known or partially known. A heat-stable enzyme known as polymerase is used to create DNA in the test tube. Polymerase chain reaction analysis revolutionized molecular biology by opening genes from small, even degraded samples of tissue or tumor to study. Analysis of certain genes is possible from archival paraffin-embedded tissue samples or small quantities of cells.

Polymorphism Variation in the exact base sequence of DNA that makes up the genome. These occurrences are normal and common in humans. Polymorphisms are used in the study of molecular genetics because they are inherited. Ones found near or within disease genes can be used to study linkage in genetics.

Primers Short DNA pieces that are complementary to portions of specific DNA sequences.

Promoter The DNA sequence of a gene to which RNA polymerase binds and initiates transcription.

Proto-oncogenes Any of a number of genes that encode various proteins involved in normal cell growth and proliferation, including growth factors, growth factor receptors, regulators of DNA synthesis, and phosphorylating modifiers of protein function. These are cellular genes that are the normal counterparts of transforming viral oncogenes.

ras gene A family of genes that encode similar cell membrane-bound proteins involved in signal transduction. Three types, K-ras, N-ras, and H-ras, are the widely studied ras genes in human tumors. Their proto-oncogene becomes activated by point mutations, most often in specific codons, of the gene sequence.

RB The first tumor suppressor gene to be discovered. It is a 4.7-kilobase gene, located on chromosome 13q14, and encodes a 110,000-dalton nuclear phosphoprotein that suppresses the cell cycle. Absence of RB is the cause of retinoblastoma, and research is revealing that it is involved in the pathogenesis of many other neoplasms.

Restriction endonucleases Enzymes that cleave DNA at specific DNA sequences.

Restriction fragment length polymorphism Variation in the DNA of different individuals that creates or destroys cleavage sites for a given restriction endonuclease.

Reverse transcriptase An enzyme discovered in retroviruses that has the unique ability to transcribe DNA from an RNA template. This is the reverse of the normal physiologic process.

Southern blot analysis A molecular biology technique in which DNA is transferred to and fixed on a nylon or nitrocellulose membrane and studied with DNA probes that can then detect, for example, the presence of an oncogene.

Splice site mutations Nucleotide substitutions that occur in the sequence adjacent to intron-exon boundaries of genes.

Splicing The process by which introns are removed from heteronuclear RNA and the exons are joined together to maintain the open reading frame of the mRNA.

Tp53 gene A tumor suppressor gene that encodes a nuclear phosphoprotein that arrests cells from entering the S-phase of the cell cycle. Located on chromosome 17(p13), Tp53 is postulated to contribute to diverse tumorigenesis.

Transcription The process of converting the DNA code into a complementary mRNA segment.

Translation The process by which specific amino acids are incorporated into a protein as dictated by the sequence of the mRNA template.

Translocation Non-homologous recombination.

Tumor suppressor gene A gene that suppresses cellular growth and proliferation. Therefore, when its protein products are absent, it contributes to tumor development or progression. Also known as antioncogenes, these normal cellular genes encode proteins that are thought to normally regulate growth in a negative fashion.

Uninformative The term used to describe the situation when the two homologous chromosomes from an individual cannot be distinguished from one another at a given locus; homozygous is an alternative term.

Vector A DNA vehicle that can be propagated in living cells (e.g., bacteria and yeast) into which foreign DNA can be inserted and propagated with the vector DNA. Examples of vectors include bacterial plasmids, cosmids, bacteriophages, and, most recently, yeast artificial chromosomes.

Wild type The term used to describe the normal gene or gene product. In contrast, a gene that has had its DNA sequence altered is referred to as a mutant gene, and its resultant product is a mutant protein. A gene that encodes a proto-oncogene, for example, is a wild-type gene because it is unaltered.

BIBLIOGRAPHY

Beadle GW: Biochemical genetics. Chem Rev 37:15, 1945.

Garrod AE: Inborn errors of metabolism. Lancet 2:1, 1908.

Mendel G: Versuche über Pflanzenhybriden. Leipzig, Engelmann, 1901.

Tatum EL: A case history of biological research. Science 129:1715, 1959.

Watson JD, Crick FHC: Molecular structure of nucleic acids: A structure for deoxyribose nucleic acid. Nature 171:737, 1953.

GENETIC ALTERATIONS IN CANCER

Callahan R, Campbell G: Mutations in human breast cancer: An overview. J Natl Cancer Inst 81:1780, 1989.

Cohen D, Chumakov I, Weissenback J: A first generation physical map of the human genome. Nature 366:698, 1993.

Coles CF et al: P53 mutations in breast cancer. Cancer Res 52:5291, 1992.

Cooper DN, Krawczak M: Cytosine methylation and the fate of CpG dinucleotides in vertebrate genomes. Hum Genet 83:181, 1989.

Cooper DN, Krawczak M: Human gene mutation, Oxford, BIOS Scientific 1993.

Fearon ER, Vogelstein B: A genetic model for colorectal tumorigenesis. Cell 61:759, 1990.

Fearon ER, Cho KR, Nigro JM et. al.: Identification of a chromosome 10q gene that is altered in colorectal cancers. Science 247: 49–51, 1990.

Fujiwara Y et al: Evidence for the presence of two tumor suppressor genes on chromosome 8p for colorectal carcinoma. Cancer Res 53:1172, 1993.

Goldgar DE et al: A large kindred with 17q-linked breast and ovarian cancer: Genetic, phenotypic and genealogical analysis. J Natl Cancer Inst 86:200, 1994.

Haas OA, Argyriou-Tirita A, Lion T: Parental origin of chromosomes involved in the translocation t(9;22). Nature 359:414, 1992.

Hashimoto K, Azuma C, Koyama M et al: Loss of imprinting in choriocarcinoma. Nat Gent 9:109, 1995.

Herman JG, Umar A, Polyak K, et. al., Incidence and functional consequences of hMLH1promoter hypermethylation in colorectal carcinoma. Proc Nat Acad of Sci USA 95:6870–6874, 1998.

Houldsworth J et al: Gene amplification in gastric and esophageal adenocarcinomas. Cancer Res 50:6417, 1990.

Kowalski LD, Mutch DC, Herzog TS et al: Mutational analysis of hMLHI and hMSH2 on 25 prospectively acquired RER and endometrial cancers. Genes Chromosomes Cancer 18:219, 1997.

Knudson AG Jr: Mutation and cancer: Statistical Study of retinoblastoma. Proc Natl Acad Sci USA 68:820, 1971.

Krawczak M, Cooper DN: Gene deletions causing human genetic disease: Mechanisms of mutagenesis and the role of local DNA sequence environment. Hum Genet 86:425, 1991.

Krawczak M, Cooper DN: The human gene mutation database. Trends Genet 13:121, 1997.

Loeb LA, Kunkel TA: Fidelity in DNA synthesis. Annu Rev Biochem 52:429, 1982.

Miki Y et al: A strong candidate for the breast and ovarian cancer susceptibility gene BRCA1. Science 266:66, 1994.

Mitelman F: Catalog of Chromosome Aberrations in Cancer, 3rd ed. New York, Alan R. Liss, 1988.

Moul JW: New medicine emerging from genes that control cancer. Contemp Ob Gyn Feb 1995.
Norris H, Klein G: Malignancy of somatic cell hybrids. Nature 224:1317, 1969.
Rainier S et al: Relaxation of imprinted genes in human cancer. Nature 362:747, 1993.
Sato T et al: Accumulation of genetic alterations and progression of primary breast cancer. Cancer Res 51:5794, 1991.
Sidransky D et al: Inherited p53 gene mutations in breast cancer. Cancer Res 52:2984, 1992.
Solomon E, Borrow J, Goddard AD: Chromosome aberrations and cancer. Science 254:1153, 1991.
Stehlin D, Varmos HE, Bishop JM, Vogt PK: DNA related to the transforming gene(s) of avian sarcoma viruses is present in normal avian DNA. Nature 260:170, 1976.
Vogelstein B: A deadly inheritance. Nature 348:681, 1990.
Vogelstein B, Fearon ER, Kern SE et al: Allelotype of colorectal carcinomas. Science 244:207, 1989.
Wu C-I, Maeda N: Inequality in mutational rates of the two strands of DNA. Nature 327:169, 1987.

ONCOGENES

Aaronson SA: Growth factors and cancer. Science 254:1146, 1991.
Adams JM, Cory S: Transgenic models of tumor development. Science 254:1161, 1991.
Baker VV, Shingleton HM, Hatch KD et al: Selective inhibition of C-myc expression by the ribonucleic acid synthesis inhibitor mithramycin. Am J Obstet Gynecol 158:762, 1988.
Bishop JM: Enemies within: The genesis of retrovirus oncogenes. Cell 23:5, 1982.
Buckley I: Oncogenes and the nature of malignancy. Adv Cancer Res 50:71, 1988.
Cantley LC, Auger KR, Carpenter C et al: Oncogenes and signal transduction. Cell 64:281, 1991.
Cline MJ, Slamon DJ, Lipsick JS: Oncogenes: Implications for the diagnosis and treatment of cancer. Ann Intern Med 101:233, 1984.
Cooper CS: Translocations in solid tumors. Curr Opin Genet Dev 6:71, 1996.
Frost P, Hart I, Kerbel RS: Transgenic mice. Cancer Metastasis Rev 14:77, 1995.
Karlan BY, Amin W, Casper SE et al: Hormonal regulation of CA-125 tumor marker expression in human ovarian carcinoma cells: Inhibition by glucocorticoids. Cancer Res 48:3502, 1988.
Lee JH, Kavanagh JJ, Wildrich JJ et al: Frequent loss of heterozygosity on chromosome 6q, 11 and 17 in human ovarian carcinomas. Cancer Res 50:2724, 1990.
Marks JR, Davidoff AM, Kerns BJ et al: Overexpression and mutation of p53 in epithelial ovarian cancer. Cancer Res 51:2979, 1991.
Meyn RE, Milas L, Stephens C: Programmed cell death in normal development and disease. Cancer Bull 46:18, 1994.
Nemunaitis J: Cytokine-mobilized peripheral blood progenitor cells. Semin Oncol 23:9, 1996.
Rous P: A sarcoma of the fowl transmissible by an agent separable from the tumor cells. Nature 13:397, 1911.
Saegusa M et al: The possible role of BCL2 expression in the progression of tumors of the uterine cervix. Cancer 76: 2297, 1995.
Schreiber G, Dubeau L: C-myc proto-oncogene amplification detected by polymerase chain reaction in archival human ovarian carcinomas. Am J Pathol 137:653, 1990.
Scrable HJ, Sapienza C, Cavenee WK: Genetic and epigenetic losses of heterozygosity in cancer predisposition and progression. Adv Cancer Res 54:25, 1990.
Sellins KS, Cohen JJ: Hyperthermia induces apoptosis in thymocytes. Radiat Res 126:88, 1991.
Tonkin KS, Berger M, Ormerod M: Epidermal growth factor receptor status in four carcinoma of the cervix cell lines. Int J Gynecol Cancer 1:185, 1991.
Wyllie AH: The biology of cell death in tumors. Anticancer Res 5:131, 1985.
Wyllie AH: Apoptosis and the regulation of cell numbers in normal and neoplastic tissues: An overview. Cancer Metastasis Rev 11:95, 1992.
Yanagihara K, Tsumuraya M: Transforming growth factor β induces apoptotic cell death in cultured human gastric carcinoma cells. Cancer Res 52:4042, 1992.
Yonish-Rouach E et al: P53-mediated cell death: Relationship to cell cycle control. Mol Cell Biol 13:1415, 1993.

MISMATCH REPAIR DEFECTS

Acharya S, Wilson T, Gradia S et al: hMSH2 forms specific mispair-binding complexes with hMSH3 and hMSH. Proc Natl Acad Sci U S A 93:13629, 1996.
Arnheim N, Shibata D: DNA mismatch repair in mammals: Role in disease and meiosis. Curr Opin Genet Dev 7:364, 1997.
Boyer JC, Umar A, Risinger JI et al: Microsatellite instability, mismatch repair deficiency and genetic defects in human cancer cell lines. Cancer Res 55:6063, 1995.
Drummond JT, Li GM, Longley MJ, Modrich P: Isolation of an hMSH2-p160 heterodimer that restores DNA mismatch repair to tumor cells. Science 268:1909, 1995.
Dunlop MG: Mutator genes and mosaicism in colorectal cancer. Curr Opin Genet Dev 6:76, 1996.
Fang WH, Modrich P: Human strand specific mismatch repair occurs by a bidirectional mechanism similar to that of the bacterial reaction. J Biol Chem 268:11838, 1993.
Fisher R, Kolodner RD: Identification of mismatch repair genes and their role in the development of cancer. Curr Opin Genet Dev 5:382, 1995.
Griffin S: DNA damage, DNA repair and disease. Curr Biol 6:497, 499, 1996.
Ionov Y, Peinado MA, Malkhosyan S et al: Ubiquitous somatic mutations in simple repeat sequences reveal a new mechanism for colonic carcinogenesis. Nature 363:558, 1993.
Kolodner RD, Alani E: Mismatch repair and cancer susceptibility. Curr Opin Biotechnol 5:585, 1994.
Kunkel TA: DNA mismatch repair: The intricacies of eukaryotic spell checking. Curr Biol 5:1091, 1995.
Li GM, Modrich P: Restoration of mismatch repair to nuclear extracts of H6 colorectal tumor-cells by heterodimer of human MutL homologs. Proc Natl Acad Sci USA 92:1950, 1995.
Loeb LA: Mutator phenotype may be required for multistage carcinogenesis. Cancer Res 51:3075, 1991.
Lynch HT, Smyrk T, Lynch JF: Overview of the natural history, pathology, molecular genetics and management of HNPCC (Lynch syndrome). Int J Cancer 69:38, 1996.
Modrich P, Lahue R: Mismatch repair in replication fidelity, genetic recombination, and cancer biology. Annu Rev Biochem 65:101, 1996.
Palombo F, Gallinari P, Laccarino I et al: GTBP, a 160 kilodalton protein essential for mismatch binding activity in human cells. 268:1912, 1995.
Palombo F, laccarino I, Nakajima E et al: hMUTs-B, a heterodimer of hMSH2 and hMSH3, binds to insertion/deletion loops in DNA. Curr Biol 6:1181, 1996.
Parsons R, Li GM, Longley M et al: Mismatch repair deficiency in phenotypically normal human cells. Science 268:738, 1995.
Thibodeau SN, Bren G, Schaid D: Microsatellite instability in cancer of the proximal colon. Science 260:816, 1993.
Umar A, Buemeyer AB, Simon JA et al: Requirement for PCNA in DNA mismatch repair at a step preceding DNA resynthesis. Cell 87:65, 1996.

TELOMERASE

Harley CB, Futcher AB, Greider CW: Telomeres shorten during aging of human fibroblasts.
Hayflick L: The limited in vitro lifetime of human diploid cell strains. Exp Cell Res 37:614, 1965.

McKenzie KE, Umbricht CB, Saraswati S: Applications of research in the fight against cancer: Review of telomerase. Mol Med 3:114, 1999.

Meeker AK, Coffey DS: Telomerase: A promising marker of biological immortality of germ, stem and cancer cells. A review. Biochemistry 62:1323, 1997.

Shay JW, Bacchetti S: A survey of telomerase activity in human cancer. Eur J Cancer 33:787, 1997. Nature 345:458, 1990.

GENE THERAPY

Brenner MK: Human somatic gene therapy: Progress and problems. J Intern Med 237:229, 1995.

Champlin RE: Peripheral blood progenitor cells: A replacement for marrow transplantation? Semin Oncol 23:15, 1996.

Fraser JK, Lill MC, Figlin RA: The biology of the cytokine sequence cascade. Semin Oncol 23:2, 1996.

Holzman D: New cancer genes crowd the horizon, create possibilities. J Natl Cancer Inst 87:1108, 1995.

Hwu P: The gene therapy of cancer. In De Vita VT et al (eds): PPO Updates, Vol 9: Cancer: Principles and Practice of Oncology, 4th ed. Philadelphia, JB Lippincott, 1995, p 1.

Jolly D: Viral vector systems for gene therapy. Cancer Gene Ther 1:51, 1994.

Krotiris TG: Oncogenes. N Engl J Med 333:303, 1995.

Mastrangelo MJ et al: A pilot study demonstrating the feasibility of using intratumoral vaccinia injections as vector for gene transfer. Vaccine Res 4:58, 1995.

Nicholas GL: Antisense oligodeoxynucleotides as therapeutic agents for chronic myelogenous leukemia. Antisense Res Dev 5:67, 1995.

Robinson A: Gene therapy-the future touches down. Can Med Assoc J 150:377, 1960.

Rosenberg SA: Gene therapy for cancer. JAMA 268:2416, 1992.

Takara H et al: Effective eradication of established murine tumors with IL-12 gene therapy using a polycistronic retroviral vector. J Immunol 154:6466, 1995.

MOLECULAR TECHNOLOGIES

Johnsson A, Zeelenberg I Min Y, Hilinski J, Berry C, Howell, SB, Los G: Identification of genes differentially expressed in association with acquired cisplatin resistance. Br J cancer 83:1047–1050, 200.

Strausberg RL, Buetow KH, Emmert-Bucki MR, Klausner RD,: the cancer genome anatomy project: building an annotated gene index. Trends in genetics 16:103–110, 2000.

Velculescu VE, Zhang L, Vogelstein B, Kinzler KW: Serial analysis of gene expression. Science 270:484–489, 1995.

Williamsson AR: the Merck Gene Index project. Drug Discovery Today 4:115, 1999.

GENETIC STUDIES IN HUMAN MALIGNANT NEOPLASMS

Alessandro R, Belluco C, Kohn EC. Proteomic approaches in colon cancer: promising tools for new cancer markers and drug target discovery. Clin Colorectal Cancer 4(6):396–402, 2005.

Amos CI et al: Age at onset for familial epithelial ovarian cancer. JAMA 268:1896, 1992.

Arca MJ, Mule JJ, Chang AE: Genetic approaches to adoptive cellular therapy for malignancy. Semin Oncol 23:108, 1996.

Baker VV et al: C-myc amplification in ovarian cancer. Gynecol Oncol 38:340, 1990.

Barbosa MS, Schlegel R: The E6 and E7 genes of HPV-18 are sufficient for inducing two-stage in vitro transformation of human keratinocytes. Oncogene 4:1529, 1989.

Breast Cancer Linkage Consortium: An evaluation of genetic heterogenicity in 145 breast ovarian cancer families. Am J Hum Genet 56:254, 1995.

Cullen AP et al: Analysis of the physical state of different human papillomavirus DNAs in intraepithelial and invasive cervical neoplasm. J Virol 65:606, 1991.

Easton DF, Bishop DT, Ford D, Crockford GP and the Breast Cancer Linkage Consortium: Genetic linkage analysis in familial breast and ovarian cancer: Results from 214 families. Am J Hum Genet 52:678, 1993.

Eschrich S, Yang I, Bloom G, Kwong KY, Boulware D, Cantor A, Coppola D, Kruhoffer M, Aaltonen L, Orntoft TF, Quackenbush J, Yeatman TJ. Molecular staging for survival prediction of colorectal cancer patients. J Clin Oncol 23:3526–3535, 2005.

Ezzell C: BRCA1 shock: Breast cancer gene encodes a secreted protein. J NIH Res 8:11, 1996.

Ferguson SE, Alshen AB, Viale A, Barakat RR, Boyd J. Stratification of intermediate-risk endometrial cancer patients into groups at high risk or low risk for recurrence based on tumor gene expression profiles. Clin Cancer Res. 11:2252–2257, 2005.

Ferguson SE, Olshen AB, Viale A, Awtrey CS, Barakat RR, Boyd J: Gene expression profiling of tamoxifen-associated uterine cancers: evidence for two molecular classes of endometrial carcinoma. Gynecologic Oncol. 92:719–25, 2004.

Fredricksen CM, Knudsen S, Laurberg S, Orntoft TF: Classification of Dukes' B and C colorectal cancers using expression arrays. J Cancer Res Clin Oncol 129:263–271, 2003.

Holt JT et al: Growth retardation and tumour inhibition by BRCA1. Nat Genet 12:298, 1996.

Kacinski BM et al: Ovarian adenocarcinomas express fms-complementary transcripts and fms antigen, often with co-expression of CSF-1. Am J Pathol 137:135, 1990.

Kacinski BM et al: Neu protein overexpression in benign, borderline, and malignant ovarian neoplasms. Gynecol Oncol 44:245, 1992.

Kastan MB et al: Participation of p53 protein in the cellular response to DNA damage. Cancer Res 51:6304, 1991.

Kessis T et al: Human papillomavirus 16 E6 disrupts the p53 mediated cellular response to DNA damage. Proc Natl Acad Sci U S A 90:3988, 1993.

Kinzler KW, Vogelstein B: Lessons from hereditary colorectal cancer. Cell 87:159, 1996.

Kuerbitz S et al: Wild type p53 is a cell cycle checkpoint determinant following irradiation. Proc Natl Acad Sci U S A 51:7491, 1992.

Lynch HT, Smyrk TC, Watson P et al: Genetics, natural history, tumor spectrum, and pathology of hereditary non-polyposis colorectal cancer: An updated review. Gastroenterology 104:1535, 1993.

Lynch HT et al: Hereditary ovarian cancer: Heterogeneity in age as a diagnosis. Cancer 67:1460, 1991.

Marks JR et al: Overexpression and mutation of p53 in epithelial ovarian cancer. Cancer Res 51:2979, 1991.

Maxwell GL, Chandramouli GV, Dainty L, Litzi TJ, Berchuk A, Barret JC, Risinger JI. Microarray analysis of endometrial carcinomas and mixed mullerian tumors reveals distinct gene expression profiles associated with different histologic types of uterine cancer. Clin Cancer Res 11:4056–66, 2005.

Mazars R et al: P53 mutations in ovarian cancer: A late event? Oncogene 6:1685, 1991.

Mok CH et al: Unifocal origin of advanced human epithelial ovarian cancers. Cancer Res 52:5119, 1992.

Munger K et al: Biochemical and biological differences between E7 oncoproteins of the high- and low-risk human papillomavirus types are determined by amino-terminal sequences. J Virol 65:3943, 1991.

Mutter GL, Baak JP, Fitzgerald JT, Gray R, Neuberg D, Kust GA, Gentleman R Gullans SR, Wei LJ, Wilcox M, Global expression changes of constituitive and hormonally regulated genes during endometrial neoplastic transformation Gynecologic Oncol. 83:177–185, 2001.

Okamoto A et al: Allelic loss on chromosome 17p and p53 mutations in human endometrial carcinoma of the uterus. Cancer Res 51:5632 1991.

Okamoto A et al: Frequent allelic losses and mutations of the p53 gene in human ovarian cancer. Cancer Res 51:5171, 1991.

Risinger JL et al: P53 gene mutations in human endometrial carcinoma. Mol Carcinog 5:250, 1992.

Risinger JI, Maxwell GL, Chandramouli GV, Aprelikova O, Litzi T, Umar A, Berchuck A Barrett JC, Gene expression profiling of microsatellite unstable and microsatellite stable endometrial cancers indicates distinct pathways of aberrant signaling. Cancer Res. 65:5031–5037, 2005.

Santin AD, Zhan F, Cane S, Bellone S, Palmeieri M, Thomas M, Burnett A, Roman JJ, Cannon MJ, Shaughnessy J Jr, Pecorelli, S. Gene expression fingerprint of uterine serous papillary carcinoma: identification of novel molecular markers for uterine serous cancer diagnosis and therapy. Br J Cancer 92: 1561–1573.

Sasano H et al: An analysis of abnormalities of the retinoblastoma gene in human ovarian and endometrial carcinoma. Cancer 66:2150, 1990.

Sasano H et al: Proto-oncogene amplification and tumor ploidy in human ovarian neoplasms. Hum Pathol 21:382, 1990.

Sato T et al: Allelotype of human ovarian cancer. Cancer Res 51: 5118, 1991.

Simpkins SB, Bocker T, Swisher EM et al: MLH1 promoter methylation and gene silencing is the primary cause of microsatellite instability in sporadic endometrial cancers. Hum Mol Genet 8:661, 1999.

Slamon DJ et al: Studies of the HER-2/neu proto-oncogene in human breast and ovarian cancer. Science 244:707, 1989.

Tsao S et al: Molecular genetic evidence of a unifocal origin for human serous ovarian carcinomas. Gynecol Oncol 48:5, 1993.

Tsao SW et al; Involvement of p53 gene in the allelic deletion of chromosome 17p in human ovarian tumors. Anticancer Res 11:1975, 1991.

Worsham MJ et al: Consistent chromosome abnormalities in squamous cell carcinomas of the vulva. Genes Chromosomes Cancer 3:420, 1991.

Zheng JP et al: Distinction of low grade from high-grade human ovarian carcinomas on the basis of losses of heterozygosity on chromosomes 3, 6 and 11 and HER-2/neu gene amplification. Cancer Res 51:4045, 1991.

21 Palliative Care and Quality of Life

Bradley J. Monk, M.D. and Lari Wenzel, Ph.D.

EVOLUTION OF PALLIATIVE CARE

Once viewed as limited and focused care during the final days of life, the scope of palliative medical care and quality of life research has evolved since the 1990s. Although several definitions of palliative care exist, it is broadly defined as interdisciplinary care, which seeks to prevent, relieve, or reduce the symptoms of a disease or disorder without affecting a cure. "Palliative care" and the related term "palliative medicine" are being used with increasing frequency in the USA and have become the labels of choice throughout the world to describe programs based on the hospice philosophy. When approaching death, including care at the end of life, the Institute of Medicine recommends:

> *"Palliative care should become, if not a medical specialty, at least a defined area of expertise, education and research."*

Palliative care overlaps with "terminal care," "death and dying," "hospice," "end-of-life care," "comfort care," and "supportive care." The term "supportive care," which is often used by oncologists, is particularly ill defined and sometimes refers to comfort care or palliative support of the critically ill patient, particularly those suffering from the adverse effects of cancer treatment. All these terms have a number of meanings and are often unfamiliar to clinicians. They outline the relationships of health care professionals with patients and family members during the terminal stages of life and the treatment of advanced malignancies (Table 21–1)

Quality of life is a concern in all areas of medicine, and of primary importance in the palliative care setting. Within the clinical setting, assessment of a patient's quality of life begins with an understanding of a patient's knowledge about his or her condition and potential management strategies, their values, and their personal cost-benefit calculations. Certain therapies have no chance of improving survival end points but may have an acceptable therapeutic index based on a reasonable balance between the toxicity of the intervention and the resolution of symptoms secondary to the condition being treated. With this concept in mind, investigators and clinicians have begun to collectively measure quality of life in clinical trials and community-based practices in an attempt to define alterations in quality of life and to prospectively ascertain interventions that might improve "survivorship." It is no longer appropriate to simply survive one's illness, but rather one must avoid the "killing cure," allowing patients to enjoy life and function productively while interacting with their environment during multimodality cancer treatment.

Table 21–1 ISSUES IN PALLIATIVE AND END-OF-LIFE CARE

Emphasis on the trajectory
Symptom control and psychological support
Comprehensive assessment
Cancer pain management
Communicating effectively
Diagnosis and prognosis
Symptoms
Negotiating goals of care
Clinical trials
Withdrawing and withholding therapy
Advanced care planning
Cancer doctors and burnout

The gynecologic oncologist is in a unique position to function collectively as a primary care provider, surgeon, radiation oncologist, and chemotherapist allowing comprehensive transfer of treatment with an emphasis on the patient's quality of life. Reports from the Institute of Medicine's Committee on Care at the End of Life and the American Society of Clinical Oncology (ASCO) Task Force on Cancer Care at the End of Life, both published in 1998, clearly acknowledge the physician's responsibility in caring for patients throughout the continuum of their illness (Table 21–2). The ASCO document asserts:

> *"In addition to appropriate anti-cancer treatment, comprehensive care includes symptom control and psychosocial support during all phases of life."*

Gynecologic oncologists are not only faced with the challenge of providing end-of-life care, but they must also explore ways to integrate palliative care throughout the continuum of illness. Indeed, recent literature suggests that gynecologic oncologists recognize the growing importance of their role as the patient's disease progresses. It is in this role, when the challenges of effective, compassionate care and communication are heightened, that an understanding of the principles and the clinical practice of palliative medicine are critical. A review of the recommendations for and barriers to effective palliative and end-of-life care as outlined by the Institute of Medicine and ASCO is listed in Table 21–2.

Palliative care is differentiated from other medical specialties by its fundamental philosophy of care delivery; care is collaboratively provided by an interdisciplinary team prompted by issues and concerns of the patient and family. "Family" as defined by the patient and staff may include friends as well as relatives. Palliative care is, by definition, care delivered through the coordinated efforts of the team that is collectively confident and skilled when assessing and addressing the physical, psychosocial, and spiritual needs of the patient and family. It differs from more traditional "multidisciplinary" care that is directed by a physician, which allows team members to simply focus on their own areas of expertise. In contrast, the palliative care "intradisciplinary" team recognizes that all information about

Table 21–2 IMPROVING END-OF-LIFE CARE: RECOMMENDATIONS OF THE INSTITUTE OF MEDICINE

1. Reliable and skilful supportive care
2. Effective use of knowledge to prevent and relieve pain and other symptoms
3. Policy makers, consumers, health practitioners, and organizations:
   - Measure quality of life (QOL) and other outcomes
   - Develop tools for improving QOL and hold health care organizations accountable
   - Revise payment mechanisms to encourage good end-of-life care
   - Reform laws and regulations that impede effective use of opioids
4. Change medical education to ensure relevant attitudes, knowledge, and skills
5. Recognition of palliative care as a defined area of expertise, education, and research
6. Research establishment to strengthen knowledge base
7. Promote public education

Barriers to optimal end-of-life care identified by the American Society of Clinical Oncology

1. Inappropriate attitudes of health care professionals and patients (e.g., reluctance to discuss death and dying)
2. Ineffective communication about the prognosis
3. Unrealistic expectations and treatment options
4. Failure of physicians to recognize and emphasize the importance of symptom management and psychosocial support
5. Social attitudes (e.g., fear of opioid addiction)
6. Economic barriers, including lack of universal access to care and underfunding of end-of-life care
7. Fear of the attending physician losing control of the patient's care; hospice teams to work more closely with attending physicians
8. Lack of systematic education for physicians about clinical and psychosocial aspects of care

Modified from the Institute of Medicine's Report and ASCO Task Force.

the patient and family is relevant. Thus, the home health aide or the pharmacist may have a point of view that would be helpful for the care plan. Common members of these multidisciplinary teams include medical social workers, pastoral care, nutritionists, radiation oncologist, medical oncologist, pain specialists, psychologists, physical therapists, and caseworkers. Early in the treatment of a gynecologic cancer, side effects of therapy should be anticipated and treated prophylactically. Later, some symptoms may be dealt with without the extensive evaluation associated with the assessment of tumor response or disease status. However, the development of symptoms often indicates disease progression, and appropriate laboratory or radiographic studies may lead to an alteration of treatment. As the cancer progresses, making cytotoxic therapy less likely to be effective, the workup of new symptoms must be tailored to the individual patient based on the prognosis as well as on the desires expressed by the patient and family. In end-of-life care, there is no room for long-term evaluation or a "wait and see" attitude. As a result, control of annoying symptoms may be pursued more aggressively, and management may resemble that given in an intensive care situation but without an extensive diagnostic evaluation. Control of symptoms is not an end in itself, but it should be sought to allow the patient time to optimize quality of life and to support the patient in reaching peace with self and closure with important people in the patient's life.

MANAGEMENT OF COMMON PHYSICAL SYMPTOMS

Even when cancer can be treated effectively and a cure or life prolongation achieved, there are always physical, psychosocial, or spiritual concerns that must be addressed to maintain function and to optimize the quality of life. Symptoms are a reminder to the patient and caregivers of the cancer and the potentially devastating effects of treatment. Symptoms related to cancer and its treatment have not attracted much notice in the past when patients and physicians alike felt that pursuing them might detract from the "real" goal of controlling the tumor. Consequently, symptoms have been taken for granted by the medical profession. Successful and appropriate management of physical symptoms can allow the care team to focus on the psychosocial closure of life and provide the patient an opportunity to participate more fully in the decisions of care and to rebuild or establish stronger relationships with family, friends, and coworkers.

Many physicians and nurses find symptom management in patients with advanced disease to be a frustrating experience, because the symptoms may persist or progress. Although the symptoms are not always completely controlled, acknowledgment of the problem and working toward its relief offer invaluable support to the patient. Reliance on medical and drug therapies has been the traditional method to control symptoms. There is increasing recognition that non-pharmacologic approaches have significant benefits for individual patients. Non-traditional approaches such as acupuncture, biofeedback, aromatherapy, massage, and herbal medicine may have a role in the management of symptoms. Each of the following four physical symptoms is addressed in detail: fatigue, pain, nausea/vomiting, and diarrhea/constipation.

Fatigue

Patients have identified fatigue with cancer as the major obstacle to normal functioning and good quality of life. Fatigue is the most prevalent (60–96%) and one of the least understood symptoms that affect cancer patients. Although almost a universal symptom of patients undergoing primary antineoplastic therapy or treatment with biologic response modifiers, it is also extremely common in populations with persistent or advanced cancer.

Table 21–3 PROPOSED CRITERIA FOR CANCER-RELATED FATIGUE

The following symptoms have been present daily or almost every day during the same 2-week period in the past month:

- Significant fatigue, diminished energy, or increased need to rest, disproportionate to any recent change in activity level

Plus five (or more) of the following:

- Complaints of generalized weakness or limb heaviness
- Diminished concentration of attention
- Decreased motivation or interest in engaging in usual activities
- Insomnia or hypersomnia
- Experience of sleep as unrefreshing or non-restorative
- Perceived need to struggle to overcome inactivity
- Marked emotional reactivity (e.g., sadness, frustration, or irritability) when feeling fatigued
- Difficulty completing daily tasks attributed to feeling fatigued
- Perceived problems with short-term memory
- Post-exertional malaise lasting several hours
- The symptoms cause clinically significant distress or impairment in social, occupational, or other important areas of functioning
- There is evidence from the history, physical examination, or laboratory findings that the symptoms are a consequence of cancer or cancer-related therapy
- The symptoms are not primarily a consequence of a comorbid psychiatric disorders, such as major depression, somatization disorder, or delirium

Adapted from Cella et al: Progress toward guidelines for the management of fatigue. Oncology 12:369–377, 1998.

Given the prevalence and impact of cancer-related fatigue, there have been remarkably few studies of the phenomenon. Its epidemiology has been poorly defined, and the variety of clinical presentations remains anecdotal. The existence of discrete fatigue syndromes linked with predisposing factors or potential etiologies has not been confirmed, and clinical trials to evaluate putative therapies for specific types of cancer-related fatigue are almost entirely lacking.

Patients and practitioners can generally differentiate "normal" fatigue experienced by the general population from clinical fatigue associated with cancer or its treatment. The term "asthenia" has been used to describe fatigue in oncology patients but has no specific meaning apart from the more common term. This condition is inherently subjective and multidimensional. Typically, it develops over time and is characterized by diminishing energy, mental capacity, and psychological condition of cancer patients (Table 21–3). It is also linked with lethargy, malaise, and asthenia in the revised National Cancer Institute Common Toxicity Criteria. These classifications may enhance awareness of fatigue and improve reporting of the condition.

When fatigue is primarily related to a treatment, there is generally a clear temporal relationship between the condition and the intervention. In patients receiving cytotoxic

Table 21–4 POTENTIAL PREDISPOSING FACTORS WITH CANCER-RELATED FATIGUE

Physiologic	
	Underlying disease
	Treatment for the disease
	Chemotherapy
	Radiotherapy
	Surgery
	Biologic response modifiers
	Intercurrent systemic disorders
	Anemia
	Infection
	Pulmonary disorders
	Hepatic failure
	Heart failure
	Renal insufficiency
	Malnutrition
	Neuromuscular disorders
	Dehydration or electrolyte disturbances
	Sleep disorders
	Immobility and lack of exercise
	Chronic pain
	Use of centrally acting drugs (e.g., opioids)
Psychosocial	
	Anxiety disorders
	Depressive disorders
	Stress-related
	Environmental reinforcers

Adapted from Portenoy RK: Principles and Practice of Supportive Oncology. Philadelphia, Lippincott-Raven, 1998, pp 109–118.

chemotherapy, for example, it often peaks within a few days and declines into the next treatment cycle. During the course of fractionated radiotherapy, it is often cumulative and may peak over a period of weeks. Occasionally, it persists for a prolonged period beyond the end of chemotherapy or radiation treatment. The relationship between fatigue and demographic characteristics, physiologic factors, and psychosocial factors is not well defined. The specific mechanisms that precipitate or sustain the syndrome are unknown. Fatigue may present a final common pathway to which many predisposing or etiologic factors contribute (Table 21–4). The pathophysiology in any individual may be multifactorial. Proposed mechanisms include abnormalities in energy metabolism related to increased nutritional requirements (e.g., due to tumor growth, infection, fever, or surgery), decreased availability of metabolic substrate (e.g., due to anemia, hypoxemia or poor nutrition), or the abnormal production of substances that impair metabolism or normal function of muscles (e.g., cytokines or antibodies). Other proposed mechanisms link fatigue to the pathophysiology of sleep disorders and major depression. Further research is necessary to determine mediating mechanisms and optimal interventions.

A detailed characterization of fatigue combined with an understanding of the most likely etiologic factors is necessary to develop a therapeutic strategy (Fig. 21–1). A comprehensive assessment includes the description of fatigue-related phenomena, a physical examination, and a review of laboratory and imaging studies that may allow a possible hypothesis concerning pathogenesis which, in turn, may suggest appropriate treatment strategies. Patients may describe fatigue in terms of decreased vitality or lack of energy, muscular weakness, dysphoric mood, insomnia, impaired cognitive functioning, or some combination of these disturbances. Although this variability suggests the existence of fatigue subtypes, this has not yet been confirmed. Regardless, the patient's history should clarify the spectrum of complaints and attempt to characterize features associated with each component. This information may suggest specific etiologies (e.g., depression) and influence the choice of therapy. Neurologic and psychological evaluation may also help further clarify potential etiologies and fatigue in some patients. Other characteristics are similarly important. Onset and duration, for example, distinguish acute and chronic fatigue. Acute fatigue of recent onset is anticipated to end in the near future. Chronic fatigue is persistent for a prolonged period (weeks to months or longer), and it is not expected to remit in a short time. Patients perceived to have chronic fatigue typically require more intensive evaluation as well as a management approach focused on both short- and long-term goals. Other important descriptors of fatigue include the severity, daily pattern, course over time, exacerbating and palliative factors, and associated distress. An assessment of cancer-related fatigue should also include consideration of broader concerns, including global quality of life, other symptoms, and disease status. Fatigue may be only one of numerous factors that influence quality of life. Among these factors are progressive physical decline, psychological disorders, social isolation, financial concerns, and spiritual distress. Optimal care of the cancer patient includes a broader assessment of these factors and should be directed toward maintaining or enhancing quality of life. Successful strategies should ameliorate fatigue within a broader approach of patient care. Evaluation of the patient regarding the nature of fatigue, options for therapy, and anticipated outcomes is an essential aspect of the therapy. Unfortunately, results of a patient survey indicate that patients and their oncologists seldom discuss fatigue.

An initial approach to cancer-related fatigue includes efforts to correct potential etiologies, if possible and appropriate. This may include elimination of non-essential centrally acting drugs, treatment of a sleep disorder, reversal of anemia or metabolic abnormalities, or management of major depression. Many of these initial interventions are relatively simple and pose minimal burdens to the patient, health care provider, and caregiver.

In patients with fatigue-associated major depression, treatment with an antidepressant is strongly indicated. As many as 25% of cancer patients develop major depression at some point during their illness. Patients at greatest risk are those with advanced disease, uncontrolled physical symptoms (e.g., pain), or a previous history of a psychiatric disorder. Although the relationship between depression and fatigue is not well understood, they often occur

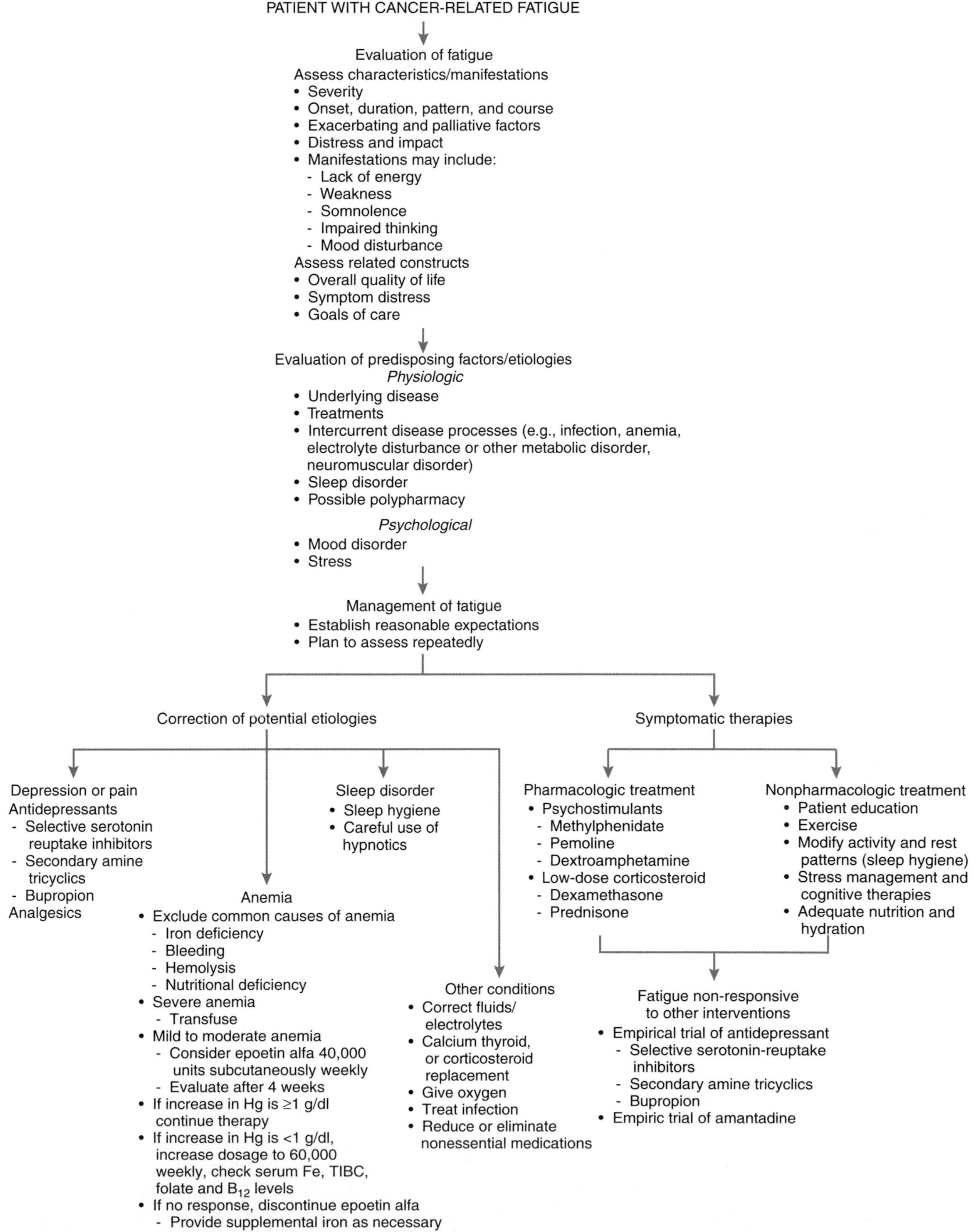

Figure 21–1 Evaluation and approach to management of the patient with cancer-related fatigue. (Adapted from Portenoy RK, Itri LM: Cancer-related fatigue: Guidelines for evaluation and management. Oncologist 4[1]:1–10, 1999.)

together and both adversely affect quality of life. Despite the high prevalence in the cancer population, depression is often underdiagnosed and consequently undertreated. A trial with an antidepressant is usually warranted in a patient with fatigue associated with any significant degree of depressed mood, and similarly can be therapeutic when concurrent anxiety or pain exists. In addition, brief, focused psychological counseling can be helpful for several reasons when a mood disorder (e.g., depression and/or anxiety) and a physical symptom (e.g., pain and/or fatigue) co-occur. First, counseling offers the patient an opportunity to identify and express her fears, which are often driving the depressed or anxious mood. Second, the depressed or anxious mood can exacerbate existing physical symptoms such as pain. Therefore, provision of counseling has the dual benefit of reducing the mood disorder, which by extension reduces fatigue and pain. Third, brief, focused counseling can offer the patient important behavioral modifications such as time and energy management strategies which permits and teaches the patient to conserve energy physically and emotionally for the priorities in their life. This is useful to address the practical challenges associated with fatigue and pain management.

Anemia may be a major factor in the development of cancer-related fatigue. Anecdotally, transfusion therapy for severe anemia has often been associated with substantial improvement in fatigue. New data demonstrate the association between chemotherapy-induced mild to moderate anemia and both fatigue and quality of life impairment. For example, combined data from 413 patients and three randomized placebo controlled trials of epoetin alfa, the recombinant form of human erythropoietin, reveal that treated patients experienced a significant increase in hematocrit, a reduced need for transfusion, and a significant improvement in overall quality of life. Those patients with an increase in hematocrit of >6% also demonstrated significant improvement in energy level and daily activities. Additional studies in patients treated with chemotherapy and radiation therapy for various gynecologic tumors confirm that epoetin alfa has positive effects on hemoglobin levels. Two large, prospective, randomized, multicenter community trials have demonstrated that patients experience significant improvement in energy levels, activity level, functional status, and overall quality of life when epoetin alfa is administered as an adjunct to cytotoxic chemotherapy.

Many of the pharmacologic therapies for fatigue associated with medical illness have not been rigorously evaluated in controlled trials. Nonetheless, there is evidence to support the use of several drug classes. Psychostimulants, such as methylphenidate, pemoline, and dextroamphetamine, have been well studied for the treatment of opioid-related somnolence and cognitive impairment and depression in elderly and medically ill patients. There are no controlled studies of these drugs for cancer-related fatigue, but empiric administration may yield favorable results in some patients.

A clinical response to one drug does not necessarily predict a response to the others, and sequential trials may be needed to identify the most beneficial therapy. Methylphenidate has been more extensively evaluated in the cancer population than other stimulant drugs and is often the first drug to be administered. Pemoline has less sympathomimetic activity than other psychostimulants but has a low risk of severe hepatotoxicity compared with similar agents. It is available in a chewable formulation that can be absorbed through the buccal mucosa for patients who are unable to swallow or take oral medications.

Adverse effects associated with the psychostimulants include anorexia, insomnia, tremulousness, anxiety, delirium, and tachycardia. To ensure safety, slow and careful dose escalation should be undertaken to minimize potential adverse effects. A regimen of methylphenidate, for example, usually begins with a dose of 5–10 mg once or twice daily (morning and, if needed, midday). If the drug is tolerated, the dose is increased. Most patients appear to require less than 60 mg/day, but some require much higher doses.

Extensive anecdotal observations and very limited data from controlled trials support the use of low-dose corticosteroid therapy in fatigued patients with advanced disease and multiple symptoms. Dexamethasone and prednisone are most commonly used. There have been no comparative trials.

The selective serotonin-reuptake inhibitors, secondary amine tricyclics (e.g., nortriptyline and desipramine), or bupropion are sometimes associated with the experience of increased energy that appears disproportionate to any change in mood. For this reason, these agents have also been tried empirically in non-depressed patients with fatigue. Given the limited experience in the use of these drugs for this indication, an empirical trial should be considered only in severe and refractory cases.

Amantadine has been used to treat fatigue in patients with multiple sclerosis, but it has not been studied in other patient populations. This drug is usually well tolerated, and an empirical trial may be warranted in selected patients with severe refractory cancer-related fatigue.

Non-pharmacologic approaches for the management of cancer-related fatigue are supported mainly by favorable anecdotal experience (Table 21–5). Patient preferences should be considered in the selection of one or more of these approaches. In particular, sleep hygiene principles should be tailored to the individual patients and might include the establishment of a specific bedtime, awake time, and routine procedures before sleep. Patients should also be instructed to avoid stimulants and central nervous system depressants before going to sleep. Regular exercise performed at least 6 hours before bedtime may improve sleep, whereas napping in the late afternoon or evening may worsen it.

Cancer and its treatment can also interfere with dietary intake. With aggressive approaches to management, the patient's weight, hydration status, and electrolyte balance should be monitored and maintained to every extent possible. Regular exercise may improve appetite and increase nutritional appetite. Referral to a dietitian for nutritional guidance and suggestions for nutritional supplements may be useful.

Table 21–5 NONPHARMACOLOGIC INTERVENTIONS FOR THE MANAGEMENT OF CANCER-RELATED FATIGUE

Patient education
Consider the patient's preferences, education level, and readiness to learn
Use of a patient's diary
Exercise
Individualize exercise program
Use of rhythmic and repetitive types of exercise
Initiate gradually
Modification of activity and rest patterns
Assess sleep hygiene
Establish routine sleep patterns
Avoid use of stimulants prior to sleep
Regular exercise
Stress management and cognitive therapies
Use of stress reduction techniques or cognitive therapies
Use of relaxation therapy, hypnosis, or distraction
Adequate nutrition and hydration
Proper diet
Monitor weight and hydration status regularly
Referral to a dietitian

Adapted from Portenoy RK: Principles and Practice of Supportive Oncology. Philadelphia, Lippincott-Raven, 1998, pp 109–118.

Pain

Cancer pain can be managed effectively through relatively simple means in up to 90% of the eight million Americans who have cancer or a history of cancer. Unfortunately, pain associated with cancer is often undertreated. Although cancer pain or associated symptoms cannot always be eliminated, proper use of available therapies can effectively relieve pain for most patients. Management of pain extends beyond pain relief and encompasses the patient's quality of life and the ability to work productively, to enjoy recreation, and to function normally in the family and society.

State and local laws often restrict the medical use of opioids to relieve cancer pain, and third party payers may not reimburse for a non-invasive pain control treatment. Thus, clinicians should work with regulators, state cancer pain initiatives, or other groups to eliminate these health care system barriers to effective pain management (Table 21–6).

Flexibility is the key to management of cancer pain. Thorough discussions with the patient and their families encouraging them to be active in pain management are critical (Table 21–7). Patients often need reassurance to report pain, because effective treatment strategies exist. Failure to assess pain is a critical factor leading to undertreatment. The goal of the initial assessment of pain is to characterize the pain by location, intensity, and etiology. This can be accomplished through a detailed history, physical examination, social assessment, and diagnostic evaluation. The mainstay of pain assessment is patient self-reporting.

Table 21–6 BARRIERS TO CANCER PAIN MANAGEMENT

Problems related to health care professionals
Inadequate knowledge of pain management
Poor assessment of pain
Concern about regulation of controlled substances
Fear of patient addiction
Concern about side effects of analgesics
Concern about patients becoming tolerant to analgesics
Problems related to patients
Reluctance to report pain
Concern about distracting physicians from treatment of underlying disease
Fear that pain means disease is worse
Concern about not being a "good" patient
Reluctance to take pain medications
Fear of addiction or of being thought of as an addict
Worries about unmanageable side effects
Concern about becoming tolerant to pain medications
Problems related to the health care system
Low priority given to cancer pain treatment
Inadequate reimbursement
The most appropriate treatment may not be reimbursed or may be too costly for patients and families.
Restrictive regulation of controlled substances
Problems of availability of treatment or access to it

Adapted from Management of Cancer Pain: Adults. Washington, D.C., U.S. Dept of Health and Human Services, March 1994.

Table 21–7 RECOMMENDED CLINICAL APPROACH

A	**Ask** about pain regularly. **Assess** pain systematically.
B	**Believe** the patient and family in their reports of pain and what relieves it.
C	**Choose** pain control options appropriate for the patient, family, and setting.
D	**Deliver** interventions in a timely, logical, coordinated fashion.
E	**Empower** patients and their families. **Enable** patients to control their course to the greatest extent possible.

Adapted from Management of Cancer Pain: Adults. Washington, D.C., U.S. Dept of Health and Human Services, March 1994.

To enhance pain management across all settings, clinicians should teach patients to use pain assessment tools in their homes. The clinicians should listen to the patient's descriptive words about the quality of the pain, inquiring about its location, severity, aggravating or relieving factors, and the patient's cognitive response to the discomfort. Finally, goals for pain control should be clear. Continued assessment of cancer pain is crucial. Changes in pain patterns and the development of new pain should trigger diagnostic evaluation and modification of the treatment plan. Persistent pain indicates the need to consider other etiologies (e.g., related to disease progression or treatment, and alternative—perhaps more invasive—treatment [see Fig. 21–2]).

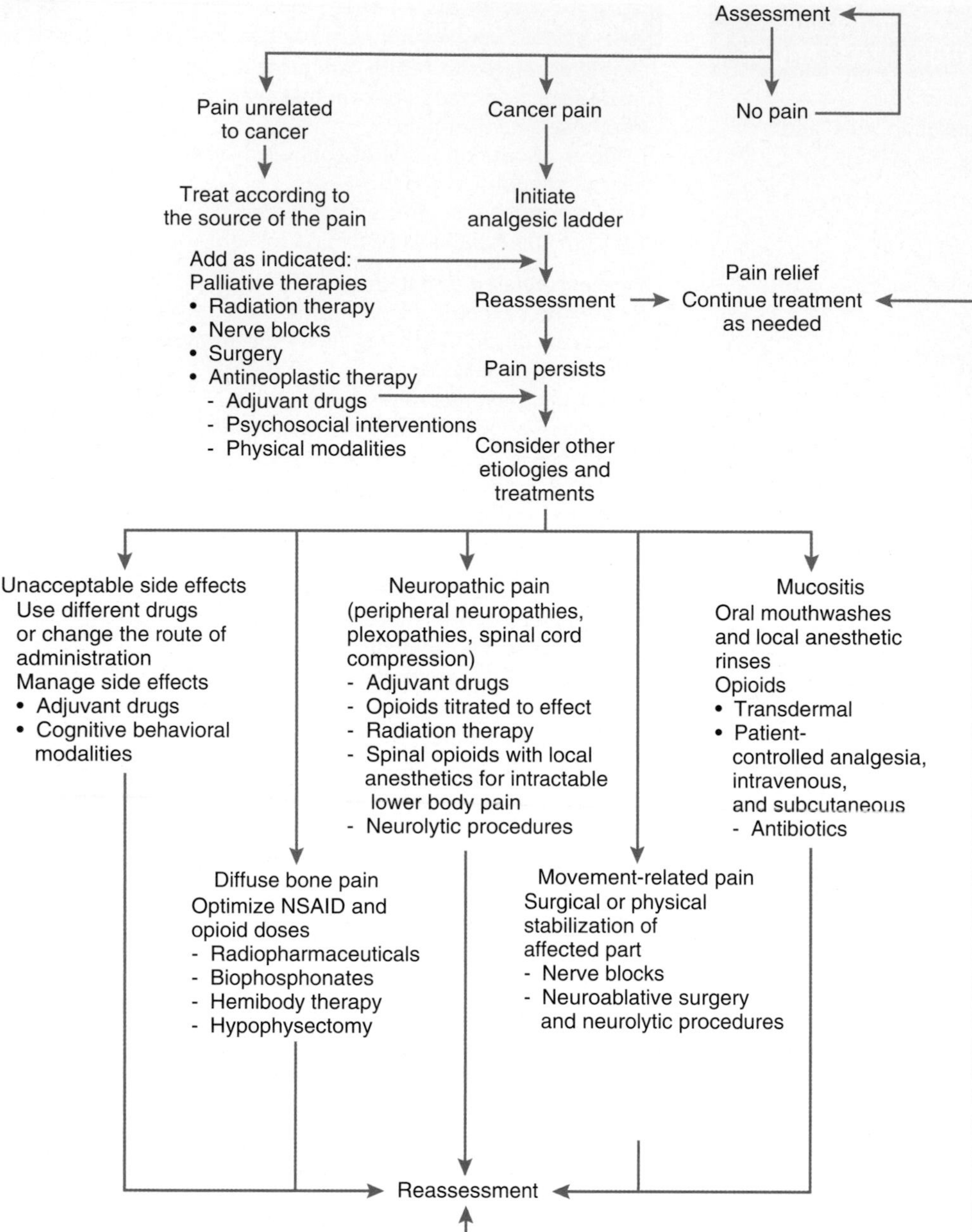

Figure 21–2 Continuing pain management. (Adapted from US Dept of Health and Human Services: Management of Cancer Pain: Adults. Washington, DC, US Dept of Health and Human Services, March 1994.)

Drug therapy is the cornerstone of cancer pain management. It is effective, relatively low risk, and inexpensive and usually works quickly. Even within the same family of analgesic drugs, individual variations in tolerability and side effects are well recognized. Recommendations for pharmacologic therapy begin with the World Health Organization (WHO) ladder (Fig. 21–3), a three-step hierarchy for analgesic pain management. Substitution of drugs within a category should be tried before switching therapy. The simplest dosage and schedule as well as the least invasive pain management modality should be attempted first. For mild to moderate pain, non-steroidal anti-inflammatory drugs (WHO ladder step 1) are often effective (Table 21–8). When pain persists or increases (Table 21–9), opioids can be added (WHO ladder step 2). Moderate to severe pain requires opioids of higher potency and dose (WHO ladder step 3) (Tables 21–10 and 21–11). Dosing should be on a regular schedule (i.e., "by the clock") to maintain a level of drugs that would help prevent the recurrence of pain. Ask for patient and family cooperation in establishing the effective level when administering medications to prevent long-term cancer pain on an around-the-clock basis with additional doses ("as needed" and usually required).

Oral administration is preferred, because it is convenient and usually cost effective. When patients cannot take oral medications, other less invasive (e.g., rectal or transdermal) routes should be offered. Parenteral methods should be used only when simpler, less demanding, less costly methods are inappropriate or ineffective. An assessment of the patient's response to several different oral opioids is usually advisable before abandoning the oral route in favor of parenteral, neurosurgical, or other invasive approaches. Rectal administration is a safe, inexpensive, and effective route for the delivery of opioids as well as non-opioids when patients

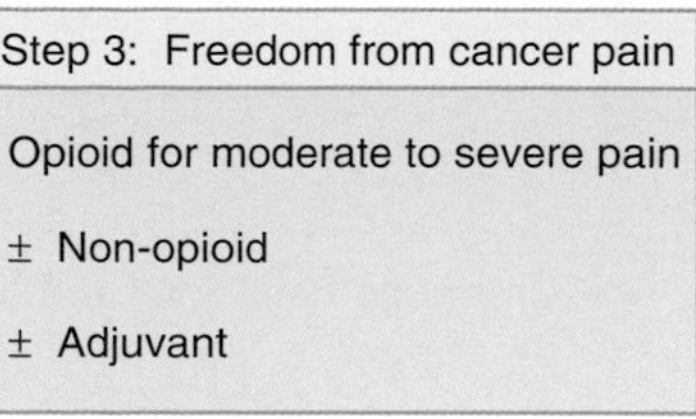

Figure 21–3 World Health Organization three-step analgesic ladder. (Adapted from World Health Organization: Cancer pain relief and palliative care. Geneva, Switzerland, World Health Organization, 1990.)

have nausea or vomiting. Rectal administration is inappropriate for the patient who has diarrhea, anal/rectal involvement, or mucositis; who is neutropenic; who is physically unable to place the suppository in the rectum; or who prefers other routes. Transdermal administration is also feasible but does not allow rapid dose titration. Patient-controlled analgesia (PCA) devices can be used both on an inpatient or outpatient basis. The opioid may be administered orally or via a dedicated portable pump to deliver the drug intravenously, subcutaneously, or epidurally (intraspinally). Intraspinal administration should be considered for the patient who develops intractable pain or intolerable side effects from other routes of administration. Use of this route requires skill and expertise that may not be available in certain settings. Table 21–11 presents the advantages and disadvantages of regional administration. This route is often efficacious because gynecologic tumors often affect the pelvis, making profound analgesia frequently possible without motor or sympathetic blockade. Drugs and routes of administration that are not recommended for the management of cancer pain are summarized in Table 21–12.

Clinicians who follow patients during long-term opioid treatment should watch for potential side effects and administer agents to counteract them. Constipation as well as nausea and vomiting, both common side effects to opioid analgesics, are discussed later. Drug-induced sedation should be treated by a reduction in dose and by increasing the frequency of opioid administration. Central nervous system stimulants as described earlier may also decrease opioid-related sedation. Patients receiving long-term opioid therapy generally develop tolerance to the respiratory depressant effects of these agents. When indicated for reversal of opioid-induced respiratory depression, administration of naloxone is indicated with titration in small increments to improve respiratory function without reversing analgesia. Careful monitoring is mandatory until the episode of respiratory depression resolves. For more subacute respiratory depression, simply withholding one or two doses until the symptoms resolve followed by restarting at 25% of the total dose is often effective. Dry mouth, urinary tension, pruritus, myoclonus, altered cognitive function, dysphoria, euphoria, sleep disturbances, sexual dysfunction, physiologic dependence, tolerance, and inappropriate secretion of antidiuretic hormone are also reported side effects of opioid agents.

Adjuvant drugs are valuable during all phases of pain management to enhance the analgesic efficacy, to treat concurrent symptoms, and to provide independent analgesia for specific types of pain. These adjuvants include corticosteroids, anticonvulsants, antidepressants, neuroleptics, local analgesics, hydroxyzine, and psychostimulants. Corticosteroids provide a range of effects, including mood elevation, anti-inflammatory activity, antiemetic activity, and appetite stimulation and may be beneficial in the management of cachexia and anorexia. They also reduce cerebral and spinal cord edema and are essential in the emergency management of elevated intracranial pressure and epidural spinal cord compression. Anticonvulsant agents are used to manage neuropathic pain, especially lancinating or burning pain. They should be used with caution when administered to patients undergoing marrow suppressant therapy such as chemotherapy and radiation. Antidepressants are useful in the pharmacologic management of neuropathic pain. These drugs have innate analgesic properties and may potentiate the analgesic effects of opioids. Perhaps the most widely reported experience has been with amitriptyline; therefore, this drug should be viewed as the tricyclic agent of choice. Neuroleptics, particularly methotrimeprazine, have been used to treat chronic pain syndromes. Methotrimeprazine lacks opioids' inhibiting effects on gut motility and may be useful for

Table 21–8 DOSING DATA FOR ACETAMINOPHEN AND COMMON NSAIDs

Drug	Usual dose for adults (≥50 kg body weight)	Usual dose for adults[1] (<50 kg body weight)
Acetaminophen and over-the-counter NSAIDs		
Acetaminophen[2]	650 mg q 4 hr 975 mg q 6 hr	10–15 mg/kg q 4 hr 15–20 mg/kg q 4 hr (rectal)
Aspirin[3]	650 mg q 4 hr 975 mg q 6 hr	10–15 mg/kg q 4 hr 15–20 mg/kg q 4 hr (rectal)
Ibuprofen (Motrin, others)	400–600 mg q 6 hr	10 mg/kg q 6–8 hr
Prescription NSAIDs		
Carprofen (Rimadyl)	100 mg t.i.d.	
Choline magnesium trisalicylate[4] (Trilisate)	1000–1500 mg t.i.d.	25 mg/kg t.i.d.
Choline salicylate (Arthropan)[4]	870 mg q 3–4 hr	
Diflunisal (Dolobid)[5]	500 mg q 12 hr	
Etodolac (Lodine)	200–400 mg q 6–8 hr	
Fenoprofen calcium (Nalfon)	300–600 mg q 6 hr	
Ketoprofen (Orudis)	25–60 mg q 6–8 hr	
Ketorolac tromethamine[6] (Toradol)	10 mg q 4–6 hr to a maximum of 40 mg/day	
Magnesium salicylate (Doan's, Magan, Mobidin, others)	650 mg q 4 hr	10 mg q 4–6 hr to a maximum of 40 mg/day
Meclofenamate sodium (Meclomen)[7]	50–100 mg q 6 hr	
Mefenamic acid (Ponstel)	250 mg q 6 hr	
Naproxen (Naprosyn)	250–275 mg q 6–8 hr	5 mg/kg q 8 hr
Naproxen sodium (Anaprox)	275 mg q 6–8 hr	
Sodium salicylate (generic)	325–650 mg q 3–4 hr	
Parenteral NSAIDs		
Ketorolac tromethamine[6, 8] (Toradol)	60 mg initially, then 30 mg q 6 hr Intramuscular dose not to exceed 5 days	
Others		

[1]Acetaminophen and NSAID dosages for adults weighing less than 50 kg should be adjusted for weight.
[2]Acetaminophen lacks the peripheral anti-inflammatory and antiplatelet activities of the other NSAIDs.
[3]The standard against which other NSAIDs are compared. May inhibit platelet aggregation for ≥ 1 week and may cause bleeding.
[4]May have minimal antiplatelet activity.
[5]Administration with antacids may decrease absorption.
[6]For short-term use only.
[7]Coombs-positive autoimmune hemolytic anemia has been associated with prolonged use.
[8]Has the same GI toxicities as oral NSAIDs
Note: Only the above NSAIDs have been approved by the Federal Drug Administration for use as simple analgesics, but clinical experience has been gained with other drugs.
q, every; t.i.d., thrice daily; NSAIDs, non-steroidal anti-inflammatory drugs.
Adapted from Management of Cancer Pain: Adults. Washington, D.C., U.S. Dept of Health and Human Services, March 1994.

treating opioid-induced intractable constipation or other dose-limiting side effects. It also has antiemetic and anxiolytic effects. Local analgesics have been used to treat neuropathic pain. Side effects for these may be greater than with other drugs used to treat neuropathic pain. Hydroxyzine is a mild anxiolytic agent with sedating and analgesic properties that is useful in treating anxious patients who are in pain. This antihistamine also has antiemetic and antipruritic properties. Psychostimulants, as discussed earlier, may be useful in reducing opioid-induced sedation when opioid dose adjustment (e.g., reduced dose and increased dose frequency) is not effective.

Patients should be encouraged to remain active and participate in self-care when possible. Non-invasive physical and psychosocial modalities can be used concurrently with drugs and other interventions to manage pain during all phases of treatment. The effectiveness of these modalities depends on the patient's participation and communication concerning which methods best alleviate pain. Generalized weakness, deconditioning, and aches and pains associated with cancer diagnosis and therapy may be treated by cutaneous stimulation such as heat or cold, massage, pressure, and vibration. Unfortunately, these modalities sometime increase pain before relief occurs. Massage should not be substituted for exercise in ambulatory patients. Exercise is useful for treating subacute and chronic pain, because it strengthens weak muscles, mobilizes stiff joints, and helps to restore coordination and balance, thus enhancing

Table 21–9 DOSE EQUIVALENTS FOR OPIOID ANALGESICS IN OPIOID-NAÏVE ADULTS ≥TO 50 KG[1]

	Approximate equianalgesic dose		Usual starting dose for moderate to severe pain	
Drug	**Oral**	**Parenteral**	**Oral**	**Parenteral**
Opioid Agonist[2]				
Morphine[3]	30 mg q 3–4 hr (repeat around-the-clock dosing) 60 mg q 3–4 hr (single dose or intermittent dosing)	10 mg q 3–4 hr	30 mg q 3–4 hr	10 mg q 3–4 hr
Morphine, controlled-release[3, 4] (MS Contin, Oramorph, others)	90–120 mg q 12 hr	N/A	90–120 mg q 12 hr	N/A
Hydromorphone[3] (Dilaudid)	7.5 mg q 3–4 hr	1.5 mg q 3–4 hr	6 mg q 3–4 hr	1.5 mg q 3–4 hr
Levorphanol (Levo-Dromoran)	30 mg q 3–4 hr (repeat around-the-	60 mg q 3–4 hr	30 mg q 3–4 hr	60 mg q 2–4 hr
Meperidine[5] (Demerol)	300 mg q 2–3 hr	100 mg q 3 hr	N/R	100 mg q 3 hr
Methadone (Dolophine, other)	20 mg q 6–8 hr	10 mg q 6–8 hr	20 mg q 6–8 hr	10 mg q 6–8 hr
Oxymorphone[3] (Numorphan)	N/A	1 mg q 3–4 hr	N/A	1 mg q 3–4 hr
Combination Opioid/NSAID Preparations[6]				
Codeine (with aspirin or acetaminophen)[7]	180–200 mg q 3–4 hr	130 mg q 3–4 hr	60 mg q 3–4 hr	60 mg q 2 hr (IM/SC)
Hydrocodone (in Lorcet, Lortab, Vicodin, others)	30 mg q 3–4 hr	N/A	10 mg q 3–4 hr	N/A
Oxycodone (Roxicodone, also in Percocet, Percodan, Tylox, others)	30 mg q 3–4 hr	N/A	10 mg q 3–4 hr	N/A

[1]Caution: Recommended doses do not apply for adult patients with body weight less than 50 kg. For recommended starting doses for adults <50 kg body weight, see Table 21-10.
[2]Caution: Recommended doses do not apply to patients with renal or hepatic insufficiency or other conditions affecting drug metabolism and kinetics.
[3]Caution: For morphine, hydromorphone, and oxymorphone, rectal administration is an alternative route for patients unable to take oral medications. Equianalgesic doses may differ from oral and parenteral doses because of pharmacokinetic differences. **Note:** A short-acting opioid should normally be used for initial therapy of moderate to severe pain.
[4]Transdermal fentanyl (Duragesic) is an alternative option. Transdermal fentanyl dosage is not calculated as equianalgesic to a single morphine dosage. See the package insert for dosing calculations. Doses above 25 μ/hr should not be used in opioid-naïve patients.
[5]Not recommended. Doses listed are for brief therapy. Switch to another opioid for long-term therapy.
[6]Caution: Doses of aspirin and acetaminophen in combination opioid/NSAID preparations must also be adjusted to the patient's bodyweight.
[7]Caution: Codeine doses above 65 mg often are not appropriate because of diminishing incremental analgesia with increasing doses but continually increasing nausea, constipation, and other side effects.
Note: Published tables vary in the suggested doses that are equianalgesic to morphine. Clinical response is the criterion that must be applied for each patient; titration to clinical responses is necessary. Because there is not complete cross-tolerance among these drugs, it is usually necessary to use a lower than equianalgesic dose when changing drugs and to retitrate to response.
q, every; N/A, not available; N/R, not recommended; IM, intramuscular; SC, subcutaneous.
Adapted from Management of Cancer Pain: Adults. Washington, D.C., U.S. Dept of Health and Human Services, March 1994.

patient comfort and providing cardiovascular conditioning. Physical therapists may be consulted to increase weightbearing exercise. Repositioning is also effective to maintain correct body alignment and prevent or alleviate pain and possibly prevent ulcers. Immobilization has only been effective to stabilize fractures or otherwise compromised limbs or joints. Finally, acupuncture, which involves inserting small solid needles into the skin, may be an effective alternative to more standard therapies.

Cognitive behavioral interventions are an important part of a multimodal approach to pain management. They help to give the patient a sense of control and to develop appropriate skills to deal with pain. These skills include relaxation and imagery, cognitive distraction and reframing, patient education, psychotherapy, biofeedback, structured support, and also support groups and pastoral counseling.

With rare exception, a less invasive analgesic approach should precede invasive palliative approaches. However, for a few patients in whom behavioral, physical, and drug therapy do not alleviate pain, invasive therapies are useful. These include radiation therapy to destructive bone metastasis, palliative surgical approaches, and nerve blocks.

Table 21–10 DOSE EQUIVALENTS FOR OPIOID ANALGESICS IN OPIOID-NAÏVE ADULTS <50 KG

	Approximate equianalgesic dose		Usual starting dose for moderate to severe pain	
Drug	**Oral**	**Parenteral**	**Oral**	**Parenteral**
Opioid Agonist[1]				
Morphine[2]	30 mg q 3–4 hr (repeat around-the-clock dosing) 60 mg q 3–4 hr (single dose or intermittent dosing)	10 mg q 3–4 hr	0.3 mg/kg q 3–4 hr	0.1 mg/kg q 3–4 hr
Morphine, controlled-release[2, 3] (MS Contin, Oramorph, others)	30 mg q 3–4 hr (repeat around	130 mg q 3–4 hr	0.3–1 mg/kg q 3–4 hr	0.105 mg/kg q 3–4)
Hydromorphone[2] (Dilaudid)	7.5 mg q 3–4 hr	1.5 mg q 3–4 hr	0.06 mg/kg q 3–4 hr	0.015 mg/kg q 3–4 hr
Levorphanol (Levo-Dromoran)	4 mg q 6–8 hr	2 mg q 6–8 hr	0.04 mg/kg q 6–8 hr	0.02 mg/kg q 6–8 hr
Meperidine[4] (Demerol)	300 mg q 2–3 hr	100 mg q 3 hr	N/R	0.75 mg/kg q 2–3 hr
Methadone (Dolophine, other)	20 mg q 6–8 hr	10 mg q 6–8 hr	0.2 mg/kg q 6–8 hr	0.1 mg/kg q 6–8 hr
Combination opioid/NSAID preparations[5]				
Codeine[6] (with aspirin or acetaminophen)[6]	180–200 mg q 3–4 hr	130 mg q 3–4 hr	0.5–1 mg/kg q 3–4 hr	N/R
Hydrocodone (in Lorcet, Lortab, Vicodin, others)	30 mg q 3–4 hr	N/A	0.2 mg/kg q 3–4 hr	N/A
Oxycodone (Roxicodone, also in Percocet, Percodan, Tylox, others)	30 mg q 3–4 hr	N/A	0.2 mg/kg q 3–4 hr	N/A

[1]Caution: Recommended doses do not apply to patients with renal or hepatic insufficiency or other conditions affecting drug metabolism and kinetics.
[2]Caution: For morphine, hydromorphone, and oxymorphone, rectal administration is an alternative route for patients unable to take oral medications. Equianalgesic doses may differ from oral and parenteral doses because of pharmacokinetic differences. **Note:** A short-acting opioid should normally be used for initial therapy of moderate to severe pain.
[3]Transdermal fentanyl (Duragesic) is an alternative option. Transdermal fentanyl dosage is not calculated as equianalgesic to a single morphine dosage. See the package insert for dosing calculations. Doses above 25 mcg?hr should not be used in opioid-naïve patients.
[4]Not recommended. Doses listed are for brief therapy. Switch to another opioid for long-term therapy.
[5]Caution: Doses of aspirin and acetaminophen in combination opioid/NSAID preparations must also be adjusted to the patient's body weight.
[6]Caution: Some clinicians recommend not exceeding 1.5 mg/kg of codeine because of an increased incidence of side effects with higher doses.
Note: Published tables vary in the suggested doses that are equianalgesic to morphine. Clinical response is the criterion that must be applied for each patient; titration to clinical responses is necessary. Because there is not complete cross-tolerance among these drugs, it is usually necessary to use a lower than equianalgesic dose when changing drugs and to retitrate to response.
q, every; N/A, not available; N/R, not recommended; NSAID, nonsteroidal anti-inflammatory drug.
Adapted from Management of Cancer Pain: Adults. Washington, D.C., U.S. Dept of Health and Human Services, March 1994.

Because vulvar cancers and occasionally ovarian or endometrial cancers occur in elderly patients, they especially require comprehensive assessment and aggressive management when cancer pain occurs. Older patients are at risk for undertreatment of pain because of underestimation of their sensitivity to pain, the expectation that they tolerate pain well, and the misconceptions about their ability to benefit from the use of opioids. Careful consideration should be given to elderly patients who are in pain and who have multiple chronic diseases that increase their risk for drug-drug and drug-disease interactions. In addition, visual, hearing, motor, and cognitive impairments may require simpler pain assessment scales and more frequent pain assessments. Non-steroidal anti-inflammatory drugs are more likely to cause gastric and renal toxicity and other drug reactions such as cognitive impairment, constipation, and headaches in older patients. Alternative non-steroidal anti-inflammatory drugs (e.g., choline magnesium trisalicylate) or co-administration of misoprostol should be considered to reduce gastric toxicity. Older persons tend to be more sensitive to the analgesic effects of opioids. In addition, the peak opioid effect is higher and the duration of pain relief is longer. Drug clearance may also be slower, thus making cautious initial dosing and subsequent titration and monitoring necessary. Elderly patients may not be able to physically place rectal suppositories or activate PCA devices.

Table 21–11 ADVANTAGES AND DISADVANTAGES OF INTRASPINAL DRUG ADMINISTRATION

System	Advantages	Disadvantages
Percutaneous temporary catheter	Used extensively both intraoperatively and postoperatively Useful when the prognosis is limited (<1 month)	Mechanical problems include catheter dislodgment, kinking, or migration
Permanent silicone-rubber epidural	Catheter implantation is a minor procedure Dislodgment and infection are less common than with temporary catheters Bolus injections, continuous infusions, or PCA (with or without continuous delivery) can be given.	
Subcutaneous implanted injection port	Increased stability, less risk of dislodgment Can deliver bolus injections or continuous infusions (with or without PCA) Useful when the prognosis is limited (<1 month)	Implantation more invasive than external catheters Approved only for epidural catheter in the U.S. Potential for infection increases with frequent injections Need for more extensive operative procedure
Subcutaneous reservoir	Potentially reduced infection in comparison with external system	Difficult to access, and fibrosis may occur after repeated injection
Implanted pumps (continuous and programmable)	Potentially decreased risk of infection	Need for more extensive operative procedure; need for specialized, costly equipment with programmable systems

PCA, patient-controlled analgesia.
Adapted from Management of Cancer Pain: Adults. U.S. Dept of Health and Human Services, March 1994.

Nausea and vomiting

Nausea and vomiting also have a high prevalence in advanced cancer patients. The cause may be divided into physiologic, treatment-related, metabolic, and psychological causes. As is the case in many symptoms of advanced cancer, the causes of nausea are often multifactorial. More than 50% of patients receiving opioids experience nausea in the first 10–14 days of therapy until they develop tolerance to this side effect. Many palliative specialists may prescribe antiemetics for the first weeks of opioid therapy. The most successful therapy is given orally and prophylactically.

An evaluation and approach to management of patients with chemotherapy-induced emesis appears in Fig. 21–4. Agents used to control nausea and vomiting have different mechanisms of action and may be used in combination for better control (Table 21–13). The management of nausea and vomiting has been advanced with the advent of 5-HT_3 serotonin antagonists. The 5-HT_3 antagonist blocks serotonin receptors of the chemoreceptor trigger zone (CTZ) to prevent vomiting. Metoclopramide has its effect locally in the gut and is excellent to control vomiting because of gastric stasis. In chemotherapy prophylaxis, it can be combined safely with steroids or benzodiazepines. Phenothiazines partially inhibit the CTZ and are the drugs of choice for radiation-induced nausea and vomiting as well as symptoms induced by mild or moderately emetogenic agents. Benzodiazepines are appropriate for refractory anticipatory vomiting that may occur with only a mention of chemotherapy. The amnesic effects of benzodiazepines are helpful to many patients. Corticosteroids are often used to enhance the effect of other agents, and yet they have an unclear antiemetic action. Dexamethasone (20 mg intravenously) is most effective when administered with a 5-HT_3 antagonist. It has been postulated that corticosteroids overcome the adrenal insufficiency that causes nausea and vomiting in patients with advanced cancer. Patients who describe around-the-clock nausea, not just intermittent with meals, may have a central nervous system lesion or a proximal small bowel obstruction that must be evaluated. Cannabinoids are best used in younger patients and have equivalent or superior activity compared with the phenothiazine and prochlorperazine agents. Vaginally induced nausea may be controlled with meclizine.

Diarrhea and constipation

Diarrhea is a common complication of pelvic radiation. It can generally be managed with anticholinergic drugs such as atropine sulfate (Lomotil). Rarely, tinctures of opium or serotonin antagonists are required for refractory or secretory diarrhea (Table 21–14). Patients who have been previously treated with antibacterial therapy or are immunocompromised should be tested for *Clostridium difficile* (e.g., enzyme-linked immunosorbent assay [ELISA]

Table 21–12 DRUGS AND ROUTES OF ADMINISTRATION NOT RECOMMENDED FOR TREATMENT OF CANCER PAIN

Class	Drug	Rationale for not recommending
Opioids	Meperidine	Short (2–3 hour) duration; repeated administration may lead to CNS toxicity (tremor, confusion, or seizures); high oral doses required to relieve severe pain, and these increase the risk of CNS toxicity
Miscellaneous	Cannabinoids	Side effects of dysphoria, drowsiness, hypotension, and bradycardia preclude its routine use as an analgesic
	Cocaine	Has demonstrated no efficacy as an analgesic or co-analgesic in combination with opioids
Opioid agonist-antagonists	Pentazocine Butorphanol Nalbuphine	Risk of precipitating withdrawal in opioid-dependent patients; analgesic ceiling; possible production of unpleasant psychomimetic effects (e.g., dysphoria, hallucinations)
Partial agonist	Buprenorphine	Analgesic ceiling; can precipitate withdrawal
Antagonist	Naloxone Naltrexone	May precipitate withdrawal; limit use to treatment of life-threatening respiratory depression
Combination preparations	Brompton's cocktail	No evidence of analgesic benefit to using Brompton's cocktail over single opioid analgesics Painful; absorption unreliable; should not be used for short (2–3 hour) duration; repeated administration may
	DPT (meperidine, promethazine, and chlorpromazine)	Efficacy poor compared with that of other analgesics; high incidence of adverse effects
Anxiolytics alone	Benzodiazepine (e.g., alprazolam)	Analgesic properties not demonstrated except for some cases of neuropathic pain; added sedation from anxiolytics may limit opioid dosing
Sedative/hypnotic drugs alone	Barbiturates Benzodiazepine	Analgesic properties not demonstrated; added sedation from sedative/hypnotic drugs limits opioid dosing
Routes of administration	*Rationale for Not Recommending*	
Intramuscular (IM)	Painful; absorption unreliable; should not be used for children or patients likely to develop dependent edema or in patients with thrombocytopenia	
Transnasal	The only drug approved by the FDA for transnasal administration at this time is butorphanol, an agonist-antagonist drug, which generally is not recommended. (See opioid agonist-antagonists above)	

Adapted from Management of Cancer Pain: Adults. Washington, D.C., U.S. Dept of Health and Human Services, March 1994.

for enterotoxin) before antidiarrheal therapy. When detected, metronidazole or vancomycin therapy is usually effective. Rarely, cholestyramine resin is needed to control the symptoms of *C. difficile* infectious diarrhea. A search for more unusual infectious etiologies such as salmonella, shigella, *Escherichia coli*, and parasites has not been cost effective among gynecologic oncology patients in the absence of foreign travel or other data, which might suggest these etiologic agents.

Constipation is highly prevalent in patients with advanced cancer. Close to 90% of patients receiving opioids have difficulty passing stool or pass stool infrequently. One cardinal rule of palliative care is "the hand that writes the opioids writes the laxative at the same time". Other causes of constipation are advanced disease, other medications such as anticholinergic agents, inability to eat a high-fiber diet, insufficient fluid intake, and lack of activity.

Metabolic causes of constipation include hypercalcemia and hypokalemia. Evaluation of complaints of constipation should include consideration of bowel obstruction and spinal cord compression. A manual rectal examination is critical when evaluating this complaint.

Several treatment options are now available for the nonsurgical candidate with bowel obstructions secondary to advanced cancer. A discussion of these treatments follows.

PSYCHOSOCIAL AND SPIRITUAL NEEDS OF PATIENTS AND FAMILIES

Management of only the physical symptoms of cancer is now considered to be an inadequate approach to oncologic care. It is well recognized that physical and psychological symptoms are intertwined, and can benefit from a

- Start before chemotherapy
  - Aprepitan 125 mg PO day 1, 80 mg PO daily days 2–3 and
  - Dexamethason 12 mg PO or IV day 1, 8 mg PO or IV daily days 2–4 and
  - 5-HT3 antagonist:
    Ordansetron 16–24 mg PO or 8-12 mg (maximum 32 mg) IV day 1
    or
    Granisetron 2 mg PO or 1 mg PO bid or 0.01 mg/kg (maximum 1 mg) IV day 1
    or
    Dolasetron 100 mg PO or 1.8 mg/kg IV day 1
    or
    Palonosetron 0.23 mg IV day 1
  - ± Larozepam 0.5–2 mg PO or IV or sublingual q 6 h days 1–4

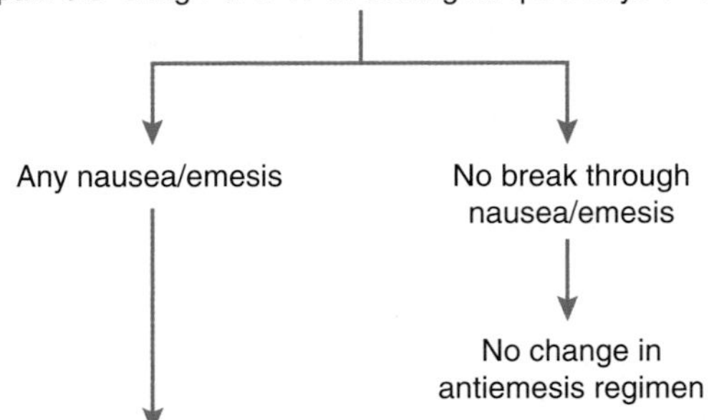

- General principle of breakthrough treatment is to give an additional agent from a different drug class
  - Prochlorperazine 23 mg supp pr q 12 h or 10 mg PO or IV q 4–6 h or 12 mg spansule PO q 8–12 h or
  - Lorazepam 0.5-2 mg PO q 4–6 h or
  - Ondansetron 8 mg PO or IV daily or
  - Graniseron 1–2 PO daily or 1 mg PO bid or 0.01 mg/kg (maximum 1 mg) IV or
  - Dolasetron 100 mg PO daily or 1.8 mg/kg IV or 100 mg IV or
  - Haloperidol 1–2 mg PO q 4–6 h or 1-3 IV q 4–6 h or
  - Dronabinol 5–10 mg PO q 3–6 h or
  - Dexamethasone 12 mg PO or IV daily, if not previously given or
  - Olanzapine 2.5–5 mg PO bid prn

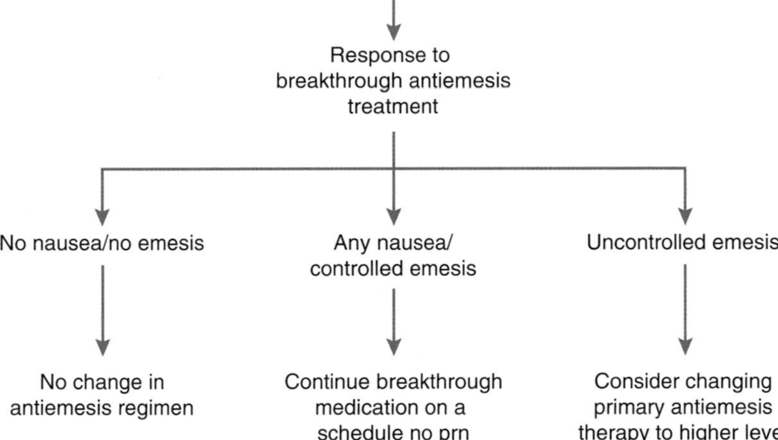

Figure 21–4 Evaluation and approach to management of patients with chemotherapy-induced emesis. (Reproduced with permission from The NCCN I. 2007 Antiemesis Guidelines: Clinical Practice Guidelines in Oncology. © 2006 National Comprehensive Cancer Network, Inc. Available at: http://www.nccn.org. Accessed December 17, 2006. To view the most recent and complete version of the guideline, go online to www.nccn.org.)

multidisciplinary approach to care. A growing body of literature suggests that tailored psychosocial interventions can enhance not only quality of life for cancer survivors, but may have the additional benefit of improving neuroendocrine and immune functioning which could positively affect disease states. If proven effective, this complementary and cost-efficient approach could significantly improve patient care, quality of life and aspects of survival. The effect of cancer on the family and patient is profound and touches every area of their lives. Effective care of the patient requires that these needs be addressed. A team of professionals is needed to foster effective communication in the patient-physician relationship; to assess the effect of disease and its treatment on the patient's psychosocial and spiritual well-being; and to achieve optimal care for the patient and family.

Strategies for breaking bad news and preserving hope

Perhaps the most important tool in caring for patients and their families is effective communication. Transferring information about the diagnosis, prognosis, risks, and

Table 21–13 ANTIEMETIC AGENTS (ADULT DOSAGES)

	Oral dosage	Intravenous dosage	Rectal dosage	Intramuscular dosage
Antidopaminergic*				
Prochlorperazine (Compazine)	5–10 mg q 6–8 hr	40 mg in divided doses/ 24 hr (5–10 mg)	25 mg q 12 hr	5–10 mg q 6–8 hr
Metoclopramide (Reglan)	10 mg q 8 hr	2 mg/kg followed by 1 mg/kg q 2–3 hr, twice	N/A	5–20 mg q 8–12 hr IM
Thiethylperazine (Torecan)	10–30 mg in divided doses/24 hr	N/A	10–30 mg in divided doses/24 hr	10 mg q 8–12 hr
Anticholinergic[†]				
Meclizine (Antivert)	50 mg q 4–6 hr	N/A	N/A	50 mg q 4–6 hr
Diphenhydramine (Benadryl)‡	25–50 mg q 6–8 hr	400 mg in divided doses/24 hr (5–50 mg)	N/A	400 mg in divided doses/ 24 hr (5–50 mg)
Trimethobenzamide (Tigan)	25–25 mg q 6–8 hr	2–16 mg q 6–12 hr	25–50 mg q 8–12 hr	2–6 mg in divided doses/ 24 hr
Antihistamine				
Hydroxyzine (Vistaril)	25 mg q 4–6 hr	N/A	N/A	25–100 mg q 4–6 hr
Promethazine (Phenergan)	25–50 mg q 8–12 hr	N/A	25–50 mg q 8–12 hr	25–50 mg q 8–12 hr
Benzodiazepines (Potentiate GABA neurotransmission)				
Lorazepam (Ativan)	2–6 mg in divided doses/24 hr (1–2 mg)	2–6 mg in divided doses/ 24 hr (1–2 mg)	N/A	2–6 mg in divided doses/ 24 hr (1–2 mg)
Diazepam (Valium)	2–10 mg q 6–12 hr	2–10 mg q 6–12 hr	N/A	2–10 mg q 6–12 hr
Glucocorticoid				
Dexamethasone (Decadron)	4–8 mg per directed q 8 hr	20 mg IV before chemotherapy	N/A	N/A
S-HT_3 antagonists				
Ondansetron (Zofran)	4–8 mg q 8 hr	32 mg before chemotherapy	N/A	N/A
Granisetron (Kytril)	1 mg q 12 hr	1–2 mg before chemotherapy	N/A	N/A
Dolasetron (Anzemet)	100 mg before chemotherapy	100 mg before chemotherapy	N/A	N/A
Palonosetron (Aloxi)	0.25 mg before chemotherapy	N/A	N/A	N/A
Substance P/NK_1 receptor antagonists				
Aprepritant (Emend)	125 mg before chemotherapy, then 80 mg on day 2 and 3	N/A	N/A	N/A
Unknown action				
Dronabinol (Marinol)	5 mg/m^2 before chemotherapy, then q 2–4 hr (maximum of 6 dosages/day)	N/A	N/A	N/A

*If extrapyramidal symptoms occur, administer 50 mg diphenhydramine IM or IV.
[†]Also Scopolamine transdermal patch—use one patch every 3 days.
‡Also has antihistamine properties.
GABA, gamma-aminobutyrate; N/A, not available; q, every

Table 21–14 ANTIDIARRHEAL AGENTS (ADULT DOSAGES)

Agent	Tablets	Mechanism of action	Adult dosage
Difenoxin/atropine (Motofen)	1 mg/0.0025 mg	Opioid/anticholinergic	2 tablets, then 1 after each loose stool; not to exceed 8 in 24 hr
Diphenoxylate/atropine (Lomotil)	262 mg or 262 mg/15 ml	Antiperistalsis	2 tablets, 4 times a day (exact mechanism 2 tablets, then 1 after each loose stool) not to exceed 8 in 24 hr
Loperamide (Imodium)	2 mg	Antiperistalsis (exact mechanism unknown)	2 tablets after each loose stool; not to exceed 8 in 24 hr
Bismuth subsalicylate (Pepto-Bismol)	262 mg or 262 mg/15 ml	Antisecretory, antimicrobial, anti-inflammatory	2 tablets q 30 to 60 minutes; not to exceed 16 tablets in 24 hr
Kaolin/pectin (Kaopectate)	750 mg or 600 mg/15 ml	Absorbent intestinal protectant	30 ml or 1500 mg after each loose stool; not to exceed 6 doses in 24 hr

benefits of treatment and progression of disease is a difficult and unavoidable responsibility. Sharing bad news and responding to the questions presented by the patient and family requires compassion, empathy, and skill. Unfortunately, development of these skills has not historically been emphasized in medical training despite the fact that powerful medical institutions and societies (e.g., ASCO, IOM, ACS, NCI) demand excellence and vigilance when caring for people with progressing cancer. The absence of an integrated formal palliative care curriculum throughout medical training continues to promote a skill set gap.

Identification of cancer progression, or progressive cancer-related symptoms, is often the catalyst for planning alterations in care and readdressing issues about the patient's and family's goals and objectives. Breaking bad news is a difficult and emotionally laden task for the physician. Thoughtful planning and delivery of such information, however, can shape the patient's subjective experience of the physician and perception of his or her degree of support and caring.

The individual's response to news is often determined by:

1. the adequacy of information given; and
2. whether the person delivering the information showed and responded to the patient's concerns.

While wishes vary from one individual to another, most patients (80%) want to know their diagnosis, their chance of cure, and adverse effects of any treatments. Significantly, patients do vary in the degree of information that they are able to assimilate at one time. Traditionally, men with advanced disease, older patients, and individuals from lower socioeconomic backgrounds are likely to want to hear fewer details and may comfortably defer to the physician and/or family with regard to decision-making. In most cases, patients want to hear the diagnosis from the physician who will be responsible for their care.

When breaking bad news, it is critical to project reasonable hope and confidence. Despite the most sensitive and effective communication style, patients are left with major concerns about their situation as it relates to their physical, social, psychological, and spiritual well-being. Open communication should be maintained, and these concerns should be explored throughout the continuum of care using expertise and support from other team members. Excessive concern about the need to preserve hope can lead to false optimism or less than full disclosure over time. This approach leads to poor coping skills and failed expectations. Lending strength does not require that the physician be less than honest but that the truth be disclosed over a period of time, in a setting where the patient has the support required, and with repetition so that information can be assimilated and understood in small amounts. Patients should be encouraged and nurtured to develop their own coping strategies and defense mechanisms in dealing with their illness. This strategy brings hope against all odds. For example, if asked, "Doctor, I know I am dying, but can there still be a miracle?" The answer is, "Yes, there can be." This suggests that the medical information is clearly understood but demonstrates confidence to overcome suffering and despair. However, it is unusual for patients to so clearly articulate their inevitable demise; more likely they would ask, "Is there still hope?" The physician's capacity to appropriately convey hope through articulation of a comprehensive care plan will help the patient to recognize that quality time is a reasonable expectation. Forcing a patient to adopt the physician's view of the odds (chance of a cure) does not take into consideration what can generally harm the personal framework that patients must deal with. It also corrodes the patient-physician relationship that must endure through the palliative therapy or future care. Thus, maintaining hope is best achieved through honesty, cautious optimism, compassion, and acceptance of the vulnerability experienced by all cancer patients.

Timing is critical to breaking bad news. Judging what portion of the information should be disclosed is an art. Conveying a balance of honesty and maintaining hope can sometimes seem impossible, often because physicians tend to project their own concerns onto patients and assume that they will give up hope. In reality, hope is an innate characteristic that is rarely abandoned by open and compassionate discussion of the prognosis and treatment options. When there are no remaining viable cytotoxic treatment options, there are still many palliative options that can achieve meaningful therapeutic ends, thus preserving hope and avoiding a sense of helplessness. It is useful for patients to hear such optimism in the face of a generally poor prognosis. As the patient's illness advances, feelings of helplessness due to loss of control and fear of dying may resurface. At this point, the physician can openly recognize the patient's fear and grief and externally acknowledge his or her own attitudes toward death. Unfortunately, doctors and other staff tend to spend less time with patients as the disease progresses and patients deteriorate into a terminal condition. This is presumably because the health care professionals feel helpless (and perhaps even threatened) when confronted with the imminence of death. Many health care professionals fail to realize the importance of compassion and active palliative care. Actively participating in symptom management and compassionate listening helps to ease the patient's mind, thus allowing the patient to ask questions that help plan realistically for the future and maintain a sense of control. Although most patients know when they are dying and can verbalize this realization, they also retain hope. The physician is uniquely poised to encourage and reinforce the patient's hope without giving false or insincere reassurance. One study that focused on end-of-life preferences of gynecologic cancer patients reported that only 5% of 108 patients would stop fighting after receiving a poor prognosis with no medically recommended treatment options left. Most (70%) of these patients expressed their resolve to continue fighting against their disease, even under the poorest prognostic circumstances. Proper management involves directing resources to assist with this fight and fostering this hope among dying patients. The involvement of other professionals familiar with care for the dying can relieve the physician of being the sole provider of hope with sensitive attention to incurable problems.

MANAGEMENT OF PSYCHOSOCIAL AND SPIRITUAL DISTRESS

Approaching "the person, not the disease" is a prerequisite to understanding the patient's experience and providing appropriate physical, psychosocial, and spiritual care. A cancer diagnosis creates a profound sense of loss of control and fear for many individuals. Changes in physical function and the effect on psychosocial issues may further compound this sense. Stressors commonly experienced by patients undergoing cancer treatment may be as problematic for the patient as the physical decline. Table 21–15 highlights the complex challenges faced by patients.

Patients are often reluctant to disclose struggles including feelings of depression and anxiety if they do not perceive this disclosure to be relevant to their physical care. Recent research has shown that many individuals are fearful of burdening their family members emotionally, physically, and financially during their final days. A recent prospective study examining the prevalence of depressed mood and request for euthanasia among terminally ill cancer patients noted that of 138 patients, 32 patients (22%) had depressed mood and made an explicit request for euthanasia. The risk to request euthanasia for patients with depressed mood was 4.1 times higher than that of patients without depressed mood at inclusion (95% CI, 2.0 to 8.5). This information heightens our awareness to formally evaluate depression in terminally ill cancer patients, and provide timely intervention as indicated.

Table 21–15 PSYCHOSOCIAL CHALLENGES EXPERIENCED BY CANCER PATIENTS

Threat of or actual:
Loss of ability to engage in employment because of side effects or symptoms
Loss of ability to participate in all social activities previously enjoyed because of symptoms of side effects or infection concerns
Guilt feeling about the impact of the diagnosis on people about whom the patient cares
Diminished sense of self-esteem and self-worth
Changes in body image
Discrimination or stigmatization by others
Role conflicts (e.g., meeting the demands of multiple responsibilities including those of being a patient)
Loss of comfort with sexual intimacy with a significant other
Fear of the dying process and concerns about symptoms that conjure up images of physical suffering (e.g., pain, cachexia, and shortness of breath)

Adapted from Portenoy RK: Principles and Practice of Supportive Oncology. Philadelphia, Lippincott-Raven, 1998, pp 109–118.

Discussions about resources available to assist patients and families, including the role and function of community agencies, support groups, and hospice programs are critical. There are many tasks that a patient should have the opportunity to accomplish in the time before death. These tasks are summarized in Table 21–16.

Identification and treatment of psychosocial problems, including depression and anxiety, should involve interventions and expertise that will offer optimal care to the patient and family. As noted earlier, pharmacologic interventions are often necessary but should be considered in combination with psychological counseling, supportive interventions and education for the patient and family. Determination of the appropriate referral depends in large part on the type and magnitude of the psychosocial or psychological disruption, as well as the extent to which this diagnosis interfaces with physical symptomatology such as pain or fatigue. Optimal programs include a team consisting of psychiatry, psychology, social work, and chaplain services. In addition, novel programs are acknowledging if not incorporating aspects of complementary and alternative medicine (CAM) based on recognition that a substantial proportion of cancer patients seek out various CAM methodologies.

Table 21–16 TASKS OF THE DYING PATIENT

Practical
Complete a family trust
Put affairs in order
Complete advanced directives
Communicate wishes regarding funeral/burial arrangements
Plan for the future of surviving family members

Psychosocial
Grieve the loss of dreams for the future
Accept the reality of the prognosis and impending death
Use medical intervention and own internal resources to cope with physical deterioration
Express thanks and love to family and friends
Find closure around interpersonal conflicts ("I forgive you, please forgive me")
Say goodbye to family and friends

Spiritual
Engage in life review, reflect on the past and present
Make meaning of one's life
Resolve existential/spiritual conflict

Adapted from Loscalzo M, Zabora J: Care of the cancer patient: Responses of family and staff. In Bruera E, Portenoy R (eds): Topics in Palliative Care, Vol 2. New York, Oxford University Press, 1998. © Oxford University Press. Reproduced by permission of Oxford University Press, Inc., www.oup.com.

Psychosocial care must continue to address the needs of the family as death imminently approaches and after death occurs. The health care team has an opportunity through the period of anticipatory grieving to assess and monitor the family and to identify risk factors indicating the need for more intensive intervention. An understanding of the spectrum of grief and the nature of "normal" grief is essential for providers to effectively support grieving families, identify abnormal reactions, and intervene. Table 21–17 illustrates the range of bereavement services that may be available for family members.

Table 21–17 INTERVENTIONS FOR BEREAVED INDIVIDUALS

Provision of information/education: offers education to surviving family members about grief response, explaining death to children, practical information to facilitate problem-solving and arranging for disposition of the body (e.g., funeral and burial arrangements) and future memorial activities

Bereavement follow-up: offers formalized contracts by the staff or volunteers at identified intervals to provide support, monitor for difficulties, and arrange for intervention as needed

Individual/family grief counseling: offers counseling for bereaved individuals experiencing grief; some individuals may require long-term psychotherapy or psychiatric care if bereavement-related depression or risk of suicide exists

Bereavement support groups: offers a forum for the mutual support among bereaved individuals; may have a special purpose (e.g., for parents who have lost a child) or have a particular religious affiliation

Memorial or remembrance services: offered by the hospital or hospice to acknowledge the grief process

Note: Families of patients who die in hospital would not necessarily have knowledge of or access to any follow-up if a bereavement program is not in place at the institution. Bereavement follow-up is typically a part of hospice services, and institutions may successfully partner with local hospices to make this service accessible for these families.
Adapted from Portenoy RK: Principles and Practice of Supportive Oncology. Philadelphia, Lippincott-Raven, 1998, pp 109–118.

QUALITY OF LIFE ISSUES IN ADVANCED AND RECURRENT OVARIAN CANCER

Small bowel obstruction

Although epithelial ovarian cancer is a surface-spreading disease that rarely invades vital organs, partial or complete bowel obstruction is often seen at the time of initial diagnosis or, more frequently, in association with recurrent disease. Obstruction may be secondary to extrinsic compression of the small bowel or hypoperistalsis due to mesenteric and bowel surface implants. The symptoms, which are almost always present, are intestinal colic, continuous abdominal pain, nausea, and vomiting. In most cases, nausea and vomiting can be relieved by conservative measures, and intestinal symptoms usually resolve after primary cytoreductive surgery and multiagent cisplatin-based cytotoxic chemotherapy. Despite the high objective response rate of primary epithelial ovarian cancer to several platinum-based combination chemotherapeutic regimens, most patients with advanced disease often develop intraperitoneal recurrences and require a salvage regimen for palliation of symptoms. Several therapeutic strategies have been used in these patients, such as including retreatment with cisplatin or carboplatin or the use of paclitaxel, hexamethylmelamine, oral etoposide, tamoxifen, gemcitabine, liposomal doxovubicin, vinorelbine, or topotecan. Multiple clinical factors must be considered when selecting the most appropriate salvage therapy. Unfortunately, in patients previously treated with cisplatin, other therapeutic agents are not likely to be effective in relieving symptoms of bowel obstruction or ascites. For most patients who present with bowel obstruction secondary to recurrent intraperitoneal cancer, initial management should include proper radiographic documentation of the obstruction, hydration, correction of any electrolyte abnormalities, parenteral alimentation, and intestinal intubation and decompression. In some patients the obstruction may be relieved with this conservative approach. However, palliative surgery is usually considered in almost every patient at some time before disease progression and death. When surgery is indicated, the type of surgery depends on the extent of the disease as well as on the number and location of obstructions. If the obstruction is mainly contained in one area, this area can be either resected (if secondary cytoreduction is indicated) or bypassed. Because the success of secondary cytoreduction depends on the chemosensitivity of the residual disease present after debulking surgery, intestinal bypass is generally preferable rather than resection because most patients present after multiple failed attempts at cytotoxic therapy resulting in chemotherapy-resistant cancer. In addition, intestinal bypass surgeries such as enterocolostomy are usually associated with reduced morbidity when compared with a radical resection. At the time of operation, the balloon at the end of a long intestinal tube can often be palpated and used to identify the small bowel proximal to the obstruction. This small bowel can then be anastomosed in a side-to-side fashion to the most appropriate area of colon, thus bypassing the site of obstruction. Obviously, it is critical to obtain a preoperative Gastrografin enema to ensure that there is no obstruction of the lower colon beyond the bypass site. In rare cases, the colon may be encased in tumor, necessitating a colostomy with or without bypass surgery.

Sadly, multiple sites of obstruction are common in patients with recurrent epithelial ovarian cancer. When multiple sites of obstruction are present, resection of several segments of intestine is usually not indicated. In such cases, an ileostomy or even a proximal jejunostomy may be necessary to provide adequate intestinal diversion. On the contrary, if the extent of disease is so great that the morbidity of intestinal surgery seems excessive, stomach decompression with a gastrostomy may be effective in palliating symptoms of obstruction and ascites such as pressure, nausea, vomiting, and pain. When the stomach or anterior abdominal wall are not involved with tumor, drainage tubes can often be placed percutaneously, thus avoiding the morbidity of a laparotomy.

With careful attention to nutrition, chemosensitivity/resistance of disease, and the sites of intestinal obstruction, some degree of palliation can generally be obtained with surgery, chemotherapy, or gastric decompression. Careful attention to each of these factors is necessary in order to avoid unnecessary morbidity and unindicated surgery in these debilitated terminal patients with recurrent or refractory ovarian cancer.

Ascites

Because malignant ascites is almost always the result of intraperitoneal cancer, treatment of these effusions generally involves therapy directed against the associated malignant neoplasm. However, treatments are occasionally directed specifically toward the palliation of symptoms related to malignant ascites, particularly when the intraperitoneal cancer is refractory to all known treatments. The traditional treatment with diuretics and salt and fluid restriction is rarely effective. Therefore, patients usually undergo therapeutic paracentesis, resulting in an imbalance of protein and electrolytes. For this reason, novel therapies such as intraperitoneal immunotherapy and drainage using a Denver peritoneal venous shunt have been proposed to palliate symptoms associated with malignant ascites. One series involved 42 patients who were treated over a 5-year period with a peritoneal venous shunt, which diverted peritoneal fluid into the vascular space. This treatment relieved symptoms with neither hematogenous metastasis nor evidence of disseminated intravascular coagulation. Interestingly, the median survival time of patients with breast and gynecologic cancer after surgery was significantly longer than that of patients with primarily gastric and intestinal neoplasms, resulting in an improvement in quality of life.

A hope for cure is no longer possible once a woman develops recurrent disease associated with symptomatic bowel obstruction and ascites. However, a sense of optimism and hope are still common, not for a cure but toward a goal of symptom relief and palliation with chemotherapy, surgery, tube drainage, or supportive care. Only through careful patient selection and insight into the toxicity associated with these therapies can hope for acceptable quality of life be realized.

Role of palliative surgical procedures

The role of surgery to palliate bowel obstruction is discussed earlier. Surgery can be useful in the palliation of pain or fistula during the terminal phase of ovarian cancer progression. The advantages and disadvantages of these procedures must be continually weighed. Cytoreductive surgery for debulking as a means to palliate pain is indicated when effective chemotherapy exists to treat unresected residua.

QUALITY OF LIFE ISSUES IN ADVANCED AND RECURRENT UTERINE/CERVICAL CANCER

Ureteral obstruction

The patient with bilateral ureteral obstruction and uremia secondary to the extension of cervical or uterine cancer presents a serious dilemma for the clinician. Management should be divided into two subsets of patients:

1. those who have not received prior radiation therapy; and
2. those who have recurrent disease after pelvic radiation.

Ureteral obstruction resulting from endometrial cancer differs from obstruction secondary to cervical cancer in that it is more frequently associated with disease outside of the pelvis and because it is more difficult to cure. In addition, adequate doses of radiation are more difficult to deliver to the corpus than to the cervix using standard brachytherapy techniques, thus contributing to the lower rate of pelvic control among patients with endometrial cancer after radiation therapy.

Patients with bilateral ureteral obstruction from untreated cancer or from recurrent pelvic disease after surgical therapy should be seriously considered for urinary diversion followed by appropriate radiation therapy. However, because the salvage rate in this clinical situation is low, supportive care alone allowing progressive uremia and demise must be considered as an alternative to more aggressive therapy. Placement of retrograde ureteral stands using cystoscopy should be attempted first if supportive care alone is declined. When this is not possible, a percutaneous nephrostomy should be placed followed by an attempt at antegrade stent placement. A third option is surgical urinary diversion such as a urinary conduit, and anastomosing both ureters into an isolated loop of ileum (Bricker procedure) or creating a continent pouch from a segment of bowel. When necessary, urinary diversion is usually performed before the radiation has begun, thus allowing for surgical assessment of the extent of the disease. If extra pelvic disease is discovered at laparotomy, therapy is altered because the chance of a cure is greatly diminished.

The patient with a bilateral ureteral obstruction after a full dose of pelvic radiation therapy presents a more complicated problem. Less than 5% of these patients will have obstruction caused by radiation fibrosis, and often this group is difficult to identify. In order to identify patients whose obstruction is a result of recurrent disease, an examination under anesthesia, cystoscopy, and proctoscopy with multiple biopsies is recommended. When recurrent cancer is absent, simple diversion of the urinary stream can be lifesaving, and, therefore, all patients must be considered to belong to this category until the recurrent malignancy is found.

When the presence of recurrent disease is established as the cause of bilateral ureteral obstruction, the decision process becomes difficult and somewhat philosophical. Numerous studies suggest that "useful life" is not achieved by urinary diversion in this subset of patients. Brin and colleagues reported on 47 cases (five with cervical cancer) with ureteral obstruction secondary to advanced pelvic malignancy undergoing diversion. The results of this report are discouraging. The average survival time was 5.3 months; only 50% of the patients were alive at 3 months and only 20% were alive at 6 months. After the diversion, 63.8% of the survival time was spent in the hospital. Delgado also reported on a group of patients with recurrent pelvic cancer and renal failure that were treated with urinary conduit diversion. Delgado's results show an insignificant increase in survival time, and he suggests that these patients should never undergo urinary diversion, because a more preferable method of expiration (uremia) is then eliminated from the patient's future. Obviously, this decision should be made in consultation with the family and even with the patient, if possible. When urinary diversion is performed, accentuation of the other clinical manifestations of recurrent pelvic cancer (i.e., severe pelvic pain, repetitive infections, and hemorrhage) is generally observed, leading to increased suffering. Pain control and progressive cachexia burden the physician and the patient. Episodes of massive pelvic hemorrhage are associated with difficult decisions concerning transfusion. An extension of the inpatient hospital stay is inevitable, and the financial impact of the patient on her family is often considerable.

Fistula

Urinary or colon fistulas are common sequelae of progressive cervical cancer and uterine corpus cancer. Because both urinary and intestinal fistulas have a great impact on quality of life, consideration should always be given to diversion of either the urinary or fecal stream in order to reduce symptomatology. Bladder drainage can often sufficiently reduce the incontinence associated with a urinary fistula without the need for surgical urinary diversion. Ureteral ligation with percutaneous nephrostomy drainage is another option. However, urinary conduit or other surgical procedures are often necessary to adequately divert the urinary stream. Surgical repair of a urinary fistula secondary to recurrent cancer or radiation is rarely successful with existing surgical techniques.

Colovaginal fistulas can generally be palliated with a colostomy. Although controversial, a loop colostomy often provides adequate fecal stream interruption to prevent further fistula drainage. However, some surgeons argue that an end colostomy with Hartmann pouch is necessary to completely interrupt the fecal stream. In either situation, a mini-laparotomy is generally all that is required to adequately accomplish the palliative goal.

Sexual dysfunction

The treatment of women with gynecologic malignancies may result in vaginal abnormalities that interfere with sexual function. Disturbances in sexuality are more common after the treatment of vulvar, vaginal, and cervical carcinoma compared with corpus and ovarian cancer. This is a result of the frequent use of radical surgery and radiotherapy to treat the three former malignancies. The reported frequency of sexual dysfunction after surgery, radiotherapy, or both varies considerably. Four per cent to 100% of women report a shortened vagina after a radical hysterectomy, whereas 17–58% have reduced lubrication. However, until recently, there were no reliable data on reductions in vaginal elasticity or genital swelling during sexual stimulation after radical hysterectomy. A report from Sweden published in the New England Journal of Medicine in 1999 demonstrated a statistically significant decrease in vaginal elasticity (23%) among women treated for early cervical cancer compared with a control group (4%). In addition, this study of 256 patients with cervical cancer, who were retrospectively surveyed and compared with 350 controls, also showed a decrease in lubrication during arousal and a reduction in perceived vaginal length after treatment. Furthermore, a large number of women indicated that these changes and their effects on sexual intercourse distressed them. Interestingly, the frequency of orgasms and orgasmic pleasure were similar in the two groups, although dyspareunia was more common in the women who had cervical cancer. Finally, this study did not show any significant difference among those women treated with radical surgery versus radiotherapy, although other retrospective comparisons have documented a significant increase in sexual dysfunction among those patients treated with radiation versus surgery. A direct comparison between radiation and surgery in the treatment of cervical cancer emphasizing not only outcome but also quality of life and sexual function is needed. Regular vaginal dilatation is widely recommended to those women treated with radiation as a way to maintain vaginal length and elasticity. Again, this intervention has never been tested in a prospective fashion. The appropriate use of hormone replacement therapy and lubricants may also improve coital function.

Dyspareunia resulting from gynecologic cancer therapy should be evaluated and treated, because dyspareunia can lead to loss of desire and can cause women to become sexually avoidant. This often leads to difficult interpersonal relationships between the woman and her partner. Loss of sexual desire in the post-cancer population is common and represents a challenging problem. Long after ordinary physical health has been regained, women may describe feeling little or no sexual desire. Counseling and support groups may be helpful in overcoming this frustration.

END-OF-LIFE DECISION-MAKING

As summarized in the American College of Obstetrics and Gynecology Committee Opinion published in May 1995, the moral character of medicine is based on three values central to the human relationship:

1. patient benefit;
2. patient self-determination; and
3. ethical integrity of the health care professional.

Patient benefit

The obligation to promote the good of the patient is a basic presumption of medical care and the defining feature of a physician's ethical responsibility. To promote the patient's good is to provide care in which benefits outweigh burdens or harms. Benefits, in turn, are understood only relative to the goals that the patient and physician hope to achieve through medical care.

Patient self-determination

The inherent value of individual autonomy or self-determination is one of the fundamental bases of democracy in the USA, and provides certain protection during end-of-life decision-making. In health care, the value of individual autonomy is as firm in the ethical and legal doctrines as in informed consent. Under this doctrine, the patient has a right to control what happens to her body. This means that:

1. no treatment may be given to the patient without her consent (or if she lacks decision-making capacity, the consent of her surrogate), and
2. the patient (or her surrogate) has the right to refuse unwanted medical treatment. This right is not contingent on the presence or absence of a terminal illness, on the agreement of family members, or on the approval of physicians or hospital administrators.

In the medical context, physician respect for patient self-determination consists of an active inclusion of the patient in decisions regarding her own care. This involves frank discussion of the diagnosis and prognosis, the relative risks and benefits of alternative treatments, and, based on these discussions, the identification or the operative goals of care.

Legal developments that bear on end-of-life decision-making

In the 1990s, several developments in the law influenced end-of-life decision-making. First, in June of 1990, in a decision on the Cruvan case, the United States Supreme Court affirmed that patients have a constitutionally protected right to refuse unwanted medical treatments. The ruling reaffirms states' authority to adopt procedural requirements for the withdrawal and withholding of life-prolonging medical interventions. A second legal development was the passage of the federal Patient Self-Determination Act (PSDA), which took effect on December 1, 1991. The PSDA requires Medicaid and Medicare participating health care institutions to inform all adult patients of their rights "to make decisions concerning medical care, including the right to accept or refuse medical or surgical treatment and the right to formulate an advance directive." Under the PSDA, institutions are legally required to provide this information to patients upon admission for care or upon enrollment in health maintenance organizations. The institution must note in the chart the existence of an advance directive and must respect such a directive to the fullest extent under state law.

An advance directive is the formal mechanism by which a patient may express her values regarding her future health status. It may take the form of a *proxy directive* or an *instructional directive,* or both. Proxy directives, such as the durable power of attorney for health care, designate a surrogate to make medical decisions on behalf of the patient who is no longer competent to express her choices. Instructional directives, such as "living wills," focus on the types of life-sustaining treatments that a person would or would not choose in various clinical circumstances.

A patient's goals of care are very likely to change with time in different clinical circumstances. As a static expression of the patient's wishes, an instructional directive may thus be a limited tool that could conceivably undermine a patient's most current desires. With this in mind, the patient's appointment of a proxy who knows her interest and accepts the role of surrogate decision-maker may be the best way of ensuring that her wishes will be carried out (proxy directive).

Surrogate decision-making

If the patient who lacks decision-making capacity has not designated a health care proxy, state law may dictate the order in which relatives should be asked to serve as surrogates. The person selected should be one who knows the patient's values and wishes and will respect them in his or her role as a surrogate decision-maker. If there is conflict regarding the decision of a surrogate, it may be appropriate to seek the advice of an ethics committee or consultant or, possibly, the courts.

In proxy decision-making for the dying patient, surrogates and health care providers should be aware that there is documentation and gender disparity in clinical medicine and research in court decisions surrounding the right to refuse life-sustaining treatment. In review of "right to die" cases, it was found that courts honored the previously stated treatment decisions of men in 75% of cases, whereas they respected the prior choices of female patients in only 14% of cases. Given the persistence and pervasiveness of social attitudes to take women's moral choices less seriously than those of men, gynecologists and patient surrogates must prevent these vices from undermining their advocacy for female patients. Likewise, this evidence should further motivate women to make a treatment decision as explicit as possible.

Futility

Treatments that offer no benefit to patients are clearly not obligatory. However, there is no single point at which all patients will conclude that they have completed a certain number of therapeutic interventions thus making further control of their disease impossible. Although the cancer is increasingly less likely to respond to second-, third-, or fourth-line agents, this is not necessarily an indication of their potential efficacy in that individual patient. Ovarian cancer, in particular, is a disease entity that requires treatment individualized to the needs and presentations of each patient in ways that other disease practices do not.

The American Medical Association (AMA) Council On Ethical and Judicial Affairs to date has not defined an approach to determine what treatment is and is not medically futile, although the council has discussed related issues concerning end-of-life care in many reports. For example, it has affirmed the ethical standing of withdrawing and withholding unwanted interventions, noted the constructive role that advanced care planning can play in pre-empting difficult and conflicting situations, and advised the use of a range of orders not to intervene. The council has also opposed physician-assisted suicide out of concern that recent calls from citizens and professionals for physician-assisted suicides are a response to experiences of excessive and futile interventions at the end of life. Because definitions of futile care are value laden, universal consensus on futile care is unlikely to be achieved. Rather, a process-based approach has been proposed that includes four distinguishable steps aimed at deliberation and resolution, two steps aimed at securing alternatives in case of irresolvable differences, and a final step aimed at closure when all alternatives have been exhausted (Fig. 21–5). This has been outlined by the report of the Council on Ethical and Judicial Affairs of the AMA published in its journal in March of 1999.

First, earnest attempts should be made to deliberate over and negotiate a prior understanding between patient, proxy, and physician about what constitutes futile care for the patient and what falls within acceptable limits for the physicians, family, and possibly also the institution. This prior understanding is best achieved before critical illness occurs. If serious disagreement is irresolvable, provisions can be made for a sensitive and orderly transfer of care at such a time that it can pre-empt later conflicts.

Second, joint decision-making should also be made at the bedside between patient or proxy and physician. This joint decision-making should:

- make use of outcome data whenever possible;
- incorporate the physician's and patient's or proxy's intent or goals for treatment; and
- abide by established standards of deliberation and informed consent.

Third, the assistance of an individual consultant or a patient representative is a further step and is often helpful to reach a resolution within all parties' acceptable limits. The role of this individual consultant is not to singlehandedly resolve the conflict but rather to facilitate discussions that help to reach that end.

Fourth, an institutional committee, such as an ethics committee, may be involved if disagreements are irresolvable. A final step may occur if the outcome of the institutional process coincides with the patient's desire, but the physician remains unpersuaded. In such a case, arrangements may be needed for transfer to another physician within the institution.

Alternatively, arrangements for transfers to another institution may be sought if the physician's position does not agree with that of the patient. Finally, if transfer is not possible because no physician and no institution can be found to follow the patient's or the proxy's wishes, it may be because the request is considered offensive to medical ethics and professional standards in the eyes of a majority of the health care profession. In such cases, by ethics standards, the intervention in question needs not to be provided, although the legal ramifications of this course of action are uncertain.

Due to the complicated nature of these proceedings, the AMA Council recommends that all health care institutions,

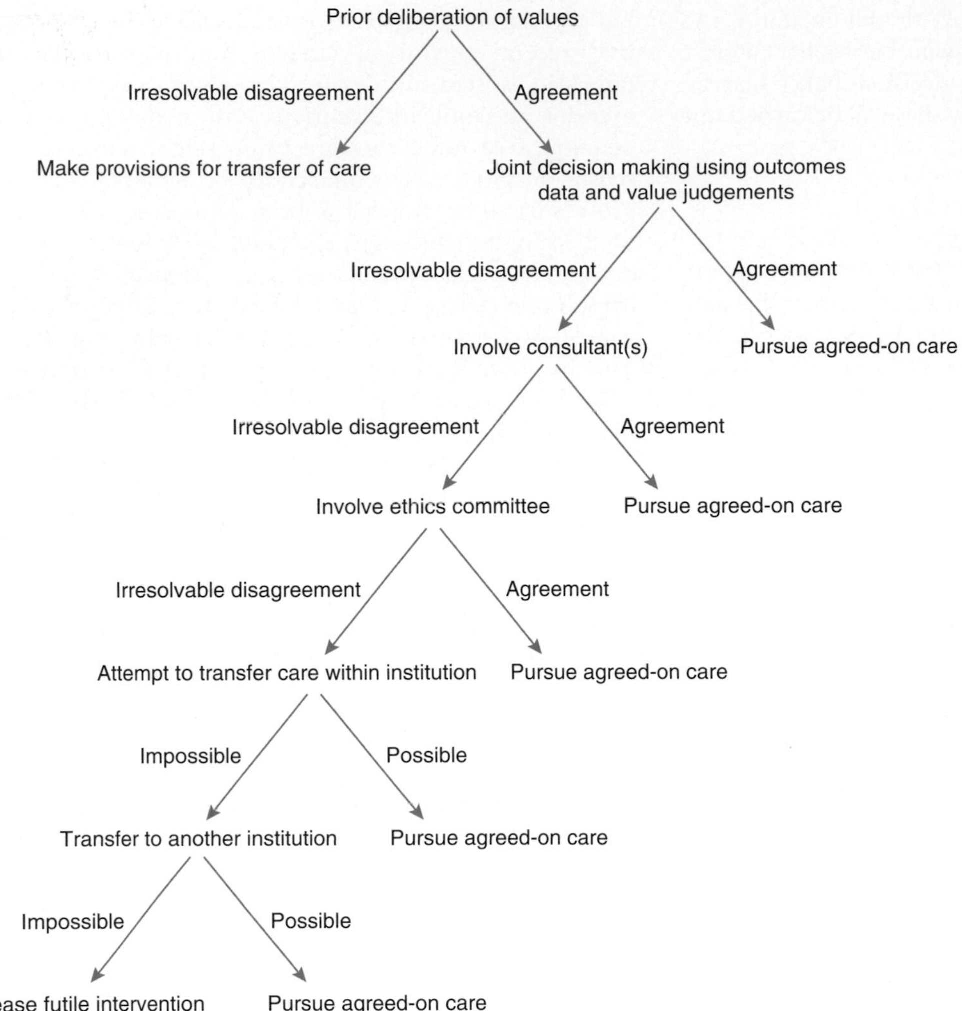

Figure 21–5 Fair process for considering futility cases. (Adapted from Medical Futility in End-of-Life Care: Report of the Council on Ethical and Judicial Affairs. JAMA 281:939, 1999.)

whether large or small, adopt the policy of medical futility and those policies on medical futility follow their process approach presented earlier.

Hospice

Palliative care programs often foster identification with hospice, and some have integrated hospice home care or inpatient programs. In the USA, hospice has come to mean primarily a government-regulated organization or program for dying persons and their families that typically focuses on home care and is limited to the following patients and situations:

1. life expectancy of 6 months or less;
2. a focus on comfort measures. This is sometimes (but not always) defined by hospice programs as a desire to forgo various "aggressive" and often expensive management approaches. These approaches may usually include cardiopulmonary resuscitation, blood product replacement, and some forms of radiotherapy, surgery, chemotherapy, and acute care hospitalization, at least insofar as these treatment modalities are used to try to cure or prolong life rather than to palliate symptoms;
3. a general preference for care at home (except where inpatient hospice is available and specifically sought);
4. A willingness to sign a form acknowledging the desire to enter a hospice program and to focus on comfort care; and
5. health insurance that covers hospice.

Many hospice programs also require a primary caregiver to be either in the home or regularly available. Another requirement reported by patients or family members is that they had to agree to forgo cardiopulmonary resuscitation, calls for emergency services, or future hospitalization. This requirement is not embodied in federal hospice regulations or the PSDA.

Although hospice staff may be perceived as more knowledgeable and empathic than conventional home care workers, hospice may actually provide much fewer hours of formal care, particularly home health aide time. This finding was recently documented for home care patients with amyotrophic lateral sclerosis. Thus, patients and families are often forced to choose between hospice care with insufficient home health aide support and a conventional home care approach that includes significantly more hours of home health aide time. Hospice programs in the USA are increasingly constricted by the eligibility require-

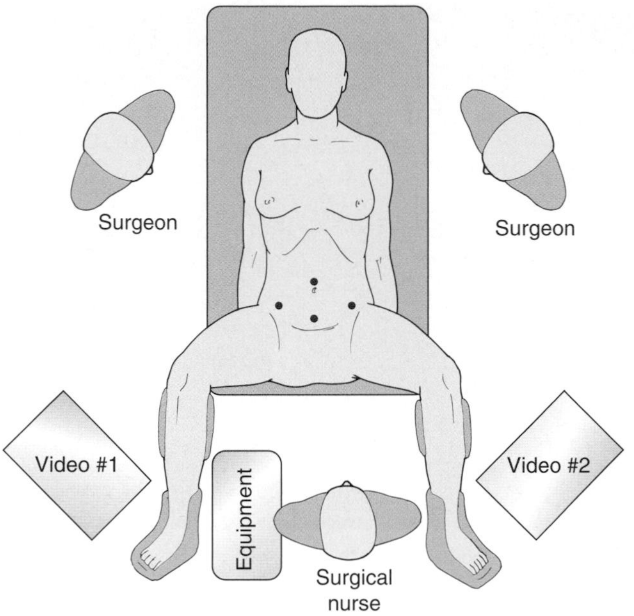

Figure 22–2 Operating room set-up for laparoscopic surgery. Positioning of patient for laparoscopic gynecologic surgery. Note: 1) Arms tucked; 2) Two video monitors towards foot of table; 3) Modified dorsal lithotomy position with adjustable stirrups.

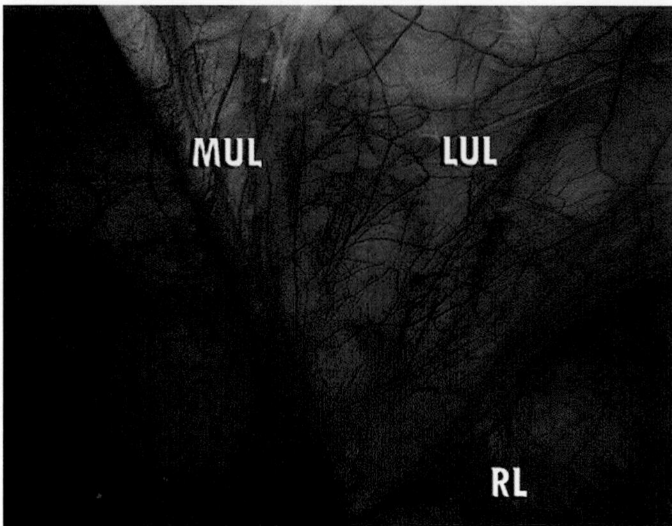

Figure 22–3 Anterior abdominal wall. LUL, lateral umbilical ligament; MUL, medial umbilical ligament; RL, round ligament.

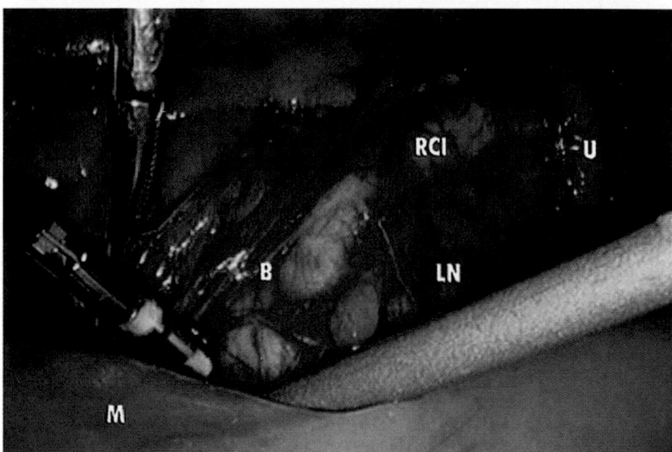

Figure 22–4 Para-aortic area. B, aortic bifurcation; M, bowel mesentery; U, ureter; LN, right para-aortic lymph nodes; RCI, right common iliac artery.

the monitors toward the patient's head can be considered in situations where extensive upper abdominal surgery will be undertaken (Fig. 22–2).

Number, position and size of trocars will depend upon the surgery anticipated. In cases that require removal of an adnexal mass or lymph nodes, a 10 mm accessory port will be needed. The surgeries can be accomplished successfully with the placement of a 5 or 10 mm port at the level of the umbilicus for camera placement, a 10 mm port suprapubically, and a 5 mm port in each of the lateral lower quadrants. Lateral ports can safely be placed in a line one-third of the distance from the anterior superior iliac spine to the umbilicus. Care should be taken when placing the lateral port to do so under direct visualization with inspection of the deep inferior epigastric vessels lying along the lateral boundary of the rectus abdominis muscles. These can be identified as the lateral umbilical ligaments (Fig. 22–3). Transillumination will not successfully reveal the location of these vessels.

Once successful insufflation and placement of the trocars is accomplished, visual inspection of the abdominal cavity is undertaken and the patient is placed in a steep Trendelenburg position. Use of steep Trendelenburg is necessary in order to achieve adequate visualization of the pelvis and lower abdominal region. Frequently a nasogastric tube needs to be placed to achieve gastric decompression. Lysis of any adhesions holding the small bowel or omentum into the pelvis or lower abdomen should occur. The small bowel is carefully placed in the upper abdomen by flipping the bowel from a caudad to a cranial position, exposing the mesentery of the small bowel and the aortic bifurcation (Fig. 22–4). In obese patients, body habitus may not allow steep Trendelenburg because of unacceptably high peak inspiratory pressure. In addition, obesity may prevent adequate mobilization of the small bowel out of the pelvis to allow for retroperitoneal dissection. Some authors have advocated use of additional port sites to help circumvent this problem.

The key to successful advanced laparoscopic surgery is the same as that for open laparotomy: access to the retroperitoneum. This is accomplished by dividing the round ligament laterally or opening the pelvic peritoneum lateral and parallel to the infundibulopelvic ligament. Dissection is then carried down to the level of the external iliac artery which is then followed in a cephalad and medial direction to the common iliac artery. At this point, the ureter can easily be found crossing the pelvic brim and a window can be created between the ovarian vessels and the ureter. Development of the pararectal space is under direct visualization after identification of the bifurcation of the common iliac vessel and the ureter. The surgeon places

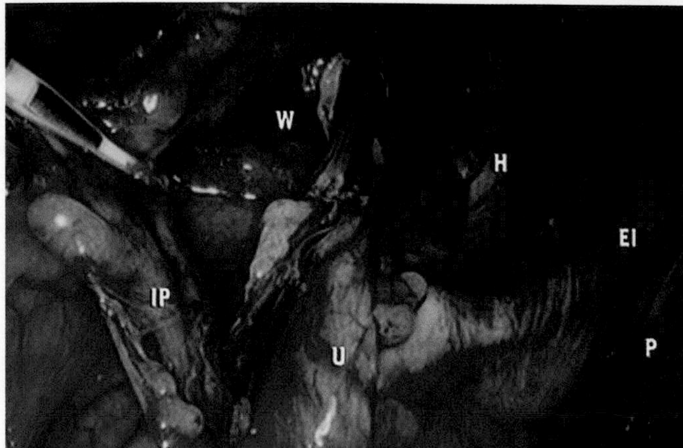

Figure 22–5 Pelvic sidewall. P, psoas muscle; IP, infundibulopelvic ligament; U, ureter; W, peritoneal window; EI, external iliac artery; H, hypogastric artery.

traction on the ureter medially developing the pararectal space between the hypogastric artery laterally and the ureter and rectum medially. Care must be taken during this dissection to avoid going too deep and disrupting the cardinal web. Because of the positive pressure environment of surgery, the boundaries of the paravesical space can be identified visually during laparoscopic surgery. The superior vesicle artery and umbilical artery are clearly visible as the medial umbilical ligament (see Fig. 22–3). Dissection is carried along the external iliac artery to the level of the superior vesicle artery. At this point the superior vesicle artery is retracted in a medial direction and the paravesical space is easily developed with the bladder and superior vesicle artery medially and external artery and obturator node bundle laterally. Once this is accomplished, the uterine artery can be clearly identified at the origin of the superior vesicle artery from the hypogastric artery. This retroperitoneal pelvic dissection is the cornerstone of any laparoscopic surgery performed in the pelvis including removal of an adnexal mass, laparoscopic-assisted vaginal hysterectomy, laparoscopic radical hysterectomy and pelvic lymph node dissection (Figs. 22–5, 22–6). Dissection can be facilitated with a variety of energy sources and clip appliers each with their own advocates.

Extension of the incision along the peritoneum overlying the right common iliac artery and then along the aorta to the level of the duodenum allows for exposure of the para-aortic retroperitoneum (Fig. 22–7). During this dissection, the peritoneum attached to the base of the cecum can be elevated in an anterior-cephalad direction providing excellent exposure to the right para-aortic lymph node region. Margins of resection are identical to an open approach and can easily be extended to the level of the renal vessels. The left-sided para-aortic lymph node dissection requires dissection underneath the inferior mesenteric artery mobilizing the descending colon and rectosigmoid off the left common iliac artery and retracting the inferior mesenteric artery and ureter laterally and cephalad. This gives excellent exposure to the left para-aortic lymph nodes inferior to the inferior mesenteric artery. Dissection can be continued above the inferior mesenteric artery in a similar manner. Some authors have advocated sacrificing the inferior mesenteric artery in order to get enhanced exposure.

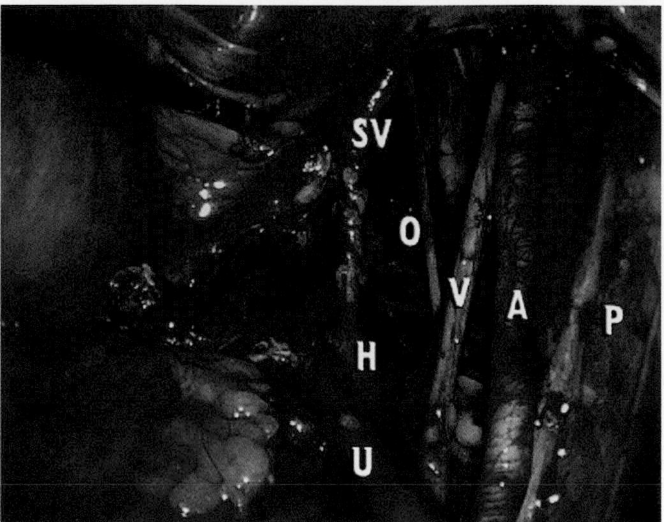

Figure 22–6 Pelvic sidewall retroperitoneal anatomy; P, psoas muscle; A, external iliac artery; V, external iliac vein; O, obturator nerve; H, hypogastric artery; U, ureter; SV, superior vesicle artery.

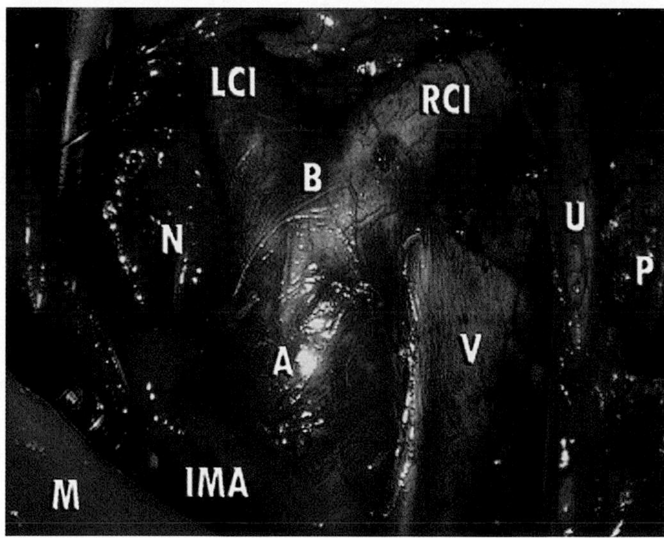

Figure 22–7 Para-aortic retroperitoneal anatomy. A, aorta; V, inferior vena cava; U, right ureter; IMA, inferior mesenteric artery; B, aortic bifurcation; P, psoas muscle; N, sympathetic nerve; M, bowel mesentery; RCI, right common iliac artery; LCI, left common iliac artery.

Adequacy of lymph node dissection

One of the cornerstones to surgical staging and treatment of gynecologic malignancies is the ability to perform a pelvic and para-aortic lymphadenectomy. In the early 1990s authors began to report the use of laparoscopic sur-

Table 22–1 LYMPH NODE COUNTS FOR LAPAROSCOPIC VERSUS OPEN LYMPHADENECTOMY

	Laparoscopic	Open	*P* value
Pelvic	18.0	18.4	n.s.
Common iliac	4.9	4.6	n.s.
Para-aortic	6.6	5.8	n.s

From Scribner et al: Laparoscopic pelvic and para-aortic lymph node dissection in the obese. Gynecol Oncol 84:426, 2002.

Table 22–2 REASONS FOR NOT COMPLETING LAPAROSCOPY

Obesity	12	(11.7%)
Adhesions	5	(4.9%)
Cancer	6	(5.9%)
IP disease	5	(4.9%)
Uterus too large	1	(0.9%)
Bleeding	4	(3.9%)
GU injury	1	(0.97%)
Catastrophic vascular injury	1	(0.97%)
Unknown	1	(0.97%)

From Scribner et al: Laparoscopic pelvic and para-aortic lymph node dissection: Analysis of the first 100 cases. Gynecol Oncol 82:498, 2001.

gery in the removal of pelvic and para-aortic lymph nodes. These early reports involved limited lymph node sampling described in case reports of surgical technique. Investigators initially reported only on right-sided para-aortic lymph node dissection but this changed with an improvement in operative skill. In 1993, Childers reported on laparoscopic pelvic and para-aortic lymphadenectomy in gynecologic malignancies including 52 right and 17 left-sided para-aortic lymphadenectomies. Several groups subsequently reported their experience with laparoscopic pelvic and para-aortic lymph node dissection including nodal count. Possover reported on 150 patients who underwent pelvic and/or para-aortic lymphadenectomy. He documented a mean of 26.8 pelvic lymph nodes and 7.3 para-aortic lymph nodes sampled. In Scribner's report of the 103 cases of attempted pelvic and bilateral para-aortic lymphadenectomy at his institution, node counts were compared between 73 patients who had successful laparoscopic completion of their surgery compared to 30 patients who required exploratory laparotomy to successfully complete the surgery. This study revealed no significant difference between pelvic, common iliac or para-aortic node counts (Table 22–1). Most authors have documented that, with an appropriate level of surgical experience, laparoscopic pelvic and para-aortic lymph node dissection will yield equivalent node counts and surgical dissection to an open approach.

Uncontrollable bleeding and obesity are the major reasons for not being able to successfully complete laparoscopic pelvic and para-aortic lymphadenectomy (Table 22–2). Numerous studies have also documented that with increased numbers of procedures performed the operative time and complication rate decrease significantly while the node count and ability to successfully complete the surgery laparoscopically increase. As with all minimally invasive surgery, there appears to be a long learning curve with several techniques not directly transferable from open laparotomy skill sets. Surgeons employing this technique need adequate training as well as an understanding that conversion to laparotomy is not a failure. Heroic laparoscopic efforts with excessively prolonged operative times are best avoided. With proper patient selection and sound surgical judgment, laparoscopic pelvic and para-aortic lymphadenectomy offers adequate surgical dissection with decreased length of stay, cost, and recovery time.

LAPAROSCOPIC MANAGEMENT OF THE ADNEXAL MASS

A major dilemma for gynecologists is the management of the adnexal mass. The only certain way to determine the etiology of the abnormality is to look at the tissue histologically after its removal. Since most masses are asymptomatic, the major reason for removing the masses is to determine if a malignancy is present. The fact that most of the masses are not malignant and are treated by general gynecologists can lead to "unexpected" findings of a malignancy with the patient and physician not prepared for the necessary cytoreductive surgery and thorough staging.

The finding of a persistent ovarian mass represents a major reason for surgery in gynecology. Killackey reported that 17% of laparotomies in gynecology are performed primarily for this indication. It has been reported that 5% of persistent premenopausal and 20–50% of postmenopausal ovarian masses will be malignant. Concerns of malignancy have prompted the recommendation that these ovarian masses be removed through a vertical midline incision. A vertical incision has been deemed necessary so that appropriate surgical debulking and staging can be performed if malignancy is found. This recommendation, however, is made with the assumption that a gynecologic oncologist or other cancer surgeon will be available to provide for adequate surgical staging and cytoreductive surgery. This surgery may include radical dissection, pelvic and para-aortic lymphadenectomy, or bowel resection. Most gynecologists do not have such assistance on standby for every surgery performed for a pelvic mass. Potential advantages of laparoscopic management of pelvic masses are cost savings and decreased morbidity in those women without cancer and early diagnosis and referral to oncologists for surgical treatment in those who are found to have malignancies.

The use of physical exam, vaginal probe ultrasound, and the CA-125 tumor marker should allow for appropriate triage of patients with an adnexal mass. Debates have been conflicting on the value of physical exam in accurately predicting the malignancy of a pelvic mass. Most authors have found exam to be less reliable than CA-125 determination and pelvic ultrasound. Schutter, however, reported that a suspicious pelvic examination had a 93% sensitivity for malignancy in postmenopausal women. This was better than CA-125 and comparable to ultrasound in their large multi-institutional study. Cul-de-sac nodularity and induration, or a fixed irregular pelvic mass, should alert the clinician to the possibility of malignancy, especially in the postmenopausal woman.

Premenopausal adnexal mass

Functional cysts such as corpus luteum and follicular cysts commonly occur in women between menarche and menopause. When a unilateral ovarian cyst less than 8 cm is found during the reproductive years the patient should have a repeat exam and ultrasound performed in six weeks. Birth control pills may be considered for ovarian suppression during this interval. Most functional cysts will resolve during this period of time. For premenopausal patients with persistent or complex ovarian masses, an ultrasound should be performed to determine the likelihood of a benign versus malignant neoplasm. Numerous scoring systems have been proposed incorporating wall thickness, percent solid components, presence and thickness of internal septa, and presence of internal papillations or nodularity. The predictive role of ultrasound has been assessed in a number of studies. The negative predictive value of transvaginal ultrasound depends upon the criteria utilized but should approach 95% (Table 22–3). Utilizing a transvaginal approach with a well defined scoring system, Sassone reported a negative predictive value of 100% in 143 patients. The negative predictive value is most important when devising a triage system that will minimize the number of unexpected malignancies found at the time of surgery. For a given set of criteria, an attempt to increase the positive predictive value may decrease the negative predictive value to an unacceptably low point.

Transvaginal color flow imaging has been reported to increase both the sensitivity and specificity of ultrasound diagnosis of malignancy of the ovary. Weiner reported on transvaginal ultrasound and blood flow impedance in 53 ovarian masses prior to laparotomy. The sensitivity and specificity of preoperative suspicious sonographic findings in detecting malignant tumors were 94 and 69% respectively. When impedance to blood flow was measured and a pulsatility index determined, the preoperative sensitivity and specificity in detecting malignant tumors increased to 94 and 97% respectively. The positive predictive value increased from 59% to 94% when the pulsatility index was used in addition to transvaginal sonography. Other authors have concluded that Doppler flow imaging provides no consistent improvement in positive predictive value over traditional transvaginal B-mode ultrasound. This may be due to the fact that neovascularization can occur in both benign and malignant neoplasms. The absence of reproducible findings that Doppler flow measurements will improve specificity and positive predictive value for determining malignancy in adnexal masses limits its application for the management of adnexal masses.

CA-125 determination appears to be of limited use in premenopausal women. This test alone has very low sensitivity and specificity for malignancy in premenopausal women with pelvic masses (Table 22–4). Common medical conditions in premenopausal women such as endometriosis, pregnancy, pelvic inflammatory disease, menses and leiomyomas can lead to a modest elevation of CA-125. An exception would be a CA-125 elevation of 500 or higher where the suspicion of a malignancy would be high. The low prevalence of malignancy in premenopausal ovarian masses combined with the common occurrence of these medical conditions in this age group markedly interferes with the ability of CA-125 to predict ovarian cancer. The

Table 22–3 ABILITY OF ULTRASOUND TO DISTINGUISH BENIGN FROM MALIGNANT OVARIAN LESIONS

Author(s)	No. of patients	Prevalence of disease (%)	Positive predictive value (%)	Negative predictive value (%)	Sensitivity (%)	Specificity (%)
Kobayashi	406	15	31	93	70.5	73
Herrmann et al	241	24	75	95	82	93
Finkler et al	102	36	88	81	62	95
Granberg et al	180	21.5	74	95	82	92
Sassone et al	143	10	37	100	100	83

Table 22–4 PREMENOPAUSAL WOMEN WITH PELVIC MASSES—VALUE OF CA-125 ASSAY

Author	No. of patients (CA-125 cutoff value)	Prevalence of malignancy	Positive predictive value	Negative predictive value	Sensitivity	Specificity
Patsner	125 (35)	40%	67%	77%	65%	78%
Malkasian	62 (> 65)	15%	49%	93%	60%	89%
Vasliev	150 (> 35)	4%	15%	100%	100%	76%
Finkler	32 (> 35)	24%	36%	82%	50%	69%

addition of CA-125 to ultrasound findings in premenopausal women does not substantially increase the predictive values of sonography.

The presence of a unilocular cystic mass in premenopausal women is very rarely malignant regardless of size. This fact is important because some of these patients are candidates for ovarian conservation with cystectomy. Cystectomy has been described using a variety of techniques through the laparoscope involving both rupture of the cyst or removal intact. The same criteria for conservative management can be utilized with laparoscopy as is already being done with laparotomy. The fact that even large unilocular cysts in this age group are almost never malignant can allow one to safely decompress these cysts prior to cystectomy or oophorectomy. Equipment such as needle aspirators and intra-abdominal bagging devices can allow for cyst decompression without spillage. Techniques have been described for either transabdominal or transvaginal cyst aspiration and removal. Large cysts can be aspirated transvaginally and removed via a posterior colpotomy with no intra-abdominal spillage. Size limits for removal of unilocular cysts seem to be related to safety of laparoscopic trocar insertion and surgical exposure. If oophorectomy is to be performed, the aspiration of the unilocular cyst will allow most of these to be removed through the anterior abdominal wall trocar site. More complex cysts that are felt to be benign can be removed through a colpotomy. Some multilocular ovarian neoplasms greater than 8 cm in size that are felt to be benign based on ultrasound have a large dominant cyst. These can be managed through a posterior colpotomy with transvaginal drainage of the dominant cyst and subsequent removal of the ovary through the colpotomy.

If known ultrasound criteria are utilized, the negative predictive value for ovarian malignancy in premenopausal women should be greater than 95%. If the schema is adhered to, those few women with malignancies should have their tumor removed with no intra-abdominal spillage (Fig. 22–8). The rare finding of malignancy will still allow for appropriate timely referral, surgical staging and treatment. Since the majority of premenopausal women will have masses with benign characteristics, this approach could substantially reduce the number of laparotomies performed for ovarian masses.

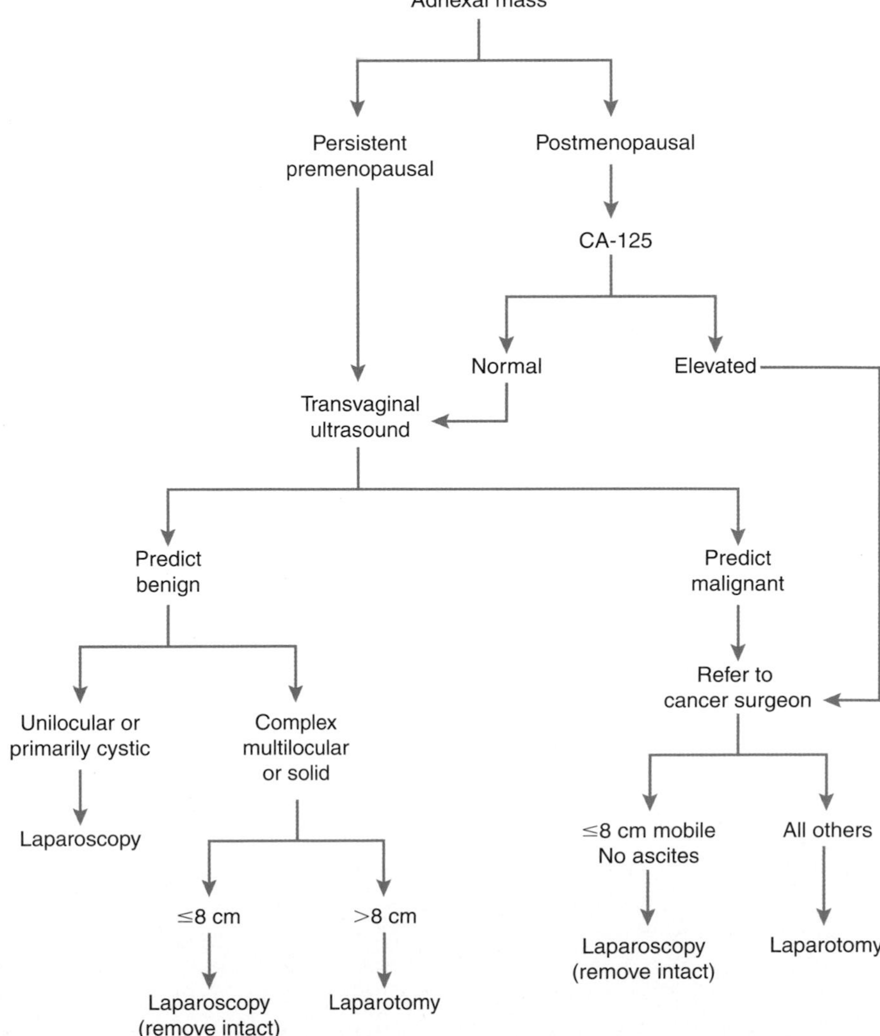

Figure 22–8 Suggested management of adnexal mass.

Suspicious premenopausal adnexal mass

When the transvaginal ultrasound is consistent with probable malignancy, a different approach is recommended (see Fig. 22–8). The positive predictive value of ultrasound alone ranges from 30 to 80%. Patients should have primary therapy by a physician trained to deal with ovarian cancer surgery and staging. These tumors can be managed with laparoscopy if they are ≤8 cm and can be removed intact through a colpotomy or mini-laparotomy. If malignancy is documented, these patients should have further surgery by appropriately trained physicians. Patients with ovarian masses greater than 8 cm that are suspicious for malignancy or those that cannot be removed unruptured by laparoscopy should undergo laparotomy by ovarian cancer specialists. Patients who are found to have disease spread beyond the ovary at time of laparoscopy should have a confirmatory biopsy and referral for definitive therapy and staging.

Postmenopausal adnexal mass

Postmenopausal women undergoing laparotomy for ovarian masses have a much greater likelihood of malignancy than premenopausal women. Killackey reported a 48% malignancy rate in women over 51 undergoing laparotomy as opposed to 8% for women aged 21–50. This series was not based on the use of screening ultrasound. Campbell et al reported on 15,977 screening ultrasounds in women 45 and older. Of these, 338 were persistently abnormal and 326 underwent exploratory laparotomy. Only 9 patients were found to have ovarian cancer. It is clear that as the use of screening ultrasound increases, a greater percentage of documented postmenopausal ovarian masses will be benign. This is particularly true of unilocular cystic masses ≤5 cm in size. Several authors have suggested that these cysts can be monitored with serial ultrasounds and not removed because of the low likelihood of malignancy. Luxman, however, reported 2 cases of malignancy in 33 postmenopausal women with unilocular cystic masses ≤5 cm. Laparoscopic removal of persistent small unilocular cystic masses in postmenopausal women should be considered until the true incidence of malignancy is established. It seems clear that laparoscopy can play a major role in the management of postmenopausal ovarian masses to limit the number of laparotomies performed.

Postmenopausal patients with ovarian masses differ from premenopausal patients with respect to the predictive value of CA-125. Table 22–5 lists studies that evaluated the positive predictive value of CA-125 in postmenopausal patients. Many of the non-malignant conditions that cause the CA-125 to be elevated in the premenopausal patient are not prevalent in the postmenopausal population, leading to an increased positive predictive value in postmenopausal patients. An elevated CA-125 has a positive predictive value for malignancy of 80 to 98% in this population. Postmenopausal patients with an adnexal mass and an elevated CA-125 are presumed to have a malignancy and should have surgery by an ovarian cancer specialist regardless of the ultrasound findings. An elevated CA-125 cannot be ignored even in the face of a benign appearing pelvic ultrasound, as demonstrated by Finkler. He reported five patients who were believed to have benign masses after an ultrasound performed by specialists where the CA-125 was found to be elevated. All five of these masses were subsequently found to be malignant. By combining the two tests, he brought the sensitivity up to 100% as well as significantly improving the negative and positive predictive values. Those postmenopausal patients with an ovarian mass and normal CA-125 are still at risk for malignancy since the sensitivity of this test is low (Table 22–5), especially in early-stage disease and non-serous ovarian adenocarcinomas. These patients should undergo diagnostic ultrasound and surgical management following the same protocol as the premenopausal patient (Fig. 22–8).

Laparoscopic management

Several authors have reported on the laparoscopic management of suspected benign masses. In 1992, Nezhat reported 1209 adnexal masses managed laparoscopically. The majority of patients had endometriosis or functional cysts. However, 64 patients had benign ovarian tumors and 4 were malignant. He reported no major complications in removing masses up to 25 cm in diameter and clearly demonstrated the technical feasibility of managing ovarian masses laparoscopically. Since then, multiple authors have reported on the use of laparoscopic oophorectomy in both pre-and postmenopausal women. The complication rates in these non-randomized reviews of laparoscopic surgery vary from 0–18% and include bowel injury, ureteral

Table 22–5 POSTMENOPAUSAL WOMEN WITH PELVIC MASSES—VALUE OF CA-125 ASSAY

Author	No. of patients (CA-125 cutoff value)	Prevalence of malignancy	Positive predictive value	Negative predictive value	Sensitivity	Specificity
Patsner	125 (35)	62%	87%	68%	77%	81%
Malkasian	92 (>65)	63%	98%	72%	78%	97%
Vasliev	31 (>35)	39%	80%	81%	66%	89%
Finkler	32 (>35)	59%	94%	80%	84%	92%

injury, wound infection, hematoma, and hemorrhage. A consensus of these retrospective reviews and small randomized trials is that laparoscopic management of adnexal masses is associated with decreased or similar operating time and decreased perioperative morbidity including pain, infection and blood loss. These studies also show a decreased length of stay and cost savings.

More recently, authors have reported on using laparoscopy in the initial management of suspicious ovarian masses. Dottino reported on 160 patients with suspicious adnexal masses that had no evidence of gross metastases or extension above the umbilicus. No distinction was made based on other risk factors for malignancy. One hundred forty-one patients were successfully managed laparoscopically. Ovarian cancer was discovered in nine patients, borderline ovarian tumors in eight, and non-gynecologic cancer in four. Dottino reported a 3% incidence of intraoperative complications requiring conversion to laparotomy and only one incidence of intra-operative spillage of tumor. This was a sex cord stromal tumor, which did recur locally. Canis reported on 230 adnexal masses suspicious or solid at ultrasound evaluated initially by laparoscopy. Twenty percent of the invasive cancers and 50% of the borderline tumors had cyst puncture or rupture at time of diagnosis. One case of tumor dissemination occurred with morcellation of an immature teratoma. These studies highlight the need to prevent tumor spill or morcellation for all suspicious masses. There is concern that the positive pressure carbon dioxide environment established during pneumoperitoneum may predispose the patient to intraperitoneal seeding. Animal studies have shown an increased seeding rate in the pneumoperitoneum group compared to controls. This may be explained by peritoneal damage and exposure of the underlying basal lamina, which could facilitate implantation. No clear conclusions can be drawn regarding the risk to humans but these studies suggest cyst rupture or spillage should be avoided in all possibly malignant adnexal masses.

LAPAROSCOPY IN OVARIAN CANCER

Diagnosis of ovarian cancer

Due to the relatively poor ability to predict malignancy with existing preoperative technology, a number of studies have looked at using laparoscopy to assess the ovary. Aspiration cytology of ovarian cyst fluid has a relatively poor negative predictive value in the range of 58–80%. Case reports have raised the possibility that aspiration or biopsy of malignant ovarian cysts may lead to peritoneal tumor implantation limiting its application for diagnostic purposes. Use of therapeutic aspiration appears to be ineffective, with a recurrence rate as high as 67%. Reports of success are likely to include functional cysts, as aspiration does nothing to interrupt the pathologic process of a neoplasm or endometriosis. When laparoscopy is highly suspicious for malignancy the surgery should be aborted, unless an appropriately trained ovarian cancer surgeon is involved.

Ovarian cyst rupture

The use of laparoscopy has been discouraged because of the potential for rupture of a malignant ovarian cyst. The impact of cyst rupture in an encapsulated stage I ovarian cancer remains controversial. Some reports indicate a decrease in survival in patients where cyst rupture occurs at the time of open oophorectomy. This has led to the incorporation of cyst rupture in the staging of early ovarian cancer. Tumors otherwise assigned to stage Ia or Ib would be upstaged to Ic if rupture occurs during surgery and this may have an impact on treatment recommendations. Other authors, however, were not able to demonstrate worsening of prognosis based on cyst rupture. Dembo reviewed over 500 cases of stage I ovarian cancer, reporting that dense ovarian adhesions, grade and ascites were predictors of relapse but not intraoperative cyst rupture. It seems likely that the majority of cysts ruptured at the time of surgery are secondary to dense adhesions and difficult surgical excision. Cyst rupture may just be an indicator of these more aggressive early ovarian malignancies rather than a surgical factor affecting prognosis. Until the true effects of spillage of cyst contents are known we should continue to attempt to remove the high-risk ovaries intact. Any spillage should be managed with copious irrigation as is the case with open surgery. Another concern has been the possible effects of a delay in referral and subsequent definitive surgery and staging. In an early report by Maiman of 42 patients referred for malignant ovarian neoplasms excised laparoscopically, the mean interval to laparotomy was 5 weeks and in more than 10% exploratory surgery was never performed. The impact of this delay on survival is not known. In a review of 48 cases of surgical staging following laparoscopic removal of malignant ovarian masses, Lehner reported that a delay of more than 17 days was associated with an increased risk of advanced stage disease for malignant and low malignant potential tumors on univariate analysis. These concerns are heightened by Kindermann's retrospective survey of 192 cases of ovarian malignancy initially diagnosed laparoscopically. Those patients with a delay of more than 8 days between laparoscopic biopsy and definitive surgery had an increased risk of port site metastasis and progression to stage III disease. In this report, only 7% of the apparent stage I tumors were removed intact due to biopsy, capsule rupture, and morcellation, making interpretation of this data difficult. These findings suggest that all efforts should be made to avoid intraoperative spillage from the ovary and to limit delay until definitive surgery. If patients are managed according to Figure 22–8, the unexpected finding of ovarian malignancy should be less than 5%. The few malignant masses that are managed laparoscopically would be removed without intra-abdominal rupture and survival should not be negatively impacted. Managing patients according to this schema should allow for appropriate and timely referral of patients with ovarian malignancy to physicians appropriately trained to manage these patients.

Early-stage ovarian cancer

The location and frequency of subclinical metastasis in patients with presumed early-stage ovarian cancer has encouraged investigation of the use of laparoscopic surgery for this patient population. Many areas traditionally evaluated during open laparotomy can be adequately assessed laparoscopically, including peritoneal cytology, diaphragm, omentum, pelvic and para-aortic lymph nodes, and pelvic peritoneum. Areas that are less likely to be fully visualized laparoscopically include the abdominal peritoneum and the bowel mesentery and serosa. Review of the literature would indicate that the most common sites of subclinical metastasis in ovarian cancer include peritoneal cytology, pelvic and para-aortic lymph nodes, the diaphragm, and the pelvic peritoneum, all of which can be evaluated laparoscopically (see Table 11–16). The inability to thoroughly evaluate the abdominal peritoneum and bowel mesentery could potentially lead to a 3% to 5% risk of understaging. Laparoscopic staging may be particularly helpful in patients who have undergone a recent exploratory laparotomy for removal of an adnexal mass found to be malignant who did not have appropriate staging. In 1995, Childers reported on the technical feasibility of laparoscopic staging of presumed stage I ovarian cancer. He found metastatic disease in eight of 14 patients including three with positive para-aortic nodes, three with pelvic disease, and two with positive cytology. Following this report, several small series of laparoscopic staging in this patient population have been published. In a case-controlled series, Chi demonstrated equivalent node counts and omental size removed in patients undergoing laparoscopic versus open procedures. There was no significant difference in rate of metastatic disease between the groups, although the numbers are too small to provide adequate power. Leblanc has recently reported on 42 patients who underwent laparoscopic restaging for ovarian and fallopian tube cancers. Eight were found to have metastatic disease. The remaining 34 patients had stage Ia grade 1–2 disease and had no follow-up chemotherapy. There were three reported recurrences in this group with a median follow-up of 54 months. To date there are no randomized trials looking at surgical or survival outcomes in early-stage ovarian cancer managed laparoscopically.

Advanced ovarian cancer

Laparoscopic surgery has had a limited role in the management of advanced ovarian cancer. Authors have reported its use in confirming the origin of abdominal carcinomatosis prior to neoadjuvant chemotherapy. Since the early 1980s, authors have reported its role in second-look laparotomy. Initial studies from the early 1980s utilizing laparoscopy followed by immediate laparotomy indicated a false negative predictive value of 29–55% for laparoscopic surgery. With advances in video equipment and surgical technology there has been a resurgence of use of laparoscopic surgery in this setting. In more recent non-randomized trials reporting on technical feasibility it appears laparoscopy is comparable to laparotomy in terms of complications, with a range of 1–5%. Unfortunately these studies were not controlled with immediate post-laparoscopy laparotomy so the false negative rate cannot be adequately assessed. Clough did report on 20 patients undergoing initial laparoscopy followed by immediate laparotomy using modern minimally invasive technology. The negative predictive value was 86%, indicating continued deficiencies in the technique. This information compounded with recent reports finding no therapeutic benefit to second-look surgery relegates this surgery to limited research applications. Some investigators have recently reported on the use of hand-assisted laparoscopy for radical intraperitoneal tumor debulking and cytoreductive surgery. These studies lack conclusive data for adequacy of surgery or comparison with open technique for morbidity and survival and should be considered investigational.

LAPAROSCOPY IN ENDOMETRIAL CANCER

Endometrial cancer provides possibly the best situation for use of minimally invasive surgery. Laparoscopic-assisted vaginal hysterectomy bilateral salpingo-oophorectomy (LAVH-BSO) can be substituted for total abdominal hysterectomy bilateral salpingo-oophorectomy (TAH-BSO) in the algorithm presented earlier in this book for the management of endometrial cancer. Likewise, laparoscopic pelvic and periaortic lymphadenectomy can be inserted for those patients traditionally selected for open lymph node dissection. Controversies surrounding when to perform lymphadenectomy in endometrial cancer patients and whether to include periaortic lymph nodes in all dissections are independent of the approach chosen by the surgeon and are covered elsewhere. According to a recent report by the American College of Surgeons commission on cancer, 80% of endometrial cancer patients in the USA have a TAH-BSO with cytology as the initial management for their endometrial cancer. Relatively few women currently undergo thorough surgical staging. Laparoscopic surgery allows for adequate visualization of the pelvis, removal of the uterus and ovaries, sampling or removal of the pelvic and periaortic lymph nodes, and washings from the abdominal pelvic cavity, thereby fulfilling the criteria for FIGO staging in endometrial cancer.

Vaginal hysterectomy has long been reported to carry less morbidity than abdominal hysterectomy. It has limitations, however, when applied to endometrial cancer. These include the inability to fully inspect the peritoneal cavity and retroperitoneum for metastatic disease, failure to perform peritoneal cytology, and potential inability to complete bilateral salpingo-oophorectomy. The addition of laparoscopy to the vaginal hysterectomy essentially eliminates these limitations. Irrespective of indications, LAVH-BSO has shown a learning curve with increased risk of urinary tract injury for less experienced surgeons. A large number of studies would indicate that LAVH-BSO allows for shorter hospital stay and a quicker return to normal activities than the traditional laparotomy approach and appears to be equivalent to a straightforward vaginal hysterectomy in this regard. These advantages of LAVH-BSO bring into question the continued use of TAH-BSO in patients in whom the uterus can be removed without morcellation.

An increasing body of literature exists supporting the use of LAVH-BSO with laparoscopic pelvic and periaortic lymphadenectomy in the management of endometrial cancer. Childers was the first to report a series with 59 patients undergoing LAVH-BSO with intraoperative assessment of depth of invasion and grade to determine need for lymphadenectomy. Twenty-nine patients had successful pelvic and periaortic lymphadenectomy. The Gynecologic Oncology Group (GOG) confirmed the feasibility of this approach with a phase II trial involving a total of 70 patients including 50 who met criteria of laparoscopic pelvic and periaortic lymphadenectomy. Based on these encouraging reports, several institutions began incorporating laparoscopy into the management of endometrial cancer. Retrospective reports have evaluated this approach with regards to feasibility, morbidity, cost, and impact on survival. Gemignani retrospectively compared 69 patients treated laparoscopically with 251 undergoing laparotomy. The laparoscopic group had significantly shortened hospitalization, fewer complications and decreased medical costs. Long-term outcome showed similar survival. The groups were poorly matched, however, as the laparoscopic group had better prognostic factors with only 11 having any form of lymph node sampling. Scribner reported on the feasibility of LAVH-BSO with laparoscopic pelvic and para-aortic lymphadenectomy in elderly patients with endometrial cancer. Sixty-seven patients managed laparoscopically were compared to 45 patients undergoing an open procedure. These groups were well matched with regard to age, obesity, and medical comorbidities. Though operating room time was increased, the laparoscopic approach decreased length of stay, postoperative ileus and infectious complications.

The Gynecologic Oncology Group has reported on the technical feasibility, complications, and quality of life data for its LAP 2 trial. In this trial, 2531 endometrial cancer patients were prospectively randomized in a two to one ratio of laparoscopy to laparotomy. Of the 1678 patients on the laparoscopy arm, 25.8% required conversion to laparotomy. Over half of these conversions were due to visualization, 16% due to metastasis, and 11% due to bleeding. Figure 22–9 graphs the likelihood of successful staging surgery as a function of body mass index. There was no significant difference in node positivity for the two groups however only 78.5% of the scope arm versus 86.4% of the open arm had nodes histologically identified from all four primary nodal regions including the right and left periaortic and pelvic lymphadenectomy specimens. Significantly fewer common toxicity criteria grade ≥ 2 complications ($p < 0.0001$) occurred on the laparoscopy arm (14.3%) compared to the open arm (21.1%) with similar transfusion rates. Consistent with other studies in the literature operative time was significantly longer for the laparoscopic arm (203 minutes) versus the laparotomy arm (136 minutes). For those patients successfully completing laparoscopic surgery the average length of hospital stay was 2 days versus 4 days for laparotomy ($p < 0.0001$). During the perioperative period the study found significantly better overall quality of life, pain scores, resumption of normal activities, and time until return to work in the laparoscopy arm. By 6 months after surgery, no significant quality of life differences were found. Survival outcome for this study has not been reported. A small prospective randomized trial of 70 endometrial cancer patients by Malur showed no difference in recurrence-free survival between a laparoscopic versus open approach. It appears that the current literature confirms the technical feasibility of the approach with probable decreased morbidity and cost and no adverse impact on survival.

Laparoscopic staging following initial hysterectomy has been reported as well. The potential advantage of this approach would be to eliminate or better define the need for postoperative adjuvant therapy. Though several small series have shown this approach to be technically feasible, it is more challenging than laparoscopic staging at the time of initial hysterectomy due to the inflammation and scarring associated with recent prior pelvic surgery.

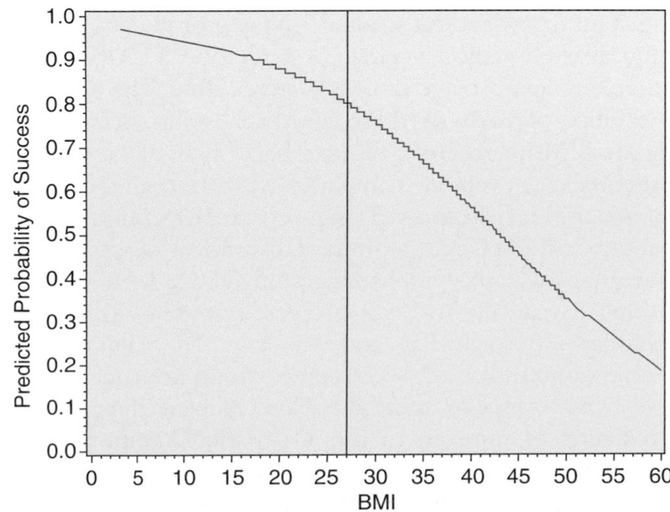

Figure 22–9 Figure comparing the likelihood of successful laparoscopic staging surgery to patient BMI.

LAPAROSCOPY IN CERVICAL CANCER

Early-stage cervical cancer

The ability to perform pelvic and para-aortic lymphadenectomy laparoscopically led to renewed interest in radical hysterectomy using the vaginal approach. Compared to endometrial or ovarian cancer, a more complete pelvic lymphadenectomy is required with cervical cancer. In a pilot study of 12 patients, Fowler followed laparoscopic lymphadenectomy with an open technique to assess adequacy of dissection. All patients were reported to have residual lymph nodes at time of laparotomy. Importantly, the laparoscopic lymph node yield increased from 63% in their first six cases to 85% in the next six cases. In a rigorously controlled study evaluating the adequacy of laparoscopic lymphadenectomy, Schlaerth reported the GOG's experience with 40 evaluable patients. Each patient had photographic record review, lymph node counts, and inspection of the laparoscopic surgical sites at the time of immediate post-laparoscopy laparotomy for completion of abdominal radical hysterectomy. Eight-five percent of these patients had no residual lymph nodes at the time of open surgery. A detailed review of the six patients who had residual lymph nodes indicated that surgeon inexperience was a contributing factor. The most common location for missed lymph nodes was lateral to the common iliac bifurcation. None of the residual nodes had evidence of metastatic disease. The authors reported a median laparoscopic operating time of 170 minutes. Other reports have confirmed the possibility of residual lymph nodes after laparoscopic pelvic lymphadenectomy though impact on clinical outcome is unknown. These studies would urge caution and development of adequate advanced laparoscopic skills before attempting to apply laparoscopic surgery for complete pelvic lymphadenectomy.

Several groups have reported case series combining laparoscopic pelvic and para-aortic lymphadenectomy with a Schauta type radical vaginal hysterectomy, laparoscopically assisted radical vaginal hysterectomy (LARVH), or complete laparoscopic radical hysterectomy. The technical feasibility of each of these approaches has been documented. More recently, reports have focused on survival outcomes as well as comparisons with the abdominal approach. Hertel reported on a prospective cohort of 200 patients with stage Ia to stage IIb cervical cancer undergoing laparoscopic lymphadenectomy with a LARVH. The overall 5-year survival was projected at 83%. This series included 26 stage Ib2 and 45 stage IIb tumors. The authors found that advanced stage, lymph node metastasis, and lymphovascular space involvement were independent predictors of survival. In the 110 patients without these risk factors, the 5-year survival was projected to be 98%. Spirtos reported a 94% 5-year survival in 78 patients with stage Ia2 to Ib2 disease who underwent total laparoscopic radical hysterectomy. In a more selective population with smaller tumors, Jackson reported an excellent overall survival of 94% for LARVH versus 96% for abdominal case-matched controls. These studies and other reports compare favorably with historical survival data for surgeons using an open laparotomy approach. To date there have been no large prospective randomized trials comparing the two approaches with regard to survival or morbidity. Reports are now describing new laparoscopic surgical techniques such as nerve-sparing radical hysterectomy and sentinel node identification. It is not currently known how these techniques will impact the standard operations.

Reports on either LARVH or laparoscopic radical hysterectomy indicate complications comparable to those seen with an open approach. Most authors stress the importance of a learning curve with decreased complications as surgeon experience increases. Commonly reported complications include cystotomy and bleeding leading to laparotomy. The argument can be made that conversion to laparotomy by itself should not be considered a complication. Some authors have reported decreased blood loss and length of stay in the laparoscopic group though these findings are not universal. Spirtos reported a length of stay of 2.9 days, which compares favorably with a 3.5-day length of stay reported by other authors for radical hysterectomy using an extended Pfannenstiel technique. There is a lack of any prospective data to compare cost and morbidity of the two approaches and retrospective data is not conclusive of an advantage for the laparoscopic approach. At the current time it appears that with appropriate training LARVH or laparoscopic radical hysterectomy with laparoscopic lymphadenectomy are comparable to the open technique with regard to cost, morbidity and survival. A significant advantage to the laparoscopic approach is yet to be confirmed in this population.

Fertility-sparing cervical cancer surgery

Adequate laparoscopic lymphadenectomy has also opened the possibility of modifying the traditional approach to the management of cervical cancer in patients desiring to maintain fertility. In an effort to define the potential number of patients who could potentially consider this fertility-sparing approach, Sonoda reported on 435 patients undergoing radical hysterectomy. Eighty-nine of these patients were under 40 years of age and had tumors that met the criteria for fertility sparing radical trachelectomy which represented 20% of their early-stage population (see Table 22–6). This study clearly shows that there is a substantial population of patients that may benefit from this approach. Several centers have now reported preliminary results on fertility-sparing radical trachelectomy with laparoscopic lymphadenectomy. Survival and fertility follow-up reports have been encouraging. To date over 300 cases have been reported with a recurrence rate of 4.1% and a death rate of 2.5%, which falls well within the range of survival data for traditional radical hysterectomy in a similar population. Plante reported on the obstetrical outcomes of 72 patients undergoing the surgery over a 12-year time span. A total

Table 22–6 SUGGESTED CLINICAL ELIGIBILITY CRITERIA FOR LAPAROSCOPIC RADICAL VAGINAL TRACHELECTOMY

1. Confirmed invasive cervical cancer: squamous, adenocarcinoma, or adenosquamous
2. FIGO stage Ia1 with lymphovascular space involvement, FIGO Ia2 to Ib1
3. Desire to preserve fertility
4. No clinical evidence of impaired fertility
5. Lesion size <2 cm
6. Patient is a candidate for a vaginal hysterectomy
7. Estimated cervical length ≥2 cm clinically
8. Adequate resolution of acute inflammation post-cone

of 50 pregnancies occurred in 31 women. Infertility rates as well as first and second trimester loss did not appear to be increased. Of the patients reaching the third trimester 22% had preterm delivery though only 8% were less than 32 weeks. There appears to be enough data now published to consider fertility-sparing radical trachelectomy a viable option for select patients.

Advanced cervical cancer

Another area of interest is the use of laparoscopic lymphadenectomy in the surgical staging of cervical cancer. The presence of metastatic disease in the para-aortic nodes or intraperitoneally may alter treatment strategies. Nonsurgical assessment of para-aortic nodes with computed tomography (CT), ultrasound or magnetic resonance imaging (MRI) has been plagued by unacceptably high false negatives. More recent studies using positron emission tomography (PET) scans are promising but have not been validated. In addition, many surgeons feel that removal of positive nodes will impact survival. Hertel reported on 109 consecutive cervical cancer patients with stage Ib2 and higher disease who underwent laparoscopic staging of the extent of disease and compared this with preoperative findings of MRI and CT. Histopathology of lymph nodes, bladder wall, and rectal pillar involvement correlated poorly with CT and MRI results, duplicating previous surgical staging studies. Overall, 25% of the patients had a change in treatment plan based on the laparoscopic findings. Complications were low and included two vascular injuries and two ureteral injuries, which were identified and managed intraoperatively.

Previous studies have confirmed the superiority of retroperitoneal assessment of para-aortic nodes compared to an open transperitoneal technique when measuring morbidity. Some investigators have recommended an extraperitoneal laparoscopic approach because of concerns for bowel morbidity associated with open transperitoneal staging. Other authors cite data that indicate fewer postoperative adhesions in animal models as well as in limited human reports when comparing transperitoneal laparoscopy to laparotomy. These authors feel that this reduction in adhesion formation will lead to fewer radiation-associated complications. To date no long-term morbidity reports are available. The conclusion that can be drawn from existing studies is that laparoscopic staging in cervical cancer patients is technically feasible with acceptable short-term complications allowing for removal of positive lymph nodes and alteration of treatment planning. Whether or not this approach translates into improved survival with acceptable long-term morbidity is unknown.

A number of case reports and small series have documented the use of laparoscopy in a number of special situations in cervical cancer. These include laparoscopic-guided interstitial implants with omental bolster, ovarian transposition prior to radiation therapy, pre-exenterative evaluation to rule out inoperable cases, and radical parametrectomy for management of occult early-stage disease found at time of simple hysterectomy. These reports confirm that laparoscopy can be substituted for laparotomy in select patients in these limited clinical scenarios.

COMPLICATIONS OF LAPAROSCOPIC SURGERY

An evaluation of minimally invasive surgery indicates that adverse events can be categorized into two broad groups—those complications that are part of laparoscopic abdominal surgery in general and those that are related to a specific technique or disease. General complications such as trocar insertion injuries to bowel or vessels, CO_2 pneumoperitoneum extravasation, and port site herniations have been discussed by other authors, including recommendation on how to lessen morbidity. The current discussion will be limited to technique and disease specific complications for gynecologic malignancies.

As noted previously in this chapter, a number of studies have reported on complications associated with laparoscopic pelvic and periaortic lymphadenectomy as well as radical pelvic dissection. In early series there appeared to be an increased number of ureteral, bladder, and vascular injuries compared to open technique. Further analysis almost uniformly indicates that there is a learning curve associated with advanced minimally invasive surgery and larger more mature series have intraoperative complication rates comparable to an open approach. Chi reported on the risk factors for complications and conversion to laparotomy in 1451 patients undergoing a wide variety of laparoscopic procedures by a gynecologic oncology division over a 10-year time frame. Significant complications occurred in 2.5% of the patients and were associated with increased age, previous radiation, and malignancy. The complication rates reported in this series fall within the accepted range using an open technique. Likewise the need to convert to laparotomy has been associated with prior abdominal surgeries, obesity, bleeding, and adhesive disease. Conversion rates decrease with increased surgery experience and should not be considered a complication but rather sound intraoperative judgment. Similar conclusions can be drawn from the experience with LAVH compared to abdominal or vaginal hysterectomy. In a recent survey of laparoscopy training among Society of Gynecologic Oncology members, 85% reported receiving none or limited laparoscopic training during their fellowship. Among active fellows, 67% report performing fewer than five laparoscopic surgeries per month. These data confirm the need for improved training during residency and fellowship programs as well as continuing medical education and mentoring for established surgeons.

Port site recurrences

Since 1978 port site recurrences have been reported in multiple carcinomas including gynecologic malignancies. Concern has been expressed that incisional seeding may be increased in laparoscopic surgery potentially leading to a reduction in overall survival. A review of the literature by Ramirez in 2003 found 31 articles describing port site metastases in 58 gynecologic cancer patients. These included 33 invasive ovarian cancers, 7 low malignant potential tumors of the ovary, 12 cervical cancers, 4 endometrial cancers, and one each of fallopian tube and vaginal cancer.

In the ovarian cancer patients, 83% had advanced stage disease with most reporting carcinomatosis and ascites. The median time to diagnosis was 17 days and it is unclear how this impacted survival. Reports of abdominal-wall metastasis after paracentesis in a similar population are common. It appears that proper preoperative assessment may have spared many of these patients a laparoscopic procedure.

The 12 cervical cancer patients reported with port site metastasis are cause for concern given that there are only a few isolated reports of metastases to an abdominal scar. Of these 12 patients, 75% had laparoscopic lymphadenectomy and the majority had positive nodes. Half the patients had recurrence in the port used for placement of the laparoscope. The median time to port site recurrence was 5 months and of the 11 patients for whom data was given, only 27% were without evidence of disease with a median 12 month follow-up.

Of the four patients reported to have port site recurrences in endometrial cancer, only one had disease limited to the uterus. The small number of port site recurrences makes it difficult to document any benefit to clipping the fallopian tubes or minimizing uterine manipulations as a way to prevent these complications.

A number of factors have been proposed to explain the etiology of port site metastasis. Studies have suggested that the risk may be increased with the use of carbon dioxide when compared to other insufflating agents. The positive pressure associated with a pneumoperitoneum has been associated with increased tumor growth and a high incidence of port site metastasis when compared to gasless laparoscopy. Some investigations have shown the potential aerosolization of viable tumor cells and efflux with gas through the trocar sites. Also theorized is a diminution of inflammatory response using minimally invasive versus open laparotomy incisions. Childers reported port site metastasis to be 0.3% per trocar site, which is comparable with the 0.1% risk of abdominal wall seeding with percutaneous biopsy of abdominal malignancies. Due to the advanced stage of most of the reported cases it is not clear whether port site metastases occur because of the aggressive nature of the disease or because of risk factors uniquely associated with laparoscopic surgery. To date, use of laparoscopy has not been associated with a decrease in survival for cancer patients. There is, however, a lack of large prospective randomized trials comparing laparotomy to laparoscopy at the current time.

BIBLIOGRAPHY

TECHNIQUE

Abu-Rustum NR, Chi DS, Sonoda Y, Di Clemente MJ, Bekker G, Gemignani M et al: Transperitoneal laparoscopic pelvic and para-aortic lymph node dissection using the argon-beam coagulator and monopolar instruments: an 8-year study and description of technique. Gynecol Oncol 89:504, 2003.

Altgassen C, Possover M, Krause N, Plaul K, Michels W, Schneider A: Establishing anew technique of laparoscopic pelvic and para-aortic lymphadenectomy. Obstet Gynecol 93:348, 2000.

Altgassen C, Possover M, Krause N, Plaul K, Michels W, Schneider A: Establishing a new technique of laparoscopic pelvic and para-aortic lymphadenectomy. Obstet Gynecol 95:348, 2000.

Chi D, Curtin J: Gynecologic cancer and laparoscopy. Obstet Gynecol Clin North Am 26:201, 1999.

Childers JM, Hatch KD, Tran AN, Surwit EA: Laparoscopic para-aortic lymphadenectomy in gynecologic malignancies. Obstet Gynecol 82:741, 1993.

Coleman RL, Muller CY: Effects of a laboratory-based skills curriculum on laparoscopic proficiency: a randomized trial. Am J Obstet Gynecol 186:836, 2002.

Coptcoat MJ: Extraperitoneal pelvic and para-aortic lymphadenectomy. Endosc Surg Allied Technol 3:9, 1995.

Dargent D, Arnould P: Percutaneous pelvic lymphadenectomy under laparoscopic guidance. In: Nichols DH, ed. Gynecologic and Obstetric Surgery. St. Louis, Mosby Yearbook, Inc., 1993, p 602.

Dargent DF: Laparoscopic surgery in gynaecologic oncology. Surg Clin North Am 81:949, 2001.

Derossis AM, Bothwell J, Sigman HH, Fried GM: The effect of practice on performance in a laparoscopic simulator. Surg Endosc 12:1117, 1998.

Djokovic JL, Hedley-Whyte J: Prediction of outcome of surgery and anesthesia in patients over 80. JAMA 242:2301, 1979.

Dottino PR, Tobias DH, Beddoe AM, Golden AL, Cohen CJ: Laparoscopic lymphadenectomy for gynecologic malignancies. Gynecol Oncol 73:383, 1999.

Eltabbakh GH: Effect of surgeon's experience on the surgical outcome of laparoscopic surgery for women with endometrial cancer. Gynecol Oncol 78:58, 2000.

Fowler JM, Carter JR, Carlson JW et al: Lymph node yield from laparoscopic lymphadenectomy in cervical cancer: A comparative study. Gynecol Oncol 51:187, 1993.

Frumovitz M, Ramirez PT, Greer M, Gregurich MA, Wolf J, Bodurka DC, Levenback C: Laparoscopic training and practice in gynecologic oncology among Society of Gynecologic Oncologists members and fellows-in-training. Gynecol Oncol 94:746, 2004.

Geisler J, Geisler H: Radical hysterectomy in the elderly female: a comparison to patients age 50 or younger. Gynecol Oncol 80:258, 2001.

Goff BA, Lentz GM, Lee DM, Mandel LS: Formal teaching of surgical skills in an obstetric-gynecologic residency. Obstet Gynecol 93:785, 1999.

Harkki-Siren P, Sjoberg J: Evaluation and the learning curve of the first one hundred laparoscopic hysterectomies. Acta Obstet Gynecol Scand 74:638, 1995.

Hatch KD: Laparoscopic lymphadenectomy and laparoscopic-assisted vaginal hysterectomy. Gynecol Oncol 90:503, 2003.

Holub Z, Jabor A, Bartos P, Hendl J, Urbanek S: Laparoscopic surgery in women with endometrial cancer: the learning curve. Eur J Obstet Gynecol Reprod Biol 107:195, 2003.

Jennings TS, Dottino P, Rahaman J, Cohen CJ: Results of selective use of operative laparoscopy in gynecologic oncology. Gynecol Oncol 70:323, 1998.

Kadar N: Laparoscopic pelvic lymphadenectomy in obese women with gynecologic malignancies. J Am Assoc Gynecol Laparosc 2:163, 1995.

Keating HJ, Lubin MF: Perioperative responsibilities of the physician/geriatrician. Clin Geriatr Med 6:459, 1990.

Kirschner CV, DeSerto TM, Isaacs JH: Surgical treatment of the elderly patient with gynecologic cancer. Surg Gynecol Obstet 170:379, 1990.

Kochli OR, Schnegg MP, Muller DJ, Surbek DV: Endobag extractor to remove masses during laparoscopy. Obstet Gynecol 95:304, 2000.

Köhler C, Klemm P, Schau A, Possover M, Krause N, Tozzi R, Schneider A: Introduction of transperitoneal lymphadenectomy in a gynecologic oncology center: analysis of 650 laparoscopic pelvic and/or para-aortic transperitoneal lymphadenectomies. Gynecol Oncol 95:52, 2004.

Köhler C, Tozzi R, Klemm P, Schneider A: Laparoscopic para-aortic left-sided transperitoneal infrarenal lymphadenectomy in patients with gynecologic malignancies: technique and results. Gynecol Oncol 91:139, 2003.

Lecuru F, Taurelle R: Transperitoneal, laparoscopic pelvic lymphadenectomy for gynaecologic malignancies (I). Technique, and results. Surg Endosc 12:1, 1998.

Lentz GM, Mandel LS, Lee D et al: Testing surgical skills of obstetric and gynecologic residents in a bench laboratory setting: validity and reliability. Am J Obstet Gynecol 184:1462, 2001.

Magrina JF: Laparoscopic surgery for gynecologic cancers: Clin Obstet Gynecol 43:619, 2000.

McGonigle K, Lagasse L, Karlan B: Ovary, uterine, and cervical cancer in the elderly woman. Clin Ger Med 1:115, 1993.

Possover M, Krause N, Plaul K, Kühne-Heid R, Schneider A: Laparoscopic para-aortic and pelvic lymphadenectomy: experience with 150 patients and review of the literature. Gynecol Oncol 78:19, 1998.

Querleu D: Laparoscopic para-aortic lymph node sampling in gynecologic oncology: a preliminary experience. Gynecol Oncol 49: 24, 1993.

Scribner DR Jr, Walker JL, Johnson GA, McMeekin DS, Gold MA, Mannel RS: Laparoscopic pelvic and para-aortic lymph node dissection in the obese. Gynecol Oncol 84:426, 2002.

Scribner DR Jr, Walker JL, Johnson GA, McMeekin SD, Gold MA, Mannel RS: Laparoscopic, pelvic and para-aortic lymph node dissection: analysis of the first 100 cases. Gynecol Oncol 82:498, 2001.

Scribner DR Jr, Walker JL, Johnson GA, McMeekin SD, Gold MA, Mannel RS: Surgical management of early-stage endometrial cancer in the elderly: Is laparoscopy feasible? Gynecol Oncol 83:563, 2001.

Spirtos NM, Schlaerth JB, Spirtos TW, Schlaerth AC, Indman PD, Kimball RE: Laparoscopic bilateral pelvic and para-aortic lymph node sampling: An evolving technique. Am J Obstet Gynecol 173:105, 1995.

Stocchi L, Nelson H, Young-Fadok TM, Larson DR, Ilstrup DM: Safety and advantages of laparoscopic vs. open colectomy in the elderly. Dis Col Rec 43:326, 2000.

Susini T, Scambia G, Margariti P, Giannice R, Signorile P, Benedetti-Panici P, Mancuso S: Gynecologic oncology surgery in the elderly: a retrospective analysis of 213 patients. Gynecol Oncol 75:437, 1999.

Trimbos J, Zola P: The present role of laparoscopy in gynaecological oncology; the EORTC point of view. Eur J Cancer 31: 803, 1995.

Vasilev SA, McGonigle KF: Extraperitoneal laparoscopic para-aortic lymph node dissection. Gynecol Oncol 61:315, 1996.

Visco AG, Barber MD, Myers ER: Early physician experience with laparoscopic-assisted vaginal hysterectomy and rates of surgical complications and conversion to laparotomy. Am J Obstet Gynecol 187:1008, 2002.

Walsh TH: Audit of outcome of major surgery in the elderly. Br J Surg 83:92, 1996.

Wise WE Jr. Padmanabhan A, Meesig DM, Arnold MW, Aguilar PS, Stewart WR: Abdominal colon and rectal operations in the elderly. Dis Col Rect 34:959, 1991.

LAPAROSCOPIC MANAGEMENT OF ADNEXAL MASS

Benacerraf BR, Finkler NJ, Wojciechowski C, Knapp RC: Sonographic accuracy in the diagnosis of ovarian masses. J Reprod Med 35:491, 1990.

Bennington JL, Ferguson BR, Haber SL: Incidence and relative frequency of benign and malignant ovarian neoplasms. Obstet Gynecol 32:627, 1968.

Bourne T, Campbell S, Steer C et al: Transvaginal color flow imaging: a possible new screening technique for ovarian cancer. Br Med J 299:1367, 1989.

Bourne TH: Transvaginal color Doppler in gynecology. Ultrasound Obstet Gynecol 1:359, 1991.

Bouvy ND, Marquet RL, Jeekel H, Bonjer HJ: Impact of gas (less) laparoscopy and laparotomy on peritoneal tumor growth and abdominal wall metastases. Ann Surg 224:694, 1996.

Brown D, Frates M, Laing F et al: Ovarian masses: can benign and malignant lesions be differentiated with color and pulsed Doppler US? Radiol 190:333, 1994.

Campbell S, Bhan V, Royston P et al: Transabdominal ultrasound screening for early ovarian cancer. BMJ 299(6713):1363–1367, 1989.

Canis M, Botchorishvili R, Manhes H, Wattiez A, Mage G, Bruhat MA: Management of adnexal masses: role and risk of laparoscopy. Sem Surg Oncol 19:28, 2000.

Canis M, Mage G, Pouly JL, Wattiez A, Manhes H, Bruhat MA: Laparoscopic diagnosis of adnexal cystic masses: A 12-year experience with long-term follow-up. Obstet Gynecol 83:707, 1994.

Canis M, Pouly JL, Wattiez A, Mage G, Manhes H, Bruhat MA: Laparoscopic management of adnexal masses suspicious at ultrasound. Obstet Gynecol 89:679, 1997.

Carvalho JP, Souen J, Pinotti JA: Trocar site metastasis after laparoscopic pelvic lymphadenectomy for cervical squamous cell carcinoma. Int J Gynaecol Obstet 67:111, 1999.

Cava A, Roman J, Gonzalez Quintela A, Martin F, Aramburo P: Subcutaneous metastasis following laparoscopy in gastric adenocarcinoma. Eur J Surg Oncol 16:63, 1990.

Chi DS, Abu-Rustum NR, Sonoda Y, Awtrey C, Hummer A, Venkatraman ES, Franklin CC, Hamilton F, Gemignani ML, Barakat RR: Ten-year experience with laparoscopy on a gynecologic oncology service: Analysis of risk factors for complications and conversion to laparotomy. Am J Obstet Gynecol 191:1138, 2004.

Chi DS, Curtin JP, Barakat RR: Laparoscopic management of adnexal masses in women with a history of non-gynecologic malignancy. Obstet Gynecol 86:964, 1995.

Childers JM, Aqua KA, Surwit EA, Hallum AV, Hatch KD: Abdominal-wall tumor implantation after laparoscopy for malignant conditions. Obstet Gynecol 84:765, 1994.

Childers JM, Nasseri A, Surwit EA: Laparoscopic management of suspicious adnexal masses. Am J Obstet Gynecol 175:1451, 1996.

Chou C, Chang C, Yao B et al: Color Doppler ultrasonography and serum CA-125 in the differentiation of benign and malignant ovarian tumors. J Clin Ultrasound 22:491, 1994.

Cohn DE, Tamimi HK, Goff BA: Intraperitoneal spread of cervical carcinoma after laparoscopic lymphadenectomy. Obstet Gynecol 89:864, 1997.

Cristalli B, Cayol A, Izard V, Levardon M: Benefit of operative laparoscopy for ovarian tumors suspected of benignity. J Laparoendo Surg 2:69, 1992.

Curtin JP: Management of the adnexal mass. Gynecol Oncol 55:542, 1994.

Daw E, Riley S: Umbilical metastasis from squamous carcinoma of the cervix: case report. Br J Obstet Gynaecol 89:1066, 1982.

Deckardt R, Saks M, Graeff H: Comparison of minimally invasive surgery and laparotomy in the treatment of adnexal masses. J Am Assoc Gynecol Lap 1:333, 1994.

Dobronte Z, Wittman T, Karacsony G: Rapid development of malignant metastases in the abdominal wall after laparoscopy. Endoscopy 10:127, 1978.

Dottino PR, Levine DA, Ripley DL, Cohen CJ: Laparoscopic management of adnexal masses in premenopausal and postmenopausal women. Obstet Gynecol 93:223, 1999.

Drouin PD-LJ, Ehlen T, Ghatage P, Heywood M, Lotocki RJ, Murphy KJ et al: Guidelines for the laparoscopic management of the adnexal mass. J Soc Obstet Gynaecol Can 20:983, 1998.

Ferrier A, Picker R, Sinosich M: A comparison of color flow Doppler and serum CA125 measurement in the preoperative evaluation of a complex pelvic mass. Int J Gynecol Cancer 8:113, 1998.

Finkler NJ, Benacerraf B, Lavin PT, Wojciechowski C, Knapp RC: Comparison of serum CA-125, clinical impression, and ultrasound in the preoperative evaluation of ovarian masses. Obstet Gynecol 72:659, 1988.

Freeman RK, Wait MA: Port site metastasis after laparoscopic staging of esophageal carcinoma. Ann Thorac Surg 71:1032, 2001.

Gal D, Lind L, Lovecchio JL, Kohn N: Comparative study of laparoscopy vs. laparotomy for adnexal surgery: Efficacy, safety, and cyst rupture. J Gynecol Surg 11:153, 1995.

Gleeson NC, Nicosia SV, Mark JE, Hoffman MS, Cavanaugh D: Abdominal wall metastases from ovarian cancer after laparoscopy. Am J Obstet Gynecol 169:522, 1993.

Goldstein SR, Subramanyam B, Snyder JR, Beller U, Raghavendra BN, Beckman EM: The postmenopausal cystic adnexal mass: The potential role of ultrasound in conservative management. Obstet Gynecol 73:8, 1989.

Granberg S, Norstrom A, Wikland M: Tumors in the lower pelvis as imaged by vaginal sonography. Gynecol Oncol 37:224, 1990.

Granberg S, Wikland M, Jansson I: Macroscopic characterization of ovarian tumors and the relation to the histologic diagnosis: criteria to be used for ultrasound evaluation. Gynecol Oncol 35:139, 1989.

Greenlee R, Chervenak F, Tovell M: Incisional recurrence of a cervical carcinoma. JAMA 246:69, 1981.

Gregor H, Sam CE, Reinthaller A, Joura EA: Port site metastases after laparoscopic lymph node staging of cervical carcinoma. J Am Assoc Gynecol Laparosc 8:591, 2001.

Hamper U, Sheth S, Abbas F et al: Transvaginal color Doppler sonography of adnexal masses: differences in blood flow impedance in benign and malignant lesions. Am J Roentgenol 160:1225, 1993.

Hasson HM: Laparoscopic management of ovarian cysts. J Reprod Med 35:863, 1990.

Havrilesky LJ, Peterson BL, Dryden DK, Soper JT, Clarke-Pearson DL, Berchuck A: Predictors of clinical outcomes in the laparoscopic management of adnexal masses. Obstet Gynecol 102:243, 2002.

Herrmann UJ Jr, Locher GW, Goldhirsch A: Sonographic patterns of ovarian tumors: Prediction of malignancy. Obstet Gynecol 69:777, 1987.

Hidlebaugh D, O'Mara P, Conboy E: Salpingo-oophorectomy: Clinical and financial analyses of laparoscopic and open techniques. J Am Assoc Gynecol Lap 1:223, 1994.

Hidlebaugh DA, Vulgaropulos S, Orr RK: Treating adnexal masses: Operative laparoscopy vs. laparotomy. J Reprod Med 42:551, 1997.

Huang KG, Wang CJ, Chang TC, Liou JD, Hsueh S, Lai CH, Huang LW: Management of port site metastasis after laparoscopic surgery for ovarian cancer. Am J Obstet Gynecol 189:16, 2003.

Jacobs I, Oram D, Fairbanks J et al: A risk of malignancy index incorporating CA-125, ultrasound and menopausal status for the accurate preoperative diagnosis of ovarian cancer. Br J Obstet Gynaecol 97:922, 1990.

Jansen FW, Kapiteyn K, Trimbos-Kemper T, Hermans J, Trimbos JB: Complications of laparoscopy: A prospective multicentre observational study. Br J Obstet Gynaecol 104:595, 1997.

Johns A: Laparoscopic oophorectomy-oophorocystectomy. Clin Obstet Gynecol 34:460, 1991.

Jones DB, Guo LW, Reinhard MK et al: Impact of pneumoperitoneum on trocar site implantation of colon cancer in hamster model. Dis Colon Rectum 38:1182, 1995.

Kadar N: Port site recurrences following laparoscopic operations for gynaecological malignancies. Br J Obstet Gynaecol 104:1308, 1997.

Kawai M, Kano T, Kikkawa F et al: Transvaginal Doppler ultrasound with color flow imaging in the diagnosis of ovarian cancer. Obstet Gynecol 79:163, 1992.

Killackey MA, Neuwirth RS: Evaluation and management of the pelvic mass: A review of 540 cases. Obstet Gynecol 71:319, 1988.

Kindermann G, Maassen V, Kuhn W: Laparoscopic management of ovarian tumors subsequently diagnosed as malignant: A survey from 127 German departments of obstetrics and gynecology. J Pelvic Surg 2:245, 1996.

Kobayashi M: Use of diagnostic ultrasound in trophoblastic neoplasms and ovarian tumors. Cancer 38:441, 1976.

Kohlberger PD, Edwards L, Collins C, Milross C, Hacker NF: Laparoscopic port site recurrence following surgery for a stage IB squamous cell carcinoma of the cervix with negative lymph nodes. Gynecol Oncol 79:324, 2000.

Koonings PP, Campbell K, Mishell DR, Grimes DA: Relative frequency of primary ovarian neoplasms: A 10-year review. Obstet Gynecol 74:921, 1989.

Kruitwagen RF, Swinkels BM, Keyser KG, Doesburg WH, Schijf CP: Incidence and effect on survival of abdominal wall metastases at trocar or puncture sites following laparoscopy or paracentesis in women with ovarian cancer. Gynecol Oncol 60:233, 1996.

Kusnetzoff D, Gnochi D, Damonte C et al: Differential diagnoses of pelvic masses: Usefulness of CA125, transvaginal sonography and echo-Doppler. Int J Gynecol Cancer 8:315, 1998.

Levine D, Felstein V, Babcook C et al: Sonography of ovarian masses: poor sensitivity of resistive index for identifying malignant lesions. Am J Roentgenol 162:1355, 1994.

Lundstedt C, Stridbeck H, Anderson R, Tranberg KG, Andren-Sandberg A: Tumor seeding occurring after fine needle biopsy of abdominal malignancies. Acta Radiol 32:518, 1991.

Luxman D, Bergman A, Sagi J, David MP: The postmenopausal adnexal mass: Correlation between ultrasonic and pathologic findings. Obstet Gynecol 77:726, 1991.

Mage G, Canis M, Manhes H, Pouly JL, Wattiez A, Bruhat MA: Laparoscopic management of adnexal cystic masses. J Gynecol Surg 6:71, 1990.

Mais V, Ajossa S, Piras B, Marongui D, Guerriero S, Melis GB: Treatment of non-endometriotic benign adnexal cysts: A randomized comparison of laparoscopy and laparotomy. Obstet Gynecol 86:770, 1995.

Malik E, Bohm W, Stoz F et al: Laparoscopic management of ovarian tumors. Surg Endosc 12:1326, 1998.

Malkasian GD Jr, Knapp RC, Lavin PT et al: Preoperative evaluation of serum CA-125 levels in premenopausal and postmenopausal patients with pelvic masses: Discrimination of benign from malignant disease. Am J Obstet Gynecol 159:341, 1988.

Mann WJ, Patsner B, Cohen H, Loesch M: Preoperative CA-125 levels in patients with surgical stage I invasive ovarian adenocarcinoma. J Natl Cancer Inst 80:208, 1988.

Manolitsas TP, Fowler JM: Role of laparoscopy in the management of the adnexal mass and staging of gynecologic cancers. Clin Obstet Gynecol 44:495, 2001.

Marana R, Caruana P, Muzii L et al: Operative laparoscopy for ovarian cysts: Excision vs. aspiration. J Reprod Med 41:435, 1996.

Mecke H, Lehmann-Willenbrock E, Ibrahim M et al: Pelviscopic treatment of ovarian cysts in premenopausal women. Gynecol Obstet Invest 34:36, 1992.

Meire HB, Farrant P, Guha T: Distinction of benign from malignant ovarian cysts by ultrasound. Br J Obstet Gynaecol 85:893, 1978.

Mettler L, Jacobs VR, Brandenburg K et al: Laparoscopic management of 641 adnexal tumors in Kiel, Germany. J Am Assoc Gynecol Laparosc 8:74, 2001.

Mettler L: The cystic adnexal mass: patient selection, surgical techniques and long-term follow-up. Endosc Surg 13:389, 2001.

Mettler L: The cystic adnexal mass: patient selection, surgical techniques and long-term follow-up. Curr Opin Obstet Gynecol 389, 2001.

Mol BW, Boll D, De Kanter M et al: Distinguishing the benign and malignant adnexal mass: an external validation of prognostic models. Gynecol Oncol 80:162, 2001.

Morice P, Viala J, Pautier P, Lhomme C, Duvillard P, Castaigne D: Port site metastasis after laparoscopic surgery for gynecologic cancer. A report of six cases. J Reprod Med 45:837, 2000.

Muntz HG, Goff BA, Madsen BL, Yon JL: Port site recurrence after laparoscopic surgery for endometrial carcinoma. Obstet Gynecol 93:807, 1999.

Neuhas SJ, Ellis T, Rofe AM, Pike GK, Jamieson GG, Watson DI: Tumor implantation following laparoscopy using different insufflation gases. Surg Endosc 12:1300, 1998.

Nezhat F, Nezhat C, Welander C et al: Four ovarian cancers diagnosed during laparoscopic management of 1011 women with adnexal masses. Am J Obstet Gynecol 167:790, 1992.

Norris HJ, Jensen RD: Relative frequency of ovarian neoplasms in children and adolescents. Cancer 30:713, 1972.

Ovadia F, Godman GA: Ovarian masses in postmenopausal women. Int J Gynecol Obstet 39:35, 1992.

Parker WH, Levine RL, Howard FM, Sansone B, Berek JS: A multicenter study of laparoscopic management of selected cystic adnexal masses in postmenopausal women. J Am Col Surg 179:733, 1994.

Parker WH: Management of adnexal by operative laparoscopy: Selection criteria. J Reprod J Med 37:603, 1992.

Patsner B, Mann WJ: The value of preoperative serum CA-125 levels in patients with a pelvic mass. Am J Obstet Gynecol 159:873, 1988.

Pittaway DE, Takacs P, Bauguess P: Laparoscopic adnexectomy: a comparison with laparotomy. Am J Obstet Gynecol 171:385, 1994.

Ramirez PT, Frumovitz M, Wolf JK, Levenback C: Laparoscopic port site metastases in patients with gynecological malignancies. Int J Gynecol Cancer 14:1070, 2004.

Roman L, Muderspach L, Stein S et al: Pelvic examination, tumor marker level, and gray-scale and Doppler sonography in the prediction of pelvic cancer. Obstet Gynecol 89:493, 1997.

Rulin MC, Preston AL: Adnexal masses in postmenopausal women. Obstet Gynecol 79:578, 1987.

Sadik S, Onoglu AS, Gokdeniz R, Turan E, Taskin O, Wheeler JM: Laparoscopic management of selected adnexal masses. J Am Assoc Gynecol Laparosc 6:313, 1999.

Sassone AM, Timor-Tritsch IE, Artner A, Westhoff C, Warren WB: Transvaginal sonographic characterization of ovarian disease: Evaluation of a new scoring system to detect ovarian malignancy. Obstet Gynecol 78:70, 1991.

Schelling M, Braun M, Kuhn W et al: Combined transvaginal B-mode and color Doppler sonography for differential diagnosis of ovarian tumors: results of a multivariate logistic regression analysis. Gynecol Oncol 77:78, 2000.

Schutter E, Kenemans P, Sohn C et al: Diagnostic value of pelvic examination, ultrasound, and serum CA-125 in postmenopausal women with a pelvic mass. An international multicenter study. Cancer 74:1398, 1994.

Shalev E, Eliyahu S, Peleg D, Tsabari A: Laparoscopic management of adnexal cystic masses in postmenopausal women. Obstet Gynecol 83:594, 1994.

Siriwardena A, Samarji WN: Cutaneous tumour seeding from a previously undiagnosed pancreatic carcinoma after laparoscopic cholecystectomy. Ann R Coll Surg Engl 75:199, 1993.

Spanos WJ: Preoperative hormonal therapy of cystic adnexal masses. Am J Obstet Gynecol 116:551, 1973.

Steege JF: Laparoscopic approach to the adnexal mass. Clin Obstet Gynecol 37:392, 1994.

Stein S, Laifer-Narin S, Johnson M et al: Differentiation of benign and malignant adnexal masses: relative value of grayscale, color Doppler, and spectral Doppler sonography. Am J Roentgenol 164:381, 1995.

Stier EA, Barakat RR, Curtin JP, Brown CL, Jones WB, Hoskins WJ: Laparotomy to complete staging of presumed early ovarian cancer. Obstet Gynecol 87:737, 1996.

Strigini F, Gadducci A, Del BB et al: Differential diagnosis of adnexal masses with transvaginal sonography, color flow imaging, and serum CA-125 assay in pre- and postmenopausal women. Gynecol Oncol 61:68, 1996.

Tseng LN, Berends FJ, Wittich P et al: Port site metastases. Impact of local tissue trauma and gas leakage. Surg Endosc 12:1377, 1998.

Ulrich U, Paulus W, Schneider A, Keckstein J: Laparoscopic surgery for complex ovarian masses. J Am Assoc Gynecol Laparosc 7:373, 2000.

VanNagell J, Ueland F: Ultrasound evaluation of pelvic masses: predictors of malignancy for the general gynecologist. Curr Opin Obstet Gynecol 11:45, 1999.

Vasliev SA, Schlaerth JB, Campeau J, Morrow CP: Serum CA-125 levels in preoperative evaluation of pelvic masses. Obstet Gynecol 71:751, 1988.

Wang PH, Yen MS, Yuan CC, Chao KC, Ng HT, Lee WL, Chao HT: Port site metastasis after laparoscopic-assisted vaginal hysterectomy for endometrial cancer: Possible mechanisms and prevention. Gynecol Oncol 66:151, 1997.

Wang PH, Yuan CC, Lin G, Ng HT, Chao HT: Risk factors contributing to early occurrence of port site metastases of laparoscopic surgery for malignancy. Gynecol Oncol 72:38, 1999.

Weiner Z, Thaler I, Beck D, Rottem S, Deutsch M, Brandes JM: Differentiating malignant from benign ovarian tumors with transvaginal color flow imaging. Obstet Gynecol 79:159, 1992.

Wexner SD, Cohen SM: Port site metastases after laparoscopic colorectal surgery for cure of malignancy. Br J Surg 82:295, 1995.

Young RC, Decker DG, Wharton JT, Piver MS et al: Staging laparotomy in early ovarian cancer. JAMA 250:3072, 1983.

LAPAROSCOPY IN OVARIAN CANCER

Abu-Rustum NR, Barakat RR, Siegel PL, Venkatraman E, Curtin JP, Hoskins WJ: Second-look operation for epithelial ovarian cancer: laparoscopy or laparotomy? Obstet Gynecol 88:549, 1996.

Abu-Rustum NR, Sonoda Y, Chi DS et al: The effects of CO_2 pneumoperitoneum on the survival of women with persistent metastatic ovarian cancer. Gynecol Oncol 90:431, 2003.

Allendorf JDF, Bessler M, Kayton MI, Oesterling SD, Treat MR, Nowygrod R et al: Increased tumor establishment and growth after laparotomy vs laparoscopy in a murine model. Arch Surg 130:649, 1995.

Amara DP, Nezhat C, Teng NNH, Nezhat F, Nezhat C, Rosati M: Operative laparoscopy in the management of ovarian cancer. Surg Laparosc Endosc 6:38, 1996.

Anaf V, Gangji D, Simon P, Saylam K: Laparoscopical insertion of intraperitoneal catheters for intraperitoneal chemotherapy. Acta Obstet Gynecol Scand 82:1140, 2003.

Bailey CL, Ueland FR, Land GL, DePriest PD, Gallion HH, Kryscio RJ et al: The malignant potential of small cystic ovarian tumors in women over 50 years of age. Gynecol Oncol 69:3, 1998.

Berek JS, Griffiths CT, Leventhal JM: Laparoscopy for second-look evaluation in ovarian cancer. Obstet Gynecol 58:192 1981.

Blanc B, Boubli L, D'ercole C, Nicoloso E: Laparoscopic management of malignant ovarian cysts: A 78-case national survey. Part 1: Pre-operative and laparoscopic evaluation. Eur J Obstet Gynecol Reprod Biol 56:177, 1994.

Canis M, Botchorishvili R, Wattiez A et al: Tumor growth and dissemination after laparotomy and CO_2 pneumoperitoneum: a rat ovarian cancer model. Obstet Gynecol 92:104, 1998.

Casey AC, Farias-Eisner R, Pisani AL, Cirisano FD, Kim YB, Muderspach L, Futoran R, Leuchter RS, Lagasse LD, Karlan BY: What is the role of reassessment laparoscopy in the management of gynecologic cancers in 1995? Gynecol Oncol 60:454, 1996.

Cass I, Li AJ, Funowicz CD, Fields AL, Goldberg GL, Leuchter RS et al: Pattern of lymph node metastases in clinically unilateral invasive stage I invasive epithelial carcinoma. Gynecol Oncol 80:56, 2001.

Chi DS, Abu-Rustum NR, Sonoda Y, Ivy J, Rhee E, Moore K, Levine DA, Barakat RR: The safety and efficacy of laparoscopic surgical staging of apparent stage I ovarian and fallopian tube cancers. Am J Obstet Gynecol 192:1614, 2005.

Childers JM, Lang J, Surwit EA, Hatch KD: Laparoscopic surgical staging of ovarian cancer. Gynecol Oncol 59:25, 1995.

Childers JM, Spirtos NM, Brainard P, Surwit EA: Laparoscopic staging of the patient with incompletely staged early adenocarcinoma of the endometrium. Obstet Gynecol 83:597, 1994.

Clough KB, Ladonne JM, Nos C, Renolleau C, Validire P, Durand JC: Second look for ovarian cancer: Laparoscopy or laparotomy? A prospective comparative study. Gynecol Oncol 72:411, 1999.

Dembo AJ, Davy M, Stenwig AE, Berle EJ, Bush RS, Kjorstad K: Prognostic factors in patients with stage I epithelial ovarian cancer. Obstet Gynecol 75:263, 1990.

Eltabbakh GH, Piver MS, Hempling RE et al: Laparoscopic management of women with a family history of ovarian cancer. J Surg Oncol 72:9, 1999.

Evrard S, Flkenrodt A, Park A, Tassetti V, Mutter D, Marescaux J: Influence of CO_2 pneumoperitoneum on systemic and peritoneal cell-mediated immunity. World J Surg 21:353, 1997.

Fruchter R, Boyce J: Delays in diagnosis and stage of disease in gynecologic cancer. Cancer Detect Prev 4:481, 1981.

Grogan R: Accidental rupture of malignant ovarian cysts during surgical removal. Obstet Gynecol 30:716, 1967.

Hempling RE, Wesolowski JA, Piver S: Second-look laparotomy in advanced ovarian cancer: a critical assessment of morbidity and impact on survival. Ann Surg Oncol 4:349, 1997.

Husain A, Chi DS, Prasad M, Abu-Rustum N, Barakat RR, Brown CL, Poynor EZ, Hoskins WJ, Curtin JP: The role of laparoscopy in second-look evaluations for ovarian cancer. Gynecol Oncol 80:44, 2001.

Jacobi CA, Sababt R, Bohm B, Zieren HU, Volk HD, Muller JM: Pneumoperitoneum with carbon dioxide stimulates growth of malignant colonic cells. Surgery 121:72, 1997.

Kindermann G, Maassen V, Kuhn W: Laparoscopic preliminary surgery of ovarian malignancies. Experiences from 127 German gynecologic clinics. Geburtshilfe Frauenheilkd 55:687, 1995.

Kindermann G, Massen V, Kuhn W: Laparoscopic management of ovarian tumors subsequently diagnosed as malignant. J Pelvic Surg 2:245, 1996.

Knolmayer TJ, Asbun HJ, Shibata G, Bowyer MW: An experimental model of cellular aerosolization during laparoscopic surgery. Surg Laparosc Endosc 7:399, 1997.

Leblanc E, Querleu D, Narducci F, Occeli B, Papageorgiou T, Sonoda Y: Laparoscopic restaging of early-stage invasive adnexal tumors: a 10-year experience. Gynecol Oncol 94:624, 2004.

Lécuru F, Agostini A, Guilbaud N, Vildé F, Taurelle R: Lack of adverse effect of pneumoperitoneum on survival in a rat ovarian carcinoma model. Eur J Gynaecol Oncol 20(Suppl):127, 1999.

Lehner R, Wenzl R, Heinzl H, Husslein P, Sevelda P: Influence of delayed staging laparotomy after laparoscopic removal of ovarian masses later found malignant. Obstet Gynecol 92:967, 1998.

Leminen A, Lehtovirta P: Spread of ovarian cancer after laparoscopic surgery: Report of eight cases. Gynecol Oncol 75:387, 1999.

Maiman M, Seltzer V, Boyce J: Laparoscopic excision of ovarian neoplasms subsequently found to be malignant. Obstet Gynecol 77:563, 1991.

Matthew G, Watson DI, Rofe AM, Baigrie CF, Ellis T, Jamieson GG: Wound metastases following laparoscopic and open surgery for abdominal cancer in a rat model. Br J Surg 83:1087, 1996.

Nezhat F, Nezhat C, Welander CE, Benigno B: Four ovarian cancers diagnosed during laparoscopic management of 1011 women with adnexal masses. Am J Obstet Gynecol 167:790, 1992.

Nicklin J, van Eijkeren M, Athanasatos P et al: A comparison of ovarian cyst aspirate cytology and histology. The case against aspiration of cystic pelvic masses. J Obstet Gynaecol 34:546, 1994.

Nicoletto MO, Tumolo S, Talamini R, Salvagno L, Franceschi S, Visona E et al: Surgical second look in ovarian cancer: a randomized study in patients with laparoscopic complete remission—a Northeastern Oncology Cooperative Group-Ovarian Cancer Cooperative Group Study. J Clin Oncol 15:994, 1997.

Piver MS, Lele SB, Barlow JJ, Gamarra M: Second-look laparoscopy prior to proposed second-look laparotomy. Obstet Gynecol 55:571, 1980.

Pomel C, Provencher D, Dauplat J, Gauthier P, Le Bouëdec G, Drouin P et al: Laparoscopic staging of early ovarian cancer. Gynecol Oncol 58(Suppl 1):301, 1995.

Querleu D, Leblanc E: Laparoscopic infrarenal para-aortic lymph node dissection for restaging of carcinoma of the ovary or fallopian tube. Cancer 73:1467, 1994.

Sainz de la Cuesta R, Goff BA, Fuller AF Jr, Nikrui N, Eichorn JH, Rice LW: Prognostic importance of intraoperative rupture of malignant ovarian epithelial neoplasms. Obstet Gynecol 84:1, 1994.

Sevelda P, Vavra N, Schemper M, Salzer H: Prognostic factors for survival in stage I epithelial ovarian carcinoma. Cancer 65:2349, 1990.

Sjövall K, Nilsson B, Einhorn N: Different types of rupture of the tumor capsule and the impact on survival in early ovarian carcinoma. Int J Gynecol Cancer 4:333, 1994.

Tozzi R, Kohler C, Ferrara A, Schneider A: Laparoscopic treatment of early ovarian cancer: surgical and survival outcomes. Gynecol Oncol 93:199, 2004.

Trimbos J, Hacker N: The case against aspirating ovarian cysts. Cancer 72:828, 1993.

Trinh H, Ott C, Fanning J: Feasibility of laparoscopic debulking with electrosurgical loop excision procedure and argon beam coagulator at recurrence in patients with previous laparotomy. Am J Obstet Gynecol 190:1394, 2004.

Vergote IB, Kaern J, Abeler VM, Pettersen EO, De Vos LN, Trope CG: Analysis of prognostic factors in stage I epithelial ovarian carcinoma: Importance of degree of differentiation and deoxyribonucleic acid ploidy in predicting relapse. Am J Obstet Gynecol 169:40, 1993.

Wang PH, Lee WL, Chao HT, Yuan CC: Disseminated carcinomatosis after laparoscopic surgery for presumably benign ruptured ovarian teratoma. Eur J Obstet Gynaecol Reprod Biol 89:89, 2000.

Webb MJ, Decker DG, Mussey E, Williams TJ: Factors influencing survival in stage I ovarian cancer. Am J Obstet Gynecol 116:222, 1972.

Wenzl R, Lehner R, Husslein P, Sevelda P: Laparoscopic surgery in cases of ovarian malignancies: An Austria-wide survey. Gynecol Oncol 63:57, 1996.

Wikborn C, Pettersson F, Moberg P: Delay in diagnosis of epithelial ovarian cancer. Int J Gynaecol Obstet 52:263, 1996.

LAPAROSCOPY IN ENDOMETRIAL CANCER

Angel C, DuBeshter D, Dawson AE, Keller J: Recurrent stage I endometrial adenocarcinoma in the non-irradiated patient: Preliminary results of surgical "staging." Gynecol Oncol 48:221, 1993.

Bloss JD, Berman ML, Bloss LP, Buller RE: Use of vaginal hysterectomy for the management of stage I endometrial cancer in the medically compromised patient. Gynecol Oncol 40:74, 1991.

Boike G, Lurain J, Burke J: A comparison of laparoscopic management of endometrial cancer with traditional laparotomy. Gynecol Oncol 52:105, 1994.

Childers JM, Brzechffa PR, Hatch KD, Surwit EA: Laparoscopically assisted surgical staging (LASS) of endometrial cancer. Gynecol Oncol 51:33, 1993.

Childers JM, Lang J, Surwit EA, Hatch KD: Laparoscopic surgical staging of ovarian cancer. Gynecol Oncol 59:25, 1995.

Childers JM, Spirtos NM, Brainard P, Surwit EA: Laparoscopic staging of the patient with incompletely staged early adenocarcinoma of the endometrium. Obstet Gynecol 83:597, 1994.

Dottino PR, Tobias DH, Beddoe AM, Golden AL, Cohen CJ: Laparoscopic lymphadenectomy for gynecologic malignancies. Gynecol Oncol 73:383, 1999.

Eltabbakh G: Effect of surgeon's experience on the surgical outcome of laparoscopic surgery for women with endometrial cancer. Gynecol Oncol 78:58, 2000.

Eltabbakh GH: Analysis of survival after laparoscopy in women with endometrial carcinoma. Cancer 95:1894, 2002.

Fram KM: Laparoscopic-assisted vaginal hysterectomy versus abdominal hysterectomy in stage I endometrial cancer. Int J Gynecol Cancer 12:57, 2002.

Gemignani M, Curtin JP, Barakat RR et al: Laparoscopic-assisted vaginal hysterectomy (LAVH) vs total abdominal hysterectomy (TAH) for endometrial carcinoma: A comparison of clinical outcomes and hospital charges. Gynecol Oncol 68:129, 1998.

Gemignani ML, Curtin JP, Zelmanovich J, Patel DA, Venkatraman E, Barakat RR: Laparoscopic-assisted vaginal hysterectomy for endometrial cancer: Clinical outcomes and hospital charges. Gynecol Oncol 73:5, 1999.

Hidlebaugh DA, Orr RK: Staging endometrioid adenocarcinoma. Clinical and financial comparison of laparoscopic and traditional approaches. J Reprod Med 42:482, 1997.

Holub Z, Bartos P, Eim J, Fischlova D, Kliment L: Laparoscopic surgery in obese woman with endometrial cancer. J Am Assoc Gynecol Laparosc 7:83, 2000.

Holub Z, Voracek J, Shomani A: A comparison of laparoscopic surgery with open procedure in endometrial cancer. Eur J Gynaecol Oncol 19:294, 1998.

Homesley HD, Boike G, Spiegel GW: Feasibility of laparoscopic management of presumed stage I endometrial carcinoma and assessment of accuracy of myoinvasion estimates by frozen section: a Gynecologic Oncology Group study. Int J Gynecol Cancer 14:341, 2004.

Kornblith A, Walker JL, Huang H, Cella D: Quality of life of patients in a randomized clinical trial of laparoscopy versus open laparotomy for the surgical resection and staging of uterine cancer: A Gynecologic Oncology Group study. Gynecol Oncol 101(S1): 22–23, 2006 [Abstract 47].

Litta P, Fracas M, Pozzan C, Merlin F, Saccardi C, Sacco G et al: Laparoscopic management of early-stage endometrial cancer. Eur J Gynaecol Oncol 24:41, 2003.

Maggino T, Romagnolo C, Landoni F et al: An analysis of approaches to the management of endometrial cancer in North America: a CTF study. Gynecol Oncol 68:274, 1998.

Magrina JF, Mutone NF, Weaver AL, Magtibay PM, Fowler RS, Cornella JL: Laparoscopic lymphadenectomy and vaginal or laparoscopic hysterectomy with bilateral salpingo-oophorectomy for endometrial cancer: morbidity and survival. Am J Obstet Gynecol 181:376, 1999.

Malur S, Possover M, Michels W, Schneider A: Laparoscopic-assisted vaginal versus abdominal surgery in patients with endometrial cancer: A prospective randomized trial. Gynecol Oncol 80:239, 2001.

Massi G, Savino L, Susini T: Vaginal hysterectomy versus abdominal hysterectomy for the treatment of stage I endometrial carcinoma. Am J Obstet Gynecol 174:1320, 1996.

Peters WD, Andersen W, Thornton WJ et al: The selective use of vaginal hysterectomy in the management of adenocarcinoma of the endometrium. Am J Obstet Gynecol 146:285, 1983.

Scribner DR Jr, Mannel RS, Walker JL, Johnson GA: Cost analysis of laparoscopy versus laparotomy for early endometrial cancer. Gynecol Oncol 75:460, 1999.

Spirtos NM, Schlaerth JB, Gross GM, Spirtos TW, Schlaerth AC, Ballon SC: Cost and quality-of-life analyses of surgery for early endometrial cancer: Laparotomy versus laparoscopy. Am J Obstet Gynecol 174:1795, 1996.

Walker J, Mannel R, Piedmonte M et al: Phase III trial of laparoscopy versus laparotomy for surgical resection and comprehensive surgical staging of uterine cancer: a Gynecologic Oncology Group study funded by the National Cancer Institute. Gynecol Oncol 101(S1):11–12, 2006 [Abstract 22].

Walker JL, Piedmonte M, Spirtos N et al: Surgical staging of uterine cancer: Randomized phase III trial of laparoscopy vs laparotomy. A Gynecologic Oncology Group Study: Preliminary results. J Clin Oncol 24:5010, 2006.

LAPAROSCOPY IN CERVICAL CANCER

Abu-Ghazeleh S, Johnston W, Creasman WT: The significance of peritoneal cytology in patients with carcinoma of the cervix. Gynecol Oncol 17:139, 1984.

Abu-Rustum NR, Gemignani ML, Moore K, Sonoda Y, Venkatraman C, Brown C et al. Total laparoscopic radical hysterectomy with pelvic lymphadenectomy using the argon-beam coagulator: pilot data and comparison to laparotomy. Gynecol Oncol 91:402, 2003.

Artman LE, Hoskins WJ, Bibro MC, Heller PB, Weiser EB, Barnhill DR et al: Radical hysterectomy and pelvic lymphadenectomy for stage Ib carcinoma of the cervix: 21-year experience. Gynecol Oncol 28:8, 1987.

Barranger E, Grahek D, Cortez A, Talbot JN, Uzan S, Darai E: Laparoscopic sentinel lymph node procedure using a combination of patent blue and radioisotope in women with cervical carcinoma. Cancer 97:3003, 2003.

Benardini M, Barrett J, Seaward G, Covens A: Pregnancy outcomes in patients after radical trachelectomy. Am J Obstet Gynecol 189:1378, 2003.

Benedetti-Panici P, Maneschi F, Cutillo G, Congiu M, Franchi M, Amoroso M, Gregg S, Mancuso S: Laparoscopic abdominal staging in locally advanced cervical cancer. Int J Gynecol Cancer 9:194, 1999.

Beretta P, Slangen T, Van Herendael BJ: Comparison between abdominal and laparoscopic lymphadenectomy. J Am Assoc Gynecol Laparosc 4:52, 1994.

Berman ML, Lagasse LD, Watring WG et al: The operative evaluation of patients with cervical carcinoma by an extraperitoneal approach. Obstet Gynecol 50:658, 1977.

Bernardini M, Barrett J, Seaward G, Covens A: Pregnancy outcome in patients post radical trachelectomy. Am J Obstet Gynecol 189:1378, 2003.

Bolger B, Lopes ADB, Ofer D et al: Comparison of laparoscopic assisted radical vaginal hysterectomy and radical abdominal hysterectomy in the treatment of early-stage cervical carcinoma. Gynecol Oncol 68:74, 1998.

Buist MR, Pijpers RJ, van Lingen A, van Diest PJ, Dijkstra J, Kenemans P et al: Laparoscopic detection of sentinel lymph nodes followed by lymph node dissection in patients with early-stage cervical cancer. Gynecol Oncol 90:290, 2003.

Burnett AF, Roman LD, O'Meara AT, Morrow CP: Radical vaginal trachelectomy and pelvic lymphadenectomy for preservation of fertility in early cervical carcinoma. Gynecol Oncol 88:419, 2003.

Canis M, Mage G, Wattiez A, Pouly JL, Chapron C, Bruhat MA: Vaginally assisted laparoscopic radical hysterectomy. J Gynecol Surg 8:103, 1992.

Chen MD, Teigen GA, Reynolds HT, Johnson PR, Fowler JM: Laparoscopy versus laparotomy: An evaluation of adhesion formation after pelvic and para-aortic lymphadenectomy in a porcine model. Am J Obstet Gynecol 178:499, 1998.

Childers JM, Brainard P, Rogoff EE, Surwit EA: Laparoscopically assisted transperineal interstitial irradiation and surgical staging for advanced cervical carcinoma. Endocur Hyper Oncol 10:83, 1994.

Childers JM, Hatch K, Surwit EA: The role of laparoscopic lymphadenectomy in the management of cervical carcinoma. Gynecol Oncol 47:38, 1992.

Choi JC, Ingenito AC, Nanda RK et al: Potential decreased morbidity of interstitial brachytherapy for gynecologic malignancies using laparoscopy: a pilot study. Gynecol Oncol 73:210, 1999.

Chu KK, Chang SD, Chen FP, Soong YK: Laparoscopic surgical staging in cervical cancer—preliminary experience among Chinese. Gynecol Oncol 64:49, 1997.

Clough KB, Goffinet F, Labib A et al: Laparoscopic unilateral ovarian transposition prior to irradiation: Prospective study of 20 cases. Cancer 77:2638, 1996.

Covens A, Shaw P, Murphy J, DePetrillo D, Lickrish G, Laframboise S et al: Is radical trachelectomy a safe alternative to radical hysterectomy for patients with stage Ia–b carcinoma of the cervix? Cancer 86:2273, 1999.

Dargent D, Ansquer Y, Mathevet P: Can laparoscopic para-aortic lymphadenectomy help to select patients with pelvic relapse of cervical cancer eligible for pelvic exenteration? Gynecol Oncol 73:172, 1999.

Dargent D, Brun JL, Remy I: Pregnancies following radical trachelectomy for invasive cervical cancer (Abstract). Gynecol Oncol 52:105, 1994.

Dargent D, Martin X, Mathevet P: Laparoscopic assessment of the sentinel lymph node in early-stage cervical cancer. Gynecol Oncol 79:411, 2000.

Dargent D, Martin X, Sacchetoni A, Mathevet P: Laparoscopic vaginal radical trachelectomy: a treatment to preserve the fertility of cervical carcinoma patients. Cancer 88:1877, 2000.

Dargent D, Mathevet P: Schauta's vaginal hysterectomy combined with laparoscopic lymphadenectomy. Baillières Clin Obstet Gynaecol 9:691, 1995.

Dargent D: A new future for Schauta's operation through presurgical retroperitoneal pelviscopy. Eur J Gynaecol Oncol 8:292, 1987.

Dargent D: Laparoscopic assisted radical vaginal hysterectomy: evolution of a concept. J Gynecol Oncol 20:102, 2003.

Downey GO, Potish RA, Adcock LL, Prem KA, Twiggs LB: Pretreatment surgical staging in cervical carcinoma: therapeutic efficacy of pelvic lymph node resection. Am J Obstet Gynecol 160:1055, 1989.

Fowler JM, Carter JR, Carlson JW, Maslonkowski R, Byers LJ, Carson LF, Twiggs LB: Lymph node yield from laparoscopic lymphadenectomy in cervical cancer: A comparative study. Gynecol Oncol 51:187, 1993.

Goff BA, Muntz HG, Paley PJ, Tamimi HK, Koh WJ, Greer BE: Impact of surgical staging in women with locally advanced cervical cancer. Gynecol Oncol 74:436, 1999.

Greggi S, Benedetti-Panici P, Amoroso M, Scambia G, Paratore MP, Salerno MG, Bezzi I, Mancuso S: Intraperitoneal tumor spread in locally advanced cervical carcinoma undergoing neoadjuvant chemotherapy. Int J Gynecol Cancer 8:207, 1998.

Hatch K, Hallum A, Nour M et al: Comparison of radical abdominal hysterectomy with laparoscopic-assisted radical vaginal hysterectomy for treatment of early-stage cervical carcinoma. Gynecol Oncol 64:293, 1997.

Hermann H, Köhler C, Michels W, Possover M, Tozzi R, Schneider A: Laparoscopic-assisted radical vaginal hysterectomy (LARVH): prospective evaluation of 200 patients with cervical cancer. Gynecol Oncol 90:505, 2003.

Hertel H, Köhler C, Elhawary T, Michels W, Possover M, Schneider A: Laparoscopic staging compared with imaging techniques in the staging of advanced cervical cancer. Gynecol Oncol 87:46, 2002.

Hertel H, Köhler C, Michels W, Possover M, Tozzi R, Schneider A: Laparoscopic-assisted radical vaginal hysterectomy (LARVH): prospective evaluation of 200 patients with cervical cancer. Gynecol Oncol 90:505, 2003.

Hertel H, Possover M, Krause N, Schneider A: Fertility after radical trachelectomy in patients with early-stage cervical cancer. Geburtsh Frauenheilk 61:117, 2001.

Holcomb K, Abulafia O, Matthews RP, Gabbur N, Lee YC, Buhl A: The impact of pretreatment staging laparotomy on survival in locally advanced cervical carcinoma. Eur J Gynaecol Oncol 20:90, 1999.

Hricak H, Quivey JM, Campos Z, Gildengorin V, Hindmarsh T, Bis KG et al: Carcinoma of the cervix: predictive value of clinical and magnetic resonance (MR) imaging assessment of prognostic factors. Int J Radiat Oncol Biol Phys 27:791, 1993.

Jackson KS, Das N, Naik R, Lopes AD, Godfrey KA, Hatem MH, Monaghan JM: Laparoscopically assisted radical vaginal hysterectomy vs. radical abdominal hysterectomy for cervical cancer: a match controlled study. Gynecol Oncol 95:655, 2004.

Kadar N, Reich H: Laparoscopically assisted radical Schauta hysterectomy and bilateral laparoscopic pelvic lymphadenectomy for the treatment of bulky stage Ib carcinoma of the cervix. Gynecol Endosc 2:135, 1993.

Kadar N: Laparoscopic vaginal radical hysterectomy: An operative technique and its evolution. Gynaecol Endosc 3:109, 1994.

Kamprath S, Possover M, Schneider A. Laparoscopic sentinel lymph node detection in patients with cervical cancer. Am J Obstet Gynecol 182:1648, 2000.

Kim DH, Moon JS: Laparoscopic radical hysterectomy with pelvic lymphadenectomy for early, invasive cervical carcinoma. J Am Assoc Gynecol Laparosc 5:411, 1998.

Kohler C, Tozzi R, Possover M, Schneider A: Explorative laparoscopy prior to exenterative surgery. Gynecol Oncol 86:311, 2002.

Lambaudie E, Collinet P, Narducci F, Sonoda Y, Papageorgiou T, Carpenter P et al: Laparoscopic identification of sentinel lymph nodes in early-stage cervical cancer: prospective study using a combination of patent blue dye injection and technetium radiocolloid injection. Gynecol Oncol 89:84, 2003.

Lee CL, Huang KG, Jain S, Lee PS, Soong YK: Comparison of laparoscopic and conventional surgery in the treatment of early cervical cancer. J Am Assoc Gynecol Laparosc 9:481, 2002.

Lee YS, Lee TH, Koo TB, Cho YL, Park IS: Laparoscopic-assisted radical vaginal parametrectomy including pelvic and/or para-aortic lymphadenectomy in women after prior hysterectomy—three cases. Gynecol Oncol 91:619, 2003.

Levenback C, Coleman RL, Burke TW, Lin WM, Erdman W, Deavers M et al: Lymphatic mapping and sentinel node identification in patients with cervix cancer undergoing radical hysterectomy and pelvic lymphadenectomy. J Clin Oncol 20:688, 2002.

Levrant SG, Bieber EJ, Barnes RB: Anterior abdominal wall adhesions after laparotomy or laparoscopy. J Am Assoc Gynecol Laparosc 4:353, 1997.

Malur S, Krause N, Köhler CH, Schneider A: Sentinel lymph node detection in patients with cervical cancer. Gynecol Oncol 80:254, 2001.

Malur S, Possover M, Schneider A: Laparoscopically assisted radical vaginal versus radical abdominal hysterectomy type II in patients with cervical cancer. Surg Endosc 15:289, 2001.

Miller B, Morris M, Rutledge F et al: Aborted exenterative procedures in recurrent cervical cancer. Gynecol Oncol 50:94, 1993.

Nam JH, Kim JH, Kim DY, Kim MK, Yoo HJ, Kim YM, Kim YT, Mok JE: Comparative study of laparoscopico-vaginal radical hysterectomy and abdominal radical hysterectomy in patients with early cervical cancer. Gynecol Oncol 92:277, 2004.

Nezhat CR, Nezhat FR, Burrell MO et al: Laparoscopic radical hysterectomy and laparoscopic assisted vaginal radical hysterectomy with pelvic and para-aortic lymph node dissection. J Gynecol Surg 9:105, 1993.

Park CT, Lim KT, Chung HW, Lee KH, Seong SJ, Shim JU et al: Clinical evaluation of laparoscopic-assisted radical vaginal hysterectomy with pelvic and/or para-aortic lymphadenectomy. J Am Assoc Gynecol Laparosc 9:49, 2002.

Plante M, Renaud MC, Harel F, Roy M: Vaginal radical trachelectomy: An oncologically safe fertility-preserving surgery. An updated series of 72 cases and review of the literature. Gynecol Oncol 94:614, 2004.

Plante M, Renaud MC, Hoskins IA, Roy M: Vaginal radical trachelectomy: A valuable fertility-preserving option in the management of early-stage cervical cancer. A series of 50 pregnancies and review of the literature. Gynecol Oncol 98:3, 2005.

Plante M, Renaud MC, Tetu B, Harel F, Roy M. Laparoscopic sentinel node mapping in early-stage cervical cancer. Gynecol Oncol 91:494, 2003.

Plante M, Roy M: Operative laparoscopy prior to a pelvic exenteration in patients with recurrent cervical cancer. Gynecol Oncol 69:94, 1998.

Pomel C, Atallah D, Le Bouedec G, Rouzier R, Morice P, Castaigne D et al: Laparoscopic radical hysterectomy for invasive cervical cancer: 8-year experience of a pilot study. Gynecol Oncol 91:534, 2003.

Pomel C, Rouzier R, Pocard M et al: Laparoscopic total pelvic exenteration for cervical relapse. Gynecol Oncol 91:616, 2003.

Pomel C, Atallah D, Bouedee Gl, Rouzier R, Morice P, Castaigne D, Dauplat J. Laparoscopic radical hysterectomy for invasive cervical cancer: 8-year experience of a pilot study. Gynecol Oncol 91:534, 2003.

Possover M, Krause N, Kühne-Heid R, Schneider A: Laparoscopic assistance for extended radicality of radical vaginal hysterectomy: description of a technique. Gynecol Oncol 70:94, 1998.

Possover M, Krause N, Schneider A: Identification of the ureter and dissection of the bladder pillar in laparoscopic-assisted radical vaginal hysterectomy. Obstet Gynecol 91:139, 1998.

Possover M, Krause N, Schneider A: Laparoscopic assistance for extended radicality of vaginal radical hysterectomy: Description of a technique. Gynecol Oncol 70:94, 1998.

Possover M, Stöber S, Plaul K, Schneider A: Identification and preservation of the motoric innervation of the bladder in radical hysterectomy type III. Gynecol Oncol 79:154, 2000.

Possover M: Technical modification of the nerve-sparing laparoscopy-assisted vaginal radical hysterectomy type 3 for better reproducibility of this procedure. Gynecol Oncol 90:245, 2003.

Querleu D, Leblanc E, Castelain B: Laparoscopic pelvic lymphadenectomy in the staging of early carcinoma of the cervix. Am J Obstet Gynecol 164:579, 1991.

Querleu D: Laparoscopic-assisted radical vaginal hysterectomy. Gynecol Oncol 51:248, 1993.

Recio FO, Piver MS, Hempling RE, Eltabbakh GH, Hahn S: Laparoscopic-assisted application of interstitial brachytherapy for locally advanced cervical carcinoma: Results of a pilot study. Int J Radiat Oncol Biol Phys 40:411, 1998.

Recio FO, Piver MS, Hempling RE: Pretreatment transperitoneal laparoscopic staging pelvic and para-aortic lymphadenectomy in large (≥ 5 cm) stage Ib2 cervical carcinoma: Report of a pilot study. Gynecol Oncol 63:333, 1996.

Renaud MC, Plante M, Roy M: Combined laparoscopic and vaginal radical surgery in cervical cancer. Gynecol Oncol 79:59, 2000.

Rose PG, Adler LP, Rodriguez M, Faulhaber PF, Abdul-Karim FW et al: Positron emission tomography for evaluating para-aortic nodal metastasis in locally advanced cervical cancer before surgical staging: a surgico-pathologic study. J Clin Oncol 17:41, 1999.

Roy M, Plante M: Pregnancies after radical vaginal trachelectomy for early-stage cervical cancer. Am J Obstet Gynecol 179:1491, 1998.

Roy M, Plante M, Renaud M-C, Têtu B: Vaginal radical hysterectomy versus abdominal radical hysterectomy in the treatment of early-stage cervical cancer. Gynecol Oncol 62:336, 1996.

Roy M, Plante M: Pregnancies after radical vaginal trachelectomy for early-stage cervical cancer. Am J Obstet Gynecol 179:1491, 1998.

Sardi J, Vidaurreta J, Bermudez A, di Paola G. Laparoscopically assisted Schauta operation: learning experience at the Gynecologic Oncology Unit, Buenos Aires University Hospital. Gynecol Oncol 75:361, 1999.

Schlaerth JB, Spirtos NM, Carson LF, Boike G, Adamec T, Stonebraker B: Laparoscopic retroperitoneal lymphadenectomy followed by immediate laparotomy in women with cervical cancer: A Gynecologic Oncology Group study. Gynecol Oncol 85:81, 2002.

Schlaerth JB, Spirtos NM, Schlaerth AC: Radical trachelectomy and pelvic lymphadenectomy with uterine preservation in the treatment of cervical cancer. Am J Obstet Gynecol 188:29, 2003.

Schneider A, Possover M, Kamprath S, Endisch U, Krause N, Noschel H: Laparoscopic-assisted radical vaginal hysterectomy modified according to Schauta-Stoeckel. Obstet Gynecol 88:1057, 1996.

Scribner DR Jr, Kamelle SA, Gould N, Tillmanns T, Wilson MA, McMeekin S, Gold MA, Mannel RS: A retrospective analysis of radical hysterectomies done for cervical cancer: Is there a role for the Pfannenstiel incision? Gynecologic Oncology 81:481, 2001.

Shepherd J, Crawford R, Oram D: Radical trachelectomy: a way to preserve fertility in the treatment of early cervical cancer. Br J Obstet Gynaecol 105:912, 1998.

Shepherd JH, Mould T, Oram DH. Radical trachelectomy in early-stage carcinoma of the cervix: outcome as judged by recurrence and fertility rates. Br J Obstet Gynaecol 108:882, 2001.

Sonoda Y, Abu-Rustum NR, Gemignani ML, Chi DS, Brown CL, Poynor EA, Barakat RR: A fertility-sparing alternative to radical hysterectomy: how many patients may be eligible? Gynecol Oncol 95:534, 2004.

Sonoda Y, Leblanc E, Querleu D, Castelain B, Papageorgiou TH, Lambaudie E et al: Prospective evaluation of surgical staging of advanced cervical cancer via a laparoscopic extraperitoneal approach. Gynecol Oncol 91:326, 2003.

Spirtos NM, Eisenkop SM, Schlaerth JB, Ballon SC: Laparoscopic radical hysterectomy (type III) with aortic and pelvic lymphadenectomy in patients with stage I cervical cancer: Surgical morbidity and intermediate follow-up. Am J Obstet Gynecol 187:340, 2002.

Spirtos NM, Schlaerth JB, Kimball RE, Leiphart VM, Ballon SC: Laparoscopic radical hysterectomy (type III) with aortic and pelvic lymphadenectomy. Am J Obstet Gynecol 174:1763, 1996.

Steed H, Rosen B, Murphy J, Laframboise S, De Petrillo D, Covens A: A comparison of laparoscopic-assisted radical vaginal hysterectomy and radical abdominal hysterectomy in the treatment of cervical cancer. Gynecol Oncol 93:588, 2004.

Su TH, Wang YC, Hong BK, Huang SH: Laparoscopic para-aortic lymph node sampling of invasive cervical carcinoma: including a comparative study of 21 laparotomy cases. Int J Gynecol Obstet 49:311, 1995.

Vergote I, Amant F, Berteloot P, Van Gramberen M: Laparoscopic lower para-aortic staging lymphadenectomy in stage Ib2, II and III cervical cancer. Int J Gynecol Cancer 12:22, 2002.

Vidaurreta J, Bermudez A, Di Paola G, Sardi J: Laparoscopic staging in locally advanced cervical carcinoma: a new possible philosophy? Gynecol Oncol 75:366, 1999.

Visco AG, Barber MD, Myers ER: Early physician experience with laparoscopically assisted vaginal hysterectomy and rates of surgical complications and conversion to laparotomy. Am J Obstet Gynecol 187:1008, 2002.

Weiser EB, Bundy BN, Hoskins WJ, Heller PB, Whittington RR, DiSaia PJ, Curry SL, Schlaerth J, Thigpen JT: Extraperitoneal versus transperitoneal selective para-aortic lymphadenectomy in the pretreatment surgical staging of advanced cervical carcinoma (A Gynecologic Oncology Group Study). Gynecol Oncol 33:283, 1989.

COMPLICATIONS

Abu-Rustum NR, Rhee EH, Chi DS et al: Subcutaneous tumor implantation after laparoscopic procedures in women with malignant disease. Obstet Gynecol 103:480, 2004.

Boike G, Miller C, Spirtos N, Mercer L, Fowler J, Summitt R, Orr J: Incisional bowel herniations after operative laparoscopy: a series of nineteen cases and review of the literature. Am J Obstet Gynecol 172:1726, 1995.

Chi DS, Abu-Rustum NR, Sonoda Y et al: Ten-year experience with laparoscopy on a gynecologic oncology service: Analysis of risk factors for complications and conversion to laparotomy. Am J Obstet Gynecol 191(4):1138–1145, 2004.

Childers JM, Aqua KA, Surwit EA, Hallum AV, Hatch KD: Abdominal-wall tumor implantation after laparoscopy for malignant conditions. Obstet Gynecol 84:765, 1994.

Chu CS, Randall TC, Bandera CA, Rubin SC: Vaginal cuff recurrence of endometrial cancer treated by laparoscopic-assisted vaginal hysterectomy. Gynecol Oncol 88:62, 2003.

Dobronte Z, Wittmann T, Karacsony G: Rapid development of malignant metastasis in the abdominal wall after laparoscopy. Endoscopy 10:127, 1978.

Harkki-Siren P, Sjoberg J, Kurki T: Major complications of laparoscopy: A follow up Finnish study. Obstet Gynecol 94:94, 1999.

Hopkins M, von GV, Gaich S: Laparoscopic port site implantation with ovarian cancer. Am J Obstet Gynecol 182:735, 2000.

Hughes ES, McDermott FT, Polglase AL, Johnson WR: Tumor recurrence in the abdominal wall scar tissue after large-bowel cancer surgery. Dis Colon Rectum 26:571, 1983.

Kadar N, Liu CY, Manko J, Gimpelson R: Incisional hernia after major laparoscopic gynecologic procedure. Am J Obstet Gynecol 168:4193, 1993.

Kadar N: Port site recurrences after laparoscopic operations for gynaecological malignancies. Br J Obstet Gynaecol 104:1308, 1997.

Kruitwagen RF, Swinkels BM, Keyser KG, Doesburg WH, Schijf CP: Incidence and effect on survival of abdominal wall metastases at trocar or puncture sites following laparoscopy or paracentesis in women with ovarian cancer. Gynecol Oncol 60:233, 1996.

Lane G, Tay J: Port site metastasis following laparoscopic lymphadenectomy for adenosquamous carcinoma of the cervix. Gynecol Oncol 74:130, 1999.

Leminen A, Lehtovirta P: Spread of ovarian cancer after laparoscopic surgery: report of eight cases. Gynecol Oncol 75:387, 1999.

Muntz HG, Goff BA, Madsen BL, Yon JL: Port site recurrence after laparoscopic surgery for endometrial carcinoma. Obstet Gynecol 93(Suppl 5):807, 1999.

Patsner B, Damien M: Umbilical metastases from stage IB cervical cancer after laparoscopy: A case report. Fertil Steril 58:1248, 1992.

Quasarano RT, Kashef M, Sherman SJ, Hagglund KH: Complications of gynecologic laparoscopy. J Am Assoc Gynecol Laparosc 6:317, 1999.

Ramirez PT, Wolf JK, Levenback C: Laparoscopic port site metastases: etiology and prevention. Gynecol Oncol 91:179, 2003.

Saida MH, Sadler RK, Vancaillie TG, Akright BD, Farhart SA, White AJ: Diagnosis and management of serious urinary complications after major operative laparoscopy. Obstet Gynecol 87:272, 1996.

Stockdale A, Pocock T: Abdominal wall metastasis after laparoscopy: a case report. Eur J Surg Oncol 11:373, 1985.

van Dam PA, DeCloedt J, Tjalma WA, Buytaert P, Becquart D, Vergote IB: Trocar implantation metastasis after laparoscopy in patients with advanced ovarian cancer: Can the risk be reduced? Am J Obstet Gynecol 181:536, 1999.

Wang PH, Yen MS, Yuan CC et al: Port site metastasis after laparoscopic-assisted vaginal hysterectomy for endometrial cancer: Possible mechanisms and prevention. Gynecol Oncol 66:151, 1997.

Wang PH, Yuan CC, Lin G, Ng HT, Chao HT: Risk factors contributing to early occurrence of port site metastases of laparoscopic surgery for malignancy. Gynecol Oncol 72:38, 1999.

23 Epidemiology of Commonly Used Statistical Terms, and Analysis of Clinical Studies

Wendy R. Brewster, M.D.

EPIDEMIOLOGY

Epidemiology is the study of distribution of disease and the factors that determine disease occurrence in populations. The focus is on groups as compared to the individual. Persons within a population do not have equal risk for disease occurrence and the risk of a disease is a function of personal characteristics and environmental exposures. Patterns of disease occurrence within specific populations can be evaluated to determine why certain groups develop illness when others do not. The impact of epidemiology is evidenced by the significance of studies such as diethylstilbestrol and vaginal adenocarcinoma, and the risk of endometrial cancer and unopposed estrogen replacement therapy. Epidemiological studies are unique in their focus on human populations and its reliance on non-experimental observations. Epidemiological methods are used in searching for causes of disease, disease surveillance, determining the cause of disease, diagnostic testing, searching for prognostic factors and testing new treatments.

Because the quality of epidemiologic evidence varies greatly among studies, the scientific community endorses the principles of Sir Austin Bradford Hill, an eminent British statistician, when attempting to identify causal associations. A cause of a specific disease is an antecedent event or characteristic that is necessary for the occurrence of the disease (Table 23–1).

EVIDENCE-BASED MEDICINE

As much as possible, medical decisions should be based on quality evidence. The best evidence is a properly designed randomized controlled trial. Evidence from non-randomized but well-designed control trials is of lesser quality. Next in reliability is well-designed cohort or case-control studies, which have been repeated by several investigators. Opinions of respected authorities and extensive clinical experience are least reliable.

Physicians are currently encouraged to practice evidence-based medicine. This means that clinical trial evidence must pass statistically valid tests for conclusions to have meaning. Good science depends on accurate (i.e., statistically significant and meaningful) data from clinical trials. The best trials are usually experimental, powered, randomized, and blinded. Patients randomly assigned to a treatment group, or a control group must have an equal probability of being assigned to either group. This prevents selection bias (e.g., putting healthier or better prognosis patients in one group and those with a poor prognosis or high likelihood of disease risk in another group). Blinding prevents patients, investigators, and statisticians from knowing who is in the control group and experimental group; thus, bias actions are avoided.

Retrospective and observational studies are descriptive and do not involve either an intervention or a manipulation, whereas an experimental study does. A prospective trial poses the question before the data are collected, thus allowing better control of confounding variables, unlike a retrospective study that poses the question after the data are collected.

MEASURES IN EPIDEMIOLOGY

In order to describe and compare groups in a meaningful manner it is important to find and enumerate appropriate denominators and statistical terms (Table 23–2).

Table 23–1 STRENGTH OF ASSOCIATION

1. Temporality. Exposure must precede the onset of the disease
2. Dose-response. Risk increases as exposure increases
3. Replication. The association is observed repeatedly
4. Coherence. The association is consistent with other scientific knowledge and does not require that established facts be ignored
5. Exclusion of the role of chance. Appropriate statistical tests demonstrate that the observed association is extremely unlikely to have arisen by chance

Adapted from Hill AB. The environment and disease: Association or causation. Proc Roy Soc Med 58:295, 1965.

Table 23–2 MATHEMATICAL DEFINITIONS OF STATISTICAL TERMS

Terminology	Mathematical definition
Prevalence rate	Number of persons with disease/total number in the group
Incidence rate	Number of new cases/total number at risk Per unit of time
Sensitivity	True positive/(True positive + False negative)
Specificity	True negative/(True negative + False positive)
Predictive value positive	True positive/(True positive + False positive)
Predictive value negative	True negative/(True negative + False negative)

Mean The average of a sample of observations.

Median The middle value when the values are arranged in order from the smallest to the largest.

Standard deviation A measure of the variability within each group. If there is a normal (bell-shaped curve) distribution, approximately 95% of the values are within two standard deviations on both sides of the average.

Prevalence rate The amount of disease in a population. Prevalence measures the proportion of diseased individuals at a particular time and represents a snapshot of the disease. Other commonly used terminology is prevalence proportion and point prevalence. It is a measure of status and includes individuals with newly diagnosed disease and those surviving with disease. The numerator is the number of affected individuals in a specific time period. The denominator is the total number of persons in the group. Prevalence rates range between 0 and 1.

Incidence rate Measures the new cases of a specific disease that develop during a defined period of time and the approximation of the risk for developing the disease. The incidence rate focuses on events. Incidence measures the probability of developing a disease.

Person time The sum of the observation period of risk for the persons in a group being studied.

Sensitivity The proportion of truly diseased persons who are classified as diseased by the test. The sensitivity of a test is therefore the probability of a test being positive when the disease is present. The sensitivity of test may also be called the true positive rate. In Fig. 23–1 it is evident that the cut off point of a test can impact the sensitivity. If the cut off point is moved to the left, more disease persons will be identified. At the same time more healthy persons will be erroneously classified as sick. However, as the cut off value for normal is moved to the right the test will become less sensitive because fewer diseased persons will be classified as such.

Specificity The proportion of a population of disease-free individuals who are classified as undiseased by a test. In contrast to the sensitivity of a test, the specificity of a test is the probability that a test being negative when the disease is absent. The cut off point of a test for normality influences the specificity. As the value of normality or cut off moves to the left the test becomes less specific because fewer health individuals are recognized as such and. In contrast, moving the cut off values to the right, increases the specificity (Fig. 23–1).

In the best scenario, a test would be able to discriminate between disease and healthy individuals without any overlap. More often the scenario is as presented in Fig. 23–1, where there is significant overlap and whatever the cut off value healthy persons may be classified as diseased and sick persons classified as healthy. When we set the cut off point for a test we must be attentive to the purpose of the test. If the disease is treatable and missing the disease has serious ramifications then we must favor sensitivity over specificity. Alternatively, if it is more important correctly identify healthy individuals then specificity is prioritized.

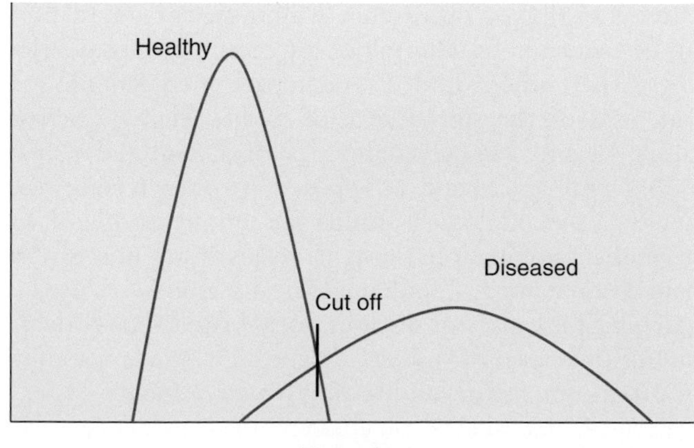

Figure 23–1 Effects of shifting cut off point on sensitivity and specificity.

Predictive value positive The proportion of positive test results that is truly positive.

Predictive value negative The proportion of negative test results that is truly negative. The predictive value of a negative test result refers to the proportion of patients with a negative test result who are free of disease. These values, unlike sensitivity and specificity, indicate the reliability of the test in the determination of presence or absence of disease.

ANALYSES OF CLINICAL TRIALS

Null hypothesis This hypothesis, symbolized by H_0, is a statement claiming that there is no difference between the experimental and population means. The alternative hypothesis (H_1) is the opposite of the null hypothesis. Often in research we need to be able to test for both the positive and adverse outcomes, therefore a two-tailed hypothesis is chosen, even though the expectation of the experiment is in a particular direction.

Significance level A level of significance termed the *alpha value* is determined before the study has begun. The alpha value is the likelihood that a difference as large or larger that occurred between the study groups could be determined by chance alone. The alpha level is established by those designing the study and becomes the level of statistical significance. The most typical alpha level is 0.05.

One-tail test A test to determine a difference in only one direction; for example, to determine if drug A is better than drug B.

Two-tail test A test to determine any difference between the variable; for example, if either drug A or drug B is superior to the other. It is usually considered that in a two-tail test more trust can be placed in the statistically significant results than with a one-tail test. When in doubt, the two-tail test is preferred.

Confidence interval (CI) The range of values that is believed to contain the true value within a specific level of certainty.

Alpha error The rejection of the null hypothesis when it is, in fact, correct. Also called a Type I error.

Beta error Failure to reject the null hypothesis when it is, in fact, incorrect. Also called a Type II error.

Power The probability that a study will be able to correctly detect a true effect of a specific magnitude. The statistical power refers to the probability of finding a difference when one truly exists or how well the null hypothesis will be rejected. The power is usually specified beforehand in prospective studies. The values of 0.8 (80%) or 0.9 (90%) are typical. The higher the value, the less chance there is of a type II error. A 0.9 value means that a type II error would be avoided 90% of the time.

Risk The proportion of unaffected individuals who, on average, will contract the disease of interest over a specified period of time. Results of a trial are often expressed as absolute or relative risk reductions. The absolute difference is the actual difference between the units of the difference. In relative risk, the differences are the percentage change. Relative risk reductions often sound much more dramatic than do the absolute values. One must consider the prevalence of a disease when evaluating risk reductions. Where there is a low prevalence of a disease process, small risk reductions become unimpressive and must be evaluated in terms of the benefits of a particular mode of therapy.

Odds ratio (OR) The ratio of the odds that an event will occur in one group compared with the odds that the event will occur in the other group. If 14 of 22 people who are thin, in an osteoporosis study, have fractures, the odds of having a fracture are 14 in 22 or 0.64. If 5 of the 33 non-thin people fracture bone, the odds are 5 in 33 or 0.15. The odds ratio is 0.64 divided by 0.15 or 4.2, meaning that thin people are 4.2 times more likely to receive fractures. An odds ratio of 1 means that both groups have a similar likelihood of having an event.

Cox proportional hazard regression analysis Cox regression analysis is a technique for assessing the association between variables and survival rate. The measure of risk provided for each variable is the risk ratio (RR). A risk ratio of 1 means that the risk is the same for each participant. A risk ratio greater than 1 indicates increased risk; a ratio less than 1 indicates less risk. A ratio of 5.4 means that the patients with a variable are 5.4 times more likely to have the outcome being studied. Confidence intervals can also be provided with risk ratios. This type of analysis is usually presented in a table.

Actuarial (life table) survival This technique uses grouped information to estimate the survival curve. The data are grouped into fixed time periods (e.g., months, years) that include the maximum follow-up. The survival curve is estimated as a continuous curve and gives an estimate of the proportions of a group of patients who will be alive at different times after the initial observation. The group includes patients with incomplete follow-up.

Chi Square (ξ^2) The primary statistical test used for studying the relationship between variables.

$$\xi^2 = (\text{observed number} - \text{expected number})^2 \div \text{expected number.}$$

This is a test used to compare proportions of categorical variables.

Multivariate analysis A technique of analysis of data that factors many variables. A mathematical model is constructed that simultaneously determines the effect of one variable while evaluating the effect of other factors that may have an influence on the variable being tested. The two most common algorithms developed to accomplish this task are the step-up and step-down procedure. Variables

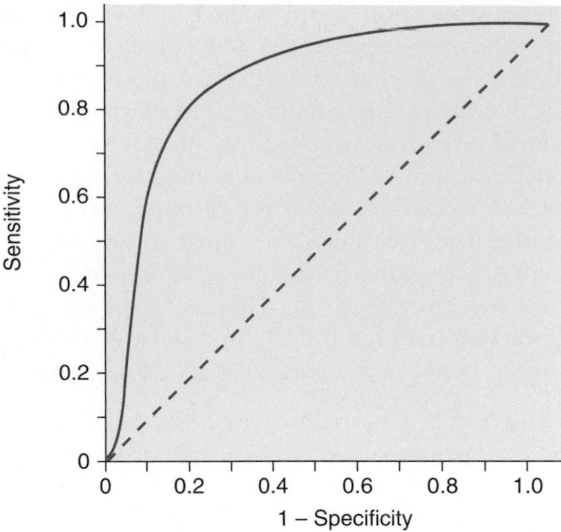

Figure 23–2 A hypothetical example of an ROC curve. The solid line represents the performance of the diagnostic test of interest; the dashed diagonal line serves as a reference of a test with no diagnostic value. (From Greenberg RS et al: Medical Epidemiology (3rd edn). Lange Medical Books/McGraw-Hill, 2001, p 84, Fig. 6-6. Reproduced by permission of The McGraw-Hill Companies.)

are added to an initial small set or deleted from an initial large set while testing repeatedly to see which new factor makes a statistical contribution to the overall model.

Univariate analysis Analyses may be univariate or multivariate as they examine one or more variables at a time, respectively.

Meta-analysis An amalgamation of studies—a complex task to avoid misleading conclusions. The goal of combining results from different sources is to delineate which features are universal. The quality of the studies included is important to the final result. Many think that only prospective randomized clinical trials should be combined for a meta-analysis because such trials are usually of the highest quality.

Receiver operator characteristics (ROC) These curves are the best way to demonstrate the relationships between sensitivity and specificity. They curves plot sensitivity (true positive rate) against the false positive rate (1-specificity) (Fig. 23–2). The closer the curve is to the upper left hand corner, the more accurate it is because the true positive rate is closer to one and the false positive rate is closer to zero. Along any particular ROC curve one can observe the impact of compromising the true positive and false positive rates. As the requirement that a test have a high true positive rate increases, the false positive rate will also increase. The closer the curve is to the 45-degree diagonal of the ROC area under the curve, the less accurate the test. (see Figure 23–2).

Clinical trials

Clinical trials are experiments in which the investigator intervenes rather than observes and is the best test of cause-and-effect relationship. A properly conducted experiment requires that when the intervention is applied to one group, there be a control group or some other suitable standard where subjects of the clinical experiment or their guardians must give informed consent. The gold standard of clinical trials is the randomized experiment. With randomization each subject has an equal chance of being in either of the arms of the trials. Randomization is important because it equalizes baseline characteristics of the subjects so that the comparison of the treatments is fair. If randomization is not feasible, possible non-random standards of comparison must include patients similar to the treated group. Randomization is the current norm for demonstrating efficacy and safety of investigational methods. The advantages of randomization are numerous:

Advantages

- Decreases investigator's bias in assigning patients to treatment groups
- Permits certain statistical methods to be used in the resulting data
- Allows for blinding of the patient and investigator
- Current norm for demonstrating efficacy and safety of investigational medicines

Unacceptable methods of randomization

- Alternate assignments
- Alternate day assignments
- Birthday assignments
- Coin tosses
- Initials of a patient

TYPES OF CLINICAL TRIALS

Single patient clinical trials are indicated only in specific situations. They are generally used to evaluate rare diseases when other types of trials are inappropriate or when only a small percentage of patients respond to a specific treatment. Single patient clinical trials are useful to determine the response of a particular patient is due to placebo or if an adverse reaction is related to a specific medication. The disease should be chronic and the disease severity must be stable during the clinical trial duration. It should be expected that the effect of the treatment should be measurable in a short period of time and the effect should be rapidly reversible once the treatment has stopped. The investigator and patient should be blinded and the patient's condition should return pre-existing baselines between treatment legs.

Multicenter trials are advantageous because they offer more rapid patient accrual and allow for greater protocol complexity. Multicenter trials reduce the opportunity for an individual's bias to influence the conduct of the trial; they increase the likelihood for the inclusion of a more representative study population and facilitate a higher standard for data processing and analysis. Disadvantages of multicenter trials are the administrative considerations that

Table 23–3 TYPES OF CLINICAL TRIALS
Single patient clinical trials
Multicenter trials
National clinical trials
Continuation trials
Compassionate plea trials
Pharmacoeconomic trials
Trials to evaluate medical devices
Pharmacokinetic trials

underlie the management and administrative arrangements for example IRB/Ethics committees. Considerations must be delineated for criteria for patient enrollment, diagnostic classification, and assessment of treatment outcome. These trials are inherently more costly (Table 23–3).

EVALUATION OF CLINICAL TRIALS

There are many factors to consider when evaluating a clinical trial. The most important is the clinical trial objective or aims. Whether the objectives of the trial are adequately assessed is dependant upon the presence and extent of *bias* and confounding factors. Bias is a non-random error in a study that can alter the outcome. Types of bias to consider when evaluating a manuscript are listed in Table 23–4.

Specifying the *sample size* or number of participants in the study needed to detect a difference or an effect of a given magnitude is dependant upon many variables. The most important is the magnitude of the effect desired or expected. Other important considerations are the desired probability of the study to identify the correct outcome (power), the variability of the variables being analyzed, the number of parts of the clinical trial, the magnitude of the placebo effect and the number of dependant parts of the clinical trials. When determining the sample size one must consider if the size of the treatment groups will be equal or non-equal (e.g. 2:1 ratio). An advantage of using groups of unequal size is that more information will be gained about patient responses in the larger arm. A disadvantage is the loss in study power, however this detraction is not usually substantial if the ratios are kept under 3:1.

Placebo treatment groups

Placebo treatment groups control for the psychological aspects of being in a treatment trial. They also control for adverse events being attributed to a medicine when they result from spontaneous changes in the disease or from other causes; and allow a stronger interpretation of the data. Placebo treatment groups are considered ethical if:

- no standard treatment exists;
- the standard treatment has been proven ineffective;
- standard treatment is inappropriate for the particular clinical trial;
- placebo has been reported to be effective in treating the condition;
- the disease is mild and lack of treatment is not considered to be medically important; or
- the disease process is characterized by frequent spontaneous exacerbations and remissions.

Table 23–4 BIAS AND CONFOUNDING FACTORS. EXAMINATION OF THE LITERATURE IN THE FIELD
Specifying and selecting the clinical trial sample
Popularity bias
Referral filter bias
Diagnostic/access bias
Wrong sample size
Migrator/non-respondent/volunteer bias
Executing the exposure
Contamination/withdrawal/compliance/therapeutic bias
Information bias
Observer bias
Interviewer bias
Use of non-validated instruments
Active control bias
Analyzing the data
Post hoc significance bias
Fishing expeditions
Interpreting the analysis
Publishing the results

Controls used in clinical trials

Control groups in clinical trials may be obtained by many different methods. Randomized control groups are the most traditional and accepted and only chance should determine who enters any of the study arms. Non-random control groups may also be used. Subjects in these non-random control groups should have similar characteristics to that of the "treatment arm" and may include historical data obtained on the same patients on no therapy, the same or different therapy. Subjects in the control arm may be assigned to a placebo, an active medication, concurrent use of non-treatment, use a different dose of the same medication or receive usual care.

Dropouts from clinical trials are inevitable. The simplest reasons may be that the subjects declined to participate after enrollment or that the clinical course during the trial required a change in therapy. Whatever the reason for non-compliance or dropout, these subjects should be followed-up, as it is essential to analyze the outcomes of the groups as intent to treat. Inclusion of these data provides a conservative estimate of the differences in treatment.

Studies of therapy

There are many different types of clinical trials and in general they are categorized into categories or phases. Phase I trials are usually to screen the safety of the intervention or drug. These trials can be inclusive of multiple doses of a new medicine or evaluation of an old medicine in a new therapeutic area. These trials usually consist of 10–100 subjects.

Phase II trials clarify and establish the protocol and elucidate the experimental conditions that will allow the most important phase of the trial to give a definitive result. These trials are valuable because they establish protocols and the experimental conditions that will allow the final phase of the trial to give a definitive result. They allow for:

1. the evaluation of a variable related to the clinical pharmacology of a medicine; and
2. development of clinical experience by research personnel under open label conditions prior to initiation of a double-blind trial.

Aims of Phase II trials are to assess how many people should be included in the final phase of testing, the end points of the trial and provides preliminary estimates of effective dose and duration of treatment.

Phase III trials are for comparison to standard therapy or placebo if ethically justifiable. These trials are more commonly randomized and are regarded as the best way to obtain unbiased data.

Blinding

Blind refers to the lack of knowledge of the investigational agent by the patients, investigators, ancillary personnel, data review committees and statisticians. Blinding is used to decrease the biases that may occur during a clinical trial. An open label trial indicates that no blind is used. Examples of open-label trials are:

- pilot trials;
- case studies in life-threatening situations;
- unusual studies in which definitive data may be obtained (e.g., coma patients); and
- clinical trials in which ethical considerations do not permit blinding.

In single-blind clinical trials, either the patient or investigator is unaware of the treatment received. Single-blind trials provide a degree of control when a double blind trial is impossible or impractical and provides a degree of assurance of the data's validity compared with open-label trials. In double-blind trials neither the investigator nor the patient is aware of what treatment the patient is receiving. This allows for strong data interpretation if all other aspects of the trial were properly designed and conducted, the blind remained intact, the protocol was not seriously breached, the power of the trial was adequate and the patients were compliant. Triple-blinds are situations in which anyone that interacts with either the patient of physician is blinded. These studies allow for the strongest interpretation of data if the conditions can be met.

Table 23–5 TYPES OF BLINDS
Open label
Single blind
Double blind
Full double blind
Keeping blind everyone who interacts with the patient
Full triple blind
Keeping blind anyone who interacts with the patients and the investigators

If blinding is to be used, then the study should be designed so that it is very difficult to break the blind. Unblinding may occur based on any of the following:

- adverse reactions;
- lack of efficacy;
- efficacy;
- changes in laboratory values;
- errors in labeling; comments from unblinded study personnel;
- information presented in correspondence or reports; and
- intentionally looking for clues (Table 23–5).

When to stop a clinical trial

The decision to stop a clinical trial has many important ramifications. The ethical dilemmas include the needs of the next eligible patient insomuch that a subject should never be randomized to an established inferior treatment. This must be balanced by the collective needs of society that terminating a trial will still result in the correct policy for the future and the need for sufficient data to change clinical practice for the better.

There are disadvantages of early termination of a trial. If the trial is stooped after recruitment of a small number of subjects, the results may lack credibility. The assumed treatment difference may be the result of chance and a false positive result. The early stopping of trials can result in imprecision and wide confidence intervals for treatment effect. Finally the treatment recommendation that result from stopping a trial early may be unduly enthusiastic.

Statistical stopping guidelines should be determined before the clinical trial begins. A sufficiently small *P* value for treatment difference on a trial's primary endpoint can be a guideline for when it is ethically desirable to stop a trial. It is most acceptable to have a limited number of preplanned interim analyses. Multiple repeated looks at the data can guard against the risk of a false positive result.

BIBLIOGRAPHY

Beresford SA, Weiss NS, Voigt LF, McKnight B: Risk of endometrial cancer in relation to use of estrogen combined with cyclic progestagen therapy in postmenopausal women. Lancet 349(9050): 458-461,1997.

Freidman G: Primer of Epidemiology (5th edn). New York, McGraw-Hill, 2004.

Giacomini MK, Cook DJ: Users' guides to the medical literature: XXIII. Qualitative research in health care A. Are the results of the study valid? Evidence-Based Medicine Working Group. JAMA, 284(3):357–362, 2000.

Hatch EE, Herbst AL, Hoover RN, Noller KL, Adam E, Kaufman RH, Palmer JR, Titus-Ernstoff L, Hyer M, Hartge P, Robboy SJ: Incidence of squamous neoplasia of the cervix and vagina in women exposed prenatally to diethylstilbestrol (United States). Cancer Causes Control 12(9):837–845, 2001.

Lasko TA, Bhagwat JG, Zou KH, Ohno-Machado L: The use of receiver operating characteristic curves in biomedical informatics. J Biomed Inform 38(5):404–415, 2005.

Montori VM, Devereaux PJ, Adhikari NK, Burns KE, Eggert CH, Briel M, Lacchetti C, Leung TW, Darling E, Bryant DM, Bucher HC, Schunemann HJ, Meade MO, Cook DJ, Erwin PJ, Sood A, Sood R, Lo B, Thompson CA, Zhou Q, Mills E, Guyatt GH: Randomized trials stopped early for benefit: a systematic review. JAMA 294(17):2203–2209, 2005.

Rothman KJ, Greenland S: Modern Epidemiology (2nd edn). Philadelphia, Lippincott-Raven, 1998.

Spilker B: Guide to Clinical Trials. Philadelphia, Lippincott, Williams and Wilkins, 1991.

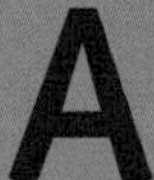

A Staging

Staging of cancer at gynecologic sites

Cervix uteri, corpus uteri, ovary, vagina, vulva, gestational trophoblastic tumors, and fallopian tube

In 1976 the American Joint Committee adopted the classification of the International Federation of Gynecology and Obstetrics (FIGO), which is the format used in the *Annual Report on the Results of Treatment in Carcinoma of the Uterus, Vagina and Ovary*, which is published every three years. This report has used the FIGO classification with periodic modifications since 1937. Numerous institutions throughout the world contribute their statistics for inclusion in this voluntary collaborative presentation of data.

The cervix and corpus uteri were among the first anatomic sites to be classified by the TNM system. This utilizes extent of primary tumor (T), nodal metastasis (N), and distant metastasis (M) status to stage cancers. This system has been approved by the American Joint Committee on Cancer (AJCC) and the International Union Against Cancer (UICC). FIGO has worked closely for many years with the AJCC and UICC in the classification of cancer at gynecologic sites. Staging of malignant tumors is essentially the same, and stages are comparable in the two (FIGO and TNM) systems regarding categories and details.

Anatomy and classification by sites of malignant tumors of the female pelvis

Cervix uteri

1.0 Anatomy

1. *Primary site:* The cervix is the lower third of the uterus. It is roughly cylindrical in shape, projects through the upper anterior vaginal wall, and communicates with the vagina through an orifice called the external os. Cancer of the cervix may originate on the vaginal surface or in the canal.
2. *Nodal stations*: The cervix is drained by preureteral, postureteral, and uterosacral routes into the following first station nodes: parametrial, hypogastric (obturator), external iliac, presacral, and common iliac. Para-aortic nodes are second station and are considered metastases.
3. *Metastatic sites:* The most common sites of distant spread include the aortic and mediastinal nodes, the lungs, and the skeleton.

2.0 Rules for classification

1. *Clinical-diagnostic staging:* Staging of cervical cancer is based on clinical evaluation; therefore, careful clinical examination should be performed in all cases by an experienced examiner, preferably with the patient under anesthesia. The clinical staging must not be changed because of subsequent findings. When there is doubt as to which stage a particular cancer should be allocated, the earlier stage is mandatory. The following examinations are permitted: palpation, inspection, colposcopy, endocervical curettage, hysteroscopy, cystoscopy, proctoscopy, intravenous urography, and X-ray examination of the lungs and skeleton. Suspected bladder or rectal involvement should be confirmed by biopsy and histologic evidence. Findings of optional examinations, such as lymphangiography, arteriography, venography, laparoscopy, computed tomography (CT) scan, and magnetic resonance imaging are valuable for planning therapy; however, because these are not generally available and the interpretation of results varies, the findings of such studies should not be the basis for changing the clinical staging.
2. *Surgical-evaluative staging:* Surgical evaluation is applicable only after laparotomy or laparoscopy and examination of tumor and nodes. Fine needle aspiration (FNA) of scan-detected suspicious lymph nodes may be helpful when planning treatment. Conization or amputation of the cervix is regarded as a clinical examination. Invasive cancers thus identified should be included in the reports (see (4), below).
3. *Postsurgical treatment-pathologic staging:* In cases treated by surgical procedures, the pathologist's findings in the removed tissues can be the basis for extremely accurate statements on the extent of disease. The findings should not be allowed to change the clinical staging but should be recorded in the manner described for the pathologic staging of disease. The TNM nomenclature is appropriate for this purpose. Infrequently, it happens that hysterectomy is carried out in the presence of unsuspected extensive invasive cervical carcinoma. Such cases cannot

be clinically staged or included in therapeutic statistics, but it is desirable that they be reported separately. Only if the rules for clinical staging are strictly observed will it be possible to present comparable results between clinics and by differing modes of therapy.

4. *Retreatment staging:* Complete examination using the procedures cited in (2) above, including a search for distant metastases, is recommended in cases known or suspected to recur. Biopsy and histologic confirmation are particularly desirable when induration and fibrosis from previously treated disease are present.
5. Only if the rules for clinical staging are strictly observed will it be possible to compare results among clinics and by differing modes of therapy.

3.0 Staging classification

FIGO nomenclature, cervix

Stage 0	Carcinoma in situ, cervical intraepithelial neoplasia grade III
Stage I	The carcinoma is strictly confined to the cervix (extension to the corpus would be disregarded)
Stage Ia	Invasive carcinoma that can be diagnosed only by microscopy. All macroscopically visible lesions—even with superficial invasion—are allotted stage Ib carcinomas. Invasion is limited to a measured stromal invasion with a maximal depth of 5 mm and a horizontal extension of no more than 7 mm. Depth of invasion should not be more than 5 mm related to the basis of the epithelium of the original tissue (superficial or glandular). The involvement of vascular spaces—venous or lymphatic—should not change the stage allotment
Stage Ia1	Measured stromal invasion of no more than 3 mm in depth and extension of no more than 7 mm
Stage Ia2	Measured stromal invasion of more than 3 mm and no more than 5 mm with an extension of no more than 7 mm
Stage Ib	Clinically visible lesions limited to the cervix, uteri, or subclinical cancers greater than stage Ia
Stage Ib1	Clinically visible lesions no larger than 4 cm
Stage Ib2	Clinically visible lesions larger than 4 cm
Stage II	The carcinoma extends beyond the cervix but has not extended to the pelvic wall. The carcinoma involves the vagina but does not extend as far as the lower third
Stage IIa	No obvious parametrial involvement
Stage IIb	Obvious parametrial involvement
Stage III	The carcinoma has extended to the pelvic wall. On rectal examination, there is no cancer-free space between the tumor and the pelvic wall. The tumor involves the lower third of the vagina. All cases with hydronephrosis or non-functioning kidney are included, unless they are known to be due to other causes
Stage IIIa	No extension to the pelvic wall
Stage IIIb	Extension to the pelvic wall and/or hydronephrosis or non-functioning kidney
Stage IV	The carcinoma has extended beyond the true pelvis or has clinically involved the mucosa of the bladder or rectum. A bullous edema as such does not permit a case to be allotted to stage IV.
Stage IVa	Spread of the growth to adjacent organs
Stage IVb	Spread to distant organs

Notes about the staging

Stage 0 comprises cases with full-thickness involvement of the epithelium with atypical cells but with no signs of invasion into the stroma. The diagnosis of stages Ia1 and Ia2 should be based on microscopic examination of removed tissue, preferably a cone, which must include the entire lesion. The depth of invasion should not be more than 5 mm, taken from the base of the epithelium—either surface or glandular—from which it originates. The second dimension, the horizontal spread, must not exceed 7 mm. Vascular space involvement, either venous or lymphatic, should not alter the staging but should be specifically recorded because it may affect treatment decisions in the future. Larger lesions should be staged as Ib. As a rule, it is impossible to estimate clinically if a cancer of the cervix has extended to the corpus. Extension to the corpus should, therefore, be disregarded.

A patient with a growth fixed to the pelvic wall by a short and indurated but not nodular parametrium should be allotted to stage IIb. It is impossible at clinical examination to decide whether a smooth and indurated parametrium is truly cancerous or only inflammatory. Therefore, the case should be placed in stage III only if the parametrium is nodular to the pelvic wall or if the growth itself extends to the pelvic wall.

The presence of hydronephrosis or non-functioning kidney resulting from stenosis of the ureter by cancer permits a case to be allotted to stage III, even if according to the other findings the case should be allotted to stages I or II.

The presence of bullous edema, as such, should not permit a case to be allotted to stage IV. Ridges and furrows into the bladder wall should be interpreted as signs of submucous involvement of the bladder if they remain fixed to the growth at palposcopy (i.e., examination from the vagina or the rectum during cystoscopy). Finding malignant cells in cytologic washings from the urinary bladder requires further examination and a biopsy from the wall of the bladder.

Histopathology

Cases should be classified as carcinomas of the cervix if the primary growth is in the cervix. All histologic types must be included. Grading by any of several methods is encouraged but is not a basis for modifying the stage groupings. When surgery is the primary treatment, the histologic findings permit the case to have pathologic staging as described in 2.0 Rules for Classification, 2. Surgical-evaluative staging, p. 594; in this section, the TNM nomenclature is to be used. All tumors are to be microscopically verified.

Histopathologic types

Cervical intraepithelial neoplasia, grade III
Squamous cell carcinoma in situ
Squamous cell carcinoma
  Keratinizing
  Non-keratinizing
Verrucous
Adenocarcinoma in situ
Adenocarcinoma in situ, endocervical type
Endometrioid adenocarcinoma
Clear cell adenocarcinoma
Adenosquamous carcinoma
Adenoid cystic carcinoma
Small cell carcinoma
Undifferentiated carcinoma

Histopathologic grade

G1: Well differentiated
G2: Moderately differentiated
G3: Poorly differentiated
G4: Undifferentiated

Stage grouping, cervix

FIGO/AJCC/UICC	T	N	M
0	Tis	N0	M0
Ia1	T1a1	N0	M0
Ia2	T1a2	N0	M0
Ib1	T1b1	N0	M0
Ib2	T1b2	N0	M0
IIa	T2a	N0	M0
IIb	T2b	N0	M0
IIIa	T3a	N0	M0
IIIb	T1	N1	M0
	T2	N1	M0
	T3	N1	M0
	T3b	any N	M0
IVa	T4	any N	M0
IVb	any T	any N	M1

Corpus

1.0 Anatomy

1.1 *Primary site:* The upper two-thirds of the uterus above the level of the internal cervical os is called the corpus. The fallopian tubes enter at the upper lateral corners of a pear-shaped body. The portion of the muscular organ that is above a line joining the tubouterine orifices is often referred to as the fundus.

1.2 *Nodal stations:* The major lymphatic trunks are the utero-ovarian (infundibulopelvic), parametrial, and presacral, which drain into the hypogastric, external iliac, common iliac, presacral, and para-aortic nodes.

1.3 *Metastatic sites:* The vagina and lung are the common metastatic sites.

2.0 Rules for classification

The FIGO committee on gynecologic oncology agreed on the system for surgical staging for carcinoma of the corpus uteri at the meeting in Rio de Janeiro in October 1988.

3.0 Surgical staging classification

FIGO nomenclature, corpus

FIGO nomenclature, corpus uteri

Stage Ia	G123	Tumor limited to endometrium
Stage Ib	G123	Invasion to less than half the myometrium
Stage Ic	G123	Invasion to more than half the myometrium
Stage IIa	G123	Endocervical glandular involvement only
Stage IIb	G123	Cervical stromal invasion
Stage IIIa	G123	Tumor invades serosa and/or adnexae and/or positive cytologic findings
Stage IIIb	G123	Vaginal metastases
Stage IIIc	G123	Metastases to pelvic and/or para-aortic lymph nodes
Stage IVa	G123	Tumor invasion of bladder and/or bowel mucosa
Stage IVb		Distant metastases, including intra-abdominal and/or inguinal lymph nodes

4.0 Notes about the staging

Histopathology—degree of differentiation

Cases of carcinoma of the corpus should be grouped with regard to the degree of differentiation of the adenocarcinoma as follows:

G1: 5% or less of a non-squamous or non-morular solid growth pattern
G2: 6%–50% of a non-squamous or non-morular solid growth pattern
G3: more than 50% of a non-squamous or non-morular solid growth pattern

Notes on pathologic grading

1. Notable nuclear atypia, inappropriate for the architectural grade, raises the grade of a grade 1 or 2 tumor by 1.
2. In serous and clear cell adenocarcinomas, nuclear grading takes precedence.
3. Adenocarcinomas with squamous differentiation are graded according to the nuclear grade of the glandular component.

Rules related to staging

1. Because corpus cancer is now surgically staged, procedures previously used for determination of stages are no longer applicable, such as the finding of fractional dilatation and curettage (D&C) to differentiate between stages I and II.

2. It is understood that there may be a few patients with corpus cancer who will be treated primarily with radiation therapy. If that is the case, the clinical staging adopted by FIGO in 1971 would still apply, but designation of that staging system would be noted.
3. Ideally, the width of the myometrium should be measured along with the width of tumor invasion.

5.0 Histopathology

The histopathologic types are:

Endometrioid carcinoma
Adenocarcinoma
Adenoacanthoma (adenocarcinoma with squamous metaplasia)
Adenosquamous carcinoma (mixed adenocarcinoma and squamous cell carcinoma)
Mucinous adenocarcinoma
Serous adenocarcinoma
Clear cell adenocarcinoma
Squamous cell adenocarcinoma
Undifferentiated adenocarcinoma

Stage grouping, uterus

FIGO/AJCC/UICC	T	N	M
0	Tis	N0	M0
Ia	T1a	N0	M0
Ib	T1b	N0	M0
Ic	T1c	N0	M0
IIa	T2a	N0	M0
IIb	T2b	N0	M0
IIIa	T3a	N0	M0
IIIb	T3b	N0	M0
IIIc	T1	N1	M0
	T2	N1	M0
	T3a	N1	M0
	T3b	N1	M0
IVa	T4	any N	M0
IVb	any T	any N	M1

Ovary

1.0 Anatomy

1.1 *Primary site:* Ovaries are a pair of solid bodies, flattened ovoids that are 2–4 cm in diameter; they are connected by a peritoneal fold to the broad ligament and by the infundibulopelvic ligament to the lateral wall of the pelvis.

1.2 *Nodal stations:* The lymphatic drainage occurs by the utero-ovarian and round ligament trunks and an external iliac accessory route into the following regional nodes: external iliac, common iliac, hypogastric, lateral sacral, and para-aortic nodes, and, rarely, to the inguinal nodes.

1.3 *Metastatic sites:* The peritoneum including the omentum and pelvic and abdominal viscera are common sites for seeding. Diaphragmatic involvement and liver metastases are common. Pulmonary and pleural involvement is often seen.

2.0 Rules for classification

Ovarian cancer is surgically staged. Operative findings prior to tumor debulking determine the stage, which may be modified by histopathologic as well as clinical or radiologic evaluation. Laparotomy and resection of the ovarian mass, as well as hysterectomy, form the basis for staging. Biopsies of all suspicious sites such as omentum, mesentery, liver, diaphragm, pelvic, and para-aortic nodes are required. The final histologic findings after surgery (and cytologic ones when available) should be considered in the staging. Clinical studies, if carcinoma of the ovary is diagnosed, include routine radiology of the chest. CT scanning may be helpful in initial staging and follow-up of tumors.

1. *Clinical-diagnostic staging:* Although clinical studies similar to those for other sites may be used, the establishment of a diagnosis most often requires a laparotomy, which is most widely accepted in surgical-pathologic staging. Clinical studies, if carcinoma of the ovary is diagnosed, include routine radiography of the chest and abdomen, liver studies, and hemograms.
2. *Surgical-evaluative staging:* Laparotomy and biopsy of all suspected sites of involvement provide the basis for this type of staging; this staging is often identical to postsurgical staging. Histologic and cytologic data are required.
3. *Postsurgical treatment-pathologic staging:* This treatment should include laparotomy and resection of ovarian masses as well as a hysterectomy. Biopsies of all suspicious sites, such as the omentum, mesentery, liver, diaphragm, and pelvic and para-aortic nodes, are required. Pleural effusions should be documented by cytology.
4. *Retreatment staging:* Second-look laparotomies and laparoscopy are being evaluated because of the limitation of routine pelvic and abdominal examinations in detecting early recurrence. Other optional and investigative procedures include ultrasound and CT scanning. All suspected recurrences need biopsy confirmation.

3.0 Staging classification

Staging is based mainly on findings seen at surgical exploration. Clinical evaluation and imaging studies should be done when appropriate. These findings may affect final staging. The histology is to be considered in the staging, as is cytology as far as effusions are concerned. It is desirable that a biopsy be taken from suspicious areas outside of the pelvis.

FIGO nomenclature, ovaries

Stage I	Growth limited to the ovaries
Stage Ia	Growth limited to one ovary; no ascites present containing malignant cells. No tumor on the external surface; capsule intact

Stage Ib	Growth limited to both ovaries; no ascites present containing malignant cells; no tumor on the external surfaces; capsules intact
Stage Ic*	Tumor stage Ia or Ib but with tumor on the surface of one or both ovaries; or with capsule ruptured; or with ascites present containing malignant cells or with positive peritoneal washings
Stage II	Growth involving one or both ovaries with pelvic extension
Stage IIa	Extension and/or metastases to the uterus and/or tubes
Stage IIb	Extension to other pelvic tissues
Stage IIc*	Tumor stage IIa or IIb but with tumor on the surface of one or both ovaries; or with capsule(s) ruptured; or with ascites present containing malignant cells or with positive peritoneal washings
Stage III	Tumor involving one or both ovaries with peritoneal implants outside the pelvis and/or positive retroperitoneal or inguinal nodes; superficial liver metastases equal to stage III; tumor limited to the true pelvis but with histologically proven malignant extension to the small bowel or omentum
Stage IIIa	Tumor grossly limited to the true pelvis with negative nodes but with histologically confirmed microscopic seeding of the abdominal peritoneal surfaces
Stage IIIb	Tumor of one or both ovaries with histologically confirmed implants of abdominal peritoneal surfaces, none exceeding 2 cm in diameter; nodes negative
Stage IIIc	Abdominal implants > 2 cm in diameter and/or positive retroperitoneal or inguinal nodes
Stage IV	Growth involving one or both ovaries with distant metastases. If pleural effusion is present, there must be positive cytology to allot a case to stage IV. Parenchymal liver metastasis equals stage IV

4.0 Histopathology

The task force of the AJC endorses the histologic typing of ovarian tumors, as presented in the WHO publication no. 9, 1973, and recommends that all ovarian epithelial tumors be subdivided according to a simplified version. The types recommended are as follows:

Serous tumors
Benign serous cystadenomas
Of borderline malignancy: Serous cystadenomas with proliferating activity of the epithelial cells and nuclear abnormalities but with no infiltrative destructive growth (carcinomas of low potential malignancy)
Serous cystadenocarcinomas
Mucinous tumors
Benign mucinous cystadenomas of borderline malignancy: Mucinous cystadenomas with proliferating activity of the epithelial cells and nuclear abnormalities but with no infiltrative destructive growth (carcinomas of low potential malignancy)
Mucinous cystadenocarcinomas
Endometrioid tumors
Benign endometrioid cystadenomas
Endometrioid tumors with proliferating activity of the epithelial cells and nuclear abnormalities but with no infiltrative destructive growth (carcinomas of low potential malignancy)
Endometrioid adenocarcinomas
Clear cell tumors
Benign clear cell tumors
Clear cell tumors with proliferating activity of the epithelial cells and nuclear abnormalities but with no infiltrative destructive growth (low potential malignancy)
Clear cell cystadenocarcinomas
Brenner
Benign Brenner
Borderline malignancy
Malignant
Transitional cell
Undifferentiated carcinomas
A malignant tumor of epithelial structure that is too poorly differentiated to be placed in any other group
Mixed epithelial tumors

These tumors consist of two or more of the five major cell types of common epithelial tumors (types should be specified).

Cases with intraperitoneal carcinoma in which the ovaries appear to be incidentally involved and not the primary origin should be labeled as extra-ovarian peritoneal carcinoma.

Stage grouping, ovaries

FIGO/AJCC/UICC	T	N	M
Ia	T1a	N0	M0
Ib	T1b	N0	M0
Ic	T1c	N0	M0
IIa	T2a	N0	M0
IIb	T2b	N0	M0
IIc	T2c	N0	
IIIa	T3a	N0	M0
IIIb	T3b	N0	M0
IIIc	T3c	N1	M0
	any T	N1	M0
IV	any T	any N	M1

Histopathologic grade (G)

Borderline
Well differentiated
Moderately differentiated
Poorly differentiated or undifferentiated

*To evaluate the impact on prognosis of the different criteria for allotting cases to stages Ic or IIc, it would be useful to know whether rupture of the capsule was spontaneous or caused by the surgeon and if the source of malignant cells was peritoneal washings or ascites.

Vagina

Classification by site

Cases should be classified as carcinoma of the vagina when the primary site of the growth is in the vagina. Tumors present in the vagina as secondary growths from genital or extragenital sites should be excluded. A growth that has extended to the portio and reached the area of the external os should always be allotted to carcinoma of the cervix. A growth limited to the urethra should be classified as carcinoma of the urethra. There should be histologic verification of the disease. The vagina is drained by lymphatics, toward the pelvic nodes in its upper two-thirds and toward the inguinal nodes in the lower third. The rules for staging are similar to those for carcinoma of the cervix.

1.0 Staging classification

FIGO nomenclature, vagina

Stage 0	Carcinoma in situ and intraepithelial carcinoma are present
Stage I	The carcinoma is limited to the vaginal wall
Stage II	The carcinoma has involved the subvaginal tissue but has not extended to the pelvic wall
Stage III	The carcinoma has extended to the pelvic wall
Stage IV	The carcinoma has extended beyond the true pelvis or has involved the mucosa of the bladder or rectum; bullous edema as such does not permit a case to be allotted to stage IV
Stage IVa	The growth spreads to adjacent organs and/or direct extension beyond the true pelvis
Stage IVb	The growth spreads to distant organs

Stage grouping, vagina

FIGO/AJCC/UICC	T	N	M
0	Tis	N0	M0
I	T1	N0	M0
II	T2	N0	M0
III	T1	N1	M0
	T2	N1	M0
	T3	N0	M0
	T3	N1	M0
IVa	T1	N2	M0
	T2	N2	M0
	T3	N2	M0
	T4	any N	M0
IVb	any T	any N	M1

Cases should be classified as carcinoma of the vulva when the primary site of growth is in the vulva. Tumors present in the vulva as secondary growths from a genital or extragenital site should be excluded. Malignant melanoma should be reported separately. A carcinoma of the vulva that extends into the vagina should be considered as a carcinoma of the vulva. There should be histologic confirmation of the cancer. The femoral, inguinal, external iliac, and hypogastric nodes are the sites of regional spread. Involvement of pelvic lymph nodes (e.g., external, internal, and common iliac) is considered as distant metastasis.

1.0 Staging classification

Definitions of the clinical stages in carcinoma of the vulva follow:

FIGO nomenclature, vulva

Stage 0	Carcinoma in situ, intraepithelial carcinoma
Stage I	Lesions 2 cm or less in size confined to the vulva or perineum with no nodal metastasis
Stage Ia	Lesions 2 cm or less in size confined to the vulva or perineum and with stromal invasion no greater than 1 mm[†]; no nodal metastasis
Stage Ib	Lesions 2 cm or less in size confined to the vulva or perineum with stromal invasion greater than 1 mm[†]; no nodal metastasis
Stage II	Tumor confined to the vulva and/or perineum; more than 2 cm in greatest dimension; no nodal metastasis
Stage III	Tumor of any size with adjacent spread to the lower urethra and/or the vagina, or the anus and/or unilateral regional lymph node metastasis
Stage IVa	Tumor invades any of the following: upper urethra, bladder mucosa, rectal mucosa, pelvic bone, and/or bilateral regional nodal metastasis
Stage IVb	Any distant metastasis, including pelvic lymph nodes

Stage grouping, vulva

T	Primary tumor
Tis	Preinvasive carcinoma (carcinoma in situ)
T1	Tumor confined to the vulva and/or perineum; 2 cm or less in greatest dimension
T1a	and with stromal invasion no greater than 1 mm
T1b	and with stromal invasion greater than 1 mm
T2	Tumor confined to the vulva and/or perineum; more than 2 cm in greatest dimension
T3	Tumor of any size with adjacent spread to the urethra and/or vagina and/or the anus
T4	Tumor of any size infiltrating the bladder mucosa and/or the rectal mucosa, including the upper part of the urethral mucosa and/or fixed to the bone
N	Regional lymph nodes
N0	No lymph node metastasis
N1	Unilateral regional lymph node metastasis
N2	Bilateral regional lymph node metastasis
M	Distant metastasis; no clinical metastasis (M0)

[†]The depth of invasion is defined as the measurement of the tumor from the epithelial-stromal junction of the adjacent most superficial dermal papilla to the deepest point of invasion.

M0 No distant metastasis
M1 Distant metastasis (including pelvic lymph node metastasis)

Stage grouping, vulva

FIGO/AJCC/UICC	T	N	M
0	Tis	N0	M0
Ia	T1a	N0	M0
Ib	T1b	N0	M0
II	T2	N0	M0
III	T1	N1	M0
	T2	N1	M0
	T3	N0	M0
	T3	N1	M0
IVa	T1	N2	M0
	T2	N2	M0
	T3	N2	M0
	T4	any N	M0
IVb	any T	any N	M1

Gestational trophoblastic tumors (GTTs)

In 1991, FIGO added non-surgical-pathologic prognostic risk factors to the classic anatomic staging system. These include β-human chorionic gonadotropin (hCG) levels of $>10^5$ and the duration of an antecedent pregnancy for longer than 6 months.

Because gestational trophoblastic tumors have a very high cure rate in almost all patients, the ultimate goal of staging is to differentiate patients who are likely to respond to less intensive chemotherapeutic protocols from those who require more intensive chemotherapy in order to achieve remission.

Staging should be based on history, clinical examination, and appropriate laboratory and radiologic studies. Because β-hCG titers accurately reflect clinical disease, histologic verification is not required for a diagnosis, although it may aid in therapy.

FIGO nomenclature, gestational trophoblastic tumors

Stage I	Disease confined to the uterus
Stage Ia	Disease confined to the uterus with no risk factors
Stage Ib	Disease confined to the uterus with one risk factor
Stage Ic	Disease confined to the uterus with two risk factors
Stage II	GTT extends outside of the uterus but is limited to the genital structures (adnexa, vagina, broad ligament)
Stage IIa	GTT involving genital structures without risk factors
Stage IIb	GTT extends outside of the uterus but is limited to genital structures with one risk factor
Stage IIc	GTT extends outside of the uterus but is limited to the genital structures with two risk factors
Stage III	GTT extends to the lungs, with or without known genital tract involvement
Stage IIIa	GTT extends to the lungs, with or without genital tract involvement and with no risk factors
Stage IIIb	GTT extends to the lungs, with or without genital tract involvement and with one risk factor
Stage IIIc	GTT extends to the lungs, with or without genital tract involvement and with two risk factors
Stage IV	All other metastatic sites
Stage IVa	All other metastatic sites, without risk factors
Stage IVb	All other metastatic sites, with one risk factor
Stage IVc	All other metastatic sites, with two risk factors

1. hCG > 100,000 U/ml
2. Duration of disease > 6 months from termination of the antecedent pregnancy

The following factors should be considered and noted in reporting:

1. Prior chemotherapy for known GTT
2. Placental site tumors should be reported separately
3. Histologic verification of disease is not required

Fallopian tube

The fallopian tube extends from the posterior superior aspect of the uterine fundus laterally and anteriorly to the ovary. Its length is approximately 10 cm. The lateral end opens to the peritoneal cavity. Carcinoma of the oviduct can metastasize to the regional lymph nodes, including the para-aortic nodes. Direct extension to surrounding organs, as well as intraperitoneal seeding, often occurs. Peritoneal implants may occur with an intact tube.

1. Carcinoma in situ of the fallopian tube is a defined entity; therefore, it is included in the staging under stage 0.
2. Because the fallopian tube is a hollow viscus and because extension into the submucosa or muscularis to and beyond the serosa can be defined (a concept similar to that of Dukes' classification for colon cancer), these are taken into consideration in stage Ia, Ib, and Ic in addition to laterality, as well as the presence or absence of ascites. As in ovarian carcinoma, peritoneal washings positive for malignant cells or malignant ascites are placed in stage Ic.
3. In stage III, the classification of the tumor is based on the size of the findings at the time of entry into the abdominal cavity and does *not* depend on the residual at the end of the debulking. In addition, surface involvement of the liver is in stage III, as is inguinal node metastasis. As in ovarian cancer, pleural effusion must have malignant cells to be called stage IV.

Laparotomy and resection of tubal masses, as well as hysterectomy, form the basis for staging. Biopsies of all suspicious sites (e.g., the omentum, mesentery, liver, diaphragm, and pelvic and para-aortic nodes) are required. The final histologic findings after surgery (and cytologic ones when available) are to be considered in the staging.

Clinical studies, if carcinoma of the tube is diagnosed, include routine radiography of chest. CT scanning may be helpful in the initial staging and follow-up of tumors.

Staging for the fallopian tube is by the surgical pathologic system. Operative findings before tumor debulking may be modified by histopathologic as well as clinical or radiologic evaluation.

FIGO nomenclature, fallopian tube carcinoma

Stage 0	Carcinoma in situ (limited to tubal mucosa)
Stage I	Growth limited to the fallopian tubes
Stage Ia	Growth limited to one tube, with extension into the submucosa and/or muscularis but not penetrating the serosal surface; no ascites
Stage Ib	Growth limited to both tubes, with extension into the submucosa and/or muscularis but not penetrating the serosal surface; no ascites
Stage Ic	Tumor either stage Ia or Ib, but with tumor extension through or onto the tubal serosa or with ascites present containing malignant cells or with positive peritoneal washings
Stage II	Growth involving one or both fallopian tubes with pelvic extension
Stage IIa	Extension and/or metastasis to the uterus and/or ovaries
Stage IIb	Extension to other pelvic tissues
Stage IIc	Tumor at either stage IIa or IIb and with ascites present containing malignant cells or with positive peritoneal washings
Stage III	Tumor involving one or both fallopian tubes, with peritoneal implants outside the pelvis and/or positive retroperitoneal or inguinal nodes; superficial liver metastasis equal to stage III; tumor apparently limited to the true pelvis but with histologically proven malignant extension to the small bowel or omentum
Stage IIIa	Tumor grossly limited to the true pelvis with negative nodes but with histologically confirmed microscopic seeding of abdominal peritoneal surfaces
Stage IIIb	Tumor involving one or both tubes with histologically confirmed implants of abdominal peritoneal surfaces, none exceeding 2 cm in diameter; lymph nodes negative
Stage IIIc	Abdominal implants greater than 2 cm in diameter and/or positive retroperitoneal or inguinal nodes
Stage IV	Growth involving one or both fallopian tubes with distant metastases; if pleural effusion is present, there must be positive cytology to be stage IV; parenchymal liver metastases equal to stage IV

B Modified from Common Terminology Criteria for Adverse Events (CTCAE)

(version 3.0)

U.S. Department of Health and Human Services

National Institutes of Health, National Cancer Institute, June 10, 2003

Full text is available by contacting:
Cancer Therapy Evaluation Program, Common Terminology Criteria for Adverse Events
Version 3.0, DCTD, NCI, NIH, DHHS
March 31, 2003 (*http://ctep.cancer.gov*), publish date: May 22, 2003

Quick reference

The NCI Common Terminology Criteria for Adverse Events v3.0 is a descriptive terminology which can be utilized for Adverse Event (AE) reporting. A grading (severity) scale is provided for each AE term.

Components and organization

Adverse event

An **adverse event** (AE) is any unfavorable and unintended sign (including an abnormal laboratory finding), symptom, or disease temporally associated with the use of a medical treatment or procedure that may or may *not* be considered related to the medical treatment or procedure. An AE is a term that is a unique representation of a specific event used for medical documentation and scientific analyses. Each AE term is mapped to a MedDRA term and code. AEs are listed alphabetically within categories.

Category

A **category** is a broad classification of AEs based on anatomy and/or pathophysiology. Within each category, AEs are listed accompanied by their descriptions of severity (grade).

Grades

Grades refer to the severity of the AE. The CTCAE v3.0 displays Grades 1 through 5 with unique clinical descriptions of severity for each AE based on these general guidelines:

Grade 1 Mid AE
Grade 2 Moderate AE
Grade 3 Severe AE
Grade 4 Life-threatening or disabling AE
Grade 5 Death related to AE

AUDITORY/EAR						
		Grade				
Adverse event	**Short name**	**1**	**2**	**3**	**4**	**5**
Hearing, patients with/without baseline audiogram and enrolled in a monitoring program	Hearing (monitoring program)	Threshold shift or loss of 15–25 dB relative to baseline, averaged at 2 or more contiguous test frequencies in at least one ear; or subjective change in the absence of a Grade 1 threshold shift	Threshold shift or loss of >25–90 dB, averaged at 2 contiguous test frequencies in at least one ear	*Adult only:* Threshold shift of >25–90 dB, averaged at 3 contiguous test frequencies in at least one ear *Pediatric:* Hearing loss (HL) sufficient to indicate therapeutic intervention, including hearing aids (e.g., ≥20 dB bilateral HL in the speech frequencies; ≥30 dB unilateral HL; and requiring additional speech-language-related services)	*Adult only:* Profound bilateral (>90 dB) *Pediatric:* Audiologic indication for cochlear implant and requiring additional speech-language-related services	—
Hearing, patients without baseline audiogram and not enrolled in a monitoring program	Hearing (without monitoring program)	—	Hearing loss not requiring hearing aid or intervention (i.e., not interfering with ADL)	Hearing loss requiring hearing aid or intervention (i.e., interfering with ADL)	Profound bilateral hearing loss (>90 dB)	—
Otitis, external ear, non-infectious	Otitis, external	External otitis with erythema or dry desquamation	External otitis with moist desquamation, edema, enhanced cerumen or discharge; tympanis membrane perforation; tympanostomy	External otitis with mastoiditis; stenosis or osteomyelitis	Necrosis of soft tissue or bone	Death
Otitis, middle ear, non-infectious	Otitis, middle	Serous otitis	Serous otitis, medical intervention indicated	Otitis with discharge; mastoiditis	Necrosis of the canal soft tissue or bone	Death
Tinnitus	Tinnitus	—	Tinnitus not interfering with ADL	Tinnitus interfering with ADL	Disabling	—

BLOOD/BONE MARROW						
		Grade				
Adverse event	Short name	1	2	3	4	5
Bone marrow cellularity	Bone marrow cellularity	Mildly hypocellular or ≤25% reduction from normal cellularity for age	Moderately hypocellular or 25–50% reduction from normal cellularity for age	Severely hypocellular or 50–75% reduction cellularity from normal for age	—	Death
CD4 count	CD4 count	<LLN–500/mm^3 <LLN–0.5 × 10	<500–200/mm^3 <0.5–0.2 × 10^9/L	<200–50/mm^3 <0.2 × 0.05–10^9/L	<50/mm^3 <0.05 × 10^9/L	Death
Haptoglobin	Haptoglobin	<LLN	—	Absent	—	Death
Hemoglobin	Hemoglobin	<LLN–10.0 g/dL <LLN–6.2 mmol/L <LLN–100 g/L	<10.0–8.0 g/dL <6.2–4.9 mmol/L <100–80g/L	<8.0–6.5 g/dL <4.9–4.0 mmol/L <80–65 g/L	<6.5 g/dL <4.0 mmol/L <65 g/L	Death
Hemolysis (e.g., immune hemolytic anemia, drug-related hemolysis)	Hemolysis	Laboratory evidence of hemolysis only, e.g., direct antiglobulin test (DAT, Coombs), schistocytes[1]	Evidence of red cell destruction and ≥2 g decrease in hemoglobin, no transfusion[1]	Transfusion or medical intervention (e.g., steroids) indicated	Catastrophic consequences of hemolysis (e.g., renal failure, hypotension, bronchospasm, emergency splenectomy)	Death
Iron overload	Iron overload	—	Asymptomatic iron overload, intervention not indicated	Iron overload, intervention indicated	Organ impairment (e.g., endocrinopathy, cardiopathy)	Death
Leukocytes (total WBC)	Leukocytes	<LLN–3000/mm^3 <LLN–3.0 × 10^9/L	<3000–2000/mm^3 <3.0–2.0 × 10^9/L	<2000–1000/mm^3 <2.0–1.0 × 10^9/L	<1000/mm^3 <1.0 × 10^9/L	Death
Lymphopenia	Lymphopenia	<LLN–800/mm^3 <LLN × 0.8–10^9/L	<800–500/mm^3 <0.8–0.5 × 10^9/L	<500–200/mm^3 <0.5–0.2 × 10^9/L	<200/mm^3 <0.2 × 10^9/L	Death
Myelodysplasia	Myelodysplasia	—	—	Abnormal marrow cytogenetics (marrow blasts <5%)	RAEB or RAEB-T (marrow blasts >5%)	Death
Neutrophils/ granulocytes (ANC/AGC)	Neutrophils	<LLN–1500/mm^3 <LLN–1.5 × 10^9/L	<1500–1000/mm^3 <1.5–1.0 × 10^9/L	<1000–500/mm^3 <1.0–0.5 × 10^9/L	<500/mm^3 <0.5 × 10^9/L	Death
Platelets	Platelets	<LLN–75,000/mm^3 <LLN–75.0 × 10^9/L	<75,000–50,000/mm^3 <50.0–25.0 × 10^9/L	<50,000–25,000/mm^3 <50.0–25.0 × 10^9/L	<25,000/mm^3 <25.0 × 10^9/L	Death

CARDIAC ARRHYTHMIA

Adverse event	Short name	Grade 1	Grade 2	Grade 3	Grade 4	Grade 5
Conduction abnormality/ atrioventricular heart block	Conduction abnormality	Asymptomatic, intervention not indicated	Non-urgent medical intervention indicated	Incompletely controlled medically or controlled with device (e.g., pacemaker)	Life-threatening (e.g., arrhythmia associated with CHF, hypotension, syncope, shock)	Death
Palpitations	Palpitations[2]	Present	Present with associated symptoms (e.g., lightheadedness, shortness of breath)	—	—	—
Prolonged QTc interval	Prolonged QTc	QTc >0.45–0.47 second	QTc >0.47–0.50 second; ≥0.06 second above baseline	QTc >0.50 second	QTc >0.50 second; life-threatening signs or symptoms (e.g., arhythmia, CHF, hypotension, shock syncope); Torsade de pointes	Death
Supraventricular and nodal arrhythmia	Supraventricular arrhythmia	Asymptomatic, intervention not indicated	Non-urgent medical intervention indicated	Symptomatic and incompletely controlled medically or controlled with device (e.g., pacemaker)	Life-threatening consequences	Death
Vasovagal episode	Vasovagal episode	—	Present without loss of consciousness	Present with loss of consciousness	Life-threatening (e.g., arrhythmia associated with CHF, hypotension, syncope, shock)	Death
Ventricular arrhythmia	Ventricular arrhythmia	Asymptomatic, no intervention indicated	Non-urgent medical intervention indicated	Symptomatic and incompletely controlled medically or controlled with device (e.g., defibrillator)	Life-threatening (e.g., arrhythmia associated with CHF, hypotension, syncope, shock)	Death
Cardiac arrhythmia, other (specify)	Cardiac arrhythmia, other (specify)	Mild	Moderate	Severe	Life-threatening; disabling	Death

CARDIAC GENERAL

Adverse event	Short name	Grade 1	Grade 2	Grade 3	Grade 4	Grade 5
Cardiac ischemia/ infarction	Cardiac ischemia/ infarction	Asymptomatic arterial narrowing without ischemia	Asymptomatic and testing suggesting ischemia; stable angina	Symptomatic and testing consistent with ischemia; unstable angina; intervention indicated	Acute myocardial infarction	Death
Cardiac troponin I (cTnI)	cTnI	—	—	Levels consistent with unstable angina as defined by the manufacturer	Levels consistent with myocardial infarction as defined by the manufacturer	Death
Cardiac troponin T (cTnT)	cTnT	0.03–<0.05 ng/mL	0.05–<0.1 ng/mL	0.1–<0.2 ng/mL	0.2 ng/mL	Death
Hypertension	Hypertension	Asymptomatic, transient (<24 hrs) increase by >20 mmHg (diastolic) or to >150/100 if previously WNL; intervention not indicated *Pediatric:* Asymptomatic, transient (<24 hrs) BP increase >ULN; intervention not indicated	Recurrent or persistent (>24 hrs) or symptomatic increase by >20 mmHg (diastolic) or to >150/100 if previously WNL; monotherapy may be indicated *Pediatric:* Recurrent or persistent (>24 hrs) BP >ULN; monotherapy may be indicated	Requiring more than one drug or more intensive therapy than previously *Pediatric:* Same as adult	Life-threatening consequences (e.g., hypertensive crisis) *Pediatric:* Same as adult	Death
Hypotension	Hypotension	Changes, intervention not indicated	Brief (<24 hrs) fluid replacement or other therapy; no physiologic consequences	Sustained (≥24 hrs) therapy, resolves without persisting physiologic consequences	Shock (e.g., academia; impairment of vital organ function)	Death
Left ventricular diastolic dysfunction	Left ventricular diastolic dysfunction	Asymptomatic diagnostic finding; intervention not indicated	Asymptomatic, intervention indicated	Symptomatic CHF responsive to intervention	Refractory CHF, poorly controlled; intervention such as ventricular assist device or heart transplant indicated	Death
Left ventricular systolic dysfunction	Left ventricular systolic dysfunction	Asymptomatic, resting ejection fraction (EF) <60 –50%; shortening fraction (SF) <30 –24%	Asymptomatic, resting EF <50–40%; SF <24–15%	Symptomatic CHF responsive to intervention; EF <40–20% SF <15%	Refractory CHF or poorly controlled; EF <20%; intervention such as ventricular assist device, ventricular reduction surgery, or heart transplant indicated	Death

Continued

CARDIAC GENERAL—CONT'D

Adverse event	Short name	Grade 1	Grade 2	Grade 3	Grade 4	Grade 5
Myocarditis	Myocarditis	—	—	CHF responsive to intervention	Severe or refractory CHF	Death
Pericardial effusion, non-malignant	Pericardial effusion	Asymptomatic effusion	—	Effusion with physiologic consequences	Life-threatening consequences (e.g., tamponade); emergency intervention indicated	Death
Pericarditis	Pericarditis	Asymptomatic, ECG or physical exam (rub) changes consistent with pericarditis	Symptomatic pericarditis (e.g., chest pain)	Pericarditis with physiologic consequences (e.g., pericardial constriction)	Life-threatening consequences; emergency intervention indicated	Death
Pulmonary hypertension	Pulmonary hypertension	Asymptomatic without therapy	Asymptomatic, therapy indicated	Symptomatic hypertension, responsive to therapy	Symptomatic hypertension, poorly controlled	Death
Restrictive cardiomyopathy	Restrictive cardiomyopathy	Asymptomatic, therapy not indicated	Asymptomatic, therapy indicated	Symptomatic CHF responsive to intervention	Refractory CHF, poorly controlled; intervention such as ventricular assist device, or heart transplant indicated	Death
Right ventricular dysfunction (cor pulmonale)	Right ventricular dysfunction	Asymptomatic without therapy	Asymptomatic, therapy indicated	Symptomatic cor pulmonale, responsive to intervention	Symptomatic cor pulmonale poorly controlled; intervention such as ventricular assist device, or heart transplant indicated	Death
Valvular heart disease	Valvular heart disease	Asymptomatic valvular thickening with or without mild valvular regurgitation or stenosis; treatment other than endocarditis prophylaxis not indicated	Asymptomatic; moderate regurgitation or stenosis by imaging	Symptomatic; severe regurgitation or stenosis; symptoms controlled with medical therapy	Life-threatening; disabling; intervention (e.g., valve replacement, valvuloplasty) indicated	Death

COAGULATION

Adverse event	Short name	Grade 1	Grade 2	Grade 3	Grade 4	Grade 5
Disseminated intravascular coagulation	DIC	—	Laboratory findings with *no* bleeding	Laboratory findings *and* bleeding	Laboratory findings, life-threatening or disabling consequences (e.g., CNS hemorrhage, organ damage, or hemodynamically significant blood loss)	Death
Fibrinogen	Fibrinogen	<1.0–0.75 × LLN or <25% decrease from baseline	<0.75–0.5 × LLN or 25–<50% decrease from baseline	<0.5–0.25 × LLN or 50–<75% decrease from baseline	<0.25 × LLN or 75% decrease from baseline or absolute value <50 mg/dL	Death
International normalized ratio of prothrombin time	INR	>1–1.5 × ULN	>1.5–2 × ULN	>2 × ULN	—	—
Partial thromboplastin time	PTT	>1–1.5 × ULN	>1.5–2 × ULN	>2 × ULN	—	—
Thrombotic microangiopathy (e.g., thrombotic thrombocytopenic purpura [TTP] or hemolytic uremic syndrome [HUS])	Thrombotic microangiopathy	Evidence of RBC destruction (schistocytosis) without clinical consequences	—	Laboratory findings present with clinical consequences (e.g., renal insufficiency, petechiae)	Laboratory findings and life-threatening or disabling consequences, (e.g., CNS hemorrhage/ bleeding or thrombosis/embolism or renal failure)	Death

CONSTITUTIONAL SYMPTOMS

		Grade				
Adverse event	**Short name**	**1**	**2**	**3**	**4**	**5**
Fatigue (lethargy, malaise, asthenia)	Fatigue	Mild fatigue over baseline	Moderate or causing difficulty performing some ADL	Severe fatigue interfering with ADL	Disabling	—
Fever (in the absence of neutropenia, where neutropenia is defined as ANC <1.0 × 10^9/L)	Fever	38.0–39.0°C (100.4–102.2°F)	>39.0–40.0°C (102.3–104.0°F)	>40.0°C (>104.0) for ≤24 hrs	>40.0°C (>104.0) for ≤24 hrs	Death
Hypothermia	Hypothermia	–	35–>32°C 95–>89.6°F	32–>28°C 89.6–>82.4°F	≤28°C 82.4°F or life-threatening consequences (e.g., coma, hypotension, pulmonary edema, academia, ventricular fibrillation)	Death
Insomnia	Insomnia	Occasional difficulty sleeping, not interfering with function	Difficulty sleeping, interfering with function but not interfering with ADL	Frequent difficulty sleeping, interfering with ADL	Disabling	—
Obesity[3]	Obesity	—	BMI* 25–29.9 kg/m^2	BMI 30–39.9 kg/m^2	BMI >40 kg/m^2	—
Odor (patient odor)	Patient odor	Mild odor	Pronounced odor	—	—	—
Rigors/chills	Rigors/chills	Mild	Moderate, narcotics indicated	Severe or prolonged, not responsive to narcotics	—	—
Sweating (diaphoresis)	Sweating	Mild and occasional	Frequent or drenching	—	—	—
Weight gain	Weight gain	5–<10% of baseline	10–<20% of baseline	≥20% of baseline	—	—
Weight loss	Weight loss	5 to <10% from baseline; intervention not indicated	10–<20% from baseline; nutritional support indicated	≥20% from baseline; tube feeding or TPN indicated	—	—
Death						
Death not associated with CTCAE term	Death not associated with CTCAE term	—	—	—	—	Death

DENTAL

Adverse event	Short name	Grade 1	Grade 2	Grade 3	Grade 4	Grade 5
Dentures or prosthesis	Dentures	Minimal discomfort, no restriction in activities	Discomfort preventing use in some activities (e.g., eating) but not others (e.g., speaking)	Unable to use dentures or prosthesis at any time	—	—
Periodontal disease	Periodontal	Gingival recession or gingivitis; limited bleeding on probing; mild local bone loss	Moderate gingival recession or gingivitis; multiple sites of bleeding on probing; moderate bone loss	Spontaneous bleeding; severe bone loss with or without tooth loss; osteonecrosis of maxilla or mandible	—	—
Teeth	Teeth	Surface stains; dental caries; restorable, without extractions	Less than full mouth extractions; tooth fracture or crown amputation or repair indicated	Full mouth extractions indicated	—	—
Teeth development	Teeth development	Hypoplasia of tooth or enamel not interfering with function	Functional impairment correctable with oral surgery	Maldevelopment with functional impairment not surgically correctable	—	—

DERMATOLOGY/SKIN						
		Grade				
Adverse event	**Short name**	**1**	**2**	**3**	**4**	**5**
Atrophy, skin	Atrophy, skin	Detectable	Marked	—	—	—
Atrophy, subcutaneous fat	Atrophy, subcutaneous fat	Detectable	Marked	—	—	—
Bruising, in absence of Grade 3 or 4 thrombocy-topenia	Bruising	Localized or in a dependent area	Generalized	—	—	—
Burn	Burn	Minimal symptoms; intervention not indicated	Medical intervention; minimal debridement indicated	Moderate to major debridement or reconstruction indicated	Life-threatening consequences	Death
Cheilitis	Cheilitis	Asymptomatic	Symptomatic, not interfering with ADL	Symptomatic, interfering with ADL	—	—
Dry skin	Dry skin	Asymptomatic	Symptomatic, not interfering with ADL	Interfering with ADL	—	—
Flushing	Flushing	Asymptomatic	Symptomatic	—	—	—
Hair loss/ alopecia (scalp or body)	Alopecia	Thinning or patchy	Complete	—	—	—
Hyperpigmen-tation	Hyperpigmen-tation	Slight or localized	Marked or generalized	—	—	—
Hypopigmen-tation	Hypopigmen-tation	Slight or localized	Marked or generalized	—	—	—
Induration/ fibrosis (skin and subcutaneous tissue)	Induration	Increased density on palpation	Moderate impairment of function not interfering with ADL; marked increase in density and firmness on palpation with or without minimal retraction	Dysfunction interfering with ADL; very marked density, retraction or fixation	—	—
Injection site reaction/ extravasation changes	Injection site reaction	Pain; itching; erythema	Pain or swelling, with inflammation or phlebitis	Ulceration or necrosis that is severe; operative intervention indicated	—	—
Nail changes	Nail changes	Discoloration; ridging (koilonychias); pitting	Partial or complete loss of nail(s); pain in nailbed(s)	Interfering with ADL	—	—
Photosensitivity	Photosensitivity	Painless erythema	Painful erythema	Erythema with desquamation	Life-threatening; disabling	Death
Pruritus/itching	Pruritus	Mild or localized	Intense or widespread	Intense or widespread and interfering with ADL	—	—
Rash/ desquamation	Rash	Macular or papular eruption or erythema without associated symptoms	Macular or papular eruption or erythema with pruritus or other associated symptoms; localized desquamation or other lesions covering <50% of body surface area (BSA)	Severe, generalized erythroderma or macular, papular or vesicular eruption; desquamation covering ≥50% BSA	Generalized exfoliative, ulcerative, or bullous dermatitis	Death

DERMATOLOGY/SKIN—CONT'D						
		Grade				
Adverse event	Short name	1	2	3	4	5
Rash, acne/acneiform	Acne	Intervention not indicated	Intervention indicated	Associated with pain, disfigurement, ulceration, or desquamation	—	Death
Rash, dermatitis associated with radiation	Dermatitis	Faint erythema or dry desquamation	Moderate to brisk erythema; patchy moist desquamation, mostly confined to skin folds and creases; moderate edema	Moist desquamation other than skin folds and creases; bleeding induced by minor trauma or abrasion	Skin necrosis or ulceration of full thickness dermis; spontaneous bleeding from involved site	Death
Rash, erythema multiforme (e.g., Stevens–Johnson syndrome, toxic epidermal necrolysis)	Erythema multiforme	—	Scattered, but not generalized eruption	Severe (e.g., generalized rash or painful stomatitis); IV fluids, tube feedings, or TPN indicated	Life–threatening; disabling	Death
Rash, hand-foot skin reaction	Hand-foot	Minimal skin changes or dermatitis (e.g., erythema) without pain	Skin changes (e.g., peeling, blisters, bleeding, edema) or pain, not interfering with function	Ulcerative dermatitis or skin changes with pain interfering with function	—	—
Skin breakdown/decubitus ulcer	Decubitus	—	Local wound care; medical intervention indicated	Operative debridement or other invasive intervention indicated (e.g., hyperbaric oxygen)	Life-threatening consequences; major invasive intervention indicated (e.g., tissue reconstruction, flap or grafting)	Death
Striae	Striae	Mild	Cosmetically significant	—	—	—
Telangiectasia	Telangiectasia	Few	Moderate number	Many and confluent	—	—
Ulceration	Ulceration	—	Superficial ulceration <2 cm size; local wound care; medical intervention indicated	Ulceration ≥2 cm size; operative debridement, primary closure or other invasive intervention indicated (e.g., hyperbaric oxygen)	Life-threatening consequences; major invasive intervention indicated (e.g., complete resection, tissue reconstruction, flap or grafting)	Death
Urticaria (hives, welts, wheals)	Urticaria	Intervention not indicated	Intervention indicated for <24 hrs	Intervention indicated for ≥24 hrs	—	—
Wound complication, non-infectious	Wound complication, non-infectious	Incisional separation of ≤25% of wound, no deeper than superficial fascia	Incisional separation >25% of wound with local care; asymptomatic hernia	Symptomatic hernia without evidence of strangulation; fascial disruption/dehiscence without evisceration; primary wound closure or revision by operative intervention indicated; hospitalization or hyperbaric oxygen indicated	Symptomatic hernia with evidence of strangulation; fascial disruption with evisceration; major reconstruction flap, grafting, resection, or amputation indicated	Death

GASTROINTESTINAL						
		Grade				
Adverse event	Short name	1	2	3	4	5
Anorexia	Anorexia	Loss of appetite without alteration in eating habits	Oral intake altered without significant weight loss or malnutrition; oral nutritional supplements indicated	Associated with significant weight loss or malnutrition (e.g., inadequate oral caloric and/or fluid intake); IV fluids, tube feedings or TPN indicated	Life-threatening consequences	Death
Ascites (non-malignant)	Ascites	Asymptomatic	Symptomatic, medical intervention indicated	Symptomatic, invasive procedure indicated	Life-threatening consequences	Death
Colitis	Colitis	Asymptomatic, pathologic or radiographic findings only	Abdominal pain; mucus or blood in stool	Abdominal pain, fever, change in bowel habits with ileus; peritoneal signs	Life-threatening consequences (e.g., perforation, bleeding, ischemia, necrosis, toxic megacolon)	Death
Constipation	Constipation	Occasional or intermittent symptoms; occasional use of stool softeners, laxatives, dietary modification, or enema	Persistent symptoms with regular use of laxatives or enemas indicated	Symptoms interfering with ADL; obstipation with manual evacuation indicated	Life-threatening consequences (e.g., obstruction, toxic megacolon)	Death
Dehydration	Dehydration	Increased oral fluids indicated; dry mucous membranes; diminished skin turgor	IV fluids indicated <24 hrs	IV fluids indicated ≥24 hrs	Life-threatening consequences (e.g., hemodynamic collapse)	Death
Diarrhea	Diarrhea	Increase of <4 stools per day over baseline; mild increase in ostomy output compared to baseline	Increase of 4–6 stools per day over baseline; IV fluids indicated <24 hrs; moderate increase in ostomy output compared to baseline; not interfering with ADL	Increase of ≥7 stools per day over baseline; incontinence; IV fluids ≥24 hrs; hospitalization; severe increase in ostomy output compared to baseline; interfering with ADL	Life-threatening consequences (e.g., hemodynamic collapse)	Death
Dry mouth/ salivary gland (xerostomia)	Dry mouth	Symptomatic (dry or thick saliva) without significant dietary alteration; unstimulated saliva flow >0.2 ml/min	Symptomatic and significant oral intake alteration (e.g., copious water, other lubricants, diet limited to purees and/or soft, moist foods); unstimulated saliva 0.1 to 0.2 ml/min	Symptoms leading to inability to adequately aliment orally; IV fluids, tube feedings, or TPN indicated; unstimulated saliva <0.1 ml/min	—	—
Dysphagia (difficulty swallowing)	Dysphagia	Symptomatic, able to eat regular diet	Symptomatic and altered eating/ swallowing (e.g., altered dietary habits, oral supplements); IV fluids indicated <24 hrs	Symptomatic and severely altered eating/swallowing (e.g., inadequate oral caloric or fluid intake); IV fluids, tube feedings, or TPN indicated ≥24 hrs	Life-threatening consequences (e.g., obstruction, perforation)	Death

GASTROINTESTINAL—CONT'D						
		Grade				
Adverse event	**Short name**	**1**	**2**	**3**	**4**	**5**
Enteritis (inflammation of the small bowel)	Enteritis	Asymptomatic, pathologic or radiographic findings only	Abdominal pain; mucus or blood in stool	Abdominal pain, fever, change in bowel habits with ileus; peritoneal signs	Life-threatening consequences (e.g., perforation, bleeding, ischemia, necrosis)	Death
Esophagitis	Esophagitis	Asymptomatic pathologic, radiographic, or endoscopic findings only	Symptomatic; altered eating/swallowing (e.g., altered dietary habits, oral supplements); IV fluids indicated <24 hrs	Symptomatic and severely altered eating/swallowing (e.g., inadequate oral caloric or fluid intake); IV fluids, tube feedings, or TPN indicated ≥24 hrs	Life-threatening consequences	Death
Fistula, GI	Fistula, GI	Asymptomatic, radiographic findings only	Symptomatic; altered GI function (e.g., altered dietary habits, diarrhea or GI fluid loss); IV fluids indicated <24 hrs	Symptomatic and severely altered GI function (e.g., altered dietary habits, diarrhea, or GI fluid loss); IV fluids, tube feedings, or TPN indicated ≥24 hrs	Life-threatening consequences	Death
Flatulence	Flatulence	Mild	Moderate	—	—	—
Gastritis (including bile reflux gastritis)	Gastritis	Asymptomatic radiographic or endoscopic findings only	Symptomatic; altered gastric function (e.g., inadequate oral caloric or fluid intake); IV fluids indicated <24 hrs	Symptomatic and severely altered gastric function (e.g., inadequate oral caloric or fluid intake); IV fluids, tube feedings or TPN indicated ≥24 hrs	Life-threatening consequences; operative intervention requiring complete organ resection (e.g., gastrectomy)	Death
Heartburn/ dyspepsia	Heartburn	Mild	Moderate	Severe	—	—
Hemorrhoids	Hemorrhoids	Asymptomatic	Symptomatic; banding or medical intervention indicated	Interfering with ADL; interventional radiology, endoscopic, or operative intervention indicated	Life-threatening consequences	Death
Ileus, GI (functional obstruction of bowel, i.e., neuro-constipation)	Ileus	Asymptomatic, radiographic findings only	Symptomatic; altered GI function (e.g., altered dietary habits); IV fluids indicated <24 hrs	Symptomatic and severely altered GI function; IV fluids, tube feeding, or TPN indicated ≥24 hrs	Life-threatening consequences	Death
Incontinence, anal	Incontinence, anal	Occasional use of pads required	Daily use of pads required	Interfering with ADL; operative intervention indicated	Permanent bowel diversion indicated	Death
Leak (including anastomotic), GI	Leak, GI	Asymptomatic radiographic findings only	Symptomatic; medical intervention indicated	Symptomatic and interfering with GI function; invasive or endoscopic intervention indicated	Life-threatening consequences	Death

Continued

GASTROINTESTINAL—CONT'D						
		Grade				
Adverse event	**Short name**	**1**	**2**	**3**	**4**	**5**
Malabsorption	Malabsorption	—	Altered diet; oral therapies indicated (e.g., enzymes, medications, dietary supplements)	Inability to aliment adequately via GI tract (i.e., TPN indicated)	Life-threatening consequences	Death
Mucositis/ stomatitis (clinical exam)	Mucositis (clinical exam)	Erythema of the mucosa	Patchy ulcerations or pseudomembranes	Confluent ulcerations or pseudomembranes; bleeding with minor trauma	Tissue necrosis; significant spontaneous bleeding; life-threatening consequences	Death
Mucositis/ stomatitis (functional/ symptomatic)	Mucositis (functional/ symptomatic)	*Upper aerodigestive tract sites:* Minimal symptoms, normal diet; minimal respiratory symptoms but not interfering with function *Lower GI sites*: Minimal discomfort, intervention not indicated	*Upper aerodigestive tract sites*: Symptomatic but can eat and swallow modified diet; respiratory symptoms interfering with function but not interfering with ADL *Lower GI sites*: Symptomatic, medical intervention indicated but not interfering with ADL	*Upper aerodigestive tract sites*: Symptomatic and unable to adequately aliment or hydrate orally; respiratory symptoms interfering with ADL *Lower GI sites*: Stool incontinence or other symptoms interfering with ADL	Symptoms associated with life-threatening consequences	Death
Nausea	Nausea	Loss of appetite without alteration in eating habits	Oral intake decreased without significant weight loss, dehydration or malnutrition; IV fluids indicated <24 hrs	Inadequate oral caloric or fluid intake; IV fluids, tube feedings, or TPN indicated ≥24 hrs	Life-threatening consequences	Death
Necrosis, GI	Necrosis, GI	—	—	Inability to aliment adequately by GI tract, (e.g., requiring enteral or parenteral nutrition); interventional radiology, endoscopic, or operative intervention indicated	Life-threatening consequences; operative intervention requiring complete organ resection (e.g., total colectomy)	Death
Obstruction, GI	Obstruction, GI	Asymptomatic radiographic findings only	Symptomatic; altered GI function (e.g., altered dietary habits, vomiting, diarrhea, or GI fluid loss); IV fluids indicated <24 hrs	Symptomatic and severely altered GI function; (e.g., altered dietary habits, vomiting, diarrhea, or GI fluid loss); IV fluids, tube feedings or TPN indicated ≥24 hrs; operative intervention indicated	Life-threatening consequences; operative intervention requiring complete organ resection (e.g., total colectomy)	Death
Perforation, GI	Perforation, GI	Asymptomatic radiographic findings only	Medical intervention indicated; IV fluids indicated <24 hrs	IV fluids, tube feedings, or TPN indicated ≥24 hrs; operative intervention indicated	Life-threatening consequences	Death

GASTROINTESTINAL—CONT'D

Adverse event	Short name	Grade 1	Grade 2	Grade 3	Grade 4	Grade 5
Proctitis	Proctitis	Rectal discomfort, intervention not indicated	Symptoms not interfering with ADL; medical intervention indicated	Stool incontinence or other symptoms interfering with ADL; operative intervention indicated	Life-threatening consequences (e.g., perforation)	Death
Prolapse of stoma, GI	Prolapse of stoma, GI	Asymptomatic	Extraordinary local care or maintenance; minor revision indicated	Dysfunctional stoma; major revision indicated	Life-threatening consequences	Death
Salivary gland changes/saliva	Salivary gland changes	Slightly thickened saliva; slightly altered taste (e.g., metallic)	Thick, ropy, sticky saliva; markedly altered taste; alteration in diet indicated; secretion-induced symptoms not interfering with ADL	Acute salivary gland necrosis; severe secretion-induced symptoms interfering with ADL	Disabling	—
Stricture/stenosis (including anastomotic), GI	Stricture, GI	Asymptomatic radiographic findings only	Symptomatic; altered GI function (e.g., altered dietary habits, vomiting, bleeding, diarrhea); IV fluids indicated <24 hrs	Symptomatic and severely altered GI function; (e.g., altered dietary habits, diarrhea, or GI fluid loss); IV fluids, tube feedings, or TPN indicated ≥24 hrs; operative intervention indicated	Life-threatening consequences; operative intervention requiring complete organ resection (e.g., total colectomy)	Death
Taste alteration (dyspepsia)	Taste	Altered taste but no change in diet	Altered taste with change in diet (e.g., oral supplements); noxious or unpleasant taste; loss of taste	—	—	—
Typhlitis (cecal inflammation)	Typhlitis	Asymptomatic pathologic or radiographic findings only	Abdominal pain; mucus or blood in stool	Abdominal pain, fever, change in bowel habits with ileus; peritoneal signs	Life-threatening consequences (e.g., perforation, bleeding, ischemia, necrosis); operative intervention indicated	Death
Ulcer, GI	Ulcer, GI	Asymptomatic, radiographic or endoscopic findings only	Symptomatic; altered GI function (e.g., altered dietary habits, oral supplements); IV fluids indicated <24 hrs	Symptomatic and severely altered GI function (e.g., inadequate oral caloric or fluid intake); IV fluids, tube feedings, or TPN indicated ≥24 hrs	Life-threatening consequences	Death
Vomiting	Vomiting	1 episode in 24 hrs	2–5 episodes in 24 hrs; IV fluids indicated <24 hrs	≥6 episodes in 24 hrs; IV fluids, or TPN indicated ≥24 hrs	Life-threatening consequences	Death

HEMORRHAGE/BLEEDING[4]

Adverse event	Short name	Grade 1	Grade 2	Grade 3	Grade 4	Grade 5
Hematoma	Hematoma	Minimal symptoms, invasive intervention not indicated	Minimally invasive evacuation or aspiration indicated	Transfusion, interventional radiology, or operative intervention indicated	Life-threatening consequences; major urgent intervention indicated	Death
Hemorrhage/ bleeding associated with surgery, intraoperative or postoperative	Hemorrhage with surgery	—	—	Requiring transfusion of 2 units non-autologous (10 cc/kg for pediatrics) pRBCs beyond protocol specification; postoperative interventional radiology, endoscopic, or operative intervention indicated	Life-threatening consequences	Death
Hemorrhage, CNS	CNS hemorrhage	Asymptomatic, radiographic findings only	Medical intervention indicated	Ventriculostomy, ICP monitoring, intraventricular thrombolysis, or operative intervention indicated	Life-threatening consequences; neurologic deficit or disability	Death
Hemorrhage, GU	Hemorrhage, GU	Minimal or microscopic bleeding; intervention not indicated	Gross bleeding, medical intervention, or urinary tract irrigation indicated	Transfusion, interventional radiology, endoscopic, or operative intervention indicated; radiation therapy (i.e., hemostasis of bleeding site)	Life-threatening consequences; major urgent intervention indicated	Death
Hemorrhage, pulmonary/ upper respiratory	Hemorrhage pulmonary	Mild, intervention not indicated	Symptomatic and medical intervention indicated	Transfusion, interventional radiology, endoscopic, or operative intervention indicated; radiation therapy (i.e., hemostasis of bleeding site)	Life-threatening consequences; major urgent intervention indicated	Death
Petechiae/ purpura (hemorrhage/ bleeding into skin or mucosa)	Petechiae	Few petechiae	Moderate petechiae; purpura	Generalized petechiae or purpura	—	—

INFECTION						
		Grade				
Adverse event	**Short name**	**1**	**2**	**3**	**4**	**5**
Colitis, infectious (e.g., *Clostridium difficile*)	Colitis, infectious	Asymptomatic, pathologic or radiographic findings only	Abdominal pain with mucus and/or blood in stool	IV antibiotics or TPN indicated	Life-threatening consequences (e.g., perforation, bleeding, ischemia, necrosis or toxic megacolon); operative resection or diversion indicated	Death
Febrile neutropenia (fever of unknown origin without clinically or microbiologically documented infection) (ANC $<1.0 \times 10^9$/L, fever ≥38.5°C)	Febrile neutropenia	—	—	Present	Life-threatening consequences (e.g., septic shock, hypotension, acidosis, necrosis)	Death
Infection (documented clinically or microbiologically) with Grade 3 or 4 neutrophils (ANC $<1.0 \times 10^9$/L)	Infection (documented clinically)	—	Localized, local intervention indicated	IV antibiotic, antifungal or antiviral intervention indicated; interventional radiology or operative intervention indicated	Life-threatening consequences (e.g., septic shock, hypotension, acidosis, necrosis)	Death
Infection with normal ANC or Grade 1 or 2 neutrophils	Infection with normal ANC	—	Localized, local intervention indicated	IV antibiotic, antifungal or antiviral intervention indicated; interventional radiology or operative intervention indicated	Life-threatening consequences (e.g., septic shock, hypotension, acidosis, necrosis)	Death
Infection with unknown ANC	Infection with unknown ANC	—	Localized, local intervention indicated	IV antibiotic, antifungal or antiviral intervention indicated; interventional radiology or operative intervention indicated	Life-threatening consequences (e.g., septic shock, hypotension, acidosis, necrosis)	Death
Opportunistic infection associates with ≥Grade 2 lymphopenia	Opportunistic infection	—	Localized, local intervention indicated	IV antibiotic, antifungal or antiviral intervention indicated; interventional radiology or operative intervention indicated	Life-threatening consequences (e.g., septic shock, hypotension, acidosis, necrosis)	Death
Viral hepatitis	Viral hepatitis	Present; transaminases and liver function normal	Transaminases abnormal, liver function normal	Symptomatic liver dysfunction; fibrosis by biopsy; compensated cirrhosis	Decompensated liver function (e.g., ascites, coagulopathy, encephalopathy, coma)	Death

LYMPHATICS

Adverse event	Short name	Grade 1	Grade 2	Grade 3	Grade 4	Grade 5
Chyle or lymph leakage	Chyle or lymph leakage	Asymptomatic, clinical or radiographic findings	Symptomatic, medical intervention indicated	Interventional radiology or operative intervention indicated	Life-threatening complications	Death
Dermal change lymphedema, phlebolym-phedema	Dermal change	Trace thickening or faint discoloration	Marked discoloration; leathery skin texture; papillary formation	—	—	—
Edema, head and neck	Edema: head and neck	Localized to dependent areas, no disability or functional impairment	Localized facial or neck edema with functional impairment	Generalized facial or neck edema with functional impairment (e.g., difficulty in turning neck or opening mouth compared to baseline)	Severe with ulceration or cerebral edema; tracheotomy or feeding tube indicated	Death
Edema, limb	Edema: limb	5–10% inter-limb discrepancy in volume or circumference at point of greatest visible difference; swelling or obscuration of anatomic architecture on close inspection; pitting edema	>10–30% inter-limb discrepancy in volume or circumference at point of greatest visible difference; readily apparent obscuration of anatomic architecture; obliteration of skin folds; readily apparent deviation from normal anatomic contour	>30% inter-limb discrepancy in volume; lymphorrhea; gross deviation from normal anatomic contour; interfering with ADL	Progression to malignancy (i.e., lymphangiosarcoma); amputation indicated; disabling	Death
Edema, trunk/genital	Edema: trunk/genital	Swelling or obscuration of anatomic architecture on close inspection; pitting edema	Readily apparent obscuration or anatomic architecture; obliteration of skin folds; readily apparent deviation from normal anatomic contour	Lymphorrhea; interfering with ADL; gross deviation from normal anatomic contour	Progression to malignancy (i.e., lymphangiosarcoma); disabling	Death
Edema, viscera	Edema: viscera	Asymptomatic; clinical or radiographic findings only	Symptomatic; medical intervention indicated	Symptomatic and unable to aliment adequately orally; interventional radiology or operative intervention indicated	Life-threatening consequences	Death
Lymphedema-related fibrosis	Lymphedema-related fibrosis	Minimal to moderate redundant soft tissue, unresponsive to elevation or compression, with moderately firm texture or spongy feel	Marked increase in density and firmness, with or without tethering	Very marked density and firmness with tethering affecting ≥40% of the edematous area	—	—
Lymphocele	Lymphocele	Asymptomatic, clinical or radiographic findings only	Symptomatic; medical intervention indicated	Symptomatic and interventional radiology or operative intervention indicated	—	—
Phlebolymphatic cording	Phlebolymphatic cording	Asymptomatic, clinical findings only	Symptomatic; medical intervention indicated	Symptomatic and leading to contracture or reduced range of motion	—	—

NEUROLOGY

Adverse event	Short name	Grade 1	Grade 2	Grade 3	Grade 4	Grade 5
Apnea	Apnea	—	—	Present	Intubation indicated	Death
Arachnoiditis/ meningismus/ radiculitis	Arachnoiditis	Symptomatic, not interfering with function; medical intervention indicated	Symptomatic (e.g., photophobia, nausea) interfering with function but not interfering with ADL	Symptomatic, interfering with ADL	Life-threatening; disabling (e.g., paraplegia)	Death
Ataxia (incoordination)	Ataxia	Asymptomatic	Symptomatic, not interfering with ADL	Symptomatic, interfering with ADL; mechanical assistance indicated	Disabling	Death
Brachial plexopathy	Brachial plexopathy	Asymptomatic	Symptomatic, not interfering with ADL	Symptomatic, interfering with ADL	Disabling	Death
CNS cerebrovascular ischemia	CNS ischemia	—	Asymptomatic, radiographic findings only	Transient ischemic event or attack (TIA) ≤24 hrs duration	Cerebral vascular accident (CVA, stroke), neurologic deficit >24 hrs	Death
CNS necrosis/ cystic progression	CNS necrosis	Asymptomatic, radiographic findings only	Symptomatic, not interfering with ADL; medical intervention indicated	Symptomatic and interfering with ADL; hyperbaric oxygen indicated	Life-threatening; disabling; operative intervention indicated to prevent or treat CNS necrosis/cystic progression	Death
Cognitive disturbance	Cognitive disturbance	Mild cognitive disability; not interfering with work/school/life performance; specialized educational services/devices not indicated	Moderate cognitive disability; interfering with work/school/life performance but capable of independent living; specialized resources on part-time basis indicated	Severe cognitive disability; significant impairment of work/school/life performance	Unable to perform ADL; full-time specialized resources or institutionalization indicated	Death
Confusion	Confusion	Transient confusion, disorientation, or attention deficit	Confusion, disorientation, or attention deficit interfering with function, but not interfering with ADL	Confusion or delirium interfering with ADL	Harmful to others or self; hospitalization indicated	Death
Dizziness	Dizziness	With head movements or nystagmus only; not interfering with function	Interfering with function, but not interfering with ADL	Interfering with ADL	Disabling	—
Encephalopathy	Encephalopathy	—	Mild signs or symptoms; not interfering with ADL	Signs or symptoms interfering with ADL; hospitalization indicated	Life-threatening; disabling	Death
Extrapyramidal/ involuntary movement/ restlessness	Involuntary movement	Mild involuntary movements not interfering with function	Moderate involuntary movements interfering with function, but not interfering with ADL	Severe involuntary movements or torticollis interfering with ADL	Disabling	Death

Continued

NEUROLOGY—CONT'D						
		Grade				
Adverse event	**Short name**	**1**	**2**	**3**	**4**	**5**
Laryngeal nerve dysfunction	Laryngeal nerve	Asymptomatic, weakness on clinical examination/testing only	Symptomatic, but not interfering with ADL; intervention not indicated	Symptomatic, interfering with ADL; intervention indicated (e.g., thyroplasty, vocal cord injection)	Life-threatening; tracheostomy indicated	Death
Leak, cerebrospinal fluid (CSF)	CSF leak	Transient headache; postural care indicated	Symptomatic, not interfering with ADL; blood patch indicated	Symptomatic, interfering with ADL; operative intervention indicated	Life-threatening; disabling	Death
Leukoence-phalopathy (radiographic findings)	Leukoence-phalopathy	Mild increase in subarachnoid space (SAS); mild ventriculomegaly; small (± multiple) focal T2 hyperintensities, involving periventricular white matter of <$\frac{1}{3}$ of susceptible areas of cerebrum	Moderate increase in SAS; moderate ventriculomegaly; focal T2 hyperintensities extending into centrum ovale or involving $\frac{1}{3}$ to $\frac{2}{3}$ of susceptible areas of cerebrum	Severe increase in SAS; severe ventriculomegaly; near total white matter T2 hyperintensities or diffuse low attenuation (CT)	—	—
Memory impairment	Memory impairment	Memory impairment not interfering with function	Memory impairment interfering with function, but not interfering with ADL	Memory impairment interfering with ADL	Amnesia	—
Mental status	Mental status	—	1–3 point below age and educational norm in Folstein Mini-Mental Status Exam (MMSE)	>3 point below age and educational norm in Folstein MMSE	—	—
Mood alteration	Mood alteration	Mild mood alteration not interfering with function	Moderate mood alteration interfering with function, but not interfering with ADL; medication indicated	Severe mood alteration interfering with ADL	Suicidal ideation; danger to self or others	Death
Myelitis	Myelitis	Asymptomatic, mild signs (e.g., Babinski's or Lhermitte's sign)	Weakness or sensory loss not interfering with ADL	Weakness or sensory loss interfering with ADL	Disabling	Death
Neuropathy, cranial	Neuropathy: cranial	Asymptomatic, detected on exam/testing only	Symptomatic not interfering with ADL	Symptomatic, interfering with ADL	Life-threatening; disabling	Death
Neuropathy, motor	Neuropathy: motor	Asymptomatic, weakness on exam/testing only	Symptomatic weakness interfering with function, but not interfering with ADL	Weakness interfering with ADL; bracing or assistance to walk (e.g., cane or walker) indicated	Life-threatening; disabling (e.g., paralysis)	Death
Neuropathy, sensory	Neuropathy: sensory	Asymptomatic; loss of deep tendon reflexes or paresthesia paresthesia (including tingling) but not interfering with function	Sensory alteration or paresthesia (including tingling), interfering with function, but not interfering with ADL	Sensory alteration or paresthesia interfering with ADL	Disabling	Death

NEUROLOGY—CONT'D						
		Grade				
Adverse event	**Short name**	**1**	**2**	**3**	**4**	**5**
Personality/ behavioral	Personality	Change, but not adversely affecting patient or family	Change, adversely affecting patient or family	Mental health intervention indicated	Change harmful to others or self; hospitalization indicated	Death
Phrenic nerve dysfunction	Phrenic nerve	Asymptomatic weakness on exam/testing only	Symptomatic but not interfering with ADL; intervention not indicated	Significant dysfunction; intervention indicated (e.g., diaphragmatic plication)	Life-threatening respiratory compromise; mechanical ventilation indicated	Death
Psychosis (hallucinations/ delusions)	Psychosis	—	Transient episode	Interfering with ADL; medication, supervision or restraints indicated	Harmful to others or self; life-threatening consequences	Death
Pyramidal tract dysfunction (e.g., ↑ tone, hyperreflexia, positive Babinski, ↓ fine motor coordination)	Pyramidal tract dysfunction	Asymptomatic, abnormality on exam or testing only	Symptomatic; interfering with function but not interfering with ADL	Interfering with ADL	Disabling; paralysis	Death
Seizure	Seizure	—	One brief generalized seizure; seizure(s) well controlled by anticonvulsants or infrequent focal motor seizures not interfering with ADL	Seizures in which consciousness is altered; poorly controlled seizure disorder, with breakthrough generalized seizures despite medical intervention	Seizures of any kind which are prolonged, repetitive, or difficult to control (e.g., status epilepticus, intractable epilepsy)	Death
Somnolence/ depressed level of consciousness	Somnolence	—	Somnolence or sedation interfering with function, but not interfering with ADL	Obtundation or stupor; difficult to arouse; interfering with ADL	Coma	Death
Speech impairment (e.g., dysphasia or aphasia)	Speech impairment	—	Awareness of receptive or expressive dysphasia, not impairing ability to communicate	Receptive or expressive dysphasia, impairing ability to communicate	Inability to communicate	—
Syncope (fainting)	Syncope (fainting)	—	—	Present	Life-threatening consequences	Death
Tremor	Tremor	Mild and brief or intermittent but not interfering with function	Moderate tremor interfering with ADL	Severe tremor interfering with ADL	Disabling	—

Adverse event	Short name	Grade 1	Grade 2	Grade 3	Grade 4	Grade 5
PAIN						
Pain	Pain (specify)	Mild pain not interfering with function	Moderate pain; pain or analgesics interfering with function, but not interfering with ADL	Severe pain; pain or analgesics severely interfering with ADL	Disabling	—
Pain, other (specify)	Pain, other (specify)	Mild pain not interfering with function	Moderate pain; pain or analgesics interfering with function, but not interfering with ADL	Severe pain; pain or analgesics severely interfering with ADL	Disabling	—
PULMONARY/UPPER RESPIRATORY						
Adult Respiratory Distress Syndrome (ARDS)	ARDS	—	—	Present, intubation not indicated	Present, intubation indicated	Death
Aspiration	Aspiration	Asymptomatic ("silent aspiration"); endoscopy or radiographic (e.g., barium swallow) findings	Symptomatic (e.g., altered eating habits, coughing or choking episodes consistent with aspiration); medical intervention indicated (e.g., antibiotics, suction or oxygen)	Clinical or radiographic signs of pneumonia or pneumonitis; unable to aliment orally	Life-threatening (e.g., aspiration pneumonia or pneumonitis)	Death
Atelectasis	Atelectasis	Asymptomatic	Symptomatic (e.g., dyspnea, cough), medical intervention indicated (e.g., bronchoscopic suctioning, chest physiotherapy, suctioning)	Operative (e.g., stent, laser) intervention indicated	Life-threatening respiratory compromise	Death
Bronchospasm, wheezing	Bronchospasm	Asymptomatic	Symptomatic, not interfering with function	Symptomatic, interfering with function	Life-threatening	Death
Carbon monoxide diffusion capacity	DLCO	90–75% of predicted value	<75–50% of predicted value	<50–25% of predicted value	<25% of predicted value	Death
Chylothorax	Chylothorax	Asymptomatic	Symptomatic; thoracentesis or tube drainage indicated	Operative intervention indicated	Life-threatening (e.g., hemodynamic instability or ventilatory support indicated)	Death
Cough	Cough	Symptomatic, non-narcotic medication only indicated	Symptomatic and narcotic medication indicated	Symptomatic and significantly interfering with sleep or ADL	—	—

PULMONARY/UPPER RESPIRATORY—CONT'D						
		Grade				
Adverse event	**Short name**	**1**	**2**	**3**	**4**	**5**
Dyspnea (shortness of breath)	Dyspnea	Dyspnea on exertion, but can walk 1 flight of stairs without stopping	Dyspnea on exertion but unable to walk 1 flight of stairs or 1 city block (0.1 km) without stopping	Dyspnea with ADL	Dyspnea at rest; intubation/ventilator indicated	Death
Edema, larynx	Edema, larynx	Asymptomatic edema by exam only	Symptomatic edema, no respiratory distress	Stridor; respiratory distress; interfering with ADL	Life-threatening airway compromise; tracheotomy, intubation, or laryngectomy indicated	Death
Forced expiratory volume in one second	FEV_1	90–75% of predicted value	<75–50% of predicted value	<50–25% of predicted value	<25% of predicted value	Death
Fistula, pulmonary/ upper respiratory	Fistula, pulmonary	Asymptomatic, radiographic findings only	Symptomatic, tube thoracostomy or medical management indicated; associated with altered respiratory function but not interfering with ADL	Symptomatic and associated with altered respiratory function interfering with ADL; or endoscopic (e.g., stent) or primary closure by operative intervention indicated	Life-threatening consequences; operative intervention with thoracoplasty, chronic open drainage or multiple thoracotomies indicated	Death
Hiccoughs (hiccups, singultus)	Hiccoughs	Symptomatic, intervention not indicated	Symptomatic, intervention indicated	Symptomatic, significantly interfering with sleep or ADL	—	—
Hypoxia	Hypoxia	—	Decreased O_2 saturation with exercise (e.g., pulse oximeter <88%); intermittent supplemental oxygen	Decreased O_2 saturation at rest; continuous oxygen indicated	Life-threatening; intubation or ventilation indicated	Death
Nasal cavity/ paranasal sinus reactions	Nasal/paranasal reactions	Asymptomatic mucosal crusting, blood-tinged secretions	Symptomatic stenosis or edema/ narrowing interfering with airflow	Stenosis with significant nasal obstruction; interfering with ADL	Necrosis of soft tissue or bone	Death
Obstruction/ stenosis of airway	Airway obstruction	Asymptomatic obstruction or stenosis on exam, endoscopy, or radiograph	Symptomatic (e.g., noisy airway breathing), but causing no respiratory distress; medical management indicated (e.g., steroids)	Interfering with ADL; stridor or endoscopic intervention indicated (e.g., stent, laser)	Life-threatening airway compromise; tracheotomy or intubation indicated	Death
Pleural effusion (non-malignant)	Pleural effusion	Asymptomatic	Symptomatic, intervention such as diuretics or up to 2 therapeutic thoracenteses indicated	Symptomatic and supplemental oxygen, >2 therapeutic thoracenteses, tube drainage, or pleurodesis indicated	Life-threatening (e.g., causing hemodynamic instability or ventilatory support indicated)	Death

Continued

PULMONARY/UPPER RESPIRATORY—CONT'D

Adverse event	Short name	Grade 1	Grade 2	Grade 3	Grade 4	Grade 5
Pneumonitis/ pulmonary infiltrates	Pneumonitis	Asymptomatic, radiographic findings only	Symptomatic, not interfering with ADL	Symptomatic, interfering with ADL; O_2 indicated	Life-threatening; ventilatory support indicated	Death
Pneumothorax	Pneumothorax	Asymptomatic, radiographic findings only	Symptomatic; intervention indicated (e.g., hospitalization for observation, tube placement without sclerosis)	Sclerosis and/or operative intervention indicated	Life-threatening, causing hemodynamic instability (e.g., tension pneumothorax); ventilatory support indicated	Death
Prolonged chest tube drainage or air leak after pulmonary resection	Chest tube drainage or leak	—	Sclerosis or additional tube thoracostomy indicated	Operative intervention indicated (e.g., thoracotomy with stapling or sealant application)	Life-threatening; debilitating; organ resection indicated	Death
Prolonged intubation after pulmonary resection (>24 hrs after surgery)	Prolonged intubation	—	Extubated within 24–72 hrs postoperatively	Extubated >72 hrs postoperatively, but before tracheostomy indicated	Tracheostomy indicated	Death
Pulmonary fibrosis (radiographic changes)	Pulmonary fibrosis	Minimal radiographic findings (or patchy or bi-basilar changes) with estimated radiographic proportion of total lung volume that is fibrotic of <25%	Patchy or bi-basilar changes with estimated radiographic proportion of total lung volume that is fibrotic of 25–<50%	Dense or widespread infiltrates/ consolidation with estimated radiographic proportion of total lung volume that is fibrotic of 50–<75%	Estimated radiographic proportion of total lung volume that is fibrotic is 75%; honeycombing	Death
Vital capacity	Vital capacity	90–75% of predicted value	<75–50% of predicted value	<50–25% of predicted value	<25% of predicted value	Death
Voice changes/ dysarthria (e.g., hoarseness, loss or alteration in voice, laryngitis)	Voice changes	Mild or intermittent hoarseness or voice change, but fully understandable	Moderate or persistent voice changes, may require occasional repetition but understandable on telephone	Severe voice changes including predominantly whispered speech; may require frequent repetition or face-to-face contact for understandability; requires voice aid (e.g., electrolarynx) for ≤50% of communication	Disabling; non-understandable voice or aphonic; requires voice aid (e.g., electrolarynx) for >50% of communication or requires >50% written communication	Death

RENAL/GENITOURINARY						
		Grade				
Adverse event	Short name	1	2	3	4	5
Bladder spasms	Bladder spasms	Symptomatic, intervention not indicated	Symptomatic, antispasmodics indicated	Narcotics indicated	Major surgical intervention indicated (e.g., cystectomy)	—
Cystitis	Cystitis	Asymptomatic	Frequency with dysuria; macroscopic hematuria	Transfusion; IV pain medications; bladder irrigation indicated	Catastrophic bleeding; major non-elective intervention indicated	Death
Fistula, GU	Fistula, GU	Asymptomatic, radiographic findings only	Symptomatic; non-invasive intervention indicated	Symptomatic interfering with ADL; invasive intervention indicated	Life-threatening consequences; operative intervention requiring partial or full organ resection; permanent urinary diversion	Death
Incontinence, urinary	Incontinence, urinary	Occasional (e.g., with coughing, sneezing, etc.), pads not indicated	Spontaneous, pads indicated	Interfering with ADL; intervention indicated (e.g., clamp, collagen injections)	Operative intervention indicated (e.g., cystectomy or permanent urinary diversion)	—
Leak (including anastomotic), GU	Leak, GU	Asymptomatic, radiographic findings only	Symptomatic; medical intervention indicated	Symptomatic, interfering with GU function; invasive or endoscopic intervention indicated	Life-threatening	Death
Obstruction, GU	Obstruction, GU	Asymptomatic, radiographic or endoscopic findings only	Symptomatic but no hydronephrosis, sepsis or renal dysfunction; dilation or endoscopic repair or stent placement indicated	Symptomatic and altered organ function (e.g., sepsis or hydronephrosis, or renal dysfunction); operative intervention indicated	Life-threatening consequences; organ failure or operative intervention requiring complete organ resection indicated	Death
Perforation, GU	Perforation, GU	Asymptomatic radiographic findings only	Symptomatic, associated with altered renal/GU function	Symptomatic; operative intervention indicated	Life-threatening consequences or organ failure; operative intervention requiring organ resection indicated	Death
Prolapse of stoma, GU	Prolapse stoma, GU	Asymptomatic; special intervention, extraordinary care not indicated	Extraordinary local care or maintenance; minor revision under local anesthesia indicated	Dysfunctional stoma; operative intervention or major stomal revision indicated	Life-threatening consequences	Death

Continued

RENAL/GENITOURINARY—CONT'D						
		Grade				
Adverse event	**Short name**	**1**	**2**	**3**	**4**	**5**
Stricture/stenosis (including anastomotic), GU	Stricture, anastomotic, GU	Asymptomatic, radiographic or endoscopic findings only	Symptomatic but no hydronephrosis, sepsis or renal dysfunction; dilation or endoscopic repair or stent placement indicated	Symptomatic and altered organ function (e.g., sepsis or hydronephrosis, or renal dysfunction); operative intervention indicated	Life-threatening consequences; organ failure or operative intervention requiring organ resection indicated	Death
Urinary electrolyte wasting (e.g., Fanconi's syndrome, renal tubular acidosis)	Urinary electrolyte wasting	Asymptomatic, intervention not indicated	Mild, reversible and manageable with replacement	Irreversible, requiring continued replacement	—	—
Urinary frequency/ urgency	Urinary frequency	Increase in frequency or nocturia up to 2 × normal; enuresis	Increase >2 × normal but, hourly	≥x /hr; urgency; catheter indicated	—	—
Urinary retention (including neurogenic bladder)	Urinary retention	Hesitancy or dribbling, no significant residual urine; retention occurring during the immediate postoperative period	Hesitancy requiring medication; or operative bladder atony requiring indwelling catheter beyond immediate postoperative period but for <6 weeks	More than daily catheterization indicated; urological intervention indicated (e.g., TURP, suprapubic tube, urethrotomy)	Life-threatening consequences; organ failure (e.g., bladder rupture); operative intervention requiring organ resection indicated	Death

SEXUAL/REPRODUCTIVE FUNCTION						
		Grade				
Adverse event	Short name	1	2	3	4	5
Breast function/ lactation	Breast function	Mammary abnormality, not functionally significant	Mammary abnormality, functionally significant	—	—	—
Breast nipple/ areolar deformity	Nipple/areolar	Limited areolar asymmetry with no change in nipple/ areolar projection	Asymmetry of nipple areolar complex with slight deviation in nipple projection	Marked deviation of nipple projection	—	—
Breast volume/ hypoplasia	Breast	Minimal asymmetry; minimal hypoplasia	Asymmetry exists, ≤⅓ of the breast volume; moderate hypoplasia	Asymmetry exists, >⅓ of the breast volume; severe hypoplasia	—	—
Irregular menses (change from baseline)	Irregular menses	1–3 months without menses	>3–6 months without menses but continuing menstrual cycles	Persistent amenorrhea for >6 months	—	—
Libido	Libido	Decrease in interest but not affecting relationship; intervention not indicated	Decrease in interest and adversely affecting relationship; intervention indicated	—	—	—
Orgasmic dysfunction	Orgasmic function	Transient decrease	Decrease in orgasmic response requiring intervention	Complete inability of orgasmic response; not responding to intervention	—	—
Vaginal discharge, non-infectious	Vaginal discharge	Mild	Moderate to heavy; pad use indicated	—	—	—
Vaginal dryness	Vaginal dryness	Mild	Interfering with sexual function; dyspareunia; intervention indicated	—	—	—
Vaginal mucositis	Vaginal mucositis	Erythema of the mucosa; minimal symptoms	Patchy ulcerations; moderate symptoms or dyspareunia	Confluent ulcerations; bleeding with trauma; unable to tolerate vaginal exam, sexual intercourse or tampon placement	Tissue necrosis; significant spontaneous bleeding; life-threatening consequences	—
Vaginal stenosis/length	Vaginal stenosis	Vaginal narrowing and/or shortening not interfering with function	Vaginal narrowing and/or shortening interfering with function	Complete obliteration; not surgically correctable	—	—
Vaginitis (not due to infection)	Vaginitis	Mild, intervention not indicated	Moderate, intervention indicated	Severe, not relieved with treatment; ulceration, but operative intervention not indicated	Ulceration and operative intervention indicated	—

SURGERY/INTRAOPERATIVE INJURY						
		Grade				
Adverse event	Short name	1	2	3	4	5
Intraoperative injury	Intraop injury	Primary repair of injured organ/ structure indicated	Partial resection of injured organ/ structure indicated	Complete resection or reconstruction of injured organ/ structure indicated	Life-threatening consequences; disabling	—
VASCULAR						
Acute vascular leak syndrome	Acute vascular leak syndrome	—	Symptomatic, fluid support not indicated	Respiratory compromise or fluids indicated	Life-threatening; pressor support or ventilatory support indicated	Death
Peripheral arterial ischemia	Peripheral arterial ischemia	—	Brief (<24 hrs) episode of ischemia managed non-surgically and without permanent deficit	Recurring or prolonged (≥24 hrs) and/or invasive intervention indicated	Life-threatening, disabling and/or associated with end organ damage (e.g., limb loss)	Death
Phlebitis, including superficial thrombosis	Phlebitis	—	Present	—	—	—
Portal vein flow	Portal flow	—	Decreased portal vein flow	Reversal/retrograde portal vein flow	—	—
Thrombosis/ embolism, vascular access-related	Thrombosis/ embolism (vascular access)	—	Deep vein thrombosis or cardiac thrombosis; intervention (e.g., anticoagulation, lysis, filter, invasive procedure) not indicated	Deep vein thrombosis or cardiac thrombosis; intervention (e.g., anticoagulation, lysis, filter, invasive procedure) indicated	Embolic event including pulmonary embolism or life-threatening thrombus	Death
Thrombosis/ thrombus/ embolism	Thrombosis/ thrombus/ embolism	—	Deep vein thrombosis or cardiac thrombosis; intervention (e.g., anticoagulation, lysis, filter, invasive procedure) not indicated	Deep vein thrombosis or cardiac thrombosis; intervention (e.g., anticoagulation, lysis, filter, invasive procedure) indicated	Embolic event including pulmonary embolism or life-threatening thrombus	Death

VASCULAR—CONT'D						
		Grade				
Adverse event	Short name	1	2	3	4	5
Vessel injury, artery	Artery injury	Asymptomatic diagnostic finding; intervention not indicated	Symptomatic (e.g., claudication); not interfering with ADL; repair or revision not indicated	Symptomatic interfering with ADL; repair or revision indicated	Life-threatening; disabling; evidence of end organ damage (e.g., stroke, MI, organ or limb loss)	Death
Vessel injury, vein	Vein injury	Asymptomatic diagnostic finding; intervention not indicated	Symptomatic (e.g., claudication); not interfering with ADL; repair or revision not indicated	Symptomatic interfering with ADL; repair or revision indicated	Life-threatening; disabling; evidence of end organ damage	Death
Visceral arterial ischemia (non-myocardial)	Visceral arterial ischemia	—	Brief (<24 hrs) episode of ischemia managed medically and without permanent deficit	Prolonged (≥24 hrs) or recurring symptoms and/or invasive intervention indicated	Life-threatening; disabling; evidence of end organ damage	Death

[1]Also consider: haptoglobin, hemoglobin

[2]Grade palpitations only in the absence of a documented arrhythmia

[3]NHLBI Obesity Task Force. Clinical guidelines on the identification, evaluation, and treatment of overweight and obesity in adults. The Evidence Report. Obes Res 6:51S–209S, 1998.

[*]BMI = (weight[kg])/height [m]^2

[4]Also consider fibrinogen, INR, platelets, PTT

ADL, activities of daily life; AGC absolute granulocyte count; ANC, absolute neutrophil count; ARDS, adult respiratory distress syndrome; BMI, body mass index; BP, blood pressure; BSA body surface1 area; CHF, congestive heart failure; CHF, congestive heart failure; CNS, central nervous system; CVA, cerebral vascular accident; DAT, direct antiglobulin test; dB, decibels; DLCO, Carbon monoxide diffusion capacity; EF, ejection fraction; FEV_1, forced expiratory volume; HL, hearing loss; HUS, hemolytic uremic syndrome INR, International normalized ratio of prothrombin time; LLN, lower limit of normal; MMSE Mini-Mental Status Exam; pRBCs, packed red blood cells; PTT, partial thromboplastin time; RBC, red blood cells; SAS, subarachnoid space ; SF, shortening fraction; TPN, total parenteral nutrition; TTP, thrombotic thrombocytopenic purpura; TURP transurethral resection of the prostate; ULN, upper limit of normal; WBC, white blood cells; WNL, within normal limits.

C Blood Component Therapy

Despite the recent increase in the use of hematopoietic growth factors, transfusion therapy plays an important role in caring for oncology patients, particularly now that more effective treatment regimens have led to longer survivals. In many instances the patient with cancer behaves like a patient with a chronic disease requiring frequent blood components caused by disorders secondary to the disease and/or treatment. Whole blood is separated into cellular and non-cellular components including red cells, platelets, and plasms.

1. Blood component: A portion of blood is separated by physical and mechanical means, such as differential centrifugation (Fig. C-1). Cell separation technology, capable of collecting platelets, plasma, granulocytes, peripheral blood stem cells and red cells, has an increasingly important role in transfusion medicine. Anticoagulants and other additives used in blood collection containers allow storage of liquid red cells for up to 42 days.
   a. Packed red blood cells (RBCs): These cells are prepared from whole blood by centrifugation and subsequent removal of plasma.
      (1) Hematocrit: 60–80%
      (2) Indications
         (a) Replacement of hemoglobin-containing cells in an anemic patient with heart failure, renal failure, burns, or bone marrow failure
         (b) Debilitated patients
         (c) Elderly patients
         (d) Patients with liver disease
      (3) Recommend to use packed RBCs for losses of blood less than 1000–1500 ml/70 kg; with greater losses, whole blood probably should be used
      (4) Therapeutic effect: In a 70 kg adult, each unit should increase the hematocrit by 3–4%.
   b. Frozen RBCs: Long-term preservation of frozen RBCs without damage can be accomplished by the addition of glycerol; before transfusion, the RBCs should be thawed and washed to remove glycerol
      (1) Advantages
         (a) Blood of rare types can be stored for long periods
         (b) 2, 3-diphosphoglycerol and adenosine triphosphate levels remain the same as they were on the day that the blood was frozen
         (c) Free of plasma protein, platelets, white blood cells, and fibrin
         (d) Has been claimed to reduce the incidence of hepatitis acquired from a blood transfusion
      (2) Disadvantages
         (a) Expensive
         (b) Outdated in 24 hours
         (c) Takes time to thaw and deglycerolize
   c. Buffy coat: poor erythrocytes; would reduce the incidence of febrile transfusion reaction
      (1) Indication
         (a) Patients with repeated febrile non-hemolytic transfusion reaction caused by leukocyte antibody
   d. Platelet concentrates
      (1) One unit of platelet concentrate contains 5.5×10^{10} platelets suspended in 30–50 ml of plasma
      (2) Shelf-life: 72 hours at room temperature
      (3) Thrombocytopenia does not usually produce serious bleeding unless the platelet count is <20,000, except if there is a platelet function defect, a coagulation defect, or local cause of hemorrhage (e.g., trauma, surgery)
      (4) A patient who has undergone trauma or requires surgery probably needs a platelet count of $100{,}000/mm^3$ to maintain adequate hemostasis
      (5) One unit of platelet concentrate will increase the platelet count by $7000–10{,}000/mm^3$
      (6) Repeated platelet transfusion can lead to immunization to HLA antigen and a refractory state
      (7) Should be administered through a 170μm filter
   e. Fresh frozen plasma
      (1) Contains albumin, globulin, active coagulation factors, complement, and electrolytes
      (2) Should be type-specific
      (3) Shelf life: 12 months at –20–30°C; should be used within 2 hours after thawing
      (4) Indications
         (a) Deficiency in coagulation factors
         (b) Situation with plasma loss
         (c) Rapid reversal of oral anticoagulant therapy
   f. Cryoprecipitate: Cold insoluble precipitate remains when fresh frozen plasma is allowed to thaw at 4°C; it contains factor VIII with fibrinogen and factor XIII

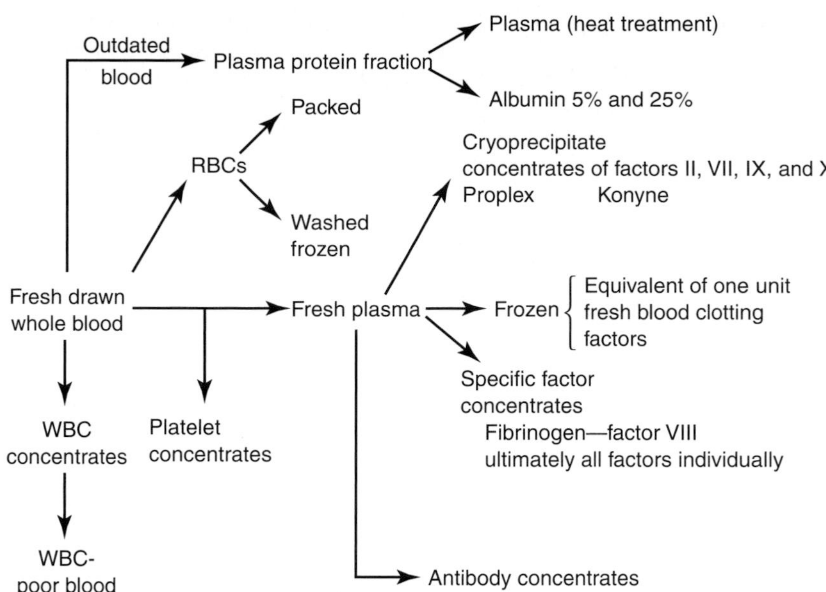

Figure C-1 Separation of a unit of whole blood into its various components.

   (1) Indications
      (a) von Willebrand disease
      (b) Replacement of fibrinogen, factor XIII

2. Plasma fraction: Derivatives of plasma are obtained by a chemical process, such as alcohol precipitation
   a. Coagulation factor concentrates
      (1) Factor VIII concentrates
      (2) Factor IX concentrates
      (3) Prothrombin complex (factor II, VII, IX, X concentrates)
      (4) Fibrinogen concentrates
   b. Immunoglobulin concentrates
   c. Albumin: Filtered and pasteurized by heating for 10 hours at 60°C to eliminate the risks of viral hepatitis
      (1) 5% albumin: isosmotic, sodium 145 mEq/L; for rapid expansion of vascular volume
      (2) 25% albumin: sodium 145 mEq/L; given intravenously; one volume of 25% albumin will draw about four volumes of additional fluid from the extravascular space into the circulation; used for treatment of hypoalbuminemia
   d. Plasma protein factor: 5% solution of selected human plasma protein in buffered saline solution; heat-treated to eliminate the risk of hepatitis; indicated for rapid expansion of vascular volume
3. Stroma-free hemoglobin solution
   a. Advantages
      (1) No need for blood typing
      (2) Longer storage capacity
      (3) Maintains better microcirculation
      (4) Potentially improved oxygenation of ischemic myocardium
      (5) No antigenicity
4. Autologous blood: The collection and reinfusion of the patient's own blood by preoperative autologous blood donation or intraoperative blood salvage. For autologous blood donation, the blood should be taken at least 2 weeks before the surgical procedure, and the patient must maintain a hemoglobin level of 11 g/dl or more. If large amounts of blood are required, frozen cells are another option. Many patients can donate as often as once a week. Intraoperative blood salvage requires the sterile collection and reinfusion of shed blood that is free of infecting agents such as malignant cells. The RBCs are collected in sterile plastic bags, washed, and concentrated before being reinfused into the patient.
5. Complications: Infection, transfusion reactions, and alloimmunization are the major complications associated with the transfusion of blood components (Table C-1).

Once in each 6000 units of blood transferred, an acute hemolytic reaction will occur with a mortality rate of 1:17. These reactions are usually due to ABO incompatibility and resultant intracellular hemolysis. Patients develop fever, chills, chest pain, nausea, hypotension, and disseminated intravascular coagulation. Mild reactions to leukocyte and platelet antigens are usually associated with a febrile episode alone. Hemolytic reactions to other blood groups such as Kidd, Duffy, and Kell can be associated with fever, anemia, hyperbilirubinemia, and a positive direct Coombs test. Some of these milder transfusions reactions manifest themselves 7–10 days after the transfusion.

Hematopoietic growth factors are designed to limit the exposure of oncology patients to blood and blood products.

Table C-1 RISK OF INFECTION

Agent risk	Unit
Hepatitis B	1:50,000
Hepatitis C	1:100,000
HIV	1:150,000–1:1,000,000
HTLV	1:50,000

HIV, human immunodeficiency virus; HTLV, human T cell lymphotropic virus
From ACOG, Technical Bulletin 199, Nov. 1994, and Management of Hepatitis C. NIH Consensus Statement Online 15(3):1, 1997.

The isolation and then synthesis of erythropoietin has been very helpful in limiting red cell transfusions. Granulocyte colony-stimulating factor (GCSF) has been proven to decrease infection rates in neutropenic patients after chemotherapy. The limitations of platelet transfusions have stimulated the research into agents that can stimulate platelet production and such products are now available. In addition, thrombopoietic growth factors have the potential to stimulate platelet apheresis donors and increase stem cell harvest yields; thus expanding progenitor cells.

BIBLIOGRAPHY

College of American Pathologists: Practice parameter for the use of fresh-frozen plasma, cryoprecipitate, and platelets. JAMA 271: 777, 1994.

Contreras, M: Consensus conference on platelet transfusion. Blood Rev 12:239, 1998.

Contreras, M: Diagnosis and treatment of patients refractory to platelet transfusions. Blood Rev 12:215, 1998.

Cumming PD, Wallace EL, Schorr JB, Dodd RY: Exposure of patients to human immunodeficiency virus through the transfusion of blood components that test antibody-negative. N Engl J Med 321:941, 1989.

Dodd RY: Will blood products be free of infectious agents? In Nanace SJ (ed): Transfusion Medicine in the 1990s. Arlington, VA, American Association of Blood Banks, 1990, p 223.

Klein, H: Standards for blood banks and transfusion services, 12th edn. Bethesda, MD, American Association of Blood Banks, 1996.

National Heart, Lungs, and Blood Institute. National Blood Resource Education Program Expert Panel: The use of autologous blood. JAMA 263:414, 1990.

Sazama K: Reports of 355 transfusion-associated deaths through 1985. Transfusion 30:583, 1990.

Stehling L, Simon TL: The red blood cell transfusion trigger: Physiology and clinical studies. Arch Pathol Lab Med 118:429, 1994.

Welch HG, Meehan KR, Goodnough LT: Prudent strategies for elective red blood cell transfusion. Ann Intern Med 116:393, 1992.

Winslow, RM: New transfusion strategies: red cell substitutes. Ann Rev Med 50:337, 1999.

D Suggested Recommendations for Routine Cancer Screening

CERVICAL CANCER

All women who are 3 years after the onset of vaginal intercourse, or no later than age 21 years should undergo an annual Papanicolaou (Pap) test and pelvic examination. ACOG recommends annual screening before age 30 years, then every 2–3 years if three consecutive tests are negative; however, Pap smears should be continued at least yearly in women with a history of in utero diethylstilbestrol (DES) exposure, human immunodeficiency virus (HIV), or immunosuppression. Pap smear screening can be stopped at age 70 years if the uterus is intact, three consecutive tests are negative, and there were no positive tests in the last 10 years. After a woman has had three or more consecutive, satisfactory annual examinations with normal findings, the Pap test may be performed less often at the discretion of her physician.

It is estimated that in the USA more than 90% of women 16 years of age or older have had at least one Pap test, and more than 60% have had a Pap test within 3 years. For the following reasons:

1. Cervical cancer has not been eradicated;
2. The incidence of cervical intraepithelial neoplasia (CIN) appears to have increased since the 1990s;
3. The Pap test has an appreciable false-negative rate; and
4. Women have a tendency to extend screening intervals; the proposed screening guidelines of annual cervical cytology for most women are prudent and warranted if early precursors to cervical cancer are to be detected and treated successfully.

BREAST CANCER

Mammography should be performed every 1–2 years for women 40–49 years of age and then annually thereafter.

Evidence from several studies indicates that there is a decrease in mortality for all women when appropriate screening by mammography is instituted and performed by qualified personnel. The efficacy of mammography is not in doubt. The question that remains is the optimal screening frequency, and the answer may be provided by data now being compiled. Safety is no longer a concern, but it is recognized that mammography is the most costly of all screening modalities. Dedicated equipment is essential, and considerable skill and experience are required to interpret the films. It is important, therefore, to determine the most prudent utilization of resources. Until the optimal screening frequency is determined, it appears reasonable to follow the recommendations of the American Cancer Society and the National Cancer Institute.

ENDOMETRIAL CANCER

Total population screening for endometrial cancer and its precursors is neither cost effective nor warranted. High-risk patients may require endometrial sampling.

The cost effectiveness of screening asymptomatic women for endometrial cancer and its precursors is very low; therefore, the practice is unwarranted. On the other hand, perimenopausal and postmenopausal women with a history or evidence of abnormal vaginal hemorrhage are at high risk for endometrial cancer, and their symptoms should be investigated by endometrial biopsy or curettage. Dilatation and curettage are recommended when endometrial hyperplasia or questionable endometrial carcinoma is present and when there is insufficient tissue for diagnosis by endometrial biopsy.

If estrogen-progestin therapy is instituted, endometrial biopsy is not required before treatment is begun unless there are reasons (e.g., abnormal bleeding) to place the patient at high risk for endometrial neoplasia. If unexpected breakthrough bleeding occurs during therapy, endometrial biopsy is recommended to rule out the development of abnormal endometrial histology. Endometrial biopsy by aspiration curettage performed in the office is diagnostically reliable and cost effective in symptomatic patients. The timing of further biopsies, if needed, is a clinical decision that should be based on previous histologic results and the patient's history.

OVARIAN CANCER

No available techniques are currently suitable for routine screening. Many different techniques, including peritoneal fluid profiles, investigation of tumor-associated antigens, and ultrasonography, have been or are being investigated as possible screening tools for ovarian cancer. To date, none of these techniques has proved to be practical or effective.

COLORECTAL CANCER

Beginning at 50 years of age, one of three screening options should be selected:

1. yearly fecal occult blood testing plus flexible sigmoidoscopy every 5 years;
2. colonoscopy every 10 years; or
3. double-contrast barium enema (DCBE) every 5–10 years.

A digital rectal examination should be performed at the time of each screening sigmoidoscopy, colonoscopy, or DCBE.

Available data do not substantiate the cost-effectiveness of various screening recommendations. Because colorectal cancer is a significant risk to women, the task force suggests that the recommendations of the American Cancer Society (ACOG) and the National Cancer Institute be used as a guide.

LUNG CANCER

No available techniques are currently suitable for routine screening. The only effective way to reduce mortality from lung cancer is to promote a "stop smoking" message to the public. Although some support is evolving for annual X-ray screening for those at risk (i.e., women 50 years and older who smoke more than one pack of cigarettes daily), neither the American Cancer Society nor the National Cancer Institute has adopted this guideline. This information is based on the ACOG Committee Opinion, No. 247, December 2000.

E Nutritional Therapy

In the cancer patient, malnutrition may appear simultaneously with the disease. Such an individual often exhibits anorexia because of decreased nutritional intake with resultant weight loss. There may be an increased nutritional requirement because of the increased demands of the patient and the tumor. Resting metabolic rates can vary greatly, but in as many as 60% of patients the rate may be elevated. The stage of malnutrition in the cancer patient can lead to cachexia with weakness and tissue wasting. The extent of malnutrition in the patient may be greater than can be explained by decreased nutritional intake. Metabolic abnormalities include an abnormal response to glucose tolerance testing, increased gluconeogenesis (which can result in decreased muscle protein synthesis), and abnormalities in protein and fat metabolism. A patient with a malignancy may need additional nutritional support while that patient undergoes intensive treatment, which can include surgery and chemotherapy. Parenteral nutrition seems to improve a patient's tolerance of the treatment and improves her nutritional state; however, parenteral nutrition has not been shown to improve survival.

The malnutrition seen in cancer patients is commonly referred to as cancer cachexia. Nutritional depletion is seen as a protein-calorie malnutrition with a loss of body cell mass. The importance of protein-calorie nutrition is its association with increases in postoperative complications, deficiencies in immune function and poorer tolerance of therapy.

Dietary nutrients required for good health include water, protein, fat, carbohydrates, vitamins, and minerals. Energy is required for normal body function, growth, and repair. Protein is necessary for growth and development to maintain body structures and function. It is the source of the essential amino acids and nitrogen needed for the synthesis of non-essential amino acids. Dietary protein replaces the essential amino acids and nitrogen that are lost through protein turnover and normal body functions. During illness, protein requirements increase. Nitrogen balance is essential for good health and requires intake of protein and energy. At higher energy intakes, less protein is needed to achieve nitrogen balance. Nitrogen is lost continuously in the body through normal body functions. Fat is the food substance with the highest concentration of calories.

Linoleic acid is the only essential fatty acid required in the diet; it is necessary for the synthesis of arachidonic acid, which is a major precursor of prostaglandin. Linoleic acid comes mainly from polyunsaturated vegetable oils. A deficiency of essential fatty acids results in poor wound healing, hair loss, and dermatitis. Fatty acids and cholesterol make up most of the fat in our diets. Carbohydrates include sugar, starch, and fibers. When carbohydrates are not included in the diet, ketosis begins to occur, and there is excessive breakdown of protein as amino acids are used for gluconeogenesis. Water-soluble and fat-soluble vitamins cannot be synthesized in adequate amounts by the body. Fat-soluble vitamins are required for absorption, transport, metabolism, and storage. They are not excreted in the urine like the water-soluble vitamins, and an excess accumulation can lead to well known toxic conditions. Major minerals, as well as trace elements, are important in human nutrition.

Lack of appetite with reduction in food intake is a key factor in cancer cachexia. The role of neurotransmitter serotonin appears to be central to appetite. Inhibition of serotonin increases appetite and food intake in animals. Cancer patients also report a loss of taste and smell with a resulting loss of appeal of most foods. Weight loss may also be greatly influenced by tumor location affecting the ability to take nutrition, e.g., a mass causing a partial bowel obstruction. Cytokines produced by the patient in response to a growing neoplasm may result in nutritional derangements. Cytokines can regulate appetite and metabolic rate so they can be very important factors. Dudrick suggests that patients who have a 10 lb weight loss or a 10% decrease in bodyweight 2 months prior to assessment, serum albumin <3.4 g/dl, anergy to 4 of 5 standard skin test antigens, and a low total lymphocyte count and who cannot or will not eat enough are candidates for nutritional assessment. Nutritional history, with a 24-hour dietary recall, can be used to assess nutritional intake. Anthropometric measurements are useful when assessing the patient's nutritional status. Relative bodyweight is probably the most useful of these measurements, because rapid weight loss is usually an indication of protein calorie undernutrition. The triceps skinfold test assesses fat stores, and mid-arm circumference tends to assess protein status. Edema, which is often seen with protein calorie deficiency, can mask true weight loss

Table E–1 TPN INDICATIONS
Severely malnourished patients undergoing surgery Patients with postoperative complications that require nutritional support Therapy-induced complications that require nutritional support

Note: Routine use of TPN in patients with cancer is *not* indicated.
TPN, total parenteral nutrition.

and muscle wasting. Serum albumin is probably the single most important test for determining protein calorie undernutrition. Albumin is the main plasma protein needed to maintain plasma osmotic pressure as well as other functions. In a patient with low albumin, morbidity and mortality are increased. Albumin can be influenced by conditions other than malnutrition and may be affected by hydration status. Transferrin binds and transports iron in the plasma and is a good indicator of protein nutritional status. The extent of malnutrition depends on the type and site of the cancer. Cancers, such as ovarian cancer with its potential effect on the gastrointestinal (GI) tract, appear to contribute to malnutrition to a greater degree than does cervical cancer. Malnutrition becomes worse, as expected, as the cancer progresses. The mechanism of cancer-related malnutrition is unknown. There are probably multiple contributing factors. Decreased food intake because of anorexia, early satiety, nausea, and vomiting can play a role. Poor absorption of nutrients can also be a contributing factor. Food aversion, particularly in patients undergoing chemotherapy or irradiation, is well known. Change of taste and smell can contribute to decreased intake. Generalized weakness may also contribute to decreased food intake. Decrease in total lymphocyte count (<1200) is also suggestive of malnutrition. Creatinine height index (CHI) may be helpful, because urinary creatinine excretion is proportional to total body muscle mass. As muscles become depleted, creatinine excretion falls. A CHI of ≥80% usually indicates a normal lean body mass. A CHI of 60–80% notes moderate depletion; a CHI of <60% indicates severe depletion.

The role of total parenteral nutrition (TPN) in the patient with cancer has yet to be determined. TPN can correct nutritional deficits that commonly occur in the cancer patient. TPN can also improve nitrogen balance and decrease catabolism. Glucose turnover and clearance rates are increased; gluconeogenesis is suppressed; and free fatty acid oxidation is increased. TPN can increase bodyweight and reverse serum markers of malnutrition; however, as an adjuvant to cancer therapy, the results have not been encouraging. TPN has not added to lean body mass or eliminated the GI or hematologic toxicity associated with chemotherapy. In patients treated with chemotherapy, response rates and survival have not been increased with TPN. Although irradiation can contribute to poor nutrition (e.g., diarrhea, enteritis, and malabsorption), particularly to the GI tract when gynecologic cancers are treated, TPN has not produced a significant improvement regarding treatment response, tolerance to treatment, local control, survival, or decreased complications of therapy. Nutritional support for the cancer patient requiring surgery is also ill defined. Malnourished patients undergoing surgery have a higher postoperative morbidity and mortality compared with well-nourished patients. Whether TPN can affect morbidity and mortality in the cancer patient is undetermined, and the concern that TPN may stimulate tumor growth is unfounded. Although routine use of TPN in the cancer patient is not warranted, it may be indicated in severely malnourished patients undergoing surgery or for those with postoperative complications. Nutritional supports are of two main types: enteric and parenteral. For the patient with a functional GI tract, enteric nutrition may be considered through the use of a nasoenteric tube. A gastrostomy or jejunostomy tube may also be used. Obviously, GI dysfunction is a contraindication to this method. Nevertheless, this method appears to be cost effective; it probably maintains the GI mucosa integrity, provides a normal sequence of intestinal and hepatic metabolism before systemic distribution, appears to preserve normal hormonal patterns, and avoids the risk of sepsis. Enteric solutions differ in composition, calorie content, and multiple other factors. These solutions are usually complete, because they contain a full supplement of nutrient requirements, or incomplete, when they are designated to contain a specific macronutrient such as fat, protein, or carbohydrate. Most solutions contain 1000 calories and 37–45 g/L of protein. Elemental diets consist mainly of amino acids and simple sugars. They are extremely hypertonic and may induce diarrhea. GI complications include diarrhea, which may be corrected with a formula of lower osmolarity. Electrolyte imbalance and glucose intolerance can also occur.

Many cancer patients who require nutritional supplementation will need TPN. In some cases, TPN can be administered through a peripheral vein, particularly if only a short amount of TPN is to be given. Although adequate protein can usually be infused peripherally, high caloric supplementation is usually given centrally. Fat solutions, which can account for a high caloric intake, can be given peripherally. A major complication of peripheral TPN is thrombophlebitis and infiltration. In most cases, TPN is given through a central vein—either the subclavian vein or a major neck vessel. The catheter can be inserted in the superior vena cava, which allows rapid infusion of hypertonic solutions without difficulty. Infusion of parenteral solution should be started slowly to prevent hyperglycemia. If glucose intolerance develops, a small amount of insulin is used to control blood sugars. Meticulous care must be taken of the central catheter, because this site can be a major source of infection. Frequent changing of IV tubing and filters and also the catheter is required routinely. TPN is usually managed as a team endeavor, with the attending physician, nutritionist, nurse, pharmacist, and dietitian. Daily requirements must be standardized regarding calories, proteins, fat, minerals, vitamins, and trace elements. These should be varied as the situation demands. Metabolic complications may include hyper- or hypoglycemia, hyperosmolarity, azotemia, hyperchloremic metabolic acidosis, mineral electrolyte disorder, liver enzyme elevations, and anemia. In many hospitals, standard hyperalimentation solutions with appropriate nutrients have been formulated, and adjustments are made for specific needs. Intense metabolic monitoring is required in these patients, and established hospital protocols are now available in many institutions.

Today, both enteric and parenteral nutritional support can be implemented successfully on an outpatient basis. Indications are not uniformly agreed on for this method of nutrition. In the cancer patient, nutritional support may be indicated to help satisfy nutritional needs while toxicity of treatment is abating. Most authorities do not believe that home nutritional support is needed for the terminally ill cancer patient.

A typical nutritional guideline for the adult patient follows. Many institutions have nutritional protocols in place. Although there may be variations on the theme, these guidelines have become relatively standardized.

Table E–2 NUTRITIONAL GUIDELINES FOR THE ADULT PATIENT

I. Daily protein needs

Maintenance	0.8–1 g/kg
Mild–moderate stress	1–1.5 g/kg
Moderate–severe stress	1.5–2 g/kg
Very high stress/burns	> 2 g/kg

II. Daily caloric needs

(consider initiating HAL with 50–75% of estimated patient needs on day 1)
Maintenance, mild stress 20–25 kcal/kg (15–20 NPC/kg)
Mild–moderate stress *(routine surgery, minor infection)* 25–30 kcal/kg (20–25 NPC/kg)
Moderate–severe stress *(major surgery, sepsis, tumor tx)* 30–35 kcal/kg (25–30 NPC/kg)

III. Body weight calculations

Total body weight (TBW) = patient's weight (kg)
Ideal body weight (IBW) (male) = 50 kg + (2.3 × no. of inches > 5 ft)
Ideal body weight (IBW) (female) = 45 kg + (2.3 × no. of inches > 5 ft)
Adjusted body weight (ABW) for the obese patient = IBW + 0.3 × (TBW – IBW)

IV. Suggested laboratory tests

Baseline and weekly: Chem 10, Chem 13
Daily: Chem 10 × 3 days or until stabilized prealbumin as clinically indicated

V. Formula

A. Standard formula

	Central	Peripheral ($D^{10}A_{3,6}$)
Amino acids (g)	55 mg/L	30 g/L
Dextrose (kcal)	555 kcal/L	280 kcal/L
Lipids (kcal)	400 kcal/L	350 kcal/L
NPC	955 NPC/L	630 NPC/L
Total kcal	1175 kcal/L	750 kcal/L
Desired total volume/day	________ ml*	________ ml*

B. Modified central formula

1. Protein:
   Daily protein needs × body weight calculations = ________ g protein/day
2. Non-protein calories (NPC):
   Daily caloric needs × body weight calculations = ________ NPC/day
3. Percentages of NPC:
   Usually 50–70% of daily NPC as CHO + usually 30–50% of daily NPC as fat = 100%
4. Infusion rate (see HAL bag for exact infusion rate)
   ☐ maximally concentrated[†] or ☐ infusion rate ________ mg/hr

VI.

Electrolytes	☐ Standard	☐ Modified	Acetate/Chloride
Sodium	80 mEq/L	________ mEq/L	________ balance
Potassium	40 mEq/L	________ mEq/L	________ maximum acetate
Calcium	5 mEq/L	________ mEq/L	________ maximum chloride
Magnesium	8 mEq/L	________ mEq/L	________ : ________ chloride : acetate

VII. Vitamins and trace elements

(MV1-12 and standard trace elements will automatically be added unless otherwise specified)
________ vitamin K 1 mg/day ________ No vitamin K

Continued

Table E–2 NUTRITIONAL GUIDELINES FOR THE ADULT PATIENT—cont'd

A. Content of MV1-12

vitamin A	3300 IU	vitamin B_5	15 mg
vitamin D	200 IU	vitamin B_6	4 mg
vitamin E	10 mg	vitamin B_{12}	5 mcg
vitamin B_1	3 mg	vitamin C	100 mg
vitamin B_2	3.6 mg	biotin	60 mcg
vitamin B_3	40 mg	folic acid	0.4 mg

B. Content of standard trace elements

chromium chloride	12 mcg
copper sulfate	1.2 mg
manganese sulfate	0.3 mg
zinc sulfate	3 mg

VIII. Other additives

_____ Humulin regular insulin _________ units/day
_____ H_2 antagonist _________ m/day
_____ Other (specify)

IX. Hyperalimentation access

_____ Central _____ Peripheral

X. Special instructions

*See HAL bag for exact infusion rate
?Calculation of volume of maximally concentrated HAL:
[1]Amino acid (AA): ______ protein/d × 10 ml/g AA = ______ ml 10% AA solution
[2]Dextrose: ______ NPC/day × ______% as CHO = ______ kcal CHO ÷ 3.4 kcal/g CHO = ______ g CHO × 1.43 ml/g = ______ ml D70
[3]Lipid: ______ NPC/day × ______% as fat = ______ kcal fat ÷ 2 kcal/ml = ______ ml 20% lipids
[4]Maximally concentrated volume = ______ (from 1 above) ml 10% AA+ ______ (from 2 above) ml D70+ ______ (from 3 above) ml 20% lipids = ______ ml/day
[5]Approximate infusion rate = ______ (from 4 above) ml/day ÷ 24 hr/day = ______ ml/hr *(Actual infusion rate may be altered by volume of additives; see HAL bag for exact infusion rate.)*
Courtesy of the nutritional and pharmacy divisions of the Medical University of South Carolina.

Additional therapies can also be considered along with nutrition support to alleviate cancer cachexia. Synthetic progestins (megestrol acetate and medroxyprogesterone acetate) in high doses decrease production of cytokines and serotonin and thus improve appetite and a sense of well-being. Responses often are seen in 15–30 days of therapy and side effects are minimal. Some authors have reported more thromboembolic events with megestrol acetate, but not in placebo controlled studies.

BIBLIOGRAPHY

Arbeit JM, Lees DE, Corsey R, Brennan MF: Resting energy expenditure in controls and cancer patients with localized and diffuse disease. Ann Surg 199:292, 1984.

Argiles JM, Lopez-Soriano FJ: the role of cytokines in cancer cachexia. Med Res Rev 19:223, 1999.

Baker JP, Detsky AS, Wesson DE et al: Nutritional assessment: A comparison of clinical judgment and objective measurements. N Engl J Med 306:969, 1982.

Bernstein LH, Leukardt-Fairfield CJ, Pleban W, Rudolph R: Usefulness of data on albumin and prealbumin concentrations in determining effectiveness of nutritional support. Clin Chem 35:271, 1989.

Brennan MF: Total parenteral nutrition in the cancer patient. N Engl J Med 305:375, 1981.

Flowers JF, Ryan JA, Gough JA: Catheter-related complications of total parenteral nutrition. In Fischer JE (ed): Total Parenteral Nutrition. Boston, Little, Brown, 1991.

Grant JP: Handbook of Total Parenteral Nutrition. Philadelphia, WB Saunders, 1980.

Grant JP, Cuter PB, Thurlow JT: Current techniques of nutritional assessment. Surg Clin North Am 61:437, 1981.

Harrison LE, Brennan MF: The role of total parenteral nutrition in the patient with cancer. Curr Probl Surg 10:833, 1995.

Kern KA, Norton JA: Cancer cachexia. J Parenter Enteral Nutr 12:286, 1988.

McGeer AJ, Detsky AS, O'Rourke K: Parenteral nutrition in patients receiving cancer chemotherapy. Ann Intern Med 110:734, 1989.

Mercadente S: Parenteral versus enteral nutrition in cancer patient practice. Supportive Care in Cancer 6:85, 1998.

Nelson KA, Walsh D, Sheehan FA: The cancer anorexia-cachexia syndrome. J Clin Oncol 12:213, 1994.

Sclafani LM, Brennan MF: Nutritional support in the cancer patient. In Fischer JE (ed): Total Parenteral Nutrition. Boston, Little, Brown, 1994.

Simons JP, Schols AM, Hoefnagels JM, et al: Effects of medroxyprogesterone acetate on food intake, body composition, and resting energy expenditure in patients with advanced, non-hormone sensitive cancer: a randomized, placebo-controlled trial. Cancer 82:553, 1998.

Smale BF, Mullen JL, Buzby GP, Rosato EF: The efficacy of nutritional assessment and support in cancer surgery. Cancer 47:2375, 1981.

Strang P: The effect of megestrol acetate on anorexia, weight loss and cachexia in cancer and AIDS patients. Anticancer Res 17:657, 1997.

Torosian MH, Mullen JL: Nutritional assessment. In Kaminski I, Mitchell V (eds): Hyperalimentation: A Guide for Clinicians. New York, Marcel Dekker, 1985.

F Basic Principles in Gynecologic Radiotherapy

Catheryn M. Yashar, M.D.

A basic understanding of the principles of radiation oncology is essential to the Gynecologic Oncologist. Radiation therapy is used in the curative treatment of locoregionally advanced cervical and vaginal carcinoma. It is often an adjuvant therapy prescribed for uterine or vulvar carcinoma and in inoperable patients may be the only definitive therapy available. Lastly, it can be used for the palliative treatment of gynecologic carcinomas.

INTRODUCTION TO ELECTROMAGNETIC RADIATION

Radiant energy or radiation is an essential component of life on earth. For example, sunlight provides heat, light, and energy for plant photosynthesis and radio waves provide a method of communication. This electromagnetic radiation physically consists of photons, or "packets" of energy without mass or charge. The primary difference between the radiations is the energy of the photons. The energy is proportional to frequency ($E = h\nu$ where h is Planck's constant and ν is frequency) and inversely proportional to wavelength (Table F–1). A common analogy is to compare wavelength with the length of a person's stride when walking; the number of strides per minute is the frequency of the wave.

Photons, a non-particulate radiation, are only one form of radiation. Another form of radiation is particulate radiation. Particulate radiation consists of subatomic particles such as electrons, protons, α particles, and neutrons.

Radiation is not harmful in ordinary quantities and is actually helpful to life processes. In fact, exposure to radiation is a constant phenomenon (Tables F–2, F–3). However, high energy, or "ionizing" radiation, is not entirely harmless, although it is commonly used for both diagnostic and therapeutic purposes. High-energy radiation can be injurious to biologic material, and its use in oncology depends on the ability of normal tissue to recover from the effects more effectively or efficiently than malignant tissue. Radiation causes both reversible and irreversible changes in normal tissue and these effects are placed into two categories, acute effects (apparent during or shortly after the radiation course) and long-term effects (apparent from 6 months to years after completion of therapy). Radiation effects may not be initially apparent except by careful chemical or microscopic study. Indeed, the effects may not be apparent for many years or may manifest only in the offspring of the irradiated organism. The accepted position regarding radiation exposure is that incidental environmental radiation, diagnostic tests, and therapeutic radiation can all be detrimental. Although in many cases the chance of injury from diagnostic or environmental radiation is slight, the possibility of damage from a known exposure must always be weighed against the importance of the information to be gained or the effect desired. Incidental exposure must be avoided through control of environmental hazards whenever possible by following the ALARA principle (*A*s *L*ow *A*s *R*easonably *A*chievable).

There are many forms and sources of radiation, including natural isotopes and manmade radiations. The natural radiation emissions (gamma and beta rays) of isotopes such as iridium, iodine, and cesium are used for therapeutic purposes in many human malignancies (Table F–4). In addition, during the past four decades increasingly sophisticated machines have been manufactured to produce high intensity, directed radiation to treat both malignant and benign conditions. Modern machines emit energies greater than 1 million electron volts (1 MeV) and are termed supervoltage or megavoltage machines. (Table F–5). The most commonly available are called linear accelerators (linacs). Even these have recently become more sophisticated to allow increasingly precise delivery of radiation in the form of *I*ntensity *M*odulated *R*adiation *T*herapy (IMRT). The newest generation models allow for real-time computed tomography for position verification. The acceleration in technology has paralleled the advances in computer technology. Newer models that combine radiation delivery planning with positron emission tomography (PET) and magnetic resonance imaging (MRI) are currently under development.

Radiation units

Those in training and in practice must familiarize themselves with the international system (SI) of weights and measures used today. The SI units and appropriate conversions are shown in Table F–6.

Table F–1 ELECTROMAGNETIC SPECTRUM

	Wavelength (m)	Frequency (Hz)	Energy (J)
Radio	$> 1 \times 10^{-1}$	$< 3 \times 10^{9}$	$< 2 \times 10^{-24}$
Microwave	1×10^{-3}–1×10^{-1}	3×10^{9}–3×10^{11}	2×10^{-24}–2×10^{-22}
Infrared	7×10^{-7}–1×10^{-3}	3×10^{11}–4×10^{14}	2×10^{-22}–3×10^{-19}
Visible	4×10^{-7}–7×10^{-7}	4×10^{14}–7.5×10^{14}	3×10^{-19}–5×10^{-19}
Ultraviolet	1×10^{-8}–4×10^{-7}	7.5×10^{14}–3×10^{16}	5×10^{-19}–2×10^{-17}
X-ray	1×10^{-11}–1×10^{-8}	3×10^{16}–3×10^{19}	2×10^{-17}–2×10^{-14}
Gamma ray	$< 1 \times 10^{-11}$	$> 3 \times 10^{19}$	$> 2 \times 10^{-14}$

Table F–2 GENERAL POPULATION RADIATION EXPOSURE

Radiation source	Average annual whole body dose (millirem/year)
Natural: Cosmic	29
Terrestrial	29
Radon	200
Internal (^{40}K, ^{14}C, etc.)	40
Manmade (diagnostic X-ray, nuclear medicine, consumer products such as smoke detectors)	64
All others (fallout, air travel, occupational)	2
Average annual total	360 mrem/year
Tobacco smokers add ~280 mrem	

Table F–3 RADIATION ASSOCIATED WITH COMMON ACTIVITIES

Activity	Typical radiation dose
Smoking	280 mrem/year
CXR	8mrem/single x-ray
Drinking water	5mrem/year
Cross country airplane trip	5mrem/year

When a radiation exposure occurs, the resultant ionizations deposit energy in the air. If a patient lies in the path of the beam, energy will be deposited in the patient. This deposition of energy by radiation exposure is called *r*adiation-*a*bsorbed *d*ose measured in the acronym rad. One rad is equivalent to depositing 100 ergs of energy in each gram of the irradiated object. The SI unit of *r*adiation *a*bsorbed *d*ose is the gray (Gy), and 1 Gy = 1 cGy =100 rads = 1 joule/kg. The erg and joule are units of energy.

RADIATION PHYSICS

Energy deposition

Radiation energy is deposited into the tissue in one of two ways, direct or indirect ionization. Ionization is when an outer shell electron is stripped from an atom leaving a positive charge. Direct ionization is the predominant mechanism of action of particles that possess charge, but photons can also cause direct ionization. Examples of directly ionizing particles include particulate radiation such as protons and neutrons. Indirect ionization produces free radicals of other molecules, namely water, which diffuse and damage critical targets (Fig. F–1). A free radical has an unpaired outer shell electron that is chemically unstable and very reactive. The hydroxyl free radical (made by the lysis of H_2O) diffuses only about 1 nm and breaks the chemical bonds in cellular proteins and other key substances such as DNA. Either form of energy deposition results in ionization of target molecules. Scientists estimate that about two-thirds of cell biologic damage is from indirect action by ionizing radiation, from sources such as X-rays or gamma rays.

The electrons generated by penetrating photons lose their energy slowly, resulting in a low energy deposition along the electron track, or low linear energy transfer (LET—defined as energy transferred per unit length of track—keV/µm). High LET radiations (neutrons, negative pi mesons, or α particles) deposit more energy per unit length, are more commonly directly ionizing, and are less susceptible to perturbations such as oxygen tension. This means that for the same reaction produced in healthy cells by all radiation modalities, high LET radiation has a higher probability (1.5 to 2.5 times that of X-rays) of killing those cells in less than ideal circumstances, i.e. hypoxic tumor cells, cells in a resistant part of the cell cycle, etc.

Sources of radiation

Gamma rays are the photons emitted from the atomic nuclear decay of radioactive isotopes, e.g., ^{137}Cs (cesium), ^{60}Co (cobalt). *X-rays* are photons electrically generated by bombarding a target such as tungsten with electrons (how a linear accelerator works). When these fast-moving electrons approach the tungsten nuclear field, they are attracted to the nucleus and thus veer from their original path. This change in direction causes deceleration and kinetic energy is converted to X-rays in the form of bremsstrahlung photons. These emitted X-rays, or photons, vary in energy from zero to a maximum determined by the kinetic energy of the bombarding electrons. Machines such as the beta-

Table F–4 RADIOACTIVE ISOTOPES USED IN RADIATION ONCOLOGY

Element	Isotope	E_{max} (MeV)	$T_{1/2}$	Clinical use
Radium	^{236}Ra	3.26	1600 y	Historical
Cesium	^{137}Cs	0.514, 1.17	30 y	Temporary intracavitary implants
Iridium	^{192}Ir	0.38_{ave}	74.2 d	Temporary interstitial implants and source for high-dose-rate machine
Iodine	^{125}I	0.028_{ave}	60.2 d	Permanent interstitial implants
Phosphorus	^{32}P	none	14.3 d	Permanent intracavitary placement

Table F–5 MODALITIES OF EXTERNAL RADIATION

Modality	Voltage	Source
Low voltage (superficial)	85–150 keV	X-ray
Medium voltage (orthovoltage)	180–400 keV	X-Ray
Supervoltage	500 keV–8 MeV	Linear accelerator, ^{60}Co machine
Megavoltage	Above supervoltage energy	Betatron, linear accelerator

Table F–6 HISTORICAL AND SI UNITS OF RADIATION

Quantity	Historical unit	SI unit	Conversion factor
Exposure	R	C/kg	2.58×10^{-4} C/kg/R
Absorbed dose	Rad	Gray (Gy)	10^{-2} Gy/rad
Dose equivalent (used in radiation protection)	Rem	Sievert (Sv)	10^{-2} Sv/rem
Activity	Curie (Ci)	Becquerel (Bq)	3.7×10^{10} Bq/Ci

tron and linear accelerator generate electrons with high kinetic energy, and thus produce high-energy X-rays. In addition to bremsstrahlung photons, characteristic photons are also produced as atoms seek to fill electron orbital vacancies (see later discussion). Gamma rays and X-rays can be collectively called *photons*, and what is of medical importance is the energy and delivery of the photon, not the source.

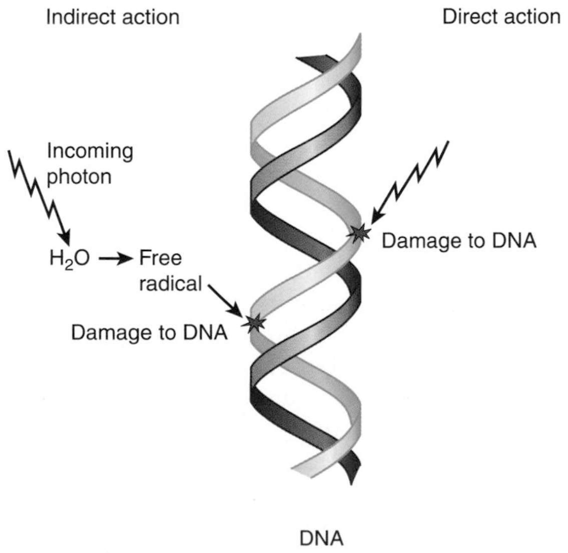

Figure F–1 Direct and indirect actions of radiation. DNA, the most lethal target of radiation, is schematically shown in the center. In direct action the incident photon displaces an electron from the target (DNA) molecule. In indirect action, another molecule, such as water, is ionized and the displaced electron diffuses to the target and damages the DNA.

Photon interactions

The interaction of photons with matter is accomplished through six mechanisms:

1. Compton scattering;
2. photoelectric absorption;
3. pair production;
4. triplet production;
5. photodisintegration; and
6. coherent scattering (no energy transfer).

The Compton effect is the major interaction of photons in tissue used in modern radiotherapy (Fig. F–2). When the photon from the linear accelerator interacts with outer orbital atomic electrons, part of the photon energy transfers to the electron as kinetic energy. The photon is deflected with reduced energy. The ejected electron is propelled forward and sets up a cascade of increasing energy deposition by displacing more electrons. As a result of this initiation and subsequent *buildup effect*, megavoltage photon beams have a skin-sparing effect not seen in older machines and therefore produce less superficial tissue change.

The photoelectric effect is seen at lower energies. This effect is the most important in diagnostic radiology. In this

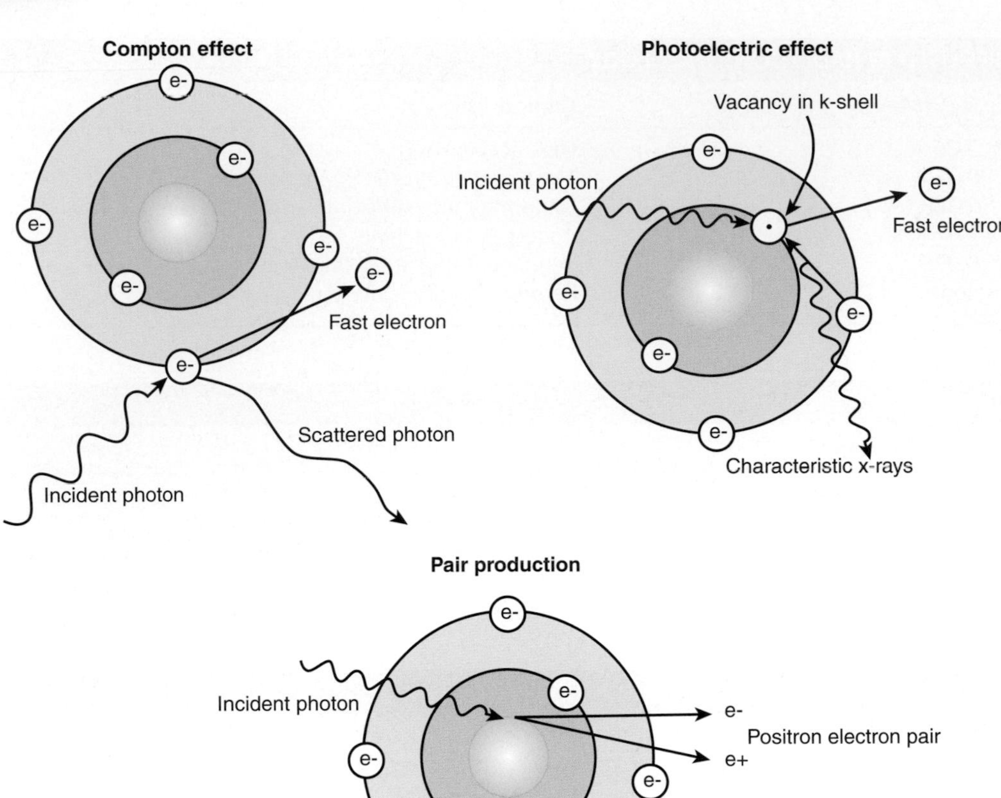

Figure F–2 The major photons interactions important in therapeutic and diagnostic radiation oncology.

interaction, the incident photon is absorbed completely by an inner shell electron. The inner shell electron is ejected with kinetic energy equal to the incident photon energy less the electron-binding energy. An outer shell electron then drops into the vacancy. As this electron changes orbit its energy is reduced and the excess energy is given off in the form a photon, called a "characteristic photon".

In pair production, photon energies >1.02 MeV interact with the strong electric field of the nucleus, and lose all incident energy. The incident photon energy is converted into matter in the form of a positron-electron pair. If this happens in the field of an orbital electron, three particles are produced in the interaction and the interaction is called triplet production.

Lastly, in photodisintegration the high energy photon enters the nucleus and ejects a neutron, proton, or alpha particle. This is important for shielding considerations in linear accelerators that operate at energies above 15 MeV.

Radioactive decay

Naturally radioactive substances decay to more stable substances by several methods:

1. beta decay (^{32}P, ^{18}F);
2. electron capture (^{125}I);
3. alpha decay (^{226}Ra); and
4. isomeric transition (gamma emission and internal conversion).

"Decay" is the manner in which an isotope releases, or gains, matter and/or energy to become a more stable substance. The rate of decay of a radionuclide is exponential and is termed the "activity." The old unit for activity was the Curie (Ci). The SI unit is the becquerel (Bq) defined by 1 Bq=1dps (disintegration per second). The half-life ($T^{1/2}$) is the time required to disintegrate to half the original activity. $T^{1/2}$ of commonly used radioactive substances are in Table F–4.

^{137}Cs (cesium-137), used in low dose rate applications, is a byproduct of the fission process in a nuclear reactor and decays via beta and gamma emission. In beta decay a neutron from the nucleus converts into a proton (positively charged) and an electron. Again, to increase stability a photon is released and the ^{137}Cs becomes the more stable ^{137}Ba. (Fig. F–3). ^{137}Cs decays approximately 2% per year.

^{192}Ir (Iridium 192) is also produced in a nuclear reactor and decays via beta decay (see above) and electron capture. In electron capture the nucleus "captures" an orbital electron and converts a proton into a neutron. ^{192}Ir then becomes the excitable ^{192m}Pt and ^{192m}Os, which release gamma rays to stabilize. ^{192}Ir is the primary isotope used for high dose rate applications and interstitial implants. It decays approximately 1% per day.

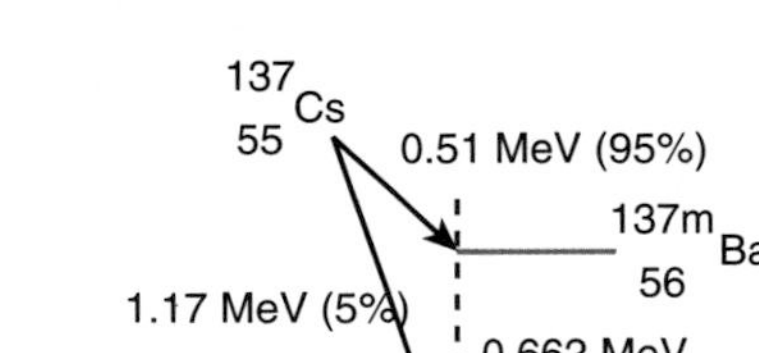

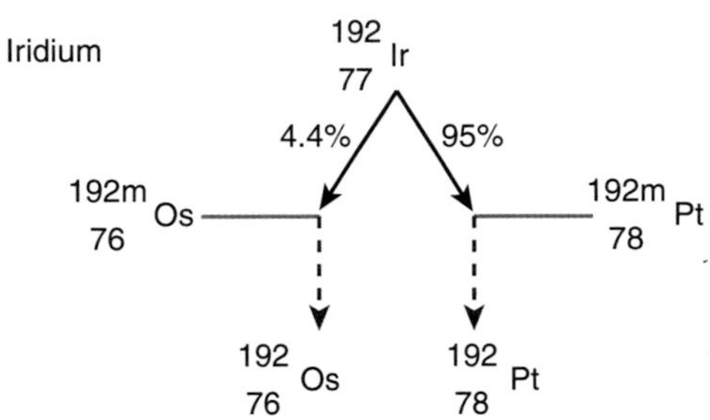

Figure F–3 Decay diagrams of ^{137}Cs and ^{192}Ir.

Inverse square law

Another important physics concept in radiotherapy is the inverse square law. This law states that the dose of radiation at a given point is inversely proportional to the square of the distance from the source of radiation (dose $\propto$/distance^2). This rapid fall off in dose is very important in brachytherapy. It underscores why the bladder and rectum can be relatively protected from the high intracavitary doses of radiation—especially with good vaginal packing to maximize the distance from the source to the normal organ. It also underscores why good geometry is critical when performing implants. Lastly, it explains the reasoning behind standing at the door (increasing the distance) while conversing with a brachytherapy patient. As a simplistic example, consider the following. The dose at point A is 4. Two feet away the dose would be 4 divided by the square of the distance (2^2) or $4/4 = 1$. Another two feet away the dose would be 1/4 ($4/4^2 = 4/16 = 1/4$).

Depth dose characteristics of radiation

The last physics concept to master is variation in radiation beam characteristics based on energy. To that end it is important to realize that the energy and penetrating power of ionizing radiation increase as the photon frequency increases and wavelength decreases. In addition, as energy increases, the depth of maximum dose increases (D_{max}—remember the *buildup effect* discussed earlier). For low energies, such as 250 keV, the maximum dose is at the skin surface. For a 4 MeV (4 million electron volts) accelerator the D_{max} is approximately 1 cm, for 6 MeV D_{max} is at 1.5 cm, and 22 MeV D_{max} at 3.5 cm, etc. Knowing this, one can see why higher energy beams are more suited to treat deeply seated tumors, such as uterine or cervix. These higher energy beams will differentially spare more superficial tissues. Depth of maximum dose curves and isodose distributions (areas receiving similar dose) for various energies are shown in Fig. F–4.

The reduced effect on skin of supervoltage radiation, compared with orthovoltage (keV range) radiation, is based on a physical characteristic of radiation. With higher energy, forward movement of the energy cascade (in the direction of the primary beam) is greater with reduced lateral scattering. As the energy increases, it becomes more penetrating and the photons and resultant liberated electrons travel a greater distance into the absorbing material. Therefore, the percentage of radiation at any specific depth, compared with the surface dose, increases as the energy increases.

In summary, above the energy of 400–800 keV, the advantages to higher energy photons are less damage to the skin at the portal of entry, greater radiation at depth relative to the surface, and reduced lateral scatter of radiation in the tissues. In addition, there is less photoelectric effect at higher energies, and therefore less absorption in bone.

RADIOBIOLOGY

The selective destruction of tissues forms the basis of therapeutic radiation. Neoplastic cells are preferentially killed by radiation compared to the surrounding normal tissues, primarily due to differences in repair capabilities. This differential radiosensitivity between normal and cancerous tissues determines in large part whether a radiated neoplasm is eradicated. The ratio that defines the dose necessary to effect tumor kill with the dose likely to cause normal tissue damage is the therapeutic ratio and modern radiotherapy is striving to maximize this ratio (Fig. F–5).

Structural changes

Deposition of radiation energy in the cell can lead to a variety of changes that alter normal function. Degradation, or breaking into smaller units, and crosslinking are examples of structural damage that can affect proteins, enzymes, and nucleic acids. The initial chemical change occurs in a fraction of a second and is rarely detected directly. Some changes are repaired almost immediately, whereas others can never be repaired. Although various morphologic and functional changes occur in irradiated cells, the bulk of direct and indirect evidence suggests that the biologic effects of radiation result principally from DNA damage. For example, it has been calculated that 1 million cGy are required to inactivate cell cytoplasmic enzyme systems, and doses of 1000 cGy are required to damage cell membranes. In contrast, chromosomal aberrations and mutations can be produced by very low doses of radiation. Because only a few hundred cGy are needed to produce a high degree of lethality in cell tissue culture, it seems logical that nuclear changes are responsible for cell death.

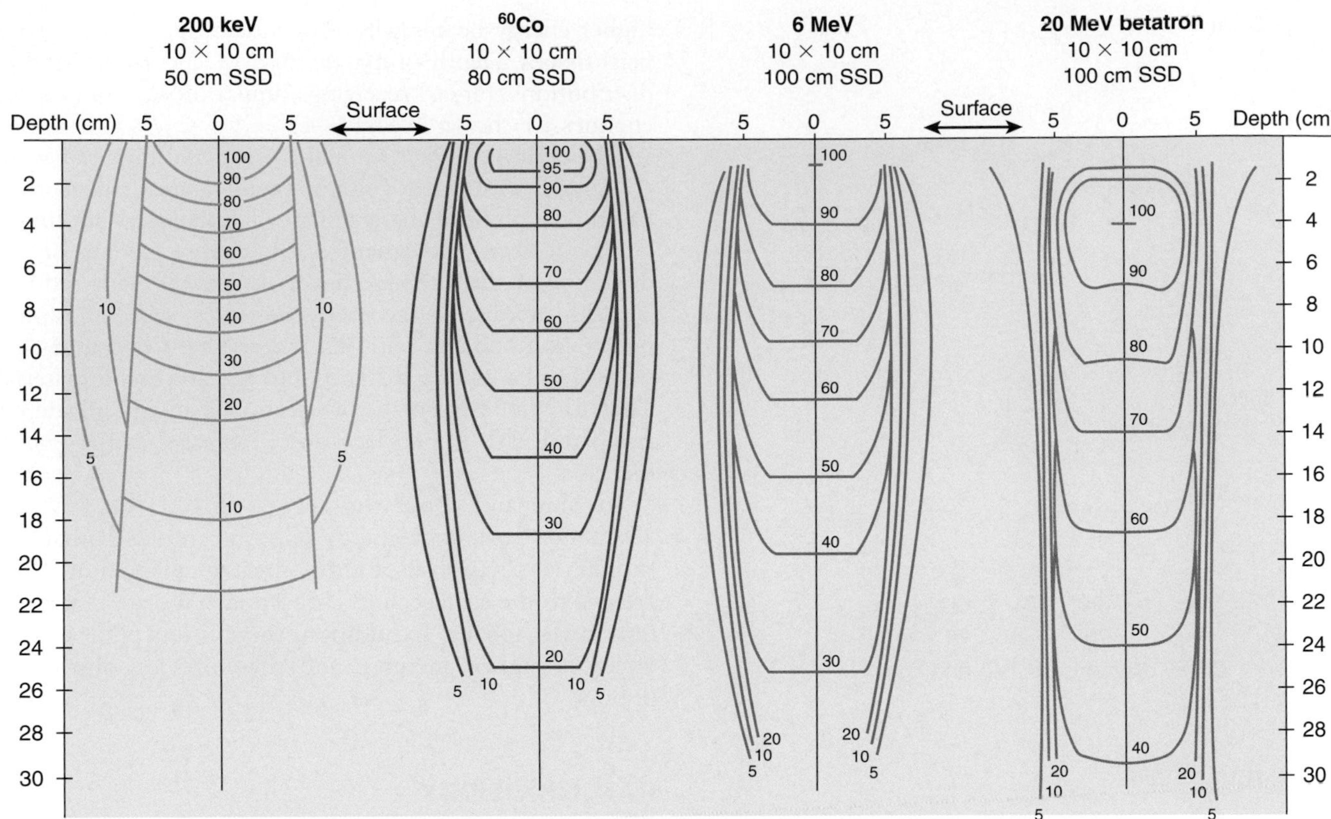

Figure F–4 Comparison isodose curves and depth-dose distribution through a single field. Each machine is delivering photons of different energies. Note that higher-energy machines deliver radiation to a greater depth for the same surface dose. Note also the skin sparing with 6 MV and 20 MV equipment. Lastly, note the difference in lateral scattering—higher energy photons are more "forward-moving" with less lateral scatter.

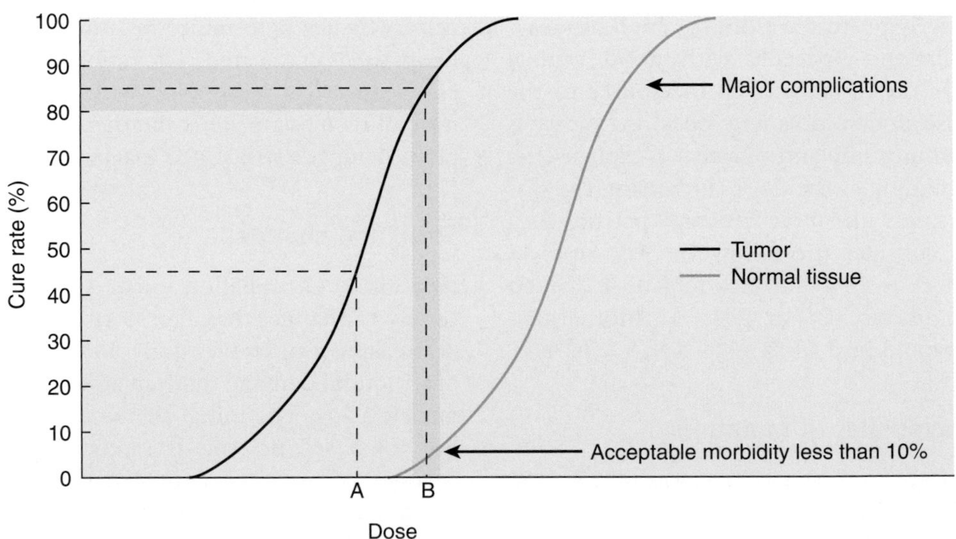

Figure F–5 Therapeutic ratio. Diagrammatic representation of a parallel tumor response and normal tissue tolerance curve demonstrating the relationship between increasing dose, increasing cure rate, and increasing morbidity. Under ideal circumstances *(B)*, an 80–90% cure rate can be achieved with 5–10% morbidity. Pushing the cure rate carries with it an increase in morbidity. On the other hand, attempts to avoid all morbidity *(A)* significantly reduce the ability to cure. Although the shape of these curves varies for various tumor types and dose rates, general concepts are valid whenever radiotherapy is used to treat malignant lesions.

Radiation-induced DNA damage destroys the cell by one of several mechanisms. It may stimulate cell apoptosis, called interphase death, which is visible by several methods including light microscopy and Western blot. Radiation may also cause mitotic death. In this form of damage the cell outwardly appears normal, but is sufficiently damaged that cell division is not possible. Actual death of the cell does not occur, however, until cell division is attempted.

This is why tumors may continue to regress after completion of radiation.

A variety of DNA lesions are produced by radiation including base damage, DNA-protein crosslinking, single strand breaks, and double strand breaks. Repairing even a single nucleotide requires many genes and a series of steps. The most toxic cellular lesion inflicted by ionizing radiation is the double strand break (DSB). In fact, the proficiency of repair of DSB correlates well with radiation-induced lethality. The repair of DSB can occur by several mechanisms. Religation of complementary DSB ends, homologous recombination (HR), is efficient and cells can usually survive. The Mre11 protein is attracted when a DSB occurs and may be the first sensor of the break as well as primarily involved in repair through nuclease activity, unwinding DNA, or removing hairpin loops. When the ends are not complementary, non-homologous end joining (NHEJ) is used and can be complicated by small DNA deletions or insertions. These errors in turn can lead to cell death or mutation. Some of the necessary proteins for NHEJ are Ku70, Ku80, DNA ligase IV, and XRCC4. The Ku70/Ku80 complex binds to the DSB and unwinds the strand while the DNA ligase IV/XRCC4 complex repairs DSBs. Mammalian cells seem to repair more by NHEJ than HR.

Radiosensitivity

Radiosensitivity is the response of the tumor to irradiation that can be measured by the extent of regression, rapidity of response, and response durability. Radiosensitivity depends on several factors. These factors include the ability to repair damage, hypoxia, cell cycle position, and growth fraction. In addition, volume of initial tumor has been demonstrated to influence the ability to eradicate tumors.

Understanding that radiosensitivity and radiocurability are not identical in meaning is essential. Relatively radioresistant tumors accessible to high-dose local radiation therapy can be cured, whereas radiosensitive tumors that are widely metastatic can only be controlled locally. An excellent example of a relatively radioresistant tumor is squamous cell carcinoma of the cervix; however, this malignancy remains one of the most curable tumors in humans because of its accessibility to high-dose irradiation and the relatively radioresistant nature of the hosting normal tissues (e.g., cervix and vagina). The ability to place radium or cesium in juxtaposition to the malignancy within dose ranges tolerable to the surrounding normal tissue is the key to success.

Many attempts have been made to develop an assay to predict tumor radiosensitivity. However, no assay yet developed accurately predicts the outcome in a given tumor. This is likely secondary to tumors containing mixed cell populations with differing sensitivities to chemotherapy and radiation. Sensitive cells are eliminated, whereas resistant cells continue to grow. This explains why many tumors initially respond to therapy but are ultimately incurable.

In vitro models have been developed to predict and study tumor cell radiosensitivity. Cellular radiosensitivity is generally quantified by measuring the loss of reproductive capacity, which can be plotted in a survival curve. Survival curves are characterized by an initial slope, α, and the terminal slope, β. Alpha (α) represents irreparable damage to the cell while β represents the repairable damage (Fig. F–6). The α/β ratio is the dose where the contribution from alpha equals the contribution from beta and is a measure of radiosensitivity. Large ratios are seen with rapidly dividing cells and help predict the response of tumors and the early effects of radiation. Low ratios characterize late responding tissues.

In addition, the size of the shoulder (Dq) on a survival curve relays valuable information as it represents the magnitude of repair of sublethal damage (SLD). Broad shoulders have small α/β ratios and good repair of SLD. This repair of sublethal damage takes several hours (2–6 hours) to complete. The ability of cells to repair SLD forms the basis for the use of fractionated doses in clinical radiation therapy, in which differential capacities between normal tissue and tumor to repair a sublethal injury can be exploited (Fig. F–7). This differential repair capacity also forms the basis for accelerated fractionation or hyperfractionation where dose is given twice a day. This approach works very well with rapidly growing tumors. Treated twice a day, the normal tissues have sufficient time to repair but the tumor tissues, less organized, efficient and accurate, are differentially killed. Some cells have almost no shoulder, indicating a limited ability to repair sublethal damage, and these cells can be eradicated with relatively low doses of radiation. For example dysgerminomas are highly curable with relatively low doses of radiation (20–30 Gy) compared with cervical cancer tumors, which may require > 70 Gy to obtain cure.

The availability of oxygen is of vital importance to the radiosensitivity of the cell, as well. As radiation enters the cell, it interacts with organic molecules (DNA). This molecule may repair itself unless an oxygen molecule becomes attached thereby "fixing" the damage. The addition of O_2 will enhance low LET radiation (photons) but does not similarly affect high LET radiation. The ability of oxygen to enhance radiation is measured by the oxygen enhancement ration, OER (OER= dose of XRT without O_2 for a given effect/dose of XRT with O_2 for the same effect). It takes at least 2% (17mm Hg) tissue O_2 to see the full oxygen effect.

Tumor cells with potentially unlimited capacity for growth are limited as they outgrow the blood supply. In fact, tumors above 200 μm have necrotic cores secondary to a limited diffusion distance for oxygen. Oxygen may effectively penetrate approximately 70 μm from the blood vessel (Fig. F-8). Outside this distance, tumor cells become deficient and enter a non-cycling phase. They may become hypoxic or even anoxic and necrotic. This is important from a radiobiologic standpoint, because non-cycling cells exhibit a greater capacity to repair radiation injury. Hypoxic cells are more resistant to the effects of radiation

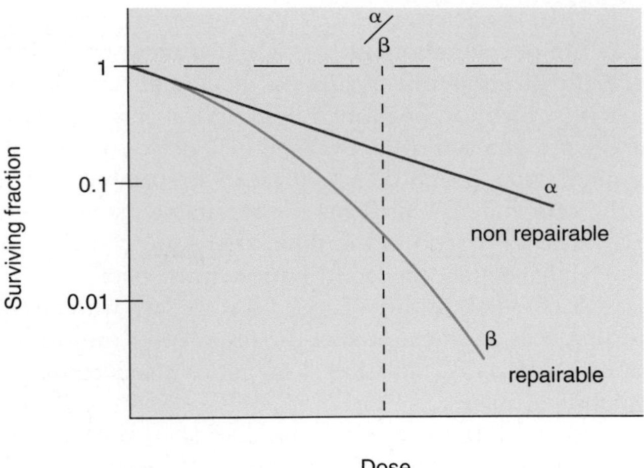

Figure F–6 Cell survival curve. The initial slope, α, represents irrepairable damage while the terminal slope, β, represents repairable damage. The α/β ratio is the point on the curve where the two are equal.

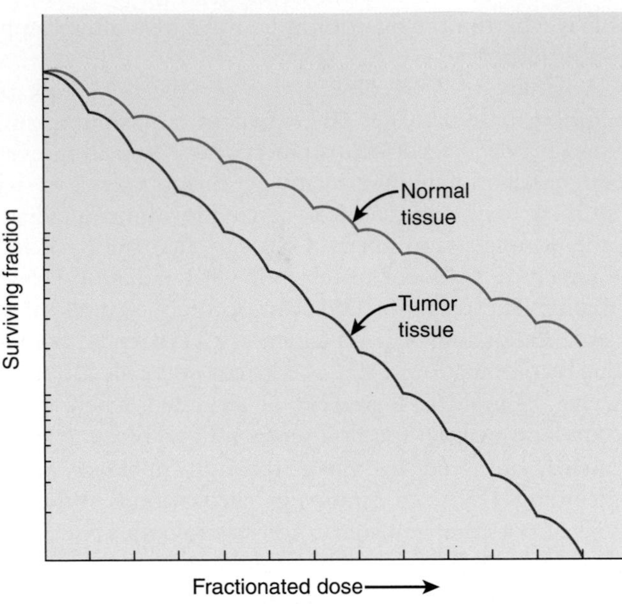

Figure F–7 Different capacities between normal tissue and tumor to accumulate and repair sublethal injury from fractionated doses result in differential survival. The normal tissue is able to repair more efficiently and effectively.

than are cells with normal oxygen tension. Thus, large tumors can be difficult to control with radiation therapy, not only because there is a greater number of cells to sterilize but also because a proportion of these cells are hypoxic, non-cycling, and radioresistant. As a clinical example, experience notes that exophytic friable cervical lesions that hemorrhage easily on contact respond better and more quickly than infiltrative lesions. The blood supply and oxygenation varies considerably between these two lesions, with the friable lesion better vascularized and oxygenated, and therefore more radiosensitive. Unfortunately attempts to overcome this differential sensitivity by mechanisms such as hyperbaric oxygen and radiosensitizers have been less than optimal to date.

Another factor important in radiosensitivity is the proportion of mitotic, or clonogenic cells in the tumor. Cycling cells are more radiosensitive. In fact, mitotic counts have been shown to correlate with the prognosis in many tumors. The position in the cell cycle is also important (Fig. F–9). Cells in late G2 and mitosis (M-phase) are the most sensitive to radiation and cells in late synthesis (S-phase) are the most resistant (Fig. F–10). This is exploited with chemotherapies such as paclitaxel, which arrests cells in mitosis and is a profound radiation sensitizer.

Finally, the initial tumor volume greatly influences the ability to sterilize a site. Generally, the smaller the tumor volume, the less radiation is required to destroy all cells. As the volume increases, the dose to obtain local control is increased. The concept of treating with "shrinking" fields is to serially reduce the size of the radiation portals to give a higher dose of radiation therapy to the central portion of the tumor where presumably more hypoxic, radioresistant cells are present.

Historically, clinicians attempted to correlate radiation tumor response and local tumor control. Generally, the

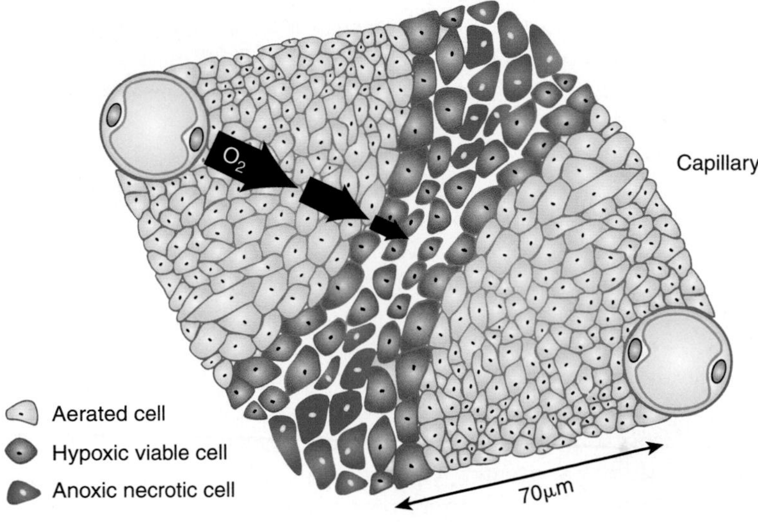

Figure F–8 As distance from blood supply increases, cells become hypoxic and even anoxic. Hypoxic cells are more radioresistant and, therefore, harder to sterilize. Oxygen diffuses about 70 μm from the capillary.

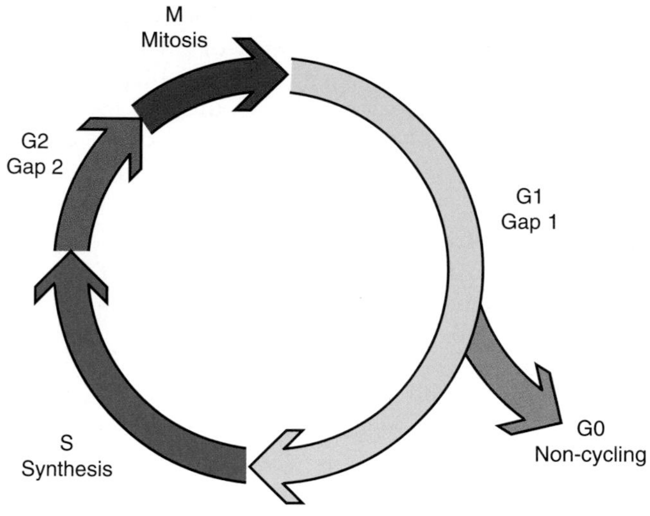

Figure F–9 Cell cycle.

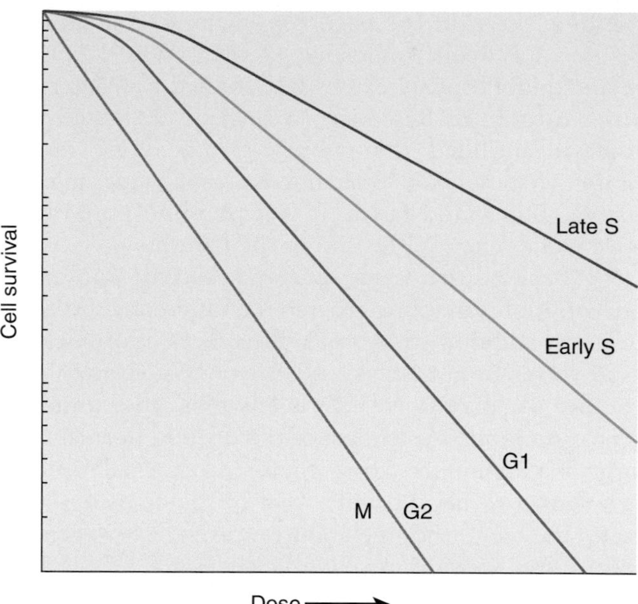

Figure F–10 The survival curve for cells in mitosis and G2 is steep and has no shoulder. The curve for cells late in S phase is shallower and has a large shoulder. G1 and early S are intermediate in sensitivity.

faster and more complete the tumor response at the completion of the therapy, the greater long-term control, assuming that no distant metastasis occurs. Although this is not uniformly true, it has been shown in cervical cancer that there is a good correlation between local tumor control and complete or partial regression of the cancer at the completion of radiation. In addition Grigsby has correlated post-treatment PET tumor response (which measures glucose metabolism) with survival.

Another factor limiting radiocurability is the normal tissue toxicity with increasing radiation doses. Normal tissue effects depend on total dose, dose fraction size, volume, and inherent tissue radiosensitivity. The ultimate goal is to obtain as high curability as possible with the least possible side effects. Combining radiation therapy with surgery or chemotherapy decreases normal tissue tolerance to a given dose. Well-established port size, total dose, and fractionation schemes have been identified but cannot remain static. Variations are being investigated to increase curability as well as decrease complications, including new chemotherapeutic radiosensitizers, technological advances in the delivery of radiation such as intensity modulated radiation therapy (IMRT, see p 789 and radioprotectors such as Ethyol).

Radiosensitizers, hypoxic cell sensitizers, and radioprotectors

Radiation sensitizers and protectors are being actively investigated to increase the effectiveness of radiation or allow dose escalation while minimizing side effects. Radiation sensitizers increase the ability of radiation to cause permanent, lethal damage. This therapeutic gain may be from a variety of mechanisms including selective uptake, targeting, or activation. To be effective sensitizers must have acceptable normal tissue side effects. Known radiation sensitizers include chemotherapeutic agents such as cisplatin, 5-fluorouracil, paclitaxel, adriamycin, and gemcitabine. Hypoxic cell sensitizers include the imidazole drugs such as misonidazole, as well as bioreductive agents such as tirapazamine. Endogenous sulfhydryl compounds and Ethyol afford radioprotection to normal tissues.

The advantages afforded by chemoradiation can be by several mechanisms. Some agents inhibit the repair of radiation damage, such as cisplatin, while others block cells in a radiosensitive cell cycle phase, such as paclitaxel. Adriamycin, docetaxel, and paclitaxel have unique effects when combined serially with radiation, as "radiation recall" is an uncommon but distressing phenomenon. After a course of radiation the normal tissue sensitization can be "recalled" when the chemotherapy is initiated—this phenomenon is a re-emergence of a prior radiation burn that conforms exactly to the prior radiation portal. The mechanism of this is unknown but well described for these chemotherapies.

The nitroimidazoles such as metronidazole, misonidazole, etanidazole, and nimorazole are electron affinic and increase the sensitivity of radioresistant hypoxic cells to XRT. They mimic oxygen and can diffuse into hypoxic areas. Unfortunately, clinical studies to date have demonstrated significant toxicity and little clinical utility with these drugs.

Tirapazamine is entering clinical trials as an adjunct to radiotherapy. GOG trial 219 randomizes chemoradiation for cervical cancer with and without tirapazamine. Tirapazamine is bioactivated intracellularly to a cytotoxic, active free radical that causes extensive chromosomal breaks and inhibits DNA repair. The reaction is driven by low tissue oxygen tension, and when combined with radiation may allow more effective destruction of tumors with hypoxic cores.

Radioprotection has been proven in several sites with the use of Ethyol. Amifostine (Ethyol; WR-2721) is an organic thiophosphate extensively studied by Walter Reed Army Institute of Research. Normal tissues noted to be protected included the salivary glands, bone marrow, immune system, skin, oral mucosa, esophagus, intestinal mucosa, kidney and testes. It is dephosphorylated to the active metabolite (WR-1065) in the tissues.

It is believed that tissue vs. tumor alkaline phosphatase concentration variations provide the differential protective effect. In addition, tissue pH differences afford selective tissue versus tumor uptake of Ethyol. When given intravenously the plasma half-life is less than 10 minutes but there is prolonged retention of the drug in normal tissue. In the first 30 minutes, drug uptake into normal tissues has been shown to be 100 times that of tumor tissues. Once inside the cell, the metabolite scavenges oxygen free radicals and provides an alternative target for alkylating agents, like cisplatin.

There have been numerous studies of the protective effect of Ethyol with no reported decrease in anti-tumor efficacy. A phase III trial in head and neck cancer unequivocally established its role in salivary gland protection confirming earlier studies. Other clinical trials have shown Ethyol protects from cisplatin-induced renal, neurologic, and bone marrow toxicity. Liu published a Phase III randomized trial in rectal cancer patients treated with pelvic radiation with and without Ethyol ($340mg/m^2$). The toxicity in the mucous membranes, genitourinary and gastrointestinal tract was reduced by 50% in the Ethyol arm. Moderate to severe late toxicities were seen in 14% of those treated without Ethyol compared to zero in the Ethyol-treated patients. Athanassiou et al randomized 205 patients with pelvic radiation plus or minus Ethyol and demonstrated a significant decrease in bladder and gastrointestinal toxicity. Complete responses to therapy and median survival were not significantly different between the arms. The RTOG (Radiation Therapy Oncology Group) has an open Phase I/II trial utilizing Ethyol with chemoradiation for pelvic and para-aortic radiation in cervical carcinoma. Toxicities with intravenous administration include hypotension, and nausea. Data on subcutaneous administration demonstrates less hypotension but treatable nausea and skin effects persist. There have been rare reports of Stevens–Johnson syndrome.

GENETIC EFFECTS

It is not possible to generalize and assign a specific mutation rate to a given radiation dose. Gene loci differ greatly in their mutability, and the random damage exerted by irradiation on any particular chromosome makes predictability impossible. The mitotic stage, cell type, sex, species, and dose rate influence the mutation rate as studied in lower animals and bacteria. Data from lower animals are difficult to extrapolate to humans and, therefore, prediction of mutation rates cannot be expected from the evidence that has been accumulated from various types of radiation exposure. Direct evidence of radiation-induced mutation in humans is lacking, although there is strong anecdotal evidence for carcinogenesis in those exposed to radiation. A few examples are excess skin cancers seen in those exposed to X-rays before safety standards were established, lung cancer in pitchblende miners, bone tumors in radium dial painters, and liver tumors in those exposed to Thorotrast contrast. The largest groups of humans available for study are survivors and descendants of those exposed in Hiroshima and Nagasaki. Although there has been no detectable effect on the frequency of prenatal or neonatal deaths or on the frequency of malformations in subsequent generations, this does not mean that no hereditary effects were produced. The number of exposed parents was small, and dosages were so low that it would have been surprising if an increase in mutation had been detected in such a brief period. There has not been sufficient time for the several generations needed to reveal recessive damage.

Radiation does not produce new and unique mutations but increases the incidence of spontaneous mutations. Based largely on experiments in mice, it is estimated that the doubling dose (i.e., the dose that will double the spontaneous mutation rate) for humans is probably 100 cGy based on low dose rate exposure. Somewhere between 1% and 6% of spontaneous mutations in humans can be ascribed to background radiation. With the use of image intensifiers, improved X-ray film, and appropriate shielding to prevent scatter, it is possible to attain satisfactory X-ray visualization of internal structures with reduced exposure. The average dose of irradiation to the gonads of some common diagnostic techniques is given in Table F–7.

In general most mutations are harmful and there is no known threshold dose for the genetic effect. Permanent

Table F–7 AVERAGE RADIATION DOSE TO THE FETUS AND TO MATERNAL GONADS FROM VARIOUS DIAGNOSTIC EXAMINATIONS (FIRST TRIMESTER)

Examination	Dose to fetus (first trimester) and maternal gonads: (mcGy)
Lower extremity X-ray	1
Cervical spine X-ray	2
Chest X-ray	8
Chest fluoroscopy	70
Lumbar spine X-ray	275
Hip X-ray	100
Intravenous pyelogram	585
Upper GI	330
Lower GI	465
Chest CT	8
Abdominal CT	800
Pelvic CT	2300

Adapted from DiSaia PJ: Basic principles in gynecologic radiotherapy. In Scott JR, DiSaia PJ, Hammond CB, Spellacy WN (eds): Danforth's Obstetrics and Gynecology, 8th edn. Philadelphia, JB Lippincott, 1999.

sterility in females is estimated to have a threshold of 250–600 cGy to acute exposure and 0.2 Gy/year for protracted exposure. The threshold dose for sterility varies based on the age of the patient, with younger patients being more resistant to the deleterious effect.

FETAL EFFECTS

The classic effects of radiation on the mammalian embryo are:

1. intrauterine and extrauterine growth retardation;
2. embryonic, fetal, or neonatal death; and
3. gross congenital malformations.

Dose, gestational age, and dose rate are all important factors influencing radiation damage. The recommendation for fetal dose during the entire gestation is = 0.5 rem (roughly 0.5 cGy). Monthly exposures should not exceed 0.05 rem. If a pregnant patient receives 10 cGy in the sensitive period of 10 days to 26 weeks, therapeutic abortion should be considered to avoid radiation effects including malformations, microcephaly, and mental retardation.

The peak incidence of gross malformations occurs during early organogenesis (10–40 days of gestation in the human) although cellular, tissue, and organ hypoplasia can be produced by radiation throughout the fetal and neonatal period with sufficient dose. Diagnostic X-ray procedures should be avoided in the pregnant woman unless there is overwhelming urgency. In women of childbearing age, possible damage to an early conceptus can be prevented by performing tests immediately after the commencement of a menstrual period and obtaining a negative pregnancy test. Compelling evidence that radiation may be a causative agent in childhood cancer after prenatal exposure comes from several studies in Great Britain and the USA.

Some concrete information is available from the Japanese survivors of the atom bomb attacks in 1945. Examination of children born to survivors demonstrates the primary effect from in utero radiation was microcephaly and mental retardation. The most sensitive phase for mental retardation was from 8 to 15 weeks of gestation. In addition, permanent growth retardation was also observed, especially in those embryos exposed less than 1500 m from the center of the explosion. Hall reached the following conclusions:

1. Moderately large doses of radiation (>200 cGy) delivered to the human embryo before 2–3 weeks' gestation are unlikely to produce severe abnormalities in most children born, although a considerable number of embryos may be reabsorbed or aborted (all-or-none phenomenon).
2. Significant irradiation between 4 and 11 weeks' gestation leads to severe abnormalities in many organs.
3. Irradiation between 11 and 16 weeks' gestation may produce some eye, skeletal, and genital organ abnormalities; however, stunted growth, microcephaly, and mental retardation are often present.
4. Irradiation of the fetus between 16 and 20 weeks' gestation may lead to a mild degree of microcephaly, mental retardation, and stunting of growth.
5. Irradiation after 30 weeks' gestation is unlikely to produce gross structural abnormalities leading to a serious handicap but could cause functional disabilities.

PRINCIPLES OF CLINICAL RADIATION THERAPY

The technical modalities used in modern radiation therapy may be divided into two major categories:

1. ***External irradiation***. This applies to irradiation from sources at a distance from the body (e.g., teletherapy with ^{60}Co, linear accelerator, betatron, or orthovoltage X-ray machines).
2. ***Local irradiation*** (brachytherapy). This applies to irradiation from sources in direct proximity to the tissue or tumor. Brachytherapy can be delivered with either a low-dose-rate (LDR) system or a high-dose-rate system (HDR). LDR systems require hospital admission to a shielded room and deliver dose at roughly 50–100 cGy/hour. HDR systems are commonly done on an outpatient basis and deliver doses at 100 cGy/minute.
   a. *Intracavitary irradiation* is delivered with applicators loaded with radioactive materials such as radium, cesium, or iridium (e.g., vaginal ovoids, vaginal cylinder, intrauterine tandem, tandem and ring, or, historically, Heyman capsules).
   b. *Interstitial irradiation* (endocurie therapy) is usually delivered in the form of removable needles containing radium, cesium, or iridium. The term also applies to permanent isotope implants, such as ^{125}I (iodine) seeds.
   c. *Direct therapy* can be delivered by means of cones from an orthovoltage machine (e.g., transvaginal) and, although useful, is no longer commonly available.
   d. *Intraperitoneal or intrapleural* instillation of radioactive colloids, such as ^{32}P is yet another local therapy, but is infrequently used.

External beam radiation (teletherapy)

External radiation is radiation therapy that is delivered from outside the body. It is most commonly delivered with protons, electrons, or photons. Machinery to deliver the radiation includes ^{60}Co units, betatrons, orthovoltage machines, or linear accelerators. Typically a patient will need planning done prior to initiation of radiation, called simulation. Marks are applied to the skin to allow for daily set up and, more and more commonly, a planning CT is performed. The use of MRI, CT, or PET images to fuse with treatment planning CT data is becoming widely available to better delineate tumor targets and normal tissue. There are three areas that must be targeted. The gross tumor volume requires the highest radiation dose. Microscopic extensions into surrounding tissues must be targeted, but generally require a lesser dose for sterilization. Subclinical disease presumed to be present in postoperative beds or regional nodes must be treated to prevent marginal failures.

Local radiation (brachytherapy)

Local application of radiation (also known as brachytherapy) permits very high doses to restricted tissue volumes. In this situation, the physical principle (inverse square law) that the intensity of irradiation rapidly decreases with distance from the radiation source is used to advantage. Brachytherapy is well suited to treat small tumors with well-defined limits and a clinical situation where it is desirable to restrict the volume of tissue irradiated. Larger volumes of tissue that need radiation therapy are best treated with external irradiation. Historically, radium (^{226}Ra) had been the most common isotope used for local application but because of storage, risk of leaks, and extremely long half-life it is rarely used in this country. Sources used today are often converted to mg-Ra-equivalents. Brachytherapy sources such as ^{125}I, ^{137}Cs, ^{192}Ir, and ^{103}Pd are more commonly used today (Table F–4).

Although conventional low-dose rate (LDR) intracavitary brachytherapy has produced very good results in cervical cancer, remote afterloading high-dose rate (HDR) intracavitary brachytherapy is becoming more widespread. The treatment results of LDR and HDR appear to be similar both for local control and survival although there are no large American randomized trials. Retrospective studies, however, mirror the results of the randomized studies. There remain concerns over potential differences in late complications due to the different biologic mechanisms between the continuous low dose rate of LDR and the intermittent high dose rate of HDR. The increased interest in HDR arises from lack of inpatient hospitalization and less radiation exposure to medical personnel. In both LDR and HDR, it is very important to keep the doses to central normal tissues as low as possible by proper use of midline blocking and packing/retraction techniques. HDR units use computer technology to "optimize" the dwell time of a single source to give the required distribution. The American Brachytherapy Society has published consensus guidelines on the administration of HDR for both cervical and uterine carcinomas.

The term *dosimetry* is applied to the measurement and calculation of dose that the patient receives. In brachytherapy as radiation intensity rapidly decreases with increasing distance from the source, tissue adjacent to the radiation source is treated to a high dose while relatively sparing surrounding tissue. The effectiveness of this distribution of irradiation depends on meticulous application of these sources. Interstitial application of radioactive sources is more difficult than intracavitary application. It is essential that the gynecologic oncologist be able to critically assess the placement of tandem and ovoids/cylinder/ring to assess the optimal placement of brachytherapy sources. (Figs F–11, F–12).

NORMAL TISSUE TOLERANCE

The tolerance of any tissue (normal or tumor) to irradiation therapy depends on several characteristics of radiation, including:

1. fractionation technique;
2. field arrangement;
3. total dose;
4. dose rate; and
5. volume irradiated.

Fractionation is the number of treatments to deliver the total dose. Pelvic radiation delivered to a patient for a total dose of 5000 cGy given in five daily fractions of 200 cGy each week for 5 weeks is well tolerated in most cases. However, if that same total dose of 5000 cGy were given in five fractions of 1000 cGy every Monday for 5 consecutive weeks, tolerance would be low.

In addition, multiple fields are used to minimize toxicity by dividing the exposure of normal tissue into multiple different regions. Three-dimensional conformal therapy (3DCF), intensity modulated radiation therapy (IMRT), and image-guided radiotherapy are areas of active investigation to further maximize dose to tumor and minimize toxicity to the surrounding normal tissues (Fig. F–13). With external irradiation, the patient is treated to all fields 5 days/wk.

As is seen in LDR brachytherapy vs HDR brachytherapy, dose rate affects tolerance. The final dose in HDR is necessarily lower to compensate for normal tissue tolerance concerns with the markedly higher dose rate in HDR.

Finally, the volume of tissue irradiated is also an integral factor in tolerance. For example, a 1 cm circular field of skin would easily tolerate the fractionation and dose rate of 1000 cGy each Monday for 5 consecutive weeks. However, for a larger volume, such as whole-pelvis radiation, such a treatment plan is intolerable.

Patient factors also impact normal tissue tolerance. Previous surgery affects the morbidity of radiation therapy. In both cervical and uterine cancer, surgery identifies adverse surgical pathologic findings that direct radiation therapy. In cervical cancer, surgical evaluation of possible lymph node metastases, particularly in advanced cancers, is often done. Transperitoneal lymph node dissection followed by pelvic and possibly para-aortic radiation increases radiation-induced complications, particularly to the bowel. Radiation complications can be severe, including fistula formation, bowel obstruction, and perforation. The retroperitoneal approach to lymph node dissection has a decreased complication rate, and is the preferred method of surgically evaluating lymph node status in cervical cancer. Medical conditions that impact blood flow such as diabetes, hypertension, and peripheral vascular disease can decrease normal tissue tolerance as well.

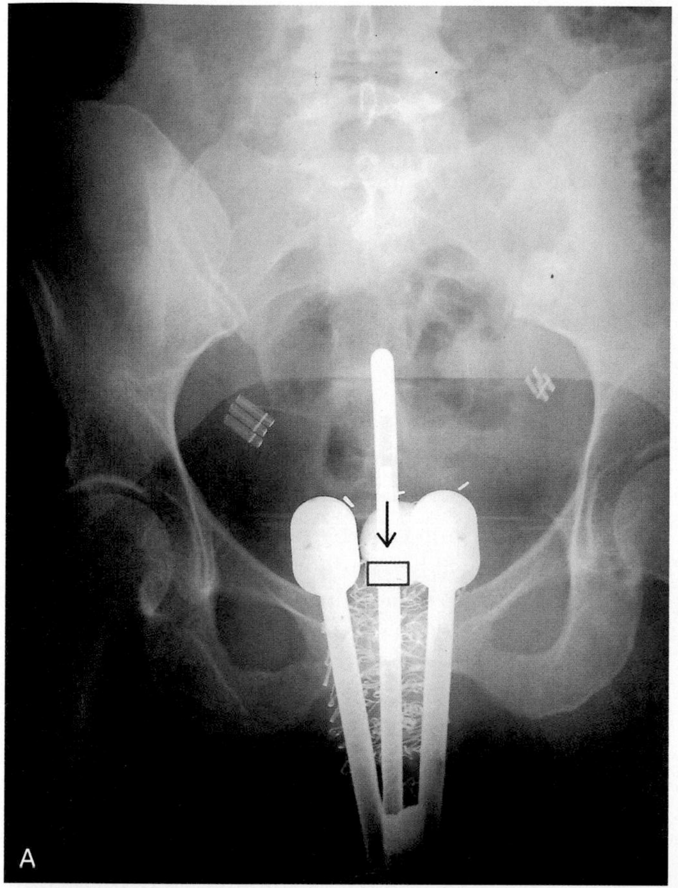

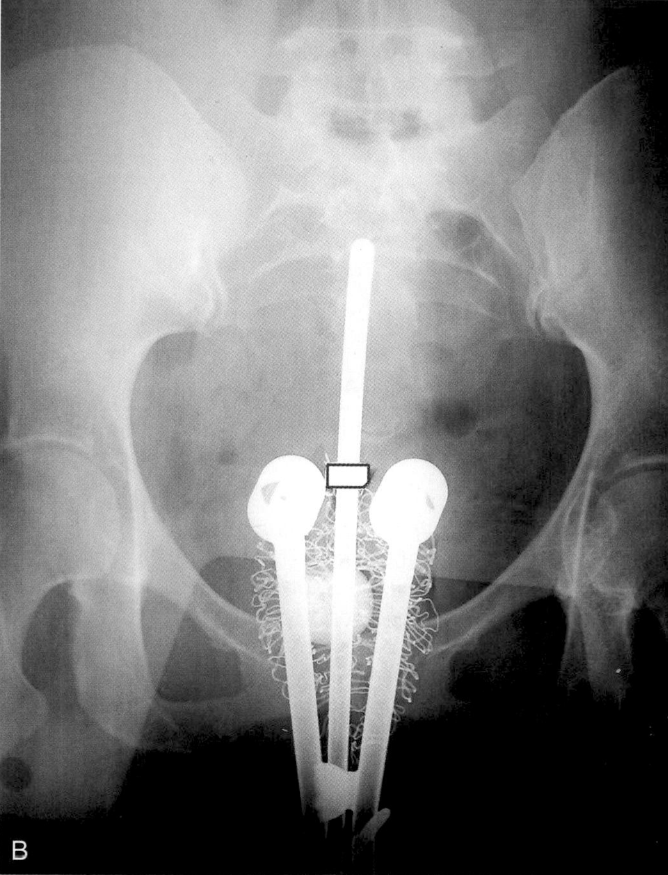

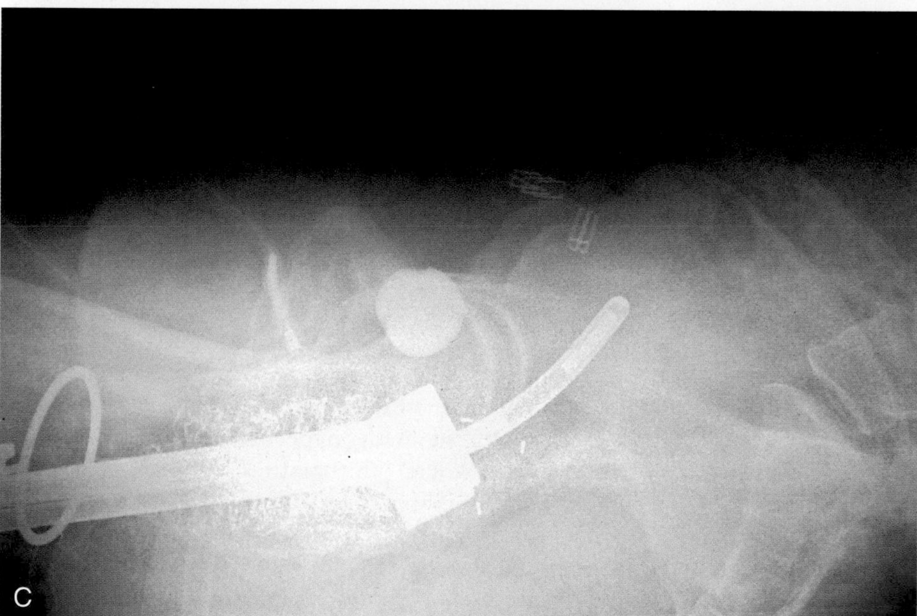

Figure F–11 Assessing proper placement of tandem and ovoids. In both photos small interstitial silver seeds mark the cervix. In *A*, the cervical stop, outlined in red, has dropped away from the cervix compromising the dose delivery to the tumor and increasing the complications. In *B*, this has been corrected. Also note the vaginal packing (delineated by radio-opaque string) lies below the ovoids and that the tandem is midline and bisects the ovoids. In *C*, a lateral radiograph, the tandem again bisects the ovoids and lies beneath the bladder (Foley balloon is filled with contrast material) and does not lie too close to the sacrum.

PELVIC ORGAN TOLERANCE

Tolerance of normal pelvic organs varies from one patient to another and is subject to the factors previously mentioned, such as volume, fractionation, and total dose of irradiation. As is illustrated in many areas of oncology, the more advanced lesions require higher doses for tumor eradication and, hence, the possibility of morbidity increases. This, combined with the fact that advanced cancer often already compromises the integrity of the bladder and rectum, means that serious sequelae can develop in patients with advanced cervical, vaginal, and corpus lesions when curative therapy is sought. New advances in radiation delivery will, hopefully, decrease these adverse effects.

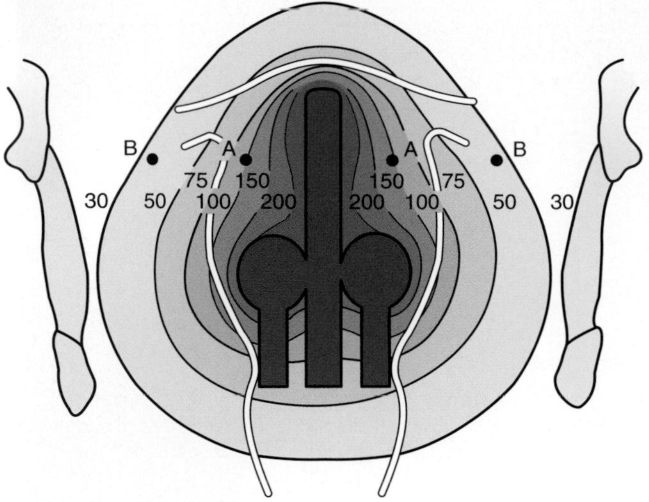

Figure F–12 Isodose curves surrounding a typical Fletcher–Suit intracavitary application (tandem plus ovoids) for cervical cancer. Note the location of points A and B and the relative dose rates at distances from the system.

The normal tissues of the cervix and the corpus of the uterus can tolerate very high doses of radiation. In fact, they withstand higher doses better than any other comparable volume of tissue in the body; surface doses of 20,000–30,000 cGy in about 2 weeks are tolerated. This remarkable tolerance level permits a large tumor dose and allows a very high percentage of central control of cervical cancer. The unusual radiation tolerance of the uterus, as well as the vagina, stemming from an unusual ability to recover from radiation injury accounts for the success of brachytherapy in the treatment of cervical lesions.

In contrast, the sigmoid, rectosigmoid, and rectum are more susceptible to radiation injury than are other pelvic organs. The frequency of injury to the large bowel often depends on the total dose administered by both the external beam and the intracavitary system. With external beam radiation alone, the large bowel is the most sensitive of pelvic structures. The bladder tolerates slightly more radiation than does the rectosigmoid according to most authorities. Acceptable maximal point doses are 75 Gy and 70 Gy to the bladder and rectum, respectively. Fletcher proposed a rule of thumb that gives the upper limits of pelvic irradiation and indirectly gives the tolerance of the bladder and rectum. The guidelines limit the sum of the central dose stating that external beam radiation dose plus the number of milligram-hours of cesium administered by brachytherapy should never exceed 10,000. There is a parallel time guideline also critical to this limit. This is a necessary precaution to prevent compact systems from exceeding vaginal/cervical tolerance. This guideline is valid only when the Fletcher–Suit brachytherapy systems are used. Most of this is applicable to therapy for the uterus, cervix, and vagina. In general, if a large dose of intracavitary irradiation is applied centrally for a small lesion, the amount of external beam applied centrally must be reduced. Conversely, if a lesion is large and the vaginal geometry poor, a smaller intracavitary dose can be given and the dose administered by external beam may be raised (6000–7000 cGy).

Pelvic radiation spares a significant portion of the small bowel, as bowel is normally in episodic motion. This tends to prevent any one segment from receiving an excessive dose. However, if loops of small bowel are immobilized as a result of adhesions caused by previous surgery, they may be held directly in the path of the radiation beam and thus be injured (Fig. F–14). The result of such an injury is usually not manifested for at least 6 months or longer after completion of radiation.

LONG-TERM EFFECTS

Finally, it is important to understand the permanent nature of radiation injury. When any area of the body is subjected to tumoricidal doses of radiation, the normal tissues of that area suffer an injury that is only partially repaired. The tumor tissue disappears but the normal tissue bed remains, and residual radiation changes must be seriously considered should other disease processes ensue. Radiobiologists estimate that in the case of injury to normal tissues, only 5–20% of the damage is repaired. If a second malignant neoplasm arises in that same area many years later, additional tumoricidal radiation is frequently impossible because of permanent radiation changes. In addition, any surgical procedures performed within a previously irradiated field are at higher risk for poor healing, fistula formation, and so forth.

Radiation-induced soft tissue necrosis can be a significant complication. This is usually due to a progressive obliterative endarteritis that leads to decreased blood flow and a resultant hypoxic tissue bed. This causes increased fibrosis, poor healing, and chronic ulceration. Local conservative management (e.g., hydrogen peroxide douche, estrogen therapy) will resolve the problem in many cases. There is a small group of patients who have significant tissue breakdown that may be painful and may lead to fistula formation. The use of hyperbaric oxygen has been shown to enhance healing in these radiation-induced injuries. Treatment with hyperbaric oxygen requires entering a tank where one breathes 100% oxygen at an increased atmospheric pressure. This increases the oxygen concentration in all body tissues up to 20 times normal. This treatment is done daily for 6–8 weeks and side effects include nausea, claustrophobia, painful pressure on the ears—similar to the changes experienced with airline pressure changes—pneumothorax, and oxygen toxicity.

Permanent changes to the genitourinary and gastrointestinal tract can cause signs and symptoms such as decreased bladder capacity, hematuria, ureteral or urethral stricture, hematochezia, bowel obstruction, chronic diarrhea, tenesmus, fecal incontinence, and fistula formation. Gynecologic changes include dryness and shortening of the vagina, dyspareunia, and decreased orgasm. The oncology team should address all these long-term effects to maximize the patient's quality of life.

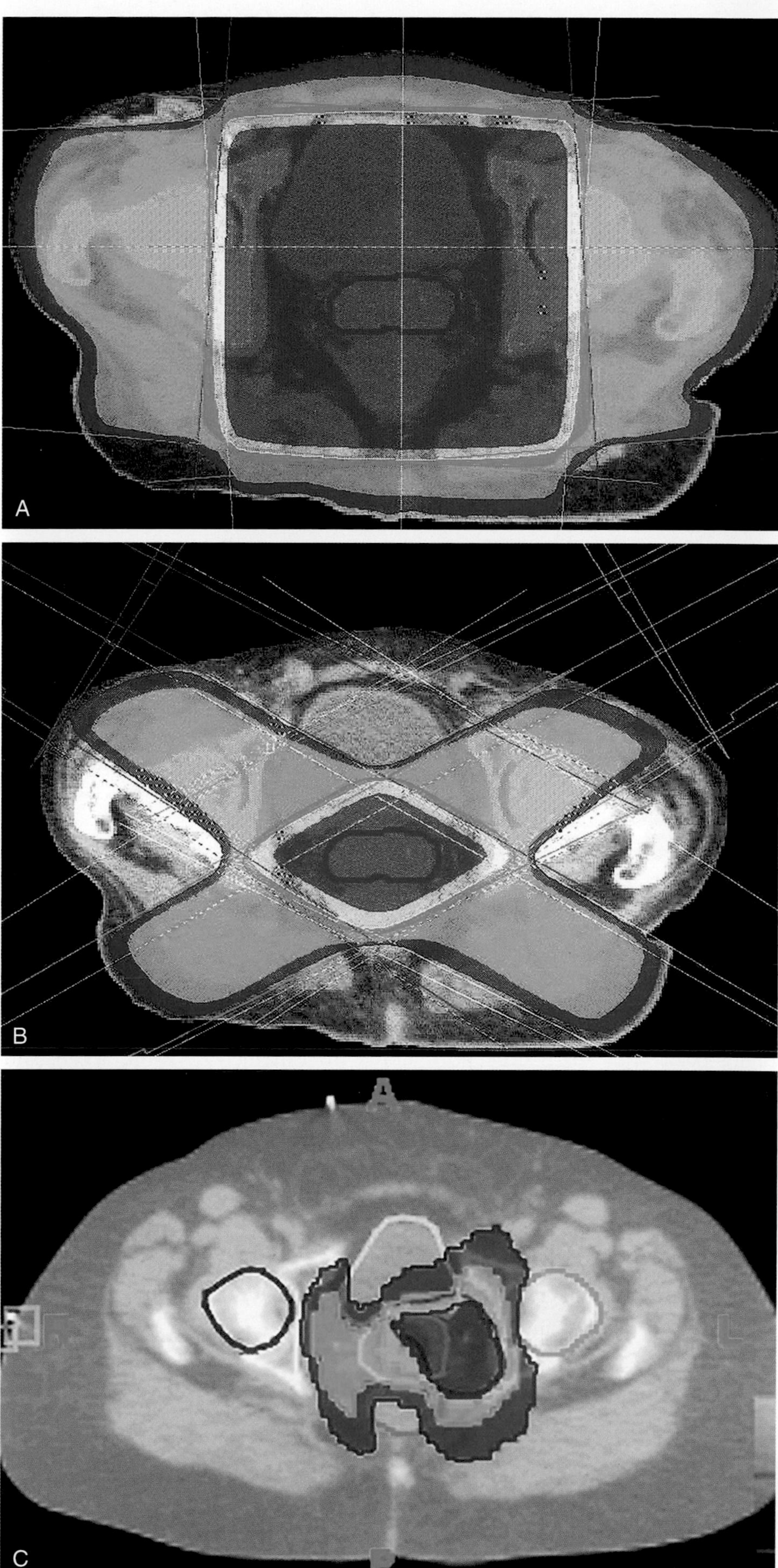

Figure F–13 Comparison of normal tissue irradiated with *A*, four field box technique, *B*, three-dimensional conformal therapy, and *C*, intensity modulated radiation therapy. The red represents areas that receive 100% of the prescription dose, yellow 90%, green 50% and blue 40%. Notice how the normal tissue volume receives less dose as the treatment is delivered more conformally.

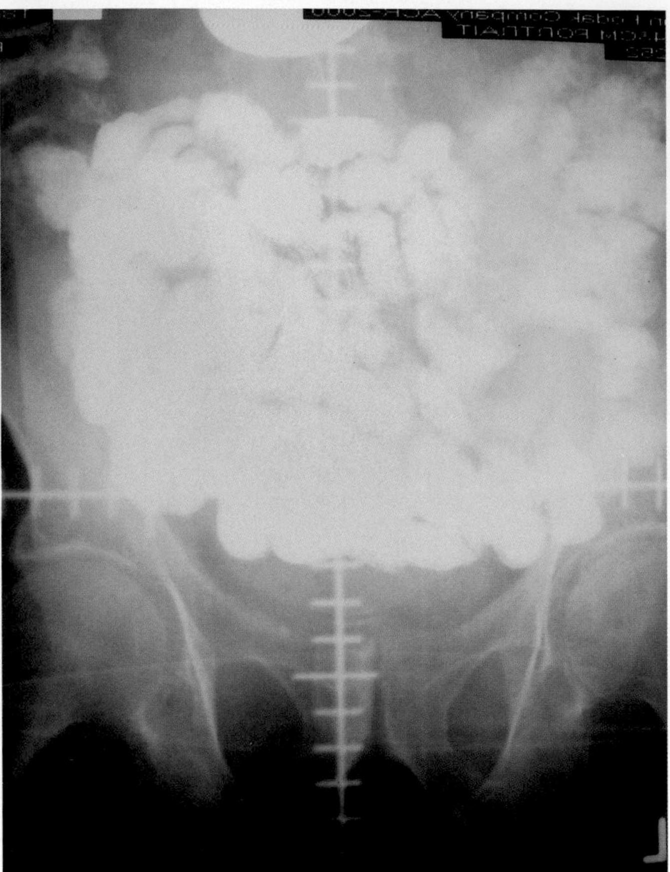

Figure F–14 Small bowel in the pelvis demonstrated by small bowel contrast.

NEW RADIATION MODALITIES

Protons

Protons result in an excellent physical dose distribution. The dose increases slowly with depth and reaches a sharp maximum near the end of the particle's range called the Bragg peak. This sharp dose peak allows for extremely precise, circumscribed delivery. Other than the physical distribution advantage, protons have biologic properties similar to X-rays. Protons are ideal for specific clinical situations, such as spinal cord tumors where a sharp dose delivery is critical to avoid normal tissue damage and to treat eye melanomas. Although useful in several clinical situations, cost of delivery from a cyclotron or special linear accelerator makes it currently available in only a few cities—Houston, Texas; Loma Linda, California; Bloomington, Illinois; and Boston, Massachusetts.

Electrons

Most modern linear accelerators can produce high-energy electron beams. Electrons lose energy rapidly as they travel in tissue and interact with tissue atoms, and ultimately their kinetic energy is reduced to zero. Therefore, unlike photons, electrons have a specific range dependent on energy and the tissue traversed. Transvaginal electron irradiation can be utilized for a copiously bleeding exophytic cervical lesion to induce hemostasis. The dosimetry is such that most of the energy delivered transvaginally is absorbed into the malignant lesions itself. Lesions of the vulva and inguinofemoral lymph nodes are also treated with electron beams in many institutions. The limitations of electron therapy are related to the strengths. Because it loses energy rapidly, it cannot be used for deep-seated tumors and the applicator must rest very close to the tumor itself, so only fairly superficial, shallow lesions are appropriately treated with electrons.

Fast neutrons

Neutrons interact in tissue to produce recoil protons, α particles, and other nuclear particles. Their potential usefulness stems from a reduced OER (oxygen enhancement ratio—this translates into decreased hypoxic cell resistance), reduced differential killing by cell cycle, reduced ability for cells to repair sublethal damage, and higher effectiveness for slowly cycling tumors.

Although randomized controlled trials demonstrated that neutron therapy provided improved local control in some tumors, its utility was limited by higher morbidity and cost. Overall, use is limited by the cost of the cyclotron, limited depth penetrations, high surface entrance dose, lack of sharp beam boundaries, and variable intensity modulation. Interest in neutron use for prostate and salivary gland tumors has been recently renewed.

Negative π mesons and other heavy ions

Negative π mesons, or pions, are negatively charged particles that have a mass 273 times that of an electron. These are produced in a cyclotron or linear accelerator using 400–800 MeV protons that bombard a beryllium target. Pions exhibit a Bragg peak produced by elicited protons, neutrons and alpha particles. Other heavy ions such as neon, argon, and carbon have been studied, but equipment to produce these special particles is expensive and not widely available. Use is limited to experimental therapy only. As with neutrons these forms of radiation have a high biologic effectiveness and a low dependence on oxygen.

NEW RADIATION DELIVERY TECHNOLOGY

Intraoperative radiation

Several centers throughout the world are attesting to the efficacy of large-fraction intraoperative external irradiation. Patients are subjected to operative procedures in which the area of involvement is carefully defined and radiation fractions of 1500–2500 cGy are delivered directly to the area identified. Applications of this technique in gynecologic oncology have been in the treatment of biopsy-proven positive para-aortic or pelvic nodes and marginally resectable recurrences. Electron beam radiation is delivered with one high-dose fraction with the bowel and other sensitive normal tissues packed to the side, thus minimizing the probability of visceral injuries. For best results, external beam radiation is often combined with intraoperative therapy. Since the intraoperative accelerators only deliver electrons it is subject to the same limitations as all electron beams (see above discussion). Experience in both primary and recurrent tumors has been reported. The results are limited but have shown increased control and survival when used selectively. The role of intraoperative radiation in gynecology is not widespread and is limited to a few institutions that are capable of providing this specialized therapy.

Hyperthermia

As discussed previously, solid tumor masses often have hypovascular centers, which are poorly penetrated by antineoplastic drugs and have hypoxic, radioresistant cell fractions. Hyperthermia is another method used to overcome these relatively radioresistant tumors. Although several anecdotal clinical observations have been made, current interest in hyperthermia is based mainly on careful biologic studies on cells and transplantable tumors performed in the 1980s. Although there is no evidence that tumor cells are consistently more sensitive to heat than normal cells, several factors may contribute to a therapeutic gain. Tumor hypoxic cell populations have an acidic pH and are nutritionally deprived. These factors increase sensitivity to heat. Therapeutic gain is also derived from selective heat retention in the tumor. The hypoxic core is maintained at a higher temperature than the normal tissues, which more efficiently remove heat secondary to better-organized vasculature. Ultimately, cell death is dependent on the temperature achieved and is time dependent. Hyperthermia is combined with radiation as each modality preferentially kills a separate part of the tumor, and in addition, heat increases the cell kill of external radiation by inhibiting sublethal and potentially lethal damage repair. Late S phase is the most sensitive phase to hyperthermia but the most resistant to low LET (photon) radiation, and thus the two modalities complement one another. The first notable use of hyperthermia in gynecologic oncology has been with interstitial hyperthermia for deep tumors of the pelvis. Increased survival has been demonstrated although reports are mixed and the therapy is not commonly available.

Three-dimensional conformal radiation therapy

Three-dimensional conformal radiation therapy (3DCF) is linked to a multiplicity of imaging modalities, especially computed tomography (CT). Beam placement using a CT simulator replaces the conventional simulator (fluoroscopic planning machine) for plan design to the extent that the term "virtual simulation" is used to describe it. The digitally reconstructed radiographs link the plan to the treatment unit in a manner that can and will likely replace the conventional simulator. 3D conformal therapy entails shaping of the beam to conform to the target as seen by CT imaging. The physician arranges the beams to maximize dose to the tumor and minimize dose to normal tissues. Patient, tumor, and normal target movement demand patient immobilization and that adequate margin be placed around the targets to prevent a "marginal miss."

Intensity modulated radiation therapy (IMRT)

Intensity modulated radiation therapy (IMRT), compared to 3DCF therapy, uses the power of computers to perform hundreds to thousands of iterations of planning to maximize and shape tumor dose and minimize normal tissue dose (Fig. F–15). This form of planning gives the computer instructions on what dose to deliver to which structures and also sets limitations on normal structures. Both 3DCF therapy and IMRT use small collimator "leaves" to finely shape the beam. These "leaves" are mobile and block portions of the generated X-rays. If the collimator "leaves" move while the radiation beam is on and vary the beam intensity, areas of tumor and normal tissue can receive a spectrum of doses, hence the term intensity modulated. These collimator "leaves" also allow for irregular shapes to be treated. This technology has demonstrated increased local control with reduced complications in several sites such as prostate and head and neck. In gynecologic cancer, decreased radiation to normal tissues including bowel, bladder and bone marrow has been demonstrated. Considerable work is being done in gynecologic cancers to identify volumes necessary to outline and treat and dose limitations for normal organs but this modality is under active investigation at this time.

Introduction of new technology such as tomotherapy (a linear accelerator linked to an online CT scanner) and cone-beam CT may allow for even more precise localization of beam and verification of dose delivered. Organ motion in the pelvis remains a challenge as constant filling and emptying of viscera leads to tumor and normal tissue movement. Concerns regarding this technology include the enormous physician and physics time employed for planning, increased cost, and the unknown long-term consequences of lower dose but increased volume of tissue exposed to radiation.

Stereotactic radiotherapy

Stereotactic radiation and Gamma Knife radiation are similar to IMRT and 3DCF radiation as they allow precise, high-dose delivery of external radiation. It is commonly used for both primary and metastatic brain tumors, and an active area of research is in "body stereotactic," allowing precisely delivered high dose radiation to other areas of the body. Stereotactic radiation uses a modification of the linear accelerator whereas Gamma Knife is a separate machine with 201 separate ^{60}Co sources used to focus on the target.

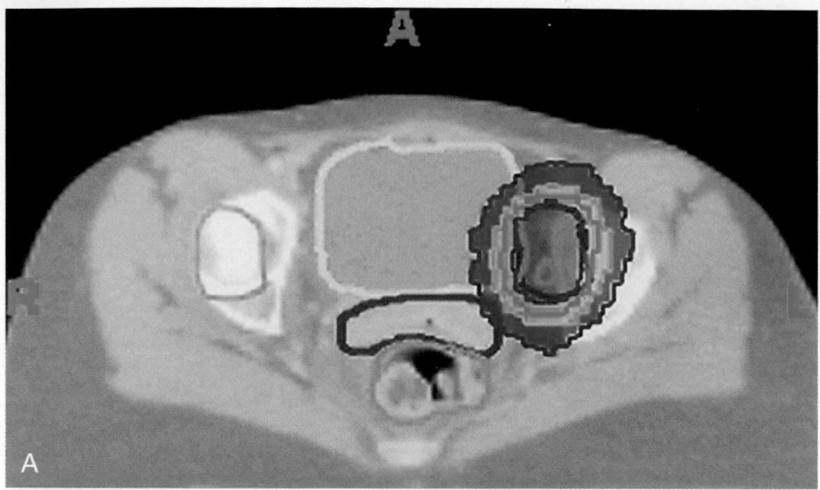

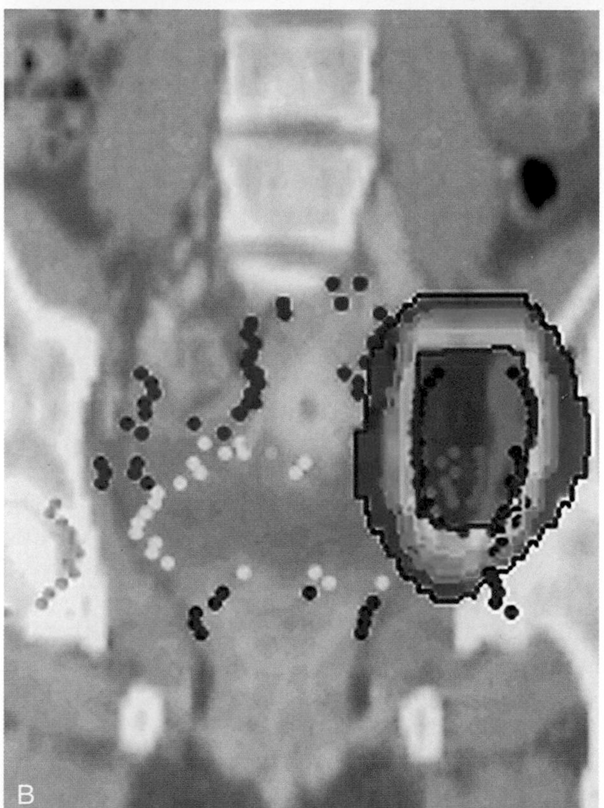

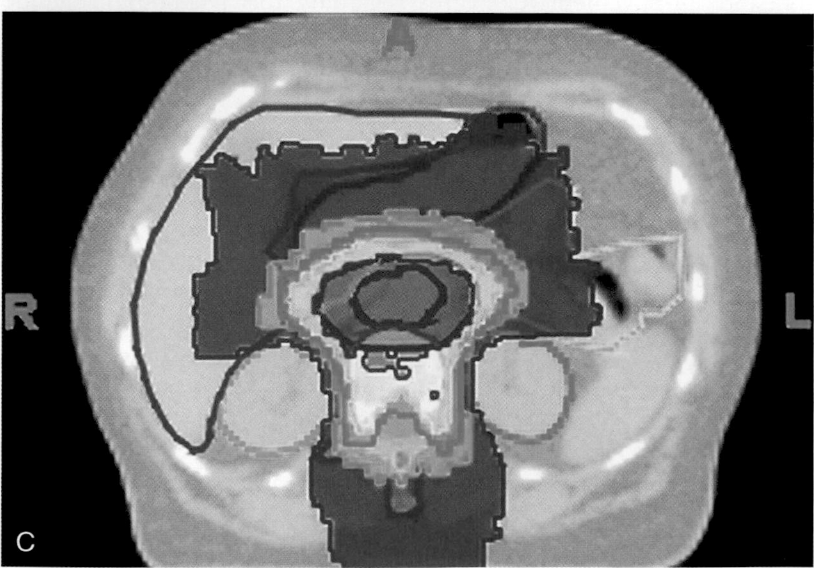

Figure F–15 In *A, B,* note how little normal tissue is treated to accomplish the sidewall nodal boost and in *C* how the renal parenchyma and spinal cord are relatively spared in treating the para-aortic recurrence.

Immune-tagged radiation therapy

Recently several products that tag a radioisotope to a monoclonal antibody have entered the market. This modality of radiation allows delivery of the radioactive isotope to the unique antibody target. It has been used successfully in lymphomas and awaits the identification of a unique target prior to development for a gynecologic use.

GLOSSARY

Absorbed dose The energy imparted to matter by ionizing radiation per unit mass of irradiated material. The unit is the gray (Gy), defined to be an energy absorption of 1 joule/kg. The old unit was the rad, which was defined as an energy absorption of 100 ergs/g.

Brachytherapy Treatment of malignant tumors by radioactive sources that are implanted close to (intracavitary) or within (interstitial) the tumor.

Dosimetry The term applied to the measurement and calculation of dose that the patient receives.

Electron volt (eV) The energy of motion acquired by an electron accelerated through a potential difference of 1 volt.

Excitation The moving of an electron to a more distant orbit within the same atom.

Gamma rays Electromagnetic irradiation (originating inside the nucleus) emitted by excited nuclei. The gamma rays from an isotope will have one or several sharply defined energies.

Gray (Gy) The special name for the unit of absorbed dose and specific energy impacted; 1 Gy = 1 joule/kg = 100 rads.

Half-life The time in which half the atoms of a radioactive species disintegrate.

Inverse square law The intensity of radiation from a point varies inversely as the square of the distance from the source. Thus, the dose rate at 2 cm from a source is one fourth that at 1 cm. At 3 cm, the dose rate is one-ninth that at 1 cm.

Ionization The removal of an electron from an atom, leaving a positively charged ion.

Ionizing radiation Radiation capable of causing ionization.

Isotope Nuclides having an equal number of protons but a different number of neutrons (excitable situation).

keV 1000 eV.

Linear energy transfer (LET) The energy lost by the particle or photon per micron of path depth. High LET radiations are more effective against hypoxic cells.

MeV 1,000,000 eV.

Oxygen enhancement ratio (OER) The ratio of the dose required for a given level of cell killing under hypoxic conditions compared with the dose needed in air.

Penumbra The radiation outside the full beam, which is often caused by scatter or incomplete collimation.

rad A unit-absorbed dose of ionizing radiation equivalent to the absorption of 100 erg per gram of irradiated material.

Relative biologic effectiveness (RBE) A ratio of the absorbed dose of a reference radiation to the absorbed dose of a test radiation to produce the same level of biologic effect, other conditions being equal.

rem The old unit of dose equivalent. It is the product of the absorbed dose in rads and modifying factor and is being replaced by the sievert.

Roentgen (R) An internationally accepted unit of radiation quantity: It is the quantity of "X-ray or gamma irradiation such that the associated corpuscular emission per 0.001293 g of air produces, in air, ions carrying 1 esu of quantity of electricity of either sign". X-rays originate outside the nucleus

Sievert (SU) The unit of dose equivalent in the SI system (1 Sv=100 rem).

X-rays Rays emitted by a particular generator will emit a spectrum of energies.

BIBLIOGRAPHY

RADIATION PHYSICS

Khan FM: The Physics of Radiation Therapy (2nd edn). Baltimore, Williams & Wilkins, 1994.

RADIOBIOLOGY

Athanassiou H, Antonadou D, Coliarakis N, Kouveli A, Synodinou M, Paraskevaidis M, Sarris G, Georgakopoulos GR, Panousaki K, Karageorgis P, Throuvalas N: Oncology Hellenic Group. Protective effect of amifostine during fractionated radiotherapy in patients with pelvic carcinomas: results of a randomized trial. Int J Radiat Oncol Biol Phys 56(4):1154–1160, 2003.

Bokemeyer C, Lampe C, Heneka M, Schabet M, Bamberg M, Kanz L: Paclitaxel-induced radiation recall dermatitis. Ann Oncol 7(7):755–756, 1996.

Brizel, DM: Phase II Randomized trial of amifostine as a radioprotector in head and neck cancer. J Clin Oncol 18(19):3339, 2000.

Budd GT, Ganapathi R, Adelstein DJ, Pelley R, Olencki T, Petrus J, McLain D, Zhang J, Capizzi R, Bukowski RM: Randomized trial of carboplatin plus amifostine versus carboplatin alone in patients with advanced solid tumors. Cancer. 80(6):1134–1140, 1997.

Buntzel J: selective cytoprotection with amifostine in concurrent radiochemotherapy for head and neck cancer. Ann Oncol 9:505, 1998.

Calabro-Jones PM: Alkaline phosphatase promotes radioprotection and accumulation of WR-1065 in V79-171 cells incubated in medium containing WR-2721. International Journal of Radiation Biology 47:23, 1985.

Chen L, Trujillo K, Sung P, Tomkinson AE: Interactions of the DNA ligase IV-XRCC4 complex with DNA ends and the DNA-dependent protein kinase. J Biol Chem 275:26196–26205, 2000.

Committee on the Biological Effects of Ionizing Radiation: The Effects on Populations of Exposure to Low Levels of Ionizing Radiation. Washington DC, National Academy of Sciences/National Research Council, 1990.

Davidson DE: Biological characteristics of some improved radioprotectors. In: Anonymous, ed. Radiation Sensitizers. New York, Masson: 309, 1980.

Dizdaroglu M: Measurement of radiation-induced damage to DNA at the molecular level. Int J Radiat Biol. 61(2):175–183, 1992.

Doll R, Wakeford R: Risk of childhood cancer from fetal irradiation. Br J Radiol. 70:130–139, 1997.

Dynan WS, Yoo S: Interaction of Ku protein and DNA-dependent protein catalytic subunit with nucleic acids. Nucleic Acids Res 26:1551–1559, 1998.

Eguchi-Kasai K, Kosaka T, Sato K, Kaneko I: Reparability of DNA double-strand breaks and radiation sensitivity in five mammalian cell lines. Int J Radiat Biol 59:97–104, 1991.

Haber JE: The many interfaces of Mre11. Cell 95(5):583–586, 1998.

Grigsby PW, Siegel BA, Dehdashti F, Mutch DG: Post-therapy surveillance monitoring of cervical cancer by FDG-PET. Int J Radiat Oncol Biol Phys 55(4):907–913, 2003.

Hall EJ, Astor M, Bedford, J, Borek C, Curtis SB, Fry M, Geard C, Hei T, Mitchell J, Oleinick N: Basic radiobiology. Am J Clin Oncol 11(3):220–252, 1988.

Hall EJ: Radiobiology for the Radiologist (5th edn). Philadelphia, Lippincott Williams & Wilkins, 2000.

Horsman MR, Overgaard J: Overcoming tumour radiation resistance rèsulting from acute hypoxia. Eur J Cancer. 28A(12):2084–2085, 1992.

Hortobagyi GN: Anthracyclines in the treatment of cancer. An overview. Drugs. 54 Suppl 4:1–7, 1997.

Jacobs AJ, Faris C, Perez CA, Kao MS, Galakatos A, Camel HM: Short-term persistence of carcinoma of the uterine cervix after radiation. An indicator of long-term prognosis. Cancer. 57(5): 944–950, 1986.

Kemp, G: Amifostine pretreatment for protection against cyclophosphamide-induced and cisplatin-induced toxicities: results of a randomized control trial in patients with advanced ovarian cancer. J Clin Oncol 14:2101, 1996.

Kerr JFR, Harmon BV: Definition and incidence of apoptosis: An historical perspective. In: Tomei LD, Cope FO, eds. Apoptosis: The Molecular Basis of Cell Death. Cold Spring Harbor, NY: Cold Harbor Laboratory Press, 1991, p 5.

Kneale GW, Stewart AM: Prenatal X-rays and cancers: further tests of data from the Oxford Survey of Childhood Cancers. Health Phys 51(3):369–376, 1986.

Koukourakis MI: Subcutaneous administration of Amifostine during fractionated radiotherapy: A randomized phase II study. J Clin Oncol 18 (11):2226, 2000.

Lee KJ, Huang J, Takeda Y, Dynan WS: DNA ligase IV and XRCC4 form a stable mixed tetramer that functions synergistically with other repair factors in a cell-free end-joining system. J Biol Chem 275:34787–34796, 2000.

Leskov, KS, Criswell T, Antonio S, Li J, Yang C, Kinsella T, Boothman DA: When X-ray-inducible proteins meet DNA double strand break repair. Sem Rad Onc 11(4):352–372, 2001.

Liu T Use of radiation with or without WR-2721 in advanced rectal cancer. Cancer 69:2820–2825, 1992.

Lorusso D, Ferrandina G, Greggi S, Gadducci A, Pignata S, Tateo S, Biamonte R, Manzione L, Di Vagno G, Ferrau' F, Scambia G: Multicenter Italian Trials in Ovarian Cancer investigators. Phase III multicenter randomized trial of amifostine as cytoprotectant in first-line chemotherapy in ovarian cancer patients. Ann Oncol 14(7):1086–1093, 2003.

Munro TR: The relative radiosensitivity of the nucleus and cytoplasm of Chinese hamster fibroblasts. Radiat Res 42(3):451–470, 1970.

Munro TR: The site of the target region for radiation-induced mitotic delay in cultured mammalian cells. Radiat Res 44(3): 747–757, 1970.

Ohhnishi ST: In vitro study on the antioxidant activities of amifostine (WR-2721). Proceedings of the American Association of Cancer Research 33:419, 1992.

Otake M, Schull WJ: Radiation-related brain damage and growth retardation among the prenatally exposed atomic bomb survivors. Int J Radiat Biol 74(2):159–171, 1998.

Paull TT, Gellert M: Nbs1 potentiates ATP-driven DNA unwinding and endonuclease cleavage by the Mre11/Rad50 complex. Genes Dev 13:1276–1288, 1999.

Preston DL, Pierce DA, Shimizu Y, Cullings HM, Fujita S, Funamoto S, Kodama K: Effect of recent changes in atomic bomb survivor dosimetry on cancer mortality risk estimates. Radiat Res 162(4):377–389, 2004.

Preston DL, Shimizu Y, Pierce DA, Suyama A, Mabuchi K: Studies of mortality of atomic bomb survivors. Report 13: Solid cancer and non-cancer disease mortality: 1950–1997. Radiat Res 160(4):381–407, 2003.

Preston DL, Pierce DA, Shimizu Y, Ron E, Mabuchi K: Dose response and temporal patterns of radiation-associated solid cancer risks. Health Phys 85(1):43–46, 2003.

Schull WJ: The children of atomic bomb survivors: a synopsis. J Radiol Prot 23(4):369–384, 2003.

Rose, PG: Amifostine cytoprotection with chemotherapy for advanced ovarian carcinoma. Semin Oncol 23 (4 Suppl 8):83, 1996.

Takahashi I: Clinical study of the radioprotective effects of amifostine (YM-08310, WR-2721) on chronic radiation injury. Int J Radiat Oncol Biol Phys 12:935, 1986.

Tanaka Y: Clinical experiences of chemical radiation protection in tumor radiotherapy in Japan. In: Brady LW, ed. Radiation Sensitizers: Their use in the clinical management of cancer. New York, Masson, 1979, p 421,

Thompson LH, Suit HD: Proliferation kinetics of x-irradiated mouse L cells studied with time-lapse photography. II. Int J Radiat Biol Relat Stud Phys Chem Med 15(4):347–362, 1969.

Utley, JF: Distribution of ^{35}S-Labeled WR-2721 in normal and malignant tissues of the mouse. Radiation Research 68:284, 1976.

Ward JF: Mechanisms of DNA repair and their potential modification for radiotherapy. Int J Radiat Oncol Biol Phys 12:1027–1032, 1986.

Washburn LC Prediction of the effective radioprotective dose of WR-2721 in humans through an interpecies tissue distribution study. Radiat Res 66:100, 1976.

Yoo S, Dynan WS Geometry of a complex formed by double strand break repair proteins at a single DNA end: recruitment of DNA-PKcs induces inward translocation of Ku protein. Nucleic Acids Res 27:4679–4686, 1999.

Yuhas JM. Active versus passive absorption kinetics as the basis for selective protection of normal tissues by S-2-(3-Aminopropylamino)-ethylphosphorothionic acid. Cancer Res 40:1519, 1980.

Yuhas JM The role of WR-2721 in radiotherapy and/or chemotherapy. Cancer Clin Trials 3:211, 1980.

PRINCIPLES OF CLINICAL RADIATION THERAPY

Ferrigno R, Nishimoto IN, Ribeiro Dos Santos Novaes PE, Pellizzon AC, Conte Maia MA, Fogarolli RC, Salvajoli JV:Comparison of low- and high-dose rate brachytherapy in the treatment of uterine cervix cancer. Retrospective analysis of two sequential series. Int J Radiat Oncol Biol Phys 62(4):1108–1116, 2005.

Fletcher GH: Textbook of Radiotherapy, 3rd edn. Philadelphia, Lea & Febiger, 1980.

Hareyama M ,Sakata K ,Oouchi A ,Nagakura H ,Shido M ,Someya M ,Koito K: High-dose-rate versus low-dose-rate intracavitary therapy for carcinoma of the uterine cervix: a randomized trial. Cancer 94(1):117–124, 2002.

Kim WC, Kim GE, Suh CO, Loh JJ: High- versus low-dose rate intracavitary irradiation for adenocarcinoma of the uterine cervix. Jpn J Clin Oncol. 31(9):432–437, 2001.

Kucera H, Potter R, Knocke TH, Baldass M, Kucera E: High-dose versus low-dose rate brachytherapy in definitive radiotherapy of cervical cancer. Wien Klin Wochenschr. 113(1–2):58–62, 2001.

Lertsanguansinchai P, Lertbutsayanukul C, Shotelersuk K, Khorprasert C, Rojpornpradit P, Chottetanaprasith T, Srisuthep A, Suriyapee S, Jumpangern C, Tresukosol D, Charoonsantikul C: Phase III randomized trial comparing LDR and HDR brachytherapy in treatment of cervical carcinoma. Int J Radiat Oncol Biol Phys 59(5):1424–1431, 2004.

Nag S, Erickson B, Thomadsen B, Orton C, Demanes JD, Petereit D: The American Brachytherapy Society recommendations for high-dose-rate brachytherapy for carcinoma of the cervix. Int J Radiat Oncol Biol Phys 48(1):201–211, 2000.

Nag S, Erickson B, Parikh S, Gupta N, Varia M, Glasgow G: The American Brachytherapy Society recommendations for high-dose-rate brachytherapy for carcinoma of the endometrium. Int J Radiat Oncol Biol Phys 48(3):779–790, 2000.

Patel FD, Sharma SC, Negi PS, Ghoshal S ,Gupta BD: Low-dose-rate vs high-dose-rate brachytherapy in the treatment of carcinoma of the uterine cervix: a clinical trial. Int J Radiat Oncol Biol Phys 28(2):335–341, 1994.

Petereit DG, Sarkaria JN, Potter DM, Schink JC: High-dose-rate versus low-dose-rate brachytherapy in the treatment of cervical cancer: analysis of tumor recurrence: the University of Wisconsin experience. Int J Radiat Oncol Biol Phys 45(5):1267–1274, 1999.

NEW RADIATION MODALITIES

Britten RA, Peters LJ, Murray D: Biological factors influencing the RBE of neutrons: implications for their past, present, and future use in radiotherapy. Radiat Res 156(2):125–135, 2001.

NEW RADIATION DELIVERY TECHNOLOGY

del Carmen MG, Eisner B, Willet CG, Fuller AF. Intraoperative radiation therapy in the management of gynecologic and genitourinary malignancies. Surg Oncol Clin N Am 12(4): 1031–1042, 2003.

Gemignani ML, Alektiar KM, Leitao M, Mychalczak B, Chi D, Venkatraman E, Barakat RR, Curtin JP: Radical surgical resection and high-dose intraoperative radiation therapy (HDR-IORT) in patients with recurrent gynecologic cancers. Int J Radiat Oncol Biol Phys 50(3):687–694, 2001.

Mundt AJ, Lujan AE, Rotmensch J, Waggoner SE, Yamada SD, Fleming G, Roeske JC: Intensity-modulated whole pelvic radiotherapy in women with gynecologic malignancies. Int J Radiat Oncol Biol Phys 52(5):1330–1337, 2002.

Roeske JC, Lujan A, Rotmensch J, Waggoner SE, Yamada D, Mundt AJ: Intensity-modulated whole pelvic radiation therapy in patients with gynecologic malignancies. Int J Radiat Oncol Biol Phys 48(5):1613–1621, 2000.

van der Zee J, Gonzalez GD. The Dutch Deep Hyperthermia Trial: results in cervical cancer. Int J Hyperthermia. 18(1):1–12, 2002.

van der Zee J, Gonzalez GD, van Rhoon GC, van Dijk JD, van Putten WL, Hart AA: Comparison of radiotherapy alone with radiotherapy plus hyperthermia in locally advanced pelvic tumours: a prospective, randomised, multicentre trial. Dutch Deep Hyperthermia Group. Lancet 355(9210):1119–1125, 2000.

Vasanthan A, Mitsumori M, Park JH, Zhi-Fan Z, Yu-Bin Z, Oliynychenko P, Tatsuzaki H, Tanaka Y, Hiraoka M: Regional hyperthermia combined with radiotherapy for uterine cervical cancers: a multi-institutional prospective randomized trial of the international atomic energy agency. Int J Radiat Oncol Biol Phys 61(1):145–153, 2005.

Index

Page numbers followed by f indicate figures, those followed by t indicate tables.

A

F

H

I

J

K

N

O

P

Q

R

S

U

V

W

X

Y

TEXTBOOK OF BIOCHEMISTRY WITH CLINICAL CORRELATIONS

FOURTH EDITION

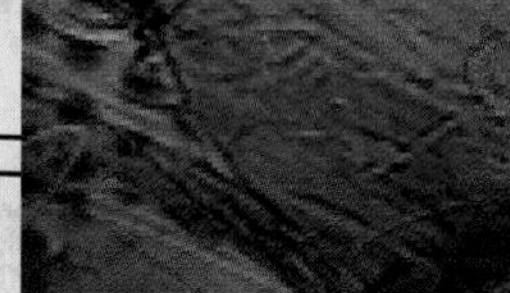

TEXTBOOK OF BIOCHEMISTRY WITH CLINICAL CORRELATIONS

Edited by

Thomas M. Devlin, Ph.D.

Professor Emeritus
Department of Biochemistry
MCP·Hahnemann School of Medicine
Allegheny University of the Health Sciences
Philadelphia, Pennsylvania

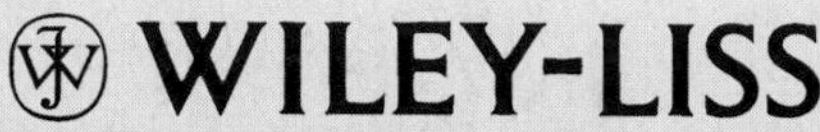

WILEY-LISS

A JOHN WILEY & SONS, INC., PUBLICATION

New York / Chichester / Weinheim / Brisbane / Singapore / Toronto

Address All Inquiries to the Publisher
Wiley-Liss, Inc., 605 Third Avenue, New York, NY 10158-0012

Printed in the United States of America.

This text is printed on acid-free paper.

Cover Illustration: An artist's conception of the initiation of the DNA transcription mechanism catalyzed by RNA polymerase and involving protein transcription factors.

Subject Editor: Stephanie Diment
Design: Laura Ierardi
Senior Managing Editor: John Sollami
Marketing Managers: David Stier and David Steltenkamp
Manufacturing Manager: Rick Mumma
Illustration Coordinator: Barbara Kennedy
Illustrations and Cover: Page Two

This book was set in ITC Garamond Light by Bi-Comp Incorporated, and was printed and bound by Von Hoffmann Press.

Library of Congress Cataloging-in-Publication Data

Textbook of biochemistry: with clinical correlations/edited by
Thomas M. Devlin. — 4th ed.
p. cm.
Includes bibliographical references and index.
ISBN 0-471-15451-2
1. Biochemistry. 2. Clinical biochemistry. I. Devlin, Thomas M.
[DNLM: 1. Biochemistry. QU 4 T355 1997]
QP514.2.T4 1997 97-1078
612′.015—dc21 CIP

10 9 8 7 6 5 4 3 2

To

Katie, Matthew, Ryan, and Laura

CONTRIBUTORS

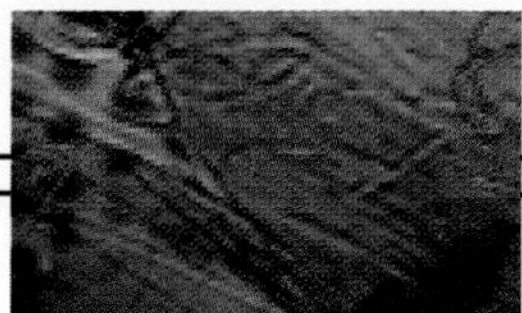

Stelios Aktipis, Ph.D.
Professor
Department of Molecular and Cellular Biochemistry
Stritch School of Medicine
Loyola University of Chicago
2160 S. First Avenue
Maywood, IL 60153

Carol N. Angstadt, Ph.D.
Professor
Department of Biomedical Sciences, M.S.# 456
Allegheny University of the Health Sciences
Broad and Vine Streets
Philadelphia, PA 19102-1192

email: angstadtc@allegheny

William Awad, JR., M.D., Ph.D.
Professor
Departments of Medicine and of Biochemistry
University of Miami School of Medicine
P.O. Box 016960
Miami, FL 33101

email: wawad@mednet.med.miami.edu

James Baggott, Ph.D.
Associate Professor
Department of Biochemistry
MCP·Hahnemann School of Medicine
Allegheny University of the Health Sciences
2900 Queen Lane
Philadelphia, PA 19129

email: baggottj@allegheny.edu

Stephen G. Chaney, Ph.D.
Professor
Departments of Biochemistry and Biophysics and of Nutrition
Mary Ellen Jones Building
University of North Carolina at Chapel Hill School of Medicine CB# 7260
Chapel Hill, NC 27599-7260

email: schaney.biochem@mhs.unc.edu

Marguerite W. Coomes, Ph.D.
Associate Professor
Department of Biochemistry and Molecular Biology
Howard University College of Medicine
520 W Street, N.W.
Washington, DC 20059-0001

email: mwcoomes@erols.com

Joseph G. Cory, Ph.D.
Professor and Chair
Department of Biochemistry
Brody Medical Sciences Building
East Carolina University School of Medicine
Greenville, NC 27858-4354

David W. Crabb, M.D.
Professor
Departments of Medicine and of Biochemistry and Molecular Biology
Emerson Hall 317
Indiana University School of Medicine
545 Barnhill Drive
Indianapolis, IN 46202-5124

email: dcrabb@medicine.dmed.iupi.edu

Thomas M. Devlin, Ph.D.
Professor Emeritus
Department of Biochemistry
MCP·Hahnemann School of Medicine
Allegheny University of the Health Sciences
Broad and Vine Streets
Philadelphia, PA 19102-1192

email: devlint@allegheny.edu

John E. Donelson, Ph.D.
Professor
Howard Hughes Medical Institute and Department of Biochemistry
University of Iowa College of Medicine
300 Eckstein Medical Research Building
Iowa City, IA 52242

email: jedonels@vaxa.weeg.viowa.edu

Robert H. Glew, Ph.D.
Professor and Chair
Department of Biochemistry
Basic Medical Science Building, Room 249
University of New Mexico
School of Medicine
915 Camino de Salud NE
Albuquerque, NM 87131

email: rglew@medusa.unm.edu

Dohn G. Glitz, Ph.D.
Professor
Department of Biological Chemistry
UCLA School of Medicine
Los Angeles, CA 90095-1737

email: dglitz@biochem.medsch.ucla.edu

Robert A. Harris, Ph.D.
Showalter Professor and Chair
Department of Biochemistry and Molecular Biology
Indiana University School of Medicine
635 Barnhill Drive
Indianapolis, IN 46202-5122

email: raharris@indyvax.dupui.edu

Ulrich Hopfer, M.D., Ph.D.
Professor
Department of Physiology and Biophysics
Case Western Reserve University
2109 Abington Road
Cleveland, OH 44106-4970

email: uxh@po.cwru.edu

Michael N. Liebman, Ph.D.
Director, Bioinformatics and Genomics
VYSIS, Inc.
3100 Woodcreek Drive
Downers Grove, IL 60515

email: mliebman@vysis.com

Gerald Litwack, Ph.D.
Professor and Chair
Department of Biochemistry and Molecular Pharmacology
Deputy Director Kimmel Cancer Institute
Jefferson Medical College
Thomas Jefferson University
233 South 10th Street
Philadelphia, PA 19107

email: litwack@lac.jci.tju.edu

Bettie Sue Siler Masters, Ph.D.
Robert A. Welch Foundation Professor in Chemistry
Department of Biochemistry
University of Texas Health Science Center at San Antonio
7703 Floyd Curl Drive
San Antonio, TX 78284-7760

email: masters@uthscsa.edu

Denis McGarry, Ph.D.
Professor
Departments of Internal Medicine and of Biochemistry
Bldg. G5, Room 210
University of Texas Southwestern Medical Center at Dallas
5323 Harry Hines Blvd
Dallas, TX 75235-9135

email: utsmc.1nparke@mednet.swmed.edu

Richard T. Okita, Ph.D.
Professor
Department of Pharmaceutical Science
105 Wegner Hall
College of Pharmacy
Washington State University
Pullman, WA 99164-6510

email: okitar@mail.wsu.edu

Merle S. Olson, Ph.D.
Professor and Chair
Department of Biochemistry
University of Texas Health Science Center
7703 Floyd Curl Drive
San Antonio, TX 78284-7760

email: olson@bioc02.uthscsa.edu

Francis J. Schmidt, Ph.D.
Professor
Department of Biochemistry
M121 Medical Sciences
University of Missouri-Columbia
Columbia, MO 65212-0001

email: bcfranks@muccmail.missouri.edu

Thomas J. Schmidt, Ph.D.
Associate Professor
Department of Physiology and Biophysics
5-610 Bowen Science Building
University of Iowa, College of Medicine
Iowa City, IA 52242-1109

email: thomas-schmidt@uiowa.edu

Richard M. Schultz, Ph.D.
Professor and Chair
Department of Molecular and Cellular Biochemistry
Stritch School of Medicine
Loyola University of Chicago
2160 South First Avenue
Maywood, IL 60153

email: rschult@luc.edu

Nancy B. Schwartz, Ph.D.
Professor
Departments of Pediatrics and of Biochemistry and Molecular Biology
University of Chicago, MC 5058
5841 S. Maryland Ave.
Chicago, IL 60637-1463

email: n-schwartz@u.chicago.edu

Thomas E. Smith, Ph.D.
Professor and Chair
Department of Biochemistry and Molecular Biology
College of Medicine
Howard University
520 W Street, N.W.
Washington, DC 20059-0001

email: tcsmith@crols.com

Gerald Soslau, Ph.D.
Professor
Department of Biochemistry and Director, IMS Program
MCP·Hahnemann School of Medicine, M.S. 344
Allegheny University of the Health Sciences
Broad and Vine Streets
Philadelphia, PA 19102-1192

email: soslaug@allegheny.edu

J. Lyndal York, Ph.D.
Professor
Department of Biochemistry and Molecular Biology
College of Medicine
University of Arkansas for Medical Science
4301 W. Markham St.
Little Rock, AR 72205-7199

email: jlyork@life.uams.edu

FOREWORD

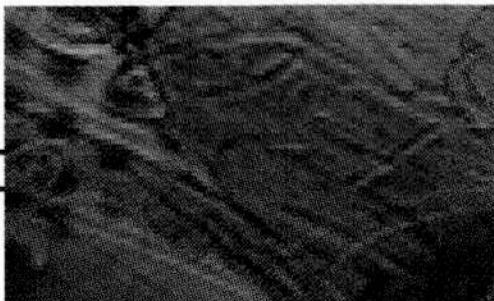

These are very exciting times for biochemistry and especially for that part that pertains to human biology and human medicine. The much discussed Human Genome Project is likely to be completed very early in the next millennium, by the time most users of *Textbook of Biochemistry With Clinical Correlations* have graduated. The Human Genome Project should provide a blueprint of the 100,000 or so genes that the human genome is estimated to contain and lead to an explosion of amazing proportions in knowledge on complex physiological processes and multigenic disorders. This mapping will reveal undreamed of interrelationships and elucidate control mechanisms of the fundamental processes of development of the human organism and of their interactions with both milieus (the internal and external). Already, one eukaryotic genome (that of brewer's yeast, comprising 14 million base pairs in 16 chromosomes) was completed just before I set out to write this Foreword, while three microbial genomes (that of *Mycoplasma genitalium*—580,070 base pairs, *Hemophilus influenzae*—1.83 million base pairs, and *Synechosystis*—a photosynthetic organism—3.57 million base pairs) have been completed within 3 to 18 months of isolation of their DNA. Work on the genomes of *Mycobacterium tuberculosis* (4.5 million base pairs) and of *Plasmodium falciparum*—the malarial parasite (27 million base pairs in 14 chromosomes)—is now being undertaken and should lead to knowledge that can produce novel approaches to the treatment and control of these two scourges of humankind. The theoretical and technical principles involved in this type of work are clearly described in Chapters 14, 15, and 18 of *Textbook of Biochemistry With Clinical Correlations,* which will ensure that readers will understand and appreciate future developments in the field.

Discoveries on the molecular basis of human disease are also being reported at an unprecedented and dizzying rate, opening wider and wider the window to many less frequent afflictions produced by mutated genes accumulating in the human gene pool. The era of molecular medicine has already arrived. Since the very first edition of *Textbook of Biochemistry With Clinical Correlations,* the correlations have been a feature that has made the book truly unique. In this new edition, the correlations are numerous, succinct, and integrated with, but also independent of, the text. They not only reflect current progress but indicate more than ever before how biochemistry, molecular biology, and human genetics have become the foundation stones of all areas of modern medicine. These previously separate disciplines have become so intimately and inextricably intertwined that little knowledge and understanding of one can occur without knowledge and understanding of others. One of the many strengths of this book is that clear examples of the convergence and integration of biological disciplines can be found in the clinical correlations.

In this fourth edition of *Textbook of Biochemistry With Clinical Correlations,* the contributors have provided an up-to-date and logical coverage of basic biochemistry, molecular biology, and normal and abnormal aspects of physiological chemistry. This material is appropriate and relevant for medical and other health science students, particularly as we approach the third millenium in the midst of amazing and pervasive progress in medical science and biotechnology. To enhance the text, a completely new series of vivid illustrations has been added, which will undoubtedly further the readers' understanding of the complexity of many of the concepts. Students of medical and health sciences should appreciate that the time and effort invested in learning the material presented here will be very well spent. This knowledge will provide the framework within which further developments will be understood and applied as the readers begin to care for the physical and mental well-being of those entrusted to them. Furthermore, the knowledge derived from this book will also provide satisfying insight into the processes that underlie human life and the amazing power of the human mind to explore and understand it. As in previous editions, the fourth edition includes many multiple choice questions (and answers) at the end of each chapter that should facilitate this learning while ensuring success in professional and other examinations.

I am happy and privileged to have watched the growth of human biochemistry (because of my teaching and research responsibilities) since my medical student days nearly half-a-century ago. It has been an amazing spectacle, full of thrills and exciting adventures into aspects of human cells that were previously shrouded in mystery and ignorance. As my knowledge has increased, so has my sense of awe and wonder at the unfolding beauty of this marvelous display of nature's secrets.

As the late Alberto Sols frequently said: "The Biochemistry of today is the Medicine of tomorrow." *Textbook of Biochemistry With Clinical Correlations* illustrates the veracity of this insight.

FRANK VELLA
University of Saskatchewan

PREFACE

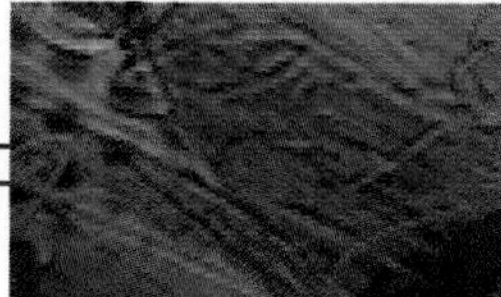

The purposes of the fourth edition of the *Textbook of Biochemistry With Clinical Correlations* remain unchanged from the earlier editions: to present a clear discussion of the biochemistry of mammalian cells; to relate the biochemical events at the cellular level to the physiological processes occurring in the whole animal; and to cite examples of deviant biochemical processes in human disease.

The continued rapid advances in knowledge, particularly due to the techniques of molecular biology, required a critical review and evaluation of the entire content of the previous edition. Every chapter has been revised and updated. Significant additions of new material, clarifications, and some deletions were made throughout. Amino acid metabolism was combined into a single chapter and DNA structure and function was divided into two chapters for better coverage of this rapidly expanding field. Topics for inclusion were selected to cover the essential areas of both biochemistry and physiological chemistry for upper-level undergraduate, graduate-level and especially professional school courses in biochemistry. Since the application of biochemistry is so important to human medicine, the text has an overriding emphasis on the biochemistry of mammalian cells.

The textbook is written such that any sequence considered most appropriate by an instructor can be presented. It is not formally divided into major sections, but related topics are grouped together. After an introductory chapter on cell structure, Chapters 2 to 5 concern the **Major Structural Components of Cells,** that is, proteins and their many functions, and cell membranes and their major roles. **Metabolism** is discussed in the following eight chapters, starting with the conservation of energy, then the synthesis and degradation of the major cellular components, and concluding with a chapter on the integration of these pathways in humans. The next section of six chapters covers **Information Transfer and Its Control,** describing the structure and synthesis of the major cellular macromolecules, that is, DNA, RNA, and protein. A separate chapter on **Biotechnology** is included because information from this area has had such a significant impact on the development of our current state of biochemical knowledge. The section concludes with a chapter on the **Regulation of Gene Expression** in which mechanisms in both prokaryotes and eukaryotes are presented. The fourth major section represents **Signal Transduction and Amplification** and includes two chapters on hormones that emphasize their biochemical functions as messengers and a chapter on **Molecular Cell Biology** describes four major mammalian signal transducing systems. The textbook concludes with six chapters on topics that comprise **Physiological Chemistry,** including cytochrome P450 enzymes and xenobiotic metabolism, iron and heme metabolism, gas transport and pH regulation, digestion and absorption, and human nutrition.

A major addition from previous editions is the extensive use of color in the **illustrations** as a means to emphasize important points. All figures were reviewed and new drawings were prepared to illustrate the narrative discussion. In many cases the adage "A picture is worth a thousand words" is appropriate and the reader is encouraged to study the illustrations because they are meant to illuminate often confusing aspects of a topic.

In each chapter the relevancy of the topic to human life processes are presented in **Clinical Correlations,** which describe the aberrant biochemistry of disease states. A number of new correlations have been included. The correlations are not intended to review all of the major diseases but rather to cite examples of disease processes where the biochemical implications are well established. In addition, we specifically avoided presenting clinical case reports because it was considered more significant to deal with the general clinical condition. References are included to facilitate exploration of the topic in more detail. In some cases similar clinical problems are presented in different chapters, but each from a different perspective. All pertinent biochemical information is presented in the main text, and an understanding of the material does not require a reading of the correlations. In a few cases, clinical discussions are part of the principal text because of the close relationship of some topics to medical conditions.

Each chapter concludes with a set of **Questions and Answers;** the multiple-choice format was retained as being valuable to students for self-assessment of their knowledge. The question type was limited to the types now occurring in national examinations. All questions were reviewed and many new ones added. The questions cover a range of topics in each chapter, and each has an annotated answer, with references to the page in the textbook covering the content of the question.

The appendix, **Review of Organic Chemistry,** is designed as a ready reference for the nomenclature and structures of organic molecules encountered in biochemistry and is not intended as a comprehensive review of organic chemistry. The material is presented in the Appendix rather than at the beginning of those chapters dealing with the metabolism of each class of organic molecules. The reader might find it valuable to become familiar with the content and then use the Appendix as a ready reference when reading related sections in the main text.

We still believe that a multicontributor textbook is the best approach to achieve an accurate and current presentation of biochemistry. Each author is involved actively in teaching biochemistry in a medical or graduate school and has an active research interest in the field in which he or she has written. Thus, each has the perspective of the classroom instructor, with the experience to select the topics and determine the emphasis required for students in a course of biochemistry. Every contributor, however, brings to the book an individual approach, leading to some differences in presentation. However, every chapter was critically edited and revised in order to have a consistent writing style and to eliminate repetitions and redundancies. A limited repetition of some topics in different chapters was permitted when it was considered that the repetition would facilitate the learning process.

The individual contributors were requested to prepare their chapters for a **teaching book.** The book is not intended as a compendium of biochemical facts or a review of the current literature, but each chapter contains sufficient detail on the subject to make it useful as a resource. Each contributor was requested not to refer to specific researchers; our apologies to those many biochemists who rightfully should be acknowledged for their outstanding research contributions to the field of biochemistry. Each chapter contains a **Bibliography** that can be used as an entry point to the research literature.

In any project one person must accept the responsibility for the final product. The decisions concerning the selection of topics and format, reviewing the drafts, and responsibility for the final checking of the book were entirely mine. I welcome comments, criticisms, and suggestions from the students, faculty, and professionals who use this textbook. It is our hope that this work will be of value to those embarking on the exciting experience of learning biochemistry for the first time and to those who are returning to a topic in which the information is expanding so rapidly.

THOMAS M. DEVLIN

ACKNOWLEDGMENTS

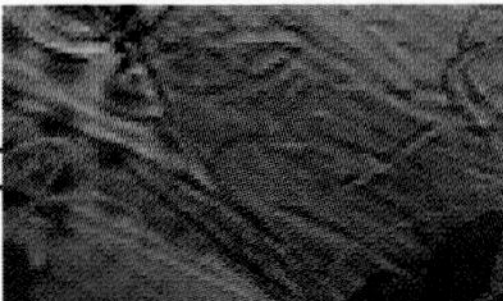

Without the encouragement and participation of many people, this project would never have been accomplished. My personal and very deep appreciation goes to each of the contributors for accepting the challenge of preparing the chapters, for sharing their ideas and making recommendations to improve the book, for accepting so readily suggestions to modify their contributions, and for cooperating throughout the period of preparation. To each I extend my sincerest thanks for a job well done.

The contributors received the support of associates and students in the preparation of their chapters, and, for fear of omitting someone, it was decided not to acknowledge individuals by name. To everyone who gave time unselfishly and shared in the objective and critical evaluation of the text, we extend a sincere thank you. In addition, every contributor has been influenced by former teachers and colleagues, various reference resources, and, of course, the research literature of biochemistry; we are deeply indebted to these many sources of inspiration.

I am particularly indebted to Dr. Frank Vella, Professor of Biochemistry at the University of Saskatchewan, Canada, who assisted me in editing the text. Dr. Vella is a distinguished biochemist who has made a major personal effort to improve the teaching of biochemistry throughout the world. He read every chapter in draft form and made significant suggestions for clarifying and improving the presentation. Dr. Vella also honored me by writing the Foreword to the fourth edition of this textbook. I extend to him my deepest appreciation and thanks for his participation and friendship.

A very special thanks to two friends and colleagues who again have been of immeasurable value to me during the preparation of this edition: My gratitude goes to Dr. James Baggott, who patiently allowed me to use him as a sounding board for ideas and who unselfishly shared with me his suggestions and criticisms of the text, and to Dr. Carol Angstadt, who reviewed many of the chapters and gave me valuable suggestions. To each I extend my deepest gratitude.

I extend my sincerest appreciation and thanks to the members of the staff of the STM Division of John Wiley & Sons who participated in the preparation of this edition. Special recognition and thanks go to Dr. Brian Crawford, Vice President and General Manager of Life Sciences and Medicine, who gave his unqualified support to the preparation of the fourth edition. I am indebted to Joe Ingram, Publisher, Life Sciences, who conscientiously guided the planning of this edition. I am very indebted to Dr. Stephanie Diment, Associate Editor, for always being available to answer questions and to make valuable suggestions, and who has patiently kept me on track. She has been a constant support; thank you. My deepest appreciation is extended to John Sollami, Senior Managing Editor, who with constant good humor meticulously oversaw the production. He kept the flow of activities reasonable, listened patiently to my suggestions and concerns, and kept us on schedule. It has been a real pleasure to work with a really knowledgeable and conscientious professional and to him I extend a very special thanks. I extend to Louise Page, New Media Editor, my deepest appreciation for her skillful organization of the CD containing the figures from the textbook. Credit for the design of the book goes to Laura Ierardi, to whom I extend my appreciation. My thanks to Christina Della Bartolomea, copyeditor, and Maria Coughlin, indexer, both of whom did an excellent job. A significant improvement in this edition is the addition of many original illustrations. My most heartfelt thanks go to Dean Gonzalez, STM Illustration Manager, and Barbara Kennedy, Illustration Supervisor, at Wiley, who handled the details and flow of illustrations. A special recognition is extended to Dr. Lisa Gardner, Production Manager and Editor of Page Two, and her staff who transformed the rough drawings of the contributors into meaningful illustrations. No book is successful without the activities of a Marketing Department; special thanks are due to Reed Elfenbein, Vice President, Marketing and Sales, David Stier, Senior Marketing Manager, David Steltenkamp, Associate Marketing Manager, and their colleagues at Wiley for their new ideas and efforts.

Finally, a very special thanks to my loving, supportive, and considerate wife, Marjorie, who had the foresight to encourage me to undertake this project, who again supported me during the days of intensive work, and who again created an environment in which I could devote the many hours required for the preparation of this textbook. To her my deepest appreciation.

THOMAS M. DEVLIN

CONTENTS IN BRIEF

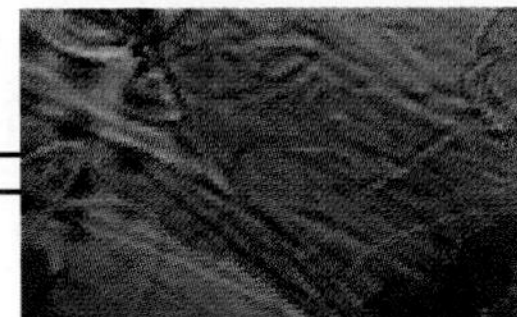

CONTENTS

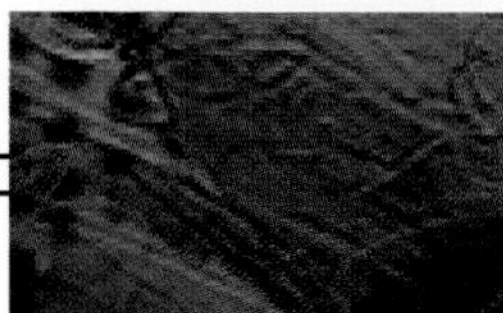

■ 9 ■

LIPID METABOLISM I: UTILIZATION AND STORAGE OF ENERGY IN LIPID FORM 361

J. Denis McGarry

■ 10 ■

LIPID METABOLISM II: PATHWAYS OF METABOLISM OF SPECIAL LIPIDS 395

Robert H. Glew

■ 11 ■

AMINO ACID METABOLISM 445

Marguerite W. Coomes

■ 12 ■

PURINE AND PYRIMIDINE NUCLEOTIDE METABOLISM 489

Joseph G. Cory

■ 13 ■

METABOLIC INTERRELATIONSHIPS 525

Robert A. Harris and David W. Crabb

■ 18 ■

RECOMBINANT DNA AND BIOTECHNOLOGY 757

Gerald Soslau

■ 19 ■

REGULATION OF GENE EXPRESSION 799

John E. Donelson

■ 20 ■

BIOCHEMISTRY OF HORMONES I: POLYPEPTIDE HORMONES 839

Gerald Litwack and Thomas J. Schmidt

■ 21 ■

BIOCHEMISTRY OF HORMONES II: STEROID HORMONES 893

Gerald Litwack and Thomas J. Schmidt

26

DIGESTION AND ABSORPTION OF BASIC NUTRITIONAL CONSTITUENTS 1055

Ulrich Hopfer

CLINICAL CORRELATIONS

27

PRINCIPLES OF NUTRITION I: MACRONUTRIENTS 1087

Stephen G. Chaney

CLINICAL CORRELATIONS

28

PRINCIPLES OF NUTRITION II: MICRONUTRIENTS 1107

Stephen G. Chaney

CLINICAL CORRELATIONS

APPENDIX

REVIEW OF ORGANIC CHEMISTRY 1137

Carol N. Angstadt

INDEX

CHAPTER QUESTIONS AND ANSWERS

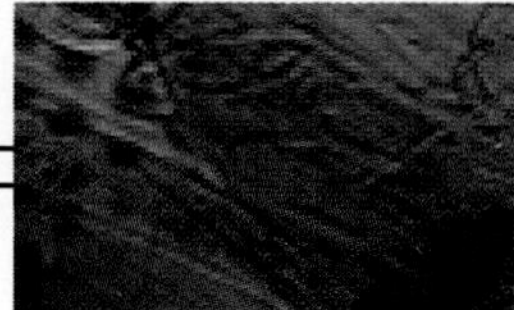

The questions at the end of each chapter are provided to help you test your knowledge and increase your understanding of biochemistry. Since they are intended to help you strengthen your knowledge, their construction does not always conform to principles for assessing your retention of individual facts. Specifically, you will sometimes be expected to draw on your knowledge of several areas to answer a single question, and some questions may take longer to analyze than the average time allowed on certain national examinations. Occasionally, you may disagree with the answer. If this occurs, we hope that after you read the commentary that accompanies the answer to the question, you will see the point and your insight into the biochemical problem will be increased.

The question types conform to those currently used in objective examinations. They are:

Type 1: Choose the one best answer

Type 2: Match the numbered statement or phrase with one of the lettered options given above.

CHAPTER

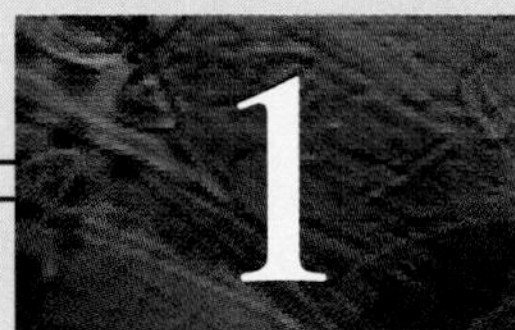

EUKARYOTIC CELL STRUCTURE

Thomas M. Devlin

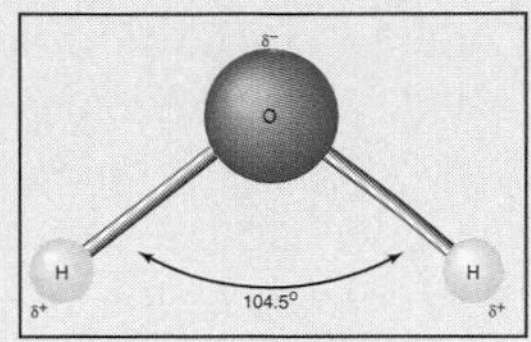

1.1 ■ OVERVIEW: CELLS AND CELLULAR COMPARTMENTS

Over three billion years ago, under conditions not entirely clear and in a time span difficult to comprehend, elements such as carbon, hydrogen, oxygen, nitrogen, sulfur, and phosphorus formed simple chemical compounds. They combined, dispersed, and recombined to form a variety of larger molecules until a combination was achieved that was capable of replicating itself. These macromolecules consisted of simpler molecules linked together by chemical bonds. With continued evolution and formation of ever more complex molecules, the water environment around some of these self-replicating molecules became enclosed by a membrane. This development gave these primordial structures the ability to control their own environment to some extent. A form of life had evolved and a unit of three-dimensional space—a cell—had been established. With the passing of time a diversity of cells evolved, and their chemistry and structure became more complex. They could extract nutrients from the environment, chemically converting these nutrients to sources of energy or to complex molecules, control chemical processes that they catalyzed, and carry out cellular replication. Thus the vast diversity of life observed today began. The cell is the basic unit of life in all forms of living organisms, from the smallest bacterium to the most complex animal.

The limiting outer membrane of cells, the **plasma membrane,** delineates the space occupied by a cell and separates the variable and potentially hostile environment outside from the relatively constant milieu within. It is the communication link between the cell and its surroundings.

On the basis of microscopic and biochemical differences, living cells are divided into two major classes: **prokaryotes,** which include bacteria, blue-green algae, and rickettsiae, and **eukaryotes,** which include yeasts, fungi, and plant and animal cells. Prokaryotes have a variety of shapes and sizes, in most cases being 1/1000 to 1/10,000 the size of eukaryotic cells. They lack intracellular membrane-bound structures that can be visualized by a microscope (Figure 1.1). The deoxyribonucleic acid (DNA) of prokaryotes is often segregated into a discrete mass, the nucleoid region, that is not surrounded by a membrane or envelope. The plasma membrane is often invaginated. In contrast, eukaryotic cells have a well-defined membrane surrounding a central nucleus and a variety of intracellular structures and organelles (Figure 1.1*b*). Intracellular membrane systems establish distinct subcellular compartments, as described in Section 1.4, that permit a unique degree of subcellular specialization. By compartmentalization different chemical reactions that require different environments can occur simultaneously. Many reactions occur in or on specific membranes, thus creating an additional environment for the diverse functions of cells.

Besides these structural variations between prokaryotic and eukaryotic cells (Figures 1*a* and 1*b*), there are differences in chemical composition and biochemical activities. Prokaryotes lack histones, a class of proteins that complex with DNA in eukaryotes. There are major structural differences in the ribonucleic acid–protein complexes involved in biosynthesis of proteins between the cell types, as well as differences in transport mechanisms across the plasma membrane and in enzyme content. The many similarities, however, are equally striking. The emphasis throughout this book is on the chemistry of eukaryotes, particularly mammalian cells, but much of our knowledge of the biochemistry of living cells has come from studies of prokaryotic and nonmammalian eukaryotic cells. The basic chemical components and fundamental chemical reactions of all living cells are very similar. Availability of certain cell populations, for example, bacteria in contrast to human liver, has led to much of our knowledge about some cells; in some areas our knowledge is derived nearly exclusively from studies of prokaryotes. The universality of many biochemical phenomena, however, permits many extrapolations from bacteria to humans.

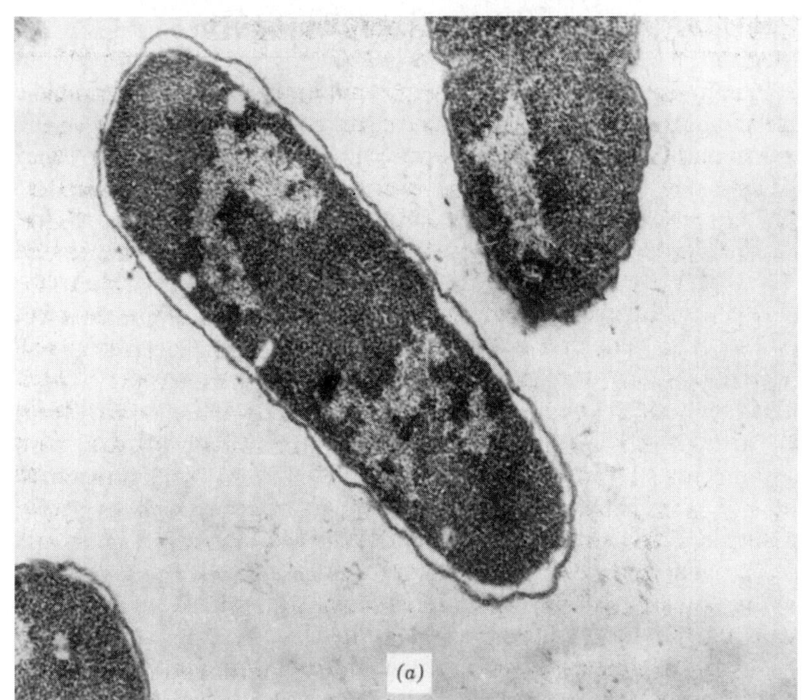

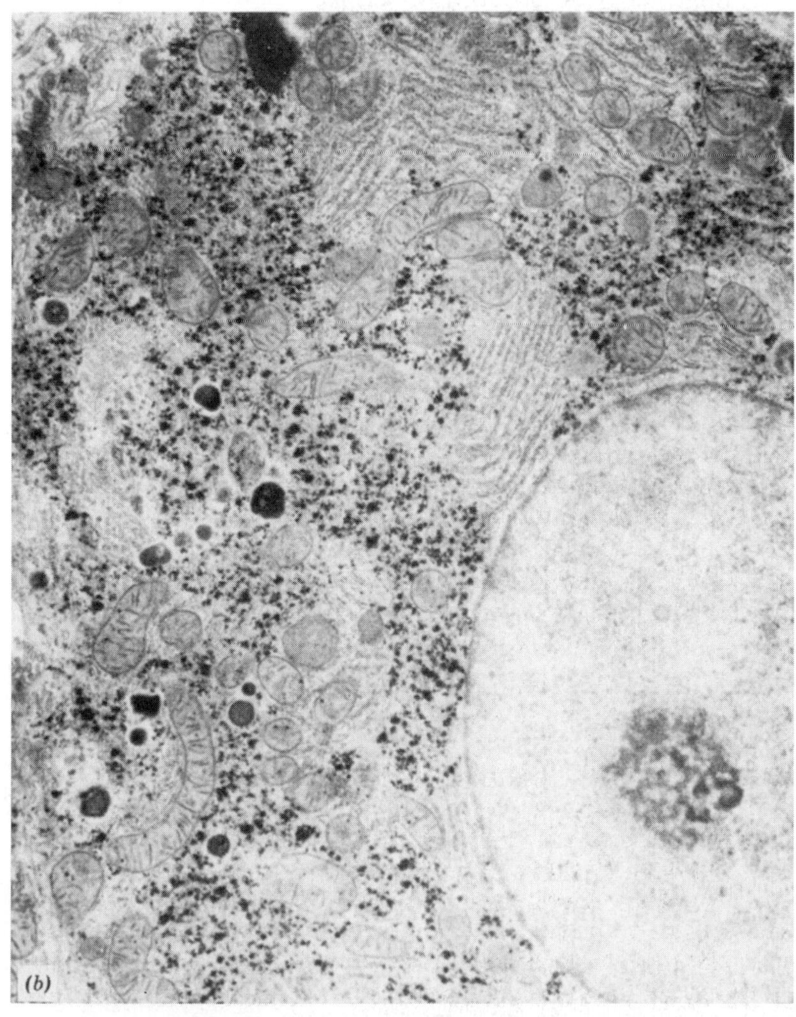

FIGURE 1.1
Cellular organization of prokaryotic and eukaryotic cells.
(*a*) Electron micrograph of *Escherichia coli*, a representative prokaryote; approximate magnification ×30,000. There is little apparent intracellular organization and no cytoplasmic organelles. Chromatin is condensed in a nuclear zone but not surrounded by a membrane. Prokaryotic cells are much smaller than eukaryotic cells. (*b*) Electron micrograph of a thin section of a liver cell (rat hepatocyte), a representative eukaryotic cell; approximate magnification ×7500. Note the distinct nuclear membrane, different membrane-bound organelles or vesicles, and extensive membrane systems. Various membranes create a variety of intracellular compartments.
Photograph (a) *generously supplied by Dr. M. E. Bayer, Fox Chase Cancer Institute, Philadelphia, PA; photograph* (b) *reprinted with permission of Dr. K. R. Porter, from Porter, K. R., and Bonneville, M. A. In:* Fine Structure of Cells and Tissues. *Philadelphia: Lea & Febiger, 1972.*

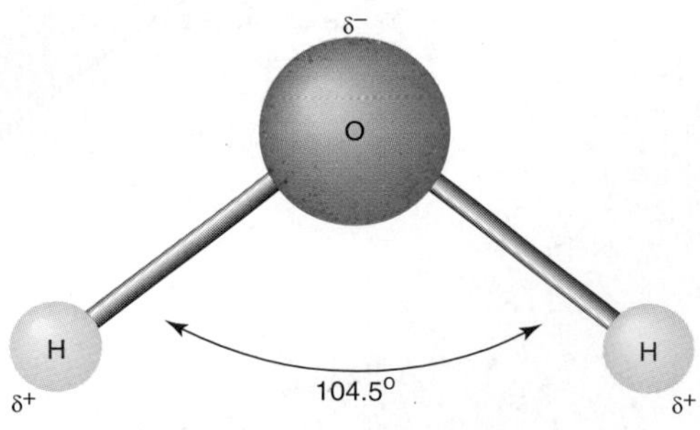

FIGURE 1.2
Structure of a water molecule.
The H—O—H bond angle is 104.5°. Both hydrogen atoms carry a partial positive charge and the oxygen a partial negative charge, creating a dipole.

Before we dissect the complexities of mammalian cells and tissues in the following chapters, it is appropriate to review some of the chemical and physical characteristics of the environment in which the various biochemical phenomena occur. This environment places many constraints on the cell's activities. The concluding section outlines the activities and roles of subcellular compartments.

1.2 ■ CELLULAR ENVIRONMENT: WATER AND SOLUTES

All biological cells contain essentially the same building blocks and types of macromolecules. The general classes of substances in cells are presented in Table 1.1. There are significant variations in concentration of specific components in different cell types and in organelles of eukaryotic cells. **Microenvironments** are also created by macromolecules and membranes in which the composition differs from that of the surrounding milieu. Cells depend on the external environment for nutrients required for replacement of components, growth, and energy needs. They have a variety of mechanisms to cope with variations in composition of the external environment. **Water** is the one common component of all environments. It is the solvent in which the substances required for the cell's existence are dissolved or suspended. The unique physicochemical properties of water make life on earth possible.

Hydrogen Bonds Form Between Water Molecules

Two hydrogen atoms share their electrons with an unshared pair of electrons of an oxygen atom to form a water molecule. The oxygen nucleus has a stronger attraction for shared electrons than hydrogen, and positively charged hydrogen nuclei are left with an unequal share of electrons, creating a partial positive charge on each hydrogen and a partial negative charge on oxygen. The bond angle between hydrogens and oxygen is 104.5°, making the molecule electrically asymmetric and producing an electric dipole (Figure 1.2). Water molecules interact because positively charged hydrogen atoms on one molecule are attracted to the negatively charged oxygen atom on another, with formation of a weak bond between two water molecules (Figure 1.3*a*). This bond, indicated by a dashed line, is a **hydrogen bond.** A detailed discussion of noncovalent interactions between molecules, including electrostatic, van der Waals, and hydrophobic, is presented on page 64. Five molecules of water form a tetrahedral structure (Figure 1.3*b*), because each oxygen shares its electrons with four hydrogen atoms and each hydrogen with another oxygen. A tetrahedral lattice structure is formed in ice and gives ice its crystalline structure. Some hydrogen bonds are broken as ice is transformed to liquid water. Each bond is relatively

(*a*)

(*b*)

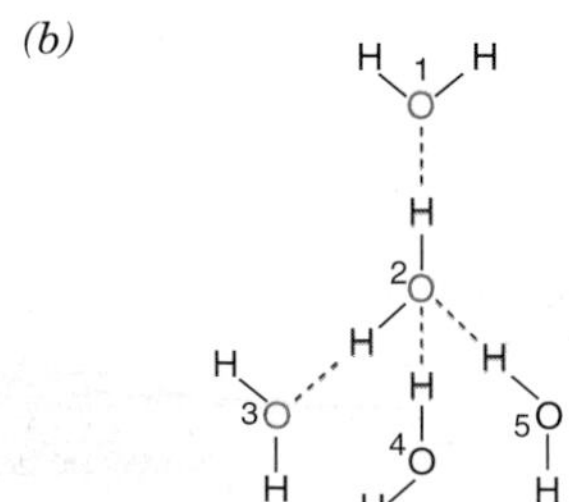

FIGURE 1.3
Hydrogen bonding.
(*a*) Hydrogen bonding, indicated by dashed lines, between two water molecules. (*b*) Tetrahedral hydrogen bonding of five water molecules. Water molecules 1, 2, and 3 are in the plane of the page, 4 is below, and 5 is above.

TABLE 1.1 Chemical Components of Biological Cells

Component	*Range of Molecular Weights*
H_2O	18
Inorganic ions	23–100
Na^+, K^+, Cl^-, SO_4^{2-},	
HCO_3^- Ca^{2+}, Mg^{2+}, etc.	
Small organic molecules	100–1200
Carbohydrates, amino acids,	
lipids, nucleotides, peptides	
Macromolecules	50,000–1,000,000,000
Proteins, polysaccharides,	
nucleic acids	

weak compared to a covalent bond but the large number of hydrogen bonds between molecules in liquid water is the reason for the stability of water. Liquid water actually has a definite structure due to hydrogen bonding that is in a dynamic state as these bonds break and reform. Hydrogen bonds in water have a half-life of less than 1×10^{-10} s. Liquid water contains a significant number of hydrogen bonds even at 100°C, which accounts for its high heat of vaporization; in the transformation from liquid to vapor state, hydrogen bonds are disrupted.

Water molecules hydrogen bond to different chemical structures. Hydrogen bonding also occurs between other molecules and within a molecule wherever electronegative oxygen or nitrogen comes in close proximity to hydrogen covalently bonded to another electronegative atom. Representative hydrogen bonds are presented in Figure 1.4. Intramolecular hydrogen bonding occurs extensively in large macromolecules such as proteins and nucleic acids and is partially responsible for their structural stability.

Many models for the structure of liquid water have been proposed, but none adequately explains all its properties.

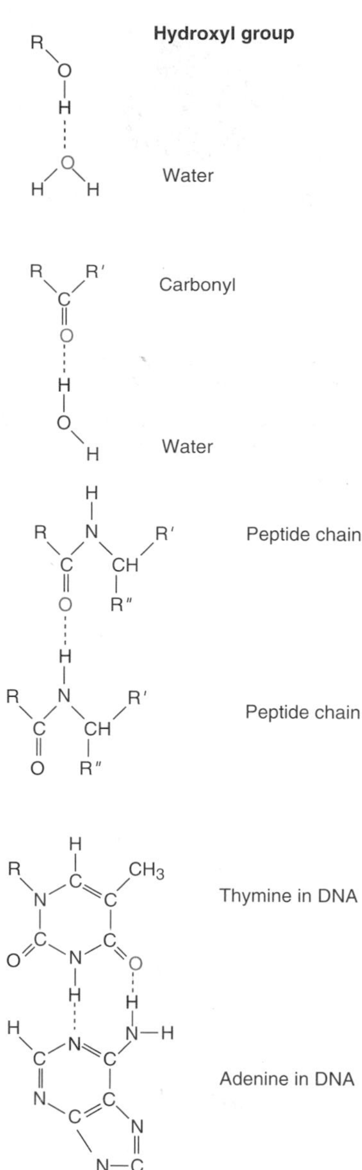

FIGURE 1.4
Representative hydrogen bonds of importance in biological systems.

Water Has Unique Solvent Properties

The polar nature and ability to form hydrogen bonds are the basis for the unique **solvent properties** of water. Polar molecules are readily dispersed in water. **Salts** in which a crystal lattice is held together by attraction of positive and negative groups dissolve in water because electrostatic forces in the crystal can be overcome by attraction of charges to the dipole of water. NaCl is an example where electrostatic attraction of individual Na^+ and Cl^- atoms is overcome by interaction of Na^+ with the negative charge on oxygen atoms, and Cl^- with positive charges on the hydrogen atoms. Thus a shell of water surrounds the individual ions. The number of weak charge–charge interactions between water and Na^+ and Cl^- ions is sufficient to separate the two charged ions.

Many organic molecules that contain nonionic but weakly polar groups are soluble in water because of attraction of these groups to molecules of water. Sugars and alcohols are readily soluble in water for this reason. **Amphipathic** molecules, compounds that contain both polar and nonpolar groups, disperse in water if attraction of the polar group for water can overcome hydrophobic interactions of nonpolar portions of the molecules. Very hydrophobic molecules, such as compounds that contain long hydrocarbon chains, however, do not readily disperse as single molecules in water but interact with one another to exclude the polar water molecules.

Some Molecules Dissociate with Formation of Cations and Anions

Substances that dissociate in water into a **cation** (positively charged ion) and an **anion** (negatively charged ion) are classified as **electrolytes.** The presence of charged ions facilitates conductance of an electrical current through an aqueous solution. Sugars or alcohols, which readily dissolve in water but do not carry a charge or dissociate into charged species, are classified as **nonelectrolytes.**

Salts of alkali metals (e.g., Li, Na, and K), dissolved in water at low concentrations, dissociate completely; at high concentrations, however, there is increased potential for interaction of anions and cations. With biological systems it is customary to consider such compounds as totally dissociated because their concentrations are low. Salts of organic acids, for example, sodium lactate, also dissociate totally and are classified as electrolytes; the dissociated anion, lactate ion, reacts to a limited extent with a proton to form undissociated acid (Figure 1.5). When such salts are dissolved in water, individual ions are present in solution rather than the undissociated salt. If a solution has been prepared with

(1) $CH_3—CHOH—CHOONa \longrightarrow$ $Na^+ + CH_3—CHOH—COO^-$

Na lactate → Lactate ion

(2) $CH_3—CHOH—COO^- + H^+ \rightleftharpoons$ $CH_3—CHOH—COOH$

Lactate ion → Lactic acid

FIGURE 1.5
Reactions that occur when sodium lactate is dissolved in water.

several different salts (e.g., NaCl, K_2SO_4, and Na lactate), the original molecules do not exist as such in solution, only the ions (e.g., Na^+, K^+, SO_4^{2-} and lactate$^-$).

Many acids, however, when dissolved in water do not totally dissociate but rather establish an equilibrium between undissociated and dissociated components. Thus lactic acid, an important metabolic intermediate, partially dissociates into lactate anions and H^+ as follows:

$$CH_3{-}CHOH{-}COOH \leftrightharpoons CH_3{-}CHOH{-}COO^- + H^+$$

Because of their partial dissociation, however, such compounds have a lower capacity to carry an electrical charge on a molar basis when compared to those that dissociate totally; they are termed **weak electrolytes.**

Weak Electrolytes Dissociate Partially

In partial dissociation of a weak electrolyte, represented by HA, the concentration of the various species can be determined from the equilibrium equation:

$$K'_{eq} = \frac{[H^+][A^-]}{[HA]}$$

A^- represents the dissociated anion and square brackets indicate concentration of each component in concentration units such as moles per liter (mol L^{-1}) or millimol L^{-1}. The **activity** of each species rather than concentration should be employed in the equilibrium equation but since most compounds of interest in biological systems are present in low concentration, the value for activity approaches that of concentration. Thus the equilibrium constant is indicated as $\boldsymbol{K'_{eq}}$ to indicate that it is an apparent constant based on concentrations. The term K'_{eq} is a function of the temperature of the system, increasing with increasing temperatures. The degree of dissociation of an electrolyte depends on the affinity of the anion for H^+. There will be more dissociation if the weak dipole forces of water interacting with the anion and cation are stronger than the electrostatic forces between anion and H^+. From the dissociation equation, it is apparent that K'_{eq} will be a small number if the degree of dissociation of a substance is small but large if the degree of dissociation is large. Obviously, for compounds that dissociate totally, a K'_{eq} cannot be determined because at equilibrium there is no remaining undissociated solute.

Water Is a Weak Electrolyte

Water dissociates as follows:

$$HOH \leftrightharpoons H^+ + OH^-$$

A proton that dissociates interacts with oxygen of another water molecule to form the hydronium ion, H_3O^+. For convenience, in this book the proton will be presented as H^+ rather than H_3O^+, even though the latter is the actual chemical species. At 25°C the value of K'_{eq} for dissociation of water is very small and is about 1.8×10^{-16}:

$$K'_{eq} = 1.8 \times 10^{-16} = \frac{[H^+][OH^-]}{[H_2O]} \quad \textbf{(1.1)}$$

With such a small K'_{eq} an insignificant number of water molecules actually dissociate relative to the number of undissociated molecules. Thus the concentration of water, which is 55.5 M, is essentially unchanged. Equation 1.1 can be rewritten as follows:

$$K'_{eq} \times [H_2O] = [H^+][OH^-] \quad \textbf{(1.2)}$$

$K'_{eq} \times [55.5]$ is a constant and is termed the **ion product of water.** Its value at 25°C is 1×10^{-14}. In pure water the concentration of H^+ equals OH^-, and by substituting $[H^+]$ for $[OH^-]$ in the equation above, $[H^+]$ is 1×10^{-7} M. Similarly,

$[OH^-]$ is also 1×10^{-7} M. The equilibrium of H_2O, H^+, and OH^- always exists in dilute solutions regardless of the presence of dissolved substances. If dissolved material alters either the H^+ or OH^- concentration, as occurs on addition of an acid or base, a concomitant change in the other ion must occur in order to satisfy the equilibrium relationship. By using the equation for the ion product, $[H^+]$ or $[OH^-]$ can be calculated if concentration of one of the ions is known.

The importance of hydrogen ions in biological systems will become apparent in subsequent chapters. For convenience $[H^+]$ is usually expressed in terms of **pH,** calculated as follows:

$$\text{pH} = \log \frac{1}{[H^+]} \qquad \textbf{(1.3)}$$

In pure water $[H^+]$ and $[OH^-]$ are both 1×10^{-7} M, and pH = 7.0. $[OH^-]$ is expressed as the pOH. For the equation describing dissociation of water, $1 \times 10^{-14} = [H^+][OH^-]$; taking negative logarithms of both sides, the equation becomes 14 = pH + pOH. Table 1.2 presents the relationship between pH and $[H^+]$.

The pH values of different **biological fluids** are presented in Table 1.3. In blood plasma, $[H^+]$ is 0.00000004 M or a pH of 7.4. Other cations are between 0.001 and 0.10 M, well over 10,000 times higher than $[H^+]$. An increase in hydrogen ion to 0.0000001 M (pH 7.0) leads to serious medical consequences and is life threatening; a detailed discussion of mechanisms by which the body maintains intra- and extracellular pH is presented in Chapter 25.

TABLE 1.2 Relationships Between $[H^+]$ and pH and $[OH^-]$ and pOH

[H⁺] (M)	*pH*	*[OH⁻] (M)*	*pOH*
1.0	0	1×10^{-14}	14
0.1 (1×10^{-1})	1	1×10^{-13}	13
1×10^{-2}	2	1×10^{-12}	12
1×10^{-3}	3	1×10^{-11}	11
1×10^{-4}	4	1×10^{-10}	10
1×10^{-5}	5	1×10^{-9}	9
1×10^{-6}	6	1×10^{-8}	8
1×10^{-7}	7	1×10^{-7}	7
1×10^{-8}	8	1×10^{-6}	6
1×10^{-9}	9	1×10^{-5}	5
1×10^{-10}	10	1×10^{-4}	4
1×10^{-11}	11	1×10^{-3}	3
1×10^{-12}	12	1×10^{-2}	2
1×10^{-13}	13	0.1 (1×10^{-1})	1
1×10^{-14}	14	1.0	0

Many Biologically Important Molecules Are Acids or Bases

The definitions of an acid and a base proposed by Lowry and Brønsted are most convenient in considering biological systems. An **acid** is a **proton donor** and a **base** is a **proton acceptor.** Hydrochloric acid (HCl) and sulfuric acid (H_2SO_4) are strong acids because they dissociate totally, and OH^- ion is a base because it accepts a proton, shifting the equilibrium

$$OH^- + H^+ \leftrightharpoons H_2O$$

When a strong acid and OH^- are combined, H^+ from the acid and OH^- interact and are in equilibrium with H_2O. Neutralization of H^+ and OH^- occurs because the ion product for water is so small.

Anions produced when strong acids dissociate totally, such as Cl^- from HCl, are not bases because they do not associate with protons in solution. When an organic acid, such as lactic acid, is dissolved in water it dissociates only partially, establishing an equilibrium between an acid (proton donor), an anion of the acid, and a proton as follows:

$$\text{Lactic acid} \leftrightharpoons \text{lactate}^- + H^+$$

Lactic acid is a **weak acid.** The anion is a base because it accepts a proton and reforms the acid. The weak acid and the base formed on dissociation are referred to as a **conjugate pair;** other examples are presented in Table 1.4. Ammonium ion (NH_4^+) is an acid because it dissociates to yield H^+ and ammonia (NH_3), an uncharged species, which is a **conjugate base.** Phosphoric acid (H_3PO_4) is an acid and PO_4^{3-} is a base, but $H_2PO_4^-$ and HPO_4^{2-} are either a base or acid depending on whether the phosphate group is accepting or donating a proton.

The tendency of a conjugate acid to dissociate H^+ can be evaluated from the K'_{eq}. The smaller the value of K'_{eq}, the less the tendency to give up a proton and the weaker the acid; the larger a K'_{eq}, the greater the tendency to dissociate a proton and the stronger the acid. Water is a very weak acid with a K'_{eq} of 1×10^{-14} at 25°C.

A convenient method of stating the K'_{eq} is in the form of $\mathbf{p}\boldsymbol{K}'$, as

$$pK' = \log \frac{1}{K'_{eq}} \qquad \textbf{(1.4)}$$

TABLE 1.3 pH of Some Biological Fluids

Fluid	*pH*
Blood plasma	7.4
Interstitial fluid	7.4
Intracellular fluid	
Cytosol (liver)	6.9
Lysosomal matrix	Below 5.0
Gastric juice	1.5–3.0
Pancreatic juice	7.8–8.0
Human milk	7.4
Saliva	6.4–7.0
Urine	5.0–8.0

TABLE 1.4 Some Conjugate Acid–Base Pairs of Importance in Biological Systems

Proton Donor (Acid)		*Proton Acceptor (Base)*
$CH_3-CHOH-COOH$ (lactic acid)	⇌	$H^+ + CH_3-CHOH-COO^-$ (lactate)
$CH_3-CO-COOH$ (pyruvic acid)	⇌	$H^+ + CH_3-CO-COO^-$ (pyruvate)
$HOOC-CH_2-CH_2-COOH$ (succinic acid)	⇌	$2H^+ + {}^-OOC-CH_2-CH_2-COO^-$ (succinate)
${}^+H_3NCH_2-COOH$ (glycine)	⇌	$H^+ + {}^+H_3N-CH_2-COO^-$ (glycinate)
H_3PO_4	⇌	$H^+ + H_2PO_4^-$
$H_2PO_4^-$	⇌	$H^+ + HPO_4^{2-}$
HPO_4^{2-}	⇌	$H^+ + PO_4^{3-}$
Glucose 6-PO_3H^-	⇌	H^+ + glucose 6-PO_3^{2-}
H_2CO_3	⇌	$H^+ + HCO_3^-$
NH_4^+	⇌	$H^+ + NH_3$
H_2O	⇌	$H^+ + OH^-$

Note the similarity of this definition with that of pH; as with pH and $[H^+]$, the relationship between pK' and K'_{eq} is an inverse one, and the smaller K'_{eq} the larger pK'. Representative values of K'_{eq} and pK' for conjugate acids of importance in biological systems are presented in Table 1.5.

A special case of a weak acid important in medicine is **carbonic acid** (H_2CO_3). Carbon dioxide when dissolved in water is involved in the following equilibrium reactions:

$$CO_2 + H_2O \overset{K'_2}{\rightleftharpoons} H_2CO_3 \overset{K'_1}{\rightleftharpoons} H^+ + HCO_3^-$$

TABLE 1.5 Apparent Dissociation Constant and pK' of Some Compounds of Importance in Biochemistry

Compound		K'_{eq} (*M*)	pK'
Acetic acid	(CH_3-COOH)	1.74×10^{-5}	4.76
Alanine	$(CH_3-CH(NH_3^+)-COOH)$	4.57×10^{-3}	2.34 (COOH)
		2.04×10^{-10}	9.69 (NH_3^+)
Citric acid	$(HOOC-CH_2-COH(COOH)-CH_2-COOH)$	8.12×10^{-4}	3.09
		1.77×10^{-5}	3.74
		3.89×10^{-6}	5.41
Glutamic acid	$(HOOC-CH_2-CH_2-CH(NH_3^+)-COOH)$	6.45×10^{-3}	2.19 (COOH)
		5.62×10^{-5}	4.25 (COOH)
		2.14×10^{-10}	9.67 (NH_3^+)
Glycine	$(CH_2(NH_3^+)-COOH)$	4.57×10^{-3}	2.34 (COOH)
		2.51×10^{-10}	9.60 (NH_3^+)
Lactic acid	$(CH_3-CHOH-COOH)$	1.38×10^{-4}	3.86
Pyruvic acid	$(CH_3-CO-COOH)$	3.16×10^{-3}	2.50
Succinic acid	$(HOOC-CH_2-CH_2-COOH)$	6.46×10^{-5}	4.19
		3.31×10^{-6}	5.48
Glucose 6-PO_3H^-		7.76×10^{-7}	6.11
H_3PO_4		1×10^{-2}	2.0
$H_2PO_4^-$		2.0×10^{-7}	6.7
HPO_4^{2-}		3.4×10^{-13}	12.5
H_2CO_3		1.70×10^{-4}	3.77
NH_4^+		5.62×10^{-10}	9.25
H_2O		1×10^{-14}	14.0

Carbonic acid is a relatively strong acid with a pK_1' of 3.77. The equilibrium equation for this reaction is

$$K_1' = \frac{[H^+][HCO_3^-]}{[H_2CO_3]} \quad \textbf{(1.5)}$$

Carbonic acid is, however, in equilibrium with dissolved CO_2 and the equilibrium equation for this reaction is

$$K_2' = \frac{[H_2CO_3]}{[CO_2][H_2O]} \quad \textbf{(1.6)}$$

Solving Eq. 1.6 for H_2CO_3 and substituting for the H_2CO_3 in Eq. 1.5, the two equilibrium reactions are combined into one equation:

$$K_1' = \frac{[H^+][HCO_3^-]}{K_2'[CO_2][H_2O]} \quad \textbf{(1.7)}$$

Rearranging to combine constants, including the concentration of H_2O, simplifies the equation and yields a new combined constant, K_3', as follows:

$$K_1'K_2'[H_2O] = K_3' = \frac{[H^+][HCO_3^-]}{[CO_2]} \quad \textbf{(1.8)}$$

It is common practice to refer to dissolved CO_2 as a conjugate acid; it is the acid anhydride of H_2CO_3. The term K_3' has a value of 7.95×10^{-7} and pK_3' = 6.1. If the aqueous system is in contact with an air phase, dissolved CO_2 will also be in equilibrium with CO_2 in the air phase. A decrease or increase of one component—that is, CO_2 (air), CO_2 (dissolved), H_2CO_3, H^+, or HCO^{3-}—will cause a change in all the other components.

The Henderson–Hasselbalch Equation Defines the Relationship Between pH and Concentrations of Conjugate Acid and Base

A change in concentration of any component in an equilibrium reaction necessitates a concomitant change in every component. For example, an increase in $[H^+]$ will decrease the concentration of conjugate base (e.g., lactate ion) with an equivalent increase in the conjugate acid (e.g., lactic acid). This relationship is conveniently expressed by rearranging the equilibrium equation and solving for H^+, as shown for the following dissociation:

$$\text{Conjugate acid} \leftrightharpoons \text{conjugate base} + H^+$$

$$K_{eq}' = \frac{[H^+][\text{conjugate base}]}{[\text{conjugate acid}]} \quad \textbf{(1.9)}$$

Rearranging Eq. 1.9 by dividing through by both $[H^+]$ and K_{eq}' leads to

$$\frac{1}{[H^+]} = \frac{1}{|K_{eq}'|} \cdot \frac{[\text{conjugate base}]}{[\text{conjugate acid}]} \quad \textbf{(1.10)}$$

Taking the logarithm of both sides gives

$$\log\frac{1}{[H^+]} = \log\frac{1}{K_{eq}'} + \log\frac{[\text{conjugate base}]}{[\text{conjugate acid}]} \quad \textbf{(1.11)}$$

Since pH = log $1/[H^+]$ and pK' = log $1/K_{eq}'$, Eq. 1.11 becomes

$$\mathbf{pH = p}K' \mathbf{+ \log\frac{[conjugate\ base]}{[conjugate\ acid]}} \quad \textbf{(1.12)}$$

Equation 1.12, developed by Henderson and Hasselbalch, is a convenient way of viewing the relationship between pH of a solution and relative amounts of conjugate base and acid present. Analysis of Eq. 1.12 demonstrates that when the ratio of [base]/[acid] is 1 : 1, pH equals the pK' of the acid because log 1 = 0,

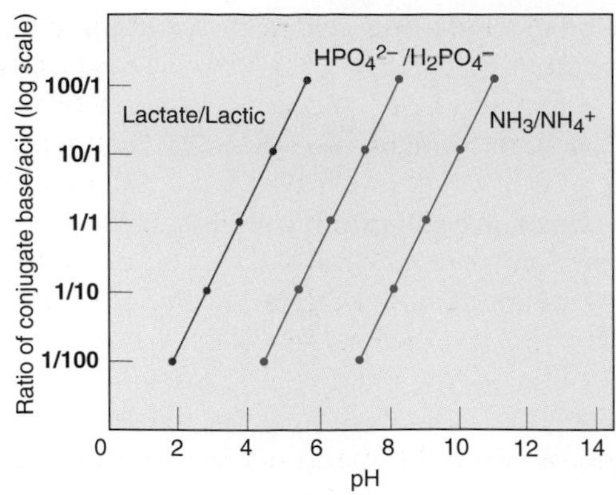

FIGURE 1.6
Ratio of conjugate [base]/[acid] as a function of the pH.
When the ratio of [base]/[acid] is 1, pH equals pK' of weak acid.

and thus pH = pK'. If pH is one unit less than pK', the [base]/[acid] ratio is 1:10, and if pH is one unit above pK', the [base]/[acid] ratio is 10:1. Figure 1.6 is a plot of ratios of conjugate base to conjugate acid versus pH of several weak acids; note that ratios are presented on a logarithmic scale.

Buffering Is Important to Control pH

When NaOH is added to a solution of a weak acid such as lactic acid, the ratio of [conjugate base]/[conjugate acid] changes. NaOH dissociates totally and the OH^- formed is neutralized by existing H^+ to form H_2O. The decrease in [H^+] will cause further dissociation of weak acid to comply with requirements of its equilibrium reaction. The amount of weak acid dissociated will be so nearly equal to the amount of OH^- added that it is considered to be equal. Thus the decrease in amount of conjugate acid is equal to the amount of conjugate base that is formed. These series of events are represented in titration curves of two weak acids presented in Figure 1.7. When 0.5 equiv of OH^- is added, 50% of the weak acid is dissociated and the [acid]/[base] ratio is 1.0; pH at this point is equal to pK' of the acid. Shapes of individual titration curves are similar but displaced due to differences in pK' values. There is a rather steep rise in pH when only 0.1 equiv of OH^- are added, but between 0.1 and 0.9 equiv of added OH^-, the pH change is only ~2. Thus a large amount of OH^- is added with a relatively small change in pH. This is called **buffering** and is defined as the ability of a solution to resist a change in pH when an acid or base is added. If weak acid were not present, the pH would be very high with only a small amount of OH^- because there would be no source of H^+ to neutralize the OH^-.

The best buffering range for a conjugate pair is in the pH range near the pK' of the weak acid. Starting from a pH one unit below to a pH one unit above pK', ~82% of a weak acid in solution will dissociate, and therefore an amount of base equivalent to about 82% of original acid can be neutralized with a change in pH of 2. The maximum buffering range for a conjugate pair is considered to be between 1 pH unit above and below the pK'. Lactic acid with pK' = 3.86 is an effective buffer in the range of pH 3 to 5 but has no buffering capacity at pH = 7.0. The $HPO_4^{2-}/H_2PO_4^-$ pair with pK' = 6.7, however, is an effective buffer at pH = 7.0. Thus at the pH of the cell's cytosol (~7.0), the lactate–lactic acid pair is not an effective buffer but the phosphate system is.

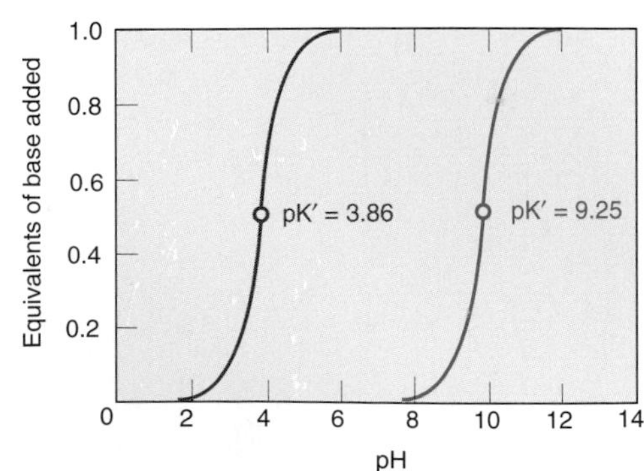

FIGURE 1.7
Acid–base titration curves for lactic acid (pK' 3.86) and NH_4^+ (pK' 9.25).
At pH equal to respective pK' values, there will be an equal amount of acid and base for each conjugate pair.

Buffering capacity also depends on the concentrations of conjugate acid and base. The higher the concentration of conjugate base, the more added H^+ with which it can react. The more conjugate acid the more added OH^- can be neutralized by the dissociation of the acid. A case in point is blood plasma at pH 7.4. For $HPO_4^{2-}/H_2PO_4^-$ the pK' of 6.7 would suggest that this conjugate pair would be an effective buffer; the concentration of the phosphate pair, however, is low compared to that of the HCO_3^-/CO_2 system with a pK' of 6.1, which is present at a 20-fold higher concentration and accounts for most of the buffering capacity. In considering the buffering capacity both the pK' and the concentration of the conjugate pair must be taken into account. Most organic acids are relatively unimportant as buffers in cellular fluids because their pK' values are more than several pH units lower than the pH of the cell, and their concentrations are too low in comparison to such buffers as $HPO_4^{2-}/H_2PO_4^-$ and the HCO_3^-/CO_2 system.

The importance of pH and buffers in biochemistry and clinical medicine will become apparent, particularly in Chapters 2, 4, and 25. Figure 1.8 presents

1. Calculate the ratio of HPO_4^{2-} / $H_2PO_4^-$ (pK=6.7) at pH 5.7, 6.7, and 8.7.

Solution:

$$\text{pH} = \text{p}K + \log \frac{[HPO_4^{2-}]}{[H_2PO_4^-]}$$

5.7 = 6.7 + log of ratio; rearranging

5.7− 6.7 = −1 = log of ratio

The antilog of −1 = 0.1 or 1/10. Thus, $HPO_4^{2-}/H_2PO_4^-$ = 1/10 at pH 5.7. Using the same procedure, the ratio at pH 6.7 = 1/1 and at pH 8.7 = 100/1.

2. If the pH of blood is 7.1 and the HCO_3^- concentration is 8 mM, what is the concentration of CO_2 in blood (pK' for HCO_3^-/CO_2 = 6.1)?

Solution:

$$\text{pH} = \text{p}K + \log \frac{[HCO_3^-]}{[CO_2]}$$

7.1 = 6.1 + log 8 mM / $[CO_2]$; rearranging

7.1 − 6.1 = 1 = log 8 mM / $[CO_2]$.

The antilog of 1 = 10. Thus, 10 = 8 mM / $[CO_2]$, or $[CO_2]$ = 8 mM/10 = 0.8 mM.

3. At a normal blood pH of 7.4, the sum of $[HCO_3^-]$ + $[CO_2]$ = 25.2 mM. What is the concentration of HCO_3^- and CO_2 (pK' for HCO_3^- /CO_2 = 6.1)?

Solution:

$$\text{pH} = \text{p}K + \log \frac{[HCO_3^-]}{[CO_2]}$$

7.4 = 6.1 + log $[HCO_3^-]$ / $[CO_2]$; rearranging

7.4 − 6.1 = 1.3 = log $[HCO_3^-]$ / $[CO_2]$.

The antilog of 1.3 is 20. Thus $[HCO_3^-]$ / $[CO_2]$ = 20. Given $[HCO_3^-]$ + $[CO_2]$ = 25.2, solve these two equations for $[CO_2]$ by rearranging the first equation:

$[HCO_3^-]$ = 20 $[CO_2]$.

Substituting in the second equation,

20 $[CO_2]$ + $[CO_2]$ = 25.2

or

CO_2 = 1.2 mM

Then substituting for CO_2, 1.2 + $[HCO_3^-]$ = 25.2, and solving, $[HCO_3^-]$ = 24 mM.

FIGURE 1.8
Typical problems of pH and buffering.

CLINICAL CORRELATION 1.1

Blood Bicarbonate Concentration in Metabolic Acidosis

Blood buffers in a normal adult control blood pH at about 7.40; if the pH should drop below 7.35, the condition is referred to as an acidosis. A blood pH of near 7.0 could lead to serious consequences and possibly death. Thus in acidosis, particularly that caused by a metabolic change, it is important to monitor the acid–base parameters of a patient's blood. Values of interest to a clinician include the pH and HCO_3^- and CO_2 concentrations. Normal values for these are pH = 7.40, $[HCO_3^-]$ = 24.0 mM, and $[CO_2]$ = 1.20 mM.

Blood values of a patient with a metabolic acidosis were pH = 7.03 and $[CO_2]$ = 1.10 mM. What is the patient's blood $[HCO_3^-]$ and how much of the normal $[HCO_3^-]$ has been used in buffering the acid causing the condition?

1. The Henderson–Hasselbalch equation is

   $$\text{pH} = \text{p}K' + \log([HCO_3^-]/[CO_2])$$

   The pK' value for $[HCO_3^-]/[CO_2]$ is 6.10.
2. Substitute the given values in the equation.

   $$7.03 = 6.10 + \log([HCO_3^-]/1.10 \text{ mM})$$

   or

   $$7.03 - 6.10 = 0.93 = \log([HCO_3^-]/1.10 \text{ mM})$$

   The antilog of 0.93 is 8.5; thus

   $$8.5 = [HCO_3^-]/1.10 \text{ mM}$$

   or

   $$[HCO_3^-] = 9.4 \text{ mM}$$
3. Since the normal value of $[HCO_3^-]$ is 24 mM, there has been a decrease of 14.6 mmol of HCO_3^- per liter of blood in this patient. If much more HCO_3^- is lost, a point would be reached when this important buffer would be unavailable to buffer any more acid in the blood and the pH would drop rapidly. In Chapter 25 there is a detailed discussion of the causes and compensations that occur in such conditions.

some typical problems using the Henderson–Hasselbalch equation and Clin. Corr. 1.1 is a representative problem encountered in clinical practice.

1.3 ■ ORGANIZATION AND COMPOSITION OF EUKARYOTIC CELLS

As described above, eukaryotic cells are organized into compartments, each delineated by a membrane (Figure 1.9). These are well-defined cellular organelles such as nucleus, mitochondria, lysosomes, and peroxisomes. Membranes also form a tubule-like network throughout the cell enclosing an interconnecting space or cisternae, as is the case of the endoplasmic reticulum or Golgi complex. As described in Section 1.4, these compartments have specific functions and activities.

The semipermeable nature of **cellular membranes** prevents the ready diffusion of many molecules from one side to the other. Specific mechanisms in membranes for translocation of large and small, charged and uncharged molecules allow membranes to modulate concentrations of substances in various compartments. Macromolecules, such as proteins and nucleic acids, do not cross biological membranes unless there is a specific mechanism for their translocation or the membrane is damaged. Thus the fluid matrix of various cellular compartments has a distinctive composition of inorganic ions, organic molecules, and macromolecules. Partitioning of activities and components in membrane-enclosed compartments and organelles has a number of advantages for the economy of the cell. These include the sequestering of substrates and cofactors where they are required, and adjustments of pH and ionic composition for maximum activity of biological processes.

The activities and composition of cellular structures and organelles have been determined with intact cells by a variety of histochemical, immunological, and fluorescent staining methods. Continuous observation in real time of cellular events in intact viable cells is possible. Examples are studies that involve changes of ionic calcium concentration in the cytosol by the use of fluorescent calcium indicators. Individual organelles, membranes, and components of the cytosol can be isolated and analyzed following disruption of the plasma membrane. Permeability of the plasma membrane can be altered to permit the release of subcellular components. Techniques for disrupting membranes include use of detergents, osmotic shock, and homogenization of tissues, where shearing forces break down the plasma membrane. In an appropriate isolation medium, cell organelles and membrane systems can be separated by centrifugation because of differences in size and density. Chromatographic procedures have been employed for isolation of individual cellular fractions and components. These techniques have permitted isolation of cellular fractions from most mammalian tissues. In addition, components of organelles such as nuclei and mitochondria can be isolated following disruption of the organelle membrane.

In many instances the isolated structures and cellular fractions appear to retain the chemical and biochemical characteristics of the structure *in situ.* But biological membrane systems are very sensitive structures, subject to damage even under very mild conditions, and alterations can occur during isolation, which can lead to change in composition of the structure. The slightest damage to a membrane alters its permeability properties, allowing substances that would normally be excluded to traverse the membrane barrier. In addition, many proteins are only loosely associated with membranes and easily dissociate when damage occurs (see p. 186).

Not unexpectedly, there are differences in structure, composition, and activities of cells from different tissues due to the diverse functions of tissues. Major biochemical activities of the cellular organelles and membrane systems, however, are fairly constant from tissue to tissue. Thus biochemical pathways in liver are often present in other tissues. The differences between cell types are

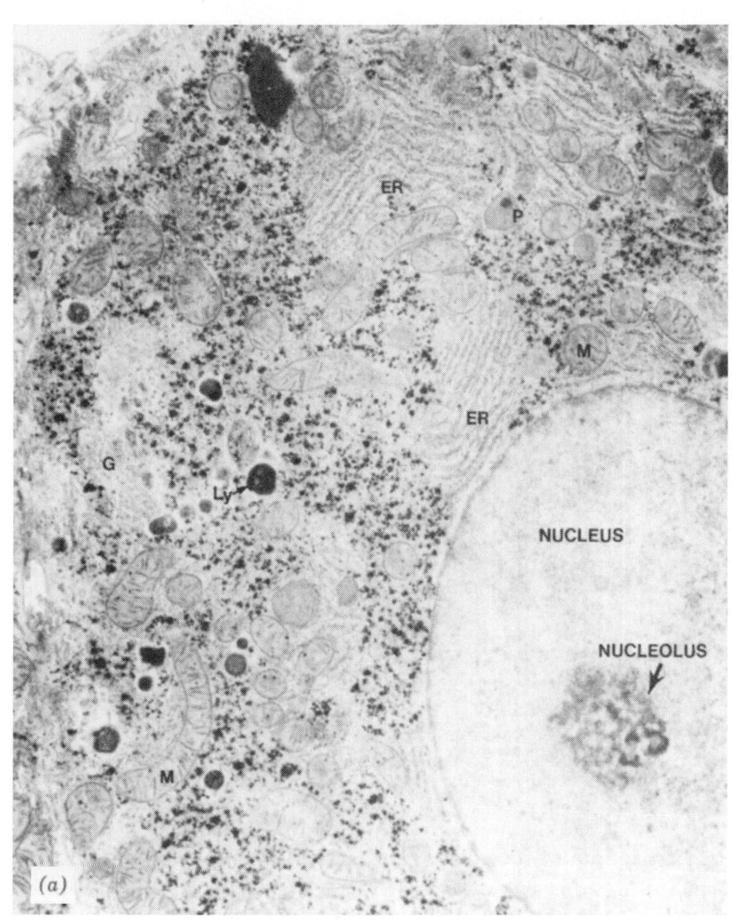

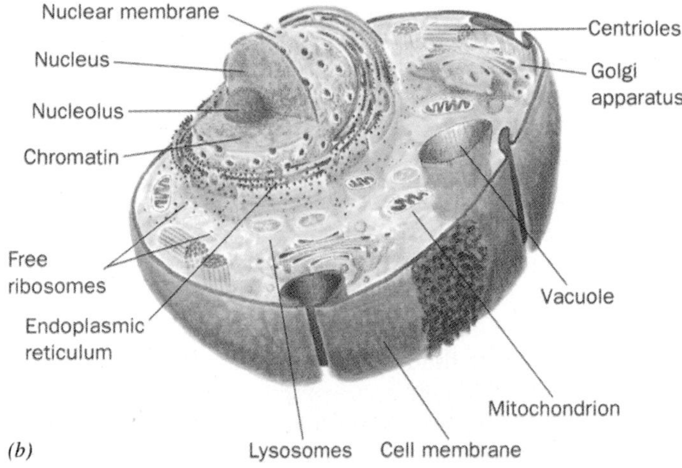

FIGURE 1.9
(*a*) Electron micrograph of a rat liver cell labeled to indicate the major structural components of eukaryotic cells and (*b*) a schematic drawing of an animal cell. Note the number and variety of subcellular organelles and the network of interconnecting membranes enclosing channels, that is, cisternae. All eukaryotic cells are not as complex in their appearance, but most contain the major structures shown in the figure. ER, endoplasmic reticulum; G, Golgi zone; Ly, lysosomes; P, peroxisomes; M, mitochondria. *Photograph* (a) *reprinted with permission of Dr. K. R. Porter from Porter, K. R., and Bonneville, M. A. In:* Fine Structure of Cells and Tissues. *Philadelphia: Lea & Febiger, 1972; schematic* (b) *reprinted with permission from Voet, D., and Voet, J. G.* Biochemistry, *2nd ed. New York: Wiley, 1995.*

usually in distinctive specialized activities. Even within one tissue, cells of different origin have qualitative and quantitative differences in cell organelle composition.

Chemical Composition of Cells

Each cellular compartment has an aqueous fluid or **matrix** that contains various ions, small molecular weight organic molecules, different proteins, and nucleic acids. Localization of specific macromolecules, such as enzymes, has been

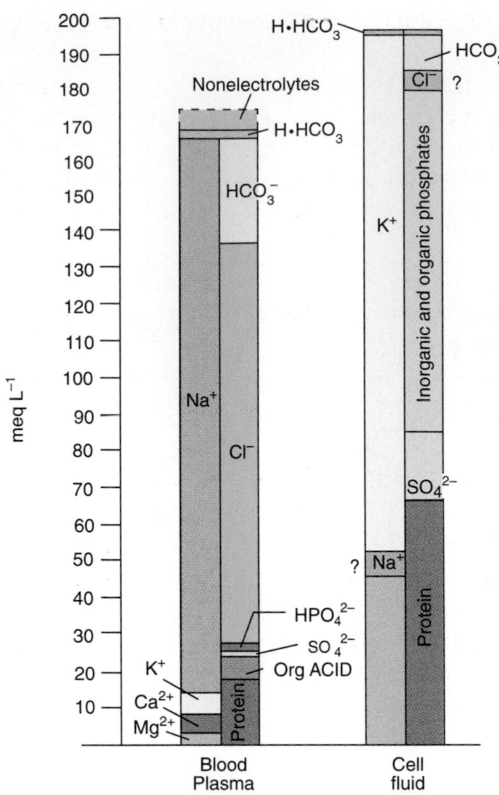

FIGURE 1.10
Major chemical constituents of blood plasma and cell fluid.
Height of left half of each column indicates total concentration of cations; that of right half, concentrations of anions. Both are expressed in milliequivalents per liter (meq L^{-1}) of fluid. Note that chloride and sodium values in cell fluid are questioned. It is probable that, at least in muscle, the cytosol contains some sodium but no chloride.
Adapted from Gregersen, M. I. In: P. Bard (Ed.), Medical Physiology, *11th ed. St. Louis, MO: Mosby, 1961, p. 307.*

determined but the exact ionic composition of the matrix of organelles is still uncertain. Each has a distinctly different ionic composition and pH. The overall ionic composition of intracellular fluid, considered to represent the cytosol primarily, compared to blood plasma is presented in Figure 1.10. **Na^+** is the major extracellular cation, with a concentration of ~140 meq L^{-1} (mM); very little Na^+ is present in intracellular fluid. **K^+** is the major intracellular cation. **Mg^{2+}** is present in both extra- and intracellular compartments at concentrations much lower than Na^+ and K^+. The major extracellular anions are **Cl^-** and **HCO_3^-** with lower amounts of phosphate and sulfate. Most proteins have a negative charge at pH 7.4 (Chapter 2), being anions at the pH of tissue fluids. Major intracellular anions are inorganic phosphate, organic phosphates, and proteins. Other inorganic and organic anions and cations are present in concentrations well below the milliequivalent per liter (millimolar) level. Except for very small differences created by membranes and leading to development of membrane potentials, the *total anion concentration equals the total cation concentration in the different fluids.*

Intracellular concentrations of most small molecular weight organic molecules, such as sugars, organic acids, amino acids, and phosphorylated intermediates, are in the range of 0.01–1.0 mM but can have significantly lower concentrations. Coenzymes, organic molecules required for activity of some enzymes, are in the same range of concentration. Substrates for enzymes are present in relatively low concentration in contrast to inorganic ions, but localization in a specific organelle or cellular microenvironment can increase their concentrations significantly.

It is not very meaningful to determine the molar concentration of individual proteins in cells. In many cases they are localized with specific structures or in combination with other proteins to create a functional unit. It is in a restricted compartment that individual proteins carry out their role, whether structural, catalytic, or regulatory.

1.4 FUNCTIONAL ROLE OF SUBCELLULAR ORGANELLES AND MEMBRANE SYSTEMS

The subcellular localization of various metabolic pathways will be described throughout this book. In some cases an entire pathway is located in a single compartment but many are divided between two locations, with the intermediates in the pathway moving or being translocated from one compartment to another. In general, organelles have very specific functions and the enzymatic activities involved are used to identify them during isolation.

The following describes briefly some major roles of eukaryotic cell structures to indicate the complexity and organization of cells. A summary of functions and division of labor within eukaryotic cells is presented in Table 1.6 and the structures are presented in Figure 1.9.

TABLE 1.6 Summary of Eukaryotic Cell Compartments and Their Major Functions

Compartment	*Major Functions*
Plasma membrane	Transport of ions and molecules Recognition Receptors for small and large molecules Cell morphology and movement
Nucleus	DNA synthesis and repair RNA synthesis
Nucleolus	RNA processing and ribosome synthesis
Endoplasmic reticulum	Membrane synthesis Synthesis of proteins and lipids for some organelles and for export Lipid synthesis Detoxification reactions
Golgi apparatus	Modification and sorting of proteins for incorporation into organelles and for export Export of proteins
Mitochondria	Energy conservation Cellular respiration Oxidation of carbohydrates and lipids Urea and heme synthesis
Lysosomes	Cellular digestion: hydrolysis of proteins, carbohydrates, lipids, and nucleic acids
Peroxisomes	Oxidative reactions involving O_2 Utilization of H_2O_2
Microtubules and microfilaments	Cell cytoskeleton Cell morphology Cell motility Intracellular movements
Cytosol	Metabolism of carbohydrates, lipids, amino acids, and nucleotides Protein synthesis

Plasma Membrane Is the Limiting Boundary of a Cell

The **plasma membrane** of every cell has a unique role in maintenance of that cell's integrity. One surface is in contact with a variable external environment and the other with a relatively constant environment provided by the cell's cytoplasm. As will be discussed in Chapter 5, the two sides of the plasma membrane, and all intracellular membranes, have different chemical compositions and functions. A major role of the plasma membrane is to permit entrance of some substances but exclude many others. With cytoskeletal elements, the plasma membrane is involved in cell shape and movements. Through this membrane cells communicate; the membrane contains many specific receptor sites for chemical signals, such as hormones (Chapter 20), released by other cells. The inner surface of plasma membranes is the site for attachment of some enzymes involved in various metabolic pathways. Plasma membranes from a variety of cells have been isolated and studied extensively; details of their structure and biochemistry and those of other membranes are presented in Chapter 5.

Nucleus Is Site of DNA and RNA Synthesis

Early microscopists divided the interior of cells into a **nucleus,** the largest membrane-bound compartment, and the **cytoplasm.** The nucleus is surrounded by two membranes, termed the **nuclear envelope,** with the outer membrane being continuous with membranes of the endoplasmic reticulum. The nuclear envelope has numerous pores about 90 Å in diameter that permit flow of all but the largest molecules between nuclear matrix and cytoplasm. The nucleus contains a subcompartment, seen clearly in electron micrographs, the **nucleolus.** The vast amount of cellular **deoxyribonucleic acid (DNA)** is located in the nucleus as a DNA–protein complex, **chromatin,** that is organized into chromosomes. DNA is the repository of genetic information and the importance of the nucleus in cell division and for controlling phenotypic expression of genetic information is well established. Biochemical reactions in the nucleus are replication of DNA during mitosis, repair of DNA following damage (Chapter 15), and transcription of the information stored in DNA into a form that can be translated into cell proteins (Chapter 16). Transcription of DNA involves synthesis of ribonucleic acid (RNA) that is processed into a variety of forms following synthesis. Part of this processing occurs in the nucleolus, which is very rich in RNA.

CLINICAL CORRELATION 1.2

Mitochondrial Diseases: Luft's Disease

A disease specifically involving mitochondrial energy transduction was first reported in 1962. A 30-year-old patient was described with general weakness, excessive perspiration, a high caloric intake without increase in body weight, and an excessively elevated basal metabolic rate (a measure of oxygen utilization). It was demonstrated that the patient had a defect in the mechanism that controls mitochondrial oxygen utilization (see Chapter 6). The condition is referred to as Luft's disease. Since that time, over 100 mitochondrial-based diseases have been identified, including those involving a variety of enzymes and transport systems required for the proper maintenance and control of energy conservation. Many involve skeletal muscle and the central nervous system. Replication of mitochondria depends on the mitochondrial DNA (mtDNA) and inheritance of mitochondria is by maternal transmission. Mutations of mtDNA as well as nuclear DNA lead to genetic diseases. Mitochondrial damage may also occur due to free-radical (superoxides) formation which can damage mtDNA. Thus age-related degenerative diseases, such as Parkinson's and Alzheimer's, and cardiomyopathies may have a component of mitochondrial damage. For details of specific diseases see Clin. Corr. 13.4 and 14.6.

Luft, R. The development of mitochondrial medicine. *Proc. Natl. Acad. Sci. USA* 91:8731,1994.

Endoplasmic Reticulum Has a Role in Many Synthetic Pathways

The cytoplasm of most eukaryotic cells contains a network of interconnecting membranes that enclose channels, **cisternae,** that thread from the perinuclear envelope to the plasma membrane. This extensive subcellular structure, termed **endoplasmic reticulum,** consists of membranes with a rough appearance in some areas and smooth in other places. The rough appearance is due to the presence of **ribonucleoprotein particles,** that is, **ribosomes,** attached on the cytosolic side of the membrane. Smooth endoplasmic reticulum does not contain bound ribosomes. During cell fractionation the endoplasmic reticulum network is disrupted, with the membrane resealing into small vesicles called **microsomes** that can be isolated by differential centrifugation. Microsomes per se do not occur in cells.

A major function of ribosomes on **rough endoplasmic reticulum** is biosynthesis of proteins for export to the outside of the cell and proteins for incorporation into cellular organelles such as the endoplasmic reticulum, Golgi apparatus, plasma membrane, and lysosomes. **Smooth endoplasmic reticulum** is involved in membrane lipid synthesis and contains an important class of enzymes termed **cytochromes P450** that catalyze hydroxylation of a variety of endogenous and exogenous compounds. These enzymes are important in biosynthesis of steroid hormones and removal of toxic substances (see Chapter 23). Endoplasmic reticulum with the Golgi apparatus has a role in formation of other cellular organelles such as lysosomes and peroxisomes.

The Golgi Apparatus Is Involved in Sequestering of Proteins

The **Golgi apparatus** is a network of flattened smooth membranes and vesicles responsible for the secretion to the external environment of a variety of proteins synthesized on the endoplasmic reticulum. Golgi membranes catalyze the transfer of carbohydrate and lipid precursors to proteins to form glycoproteins and lipoproteins and is a major site of new membrane formation. Membrane vesicles are formed in the Golgi apparatus in which various proteins and enzymes are encapsulated to be secreted from the cell after an appropriate signal. Digestive enzymes synthesized by the pancreas are stored in intracellular vesicles formed by the Golgi apparatus and released when needed in the digestive process (see p. 1059). The role in membrane synthesis also includes the formation of intracellular organelles such as lysosomes and peroxisomes.

Mitochondria Supply Most Cell Needs for ATP

Mitochondria appear as spheres, rods, or filamentous bodies that are usually about 0.5–1 mm in diameter and up to 7 mm in length. The internal matrix, the **mitosol,** is surrounded by two membranes, distinctively different in appearance and biochemical function. The inner membrane convolutes into the matrix to form **cristae** and contains numerous small spheres attached by stalks on the inner surface. Outer and inner membranes contain different enzymes. The components of the respiratory chain and the mechanism for ATP synthesis are part of the inner membrane and are described in detail in Chapter 6. Major metabolic pathways involved in oxidation of carbohydrates, lipids, and amino acids, and parts of special biosynthetic pathways involving urea and heme synthesis are located in the mitosol. The outer membrane is relatively permeable but the inner membrane is highly selective and contains a variety of transmembrane transport systems.

Mitochondria contain a specific DNA, with genetic information for some of the mitochondrial proteins, and the biochemical equipment for limited protein synthesis. The presence of this biosynthetic capacity indicates the unique role that mitochondria have in their own destiny. See Clin. Corr. 1.2 for descriptions of diseases attributed to deficits in mitochondrial function.

Lysosomes Are Required for Intracellular Digestion

Intracellular digestion of a variety of substances occurs inside structures designated as **lysosomes.** They have a single limiting membrane and maintain a pH lower in the lysosomal matrix than that of the cytosol. Encapsulated in lysosomes is a group of glycoprotein enzymes—hydrolases—that catalyze hydrolytic cleavage of carbon-oxygen, carbon–nitrogen, carbon–sulfur, and oxygen–phosphorus bonds in proteins, lipids, carbohydrates, and nucleic acids. A partial list of lysosomal enzymes is presented in Table 1.7. As in gastrointestinal digestion, lysosomal enzymes split complex molecules into simple low molecular weight compounds that can be utilized by metabolic pathways of the cell. Enzymes of the lysosome are characterized by being most active when the pH of the medium is acidic, that is, pH 5 and below. The relationship between pH and enzyme activity is discussed in Chapter 4. The pH of the cytosol is close to pH 7.0 and lysosomal enzymes have little activity at this pH.

TABLE 1.7 Representative Lysosomal Enzymes and Their Substrates

Type of Substrate and Enzyme	*Specific Substrate*
POLYSACCHARIDE-HYDROLYZING ENZYMES	
α-Glucosidase	Glycogen
α-Flucosidase	Membrane fucose
	Galactosides
β-Galactosidase	Mannosides
α-Mannosidase	Glucuronides
β-Glucuronidase	Hyaluronic acid
Hyaluronidase	and chondroitin sulfates
Arylsulfatase	Organic sulfates
Lysozyme	Bacterial cell walls
PROTEIN-HYDROLYZING ENZYMES	
Cathepsins	Proteins
Collagenase	Collagen
Elastase	Elastin
Peptidases	Peptides
NUCLEIC ACID-HYDROLYZING ENZYMES	
Ribonuclease	RNA
Deoxyribonuclease	DNA
LIPID-HYDROLYZING ENZYMES	
Lipases	Triglyceride and cholesterol esters
Esterase	Fatty acid esters
Phospholipase	Phospholipids
PHOSPHATASES	
Phosphatase	Phospho-monoesters
Phosphodiesterase	Phosphodiesters
SULFATASES	
Heparan sulfate	
Dermatan sulfate	

The enzyme content of lysosomes in different tissues varies and depends on specific needs of individual tissues. The lysosomal membrane is impermeable to both small and large molecules and specific protein mediators in the membrane are necessary for translocation of substances. Carefully isolated lysosomes do not catalyze hydrolysis of substrates until this membrane is disrupted. The activities of lysosomal enzymes are termed **"latent."** Membrane disruption *in situ* can lead to cellular digestion, and various pathological conditions have been attributed to release of lysosomal enzymes, including arthritis, allergic responses, several muscle diseases, and drug-induced tissue destruction (see Clin. Corr. 1.3).

Lysosomes are involved in normal digestion of intra- and extracellular substances that must be removed by a cell. Through **endocytosis,** external material is taken into cells and encapsulated in membrane-bound vesicles (Figure 1.11). The plasma membrane invaginates around formed foreign substances, such as microorganisms, by **phagocytosis** and takes up extracellular fluid containing suspended material by **pinocytosis.** Vesicles containing external material fuse with lysosomes to form organelles that contain the materials to be digested and enzymes capable of carrying out the digestion. These vacuoles are identified microscopically by their size and often by the presence of partially formed structures in the process of being digested. Lysosomes in which the

CLINICAL CORRELATION 1.3

Lysosomal Enzymes and Gout

Catabolism of purines, nitrogen-containing heterocyclic compounds found in nucleic acids, leads to formation of uric acid, which is excreted in the urine (see Chapter 12 for details). Gout is an abnormality in which there is excessive uric acid production with an increase in uric acid in blood and deposition of urate crystals in joints. The consequences are clinical manifestations in the joint, particularly the big toe, including inflammation, pain, swelling, and increased warmth. Uric acid is not very soluble and some of the clinical symptoms of gout can be attributed to damage done by urate crystals. Crystals are phagocytosed by cells in the joint and accumulate in digestive vacuoles that contain lysosomal enzymes. Crystals cause physical damage to the vacuoles, releasing lysosomal enzymes into the cytosol. Even though the pH optima of lysosomal enzymes are lower than the pH of the cytosol, they have some hydrolytic activity at the higher pH. This activity causes digestion of cellular components, release of substances from the cell and autolysis.

Weissmann, G. Crystals, lysosomes and gout. *Adv. Intern. Med.* 19:239, 1974; and Burt, H. M., Kalkman, P. H., and Mauldin, D. Membranolytic effects of crystalline monosodium urate monohydrate. *J. Rheumatol.* 10:440, 1983.

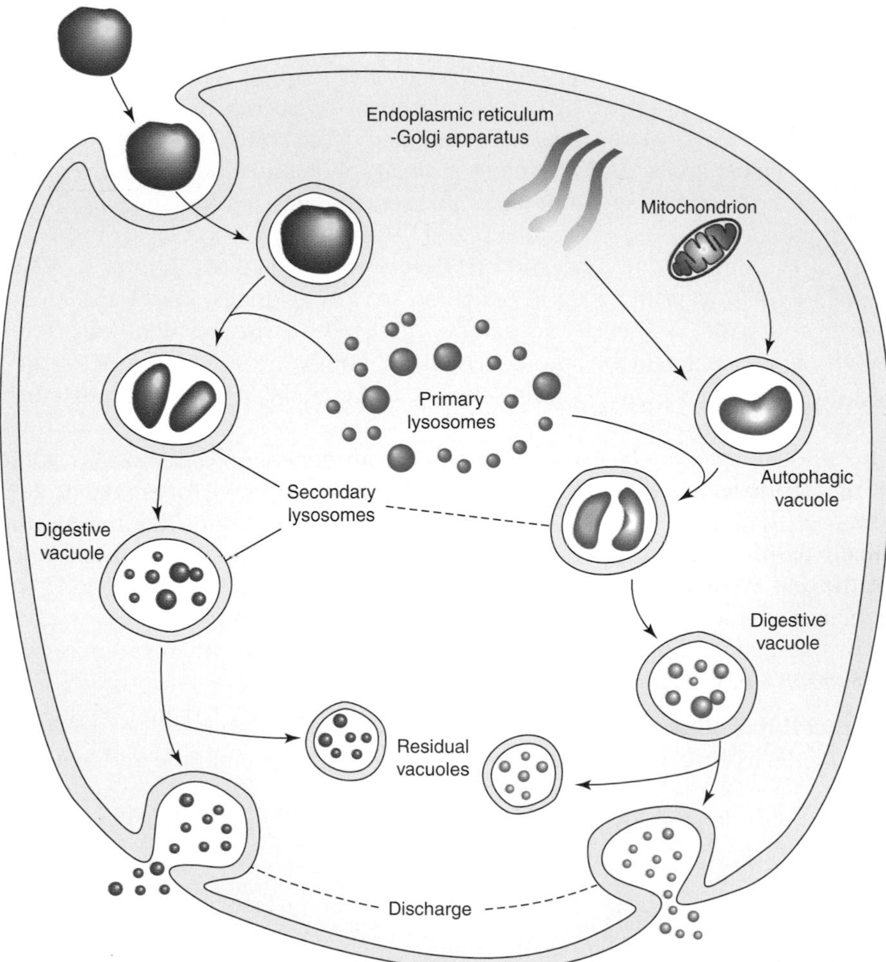

FIGURE 1.11
Diagrammatic representation of the role of lysosomes in intracellular digestion of substances internalized by phagocytosis (heterophagy) and of cellular components (autophagy).
In both processes substances to be digested are enclosed in a membrane vesicle, followed by fusing with a primary lysosome to form a secondary lysosome.

enzymes are not as yet involved in the digestive process are termed **primary lysosomes,** whereas those in which digestion of material is under way are **secondary lysosomes** or **digestive vacuoles** that will vary in size and appearance.

Cell constituents are synthesized and degraded continuously, and lysosomes function in digesting this cellular debris. The dynamic synthesis and degradation includes proteins and nucleic acids, as well as structures such as mitochondria and endoplasmic reticulum. During this normal self-digestion process, that is, **autolysis,** cell substances are encapsulated within a membrane vesicle that fuses with a lysosome to complete the degradation. The overall process is termed **autophagy** and is also represented in Figure 1.11.

Products of lysosomal digestion diffuse across lysosomal membranes and are reutilized by the cell. Indigestible material accumulates in vesicles referred to as residual bodies, whose contents are removed from the cell by exocytosis. In some cases, residual bodies that contain a high concentration of lipid persist for long periods of time. Lipid is oxidized and a pigmented substance, which is chemically heterogeneous and contains polyunsaturated fatty acids and proteins, accumulates in the cell. This material, **lipofuscin,** is also called the **"age pigment"** or **"wear and tear pigment"** because it accumulates in cells of older individuals. It occurs in all cells but particularly in neurons and muscle cells and has been implicated in the aging process.

Under controlled conditions lysosomal enzymes are secreted from the cell for the digestion of extracellular material; an extracellular role for some lysosomal enzymes has been demonstrated in connective tissue and prostate gland and in the process of embryogenesis. Thus they have a role in programmed cell death or **apoptosis.**

Absence of specific lysosomal enzymes occurs in a number of genetic diseases in which there is accumulation in the cell of specific cellular components that cannot be digested. Lysosomes of affected cells become enlarged with undigested material, which interferes with normal cell processes. Lysosomal storage diseases are discussed in Chapter 10 (see p. 427); see Clin. Corr. 1.4 for a description of a deficiency of lysosomal lipase.

CLINICAL CORRELATION 1.4

Lysosomal Acid Lipase Deficiency

Two phenotypic forms of a genetic deficiency of lysosomal acid lipase are known. Wolman's disease occurs in infants and is usually fatal by age 1, while cholesterol ester-storage disease usually is diagnosed in adulthood. Both are autosomal recessive disorders. There is deposition of triacylglycerols and cholesterol esters in tissues, particularly the liver. In the latter disease there is early onset of severe atherosclerosis. Acid lipase catalyzes hydrolysis of mono-, di-, and triglycerols as well as cholesterol esters. It is a critical enzyme in cholesterol metabolism, serving to make available free cholesterol for cell needs.

Hegele, R. A., Little, J. A., Vezina, C., et al., Hepatic lipase deficiency: clinical, biochemical, and molecular genetic characteristics. *Atherosclerosis and Thrombosis* 13:720, 1993.

Peroxisomes Contain Oxidative Enzymes Involving Hydrogen Peroxide

Most eukaryotic cells of mammalian origin and those of protozoa and plants have organelles, designated **peroxisomes** or **microbodies,** which contain enzymes that either produce or utilize **hydrogen peroxide** (H_2O_2). They are small (0.3–1.5 mm in diameter), spherical or oval in shape, with a granular matrix and in some cases a crystalline inclusion termed a nucleoid. Peroxisomes contain enzymes that oxidize D-amino acids, uric acid, and various 2-hydroxy acids using molecular O_2 with formation of H_2O_2. Catalase, an enzyme present in peroxisomes, catalyzes the conversion of H_2O_2 to water and oxygen and oxidation by H_2O_2 of various compounds (Figure 1.12). By having both peroxide-producing and peroxide-utilizing enzymes in one compartment, cells protect themselves from the toxicity of H_2O_2.

Peroxisomes also contain enzymes involved in lipid metabolism, particularly oxidation of very long-chain fatty acids, and synthesis of glycerolipids and glycerol ether lipids (plasmalogens) (see Chapter 10). See Clin. Corr. 1.5 for a discussion of Zellweger syndrome in which there is an absence of peroxisomes.

Peroxisomes of different tissues contain different complements of enzymes, and the peroxisome content of cells can vary depending on cellular conditions.

(1) $2H_2O_2 \longrightarrow 2H_2O + O_2$

(2) $RH_2 + H_2O_2 \longrightarrow R + 2H_2O$

FIGURE 1.12
Reactions catalyzed by catalase.

Cytoskeleton Organizes the Intracellular Contents

Eukaryotic cells contain microtubules and actin filaments (microfilaments) as parts of the cytoskeletal network. The **cytoskeleton** has a role in maintenance

CLINICAL CORRELATION 1.5

Zellweger Syndrome and the Absence of Functional Peroxisomes

Zellweger syndrome is a rare, autosomal recessive disease characterized by abnormalities of the liver, kidney, brain, and skeletal system. It usually results in death by age 6 months. A number of seemingly unrelated biochemical abnormalities have been described including decreased levels of glycerol-ether lipids (plasmalogens) and increased levels of very long-chain fatty acids (C-24 and C-26) and cholestanoic acid derivatives (precursors of bile acids). These abnormalities are due to the absence of functional peroxisomes in the afflicted children. Peroxisomes are responsible for synthesis of glycerol ethers, for shortening very long-chain fatty acids so that mitochondria can completely oxidize them, and for oxidation of the side chain of cholesterol needed for bile acid synthesis. Evidence indicates that there is a defect in the transport of peroxisomal enzymes between the cytosol and the interior of peroxisomes during synthesis. Cells of afflicted individuals contain empty ghosts of peroxisomes. The disease can be diagnosed prenatally by assaying amniotic fluid cells for peroxisomal enzymes or analyzing the fatty acids in the fluid.

Datta, N. S., Wilson, G. N., and Hajra, A. K. Deficiency of enzymes catalyzing the biosynthesis of glycerol-ether lipids in Zellweger syndrome. *N. Engl. J. Med.* 311:1080, 1984; Moser, A. E., Singh, I., Brown, F. R., Solish, G. I., Kelley, R. I., Benke, P. J., and Moser, H. W. The cerebrohepatorenal (Zellweger) syndrome. Increased levels and impaired degradation of very long chain fatty acids and their use for prenatal diagnosis. *N. Engl. J. Med.* 310:1141, 1984; and Wanders, R. J., Schutgens, R.B., and Barth, P. G. Peroxisomal disorders: a review. *J. Neuropathol. Exp. Neurol.* 54:726,1995.

of cellular morphology, intracellular transport, cell motility, and cell division. **Microtubules,** multimers of the protein **tubulin,** can be rapidly assembled and disassembled depending on the cell's needs. Two very important cellular filaments, actin and myosin, occur in striated muscle and are responsible for muscular contraction (see Chapter 22). Three **mechanochemical proteins—myosin, dynein,** and **kinesin**—convert chemical energy into mechanical energy for movement of cellular components. These molecular motors are associated with the cytoskeleton; the actual mechanism for the energy conversion, however, has not been defined completely. Dynein is involved in ciliary and flagellar movement, whereas kinesin is a driving force for the movement of vesicles and organelles along microtubules.

Cytosol Contains Soluble Cellular Components

The least complex in structure, but not in chemistry, is the organelle-free cell sap, or **cytosol.** It is here that many of the chemical reactions of metabolism occur and where substrates and cofactors interact with various enzymes. Although there is no apparent structure to the cytosol, the high protein content precludes it from being a truly homogeneous mixture of soluble components. Many reactions are localized in selected areas where substrate availability is more favorable. The actual physicochemical state of the cytosol is poorly understood. A major role of the cytosol is to support synthesis of proteins on the rough endoplasmic reticulum by supplying cofactors and energy. The cytosol also contains free ribosomes, often in a polysome form, for synthesis of intracellular proteins.

Studies with isolated cytosol suggest that many reactions are catalyzed by soluble enzymes, but in the intact cell some of these enzymes may be loosely attached to one of the many membrane structures or to cytoskeletal components and are readily released upon cell disruption.

Conclusion

A eukaryotic cell is a complex structure whose purpose is to replicate itself when necessary, maintain an intracellular environment to permit a myriad of complex reactions to occur as efficiently as possible, and to protect itself from the hazards of its surrounding environment. Cells of multicellular organisms also participate in maintaining the well-being of the whole organism by exerting influences on each other to maintain all tissue and cellular activities in balance. Thus, as we proceed to study the separate chemical components and activities of cells in subsequent chapters, it is important to keep in mind the concurrent and surrounding activities, constraints, and influences of the environment. Only by bringing together all the parts and activities of a cell, that is, reassembling the puzzle, will we appreciate the wonder of living cells.

BIBLIOGRAPHY

Water and Electrolytes

Dick, D. A. T. *Cell Water.* Washington, DC: Butterworths, 1966.

Eisenberg, D., and Kauzmann, W. *The Structures and Properties of Water.* Fairlawn, NJ: Oxford University Press, 1969.

Morris, J. G. *A Biologist's Physical Chemistry.* Reading, MA: Addison-Wesley, 1968.

Stillinger, F. H. Water revisited. *Science* 209:451, 1980.

Westof, E., *Water and Biological Macromolecules.* Boca Raton, FL: CRC Press, 1993.

Cell Structure

Alberts, B., Bray, D., Lewis, J., Raff, M., Roberts, K., and Watson, J. D. *Molecular Biology of the Cell.* New York: Garland, 1989.

Becker, W. M., and Deamer, D. W. *The World of the Living Cell,* 2nd. ed. Redwood City, CA: Benjamin, 1991.

DeDuve, C. *Guided Tour of the Living Cell,* Vols. 1 and 2. New York: Scientific American Books, 1984.

Dingle, J. T., Dean, R. T., and Sly, W. S. (Eds.). *Lysosomes in Biology and Pathology.* Amsterdam: Elsevier (a serial publication covering all aspects of lysosomes).

Fawcett, D. W. *The Cell.* Philadelphia: Saunders, 1981.

Holtzman, E., and Novikoff, A. B. *Cells and Organelles,* 3rd ed. New York: Holt, Rinehart & Winston, 1984.

Porter, K. R., and Bonneville, M. A. Fine Structure of Cells and Tissues. Philadelphia: Lea & Febiger, 1972.

Vale, R. D. Intracellular transport using microtubule-based motors. *Annu. Rev. Cell Biol.* 3:347, 1987.

Cell Organelles

Attardi, G., and Chomyn, A. *Mitochondrial Biogenesis and Genetics.* San Diego, CA: Academic Press, 1995.

Holtzman, E. *Lysosomes.* New York: Plenum Press, 1989.

Latruffe, N., and Bugaut, M. *Peroxisomes.* New York: Springer-Verlag, 1994.

Pavelka, M. *Functional Morphology of the Golgi Apparatus.* New York: Springer-Verlag, 1987.

Preston, T. M., King, C. A., and Hyams, J. S. *The Cytoskeleton and Cell Motility.* New York: Chapman and Hall, 1990.

Strauss, P. R., and Wilson, S. H. *The Eukaryotic Nucleus: Molecular Biochemistry and Macromolecular Assemblies.* Caldwell, NJ: Telford Press, 1990.

Tyler, D. D. *Mitochondrion in Health and Disease.* New York: VCH, 1992.

Tzagoloff, A. *Mitochondria.* New York: Plenum Press, 1982.

QUESTIONS ■ J. BAGGOTT AND C. N. ANGSTADT

1. Prokaryotic cells, but not eukaryotic cells, have:
   A. endoplasmic reticulum.
   B. histones.
   C. nucleoid.
   D. a nucleus.
   E. a plasma membrane.

2. Factors responsible for the polarity of the water molecule include:
   A. the similarity in electron affinity of hydrogen and oxygen.
   B. the tetrahedral structure of liquid water.
   C. the magnitude of the H—O—H bond angle.
   D. the ability of water to hydrogen bond to various chemical structures.
   E. the difference in bond strength between hydrogen bonds and covalent bonds.

3. Hydrogen bonds can be expected to form only between electronegative atoms such as oxygen or nitrogen and a hydrogen atom bonded to:
   A. carbon.
   B. an electronegative atom.
   C. hydrogen.
   D. iodine.
   E. sulfur.

4. Which of the following is least likely to be soluble in water?
   A. nonpolar compound
   B. weakly polar compound
   C. strongly polar compound
   D. weak electrolyte
   E. strong electrolyte

5. Which of the following is most likely to be partly associated in weak aqueous solution?
   A. alcohol
   B. lactic acid
   C. potassium sulfate (K_2SO_4)
   D. sodium chloride (NaCl)
   E. sodium lactate

6. The ion product of water:
   A. is independent of temperature.
   B. has a numerical value of 10^{-14} at 25°C.
   C. is the equilibrium constant for the reaction HOH $\rightleftharpoons$ H^+ + OH^-
   D. requires that $[H^+]$ and $[OH^-]$ always be identical.
   E. is an approximation that fails to take into account the presence of the hydronium ion, H_3O^+.

7. Which of the following is both a Brønsted acid and a Brønsted base in water?
   A. $H_2PO_4^-$
   B. H_2CO_3
   C. NH_3
   D. NH_4^+
   E. Cl^-

Refer to the following information for Questions 8 and 9.

A. pyruvic acid	$pK' = 2.50$
B. acetoacetic acid	$pK' = 3.6$
C. lactic acid	$pK' = 3.86$
D. β-hydroxybutyric acid	$pK' = 4.7$
E. propionic acid	$pK' = 4.86$

8. Which weak acid will be 91% neutralized at pH 4.86?

9. Assuming that the sum of [weak acid] + [conjugate base] is identical for buffer systems based on the acids listed above, which has the greatest buffer capacity at pH 4.86?

10. All of the following subcellular structures can be isolated essentially intact EXCEPT:
    A. endoplasmic reticulum.
    B. lysosomes.
    C. mitochondria.
    D. nuclei.
    E. peroxisomes.

11. Biological membranes are associated with all of the following EXCEPT:
    A. prevent free diffusion of ionic solutes.
    B. release of proteins when damaged.
    C. contain specific systems for the transport of uncharged molecules.
    D. sites for biochemical reactions.
    E. proteins and nucleic acids cross freely.

12. Mitochondria are associated with all of the following EXCEPT:
    A. ATP synthesis.
    B. DNA synthesis.
    C. protein synthesis.
    D. hydrolysis of various macromolecules at low pH.
    E. two different membranes.

13. Analysis of the composition of the major fluid compartments of the body shows that:
    A. the major blood plasma cation is K^+.
    B. the major cell fluid cation is Na^+.
    C. one of the major intracellular anions is Cl^-.
    D. one of the major intracellular anions is phosphate.
    E. plasma and the cell fluid are all very similar in ionic composition.

Refer to the following for Questions 14–17.

A. peroxisome
B. nucleus
C. cytoskeleton
D. endoplasmic reticulum
E. Golgi apparatus

14. Consists of microtubules and actin fibers.

15. Oxidizes very long-chain fatty acids.

16. Connected to the plasma membrane by a network of membranous channels.

17. Transfers carbohydrate precursors to proteins during glycoprotein synthesis.

ANSWERS

1. C Prokaryotic DNA is organized into a structure that also contains RNA and protein, called nucleoid. A, B, and D are found in eukaryotic cells, and E is an element of both prokaryotic and eukaryotic cells (p. 2).
2. C Water is a polar molecule because the bonding electrons are attracted more strongly to oxygen than to hydrogen. The bond angle gives rise to asymmetry of the charge distribution; if water were linear, it would not be a dipole (p. 4). A: Hydrogen and oxygen have very different electron affinity. B and D are consequences of water's structure, not factors responsible for it.
3. B Only hydrogen atoms bonded to one of the electronegative elements (O, N, F) can form hydrogen bonds (p. 5). A hydrogen atom participating in hydrogen bonding must have an electronegative element on both sides of it.
4. A In general, compounds that interact with the water dipoles are more soluble than those that do not. Thus ionized compounds and polar compounds tend to be soluble. Nonpolar compounds prefer to interact with one another rather than with polar solvents such as water (p. 5).
5. B Lactic acid is a weak acid, and weak acids dissociate only partially in aqueous solution (p. 6) A: Alcohol is fully associated. C–E: These are salts and are considered to be fully dissociated under physiological conditions, although at high concentration some association occurs.
6. B The constant is a function of temperature and is numerically equal to the equilibrium constant for the dissociation of water divided by the molar concentration of water (p. 6). D: $[H^+] = [OH^-]$ in pure water, but not in solutions of solutes that contribute H^+ or OH^-.
7. A $H_2PO_4^-$ can donate a proton to become HPO_4^{2-}. It can also accept a proton to become H_3PO_4. B and D are Brønsted acids; C is a Brønsted base. The Cl^- ion in water is neither (p. 8).
8. C If weak acid is 91% neutralized, 91 parts are present as conjugate base and 9 parts remain as the weak acid. Thus the conjugate base/acid ratio is 10 : 1. Substituting into the Henderson–Hasselbalch equation, $4.86 = pK + \log(10/1)$, and solving for pH gives the answer (p. 9).
9. E The buffer capacity of any system is maximal at pH = pK (p. 10). Buffer concentration also affects buffer capacity, but in this case concentrations are equal.
10. A Gentle disruption of cells will not destroy B–E. The tube-like endoplasmic reticulum, however, is disrupted and forms small vesicles. These vesicles, not the original structure from which they were derived, may be isolated (pp. 12, 16).
11. E (p. 17).
12. D This is a lysosomal function (p. 17). Mitochondrial properties are described on p. 17.
13. D Phosphate and protein are the major intracellular anions. A, B, and E: Plasma and cell fluid are strikingly different. The Na^+ ion is the major cation of plasma. C: Most chloride is extracellular (p. 14, Figure 1.10).
14. C (p. 19).
15. A Fatty acid oxidation occurs in the mitochondria, but the oxidation of very long-chain fatty acids involves the peroxisomes (p. 19).
16. B This describes only the nucleus (p. 16).
17. E Lipids, too, are attached covalently to certain proteins in the Golgi apparatus (p. 17).

CHAPTER

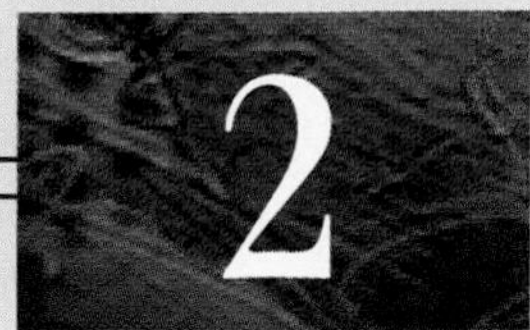

PROTEINS I: COMPOSITION AND STRUCTURE

Richard M. Schultz and Michael N. Liebman

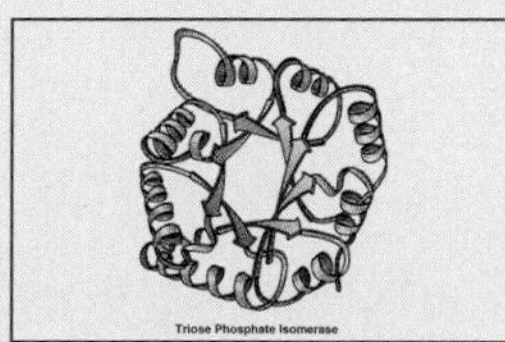

2.1 ■ FUNCTIONAL ROLES OF PROTEINS IN HUMANS

Proteins perform a surprising variety of essential functions in mammalian organisms. These may be grouped into dynamic and structural. Dynamic functions include transport, metabolic control, contraction, and catalysis of chemical transformations. In their structural functions, proteins provide the matrix for bone and connective tissue, giving structure and form to the human organism.

An important class of dynamic proteins are the enzymes. They catalyze chemical reactions, converting a substrate to a product at the enzyme's active site. Almost all of the thousands of chemical reactions that occur in living organisms require a specific enzyme catalyst to ensure that reactions occur at a rate compatible with life. The character of any cell is based on its particular chemistry, which is determined by its specific enzyme composition. Genetic traits are expressed through synthesis of enzymes, which catalyze reactions that establish the phenotype. Many genetic diseases result from altered levels of enzyme production or specific alterations to their amino acid sequence. Transport is another major function for proteins. Particular examples discussed in greater detail in this text are hemoglobin and myoglobin, which transport oxygen in blood and in muscle, respectively. Transferrin transports iron in blood. Transport proteins bind and carry steroid hormones in blood from their site of synthesis to their site of action. Many drugs and toxic compounds are transported bound to proteins. Proteins participate in contractile mechanisms. Myosin and actin function in muscle contraction.

Proteins have a protective role through a combination of dynamic functions. Immunoglobulins and interferon are proteins that protect the human against bacterial or viral infection. Fibrin stops the loss of blood on injury to the vascular system.

Many hormones are proteins or peptides. Protein hormones include insulin, thyrotropin, somatotropin (growth hormone), luteinizing hormone, and follicle-stimulating hormone. Many diverse polypeptide hormones have a low molecular weight (<5000) and are referred to as peptides. In general, the term **protein** is used for molecules composed of over 50 amino acids and the term **peptide** is used for molecules of less than 50 amino acids. Important peptide hormones include adrenocorticotropin hormone, antidiuretic hormone, glucagon, and calcitonin.

Proteins control and regulate gene transcription and translation. These include histones that are closely associated with DNA, repressor and enhancer transcription factors that control gene transcription, and proteins that form a part of the heteronuclear RNA particles and ribosomes.

Structural proteins function in "brick-and-mortar" roles. They include collagen and elastin, which form the matrix of bone and ligaments and provide structural strength and elasticity to organs and the vascular system. α-Keratin forms the structure of epidermal tissue.

An understanding of both the normal functioning and the pathology of the mammalian organism requires a clear understanding of the properties of the proteins.

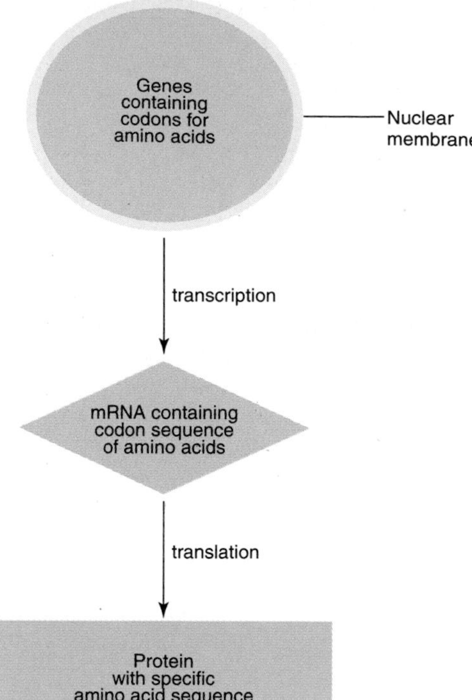

FIGURE 2.1
Genetic information is transcribed from a DNA sequence into mRNA and then translated to the amino acid sequence of a protein.

2.2 AMINO ACID COMPOSITION OF PROTEINS

Proteins Are Polymers of α-Amino Acids

It is notable that all the different types of proteins are initially synthesized as polymers of only 20 amino acids. These **common amino acids** are defined as those for which at least one specific codon exists in the DNA genetic code. There are 20 amino acids for which DNA codons are known. Transcription and translation of the DNA code result in polymerization of amino acids into a specific linear sequence characteristic of a protein (Figure 2.1). In addition to the common amino acids, proteins may contain **derived amino acids,** which are usually formed by an enzyme-facilitated reaction on a common amino acid after that amino acid has been incorporated into a protein structure. Examples of derived amino acids are cystine (see p. 30), desmosine and isodesmosine found in elastin, hydroxyproline and hydroxylysine found in collagen, and γ-carboxyglutamate found in prothrombin.

Common Amino Acids Have a General Structure

Common amino acids have the general structure depicted in Figure 2.2. They contain in common a central ***alpha* (α)-carbon** atom to which a carboxylic acid group, an amino group, and a hydrogen atom are covalently bonded. In addition, the α-carbon atom is bound to a specific chemical group, designated R and called the side chain, that uniquely defines each of the 20 common amino acids. Figure 2.2 depicts the ionized form of a common amino acid in solution at pH 7. The α-amino group is protonated and in its ammonium ion form; the carboxylic acid group is in its unprotonated or carboxylate ion form.

Side Chains Define Chemical Nature and Structures of Different Amino Acids

Structures of the common amino acids are shown in Figure 2.3. Alkyl amino acids have alkyl group side chains and include glycine, alanine, valine, leucine, and isoleucine. **Glycine** has the simplest structure, with R = H. **Alanine** contains a methyl (CH_3—) side chain group. **Valine** has an isopropyl R group (Figure 2.4). The leucine and isoleucine R groups are butyl groups that are structural isomers of each other. In **leucine** the branching in the isobutyl side chain occurs on the *gamma* (γ)-carbon of the amino acid. In isoleucine it is branched at the *beta* (β)-carbon.

The aromatic amino acids are phenylalanine, tyrosine, and tryptophan. The **phenylalanine** R group contains a benzene ring, **tyrosine** contains a phenol group, and the **tryptophan** R group contains the heterocyclic structure, indole.

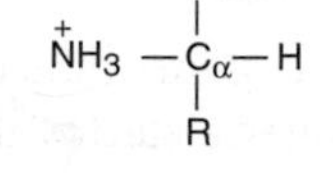

FIGURE 2.2
General structure of the common amino acids.

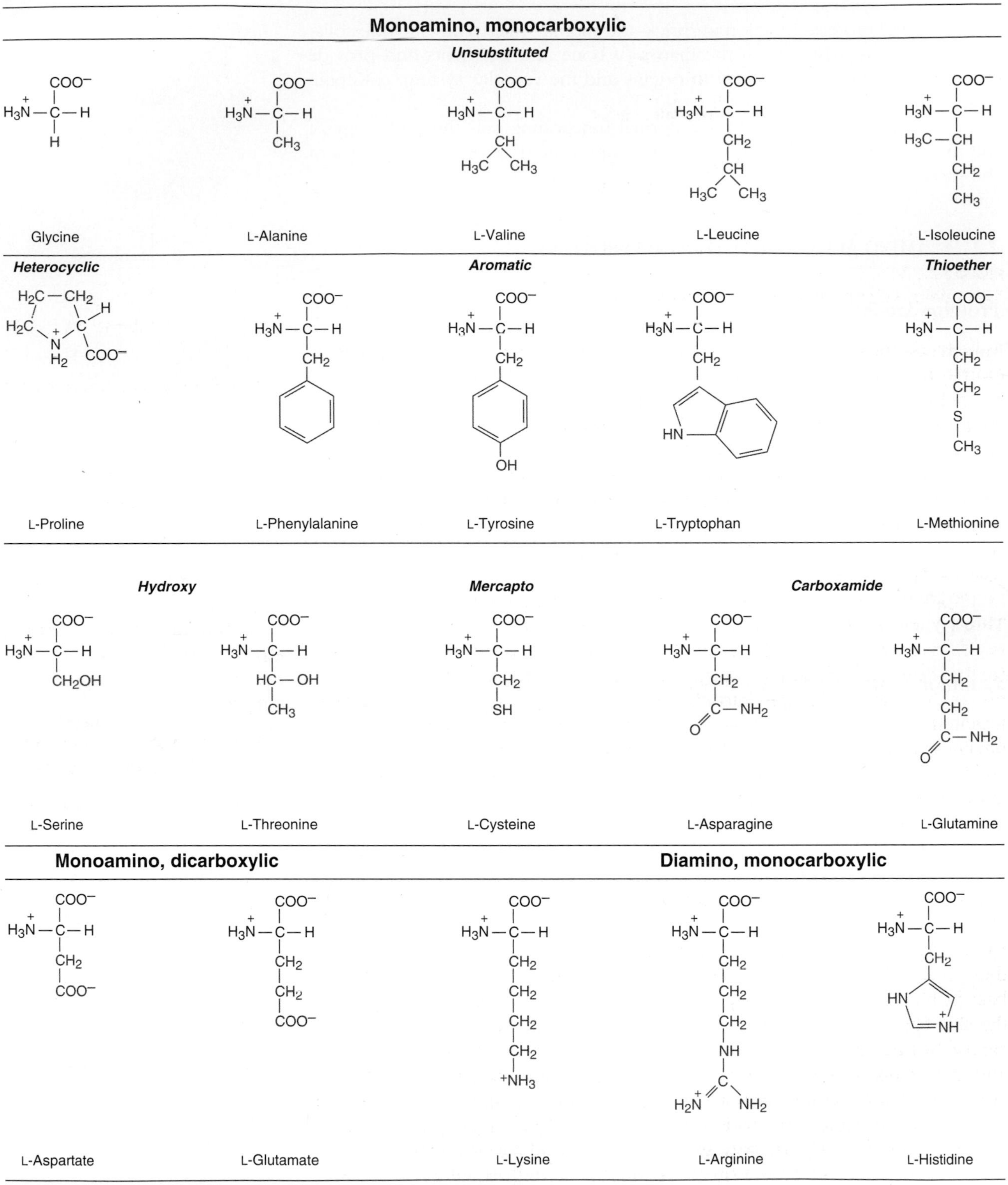

FIGURE 2.3
Structures of the common amino acids.
Charge forms are those present at pH 7.0.

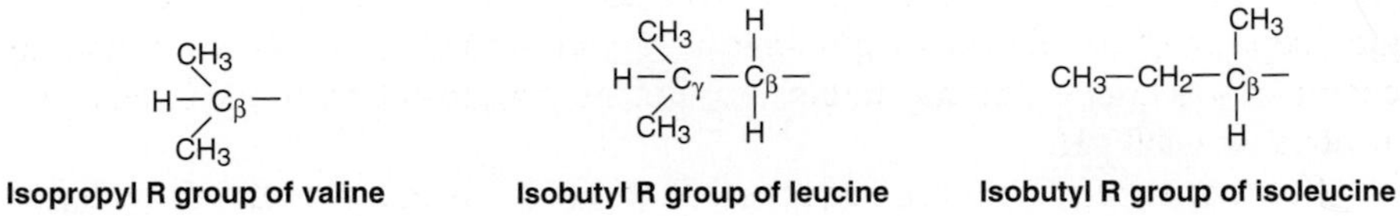

FIGURE 2.4
Alkyl side chains of valine, leucine, and isoleucine.

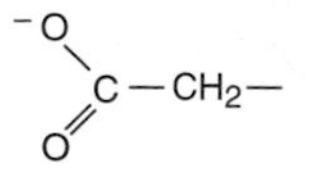

Aspartate R group

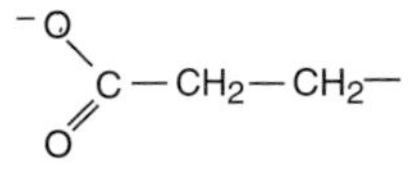

Glutamate R group

FIGURE 2.5
Side chains of aspartate and glutamate.

In each case the aromatic moiety is attached to the α-carbon through a methylene (—CH_2—) carbon (Figure 2.3).

Sulfur-containing common amino acids are cysteine and methionine. The **cysteine** side chain group is a thiolmethyl ($HSCH_2$—). In **methionine** the side chain is a methyl ethyl thiol ether ($CH_3SCH_2CH_2$—).

There are two hydroxy (alcohol)-containing common amino acids, serine and threonine. The **serine** side chain is a hydroxymethyl ($HOCH_2$—). In **threonine** an ethanol structure is connected to the α-carbon through the carbon containing the hydroxyl substituent, resulting in a secondary alcohol structure (CH_3—CHOH—CH_α—).

The **proline** side chain is unique in that it incorporates the α-amino group. Thus proline is more accurately classified as an α-imino acid, since its α-amine is a secondary amine with its α-nitrogen having two covalent bonds to carbon (to the α-carbon and side chain carbon), rather than a primary amine. Incorporation of the α-amino nitrogen into a five-membered ring constrains the rotational freedom around the —N_α—C_α— bond in proline to a specific rotational angle, which limits participation of proline in polypeptide chain conformations.

The amino acids discussed so far contain side chains that are uncharged at physiological pH. The **dicarboxylic monoamino acids** contain a carboxylic group in their side chain. **Aspartate** contains a carboxylic acid group separated by a methylene carbon (—CH_2—) from the α-carbon (Figure 2.5). In **glutamate** (Figure 2.5), the carboxylic acid group is separated by two methylene (—CH_2—CH_2—) carbon atoms from the α-carbon (Figure 2.2). At physiological pH, side chain carboxylic acid groups are unprotonated and negatively charged. **Dibasic monocarboxylic acids** include lysine, arginine, and histidine (Figure 2.3). In these structures, the R group contains one or two nitrogen atoms that act as a base by binding a proton. The **lysine** side chain is a *N*-butyl amine. In **arginine,** the side chain contains a guanidino group (Figure 2.6) separated from the α-carbon by three methylene carbon atoms. Both the guanidino group of arginine and the ε-amino group of lysine are protonated at physiological pH (pH~7) and in their charged form. In **histidine** the side chain contains a five-membered heterocyclic structure, the imidazole (Figure 2.6). The pK_a' of the imidazole group is approximately 6.0 in water; physiological solutions contain relatively high concentrations of both basic (imidazole) and acidic (imidazolium) forms of the histidine side chain (see Section 2.3).

The last two common amino acids are glutamine and asparagine. They contain an amide moiety in their side chain. **Glutamine** and **asparagine** are structural analogs of glutamic acid and aspartic acid with their side chain carboxylic acid groups amidated. Unique DNA codons exist for glutamine and asparagine separate from those for glutamic acid and aspartic acid. The amide side chains of glutamine and asparagine cannot be protonated and are uncharged at physiological pH.

In order to represent the sequence of amino acids in a protein, three-letter and one-letter abbreviations for the common amino acids have been established (Table 2.1). These abbreviations are universally accepted and will be used

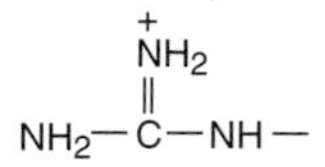

Guanidinium group (charged form) of arginine

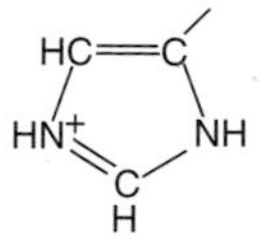

Imidazolium group of histidine

FIGURE 2.6
Guanidinium and imidazolium groups of arginine and histidine.

TABLE 2.1 Abbreviations for the Amino Acids

Amino Acid	*Abbreviation* Three Letter	One Letter
Alanine	Ala	A
Arginine	Arg	R
Asparagine	Asn	N
Aspartic	Asp	D
Asparagine or aspartic	Asx	B
Cysteine	Cys	C
Glycine	Gly	G
Glutamine	Gln	Q
Glutamic	Glu	E
Glutamine or glutamic	Glx	Z
Histidine	His	H
Isoleucine	Ile	I
Leucine	Leu	L
Lysine	Lys	K
Methionine	Met	M
Phenylalanine	Phe	F
Proline	Pro	P
Serine	Ser	S
Threonine	Thr	T
Tryptophan	Trp	W
Tyrosine	Tyr	Y
Valine	Val	V

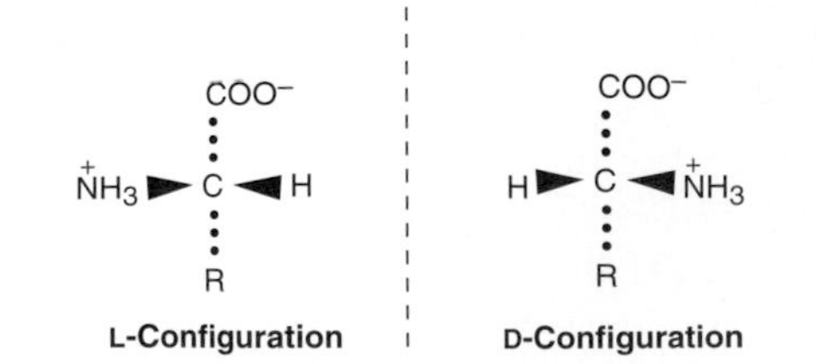

L-Configuration D-Configuration

FIGURE 2.7
Absolute configuration of an amino acid.

throughout the book. The three-letter abbreviations of aspartic acid (Asp) and glutamic acid (Glu) should not be confused with those for asparagine (Asn) and glutamine (Gln). In experimentally determining the amino acids of a protein by chemical procedures, one cannot easily differentiate between Asn and Asp, or between Gln and Glu, because the side chain amide groups in Asn and Gln are hydrolyzed and generate Asp and Glu (see Section 2.9). In these cases, the symbols of Asx for Asp or Asn, and Glx for Glu or Gln indicate this ambiguity. A similar scheme is used with the one-letter abbreviations to symbolize Asp or Asn, and Glu or Gln.

Amino Acids Have an Asymmetric Center

The common amino acids with the general structure in Figure 2.2 have four substituents (R, H, COO^-, NH_3^+) covalently bonded to the α-carbon atom in the α-amino acid structure. A carbon atom with four different substituents arranged in a tetrahedral configuration is asymmetric and exists in two enantiomeric forms. Thus each of the amino acids exhibits optical isomerism except glycine, in which R = H and thus two of the four substituents on the α-carbon atom are hydrogen. The absolute configuration for an amino acid is depicted in Figure 2.7 using the Fischer projection to show the direction in space of the tetrahedrally arranged α-carbon substituents. The α-COO^- group is directed up and behind the plane of the page, and the R group is directed down and behind the plane of the page. The α-H and α-NH_3^+ groups are directed toward the reader. An amino acid held in this way projects its α-NH_3^+ group either to the left or right of the α-carbon atom. By convention, if the α-NH_3^+ is projected to the left, the amino acid has an L absolute configuration. Its optical enantiomer, with α-NH_3^+ projected toward the right, has a D absolute configuration. In mammalian proteins only amino acids of L configuration are found. The L and D designations refer to the ability to rotate polarized light to the left (L, levo) or right (D, dextro) from its plane of polarization. As the amino acids in proteins are asymmetric, the proteins that contain them also exhibit asymmetric properties.

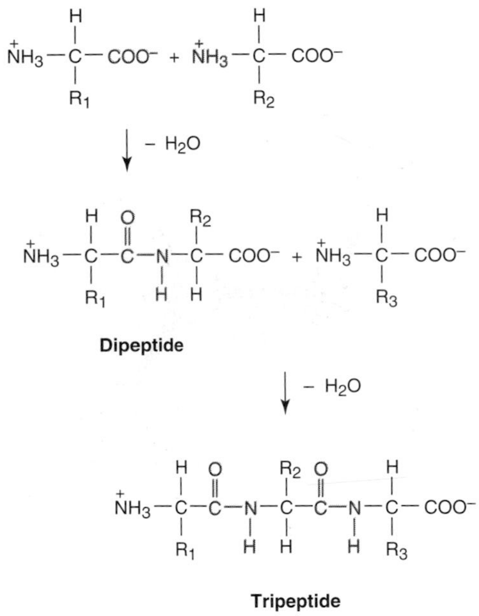

Dipeptide

Tripeptide

FIGURE 2.8
Peptide bond formation.

Amino Acids Are Polymerized into Peptides and Proteins

Polymerization of the 20 common amino acids into polypeptide chains in cells is catalyzed by enzymes and is associated with the ribosomes (Chapter 15). Chemically, this polymerization is a dehydration reaction (Figure 2.8). The α-carboxyl group of an amino acid with side chain R_1 forms a covalent **peptide bond** with the α-amino group of the amino acid with side chain R_2 by elimination of a molecule of water. The **dipeptide** (two amino acid residues joined by a single peptide bond) can then form a second peptide bond through its terminal carboxylic acid group and the α-amino of a third amino acid (R_3), to generate a tripeptide (Figure 2.8). Repetition of this process generates a **polypeptide** or protein of specific amino acid sequence (R_1-R_2-R_3-R_4-$\cdots R_n$). The amino acid sequence of the polypeptide chains is the **primary structure** of the protein, and it is predetermined by the DNA sequence of its gene (Chapter 14). It is the unique primary structure that enables a polypeptide chain to fold into a specific three-dimensional structure that gives the protein its chemical and physiological properties.

A peptide bond can be represented using two **resonance isomers** (Figure 2.9). In structure I, a double bond is located between the carbonyl carbon and carbonyl oxygen (C′=O), and the carbonyl carbon to nitrogen (C′—N) linkage is a single bond. In structure II, the carbonyl carbon to oxygen bond (C′—O^-) is a single bond and the bond located between the carbonyl carbon and nitrogen is a double bond (C′=N). In structure II there is a negative charge on the oxygen and a positive charge on the nitrogen. Actual peptide bonds are a

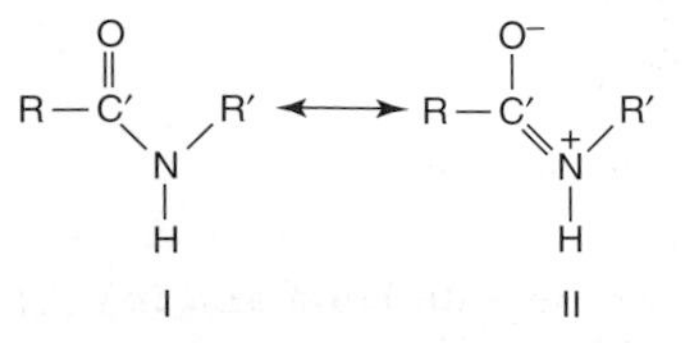

I II

FIGURE 2.9
Electronic isomer structures of a peptide bond.

resonance hybrid of these two electron isomer structures, the carbonyl carbon to nitrogen bond having a 50% double-bond character. The hybrid bond is supported by spectroscopic measurements and X-ray diffraction studies, the latter showing that the carbonyl carbon to nitrogen peptide bond length (1.33 Å) is approximately half-way between that found for a C—N single bond (~1.45 Å) and a C=N double bond (~1.25 Å).

A consequence of this partial double-bond character is that, as for normal double-bond structures, rotation does not occur about the carbonyl carbon to nitrogen of a peptide bond at physiological temperatures. Also, a consequence of the C′=N double-bond's chemistry is that the atoms attached to C′ and N

$$\mathrm{-C-C'(O^-)=N^+(H)-C-}$$

all lie in a common plane. Thus a polypeptide chain is a polymer of peptide-bond planes interconnected at the α-carbon atoms. The α-carbon interconnects peptide bonds through single bonds that allow rotation of adjacent peptide planes with respect to each other. Each **amino acid residue** contributes one α-carbon (two single bonds and a peptide bond, Figure 2.10) to the polypeptide chain. The term residue refers to the atoms contributed by an amino acid to a polypeptide chain including the atoms of the side chain.

The peptide bond in Figure 2.11*a* shows a ***trans* configuration** between the oxygen (O) and the hydrogen (H) atoms of the peptide bond. This is the most stable configuration for the peptide bond with the two side chains (R and R′) also in *trans*. The ***cis* configuration** (Figure 2.11*b*) brings the two side chain groups to the same side of the C′=N bond, where unfavorable repulsive steric forces occur between the two side chain (R) groups. Accordingly, *trans*-peptide bonds are always found in proteins except where there are proline residues. In proline the side chain is linked to its α-amino group, and the *cis*- and *trans*-peptide bonds with the proline α-imino group have near equal energies. The configuration of the peptide bond actually found for a proline in a protein will depend on the specific forces generated by the unique folded three-dimensional structure of the protein molecule.

One of the largest natural polypeptide chains in humans is that of apolipoprotein B-100, which contains 4536 amino acid residues in one polypeptide chain. Chain length alone, however, does not determine the function of a polypeptide. Many small peptides with less than ten amino acids perform important biochemical and physiological functions in humans (Table 2.2). Primary structures are written in a standard convention and sequentially numbered from their NH_2-terminal end toward their COOH-terminal end, consistent with the order of addition of the amino acid to the chain during biosynthesis. Accordingly, for thyrotropin-releasing hormone (Table 2.2) the glutamic acid residue written on the left is the NH_2-terminal amino acid of the tripeptide and is designated amino acid residue 1 in the sequence. The proline is the COOH-terminal amino acid and is designated residue 3. The defined direction of the polypeptide chain is from Glu to Pro (NH_2-terminal amino acid to COOH-terminal amino acid).

FIGURE 2.10
Amino acid residue.
Each amino acid residue of a polypeptide contributes two single bonds and one peptide bond to the chain. The single bonds are those between the C_α and carbonyl C′ atoms, and the C_α and N atoms. See p. 43 for definition of ϕ and ψ.

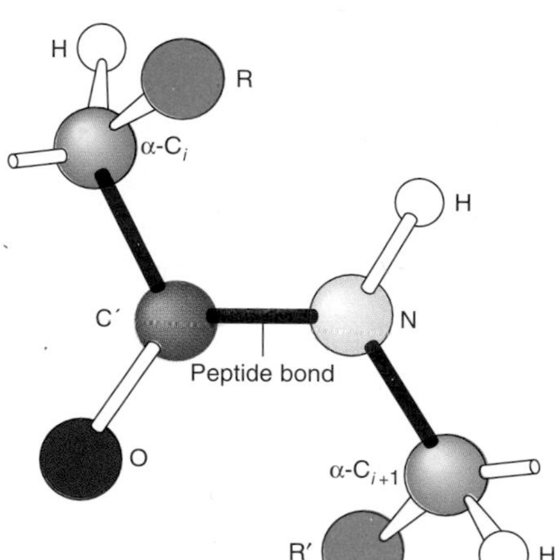

(*a*) *trans* configuration

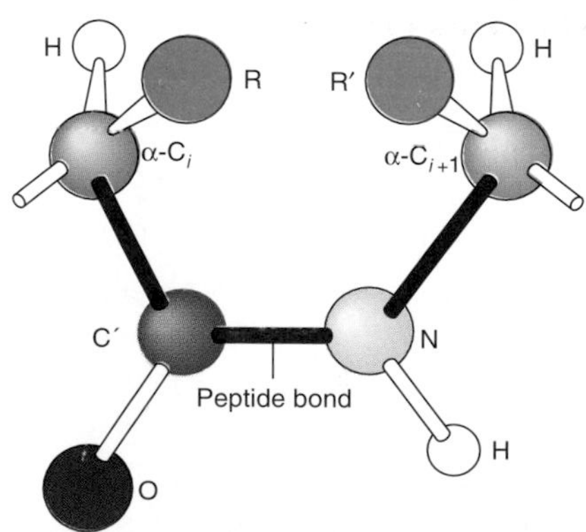

(*b*) *cis* configuration

FIGURE 2.11
(*a*) *Trans*-peptide bond and (*b*) the rare *cis*-peptide bond.
The C′—N have a partial double-bond character.

TABLE 2.2 Some Examples of Biologically Active Peptides

Amino Acid Sequence	*Name*	*Function*
1 3 pyroGlu-His-Pro(NH_2)[a]	Thyrotropin-releasing hormone	Secreted by hypothalamus; causes anterior pituitary gland to release thyrotropic hormone
1 9 H-Cys-Tyr-Phe-Gln-Asn-Cys-Pro-Arg-Gly(NH_2)[b] S————S	Vasopressin (antidiuretic hormone)	Secreted by posterior pituitary gland; causes kidney to retain water from urine
1 5 H-Tyr-Gly-Gly-Phe-Met-OH	Methionine enkephalin	Opiate-like peptide found in brain that inhibits sense of pain
1 10 pyroGlu-Gly-Pro-Trp-Leu-Glu-Glu-Glu-Glu-Glu- 11 17 Ala-Tyr-Gly-Trp-Met-Asp-Phe(NH_2)[a,c] SO_3	Little gastrin (human)	Hormone secreted by mucosal cells in stomach; causes parietal cells of stomach to secrete acid
1 10 H-His-Ser-Gln-Gly-Thr-Phe-Thr-Ser-Asp-Tyr- 11 20 Ser-Lys-Tyr-Leu-Asp-Ser-Arg-Arg-Ala-Gln- 21 29 Asp-Phe-Val-Gln-Trp-Leu-Met-Asn-Thr-OH	Glucagon (bovine)	Pancreatic hormone involved in regulating glucose metabolism
1 8 H-Asp-Arg-Val-Tyr-Ile-His-Pro-Phe-OH	Angiotensin II (horse)	Pressor or hypertensive peptide; also stimulates release of aldosterone from adrenal cortex
1 9 H-Arg-Pro-Pro-Gly-Phe-Ser-Pro-Phe-Arg-OH	Plasma bradykinin (bovine)	Vasodilator peptide
1 10 H-Arg-Pro-Lys-Pro-Gln-Phe-Phe-Gly-Leu-Met(NH_2)	Substance P	Neurotransmitter

[a] The NH_2 terminal Glu is in the pyro form in which its γ-COOH is covalently joined to its α-NH_2 via amide linkage; the COOH terminal amino acid is amidated and thus also not free.
[b] Cysteine-1 and cysteine-6 are joined to form a disulfide bond structure within the nonapeptide.
[c] The Tyr 12 is sulfonated on its phenolic side chain OH.

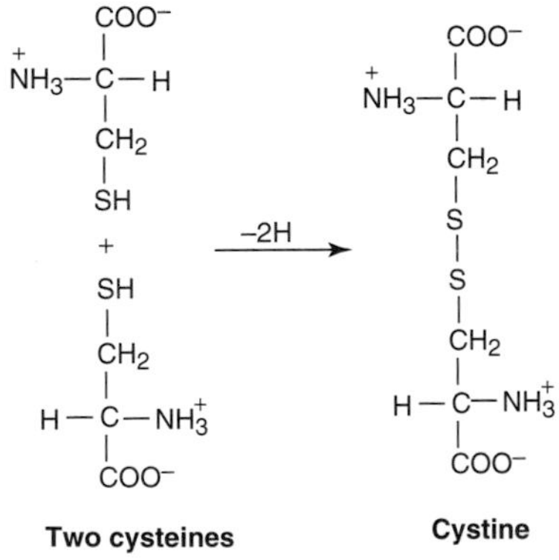

FIGURE 2.12
Cystine bond formation.

Cystine Is a Derived Amino Acid

A derived amino acid found in many proteins is cystine. It is formed by the oxidation of two cysteine thiol side chains, joined to form a disulfide covalent bond (Figure 2.12). Within proteins disulfide links of cystine formed from cysteines, separated from each other in the primary structure, have an important role in stabilizing the folded conformation of proteins.

2.3 ■ CHARGE AND CHEMICAL PROPERTIES OF AMINO ACIDS AND PROTEINS

Ionizable Groups of Amino Acids and Proteins Are Critical for Biological Function

Ionizable groups common to proteins and amino acids are shown in Table 2.3. The acid forms are on the left of the equilibrium sign and the base forms on the right side. In forming its conjugate base, the acid form releases a proton. In reverse, the base form associates with a proton to form the respective acid. The proton dissociation of an acid is characterized by an acid **dissociation constant (K_a')** with its corresponding pK_a' value: p$K_a' = \log_{10}(1/K_a')$. Table 2.3 shows a range of pK_a' values for each acid group, as the actual pK_a' depends on the environment in which an acid group is placed. For example, when a

TABLE 2.3 Characteristic pK'_a Values for the Common Acid Groups in Proteins

Where Acid Group Is Found	*Acid Form*		*Base Form*	*Approximate pK_a Range for Group*
NH_2-terminal residue in peptides, lysine	$R{-}NH_3^+$ Ammonium	⇌	$R{-}NH_2 + H^+$ Amine	7.6–10.6
COOH-terminal residue in peptides, glutamate, aspartate	R—COOH Carboxylic acid	⇌	$R{-}COO^- + H^+$ Carboxylate	3.0–5.5
Arginine	$R{-}NH{-}\overset{+}{C}(NH_2){\cdots}NH_2$ Guanidinium	⇌	$R{-}NH{-}C(NH_2){=}NH + H^+$ Guanidino	11.5–12.5
Cysteine	R—SH Thiol	⇌	$R{-}S^- + H^+$ Thiolate	8.0–9.0
Histidine	R—C=CH, HN, +NH, C, H Imidazolium	⇌	R—C=CH, HN, N + H^+, C, H Imidazole	6.0–7.0
Tyrosine	R—(benzene ring)—OH Phenol	⇌	R—(benzene ring)—$O^- + H^+$ Phenolate	9.5–10.5

positive-charged ammonium group ($—NH_3^+$) is placed near a negatively charged group within a protein, the negative charge stabilizes the positively charged acid form of the amino group, making it more difficult to dissociate its proton. The pK'_a of the $—NH_3^+$ will have a higher value than normal for an ammonium group in the absence of a nearby negative charge stabilization. Factors other than charge that affect the pK'_a of an acid group include polarity of the environment, the absence or presence of water, and the potential for formation of hydrogen bonding. Also, the acid groups (α-COOH or α-NH_3^+) at the ends of polypeptide chains typically have lower pK'_a values than the same types of acid groups in the side chains (Table 2.4). The amino acids whose R groups contain nitrogen atoms (Lys and Arg) are the **basic amino acids,** since their side chains have relatively high pK'_a values and function as bases at physiological pH. They are usually in their acid form and positively charged at physiological pH. Amino acids whose side chains contain a carboxylic acid group have relatively low pK'_a values and are called **acidic amino acids.** They are predominantly in their unprotonated forms and are negatively charged at physiological pH. Proteins in which the ratio (ΣLys + ΣArg)/(ΣGlu + ΣAsp) is greater than 1 are referred to as **basic proteins.** Proteins in which the above ratio is less than 1 are referred to as **acidic proteins.**

TABLE 2.4 pK'_a of Side Chain and Terminal Acid Groups in Protein Ribonuclease

	$—NH_3^+$	*—COOH*
Side chain	Lysines $\simeq$ 10.2	Glu and Asp $\simeq$ 4.6
Chain end	N-terminal = 7.8	C-terminal = 3.8

$$pH = pKa + \log \frac{[\text{conjugate base}]}{[\text{conjugate acid}]}$$

or

$$pH - pKa = \log \frac{[\text{conjugate base}]}{[\text{conjugate acid}]}$$

FIGURE 2.13
Henderson–Hasselbalch equation.
For a more detailed discussion of this equation, see p. 9.

Ionic Form of an Amino Acid or Protein Can Be Determined at a Given pH

From a knowledge of the pK'_a for each ionizable acid group in an amino acid or protein and the Henderson–Hasselbalch equation (Figure 2.13), the ionic form of the molecule can be calculated at a given pH. This is an important relationship as it shows the change in ionization state and charge of a molecule with pH. A molecule will have different physiological activities with changes in pH and ionization state. For example, an enzyme may require a histidine imidazole in its base form for catalytic activity. If the pK'_a of the catalytically essential histidine in the enzyme is 6.0, at pH 6.0 one-half of the enzyme molecules are in the active base (imidazole) form and one-half in the inactive acid (imidazolium) form. Accordingly, the enzyme exhibits 50% of its potential activity. At pH 7.0, the pH is one unit above the imidazolium pK'_a and the ratio of [imidazole]/[imidazolium] is 10 : 1 (Table 2.5). Based on this ratio, the enzyme exhibits $10/(10 + 1) \times 100 = 91\%$ of its maximum potential activity. Thus a change in pH has a dramatic effect on the enzyme's activity. Most protein activities demonstrate similar pH dependency due to their acid and base group(s).

Titration of a Monoamino Monocarboxylic Acid: Determination of the Isoelectric pH

An understanding of a protein's acid and base forms and their relation to charge is made more clear by following the titration of the ionizable groups for a simple amino acid. As presented in Figure 2.14, leucine contains an α-COOH with p$K'_a = 2.4$ and an α-NH_3^+ group with p$K'_a = 9.6$. At pH 1.0 the predominant ionic form (form I) has a charge of +1 and migrates toward the cathode in an

TABLE 2.5 Relationship Between the Difference of pH and Acid pK'_a and the Ratio of the Concentrations of Base to Its Conjugate Acid

pH − pK′ₐ (Difference Between pH and pK′ₐ)	*Ratio of Concentration of Base to Conjugate Acid*
0	1
1	10
2	100
3	1000
−1	0.1
−2	0.01
−3	0.001

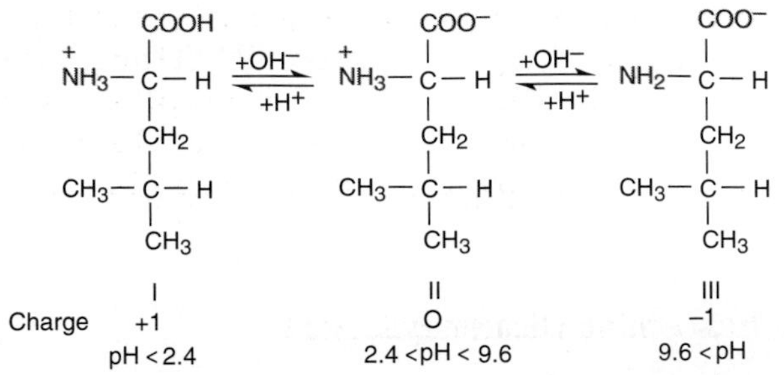

$$\underset{\substack{\text{I} \\ \text{Charge } +1 \\ \text{pH} < 2.4}}{\overset{+}{N}H_3-\underset{\substack{|\\CH_2\\|\\CH_3-C-H\\|\\CH_3}}{\overset{\substack{COOH\\|}}{C}}-H} \underset{+H^+}{\overset{+OH^-}{\rightleftharpoons}} \underset{\substack{\text{II} \\ 0 \\ 2.4 < \text{pH} < 9.6}}{\overset{+}{N}H_3-\underset{\substack{|\\CH_2\\|\\CH_3-C-H\\|\\CH_3}}{\overset{\substack{COO^-\\|}}{C}}-H} \underset{+H^+}{\overset{+OH^-}{\rightleftharpoons}} \underset{\substack{\text{III} \\ -1 \\ 9.6 < \text{pH}}}{NH_2-\underset{\substack{|\\CH_2\\|\\CH_3-C-H\\|\\CH_3}}{\overset{\substack{COO^-\\|}}{C}}-H}$$

FIGURE 2.14
Ionic forms of leucine.

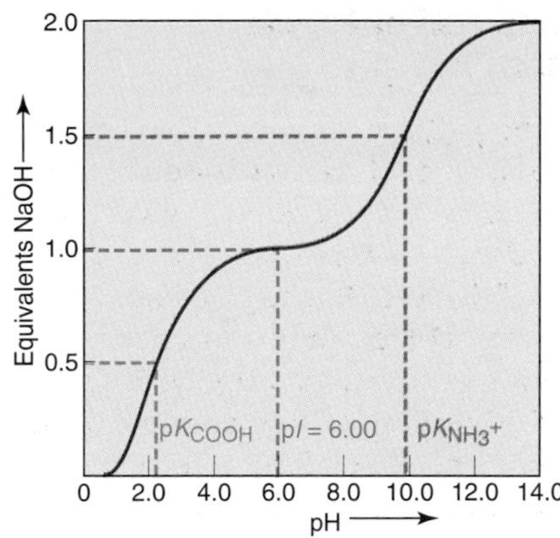

FIGURE 2.15
Titration curve of leucine.

electrical field. The addition of 0.5 equivalent of base half-titrates the α-COOH group of the leucine; that is, the ratio of $[COO^-]/[COOH]$ will equal 1. The Henderson–Hasselbalch equation, with the second term on the right side of the equation $\log_{10}[(\text{base})/(\text{acid})] = \log_{10}[1] = 0$ at a ratio of conjugate base to acid of 1 : 1, shows that the pH (when the α-COOH is half-titrated) is directly equal to the $pK_{a(\alpha\text{-COOH})}$ (Figure 2.15).

Addition of 1 equivalent of base completely titrates the α-COOH but leaves the α-NH_3^+ group intact. In the resulting form (II), the negatively charged α-COO^- and positively charged α-NH_3^+ cancel each other and the net charge of this ionic form is zero. Form II is thus the **zwitterion** form, that is, the ionic form in which the total of positive charges is exactly equal to the total of the negative charges. As the net charge on a zwitterion molecule is zero, it will not migrate toward either the cathode or anode in an electric field. Further addition of 0.5 equivalent of base to the zwitterion form of leucine (total base added is 1.5 equivalents) will then half-titrate the α-NH_3^+ group. At this point in the titration, the ratio of $[NH_2]/[NH_3^+] = 1$, and the pH is equal to the value of the pK_a' for the α-NH_3^+ group (Figure 2.15). Addition of a further 0.5 equivalent of base (total of 2 full equivalents of base added; Figure 2.15) completely titrates the α-NH_3^+ group to its base form (α-NH_2). The solution pH is greater than 11, and the predominant molecular species has a negative charge of -1 (form III).

It is useful to calculate the exact pH at which an amino acid is electrically neutral and in its zwitterion form. This pH is known as the **isoelectric pH** for the molecule, and the symbol is ***pI***. The p*I* value is a constant of a compound at a particular ionic strength and temperature. For simple molecules, such as leucine, p*I* is directly calculated as the average of the two pK_a' values that regulate the boundaries of the zwitterion form. Leucine has two ionizable groups that regulate the zwitterion form boundaries, and the p*I* is calculated as follows:

$$pI = \frac{pK_a'\text{COOH} + pK_a'\text{NH}_3^+}{2} = \frac{2.4 + 9.6}{2} = 6.0$$

At pH > 6.0, leucine assumes a partial negative charge that formally rises at high pH to a full negative charge of -1 (form III) (Figure 2.14). At pH < 6, leucine has a partial positive charge until at very low pH it has a charge of $+1$ (form I) (Figure 2.14). The partial charge at any pH can be calculated from the Henderson–Hasselbalch equation or from extrapolation from the titration curve of Figure 2.15.

Titration of a Monoamino Dicarboxylic Acid

A more complicated example of the relationship between molecular charge and pH is provided by glutamic acid. Its ionized forms and titration curve are

	$^{+}NH_3-CH(COOH)-CH_2-CH_2-COOH$	$\underset{+H^+}{\overset{+OH^-}{\rightleftharpoons}}$	$^{+}NH_3-CH(COO^-)-CH_2-CH_2-COOH$	$\underset{+H^+}{\overset{+OH^-}{\rightleftharpoons}}$	$^{+}NH_3-CH(COO^-)-CH_2-CH_2-COO^-$	$\underset{+H^+}{\overset{+OH^-}{\rightleftharpoons}}$	$NH_2-CH(COO^-)-CH_2-CH_2-COO^-$
Charge	+1		0		−1		−2
	pH < 2.2		2.2 < pH < 4.3		4.3 < pH < 9.7		9.6 < pH

FIGURE 2.16
Ionic forms of glutamic acid.

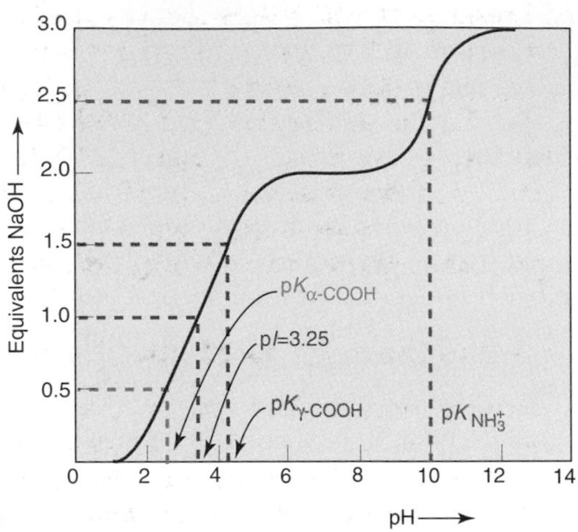

FIGURE 2.17
Titration curve of glutamic acid.

shown in Figures 2.16 and 2.17. In glutamic acid the α-COOH $pK'_a = 2.2$, the γ-COOH $pK'_a = 4.3$, and the α-NH_3^+ $pK'_a = 9.7$. The zwitterion form is generated after 1.0 equivalent of base is added to the low pH form, and the isoelectric pH (pI) is calculated from the average of the two pK'_a values that control the boundaries of the zwitterion form:

$$pI = \frac{2.2 + 4.3}{2} = 3.25$$

Accordingly, at values above pH 3.25 the molecule assumes a net negative charge until at high pH the molecule has a net charge of -2. At pH < 3.25 glutamic acid is positively charged, and at extremely low pH it has a net positive charge of $+1$.

General Relationship Between Charge Properties of Amino Acids and Proteins and pH

Analysis of charge forms present in other common amino acids shows that the relationship observed between pH and charge for leucine and glutamate is generally true. That is, at a solution pH less than pI, the amino acid is positively charged. At a solution pH greater than pI, the amino acid is negatively charged. The degree of positive or negative charge is a function of the magnitude of the difference between pH and pI. As a protein is a complex polyelectrolyte containing multiple ionizable acid groups that regulate the boundaries of its zwitterion form, calculation of a protein's isoelectric pH from its acid pK'_a values utilizing the Henderson–Hasselbalch relationship would be difficult. Accordingly, the pI values for proteins are always experimentally measured by determining the pH value at which the protein does not move in an electrical field. pI values for some representative proteins are given in Table 2.6.

TABLE 2.6 p*I* Values for Some Representative Proteins

Protein	*pI*
Pepsin	~1
Human serum albumin	5.9
α_1-Lipoprotein	5.5
Fibrinogen	5.8
Hemoglobin A	7.1
Ribonuclease	7.8
Cytochrome-*c*	10.0
Thymohistone	10.6

pH > p*I*, then protein charge negative
pH < p*I*, then protein charge positive

FIGURE 2.18
Relationship between solution pH, protein p*I*, and protein charge.

As with the amino acids, at a pH greater than the p*I*, a protein has a net negative charge. At a pH less than the p*I*, a protein has a net positive charge (Figure 2.18). The magnitude of the net charge of a protein increases as the difference between pH and p*I* increases. An example is human plasma albumin with 585 amino acid residues of which there are 61 glutamates, 36 aspartates, 57 lysines, 24 arginines, and 16 histidines. The titration curve for this complex molecule is shown in Figure 2.19. Albumin's p*I* = 5.9, at which pH its net charge is zero. At pH 7.5 the imidazolium groups of histidines have been partially titrated and albumin has a negative charge of −10. At pH 8.6 additional groups have been titrated to their base forms, and the net charge is approximately −20. At pH 11 the net charge is approximately −60. On the acid side of the p*I* value, at pH 3, the approximate net charge of albumin is +60.

Amino Acids and Proteins Can Be Separated Based on p*I* Values

The techniques of electrophoresis, isoelectric focusing, and ion-exchange chromatography separate and characterize biological molecules on the basis of differences in their p*I* (see p. 34). In clinical medicine, separation of plasma proteins by electrophoresis has led to the classification of the proteins based on their relative electrophoretic mobility. The separation is commonly carried out at pH 8.6, which is higher than the p*I* values of the major plasma proteins.

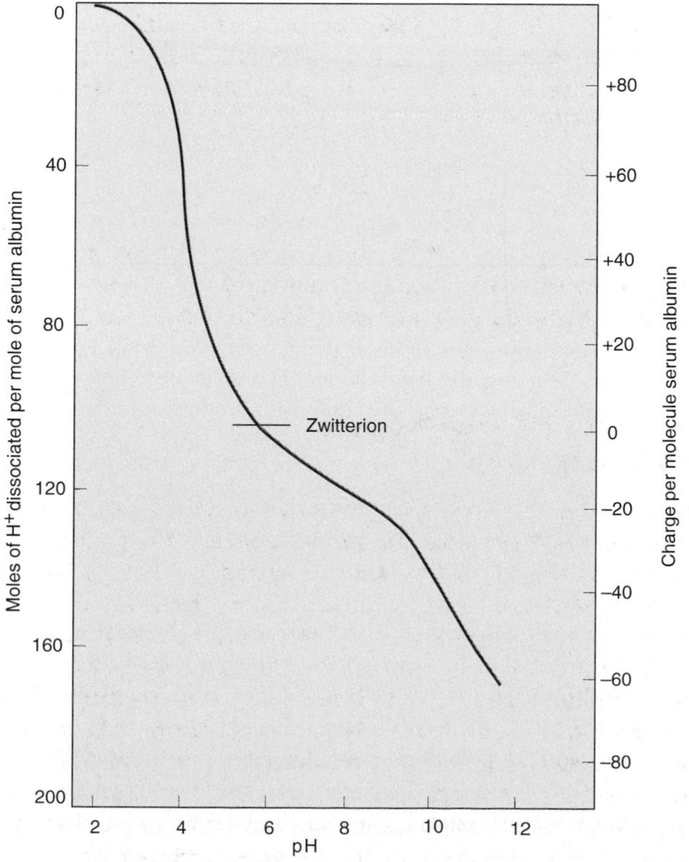

FIGURE 2.19
Titration curve of human serum albumin at 25°C and an ionic strength of 0.150.
Redrawn from Tanford, C. J. Am. Chem. Soc. *72:441, 1950.*

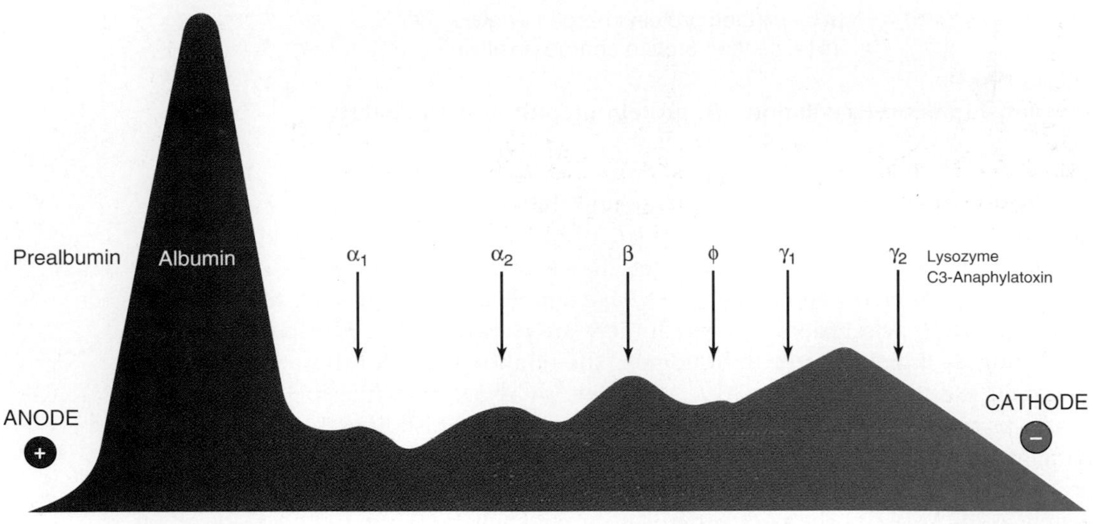

α_1

- α_1-Acid glycoprotein
- α_1-T Glycoprotein
- α_1-Antitrypsin
- Transcortin
- α_1-Antichymotrypsin
- α_1-B Glycoprotein
- 9,5 S-α_1-glycoprotein
- Vitamin D-binding protein
- α_1-Lipoproteins

α_1/α_2

- Thyroxine-binding globulin
- Zn-α_2-glycoprotein
- Gc globulin
- Ceruloplasmin
- Inter-α-trypsin inhibitor
- Antithrombin III
- Factor X (Stuart-Prower)
- Transcobalamin I
- C9

α_2

- Retinol-binding protein
- α_2 HS glycoprotein
- Histidine-rich 3,8 S-α_2-glycoprotein
- Haptoglobin
- Pregnancy zone protein
- α_2-Macroglobulin
- Prothrombin
- Antihemophilic factor
- C1 inactivator
- C1s

α_2/β_1

- Serum cholinesterase
- 8 S-α_3-glycoprotein
- 4 S-α_2, β_1-glycoprotein
- Transcobalamin III

β_1

- Hemopexin
- Steroid-binding β-globulin
- Transferrin
- Pregnancy-specific β_1-glycoprotein
- Cold insoluble globulin
- Factor V (Accelerin)
- Factor VII (Proconvertin)
- Factor IX (Christmas)
- Plasminogen
- C3 Proactivator
- Transcobalamin II
- β-Lipoproteins
- C1r, C2
- C4, C5

β_2

- β_2-Microglobulin
- β_2-Glycoprotein III
- β_2-Glycoprotein I
- Fibrinogen
- Factor XI (PTA)
- Factor XII (Hageman)
- Factor XIII (FSF)
- C3, C6, C7
- C3 Activator (β_2II)

γ_1

- IgG
- IgA
- IgD
- IgE
- IgM
- Amylase

γ_2

- IgG
- Clq
- Properdin

FIGURE 2.20
Electrophoresis pattern for plasma proteins at pH 8.6.
Plot shows the order of migration along the horizontal axis with proteins of highest mobility closest to the anode. Height of the band along the vertical axis shows the protein concentration. Different major proteins are designated underneath their electrophoretic mobility peaks.
Reprinted with permission from Heide, K., Haupt, H., and Schwick, H. G. In: F. W. Putnam (Ed.), The Plasma Proteins, *2nd ed., Vol. III. New York: Academic Press, 1977, p. 545.*

Accordingly, the proteins are negatively charged and move toward the anode at a rate dependent on their net charge. Major peaks observed in order of their migration are those of albumin, α_1-, α_2-, and β-globulins, fibrinogen, and the γ_1- and γ_2-globulins (Figure 2.20). Some of these peaks represent tens to hundreds of different plasma proteins that have a similar migration rate at pH 8.6. However, certain proteins predominate in each peak and variation in their relative amounts is characteristic of certain diseases (Figures 2.20 and 2.21; see Clin. Corr. 2.1).

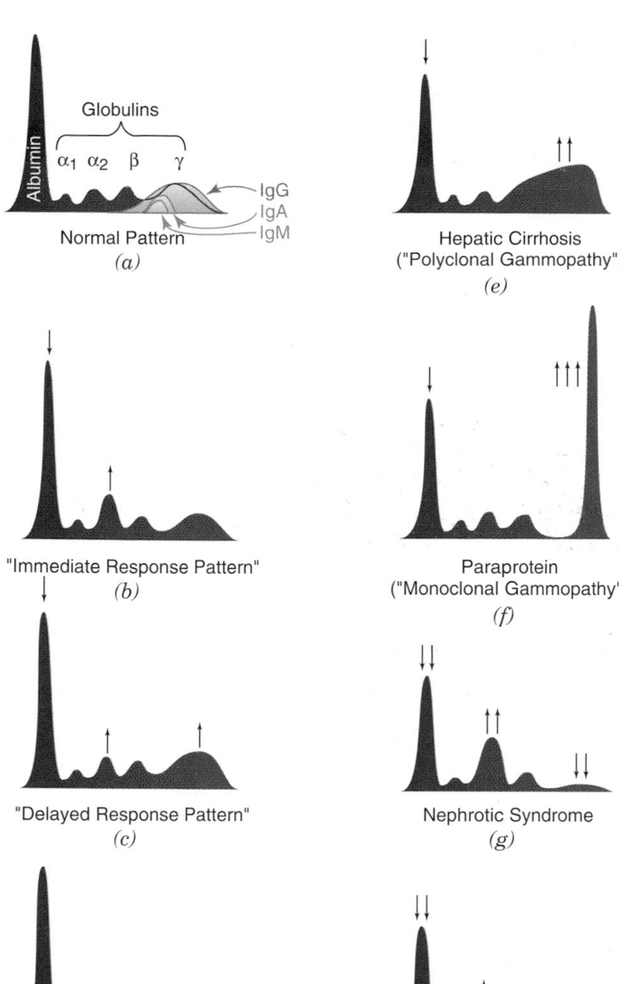

FIGURE 2.21
Examples of the electrophoretic mobility patterns observed for a normal individual and patients with abnormal concentrations of serum proteins, analyzed by agarose gel electrophoresis.
Redrawn from McPherson, R. A. Specific proteins. In: J. B. Henry (Ed.), Clinical Diagnosis and Management, *17th ed. Philadelphia: Saunders Co, 1984.*

CLINICAL CORRELATION 2.1

Plasma Proteins in Diagnosis of Disease

Electrophoretic analysis of the plasma proteins is commonly used in diagnosis of disease. Electrophoresis of plasma buffered at pH 8.6 separates the major plasma proteins as they migrate to the anode in the electric field into bands or peaks, based on their charge differences (see text). Examples of abnormal electrophoresis patterns are shown in Figure 2.21. An "immediate response" that occurs with stress or inflammation caused by infection, injury, or surgical trauma is shown in pattern (*b*) in which haptoglobins in the α_2 mobility band are selectively increased. A "late response" shown in pattern (*c*) is correlated with infection and shows an increase in the τ-globulin peaks due to an increase in immunoglobulins. An example of a hypogammaglobulinemia due to an immunosuppressive disease is shown in pattern (*d*). In hepatic cirrhosis there is a broad elevation of the τ-globulins with reduction of albumin, as in pattern (*e*). Monoclonal gammopathies are due to the clonal synthesis of a unique immunoglobulin and give rise to a sharp τ-globulin band, as in pattern (*f*). Nephrotic syndrome shows a selective loss of lower molecular weight proteins from plasma, as in pattern (*g*). The pattern shows a decrease in albumin (65 kDa), but a retention of the bands composed of the higher molecular weight proteins α_2-macroglobulin (725 kDa) and β-lipoproteins (2000 kDa) in the α_2 band. Pattern (*h*) is from a patient with a protein-losing enteropathy. The slight increase in the α_2-band in pattern (*h*) is due to an immediate or late response from a stressful stimulus, as previously observed in patterns (*b*) and (*c*).

Ritzmann, S. E., and Daniels, J. C. Serum protein electrophoresis and total serum proteins. In: S. E. Ritzmann and J. C. Daniels (Eds.), *Serum Protein Abnormalities, Diagnostic and Clinical Aspects.* Boston: Little, Brown and Co., 1975, pp. 3–25; and McPherson, R. A. Specific proteins. In: J. B. Henry (Ed.), *Clinical Diagnosis and Management by Laboratory Methods,* 17th ed. Philadelphia: Saunders, 1984, pp. 204–215.

Amino Acid Side Chains Have Polar or Apolar Properties

The relative **hydrophobicity** of amino acid side chains is critical for the folding of a protein to its native structure and for the stability of the folded protein. Figure 2.22 plots the values of relative hydrophobicity of the common amino acids based on the tendency of each amino acid to partition itself in a mixture of water and a nonpolar solvent. The scale is based on a value of zero for glycine. The side chains that preferentially dissolve in the nonpolar solvent relative to glycine show a positive (+) hydrophobicity value, the more positive the greater the preference for the nonpolar solvent. Most hydrophobic are those amino acids found buried in folded protein structures away from the water solvent that interacts with the surface of a soluble protein. However, the general correlation is not perfect due to the amphoteric nature of many of the hydrophobic amino acids that place the more polar portions of their side chain structure near the surface to interact with the polar solvent water on the outside. In addition, contrary to expectation, not all hydrophobic side chains are in a buried position in a folded three-dimensional structure of a globular protein. When on the surface, the hydrophobic groups are generally dispersed among the polar side chains. When clustering of nonpolar side chains occurs on the surface, it is usually associated with a function of the protein, such as to provide a site for binding of substrate molecules through hydrophobic interactions.

Most charged side chains are found on the surface of soluble globular proteins where they are stabilized by favorable energetic interactions with the water solvent. The rare positioning of a charged side chain in the interior of a globular protein usually implies an important functional role for that "buried" charge within the nonpolar interior in stabilizing conformation of the folded protein or participation in a catalytic mechanism.

Amino Acids Undergo a Variety of Chemical Reactions

Amino acids in proteins undergo a variety of chemical reactions with reagents that may be used to investigate the function of specific side chains. Some common chemical reactions are presented in Table 2.7. Reagents for amino acid side chain modification have also been synthesized that bind to specific sites in a folded protein's structure, like the substrate-binding site. The strategy

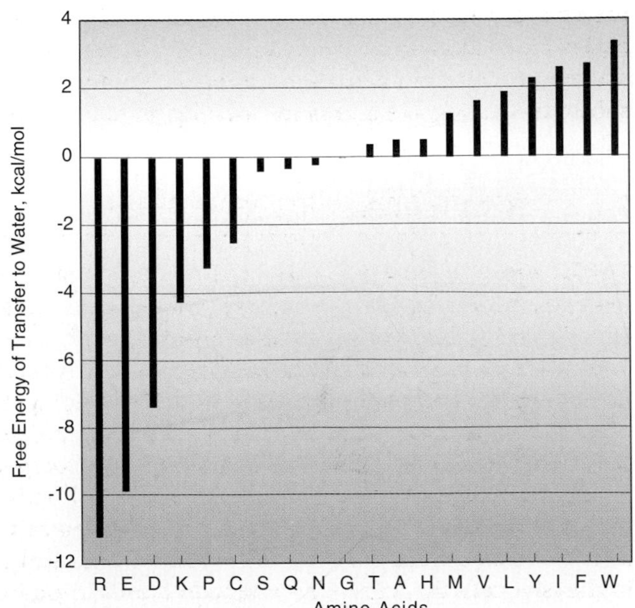

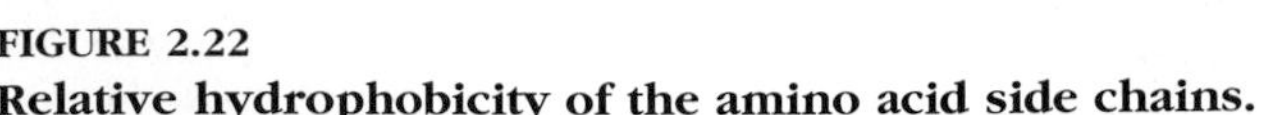

FIGURE 2.22
Relative hydrophobicity of the amino acid side chains.
Based on the partition of the amino acid between organic solvent and water. Negative values indicate preference for water and positive values preference for nonpolar solvent (ethanol or dioxane) relative to glycine (see text).
Based on data from Von Heijne, G., and Blomberg, C. Eur. J. Biochem. *97:175, 1979; and from Nozaki, Y., and Tanford, C.* J. Biol. Chem. *246:2211, 1971.*

TABLE 2.7 Some Chemical Reactions of the Amino Acids

Reactive Group	*Reagent or Reaction*	*Product*
Amine ($-NH_2$) groups	Ninhydrin	Blue colored product that absorbs at 540 nm[a]
	Fluorescamine	Product that fluoresces
Carboxylic acid groups	Alcohols	Ester products
	Amines	Amide products
	Carbodiimide	Activates for reaction with nucleophiles
$-NH_2$ of Lys	2,3,6-Trinitrobenzene sulfonate	Product that absorbs at 367 nm
	Anhydrides	Acetylates amines
	Aldehydes	Forms Shiff base adducts
Guanidino group of Arg	Sakaguchi reaction	Pink-red product that can be used to assay Arg
Phenol of Tyr	I_2	Iodination of positions ortho to hydroxyl group on aromatic ring
	Acetic anhydride	Acetylation of $-OH$
S atom of Met side chain	CH_3I	Methyl sulfonium product
	$[O^-]$ or H_2O_2	Methionine sulfoxide or methionine sulfone
$-SH$ of Cys	Iodoacetate	Carboxymethyl thiol ether product
	N-Ethylmaleimide	Addition product with S
	Organic mercurials	Mercurial adducts
	Performic acid	Cysteic acid ($-SO_3H$) product
	Dithionitrobenzoic acid	Yellow product that can be used to quantitate $-SH$ groups
Imidazole of His and phenol of Tyr	Pauly's reagent	Yellow to reddish product

[a] Proline imino group reacts with ninhydrin to form product that absorbs light at 440 nm (yellow color).

is to model the structural features of the enzyme's natural substrate into the modifying reagent. The reagent binds to the active site like a natural substrate and, while within the active site, reacts with a specific side chain in the enzyme active site. This identifies the modified amino acid as being located in the substrate-binding site and helps identify its role in the catalytic mechanism.

2.4 ■ PRIMARY STRUCTURE OF PROTEINS

The **primary structure** (amino acid sequence) of a protein is required for an understanding of a protein's structure, its mechanism of action at a molecular level, and its relationship to other proteins with similar physiological roles. The primary structure of **insulin** illustrates the value of this knowledge for understanding a protein's biosynthesis and physiological forms. Insulin is produced in pancreatic islet cells as a single chain precursor, **proinsulin,** with the primary structure shown in Figure 2.23. The polypeptide chain contains 86 amino acids and 3 intrachain cystine disulfide bonds. It is transformed into biologically active insulin by proteolytic modifications in its primary structure as it is secreted from the islet cells. Proinsulin is cleaved by proteases present in the islet cells that cleave two peptide bonds in proinsulin between residues 30 and 31 and 65 and 66. This releases a 35 amino acid segment (the **C-peptide**)

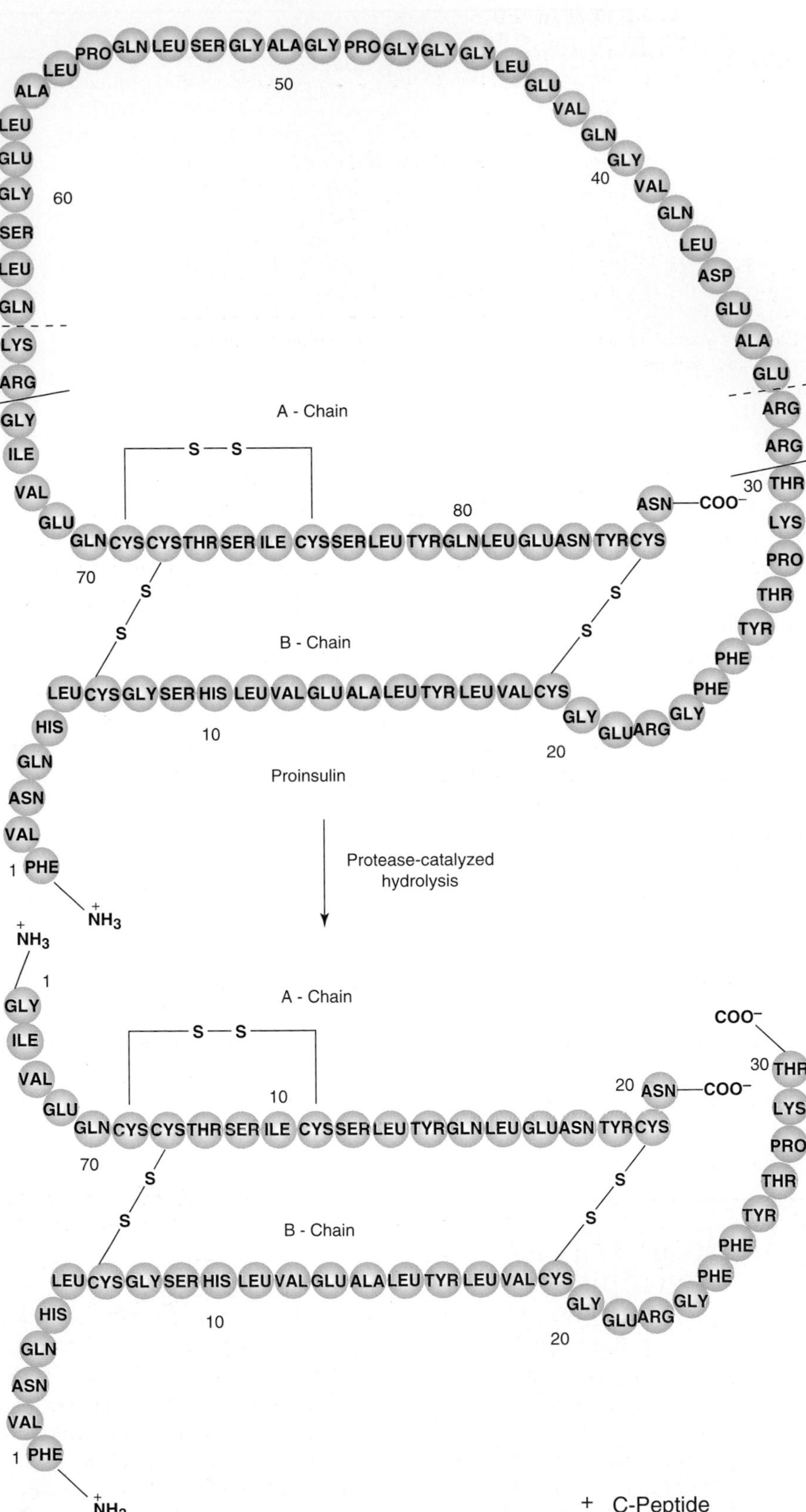

FIGURE 2.23
Primary structures of human proinsulin, insulin, and C-peptide.
In proinsulin, the B-chain peptide extends from Phe at position 1 to Thr at position 30, the C-peptide from Arg at position 31 to Arg at position 65, and the A-chain peptide from Gly at position 66 to Asn at position 86. Cystine bonds from positions 7 to 72, 19 to 85, and 71 to 76 are found in proinsulin.
Redrawn from Bell, G. I., Swain, W. F., Pictet, R., Cordell, B., Goodman, H. M., and Rutter, W. J. Nature *282:525, 1979.*

and the active insulin molecule. The active insulin consists of two polypeptide chains (A and B) of 21 amino acids and 30 amino acids, respectively, covalently joined by the same disulfide bonds present in proinsulin (Figure 2.23). The C-

TABLE 2.8 Variation in Positions A8, A9, A10, and B30 of Insulin

Species	*A8*	*A9*	*A10*	*B30*
Human	Thr	Ser	Ile	Thr
Cow	Ala	Ser	Val	Ala
Pig	Thr	Ser	Ile	Ala
Sheep	Ala	Gly	Val	Ala
Horse	Thr	Gly	Ile	Ala
Dog	Thr	Ser	Ile	Ala
Chicken[a]	His	Asn	Thr	Ala
Duck[a]	Glu	Asn	Pro	Thr

[a] Positions 1 and 2 of B chain are both Ala in chicken and duck; whereas in the other species in the table, position 1 is Phe and position 2 is Val in B chain.

peptide is further processed in the pancreatic islet cells by proteases that hydrolyze a dipeptide from the COOH terminal and a second dipeptide from the NH_2 terminal of the C-peptide. The modified C-peptide is secreted into the blood with the active insulin. Besides giving information on the pathway for formation of active insulin, knowledge of primary structures shows the role of particular amino acids in the structure of insulin through comparison of the primary structures of the insulins from different animal species. The aligned primary structures show a residue identity in most amino acid positions, except for residues 8, 9, and 10 of the A chain and residue 30 of the B chain. Amino acids in these positions vary widely in different animal insulins (Table 2.8) and apparently do not affect the biological properties of the insulin molecule (see Clin. Corr. 2.2). Other amino acids of the primary structure are rarely substituted, suggesting that they have an essential role in insulin function.

Comparison of primary structures is commonly used to predict the similarity in structure and function between proteins. Sequence comparisons typically require aligning sequences to maximize the number of identical residues while minimizing the number of insertions or deletions required to achieve this alignment. Two sequences are termed **homologous** when their sequences are highly alignable. In its correct usage homology only refers to proteins that have evolved from the same gene. **Analogy** is used to describe sequences from proteins that are structurally similar but for which no evolutionary relationship has been demonstrated. Substitution of an amino acid by another amino acid of similar

CLINICAL CORRELATION 2.2

Differences in Primary Structure of Insulins Used in Treatment of Diabetes Mellitus

Both pig (porcine) and cow (bovine) insulins are commonly used in the treatment of human diabetics. Because of the differences in amino acid sequence from the human insulin, some diabetic individuals will have an initial allergic response to the injected insulin as their immunological system recognizes the insulin as foreign, or develop an insulin resistance due to a high anti-insulin antibody titer at a later stage in treatment. However, the number of diabetics who have a deleterious immunological response to pig and cow insulins is small; the great majority of human diabetics can utilize the nonhuman insulins without immunological complication. The compatibility of cow and pig insulins in humans is due to the small number and the conservative nature of the changes between the amino acid sequences of the insulins. These changes do not significantly perturb the three-dimensional structure of the insulins from that of human insulin. Pig insulin is usually more acceptable than cow insulin in insulin-reactive individuals because it is more similar in sequence to human insulin (see Table 2.8). Human insulin is now available for clinical use. It can be made using genetically engineered bacteria or by modifying pig insulin.

Brogdon, R. N., and Heel, R. C. Human insulin: a review of its biological activity, pharmacokinetics, and therapeutic use. *Drugs* 34:350, 1987.

CLINICAL CORRELATION 2.3

A Nonconservative Mutation Occurs in Sickle Cell Anemia

Hemoglobin S (HbS) is a variant form of the normal adult hemoglobin in which a nonconservative substitution occurs in the sixth position of the β-polypeptide chain of the normal hemoglobin (HbA_1). Whereas in HbA_1 this position is taken by a glutamic acid residue, in HbS the position is occupied by a valine. Consequently, in HbS a polar side chain group on the molecule's outside surface has been replaced with a nonpolar hydrophobic side chain (a nonconservative mutation). Through hydrophobic interactions with this nonpolar valine, HbS in its deoxy conformation polymerizes with other molecules of deoxy-HbS, leading to a precipitation of the hemoglobin within the red blood cell. This precipitation makes the red blood cell assume a sickle shape that results in a high rate of hemolysis and a lack of elasticity during circulation through the small capillaries, which become clogged by the abnormal shaped cells.

Only individuals homozygous for HbS exhibit the disease. Individuals heterozygous for HbS have approximately 50% HbA_1 and 50% HbS in their red blood cells and do not exhibit symptoms of the sickle cell anemia disease except under extreme conditions of hypoxia.

Individuals heterozygous for HbS have a resistance to the malaria parasite, which spends a part of its life cycle in red blood cells. This is a factor selecting for the HbS gene in malarial regions of the world and is the reason for the high frequency of this lethal gene in the human genetic pool. Approximately 10% of American blacks are heterozygous for HbS, and 0.4% of American blacks are homozygous for HbS and exhibit sickle cell anemia.

HbS is detected by gel electrophoresis. Because it lacks a glutamate, it is less acidic than HbA. HbS therefore does not migrate as rapidly toward the anode as does HbA. It is also possible to diagnose sickle cell anemia by recombinant DNA techniques.

Embury, S. H. The clinical pathophysiology of sickle-cell disease. *Annu. Rev. Med.* 37:361, 1986.

polarity (i.e., Val for Ile in position 10 of insulin) is called a **conservative** substitution and is commonly observed in amino acid sequences of the same protein from different animal species. If a particular amino acid is always found at the same position in these comparisons, then these are designated **invariant residues** and it can be assumed that these residues have an essential role in the structure or function of the protein. In contrast, a **nonconservative** substitution involves replacement of an amino acid by another of dramatically different polarity. This may produce severe changes in the properties of the resultant protein or occur in regions that are apparently unimportant functionally (see Clin. Corr. 2.3). Polarity is only one physical property of amino acids that determines whether a substitution will significantly alter the protein's function. Other physical properties of importance are the volume and surface area.

2.5 ■ HIGHER LEVELS OF PROTEIN ORGANIZATION

Primary structure of a protein refers to the covalent structure of a protein. It includes amino acid sequence and location of disulfide (cystine) bonds. Higher levels of protein organization refer to noncovalently generated conformational properties of the primary structure. These higher levels of protein conformation and organization are defined as the secondary, tertiary, and quaternary structures of a protein. **Secondary structure** refers to the local three-dimensional folding of the polypeptide chain in the protein. The polypeptide chain in this context is the covalently interconnected atoms of the peptide bonds and α-carbon linkages that sequentially link the amino acid residues of the protein. Side chains are not considered at the level of secondary structure. **Tertiary structure** refers to the three-dimensional structure of the polypeptide. It includes the conformational relationships in space of the side chains and the geometric relationship between distant regions of the polypeptide chain. **Quaternary structure** refers to the structure and interactions of the noncovalent association of discrete polypeptide subunits into a multisubunit protein. Not all proteins have a quaternary structure.

Proteins generally assume unique secondary, tertiary, and quaternary conformations as determined by their particular amino acid sequence and termed the **native conformation.** Folding of the primary structure into the native conformation occurs, in most cases, spontaneously through noncovalent interactions. This unique conformation is the one of lowest total Gibbs free energy kinetically accessible to the polypeptide chain(s) for the particular conditions of ionic strength, pH, and temperature of the solvent in which the folding occurs. Chaperone proteins may facilitate the rate of protein folding.

Proteins Have a Secondary Structure

The conformation of a polypeptide chain may be described by the rotational angles of the covalent bonds that contribute to the polypeptide chain. These are the bonds contributed by each of the amino acids between (1) the nitrogen and α-carbon and (2) the α-carbon and the carbonyl carbon. The first of these is designated the **phi (ϕ) bond** and the second is called the **psi (ψ) bond** for an amino acid residue in a polypeptide chain (Figure 2.24). The third bond contributed by each amino acid to the polypeptide chain is the peptide bond. As previously discussed, due to the partial double-bond character of the C′⋯N bonds, there is a barrier to free rotation about this peptide bond.

Regular secondary structure conformations in segments of a polypeptide chain occur when all ϕ bond angles in that polypeptide segment are equal, and all the ψ bond angles are equal. The rotational angles for ϕ and ψ bonds for common regular secondary structures are given in Table 2.9.

The α-helix and β-structure conformations for polypeptide chains are the most thermodynamically stable of the regular secondary structures. However, a particular sequence may form regular conformations other than α-helical or β-structure. There are also regions of unordered secondary structure, in which neither the ϕ bond angles nor the ψ bond angles are equal. Proline interrupts α-helical conformations since the pyrrolidine side chain of proline sterically interacts with the amino acid preceding it in the polypeptide sequence when in an α-helical structure. This repulsive steric interaction tends to prevent formation of α-helical structure in sections of a polypeptide chain that contain proline.

Helical structures of polypeptide chains are characterized by the number of amino acid residues per turn of helix (n) and the distance between α-carbon atoms of adjacent amino acids measured parallel to the axis of the helix (d). The **helix pitch** (p), defined as the product of $n \times d$, then measures the distance between repeating turns of the helix on a line drawn parallel to the helix axis (Figure 2.25):

$$p = n \times d$$

α-Helical Structure

An amino acid sequence in an α-helical conformation is shown in Figure 2.26. Characteristic of the α-helical conformation are 3.6 amino acid residues per

TABLE 2.9 Helix Parameters of Regular Secondary Structures

Structure	*Approximate Bond Angles (°)* ϕ	ψ	*Residues per turn, n*	*Helix Pitch,[a] p (Å)*
Right-handed α-helix [3.6_{13}-helix)	−57	−47	3.6	5.4
3_{10}-helix	+49	−26	3.0	6.0
Parallel β-strand	−119	+113	2.0	6.4
Antiparallel β-strand	−139	+135	2.0	6.8
Polyproline type II[b]	−78	+149	3.0	9.4

[a] Distance between repairing turns on a line drawn parallel to helix axis.
[b] Helix type found for polypeptide chains of collagen.

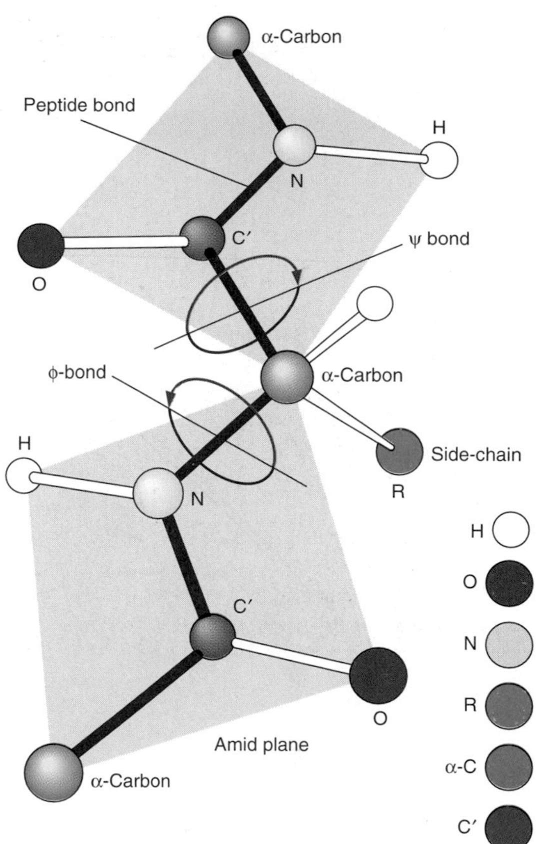

FIGURE 2.24
Polypeptide chain showing ϕ, ψ, and peptide bonds for residue R_i within a polypeptide chain.
Redrawn with permission from Dickerson, R. E., and Geis, I. The Structure and Action of Proteins. *Menlo Park, CA: Benjamin, 1969, p. 25.*

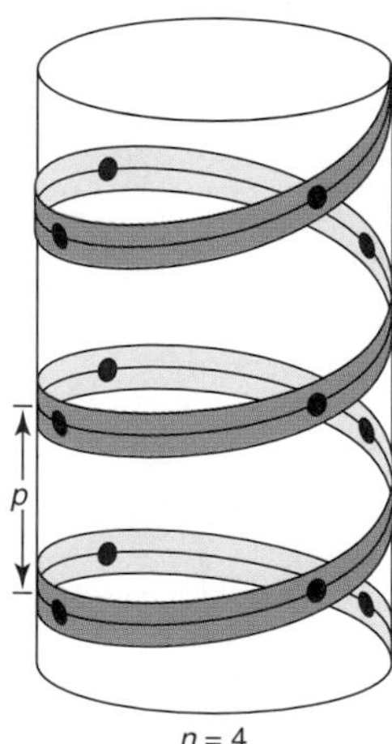

FIGURE 2.25
The helix pitch (p) for a helix with $n = 4$.
Each circle on a line represents an α-carbon from an amino acid residue. The rise per residue would be p/n (see equation in text).
From Dickerson, R. E,. and Geis, I. The Structure and Action of Proteins. *Menlo Park, CA: Benjamin, 1969, p. 26.*

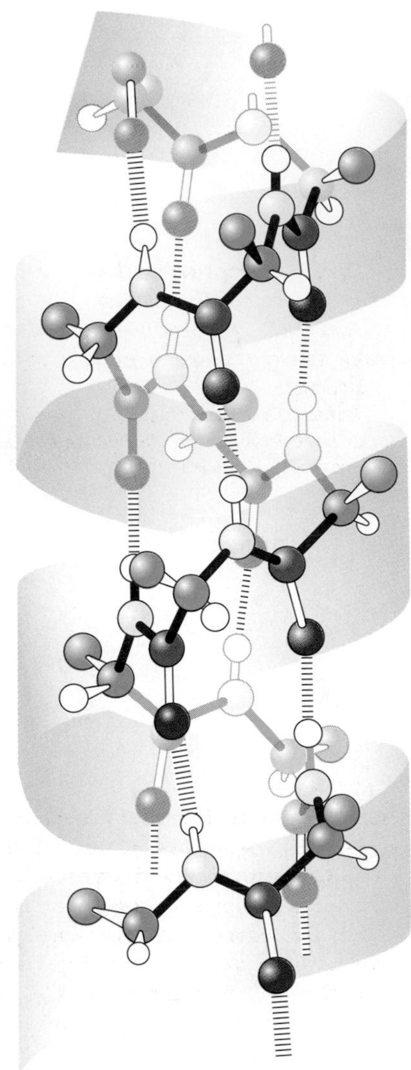

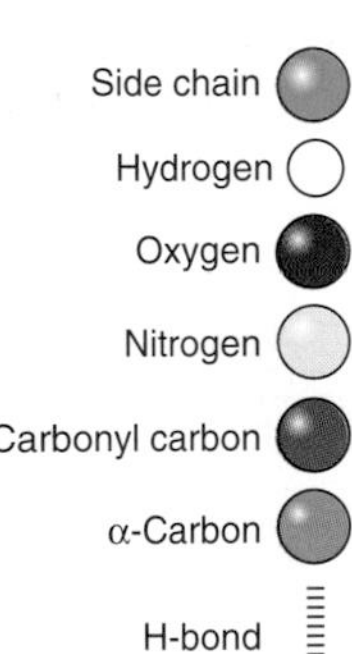

FIGURE 2.26
An α-helix.
Redrawn with permission, based on figure from Pauling, L. The Nature of the Chemical Bond, *3rd ed. Ithaca, NY: Cornell University Press, 1960.*

360° turn ($n = 3.6$). The peptide bond planes in the α-helix are parallel to the axis of the helix. In this geometry each peptide forms two hydrogen bonds, one to the peptide bond of the fourth amino acid above and the second to the peptide bond of the fourth amino acid below in the primary structure. Other α-helix parameters, such as the pitch (p), are given in Table 2.9. In the hydrogen bonds between the peptide groups of an α-helical structure, the distance between the hydrogen-donor atom and the hydrogen-acceptor atom is 2.9 Å. Also, the donor, acceptor , and hydrogen atoms are approximately collinear, in that they determine a straight line. This is an optimum geometry and distance for maximum hydrogen-bond strength (see Section 2.7).

The side chains in an α-helical conformation are on the outside of the spiral structure generated by the polypeptide chain. Due to the characteristic 3.6 residues per turn, the first and every third and fourth R group of the amino acid sequence in the helix come close to the other. Helices often present separable polar and nonpolar faces based on their amino acid sequences, which place polar or nonpolar side chains three or four amino acids apart in the sequence, which folds into the α-helix. This will give rise to unique functional characteristics of the helix. However, if every third or fourth side chain that come close together have the same charge sign or are branched at their β-carbon (valine and isoleucine), their unfavorable ionic or steric interactions destabilize the helix structure. The α-helix may theoretically form its spiral in either a left-handed or right-handed sense, giving the helix asymmetric properties and correlated optical activity. In the structure shown, a right-handed α-helix is depicted; this is more stable than the left-handed helix.

β-Structure

A polypeptide chain in a β-strand conformation (Figure 2.27) is hydrogen bonded to another similar strand aligned either in a parallel or antiparallel direction (Figure 2.28). Hydrogen-bonded β-strands appear like a pleated sheet (Figure 2.29). The side chains project above and below the pleated sheet-like structure.

Supersecondary Structures

Certain combinations of secondary structure can be observed in different folded protein structures. They are referred to as **structural motifs** and include helix-turn-helix (see p. 108), leucine zipper (see p. 110), calcium binding EF hand (see p. 209), and zinc finger (see p. 108). Even longer orderings may occur to form a domain (see below) such as the β-barrel and the immunoglobulin fold. These longer pattern lengths of secondary structure may include multiple structural motifs and when commonly observed in more than one protein are referred to as **supersecondary structures.**

Proteins Fold into a Three-Dimensional Structure Called the Tertiary Structure

The **tertiary structure** of a protein is the three-dimensional structure of a protein. It includes the geometric relationship between distant segments of primary structure and the relationship of the side chains with one another in three-dimensional space. As an example of a protein's tertiary structure, the structure for trypsin is shown in Figure 2.30. In Figure 2.30*a* the ribbon structure shows the conformation of polypeptide strands and the overall pattern of polypeptide chain folding (supersecondary structure). The tertiary structure is then further built upon in Figure 2.30*b* by showing the side chain groups and their interconnections with a stick model. Active site catalytic side chains are shown in yellow, which include the hydroxymethyl group of serine (residue 177 in the sequence), the imidazole of histidine (residue 40), and the carboxylate-containing side chain of aspartate (residue 85). Although these catalytic residues

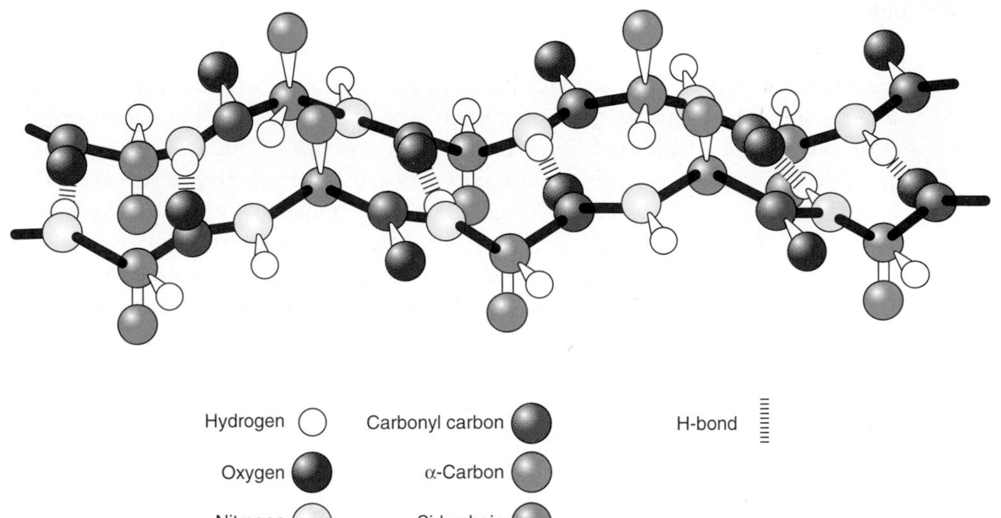

FIGURE 2.27
Two polypeptide chains in a β-structure conformation.
Additional polypeptide chains may be added to generate more extended structure.
Redrawn with permission from Fersht, A. Enzyme Structure and Mechanism, *San Francisco: Freeman, 1977, p. 10.*

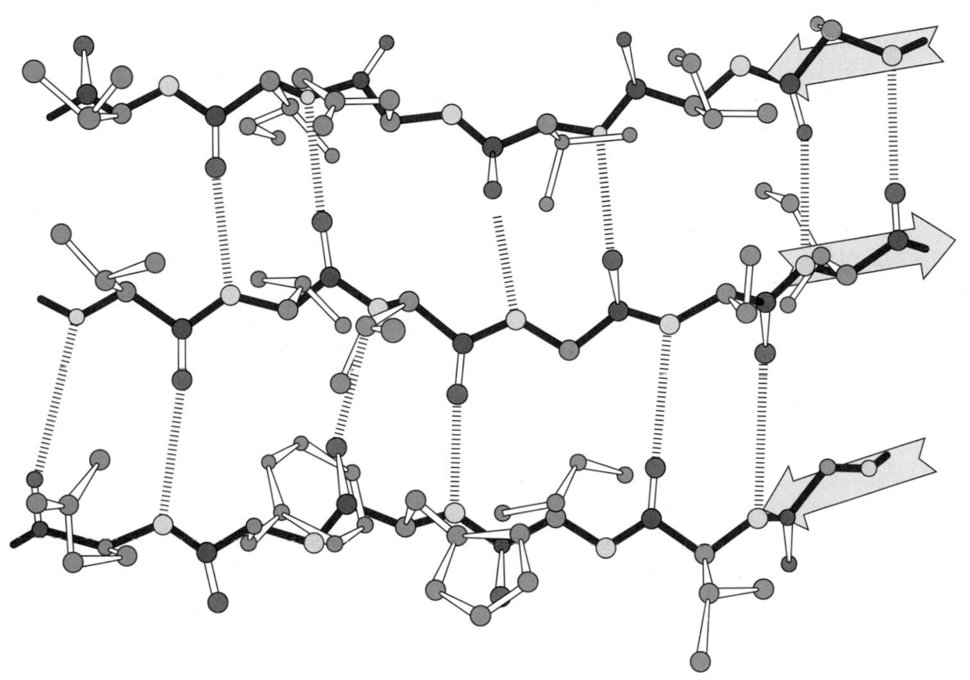

FIGURE 2.28
Example of antiparallel β-structure (residues 93–98, 28–33, and 16–21 of Cu,Zn superoxide dismutase).
Dashed line shows hydrogen bonds between carbonyl oxygen atoms and peptide nitrogen atoms; arrows show direction of polypeptide chains from N terminal to C terminal. In the characteristic antiparallel β-structure, pairs of closely spaced interchain hydrogen bonds alternate with widely spaced hydrogen bond pairs.
Redrawn with permission from Richardson, J. S. Adv. Protein Chem. *34:168, 1981.*

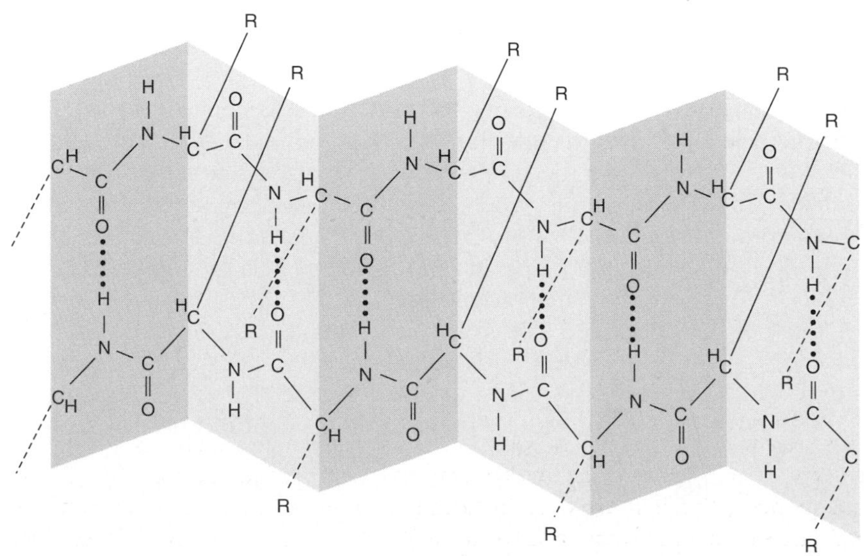

FIGURE 2.29
β-Pleated sheet structure between two polypeptide chains.
Additional polypeptide chains may be added above and below to generate a more extended structure.

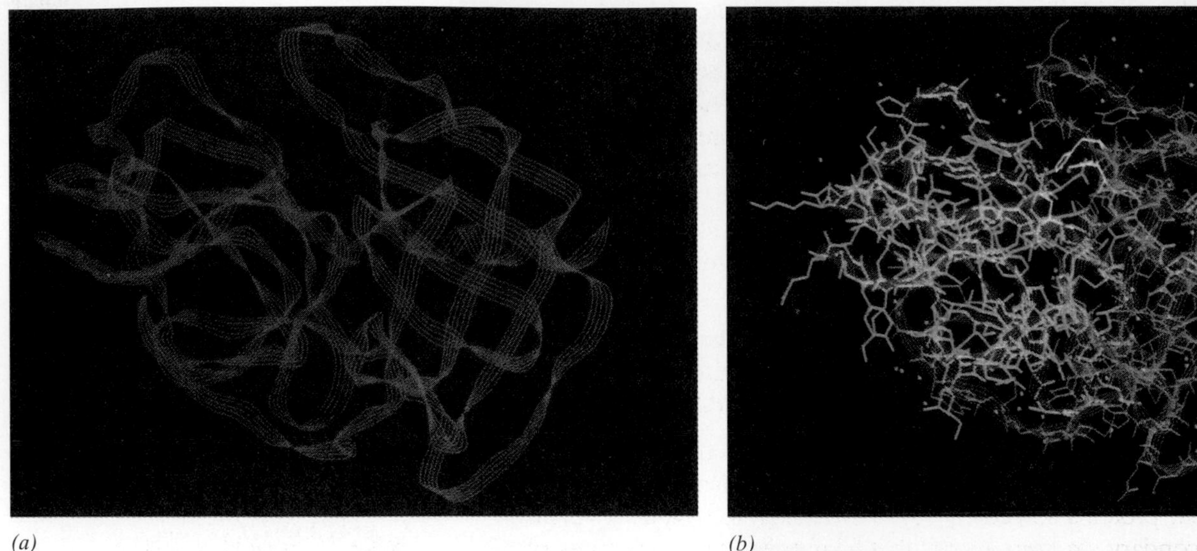

(a) (b)

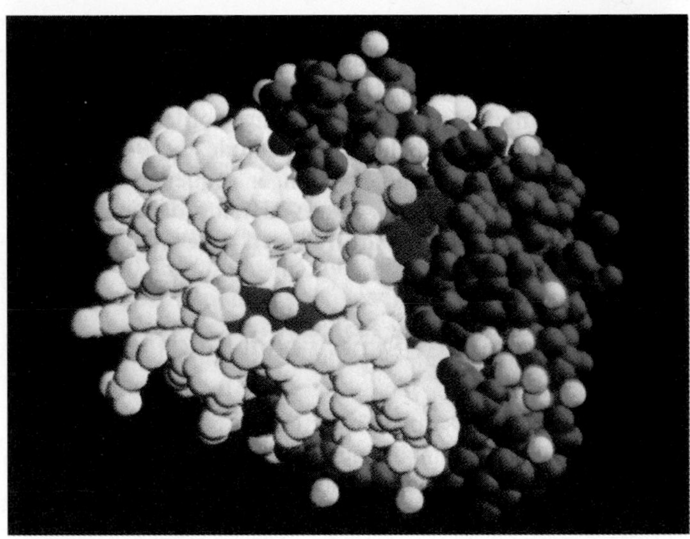

(c)

FIGURE 2.30
Tertiary structure of trypsin.
(*a*) Ribbon structure outlines the conformation of the polypeptide chain. (*b*) Structure shows side chains including active site residues (in yellow) with outline of polypeptide chain (ribbon) superimposed. (*c*) Space-filling structure in which each atom is depicted as the size of its van der Waals radius. Hydrogen atoms are not shown. Different domains are shown in dark blue and white. The active site residues are in yellow and intrachain disulfide bonds of cystine in red. Light blue spheres represent water molecules associated with the protein. This structure shows the density of packing within the interior of the protein.

are widely separated in the primary structure, the folded tertiary structure brings them together in space to form the catalytic site. In Figure 2.30*c* a space-filling model shows C, N, and O atoms represented by balls of radius proportional to their van der Waals radius.

The tertiary structure of trypsin conforms to the general rules of folded proteins (see Section 2.2). Hydrophobic side chains are generally in the interior of the structure, away from the water interface. Ionized side chains occur on the outside of a protein structure, where they are stabilized by water of solvation. Within the protein structure (not shown) are buried water molecules, noncovalently associated, which exhibit specific arrangements. A large number of water molecules form a solvation shell around the outside of the protein.

A long polypeptide strand often folds into multiple compact semi-independent folded regions or **domains,** each domain having a characteristic compact geometry with a hydrophobic core and polar outside. They typically contain 100–150 contiguous amino acids. The domains of a **multidomain protein** may be connected by a segment of the polypeptide chain lacking regular secondary structure. Alternatively, the dense spherical folded regions are separated by a cleft or less dense region of tertiary structure (Figure 2.31). There are two folded domains in the trypsin molecule with a cleft between the domains that includes the substrate-binding catalytic site of the protein. An active site within an interdomain interface is an attribute of many enzymes. Different domains within a protein can move with respect to each other. Hexokinase (Figure 2.32), which catalyzes phosphorylation of a glucose molecule by adenosine triphosphate (ATP), has the glucose-binding site in a region between two domains. When the glucose binds in the active site, the surrounding domains move to enclose the substrate to trap it for phosphorylation (Figure 2.32). In enzymes with more than one substrate or allosteric effector site (see Chapter 4), the different sites may be located within different domains. In multifunctional proteins, each domain performs a different task.

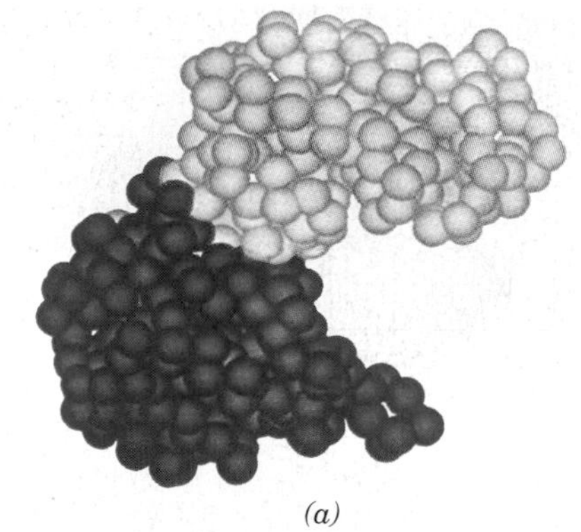

(a)

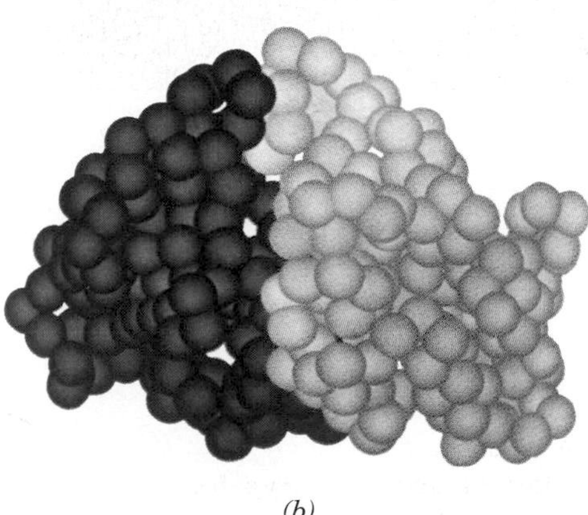

(b)

FIGURE 2.31
Globular domains within proteins.
(*a*) Phosphoglycerate kinase has two domains with a relatively narrow neck in between. (*b*) Elastase has two tightly associated domains separated by a narrow cleft. Each sphere in the space-filling drawing represents the α-carbon position for an amino acid within the protein structure.
Reprinted with permission from Richardson, J. S. Adv. Protein Chem. *34:168, 1981.*

Homologous Three-Dimensional Domain Structures Are Often Formed from Common Arrangements of Secondary Structures

A protein can adopt a range of conformations for a particular amino acid sequence. Although each native structure is unique, a comparison of the tertiary structures of different proteins solved by X-ray crystallography shows similar arrangements of secondary structure motifs that form the tertiary structures of domains. Thus proteins unrelated by function, sequence, or evolution show similar patterns of arrangement of their secondary structures or supersecondary

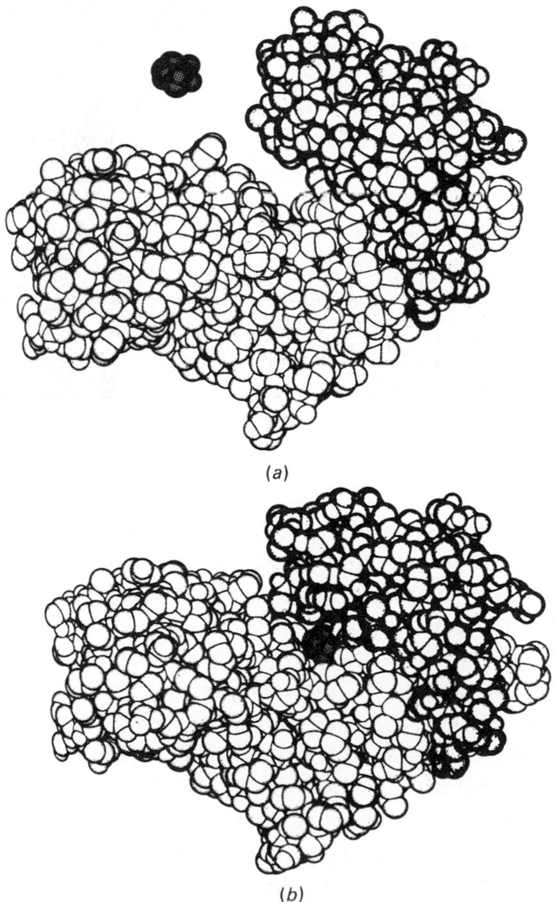

(a)

(b)

FIGURE 2.32
Drawings of (*a*) unliganded form of hexokinase and free glucose and (*b*) the conformation of hexokinase with glucose bound.
In this space-filling drawing each circle represents the van der Waals radius of an atom in the structure. Glucose is black, and each domain is differently shaded.
Reprinted with permission from Bennett, W. S., and Huber, R. CRC Rev. Biochem. *15:291, 1984. Copyright © CRC Press, Inc., Boca Raton, FL.*

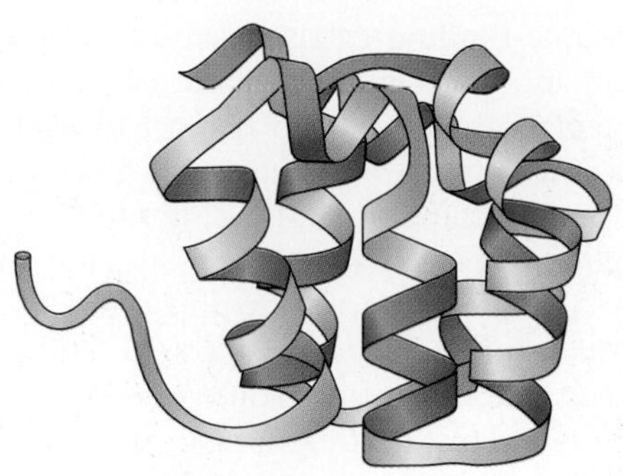

FIGURE 2.33
An example of an all α-folded domain.
In this drawing and those that follow (Figures 2.34–2.36), only the outline of the polypeptide chain is shown. β-Structure strands are shown by arrows with the direction of the arrow showing the N→C terminal direction of the chain; lightning bolts represent disulfide bonds, and circles represent metal ion cofactors (when present).
Redrawn with permission from Richardson, J. S. Adv. Protein Chem. *34:168, 1981.*

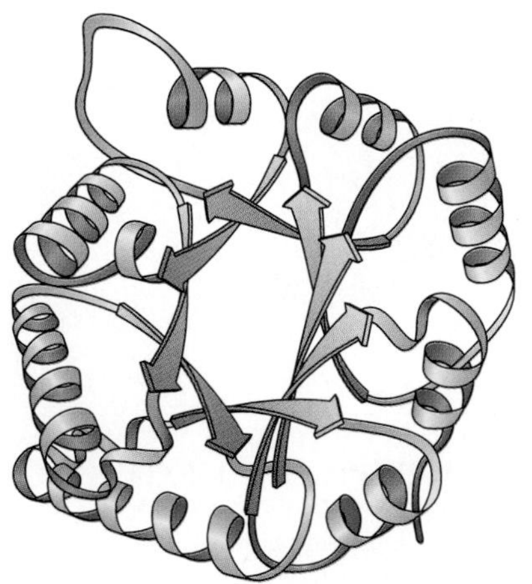

Triose Phosphate Isomerase

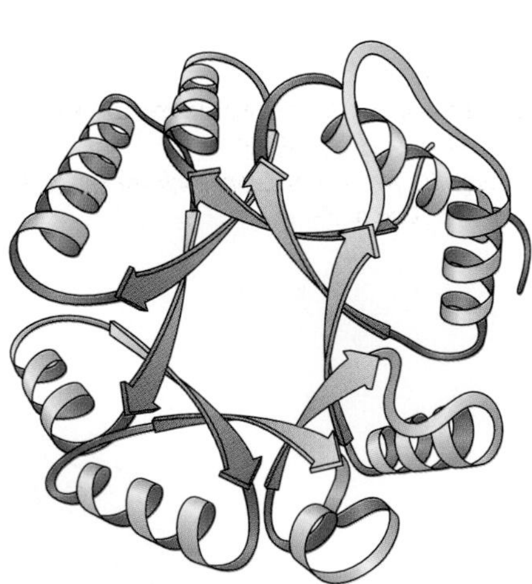

Pyruvate Kinase domain 1

FIGURE 2.34
Examples of α,β-folded domains in which β-structural strands form a β-barrel in the center of the domain (see legend to Figure 2.33).
Redrawn with permission from Richardson, J. S. Adv. Protein Chem. *34:168, 1981.*

structures. A classification system for supersecondary patterns places common folding patterns for secondary structures into structural families. The key supersecondary structures are formed because of the thermodynamic stability of their folding patterns.

A common all-α structure is found in the enzyme lysozyme (Figure 2.33). Other examples of all-α structure are in myoglobin and the subunits of hemoglobin, whose structures are discussed in Chapter 3. In this supersecondary folding pattern, seven or eight sections of α-helices are joined by smaller segments of polypeptide chains that allow the helices to fold back upon themselves to form a characteristic globular shape. Another common supersecondary structure is the **α,β-domain structure** shown by triose phosphate isomerase (Figure 2.34) in which the strands (designated by arrows) are wound into a **β-barrel.** Each β-strand in the interior of the β-barrel is interconnected by α-helical regions of the polypeptide chain on the outside of the molecule. A similar supersecondary structure is found in pyruvate kinase (Figure 2.34). A different type of α,β-domain supersecondary structure is seen in lactate dehydrogenase and phosphoglycerate kinase (Figure 2.35). In these the interior polypeptide sections participate in a **twisted-sheet** β-structure. The β-structure segments are joined by α-helix regions positioned on the outside of the molecule to give a characteristic α,β-domain folding pattern. An **all-β-domain** supersecondary structure is present in Cu,Zn superoxide dismutase, in which the antiparallel β-sheet forms a **Greek key β-barrel** (Figure 2.36). A similar pattern occurs in each of the domains of the immunoglobulins, discussed in Chapter 3. Concanavalin A (Figure 2.36) shows an all-β-domain structure in which the antiparallel β-strands form a β-barrel pattern called a "jellyroll." Protein structures used to define these classes have been observed by X-ray crystallographic analysis (Section 2.9), primarily of globular proteins that are water soluble. Proteins that are not water soluble may contain different supersecondary patterns (see Section 2.6).

A Quaternary Structure Occurs When Several Polypeptide Chains Form a Specific Noncovalent Association

Quaternary structure refers to the arrangement of polypeptide chains in a multichain protein. The subunits in a quaternary structure must be in noncovalent association. α-Chymotrypsin contains three polypeptide chains covalently joined together by interchain disulfide bonds into a single covalent unit and therefore does not have a quaternary structure. Myoglobin consists of a single polypeptide chain and has no quaternary structure. However, hemoglobin A

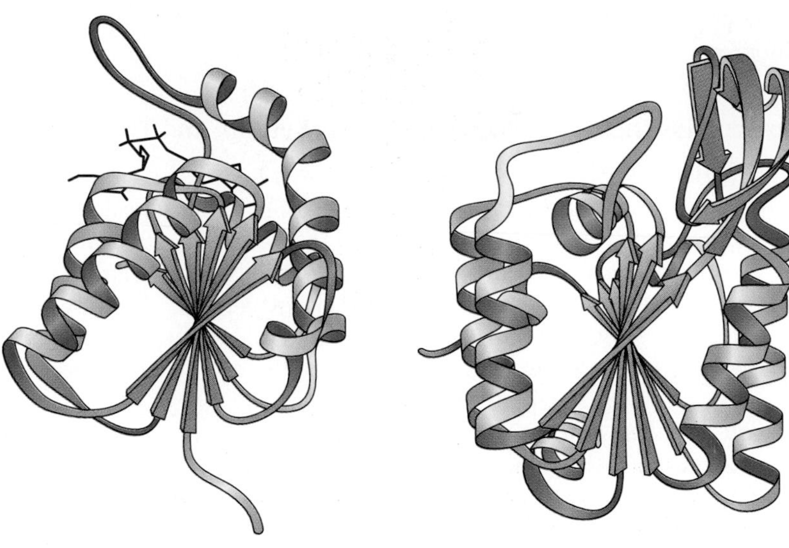

FIGURE 2.35
Examples of α,β-folded domains in which β-structure strands are in the form of a classical twisted β-sheet (see legend to Figure 2.33).
Redrawn with permission from Richardson, J. S. Adv. Protein Chem. *34:168, 1981.*

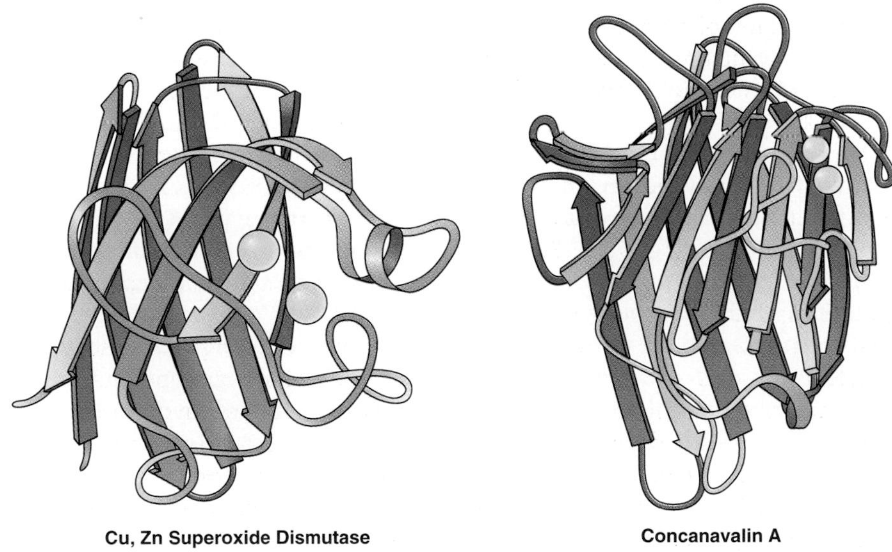

FIGURE 2.36
Examples of all β-folded domains (see legend to Figure 2.33).
Redrawn with permission from Richardson, J. S. Adv. Protein Chem. *34:168, 1981.*

contains four polypeptide chains ($\alpha_2\beta_2$) held together noncovalently in a specific conformation as required for its function (see Chapter 3). Thus hemoglobin has a quaternary structure. Aspartate transcarbamylase (see Chapter 13) has a quaternary structure comprised of 12 polypeptide subunits. The poliovirus protein coat contains 60 polypeptide subunits, and the tobacco mosaic virus protein has 2120 polypeptide subunits held together noncovalently in a specific structural arrangement.

2.6 ■ OTHER TYPES OF PROTEINS

The characteristics of protein structure, discussed above, are based on observations on globular, water-soluble proteins. Other proteins, such as the fibrous proteins, are nonglobular and have a low water solubility; lipoproteins and glycoproteins have a heterogeneous composition and may or may not be water soluble.

Fibrous Proteins Include Collagen, Elastin, α-Keratin, and Tropomyosin

Globular proteins have a spheroidal shape, variable molecular weights, relatively high water solubility, and a variety of functional roles as catalysts, transporters, and control proteins for the regulation of metabolic pathways and gene expression. In contrast, fibrous proteins characteristically contain larger amounts of regular secondary structure, a long cylindrical (rod-like) shape, a low solubility in water, and a structural rather than a dynamic role in the cell or organism. Examples of fibrous proteins are collagen, α-keratin, and tropomyosin.

Distribution of Collagen in Humans

Collagen is present in all tissues and organs where it provides the framework that gives the tissues their form and structural strength. Its importance is shown by its high concentration in all organs; the percentage of collagen by weight for some representative human tissues and organs is 4% of the liver, 10% of lung, 12–24% of the aorta, 50% of cartilage, 64% of the cornea, 23% of whole cortical bone, and 74% of skin (see Clin. Corr. 2.4).

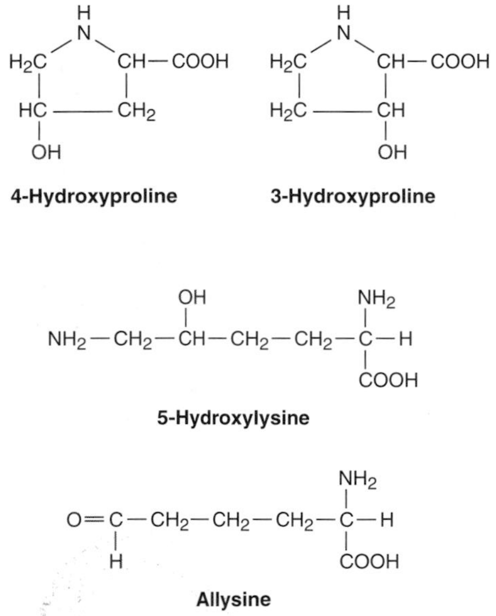

Amino Acid Composition of Collagen

The amino acid composition of collagen is quite different from that of a typical globular protein. The amino acid composition of type I skin collagen and of globular proteins ribonuclease and hemoglobin are given in Table 2.10. Skin collagen is comparatively rich in glycine (33% of its amino acids), proline (13%), the derived amino acid 4-hydroxyproline (9%), and another derived amino acid 5-hydroxylysine (0.6%) (Figure 2.37). Hydroxyproline is unique to collagens being formed enzymatically from prolines within a collagen polypeptide chain. The enzyme-catalyzed hydroxylation of proline requires the presence of ascorbic acid (vitamin C); thus in vitamin C deficiency (scurvy) there is poor synthesis of new collagen. Most hydroxyprolines in a collagen have the hydroxyl group in the 4-position (γ-carbon) of the proline structure, although a small amount of 3-hydroxyproline is also formed (Table 2.10). Collagens are glycoproteins with carbohydrate covalently joined to the derived amino acid, 5-hydroxylysine, by an *O*-glycosidic bond through the δ-carbon hydroxyl group. Formation of 5-hydroxylysine from lysines and addition of the carbohydrate to the 5-hydroxylysine occur after polypeptide chain formation but prior to the folding of the collagen chains into their unique supercoiled structure.

4-Hydroxyproline 3-Hydroxyproline

5-Hydroxylysine

Allysine

FIGURE 2.37
Derived amino acids found in collagen. Carbohydrate is attached to 5-OH in 5-hydroxylysine by a type III glycosidic linkage (see Figure 2.45).

Amino Acid Sequence of Collagen

The molecular unit of mature collagen or tropocollagen contains three polypeptide chains. Various distinct collagen chains exist that make up the different

CLINICAL CORRELATION 2.4

Symptoms of Diseases of Abnormal Collagen Synthesis

Collagen is present in virtually all tissues and is the most abundant protein in the body. Certain organs depend heavily on normal collagen structure to function physiologically. Abnormal collagen synthesis or structure causes dysfunction of cardiovascular organs (aortic and arterial aneurysms and heart valve malfunction), bone (fragility and easy fracturing), skin (poor healing and unusual distensibility), joints (hypermobility and arthritis), and eyes (dislocation of the lens). Examples of diseases caused by abnormal collagen synthesis include Ehlers–Danlos syndrome, osteogenesis imperfecta, and scurvy. These diseases may result from abnormal collagen genes, abnormal posttranslational modification of collagen, or deficiency of cofactors needed by the enzymes that carry out posttranslational modification of collagen.

Byers, P. H. Disorders of collagen biosynthesis and structure. In: C. R. Scriver, A. L. Beaudet, W. S. Sly, and D. Valle (eds.), *The Metabolic and Molecular Bases of Inherited Disease,* 7th ed. McGraw-Hill, 1995, Chap. 134.

TABLE 2.10 Comparison of the Amino Acid Content of Human Skin Collagen (Type I) and Mature Elastin with That of Two Typical Globular Proteins[a]

Amino Acid	*Collagen (Human Skin)*	*Elastin (Mammalian)*	*Ribonuclease (Bovine)*	*Hemoglobin (Human)*
COMMON AMINO ACIDS		PERCENT OF TOTAL		
Ala	11	22	8	9
Arg	5	0.9	5	3
Asn			8	3
Asp	5	1	15	10
Cys	0	0	0	1
Glu	7	2	12	6
Gln			6	1
Gly	33	31	2	4
His	0.5	0.1	4	9
Ile	1	2	3	0
Leu	2	6	2	14
Lys	3	0.8	11	10
Met	0.6	0.2	4	1
Phe	1	3	4	7
Pro	13	11	4	5
Ser	4	1	11	4
Thr	2	1	9	5
Trp	2	1	9	2
Tyr	0.3	2	8	3
Val	2	12	8	10
DERIVED AMINO ACIDS				
Cystine	0	0	7	0
3-Hydroxyproline	0.1		0	0
4-Hydroxyproline	9	1	0	0
5-Hydroxylysine	0.6	0	0	0
Desmosine and isodesmosine	0	1	0	0

[a] Boxed numbers emphasize important differences in amino acid composition between the fibrous proteins (collagen and elastin) and typical globular proteins.

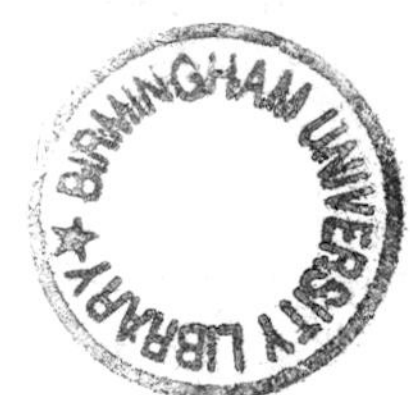

collagen types, each with their own genes. In some types, the three polypeptide chains have an identical amino acid sequence. In others such as type I (Table 2.11), two of the chains are identical while the amino acid sequence of the third chain is slightly different. In type I collagen, the identical chains are designated α1(I) chains and the third nonidentical chain, α2(I). In type V collagen all three chains are different, designated α1(V), α2(V), and α3(V). Different types of collagen differ in their physical properties due to differences in the amino acid sequence among chains, even though there are large regions of homologous sequence among the different chain types. Collagen has covalently attached carbohydrate and the collagen types differ in their carbohydrate component. Table 2.11 describes some characteristics of collagen types I–VI; additional collagen types (designated up through type XVI) have been reported.

The amino acid sequence of the chains of collagens is unusual. In long segments of all the collagen types glycine occurs as every third residue and proline or hydroxyproline also occurs three residues apart in these same regions. Accordingly, the amino acid sequences Gly-Pro-Y and Gly-X-Hyp (where X and Y are any of the amino acids) are repeated in tandem several hundred times. In type I collagen, the triplet sequences are reiterated over 200 times, encompassing over 600 amino acids within a chain of approximately 1000 amino acids.

TABLE 2.11 Classification of Collagen Types

Type	Chain Designations	Tissue Found	Characteristics
I	$[\alpha1(I)]_2\alpha2(I)$	Bone, skin, tendon, scar tissue, heart valve, intestinal, and uterine wall	Low carbohydrate; <10 hydroxylysines per chain; two types of polypeptide chains
II	$[\alpha1(II)]_3$	Cartilage, vitreous	10% carbohydrate; >20 hydroxylysines per chain
III	$[\alpha1(III)]_3$	Blood vessels, newborn skin, scar tissue, intestinal, and uterine wall	Low carbohydrate; high hydroxyproline and Gly; contains Cys
IV	$[\alpha1(IV)]_3$ $[\alpha2(IV)]_3$	Basement membrane, lens capsule	High 3-hydroxyproline; >40 hydroxylysines per chain; low Ala and Arg; contains Cys; high carbohydrate (15%)
V	$[\alpha1(V)]_2\alpha2(V)$ $[\alpha1(V)]_3$ $\alpha1(V)\alpha2(V)\alpha3(V)$	Cell surfaces or exocytoskeleton; widely distributed in low amounts	High carbohydrate, relatively high glycine, and hydroxylysine
VI	—	Aortic intima, placenta, kidney, and skin in low amounts	Relatively large globular domains in telopeptide region; high Cys and Tyr; molecular weight relatively low (~160,000); equimolar amounts of hydroxylysine and hydroxyproline

Structure of Collagen

Polypeptides that contain only proline can be synthesized in the laboratory. These polyproline chains assume a regular secondary structure in aqueous solution in which the chain is in a tightly twisted extended helix with three residues per turn of the helix ($n = 3$). This helix with all *trans*-peptide bonds is designated the **polyproline type II** helix (see Figure 2.11 for differences between *cis*- and *trans*-peptide bonds). The polyproline helix has the same characteristics as the helix found in collagen chains in regions of the primary structure that contain a proline or hydroxyproline at approximately every third position. Since the helix structure in collagen is the same as that of polyproline, the thermodynamic forces leading to formation of the collagen helix structure are due to the properties of proline. In proline, the ϕ angle contributed to the polypeptide chain is part of the five-member cyclic side chain. The five-member ring constrains the C_α—N bond to an angle compatible with the polyproline helix structure.

In polyproline type II helix, the plane of each peptide bond is perpendicular to the axis of the helix. In this geometry the peptide carbonyl groups are pointed toward neighboring chains and are correctly oriented to form strong interchain hydrogen bonds with other chains of the collagen molecule. This is in contrast to the α-helix, in which the plane containing the atoms of the peptide bond is

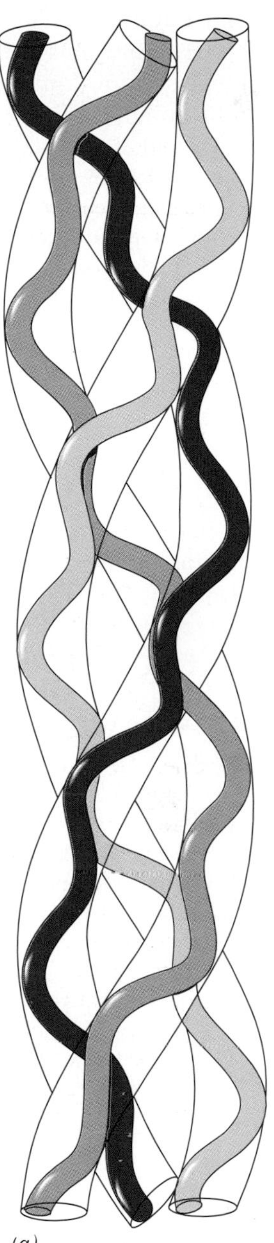
(a)

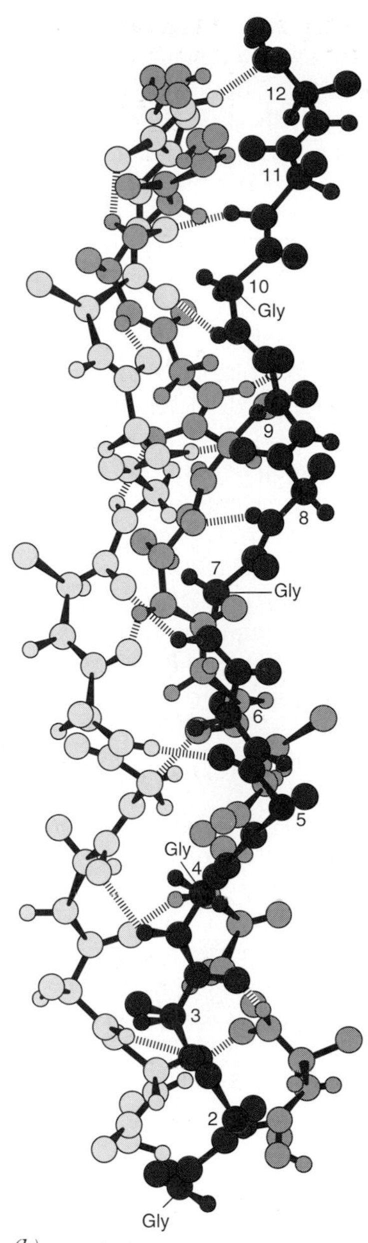

(b)

FIGURE 2.38
Diagram of collagen demonstrating necessity for glycine in every third residue to allow the different chains to be in close proximity in the structure.
(*a*) Ribbon model for supercoiled structure of collagen with each individual chain in a polyproline type II helix. (*b*) More detailed model of supercoiled conformation. All α-carbon atoms are numbered and proposed hydrogen bonds are shown by dashed lines.
Redrawn with permission from Dickerson, R. E., and Geis, I. The Structure and Actions of Proteins, *Menlo Park, CA: Benjamin, 1969, pp. 41, 42.*

parallel to the α-helix axis and the peptide bonds form only intrachain hydrogen bonds with peptide bonds in the same polypeptide chain. The three chains of a collagen molecule, where each of the chains is in a polyproline type II helix conformation, are wound about each other in a defined way to form a **superhelical structure** (Figure 2.38). The three-chain superhelix has a characteristic rise (d) and pitch (p) as does the single-chain helix. The collagen superhelix forms because glycines have a side chain of low steric bulk (R = H). As the polyproline type II helix has three residues per turn (n = 3) and glycine is at every third position, the glycines in each of the polypeptide chains are aligned along one side of the helix, forming an **apolar edge** of the chain. The glycine edges from the three polypeptide chains associate noncovalently in a close arrangement, held together by hydrophobic interactions, to form the superhelix structure of collagen. A larger side chain than that of glycine would impede the adjacent chains from coming together in the superhelix structure (Figure 2.38).

In collagen molecules the superhelix conformation may propagate for long stretches of the sequence, which is especially true for type I collagen where only the COOH-terminal and NH_2-terminal segments (known as the **telopeptides**) are not in a superhelical conformation. The type I collagen molecule has a length of 3000 Å and a width of only 15 Å, a very long cylindrical structure. In other collagen types, the superhelical regions may be broken periodically by regions of the chain that fold into globular domains.

Formation of Covalent Cross-links in Collagen

An enzyme present in extracellular space acts on the secreted collagen molecules (see p. 747) to convert some of the ε-amino groups of lysine side chains to δ-aldehydes (Figure 2.39). The resulting amino acid, containing an aldehydic R group, is the derived amino acid **allysine.** The newly formed aldehyde side chain spontaneously undergoes nucleophilic addition reactions with nonmodified lysine ε-amino groups and with the δ-carbon atoms of other allysine aldehydic groups to form linking covalent bonds (Figure 2.39). These covalent linkages can be between chains within the superhelical structure or between adjacent superhelical collagen molecules in a collagen fibril.

Elastin Is a Fibrous Protein with Allysine-Generated Cross-links

Elastin gives tissues and organs the capacity to stretch without tearing. It is classified as a fibrous protein because of its structural function and relative insolubility. It is abundant in ligaments, lungs, walls of arteries, and skin. Elastin does not contain repeating sequences of Gly-Pro-Y or Gly-X-Hyp and does not fold into either a polyproline helix or a superhelix. It appears to lack a regular secondary structure, but rather contains an unordered coiled structure in which amino acid residues within the folded structure are highly mobile. The highly mobile, kinetically free, though extensively cross-linked structure gives the

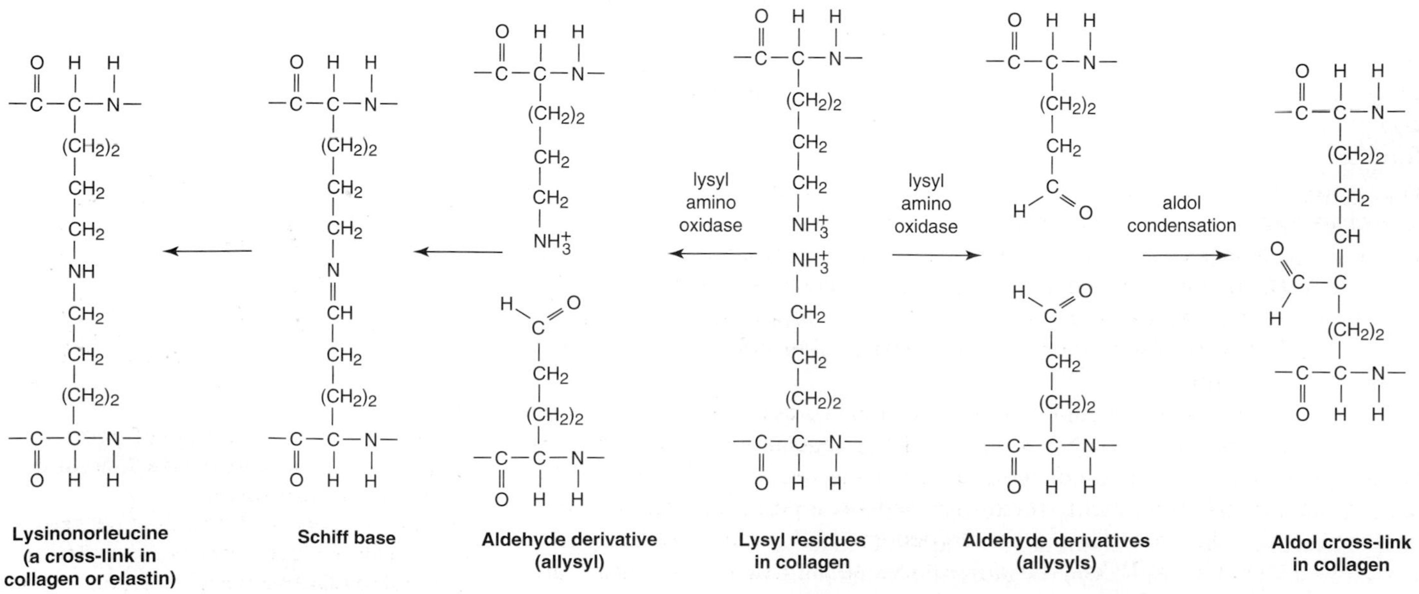

FIGURE 2.39
Covalent cross-links formed in collagen through allysine intermediates. Formation of allysines is catalyzed by lysyl amino oxidase.

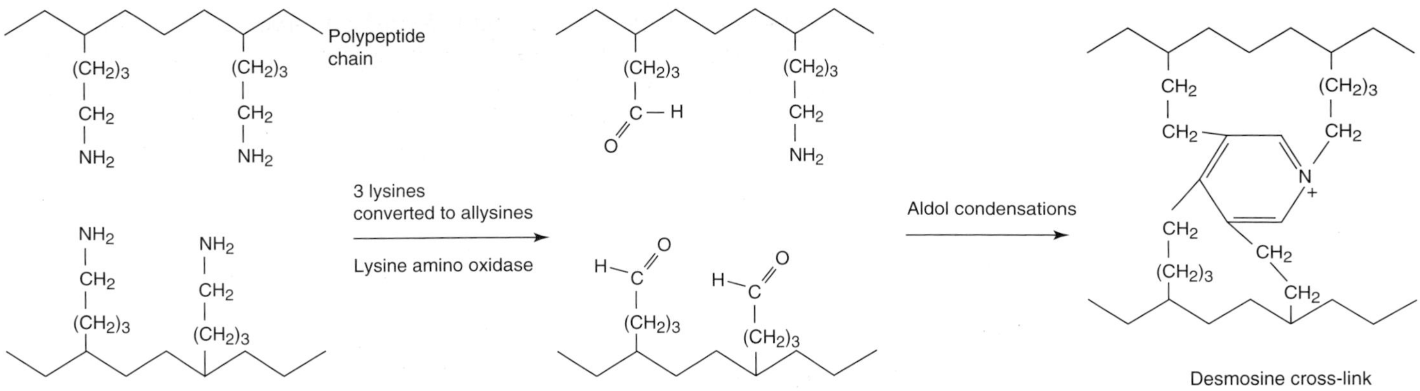

Polypeptide chain
$(CH_2)_3$ $(CH_2)_3$
CH_2 CH_2
NH_2 NH_2
NH_2 NH_2
CH_2 CH_2
$(CH_2)_3$ $(CH_2)_3$
3 lysines converted to allysines
Lysine amino oxidase
Aldol condensations
Desmosine cross-link

FIGURE 2.40
Formation of desmosine covalent cross-link in elastin from lysine and allysines.
Polypeptide chain drawn schematically with intersections of lines representing the placement of α-carbons.

protein a rubber-like elasticity. As in collagen, allysines form cross-links in **elastin.** An extracellular **lysine amino oxidase** converts lysine side chains of elastin to allysines. The amino oxidase is specific for lysines in the sequence -Lys-Ala-Ala-Lys- and -Lys-Ala-Ala-Ala-Lys-. Three allysines and an unmodified lysine in these sequences, from different regions in the polypeptide chains, react to form the heterocyclic structure of **desmosine** or **isodesmosine.** The desmosines covalently cross-link the polypeptide chains in elastin fibers (Figure 2.40).

α-Keratin and Tropomyosin

α-Keratin and tropomyosin are fibrous proteins in which each chain has an α-helical conformation. α-Keratin is found in the epidermal layer of skin, in nails, and in hair. Tropomyosin is a component of the thin filament in muscle tissue. Analysis of the α-helical sequences in both these proteins shows the tandem repetition of seven amino acid segments, in which the first and fourth amino acids have hydrophobic side chains and the fifth and seventh polar side chains. The reiteration of hydrophobic and polar side chains in seven amino acid segments is symbolically represented by the formulation $(\text{a-b-c-d-e-f-g})_i$, where residues a and d are hydrophobic amino acids, and residues e and g are polar or ionized side chain groups. Since a seven amino acid segment represents two complete turns of an α-helix ($n = 3.6$), the apolar residues at a and d align to form an apolar edge along one side of the α-helix (Figure 2.41). This apolar edge in α-keratin interacts with polypeptide apolar edges of other α-keratin chains to form a superhelical structure containing two or three polypeptide chains. Each strand also contains a polar edge, due to residues e and g, that interacts with the water solvent on the outside of the superhelix and also stabilizes the superhelical structure. Similarly, two tropomyosin polypeptide strands in α-helical conformation wind around each other to form a tropomyosin superhelical structure.

Thus collagen, α-keratin, and tropomyosin molecules are multistrand structures in which polypeptide chains with a highly regular secondary structure (polyproline type II helix in collagen, α-helix in α-keratin and tropomyosin) are wound around each other to form a rod-shaped supercoiled conformation. In turn, the supercoiled molecules are aligned into multimolecular fibrils stabilized by covalent cross-links. The amino acid sequences of the chains are repetitive, generating edges on the cylindrical surfaces of each of the chains that stabilize a hydrophobic interaction between the chains required for generation of the supercoiled conformation.

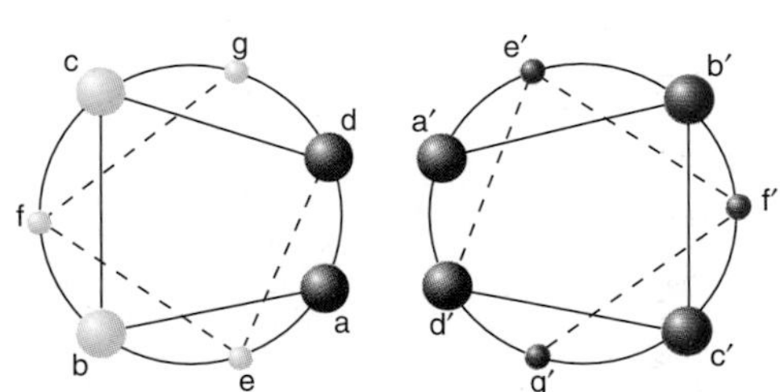

FIGURE 2.41
Interaction of an apolar edge of two chains in α-helical conformation as in α-keratin and tropomyosin.
Interaction of apolar a–d′ and d–a′ residues of two α-helices aligned parallel in an NH_2-terminal (top) to COOH-terminal direction is presented.
Redrawn from McLachlan, A. D., and Stewart, M. J. Mol. Biol. *98:293, 1975.*

Lipoproteins Are Complexes of Lipids with Proteins

Lipoproteins are multicomponent complexes of proteins and lipids that form distinct molecular aggregates with an approximate stoichiometry between protein and lipid components within the complex. Each type of lipoprotein has a characteristic molecular mass, size, chemical composition, density, and physiological role. The protein and lipid in the complex are held together by noncovalent forces.

Plasma lipoproteins are extensively characterized and changes in their relative amounts are predictive of atherosclerosis, a major human disease (see Clin. Corr. 2.5). They have a wide variety of roles in blood including transport of lipids from tissue to tissue and participating in lipid metabolism (see Chapter 9). Four classes of plasma lipoproteins exist in normal fasting humans (Table 2.12); in the postabsorptive period a fifth type, **chylomicrons,** is also present. Lipoprotein classes are identified by their density, as determined by ultracentrifugation and by electrophoresis (Figure 2.42). The protein components of a lipoprotein particle are the **apolipoproteins.** Each type of lipoprotein has a

TABLE 2.12 Hydrated Density Classes of Plasma Lipoproteins

Lipoprotein Fraction	*Density* ($g\ mL^{-1}$)	*Flotation Rate, S_f (Svedberg units)*	*Molecular Weight (daltons)*	*Particle Diameter (Å)*
HDL	1.063–1.210		HDL_2, 4×10^5	70–130
			HDL_3, 2×10^5	50–100
LDL (or LDL_2)	1.019–1.063	0–12	2×10^6	200–280
IDL (or LDL_1)	1.006–1.019	12–20	4.5×10^6	250
VLDL	0.95–1.006	20–400	5×10^6–10^7	250–750
Chylomicrons	<0.95	>400	10^9–10^{10}	10^3–10^4

Source: Data from Soutar, A. K., and Myant, N. B. In: R. E. Offord (Ed.), *Chemistry of Macromolecules,* IIB. Baltimore, MD: University Park Press, 1979.

CLINICAL CORRELATION 2.5

Hyperlipidemias

Hyperlipidemias are disorders of the rates of synthesis or clearance of lipoproteins from the bloodstream. Usually they are detected by measuring plasma triacylglycerol and cholesterol and are classified on the basis of which class of lipoproteins is elevated.

Type I hyperlipidemia is due to accumulation of chylomicrons. Two genetic forms are known: lipoprotein lipase deficiency and ApoCII deficiency. ApoCII is required by lipoprotein lipase for full activity. Patients with type I hyperlipidemia have exceedingly high plasma triacylglycerol levels (over 1000 mg dL^{-1}) and suffer from eruptive xanthomas (triacylglycerol deposits in the skin) and pancreatitis.

Type II hyperlipidemia is characterized by elevated LDL levels. Most cases are due to genetic defects in the synthesis, processing, or function of the LDL receptor. Heterozygotes have elevated LDL levels; hence the trait is dominantly expressed. Homozygous patients have very high LDL levels and may suffer myocardial infarctions before age 20.

Type III hyperlipidemia is due to abnormalities of ApoE, which interfere with the uptake of chylomicron and VLDL remnants. Hypothyroidism can produce a very similar hyperlipidemia. These patients have an increased risk of atherosclerosis.

Type IV hyperlipidemia is the commonest abnormality. The VLDL levels are increased, often due to obesity, alcohol abuse, or diabetes. Familial forms are also known but the molecular defect is unknown.

Type V hyperlipidemia is, like type I, associated with high chylomicron triacylglycerol levels, pancreatitis, and eruptive xanthomas.

Hypercholesterolemia also occurs in certain types of liver disease in which biliary excretion of cholesterol is reduced. An abnormal lipoprotein called lipoprotein X accumulates. This disorder is not associated with increased cardiovascular disease from atherosclerosis.

Havel, R. J., and Kane, J. P. Introduction: structure and metabolism of plasma lipoproteins. In: C. R. Scriver, A. L. Beaudet, W. S. Sly, and D. Valle (Eds.), *The Metabolic and Molecular Basis of Inherited Disease,* 7th ed. New York: McGraw-Hill, 1995, Chap. 56; and Goldstein, J. L., Hobbs, H. H., and Brown, M. S. Familial hypercholesterolemia. In: C. R. Scriver, A. L. Beaudet, W. S. Sly, and D. Valle (Eds.), *The Metabolic and Molecular Bases of Inherited Disease,* 7th ed., New York: McGraw Hill, 1995, Chap. 62.

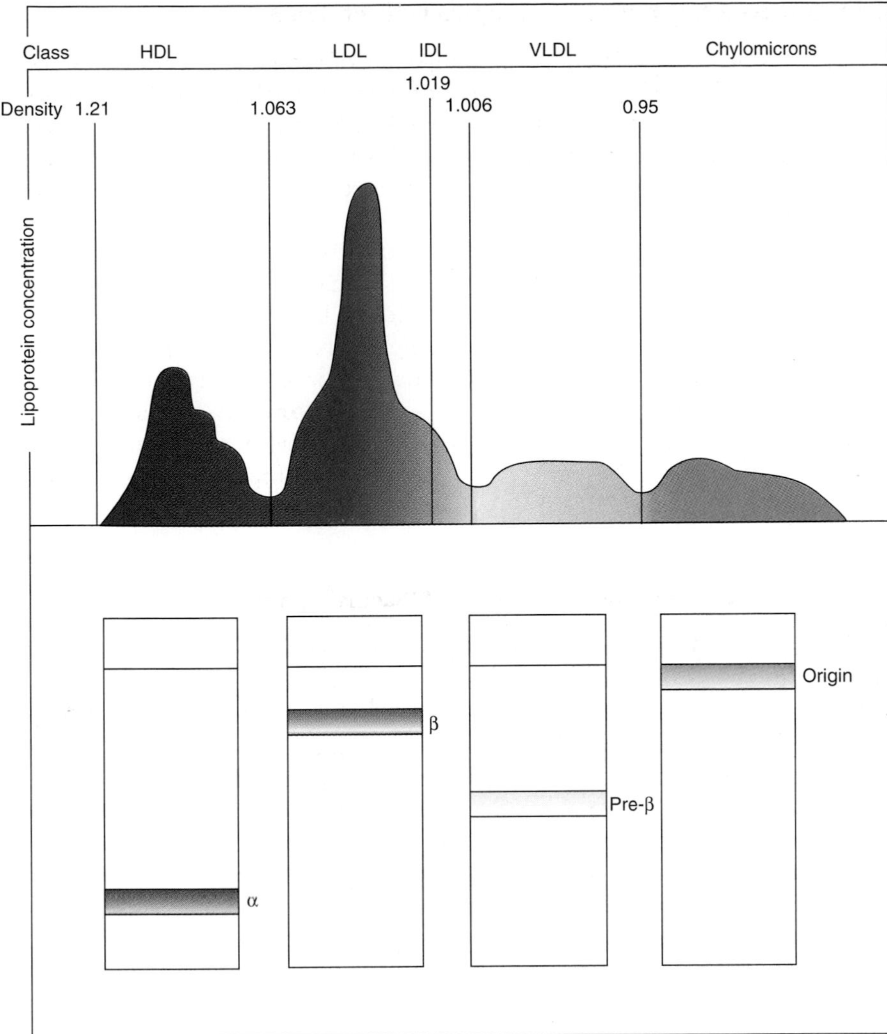

FIGURE 2.42
Correspondence of plasma lipoprotein density classes with electrophoretic mobility in a plasma electrophoresis.
In the upper diagram an ultracentrifugation Schlieren pattern is shown. At the bottom, electrophoresis on a paper support shows the mobilities of major plasma lipoprotein classes with respect to α- and β-globulin bands.
Reprinted with permission from Soutar, A. K., and Myant, N. B. In: R. E. Offord (Ed.), Chemistry of Macromolecules, *IIB. Baltimore, MD: University Park Press, 1979.*

characteristic apolipoprotein composition, the different apolipoproteins often being present in a set ratio. The most prominent apolipoprotein in **high density lipoproteins (HDLs)** is apolipoprotein A-I (ApoA-I) (Table 2.13). In **low den-**

TABLE 2.13 Apolipoproteins of Human Plasma Lipoproteins (Values in Percentage of Total Protein Present)[a]

Apolipoprotein	*HDL_2*	*HDL_3*	*LDL*	*IDL*	*VLDL*	*Chylomicrons*
ApoA-I	85	70–75	Trace	0	0–3	0–3
ApoA-II	5	20	Trace	0	0–0.5	0–1.5
ApoD	0	1–2			0	1
ApoB	0–2	0	95–100	50–60	40–50	20–22
ApoC-I	1–2	1–2	0–5	<1	5	5–10
ApoC-II	1	1	0.5	2.5	10	15
ApoC-III	2–3	2–3	0–5	17	20–25	40
ApoE	Trace	0–5	0	15–20	5–10	5
ApoF	Trace	Trace				
ApoG	Trace	Trace				

Source: Data from Soutar, A. K., and Myant, N. B. In: R. E. Offord (Ed.), *Chemistry of Macromolecules,* IIB. Baltimore, MD: University Park Press, 1979; Kostner, G. M. *Adv. Lipid Res.* **20**:1, 1983.

[a] Values show variability from different laboratories.

sity lipoproteins (LDLs) the prominent apolipoprotein is ApoB, which is also present in the **intermediate density lipoproteins (IDLs)** and **very low density lipoproteins (VLDLs).** The ApoC family is also present in high amounts in IDLs and VLDLs. Each apolipoprotein class (A, B, etc.) is distinct (see Clin. Corr. 2.6). Proteins within a class do not cross-react with antibodies to another class. The molecular weights of the apolipoproteins of the plasma lipoproteins vary from 6 kDa (ApoC-I) to 550 kDa for ApoB-100. This latter is one of the longest single-chain polypeptides known (4536 amino acids).

A model for a VLDL particle is shown in Figure 2.43. On the inside are neutral lipids such as cholesterol esters and triacylglycerols. Surrounding this inner core of neutral lipids, in a shell ~20 Å thick, reside the proteins and the

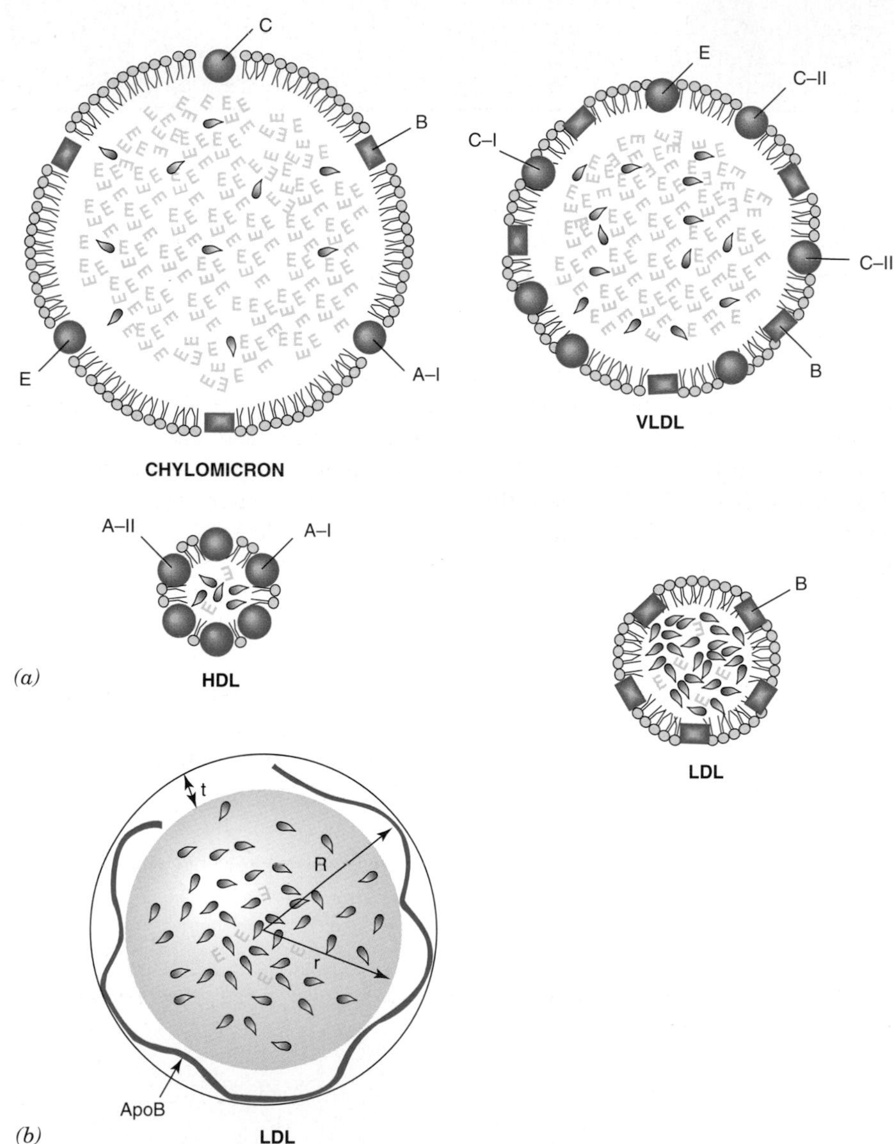

FIGURE 2.43
Generalized structure of plasma lipoproteins.
(*a*) Spherical particle model consisting of a core of triacylglycerols (yellow E's) and cholesterol esters (orange drops) with a shell ~20 Å thick of apolipoproteins (lettered), phospholipids, and unesterified cholesterol. Apolipoproteins are embedded with their hydrophobic edges oriented toward the core and their hydrophilic edges toward the outside.
From Segrest, J. P., et al. Adv. Protein Chem. *45:303, 1994.*
(*b*) LDL particle showing ApoB-100 imbedded in outer shell of particle.
From Schumaker, V. N., et al., Protein Chem. *45:205, 1994.*

CLINICAL CORRELATION 2.6

Hypolipoproteinemias

Abetalipoproteinemia is a genetic disease that is characterized by absence of chylomicrons, VLDLs, and LDLs due to an inability to synthesize apolipoprotein B-100. Patients show accumulation of lipid droplets in small intestinal cells, malabsorption of fat, acanthocytosis (spiny shaped red cells), and neurological disease (retinitis pigmentosa, ataxia, and retardation).

Tangier disease, an α-lipoprotein deficiency, is a rare autosomal recessive disease in which the HDL level is 1–5% of its normal value. Clinical features are due to the accumulation of cholesterol in the lymphoreticular system, which may lead to hepatomegaly and splenomegaly. In this disease the plasma cholesterol and phospholipids are greatly reduced.

Deficiency of the enzyme lecithin:cholesterol acyltransferase is a rare disease that results in the production of lipoprotein X (see Clin. Corr. 2.5). Also characteristic of this disease is the decrease in the α-lipoprotein and pre-β-lipoprotein bands, with the increase in the β-lipoprotein (lipoprotein X) in electrophoresis.

Kane, J. P., and Havel, R. J. Disorders of the biogenesis and secretion of lipoproteins containing the β apolipoproteins. In: C. R. Scriver, A. L. Beaudet, W. S. Sly, and D. Valle (Eds.), *The Metabolic and Molecular Basis of Inherited Disease,* 7th ed. New York: McGraw-Hill, 1995, Chap. 57; and Assmann, G., von Eckardstein, A., and Brewer, H. B. Jr. Familial high density lipoprotein deficiency: Tangier disease. In: C. R. Scriver, A. L. Beaudet, W. S. Sly, and D. Valle (Eds.), *The Metabolic and Molecular Bases of Inherited Disease,* 7th ed. New York: McGraw-Hill, 1995, Chap. 64.

charged amphoteric lipids such as unesterified cholesterol and the phosphatidylcholines (see Chapter 10). Amphoteric lipids and proteins in the outer shell place their hydrophobic apolar regions toward the inside of the particle and their charged groups toward the outside where they interact with each other and with water.

This spherical structural model with a hydrophobic inner core of neutral lipids and amphoteric lipids and proteins in the outer shell applies to all plasma lipoproteins, irrespective of their density class and particle size. The smaller lipoprotein particles, such as HDLs, have a smaller diameter. As the diameter of a spherical particle decreases, the molecules in the outer shell make up a greater percentage of the total molecules in the particle. The smaller HDL particles would therefore be theoretically predicted to have a higher percentage of surface proteins and amphoteric lipids than the larger VLDL particles. Thus the HDL particle is 45% protein and 55% lipid, while the larger VLDL particle is only 10% protein with 90% lipid (Table 2.14).

The apolipoproteins, with the exception of ApoB, have a high α-helical content when in association with lipid. The helical regions have amphipathic properties. Every third or fourth amino acid in the helix is charged and forms a polar edge along the helix that associates with the polar heads of phospholipids and the aqueous solvent on the outside. The opposite side of the helix has hydrophobic side chains that associate with the nonpolar neutral lipid core of the phospholipid particle. The α-helical structure of part of ApoC-I is shown

TABLE 2.14 Chemical Composition of the Different Plasma Lipoprotein Classes

			Percent Composition of Lipid Fraction			
Lipoprotein Class	*Total Protein (%)*	*Total Lipid (%)*	*Phospholipids*	*Esterified Cholesterol*	*Unesterified Cholesterol*	*Triacylglycerols*
HDL_2[a]	40–45	55	35	12	4	5
HDL_3[a]	50–55	50	20–25	12	3–4	3
LDL	20–25	75–80	15–20	35–40	7–10	7–10
IDL	15–20	80–85	22	22	8	30
VLDL	5–10	90–95	15–20	10–15	5–10	50–65
Chylomicrons	1.5–2.5	97–99	7–9	3–5	1–3	84–89

Source: Data from Soutar, A. K., and Myant, N. B. In: R. E. Offord (Ed.), *Chemistry of Macromolecules,* IIB. Baltimore, MD: University Park Press, 1979.

[a] Subclasses of HDL.

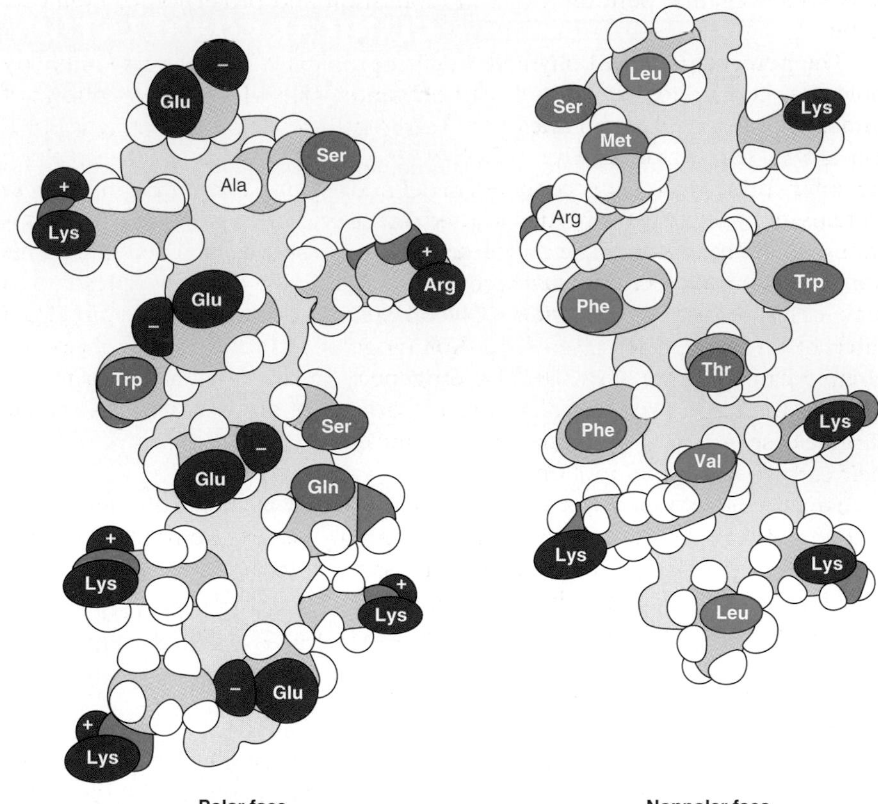

FIGURE 2.44
Illustration showing side chains of a helical segment of apolipoprotein C-1 between residues 32 and 53.
The polar face shows ionizable acid residues in the center and basic residues at the edge. On the other side of the helix, the hydrophobic residues form a nonpolar longitudinal face.
Redrawn with permission from Sparrow, J. T., and Gotto, A. M., Jr. CRC Crit. Rev. Biochem. *13:87, 1983. Copyright © CRC Press, Inc., Boca Raton, FL.*

in Figure 2.44. ApoB appears to have both α-helical and β-structural regions embedded in the phospholipid outer core. The long 4536 amino acid polypeptide chain of ApoB-100 surrounds the circumference of the LDL particle like a belt weaving in and out of the monolayer phospholipid outer shell (Figure 2.43). One ApoB molecule associates per LDL particle.

Glycoproteins Contain Covalently Bound Carbohydrate

Glycoproteins participate in many normal and disease-related functions of clinical relevance. Many plasma membrane proteins are glycoproteins. Some may be antigens, which determine the blood antigen system (A, B, O) and the histocompatibility and transplantation determinants of an individual. Immunoglobulin antigenic sites and viral and hormone receptor sites in plasma membranes are often glycoproteins. The carbohydrate portions of glycoproteins in membranes provide a surface code for identification by other cells and for contact inhibition in the regulation of cell growth. Changes in membrane glycoproteins can be correlated with tumorigenesis and malignant transformation in cancer. Most plasma proteins, except albumin, are glycoproteins including blood-clotting proteins, immunoglobulins, and many of the complement proteins. Some protein hormones, such as follicle-stimulating hormone (FSH) and thyroid-stimulating hormone (TSH), are glycoproteins. The structural proteins collagen, laminin, and fibronectin contain carbohydrate, as do proteins of mucous secretions that perform a role in lubrication and protection of epithelial tissue.

The percentage of carbohydrate in glycoproteins is variable. IgG antibody molecules contain low amounts of carbohydrate (4%), whereas glycophorin of human red blood cell membranes is 60% carbohydrate. Human gastric glycoprotein is 82% carbohydrate. The carbohydrate can be distributed evenly along the polypeptide chain or concentrated in defined regions. For plasma membrane proteins, typically only the portion located on the outside of the cell has carbohydrate covalently attached. The carbohydrate attached at one or at multiple points along a polypeptide chain usually contains less than 15 sugar residues and in some cases only one sugar residue. Glycoproteins with the same function from different animal species often have homologous amino acid sequences but variable carbohydrate structures. Heterogeneity in carbohydrate content can occur in the same protein within a single organism. For example, pancreatic ribonuclease A and B forms have an identical primary structure but differ in their carbohydrate composition.

Functional glycoproteins are also found in different stages of completion. Addition of complex carbohydrate units occurs in a series of enzyme-catalyzed reactions as the polypeptide chain is transported through the endoplasmic reticulum and Golgi network (see Chapter 17). Immature glycoproteins are sometimes expressed with intermediate stages of carbohydrate additions.

Types of Carbohydrate–Protein Covalent Linkages

Different types of covalent linkages join the sugar moieties and protein in a glycoprotein. The two most common are the ***N*-glycosidic linkage** (type I linkage) between an asparagine amide group and a sugar, and the ***O*-glycosidic linkage** (type II linkage) between a serine or threonine hydroxyl group and a sugar (Figure 2.45). In type I linkage the bond to asparagine is within the sequence Asn-X-Thr(Ser). Another linkage found in mammalian glycoproteins is an *O*-glycosidic bond to a 5-hydroxylysine residue (type III linkage) found in collagens and in the serum complement protein C1q. Less common linkages include attachment to the hydroxyl group of 4-hydroxyproline (type IV linkage), to a cysteine thiol side chain (type V linkage), and to a NH_2-terminal α-amino group of a polypeptide chain (type VI linkage). High concentrations of type VI linkages are spontaneously formed with hemoglobin and blood glucose in uncontrolled diabetics. Assay of the concentration of glycosylated hemoglobin is used to follow changes in blood glucose concentration (see Clin. Corr. 2.7).

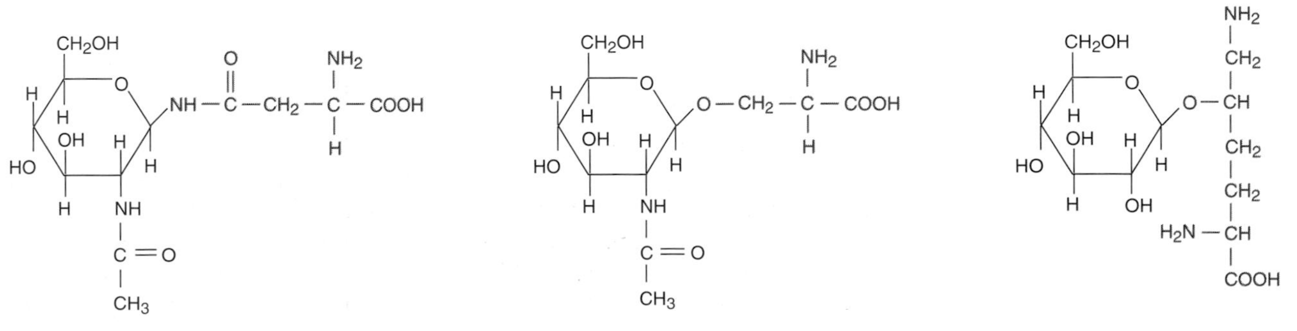

Type I *N*-Glycosyl linkage to asparagine

Type II *O*-Glycosyl linkage to serine

Type III *O*-Glycosyl linkage to 5-hydroxylysine

FIGURE 2.45
Examples of glycosidic linkages to amino acids in proteins.
Type I is an *N*-glycosidic linkage through an amide nitrogen of Asn; type II is an *O*-glycosidic linkage through the OH of Ser or Thr; and type III is an *O*-glycosidic linkage to the 5-OH of 5-hydroxylysine.

CLINICAL CORRELATION 2.7

Glycosylated Hemoglobin, HbA_{1c}

A glycosylated hemoglobin, designated HbA_{1c}, is formed spontaneously in red blood cells by combination of the NH_2-terminal amino groups of the hemoglobin β-chain and glucose. The aldehyde group of the glucose first forms a Schiff base with the NH_2-terminal amino group,

$$-N{=}\underset{\displaystyle H}{\underset{|}{C}}-\underset{\displaystyle H}{\underset{|}{\overset{\overset{\displaystyle OH}{|}}{C}}}-$$

which then rearranges to a more stable amino ketone linkage,

$$-\underset{\displaystyle H}{\underset{|}{N}}-\underset{\displaystyle H}{\underset{|}{\overset{\overset{\displaystyle H}{|}}{C}}}-\overset{\overset{\displaystyle O}{\|}}{C}-$$

by a spontaneous (nonenzymatic) reaction known as the Amadori rearrangement. The concentration of HbA_{1c} is dependent on the concentration of glucose in the blood and the duration of hyperglycemia. In prolonged hyperglycemia the concentration may rise to 12% or more of the total hemoglobin. Patients with diabetes mellitus have high concentrations of blood glucose and therefore high amounts of HbA_{1c}. The changes in the concentration of HbA_{1c} in diabetic patients can be used to follow the effectiveness of treatment for the diabetes.

Bunn, H. F. Evaluation of glycosylated hemoglobin in diabetic patients. *Diabetes* 30:613, 1980; and Brown, S. B., and Bowes, M. A. Glycosylated haemoglobins and their role in management of diabetes mellitus. *Biochem. Educ.* 13:2, 1985.

2.7 ■ FOLDING OF PROTEINS FROM RANDOMIZED TO UNIQUE STRUCTURES: PROTEIN STABILITY

The Protein Folding Problem: A Possible Pathway

The ability of a primary protein structure to fold spontaneously to its native secondary or tertiary conformation, without any information other than the amino acid sequence and the noncovalent forces that act on the sequence, has been demonstrated. RNase will spontaneously refold to its native conformation after being denatured with loss of native structure but without the hydrolysis of peptide bonds. Such observations led to the hypothesis that a polypeptide sequence contains the properties sufficient to promote spontaneous protein folding to its unique active conformation under the correct solvent conditions and in the presence of prosthetic groups that may be a part of its structure. As described below chaperone proteins may facilitate the rate of protein folding. Quaternary structures also assemble spontaneously, after the tertiary structure of the individual polypeptide subunits are formed.

It may appear surprising that a protein folds into a single unique conformation given all the possible *a priori* rotational conformations available around single bonds in the primary structure. For example, the α-chain of hemoglobin contains 141 amino acids in which there are at least four single bonds per amino acid residue around which free rotation can occur. If each bond about which free rotation occurs has two or more stable rotamer conformations accessible to it, then there are a minimum of 4^{141} or 5×10^{86} possible conformations for the α-chain amino acid sequence.

The **conformation of a protein** is that conformation of the lowest Gibbs free energy accessible to the amino acid sequence within a physiological time frame. Thus folding is under thermodynamic and kinetic control. Although an exact knowledge of *de novo* folding of a polypeptide is at present an unattainable goal, certain processes appear reasonable. There is evidence that folding is initiated by short-range interactions forming secondary structures in small regions of the polypeptide. Short-range interactions are noncovalent interactions that occur between a side chain and its nearest neighbors. Particular side chains have a propensity to promote the formation of α-helices, β-structure, and sharp turns or bends (β-turns) in the polypeptide. The interaction of a side chain with its nearest neighbors in the polypeptide determines the secondary structure into which that section of the polypeptide strand folds. Sections of polypeptide, called **initiation sites,** thus spontaneously fold into small regions of secondary structure. The partially folded structures then condense with each other to form a **molten-globular** state. This is a condensed intermediate on the folding pathway that contains much of the secondary structure elements of the native structure, but a large number of incorrect tertiary structure interactions. Segments of secondary structure in the molten-globular state are highly mobile relative to one another, and the molten-globular structure is in rapid equilibrium with the fully unfolded denatured state. The correct medium- and long-range interactions between different initiation sites are found by rearrangements within the molten-globule and the low free energy, native tertiary structure for the polypeptide chain is formed. With formation of the native tertiary structure, the correct disulfide bonds (cystine) are formed. The rate-determining step for folding and unfolding of the native conformation lies between the molten-globular state and the native structure.

Chaperone Proteins May Assist the Protein Folding Process

Cells contain proteins that facilitate the folding process. These include *cis-trans*-prolyl isomerases, protein disulfide isomerases, and chaperone proteins. ***cis-trans*-Prolyl isomerases** increase the rate of folding by catalyzing interconversion of *cis*- and *trans*-peptide bonds of proline residues within the polypeptide chain. This allows the correct proline peptide bond conformation to form for each proline as required by the folded native structure. **Protein disulfide isomerases** catalyze the breakage and formation of disulfide cystine linkages so incorrect linkages are not stabilized and the correct arrangement of cystine linkages for the folded conformation is rapidly achieved.

Chaperone proteins were discovered as **heat shock proteins (hsps),** a family of proteins whose synthesis is increased at elevated temperatures. The chaperones do not change the final outcome of the folding process but act to prevent protein aggregation prior to the completion of folding and to prevent formation of metastable dead-end or nonproductive intermediates during folding. They increase the rate of the folding process by limiting the number of unproductive folding pathways available to a polypeptide. Chaperones of the hsp 70-kDa family bind to polypeptide chains as they are synthesized on the ribosomes, shielding the hydrophobic surfaces that would normally be exposed to solvent. This protects the protein from aggregation until the full chain is synthesized and folding can occur. Some proteins, however, cannot complete their folding process while in the presence of hsp70 chaperones and are delivered to the hsp60 family (GroEL in *Escherichia coli*) of chaperone proteins, also called **chaperonins.** The chaperonins form long cylindrical multisubunit quaternary structures that bind unfolded proteins in their molten-globular state within their central hydrophobic cavity. Chaperonins have an ATPase activity, hydrolyzing ATP as they facilitate folding. The folding process in *E. coli* is presented in Figure 2.46. Chaperone proteins are also required for refolding of proteins after they cross cellular membranes. A system of chaperones exists to facilitate protein transport into mitochondria and into and through the endoplasmic reticulum. Proteins cross the lipid bilayer of the mitochondrial and endoplasmic reticulum membranes in an unfolded conformation, and local chaperones are required to facilitate their folding.

Noncovalent Forces Lead to Protein Folding and Contribute to a Protein's Stability

Noncovalent forces cause a polypeptide to fold into a unique conformation and then stabilize the native structure against denaturation. Noncovalent forces are weak bonding forces with strengths of 1–7 kcal mol^{-1} (4–29 kJ mol^{-1}). This may be compared to the strength of covalent bonds that have a bonding strength

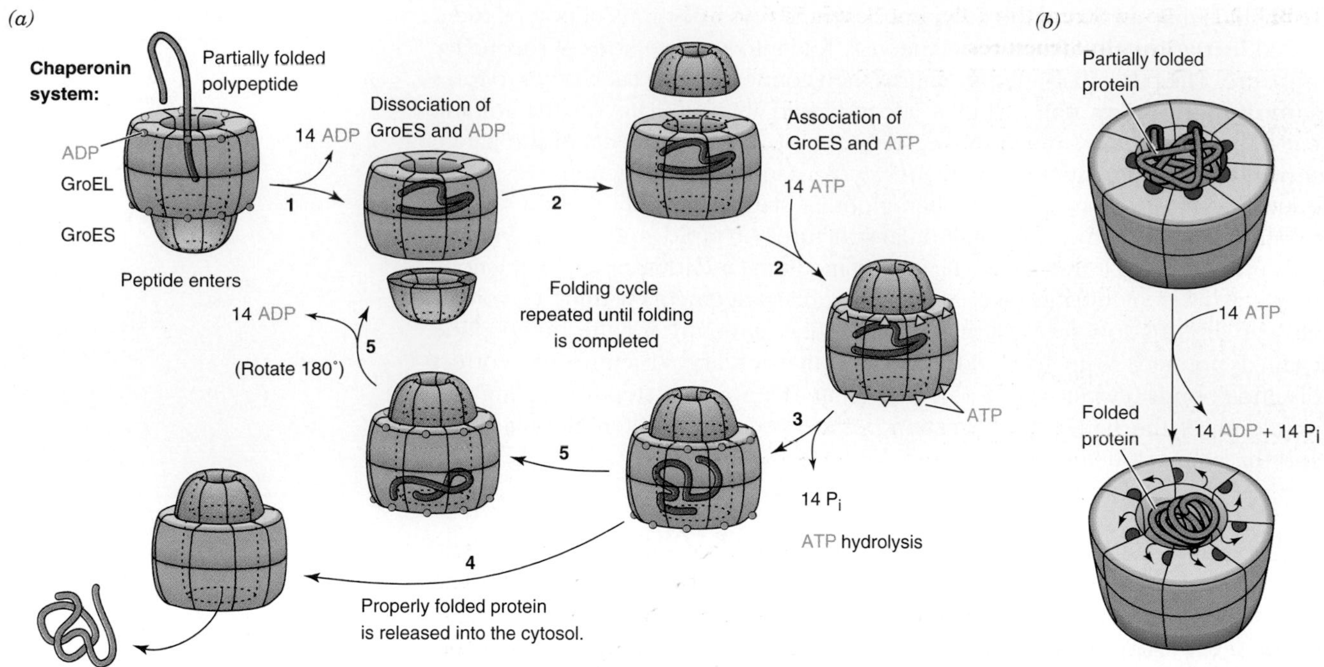

FIGURE 2.46
Chaperonin directed protein folding in *E. coli*.
(*a*) A proposed reaction cycle of the *E. coli* chaperonins GroEL and GroES in protein folding. (1) GroEL is a complex of 14 subunits, each with ADP attached. An associated ring of 8 GroES subunits binds an unfolded polypeptide in its central cavity and ADP and GroES are released. (2) Each GroEL subunit binds an ATP, weakening the interaction between unfolded polypeptide and GroEL. GroES is rebound on the opposite face of GroEL. (3) The 14 ATP are simultaneously hydrolyzed, releasing the bound polypeptide inside GroEL. The polypeptide, which is probably in its molten-globular state, folds in a protected microenvironment, preventing aggregation with other partially folded polypeptides. (4) The polypeptide is released from GroEL after folding into its native conformation. (5) If the polypeptide fails to attain its native fold, it remains bound to GroEL and reenters the reaction cycle at step 2. In the diagram GroEL turns over by 180°. GroES binds but does not hydrolyze ATP and facilitates the binding of ATP to GroEL. It coordinates simultaneous hydrolysis of ATP and prevents escape of a partially folded polypeptide from the GroEL cavity. (*b*) A model for the ATP-dependent release of an unfolded polypeptide from its multiple attachment sites in GroEL. ATP binding and hydrolysis mask the hydrophobic sites of GroEL (darker areas) that bind to the unfolded polypeptide, thus permitting it to fold in an isolated environment.
Adapted from Hartl, R.-U, Hlodan, R., and Langer, T. Trends Biochem. Sci. *19:23, 1994. Figure reproduced with permission from Voet, D., and Voet, J.* Biochemistry, *2nd ed., New York: John Wiley, 1995.*

of at least 50 kcal mol^{-1} (Table 2.15). Even though individually weak, the large number of individually weak noncovalent contacts within a protein add up to a large energy factor that promotes protein folding.

Hydrophobic Interaction Forces

The most important noncovalent forces that cause a randomized polypeptide conformation to lose rotational freedom and fold into its native structure are **hydrophobic interaction forces.** The strength of a hydrophobic interaction is not due to an intrinsic attraction between nonpolar groups, but rather to the properties of the water solvent in which the nonpolar groups are dissolved. A nonpolar molecule or a region of a protein molecule dissolved in water induces a solvation shell of water in which water molecules are highly ordered. When two nonpolar side chains come together on folding of a polypeptide, the surface area exposed to solvent is reduced and some of the highly ordered water

TABLE 2.15 Bond Strength of Typical Bonds Found in Protein Structures

Bond Type	*Bond Strength (kcal mol^{-1})*
Covalent bonds	>50
Noncovalent bonds	0.6–7
Hydrophobic bond (i.e., two benzyl side chain groups of Phe)	2–3
Hydrogen bond	1–7
Ionic bond (low dielectric environment)	1–6
van der Waals	<1
Average energy of kinetic motion (37°C)	0.6

molecules in the solvation shell are released to bulk solvent. Accordingly, the entropy of the system (i.e., net disorder of the water molecules in the system) is increased. The increase in entropy is thermodynamically favorable and is the driving force causing nonpolar moieties to come together in aqueous solvent. A favorable free energy change of -2 kcal mol^{-1} for association of two phenylalanine side chain groups in water is due to this favorable water solvent entropy gain (Figure 2.47).

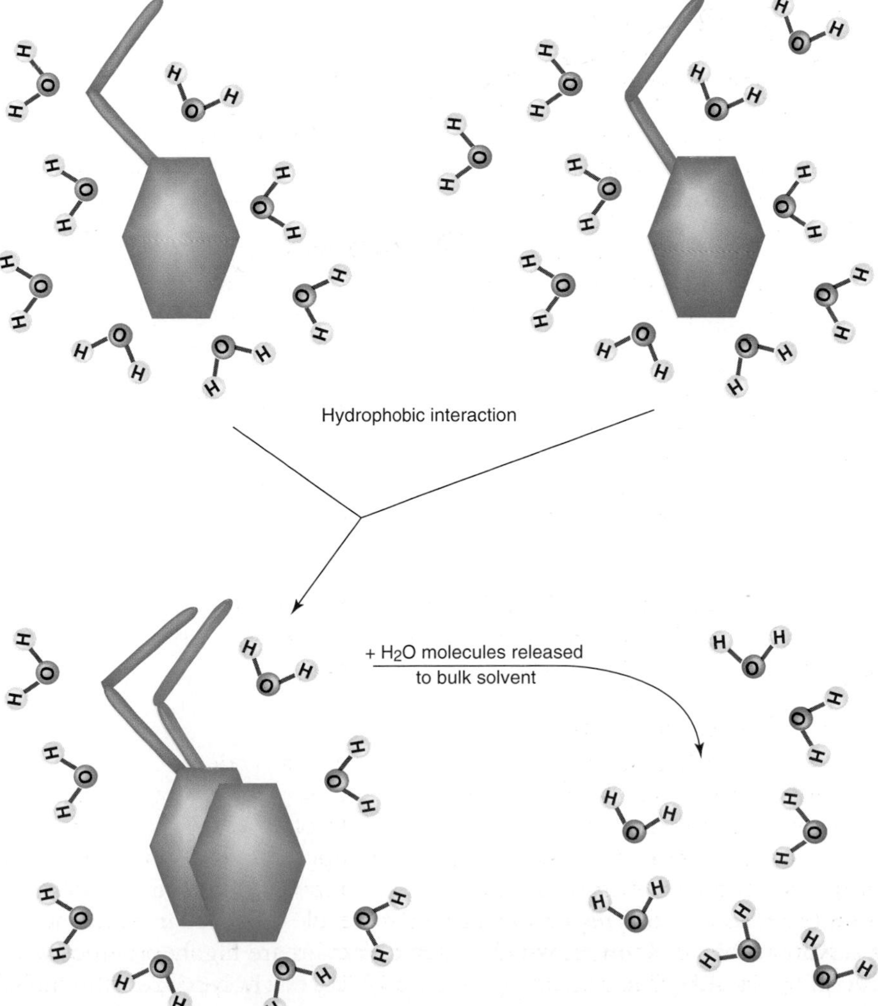

FIGURE 2.47
Formation of hydrophobic interaction between two phenylalanine side chain groups.

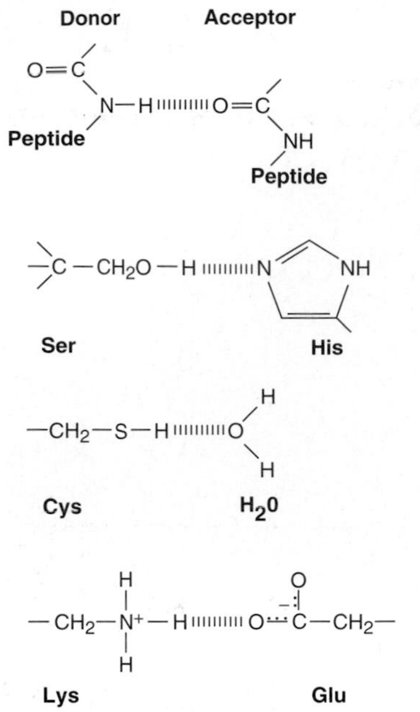

In transition from a random into a regular secondary conformation such as an α-helix or β-structure, approximately one-third of the ordered water of solvation about the unfolded polypeptide is lost to bulk solvent. This approximates 0.5–0.9 kcal mol^{-1} for each peptide residue. An additional one-third of the original solvation shell is lost when a protein that has folded into a secondary structure folds into a tertiary structure. The tertiary folding brings different segments of folded polypeptide chains into close proximity with the release of water of solvation between the polypeptide chains.

Hydrogen Bonds

Another noncovalent force in proteins is hydrogen bonding. **Hydrogen bonds** are formed when a hydrogen atom covalently bonded to an electronegative atom is shared with a second electronegative atom. The atom to which the hydrogen atom is covalently bonded is designated the hydrogen-**donor atom.** The atom with which the hydrogen atom is shared is the hydrogen-**acceptor atom.** Typical hydrogen bonds found in proteins are shown in Figure 2.48. α-Helical and β-structure conformations are extensively hydrogen bonded.

FIGURE 2.48
Some common hydrogen bonds found in proteins.

The strength of a hydrogen bond is dependent on the distance between the donor and acceptor atoms. High bonding energies occur when the distance is between 2.7 and 3.1 Å. Of lesser importance, but not negligible, to bonding strength is the dependence of hydrogen-bond strength on geometry. Bonds of higher energy are geometrically collinear, with donor, hydrogen, and acceptor atoms lying in a straight line. The dielectric constant of the medium around the hydrogen bond may also be reflected in the bonding strength. Typical hydrogen-bond strengths in proteins are 1–7 kcal mol^{-1}. Although hydrogen bonds contribute to thermodynamic stability of a protein's conformation, their formation may not be as major a driving force for folding as we might at first believe. This is because peptide bonds and other hydrogen-bonding groups in proteins form hydrogen bonds to the water solvent in the denatured state, and these bonds must be broken before the protein folds. The energy required to break the hydrogen bonds to water must be subtracted from the energy gained from formation of new hydrogen bonds between atoms in the folded protein in calculating the net contribution of hydrogen-bonding forces to the folding.

Electrostatic Interactions

Electrostatic interactions (also referred to as **ionic** or **salt linkages**) between charged groups are important in the stabilization of protein structure and in binding of charged ligands and substrates to proteins. Electrostatic forces are repulsive or attractive depending on whether the interacting charges are of the same or opposite sign. The strength of an electrostatic force (ΔE_{el}) is directly dependent on the charge (Z) of each ion and is inversely dependent on the dielectric constant (D) of the solvent and the distance between the charges (r_{ab}) (Figure 2.49).

$$E_{el} \approx \frac{Z_A \cdot Z_B \cdot \varepsilon^2}{D \cdot r_{ab}}$$

FIGURE 2.49
Strength of electrostatic interactions.

Water has a high dielectric constant (D = 80), and interactions in water are relatively weak in comparison to the strength of charge interactions in the interior of a protein where the dielectric constant is low. However, most charged groups of proteins remain on the surface of the protein where they do not interact with other charged groups from the protein because of the high dielectric constant of the water solvent, but are stabilized by hydrogen bonding and polar interactions to the water. These water interactions generate the dominant forces that lead to placement of most charged groups of a protein on the outside of the folded structures.

Van der Waals–London Dispersion Forces

Van der Waals and **London dispersion forces** are the weakest of the noncovalent forces. They have an attractive term (A) inversely dependent on the 6th power of the distance between two interacting atoms (r_{ab}), and a repulsive term (B) inversely dependent on the 12th power of r_{ab} (Figure 2.50). The A term contributes at its optimum distance an attractive force of less than 1 kcal mol^{-1} per atomic interaction due to the induction of complementary partial charges or dipoles in the electron density of adjacent atoms when the electron orbitals of the two atoms approach to a close distance. As the atoms come even closer, however, the repulsive component (term B) of the van der Waals force predominates as the electron orbitals of the adjacent atoms begin to overlap. The repulsive force is commonly called **steric hindrance.**

The distance of maximum favorable interaction between two atoms is the **van der Waals contact distance,** which is the sum of the van der Waals radii for the two atoms (Figure 2.51). The van der Waals radii for atoms found in proteins are given in Table 2.16.

The van der Waals repulsive forces between atoms attached to a peptide bond are weakest at the specific ϕ and ψ angles compatible with the α-helix and β-strand structures. Thus van der Waals forces are critical for secondary structure formation in proteins. In folding into a tertiary structure, the number of weak van der Waals interactions that occur are in the thousands. Thus the total contribution of van der Waals–London dispersion forces to the stability of a folded structure is substantial, even though a single interaction between any two atoms is less than 1 kcal mol^{-1}.

A special type of interaction (π-electron–π-electron) occurs when two aromatic rings approach each other with electrons of their aromatic rings favorably interacting (Figure 2.52). This interaction can result in attractive forces of up to 6 kcal mol^{-1}. A number of π–π aromatic interactions occur in a typical folded protein, contributing to the stability of the folded structure.

$$E_{VDW} = -\frac{A}{r_{ab}^{6}} + \frac{B}{r_{ab}^{12}}$$

FIGURE 2.50
Strength of van der Waals interactions.

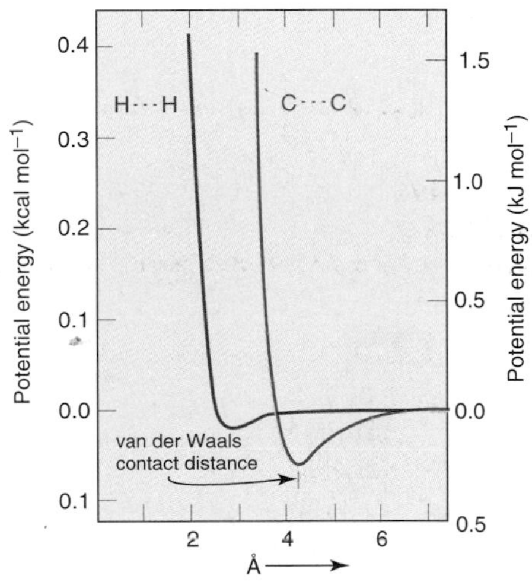

FIGURE 2.51
Van der Waals–London dispersion interaction energies between two hydrogen atoms and two (tetrahedral) carbon atoms.
Negative energies are favorable and positive energies unfavorable.
Redrawn from Fersht, A. Enzyme Structure and Mechanism. *San Francisco: Freeman, 1977, p. 228.*

Denaturation of Proteins Leads to Loss of Native Structure

Denaturation occurs when a protein loses its native secondary, tertiary, and/or quaternary structure. The primary structure is not necessarily broken by denaturation. The **denatured state** is always correlated with the loss of a protein's function. Loss of a protein's function is not necessarily synonymous with denaturation, however, because small conformational changes can lead

TABLE 2.16 Covalent Bond Radii and van der Waals Radii for Selected Atoms

Atom	*Covalent Radius (Å)*	*van der Waals Radius (Å)*[a]
Carbon (tetrahedral)	0.77	2.0
Carbon (aromatic)	0.69 along=bond 0.73 along—bond	1.70
Carbon (amide)	0.72 to amide N 0.67 to oxygen 0.75 to chain C	1.50
Hydrogen	0.33	1.0
Oxygen (—O—)	0.66	1.35
Oxygen (=O)	0.57	1.35
Nitrogen (amide)	0.60 to amide C 0.70 to hydrogen bond H 0.70 to chain C	1.45
Sulfur, diagonal	1.04	1.70

Source: Fasman, G. D. (Ed.), *CRC Handbook of Biochemistry and Molecular Biology,* 3rd ed., Sect. D, Vol. II, Boca Raton, FL: CRC Press, 1976, p. 221.

[a] The van der Waals contact distance is the sum of the two van der Waals radii for the two atoms in proximity.

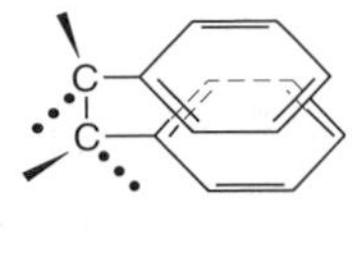

FIGURE 2.52
π-Electron–π-electron interactions between two aromatic rings.

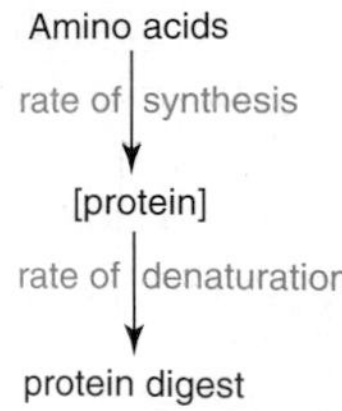

FIGURE 2.53
Steady-state concentration of a protein is due to its rates of synthesis and denaturation.

to loss of function. A change in conformation of a single side chain in the active site of an enzyme or a change in protonation of a side chain can result in loss of activity, but does not lead to a complete loss of the native protein structure.

Even though conformational differences between denatured and native structures may be substantial, the free energy difference between such structures can in some cases be as low as the free energy of three or four noncovalent bonds. Thus the loss of a single hydrogen bond or electrostatic or hydrophobic interaction can lead to destabilization of a folded structure. A change in stability of a noncovalent bond can, in turn, be caused by a change in pH, ionic strength, or temperature. Binding of prosthetic groups, cofactors, and substrates also affects stability of the native conformation.

The statement that the breaking of a single noncovalent bond in a protein can cause denaturation apparently conflicts with the observation that the amino acid sequence can often be extensively varied without loss of a protein's structure. The key to the resolution of this apparent conflict is the word "essential." Many noncovalent interactions are not essential to the structural stability of the native conformation of a protein. However, substitution or modification of an essential amino acid that provides a critical noncovalent interaction dramatically affects the stability of a native protein structure.

The concentration of a protein in a cell is controlled by its rate of synthesis and degradation (Figure 2.53). Understanding the processes that control protein degradation is therefore as equally important as an understanding of the processes that regulate protein synthesis. Under many circumstances the denaturation of a protein is the rate-controlling step in its degradation. Cellular enzymes and organelles that digest proteins "recognize" denatured protein conformations and eliminate them rapidly. In experimental situations, protein denaturation occurs on addition of urea or detergents (sodium dodecyl sulfate or guanidine hydrochloride) that weaken hydrophobic bonding in proteins. These reagents stabilize the denatured state and shift the equilibrium toward the denatured form of the protein. Addition of strong base, acid, or organic solvent, or heating to temperatures above 60°C are also common ways to denature a protein.

2.8 ■ DYNAMIC ASPECTS OF PROTEIN STRUCTURE

While high-resolution X-ray diffraction experiments yield atomic coordinates for each atom in a protein structure, experimental evidence from NMR, fluorescence spectroscopy, and the temperature dependence of the X-ray diffraction reveals that the atoms in a folded protein molecule have a fluid-like dynamic motion and do not exist in a single static position. Rather than an exact location, the atomic coordinates obtained by X-ray diffraction represent the time-averaged position for each atom. The time frame for position averaging is the length of time for data collection, which may be several days. Thus the active conformation may differ from the average conformation. An X-ray structure also shows small "defects" in packing of the folded structure, indicating the existence of "holes" in the structure that will allow the protein space for flexibility. The concept that each atom in a protein is in constant motion such as molecules within a fluid, although constrained by its covalent bonds and the secondary and tertiary structure, is an important aspect of protein structure.

Theoretical **molecular dynamics** calculations describe the changes in coordinates of atoms in a folded protein structure, with corresponding changes in position of regions of the structure due to summation of the movements of atoms in that region. The dynamic motion computation is based on the solving of Newton's equations of motion simultaneously for all the atoms of the protein and the solvent that interacts with the protein. The energy functions used in the equation include representations of covalent and noncovalent bonding energies due to electrostatic forces, hydrogen bonding, and van der Waals

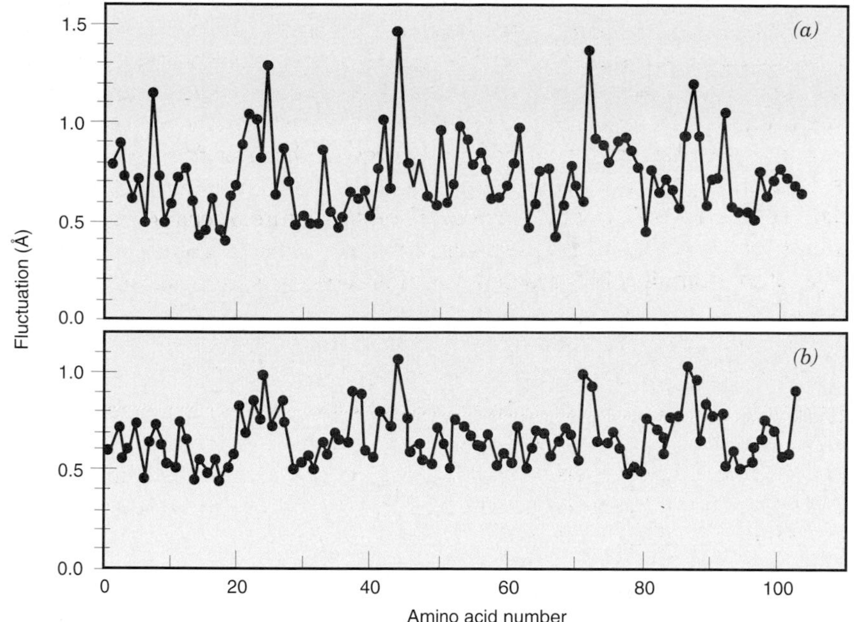

FIGURE 2.54
Fluctuation of structure of cytochrome *c*. (*a*) Calculated fluctuation on a picosecond time scale of α-carbons within each amino acid residue in the folded structure of cytochrome-*c* and (*b*) experimentally observed fluctuation of each α-carbon of the amino acid residues determined from the temperature dependency of the X-ray diffraction pattern for the protein. Cytochrome-*c* has 103 amino acid residues. The *x*-axis plots the amino acid residues in cytochrome-*c* from 1 to 103, and the *y*-axis the fluctuation distances in angstroms.
Redrawn from Karplus, M., and McCammon, J. A. Annu. Rev. Biochem. *53:263, 1983.*

forces. Individual atoms are randomly assigned a velocity from a theoretical distribution and Newton's equations are used to "relax" the system at a given "temperature." The calculation is a computationally intensive activity, even when limited to less than several hundred picoseconds (1 ps $= 10^{-12}$ s) of protein dynamic time, and frequently requires supercomputers. These calculations indicate that the average atom within a typical protein is oscillating over a distance of 0.7 Å on the picosecond scale. Some atoms or groups of atoms move smaller or larger distances than this calculated average (Figure 2.54).

Net movement of any segment of a polypeptide over time represents the sum of forces due to rapid atomic oscillations and the local jiggling and elastic movements of covalently attached groups of atoms. These movements within the closely packed interior of a protein molecule are frequently large enough to allow the planar aromatic rings of buried tyrosines to flip. Furthermore, the small amplitude fluctuations provide the "lubricant" for large motions in proteins such as domain motions and quaternary structure changes, like those observed in hemoglobin on O_2 binding (see Chapter 3). The dynamic behavior of proteins is implicated in conformational changes induced by substrate, inhibitor, or drug binding to enzymes and receptors, generation of allosteric effects in hemoglobins, electron transfer in cytochromes, and in the formation of supramolecular assemblies such as viruses. The movements may also have a functional role in the protein's mechanism of action.

2.9 METHODS FOR CHARACTERIZATION, PURIFICATION, AND STUDY OF PROTEIN STRUCTURE AND ORGANIZATION

Separation of Proteins on Basis of Charge

In **electrophoresis,** the protein dissolved in a solution buffered at a particular pH is placed in an electric field. Depending on the relationship of the buffer pH to the p*I* of the protein, the molecule moves toward the cathode (−) or the anode (+) or remains stationary (pH = p*I*). Procedures for electrophoresis use supports such as polymer gels (e.g., polyacrylamide), starch, or paper. The inert supports are saturated with buffer solution, a sample of protein is placed

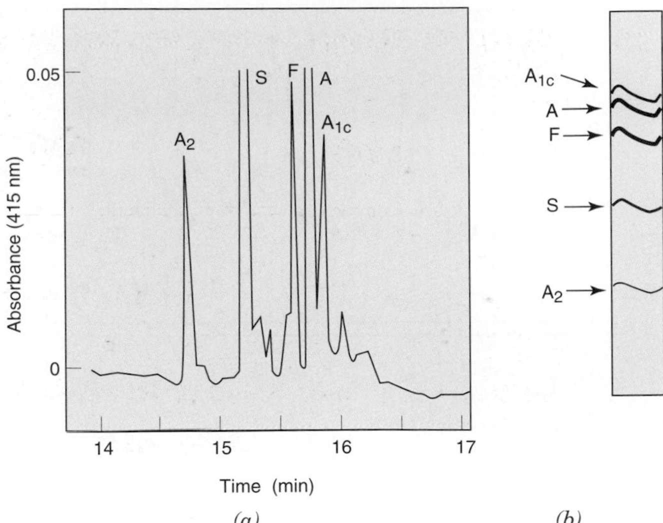

FIGURE 2.55
Isoelectric focusing of hemoglobins from patient heterozygous for HbS and β-thalassemia.
Figure shows separation by isoelectric focusing of HbA_{1c} (HbA glycosylated on NH_2 end, see Clin. Corr. 2.7), normal adult HbA, fetal HbF, sickle cell HbS (see Clin. Corr. 2.3), and the minor adult HbA_2. (*a*) Isoelectric focusing carried out by capillary electrophoresis with ampholyte pH range between 6.7 and 7.7 and detection of bands at 415 nm. (*b*) Isoelectric focusing carried out on gel with Pharmacia PhastSystem; ampholyte pH range is between 6.7 and 7.7.
From Molteni, S., Frischknecht, H., and Thormann, W. Electrophoresis *15:22, 1994 (Figure 4, parts A and B).*

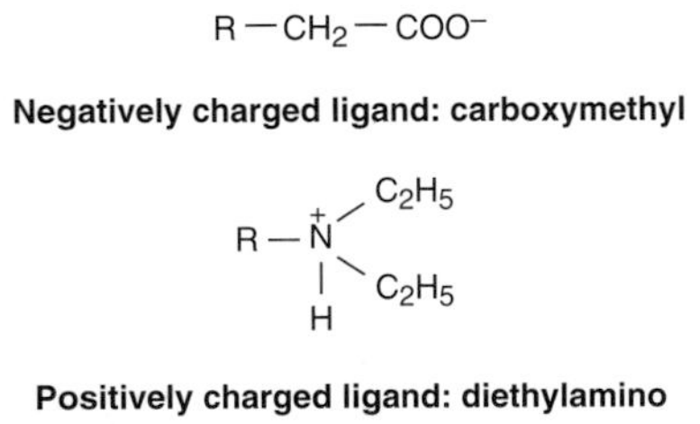

$R-CH_2-COO^-$

Negatively charged ligand: carboxymethyl

$R-\overset{+}{N}H(C_2H_5)_2$

Positively charged ligand: diethylamino

FIGURE 2.56
Two examples of charged ligands used in ion-exchange chromatography.

on the support, an electric field is applied across the support, and the charged proteins migrate in the support toward the oppositely charged pole.

An electrophoresis technique with extremely high resolution is **isoelectric focusing,** in which mixtures of polyamino–polycarboxylic acid ampholytes with a defined range of p*I* values are used to establish a pH gradient across the applied electric field. A charged protein migrates through the pH gradient in the electric field until it reaches a pH region in the gradient equal to its p*I* value. At this point the protein becomes stationary and may be visualized (Figure 2.55). Proteins that differ by as little as 0.0025 in p*I* values are separated on the appropriate pH gradient.

Ion-exchange column chromatography is used for preparative separation of proteins by charge. Ion-exchange resins consist of insoluble materials (agarose, polyacrylamide, cellulose, and glass) that contain negatively or positively charged groups (Figure 2.56). Negatively charged resins bind cations strongly and are **cation-exchange resins.** Positively charged resins bind anions strongly and are **anion-exchange resins.** The degree of retardation of a protein (or an amino acid) by a resin depends on the magnitude of the charge on the protein at the particular pH of the experiment. Molecules of the same charge as the resin are eluted first in a single band, followed by proteins with an opposite charge to that of the resin, in an order based on the protein's charge density (Figure 2.57). When it is difficult to remove a molecule from the resin because of the strength of the attractive interaction between the bound molecule and resin, systematic changes in pH or in ionic strength are used to weaken the interaction. For example, an increasing pH gradient through a cation-exchange resin reduces the difference between the solution pH and the p*I* of the bound protein. This decrease between pH and p*I* reduces the magnitude of the net charge on the protein and decreases the strength of the charge interaction between the protein and the resin. An increasing gradient of ionic strength also decreases the strength of charge interactions and elutes tightly bound electrolytes from the resin.

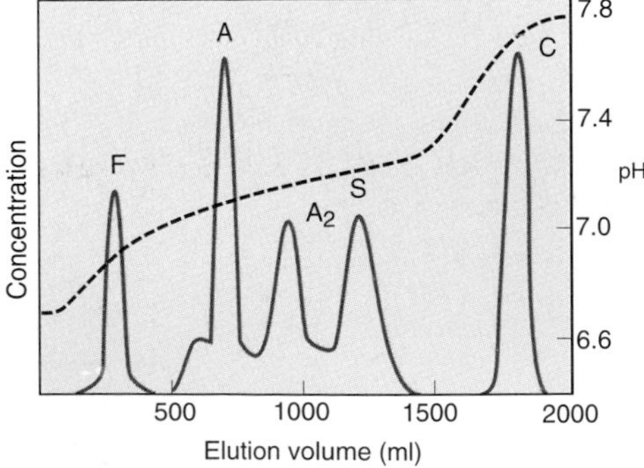

FIGURE 2.57
Example of ion-exchange chromatography.
Elution diagram of an artificial mixture of hemoglobins F, A, A_2, S, and C on carboxymethyl–Sephadex C-50.
From Dozy, A. M., and Juisman, T. H. J. J. Chromatog. *40:62, 1969.*

Capillary Electrophoresis

Electrophoresis within a fused silica capillary tube has a high separation efficiency, utilizes very small samples, and requires only several minutes for an assay. A long capillary tube is filled with the electrophoretic medium, the sample is injected in a narrow band near the anode end of the tube, and the molecules of the sample are separated by their mobility toward the negatively charged pole. The fused silica wall of the capillary has a negatively charged surface to

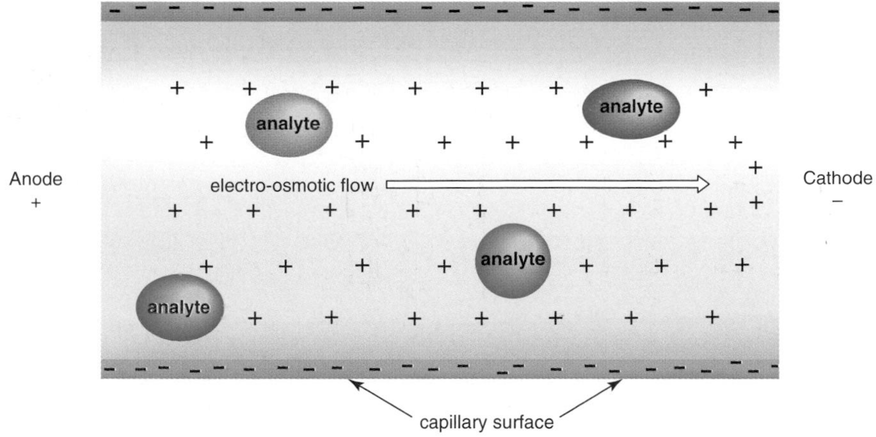

FIGURE 2.58
Generation of electro-osmotic flow toward cathode in capillary electrophoresis.

which an immobile cationic layer is fixed. An adjacent diffuse layer of cations moves toward the cathode in the applied electric field and causes a flow of solvent toward the cathode. This electro-osmotic flow creates a "current" that carries analyte molecules toward the cathode, irrespective of the analyte's charge (Figure 2.58). Molecules with a high positive charge to mass ratio "swim" with the current and have the highest mobility, followed by neutral molecules. Anionic molecules will be repelled by the cathode and will "swim" against the electro-osmotic flow. However, the electro-osmotic current toward the cathode overcomes any negative migration, and anions also migrate toward the cathode but at a slower rate than the cationic or neutral molecules.

In addition to zone electrophoresis, in which the separations are run in the presence of a single buffer, capillary electrophoresis may be performed in the presence of ampholytes to separate proteins by isoelectric focusing, in the presence of a porous gel to separate proteins by molecular weight, or in the presence of a micellar component to separate by hydrophobicity. Detectors that utilize UV light, fluorescence, Raman spectroscopy, electrochemical detection, or mass spectroscopy make the capillary method sensitive and versatile.

Separation of Proteins Based on Molecular Mass or Size

Ultracentrifugation: Definition of Svedberg Coefficient

A protein subjected to centrifugal force moves in the direction of the force at a velocity dependent on its mass. The rate of movement is measured with an appropriate optical detection system, and from the rate the sedimentation coefficient is calculated in **Svedberg units** (units of 10^{-13} s). In the equation (Figure 2.59), v is the measured velocity of protein movement, ω the angular velocity of the centrifuge rotor, and r the distance from the center of the tube in which the protein is placed to the center of rotation. Sedimentation coefficients between 1 and 200 Svedberg units (S) have been found for proteins (Table 2.17). Equations have been derived to relate the sedimentation coefficient to the molecular mass of a protein. One of the more simple equations is shown in Figure 2.60, in which R is the gas constant, T the temperature, s the sedimentation coefficient, D the diffusion coefficient of the protein, $\bar{v}$ the partial specific volume of the protein, and ρ the density of the solvent. The quantities D and $\bar{v}$ must be measured in independent experiments. The equation assumes a spheroidal geometry for the protein. Because this assumption may not be true and independent measurements of D and $\bar{v}$ are difficult, usually only the sedimentation coefficient for a molecule is reported. A protein's sedimentation coefficient is a qualitative measurement of molecular mass.

$$s = \frac{v}{\omega^2 r}$$

FIGURE 2.59
Equation for calculation of the Svedberg coefficient.

$$\text{Molecular weight} = \frac{RTs}{D(1 - \bar{v}\rho)}$$

FIGURE 2.60
An equation relating the Svedberg coefficient to molecular weight.

TABLE 2.17 Svedberg Coefficients for Some Plasma Proteins of Different Molecular Weights

Protein	*s_{20}, × 10^{-13} (cm s^{-1} dyn^{-1})[a]*	*Molecular Weight*
Lysozyme	2.19	15,000–16,000
Albumin	4.6	69,000
Immunoglobulin G	6.6–7.2	153,000
Fibrinogen	7.63	341,000
C1q (factor of complement)	11.1	410,000
α_2-Macroglobulin	19.6	820,000
Immunoglobulin M	18–20	1,000,000
Factor VIII of blood coagulation	23.7	1,120,000

Source: Fasman, G. D. (Ed.), *CRC Handbook of Biochemistry and Molecular Biology,* 3rd ed., Sect. A, Vol. II. Boca Raton, FL: CRC Press, 1976, p. 242.

[a] s_{20}, × 10^{-13} is sedimentation coefficient in Svedberg units, referred to water at 20°C, and extrapolated to zero concentration of protein.

Molecular Exclusion Chromatography

A porous gel in the form of small insoluble beads is commonly used to separate proteins by size in column chromatography. Small protein molecules penetrate the pores of the gel and have a larger solvent volume through which to travel in the column than large proteins, which are sterically excluded from the pores. Accordingly, a protein mixture is separated by size. The larger proteins are eluted first, followed by the smaller proteins, which are retarded by their accessibility to a larger solvent volume (Figure 2.61). As with ultracentrifugation, an assumption is made as to the geometry of an unknown protein in the determination of molecular mass. Elongated nonspheroidal proteins give anomalous molecular masses when analyzed using a standard curve determined with proteins of spheroidal geometry.

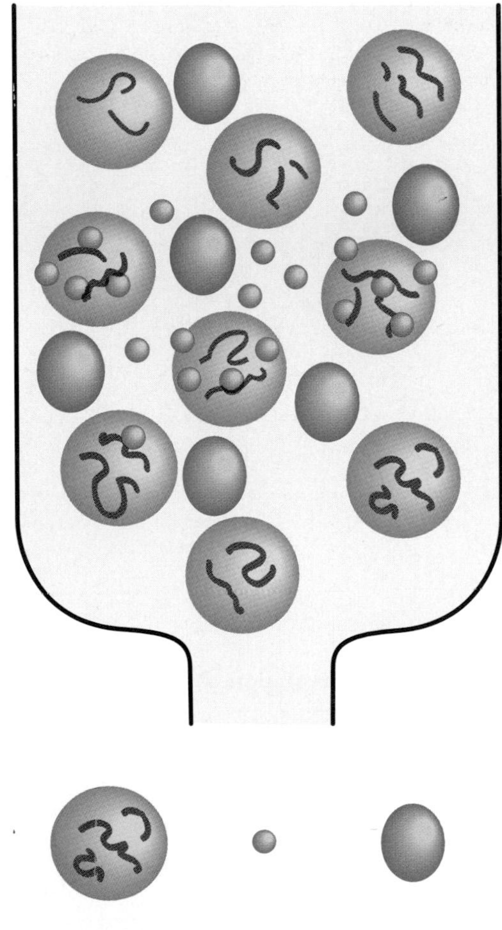

FIGURE 2.61
Molecular exclusion chromatography.
A small protein can enter the porous gel particles and will be retarded on the column with respect to a larger protein that cannot enter the porous gel particles.

Polyacrylamide Gel Electrophoresis in the Presence of a Detergent

If a charged detergent is added to a protein electrophoresis assay and electrophoresis occurs through a sieving support, the separation of proteins is based on protein size and not charge. A common detergent is **sodium dodecyl sulfate (SDS)** and a common sieving support is **cross-linked polyacrylamide.** The dodecyl sulfates are amphophilic C12 alkyl sulfate molecules, which stabilize a denatured protein by forming a charged micellar SDS solvation shell around its polypeptide chain. The inherent charge of the polypeptide chain is obliterated by the negatively charged micelle of SDS molecules, and each protein–SDS solubilized aggregate has an identical charge per unit volume. Negatively charged micelle particles move through the polyacrylamide gel toward the anode. Polyacrylamide acts as a molecular sieve and the protein–micelle complexes are separated by size; proteins of larger mass are retarded. A single band in an SDS polyacrylamide electrophoresis experiment is often used to demonstrate the purity of a protein. The conformation of the native structure is not a factor in the calculation of molecular mass, which is determined by comparison to known standards that are similarly denatured. The detergent dissociates quaternary structure into its constituent subunits. Only the molecular masses of the covalent polypeptide subunits within a protein are determined by this method.

HPLC Chromatographic Techniques Separate Amino Acids, Peptides, and Proteins

In high-performance liquid chromatography (HPLC), a liquid solvent containing a mixture of components to be identified is passed through a column densely

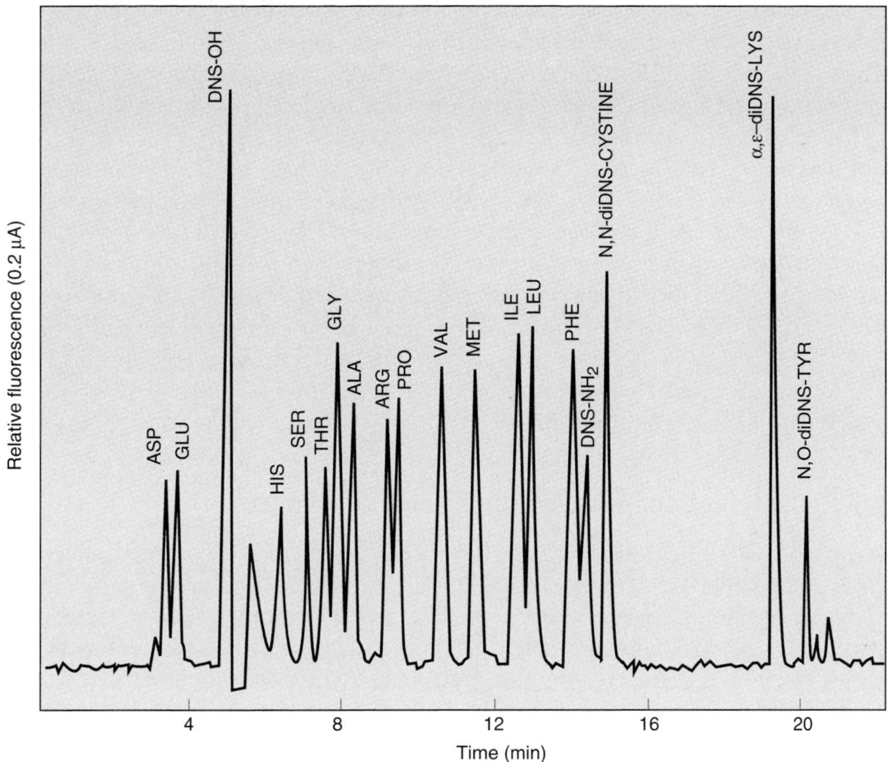

FIGURE 2.62
Separation of amino acids utilizing reverse-phase HPLC.
The x-axis is time of elution from column. Amino acids are derivatized by reaction with dansyl chloride (DNS) so that they emit a fluorescence that is used to assay them as they are eluted from the column.
Reprinted with permission from Hunkapiller, M. W., Strickler, J. E., and Wilson, K. J. Science *226:304, 1984. Copyright © 1984 by American Association for the Advancement of Science.*

packed with a small-diameter insoluble bead-like resin. In column chromatography, the smaller and more tightly packed the resin beads, the greater the resolution of the separation technique. In HPLC, the resin is so tightly packed that in order to overcome the resistance the liquid must be pumped through the column at high pressure. Therefore HPLC uses precise high-pressure pumps with metal plumbing and columns rather than glass and plastics as used in gravity chromatography. Resin beads are coated with charged chemical groups to separate compounds by ion exchange or with hydrophobic groups to retard hydrophobic nonpolar molecules. In hydrophobic chromatography, tightly associated nonpolar compounds are eluted from the hydrophobic beads in aqueous solvents containing various percentages of an organic reagent. The higher the percentage of organic solvent in the eluent, the faster the nonpolar component is eluted from the hydrophobic resin. This latter type of chromatography over nonpolar resin beads is called **reverse-phase HPLC** (Figure 2.62). The HPLC separations have extremely high resolution and reproducibility.

Affinity Chromatography

Proteins have a high affinity for their substrates, prosthetic groups, membrane receptors, specific noncovalent inhibitors, and antibodies made against them. These high-affinity compounds can be covalently attached to an insoluble resin and the modified resin used to purify its conjugate protein in column chromatography. In a mixture of proteins eluted through the resin, the one of interest is selectively retarded.

General Approach to Protein Purification

A protein must be purified prior to a meaningful characterization of its chemical composition, structure, and function. As living cells contain thousands of genetically distinct proteins, the purification of a single protein from the other cellular constituents may be difficult. The first task in the purification of a protein is

CLINICAL CORRELATION 2.8

Use of Amino Acid Analysis in Diagnosis of Disease

There are a number of clinical disorders in which a high concentration of amino acids is found in plasma and urine. An abnormally high concentration of an amino acid in urine is called an aminoaciduria. In phenylketonuria patients lack sufficient amounts of the enzyme phenylalanine hydroxylase, which catalyzes the transformation of phenylalanine to tyrosine. As a result, large concentrations of phenylalanine, phenylpyruvate, and phenyllactate accumulate in the plasma and urine. Phenylketonuria occurs clinically in the first few weeks after birth, and if the infant is not placed on a special diet, severe mental retardation will occur (see Clin. Corr. 11.5). Cystinuria is a genetically transmitted defect in the membrane transport system for cystine and the basic amino acids (lysine, arginine, and the derived amino acid ornithine) in epithelial cells. Large amounts of these amino acids are excreted in urine. Other symptoms of this disease may arise from the formation of renal stones composed of cystine precipitated within the kidney (see Clin. Corr. 11.9). Hartnup disease is a genetically transmitted defect in epithelial cell transport of neutral amino acids (monoamino monocarboxylic acids), and high concentrations of these amino acids are found in the urine. The physical symptoms of the disease are primarily caused by a deficiency of tryptophan. These symptoms may include a pellagra-like rash (nicotinamide is partly derived from tryptophan) and cerebellar ataxia (irregular and jerky muscular movements) due to the toxic effects of indole derived from the bacterial degradation of unabsorbed tryptophan present in large amounts in the gut. Fanconi's syndrome is a generalized aminoaciduria associated with hypophosphatemia and a high excretion of glucose. Abnormal reabsorption of amino acids, phosphate, and glucose by the tubular cells is the underlying defect.

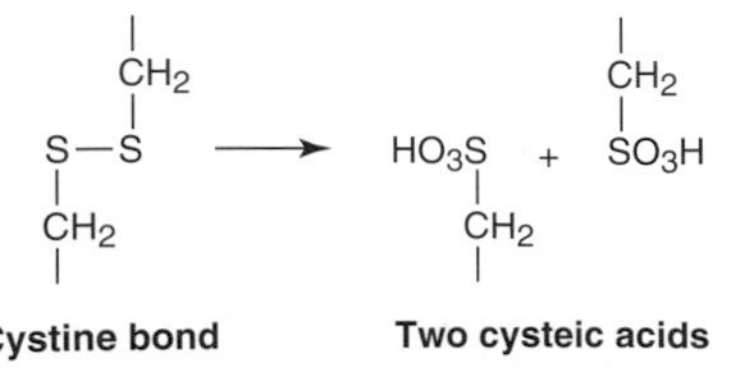

$$\begin{matrix} | \\ CH_2 \\ | \\ S-S \\ | \\ CH_2 \\ | \end{matrix} \longrightarrow \begin{matrix} HO_3S \\ | \\ CH_2 \\ | \end{matrix} + \begin{matrix} | \\ CH_2 \\ | \\ SO_3H \end{matrix}$$

Cystine bond — Two cysteic acids

FIGURE 2.63
Breaking of disulfide bonds by oxidation to cysteic acids.

the development of a simple assay for the protein. Whether it utilizes the rate of a substrate transformation to a product, an antibody–antigen reaction, or a physiological response in an animal assay system, a protein assay must give a quantitative measurement of activity per unit of protein concentration. This quantity is known as the sample's **specific activity.** The purpose of a purification procedure is to increase a sample's specific activity to the value expected for the pure protein. A typical protocol for purification of a soluble cellular protein involves the disruption of the cellular membrane, followed by a differential centrifugation in a density gradient to isolate the protein from subcellular particles and high molecular weight aggregates. Further purification may utilize selective precipitation by addition of inorganic salts (salting out) or addition of miscible organic solvent to the solution containing the protein. Final purification will include a combination of techniques that separate based on molecular charge, molecular size, and affinity.

Determination of Amino Acid Composition of a Protein

Determination of the amino acid composition is an essential component in the study of a protein's structure and physiological properties. Analysis of the amino acid composition of physiological fluids (i.e., blood and urine) is utilized in diagnosis of disease (see Clin. Corr. 2.8). A protein is hydrolyzed to its constituent amino acids by heating the protein at 110°C in 6 N HCl for 18–36 h, in a sealed tube under vacuum to prevent degradation of oxidation-sensitive amino acid side chains by oxygen in air. Tryptophan is destroyed in this method and alternative procedures are used for its analysis. Asparagine and glutamine side chain amides are hydrolyzed to unsubstituted carboxylic acid side chains and free ammonia; thus they are counted within the glutamic acid and aspartic acid content in the analysis.

Common procedures for amino acid identification use cation-exchange chromatography or reverse-phase HPLC to separate the amino acids, which are then reacted with ninhydrin, fluorescamine, dansyl chloride, or similar chromophoric or fluorophoric reagents to quantitate the separated amino acids (Figure 2.62). With some types of derivatization, amino acids are identified at concentrations as low as 0.5×10^{-12} mol (pmol).

Techniques to Determine Amino Acid Sequence of a Protein

The ability to clone genes for proteins has led to the determination of the amino acid sequence of a protein as derived from the DNA or RNA sequences (see Chapter 18). This is a much faster method for obtaining an amino acid sequence. Sequencing of a protein, however, is required for the determination of modifications to the protein structure that occur after its biosynthesis, to identify a part of the protein sequence in order that its gene can be cloned, and to identify a protein as the product of a particular gene (see Chapter 17). Determination of the primary structure of a protein requires a purified protein. Many proteins contain several polypeptide chains and it is necessary to determine the number of chains in the protein. Individual chains are purified by the same techniques used in purification of the whole protein. If disulfide bonds covalently join the chains, these bonds have to be broken (Figure 2.63).

Polypeptide chains are most commonly sequenced by the **Edman reaction** (Figure 2.64) in which the polypeptide chain is reacted with phenylisothiocyanate, which forms a covalent bond to the NH_2-terminal amino acid. In this derivative, acidic conditions catalyze an intramolecular cyclization that results in cleavage of the NH_2-terminal amino acid from the polypeptide chain as a phenylthiohydantoin derivative. This NH_2-terminal amino acid derivative may be separated chromatographically and identified against standards. The polypeptide chain minus the NH_2-terminal amino acid is then isolated, and the

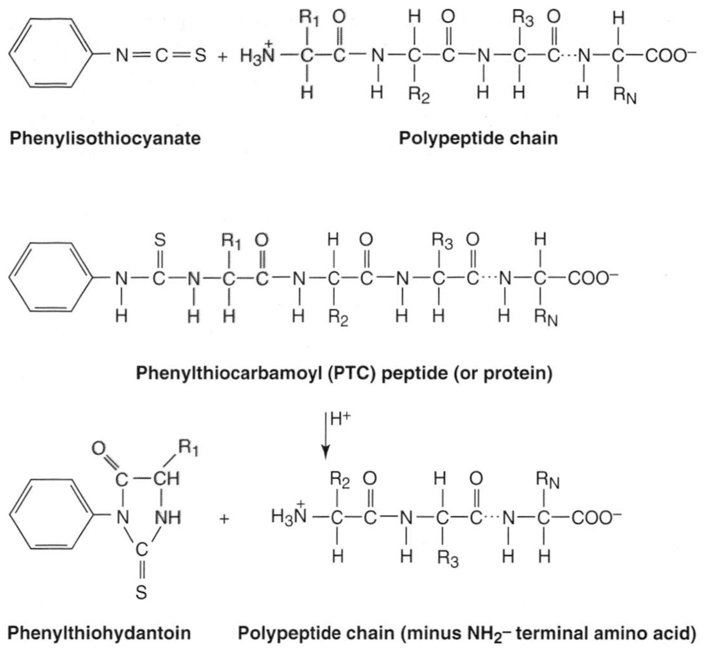

Phenylisothiocyanate

Polypeptide chain

Phenylthiocarbamoyl (PTC) peptide (or protein)

Phenylthiohydantoin

Polypeptide chain (minus NH_2– terminal amino acid)

FIGURE 2.64
Edman reaction.

Edman reaction is repeated to identify the next NH_2-terminal amino acid. This series of reactions can theoretically be repeated until the sequence of the entire polypeptide chain is determined but under favorable conditions can only be carried out for 30 or 40 amino acids into the polypeptide chain. At this point in the analysis, impurities generated from incomplete reactions in the reaction series make further **Edman cycles** unfeasible. Since most polypeptide chains in proteins contain many more than 30 or 40 amino acids, they have to be hydrolyzed into smaller fragments and sequenced in sections.

Enzymatic and chemical methods are used to break polypeptide chains into smaller polypeptide fragments for sequencing. The enzyme **trypsin** preferentially catalyzes hydrolysis of the peptide bond on the COOH-terminal side of the basic amino acid residues of lysine and arginine within polypeptide chains. **Chymotrypsin** hydrolyzes peptide bonds on the COOH-terminal side of residues with large apolar side chains. Other proteolytic enzymes cleave polypeptide chains on the COOH-terminal side of glutamic and aspartic acid (Figure 2.65). **Cyanogen bromide** specifically cleaves peptide bonds on the COOH-terminal side of methionine residues within polypeptide chains (Figure

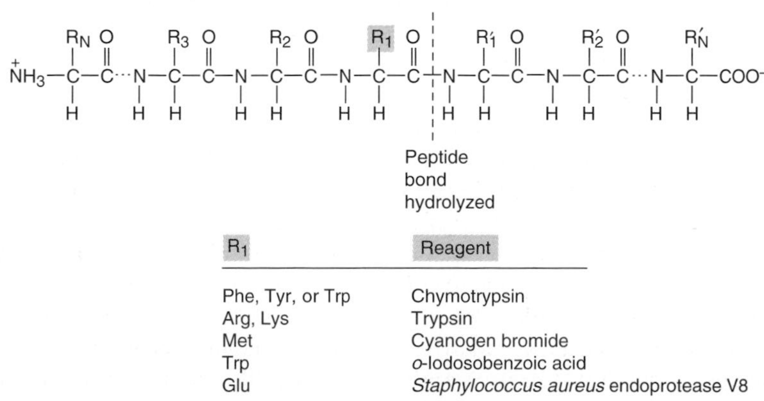

R_1	Reagent
Phe, Tyr, or Trp	Chymotrypsin
Arg, Lys	Trypsin
Met	Cyanogen bromide
Trp	*o*-Iodosobenzoic acid
Glu	*Staphylococcus aureus* endoprotease V8

FIGURE 2.65
Specificity of some polypeptide cleaving reagents.

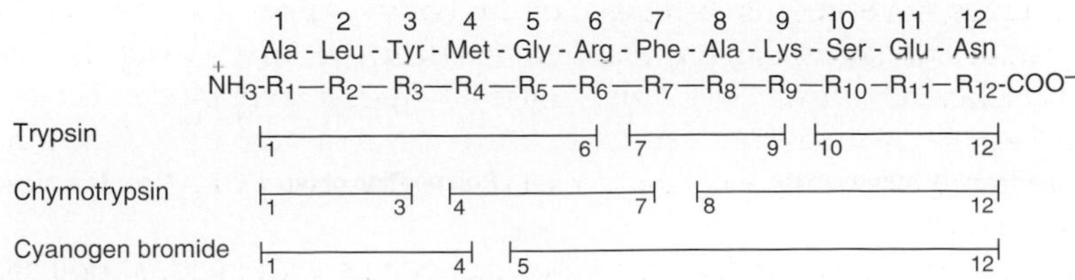

FIGURE 2.66
Ordering of peptide fragments from overlapping sequences produced by specific proteolysis of a peptide.

2.65). To establish the amino acid sequence of a large polypeptide, it is subjected to **partial hydrolysis** by one of the specific cleaving reagents, the polypeptide segments are separated, and the amino acid sequence of each of the small segments is determined by the Edman reaction. To place the sequenced peptides correctly into the complete sequence of the original polypeptide, a sample of the original polypeptide is subjected to a second partial hydrolysis by a different hydrolytic reagent from that used initially. This generates overlapping sequences to the first set of sequences, leading to the complete sequence (Figure 2.66).

X-Ray Diffraction Techniques Are Used to Determine the Three-Dimensional Structure of Proteins

X-ray diffraction enables determination of the three-dimensional structure of proteins at near atomic resolution. The approach requires formation of a protein crystal, which contains solvent and is thus a concentrated solution, for use as the target. Our present understanding of the detailed components of protein structure derived from experiments performed in this crystalline state correlate well with other physical measurements of protein structure in solution such as those made using NMR spectroscopy (see p. 81).

Generation of the protein crystal can be the most time-consuming aspect of the process. A significant factor in both experimental and computational handling of protein crystals, in contrast with most small molecule crystals, stems from the content of the protein crystalline material. Proteins exhibit molecular dimensions an order of magnitude greater than small molecules, and the packing of large protein molecules into the crystal lattice generates a crystal with large "holes" or solvent channels. A protein crystal typically contains 40–60% solvent and may be considered a concentrated solution rather than the hard crystalline solid associated with most small molecules. This attribute proves both beneficial and detrimental. The presence of solvent and unoccupied volume in the crystal allows the infusion of inhibitors and substrates into the protein molecules in the "crystalline state" but also permits a **dynamic flexibility** within regions of the protein structure. The flexibility may be seen as "disorder" in the X-ray diffraction experiment. Disorder is used to describe the situation in which the observed electron density can be fitted by more than a single local conformation. Two explanations for the disorder exist and must be distinguished. The first involves the presence of two or more static molecular conformations, which are present in a stoichiometric relationship. The second involves the actual dynamic range of motion exhibited by atoms or groups of atoms in localized regions of the molecule. An experimental distinction between the two explanations can be made by lowering the environmental temperature of the crystal to a point where dynamic disorder is "frozen out"; in contrast, the static disorder is not temperature dependent and persists. Analysis of dynamic disorder by its temperature dependency using X-ray diffraction determinations is an important method for studying protein dynamics (see Section 2.8). Crystallization techniques have advanced so that crystals are now obtainable from less abundant proteins. Interesting structures are reported for proteins in which specific amino acid residues have been substituted, of antibody–antigen complexes, and of viral products such as the protease required for the infection of the human immunodeficiency virus (HIV) that causes acquired immunodeficiency syndrome (AIDS). Many structures have been solved by X-ray diffraction and the details are stored in a database called the **Protein Data Bank,** which is readily accessible.

Diffraction of X-ray radiation by a crystal occurs with incident radiation of a characteristic wavelength (e.g., copper, K_α = 1.54 Å). The X-ray beam is diffracted by the electrons surrounding the atomic nuclei in the crystal, with an intensity proportional to the number of electrons around the nucleus. Thus the technique establishes the **electron distribution** of the molecule and infers the nuclear distribution. The actual positions of atomic nuclei can be determined directly by diffraction with **neutron beam radiation,** an interesting but very expensive technique as it requires a source of neutrons (nuclear reactor or particle accelerator). With the highest resolution now available for X-ray diffraction determinations of protein structures, the electron diffraction from C, N, O, and S atoms can be observed. The diffraction from hydrogen atoms is not observed due to the low density of electrons—that is, a single electron—around a hydrogen nucleus. Detectors of the diffracted beam, typically photographic film or electronic area detectors, permit the recording of the amplitude (intensity) of radiation diffracted in a defined orientation. However, the data do not give information about phases of the radiation, which are essential to the solution of a protein's structure. Determination of the **phase angles** historically required the placement of heavy atoms (such as iodine, mercury, or lead) in the protein structure. Modern procedures, however, can often solve the phase problem without use of a heavy atom.

It is convenient to consider an analogy between X-ray crystallography and light microscopy to understand the processes involved in carrying out the three-dimensional structure determination. In light microscopy, incident radiation is reflected by an object under study and the reflected beam is recondensed by the objective lens to form an image of the object. The analogy is appropriate to incident X rays with the notable exception that no known material exists that can serve as an objective lens for X-ray radiation. To replace the objective lens, amplitude and phase angle measurements of the diffracted radiation are mathematically reconstructed by **Fourier synthesis** to yield a three-dimensional **electron-density map** of the diffracted object. Initially a few hundred reflections are obtained to construct a low-resolution electron-density map. For example, in one of the first protein crystallographic structures, 400 reflections were utilized to obtain a 6-Å map of myoglobin. At this level of resolution it is possible to locate clearly the molecule within the unit cell of the crystal and study the overall packing of the subunits in a protein with a quaternary structure. A trace of the polypeptide chain of an individual protein molecule is made with difficulty. Utilizing the low-resolution structure as a base, further reflections may be used to obtain higher-resolution maps. For myoglobin, where 400 reflections were utilized to obtain the 6-Å map, 10,000 reflections were needed for a 2-Å map, and 17,000 reflections for an extremely high-resolution 1.4-Å map. Many of these steps are now partially automated using computer graphics. A two-dimensional slice through a three-dimensional electron-density map of trypsinogen is shown in Figure 2.67. The known primary structure of the protein is fitted to the electron-density pattern by refinement. **Refinement** is the computer-intensive process of aligning a protein's amino acid sequence to the electron-density map until the best fit is obtained.

Whereas X-ray diffraction has provided extensive knowledge on protein structure, such a structure provides incomplete evidence for a protein's mechanism of action. The X-ray determined structure is an average structure of a molecule in which atoms are normally undergoing rapid fluctuations in solution (see Section 2.8). Thus the average crystalline structure determined by X-ray

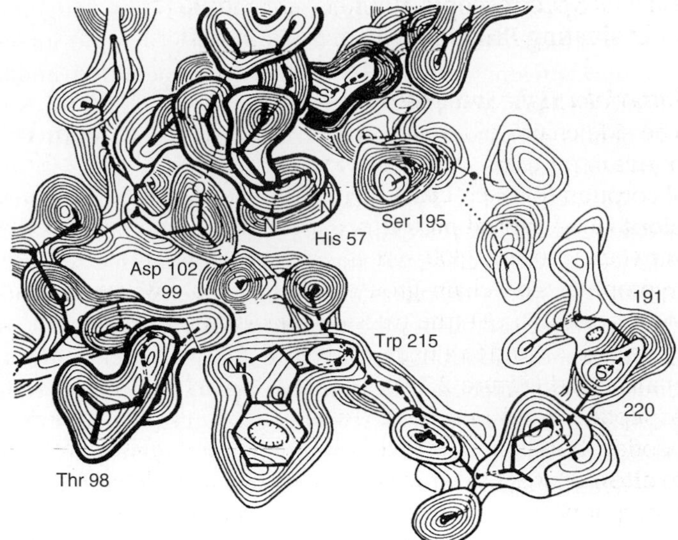

FIGURE 2.67
Electron-density map at 1.9-Å resolution of active site region of proenzyme form of trypsin.
Active site amino acid residues are fitted onto density map.
Reprinted with permission from Kossiakoff, A. A., Chambers, J. L., Kay, L. M., and Stroud, R. M. Biochemistry *16:654, 1977. Copyright © 1977 by American Chemical Society.*

diffraction may not be the active structure of a particular protein in solution. A second important consideration is that it currently takes at least a day to collect data in order to determine a structure. On this time scale, the structures of reactive enzyme–substrate complexes, intermediates, and reaction transition states of an enzyme can not be observed. Rather, these structures must be inferred from the static pictures of an inactive form of the protein or from complexes with inactive analogs of the substrates of the protein (Figure 2.68). Newer methods for X-ray diffraction using synchrotron radiation to generate a X-ray beam at least 10,000 times brighter than that of standard X-ray generators will enable collection of diffraction data to solve a protein structure on a millisecond time scale. Application of the later X-ray techniques will enable scientists to determine short-lived structures and solve mechanistic and dynamic structural questions not addressable by current technology.

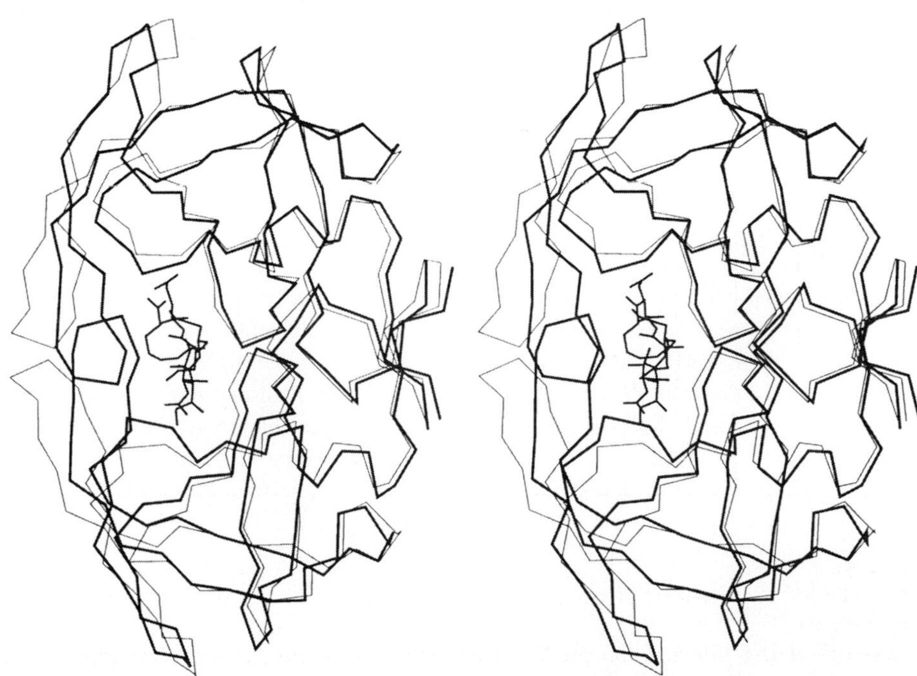

FIGURE 2.68
Stereo tracing of superimposed α-carbon backbone structure of HIV protease with inhibitor bound (thick lines) and the native structure of HIV protease without inhibitor bound (thin lines).
Redrawn with permission from Miller, M., Schneider, J., Sathyanarayana, B. K., Toth, M. V., Marshall, G. R., Clawson, L., Selk, L., Kent, S. B. H., and Wlodawer, A. Science *246:1149, 1989.*

Various Spectroscopic Methods Are Employed in Evaluating Protein Structure and Function

Ultraviolet Light Spectroscopy

The side chains of tyrosine, phenylalanine, and tryptophan, as well as peptide bonds in proteins, absorb **ultraviolet (UV) light.** The efficiency of light energy absorption for each **chromophore** is related to its **molar extinction coefficient** (ε). A typical protein spectrum is shown in Figure 2.69. The absorbance between 260 and 300 nm is primarily due to phenylalanine, tyrosine, and tryptophan side chain groups (Figure 2.70). When the tyrosine side chain is ionized at high pH (the tyrosine R group has a $pK'_a \approx 10$), the absorbance for tyrosine is shifted to a higher wavelength (red shifted) and its molar absorptivity is increased (Figure 2.70). Peptide bonds absorb in the far-UV (180–230 nm). A peptide bond in α-helix conformation interacts with the electrons of other peptide bonds above and below it in the spiral conformation to create an **exciton system** in which electrons are delocalized. The result is a shift of the absorption maximum from that of an isolated peptide bond to either a lower or higher wavelength (Figure 2.71). Thus UV spectroscopy can be used to study changes in a protein's secondary and tertiary structure. As a protein is denatured (helix unfolded), differences are observed in the absorption characteristics of the peptide bonds due to the disruption of the exciton system. In addition, the absorption maximum for an aromatic chromophore appears at a lower wavelength in an aqueous environment than in a nonpolar environment.

The **molar absorbency** of a chromophoric substrate often changes on binding to a protein. This change in the binding molecule's extinction coefficient can be used to measure its binding constant. Changes in chromophore extinction coefficients during the enzyme catalysis of a chemical reaction are used to obtain the kinetic parameters for the reaction.

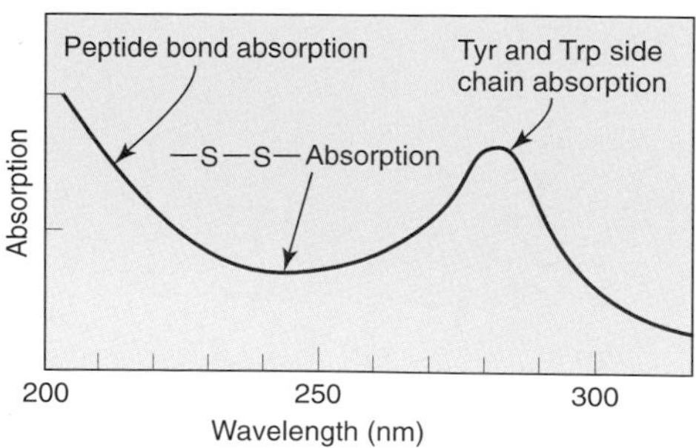

FIGURE 2.69
Ultraviolet absorption spectrum of the globular protein α-chymotrypsin.

Fluorescence Spectroscopy

The energy of an excited electron produced by light absorption is lost by various mechanisms and most commonly as thermal energy in a collision process. In some chromophores the excitation energy is dissipated by fluorescence. The **fluorescent emission** is always at a longer wavelength of light (lower energy) than the absorption wavelength of the fluorophore. Higher vibrational energy

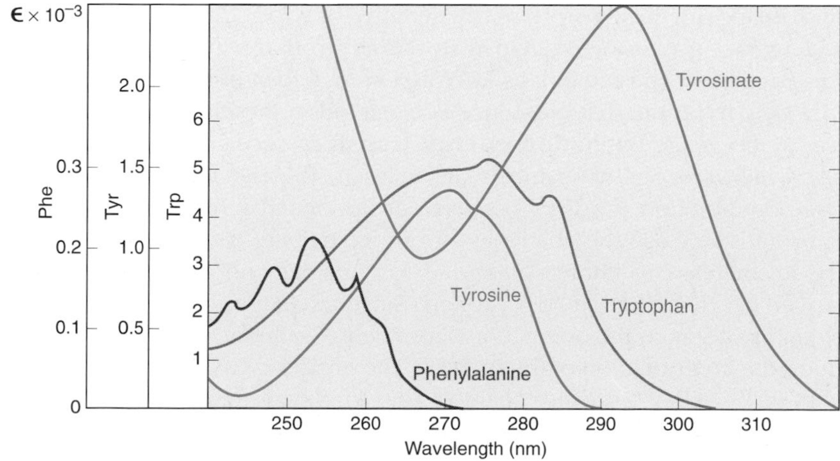

FIGURE 2.70
Ultraviolet absorption for the aromatic chromophores in Phe, Tyr, Trp, and tyrosinate.
Note differences in extinction coefficients on left axis for the different chromophores.
Redrawn from d'Albis, A., and Gratzer, W. B. In: A. T. Bull, J. R. Lagmado, J. O. Thomas, and K. F. Tipton (Eds.), Companion to Biochemistry. *London: Longmans, 1974, p. 170.*

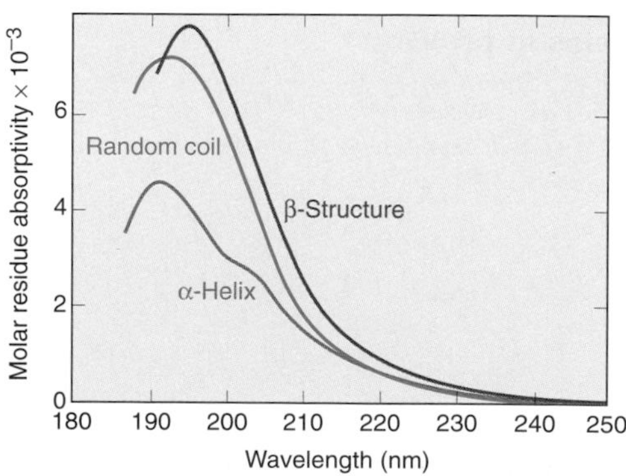

FIGURE 2.71
Ultraviolet absorption of the peptide bonds of a polypeptide chain in α-helix, random coil, and antiparallel β-structure conformations.
Redrawn from d'Albis, A., and Gratzer, W. B. In: A. T. Bull, J. R. Lagmado, J. O. Thomas, and K. F. Tipton (Eds.), Companion to Biochemistry. *London: Longmans, 1970, p. 175.*

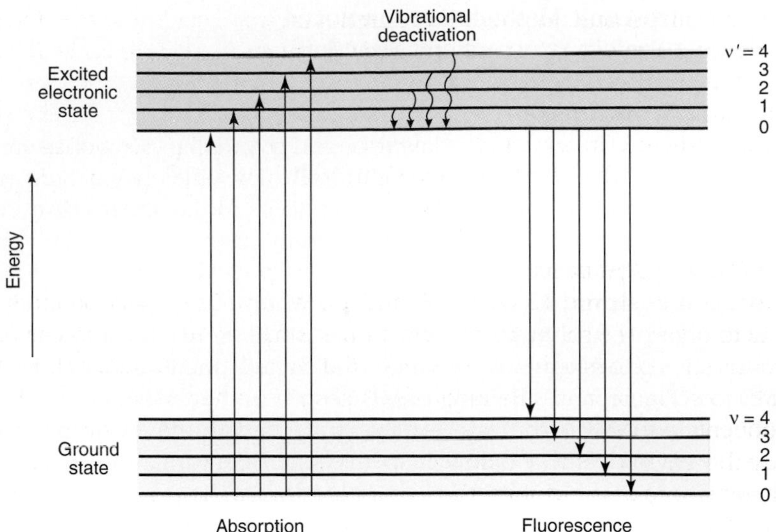

FIGURE 2.72
Absorption and fluorescence electronic transitions.
Excitation is from zero vibrational level in ground state to various higher vibrational levels in the excited state. Fluorescence is from zero vibrational level in excited electronic state to various vibrational levels in the ground state.
Redrawn from d'Albis, A., and Gratzer, W. B. In: A. T. Bull, J. R. Lagmado, J. O. Thomas, and K. F. Tipton (Eds.), Companion to Biochemistry. *London: Longmans, 1970, p. 166.*

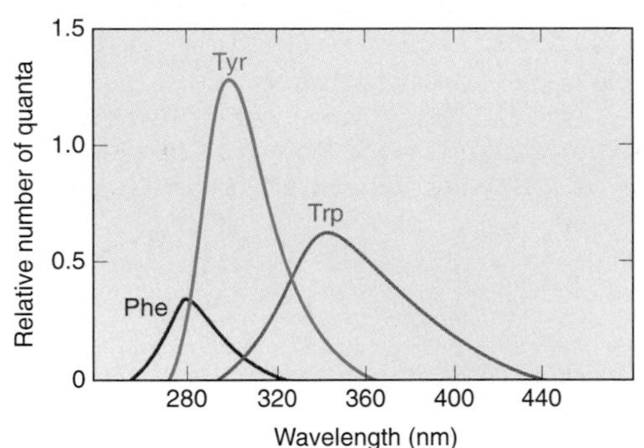

FIGURE 2.73
Characteristic fluorescence of aromatic groups in proteins.
Redrawn from d'Albis, A., and Gratzer, W. B. In: A. T. Bull, J. R. Lagmado, J. O. Thomas, and K. F. Tipton (Eds.), Companion to Biochemistry. *London: Longmans, 1970, p. 478.*

levels, formed in the excited electron state during the excitation event, are lost prior to the fluorescent event (Figure 2.72). If a chromophoric molecule is present that absorbs light energy emitted by the **fluorophore,** the emitted fluorescence is not observed. Rather, the fluorescence energy is transferred to the absorbing molecule. The **acceptor molecule,** in turn, either emits its own characteristic fluorescence or loses its excitation energy by an alternative process. If the acceptor molecule loses its excitation energy by a nonfluorescent process, it is acting as a **quencher** of the **donor molecule's** fluorescence. The efficiency of the **excitation transfer** is dependent on the distance and orientation between donor and acceptor molecules.

Fluorescence emission spectra for phenylalanine, tyrosine, and tryptophan side chains are shown in Figure 2.73. The emission wavelengths for phenylalanine overlap with the absorption wavelengths for tyrosine. In turn, the emission wavelengths for tyrosine overlap with the absorption wavelengths for tryptophan. Because of these overlaps in emission and absorption wavelengths, primarily only tryptophan fluorescence is observed in proteins that contain all of these amino acids. **Excitation energy transfers** occur over distances up to 80 Å, which are typical diameter distances in folded globular proteins. On protein denaturation, the distances between donor and acceptor groups become greater and decrease the efficiency of energy transfer to tryptophan. Accordingly, an increase in fluorescence due to tyrosines and/or phenylalanines is observed on denaturation of a protein. Since excitation transfer processes in proteins are distance and orientation dependent, the fluorescence yield is dependent on the conformation of the protein. The greatest sensitivity of this analysis occurs in its ability to detect changes due to solvent or binding interactions rather than establish absolute structure.

Optical Rotatory Dispersion and Circular Dichroism Spectroscopy

Optical rotation is caused by differences in the refractive index and **circular dichroism** (CD) is caused by differences in the light absorption between the clockwise and counterclockwise component vectors of a beam of polarized light as it travels through a solution containing an optically active molecule such as an L-amino acid. In proteins the aromatic amino acids and the polypeptide chain generate an optical rotation and CD spectrum (Figure 2.74). Because of the differences between α-helical, β-structure, and random polypeptide spectra, circular dichroism has been a sensitive assay for the amount and type of secondary structure in a protein. Newer developments in vibrational circular dichroism examine the CD in regions of the spectrum more sensitive to protein backbone conformation.

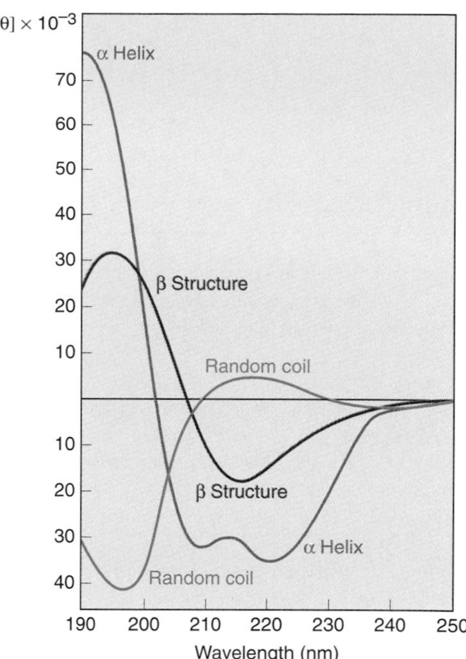

FIGURE 2.74
Circular dichroism spectra for polypeptide chains in α-helix, β-structure, and random coil conformations.
Redrawn from d'Albis, A., and Gratzer, W. B. In: A. T. Bull, J. R. Lagnado, J. O. Thomas, and K. F. Tipton (Eds.), Companion to Biochemistry. *London: Longmans, 1970, p. 190.*

Nuclear Magnetic Resonance

With **two-dimensional** (2-D) **NMR** and powerful NMR spectrometers it is possible to obtain the solution conformation of small proteins of approximately 150 amino acids or less. Multidimensional NMR and triple resonance can extend the NMR to solve protein structures with up to 250 amino acids.

Conventional NMR techniques involve use of radiofrequency (rf) radiation to study the environment of atomic nuclei that are magnetic. The requirement for magnetic nuclei is absolute and is based on an unpaired spin state in the nucleus. Thus the naturally abundant carbon (^{12}C), nitrogen (^{14}N), and oxygen (^{16}O) do not absorb, while ^{13}C, ^{15}N, and ^{17}O do absorb. The absorption bands in an NMR spectrum are characterized by (1) a position or chemical shift value, reported as the frequency difference between that observed for a specific absorption band and that for a standard reference material; (2) the intensity of the peak or integrated area, which is proportional to the total number of absorbing nuclei; (3) the half-height peak width, which reflects the degree of motion in solution of the absorbing species; and (4) the coupling constant, which measures the extent of direct interaction or influence of neighboring nuclei on the absorbing nuclei. These four measurements enable the determination of the identity and number of nearest-neighbor groups that can affect the response of absorbing species through bonded interactions. They give no information on through-space (nonbonded) interaction due to the three-dimensional structure of the protein. To determine through-space interactions and protein tertiary structure requires the use of **nuclear Overhauser effects** (NOEs) and the application of the two-dimensional technique.

The major difference in two-dimensional versus one-dimensional (1-D) NMR is the addition of a second time delay rf pulse. The technique first requires the identification in the spectrum of a proton absorbance from a particular position in the protein structure. A maximum distance of approximately 5 Å is the limit for which these through-space interactions can be observed. Upon the generation of distance information for interresidue pairs through the protein structure, three-dimensional protein conformations consistent with the spectra are generated. In this calculation, a distance matrix is constructed containing ranges of distances (minimum and maximum) for as many interresidue interactions as may be measured. Possible structures are generated from the data consistent with the constraints imposed by the NMR spectra. Computational refinements of the initially calculated structures can be made to optimize covalent bond distances and bond angles. The method generates a family of structures, the variability showing either the imprecision of the technique or the dynamic "disorder" of the folded structure (Figure 2.75). Such computations based on NMR experiments have yielded structures for proteins that do not significantly differ from the time-averaged structure observed with X-ray diffraction methods.

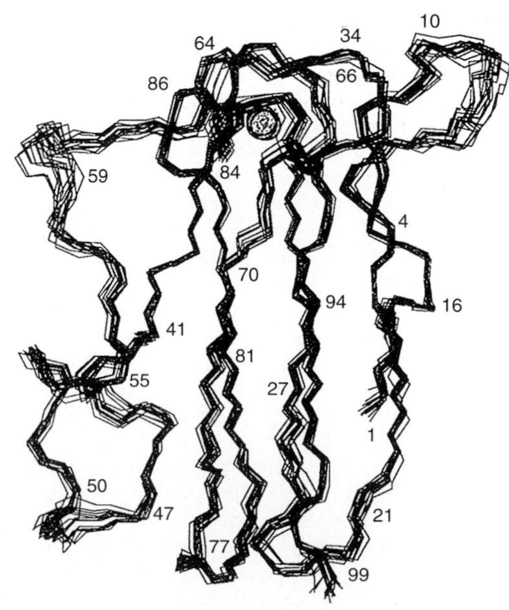

FIGURE 2.75
NMR structure of the protein plastocyanin from the French bean.
The structure shows superposition of eight structures of the polypeptide backbone for the protein, calculated from the constraints of the NMR spectrum.
From Moore, J. M., Lepre, C. A., Gippert, G. P., Chazin, W. J., Case, D. A., and Wright, P. E. J. Mol. Biol. *221:533, 1991. Figure generously supplied by P. E. Wright.*

Other enhancements to NMR, which are applicable to the determination of protein structure, include the ability to synthesize proteins containing isotopically enriched (e.g., containing ^{13}C or ^{15}N) amino acids, and development of paramagnetic shift reagents to study localized environments on paramagnetic resonances, such as the lanthanide ion reporting groups.

BIBLIOGRAPHY

Physical and Structural Properties of Proteins

Bowie, J. U., Luethy, R., and Eisenberg, D. A method to identify protein sequences that fold into a known three-dimensional structure. *Science* 253:164, 1991.

Bryson, J. W., Betz, S. F., Lu, H. S., Suich, D. H., Zhou, H. X., O'Neil, K. T., and DeGrado, W. F. Protein design: a hierarchic approach. *Science* 270:935, 1995.

Chothia, C. Principles that determine the structure of proteins. *Annu. Rev. Biochem.* 53:537, 1984.

Doolittle, R. F. The multiplicity of domains in proteins. *Annu. Rev. Biochem.* 64:287, 1995.

Eisenberg, D., and McLachlan, A. D. Solvation energy in protein folding and binding. *Nature* 319:199, 1986.

Fasman, G. D. Protein conformational prediction. *Trends Biochem. Sci.* 14:295, 1989.

Finkelstein, A. V., Gutun, A. M., and Badretdinov, A. Ya. Why are the same protein folds used to perform different functions? *FEBS Lett.* 325:23, 1993.

Flöckner, H., Braxenthaler, M., Lackner, P., Jaritz, M., Ortner, M., and Sippl, M. J. Progress in fold recognition. *Proteins* 23:376, 1995.

Mosimann, S., Meleshko, R., and James, M. N. G. A critical assessment of comparative molecular modeling of tertiary structures of proteins. *Proteins* 23:301, 1995.

Orengo, C. A., Jones, D. T., and Thornton, J. M. Protein superfamilies and domain superfolds. *Nature* 372:631, 1994.

Richardson, J. S. The anatomy and taxonomy of protein structure. *Adv. Protein Chem.* 34:168, 1981.

Rose, G. D., and Wolfenden, R. Hydrogen bonding, hydrophobicity, packing, and protein folding. *Annu. Rev. Biophys. Biomol. Struct.* 22:381, 1993.

Protein Folding

Anfinsen, C. B., and Scheraga, H. Experimental and theoretical aspects of protein folding. *Adv. Protein Chem.* 29:205, 1975.

Baldwin, R. L. How does protein folding get started? *Trends Biochem. Sci.* 14:291, 1989.

Bychkova, V. E., and Ptitsyn, O. B. The molten globule state is involved in genetic disease? *FEBS Lett.* 359:6, 1995.

Chen, S., Roseman, A. M., Hunter, A. S., Wood, S. P. Burston, S. G., Ranson, N. A., Clarke, A. R., and Saibil, H. R. Location of a folding protein and shape changes in GroEL–GroES complexes imaged by cryo-electron microscopy. *Nature* 371:261, 1994.

Dobson, C. M., Evans, P. A., and Radford, S. E. Understanding how proteins fold: the lysozyme story so far. *Trends Biochem. Sci.* 19:31, 1994.

Hendrick, J. P., and Hartl, F. U. The role of molecular chaperones in protein folding. *FASEB J.* 9:1559, 1995.

Jaenicke, R. Protein folding: local structures, domains, subunits and assemblies. *Biochemistry* 30:3147, 1991.

Lins, L., and Brasseur, R. The hydrophobic effect in protein folding. *FASEB J.* 9:535, 1995.

Ptitsyn, O. B. How the molten globule became. *Trends Biochem. Sci.* 20:376, 1995.

Shakhnovich, E., Abkevich, V., and Ptitsyn, O. Conserved residues and the mechanism of protein folding. *Nature* 379:96, 1996.

Sosnick, T. R., Mayne, L., Hiller, R., and Englander, S. W. The barriers in protein folding. *Nature Struct. Biol.* 1:149, 1994.

Wolynes, P. G., Onuchic, J. N., and Thirumalai, D. Navigating the folding routes. *Science* 267:1619, 1995.

Techniques for the Study of Proteins

Bax, A., and Grzesiek, S. Methodological advances in protein NMR. *Acc. Chem. Res.* 26:131, 1993.

Clauser, K. R., Hall, S. C., Smith, D. M., Webb, J. W., Andrews, L. E., Tran, H. M., Epstein, L. B., and Burlingame, A. L. Rapid mass spectrometric peptide sequencing and mass matching for characterization of human melanoma proteins isolated by two dimensional PAGE. *Proc. Natl. Acad. Sci. U.S.A.* 92:4801, 1995.

Farrow, N. A., Muhandiram, D. R., Singer, A. U., Pascal, S. M., Kay, C. M., Gish, G., Shoelson, S. E., Pawson, T., and Forman-Kay, L. E. Back-bone dynamics of a free and phosphopeptide-complexed Src homology 2 domain studied by ^{15}N NMR relaxation. *Biochemistry* 33:5984, 1994.

Nikolov, C. B., Chen, H., Halay, E. D., Usheva, A. A., Hisatake, K., Lee, D. K., Roeder, R. G., and Burley, S. K. Crystal structure of a TFIIB-TBP-TATA-element ternary complex. *Nature* 377:119, 1995.

Reif, O. W., Lausch, R., and Fritag, R. High-performance capillary electrophoresis of human serum and plasma proteins. *Adv. Chromatogr.* 34:1, 1994.

Shively, J. E., Paxton, R. J., and Lee, T. D. Highlights of protein structural analysis. *Trends Biochem. Sci.* 14:246, 1989.

Dynamics in Folded Proteins

Daggett, V., and Levitt, M. Realistic simulations of native-protein dynamics in solution and beyond. *Annu. Rev. Biophys. Biomol. Struct.* 22:353, 1993.

Joseph, D., Petsko, G. A., and Karplus, M. Anatomy of a conformational change: hinged lid motion of the triosephosphate isomerase loop. *Science* 249:1425, 1990.

Karplus, M., and McCammon, J. A. Dynamics of proteins: elements and function. *Annu. Rev. Biochem.* 53:263, 1983.

Karplus, M., and McCammon, J. A. The dynamics of proteins. *Sci. Am.* 254:42, 1986.

Smith, P. E., van Schaik, R. C., Szyperski, T., Würthrick, K., and van Gunsteren, W. F. Internal mobility of the basic pancreatic trypsin inhibitor in solution: a comparison of NMR spin relaxation measurements and molecular dynamics simulations. *J. Mol. Biol.* 246:356, 1995.

Glycoproteins

Brockhausen, I. Clinical aspects of glycoprotein biosynthesis. *Crit. Rev. Clin. Lab. Sci.* 30:65, 1993.

Lis., H., and Sharon, N. Protein glycosylation. Structural and functional aspects. *Eur. J. Biochem.* 218:1, 1993.

Paulson, J. C. Glycoproteins: what are the sugar chains for? *Trends Biochem. Sci.* 14:272, 1989.

Lipoproteins

Gotto, A. M. Jr. Plasma lipoproteins. In: A. Neuberger and L. L. M. van Deenen (Eds.), *New Comprehensive Biochemistry*. Amsterdam: Elsevier, 1987.

Myers, G. L., Cooper, G. R., and Sampson, E. J. Traditional lipoprotein profile: clinical utility, performance requirement, and standardization. *Atherosclerosis* 108:S157, 1994.

Schumaker, V. N., Phillips, M. L., and Chatterton, J. E. Apolipoprotein B and low-density lipoprotein structure: implications for biosynthesis of triglyceride-rich lipoproteins. *Adv. Protein Chem.* 45:205, 1994.

Schuster, B., Prassl, R., Nigon, F., Chapman, M. J., and Laggner, P. Core lipid structure is a major determinant of the oxidative resistance of low density lipoprotein. *Proc. Natl. Acad. Sci. U.S.A.* 92:2509, 1995.

Segrest, J. P., Garber, D. W., Brouillette, C. G., Harvey, S. C., and Anantharamaiah, G. M. The amphipathic α helix: a multifunctional structural motif in plasma apolipoproteins. *Adv. Protein Chem.* 45:303, 1994.

Collagen

Brodsky, B., and Shah, N. K. The triple-helix motif in proteins. *FASEB J.* 9:1537, 1995.

Kuivaniemi, H., Tromp, G., and Prockop, D. J. Mutations in collagen genes: causes of rare and some common diseases in humans. *FASEB J.* 5:2052, 1991.

Prockop, D. J., and Kivirikko, K. I. Collagens: molecular biology, diseases, and potentials for therapy. *Annu. Rev. Biochem.* 64:403, 1995.

QUESTIONS ■ J. BAGGOTT AND C. N. ANGSTADT

Refer to the following structure for Questions 1 and 2.

Gly—Ser—Cys—Glu—Asp—Asn—Cys—Arg (disulfide bond S—S between the two Cys residues)

1. The peptide shown above:
   A. has arginine in position 1 of the sequence.
   B. contains a derived amino acid.
   C. is basic.
   D. consists entirely of amino acids with charged or nonpolar side chains.
   E. contains more amino acids with side chains that are charged than ones with electrically neutral side chains at pH 7.0.

2. The charge on the peptide shown above is about:
   A. -2 at pH > 13.5.
   B. -1 at pH ~ 11.5.
   C. $+1$ at pH ~ 6.5.
   D. $+2$ at pH ~ 5.5.
   E. 0 at pH ~ 4.5.

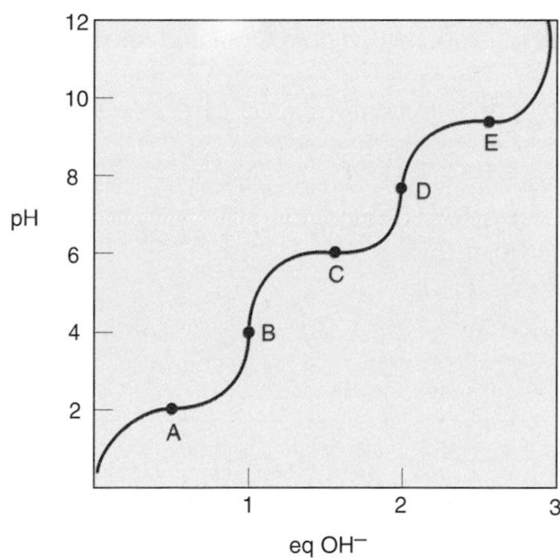

3. The figure above shows the titration curve of one of the common amino acids. From this curve we can conclude:
   A. the amino acid contains two carboxyl groups.
   B. at point B the amino acid is zwitterionic.
   C. the amino acid contains an aromatic hydroxyl group.
   D. point D corresponds to the pK_a' of an ionizable group.
   E. at point E the amino acid has a net negative charge.

4. Which of the following can be used for a quantitative determination of amino acids in general?
   A. acetic anhydride
   B. iodoacetate
   C. ninhydrin
   D. Pauly's reagent
   E. the Sakaguchi reaction

5. Which of the following is a conservative substitution?
   A. Val for Ile
   B. His for Pro
   C. Asp for Ala
   D. Lys for Leu
   E. Ser for Ala

6. Which of the following has quaternary structure?
   A. α-chymotrypsin
   B. hemoglobin
   C. insulin
   D. myoglobin
   E. trypsin

Refer to the drawing for Questions 7 and 8.

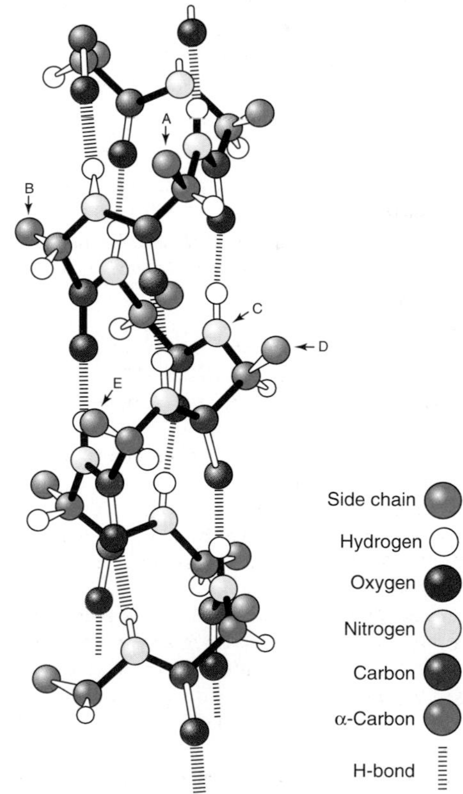

7. When group E contains a negatively charged carboxyl function, the structure is destabilized by:
   A. alanine at position A.
   B. arginine at position B.
   C. serine at position B.
   D. proline at position D.
   E. aspartate at position D.

8. The properties of atom C are essential to which stabilizing force in the structure?
   A. hydrogen bonding
   B. steric effects
   C. ionic attraction
   D. disulfide bridge
   E. none of the above

Refer to the following for Questions 9–11.
   A. disulfide bond formation
   B. hydrogen bonding
   C. hydrophobic interaction
   D. electrostatic interactions
   E. van der Waals forces

9. Which interaction is NOT formed when protein subunits combine to form a quaternary structure?

10. Driven by the entropy of water.

11. Repulsive forces between atoms attached to a peptide bond are weakest when the ϕ and φ angles are compatible with the α-helix and β-structures.

12. In collagen:
   A. intrachain hydrogen bonding stabilizes the native structure.
   B. three chains with polyproline type II helical conformation can wind about one another to form a superhelix because of the structure of glycine.
   C. the ϕ angles contributed by proline are free to rotate, but the φ angles are constrained by the ring.
   D. regions of superhelicity comprise the entire structure except for the N and C termini.
   E. cross-links between triple helices form after an intracellular enzyme converts some of the lysine to allysine.

13. Chaperone proteins:
   A. all require ATP to exert their effect.
   B. cleave incorrect disulfide bonds, allowing correct ones to subsequently form.
   C. guide the folding of polypeptide chains into patterns that would be thermodynamically unstable without the presence of chaperones.
   D. are involved in transport of proteins across mitochondrial and endoplasmic reticulum membranes.
   E. act primarily on fully synthesized polypeptide chains, unfolding incorrect structures so they can refold correctly.

14. Proteins may be separated according to size by:
   A. isoelectric focusing.
   B. polyacrylamide gel electrophoresis.
   C. ion-exchange chromatography.
   D. molecular exclusion chromatography.
   E. reverse-phase HPLC.

Refer to the following for Questions 15–18.
   A. primary structure
   B. secondary structure
   C. tertiary structure
   D. quaternary structure
   E. random conformation

15. All ϕ angles are equal and all φ angles are equal.

16. May bring distant segments of a single polypeptide chain into close juxtaposition.

17. Unaffected by binding of a charged detergent, such as SDS.

18. Exemplified by the β-structure (pleated sheet).

19. Changes in protein conformation can be detected rapidly by:
   A. ultraviolet absorbance spectroscopy.
   B. fluorescence emission spectroscopy.
   C. optical rotatory dispersion.
   D. circular dichroism.
   E. all of the above.

ANSWERS

1. B Cystine, formed by joining two cysteine residues through a disulfide bridge, is a derived amino acid (p. 30). A: The convention is to write the N terminal to the left. Numbering begins at the N terminal, so glycine is in position 1 (p. 29). C: The peptide contains two acidic amino acids, glutamate and aspartate, and only one basic amino acid, arginine, so it is acidic (p. 31). D and E: Cysteine is nonpolar and uncharged, and glutamate, aspartate, and arginine are charged at physiological pH; serine and asparagine are polar but are not charged (p. 26).
2. E At pH 4.5 the peptide is in the following ionic state: the N-terminal amino group is +1, the side chain carboxyls of glutamate and aspartate each average about −0.5 (since this pH is about at their pK values), the side chain of arginine is +1, and its terminal carboxyl group is −1. The sum is zero (pp. 30–33).
3. E The axes of this titration curve are reversed from the presentation in the text. The abscissa shows that three ionizable groups are present. The pK values, where the groups are 50% titrated, are at points A (pH ~ 2), C (pH ~ 6.5), and E (pH ~ 9.5). Histidine is the only common amino acid with these pK values. At point B, its net charge is $-1 + 1 + 1 = +1$. At point E, the net charge is $-1 + 0 + 0.5 = -0.5$ (pp. 31–34).
4. C A: Acetic anhydride acetylates tyrosyl residues. B: Iodoacetate reacts with the —SH of cysteine. D: Pauly's reagent reacts only with histidine and tyrosine. E: The Sakaguchi reaction is for arginine. (See Table 2.7.)
5. A B: His and Pro both have rings in their side chains, but the rings are very different. C–E: In each of these pairs the first amino acid is charged or polar, and the second has an aliphatic R group (p. 26).
6. B Quaternary structure consists of a specific noncovalent association of subunits having their own tertiary structures (p. 44). Myoglobin is a single polypeptide chain (p. 48). Insulin, trypsin (p. 40), and α-chymotrypsin (p. 46) are multichain proteins covalently joined by cystine bonds, and, each chain having arisen from a single polypeptide chain by proteolytic cleavage.

7. D Like charges in the third or fourth position in either direction from the designated position destabilize the helix due to charge repulsion. Thus aspartate at position D is harmless, whereas glutamate at position A or B would destabilize. Alanine has a small side chain. Proline destabilizes the α-helix conformation and is usually not found in either α-helix or β-structure (p. 44).
8. A Atom C is an amide nitrogen. The attached hydrogen atom participates in hydrogen bonding (pp. 43–44). Hydrogen bonds contribute to the stability of the structure (p. 43).
9. A Quaternary structure is stabilized exclusively by noncovalent interactions. Disulfide bonds are covalent (p. 48).
10. C Hydrophobic groups in contact with water result in formation of a relatively highly ordered solvation shell of water around the group. If the hydrophobic groups come together, eliminating the bound water, the water becomes more random, a favorable process (pp. 64–66).
11. E Van der Waals repulsive forces (as opposed to the attractive element of van der Waals forces) are weakest at these angles (p. 66).
12. B The close contacts in the interior of the triple helix are possible only when the R group of the amino acid at that position is very small, that is, hydrogen. A: The hydrogen bonding in collagen is interchain. C: The ϕ angle is part of the proline ring and is not free to rotate. D: Although the statement is true of type I collagen, the superhelical regions in other collagen types may be broken by regions of globular domains (p. 52). E: The conversion and cross-linking are extracellular.
13. D A: The hsp60 family of chaperones is ATP-linked, but the hsp70 family is not. B: Disulfide isomerases catalyze this reaction. C: The final product is thermodynamically stable; chaperones merely prevent unfavorable intermediate interactions. E: Hsp70 chaperones react with nascent polypeptide chains as they are synthesized by the ribosome. The protein may then be delivered to a hsp60 chaperone for facilitation of final folding (pp. 62–63).
14. D A–C separate molecules on the basis of charge (p. 72). E: Reverse-phase HPLC effects separations on the basis of polarity (p. 73).
15. B This statement is a definition of secondary structure (p. 43).
16. C This is a consequence of folding into a compact structure (p. 44).
17. A SDS binding produces an extended conformation of a polypeptide chain due to charge repulsion, but no peptide bonds are broken (p. 72).
18. B β-Structure is an important type of secondary structure (p. 44).
19. E A: Peptide bond absorption (180–230 nm) in the α-helical conformation differs from that in other conformations (p. 79). B: Excitation transfers become less efficient as donor and acceptor groups become further apart, as in denaturation. C and D: These effects of optically active chromophors upon polarized light are sensitive to environment; in addition, the peptide bond itself becomes part of an optically active system when it forms an asymmetric structure like the α-helix (p. 80).

CHAPTER

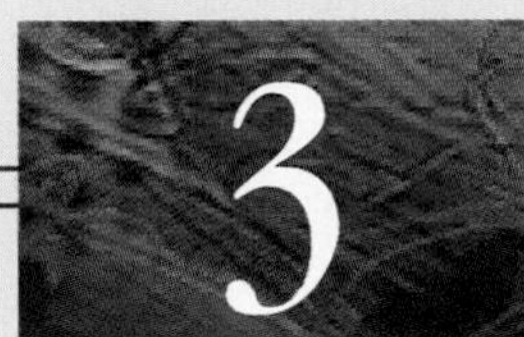

PROTEINS II: STRUCTURE–FUNCTION RELATIONSHIPS IN PROTEIN FAMILIES

Richard M. Schultz and Michael N. Liebman

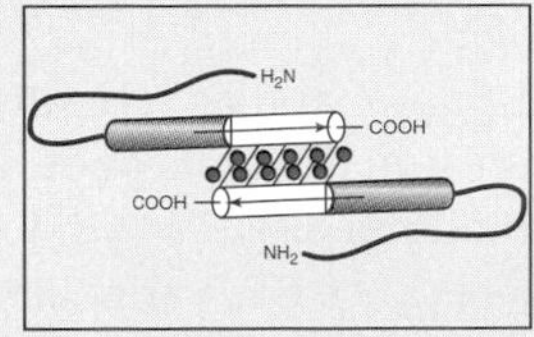

3.1 ■ OVERVIEW

In Chapter 2 we discussed the fundamentals of protein architecture, including structural organization and physical properties of the amino acid constituents, hierarchical organization of primary, secondary, supersecondary, tertiary, and quaternary structure, and energetic forces that hold these molecules together and provide the flexibility observed in their dynamic motion. Computational and experimental tools were introduced that enable the analysis of high-resolution structural features and their conformational response to perturbations, which may be a simple alteration of the solution environment or aspects of their interactions with other molecules that define their biological function. The concept that structure and function are interrelated was introduced through examples of conservation of primary structure with function, and the reoccurrence of elements of secondary, supersecondary, tertiary, and quaternary structural patterns in molecules that may not share similar functional or evolutionary origin.

In this chapter we examine the specific relationships between structure and function in four **protein families**: immunoglobulins, serine proteases, DNA-binding proteins, and hemoglobins. We pursue this study through the examination of the variability in amino acid sequence, structural organization, and biological function. The significance of the structure–function relationship can best be appreciated through observation of the range of such variations within specific protein families.

The **immunoglobulin family** provides examples of multidomain architecture that supports recognition and binding to foreign molecules and leads to their sequestration. Diversity among family members is the source of specific molecular recognition and individual binding capabilities.

The **serine proteases** provide examples of a family of enzymes that appear to have diverged to perform unique physiological functions, frequently highly organized within enzyme cascade processes. Their inherent similarities in catalytic mechanism and three-dimensional structure are a common link.

DNA-binding proteins are multifamilies of proteins that bind to regulatory sites in DNA and regulate gene expression, an amazing feat as the mammalian genome contains approximately 100,000 unique genes. These proteins contain unusual supersecondary structure motifs that allow them to selectively bind regulatory sites of specific genes.

The **hemoglobin** family offers examples of a highly fine-tuned system that can accommodate small substitutions or mutations, many of which have been studied as to their clinical implications. This family reveals the potential diversity of amino acid sequence substitutions that can be tolerated and allow the protein to function in an acceptable physiological manner.

3.2 ■ ANTIBODY MOLECULES: THE IMMUNOGLOBULIN SUPERFAMILY

Antibody molecules are produced in response to invasion by foreign compounds that can be proteins, carbohydrates, and nucleic acid polymers. An antibody molecule noncovalently associates with the foreign substance, initiating a process by which the foreign substance can be eliminated from the organism.

Molecules that induce antibody production are **antigens** and may contain multiple antigenic determinants, small regions of the antigen molecule that elicit the production of a specific antibody to which the antigen binds. In proteins, an antigenic determinant may comprise only six or seven amino acids.

A **hapten** is a small molecule that cannot alone elicit production of specific antibodies but when covalently attached to a larger molecule it acts as an antigenic determinant and induces antibody synthesis. Whereas hapten molecules need attachment to a larger molecule to elicit antibody synthesis, when detached from their carrier, they will retain the ability to bind strongly to antibody.

It is estimated that each human can potentially produce about 1×10^8 different antibody structures. All antibodies, however, have a similar structure. The determination of the structure has been accomplished from studies of immunoglobulin primary structures and X-ray diffraction that show the three-dimensional structure of the antibody molecule alone and in complex with antigen.

Structural studies of proteins require pure homogeneous preparations. Such samples of antibodies are extremely difficult to isolate from blood because of the wide diversity of antibody molecules present. Homogeneous antibodies can be obtained, however, by the monoclonal hybridoma technique in which mouse myeloma cells are fused with mouse antibody-producing B lymphocytes to construct immortalized hybridoma cells that express a single antibody.

Antibody (Immunoglobulin) Molecules Consist of Four Polypeptide Chains

Antibody molecules are glycoproteins with four polypeptide chains, two identical copies of each of two nonidentical polypeptide chains. Two light chains (L) of identical sequence combine with two heavy chains (H) of identical sequence to form the structure $(LH)_2$. In the most common immunoglobulin type, IgG, the H chains have approximately 440 amino acids (50 kDa). The smaller L polypeptide chains contain about 220 amino acids (25 kDa). The four chains are covalently interconnected by disulfide bonds (Figures 3.1 and 3.2). Each H chain is associated with an L chain such that the NH_2-terminal ends of both chains are near each other. Since the L chain is half the size of the H chain, only the NH_2-terminal half of the H chain is associated with the L chain.

In the other classes of immunoglobulins (Table 3.1) the H chains are slightly longer than those of the IgG class. A variable amount of carbohydrate (2–12%, depending on immunoglobulin class) is attached to the H chain.

Constant and Variable Regions of Primary Structure

Comparison of amino acid sequences of antibody molecules elicited by different antigens shows regions of sequence homology and other regions of sequence variability. In particular, sequences of the NH_2-terminal half of L chains and the

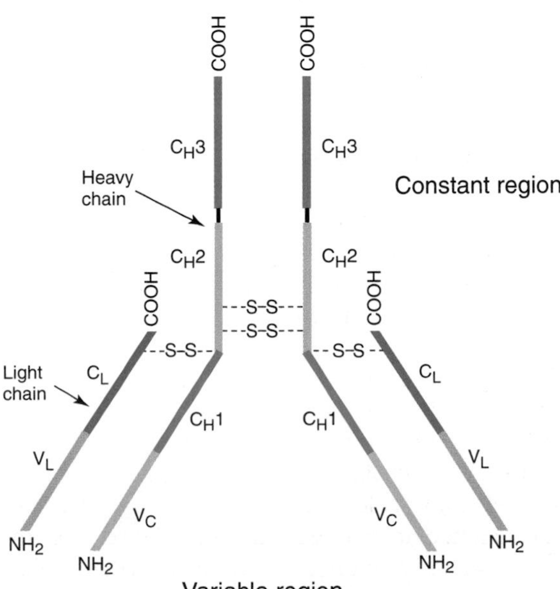

FIGURE 3.1
Linear representation of four-chain IgG antibody molecule.
Two H chains and two L chains are co-oriented in their COOH-terminal to NH_2-terminal directions, as shown. Interchain disulfide bonds link heavy (H) chains, and light (L) chains to the H chains. Domains of the constant (C) region of the H chain are C_H1, C_H2, and C_H3. The constant region of the L chain is designated C_L, and variable (V) regions are V_H and V_L of H and L chains, respectively.
Based on figure by Burton, D. R. In: F. Calabi and M. S. Neuberger (Eds.), Molecular Genetics of Immunoglobulin. *Amsterdam: Elsevier, 1987, pp. 1–50.*

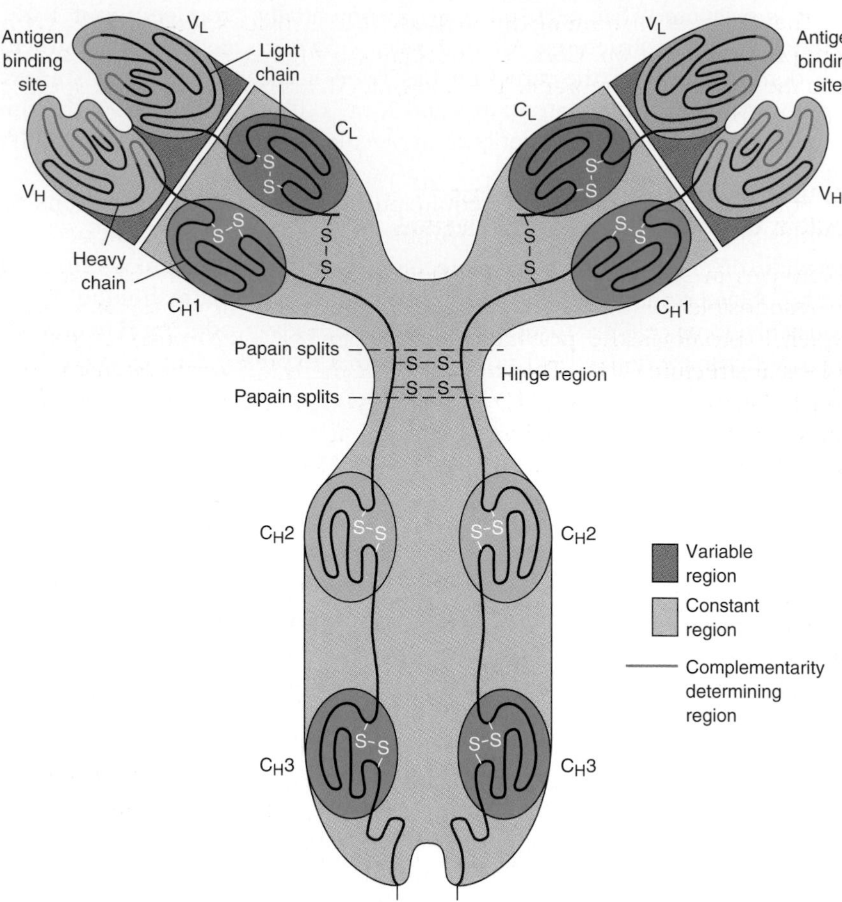

FIGURE 3.2
Diagrammatic structure for IgG.
Light chains (L) are divided into domains V_L (variable amino acid sequence) and C_L (constant amino acid sequence). Heavy chains (H) are divided into domains V_H (variable amino acid sequence) and C_H1, C_H2, and C_H3. Antigen-binding sites are V_H–V_L. "Hinge" polypeptides interconnect domains. Positions of inter- and intrachain cystine bonds are shown.
From Cantor, C. R. and Schimmel, P. R. Biophysical Chemistry, *Part I. San Francisco: Freeman, 1980. Reprinted with permission of Mr. Irving Geis, New York.*

NH_2-terminal quarter of H chains are highly variable between different antibody molecules. These NH_2-terminal segments are the **variable (V) regions** and designated V_H and V_L domains of H and L chains, respectively. Within these V domains certain segments are "hypervariable." Three **hypervariable regions** of between 5 and 7 residues in the V_L domain and three or four hypervariable regions of between 6 and 17 residues in the V_H domain are commonly found. The hypervariable sequences are also termed the **complementarity-determining regions (CDRs)** as they form the antigen-binding site complementary to the topology of the antigen structure.

In contrast, the COOH-terminal three-quarters of H chains and the COOH-terminal half of L chains are homologous in sequence with other H or L chains

TABLE 3.1 Immunoglobulin Classes

Classes of Immunoglobulin	*Approximate Molecular Mass*	*H Chain Isotype*	*Carbohydrate by Weight (%)*	*Concentration in Serum (mg 100 mL^{-1})*
IgG	150,000	γ, 53,000	2–3	600–1800
IgA	170,000–720,000[a]	α, 64,000	7–12	90–420
IgD	160,000	δ, 58,000		0.3–40
IgE	190,000	ε, 75,000	10–12	0.01–0.10
IgM	950,000[a]	μ, 70,000	10–12	50–190

[a] Forms polymer structures of basic structural unit.

of the same class. These **constant (C) regions** with a homologous primary structure are designated C_H and C_L in the H and L chains, respectively.

The C_H regions determine the antibody class, provide for binding of complement proteins (see Clin. Corr. 3.1), and are the site necessary for antibodies to cross the placental membrane. The V regions determine the antigen specificity of the antibody molecule.

Immunoglobulins in a Single Class Contain Common Homologous Regions

Differences in sequence of the C_H regions between immunoglobulin classes are responsible for the characteristics of each class. In some cases, the C_H sequence promotes the polymerization of antibody molecules of the basic molecular structure $(LH)_2$. Thus antibodies of the IgA class are often covalently linked dimeric structures $[(LH)_2]_2$. Similarly, IgM molecules are pentamers $[(LH)_2]_5$. The different H chains, designated τ, α, δ, ε, and μ, occur in IgG, IgA, IgM, IgD, and IgE classes, respectively (Table 3.1; see Clin. Corr. 3.2). Two types of L chain sequences are synthesized, designated lambda (λ) and kappa (κ) chains, either of which are found combined with the five classes of H chains.

IgG is the major immunoglobulin in plasma. Biosynthesis of a specific IgG in significant concentrations takes about 10 days after exposure to a new antigen (see Clin. Corr. 3.3). In the absence of an initially high concentration of IgG to a specific antigen, antibodies of the IgM class, which are synthesized at faster

CLINICAL CORRELATION 3.1

The Complement Proteins

At least 11 distinct complement proteins exist in plasma. They are activated by IgG or IgM antibody binding to antigens on the outer cell membrane of invading bacterial cells, protozoa, or tumor cells. After the immunoglobulin-binding event, the 11 complement proteins are sequentially activated and associate with the cell membrane to cause a lysis of the membrane and death of the target cell.

Many complement proteins are precursors of proteolytic enzymes that are present in a nonactive form prior to activation. Upon their activation, they will, in turn, activate a succeeding protein of the pathway by the hydrolysis of a specific peptide bond in the second protein, leading to a cascade phenomenon. Activation of enzymes by specific proteolysis (i.e., hydrolysis of a specific peptide bond) is an important general method for activating extracellular enzymes. For example, the enzymes that catalyze blood clot formation, induce fibrinolysis of blood clots, and digest dietary proteins in the gut are all activated by a specific proteolysis catalyzed by a second enzyme (see pp. 964, 1071).

Upon association to a cellular antigen the exposure of a complement-binding site in the antibody's Fc region occurs and causes the binding of the C1 complement proteins, which are a protein complex composed of three individual proteins: Clq, Clr, and Cls. Clr and Cls undergo a conformational change and become active enzymes on the cell surface. The activated C1 complex (Cla) hydrolyzes a peptide bond in complement proteins C2 and C4, which then also associate on the cell surface. The now active C2–C4 complex has a proteolytic activity that hydrolyzes a peptide bond in complement protein C3. Activated C3 protein binds to the cell surface and the activated C2–C4–C3 complex activates protein C5. Activated protein C5 will associate with complement proteins C6, C7, C8, and six molecules of complement protein C9. This multiprotein complex binds to the cell surface and initiates membrane lysis.

The mechanism is a cascade in which amplification of the trigger event occurs. In summary, activated C1 can activate a number of molecules of C4–C2–C3, and each activated C4–C2–C3 complex can, in turn, activate many molecules of C5 to C9. The reactions of the classical complement pathway are summarized below, where "a" and "b" designate the proteolytically modified proteins and a line above a protein indicates an enzyme activity.

$$\text{IgG or IgM} \xrightarrow{\text{Clq, Clr, Cls}} \overline{\text{Cla}} \xrightarrow{\text{C2,C4}}$$

$$\text{C4b.}\overline{\text{C2a}} \xrightarrow{\text{C3}}$$

$$\text{C4b.}\overline{\text{C2a}}\text{.C3b} \xrightarrow{\text{C5,C6,C7,C8,C9}}$$

There is an "alternative pathway" for C3 complement activation, initiated by aggregates of IgA or by bacterial polysaccharide in the absence of immunoglobulin binding to cell membrane antigens. This pathway involves the proteins properdin, C3 proactivator convertase, and C3 proactivator.

A major role of the complement systems is to generate opsonins—an old term for proteins that stimulate phagocytosis by neutrophils and macrophages. The major opsonin is C3b; macrophages have specific receptors for this protein. Patients with inherited deficiency of C3 are subject to repeated bacterial infections.

Colten, H. R., and Rosen, F. S. Complement deficiencies. *Annu. Rev. Immunol.* 10:809, 1992; and Morgan, B. P. Physiology and pathophysiology of complement: progress and trends. *Crit. Rev. Clin. Lab. Sci.* 32:265, 1995.

CLINICAL CORRELATION 3.2

Functions of Different Antibody Classes

The IgA class of immunoglobulins is found primarily in the mucosal secretions (bronchial, nasal, and intestinal mucous secretions, tears, milk, and colostrum). These immunoglobulins are the initial defense against invading viral and bacterial pathogens prior to their entry into plasma or other internal space.

The IgM class is found primarily in plasma. They are the first antibodies elicited in significant quantity on the introduction of a foreign antigen into a host's plasma. IgM antibodies promote phagocytosis of microorganisms by macrophage and polymorphonuclear leukocytes and are also potent activators of complement (see Clin. Corr. 3.1). IgM antibodies occur in many external secretions but at levels lower than those of IgA.

The IgG class occurs in high concentration in plasma. Their response to foreign antigens takes a longer period of time than that of IgM. At maximum concentration they are present in significantly higher concentration than IgM. Like IgM, IgG antibodies promote phagocytosis in plasma and activate complement.

The normal biological functions of the IgD and IgE classes of immunoglobulins are not known; however, the IgE antibodies play an important role in allergic responses such as anaphylactic shock, hay fever, and asthma.

Immunoglobulin deficiency usually causes increased susceptibility to infection. X-linked agammaglobulinemia and common variable immunodeficiency are two examples. The commonest disorder is selective IgA deficiency, which results in recurrent infections of sinuses and the respiratory tract.

Rosen, F. S., Cooper, M. D., and Wedgewood, R. J. P. The primary immunodeficiencies. *N. Engl. J. Med.* 311:235 (Part 1); 300 (Part II), 1984.

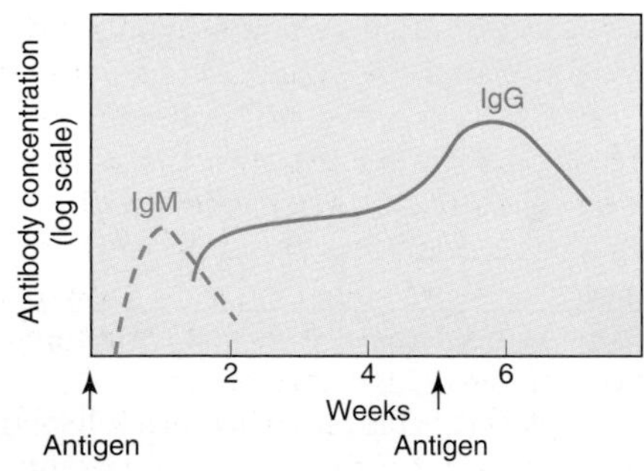

FIGURE 3.3
Time course of specific antibody IgM and IgG response to added antigen.
Based on a figure in Stryer, L. Biochemistry. *San Francisco: Freeman, 1988, p. 890.*

rates, will associate with the antigen and serve as the first line of defense until large quantities of IgG are produced (Figure 3.3; see Clin. Corr. 3.3).

Repeating Amino Acid Sequences and Homologous Three-Dimensional Domains Occur Within an Antibody

Within each of the polypeptide chains of an antibody molecule is a repeating pattern of amino acid sequences. For the IgG class, the repetitive pattern is observed between segments of approximately 110 amino acids within both L and H chains. This homology is far from exact, but clearly a number of amino acids match identically following alignment of 110 amino acid segments. Other amino acids are matched in the sequence by having similar nonpolar or polar side chains. As the H chains are about 440 amino acids in length, the repetition of the homologous sequence occurs four times along an immunoglobulin H chain. Based on this sequence pattern, the chain is divided into one V_H region and three C_H regions (designated C_H1, C_H2, and C_H3) (see Figures 3.1 and 3.2). The L chain of about 220 amino acids is divided into one V_L region and one

CLINICAL CORRELATION 3.3

Immunization

An immunizing vaccine can consist of killed bacterial cells, inactivated viruses, killed parasites, a nonvirulent form of live bacterium related to a virulent bacterium, a denatured bacterial toxin or recombinant protein. The introduction of a vaccine into a human can lead to protection against virulent forms of microorganisms or toxic agents that contain the same antigen. Antigens in nonvirulent material not only cause the differentiation of lymphoid cells so that they produce antibody toward the foreign antigen but also cause differentiation of some lymphoid cells into memory cells. Memory cells do not secrete antibody but place antibodies to the antigen onto their outer surface, where they act as future sensors for the antigen. These memory cells are like a longstanding radar for the potentially virulent antigen. On reintroduction of the antigen at a later time, the binding of the antigen to the cell surface antibody in the memory cells stimulates the memory cell to divide into antibody-producing cells as well as new memory cells. This reduces the time for antibody production that is required on introduction of an antigen and increases the concentration of antigen-specific antibody produced. It is the basis for the protection provided by immunization.

Recently introduced vaccines for adults include pneumococcal vaccine (to prevent pneumonia due to *Diplococcus pneumoniae*), hepatitis B vaccine, and influenza vaccine. The latter changes each year to account for antigenic variation in the influenza virus.

Flexner, C. New approaches to vaccination. *Adv. Pharmacol.* 21:51, 1990; and Sparling, P. F., Elkins, C., Wyrick, P. B., and Cohen, M. S. Vaccines for bacterial sexually transmitted infections: a realistic goal? *Proc. Natl. Acad. Sci. U.S.A.* 91:2456, 1994.

C_L region. Each of these sequence repeats contains an intrachain disulfide bond linking two cysteines (Figure 3.2).

Each of the 110 amino acid segments form separate structural domains of similar tertiary structure as shown by X-ray diffraction studies. Each 110 segment of the H and L chains folds into a supersecondary structure with a unique but similar arrangement of antiparallel β-strands, which generates a motif known as an **immunoglobulin fold** (Figure 3.4). This motif consists of 7 to 9 polypeptide strands that form two antiparallel β-sheets that are aligned face-to-face. Globular domains result from the strong interaction between two immunoglobulin folds on two separate chains (Figure 3.5). The associations are between domains V_L–V_H and C_L–C_H1 in the H and L chains. In the C-terminal half of the H chains, the two chains associate to generate domains C_H2–C_H2 and C_H3–C_H3 (Figure 3.2). A "hinge" polypeptide sequence interconnects the two C_L–C_H1 domains with the C_H2–C_H2 domain in the antibody structure. Thus the antibody structure

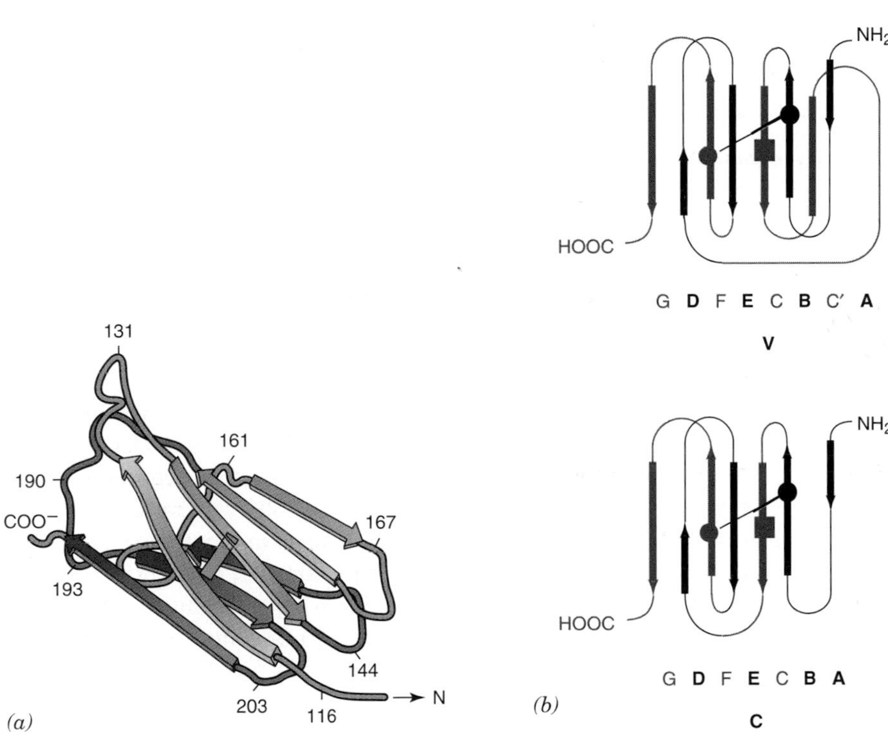

FIGURE 3.4
Immunoglobulin fold.
(*a*) Schematic diagram of folding of a C_L domain, showing β-pleated sheet structure. Arrows show strands of β-sheet and bar (blue) shows position of cystine bond. Light arrows are for β-strands in plane above and dark arrows are β-strands in plane below. (*b*) Diagrammatic outline of arrangement of β-strands in immunoglobulin fold motif. Examples are for IgG variable and constant regions. Thick arrows indicate β-strands and thin lines loops that interconnect the β-strands. Circles indicate cysteines that form intradomain disulfide bond. Squares show positions of tryptophan residues that are an invariant component of the core of the immunoglobulin fold. Boldface black letters indicate strands that form one plane of the sheet, while other letters form the parallel plane behind the first plane.
(a) From Edmundson, A. B., Ely, K. R., Abola, E. E., Schiffer, M., and Pavagiotopoulos, N. Biochemistry 14:3953, 1975. Copyright © 1975 by American Chemical Society. Reprinted with permission.
(b) Based on a figure by Calabi, F. In: F. Calabi and M. S. Neuberger (Eds.), Molecular Genetics of Immunoglobulin. *Amsterdam: Elsevier, 1987, pp. 203–239.*

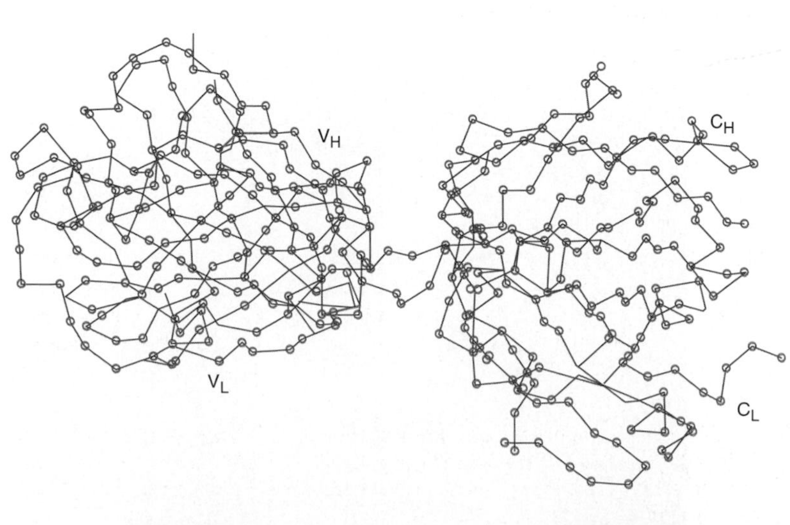

FIGURE 3.5
α-Carbon (○) structure of Fab fragment of IgG KOL showing V_L–V_H and C_L–C_H1 domains interconnected by the hinge polypeptides.
From Huber, R., Deisenhofer, J., Coleman, P. M., Matsushima, M., and Palm, W. In The Immune System, *27th Mosbach Colloquium. Berlin: Springer-Verlag, 1976, p. 26.*

exhibits six domains, each domain due to the association of two immunoglobulin folds (Figures 3.2 and 3.6). The NH_2-terminal V_L–V_H domains contain a shallow crevice in the center of a hydrophobic core that binds the antigen. Hypervariable sequences in the V domain crevices form loops that come close together and are the complementarity binding site for the antigen (see Figures 3.6 and 3.7). The sequences of the hypervariable loops give a unique three-dimensional conformation for each antibody that makes it specific to its antigenic determinant. Small changes in conformation of the CDRs occur on antigen binding to V_L–V_H domains, indicating that antigen binding induces an optimum complementary fit to the variable CDR site. Antigen binding may also induce conformational changes between V_L–V_H domains and the other domains that activate effector sites, such as for complement binding to the C_H2–C_H2 domain. The strength of association between antibody and antigen is due to noncovalent forces (see Chapter 2). Complementarity of the structures of the antigenic determinant and antigen-binding site results in extremely high equilibrium affinity constants, between 10^5 and 10^{10} M^{-1} (strength of 7–14 kcal mol^{-1}) for this noncovalent association.

There Are Two Antigen-Binding Sites per Antibody Molecule

The NH_2-terminal variable (V) domains of each pair of L and H chains (V_L–V_H) comprise an antigen-binding site; thus there are two antigen-binding sites per antibody molecule. The existence of an antigen-binding site in each LH pair is demonstrated by treating antibody molecules with the proteolytic enzyme papain, which hydrolyzes a peptide bond in the hinge peptide of each H chain (see Figures 3.2 and 3.8). The antibody molecule is cleaved into three products. Two are identical and consist of the NH_2-terminal half of the H chain (V_H–C_H1) associated with the full L chain (Figure 3.8). Each of these fragments binds antigen with a similar affinity to that of the intact antibody molecule and is designated an **Fab** (antigen binding) **fragment.** The other product from the papain hydrolysis is the COOH-terminal half of the H chains (C_H2–C_H3) joined together in a single covalent fragment by cystine bonds. This is the **Fc** (crystallizable) **fragment,** which exhibits no binding affinity for the antigen. The L chain can be dissociated from its H chain segment within the Fab fragment by oxidation of disulfide bonds, which eliminates antigen binding. Accordingly, each antigen-binding site must be formed from components of both the L chain (V_L) and the H chain (V_H) domains acting together.

In summary, the major features of antibody structure and antibody–antigen interactions include the following: (1) The polypeptide chains fold into multiple

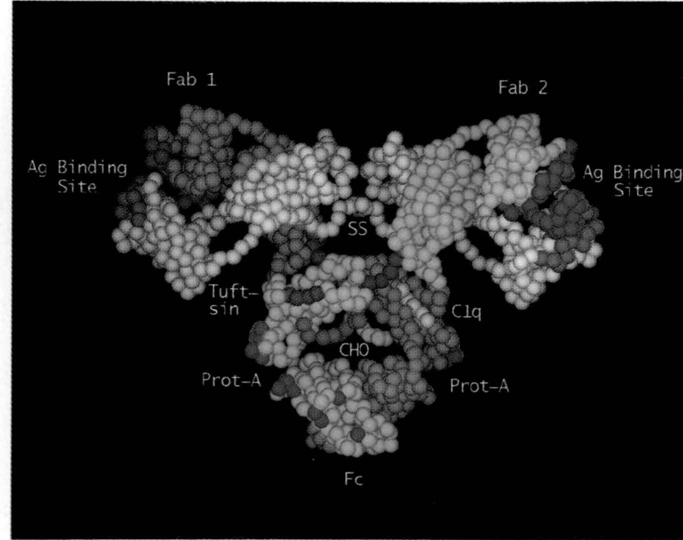

FIGURE 3.6
Model of an IgG antibody molecule.
Only the α-carbons of the structure appear. The two L chains are represented by light gray spheres and the H chains by lavender spheres. Carbohydrates attached to the two C_H2 domains are green and orange. The CDR regions of the V_H–V_L domains are dark red in the H chains and pink in the L chains. The interchain disulfide bond between the L and H chains is a magenta ball-and-stick representation (partially hidden). The heptapeptide hinge between C_H1 and C_H2 domains, connecting the Fab and Fc units, are dark red. The center of the C1q complement site in the C_H2 domains is yellow-green the protein A docking sites at the junction of C_H2 and C_H3 are magenta, and the tuftsin binding site in C_H2 is gray. Tuftsin is a natural tetrapeptide that induces phagocytosis by macrophages and may be transported bound to an immunoglobulin. Protein A is a bacterial protein with a high affinity to immunoglobulins.
Photograph generously supplied by Dr. Allen B. Edmundson, from Guddat, L. W., Shan, L., Fan, Z-C., et al. FASEB J. *9:101, 1995.*

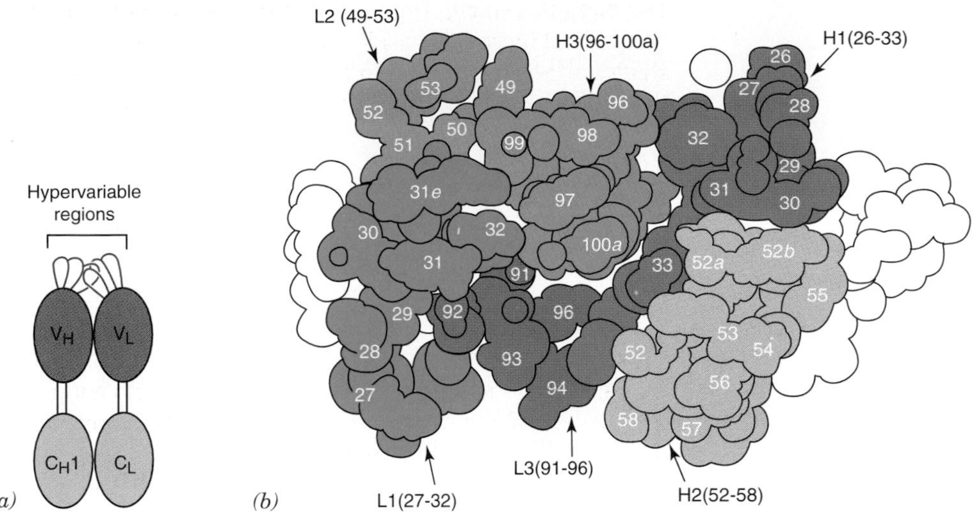

FIGURE 3.7
Hypervariable loops in immunoglobin.
(*a*) Schematic diagram showing hypervariable loops (CDRs) in V_L–V_H domain that form the antigen-binding site. (*b*) A cut through an antigen-binding site showing contributions of different CDRs using CPK space-filling models of the atoms.

(a) From Branden, C. and Tooze, J. Introduction to Protein Structure. *New York: Garland Publishing, 1991, p. 187.*
(b) From Branden, C., and Tooze, J. Introduction to Protein Structure. *New York: Garland Publishing, 1991, p. 189, and attributed to Chothia, C. and Lesk, A.* J. Mol. Biol. *196:914, 1987.*

domains, each domain having an immunoglobulin fold supersecondary structure motif. (2) Two immunoglobulin folds on separate chains associate to form the six domains of the basic immunoglobulin structure. The V_L and V_H associate to form the two NH_2-terminal domains that bind to antigen. (3) The antigen-binding site of the V_L–V_H domains is generated by hypervariable loops (CDRs), which form a continuous surface with a complementary topology to the antigenic determinant. (4) The strong interactions between antigen and antibody CDRs are noncovalent and include van der Waals, hydrogen bonding, and hydrophobic interactions. Ionic salt bridges participate in antigen–antibody associations to a much lesser extent. (5) Small conformational changes occur in the V_L–V_H domain upon association of antigen, indicating an "induced-fit" mechanism in association of antigen to antibody. (6) The binding of antigen to the V_L–V_H domains induces conformational changes between binding and distant domains of the antibody. These allosteric movements alter the binding affinity of effector sites in the constant domains such as that for binding of complement protein C1q to the C_H2–C_H2 domain (see Clin. Corr. 3.1).

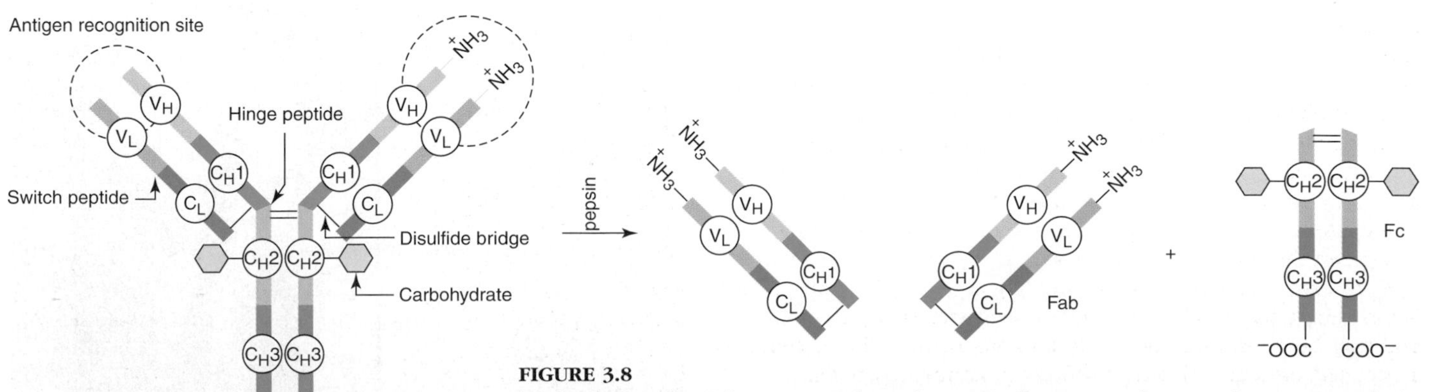

FIGURE 3.8
Hydrolysis of IgG into two Fab and one Fc fragments by papain, a proteolytic enzyme.

The Genetics of the Immunoglobulin Molecule Have Been Determined

Genes that code for amino acid sequences of human IgG L chains are located on different chromosomes than those for IgG H. The V and C regions of the L and H chains are specified by distinct genes. There are four unique genes that code for the C domains of the H chain in the IgG antibody class. Each gene codes for a complete constant region, thus coding for all the amino acids of the H chain except for the V_H region sequence. These four genes are known as gamma (γ) genes—that is, γ_1, γ_2, γ_3, and γ_4—that give rise to **IgG isotypes** IgG_1, IgG_2, IgG_3, and IgG_4. Figure 3.9 presents the amino acid sequences of three γ-gene proteins. There is a 95% homology in amino acid sequence among the genes.

It is likely that a primordial gene coded for a single segment of approximately 110 amino acids, and **gene duplication** events resulted in the three repeating units within the same gene. Mutations modified the individual sequences so that an exact correspondence in sequence no longer exists. Each

Constant Region C1:

$C\gamma_1$:	AlaSerThrLysGlyProSerValPheProLeuAlaProSerSerLysSerThrSerGlyGlyThrAlaAlaLeuGly
$C\gamma_2$	C R E S
$C\gamma_4$	
$C\gamma_1$	CysLeuValLysAspTyrPheProGluProValThrValSerTrpAsnSerGlyAlaLeuThrSerGlyValHisThr
$C\gamma_2$	
$C\gamma_4$	
$C\gamma_1$	PheProAlaValLeuGlnSerSerGlyLeuTyrSerLeuSerSerValValThrValProSerSerSerLeuGly
$C\gamma_2$	N F
$C\gamma_4$	
$C\gamma_1$	ThrGlnThrTyrIleCysAsnValAsnHisLysProSerAsnThrLysValAspLysLysVal
$C\gamma_2$	T D T
$C\gamma_4$	K R

Hinge Region H:

$C\gamma_1$	GluProLysSerCysAspLysThrHisThrCysProProCysPro
$C\gamma_2$	R C V E C P P – – –
$C\gamma_4$	S Y G P P S – – –

Constant Region C2:

$C\gamma_1$	AlaPro GluLeuLeuGlyGlyProSerValPheLeuPheProProLysProLysAspThrLeuMetIleSerArg
$C\gamma_2$	– P V A
$C\gamma_4$	E F G
$C\gamma_1$	ThrProGluValThrCysValValValAspValSerHisGluAspProGluValLysPheAsnTrpTyrValAspGly
$C\gamma_2$	Q
$C\gamma_4$	Q
$C\gamma_1$	ValGluValHisAsnAlaLysThrLysProArgGluGluGlnTyrAsnSerThrThrArgValValSerValLeuThr
$C\gamma_2$	F F
$C\gamma_4$	Y
$C\gamma_1$	ValLeuHisGlnAspTrpLeuAsnGlyLysGluTyrLysCysLysValSerAsnLysAlaLeuProAlaProIleGlu
$C\gamma_2$	V G
$C\gamma_4$	S S
$C\gamma_1$	LysThrIleSerLysAlaLys
$C\gamma_2$	T
$C\gamma_4$	

Constant Region C3:

$C\gamma_1$	GlyGlnProArgGluProGlnValTyrThrLeuProProSerArgAspGluLeuThrLysAsnGlnValSerLeuThr
$C\gamma_2$	E M
$C\gamma_4$	Q
$C\gamma_1$	CysLeuValLysGlyPheTyrProSerAspIleAlaValGluTrpGluSerAsnGlyGlnProGluAsnAsnTyrLys
$C\gamma_2$	
$C\gamma_4$	
$C\gamma_1$	ThrThrProProValLeuAspSerAspGlySerPhePheLeuTyrSerLysLeuThrValAspLysSerArgTrpGln
$C\gamma_2$	M
$C\gamma_4$	R
$C\gamma_1$	GlnGlyAsnValPheSerCysSerValMetHisGluAlaLeuHisAsnHisTyrThrGlnLysSerLeuSerLeuSer
$C\gamma_2$	
$C\gamma_4$	E
$C\gamma_1$	ProGlyLysStop
$C\gamma_2$	
$C\gamma_4$	L

FIGURE 3.9
Amino acid sequence of the heavy chain constant regions of the IgG heavy chain γ_1, γ_2, and γ_4 genes. Domains of constant domain C_H1, hinge region H, constant domain C_H2, and constant domain C_H3 are presented. Sequence for γ_1 is fully given and differences in γ_2 and γ_4 from γ_1 sequence are shown using single-letter amino acid abbreviations. Dashed line (–) indicates absence of an amino acid in position correlated with γ_1, in order to better align sequences to show maximum homology.
Sequence of γ_1 chain from Ellison, J. W., Berson, B. J., and Hood, L. E. Nucleic Acid Res. *10:4071, 1982; and sequences of the γ_2 and γ_4 genes from Ellison, J. and Hood, L.* Proc. Natl. Acad. Sci. U.S.A. *79:1984, 1982.*

immunoglobulin domain has a similar domain length and immunoglobulin folding pattern stabilized by a cystine linkage. Later in evolution gene duplications led to the multiple genes (γ_1, γ_2, γ_3, and γ_4) that code for the constant regions of the IgG class H chains.

The Immunoglobulin Fold Is a Tertiary Structure Found in a Large Family of Proteins with Different Functional Roles

The immunoglobulin fold motif is present in many nonimmunological proteins, which exhibit widely different functions. Based on their structural homology they are grouped into a **protein superfamily** (Figure 3.10). For example, the Class I major histocompatibility complex proteins are in this superfamily; they have immunoglobulin fold motif structures consisting of two stacked antiparallel β-sheets enclosing an internal space filled mainly by hydrophobic amino acids. Two cysteines in the structure form a disulfide bond linking the facing β-sheets. Transcription factors NF-κB and p53 also contain an immunoglobulin fold motif. It can be speculated that gene duplication during evolution led to distribution of the structural motif in the functionally diverse protein superfamily.

3.3 PROTEINS WITH A COMMON CATALYTIC MECHANISM: SERINE PROTEASES

Serine proteases are a family of enzymes that utilize a single uniquely activated serine residue in their substrate-binding site to catalytically hydrolyze peptide bonds. This serine can be characterized by the irreversible reaction of its side chain hydroxyl group with diisopropylfluorophosphate (DFP) (Figure 3.11). Of

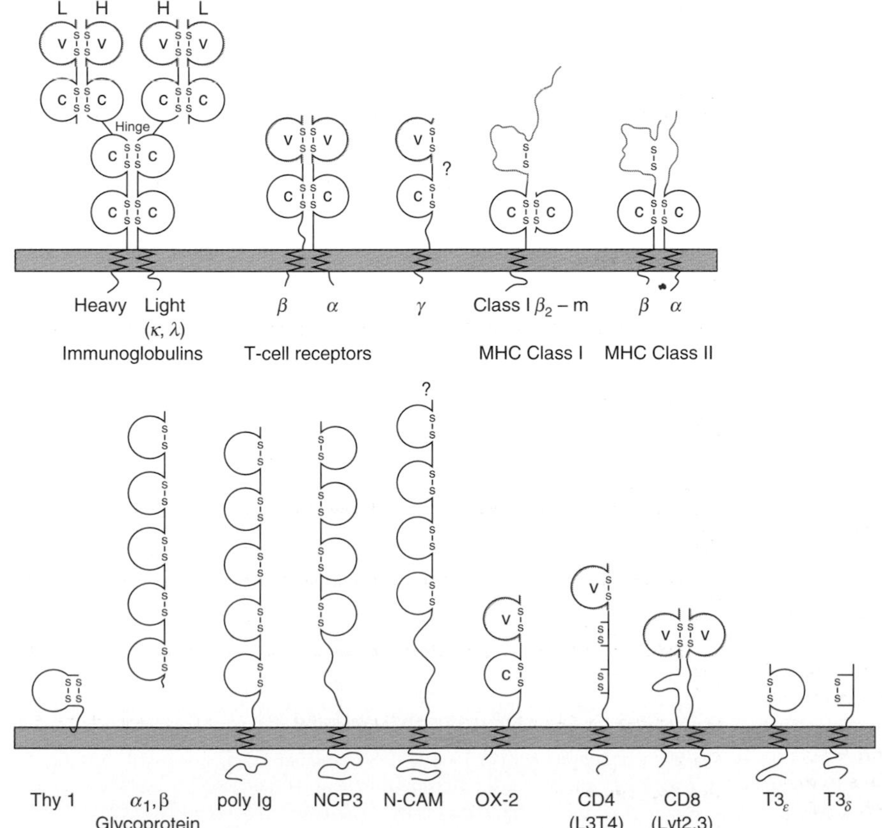

FIGURE 3.10
Diagrammatic representation of immunoglobulin domain structures from different proteins of immunoglobulin gene superfamily.
Proteins presented include heavy and light chains of immunoglobulins, T-cell receptors, major histocompatibility complex (MHC) Class I and Class II proteins, T-cell accessory proteins involved in Class I (CD8) and Class II (CD4) MHC recognition and possible ion channel formation, a receptor responsible for transporting certain classes of immunoglobulin across mucosal membranes (poly-Ig), $\beta_2$microglobulin, which associates with class I molecules, a human plasma protein with unknown function (α_1/β-glycoprotein), two molecules of unknown function with a tissue distribution that includes lymphocytes and neurons (Thy-1, OX-2), and two brain-specific molecules, neuronal cell adhesion molecule (N-CAM) and neurocytoplasmic protein 3 (NCP3).
Reprinted with permission from Hunkapiller, T., and Hood, L. Nature *323:15, 1986.*

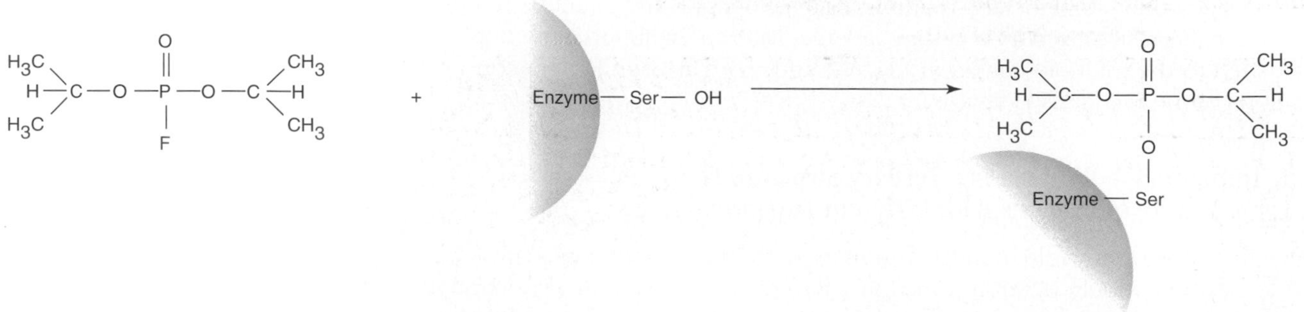

FIGURE 3.11
Reaction of diisopropylfluorophosphate (DFP) with the active-site serine in a serine protease.

all the serines in the protein, DFP reacts only with the catalytically active serine to form a phosphate ester.

Proteolytic Enzymes Are Classified Based on Their Catalytic Mechanism

Proteolytic enzymes are classified according to their catalytic mechanism. Besides serine proteases, other classes utilize cysteine **(cysteine proteases),** aspartate **(aspartate proteases),** or metal ions **(metallo proteases)** to perform their catalytic function. Proteases that hydrolyze peptide bonds within a polypeptide chain are classified as **endopeptidases** and those that cleave the peptide bond of either the COOH- or NH_2-terminal amino acid are classified as **exopeptidases.**

Serine proteases often activate other serine proteases from their inactive precursor form, termed a **zymogen,** by the catalytic cleavage of a specific peptide bond in their structure. Serine proteases participate in carefully controlled physiological processes such as blood coagulation (see Clin. Corr. 3.4),

CLINICAL CORRELATION 3.4

Fibrin Formation in a Myocardial Infarct and the Action of Recombinant Tissue Plasminogen Activator (rt-PA)

Coagulation is an enzyme cascade process in which inactive serine protease enzymes (zymogens) are catalytically activated by other serine proteases in a stepwise manner (the coagulation pathway is described in Chapter 22). These multiple activation events generate catalytic products with a dramatic amplification of the initial signal of the pathway. The end product of the coagulation pathway is a cross-linked fibrin clot. The zymogen of the serine protease components of coagulation include factor II (prothrombin), factor VII (proconvertin), factor IX (Christmas factor), factor X (Stuart factor), factor XI (plasma thromboplastin antecedent), and factor XII (Hageman factor). The roman numeral designation was assigned in the order of their discovery and not from their order of action within the pathway. Upon activation of their zymogen forms, the activated enzymes are noted with the suffix "a." Thus prothrombin is denoted as factor II, and the activated enzyme, thrombin, is factor IIa.

The main function of coagulation is to maintain the integrity of the closed circulatory system after blood vessel injury. The process, however, can be dangerously activated in a myocardial infarction and decrease blood flow to heart muscle. About 1.5 million individuals suffer heart attacks each year, resulting in 600,000 deaths. A fibrinolysis pathway also exists in blood to degrade fibrin clots. This pathway also utilizes zymogen factors that are activated to serine proteases. The end reaction is the activation of plasmin, a serine protease. Plasmin acts directly on fibrin to catalyze the degradation of the fibrin clot. Tissue plasminogen activator (t-PA) is one of the plasminogen activators that activates plasminogen to form plasmin. Recombinant t-PA (rt-PA) is produced by gene cloning technology (see Chapter 18). Clinical studies show that the administration of rt-PA shortly after a myocardial infarct significantly enhances recovery. Other plasminogen activators such as urokinase and streptokinase are also effective.

The GUSTO investigators (authors). An international randomized trial comparing four thrombolytic strategies for acute myocardial infarction. *N. Engl. J. Med.* 329:673, 1993; International Study Group (authors). In hospital mortality and clinical course of 20,891 patients with suspected acute myocardial infarction randomized between alteplase and streptokinase with or without heparin. *Lancet* 336:71, 1990; and Gillis, J. C., Wagstaff, A. J., and Goa, K. L. Alteplase. A reappraisal of its pharmacological properties and therapeutic use in acute myocardial infarction. *Drugs* 50:102, 1995.

TABLE 3.2 Some Serine Proteases and Their Biochemical and Physiological Roles

Protease	*Action*	*Possible Disease Due to Deficiency or Malfunction*
Plasma kallikrein Factor XIIa Factor XIa Factor IXa Factor VIIa Factor Xa Factor IIa (thrombin) Activated protein C	Coagulation (see Clin. Corr. 3.4)	Cerebral infarction (stroke), coronary infarction, thrombosis, bleeding disorders
Factor $C\bar{1}r$ Factor $C\bar{1}s$ Factor D Factor B C3 convertase	Complement (see Clin. Corr. 3.1)	Inflammation, rheumatoid arthritis, autoimmune disease
Trypsin Chymotrypsin Elastase (pancreatic) Enteropeptidase	Digestion	Pancreatitis
Urokinase plasminogen activator Tissue plasminogen activator Plasmin	Fibrinolysis, cell migration, embryogenesis, menstruation	Clotting disorders, tumor metastasis (see Clin. Corr. 3.5)
Tissue kallikreins	Hormone activation	
Acrosin	Fertilization	Infertility
α-Subunit of nerve growth factor γ-Subunit of nerve growth factor	Growth factor activation	
Granulocyte elastase Cathepsin G Mast cell chymases Mast cell tryptases	Extracellular protein and peptide degradation, mast cell function	Inflammation, allergic response

fibrinolysis, complement activation (see Clin. Corr. 3.1), fertilization, and hormone production (Table 3.2). The protein activations catalyzed by serine proteases are examples of "limited proteolysis" because only one or two specific peptide bonds of the hundreds in a protein substrate are hydrolyzed. Under denaturing conditions, however, these same enzymes hydrolyze multiple peptide bonds and lead to digestion of peptides, proteins, and even self-digestion (autolysis). Several diseases, such as emphysema, arthritis, thrombosis, cancer metastasis (see Clin. Corr. 3.5), and some forms of hemophilia, are thought to result from the lack of regulation of serine protease activities.

Serine Proteases Exhibit Remarkable Specificity for Site of Peptide Bond Hydrolysis

Many serine proteases exhibit preference for hydrolysis of peptide bonds adjacent to a particular class of amino acid. The serine protease trypsin cleaves following basic amino acids such as arginine and lysine, and chymotrypsin cleaves peptide bonds following large hydrophobic amino acid residues such

CLINICAL CORRELATION 3.5

Involvement of Serine Proteases in Tumor Cell Metastasis

The serine protease urokinase is believed to be required for the metastasis of cancer cells. Metastasis is the process by which a cancer cell leaves a primary tumor and migrates through the blood or lymph system to a new tissue or organ, where a secondary tumor grows. Increased synthesis of urokinase has been correlated with an increased ability to metastasize in many cancers. Urokinase activates plasminogen to form plasmin. Plasminogen is ubiquitously located in extracellular space and its activation to plasmin can cause the catalytic degradation of the proteins in the extracellular matrix through which the metastasizing tumor cells migrate. Plasmin can also activate procollagenase to collagenase, promoting the degradation of collagen in the basement membrane surrounding the capillaries and lymph system. This promotion of proteolytic degradative activity by the urokinase secreted by tumor cells allows the tumor cells to invade the target tissue and form secondary tumor sites.

Dano, K., Andreasen, P. A., Grondahl-Hansen, J., Kristensen, P., Nielsen, L. S., and Skriver, L. Plasminogen activators, tissue degradation and cancer. *Adv. Cancer Res.* 44:139, 1985; Yu, H., and Schultz, R. M. Relationship between secreted urokinase plasminogen activator activity and metastatic potential in murine B16 cells transfected with human urokinase sense and antisense genes. *Cancer Res.* 50:7623, 1990; and Fazioli, F., and Blasi, F. Urokinase-type plasminogen activator and its receptor: new targets for anti-metastatic therapy? *Trends Pharmacol. Sci.* 15:25, 1994.

as tryptophan, phenylalanine, tyrosine, and leucine. Elastase cleaves peptide bonds following small hydrophobic residues such as alanine. A serine protease may be called trypsin-like if it prefers to cleave peptide bonds of lysine and arginine, chymotrypsin-like if it prefers aromatic amino acids, and elastase-like if it prefers amino acids with small side chain groups like alanine. The specificity for a certain type of amino acid only indicates its relative preference. Trypsin can also cleave peptide bonds following hydrophobic amino acids, but at a much slower rate than for the basic amino acids. Thus specificity for hydrolysis of the peptide bond of a particular type of amino acid may not be absolute, but may be more accurately described as a range of most likely targets. Each of the identical amino acid hydrolysis sites within a protein substrate is not equally susceptible. Trypsin hydrolyzes each of the multiple arginine peptide bonds in a particular protein at a different catalytic rate, and some may require a conformational change to make them accessible.

Detailed studies of the specificity of serine proteases for a particular peptide bond have been performed with synthetic substrates with fewer than 10 amino acids (Table 3.3). Because these substrates are significantly smaller than the

TABLE 3.3 Reactivity of α-Chymotrypsin and Elastase Toward Substrates of Various Structures

Structure	*Variation in Side Chain Group (Chymotrypsin)*	*Relative Reactivity*[a]
Glycyl	H—	1
Leucyl	$(H_3C)_2CH-CH_2-$	1.6×10^4
Methionyl	$CH_3-S-CH_2-CH_2-$	2.4×10^4
Phenylalaninyl	$C_6H_5-CH_2-$ (phenyl ring)	4.3×10^6
Hexahydrophenylalaninyl	(S ring)$-CH_2-$	8.2×10^6
Tyrosyl	$HO-C_6H_4-CH_2-$	3.7×10^7
Tryptophanyl	(indolyl, N–H)$-CH_2-$	4.3×10^7
Variation in chain length (elastase hydrolysis of Ala N-terminal amide)[b]		
Ac-Ala-NH_2		
Ac-Pro-Ala-NH_2		1
Ac-Ala-Pro-Ala-NH_2		1.4×10^1
Ac-Pro-Ala-Pro-Ala-NH_2		4.2×10^3
Ac-Ala-Pro-Ala-Pro-Ala-		4.4×10^5
NH_2		2.7×10^5

[a] Calculated from values of k_{cat}/K_m found for *N*-acetyl amino acid methyl esters in chymotrypsin substrates.

[b] Calculated from values of k_{cat}/K_m in Thompson, R. C., and Blout, E. R. *Biochemistry* 12:57, 1973.

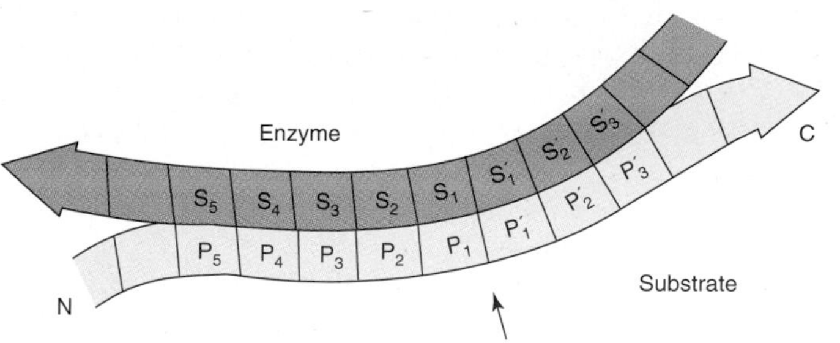

FIGURE 3.12
Schematic diagram of binding of a polypeptide substrate to binding site in a proteolytic enzyme.
$P_5, P_4, \ldots, P'_3$ are amino acid residues in the substrate that are binding to subsites $S_5, S_4, \ldots, S'_3$ in the enzyme with peptide hydrolysis occurring between P_1–P'_1 (arrow). NH_2-terminal direction of substrate polypeptide chain is indicated by N, and COOH-terminal direction by C.
Redrawn from Polgar, L. In: A. Neuberger and K. Brocklehurst (Eds.), Hydrolytic Enzymes. *Amsterdam: Elsevier, 1987, p. 174.*

natural ones, they interact only with the catalytic site (primary binding site S_1, see below) and are said to be **active-site directed.** Studies with small substrates and inhibitors indicate that the site of hydrolysis is flanked by approximately four amino acid residues in both directions that bind to the enzyme and impact on the reactivity of the bond hydrolyzed. The two amino acids in the substrate that contribute the hydrolyzable bond are designated $\mathbf{P_1}$**—**$\mathbf{P'_1}$**.** Thus in trypsin-like substrates P_1 will be lysine or arginine and in chymotrypsin-like substrates P_1 will be a hydrophobic amino acid. The other interacting residues in the substrate are labeled P_4—P_2 on the NH_2-terminal side of P_1—P'_1 and the COOH-terminal residues to the scissile bond are substrate residues P'_2—P'_4. Thus the residues in the substrate that interact with the **extended active site** in the serine protease will be P_4—P_3—P_2—P_1—P'_1—P'_2—P'_3—P'_4. The complementary regions in the enzyme that bind the amino acid residues in the substrate are designated subsites $\mathbf{S_4 \cdots S'_4}$ (Figure 3.12). It is the **secondary interactions,** outside S_1—S'_1, with the substrate that ultimately determines a protease's specificity toward a particular protein substrate. Thus the serine protease in coagulation, factor Xa, only cleaves a particular arginine peptide bond in prothrombin, activating prothrombin to thrombin. It is the secondary interaction that allows factor Xa to recognize the particular arginine in the structure of prothrombin to be cleaved. The interaction of the substrate residues $P_4 \cdots P'_4$ with the enzyme-binding subsites $S_4 \cdots S'_4$ are due to noncovalent interactions. The substrate interacts with the enzyme-binding site to extend a β-sheet structure between the polypeptide chain in the enzyme and the polypeptide chain of the substrate, which places the scissile peptide bond of the substrate into S_1—S'_1 (Figure 3.13).

Serine Proteases Are Synthesized in a Zymogen Form

Serine proteases are synthesized in an inactive **zymogen** form, which requires limited proteolysis to produce the active enzyme. Those for coagulation are synthesized in liver cells and are secreted into the blood for subsequent activation by other serine proteases following vascular injury. Zymogen forms are usually designated by the suffix *-ogen* after the enzyme name; the zymogen form of trypsin is termed trypsin*ogen* and for chymotrypsin is termed chymotrypsin*ogen.* In some cases the zymogen form is referred to as a **proenzyme;** the zymogen form of thrombin is prothrombin.

Several plasma serine proteases secrete zymogen forms that contain **multiple nonsimilar domains.** Protein C, involved in a fibrinolysis pathway in blood, has four distinct domains (Figure 3.14). The NH_2-terminal domain con-

FIGURE 3.13
Schematic drawing of binding of pancreatic trypsin inhibitor to trypsinogen based on X-ray diffraction data.
Binding-site region of trypsinogen in the complex assumes a conformation like that of active trypsin with inhibitor, which is believed to bind in a similar manner to a substrate in the active enzyme-binding site. One cannot obtain X-ray structures of a natural enzyme–substrate complex because substrate is used up at a rate faster than the time of the X-ray diffraction experiment (see p. 76). Note that inhibitor has an extended conformation so that amino acids P_9, P_7, P_5, P_3, P_1 . . . , P_3' interact with binding subsites S_5, . . . , S_3'. Potentially hydrolyzable bond in inhibitor is between P_1–P_1'.
Reprinted with permission from Bolognesi, M., Gatti, B., Menegatti, E., Guarneri, M., Papamokos, E., and Huber, R. J. Mol. Biol. *162:839, 1983.*

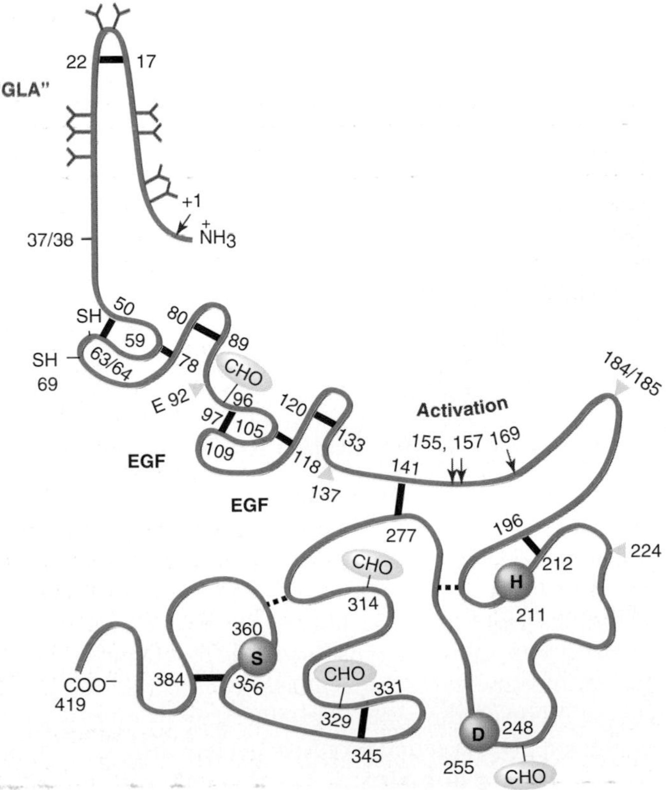

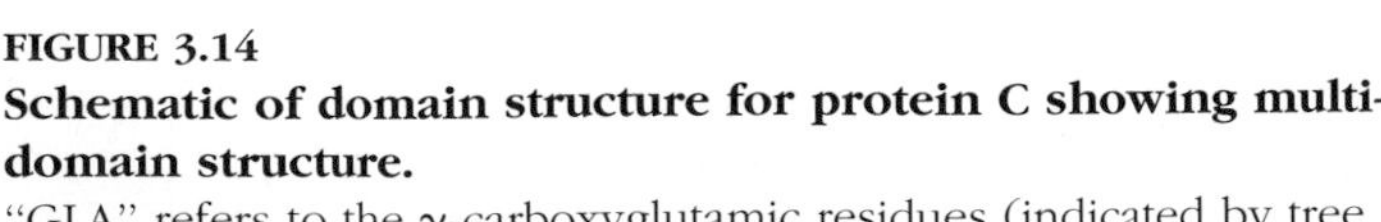

FIGURE 3.14
Schematic of domain structure for protein C showing multidomain structure.
"GLA" refers to the γ-carboxyglutamic residues (indicated by tree structures) in the NH_2-terminal domain, disulfide bridges are indicated by thick bars, EGF indicates positions of epidermal growth factor-like domains, and CHO indicates positions where sugar residues are joined to the polypeptide chain. Proteolytic cleavage sites leading to catalytic activation are shown by arrows. Amino acid sequence is numbered from NH_2-terminal end, and catalytic sites of serine, histidine, and aspartate are shown by circled one-letter abbreviations S, H, and D, respectively.
Redrawn from a figure in Long, G. L. J. Cell. Biochem. *33:185, 1987.*

tains the derived amino acid, **γ-carboxyglutamic acid** (Figure 3.15), which is enzymatically formed by carboxylation of glutamic acid residues in a vitamin K-dependent reaction. The γ-carboxyglutamic acids chelate calcium ions and form part of a binding site to membranes. The COOH-terminal segment contains the catalytic domains. Activation of these zymogens requires specific proteolysis outside the catalytic domains (Figure 3.14) and is controlled by the binding through the nine γ-carboxyglutamic acid residues at the NH_2-terminal end to a membrane.

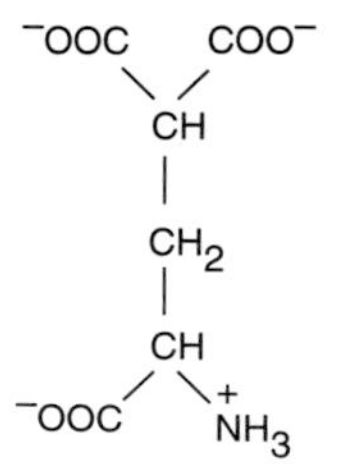

$$\begin{array}{c} ^{-}OOC\quad COO^{-} \\ \diagdown\ \diagup \\ CH \\ | \\ CH_2 \\ | \\ CH \\ \diagup\ \diagdown \\ ^{-}OOC\quad \overset{+}{N}H_3 \end{array}$$

FIGURE 3.15
Structure of the derived amino acid γ-carboxyglutamic acid (abbreviation Gla), found in NH_2-terminal domain of many clotting proteins.

There Are Specific Protein Inhibitors of Serine Proteases

Evolutionary selection of this enzyme family for participation in physiological processes requires a parallel evolution of control factors. Specific proteins inhibit the activities of serine proteases after their physiological role has ended (Table 3.4). Thus coagulation is limited to the site of vascular injury and complementation activation leads to lysis only of cells exhibiting foreign antigens. Inability to control these protease systems, which may be caused by a deficiency of a specific inhibitor, can lead to undesirable consequences, such as thrombi formation in myocardial infarction and stroke or uncontrolled reactions of complement in autoimmune disease. Natural inhibitors of serine proteases, termed **serpins** for *ser*ine *p*rotease *in*hibitors, have evolved. This family of inhibitors occurs in animals that have the proteases, but surprisingly these inhibitors are also found in plants that lack proteases.

Serine Proteases Have Similar Structure–Function Relationships

The complex relationships between structure and physiological function in the serine proteases require analysis of a number of observations. (1) Only one serine residue is catalytically active and participates in peptide bond hydrolysis. Bovine trypsin contains 34 serine residues with only one catalytically active or able to react with the inhibitor DFP (see Figure 3.11). (2) X-ray diffraction and amino acid sequence homology studies demonstrate that there are two residues, a histidine and an aspartate, that are always associated with the activated serine

TABLE 3.4 Some Human Proteins that Inhibit Serine Proteases

Inhibitor	*Action*
α_1-Proteinase inhibitor	Inhibits tissue proteases including neutrophil elastase; deficiency leads to pulmonary emphysema
α_1- Antichymotrypsin	Inhibits proteases of chymotrypsin-like specificity from neutrophils, basophils, and mast cells including cathepsin G and chymase
Inter-α-trypsin inhibitor	Inhibits broad range of serine protease activities in plasma
α_2-Antiplasmin	Inhibits plasmin
Antithrombin III	Inhibits thrombin and other coagulation proteases
C_1 Inhibitor	Inhibits complement reaction
α_2-Macroglobulin	General protease inhibitor
Protease nexin I	Inhibits thrombin, urokinase, and plasmin
Protease nexin II	Inhibits growth factor-associated serine proteases, identical to NH_2-terminal domain of amyloid protein secreted in Alzheimer's disease
Plasminogen activator inhibitor I	Inhibits plasminogen activators
Plasminogen activator inhibitor II	Inhibits urokinase plasminogen activator

in the catalytic site. Based on their positions in chymotrypsinogen, these three invariant active site residues of serine proteases are named Ser 195, His 57, and Asp 102. This numbering, based on their sequence number in chymotrypsinogen, is used to identify these residues irrespective of their exact position in the primary structure of any serine protease. (3) Eukaryotic serine proteases exhibit a high sequence and structural similarity with each other. (4) Genes that code for serine proteases are organized similarly (Figure 3.16). In eukaryotic genes, exons are segments of the genomic DNA that are combined into the final messenger RNA that carries the information for the protein. The exons are separated by introns, which are spliced out of RNA and not present in the final messenger RNA (see p. 703). The **exon–intron patterns** of serine proteases show that each of the catalytically essential amino acid residues (Ser 195 , His 57, and Asp 102) are on different exons. The catalytically essential histidine and serine are all almost adjacent to their exon boundary. The similarity in exon–intron organization exists for the serine protease family of enzymes among eukaryotic species. The cross-species homology in serine protease gene structure further supports the concept that the serine proteases evolved from a common primordial gene. (5) The catalytic unit of serine proteases exhibits two structural domains, of approximately equal size. The catalytic site is within the interface (crevice) between the two domains. (6) Serine proteases that function through direct interaction with membranes typically have an additional domain to provide this specific function. (7) Natural protein substrates and inhibitors of serine proteases bind through an extended specificity site. (8) Specificity for natural protein inhibitors is marked by extremely tight binding. The binding constant for trypsin to pancreatic trypsin inhibitor is on the order of 10^{13} M^{-1}, reflecting a binding free energy of approximately 18 kcal mol^{-1}. (9) Natural protein inhibitors are usually poor substrates with strong inhibition by the inhibitor requiring hydrolysis of a peptide bond in the inhibitor by the

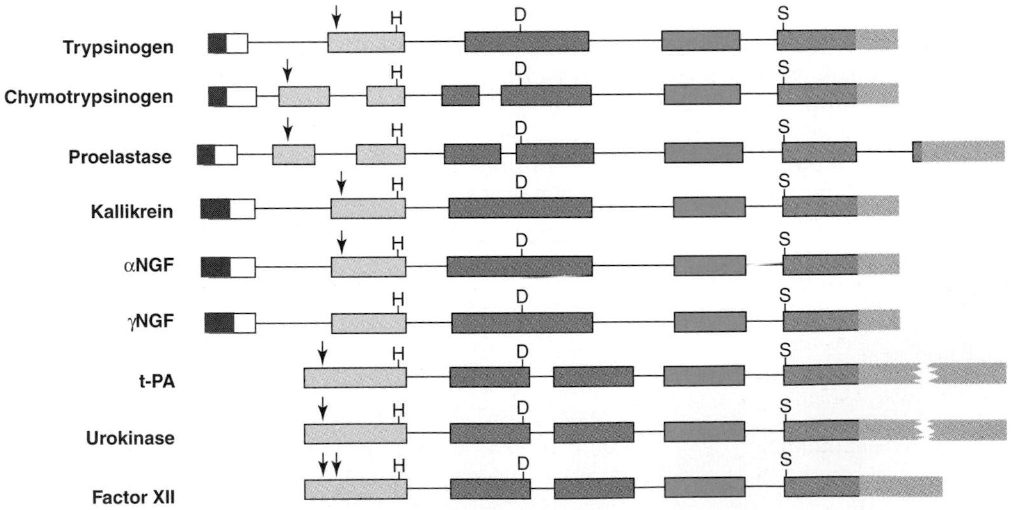

FIGURE 3.16
Organization of exons and introns in genes that code for serine proteases. t-PA is tissue plasminogen activator and NGF is nerve growth factor. Exons are shown by boxes and introns by connecting lines. Position of the nucleotide codons for active-site serine, histidine, and aspartate are denoted by S, H, and D, respectively. Red boxes, on left, show regions that code for NH_2-terminal part of polypeptide chain (signal peptide) cleaved before protein is secreted. Light-colored boxes, on right, represent part of gene sequence transcribed into messenger RNA (mRNA), but not translated into protein. Arrows show codons for residues at which proteolytic activation of zymogen forms occurs.
Based on a figure in Irwin, D. M., Roberts, K. A., and MacGillivray, R. T. J. Mol. Biol. *200:31, 1988.*

protease. (10) Serine proteases in eukaryotes are synthesized in zymogen forms to permit their production and transport in an inactive state to their sites of action. (11) Zymogen activation frequently involves hydrolysis by another serine protease. (12) Several serine proteases undergo **autolysis** or self-hydrolysis. Sometimes the self-reaction leads to specific peptide bond cleavage and activation of the catalytic activity. At other times autolysis leads to inactivation of the protease.

Amino Acid Sequence Homology Occurs in the Serine Protease Family

Much of our early knowledge of the serine protease family came from trypsin and chymotrypsin purified from bovine materials obtained from a slaughterhouse. This has yielded a useful but nonintuitive nomenclature, which uses a sequence alignment against the amino acid sequence of chymotrypsin, to name and number residues of other serine proteases. As mentioned previously, the catalytically essential residues are Ser 195, His 57, and Asp 102. Insertions and deletions of the amino acids in another serine protease are compared to the numbering of residues in chymotrypsin. Alignment is made by algorithms that maximize sequence homology, with exact alignment of the essential serine, histidine, and aspartate residues. These three residues are invariant in all serine proteases and the sequences surrounding them are invariant among the serine proteases of the chymotrypsin family (Table 3.5).

Members of the chymotrypsin family also occur in prokaryotes. Thus bacterial serine proteases from *Streptomyces griseus* and *Myxobacteria* 450 have a structural and functional homology with chymotrypsin. A separate class of serine protease enzymes has been isolated, however, from bacteria that has no structural homology to the mammalian chymotrypsin family. The serine protease subtilisin, isolated from *Bacillus subtilis,* hydrolyzes peptide bonds and contains an activated serine with a histidine and aspartate in its active site but the active

TABLE 3.5 Invariant Sequences Found Around the Catalytically Essential Serine (S) and Histidine (H)

Enzyme	*Sequence (Identical Residues to Chymotrypsin Are in Bold)*
	Residues Around Catalytically Essential Histidine
Chymotrypsin A	F **H F C G G S L I N E N W V V T A A H C** G V T T S D
Trypsin	Y **H F C G G S L I N** S Q **W V V** S **A A H C** Y K S G I Q
Pancreatic elastase	A **H** T **C G G** T **L I** R Q **N W V** M **T A A H C** V D R E L T
Thrombin	E L L **C G** A **S L I** S D R **W V** L **T A A H C** L L Y P P W
Factor X	E G **F C G G** T I L **N E** F Y **V** L **T A A H C** L H Q A K R
Plasmin	M **H F C G G** T **L I** S P E **W V** L **T A A H C** L E K S P R
Plasma kallikrein	S F Q **C G G** V **L** V **N** P K **W V** L **T A A H C** K N D N Y E
Streptomyces trypsin	– – – **C G G** A **L** Y A Q D I **V** L **T A A H C** V S G S G N
Subtilisin	V G G A S F V A G E A Y N T D G N G **H** G T H V A G T
	Residues Around Catalytically Essential Serine
Chymotrypsin A	**C A G** – – – A S **G V** – – **S S C M G D S G G P L V**
Trypsin	**C A G** Y – – L E **G** G K – D **S C** Q ***G D S G G P*** V **V**
Pancreatic elastase	**C A G** – – – G N **G V** R – **S** G **C** Q **G D S G G P L H**
Thrombin	**C A G** Y K P G E **G** K R G D A **C** E **G D S G G P** F **V**
Factor X	**C A G** Y – – D T **Q** P E – D A **C** Q **G D S G G P** H **V**
Plasmin	**C A G** H – – L A **G** G T – D **S C** Q **G D S G G P L V**
Pl. kallikrein	**C A G** Y – – L P **G** G K – D T **C M G D S G G P L** I
Streptomyces trypsin	**C A G** Y – P D T **G** G V – D T **C** Q **G D S G G P** M F
Subtilisin	A G V Y S T Y P T N T Y A T L N **G** T **S** M A S P H

Source: From Barrett, A. J. In: A. J. Barrett and G. Salvesen (Eds.), *Proteinase Inhibitors*. Amsterdam: Elsevier, 1986, p. 7.

site arises from structural regions of the protein that bear no sequence or structural homology with the chymotrypsin serine proteases. This serine protease is an example of **convergent evolution** of an enzyme catalytic mechanism. Apparently a gene completely different from those that code for chymotrypsin-like serine proteases evolved the same catalytic mechanism utilizing an active-site serine. The primary and tertiary structure , however, is different from that of the trypsin- and chymotrypsin-like structure.

Tertiary Structures of Serine Proteases Are Similar

Ser 195 in chymotrypsin reacts with diisopropylfluorophosphate (DFP), with a 1 : 1 enzyme : DFP stoichiometry, that inhibits the enzyme. The three-dimensional structure of chymotrypsin reveals that the Ser 195 is situated within an internal pocket, with access to the solvent interface. His 57 and Asp 102 are oriented so that they participate with the Ser 195 in the catalytic mechanism of the enzyme (see Chapter 4).

Structure determinations by X-ray crystallography have been carried out on many members of this class of proteins (Table 3.6). Structural data are available for catalytically active enzyme forms, zymogens, the same enzyme in multiple species, enzyme–inhibitor complexes, and a particular enzyme at different temperatures and in different solvents. The most complete analysis has been that of trypsin. Its X-ray diffraction analysis has yielded a three-dimensional structure at better than 1.7-Å resolution, which can resolve atoms at a separation of 1.3 Å such as the C=O separation of the carbonyl group (1.2 Å). This resolution, however, is not uniform over the entire trypsin structure. Different regions of the molecule have a variable tendency to be localized in space during the time course of the X-ray diffraction experiment, and for some atoms in the structure their exact position cannot be as precisely defined as for others. The structural disorder is especially apparent in surface residues not in contact with neighboring molecules. Rapid methods for X-ray data acquisition (see Chapter 2) further support this observation of dynamic fluctuation. Trypsin is globular in its overall shape and consists of two domains of approximately equal size (Figure 3.17), which do not penetrate one another. The secondary structure of trypsin has little α-helix, except in the COOH-terminal region of the molecule. The structure is predominantly β-structure, with each of the

TABLE 3.6 Serine Protease Structures Determined by X-Ray Crystallography

Enzyme	*Species Source*	*Inhibitors Present*	*Resolution (Å)*
Chymotrypsin[a]	Bovine	Yes[b]	1.67[c]
Chymotrypsinogen	Bovine	No	2.5
Elastase	Porcine	Yes	2.5
Kallikrein	Porcine	Yes	2.05
Proteinase A	*S. griseus*	No	1.5
Proteinase B	*S. griseus*	Yes	1.8
Proteinase II	Rat	No	1.9
Trypsin[a]	Bovine	Yes[b]	1.4[c]
Trypsinogen[a]	Bovine	Yes[b]	1.65[c]

[a] Structure of this enzyme molecule independently determined by two or more investigators.

[b] Structure obtained with no inhibitor present (native structure) and with inhibitors. Inhibitors used include low molecular weight inhibitors (i.e., benzamidine, DFP, and tosyl) and protein inhibitors (i.e., bovine pancreatic trypsin inhibitor).

[c] Highest resolution for this molecule of the multiple determinations.

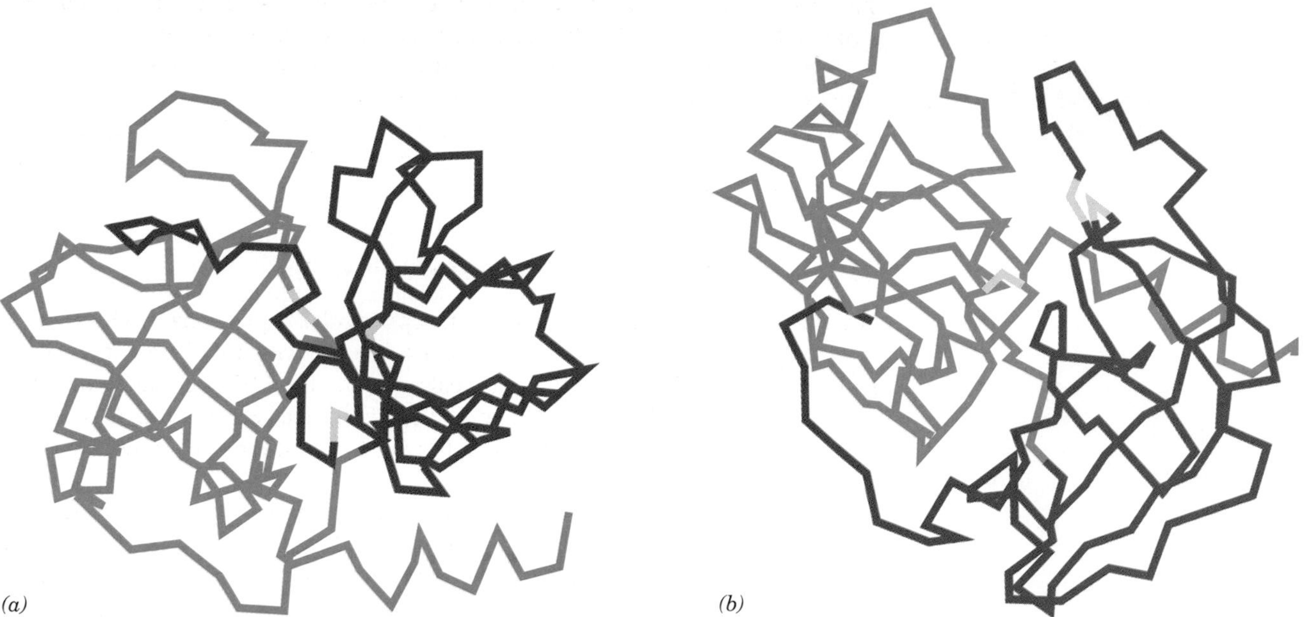

FIGURE 3.17
Two views of the structure of trypsin showing tertiary structure of two domains. Active-site serine, histidine, and aspartate are indicated in yellow.

domains in a "deformed" β-barrel. Loop regions protrude from the barrel ends, being almost symmetrically presented by each of the two folded domains. These loop structures combine to form a surface region of the enzyme that extends outward, above the catalytic site. These loops have a structural and functional similarity to the CDRs of immunoglobulins.

Alignment of three-dimensional structures can be performed on serine proteases using a mathematical function that compares structural equivalence and allows for insertion and deletion of amino acids in a particular sequence. The data of Table 3.7 contrast the extent of structural superimposability with the homology of sequences brought into coincidence by the structural superposition. This table shows the total number of amino acids and the number that are statistically identical in each structure, by X-ray diffraction, in their topological position, even if they are chemically different amino acids. Topologically equivalent amino acids have the same relationship in three-dimensional space to the point where they cannot be distinguished from one another by X-ray diffraction. The last column presents the number of amino acids that are chemically identical. In these structural alignments the regions of greatest difference appear to be localized to the CDR-like loop regions, which extend from the β-barrel domains to form the surface region out from the catalytic site. The effect of

TABLE 3.7 Structural Superposition of Selected Serine Proteases and the Resultant Amino Acid Sequence Comparison

Comparison	*Number of Amino Acids in Sequence*		*Number of Structurally Equivalent Residues*	*Number of Chemically Identical Residues*
	Protease 1	*Protease 2*		
Trypsin–elastase	223	240	188	81
Trypsin–chymotrypsin	223	241	185	93
Trypsin–mast cell protease	223	224	188	69
Trypsin–prekallikrein	223	232	194	84
Trypsin–*S. griseus* protease	223	180	121	25

altering the amino acids in these loops is to alter the **macromolecular binding specificity** of the protease. It is the structure of the loop in factor Xa, for example, that allows it to specifically bind to prothrombin. Serpins interact with different proteases based on their affinity for the loop structures. Bacterial proteases related to the eukaryotic serine protease family contain the same two domains as do the eukaryotic family but lack most of the loop structures. This agrees with the lack of a requirement of bacterial proteases for complex interactions that the eukaryotic protease must carry out and the observation that bacterial proteases are not produced in a zymogen form.

Thus the serine protease family constitutes a structurally related series of proteins that use a catalytically active serine. During evolution, the basic two-domain structure and the catalytically essential residues have been maintained, but the region of the secondary interactions (loop regions) have changed to give the different proteins of the family their different specificities toward substrates, activators, and inhibitors, characteristic of their important physiological functions.

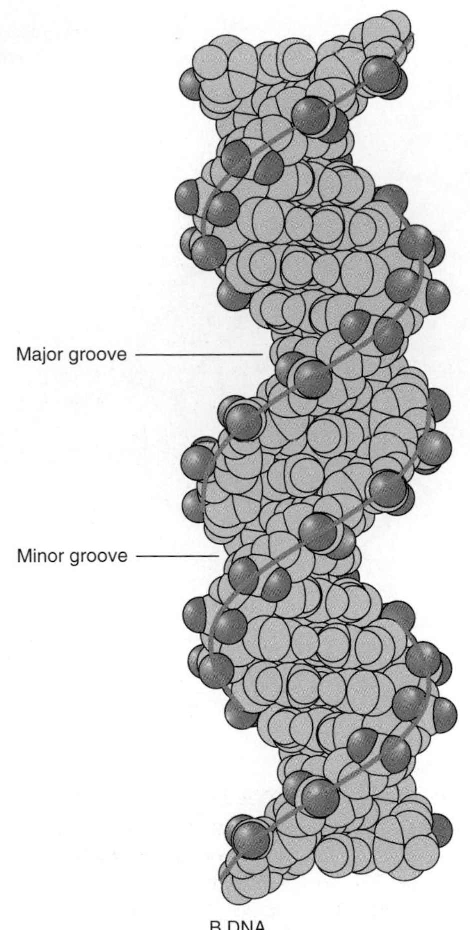

FIGURE 3.18
Space-filling model of DNA in B conformation showing major and minor grooves.
Reprinted with permission from Rich, A. J. Biomol. Struct. Dyn. *1:1, 1983.*

3.4 ■ DNA-BINDING PROTEINS

Regulatory sites exist in DNA that bind proteins that control gene expression. These sites contain a nucleotide sequence that binds regulatory proteins known as transcription factors. The specific DNA sequence, or **transcription factor binding element,** is usually less than 10 nucleotides long. Noncovalent interactions between the protein and DNA allow the protein to recognize the nucleotide sequence and bind to a specific regulatory site. This is a highly selective feat as the human genome has up to 100,000 genes, each with its own regulatory sequences. While there are huge gaps in our knowledge of how proteins regulate gene expression, some common structural motifs of DNA-binding proteins are apparent.

Three Major Structural Motifs of DNA-Binding Proteins

Along the helical spiral of a DNA molecule in its most common form (B form) are two grooves, the major and minor grooves (Figure 3.18) (see Chapter 14) to which the proteins must associate. A structural motif found in many DNA-binding proteins is the **helix–turn–helix (HTH).** An HTH places one of its α-helices, designated the **recognition helix,** across the major groove where side chain residues of the helix form specific noncovalent interactions with the base sequence of the target DNA. The interaction appears to induce distortions in conformation of the B-DNA binding site that better accommodate the interactions with protein. Nonspecific interactions are made between the protein and sugar–phosphate backbone of DNA. HTH proteins bind as dimers; thus there are two helix–turn–helix motifs per active regulatory protein. X-ray structures show the two helix–turn–helix motifs protruding from the structure of each monomer domain binding at two adjacent turns of the major groove in the DNA, making a strong protein–DNA interaction (Figures 3.19–3.21).

The **zinc-finger** motif is another structure found in some DNA-binding proteins. Zinc-finger proteins contain repeating motifs of a Zn^{2+} atom bonded to two cysteine and two histidine side chains (Figure 3.22). In some cases the histidines may be substituted by cysteines. The primary structure for the motif contains two close cysteines separated by about 12 amino acids from a second pair of Zn^{2+} liganding amino acids (histidine or cysteine). The three-dimensional structure of one zinc finger has been deduced by ^{1}H-NMR (Figure 3.23). The motif contains an α-helix segment that can bind within the major groove at its target site in DNA and makes specific interactions with the nucleotide base sequence.

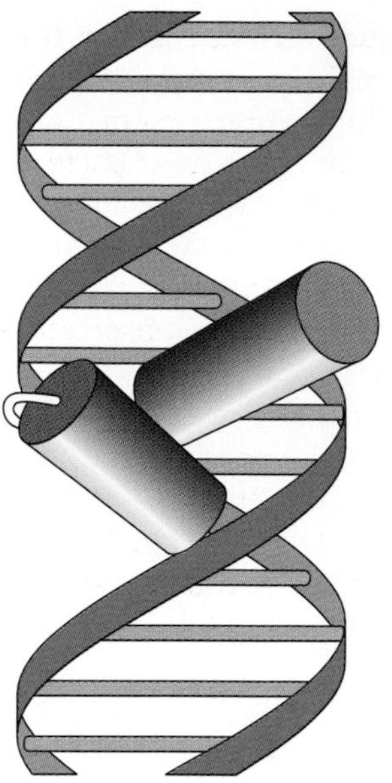

FIGURE 3.19
Binding of a helix–turn–helix motif into the major groove of B-DNA.
The recognition helix lies across the major groove.
Redrawn from Schleif, R. Science *241:241, 1988.*

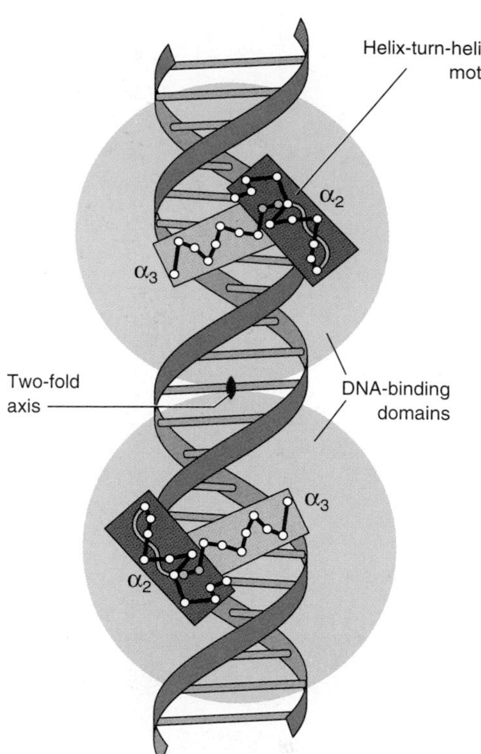

FIGURE 3.20
Association of a DNA-binding protein (dimer) with two helix–turn–helix motifs into adjacent major grooves of B-DNA.
Redrawn from Brennan, R. G., and Matthews, B. W. Trends Biochem. Sci. *14:287, 1989 (Fig. 1b).*

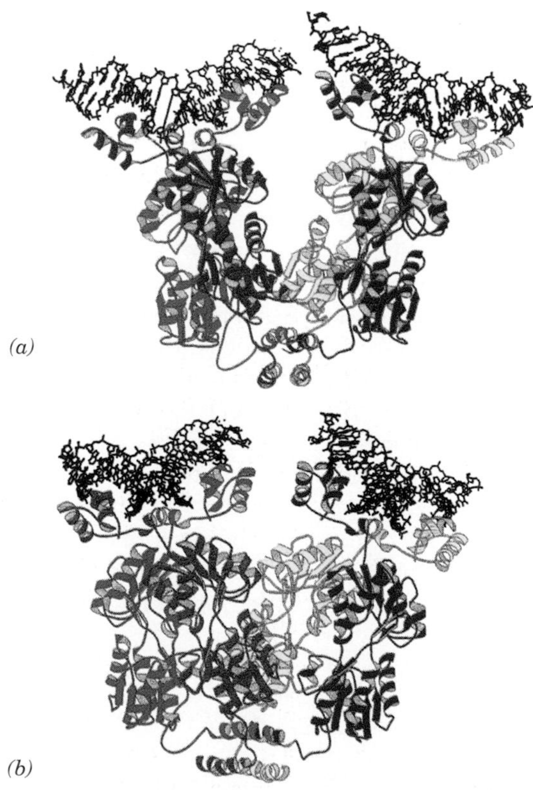

FIGURE 3.21
X-ray crystallographic structure of helix–turn–helix motif *lac* repressor protein in association with target DNA.
(*a*) Repressor is a tetramer protein with individual monomers colored green and violet (left), red and yellow (right). The DNA targets are colored blue (top). Recognition helices from dimer of tetramer are shown to interact in adjacent major grooves of target DNAs. Each dimer in tetramer interacts with a discrete (separated) target consensus sequence present in DNA. (*b*) A different view of the same tetramer.
Reprinted with permission from Lewis, M., Chang, G., Horton, N. C., Kercher, M. A., Pace, H. C., Schumacher, M. A., Brennan, R. G., and Lu, P. Science *271:1247, 1996. Copyright 1996 American Association for the Advancement of Science.*

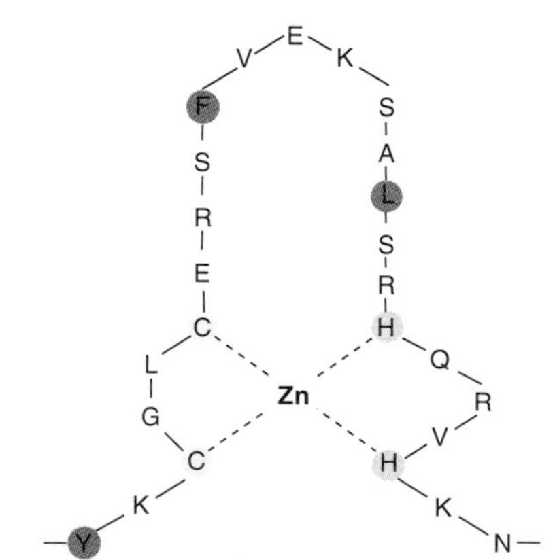

FIGURE 3.22
Primary sequence of a zinc-finger motif found in DNA-binding protein Xfin from *Xenopus*.
Invariant and highly conserved amino acids in structure are circled in dark red.
Redrawn from Lee, M. S., Gippert, G. P., Soman, K. V., Case, D. A., and Wright, P. E. Science *245:635, 1989.*

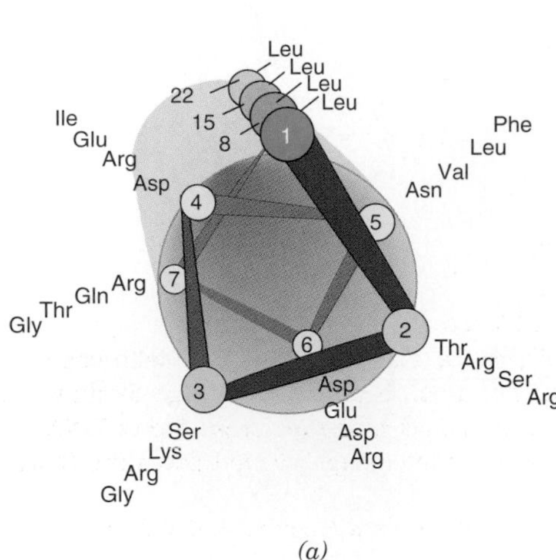

(a)

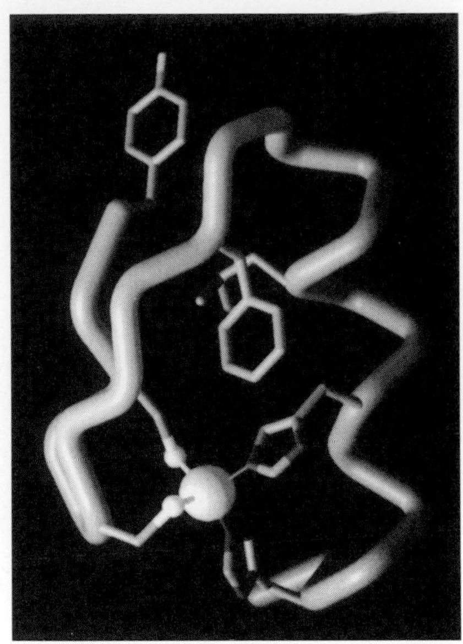

FIGURE 3.23

Three-dimensional structure obtained by ^{1}H-NMR of zinc-finger motif from *Xenopus* protein Xfin (sequence shown in Figure 3.22).

Superposition of 37 possible structures derived from calculations based on the ^{1}H-NMR. NH_2 terminal is at upper left and COOH terminal is at bottom right. Zinc is sphere at the bottom with Cys residues to the left and His residues to the right.

Photograph provided by Michael Pique, and Peter E. Wright, Department of Molecular Biology, Research Institute of Scripps Clinic, La Jolla, California.

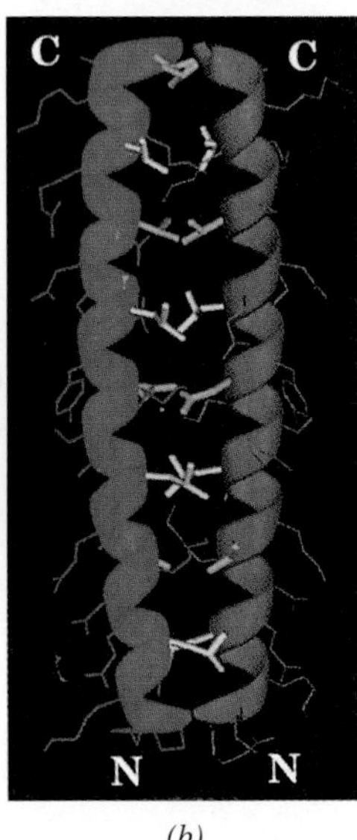

(b)

FIGURE 3.24

Leucine zipper motif of DNA-binding proteins.

(a) Helical wheel analysis of the leucine-zipper motif in DNA enhancer-binding protein. The amino acid sequence in the wheel analysis is displayed end-to-end down the axis of a schematic α-helix structure. The leucines (Leu) are observed in alignment along one edge of the helix (residues 1, 8, 15, and 22 in the sequence). (b) The X-ray structure, in side view, in which the helices are presented in ribbon form and side chains in stick form. Contacting leucine residues in yellow and green.

(a) Redrawn from Landschulz, W. H., Johnson, P. F., and McKnight, S. L. Science *240:1759, 1988. (b) Figure reproduced with permission from D. Voet and J. Voet,* Biochemistry, 2nd ed. *New York: Wiley, 1995 and based on an X-ray structure by Peter Kim, MIT, and Tom Alber, University of Utah School of Medicine.*

A third structural motif found in some of the DNA-binding proteins is the **leucine zipper.** Leucine zippers are formed from a region of α-helix that contain at least four leucines, each leucine separated by six amino acids from one another (i.e., Leu-X_6-Leu-X_6-Leu-X_6-Leu, where X is any common amino acid). With 3.6 residues per turn of the α-helix, the leucines align on one edge of the helix, with a leucine at every second turn of the helix (Figure 3.24). The leucine-rich helix forms a hydrophobic interaction with a second leucine helix on another polypeptide chain subunit, to "zipper" the two subunits together to form a dimer (Figure 3.25). The leucine-zipper motif does not directly interact with the DNA, as do the zinc-finger or helix–turn–helix motifs. Mutations in the zipper motif show that if the dimer is not formed by association of the monomers through the zipper, the protein will not bind to DNA strongly. However, just adjacent to the α-helix of the zipper motif in the primary structures

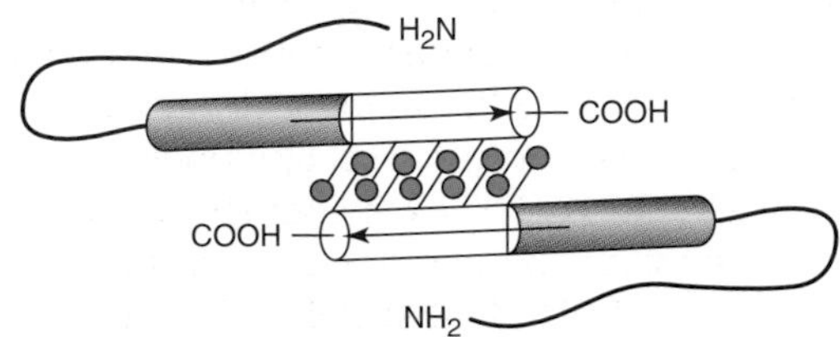

FIGURE 3.25

Schematic diagram of two proteins with leucine zippers in antiparallel association.

DNA-binding domains containing a high content of basic amino acids (arginines and lysines) are shown in pink.

Redrawn from Landschulz, W. H., Johnson, P. F., and McKnight, S. L. Science *240:1759, 1988.*

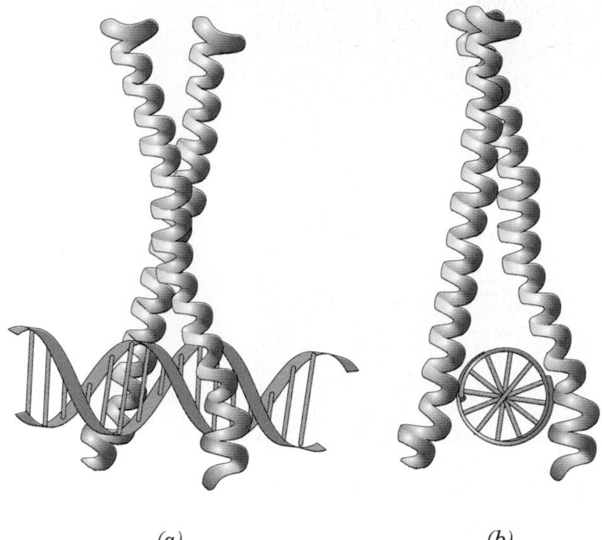

FIGURE 3.26
Structure of the bZIP GCN4–DNA complex.
(*a*) bZIP protein is a dimer (polypeptide chains colored blue) with each monomer joined by a leucine-zipper motif. NH_2 termini diverge to allow the basic region of the sequence to interact in the major groove of DNA target site (DNA colored red). (*b*) Same interaction viewed down the DNA axis.
From Ellenberger, T. E., Brandl, C. J., Struhl, K., and Harrison, S. C. Cell *71:1223, 1992.*

there is a sequence containing a high concentration of basic amino acids, arginine and lysine. This evolutionary conserved basic region interacts with the DNA. The positive charges of the arginine and lysine side chains are drawn to the negatively charged DNA phosphate groups.

The yeast transcription factor GCN4 is one eukaryotic DNA-binding protein that contains the leucine-zipper (bZIP) motif. It is a dimer of two continuous α-helical subunits joined by a leucine-zipper interface. The α-helices cross at this interface and then diverge with their two N-terminal ends separated to pass directly through different sides of the same major groove of the DNA target site (Figure 3.26). Amazingly, there are no bends or kinks in the linear helical structure of each subunit of the dimer. As discussed above, the DNA contact regions contain many positively charged amino acid residues that interact with negatively charged phosphate groups in the DNA.

Many regulatory proteins with the leucine-zipper motif have been shown to be oncogene products (Myc, Jun, and Fos). Fos forms a heterodimer with Jun through a leucine-zipper interaction, and the Fos/Jun dimers bind to gene regulatory sites. If these regulatory proteins are mutated or produced in an unregulated manner, the cell can be transformed to a cancer cell.

DNA-Binding Proteins Utilize a Variety of Strategies for Interaction with DNA

The helix–loop–helix motif was the first motif to be identified for interaction with DNA. X-ray structural studies of protein–DNA complexes show a great variety of other mechanisms for protein–DNA association. The TATA box-binding protein (TBP) associates with the TATA sequence of gene promoters. Association of TBP with the TATA sequence forms the foundation for a large protein complex that initiates gene transcription by RNA polymerase. The X-ray structure of the C-terminal domain of the TBP bound to a TATA sequence shows that TBP contains two domains, each composed of a curved antiparallel β-sheet with a concave surface. The two-domain structure forms the shape of a "saddle" that sits over the DNA double helix. The concave surface of the "saddle" distorts the B-DNA structure and partially unwinds the DNA helix. This distortion, in turn, produces a wide open, though shallow, minor groove that interacts extensively with the under portion of the TBP saddle (Figure 3.27*a*). One critical protein that forms a part of the initiation complex for RNA transcription is TFIIB. An X-ray structure shows TFIIB associates with one of the "stirrups" of the TBP "saddle" in the TATA sequence complex (Figure 3.27*b*).

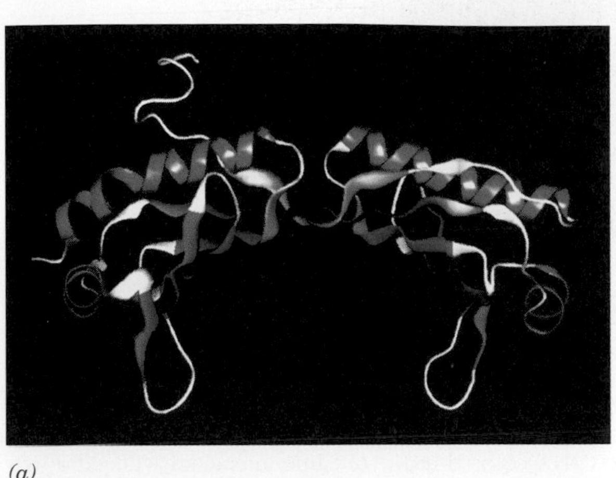

(a)

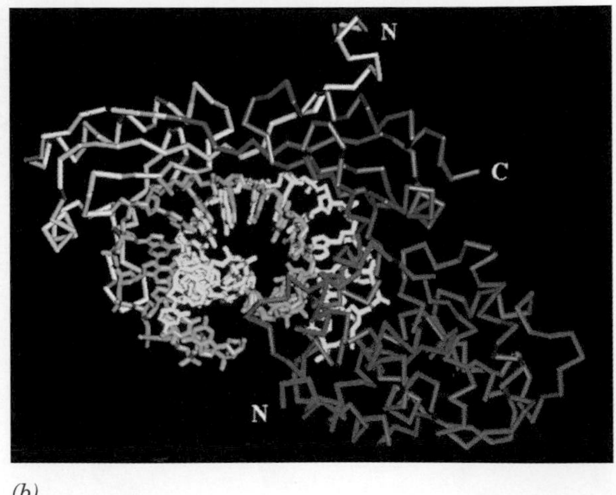

(b)

FIGURE 3.27
Structures of TBP–DNA binary and TBP–TFIIB–DNA ternary complexes.
(*a*) Computer model generated from X-ray structure of TBP interaction with DNA; α-helices and β-strands are shown in red and blue, respectively, with the remainder in white. (*b*) TBP–TFIIB–DNA complex. Proteins are depicted as α-carbon traces while the DNA is shown as an atomic stick model. TFIIB first repeat is colored red and the second repeat magenta. One domain of TBP is light blue while the second is dark blue. DNA-coding strand is colored green and noncoding strand is in yellow. N and C termini of TBP and TFIIB are labeled when visible.
Courtesy of S. K. Burley. Reprinted with permission from (a) Nikolov, D. B., Hu, S.-H., Lin, J., Gasch, A., Hoffmann, A., Horikoshi, M., Chua, N.-H., Roeder, R. G., and Burley, S. K. Nature *360:40, 1992; and (b) Nikolov, D. B., Chen, H., Halay, E. D., Usheva, A. A., Hisatake, K., Lee, D. K., Roeder, R. G., and Burley, S. K.* Nature *377:119, 1995. Copyright 1992 and 1995 Macmillan Magazines Limited.*

The p53 protein is a transcription factor that, on sensing damaged DNA, upregulates the expression of genes that inhibit cell division, giving the cell time to repair the damaged DNA. Alternatively, it can instruct the cell to undergo apoptosis (programmed cell death) if the DNA damage is too extensive for repair. This transcription factor is a key tumor suppressor protein and mutant forms of p53 are found in the majority of human cancers. The DNA-binding domain of p53 consists of two sheets of antiparallel β-strands like an immunoglobulin fold. This central fold provides the scaffolding for the **loop–sheet–helix motif** and for the two large loops (15 and 32 residues) that interact with the DNA. The α-helix (designated H2) of the loop–sheet–helix motif fits into a major groove with loop 1 (L1), while loop 3 (L3) interacts strongly with the adjacent minor groove (Figure 3.28*a*). Figure 3.28*b* shows the side chains of the amino acids commonly found mutated in human cancers. Many mutations are in residues that interact directly with the DNA, such as Arg 248, which is a part of loop 3. Other common mutations are in residues within the domain core required for protein stability. p53 binds as a tetramer to DNA (Figure 3.28*c*).

NF-κB transcription factors are ubiquitous transcription factors of the Rel family. They regulate a variety of genes, especially genes with roles in cellular defense mechanisms against infection and in differentiation. The NF-κB p50 protein has two domains interconnected by a 10 amino acid linker region (Figure 3.29*a*). Each domain contains a β-barrel core with antiparallel strands that have structural homology to the immunoglobulin fold motif. The C-terminal domains provide the dimer interface, in which one surface of each immunoglobulin fold pack together to form the subunit interface. Both N-terminal and C-terminal domains, as well as the loop that connects them, bind to the DNA surface, contributing 10 loops (5 from each subunit in the dimer) that fill the entire major groove in the target DNA (Figure 3.29). N-terminal domains also have an α-helical segment that forms a strong interaction in the minor groove near the center of the target element. In contrast to many other DNA-binding proteins, the NF-κB p50 dimer does not make contact with two separated sites

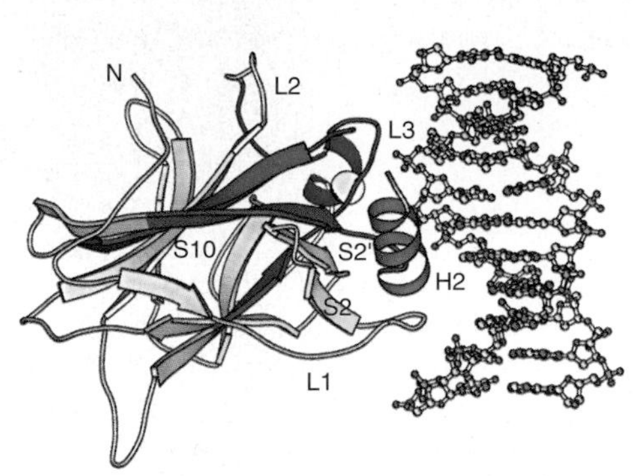

(a)

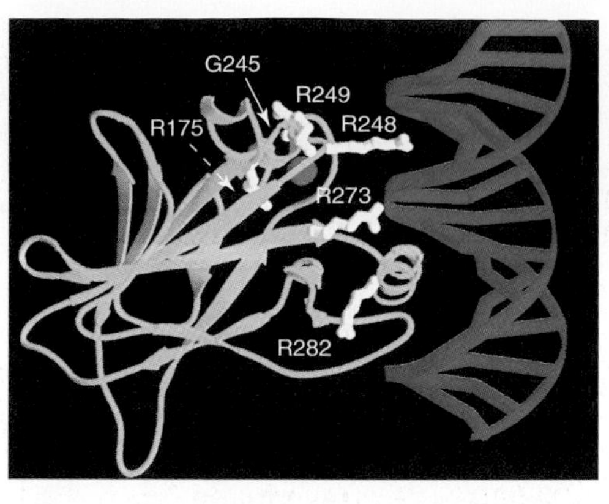

(b)

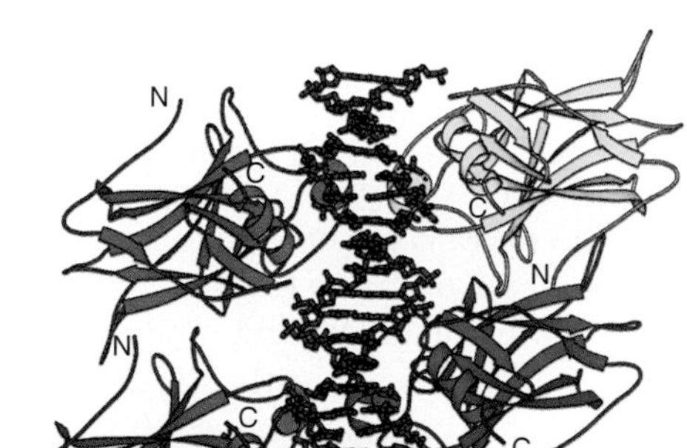

(c)

FIGURE 3.28
Structure of p53–DNA complex.
(*a*) Structure of p53 core domain complexed with DNA. β-Strands (S), α-helices (H), loops (L), and zinc atom (sphere) are lettered and numbered. Helix (H2), loop 1 (L1), and loop 3 (L3) associate in major and minor grooves of target DNA. (*b*) Frequently mutated amino acid side chains commonly found in human cancers are colored yellow. Zinc atom is colored red. (*c*) Structure of tetramer p53 in association with DNA. Each monomer of tetramer binds to a discrete consensus binding site in the target DNA. Four core domains of the tetramer are colored green, purple, yellow, and red, and DNA is colored blue.
Reprinted with permission from Cho, Y., Gorina, S., Jeffrey, P. D., and Pavletich, N. P. Science *265:346, 1994. Copyright 1994 American Association for the Advancement of Science.*

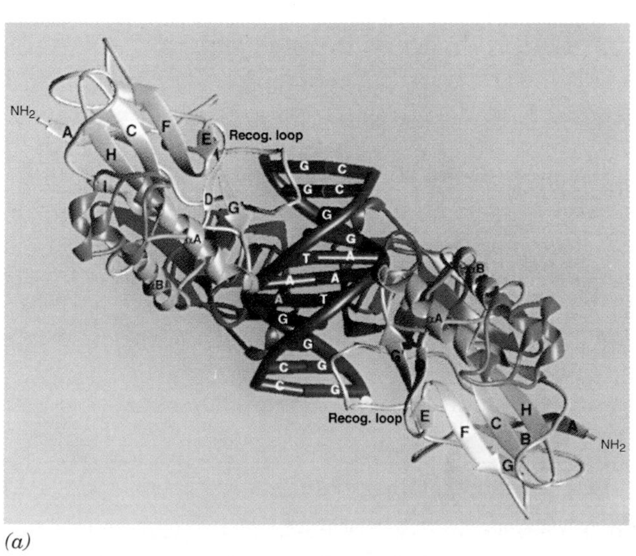

(a)

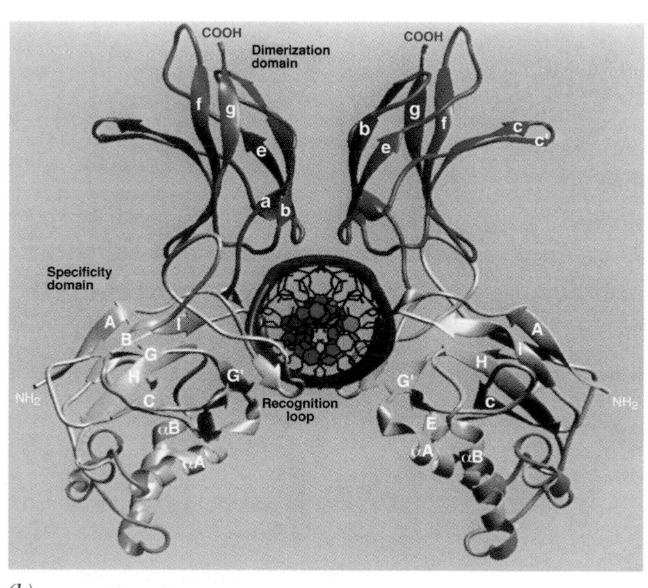

(b)

FIGURE 3.29
Structure of the NF-κB p50 homodimer to DNA.
Only residues 43 through 352 of both subunits are shown in structures. NF-κB p50 protein binds as a dimer. In each monomer, the N-terminal domain is colored yellow and the C-terminal domain is colored red. Orange insert in N-terminal domain is a region unique to p50 and not present in other structures of Rel family of transcription factors. (*a*) View along DNA axis. (*b*) Alternative view of same complex.
Reprinted with permission from Müller, C. W., Rey, F. A., Sodeoka, M., Verdine, G. L., and Harrison, S. C. Nature *373:311, 1995. Copyright 1995 Macmillan Magazines Limited.*

on the DNA target. Rather, the contacts from one monomer combine with those of the second monomer to form a continuous interaction through the single binding site in the DNA.

3.5 ■ HEMOGLOBIN AND MYOGLOBIN

Hemoglobins are globular proteins, present in high concentrations in red blood cells, that bind oxygen in the lungs and transport the oxygen in blood to tissues and cells around the capillary beds of the vascular system. Hemoglobins also transport carbon dioxide and protons from the tissues to the lungs. Hemoglobins carry and release nitric oxide (NO), a potent vasodilator and inhibitor of platelet aggregation (see p. 995). In this section the structural and molecular aspects of hemoglobin and myoglobin are described. The physiological roles of these proteins are discussed in Chapter 25.

Human Hemoglobin Occurs in Several Forms

A hemoglobin molecule consists of four polypeptide chains, two each of two different amino acid sequences. The major form of human adult hemoglobin, **HbA_1,** consists of two α chains and two β chains ($\alpha_2\beta_2$). The α polypeptide has 141 and the β polypeptide has 146 amino acids. Other forms of hemoglobin predominate in the blood of the human fetus and early embryo (Figure 3.30). The fetal form **(HbF)** contains the same α chains found in HbA_1, but a second type of chain (γ chain) occurs in the tetramer molecule and differs in amino acid sequence from that of the β chain of adult HbA_1 (Table 3.8). Additional forms appear in the first months after conception (embryonic) in which the α chains are substituted by *zeta* (ζ) chains of different amino acid sequence and the ε chains serve as the β chains. A minor form of adult hemoglobin, HbA_2, comprises about 2% of normal adult hemoglobin and contains two α chains and two chains designated delta (δ) (Table 3.8).

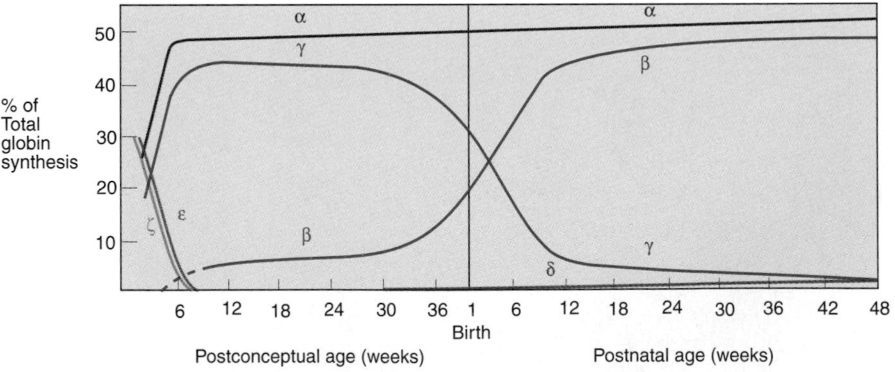

FIGURE 3.30
Changes in globin chain production during development.
Based on a figure in Nienhuis, A. W. and Maniatis, T. In: G. Stamatoyannopoulos, A. W. Nienhuis, P. Leder, and P. W. Majerus (Eds.), The Molecular Basis of Blood Diseases. *Philadelphia: Saunders, 1987, p. 68, in which reference of Weatherall, D. J., and Clegg, J. B.,* The Thalassemia Syndromes, *3rd ed. Oxford: Blackwell Scientific Publications, 1981, is acknowledged.*

TABLE 3.8 Chains of Human Hemoglobin

Developmental Stage	*Symbol*	*Chain Designations*
Adult	HbA_1	$\alpha_2\beta_2$
Adult	HbA_2	$\alpha_2\delta_2$
Fetus	HbF	$\alpha_2\gamma_2$
Embryo	Hb Gower-1	$\zeta_2\varepsilon_2$
Embryo	Hb Portland	$\zeta_2\gamma_2$

Myoglobin: A Single Polypeptide Chain with One O_2-Binding Site

Myoglobin (Mb) is an O_2-carrying protein that binds and releases O_2 with changes in the oxygen concentration in the sarcoplasm of skeletal muscle cells. In contrast to hemoglobin, which has four polypeptide chains and four O_2-binding sites, myoglobin contains only a single polypeptide chain and one O_2-binding site. Myoglobin is a model for what occurs when a single protomer molecule acts alone without the interactions exhibited among the four O_2-binding sites in the more complex tetramer molecule of hemoglobin.

A Heme Prosthetic Group Is at the Site of O_2 Binding

The four polypeptides of globin subunits in hemoglobin and the one of myoglobin each contain a heme prosthetic group. A **prosthetic group** is a nonpolypeptide moiety that forms a functional part of a protein. Without its prosthetic group, a protein is designated an **apoprotein.** With its prosthetic group it is a **holoprotein**.

Heme contains protoporphyrin IX (see Chapter 24) with an iron atom in its center (Figure 3.31). The iron atom is in the ferrous (2+ charge) oxidation state in functional hemoglobin and myoglobin. The ferrous atom in the heme can form five or six ligand bonds, depending on whether or not O_2 is bound to the molecule. Four bonds are to the pyrrole nitrogen atoms of the porphyrin. Since all pyrrole rings of porphyrin lie in a common plane, the four ligand bonds from the porphyrin to the iron atom will have a tendency to lie in the plane of the porphyrin ring. The fifth and the potentially sixth ligand bonds to the ferrous atom are directed along an axis perpendicular to the plane of the porphyrin ring (Figure 3.32). The fifth coordinate bond of the ferrous atom is to a nitrogen of a histidine imidazole. This is designated the **proximal histidine** in hemoglobin and myoglobin structures (Figures 3.32 and 3.33). O_2 forms a sixth coordinate bond to the ferrous atom when bound to hemoglobin. In this bonded position the O_2 is placed between the ferrous atom to which it is liganded and a second histidine imidazole, designated the **distal histidine.** In deoxyhemoglobin, the sixth coordination position of the ferrous atom is unoccupied.

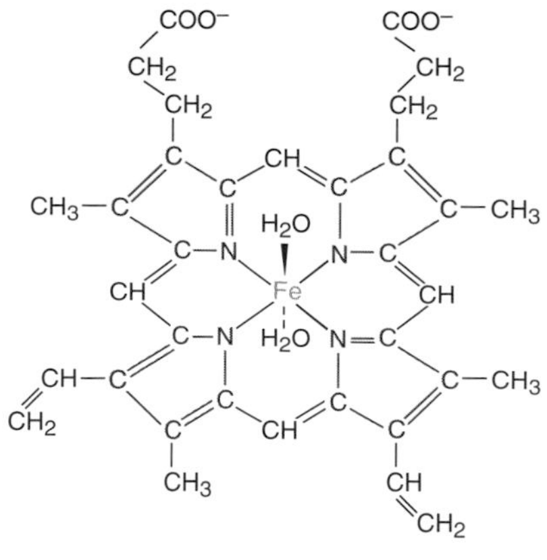

Heme

FIGURE 3.31
Structure of heme.

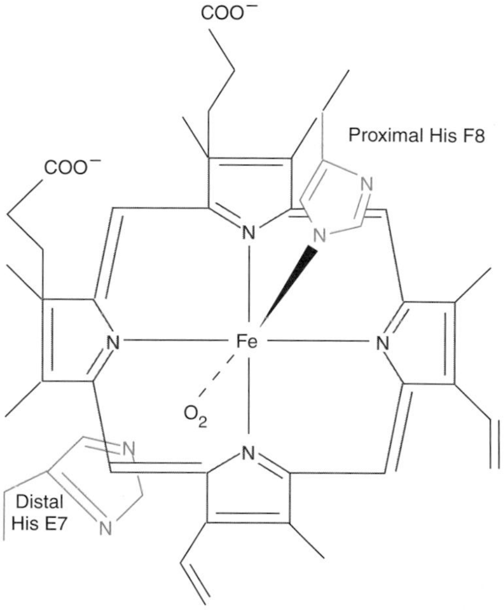

FIGURE 3.32
Ligand bonds to ferrous atom in oxyhemoglobin.

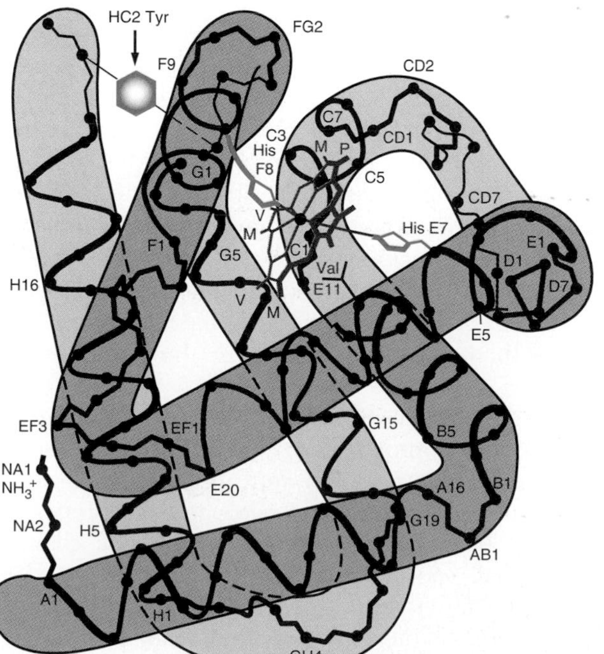

FIGURE 3.33
Secondary and tertiary structure characteristics of chains of hemoglobin.
Proximal His F8, distal His E7, and Val E11 side chains are shown. Other amino acids of polypeptide chain are represented by α-carbon positions only; the letters M, V, and P refer to the methyl, vinyl, and propionate side chains of the heme.
Reprinted with permission from Perutz, M. Br. Med. Bull. *32:195, 1976.*

The porphyrin part of the heme is positioned within a hydrophobic pocket of each globin subunit. In the heme pocket X-ray diffraction studies show that approximately 80 interactions are provided by approximately 18 residues to the heme. Most of these noncovalent interactions are between apolar side chains of amino acids and the apolar regions of the porphyrin. As discussed in Chapter 2, the driving force for these interactions is the expulsion of water of solvation on association of the hydrophobic heme with the apolar amino acid side chains in the heme pocket. In myoglobin additional noncovalent interactions are made between the negatively charged propionate groups of the heme and positively charged arginine and histidine side chains of the protein. However, in hemoglobin chains a difference in the amino acid sequence in this region of the heme-binding site leads to stabilization of the porphyrin propionates by interaction with an uncharged histidine imidazole and with water molecules of solvent toward the outer surface of the molecule.

X-Ray Crystallography Has Assisted in Defining the Structure of Hemoglobin and Myoglobin

The structure of deoxy and oxy forms of hemoglobin and myoglobin have been resolved by X-ray crystallography. In fact, sperm whale myoglobin was the first globular protein whose full three-dimensional structure was determined by this technique. This was followed by the X-ray structure of the more complex horse hemoglobin molecule. These structures show that each globin polypeptide in the hemoglobins and the single subunit of myoglobin are composed of multiple α-helical regions connected by turns of the polypeptide chain that allow the protein to fold into a spheroidal shape (Figure 3.33). The mechanism of cooperative associations of O_2, discussed below, is based on the X-ray structures of oxyhemoglobin, deoxyhemoglobin, and a variety of hemoglobin derivatives.

Primary, Secondary, and Tertiary Structures of Myoglobin and the Individual Hemoglobin Chains

The amino acid sequences of the polypeptide chain of myoglobin of 23 different animal species have been determined. All myoglobins contain 153 amino acids in their polypeptide chains, of which 83 are invariant. Only 15 of these invariant residues in the myoglobin sequence are identical to the invariant residues of the sequenced mammalian globins of hemoglobin. However, the changes are, in the great majority of cases, conservative and preserve the general physical properties of the residues (Table 3.9). Since myoglobin is active as a monomer, many of its surface positions interact with water and prevent another molecule of myoglobin from associating. In contrast, surface residues of the individual subunits in hemoglobin are designed to provide hydrogen bonds and nonpolar contacts with other subunits in the hemoglobin quaternary structure. Proximal and distal histidines are preserved in the sequences of all the polypeptide chains. Other invariant residues are in the hydrophobic heme pocket and form essential nonpolar contacts with the heme that stabilize the heme–protein complex.

While there is surprising variability in amino acid sequences among the different polypeptide chains, to a first approximation the secondary and tertiary structures of each of the subunits of hemoglobin and myoglobin are almost identical (Figure 3.34). Significant differences in physiological properties between α, β, γ, and δ chains of hemoglobins and the polypeptide chain of myoglobin are due to rather small specific changes in their structures. The similarity in tertiary structure, resulting from widely varied amino acid sequences, shows that the same tertiary structure for a protein can be arrived at by many different sequences.

TABLE 3.9 Amino Acid Sequences of Human Hemoglobin Chains and of Sperm Whale Myoglobin[a]

	NA 1	2	3	A 1	2	3	4	5	6	7	8	9	10	11	12	13	14	15	A 16	AB 1	B 1	2	3	4	5	6
MYOGLOBIN	Val	....	Leu	Ser	Glu	Gly	Glu	Trp	Gln	Leu	Val	Leu	His	Val	Trp	Ala	Lys	Val	Glu	Ala	Asp	Val	Ala	Gly	His	Gly
HEMOGLOBIN Horse α	Val	....	Leu	Ser	Ala	Ala	Asp	Lys	Thr	Asn	Val	Lys	Ala	Ala	Trp	Ser	Lys	Val	Gly	Gly	His	Ala	Gly	Glu	Tyr	Gly
β	Val	Gln	Leu	Ser	Gly	Glu	Glu	Lys	Ala	Ala	Val	Leu	Ala	Leu	Trp	Asp	Lys	Val	Asn	....	....	Glu	Glu	Glu	Val	Gly
Human α	Val	....	Leu	Ser	Pro	Ala	Asp	Lys	Thr	Asn	Val	Lys	Ala	Ala	Trp	Gly	Lys	Val	Gly	Ala	His	Ala	Gly	Glu	Tyr	Gly
β	Val	His	Leu	Thr	Pro	Glu	Glu	Lys	Ser	Ala	Val	Thr	Ala	Leu	Trp	Gly	Lys	Val	Asn	....	....	Val	Asp	Glu	Val	Gly
γ	Gly	His	Phe	Thr	Glu	Glu	Asp	Lys	Ala	Thr	Ilu	Thr	Ser	Leu	Trp	Gly	Lys	Val	Asn	....	....	Val	Glu	Asp	Ala	Gly
δ	Val	His	Leu	Thr	Pro	Glu	Glu	Lys	Thr	Ala	Val	Asn	Ala	Leu	Trp	Gly	Lys	Val	Asn	....	....	Val	Asp	Ala	Val	Gly

	7	8	9	10	11	12	13	14	15	16	C 1	2	3	4	5	6	7	CD 1	2	3	4	5	6	7	8	D 1
MYOGLOBIN	Gln	Asp	Ilu	Leu	Ilu	Arg	Leu	Phe	Lys	Ser	His	Pro	Glu	Thr	Leu	Glu	Lys	Phe	Asp	Arg	Phe	Lys	His	Leu	Lys	Thr
HEMOGLOBIN Horse α	Ala	Glu	Ala	Leu	Glu	Arg	Met	Phe	Leu	Gly	Phe	Pro	Thr	Thr	Lys	Thr	Tyr	Phe	Pro	His	Phe	....	Asp	Leu	Ser	His
β	Gly	Glu	Ala	Leu	Gly	Arg	Leu	Leu	Val	Val	Tyr	Pro	Trp	Thr	Gln	Arg	Phe	Phe	Asp	Ser	Phe	Gly	Asp	Leu	Ser	Gly
Human α	Ala	Glu	Ala	Leu	Glu	Arg	Met	Phe	Leu	Ser	Phe	Pro	Thr	Thr	Lys	Thr	Tyr	Phe	Pro	His	Phe	....	Asp	Leu	Ser	His
β	Gly	Glu	Ala	Leu	Gly	Arg	Leu	Leu	Val	Val	Tyr	Pro	Trp	Thr	Gln	Arg	Phe	Phe	Glu	Ser	Phe	Gly	Asp	Leu	Ser	Thr
γ	Gly	Glu	Thr	Leu	Gly	Arg	Leu	Leu	Val	Val	Tyr	Pro	Trp	Thr	Gln	Arg	Phe	Phe	Asp	Ser	Phe	Gly	Asn	Leu	Ser	Ser
δ	Gly	Glu	Ala	Leu	Gly	Arg	Leu	Leu	Val	Val	Tyr	Pro	Trp	Thr	Gln	Arg	Phe	Phe	Glu	Ser	Phe	Gly	Asp	Leu	Ser	Ser

	2	3	4	5	6	7	E 1	2	3	4	5	6	7	8	9	10	11	12	13	14	E 15	16	17	18	19	20
MYOGLOBIN	Glu	Ala	Glu	Met	Lys	Ala	Ser	Glu	Asp	Leu	Lys	Lys	His	Gly	Val	Thr	Val	Leu	Thr	Ala	Leu	Gly	Ala	Ilu	Leu	Lys
HEMOGLOBIN Horse α	....	....	....	....	....	Gly	Ser	Ala	Gln	Val	Lys	Ala	His	Gly	Lys	Lys	Val	Ala	Asp	Gly	Leu	Thr	Leu	Ala	Val	Gly
β	Pro	Asp	Ala	Val	Met	Gly	Asn	Pro	Lys	Val	Lys	Ala	His	Gly	Lys	Lys	Val	Leu	His	Ser	Phe	Gly	Glu	Gly	Val	His
Human α	....	....	....	....	....	Gly	Ser	Ala	Gln	Val	Lys	Gly	His	Gly	Lys	Lys	Val	Ala	Asp	Ala	Leu	Thr	Asn	Ala	Val	Ala
β	Pro	Asp	Ala	Val	Met	Gly	Asn	Pro	Lys	Val	Lys	Ala	His	Gly	Lys	Lys	Val	Leu	Gly	Ala	Phe	Ser	Asp	Gly	Leu	Ala
γ	Ala	Der	Ala	Ilu	Met	Gly	Asn	Pro	Lys	Val	Lys	Ala	His	Gly	Lys	Lys	Val	Leu	Thr	Ser	Leu	Gly	Asp	Ala	Ilu	Lys
δ	Pro	Asp	Ala	Val	Met	Gly	Asn	Pro	Lys	Val	Lys	Ala	His	Gly	Lys	Lys	Val	Leu	Gly	Ala	Phe	Ser	Asp	Gly	Leu	Ala

	EF 1	2	3	4	5	6	7	8	F 1	2	3	4	F 5	6	7	8	9	FG 1	2	3	4	5	G 1	2	3	4
MYOGLOBIN	Lys	Lys	Gly	His	His	Glu	Ala	Glu	Leu	Lys	Pro	Leu	Ala	Gln	Ser	His	Ala	Thr	Lys	His	Lys	Ilu	Pro	Ilu	Lys	Tyr
HEMOGLOBIN Horse α	His	Leu	Asp	Asp	Leu	Pro	Gly	Ala	Leu	Ser	Asp	Leu	Ser	Asn	Leu	His	Ala	His	Lys	Leu	Arg	Val	Asp	Pro	Val	Asn
β	His	Leu	Asp	Asn	Leu	Lys	Gly	Thr	Phe	Ala	Ala	Leu	Ser	Glu	Leu	His	Cys	Asp	Lys	Leu	His	Val	Asp	Pro	Glu	Asn
Human α	His	Val	Asp	Asp	Met	Pro	Asn	Ala	Leu	Ser	Ala	Leu	Ser	Asp	Leu	His	Ala	His	Lys	Leu	Arg	Val	Asp	Pro	Val	Asn
β	His	Leu	Asp	Asn	Leu	Lys	Gly	Thr	Phe	Ala	Thr	Leu	Ser	Glu	Leu	His	Cys	Asp	Lys	Leu	His	Val	Asp	Pro	Glu	Asn
γ	His	Leu	Asp	Asp	Leu	Lys	Gly	Thr	Phe	Ala	Gln	Leu	Ser	Glu	Leu	His	Cys	Asp	Lys	Leu	His	Val	Asp	Pro	Glu	Asn
δ	His	Leu	Asp	Asn	Leu	Lys	Gly	Thr	Phe	Ser	Gln	Leu	Ser	Glu	Leu	His	Cys	Asp	Lys	Leu	His	Val	Asp	pro	Glu	Asn

	5	6	7	8	G 9	10	11	12	13	14	15	16	17	18	19	GH 1	2	3	4	5	6	H 1	2	H 3	4	5
MYOGLOBIN	Leu	Glu	Phe	Ilu	Ser	Glu	Ala	Ilu	Ilu	His	Val	Leu	His	Ser	Arg	His	Pro	Gly	Asn	Phe	Gly	Ala	Asp	Ala	Gln	Gly
HEMOGLOBIN Horse α	Phe	Lys	Leu	Leu	Ser	His	Cys	Leu	Leu	Ser	Thr	Leu	Ala	Val	His	Leu	Pro	Asn	Asp	Phe	Thr	Pro	Ala	Val	His	Ala
β	Phe	Arg	Leu	Leu	Gly	Asn	Val	Leu	Ala	Leu	Val	Val	Ala	Arg	His	Phe	Gly	Lys	Asp	Phe	Thr	Pro	Glu	Leu	Gln	Ala
Human α	Phe	Lys	Leu	Leu	Ser	His	Cys	Leu	Leu	Val	Thr	Leu	Ala	Ala	His	Leu	Pro	Ala	Glu	phe	Thr	Pro	Ala	Val	His	Ala
β	Phe	Srg	Leu	Leu	Gly	Asn	Val	Leu	Val	Cys	Val	Leu	Ala	His	His	Phe	Gly	Lys	Glu	Phe	Thr	Pro	Pro	Val	Gln	Ala
γ	Phe	Lys	Leu	Leu	Gly	Asn	Val	Leu	Val	Thr	Val	Leu	Ala	Ilu	His	Phe	Gly	Lys	Glu	Phe	Thr	Pro	Glu	Val	Gln	Ala
δ	Phe	Arg	Leu	Leu	Gly	Asn	Val	Leu	Val	Cys	Val	Leu	Ala	Arg	Asn	Phe	Gly	Lys	Glu	Phe	Thr	Pro	Gln	Met	Gln	Ala

	6	7	8	9	10	11	12	13	14	15	16	17	18	19	20	H 21	22	23	2	HC 1	2	3	4	5
MYOGLOBIN	Ala	Met	Asn	Lys	Ala	Leu	Glu	Leu	Phe	Arg	Lys	Asp	ilu	Ala	Ala	Lys	Tyr	Lys	Glu	Leu	Gly	Tyr	Gin	Gly
HEMOGLOBIN Horse α	Ser	Leu	Asp	Lys	Phe	Leu	Ser	Ser	Val	Ser	Thr	Val	Leu	Thr	Ser	Lys	Tyr	Arg						
β	Ser	Tyr	Gln	Lys	Val	Val	Ala	Gly	Val	Ala	Asn	Ala	Leu	Ala	His	Lys	Tyr	His						
Human α	Ser	Leu	Asp	Lys	Phe	Leu	Ala	Ser	Val	Ser	Thr	Val	Leu	Thr	Ser	Lys	Tyr	Arg						
β	Ala	Tyr	Gln	Lys	Val	Val	Ala	Gly	Val	Ala	Asn	Ala	Leu	Ala	His	Lys	Tyr	His						
γ	Ser	Trp	Gln	Lys	Met	Val	Thr	Gly	Val	Ala	Ser	Ala	Leu	Ser	Ser	Arg	Tyr	His						
δ	Ala	Tyr	Gln	Lys	Val	Val	Ala	Gly	Val	Ala	Asn	Ala	Leu	Ala	His	Lys	Tyr	His						

Source: Based on diagram in Dickerson, R. E., and Geis, I. *The Structure and Function of Proteins.* New York: Harper & Row, 1969, p. 52.

[a] Residues that are identical are enclosed in box. A, B, C, . . . designate different helices of tertiary structure (see text).

Approximately 70% of the residues participate in the α-helical secondary structures generating seven helical segments in the α chain and eight in the β chain. These latter eight helical regions are commonly lettered A–H, starting from the first (A) helix at the NH_2-terminal end. The interhelical regions are designated as AB, BC, CD, . . . , GH, respectively. The nonhelical region between the NH_2-terminal end and the A helix is designated the NA region; and the region between the COOH-terminal end and the H helix is designated the HC region (Figure 3.33). This naming system allows discussion of particular residues that have similar functional and structural roles in hemoglobin and myoglobin.

A Simple Equilibrium Defines O_2 Binding to Myoglobin

The association of oxygen to myoglobin is characterized by a simple equilibrium constant (Eqs. 3.1 and 3.2). In Eq. 3.2 [MbO_2] is the solution concentration of oxymyoglobin, [Mb] is that of deoxymyoglobin, and [O_2] is the concentration

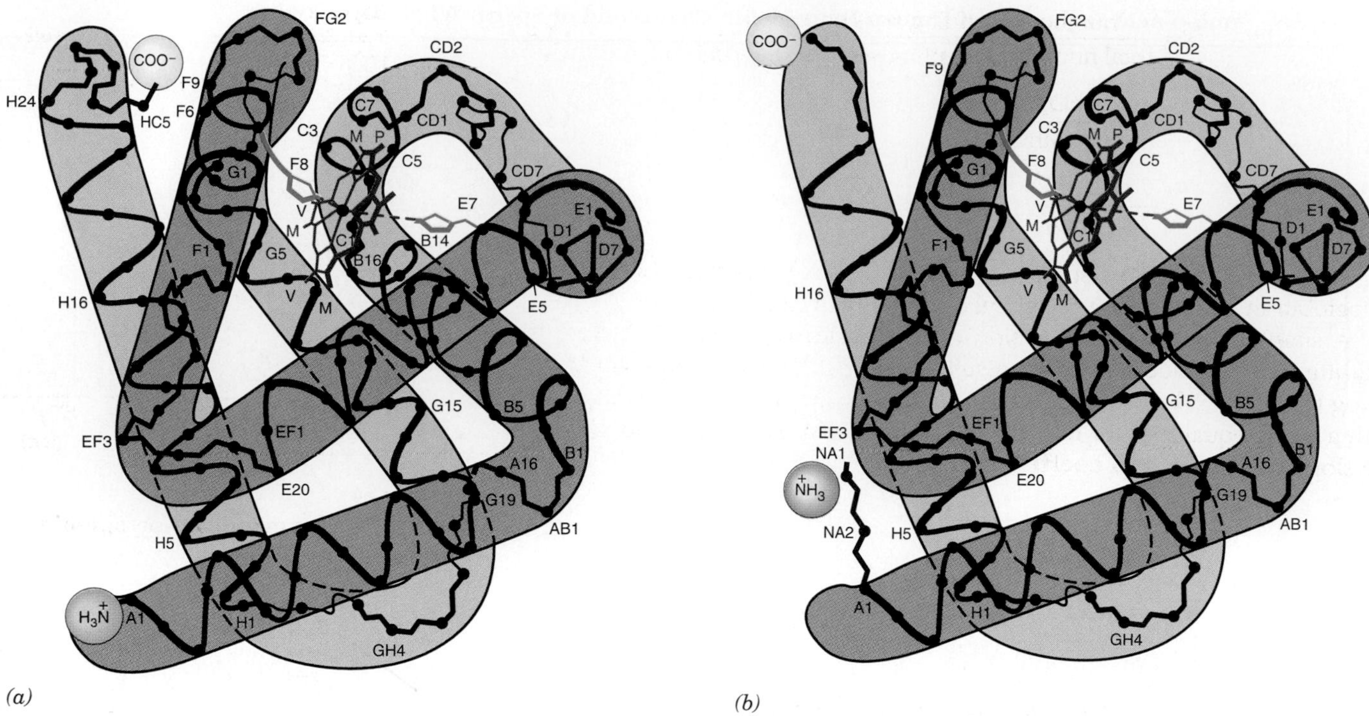

FIGURE 3.34
Comparison of conformation of (*a*) myoglobin and (*b*) β chain of HbA_1.
Overall structures are very similar, except at NH_2-terminal and COOH-terminal ends. *Reprinted with permission from Fersht, A.* Enzyme Structure and Mechanism. *San Francisco: Freeman, 1977, pp. 12, 13.*

of oxygen, in moles per liter. The equilibrium constant, K_{eq}, will also have the units of moles per liter. As for any true equilibrium constant, the value of K_{eq} is dependent on pH, ionic strength, and temperature.

$$Mb + O_2 \overset{K_{eq}}{\rightleftharpoons} MbO_2 \quad \textbf{(3.1)}$$

$$K_{eq} = \frac{[Mb][O_2]}{[MbO_2]} \quad \textbf{(3.2)}$$

Since oxygen is a gas, it is more convenient to express its concentration as the pressure of oxygen in torr (1 torr is equal to the pressure of 1 mmHg at 0°C and standard gravity). In Eq. 3.3 this conversion of units has been made: P_{50}, the equilibrium constant, and pO_2, the concentration of oxygen, being expressed in torr.

$$P_{50} = \frac{[Mb] \cdot pO_2}{[MbO_2]} \quad \textbf{(3.3)}$$

An oxygen-saturation curve characterizes the properties of an oxygen-binding protein. In this plot the fraction of oxygen-binding sites in solution that contain oxygen (Y, Eq. 3.4) is plotted on the ordinate *versus* pO_2 (oxygen concentration) on the abscissa. The Y value is simply defined for myoglobin by Eq. 3.5. Substitution into Eq. 3.5 of the value of $[MbO_2]$ obtained from Eq. 3.3, and then dividing through by [Mb], results in Eq. 3.6, which shows the dependence of Y on the value of the equilibrium constant P_{50} and the oxygen concentration. It is seen from Eqs. 3.3 and 3.6 that the value of P_{50} is equal to the oxygen concentration, pO_2, when $Y = 0.5$ (50% of the available sites occupied)—hence the designation of the equilibrium constant by the subscript 50.

$$Y = \frac{\text{number of binding sites occupied}}{\text{total number of binding sites in solution}} \quad (3.4)$$

$$Y = \frac{[MbO_2]}{[Mb] + [MbO_2]} \quad (3.5)$$

$$Y = \frac{pO_2}{P_{50} + pO_2} \quad (3.6)$$

A plot of Eq. 3.6 of Y versus pO_2 generates an oxygen-saturation curve for myoglobin in the form of a rectangular hyperbola (Figure 3.35).

A simple algebraic manipulation of Eq. 3.6 leads to Eq. 3.7. Taking the logarithm of both sides of Eq. 3.7 results in Eq. 3.8, the **Hill equation.** A plot of log ([$Y/(1 - Y)$] versus log pO_2, according to Eq. 3.8, yields a straight line with a slope equal to 1 for myoglobin (Figure 3.36). This is the Hill plot, and the slope (n_H) is the **Hill coefficient** (see Eq. 3.9).

$$\frac{Y}{1 - Y} = \frac{pO_2}{P_{50}} \quad (3.7)$$

$$\log \frac{Y}{1 - Y} = \log pO_2 - \log P_{50} \quad (3.8)$$

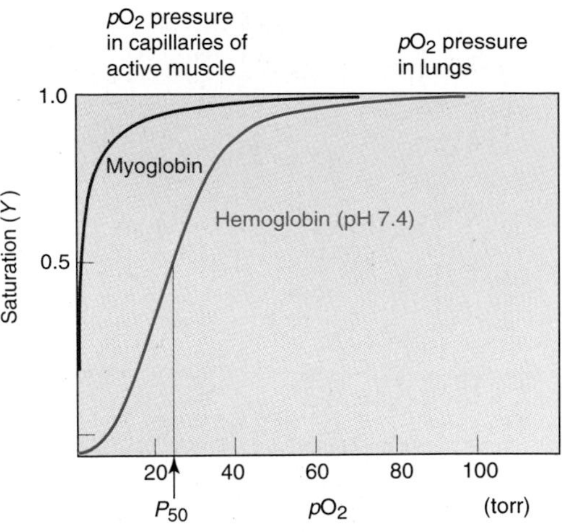

FIGURE 3.35
Oxygen-binding curves for myoglobin and hemoglobin.

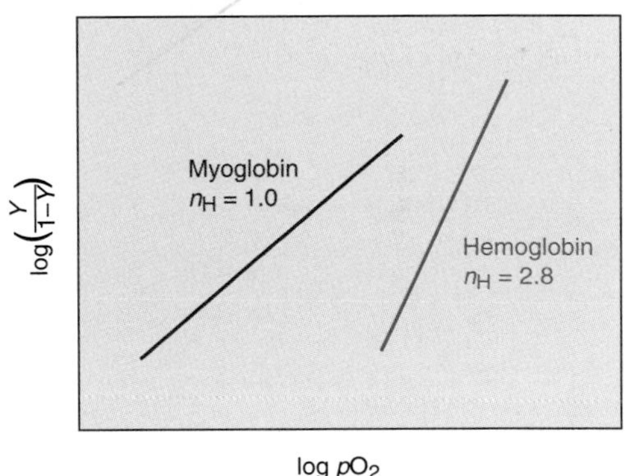

FIGURE 3.36
Hill plots for myoglobin and hemoglobin HbA$_1$.

Binding of O_2 to Hemoglobin Involves Cooperativity Between the Hemoglobin Subunits

Whereas myoglobin has a single O_2-binding site per molecule, hemoglobins, with four monomeric subunits, have four heme-binding sites for O_2. Binding of the four O_2 molecules in hemoglobin is found to be **positively cooperative,** so that the binding of the first O_2 to deoxyhemoglobin facilitates the binding of O_2 to the other subunits in the molecule. Conversely, dissociation of the first O_2 from fully oxygenated hemoglobin, $Hb(O_2)_4$, will make the dissociation of O_2 from the other subunits of the tetramer easier.

Because of cooperativity in oxygen association and dissociation, the oxygen saturation curve for hemoglobin differs from that for myoglobin. A plot of Y versus pO_2 for hemoglobin is a sigmoidal line, indicating cooperativity in oxygen association (Figure 3.35). A plot of the Hill equation (Eq. 3.9) gives a value of the slope (n_H) equal to 2.8 (Figure 3.36).

$$\log \frac{Y}{1 - Y} = n_H \log pO_2 - \text{constant} \quad (3.9)$$

The meaning of the Hill coefficient to cooperative O_2 association can be evaluated quantitatively as presented in Table 3.10. A parameter known as the **cooperativity index,** R_x, is calculated, which shows the ratio of pO_2 required to change Y from a value of $Y = 0.1$ (10% of sites filled) to a value of $Y = 0.9$ (90% of sites filled) for designated Hill coefficient values found experimentally. For myoglobin, $n_H = 1$, and an 81-fold change in oxygen concentration is required to change from $Y = 0.1$ to $Y = 0.9$. For hemoglobin, where positive cooperativity is observed, $n_H = 2.8$ and only a 4.8-fold change in oxygen concentration is required to change the fractional saturation from 0.1 to 0.9.

TABLE 3.10 Relationship Between Hill Coefficient (n_H) and Cooperativity Index (R_x)

n_H	R_x	*Observation*
0.5	6560	Negative substrate cooperativity
0.6	1520	
0.7	533	
0.8	243	
0.9	132	
1.0	81.0	Noncooperativity
1.5	18.7	
2.0	9.0	
2.8	4.8	Positive substrate cooperativity
3.5	3.5	
6.0	2.1	
10.0	1.6	
20.0	1.3	

Source: Based on Table 7.1 in Cornish-Bowden, A. *Principles of Enzyme Kinetics*. London: Butterworths Scientific Publishers, 1976.

The Molecular Mechanism of Cooperativity in O_2 Binding

X-ray diffraction data on deoxyhemoglobin show that the ferrous atoms actually sit out of the plane of their porphyrins by about 0.4–0.6 Å. This is thought to occur because of two factors. The electronic configuration of the five-coordinated ferrous atom in deoxyhemoglobin has a slightly larger radius than the distance from the center of the porphyrin to each of the pyrrole nitrogen atoms.

Accordingly, the iron can be placed in the center of the porphyrin only with some distortion of the porphyrin conformation. Probably a more important consideration is that if the iron atom sits in the plane of the porphyrin, the proximal His F8 imidazole will interact unfavorably with atoms of the porphyrin. The strength of this unfavorable steric interaction is due, in part, to conformational constraints on the His F8 and the porphyrin in the deoxyhemoglobin conformation that forces the approach of the His F8 toward the porphyrin to a particular path (Figure 3.37). These constraints become less significant in the oxy conformation of hemoglobin.

The conformation with the iron atom out of the plane of the porphyrin is unstrained and energetically favored for the five-coordinate ferrous atom. When O_2 binds the sixth coordinate position of the iron, however, this conformation becomes strained. A more energetically favorable conformation for the O_2 liganded iron is one in which the iron atom is within the plane of the porphyrin structure.

On binding of O_2 to a ferrous atom the favorable free energy of bond formation overcomes the repulsive interaction between His F8 and porphyrin, and the ferrous atom moves into the plane of the porphyrin ring. This is the most thermodynamically stable position for the now six-bonded iron atom; one axial ligand is on either side of the plane of the porphyrin ring, and the steric repulsion of one of the axial ligands with the porphyrin is balanced by the repulsion of the second axial ligand on the opposite side when the ferrous atom is in the center. If the iron atom is displaced from the center, the steric interactions of the two axial ligands with the porphyrin in the deoxy conformation are unbalanced, and the stability of the unbalanced structure will be lower than that of the equidistant conformation. Also, the radius of the iron atom with six ligands is reduced so that it can just fit into the center of the porphyrin without distortion of the porphyrin conformation.

Since steric repulsion between porphyrin and His F8 in the deoxy conformation must be overcome on O_2 association, binding of the first O_2 is characterized by a relatively low affinity constant. However, when O_2 association occurs to the first heme in deoxyhemoglobin, the change in position of the iron atom from above the plane of the porphyrin into the center of the porphyrin triggers

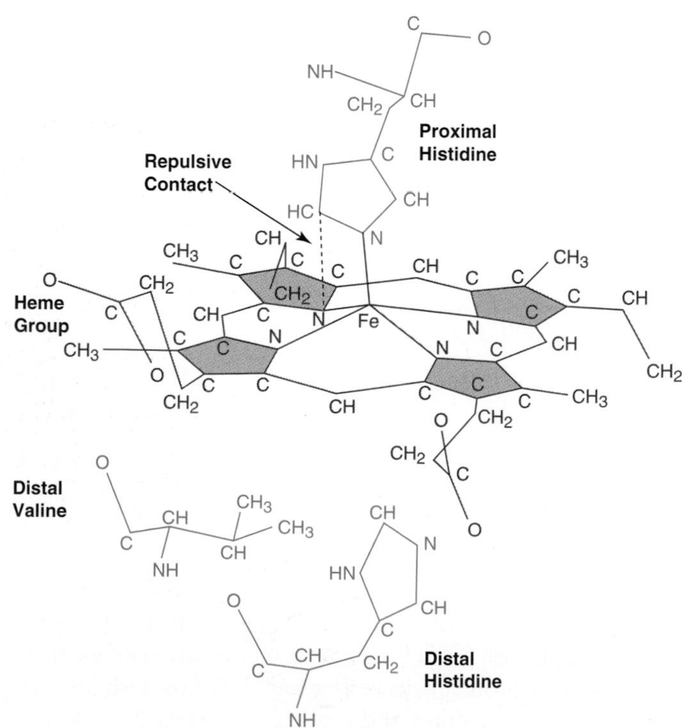

FIGURE 3.37
Steric hindrance between proximal histidine and porphyrin in deoxyhemoglobin.
From Perutz, M. Sci. Am.*, 239:92, 1978 Copyright © 1978 by Scientific American, Inc. All rights reserved.*

a conformational change in the whole molecule. The change in conformation results in a greater affinity of O_2 to the other heme sites after the first O_2 has bound.

The conformation of deoxyhemoglobin is stabilized by noncovalent interactions of the quaternary structure at the interface between α and β subunits in which the FG corner of one subunit noncovalently binds to the C helix of the adjacent subunit (Figure 3.38). In addition, ionic interactions stabilize the deoxy

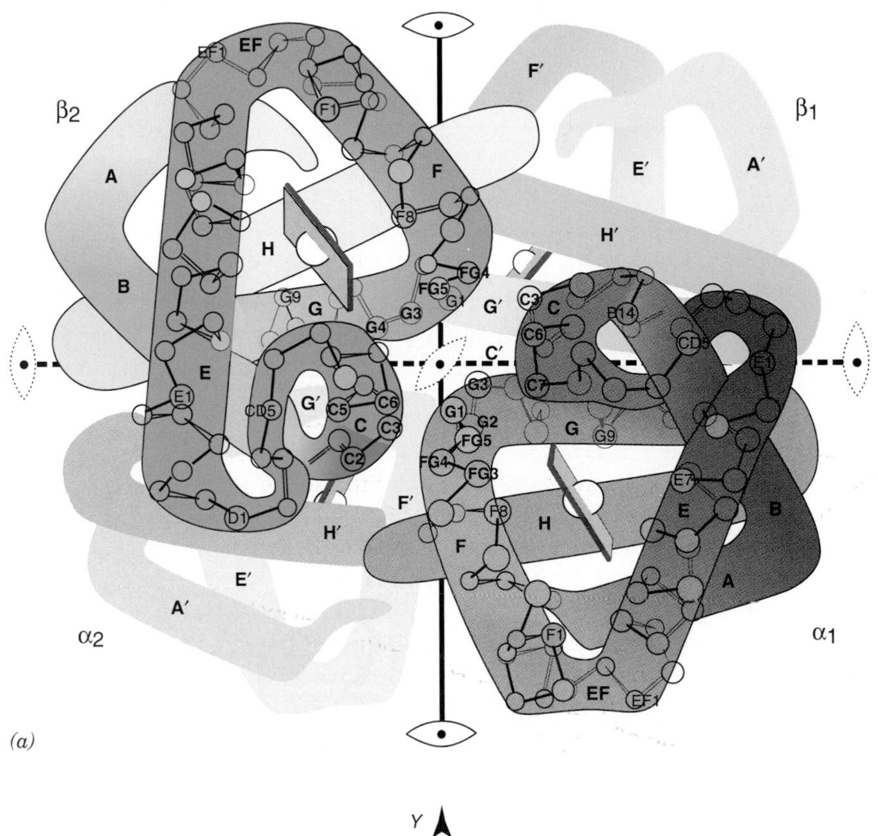

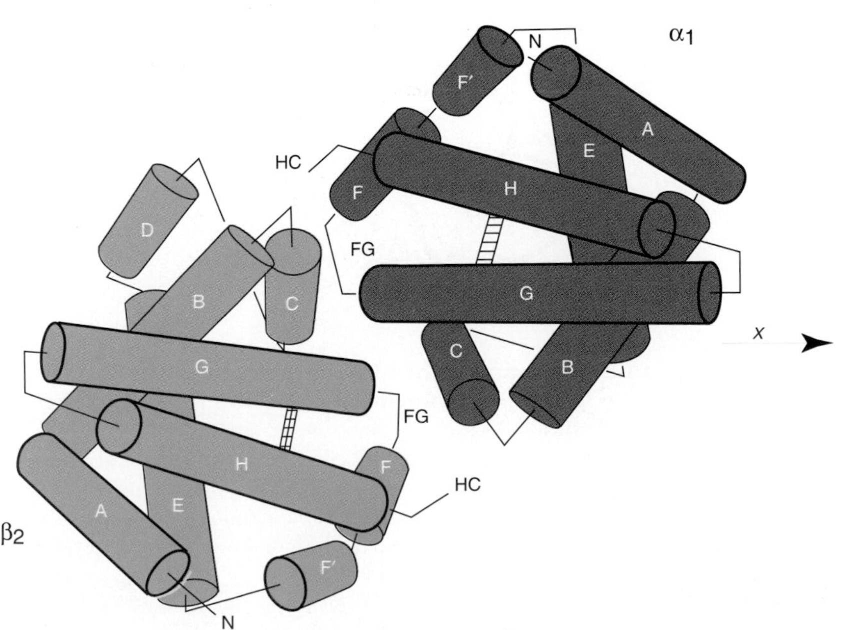

FIGURE 3.38
Quaternary structure of hemoglobin.
(*a*) $\alpha_1\beta_2$ interface contacts between FG corners and C helix are shown. (*b*) Cylinder representation of α_1 and β_2 subunits in hemoglobin molecule showing α_1 and β_2 interface contacts between FG corner and C helix, viewed from opposite side of *x–y* plane from (*a*).
(a) Reprinted with permission from Dickerson, R. E., and Geis, I. The Structure and Action of Proteins. *Menlo Park, CA: Benjamin, Inc., 1969, p. 56.*
(b) Reprinted with permission from Baldwin, J., and Chothia, C. J. Mol. Biol. *129:175, 1979. Copyright © 1979 by Academic Press, Inc. (London) Ltd.*

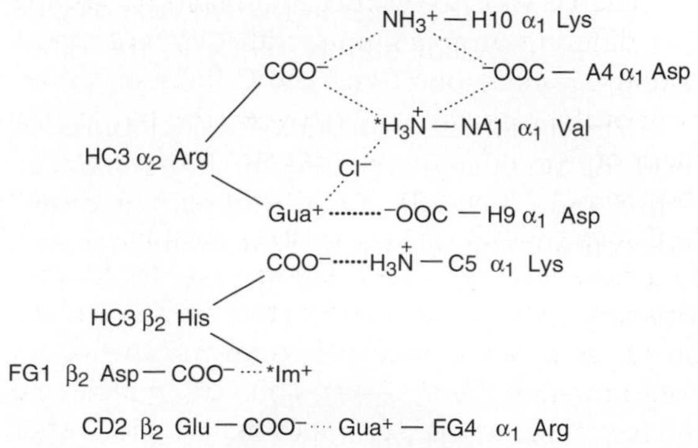

NH$_3^+$ — H10 α_1 Lys
COO$^-$ ⋯ $^-$OOC — A4 α_1 Asp
HC3 α_2 Arg
*H$_3\overset{+}{N}$ — NA1 α_1 Val
Cl$^-$
Gua$^+$ ⋯ $^-$OOC — H9 α_1 Asp
COO$^-$ ⋯ H$_3\overset{+}{N}$ — C5 α_1 Lys
HC3 β_2 His
FG1 β_2 Asp — COO$^-$ ⋯ *Im$^+$
CD2 β_2 Glu — COO$^-$ ⋯ Gua$^+$ — FG4 α_1 Arg

FIGURE 3.39
Salt bridges between subunits in deoxyhemoglobin.
Im$^+$ is imidazolium; Gua$^+$ is guanidinium; starred residues account for approximately 60% of alkaline Bohr effect.
Redrawn from Perutz, M. Br. Med. Bull. *32:195, 1976.*

conformation of the protein (Figure 3.39). These interactions of the deoxy conformation are now destabilized on the binding of O_2 to one of the heme subunits of a deoxyhemoglobin molecule. The binding of O_2 pulls the Fe^{2+} atom into the porphyrin plane and moves the His F8 toward the porphyrin and with it the F helix of which the His F8 is a part. Movement of the F helix, in turn, moves the FG corner of its subunit, destabilizing the FG noncovalent interaction with the C helix of the adjacent subunit at an $\alpha_1\beta_2$ or $\alpha_2\beta_1$ subunit interface (Figures 3.38 and 3.40).

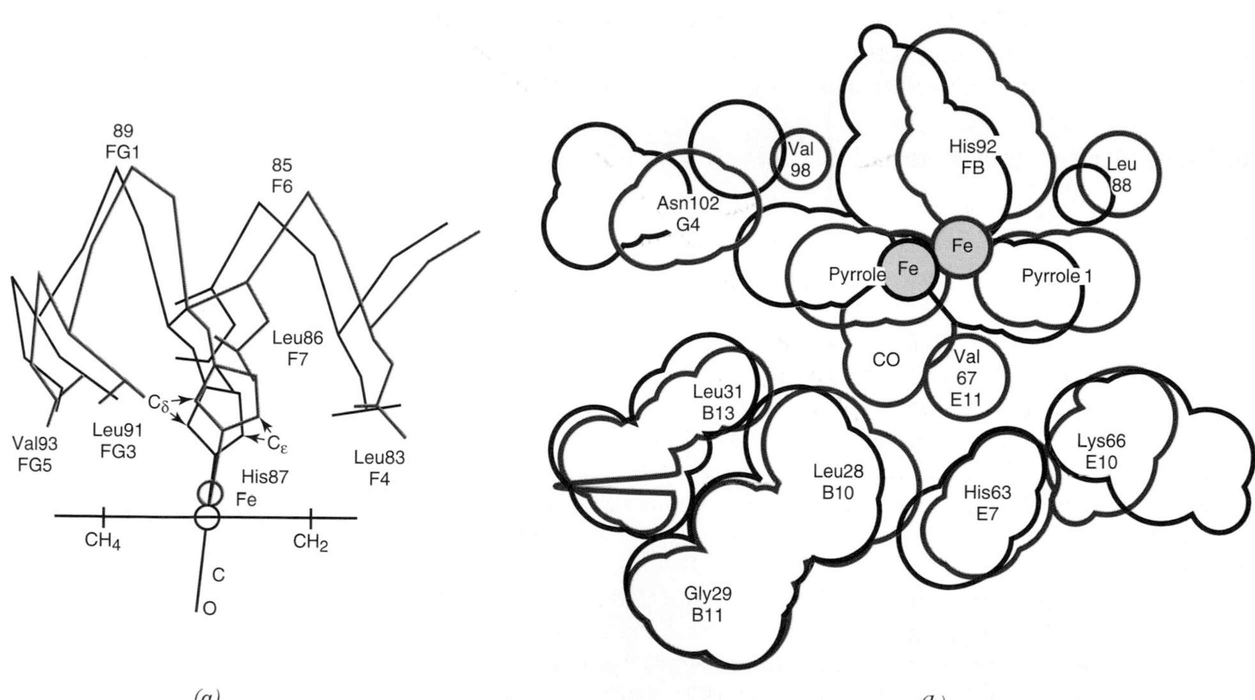

FIGURE 3.40
Stick and space-filling diagrams drawn by computer graphics showing movements of residues in heme environment on transition from deoxyhemoglobin to oxyhemoglobin.
(*a*) Black line outlines position of polypeptide chain and His F8 in carbon monoxide hemoglobin, a model for oxyhemoglobin. Red line outlines the same for deoxyhemoglobin. Position of iron atom shown by circle. Movements are for an α subunit. (*b*) Similar movements in a β subunit using space-filling diagram shown. Residue labels centered in density for the deoxyconformation.
Redrawn with permission from Baldwin, J., and Chothia, C. J. Mol. Biol. *129:175, 1979. Copyright © 1979 by Academic Press, Inc. (London) Ltd.*

The FG to C intersubunit contacts act as a "switch," because they exist in two different arrangements with different modes of contact between the FG corner of one subunit and the C helix of the adjacent subunit. The switch in noncovalent interactions between the two positions involves a relative movement of FG and C in adjacent subunits of about 6 Å. In the second position of the "switch," the tertiary conformation of the subunits participating in the FG to C intersubunit contact is less constrained and the adjacent subunit changes to a new tertiary conformation (oxy conformation) even without O_2 bound. This oxy conformation allows the His F8 residues to approach their porphyrins on O_2 association with a less significant steric repulsion than in the deoxy conformation (Figure 3.40). Thus an O_2 molecule binds to the empty hemes in the less constrained oxy conformation more easily than to a subunit conformation held by the quaternary interactions in the deoxy conformation.

In addition, Val E11 in the deoxy conformation of β subunits is at the entrance to the O_2-binding site, where it sterically impedes O_2 association to heme (see Figure 3.33). In the oxy conformation the heme in β subunits moves approximately 1.5 Å further into the heme-binding site, changing the geometric relationship of the O_2-binding site to the Val El1 side chain, so that the Val El1 no longer sterically interferes with O_2 binding. This is an important additional factor that increases affinity of O_2 for the oxy conformation of the β chain over that for the deoxy conformation.

The deoxy conformation of hemoglobin is referred to as the "tense" or **T conformational state.** The oxyhemoglobin conformational form is referred to as the "relaxed" or **R conformational state.** The allosteric mechanism shows how initial binding of the oxygen to one of the heme subunits of the tetrameric molecule pushes the molecular conformation from the T to R conformational state. The affinity constant of O_2 is greater for the R state hemes than the T state by a factor of 150–300, depending on the solution conditions.

The Bohr Effect Involves Dissociation of a Proton on Binding of Oxygen

The equilibrium expression for oxygen association to hemoglobin includes a term that indicates participation of H^+ in the equilibrium.

$$\underset{T}{Hb} + 4O_2 \rightleftharpoons \underset{R}{Hb(O_2)_4} + xH^+ \qquad \textbf{(3.10)}$$

Equation 3.10 shows that the R form is more acidic, and the H^+ dissociate when hemoglobin is changed to the R form. The equivalents of H^+ that dissociate per mole of hemoglobin depends on the pH of the solution and the concentration of other factors that can bind to hemoglobin, such as Cl^- and bisphosphoglycerate (see Chapter 25). At pH 7.4, the value of x may vary from 1.8 to 2.8, depending on the solution conditions. This production of H^+ at an alkaline pH (pH > 6), when deoxyhemoglobin is transformed to oxyhemoglobin, is known as the alkaline **Bohr effect.**

The H^+ are derived from the partial dissociation of acid residues with pK'_a values within 1.5 pH units of the solution pH, which change from a higher to lower pK'_a, on the change of the T to R conformation. For example, the HC3 His 146(β) in the deoxy (T) conformation is predominantly in its imidazolium form (positively charged acid form), which is stabilized by a favorable interaction with the negatively charged side chain of the FG1 Asp 94(β) (Figure 3.39). This ion pair makes it more difficult to remove the imidazolium proton and thus raises the pK'_a of the imidazolium to a higher value than normally found for a free imidazolium ion in solution, where a stabilization by a proximal negatively charged group does not normally occur. However, on conversion of the protein to the R conformation, the strength of this ionic interaction is broken and the imidazolium assumes a lower pK'_a. The decrease in pK'_a of histidine at blood pH results in conversion of some of its acid form to its conjugate base (imidazole) form, with dissociation of H^+ that forms a part of the Bohr effect. Breakage of this ion pair with release of protons accounts for 50% of the H^+ released on conversion to the R conformation. Other acid groups in the protein contribute the additional H^+ due to analogous decreases in their pK'_a values on changing from the T to R conformation.

The equilibrium involving hydrogen ions produced by the Bohr effect has important physiological consequences. Cells metabolizing at high rates, with high requirements for molecular oxygen, produce carbonic acid and lactic acid, which act to increase the hydrogen ion concentration in the cell's environment. As the increase in hydrogen ion concentration forces the equilibrium of Eq. 3.10 to the left, from the higher O_2 affinity conformation (R) to the lower affinity conformation (T), an increased amount of oxygen is dissociated from the hemoglobin molecule.

BIBLIOGRAPHY

Immunoglobulins

Alzari, P. M., Lascombe, M.-B., and Poljak, R. J. Structure of antibodies. *Annu. Rev. Immunol.* 6:555, 1988.

Chothia, C., Lesk, A. M., Tramontano, A., Levitt, M., Smith-Gill, S. J., Air, G., Sheriff, S., Padlan, E. A., Davies, D., Tulip, W. R., Colman, P. M., Spinelli, S., Alzari, P. M., and Poljak, R. J. Conformations of immunoglobulin hypervariable regions. *Nature* 342:877, 1989.

Davies, D. R., Padlan, E. A., and Sheriff, S. Antibody–antigen complexes. *Acc. Chem. Res.* 26:421, 1993.

Guddat, L. W., Shan, L., Fan, Z.-C., Andersen, K. N., Rosauer, R., Linthicum, D. S., and Edmundson, A. B. Intramolecular signaling upon complexation. *FASEB J.* 9:101, 1995.

Hunkapiller, T., and Hood, L. Diversity of the immunoglobulin gene superfamily. *Adv. Immunol.* 44:1, 1989.

Padlan, E. A. Anatomy of the antibody molecule. *Mol. Immunol.* 31:169, 1994.

Rini, J. M., Schultze-Gahmen, U., Wilson, I. A. Structural evidence for induced fit as a mechanism for antibody–antigen recognition. *Science* 255:959, 1992.

Stanfield, R. L., Takimoto-Kaminmura, M., Rini, J. M., Profy, A. T., and Wilson, I. A. Major antigen-induced domain rearrangements in an antibody. *Structure* 1:83, 1993.

Serine Proteases

Birk, Y. Proteinase inhibitors. In: A. Neuberger and K. Brocklehurst (Eds.), *Hydrolytic Enzymes*. Amsterdam: Elsevier, 1987, p. 257.

Dufton, M. J. Could domain movements be involved in the mechanism of trypsin-like serine proteases? *FEBS Lett.* 271:9, 1990.

Greer, J. Comparative modeling methods: application to the family of the mammalian serine proteases. *Proteins* 7:317, 1990.

Liebman, M. N. Structural organization in the serine proteases. *Enzyme* 36:115, 1986.

Neurath, H. Proteolytic processing and physiological regulation. *Trends Biochem. Sci.* 14:268, 1989.

Perona, J. J., and Craik, C. S. Structural basis of substrate specificity in the serine proteases. *Protein Sci.* 4:337, 1995.

Polgar, L. Structure and function of serine proteases. In: A. Neuberger and K. Brocklehurst (Eds.), *Hydrolytic Enzymes,* series in *New Comprehensive Biochemistry,* Vol. 16. Amsterdam: Elsevier, 1987, p. 159.

Zwaal, R. F. A., and Hemker, H. C. (Eds.). *Blood Coagulation,* series in *New Comprehensive Biochemistry,* Vol. 13. Amsterdam: Elsevier, 1986.

DNA-Binding Proteins

Berger, J. M., Gamblin, S. J., Harrison, S. C., and Wang, J. C. Structure and mechanism of DNA topoisomerase II. *Nature* 379:225, 1996.

Cho, Y., Gorina, S., Jeffrey, P. D., Pavletich, N. P. Crystal structure of a p53 tumor suppressor–DNA complex: understanding tumorigenic mutations. *Science* 265:346, 1994.

Ellenberger, T. E., Brandl, C. J., Struhl, K., and Harrison, S. C. The GCN4 basic region leucine zipper binds DNA as a dimer of uninterrupted α helices: crystal structure of the protein–DNA complex. *Cell* 71:1223, 1992.

Ghosh, G., Van Duyne, G., Ghosh, S., and Sigler, P. B. Structure of NF-κB p50 homodimer bound to a κB site. *Nature* 373:303, 1995.

Landschulz, W. H., Johnson, P. F., and McKnight, S. L. The leucine zipper: a hypothetical structure common to a new class of DNA binding proteins. *Science* 240:1759, 1988.

Lee, M. S., Gippert, G. P., Soman, K. V., Case, D. A., and Wright, P. E. Three-dimensional solution structure of a single zinc finger DNA-binding domain. *Science* 245:635, 1989.

Lewis, M., Chang, G., Horton, N. C., Kercher, M. A., Pace, H. C., Schumacher, M. A., Brennan, R. G., and Lu, P. Crystal structure of the lactose operon repressor and its complexes with DNA and inducer. *Science* 271:1247, 1996.

Müller, C. W., Rey, F. A., Sodeoka, M., Verdine, G. L., and Harrison, S. C. Structure of the NF-κB p50 homodimer bound to DNA. *Nature* 373:311, 1995.

Nikolov, D. B., Chen, H., Halay, E. D., Usheva, A. A., Hisatake, K., Lee, D. K., Roeder R. G., and Burley, S. K. Crystal structure of a TFIIB-TBP-TATA-element ternary complex. *Nature* 377:119, 1995.

Pavletich, N. P., and Pabo, C. O. Zinc finger—DNA recognition: crystal structure of a Zif-268-DNA complex at 2.1 Å. *Science* 252:809, 1991.

Pellegrini, L., Tan, S., and Richmond, T. J. Structure of serum response factor core bound to DNA. *Nature* 376:490, 1995.

Hemoglobin

Baldwin, J., and Chothia, C. Haemoglobin: the structural changes related to ligand binding and its allosteric mechanism. *J. Mol. Biol.* 129:175, 1979.

Busch, M. R., Mace, J. E., Ho, N. T., and Ho, C. Roles of the *beta*-146 histidyl residue in the molecular basis of the Bohr effect of hemoglobin: a protein nuclear magnetic resonance study. *Biochemistry* 30:1865, 1991.

Dickerson, R. E., and Geis, I. *Hemoglobin: Structure, Function, Evolution and Pathology*. Menlo Park, CA: Benjamin-Cummings, 1983

Ho, C. Proton nuclear magnetic resonance studies on hemoglobin: cooperative interactions and partially ligated intermediates. *Adv. Protein Chem.* 43:154, 1992.

Jayaraman, V., Rodgers, K. R., Mukerji, I., and Spiro, T. G. Hemoglobin allostery: resonance Raman spectroscopy of kinetic intermediates. *Science* 269:1843, 1995.

Jia, L., Bonaventura, C., Bonaventura, J., and Stamler, J. S. *S*-Nitrosohaemoglobin: a dynamic activity of blood involved in vascular control. *Nature* 380:221, 1996.

Mathews, A. J., Rohlfs, R. J., Olson, J. S., Tame, J., Renaud, J. P., and Nagai, K. The effects of E7 and E11 mutations on the kinetics of ligand binding to R state human hemoglobin, *J. Biol. Chem.* 264:16573, 1989.

Perutz, M. Hemoglobin structure and respiratory transport. *Sci. Am.* 239:92, 1978.

Perutz, M. F., Fermi, G., and Shih, T.-B. Structure of deoxy cowtown [His HC3(146)beta to Leu]: origin of the alkaline Bohr effect. *Proc. Natl. Acad. Sci. U.S.A.* 81:4781, 1984.

Srinivasan, R., and Rose, G. D. The T-to-R transformation in hemoglobin: a reevaluation. *Proc. Natl. Acad. Sci. U.S.A.* 91:11113, 1994.

QUESTIONS ■ J. Baggott and C. N. Angstadt

1. Haptens:
   A. can function as antigens.
   B. strongly bind to antibodies specific for them.
   C. may be macromolecules.
   D. never act as antigenic determinants.
   E. can directly elicit the production of specific antibodies.

2. IgG:
   A. is found primarily in mucosal secretions.
   B. is one of the less common immunoglobulin types.
   C. has the highest molecular weight of all the immunoglobulins.
   D. contains carbohydrate covalently attached to the H chain.
   E. plays an important role in allergic responses.

3. In the three-dimensional structure of immunoglobulins:
   A. β-sheets align edge to edge.
   B. in each chain (H and L) the C and V regions fold onto one another, forming C–V associations.
   C. C_L–V_L associations form the complementary sites for binding antigens.
   D. free —SH groups are preserved to function in tight binding of antigens.
   E. hinge domains connect globular domains

4. Study of the papain hydrolysis products of an antibody indicates:
   A. antibodies are bivalent.
   B. the products have decreased affinity for antigens.
   C. each antibody molecule is hydrolyzed into many small peptides.
   D. the hypervariable sequences are in the hinge region of the intact molecule.
   E. none of the above is true.

5. In immunoglobulins all of the following are true EXCEPT:
   A. there are four polypeptide chains.
   B. there are two copies of each type of chain.
   C. all chains are linked by disulfide bonds.
   D. carbohydrate is covalently bound to the protein.
   E. immunoglobulin class is determined by the C_L regions.

6. Serine proteases:
   A. hydrolyze peptide bonds involving the carboxyl groups of serine residues.
   B. are characterized by having several active sites per molecule, each containing a serine residue.
   C. are inactivated by reacting with one molecule of diisopropylfluorophosphate per molecule of protein.
   D. are exopeptidases.
   E. are synthesized in an active form in eukaryotes.

7. The active sites of all serine proteases contain which of the following amino acid residues?
   A. asparagine
   B. γ-carboxyglutamate
   C. histidine
   D. lysine or arginine
   E. threonine

8. All of the following are characteristic of serine proteases as a class EXCEPT:
   A. only one serine residue is catalytically active.
   B. natural protein substrates and inhibitors bind very tightly to the protease.
   C. the genes that code for them are analogously organized.
   D. catalytic units exhibit two structural domains of dramatically different size.
   E. in eukaryotes, the serine proteases are produced initially as zymogens.

9. All of the following serine proteases exhibit sequence homology EXCEPT:
   A. chymotrypsin.
   B. elastase.
   C. *Streptomyces griseus* protease.
   D. subtilisin.
   E. trypsin.

Refer to the following for Questions 10–13.
   A. helix–turn–helix
   B. leucine zipper
   C. zinc finger
   D. all of the above
   E. none of the above

10. Not a DNA-binding motif.

11. Contains a single α-helix.

12. Two domains form a β-pleated sheet, which fits over the DNA double helix.

13. Found in proteins which bind to DNA.

14. The α-chain appears in all normal human hemoglobins EXCEPT:
   A. HbA_1.
   B. HbA_2.
   C. HbF.
   D. Hb Gower-1.

15. Hemoglobin and myoglobin both have all of the following characteristics EXCEPT:
   A. consist of subunits designed to provide hydrogen bonds to and nonpolar interaction with other subunits.
   B. highly α-helical.
   C. bind one molecule of heme per globin chain.
   D. bind heme in a hydrophobic pocket.
   E. can bind one O_2 per heme.

16. Hemoglobin, but not myoglobin, when it binds oxygen, exhibits:
    A. a hyperbolic saturation curve.
    B. a Hill coefficient of 1.
    C. positive cooperativity.
    D. a cooperativity index of 81.

17. All of the following are believed to contribute to the stability of the deoxy or T conformation of hemoglobin EXCEPT:
    A. the larger ionic radius of the six-coordinated ferrous ion as compared to the five-coordinated ion.
    B. steric interaction of His F8 with the porphyrin ring.
    C. interactions between the FG corner of one subunit and the C helix of the adjacent subunit.
    D. a valyl residue that tends to block O_2 from approaching the hemes of the β-chains.

18. In the Bohr effect:
    A. oxygen is released with increasing difficulty as the pH decreases.
    B. the R form of hemoglobin is more acidic than the T form.
    C. histidine 146 (β) interacts with a nearby Cl^-.
    D. cells with higher voluntary oxygen demand are deprived to ensure adequate oxygen for other tissues.
    E. bisphosphoglycerate decreases the oxygen affinity of hemoglobin.

ANSWERS

1. B Haptens are small molecules and cannot alone elicit antibody production; thus they are not antigens. They can act as antigenic determinants if covalently bound to a larger molecule, and free haptens may bind strongly to the antibodies thereby produced (p. 88).
2. D All immunoglobulins are glycoproteins. A: IgA is associated with mucosal secretions. B: IgG is the most common immunoglobulin type. C: IgM has the highest molecular weight (Table 3.1, p. 90) E: IgE plays an important role in allergic responses (Clin. Corr. 3.2, p. 92).
3. E See Figures 3.4–3.7, p. 93. A: The β-sheets align face-to-face. D: Antigen binding is noncovalent.
4. A In these hydrolysis experiments, three fragments are produced: two identical Fab fragments, each of which binds antigen with an affinity similar to that of the whole antibody molecule, and one Fc fragment, which does not bind antigens (p. 92).
5. E There are two copies of each of two types of polypeptide chain (p. 89).
6. C This is the distinguishing characteristic of the serine proteases, and of the serine hydrolases in general. A: They have various specificities (p. 99). B: There is only one active site per molecule (p. 103). D: They are all endopeptidases (p. 98). E: In eukaryotes they are synthesized as inactive precursors, zymogens, or proenzymes (p. 105).
7. C (p. 103). A: Aspartate, not asparagine, is involved. B: γ-Carboxyglutamate is essential to some of the serine proteases, but it is not at the active site. D: These are the substrate specificities of the trypsin-like proteases.
8. D The domains are of about equal size (p. 105).
9. D The bacterial protease subtilisin may be an example of converging evolution (p. 106). See also Table 3.7, p. 107.
10. B The leucine zipper binds two subunits in a head-to-head manner but does not itself interact with DNA (p. 110).
11. C See p. 108 and Figure 3.23.
12. E This describes the TATA box-binding protein (p. 112).
13. D
14. D Hb Gower-1 has the structure $\zeta_2\varepsilon_2$ (p. 114, Table 3.8).
15. A Hemoglobin has four chains and four oxygen-binding sites, whereas myoglobin has one chain and one oxygen-binding site. Each oxygen-binding site is a heme (p. 115).
16. C Hemoglobin's Hill coefficient of 2.8 indicates positive cooperativity (p. 119). A: See p. 118, Figure 3.35. B: Myoglobin has a Hill coefficient of 1. D: A cooperativity index of 81 indicates noncooperativity; hemoglobin's lower value of 4.8 reflects cooperative oxygen binding (p. 119).
17. A Six-coordinated ferrous ion has a smaller ionic radius than the five-coordinated species and just fits into the center of the porphyrin ring without distortion (p. 120).
18. B His 146 (β) is a major contributor to the Bohr effect. Thus its pK_a' will be lower (it will be a stronger acid) in oxyhemoglobin (p. 123). E: This is true but is unrelated to the Bohr effect.

CHAPTER

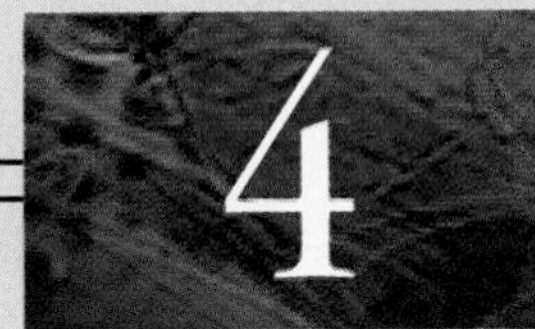

ENZYMES: CLASSIFICATION, KINETICS, AND CONTROL

J. Lyndal York

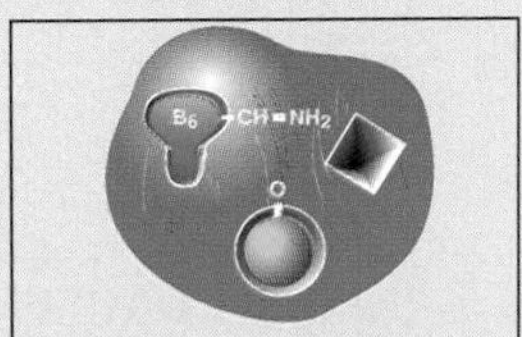

4.1 ■ GENERAL CONCEPTS

Enzymes are specialized proteins that function in the acceleration of chemical reactions. Many reactions required for normal activity of cells would not proceed fast enough at the pH and temperature of the body without these specialized proteins. The term defining the speed of a chemical reaction, whether catalyzed or uncatalyzed, is **rate** or **velocity.** Rate (velocity) is the change in amount (moles, grams) of starting materials or products per unit time. Enzymes increase the rate by acting as catalysts. A **catalyst** increases the rate of a chemical reaction but is not itself changed in the process. An enzyme may become temporarily covalently bound to a molecule being transformed during intermediate stages of the reaction but at the end of the reaction the enzyme will again be in its original form as the product is released.

Two important characteristics of enzyme catalysts are that the enzyme is not changed as a result of catalysis and the enzyme does not change the equilibrium constant of the reaction but simply increases the rate at which the reaction approaches equilibrium. As will be discussed later, it accomplishes the rate increase by lowering the barrier to reaction; that is, it lowers the energy of activation. Therefore a catalyst increases the rate but does not change the thermodynamic properties of the system with which it is interacting.

Several terms need to be defined before we enter into a discussion of the mechanism of enzyme action. An **apoenzyme** is the protein part of an enzyme without any cofactors or prosthetic groups that may be required for the enzyme to be functional. The apoenzyme is catalytically inactive. Not all enzymes require cofactors or prosthetic groups. **Cofactors** are small organic or inorganic molecules that an apoenzyme requires for its activity. For example, in lysine oxidase copper is loosely bound but is required for the enzyme to be active. A **prosthetic** group is similar to a cofactor but is tightly bound to an apoenzyme. For example, in the cytochromes, the heme prosthetic group is very tightly bound and requires strong acids to disassociate it from the apocytochrome. Addition of a cofactor or prosthetic group to the apoprotein yields the **holoenzyme,** that is, the active enzyme. The molecule acted upon by the enzyme to form product is the **substrate.** Since most reactions are reversible, the products of the forward reaction become substrates for the reverse reaction.

Enzymes have a great deal of specificity. For example, glucose oxidase will oxidize glucose but not galactose. The specificity resides in a particular region on the enzyme surface, the **substrate-binding site,** a particular arrangement of amino acid side chains in the polypeptide that is specially formulated to bind a specific substrate. Some enzymes have broad specificity; glucose, mannose, and fructose are phosphorylated by hexokinase, whereas glucokinase is specific for glucose. The substrate-binding site may contain the **active site.** In some cases, however, the active site may not be within the substrate-binding site but may be contiguous to it in the primary sequence. In other instances the active-site residues lie in distant regions of the primary sequence but are brought adjacent to the substrate-binding site by folding in the tertiary structure. The **active site** contains the machinery, in the form of particular amino acid side chains, involved in catalyzing the reaction.

Some enzymes have variants called **isoenzymes** (isozymes) that catalyze the same chemical reaction. Isoenzymes are electrophoretically distinguishable because of mutations in one or more amino acids in noncritical areas of the protein.

Some enzymes have a region of the molecule, the **allosteric** site, that is not at the active site or substrate-binding site but is a unique site where small molecules bind and effect a change in the substrate-binding site or the activity occurring in the active site. The binding of a specific small molecule at the allosteric site causes a change in the conformation of the enzyme. This can cause the active site to become either more active or less active by increasing or decreasing the affinity of the binding site for substrate. Such interactions regulate the enzyme's activity and are discussed in detail on page 151.

4.2 CLASSIFICATION OF ENZYMES

The International Union of Biochemistry and Molecular Biology (IUBMB) has established a system whereby all enzymes are classified into six major classes, each subdivided into subclasses that are further subdivided. In naming an enzyme, the substrates are stated first, followed by the reaction type to which the ending -ase is affixed. For example, alcohol dehydrogenase is alcohol:NAD^+ oxidoreductase because it catalyzes an oxidation–reduction reaction and the electron donor is an alcohol and the acceptor is NAD^+. Many common names persist but are not very informative. For example, "aldolase" does not tell much about the substrates, although it does identify the reaction type. We will use trivial names recognized by the IUBMB and that are in common usage. Table 4.1 summarizes the six major classes and subclasses of enzymes.

Class 1: Oxidoreductases

These enzymes catalyze **oxidation–reduction reactions.** For example, alcohol:NAD^+ oxidoreductase (alcohol **dehydrogenase**) catalyzes the oxidation of an alcohol to an aldehyde. It removes two electrons and two hydrogen atoms from the alcohol to yield an aldehyde, and, in the process, the two electrons originally in the carbon–hydrogen bond of the alcohol are transferred to the NAD^+, which is reduced (Figure 4.1). NAD^+, whose structure is presented in Figure 4.19, is a cofactor that mediates many biological oxidation–reduction reactions. The redox site in NAD^+ is shown in Figure 4.20. In addition to the alcohol and aldehyde functional groups, dehydrogenases also act on the following functional groups as electron donors: $-CH_2-CH_2-$, $-CH_2-NH_2$, and $-CH{=}NH$, as well as the cofactors NADH and NADPH.

There are other subclasses of the oxidoreductases. **Oxidases** transfer two electrons from the donor to oxygen, resulting usually in hydrogen peroxide (H_2O_2) formation. For example, **glucose oxidase** catalyzes the reaction shown in Figure 4.2. **Cytochrome oxidase** produces H_2O rather than H_2O_2. **Oxygenases** catalyze the incorporation of oxygen into a substrate. With dioxygenases both atoms of O_2 are incorporated in a single product, whereas with the monooxygenases a single oxygen atom is incorporated as a hydroxyl group

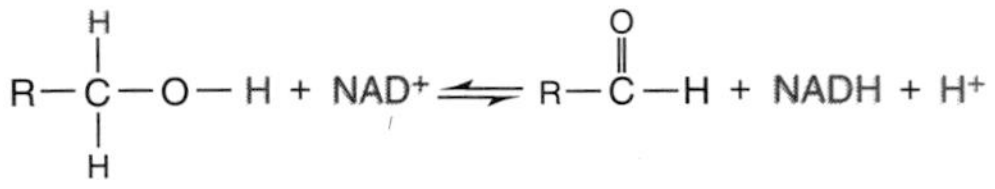

$$R-CH_2-O-H + NAD^+ \rightleftharpoons R-CHO + NADH + H^+$$

FIGURE 4.1
Oxidation of ethanol by alcohol dehydrogenase.

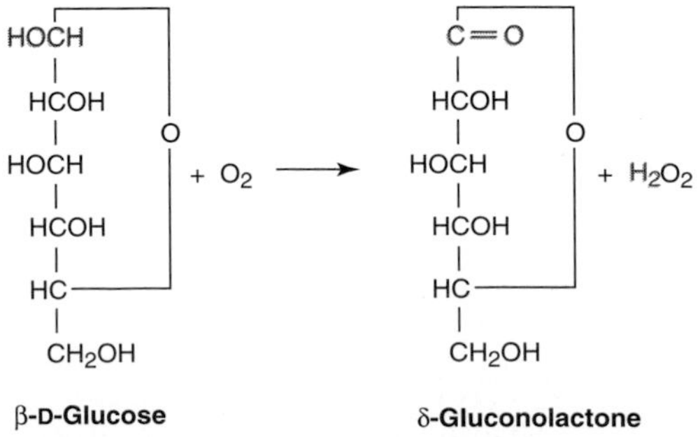

FIGURE 4.2
Oxidation of glucose by glucose oxidase.

TABLE 4.1 Summary of the Enzyme Classes and Major Subclasses

1. Oxidoreductases	2. Transferases
Dehydrogenases	Transaldolase and transketolase
Oxidases	Acyl, methyl, glucosyl, and phosphoryltransferase
Reductases	Kinases
Peroxidases	Phosphomutases
Catalase	4. Lyases
Oxygenases	Decarboxylases
Hydroxylases	Aldolases
3. Hydrolases	Hydratases
Esterases	Dehydratases
Glycosidases	Synthases
Peptidases	Lyases
Phosphatases	
Thiolases	
Phospholipases	
Amidases	
Deaminases	
Ribonucleases	
5. Isomerases	6. Ligases
Racemases	Synthetases
Epimerases	Carboxylases
Isomerases	
Mutases (not all)	

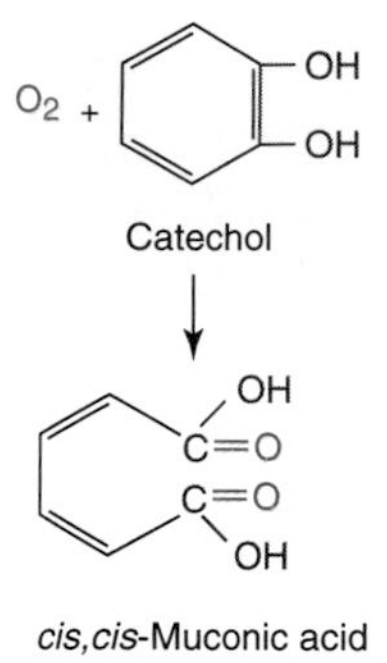

FIGURE 4.3
Oxygenation of catechol by an oxygenase.

and the other oxygen atom is reduced to water by electrons from the substrate or from a second substrate that is not oxygenated. **Catechol oxygenase** catalyzes the dioxygenase reaction (Figure 4.3); steroid hydroxylase illustrates a monooxygenase (mixed function oxygenase) reaction (Figure 4.4). **Peroxidases** utilize H_2O_2 rather than oxygen as the oxidant. NADH peroxidase catalyzes the reaction

$$\text{NADH} + \text{H}^+ + \text{H}_2\text{O}_2 \leftrightharpoons \text{NAD}^+ + 2\text{H}_2\text{O}$$

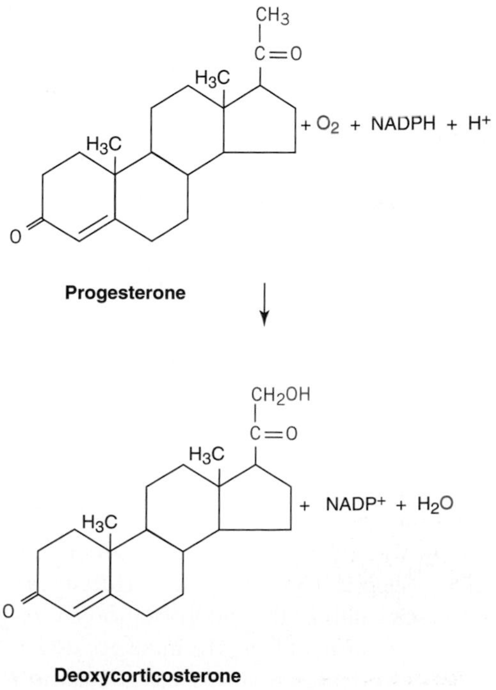

FIGURE 4.4
Hydroxylation of progesterone by a monooxygenase.

Catalase is unique in that H_2O_2 serves as both donor and acceptor. Catalase functions in the cell to detoxify H_2O_2:

$$H_2O_2 + H_2O_2 \leftrightharpoons O_2 + 2H_2O$$

Class 2: Transferases

These enzymes transfer functional groups between donors and acceptors. The amino, acyl, phosphate, one-carbon, and glycosyl groups are the major moieties that are transferred. **Aminotransferases (transaminases)** transfer an amino group from one amino acid to an α-keto acid acceptor, resulting in the formation of a new amino acid and a new keto acid (Figure 4.5). **Kinases** are the phosphorylating enzymes that catalyze the transfer of the γ phosphoryl group from ATP or another nucleoside triphosphate to alcohol or amino group acceptors. For example, glucokinase catalyzes the phosphorylation of glucose (Figure 4.6).

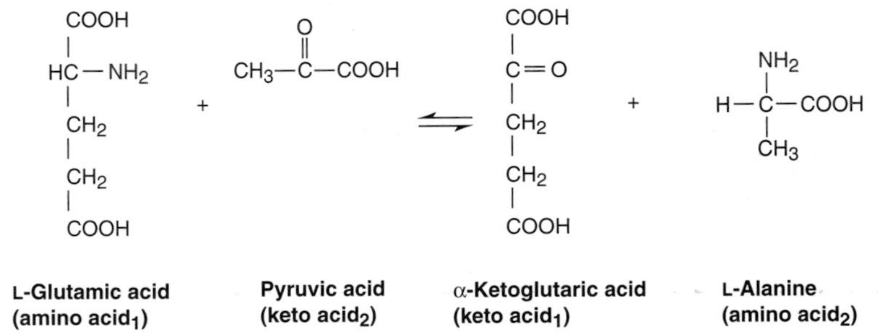

L-Glutamic acid (amino acid$_1$) + Pyruvic acid (keto acid$_2$) ⇌ α-Ketoglutaric acid (keto acid$_1$) + L-Alanine (amino acid$_2$)

FIGURE 4.5
Examples of a reaction catalyzed by an aminotransferase.

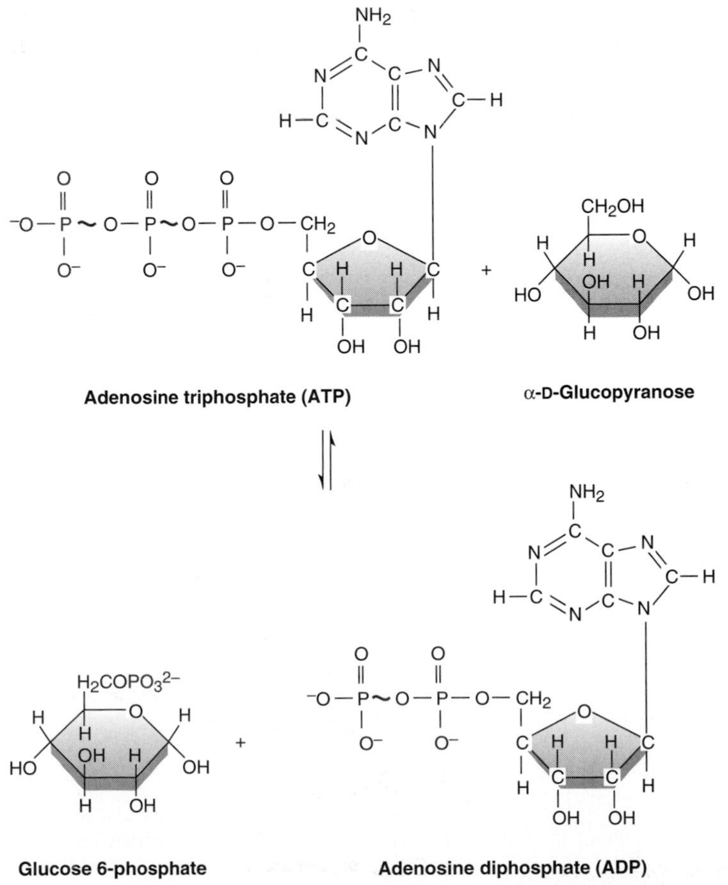

Adenosine triphosphate (ATP) + α-D-Glucopyranose ⇌ Glucose 6-phosphate + Adenosine diphosphate (ADP)

FIGURE 4.6
Phosphorylation of glucose by a kinase.

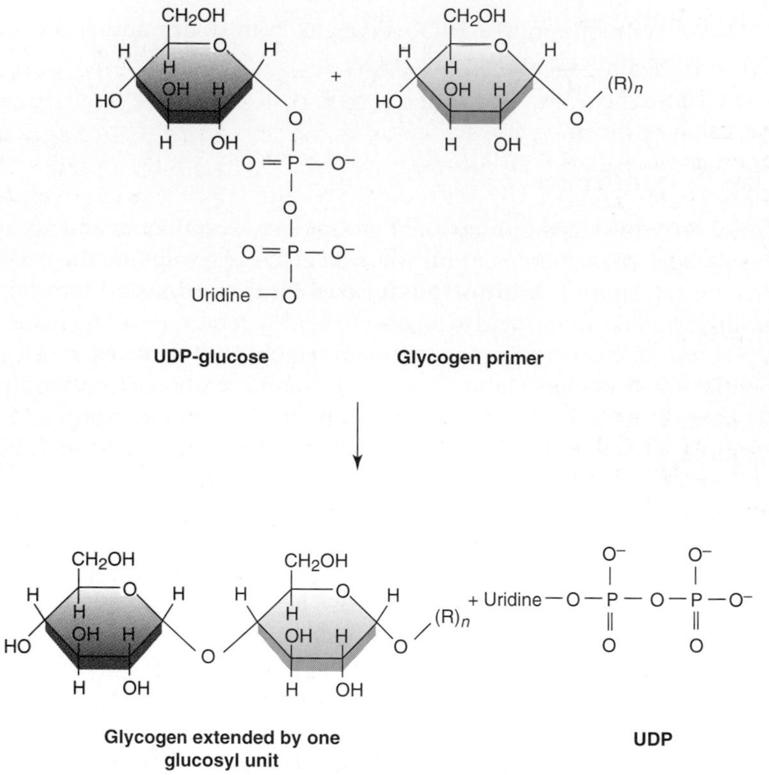

UDP-glucose + Glycogen primer

↓

Glycogen extended by one glucosyl unit + UDP

FIGURE 4.7
A transferase reaction—synthesis of glycogen.

Glycogen synthesis depends on **glucosyltransferases,** which transfer an activated glucosyl residue to a glycogen primer. The phosphoester bond in uridine diphosphoglucose is labile, which allows the glucose to be transferred to the growing end of the glycogen primer as indicated in Figure 4.7.

Although a polymer is synthesized, the reaction is not of the ligase type reaction; see Class 6.

Class 3: Hydrolases

This group of enzymes can be considered as a special class of the transferases in which the donor group is transferred to water. The generalized reaction involves the hydrolytic cleavage of C—O, C—N, O—P, and C—S bonds. The cleavage of a peptide bond is a good example of this reaction:

$$R_1-\overset{\overset{\displaystyle O}{\|}}{C}-NH-R_2 + H_2O \longrightarrow R_1-\overset{\overset{\displaystyle O}{\|}}{C}-O^- + H_3\overset{+}{N}-R_2$$

Proteolytic enzymes are a special class of hydrolases called **peptidases.**

Class 4: Lyases

Lyases add or remove the elements of water, ammonia, or carbon dioxide. **Decarboxylases** remove the element of CO_2 from α- or β-keto acids or amino acids:

$$R-\overset{\overset{\displaystyle O}{\|}}{C}-\overset{\overset{\displaystyle O}{\|}}{C}-O^- + H^+ \longrightarrow R-\overset{\overset{\displaystyle O}{\|}}{C}-H + CO_2$$

Dehydratases remove H_2O in a dehydration reaction. Fumarase converts fumarate to malate (Figure 4.8).

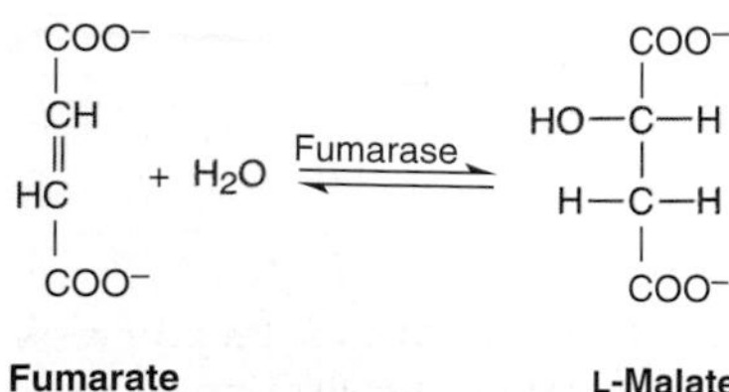

FIGURE 4.8
The fumarase reaction.

Class 5: Isomerases

This very heterogeneous group of enzymes catalyze isomerizations of several types. These include cis–trans and aldose–ketose interconversions. Isomerases that catalyze inversion at asymmetric carbon atoms are either **epimerases** or **racemases** (Figure 4.9). **Mutases** involve intramolecular transfer of a group such as a phosphoryl. The transfer may be direct but can involve a phosphorylated enzyme as an intermediate. Phosphoglycerate mutase catalyzes conversion of 2-phosphoglycerate to 3-phosphoglycerate (Figure 4.10).

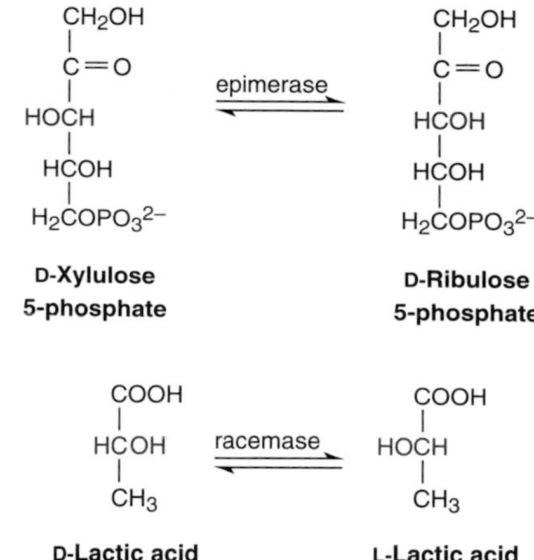

FIGURE 4.9
Examples of reactions catalyzed by an epimerase and a racemase.

Class 6: Ligases

Since to ligate means to bind, these enzymes are involved in synthetic reactions where two molecules are joined at the expense of a "high-energy phosphate bond" of ATP. The term **synthetase** is reserved for this particular group of enzymes. The formation of aminoacyl tRNAs, acyl coenzyme A, and glutamine and the addition of CO_2 to pyruvate are reactions catalyzed by ligases. Pyruvate carboxylase is a good example of a ligase enzyme (Figure 4.11). The substrates bicarbonate and pyruvate are ligated to form a four-carbon (C4) α-keto acid.

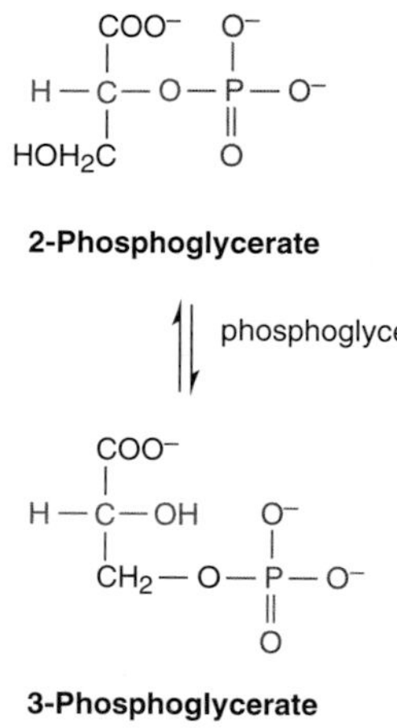

2-Phosphoglycerate

phosphoglyceromutase

3-Phosphoglycerate

FIGURE 4.10
Interconversion of the 2- and 3-phosphoglycerates.

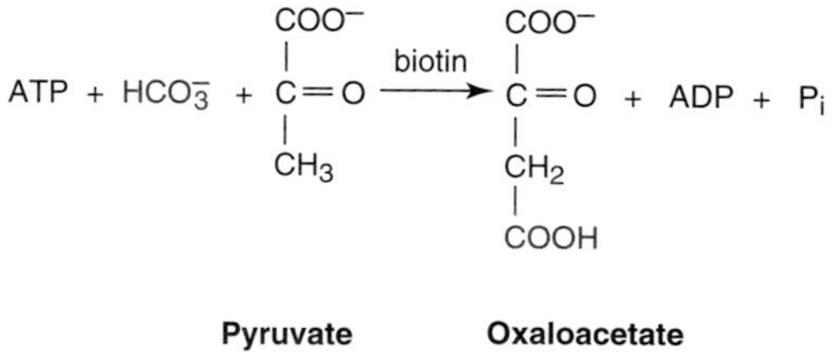

ATP + HCO_3^- + Pyruvate $\xrightarrow{\text{biotin}}$ Oxaloacetate + ADP + P_i

FIGURE 4.11
Pyruvate carboxylase reaction.

4.3 KINETICS

Kinetics Studies the Rate of Change of Reactants to Products

Since enzymes affect the rate of chemical reactions, it is important to understand basic chemical kinetics and how kinetic principles apply to enzyme-catalyzed reactions. **Kinetics** is a study of the rate of change of reactants to products. **Velocity** is expressed in terms of change in the *concentration* of substrate or product per unit time, whereas **rate** refers to changes in *total quantity* (moles or grams) per unit time. Biochemists tend to use these terms interchangeably.

The velocity of a reaction A → P is determined from a progress curve or velocity profile of a reaction. The progress curve can be determined by following the disappearance of reactants or the appearance of product at several different times. In Figure 4.12, product appearance is plotted against time. The slope of tangents to the progress curve yields the instantaneous velocity at that point in time. The initial velocity is an important parameter in the assay of enzyme concentration. Note that the velocity changes constantly as the reaction proceeds to equilibrium, where it becomes zero. Mathematically, the velocity is expressed as

$$\text{Velocity} = v = \frac{-d[\text{A}]}{dt} = \frac{d[\text{P}]}{dt} \quad \textbf{(4.1)}$$

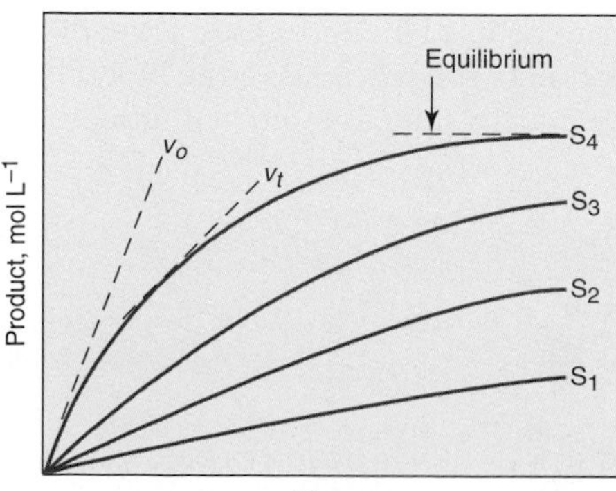

FIGURE 4.12
Progress curves for an enzyme-catalyzed reaction.
The initial velocity (v_0) of the reaction is determined from the slope of the progress curve at the beginning of the reaction. The initial velocity increases with increasing substrate concentration (S_1–S_4) but reaches a limiting value characteristic of each enzyme. The velocity at any time, t, is denoted as v_t.

and represents the change in concentration of reactants or products per unit time.

The Rate Equation

Determination of the velocity of a reaction reveals nothing about the stoichiometry of the reactants and products or about the reaction mechanism. An equation is needed that relates the experimentally determined initial velocity to the concentration of reactants. This is the velocity or rate equation. In the reaction A → P, the velocity equation is

$$\frac{-d[\mathrm{A}]}{dt} = v = k[\mathrm{A}]^n \qquad \textbf{(4.2)}$$

Thus the observed initial velocity depends on the starting concentration of A to the nth power multiplied by a proportionality constant (***k***). The latter is known as the **rate constant.** The exponent n is usually an integer from 1 to 3 that is required to satisfy the mathematical identity of the velocity expression.

Characterization of Reactions Based on Order

Another term useful in describing a reaction is the **order of reaction.** Empirically the order is determined as the sum of the exponents on each concentration term in the rate expression. In the case under discussion the reaction is **first order,** since the velocity depends on the concentration of A to the first power, $v = k[\mathrm{A}]^1$. In the reaction A + B → C, if the order with respect to A and B is 1, that is, $v = k[\mathrm{A}]^1[\mathrm{B}]^1$, overall the reaction is second order. Note that the order of reaction is independent of the stoichiometry of the reaction; that is, if the reaction were third order, the rate expression could be either $v = k[\mathrm{A}][\mathrm{B}]^2$ or $v = k[\mathrm{A}]^2[\mathrm{B}]$, depending on the order in A and B. Since the velocity of the reaction is constantly changing as the reactant concentration changes, first-order reaction conditions would not be ideal for assaying an enzyme-catalyzed reaction because one would have two variables, the changing substrate concentration and the unknown enzyme concentration.

If the differential first-order rate expression Eq. 4.2 is integrated, one obtains

$$k_1 \cdot t = 2.3 \log\left(\frac{[\mathrm{A}]}{[\mathrm{A}] - [\mathrm{P}]}\right) \qquad \textbf{(4.3)}$$

where [A] is the initial reactant concentration and [P] is the concentration of product formed at time t. The first-order rate constant k_1 has the units of reciprocal time. If the data shown in Figure 4.12 were replotted as log [P] versus time for any one of the substrate concentrations, a straight line would be obtained whose slope is equal to $k_1/2.303$. The rate constant k_1 should not be confused with the rate or velocity of the reaction.

Many biological processes proceed under first-order conditions. The clearance of many drugs from the blood by peripheral tissues is a first-order process. A specialized form of the rate equation can be used in these cases. If we define $t_{1/2}$ as the time required for the concentration of the reactants or the blood level of a drug to be reduced by one-half the initial value, then Eq. 4.3 reduces to

$$k_1 \cdot t_{1/2} = 2.3 \log\left(\frac{1}{1 - \frac{1}{2}}\right) = 2.3 \log 2 = 0.69 \qquad \textbf{(4.4)}$$

or

$$t_{1/2} = \frac{0.69}{k_1} \qquad \textbf{(4.5)}$$

Note that $t_{1/2}$ is not one-half the time required for the reaction to be completed. The term $t_{1/2}$ is referred to as the half-life of the reaction.

Many **second-order** reactions that involve water or any one of the reactants in large excess can be treated as pseudo-first-order reactions. In the hydrolysis of an ester,

$$\text{R—}\overset{\overset{\text{O}}{\|}}{\text{C}}\text{—O—CH}_3 + \text{H}_2\text{O} \rightleftharpoons \text{R—}\overset{\overset{\text{O}}{\|}}{\text{C}}\text{—OH} + \text{CH}_3\text{OH}$$

the second-order rate expression is

$$\text{velocity} = v = k_2[\text{ester}]^1[\text{H}_2\text{O}]^1 \qquad \textbf{(4.6)}$$

but since water is in abundance (55.5 M) compared to the ester (10^{-3}–10^{-2} M), the system obeys the first-order rate law Eq. 4.2, and the reaction appears to proceed as if it were a first-order reaction. Reactions in the cell that involve hydration, dehydration, or hydrolysis are pseudo-first-order.

The rate expression for the **zero-order** reaction is $v = k_0$. Note that there is no concentration term for reactants; therefore the addition of more reactant does not augment the rate. The disappearance of reactant or the appearance of product proceeds at a constant velocity irrespective of reactant concentration. The units of the rate constant are concentration per unit time. Zero-order reaction conditions only occur in catalyzed reactions where the concentration of reactants is large enough to saturate all the catalytic sites. Under these conditions the catalyst is operating at maximum velocity, and all catalytic sites are filled; therefore addition of more reactant cannot increase the rate.

Reversibility of Reactions

Although most chemical reactions are reversible, some directionality is imposed on particular steps in a metabolic pathway by rapid removal of end product by subsequent reactions in the pathway. Many ligase reactions involving the nucleoside triphosphates result in release of pyrophosphate (PP_i). These reactions are rendered irreversible by the hydrolysis of the pyrophosphate to 2 moles of inorganic phosphate, P_i. Schematically,

$$\text{A} + \text{B} + \text{ATP} \longrightarrow \text{A—B} + \text{AMP} + \text{PP}_i$$
$$\text{PP}_i + \text{H}_2\text{O} \longrightarrow 2\text{P}_i$$

Conversion of the "high-energy" pyrophosphate to inorganic phosphate imposes irreversibility on the system by virtue of the thermodynamic stability of the products.

For reactions that are reversible, the equilibrium constant for

$$\text{A} + \text{B} \rightleftharpoons \text{C}$$

is

$$K_{eq} = \frac{[\text{C}]}{[\text{A}][\text{B}]} \qquad \textbf{(4.7)}$$

and can also be expressed in terms of rate constants of the forward and reverse reactions:

$$\text{A} + \text{B} \underset{k_2}{\overset{k_1}{\rightleftharpoons}} \text{C}$$

where

$$\frac{k_1}{k_2} = K_{eq} \qquad \textbf{(4.8)}$$

Equation 4.8 shows the relationship between thermodynamic and kinetic quantities. The term K_{eq} is a thermodynamic expression of the state of the system, while k_1 and k_2 are kinetic expressions that are related to the speed at which that state is reached.

Enzymes Show Saturation Kinetics

Terminology

Enzyme activity is usually expressed as micromoles (μmol) of substrate converted to product per minute under specified assay conditions. One standard unit of enzyme activity (U) is that activity that catalyzes transformation of 1 μmol min^{-1}. **Specific activity** of an enzyme preparation is defined as the number of enzyme units per milligram of protein (μmol min^{-1} mg of protein^{-1} or U/mg of protein). This expression, however, does not indicate whether the sample tested contains only the enzyme protein; during enzyme purification the value will increase as contaminating protein is removed. The **catalytic constant,** or **turnover number,** of an enzyme is equal to the units of activity per mole of enzyme (μmol/min/mol of enzyme). Where the enzyme has more than one catalytic center, the catalytic constant is often given on the basis of the particle weight of the subunit rather than the molecular weight of the entire protein. The Commission on Enzyme Nomenclature of the International Union of Biochemistry and Molecular Biology recommends that enzyme activity be expressed in units of moles per second, instead of micromoles per minute, to conform with the rate constants used in chemical kinetics. A new unit, the **katal** (abbreviated kat), is proposed where 1 kat denotes conversion of 1 mol substrate per second. Activity can be expressed, however, as millikatals (mkat), microkatals (μkat), and so forth. The specific activity and catalytic constant can also be expressed in katals.

The catalytic constant or turnover number allows direct comparison of relative catalytic ability between enzymes. For example, the constants for catalase and α-amylase are 5×10^6 and 1.9×10^4, respectively, indicating that catalase is about 2500 times more active than amylase.

Maximum velocity, V_{max}, is the velocity obtained under conditions of substrate saturation of the enzyme under specified conditions of pH, temperature, and ionic strength. V_{max} is a constant for a given enzyme.

Interaction of Enzyme and Substrate

The initial velocity of an enzyme-catalyzed reaction is dependent on the concentration of substrate (S) (Figure 4.12). As concentration of substrate increases (S_1–S_4), initial velocity increases until the enzyme is completely saturated with substrate. If initial velocities obtained at given substrate concentrations are plotted (Figure 4.13), a rectangular hyperbola is obtained like that obtained for binding of oxygen to myoglobin as a function of increasing oxygen pressure. In general, a rectangular hyperbola is obtained for any process that involves interaction or binding of reactants or other substances at a specific but limited number of sites. The velocity of the reaction reaches a maximum at the point at which all the available sites are saturated. The curve in Figure 4.13 is referred

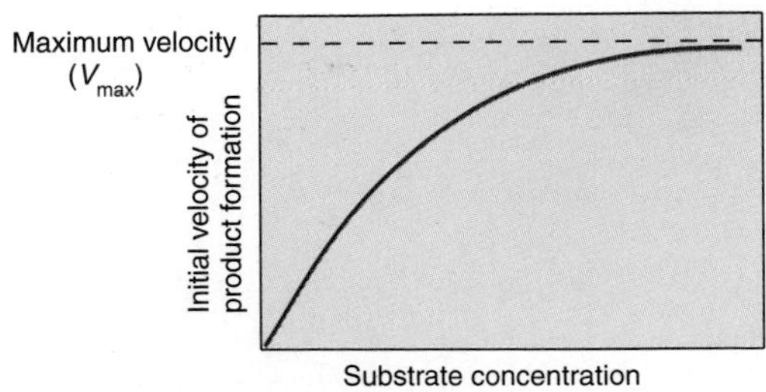

FIGURE 4.13
Plot of velocity versus substrate for an enzyme-catalyzed reaction.
Initial velocities are plotted against the substrate concentration at which they were determined. The curve is a rectangular hyperbola, which asymptotically approaches the maximum velocity possible with a given amount of enzyme.

to as the substrate saturation curve of an enzyme-catalyzed reaction and reflects the fact that an enzyme has a specific binding site for the substrate. Enzyme (E) and substrate must interact in some way if the substrate is to be converted to products. Initially there is formation of a complex between the enzyme and substrate:

$$E + S \underset{k_2}{\overset{k_1}{\rightleftharpoons}} ES \qquad \textbf{(4.9)}$$

The rate constant for formation of the ES complex is defined as k_1, and the rate constant for disassociation of the ES complex is defined as k_2. So far, we have described only an equilibrium binding of enzyme and substrate. The chemical event in which bonds are made or broken occurs in the ES complex. The conversion of substrate to products (P) then occurs from the ES complex with a rate constant k_3. Therefore, Eq. 4.9 is transformed to

$$E + S \underset{k_2}{\overset{k_1}{\rightleftharpoons}} ES \xrightarrow{k_3} E + P \qquad \textbf{(4.10)}$$

Equation 4.10 is a general statement of the mechanism of enzyme action. The equilibrium between E and S can be expressed as an affinity constant, K_a, only if the rate of the chemical phase of the reaction, k_3, is small compared to k_2; then $K_a = k_1/k_2$. Earlier we used K_{eq} to describe chemical reactions. In enzymology the association or affinity constant K_a is preferred.

The **initial velocity,** v_0, of an enzyme-catalyzed reaction is dependent on amount of substrate present and on enzyme concentration. Figure 4.14 shows progress curves for increasing concentrations of enzyme, where there is enough substrate initially to saturate the enzyme at all levels. The initial velocity doubles as the concentration of enzyme doubles. At the lower concentrations of enzyme, equilibrium is reached more slowly than at higher concentrations, but the final equilibrium position is the same.

From this discussion, we can conclude that the velocity of an enzyme reaction is dependent on both substrate and enzyme concentrations.

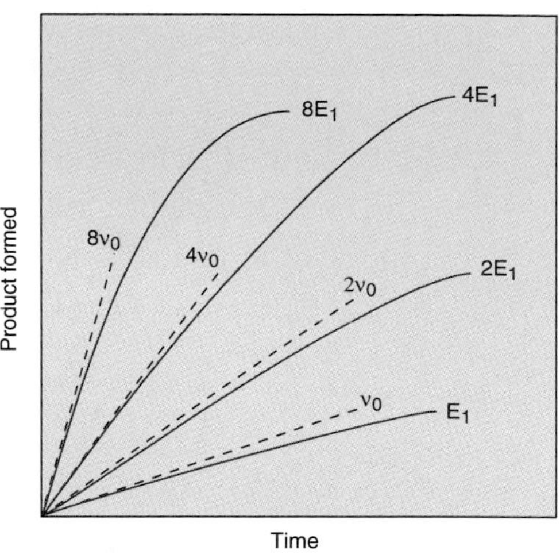

FIGURE 4.14
Progress curves at variable concentrations of enzyme and saturating levels of substrate.
The initial velocity (v_0) doubles as the enzyme concentration doubles. Since the substrate concentrations are the same, the final equilibrium concentrations of product will be identical in each case; however, equilibrium will be reached at a slower rate in those assays containing small amounts of enzyme.

Formulation of the Michaelis–Menten Equation

In the discussion of chemical kinetics, rate equations were developed so that velocity of the reaction could be expressed in terms of substrate concentration. This approach also holds for enzyme-catalyzed reactions, where the goal is to develop a relationship that will allow the velocity of a reaction to be correlated with the amount of enzyme. First, a rate equation must be developed that relates the velocity of the reaction to the substrate concentration.

Development of this rate equation, known as the **Michaelis–Menten equation,** requires three basic assumptions. The first is that the ES complex is in a **steady state;** that is, during the initial phases of the reaction, the concentration of the ES complex remains constant, even though many molecules of substrate are converted to products via the ES complex. The second assumption is that under saturating conditions all of the enzyme is converted to ES complex, and none is free. This occurs when the substrate concentration is high. The third assumption is that if all the enzyme is in the ES complex, then the rate of formation of products will be maximal; that is,

$$V_{max} = k_3[ES] \qquad \textbf{(4.11)}$$

If we then write the steady-state expression for formation and breakdown of the ES complex as

$$K_m = \frac{k_2 + k_3}{k_1} \qquad \textbf{(4.12)}$$

CLINICAL CORRELATION 4.1

A Case of Gout Demonstrates Two Phases in the Mechanism of Enzyme Action

The two phases of the Michaelis–Menten model of enzyme action, binding followed by modification of substrate, are illustrated by studies on a family with gout. The patient excreted three times the normal amount of uric acid per day and had markedly increased levels of 5′-phosphoribosyl-α-pyrophosphate (PRPP) in his red blood cells. PRPP is an intermediate in the biosynthesis of AMP and GMP, which are converted to ATP and GTP. Uric acid arises directly from degradation of AMP and GMP. Assays *in vitro* revealed that the patient's red cell PRPP synthetase activity was increased threefold. The pH optimum and the K_m of the enzyme for ATP and ribose 5-phosphate were normal, but V_{max} was increased threefold! This increase was not due to an increase in the amount of enzyme; immunologic testing with a specific antibody to the enzyme revealed similar quantities of the enzyme protein as in normal red cells. This finding demonstrates that the binding of substrate as reflected by K_m and the subsequent chemical event in catalysis, which is reflected in V_{max}, are separate phases of the overall catalytic process. This situation holds only for those enzyme mechanisms in which $k_3 \gg k_2$.

Becker, M. A., Kostel, P. J., Meyer, L. J., and Seegmiller, J. E. Human phosphoribosylpyrophosphate synthetase: increased enzyme specific activity in a family with gout and excessive purine synthesis. *Proc. Natl. Acad. Sci. U.S.A.* 70:2749, 1973.

the rate expression obtained by suitable algebraic manipulation becomes

$$\text{Velocity} = v = \frac{V_{max} \cdot [S]}{K_m + [S]} \qquad \textbf{(4.13)}$$

The complete derivation of this equation is at the end of this section. The two constants in this rate equation, V_{max} and K_m, are unique to each enzyme under specific conditions of pH and temperature. For enzymes in which $k_3 \ll k_2$, K_m becomes the reciprocal of the enzyme–substrate binding constant, and V_{max} reflects the catalytic phase of the enzyme mechanism as suggested by Eq. 4.11. Thus, in this model, activity of the enzyme can be separated into two phases: binding of substrate followed by chemical modification of the substrate. This biphasic nature of the enzyme mechanism is reinforced in the clinical example discussed in Clin. Corr. 4.1.

Significance of K_m

The concept of K_m may appear to have no physiological or clinical relevance. The truth is quite the contrary. As discussed in Section 4.9, all valid enzyme assays performed in the clinical laboratory are based on knowledge of K_m values for each substrate. In terms of the physiological control of glucose and phosphate metabolism, two **hexokinases** have evolved, one with a high K_m and one with a low K_m for glucose. Together, they contribute to maintaining steady-state levels of blood glucose and phosphate, as discussed on page 284.

In general, K_m values are near the concentrations of substrate found in cells. Perhaps enzymes have evolved substrate-binding sites with affinities comparable to *in vivo* levels of their substrates. Occasionally, mutation of an enzyme-binding site occurs, or an isoenzyme with an altered K_m is expressed. Either of these events can result in an abnormal physiology. An interesting example (Clin. Corr. 4.2) is the expression of only the atypical form of **aldehyde dehydrogenase** in people of Asiatic origin.

Note that if one allows the initial velocity, v_0, to be equal to $\frac{1}{2}V_{max}$ in Eq. 4.13, K_m will be equal to [S]:

$$\frac{1}{2}V_{max} = \frac{V_{max} \cdot [S]}{K_m + [S]}$$

$$K_m + [S] = \frac{2\,V_{max} \cdot [S]}{V_{max}}$$

$$K_m = [S]$$

Thus, from a substrate saturation curve, the numerical value of K_m can be derived by graphical analysis (Figure 4.15). Here the K_m is equal to the substrate concentration that gives one-half the maximum velocity.

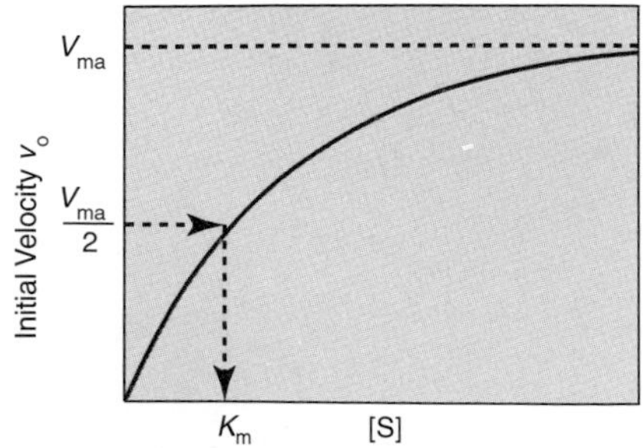

FIGURE 4.15
Graphic estimation of K_m for the v_0 versus [S] plot.
K_m is the substrate concentration at which the enzyme has half-maximal activity.

Linear Form of the Michaelis–Menten Equation

In practice the determination of K_m from the substrate saturation curve is not very accurate, because V_{max} is approached asymptotically. If one takes the reciprocal of Eq. 4.13 and separates the variables into a format consistent with the equation of a straight line ($y = mx + b$), then

$$\frac{1}{v_0} = \frac{K_m}{V_{max}} \times \frac{1}{[S]} + \frac{1}{V_{max}}$$

A plot of the reciprocal of the initial velocity versus the reciprocal of the initial substrate concentration yields a line whose slope is K_m/V_{max} and whose y-intercept is $1/V_{max}$. Such a plot is shown in Figure 4.16. It is often easier to obtain the K_m from the intercept on the x-axis, which is $-1/K_m$.

This linear form of the Michaelis–Menten equation is often referred to as the **Lineweaver–Burk** or **double-reciprocal plot.** Its advantage is that

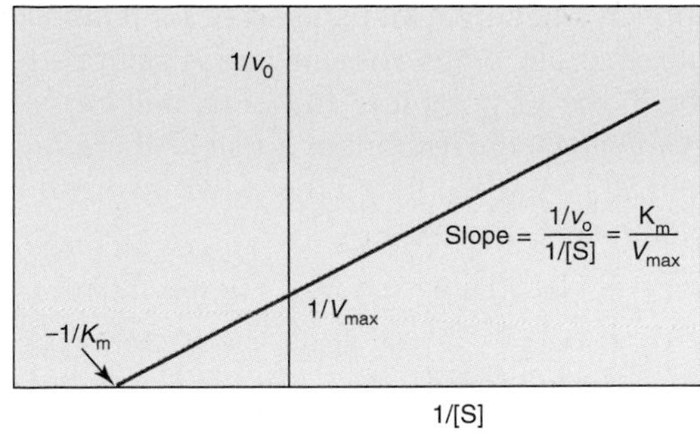

FIGURE 4.16
Determination of K_m and V_{max} from the Lineweaver–Burk double-reciprocal plot.
Plots of the reciprocal of the initial velocity versus the reciprocal of the substrate concentration used to determine the initial velocity yield a line whose *x*-intercept is $-1/K_m$.

statistically significant values of K_m and V_{max} can be obtained directly with six to eight data points.

Derivation of the Michaelis–Menten Equation

The generalized statement of the mechanism of enzyme action is

$$E + S \underset{k_2}{\overset{k_1}{\rightleftharpoons}} ES \xrightarrow{k_3} E + P \qquad \textbf{(4.10)}$$

If we assume that the rate of formation of the ES complex is balanced by its rate of breakdown (the steady-state assumption), then we can write

$$v_{\text{formation}} = k_1[S][E]$$
$$v_{\text{breakdown}} = k_2[ES] + k_3[ES] = [ES](k_2 + k_3)$$

If we set the rate of formation equal to the rate of breakdown, then

$$k_1[S][E] = [ES](k_2 + k_3)$$

After dividing both sides of the equation by k_1, we have

$$[S][E] = [ES]\left[\frac{k_2 + k_3}{k_1}\right] \qquad \textbf{(4.14)}$$

If we now define the ratio of the rate constants $(k_2 + k_3)/k_1$ as K_m, the Michaelis constant, and substitute it into Eq. 4.14, then

$$[S][E] = [ES]K_m \qquad \textbf{(4.15)}$$

Since [E] is equal to the free enzyme, we must express its concentration in terms of the total enzyme added to the system minus any enzyme in the [ES] complex; that is,

$$[E] = ([E_t] - [ES])$$

Upon substitution of the equivalent expression for [E] into Eq. 4.15 we have

$$[S]([E_t] - [ES]) = [ES]K_m$$

Dividing through by [S] yields

$$[E_t] - [ES] = \frac{[ES]K_m}{[S]}$$

and dividing through by [ES] yields

$$\frac{[E_t]}{[ES]} - 1 = \frac{K_m}{[S]} \quad \text{or} \quad \frac{[E_t]}{[ES]} = \frac{K_m}{[S]} + 1 = \frac{K_m + [S]}{[S]} \qquad \textbf{(4.16)}$$

CLINICAL CORRELATION 4.2

The Physiological Effect of Changes in Enzyme K_m Values

The unusual sensitivity of Asians to alcoholic beverages has a biochemical basis. In some Japanese and Chinese, much less ethanol is required to produce vasodilation that results in facial flushing and rapid heart rate than is required to achieve the same effect in Europeans. The physiological effects are due to acetaldehyde generated by liver alcohol dehydrogenase.

$$CH_3CH_2OH + NAD^+ \leftrightharpoons CH_3CHO + H^+ + NADH$$

Acetaldehyde is normally removed by a mitochondrial aldehyde dehydrogenase that converts it to acetate. In some Asians, the normal form of the mitochondrial aldehyde dehydrogenase, with a low K_m for acetaldehyde, is missing. These individuals have only the cytosolic high K_m (lower affinity) form of the enzyme, which leads to a high steady-state level of acetaldehyde in the blood after alcohol consumption. This accounts for the increased sensitivity to alcohol.

Crabb, D. W., Edenberg, H. J., Bosron, W. F., and Li, T.-K. Genotypes for aldehyde dehydrogenase deficiency and alcohol sensitivity: The ALDH22 allele is dominant. *J. Clin. Invest.* 83:314, 1989.

We now need to obtain an alternative expression for $[E_t]/[ES]$, since [ES] cannot be measured easily, if at all. When the enzyme is saturated with substrate all the enzyme will be in the ES complex, and none will be free, $[E_t] = [ES]$, and the velocity observed will be the maximum possible; therefore, $V_{max} = k_3$. When $[E_t]$ is not equal to [ES], $v = k_3[ES]$. From these two expressions we can obtain the ratio of $[E_t]/[ES]$; that is,

$$\frac{[E_t]}{[ES]} = \frac{V_{max}/k_3}{v/k_3} = \frac{V_{max}}{v} \tag{4.17}$$

Substituting this value of $[E_t]/[ES]$ into Eq. 4.16 yields a form of the Michaelis–Menten equation:

$$\frac{V_{max}}{v} = \frac{K_m + [S]}{[S]}$$

or

$$v = \frac{V_{max}[S]}{K_m + [S]}$$

An Enzyme Catalyzes Both Forward and Reverse Directions of a Reversible Reaction

As indicated previously, enzymes do not alter the equilibrium constant of a reaction; consequently, in the reaction

$$S \underset{k_2}{\overset{k_1}{\rightleftharpoons}} P$$

the direction of flow of material, either in the forward or the reverse direction, will depend on the concentration of S relative to P and the equilibrium constant of the reaction. Since enzymes catalyze the forward and reverse reactions, a problem may arise if product has an affinity for the enzyme that is similar to that of substrate. In this case the product can easily rebind to the active site of the enzyme and will compete with the substrate for that site. In such cases the product inhibits the reaction as concentration of product increases. The Lineweaver–Burk plot will not be linear in those cases where the enzyme is susceptible to **product inhibition.** If the subsequent enzyme in a metabolic pathway removes the product rapidly, then product inhibition should not occur.

Product inhibition in a metabolic pathway provides a limited means of controlling or modulating flux of substrates through the pathway. As the end product of a pathway increases, each intermediate will also increase by mass action. If one or more enzymes are particularly sensitive to product inhibition, output of end product of the pathway will be suppressed. Reversibility of a pathway or a particular enzyme-catalyzed reaction is dependent on the rate of product removal. If the end product is quickly removed, then the pathway may be physiologically unidirectional.

Multisubstrate Reactions Follow Either a Ping–Pong or Sequential Mechanism

Most enzymes utilize more than one substrate, or act upon one substrate plus a coenzyme and generate one or more products. In any case, a K_m must be determined for each substrate and coenzyme involved in the reaction when establishing an enzyme assay.

Mechanistically, enzyme reactions are divided into two major categories, ping–pong or sequential. There are many variations on these major mechanisms. The **ping–pong mechanism** can be represented as follows:

$$E + A \longrightarrow EA \xrightarrow{\uparrow P_1} E' \xrightarrow{\downarrow B} E'B \longrightarrow P_2 + E$$

where substrate A reacts with E to produce product P_1, which is released before the second substrate B binds to the modified enzyme E′. Substrate B is then converted to product P_2 and the enzyme is regenerated. A good example of this mechanism is the transaminase-catalyzed reaction (see p. 448) in which the α-amino group of amino $acid_1$ is transferred to the enzyme and the newly formed α-keto $acid_1$ is released, as the first product, followed by the binding of the acceptor α-keto $acid_2$ and release of amino $acid_2$. This reaction is outlined in Figure 4.17.

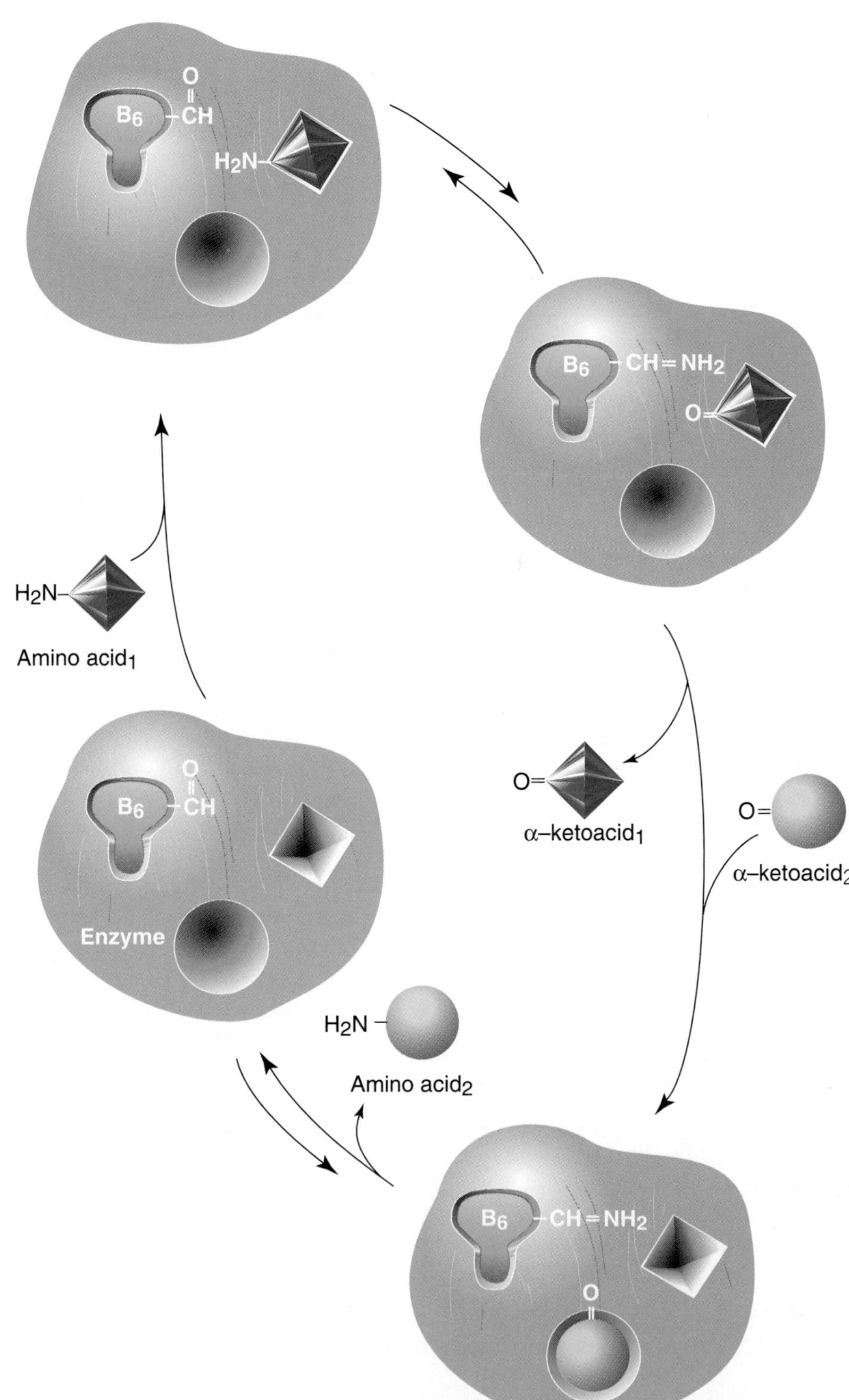

FIGURE 4.17
Schematic representation of the transaminase reaction mechanism: an example of a ping-pong mechanism.
Enzyme-bound pyridoxal phosphate (vitamin B_6 coenzyme) accepts the α-amino group from the first amino acid (AA_1), which is then released from the enzyme as an α-keto acid. The acceptor α-keto acid (AA_2) is then bound to the enzyme, and the bound amino group is transferred to it, forming a new amino acid, which is then released from the enzyme. The terms "oxy" and "keto" are used interchangeably.

CLINICAL CORRELATION 4.3

Mutation of a Coenzyme-Binding Site Results in Clinical Disease

Cystathioninuria is a genetic disease in which γ-cystathionase is either deficient or inactive. Cystathionase catalyzes the reaction:

Cystathionine ⇆ cysteine + α-ketobutyrate

Deficiency of the enzyme leads to accumulation of cystathionine in the plasma. Since cystathionase is a pyridoxal phosphate-dependent enzyme, vitamin B_6 was administered to patients whose fibroblasts contained material that cross-reacted with antibody against cystathionase. Many responded to B_6 therapy with a fall in plasma levels of cystathionine. These patients produce the apoenzyme that reacted with the antibody. In one patient the enzyme activity was undetectable in fibroblast homogenates but increased to 31% of normal with the addition of 1 mM of pyridoxal phosphate to the assay mixture. It is thought that the K_m for pyridoxal phosphate binding to the enzyme was increased because of a mutation in the binding site. Activity is partially restored by increasing the concentration of coenzyme. Apparently these patients require a higher steady-state concentration of coenzyme to maintain γ-cystathionase activity.

Pascal, T. A., Gaull, G. E., Beratis, N. G., Gillam, B. M., Tallan, H. H., and Hirschhorn, K. Vitamin B_6-responsive and unresponsive cystathionuria: two variant molecular forms. *Science* 190:1209, 1975.

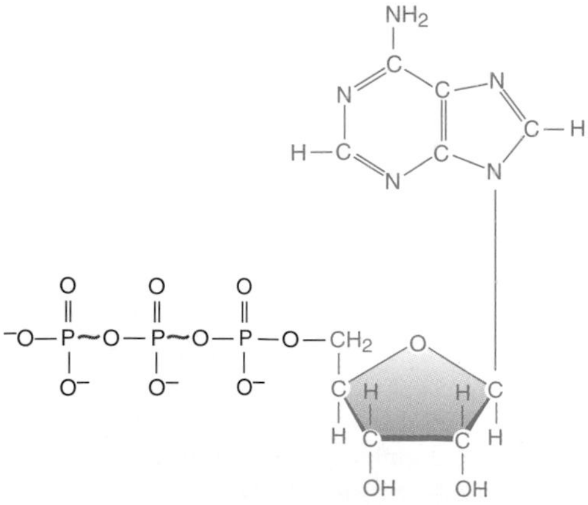

In the **sequential mechanism,** if two substrates A and B can bind in any order, it is a random mechanism; if binding of A is required before B can be bound, then it is an ordered mechanism. In either case the reaction is bimolecular; that is, both A and B must be bound before reaction occurs. Examples of these mechanisms are found among the dehydrogenases in which the second substrate is a coenzyme (NAD^+, FAD, etc.; see p. 143). Release of products may or may not be ordered in either mechanism.

4.4 ■ COENZYMES: STRUCTURE AND FUNCTION

Coenzymes are small organic molecules, often derivatives of vitamins, that function with the enzyme in the catalytic process. Often the coenzyme has an affinity for the enzyme that is similar to that of the substrate; consequently, the coenzyme can be considered to be a second substrate. In some cases, the coenzyme is covalently bound to the apoenzyme and functions at or near the active site in catalysis. In other enzymes the role of the coenzyme falls between these two extremes.

Several coenzymes are derived from the B vitamins. Vitamin B_6, pyridoxine, requires little modification to form the active coenzyme, pyridoxal phosphate (see p. 1121). Clinical Correlation 4.3 points out the importance of the coenzyme-binding site and how alterations in this site cause metabolic dysfunction.

In contrast to vitamin B_6, niacin requires major alteration in mammalian cells to form a coenzyme, as outlined in Section 12.9.

The structures and functions of the coenzymes of only two B vitamins, niacin and riboflavin, and of ATP are discussed in this chapter. The structures and functions of coenzyme A (CoA) (see p. 514), thiamine (see p. 1119), biotin, and vitamin B_{12} are included in those chapters dealing with enzymes dependent on the given coenzyme for activity.

Adenosine Triphosphate May Be a Second Substrate or a Modulator of Activity

Adenosine triphosphate (ATP) often functions as a second substrate but can also serve as a cofactor in modulation of the activity of specific enzymes. This compound is central in biochemistry (Figure 4.18) and it is synthesized *de novo* in all mammalian cells. The nitrogenous heterocyclic ring is adenine. The combination of the base, adenine, plus ribose is known as adenosine; hence ATP is adenosine that has at the 5′-hydroxyl a triphosphate. The biochemically functional end is the reactive triphosphate. The terminal phosphate–oxygen bond has a high free energy of hydrolysis, which means that the phosphate can be transferred from ATP to other acceptor groups. For example, as a cosubstrate ATP is utilized by the kinases for the transfer of the terminal phosphate to various acceptors. A typical example is the reaction catalyzed by **glucokinase:**

Glucose + ATP → glucose 6-phosphate + ADP

ADP is adenosine diphosphate.

ATP also serves as a modulator of the activity of some enzymes. These enzymes have binding sites for ATP, occupancy of which changes the affinity or reactivity of the enzyme toward its substrates. In these cases, ATP acts as an **allosteric effector** (see p. 151).

FIGURE 4.18
Adenosine triphosphate (ATP).

NAD and NADP Are Coenzyme Forms of Niacin

Niacin is pyridine-3-carboxylic acid. It is converted to two coenzymes involved in oxidoreductase reactions. They are **NAD (nicotinamide adenine dinucleo-**

tide) and **NADP (nicotinamide adenine dinucleotide phosphate).** The abbreviations NAD and NADP are convenient to use when referring to the coenzymes regardless of their state of oxidation or reduction. NAD^+ and $NADP^+$ represent the oxidized forms, and NADH and NADPH represent the reduced forms. Some dehydrogenases are specific for NADP and others for NAD; some function with either coenzyme. This arrangement allows for specificity and control over dehydrogenases that reside in the same subcellular compartment.

NAD^+ consists of adenosine and *N*-ribosyl-nicotinamide linked by a pyrophosphate linkage between the 5′-OH groups of the two ribosyl moieties (Figure 4.19). NADP differs structurally from NAD in having an additional phosphate esterified to the 2′-OH group of the adenosine moiety. Both coenzymes function as intermediates in transfer of two electrons between an electron donor and an acceptor. The donor and acceptor need not be involved in the same metabolic pathway. Thus the reduced form of these nucleotides acts as a common "pool" of electrons that arise from many oxidative reactions and can be used for various reductive reactions.

The adenine, ribose, and pyrophosphate components of NAD are involved in binding of NAD to the enzyme. Enzymes requiring NADP do not have a conserved aspartate residue present in the NAD-binding site. If the aspartate were present, a charge–charge interaction between the negative charged aspartate and the 2′-phosphate of NADP would prevent binding. Since there is no negatively charged phosphate on the 2′-OH in NAD, there is discrimination between NAD and NADP binding. The nicotinamide reversibly accepts and donates two electrons at a time. It is the active center of the coenzyme. In oxidation of deuterated ethanol by alcohol dehydrogenase, NAD^+ accepts two electrons and the deuterium from the ethanol. The other hydrogen is released as a H^+ (Figure 4.20).

The binding of NAD^+ to the enzyme surface confers a chemically recognizable "top side" and "bottom side" to the planar nicotinamide. The former is known as the **A** face and the latter as the **B** face. In the case of alcohol dehydrogenase, the proton or deuterium ion that serves as a tracer is added to the **A** face. Other dehydrogenases utilize the **B** face. This particular effect demonstrates how enzymes can induce **stereospecificity** in chemical reactions by virtue of the asymmetric binding of coenzymes and substrates.

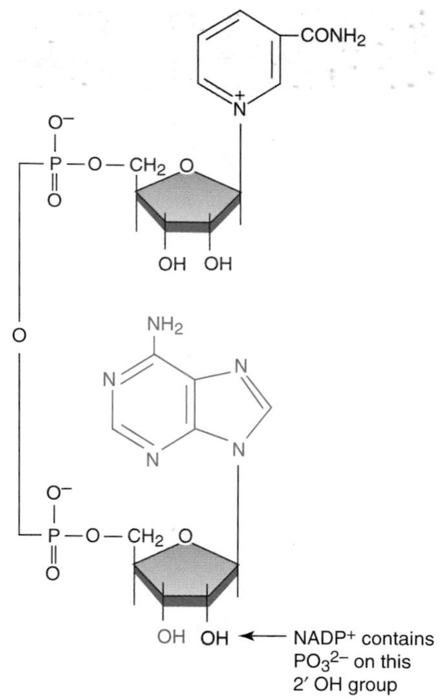

FIGURE 4.19
Nicotinamide adenine dinucleotide (NAD^+).

FMN and FAD Are Coenzyme Forms of Riboflavin

The two coenzyme forms of riboflavin are **FMN (flavin mononucleotide)** and **FAD (flavin adenine dinucleotide).** The vitamin riboflavin consists of the heterocyclic ring, isoalloxazine (flavin) connected through N-10 to the alcohol ribitol (Figure 4.21). FMN has a phosphate esterified to the 5′-OH group of ribitol. FAD is structurally analogous to NAD in having adenosine linked by a pyrophosphate linkage to a heterocyclic ring, in this case riboflavin (Figure 4.22). Both FAD and FMN function in oxidoreduction reactions by accepting and donating $2e^-$ in the isoalloxazine ring. A typical example of FAD participation in an enzyme reaction is the oxidation of succinate to fumarate by succinate

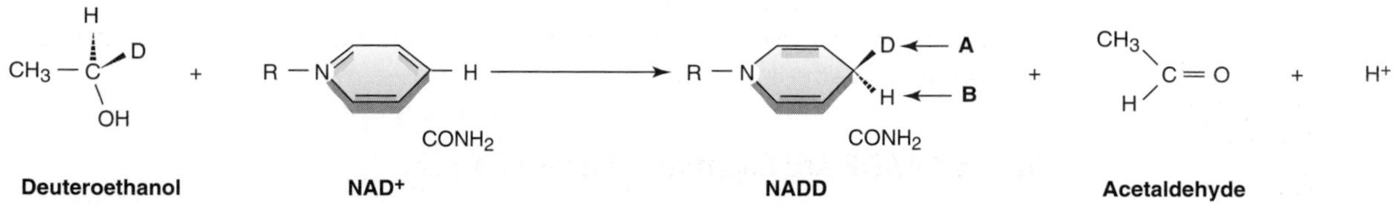

FIGURE 4.20
Stereo specific transfer of deuterium from deuterated ethanol to NAD^+.

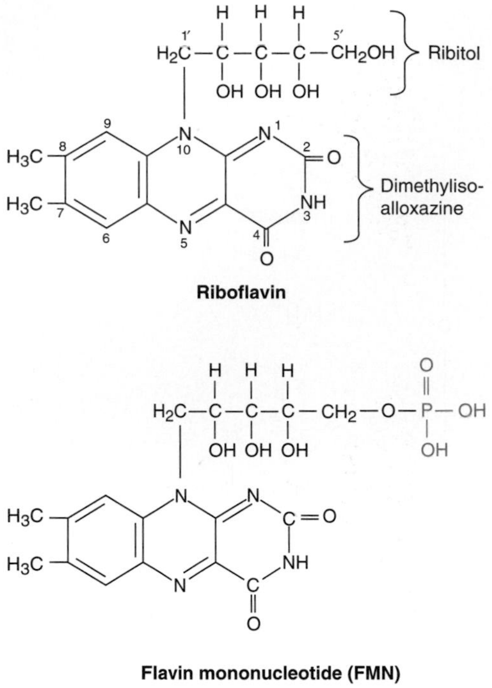

Riboflavin

Flavin mononucleotide (FMN)

FIGURE 4.21
Riboflavin and flavin mononucleotide.

Flavin adenine dinucleotide (FAD)

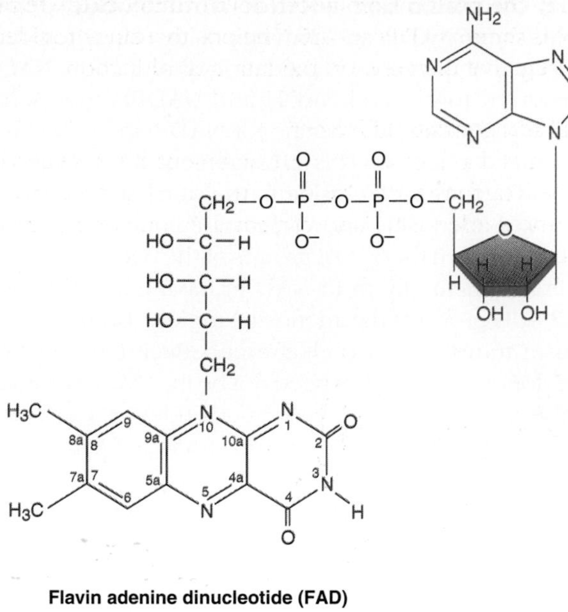

FIGURE 4.22
Flavin adenine dinucleotide (FAD).

Succinic acid — FAD

Fumaric acid — $FADH_2$

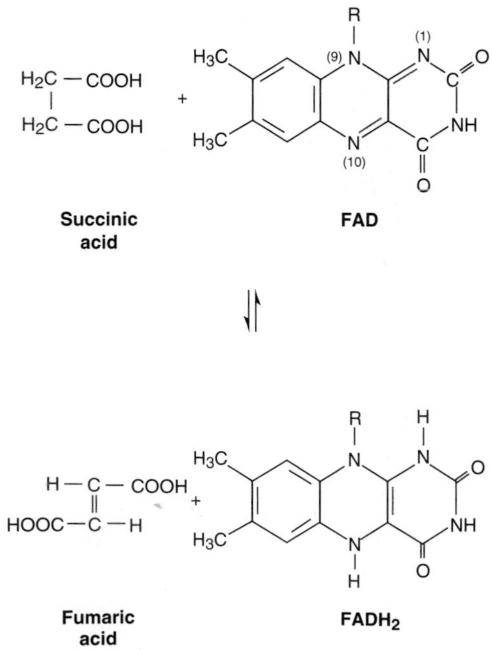

FIGURE 4.23
FAD as a coenzyme in the succinic dehydrogenase reaction.

dehydrogenase (see p. 236) (Figure 4.23). In some cases, these coenzymes are $1e^-$ acceptors, which lead to flavin semiquinone formation (a free radical).

Flavin coenzymes tend to be bound much tighter to their apoenzymes than the niacin coenzymes and often function as prosthetic groups rather than as cofactors.

Metal Cofactors Have Various Functions

Metals are not coenzymes in the same sense as FAD, FMN, NAD^+, and $NADP^+$ but are required as cofactors in approximately two-thirds of all enzymes. Metals participate in enzyme reactions by acting as Lewis acids and by various modes of chelate formation. **Chelates** are organometallic coordination complexes. A good example of a chelate is the complex between iron and protoporphyrin IX to form a heme (see p. 115). Metals that act as Lewis acid catalysts are found among the transition metals like Zn, Fe, Mn, and Cu, which have empty *d* electron orbitals that act as electron sinks. The alkaline earth metals such as K and Na do not possess this ability. A good example of a metal functioning as a Lewis acid is found in **carbonic anhydrase,** a zinc enzyme that catalyzes the reaction

$$CO_2 + H_2O \leftrightharpoons H_2CO_3$$

The first step (Figure 4.24) can be visualized as the *in situ* generation of a proton and a hydroxyl group from water binding to the zinc (Lewis acid function of zinc). The proton and hydroxyl group are then added to the carbon dioxide and carbonic acid is released. Actually, the reactions presented in sequence may occur in a concerted fashion, that is, all at one time.

Metals can also promote catalysis either by binding substrate and promoting electrophilic catalysis at the site of bond cleavage or by stabilizing intermediates in the reaction pathway. In the case of **carboxypeptidase** and **thermolysin, zinc proteases** with identical active sites, the zinc functions to generate a hydroxyl group from water, and then to stabilize the transition state resulting from attack of the hydroxyl on the peptide bond. Figure 4.25 depicts the generation of the active-site hydroxyl by zinc. As shown, Glu 270 functions as a base in plucking the proton from water. Stabilization of the tetrahedral transition state by zinc is shown in Figure 4.26. The positive zinc provides a counterion to stabilize the negative oxygens on the tetrahedral carbon.

Role of the Metal as a Structural Element

The function of a metal as a Lewis acid in carbonic anhydrase and carboxypeptidase requires chelate formation. Various modes of chelation occur between metal, enzyme, and substrate that are structural in nature, but in which no acid catalysis occurs.

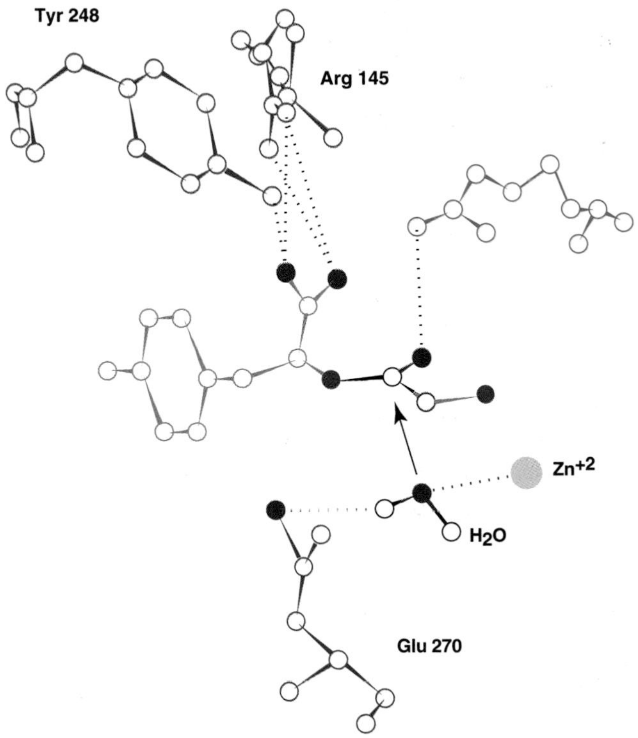

FIGURE 4.25
Zinc in the mechanism of reaction of carboxypeptidase A.
Enzyme-bound zinc generates a hydroxyl nucleophile from bound water, which attacks the carbonyl of the peptide bond as indicated by the arrows. Glu 270 assists by pulling the proton from the zinc-bound water.
Redrawn from Lipscomb, W. N. Robert A. Welch Found. Conf. Chem. Res. *15:140,1971.*

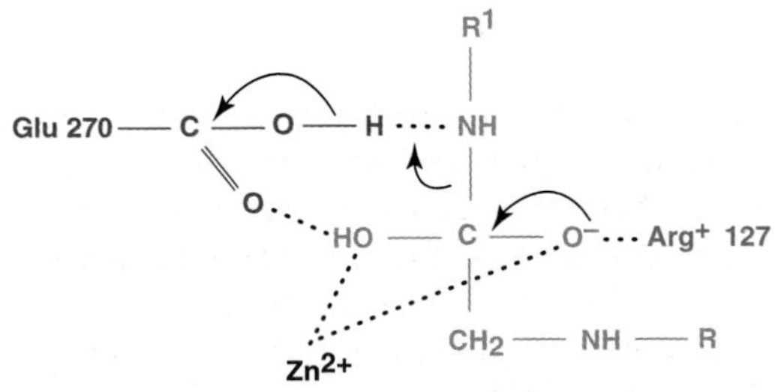

FIGURE 4.26
Stabilization of the transition state of the tetrahedral intermediate by zinc.
Positive charge on the zinc stabilizes the negative charge that develops on the oxygens of the tetrahedral carbon in the transition state. The tetrahedral intermediate then collapses as indicated by the arrows, resulting in breakage of the peptide bond.

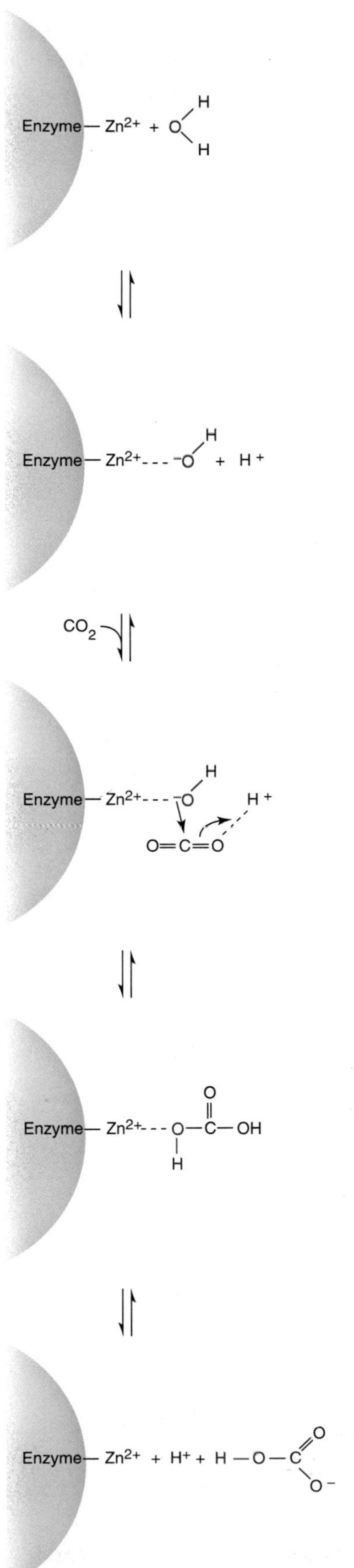

FIGURE 4.24
Zinc functions as a Lewis acid in carbonic anhydrase.

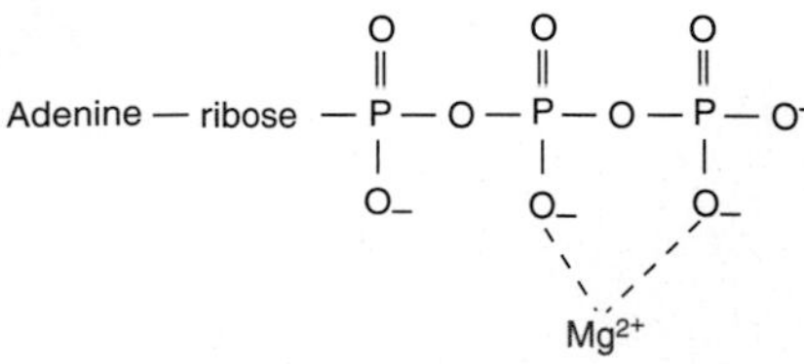

Adenine — ribose — P(=O)(O⁻) — O — P(=O)(O⁻) — O — P(=O)(O⁻) — O⁻ ··· Mg^{2+}

FIGURE 4.27
Mg^{2+}–ATP.

In several kinases, creatine kinase being the best example, the true substrate is not ATP but Mg^{2+}–ATP (Figure 4.27). In this case, Mg^{2+} does not interact directly with the enzyme. It may serve to neutralize the negative charge density on ATP and facilitate binding to the enzyme. Ternary complexes of this conformation are known as "substrate-bridged" complexes and can be schematically represented as Enz–S–M. A hypothetical scheme for the binding of Mg^{2+}–ATP and glucose in the active site of hexokinase is presented in Figure 4.28. All kinases except muscle pyruvate kinase and phosphoenolpyruvate carboxykinase are substrate-bridged complexes. In pyruvate kinase, Mg^{2+} chelates ATP to the enzyme as shown in Figure 4.29. Absence of the metal cofactor results in failure of ATP to bind to the enzyme. Enzymes of this class are "metal-bridged" ternary complexes, Enz–S–M. All **metalloenzymes** are of this type and contain a tightly bound transition metal such as Zn^{2+} or Fe^{2+}. Several enzymes that catalyze enolization and elimination reactions are metal-bridged complexes.

In addition to the role of binding enzyme and substrate, metals may also bind directly to the enzyme to stabilize it in the active conformation or perhaps to induce the formation of a binding site or active site. Not only do the strongly chelated metals like Mn^{2+} play a role in this regard, but the weakly bound alkali metals (Na^+ or K^+) are also important. In **pyruvate kinase,** K^+ induces an initial conformation change, which is necessary, but not sufficient, for ternary complex formation. Upon substrate binding, K^+ induces a second conformational change to the catalytically active ternary complex as indicated in Figure 4.29. Thus Na^+ and K^+ stabilize the active conformation of the enzyme but are passive in catalysis.

Role of Metals in Oxidation and Reduction

Iron–sulfur proteins, often referred to as nonheme iron proteins, are a unique class of metalloenzymes in which the active center consists of one or more clusters of sulfur-bridged iron chelates. The structures are presented on page 252. In some cases the sulfur comes only from cysteine and in others from both cysteine and free ionic sulfur. The free sulfur is released as hydrogen

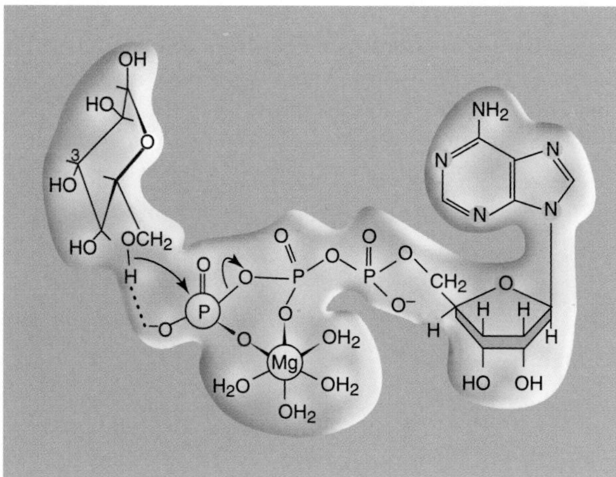

FIGURE 4.28
Role of Mg^{2+} as a substrate-bridged complex in the active site of the kinases. In hexokinase the terminal phosphate of ATP is transferred to glucose, yielding glucose 6-phosphate. Mg^{2+} coordinates with the ATP to form the true substrate and in addition may labilize the terminal P—O bond of ATP to facilitate transfer of the phosphate to glucose. There are specific binding sites (light blue) on the enzyme (darker blue) for glucose (upper left) in red as well as the adenine and ribose moieties of ATP (black).

sulfide upon acidification. These nonheme iron enzymes have reasonably low reducing potentials (E_0') and function in electron-transfer reactions (see p. 251).

Cytochromes are heme iron proteins that function as cosubstrates for their respective reductases (see p. 252). Iron in hemes of cytochromes undergoes reversible 1e$^-$ transfers. Heme is bound to the apoprotein by coordination of an amino acid side chain to iron of heme. Thus the metal serves not only a structural role but also participates in the chemical event.

Metals, specifically copper and iron, also have a role in activation of molecular oxygen. Copper is an active participant in several oxidases and hydroxylases. For example, **dopamine β-hydroxylase** catalyzes the introduction of one oxygen atom from O_2 into dopamine to form norepinephrine (Figure 4.30). The active enzyme contains one atom of cuprous ion that reacts with oxygen to form an activated oxygen–copper complex. The copper–hydroperoxide complex shown in Figure 4.30 is thought to be converted to a copper(II)–O$^-$ species that serves as the "active oxygen" in the hydroxylation of DOPA. In other metalloenzymes other species of "active oxygen" are generated and used for hydroxylation.

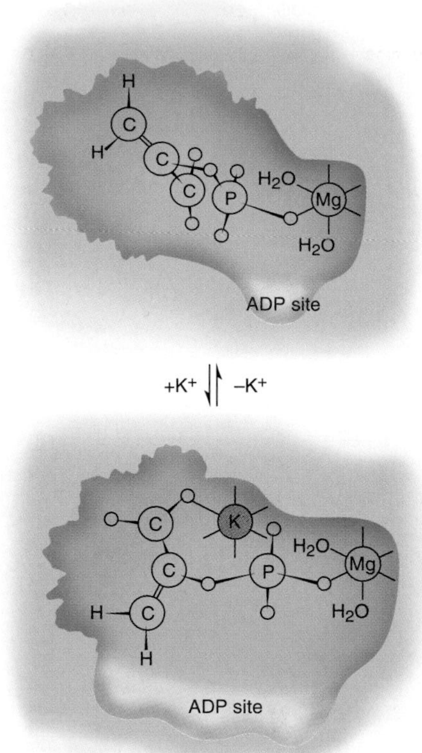

FIGURE 4.29
Model of the role of K$^+$ in the active site of pyruvate kinase.
Pyruvate kinase catalyzes the reaction: phosphoenolpyruvate + ADP → ATP + pyruvate. Initial binding of K$^+$ induces conformational changes in the kinase, which result in increased affinity for phosphoenolpyruvate. In addition, K$^+$ orients the phosphoenolpyruvate in the correct position for transfer of its phosphate to ADP, the second substrate. Mg^{2+} coordinates the substrate to the enzyme active site.
Modified with permission from Mildvan, A. S. Annu. Rev. Biochem. *43:365, 1974. Copyright © 1974 by Annual Reviews, Inc.*

4.5 ■ INHIBITION OF ENZYMES

Mention was made of product inhibition of enzyme activity and how an entire pathway can be controlled or modulated by this mechanism (see p. 140). In addition to inhibition by the immediate product, products of other enzymes can also inhibit or activate a particular enzyme. Much of current drug therapy is based on inhibition of specific enzymes by a substrate analog.

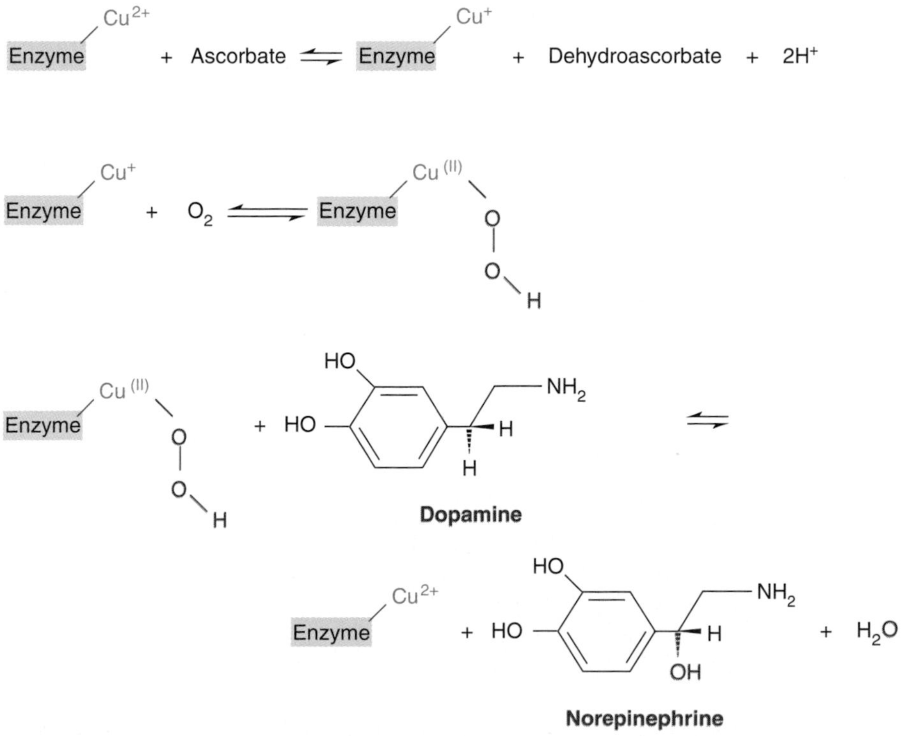

$$\text{Enzyme–}Cu^{2+} + \text{Ascorbate} \rightleftharpoons \text{Enzyme–}Cu^{+} + \text{Dehydroascorbate} + 2H^+$$

$$\text{Enzyme–}Cu^{+} + O_2 \rightleftharpoons \text{Enzyme–}Cu^{(II)}\text{–O–O–H}$$

$$\text{Enzyme–}Cu^{(II)}\text{–O–O–H} + \text{Dopamine} \rightleftharpoons \text{Enzyme–}Cu^{2+} + \text{Norepinephrine} + H_2O$$

Dopamine

Norepinephrine

FIGURE 4.30
Role of copper in activation of molecular oxygen by dopamine hydroxylase.
The normal cupric form of the enzyme is not reactive with oxygen but on reduction by the cosubstrate, ascorbate, generates a reactive enzyme–copper bound oxygen radical that then reacts with dopamine to form norepinephrine and an inactive cupric enzyme.

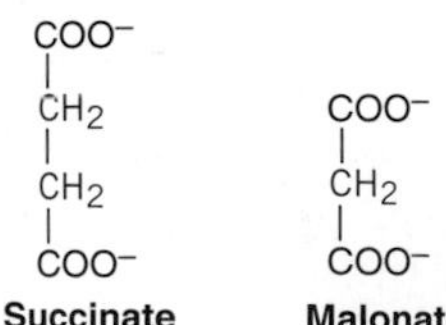

FIGURE 4.31
Substrate and inhibitor of succinate dehydrogenase.

There are three major classes of inhibitors: competitive, noncompetitive, and uncompetitive.

Competitive Inhibition May Be Reversed by Increased Substrate

Competitive inhibitors are inhibitors whose action can be reversed by increasing amounts of substrate. Competitive inhibitors are structurally similar to the substrate and bind at the substrate-binding site, thus competing with the substrate for the enzyme. Once bound, the enzyme cannot convert the inhibitor to products. Increasing substrate concentrations will displace the reversibly bound inhibitor by the law of mass action. For example, in the **succinate dehydrogenase** reaction, malonate is structurally similar to succinate and is a competitive inhibitor (Figure 4.31).

Since substrate and inhibitor compete for the same binding site, the K_m for the substrate shows an apparent increase in the presence of inhibitor. This can be seen in a double-reciprocal plot as a shift in the x-intercept ($-1/K_m$) and in the slope of the line (K_m/V_{max}). If we first establish the velocity at several levels of substrate and then repeat the experiment with a given but constant amount of inhibitor at various substrate levels, two different straight lines will be obtained (Figure 4.32). V_{max} does not change; hence the intercept on the y-axis remains the same. In the presence of inhibitor, the x-intercept is no longer the negative reciprocal of the true K_m, but of an apparent value, $K_{m,app}$ where

$$K_{m,app} = K_m \cdot \left(1 + \frac{[I]}{K_I}\right)$$

Thus the inhibitor constant, K_I, can be determined from the concentration of inhibitor used and the K_m, which was obtained from the x-intercept of the line obtained in the absence of inhibitor.

Noncompetitive Inhibitors Do Not Prevent Substrate from Binding

A **noncompetitive inhibitor** binds at a site other than the substrate-binding site. Inhibition is not reversed by increasing concentration of substrate. Both binary (EI) and ternary (EIS) complexes form, which are catalytically inactive

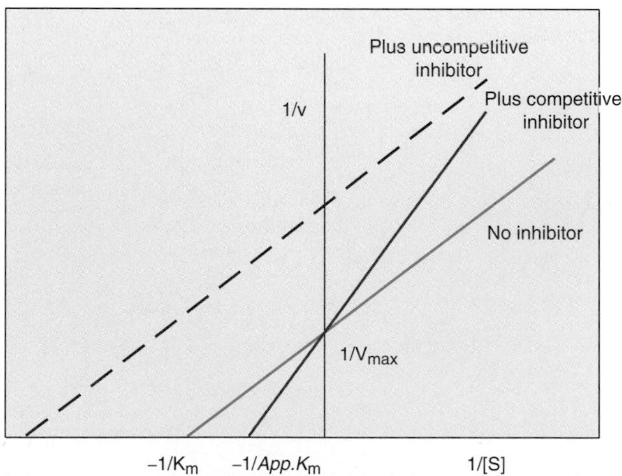

FIGURE 4.32
Double-reciprocal plots for competitive and uncompetitive inhibition.
A competitive inhibitor binds at the substrate-binding site and effectively increases the K_m for the substrate. An uncompetitive inhibitor causes an equivalent shift in both V_{max} and K_m, resulting in a line parallel to that given by the uninhibited enzyme.

and are therefore dead-end complexes. A noncompetitive inhibitor behaves as though it were removing active enzyme from the solution, resulting in a decrease in V_{max}. This is seen graphically in the double-reciprocal plot (Figure 4.33), where K_m does not change but V_{max} does change. Inhibition can often be reversed by exhaustive dialysis of the inhibited enzyme provided that the inhibitor has not reacted covalently with the enzyme as discussed under irreversible inhibitors.

An **uncompetitive inhibitor** binds only with the ES form of the enzyme in the case of a one-substrate enzyme. The result is an apparent equivalent change in K_m and V_{max}, which is reflected in the double-reciprocal plot as a line parallel to that of the uninhibited enzyme (Figure 4.32). In the case of multisubstrate enzymes the interpretation is complex and will not be considered further.

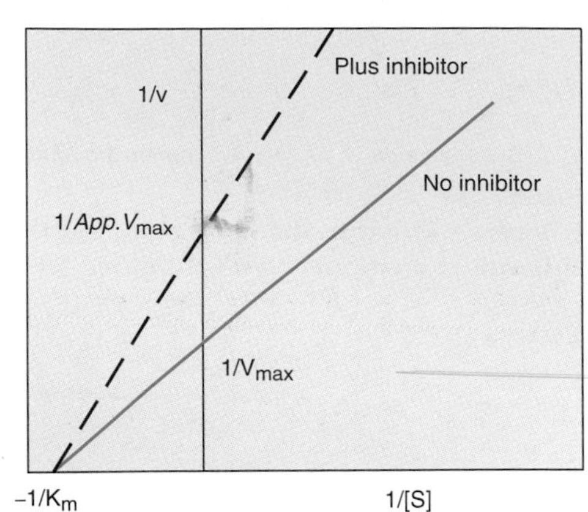

FIGURE 4.33
Double-reciprocal plot for an enzyme subject to reversible noncompetitive inhibition.
A noncompetitive inhibitor binds at a site other than the substrate-binding site; therefore the effective K_m does not change, but the apparent V_{max} decreases.

Irreversible Inhibition Involves Covalent Modification of an Enzyme Site

When covalent modification occurs at the binding site or the active site, inhibition will not be reversed by dialysis unless the linkage is chemically labile like that of an ester or thioester. The active-site thiol group in glyceraldehyde-3-phosphate dehydrogenase reacts with ***p*-chloromercuribenzoate** to form a mercuribenzoate adduct of the enzyme (Figure 4.34). Such adducts are not reversed by dialysis or by addition of substrate. Double-reciprocal plots show the characteristic pattern for noncompetitive inhibition (Figure 4.33).

Many Drugs Are Enzyme Inhibitors

Most modern drug therapy is based on the concepts of enzyme inhibition that were described in the previous section. Drugs are designed to inhibit a specific enzyme in a metabolic pathway. This application is most easily appreciated with antiviral, antibacterial, and antitumor drugs that are administered to the patient under conditions of limited toxicity. Such toxicity is often unavoidable because, with the exception of cell wall biosynthesis in bacteria, there are few critical metabolic pathways that are unique to tumors, viruses, or bacteria. Hence drugs that kill these organisms will often kill host cells. The one characteristic that can be taken advantage of is the comparatively short generation time of the undesirable organisms. They are much more sensitive to antimetabolites and in particular those that inhibit enzymes involved in replication. Antimetabolites are compounds with some structural difference from the natural substrate. In subsequent chapters, numerous examples of **antimetabolites** will be described. Here we will present a few examples that illustrate the concept.

Sulfa Drugs

Modern chemotherapy had its beginning in compounds of the general formula R—SO_2—NHR′. Sulfanilamide, the simplest member of the class, is an antibacterial agent because of its competition with ***p*-aminobenzoic acid** (PABA), which

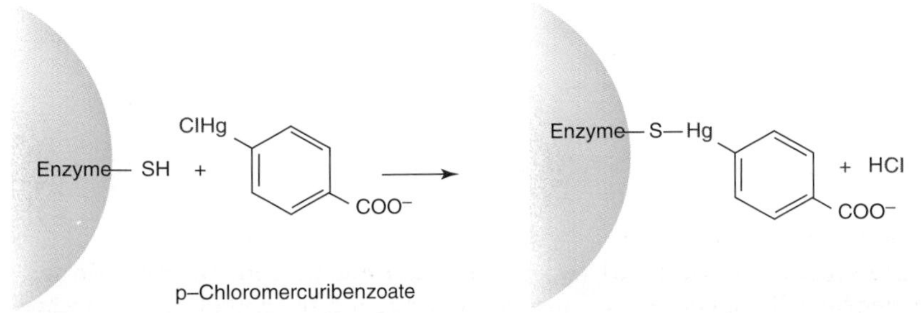

FIGURE 4.34
Enzyme inhibition by a covalent modification of an active center cysteine.

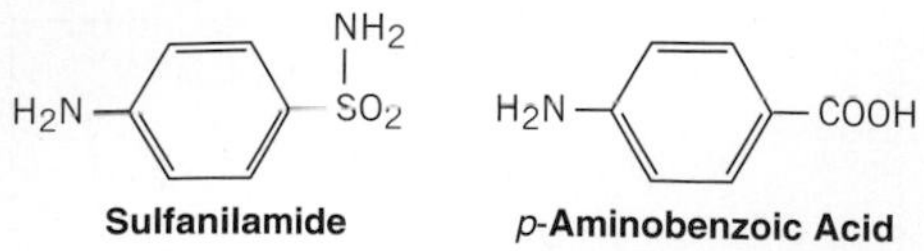

Sulfanilamide　　*p*-Aminobenzoic Acid

FIGURE 4.35
Structure of *p*-aminobenzoic acid and sulfanilamide, a competitive inhibitor.

is required for bacterial growth. Structures of these compounds are shown in Figure 4.35.

Bacteria cannot absorb folic acid, a required vitamin for the host, but must synthesize it. Since sulfanilamide is a structural analog of *p*-aminobenzoate, the bacterial dihydropteroate synthetase is tricked into making an intermediate, containing sulfanilamide, that cannot be converted to folate. Figure 4.36*b* shows the fully reduced or coenzyme form of folate. Thus the bacterium is starved of the required folate and cannot grow or divide. Since humans require folate from dietary sources, the sulfanilamide is not harmful at the doses that kill bacteria.

Methotrexate

Biosynthesis of purines and pyrimidines, heterocyclic bases required for synthesis of RNA and DNA, requires folic acid, which serves as a coenzyme in transfer of one-carbon units from various amino acid donors (see p. 460). Methotrexate (Figure 4.36*a*), a structural analog of folate, has been used with great success in childhood leukemia. Its mechanism of action is based on competition with dihydrofolate for dihydrofolate reductase. It binds 1000-fold more strongly than the natural substrate and is a powerful competitive inhibitor of the enzyme. The synthesis of thymidine monophosphate stops in the presence of methotrexate because of failure of the one-carbon transfer reaction. Since cell division depends on thymidine monophosphate as well as the other nucleotides, the leukemia cell cannot multiply. One problem is that rapidly dividing human cells such as those in bone marrow and intestinal mucosa are sensitive to the drug for the same reasons. Also, prolonged usage leads to amplification of the gene for dihydrofolate reductase, with increased levels of the enzyme and preferential growth of methotrexate-resistant cells.

Nonclassical Antimetabolites

A nonclassical antimetabolite is a substrate for an enzyme that upon action of the enzyme generates a highly reactive species. This species forms a covalent adduct with an amino acid at the active site, leading to irreversible inactivation of the enzyme. These inhibitors are referred to as suicide substrates and are very specific. Another group of inhibitors contains a reactive functional group. For example, the compound shown in Figure 4.37 is an irreversible inhibitor of **dihydrofolate reductase** because it is specifically bound at the active site and the reactive benzylsulfonyl fluoride is positioned to react with a serine hydroxyl group in the substrate-binding site. Covalent binding of this substrate analog to the enzyme prevents binding of the normal substrate and inhibits the enzyme.

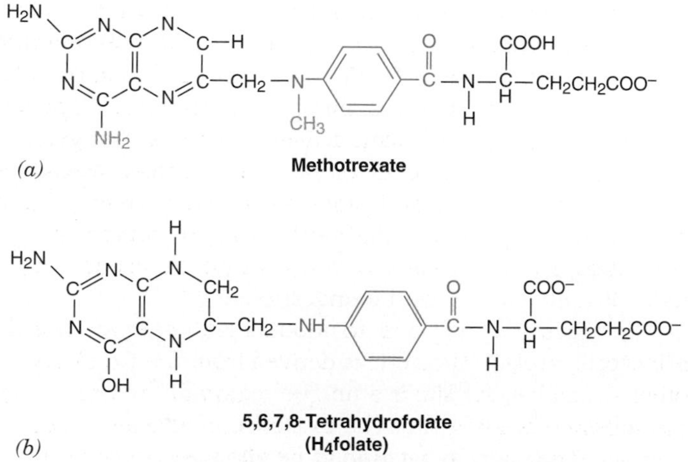

(a) Methotrexate

(b) 5,6,7,8-Tetrahydrofolate (H_4folate)

FIGURE 4.36
Methotrexate (4-amino-N^{10}-methyl folic acid) and tetrahydrofolic acid.
Contribution from *p*-aminobenzoate is shown in green.

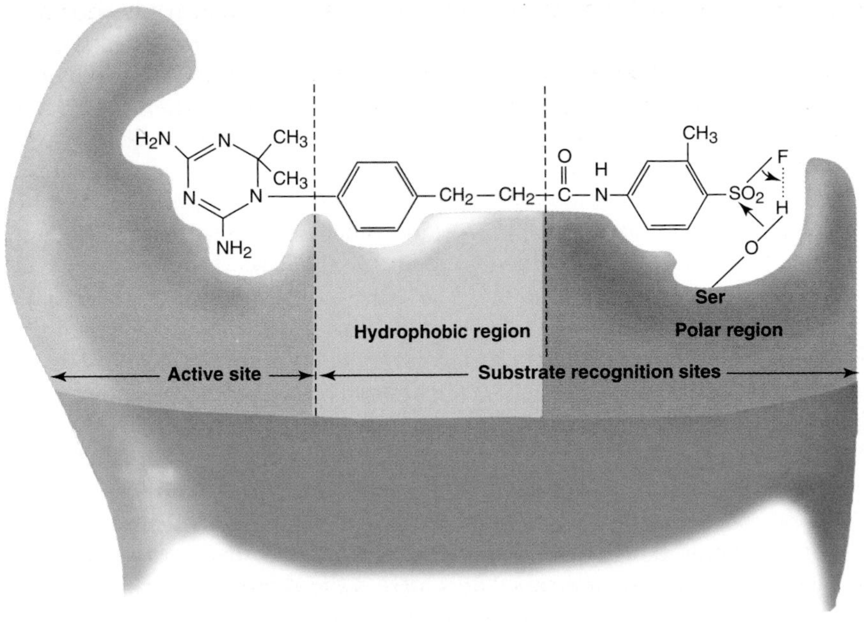

FIGURE 4.37
Site-directed inactivation of tetrahydrofolate reductase.
The irreversible inhibitor, a substituted dihydrotriazine, structurally resembles dihydrofolate and binds specifically to the dihydrofolate site on dihydrofolate reductase. The triazine portion of the inhibitor resembles the pterin moiety and therefore binds to the active site. The ethylbenzene group (in red) binds to the hydrophobic site normally occupied by the *p*-aminobenzoyl group. The reactive end of the inhibitor contains a reactive sulfonyl fluoride that forms a covalent linkage with a serine hydroxyl on the enzyme surface. Thus this inhibitor irreversibly inhibits the enzyme by blocking access of dihydrofolate to the active site.

Other Antimetabolites

Two other analogs of the purines and pyrimidines will be mentioned to emphasize the structural similarity of chemotherapeutic agents to normal substrates. **Fluorouracil** (Figure 4.38) is a thymine analog in which the ring-bound methyl is substituted by fluorine. The deoxynucleotide of this compound is an irreversible inhibitor of thymidylate synthetase. **6-Mercaptopurine** (Figure 4.38) is an analog of hypoxanthine, adenine, and guanine, which is converted to the 6-mercaptopurine nucleotide in cells. This nucleotide is a broad spectrum antimetabolite because of its competition in reactions involving adenine and guanine nucleotides. The antimetabolites discussed relate to purine and pyrimidine metabolism but the general concepts can be applied to any enzyme or metabolic pathway.

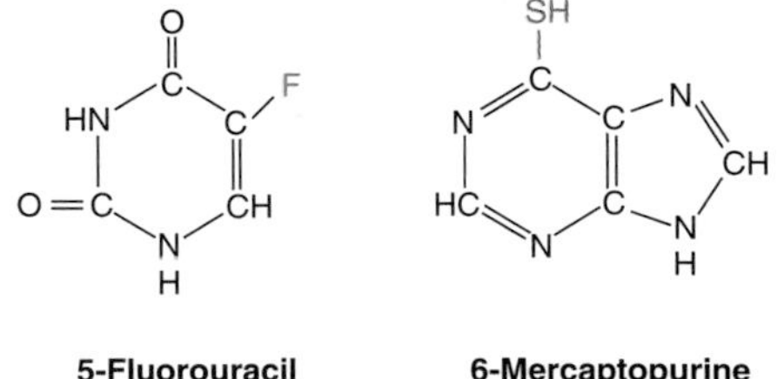

FIGURE 4.38
Structures of two antimetabolites.

4.6 ■ ALLOSTERIC CONTROL OF ENZYME ACTIVITY

Allosteric Effectors Bind at Sites Different from Substrate-Binding Sites

Although the substrate-binding and active site of an enzyme are well-defined structures, the activity of many enzymes can be modulated by ligands acting in ways other than as competitive or noncompetitive inhibitors. A **ligand** is any molecule that is bound to a macromolecule; the term is not limited to small organic molecules, such as ATP, but includes low molecular weight proteins. Ligands can be activators, inhibitors, or even the substrates of enzymes. Those ligands that change enzymatic activity, but are unchanged as a result of enzyme action, are referred to as effectors, modifiers, or modulators. Most of the enzymes subject to modulation by ligands are rate-determining enzymes in metabolic pathways. To appreciate the mechanisms by which metabolic pathways are controlled, the principles governing the allosteric and cooperative behavior of individual enzymes must be understood.

Enzymes that respond to modulators have additional site(s) known as **allosteric site(s).** Allosteric is derived from the Greek root *allo,* meaning "the other." An allosteric site is a unique region of the enzyme quite different from the substrate-binding site. The existence of allosteric sites is illustrated in Clin. Corr. 4.4. The ligands that bind at the allosteric site are called allosteric effectors

CLINICAL CORRELATION 4.4

A Case of Gout Demonstrates the Difference Between an Allosteric and Substrate-Binding Site

The realization that allosteric inhibitory sites are separate from allosteric activator sites as well as from the substrate-binding and the catalytic sites is illustrated by a study of a gouty patient whose red blood cell PRPP level was increased (see Clin. Corr. 4.1). It was found that the patient's PRPP synthetase had normal K_m and V_{max} values, and sensitivity to activation by phosphate. The increased PRPP levels and hyperuricemia arose because the end products of the pathway (ATP, GTP) were not able to inhibit the synthetase through the allosteric inhibitory site (I). It was suggested that a mutation in the inhibitory site or in the coupling mechanism between the inhibitory and catalytic site led to failure of the feedback control mechanism.

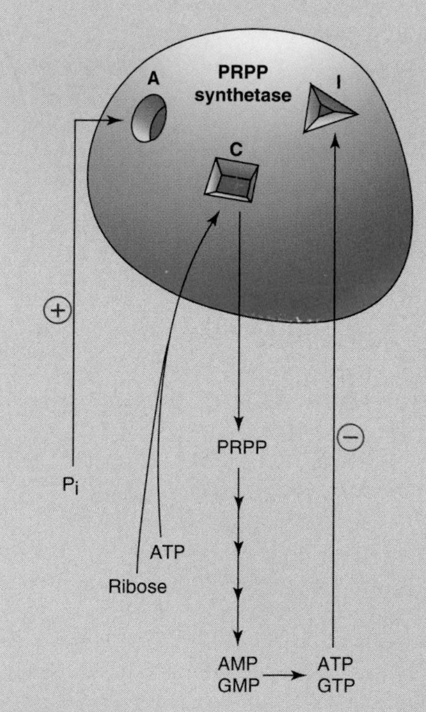

Sperling, O., Persky-Brosh, S., Boen, P., and DeVries, A. Human erythrocyte phosphoribosylpyrophosphate synthetase mutationally altered in regulatory properties. *Biochem. Med.* 7:389, 1973.

or modulators. Binding of an allosteric effector causes a conformational change of the enzyme so that the affinity for the substrate or other ligands also changes. Positive (+) allosteric effectors increase the enzyme affinity for substrate or other ligand. The reverse is true for negative (−) allosteric effectors. The allosteric site at which the positive effector binds is referred to as an activator site; the negative effector binds at an inhibitory site.

Allosteric enzymes are divided into two classes based on the effect of the allosteric effector on the K_m and V_{max}. In the **K class** the effector alters the K_m but not V_{max}, whereas in the **V class** the effector alters V_{max} but not K_m. K class enzymes give double-reciprocal plots like those of competitive inhibitors (Figure 4.32) and V class enzymes give double-reciprocal plots like those of noncompetitive inhibitors (Figure 4.33). The terms competitive and noncompetitive are inappropriate for allosteric enzyme systems because the mechanism of the effect of an allosteric inhibitor on a V or K enzyme is different from that of a simple competitive or noncompetitive inhibitor. For example, in the K class, the negative effector binding at an allosteric site affects the affinity of the substrate-binding site for the substrate, whereas in simple competitive inhibition the inhibitor competes directly with substrate for the site. In V class enzymes, positive and negative allosteric modifiers increase or decrease the rate of breakdown of the ES complex to products. The catalytic rate constant, k_3, is affected and not the substrate-binding constant. There are a few enzymes in which both K_m and V_{max} are affected.

In theory, a monomeric enzyme can undergo an allosteric transition in response to a modulating ligand. In practice, only two monomeric allosteric enzymes are known, ribonucleoside diphosphate reductase and pyruvate-UDP-*N*-acetylglucosamine transferase. Most allosteric enzymes are **oligomeric;** that is, they consist of several subunits. Identical subunits are designated as **protomers,** and each protomer may consist of one or more polypeptide chains. As a consequence of the oligomeric nature of allosteric enzymes, binding of ligand to one protomer can affect the binding of ligands on the other protomers in the oligomer. Such ligand effects are referred to as **homotropic** interactions. Transmission of the homotropic effects between protomers is one aspect of cooperativity, considered later. Substrate influencing substrate, activator influencing activator, or inhibitor influencing inhibitor binding are homotropic interactions. Homotropic interactions are almost always positive.

A **heterotropic** interaction is the effect of one ligand on the binding of a different ligand. For example, the effect of a negative effector on the binding of substrate or on binding of an allosteric activator are heterotropic interactions. Heterotropic interactions can be positive or negative and can occur in monomeric allosteric enzymes. Heterotropic and homotropic effects in oligomeric enzymes are mediated by cooperativity between subunits.

Based on the foregoing descriptions of allosteric enzymes, two models are pictured in Figure 4.39. In (*a*) a monomeric enzyme is shown, and in panel (*b*) an oligomeric enzyme consisting of two protomers is visualized. In both models heterotropic interactions can occur between the activator and substrate sites. In model (*b*), homotropic interactions can occur between the activator sites or between the substrate sites.

Allosteric Enzymes Exhibit Sigmoidal Kinetics

As a consequence of interaction between substrate site, activator site, and inhibitor site, a characteristic sigmoid or S-shaped curve is obtained in [S] versus v_0 plots of allosteric enzymes, as shown in Figure 4.40 (curve A). Negative allosteric effectors move the curve toward higher substrate concentrations and enhance the sigmoidicity of the curve. If we use $\frac{1}{2}v_{max}$ as a guideline, Figure 4.40 shows that a higher concentration of substrate would be required to achieve $\frac{1}{2}v_{max}$ in the presence of a negative effector (curve C) than required in the absence

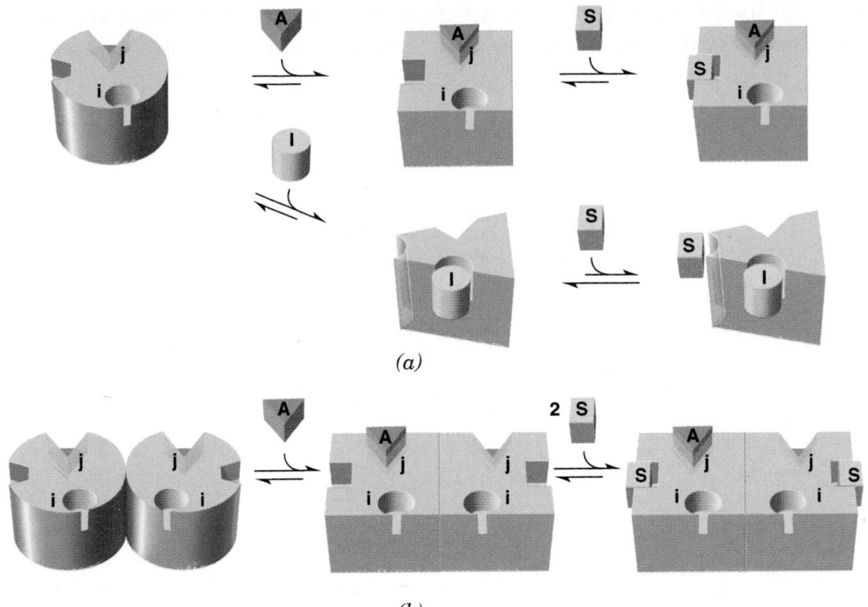

FIGURE 4.39
Models of allosteric enzyme systems.
(*a*) Model of a monomeric enzyme. Binding of a positive allosteric effector, A (green), to the activator site, j, induces a new conformation to the enzyme, one that has a greater affinity for the substrate. Binding of a negative allosteric effector (purple) to the inhibitor site, i, results in an enzyme conformation having a decreased affinity for substrate (orange). (*b*) A model of a polymeric allosteric enzyme. Binding of the positive allosteric effector, A, at the j site causes an allosteric change in the conformation of the protomer to which the effector binds. This change in the conformation is transmitted to the second protomer through cooperative protomer–protomer interactions. The affinity for the substrate is increased in both protomers. A negative effector decreases the affinity for substrate of both protomers.

of negative effector (curve A). In the presence of a positive modulator (curve B), $\frac{1}{2}v_{max}$ can be reached at a lower substrate concentration than is required in the absence of the positive modulator (curve A). Positive modulators shift the v_0 versus [S] plots toward the hyperbolic plots observed in Michaelis–Menten kinetics.

The rates of allosteric-controlled enzymes can be finely controlled by small fluctuations in the level of substrate; often the *in vivo* concentration of substrate corresponds with the sharply rising segment of the sigmoid v_0 versus [S] plot; thus large changes in enzyme activity are effected by small changes in substrate concentration (see Figure 4.40). It is also possible to "turn an enzyme off" with small amounts of a negative allosteric effector by having the apparent K_m shifted to values well above the *in vivo* level of substrate. Note that at a given *in vivo* concentration of substrate the initial velocity, v_0, is decreased in the presence of a negative effector (compare curves A and C).

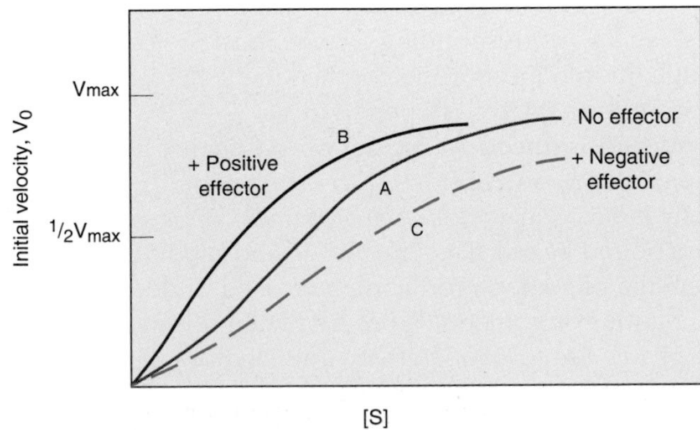

FIGURE 4.40
Kinetic profile of a K class allosteric enzyme.
The enzyme shows sigmoid V_0 versus [S] plots. Negative effectors shift the curve to the right, resulting in an increase in K_m. Positive effectors shift the curve to the left and effectively lower the apparent K_m. The V_{max} is not changed.

Cooperativity Explains Interaction Between Ligand Sites in an Oligomeric Protein

Since allosteric enzymes are usually oligomeric with sigmoid [S] versus v_0 plots, the concept of cooperativity was proposed to explain the interaction between ligand sites in oligomeric enzymes. **Cooperativity** is the influence that the binding of a ligand to one protomer has on the binding of ligand to another protomer in an oligomeric protein. It should be emphasized that kinetic mechanisms other than cooperativity can also produce sigmoid v_0 versus [S] plots; consequently, sigmoidicity is not diagnostic of cooperativity in a v_0 versus [S] plot. The relationship between allosterism and cooperativity has frequently been confused. Conformational change occurring in a given protomer in response to ligand binding at an allosteric site is an allosteric effect. Cooperativity generally involves a change in conformation of an effector-bound protomer that in turn transforms an adjacent protomer into a new conformation with an altered affinity for the effector ligand or for a second ligand. The conformation change may be induced by an allosteric effector or it may be induced by substrate, as it is in the case of hemoglobin where the oxygen-binding site on each protomer corresponds to the substrate site on an enzyme rather than to an allosteric site. Therefore the oxygen-induced conformational change in the hemoglobin protomers is technically not an allosteric effect, although some authors describe it as such. It is a homotropic cooperative interaction. Those who consider the oxygen-induced changes in hemoglobin to be "allosteric" are using the term in a much broader sense than the original definition allows; however, "allosteric" is now used by many to describe any ligand-induced change in the tertiary structure of a protomer.

An allosteric effect can occur in the absence of any cooperativity. For example, in **alcohol dehydrogenase,** conformational changes occur independently in each of the protomers upon the addition of positive allosteric effectors. The active site of each protomer is completely independent of the other and there is no cooperativity between protomers; that is, induced conformational changes in one protomer are not transmitted to adjacent protomers.

To describe experimentally observed ligand saturation curves mathematically, several models of cooperativity have been proposed. The two most prominent are the concerted model and the sequential induced-fit model. Although the **concerted model** is rather restrictive, most of the nomenclature associated with allosterism and cooperativity arose from it. The model proposes that the enzyme exists in only two states, the T (tense or taut) and the R (relaxed) (Figure 4.41*a*). The T and R states are in equilibrium. Activators and substrates favor the R state and shift the preexisting equilibrium toward the R state by the law of mass action. Inhibitors favor the T state. A conformational change in one protomer causes a corresponding change in all protomers. No hybrid states occur. Although this model accounts for the kinetic behavior of many enzymes, it cannot account for negative cooperativity.

The **sequential induced-fit model** proposes that ligand binding induces a conformational change in a protomer. A corresponding conformational change is then partially induced in an adjacent protomer contiguous with the protomer containing the bound ligand. The effect of ligand binding is sequentially transmitted through the oligomer, producing increased or decreased affinity for the ligand by contiguous protomers (Figure 4.41*b*). In this model numerous hybrid states occur, giving rise to cooperativity and sigmoid [S] versus v_0 plots. Both positive and negative cooperativity can be accommodated by the model. A positive modulator induces a conformation in the protomer, which has an increased affinity for the substrate. A negative modulator induces a different conformation in the protomer, one that has a decreased affinity for substrate. Both effects are cooperatively transmitted to adjacent protomers. For the V class enzymes the effect is on the catalytic event (k_3) rather than on K_m.

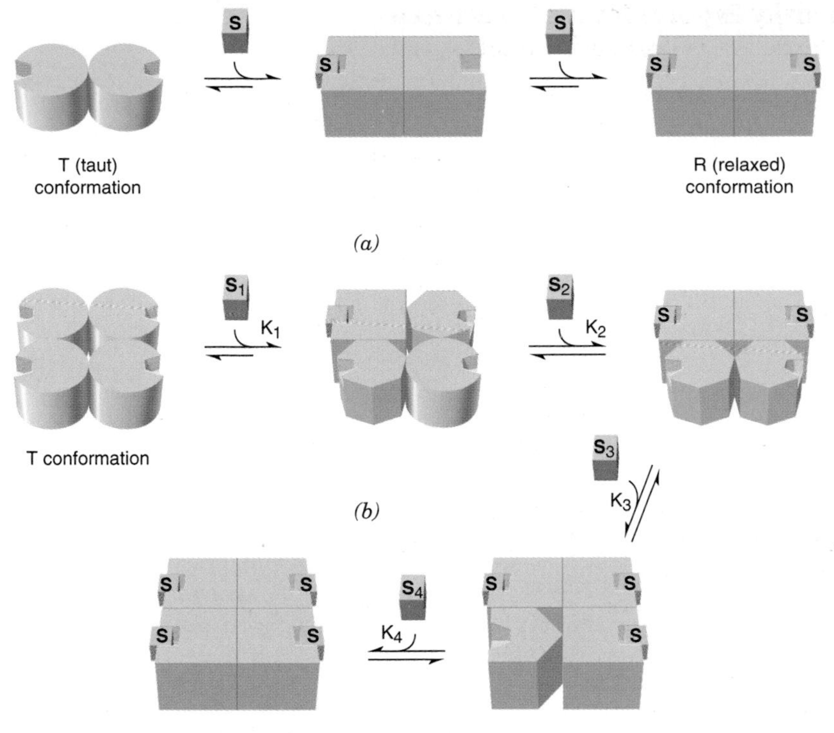

FIGURE 4.41
Models of cooperativity.
(*a*) The concerted model. The enzyme exists in only two states, the T (tense or taut) and R (relaxed) conformations. Substrates and activators have a greater affinity for the R state and inhibitors for the T state. Ligands shift the equilibrium between the T and R states. (*b*) The sequential induced-fit model. Binding of a ligand to any one subunit induces a conformational change in that subunit. This conformational change is transmitted partially to adjoining subunits through subunit–subunit interaction. Thus the effect of the first ligand bound is transmitted cooperatively and sequentially to the other subunits (protomers) in the oligomer, resulting in a sequential increase or decrease in ligand affinity of the other protomers. The cooperativity may be either positive or negative, depending on the ligand.

Regulatory Subunits Modulate the Activity of Catalytic Subunits

In the foregoing an allosteric site was considered to reside on the same protomer as the catalytic site and all protomers were considered to be identical. In several very important enzymes a distinct regulatory protomer exists. These **regulatory subunits** have no catalytic function, but their binding with the catalytic protomer modulates the activity of the catalytic subunit through an induced conformational change. One strategy for regulation by regulatory subunits is outlined in Figure 4.42 for the **protein kinase A (PKA)** complex. Each regulatory subunit (R) has a segment of its primary sequence that is a pseudosubstrate for the catalytic subunit (C). In the absence of cAMP, the R subunit binds to the C subunit at its active site through the pseudosubstrate sequence, which inhibits the protein kinase activity. When cellular cAMP levels rise, cAMP binds to a site on the R subunits, causing a conformational change. This removes the pseudosubstrate sequence from the active site of the C subunit. The C subunits are released and can accept other protein substrates containing the pseudosubstrate sequence.

Calmodulin, a 17-kDa Ca^{2+}-binding protein, is a regulatory subunit for enzymes using Ca^{2+} as a modulator of their activity. Binding of calcium to calmodulin induces a conformational change in calmodulin allowing it to bind to the Ca^{2+}-dependent enzyme. This binding induces a conformational change in the enzyme, restoring enzymatic activity.

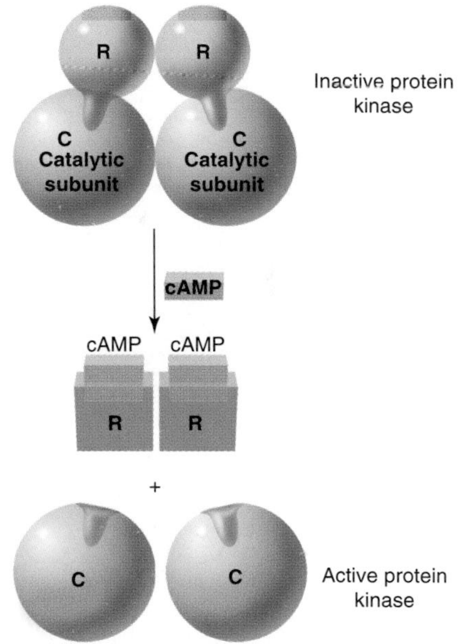

FIGURE 4.42
Model of allosteric enzyme with separate catalytic (C) and regulatory (R) subunits.
The regulatory subunit of protein kinase A contains a pseudosubstrate region in its primary sequence that binds to the substrate site of the catalytic subunit. In the presence of cAMP the conformation of the R subunit changes so that the pseudosubstrate region can no longer bind, resulting in release of active C subunits.

4.7 ■ ENZYME SPECIFICITY: THE ACTIVE SITE

Enzymes are the most specific catalysts known, as regards the substrate and the type of reaction undergone by substrate. Specificity resides in the **substrate-binding site** on the enzyme surface. The tertiary structure of the enzyme is folded in such a way as to create a region that has the correct molecular dimensions, the appropriate topology, and the optimal alignment of counter-

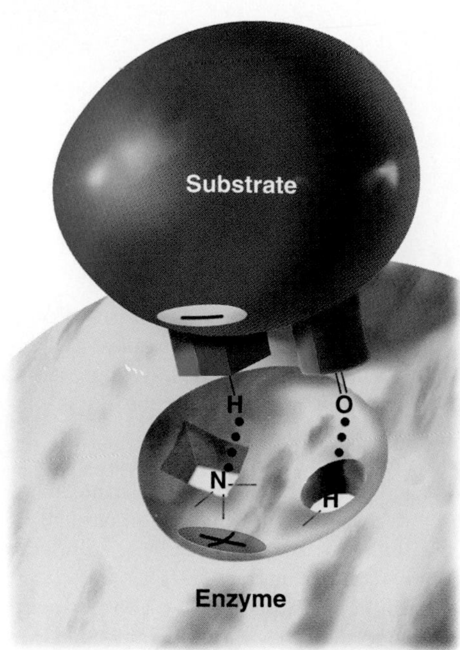

FIGURE 4.43
Lock-and-key model of the enzyme-binding site.
The enzyme contains a negative impression of the molecular features of the substrate, thus allowing specificity of the enzyme for a particular substrate. Specific ion pair formation can contribute to recognition of the substrate.

ionic groups and hydrophobic regions to accommodate a specific substrate. The tolerances in the active site are so small that usually only one isomer of a diastereomeric pair will bind. For example, D-amino acid oxidase will bind only D-amino acids but not L-amino acids. Some enzymes show absolute specificity for substrate. Others have broader specificity and will accept several different analogs of a specific substrate. For example, hexokinase catalyzes the phosphorylation of glucose, mannose, fructose, glucosamine, and 2-deoxyglucose, but at different rates. Glucokinase, on the other hand, is specific for glucose.

The specificity of the reaction rests in the active site and the amino acids that participate in the bond-making and bond-breaking phase of catalysis (see Section 4.8).

Complementarity of Substrate and Enzyme Explains Substrate Specificity

Various models have been proposed to explain the substrate specificity of enzymes. The first proposal was the **"lock-and-key" model** (Figure 4.43), in which a negative impression of the substrate is considered to exist on the enzyme surface. Substrate fits in this binding site just as a key fits into the proper lock or a hand into the proper sized glove. Hydrogen and ionic bonding and hydrophobic interactions contribute in binding substrate to the binding site. This model gives a rigid picture of the enzyme and cannot account for the effects of allosteric ligands.

A more flexible model of the binding site is provided by the **induced fit model** in which the binding and active sites are not fully preformed. The essential elements of the binding site are present to the extent that the correct substrate can position itself properly. Interaction of substrate with enzyme induces a conformational change in the enzyme, resulting in the formation of a stronger binding site and the repositioning of the appropriate amino acids to form the active site. There is excellent X-ray evidence for this model with carboxypeptidase A. A schematic of the induced-fit model is shown in Figure 4.44*a*. Figure 4.45 shows a significant movement of the lower lobe of **hexokinase** on binding glucose. The hexokinase essentially closes around the glucose to bring the active-site residues into proximity with the glucose.

Induced fit combined with **substrate strain** accounts for more experimental observations concerning enzyme action than other models. In this model (Figure 4.44*b*), substrate is "strained" toward product formation by an induced conformational transition of the enzyme. A good example of enzyme-induced

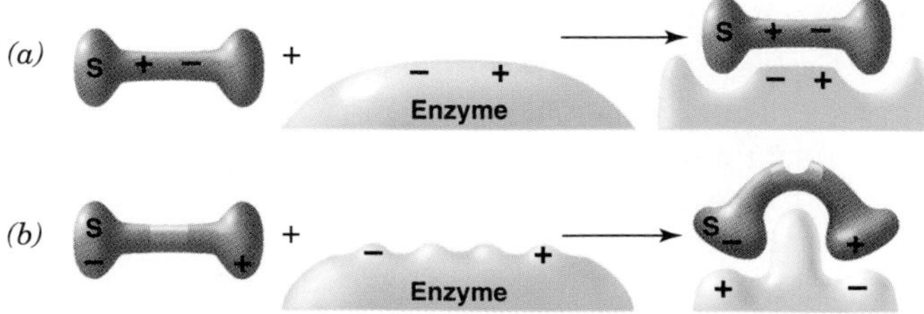

FIGURE 4.44
Models for induced fit and substrate strain.
(*a*) Approach of substrate to the enzyme induces the formation of the active site. (*b*) Substrate strain, induced by substrate binding to the enzyme, contorts normal bond angles and "activates" the substrate.
Reprinted with permission from Koshland, D. Annu. Rev. Biochem. *37:374, 1968. Copyright © 1968 by Annual Reviews, Inc.*

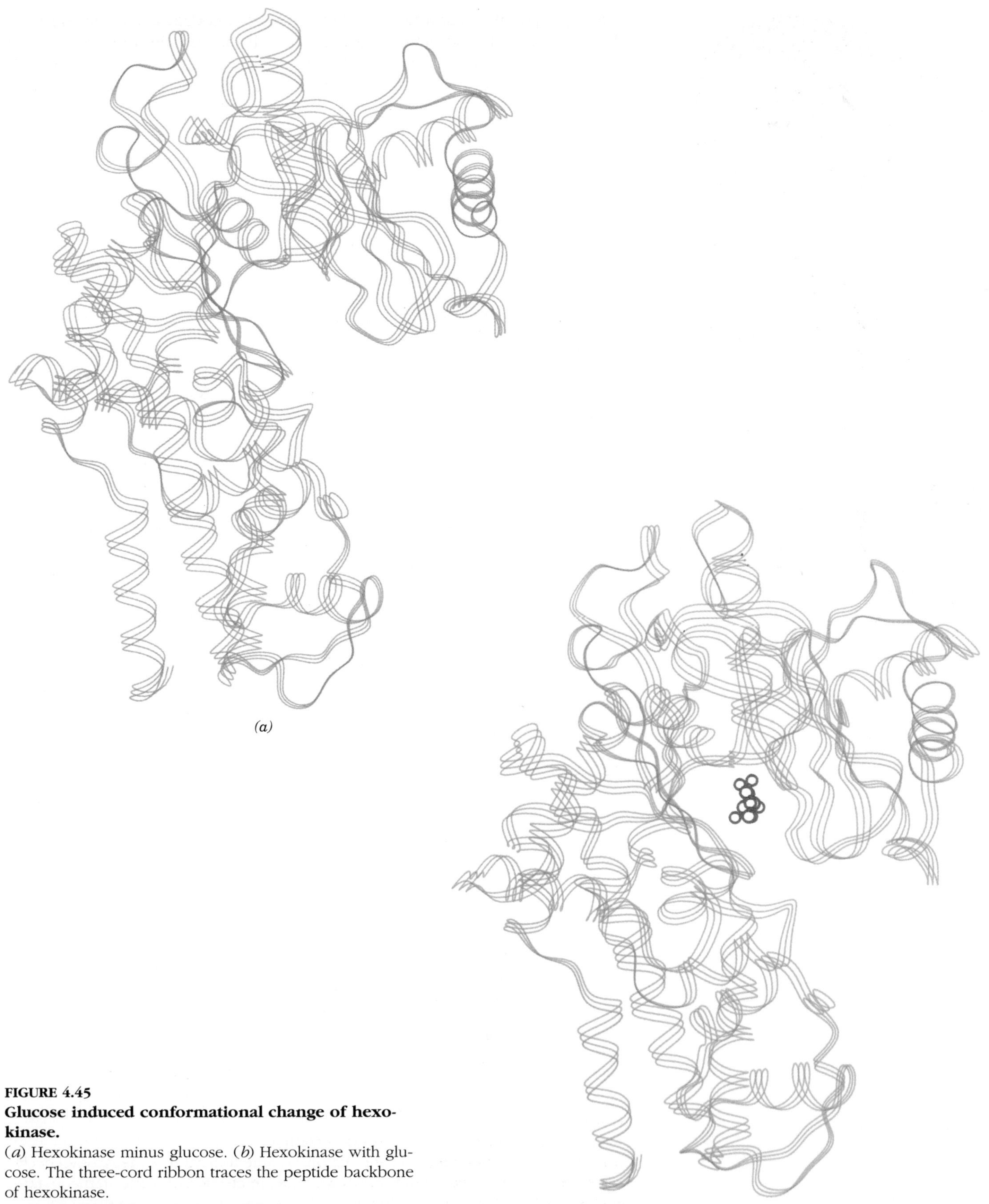

FIGURE 4.45
Glucose induced conformational change of hexokinase.
(*a*) Hexokinase minus glucose. (*b*) Hexokinase with glucose. The three-cord ribbon traces the peptide backbone of hexokinase.
Drawn from PDB files 1HKG and 2YHX; Bennett, W. S. Jr., and Steitz, T. A. J. Mol. Biol. *140: 211, 1980.*

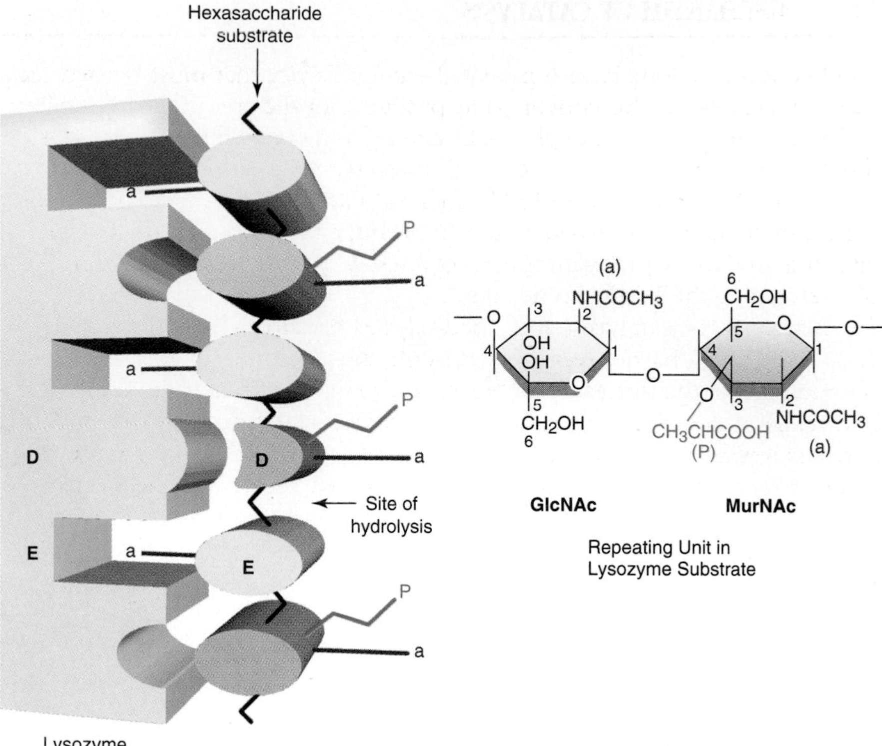

FIGURE 4.46
Hexasaccharide binding at active site of lysozyme.
In the model substrate pictured, the ovals represent individual pyranose rings of the repeating units of the lysozyme substrate shown to the right. Ring D is strained by the enzyme to the half-chair conformation and hydrolysis occurs between the D and E rings. Six subsites on the enzyme bind substrate. Alternate sites are specific for acetamido groups (a) but are unable to accept the lactyl (P) side chains, which occur on the *N*-acetylmuramic acid residues. Thus the substrate can bind to the enzyme in only one orientation.
Redrawn based on model proposed by Imoto, T., et al. In P. Boyer (Ed.), The Enzymes, *3rd ed., Vol. 7. New York: Academic Press, 1972, p. 713.*

substrate strain is that of **lysozyme** (Figure 4.46) in which the conformation of the sugar residue "D" at which bond breaking occurs is strained from the stable chair to the unstable half-chair conformation upon binding. These conformations of glucose are shown in Figure 4.47. The concept of substrate strain explains the role of the enzyme in increasing the rate of reaction (see Section 4.8).

Asymmetry of the Binding Site

Not only are enzymes able to distinguish between isomers of the substrate, but they are able to distinguish between two equivalent atoms in a symmetrical molecule. For example, glycerol kinase distinguishes between configurations of H and OH on C-2 in the symmetric substrate glycerol, so that only the asymmetric product L-glycerol 3-phosphate is formed. These **prochiral substrates** have two identical substituents and two additional but dissimilar groups on the same carbon ($C_{aa'bd}$).

$$\begin{array}{lcl} (a)\ CH_2OH & & CH_2OH \\ \quad\ CHOH\ (b,d) & \xrightarrow[ATP]{\text{glycerol kinase}} & HOCH \quad + ADP \\ (a')\ CH_2OH & & CH_2OPO_3^{2-} \\ \text{Glycerol} & & \text{L-Glycerol 3-phosphate} \end{array}$$

Prochiral substrates possess no optical activity but can be converted to chiral compounds, that is, ones that possess an asymmetric center. The explanation for this enigma is provided if the enzyme binds the two dissimilar groups at specific sites and only one of the two similar substituents is able to bind at the active site (Figure 4.48). Thus the enzyme is able to recognize only one specific orientation of the symmetrical molecule. Asymmetry is produced in the product by modification of one side of the bound substrate. A minimum of three different binding sites on the enzyme surface is required to distinguish between identical groups on a prochiral substrate.

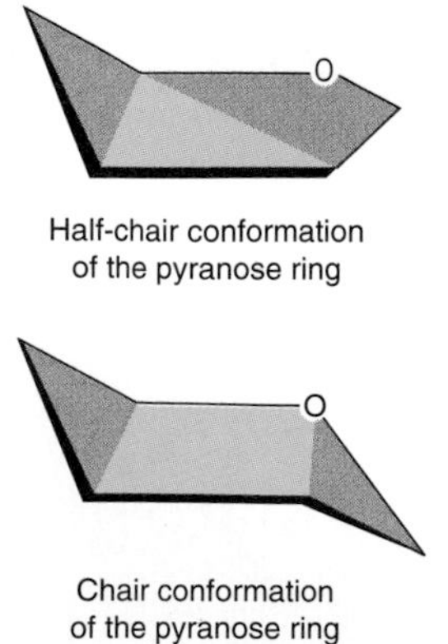

FIGURE 4.47
Two possible conformations of glucose.

4.8 ■ MECHANISM OF CATALYSIS

All chemical reactions have a potential energy barrier that must be overcome before reactants can be converted to products. In the gas phase the reactant molecules can be given enough kinetic energy by heating them so that collisions result in product formation. The same is true with solutions. However, a well-controlled body temperature of 37°C does not allow temperature to be increased to accelerate the reaction, and 37°C is not warm enough to provide the reaction rates required for fast-moving species of animals. Enzymes employ other means of overcoming the barrier to reaction.

Diagrams for catalyzed and noncatalyzed reactions are shown in Figure 4.49. The energy barrier represented by the uncatalyzed curve in Figure 4.49 is a measure of the **activation energy,** E_a, required for the reaction to occur. The reaction coordinate is simply the pathway in terms of bond stretching between reactants and products. At the apex of the energy barrier is the activated complex known as the **transition state,** Ts, that represents the reactants in their activated state. In this state reactants are in an intermediate stage along the reaction pathway and cannot be identified as starting material or products. For example, in the hydrolysis of ethyl acetate:

$$CH_3{-}\overset{\overset{\large O}{\|}}{C}{-}O{-}CH_2{-}CH_3 \xrightarrow{H_2O} CH_3{-}CH_2{-}OH + CH_3{-}\overset{\overset{\large O}{\|}}{C}{-}OH$$

the Ts might look like

$$\left[CH_3{-}\overset{\overset{\large O^-}{|}}{C}\cdots O{-}CH_2{-}CH_3 \quad \text{with } \vdots\ \overset{\cdot\cdot}{O} \text{ (H}_2\text{O, } H \diagup \ \diagdown H\text{) bonding to C} \right]$$

The transition state complex can break down to products or go back to reactants. The Ts is not an intermediate and cannot be isolated! In the case of the enzyme-catalyzed reaction (Figure 4.49) the energy of the reactants and products is no different than in the uncatalyzed reaction. Enzymes do not change the thermodynamics of the system but they do change the pathway for reaching the final state.

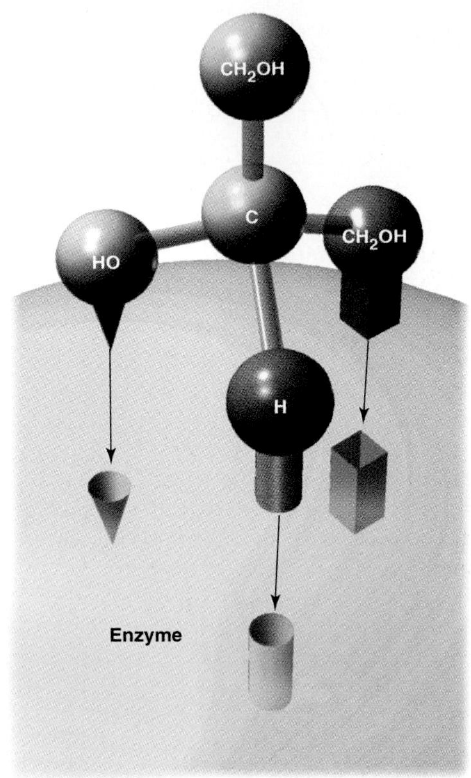

FIGURE 4.48
Three-point attachment of a symmetrical substrate to an asymmetric substrate-binding site.
Glycerol kinase by virtue of dissimilar binding sites for the —H and —OH group of glycerol binds only the α′-hydroxymethyl group to the active site. One stereoisomer results from the kinase reaction, L-glycerol 3-phosphate.

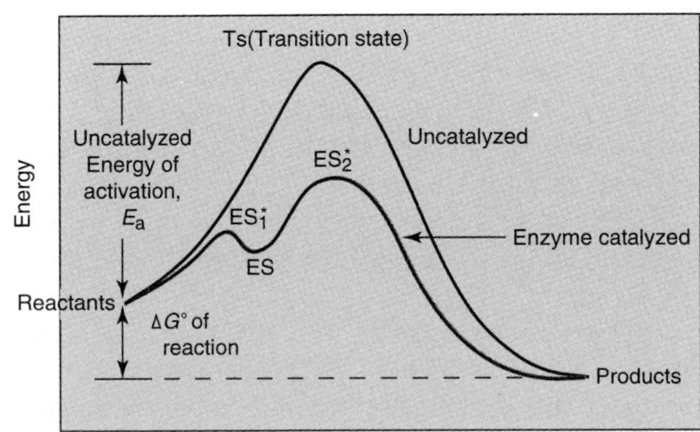

FIGURE 4.49
Energy diagrams for catalyzed versus noncatalyzed reactions.
The overall energy difference between reactants and products is the same in catalyzed and noncatalyzed reactions. The enzyme-catalyzed reaction proceeds at a faster rate because the energy of activation is lowered.

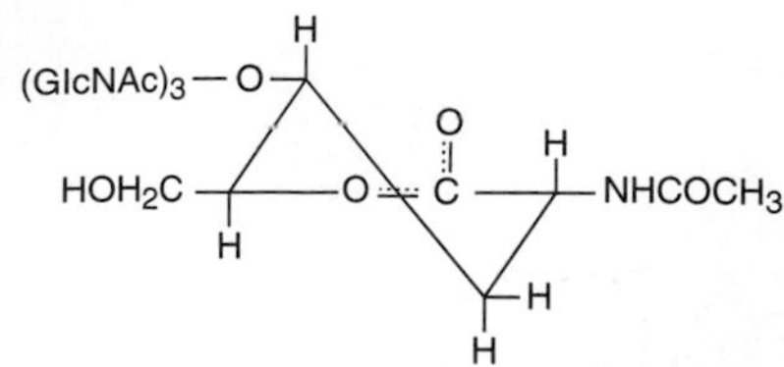

FIGURE 4.50
A transition state analog (tetra-*N*-acetyl-chitotetrose-*d*-lactone) of ring D of the substrate for lysozyme.

As noted on the energy diagram, there may be several plateaus or valleys on the energy contour for an enzyme reaction. At these points metastable intermediates exist. An important point is that each valley may be reached with the heat input available in 37°C. The enzyme allows the energy barrier to be scaled in increments. The Michaelis–Menten ES complex is not the transition state but may be found in one of the valleys because in the ES complex substrates are properly oriented and may be "strained." The bonds to be broken lie further along the reaction coordinate.

If our concepts of the transition state are correct, one would expect that compounds designed to resemble closely the transition state would bind more tightly to the enzyme than the natural substrate. This has proved to be the case. In such substrate analogs one finds affinities 10^2–10^5 times greater than those for substrate. These compounds are called **transition state analogs** and are potent enzyme inhibitors. Previously, lysozyme was discussed in terms of substrate strain, and mention was made of the conversion of sugar ring D from a chair to a strained half-chair conformation. Synthesis of a transition state analog in the form of the δ-lactone of tetra-*N*-acetylchitotetrose (Figure 4.50), which has a distorted half-chair conformation, followed by binding studies, showed that this transition state analog was bound 6000 times tighter than the normal substrate.

Enzymes Decrease Activation Energy

Enzymes can enhance the rates of reaction by a factor of 10^9–10^{12} times that of the noncatalyzed reaction. Most of this rate enhancement can be accounted for by four processes: acid–base catalysis, substrate strain (transition state stabilization), covalent catalysis, and entropy effects.

Acid–Base Catalysis

Specific acids and bases are H^+ and OH^-, respectively. Free protons and hydroxide ions are not encountered in most enzyme reactions and then only in some metal-dependent enzymes (see p. 144). A **general acid** or base is a compound that is weakly ionizable. In the physiological pH range, the protonated form of histidine is the most important general acid and its conjugate base is an important general base (Figure 4.51). Other acids are the thiol —SH of cysteine, tyrosine —OH, and the ε-amino group of lysine. Other bases are carboxylic acid anions and the conjugate bases of the general acids.

Ribonuclease (RNase) exemplifies the role of acid and base catalysis at the enzyme active site. RNase cleaves an RNA chain at the 3′-phosphodiester linkage of pyrimidine nucleotides with an obligatory formation of a cyclic 2′,3′-phosphoribose on a pyrimidine nucleotide as intermediate. In the mechanism outlined in Figure 4.52, His 119 acts as a general acid to protonate the phosphodiester bridge, whereas His 12 acts as a base in generating an alkoxide on the ribose-3′-hydroxyl. The latter then attacks the phosphate group, forming a cyclic phosphate and breakage of the RNA chain at this locus. The cyclic phosphate is then cleaved in phase 2 by a reversal of the reactions in phase 1, but with water replacing the leaving group. The active-site histidines revert to their original protonated state.

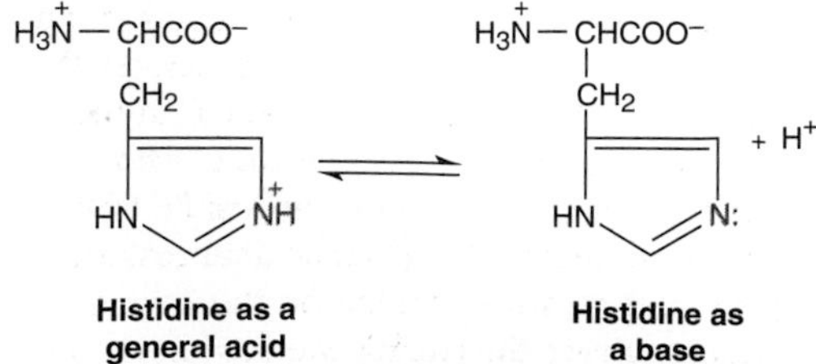

FIGURE 4.51
Acid and base forms of histidine.

Substrate Strain

Previous discussion of this topic related to induced fit of enzymes to substrate. Binding of substrate to a preformed site on the enzyme can induce strain in the substrate. Irrespective of the mechanism of strain induction, the energy level of the substrate is raised, and the bond lengths and angles of the substrate more closly resemble those found in the transition state.

A combination of substrate strain and acid–base catalysis is observed in the action of lysozyme (Figure 4.53). X-ray evidence shows that ring D of the

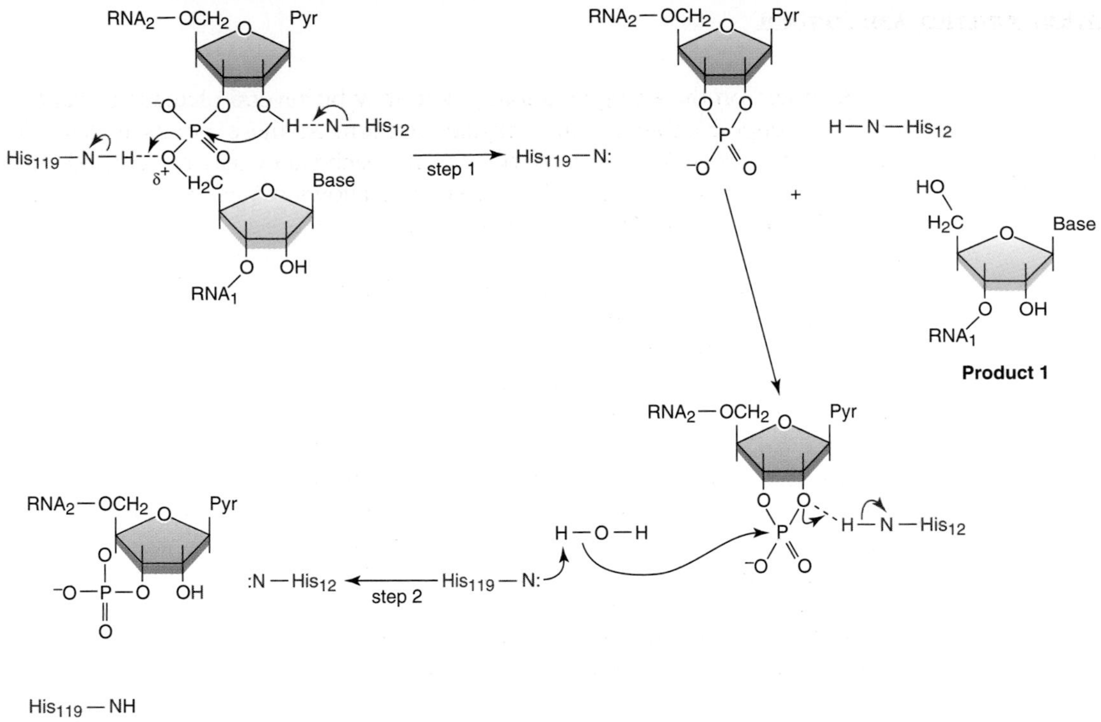

FIGURE 4.52
Role of acid and base catalysis in the active site of ribonuclease.
RNase cleaves the phosphodiester bond in a pyrimidine locus in RNA. Histidine residues 12 and 119, respectively, at the ribonuclease active site function as acid and base catalysts in enhancing the formation of an intermediate 2′,3′-cyclic phosphate and release of a shorter fragment of RNA (product 1). These same histidines then play a reverse role in the hydrolysis of the cyclic phosphate and release of the other fragment of RNA (product 2) that ends in a pyrimidine nucleoside 3′-phosphate. As a result of the formation of product 2, the active site of the enzyme is regenerated.

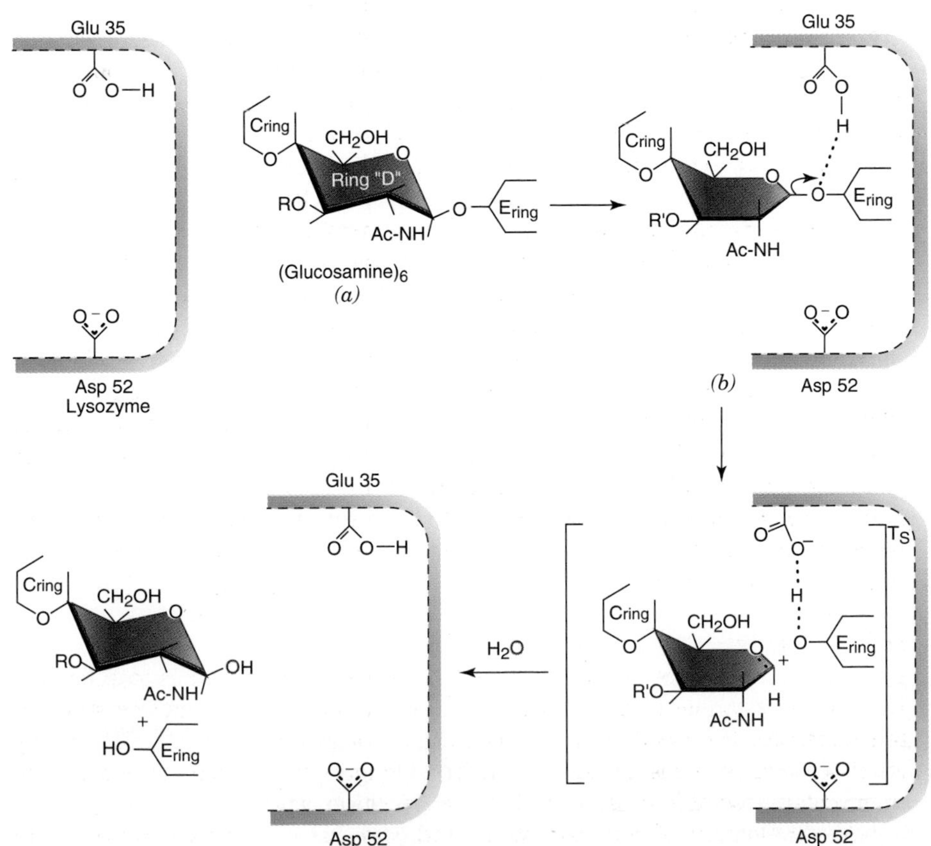

FIGURE 4.53
Mechanism for lysozyme action: substrate strain.
Binding of the stable chair (*a*) conformation of the substrate to the enzyme generates the strained half-chair conformation (*b*) in the ES complex. In the transition state, acid-catalyzed hydrolysis of the glycosidic linkage by an active-site glutamic acid residue generates a carbonium ion on the D ring, which relieves the strain generated in the initial ES complex and results in collapse of the transition state to products.

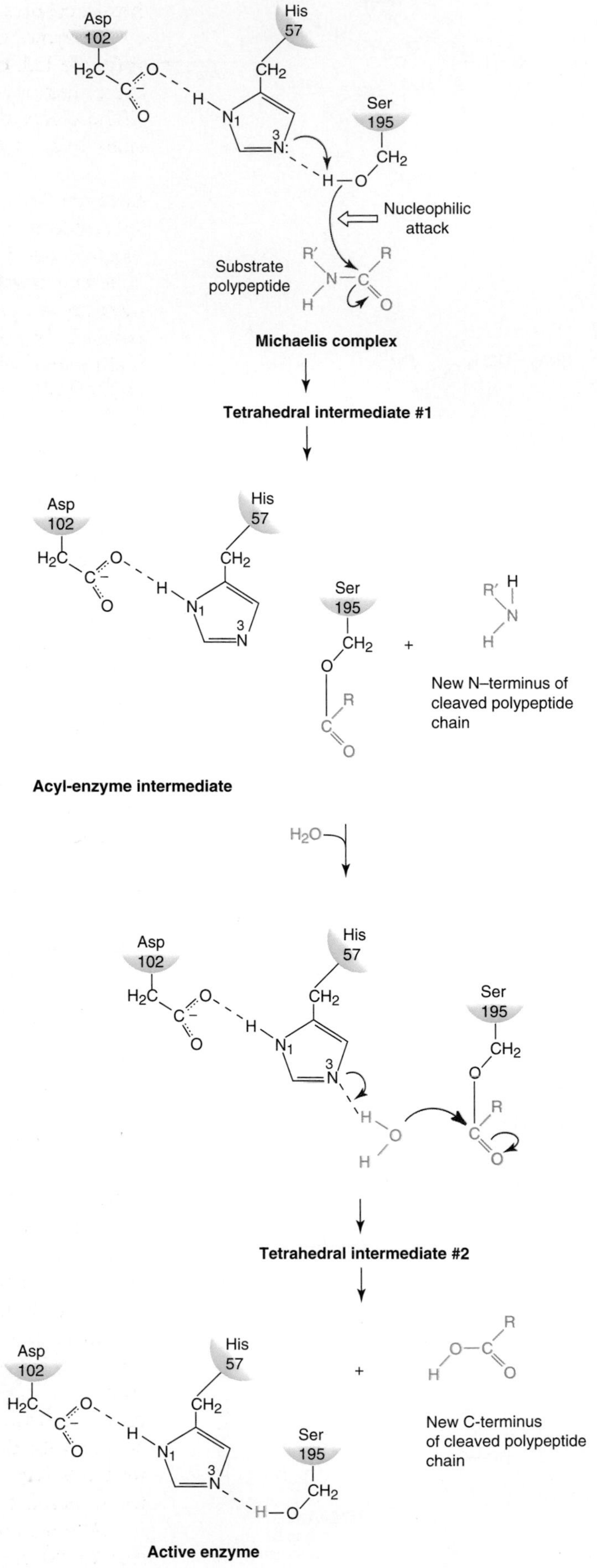

Asp 102
His 57
Ser 195
Nucleophilic attack
Substrate polypeptide
Michaelis complex
Tetrahedral intermediate #1
Acyl-enzyme intermediate
New N–terminus of cleaved polypeptide chain
Tetrahedral intermediate #2
New C-terminus of cleaved polypeptide chain
Active enzyme

FIGURE 4.54
Covalent catalysis in active site of chymotrypsin.
Through acid-catalyzed nucleophilic attack, as shown by red arrows, the stable amide linkage of the peptide substrate is converted into an unstable acylated enzyme through serine-195 of the enzyme. The latter is hydrolyzed in the rate-determining step. The new amino-terminal peptide, shown in blue, is released concomitant with formation of the acylated enzyme.

hexasaccharide substrate is strained to the half-chair conformation upon binding to lysozyme. General acid catalysis by active-site glutamic acid promotes the unstable half-chair into the transition state. The oxycarbonium ion formed in the transition state is stabilized by the negatively charged aspartate. Breakage of the glycosidic linkage between rings D and E relieves the strained transition state by allowing ring D to return to the stable chair conformation.

Covalent Catalysis

In **covalent catalysis,** the attack of a nucleophilic (negatively charged) or electrophilic (positively charged) group in the enzyme active site upon the substrate results in covalent binding of the substrate to the enzyme as an intermediate in the reaction sequence. Enzyme-bound coenzymes often form covalent bonds with the substrate. For example, in the **transaminases,** the amino acid substrate forms a Schiff base with enzyme-bound pyridoxal phosphate (see p. 449). In all cases of covalent catalysis, the enzyme- or coenzyme-bound substrate is more labile than the original substrate. The enzyme–substrate adduct represents one of the valleys on the energy profile.

Serine proteases, such as trypsin, chymotrypsin, and thrombin, are good representatives of the covalent catalytic mechanism (see p. 97). Acylated enzyme has been isolated in the case of chymotrypsin. Covalent catalysis is assisted by acid–base catalysis in these particular enzymes (Figure 4.54). In chymotrypsin the attacking nucleophile is Ser 195, which is not dissociated at pH 7.4 and a mechanism for ionizing this very basic group is required. It is now thought that in the anhydrous milieu of the active site, Ser 195 and His 57 have similar pK values and that the negative charge on Asp 102 stabilizes the transfer of the proton from the OH of Ser 195 to N3 of His 57 (Figure 4.54). The resulting serine alkoxide attacks the carbonyl carbon of the peptide bond, releasing the amino terminal end of the protein and forming an **acylated enzyme** intermediate (through Ser 195). The acylated enzyme is then cleaved by reversal of the reaction sequence, but with water as the nucleophile rather than Ser 195. Chemical evidence indicates the formation of two tetrahedral intermediates, one preceding the formation of the acylated enzyme and one following the attack of water on the acyl-enzyme (Figure 4.55).

Transition State Stabilization

The previously mentioned effects promote the substrate to enter the transition state. Since the active site binds the transition state with a much greater affinity than the substrate, that small fraction of substrate molecules existing in a transition state geometry will be converted to products quickly. Thus, by mass action, all the substrate can be rapidly converted to products. Any factor that increases the population of substrate molecules resembling the transition state will contribute to catalysis.

Entropy Effect

Entropy is a thermodynamic term, ΔS, which defines the extent of disorder in a system. At equilibrium, entropy is maximal. For example, in solution two reactants A and B exist in many different orientations. The chances of A and B coming together with the correct geometric orientation and with enough energy to react is small at 37°C and in dilute solution. However, if an enzyme with two high-affinity binding sites for A and B is introduced into the dilute solution of these reactants, as suggested in Figure 4.56, A and B will be bound to the enzyme in the correct orientation for the reaction to occur. They will be bound with the correct stoichiometry, and the effective concentration of the reactants will be increased on the enzyme surface, all of which will contribute to an increased rate of reaction.

When correctly positioned and bound on the enzyme surface, the substrates may be "strained" toward the transition state. At this point the substrates have

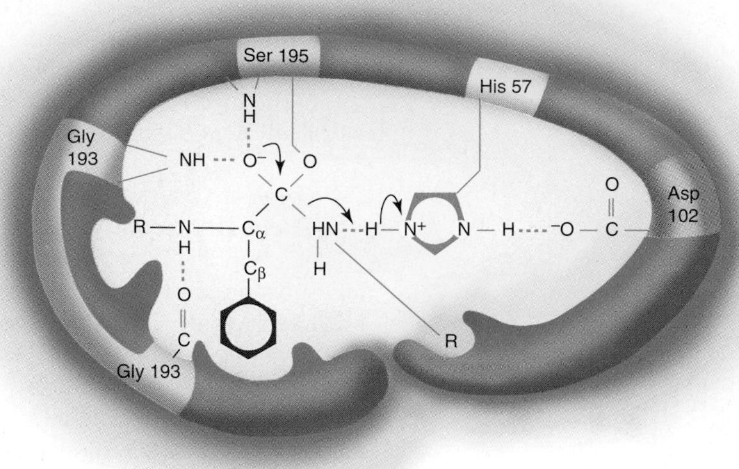

Tetrahedral intermediate #1

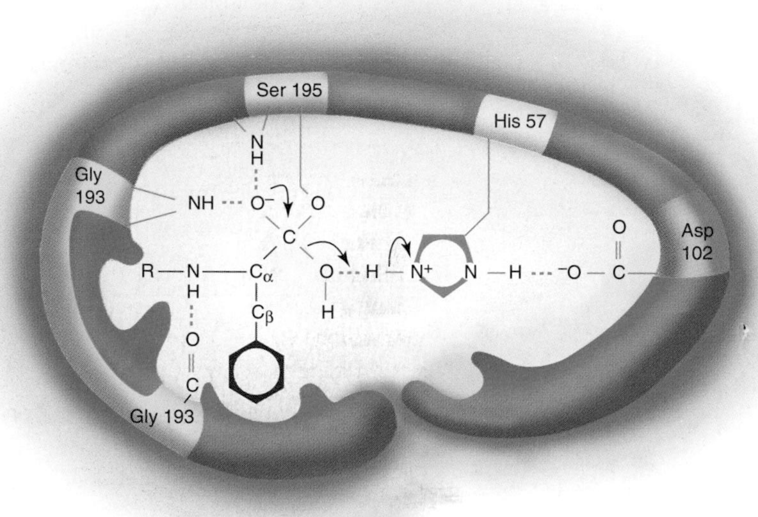

Tetrahedral intermediate #2

FIGURE 4.55
Tetrahedral intermediates.
(*a*) Model of tetrahedral intermediate #1 that precedes formation of the acyl-enzyme intermediate. (*b*) Model of tetrahedral intermediate #2 resulting from the attack of water on acyl-enzyme intermediate.

been "set up" for acid–base and/or covalent catalysis. Proper orientation and the nearness of the substrate with respect to the catalytic groups, which has been dubbed the "proximity effect," contribute 10^3–10^5-fold to the rate enhancement observed with enzymes. It is estimated that the decrease in entropy contributes a factor of 10^3 to the rate enhancement.

Abzymes Are Artificially Synthesized Antibodies with Catalytic Activity

If the principles discussed above for enzyme catalysis are correct, then one should be able to design an artificial enzyme. This feat has been accomplished by the use of several different approaches, but only the synthesis of antibodies that have catalytic activity will be considered in this discussion. These antibodies are called **abzymes.** Design of abzymes is based on two principles. The first principle is the ability of the immune system to recognize any arrangement

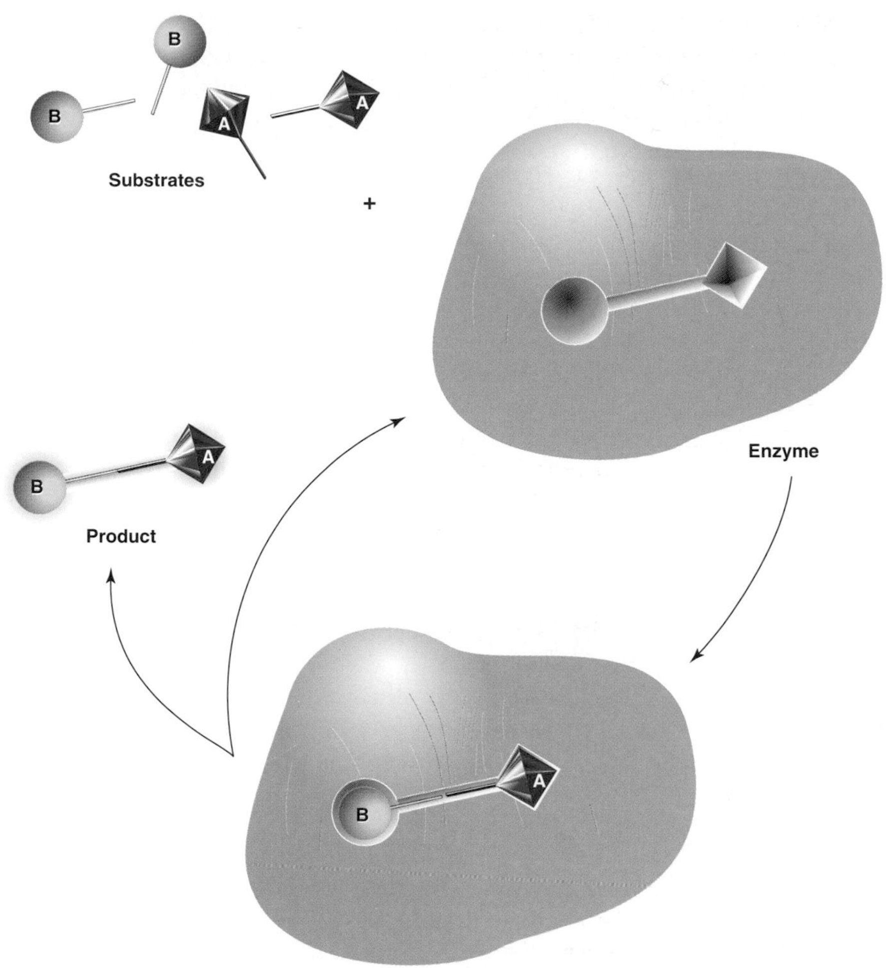

FIGURE 4.56
Role of the enzyme in enhancing reaction rate by decreasing entropy.
Substrates in dilute solution are concentrated and oriented on the enzyme surface so as to enhance the rate of the reaction.

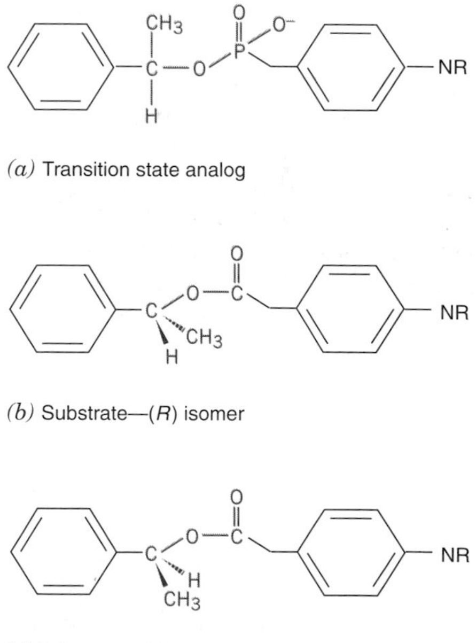

of atoms in the foreign antigen and to make a binding site on the resulting immunoglobulin that is exquisitely suited to binding that antigen. The second principle is that strong binding of transition state-like substrates reduces the energy barrier along the reaction pathway (see discussion on p. 160).

In abzymes a transition state analog serves as the hapten. For a lipase abzyme, a racemic phosphonate (Figure 4.57) serves as a hapten. Two enantiomeric fatty acid ester substrates are shown in Figure 4.57*b*,*c*. See page 159 for the transition state structure expected for ester hydrolysis. Among many antibodies produced by rabbits on challenge with the protein-bound transition state analog (Figure 4.57*a*), one hydrolyzed only the (*R*) isomer (Figure 4.57*b*) and another only the (*S*) isomer. These abzymes enhanced the rate of hydrolysis of substrates (*a*) and (*b*) 10^3–10^5-fold above the background rate in a stereospecific manner. Acceleration of 10^6-fold, which is close to the enzymatic rate, has been achieved in another esterase-like system.

(*a*) Transition state analog

(*b*) Substrate—(*R*) isomer

(*c*) Substrate—(*S*) isomer

FIGURE 4.57
Hapten and substrate for a catalytic antibody (abzyme).
Phosphonate (*a*) is the transition state analog used as the hapten to generate antibodies with lipase-like catalytic activity. Specific abzymes can be generated for either the (*R*) isomer (*b*) or the (*S*) isomer (*c*) of methyl benzyl esters.

Environmental Parameters Influence Catalytic Activity

A number of external parameters, including pH, temperature, and salt concentration, affect enzyme activity. These effects are probably not important *in vivo* under normal conditions but are very important in setting up enzyme assays *in vitro* to measure enzyme activity in samples of a patient's plasma or tissue.

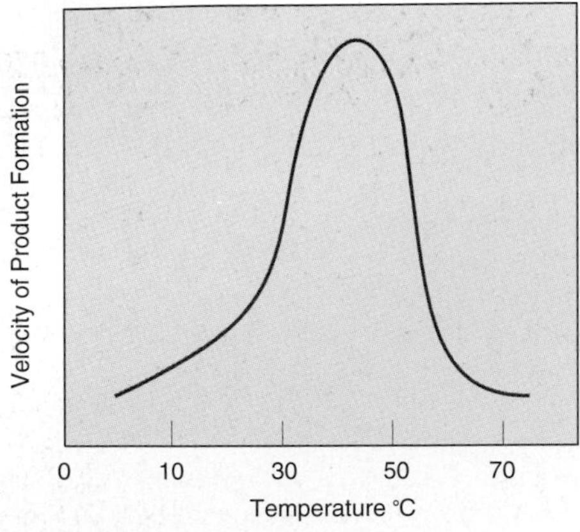

FIGURE 4.58
Temperature dependence of a typical mammalian enzyme.
To the left of the optimum, the rate is low because the environmental temperature is too low to provide enough kinetic energy to overcome the energy of activation. To the right of the optimum, the enzyme is inactivated by heat denaturation.

Temperature

Plots of velocity versus temperature for most enzymes reveal a bell-shaped curve with an optimum between 40°C and 45°C for mammalian enzymes, as indicated in Figure 4.58. Above this temperature, heat denaturation of the enzyme occurs. Between 0°C and 40°C, most enzymes show a twofold increase in activity for every 10°C rise. Under conditions of hypothermia, most enzyme reactions are depressed, which accounts for the decreased oxygen demand of living organisms at low temperature. Mutation of an enzyme to a thermolabile form can have serious consequences (see Clin. Corr. 4.5).

pH

Nearly all enzymes show a bell-shaped pH–velocity profile, but the maximum **(pH optimum)** varies greatly with different enzymes. Alkaline and acid phosphatases with very different pH optima are both found in humans, as shown in Figure 4.59. The bell-shaped curve and its position on the x-axis are dependent on the particular ionized state of the substrate that will be optimally bound to the enzyme. This in turn is related to the ionization of specific amino acid residues that constitute the substrate-binding site. In addition, amino acid residues involved in catalyzing the reaction must be in the correct charge state to be functional. For example, if aspartic acid is involved in catalyzing the reaction, the pH optimum may be in the region of 4.5 at which the α-carboxyl of aspartate ionizes; whereas if the ε-amino of lysine is the catalytic group, the pH optimum may be around 9.5, the pK_a of the ε-amino group. Studies of the pH dependence of enzymes are useful for suggesting which amino acid(s) may be operative in catalysis.

Clinical Correlation 4.6 points out the effect of a mutation leading to a change in the pH optimum of a physiologically important enzyme. Such a mutated enzyme may function on the shoulder of the pH-rate profile, but not be optimally active, even under normal physiological conditions. When an abnormal condition such as alkalosis (observed in vomiting) or acidosis (observed in pneumonia and often in surgery) occurs, the enzyme activity may disappear because the pH is inappropriate. Thus under normal conditions, the enzyme may be active enough to meet normal requirements, but under stress conditions the enzyme may be less active.

CLINICAL CORRELATION 4.5

Thermal Lability of Glucose-6-Phosphate Dehydrogenase Results in Hemolytic Anemia

In red cells, glucose-6-phosphate (G6PD) is an important enzyme in the red cell for the maintenance of the membrane integrity. A deficiency or inactivity of this enzyme leads to a hemolytic anemia. In other cases, a variant enzyme is present that normally has sufficient activity to maintain the membrane but fails under conditions of oxidative stress. A mutation of this enzyme leads to a protein with normal kinetic constants but a decreased thermal stability. This condition is especially critical to the red cell, since it is devoid of protein-synthesizing capacity and cannot renew enzymes as they denature. The end result is a greatly decreased lifetime for those red cells that have an unstable G6PD. These red cells are also susceptible to drug-induced hemolysis. See Clin. Corr. 8.1.

Lazzatio, L., and Meta, A., Glucose-6-phosphate dehydrogenase deficiency. In: C. R. Scriver, A. L. Beaudet, W. S. Sly, and D. Valle (Eds.), *The Metabolic and Molecular Bases of Inherited Disease,* 7th ed. New York: McGraw-Hill, 1995, p. 3369.

4.9 ■ CLINICAL APPLICATIONS OF ENZYMES

The principles of enzymology outlined in previous sections are applied in the clinical laboratory in measurement of plasma or tissue enzyme activities and concentrations of substrates in patients. The rationale for measuring plasma enzyme activities is based on the premise that changes in activities reflect changes that have occurred in a specific tissue or organ. Plasma enzymes are of two types: (1) one type is present in the highest concentration, is specific to plasma, and has a functional role in plasma; and (2) the second is normally present at very low levels and plays no functional role in the plasma. The former includes the enzymes associated with blood coagulation (e.g., thrombin), fibrin dissolution (plasmin), and processing of chylomicrons (lipoprotein lipase).

In disease of tissues and organs, the nonplasma-specific enzymes are most important. Normally, the plasma levels of these enzymes are low to absent. A disease process may cause changes in cell membrane permeability or increased cell death, resulting in release of intracellular enzymes into the plasma. When permeability changes, those enzymes of lower molecular weight will appear in the plasma first and the greater the concentration gradient between intra- and extracellular levels, the more rapidly the enzyme diffuses out. Cytosolic enzymes will appear in the plasma before mitochondrial enzymes, and the

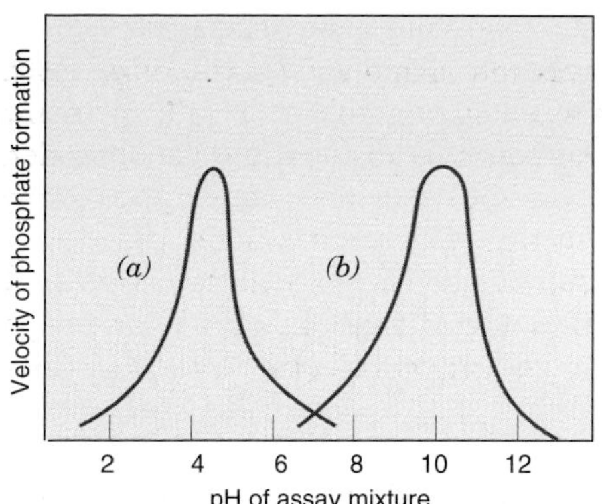

FIGURE 4.59
The pH dependence of (*a*) acid and (*b*) alkaline phosphatase reactions.
In each case the optimum represents the ideal ionic state for binding of enzyme and substrate and the correct ionic state for the amino acids involved in the catalytic event.

greater the quantity of tissue damaged, the larger the increase in plasma level. The nonplasma-specific enzymes will be cleared from the plasma at varying rates, which depend on the stability of the enzyme and its uptake by the reticuloendothelial system.

In the diagnosis of specific organ involvement in a disease process it would be ideal if enzymes unique to each organ could be identified. This is unlikely because the metabolic processes of various organs are very similar. Alcohol dehydrogenase of the liver and acid phosphatase of the prostate are useful for specific identification of disease in these organs. Other than these two examples, there are few enzymes that are tissue or organ specific. However, the ratio of various enzymes does vary from tissue to tissue. This fact, combined with a study of the kinetics of appearance and disappearance of particular enzymes in plasma, allows a diagnosis of specific organ involvement to be made. Figure 4.60 illustrates the time dependence of the plasma activities of enzymes released

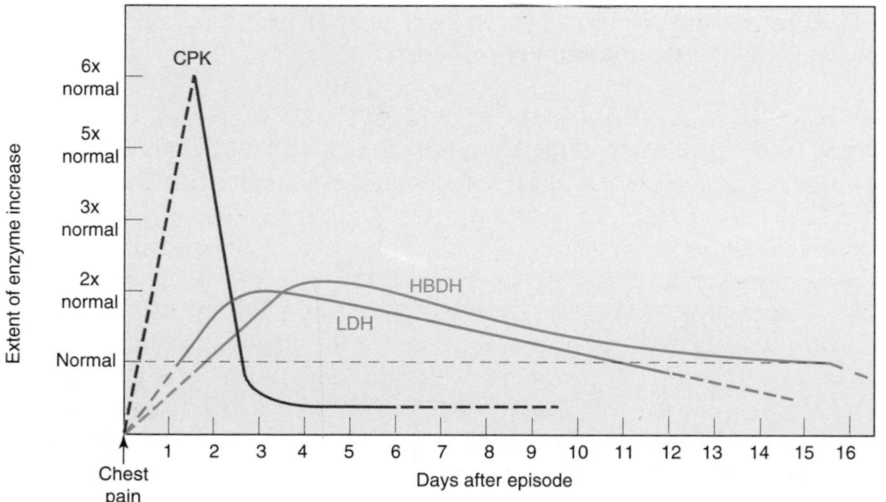

FIGURE 4.60
Kinetics of release of cardiac enzymes into serum following a myocardial infarction.
CPK, creatine kinase; LDH, lactic dehydrogenase; HBDH, α-hydroxybutyric dehydrogenase. Such kinetic profiles allow one to determine where the patient is with respect to the infarct and recovery. Note: CPK rises sharply but briefly; HBDH rises slowly but persists.
Reprinted with permission from Coodley, E. L. Diagnostic Enzymes. *Philadelphia: Lea & Febiger, 1970, p. 61.*

CLINICAL CORRELATION 4.6

Alcohol Dehydrogenase Isoenzymes with Different pH Optima

In addition to the change in aldehyde dehydrogenase isoenzyme composition in some Asians (see Clin. Corr. 4.2), different alcohol dehydrogenase isoenzymes are also observed. Alcohol dehydrogenase (ADH) is encoded by three genes, which produce three different polypeptides: α, β, and γ. Three alleles are found for the β-gene that differ in a single nucleotide base, which causes substitutions for arginine. The substitutions are shown below:

	Residue 47	*Residue 369*
β_1	Arg	Arg
β_2	His	Arg
β_3	Arg	Cys

The liver β_3 form has ADH activity with a pH optimum near 7, compared with 10 for β_1, and 8.5 for β_2. The rate-determining step in alcohol dehydrogenase is the release of NADH. NADH is held on the enzyme by ionic bonds between the phosphates of the coenzyme and the arginines at positions 47 and 369. In the β_1 isozyme this ionic interaction is not broken until the pH is quite alkaline and the guanidinium group of arginine starts to dissociate H^+. Substitution of amino acids with lower pK values, as in β_2 and β_3, weakens the interaction and lowers the pH optimum. Since the release of NADH is facilitated, the V_{max} values for β_2 and β_3 are also higher than for β_1.

Burnell, J. C., Carr, L. G., Dwulet, F. E., Edenberg, H. J., Li, T-K., and Bosron, W. F. The human β_3 alcohol dehydrogenase subunit differs from β_1 by a cys- for arg-369 substitution which decreased NAD(H) binding. *Biochem. Biophys. Res. Commun.* 146:1227, 1987.

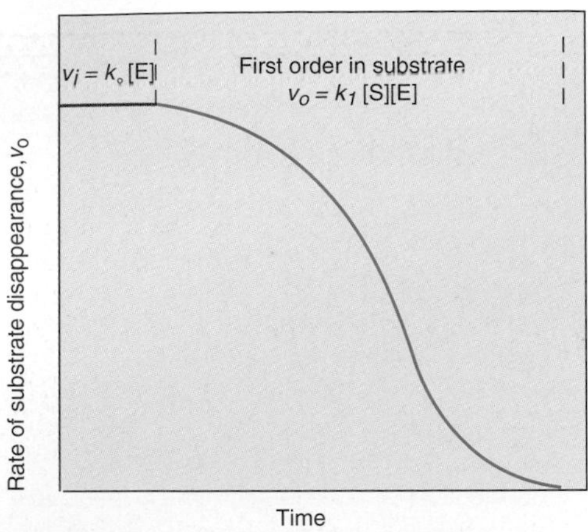

FIGURE 4.61
Relation of substrate concentration to order of the reaction.
When the enzyme is completely saturated, the kinetics are zero order with respect to substrate and are first order in the enzyme; that is, the rate depends only on enzyme concentration. When the substrate level falls below saturating levels, the kinetics are first order in both substrate and enzyme and are therefore second order; that is, the observed rate is dependent on both enzyme and substrate.

from the myocardium following a heart attack. Such profiles allow one to establish when the attack occurred and whether treatment is effective. Clinical Correlation 4.7 demonstrates how diagnosis of a specific enzyme defect led to a rational clinical treatment that restored the patient to health.

Studies of the kinetics of appearance and disappearance of plasma enzymes require a valid enzyme assay. A good assay is based on temperature and pH control, as well as saturating levels of all substrates, cosubstrates, and cofactors. To accomplish the latter, the K_m must be known for those particular conditions of pH, ionic strength, and so on, that are to be used in the assay. Recall that K_m is the substrate concentration at half-maximal velocity ($\frac{1}{2} V_{max}$). To assure that the system is saturated, substrate concentration is generally increased five- to tenfold over the K_m. With saturation of the enzyme with substrate, the reaction is zero order. This fact is emphasized in Figure 4.61. Under zero-order conditions changes in velocity are proportional to enzyme concentration alone. Under first-order conditions, the velocity is dependent on both the substrate and enzyme concentrations. Clinical Correlation 4.8 demonstrates the importance of determining if the assay conditions accurately reflect the amount of enzyme actually present. Clinical laboratory assay conditions are optimized for the properties of the normal enzyme and may not correctly measure levels of mutated enzyme. pH dependence and/or the K_m for substrate and cofactors may drastically change in a mutated enzyme. Under optimal conditions a valid enzyme assay reflects a linear dependence of velocity and amount of enzyme. This can be tested by determining if the velocity of the reaction doubles when the plasma sample size is doubled, while keeping the total volume of the assay constant (Figure 4.62).

Coupled Assays Utilize the Optical Properties of NAD, NADP, or FAD

Enzymes that employ the coenzymes NAD^+, $NADP^+$, and FAD are easily measured because of the optical properties of NADH, NADPH, and FAD. The absorption spectra of NADH and FAD in the ultraviolet and visible light regions are shown in Figure 4.63. Oxidized FAD absorbs strongly at 450 nm, while NADH has maximal absorption at 340 nm. The concentrations of both FAD and NADH are related to their absorption of light at the respective absorption maximum by the **Beer–Lambert relation**

$$A = \varepsilon \cdot c \cdot l$$

where l is the pathlength of the spectrophotometer cell in centimeters (usually 1 cm), ε is absorbance of a molar solution of the substance being measured at

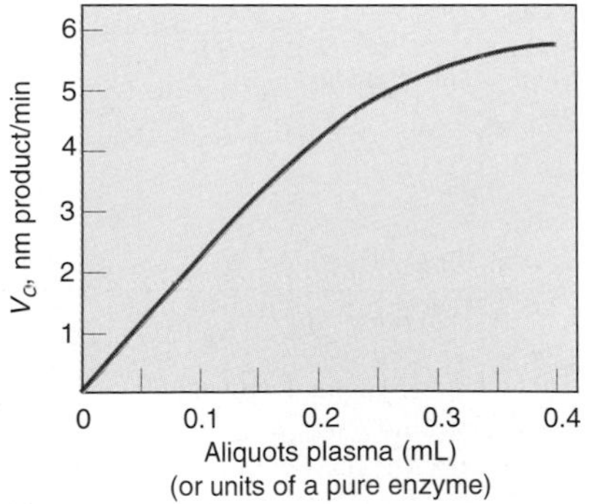

FIGURE 4.62
Assessing the validity of an enzyme assay.
The line shows what is to be expected for any reaction where the concentration of substrate is held constant and the aliquots of enzyme are increased. In this example linearity between initial velocity observed and amount of enzyme, whether pure or in a plasma sample, is only observed up to 0.2 mL of plasma or 0.2 units of pure enzyme. If more than 0.2 mL is used, the actual amount of enzyme in the sample would be underestimated.

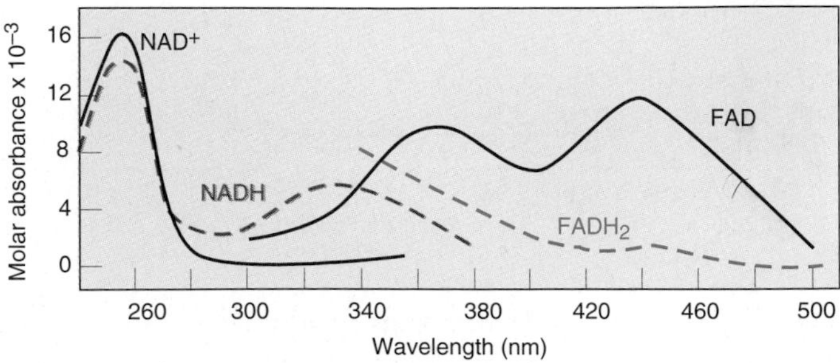

FIGURE 4.63
Absorption spectra of niacin and flavin coenzymes.
The reduced form of NAD (NADH) absorbs strongly at 340 nm. The oxidized form of flavin coenzymes absorbs strongly at 450 nm. Thus one can follow the rate of reduction of NAD^+ by observing the increase in the absorbance at 340 nm and the formation of $FADH_2$ by following the decrease in absorbance at 450 nm.

CLINICAL CORRELATION 4.7

Identification and Treatment of an Enzyme Deficiency

Enzyme deficiencies usually lead to increased accumulation of specific intermediary metabolites in plasma and hence in urine. Recognition of the intermediates that accumulate in biological fluids is useful in pinpointing possible enzyme defects. After the enzyme deficiency is established, metabolites that normally occur in the pathway but are distal to the block may be supplied exogenously in order to overcome the metabolic effects of the enzyme deficiency.

In hereditary orotic aciduria there is a double enzyme deficiency in the pyrimidine biosynthetic pathway leading to accumulation of orotic acid. Both orotate phosphoribosyltransferase and orotidine 5′-phosphate decarboxylase are deficient, causing decreased *in vivo* levels of CTP and TTP. The two activities are deficient because they reside in separate domains of a bifunctional polypeptide of 480 amino acids. dCTP and dTTP, which arise from CTP and TTP, are required for cell division. In these enzyme deficiency diseases the patients are pale, weak, and fail to thrive. Administration of the missing pyrimidines as uridine or cytidine promotes growth and general well-being and also decreases orotic acid excretion. The latter occurs because the TTP and CTP formed from the supplied uridine and cytidine repress carbamoyl-phosphate synthetase, the committed step, by feedback inhibition, resulting in a decrease in orotate production.

Webster, D. R., Becroft, D. M. O., and Suttie, D. P. Hereditary orotic aciduria and other diseases of pyrimidine metabolism. In C. R. Scriver, A. L. Beaudet, W. S. Sly, and D. Valle (Eds.), *The Metabolic and Molecular Bases of Inherited Disease,* 7th ed. McGraw-Hill, 1995, p. 1799.

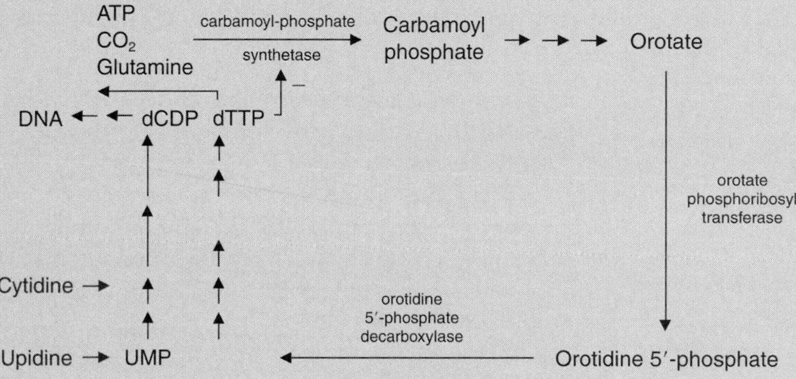

CLINICAL CORRELATION 4.8

Ambiguity in the Assay of Mutated Enzymes

Structural gene mutations leading to production of enzymes with increases or decreases in K_m are frequently observed. A case in point is a patient with hyperuricemia and gout, whose red blood cell hypoxanthine–guanine–phosphoribosyltransferase (HGPRT) showed little activity in assays *in vitro*. This enzyme is involved in the salvage of purine bases and catalyzes the reaction

$$\text{Hypoxanthine} + \text{PRPP} \rightarrow \text{inosine monophosphate} + \text{PP}_i$$

where PRPP is phosphoribosylpyrophosphate.

The absence of HGPRT activity results in a severe neurological disorder known as Lesch–Nyhan syndrome (see p. 499), yet this patient did not have the clinical signs of this disorder. Immunological testing with a specific antibody to the enzyme revealed as much cross-reacting material in the patient's red blood cells as in normal controls. The enzyme was therefore being synthesized but was inactive in the assay *in vitro*. Increasing the substrate concentration in the assay restored full activity in the patient's red cell hemolysate. This anomaly is explained as a mutation in the substrate-binding site of HGPRT, leading to an increased K_m. Neither the substrate concentration in the assay nor in the red blood cells was high enough to bind to the enzyme. This case reinforces the point that an accurate enzyme determination is dependent on zero-order kinetics, that is, the enzyme being saturated with substrate.

Sorenson, L., and Benke, P. J. Biochemical evidence for a distinct type of primary gout. *Nature* 213:1122, 1967.

a specific wavelength of light, A is absorbance, and c is concentration. Absorbance is the log of transmittance (I_0/I). The term ε is a constant that varies from substance to substance; its value can be found in a handbook of biochemistry. In an optically clear solution, the concentration c can be calculated after determination of the absorbance A and substituting into the Beer–Lambert equation.

Many enzymes do not employ NAD^+ or FAD but do generate products that can be utilized by a NAD^+- or FAD-linked enzyme. For example, glucokinase catalyzes the reaction

$$\text{Glucose} + \text{ATP} \leftrightharpoons \text{glucose 6-phosphate} + \text{ADP}$$

ADP and glucose 6-phosphate (G6P) are difficult to measure directly; however, glucose-6-phosphate dehydrogenase catalyzes the reaction

$$\text{Glucose 6-phosphate} + \text{NADP}^+ \leftrightharpoons \text{6-phosphogluconolactone} + \text{NADPH} + \text{H}^+$$

Thus by adding an excess of G6P dehydrogenase and $NADP^+$ to the assay mixture, the velocity of production of G6P by glucokinase is proportional to the rate of reduction of $NADP^+$, which can be measured directly in the spectrophotometer.

Clinical Analyzers Use Immobilized Enzymes as Reagents

Enzymes are used as chemical reagents in desk-top clinical analyzers in offices or for screening purposes in shopping centers and malls. For example, screening tests for cholesterol and triacylglycerols can be completed in a few minutes using 10 μL of plasma. The active components in the assay system are cholesterol oxidase for the cholesterol determination and lipase for the triacylglycerols. The enzymes are immobilized in a bilayer along with the necessary buffer salts, cofactors or cosubstrates, and indicator reagents. The ingredients are arranged in a multilayered vehicle the size and thickness of a 35-mm slide. The plasma sample provides the substrate and water necessary to activate the system. In the case of cholesterol oxidase, hydrogen peroxide is a product that subsequently oxidizes a colorless dye to a colored product that is measured by reflectance spectroscopy. Peroxidase is included in the reagents to catalyze the latter reaction.

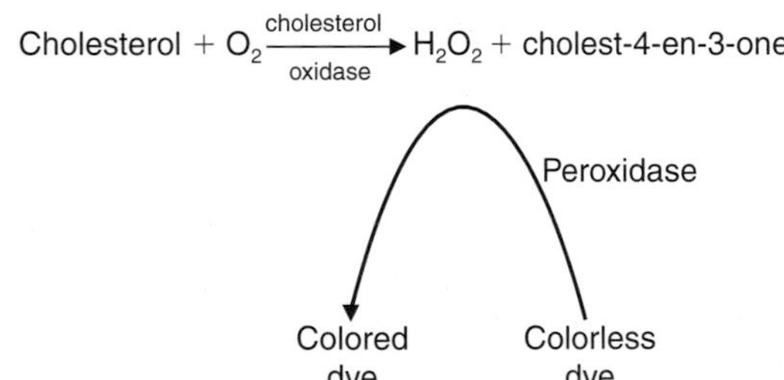

Each slide packet is constructed to measure a specific substance or enzyme and is stored in the cold for use as needed. In many cases the slide packet contains several enzymes in a coupled assay system that eventually generates a reduced nucleotide or a colored dye that can be measured spectroscopically. This technology has been made possible, in part, by the fact that the enzymes involved are stabilized when bound to immobilized matrices and are stored in the dry state or in the presence of a stabilizing solvent such as glycerol.

Enzyme-Linked Immunoassays Employ Enzymes as Indicators

Modern clinical chemistry has benefited from the marriage of enzyme chemistry and immunology. Antibodies specific to a protein antigen are coupled to an indicator enzyme such as horseradish peroxidase to generate a very specific and sensitive assay. After binding of the peroxidase-coupled antibody to the antigen, the peroxidase is used to generate a colored product that is measurable and whose concentration is related to the amount of antigen in a sample. Because of the catalytic nature of the enzyme the system greatly amplifies the signal. This assay has been given the acronym **ELISA** for enzyme-linked immunoadsorbent assay.

Application of these principles is demonstrated by an assay for **human immunodeficiency virus (HIV)** coat protein antigens. This virus can lead to development of **acquired immunodeficiency syndrome (AIDS).** Antibodies are prepared in a rabbit against HIV coat proteins. In addition, a reporter antibody is prepared in a goat against rabbit IgG directed against the HIV protein. To this goat anti-rabbit IgG is linked the enzyme, horseradish peroxidase. The test for the virus is performed by incubating patient serum in a polystyrene dish that binds the proteins in the serum sample. Any free protein-binding sites remaining on the dish after incubation with patient serum are then covered by incubating with a nonspecific protein like bovine serum albumin. Next, the rabbit IgG antibody against the HIV protein is incubated in the dish during which time the IgG attaches to any HIV coat proteins that are attached to the polystyrene dish. All unbound rabbit IgG is washed out with buffer. The goat anti-rabbit IgG–peroxidase is now placed in the dish where it binds to any rabbit IgG attached to the dish via the HIV viral coat protein. Unattached antibody–peroxidase is washed out. Peroxidase substrates are added and the amount of color developed in a given time period is a measurement of the amount of HIV coat protein present in a given volume of patient plasma when compared against a standard curve. This procedure is schematically diagrammed in Figure 4.64. This assay amplifies the signal because of the catalytic nature of the reporter group, the enzyme peroxidase. Such amplified enzyme assays allow the measurement of remarkably small amounts of antigens.

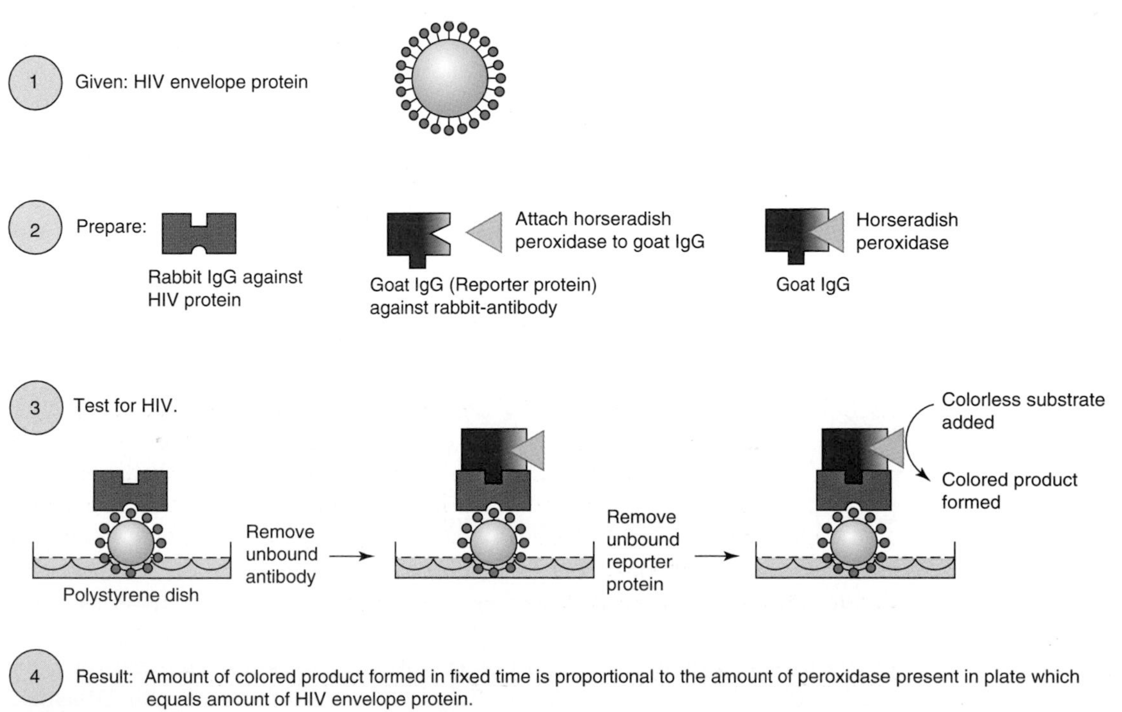

FIGURE 4.64
Schematic of ELISA (enzyme-linked immunoadsorbent assay) for detecting the human immunodeficiency virus (HIV) envelope proteins.

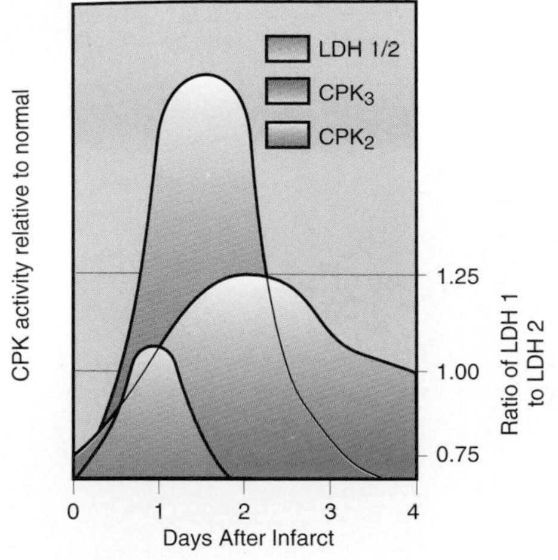

FIGURE 4.65
Characteristic changes in serum CPK and LDH isozymes following a myocardial infarction.
CPK_2 (MB) isozyme increases to a maximum within 1 day of the infarction. CPK_3 lags behind CPK_2 by about 1 day. Total LDH level increases more slowly. The increase of LDH_1 and LDH_2 within 12–24 h coupled with an increase in CPK_2 is diagnostic of myocardial infarction.

Measurement of Isozymes Is Used Diagnostically

Isozymes (or isoenzymes) are enzymes that catalyze the same reaction but migrate differently on electrophoresis. Their physical properties may also differ, but not necessarily. The most common mechanism for the formation of isozymes involves the arrangement of subunits arising from two different genetic loci in different combinations to form the active polymeric enzyme. Isozymes that have wide clinical application are lactate dehydrogenase, creatine kinase, and alkaline phosphatase. **Creatine kinase (CPK)** (see p. 955) occurs as a dimer with two types of subunits, M (muscle type) and B (brain type). In brain both subunits are electrophoretically the same and are designated B. In skeletal muscle the subunits are both of the M type. The isozyme containing both M and B type subunits (MB) is found only in the myocardium. Other tissues contain variable amounts of the MM and BB isozymes. The isozymes are numbered beginning with the species migrating the fastest to the anode on electrophoresis—thus, CPK_1 (BB), CPK_2 (MB), and CPK_3 (MM).

Lactate dehydrogenase is a tetrameric enzyme containing only two distinct subunits: those designated H for heart (myocardium) and M for muscle. These two subunits are combined in five different ways. The lactate dehydrogenase isozymes, subunit compositions, and major locations are as follows:

Type	*Composition*	*Location*
LDH_1	HHHH	Myocardium and RBC
LDH_2	HHHM	Myocardium and RBC
LDH_3	HHMM	Brain and kidney
LDH_4	HMMM	
LDH_5	MMMM	Liver and skeletal muscle

To illustrate how kinetic analyses of plasma enzyme activities are useful in medicine, activities of some CPK and LDH isozymes are plotted in Figure 4.65 as a function of time after infarction. After damage to heart tissue the cellular breakup releases CPK_2 into the blood within the first 6–18 h after an infarct, but LDH release lags behind the appearance of CPK_2 by 1 to 2 days. Normally, the activity of the LDH_2 isozyme is higher than that of LDH_1; however, in the case of infarction the activity of LDH_1 becomes greater than LDH_2, at about the time CPK_2 levels are back to baseline (48–60 h). Figure 4.66 shows the fluctuations of all five LDH isozymes after an infarct. The increased ratio of LDH_2 and LDH_1 can be seen in the 24-h tracing. The LDH isozyme "switch" coupled with increased CPK_2 is diagnostic of myocardial infarct (MI) in virtually 100% of the cases. Increased activity of LDH_5 is an indicator of liver congestion. Thus secondary complications of heart failure can be monitored.

The electrophoresis method for determining cardiac enzymes is too slow and insensitive to be of value in the emergency room situation. ELISAs assays based on monoclonal antibodies to CPK_2 are both quick (30 min) and sensitive enough to detect CPK_2 in the serum within an hour or so of a heart attack.

Some Enzymes Are Used as Therapeutic Agents

In a few cases enzymes have been used as drugs in the therapy of specific medical problems. **Streptokinase,** an enzyme mixture prepared from a streptococcus, is useful in clearing blood clots that occur in myocardial infarcts and in the lower extremities. It activates the fibrinolytic proenzyme plasminogen that is normally present in plasma. The activated enzyme is plasmin. **Plasmin** is a serine protease that cleaves the insoluble fibrin in blood clots into several soluble components (see p. 975). Another serine protease, human **tissue plasminogen activator, t-PA,** is being commercially produced by bioengineered

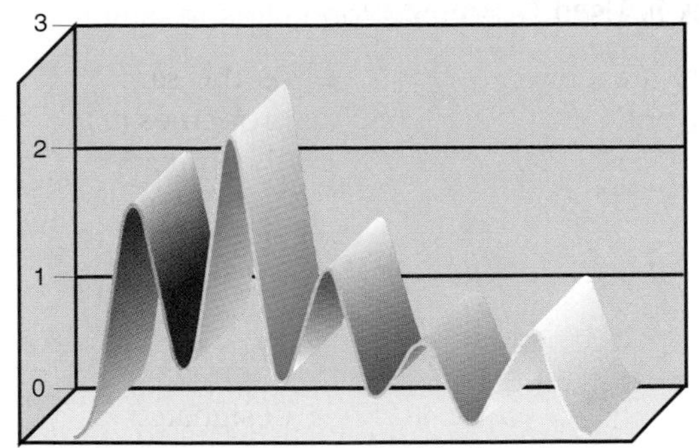

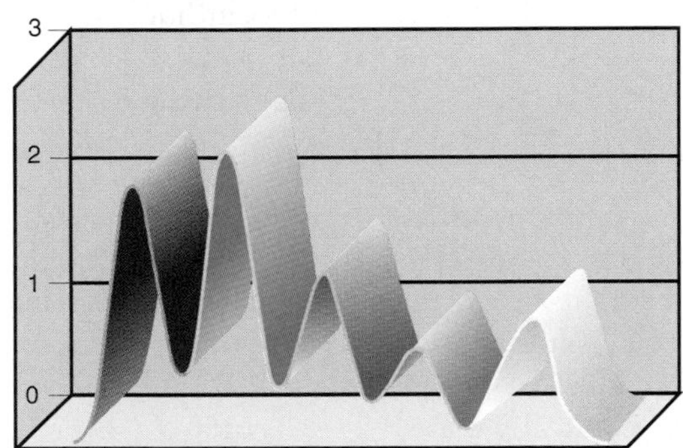

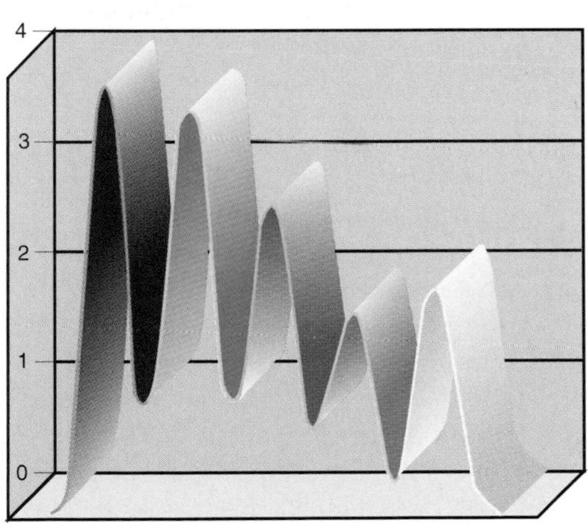

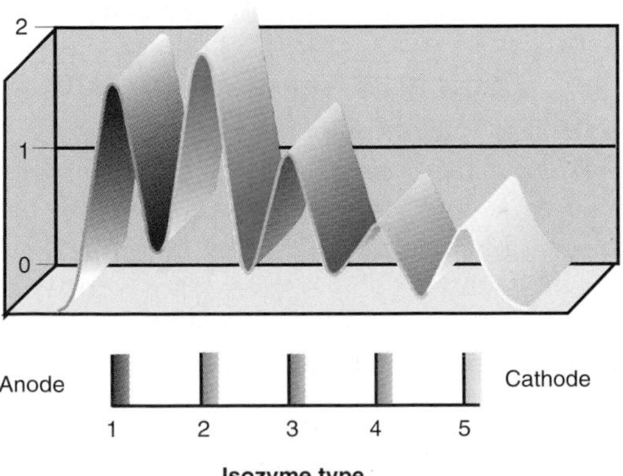

FIGURE 4.66
Tracings of densitometer scans of LDH isozymes at time intervals following a myocardial infarction. Total LDH increases and LDH_1 becomes greater than LDH_2 between 12 and 24 h. Increase in LDH_5 is diagnostic of a secondary congestive liver involvement. Note the Y axis scales are not identical. After electrophoresis on agarose gels, the LDH activity is assayed by measuring the fluorescence of the NADH formed in LDH-catalyzed reaction. *Courtesy of Dr. A. T. Gajda, Clinical Laboratories, The University of Arkansas for Medical Science.*

Escherichia coli (*E. coli*) for use in dissolving blood clots in patients suffering myocardial infarction (see p. 98). t-PA also functions by activating the patient's plasminogen.

Asparaginase therapy is used for some types of adult leukemia. Tumor cells have a requirement for asparagine and must scavenge it from the host's plasma. Intravenous (i.v.) administration of asparaginase lowers the host's plasma level of asparagine, which results in depressing the viability of the tumor.

Most enzymes have a short half-life in blood; consequently, unreasonably large amounts of enzyme are required to maintain therapeutic levels. Work is in progress to enhance enzyme stability by coupling enzymes to solid matrices and implanting these materials in areas that are well perfused. In the future, enzyme replacement in individuals that are genetically deficient in a particular enzyme may be feasible.

Enzymes Linked to Insoluble Matrices Are Used as Chemical Reactors

Specific enzymes linked to insoluble matrices are used in the pharmaceutical industry as highly specific chemical reactors. For example, immobilized β-galactosidase is used to decrease the lactose content of milk for lactose-intolerant people. In production of prednisolone, immobilized steroid 11-β-hydroxylase and a δ-1,2-dehydrogenase convert a cheap precursor to prednisolone in a rapid, stereospecific, and economical manner.

4.10 ■ REGULATION OF ENZYME ACTIVITY

Our discussion up to this point has centered on the chemical and physical characteristics of individual enzymes, but we must be concerned with the physiological integration of many enzymes into a metabolic pathway and the interrelationship of the products of one pathway with the metabolic activity of other pathways. Control of a pathway occurs through modulation of the activity of one or more key enzymes in the pathway. One of the key enzymes is the **rate-limiting** enzyme, which is the enzyme with the lowest V_{max}. It usually occurs early in the pathway. Another is that catalyzing the **committed step** of the pathway, the first irreversible reaction that is unique to a metabolic pathway. The rate-limiting enzyme is not necessarily the enzyme associated with the committed step. Specific examples of these regulatory enzymes will be pointed out in the sections on metabolism.

The activity of the enzyme associated with the committed step or with the rate-limiting step can be regulated in a number of ways. First, the absolute amount of the enzyme can be regulated by change in *de novo* synthesis of the enzyme. Second, the activity of the enzyme can be modulated by activators, by inhibitors, and by covalent modification through mechanisms previously discussed. Finally, the activity of a pathway can be regulated by physically partitioning the pathway from its initial substrate and by controlling access of the substrate to the enzymes of the pathway. This is referred to as **compartmentation.**

Anabolic and catabolic pathways are usually segregated into different organelles in order to maximize the cellular economy. There would be no point to oxidation of fatty acids occurring at the same time and in the same compartment as biosynthesis of fatty acids. If such occurred, a futile cycle would exist. By maintaining fatty acid biosynthesis in the cytoplasm and oxidation in the mitochondria, control can be exerted by regulating transport of common intermediates across the mitochondrial membrane. Table 1.6 (p. 15) contains a compilation of some of the metabolic pathways and their intracellular distribution.

As indicated earlier, the velocity of any reaction is dependent on the amount of enzyme present. Many rate-controlling enzymes are present in very low concentrations. More enzyme may be synthesized or existing rates of synthesis repressed through hormonally instituted activation of the mechanisms controlling gene expression. In some instances substrate can repress the synthesis of enzyme. For example, glucose represses the *de novo* synthesis of pyruvate carboxykinase, which is the rate-limiting enzyme in the conversion of pyruvate to glucose. If there is plenty of glucose available there is no point in synthesizing glucose. This effect of glucose may be mediated via insulin and is not direct feedback inhibition.

Many rate-controlling enzymes have relatively short half-lives; for example, that of pyruvate carboxykinase is 5 h. Teleologically this is reasonable because it provides a mechanism for effecting much larger fluctuations in the activity of a pathway than would be possible by inhibition or activation of existing levels of enzyme.

Short-term regulation occurs through modification of the activity of existing enzyme. For example, when the cellular concentration of deoxyribonucleotides builds up such that the cell has sufficient amounts for synthesis of DNA, the key enzyme of the synthetic pathway is inhibited by the end products, resulting in shutdown of the pathway. This is referred to as **feedback inhibition.** The inhibition may take the form of competitive inhibition or allosteric inhibition. In any case, the apparent K_m may be raised above the *in vivo* levels of substrate, and the reaction ceases or decreases in velocity.

In addition to feedback within the pathway, feedback on other pathways also occurs. This is referred to as **cross-regulation.** In cross-regulation a product of one pathway serves as an inhibitor or activator of an enzyme occurring early in another pathway as depicted in Figure 4.67. A good example, considered in detail in Chapter 12, is the cross-regulation of the production of the four deoxyribonucleotides for DNA synthesis.

An example of reversible covalent modification is glycogen phosphorylase, in which the interconvertible active and inactive forms are phosphorylated and dephosphorylated proteins, respectively. Protein kinases and protein phosphatases are also regulated by phosphorylation and dephosphorylation. Other examples of reversible covalent modification include acetylation–deacetylation, adenylylation–deadenylylation, uridylylation–deuridylylation, and methylation–demethylation.The phosphorylation-dephosphorylation scheme is most common.

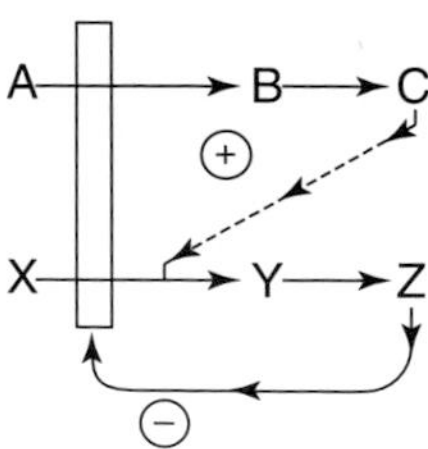

FIGURE 4.67
Model of feedback inhibition and cross-regulation.
Open bar indicates inhibition and broken line indicates activation. Product Z cross-regulates production of C by its inhibitory effect on the enzyme responsible for the conversion of A to B in the A → B pathway. C in turn cross-regulates the production of Z. The product Z inhibits its own formation by feedback inhibition of the conversion of X to Y.

BIBLIOGRAPHY

Blackburn, G. M., Kang, A. S., Kingsbury, G. A., and Burton, D. R. Review of abzymes. *Biochem. J.* 262:381, 1989.

Boyer, P. D. (Ed.). *The Enzymes,* 3rd ed. (28 vols.). New York: Academic Press, 1970–1987.

Dixon, M., and Webb, E. C. *Enzymes,* 3rd ed. New York: Academic Press, 1979.

Fersht, A. *Enzyme Structure and Mechanism,* 2nd ed. New York: Freeman, 1985.

Kyte, J. *Mechanism in Protein Chemistry*. New York: Garland Publishing, 1995.

Keffer, J. H. Myocardial Markers of Injury. *Am. J. Clin. Path.* 105:305, 1996.

Knowles, J. R., and Alberty, W. J. Evolution of enzyme function and the development of catalytic efficiency. *Biochemistry* 15:5631, 1976.

Kraut, J. How do enzymes work? *Science* 242:533, 1988.

Lerner, R. A., Benkovic, S. J., and Schultz. P. G. At the crossroads of chemistry and immunology: catalytic antibodies. *Science* 252:659, 1991.

Lolis, E., and Petsko, G. A. Transition-state analogues in protein crystallography: probes of the structural source of enzyme catalysis. *Annu. Rev. Biochem*. 59:597,1990.

Meister, A. (Ed.). *Advances in Enzymology*. New York: Wiley-Interscience, issued annually.

Neurath, H. Evolution of proteolytic enzymes. *Science* 234:350, 1984.

Page, M. I. and Williams, A. (Eds.). *Enzyme Mechanisms*. London: Royal Society of Chemistry, 1987.

Richardson, C. C. (Ed.). *Annual Reviews of Biochemistry*. Palo Alto, CA: Annual Reviews, issued annually.

Segel, I. H. *Enzyme Kinetics*. New York: Wiley, 1975.

Walsh, C. *Enzyme Reaction Mechanisms*. New York: Freeman. 1979.

Weber, G. (Ed.). *Advances in Enzyme Regulation,* Elmsford, NY: Pergamon, issued annually.

QUESTIONS ■ J. BAGGOTT AND C. N. ANGSTADT

1. In all enzymes the active site:
   A. contains the substrate-binding site.
   B. is contiguous with the substrate-binding site in the primary sequence.
   C. lies in a region of the primary sequence distant from the substrate-binding site.
   D. contains a metal ion as a prosthetic group.
   E. contains the amino acid side chains involved in catalyzing the reaction.

2. Which of the following types of oxidoreductase enzymes usually form hydrogen peroxide (H_2O_2) as one of their products?
   A. dehydrogenases
   B. oxidases
   C. oxygenases
   D. peroxidases
   E. none of the above

3. The following reaction is catalyzed by:

$$\mathrm{HO{-}C(CH_2{-}COOH)_2{-}COOH} + \mathrm{CoA{-}SH} \rightleftharpoons \mathrm{HOOC{-}CH_2{-}\overset{O}{\overset{\|}{C}}{-}COOH} + \mathrm{CH_3{-}\overset{O}{\overset{\|}{C}}{-}S{-}CoA} + \mathrm{H_2O}$$

   A. an oxidoreductase.
   B. a transferase.
   C. a hydrolase.
   D. a lyase.
   E. a ligase.

4. In the enzyme-catalyzed reaction

$$2\ \mathrm{A} + \mathrm{B} \rightleftharpoons \mathrm{B} + \text{products}$$

   where B is the enzyme, when the concentration of A is very high the reaction order is:
   A. zero order.
   B. first order.
   C. second order.
   D. third order.
   E. a fractional order between first and second.

5. Although enzymic catalysis is reversible, a given reaction may appear irreversible:
   A. if the products are thermodynamically far more stable than the reactants.
   B. under equilibrium conditions.
   C. if a product accumulates.
   D. at high enzyme concentrations.
   E. at high temperatures.

6. K_m of an enzyme is always:
   A. one-half of the V_{max}.
   B. a dissociation constant.
   C. the normal physiological substrate concentration.
   D. the substrate concentration that gives half-maximal velocity.
   E. numerically identical for all isozymes that catalyze a given reaction.

7. Cofactors containing the adenosyl group include all of the following EXCEPT:
   A. ATP.
   B. NAD.
   C. NADP.
   D. FAD.
   E. FMN.

8. Which of the following inhibitor types can be expected to change the K_m of an enzyme but not its V_{max}?
   A. competitive
   B. noncompetitive
   C. uncompetitive
   D. irreversible
   E. V class allosteric

9. Metal cations may do all of the following EXCEPT:
   A. donate electron pairs to functional groups found in the primary structure of the enzyme protein.
   B. serve as Lewis acids in enzymes.
   C. participate in oxidation–reduction processes.
   D. stabilize the active conformation of an enzyme.
   E. form chelates with the substrate, with the chelate being the true substrate.

10. Drugs that act as enzyme inhibitors:
    A. may function as competitive inhibitors.
    B. are clinically useful only when directed against an enzyme unique to a cell that is to be killed.
    C. unlike antibiotics, are free of the danger of drug resistance.
    D. must be harmless to the patient.
    E. generally mimic the three-dimensional structure of the enzyme's active site.

11. Enzymes may be specific with respect to all of the following EXCEPT:
    A. chemical identity of the substrate.
    B. the atomic mass of the elements in the reactive group (e.g., ^{12}C but not ^{14}C).
    C. optical activity of product formed from a symmetrical substrate.
    D. type of reaction catalyzed.
    E. which of a pair of optical isomers will react.

12. All of the following can be chemically isolated EXCEPT:
    A. enzymes.
    B. enzyme–substrate complexes.
    C. enzyme–inhibitor complexes.
    D. enzyme–substrate covalent intermediates.
    E. transition states.

13. Which of the following necessarily results in formation of an enzyme–substrate intermediate?
    A. substrate strain
    B. acid–base catalysis
    C. entropy effects
    D. allosteric regulation
    E. covalent catalysis

14. An enzyme with histidyl residues that participate in both general acid and general base catalysis would be most likely to have a pH–activity profile resembling which curve on the following drawing?

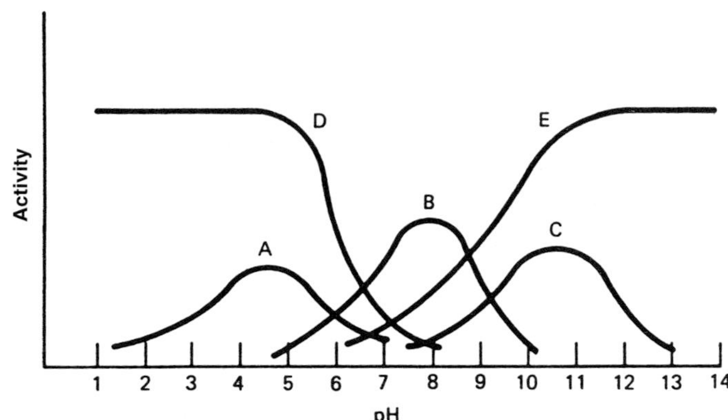

A. Curve A
B. Curve B
C. Curve C
D. Curve D
E. Curve E

15. In the reaction sequence below the best point for controlling production of Compound 6 is reaction:

Cpd 3 ⇅ (B)
Cpd 1 —A→ Cpd 2 ⇌(C) Cpd 4 —D→ Cpd 5 ⇌(E) Cpd 6

A. A.
B. B.
C. C.
D. D.
E. E.

16. If the plasma activity of an intracellular enzyme is abnormally high, all of the following may be a valid explanation EXCEPT:
A. the rate of removal of the enzyme from plasma may be depressed.
B. tissue damage may have occurred.
C. the enzyme may have been activated.
D. determination of the isozyme distribution may yield useful information.
E. the rate of synthesis of the enzyme may have increased.

17. Types of physiological regulation of enzyme activity include all of the following EXCEPT:
A. covalent modification.
B. changes in rate of synthesis of the enzyme.
C. allosteric activation.
D. suicide inhibition.
E. competitive inhibition.

ANSWERS

1. E The active site contains all the machinery, including the amino acid side chains, involved in catalyzing the reaction. A–D are all possible, but none is necessarily true (p. 129).
2. B Most oxidases produce H_2O_2 as a product of the transfer of two electrons from the donor to oxygen. Typical oxidases are flavoenzymes; the cytochrome oxidase complex is a striking exception (p. 129).
3. D This is an unusually complicated lyase reaction, since secondary reactions are involved. It is a lyase because it removes a group (the acetyl group) with formation of a double bond (the C=O bond of the C4 product, oxalacetate). The common name of this enzyme is citrate synthase (p. 132).
4. A At very high concentration of substrate the enzyme is saturated, and the rate of the reaction is independent of reactant (A) concentration. One could argue that the reaction rate depends on enzyme concentration, but in this situation, where enzyme is regenerated, the system would follow a zero-order rate law (p. 136).
5. A Stable products do not react in the reverse direction at an appreciable rate (p. 135). At equilibrium the forward and reverse reactions proceed at identical rates. Product accumulation would tend to reverse the reaction. Enzymes merely catalyze reactions and do not affect the equilibrium of the reaction (p. 128). Temperature affects the rates of reactions, and may also affect the position of the equilibrium, but does not interconvert reversible and irreversible reactions (p. 135).
6. D This is the experimental definition of K_m. The value can be interpreted as a dissociation constant under certain conditions (p. 139), and often it makes sense that K_m be within the physiological range of substrate concentrations (p. 138).
7. E The A in ATP, NAD, NADP, and FAD refers to an adenylate moiety. It is curious that all these different cofactors incorporate the same group, a group that plays no role in the catalytic process. Presumably its role is in cofactor binding (p. 143).
8. A In the presence of a competitive inhibitor the same V_{max} can be reached, but only if the substrate concentration is increased sufficiently. Effectors of K class allosteric enzymes act like competitive inhibitors, changing K_m but not V_{max}; the opposite is true of V class enzymes (pp. 145 and 152).
9. A Metal cations are electron deficient and may accept electron pairs, serving as Lewis acids, but they do not donate electrons to other functional groups. On the contrary, they sometimes accept electron pairs from groups in amino acid side chains. In doing so they may become chelated (p. 143). Sometimes they are chelated by the substrate, with the chelate being the true substrate (p. 144).
10. A Drugs may serve as competitive inhibitors, such as sulfanilamide (p. 149), or as irreversible inhibitors, such as fluorouracil (p. 151). Pathways unique to pathogenic bacteria, viruses, and so on are rare, so drugs are often developed that are merely less harmful to the host than the target cell because of differences in cell permeability, metabolic rate, and so on (p. 149). Drug resistance can arise through gene amplification in the patient; this can occur with methotrexate (p. 150). Methotrexate is also an example of a drug that is toxic to the patient and must be used with care. Enzyme inhibitors do

not mimic the structure of the active site; rather, they often complement it (p. 156), so that they bind in place of the substrate (p. 148).

11. B Enzymes are specific for the substrate and the type of reaction (p. 154). The asymmetry of the binding site generally permits only one of a pair of optical isomers to react, and only one optical isomer is generated when a symmetric substrate yields an asymmetric product (p. 155). Enzymes do not distinguish among different nuclides of an element, although the rate of reaction of a heavier nuclide might be less than that of a lighter one.

12. E The transition state is not an intermediate and cannot be isolated (p. 159). Rather, it can be thought of as a state in which old bonds are partly broken and new bonds partly formed. All the other species (A–D) can be isolated under suitable experimental conditions.

13. E All enzyme-catalyzed reactions involve an enzyme–substrate complex. There is always at least one transition state involved, but only in covalent catalysis is a covalent bond between enzyme and a portion of the substrate involved (p. 163).

14. B A group must be in the correct ionization state to act catalytically. For a histidyl group to serve as a general acid and a general base (as it does in chymotrypsin), the pH must be compatible with both ionization states of histidine. Since the p*K* of the histidyl side chain is about 6.8, the maximum activity is likely to be near that pH. Chymotrypsin's pH optimum is in the 7–9 range (pp. 160 and 166).

15. D Control of reaction A would control production of Cpd 3 and Cpd 6. Reaction B is not on the direct route. Reaction C is freely reversible, so it does not need to be controlled. Reaction D is irreversible; if it were not controlled, Cpd 5 might build up to toxic levels (p. 174).

16. E Intracellular enzymes may appear in abnormal amounts when tissues are damaged. Different tissues have characteristic distributions of isozymes. Since appearance of intracellular enzymes in plasma arises from leakage, typically from damaged or destroyed cells, changes in their rates of synthesis within the cell would not be expected to affect plasma concentration (p. 166).

17. D Covalent modification includes zymogen activation and phospho–dephospho protein conversions (p. 175). Enzyme levels may be controlled (p. 174). Allosteric activation is common. End products of a reaction or reaction sequence may inhibit their own formation by competitive inhibition (p. 140). Suicide inhibitors are sometimes used as drugs (p. 150).

CHAPTER

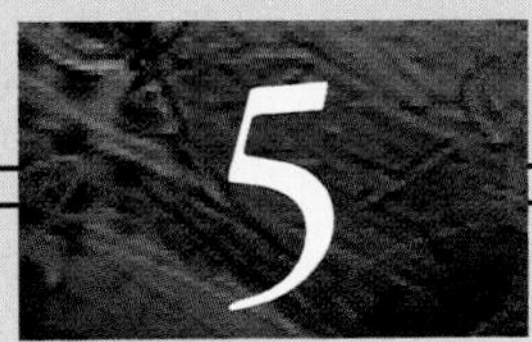

BIOLOGICAL MEMBRANES: STRUCTURE AND MEMBRANE TRANSPORT

Thomas M. Devlin

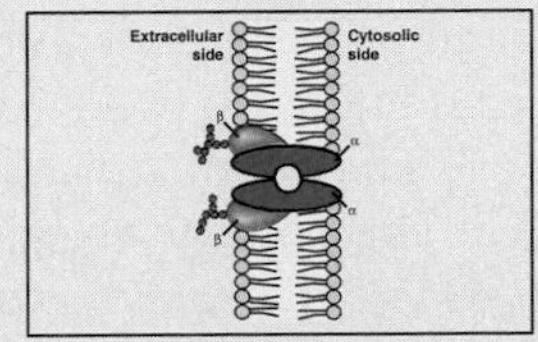

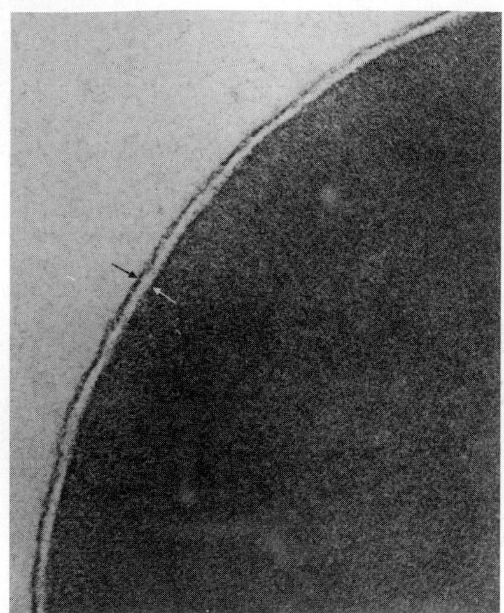

FIGURE 5.1
Electron micrograph of the erythrocyte plasma membrane showing the trilaminar appearance.
A clear space separates the two electron-dense lines. Electron microscopy has demonstrated that the inner dense line is frequently thicker than the outer line. Magnification about ×150,000.
Courtesy of Dr. J. D. Robertson, Duke University, Durham, North Carolina.

5.1 ■ OVERVIEW

Biological membranes from either eukaryotic or prokaryotic cells have the same classes of chemical components, a similarity in structural organization, and many properties in common. There are major differences in specific lipid, protein, and carbohydrate components but not in physicochemical interaction of these molecules. Membranes have a trilaminar appearance when viewed by electron microscopy (Figure 5.1), with two dark bands on each side of a light band. The overall width of most mammalian membranes is 7–10 nm but some have significantly smaller widths. Intracellular membranes are usually thinner than plasma membranes. Many do not appear symmetrical, with an inner dense layer often thicker than an outer dense layer; there is a chemical asymmetry of membranes. With development of sophisticated techniques for preparation of tissue samples and staining, including negative staining and freeze fracturing, surfaces of membranes have been viewed; at the molecular level surfaces are not smooth but dotted with protruding globular-shaped masses.

Membranes are very dynamic structures with a movement that permits cells as well as subcellular structures to adjust their shapes and to change position. Chemical components of membranes, that is, lipids and protein, are ideally suited for their dynamic role. Membranes are an organized sea of lipid in a fluid state, a nonaqueous compartment of cells, in which various components are able to move and interact.

Cellular membranes control the composition of space that they enclose by excluding a variety of molecules and by selective transport systems allowing movement of specific molecules from one side to the other. These transporters are proteins. By controlling translocation of substrates, cofactors, ions, and so on, membranes modulate the concentration of substances in cellular compartments, thereby exerting an influence on metabolic pathways. Hormones, and growth and metabolic regulators bind to specific protein receptors on plasma membranes (Chapter 20) and the information to be imparted to the cell is transmitted by the membrane component to the appropriate metabolic pathway by a series of intracellular intermediates, termed second messengers. Plasma membranes of eukaryotic cells also have a role in cell–cell recognition, maintenance of the shape of cells, and cell locomotion.

The discussion that follows is directed to the chemistry and transport functions of membranes primarily of mammalian cells but the observations and activities described are applicable to all biological membranes.

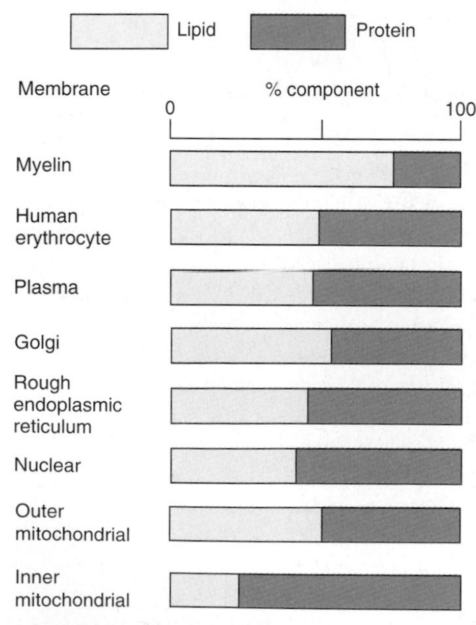

FIGURE 5.2
Representative values for the percentage of lipid and protein in various cellular membranes.
Values are for rat liver, except for the myelin and human erythrocyte plasma membrane. Values for liver from other species, including human, indicate a similar pattern.

5.2 ■ CHEMICAL COMPOSITION OF MEMBRANES

Lipids and proteins are the two major components of all membranes. The amount of each varies greatly between different membranes (Figure 5.2). Protein ranges from about 20% in the myelin sheath to over 70% in the inner membrane of the mitochondria. Intracellular membranes have a high percentage of protein because of the large number of enzymic activities of these membranes. Membranes also contain a small amount of various polysaccharides in the form of glycoprotein and glycolipid; there is no free carbohydrate in membranes.

Lipids Are a Major Component of Membranes

The three major lipid components of eukaryotic cell membranes are glycerophospholipids, sphingolipids, and cholesterol. Glycerophospholipids and sphingomyelin, a sphingolipid containing phosphate, are classified as **phospholipids.** Bacteria and blue-green algae contain glycerolipids where a carbohydrate is attached directly to the glycerol. Individual cellular membranes also contain small quantities of other lipids, such as triacylglycerol and diol derivatives (see the Appendix).

Glycerophospholipids Are the Most Abundant Lipids of Membranes

Glycerophospholipids (phosphoglycerides) have a glycerol molecule as the basic component to which phosphoric acid is esterified at the α carbon (Figure 5.3) and two long-chain fatty acids are esterified at the remaining carbon atoms (Figure 5.4). Glycerol does not contain an asymmetric carbon, but the α-carbon atoms are not stereochemically identical. Esterification of a phosphate to an α carbon makes the molecule asymmetric. The naturally occurring glycerophospholipids are designated by the stereospecific numbering system (*sn*)(Figure 5.3) discussed on p. 397.

1,2-Diacylglycerol 3-phosphate, **phosphatidic acid,** is the parent compound of a series of glycerophospholipids, where different hydroxyl-containing compounds are esterified to the phosphate. The major compounds attached by a phosphodiester bridge to glycerol are choline, ethanolamine, serine, glycerol, and inositol. These structures are presented in Figure 5.5. **Phosphatidylethanolamine** (ethanolamine glycerophospholipids or the trivial name cephalin) and **phosphatidylcholine** (choline glycerophospholipid or lecithin) are the most common glycerophospholipids in membranes (Figure 5.6). **Phosphatidylglycerol phosphoglyceride** (Figure 5.7) (diphosphatidylglycerol or cardiolipin) contains two phosphatidic acids linked by a glycerol and is found nearly exclusively in mitochondrial inner membranes and bacterial membranes.

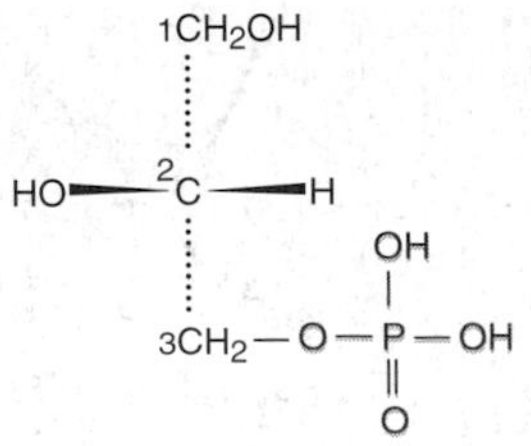

$$\begin{array}{c} {}^{1}CH_2OH \\ \vdots \\ HO-{}^{2}C-H \\ \vdots \\ {}^{3}CH_2-O-\underset{\underset{O}{\|}}{\overset{\overset{OH}{|}}{P}}-OH \end{array}$$

FIGURE 5.3
Stereochemical configuration of L-glycerol 3-phosphate (*sn*-glycerol 3-phosphate).
The H and OH attached to C-2 are above and C-1 and C-3 are below the plane of the page.

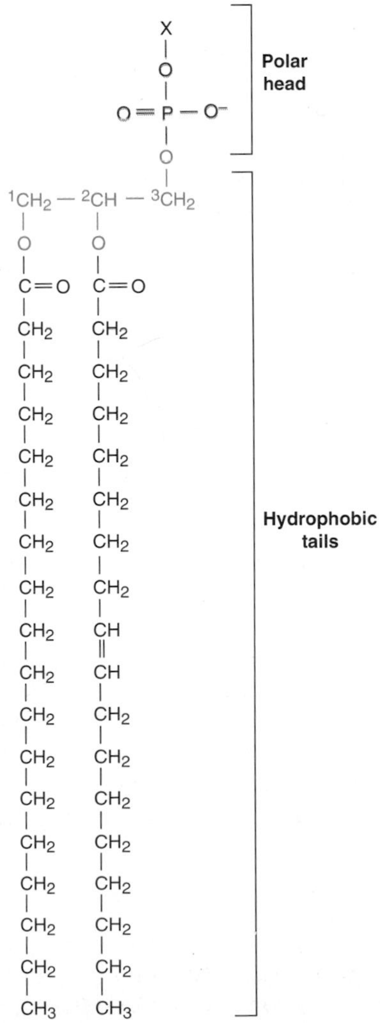

Polar head: X–O–P(=O)(O⁻)–O–

$^{1}CH_2-{}^{2}CH-{}^{3}CH_2$; C-1 and C-2 each –O–C(=O)–(CH₂)ₙ–CH₃

Hydrophobic tails

FIGURE 5.4
Structure of glycerophospholipid.
Long-chain fatty acids are esterified at C-1 and C-2 of the L-glycerol 3-phosphate. X can be a H (phosphatidic acid) or one of several alcohols presented in Figure 5.5.

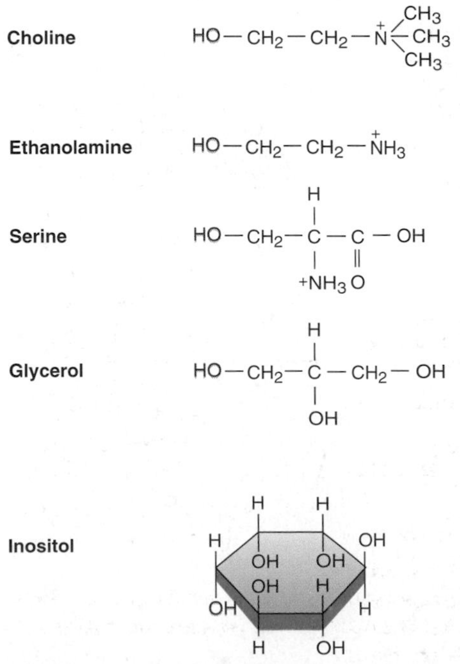

Choline	$HO-CH_2-CH_2-\overset{+}{N}(CH_3)_3$
Ethanolamine	$HO-CH_2-CH_2-\overset{+}{N}H_3$
Serine	$HO-CH_2-CH(^{+}NH_3)-C(=O)-OH$
Glycerol	$HO-CH_2-CH(OH)-CH_2-OH$
Inositol	(ring structure)

FIGURE 5.5
Structures of the major alcohols esterified to phosphatidic acid to form the glycerophospholipid.

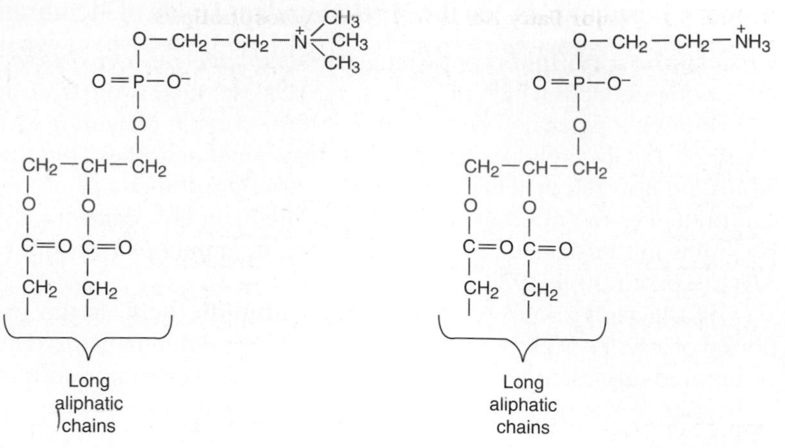

Phosphatidylcholine   Phosphatidylethanolamine

FIGURE 5.6
Structures of the two most common glycerophospholipids—phosphatidylcholine and phosphatidylethanolamine.

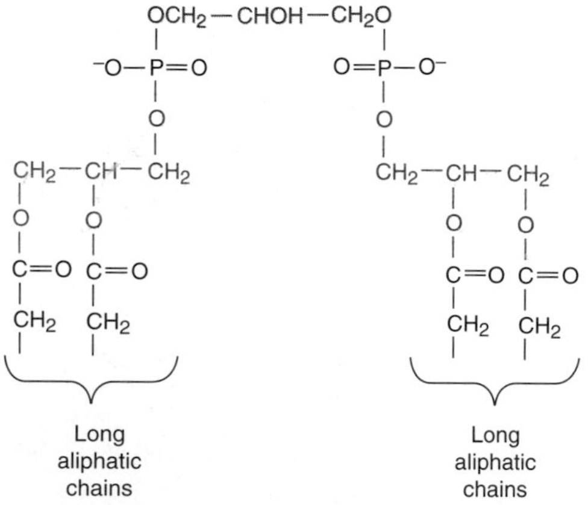

FIGURE 5.7
Phosphatidylglycerol phosphoglyceride (cardiolipin).

Inositol, a hexahydroxy alcohol, is esterified to phosphate in phosphatidylinositol (Figure 5.8). 4-Phospho- and **4,5-bisphosphoinositol glycerophospholipids** (Figure 5.8) are present in plasma membranes; the latter is the source of **inositol trisphosphate** and diacylglycerol that are involved in hormone action (see p. 865).

Glycerophospholipids contain two fatty acyl groups esterified to carbon atoms 1 and 2 of glycerol; some of the major fatty acids found in glycerophospholipids are presented in Table 5.1. A saturated fatty acid is usually found on C-1 of the glycerol and an unsaturated fatty acid on C-2. Designation of different glycerophospholipids does not specify which fatty acids are present. Phosphatidylcholine usually contains palmitic or stearic in the *sn*-1 position and a C18 unsaturated fatty acid, oleic, linoleic, or linolenic, on the *sn*-2 carbon. Phosphatidylethanolamine contains palmitic or oleic on *sn*-1 but a long-chain polyunsaturated fatty acid, such as arachidonic, on the *sn*-2 position.

A saturated fatty acid is a straight chain, as is a fatty acid with an unsaturation in the *trans* position. A *cis* double bond, however, creates a kink in the hydrocar-

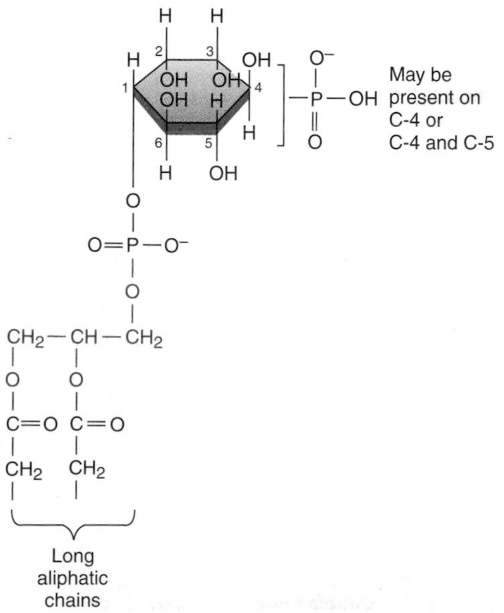

FIGURE 5.8
Phosphatidylinositol.
Phosphate groups are also found on C-4 or C-4 and C-5 of the inositol. The additional phosphate groups increase the charge on the polar head of this glycerophospholipid.

TABLE 5.1 Major Fatty Acids in Glycerophospholipids

Common Name	Systematic Name	Structural Formula
Myristic acid	*n*-Tetradecanoic	$CH_3-(CH_2)_{12}-COOH$
Palmitic acid	*n*-Hexadecanoic	$CH_3-(CH_2)_{14}-COOH$
Palmitoleic acid	*cis*-9-Hexadecenoic	$CH_3-(CH_2)_5-CH=CH-(CH_2)_7-COOH$
Stearic acid	*n*-Octadecanoic	$CH_3-(CH_2)_{16}-COOH$
Oleic acid	*cis*-9-Octadecenoic acid	$CH_3-(CH_2)_7-CH=CH-(CH_2)_7-COOH$
Linoleic acid	*cis,cis*-9,12-Octadecadienoic	$CH_3-(CH_2)_3-(CH_2-CH=CH)_2-(CH_2)_7-COOH$
Linolenic acid	*cis,cis,cis*-9,12,15-Octadecatrienoic	$CH_3-(CH_2-CH=CH)_3-(CH_2)_7-COOH$
Arachidonic acid	*cis,cis,cis,cis*-5,8,11,14-Icosatetraenoic	$CH_3-(CH_2)_3-(CH_2-CH=CH)_4-(CH_2)_3-COOH$

bon chain (Figure 5.9). A straight chain diagram, as shown in Figures 5.4 and 5.9, does not adequately represent the chemical configuration of a long-chain fatty acid. Actually, there is a high degree of coiling of the hydrocarbon chain in a glycerophospholipid that is disrupted by a double bond. The presence of unsaturated fatty acids has a marked effect on the physicochemical state of the membrane (see p. 195).

Glycerol ether phospholipids contain a long aliphatic chain in ether linkage to the glycerol at the *sn*-1 position (Figure 5.10). Ether phospholipids contain an alkyl group (alkyl acylglycerophospholipid) or an α, β-unsaturated ether, termed a **plasmalogen.** The latter groups are more prevalent in membranes. Plasmalogens containing ethanolamine (ethanolamine plasmalogen) and choline (choline plasmalogen) esterified to the phosphate are abundant in nervous tissue and heart but not in liver. In human hearts more than 50% of the ethanolamine glycerophospholipids are plasmalogens.

Glycerophospholipids are **amphipathic,** containing both a polar end, or head group, due to the charged phosphate and substitutions on the phosphate, and a nonpolar tail due to hydrophobic hydrocarbon chains of the fatty acyl

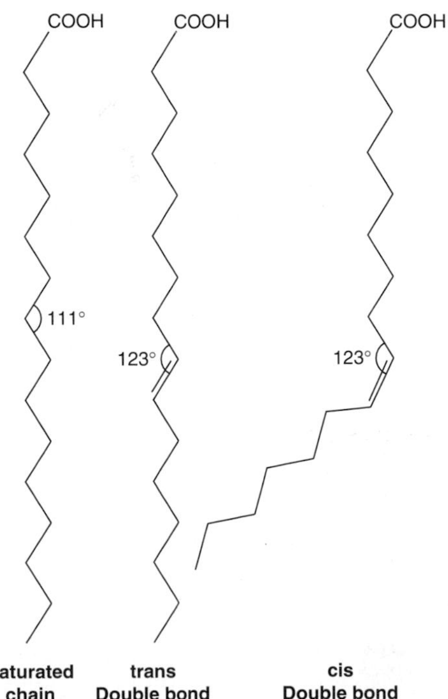

FIGURE 5.9
Conformation of fatty acyl groups in phospholipids.
The saturated and unsaturated fatty acids with trans double bonds are straight chains in their minimum energy conformation, whereas a chain with a cis double bond has a bend. The trans double bond is rare in naturally occurring fatty acids.

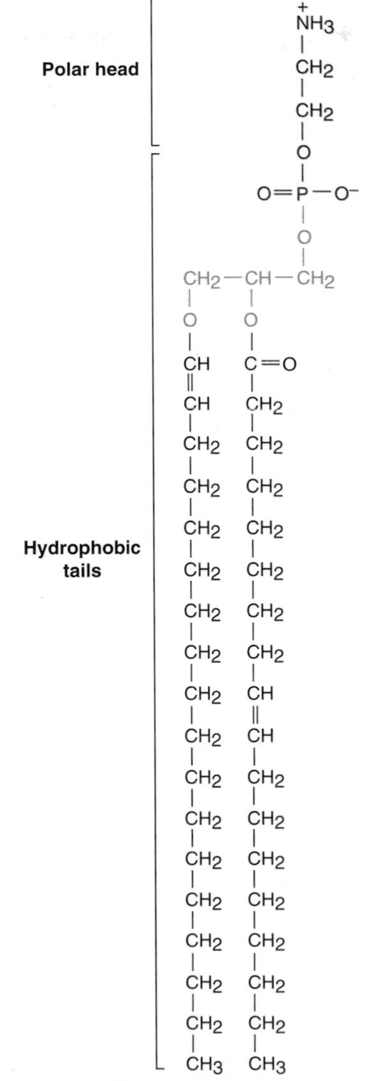

FIGURE 5.10
Ethanolamine plasmalogen.
Note the ether linkage of the aliphatic chain on C-1 of glycerol.

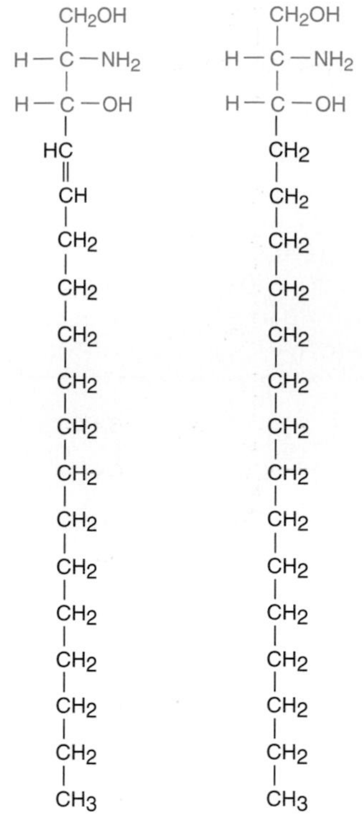

Sphingosine (D-4-sphingenine) Dihydrosphingosine (D-sphingenine)

FIGURE 5.11
Structures of sphingosine and dihydrosphingosine.

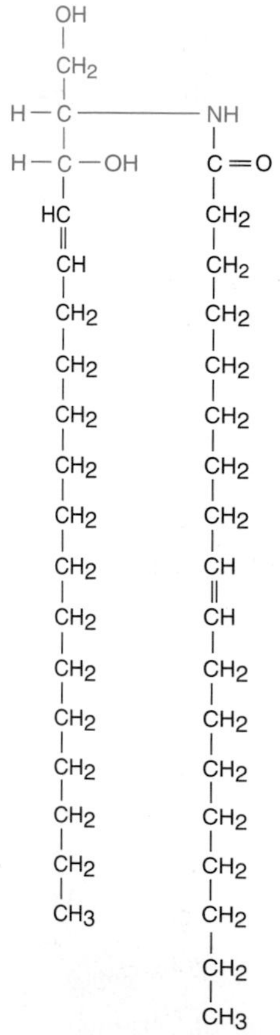

FIGURE 5.12
Structure of a ceramide.

TABLE 5.2 Predominant Charge on Glycerophospholipids and Sphingomyelin at pH 7.0

Lipid	*Phosphate Group*	*Base*	*Net Charge*
Phosphatidylcholine	−1	+1	0
Phosphatidylethanolamine	−1	+1	0
Phosphatidylserine	−1	+1, −1	−1
Phosphatidylglycerol	−1	0	−1
Diphosphatidylglycerol (cardiolipin)	−2	0	−2
Phosphatidylinositol	−1	0	−1
Sphingomyelin	−1	+1	0

groups. The polar groups are charged at pH 7.0 with a negative charge due to ionization of the phosphate group (p$K \approx 2$) and charges from groups esterified to phosphate (Table 5.2). Choline and ethanolamine glycerophospholipids are zwitterions at pH 7.0, with both a negative charge from phosphate and a positive charge on nitrogen. Phosphatidylserine has two negative charges, one on phosphate and one on the carboxyl group of serine, and a positive charge on the α-amino group of serine, with a net charge of −1 at pH 7.0. In contrast, glycerophospholipids containing inositol and glycerol have only a single negative charge on phosphate; 4-phospho- and 4,5-bisphosphoinositol derivatives are very polar compounds with additional negative charges on the phosphate groups.

Every tissue and cellular membrane has a distinctive composition of glycerophospholipids and a definite pattern in fatty acid composition. There is a greater variability in the fatty acyl groups of different tissues in a single species than in the fatty acyl groups of the same tissue in a variety of species. In addition, the fatty acid content of the glycerophospholipids can vary, depending on the physiological or pathophysiological state of the tissue.

Sphingolipids Are Also Present in Membranes

The amino alcohols **sphingosine** (D-4-sphingenine) and **dihydrosphingosine** (Figure 5.11) are the basis for another series of membrane lipids, the **sphingolipids.** A **ceramide** is sphingosine with a saturated or unsaturated long-chain fatty acyl group in amide linkage on the amino group (Figure 5.12). With two nonpolar tails a ceramide is similar in structure to diacylglycerol. Various substitutions are found on the hydroxyl group at position 1. The sphingomyelin series has phosphorylcholine esterified to the 1-OH (Figure 5.13) and is the most abundant sphingolipid in mammalian tissues. The similarity of this structure to choline glycerophospholipids is apparent, and they have many properties in common; note that the sphingomyelins are amphipathic compounds with a charged head group. Sphingomyelins and glycerophospholipids are classified as phospholipids. The sphingomyelin of myelin contains predominantly the longer chain fatty acids, with carbon lengths of 24; as with glycerophospholipids, there is a specific fatty acid composition of the sphingomyelin, depending on the tissue.

Glycosphingolipids do not contain phosphate and have a sugar attached by a β-glycosidic linkage to the 1-OH group of the sphingosine in a ceramide. One subgroup is the **cerebrosides,** which contain either a glucose **(glucocerebrosides)** or galactose **(galactocerebrosides)** attached to a ceramide (Figure 5.14). Cerebrosides are neutral compounds. Galactocerebrosides are found predominantly in brain and nervous tissue, whereas the small quantities of cerebrosides in nonneural tissues usually contain glucose. **Phrenosin,** a specific galactocerebroside, contains a 2-OH C_{24} fatty acid. Galactocerebrosides may contain a sulfate group esterified on the 3 position of the sugar. They are called **sulfatides** (Figure 5.15). Cerebrosides and sulfatides usually contain fatty acids with 22–26 carbon atoms.

In place of monosaccharides, neutral glycosphingolipids often have 2 (dihexosides), 3 (trihexosides), or 4 (tetrahexosides) sugar residues attached to the 1-OH group of sphingosine. Diglucose, digalactose, *N*-acetylglucosamine, and *N*-acetyldigalactosamine are the usual sugars.

The most complex group of glycosphingolipids, the **gangliosides,** contain oligosaccharide head groups with one or more residues of sialic acid; these are amphipathic compounds with a negative charge at pH 7.0. The gangliosides represent 5–8% of the total lipids in brain, and some 20 different types have been identified differing in the number and relative position of the hexose and sialic acid residues. This is the basis of their classification; a detailed description of the nomenclature and structures of gangliosides is presented on p. 426.

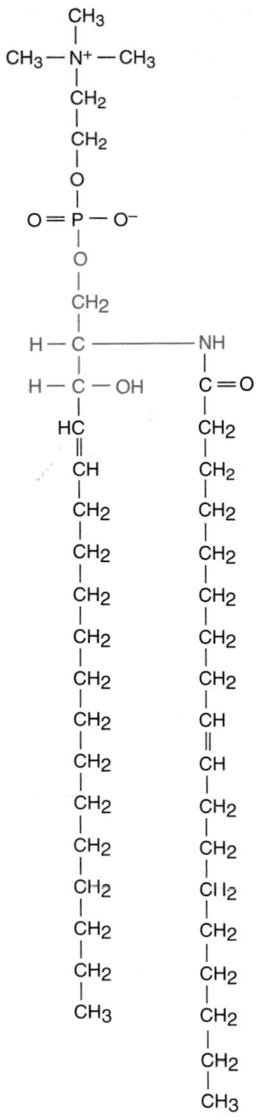

FIGURE 5.13
Structure of a choline containing sphingomyelin.

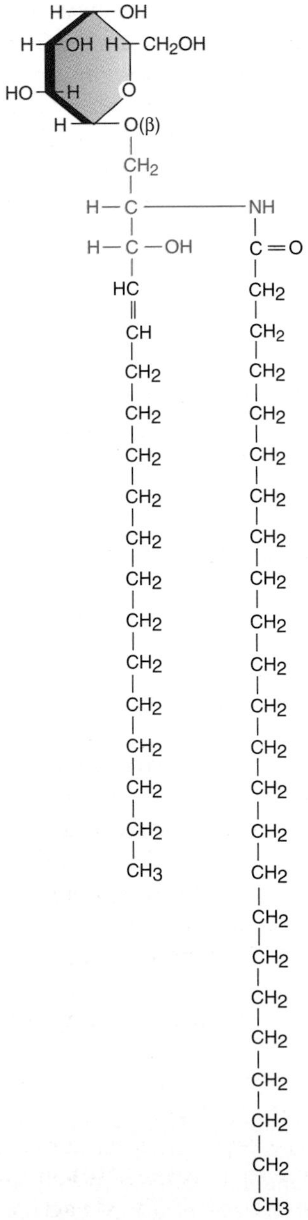

FIGURE 5.14
Structure of a galactocerebroside containing a C24 fatty acid.

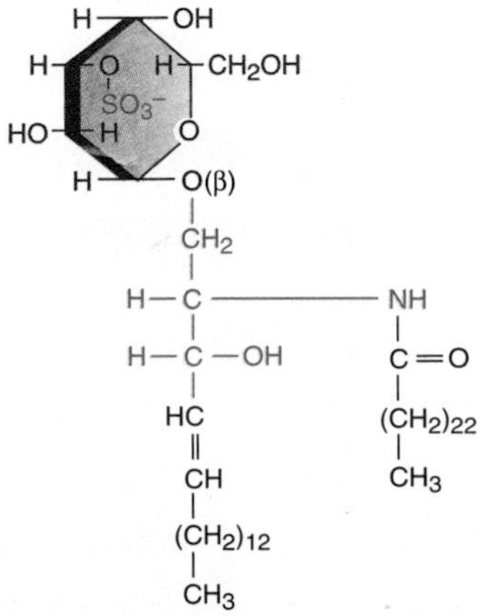

FIGURE 5.15
Structure of a sulfatide.

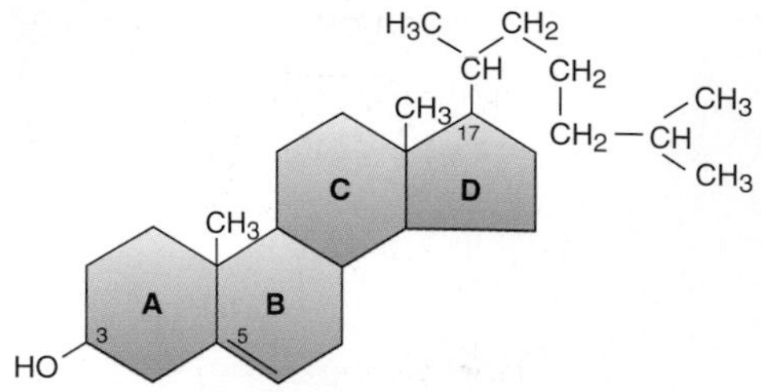

FIGURE 5.16
Structure of cholesterol.

Most Membranes Contain Cholesterol

Cholesterol is the third major lipid in membranes. With four fused rings and an eight-member branched hydrocarbon chain attached to the D ring at position 17, cholesterol is a compact, rigid, hydrophobic molecule (Figure 5.16). It also has a polar hydroxyl group at C-3.

Lipid Composition Varies in Different Membranes

There are quantitative differences between the classes of lipids and individual lipids in various cell membranes (Figure 5.17). The lipid composition is very similar in the same intracellular membrane of a specific tissue in different species. The plasma membrane exhibits the greatest variation in percentage composition because the amount of cholesterol is affected by the nutritional state of the animal. Plasma membranes have the highest concentration of neutral lipids and sphingolipids; myelin membranes of axons of neural tissue are rich in sphingolipids, with a high proportion of glycosphingolipids. Intracellular membranes primarily contain glycerophospholipids with little sphingolipids or cholesterol. The membrane lipid composition of mitochondria, nuclei, and rough endoplasmic reticulum are similar, with Golgi membrane being somewhere between other intracellular membranes and the plasma membrane. As indicated previously, cardiolipin is found nearly exclusively in the inner mitochondrial membrane. Choline containing lipids, phosphatidylcholine, and sphingomyelin, are predominant, with ethanolamine glycerophospholipid second. The constancy of composition of various membranes indicates the relationship between lipids and the specific functions of individual membranes.

Membrane Proteins Are Classified Based on Their Ease of Removal

Membrane proteins are classified on the basis of ease of removal from isolated membrane fractions. **Peripheral (or extrinsic) proteins** are released from a

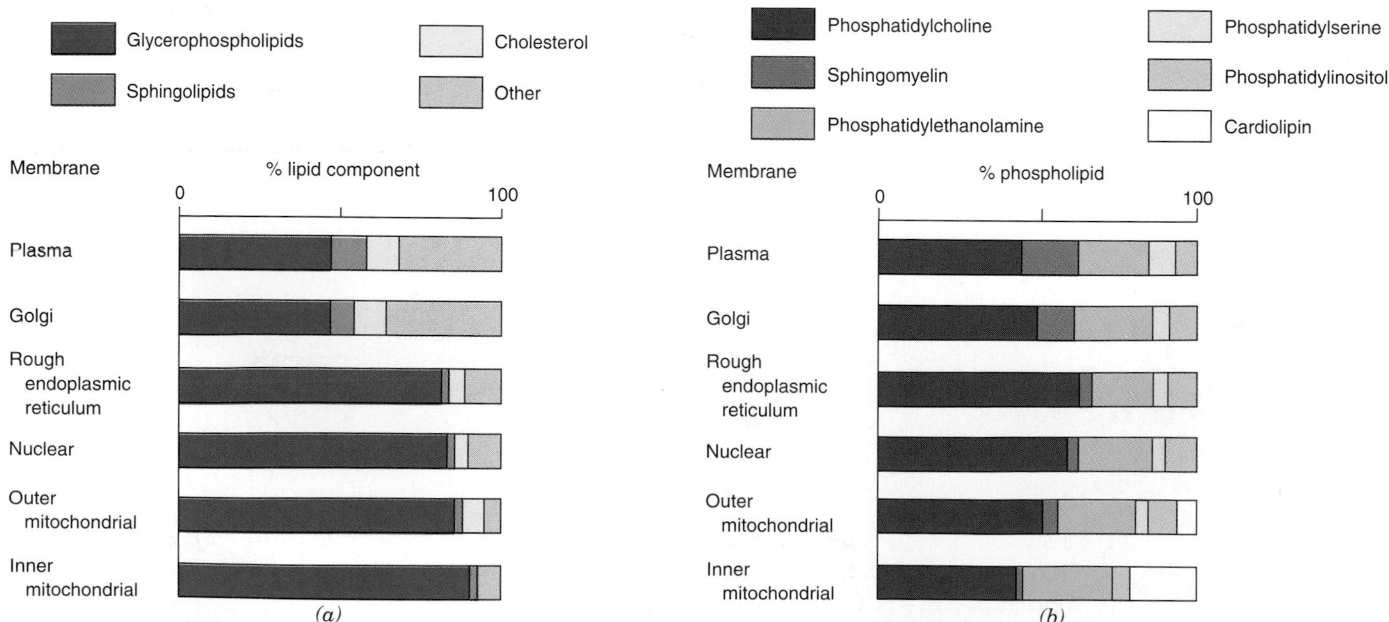

FIGURE 5.17
Lipid composition of cellular membranes isolated from rat liver.
(*a*) Amount of major lipid components as percentage of total lipid. The area labeled "Other" includes mono-, di-, and triacylglycerol, fatty acids, and cholesterol esters. (*b*) Phospholipid composition as a percentage of total phospholipid.
Values from R. Harrison and G. G. Lunt, Biological Membranes. *New York: Wiley, 1975.*

membrane by treatment with salt solutions of different ionic strength or extremes of pH, and named to imply a physical location on the surface of the membrane. Peripheral proteins, many of which are enzymes, are usually soluble in water and free of lipids. **Integral (or intrinsic) proteins** require rather drastic treatment, such as use of detergents or organic solvents, to be separated from a membrane They usually contain tightly bound lipid, which if removed leads to denaturation of the protein and loss of biological function. Integral proteins have sequences of hydrophobic amino acids, which create hydrophobic domains in the tertiary structure. These hydrophobic regions interact with the hydrophobic hydrocarbons of the lipids stabilizing the protein–lipid complex. Removal of integral proteins leads to disruption of the membrane, whereas peripheral proteins can be removed with little or no change in the integrity of the membrane.

Proteolipids are hydrophobic **lipoproteins** soluble in chloroform and methanol but insoluble in water. They are present in many membranes but particularly in myelin, where they represent about 50% of the protein component. An example is lipophilin, a major lipoprotein of brain myelin that contains over 65% hydrophobic amino acids and covalently bound fatty acids.

Another class of integral membrane proteins is the **glycoproteins;** plasma membranes of cells contain a number of different glycoproteins, each with its own unique carbohydrate content.

The complexity, variety, and interaction of membrane proteins with lipids are just being resolved. Many of the proteins are enzymes located within or on the cellular membranes. Membrane proteins have a role in transmembrane movement of molecules and as receptors for the binding of hormones and growth factors. In many cells, such as neurons and erythrocytes, membrane proteins have a structural role to maintain the shape of the cell. Thus individual membrane proteins can have a *catalytic, transport, receptor, structural,* or *recognition role.* It is not surprising to find a high protein content in a membrane being correlated with the complexity and variety of functions of a membrane.

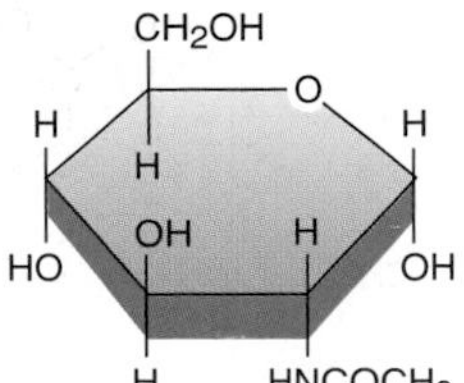

N-Acetyl-α-D-glucosamine

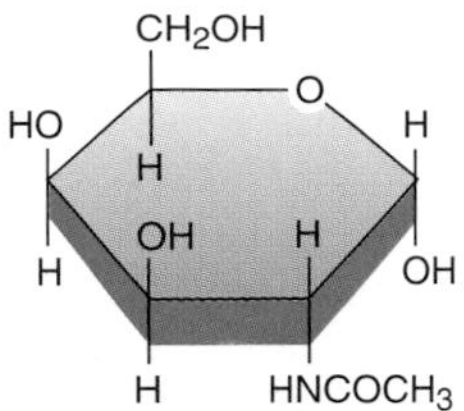

N-Acetyl-α-D-galactosamine

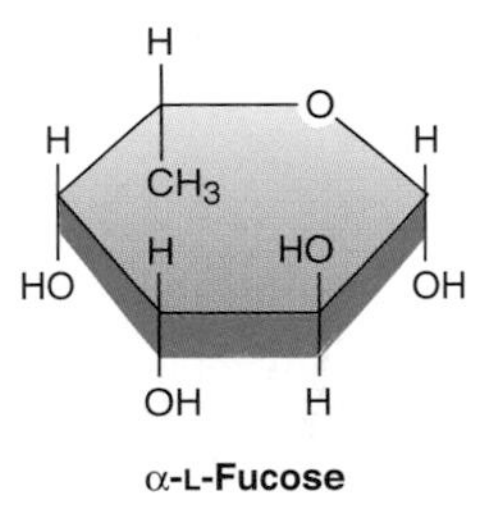

α-L-Fucose

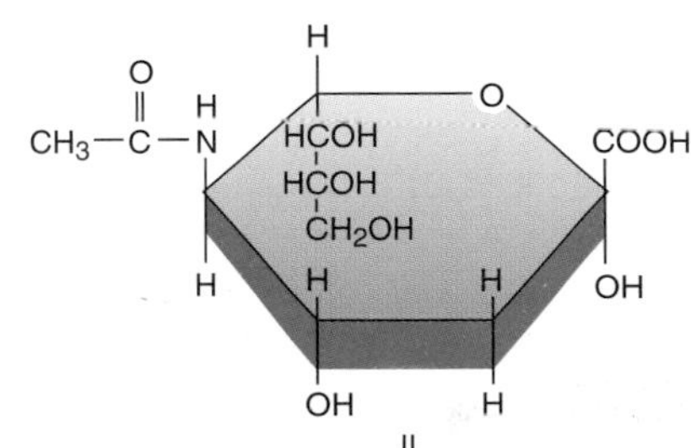

N-Acetyl-D-neuraminic acid

FIGURE 5.18
Structures of some membrane carbohydrates.

Carbohydrates of Membranes Are Present as Glycoproteins or Glycolipids

Carbohydrates present in membranes are **oligosaccharides** covalently attached to proteins to form glycoproteins and to a lesser amount to lipids to form glycolipids. The sugars found in glycoproteins and glycolipids include glucose, galactose, mannose, fucose, *N*-acetylgalactosamine, *N*-acetylglucosamine, and sialic acid (see Figure 5.18 and the Appendix for structures). Structures of glycoproteins and glycolipids are presented on pages 348 and 422, respectively. The carbohydrate is on the exterior side of the plasma membrane or the luminal side of the endoplasmic reticulum. Roles for membrane carbohydrates include cell–cell recognition, adhesion, and receptor action.

5.3 ■ MICELLES AND LIPOSOMES

Lipids Form Vesicular Structures

The basic structural characteristic of membranes is derived from the physicochemical properties of the major lipid components, the glycerophospholipids and sphingolipids. These amphipathic compounds, with a hydrophilic head and a hydrophobic tail (Figure 5.19*a*), will at appropriate concentrations interact in an aqueous system to form spheres, termed **micelles** (Figure 5.19*b*). The hydrophobic tails interact to exclude water and charged polar head groups will be on the outside of the sphere. The specific concentration of lipid required for micelle formation is referred to as the **critical micelle concentration.** Micelles with a single lipid or a mixture of lipids can be made. Formation of

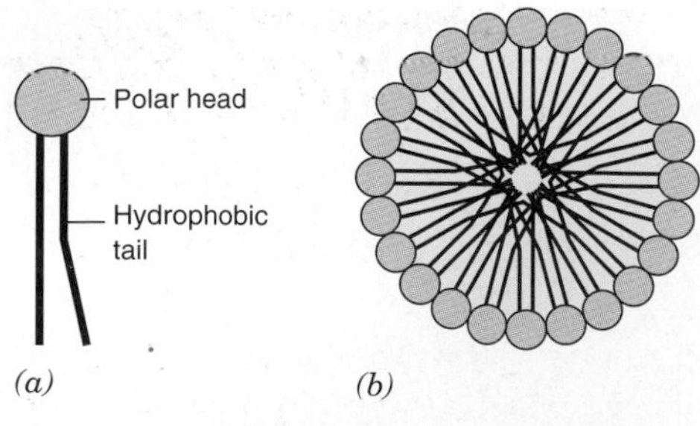

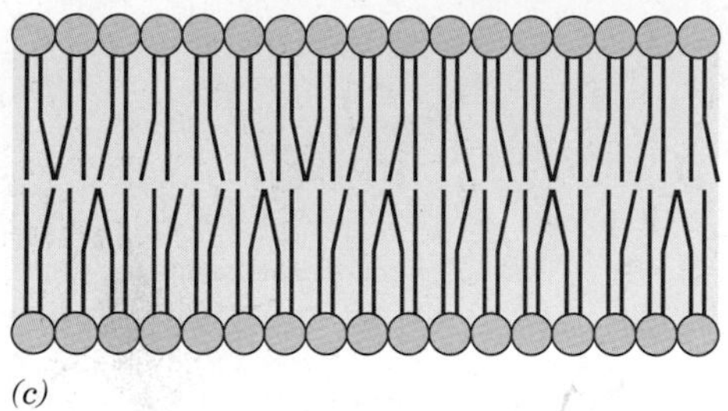

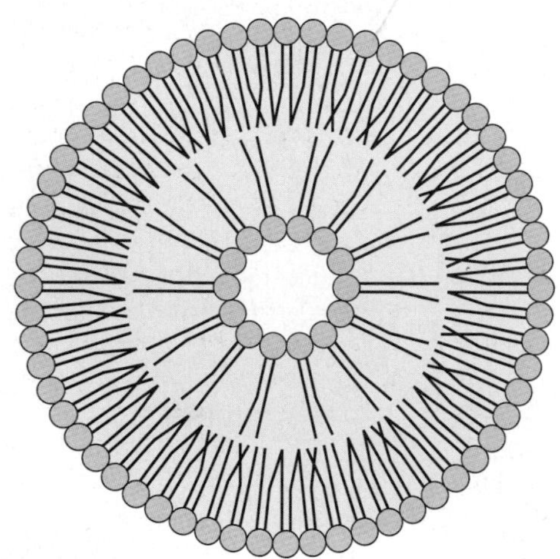

FIGURE 5.19
Representations of the interactions of phospholipids in an aqueous medium. (*a*) Representation of an amphipathic lipid. (*b*) Cross-sectional view of the structure of a micelle. (*c*) Cross-sectional view of the structure of lipid bilayer. (*d*) Cross section of a liposome. Each structure has an inherent stability due to the hydrocarbon chains and the attraction of the polar head groups to water.

micelles depends also on the temperature of the system and, if a mixture of lipids are used, on the ratio of concentrations of the different lipids in the mixture (see p. 1079). The micelle structure is very stable because of hydrophobic interaction of hydrocarbon chains and attraction of polar groups to water. Micelles are important in the digestion of lipids (see p. 1081).

Liposomes Have a Membrane Structure Similar to Biological Membranes

Depending on conditions, amphipathic lipids such as glycerophospholipids will form a bimolecular leaf structure with two layers of lipid. The polar head groups will be at the interface between the aqueous medium and the lipid, and the hydrophobic tails will interact to form an environment that excludes water (Figure 5.19*c*). This bilayer conformation is the basic lipid structure of all biological membranes.

Lipid bilayers are extremely stable structures held together by noncovalent interactions of the hydrocarbon chains and ionic interactions of charged head groups with water. Hydrophobic interactions of the hydrocarbon chains lead to the smallest possible area for water to be in contact with the chains, and water is essentially excluded from the interior of the bilayer. If disrupted, bilayers will self-seal because hydrophobic groups will seek to establish a structure in which there is minimal contact of the hydrocarbon chains with water, a condition that is most favorable thermodynamically. A lipid bilayer will close in on itself, forming a spherical vesicle separating the external environment from an internal compartment. Such vesicles are termed **liposomes.** Because individual lipid–lipid interactions have low energies of activation, lipids in a bilayer have a circumscribed mobility, breaking and forming interactions with surrounding molecules but not readily escaping from the lipid bilayer (Figure 5.19*d*). Self-assembly of amphipathic lipids into bilayers is an important characteristic and is involved in formation of cell membranes.

Individual phospholipid molecules exchange places with neighboring molecules in a bilayer, leading to rapid lateral diffusion in the plane of the membrane (Figure 5.20). There is rotation around the carbon–carbon bonds in fatty acyl chains; in fact, there is a greater degree of rotation nearer the methyl end,

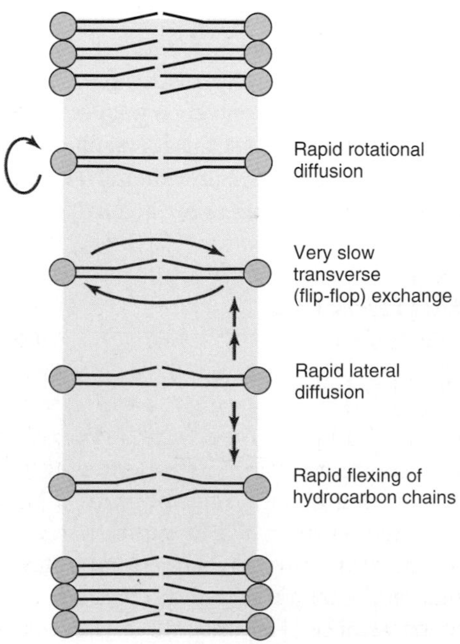

FIGURE 5.20
Mobility of lipid components in membranes.

leading to greater motion at the center than the peripheral region of the lipid bilayer. Individual lipid molecules, however, do not migrate readily from one monolayer to the other, a transverse movement, termed flip-flop, because of the thermodynamic constraints on movement of a charged head group through the lipophilic core. Thus lipid bilayers have an inherent stability and a fluidity in which individual molecules move rapidly in their own monolayer but do not readily exchange with an adjoining monolayer. In artificial bilayer membranes composed of different lipids, the components will be distributed randomly.

Artificial membrane systems have been studied extensively in order to understand the properties of biological membranes. A variety of techniques are available to prepare liposomes, using synthetic phospholipids and lipids extracted from natural membranes. Depending on the procedure, unilamellar and multilamellar (vesicles within vesicles) vesicles of various sizes (20 nm to 1 μm diameter) can be prepared. Figure 5.19*d* contains a representation of a liposome structure. The interior of the vesicle is an aqueous environment, and it is possible to prepare liposomes with different substances entrapped. Both the external and internal environments of liposomes can be manipulated and properties—including ability to exclude molecules, interaction with various substances, and stability under different conditions—of these synthetic membranes have been studied. Na^+, K^+, Cl^-, and most polar molecules do not readily diffuse across lipid bilayers of liposomes, whereas the bilayer presents no barrier to water. Lipid-soluble nonpolar substances such as triacylglycerol and undissociated organic acids readily diffuse into the membrane remaining in the hydrophobic environment of the hydrocarbon chains. Proteins have been incorporated into liposomes to mimic a natural membrane. Membrane-bound enzymes and proteins involved in translocating ions have been isolated from various tissues and incorporated into the membrane of liposomes for evaluation of the protein's function. With liposomes it is easier to manipulate the various parameters of membrane systems and thus study various activities free of interfering reactions present in cell membranes. Liposomes are used in delivery of drugs in humans (see Clin. Corr. 5.1).

5.4 ■ STRUCTURE OF BIOLOGICAL MEMBRANES

Fluid Mosaic Model of Biological Membranes

Based on evidence from physicochemical, biochemical, and electron microscopic investigations, knowledge of membrane structure has evolved. All biological membranes have a **bimolecular leaf** arrangement of lipids, as in liposomes. The amphipathic lipids and cholesterol are oriented so that hydrophobic portions of the molecules interact, minimizing their contact with water or other polar groups, and polar head groups of lipids are at the interface with the aqueous environment. J. D. Davson and J. Danielli in 1935 proposed this model for a membrane; their proposal was later refined by J. D. Robertson. A major question with the earlier models was how to explain the interaction of membrane proteins with the lipid bilayer. In the early 1970s, S. J. Singer and G. L. Nicolson proposed the mosaic model for membranes in which some proteins (intrinsic) are actually immersed in the lipid bilayer while others (extrinsic) are loosely attached to the surface of the membrane. It was suggested that some proteins spanned the lipid bilayer being in contact with the aqueous environment on both sides. Figure 5.21 is a current representation of a biological membrane and is referred to as the **fluid mosaic model** to indicate the movement of both lipids and proteins in the membrane. The characteristics of the lipid bilayer explain many of the observed cellular membrane properties, including fluidity, flexibility that permits changes of shape and form, ability to self-seal, and impermeability. The model continues to undergo modification and refinement;

CLINICAL CORRELATION 5.1

Liposomes as Carriers of Drugs and Enzymes

A major obstacle in the use of many drugs is lack of tissue specificity in the action of the drug. Administration of drugs orally or intravenously leads to a drug acting on many tissues and not exclusively on a target organ, resulting in toxic side effects. An example is the commonly observed suppression of bone marrow cells by anticancer drugs. Some drugs are metabolized rapidly and their period of effectiveness is relatively short. Liposomes have been prepared with drugs, enzymes, and DNA encapsulated inside and used as carriers for these substances to target organs. Liposomes prepared from purified phospholipids and cholesterol are nontoxic and biodegradable. Alteration of surface charge enhances drug incorporation and release. Attempts have been made to prepare liposomes for interaction at a specific target organ. Antibiotic, antineoplastic, antimalarial, antiviral, antifungal, and anti-inflammatory agents have been found to be effective when administered in liposomes. Some drugs have a longer period of effectiveness when administered encapsulated in liposomes. It may be possible to prepare liposomes with a high degree of tissue specificity so that drugs and perhaps even enzyme replacement can be carried out with this technique.

Ranade, V. V. Drug delivery systems. 1. Site-specific drug delivery using liposomes as carriers. *J. Clin. Pharmacol.* 29:685, 1989; Caplen, N. J., Gao, X., Hayes, P., et al. Gene therapy for cystic fibrosis in humans by liposome-mediated DNA transfer: the production of resources and the regulatory process. *Gene Ther.* 1:139, 1994; and Gregoriadis, G. Engineering liposomes for drug delivery: progress and problems. *Trends Biotechnol.* 13:527, 1995.

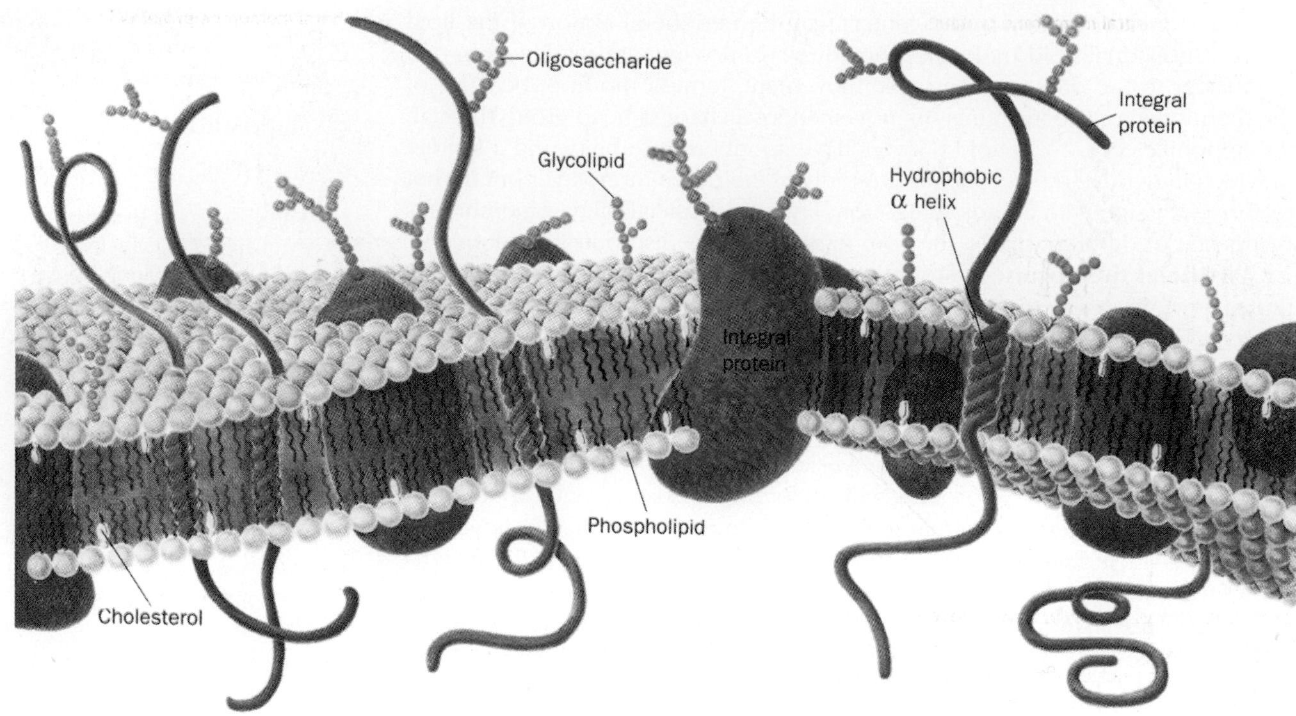

FIGURE 5.21
Fluid mosaic model of biological membranes.
Figure reproduced with permission from D. Voet and J. Voet, Biochemistry, *2nd ed. New York: Wiley, 1995.*

as an example, under some conditions membrane lipids can assume structural variations other than the bimolecular leaf arrangement.

Integral Membrane Proteins Are Immersed in Lipid Bilayer

The development of techniques for isolation of integral membrane proteins, for determination of their primary structure, and for identification of specific functional domains in the protein has led to an understanding of the structural relationship between the hydrophobic lipid bilayer and membrane proteins. Figure 5.22 illustrates the various ways of attachment of proteins to a biological membrane. Some integral membrane proteins (see p. 187) span the membrane, whereas others may only be immersed partially in the lipid. Based on measurements of the hydrophobicity of the amino acid residues and partial proteolytic digestion of proteins, sequences of amino acids embedded in the membrane have been determined. Some proteins contain an α-helical structure consisting primarily of hydrophobic amino acids (such as leucine, isoleucine, valine, and phenylalanine), which is the transmembrane sequence. This is illustrated in Figure 5.22*a*. An example is **glycophorin** present in the plasma membrane of human erythrocytes; amino acid residues 73–91, of the 131 total amino acids, are the transmembrane sequence and are predominantly hydrophobic. Glycophorin has three domains: a sequence exterior to the cell containing the amino terminal end, the transmembrane sequence, and a sequence extending into the cell with the carboxyl-terminal end. In other transmembrane proteins the amino acid chain loops back and forth across the membrane (Figure 5.22*b*). In some cases there are 12 loops snaking across the lipid bilayer. Often these multiple α helices spanning the membrane are organized to form a tubular structure. The **anion channel** of human erythrocytes, which has 926 amino acids and is responsible for the exchange of Cl^- and HCO_3^- across the membrane, is an example (see p. 204). Secondary and tertiary structures of proteins are critical

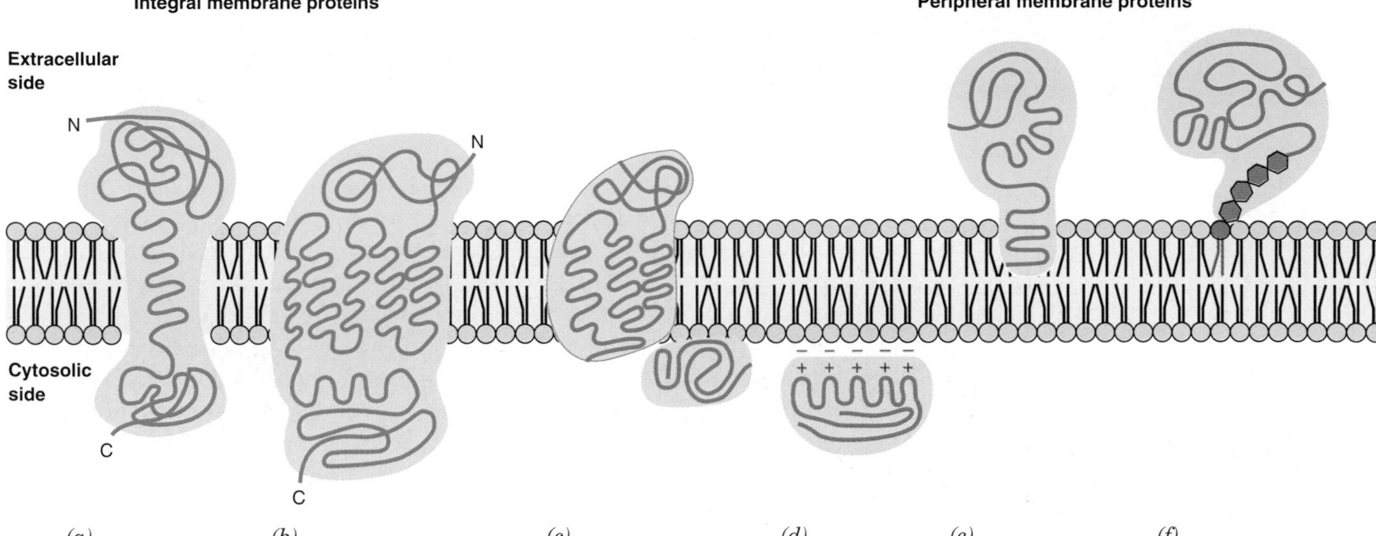

FIGURE 5.22
Interactions of membrane proteins with the lipid bilayer.
Diagram illustrates the multiple types of binding of proteins in or to the lipid bilayer: (*a*) a single transmembrane segment; (*b*) multiple transmembrane segments; (*c*) bound to an integral protein; (*d*) bound electrostatically to the lipid bilayer; (*e*) attached by a short terminal hydrophobic sequence of amino acids; and (*f*) attached by covalently bound lipid.

in the topography of the protein in the membrane. Some proteins in membranes form a quaternary structure with multiple subunits.

Integral membrane proteins have specific domains, for ligand binding, catalytic activity, and attachment of carbohydrate or lipid. The anion channel of the erythrocyte has two major domains: a hydrophilic amino-terminal domain on the cytosolic side of the membrane with binding sites for ankyrin, a protein that anchors the cytoskeleton and other cytosolic proteins, and a domain with 509 amino acids that traverses the membrane and mediates the exchange of Cl^- and HCO_3^-. Glycophorin contains 60% carbohydrate, all of which is attached to the protein domain on the extracellular side of the membrane. With such well-defined domains, integral membrane proteins have a defined orientation in the membrane rather than a random one. Specific structural orientation demonstrates another important aspect of membrane structure; biological membranes are asymmetric, with each surface having specific characteristics. The orientation of proteins is fixed during the synthesis of the membrane or replacement of the protein; the bulkiness of the proteins, as well as thermodynamic restrictions, prevents transverse (flip-flop) movement.

Many enzymes that are integral membrane proteins require the presence of the membrane lipid for activity. As an example, D-β-hydroxybutyrate dehydrogenase, located in the inner mitochondrial membrane, requires phosphatidylcholine for activity. Cholesterol has been implicated in the activity of various membrane ion pumps, including Na^+,K^+– and Ca^{2+}–ATPases (see p. 206), and acetylcholine receptors. Some of these modulating effects of lipids may be a reflection of a change in ordering and fluidity of the membrane but the lipid may also have a direct influence on the activity.

Peripheral Membrane Proteins Have Various Modes of Attachment

Peripheral membrane proteins are loosely attached to membranes and if removed do not disrupt lipid bilayers. Some apparently bind to integral membrane proteins, such as **ankyrin** binding to the anion channel protein in erythro-

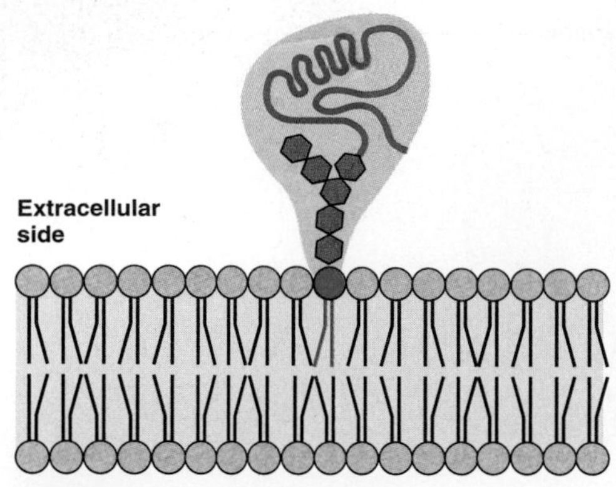

FIGURE 5.23
Attachment of a protein to a membrane by a glycosyl phosphatidylinositol anchor.

cytes (Figure 5.22*c*). Negatively charged phospholipids of membranes interact with positively charged regions of proteins allowing electrostatic binding (Figure 5.22*d*). Some peripheral proteins have sequences of hydrophobic amino acids at one end of the peptide chain that serve as an anchor in the membrane lipid (Figure 5.22*e*); cytochrome b_5 is attached to the endoplasmic reticulum by such an anchor.

Phosphatidylinositol has a role in anchoring proteins to membranes (Figures 5.22*f* and 5.23). A **glycan,** consisting of ethanolamine, phosphate, mannose, mannose, mannose, and glycosamine is covalently bound to the carboxyl terminal of the protein. This glycan has been conserved throughout evolution because it is found in different species attached to carboxyl-terminal amino acid residues of various membrane-bound proteins. Additional carbohydrate can be attached to the last mannose. The glycosamine of the glycan is covalently bonded to phosphatidylinositol. The fatty acids of this glycerophospholipid are inserted into the lipid membrane, thus anchoring the protein. These molecules are now referred to as **glycosyl phosphatidylinositol** (GPI) **anchors.** Various proteins are attached in this manner including enzymes, antigens, and cell adhesion proteins; a partial list is presented in Table 5.3. Fatty acyl groups of phosphatidylinositol are apparently specific for different proteins. To date, proteins found to be attached by a GPI anchor are on the external surface of plasma membranes. The significance of this form of anchoring has yet to be determined but it may be important for localization of the protein on a membrane, control of function of the protein, and controlled release of the protein from the membrane. A specific phosphatidylinositol-specific phospholipase C catalyzes the hydrolysis of the phosphate–inositol bond leading to release of the protein.

Myristic and **palmitic acids** can also be covalently linked to proteins and serve to anchor proteins by insertion of the acyl chain into the lipid bilayer (Figure 5.22*f*). Myristic acid (C_{14}) is attached by an amide linkage to an amino-terminal glycine, and palmitic acid (C_{16}) is most often attached by a thioester linkage to cysteine or by a hydroxyester bond to serine or threonine.

Even though membrane models suggest that proteins are randomly distributed throughout and on the membrane, there is a high degree of functional organization with definite restrictions on the localization of some proteins. As an example, proteins participating in electron transport in the inner membrane of mitochondria function in consort and are organized into functional units both laterally and transversely. The location of specific proteins on the surface of plasma membranes is also controlled. Cells lining the lumen of kidney nephrons have specific plasma membrane enzymes on the luminal surface but not on the contraluminal surface of cells; enzymes restricted to a particular region of the membrane are located to meet specific functions of these cells. Thus there is a high degree of molecular organization of biological membranes that is not apparent from diagrammatic models.

TABLE 5.3 Proteins with a Glycosyl Phosphatidylinositol Anchor

Alkaline phosphatase
5′-Nucleotidase
Acetylcholinesterase
Trehalase
Renal dipeptidase
Lipoprotein lipase
Carcinoembryonic antigen
Neural cell adhesion molecule
Scrapie prion protein
Oligodendrocyte–myelin protein

Source: M. G. Low, Glycosyl-phosphatidylinositol: a versatile anchor for cell surface proteins. *FASEB J.* 3:1600, 1989.

Human Erythrocytes Are Ideal for Studying Membrane Structure

The structure of the plasma membrane of the human erythrocyte has been investigated extensively because of the ease with which the membrane can be purified from other cellular components. Figure 5.24 is a representation of the interaction of some of the many proteins in this membrane.

Lipids Are Distributed in an Asymmetric Manner in Membranes

There is an **asymmetric distribution of lipid** components across biological membranes in contrast to the random distribution of lipids between the outer and inner lipid monolayers of liposomes. Each layer of the bilayer has a different composition with respect to individual glycerophospholipids and sphingolipids. An example is the asymmetric distribution of lipids in the human erythrocyte

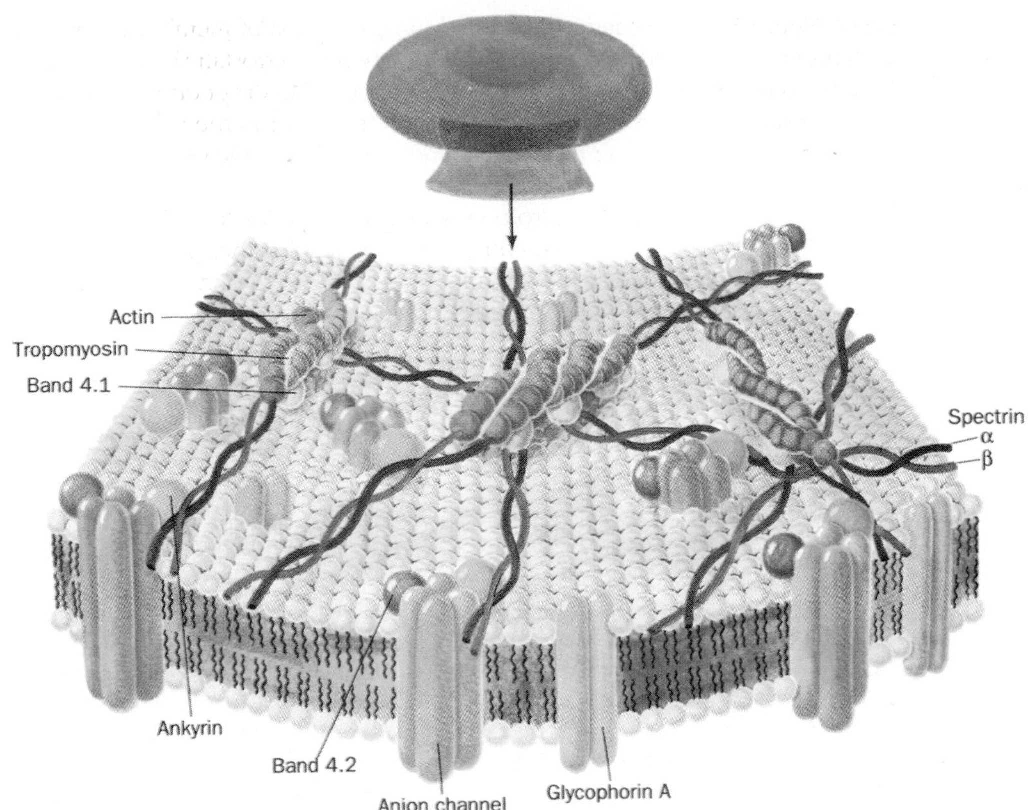

FIGURE 5.24
Schematic diagram of the erythrocyte membrane.
Diagram indicates the relationship of four membrane-associated proteins with the lipid bilayer. Glycophorin is a glycoprotein that contains 131 amino acids but whose function is unknown. Band 3, so designated because of its mobility in electrophoresis, contains over 900 amino acids and is involved in interacting with ankyrin and possibly in the facilitated diffusion of Cl^- and HCO_3^- (see Section 5.1). Ankyrin and spectrin are part of the cytoskeleton and are peripheral membrane proteins. Ankyrin binds to band 3 and spectrin is anchored to the membrane by ankyrin.
Figure reproduced with permission from D. Voet and J. Voet, Biochemistry, *2nd ed., New York: Wiley, 1995.*

membrane (Figure 5.25). Sphingomyelin is predominantly in the outer layer, whereas phosphatidylethanolamine is predominantly in the inner lipid layer. In contrast, cholesterol is equally distributed on both sides of the plasma membrane.

Asymmetry of lipids may be maintained by specific membrane proteins that promote the transverse movement of specific lipids from one side to the other. Metabolic energy may be involved in this process. Uncatalyzed transverse movement from one side to the other (i.e., flip-flop movement) of the glycerophospholipids and sphingolipids is slow. The asymmetry of lipids in erythrocyte membranes is an example of how slow is the transverse movement of membrane lipids. Mature erythrocytes have a lifetime of about 120 days, during which there is no new membrane synthesis or even significant repair. Even so, there appears to be little mixing of phospholipids between molecular layers. Individual lipids can exchange with lipids in the cell matrix, as well as with lipids of other membranes. Specific mechanisms to maintain both the composition and asymmetry of lipids in membranes apparently exist.

Proteins and Lipids Diffuse in Membranes

Interactions among different lipids and between lipids and proteins are very complex and dynamic. There is a **fluidity** in the lipid portion of

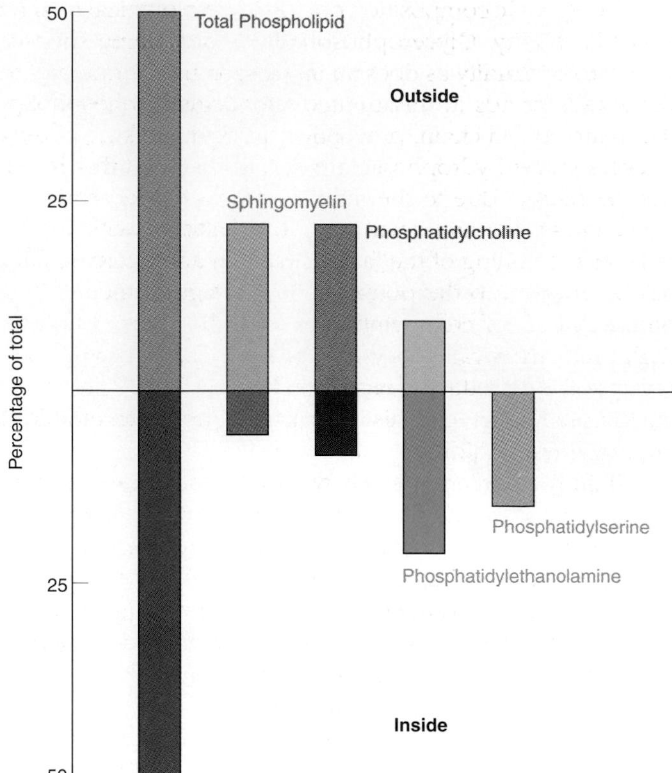

FIGURE 5.25
Distribution of phospholipids between inner and outer layers of the human erythrocyte membrane.
Values are percentage of each phospholipid in the membrane. *Redrawn from A. J. Verkeij, R. F. A. Zwaal, B. Roelofsen, P. Comfurius, D. Kastelijn, and L. L. M. Van Deenan. The asymmetric distribution of phospholipids in the human red cell membrane.* Biochim. Biophys. Acta *323:178, 1973.*

membranes in which both the lipids and proteins move. The degree of fluidity is dependent on the temperature and composition of the membrane. At low temperatures, lipids are in a gel–crystalline state, with lipids restricted in their mobility. As temperature is increased, there is a phase transition into a liquid–crystalline state, with an increase in fluidity (Figure 5.26). With liposomes prepared from a single pure phospholipid, the **phase transition temperature, T_m,** is rather precise; but with liposomes prepared from a mixture of lipids, T_m becomes less precise because individual clusters of lipids may be in either the gel–crystalline or liquid–crystalline state. T_m is not precise for biological membranes because of their heterogeneous chemical composition. Interactions between lipids and proteins lead to variations in the gel–liquid state throughout the membrane and differences in fluidity in different areas of the membrane.

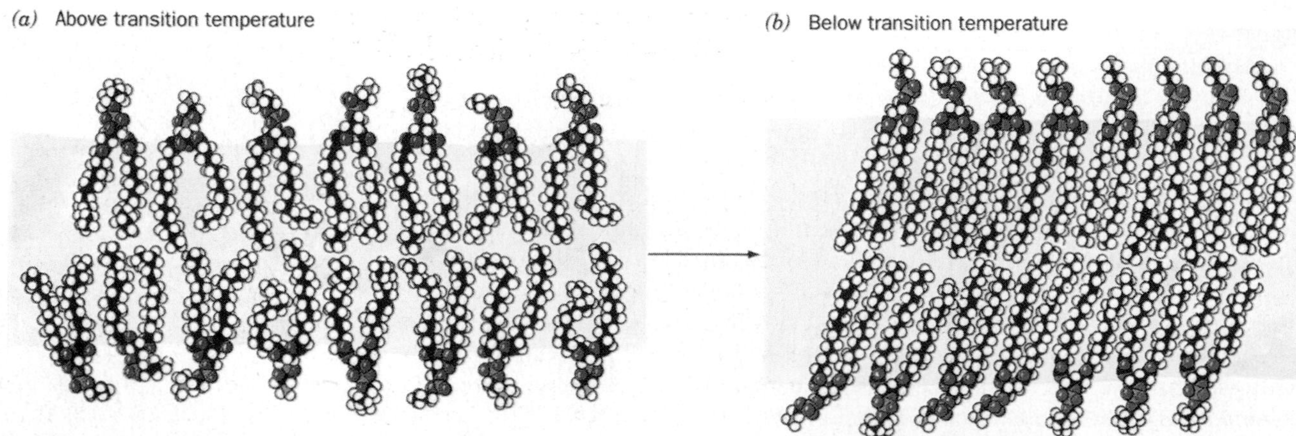

FIGURE 5.26
Structure of lipid bilayer above and below transition temperature.
Figure reproduced with permission from D. Voet and J. Voet, Biochemistry, *2nd ed. New York: Wiley, 1995. (After Robertson, R. N.,* The Lively Membranes, *Cambridge, MA: Cambridge University Press, 1983.)*

The specific composition of individual biological membranes leads to differences in fluidity. Glycerophospholipids containing short-chain fatty acids will increase the fluidity as does an increase in unsaturation of the fatty acyl groups. Cis double bonds in unsaturated fatty acids of phospholipids lead to kinks in the hydrocarbon chain, preventing the tight packing of the chains and creating pockets in the hydrophobic areas. It is assumed that these spaces, which will also be mobile due to the mobility of the hydrocarbon chains, are filled with water molecules and small ions. **Cholesterol** with its flat stiff ring structure reduces the coiling of the fatty acid chain and decreases fluidity. Consideration has been given to the potential clinical significance of high blood cholesterol on the fluidity of cell membranes (see Clin. Corr. 5.2). **Ca^{2+}** ion decreases the fluidity of membranes because of its interaction with the negatively charged phospholipids, reducing repulsion between polar groups and increasing packing of lipid molecules. This ion causes aggregation of lipids into clusters, reducing membrane fluidity.

Fluidity at different levels within the membrane also varies. The hydrocarbon chains of the lipids have a motion, which produces a fluidity in the hydrophobic core. The central area of a bilayer is occupied by ends of the hydrocarbon chains and is more fluid than areas closer to the two surfaces, where there are more constraints due to stiffer portions of the hydrocarbon chains. Cholesterol makes membranes more rigid toward the periphery because it does not reach into the central core of membranes.

Individual lipids and proteins move rapidly in a lateral motion along the surface of membranes. Electrostatic interactions of polar head groups, hydrophobic interactions of cholesterol with selected phospholipids or glycolipids, and protein–lipid interactions, however, lead to constraints on movement. There are lipid domains in which lipids move together as a unit.

Movement of integral membrane proteins in the lipid environment has been demonstrated by fusion of human and rat cells. When antigenic membrane proteins on cells of each species were labeled with different antibody markers, the markers indicated the localization of the proteins on the membrane. Immediately following fusion of the cells, proteins on the membranes of the human and rat cells were segregated in different hemispheres of the new cell, but within 40 minutes the two groups of proteins were evenly distributed over the membrane of the new cell. Movement of protein is slower than that of lipids and may be restricted by other membrane proteins, matrix proteins, or cellular structural elements such as microtubules or microfilaments to which they may be attached.

CLINICAL CORRELATION 5.2

Abnormalities of Cell Membrane Fluidity in Disease States

Membrane fluidity can control the activity of membrane-bound enzymes, membrane functions such as phagocytosis, and cell growth. A major factor in controlling the fluidity of the plasma membrane in higher organisms and mammals is the presence of cholesterol. With increasing cholesterol content the lipid bilayers become less fluid on their outer surface but more fluid in the hydrophobic core. Erythrocyte membranes of individuals with spur cell anemia have an increased cholesterol content. This condition occurs in severe liver disease such as cirrhosis of the liver in alcoholics. Erythrocytes have a spiny shape and are destroyed prematurely in the spleen. The cholesterol content is increased 25–65%, and the fluidity of the membrane is decreased. The erythrocyte membrane requires a high degree of fluidity for its function and any decrease would have serious effects on the cell's ability to pass through the capillaries. The increased plasma membrane cholesterol in other cells leads to an increase in intracellular membrane cholesterol, which also affects their fluidity. The intoxicating effect of ethanol on the nervous system is probably due to modification of membrane fluidity and alteration of membrane receptors and ion channels. Individuals with abetalipoproteinemia have an increase in sphingomyelin content and a decrease in phosphatidylcholine, thus causing a decrease in fluidity. The ramifications of these changes in fluidity are not completely understood, but it is presumed that, as techniques for the measurement and evaluation of cellular membrane fluidity improve, some of the pathological manifestations in disease states will be explained on the basis of changes in membrane structure and function.

Cooper, R. A. Abnormalities of cell membrane fluidity in the pathogenesis of disease. *N. Engl. J. Med.* 297:371, 1977.

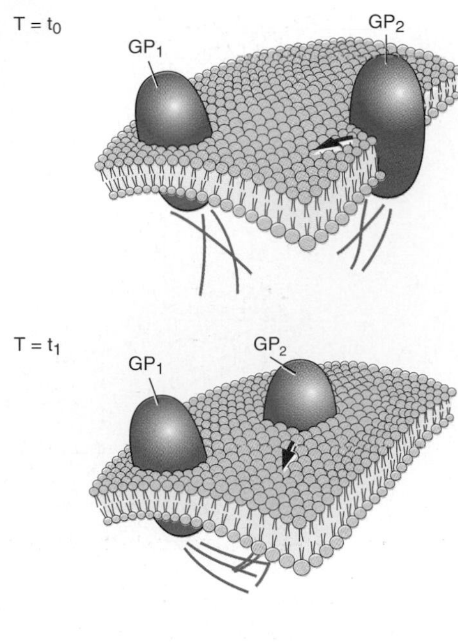

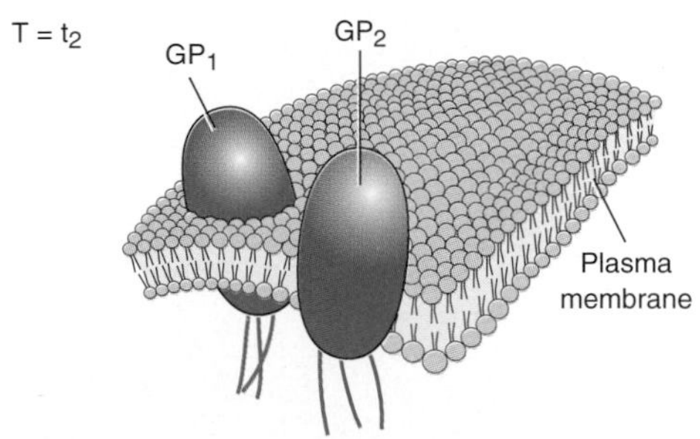

FIGURE 5.27
Modified version of the fluid mosaic model of biological membranes to indicate the mobility of membrane proteins. t_0, t_1, and t_2 represent successive points in time. Some integral proteins (GP_2) are free to diffuse laterally in the plane of the membrane directed by the cytoskeletal components, whereas others (GP_1) may be restricted in their mobility.

Evidence is accumulating that the fluidity of cellular membranes can change in response to changes in diet or physiological state. Fatty acid and cholesterol content of membranes is modified by a variety of factors. In addition, pharmacological agents may have a direct effect on membrane fluidity. Anesthetics that induce sleep and muscular relaxation may have their action because of their effect on membrane fluidity of specific cells. A number of structurally unrelated compounds induce anesthesia, but their common feature is lipid solubility. Anesthetics increase membrane fluidity *in vitro*.

Thus cellular membranes are in a constantly changing state, with not only movement of proteins and lipids laterally on the membrane but with molecules moving into and out of the membrane. The membrane creates a number of microenvironments, from the hydrophobic portion of the core of the membrane to the interface with the surrounding environments. It is difficult to express in words or pictures the very fluid and dynamic state, in that neither captures the time-dependent changes that occur in the structure of biological membranes. Figure 5.27 attempts to illustrate the structural and movement aspects of cellular membranes.

5.5 ■ MOVEMENT OF MOLECULES THROUGH MEMBRANES

The lipid nature of biological membranes severely restricts the type of molecules that diffuse readily from one side to another. Inorganic ions or charged organic molecules do not diffuse at a significant rate because of their attraction to water molecules and exclusion of charged species by the hydrophobic environment of lipid membranes. The diffusion rate of carbohydrates, amino acids, and inorganic ions, however, is not zero but may be too slow to accommodate a cell's requirements for the substance. Where there is a need to move a substance across a cell membrane, specific mechanisms are available for its translocation.

The basic mechanisms by which molecules cross cellular membranes is presented in the following sections with examples of the processes for illustrative purposes. Specific systems are described in the context of individual metabolic processes in later chapters.

Some Molecules Can Diffuse Through Membranes

Diffusion of a substance through a membrane involves three major steps: (1) solute must leave the aqueous environment on one side and enter the membrane; (2) solute must traverse the membrane; and (3) solute must leave the membrane to enter a new environment on the opposite side (Figure 5.28). Each step involves an equilibrium of solute between two states. Thermodynamic and kinetic constraints control the concentration equilibrium of a substance on two sides of a membrane and the rate at which it can attain equilibrium. Diffusion of gases such as O_2, N_2, CO_2, and NO occur rapidly and depend entirely on the concentration gradient. **Water** diffuses readily through biological membranes; its movement occurs via gaps in the hydrophobic environment created by random movement of fatty acyl chains of lipids. Water and other small molecules move into these **transitory spaces** and equilibrate across the membrane from one gap to another. For diffusion of a solute with strong interaction with water molecules, the shell of water surrounding the solute must be stripped away before it enters the lipid milieu and then regained on leaving the membrane. Distribution of hydrophobic substances between the aqueous phase and lipid membrane will depend on the degree of lipid solubility of the substance; very lipid-soluble materials will dissolve in the membrane.

The **rate of diffusion** of a lipophilic substance is directly proportional to its lipid solubility and diffusion coefficient in lipids; the latter is a function of the size and shape of the substance. Uncharged lipophilic molecules, for example, fatty acids and steroids, diffuse relatively rapidly but water-soluble substances, for example, sugars and inorganic ions, diffuse very slowly.

Direction of movement of solutes by diffusion is always from a higher to a lower concentration and the rate is described by **Fick's first law of diffusion:**

$$J = -D\left(\frac{\delta c}{\delta x}\right)$$

where J is the net amount of substance moved per time, D is the diffusion coefficient, and $\delta c/\delta x$ is the chemical gradient of substance. As the concentration of solute on one side of the membrane is increased, there will be an increasing *initial rate* of diffusion as illustrated in Figure 5.29. A *net movement* of molecules from one side to another will continue until the concentration in each is at chemical equilibrium. A continued exchange of solute molecules from one side to another occurs after equilibrium is attained but no net accumulation on one side can occur because this would recreate a concentration gradient if it occurred.

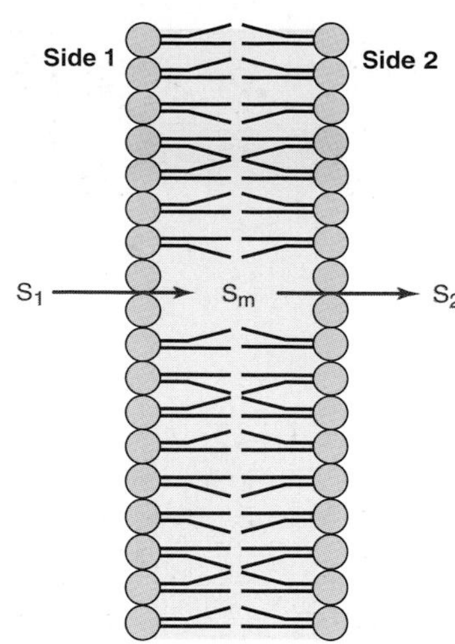

FIGURE 5.28
Diffusion of a solute molecule through a membrane.
S_1 and S_2 are solutes on each side of the membrane, and S_m is a solute in the membrane.

Movement of Molecules Across Membranes Can Be Facilitated

Mechanisms for membrane translocation of various substances including sugars, amino acids, metabolic intermediates, inorganic ions, and even H^+ have been determined. The plasma membrane of both prokaryotic and eukaryotic cells, as well as membranes of subcellular organelles, contain **transport systems** that have an important role in the uptake of nutrients, maintenance of ion concentrations, and control of metabolism. These systems involve intrinsic membrane proteins and are classified on the basis of their mechanism of translocation of substrate across the membrane and the energetics of the system. A classification of transport systems is presented in Table 5.4. Each will be discussed in more detail in subsequent sections but for now it is important to distinguish the three main types.

Membrane Channels

Membranes of most cells contain specific **channels,** in some cases referred to as **pores,** which permit the rapid movement of specific molecules or ions from one side of a membrane to the other. The tertiary and quaternary structures of these intrinsic membrane proteins create an aqueous hole in the membrane that permits diffusion of substances in both directions through the membrane. Like diffusion, the substances will move only in the direction of lower concentration, that is, down a concentration gradient. In contrast to transporters, the channel proteins do not bind the molecules or ions to be transported. The

TABLE 5.4 Classification of Membrane Translocation Systems

Type	*Class*	*Example*
Channel	1. Voltage regulated	Na^+ channel
	2. Chemically regulated	Acetylcholine receptor
	3. cAMP regulated	Cl^- channel
	4. Other	Pressure sensitive
Transporter	1. Passive mediated	Glucose transporter
	2. Active mediated	
	a. Primary-redox coupled	Respiratory chain linked
	Primary-ATPases	Na^+,K^+–ATPase
	b. Secondary	Na^+-dependent glucose transport
Group translocation		Amino acid translocation

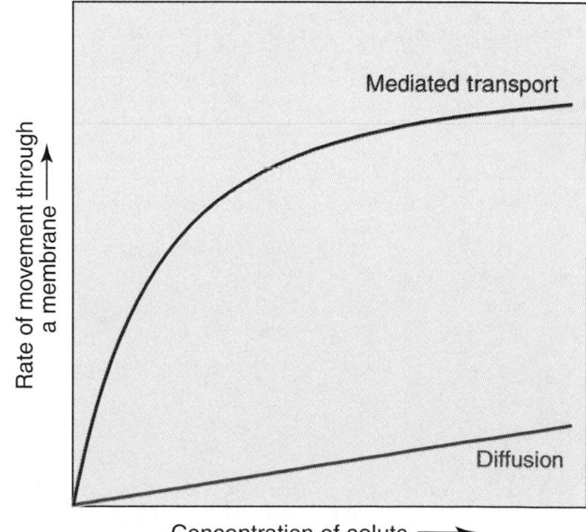

FIGURE 5.29
Kinetics of movement of a solute molecule through a membrane.
The initial rate of diffusion is directly proportional to the concentration of the solute. In mediated transport, the rate will reach a V_{max} when the carrier is saturated.

channels have some degree of specificity, however, based on the size and charge of the substance. Flow through the channel can be regulated by opening and shutting the passageway, like a gate to a garden.

Transporters

Transporters actually translocate the molecule or ion across the membrane by binding and physically moving the substance. The activity can be evaluated in the same kinetic terms as an enzyme-catalyzed reaction except no chemical reaction occurs. Transporters have specificity for the substance to be transported, frequently referred to as the substrate, have defined reaction kinetics, and can be inhibited by both competitive and noncompetitive inhibitors. Some transporters only move substrates down their concentration gradient (referred to as passive transport), while others can move the substrate against its concentration gradient (active transport) requiring the expenditure of some form of energy. With both channels and transporters the molecule is unchanged following translocation across the membrane.

A major difference between membrane channels and transporters is the rate of substrate translocation; for a channel, rates in the range of 10^7 ions s^{-1} are usual, whereas with a transporter the rate is in the range of 10^2–10^3 molecules s^{-1}. The activity of all translocation systems can be modulated, permitting cells and tissues to control the movement of substances across membranes. Drugs for specific channels and transporters have been developed to control these processes.

Group Translocation

Group translocation involves not only movement of the substance across the membrane but also chemical modification of the substance during the process. One mechanism of uptake of sugars by bacteria involves transport and then phosphorylation of the sugar before release into the cytosol of the cell. In some mammalian cells uptake of amino acids involves a group translocation mechanism.

Membrane Transport Systems Have Common Characteristics

Membranes of all cells contain highly specific transporters for the movement of inorganic anions and cations (e.g., Na^+, K^+, Ca^{2+}, HPO_4^{2+}, Cl^-, and HCO_3^-), and uncharged and charged organic compounds (e.g., amino acids and sugars). Different cellular membranes have different transport systems; as an example, the mitochondrial membrane has a specific mechanism to translocate ADP and ATP that is not present in other cellular membranes. Transport systems involve integral membrane proteins with a high degree of specificity for the substances transported. These proteins or protein complexes have been designated by a variety of names, including **transporter, translocase, translocator, permease,** and **pump,** or termed **transporter system, translocation mechanism,** and **mediated transport system.** The designations above are used interchangeably, but for convenience we will use transporter or translocase when referring to the proteins involved in translocation.

Membrane transporters have a number of characteristics in common. Each facilitates the movement of a molecule or molecules through the lipid bilayer at a rate that is significantly faster than can be accounted for by simple diffusion. If S_1 is the solute on side 1 and S_2 on side 2, then the transporter promotes establishment of an equilibrium as follows:

$$[S_1] \rightleftharpoons [S_2]$$

where the brackets represent the concentration of solute. If the transporter (T) is included in the equilibrium the rection is

$$[S_1] + T \rightleftharpoons [S - T] \rightleftharpoons [S_2] + T$$

TABLE 5.5 Characteristics of Membrane Transporters

Passive Mediated	*Active Mediated*
1. Saturation kinetics	1. Saturation kinetics
2. Specificity for solute transported	2. Specificity for solute transported
3. Can be inhibited	3. Can be inhibited
4. Solute moves down concentration gradient	4. Solute can move against concentration gradient
5. No expenditure of energy	5. Requires coupled input of energy

If no energy is put into the system, the concentration on both sides of the membrane will be equal at equilibrium; but if there is an expenditure of energy, a concentration gradient can be established. Note the similarity of the role of a transporter to that of an enzyme; in both cases the protein increases the rate but does not determine the final equilibrium.

Table 5.5 lists major characteristics of membrane transport systems. As presented in Figure 5.29, they demonstrate **saturation kinetics;** as the concentration of the substance to be translocated increases, the initial rate of transport increases but reaches a maximum when the substance saturates the protein transporter. Simple diffusion does not have saturation kinetics. Constants such as V_{max} and K_m can be calculated for transporters. As with enzymes, transporters can catalyze movement of a solute in both directions across the membrane depending on the $\Delta G'$ for the reaction.

Most transporters have a high degree of structural and stereo specificity for the substance transported. An example is mediated transport of D-glucose in erythrocytes, where the K_m for D-galactose is 10 times larger and for L-glucose 1000 times larger than for D-glucose. The transporter has essentially no activity with D-fructose or disaccharides. Competitive and noncompetitive inhibitors have been found for many transporters. Structural analogs of the substrate inhibit competitively and reagents that react with specific groups on proteins are noncompetitive inhibitors.

Recognition: $S_1 + T_1 \rightleftharpoons S-T_1$
Transport: $S-T_1 \rightleftharpoons S-T_2$
Release: $S-T_2 \rightleftharpoons T_2 + S_2$
Recovery: $T_2 \rightleftharpoons T_1$

FIGURE 5.30
Reactions involved in mediated transport across a biological membrane.
S_1 and S_2 are the solutes on sides 1 and 2 of the membrane, respectively; T_1 and T_2 are the binding sites on the transporter on sides 1 and 2, respectively.

There Are Four Common Steps in the Transport of Solute Molecules

We need to expand the equation above and consider four aspects of mediated transport (Figure 5.30). These are (1) *recognition by transporter of appropriate solute from a variety of solutes in the aqueous environment,* (2) *translocation of solute across membrane,* (3) *release of solute by transporter,* and (4) *recovery of transporter to its original condition to accept another solute molecule.*

The first step, **recognition** of a specific substrate by the transporter, is explained on the same basis as that described for recognition of a substrate by an enzyme. The presence of very specific binding sites on the protein permits the transporter to recognize the correct structure of the solute to be translocated.

The second step, **translocation,** is not completely understood. A reasonable mechanism (Figure 5.31) is one in which the protein transporter creates a channel between the environments on each side of the membrane with access through the channel being controlled by a gating mechanism in order to control which solutes can move into the channel. Transporters have receptor sites to which the solute attaches. After binding of solute and transporter, a conformational change of the protein moves the solute molecule a short distance, perhaps only 2 or 3 Å, but into the environment of the opposite side of the membrane. In this manner, it is not necessary for the transporter to move the molecule the entire distance across the membrane. Earlier suggestions for the translocation step included the possibility of a diffusible or rotating carrier, but both are improbable considering that transporters are large integral membrane proteins that do not diffuse transversely.

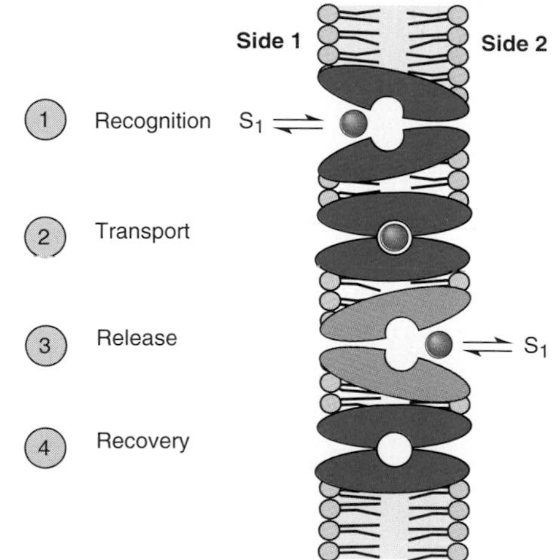

FIGURE 5.31
Model for a mediated transport system in a biological membrane.
Model is based on the concept of specific sites for binding of substrate and a conformational change in the transporter to move the bound solute a short distance but into the environment of the other side of the membrane. Once moved, the solute is released from the transporter.

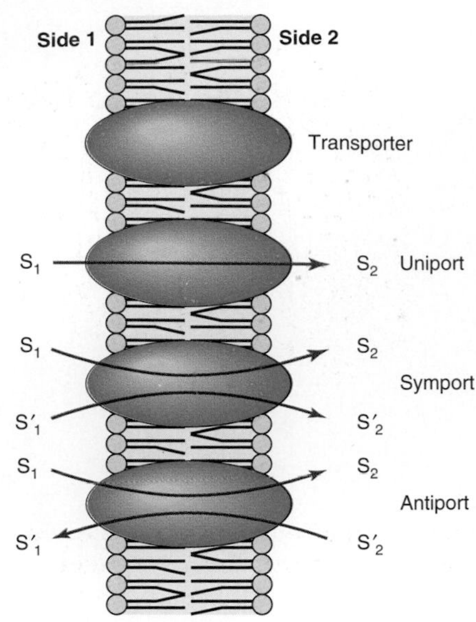

FIGURE 5.32
Uniport, symport, and antiport mechanisms for translocation of substances. S and S′ represent different molecules.

Release, step 3, of the solute can occur readily if the concentration of solute is lower in the new compartment than on the initial side of binding. Without a change in the affinity (K_{eq}), there would be a shift in the equilibrium and release of a portion of the solute. For those transporters that move a solute against a concentration gradient, release of the solute at the higher concentration requires a decrease in the affinity for the solute by the transporter. A change in the conformation of the transporter decreases the affinity. In group translocation (p. 210) the solute is chemically altered while attached to the transporter and the modified molecule has a lower affinity for the transporter.

Finally, in **recovery,** step 4, the transporter must return to its original state. If a conformational change has occurred, the transporter reverts to the original conformation.

The discussion above has centered on the movement of a single solute molecule by the transporter. There are systems that move two molecules simultaneously in one direction **(symport mechanisms),** two molecules in opposite directions **(antiport mechanism),** as well as a single molecule in one direction **(uniport mechanism)** (Figure 5.32). When a charged substance, such as K^+, is translocated and no ion of the opposite charge is moved, a charge separation occurs across the membrane. This mechanism is termed electrogenic and leads to development of a membrane potential. If an oppositely charged ion is moved to balance the charge, the mechanism is called neutral or electrically silent.

Energetics of Membrane Transport Systems

The change in **free energy** when an uncharged molecule moves from a concentration of C_1 to a concentration of C_2 on the other side of a membrane is given by Eq. 5.1:

$$\Delta G' = 2.3RT\log\left(\frac{C_2}{C_1}\right) \qquad \textbf{(5.1)}$$

When $\Delta G'$ is negative—that is, there is release of free energy—movement of solute will occur without the need for a driving force. When $\Delta G'$ is positive, as would be the case if C_2 is larger than C_1, then there needs to be an input of energy to drive the transport. For a charged molecule (e.g., Na^+) both the electrical potential and concentrations of solute are involved in calculating the change in free energy as indicated in Eq. 5.2:

$$\Delta G' = 2.3RT\log\left(\frac{C_2}{C_1}\right) + Z\mathcal{F}\Psi \qquad \textbf{(5.2)}$$

where Z is the charge of the species moving, $\mathcal{F}$ is the Faraday constant (23.062 kcal V^{-1} mol^{-1}), and Ψ is the difference in electrical potential in volts across the membrane. The electrical component is the membrane potential and $\Delta G'$ is the electrochemical potential.

A **passive transport** system is one in which $\Delta G'$ is negative and the movement of solute occurs spontaneously. When $\Delta G'$ is positive, coupled input of energy from some source is required for movement of the solute and the process is called active transport. **Active transport** is driven by either hydrolysis of ATP to ADP or utilization of an electrochemical gradient of Na^+ or H^+ across the membrane. In the first the chemical energy released on hydrolysis of a pyrophosphate bond drives the reaction, whereas in the latter an electrochemical gradient is dissipated to transport the solute.

Transport systems that can maintain very large concentration gradients are present in various membranes. An example is the plasma membrane transport system that maintains the Na^+ and K^+ gradients. One of the most striking examples of an active transport system is that present in the parietal cells of gastric glands, which are responsible for secretion of HCl into the lumen of the stomach (see p. 1069). The pH of plasma is about 7.4 (4×10^{-8} M H^+), and the luminal pH of the stomach can reach 0.8 (0.15 M H^+). The cells transport H^+ against a concentration gradient of $1 \times 10^{6.6}$. Assuming there is no electrical component, the energy for H^+ secretion under these conditions can be calculated from Eq. 5.1 and is 9.1 kcal mol^{-1} of HCl.

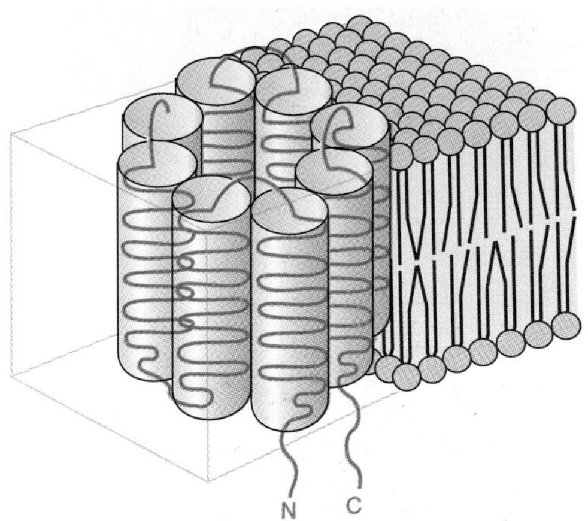

FIGURE 5.33
Arrangement of protein subunits or domains to form a membrane channel.

5.6 ■ CHANNELS AND PORES

Channels and Pores in Membranes Function Differently

Membrane channels are differentiated from membrane pores on the basis of their degree of specificity for molecules crossing the membrane. **Channels** are selective for specific inorganic cations and anions, whereas pores are not selective, permitting inorganic and organic molecules to pass through the membrane. The Na^+ channel of plasma membranes of eukaryotic cells, for example, permits movement of Na^+ at a rate more than ten times greater than that for K^+. This difference between channels and pores is due to differences in size of the aqueous area created in the protein structure as well as amino acid residues lining the channel area. Channels and pores are intrinsic membrane proteins and amino acid sequences in the proteins of many channels suggest existence of structurally related superfamilies of proteins in which similar amino acid sequences occur. A common motif is a structure formed by amphipathic α-helices of associated protein subunits or from domains within a single polypeptide chain creating a central aqueous space as pictured in Figure 5.33. Exceptions to the α-helical structure are the porins (see below) of Gram-negative bacteria, which have α,β-sheet structure lining the central pore. The opening and closing of membrane channels involve a conformational change in the channel protein.

Opening and Closing of Channels Are Controlled

As indicated in Table 5.4, the opening and closing of some channels can be controlled by changes in the **transmembrane potential.** These are referred to as **voltage-gated channels.** In the case of the Na^+ channel, depolarization of the membrane leads to an opening of the channel. Voltage-gated channels for Na^+, K^+, and Ca^{2+} are present in the plasma membrane of most cells. Clinical Correlation 22.8 (p. 956) describes changes in voltage-gated channels in myotonic muscle disorders. Mitochondria have a voltage-dependent channel for anions. Binding of a specific agent, termed an **agonist,** can also control the opening of a channel. A channel opens in the **nicotinic–acetylcholine receptor** on binding of acetylcholine allowing the flow of Na^+ into the cell. This mechanism is important to neuronal electrical signal transmission (see p. 928). In addition, some channels are controlled by cAMP (see p. 862); Clin. Corr. 5.3 describes the modification of the Cl^- channel in cystic fibrosis. These forms of control for opening channels are very fast, permitting bursts of ion flow through the membrane at rates of over 10^7 ions s^{-1}, which is near the diffusion rate of these ions in water. This rate is necessary because these channels are involved in nerve conduction and muscle contraction. A number of pharmacological agents that modulate these channels are used therapeutically.

Sodium Channel

Voltage-sensitive **sodium channels** mediate rapid increase in intracellular Na^+ following depolarization of the plasma membrane in nerve and muscle cells. The channel consists of a single large glycopolypeptide and several smaller glycoproteins. The genes for some of the Na^+ channels have been cloned and the amino acid sequences have been determined. There are four repeat homology units, each with six transmembrane α-helices. A model for this trans-

CLINICAL CORRELATION 5.3

Cystic Fibrosis and the Cl^- Channel

Cystic fibrosis (CF), an autosomal recessive disease, is the commonest, fatal, inherited disease of caucasians, occurring with a frequency of 1 in 2000 live births. It is a multiorgan disease, with a principal manifestation being pulmonary obstruction; thick mucous secretions obstruct the small airways allowing recurrent bacterial infections. Exocrine pancreatic dysfunction occurs early and leads to steatorrhea (fatty stool) in CF patients; see page 1059 for a discussion of the role of the pancreas in fat digestion and absorption. CF patients have reduced Cl^- permeability, which impairs fluid and electrolyte secretion, leading to luminal dehydration. Diagnosis of CF is confirmed by a significant increase of Cl^- in sweat of affected in comparison to normal individuals.

The gene responsible for CF was identified in 1989 and over 400 mutations leading to CF have been found. The most common mutation (about 70%) leads to a deletion of a single phenylalanine at position 508 on the protein, but missense, nonsense, frameshift, and splice-junction mutations (see p. 628) have also been reported. The CF gene product is the cystic fibrosis transmembrane conductance regulator (CFTR), which is a cAMP-dependent Cl^- channel. CFTR is composed of 1480 amino acids with structural homology to a family of transport proteins termed the transport ATPases. The gene has been cloned (see p. 765) and a major effort is under way to treat the disease by gene therapy, using both viral and nonviral vectors including liposomes (see Clin. Corr. 5.1).

Alton, E. W., and Geddes, D. M. Gene therapy for cystic fibrosis; a clinical perspective. *Gene Ther.* 2:88, 1995; Frizzell, R. A. Functions of the cystic fibrosis transmembrane conductance regulator protein. *Am. J. Respir. Crit. Care Med.* 151:54, 1995; and Wagner, J. A., Chao, A. C., and Gardner, P. Molecular strategies for therapy of cystic fibrosis. *Annu. Rev. Pharmacol. Toxicol.* 35:257, 1995.

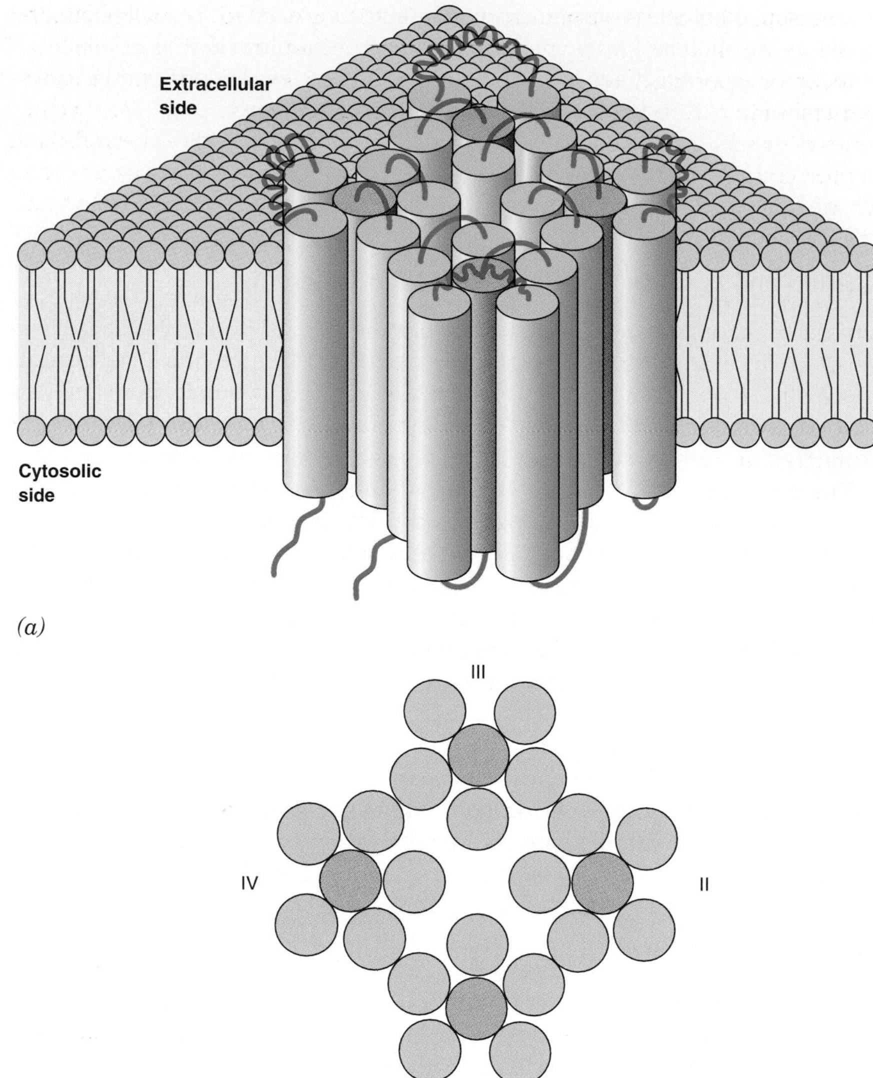

FIGURE 5.34
Possible model of the Na^+ channel.
(*a*) The single peptide consists of four repeating units with each unit folding into six transmembrane helices. (*b*) Proposed arrangement of the transmembrane sequences as viewed down on the membrane.
Redrawn from M. Noda et al., Nature *320:188, 1986.*

porter is presented in Figure 5.34*a* and a possible arrangement of the helices in the membrane as viewed down on a membrane is presented in Figure 5.34*b*. One transmembrane segment, labeled S4, has a positively charged amino acid at every third position and may serve as a voltage sensor. A mechanical shift of this region due to a change in the membrane potential may lead to a conformational change in the protein, resulting in the opening of the channel. The channel size created by the protein, however, cannot totally explain the specificity for Na^+.

Nicotinic–Acetylcholine Channel (nAChR)

The **nicotinic–acetylcholine channel,** also referred to as the **acetylcholine receptor,** is an example of a chemically regulated channel, where the binding of acetylcholine (Figure 5.35) opens the channel. The dual name is used to differentiate this receptor from other acetylcholine receptors, which function in a different manner. **Acetylcholine,** a neurotransmitter, is released at the

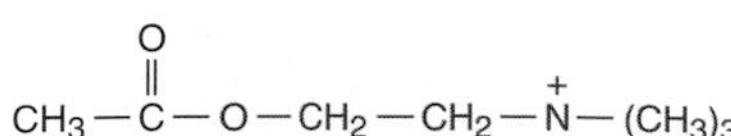

FIGURE 5.35
Structure of acetylcholine.

neuromuscular junction by a neuron when electrically excited. The acetylcholine diffuses to the skeletal muscle membrane where it interacts with the acetylcholine receptor, opening the channel and allowing selective cations to move across the membrane (see p. 928). The change in transmembrane potential leads to a series of events culminating in muscle contraction. The nicotinic–acetylcholine receptor consists of five polypeptide subunits, with two α subunits and one each of β, γ, and δ; each α subunit is phosphorylated and glycosylated and two others contain covalently bound lipid. The channel opens when two acetylcholine molecules bind to α subunits and cause a change in protein conformation; reclosure of the channel occurs within a millisecond due to hydrolysis of acetylcholine to acetate and choline and release of bound ligand. A desensitized state of the receptor has been reported that does not open when acetylcholine binds. In the open conformation, cations and small nonelectrolytes can flow through the channel but not anions; negatively charged amino acid residues in the channel are sufficient to repel negatively charged ions from passing.

The nicotinic–acetylcholine receptor is inhibited by a number of deadly neurotoxins including ***d*-tubocurarine,** the active ingredient of curare, and several toxins from snakes including **α-bungarotoxin, erabutoxin,** and **cobratoxin,** the latter from the cobra. **Succinylcholine,** a muscle relaxant, activates the channel leading to depolarization of the membrane; succinyl choline is used in surgical procedures because its activity is reversible due to the rapid hydrolysis of the compound after cessation of administration.

Examples of Pores Are Gap Junctions and Nuclear Pores

Plasma membrane gap junctions and **nuclear membrane pores** are relatively large aqueous openings in the membrane created by specific proteins. **Gap junctions** are clusters of membrane channels lined by proteins spanning two plasma membranes that create aqueous connections between two cells. They permit the exchange between cells of ions and metabolites but not large molecular weight compounds such as proteins. The diameter of the opening ranges from 12 to 20 Å. Oligomers of the gap junction polypeptide (32 kDa), referred to as **connexin,** form the channel. Twelve subunits, six from each cell, form a hexameric structure in each membrane as shown in Figure 5.36. The channels are normally open but increases in cytosolic Ca^{2+}, a change in metabolism, a drop in transmembrane potential, or acidification of the cytosol cause closure. When the channel is open subunits appear to be slightly tilted

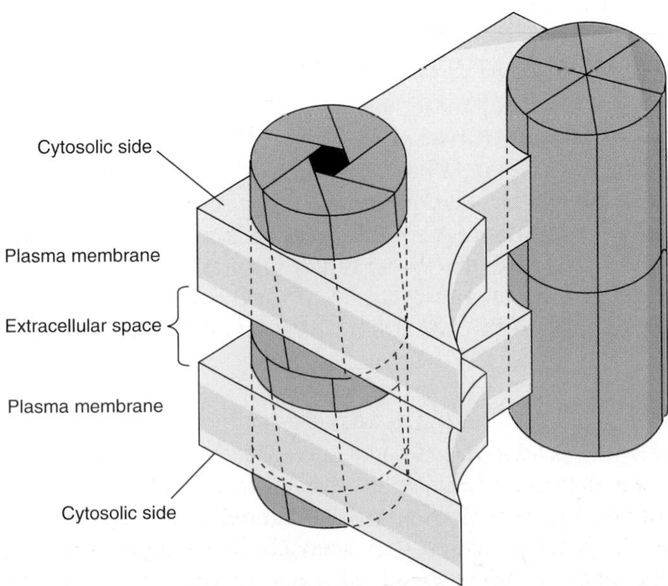

FIGURE 5.36
Model for a channel in the gap junction.

Phloretin

2,4,6-Trihydroxyacetosphenone

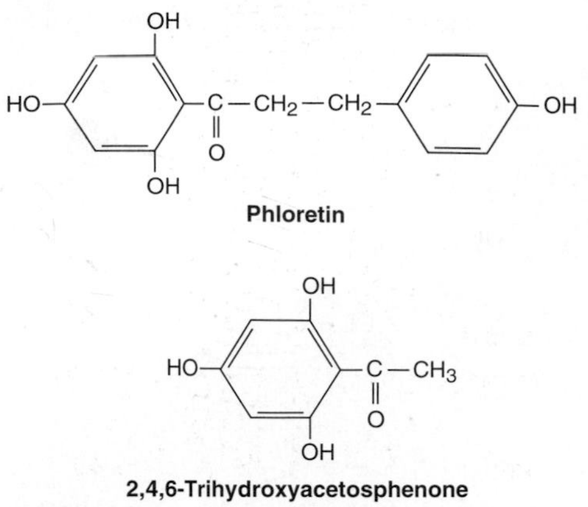

FIGURE 5.37
Inhibitors of passive mediated transport of D-glucose in erythrocytes.

but when closed they appear to be more nearly parallel to a perpendicular to the membrane, suggesting that subunits slide over each other. The detailed mechanism of opening and closing, however, is unknown.

Like gap junctions **nuclear pores** cover two membranes, creating aqueous channels in the nuclear envelope. Pores are about 90 Å in diameter and permit the movement of large macromolecules. They are presumably lined with protein. The plasma membranes of Gram-negative bacteria also contain protein pores, termed **porins.** Over 40 different porins have been isolated and they range in size from 28 to 48 kDa. In contrast to most mammalian channels, these transmembrane segments are β-sheets not α-helices and exist in the membrane as trimers. Porins are water-filled transmembrane channels and range in diameter from 6 to 23 Å with some degree of selectivity for inorganic ions; some, however, permit the uptake of sugars.

5.7 ■ PASSIVE MEDIATED TRANSPORT SYSTEMS

Passive mediated transport, also referred to as **facilitated diffusion,** leads to translocation of solutes through cell membranes without expenditure of metabolic energy (see Table 5.5, p. 199). As with nonmediated diffusion the direction of flow is always from a higher to a lower concentration. The distinguishing differences between measurements of simple diffusion and passive mediated transport are the demonstration of saturation kinetics, a structural specificity for the class of molecule moving across the membrane, and specific inhibition of solute movement.

Glucose Transport Is Facilitated

A family of passive mediated transporters for D-glucose, frequently referred to as **glucose permeases,** has been identified in the plasma membrane of mammalian cells. Six members have been described and are termed GLUT-1, GLUT-2, and so on. All have 12 hydrophobic segments considered to be the transmembrane regions. The physiological direction of movement is into the cell because the extracellular level of glucose is about 5 mM and most cells metabolize glucose rapidly, thus maintaining low intracellular concentrations. The transporter catalyzes a uniport mechanism and is most active with D-glucose. D-Galactose, D-mannose, D-arabinose, and several other D-sugars as well as glycerol are translocated by the same transporter. L-Isomers are not transported. It has been proposed that the β-D-glucopyranose is transported with carrier interaction at the hydrogen atoms on at least C-1, C-3, and C-6 of the sugar. The affinity of erythrocyte translocase for D-glucose is highest with a K_m of ~6.2 mM, whereas for other sugars K_m values are much higher. The transporter has a very low affinity for D-fructose, precluding a role in cellular uptake of fructose; a separate carrier for fructose has been proposed. With isolated erythrocytes, glucose will move either into or out of the erythrocyte, depending on the direction of the experimentally established concentration gradient, demonstrating the reversibility of the system. Several sugar analogs as well as phoretin and 2,4,6-trihydroxyacetophenone (Figure 5.37) are competitive inhibitors. Some physiological aspects of the glucose translocase are presented on p. 881.

Side 1 Side 2

Cl^- HCO_3^- Cl^- HCO_3^-

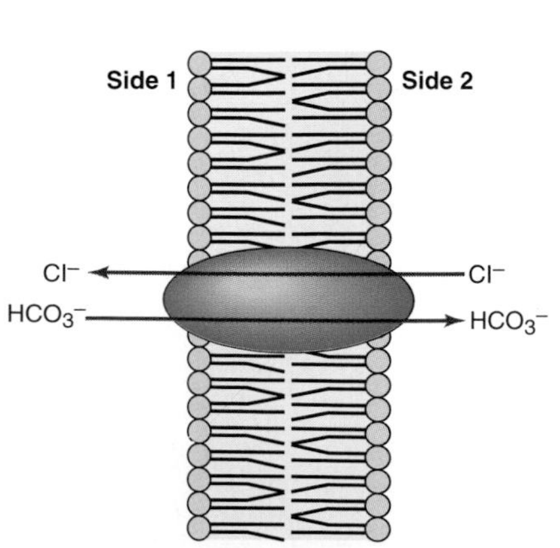

FIGURE 5.38
Passive anion antiport mechanism for movement of Cl^- and HCO_3^- across the erythrocyte plasma membrane.

Cl^- and HCO_3^- Are Transported by an Antiport Mechanism

An anion transporter in erythrocytes involves the antiport movement of Cl^- and HCO_3^- (Figure 5.38). The transporter is referred to as the **Cl^-–HCO_3^- exchanger, anion exchange protein,** or **band 3,** the latter because of its position in SDS polyacrylamide gel electrophoresis of erythrocyte membrane proteins. The direction of ion flow is reversible and depends on the concentration gradients of the ions across the membrane. The transporter has an important role in adjusting the erythrocyte HCO_3^- concentration in arterial and venous blood (see p. 1035).

Mitochondria Contain a Number of Transport Systems

The inner mitochondrial membrane contains several antiport systems for the exchange of anions between the cytosol and mitochondrial matrix. These include (1) a transporter for exchange of ADP and ATP, (2) a transporter for exchange of phosphate and OH^-, (3) a dicarboxylate carrier that catalyzes an exchange of malate for phosphate, and (4) a translocator for exchange of aspartate and glutamate (Figure 5.39). The relationship of these translocases and energy coupling are discussed on page 243. In the absence of an input of energy these transporters will catalyze a passive exchange of metabolites down their concentration gradient to achieve a thermodynamic equilibrium of all intermediates. As an antiport mechanism, a concentration gradient of one compound can drive the movement of the other solute. In several cases, the transporter catalyzes the antiport movement of an equal number of charges on the substrate; in such movement the mitochondrial membrane potential influences the equilibrium and the anions can be moved against their concentration gradients. ADP–ATP and the phosphate transporters, as well as an uncoupling protein that translocates H^+, have significant amino acid homology and are presumably derived from a common ancestor. It has been suggested that each subunit has six transmembrane α-helices. The **uncoupling protein,** found in mitochondria of brown adipose tissue, has been proposed to be involved in generation of heat.

The **ATP–ADP translocase** is very specific for ATP and ADP and deoxyribose derivatives, dATP and dADP, but does not transport AMP or other nucleotides. It is a dimer containing two subunits of 33 kDa each and represents about 12% of the total protein in heart mitochondria. It is very hydrophobic and can exist in two conformations. Atractyloside and bongkrekic acid (Figure 5.40) are

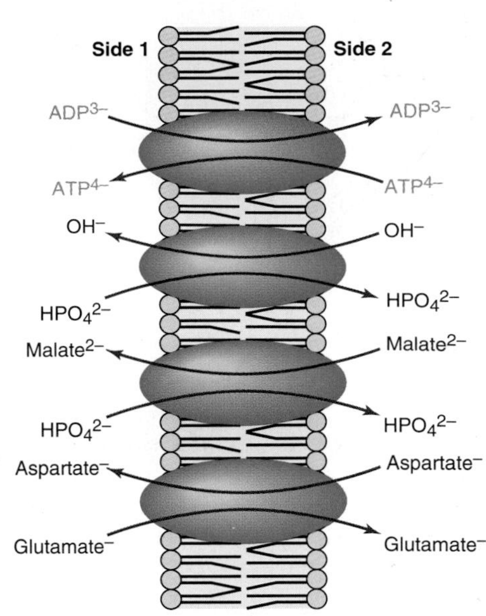

FIGURE 5.39
Representative anion transport systems in liver mitochondria.
Note that each is an antiport mechanism. Several other transport systems are known and are discussed in Chapter 6.

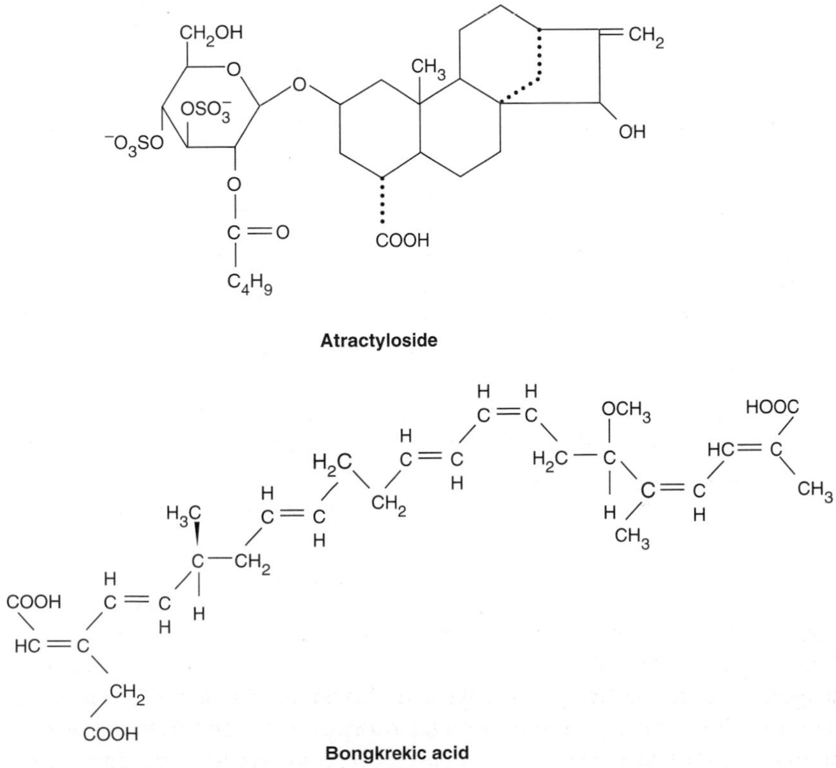

Atractyloside

Bongkrekic acid

FIGURE 5.40
Structure of two inhibitors of the ATP–ADP transport system of liver mitochondria.

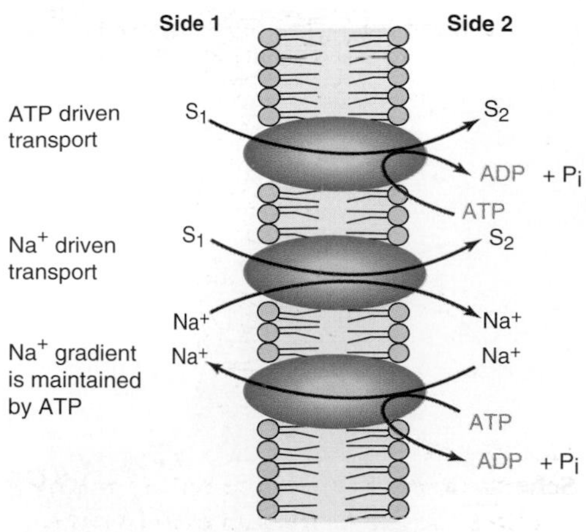

FIGURE 5.41
Involvement of metabolic energy (ATP) in active mediated transport systems. The chemical energy released on the hydrolysis of ATP to ADP and inorganic phosphate is used to drive the active transport of various substances, including Na^+. The transmembrane concentration gradient of Na^+ is also used for the active transport of substances.

specific inhibitors, each apparently reacting with a different conformation of the protein. The mitochondrial membrane potential can drive the movement of the nucleotides by this translocator, but in the absence of the membrane potential it functions as a passive mediated transporter.

It is sometimes difficult to differentiate passive mediated transport from simple diffusion, but inhibition of the process is good evidence of a carrier.

5.8 ■ ACTIVE MEDIATED TRANSPORT SYSTEMS

Active mediated transporters have the same three characteristics as passive transporters, that is, saturation kinetics, substrate specificity, and inhibitability (see Table 5.5, p. 199). They also require the utilization of energy to translocate solutes and if the energy source is removed or inhibited, the transport system will not function. These active transporters can be classified as either **primary active transporters,** if they utilize ATP directly, or **secondary active transporters** if a transmembrane chemical gradient of Na^+ or H^+ is utilized (Figure 5.41). The transporters that utilize ATP are also referred to as an **ATPase** because during the translocation ATP is hydrolyzed to ADP and phosphate. They are classified as either **P, V, or F type transporters or ATPases.** P type translocases are phosphorylated and dephosphorylated during the transport activity; the Na^+,K^+-translocase is an example of a P type. V, for vacuole, type are present in membranes of lysosomes, endosomes, Golgi vesicles, and secretory vesicles and are responsible for acidification of the interior of these vesicles. F type translocases, present in mitochondria and chloroplasts, are involved in ATP synthesis (see p. 263). A special case of active transport is the translocation of protons across the inner mitochondrial membrane during electron transport; this mechanism is discussed in detail on page 262 and will not be reviewed here. Active mediated transporters, which use the transmembrane Na^+ or H^+ gradient, require maintenance of the gradient; for Na^+ this is achieved by expenditure of ATP (Figure 5.41). Inhibition of ATP synthesis leads to a dissipation of the Na^+ gradient, which in turn causes a cessation of transport activity.

Translocation of Na^+ and K^+ Is a Primary Active Transport System

All mammalian cells contain a Na^+,K^+ antiporter, type P, which utilizes ATP to drive the movement of the ions. Knowledge of this transporter has developed along two paths: (1) from studies of a membrane enzyme, the **Na^+,K^+–ATPase,** that catalyzes ATP hydrolysis and has a requirement for Na^+ and K^+ ions, and (2) from measurements of Na^+ and K^+ movements across intact plasma membranes by a protein referred to as the **Na^+,K^+ pump.** The two activities are catalyzed by the same protein.

All Plasma Membranes Contain a Na^+,K^+-Activated ATPase

All mammalian plasma membranes catalyze the reaction

$$\text{ATP} \xrightarrow[\text{Mg}^{2+}]{\text{Na}^+ + \text{K}^+} \text{ADP} + \text{P}_i$$

The enzyme, officially termed the **Na^+,K^+-exchanging ATPase,** has a requirement for both Na^+ and K^+ ions, as well as Mg^{2+}, which is a cofactor for ATP-requiring reactions. The level of the ATPase in plasma membranes correlates with the Na^+,K^+ transport activity. Excitable tissues, such as muscle and nerve, and cells actively involved in the movement of Na^+ ion, such as those in the salivary gland and kidney cortex, have high activities of both Na^+,K^+-ATPase and Na^+,K^+ transport system. The protein responsible for the Na^+,K^+–ATPase activity is an oligomer containing two α subunits of about 110 kDa each and two β subunits of about 55 kDa each. The smallest subunits are glycoproteins, and the complex has the characteristics of an integral membrane protein. Figure 5.42 is a schematic diagram of the Na^+,K^+-exchanging ATPase. The ATPase activity has a requirement for phospholipids indicating its close relationship to the membrane. During transport the larger subunit is *cyclically phosphorylated* and *dephosphorylated* on a specific aspartic acid residue forming a β-aspartyl phosphate. Phosphorylation of the protein requires Na^+ and Mg^{2+} but not K^+, whereas dephosphorylation of the protein requires K^+ but not Na^+ or Mg^{2+}. The isolated enzyme has an absolute requirement for Na^+, but K^+ can be replaced with NH_4^+ or Rb^+. Two distinguishable conformations of the protein complex have been observed and thus it is classified as an **E_1–E_2 type transporter.** A possible sequence of reactions for the enzyme is presented in Figure 5.43.

Of significance to its physiological role as a transporter, the enzyme is inhibited by a series of **cardiotonic steroids.** These pharmacological agents, which include **digitalis,** increase the force of contraction of heart muscle by altering the excitability of the tissue, which is a function of the Na^+–K^+ concentrations across the membrane. **Ouabain** (Figure 5.44) is one of the most active Na^+,K^+–ATPase inhibitors of the series; its site of binding is on the smaller subunit of the enzyme complex and at some distance from the ATP-binding site on the larger monomer. An inhibitor in human serum of the transporter competes with ouabain binding and may be involved in the control of Na^+,K^+ transport.

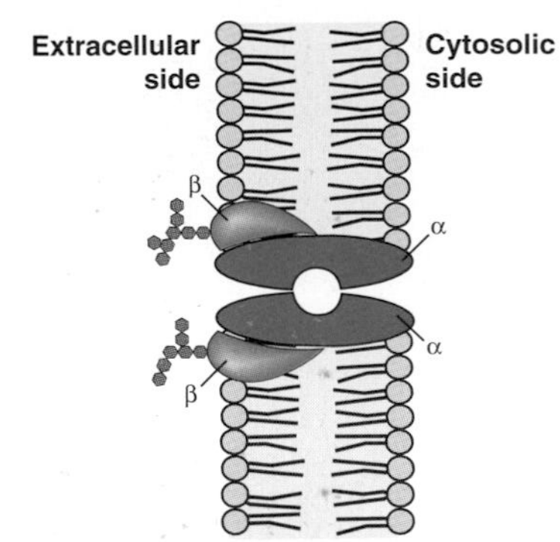

FIGURE 5.42
Schematic drawing of the Na^+,K^+-transporting ATPase of plasma membranes.

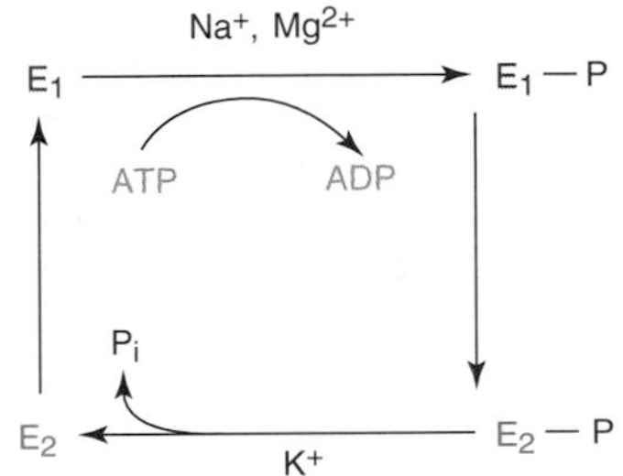

FIGURE 5.43
Proposed sequence of reactions and intermediates in hydrolysis of ATP by the Na^+,K^+–ATPase.
E_1 and E_2 are different conformations of the enzyme. Phosphorylation of the enzyme requires Na^+ and Mg^{2+} and dephosphorylation involves K^+.

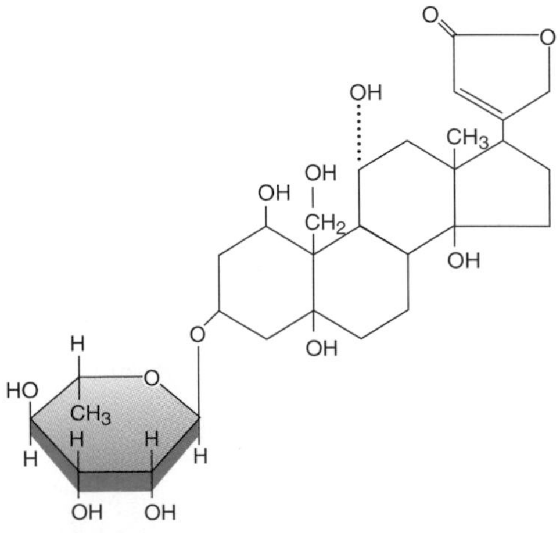

Erythrocyte Ghosts Are Used to Study Na^+,K^+ Translocation

Studies of the **Na^+,K^+ transporter** activity have been facilitated by use of erythrocyte preparations free of hemoglobin, referred to as **erythrocyte ghosts.** By carefully adjusting the tonicity of the medium, erythrocytes will swell with breaks in the phospholipid bilayer, permitting leaking from cells of cytosolic material, including hemoglobin. The cytosol can be replaced with a defined medium by readjusting the tonicity so that the membrane reseals, trapping isolation medium inside. In this manner intracellular ionic and substrate composition and even protein content can be altered. With erythrocyte ghosts intra- and extracellular Na^+ and K^+ can be manipulated as well as ATP or inhibitor content. Movement of Na^+ and K^+ is an antiport vectorial process, with Na^+ moving out and K^+ moving into the cell. This transporter is responsible for maintaining the high K^+ and low Na^+ concentrations in a mammalian cell (see p. 14). ATP-binding site on the protein is on the inner surface of the membrane in that hydrolysis occurs only if ATP, Na^+, and Mg^{2+} are inside the cell. K^+ ion is required externally for internal dephosphorylation of protein. Ouabain inhibits translocation of Na^+ and K^+ but only if present externally. There are between 100 and 200 transporter molecules per erythrocyte, but the number is significantly larger for other tissues.

ATP hydrolysis by the translocase occurs only if Na^+ and K^+ are translocated, demonstrating that the enzyme is not involved in dissipation of energy in a useless activity. For each ATP hydrolyzed, three ions of Na^+ are moved out of the cell but only two ions of K^+ in, which leads to an increase in external positive charges. This electrogenic movement of Na^+ and K^+ is part of the mechanism for the maintenance of the transmembrane potential in tissues. Even though the energetics of the system dictate that it functions in only one direction, the translocator can be reversed *in vitro* by adjusting the Na^+ and K^+ levels; a small net synthesis of ATP has been observed when transport is forced to run in the reverse direction.

A hypothetical model for movement of Na^+ and K^+ is presented in Figure 5.45. The protein goes through conformational changes during which the Na^+ and K^+ are moved short distances. During the transition a change in the affinity

FIGURE 5.44
Structure of ouabain, a cardiotonic steroid, which is a potent inhibitor of the Na^+,K^+–ATPase and of active Na^+ and K^+ transport.

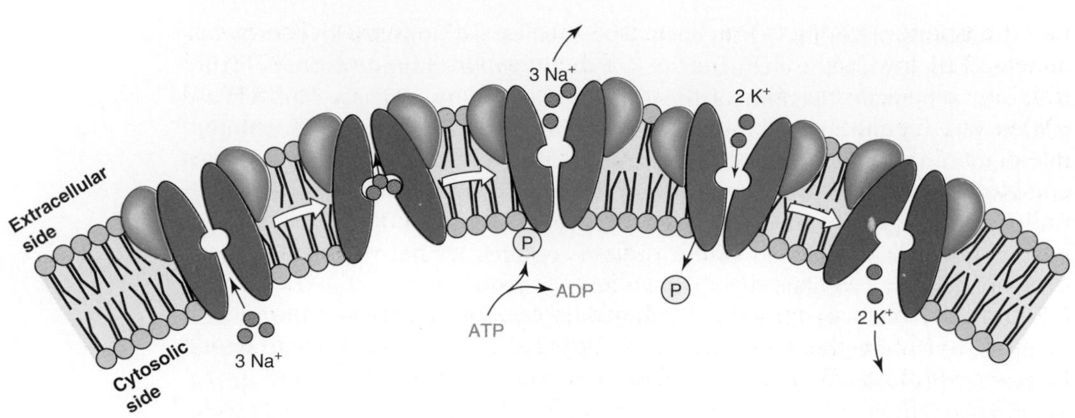

FIGURE 5.45
Hypothetical model for the translocation of Na^+ and K^+ across the plasma membrane by the Na^+,K^+–ATPase.
(1) Transporter in conformation 1 picks up Na^+. (2) Transporter in conformation 2 translocates and releases Na^+. (3) Transporter in conformation 2 picks up K^+. (4) Transporter in conformation 1 translocates and releases K^+.

of the binding protein for the cations can occur such that there is a decrease in affinity constants, resulting in the release of the cation into a milieu where the concentration is higher than that from which it was transported.

As an indication of the importance of this enzyme, it has been estimated that Na^+,K^+–ATPase uses about 60–70% of the ATP synthesized by cells in nerve and muscle, and may utilize about 35% of ATP generated in a resting individual.

Ca^{2+} Translocation Is Another Example of a Primary Active Transport System

Ca^{2+} is an important **intracellular messenger** regulating cellular processes as varied as muscle contraction and carbohydrate metabolism. The signal initiated by some hormones, the primary messenger to direct cells to alter their function, is transmitted by changes in cytosolic Ca^{2+}; for this reason Ca^{2+} is referred to as a **second messenger.** Cytosolic Ca^{2+} is in the range of 0.10 μM, over 10,000 times lower than extracellular Ca^{2+}. Intracellular Ca^{2+} concentrations can be increased rapidly by (1) transient opening of Ca^{2+} channels in the plasma membrane, permitting flow of Ca^{2+} down the large concentration gradient, or (2) by release from stores of Ca^{2+} in endoplasmic or sarcoplasmic reticulum. In order to reestablish low cytosolic levels, Ca^{2+} is actively transported out of cells across the plasma membrane or into the endoplasmic or sarcoplasmic reticulum. With both membrane systems, a **Ca^{2+} transporter** of the E_1–E_2 type is involved in which ATP is hydrolyzed during translocation. The transporter catalyzes a Ca^{2+}-stimulated ATPase activity.

Ca^{2+}–ATPase of sarcoplasmic reticulum of muscle, which is involved in the contraction–relaxation cycles of muscle, represents 80% of the integral membrane protein of the sarcoplasmic reticulum and occupies one-third of the surface area (see p. 954); it has many properties similar to Na^+,K^+–ATPase. The protein has ten membrane-spanning helices and is phosphorylated on an aspartyl residue during the Ca^{2+} translocation reaction. Two Ca^{2+} ions are translocated for each ATP hydrolyzed and it can move Ca^{2+} against a very large concentration gradient.

The Ca^{2+} transporter of plasma membranes has properties similar to the enzyme of sarcoplasmic reticulum. In eukaryotic cells, the transporter is regulated by cytosolic Ca^{2+} levels through a calcium-binding protein termed **calmodulin.** As cellular Ca^{2+} levels rise, Ca^{2+} is bound to calmodulin, which has a dissociation constant of ~1 μM. The Ca^{2+}–calmodulin complex binds to the

Ca^{2+} transporter, leading to an increased rate in Ca^{2+} transport. The rate is increased by lowering the K_m for Ca^{2+} of the transporter from about 20 to 0.5 μM. Increased activity reduces cytosolic Ca^{2+} to its normal resting level (~0.10 μM) at which concentration the Ca^{2+}–calmodulin complex dissociates and the rate of the Ca^{2+} transporter returns to a lower value. Thus the Ca^{2+}–calmodulin complex exerts fine control on the Ca^{2+} transporter. Calmodulin is one of several Ca^{2+}-binding proteins, including **parvalbumin** and **troponin C,** all of which have very similar structures. The Ca^{2+}–calmodulin complex is also involved in control of other cellular processes, which are affected by Ca^{2+}. The protein (17 kDa) has the shape of a dumbbell with two globular ends connected by a seven-turn α-helix; there are four Ca^{2+}-binding sites, two high affinity on one lobe and two low affinity on the other. It is believed that the binding of Ca^{2+} to the lower affinity binding sites causes a conformational change in the protein, revealing a hydrophobic area that can interact with a protein that it controls. Each Ca^{2+}-binding site consists of a helix–loop–helix structural motif (Figure 5.46) and Ca^{2+} is bound in the loop connecting the helices. A similar structure is found in other Ca^{2+}-binding proteins. The motif is referred to as the **EF hand,** based on studies with parvalbumin where the Ca^{2+} is bound between helices E and F of the protein.

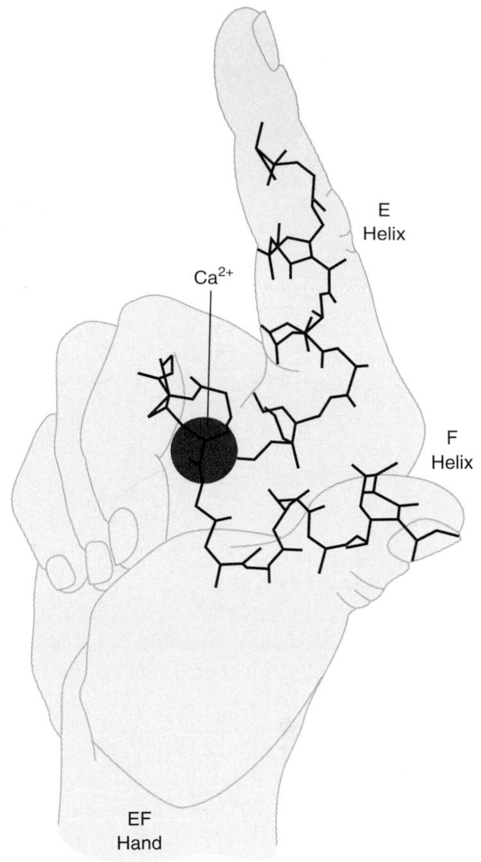

FIGURE 5.46
Binding site for Ca^{2+} in calmodulin.
Calmodulin contains four Ca^{2+}-binding sites, each with a helix–loop–helix motif. The Ca^{2+} ion is bound in the loop that connects two helices. This motif occurs in various Ca^{2+}-binding proteins and is referred to as the EF hand.

Na^+-Dependent Transport of Glucose and Amino Acids Are Secondary Active Transport Systems

The mechanisms described above for the active transport of cations involve the direct hydrolysis of ATP as the driving force. *Cells have another energy source, the gradient of Na^+ ion across the plasma membrane, which is utilized to move sugars, amino acids, and Ca^{2+} actively.* A symport translocation system involving simultaneous movement of both a Na^+ ion and glucose in the same direction is present in plasma membranes of cells of kidney tubule and intestinal epithelium. The general mechanism is presented in Figure 5.47. The diagram represents the **transport of D-glucose** driven by the movement of Na^+ ion down its concentration gradient. During transport of the sugar no hydrolysis of ATP occurs. There is an absolute requirement for Na^+, and in the process of translocation one Na^+ is moved with each glucose molecule. It can be considered that Na^+ is moving by passive facilitated transport down its chemical gradient and glucose carried along even against its concentration gradient. It is obligatory that the transporter translocates a glucose with the Na^+ ion. In the transport the chemical gradient of Na^+ ion is dissipated and unless the Na^+ ion gradient is continuously regenerated, transport of glucose will cease. The Na^+ gradient is maintained by the Na^+,K^+-exchanging ATPase described above and also represented in Figure 5.47. Thus metabolic energy in the form of ATP is indirectly involved in glucose transport because it is utilized to maintain the Na^+ ion gradient. Inhibition of ATP synthesis and a subsequent decrease in ATP will alter the Na^+ ion gradient and inhibit glucose uptake. Ouabain, the inhibitor of the Na^+,K^+ transporter, inhibits uptake of glucose by preventing the cell from maintaining the Na^+–K^+ gradient. Each glucose molecule requires only one-third of an ATP to be translocated because three Na^+ ions are translocated for the hydrolysis of each ATP in the Na^+,K^+-exchanging ATPase.

Amino acids are also translocated by the luminal epithelial cells of the intestines by Na^+-dependent pathways similar to the Na^+-dependent glucose transporter. At least seven different translocators have been identified for different classes of amino acids (see p. 1072 for details). The Na^+ gradient is also utilized to drive the transport of other ions, including a symport mechanism in the small intestines for the uptake of Cl^- with Na^+ and an antiport mechanism for the excretion of Ca^{2+} out of the cell.

The chemical mechanism for the symport movement of molecules utilizing the Na^+ ion gradient involves a cooperative interaction of the Na^+ ion and the other molecule translocated on the protein. A conformational change of

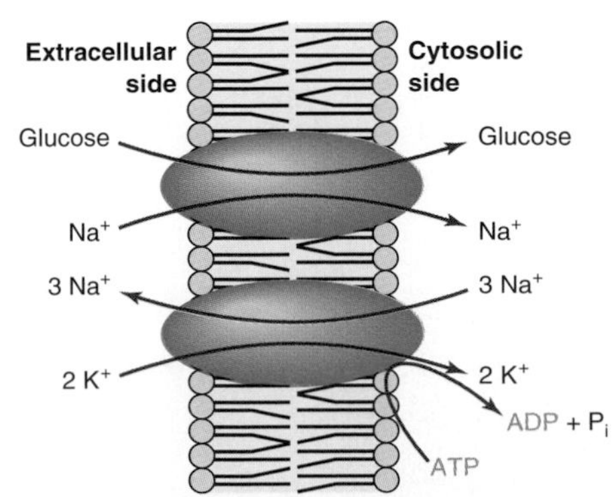

FIGURE 5.47
Na^+-dependent symport transport of glucose across the plasma membrane.

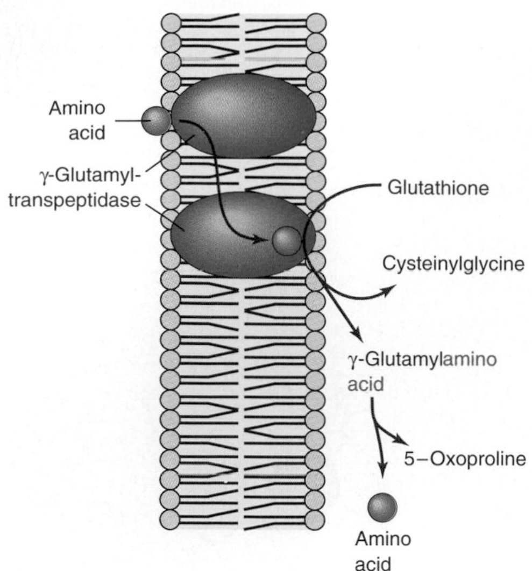

FIGURE 5.48
The γ-glutamyl cycle.
Represented are the key reactions involved in the group translocation of amino acids across liver cell plasma membranes. The continued uptake of amino acids requires the constant resynthesis of glutathione via a series of ATP-requiring reactions described in Chapter 11, page 485.

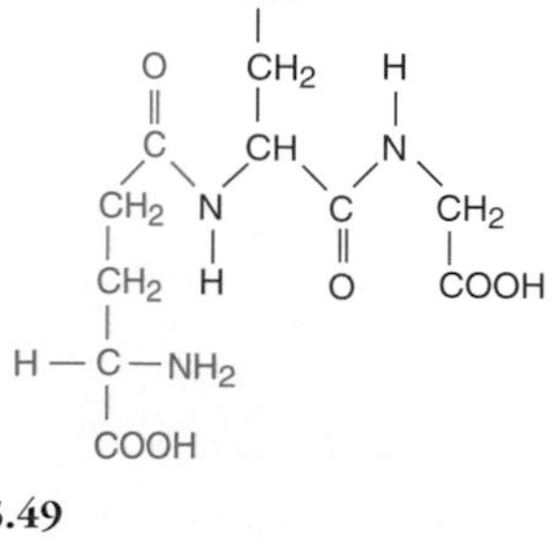

FIGURE 5.49
Glutathione (γ-glutamylcysteinylglycine).

the protein occurs following association of the two ligands, which moves them the necessary distance to bring them into contact with the cytosolic environment. Dissociation of Na^+ ion from the transporter because of the low Na^+ ion concentration inside the cell leads to a return of the protein to its original conformation, a decrease in affinity for the other ligand, and release of ligand into the cytosol.

Group Translocation Involves Chemical Modification of the Substrate Transported

As discussed previously, a major hurdle for any active transport system is release of the transported molecule from the binding site after translocation. If affinity of the transporter for the translocated molecule does not change, there cannot be movement against a concentration gradient. In the active transport systems described above a change in affinity for the substance by the transporter occurs by a conformational change of the protein. An alternate mechanism for release of a substrate is chemical change of the molecule after translocation but before release from the transporter, leading to a new compound bound to the transporter with a lower affinity for the transporter. The process is termed **group translocation.** The **γ-glutamyl cycle** for the transport of amino acids across the plasma membrane of some tissues is an example where the substrate is altered during transport and released into the cell as a different molecule. Reactions of the transport mechanism are presented in Figure 5.48. The pathway involves the enzyme **γ-glutamyltranspeptidase,** a membrane-bound enzyme. This leads to formation of a dipeptide with the amino acid transported. The amino acid transported is the substrate to which the γ-glutamyl residue of **glutathione** (Figure 5.49; see p. 485) is transferred. The new dipeptide is not part of the chemical gradient across the membrane of the amino acid. The γ-glutamyl derivative is then hydrolyzed by a separate enzyme, not on the membrane, leaving the free amino acid and oxoproline.

All the amino acids except proline can be transported by group translocation. The energy for transport comes from the hydrolysis of a peptide bond in glutathione. For the system to continue, glutathione must be resynthesized, which requires the expenditure of three ATP molecules (see p. 485). Thus for each amino acid translocated, three ATPs are required. Recall that the expenditure of only one-third of an ATP is required for each amino acid transported in the Na^+-dependent translocase system. Group translocation is an expensive energetic mechanism for transport of amino acids. The pathway is present in many tissues but some doubt has been raised about its physiological significance in that individuals have been identified with a genetic absence of the γ-glutamyl-transpeptidase without any apparent difficulty in amino acid transport. Cells may have several alternate methods for the transport of amino acids and are not dependent on one mechanism.

A group translocation mechanism for uptake of sugars is found in bacteria. This pathway involves phosphorylation of the sugar, using phosphoenolpyruvate as the phosphate donor. The mechanism is referred to as the **phosphoenolpyruvate-dependent phosphotransferase system** (PTS).

Summary of Transport Systems

The foregoing has presented the major mechanisms for movement of molecules across cellular membranes, particularly the plasma membrane. Cell organelles and membrane systems have a variety of transport systems. Mitochondria have transport mechanisms utilizing a proton gradient (see p. 243). Bacteria have transport systems analogous to those observed in mammalian cells. Table 5.6 summarizes characteristics of some major transport systems found in mammalian cells (see Clin. Corr. 5.4).

TABLE 5.6 Major Transport Systems in Mammalian Cells[a]

Substance Transported	*Mechanism of Transport*	*Tissues*
Sugars		
Glucose	Passive	Widespread
	Active symport with Na^+	Small intestines and renal tubular cells
Fructose	Passive	Intestines and liver
Amino acids		
Amino acid-specific transporters	Active symport with Na^+	Intestines, kidney, and liver
All amino acids except proline	Active group translocation	Liver
Specific amino acids	Passive	Small intestine
Other organic molecules		
ATP–ADP	Antiport transport of nucleotides; can be active transport	Mitochondria
Ascorbic acid	Active symport with Na^+	Widespread
Biotin	Active symport with Na^+	Liver
Cholic acid, deoxycholic acid, and taurocholic acid	Active symport with Na^+	Intestines
Dicarboxylic acids	Active symport with Na^+	Kidney
Folate	Active	Widespread
Lactate and monocarboxylic acids	Active symport with H^+	Widespread
Neurotransmitters (e.g., γ-amino butyric acid, norepinephrine, glutamate, dopamine)	Active symport with Na^+	Brain
Organic anions (e.g., malate, α-ketoglutarate, glutamate)	Antiport with counterorganic anion	Mitochondria
Peptides (2 to 4 amino acids)	Active symport with H^+	Intestines
Urea	Passive	Erythrocytes and kidney
Inorganic ions		
H^+	Active	Mitochondria
H^+	Active; vacuolar ATPase	Widespread; lysosomes, endosomes, and Golgi complex
Na^+	Passive	Distal renal tubular cells
Na^+, H^+	Active antiport	Proximal renal tubular cells and small intestines
Na^+, K^+	Active: ATP driven	Plasma membrane of all cells
Na^+, HPO_4^{2-}	Active cotransport	Kidney
Ca^{2+}	Active: ATP driven	Plasma membrane and endoplasmic (sarcoplasmic) reticulum
Ca^{2+}, Na^+	Active antiport	Widespread
H^+, K^+	Active antiport	Parietal cells of gastric mucosa secreting H^+
Cl^-/HCO_3^-	Passive antiport	Erythrocytes and other cells

[a] The transport systems are only indicative of the variety of transporters known; others responsible for a variety of substances have been proposed. Most systems have been studied in only a few tissues and their localization may be more extensive than indicated.

5.9 ■ IONOPHORES

An interesting class of antibiotics of bacterial origin facilitates the movement of monovalent and divalent inorganic ions across biological and synthetic lipid membranes. These molecules, called **ionophores,** are not large macromolecules such as proteins but are relatively small molecular weight compounds (up to several thousand daltons). Ionophores are divided into two major groups:

CLINICAL CORRELATION 5.4

Diseases Due to Loss of Membrane Transport Systems

A number of pathological conditions are due to an alteration in the transport systems for specific cellular components. Some of these are discussed in the appropriate sections describing the metabolism of the intermediates. Individuals have been observed with a decrease in glucose uptake from the intestinal tract due to a loss of the specific sodium-coupled glucose–galactose transporter. Fructose malabsorption syndromes have been observed, which are due to an alteration in the activity of the transport system for fructose. In Hartnup's disease there is a decrease in the transport of neutral amino acids in the epithelial cells of the intestine and renal tubules.

In cystinuria, renal reabsorption of cystine and the basic amino acids lysine and arginine is abnormal, resulting in formation of cystine kidney stones. In hypophosphatemic, vitamin D resistant rickets, renal absorption of phosphate is abnormal. Little is known concerning possible changes of transport activities in tissues such as muscle, liver, and brain but it has been suggested that there may be a number of pathological states due to the loss of specific transport mechanisms.

Evans, L., Grasset, E., Heyman, M., et. al. Congenital selective malabsorption of glucose and galactose. *J. Pediatr. Gastroenterol. Nutr.* 4:878, 1985.

TABLE 5.7 Major Ionophores

Compound	*Major Cations Transported*	*Action*
Valinomycin	K^+ or Rb^+	Uniport, electrogenic
Nonactin	NH_4^+, K^+	Uniport, electrogenic
A23187	$Ca^{2+}/2\ H^+$	Antiport, electroneutral
Nigericin	K^+/H^+	Antiport, electroneutral
Monensin	Na^+/H^+	Antiport, electroneutral
Gramicidin	H^+, Na^+, K^+, Rb^+	Forms channels
Alamethicin	K^+, Rb^+	Forms channels

(1) **mobile carriers** are those ionophores that diffuse back and forth across the membrane carrying the ion from one side of the membrane to the other, and (2) ionophores that form a **channel** that transverses the membrane and through which ions can diffuse. With both types, ions are translocated by a passive mediated transport mechanism. The ionophores that diffuse back and forth across the membrane are more affected by changes in the fluidity of the membrane than those that form a channel. Some major ionophores are listed in Table 5.7.

Each ionophore has a definite ion specificity; **valinomycin,** whose structure is given in Figure 5.50, has an affinity for K^+ that is 1000 times greater than that for Na^+, and the antibiotic A23187 (Figure 5.51) translocates Ca^{2+} 10 times more actively than Mg^{2+}. Several of the diffusion type ionophores have a cyclic structure. The metal ion is coordinated to several oxygen atoms in the core of the ionophore; the periphery of the molecule consists of hydrophobic groups. The interaction of the ionophore leads to a chelation of the ion, stripping away its surrounding water shell and encompassing the ion by a hydrophobic shell. The ionophore–ion complex freely diffuses across the membrane. Since the interaction of ion and ionophore is an equilibrium reaction, a steady state develops in the concentration of ions on both sides of the membrane. The specificity of the ionophore is due in part to the size of the pore into which the ion fits and to the attraction of the ionophore for the ion in competition with water molecules.

Valinomycin transports K^+ by an electrogenic uniport mechanism and can create an electrochemical gradient across a membrane as it carries a positively charged K^+ across the membrane. **Nigericin** is an electrically neutral antiporter; its carboxyl group when dissociated binds a positive ion, such as K^+, leading to a neutral molecule that crosses a membrane. On diffusion back through the

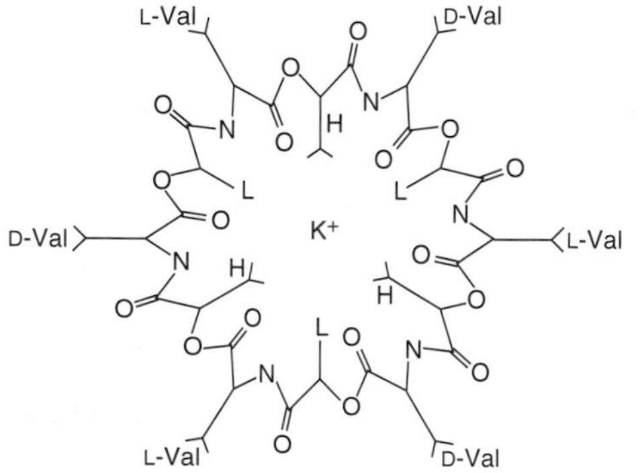

FIGURE 5.50
Structure of the valinomycin–K^+ complex.
Abbreviations: D-Val, D-valine; L-Val, L-valine; L, L-lactate; and H, D-hydroxyisovalerate.

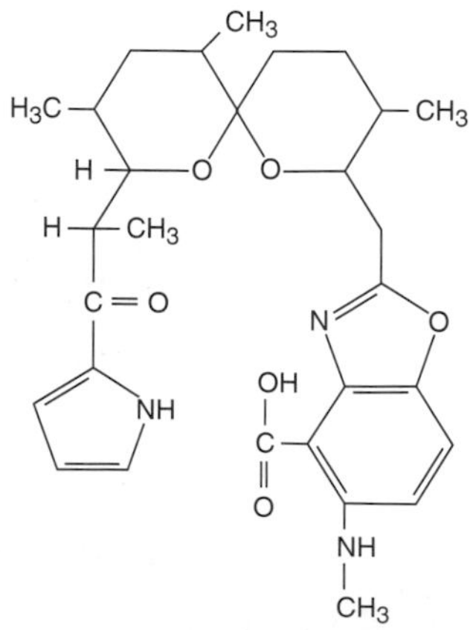

FIGURE 5.51
Structure of A23187, a Ca^{2+} ionophore.

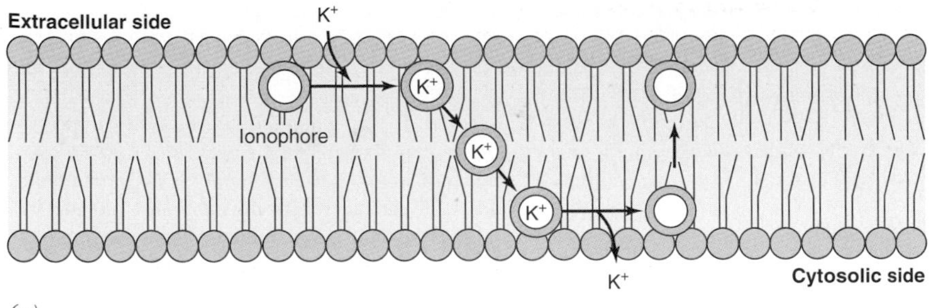

(a)

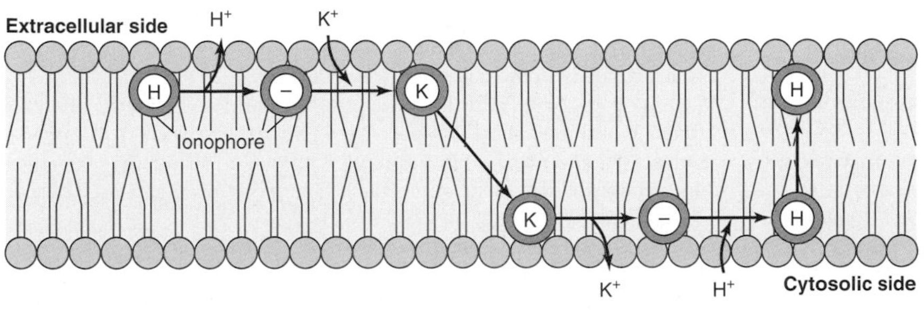

(b)

FIGURE 5.52
Proposed mechanism for the ionophoretic activities of valinomycin and nigericin. (*a*) Transport by valinomycin. (*b*) Transport by nigericin. The valinomycin–K^+ complex is positively charged and translocation of K^+ is electrogenic, leading to the creation of a charge separation across the membrane. Nigericin translocates K^+ in exchange for a H^+ across the membrane and the mechanism is electrically neutral.
Diagram adopted from B. C. Pressman, Annu. Rev. Biochem. *45:501, 1976.*

membrane it transports a proton; overall K^+ exchanges for H^+. These mechanisms are presented in Figure 5.52.

Gramicidin A is an example of an ionophore that creates a pore in the membrane. This type of ionophore has a low ion selectivity because ions are diffusing through a hole in the membrane. Two molecules of gramicidin A form a channel and the dimer is in constant equilibrium with the free monomer form. By association and dissociation of the monomers in the membrane, channels can be formed and broken; the rate of interaction of two molecules of gramicidin A controls the rate of ion flux. The structure of the molecule suggests that polar peptide groups line the channel and hydrophobic groups are on the periphery of the channel interacting with the lipid membrane.

The antibiotic ionophores have been a valuable experimental tool in studies involving ion translocation in biological membranes and for the manipulation of the ionic compositions of cells. There have been reports that proteolipids, prostaglandins, and perhaps other lipids present in mammalian tissues may function as ionophores.

BIBLIOGRAPHY

General

Bonner, F. *Current Topics in Membranes and Transport.* A series published regularly. New York: Academic Press.

Caplen, M. *Cell Biology and Membrane and Transport Processes.* San Diego: Academic Press, 1994.

Davis, L. I. The nuclear pore complex. *Annu. Rev. Biochem.* 64:865, 1995.

Dobler, M. *Ionophores and Their Structure.* New York: Wiley-Interscience, 1981.

Gennis, R. B. *Biomembranes: Molecular Structure and Function.* New York: Springer-Verlag, 1989.

Gregoriadas, G. Engineering liposomes for drug delivery: progress and problems. *Trends Biotechnol.* 13:527, 1995.

Harwood, J. L. Understanding liposomal properties to aid in their clinical usage. *Trends Biochem. Sci.* 17:203, 1992.

Hockstra, D. *Cell Lipids.* San Diego: Academic Press, 1994.

Jain, M. K. *Introduction to Biological Membranes,* 2nd ed. New York: Wiley, 1988.

Jones, M. N. *Micelles, Monolayers, and Biomembranes.* New York: Wiley-Liss, 1995.

Lipowsky, R., and Sackmann, E. *Structure and Dynamics of Membranes.* New York: Elsevier Science, 1995.

Papa, S., and Tager, J. M. *Biochemistry of Cell Membranes.* Basel: Birkhauser Verlag, 1995.

Shohet, S. B., and Lux, S. E. The erythrocyte membrane skeleton: biochemistry and pathophysiology. *Hosp. Pract.* 19:77–83 and 89–108, 1984.

Stein, W. D. *Channels, Carriers, and Pumps: An Introduction to Membrane Transport.* San Diego: Academic Press, 1990.

Watts, A. *Protein–Lipid Interactions.* New York: Elsevier, 1993.

Yeagle, P. *The Membranes of Cells.* San Diego: Academic Press, 1993.

Membrane Structure

Devaux, P. F. Static and dynamic lipid asymmetry in cell membranes. *Biochemistry 30:1163, 1991.*

Low, M., and Saltiel, A. R. Structural and functional roles of glycosylphosphatidyl inositol in membranes. *Science* 239:268, 1988.

McMurchie, E. J. Dietary lipids and the regulation of membrane fluidity and function. In: *Physiological Regulation of Membrane Fluidity*. New York: Liss, 1988, p. 189.

Singer, S. J., and Nicolson, G. L. The fluid mosaic model of the structure of cell membranes. *Science* 175:720, 1972.

Stubbs, C. D. Membrane fluidity: structure and dynamics of membrane lipids. In: P. N. Campbell and R. D. Marshall (Eds.), *Essays in Biochemistry,* Vol. 19. London: Academic Press, 1983, p. 1.

Yeagle, P. L. Lipid regulation of cell membrane structure and function. *FASEB J.* 3:1833, 1989.

Transport Processes

Agutter, P. S. Intracellular structure and nucleocytoplasmic transport. *Int. Rev. Cytol.* 162B:183, 1995.

Bamberg, E., and Passow, H. *The Band 3 Proteins: Anion Transporters, Binding Proteins and Senescent Antigens.* New York: Elsevier, 1992.

Carafoli, E. The Ca^{2+} pump of the plasma membrane. *J. Biol. Chem.* 267: 2115, 1992.

Catterall, W. A. Structure and function of voltage-gated ion channels. *Annu. Rev. Biochem.* 64:493, 1995.

Eisenman, G., and Dani, J. A. An introduction to molecular architecture and permeability of ion channels. *Annu. Rev. Biophys. Chem.* 16:205, 1987.

Gould, G. W., and Holman, G. D. The glucose transporter family: structure, function and tissue specific expression. *Biochem. J.* 295:329, 1993.

Hediger, M. A., Kanai, U., You, G., and Nussberger, S. Mammalian ion-coupled solute transporters. *J. Physiol. (Lond)* 482:75, 1995.

Horne, D. W. Transport of folates and antifolates in liver. *Proc. Soc. Exp. Biol. Med.* 202:385, 1993.

Kakuda, D. K., and MacLeod, C. L. Na^+-independent transport (uniport) of amino acids and glucose in mammalian cells. *J. Exp. Biol.* 196:93, 1994.

Kanai, Y., Smith, C. P., and Hediger, M. A. A new family of neurotransmitter transporters: the high affinity glutamate transporters. *FASEB J.* 7:1450, 1993.

Kanner, B. I. Sodium-coupled neurotransmitter: structure, function and regulation. *J. Exp. Biol.* 196:237, 1994.

Katz, A. M. Cardiac ion channels. *N. Engl. J. Med.* 328:1244, 1993.

Maeckler, M. Facilitative glucose transporters. *Eur. J. Biochem.* 219:713, 1994.

Marsh, D. Peptide models for membrane channels. *Biochem. J.* 315:345, 1996.

Martonosi, A. (Ed.). *The Enzymes of Biological Membranes: Membrane Transport,* Vol. 3, New York: Plenum Press, 1985.

McGiven, J. D., and Pastor-Anglada, M. Regulatory and molecular aspects of mammalian amino acid transport. *Biochem. J.* 299:321, 1994.

Miller, M., Park, N. K., and Hanover, J. A. Nuclear pore complex: structure, function and regulation. *Physiol. Rev.* 71:909, 1991.

Pederson, P., and Carafoli, E. Ion motive ATPases. I. Ubiquity, properties, and significance to cell function, and II. Energy coupling and work output. *Trends Biochem. Sci.* 12:146 and 186, 1987.

Poole, R. C., and Halestrap, A. P. Transport of lactate and other monocarboxylates across mammalian plasma membranes. *Am. J. Physiol.* 264:C761, 1993.

Skou, J. C., and Norby, D. G. (Eds.). *Na^+,K^+–ATPase: Structure and Kinetics.* New York: Academic Press, 1979.

Worrall, D. M., and Williams, D. C. Sodium ion-dependent transporters for neurotransmitters: a review of recent developments. *Biochem. J.* 297: 425, 1994.

QUESTIONS ■ C. N. ANGSTADT AND J. BAGGOTT

1. Cell membranes typically:
   A. are about 90% phospholipid.
   B. have both integral and peripheral proteins.
   C. contain cholesteryl esters.
   D. contain free carbohydrate such as glucose.
   E. contain large amounts of triacylglycerols.

Refer to the following for Questions 2–5:
   A. cerebrosides
   B. gangliosides
   C. phosphatidylcholines
   D. phosphatidylinositols
   E. sphingomyelins

2. Sphingolipids containing phosphorus.

3. Incorporate an oligosaccharide containing sialic acid.

4. Belong to the class of neutral glycosphingolipids.

5. Contain a hexahydroxy alcohol.

6. According to the fluid mosaic model of a membrane:
   A. proteins are always completely embedded in the lipid bilayer.
   B. transverse movement (flip-flop) of a protein in the membrane is thermodynamically favorable.
   C. the transmembrane domain has largely hydrophobic amino acids.
   D. proteins are distributed symmetrically in the membrane.
   E. peripheral proteins are attached to the membrane only by noncovalent forces.

7. Characteristics of a mediated transport system include:
   A. nonspecific binding of solute to transporter.
   B. release of the transporter from the membrane following transport.
   C. a rate of transport directly proportional to the concentration of solute.
   D. release of the solute only if the concentration on the new side is lower than that on the original side.
   E. a mechanism for translocating the solute from one side of the membrane to the other.

8. Membrane channels:
   A. have a large aqueous area in the protein structure so are not very selective.
   B. commonly contain amphipathic α-helices.
   C. are opened or closed only as a result of a change in the transmembrane potential.
   D. are the same as gap junctions.
   E. allow substrates to flow only from the outside to inside of the cell.

9. Which of the following require(s) a transporter that specifically binds a solute?
   A. active mediated transport
   B. gap junction
   C. membrane channel
   D. simple diffusion
   E. all of the above

10. Which of the following can transport a solute against its concentration gradient?
    A. active mediated transport
    B. passive mediated transport
    C. both of the above systems
    D. neither of the above systems

11. The transport system that maintains the Na^+ and K^+ gradients across the plasma membrane of cells:
    A. involves an enzyme that is an ATPase.
    B. is a symport system.
    C. moves Na^+ either into or out of the cell.
    D. is an electrically neutral system.
    E. in the membrane, hydrolyzes ATP independently of the movement of Na^+ and K^+.

12. A mediated transport system would be expected to:
    A. show a continuously increasing initial rate of transport with increasing substrate concentration.
    B. exhibit structural and/or stereospecificity for the substance transported.
    C. be slower than that of a simple diffusion system.
    D. establish a concentration gradient across the membrane.
    E. exist only in plasma membranes.

The answers to Questions 13 and 14 are based on the following figure:

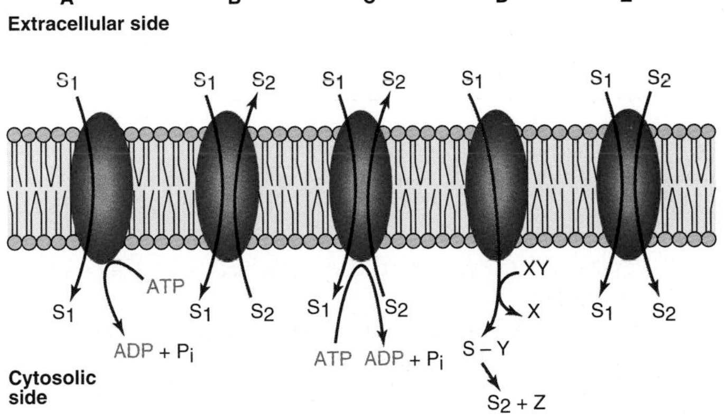

13. Represents a passive mediated antiport system.

14. Could represent the Na^+-driven uptake of glucose.

15. The translocation of Ca^{2+} across a membrane:
    A. is a passive mediated transport.
    B. is an example of a symport system.
    C. involves the phosphorylation of a serine residue by ATP.
    D. may be regulated by the binding of a Ca^{2+}–calmodulin complex to the transporter.
    E. maintains $[Ca^{2+}]$ very much higher in the cell than in extracellular fluid.

16. The group translocation type of transport system:
    A. does not require metabolic energy.
    B. involves the transport of two different solute molecules simultaneously.
    C. has been demonstrated for fatty acids.
    D. results in the alteration of the substrate molecule during the transport process.
    E. uses ATP to maintain a concentration gradient.

17. All of the following are correct about an ionophore EXCEPT it:
    A. requires the input of metabolic energy for mediated transport of an ion.
    B. may diffuse back and forth across a membrane.
    C. may form a channel across a membrane through which an ion may diffuse.
    D. may catalyze electrogenic mediated transport of an ion.
    E. will have specificity for the ion it moves.

ANSWERS

1. B (Figures 5.2 and 5.17). A: This is more than the total lipid. C: Cholesterol in membranes is unesterified. D: All carbohydrate in membranes is in the form of glycoproteins and glycolipids. E: This is a minor component, if present (pp. 180 and 187).
2. E A sphingomyelin is the only type of sphingolipid-containing phosphate (Figures 5.13).
3. B By definition, gangliosides contain sialic acid (p. 185).
4. A Cerebrosides are neutral; no phosphate; uncharged sugar. Gangliosides, by virtue of the presence of sialic acid, are acidic. Note: Sulfatides, which are acidic, are derived from cerebrosides but are not themselves classified as cerebrosides (pp. 184 and 185).
5. D The alcohol is inositol, which is often phosphorylated (p. 182).
6. C Hydrophobic domains will be in the interior; hydrophilic domains will be at either surface of the membrane (p. 189, Figure 5.19). A: Proteins may also be on the surface. B: Transverse motion of proteins is even less than that of lipids (p. 195). D: Both proteins and lipids are distributed asymmetrically. E: Glycans bind covalently to an amino acid as part of GPI anchors (p. 192).
7. E A: Specificity of binding is an integral part of the process. B: Recovery of the transporter to its original condition is one of the characteristics of mediated transport. C: Only at low concentrations of solute; transporters show saturation kinetics. D: Active transport, movement against a gradient, is also mediated transport (p. 198).
8. B A: This describes a pore; channels are quite specific. C: Voltage-gated channels, like that for Na^+, are controlled this way but others, like the nicotinic–acetylcholine channel, are chemically regulated. D: Clusters of membrane channels

work together to form a gap junction. E: Substances may move in either direction as dictated by the concentration gradient (p. 201).

9. A Specific binding by the transporter is a characteristic of mediated systems. B–D: These do not require a transporter (p. 196).
10. A Transportation against a gradient requires the input of energy (p. 204).
11. A The Na^+,K^+ transporter is the Na^+,K^+–ATPase. It is an antiport, vectorial (Na^+ out), electrogenic (3 Na^+, 2 K^+) system. ATP hydrolysis is not useless (p. 206).
12. B A and B: Mediated transport systems show saturation kinetics and substrate specificity (p. 199). C: The purpose of the transporter is to aid the transport of water-soluble substances across the lipid membrane (p. 197). D: This would be true only if the system were an active one. E: Mediated systems are also present in other membranes, for example, mitochondrial membrane (p. 199).
13. B The figure is a modified composite of Figures 5.32, 5.38, 5.39, and 5.48.
14. E All systems are mediated. A: An active uniport. B: A passive antiport; for example, Cl^-–HCO_3^-. C: An *active* antiport; for example, Na^+,K^+–ATPase. D: A group translocation representing a change in S_1 during transport. E: A symport system; in this case, S_1 could be glucose and S_2 could be Na^+.
15. D This occurs with the eukaryotic plasma membrane (p. 208). A and B: Ca^{2+} translocation is an active uniport. C: Like Na^+,K^+–ATPase, phosphorylation occurs on an aspartyl residue. E: Extracellular is about 10,000 times higher.
16. D In eukaryotic cells, amino acids are transported by group translocation in which they are converted to a γ-glutamyl amino acid during transport (Figure 5.48). A and E: It is an active system with the ATP used to resynthesize the intermediate, glutathione. B and C: The system transports a single amino acid at a time (p. 210).
17. A Ionophores transport by passive mediated mechanisms (p. 212). B and C: These are the two major types of ionophores. D: Valinomycin transports K^+ by a uniport mechanism. There are also antiport systems that are electroneutral. E: For example, valinomycin has an affinity for K^+ 1000 times greater than for Na^+.

CHAPTER

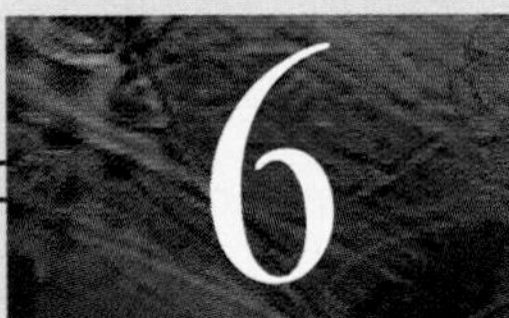

BIOENERGETICS AND OXIDATIVE METABOLISM

Merle S. Olson

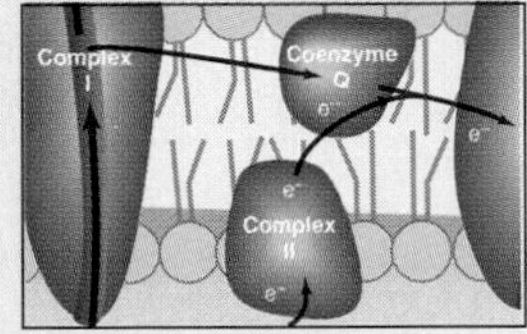

6.1 ENERGY-PRODUCING AND ENERGY-UTILIZING SYSTEMS

Living cells are composed of a complex, intricately regulated system of energy-producing and energy-utilizing chemical reactions. Metabolic reactions involved in energy generation break down ingested or stored fuels such as carbohydrate, lipid, or protein in what are termed **catabolic** pathways. These reactions usually result in the conversion of large complex molecules to smaller molecules (ultimately CO_2 and H_2O), with production of storable or conservable energy, and often require the consumption of oxygen during this process. Such reactions are accelerated during periods of fuel deprivation or stress to an organism.

Energy-utilizing reactions perform various necessary, and in many instances tissue-specific, cellular functions, for example, nerve impulse conduction, muscle contraction, growth, and cell division. Metabolic pathways involved in the biosynthesis of large, complex molecules from smaller precursors are termed **anabolic** pathways and require the expenditure of energy. Such reactions are accelerated when energy is readily available, when precursor molecules are in abundance, or during periods of growth or regeneration of cellular material.

ATP Links Energy-Producing and Energy-Utilizing Systems

The relationship between energy-producing and energy-utilizing functions of the cell is illustrated in Figure 6.1. Energy may be derived from oxidation of metabolic fuels presented to the organism usually in the form of carbohydrate, lipid, and protein. The proportion of each fuel utilized as an energy source depends on the tissue and the dietary and hormonal state of the organism. For example, mature erythrocytes and adult brain in the fed state use only carbohydrate as a source of energy, whereas the liver of a diabetic or fasted individual metabolizes primarily lipid to meet the energy demands. Energy may be consumed during performance of various energy-linked (work) functions, some of which are indicated in Figure 6.1. Note that the liver and the pancreas are primarily involved in biosynthetic and secretory work functions, whereas the primary function of cardiac and skeletal muscle involves converting metabolic energy into mechanical energy during muscle contraction.

The essential link between energy-producing and energy-utilizing pathways is the nucleoside triphosphate, **adenosine 5′-triphosphate (ATP)** (Figure 6.2). The ATP molecule is a purine (adenine) nucleotide in which the adenine is attached in a glycosidic linkage to D-ribose. Three phosphoryl groups are esterified to the 5 position of the ribose moiety in **phosphoanhydride bonds.** The

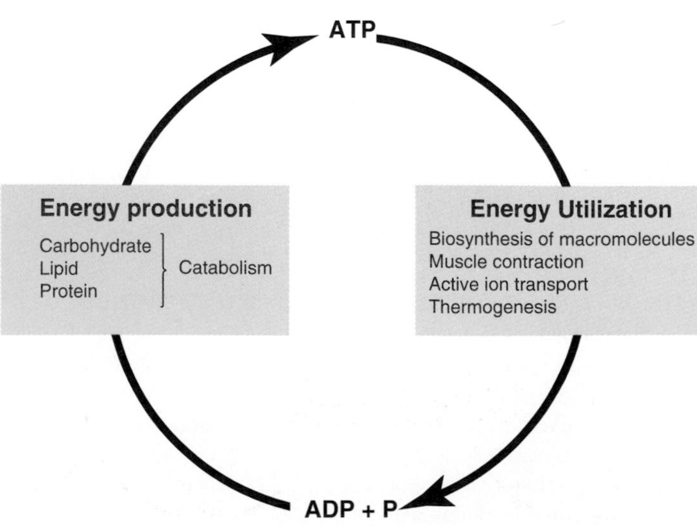

FIGURE 6.1
Relationship between energy production and energy utilization.

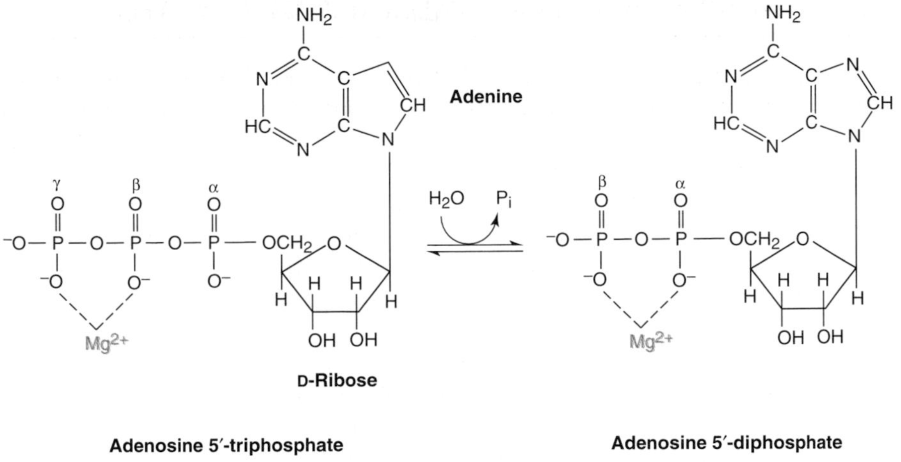

Adenine

D-Ribose

Adenosine 5′-triphosphate

H_2O P_i

Adenosine 5′-diphosphate

FIGURE 6.2
Structure of ATP and ADP complexed with Mg^{2+}.

two terminal phosphoryl groups (i.e., β and γ) are involved in the phosphoric acid anhydride bonding and are designated as energy-rich or **high-energy bonds.** Synthesizing ATP as a result of a catabolic process or consuming ATP in an energy-linked cellular function involves formation and either hydrolysis or transfer of the terminal phosphate group of ATP. The physiological form of this nucleotide is chelated with a divalent metal cation such as magnesium. Adenosine diphosphate also chelates magnesium, but the affinity of the metal cation for ADP is considerably less than for ATP. Although adenine nucleotides are mainly involved in energy generation or conservation, various nucleoside triphosphates, including ATP, are involved in transferring energy during biosynthetic processes. As indicated in Figure 6.3, the guanine nucleotide **GTP** serves as the source of energy in gluconeogenesis and protein synthesis, whereas

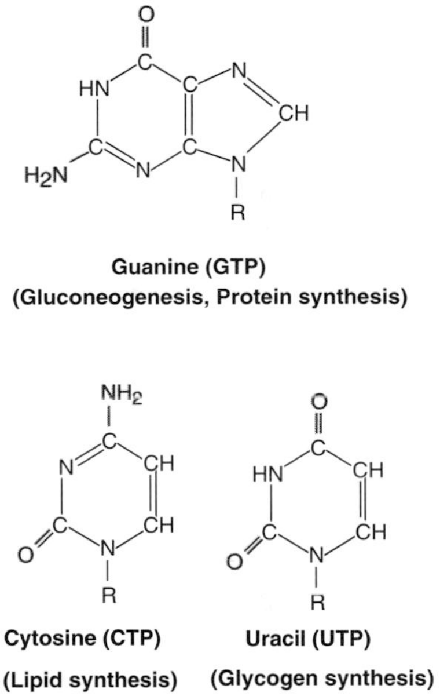

Guanine (GTP)
(Gluconeogenesis, Protein synthesis)

Cytosine (CTP)
(Lipid synthesis)

Uracil (UTP)
(Glycogen synthesis)

FIGURE 6.3
Structures of purine and pyrimidine bases involved in various biosynthetic pathways.

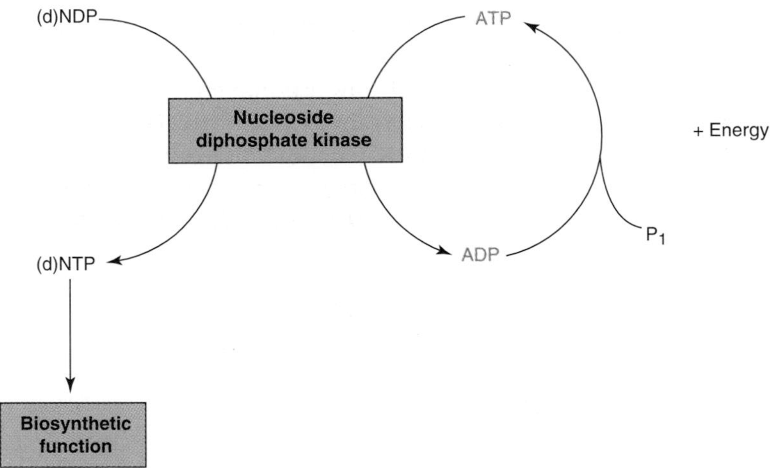

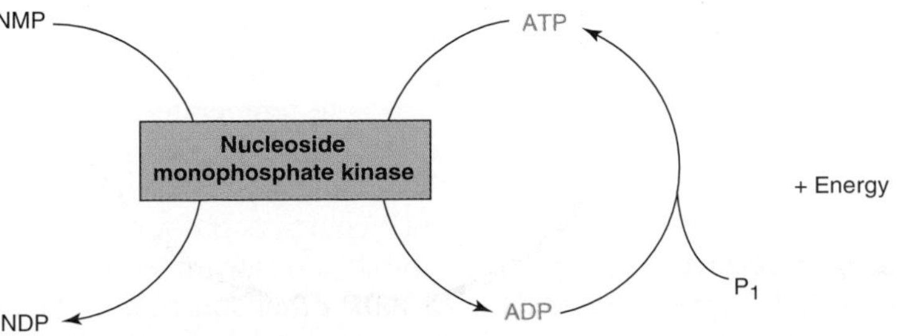

FIGURE 6.4
Nucleoside diphosphate kinase and nucleoside monophosphate kinase reactions.
N represents any purine or pyrimidine base; (d) indicates a deoxyribonucleotide.

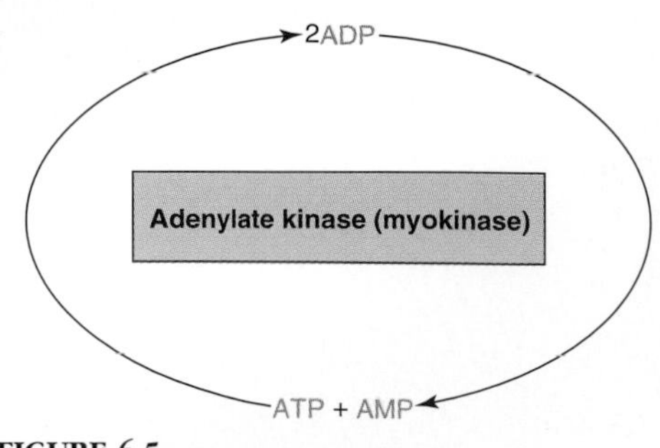

FIGURE 6.5
Adenylate kinase (myokinase) reaction.

UTP (uracil) and **CTP** (cytosine) are utilized in glycogen and lipid synthesis, respectively. The energy in the terminal phosphate bonds of ATP may be transferred to the other nucleotides, using either the **nucleoside diphosphate kinase** or the **nucleoside monophosphate kinase** reactions illustrated in Figure 6.4 (p. 219). Two nucleoside diphosphates can be converted to a nucleoside triphosphate and a nucleoside monophosphate in various nucleoside **monophosphate kinase** reactions, such as the adenylate kinase reaction (Figure 6.5). The utility of these types of enzymes is that the terminal energy-rich phosphate bonds of ATP may be transferred to the appropriate nucleotides and utilized in a variety of biosynthetic processes.

6.2 ■ THERMODYNAMIC RELATIONSHIPS AND ENERGY-RICH COMPONENTS

Because living cells interconvert different forms of energy and may exchange energy with their surroundings, it is necessary to review the principles of **thermodynamics,** which govern reactions of this type. Knowledge of these principles will facilitate a perception of how energy-producing and energy-utilizing metabolic reactions are permitted to occur within the same cell and how an organism is able to accomplish various work functions.

The **first law of thermodynamics** states that energy can neither be created nor destroyed. This law of energy conservation stipulates that, although energy may be converted from one form to another, the total energy in a system must remain constant. For example, chemical energy available in a metabolic fuel such as glucose can be converted in the process of glycolysis to another form of chemical energy, ATP. In skeletal muscle chemical energy involved in the energy-rich phosphate bonds of ATP may be converted to mechanical energy during the process of muscle contraction. The energy involved in an osmotic electropotential gradient of protons across the mitochondrial membrane may be converted to chemical energy using the proton gradient to drive ATP synthesis.

To discuss the **second law of thermodynamics** the term **entropy** must be defined. Entropy, designated by S, is a measure or indicator of the degree of disorder or randomness in a system. Entropy can be viewed as the energy in a system that is unavailable to perform useful work. All processes, whether chemical or biological, tend to progress toward a situation of maximum entropy. Equilibrium in a system will result when the randomness or disorder (entropy) is at a maximum. However, it is nearly impossible to quantitate entropy changes in biochemical systems and such systems are rarely at equilibrium. For simplicity and because of its inherent utility in these considerations, a quantity termed **free energy** is employed.

Free Energy Is the Energy Available for Useful Work

Free energy (denoted by G) of a system is that portion of the total energy in a system that is available for useful work. It can be further defined by

$$\Delta G = \Delta H - T\Delta S$$

In this expression for a system proceeding toward equilibrium at a constant temperature and pressure, ΔG is the change in free energy, ΔH is the change in enthalpy or the heat content, T is the absolute temperature, and ΔS is the change in entropy of the system. It can be deduced from this relationship that at equilibrium $\Delta G = 0$. Furthermore, any process that exhibits a negative free-energy change proceeds to equilibrium, since energy is given off, and is called an **exergonic reaction.** A process that exhibits a positive free-energy change will not occur independently; energy from some other source must be applied to this process to allow it to proceed toward equilibrium, and this type of process is termed an **endergonic reaction.** It should be noted that the change in free energy in a biochemical process is the same regardless of the pathway or mechanism employed to attain the final state. Whereas the rate of a given reaction depends on the free energy of activation, the magnitude of the ΔG is not related to the rate of the reaction. The change in free energy for a chemical reaction is related to the equilibrium constant of that reaction. For example, an enzymatic reaction may be described as

$$A + B \rightleftharpoons C + D$$

And an expression for the equilibrium constant may be written as

$$K_{eq} = \frac{[C][D]}{[A][B]}$$

The free-energy change (ΔG) at a constant temperature and pressure is defined as

$$\Delta G = \Delta G^\circ + RT \ln\left(\frac{[C][D]}{[A][B]}\right)$$

where ΔG is the free-energy change; ΔG° is the standard free-energy change, which is a constant for each individual reaction; reactants and products in the reaction are present at concentrations of 1.0 M; R is the gas constant, which is 1.987 cal mol^{-1} K^{-1} or 8.134 J mol^{-1} K^{-1}, depending on whether the resultant free-energy change is expressed in calories (cal) or joules (J) per mole; and T is the absolute temperature in degrees Kelvin (K).

Because at equilibrium $\Delta G = 0$, the expression reduces to

$$\Delta G^\circ = -RT \ln K_{eq}$$

or

$$\Delta G^\circ = -2.3RT \log K_{eq}$$

Hence, if the **equilibrium constant** for a reaction can be determined, the standard free-energy change (ΔG°) for that reaction also can be calculated. The relationship between ΔG° and K_{eq} is illustrated in Table 6.1. When the equilibrium constant of a reaction is less than unity, the reaction is endergonic, and ΔG° is positive. When the equilibrium constant is greater than unity, the reaction is exergonic, and ΔG° is negative.

In energy-producing and energy-utilizing metabolic pathways in cellular systems, free-energy changes characteristic of individual enzymatic reactions in an entire pathway are additive, for example,

$$A \rightarrow B \rightarrow C \rightarrow D$$

$$\Delta G^\circ_{A\rightarrow D} = \Delta G^\circ_{A\rightarrow B} + \Delta G^\circ_{B\rightarrow C} + \Delta G^\circ_{C\rightarrow D}$$

Although any given enzymatic reaction in a sequence may have a characteristic positive free-energy change, as long as the sum of all the free-energy changes is negative, the pathway will proceed.

Another way of expressing this principle is that enzymatic reactions with positive free-energy changes may be coupled to or driven by reactions with negative free-energy changes associated with them. In a metabolic pathway such as glycolysis, various individual reactions either have positive ΔG° values or ΔG° values that are close to zero. On the other hand, there are other reactions that have large and negative ΔG° values, which drive the entire pathway. The crucial consideration is that the sum of the ΔG° values for the individual reactions in a pathway must be negative in order for such a metabolic sequence to be thermodynamically feasible. Also, as for all chemical reactions, individual enzymatic reactions in a metabolic pathway or the pathway as a whole would

TABLE 6.1 Tabulation of Values of K_{eq} and ΔG°

K_{eq}	ΔG° (kcal mol^{-1})
10^{-4}	5.46
10^{-3}	4.09
10^{-2}	2.73
10^{-1}	1.36
1	0
10	−1.36
10^2	−2.73
10^3	−4.09
10^4	−5.46

TABLE 6.2 Free-Energy Changes and Caloric Values Associated with the Total Metabolism of Various Metabolic Fuels

Compound	*Molecular Weight*	*$\Delta G°$ (kcal mol^{-1})*	*Caloric Value (kcal g^{-1})*
Glucose	180	−686	3.81
Lactate	90	−326	3.62
Palmitate	256	−2380	9.30
Tripalmitin	809	−7510	9.30
Glycine	75	−234	3.12

be facilitated if the concentrations of the reactants (substrates) of the reaction exceed the concentrations of the products of the reaction.

The Caloric Value of Dietary Substances

During complete stepwise oxidation of glucose, a primary metabolic fuel in cells, a large quantity of energy is available. The free energy released during the oxidation of glucose in a functioning cell is illustrated in the following equation:

$$C_6H_{12}O_6 + 6\ O_2 \rightarrow 6\ CO_2 + 6\ H_2O \qquad \Delta G° = -686{,}000\ \text{cal mol}^{-1}$$

When this process occurs under aerobic conditions in most cells, it is possible to conserve less than one half of this "available" energy as 38 molecules of ATP. The $\Delta G°$ values for oxidation of other metabolic fuels are listed in Table 6.2. Carbohydrates and proteins (amino acids) have a caloric value of 3–4 kcal g^{-1}, while lipid (i.e., palmitate, a long-chain fatty acid, or a triacylglycerol) exhibits a caloric value nearly three times greater. The reason that more energy can be derived from lipid than from carbohydrate or protein relates to the average oxidation state of the carbon atoms in these substances. Carbon atoms in carbohydrates are considerably more oxidized (or less reduced) than those in lipids (Figure 6.6). Hence during sequential breakdown of lipid nearly three times as many **reducing equivalents** (a reducing equivalent is defined as a proton plus an electron, i.e., $H^+ + e^-$) can be extracted than from carbohydrate. Reducing equivalents may be utilized for ATP synthesis in the mitochondrial energy transduction sequence.

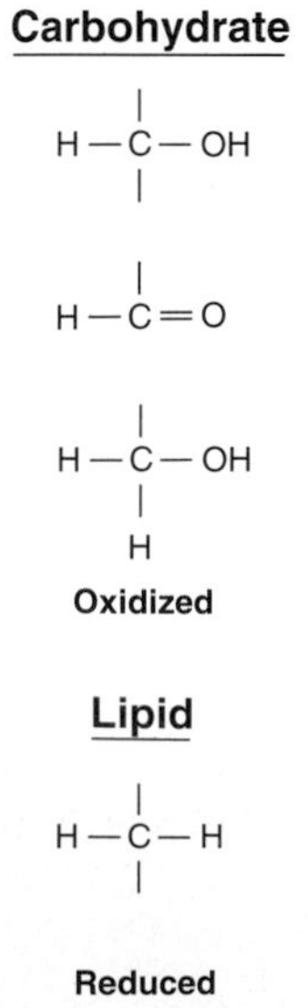

Carbohydrate

H—C—OH

H—C=O

H—C—OH
H

Oxidized

Lipid

H—C—H

Reduced

FIGURE 6.6
Oxidation states of typical carbon atoms in carbohydrates and lipids.

Compounds Are Classified on the Basis of Energy Released on Hydrolysis of Specific Groups

The two terminal phosphoryl groups of ATP contain energy-rich or high-energy bonds. What this description is intended to convey is that the free energy of hydrolysis of an energy-rich phosphoanhydride bond is much greater than would be obtained for a simple phosphate ester. High-energy is not synonymous with stability of the bonding arrangement in question, nor does it refer to the energy required to break such bonds. The concept of high-energy compounds implies that the products of the hydrolytic cleavage of the energy-rich bond are in more stable forms than the original compound. As a rule, simple phosphate esters (low-energy compounds) exhibit negative $\Delta G°$ values of hydrolysis in the range 1–3 kcal mol^{-1}, whereas high-energy bonds have negative $\Delta G°$ values in the range 5–15 kcal mol^{-1}. Phosphate esters such as glucose 6-phosphate and glycerol 3-phosphate are examples of low-energy compounds. Table 6.3 lists various types of energy-rich compounds with approximate values for their $\Delta G°$ values of hydrolysis.

There are various reasons why certain compounds or bonding arrangements

TABLE 6.3 Examples of Energy-Rich Compounds

Type of Bond	*ΔG° of Hydrolysis (kcal mol⁻¹)*	*Example*
Phosphoric acid anhydrides	−7.3	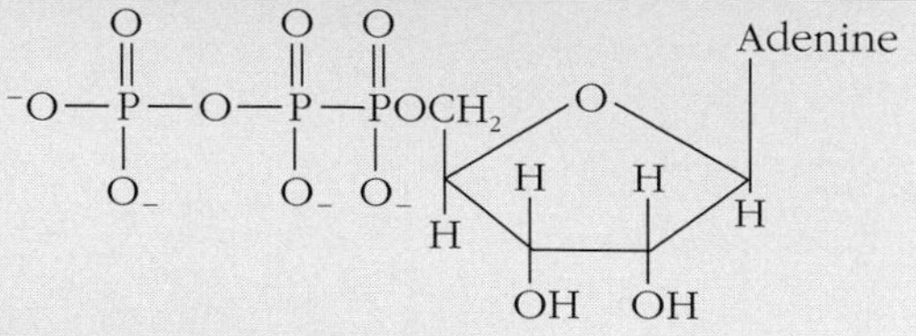 ATP
	−11.9	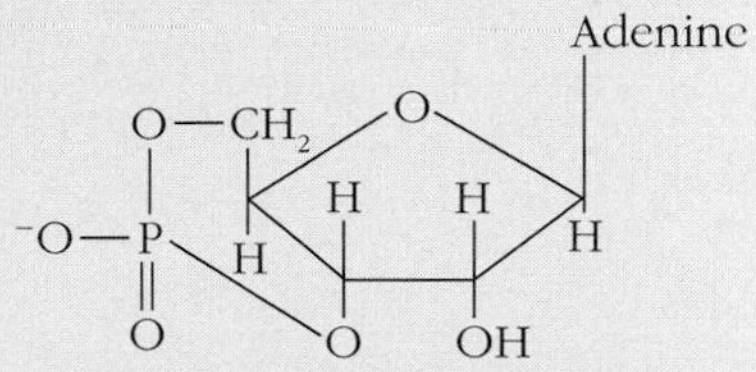 3′5′ cyclic AMP
Phosphoric–carboxylic acid anhydrides	−10.1	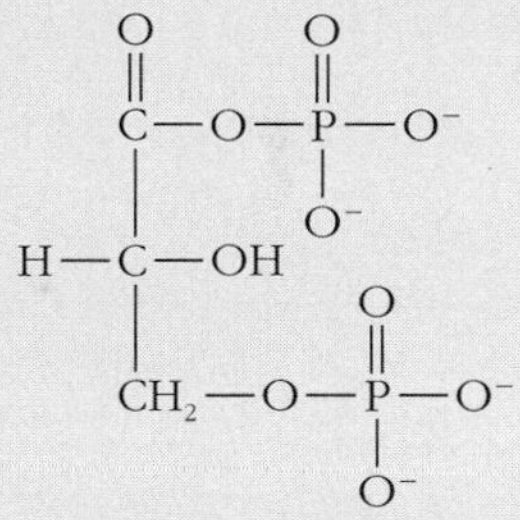 1,3-Bisphosphoglycerate
	−10.3	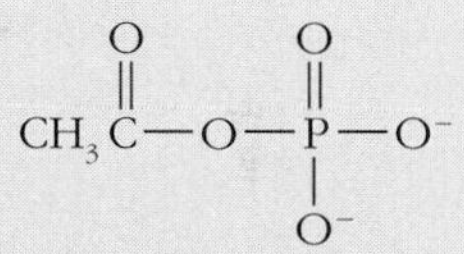 Acetyl phosphate
Phosphoguanidines	−10.3	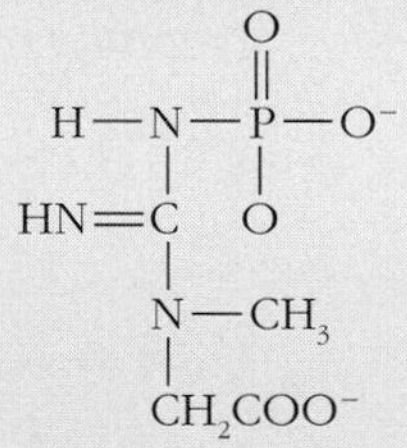 Creatine phosphate
Enol phosphates	−14.8	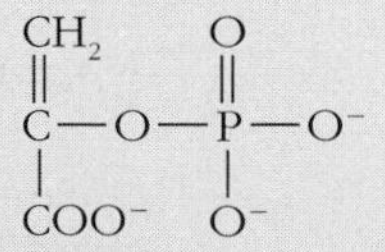 Phosphoenolpyruvate
Thiol esters	−7.7	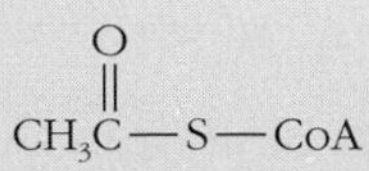 Acetyl CoA

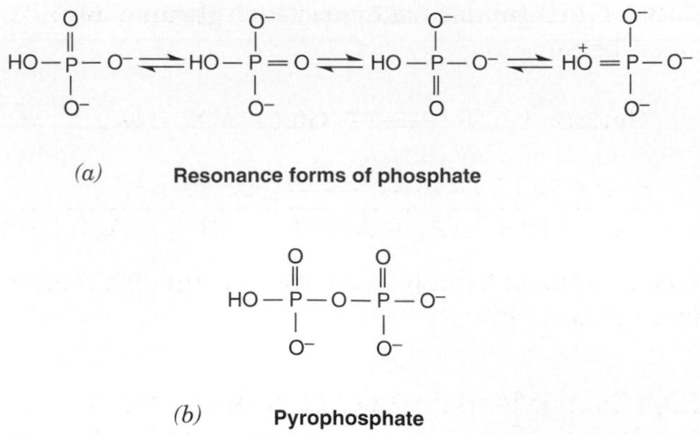

(a) Resonance forms of phosphate

(b) Pyrophosphate

FIGURE 6.7
(a) Resonance forms of phosphate. (b) Structure of pyrophosphate.

are energy rich. First, products of the hydrolysis of an energy-rich bond may exist in more **resonance forms** than the precursor molecule. The more possible resonance forms in which a molecule can exist stabilize that molecule. The resonance forms for inorganic phosphate (P_i) can be written as indicated in Figure 6.7.

Fewer resonance forms can be written for ATP or **pyrophosphate** (PP_i) (Figure 6.7) than for phosphate (P_i).

Second, many high-energy bonding arrangements have groups of similar electrostatic charges located in close proximity to each other in such compounds. Because like charges repel one another, hydrolysis of energy-rich bonds alleviates this situation and, again, lends stability to the products of hydrolysis. Third, hydrolysis of certain energy-rich bonds results in the formation of an unstable compound, which may isomerize spontaneously to form a more stable compound. Hydrolysis of phosphoenolpyruvate is an example of this type of compound (Figure 6.8). The ΔG° for isomerization is considerable, and the final product, in this case pyruvate, is much more stable. Finally, if a product of the hydrolysis of a high-energy bond is an undissociated acid, dissociation of the proton and its subsequent buffering may contribute to the overall ΔG° of the hydrolytic reaction. In general, any property or process that lends stability to products of hydrolysis tends to confer a high-energy character to that compound.

The high-energy character of **3′,5′-cyclic adenosine monophosphate (cAMP)** has been attributed to the fact that the phosphoanhydride bonding character in this compound is strained as it bridges the 3′ and 5′ positions on the ribose. The energy-rich character of thiol ester compounds such as acetyl CoA or succinyl CoA results from the relatively acidic character of the thiol group. Hence **acetyl CoA** is nearly equivalent to an anhydride rather than a simple thioester.

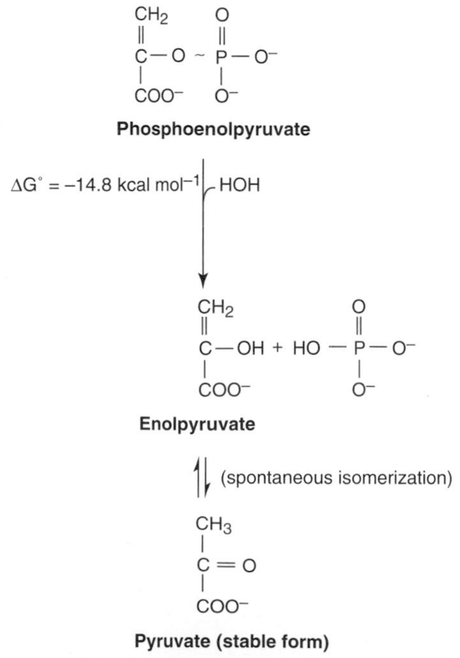

Phosphoenolpyruvate

$\Delta G^\circ = -14.8$ kcal mol^{-1} HOH

Enolpyruvate

(spontaneous isomerization)

Pyruvate (stable form)

FIGURE 6.8
Hydrolysis of phosphoenolpyruvate.

Free-Energy Changes Can Be Determined in Coupled Enzyme Reactions

The ΔG° value of hydrolysis of the terminal phosphate of ATP is difficult to determine by simply utilizing the K_{eq} of the hydrolytic reaction because of the position of the equilibrium.

$$\text{ATP} + \text{HOH} \rightleftharpoons \text{ADP} + \text{P}_i + \text{H}^+$$

However, the ΔG° of hydrolysis of ATP can be determined indirectly because of the additive nature of free-energy changes. Hence free energy of hydrolysis of ATP can be determined by adding ΔG° of an ATP-utilizing reaction such as hexokinase to ΔG° of a reaction that cleaves the phosphate from the product of the **hexokinase** reaction, **glucose 6-phosphate** (G6P), as indicated below:

$$\text{Glucose} + \text{ATP} \xrightleftharpoons{\text{hexokinase}} \text{G6P} + \text{ADP} + \text{H}^+ \qquad \Delta G^\circ = -4.0\ \text{kcal mol}^{-1}$$

$$\text{G6P} + \text{HOH} \xrightleftharpoons{\text{glucose 6-phosphate}} \text{glucose} + \text{P}_\text{i} \qquad \Delta G^\circ = -3.3\ \text{kcal mol}^{-1}$$

$$\text{ATP} + \text{HOH} \rightleftharpoons \text{ADP} + \text{P}_\text{i} + \text{H}^+ \qquad \Delta G^\circ = -7.3\ \text{kcal mol}^{-1}$$

Free energies of hydrolysis for other energy-rich compounds can be determined in a similar fashion.

High-Energy Bond Energies of Various Groups Can Be Transferred from One Compound to Another

Energy-rich compounds can transfer various groups from the parent (donor) compound to an acceptor compound in a thermodynamically feasible fashion as long as an appropriate enzyme is present to facilitate the transfer. The energy-rich intermediates in the glycolytic pathway such as **1,3-bisphosphoglycerate** and phosphoenolpyruvate can transfer their high-energy phosphate moieties to ATP in the **phosphoglycerate kinase** and **pyruvate kinase** reactions, respectively (Figure 6.9*a*). The ΔG° values of these two reactions are -4.5 and -7.5 kcal mol^{-1}, respectively, and hence transfer of "high-energy" phosphate is thermodynamically possible, and ATP synthesis is the result. ATP can transfer its terminal high-energy phosphoryl groups to form compounds of relatively similar high-energy character [i.e., **creatine phosphate** in the **creatine kinase** reaction (Figure 6.9*b*)] or compounds that are of considerably lower energy, such as glucose 6-phosphate formed in the hexokinase reaction (Figure 6.9*c*).

Thus phosphate or other transferable groups can be transferred from compounds that contain energy-rich bonding arrangements to compounds that have bonding characteristics of a lower energy in thermodynamically permissible enzymatic reactions. This principle is a major premise of the interaction between energy-producing and energy-utilizing metabolic pathways in living cells.

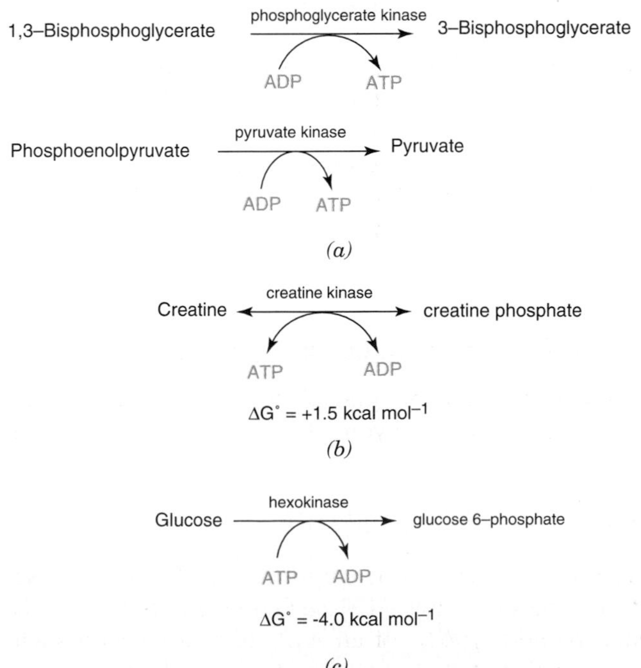

FIGURE 6.9
Examples of reactions involved in transfer of "high-energy" phosphate.

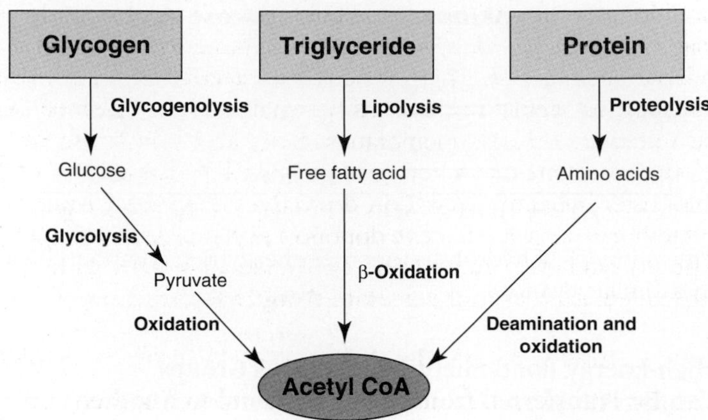

FIGURE 6.10
General precursors of acetyl CoA.

6.3 ■ SOURCES AND FATES OF ACETYL COENZYME A

Most of the major energy-generating metabolic pathways of cells eventually result in production of the two-carbon unit **acetyl coenzyme A** (CoA). As illustrated in Figure 6.10, the catabolic breakdown of ingested or stored carbohydrate in the glycolytic pathway, of long-chain fatty acids in the ***β*-oxidation sequence,** or certain amino acids following **transamination** or **deamination** and subsequent oxidation provide precursors for the formation of acetyl CoA.

The structure of acetyl CoA is shown in Figure 6.11. This complex coenzyme, abbreviated either as CoA or CoASH, is composed of *β*-mercaptoethylamine, the vitamin **pantothenic acid,** and the adenine nucleotide, adenosine 3′-phosphate 5′-diphosphate. Coenzyme A exists as the reduced thiol (CoASH) and is involved in a variety of acyl group transfer reactions, where CoA alternately serves as the acceptor, then the donor, of the acyl group. Various metabolic pathways involve only acyl CoA derivatives, for example, *β*-oxidation of fatty acids and **branched-chain amino acid** degradation. Information on the

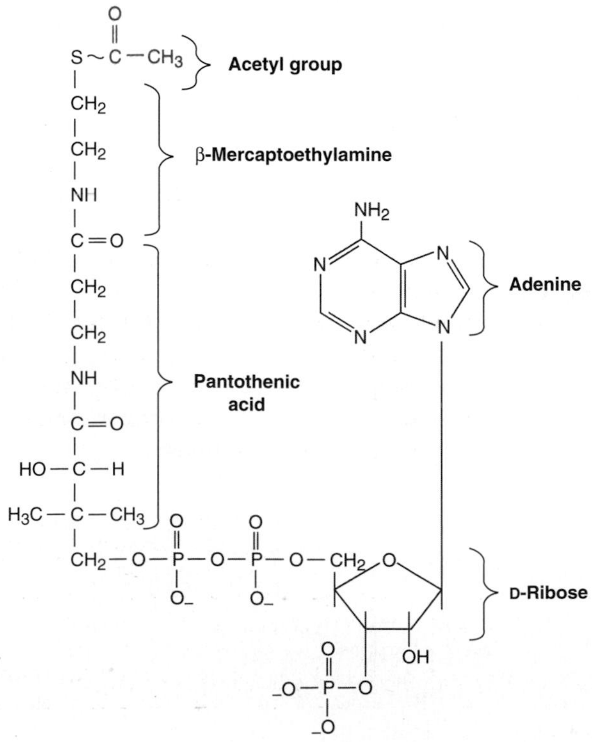

FIGURE 6.11
Structure of acetyl CoA.

nutritional aspects of the pantothenic acid will be described in Chapter 28. Like many other nucleotide species, CoA derivatives are not freely transported across cellular membranes. This property has necessitated the evolution of certain transport or shuttle mechanisms by which various intermediates or groups can be transferred across membranes. Such acyl transferase reactions for acetyl groups and long-chain acyl groups will be discussed in Chapter 9. Since the thiol ester linkage in acyl CoA derivatives is an energy-rich bond, these compounds can serve as effective donors of acyl groups in acyl transferase reactions. Also, to synthesize an acyl CoA derivative a high-energy bond of ATP must be expended, such as in the **acetate thiokinase** reaction,

$$\text{Acetate} + \text{CoASH} + \text{ATP} \xrightleftharpoons{\text{acetate kinase}} \text{acetyl CoA} + \text{AMP} + \text{PP}_i$$

The β-oxidation of fatty acids is a primary source of acetyl CoA in many tissues; a detailed description of the mobilization, transport, and oxidation of fatty acids is presented in Chapter 9. Note, however, that the products of the β-oxidation sequence are acetyl CoA and reducing equivalents (i.e., **NADH**). In certain tissues (e.g., cardiac muscle) and under somewhat special metabolic conditions in other tissues (e.g., in brain during prolonged starvation), acetyl CoA for energy generation may be derived from the **ketone bodies, acetoacetate** and **β-hydroxybutyrate.**

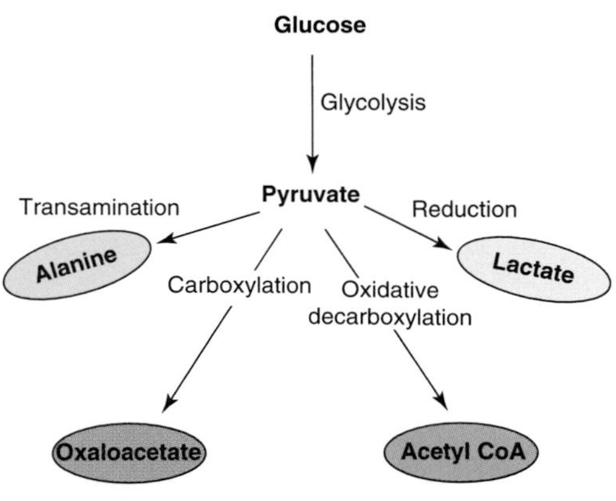

FIGURE 6.12
Metabolic fates of pyruvate.

Metabolic Sources and Fates of Pyruvate

During aerobic glycolysis (Chapter 7), glucose or other monosaccharides are converted to pyruvate, the end product of this cytosolic pathway. Also, degradation of amino acids such as alanine, serine, and cysteine results in the production of **pyruvate** (see p. 447). Pyruvate has a variety of metabolic fates, depending on the tissue and the metabolic state of that tissue. The major types of reactions in which pyruvate participates are indicated in Figure 6.12. The oxidative decarboxylation of pyruvate in the **pyruvate dehydrogenase** reaction is discussed next; the other reactions involving pyruvate are discussed in Chapter 7.

Pyruvate Dehydrogenase Is a Multienzyme Complex

Pyruvate is converted to acetyl CoA by the pyruvate dehydrogenase multienzyme complex.

$$\text{Pyruvate} + \text{NAD}^+ + \text{CoASH} \xrightarrow{\text{pyruvate dehydrogenase}} \text{acetyl CoA} + \text{CO}_2 + \text{NADH} + \text{H}^+ \qquad \Delta G^\circ = -8 \text{ kcal mol}^{-1}$$

This enzyme is located exclusively in the mitochondrial matrix and is present in high concentrations in tissues such as cardiac muscle and kidney. Because of the large negative ΔG° of the pyruvate dehydrogenase reaction, under physiological conditions the reaction is irreversible. This fact is the primary reason that a net conversion of fatty acid carbon to carbohydrate cannot occur; for example, acetyl CoA from fatty acids cannot be converted to pyruvate. Molecular weights of the multienzyme complex derived from kidney, heart, or liver range from 7 to 8.5 × 10^6. The mammalian pyruvate dehydrogenase enzyme complex consists of three different types of catalytic subunits:

Number of Subunits/Complex	*Type*	*Molecular Weight*	*Subunit Structure*
20 or 30[a]	Pyruvate dehydrogenase	154,000	$\alpha_2\beta_2$ Tetramer
60	Dihydrolipoyl transacetylase	52,000	Identical
6	Dihydrolipoyl dehydrogenase	110,000	α_2 Dimer

[a] Depending on source.

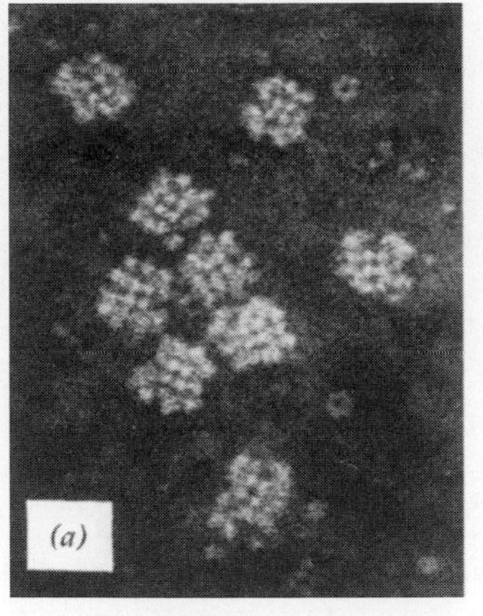

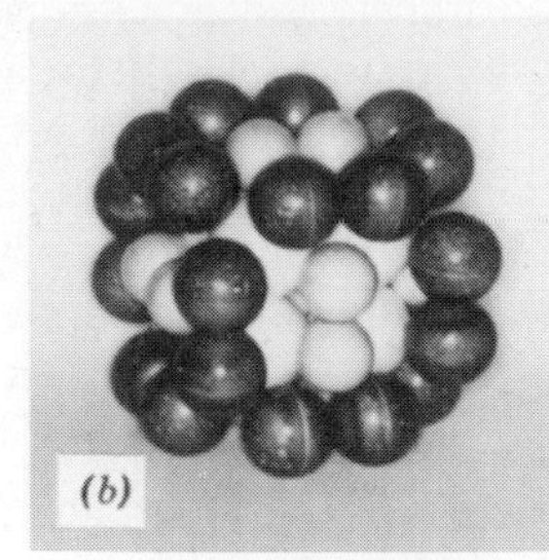

FIGURE 6.13
Pyruvate dehydrogenase complex from *E. coli.*
(*a*) Electron micrograph. (*b*) Molecular model. The enzyme complex was negatively stained with phosphotungstate (×200,000).
Courtesy of Dr. Lester J. Reed, University of Texas, Austin.

The structure of the pyruvate dehydrogenase complex derived from *Escherichia coli* (particle weight, 4.6×10^6) is somewhat different from that of the mammalian enzyme. Electron micrographs of the bacterial enzyme complex (Figure 6.13) indicate that the transacetylase, which consists of 24 identical polypeptide chains (mol wt = 64,500), forms the cube-like core of the complex (white spheres in the model shown in Figure 6.11). Twelve pyruvate dehydrogenase dimers (black spheres; mol wt = 90,500) are distributed symmetrically on the 12 edges of the transacetylase cube. Six dihydrolipoyl dehydrogenase dimers (gray spheres; mol wt = 56,000) are distributed on the six faces of the cube. Five different coenzymes or prosthetic groups are involved in the pyruvate dehydrogenase reaction (Table 6.4 and Figure 6.14). The mechanism of the pyruvate dehydrogenase reaction occurs as illustrated in Figure 6.15.

Because of active participation of thiol groups in the catalytic mechanism, agents that either oxidize or complex with thiol groups are strong inhibitors of the enzyme complex. **Arsenite** is such an inhibitor.

Pyruvate Dehydrogenase Is Strictly Regulated

Two types of regulation of the pyruvate dehydrogenase complex have been characterized. First, two products of the pyruvate dehydrogenase reaction, acetyl

TABLE 6.4 Function of Coenzymes and Prosthetic Groups of the Pyruvate Dehydrogenase Reaction

Coenzyme or Prosthetic Group	*Location*	*Function*
Thiamine pyrophosphate	Bound to pyruvate dehydrogenase	Reacts with substrate, pyruvate
Lipoic acid	Covalently attached to a lysine residue on the dihydrolipoyl transacetylase	Accepts acetyl group from thiamine pyrophosphate
Coenzyme A	Free in solution	Accepts acetyl group from lipoamide group on the transacetylase
Flavin adenine dinucleotide (FAD)	Tightly bound to dihydrolipoyl dehydrogenase	Accepts reducing equivalents from reduced lipoamide group
Nicotinamide adenine dinucleotide	Free in solution	Terminal acceptor of reducing equivalents from the reduced flavoprotein

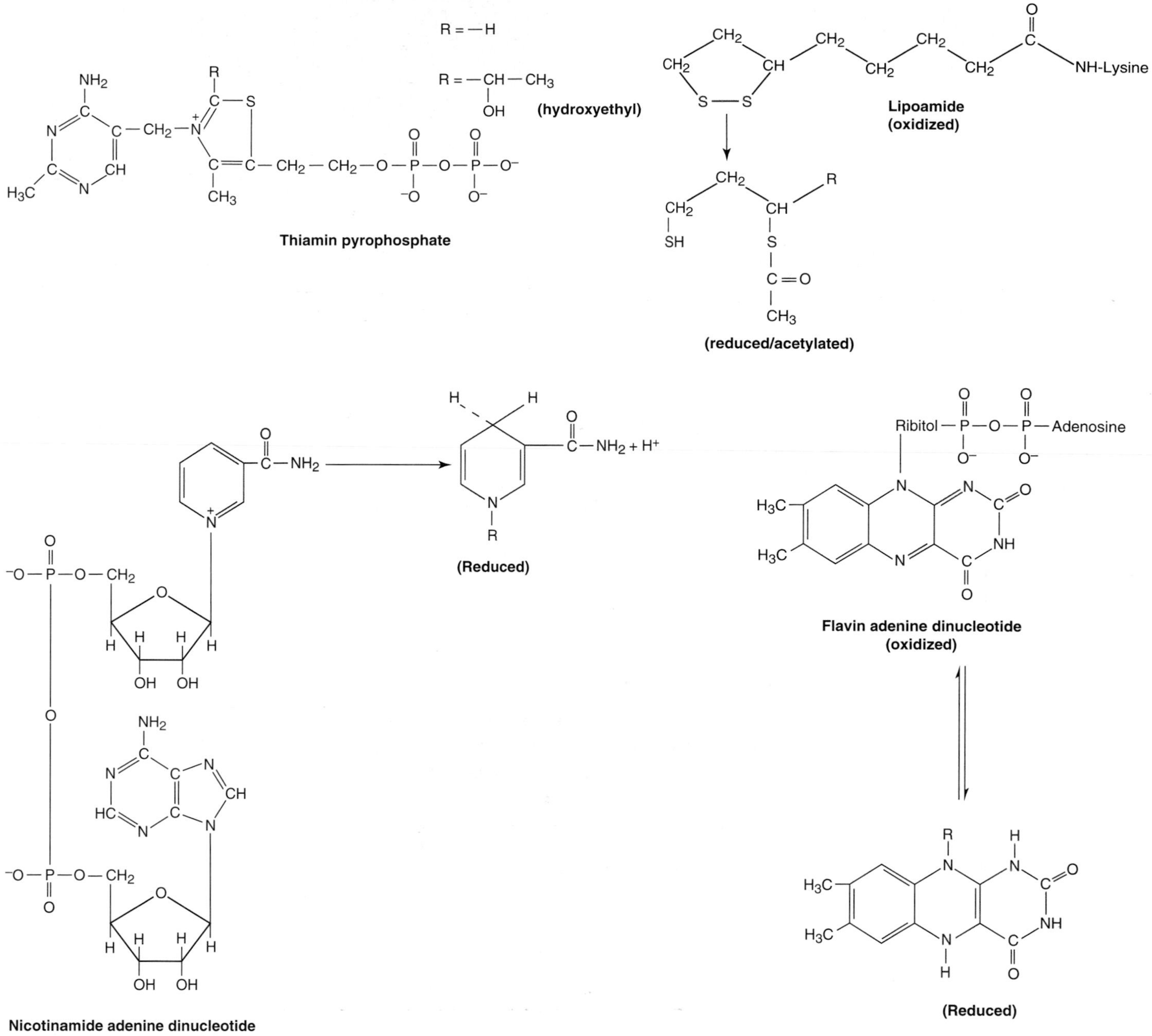

FIGURE 6.14
Structures of coenzymes involved in the pyruvate dehydrogenase reaction. See Figure 6.11 for the structure of CoA.

CoA and NADH, inhibit the complex in a competitive fashion. Second, the pyruvate dehydrogenase complex exists in two forms: (1) an active, dephosphorylated complex and (2) an inactive, phosphorylated complex. Inactivation of the complex is accomplished by a Mg^{2+}–ATP-dependent **protein kinase,** which is tightly bound to the enzyme complex. Reactivation is accomplished by a **phosphoprotein phosphatase,** which dephosphorylates the complex in a Mg^{2+}- and Ca^{2+}-dependent reaction. Three separate serine residues on the α subunit of pyruvate dehydrogenase are phosphorylated by the protein kinase but the phosphorylation of only one serine is related to the activity of the complex. The differential regulation of the pyruvate dehydrogenase kinase and phosphatase is the key to the regulation of the pyruvate dehydrogenase complex. Essential features of this complex regulatory system are illustrated in Figure 6.16. Acetyl CoA and NADH, products of pyruvate dehydrogenase, inhibit the

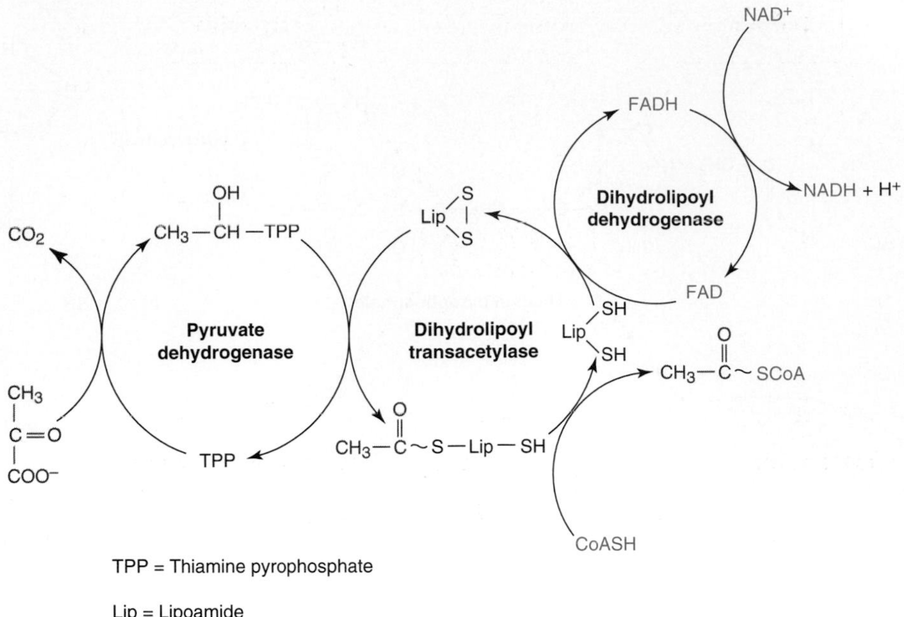

FIGURE 6.15
Mechanism of the pyruvate dehydrogenase reaction; the pyruvate dehydrogenase multienzyme complex.

dephospho (active) form of the enzyme, but these two compounds stimulate the protein kinase reaction, leading to an interconversion of the complex to its inactive form. In addition, free CoASH and NAD$^+$ inhibit the protein kinase. Hence, with any increase of the mitochondrial NADH/NAD$^+$ or acetyl CoA/CoASH ratio, such as during rapid β-oxidation of fatty acids, pyruvate dehydrogenase will be inactivated by the kinase reaction. In addition, pyruvate, the substrate of the enzyme, is a potent inhibitor of the protein kinase, and therefore in the presence of elevated tissue pyruvate levels the kinase will be inhibited and the complex maximally active. Finally, **insulin** administration activates

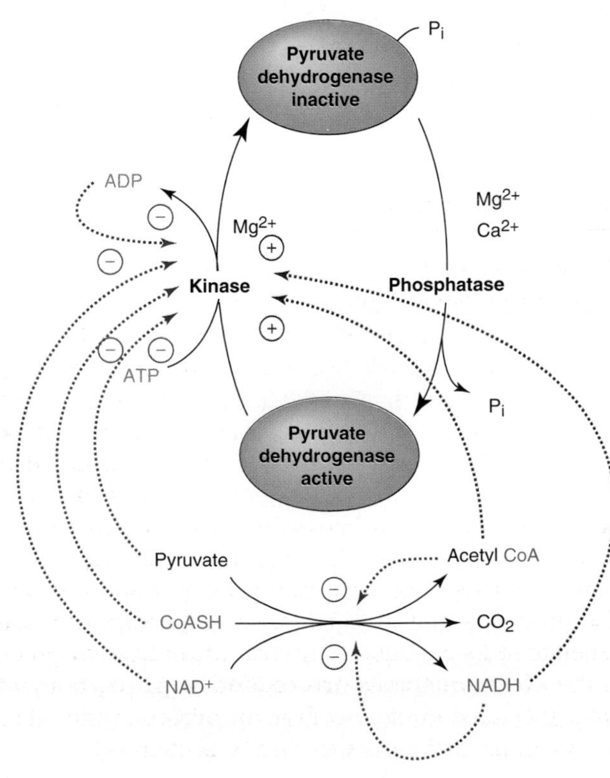

FIGURE 6.16
Regulation of the pyruvate dehydrogenase multienzyme complex.

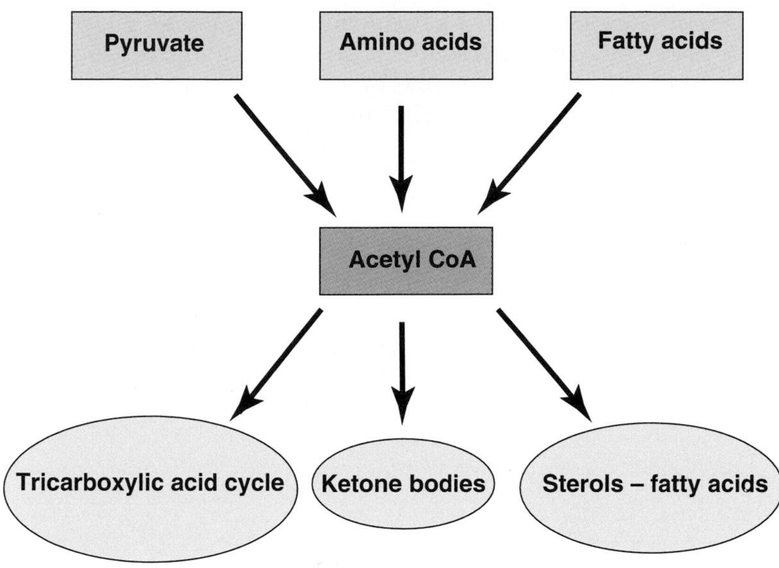

FIGURE 6.17
Sources and fates of acetyl CoA.

pyruvate dehydrogenase in adipose tissue, and catecholamines, such as **epinephrine,** activate pyruvate dehydrogenase in cardiac tissue. The mechanisms of these hormonal effects are not well understood, but alterations of the intracellular distribution of Ca^{2+}, such that the phosphoprotein phosphatase reaction is stimulated in the mitochondrial matrix, may be involved in these effects. These hormonal effects are not mediated directly by alterations in the tissue cAMP levels because the pyruvate dehydrogenase protein kinase and phosphatase are cAMP-independent or insensitive (see Clin. Corr. 6.1).

Acetyl CoA Is Used by Several Different Pathways

The various fates of acetyl CoA generated in the mitochondrial matrix include (1) complete oxidation of the acetyl group in the tricarboxylic acid cycle for energy generation; (2) in the liver, conversion of excess acetyl CoA into ketone bodies, acetoacetate and β-hydroxybutyrate; and (3) transfer of the acetyl units to the cytosol with subsequent biosynthesis of such molecules as sterols (see Chapter 10) and long-chain fatty acids (see Chapter 9) (Figure 6.17).

6.4 ■ THE TRICARBOXYLIC ACID CYCLE

The primary metabolic fate of acetyl CoA produced in the various energy-generating catabolic pathways of most cells is its complete oxidation in a cyclic series of reactions termed the **tricarboxylic acid (TCA) cycle.** This metabolic cycle is also commonly referred to as the **citric acid cycle** or the **Krebs cycle** after Sir Hans Krebs who postulated the essential features of this pathway in 1937. Various investigators defined many of the enzymes and di- and tricarboxylic acid intermediates but it was Krebs who pieced them together. The primary location of the enzymes of the TCA cycle is in the mitochondrion, although isozymes of some are found in the cytosol. This type of distribution is appropriate because the pyruvate dehydrogenase multienzyme complex and the fatty acid β-oxidation sequence, the two primary sources for generating acetyl CoA, are also located in the mitochondrion. A primary function of the TCA cycle is to generate reducing equivalents that are utilized to generate energy, that is, ATP, in the **electron transport–oxidative phosphorylation** sequence, another process contained exclusively in the mitochondrion (Figure 6.18). Mitochondrial energy transduction is discussed in Section 6.7.

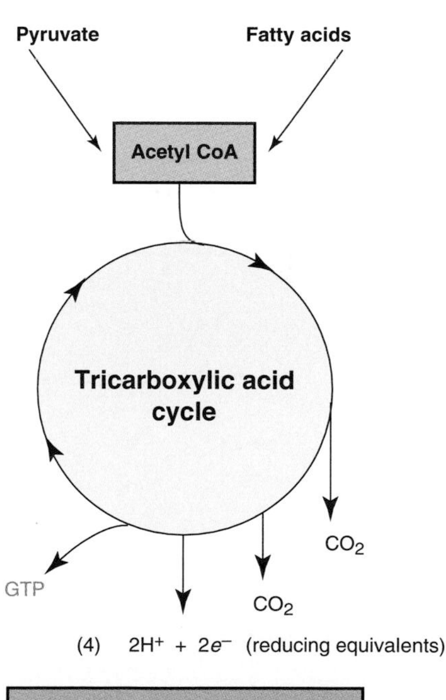

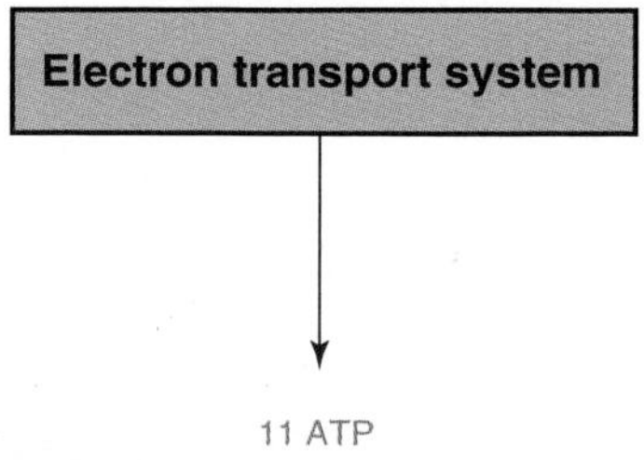

FIGURE 6.18
General description of mitochondrial ATP synthesis.

Figure 6.18 illustrates the essential process involved in the TCA cycle. The substrate of the cycle is the two-carbon unit acetyl CoA and the products of a complete turn of the cycle are two CO_2 plus one high-energy phosphate bond (as GTP) and four reducing equivalents (i.e., three NADH and one $FADH_2$).

Reactions of the Tricarboxylic Acid Cycle

The individual enzymatic reactions are presented in Figure 6.19. The initial step of the cycle is catalyzed by **citrate synthase.** This is a highly exergonic reaction and commits acetyl groups to **citrate** formation and complete oxidation in the Krebs cycle. As shown below citrate synthase involves condensation of an acetyl moiety and the α-keto function of the dicarboxylic acid **oxaloacetate.** Citrate synthase (mol wt 100,000) is in the mitochondrial matrix.

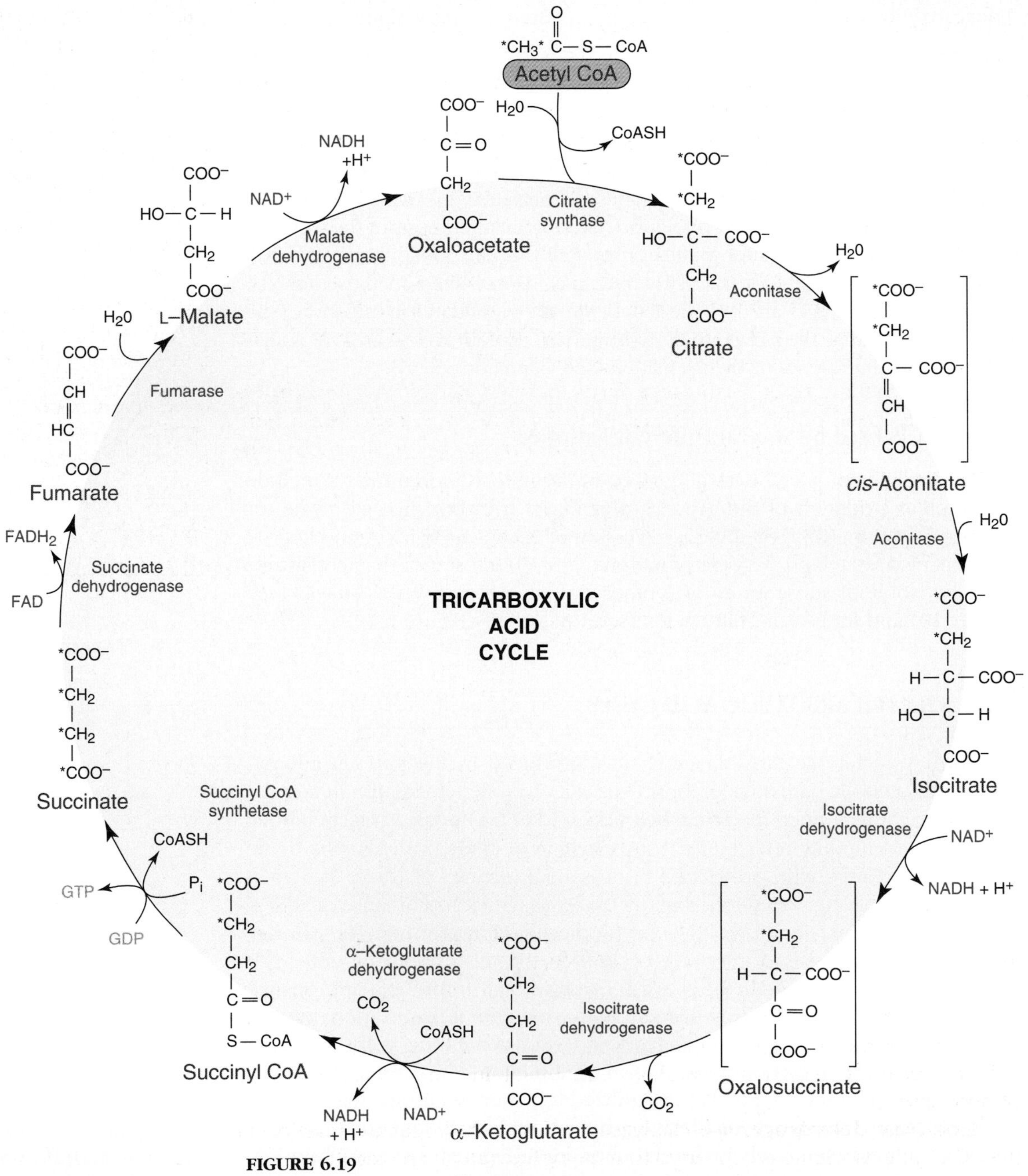

FIGURE 6.19
The tricarboxylic acid cycle.
Asterisked carbons indicate the fate of the carbons of the acetyl group.

$$\mathrm{CH_3C(=O)\text{—}SCoA}\ (\text{Acetyl CoA}) + \mathrm{O{=}C(COO^-)\text{—}CH_2COO^-}\ (\text{Oxaloacetate}) \rightarrow [\text{Enzyme Bound Citroyl-SCoA}] \xrightarrow{H_2O} \text{CoASH} + \text{Citrate}$$

Acetyl CoA

Oxaloacetate

Enzyme Bound

Citroyl-SCoA

Citrate

CITRATE SYNTHASE

The equilibrium of this reaction is far toward citrate formation with a ΔG° near -9 kcal mol^{-1}. The citroyl-SCoA intermediate is not released from the enzyme during the reaction and remains bound to the catalytic site on citrate synthase. The citrate synthase reaction is considerably displaced from equilibrium under *in situ* conditions, which makes this step a primary candidate for regulatory modulation. The purified enzyme is regulated (inhibited) by ATP, NADH, succinyl CoA, and long-chain acyl CoA derivatives, but these effects have not been demonstrated in intact metabolic systems under physiological conditions.

The most probable means for regulating the citrate synthase reaction is availability of its two substrates, acetyl CoA and oxaloacetate. Note the many important fates and effects of citrate in energy and biosynthetic metabolism indicated in Figure 6.20; citrate is a regulatory effector of other metabolic pathways and a source of carbon and reducing equivalents for various synthetic purposes (see Chapters 7 and 9 for further details).

Citrate synthase reacts with **monofluoroacetyl CoA** to form **monofluorocitrate,** a potent inhibitor of the next step in the cycle, the **aconitase** reaction. In fact, whether monofluorocitrate is synthesized *in situ* as a result of **fluoroacetate** poisoning or administered experimentally, a nearly complete block of TCA cycle activity is observed.

Citrate is converted to isocitrate in the aconitase reaction:

$$\text{Citrate} \underset{}{\overset{H_2O}{\rightleftharpoons}} [\textit{cis}\text{-Aconitate}] \overset{H_2O}{\rightleftharpoons} \text{Isocitrate}$$

Citrate

cis-Aconitate

Isocitrate

ACONITASE

This reaction involves generation of an enzyme-bound intermediate, ***cis*-aconitate.** At equilibrium there exist 90% citrate, 3% *cis*-aconitate, and 7% isocitrate; hence the equilibrium of aconitase lies toward citrate formation. Although the aconitase reaction does not require cofactors, it requires ferrous (Fe^{2+}) iron in its catalytic mechanism. This Fe^{2+} is involved in an **iron–sulfur center,** which is an essential component in the hydratase activity of aconitase.

Isocitrate dehydrogenase catalyzes the first dehydrogenase reaction in the TCA cycle. Isocitrate is converted to **α-ketoglutarate** in an oxidative decarboxylation reaction. In this step of the cycle the initial (of two) CO_2 is produced and the initial (of three) NADH + H^+ are generated. Isocitrate dehydrogenase

CLINICAL CORRELATION 6.1

Pyruvate Dehydrogenase Deficiency

A variety of disorders in pyruvate metabolism have been detected in children. Some involve deficiencies of the different catalytic or regulatory subunits of the pyruvate dehydrogenase multienzyme complex. Children diagnosed with pyruvate dehydrogenase deficiency usually exhibit elevated serum levels of lactate, pyruvate, and alanine, which produce a chronic lactic acidosis. Such patients frequently exhibit severe neurological defects, and in most situations this type of enzymatic defect results in death. The diagnosis of pyruvate dehydrogenase deficiency is usually made by assaying the enzyme complex and/or its various enzymatic subunits in cultures of skin fibroblasts taken from the patient. In certain instances patients respond to dietary management in which a ketogenic diet is administered and carbohydrates are minimized. Patients in shock have lactic acidosis because decreased delivery of O_2 to tissues inhibits pyruvate dehydrogenase and increases anaerobic metabolism. This situation has been treated with dichloro acetate, an inhibitor of pyruvate dehydrogenase kinase and therefore an activator of the enzyme complex.

Patel, M. S., and Harris, R. A. Mammalian α-keto acid dehydrogenase complexes: gene regulation and genetic defects. *FASEB J.* 9:1164, 1995.

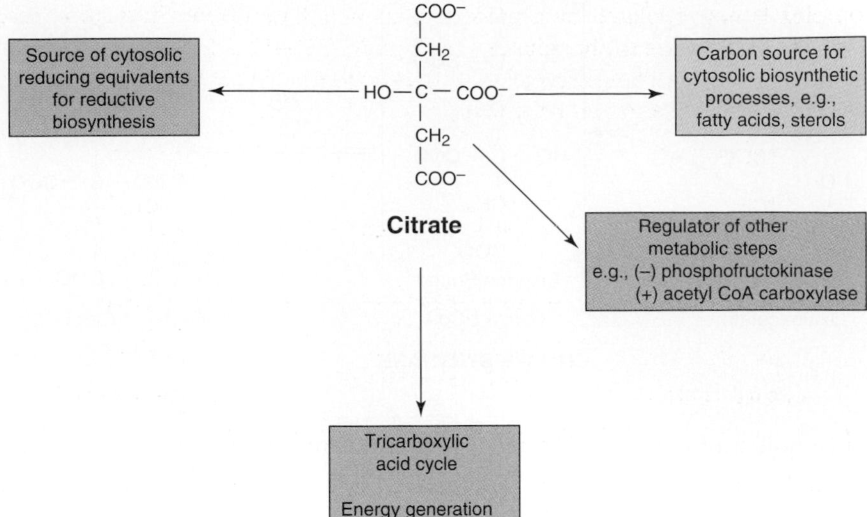

FIGURE 6.20
Fates and functions of citrate.

involved in mitochondria from mammalian tissues requires NAD^+ as the acceptor of reducing equivalents.

$$\underset{\text{Isocitrate}}{{}^*COO^- - {}^*CH_2 - HC(COO^-) - HO{-}C{-}H - COO^-} \underset{}{\overset{NAD^+ \quad NADH + H^+}{\rightleftharpoons}} \left[\underset{\text{Oxalosuccinate}}{{}^*COO^- - {}^*CH_2 - H{-}C{-}COO^- - C{=}O - COO^-}\right] \overset{CO_2}{\rightleftharpoons} \underset{\alpha\text{-Ketoglutarate}}{{}^*COO^- - {}^*CH_2 - CH_2 - C{=}O - COO^-}$$

ISOCITRATE DEHYDROGENASE

Mitochondria possess an isocitrate dehydrogenase that requires $\mathbf{NADP^+}$. The $NADP^+$-linked enzyme is also found in the cytosol, where it is involved in providing reducing equivalents for cytosolic reductive processes. The equilibrium of this reaction lies strongly toward **α-ketoglutarate** formation with a ΔG° of nearly -5 kcal mol^{-1}. NAD^+-linked isocitrate dehydrogenase has a molecular weight of 380,000 and consists of eight identical subunits. The reaction requires a divalent metal cation (e.g., Mn^{2+} or Mg^{2+}) in decarboxylation of the β position of oxalosuccinate. NAD^+-linked isocitrate dehydrogenase is stimulated by ADP and in some cases AMP and is inhibited by ATP and NADH. Hence, under high-energy conditions (i.e., high ATP/ADP + P_i and high NADH/NAD^+ ratios), NAD^+-linked isocitrate dehydrogenase of the TCA cycle is inhibited. During periods of low energy the activity of this enzyme is stimulated in order to accelerate energy generation by the TCA cycle.

Conversion of α-ketoglutarate to **succinyl CoA** is catalyzed by the **α-ketoglutarate dehydrogenase** multienzyme complex, which is nearly identical to the pyruvate dehydrogenase complex in terms of reactions catalyzed and some of its structural features. Again, **thiamine pyrophosphate, lipoic acid,** CoASH, **FAD,** and NAD^+ participate in the catalytic mechanism. The multienzyme complex consists of α-ketoglutarate dehydrogenase, **dihydrolipoyl transsuccinylase,** and dihydrolipoyl dehydrogenase as three catalytic subunits. The equilibrium of the α-ketoglutarate dehydrogenase reaction lies strongly toward succinyl CoA formation with a ΔG° of -8 kcal mol^{-1}. In this reaction the second molecule of CO_2 and the second reducing equivalent (i.e., NADH + H^+) of the cycle are produced. Another product of this reaction, succinyl CoA, is an energy-rich thiol ester compound similar to acetyl CoA. Unlike the pyruvate dehydrogenase complex, α-ketoglutarate dehydrogenase complex is not regulated by a protein kinase-mediated phosphorylation reaction. The nucleoside triphosphates—ATP and GTP—NADH, and succinyl CoA inhibit this enzyme complex while Ca^{2+} has been shown to activate α-ketoglutarate dehydrogenase in certain tissues.

$$\underset{\alpha\text{-Ketoglutarate}}{{}^{*}COO^- - {}^{*}CH_2 - CH_2 - C(=O) - COO^-} \xrightarrow[NAD^+ \;\to\; NADH + H^+]{CoASH \;\to\; CO_2} \underset{\text{Succinyl CoA}}{{}^{*}COO^- - {}^{*}CH_2 - CH_2 - C(=O) - S - CoA}$$

α-KETOGLUTARATE DEHYDROGENASE

It is at the level of α-ketoglutarate that an intermediate may leave the TCA cycle to be reductively aminated in the glutamate dehydrogenase reaction. This mitochondrial enzyme converts α-ketoglutarate to glutamate in the presence of NADH or NADPH and ammonia. Using various transamination reactions the amino group incorporated into glutamate can be transferred to a variety of amino acids. These enzymes and the relevance of the incorporation or release of ammonia into or from α-keto acids are discussed in Chapter 11.

$$\overset{+}{N}H_4 + \underset{\alpha\text{-Ketoglutarate}}{COO^- - C(=O) - CH_2 - CH_2 - COO^-} \xrightleftharpoons{NAD(P)H \;\to\; NAD(P)^+} \underset{\text{Glutamate}}{COO^- - CH(\overset{+}{N}H_3) - CH_2 - CH_2 - COO^-}$$

GLUTAMATE DEHYDROGENASE

$$\underset{\text{Glutamate}}{COO^- - CH(\overset{+}{N}H_3) - CH_2 - CH_2 - COO^-} + \underset{\text{Oxaloacetate}}{COO^- - C(=O) - CH_2 - COO^-} \rightleftharpoons \underset{\text{Aspartate}}{COO^- - CH(\overset{+}{N}H_3) - CH_2 - COO^-} + \underset{\alpha\text{-Ketoglutarate}}{COO^- - C(=O) - CH_2 - CH_2 - COO^-}$$

GLUTAMATE-OXALOACETATE TRANSAMINASE

The energy-rich character of the thiol ester linkage of succinyl CoA is conserved in a substrate-level phosphorylation reaction in the next step of the TCA cycle. **Succinyl-CoA synthetase** (or succinate thiokinase) converts succinyl CoA to succinate and in mammalian tissues results in phosphorylation of GDP to GTP.

$$\underset{\text{Succinyl CoA}}{{}^{*}COO^- - {}^{*}CH_2 - {}^{*}CH_2 - C(=O) - S - CoA} \xrightleftharpoons{GDP + P_i \;\to\; GTP} \underset{\text{Succinate}}{{}^{*}COO^- - {}^{*}CH_2 - {}^{*}CH_2 - {}^{*}COO^-} + CoASH$$

SUCCINYL CoA SYNTHETASE

This reaction is freely reversible with a $\Delta G^{\circ\prime} = -0.7$ kcal mol^{-1} and the catalytic mechanism involves an enzyme–succinyl phosphate intermediate.

$$\text{Succinyl CoA} + P_i + \text{Enz} \rightleftharpoons \text{Enz–succinyl phosphate} + \text{CoASH}$$

$$\text{Enz–succinyl phosphate} \rightleftharpoons \text{Enz–phosphate} + \text{succinate}$$

$$\text{Enz–phosphate} + \text{GDP} \rightleftharpoons \text{Enz} + \text{GTP}$$

The enzyme is phosphorylated on the 3 position of a histidine residue during the succinyl-CoA synthetase reaction. Hence, in this step of the TCA cycle, a high-energy bond is conserved as GTP. Because of the presence of the nucleoside diphosphate kinase discussed earlier in this chapter, the γ-phosphate of GTP can be transferred to ADP to generate ATP.

Succinyl CoA represents a metabolic branch point in that intermediates may enter or exit the TCA cycle at this point (Figure 6.21). Succinyl CoA may be formed either from α-ketoglutarate in the cycle or from **methylmalonyl CoA** in the final steps of breakdown of odd-chain length fatty acids or the branched-chain amino acids valine and isoleucine. Metabolic fates of succinyl CoA include its conversion to succinate in the succinyl-CoA synthetase reaction of the Krebs cycle and its condensation with glycine to form **δ-aminolevulinate** by **δ-aminolevulinate synthase,** the initial reaction in **porphyrin** biosynthesis (see p. 1011).

$$\underset{\text{Succinate}}{{}^-OOC{-}CH_2{-}CH_2{-}COO^-} \xrightleftharpoons[]{\text{FAD} \;\to\; \text{FADH}_2} \underset{\text{Fumarate}}{{}^-OOC{-}CH{=}CH{-}COO^-}$$

SUCCINATE DEHYDROGENASE

Succinate is oxidized to **fumarate** by **succinate dehydrogenase,** which is tightly bound to the inner mitochondrial membrane and is composed of two

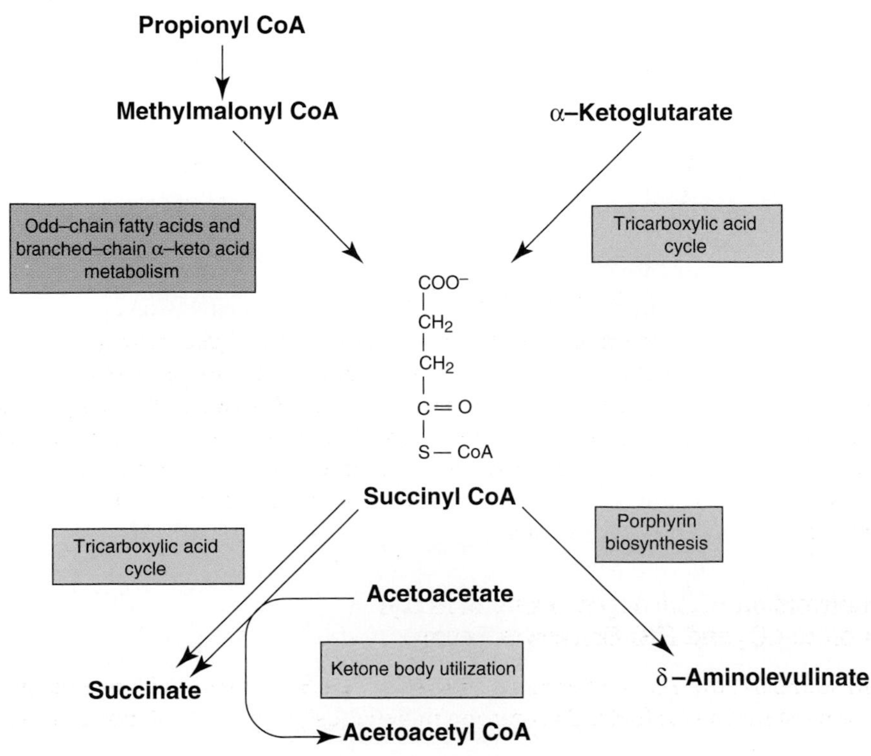

FIGURE 6.21
Sources and fates of succinyl CoA.

subunits with mol wt 70,000 and 30,000. The 70,000 mol wt subunit contains the substrate-binding site, covalently bound FAD (to a lysine residue), four nonheme iron atoms, and four acid-labile sulfur atoms, whereas the 30,000 mol wt subunit contains four nonheme irons and four acid-labile sulfur atoms. This enzyme is a typical example of an **iron–sulfur protein** in which nonheme iron undergoes valence changes (e.g., $Fe^{2+} \rightarrow Fe^{3+}$) during removal of electrons and protons from succinate and subsequent transfer of these reducing equivalents through covalently bound FAD to the mitochondrial electron-transfer chain at the coenzyme Q–cytochrome *b* level.

Succinate dehydrogenase is strongly inhibited by malonate and oxaloacetate and is activated by ATP, P_i, and succinate. **Malonate** inhibits succinate dehydrogenase competitively with respect to succinate. This inhibitory characteristic of malonate is due to a very close structural similarity between malonate and succinate (Figure 6.22). Malonate is used experimentally as a very effective inhibitor of the TCA cycle in complex metabolic systems. In fact, the ability of malonate to inhibit the cycle was used by Krebs as evidence for the cyclic nature of this oxidative metabolic pathway.

Fumarate is hydrated to form **L-malate** in the next step in the TCA cycle by the enzyme fumarase.

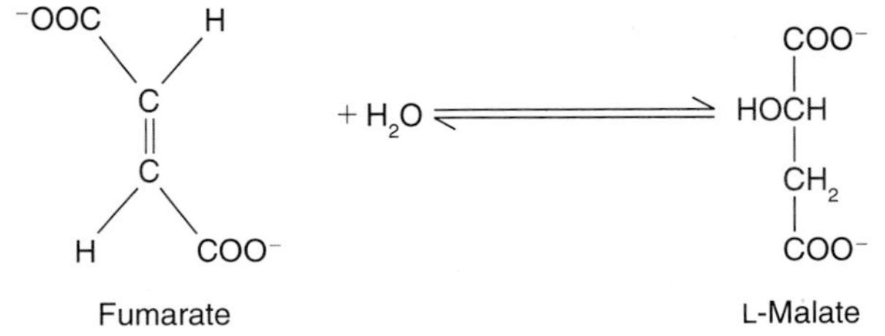

$$\text{Fumarate } ({}^-OOC\text{–CH=CH–COO}^-) + H_2O \rightleftharpoons \text{L-Malate } (COO^-\text{–HOCH–}CH_2\text{–}COO^-)$$

FUMARASE

Fumarase is a tetramer (mol wt 200,000) and is stereospecific for the trans form of substrate (the cis form, maleate, is not a substrate; Figure 6.22). The product of the reaction is L-malate and the reaction is freely reversible under physiological conditions. See Clin. Corr. 6.2 concerning a genetic deficiency of fumarase.

The final reaction in the TCA cycle is catalyzed by malate dehydrogenase with the final (of three) reducing equivalents as NADH + H^+ being removed from the cycle intermediates.

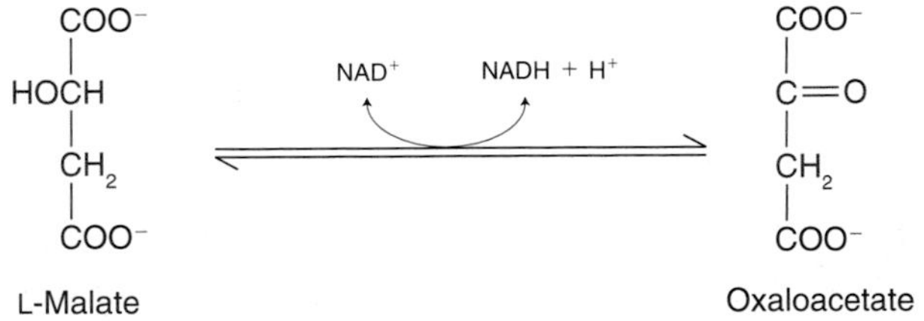

$$\text{L-Malate } (COO^-\text{–HOCH–}CH_2\text{–}COO^-) + NAD^+ \rightleftharpoons \text{Oxaloacetate } (COO^-\text{–C=O–}CH_2\text{–}COO^-) + NADH + H^+$$

MALATE DEHYDROGENASE

The equilibrium of the **malate dehydrogenase** reaction lies far toward L-malate formation, because $\Delta G^{\circ} = +7.0$ kcal mol^{-1}. Thus the reaction is an endothermic reaction when considered in the forward direction. However, **citrate synthase** and other reactions of the cycle pull malate dehydrogenase toward **oxaloacetate** formation by removing oxaloacetate. In addition, NADH produced in various cycle NAD^+-linked dehydrogenases is oxidized rapidly to NAD^+ by the mitochondrial respiratory chain.

Conversion of the Acetyl Group of Acetyl CoA to CO_2 and H_2O Conserves Energy

In summary, the TCA cycle (Figure 6.18) serves as a terminal oxidative pathway for most metabolic fuels. Two-carbon moieties as acetyl CoA are taken into the

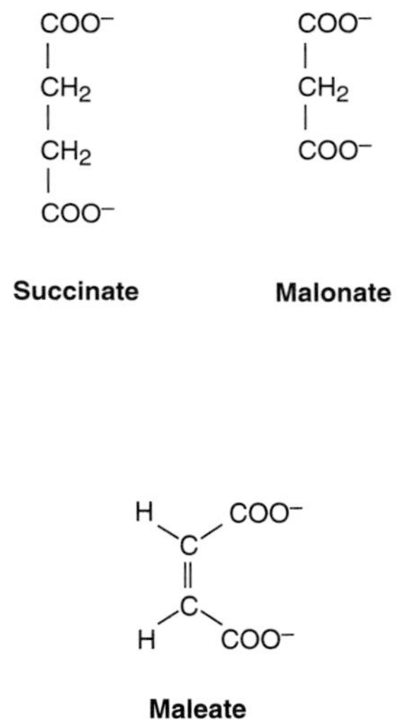

Succinate: COO^-–CH_2–CH_2–COO^-; Malonate: COO^-–CH_2–COO^-; Maleate: H(COO$^-$)C=C(COO$^-$)H

FIGURE 6.22
Structures of succinate, a TCA cycle intermediate; malonate, a cycle inhibitor; and maleate, a compound not involved in the cycle.

CLINICAL CORRELATION 6.2

Fumarase Deficiency

Deficiencies of enzymes of the TCA cycle are rarely found. Several cases, however, are on record in which there is a severe deficiency of fumarase in both mitochondria and cytosol of tissues (e.g., blood lymphocytes). The condition is characterized by severe neurological impairment, encephalopathy, and dystonia developing soon after birth. Urine contains abnormal amounts of fumarate and one or more of succinate, α-ketoglutarate, citrate, and malate. Both enzymes are derived from a single gene and both parents had half-normal levels of enzyme activity but are clinically normal, as is appropriate for an autosomal recessive disorder. The first description of a mutation in the gene reported that glutamate at residue 319 was replaced by glutamine.

Bourgeron, T., Chretien, D., Poggi-Bach, J., et al. Mutation of the fumarase gene in two siblings with progressive encephalopathy and fumarase deficiency. *J. Clin. Invest.* 93:2514, 1994.

cycle and are oxidized completely to CO_2 and H_2O. During this process 4 reducing equivalents (3 as NADH + H^+ and 1 as $FADH_2$) are produced, which are used subsequently for energy generation. Oxidation of each NADH + H^+ results in formation of 3 ATP molecules in **oxidative phosphorylation,** while oxidation of $FADH_2$ formed in the succinate dehydrogenase reaction yields 2 molecules of ATP. Also, a high-energy bond is formed as GTP in the succinyl-CoA synthetase reaction. Hence the net yield of ATP or its equivalent (i.e., GTP) for the complete oxidation of an acetyl group in the Krebs cycle is 12.

During complete oxidation of glucose to CO_2 and H_2O, there is a net formation of (1) 2 molecules of ATP per glucose in the conversion of glucose to 2 molecules of pyruvate; (2) 6 molecules of ATP per glucose as a result of the translocation and subsequent oxidation in the mitochondrial matrix of 2 molecules of NADH + H^+ formed in the glyceraldehyde-3-phosphate dehydrogenase reaction of glycolysis; and (3) 30 molecules of ATP per glucose from the oxidation of the 2 molecules of pyruvate in the pyruvate dehydrogenase reaction and subsequent conversion of 2 molecules of acetyl CoA to CO_2 and H_2O in the TCA cycle. Hence the net ATP yield during the complete oxidation of glucose to 6 CO_2 + 6 H_2O is 38 molecules of ATP.

The Activity of the Tricarboxylic Acid Cycle Is Carefully Regulated

A variety of factors are involved in the regulation of the activity of the TCA cycle. First, the supply of acetyl units, whether derived from pyruvate (i.e., carbohydrate) or fatty acids, is a crucial factor in determining the rate of the cycle. Regulatory influences on the pyruvate dehydrogenase complex have an important effect on the cycle. Likewise, any control exerted on the processes of transport and β-oxidation of fatty acids would be an effective determinant of the cycle activity.

Second, because the primary dehydrogenase reactions of the Krebs cycle are dependent on a continuous supply of both NAD^+ and FAD, their activities are very stringently controlled by the mitochondrial respiratory chain, which is responsible for oxidizing the NADH and $FADH_2$ produced by substrate oxidation in the cycle. Because the activity of the respiratory chain is coupled obligatorily to the generation of ATP in the reactions of oxidative phosphorylation, the activity of the Krebs cycle is very much dependent on a respiratory control, which is strongly affected by the availability of ADP + phosphate and oxygen. Hence an inhibitory agent or metabolic condition that interrupts the supply of oxygen, the continuous supply of ADP, or the source of reducing equivalents (e.g., substrate for the cycle) would shut down cycle activity. This type of control of the cycle is generally considered to be a coarse control of the cycle. There are a variety of postulated effector-mediated regulatory interactions between various intermediates or nucleotides and the individual enzymes of the cycle, which may serve to exert a fine control on the activity of the cycle. Illustrations of these interactions are shown in Figure 6.23 and have been noted during the discussions of individual enzymes of the Krebs cycle. The physiological relevance of many of these types of individual regulatory interactions has not been established rigorously in intact metabolic systems.

6.5 ■ STRUCTURE AND COMPARTMENTATION BY MITOCHONDRIAL MEMBRANES

Because the metabolic pathways for oxidation of pyruvate, the end product of glycolysis, and fatty acids are located in mitochondria, a major portion of the energy-generating capacity of most cells resides in the mitochondrial compartment of the cell. The number of mitochondria in various tissues (Figure 6.24*a, b*) reflects the physiological function of the tissue and determines its capacity

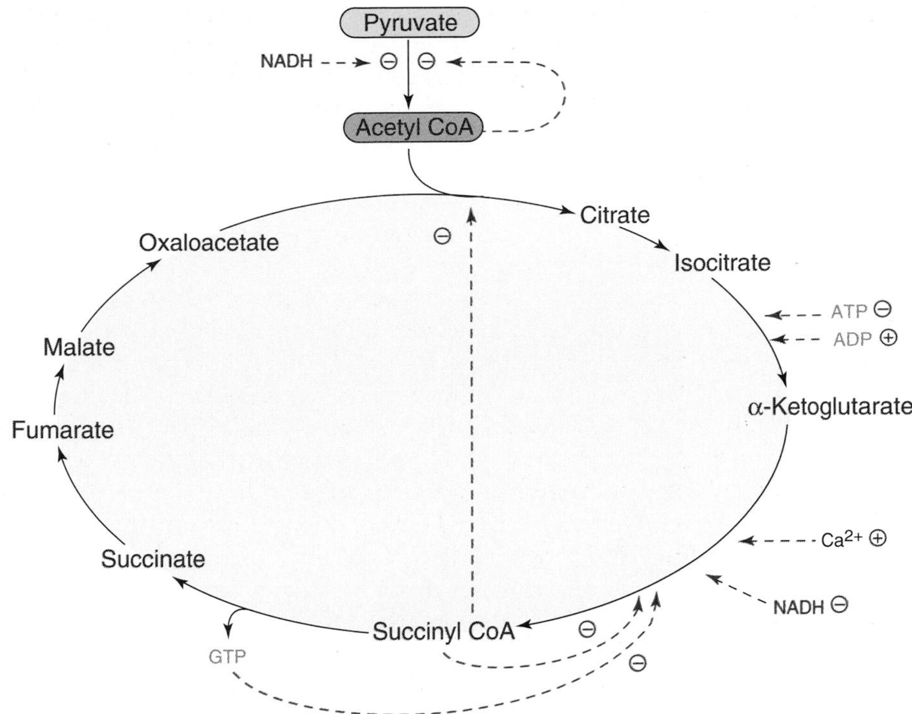

FIGURE 6.23
Representative examples of regulatory interactions in the TCA cycle.

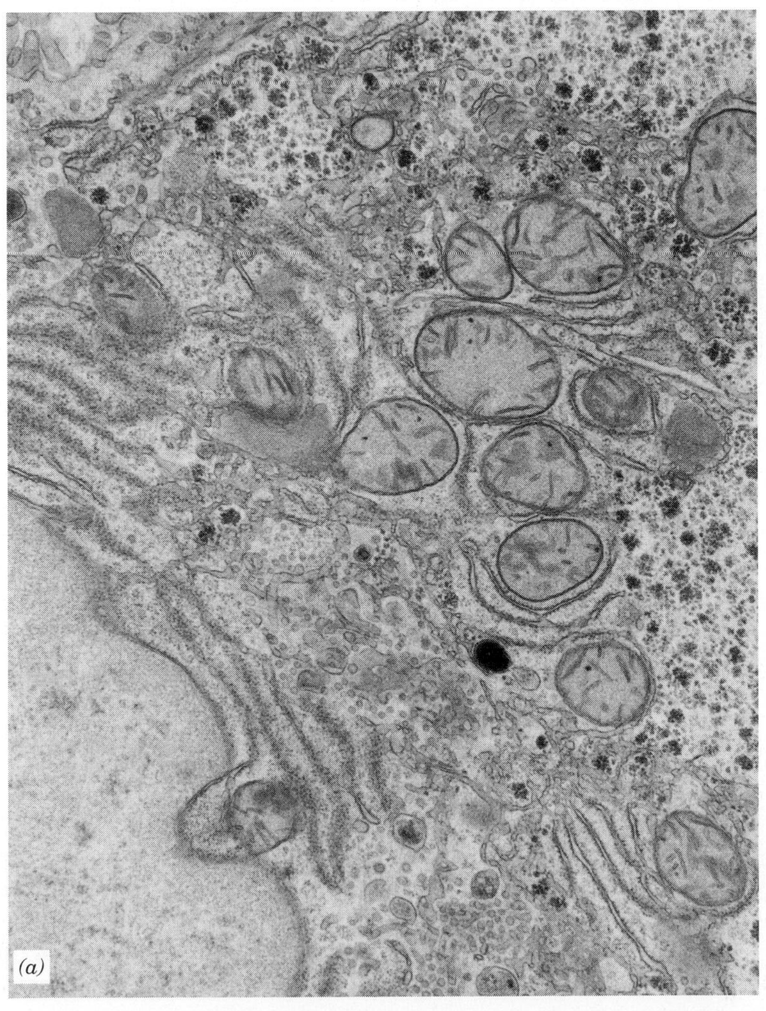

FIGURE 6.24 (*a*)
Electron micrograph of mitochondria in hepatocytes from rat liver (×39,600).
Courtesy of Dr. W. B. Winborn, Department of Anatomy, The University of Texas Health Science Center at San Antonio, and the Electron Microscopy Laboratory, Department of Pathology, The University of Texas Health Science Center at San Antonio.

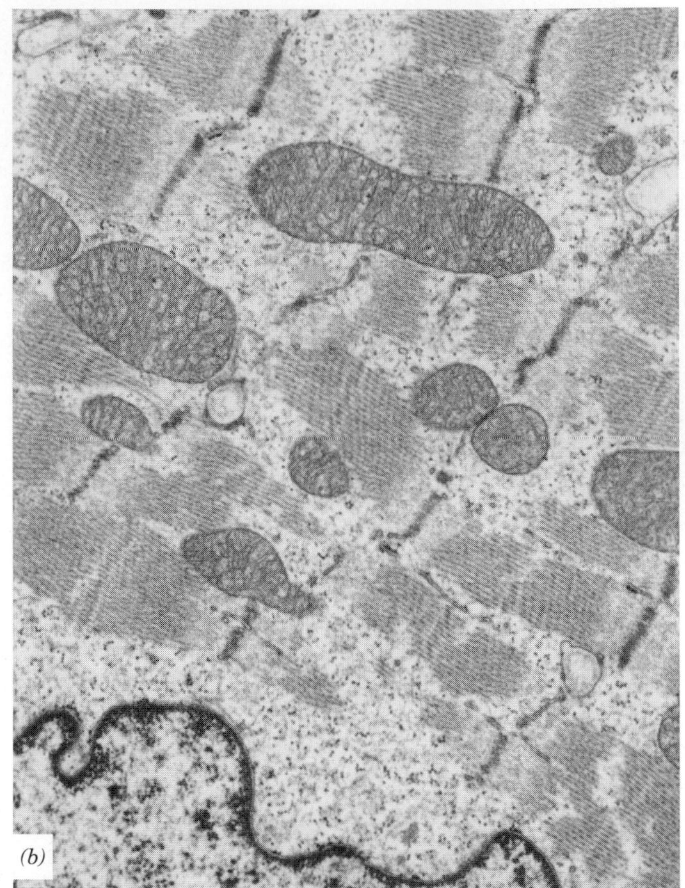

FIGURE 6.24 (*b*)
Electron micrograph of mitochondria in muscle fibers from rabbit heart (×39,600).
Courtesy of Dr. W. B. Winborn, Department of Anatomy, The University of Texas Health Science Center at San Antonio, and the Electron Microscopy Laboratory, Department of Pathology, The University of Texas Health Science Center at San Antonio.

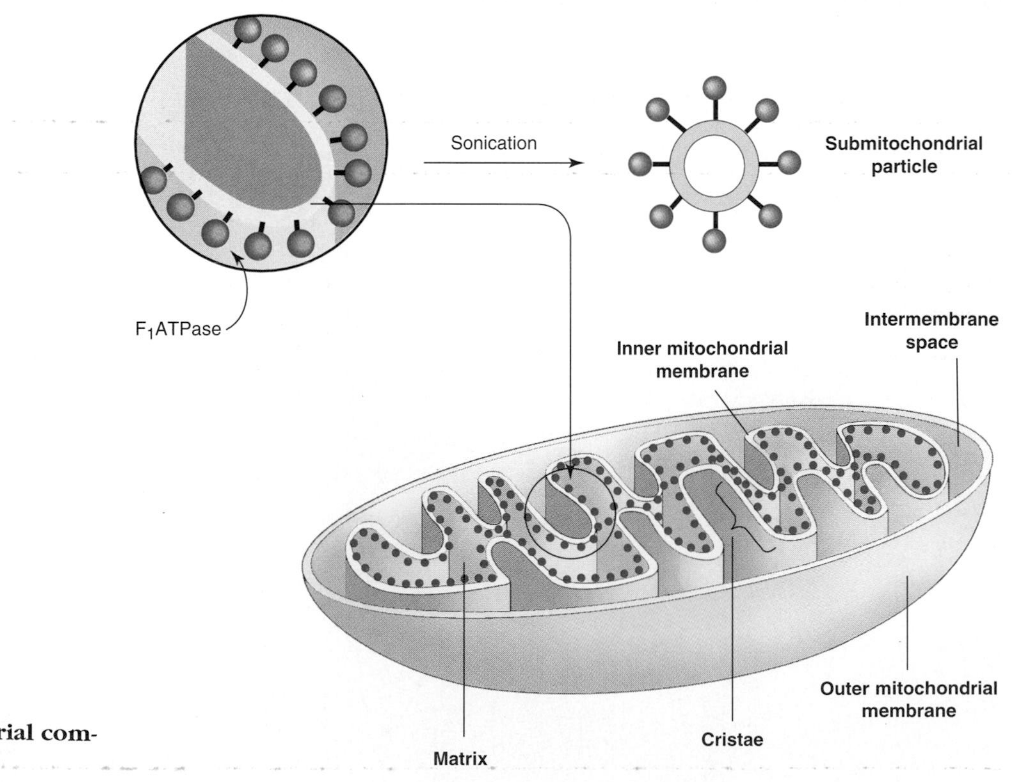

FIGURE 6.25
Diagram of various submitochondrial compartments.

to perform aerobic metabolic functions. For example, the erythrocyte has no mitochondria and does not possess the capacity to generate energy using oxygen as a terminal electron acceptor. On the other hand, cardiac tissue is a highly aerobic tissue, and it has been estimated that about one-half of the cytoplasmic volume of cardiac cells is composed of mitochondria. The liver is also highly dependent on aerobic metabolic processes for its various functions, and it has been estimated that mammalian hepatocytes contain between 800 and 2000 mitochondria. Mitochondria exist in a variety of different shapes, depending on the cell type from which they are derived. As can be seen in Figure 6.24 mitochondria from liver are nearly spherical in shape, whereas those found in cardiac muscle are oblong or cylindrical.

Inner and Outer Mitochondrial Membranes Have Different Compositions and Functions

Mitochondria are composed of two membranes, an outer and a highly invaginated inner membrane (Figure 6.25). The outer membrane is considered a rather simple membrane, composed of about 50% lipid and 50% protein, with relatively few enzymatic or transport functions. Table 6.5 defines some of the enzymatic components of the outer membrane.

The inner membrane is structurally and functionally much more complex than the outer membrane. Roughly 80% of the inner membrane is protein. It contains most of the enzymes involved in **electron transport** and oxidative phosphorylation, various dehydrogenases and several transport systems, which are involved in transferring substrates, metabolic intermediates and adenine nucleotides between the cytosol and the mitochondrial matrix (Table 6.5).

Some enzymatic components are loosely associated with the inner membrane, whereas others are either tightly bound or are actual structural elements of the membrane. Hence there is a wide variability in the extent to which physical (ultrasonic irradiation or freezing and thawing), chemical (organic solvent or detergent treatment), or enzymatic (protease or lipase) treatments remove, release, or inactivate the enzymes associated with the inner membrane.

TABLE 6.5 Enzymatic Composition of the Various Mitochondrial Subcompartments

Outer Membrane	*Intermembrane Space*	*Inner Membrane*	*Matrix*
Monoamine oxidase	Adenylate kinase	Succinate dehydrogenase	Pyruvate dehydrogenase
Kynurenine hydroxylase	Nucleoside diphosphate kinase	F_1-ATPase	Citrate synthase
Nucleoside diphosphate kinase		NADH dehydrogenase	Isocitrate dehydrogenase
Phospholipase A		β-Hydroxybutyrate dehydrogenase	α-Ketoglutarate dehydrogenase
Fatty acyl-CoA synthetases		Cytochromes b, c_1, c, a, a_3	Aconitase
NADH: cytochrome-*c* reductase (rotenone-insensitive)		Carnitine: acyl-CoA transferase	Fumarase
Choline phosphotransferase		Adenine nucleotide translocase	Succinyl-CoA synthetase
		Mono-, di-, and tricarboxylate translocase	Malate dehydrogenase
		Glutamate–aspartate translocase	Fatty acid β-oxidation system
			Glutamate dehydrogenase
			Glutamate–oxaloacetate transaminase
			Ornithine transcarbamoylase

Experimental procedures permit separation of inner from outer mitochondrial membranes. The outer membrane may be stripped off and isolated, using digitonin (a detergent), osmotic shock, or ultrasonic irradiation followed by density-gradient ultracentrifugation (Figure 6.26). The resulting inner membrane plus matrix fraction is referred to as a **mitoplast.** The contents of the matrix can be released from the mitoplast, by treatment with a nonionic detergent or vigorous sonication. Once the various subcompartments of the mitochondrion have been separated, analyses may be performed to determine the location of the various characteristic marker enzymes, several of which are listed in Table 6.5. Enzymatic markers have been used effectively to detect the presence of mitochondria or even a particular portion of mitochondria in membrane preparations of diverse derivation.

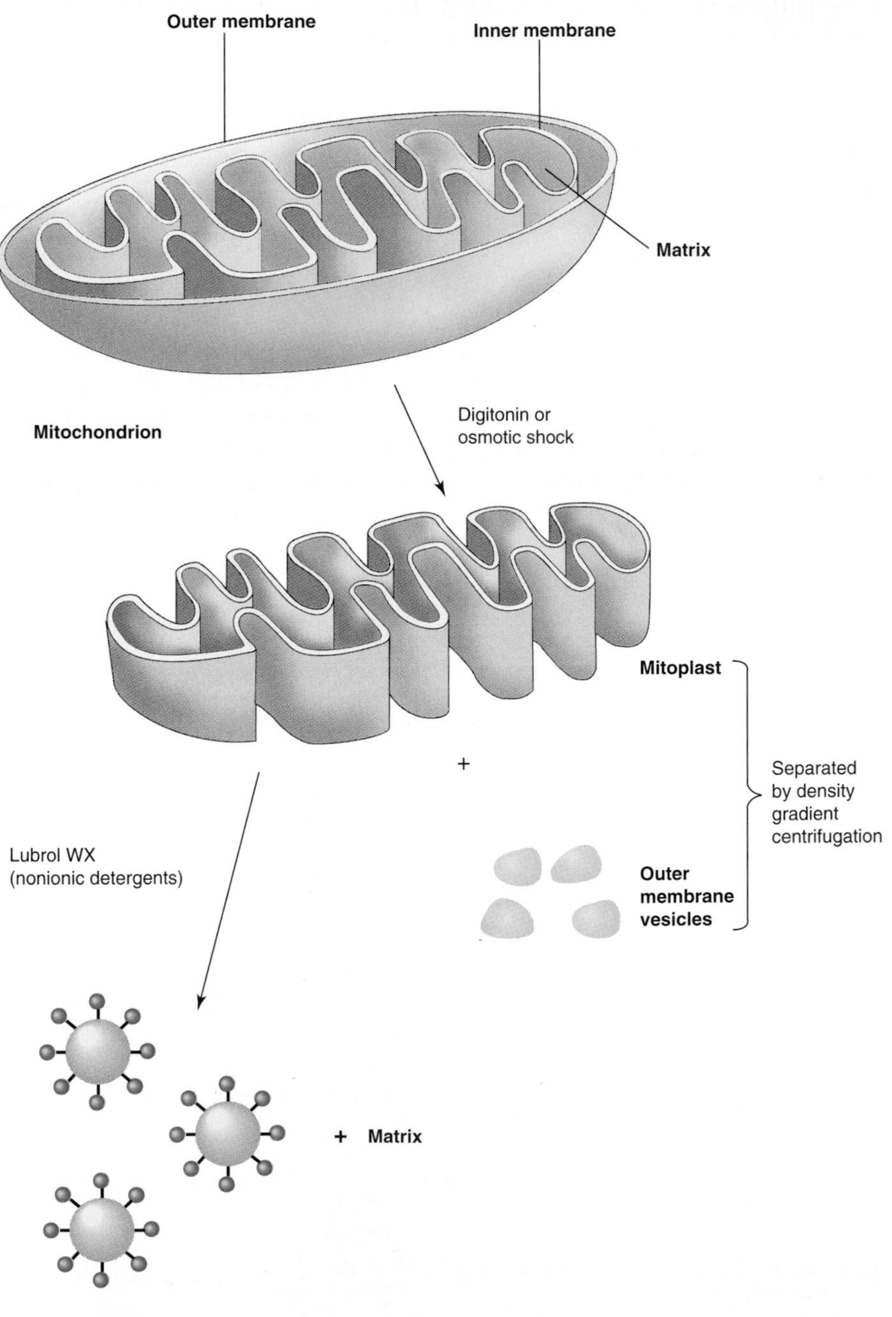

FIGURE 6.26
Separation of mitochondrial membranes.

Mitochondrial Inner Membranes Contain Substrate Transport Systems

Whereas the outer membrane presents little or no permeability barrier to substrate or nucleotide molecules of interest in energy metabolism, the inner membrane limits the types of substrates, intermediates, and nucleotides that can diffuse from the cytosol into the matrix compartment.

Various transport systems have been described in mitochondria (Figure 6.27), some of which have been thoroughly characterized. The primary function of these transport systems is to facilitate the selective movement of various substrates and intermediates back and forth across the inner mitochondrial membrane from the cytosol to the mitochondrial matrix. Through the action of these transporters, various substrates and other molecules can be accumulated in the mitochondrial matrix since the transporters can facilitate the movement of the substrate against a concentration gradient. The importance of a mitochondrial transporter derives from involvement of the substance transported in a variety of mitochondrial metabolic processes.

Substrate Shuttles Transport Reducing Equivalents Across the Inner Mitochondrial Membrane

The various nucleotides involved in cellular oxidation–reduction reactions (e.g., NAD^+, NADH, $NADP^+$, NADPH, FAD, and $FADH_2$) and CoA and its derivatives are not permeable to the inner mitochondrial membrane. Hence, for example, to transport reducing equivalents (e.g., protons and electrons) from cytosol to mitochondrial matrix or vice versa, "**substrate shuttle** mechanisms" involving the reciprocal transfer of reduced and oxidized members of various oxidation–reduction couples are used to accomplish the net transfer of reducing equivalents across the membrane. Two examples of how this transfer of reducing equivalents from the cytosol to the matrix occurs are shown in Figure 6.28. The **malate–aspartate shuttle** and the **α-glycerol phosphate shuttle** are

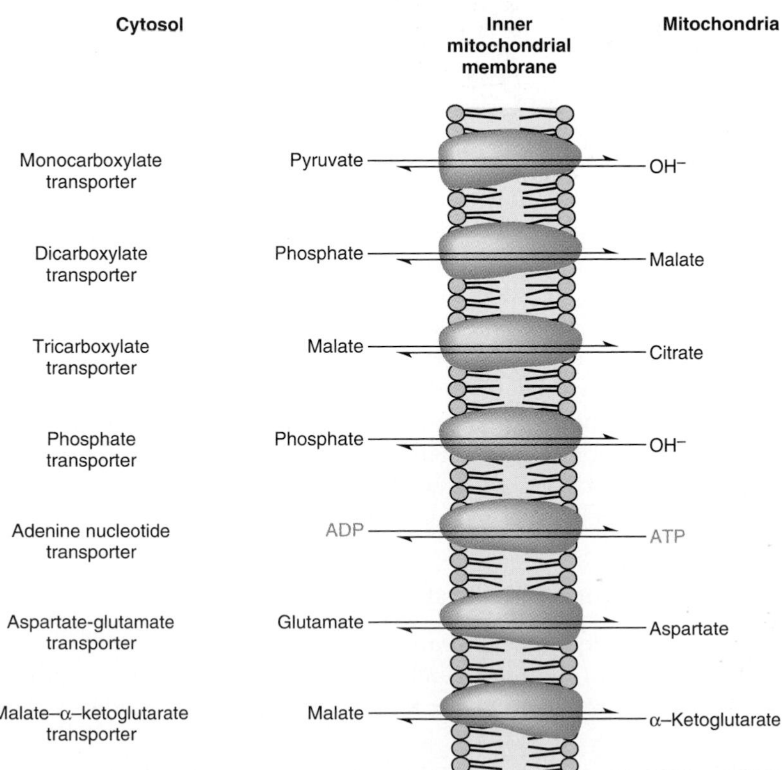

FIGURE 6.27
Mitochondrial metabolite transporters.

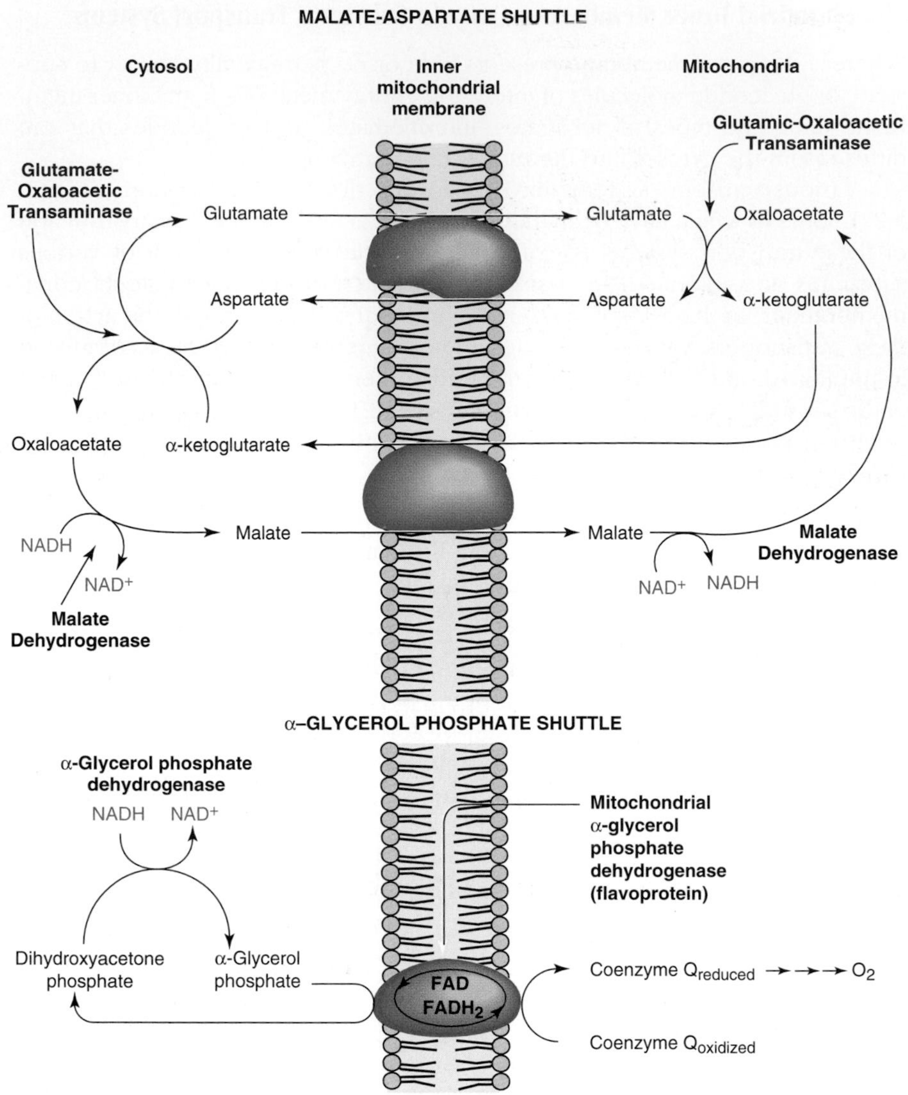

FIGURE 6.28
Transport shuttles for reducing equivalents.

employed in various tissues to translocate reducing equivalents from the cytosol to the mitochondrial matrix, where they are oxidized to yield energy. The operation of such substrate shuttles requires that the appropriate enzymes are localized on the correct side of the membrane and that appropriate transporters or translocases be present on/in the membrane. The operation of the malate–aspartate shuttle depends on the fact that NADH, NAD^+, and oxaloacetate are not permeable to the inner mitochondrial membrane, on the distribution of malate dehydrogenase and aspartate aminotransferase on both sides of the inner mitochondrial membrane, and on the existence of membrane transporters that exchange intramitochondrial aspartate for cytosolic glutamate and cytosolic malate for intramitochondrial α-ketoglutarate.

Acetyl Units Are Transported by Citrate

Acetyl CoA is impermeable to the inner mitochondrial membrane but the acetyl group can be transferred from the mitochondrial compartment to the cytosol, where acetyl moieties are required for fatty acid or sterol biosynthesis (Figure 6.29).

Intramitochondrial acetyl CoA is converted to citrate by citrate synthase of the TCA cycle. Subsequently, the citrate is exported to the cytosol by a

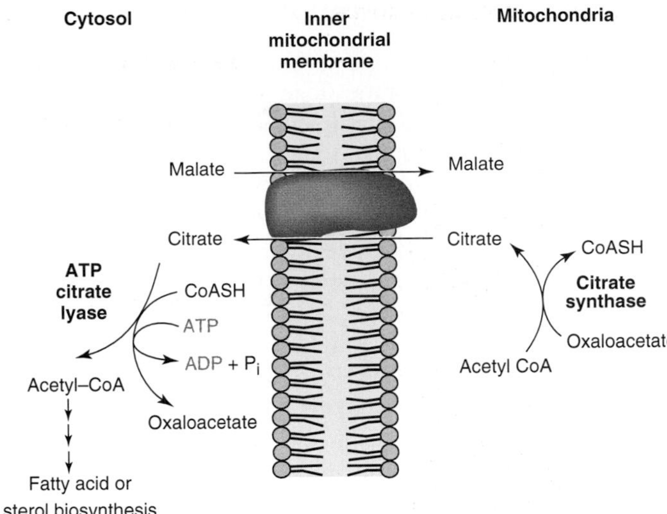

FIGURE 6.29
Export of intramitochondrially generated citrate to the cytosol to serve as a source of acetyl CoA for biosynthesis of fatty acids or sterols.

tricarboxylate transporter in exchange for a dicarboxylate such as malate. Cytosolic citrate is then cleaved to acetyl CoA and oxaloacetate at the expense of an ATP by ATP : citrate lyase (see p. 371). Substrate shuttle mechanisms in liver are involved in movement of appropriate substrates and intermediates in both directions across the inner mitochondrial membranes during periods of active **gluconeogenesis** (see p. 302) and **ureagenesis** (see p. 454).

Transport of Adenine Nucleotides and Phosphate

Adenine nucleotides are transported across the inner mitochondrial membrane by a very specific **adenine nucleotide translocator.** Nucleotide species such as the guanine, uridine, or cytosine nucleotides are neither exchanged across the inner membrane on the adenine nucleotide-specific translocator nor transported by a comparable carrier specific for nonadenine nucleotides. Cytosolic ADP, formed during energy-consuming reactions, is exchanged for mitochondrial ATP, generated in the process of oxidative phosphorylation (Figure 6.30). At pH 7 ADP has three negative charges and ATP has four, so that a 1 : 1 exchange of ADP:ATP would cause a charge imbalance across the membrane. Hence the ADP for ATP exchange across the mitochondrial membrane is an electrogenic process, requiring that the charge imbalance be compensated for by the movement of a proton or another charged species. The adenine nucleotide carrier was isolated due to its capacity to bind very tightly to atractyloside, a specific inhibitor of the carrier. It is a dimer with a subunit molecular weight of 30,000. It is unlikely that the rate of transport of adenine nucleotides across the mitochondrial membrane is ever limiting to the overall process of mitochondrial ATP synthesis. Low concentrations of long-chain fatty acyl CoA derivatives inhibit (i.e., $K_i = 1\ \mu$M) the transport of ATP and ADP in isolated liver mitochondria. However, experimental results obtained under *in vivo* conditions in intact liver cells indicate that there occurs little, if any, inhibition of the adenine nucleotide transporter under metabolic conditions in which a large concentration of long-chain fatty acyl CoA accumulates.

A specific transporter transports cytosolic phosphate into the mitochondrial matrix for negatively charged hydroxyl ions in an electroneutral exchange (Figure 6.30). Also, phosphate transport may be accomplished in a proton-compensated mechanism; for example, phosphate and protons are transported in a 1 : 1 ratio. Phosphate transport is strongly inhibited by mersalyl and various mercurial reagents.

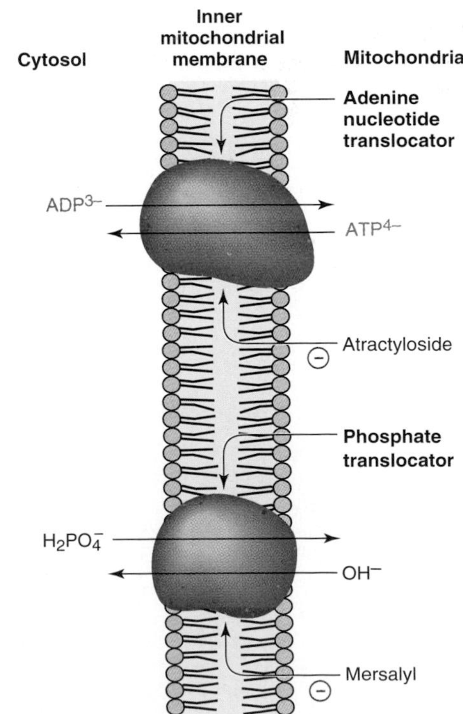

FIGURE 6.30
The adenine nucleotide and phosphate translocators.

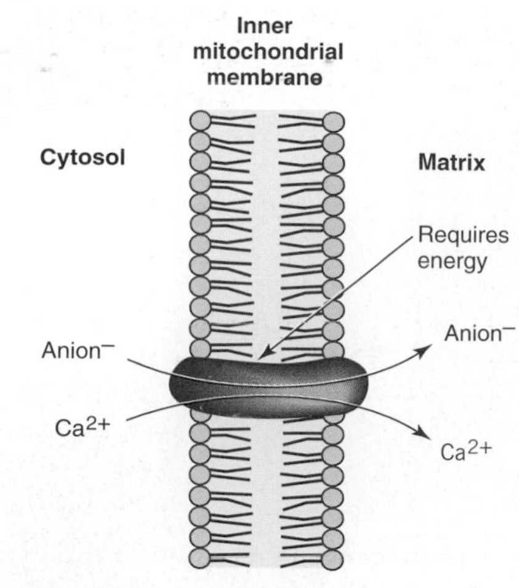

FIGURE 6.31
Mitochondrial calcium carrier.
The energy requirement can be met from ATP, ΔpH, or membrane potential.

Mitochondria Have a Specific Calcium Transport Mechanism

Mitochondria from most tissues possess a transport system for translocating Ca^{2+} across the mitochondrial inner membrane. It is difficult to overestimate the importance of the distribution/redistribution of cellular calcium pools in different cell functions, such as muscle contraction, neural transmission, secretion, and hormone action. Calcium exists in distinct pools in the cell. The cytosol, mitochondria, endoplasmic reticulum, nuclei, and Golgi complex have their own pools of calcium. Some of the intracellular calcium is bound to nucleotides, metabolites, or membrane ligands, while a portion of the intracellular calcium is free in solution. A gradient of Ca^{2+} exists from outside to inside a cell. Estimates of intracellular cytosolic calcium are in the range of 10^{-7} M, whereas extracellular calcium is at least four orders of magnitude greater. Total intramitochondrial calcium has been estimated to be $\sim 10^{-4}$ M but the free ionic calcium concentration in the mitochondrion is in the range of 10^{-7} M. Hence processes involved in the alternate sequestering and release of an intracellular store of calcium can greatly influence intracellular calcium pools and various cell functions. Mitochondria accumulate rather large quantities of calcium at the expense of ATP hydrolysis, respiration, or the electrochemical gradient created across the mitochondrial membrane. Mitochondrial calcium transport is inhibited by low concentrations of lanthanides (trivalent metal cations) and by ruthenium red. Mg^{2+} competes with Ca^{2+} for the carrier in certain types of mitochondria. The current view is that there is a specific carrier in the inner mitochondrial membrane, which is likely a glycoprotein (Figure 6.31). The mitochondrial calcium carrier exhibits saturation kinetics, has a high affinity for calcium, and is highly specific for calcium. Permeant counterions such as phosphate or acetate stimulate calcium transport and allow the cation to be retained in the matrix. The most probable utility of the ability of mitochondria to accumulate calcium occurs during cellular injury when extracellular calcium enters the cell. Mitochondria can sequester the calcium to minimize the change in the cytosolic calcium level. Certain hormones may affect intracellular calcium distribution (e.g., epinephrine or vasopressin) as part of the mechanism of the hormone response; it is unlikely that the mitochondrial calcium pool contributes to the hormone-sensitive pool of calcium.

In summary, the inner mitochondrial membrane possesses a variety of transport systems involved in the movement of nucleotides, substrates, metabolites, and metal cations into and out of the mitochondrial matrix. These transport functions are essential for the complex cellular metabolic pathways and their regulation (see Clin. Corr. 6.3).

6.6 ■ ELECTRON TRANSFER

During the enzymatic reactions involved in glycolysis, fatty acid oxidation, and the TCA cycle, reducing equivalents are derived from the sequential breakdown of the initial metabolic fuel. In glycolysis, NADH is produced by glyceraldehyde-3-phosphate dehydrogenase and must be reoxidized in the cytosol (e.g., by lactate dehydrogenase as is the case in the red blood cell) or the reducing equivalents of NADH must be transported to the mitochondrial matrix via one of the substrate shuttles. The latter mechanism will yield the maximum energy from the metabolism of glucose. In fatty acid oxidation and the TCA cycle, reducing equivalents as both NADH and $FADH_2$ are produced in the mitochondrial matrix. To transduce this reducing power into utilizable energy, mitochondria have a system of electron carriers in or associated with the inner mitochondrial membrane, which in the presence of oxygen convert reducing equivalents into utilizable energy. This process is called **electron transport.** As will be seen, NADH and $FADH_2$ oxidation in this process results in production of

3 and 2 mol of ATP per mole of reducing equivalent transferred to oxygen, respectively.

Oxidation–Reduction Reactions

Prior to the presentation of a description of the many components and the mechanism of the electron transport sequence, it is important to discuss some basic information concerning oxidation–reduction reactions. The mitochondrial electron transport system is little more than a sequence of linked oxidation–reduction reactions, for example,

$$AH_2 + B \rightleftharpoons A + BH_2$$

Oxidation–reduction reactions occur when there is a transfer of electrons from a suitable electron donor (the reductant) to a suitable electron acceptor (the oxidant). In some oxidation–reduction reactions only electrons are transferred from the reductant to the oxidant (i.e., electron transfer between cytochromes),

$$\text{Cytochrome } c\ (Fe^{2+}) + \text{cytochrome } a\ (Fe^{3+}) \rightleftharpoons \text{cytochrome } c\ (Fe^{3+}) + \text{cytochrome } a\ (Fe^{2+})$$

whereas in other types of reactions, both electrons and protons (hydrogen atoms) are transferred (e.g., electron transfer between NADH and FAD).

$$NADH + H^+ + FAD \rightleftharpoons NAD^+ + FADH_2$$

Oxidized and reduced forms of compounds or groups operating in oxidation–reduction reactions are referred to as **redox couples** or pairs. The facility with which a given electron donor (reductant) gives up its electrons to an electron acceptor (oxidant) is expressed quantitatively as the oxidation–reduction potential of the system. An **oxidation–reduction potential** is measured in volts as an **electromotive force** (emf) of a half-cell made up of both members of an oxidation–reduction couple when compared to a standard reference half-cell (usually the hydrogen electrode reaction). The potential of the standard hydrogen electrode is set by convention at 0.0 V at pH 0.0. However, when this standard potential is corrected for pH 7.0 the reference electrode potential becomes −0.42 V. The oxidation–reduction potentials for a variety of important biochemical reactions are tabulated in Table 6.6. The reductant of an oxidation–reduction pair with large negative potential will give up its electrons more readily than pairs with smaller negative or positive redox potentials. On the

TABLE 6.6 Standard Oxidation–Reduction Potentials for Various Biochemical Reactions

Oxidation–Reduction System	*Standard Oxidation–Reduction Potential E'_0 (V)*
Acetate + $2H^+ + 2e^- \rightleftharpoons$ acetaldehyde	−0.60
$2H^+ + 2e^- \rightleftharpoons H_2$	−0.42
Acetoacetate + $2H^+ + 2e^- \rightleftharpoons$ β-hydroxybutyrate	−0.35
$NAD^+ + 2H^+ + 2e^- \rightleftharpoons NADH + H^+$	−0.32
Acetaldehyde + $2H^+ + 2e^- \rightleftharpoons$ ethanol	−0.20
Pyruvate + $2H^+ + 2e^- \rightleftharpoons$ lactate	−0.19
Oxaloacetate + $2H^+ + 2e^- \rightleftharpoons$ malate	−0.17
Coenzyme $Q_{ox} + 2e^- \rightleftharpoons$ coenzyme Q_{red}	+0.10
Cytochrome b (Fe^{3+}) + $e^- \rightleftharpoons$ cytochrome b (Fe^{2+})	+0.12
Cytochrome c (Fe^{3+}) + $e^- \rightleftharpoons$ cytochrome c (Fe^{2+})	+0.22
Cytochrome a (Fe^{3+}) + $e^- \rightleftharpoons$ cytochrome a (Fe^{2+})	+0.29
$\frac{1}{2}O_2 + 2H^+ + 2e^- \rightleftharpoons H_2O$	+0.82

CLINICAL CORRELATION 6.3

Mitochondrial Myopathies

Diseases that involve defects in various metabolic functions of muscle have been described. Clinically, patients with myopathy complain of weakness and cramping of the affected muscles; infants have difficulty feeding and crawling; severe fatigue results from minimal exertion; and there is usually evidence of muscle wasting. On the basis of electron microscopic examination and enzymatic characterization of muscle biopsy material, many myopathies have been found that have a primary lesion in mitochondrial function.

Deficiencies in mitochondrial transport functions (i.e., carnitine : palmitoyl-CoA transferase) and in components of the mitochondrial electron transport chain (NADH dehydrogenase, cytochrome b, cytochrome a,a_3, or the mitochondrial F_1F_0-ATPase) have been described. In many mitochondrial myopathies large paracrystalline inclusions occur within the mitochondrial matrix (see figure). It is not known whether this crystalline material is inorganic or organic in composition. In certain mitochondrial myopathies electron transport is only loosely coupled to ATP production; in other cases these processes exhibit normal tight coupling. Because some of these disorders involve defects in enzymes encoded by mitochondrial genes, they have the unique pattern of inheritance from the mother, since all mitochondria are derived from mitochondria in the ovum.

Petty, R. K. H., Harding, A. E., and Morgan-Hughes, J. A. The clinical features of mitochondrial myopathy. *Brain* 109:915, 1986; and Shoffner, J. M., and Wallace, D. C. Oxidative phosphorylation diseases and mitochondrial mutations: diagnosis and treatment. *Annu. Rev. Nutr.* 14:535, 1994.

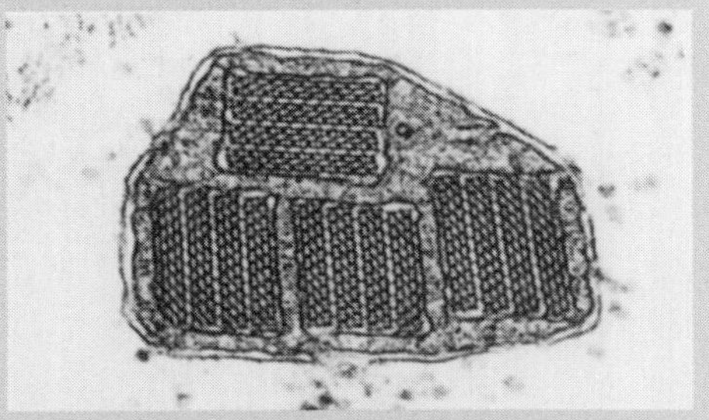

Example of paracrystalline inclusions in mitochondria from muscles of ocular myopathic patients (×36,000).
Courtesy of Dr. D. N. Landon, Institute of Neurology, University of London.

other hand, a strong oxidant (e.g., characterized by a large positive potential) has a very high affinity for electrons.

The **Nernst equation** characterizes the relationship between the standard oxidation–reduction potential of a particular redox pair (E_0'), the observed potential (E), and the ratio of the concentrations of oxidant and reductant in the system:

$$E = E_0' + \frac{2.3\ RT}{nF} \log \left(\frac{[\text{oxidant}]}{[\text{reductant}]} \right)$$

E is the observed potential with all concentrations at 1 M. E_0' is the standard potential at pH 7.0. R is the gas constant of 8.3 J deg^{-1} mol^{-1}. T is the absolute temperature in kelvin units (K). n is the number of electrons being transferred. F is the Faraday constant of 96,500 J V^{-1}.

When an observed potential is equal to the standard potential, a potential is defined that is referred to as the midpoint potential. At the midpoint potential the concentration of oxidant is equal to that of reductant. Knowing standard oxidation–reduction potentials of a diverse variety of biochemical reactions allows one to predict the direction of electron flow or transfer when more than one redox pair is linked together by the appropriate enzyme that causes a reaction to occur. For example, as shown in Table 6.6 the NAD^+–NADH pair has a standard potential of −0.32 V, and the pyruvate–lactate pair possesses a potential of −0.19. This means that electrons will flow from the NAD^+–NADH system to the pyruvate–lactate system as long as the enzyme (lactate dehydrogenase) is present; for example,

$$\text{Pyruvate} + \text{NADH} + H^+ \rightleftharpoons \text{lactate} + NAD^+$$

Hence in the mitochondrial electron-transfer system electrons or reducing equivalents are produced in NAD^+- and FAD-linked dehydrogenase reactions, which have standard potentials at or close to that of NAD^+–NADH and are passed through the electron-transfer chain, which has as its terminal acceptor the oxygen–water couple.

Free-Energy Changes in Redox Reactions

Oxidation–reduction potential differences between two redox pairs are similar to free-energy changes in chemical reactions, in that both quantities depend on the concentration of reactants and products of the reaction and the following relationship exists:

$$\Delta G^{\circ\prime} = -nF\,\Delta E_0'$$

Using this expression, the free-energy change for electron-transfer reactions can be calculated if the potential difference between two oxidation–reduction pairs is known. Hence, for the mitochondrial electron-transfer process in which electrons are transferred between the NAD^+–NADH couple (E_0' = −0.32 V) and the $\frac{1}{2}O_2$–H_2O couple (E_0' = +0.82 V), the free-energy change for this process can be calculated:

$$\Delta G^{\circ} = -nF\Delta E_0' = -2 \times 23.062 \times 1.14\ \text{V}$$

$$\Delta G^{\circ} = -52.6\ \text{kcal mol}^{-1}$$

where 23.062 is the Faraday constant in kcal V^{-1} and n is the number of electrons transferred; for example, in the case of NADH → O_2, n = 2. The free energy available from the potential span between NADH and oxygen in the electron-transfer chain is capable of generating more than enough energy to synthesize three molecules of ATP per two reducing equivalents or two electrons transported to oxygen. In addition, because of the negative sign of the free energy available in the mitochondrial electron transfer, this process is exergonic and will proceed provided that the necessary enzymes are present.

Mitochondrial Electron Transport Is a Multicomponent System

Before defining the mechanistic details of the mitochondrial electron transport chain it is necessary to describe the various components that participate in the transfer of electrons in this system. The major enzymes or proteins functioning as electron-transfer components involved in the mitochondrial electron-transfer system are as follows: (1) NAD^+-linked dehydrogenases, (2) flavin-linked dehydrogenases, (3) iron–sulfur proteins, and (4) **cytochromes.**

NAD-Linked Dehydrogenases

The initial stage in the mitochondrial electron transport sequence consists of the generation of reducing equivalents in the TCA cycle, the fatty acid β-oxidation sequence, and various other dehydrogenase reactions. The NAD-linked dehydrogenase reactions of these pathways reduce NAD^+ to NADH while converting the reduced member of an oxidation–reduction couple to the oxidized form; for example, for the isocitrate dehydrogenase reaction,

$$\text{Isocitrate} + NAD^+ \rightleftharpoons \alpha\text{-ketoglutarate} + CO_2 + NADH + H^+$$

Two nicotinamide nucleotides are involved in various metabolic reactions, NAD and NADP (Figure 6.32). Nicotinamide adenine dinucleotide phosphate has a phosphate esterified to the 2 position of the ribose in the adenosine portion of

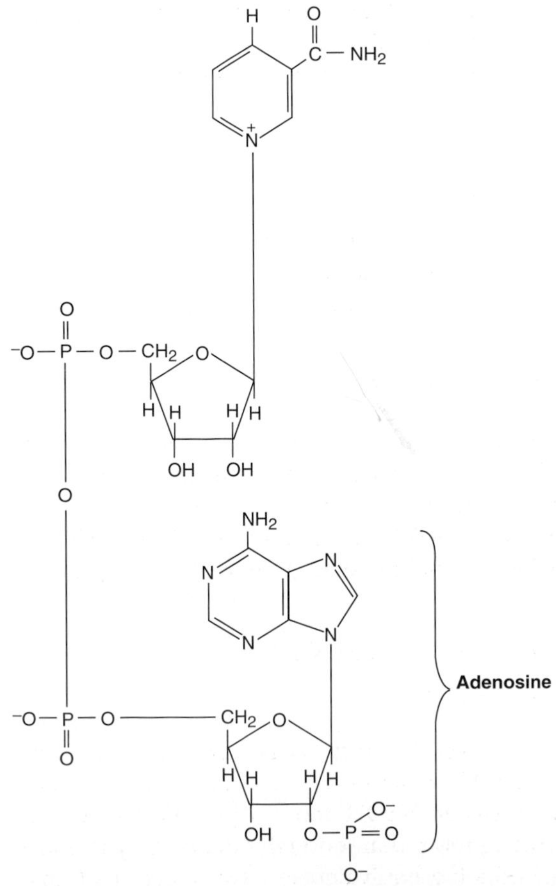

FIGURE 6.32
Structure of nicotinamide adenine dinucleotide phosphate: NADP.

TABLE 6.7 The Stereospecificity of NAD(P)-Linked Dehydrogenases

NAD(P)-Linked Dehydrogenase	*Specificity*
Alcohol dehydrogenase	A
Malate dehydrogenase	A
Lactate dehydrogenase	A
Isocitrate dehydrogenase ($NADP^+$)	A
Hydroxyacyl-CoA dehydrogenase	B
Glyceraldehyde-3-phosphate dehydrogenase	B
Glucose-6-phosphate dehydrogenase ($NADP^+$)	B

the dinucleotide. Each NAD(P)-linked dehydrogenase catalyzes a stereospecific transfer of the reducing equivalent from the substrate to the nucleotide (see p. 143).

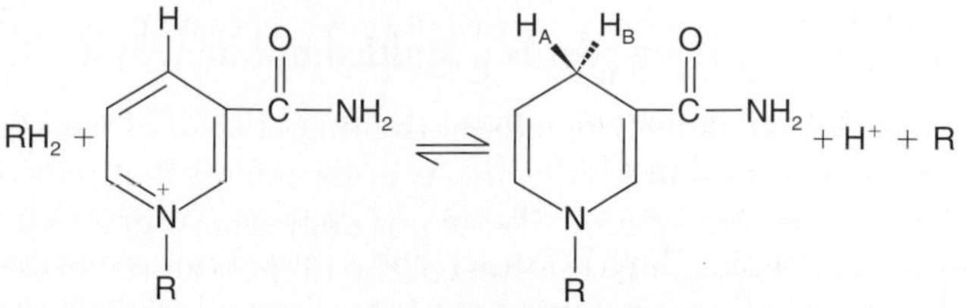

NAD(P)-linked dehydrogenases are either A specific or B specific. Table 6.7 lists examples of the stereospecificity of NAD(P)-linked dehydrogenases. Once formed, NAD(P)H is released from the dehydrogenase and serves as the substrate for the mitochondrial electron transport system. NADPH is not a substrate for the mitochondrial respiratory chain but is used in reductive biosynthetic reactions of such processes as fatty acid and sterol synthesis. When $NAD(P)^+$ is converted to NAD(P)H, there is a characteristic change in the absorbance and fluorescence properties of these nucleotides, which occurs as a result of the reduction of $NAD(P)^+$. The reduced form of the nicotinamide coenzyme has an absorbance maximum at 340 nm (Figure 6.33) not present in the oxidized $NAD(P)^+$ form. Furthermore, when the reduced form of the nicotinamide coenzyme is excited by light at 340 nm a fluorescence emission maximum is seen at 465 nm. These absorbance and fluorescence properties of the nicotinamide coenzymes have been employed extensively in developing assays for dehydrogenase reactions (see p. 168) and have been utilized to monitor the oxidation–reduction state of a tissue or a preparation of intact mitochondria. With an appropriate spectrophotometer (e.g., dual wavelength), capable of measuring small absorbance changes in turbid cell or mitochondrial suspensions, the relative changes in the oxidized–reduced nicotinamide coenzymes may be determined as a function of the metabolic condition of the cell or subcellular suspension (e.g., changes in substrate, oxygen concentration, or upon drug or hormone addition). This type of spectrophotometric technique and more sophisticated techniques—in which a light guide is used to direct a beam of excitation light to the surface of an intact organ or tissue, and another light guide is employed to observe the reflected fluorescence emission at a longer wavelength—have been valuable tools in understanding the very complicated relationships that exist between the mitochondrial respiratory chain and the metabolic characteristics of various tissues.

Another effective method for monitoring the oxidation–reduction state of the cytosolic or mitochondrial compartments is to measure the oxidized and reduced members of various redox couples in tissue extracts, in the bathing solution of a tissue, or in the effluent perfusate of an isolated, perfused organ. Because lactate dehydrogenase is exclusively a cytosolic enzyme the pyruvate/lactate ratio in the tissue or organ perfusate should accurately reflect the cytosolic $NAD^+/NADH$ ratio under a variety of metabolic conditions. Similarly, the **β-hydroxybutyrate dehydrogenase** is exclusively mitochondrial, and hence the ratio of acetoacetate/β-hydroxybutyrate should reflect the oxidation–reduction state of the mitochondrial NAD^+–NADH system. If the ratio of acetoacetate/β-hydroxybutyrate and the equilibrium constant for β-hydroxybutyrate dehydrogenase are known, the $NAD^+/NADH$ ratio under any condition can be calculated:

$$\text{Acetoacetate} + \text{NADH} + \text{H}^+ \rightleftharpoons \beta\text{-hydroxybutyrate} + \text{NAD}^+$$

$$K_{eq} = \frac{[\beta\text{-hydroxybutyrate}][\text{NAD}^+]}{[\text{acetoacetate}][\text{NADH}][\text{H}^+]}$$

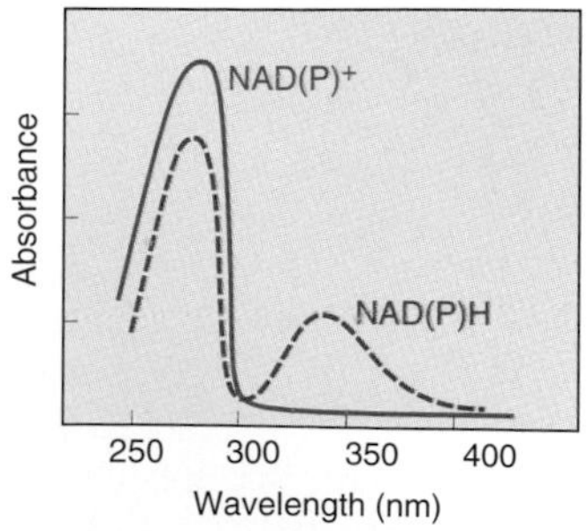

FIGURE 6.33
Absorbance properties of NAD^+ and NADH.

Flavin-Linked Dehydrogenases

The second type of oxidation–reduction reaction essential in mitochondrial electron transport employs a **flavin** (e.g., derived from riboflavin) as electron acceptor as part of flavin-linked dehydrogenases. The two flavins commonly utilized in oxidation–reduction reactions are FAD (flavin adenine dinucleotide) and FMN (flavin mononucleotide) (Figure 6.34).

Five flavin-containing enzymes play an essential role in energy metabolism in mammalian mitochondria (Table 6.8). In the pyruvate and α-ketoglutarate dehydrogenase multienzyme complexes, the final reaction catalyzed involves the flavoprotein enzyme, dihydrolipoyl dehydrogenase, in which the bound FAD moiety accepts electrons from reduced lipoamide on the transacylase subunit and then transfers the reducing equivalents to NAD^+. Also, in the TCA cycle, succinate dehydrogenase is a flavin-linked protein, which oxidizes succinate to fumarate and converts FAD to $FADH_2$. The first dehydrogenation reaction in β-oxidation of fatty acids is catalyzed by the acyl-CoA dehydrogenase, another flavin-linked enzyme. Finally, oxidation of NADH in the mitochondrial respiratory chain is catalyzed by a FMN-containing enzyme, NADH dehydrogenase, and the reducing equivalents are transferred to another flavoprotein called the electron-transferring flavoprotein.

The flavins FAD and FMN either may be bound very tightly noncovalently (i.e., with dissociation constants in the range of 10^{-10} M) to their respective enzymes, as is the case for NADH dehydrogenase, or may be bound covalently to the protein (e.g., to a histidine residue), as is the case with succinate dehydrogenase. Flavoproteins are classified into two groups: (1) dehydrogenases in which the reduced flavin is reoxidized by electron carriers other than oxygen (e.g., coenzyme Q and other flavins, or *in vitro* with chemical agents such as ferricyanide, methylene blue, or phenazine methosulfate) and (2) oxidases in which the flavin may be reoxidized using molecular oxygen, O_2, as the electron acceptor, and yielding H_2O_2 as the product. The H_2O_2 may then be broken down to water and oxygen by the enzyme **catalase,**

$$2H_2O_2 \xrightleftharpoons{\text{catalase}} 2H_2O + O_2$$

Iron–Sulfur Centers

A number of flavin-linked enzymes contain nonheme iron (i.e., an iron–sulfur center; see p. 1004) involved in the catalytic mechanism. In these enzymes iron is converted from the oxidized (Fe^{3+}) to reduced (Fe^{2+}) form during the transfer of reducing equivalents on and off the flavin moiety. Both succinate dehydroge-

TABLE 6.8 Various Flavin-Linked Dehydrogenases

Enzyme	*Function*	*Flavin Nucleotide*
Succinate dehydrogenase	Tricarboxylic acid cycle	FAD
Dihydrolipoyl dehydrogenase	Component in pyruvate and α-ketoglutarate dehydrogenase complexes	FAD
NADH dehydrogenase	Electron transport chain	FMN
Electron-transferring flavoprotein	Electron transport chain	FAD
Acyl-CoA dehydrogenase	Fatty acid β-oxidation	FAD
D-Amino acid oxidase	Amino acid oxidation	FAD
Monoamine oxidase	Oxidation of monoamines	FAD

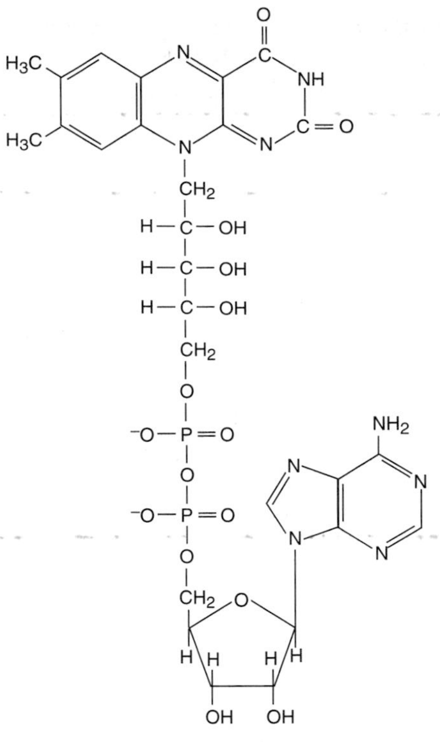

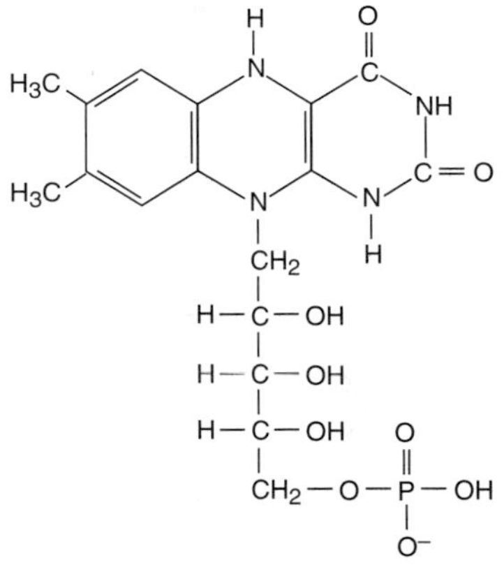

FIGURE 6.34
Structures of flavin adenine dinucleotide (FAD) and flavin mononucleotide (FMN).

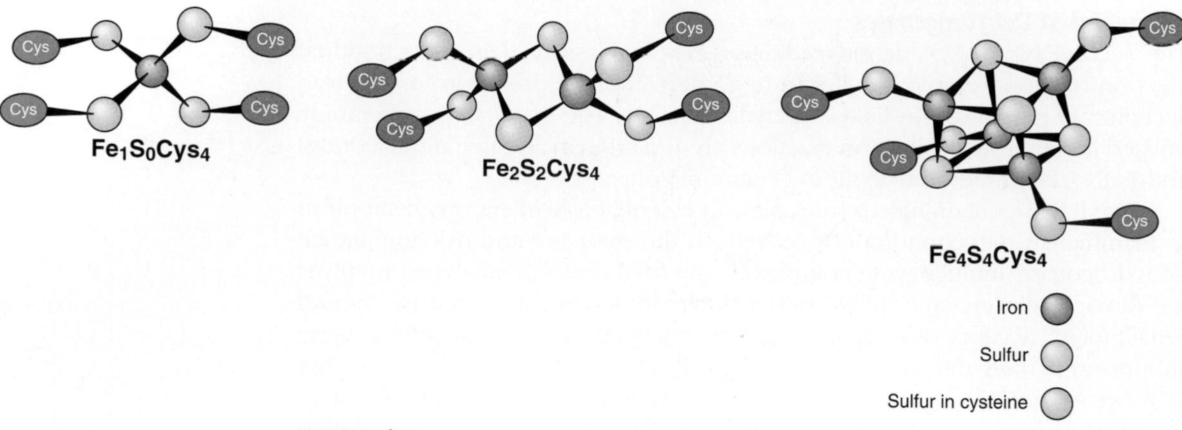

FIGURE 6.35
The structures of iron–sulfur centers.
White, sulfur; gray, sulfur in cysteine; and black, iron.

nase and NADH dehydrogenase contain iron–sulfur centers. The iron component of the iron–sulfur center is bound in various arrangements to cysteine residues in the protein and to acid-labile sulfur, for example, $Fe_4S_4Cys_4$, $Fe_2S_2Cys_4$, and $Fe_1S_0Cys_4$ (Figure 6.35). Iron–sulfur proteins are found in abundance in all species from the simplest microorganism to mammals. Certain flavin-linked enzymes (e.g., xanthine oxidase) contain one or two molybdenum atoms associated with their catalytic mechanism. The tightly bound molybdenum undergoes a valence change during transfer of electrons: $Mo^{6+} \rightarrow Mo^{5+}$.

Cytochromes

Organisms that require oxygen (i.e., aerobic organisms) in their energy-generating functions possess various cytochromes that are involved in electron-transfer systems. Cytochromes are a class of proteins characterized by the presence of an iron-containing heme group bound to the protein. Unlike the heme group in hemoglobin or myoglobin in which the heme iron remains in the Fe^{2+} state,

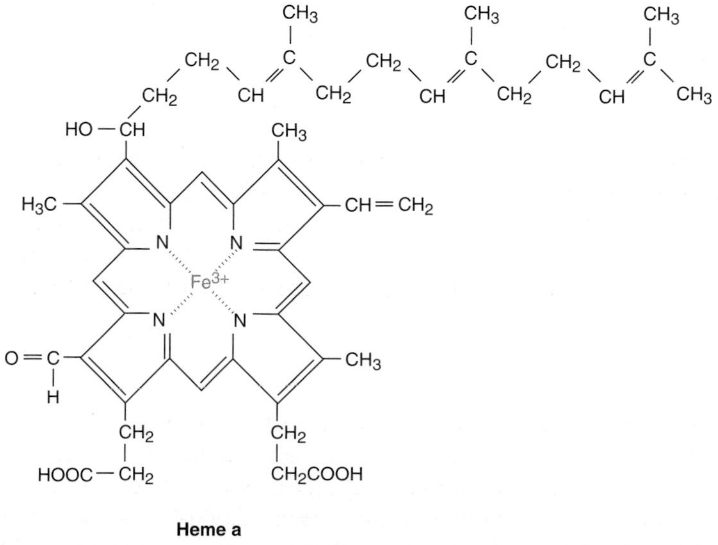

Heme a

FIGURE 6.36
Structures of heme a and heme c.

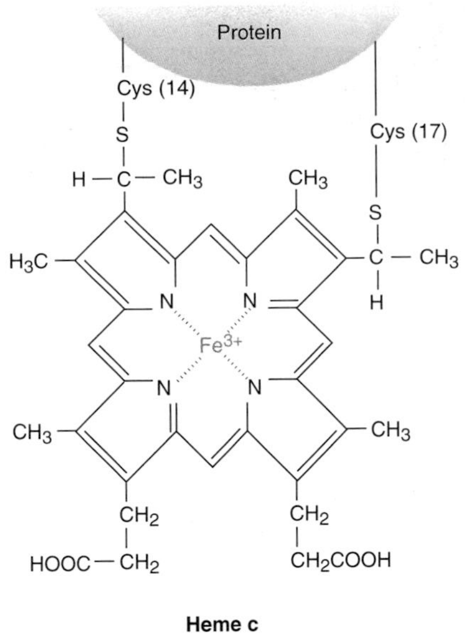

Heme c

FIGURE 6.36
Continued.

the iron in the heme of a cytochrome is alternately oxidized (Fe^{3+}) or reduced (Fe^{2+}) as it functions in the electron transport chain.

Cytochromes of mammalian mitochondria are designated as *a*, *b*, and *c* on the basis of the α band of their absorption spectrum and the type of heme group (Figure 6.36). Cytochrome *c* is a small protein (104 amino acid residues) with mol wt = 13,000. Amino acid sequences of cytochrome *c* from a great many species have been described and show that 20 out of 104 amino acid residues are invariant. The iron of the heme group in cytochrome *c* is coordinated between the four nitrogen atoms of the tetrapyrrole structure of the porphyrin group, whereas the fifth and sixth coordination positions are occupied by the methionine residue at position 80 and the histidine residue at position 18 of the protein (Figure 6.37). Since all six coordination positions are filled in most of the cytochromes, binding of oxygen directly to the iron is prevented as is binding of respiratory inhibitors such as cyanide, azide, and carbon monoxide. The notable exception is cytochrome a_3, which is involved in the terminal step in mitochondrial electron transport. The heme group in cytochrome *c* is attached to the protein, not only by the fifth and sixth coordination positions of the heme iron, but also by the vinyl side chains of the protoporphyrin IX structure, from which hemes in cytochromes *a* and *c* are derived. These vinyl side chains are reduced by the addition of reduced sulfhydryls from cysteine residues at positions 14 and 17 in cytochrome c apoprotein. Hence the heme is covalently linked to the protein as well as being coordinated through the Fe^{2+} group in the heme. The three-dimensional structure of cytochrome c is shown in Figure 6.38.

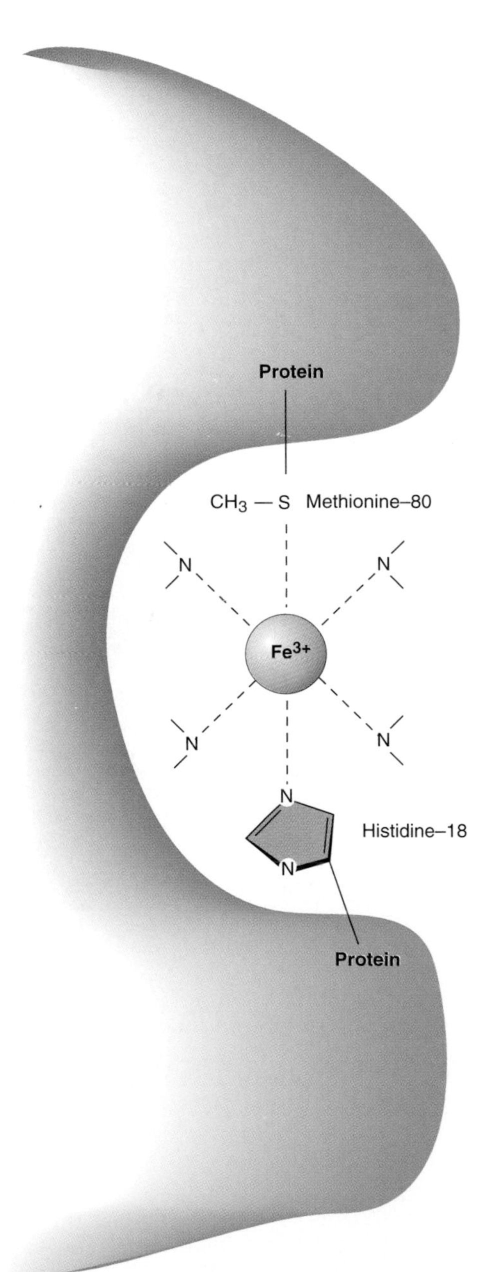

FIGURE 6.37
The six coordination positions of cytochrome *c*.

Coenzyme Q

Coenzyme Q, also called **ubiquinone,** is neither a nucleotide nor a protein but a lipophilic electron carrier. Like the nicotinamide coenzymes and to a certain extent cytochrome *c*, coenzyme Q serves as a "mobile" electron transport component that operates between the various flavin-linked dehydrogenases (e.g., NADH dehydrogenase, succinate dehydrogenase, and fatty acyl-CoA dehydrogenase) and cytochrome *b* of the electron transport chain. The quinone portion of the coenzyme Q molecule is alternately oxidized and reduced by

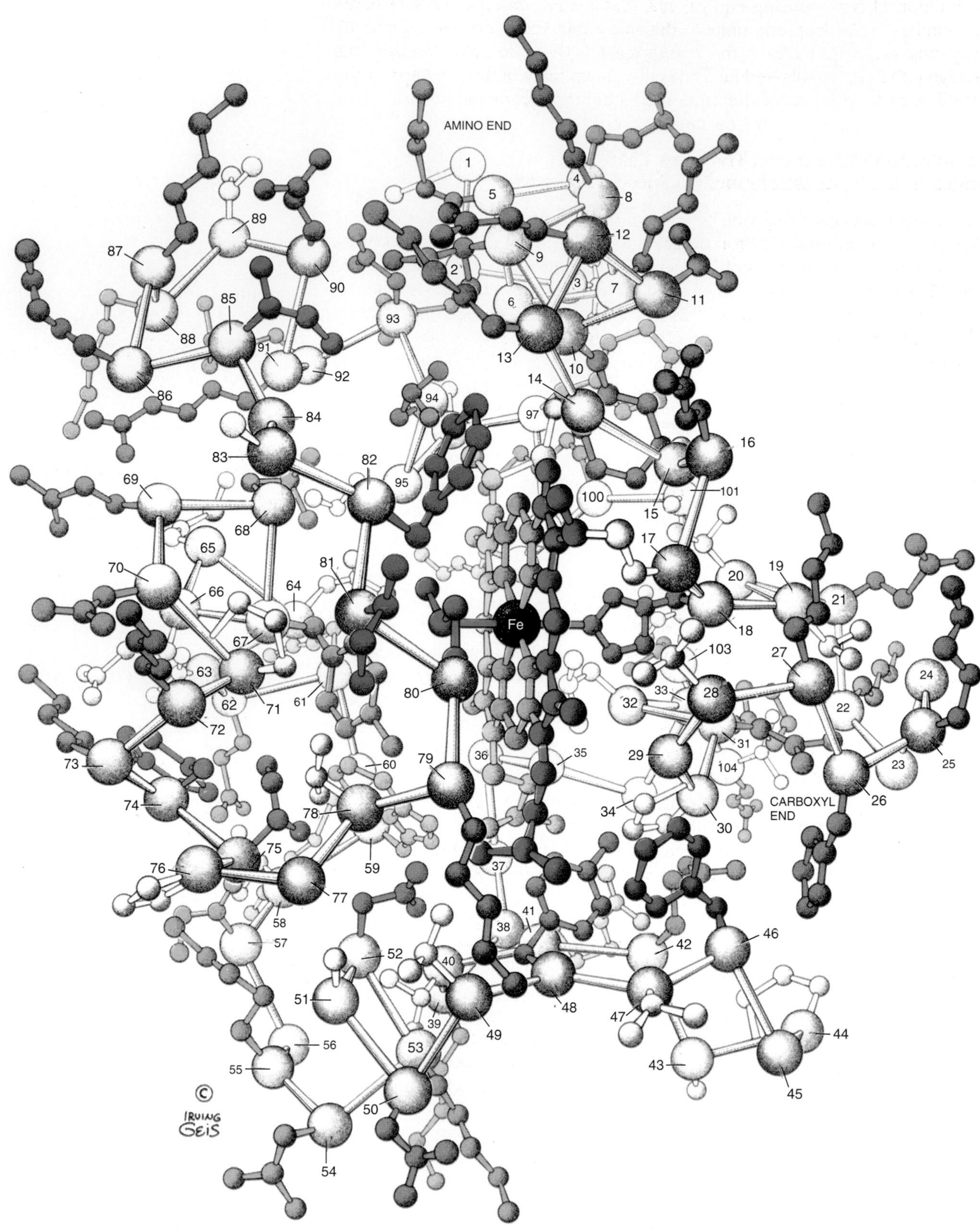

FIGURE 6.38
The three-dimensional structure of cytochrome *c*.
Copyright © 1992 Irving Geis.

the addition of two reducing equivalents, that is 2 H^+, and 2 e^- (Figure 6.39). The number (n) of isoprene units in the side chain varies between 6 and 10, depending on the source of the coenzyme Q. The side chain renders the coenzyme Q lipid soluble and facilitates the accessibility of this electron carrier to the lipophilic portions of the inner mitochondrial membrane.

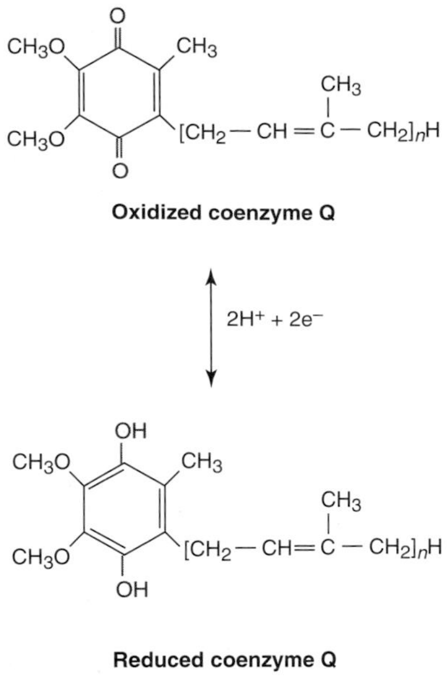

FIGURE 6.39
Oxidation–reduction of coenzyme Q.

The Mitochondrial Electron Transport Chain Is Located in the Inner Membrane in a Specific Sequence

The various electron-transferring proteins and other electron carriers that comprise the mitochondrial electron-transfer chain are arranged in a sequential pattern in the inner mitochondrial membrane. Reducing equivalents are extracted from substrates in the TCA cycle, the fatty acid β-oxidation sequence, and indirectly from glycolysis and passed sequentially through the electron transport chain to molecular oxygen. The arrangement of carriers is illustrated in Figure 6.40. Electrons or reducing equivalents are fed into the electron transport chain at the level of NADH or coenzyme Q from the primary NAD^+- and FAD-linked dehydrogenase reactions and are transported to molecular oxygen through the cytochrome chain. This electron transport system is constructed so that the reduced member of one redox couple is oxidized by the oxidized member of the next component in the system:

$$\text{NADH} + \text{H}^+ + \text{FMN} \leftrightarrow \text{FMNH}_2 + \text{NAD}^+$$

or

$$\text{Cytochrome } b\,(\text{Fe}^{2+}) + \text{cytochrome } c_1\,(\text{Fe}^{3+}) \leftrightarrow \text{cytochrome } b\,(\text{Fe}^{3+}) + \text{cytochrome } c_1\,(\text{Fe}^{2+})$$

Note that electron transfer from NADH through coenzyme Q involves 2 e^-, whereas the reactions between coenzyme Q and oxygen involving the various cytochromes are 1 e^- transfer reactions.

The components of the respiratory chain have characteristic absorption spectra that can be determined in suspensions of isolated mitochondria or submitochondrial particles using a dual-beam spectrophotometer. The different absorption bands are shown in Figure 6.41. One of the light beams of the spectrophotometer was passed through a suspension of liver mitochondria, which was maintained under fully reduced conditions (e.g., substrate plus no oxygen), and the other beam was passed through an identical suspension in the presence of oxygen. The resulting spectrum is a difference spectrum of the reduced minus the oxidized states of the mitochondrial respiratory chain.

During transfer of electrons from the NADH–NAD^+ couple ($E_0' = -0.32$) to molecular oxygen ($E_0' = +0.82$) there occurs an oxidation–reduction potential decrease of 1.14 V. This drop in potential occurs in discrete steps as reducing equivalents or electrons are passed between the different segments of the chain (Figure 6.42). There is at least a 0.3-V decrease in potential between each of the three coupling or phosphorylation sites. A potential drop of 0.3 V is more than sufficient to accommodate synthesis of a high-energy phosphate bond of ATP. For example,

$$\Delta E_0' = 0.3\text{ V}$$

$$\Delta G^\circ = -nF\Delta E_0'$$

$$\Delta G^\circ = -2 \times 23.062 \times 0.3$$

$$\Delta G^\circ = -13.8\text{ kcal mol}^{-1}$$

Various components of the electron transport chain are located asymmetrically in the mitochondrial membrane. **Cytochrome-*c* oxidase,** which catalyzes the

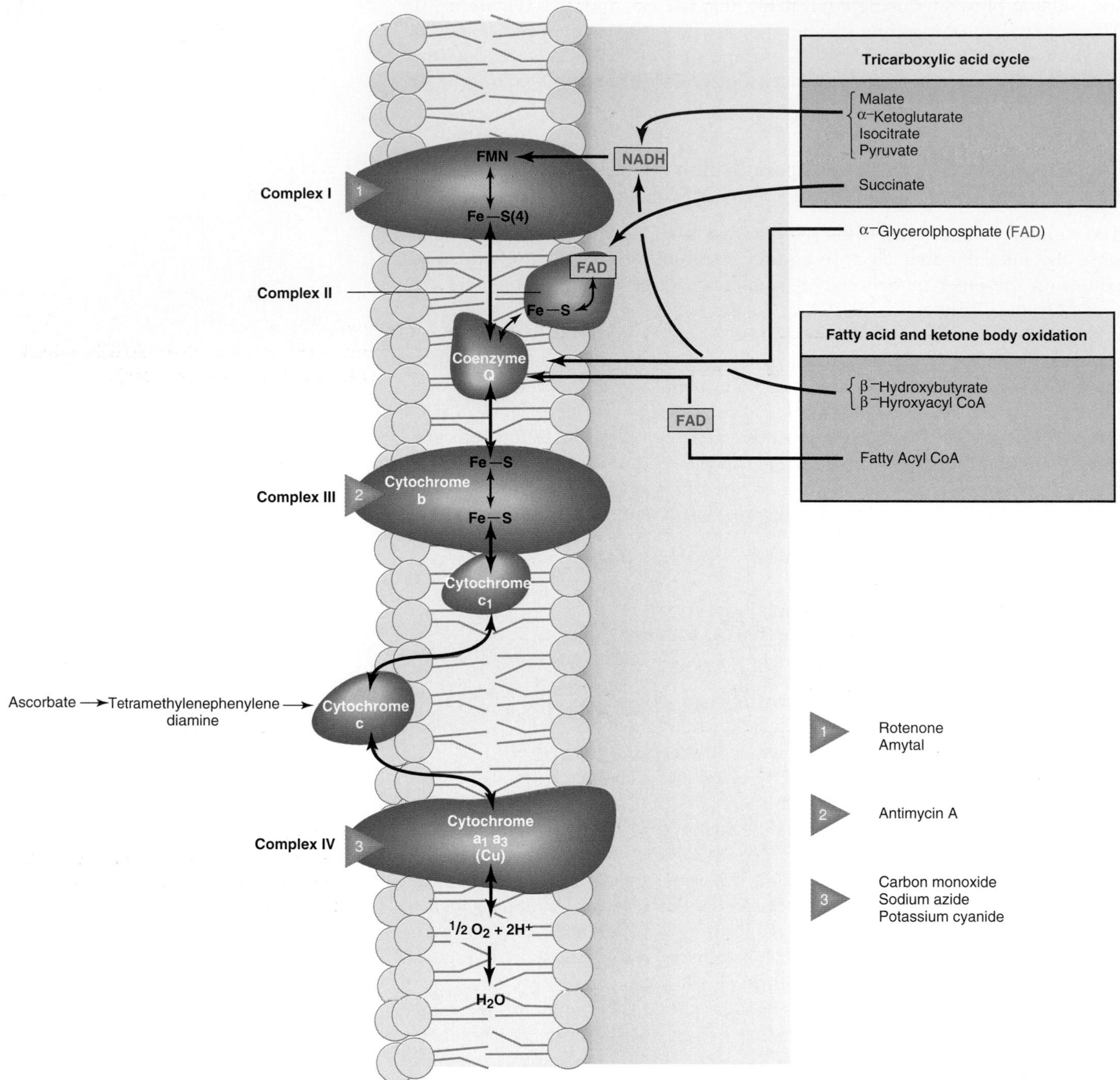

FIGURE 6.40
Mitochondrial electron transport chain.

terminal step in the electron-transfer chain, spans the membrane between the matrix and the intermembrane space (Figure 6.43). This protein is a dimeric complex of 13 polypeptides that contains heme a, heme a_3, and three copper atoms. Cytochrome *c* binds to the oxidase from the cytosolic side of the membrane, whereas oxygen binds from the matrix side of the membrane during the electron-transferring event.

Figure 6.44 depicts the organization of the entire electron transport sequence in the inner mitochondrial membrane. The initial reaction is catalyzed by the NADH dehydrogenase complex, designated **Complex I,** which accepts

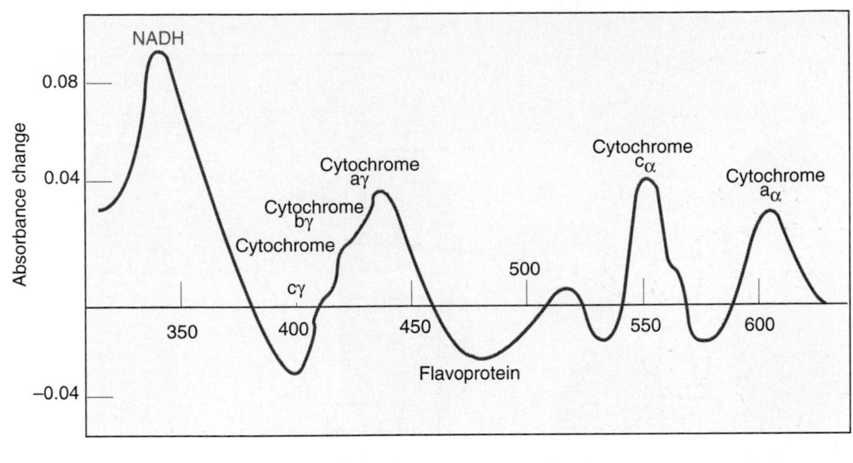

FIGURE 6.41
Difference spectrum of liver mitochondrial suspension (oxidized − reduced).

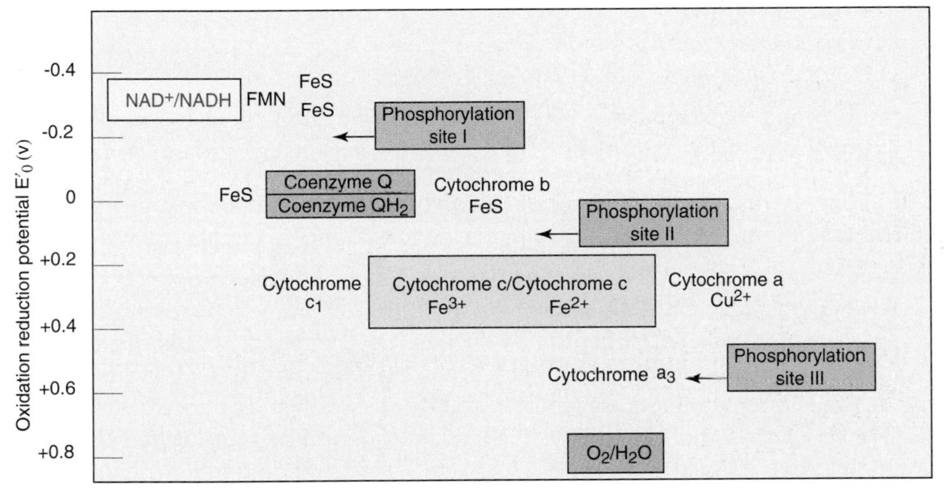

FIGURE 6.42
Oxidation–reduction potentials of the mitochondrial electron transport chain carriers.

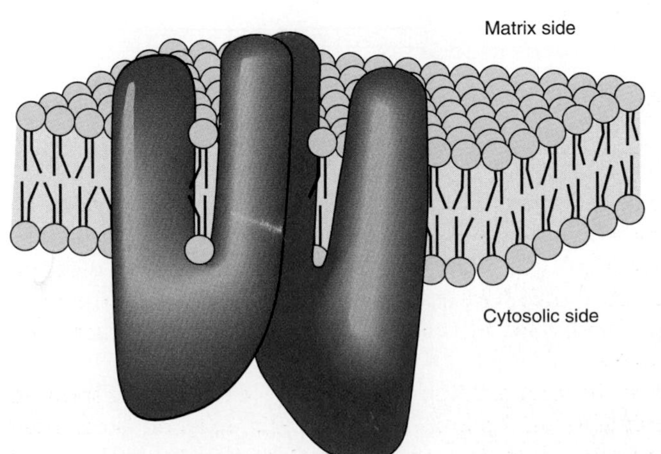

FIGURE 6.43
Model of cytochrome-*c* oxidase dimer in the mitochondrial inner membrane.
Redrawn with permission from Frey, T. G., Costello, M. J., Karlsson, B., Haselgrove, J. C., and Leigh, J. S. J. Mol. Biol. *162:113, 1982.*

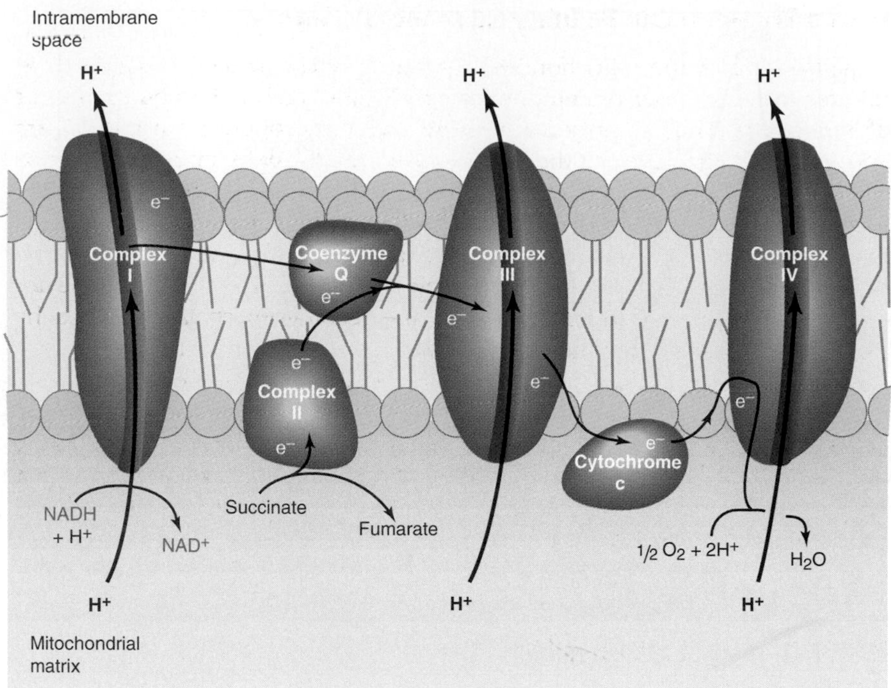

FIGURE 6.44
The four electron transport complexes of the mitochondrial electron transport sequence.

protons and electrons from NADH + H^+ and transfers them to coenzyme Q. **Complex II** consists of the succinate dehydrogenase flavoprotein component, which accepts reducing equivalents from succinate, again for passage to coenzyme Q. Being a highly lipophilic molecule, coenzyme Q is quite mobile in the mitochondrial membrane, which facilitates its ability to transfer electrons from both Complex I and Complex II to the cytochrome bc_1 complex **(Complex III).** Cytochrome *c* then accepts electrons from Complex III for transport to cytochrome oxidase **(Complex IV)** where molecular oxygen is the terminal electron acceptor. Protons (e.g., H^+) are ejected from the mitochondrial matrix into the intramembrane space at three points in this sequence of reactions (Figure 6.44). As described below, these protons will be translocated back into the matrix by the F_1F_0-ATPase present in the mitochondrial inner membrane as part of the oxidative phosphorylation phase of this energy-transducing system. Clinical Correlation 6.4 describes clinical conditions in which there are genetic dysfunctions of some of the Complexes.

CLINICAL CORRELATION 6.4

Subacute Necrotizing Encephalomyelopathy

This condition is also called Leigh disease. It manifests in infants and young children as severe lactic acidosis and neurological abnormalities. It is characterized by symmetrical lesions in basal ganglia, brain stem, and spinal cord that are detectable by computerized tomography (CT) scanning. The condition is frequently fatal. Dysfunction in oxidative phosphorylation especially in Complex IV (cytochrome-*c* oxidase) is common. Dysfunction in Complex I (NADH dehydrogenase), Complex II (succinate dehydrogenase), F_1F_0-ATPase, or pyruvate dehydrogenase complex can also produce the same clinical picture. It is clear that the condition is genetically heterogeneous and can arise from a variety of mutations either in nuclear genes that code for proteins of the mitochondrial matrix or inner membrane, or in mitochondrial genes. Leigh disease may occur without a family history of a similar disease or be transmitted as an autosomal recessive defect when the mutation is in a nuclear gene or by maternal inheritance when the mutation is in a mitochondrial gene.

Shoffner, J. M., and Wallace, D. C. In: C. R. Scriver, A. L. Beaudet, W. S. Sly, and D. Valle (Eds.), *The Metabolic and Molecular Bases of Inherited Disease,* 7th ed. New York: McGraw-Hill, 1995, p. 1535.

Electron Transport Can Be Inhibited at Specific Sites

The illustration of the mitochondrial respiratory chain shown in Figure 6.40 indicates that a number of compounds specifically inhibit electron transfer at different points. The fish poison **rotenone** and the barbiturate **amytal** (Figure 6.45) inhibit at the level of the flavoprotein, NADH dehydrogenase. Hence electrons or reducing equivalents derived from NAD^+-linked dehydrogenases are not oxidized by the respiratory chain in the presence of rotenone, whereas those derived from flavin-linked dehydrogenases are freely oxidized. The antibiotic **antimycin A** (Figure 6.45) inhibits electron transfer at the level of cytochrome *b*, whereas the terminal step in the respiratory chain catalyzed by cytochrome oxidase is inhibited by cyanide, azide, or carbon monoxide (see Clin. Corr. 6.5). Cyanide and azide combine with the oxidized heme iron (Fe^{3+}) in cytochromes *a* and a_3 and prevent the reduction of heme iron by electrons derived from reduced cytochrome *c*. Carbon monoxide binds to the reduced iron (Fe^{2+}) of cytochrome oxidase. Hence inhibition of mitochondrial electron transport results in an impairment of normal energy-generating function and death of the organism.

Electron Transport Is Reversible

The various events in the mitochondrial electron transport system and the closely coupled reactions of oxidative phosphorylation are reversible, provided an appropriate amount of energy is supplied to drive the system. In mitochondrial systems, reducing equivalents derived from succinate can be transferred to NADH with the concomitant hydrolysis of ATP (Figure 6.46). Electron transport across the other two phosphorylation sites can be reversed in a similar fashion.

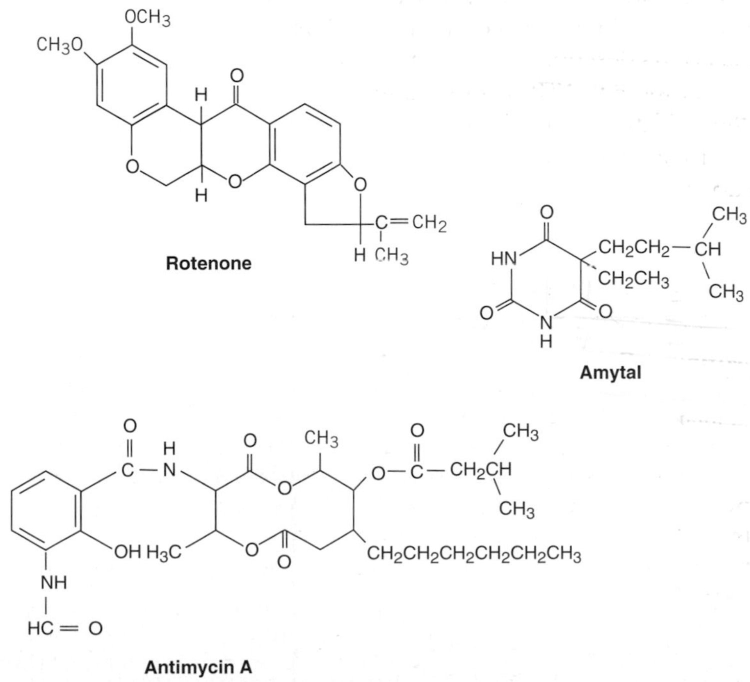

Rotenone

Amytal

Antimycin A

FIGURE 6.45
Structures of respiratory chain inhibitors.

CLINICAL CORRELATION 6.5

Cyanide Poisoning

Inhalation of hydrogen cyanide gas or ingestion of potassium cyanide causes a rapid and extensive inhibition of the mitochondrial electron transport chain at the cytochrome oxidase step. Cyanide is one of the most potent and rapidly acting poisons known. Cyanide binds to the Fe^{3+} in the heme of the cytochrome a,a_3 component of the terminal step in the electron transport chain and prevents oxygen from reacting with cytochrome a,a_3 and serving as the final electron acceptor. Mitochondrial respiration and energy production cease, and cell death occurs rapidly. Death due to cyanide poisoning occurs from tissue asphyxia, most notably of the central nervous system. If cyanide poisoning is diagnosed very rapidly, a patient who has been exposed to cyanide is given various nitrites that convert oxyhemoglobin to methemoglobin, which merely involves converting the Fe^{2+} of hemoglobin to Fe^{3+} in methemoglobin. Methemoglobin (Fe^{3+}) competes with cytochrome a,a_3 (Fe^{3+}) for cyanide, forming a methemoglobin–cyanide complex. Administration of thiosulfate causes the cyanide to react with the enzyme rhodanese, forming the nontoxic compound thiocyanate.

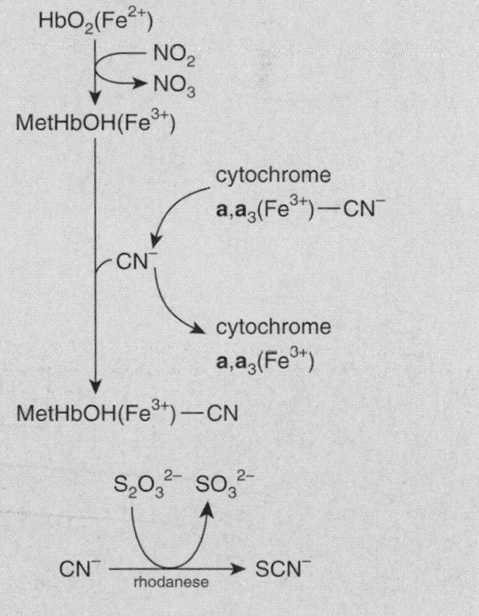

$HbO_2(Fe^{2+})$ → (NO_2^- → NO_3^-) → $MetHbOH(Fe^{3+})$ → (CN^- from cytochrome $a,a_3(Fe^{3+})$—CN^-, giving cytochrome $a,a_3(Fe^{3+})$) → $MetHbOH(Fe^{3+})$—CN

CN^- → ($S_2O_3^{2-}$ → SO_3^{2-}; rhodanese) → SCN^-

Holland, M. A., and Kozlowski, L. M. Clinical features and management of cyanide poisoning. *Clin. Pharmacol.* 5:737, 1986.

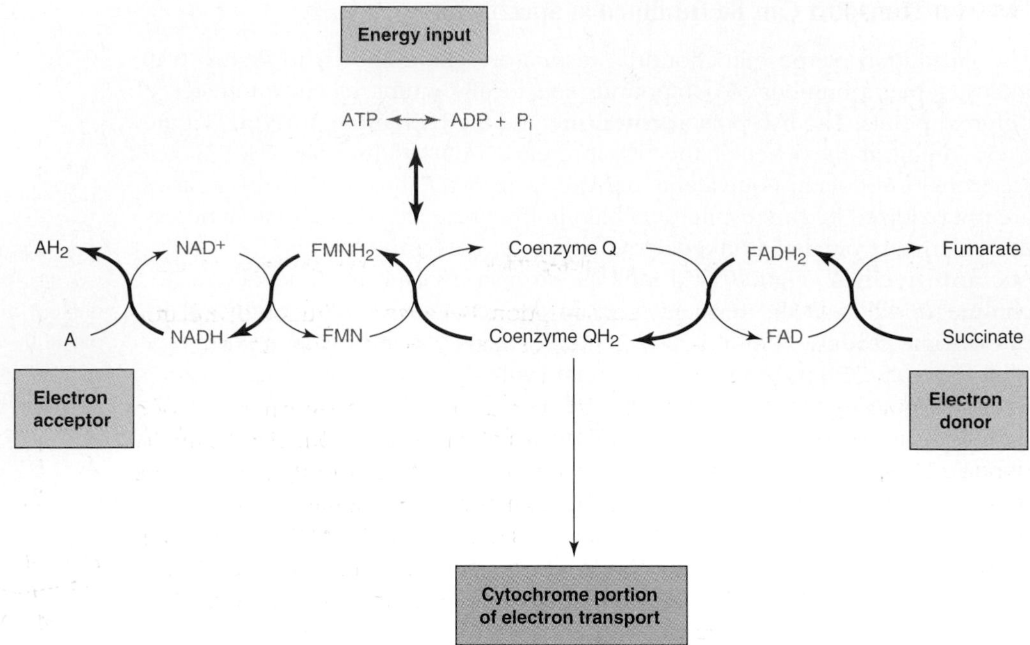

FIGURE 6.46
Reversal of mitochondrial electron transfer.

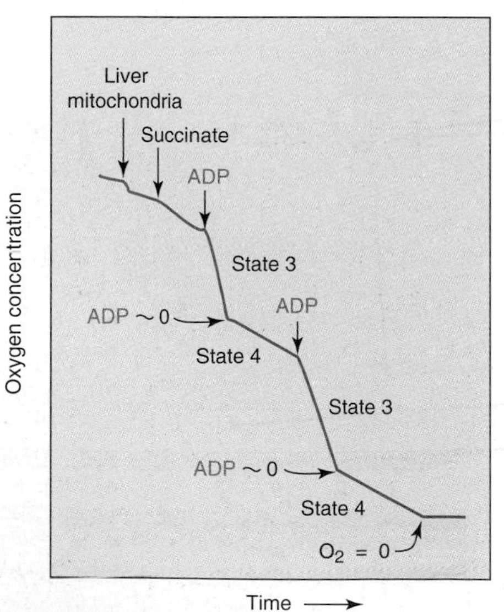

FIGURE 6.47
Demonstration of the coupling of electron transport to oxidative phosphorylation in a suspension of liver mitochondria.
State 3/state 4 = respiratory control ratio.

Oxidative Phosphorylation Is Coupled to Electron Transport

The obligatory coupling between the electron-transferring reactions and oxidative phosphorylation can best be illustrated in the experiment shown in Figure 6.47. Mitochondrial electron transport monitored by measuring the rate of oxygen consumption by a suspension of liver mitochondria can occur at a rapid rate only following the addition of an oxidizable substrate (the electron donor) and ADP (a phosphate acceptor) plus P_i. The "active" state in the presence of substrate and ADP has been designated State 3 and is a situation in which there occurs rapid electron transfer, oxygen consumption, and rapid synthesis of ATP. Following conversion of all the added ADP to ATP, the rate of electron transfer subsides back to the rate observed prior to ADP addition. Hence respiration is tightly coupled to ATP synthesis and this relationship has been termed respiratory control or phosphate acceptor control. The ratio of the active **(State 3)** rate to the resting **(State 4)** rate of respiration is referred to as the respiratory control ratio and is a measure of the "tightness" of coupling between electron transfer and oxidative phosphorylation. Damaged mitochondrial preparations and preparations to which various uncoupling compounds (see below) have been added exhibit low respiratory control ratios, indicating that the integrity of the mitochondrial membrane is required for tight coupling.

The effect of **uncouplers** and inhibitors of the electron transport–oxidative phosphorylation sequence is illustrated in Figure 6.48. Following the addition of ADP, which initiates a rapid State 3 rate of respiration, an inhibitor of the oxidative phosphorylation sequence (actually the mitochondrial F_1F_0-ATPase), **oligomycin,** is added. Oligomycin stops ATP synthesis, and because electron transport and ATP synthesis are tightly coupled, respiration or electron transport is inhibited nearly completely. Following inhibition of both oxygen consumption and ATP synthesis, addition of an uncoupler of these two processes such as **2,4-dinitrophenol** or **carbonylcyanide-*p*-trifluoromethoxy phenylhy-**

drazone (FCCP),

2,4-Dinitrophenol

Carbonylcyanide-*p*-trifluoromethoxy phenylhydrazone (FCCP)

causes a rapid initiation of oxygen consumption. Because respiration or electron transport is now uncoupled from ATP synthesis, electron transport may continue but without ATP synthesis.

Note that regulation of the respiration rate of a tissue by provision of a phosphate acceptor, ADP, is a normal physiological situation. For example, when a muscle is exercised, ATP is broken down to ADP and P_i, and creatine phosphate is converted to creatine as the high-energy phosphate bond is transferred to ATP by creatine phosphokinase (see p. 957). As ADP accumulates during the muscular activity, respiration or oxygen consumption is activated, and the energy generated in this fashion allows the ATP and creatine phosphate levels to be replenished (see Clin. Corr. 6.6).

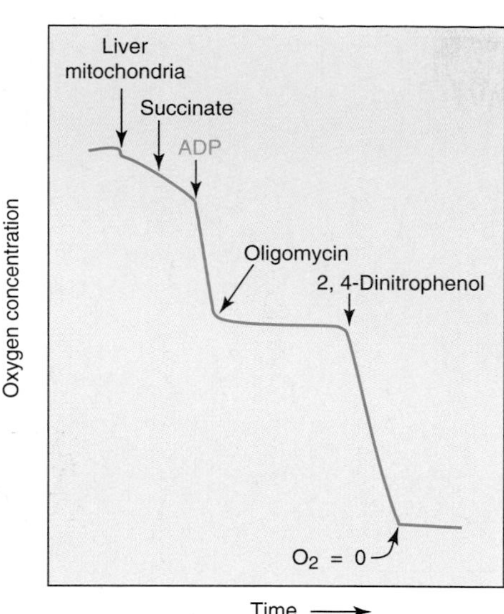

FIGURE 6.48
Inhibition and uncoupling of oxidative phosphorylation in liver mitochondria.

6.7 OXIDATIVE PHOSPHORYLATION

One of the most vexing problems that confronted biochemists during the last four decades was the delineation of the mechanism of oxidative phosphorylation. After years of experimental consideration were expended to define the mechanism of mitochondrial energy conservation, consensus was reached on many of the details of the mechanism by which energy derived from the passage of electrons sequentially along the electron transport chain is transduced into the chemical energy involved in the phosphoanhydride bonds of ATP.

Several hypotheses for the mechanism of oxidative phosphorylation were tested including the **chemical-coupling hypothesis** developed in the early

CLINICAL CORRELATION 6.6

Hypoxic Injury

Acute hypoxic tissue injury has been studied in a variety of human tissues. The occlusion of a major coronary artery during myocardial infarction produces a large array of biochemical and physiological sequelae. When a tissue is deprived of its oxygen supply, the mitochondrial electron transport–oxidative phosphorylation sequence is inhibited, resulting in the decline of cellular levels of ATP and creatine phosphate. As cellular ATP levels diminish, anaerobic glycolysis is activated in an attempt to maintain normal cellular functions. Glycogen levels are rapidly depleted and lactic acid levels in the cytosol increase, reducing the intracellular pH. Hypoxic cells in such an energy deficit begin to swell as they can no longer maintain their normal intracellular ionic environments. Mitochondria swell and begin to accumulate calcium, which may be deposited in the matrix compartment as calcium phosphate. The cell membranes of swollen cells become more permeable, leading to the leakage of various soluble enzymes, coenzymes, and other cell constituents from the cell. As the intracellular pH falls, damage occurs to lysosomal membranes, which release various hydrolytic proteases, lipases, glucosidases, and phosphatases into the cell. Such lysosomal enzymes begin an autolytic digestion of cellular components.

Cells that have been exposed to short periods of hypoxia can recover, without irreversible damage, upon reperfusion with an oxygen-containing medium. The exact point at which hypoxic cell damage becomes irreversible is not precisely known. This process is of great practical importance for transplantation of organs (heart, kidney, and liver), which always undergo a period of hypoxia between the time they are removed from the donor and implanted into the recipient.

Kehrer, J. P. Concepts related to the study of reactive oxygen and cardiac reperfusion injury. *Free Radic Res. Commun.* 5:305, 1986; and Granger, D. N. Role of xanthine oxidase and granulocytes in ischemia—reperfusion injury. *Am. J. Physiol.* 255:H1269, 1988.

1950s. This mechanism was based on an analogy with the mechanism of **substrate-level phosphorylation** in the glyceraldehyde-3-phosphate dehydrogenase reaction (see p. 276) of glycolysis. In this reaction glyceraldehyde 3-phosphate is oxidized and a high-energy phosphoric–carboxylic acid anhydride bond is generated in the product of the reaction, 1,3-bisphosphoglycerate. An enzyme-bound high-energy intermediate is generated in this reaction, which is utilized to form the intermediate high-energy compound 1,3-bisphosphoglycerate and ultimately to form ATP in the next reaction in the glycolytic pathway, that of phosphoglycerate kinase (see p. 276). Another example of a substrate-level phosphorylation reaction, which was defined in the 1960s, is the succinyl-CoA synthetase reaction of the TCA cycle. Here the high-energy character of succinyl CoA is converted to the phosphoric acid anhydride bond in GTP with the intermediate participation of a high-energy, phosphorylated histidine moiety on the enzyme. Because of these types of substrate-level phosphorylation reactions, it was proposed that the mechanism of mitochondrial energy transduction involved a series of high-energy intermediates generated in the mitochondrial membrane as a consequence of electron transport. No high-energy intermediates have ever been defined or isolated.

A second proposal for the mechanism of oxidative phosphorylation was the **conformational-coupling hypothesis.** This hypothesis has an analogy in the process of muscle contraction in which ATP hydrolysis is used to drive conformational changes in myosin head groups, which result in the disruption of cross-bridges to actin thin filaments. The conformational-coupling hypothesis proposed that as a consequence of electron transport in the inner mitochondrial membrane a conformational change in a membrane protein occurred. ATP could be synthesized by a mechanism that allowed the membrane protein in its high-energy conformation to revert to its low-energy or random state, with the resultant formation of ATP from ADP and P_i. Hence the high-energy state of the membrane protein is transduced into the bond energy of the γ-phosphate group of ATP. There are various experimental observations indicating that mitochondrial membrane proteins undergo conformational changes during the process of active electron transport. However, there is relatively little evidence demonstrating conclusively that such conformational changes are actually involved in the mechanism of ATP synthesis.

The Chemiosmotic-Coupling Mechanism Involves the Generation of a Proton Gradient and Reversal of an ATP-Dependent Proton Pump

The **chemiosmotic-coupling mechanism** proposed by Peter Mitchell is the mechanism for energy transduction in mitochondria, as well as other biological systems. Mitchell's original proposition compared the energy-generating systems in biological membranes to a common storage battery. Just as energy can be stored in batteries because of the separation of positive and negative charges in the different components of the battery, energy may be generated as a consequence of the separation of charges in complex membrane systems. In the chemiosmotic mechanism (Figure 6.49) an electrochemical gradient (protons) is established across the inner mitochondrial membrane during electron transport. This proton gradient is formed by pumping protons from the mitochondrial matrix side of the inner membrane to the cytosolic side of the membrane. Once a substantial electrochemical gradient is established, the subsequent dissipation of the gradient is coupled to the synthesis of ATP by the **mitochondrial F_1F_0-ATPase.** The electron transport carriers and the F_1F_0-ATPase are localized in such a fashion in the inner mitochondrial membrane that protons are pumped out of the matrix compartment during the electron transport phase of the process and allowed back through the membrane during the ATP synthetase aspect of the process.

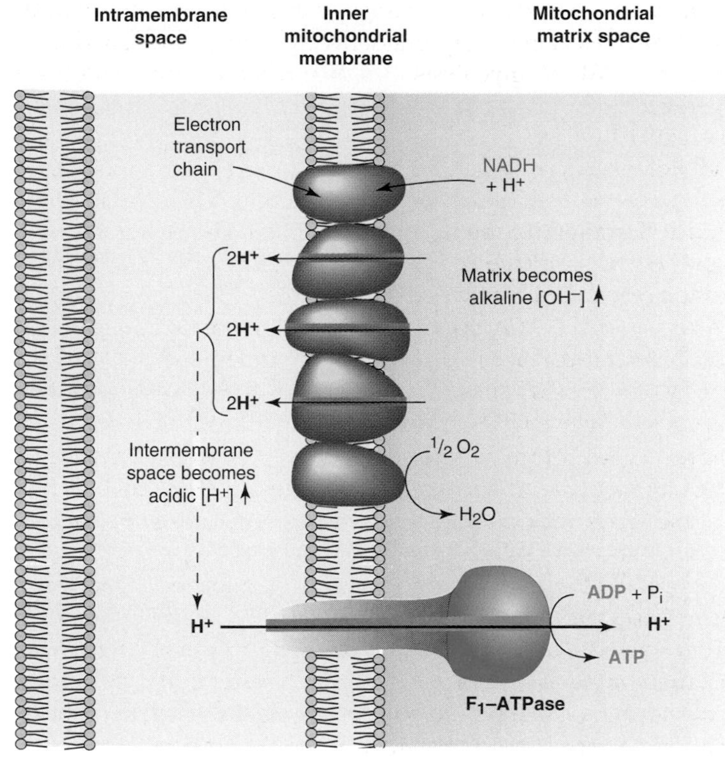

FIGURE 6.49
The mechanism of chemiosmotic coupling of electron transport and oxidative phosphorylation.

Uncouplers of the processes of respiration and phosphorylation are relatively lipophilic weak acids and act to dissipate the proton gradient by transporting protons through the membrane from the intermembrane space to the matrix. This short-circuits the normal flow of protons through the F_1F_0-ATPase. F_1F_0-ATPase can be purified and when incorporated into artificial membrane vesicles is able to synthesize ATP when an electrochemical gradient is established across the membrane. Proton-translocating ATPases are present and can be purified from a variety of mammalian tissues, bacteria, and yeast. The ATPase is a multicomponent complex with a suggested molecular weight of 480,000–500,000 (Figure 6.50). These ATPases can be incorporated into artificial membranes and can catalyze ATP synthesis. The F_1F_0-ATPase complex consists of a water-soluble portion called F_1 and a hydrophobic portion called F_0. The F_1 consists of five nonidentical subunits (α, β, γ, δ, and ε) with a subunit stoichiometry of $\alpha_3\beta_3\gamma\delta\varepsilon$ and a molecular weight of 350,000–380,000. Nucleotide-binding sites of the enzyme have been localized on the α and β subunits. The γ subunit has been proposed to function as a gate to the proton-translocating activity of the complex, while the δ subunit has been suggested to be necessary for the attachment of the F_1 portion to the membrane. The ε subunit has been proposed to regulate the F_1-ATPase. The F_0 portion consists of three or four nonidentical subunits that are an integral part of the membrane from which the ATPase is derived. When purified F_0 is incorporated into an artificial membrane, it renders the membrane permeable to protons. In addition, the F_0 contains a subunit called the oligomycin-sensitivity-conferring protein, which, as the name implies, causes the ATPase complex to be sensitive to the inhibitory action of oligomycin.

A number of questions relating to the details of the mechanism by which this important biochemical process occurs have been resolved. Such questions relate to the mechanism by which protons are pumped out of the mitochondrial matrix during electron transport, the stoichiometry of protons translocated per ATP synthesized, and the mechanism by which protons are pumped back into the matrix through the F_1F_0-ATPase.

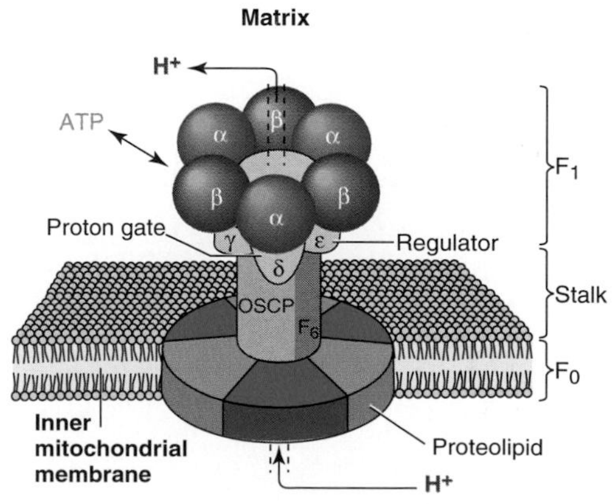

FIGURE 6.50
A model for the mitochondrial F_1F_0-ATPase.

BIBLIOGRAPHY

Energy-Producing and Energy-Utilizing Systems

Atkinson, D. E. *Cellular Energy Metabolism and Its Regulation*. New York: Academic Press, 1977.

Bock, R. M. Adenosine nucleotides and properties of pyrophosphate compounds. In: P. D. Boyer, H. Lardy, and K. Myrback (Eds.), *The enzymes*, 2nd ed., Vol. 2. New York: Academic Press, 1960, p. 3.

Hanson, R. W. The role of ATP in metabolism. *Biochem. Educ.* 17:86, 1989.

Lipmann, F. Metabolic generation and utilization of phosphate bound energy. *Adv. Enzymol.* 1:99, 1941.

Sources and Fates of Acetyl Coenzyme A

Behal, R. H., Buxton, D. B., Robertson, J. G., and Olson, M. S. Regulation of the pyruvate dehydrogenase multienzyme complex, *Annu. Rev. Nutr.* 13:497, 1993.

Denton, R. M., and Halestrap, A. Regulation of pyruvate metabolism in mammalian tissues. *Essays Biochem.* 15:37, 1979.

Patel, M. S., and Harris, R. A. Mammalian α-keto acid dehydrogenase complexes: gene regulation and genetic defects. *FASEB J.* 9:1164, 1995.

Reed, L. J., and Hackert, M. L. Structure–function relationships in dihydrolipoamide acyl transferases. *J. Biol. Chem.* 265:8971, 1990.

Roche, T. E., and Patel, M. S. α-Keto acid dehydrogenase complexes: organization, regulation and biomedical ramifications. *Ann. N. Y. Acad. Sci.* 573:1, 1989.

The Tricarboxylic Acid Cycle

Hansford, R. G. Control of mitochondrial substrate oxidation. *Curr. Top. Bioenerg.* 10:217, 1980.

Krebs, H. A. The history of the tricarboxylic acid cycle. *Perspect. Biol. Med.* 14:154, 1970.

Kornberg, H. L. Tricarboxylic acid cycles. *BioEssays* 7:236, 1987.

Lowenstein, J. M. (Ed.). *Cittric Acid Cycle: Control and Compartmentation*. New York: Marcel Dekker, 1969.

McCormack, J. G., and Denton, R. M. Ca^{2+} as a second messenger within mitochondria. *Trends Biochem. Sci.* 11:258, 1986.

Srere, P. M. The enzymology of the formation and breakdown of citrate. *Adv. Enzymol.* 43:57, 1975.

Williamson, J. R., and Copper, R. V. Regulation of the citric acid cycle in mammalian systems. *FEBS Lett.* 117 (Suppl.), K73, 1980.

Structure and Compartmentation of Mitochondrial Membranes

Ernster, L. (Ed.). *Bioenergetics*. Amsterdam: Elsevier, 1984.

Klingenberg, M. The ATP–ADP carrier in mitochondrial membranes. In: A. N. Martinosi (Ed.), *The Enzymes of Biological Membranes*. New York: Plenum Press, 1976, p. 383.

LaNoue, K. F., and Schoolwerth, A. C. Metabolite transport in mitochondria. *Annu. Rev. Biochem.* 48:871, 1979.

Tzagoloff, A. *Mitochondria*. New York: Plenum Press, 1982.

Yaffe, M., and Schatz, G. The future of mitochondrial research. *Trends Biochem. Sci.* 9:179, 1984.

Electron Transport

Babcock, G. T., and Wickstrom, M. Oxygen activation and the conservation of energy in cell respiration. *Nature* 356:301, 1992.

Brand, M. D., and Murphy, M. P. Control of electron flux through the respiratory chain in mitochondria and cells. *Biol. Rev. Camb. Philos. Soc.* 62:141, 1987.

Calhoun, M. W., Thomas, J. W., and Gennis, R. B. The cytochrome oxidase superfamily of redox-driven proton pumps. *Trends Biochem. Sci.* 19:325, 1994.

Hatefi, Y. The mitochondrial electron transport and oxidative phosphorylation system. *Annu. Rev. Biochem.* 54:1015, 1985.

Trumpower, B. L., and Gennis, R. B. Energy transduction by cytochrome complexes in mitochondrial and bacterial respiration. *Annu. Rev. Biochem.* 63:675, 1994.

Wikstrom, M., Krab, K., and Saraste, M. Proton-translocating cytochrome complexes. *Annu. Rev. Biochem.* 50:623, 1981.

Oxidative Phosphorylation

Boyer, P. D. A perspective of the binding change mechanism for ATP synthesis. *FASEB J.* 3:2164, 1989.

Boyer, P. D., Chance, B., Ernster, L., Mitchell, P., Racker, E., and Slater, E. Oxidative phosphorylation and photophosphorylation. *Annu. Rev. Biochem.* 49:955, 1977.

Chernyak, B. V., and Kozlov, I. A. Regulation of H^+-ATPases in oxidative and photophosphorylation. *Trends Biochem. Sci.* 11:32, 1986.

Mitchell, P. Vectorial chemistry and the molecular mechanism of chemiosmotic coupling: power transmission by proticity. *Biochem. Soc. Trans.* 4:398, 1976.

Mitchell, P. Keilin's respiratory chain concept and its chemiosmotic consequences. *Science* 206:1148, 1979.

Pedersen, P. L., and Carafoli, E. Ion motive ATPases. I. Ubiquity, properties and significance to cell function. *Trends Biochem. Sci.* 12:145, 1987; II Energy coupling and work output. *Trends Biochem. Sci.* 12:186, 1987.

Racker, E. From Pasteur to Mitchell: a hundred years of bioenergetics. *Fed. Proc.* 39:210, 1980.

Senior, A. E. ATP synthesis by oxidative phosphorylation. *Physiol. Rev.* 68:177, 1988.

Shoffner, J. M., and Wallace, D. C. Oxidative phosphorylation diseases and mitochondrial DNA mutations. *Annu. Rev. Nutr.* 14:535, 1994.

QUESTIONS ■ J. BAGGOTT AND C. N. ANGSTADT

1. At 37°C, $-2.303RT = -1.42$ kcal mol^{-1}. For the reaction A $\leftrightarrow$ B, if $\Delta G° = -7.1$ kcal mol^{-1}, what is the equilibrium ratio of B/A?
   A. 10,000,000/1
   B. 100,000/1
   C. 1000/1
   D. 1/1000
   E. 1/100,000

2. A bond may be "high energy" for any of the following reasons EXCEPT:
   A. products of its cleavage are more resonance stabilized than the original compound.
   B. the bond is unusually stable, requiring a large energy input to cleave it.
   C. electrostatic repulsion is relieved when the bond is cleaved.
   D. a cleavage product may be unstable, tautomerizing to a more stable form.
   E. the bond may be strained.

3. The active form of pyruvate dehydrogenase is favored by the influence of all of the following on pyruvate dehydrogenase kinase EXCEPT:
   A. low $[Ca^{2+}]$.
   B. low acetyl CoA/CoASH.
   C. high [pyruvate].
   D. low $NADH/NAD^+$.

4. At which of the following enzyme-catalyzed steps of the tricarboxylic acid cycle does net incorporation of the elements of water into an intermediate of the cycle occur?
   A. aconitase
   B. citrate synthase
   C. malate dehydrogenase
   D. succinate dehydrogenase
   E. succinyl-CoA synthase

5. A freely reversible reaction of the tricarboxylic acid cycle is catalyzed by:
   A. citrate synthase.
   B. isocitrate dehydrogenase.
   C. α-ketoglutarate dehydrogenase.
   D. pyruvate dehydrogenase.
   E. succinyl-CoA synthetase.

6. All of the following tricarboxylic acid cycle intermediates may be added or removed by other metabolic pathways EXCEPT:
   A. citrate.
   B. fumarate.
   C. isocitrate.
   D. α-ketoglutarate.
   E. oxaloacetate.

7. Regulation of tricarboxylic acid cycle activity *in vivo* may involve the concentration of all of the following EXCEPT:
   A. acetyl CoA.
   B. ADP.
   C. ATP.
   D. CoA.
   E. oxygen.

8. The mitochondrial membrane contains a transporter for:
   A. NADH.
   B. acetyl CoA.
   C. GTP.
   D. ATP.
   E. NADPH.

9. Which line of the accompanying table correctly describes the indicated properties of BOTH the malate shuttle and the α-glycerophosphate shuttle?

Table for Question 9

Property	*Malate Shuttle*	*α-Glycerophosphate Shuttle*
A. Location	Inner mitochondrial membrane	Outer mitochondrial membrane
B. ATP generated per cytoplasmic NADH	3	2
C. Transporter	Malate dehydrogenase	α-Glycerophosphate dehydrogenase
D. Species transported	Malate	α-Glycerophosphate
E. Matrix electron acceptor	Oxaloacetate	Cytochrome *b*

Refer to the following for Questions 10–12.
   A. FAD
   B. FMN
   C. NAD^+
   D. NADPH
   E. none of the above

10. Prosthetic group of NADH dehydrogenase.

11. The usual source of reducing equivalents for anabolic processes.

12. Irradiation with light of 340-nm wavelength causes fluorescence emission at 465 nm.

13. If rotenone is added to the mitochondrial electron transport chain:
   A. the P/O ratio of NADH is reduced from 3 : 1 to 2 : 1.
   B. the rate of NADH oxidation is diminished to two-thirds of its initial value.
   C. succinate oxidation remains normal.
   D. oxidative phosphorylation is uncoupled at site I.
   E. electron flow is inhibited at site II.

14. If cyanide is added to tightly coupled mitochondria that are actively oxidizing succinate:
   A. subsequent addition of 2,4-dinitrophenol will cause ATP hydrolysis.
   B. subsequent addition of 2,4-dinitrophenol will restore succinate oxidation.
   C. electron flow will cease, but ATP synthesis will continue.
   D. electron flow will cease, but ATP synthesis can be restored by subsequent addition of 2,4-dinitrophenol.
   E. subsequent addition of 2,4-dinitrophenol and the phosphorylation inhibitor oligomycin will cause ATP hydrolysis.

15. The heme iron of which of the following is bound to the protein by only one coordination linkage?
   A. cytochrome *a*
   B. cytochrome a_3
   C. cytochrome *b*
   D. cytochrome *c*
   E. none of the above

16. In substrate level phosphorylation:
   A. the substrate reacts to form a product containing a high-energy bond.
   B. ATP synthesis is linked to dissipation of a proton gradient.
   C. high-energy intermediate compounds cannot be isolated.
   D. oxidation of one molecule of substrate is linked to synthesis of more than one ATP molecule.
   E. mitochondria participate, but not cytoplasm.

17. The chemiosmotic hypothesis involves all of the following EXCEPT:
   A. a membrane impermeable to protons.
   B. electron transport by the respiratory chain pumps protons out of the mitochondrion.
   C. proton flow into the mitochondria depends on the presence of ADP and P_i.
   D. ATPase activity is reversible.
   E. only proton transport is strictly regulated; other positively charged ions can diffuse freely across the mitochondrial membrane.

ANSWERS

1. B $\Delta G° = -2.3RT \log K$. log 100,000 = 5. Substitution gives $\Delta G° = -7.1$ (p. 221).
2. B A "high-energy" bond is so designated because it has a high free energy of hydrolysis. This could arise for reasons A, C, D, or E. High-energy does not refer to a high energy of formation (bond stability) (p. 222).
3. A High [Ca^{2+}] favors the active dehydrogenase but by activating the phosphatase. NADH and acetyl CoA activate pyruvate dehydrogenase kinase, thus inactivating pyruvate dehydrogenase. Pyruvate inhibits the kinase, favoring the active dehydrogenase (p. 230, Figure 6.16).
4. B Water is required to hydrolyze the thioester bond of acetyl CoA. A: Aconitase removes water, then adds it back. C and D: The dehydrogenases remove two protons and two electrons. E. Here the thioester undergoes phosphorolysis, not hydrolysis; the phosphate is subsequently transferred from the intermediate succinyl phosphate to GDP. (See p. 232, Figure 6.19).
5. E There are high-energy compounds on both sides of the reaction, namely, GTP and succinyl CoA (p. 235). A is irreversible due to cleavage of the thioester link, a high-energy bond. In B and C, CO_2 is released. D: Pyruvate dehydrogenase is not a part of the tricarboxylic acid cycle; it is, however, irreversible.
6. C A: Citrate is transported out of the mitochondria to be used as a source of cytoplasmic acetyl CoA. B: Fumarate is produced during phenylalanine and tyrosine degradation. D can be formed from glutamate. E: Oxaloacetate is produced by pyruvate carboxylase and is used in gluconeogenesis. Clearly, most of the tricarboxylic acid cycle intermediates play multiple roles in the body.
7. D CoA is not a regulator, though admittedly there is a reciprocal relationship between CoA and acetyl CoA concentrations in the short term. A is the substrate (p. 232). B activates isocitrate dehydrogenase, and C inhibits it (p. 239, Figure 6.23). E: The cycle requires oxygen to oxidize NADH and ADP to be converted to ATP (respiratory control) (p. 231).
8. D A and B: Reducing equivalents from NADH are shuttled across the membrane, as is the acetyl group of acetyl CoA, but NADH and acetyl CoA themselves cannot cross (p. 243, Figures 6.28 and 6.29). C and D: Of the nucleotides, only ATP and ADP are transported. The translocator is inhibited by atractyloside (p. 245). E: Like NADH, NADPH does not cross the membrane.
9. B A: Both shuttles operate across the inner membrane. C: Two transporters are used by the malate shuttle, the malate α-ketoglutarate antiporter and the aspartate–glutamate antiporter. D: α-Glycerophosphate is not translocated; only reducing equivalents are. E: Oxaloacetate is a reaction product. NAD^+ is the electron acceptor (p. 244, Figure 6.28).
10. B See Figure 6.40, p. 256.
11. D NADPH is not a substrate for mitochondrial electron transport (p. 250).
12. D Fluorescence excitation of the reduced pyridine ring occurs in a wavelength range where it absorbs light, about 340 nm. Absorbance is a minimum at 300 nm (p. 250, Figure 6.33).
13. C Rotenone inhibits at the level of NADH dehydrogenase (site I), preventing all electron flow and all ATP synthesis from NADH. Flavin-linked dehydrogenases feed in electrons below site I and are unaffected by site I inhibitors (pp. 259, 256, Figure 6.40).
14. A Cyanide inhibits electron transport at site III, blocking electron flow throughout the system. In coupled mitochondria, ATP synthesis ceases too. Addition of an uncoupler permits the mitochondrial ATPase (which is normally driven in the synthetic direction) to operate, and it catalyzes the favorable ATP hydrolysis reaction unless it is inhibited by a phosphorylation inhibitor such as oligomycin (p. 260).
15. B Fe^{2+} has six coordination positions. In heme, four are filled by the porphyrin ring. In cytochromes *a*, *b*, and *c* the other two are filled by the protein. But in cytochrome a_3, one position must be left vacant to provide an oxygen-binding site (p. 252).
16. A A good example of substrate-level phosphorylation is seen in the glyceraldehyde-3-phosphate dehydrogenase reaction, where a phosphoric–carboxylic acid anhydride intermediate forms (p. 262). This is a cytoplasmic process, part of glycolysis. The intermediate can be isolated.
17. E If the charge separation could be dissipated by free diffusion of other ions, the energy would be lost, and no ATP could be synthesized.

CHAPTER

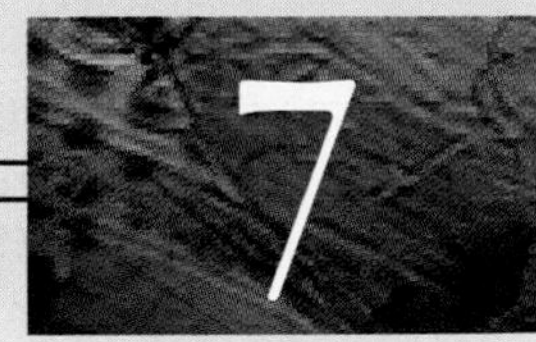

CARBOHYDRATE METABOLISM I: MAJOR METABOLIC PATHWAYS AND THEIR CONTROL

Robert A. Harris

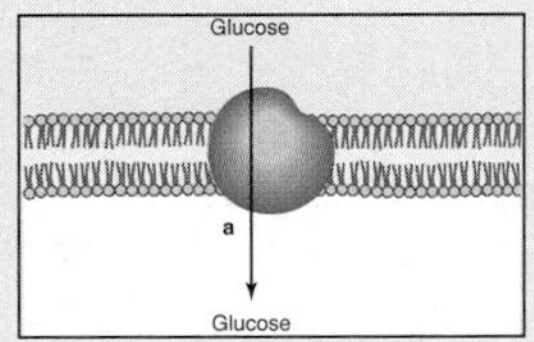

7.1 OVERVIEW

The major pathways of carbohydrate metabolism either begin or end with glucose (Figure 7.1). This chapter describes the utilization of glucose as a source of energy, formation of glucose from noncarbohydrate precursors, storage of glucose in the form of glycogen for later use, and release of glucose from glycogen for use by cells. An understanding of the pathways and their regulation is necessary because of the important role played by glucose in the body. Glucose is the major form in which carbohydrate absorbed from the intestinal tract is presented to cells of the body. Glucose is the only fuel used to any significant extent by a few specialized cells and the major fuel used by the brain. Indeed, glucose is so important to these specialized cells and the brain that several of the major tissues of the body work together to ensure a continuous supply of this essential substrate. Glucose metabolism is defective in two very common metabolic diseases, obesity and diabetes, which contribute in development of a number of major medical problems, including atherosclerosis, hypertension, small vessel disease, kidney disease, and blindness.

The discussion begins with **glycolysis,** a pathway used by all cells of the body to extract part of the chemical energy inherent in the glucose molecule. This pathway also converts glucose to pyruvate and sets the stage for complete oxidation of glucose to CO_2 and H_2O. The *de novo* synthesis of glucose, that is, gluconeogenesis, is a function of the liver and kidneys and can conveniently be discussed following glycolysis because it makes use of some of the same enzymes used in the glycolytic pathway, although the reactions catalyzed are in the opposite direction. In contrast to glycolysis, which produces ATP, gluconeogenesis requires ATP and is therefore an energy-requiring process. The consequence is that only some of the enzyme-catalyzed steps can be common to both the glycolytic and gluconeogenic pathways. Indeed, additional enzymes including some in mitochondria become involved to make the overall process of gluconeogenesis exergonic. Regulation of the rate-limiting and key enzyme-catalyzed steps will be stressed throughout the chapter. This will be particularly

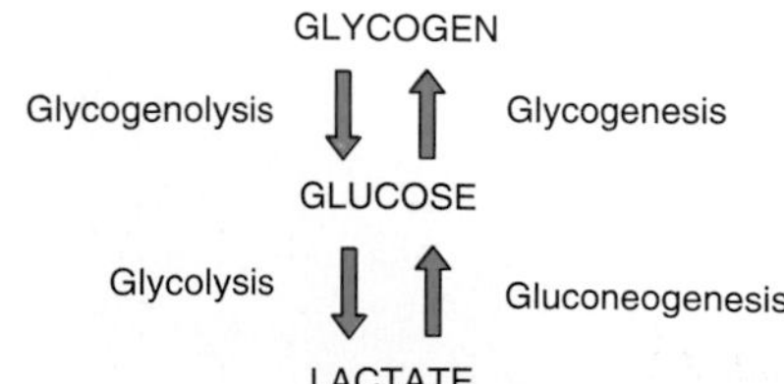

FIGURE 7.1
Relationship of glucose to the major pathways of carbohydrate metabolism.

true for glycogen synthesis **(glycogenesis)** and degradation **(glycogenolysis).** Many cells store glycogen for the purpose of having glucose available for later use. The liver is less selfish, storing glycogen not for its own use, but for maintenance of blood glucose levels that ensure that other tissues, especially the brain, have an adequate supply of this important substrate. Regulation of the synthesis and degradation of glycogen is a model for our understanding of how hormones work and how other metabolic pathways may be regulated. This subject contributes to our understanding of the diabetic condition, starvation, and how tissues of the body respond to stress, severe trauma, and injury. The Appendix presents the nomenclature and chemistry of the carbohydrates.

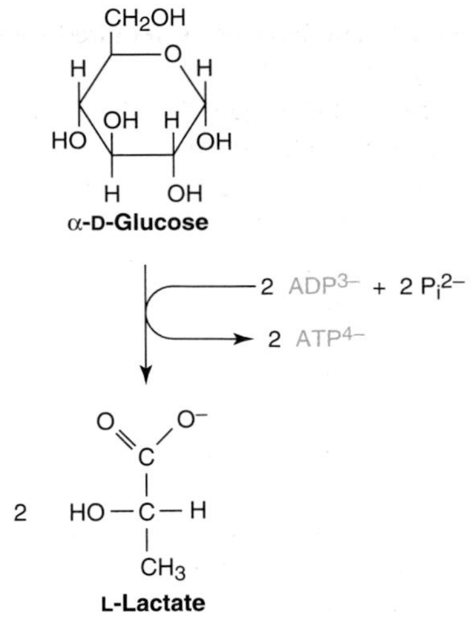

7.2 GLYCOLYSIS

Glycolysis Occurs in All Human Cells

The Embden–Meyerhof or glycolytic pathway represents an ancient process, possessed by all cells of the human body, in which anaerobic degradation of glucose to lactate occurs. This is one example of anaerobic **fermentation,** a term used to refer to pathways by which organisms extract chemical energy from high-energy fuels in the absence of molecular oxygen. For many tissues glycolysis is an emergency energy-yielding pathway, capable of yielding 2 mol of ATP from 1 mol of glucose in the absence of molecular oxygen (Figure 7.2). Thus when the oxygen supply to a tissue is shut off, ATP levels can still be maintained by glycolysis for at least a short period of time. Many examples could be given, but the capacity to use glycolysis as a source of energy is particularly important to the human being at birth. With the exception of the brain, circulation of blood decreases to most parts of the body of the neonate during delivery. The brain is not normally deprived of oxygen during delivery, but other tissues must depend on glycolysis for their supply of ATP until circulation returns to normal and oxygen becomes available again. This conserves oxygen for use by the **brain,** illustrating one of many mechanisms that have evolved to assure survival of brain tissue in times of stress. Glycolysis sets the stage for aerobic oxidation of carbohydrate. Oxygen is not necessary for glycolysis, and the presence of oxygen can indirectly suppress glycolysis, a phenomenon called the **Pasteur effect** that is considered later. Nevertheless, glycolysis can and does occur in cells with an abundant supply of molecular oxygen. Provided cells also contain mitochondria, the end product of glycolysis in the presence of oxygen is pyruvate rather than lactate. Pyruvate can then be completely oxidized to CO_2 and H_2O by enzymes housed within the mitochondria. The overall process of glycolysis plus the subsequent mitochondrial oxidation of pyruvate to CO_2 and H_2O has the following equation:

$$\text{D-Glucose} + 6\,O_2 + 38\,ADP^{3-} + 38P_i^{2-} + 38\,H^+ \rightarrow 6\,CO_2 + 6\,H_2O + 38\,ATP^{4-}$$
$$(C_6H_{12}O_6)$$

Much more ATP is produced in complete oxidation of glucose to CO_2 and H_2O than in the conversion of glucose to lactate. This has important consequences, which are considered in detail later. For glucose to be completely oxidized to CO_2 and H_2O, it must first be converted to pyruvate by glycolysis (Figure 7.3). The importance of glycolysis as a preparatory pathway is best exemplified by

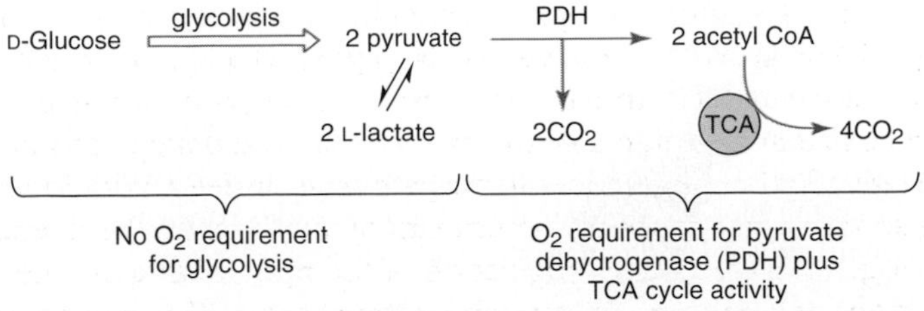

FIGURE 7.2
Overall balanced equation for the sum of the reactions of the glycolytic pathway.

FIGURE 7.3
Glycolysis is a preparatory pathway for aerobic metabolism of glucose.
TCA refers to the tricarboxylic acid cycle.

the brain. This tissue has an absolute need for glucose and processes most of it via glycolysis. Pyruvate produced is then oxidized to CO_2 and H_2O in mitochondria. An adult human **brain** uses approximately 120 g of glucose each day in order to meet its need for ATP. In contrast, glycolysis with lactate as the end product is the major mechanism of ATP production in a number of other tissues. **Red blood cells** lack mitochondria and therefore are unable to convert pyruvate to CO_2 and H_2O. The **cornea, lens,** and regions of the **retina** have a limited blood supply and also lack mitochondria (because mitochondria would absorb and scatter light) and depend on glycolysis as the major mechanism for ATP production. **Kidney medulla, testis, leukocytes,** and white **muscle fibers** are almost totally dependent on glycolysis as a source of ATP, because these tissues have relatively few mitochondria. Tissues dependent primarily on glycolysis for ATP production consume about 40 g of glucose per day in a normal adult.

Major dietary sources of glucose are indicated in Chapter 26. **Starch** is the storage form of glucose in plants and contains α-1,4-glycosidic linkages along with α-1,6-glycosidic branches. **Glycogen** is the storage form of glucose in animal tissues and contains the same type of glycosidic linkages and branches. Exogenous glycogen refers to that which we eat and digest; endogenous glycogen is that synthesized or stored in our tissues. Exogenous starch or glycogen is hydrolyzed in the intestinal tract with the production of glucose, whereas stored glycogen endogenous to our tissues is converted to glucose or glucose 6-phosphate by enzymes present within the cells. Disaccharides that serve as important sources of glucose in our diet include milk sugar (lactose) and grocery store sugar (sucrose). Hydrolysis of these sugars by enzymes of the brush border of the intestinal tract is discussed on page 1075. Glucose can be used as a source of energy for cells of the intestinal tract. However, these cells do not depend on glucose to any great extent; most of their energy requirement is met by glutamine catabolism (see p. 450). Most of the glucose passes through the cells of the intestinal tract into the portal blood, then the general circulation, to be used by other tissues. Liver is the first major tissue to have an opportunity to remove glucose from the portal blood. When blood glucose is high, the liver removes glucose for the glucose-consuming processes of glycogenesis and glycolysis. When blood glucose is low, the liver supplies the blood with glucose by the glucose-producing processes of glycogenolysis and gluconeogenesis. The liver is also the first organ exposed to the blood flowing from the pancreas and therefore is exposed to the highest concentrations of the hormones released from this endocrine tissue—**glucagon** and **insulin.** These important hormonal regulators of blood glucose levels have effects on enzyme-catalyzed steps in the liver.

Glucose Is Metabolized Differently in Various Cells

After penetrating the plasma membrane by mediated transport on the **glucose transport protein GLUT-1,** glucose is metabolized mainly by glycolysis in red blood cells (Figure 7.4*a*). Since red blood cells lack mitochondria, the end

FIGURE 7.4
Overviews of the major ways in which glucose is metabolized within cells of selected tissues of the body.
(*a*) Glucose transport into the cell by a glucose transport protein (GLUT); (*b*) glucose phosphorylation by hexokinase; (*c*) the pentose phosphate pathway; (*d*) glycolysis; (*e*) lactic acid transport out of the cell; (*f*) pyruvate decarboxylation by pyruvate dehydrogenase; (*g*) TCA cycle; (*h*) glycogenesis; (*i*) glycogenolysis; (*j*) lipogenesis; (*k*) gluconeogenesis; (*l*) hydrolysis of glucose 6-phosphate and release of glucose from the cell into the blood; (*m*) formation of glucuronides (drug and bilirubin detoxification by conjugation) by the glucuronic acid pathway.

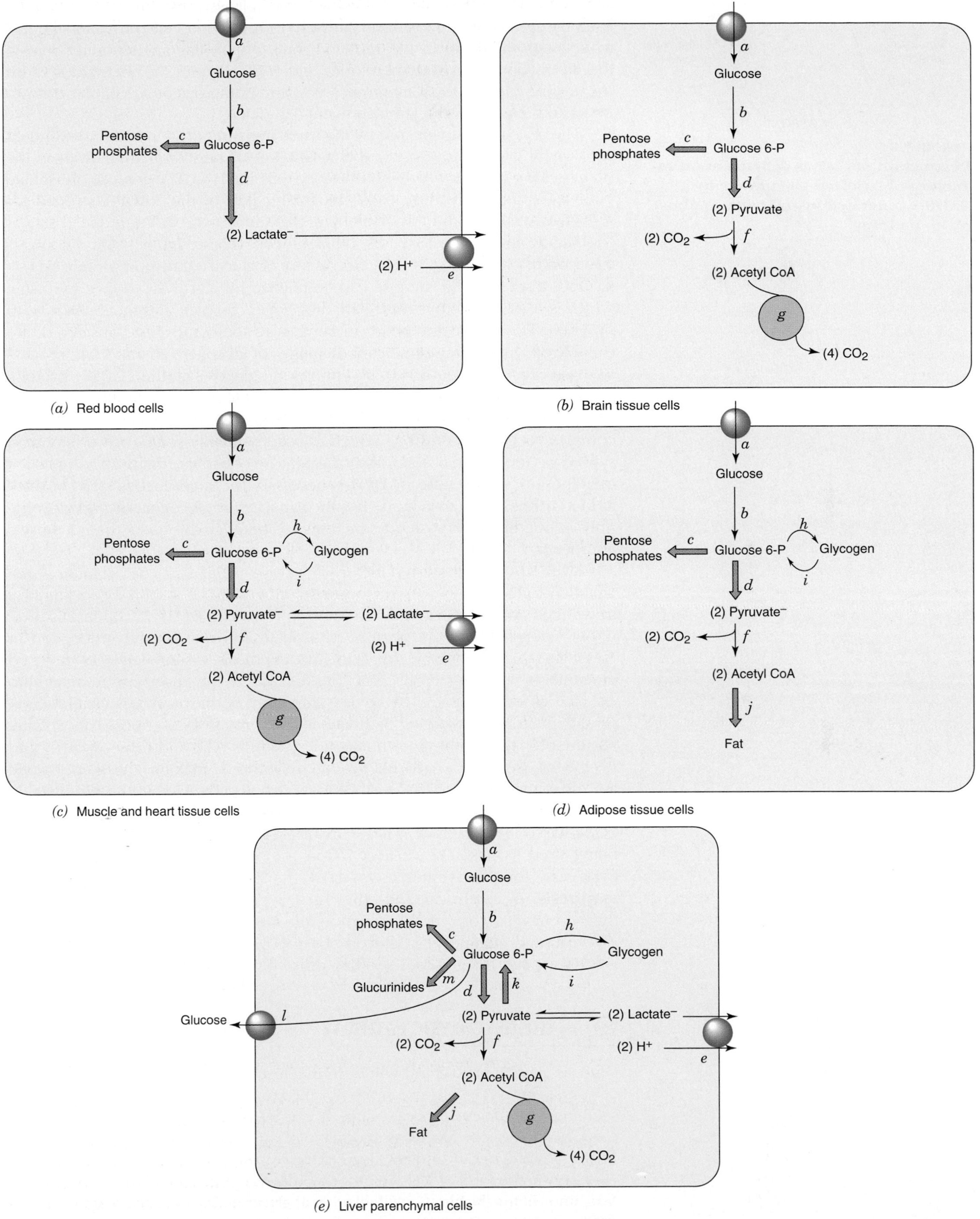

a
Glucose
b
Pentose phosphates
c
Glucose 6-P
d
(2) Lactate⁻
(2) H⁺
e
(a) Red blood cells
a
Glucose
b
Pentose phosphates
c
Glucose 6-P
d
(2) Pyruvate
(2) CO_2
f
(2) Acetyl CoA
g
(4) CO_2
(b) Brain tissue cells
a
Glucose
b
h
Pentose phosphates
c
Glucose 6-P
Glycogen
i
d
(2) Pyruvate⁻
(2) Lactate⁻
(2) CO_2
f
(2) H⁺
e
(2) Acetyl CoA
g
(4) CO_2
(c) Muscle and heart tissue cells
a
Glucose
b
h
Pentose phosphates
c
Glucose 6-P
Glycogen
i
d
(2) Pyruvate⁻
(2) CO_2
f
(2) Acetyl CoA
j
Fat
(d) Adipose tissue cells
a
Glucose
Pentose phosphates
b
h
c
Glucose 6-P
Glycogen
i
Glucurinides
m
d
k
Glucose
l
(2) Pyruvate
(2) Lactate⁻
(2) CO_2
f
(2) H⁺
e
(2) Acetyl CoA
j
Fat
g
(4) CO_2
(e) Liver parenchymal cells

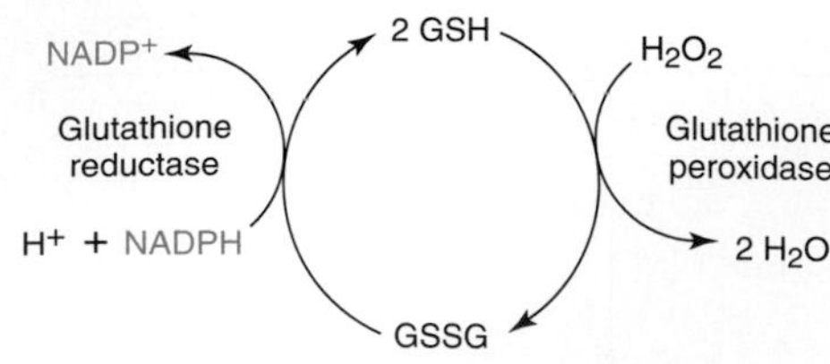

FIGURE 7.5
Destruction of H_2O_2 is dependent on reduction of oxidized glutathione by NADPH generated by the pentose phosphate pathway.

product of glycolysis is lactic acid, which is released into the blood. Glucose used by the pentose phosphate pathway in red blood cells provides NADPH to keep **glutathione** in the reduced state, which has an important role in the destruction of organic peroxides and H_2O_2 (Figure 7.5). Peroxides cause irreversible damage to membranes, DNA, and numerous other cellular components and must be removed to prevent cell death.

The brain takes up glucose by mediated transport in an insulin-independent manner by glucose transport protein **GLUT-3** (Figure 7.4*b*). Glycolysis in the brain yields pyruvate, which is oxidized to CO_2 and H_2O. The pentose phosphate pathway is active in these cells, generating part of the NADPH needed for reductive synthesis and the maintenance of glutathione in the reduced state.

Muscle and heart cells readily utilize glucose (Figure 7.4*c*). Insulin stimulates transport of glucose into these cells by way of glucose transport protein **GLUT-4.** Once in these cells, glucose can be utilized by glycolysis to give pyruvate, which is used by the pyruvate dehydrogenase complex and the TCA cycle to provide ATP. Muscle and heart, in contrast to the tissues just considered, are capable of synthesizing significant quantities of glycogen, an important process in these cells. Adipose tissue also transports glucose by the GLUT-4 protein, again in an insulin-dependent mechanism (Figure 7.4*d*). Pyruvate, as in other cells, is generated by glycolysis and is oxidized by the pyruvate dehydrogenase complex to give acetyl CoA, which is used primarily for *de novo* fatty acid synthesis. Generation of NADPH by the pentose phosphate pathway is important in adipose tissue because NADPH is necessary for the reductive steps of **fatty acid synthesis.** Adipose tissue has the capacity for glycogenesis and glycogenolysis, but these processes are much more limited in this tissue than in muscle and heart.

Liver has the greatest number of ways to utilize glucose (Figure 7.4*e*). Uptake of glucose by the liver occurs independent of insulin by means of a low-affinity, high-capacity glucose transport protein, **GLUT-2.** Glucose is used rather extensively by the pentose phosphate pathway for the production of NADPH, which is needed for reductive synthesis, maintenance of reduced glutathione, and numerous reactions catalyzed by endoplasmic reticulum enzyme systems. A quantitatively less important but nevertheless vital function of the pentose phosphate pathway is the provision of ribose phosphate, required for the synthesis of nucleotides such as ATP and those in DNA and RNA. Glucose is also used for glycogen synthesis, making glycogen storage an important feature of the liver. Glucose can also be used in the **glucuronic acid pathway,** which is important in **drug** and **bilirubin detoxification** (see Chapter 23). The liver is also capable of glycolysis, the pyruvate produced being used as a source of acetyl CoA for complete oxidation by the TCA cycle and for the synthesis of fat by the process of *de novo* **fatty acid synthesis.** In contrast to the other tissues, the liver is unique in that it has the capacity to convert three-carbon precursors, such as lactate, pyruvate, glycerol, and alanine, into glucose by the process of **gluconeogenesis,** to meet the need for glucose of other cells.

7.3 THE GLYCOLYTIC PATHWAY

Glucose is combustible and will burn in a test tube to yield heat and light but, of course, no ATP. Cells use some 30 steps to take glucose to CO_2 and H_2O, a seemingly inefficient process, since it can be done in a single step in a test tube. However, side reactions and some of the actual steps used by the cell to "burn" glucose to CO_2 and H_2O lead to the conservation of a significant amount of energy in the form of ATP. In other words, ATP is produced by the controlled "burning" of glucose in the cell, glycolysis representing only the first few steps, shown in Figure 7.6, in the overall process.

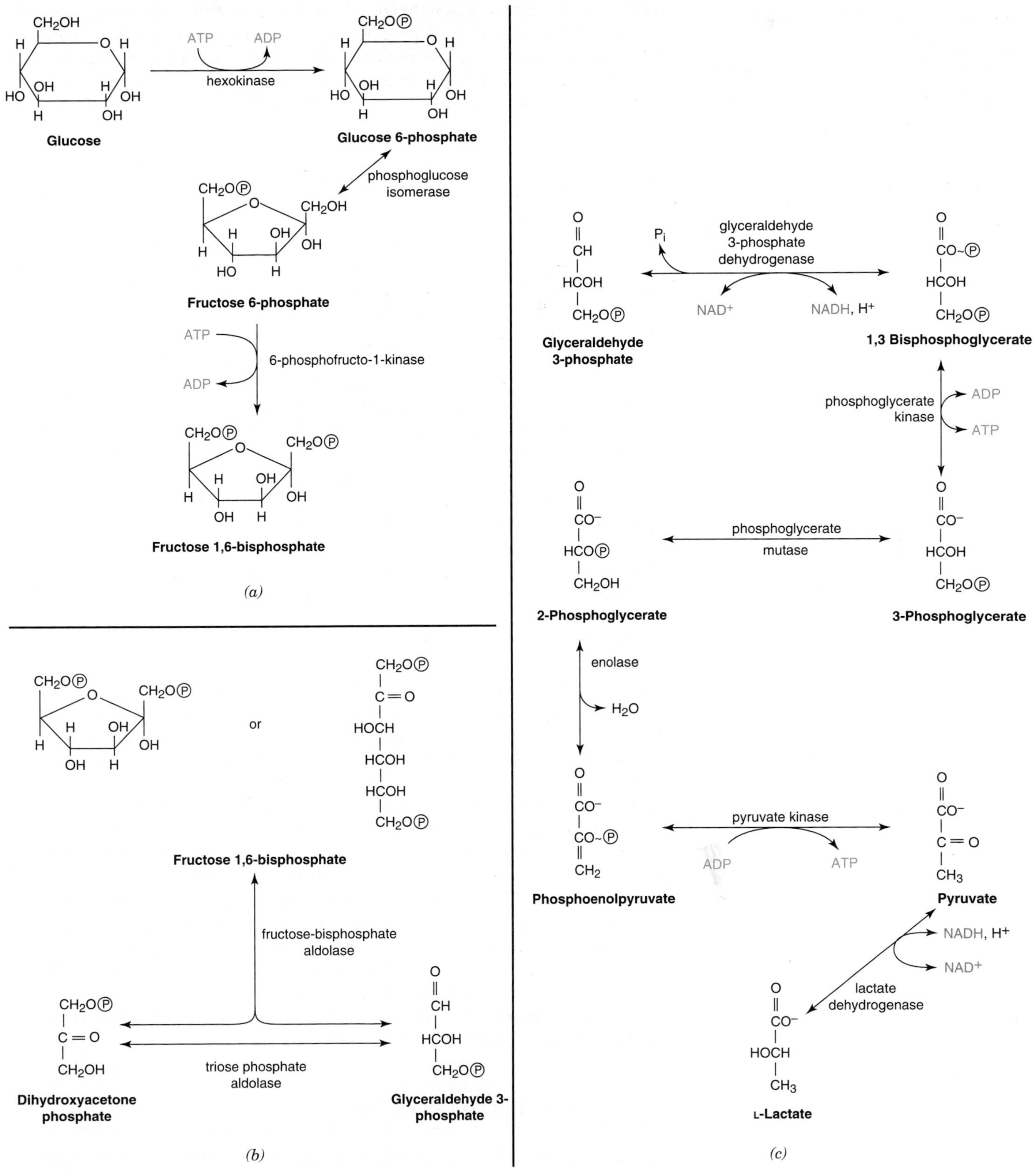

Glucose — ATP, ADP; hexokinase → Glucose 6-phosphate

Glucose 6-phosphate ⇌ (phosphoglucose isomerase) Fructose 6-phosphate

Fructose 6-phosphate — ATP, ADP; 6-phosphofructo-1-kinase → Fructose 1,6-bisphosphate

(a)

Fructose 1,6-bisphosphate (ring form) or Fructose 1,6-bisphosphate (open chain)

fructose-bisphosphate aldolase

Dihydroxyacetone phosphate ⇌ (triose phosphate aldolase) Glyceraldehyde 3-phosphate

(b)

Glyceraldehyde 3-phosphate ⇌ (P_i; glyceraldehyde 3-phosphate dehydrogenase; NAD^+, NADH, H^+) 1,3 Bisphosphoglycerate

1,3 Bisphosphoglycerate ⇌ (phosphoglycerate kinase; ADP, ATP) 3-Phosphoglycerate

2-Phosphoglycerate ⇌ (phosphoglycerate mutase) 3-Phosphoglycerate

2-Phosphoglycerate ⇌ (enolase; H_2O) Phosphoenolpyruvate

Phosphoenolpyruvate ⇌ (pyruvate kinase; ADP, ATP) Pyruvate

Pyruvate ⇌ (lactate dehydrogenase; NADH, H^+, NAD^+) L-Lactate

(c)

FIGURE 7.6

The glycolytic pathway, divided into its three stages.

The symbol P refers to the phosphoryl group PO_3^{2-}; ~ indicates a high-energy phosphate bond. (*a*) Priming stage. (*b*) Splitting stage. (*c*) Oxidoreduction–phosphorylation stage.

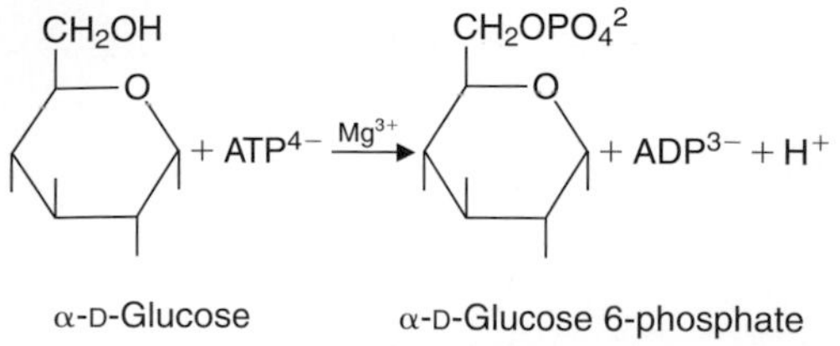

CH_2OH … + ATP^{4-} $\xrightarrow{Mg^{2+}}$ $CH_2OPO_3^{2-}$ … + ADP^{3-} + H^+

α-D-Glucose α-D-Glucose 6-phosphate

Step 1

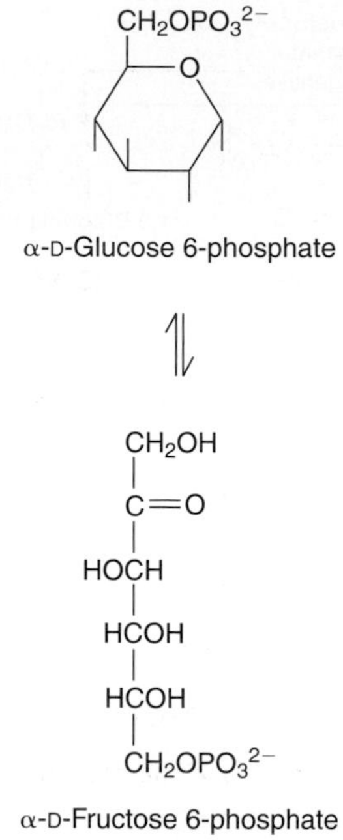

α-D-Glucose 6-phosphate ⇌ α-D-Fructose 6-phosphate

Step 2

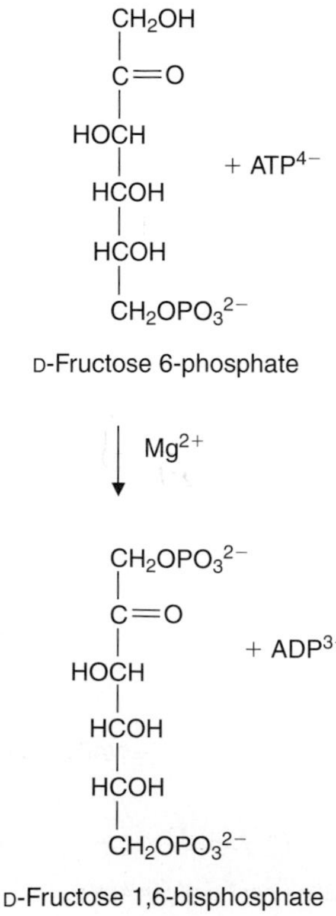

D-Fructose 6-phosphate + ATP^{4-} $\xrightarrow{Mg^{2+}}$ D-Fructose 1,6-bisphosphate + ADP^{3-} + H^+

Step 3

Glycolysis Occurs in Three Stages

Glycolysis can conveniently be pictured as occurring in three major stages (also see Figure 7.6).

Priming stage:

$$\text{D-Glucose} + 2\ ATP^{4-} \rightarrow \text{D-fructose 1,6-bisphosphate}^{4-} + 2\ ADP^{3-} + 2\ H^+$$

Splitting stage:

$$\text{D-Fructose 1,6-bisphosphate}^{4-} \rightarrow 2\ \text{D-glyceraldehyde 3-phosphate}^{2-}$$

Oxidoreduction–phosphorylation stage:

$$2\ \text{D-Glyceraldehyde 3-phosphate}^{2-} + 4\ ADP^{3-} + 2\ P_i^{2-} + 2\ H^+ \rightarrow 2\ \text{L-lactate}^- + 4\ ATP^{4-}$$

Sum:

$$\text{D-Glucose} + 2\ ADP^{3-} + 2\ P_i^{2-} \rightarrow 2\ \text{L-lactate}^- + 2\ ATP^{4-}$$

Priming stage involves input of two molecules of ATP to convert glucose into a molecule of fructose 1,6-bisphosphate. ATP is therefore "invested" in the priming stage of glycolysis. However, ATP beyond this investment is gained from the glycolytic process. The **splitting stage** "splits" the six-carbon molecule fructose 1,6-bisphosphate into two molecules of glyceraldehyde 3-phosphate. In the **oxidoreduction–phosphorylation stage** two molecules of glyceraldehyde 3-phosphate are converted into two molecules of lactate with the production of four molecules of ATP. The overall process of glycolysis generates two molecules of lactate and two molecules of ATP at the expense of one molecule of glucose.

Stage One Primes the Glucose Molecule

Hexokinase catalyzes the first step of glycolysis (see Figure 7.6*a* and Step 1). Although this reaction consumes ATP, it gets glycolysis off to a good start by trapping glucose as glucose 6-phosphate (G6P) within the cytosol of the cell where all of the glycolytic enzymes are located. Phosphate esters are charged hydrophilic compounds that do not readily penetrate cell membranes. The phosphorylation of glucose with ATP is a thermodynamically favorable reaction, requiring the use of one high-energy phosphate bond. It is irreversible under cellular conditions. It is not, however, a way to synthesize ATP or to hydrolyze G6P to give glucose by the reverse reaction. Hydrolysis of G6P is accomplished by a different reaction, catalyzed by **glucose 6-phosphatase:**

$$\text{Glucose 6-phosphate}^{2-} + H_2O \rightarrow \text{glucose} + P_i^{2-}$$

This reaction is thermodynamically favorable in the direction written and cannot be used in cells for the synthesis of G6P from glucose. (A common mistake is to note that ATP and ADP are involved in the hexokinase reaction but not to note that they are not involved in the glucose 6-phosphatase reaction.) Glucose 6-phosphatase is an important enzyme in liver, functioning to produce free glucose from G6P in the last step of both gluconeogenesis and glycogenolysis; it has no role in glycolysis.

The next reaction is a readily reversible step of the glycolytic pathway, catalyzed by **phosphoglucose isomerase** (Step 2). This step is not subject to regulation and, since it is readily reversible, functions in both glycolysis and gluconeogenesis.

6-Phosphofructo-1-kinase (or phosphofructokinase-1) catalyzes the next reaction, an ATP-dependent phosphorylation of fructose 6-phosphate (F6P) to give fructose 1,6-bisphosphate (FBP) (Step 3). This is a favorite enzyme of many students of biochemistry, being subject to regulation by several effectors and often considered the rate-limiting enzyme of the glycolytic pathway. The reaction is irreversible under intracellular conditions; that is, it represents a way to produce FBP but not a way to produce ATP or F6P by the reverse reaction. This reaction utilizes the second ATP needed to "prime" glucose, thereby completing the first stage of glycolysis.

Stage Two Is Splitting of a Phosphorylated Intermediate

Fructose 1,6-bisphosphate **aldolase** catalyzes the cleavage of fructose 1,6-bisphosphate into a molecule each of dihydroxyacetone phosphate and glyceraldehyde 3-phosphate (GAP) (Figure 7.6*b*) (Step 4). This is a reversible reaction, the enzyme being called aldolase because the overall reaction is a variant of an aldol cleavage in one direction and an aldol condensation in the other. **Triose phosphate isomerase** then catalyzes the reversible interconversion of dihydroxyacetone phosphate and GAP to complete the splitting stage of glycolysis (Step 5). With the transformation of dihydroxyacetone phosphate (DHAP) into GAP, one molecule of glucose is converted into two molecules of GAP.

Stage Three Involves Oxidoreduction Reactions and the Synthesis of ATP

The first reaction of the last stage of glycolysis (Figure 7.6*c*) is catalyzed by **glyceraldehyde-3-phosphate dehydrogenase** (Step 6). This reaction is of considerable interest because of what is accomplished in a single enzyme-catalyzed step. An aldehyde (glyceraldehyde 3-phosphate) is oxidized to a carboxylic acid with the reduction of NAD^+ to NADH. In addition to NADH, the reaction produces 1,3-bisphosphoglycerate, a mixed anhydride of a carboxylic acid and phosphoric acid. 1,3-Bisphosphoglycerate has a large negative free energy of hydrolysis, enabling it to participate in a subsequent reaction that yields ATP. The overall reaction catalyzed by glyceraldehyde-3 phosphate dehydrogenase can be visualized as the coupling of a very favorable exergonic reaction with an unfavorable endergonic reaction. The exergonic reaction can be thought of as being composed of a half-reaction in which an aldehyde is oxidized to a carboxylic acid, which is then coupled with a half-reaction in which NAD^+ is reduced to NADH:

$$R{-}\overset{\overset{O}{\|}}{C}H + H_2O \longrightarrow R{-}\overset{\overset{O}{\|}}{C}OH + 2H^+ + 2e^-$$

$$NAD^+ + 2H^+ + 2e^- \longrightarrow NADH + H^+$$

The overall reaction (sum of the half-reactions) is quite exergonic, with the aldehyde being oxidized to a carboxylic acid and NAD^+ being reduced to NADH:

$$R{-}\overset{\overset{O}{\|}}{C}H + NAD^+ + H_2O \longrightarrow R{-}\overset{\overset{O}{\|}}{C}OH + NADH + H^+, \quad \Delta G^{\circ\prime} = -10.3\ \text{kcal mol}^{-1}$$

The endergonic component of the reaction corresponds to the formation of a mixed anhydride between the carboxylic acid and phosphoric acid:

$$R{-}\overset{\overset{O}{\|}}{C}OH + P_i^{2-} \longrightarrow R{-}\overset{\overset{O}{\|}}{C}{-}OPO_3^{2-} + H_2O, \ \Delta G^{\circ\prime} = +\ 11.8\ \text{kcal mol}^{-1}$$

The overall reaction involves coupling of the endergonic and exergonic components to give an overall standard free-energy change of $+1.5$ kcal mol^{-1}.

$$\text{Sum: } R{-}\overset{\overset{O}{\|}}{C}H + NAD^+ + P_i^{2-} \longrightarrow$$

$$R{-}\overset{\overset{O}{\|}}{C}OPO_3^{2-} + NADH + H^+, \ \Delta G^{\circ\prime} = +\ 1.5\ \text{kcal mol}^{-1}$$

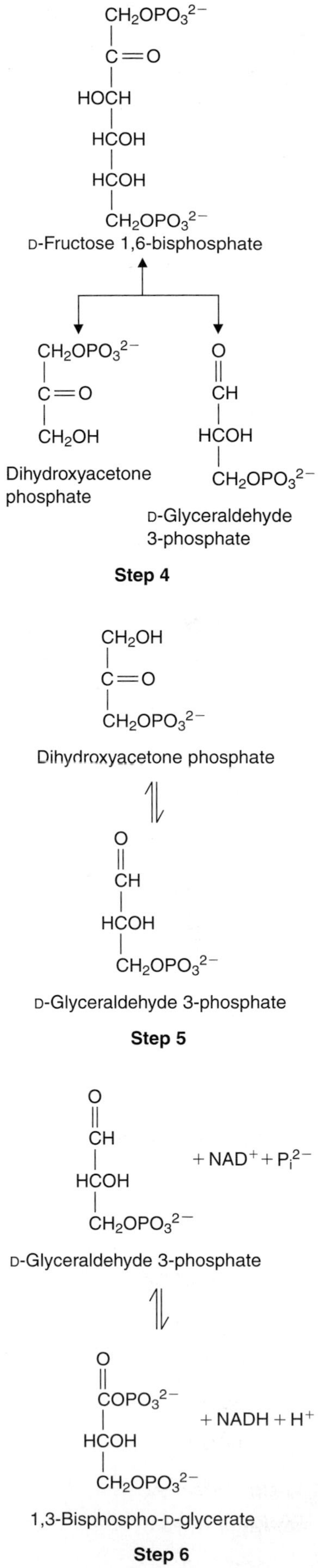

$$\begin{array}{c} CH_2OPO_3^{2-} \\ | \\ C{=}O \\ | \\ HOCH \\ | \\ HCOH \\ | \\ HCOH \\ | \\ CH_2OPO_3^{2-} \end{array}$$

D-Fructose 1,6-bisphosphate

$$\begin{array}{c} CH_2OPO_3^{2-} \\ | \\ C{=}O \\ | \\ CH_2OH \end{array} \qquad \begin{array}{c} O \\ \| \\ CH \\ | \\ HCOH \\ | \\ CH_2OPO_3^{2-} \end{array}$$

Dihydroxyacetone phosphate

D-Glyceraldehyde 3-phosphate

Step 4

$$\begin{array}{c} CH_2OH \\ | \\ C{=}O \\ | \\ CH_2OPO_3^{2-} \end{array}$$

Dihydroxyacetone phosphate

$$\rightleftharpoons$$

$$\begin{array}{c} O \\ \| \\ CH \\ | \\ HCOH \\ | \\ CH_2OPO_3^{2-} \end{array}$$

D-Glyceraldehyde 3-phosphate

Step 5

$$\begin{array}{c} O \\ \| \\ CH \\ | \\ HCOH \\ | \\ CH_2OPO_3^{2-} \end{array} + NAD^+ + P_i^{2-}$$

D-Glyceraldehyde 3-phosphate

$$\rightleftharpoons$$

$$\begin{array}{c} O \\ \| \\ COPO_3^{2-} \\ | \\ HCOH \\ | \\ CH_2OPO_3^{2-} \end{array} + NADH + H^+$$

1,3-Bisphospho-D-glycerate

Step 6

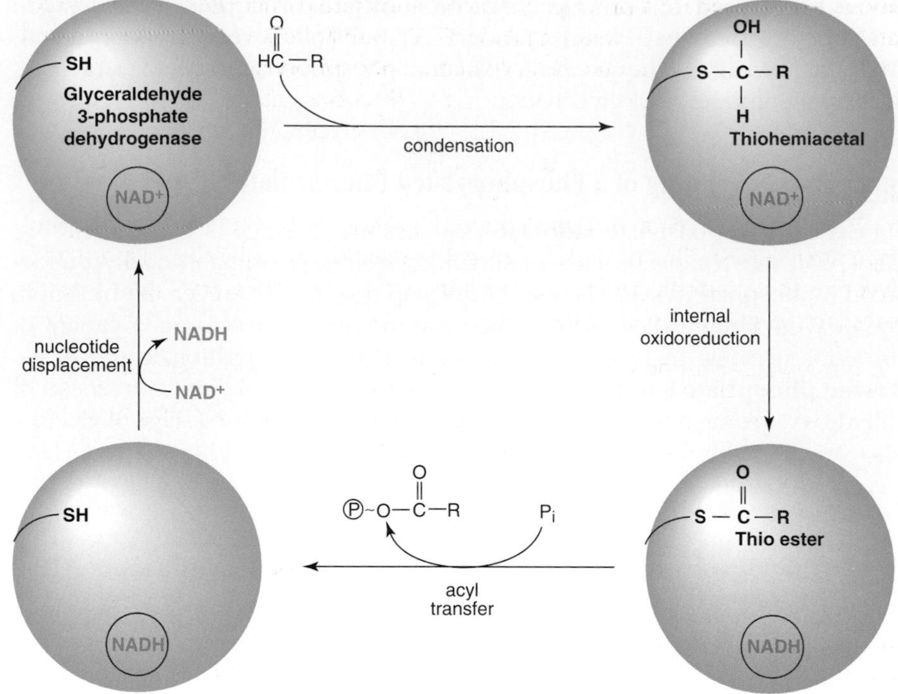

FIGURE 7.7
Mechanism of action of glyceraldehyde-3-phosphate dehydrogenase.
Large sphere represents the enzyme; small circle, the binding site for NAD^+; $R\overset{\overset{O}{\|}}{C}H$, glyceraldehyde 3-phosphate; —SH, the sulfhydryl group of the cysteine residue located at the active site; and ~P, the high-energy phosphate bond of 1,3-bisphosphoglycerate.

The reaction is freely reversible in cells and is used in both the glycolytic and gluconeogenic pathways. The proposed mechanism for the enzyme-catalyzed reaction is shown in Figure 7.7. Glyceraldehyde 3-phosphate reacts with a sulfhydryl group of a cysteine residue of the enzyme to generate a thiohemiacetal. An internal oxidation–reduction reaction occurs in which bound NAD^+ is reduced to NADH and the thiohemiacetal is oxidized to give a high-energy thiol ester. The high-energy thiol ester reacts with P_i to form the mixed anhydride and regenerate the free sulfhydryl group. The mixed anhydride dissociates from the enzyme. Exogenous NAD^+ then replaces the bound NADH. Note that a carboxylic acid (RCOOH) is not an intermediate in the actual reaction. Instead, the enzyme generates a high-energy thiol ester, which is converted into another high-energy compound, a mixed anhydride of carboxylic and phosphoric acids.

The reaction catalyzed by glyceraldehyde-3-phosphate dehydrogenase requires NAD^+ and produces NADH. Since the cytosol has only a limited amount of NAD^+, it is imperative for continuous glycolytic activity that the NADH be reoxidized to NAD^+, otherwise glycolysis will stop for want of NAD^+. The options that cells have for accomplishing the regeneration of NAD^+ are considered later (see p. 281).

The next reaction, catalyzed by **phosphoglycerate kinase,** produces ATP from the high-energy compound 1,3-bisphosphoglycerate (Figure 7.6*c*; Step 7). This is the first site of ATP production in the glycolytic pathway. Because two ATP molecules were invested for each glucose molecule in the priming stage, and because two molecules of 1,3-bisphosphoglycerate are produced from each glucose, all of the ATP "invested" in the priming stage is recovered in this step of glycolysis. Since ATP production occurs in the forward direction and ATP utilization in the reverse direction, it may seem surprising that the reaction is freely reversible and can be used in both the glycolytic and gluconeogenic pathways. The reaction provides a means for the generation of ATP in the glycolytic pathway but, when needed for glucose synthesis, can also be used in the reverse direction for the synthesis of 1,3-bisphosphoglycerate at the expense of ATP. The glyceraldehyde-3-phosphate dehydrogenase–phosphoglycerate kinase system is an example of **substrate-level phosphory-**

$$\begin{array}{l} \overset{O}{\|} \\ COPO_3^{2-} \\ | \\ HCOH \\ | \\ CH_2OPO_3^{2-} \end{array} + ADP^{3-}$$

1,3-Bisphospho-D-glycerate

$$\Big\Updownarrow Mg^{2+}$$

$$\begin{array}{l} \overset{O}{\|} \\ CO^- \\ | \\ HCOH \\ | \\ CH_2OPO_3^{2-} \end{array} + ATP^{4-}$$

3-Phospho-D-glycerate

Step 7

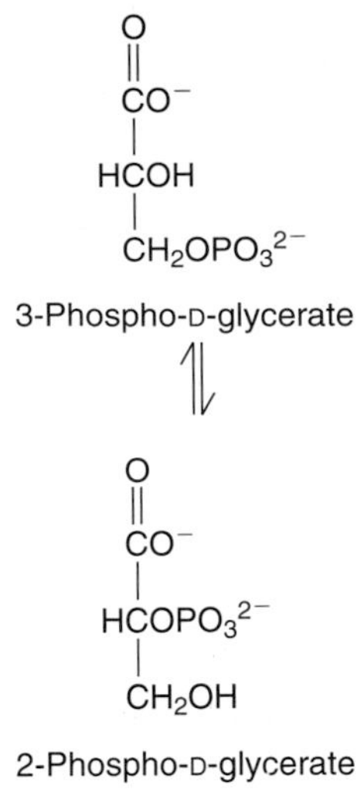

lation, a term used for a process in which a substrate participates in an enzyme-catalyzed reaction that yields ATP or GTP. Substrate-level phosphorylation stands in contrast to mitochondrial oxidative phosphorylation (see Chapter 6). Note, however, that the combination of the reactions catalyzed by glyceraldehyde-3-phosphate dehydrogenase and phosphoglycerate kinase accomplishes the coupling of an oxidation (an aldehyde goes to a carboxylic acid) to a phosphorylation.

Phosphoglycerate mutase converts 3-phosphoglycerate to 2-phosphoglycerate (Step 8). This is a freely reversible reaction in which 2,3-bisphosphoglycerate (or 2,3-diphosphoglycerate) functions as an obligatory intermediate at the active site of the enzyme (E):

E-phosphate + 3-phosphoglycerate $\rightleftharpoons$ E + 2,3-bisphosphoglycerate

E + 2,3-bisphosphoglycerate $\rightleftharpoons$ E-phosphate + 2-phosphoglycerate

Sum: 3-phosphoglycerate $\rightleftharpoons$ 2-phosphoglycerate

The involvement of 2,3-bisphosphoglycerate as an intermediate creates an absolute requirement for the presence of a catalytic amount of this compound in cells. This can be appreciated by noting that E-phosphate in this reaction cannot be generated without 2,3-bisphosphoglycerate. Cells synthesize 2,3-bisphosphoglycerate, independent of the reaction catalyzed by phosphoglycerate mutase, by a reaction catalyzed by 2,3-bisphosphoglycerate mutase:

$$\begin{array}{c} O \\ \| \\ COPO_3^{2-} \\ | \\ HCOH \\ | \\ CH_2OPO_3^{2-} \end{array} \longrightarrow \begin{array}{c} O \\ \| \\ CO^- \\ | \\ HCOPO_3^{2-} \\ | \\ CH_2OPO_3^{2-} \end{array} + H^+$$

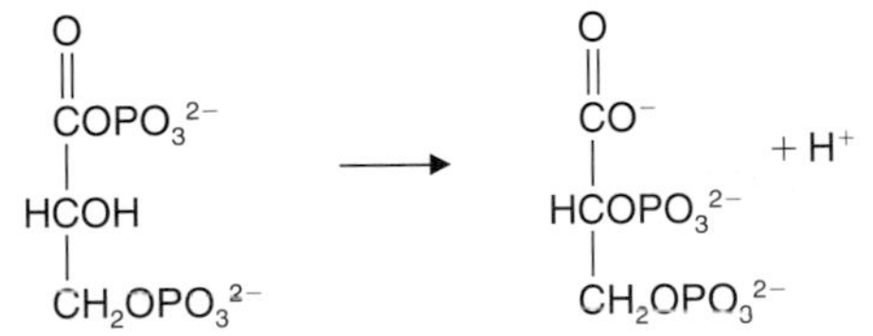

1,3-Bisphospho-D-glycerate 2,3-Bisphospho-D-glycerate

The mutase is unusual in that it is a bifunctional enzyme, serving also as a phosphatase that converts 2,3-bisphosphoglycerate to 3-phosphoglycerate and P_i. All cells contain at least minute quantities of **2,3-bisphosphoglycerate** for no apparent purpose other than to produce the phosphorylated form of newly synthesized phosphoglycerate mutase. The amounts needed are small because phosphoglycerate mutase has to be phosphorylated only once, the phosphorylated enzyme being regenerated during each reaction cycle. Red blood cells contain very high 2,3-bisphosphoglycerate concentrations because it serves as an important allosteric effector of the association of oxygen with the hemoglobin (see Chapter 25). From 15% to 25% of the glucose converted to lactate in red blood cells goes by way of the **"BPG shunt"** (Figure 7.8). Catabolism of glucose by the BPG shunt generates no net ATP since the reaction catalyzed by the phosphoglycerate kinase is bypassed.

Enolase catalyzes elimination of water from 2-phosphoglycerate to form phosphoenolpyruvate (PEP) in the next reaction (Step 9; Figure 7.6*c*). This is a remarkable reaction from the standpoint that a high-energy phosphate compound is generated from one of markedly lower energy level. The standard free-energy change ($\Delta G^{\circ\prime}$) for the hydrolysis of phosphoenolpyruvate is -14.8 kcal mol^{-1}, a much greater value than the standard free energy for 2-phosphoglycerate hydrolysis (-4.2 kcal mol^{-1}). Although the reaction catalyzed by enolase is freely reversible, a large change in the distribution of energy occurs as a consequence of its action on 2-phosphoglycerate. The free-energy levels of PEP and 2-phosphoglycerate are not markedly different; however, the free-energy levels of their products of hydrolysis (pyruvate and glycerate, respectively) are quite different. Since $\Delta G^{\circ\prime} = \Delta G^{\circ\prime}_{\text{products}} - G^{\circ\prime}_{\text{substrates}}$, this accounts for the marked differences in the standard free energy of hydrolysis of these two compounds.

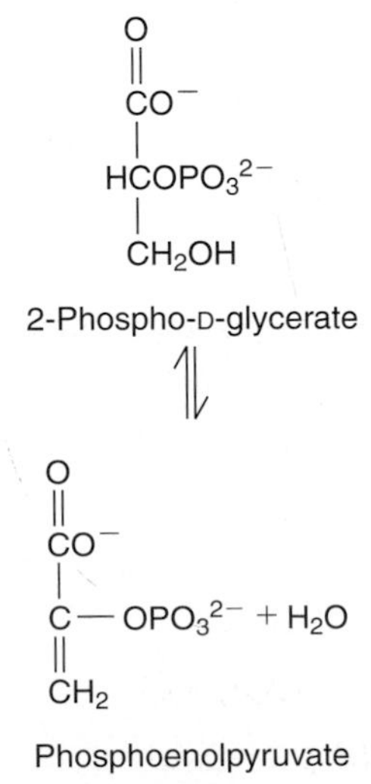

$$\begin{array}{c} O \\ \| \\ CO^- \\ | \\ HCOH \\ | \\ CH_2OPO_3^{2-} \end{array}$$

3-Phospho-D-glycerate

$$\rightleftharpoons$$

$$\begin{array}{c} O \\ \| \\ CO^- \\ | \\ HCOPO_3^{2-} \\ | \\ CH_2OH \end{array}$$

2-Phospho-D-glycerate

Step 8

$$\begin{array}{c} O \\ \| \\ CO^- \\ | \\ HCOPO_3^{2-} \\ | \\ CH_2OH \end{array}$$

2-Phospho-D-glycerate

$$\rightleftharpoons$$

$$\begin{array}{c} O \\ \| \\ CO^- \\ | \\ C-OPO_3^{2-} \\ \| \\ CH_2 \end{array} + H_2O$$

Phosphoenolpyruvate

Step 9

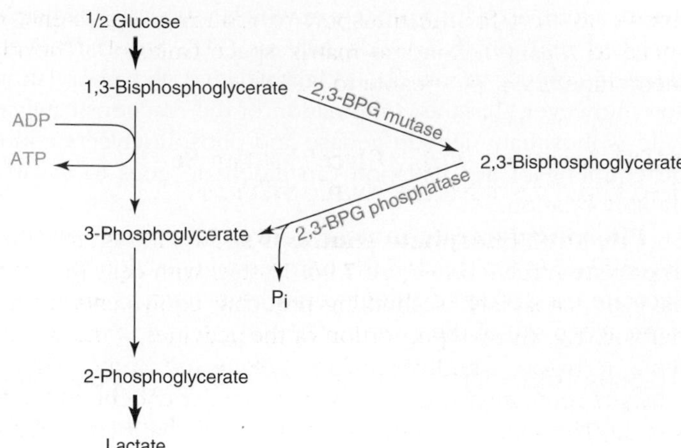

FIGURE 7.8
The 2,3-bisphosphoglycerate (2,3-BPG) shunt consists of reactions catalyzed by the bifunctional enzyme, 2,3-BPG mutase/phosphatase.

COO^-—$C(OPO_3^{2-})$=CH_2 + ADP^{3-} + H^+

Phosphoenolpyruvate

↓ + Mg^{2+}

COO^-—C=O—CH_3 + ATP^{4-}

Pyruvate

Step 10

COO^-—C=O—CH_3 + NADH + H^+

Pyruvate

⇅

COO^-—HOCH—CH_3 + NAD^+

L-Lactate

Step 11

Pyruvate kinase (Step 10; Figure 7.6*c*) accomplishes another **substrate-level phosphorylation:** that is, the synthesis of ATP with the conversion of the high-energy compound PEP into pyruvate. It constitutes a way to synthesize ATP but, in contrast to the phosphoglycerate kinase reaction, is not reversible under conditions that exist in cells and cannot be used for the synthesis of PEP when needed for glucose synthesis.

The last step of the glycolytic pathway is an oxidoreduction reaction catalyzed by **lactate dehydrogenase** (Step 11; Figure 7.6*c*). Pyruvate is reduced to give L-lactate and NADH is oxidized to NAD^+. This is a freely reversible reaction and the only reaction that can result in L-lactate formation or L-lactate utilization.

A Balance of Reduction of NAD^+ and Reoxidation of NADH Is Required: Role of Lactate Dehydrogenase

There is a perfect coupling between the generation of NADH and its utilization in glycolysis (Figure 7.6*c*). Two molecules of NADH are generated at the level of glyceraldehyde-3-phosphate dehydrogenase and two molecules of NADH are utilized by lactate dehydrogenase in the conversion of one molecule of glucose into two molecules of lactate. NAD^+, a soluble molecule present in the cytosol, is available in only limited amounts and must be regenerated from NADH for glycolysis to continue unabated. The overall reaction catalyzed by the combined actions of glyceraldehyde-3-phosphate dehydrogenase and lactate dehydrogenase is the conversion of pyruvate, glyceraldehyde 3-phosphate, and P_i into lactate and 1,3-bisphosphoglycerate. The two reactions are

D-Glyceraldehyde 3-phosphate + NAD^+ + P_i →
1,3-bisphospho-D-glycerate + NADH + H^+

Pyruvate + NADH + H^+ → L-lactate + NAD^+

Sum: D-Glyceraldehyde 3-phosphate + pyruvate + P_i →
1,3-bisphosphoglycerate + L-lactate

This perfect coupling of reducing equivalents in the glycolytic pathway has to occur under conditions of anaerobiosis or in cells that lack mitochondria. With the availability of oxygen and mitochondria, reducing equivalents in the form of NADH generated at the level of glyceraldehyde-3-phosphate dehydrogenase can be shuttled into the mitochondria for the synthesis of ATP, leaving pyruvate rather than lactate as the end product of glycolysis. Two shuttle systems are known to exist for the transport of reducing equivalents from the cytosolic space to the mitochondrial matrix space (mitosol). The mitochondrial inner membrane is not permeable to NADH.

NADH Generated During Glycolysis Can Be Reoxidized via Substrate Shuttle Systems

The **glycerol phosphate shuttle** is shown in Figure 7.9*a* and the **malate–aspartate shuttle** in Figure 7.9*b*. Tissues with cells that contain mitochondria have the capability of shuttling reducing equivalents from the cytosol to the mitosol. The relative proportion of the activities of the two shuttles varies from tissue to tissue, with liver making greater use of the malate–aspartate shuttle, whereas some muscle cells may be more dependent on the glycerol phosphate shuttle. The shuttle systems are irreversible; that is, they represent mechanisms for moving reducing equivalents into the mitosol, but not mechanisms for moving mitochondrial reducing equivalents into the cytosol.

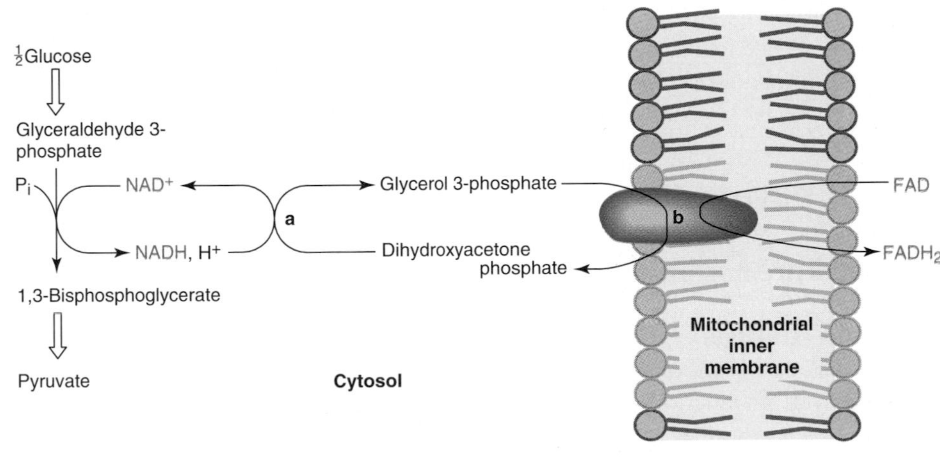

(*a*)

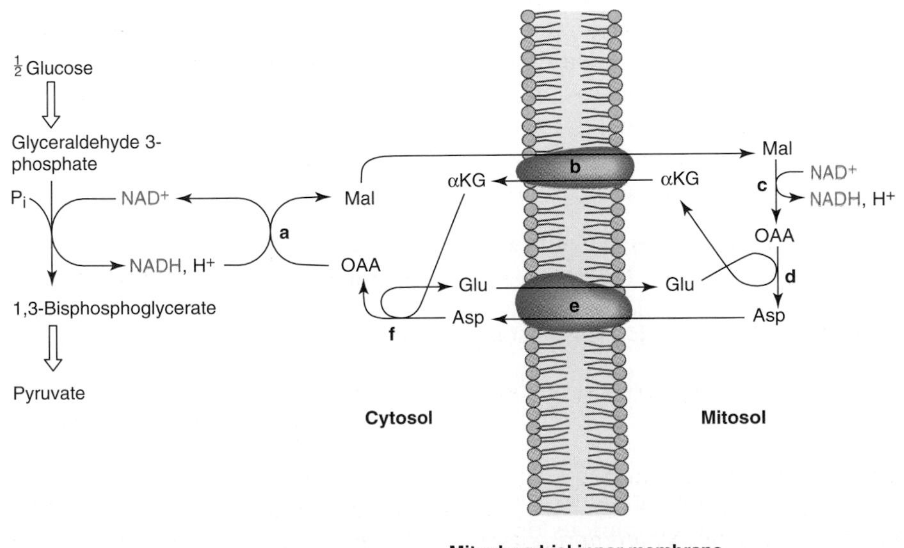

(*b*)

FIGURE 7.9
Shuttles for the transport of reducing equivalents from the cytosol to the mitochondrial electron-transfer chain.
(*a*) Glycerol phosphate shuttle: **a,** cytosolic glycerol 3-phosphate dehydrogenase oxidizes NADH; **b,** mitochondrial glycerol-3-phosphate dehydrogenase of the outer surface of the inner membrane reduces FAD. (*b*) Malate–aspartate shuttle: **a,** cytosolic malate dehydrogenase reduces oxaloacetate (OAA) to malate; **b,** dicarboxylic acid antiport of the mitochondrial inner membrane catalyzes electrically silent exchange of malate for α-ketoglutarate (α-KG); **c,** mitochondrial malate dehydrogenase produces intramitochondrial NADH; **d,** mitochondrial aspartate aminotransferase transaminates glutamate and oxaloacetate; **e,** glutamate–aspartate antiport of the mitochondrial inner membrane catalyzes electrogenic exchange of glutamate for aspartate; **f,** cytosolic aspartate aminotransferase transaminates aspartate and α-ketoglutarate.

The transport of aspartate out of mitochondria in exchange for glutamate is the irreversible step in the malate–aspartate shuttle. The mitochondrial inner membrane has a large number of transport systems (see Chapter 6) but lacks one that is effective for oxaloacetate. For this reason oxaloacetate transaminates with glutamate to produce aspartate, which then exits irreversibly from the mitochondrion in exchange for glutamate. The aspartate entering the cytosol transaminates with α-ketoglutarate to give oxaloacetate and glutamate. The oxaloacetate accepts the reducing equivalents of NADH and becomes malate. Malate then penetrates the mitochondrial inner membrane, where it is oxidized by the mitochondrial **malate dehydrogenase.** This produces NADH within the mitosol and regenerates oxaloacetate to complete the cycle. The overall balanced equation for the sum of all the reactions of the malate–aspartate shuttle is simply

$$\text{NADH}_{\text{cytosol}} + \text{H}^+_{\text{cytosol}} + \text{NAD}^+_{\text{mitosol}} \rightarrow \text{NAD}^+_{\text{cytosol}} + \text{NADH}_{\text{mitosol}} + \text{H}^+_{\text{mitosol}}$$

The glycerol phosphate shuttle is simpler, in the sense that fewer reactions are involved, but $FADH_2$ is generated within the mitochondrial inner membrane rather than NADH within the mitosolic compartment. The irreversible step of the shuttle is catalyzed by the mitochondrial **glycerol-3-phosphate dehydrogenase.** The active site of this enzyme is exposed on the cytosolic surface of the mitochondrial inner membrane, making it unnecessary for glycerol 3-phosphate to penetrate into the mitosol for oxidation. The overall balanced equation for the sum of the reactions of the glycerol phosphate shuttle is

$$\text{NADH}_{\text{cytosol}} + \text{H}^+_{\text{cytosol}} + \text{FAD}_{\text{inner membrane}} \rightarrow \text{NAD}^+_{\text{cytosol}} + \text{FADH}_{2\text{ inner membrane}}$$

Shuttles Are Important in Other Oxidoreductive Pathways

Alcohol Oxidation

The first step of **alcohol** (i.e., ethanol) metabolism is its oxidation to **acetaldehyde** with production of NADH by **alcohol dehydrogenase.**

$$\underset{\text{Ethanol}}{\text{CH}_3\text{CH}_2\text{OH}} + \text{NAD}^+ \longrightarrow \underset{\text{Acetaldehyde}}{\text{CH}_3\overset{\overset{\displaystyle\text{O}}{\|}}{\text{C}}\text{H}} + \text{NADH} + \text{H}^+$$

This enzyme is located almost exclusively in the cytosol of liver parenchymal cells. The acetaldehyde generated traverses the mitochondrial inner membrane for oxidation by a mitosolic **aldehyde dehydrogenase.**

$$\underset{\text{Acetaldehyde}}{\text{CH}_3\overset{\overset{\displaystyle\text{O}}{\|}}{\text{C}}\text{H}} + \text{NAD}^+ \longrightarrow \underset{\text{Acetate}}{\text{CH}_3\overset{\overset{\displaystyle\text{O}}{\|}}{\text{C}}\text{O}^-} + \text{NADH} + 2\text{H}^+$$

The NADH generated by the last step can be used directly by the mitochondrial electron-transfer chain. However, NADH generated by cytosolic alcohol dehydrogenase must be oxidized back to NAD^+ by one of the shuttles. Thus the capacity of a human being to oxidize alcohol is dependent on the ability of the liver to transport reducing equivalents from the cytosol to the mitosol by these shuttle systems.

Glucuronide Formation

The shuttles play an important role in the formation of water-soluble **glucuronides** of bilirubin and various drugs (see p. 1018) so that these compounds can be eliminated from the body in the urine and bile. In this process **UDP-glucose** (structure on p. 343) is oxidized to **UDP-glucuronic acid** (structure on p. 344).

$$\text{UDP-D-glucose} + 2\,\text{NAD}^+ + \text{H}_2\text{O} \rightarrow \text{UDP-D-glucuronic acid} + 2\,\text{NADH} + 2\,\text{H}^+$$

CLINICAL CORRELATION 7.1

Alcohol and Barbiturates

Acute alcohol intoxication causes increased sensitivity of an individual to the general depressant effects of barbiturates. Barbiturates and alcohol both interact with the γ-aminobutyrate (GABA)-activated chloride channel. Activation of the chloride channel inhibits neuronal firing, which may explain the depressant effects of both compounds. This drug combination is very dangerous and normal prescription doses of barbiturates have potentially lethal consequences in the presence of ethanol. In addition to the depressant effects of both ethanol and barbiturates on the central nervous system (CNS), ethanol inhibits the metabolism of barbiturates, thereby prolonging the time barbiturates remain effective in the body. Hydroxylation of barbiturates by the endoplasmic reticulum of the liver is inhibited by ethanol. This reaction, catalyzed by the NADPH-dependent cytochrome system, forms water-soluble derivatives of the barbiturates that are eliminated readily from the circulation by the kidneys. Blood levels of barbiturates remain high when ethanol is present, causing increased CNS depression.

Surprisingly, the alcoholic when sober is less sensitive to barbiturates. Chronic ethanol consumption apparently causes adaptive changes in the sensitivity of the CNS to barbiturates (cross-tolerance). It also results in the induction of the enzymes of liver endoplasmic reticulum involved in drug hydroxylation reactions. Consequently, the sober alcoholic is able to metabolize barbiturates more rapidly. This sets up the following scenario. A sober alcoholic has trouble falling asleep, even after taking several sleeping pills, because his/her liver has increased capacity to hydroxylate the barbiturate contained in the pills. In frustration he/she consumes more pills and then alcohol. Sleep results, but may be followed by respiratory depression and death because the alcoholic, although less sensitive to barbiturates when sober, remains sensitive to the synergistic effect of alcohol.

Misra, P. S., Lefevre, A., Ishii, H., Rubin, E., and Lieber, C. S. Increase of ethanol, meprobamate and pentobarbital metabolism after chronic ethanol administration in man and in rats. *Am. J. Med.* 51:346, 1971.

In a reaction that occurs primarily in the liver, the "activated" glucuronic acid molecule is then transferred to a nonpolar acceptor molecule, such as **bilirubin** or a compound foreign to the body:

$$\text{UDP-D-glucuronic acid} + \text{R—OH} \rightarrow \text{R—O—glucuronic acid} + \text{UDP}$$

Excess NADH generated by the first reaction has to be reoxidized by the shuttles for this process to continue. Since ethanol oxidation and drug conjugation are properties of the liver, the two of them occurring together may overwhelm the combined capacity of the shuttles. A good thing to tell patients is not to mix the intake of pharmacologically active compounds and alcohol (see Clin. Corr. 7.1).

Two Shuttle Pathways Yield Different Amounts of ATP

The mitosolic NADH formed by the malate–aspartate shuttle activity can be used by the mitochondrial respiratory chain for the production of three molecules of ATP by oxidative phosphorylation:

$$\text{NADH}_{\text{mitosol}} + \text{H}^+ + \tfrac{1}{2}\,\text{O}_2 + 3\ \text{ADP} + 3\ \text{P}_i \rightarrow \text{NAD}^+_{\text{mitosol}} + 3\ \text{ATP} + \text{H}_2\text{O}$$

In contrast, the $FADH_2$ obtained by the glycerol phosphate shuttle yields only two ATP molecules:

$$\text{FADH}_{2\ \text{inner membrane}} + \tfrac{1}{2}\,\text{O}_2 + 2\ \text{ADP} + 2\ \text{P}_i \rightarrow \text{FAD}_{\text{inner membrane}} + 2\ \text{ATP} + \text{H}_2\text{O}$$

Without the intervention of the shuttle systems, conversion of one molecule of glucose to two molecules of lactate by glycolysis results in the net formation of two molecules of ATP. Two molecules of ATP are used in the priming stage to set glucose up so that it can be cleaved. However, subsequent steps then yield four molecules of ATP so that the overall net production of ATP by the glycolytic pathway is two molecules of ATP. Biological cells have only a limited amount of ADP and P_i. Therefore flux through the glycolytic pathway is also dependent on an adequate supply of these substrates. If the ATP is not utilized for performance of work, glycolysis will stop for want of ADP and/or P_i. Consequently, the ATP generated has to be used, that is, turned over, in normal work-related processes in order for glycolysis to occur. The equation for the use of ATP for any work-related process is simply

$$\text{ATP}^{4-} \rightarrow \text{ADP}^{3-} + \text{P}_i^{2-} + \text{H}^+ + \text{“work”}$$

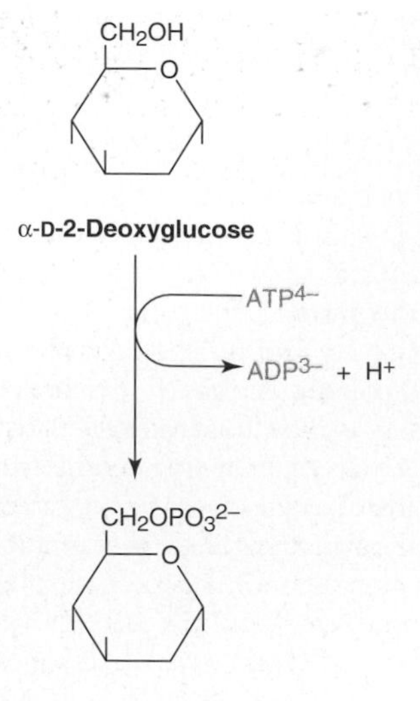

α-D-2-Deoxyglucose 6-phosphate

FIGURE 7.10
Hexokinase catalyzes the phosphorylation of 2-deoxyglucose.

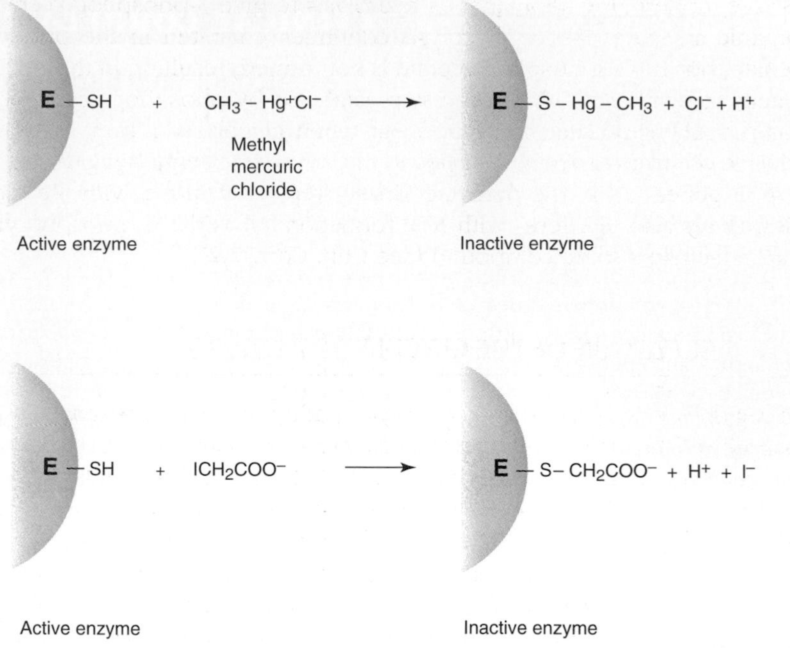

$$E{-}SH + CH_3{-}Hg^+Cl^- \longrightarrow E{-}S{-}Hg{-}CH_3 + Cl^- + H^+$$

Methyl mercuric chloride

Active enzyme — Inactive enzyme

$$E{-}SH + ICH_2COO^- \longrightarrow E{-}S{-}CH_2COO^- + H^+ + I^-$$

Active enzyme — Inactive enzyme

FIGURE 7.11
Mechanism responsible for inactivation of glyceraldehyde-3-phosphate dehydrogenase by sulfhydryl reagents.

When this equation is added to that given above for glycolysis, excluding the work accomplished, the overall balanced equation becomes

$$\text{D-Glucose} \rightarrow 2\ \text{lactate}^- + 2\ H^+$$

Glycolysis Can Be Inhibited at Different Stages

The best known inhibitors of the glycolytic pathway are **2-deoxyglucose,** sulfhydryl reagents, and **fluoride.** 2-Deoxyglucose is a substrate for hexokinase, being converted to its 6-phosphate ester (Figure 7.10). Like glucose 6-phosphate, 2-deoxyglucose 6-phosphate is an effective inhibitor of the reaction catalyzed by hexokinase but, unlike glucose 6-phosphate, will not function as a substrate for the reaction catalyzed by phosphoglucose isomerase. Thus it will accumulate in cells.

Sulfhydryl reagents inhibit **glyceraldehyde-3-phosphate dehydrogenase.** This enzyme has a cysteine residue at the active site. The sulfhydryl group combines with glyceraldehyde 3-phosphate to give a thiohemiacetal (Figure 7.7). Sulfhydryl reagents are usually mercury-containing compounds or alkylating compounds, such as **iodoacetate,** which readily react with the sulfhydryl group of glyceraldehyde-3-phosphate dehydrogenase to prevent the formation of the thiohemiacetal (Figure 7.11).

Fluoride is a potent inhibitor of enolase. Mg^{2+} and P_i form an ionic complex with fluoride ion, which is responsible for inhibition of enolase by interfering with binding of its substrate (Mg^{2+} 2-phosphoglycerate).

Pentavalent arsenic or arsenate is special with respect to its effects on glycolysis. It is not an inhibitor of the process, and under some conditions can even stimulate glycolytic flux. Arsenate prevents net synthesis of ATP by causing arsenolysis in the glyceraldehyde-3-phosphate dehydrogenase reaction. Arsenate looks like P_i and is able to substitute for P_i in enzyme-catalyzed reactions. The result is the formation of a mixed anhydride of arsenic acid and the carboxyl group of 3-phosphoglycerate during the reaction catalyzed by glyceraldehyde-3-phosphate dehydrogenase (Figure 7.12). 1-Arsenato 3-phosphoglycerate is

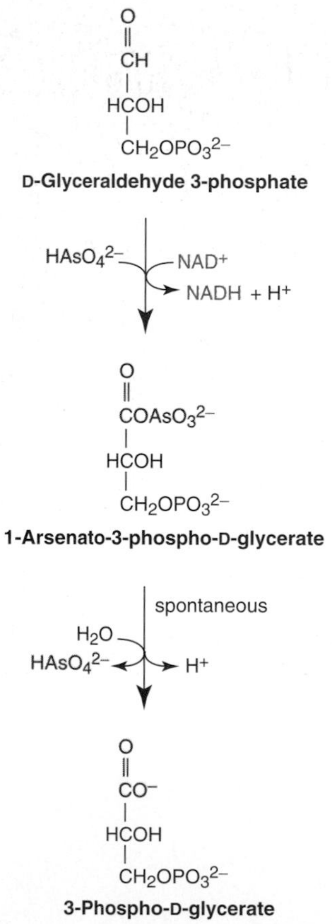

O=CH–HCOH–$CH_2OPO_3^{2-}$

D-Glyceraldehyde 3-phosphate

$HAsO_4^{2-}$, NAD^+ → NADH + H^+

O=$COAsO_3^{2-}$–HCOH–$CH_2OPO_3^{2-}$

1-Arsenato-3-phospho-D-glycerate

spontaneous; H_2O, $HAsO_4^{2-}$, H^+

O=CO^-–HCOH–$CH_2OPO_3^{2-}$

3-Phospho-D-glycerate

FIGURE 7.12
Arsenate uncouples oxidation from phosphorylation at the step catalyzed by glyceraldehyde-3-phosphate dehydrogenase.

unstable, undergoing spontaneous hydrolysis to give 3-phosphoglycerate and inorganic arsenate. Hence glycolysis continues unabated in the presence of arsenate, but 1,3-bisphosphoglycerate is not formed, resulting in the loss of the capacity to synthesize ATP at the step catalyzed by phosphoglycerate kinase. Thus net ATP synthesis does not occur when glycolysis is carried out in the presence of arsenate, the ATP invested in the priming stage being balanced by the ATP generated in the pyruvate kinase step. This, along with the fact that **arsenolysis** also interferes with ATP formation by oxidative phosphorylation, makes arsenate a toxic compound (see Clin. Corr. 7.2).

7.4 REGULATION OF THE GLYCOLYTIC PATHWAY

The regulatory enzymes of the glycolytic pathway are **hexokinase, 6-phosphofructo-1-kinase,** and **pyruvate kinase.** A summary of the important regulatory features of these enzymes is presented in Figure 7.13. A regulatory enzyme is controlled by either allosteric effectors or covalent modification (see p. 151). Both mechanisms are used by cells to control the most important of the regulatory enzymes. A regulatory enzyme can often be identified by determining whether the concentrations of the substrates and products within a cell indicate that the reaction catalyzed by the enzyme is close to equilibrium. An enzyme

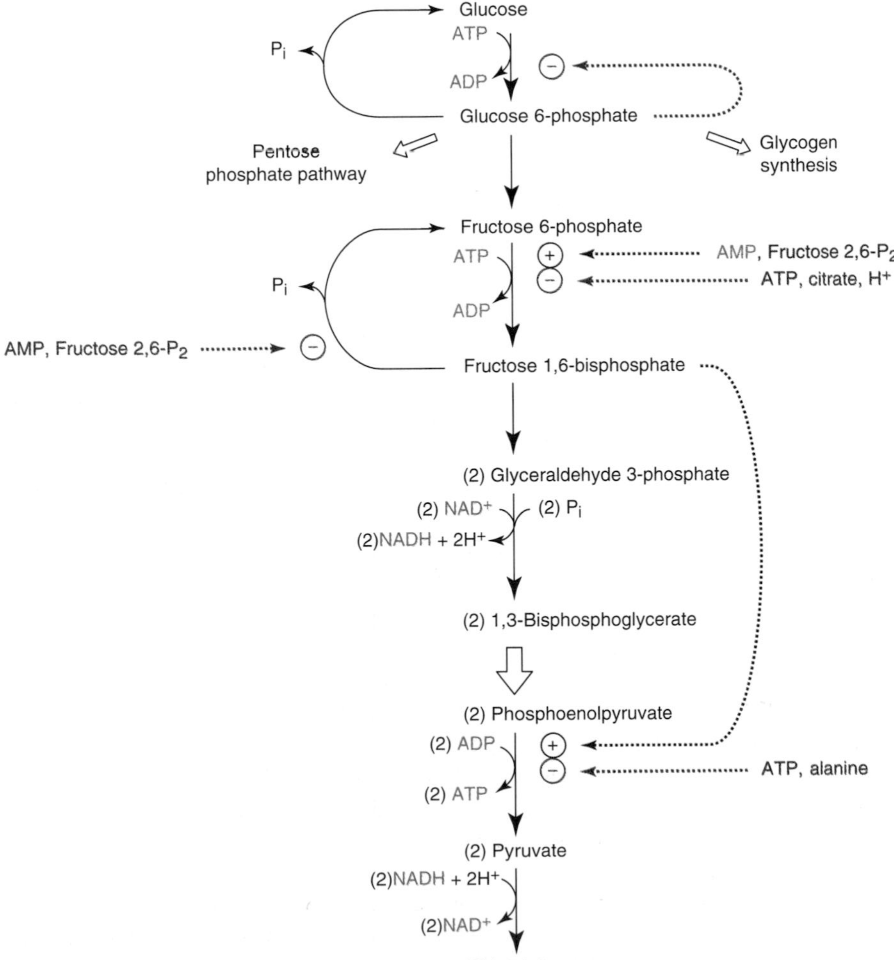

FIGURE 7.13
Important regulatory features of the glycolytic pathway.
Because of differences in isoenzyme distribution, not all tissues of the body have all of the regulatory mechanisms shown here.

CLINICAL CORRELATION 7.2

Arsenic Poisoning

Most forms of arsenic are toxic, but the trivalent form (arsenite as AsO_2^-) is much more toxic than the pentavalent form (arsenate or $HAsO_4^{2-}$). Less ATP is produced whenever arsenate substitutes for P_i in biological reactions. Arsenate competes for P_i-binding sites on enzymes, resulting in the formation of arsenate esters that are unstable. Arsenite works by a completely different mechanism, involving the formation of a stable complex with enzyme-bound lipoic acid:

SH SH $(CH_2)_4C(=O)$—enzyme $+ ASO_2^- + H^+$

↓

S—As(OH)—S $(CH_2)_4C(=O)$—enzyme $+ H_2O$

For the most part arsenic poisoning is explained by inhibition of those enzymes that require lipoic acid as a coenzyme. These include pyruvate dehydrogenase, α-ketoglutarate dehydrogenase, and branched-chain α-keto acid dehydrogenase. Chronic arsenic poisoning from well water contaminated with arsenical pesticides or through the efforts of a murderer is best diagnosed by determining the concentration of arsenic in the hair or fingernails of the victim. About 0.5 mg of arsenic would be found in a kilogram of hair from a normal individual. The hair of a person chronically exposed to arsenic could have 100 times as much.

Hindmarsh, J. T., and McCurdy, R. F. Clinical and environmental aspects of arsenic toxicity. *CRC Crit. Rev. Clin. Lab. Sci.* 23:315, 1986.

that is not subject to regulation will catalyze a **"near-equilibrium reaction,"** whereas a regulatory enzyme will catalyze a **"nonequilibrium reaction"** under intracellular conditions. This makes sense because flux through the regulated enzyme is restricted by controls imposed on that enzyme. A nonregulatory enzyme is so active that it readily brings its substrates and products to equilibrium concentrations. Whether an enzyme-catalyzed reaction is near equilibrium or nonequilibrium can be determined by comparing the established equilibrium constant for the reaction with the mass–action ratio as it exists within a cell. The **equilibrium constant** for the reaction A + B ⇌ C + D is defined as

$$K_{eq} = \frac{[C][D]}{[A][B]}$$

where the brackets indicate the concentrations at equilibrium. The **mass–action ratio** is calculated in a similar manner, except that the steady-state (ss) concentrations of reactants and products within the cell are used in the equation:

$$\text{Mass–action ratio} = \frac{[C]_{ss}[D]_{ss}}{[A]_{ss}[B]_{ss}}$$

If the mass–action ratio is approximately equal to the K_{eq}, the enzyme is said to be active enough to catalyze a near-equilibrium reaction and the enzyme is not considered subject to regulation. When the mass–action ratio is considerably different from the K_{eq}, the enzyme is said to catalyze a nonequilibrium reaction and usually will be found subject to regulation by one or more mechanisms. Mass–action ratios and equilibrium constants are compared for the glycolytic enzymes of liver in Table 7.1. The reactions catalyzed by **glucokinase** (liver isoenzyme of hexokinase), 6-phosphofructo-1-kinase, and pyruvate kinase in the intact liver are considered far enough from equilibrium to indicate that these enzymes are "regulatory" in this tissue.

Hexokinase and Glucokinase Have Different Properties

Different isoenzymes of **hexokinase** occur in different tissues. The hexokinase isoenzymes found in most tissues have a low K_m for glucose (<0.1 mM) relative

TABLE 7.1 Apparent Equilibrium Constants and Mass–Action Ratios for the Reactions of Glycolysis and Gluconeogenesis in Liver

	Reaction in the Pathway of		*Apparent Equilibrium*		*Considered Near-Equilibrium*
Reaction Catalyzed by	***Glycolysis***	***Gluconeogenesis***	***Constant*** (K'_{eq})	***Mass–Action Ratios***	***Reaction?***
Glucokinase	Yes	No	2×10^3	0.02	No
Glucose 6-phosphatase	No	Yes	850 M	120 M	No
Phosphoglucoisomerase	Yes	Yes	0.36	0.31	Yes
6-Phosphofructo-1-kinase	Yes	No	1×10^3	0.09	No
Fructose 1,6-bisphosphatase	No	Yes	530 M	19 M	No
Aldolase	Yes	Yes	13×10^{-5} M	12×10^{-7} M	Yes[a]
Glyceraldehyde-3-phosphate dehydrogenase + phosphoglycerate kinase	Yes	Yes	2×10^3 M^{-1}	0.6×10^3 M^{-1}	Yes
Phosphoglycerate mutase	Yes	Yes	0.1	0.1	Yes
Enolase	Yes	Yes	3.0	2.9	Yes
Pyruvate kinase	Yes	No	2×10^4	0.7	No
Pyruvate carboxylase + phosphoenolpyruvate carboxykinase	No	Yes	7.0 M	1×10^{-3} M	No

[a] Reaction catalyzed by aldolase appears to be out of equilibrium by two orders of magnitude. However, *in vivo* concentrations of fructose 1,6-micromolar bisphosphate and glyceraldehyde 3-phosphate are so low (micromolar concentration range) that significant enzyme binding of both metabolites is believed to occur. Although only the total concentration of any metabolite of a tissue can be measured, only that portion of the metabolite that is not bound should be used in the calculations of mass–action ratios. This is usually not possible, introducing uncertainty in the comparison of *in vitro* equilibrium constants to *in vivo* mass–action ratios.

CLINICAL CORRELATION 7.3

Fructose Intolerance

Patients with hereditary fructose intolerance are deficient in the liver aldolase responsible for splitting fructose 1-phosphate into dihydroxyacetone phosphate and glyceraldehyde. Consumption of fructose by these patients results in the accumulation of fructose 1-phosphate and depletion of P_i and ATP in the liver. The reactions involved are those catalyzed by fructokinase and the enzymes of oxidative phosphorylation:

Fructose + ATP → fructose 1-phosphate + ADP

ADP + P_i + "energy provided by electron transport chain" → ATP

Net: P_i + fructose → fructose 1-phosphate

Tying up P_i in the form of fructose 1-phosphate makes it impossible for liver mitochondria to generate ATP by oxidative phosphorylation. The ATP levels fall precipitously, making it also impossible for the liver to carry out its normal work functions. Damage results to the cells in large part because they are unable to maintain normal ion gradients by means of the ATP-dependent cation pumps. The cells swell and eventually lose their internal contents by osmotic lysis (see Clin. Corr. 6.6).

Although patients with fructose intolerance are particularly sensitive to fructose, humans in general have a limited capacity to handle this sugar. The capacity of the normal liver to phosphorylate fructose greatly exceeds its capacity to split fructose 1-phosphate. This means that fructose use by the liver is poorly controlled and that excessive fructose could deplete the liver of P_i and ATP. Fructose was actually tried briefly in hospitals as a substitute for glucose in patients being maintained by parenteral nutrition. The rationale was that fructose would be a better source of calories than glucose because fructose utilization is relatively independent of the insulin status of a patient. Delivery of large amounts of fructose by intravenous feeding was soon found to result in severe liver damage. Similar attempts have been made to substitute sorbitol and xylitol for glucose. These sugars also tend to deplete the liver of ATP and, like fructose, should not be used for parenteral nutrition.

Gitzelmann, R., Steinmann, B., and Van den Berghe, G. Disorders of fructose metabolism. In: C. R. Scriver, A. L. Beaudet, W. S. Sly, and D. Valle (Eds.), *The Metabolic and Molecular Bases of Inherited Disease,* 7th ed. New York: McGraw-Hill, 1995, pp. 905–934.

to its concentration in blood (~5 mM) and are strongly inhibited by the product of the reaction, glucose 6-phosphate. The latter is an important regulatory feature because it prevents hexokinase from tying up all of the P_i of a cell in the form of phosphorylated hexoses (see Clin. Corr. 7.3). Thus the reaction catalyzed by hexokinase may not be at equilibrium within cells that contain this enzyme because of the inhibition imposed by G6P. Liver parenchymal cells are unique in that they contain glucokinase, an isoenzyme of hexokinase with strikingly different kinetic properties from the other hexokinases. This isoenzyme catalyzes an ATP-dependent phosphorylation of glucose but has a much higher K_m for glucose and is not subject to product inhibition by G6P. It is, however, inhibited by fructose 6-phosphate and activated by fructose 1-phosphate. These effects depend on an inhibitory protein that inhibits by binding tightly to glucokinase. Fructose 6-phosphate promotes but fructose 1-phosphate inhibits binding of the inhibitory protein to glucokinase. The high K_m of glucokinase for glucose contributes to the capacity of the liver to "buffer" blood glucose levels. Glucose equilibrates readily across the plasma membrane of the liver on the glucose transport protein GLUT-2, the concentration of glucose within the liver reflecting that of the blood. Since the K_m of glucokinase for glucose (~10 mM) is considerably greater than normal blood glucose concentrations (~5 mM), any increase in glucose concentration leads to a proportional increase in the rate of glucose phosphorylation by glucokinase (Figure 7.14). Likewise, any decrease in glucose concentration leads to a proportional decrease in the rate of glucose phosphorylation. Thus liver uses glucose at a significant rate only when blood glucose levels are greatly elevated. This buffering effect of liver glucokinase on blood glucose levels would not occur if glucokinase had the low K_m for glucose characteristic of other hexokinases and was therefore completely saturated at physiological concentrations of glucose (Figure 7.14). On the other hand, a low K_m form of hexokinase is a good choice for tissues such as the brain in that it allows phosphorylation of glucose even when blood and tissue glucose concentrations are dangerously low.

The reaction catalyzed by glucokinase is not at equilibrium under the intracellular conditions of liver cells (Table 7.1). Part of the explanation lies in the rate restriction imposed by the high K_m of glucokinase for glucose and part

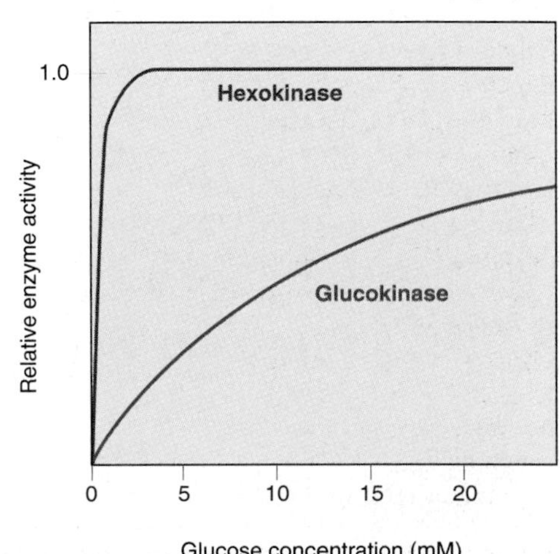

FIGURE 7.14
Comparison of the substrate saturation curves for hexokinase and glucokinase.

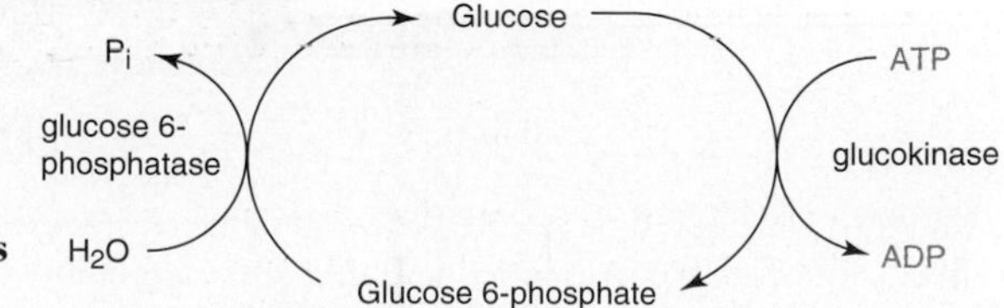

FIGURE 7.15
Phosphorylation of glucose followed by dephosphorylation constitutes a futile cycle in parenchymal cells of the liver.

is due to the inhibitory protein mentioned above. Yet another important factor is that the activity of glucokinase is opposed in liver by that of **glucose 6-phosphatase.** Like glucokinase, this enzyme has a high K_m (3 mM) with respect to the normal intracellular concentration (~0.2 mM) of its primary substrate, glucose 6-phosphate. Thus the flux through this step is almost directly proportional to the intracellular concentration of glucose 6-phosphate. As shown in Figure 7.15, the combined action of glucokinase and glucose 6-phosphatase constitutes a futile cycle; that is, the sum of their reactions is hydrolysis of ATP to give ADP and P_i without the performance of any work. When blood glucose concentrations are about 5 mM, the activity of glucokinase is almost exactly balanced by the opposing activity of glucose 6-phosphatase. The result is that no net flux occurs in either direction. This futile cycling between glucose and glucose 6-phosphate is wasteful of ATP but, combined with the process of gluconeogenesis, contributes significantly to the "buffering" action of the liver on blood glucose levels. Furthermore, it provides a mechanism for preventing glucokinase from tying up all of the P_i of the liver (see Clin. Corr. 7.3).

Fructose, a component of many vegetables, fruits, and sweeteners, promotes hepatic glucose utilization by an indirect mechanism. It is converted in liver to fructose 1-phosphate (see Clin. Corr. 7.3), which activates glucokinase activity by promoting dissociation of the inhibitory protein. This may be a factor in the adverse effects (e.g., **hypertriglyceridemia**) sometimes associated with excessive dietary fructose consumption.

Glucokinase is an inducible enzyme. Under various physiological conditions the amount of the enzyme protein increases or decreases. Induction of synthesis and repression of synthesis of an enzyme are relatively slow processes, usually requiring several hours before significant changes occur. **Insulin** increases the amount of glucokinase by promoting transcription of the glucokinase gene. An increase in blood glucose levels signals an increase in insulin release from the β cells of the pancreas. This results in an increase in blood insulin levels, which promotes transcription of the glucokinase gene and increases the amount of liver glucokinase enzyme protein. Thus the amount of glucokinase in liver reflects how much glucose is being delivered to the liver via the portal vein. In other words, a person consuming large meals rich in carbohydrate will have greater amounts of glucokinase in the liver than one who is not. The liver in which glucokinase has been induced can make a greater contribution to the lowering of elevated blood glucose levels. The absence of insulin makes the liver of the diabetic patient deficient in glucokinase, in spite of high blood glucose levels, and this is one of the reasons why the liver of the diabetic has less blood glucose "buffering" action (see Clin. Corr. 7.4).

6-Phosphofructo-1-kinase Is the Major Regulatory Site

Evidence suggests that **6-phosphofructo-1-kinase** is the rate-limiting enzyme and most important regulatory site of glycolysis in most tissues. Usually we think of the first step of a pathway as the most logical choice for the rate-limiting step. However, the first committed step of a pathway is most appropriate for the site of the greatest degree of control, and 6-phosphofructo-1-kinase catalyzes the first committed step of the glycolytic pathway. The phosphoglucose isomerase catalyzed reaction is reversible, and most cells can use glucose

CLINICAL CORRELATION 7.4

Diabetes Mellitus

Diabetes mellitus is a chronic disease characterized by derangements in carbohydrate, fat, and protein metabolism. Two major types are recognized clinically—the juvenile-onset or insulin-dependent type (see Clin. Corr. 14.7) and the maturity-onset or insulin-independent type (see Clin. Corr. 14.8).

In patients who do not have fasting hyperglycemia, the oral glucose tolerance test can be used for the diagnosis of diabetes. It consists of determining the blood glucose level in the fasting state and at intervals of 30–60 min for 2 h or more after consuming a 100-g carbohydrate meal. In a normal individual blood glucose returns to normal levels within 2 h after ingestion of the carbohydrate meal. In the diabetic patient, blood glucose will reach a higher level and remain elevated for longer periods of time, depending on the severity of the disease. However, many factors may contribute to an abnormal glucose tolerance test. The patient must have consumed a high carbohydrate diet for the preceding 3 days, presumably to allow for induction of enzymes of glucose-utilizing pathways, for example, glucokinase, fatty acid synthase, and acetyl-CoA carboxylase. In addition, almost any infection (even a cold) and less well-defined "stress" (presumably by effects on the sympathetic nervous system) can result in (transient) abnormalities of the glucose tolerance test. Because of problems with the glucose tolerance test, elevation of the fasting glucose level should probably be the *sine qua non* for the diagnosis of diabetes. Glucose uptake by cells of insulin-sensitive tissues, that is, muscle and adipose, is decreased in the diabetic state. Insulin is required for glucose uptake by these tissues, and the diabetic patient either lacks insulin or has developed "insulin resistance" in these tissues. Resistance to insulin is an abnormality of the insulin receptor or in subsequent steps mediating the metabolic effects of insulin. Parenchymal cells of the liver do not require insulin for glucose uptake. Without insulin, however, the liver has diminished enzymatic capacity to remove glucose from the blood. This is explained in part by decreased glucokinase activity plus the loss of insulin's action on key enzymes of glycogenesis and the glycolytic pathway.

Taylor, S. I. Diabetes mellitus. In: C. R. Scriver, A. L. Beaudet, W. S. Sly, and D. Valle (Eds), *The Metabolic and Molecular Bases of Inherited Disease,* 7th ed. New York: McGraw-Hill, 1995, pp. 843–896.

6-phosphate for glycogen synthesis and in the pentose phosphate pathway. The reaction catalyzed by 6-phosphofructo-1-kinase commits the cell to the metabolism of glucose by glycolysis and is therefore a logical site for the step of the pathway that is rate limiting and subject to the greatest degree of regulation by allosteric effectors. Citrate, ATP, and hydrogen ions (low pH) are the most important negative allosteric effectors, whereas **AMP** and **fructose 2,6-bisphosphate** are the most important positive allosteric effectors (Figure 7.13). Through their actions as strong inhibitors or activators of 6-phosphofructo-1-kinase, these compounds signal different rates of glycolysis in response to changes in (1) energy state of the cell (ATP and AMP), (2) internal environment of the cell (hydrogen ions), (3) availability of alternate fuels such as fatty acids and ketone bodies (citrate), and (4) insulin/glucagon ratio in the blood (fructose 2,6-bisphosphate). Evidence for the physiological importance of these effectors comes in part from application of the crossover theorem to the glycolytic pathway.

Crossover Theorem Explains Regulation of 6-Phosphofructo-1-kinase by ATP and AMP

For the hypothetical pathway $A \rightarrow B \rightarrow C \rightarrow D \rightarrow E \rightarrow F \rightarrow$, the **crossover theorem** proposes that an inhibitor that partially inhibits conversion of C to D will cause a "crossover" in the metabolite profile between C and D. Thus when the steady-state concentrations of intermediates in the presence and absence of an inhibitor are compared, the concentrations of intermediates before the site of inhibition should increase in response to the inhibitor, whereas those after the site should decrease. Crossover plots are constructed by setting the concentrations of all intermediates without some effector of the pathway equal to 100%. Concentrations of intermediates observed in the presence of the effector are then expressed as percentages of these values. The expected result with a negative effector is shown in Figure 7.16*a*. The effect of returning the perfused rat heart from an anoxic condition to a well-oxygenated state is also shown (Figure 7.16*b*). This transition with the perfused rat heart is known to

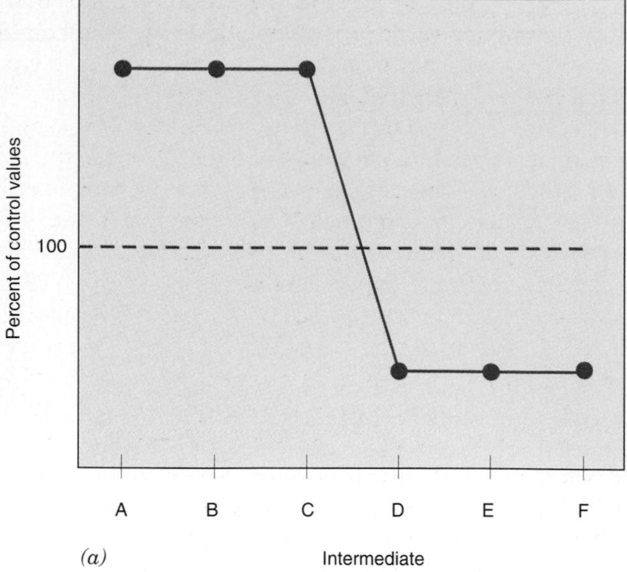

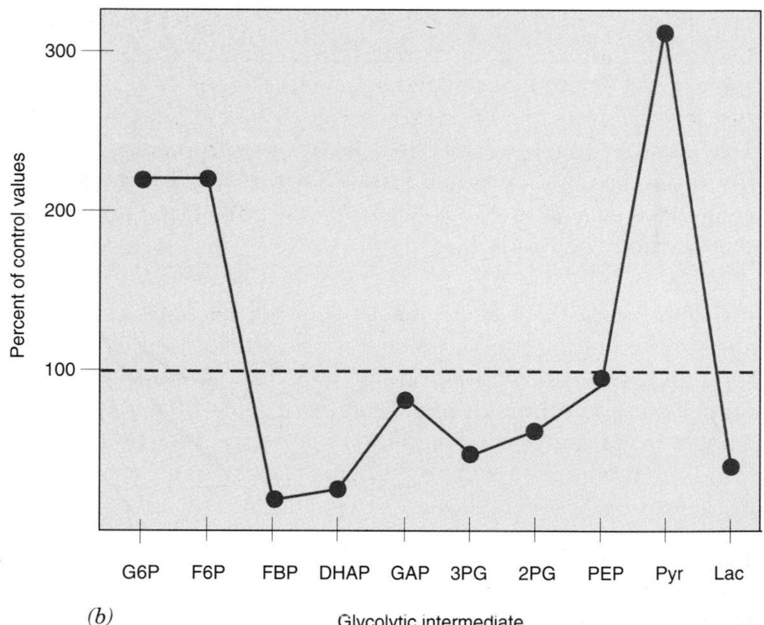

FIGURE 7.16
Crossover analysis is used to locate sites of regulation of a metabolic pathway.
(*a*) Theoretical effect of an inhibitor of the C to D step in the pathway of A → B → C → D → E → F →. Steady-state concentrations of all intermediates of the pathway without the inhibitor present are arbitrarily set equal to 100%. Steady-state concentrations of all intermediates when the inhibitor is present are then expressed as percentages of the control values. (*b*) Effect of oxygen on the relative steady-state concentrations of the intermediates of the glycolytic pathway in the perfused rat heart. The changes in concentrations of metabolites caused by perfusion with oxygen are recorded as percentages of anoxic values. Oxygen strongly inhibits glucose utilization and lactate production under such conditions. The dramatic increase in pyruvate concentration occurs as a consequence of greatly increased utilization of cytosolic NADH by the shuttle systems. Abbreviations: G6P, glucose 6-phosphate; F6P, fructose 6-phosphate; FBP, fructose 1,6-bisphosphate; DHAP, dihydroxyacetone phosphate; GAP, glyceraldehyde 3-phosphate; 3PG, 3-phosphoglycerate; 2PG, 2-phosphoglycerate; PEP, phosphoenolpyruvate; Pyr, pyruvate; Lac, lactate.
Redrawn with permission from Williamson, J. R. J. Biol. Chem. *241:5026, 1966. © The American Society of Biological Chemists, Inc.*

establish new steady-state concentrations of glycolytic intermediates, the flux being much greater through the glycolytic pathway in the absence of oxygen. Under the experimental conditions used, perfused hearts consumed glucose at rates some 20 times greater in the absence than in the presence of oxygen. This illustrates what is known as the **Pasteur effect,** defined as the inhibition of glucose utilization and lactate accumulation by the initiation of respiration (oxygen consumption). This is readily understandable on a thermodynamic basis, the complete oxidation of glucose to CO_2 and H_2O yielding much more ATP than anaerobic glycolysis:

Glycolysis: $\text{D-Glucose} + 2\,ADP^{3-} + 2\,P_i^{2-} \rightarrow 2\,\text{L-lactate}^- + 2\,ATP^{4-}$

Complete oxidation: $\text{D-Glucose} + 6\,O_2 + 38\,ADP^{3-} + 38\,P_i^{2-} + 38\,H^+ \rightarrow 6\,CO_2 + 6\,H_2O + 38\,ATP^{4-}$

ATP is used by a cell only to meet its metabolic demand, that is, to provide the necessary energy for work processes inherent to that cell. Since so much more ATP is produced from glucose in the presence of oxygen, much less glucose is consumed to meet the metabolic demand of the cell. The "crossover" at the conversion of fructose 6-phosphate to fructose 1,6-bisphosphate argues that oxygen imposes an inhibition at the level of 6-phosphofructo-1-kinase. This can readily be rationalized since **ATP** is a well-recognized inhibitor of 6-phosphofructo-1-kinase, and more ATP is generated in the presence than in the absence of oxygen. However, ATP levels do not change greatly between these two conditions (in the experiment of Figure 7.16*b*, ATP increased from 4.7 μmol/g of wet weight in the absence of oxygen to 5.6 μmol/g of wet weight in the presence of oxygen). Since 6-phosphofructo-1-kinase is severely inhibited at concentrations of ATP (2.5–6 mM) normally present in cells, such a small difference in ATP concentration cannot account completely for the change in flux through 6-phosphofructo-1-kinase. However, much greater changes, percentage wise, occur in the concentrations of **AMP,** a positive allosteric effector of 6-phosphofructo-1-kinase. The change that occurs in steady-state concentrations of AMP when oxygen is introduced into the system is exactly what might have been predicted; that is, the level goes down dramatically. This results in less 6-phosphofructo-1-kinase activity. This greatly suppresses glycolysis and accounts in part for the Pasteur effect. Levels of AMP automatically go down in a cell when ATP levels increase. The reason is simple. The sum of the adenine nucleotides in a cell, that is, ATP + ADP + AMP, is nearly constant under most physiological conditions, but the relative concentrations are such that the ATP concentration is always much greater than the AMP concentration. Furthermore, adenine nucleotides are maintained in equilibrium in the cytosol through action of **adenylate kinase** (also referred to as **myokinase**), which catalyzes the reaction 2ADP $\rightleftharpoons$ ATP + AMP. The equilibrium constant (K'_{eq}) for this reaction is given by

$$K'_{eq} = \frac{[\mathrm{ATP}][\mathrm{AMP}]}{[\mathrm{ADP}]^2}$$

Since this reaction is "near equilibrium" under intracellular conditions, the concentration of AMP is given by

$$[\mathrm{AMP}] = \frac{K'_{eq}[\mathrm{ADP}]^2}{[\mathrm{ATP}]}$$

Because intracellular [ATP] $\gg$ [ADP] $\gg$ [AMP], a small decrease in [ATP] causes a substantially greater percentage increase in [ADP]; and, since [AMP] is related to the square of [ADP], an even greater percentage increase in [AMP]. Because of this relationship, a small decrease in ATP concentration leads to a greater percent increase in [AMP] than in the percent decrease in [ATP]. This makes the [AMP] an excellent signal of the energy status of the cell and allows it to function as an important allosteric effector of 6-phosphofructo-1-kinase activity. Furthermore, [AMP] influences in yet another way the effectiveness of 6-phosphofructo-1-kinase. The enzyme **fructose 1,6-bisphosphatase** catalyzes an irreversible reaction, which opposes that of 6-phosphofructo-1-kinase:

$$\text{Fructose 1,6-bisphosphate} + H_2O \rightarrow \text{fructose 6-phosphate} + P_i$$

This enzyme sits "cheek by jowl" with 6-phosphofructo-1-kinase in the cytosol of many cells. Together they catalyze a futile cycle (ATP $\rightarrow$ ADP + P_i + "heat"), and, at the very least, they decrease "effectiveness" of one another. AMP concentration is a perfect signal of the energy status of the cell— not only because AMP activates 6-phosphofructo-1-kinase but also because AMP inhibits fructose 1,6-bisphosphatase. Thus a small decrease in ATP concentration triggers, via the increase in AMP concentration, a large increase in net conversion of fructose 6-phosphate into fructose 1,6-bisphosphate. This increases glycolytic flux by increasing the amount of substrate available for the splitting stage. In cells containing hexokinase, it also results in greater phosphorylation of glucose because a decrease in fructose 6-phosphate automatically causes a decrease in glucose 6-phosphate, which in turn results in less inhibition of hexokinase.

The decrease in lactate production in response to onset of respiration is another feature of the Pasteur effect that can readily be explained. The most important factor is decreased glycolytic flux caused by oxygen. Other factors include competition between lactate dehydrogenase and mitochondrial pyruvate dehydrogenase complex for pyruvate, as well as competition between lactate dehydrogenase and shuttle systems for NADH. For the most part, lactate dehydrogenase loses the competition in the presence of oxygen.

Intracellular pH Can Regulate 6-Phosphofructo-1-kinase

It would make sense that lactate, as the end product of glycolysis, should inhibit the rate-limiting enzyme of glycolysis. It does not. However, **hydrogen ions,** the other glycolytic end product, do inhibit 6-phosphofructo-1-kinase. As shown in Figure 7.17, glycolysis in effect generates **lactic acid,** and the cell must dispose of it as such. This explains why excessive glycolysis in the body lowers blood pH and leads to an emergency medical situation termed **lactic acidosis** (see Clin. Corr. 7.5). Plasma membranes of cells contain a symport for lactate and hydrogen ions. That allows release of lactic acid into the bloodstream. This is a defense mechanism, preventing pH from getting so low that everything becomes pickled (see Clin. Corr. 7.6). The sensitivity of 6-phosphofructo-1-kinase to hydrogen ions is also part of this mechanism. Hydrogen ions are able to shut off glycolysis, the process responsible for decreasing pH. Transport of lactic acid out of a cell requires that blood be available to carry it away. When

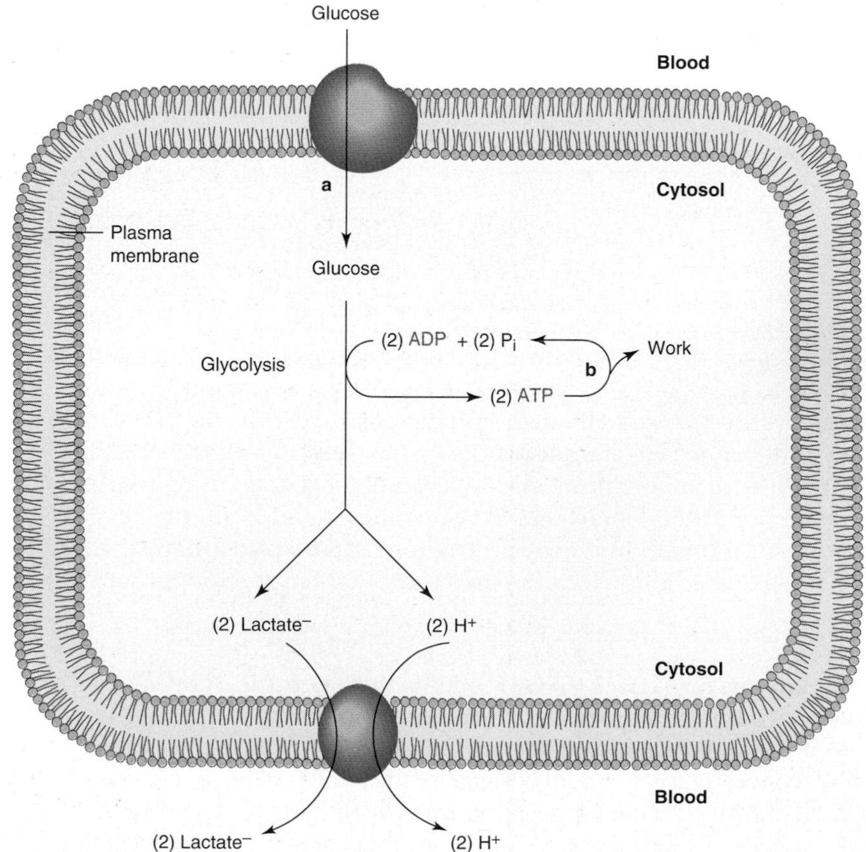

FIGURE 7.17
Unless lactate formed by glycolysis is transported out of the cell, the intracellular pH will be decreased by the accumulation of intracellular lactic acid.
The low pH decreases 6-phosphofructo-1-kinase activity so that further lactic acid production by glycolysis is shut off. (*a*) Glucose transport into the cell. (*b*) All work performances that convert ATP back to ADP and P_i. (*c*) Lactate–hydrogen ion symport (actual stoichiometry of one lactate$^-$ and one H^+ transported by the symport).

CLINICAL CORRELATION 7.5

Lactic Acidosis

This problem is characterized by elevated blood lactate levels, usually greater than 5 mM, along with decreased blood pH and bicarbonate concentrations. Lactic acidosis is the most commonly encountered form of metabolic acidosis and can be the consequence of overproduction of lactate, underutilization of lactate, or both. Lactate production is normally balanced by lactate utilization, with the result that lactate is usually not present in the blood at concentrations greater than 1.2 mM. All tissues of the body have the capacity to produce lactate by anaerobic glycolysis, but most tissues do not produce large quantities because much more ATP can be gained by the complete oxidation of the pyruvate produced by glycolysis. However, all tissues respond with an increase in lactate generation when oxygenation is inadequate. A decrease in ATP resulting from reduced oxidative phosphorylation allows the activity of 6-phosphofructo-1-kinase to increase. These tissues have to rely on anaerobic glycolysis for ATP production under such conditions and this results in lactic acid production. A good example is muscle exercise, which can deplete the tissue of oxygen and cause an overproduction of lactic acid. Tissue hypoxia occurs, however, in all forms of shock, during convulsions, and in diseases involving circulatory and pulmonary failure.

The major fate of lactate in the body is either complete combustion to CO_2 and H_2O or conversion back to glucose by the process of gluconeogenesis. Both require oxygen. Decreased oxygen availability therefore increases lactate production and decreases lactate utilization. The latter can also be decreased by liver diseases, ethanol, and a number of other drugs. Phenformin, a drug that was once used to treat the hyperglycemia of insulin-independent diabetes, was well-documented to induce lactic acidosis in certain patients.

Bicarbonate is usually administered in an attempt to control the acidosis associated with lactic acid accumulation. The key to successful treatment, however, is to find and eliminate the cause of the overproduction and/or underutilization of lactic acid and most often involves the restoration of circulation of oxygenated blood.

Newsholme, E. A., and Leech, A. R. *Biochemistry for the Medical Sciences*. New York: Wiley, 1983; and Kruse, J. A., and Carlson, R. W. Lactate metabolism. *Crit. Care Clin.* 3:725, 1985.

blood flow is inadequate, for example, in heavy exercise of a skeletal muscle or an attack of **angina pectoris** in the case of the heart, hydrogen ions cannot escape from cells fast enough. Yet, the need for ATP within such cells, because of lack of oxygen, may partially override inhibition of 6-phosphofructo-1-kinase by hydrogen ions. Unabated accumulation of hydrogen ions then results in pain, which, in the case of skeletal muscle, can be relieved by simply terminating

CLINICAL CORRELATION 7.6

Pickled Pigs and Malignant Hyperthermia

In patients with malignant hyperthermia, a variety of agents, especially the widely used general anesthetic halothane, will produce a dramatic rise in body temperature, metabolic and respiratory acidosis, hyperkalemia, and muscle rigidity. This gentic abnormality occurs in about 1 in 15,000 children and 1 in 50,000–100,000 adults. It is dominantly inherited. Death may result the first time a susceptible person is anesthetized. Onset occurs within minutes of drug exposure and the hyperthermia must be recognized immediately. Packing the patient in ice is effective and should be accompanied by measures to combat acidosis. The drug dantrolene is also effective.

A phenomenon similar, if not identical, to malignant hyperthermia is known to occur in pigs. Pigs with this problem, called porcine stress syndrome, respond poorly to stress. This genetic disease usually manifests itself as the pig is being shipped to market. Pigs with the syndrome can be identified by exposure to halothane, which triggers the same response seen in patients with malignant hyperthermia. The meat of pigs that have died as a result of the syndrome is pale, watery, and of very low pH (i.e., nearly pickled).

Muscle is the site of the primary lesion in both malignant hyperthermia and porcine stress syndrome. In response to halothane the skeletal muscles become rigid and generate heat and lactic acid. The sarcoplasmic reticulum of such pigs and patients have a genetic abnormality in the ryanodine receptor, a Ca^{2+} release channel, that plays an important function in excitation–contraction coupling in muscle. Because of a defect in this protein, the anesthetic triggers inappropriate release of Ca^{2+} from the sarcoplasmic reticulum. This results in uncontrolled stimulation of a number of heat-producing processes, including myosin ATPase, glycogenolysis, glycolysis, and cyclic uptake and release of Ca^{2+} by mitochondria and sarcoplasmic reticulum. Muscle cells become irreversibly damaged as consequence of excessive heat production, lactic acidosis, and ATP loss.

Kalow, W., and Grant, D. M. Pharmacogenetics. In: C. R. Scriver, A. L. Beaudet, W. S. Sly, and D. Valle (Eds.), *The Metabolic and Molecular Bases of Inherited Disease,* 7th ed. New York: McGraw-Hill, 1995, pp. 293–326.

CLINICAL CORRELATION 7.7

Angina Pectoris and Myocardial Infarction

Chest pain associated with reversible myocardial ischemia is termed angina pectoris (literally, strangling pain in the chest). The pain is the result of an imbalance between demand for and supply of blood flow to cardiac muscles and is most commonly caused by narrowing of the coronary arteries. The patient experiences a heavy squeezing pressure or ache substernally, often radiating to either the shoulder and arm or occasionally to the jaw or neck. Attacks occur with exertion, last from 1 to 15 min, and are relieved by rest. The coronary arteries involved are obstructed by atherosclerosis (i.e., lined with characteristic fatty deposits) or less commonly narrowed by spasm. Myocardial infarction occurs if the ischemia persists long enough to cause severe damage (necrosis) to the heart muscle. Commonly, a blood clot forms at the site of narrowing and completely obstructs the vessel. In myocardial infarction, tissue death occurs and the characteristic pain is longer lasting, and often more severe.

Nitroglycerin and other nitrates are frequently prescribed to relieve the pain caused by the myocardial ischemia of angina pectoris. These drugs can be used prophylactically, enabling patients to participate in activities that would otherwise precipitate an attack of angina. Nitroglycerin may work in part by causing dilation of the coronary arteries, improving oxygen delivery to the heart and washing out lactic acid. Probably more important is the effect of nitroglycerin on the peripheral circulation. Breakdown of nitroglycerin produces nitric oxide (NO), a compound that relaxes smooth muscle, causing venodilation throughout the body. This reduces arterial pressure and allows blood to accumulate in the veins. The result is decreased return of blood to the heart, and a reduced volume of blood the heart has to pump, which reduces the energy requirement of the heart. In addition, the heart empties itself against less pressure, which also spares energy. The overall effect is a lowering of the oxygen requirement of the heart, bringing it in line with the oxygen supply via the diseased coronary arteries. Other useful agents are calcium channel blockers, which are coronary vasodilators, and β-adrenergic blockers. The β-blockers prevent the increase in myocardial oxygen consumption induced by sympathetic nervous system stimulation of the heart, as occurs with physical exertion.

The coronary artery bypass operation is used in severe cases of angina that cannot be controlled by medication. In this operation veins are removed from the leg and interposed between the aorta and coronary arteries of the heart. The purpose is to bypass the portion of the artery diseased by atherosclerosis and provide the affected tissue with a greater blood supply. Remarkable relief from angina can be achieved by this operation, with the patient being able to return to normal productive life in some cases.

Hugenholtz, P. G. Calcium antagonists for angina pectoris. *Ann. N.Y. Acad. Sci.* 522:565, 1988; Feelishch, M., and Noack, E. A. Correlation between nitric oxide formation during degradation of organic nitrates and activation of guanylate cyclase. *Eur. J. Pharmacol.* 139:19, 1987; and Ignarro, L. J. Biological actions and properties of endothelium-derived nitric oxide formed and released from artery and vein. *Circ. Res.* 65:1, 1989.

the exercise. In the case of the heart, rest or pharmacologic agents that increase blood flow or decrease the need for ATP within myocytes may be effective (see Clin. Corr. 7.7).

Intracellular Citrate Levels Regulate 6-Phosphofructo-1-kinase

Many tissues prefer to use fatty acids and ketone bodies as oxidizable fuels in place of glucose. Most of these tissues can use glucose but actually prefer to oxidize fatty acids and ketone bodies. This helps preserve glucose for tissues, such as brain, that are absolutely dependent on glucose as an energy source. Oxidation of both fatty acids and ketone bodies elevates levels of cytosolic **citrate,** which inhibits 6-phosphofructo-1-kinase. The result is decreased glucose utilization by the tissue when fatty acids or ketone bodies are available.

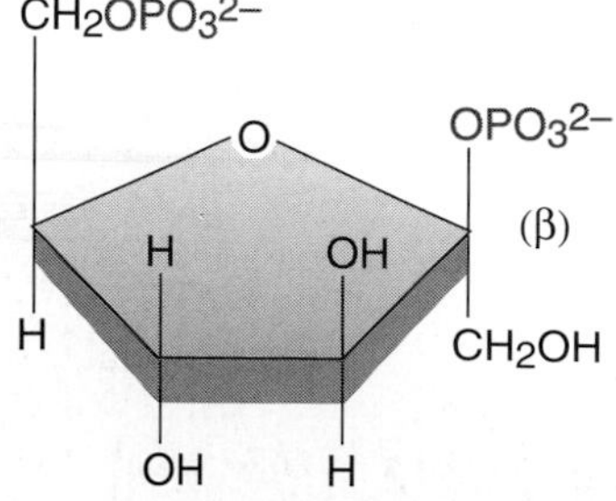

FIGURE 7.18
Structure of fructose 2,6-bisphosphate.

Hormonal Control of 6-Phosphofructo-1-kinase by cAMP and Fructose 2,6-bisphosphate

Fructose 2,6-bisphosphate (Figure 7.18), like AMP, functions as a positive allosteric effector of 6-phosphofructo-1-kinase and as a negative allosteric effector of fructose 1,6-bisphosphatase. Indeed, without the presence of this compound, glycolysis could not occur in liver because 6-phosphofructo-1-kinase would have insufficient activity and fructose 1,6-bisphosphatase would have too much activity for net conversion of fructose 6-phosphate to fructose 1,6-bisphosphate.

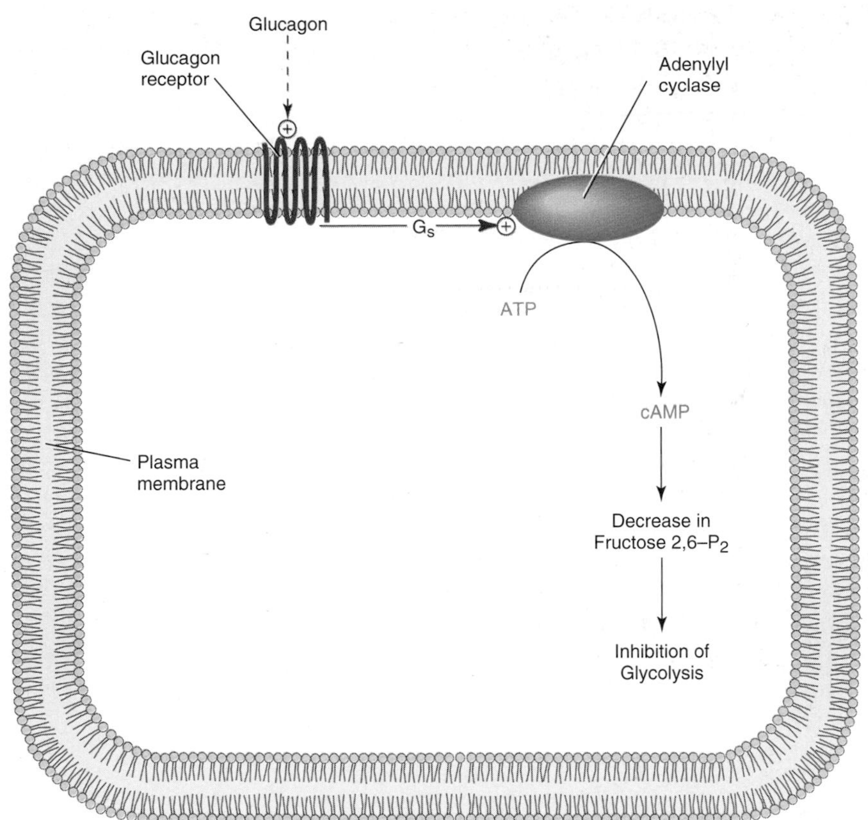

FIGURE 7.19
Overview of the mechanism responsible for glucagon inhibition of hepatic glycolysis. Binding of glucagon to its receptor (a protein that spans the membrane seven times) activates adenylate cyclase (an intrinsic membrane protein) activity through the action of a stimulatory G-protein (G_s). The (+) symbol indicates activation.

Figure 7.19 gives a brief overview of the role of fructose 2,6-bisphosphate in hormonal control of hepatic glycolysis. Understanding this mechanism requires an appreciation of the role of **cAMP** (Figure 7.20) as the "second messenger" of hormone action. As discussed in more detail in Chapters 14 and 20, **glucagon** is released from α cells of pancreas and circulates in blood until it comes in contact with glucagon receptors located on the outer surface of liver plasma membrane (Figure 7.19). Binding of glucagon to these receptors is sensed by **adenylate** (adenylyl) **cyclase,** an enzyme located on the inner surface of the plasma membrane, stimulating it to convert ATP into cAMP. Cyclic AMP triggers a series of intracellular events that result ultimately in a decrease in fructose 2,6-bisphosphate levels. A decrease in this compound makes 6-phosphofructo-1-kinase less effective but makes fructose 1,6-bisphosphatase more effective, thereby severely restricting flux from fructose 6-phosphate to fructose 1,6-bisphosphate in glycolysis.

Fructose 2,6-bisphosphate is not an intermediate of glycolysis. As shown in Figure 7.21, fructose 2,6-bisphosphate is produced from F6P by the enzyme **6-phosphofructo-2-kinase.** We now have two "phosphofructokinases" to contend with: one produces an intermediate (FBP) of glycolysis and the other

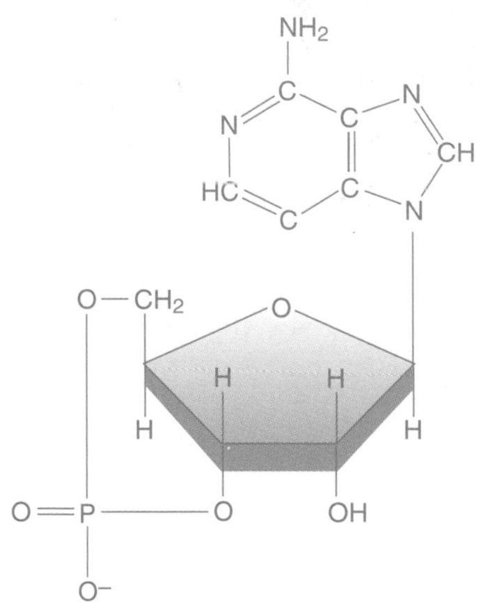

FIGURE 7.20
Structure of cAMP.

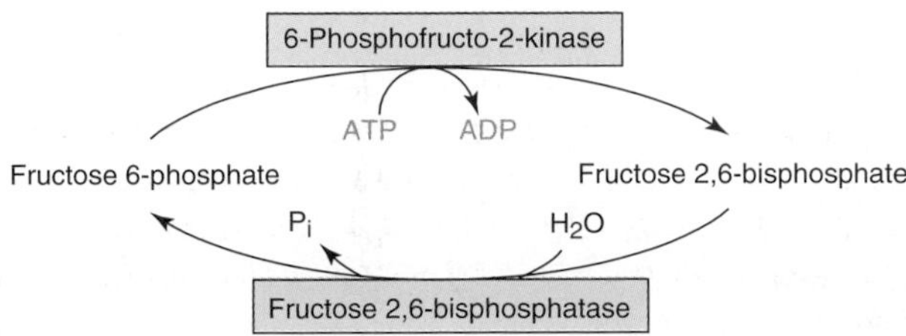

FIGURE 7.21
Reactions involved in the formation and degradation of fructose 2,6-bisphosphate.

produces a positive allosteric effector (fructose 2,6-bisphosphate) of the first enzyme. Fructose 2,6-bisphosphate can be destroyed by being converted back to F6P by fructose 2,6-bisphosphatase (Figure 7.21). This is a simple hydrolysis, with no ATP or ADP being involved. Synthesis and degradation of fructose 2,6-bisphosphate are catalyzed by a **bifunctional enzyme;** that is, 6-phosphofructo-2-kinase and fructose 2,6-bisphosphatase are part of the same protein. Because of its bifunctional nature, the combined name of 6-phosphofructo-2-kinase/fructose 2,6-bisphosphatase is used to refer to this enzyme that makes and degrades fructose 2,6-bisphosphate. cAMP regulates fructose 2,6-bisphosphate levels in liver. How is this possible when the same enzyme carries out both synthesis and degradation of the molecule? The answer is that a mechanism exists whereby cAMP inactivates the kinase function and, at the same time, activates the phosphatase function of this bifunctional enzyme.

cAMP Activates Protein Kinase A

Cyclic AMP activates **protein kinase A** (also called **cAMP-dependent protein kinase**). In its inactive state, this enzyme consists of two regulatory subunits plus two catalytic subunits. Binding of cAMP to regulatory subunits causes conformational changes with release of catalytic subunits, which are active only when dissociated from regulatory subunits. Liberated protein kinase then catalyzes phosphorylation of specific serine residues of several different enzymes (Figure 7.22).

Phosphorylation of an enzyme can conveniently be abbreviated as

$$\boxdot + \text{ATP} \rightarrow \odot\text{-P} + \text{ADP}$$

where $\boxdot$ and $\odot$-P are used to indicate dephosphorylated and phosphorylated enzymes, respectively. Circle and square symbols are used because **phosphorylation** of enzymes subject to regulation by covalent modification causes a change in their conformation, which affects the active site. The change in conformation due to phosphorylation increases catalytic activity of some enzymes but decreases catalytic activity of others. Direction of change in activity depends on the enzyme involved. Many enzymes are subject to this type of regulation, an important type of **covalent modification.** Regardless of whether phosphorylation or dephosphorylation activates the enzyme, the active form of the enzyme is called the *a* form and the inactive form the *b* form. Likewise, regardless of the effect of phosphorylation on catalytic activity, the action of a protein kinase is always opposed by that of a phosphoprotein phosphatase, which catalyzes the reaction of

$$\odot\text{-P} + H_2O \rightarrow \boxdot + P_i$$

Putting these together creates a **cyclic control system** (see Figure 7.23), such that the ratio of phosphorylated enzyme to dephosphorylated enzyme is a function of the relative activities of protein kinase and phosphoprotein phosphatase. If the kinase has greater activity than the phosphatase, more enzyme will be in the phosphorylated mode, and vice versa. Since activity of an interconvertible enzyme (i.e., an enzyme subject to covalent modification) is determined by whether it is in the phosphorylated or dephosphorylated mode, the relative

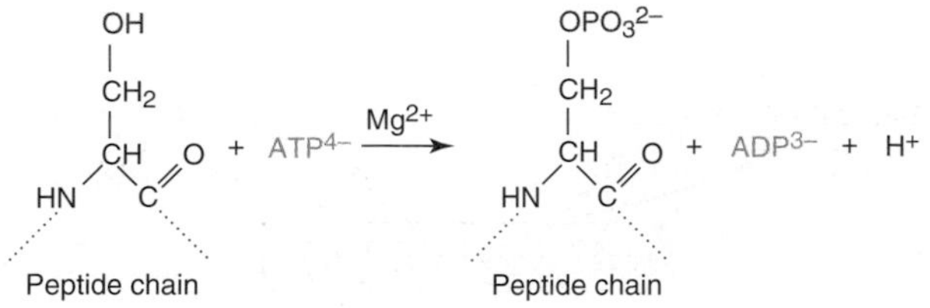

FIGURE 7.22
Enzymes subject to covalent modification are usually phosphorylated on specific serine residues.
Tyrosine and threonine residues are also important sites of covalent modification by phosphorylation.

activities of kinase and phosphatase determine the amount of a particular enzyme that is in the catalytically active state.

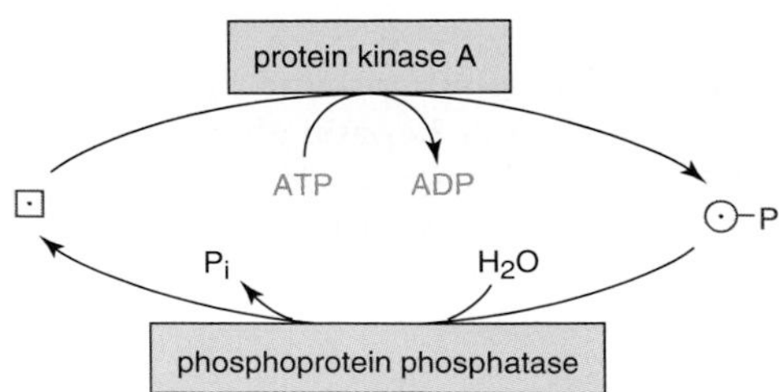

FIGURE 7.23
General model of the mechanism responsible for regulation of enzymes by phosphorylation–dephosphorylation.
The symbols ⊡ and ⊙-P indicate that different conformational and activity states of the enzyme are produced as a result of phosphorylation–dephosphorylation.

6-Phosphofructo-2-kinase and Fructose 2,6-bisphosphatase Are Domains of a Bifunctional Polypeptide Regulated by Phosphorylation–Dephosphorylation

Most enzymes are either turned on or off by phosphorylation but with **6-phosphofructo-2-kinase** and **fructose 2,6-bisphosphatase,** advantage is taken of the bifunctional nature of the enzyme. In the case of the isoenzyme present in liver, phosphorylation causes inactivation of the active site responsible for synthesis of fructose 2,6-bisphosphate but activation of the active site responsible for hydrolysis of fructose 2,6-bisphosphate (Figure 7.24). Dephosphorylation of the enzyme has the opposite effects. A sensitive mechanism has therefore evolved to set the intracellular concentration of **fructose 2,6-bisphosphate** in liver cells in response to changes in blood levels of **glucagon** or **epinephrine** (Figure 7.25). Increased levels of glucagon or epinephrine, acting through plasma membrane glucagon receptors and β-adrenergic receptors, respectively, have the common effect of inducing an increase in intracellular levels of **cAMP.** This second messenger activates **protein kinase A,** which phosphorylates a single serine residue of 6-phosphofructo-2-kinase/fructose 2,6-bisphosphatase (Figure 7.26). This inhibits fructose 2,6-bisphosphate synthesis and promotes its degradation. The resulting decrease in fructose 2,6-bisphosphate makes 6-phosphofructo-1-kinase less effective and fructose 1,6-bisphosphatase more effective. The result is inhibition of glycolysis at the level of the conversion of fructose 6-phosphate to fructose 1,6-bisphosphate. Decreased levels of either glucagon or epinephrine in blood result in less cAMP in liver because adenylate cyclase is less active and cAMP that had accumulated is converted to AMP by the action of **cAMP phosphodiesterase.** Loss of the cAMP signal results in inactivation of protein kinase A and a corresponding decrease in phosphorylation of 6-phosphofructo-2-kinase/fructose 2,6-bisphosphatase by protein kinase A. A **phosphoprotein phosphatase** removes phosphate from the bifunctional enzyme to produce active 6-phosphofructo-2-kinase and inactive fructose 2,6-bisphosphatase. Fructose 2,6-bisphosphate can now accumulate to a higher steady-state concentration and, by activating 6-phosphofructo-1-kinase and inhibiting fructose 1,6-bisphosphatase, greatly increases glycolysis. Thus glucagon and epinephrine are extracellular signals that stop liver from using glucose, whereas fructose 2,6-bisphosphate is an intracellular signal that promotes glucose utilization by this tissue.

Insulin opposes the actions of glucagon and epinephrine, but exactly how insulin works after binding to the plasma membrane remains a subject of intense investigation (see Chapter 20). There is evidence that insulin promotes formation of a second messenger, much as glucagon promotes formation of cAMP. Obvious enzyme targets that a second messenger might influence include cAMP phosphodiesterase, protein kinase A, and phosphoprotein phosphatase (Figure 7.27). There also is evidence, however, that insulin signals a cascade of events that depends upon activation of a number of protein kinases (see Chapter 20).

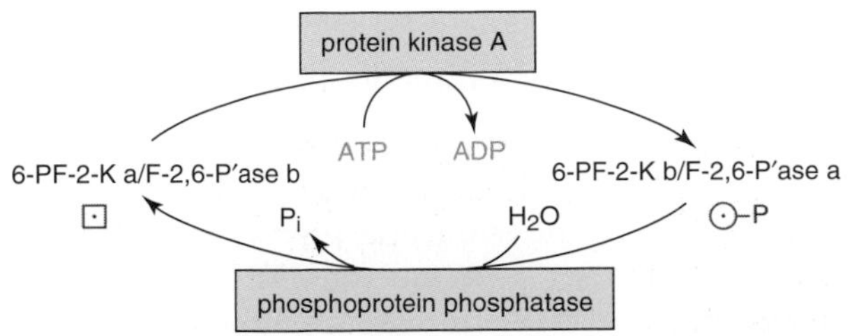

FIGURE 7.24
Mechanism responsible for covalent modification of the bifunctional enzyme 6-phosphofructo-2-kinase/fructose 2,6-bisphosphatase.
Name of the enzyme is abbreviated as 6-PF-2-K/F-2,6-P'ase. Letters *a* and *b* indicate the active and inactive forms of the enzymes, respectively.

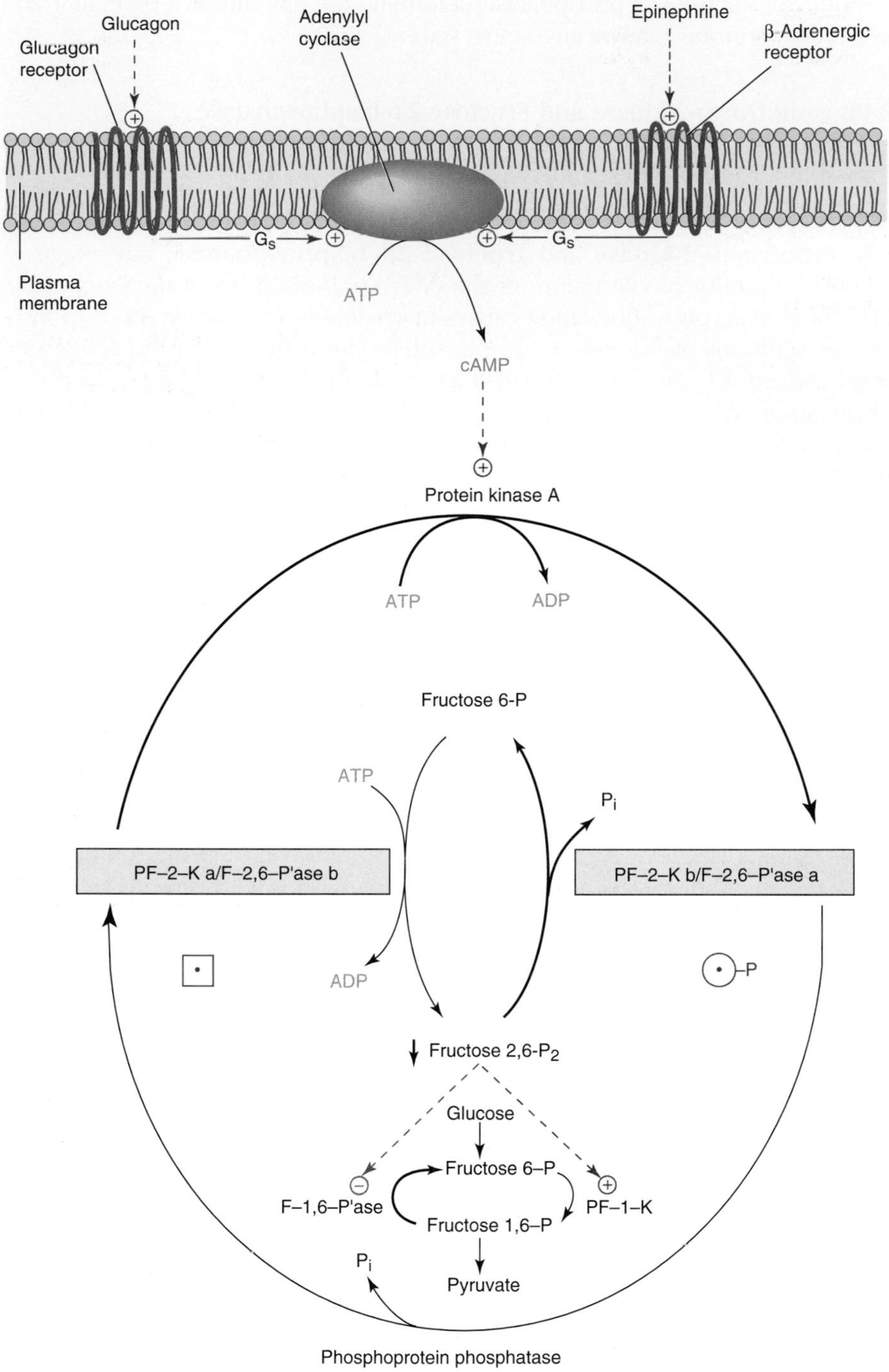

FIGURE 7.25
Mechanism of glucagon and epinephrine inhibition of hepatic glycolysis via cAMP-mediated decrease in fructose 2,6-bisphosphate concentration.
See legend for Figure 7.19. The heavy arrows indicate the reactions that predominate in the presence of glucagon. Small arrow before fructose 2,6-bisphosphate indicates a decrease in concentration of this compound.

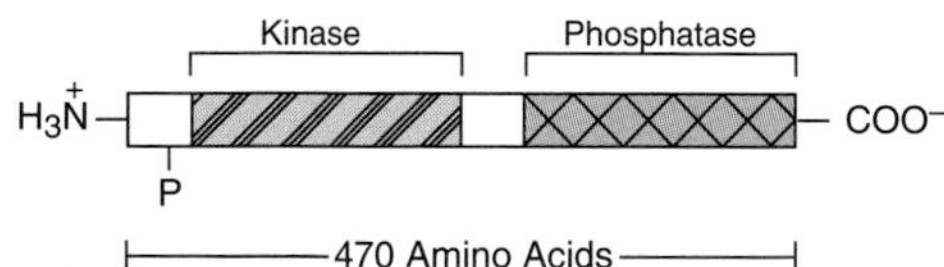

FIGURE 7.26
Schematic diagram of the primary structure of the liver isoenzyme of 6-phosphofructo-2-kinase/fructose-2,6-bisphosphatase.
NH_2 and CO_2H designate the N-terminal and C-terminal ends of the enzyme, respectively. Domain with kinase activity is located in the N-terminal half of the enzyme; domain with phosphatase activity in the C-terminal half of the enzyme. The letter P indicates the site (serine 32) phosphorylated by protein kinase A.

Regardless of its exact mechanism, insulin acts in the opposite direction from that of glucagon and epinephrine in determining the levels of fructose 2,6-bisphosphate in liver cells and, therefore, the rate of glycolysis.

Heart Contains a Different Isoenzyme of the Bifunctional Enzyme

An increase in blood level of **epinephrine** has a markedly different effect on glycolysis in **heart** from that in liver. Glycolysis is inhibited in liver to conserve glucose for use by other tissues. Epinephrine stimulates glycolysis in heart as part of a mechanism to meet the increased demand for ATP caused by an epinephrine-signaled increase in work load. As in liver, epinephrine acts on

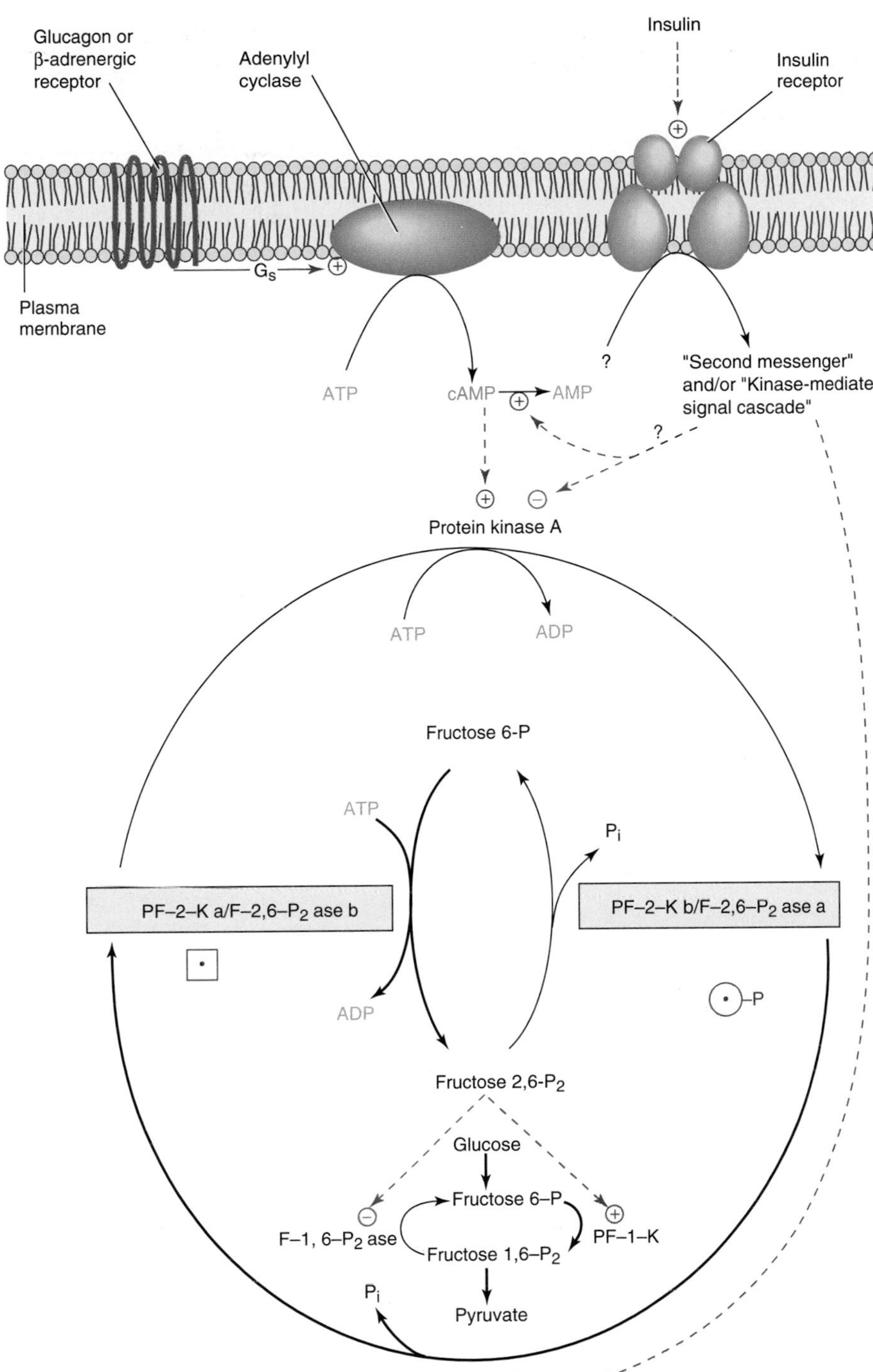

FIGURE 7.27
Mechanism responsible for accelerated rates of hepatic glycolysis when the concentration of glucagon and epinephrine are low and that of insulin is high in the blood.
See legends for Figures 7.19 and 7.25. The insulin receptor is an intrinsic component of the plasma membrane. Small arrow before fructose 2,6-bisphosphate indicates an increase in concentration. The question marks indicate that the details of the mechanism of action of insulin are unknown at this time.

the heart by way of a β-adrenergic receptor on the plasma membrane, promoting formation of cAMP by adenylate cyclase (Figure 7.28). This results in the activation of protein kinase A, which in turn phosphorylates 6-phosphofructo-2-kinase/fructose 2,6-bisphosphatase. In contrast, however, to what happens in liver, phosphorylation of the bifunctional enzyme in heart produces an increase rather than a decrease in fructose 2,6-bisphosphate levels. This is because heart expresses a different isoenzyme of the bifunctional enzyme. Although still a bifunctional enzyme that carries out exactly the same reactions as the liver enzyme, the amino acid sequence of the heart isoenzyme is different, and phosphorylation by protein kinase A occurs at a site that activates rather than inhibits 6-phosphofructo-2-kinase (Figure 7.29). Increased fructose 2,6-bisphos-

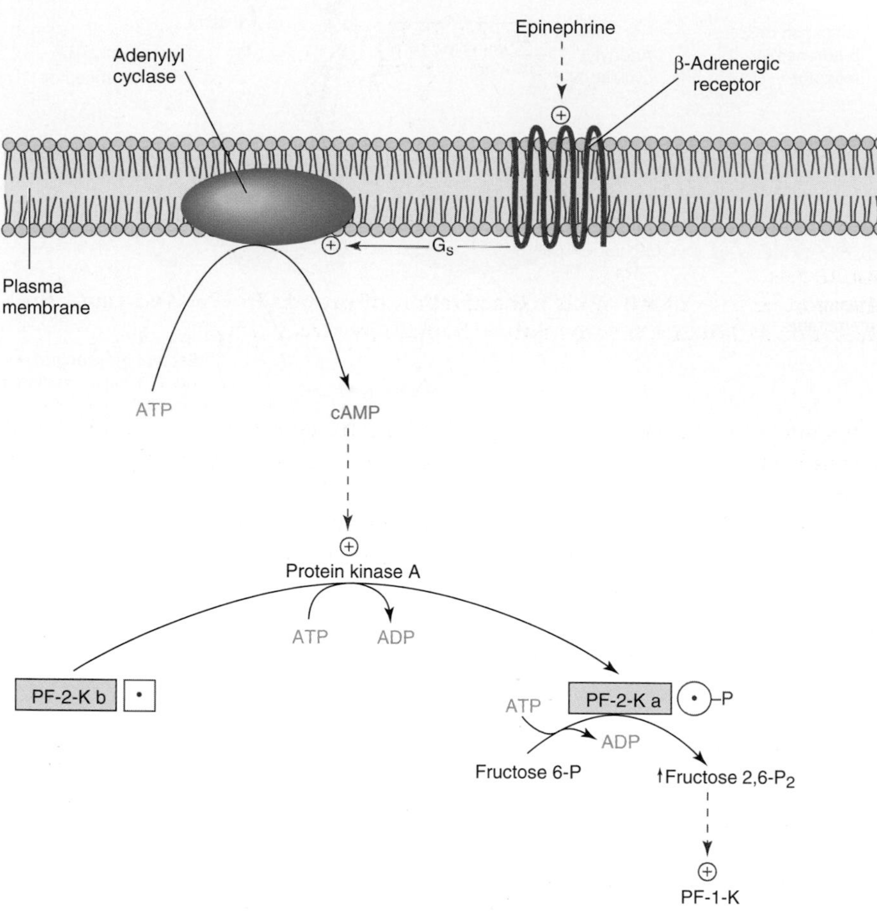

FIGURE 7.28
Mechanism responsible for accelerated rates of glycolysis in the heart in response to epinephrine.
See legends for Figures 7.19 and 7.27.

phate results in increased 6-phosphofructo-1-kinase activity and increased glycolytic flux in response to epinephrine in heart.

Pyruvate Kinase Is a Regulated Enzyme of Glycolysis

Pyruvate kinase is another regulatory enzyme of glycolysis (see Clin. Corr. 7.8). This enzyme is drastically inhibited by physiological concentrations of ATP, so much so that its potential activity is never fully realized under physiological conditions. The isoenzyme found in liver is greatly activated by fructose 1,6-bisphosphate, thereby linking regulation of pyruvate kinase to what is happening to 6-phosphofructo-1-kinase. Thus, if conditions favor increased flux through 6-phosphofructo-1-kinase, the level of FBP increases and acts as a feed-forward activator of pyruvate kinase. The liver enzyme is also subject to covalent modification, being active in the dephosphorylated state and inactive in the phosphorylated state (Figure 7.30); phosphorylation is catalyzed by protein kinase A in liver. Thus glucagon inhibition of hepatic glycolysis and stimulation

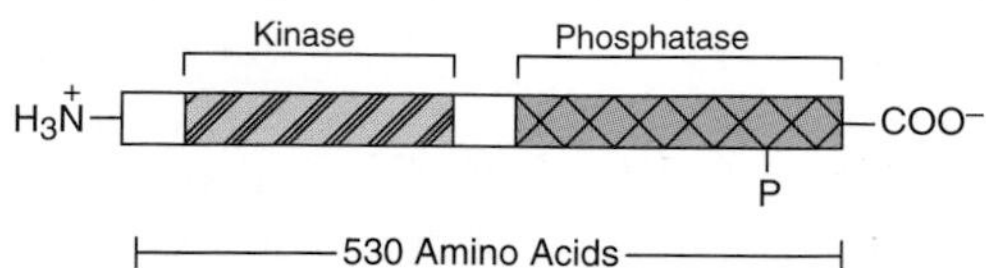

FIGURE 7.29
Schematic diagram of the primary structure of the heart isoenzyme of 6-phosphofructo-2-kinase/fructose 2,6-bisphosphatase that is present in the heart.
See legend for Figure 7.26. The letter P indicates the site (serine 466) phosphorylated by protein kinase A.

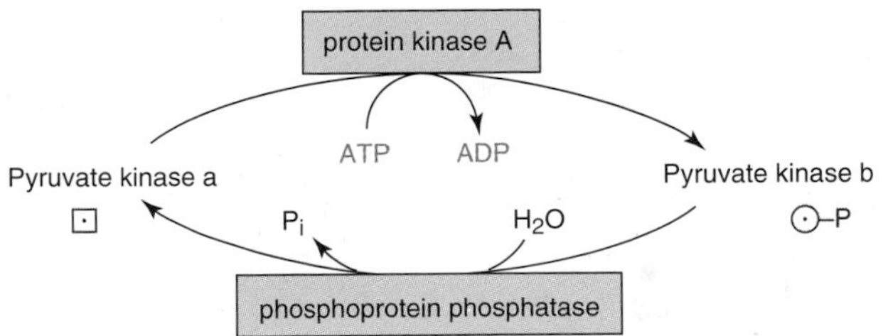

FIGURE 7.30
Glucagon acts via cAMP-mediated activation of protein kinase A to cause the phosphorylation and inactivation of hepatic pyruvate kinase.

of hepatic gluconeogenesis are explained in part by elevation of cAMP levels caused by this hormone. This aspect is explored more thoroughly in Section 7.5 in the discussion of gluconeogenesis.

Pyruvate kinase, like glucokinase, is induced to higher steady-state concentrations in liver by combination of high carbohydrate intake and high insulin levels. This increase in enzyme concentration is a major reason why liver of the well-fed individual has much greater capacity for utilizing carbohydrate than a fasting or diabetic person (see Clin. Corr. 7.4).

7.5 GLUCONEOGENESIS

Glucose Synthesis Is Required for Survival

Net synthesis or formation of glucose from various substrates is termed **gluconeogenesis.** This includes use of various amino acids, lactate, pyruvate, propionate, and glycerol, as sources of carbon for the pathway (see Figure 7.31). Glucose is also synthesized from galactose and fructose. **Glycogenolysis,** that is, formation of glucose or glucose 6-phosphate from glycogen, should be differentiated from gluconeogenesis; glycogenolysis refers to

$$\text{Glycogen or (glucose)}_n \rightarrow \text{molecules of glucose}$$

and thus does not correspond to *de novo* synthesis of glucose, the hallmark of the process of gluconeogenesis.

The capacity to synthesize glucose is crucial for survival of humans and other animals. Blood glucose levels have to be maintained to support metabolism of tissues that use glucose as their primary substrate (see Clin. Corr. 7.9). These include brain, red blood cells, kidney medulla, lens, cornea, testis, and a number of other tissues. Gluconeogenesis enables the maintenance of blood glucose levels long after all dietary glucose has been absorbed and completely oxidized.

The Cori and Alanine Cycles

Two important cycles between tissues that involve gluconeogenesis are recognized. The **Cori cycle** and the alanine cycle (Figure 7.32) depend on gluconeo-

CLINICAL CORRELATION 7.8

Pyruvate Kinase Deficiency and Hemolytic Anemia

Mature erythrocytes are absolutely dependent on glycolytic activity for ATP production. ATP is needed for the ion pumps, especially the Na^+,K^+–ATPase, which maintain the biconcave disk shape of erythrocytes, a characteristic that helps erythrocytes slip through the capillaries as they deliver oxygen to the tissues. Without ATP the cells swell and lyse. Anemia due to excessive erythrocyte destruction is referred to as hemolytic anemia. Pyruvate kinase deficiency is rare but is by far the most common genetic defect of the glycolytic pathway known to cause hemolytic anemia. Most pyruvate kinase-deficient patients have 5–25% of normal red blood cell pyruvate kinase levels and flux through the glycolytic pathway is restricted severely, resulting in markedly lower ATP concentrations. The expected crossover of the glycolytic intermediates is observed; that is, those intermediates proximal to the pyruvate kinase-catalyzed step accumulate, whereas pyruvate and lactate concentrations decrease. Normal ATP levels are observed in reticulocytes of patients with this disease. Although deficient in pyruvate kinase, these "immature" red blood cells have mitochondria and can generate ATP by oxidative phosphorylation. Maturation of reticulocytes into red blood cells results in the loss of mitochondria and complete dependence on glycolysis for ATP production. Since glycolysis is defective, the mature cells are lost rapidly from the circulation. Anemia results because the cells cannot be replaced rapidly enough by erythropoiesis.

Valentine, W. N. The Stratton lecture: hemolytic anemia and inborn errors of metabolism. *Blood* 54:549, 1979; and Tanaka, K. R., and Paglia, D. E. Pyruvate kinase and other enzymopathies of the erythrocyte. In: C. R. Scriver, A. L. Beaudet, W. S. Sly, and D. Valle (Eds.), *The Metabolic and Molecular Bases of Inherited Disease,* 7th ed. New York: McGraw-Hill, 1995, pp. 3485–3511.

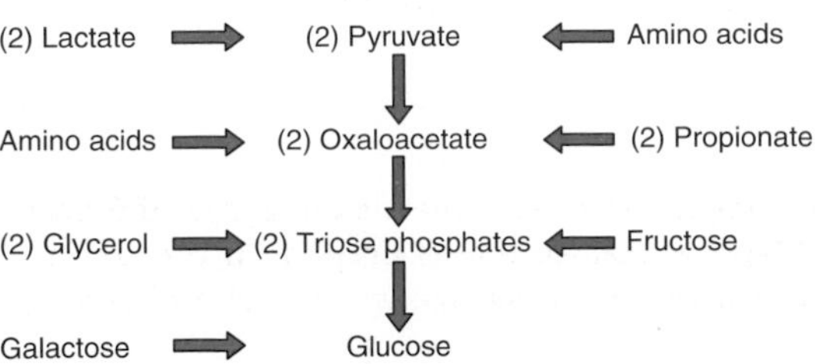

FIGURE 7.31
Abbreviated pathway of gluconeogenesis, illustrating the major substrate precursors for the process.

CLINICAL CORRELATION 7.9

Hypoglycemia and Premature Infants

Premature and small-for-gestational-age neonates have a greater susceptibility to hypoglycemia than full-term, appropriate-for-gestational-age infants. Several factors appear to be involved. Children in general are more susceptible than adults to hypoglycemia, simply because they have larger brain/body weight ratios and the brain utilizes disproportionately greater amounts of glucose than the rest of the body. Newborn infants have a limited capacity for ketogenesis, apparently because the transport of long-chain fatty acids into liver mitochondria of the neonate is poorly developed. Since ketone body use by the brain is directly proportional to the circulating ketone body concentration, the neonate is unable to spare glucose to any significant extent by using ketone bodies. The consequence is that the neonate's brain is almost completely dependent on glucose obtained from liver glycogenolysis and gluconeogenesis.

The capacity for hepatic glucose synthesis from lactate and alanine is also limited in newborn infants. This is because the rate-limiting enzyme phosphoenolpyruvate carboxykinase is present in very low amounts during the first few hours after birth. Induction of this enzyme to the level required to prevent hypoglycemia during the stress of fasting requires several hours. Premature and small-for-gestational-age infants are believed to be more susceptible to hypoglycemia than normal infants because of smaller stores of liver glycogen. Fasting depletes their glycogen stores more rapidly, making these neonates more dependent on gluconeogenesis than normal infants.

Ballard, F. J. The development of gluconeogenesis in rat liver: controlling factors in the newborn. *Biochem. J.* 124:265, 1971; and Newsholme, E. A., and Leech, A. R. *Biochemistry for the Medical Sciences*. New York: Wiley, 1983.

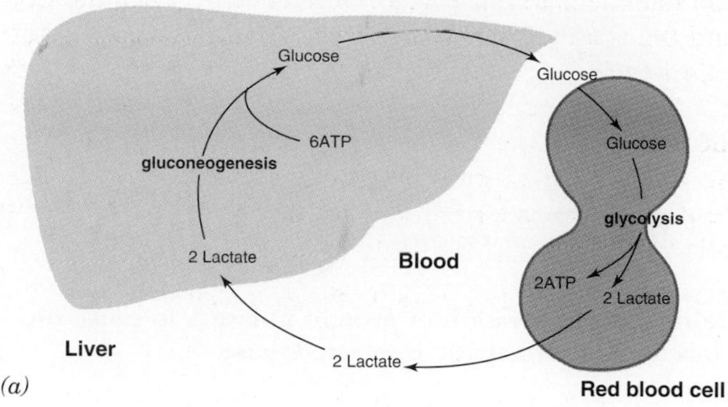

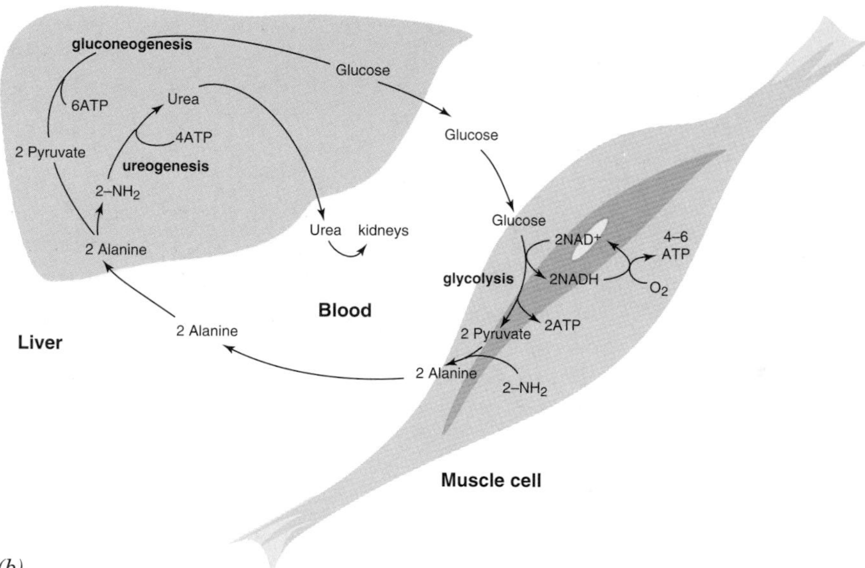

FIGURE 7.32
Relationship between gluconeogenesis in the liver and glycolysis in the rest of the body.
(*a*) Cori cycle. (*b*) Alanine cycle.

genesis in liver followed by delivery of glucose and its use in a peripheral tissue. Both cycles provide a mechanism for continuously supplying tissues that require glucose as their primary energy source. The cycles are only functional between liver and tissues that do not completely oxidize glucose to CO_2 and H_2O. In order to participate in these cycles, peripheral tissues must release either alanine or lactate as the end product of glucose metabolism. The type of recycled three-carbon intermediate is the major difference between the Cori cycle (Figure 7.32*a*) and the alanine cycle (Figure 7.32*b*), carbon returning to liver as lactate in the Cori cycle but as alanine in the alanine cycle. Another major difference is that NADH generated by glycolysis in the alanine cycle cannot be used to reduce pyruvate to lactate. In tissues that have mitochondria, electrons of NADH can be transported into the mitochondria by the malate–aspartate shuttle or the glycerol phosphate shuttle for the synthesis of ATP by oxidative phosphorylation:

$$\text{NADH} + \text{H}^+ + \tfrac{1}{2}\,\text{O}_2 + 3\ \text{ADP} + 3\ \text{P}_i \rightarrow \text{NAD}^+ + 3\ \text{ATP} + \text{H}_2\text{O}$$

or

$$\text{FADH}_2 + \tfrac{1}{2}\,\text{O}_2 + 2\ \text{ADP} + 2\ \text{P}_i \rightarrow \text{FAD} + 2\ \text{ATP} + \text{H}_2\text{O}$$

The consequence is that six to eight molecules of ATP can be formed per glucose molecule in peripheral tissues that participate in the alanine cycle. This stands in contrast to the Cori cycle in which only two molecules of ATP per molecule of glucose are produced. Overall stoichiometry for the Cori cycle is

$$6\ \text{ATP}_{\text{liver}} + 2\ (\text{ADP} + \text{P}_i)_{\text{red blood cells}} \rightarrow 6\ (\text{ADP} + \text{P}_i)_{\text{liver}} + 2\ \text{ATP}_{\text{red blood cells}}$$

Six molecules of ATP are needed in liver to provide the energy necessary for glucose synthesis. The alanine cycle also transfers the energy from liver to peripheral tissues and, because of the six to eight molecules of ATP produced per molecule of glucose, is an energetically more efficient cycle. Participation of alanine in the cycle presents liver with amino nitrogen, which must be disposed of as urea (Figure 7.32*b* and p. 453). Urea synthesis is expensive since four ATP molecules are consumed per urea molecule. The concurrent need for urea synthesis results in more ATP being needed per glucose molecule synthesized in liver. Overall stoichiometry for the alanine cycle is

$$10\ \text{ATP}_{\text{liver}} + 6\text{–}8\ (\text{ADP} + \text{P}_i)_{\text{muscle}} + \text{O}_{2\,\text{muscle}} \rightarrow 10\ (\text{ADP} + \text{P}_i)_{\text{liver}} + 6\text{–}8\ \text{ATP}_{\text{muscle}}$$

In contrast to the Cori cycle, oxygen and mitochondria are required in peripheral tissue for participation in the alanine cycle.

Pathway of Glucose Synthesis from Lactate

Gluconeogenesis from lactate is an ATP-requiring process with the overall equation of

$$2\ \text{L-Lactate}^- + 6\ \text{ATP}^{4-} \rightarrow \text{glucose} + 6\ \text{ADP}^{3-} + 6\ \text{P}_i^{2-} + 4\ \text{H}^+$$

Many enzymes of glycolysis are common to the gluconeogenic pathway. Additional reactions have to be involved because glycolysis produces 2 ATPs and gluconeogenesis requires 6 ATPs per molecule of glucose. Also, certain steps of glycolysis are irreversible under intracellular conditions and are replaced by irreversible steps of the gluconeogenic pathway. The reactions of gluconeogenesis from lactate are given in Figure 7.33. The initial step is conversion of lactate to pyruvate by **lactate dehydrogenase.** NADH is generated and is also needed for a subsequent step in the pathway. Pyruvate cannot be converted to phosphoenolpyruvate (PEP) by **pyruvate kinase** because the reaction is irreversible under intracellular conditions. Pyruvate is converted into the high-energy phosphate compound PEP by coupling of two reactions requiring high-energy phosphate compounds (an ATP and a GTP). The first is catalyzed by pyruvate carboxylase and the second by PEP carboxykinase (see Figure 7.34).

Pyruvate Carboxylase and Phosphoenolpyruvate Carboxykinase

GTP, required for the **PEP carboxykinase,** is equivalent to an ATP through the action of **nucleoside diphosphate kinase** (GDP + ATP $\rightleftharpoons$ GTP + ADP),

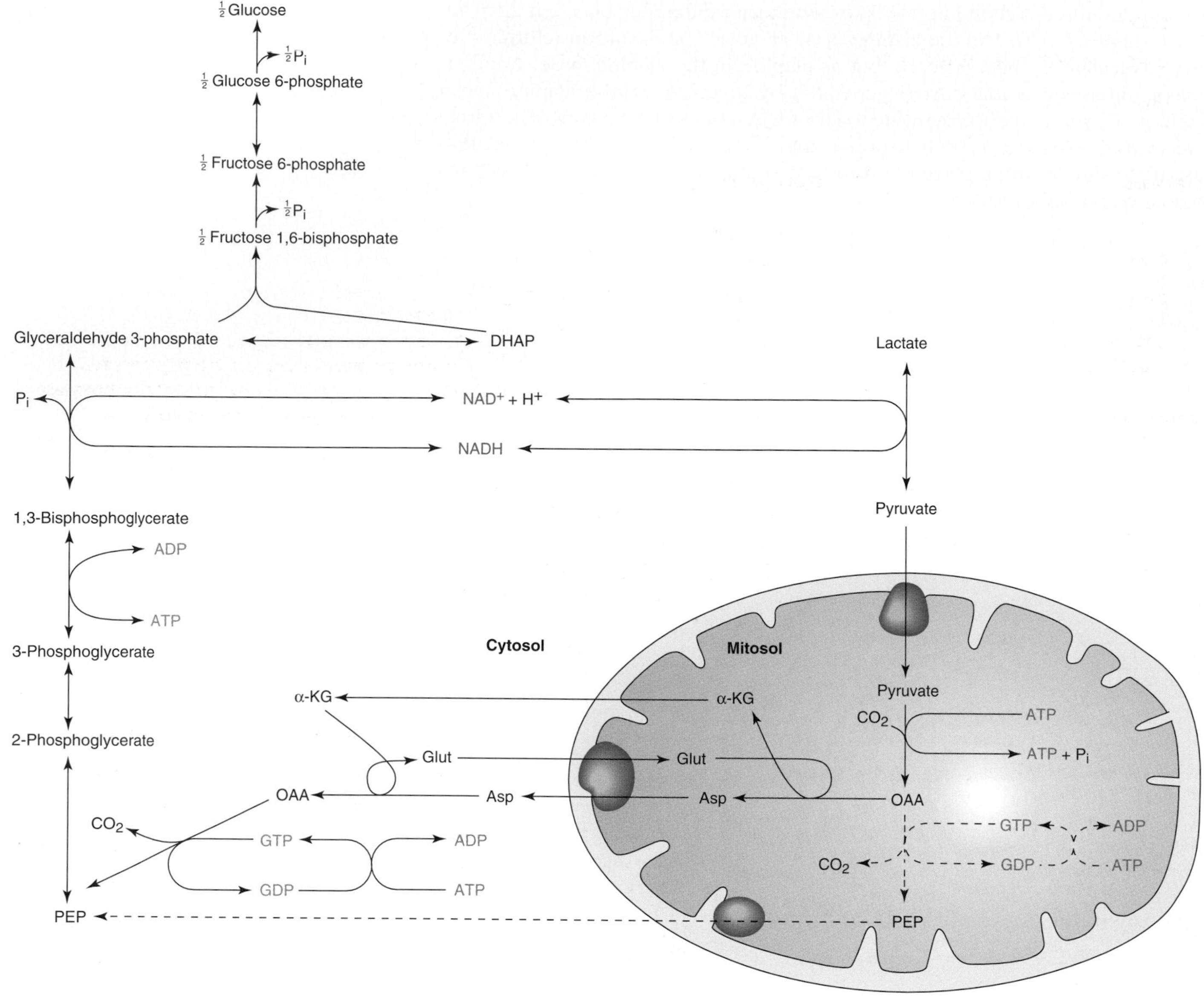

FIGURE 7.33
Pathway of gluconeogenesis from lactate.
The involvement of the mitochondrion in the process is indicated. Dashed arrows refer to an alternate route, which employs mitosolic PEP carboxykinase rather than the cytosolic isoenzyme. Abbreviations: OAA, oxaloacetate; α-KG, α-ketoglutarate; PEP, phosphoenolpyruvate; DHAP, dihydroxyacetone phosphate.

and CO_2 and HCO_3^- readily equilibrate by action of **carbonic anhydrase** ($CO_2 + H_2O \rightleftharpoons H_2CO_3 \rightleftharpoons H+ + HCO_3^-$). Thus the sum of these reactions is

$$\text{Pyruvate}^- + 2\ \text{ATP}^{4-} \rightarrow \text{phosphoenolpyruvate}^{3-} + 2\ \text{ADP}^{3-} + 2\ \text{Pi}^{2-} + 4\ \text{H}^+$$

Thus conversion of pyruvate into PEP during gluconeogenesis costs the cell two molecules of ATP whereas conversion of PEP to pyruvate during glycolysis yields the cell one molecule of ATP.

The intracellular location of **pyruvate carboxylase** makes the mitochondrion mandatory for conversion of cytosolic pyruvate into cytosolic PEP (Figure 7.33). There are two routes that oxaloacetate can then take to glucose. This

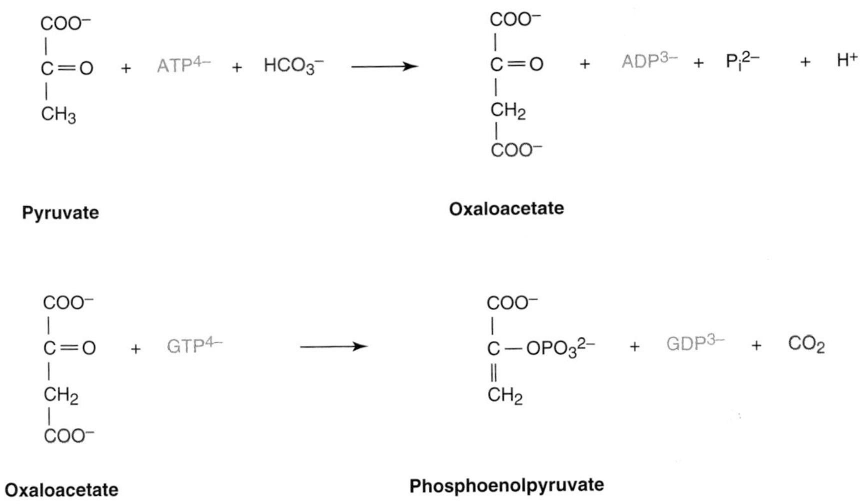

$$\begin{array}{c} COO^- \\ | \\ C{=}O \\ | \\ CH_3 \end{array} + ATP^{4-} + HCO_3^- \longrightarrow \begin{array}{c} COO^- \\ | \\ C{=}O \\ | \\ CH_2 \\ | \\ COO^- \end{array} + ADP^{3-} + P_i^{2-} + H^+$$

Pyruvate **Oxaloacetate**

$$\begin{array}{c} COO^- \\ | \\ C{=}O \\ | \\ CH_2 \\ | \\ COO^- \end{array} + GTP^{4-} \longrightarrow \begin{array}{c} COO^- \\ | \\ C{-}OPO_3^{2-} \\ \| \\ CH_2 \end{array} + GDP^{3-} + CO_2$$

Oxaloacetate **Phosphoenolpyruvate**

FIGURE 7.34
Energy-requiring steps involved in phosphoenolpyruvate formation from pyruvate. Reactions are catalyzed by pyruvate carboxylase and PEP carboxykinase, respectively.

happens because PEP carboxykinase is present in both cytosolic and mitosolic compartments. The simplest pathway involves the mitochondrial PEP carboxykinase. Oxaloacetate is converted within the mitochondrion into PEP, which then traverses the mitochondrial inner membrane. The second pathway would be just as simple if oxaloacetate could traverse the mitochondrial inner membrane. However, oxaloacetate cannot be transported out of mitochondria for want of a transporter (Figure 7.9*b*). Thus oxaloacetate is converted into aspartate, which is transported out by the **glutamate–aspartate antiport.** In the cytosol, transamination with α-ketoglutarate converts aspartate back to oxaloacetate.

Gluconeogenesis Uses Many Glycolytic Enzymes but in the Reverse Direction

The steps from PEP to fructose 1,6-bisphosphate are steps of the glycolytic pathway in reverse. NADH generated by lactate dehydrogenase is utilized by glyceraldehyde-3-phosphate dehydrogenase, establishing an equal balance of generation and utilization of reducing equivalents.

6-Phosphofructo-1-kinase catalyzes an irreversible step in glycolysis and cannot be used for conversion of FBP to fructose 6-phosphate. A way around this step is provided by **fructose 1,6-bisphosphatase,** which catalyzes irreversible hydrolysis of fructose 1,6-bisphosphate (Figure 7.35). This reaction produces F6P but, since the reaction is irreversible, it cannot be used in glycolysis to produce FBP.

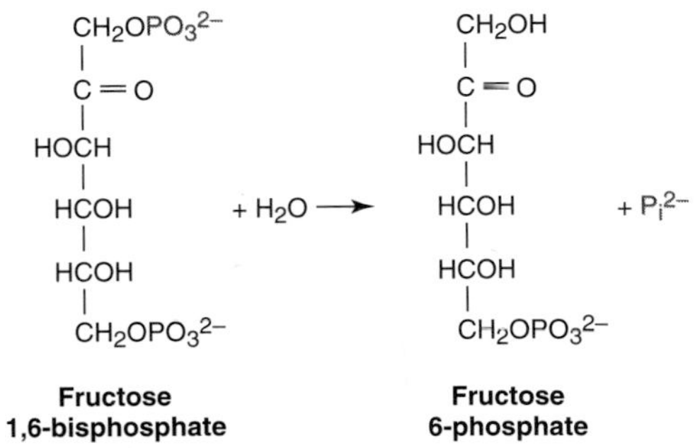

Phosphoglucose isomerase is freely reversible and functions in both glycolytic and gluconeogenic pathways. **Glucose 6-phosphatase,** which is used instead of glucokinase for the last step, catalyzes an irreversible hydrolytic reaction under intracellular conditions (Figure 7.36). Nucleotides have no role in this reaction; the function of this enzyme is to generate glucose, not to convert glucose into glucose 6-phosphate. Glucose 6-phosphatase is a membrane-bound enzyme, within the endoplasmic reticulum, with its active site available for G6P hydrolysis on the cisternal surface of the tubules (see Figure 7.37). A translocase for G6P is required to move G6P from the cytosol to its site of

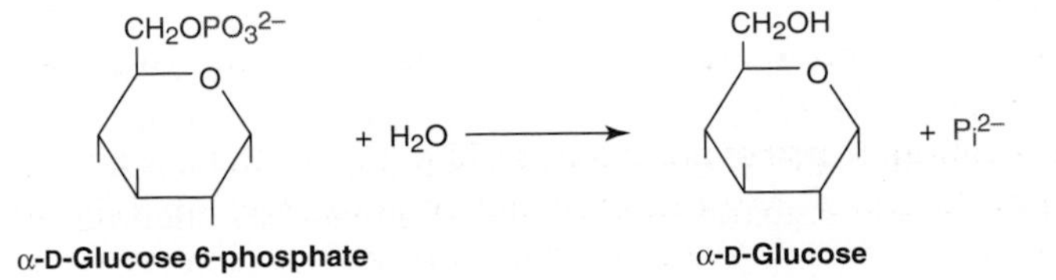

$$\begin{array}{c} CH_2OPO_3^{2-} \\ | \\ C{=}O \\ | \\ HOCH \\ | \\ HCOH \\ | \\ HCOH \\ | \\ CH_2OPO_3^{2-} \end{array} + H_2O \longrightarrow \begin{array}{c} CH_2OH \\ | \\ C{=}O \\ | \\ HOCH \\ | \\ HCOH \\ | \\ HCOH \\ | \\ CH_2OPO_3^{2-} \end{array} + P_i^{2-}$$

Fructose 1,6-bisphosphate **Fructose 6-phosphate**

FIGURE 7.35
Reaction catalyzed by fructose 1,6-bisphosphatase.

$CH_2OPO_3^{2-}$ … O … $+ H_2O \longrightarrow$ CH_2OH … O … $+ P_i^{2-}$

α-D-Glucose 6-phosphate **α-D-Glucose**

FIGURE 7.36
Reaction catalyzed by glucose 6-phosphatase.

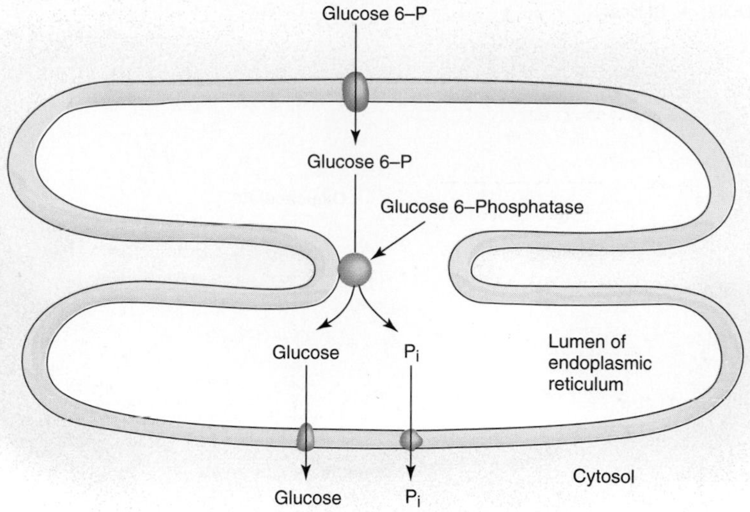

FIGURE 7.37
Glucose 6-phosphate is hydrolyzed by glucose 6-phosphatase located on the cisternal surface of the endoplasmic reticulum. Three transporters are involved: one moves glucose 6-phosphate into the lumen, a second moves P_i back to the cytosol, and a third moves glucose back into the cytosol.

hydrolysis within the endoplasmic reticulum. A genetic defect in either the translocase or the phosphatase interferes with gluconeogenesis and results in accumulation of glycogen in liver, as discussed later for glycogen metabolism (Section 7.6).

Glucose Is Synthesized from the Carbon Chains of Some Amino Acids

All **amino acids** except **leucine** and **lysine** can supply carbon for net synthesis of glucose by gluconeogenesis (see Chapter 11). If catabolism of an amino acid can yield either net pyruvate or net oxaloacetate formation, then net glucose synthesis can occur from that amino acid. Oxaloacetate is an intermediate in gluconeogenesis and pyruvate is readily converted to oxaloacetate by action of pyruvate carboxylase (Figure 7.34). The abbreviated pathway given in Figure 7.31 shows where amino acid catabolism fits with the process of gluconeogenesis. Catabolism of amino acids feeds carbon into the tricarboxylic cycle at more than one point. As long as net synthesis of a TCA cycle intermediate occurs as a consequence of catabolism of a particular amino acid, net synthesis of oxaloacetate will follow. Reactions that lead to net synthesis of TCA cycle intermediates are called **anaplerotic reactions (anaplerosis)** and support gluconeogenesis because they provide for net synthesis of oxaloacetate. Reactions catalyzed by pyruvate carboxylase and glutamate dehydrogenase are good examples of anaplerotic reactions :

$$\text{Pyruvate}^- + \text{ATP}^{4-} + \text{HCO}_3^- \rightarrow \text{oxaloacetate}^{2-} + \text{ADP}^{3-} + \text{P}_i^{2-} + \text{H}^+$$

$$\text{Glutamate}^- + \text{NAD(P)}^+ \rightleftharpoons \alpha\text{-ketoglutarate}^{2-} + \text{NAD(P)H} + \text{NH}_4^+ + \text{H}^+$$

On the other hand, the reaction catalyzed by glutamate–oxaloacetate transaminase (α-ketoglutarate + aspartate $\rightleftharpoons$ glutamate + oxaloacetate) is not anaplerotic because net synthesis of a TCA cycle intermediate is not accomplished. An intermediate of the TCA cycle is utilized in the reaction.

Since gluconeogenesis from amino acids imposes a nitrogen load on liver, a close relationship exists between urea synthesis and glucose synthesis from amino acids. This relationship is illustrated in Figure 7.38 for alanine. Two alanine molecules are shown being metabolized, one yielding NH_4^+ and the other aspartate, the primary substrates for the urea cycle. Aspartate leaves the mitochondrion and becomes part of the urea cycle after reacting with citrulline. Carbon of aspartate is released from the urea cycle as fumarate, which is then converted to malate by cytosolic fumarase. Both this malate and another malate

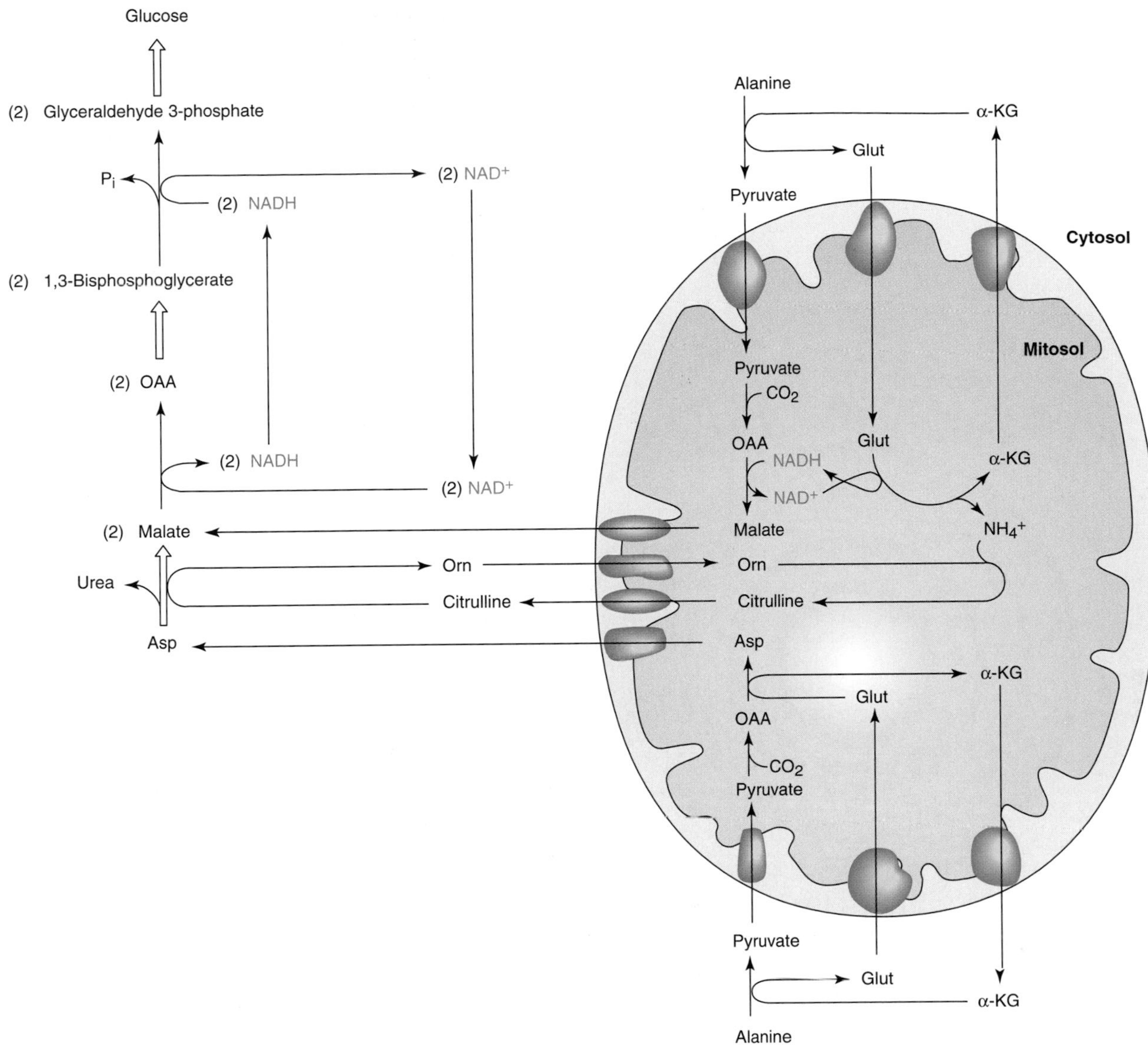

FIGURE 7.38
Pathway of gluconeogenesis from alanine and its relationship to urea synthesis.

exiting from the mitochondria are converted to glucose by cytosolic enzymes of gluconeogenesis. A balance is achieved between reducing equivalents (NADH) generated and those required in the cytosol and mitosol.

Leucine and **lysine** are the only amino acids that cannot function as carbon sources for net synthesis of glucose. These amino acids are **ketogenic** but not **glucogenic.** As shown in Table 7.2, all other amino acids are classified as glucogenic, or at least both glucogenic and ketogenic. Glucogenic amino acids give rise to net synthesis of either pyruvate or oxaloacetate, whereas amino acids that are both glucogenic and ketogenic also yield the ketone body acetoacetate, or acetyl CoA, which is readily converted into ketone bodies. Acetyl CoA is the end product of lysine metabolism, and acetoacetate and acetyl CoA are end products of leucine metabolism. No pathway exists for converting acetoacetate or acetyl CoA into pyruvate or oxaloacetate in humans and other animals. Acetyl CoA cannot be used for net synthesis of glucose because the reaction catalyzed by the **pyruvate dehydrogenase** complex is irreversible:

$$\text{Pyruvate} + \text{NAD}^+ + \text{CoASH} \rightarrow \text{acetyl CoA} + \text{NADH} + \text{CO}_2$$

TABLE 7.2 Glucogenic and Ketogenic Amino Acids

Glucogenic	*Ketogenic*	*Both*
Glycine	Leucine	Threonine
Serine	Lysine	Isoleucine
Valine		Phenylalanine
Histidine		Tyrosine
Arginine		Tryptophan
Cysteine		
Proline		
Hydroxyproline		
Alanine		
Glutamate		
Glutamine		
Aspartate		
Asparagine		
Methionine		

It might be argued that oxaloacetate is generated from acetyl CoA by the TCA cycle:

$$\text{Acetyl CoA} \rightarrow \text{citrate} \rightarrow\rightarrow 2\ CO_2 + \text{oxaloacetate}$$

However, this is a fallacious argument because it ignores the requirement for oxaloacetate in formation of citrate from acetyl CoA by **citrate synthase:**

$$\text{Acetyl CoA} + \text{oxaloacetate} \rightarrow \text{citrate} + \text{CoA}$$

The TCA cycle then catalyzes

$$\text{Citrate} \rightarrow\rightarrow 2\ CO_2 + \text{oxaloacetate}$$

The true sum reaction is then

$$\text{Acetyl CoA} \rightarrow 2CO_2 + \text{CoA}$$

Since net synthesis of a **TCA cycle** intermediate does not occur during oxidation of acetyl CoA, it is impossible for animals to synthesize glucose from acetyl CoA.

Glucose Can Be Synthesized from Odd-Chain Fatty Acids

Lack of an anaplerotic pathway from acetyl CoA also means that in general it is impossible to synthesize glucose from fatty acids. Most fatty acids found in humans have straight chains with an even number of carbon atoms. Their catabolism by fatty acid oxidation followed by ketogenesis or complete oxidation to CO_2 can be abbreviated as in Figure 7.39. Since acetyl CoA and other intermediates of even-numbered fatty acid oxidation cannot be converted to oxaloacetate or any other intermediate of gluconeogenesis, it is impossible to synthesize glucose from fatty acids. An exception to this general rule applies to fatty acids with methyl branches (e.g., **phytanic acid,** a breakdown product of chlorophyll; see discussion of **Refsum's disease,** Clin. Corr. 9.6) and fatty acids with an odd number of carbon atoms. Catabolism of such compounds yields propionyl CoA:

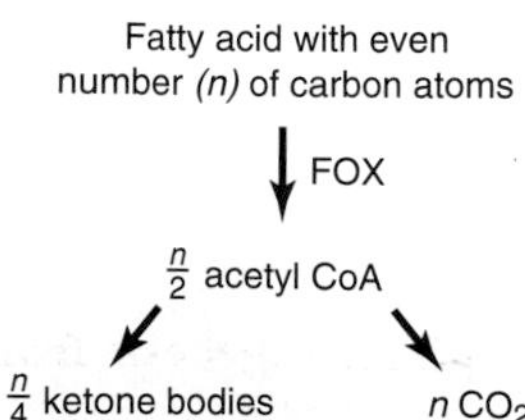

FIGURE 7.39
Overview of the catabolism of fatty acids to ketone bodies and CO_2.

Fatty acid with an odd number (n) of carbon atoms $\rightarrow$

$$\frac{(n-3)}{2}\ \text{acetyl CoA} + 1\ \text{propionyl CoA}$$

Propionate is a good precursor for gluconeogenesis, generating oxaloacetate by the anaplerotic pathway shown in Figure 7.40. The coenzyme A ester of propionate is also produced in catabolism of valine and isoleucine and conversion of cholesterol into bile acids.

It is sometimes loosely stated that fat *cannot* be converted into carbohydrate (glucose) by liver. In a sense this is certainly true since catabolism of fatty acids with an even number of carbon atoms cannot give rise to net synthesis of glucose. However, the term "fat" refers to triacylglycerols, which are composed of three *O*-acyl groups combined with one glycerol molecule. Hydrolysis of a triacylglycerol yields three fatty acids and glycerol, the latter compound being an excellent substrate for gluconeogenesis (Figure 7.41). Phosphorylation of glycerol by **glycerol kinase** produces glycerol 3-phosphate, which can be converted by glycerol-3-phosphate dehydrogenase into dihydroxyacetone phosphate, an intermediate of the gluconeogenic pathway (see Figure 7.33). The last stage of glycolysis can compete with the gluconeogenic pathway and convert dihydroxyacetone phosphate into lactate (or into pyruvate for subsequent complete oxidation to CO_2 and H_2O).

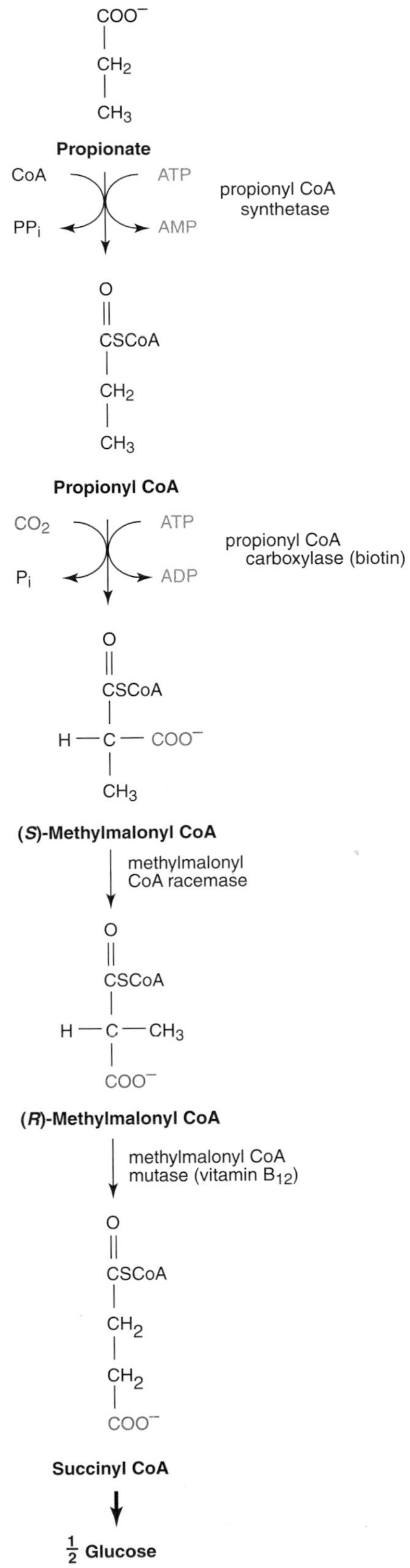

Glucose Is Synthesized from Other Sugars

Fructose

Humans consume considerable quantities of fructose in the form of sucrose hydrolyzed in the small bowel. In the liver, fructose is phosphorylated by a special ATP-linked kinase (Figure 7.42), yielding fructose 1-phosphate (see Clin. Corr. 7.3). A special aldolase then cleaves **fructose 1-phosphate** to yield one molecule of dihydroxyacetone phosphate and one of glyceraldehyde. The latter is reduced to glycerol and used by the same pathway given in the previous figure. Two molecules of dihydroxyacetone phosphate obtainable from one molecule of fructose can be converted to glucose by enzymes of gluconeogenesis or, alternatively, into pyruvate or lactate by the last stage of glycolysis. In analogy to glycolysis, conversion of fructose into lactate is called **fructolysis.**

The major energy source of spermatozoa is fructose, formed from glucose by cells of seminal vesicles as shown in Figure 7.43. An NADPH-dependent reduction of glucose to sorbitol is followed by an NAD^+-dependent oxidation of sorbitol to fructose. Fructose is secreted from seminal vesicles in a fluid that becomes part of semen. Although the fructose concentration in human semen can exceed 10 mM, tissues that come in contact with semen utilize fructose poorly, allowing this substrate to be conserved to meet the energy demands of spermatozoa in their search for ova. Spermatozoa contain mitochondria and thus can metabolize fructose completely to CO_2 and H_2O by the combination of fructolysis and TCA cycle activity.

Galactose

Milk sugar or **lactose** is an important source of **galactose** in the human diet. Glucose formation from galactose follows the pathway shown in Figure 7.44. **UDP-glucose** serves as a recycling intermediate in the overall process of converting galactose into glucose. Absence of the enzyme **galactose 1-phosphate uridylyltransferase** accounts for most cases of **galactosemia** (see Clin. Corr. 8.3).

Mannose

Mannose is found in very limited quantities in our diet. It is phosphorylated by hexokinase and then converted into fructose 6-phosphate by mannose phosphate isomerase:

$$\text{D-Mannose} + \text{ATP} \rightarrow \text{D-mannose 6-phosphate} + \text{ADP}$$

$$\text{D-Mannose 6-phosphate} \rightarrow \text{D-fructose 6-phosphate}$$

The latter compound can then be used in either glycolysis or gluconeogenesis.

COO^-–CH_2–CH_3

Propionate

CoA, ATP → PP_i, AMP (propionyl CoA synthetase)

CH_3–CH_2–C(=O)SCoA

Propionyl CoA

CO_2, ATP → P_i, ADP (propionyl CoA carboxylase (biotin))

H–C(CH_3)(COO^-)–C(=O)SCoA

(*S*)-Methylmalonyl CoA

↓ methylmalonyl CoA racemase

H–C(CH_3)(COO^-)–C(=O)SCoA

(*R*)-Methylmalonyl CoA

↓ methylmalonyl CoA mutase (vitamin B_{12})

COO^-–CH_2–CH_2–C(=O)SCoA

Succinyl CoA

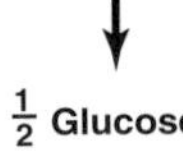

$\frac{1}{2}$ Glucose

FIGURE 7.40
Pathway of gluconeogenesis from propionate.
The large arrow refers to steps of the tricarboxylic acid cycle plus steps of lactate gluconeogenesis (see Figure 7.33).

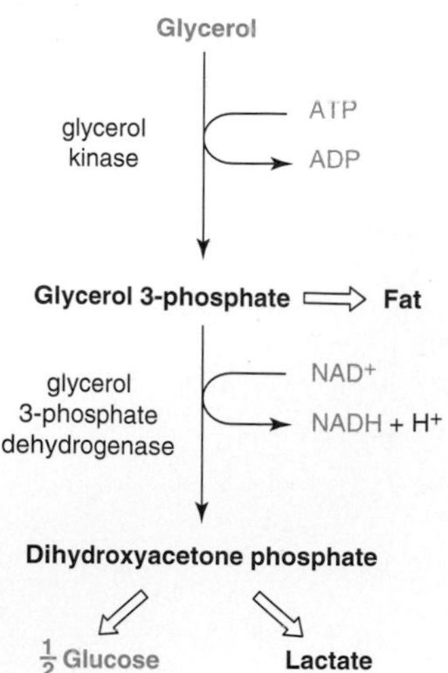

FIGURE 7.41
Pathway of gluconeogenesis from glycerol, along with competing pathways.
Large arrows indicate steps of the glycolytic and gluconeogenic pathways that have been given in detail in Figures 7.6 and 7.33, respectively. The large arrow pointing to fat refers to the synthesis of triacylglycerols and glycerophospholipids.

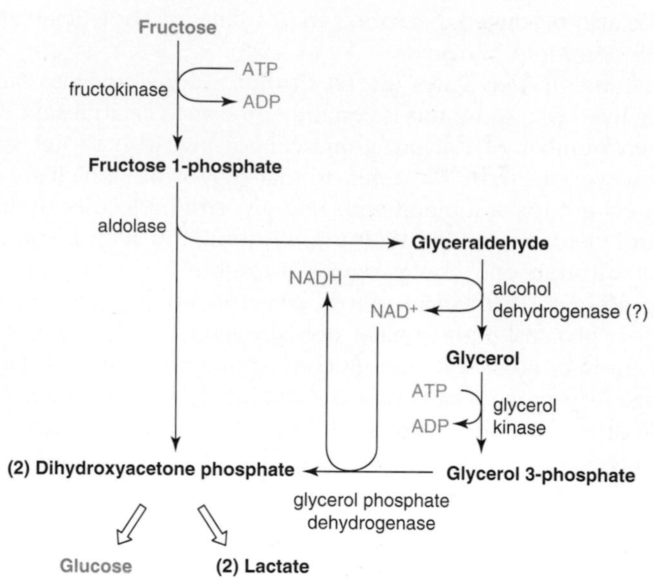

FIGURE 7.42
Pathway of glucose formation from fructose, along with the competing pathway of fructolysis.
Large arrows indicate steps of the glycolytic and gluconeogenic pathways that have been given in detail in Figures 7.6 and 7.33, respectively.

Gluconeogenesis Requires Expenditure of ATP

Synthesis of glucose is costly in terms of ATP. Six molecules are required for synthesis of one molecule of glucose from two molecules of lactate. ATP needed by liver cells for glucose synthesis is provided in large part by fatty acid oxidation. Metabolic conditions under which liver is required to synthesize glucose generally favor increased availability of fatty acids in blood. These fatty acids are oxidized by liver mitochondria to ketone bodies with concurrent production of large amounts of ATP. This ATP is used to support the energy requirements of gluconeogenesis, regardless of the substrate being used as carbon source for the process.

Gluconeogenesis Has Several Sites of Regulation

Sites of regulation of the gluconeogenesis pathway are apparent from the mass–action ratios and equilibrium constants in Table 7.1 and are further indicated in Figure 7.45. Those enzymes that are used to "go around" the irreversible steps of glycolysis are primarily involved in regulation of the pathway, that is, pyruvate carboxylase, PEP carboxykinase, fructose 1,6-bisphosphatase, and glucose 6-phosphatase. Regulation of hepatic gluconeogenesis is almost the

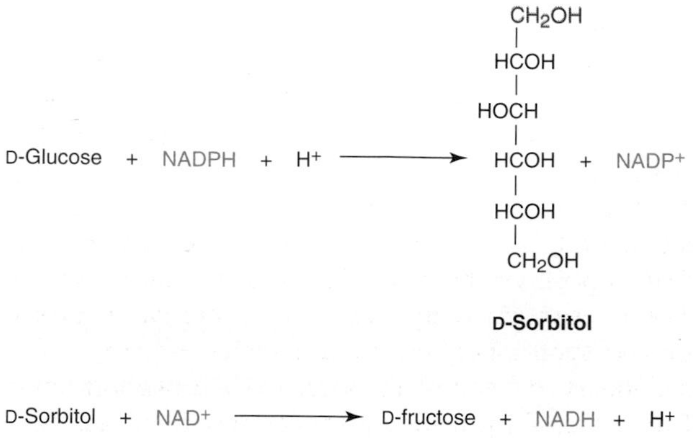

D-Glucose + NADPH + H^+ ⟶ D-Sorbitol (CH_2OH–HCOH–HOCH–HCOH–HCOH–CH_2OH) + $NADP^+$

D-Sorbitol + NAD^+ ⟶ D-fructose + NADH + H^+

FIGURE 7.43
The pathway responsible for the formation of sorbitol and fructose from glucose.

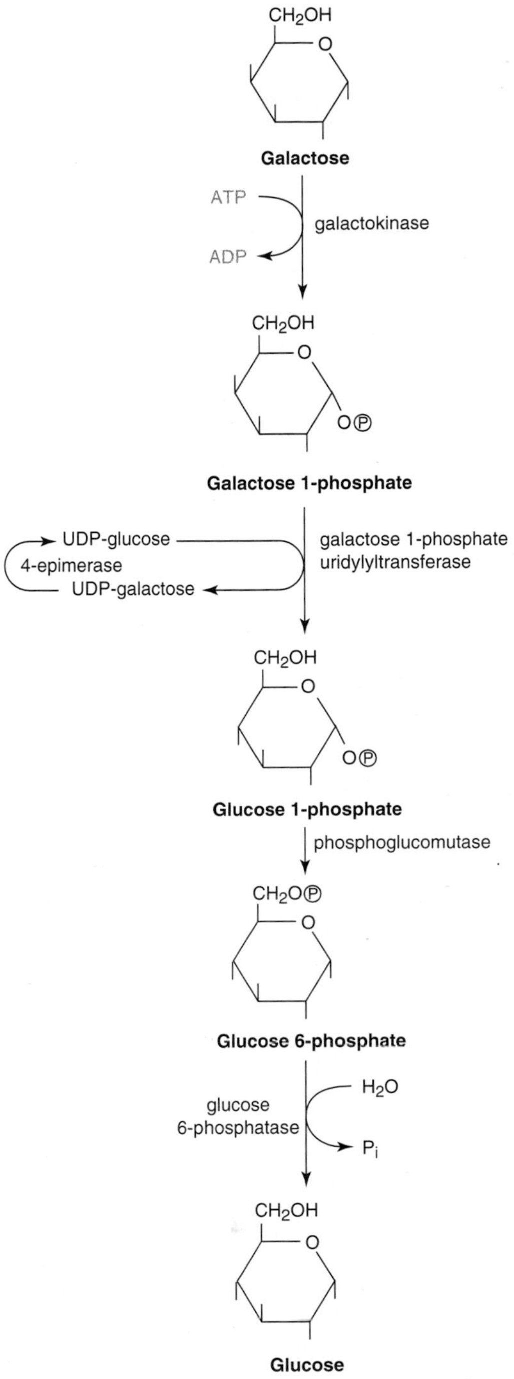

Galactose

ATP → ADP (galactokinase)

Galactose 1-phosphate

UDP-glucose → UDP-galactose (galactose 1-phosphate uridylyltransferase; 4-epimerase)

Glucose 1-phosphate

phosphoglucomutase

Glucose 6-phosphate

glucose 6-phosphatase (H_2O → P_i)

Glucose

FIGURE 7.44
Pathway of glucose formation from galactose.

same as regulation of hepatic glycolysis. Inhibition of glycolysis at its chief regulatory sites, or repressing synthesis of enzymes involved at these sites (glucokinase, 6-phosphofructo-1-kinase, and pyruvate kinase), greatly increases effectiveness of opposing gluconeogenic enzymes. Turning on gluconeogenesis is therefore accomplished in large part by shutting off glycolysis. Fatty acid oxidation does more than just supply ATP for the process. It promotes glucose synthesis by increasing the steady-state concentration of mitochondrial acetyl CoA, a positive allosteric effector of the mitochondrial **pyruvate carboxylase.** The increase in acetyl CoA and in pyruvate carboxylase activity results in a greater synthesis of citrate, a negative effector of 6-phosphofructo-1-kinase. A secondary effect of inhibition of 6-phosphofructo-1-kinase is a decrease in fructose 1,6-bisphosphate concentration, an activator of pyruvate kinase. This

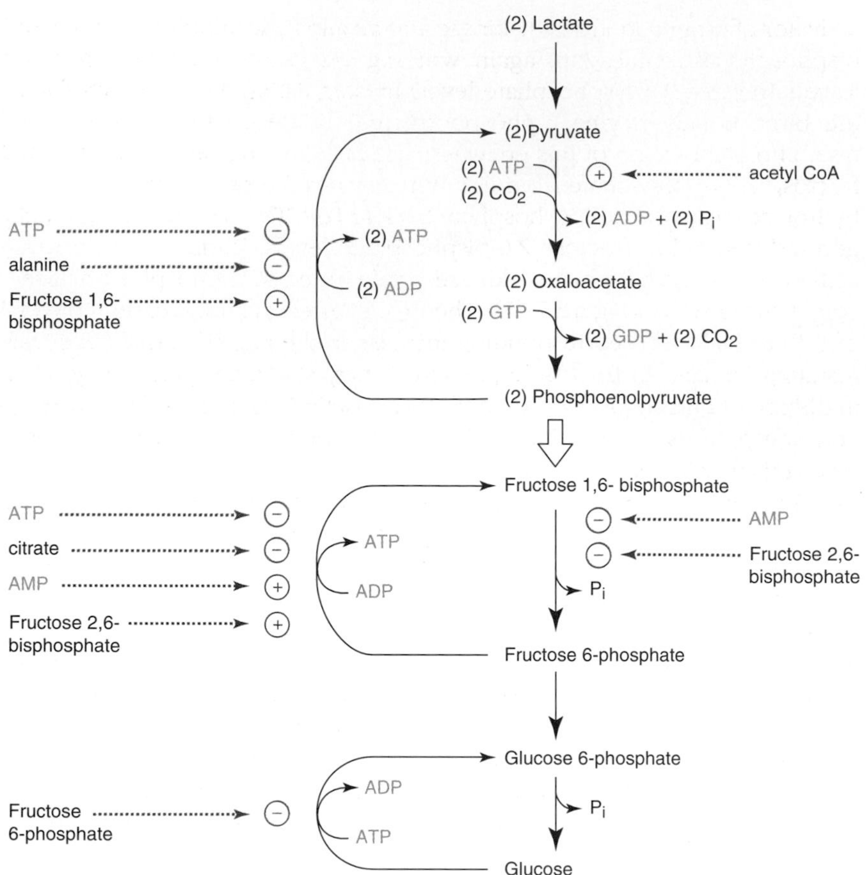

FIGURE 7.45
Important allosteric regulatory features of the gluconeogenic pathway.

decreases the flux of PEP to pyruvate by pyruvate kinase and increases effectiveness of the combined efforts of pyruvate carboxylase and PEP carboxykinase in conversion of pyruvate to PEP. An increase in ATP levels with the consequential decrease in AMP levels would favor gluconeogenesis by way of inhibition of 6-phosphofructo-1-kinase and pyruvate kinase and activation of fructose 1,6-bisphosphatase (see Figure 7.45 and the discussion of regulation of glycolysis, p. 283). A shortage of oxygen for respiration, a shortage of fatty acids for oxidation, or any inhibition or uncoupling of oxidative phosphorylation would be expected to cause liver to turn from gluconeogenesis to glycolysis.

Hormonal Control of Gluconeogenesis Is Critical for Homeostasis

Hormonal control of gluconeogenesis is a matter of regulating the supply of fatty acids to liver and the enzymes of both the glycolytic and gluconeogenic pathways. Glucagon increases plasma fatty acids by promoting lipolysis in adipose tissue, an action opposed by insulin. The greater availability of fatty acids results in more fatty acid oxidation by liver, which promotes glucose synthesis. Insulin has the opposite effect. Glucagon and insulin also regulate gluconeogenesis by influencing the state of phosphorylation of hepatic enzymes subject to covalent modification. As discussed previously (Figure 7.30), pyruvate kinase is active in the dephosphorylated mode and inactive in the phosphorylated mode. Glucagon activates adenylate cyclase to produce cAMP, which activates protein kinase A, which, in turn, phosphorylates and inactivates pyruvate kinase. Inactivation of this glycolytic enzyme stimulates the opposing pathway gluconeogenesis, by blocking the futile conversion of PEP to pyruvate. Glucagon also stimulates gluconeogenesis at the conversion of fructose 1,6-bisphosphate to fructose 6-phosphate by decreasing the concentration of fructose 2,6-bisphosphate in liver. **Fructose 2,6-bisphosphate** is an allosteric activator of 6-phosphofructo-1-kinase and an allosteric inhibitor of fructose 1,6-bisphosphatase. Glucagon, again working via its second messenger cAMP, lowers fructose 2,6-bisphosphate levels by stimulating the phosphorylation of the bifunctional enzyme 6-phosphofructo-2-kinase/fructose 2,6-bisphosphatase. Phosphorylation of this enzyme inactivates the kinase activity that makes fructose 2,6-bisphosphate from F6P but activates the phosphatase activity that hydrolyzes fructose 2,6-bisphosphate back to F6P. The consequence is a glucagon-induced fall in fructose 2,6-bisphosphate levels, leading to a decrease in activity of 6-phosphofructo-1-kinase while fructose 1,6-bisphosphatase becomes more active (Figure 7.45). The overall effect is an increased conversion of FBP to F6P and a corresponding increase in the rate of gluconeogenesis. A resulting increase in fructose 6-phosphate may also favor gluconeogenesis by inhibition of glucokinase via an inhibitory protein (see discussion of the regulation of glycolysis, p. 283). Insulin has effects opposite to those of glucagon by mechanisms not completely defined.

Glucagon and insulin also have long-term effects on hepatic glycolysis and gluconeogenesis by induction and repression of synthesis of key enzymes of the pathways. A high glucagon/insulin ratio in blood increases the enzymatic capacity for gluconeogenesis and decreases enzymatic capacity for glycolysis in liver. A low glucagon/insulin ratio has the opposite effects. The glucagon/insulin ratio increases when gluconeogenesis is needed and decreases when glucose is plentiful from the gastrointestinal tract. Glucagon signals induction of synthesis of greater quantities of PEP carboxykinase, fructose 1,6-bisphosphatase, glucose 6-phosphatase, and various aminotransferases. A model for how this occurs is given in Figure 7.46. Binding of glucagon to its plasma membrane receptor increases cAMP, which activates protein kinase A. Protein kinase A

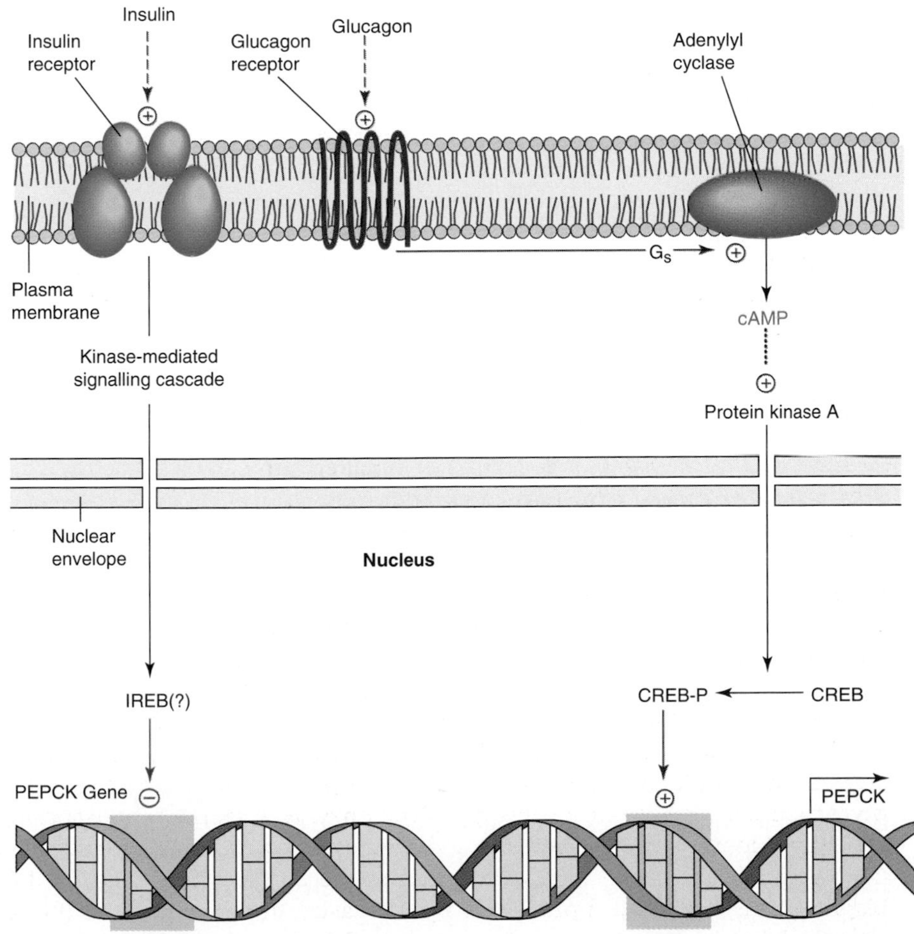

FIGURE 7.46
Glucagon promotes transcription of the gene that encodes PEP carboxykinase.
Abbreviations: PEPCK, PEP carboxykinase; CRE, cAMP-response element; CREB, cAMP-response element binding protein; IRE, insulin-response element; IREB, insulin-response element binding protein.

CLINICAL CORRELATION 7.10

Hypoglycemia and Alcohol Intoxication

Consumption of alcohol, especially by an undernourished person, can cause hypoglycemia. The same effect can result from drinking alcohol after strenuous exercise. In both cases the hypoglycemia results from the inhibitory effects of alcohol on hepatic gluconeogenesis and thus occurs under circumstances of hepatic glycogen depletion. The problem is caused by the NADH produced during the metabolism of alcohol. The liver simply cannot handle the reducing equivalents provided by ethanol oxidation fast enough to prevent metabolic derangements. The extra reducing equivalents block the conversion of lactate to glucose and promote the conversion of alanine into lactate, resulting in considerable lactate accumulation in the blood. Since lactate has no place to go, lactic acidosis (see Clin. Corr. 7.5) can develop, although it is usually mild.

Low doses of alcohol cause impaired motor and intellectual performance; high doses have a depressant effect that can lead to stupor and anesthesia. Low blood sugar can contribute to these undesirable effects of alcohol. What is more, a patient may be thought to be inebriated when in fact the patient is suffering from hypoglycemia that may lead to irreversible damage to the central nervous system. Children are highly dependent on gluconeogenesis while fasting, and accidental ingestion of alcohol by a child can produce severe hypoglycemia (see Clin. Corr. 7.9).

Krebs, H. A., Freedland, R. A., Hems, R., and Stubbs, M. Inhibition of hepatic gluconeogenesis by ethanol. *Biochem. J.* 112:117, 1969; and Service, F. J. Hypoglycemia. *Med. Clin. North Am.* 79:1, 1995.

then phosphorylates a protein called the **cAMP-response element binding protein (CREB),** a trans-acting factor that in its phosphorylated form can bind to a **cAMP-response element (CRE),** a cis acting element within the regulatory region of genes that respond to cAMP. This promotes transcription of genes encoding key gluconeogenic enzymes such as **PEP carboxykinase** (Figure 7.46). By a similar mechanism, but one that causes repression of **gene transcription,** glucagon acts to decrease the amounts of glucokinase, 6-phosphofructo-1-kinase, and pyruvate kinase. Insulin opposes the action of glucagon (Figure 7.46), acting through a signal cascade that results in activation of an insulin-response element binding protein (IREB), which inhibits transcription of genes encoding key gluconeogenic enzymes by binding to an **insulin-response element (IRE)** in the regulatory region of such genes. When glucose synthesis is not needed, synthesis of key gluconeogenic enzymes is turned off and synthesis of key glycolytic enzymes is turned on as a consequence of a decrease in the blood glucagon/insulin ratio.

Ethanol Ingestion Inhibits Gluconeogenesis

Ethanol inhibits gluconeogenesis by liver (see Clin. Corr. 7.10). It is oxidized primarily in liver with production of a large load of reducing equivalents that must be transported into the mitochondria by the **malate–aspartate shuttle.** This excess NADH in the cytosol creates problems for liver gluconeogenesis because it forces the equilibrium of the lactate dehydrogenase- and malate dehydrogenase-catalyzed reactions in the directions of lactate and malate formation, respectively:

$$\underset{\text{Ethanol}}{CH_3CH_2OH} + NAD^+ \rightarrow \underset{\text{Acetaldehyde}}{CH_3\overset{\overset{O}{\|}}{C}H} + NADH + H^+$$

$$\text{Pyruvate} + NADH + H^+ \rightarrow \text{lactate} + NAD^+$$

$$\text{Sum:}\quad \text{Ethanol} + \text{pyruvate} \rightarrow \text{acetaldehyde} + \text{lactate}$$

or

$$\text{Oxaloacetate} + NADH + H^+ \rightarrow \text{malate} + NAD^+$$

$$\text{Sum:}\quad \text{Ethanol} + \text{oxaloacetate} \rightarrow \text{acetaldehyde} + \text{malate}$$

Forcing these reactions in the directions shown above inhibits glucose synthesis by limiting the amounts of pyruvate and oxaloacetate available for the reactions catalyzed by pyruvate carboxylase and PEP carboxykinase, respectively.

7.6 ■ GLYCOGENOLYSIS AND GLYCOGENESIS

Glycogen, a Storage Form of Glucose, Is Required as a Ready Source of Energy

Glycogenolysis refers to breakdown of glycogen to glucose or glucose 6-phosphate; and **glycogenesis** refers to synthesis of glycogen. These processes are of some importance in almost every tissue but especially in muscle and liver. The liver has tremendous capacity for storing glycogen. In the well-fed human, liver glycogen content can account for as much as 10% of wet weight of this organ. Muscle stores less when expressed on the same basis–a maximum of only 1–2% of its wet weight. However, since the average person has more muscle than liver, there is about twice as much total muscle glycogen as liver glycogen.

Muscle and liver **glycogen stores** serve completely different roles. Glycogen serves as a fuel reserve for the synthesis of ATP within muscle, whereas liver glycogen functions as a glucose reserve for the maintenance of blood glucose concentrations. Liver glycogen levels vary greatly in response to the intake of food, accumulating to high levels shortly after a meal and then decreasing slowly as it is mobilized to help maintain a nearly constant blood glucose level (see Figure 7.47). Liver glycogen is called into play between meals and to a greater extent during the nocturnal fast. In both humans and the rat, the store of liver glycogen lasts somewhere between 12 and 24 h during fasting, depending greatly, of course, on whether the individual under consideration is caged or running wild.

Muscle glycogen is a source of ATP for increased muscular activity. Most of the glucose of glycogen is consumed within muscle cells without formation of free glucose as an intermediate. However, because of a special feature of glycogen catabolism to be discussed below, about 8% of muscle glycogen is converted into free glucose within the tissue. Some of this glucose may be released into the bloodstream, but most gets metabolized by glycolysis in muscle. Since muscle lacks glucose 6-phosphatase, and most free glucose formed during glycogen breakdown is further catabolized, muscle glycogen is not of quantitative importance in maintenance of blood glucose levels in the fasting state. Liver glycogen converted to glucose by glycogenolysis and glucose 6-phosphatase is of much greater importance as a source of blood glucose in the fasting state. Conversion of glucose to glycogen in muscle plays an important role in lowering blood glucose levels elevated by a high carbohydrate meal. Glycogenesis in liver contributes to the lowering of blood glucose but is of less importance than glycogen synthesis in muscle.

Exercise of a muscle triggers mobilization of muscle glycogen for formation of ATP. The yield of ATP and the fate of the carbon of glycogen depend on whether a "white" or "red" muscle is under consideration. Red muscle fibers are supplied with a rich blood flow, contain large amounts of myoglobin, and are packed with mitochondria. Glycogen mobilized within these cells is converted into pyruvate, which, because of the availability of O_2 and mitochondria, can be converted into CO_2 and H_2O. In contrast, white muscle fibers have a poorer blood supply and fewer mitochondria. **Glycogenolysis** within this tissue supplies substrate for glycolysis, with the end product being primarily lactate. **White muscle fibers** have enormous capacity for glycogenolysis and glycolysis, much more than **red muscle fibers.** Since their glycogen stores are limited, however, muscles of this type can only function at full capacity for relatively short periods of time. Breast muscle and the heart of chicken are good examples of white and red muscles, respectively. The heart has to beat

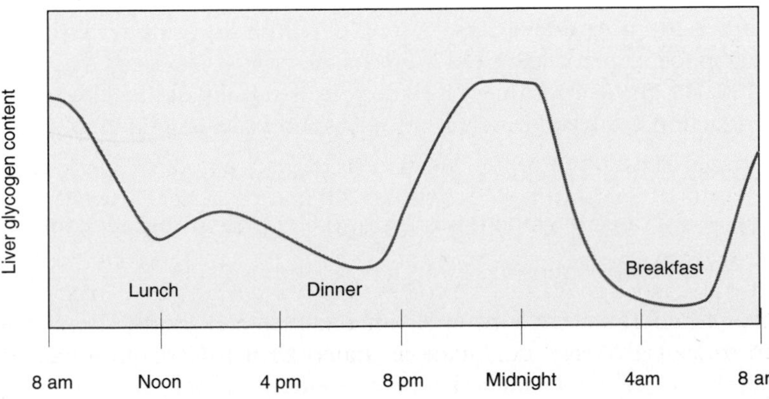

FIGURE 7.47
Variation of liver glycogen levels between meals and during the nocturnal fast.

continuously and has many mitochondria and a rich supply of blood via the coronary arteries. The heart stores glycogen to be used when a greater work load is imposed. Breast muscle of chicken is not continuously carrying out work. Its important function is to enable the chicken to fly rapidly for short distances, as in fleeing from predators (or amorous roosters). Because glycogen can be mobilized so rapidly, breast muscle is designed for maximal activity for a relatively short period of time. Although it was easy to point out readily recognizable white and red muscles in the chicken, most skeletal muscles of the human body are composed of a mixture of red and white fibers in order to provide for both rapid and sustained muscle activity. The distribution of white and red muscle fibers in cross sections of a human skeletal muscle can be shown by using special staining procedures (see Figure 7.48).

Glycogen granules are abundant in **liver** of the well-fed animal but are virtually absent from liver of the 24-h-fasted animal (Figure 7.49). Heavy exercise causes the same loss of glycogen granules in muscle fibers. These granules of glycogen correspond to clusters of glycogen molecules, the molecular weights of which can approach 2×10^7 Da. Glycogen is composed entirely of glucosyl residues, the majority of which are linked together by α-1,4-glycosidic linkages (Figure 7.50). Branches also occur in the glycogen molecule, however, because of frequent α-1,6-glycosidic linkages (Figure 7.50). A limb of the glycogen "tree" (see Figure 7.51) is characterized by branches at every fourth glucosyl residue within the more central core of the molecule. These branches occur much less frequently in outer regions of the molecule. An interesting question, which we shall attempt to answer below, is why this polymer is constructed with so many intricate branches and loose ends. Glycogen certainly stands in contrast to proteins and nucleic acids in this regard but, of course, it is a storage form of fuel and never has to catalyze a reaction or convey information within a cell.

Glycogen Phosphorylase Catalyzes the First Step in Glycogen Degradation

Glycogen phosphorylase catalyzes **phosphorolysis** of glycogen, a reaction in which P_i is used in the cleavage of an α-1,4-glycosidic linkage to yield glucose 1-phosphate (Figure 7.52). This always occurs at a terminal, nonreducing end of a glycogen molecule:

The reaction catalyzed by glycogen phosphorylase should be distinguished from that catalyzed by α-amylase, which degrades glycogen and starch in the gut (see Chapter 26). ***α*-Amylase** acts by simple hydrolysis, using water rather than inorganic phosphate to cleave α-1,4-glycosidic bonds. Glycogen may contain up to 100,000 glucose residues; its structure is usually abbreviated (glucose)$_n$. The reaction catalyzed by glycogen phosphorylase is written as

$$(\text{Glucose})_n + P_i^{2-} \rightarrow (\text{glucose})_{n-1} + \alpha\text{-D-glucose 1-phosphate}^{2-}$$

The next step of glycogen degradation is catalyzed by **phosphoglucomutase:**

$$\text{Glucose 1-phosphate} \rightarrow \text{glucose 6-phosphate}$$

This is a near-equilibrium reaction under intracellular conditions, allowing it to function in both glycogen degradation and synthesis. Like phosphoglycerate mutase (see p. 277), a bisphosphate compound is an obligatory interme-

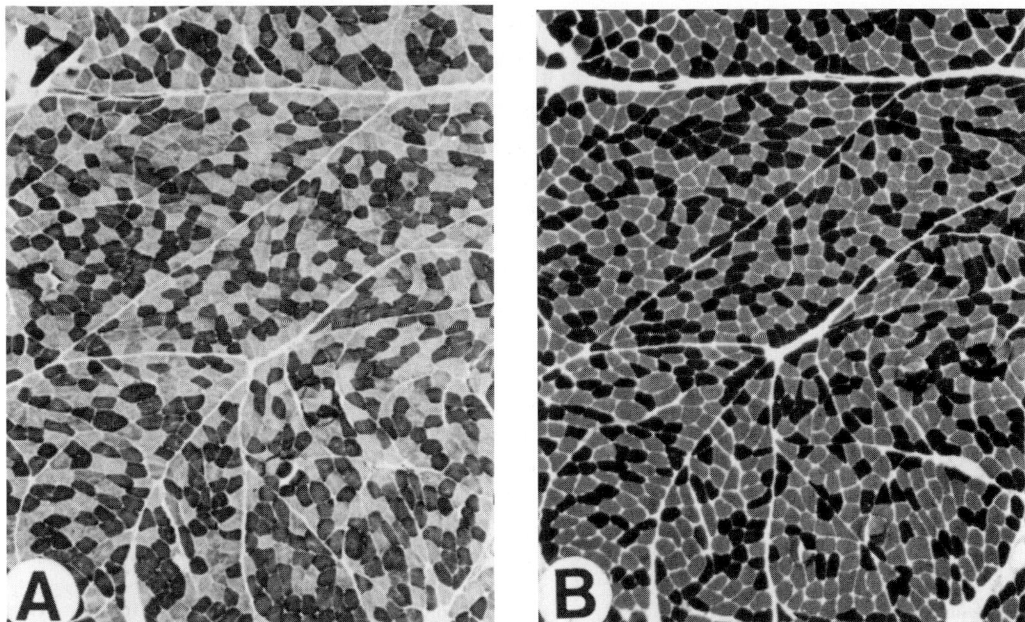

FIGURE 7.48
Cross section of human skeletal muscle showing red and white muscle fibers.
Sections were stained for NADH diaphorase activity in (*a*); for ATPase activity in (*b*). The red fibers are dark and the white fibers are light in (*a*); vice versa in (*b*).
Pictures generously provided by Dr. Michael H. Brooke of the Jerry Lewis Neuromuscular Research Center, St. Louis, Missouri.

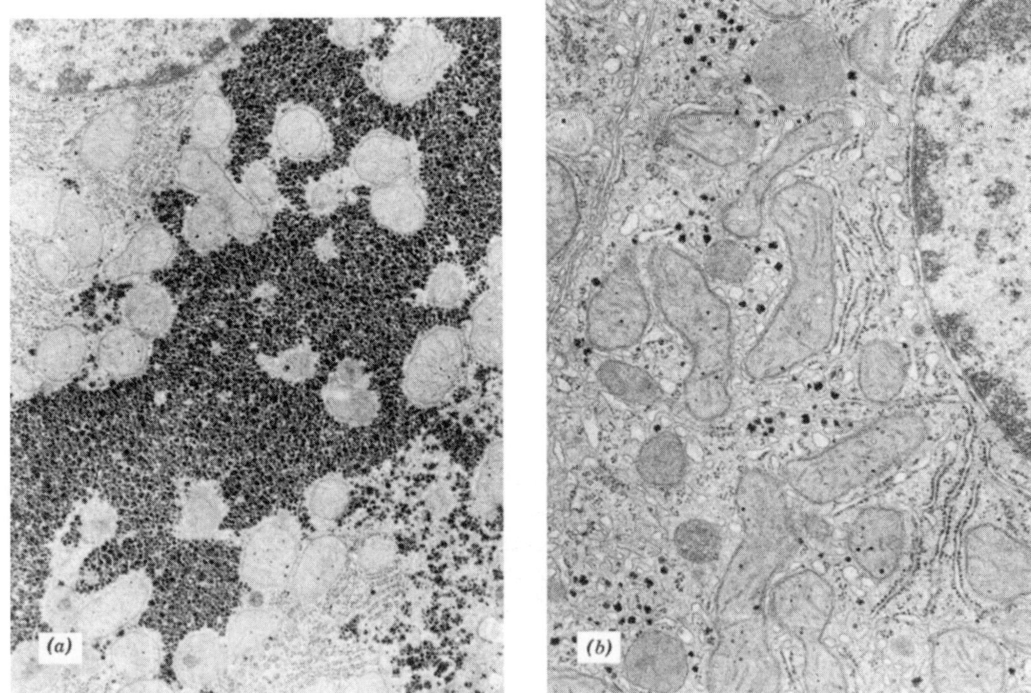

FIGURE 7.49
Electron micrographs showing glycogen granules (darkly stained material) in the liver of a well-fed rat (*a*) and the relative absence of such granules in the liver of a rat starved for 24 h (*b*).
Micrographs generously provided by Dr. Robert R. Cardell of the Department of Anatomy at the University of Cincinnati.

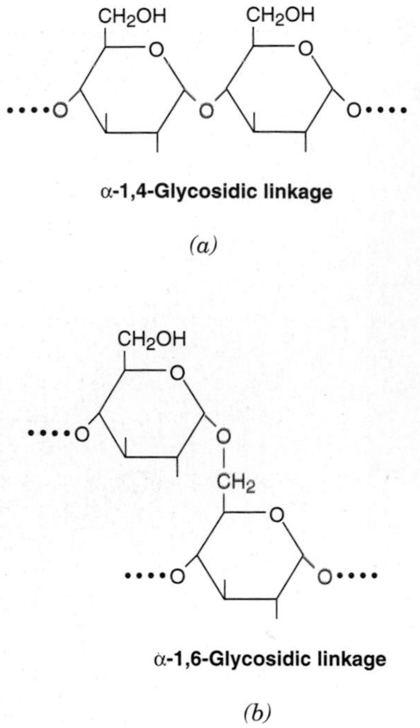

α-1,4-Glycosidic linkage

(a)

α-1,6-Glycosidic linkage

(b)

FIGURE 7.50
Two types of linkage between glucose molecules are present in glycogen.

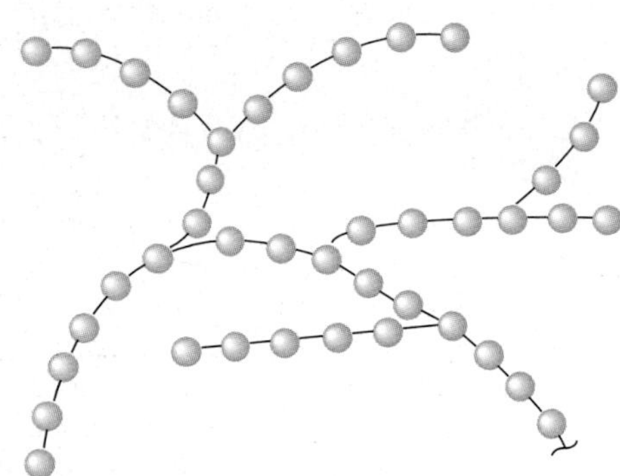

FIGURE 7.51
The branched structure of glycogen.

diate:

$$\text{E-P} + \text{glucose 1-phosphate} \rightleftharpoons \text{E} + \text{glucose 1,6-bisphosphate}$$

$$\text{E} + \text{glucose 1,6-bisphosphate} \rightleftharpoons \text{E-P} + \text{glucose 6-phosphate}$$

$$\text{Sum:}\quad \text{Glucose 1-phosphate} \rightleftharpoons \text{glucose 6-phosphate}$$

A catalytic amount of glucose 1,6-bisphosphate must be present for the reaction to occur. It is produced in small quantities for this specific purpose by an enzyme called **phosphoglucokinase:**

$$\text{Glucose 6-phosphate} + \text{ATP} \rightarrow \text{glucose 1,6-bisphosphate} + \text{ADP}$$

The next enzyme involved in glycogenolysis depends on the tissue under consideration (Figure 7.52). In liver, glucose 6-phosphate produced by glycogenolysis is hydrolyzed by **glucose 6-phosphatase** to give free glucose:

$$\text{Glucose 6-phosphate}^{2-} + H_2O \rightarrow \text{glucose} + P_i^{2-}$$

Lack of this enzyme or of the translocase that transports G6P into the endoplasmic reticulum (Figure 7.37) results in type I **glycogen storage disease** (see Clin. Corr. 7.11). The overall balanced equation for removal of one glucosyl residue from glycogen in liver by glycogenolysis is then

$$(\text{Glucose})_n + H_2O \rightarrow (\text{glucose})_{n-1} + \text{glucose}$$

In other words, glycogenolysis in liver involves phosphorolysis but, because the phosphate ester is cleaved by a phosphatase, the overall reaction adds up to hydrolysis of glycogen. No ATP is used or formed in glycogenolysis.

In peripheral tissues the G6P generated by glycogenolysis is used by glycolysis, leading primarily to the generation of lactate in white muscle fibers and primarily to complete oxidation to CO_2 in red muscle fibers. Since no ATP had to be invested to produce G6P obtained from glycogen, the overall equation

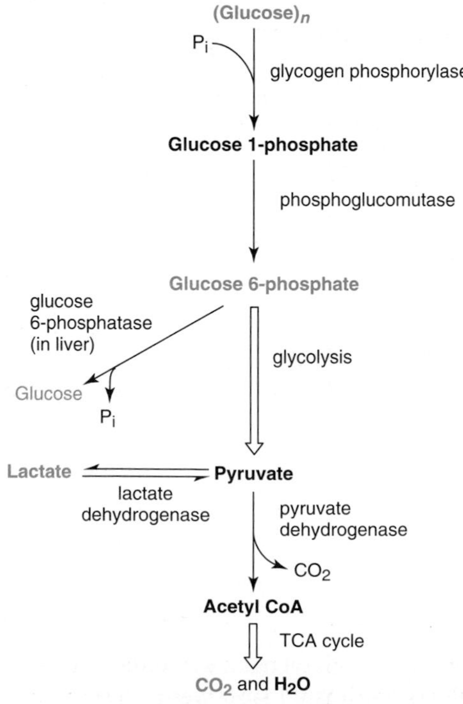

FIGURE 7.52
Glycogenolysis and the fate of glycogen degraded in liver versus its fate in peripheral tissues.

CLINICAL CORRELATION 7.11

Glycogen Storage Diseases

There are a number of well-characterized glycogen storage diseases, all due to inherited defects of one or more of the enzymes involved in the synthesis and degradation of glycogen. The liver is usually the tissue most affected, but heart and muscle glycogen metabolism can also be defective.

Chen, Y.-T., and Burchell, A. Glycogen storage diseases. In: C. R. Scriver, A. L. Beaudet, W. S. Sly, and D. Valle (Eds.), *The Metabolic and Molecular Bases of Inherited Disease,* 7th ed. New York: McGraw-Hill, 1995, pp. 935–965.

Von Gierke's Disease

The most common glycogen storage disease, referred to as type I or von Gierke's disease, is caused by a deficiency of liver, intestinal mucosa, and kidney glucose 6-phosphatase. Thus diagnosis by small bowel biopsy is possible. Patients with this disease can be further subclassified into those lacking the glucose 6-phosphatase enzyme per se (type Ia) and those lacking the glucose 6-phosphatase translocase (type Ib) (see Figure 7.37). A genetic abnormality in glucose 6-phosphate hydrolysis occurs in only about 1 person in 200,000 and is transmitted as an autosomal recessive trait. Clinical manifestations include fasting hypoglycemia, lactic acidemia hyperlipidemia, and hyperuricemia with gouty arthritis. The fasting hypoglycemia is readily explained as a consequence of the glucose 6-phosphatase deficiency, the enzyme required to obtain glucose from liver glycogen and gluconeogenesis. The liver of these patients does release some glucose by the action of the glycogen debranching enzyme. The lactic acidemia occurs because the liver cannot use lactate effectively for glucose synthesis. In addition, the liver inappropriately produces lactic acid in response to glucagon. This hormone should trigger glucose release without lactate production; however, the opposite occurs because of the lack of glucose 6-phosphatase. Hyperuricemia results from increased purine degradation in the liver; hyperlipidemia results because of increased availability of lactic acid for lipogenesis and lipid mobilization from the adipose tissue caused by high glucagon levels in response to hypoglycemia. The manifestations of von Gierke's disease can greatly be diminished by providing carbohydrate throughout the day to prevent hypoglycemia. During sleep this can be done by infusion of carbohydrate into the gut by a nasogastric tube.

Cori, G. T., and Cori, C. F. Glucose-6-phosphatase of the liver in glycogen storage disease. *J. Biol. Chem.* 199:661, 1952.

Pompe's Disease

Type II glycogen storage disease or Pompe's disease is caused by the absence of α-1,4-glucosidase (or acid maltase), an enzyme normally found in lysosomes. The absence of this enzyme leads to the accumulation of glycogen in virtually every tissue. This is somewhat surprising, but lysosomes take up glycogen granules and become defective with respect to other functions if they lack the capacity to destroy the granules. Because other synthetic and degradative pathways of glycogen metabolism are intact, metabolic derangements such as those in von Gierke's disease are not seen. The reason for extralysosomal glycogen accumulation is unknown. Massive cardiomegaly occurs and death results at an early age from heart failure.

Hers, H. G. α-Glucosidase deficiency in generalized glycogen storage disease (Pompe's disease). *Biochem. J.* 86:11, 1963.

Cori's Disease

Also called type III glycogen storage disease, Cori's disease is caused by a deficiency of the glycogen debranching enzyme. Glycogen accumulates because only the outer branches can be removed from the molecule by phosphorylase. Hepatomegaly occurs but diminishes with age. The clinical manifestations are similar to but much milder than those seen in von Gierke's disease, because gluconeogenesis is unaffected, and hypoglycemia and its complications are less severe.

Van Hoff, F., and Hers, H. G. The subgroups of type III glycogenesis. *Eur. J. Biochem.* 2:265, 1967.

McArdle's Disease

Also called the type V glycogen storage disease, McArdle's disease is caused by an absence of muscle phosphorylase. Patients suffer from painful muscle cramps and are unable to perform strenuous exercise, presumably because muscle glycogen stores are not available to the exercising muscle. Thus the normal increase in plasma lactate (released from the muscle) following exercise is absent. The muscles are probably damaged because of inadequate energy supply and glycogen accumulation. Release of muscle enzymes creatine kinase and aldolase and of myoglobin is common; elevated levels of these substances in the blood suggests a muscle disorder.

McArdle, B. Myopathy due to a defect in muscle glycogen breakdown. *Clin. Sci.* 10:13, 1951.

for glycogenolysis followed by glycolysis is

$$(\text{Glucose})_n + 3\ \text{ADP}^{3-} + 3\ \text{P}_i^{2-} + \text{H}^+ \rightarrow (\text{glucose})_{n-1} + 2\ \text{lactate}^- + 3\ \text{ATP}^{4-}.$$

Debranching Enzyme Is Required for Complete Hydrolysis of Glycogen

The first enzyme involved in glycogen degradation, glycogen phosphorylase, is specific for α-1,4-glycosidic linkages. However, it stops attacking α-1,4-glucosidic linkages four glucosyl residues from an α-1,6-branch point. A glycogen molecule that has been degraded by phosphorylase to the limit caused by the branches is called phosphorylase-**limit dextrin.** The action of a **debranching**

enzyme is what allows glycogen phosphorylase to continue to degrade glycogen. Debranching enzyme is a bifunctional enzyme that catalyzes two reactions necessary for debranching of glycogen. The first is a 4-α-D-glucanotransferase activity in which a strand of three glucosyl residues is removed from a four glucosyl residue branch of the glycogen molecule (Figure 7.53). The strand remains covalently attached to the enzyme until it can be transferred to a free 4-hydroxyl of a glucosyl residue at the end of the same or an adjacent glycogen molecule. The result is a longer amylose chain with only one glucosyl residue remaining in α-1,4-linkage. This linkage is broken hydrolytically by the second enzyme activity of debranching enzyme, which is its **amylo-α-1,6-glucosidase** activity:

Glycogen $\xrightarrow{H_2O}$ α-D-Glucose + Glycogen

The cooperative and repetitive action of phosphorylase and debranching enzyme results in complete phosphorolysis and hydrolysis of glycogen. **Glycogen**

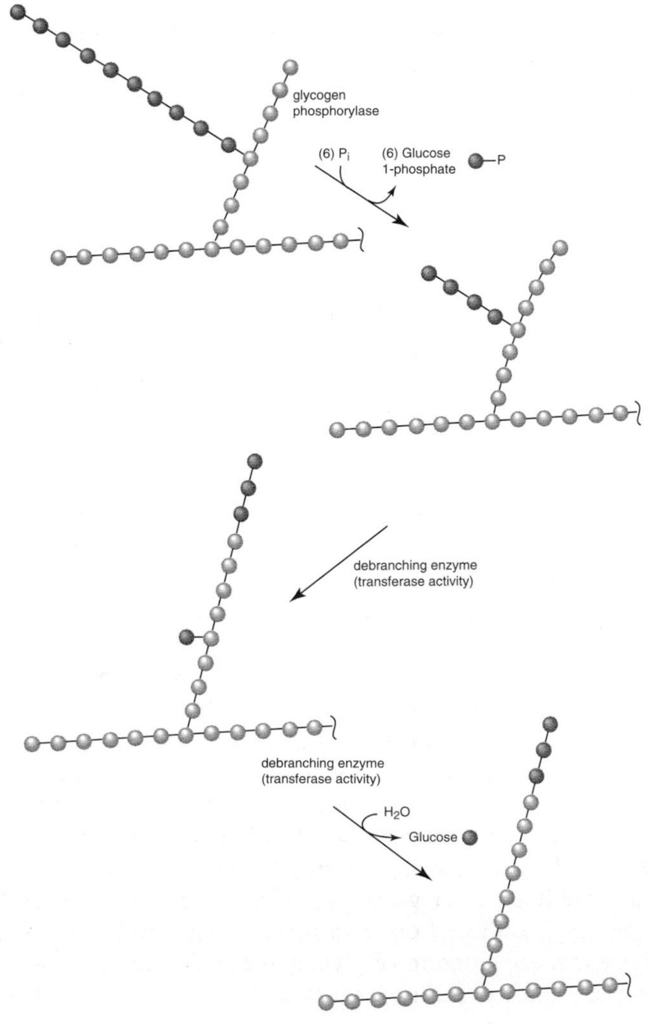

FIGURE 7.53
Action of the glycogen debranching enzyme.

storage diseases result when either of these enzymes is defective. The average molecule of glycogen yields about 12 molecules of glucose 1-phosphate by action of phosphorylase for every molecule of free glucose produced by action of debranching enzyme.

There is another, albeit quantitatively less important, pathway for glycogen degradation. A defect in this minor pathway, however, creates a major problem. As pointed out in Clin. Corr. 7.11, a **glucosidase** present in lysosomes degrades glycogen that enters these organelles during normal turnover of intracellular components.

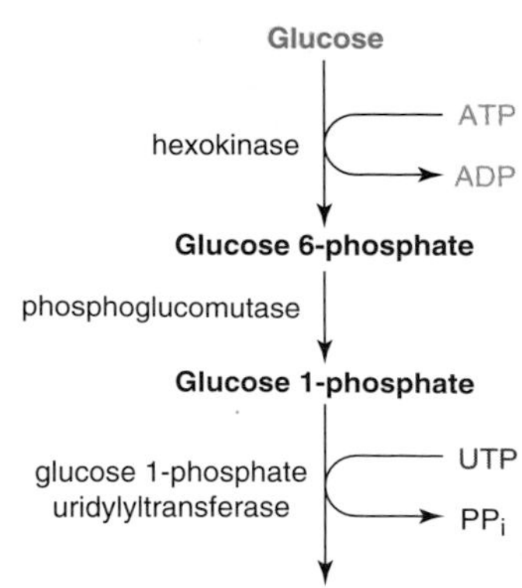

FIGURE 7.54
Pathway of glycogen synthesis.

Synthesis of Glycogen Requires Unique Enzymes

The first reaction involved in **glycogen synthesis** (Figure 7.54) is already familiar, being catalyzed by glucokinase in hepatic tissue and hexokinase in peripheral tissues:

$$\text{Glucose} + \text{ATP} \rightarrow \text{glucose 6-phosphate} + \text{ADP}$$

Phosphoglucomutase, discussed in relation to glycogen degradation, catalyzes a readily reversible reaction as follows:

$$\text{Glucose 6-phosphate} \rightarrow \text{glucose 1-phosphate}$$

A unique reaction found at the next step involves formation of UDP-glucose by action of **glucose 1-phosphate uridylyltransferase:**

$$\textbf{Glucose 1-phosphate + UTP} \rightarrow \textbf{UDP-glucose + PP}_i$$

This reaction generates UDP-glucose, sometimes called **"activated glucose"** because of its large negative free energy of hydrolysis, which is used to build the glycogen molecule. Formation of UDP-glucose is made energetically favorable and irreversible by hydrolysis of pyrophosphate by **pyrophosphatase:**

$$PP_i^{4-} + H_2O \rightarrow 2\ P_i^{2-}$$

Glycogen Synthase

Glycogen synthase catalyzes transfer of the activated glucosyl moiety of UDP-glucose to a glycogen molecule to form a new glycosidic bond between the hydroxyl group of C-1 of the activated sugar and C-4 of a glucosyl residue of the growing glycogen chain. The reducing end of glucose (C-1 of glucose is an aldehyde that can reduce other compounds) is always added to a nonreducing end of the glycogen chain. The glycogen molecule, regardless of its size, theoretically has only one free reducing end tucked away within its core. UDP formed as a product of glycogen synthase is converted back to UTP by action of **nucleoside diphosphate kinase:**

$$\text{UDP} + \text{ATP} \rightarrow \text{UTP} + \text{ADP}$$

Glycogen synthase creates chains of glucose molecules with α-1,4-glycosidic linkages, but does not form the α-1,6-glycosidic branches found in glycogen. Its action alone would only produce α-amylose, a straight-chain polymer of glucose with α-1,4-glycosidic linkages. Once an amylose chain of at least 11 residues has been formed, a **"branching" enzyme** comes into play. Its name is **1,4-α-glucan branching enzyme** because it removes a block of about seven glucosyl residues from a growing chain and transfers it to another chain to produce an α-1,6 linkage (see Figure 7.55). The new branch has to be introduced at least four glucosyl residues from an adjacent branch point. Thus the creation of the highly branched structure of glycogen requires the concerted efforts of glycogen synthase and branching enzyme. The overall balanced equation for

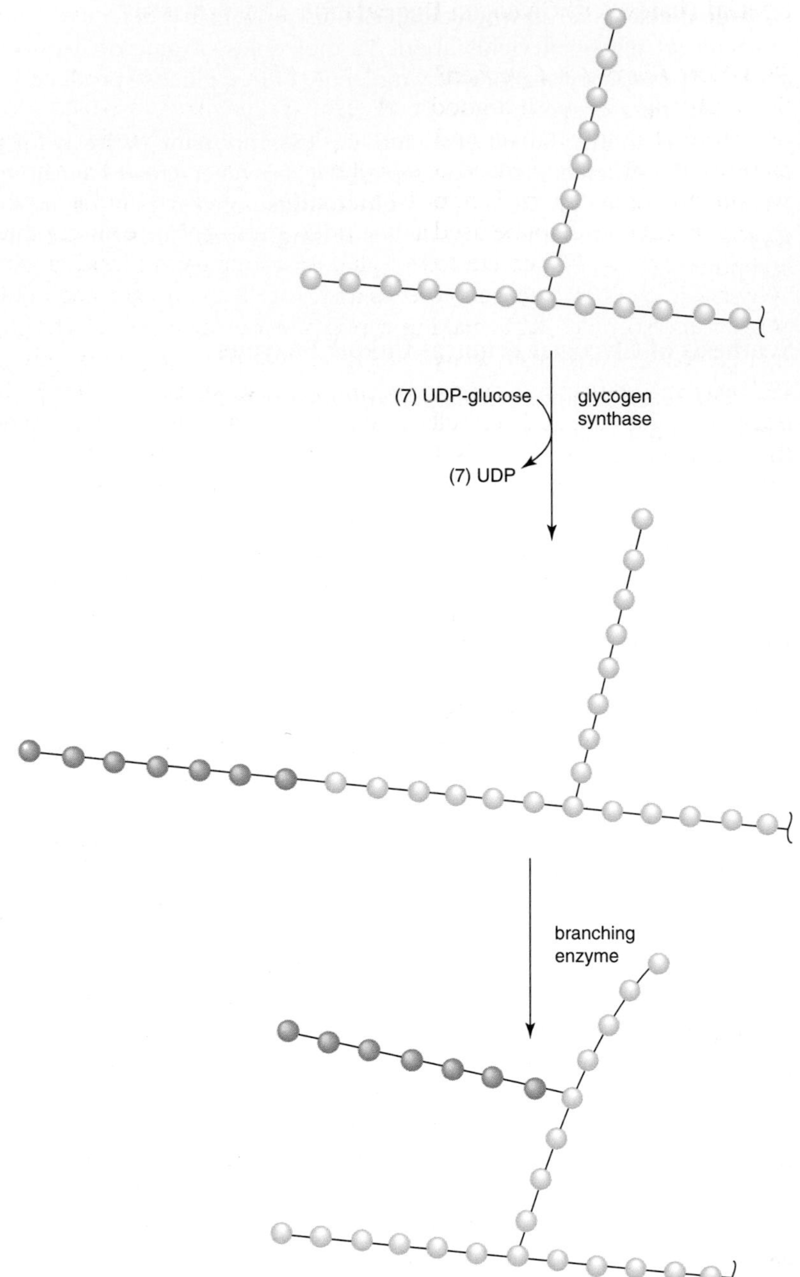

FIGURE 7.55
Action of the glycogen branching enzyme.

glycogen synthesis by the pathway just outlined is

$$(\text{Glucose})_n + \text{glucose} + 2\ \text{ATP} \rightarrow (\text{glucose})_{n+1} + 2\ \text{ADP} + 2\ \text{P}_\text{i}$$

As noted above, the combination of glycogenolysis and glycolysis yields only three molecules of ATP per glucosyl residue:

$$(\text{Glucose})_n + 3\ \text{ADP} + 3\ \text{P}_\text{i} \rightarrow (\text{glucose})_{n-1} + 2\ \text{lactate} + 3\ \text{ATP}$$

Thus the combination of glycogen synthesis plus glycogen degradation to lactate actually yields only one ATP. However, glycogen synthesis and degradation are normally carried out at different times in a cell. For example, white muscle fibers synthesize glycogen at rest when glucose is plentiful and less ATP is needed for muscle contraction. Glycogen is then used during periods of exertion. Although in such terms glycogen storage is not a very efficient process, it provides cells with a fuel reserve that can be very quickly and efficiently mobilized.

Special Features of Glycogen Degradation and Synthesis

Why Store Glucose as Glycogen?

Since **glycogen** is such a good fuel reserve, it is obvious why we synthesize and store glycogen in liver and muscle. But why not store our excess glucose calories entirely as fat instead of glycogen? The answer is at least threefold: (1) we do store **fat,** but fat cannot be mobilized nearly as rapidly in muscle as glycogen; (2) fat cannot be used as a source of energy in the absence of oxygen; and (3) fat cannot be converted to glucose to maintain blood glucose levels. Why not just pump glucose into cells and store it as free glucose until needed? Why waste so much ATP making a polymer out of glucose? The problem is that glucose is osmotically active. It would cost ATP to "pump" glucose into a cell against a concentration gradient, and glucose would have to reach concentrations of 400 mM in liver cells to match the "glucose reserve" provided by the usual liver glycogen levels. Unless balanced by outward movement of some other osmotically active compound, accumulation of such concentrations of glucose would cause uptake of considerable water and osmotic lysis of the cell. Assuming the molecular mass of a glycogen molecule is of the order of 10^7 Da, 400 mM glucose is in effect stored at an intracellular glycogen concentration of 0.01 μM. Storage of glucose as glycogen therefore creates no osmotic pressure problem for the cell.

Glycogenin Is Required as a Primer for Glycogen Synthesis

Like DNA synthesis, a primer is needed for glycogen synthesis. No template, however, is required. Glycogen itself is the usual **primer,** in that glycogen synthesis can take place by addition of glucosyl units to glycogen "core" molecules, which are almost invariably present in the cell. The outer regions of the glycogen molecule get removed and resynthesized more rapidly than the inner core. Glycogen within a cell is frequently sheared by the combined actions of glycogen phosphorylase and debranching enzyme but is seldom obliterated before glycogen synthase and branching enzyme rebuild the molecule. This begs the question why glycogen is a branched molecule with only one real beginning (the reducing end) and many branches terminating with nonreducing glucosyl units. The answer is that this gives numerous sites of attack for glycogen phosphorylase on a mature glycogen molecule and the same number of sites that function as primers for the addition of glucosyl units by glycogen synthase. If cells synthesized ***α*-amylose,** that is, an unbranched glucose polymer, there would only be one nonreducing end per molecule. This would surely make glycogen degradation and synthesis much slower. As it is, glycogen phosphorylase and glycogen synthase are found in tight association with glycogen granules in a cell. By taking up residence in the branches of the glycogen tree, both enzymes have ready access to a multitude of nonreducing sugars at the ends of the limbs.

But why is a primer needed for glycogen synthesis? It turns out to be impossible to initiate glycogen synthesis with simply a glucose molecule as the acceptor of an activated glucosyl residue from UDP-glucose. Glycogen synthase has a very low K_m for very large glycogen molecules and therefore readily adds glucosyl residues to make even larger glycogen molecules. However, the K_m gets larger and larger as the glycogen molecule gets smaller and smaller. This phenomenon is so pronounced that glucose, at its physiological concentration, could never function as a primer. This led for some time to the notion that glycogen must be immortal; that is, some glycogen must be handed down from one cell generation to the next in order for glycogen to be synthesized. However, it is now known that a polypeptide of 332 amino acids called **glycogenin** functions as a primer for glycogen synthesis. Glycogenin is a self-glucosylating enzyme that uses UDP-glucose to link glucose to one of its own tyrosine residues (Figure 7.56). Glycosylated glycogenin then serves as a primer for synthesis of glycogen. Alas, glycogen is not immortal.

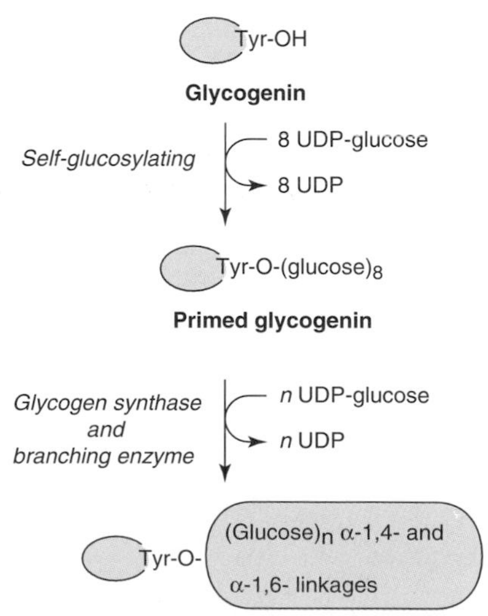

FIGURE 7.56
Glycogenin provides a primer for glycogen synthesis by glycogen synthase. Tyr designates a tyrosine residue of glycogenin.

Glycogen Limits Its Own Synthesis

If glycogen synthase becomes more efficient as the glycogen molecule gets bigger, how is synthesis of this ball of sugar curtailed? Fat cells have an almost unlimited capacity to pack away fat— but then fat cells have nothing else to do. Muscle cells participate in mechanical activity and liver cells carry out many processes other than glycogen synthesis. Even in the face of excess glucose, there has to be a way to limit the intracellular accumulation of glycogen. Glycogen itself inhibits glycogen synthase by a mechanism discussed later (see p. 326).

Glycogen Synthesis and Degradation Are Highly Regulated Pathways

Glycogen synthase and glycogen phosphorylase are regulatory enzymes of glycogen synthesis and degradation, respectively. Both catalyze nonequilibrium reactions, and both are subject to control by allosteric effectors and covalent modification.

Regulation of Glycogen Phosphorylase

Glycogen phosphorylase is subject to allosteric activation by AMP and allosteric inhibition by glucose and ATP (Figure 7.57). Control by these effectors is integrated with a very elaborate control by covalent modification. Phosphorylase exists in an *a* form, which is active, and a *b* form, which is inactive. These forms are interconverted by the actions of **phosphorylase kinase** and **phosphoprotein phosphatase** (Figure 7.57). A conformational change caused by phosphorylation transforms the enzyme into a more active catalytic state. Phosphorylase *b* has some catalytic activity and can be greatly activated by AMP. This allosteric effector has little activating effect, however, on the already active phosphorylase *a*. Hence the covalent modification mechanism can be bypassed by the allosteric mechanism and vice versa.

Phosphorylase kinase is responsible for phosphorylation and activation of phosphorylase (Figure 7.57). Moreover, phosphorylase kinase itself is also sub-

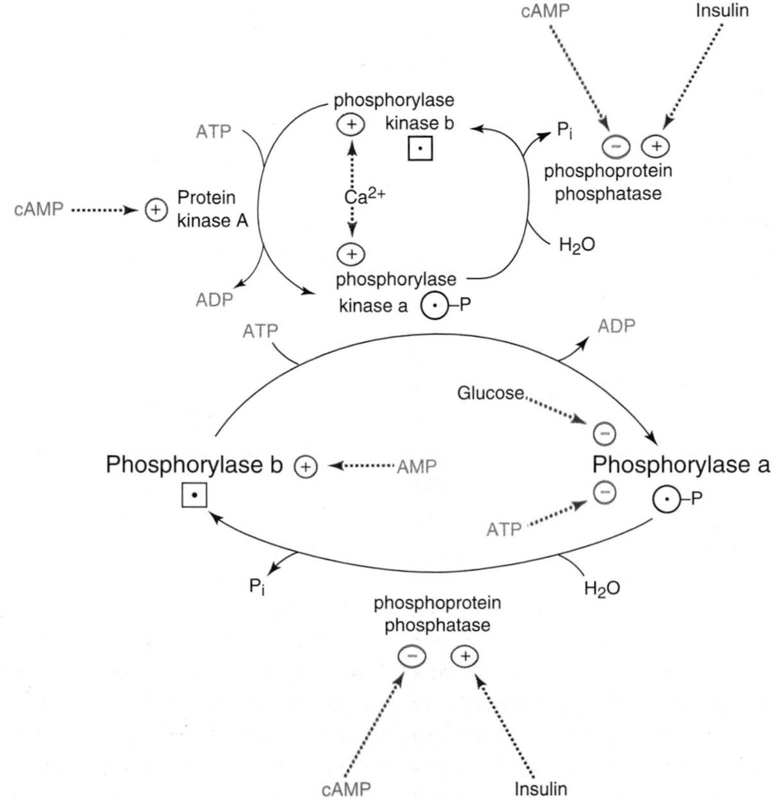

FIGURE 7.57
Regulation of glycogen phosphorylase by covalent modification.
Phosphorylation converts glycogen phosphorylase and phosphorylase kinase from their inactive *b* forms to their active *a* forms.

ject to regulation by a cyclic phosphorylation–dephosphorylation mechanism. Protein kinase A phosphorylates and activates phosphorylase kinase; phosphoprotein phosphatase in turn dephosphorylates and inactivates phosphorylase kinase. Phosphorylase kinase is a large enzyme complex (1.3×10^6 Da), composed of four subunits with four molecules of each subunit in the complex ($\alpha_4\beta_4\gamma_4\delta_4$). Catalytic activity resides with the γ subunit; α, β, and δ subunits exert regulatory control. The α and β subunits are phosphorylated in the transition from the inactive *b* form to the active *a* form of the enzyme. Protein kinase A can only exert an effect on phosphorylase via its ability to phosphorylate and activate phosphorylase kinase. Thus a bicyclic system is required for activation of phosphorylase in response to cAMP-mediated signals.

The δ subunit of phosphorylase kinase also plays a regulatory role. It corresponds to a Ca^{2+}-binding regulatory protein, called **calmodulin.** Not unique to phosphorylase kinase, calmodulin is found in cells as the free molecule and also bound to other enzyme complexes. It functions as a **Ca^{2+}** receptor in the cell, responding to changes in intracellular Ca^{2+} concentration and affecting the relative activities of a number of enzyme systems. Binding of Ca^{2+} to the calmodulin subunit of phosphorylase kinase changes the conformation of the complex, making the enzyme more active with respect to the phosphorylation of phosphorylase. As shown in Figure 7.57, Ca^{2+} is an activator of both phosphorylase kinase *a* and phosphorylase kinase *b.* Maximum activation of phosphorylase kinase requires both phosphorylation of specific serine residues of the enzyme and interaction of Ca^{2+} with the calmodulin subunit of the enzyme. This is one mechanism by which Ca^{2+} functions as an important "second messenger" of hormone action, as will be discussed below.

Activation of phosphorylase kinase by phosphorylation and Ca^{2+} will have a substantial effect on the activity of glycogen phosphorylase. It is equally obvious, however, that turning off the phosphoprotein phosphatase that modulates the phosphorylation states of both phosphorylase kinase and glycogen phosphorylase (Figure 7.57) could achieve the same effect. Ultimate control of glycogen phosphorylase would involve the reciprocal regulation of phosphoprotein phosphatase and phosphorylase kinase activities. Although numerous details remain to be understood, there is evidence that activities of phosphoprotein phosphatase and phosphorylase kinase are controlled in a reciprocal manner. Regulation of phosphoprotein phosphatase activity is linked to cAMP (see p. 325). The important point in Figure 7.57 is that hormones that increase cAMP levels, such as **glucagon** and **epinephrine,** promote activation of glycogen phosphorylase by signaling activation of phosphorylase kinase and inactivation of phosphoprotein phosphatase. On the other hand, **insulin,** which acts either though a second messenger or a kinase-mediated signal cascade (see p. 879), exerts the opposite effect on phosphorylase by promoting activation of phosphoprotein phosphatase activity.

The Cascade that Regulates Glycogen Phosphorylase Amplifies a Small Signal into a Very Large Effect

There is a good reason for the existence of the bicyclic control system for phosphorylation of glycogen phosphorylase. It provides a tremendous amplification mechanism of a very small initial signal. Activation of **adenylate cyclase** by one molecule of epinephrine causes formation of many molecules of cAMP. Each cAMP molecule activates a protein kinase A molecule, which in turn activates many molecules of phosphorylase kinase as well as many molecules of phosphoprotein phosphatase. In turn, phosphorylase kinase phosphorylates many molecules of glycogen phosphorylase, which in turn catalyze phosphorolysis of many glycosidic bonds of glycogen. A very elaborate amplification system is therefore provided in which the signal provided by just a few molecules of hormone is amplified into production of an enormous number of glucose 1-phosphate molecules. If each step represents, for argument's sake, an amplification factor of 100, then a total of four steps would result in an amplification of 100 million! This system is so rapid, in large part because of this **amplification mechanism,** that all of the stored glycogen of white muscle fibers could be completely mobilized within just a few seconds.

Regulation of Glycogen Synthase

Glycogen synthase has to be active for glycogen synthesis and inactive for glycogen degradation. The combination of the reactions catalyzed by glycogen synthase, glycogen phosphorylase, glucose 1-phosphate uridylyltransferase, and nucleoside diphosphate kinase adds up to a futile cycle with the overall equation ATP $\rightarrow$ ADP + P_i. Hence glycogen synthase needs to be turned off when glycogen phosphorylase is turned on, and vice versa.

Activation of **glycogen synthase** by glucose 6-phosphate, an allosteric effector, is probably of physiological significance under some circumstances (Figure 7.58). However, as with glycogen phosphorylase, this mode of control is integrated with regulation by covalent modification (Figure 7.58). Glycogen synthase exists in two forms. One is designated the D form because it is dependent on the presence of G6P for activity. The other is designated the I form because its activity is independent of the presence of G6P. The D form corresponds to the *b* or inactive form of the enzyme, the I form to the *a* or active form of the enzyme. Phosphorylation of glycogen synthase is catalyzed by several different kinases, which in turn are regulated by second messengers of

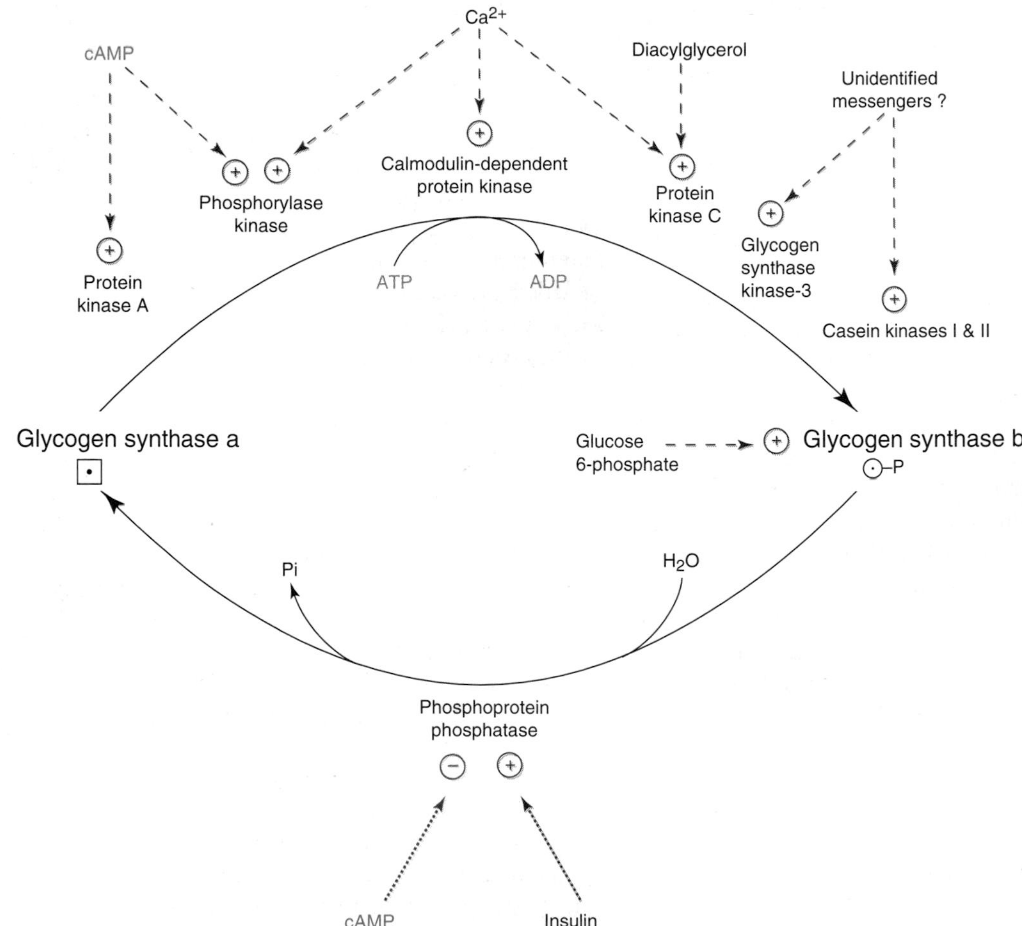

FIGURE 7.58
Regulation of glycogen synthase by covalent modification.
Phosphorylation converts glycogen synthase from its active *a* form to its inactive *b* form.

hormone action, including cAMP, Ca^{2+}, **diacylglycerol,** and probably yet to be identified compounds. Each of the protein kinases shown in Figure 7.58 is capable of catalyzing the phosphorylation and contributing to inactivation of glycogen synthase. Although glycogen synthase is a simple tetramer (α_4) of only one subunit type (mol wt 85,000 Da), it can be phosphorylated on at least nine different serine residues. Eleven different protein kinases have been identified that can phosphorylate glycogen synthase. This stands in striking contrast to glycogen phosphorylase, which is regulated by phosphorylation of one site by one specific kinase.

Cyclic AMP is an extremely important intracellular signal for reciprocally controlling glycogen synthase (Figure 7.58) and glycogen phosphorylase (Figure 7.57). An increase in cAMP signals activation of glycogen phosphorylase and inactivation of glycogen synthase via activation of protein kinase A and inhibition of phosphoprotein phosphatase. Ca^{2+} likewise can influence the phosphorylation state of both enzymes and reciprocally regulate their activity via its effects on phosphorylase kinase. Two cAMP-independent, Ca^{2+}-activated protein kinases have been identified that also may have physiological significance. One of these is a calmodulin-dependent protein kinase and the other a Ca^{2+}- and phospholipid-dependent protein kinase (protein kinase C). Both enzymes phosphorylate glycogen synthase, but neither can phosphorylate glycogen phosphorylase. Protein kinase C requires phospholipid, diacylglycerol, and Ca^{2+} for full activity. There is considerable interest in protein kinase C because **tumor-promoting agents** called **phorbol esters** have been found to mimic diacylglycerol as activators of this enzyme. Diacylglycerol is considered an important "second messenger" of hormone action, acting via protein kinase C to regulate numerous cellular processes (see p. 865).

Glycogen synthase is also phosphorylated by glycogen synthase kinase-3, casein kinase I, and casein kinase II. These kinases are not subject to regulation by cAMP or Ca^{2+}. It is likely, however, that special regulatory mechanisms exist to regulate these kinases. Herein may lie solutions to unsolved problems such as the mechanism of action of insulin and other hormones.

The phosphoprotein phosphatase that converts glycogen synthase *b* back to glycogen synthase *a* (Figure 7.58) is regulated in a manner analogous to that described in the discussion of glycogen phosphorylase regulation (Figure 7.57). Cyclic AMP promotes inactivation whereas insulin promotes activation of glycogen synthase through opposite effects on phosphoprotein phosphatase activity.

Regulation of Phosphoprotein Phosphatases

About a dozen different **phosphoprotein phosphatases** with specificity for removal of phosphate from serine residues of proteins are currently being studied. In general, phosphoprotein phosphatases occur as catalytic subunits associated with a number of different regulatory subunits that control the activity of the catalytic subunit, determine which substrate(s) the catalytic subunit can interact with and dephosphorylate, and target the association of a catalytic subunit with a specific structure or component within a cell. One such regulatory protein important for glycogen metabolism has been given the name **G subunit,** denoting a glycogen-binding protein. G subunit binds both glycogen and a phosphatase catalytic subunit (Figure 7.59). This association makes the phosphatase ten times more active toward glycogen synthase and glycogen phosphorylase and thereby greatly promotes their dephosphorylation. However, phosphorylation of the G subunit by protein kinase A results in release of the phosphatase catalytic subunit, which is then less active. Interaction of the free catalytic subunit with yet another regulatory protein (called **inhibitor 1**) then causes further inhibition of phosphatase activity. Effective inhibition of the residual phosphatase activity of the catalytic subunit requires phosphorylation of inhibitor 1 by protein kinase A, thereby creating yet another link to hormones that increase cAMP levels. **Insulin** has effects opposite to those of cAMP;

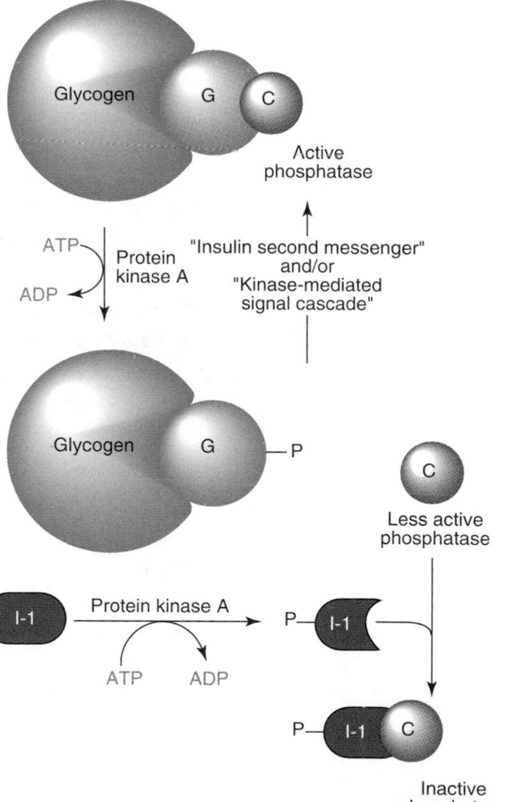

FIGURE 7.59
Mechanism for regulation of a phosphatase that binds to glycogen.
The glycogen-binding subunit G binds directly to glycogen; the phosphoprotein phosphatase catalytic subunit C binds to glycogen via the G subunit; and the phosphorylated inhibitor 1 (I-1) binds the free catalytic subunit.

that is, insulin promotes activation of the catalytic subunit of phosphoprotein phosphatase. This presumably involves reversal of the steps promoted by cAMP, but details of how this is accomplished remain to be established.

Effector Control of Glycogen Metabolism

Certain muscles are known to mobilize their glycogen stores rapidly in response to anaerobic conditions without marked conversion of phosphorylase *b* to phosphorylase *a* or glycogen synthase *a* to glycogen synthase *b*. Presumably this is accomplished by effector control in which ATP levels decrease, causing less inhibition of phosphorylase; glucose 6-phosphate levels decrease, causing less activation of glycogen synthase; and AMP levels increase, causing activation of phosphorylase. This enables muscle to keep working, for at least a short period of time, by using ATP produced by glycolysis of glucose 6-phosphate obtained from glycogen.

Proof that effector control can operate has also been obtained in studies of a special strain of mice that are deficient in muscle phosphorylase kinase. Phosphorylase *b* in muscle of such mice cannot be converted into phosphorylase *a*. Nevertheless, heavy exercise of these mice results in depletion of muscle glycogen, presumably because of stimulation of phosphorylase *b* by effectors.

Negative Feedback Control of Glycogen Synthesis by Glycogen

Glycogen exerts feedback control over its own formation. The portion of glycogen synthase in the active *a* form decreases as glycogen accumulates in a particular tissue. The mechanism is not well understood, but glycogen may make the *a* form a better substrate for one of the protein kinases, or, alternatively, glycogen may inhibit dephosphorylation of glycogen synthase *b* by phosphoprotein phosphatase. Either mechanism would account for the shift in the steady state in favor of glycogen synthase *b* that occurs in response to glycogen accumulation.

Phosphorylase a *Functions as a "Glucose Receptor" in the Liver*

Consumption of a carbohydrate-containing meal results in an increase in blood and liver glucose, which signals an increase in glycogen synthesis in the latter tissue. The mechanism involves glucose stimulation of insulin release from the pancreas and its effects on hepatic glycogen phosphorylase and glycogen synthase. However, hormone-independent mechanisms also appear to be important in liver (Figure 7.60). Direct inhibition of phosphorylase *a* by glucose is probably of importance. Binding of glucose to phosphorylase makes the *a* form of phosphorylase a better substrate for dephosphorylation by phosphoprotein phosphatase. Therefore phosphorylase *a* functions as a glucose receptor in liver. Binding of glucose to phosphorylase *a* promotes inactivation of phosphorylase *a*, with the overall result being inhibition of glycogen degradation by glucose. This "negative feedback" control of glycogenolysis by glucose would not necessarily promote glycogen synthesis. However, there also is evidence that phosphorylase *a* is an inhibitor of the dephosphorylation of glycogen synthase *b* by phosphoprotein phosphatase. This inhibition is lost once phosphorylase *a* has been converted to phosphorylase *b* (Figure 7.60). In other words, phosphoprotein phosphatase can turn its attention to glycogen synthase *b* only following dephosphorylation of phosphorylase *a*. Thus, as a result of interaction of glucose with phosphorylase *a*, phosphorylase becomes inactivated, glycogen synthase becomes activated, and glycogen is synthesized rather than degraded in liver. Phosphorylase *a* can serve this function of "glucose receptor" in liver because the concentration of glucose in liver always reflects the blood concentration of glucose. This is not true for extrahepatic tissues. Liver cells have a very high-capacity transport system for glucose and a high K_m enzyme for glucose phosphorylation (glucokinase). Cells of extrahepatic

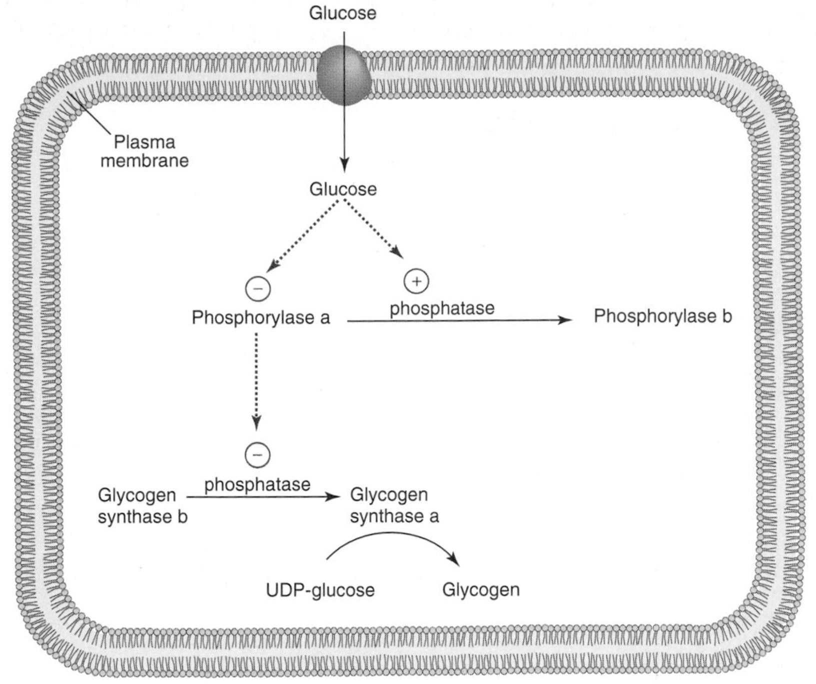

FIGURE 7.60
Overview of the mechanism responsible for glucose stimulation of glycogen synthesis in the liver.

tissues as a general rule have glucose transport and phosphorylation systems that maintain intracellular glucose at concentrations too low for phosphorylase *a* to function as a "glucose receptor."

Glucagon Stimulates Glycogen Degradation in the Liver

Glucagon is released from α cells of pancreas in response to low blood glucose levels. One of glucagon's primary jobs during periods of low food intake (fasting or starvation) is to mobilize **liver glycogen,** that is, stimulate glycogenolysis, in order to ensure that adequate blood glucose is available to meet the needs of glucose-dependent tissues. Glucagon circulates in blood until it interacts with glucagon receptors such as those located on the plasma membrane of liver cells (see Figure 7.61). Binding of glucagon to these receptors activates adenylate cyclase and triggers the cascades that result in activation of glycogen phosphorylase and inactivation of glycogen synthase by the mechanisms given in Figures 7.57 and 7.58, respectively. Glucagon also inhibits glycolysis at the level of 6-phosphofructo-1-kinase and pyruvate kinase by the mechanisms given in Figures 7.25 and 7.30, respectively. The net result of these effects of glucagon, all mediated by the second messenger cAMP and covalent modification, is a very rapid increase in blood glucose levels. Hyperglycemia might be expected but does not occur because less glucagon is released from the pancreas as blood glucose levels increase.

Epinephrine Stimulates Glycogen Degradation in the Liver

Epinephrine is released into blood from chromaffin cells of the adrenal medulla in response to stress. This hormone is our "fright, flight, or fight" hormone, preparing the body for either combat or escape.

Epinephrine interacts directly with receptors in the plasma membrane of liver cells to activate **adenylate cyclase** (Figure 7.61). The resulting increase in cAMP has the same effect as that caused by glucagon, that is, activation of glycogenolysis and inhibition of glycogenesis and glycolysis to maximize the release of glucose from liver. The plasma membrane receptor for epinephrine,

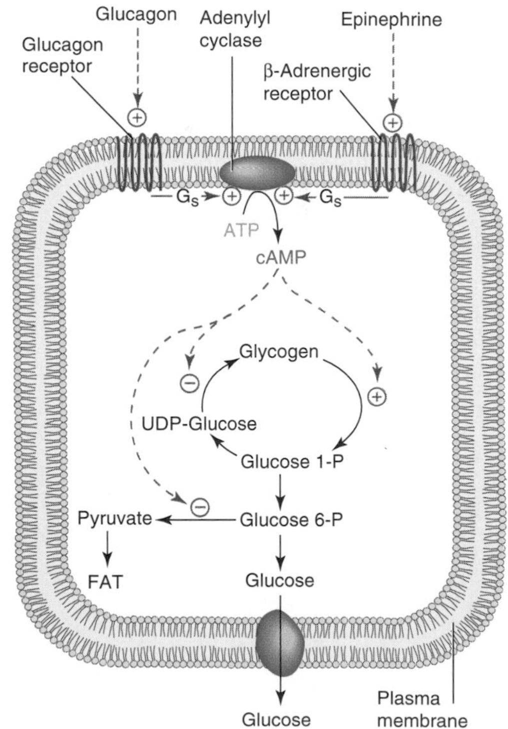

FIGURE 7.61
Cyclic AMP mediates the stimulation of glycogenolysis in liver by glucagon and β agonists (epinephrine).
See legends for Figures 7.19 and 7.25.

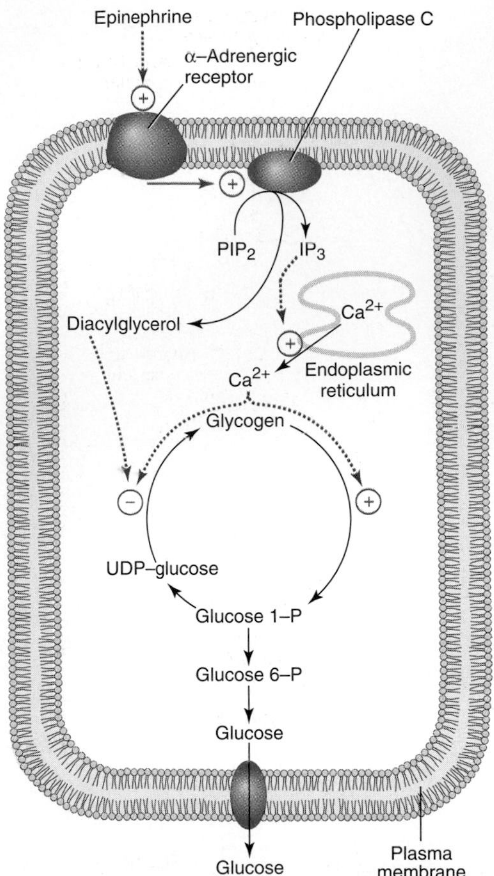

FIGURE 7.62
Inositol trisphosphate (IP_3) and Ca^{2+} mediate the stimulation of glycogenolysis in liver by α agonists.
The α-adrenergic receptor and glucose transporter are intrinsic components of the plasma membrane. Although not indicated, phosphatidylinositol 4,5-bisphosphate (PIP_2) is also a component of the plasma membrane.

which is in communication with adenylate cyclase, is the β-adrenergic receptor. The plasma membrane of liver cells also has another binding protein for epinephrine, called the **α-adrenergic receptor.** Interaction of epinephrine with α-adrenergic receptors leads to formation of **inositol 1,4,5-trisphosphate** (IP_3) and **diacylglycerol** (Figure 7.62). These compounds are second messengers, produced in the plasma membrane by the action of a phospholipase C on phosphatidylinositol 4,5-bisphosphate (Figure 7.63). Inositol 1,4,5-trisphosphate stimulates the release of Ca^{2+} from the endoplasmic reticulum (Figure 7.62). As previously discussed (Figure 7.57), the increase in Ca^{2+} activates phosphorylase kinase, which in turn activates glycogen phosphorylase. Likewise (Figure 7.58), Ca^{2+}-mediated activation of phosphorylase kinase, calmodulin-dependent protein kinase, and protein kinase C, as well as diacylglycerol-mediated activation of protein kinase C, may all be important for inactivation of glycogen synthase.

The consequences of epinephrine action is an increased release of glucose into the blood from the glycogen stored in liver. This makes more blood glucose available to tissues that are called upon to meet the challenge of the stressful situation that triggered the release of epinephrine from adrenal medulla.

Epinephrine Stimulates Glycogen Degradation in Heart and Skeletal Muscle

Epinephrine also stimulates glycogen degradation in heart and skeletal muscle. Cyclic AMP, produced in response to epinephrine stimulation of adenylate cyclase via **β-adrenergic** receptors (Figure 7.64), signals concurrent activation of glycogen phosphorylase and inactivation of glycogen synthase by mechanisms given previously in Figures 7.57 and 7.58, respectively. This does not lead, however, to glucose release into blood from these tissues. In contrast to liver, heart and skeletal muscle lack glucose 6-phosphatase, and in these tissues cAMP does not inhibit but rather stimulates glycolysis (see Figure 7.28). Thus the role of epinephrine on glycogen metabolism in heart and skeletal muscle is to make more glucose 6-phosphate available for glycolysis. ATP generated by glycolysis can then be used to meet the metabolic demand imposed on these muscles by the stress that triggered epinephrine release.

Neural Control of Glycogen Degradation in Skeletal Muscle

Nervous excitation of muscle activity is mediated via changes in intracellular Ca^{2+} concentrations (Figure 7.65). A **nerve impulse** causes **membrane depo-**

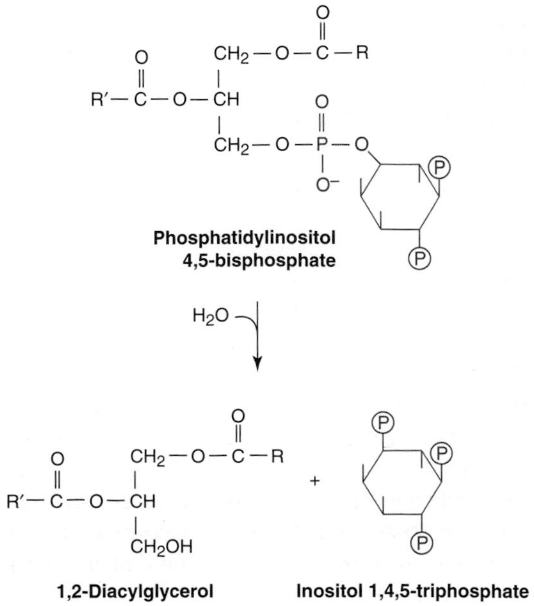

Phosphatidylinositol 4,5-bisphosphate

H_2O

1,2-Diacylglycerol

Inositol 1,4,5-triphosphate

FIGURE 7.63
Phospholipase C cleaves phosphatidylinositol 4,5-bisphosphate to produce 1,2-diacylglycerol and inositol 1,4,5-trisphosphate.

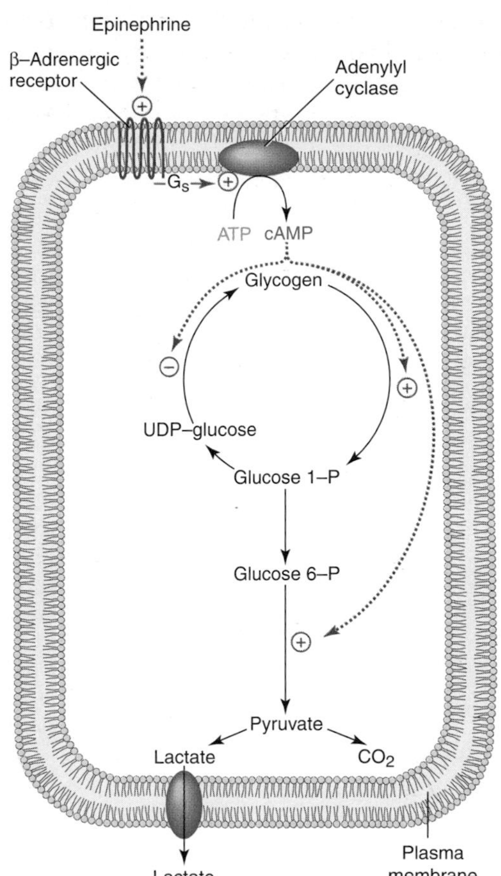

FIGURE 7.64
Cyclic AMP mediates the stimulation of glycogenolysis in muscle by β agonists (epinephrine).
The β-adrenergic receptor is an intrinsic component of the plasma membrane that acts to stimulate adenylate cyclase via a stimulatory G-protein (G_s).

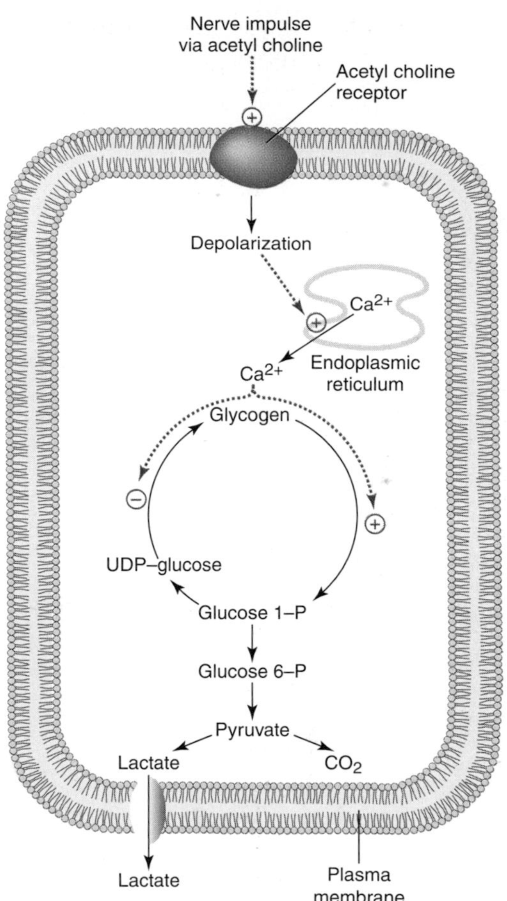

FIGURE 7.65
Ca^{2+} mediates the stimulation of glycogenolysis in muscle by nervous excitation.

larization, which in turn causes Ca^{2+} release from the **sarcoplasmic reticulum** into the sarcoplasm of muscle cells. This release of Ca^{2+} triggers muscle contraction, whereas reaccumulation of Ca^{2+} by the sarcoplasmic reticulum causes relaxation. The same change in Ca^{2+} concentration effective in causing muscle contraction (from 10^{-8} to 10^{-6} M) also greatly affects the activity of phosphorylase kinase. As Ca^{2+} concentrations increase there is more muscle activity and a greater need for ATP. Activation of phosphorylase kinase by Ca^{2+} leads to the subsequent activation of glycogen phosphorylase and perhaps the inactivation of glycogen synthase. The result is that more glycogen is converted to glucose 6-phosphate so that more ATP can be produced to meet the greater energy demand of muscle contraction.

Insulin Stimulates Glycogen Synthesis in Muscle and Liver

An increase in blood glucose signals release of insulin from β cells of the pancreas. Insulin circulates in blood, serving as a first messenger to inform several tissues that excess glucose is present. Insulin receptors, located on the plasma membranes of insulin-responsive cells, respond to insulin binding by either producing a second messenger of insulin action or inducing a protein kinase cascade that promotes glucose use within these tissues (Figures 7.66 and 7.67). The pancreas responds to a decrease in blood glucose with less release of insulin but greater release of glucagon. These hormones have opposite effects on glucose utilization by liver, thereby establishing the pancreas as a fine-tuning device that prevents dangerous fluctuations in blood glucose levels.

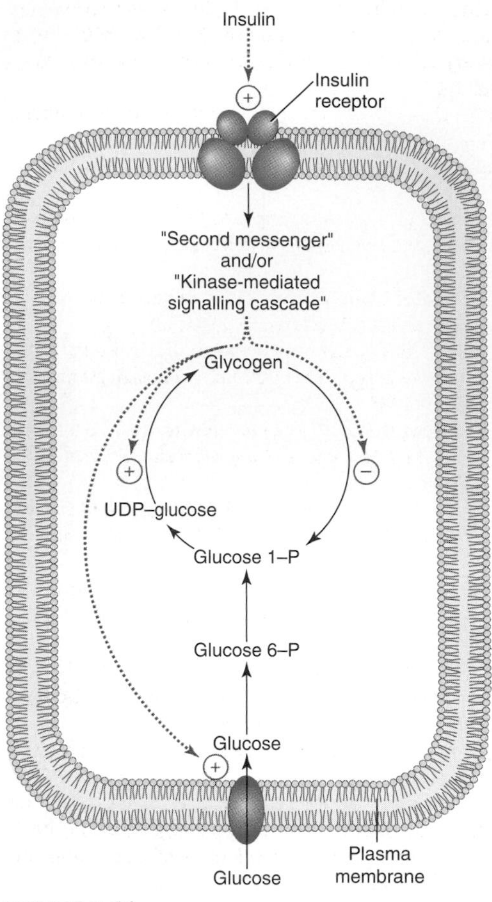

FIGURE 7.66
Insulin acts via a plasma membrane receptor to promote glycogen synthesis in muscle.

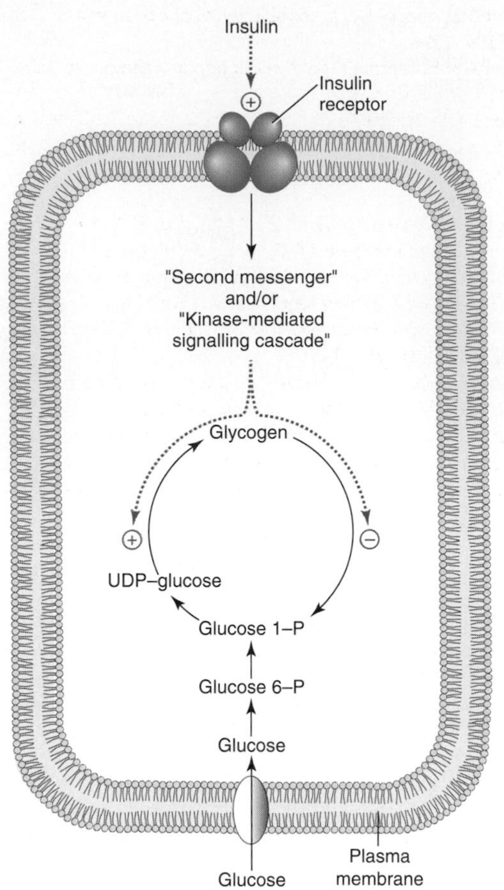

FIGURE 7.67
Insulin acts via a plasma membrane receptor to promote glycogen synthesis in liver.

Insulin increases glucose utilization in part by promoting glycogenesis and inhibiting glycogenolysis in muscle (Figure 7.66) and liver (Figure 7.67). Insulin stimulation of glucose transport at the plasma membrane is essential for these effects in muscle but not liver. Hepatocytes have a high-capacity, **insulin-insensitive glucose transport system** (GLUT-2), whereas muscle cells and adipocytes are equipped with a **glucose transport system** (GLUT-4) that requires insulin for maximum rates of glucose uptake. Insulin stimulates muscle and adipose tissue glucose transport by signaling an increase in the number of functional GLUT-4 proteins associated with the plasma membrane. This is accomplished by promoting translocation of GLUT-4 from an intracellular pool to the plasma membrane (see Chapter 20). Insulin further promotes glycogen accumulation in both tissues by activating glycogen synthase and inhibiting glycogen phosphorylase as discussed previously (Figures 7.57, 7.58, and 7.59).

BIBLIOGRAPHY

Arion, W. J., Lange, A. J., Walls, H. E., and Ballas, L. M. Evidence for the participation of independent translocases for phosphate and glucose 6-phosphate in the microsomal glucose 6-phosphatase system. *J. Biol. Chem.* 255:10396, 1980.

Berridge, M. J. Review article: inositol trisphosphate and diacylglycerol as second messengers. *Biochem. J.* 220:345, 1984.

Brooke, M. H., and Kaiser, K. K. The use and abuse of muscle histochemistry. *Ann. N.Y. Acad. Sci.* 228:121, 1974.

Cheatham, B., and Kahn, C. R. Insulin action and the insulin signaling network. *Endocr. Rev.* 16:117, 1995.

Cohen, P. Dissection of the protein phosphorylation cascades involved in insulin and growth factor action. *Biochem. Soc. Trans.* 21:555, 1993.

DeFronzo, R. A., and Ferrannini, E. Regulation of hepatic glucose metabolism in humans. *Diabetes Metab. Reviews* 3:415, 1987.

DePaoli-Roach, A. A., Park, I.-K., Cerovsky, V., Csortos, C., Durbin, S. D., Kuntz, M. J., Sitikov, A., Tang, P. M., Verin, A., and Zolnierowicz, S.

Serine/threonine protein phosphatases in the control of cell function. *Adv. Enzyme Regul.* 34:199, 1994.

Exton, J. H. Mechanisms of hormonal regulation of hepatic glucose metabolism. *Diabetes Metab. Rev.* 3:163, 1987.

Garcia, C. K., Goldstein, J. L., Pathak, R. K., Anderson, R. G. W., and Brown, M. S. Molecular characterization of a membrane transporter for lactate, pyruvate, and other monocarboxylates: implications for the Cori cycle. *Cell* 76:865, 1994.

Geelen, M. J. H., Harris, R. A., Beynen, A. C., and McCune, S. A. Short-term hormonal control of hepatic lipogenesis. *Diabetes* 29:1006, 1980.

Gitzelmann, R., Steinmann, B., and Van den Berghe, G. Disorders of fructose metabolism. In: C. R. Scriver, A. L. Beaudet, W. S. Sly, and D. Valle (Eds.), *The Metabolic and Molecular Bases of Inherited Disease,* 7th ed. New York: McGraw-Hill, 1995, pp. 905–934.

Gould, G. W., and Holman, G. D. The glucose transporter family: structure, function and tissue-specific expression. *Biochem. J.* 295:329, 1993.

Greene, H. L., Slonin, A. E., and Burr, I. M. Type I glycogen storage disease: a metabolic basis for advances in treatment. In: L. A. Barness (Ed.), *Advances in Pediatrics,* Vol. 26. Chicago: Year Book Publishers, 1979, p. 63.

Gurney, A. L., Park, E. A., Liu, J., Giralt, M., McGrane, M. M., Patel, Y. M., Crawford, D. R., Nizielski, S. E., Savon, S., and Hanson, R. W. Metabolic regulation of gene transcription. *J. Nutr.* 124:1533S, 1994.

Hallfrisch, J. Metabolic effects of dietary fructose. *FASEB J.* 4:2652, 1990.

Hanson, R. W., and Mehlman, M. A. (Eds.). *Gluconeogenesis, Its Regulation in Mammalian Species.* New York: Wiley, 1976.

Hunter, T. Protein kinases and phosphatases: the yin and yang of protein phosphorylation and signaling. *Cell* 80:225, 1995.

Ingebritsen, T. S., and Cohen, P. Protein phosphatases: properties and role in cellular regulation. *Science* 221:331, 1983.

Isselbacher, K. J., Adams, R. D., Braundwald, E., Petersdorf, R. B., and Wilson, J. D. (Eds.). *Harrison's principles of internal medicine,* 9th ed. New York: McGraw-Hill, 1980.

Lalli, E., and Sassone-Corsi, P. Signal transduction and gene regulation: the nuclear response to cAMP. *J. Biol. Chem.* 269:17359, 1994.

Lieber, C. S. The metabolism of alcohol. *Sci. Am.* 234:25, 1976.

Lomako, J., Lomako, W. M., and Whelan, W. J. A self-glucosylating protein is the primer for rabbit muscle glycogen biosynthesis. *FASEB J.* 2:3097, 1988.

Metzler, D. E. *Biochemistry, The Chemical Reactions of Living Cells.* New York: Academic Press, 1977.

Newsholme, E. A., and Leech, A. R. *Biochemistry for the Medical Sciences.* New York: Wiley, 1983.

Newsholme, E. A., and Start, C. *Regulation in Metabolism.* New York: Wiley, 1973.

Pilkis, S. J., Claus, T. H., Kurland, I. J., and Lange, A. J. 6-Phosphofructo-2-kinase/fructose-2,6-bisphosphatase: a metabolic signaling enzyme. *Annu. Rev. Biochem.* 64:799, 1995.

Pilkis, S. J., and El-Maghrabi, M. R. Hormonal regulation of hepatic gluconeogenesis and glycolysis. *Annu. Rev. Biochem.* 57:755, 1988.

Roach, P. J. Hormonal control of glycogen metabolism. In: H. Rupp (Ed.), *Regulation of Heart Function: Basic Concepts and Clinical Applications.* New York: Thieme-Stratton, 1985.

Roach, P. J. Principles of the regulation of enzyme activity. In: L. Goldstein and D. M. Prescott (Eds.), *Cell Biology, A Comprehensive Treatise,* Vol. IV. New York: Academic Press, 1980.

Scriver, C. R., Beaudet, A. L., Sly, W. S., and Valle, D. (Eds.). *The Metabolic and Molecular Bases of Inherited Disease,* 7th ed. New York: McGraw-Hill, 1995.

Stanley, C. A., Anday, E. K., Baker, L., and Delivoria-Papadopolous, M. Metabolic fuel and hormone responses to fasting in newborn infants. *Pediatrics* 64:613, 1979.

Taylor, S. I. Diabetes mellitus. In: C. R. Scriver, A. L. Beaudet, W. S. Sly, and D. Valle (Eds.), *The Metabolic and Molecular Bases of Inherited Disease,* 7th ed. New York: McGraw-Hill, 1995, pp. 843–896.

van de Werve, G., and Jeanrenaud, B. Liver glycogen metabolism: an overview. *Diabetes Metab. Rev.* 3:47, 1987.

van Schaftingen, E., Vandercammen, A., Detheux, M., and Davies, D. R. The regulatory protein of liver glucokinase. *Adv. Enzyme Regul.* 32:133, 1992.

Vaulont, S., and Kahn, A. Transcriptional control of metabolic regulation genes by carbohydrates. *FASEB J.* 8:28, 1994.

Viskupic, E., Cao, Y., Zhang, W., Cheng, C., DePaoli-Roach, A. A., and Roach, P. J. Rabbit skeletal muscle glycogenin. *J. Biol. Chem.* 267:25759, 1992.

QUESTIONS ■ J. BAGGOTT AND C. N. ANGSTADT

1. In glycolysis ATP synthesis is catalyzed by:
   A. hexokinase.
   B. 6-phosphofructo-1-kinase.
   C. glyceraldehyde-3-phosphate dehydrogenase.
   D. phosphoglycerate kinase.
   E. none of the above.

2. The irreversible reactions of glycolysis include that catalyzed by:
   A. phosphoglucose isomerase.
   B. 6-phosphofructo-1-kinase.
   C. fructose-bisphosphate aldolase.
   D. glyceraldehyde-3-phosphate dehydrogenase.
   E. phosphoglycerate kinase.

3. NAD^+ can be regenerated in the cytoplasm if NADH reacts with any of the following EXCEPT:
   A. pyruvate.
   B. dihydroxyacetone phosphate.
   C. oxaloacetate.
   D. the flavin bound to NADH dehydrogenase.

4. Glucokinase:
   A. has a K_m considerably greater than the normal blood glucose concentration.
   B. is found in muscle.
   C. is inhibited by glucose 6-phosphate.
   D. is also known as the GLUT-2 protein.
   E. has glucose 6-phosphatase activity as well as kinase activity.

5. The primary short-term regulation of glucokinase activity in the liver is effected by:
   A. substrate concentration.
   B. fructose 1-phosphate concentration.
   C. induction of glucokinase synthesis by high intracellular glucose concentrations.
   D. insulin-induced increase in transcription of the glucokinase gene.
   E. allosteric activation by ADP.

6. 6-Phosphofructo-1-kinase activity can be decreased by all of the following EXCEPT:
   A. ATP at high concentrations.
   B. citrate.
   C. AMP.
   D. low pH.
   E. decreased concentration of fructose 2,6-bisphosphate.

7. Which of the following supports gluconeogenesis?
   A. α-ketoglutarate + aspartate = glutamate + oxaloacetate
   B. pyruvate + ATP + HCO_3^- $\rightleftharpoons$ oxaloacetate + ADP + P_i + H^+
   C. acetyl CoA + oxaloacetate + H_2O $\rightleftharpoons$ citrate + CoA
   D. leucine degradation
   E. lysine degradation

8. In the Cori cycle:
   A. only tissues with aerobic metabolism (i.e., mitochondria and O_2) are involved.
   B. a three-carbon compound arising from glycolysis is converted to glucose at the expense of energy from fatty acid oxidation.
   C. glucose is converted to pyruvate in anaerobic tissues, and this pyruvate returns to the liver, where it is converted to glucose.
   D. the same amount of ATP is used in the liver to synthesize glucose as is released during glycolysis, leading to no net effect on whole-body energy balance.
   E. nitrogen from alanine must be converted to urea, increasing the amount of energy required to drive the process.

9. The uncontrolled production of NADH from NAD^+ during ethanol metabolism blocks gluconeogenesis from all of the following EXCEPT:
   A. galactose.
   B. glycerol.
   C. α-ketoglutarate.
   D. oxaloacetate.
   E. pyruvate.

10. Gluconeogenic enzymes include all of the following EXCEPT:
    A. fructose 1,6-bisphosphatase.
    B. glucose 6-phosphatase.
    C. phosphoenolpyruvate carboxykinase.
    D. phosphoglucomutase.
    E. pyruvate carboxylase.

11. When blood glucagon rises, which of the following hepatic enzyme activities FALLS?
    A. adenylate cyclase
    B. protein kinase
    C. 6-phosphofructo-2-kinase
    D. fructose 1,6-bisphosphatase
    E. hexokinase

12. Phospho–dephospho regulation of 6-phosphofructo-1-kinase, 6-phosphofructo-2-kinase, and pyruvate kinase is an important regulatory mechanism in:
    A. brain.
    B. erythrocytes.
    C. intestine.
    D. liver.
    E. skeletal muscle.

Refer to the following for Questions 13–15.
   A. glycogen phosphorylase
   B. phosphoglucomutase
   C. phosphoglucokinase
   D. glucose 6-phosphatase
   E. debranching enzyme

13. A bifunctional enzyme.

14. Lacking in muscle, but present in normal liver.

15. Catalyzes phosphorolysis of glycogen.

16. Phosphorylation activates all of the following EXCEPT:
    A. glycogen phosphorylase.
    B. inhibitor 1.
    C. phosphorylase kinase.
    D. protein kinase.

17. cAMP activates:
    A. glycogen phosphorylase.
    B. hexokinase.
    C. 6-phosphofructo-1-kinase.
    D. protein kinase.
    E. protein kinase C.

ANSWERS

1. D Phosphoglycerate kinase synthesizes ATP in the forward direction (p. 276). A and B use ATP. C synthesizes 1,3-bisphosphoglycerate.
2. B E: The phosphoglycerate kinase reaction is reversible because the product contains a high energy carboxylic acid–phosphoric acid anhydride link. Many other kinases, including 6-phosphofructo-1-kinase, form phosphate esters, which have low-energy bonds.
3. D The flavin is mitochondrial (p. 279). A may be converted to lactate. B and C are the cytoplasmic acceptors for shuttle systems.
4. A Blood glucose is ~5 mM. K_m of glucokinase is ~10 mM. B: Glucokinase is hepatic, and, unlike the muscle hexokinase, it is not inhibited by glucose 6-phosphate (p. 285).
5. A B, C, and D affect glucokinase activity, but they are not the primary short-term regulators (pp. 285–286). E: ADP is not a known effector of glucokinase.
6. C AMP is an allosteric regulator that relieves inhibition by ATP (p. 287). B and D are probably important physiological regulators in muscle, and E is critical in liver.

7. B This reaction is on the direct route of conversion of pyruvate to glucose. A :α-Ketoglutarate and oxaloacetate both give rise to glucose; interconversion of one to the other accomplishes nothing (p. 304). C: Citrate ultimately gives rise to oxaloacetate, losing two carbon atoms in the process; again nothing is gained (p. 306). D and E involve the two amino acids that are strictly ketogenic.
8. B The liver derives the energy required for gluconeogenesis from aerobic oxidation of fatty acids. A: The liver is an essential organ in the Cori cycle; it is aerobic. C: In anaerobic tissues the end product of glycolysis is lactate; in aerobic tissues it is pyruvate, but there the pyruvate would likely be oxidized aerobically. D: Gluconeogenesis requires six ATP molecules per glucose synthesized; glycolysis yields two ATP molecules per glucose metabolized. E: Alanine is not part of the Cori cycle. See Figure 7.32, p. 300.
9. A Gluconeogenesis from galactose is not affected by the redox state of the cell (p. 309, Figure 7.44). B is converted to α-glycerophosphate, which cannot be oxidized to dihydroxyacetone phosphate when $NADH/NAD^+$ is high. For the same reason, C and D will be trapped as malate, since the interconversion of malate and oxaloacetate strongly favors malate even under normal conditions. E will be converted to lactate. Clearly, very high NADH blocks gluconeogenesis at many points (p. 312). If an inebriated person has depleted glycogen stores and has not been ingesting carbohydrates, sources of blood glucose are seriously compromised, and hypoglycemia could become life-threatening (Clin. Corr 7.10). The oft-heard statement that alcohol is metabolized as a carbohydrate is false.
10. D Phosphoglucomutase is on the pathway of glycogen metabolism (p. 314). A–C and E are the so-called gluconeogenic enzymes; they get around the irreversible steps of glycolysis (p. 303).
11. C As blood glucagon rises, A is activated, producing cAMP; cAMP activates B, and B inactivates C. Low levels of fructose 2,6-bisphosphate increase the activity of D (p. 310). E is not an important hepatic enzyme; its role is filled in liver by glucokinase.
12. D Regulation of these enzymes by hormonally controlled phosphorylation and dephosphorylation is of central importance in liver. 6-Phosphofructo-2-kinase is present in other tissues but does not appear to change its activity in response to hormones except in liver. Other enzymes in extrahepatic tissues, such as those of glycogen metabolism in muscle, are under phospho–dephospho regulation.
13. E Debranching enzyme has 4-α-D-glucanotransferase activity, which moves a strand of three glucosyl units from a branch to an end of a glucosyl chain. It also has amylo-α-[1,6]-glucosidase activity, which hydrolyzes the last glucosyl residue from the branch, yielding free glucose (p. 318).
14. D This is why muscle glycogen cannot contribute directly to blood glucose (p. 316).
15. A Note that it is phosphorolysis, not hydrolysis; the product is glucose 1-phosphate, not glucose (p. 314).
16. D A, B, and C are activated by phosphorylation (p. 322, Figure 7.57). Protein kinase (sometimes referred to as protein kinase A) is not a phospho–dephospho enzyme (p. 323).
17. D A (p. 322) and C (p. 287) are allosterically activated by AMP. B is controlled by glucose 6-phosphate. E is activated by Ca^{2+}, phospholipid, and diacylglycerol (p. 325).

CHAPTER

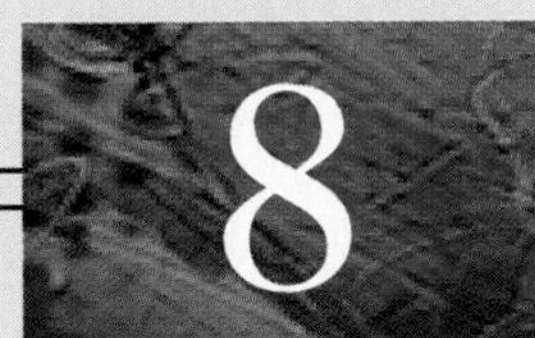

CARBOHYDRATE METABOLISM II: SPECIAL PATHWAYS

Nancy B. Schwartz

—IdUA $\frac{(2)}{\alpha}$ GalNAc $\frac{(4)}{\beta}$ GlcUA
| (1) | (3)
OSO_3H OSO_3H
—IdUA $\frac{(2)}{\alpha}$ GlcN $\frac{(7)}{\alpha}$ GlcUA
| (1) | (6)
OSO_3H OSO_3H

8.1 OVERVIEW

In addition to catabolism of glucose for the specific purpose of energy production in the form of ATP, several other pathways involving sugar metabolism exist in cells. One, the **pentose phosphate pathway,** known also as the **hexose monophosphate shunt** or the **6-phosphogluconate pathway,** is particularly important in animal cells. It functions side by side with glycolysis and the tricarboxylic acid cycle for production of reducing power in the form of NADPH and pentose intermediates. It has previously been mentioned that NADPH serves as a hydrogen and electron donor in reductive biosynthetic reactions, while in most biochemical reactions NADH is oxidized by the respiratory chain to produce ATP (Chapter 6). The enzymes involved in this pathway are located in the cytosol, indicating that the oxidation that occurs is not dependent on mitochondria or the tricarboxylic acid cycle. Another important function is to convert hexoses into pentoses, particularly ribose 5-phosphate. This C_5 sugar or its derivatives are components of ATP, CoA, NAD, FAD, RNA, and DNA. The pentose phosphate pathway also catalyzes the interconversion of C_3, C_4, C_6, and C_7 sugars, some of which can enter glycolysis.

There are also specific pathways for synthesis and degradation of monosaccharides, oligosaccharides, and polysaccharides (other than glycogen) and a profusion of chemical **interconversions,** whereby one sugar can be changed into another. All monosaccharides, and most oligo- and polysaccharides synthesized from the monosaccharides, can originate from glucose. The interconversion reactions by which one sugar is changed into another can occur directly or at the level of nucleotide-linked sugars. In addition to their important role in sugar transformation, nucleotide sugars are the obligatory activated form for polysaccharide synthesis. Monosaccharides are also often found as components of more complex macromolecules like oligo- and polysaccharides, glycoproteins, glycolipids, and proteoglycans. In higher animals these complex carbohydrate molecules are predominantly structural elements filling the extracellular space in tissues and associated with cell membranes. However, more dynamic functions for these complex macromolecules, such as recognition markers and determinants of biological specificity, have been discovered. The discussion of complex carbohydrates in this chapter is limited to the chemistry and biology of those complex carbohydrates found in animal tissues and fluids. The Appendix discusses the nomenclature and chemistry of the carbohydrates.

8.2 PENTOSE PHOSPHATE PATHWAY

The Pentose Phosphate Pathway Has Two Phases

The oxidative pentose phosphate pathway provides a means for cutting the carbon chain of a sugar molecule one carbon at a time. However, in contrast to glycolysis and the tricarboxylic acid cycle, the operation of this pathway does not occur as a consecutive set of reactions leading directly from glucose 6-phosphate (G6P) to six molecules of CO_2. The pathway can be visualized as occurring in two stages. In the first stage, hexose is decarboxylated to pentose, followed by two oxidation reactions that lead to formation of NADPH. The pathway then continues and, by a series of transformations, six molecules of pentose undergo rearrangements to yield five molecules of hexose. To understand this pathway, it is necessary to examine each reaction individually.

Glucose 6-Phosphate Is Oxidized and Decarboxylated to a Pentose Phosphate

The first reaction of the pentose phosphate pathway (Figure 8.1) is **dehydrogenation** of G6P at C-1 to form **6-phosphoglucono-δ-lactone** and **NADPH.**

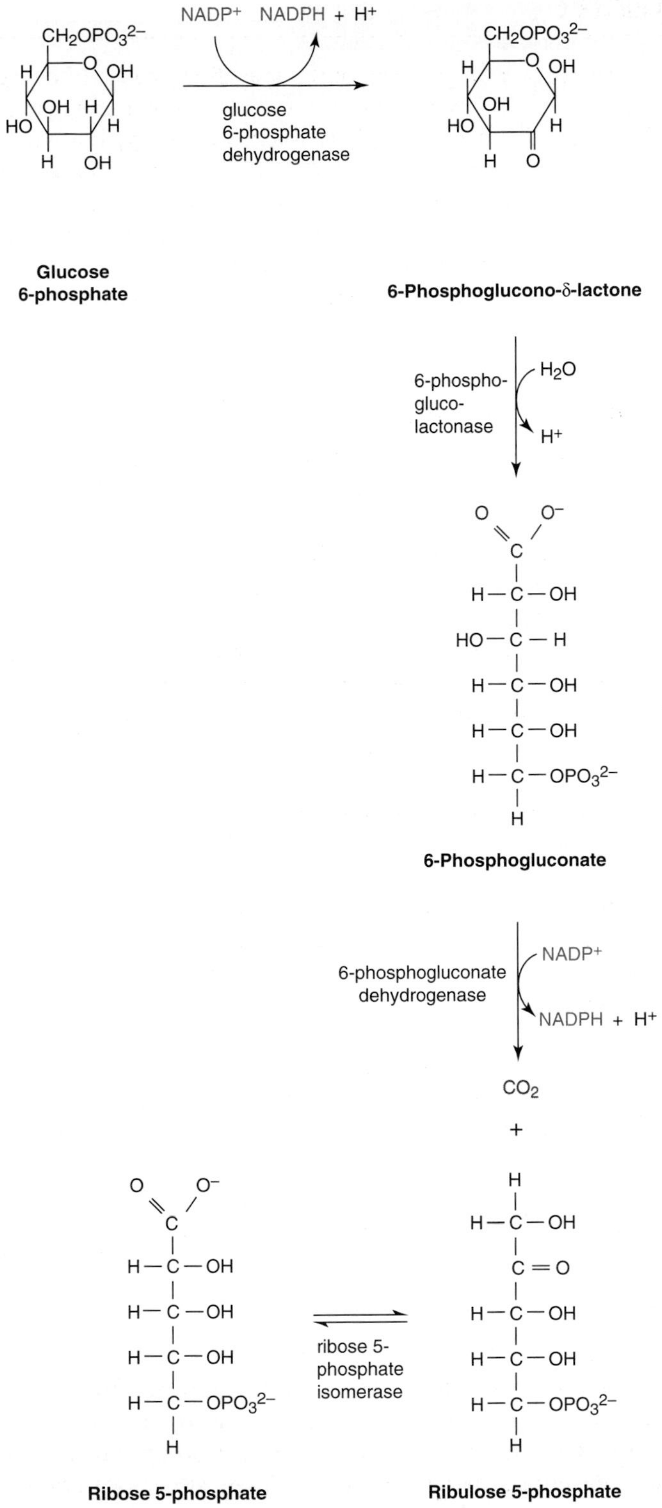

FIGURE 8.1
Formation of pentose phosphate.

The enzyme catalyzing this reaction is **G6P dehydrogenase,** the first enzyme found to be specific for $NADP^+$ and the major regulatory site for the pathway. Special interest in this enzyme stems from the severe anemia that may result from the absence of G6P dehydrogenase in erythrocytes or from the presence of one of several genetic variants of the enzyme (see Clin. Corr. 8.1). The intermediate product of this reaction, a lactone, is a substrate for gluconolacto-

CLINICAL CORRELATION 8.1

Glucose 6-Phosphate Dehydrogenase: Genetic Deficiency or Presence of Genetic Variants in Erythrocytes

When certain seemingly harmless drugs, such as antimalarials, antipyretics, or sulfa antibiotics, are administered to susceptible patients, an acute hemolytic anemia may result in 48–96 h. Susceptibility to drug-induced hemolytic disease may be due to a deficiency of G6P dehydrogenase activity in erythrocytes and was one of the early indications that X-linked genetic deficiencies of this enzyme exist. This enzyme, which catalyzes the oxidation of G6P to 6-phosphogluconate and the reduction of $NADP^+$, is particularly important, since the pentose phosphate pathway is the major pathway of NADPH production in the red cell. For example, red cells with the relatively mild A-type of glucose-6-phosphate dehydrogenase deficiency can oxidize glucose at a normal rate when the demand for NADPH is normal. However, if the rate of NADPH oxidation is increased, the enzyme-deficient cells cannot increase the rate of glucose oxidation and carbon dioxide production adequately. In addition, cells lacking glucose-6-phosphate dehydrogenase do not reduce enough NADP to maintain glutathione in its reduced state. Reduced glutathione is necessary for the integrity of the erythrocyte membrane, thus rendering enzyme-deficient red cells more susceptible to hemolysis by a wide range of compounds. Therefore the basic abnormality in G6P deficiency is the formation of mature red blood cells that have diminished glucose-6-phosphate dehydrogenase activity. Young red blood cells may have significantly higher enzyme activity than older cells, because of an unstable enzyme variant; following an episode of hemolysis, young red cells predominate and it may not be possible to diagnose this genetic deficiency until the red cell population ages. This enzymatic deficiency, which is usually undetected until administration of certain drugs, illustrates the interplay of heredity and environment on the production of disease. Enzyme defects are only one of several abnormalities that can affect enzyme activity, and others have been detected independent of drug administration. There are more than 300 known genetic variants of this enzyme that contains 516 amino acids, accounting for a wide range of symptoms. These variants can be distinguished from one another by clinical, biochemical, and molecular differences (see Clin. Corr. 4.5).

nase, which ensures that the reaction goes to completion. The overall equilibrium of these two reactions lies far in the direction of NADPH maintaining a high $NADPH/NADP^+$ ratio within cells. A second **dehydrogenation** and decarboxylation is catalyzed by **6-phosphogluconate dehydrogenase** and produces the pentose phosphate, **ribulose 5-phosphate,** and a second molecule of NADPH. The final step in synthesis of ribose 5-phosphate is the **isomerization,** through an enediol intermediate, of ribulose 5-phosphate by **ribose isomerase.**

These first reactions result in decarboxylation and production of NADPH and are considered to be the most important. Under certain metabolic conditions, the pentose phosphate pathway can end at this point, with utilization of NADPH for reductive biosynthetic reactions and ribose 5-phosphate as a precursor for nucleotide synthesis. The overall equation may be written as

$$\text{Glucose 6-phosphate} + 2\ NADP^+ + H_2O \rightleftharpoons \text{ribose 5-phosphate} + 2\ NADPH + 2\ H^+ + CO_2$$

Interconversions of Pentose Phosphates Lead to Glycolytic Intermediates

In certain cells more NADPH is needed for **reductive biosynthesis** than ribose 5-phosphate for incorporation into nucleotides. A **sugar rearrangement** system (Figure 8.2) forms triose, tetrose, hexose, and heptose sugars from the pentoses, thus creating a **disposal mechanism** for ribose 5-phosphate and providing a **reversible link** between the pentose phosphate pathway and glycolysis via intermediates common to both pathways. For the interconversions, another pentose phosphate, **xylulose 5-phosphate,** must first be formed through **isomerization of ribulose 5-phosphate** by the action of **phosphopentose epimerase.** As a consequence, these three pentose phosphates exist as an equilibrium mixture and can then undergo further transformations catalyzed by **transketolase** and **transaldolase.** Both enzymes catalyze chain cleavage and transfer reactions involving the same group of substrates.

Transketolase requires thiamine pyrophosphate (TPP) and Mg^{2+}, transfers a C_2 unit designated **"active glycolaldehyde"** from **xylulose 5-phosphate**

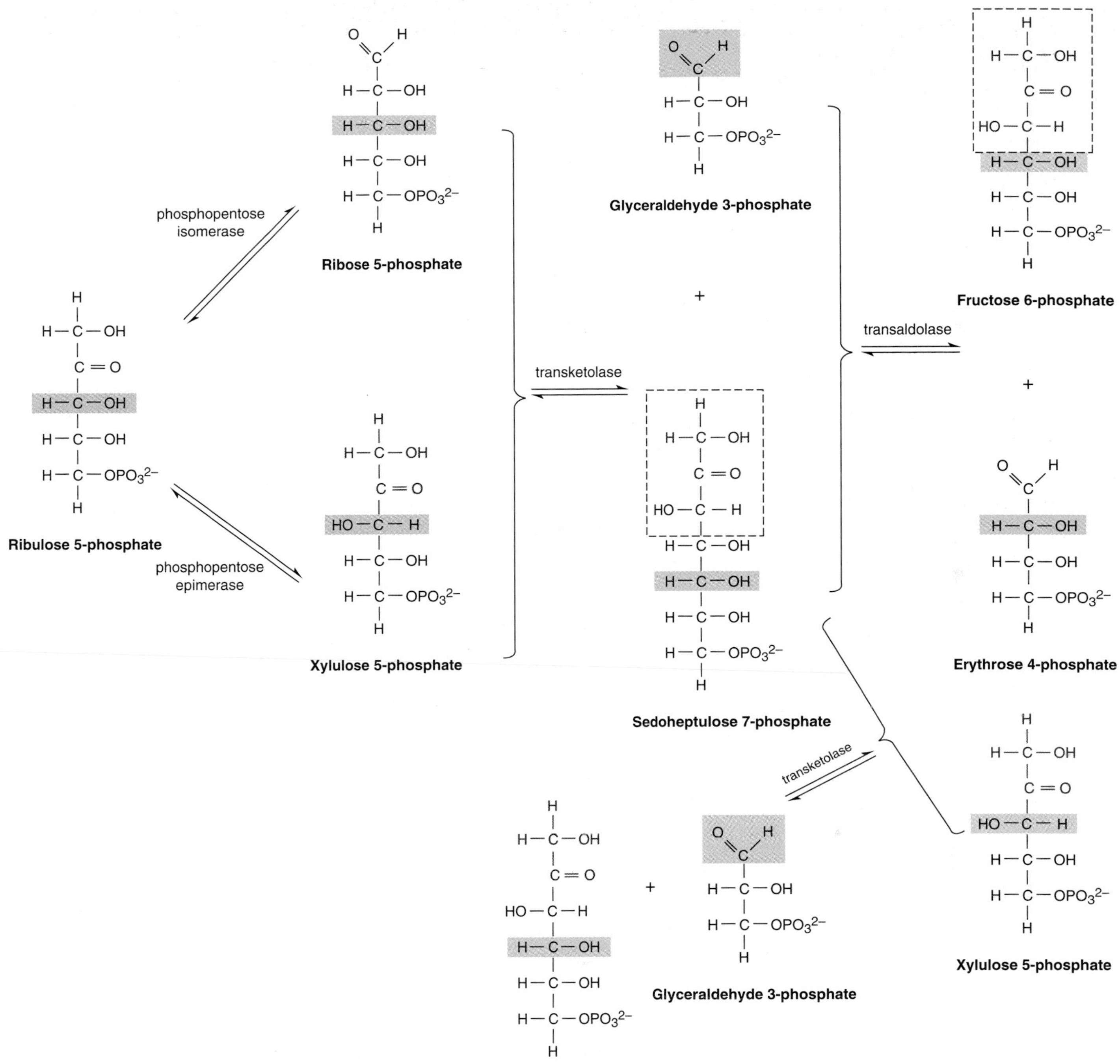

FIGURE 8.2
Interconversions of pentose phosphates.

to **ribose 5-phosphate,** and produces the C_7 sugar **sedoheptulose** and **glyceraldehyde 3-phosphate,** an intermediate of glycolysis. A further transfer reaction, catalyzed by transaldolase, results in the recovery of the first hexose phosphate. In this reaction a C_3 unit **(dihydroxyacetone)** from sedoheptulose 7-phosphate is transferred to glyceraldehyde 3-phosphate, forming the tetrose, **erythrose 4-phosphate,** and fructose 6-phosphate, another intermediate of glycolysis. In a third reaction, transketolase catalyzes the synthesis of fructose 6-phosphate and glyceraldehyde 3-phosphate from erythrose 4-phosphate and a second molecule of xylulose 5-phosphate. In this case, the C_2 unit is transferred from xylulose 5-phosphate to an acceptor C_4 sugar, forming two glycolytic intermediates. The sum of these reactions is

$$2 \text{ Xylulose 5-phosphate} + \text{ribose 5-phosphate} \rightleftharpoons 2 \text{ fructose 6-phosphate} + \text{glyceraldehyde 3-phosphate}$$

Since xylulose 5-phosphate is derived from ribose 5-phosphate, the net reaction starting from ribose 5-phosphate is

$$3 \text{ Ribose 5-phosphate} \rightleftharpoons 2 \text{ fructose 6-phosphate} + \text{glyceraldehyde 3-phosphate}$$

Therefore excess ribose 5-phosphate, whether it arises from the initial oxidation of G6P or from the degradative metabolism of nucleic acids, is effectively scavenged by conversion to intermediates that can enter the carbon flow of glycolysis.

Glucose 6-Phosphate Can Be Completely Oxidized to CO_2

In certain tissues, like lactating mammary gland, a pathway for complete **oxidation** of **G6P** to CO_2, with concomitant reduction of $NADP^+$ to NADPH, also exists (Figure 8.3). By a complex sequence of reactions, ribulose 5-phosphate produced by the pentose phosphate pathway is recycled into G6P by transketolase, transaldolase, and certain enzymes of the gluconeogenic pathway. Hexose continually enters this system, and CO_2 evolves as the only carbon compound. A balanced equation for this process would involve the oxidation of six molecules of G6P to six molecules of ribulose 5-phosphate and six molecules of CO_2. This represents essentially the first part of the pentose phosphate pathway and results in transfer of 12 pairs of electrons to $NADP^+$, the requisite

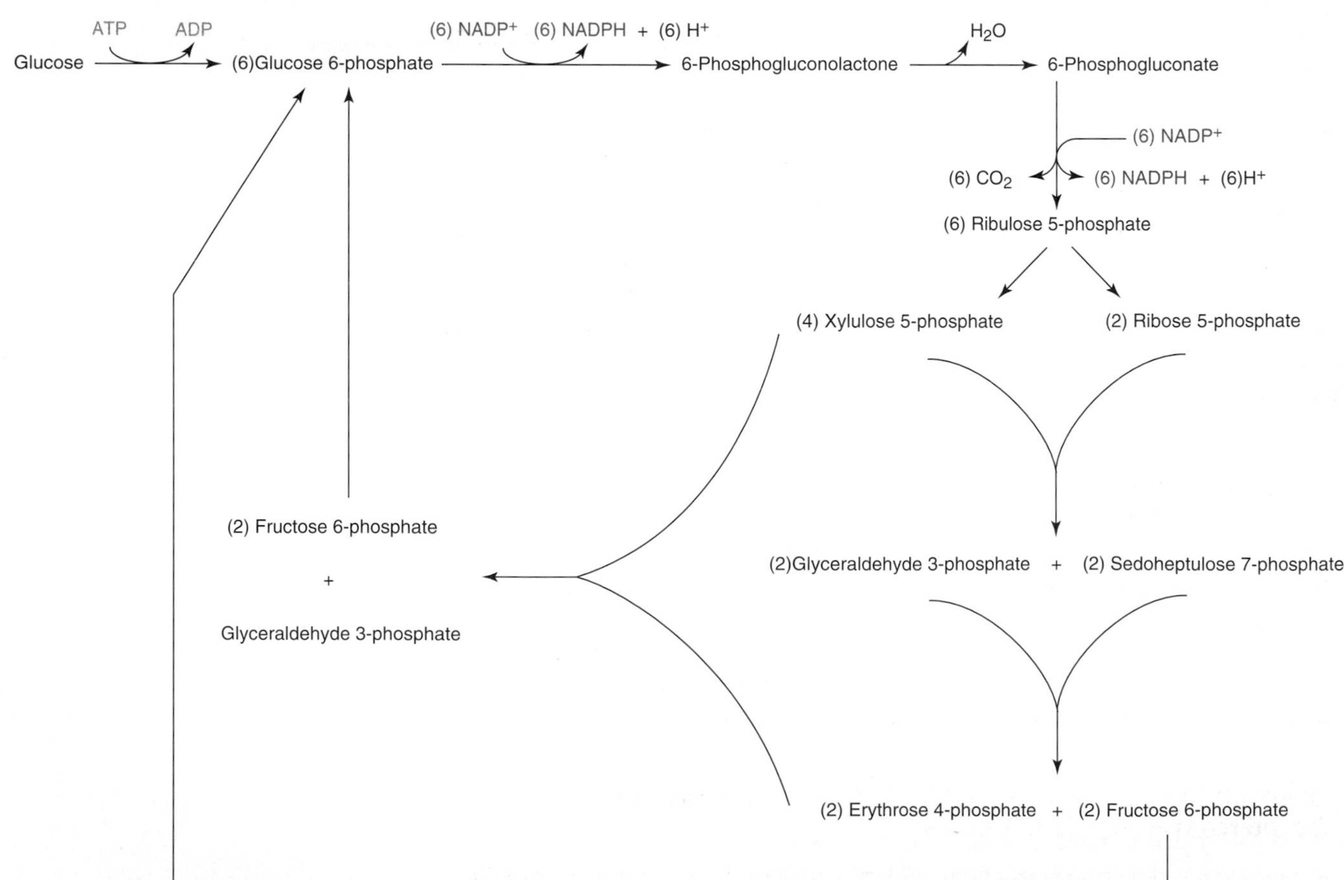

FIGURE 8.3
Pentose phosphate pathway.

amount for total oxidation of one glucose to six CO_2. The remaining six molecules of ribulose 5-phosphate are then rearranged by the pathway described above to regenerate five molecules of G6P. The overall equation can be written as

$$6 \text{ Glucose 6-phosphate} + 12 \text{ NADP}^+ + 7 \text{ H}_2\text{O} \rightleftharpoons 5 \text{ glucose 6-phosphate} + 6 \text{ CO}_2 + 12 \text{ NADPH} + 12 \text{ H}^+ + \text{P}_i$$

The net reaction is therefore

$$\text{Glucose 6-phosphate} + 12 \text{ NADP}^+ + 7 \text{ H}_2\text{O} \rightleftharpoons 6 \text{ CO}_2 + 12 \text{ NADPH} + 12 \text{ H}^+ + \text{P}_i$$

Pentose Phosphate Pathway Produces NADPH

The pentose phosphate pathway serves several purposes, including synthesis and degradation of sugars other than hexoses, particularly pentoses necessary for nucleotides and nucleic acids, and other glycolytic intermediates. Most important is the ability to synthesize NADPH, which has a unique role in biosynthetic reactions. The direction of flow and path taken by G6P after entry into the pathway is determined largely by the needs of the cell for NADPH or sugar intermediates. When more NADPH than ribose 5-phosphate is required, the pathway leads to complete oxidation of G6P to CO_2 and resynthesis of G6P from ribulose 5-phosphate. Alternatively, if more ribose 5-phosphate than NADPH is required, G6P is converted to fructose 6-phosphate and glyceraldehyde 3-phosphate by the glycolytic pathway. Two molecules of fructose 6-phosphate and one molecule of glyceraldehyde 3-phosphate are converted into three molecules of ribose 5-phosphate by reversal of the transaldolase and transketolase reactions.

The **distribution** of the **pentose phosphate pathway** in tissues is consistent with its functions. It is present in erythrocytes for production of NADPH, used to generate reduced glutathione, which is essential for maintenance of normal red cell structure. It is also active in liver, mammary gland, testis, and adrenal cortex, sites of fatty acid or steroid synthesis, which also require the reducing power of NADPH. In contrast, in mammalian striated muscle, which exhibits little fatty acid or steroid synthesis, all catabolism proceeds via glycolysis and the TCA cycle and no direct oxidation of glucose 6-phosphate occurs through the pentose phosphate pathway. In some other tissues like liver, 20–30% of the CO_2 produced may arise from the pentose phosphate pathway, and the balance between glycolysis and the pentose phosphate pathway depends on the metabolic requirements of the cell.

8.3 ■ SUGAR INTERCONVERSIONS AND NUCLEOTIDE SUGAR FORMATION

In considering the general principles of carbohydrate metabolism, certain aspects of the origin and fate of other monosaccharides, oligosaccharides, and polysaccharides should be included. Most monosaccharides found in biological compounds derive from glucose. The most common reactions for sugar transformations in mammalian systems are summarized in Figure 8.4.

Isomerization and Phosphorylation Are Common Reactions for Interconverting Carbohydrates

Formation of some sugars can occur directly, starting from glucose via modification reactions, such as the conversion of G6P to fructose 6-phosphate by phosphoglucose isomerase in the glycolytic pathway. A similar **aldose–ketose**

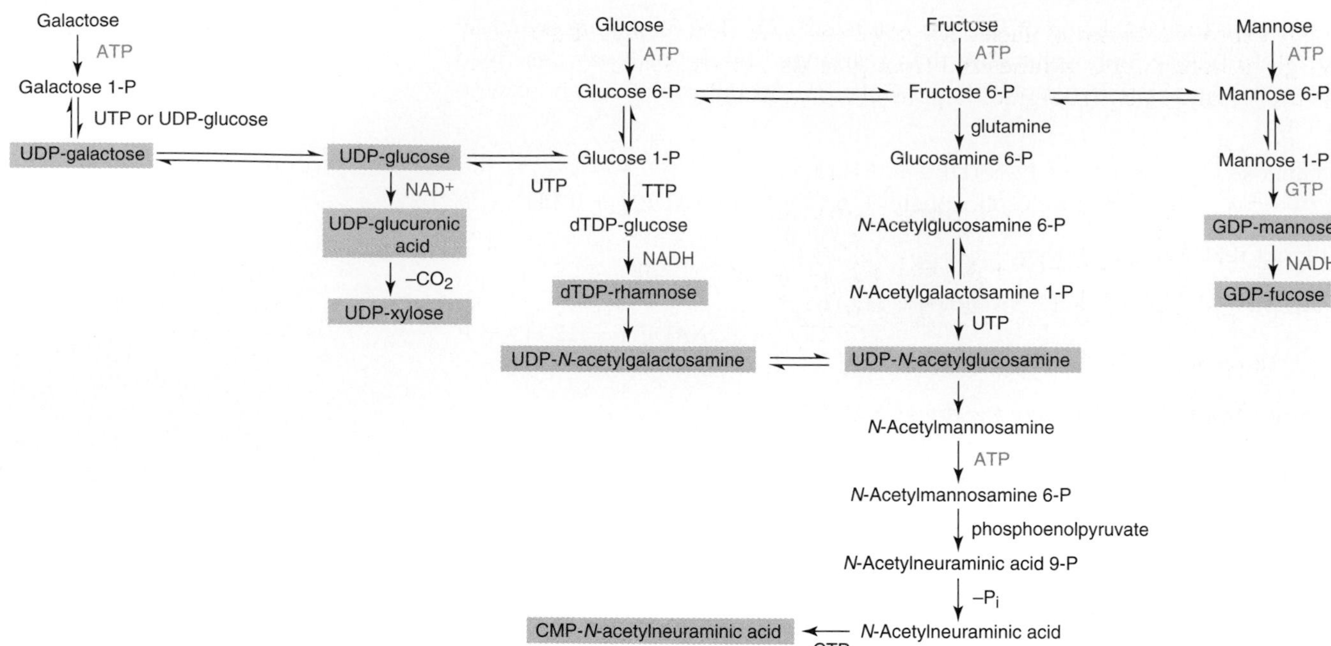

FIGURE 8.4
Pathways of formation of nucleotide sugars and interconversions of some hexoses.

CLINICAL CORRELATION 8.2

Essential Fructosuria and Fructose Intolerance: Deficiency of Fructokinase and Fructose 1-Phosphate Aldolase

Fructose may account for 30–60% of the total carbohydrate intake of mammals. It is predominantly metabolized by a specific fructose pathway. The first enzyme in this pathway, fructokinase, is deficient in essential fructosuria. This disorder is a benign asymptomatic metabolic anomaly, which appears to be inherited as an autosomal recessive. Following intake of fructose, blood levels and urinary fructose are unusually high; however, 90% of fructose is eventually metabolized. In contrast, hereditary fructose intolerance is characterized by severe hypoglycemia after ingestion of fructose. Prolonged ingestion in young children may lead to death. In this disorder fructose 1-phosphate aldolase is deficient, and fructose 1-phosphate accumulates intracellularly (see Clin. Corr. 7.3).

Steinitz, H., and Mizrohy, O. Essential fructosuria and hereditary fructose intolerance. *N. Eng. J. Med.* 280:222, 1969.

isomerization catalyzed by **phosphomannose isomerase** results in synthesis of mannose 6-phosphate.

Internal transfer of a phosphate group on the same sugar molecule from one hydroxyl group to another is a common modification. Glucose 1-phosphate, resulting from enzymatic phosphorolysis of glycogen, is converted to G6P by phosphoglucomutase. Galactose can be phosphorylated directly to galactose 1-phosphate by a galactokinase and mannose to mannose 6-phosphate by a mannokinase. Free fructose, an important dietary constituent, can be phosphorylated in the liver to fructose 1-phosphate by a special fructokinase. However, no mutase exists to interconvert fructose 1-phosphate and fructose 6-phosphate, nor can phosphofructokinase synthesize fructose 1,6-bisphosphate from fructose 1-phosphate. Rather, a fructose 1-phosphate aldolase cleaves fructose 1-phosphate to dihydroxyacetone phosphate (DHAP), which enters the glycolytic pathway directly, and glyceraldehyde, which must first be reduced to glycerol, phosphorylated, and then reoxidized to DHAP. Lack of this aldolase leads to fructose intolerance (see Clin. Corr. 8.2).

Nucleotide-Linked Sugars Are Intermediates in Many Sugar Transformations

Most other sugar transformation reactions require prior conversion into **nucleotide-linked sugars.** Formation of nucleoside diphosphate (NDP)-sugar involves the reaction of hexose 1-phosphate and nucleoside triphosphate (NTP), catalyzed by a pyrophosphorylase. While these reactions are readily reversible, *in vivo* pyrophosphate is rapidly hydrolyzed by pyrophosphatase, thereby driving the synthesis of nucleotide sugars. These reactions are summarized as follows:

$$\begin{array}{c} \text{NTP} + \text{sugar 1-phosphate} + H_2O \rightleftharpoons \text{NDP-sugar} + PP_i \\ PP_i + H_2O \rightleftharpoons 2\,P_i \\ \hline \text{NTP} + \text{sugar 1-phosphate} + H_2O \rightleftharpoons \text{NDP-sugar} + 2\,P_i \end{array}$$

UDP-glucose is a common nucleotide sugar involved in synthesis of glycogen and glycoproteins. It is synthesized from glucose 1-phosphate and UTP in a reaction catalyzed by UDP-glucose pyrophosphorylase.

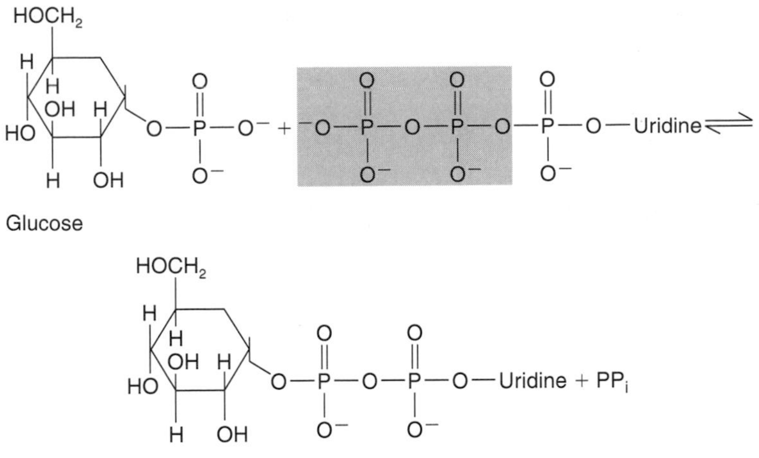

Glucose

UDP-Glucose

Nucleoside diphosphate-sugars contain two phosphoryl bonds, with a large negative ΔG of hydrolysis, that contribute to the energized character of these compounds as glycosyl donors in further transformation and transfer reactions, as well as conferring specificity on the enzymes catalyzing these reactions. For instance, uridine diphosphate usually serves as the glycosyl carrier, while ADP, GDP, and CMP act as carriers in other reactions. Many sugar transformation reactions, including epimerization, oxidation, decarboxylation, reduction, and rearrangement, occur only at the level of nucleotide sugars.

Epimerization Interconverts Glucose and Galactose

Epimerization is a common type of reaction in carbohydrate metabolism. Reversible conversion of glucose to galactose in animals occurs by epimerization of UDP-glucose to UDP-galactose, catalyzed by UDP-glucose epimerase. UDP-galactose is also an important intermediate in metabolism of free galactose, derived from the hydrolysis of lactose in the intestinal tract. Galactose is phosphorylated by galactokinase and ATP to yield galactose 1-phosphate. Then galactose 1-phosphate uridylyltransferase transforms galactose 1-phosphate into UDP-galactose by displacing glucose 1-phosphate from UDP-glucose. These reactions are summarized as follows:

$$\text{Galactose} + \text{ATP} \rightleftharpoons \text{galactose 1-phosphate} + \text{ADP}$$

$$\text{UDP-glucose} + \text{galactose 1-phosphate} \rightleftharpoons \text{UDP-galactose} + \text{glucose 1-phosphate}$$

A hereditary disorder, galactosemia, results from the absence of this uridylyltransferase (see Clin. Corr. 8.3).

A combination of these reactions allows an efficient transformation of dietary galactose into glucose 1-phosphate, which can then be further metabolized by previously described pathways. Alternatively, the 4-epimerase can operate in the reverse direction when UDP-galactose is needed for biosynthesis. Epimerization reactions are not exclusively restricted to nucleotide-linked sugars but also occur at the polymer level; D-glucuronic acid is epimerized to L-iduronic acid after incorporation into heparin and dermatan sulfate (see Section 8.6).

CLINICAL CORRELATION 8.3

Galactosemia: Inability to Transform Galactose into Glucose

Reactions of galactose are of particular interest because in humans they are subject to genetic defects resulting in the hereditary disorder galactosemia. When a defect is present, individuals are unable to metabolize the galactose derived from lactose (milk sugar) to glucose metabolites, often with resultant cataract formation, growth failure, mental retardation, or eventual death from liver damage. The genetic disturbance is expressed as a cellular deficiency of either galactokinase, causing a relatively mild disorder characterized by early cataract formation, or of galactose 1-phosphate uridylyltransferase, resulting in severe disease.

Galactose is reduced to galactitol in a reaction similar to the reduction of glucose to sorbitol. Galactitol is the initiator of cataract formation in the lens and may play a role in the central nervous system damage. Accumulation of galactose 1-phosphate is responsible for liver failure; the toxic effects of galactose metabolites disappear when galactose is removed from the diet.

Segal, S., Blair, A., and Roth, H. The metabolism of galactose by patients with congenital galactosemia. *Am. J. Med.* 83:62, 1965.

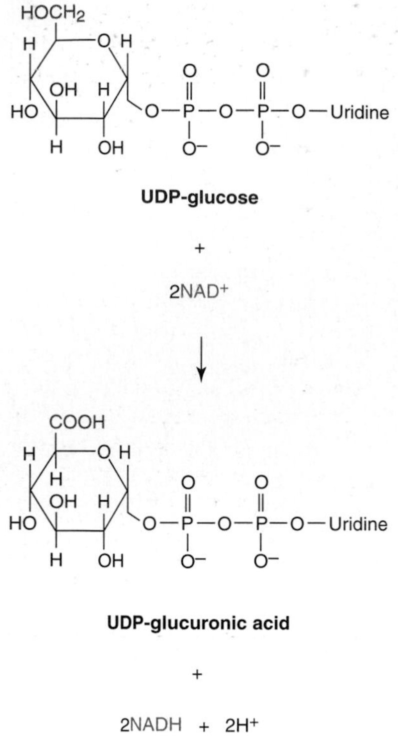

Glucuronic Acid Is Formed by Oxidation of UDP-Glucose

Oxidation and reduction interconversions result in formation of several additional sugars. **Glucuronic acid** is formed by oxidation of UDP-glucose catalyzed by **UDP-glucose dehydrogenase** (Figure 8.5) and most likely follows the outline in Figure 8.6. In humans glucuronic acid is converted to L-xylulose, the ketopentose excreted in **essential pentosuria** (see Clin. Corr. 8.4), and participates in detoxification by production of glucuronide conjugates (see Clin. Corr. 8.5).

Glucuronic acid is a precursor of **L-ascorbic acid** in those animals that synthesize vitamin C. Free glucuronic acid can be metabolized by reduction with NADPH to L-gulonic acid (Figure 8.7), which is then converted by a two-step process through L-gulonolactone to L-ascorbic acid (vitamin C) in plants and most higher animals. Humans, other primates, and the guinea pig lack the enzyme that converts L-gulonolactone to L-ascorbic acid and therefore must satisfy their needs for ascorbic acid by its ingestion. Gulonic acid can also be oxidized to 3-ketogulonic acid and decarboxylated to L-xylulose. L-Xylulose is reduced to xylitol, reoxidized to D-xylulose, and phosphorylated with ATP and an appropriate kinase to xylulose 5-phosphate. The latter compound can then reenter the pentose phosphate pathway described previously. The glucuronic acid pathway represents another pathway for oxidation of glucose. This pathway operates in adipose tissue, and its activity can be increased in tissue from starved or diabetic animals.

UDP-glucose + $2NAD^+$ → UDP-glucuronic acid + 2NADH + $2H^+$

FIGURE 8.5
Formation of UDP-glucuronic acid from UDP-glucose.

Decarboxylation, Oxidoreduction, and Transamination of Sugars Produce Necessary Products

Although **decarboxylation,** which degrades sugars one carbon atom at a time, has been encountered previously in the major metabolic pathways, the only known decarboxylation of a nucleotide sugar is the conversion of UDP-glucuronic acid to UDP-xylose. UDP-xylose is necessary for synthesis of proteoglycans (Section 8.6) and is a potent inhibitor of UDP-glucose dehydrogenase, the enzyme that oxidizes UDP-glucose to UDP-glucuronic acid (Figure 8.5). Thus the level of these nucleotide sugar precursors is regulated by this sensitive feedback mechanism.

Deoxyhexoses and **dideoxyhexoses** are also synthesized while the sugars are attached to nucleoside diphosphates, by a multistep process. For example, L-rhamnose is synthesized from glucose by a series of oxidation–reduction reactions starting with dTDP-glucose and yielding dTDP-rhamnose, catalyzed by oxidoreductases. Presumably, similar reactions account for synthesis of GDP-fucose from GDP-mannose and for various dideoxyhexoses.

Formation of amino sugars, major components of human oligo- and polysaccharides and as constituents of antibiotics, occurs by **transamidation.** For example, synthesis of glucosamine 6-phosphate occurs by reaction of fructose 6-phosphate with glutamine.

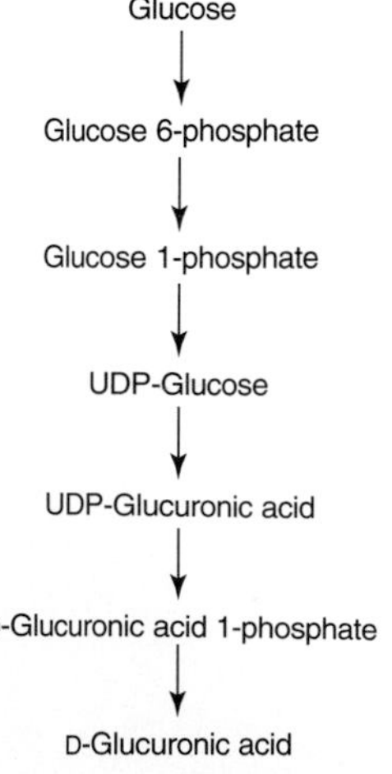

FIGURE 8.6
Biosynthesis of D-glucuronic acid from glucose.

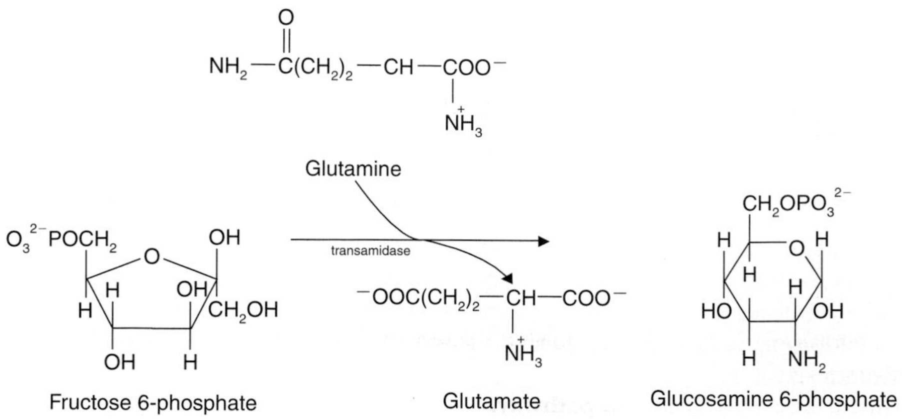

Glutamine ($NH_2—C(=O)(CH_2)_2—CH(NH_3^+)—COO^-$) + Fructose 6-phosphate —transamidase→ Glutamate ($^-OOC(CH_2)_2—CH(NH_3^+)—COO^-$) + Glucosamine 6-phosphate

Glucosamine 6-phosphate can be *N*-acetylated, forming N-acetylglucosamine 6-phosphate, followed by isomerization to *N*-acetylglucosamine 1-phosphate. This latter sugar is converted to UDP-*N*-acetylglucosamine by reactions similar to those of UDP-glucose synthesis. UDP-*N*-acetylglucosamine, a precursor of glycoprotein synthesis, can be epimerized to UDP-*N*-acetylgalactosamine, necessary for proteoglycan synthesis. The fructose 6-phosphate–glutamine transamidase reaction is under negative feedback control by UDP-*N*-acetylglucosamine; thus synthesis of both nucleotide sugars is regulated (Figure 8.4). This regulation is meaningful in certain tissues such as skin, in which this pathway can involve up to 20% of glucose flux.

Sialic Acids Are Derived from *N*-Acetylglucosamine

Another product derived from UDP-*N*-acetylglucosamine is **acetylneuraminic acid,** one of a family of C_9 sugars, called **sialic acids** (Figure 8.8). The first

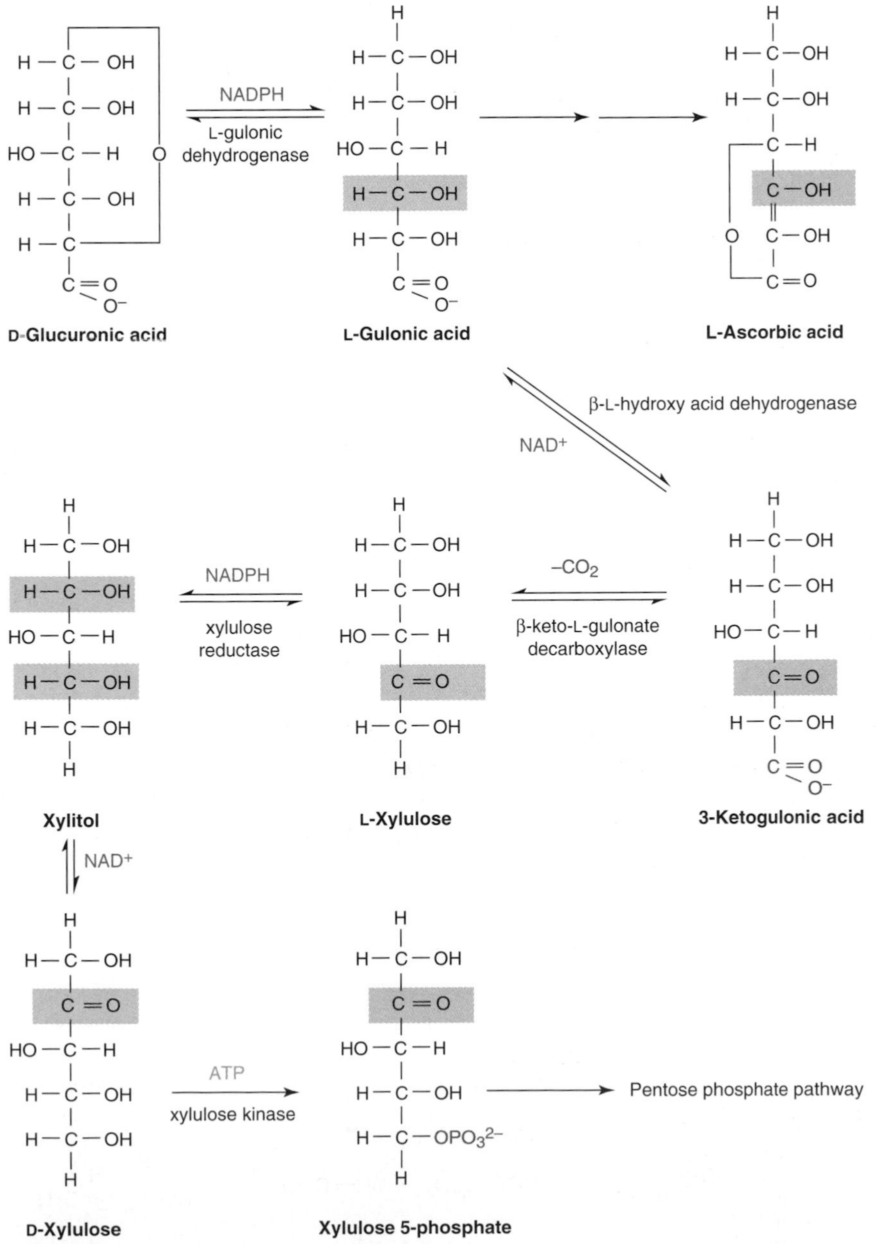

D-Glucuronic acid ⇌ (NADPH; L-gulonic dehydrogenase) L-Gulonic acid → → L-Ascorbic acid

L-Gulonic acid ⇌ (NAD⁺; β-L-hydroxy acid dehydrogenase) 3-Ketogulonic acid

3-Ketogulonic acid ⇌ ($-CO_2$; β-keto-L-gulonate decarboxylase) L-Xylulose

L-Xylulose ⇌ (NADPH; xylulose reductase) Xylitol

Xylitol ⇌ (NAD⁺) D-Xylulose

D-Xylulose → (ATP; xylulose kinase) Xylulose 5-phosphate → Pentose phosphate pathway

FIGURE 8.7
Glucuronic acid oxidation pathway.

> **CLINICAL CORRELATION 8.4**
>
> **Pentosuria: Deficiency of Xylitol Dehydrogenase**
>
> The glucuronic acid oxidation pathway presumably is not essential for human carbohydrate metabolism, since individuals in whom the pathway is blocked suffer no ill effects. A metabolic variation, called idiopathic pentosuria, results from reduced activity of NADP-linked L-xylulose reductase, the enzyme that catalyzes the reduction of xylulose to xylitol. Hence affected individuals excrete large amounts of pentose into the urine especially following intake of glucuronic acid.
>
> Wang, Y. M., and van Eys, J. The enzymatic defect in essential pentosuria. *N. Engl. J. Med.* 282:892, 1970.

reaction involves epimerization of UDP-*N*-acetylglucosamine by a 2-epimerase to *N*-acetylmannosamine, concomitant with elimination of UDP. Since the monosaccharide product is no longer bound to nucleotide, this epimerization is clearly different from those previously encountered. Most likely, this 2-epimerase reaction proceeds by a trans elimination of UDP, with formation of the unsaturated intermediate, 2-acetamidoglucal. In mammalian tissues *N*-acetylmannosamine is phosphorylated by ATP to *N*-acetylmannosamine 6-phosphate, which then condenses with phosphoenolpyruvate to form *N*-acetylneuraminic acid 9-phosphate. This product is cleaved by a phosphatase and activated by CTP to form the CMP derivative, CMP-*N*-acetylneuraminic acid. This is an unusual nucleotide sugar, containing only one phosphate group, and is formed by an irreversible reaction. *N*-Acetylneuraminic acid is a precursor of other sialic acid derivatives, some of which evolve by modification of *N*-acetyl to *N*-glycolyl or *O*-acetyl after incorporation into glycoprotein.

8.4 ■ BIOSYNTHESIS OF COMPLEX CARBOHYDRATES

In complex carbohydrate-containing molecules, sugars are linked to other sugars by glycosidic bonds, formed by specific **glycosyltransferases.** Energy is required for synthesis of a glycosidic bond and is derived from nucleotide sugars as donor substrates. A glycosyltransferase reaction proceeds by donation of the glycosyl unit from the nucleotide derivative to the nonreducing end of an acceptor sugar. The nature of the bond formed is determined by the specificity of the glycosyltransferase, which is unique for the sugar acceptor, the sugar transferred, and the linkage formed. Thus polysaccharide synthesis is controlled by a nontemplate mechanism directed by specific glycosyltransferases. A glycosyltransferase reaction is summarized as follows:

$$\underset{\text{(donor)}}{\text{Nucleoside diphosphate-glycose}} + \underset{\text{(acceptor)}}{\text{glycose}} \xrightleftharpoons{\text{glycosyltransferase}} \underset{\text{(glycoside)}}{\text{glycosyl}_1\text{-}O\text{-glycose}_2} + \text{nucleoside diphosphate}$$

At least 40 different glycosidic bonds have been identified in mammalian oligosaccharides and about 15 more in connective tissue polysaccharides. The number of possible linkages is even greater and arises both from the diversity of monosaccharides covalently bonded and from the formation of both α and β

CLINICAL CORRELATION 8.5

Glucuronic Acid: Physiological Significance of Glucuronide Formation

The biological significance of glucuronic acid extends to its ability to be conjugated with certain endogenous and exogenous substances, forming a group of compounds collectively termed glucuronides in a reaction catalyzed by UDP-glucuronyltransferase. Conjugation of a compound with glucuronic acid produces a strongly acidic compound that is more water soluble at physiological pH than its precursor and therefore may alter the metabolism, transport, or excretion properties. Glucuronide formation is important in drug detoxification, steroid excretion, and bilirubin metabolism. Bilirubin is the major metabolic breakdown product of heme, the prosthetic group of hemoglobin. The central step in excretion of bilirubin is conjugation with glucuronic acid by UDP-glucuronyltransferase. Development of this conjugating mechanism occurs gradually and may take several days to 2 weeks after birth to become fully active in humans. So-called physiological jaundice of the newborn results in most cases from the inability of the neonatal liver to form bilirubin glucuronide at a rate comparable to that of bilirubin production. A defect in glucuronide synthesis has been found in a mutant strain of Wistar ("Gunn") rats, due to a deficiency of UDP-glucuronyltransferase and results in hereditary hyperbilirubinemia. In humans a similar defect is found in congenital familial nonhemolytic jaundice (Crigler–Najjar syndrome). Patients with this condition are also unable to conjugate foreign compounds efficiently with glucuronic acid.

Crigler, J. F., and Najjar, V. A. Congenital familial non-hemolytic jaundice with kernicterus. *Pediatrics* 10:169, 1952; Gunn, C. H. Hereditary acholuric jaundice in a new mutant strain of rats. *J. Hered.* 29:137, 1938; and Ostrow, J. D. (Ed.). *Bile Pigments and Jaundice.* New York: Marcel Dekker, 1986.

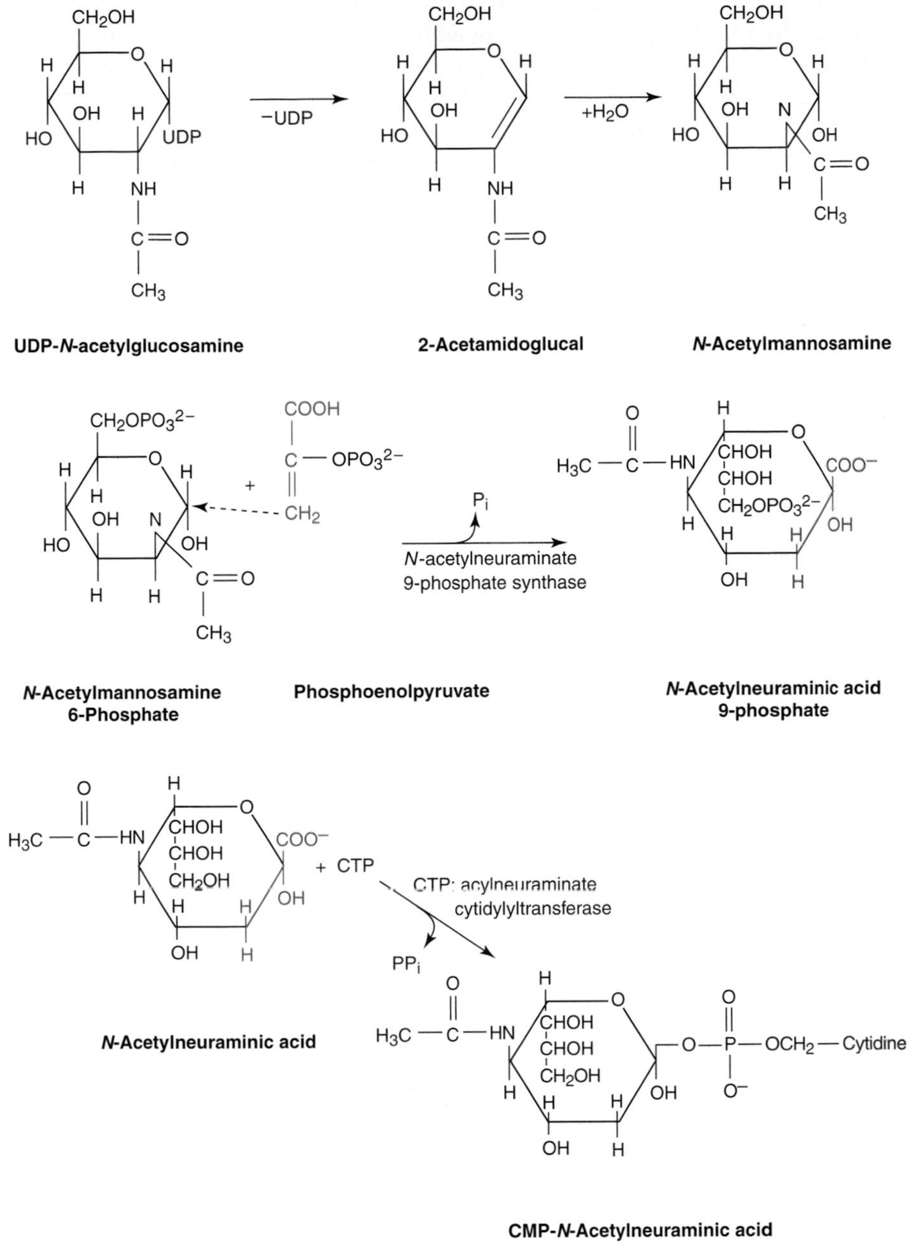

FIGURE 8.8
Biosynthesis of CMP-*N*-acetylneuraminic acid.

linkages, with each of the available hydroxyl groups on the acceptor saccharide. The large and diverse number of molecules that can be generated suggests that oligosaccharides have the potential for great informational content. In fact, it is known that the specificity of many biological molecules is determined by the nature of the composite sugar residues. For example, the specificity of the major blood types is determined by sugars (see Clin. Corr. 8.6). *N*-Acetylgalactosamine is the immunodeterminant of blood type A and galactose of blood type B. Removal of *N*-acetylgalactosamine from type A erythrocytes, or of galactose from type B erythrocytes, converts both to type O erythrocytes. Increasingly, other examples of sugars as determinants of specificity for cell surface receptor and lectin interactions, targeting of cells to certain tissues, and survival or clearance from the circulation of certain molecules are being recognized. All glycosidic bonds identified in biological compounds are degraded by specific hydrolytic enzymes, glycosidases. In addition to being valuable tools for the

CLINICAL CORRELATION 8.6

Blood Group Substances

The surface of human erythrocytes is covered with a complex mosaic of specific antigenic determinants, many of which are polysaccharides. There are about 100 blood group determinants, belonging to 21 independent human blood group systems. The most widely studied are the antigenic determinants of the ABO blood group system and the closely related Lewis system. From the study of these systems, a definite correlation was established between gene activity as it relates to specific glycosyltransferase synthesis and oligosaccharide structure. The genetic variation is achieved through specific glycosyltransferases responsible for synthesis of the heterosaccharide determinants. For example, the *H* gene codes for a fucosyltransferase, which adds fucose to a peripheral galactose in the heterosaccharide precursor. The *A*, *B*, and *O* genes are located on chromosome 9. The *A* gene encodes an *N*-acetylgalactosamine glycosyltransferase, the *B* gene encodes a galactosyltransferase, and the *O* gene encodes an inactive enzyme. The sugars are added to the *H*-specific oligosaccharide. The Lewis (*Le*) gene codes for another fucosyltransferase, which adds fucose to a peripheral *N*-acetylglucosamine residue in the precursor. Absence of the *H* gene gives rise to the Le^a-specific determinant, whereas in the absence of both the *H* and *Le* genes, the interaction product responsible for the Le^b specificity is found. The elucidation of the structures of these oligosaccharide determinants represents a milestone in carbohydrate chemistry. This knowledge is essential to blood transfusion practices and for legal and historical purposes. For example, tissue dust containing complex carbohydrates has been used in serological analysis to establish the blood group of Tutankhamen and his probable ancestral background.

Watkins, W. M. Blood group substances. *Science* 152:172, 1966.

structural elucidation of oligosaccharides, interest in this class of enzymes exists because many genetic diseases of complex carbohydrate metabolism result from defects in glycosidases (see Clin. Corr. 8.7 and 8.8).

8.5 ■ GLYCOPROTEINS

Glycoproteins have been restrictively defined as conjugated proteins that contain, as a prosthetic group, one or more saccharides lacking a serial repeat unit and bound covalently to a peptide chain. This definition excludes proteoglycans, which are discussed in Section 8.6.

The functions of glycoproteins in the human are of great interest. Glycoproteins in cell membranes may have an important role in the group behavior of cells and other important biological functions of the membrane. Glycoproteins form a major part of the mucus that is secreted by epithelial cells, where they perform an important role in lubrication and in the protection of tissues lining the body's ducts. Many other proteins secreted from cells into extracellular fluids are glycoproteins. These proteins include hormones found in blood, such as follicle-stimulating hormone, luteinizing hormone, and chorionic gonadotropin; and plasma proteins such as the orosomucoids, ceruloplasmin, plasminogen, prothrombin, and immunoglobulins (see Clin. Corr. 2.7).

Glycoproteins Contain Variable Amounts of Carbohydrate

The percentage of carbohydrate in glycoproteins is highly variable. Some glycoproteins such as IgG contain low amounts (4%) of carbohydrate by weight, while glycophorin, the human red cell membrane glycoprotein, contains 60% carbohydrate. Human ovarian cyst glycoprotein contains 70% carbohydrate, and human gastric glycoprotein is 82% carbohydrate. The carbohydrate can be distributed fairly evenly along the polypeptide chain or concentrated in defined regions. For example, in human glycophorin A the carbohydrate is found in the NH_2-terminal half of the polypeptide chain that lies on the outside of the cellular membrane.

The carbohydrate attached at one or at multiple points along a polypeptide chain usually contains less than 12–15 sugar residues. In some cases the carbohydrate component consists of a single sugar moiety, as in the submaxillary gland glycoprotein (single *N*-acetyl-α-D-galactosaminyl residue) and in some types of

CLINICAL CORRELATION 8.7

Aspartylglycosylaminuria: Absence of 4-L-Aspartylglycosamine Amidohydrolase

A group of human inborn errors of metabolism involving storage of glycolipids, glycopeptides, mucopolysaccharides, and oligosaccharides exists. These diseases are caused by defects in lysosomal glycosidase activity, which prevents the catabolism of oligosaccharides. The disorders involve gradual accumulation in tissues and urine of compounds derived from incomplete degradation of the oligosaccharides and may be accompanied by skeletal abnormalities, hepatosplenomegaly, cataracts, or mental retardation. One disorder resulting from a defect in catabolism of asparagine-*N*-acetylglucosamine-linked oligosaccharides is aspartylglycosylaminuria. A deficiency in the enzyme 4-L-aspartylglycosylamine amidohydrolase allows accumulation of aspartylglucosamine-linked structures. (See accompanying table.)

Other disorders have been described involving accumulation of oligosaccharides derived from both glycoproteins and glycolipids, which may share common oligosaccharide structures (see table). Examples of genetic diseases include mannosidosis (α-mannosidase), the GM_2 gangliosidosis variant O (Sandhoff–Jatzkewitz disease; β-*N*-acetylhexosaminidases A and B), and GM_1 gangliosidosis (β-galactosidase). Mucolipidosis II ("I-Cell Disease") is a generalized degradative disorder resulting from a deficiency of UDP-GlcNAc: lysosomal enzyme precursor GlcNAc phosphotransferase, which attacks Man-6-PO_4 (see also Chapter 10).

Sewell, A. C. Urinary oligosaccharide excretion in disorders of glycolipid, glycoprotein, and glycogen metabolism: a review of screening for differential diagnosis. *Eur. J. Pediatr.* 134:183, 1980.

Enzymic Defects in Degradation of Asn-GlcNAc Type Glycoproteins[a]

Disease	*Deficient Enzyme*[b]
Aspartylglycosylaminuria	4-L-Aspartylglycosylamine amidohydrolase (a)
β-Mannosidosis	β-Mannosidase (7)
α-Mannosidosis	α-Mannosidase (3)
GM_2 Gangliosidosis variant O (Sandhoff–Jatzkewitz disease)	β-*N*-Acetylhexosaminidases (A and B) (4)
GM_1 Gangliosidosis	β-Galactosidase (5)
Mucolipidosis I (Sialidosis)	Sialidase (6)
Fucosidosis	α-Fucosidase (8)

[a] A typical Asn-GlcNAc oligosaccharide structure.

Dermatan sulfate —IdUA $\xrightarrow[\alpha]{(2)}$ GalNAc $\xrightarrow[\beta]{(4)}$ GlcUA $\xrightarrow[\beta]{(4)}$ GalNAc $\xrightarrow[\beta]{}$
IdUA (1) OSO_3H; GalNAc (3) OSO_3H; GalNAc OSO_3H

Heparan sulfate —IdUA $\xrightarrow[\alpha]{(2)}$ GlcN $\xrightarrow[\alpha]{(7)}$ GlcUA $\xrightarrow[\beta]{(5)}$ GlcNAc $\xrightarrow[\alpha]{(9)}$
IdUA (1) OSO_3H; GlcN (6) OSO_3H; GlcNAc (8) OSO_3H

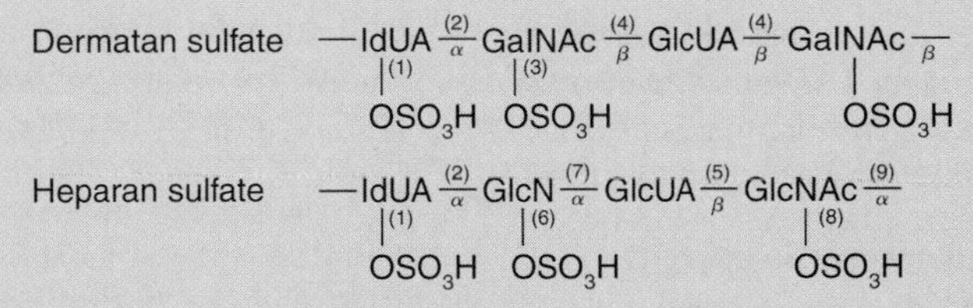

[b] The numbers in parentheses refer to the enzymes that hydrolyze those bonds.

mammalian collagens (single α-D-galactosyl residue). In general, glycoproteins contain sugar residues in the D form, except for L-fucose, L-arabinose, and L-iduronic acid. A glycoprotein from different animal species often has an identical primary structure in the protein component, but a variable carbohydrate component. This heterogeneity of a given protein may even be true within a single organism. For example, pancreatic ribonuclease A and B forms have identical amino acid sequences and a similar kinetic specificity toward substrates, but they differ significantly in their carbohydrate composition.

Carbohydrates Are Covalently Linked to Glycoproteins by *N*- or *O*-Glycosyl Bonds

At present, the structures of a limited number of oligosaccharide components have been elucidated completely. **Microheterogeneity** of glycoproteins, arising from incomplete synthesis or partial degradation, makes structural analyses

CLINICAL CORRELATION 8.8

Heparin Is an Anticoagulant

Heparin is a naturally occurring sulfated polysaccharide that is used to reduce the clotting tendency of patients. Both *in vivo* and *in vitro* heparin prevent the activation of clotting factors but do not act directly on the clotting factors. Rather, the anticoagulant activity of heparin is brought about by the binding interaction of heparin with an inhibitor of the coagulation process. Presumably, heparin binding induces a conformational change in the inhibitor that generates a complementary interaction between the inhibitor and the activated coagulation factor, thereby preventing the factor from participating in the coagulation process. The inhibitor that interacts with heparin is antithrombin III, a plasma protein inhibitor of serine proteases. In the absence of heparin, antithrombin III slowly (10–30 min) combines with several clotting factors, yielding complexes devoid of proteolytic activity. In the presence of heparin, inactive complexes are formed within a few seconds. Antithrombin III contains an arginine residue that combines with the active site serine of factors Xa and IXa; thus the inhibition is stoichiometric. Heterozygous antithrombin III deficiency results in an increased risk of thrombosis in the veins and resistance to the action of heparin.

Rosenberg, R. D., and Rosenberg, J. S. Natural anticoagulant mechanisms. *J. Clin. Invest.* 74:1, 1984.

extremely difficult. However, certain generalities about the structure of glycoproteins have emerged. Covalent linkage of sugars to the peptide chain is a central part of glycoprotein structure, and only a limited number of bonds are found (see Chapter 2). The three major types of **glycopeptide bonds,** as shown in Figure 8.9 and Figure 2.45, are *N*-glycosyl to **asparagine** (Asn), *O*-glycosyl to **serine** (Ser) or **threonine** (Thr), and *O*-glycosyl to **5-hydroxylysine.** The latter linkage, representing the carbohydrate side chains of either a single galactose or the disaccharide glucosylgalactose covalently bonded to hydroxylysine, is generally confined to the collagens. The other two linkages occur in a wide variety of glycoproteins. Of the three major types, only the *O*-glycosidic linkage to serine or threonine is labile to alkali cleavage. By this procedure two types of oligosaccharides (simple and complex) are released. Examination of the simple class from porcine submaxillary mucins reveals some general structural features. A core structure exists, consisting of galactose (Gal) linked $\beta(1 \rightarrow 3)$ to *N*-acetylgalactosamine (GalNAc) *O*-glycosidically linked to serine or threonine residues. Residues of L-fucose (Fuc), sialic acid (NeuAc), and another *N*-acetylgalactosamine are found at the nonreducing periphery of this class of glycopeptides. The general structure of this type of glycopeptide is as follows:

$$\begin{array}{ccccccc} \text{GalNAc} & \xrightarrow{1,3} & \text{Gal} & \xrightarrow{1,3} & \text{GalNAc} & \rightarrow & O\text{-Ser/Thr} \\ & & \uparrow{\scriptstyle 1,2} & & \uparrow{\scriptstyle 2,6} & & \\ & & \text{Fuc} & & \text{NeuAc} & & \end{array}$$

More complex heterosaccharides are also linked to peptides via serine or threonine residues and are exemplified by the blood group substances. Study of these determinants has shown how complex and variable these structures are, as well as how the oligosaccharides of cell surfaces are assembled and how that assembly pattern is genetically determined. An example of how oligosaccharide structures on the surface of red blood cells determine blood group specificity is presented in Clin. Corr. 8.6. Certain common structural features of the oligosaccharide *N*-glycosidically linked to asparagine have also emerged. These glycoproteins commonly contain a core structure consisting of mannose (Man) residues linked to *N*-acetylglucosamine (GlcNAc) in the following structure:

$$(\text{Man})_n \xrightarrow[1,4]{} \text{Man} \xrightarrow[1,4]{} \text{GlcNAc} \xrightarrow[1,4]{} \text{GlcNAc} \rightarrow \text{Asn}$$

Synthesis of *N*-Linked Glycoproteins Involves Dolichol Phosphate

While the synthesis of *O*-glycosidically linked glycoproteins involves the sequential action of a series of glycosyltransferases, the synthesis of *N*-glycosidically linked peptides involves a somewhat different and more complex mechanism (Figure 8.10). A common core is preassembled as a **lipid-linked oligosaccharide** prior to incorporation into the polypeptide. During synthesis, the oligosaccharide intermediates are bound to derivatives of **dolichol phosphate**.

$$(CH_2{=}\overset{\overset{\displaystyle CH_3}{|}}{C}{-}CH{=}CH)_n{-}CH_2{-}\overset{\overset{\displaystyle CH_3}{|}}{CH}{-}CH_2{-}CH_2O{-}PO_3H_2$$

Dolichol phosphate

Dolichols are polyprenols (C_{80}–C_{100}) containing 16–20 isoprene units, in which the final isoprene unit is saturated. These lipids participate in two types of reactions in core oligosaccharide synthesis. The first reaction involves formation of *N*-acetylglucosaminylpyrophosphoryldolichol with release of UMP from the respective nucleotide sugar. The second *N*-acetylglucosamine and the mannose transferase reactions proceed by sugar transfer from the nucleotide without formation of intermediates. Subsequent addition of mannose units occurs via a dolichol-linked mechanism. In the final step, the oligosaccharide is transferred from the dolichol pyrophosphate to an asparagine residue in the polypeptide chain.

After synthesis of the specific core region, the oligosaccharide chains are completed by action of glycosyltransferases without further participation of lipid intermediates. Extensive processing in the Golgi body, involving addition and subsequent removal of certain glycosyl residues, occurs during the course of synthesis of asparagine-*N*-acetylglucosamine-linked glycoproteins. Just as the synthesis of oligosaccharides requires specific glycosyltransferases, degradation requires specific glycosidases. Exoglycosidases remove sugars sequentially from the nonreducing end, exposing the substrate for the subsequent glycosidase. The absence of a particular glycosidase prevents the action of the next enzyme, resulting in cessation of catabolism and accumulation of the product (see Clin. Corr. 8.7). Endoglycosidases with broader specificity also exist and the action of endo- and exoglycosidases results in catabolism of glycoproteins. Although the primary degradation process occurs in lysosomes, there are specific endoplasmic reticulum glycosidases involved in processing of glycoproteins during synthesis as well.

8.6 PROTEOGLYCANS

In addition to glycoproteins, which usually contain proportionally less carbohydrate than protein by weight, there is another class of complex macromolecules, which can contain as much as 95% or more carbohydrate. Their properties resemble polysaccharides more than proteins. To distinguish these compounds

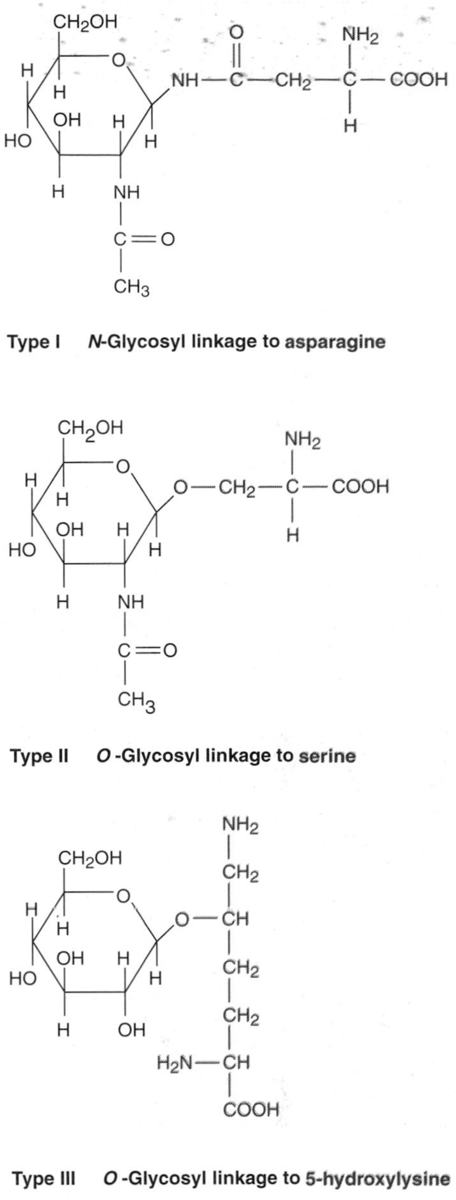

Type I *N*-Glycosyl linkage to asparagine

Type II *O*-Glycosyl linkage to serine

Type III *O*-Glycosyl linkage to 5-hydroxylysine

FIGURE 8.9
Structure of three major glycopeptide bonds.

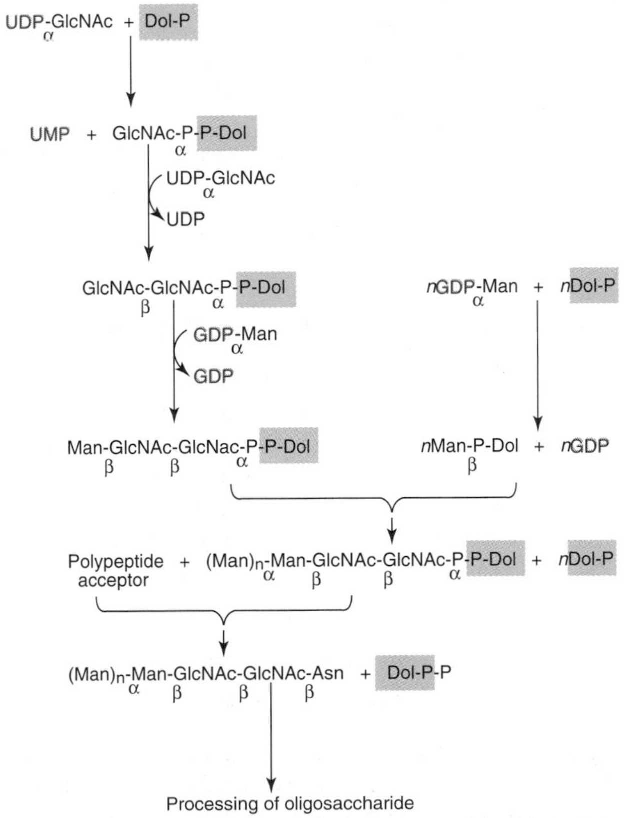

UDP-GlcNAc (α) + Dol-P → UMP + GlcNAc-P-P-Dol (α)

GlcNAc-P-P-Dol (α) + UDP-GlcNAc (α) → UDP + GlcNAc-GlcNAc-P-P-Dol (β, α)

GlcNAc-GlcNAc-P-P-Dol + GDP-Man (α) → GDP + Man-GlcNAc-GlcNac-P-P-Dol (β, β, α)

*n*GDP-Man (α) + *n*Dol-P → *n*Man-P-Dol (β) + *n*GDP

Polypeptide acceptor + (Man)$_n$-Man-GlcNAc-GlcNAc-P-P-Dol (α, β, β, α) + *n*Dol-P

(Man)$_n$-Man-GlcNAc-GlcNAc-Asn (α, β, β, β) + Dol-P-P

Processing of oligosaccharide

FIGURE 8.10
Biosynthesis of the oligosaccharide core in asparagine-*N*-acetylgalactosamine-linked glycoproteins.
Dol, dolichol.

from other glycoproteins, they are referred to as **proteoglycans** and their carbohydrate chains as **glycosaminoglycans.** An older name, mucopolysaccharides, is still in use, especially in reference to the group of storage diseases, mucopolysaccharidoses, which result from an inability to degrade these molecules (see Clin. Corr. 8.9).

Proteoglycans are high molecular weight polyanionic substances consisting of many different glycosaminoglycan chains linked covalently to a protein core. Although six distinct classes of glycosaminoglycans are now recognized,

CLINICAL CORRELATION 8.9

Mucopolysaccharidoses

A group of human genetic disorders characterized by excessive accumulation and excretion of the oligosaccharides of proteoglycans exists, collectively called mucopolysaccharidoses. These disorders result from a deficiency of one or more lysosomal hydrolases responsible for the degradation of dermatan and/or heparan sulfate. The enzymes lacking in specific mucopolysaccharidoses that have been identified are presented in the accompanying table.

Although the chemical basis for this group of disorders is similar, their mode of inheritance as well as clinical manifestations may vary. Hurler's syndrome and Sanfilippo's syndrome are transmitted as autosomal recessives, whereas Hunter's syndrome is X-linked. Both Hurler's syndrome and Hunter's syndrome are characterized by skeletal abnormalities and mental retardation, which in severe cases may result in early death. In contrast, in the Sanfilippo syndrome, the physical defects are relatively mild, while the mental retardation is severe. Collectively, the incidence for all mucopolysaccharidoses is 1 per 30,000 births.

In addition to those listed in the table, some others exist. Morquio's syndrome involves impaired degradation of keratan sulfate, and two types have been identified: type A due to deficiency of galactose 6-sulfatase and type B due to deficiency of β-galactosidase. Multiple sulfatase deficiency (MSD) is characterized by decreased activity of all known sulfatases. Recent evidence suggests that a co- or posttranslational modification of a cysteine to a 2-amino 3-oxopropionic acid is required for active sulfatases and that a lack of this modification results in MSD.

These disorders are amenable to prenatal diagnosis, since the pattern of metabolism by affected cells obtained from amniotic fluid is strikingly different from normal.

McKusick, V., and Neufeld, E. F. The mucopolysaccharide storage diseases. In: J. B. Stansbury, J. B. Wyngaarden, D. S. Frederickson, J. L. Goldstein, and M. S. Brown (Eds.). *The Metabolic Basis of Inherited Disease,* 5th ed. New York: McGraw-Hill, 1983, p. 751.

Enzymic Defects in the Mucopolysaccharidoses

Disease	***Accumulated Products***[a]	***Deficient Enzyme***[b]
Hunter	Heparan sulfate Dermatan sulfate	Iduronate sulfatase (1)
Hurler + Scheie	Heparan sulfate Dermatan sulfate	α-L-Iduronidase (2)
Maroteaux–Lamy	Dermatan sulfate	*N*-Acetylgalactosamine (3) sulfatasc
Mucolipidosis VII	Heparan sulfate Dermatan sulfate	β-Glucuronidase (5)
Sanfilippo A	Heparan sulfate	Heparan sulfamidase (6)
Sanfilippo B	Heparan sulfate	*N*-Acetylglucosaminidase (9)
Sanfilippo D	Heparan sulfate	*N*-Acetylglucosamine 6-sulfatase (8)

[a] Structures of dermatan sulfate and heparan sulfate.

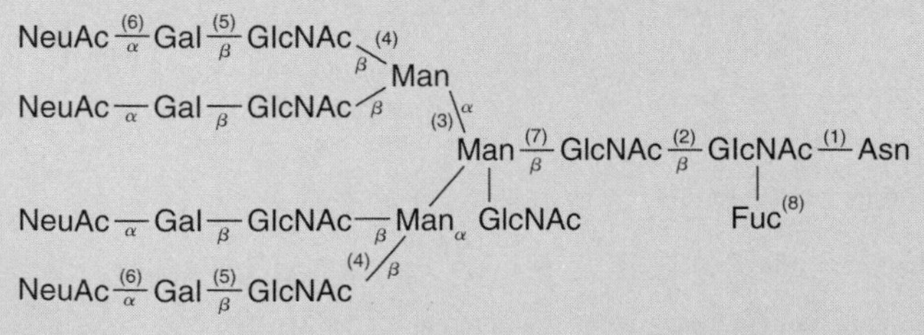

```
NeuAc -(6)α- Gal -(5)β- GlcNAc \ (4)
                               β Man
NeuAc -α- Gal -β- GlcNAc / β       (3) \ α
                                        Man -(7)β- GlcNAc -(2)β- GlcNAc -(1)- Asn
                                       /  |                        |
NeuAc -α- Gal -β- GlcNAc -β- Man α  GlcNAc                    Fuc(8)
                          (4) / β
NeuAc -(6)α- Gal -(5)β- GlcNAc
```

[b] The numbers in parentheses refer to the enzymes that hydrolyze those bonds.

certain features are common to all classes. The long unbranched heteropolysaccharide chains are made up largely of disaccharide repeating units, in which one sugar is a hexosamine and the other a uronic acid. Other common constituents of glycosaminoglycans are sulfate groups, linked by ester bonds to certain monosaccharides or by amide bonds to the amino group of glucosamine. An exception, hyaluronate, is not sulfated and has not been shown to exist covalently attached to protein. The carboxyl from uronic acids and sulfate groups contribute to the highly charged polyanionic nature of glycosaminoglycans. Both their electrical charge and macromolecular structure aid in their biological role as lubricants and support elements in connective tissue. Proteoglycans form solutions with high viscosity and elasticity by absorbing large volumes of water. This allows them to act in stabilizing and supporting fibrous and cellular elements of tissues, as well as contributing to the maintenance of water and salt balance in the body. Increasingly more dynamic roles as receptors for growth factors, transport proteins, and viruses are being elucidated for the proteoglycans.

Hyaluronate Is a Copolymer of *N*-Acetylglucosamine and Glucuronic Acid

Hyaluronate is very different from the other five types of glycosaminoglycans. It is unsulfated, not covalently complexed with protein, and the only glycosaminoglycan not limited to animal tissue; it is also produced by bacteria. It is classified as a glycosaminoglycan because of its structural similarity to these other polymers, since it consists solely of repeating disaccharide units of *N*-acetylglucosamine and glucuronic acid (Figure 8.11). Although hyaluronate has the least complex chemical structure of all the glycosaminoglycans, the chains can reach molecular weights of 10^5–10^7. The large molecular weight, polyelec-

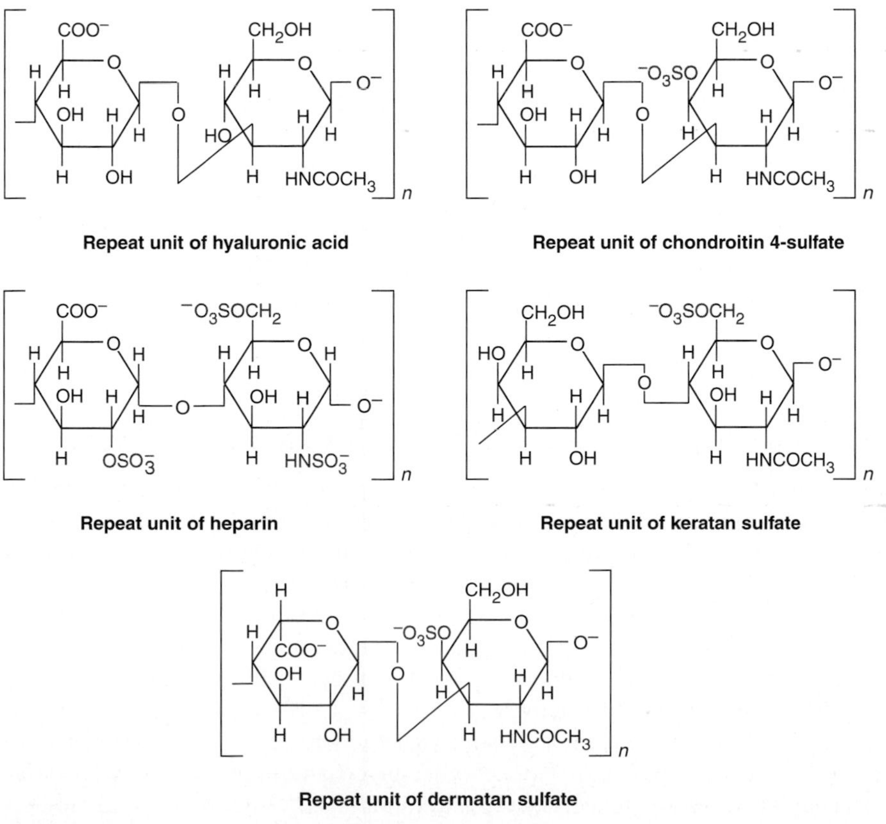

Repeat unit of hyaluronic acid

Repeat unit of chondroitin 4-sulfate

Repeat unit of heparin

Repeat unit of keratan sulfate

Repeat unit of dermatan sulfate

FIGURE 8.11
Major repeat units of glycosaminoglycan chains.

trolyte character, and large volume it occupies in solution all contribute to the properties of hyaluronate as a lubricant and shock absorbent. Hence it is found predominantly in synovial fluid, vitreous humor, and umbilical cord.

Chondroitin Sulfates Are the Most Abundant Glycosaminoglycans

The most abundant glycosaminoglycans in the body are the chondroitin sulfates. Individual polysaccharide chains are attached to specific serine residues in a protein core of variable molecular weight through a tetrasaccharide linkage region.

$$\text{GlcUA} \xrightarrow[1,3]{} \text{Gal} \xrightarrow[1,3]{} \text{Gal} \xrightarrow[1,4]{} \text{Xyl} \rightarrow O\text{-Ser}$$

The characteristic repeating disaccharide units of *N*-acetylgalactosamine and glucuronic acid are covalently attached to this linkage region (Figure 8.11). The disaccharides can be sulfated in either the 4 or 6 position of *N*-acetylgalactosamine. Each polysaccharide chain contains between 30 and 50 such disaccharide units, corresponding to molecular weights of 15,000–25,000. An average chondroitin sulfate proteoglycan molecule has approximately 100 chondroitin sulfate chains attached to the protein core, giving a molecular weight of $1.5–2 \times 10^6$. Proteoglycan preparations are, however, extremely heterogeneous, differing in length of protein core, degree of substitution, distribution of polysaccharide chains, length of chondroitin sulfate chains, and degree of sulfation. Chondroitin sulfate proteoglycans have also been shown to aggregate noncovalently with hyaluronate, forming much larger structures. They are prominent components of cartilage tendons, ligaments, and aorta and have also been isolated from brain, kidney, and lung.

Dermatan Sulfate Contains L-Iduronic Acid

Dermatan sulfate differs from chondroitin 4- and 6-sulfates in that its predominant uronic acid is L-iduronic acid, although D-glucuronic acid is also present in variable amounts. The glycosidic linkages have the same position and configuration as in chondroitin sulfates, with average polysaccharide chains of molecular weights of $2–5 \times 10^4$. Unlike the chondroitin sulfates, dermatan sulfate is antithrombic like heparin, but in contrast to heparin, it shows only minimal whole-blood anticoagulant and blood lipid-clearing activities. As a connective tissue macromolecule, dermatan sulfate is found in skin, blood vessels, and heart valves.

Heparin and Heparan Sulfate Differ from Other Glycosaminoglycans

Heparin differs from other glycosaminoglycans in a number of important respects. Glucosamine and D-glucuronic acid or L-iduronic acid form the characteristic disaccharide repeat unit, as in dermatan sulfate (Figure 8.11). In contrast to most other glycosaminoglycans, heparin contains α-glycosidic linkages. Almost all glucosamine residues contain sulfamide linkages, but a small number of glucosamine residues are *N*-acetylated. The sulfate content of heparin, although variable, approaches 2.5 sulfate residues per disaccharide unit in preparations with the highest biological activity. In addition to *N*-sulfate and *O*-sulfate on C-6 of glucosamine, heparin can also contain sulfate on C-3 of the hexosamine and C-2 of the uronic acid. Unlike other glycosaminoglycans, heparin is an intracellular component of mast cells and functions predominantly as an anticoagulant and lipid-clearing agent (see Clin. Corr. 8.8 on p. 350).

Heparan sulfate contains a similar disaccharide repeat unit but has more *N*-acetyl groups, fewer *N*-sulfate groups, and a lower degree of *O*-sulfate groups. Heparan sulfate may be extracellular or an integral and ubiquitous component of the cell surface in many tissues including blood vessel walls, amyloid, and brain.

Keratan Sulfate Exists in Two Forms

Keratan sulfate is composed principally of the repeating disaccharide unit of *N*-acetylglucosamine and galactose, with no uronic acid in the molecule (Figure 8.11). Sulfate content is variable, with ester sulfate present on C-6 of both galactose and hexosamine. Two types of keratan sulfate differ in overall carbohydrate content and tissue distribution. Both contain as additional monosaccharides, mannose, fucose, sialic acid, and *N*-acetylgalactosamine. Keratan sulfate I, isolated from cornea, is linked to protein by an *N*-acetylglucosamine–asparaginyl bond, typical of glycoproteins. Keratan sulfate II, isolated from cartilage, is attached to protein through *N*-acetylgalactosamine in *O*-glycosidic linkage to either serine or threonine. Skeletal keratan sulfates are often found covalently attached to the same core protein as are the chondroitin sulfate chains.

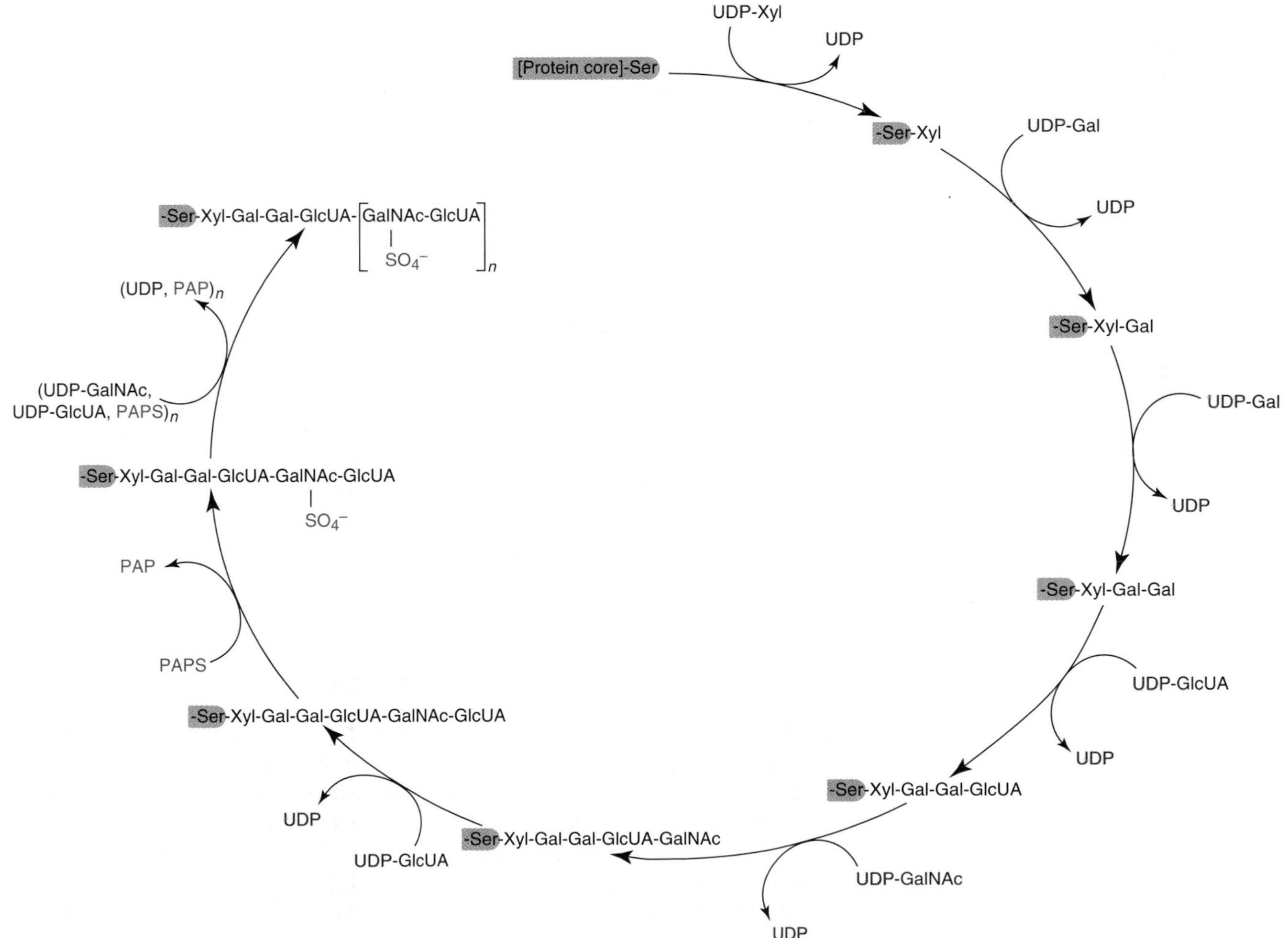

FIGURE 8.12
Synthesis of chondroitin sulfate proteoglycan.
Xyl, xylose; Gal, galactose; GlcUA, glucuronic acid; GalNAc, *N*-acetylgalactosamine; PAPS, 3′-phosphoadenosine 5′-phosphosulfate.

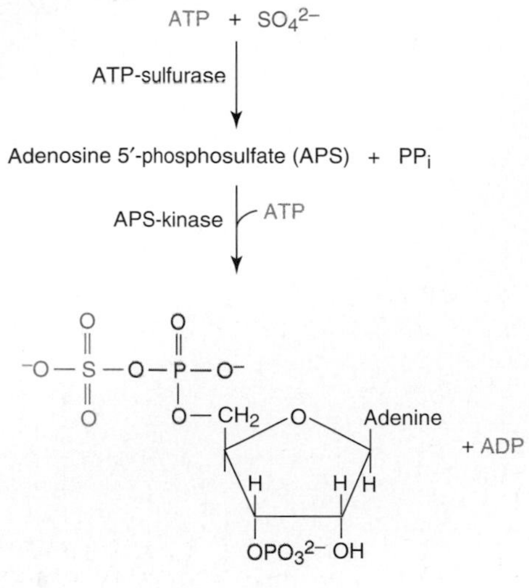

$$ATP + SO_4^{2-} \xrightarrow{\text{ATP-sulfurase}} \text{Adenosine 5'-phosphosulfate (APS)} + PP_i$$

$$\text{APS} \xrightarrow[\text{APS-kinase}]{ATP} \text{PAPS} + ADP$$

3′-Phosphoadenosine 5′-phosphosulfate (PAPS)

FIGURE 8.13
Biosynthesis of 3′-phosphoadenosine 5′-phosphosulfate (PAPS).

Biosynthesis of Chondroitin Sulfate Is Typical of Glycosaminoglycan Formation

The polysaccharide chains of proteoglycans are assembled by sequential action of a series of glycosyltransferases in the endoplasmic reticulum, which catalyze the transfer of a monosaccharide from a nucleotide sugar to an appropriate acceptor, either the nonreducing end of another sugar or a polypeptide. Since the biosynthesis of the chondroitin sulfates is most thoroughly understood, this pathway will be discussed as the prototype for glycosaminoglycan formation (Figure 8.12 on p. 355).

Formation of the core protein of the chondroitin sulfate proteoglycan is the first step in this process, followed by assembly of the polysaccharide chains catalyzed by six different glycosyltransferases in the lumen of the endoplasmic reticulum. Strict substrate specificity is required for completion of the unique tetrasaccharide linkage region. Polymerization then results from the concerted action of two glycosyltransferases, an *N*-acetylgalactosaminyltransferase and a glucuronosyltransferase, which alternately add the two monosaccharides, forming the characteristic repeating disaccharide units. Sulfation of *N*-acetylgalactosamine residues in either the 4 or 6 position apparently occurs along with chain elongation. The sulfate donor, as in other biological systems, is 3′-phosphoadenosine 5′-phosphosulfate (PAPS), which is formed from ATP and sulfate in two steps (Figure 8.13).

Synthesis of other glycosaminoglycans requires additional transferases specific for the sugars and linkages found in these molecules. Completion often involves modifications in addition to *O*-sulfation, including epimerization, acetylation, and *N*-sulfation. Interestingly, the epimerization of D-glucuronic acid to L-iduronic acid occurs after incorporation into the polymer chain and is coupled with the process of sulfation.

Synthesis of both proteoglycans and glycoproteins is regulated by the same mechanism at the level of hexosamine synthesis. The fructose 6-phosphate–glutamine transamidase reaction (Figure 8.4) is subject to feedback inhibition by UDP-*N*-acetylglucosamine, which is in equilibrium with UDP-*N*-acetylgalactosamine. More specific to proteoglycan synthesis, the levels of UDP-xylose and UDP-glucuronic acid are stringently controlled by the inhibition by UDP-xylose of the UDP-glucose dehydrogenase conversion of UDP-glucose to UDP-glucuronic acid (Figure 8.4). Since xylose is the first sugar added during synthesis of chondroitin sulfate, dermatan sulfate, heparin, and heparan sulfate, the earliest effect of decreased core protein synthesis would be accumulation of UDP-xylose, which aids in maintaining a balance between synthesis of protein and polysaccharide moieties of these complex macromolecules.

Proteoglycans, like glycoproteins, are degraded by the sequential action of proteases and **glycosidases,** as well as **deacetylases** and **sulfatases.** Much of the information about metabolism and degradation of proteoglycans has been derived from the study of **mucopolysaccharidoses** (see Clin. Corr. 8.9). This group of human genetic disorders is characterized by accumulation in tissues and excretion in urine of oligosaccharide products derived from incomplete breakdown of the proteoglycans, due to a deficiency of one or more lysosomal hydrolases. In the diseases for which the biochemical defect has been identified, a product accumulates that has a nonreducing terminus that would have been the substrate for the deficient enzyme.

Although proteoglycans continue to be defined on the basis of the glycosaminoglycan chain they contain, new ones are increasingly being described based largely on functional properties or location. Aggrecan and versican are the predominant extracellular species; syndecan, CD44, and thrombomodulin are integral membrane proteins; neurocan, brevican, cerebrocan, and phosphacan are largely restricted to the nervous system; while many proteoglycans (i.e., aggrecan, syndecan, and betaglycan) carry two types of glycosaminoglycan chains, whose size and ratio may change with development, age, or disease. Thus it appears that the versatile structure of these abundant carbohydrate-containing molecules is well exploited by cells in many as yet undiscovered ways.

BIBLIOGRAPHY

Dutton, G. J. (Ed.). *Glucuronic Acid, Free and Combined.* New York: Academic Press, 1966.

Ginsburg, V., and Robbins, P. (Eds.). *Biology of Carbohydrates.* New York: Wiley, 1984.

Horecker, B. L. *Pentose Metabolism in Bacteria.* New York: Wiley, 1962.

Kornfeld, R., and Kornfeld, S. Assembly of Asn-linked oligosaccharides. *Annu. Rev. Biochem.* 54:631, 1985.

Lennarz, W. J. (Ed.). *The Biochemistry of Glycoproteins.* New York: Plenum Press, 1980.

Menkes, J. A. Metabolic diseases of the nervous system. In: *Textbook of Child Neurology,* 4th ed. Philadelphia: Lea & Febiger, 1990, p. 28.

Nyhan, W. L., and Sakati, N. A. Mucopolysaccharidoses and related disorders. In: *Diagnostic Recognition of Genetic Disease.* Philadelphia: Lea & Febiger, 1987, p. 371.

Rademacker, T. W., Parck, R. B., and Dwek, R. A. Glycobiology. *Annu. Rev. Biochem.* 57:285, 1988.

Schwartz, N. B., and Smalheiser, N. Biosynthesis of glycosaminoglycans and proteoglycans. In: *Neurobiology of Glycoconjugates.* New York: Plenum Press, 1989, p. 151.

Scriver, C. R., Beaudet, A. L., Sly, W. S. and Valle, D. (Eds.) *The Metabolic and Molecular Bases of Inherited Disease,* 7th ed. New York: McGraw-Hill, 1995.

QUESTIONS ■ C. N. ANGSTADT AND J. BAGGOTT

1. [NADPH/NADP$^+$] is maintained at a high level in cells primarily by:
   A. lactate dehydrogenase.
   B. the combined actions of glucose-6-phosphate dehydrogenase and gluconolactonase.
   C. the action of the electron transport chain.
   D. shuttle mechanisms such as the α-glycerophosphate dehydrogenase shuttle.
   E. the combined actions of transketolase and transaldolase.

2. Transketolase:
   A. transfers a C_2 fragment to an aldehyde acceptor.
   B. transfers a C_3 ketone-containing fragment to an acceptor.
   C. converts the ketose sugar ribulose 5-phosphate to ribose 5-phosphate.
   D. is part of the irreversible oxidative phase of the pentose phosphate pathway.
   E. converts two C_5 sugar phosphates to fructose 6-phosphate and erythrose 4-phosphate.

3. If a cell requires more NADPH than ribose 5-phosphate:
   A. only the first phase of the pentose phosphate pathway would occur.
   B. glycolytic intermediates would flow into the reversible phase of the pentose phosphate pathway.
   C. there would be sugar interconversions but no net release of carbons from glucose 6-phosphate.
   D. the equivalent of the carbon atoms of glucose 6-phosphate would be released as 6 CO_2.
   E. only part of this need could be met by the pentose pathway, and the rest would have to be supplied by another pathway.

4. All of the following interconversions of monosaccharides (or derivatives) require a nucleotide-linked sugar intermediate EXCEPT:
   A. galactose 1-phosphate to glucose 1-phosphate.
   B. glucose 6-phosphate to mannose 6-phosphate.
   C. glucose to glucuronic acid.
   D. glucuronic acid to xylose.
   E. glucosamine 6-phosphate to *N*-acetylneuraminic acid (a sialic acid).

5. Fructose:
   A. unlike glucose, cannot be catabolized by the glycolytic pathway.
   B. in the liver, enters directly into glycolysis as fructose 6-phosphate.
   C. must be isomerized to glucose before it can be metabolized.
   D. is converted to a UDP-linked form and then epimerized to UDP-glucose.
   E. catabolism in liver uses fructokinase and a specific aldolase that recognizes fructose 1-phosphate.

6. Galactosemia:
   A. is a genetic deficiency of a uridylyltransferase that exchanges galactose 1-phosphate for glucose on UDP-glucose.
   B. results from a deficiency of an epimerase.
   C. is not apparent at birth but symptoms develop in later life.
   D. is an inability to form galactose 1-phosphate.
   E. would be expected to interfere with the use of fructose as well as galactose because the deficient enzyme is common to the metabolism of both sugars.

7. All of the following are true about glucuronic acid EXCEPT:
   A. it enhances the water solubility of compounds to which it is conjugated.
   B. as a UDP derivative, it can be decarboxylated to a component used in proteoglycan synthesis.
   C. it is a precursor of ascorbic acid in humans.
   D. its formation from glucose is under feedback control by a UDP-linked intermediate.
   E. it can ultimately be converted to xylulose 5-phosphate and thus enter the pentose phosphate pathway.

8. The conversion of fructose 6-phosphate to glucosamine 6-phosphate:
   A. is a transamination reaction with glutamate as the nitrogen donor.
   B. is stimulated by UDP-*N*-acetylglucosamine.
   C. requires that fructose 6-phosphate first be linked to a nucleotide.
   D. is a first step in the formation of *N*-acetylated amine sugars.
   E. occurs only in the liver.

9. Roles for the complex carbohydrate moiety of glycoproteins include all of the following EXCEPT:
   A. determinant of blood type.
   B. template for the synthesis of glycosaminoglycans.
   C. cell surface receptor specificity.
   D. determinant of the rate of clearance from the circulation of certain molecules.
   E. targeting of cells to certain tissues.

10. Glycoproteins:
   A. may contain 95% or more carbohydrate.
   B. always contain a serially repeating carbohydrate unit.
   C. are found only intracellularly.
   D. from different animal species may have a different primary sequence in the protein but have identical carbohydrate chains.
   E. have the carbohydrate linked to the protein by either *N*- or *O*-glycosidic bonds.

11. The carbohydrate core structure is assembled on dolichol phosphate before transfer to the protein for:
   A. *N*-linked glycoproteins.
   B. *O*-linked glycoproteins.
   C. proteoglycans.
   D. glycosaminoglycans.
   E. all of the above.

12. Fucose and sialic acid:
   A. are found most commonly in *N*-linked glycoproteins.
   B. are the parts of the carbohydrate chain that are covalently linked to the protein.
   C. can be found in the core structure of certain *O*-linked glycoproteins.
   D. are transferred to a carbohydrate chain when it is attached to dolichol phosphate.
   E. are the repeating unit of proteoglycans.

13. Glycosaminoglycans:
   A. are the carbohydrate portion of glycoproteins.
   B. contain large segments of a repeating unit typically consisting of a hexosamine and a uronic acid.
   C. are low molecular weight cations.
   D. exist in only two forms.
   E. are bound to protein by ionic interaction.

Refer to the following for Questions 14–16.
   A. chondroitin sulfate
   B. dermatan sulfate
   C. heparin
   D. hyaluronate
   E. keratan sulfate

14. Differs from other glycosaminoglycans in being predominantly intracellular rather than extracellular.

15. Only glycosaminoglycan not covalently linked to protein.

16. The most abundant glycosaminoglycan in the body.

17. All of the following are true of proteoglycans EXCEPT:
   A. specificity is determined, in part, by the action of glycosyltransferases.
   B. synthesis is regulated, in part, by UDP-xylose inhibition of the conversion of UDP-glucose to UDP-glucuronic acid.
   C. synthesis involves sulfation of carbohydrate residues by PAPS.
   D. synthesis of core protein is balanced with synthesis of the polysaccharide moieties.
   E. degradation is catalyzed in the cytosol by nonspecific glycosidases.

ANSWERS

1. B Although the glucose-6-phosphate dehydrogenase reaction, specific for NADP, is reversible, hydrolysis of the lactone assures that the overall equilibrium lies far in the direction of NADPH. A, C, and D: These all use NAD, not NADP. E: These enzymes are part of the pentose phosphate pathway but catalyze freely reversible reactions that do not involve NADP (pp. 337–338).
2. A Both reactions catalyzed by transketolase are of this type. B and E describe transaldolase. C describes an isomerase. D: Transketolase is part of the reversible phase of the pentose phosphate pathway that also allows glycolytic intermediates to be converted to pentose sugars, if necessary (p. 338).
3. D A, C, D, E: Glucose 6-phosphate yields ribose 5-phosphate + CO_2 in the oxidative phase. If this is multiplied by six, the six ribose 5-phosphates can be rearranged to five glucose 6-phosphates by the second, reversible phase. B: If more ribose 5-phosphate than NADPH were required, the flow would be in this direction to supply the needed pentoses (pp. 338–340).
4. B The glucose and mannose phosphates are both in equilibrium with fructose 6-phosphate by phosphohexose isomerases. A: This occurs via an epimerase at the UDP-galactose level. C and D: This oxidation of glucose is catalyzed by UDP-glucose dehydrogenase and the product can be decarboxylated to UDP-xylose. E: Again, an epimerization occurs on the nucleotide intermediate (p. 342, Fig. 8.4).
5. E A, C, E: Fructokinase produces fructose 1-phosphate. Since this cannot be converted to fructose 1,6-bisphosphate, a specific aldolase cleaves it to dihydroxyacetone phosphate and glyceraldehyde. The first product is a glycolytic intermediate; the second requires modification to enter glycolysis. D: Glucose and fructose are not epimers (p. 342, Clin. Corr. 8.2).
6. A B: The epimerase is normal. C: Galactose is an important sugar for infants. E: Fructose metabolism does not use the uridylyltransferase that is deficient in galactosemia (p. 353, Clin. Corr. 8.3).
7. C Humans do not make ascorbic acid. A: Enhancing water solubility is a major physiological role for glucuronic acid,

for example, bilirubin metabolism. B and D: Decarboxylation of UDP-glucuronic acid gives UDP-xylose, which is a potent inhibitor of the oxidation of UDP-glucose to the acid. E: The reduction of D-glucuronic acid to L-gulonic acid leads to ascorbate as well as xylulose 5-phosphate for the pentose phosphate pathway (p. 345, Figure 8.7).

8. D Glucosamine 6-phosphate is acetylated. UDP-*N*-acetylglucosamine is formed, and the UDP derivative can be epimerized to the galactose derivative. A and C: This conversion is a transamidation of the amide nitrogen of glutamine and does not involve nucleotide intermediates. B: This is a feedback inhibitor of the transamidase reaction, thus controlling formation of the nucleotide sugars. E: May account for 20% of the glucose flux in skin (p. 344).

9. B Synthesis of complex carbohydrates is not template directed but determined by the specificity of individual enzymes. A, C, D, and E: Because of the diversity possible with oligosaccharides, they play a significant role in determining the specificity of many biological molecules (pp. 345–347).

10. E A and B: This is true of proteoglycans. C: Some hormones in blood are glycoproteins. D: Heterogeneity of carbohydrates is common (pp. 348–350).

11. A This is characteristic of *N*-linked glycoproteins. B, C, and D: Synthesis of *O*-linked glycoproteins involves the sequential addition to the *N*-acetylgalactosamine linked to serine or threonine (p. 350).

12. C Core also contains galactose and *N*-acetylgalactosamine. A and D: Core structure of *N*-linked carbohydrates contains mannose and *N*-acetylglucosamine. B: Usually found at the periphery of the carbohydrate. E: Repeating unit is hexosamine and uronic acids (pp. 350 and 353).

13. B This is a major distinction from glycoproteins, which, by definition, do not have a serial repeating unit. A: These are carbohydrate of proteoglycans. C: They have anionic character contributed by carboxyl and sulfate (another common feature) groups. D: There are at least six different classes. E: Carbohydrates are bound by covalent links (p. 353).

14. C (p. 354).

15. D Classified as a glycosaminoglycan because of its structural similarity to the others (p. 353).

16. A (p. 354).

17. E Degradation is lysosomal; deficiencies of one or more lysosomal hydrolases lead to accumulation of proteoglycans in the mucopolysaccharidoses. A: Strict substrate specificity of the enzymes is important in determining the type and quantity of proteoglycans synthesized. Formation of specific protein acceptors for the carbohydrate is also important. B and D: Both xylose and glucuronic acid levels are controlled by this; xylose is the first sugar added in the synthesis of four of the six types and would accumulate if core protein synthesis is decreased. C: This is necessary for the formation of all proteoglycans (hyaluronic acid is not part of a proteoglycan) (p. 356).

CHAPTER

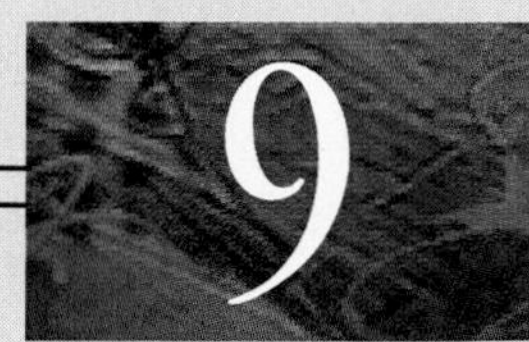

LIPID METABOLISM I: UTILIZATION AND STORAGE OF ENERGY IN LIPID FORM

J. Denis McGarry

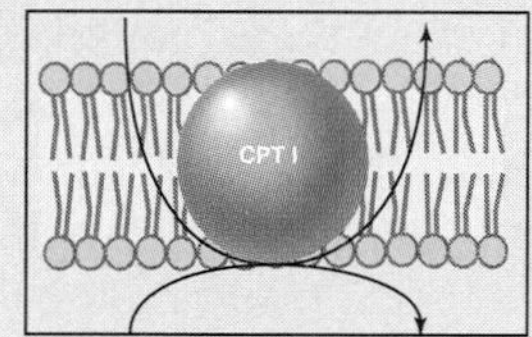

9.1 ■ OVERVIEW

As the human body builds and renews its structures, obtains and stores energy, and performs its various functions, there are many circumstances in which it is essential to use molecules or parts of molecules that do not associate with water. This property of being **nonpolar** and **hydrophobic** is the defining characteristic of substances classed as **lipids.** Most of these are molecules that contain or are derived from **fatty acids.** In the early stages of biochemical research, lipids were not investigated as intensively as other body constituents, largely because techniques for studying aqueous systems were easier to develop. This benign neglect led to assumptions that lipids were relatively inert and their metabolism was of lesser importance than that of carbohydrates, for instance.

As the methodology for analyzing lipid metabolism developed, it became evident that fatty acids and their derivatives had at least two major roles in the body. On the one hand, oxidation of fatty acids was shown to be a major means of metabolic energy production. It also became clear that their storage in the form of **triacylglycerols** was more efficient and quantitatively more important than storage of carbohydrates as glycogen. On the other hand, as details of the chemistry of biological structures were defined, hydrophobic structures were found to be largely composed of fatty acids and their derivatives. Thus the major separation of cells and subcellular structures into separate aqueous compartments is accomplished with membranes whose hydrophobic characteristics are largely supplied by the fatty acid moieties of complex lipids. These latter compounds contain constituents other than fatty acids and glycerol. They frequently have significant covalently bound hydrophilic moieties, notably carbohydrates in the glycolipids and organic phosphate esters in phospholipids.

Lipids have several other quantitatively less important roles, which are nonetheless of great functional significance. These include the use of surface active properties of some complex lipids for specific functions, such as maintenance of lung alveolar integrity and solubilization of nonpolar substances in body fluids. In addition, several classes of lipids, for example, steroid hormones and prostaglandins, have highly potent and specific physiological roles in control of metabolic processes. The interrelationships of some processes involved in lipid metabolism are outlined in Figure 9.1. The metabolism of fatty acids and triacylglycerols is so crucial to proper functioning of the human body that imbalances and deficiencies in these processes can have serious pathological consequences. Disease states related to fatty acid and triacylglycerol metabolism include obesity, diabetes, ketoacidosis, and abnormalities in transport of lipids in blood. In addition, some unique deficiencies have been found, such as Refsum's disease and familial hypercholesterolemia, which have helped to elucidate some pathways in lipid metabolism.

This chapter is concerned primarily with the structure and metabolism of fatty acids and of their major storage form, triacylglycerols. After a discussion of the structures of the more important fatty acids found in humans, how they

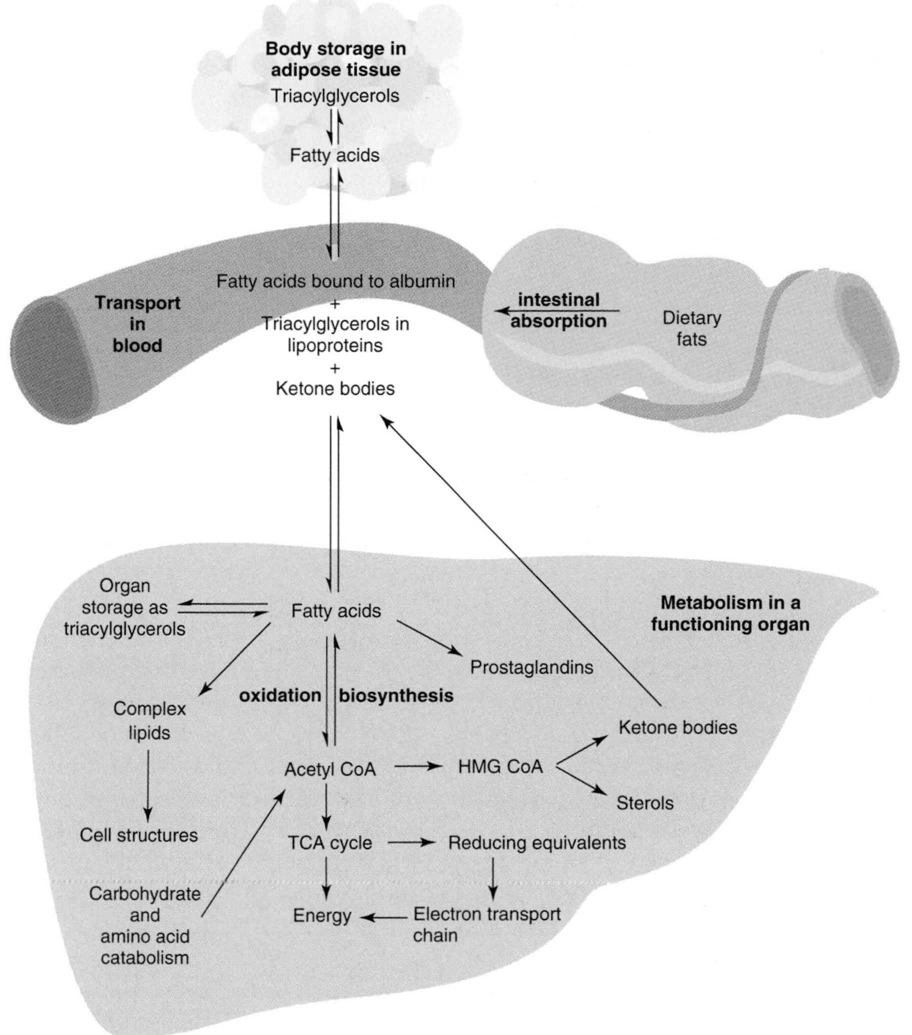

FIGURE 9.1
Metabolic interrelationships of fatty acids in the human.

are supplied from the diet or by biosynthesis is described. The mechanism for storage as triacylglycerols and how fatty acids are mobilized and transported throughout the body to sites where they are needed are discussed. The central process of energy production from fatty acids is then examined, and finally the mechanisms by which the ketone bodies are synthesized and used are presented.

The Appendix includes the nomenclature and chemistry of lipids and in Chapter 26 there is a discussion of digestion and absorption of lipids.

9.2 ■ CHEMICAL NATURE OF FATTY ACIDS AND ACYLGLYCEROLS

Fatty Acids Are Alkyl Chains Terminating in a Carboxyl Group

Fatty acids consist of an **alkyl chain** with a terminal carboxyl group, the basic formula of completely saturated species being CH_3—$(CH_2)_n$—COOH. The important fatty acids for humans have relatively simple structures, although in some organisms they may be quite complex, containing cyclopropane rings or extensive branching. Unsaturation occurs commonly in human fatty acids, with up to six double bonds per chain, these being almost always of the cis configuration. If there is more than one double bond per molecule, they are always separated by a **methylene** (—CH_2—) **group.** The most common fatty acids

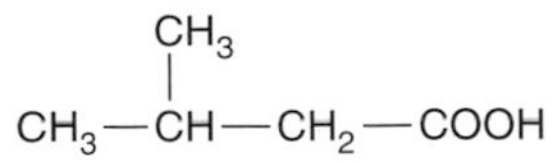

$$CH_3-CH(CH_3)-CH_2-COOH$$

FIGURE 9.2
Isovaleric acid.

in biological systems have an even number of carbon atoms, although some organisms do synthesize those with an odd number of carbon atoms. Humans can use the latter for energy but incorporate them into complex lipids to a minimal degree.

A few fatty acids with an α-OH group are produced and used structurally by humans. However, more oxidized forms are normally produced only as metabolic intermediates during energy production or for specific physiological activity in the case of prostaglandins and thromboxanes. Some animals, including humans, also produce relatively simple **branched-chain acids,** branching being limited to methyl groups along the chain at one or more positions. These are apparently produced to contribute specific physical properties to some secretions and structures. For instance, large amounts of branched-chain fatty acids, particularly isovaleric acid (Figure 9.2), occur in lipids of echo-locating structures in marine mammals. Elucidation of the role of these compounds in sound focusing should be fascinating.

Most fatty acids in humans have C16, C18, or C20 atoms, but there are several with longer chains that occur principally in lipids of the nervous system. These include nervonic acid and a C22 acid with six double bonds (Figure 9.3).

$$CH_3-(CH_2)_7-CH=CH-(CH_2)_{13}-COOH$$

Nervonic acid

$$CH_3-(CH_2-CH=CH)_6-(CH_2)_2-COOH$$

All-*cis*-4,7,10,13,16,19,-docosahexaenoic acid

FIGURE 9.3
Long-chain fatty acids.

Nomenclature of Fatty Acids

The most abundant fatty acids have common names that have been accepted for use in the official nomenclature. Examples are given in Table 9.1 with official systematic names. The approved abbreviations consist of the number of carbon atoms followed, after a colon, by the number of double bonds. Carbon atoms are numbered with the carboxyl carbon as number 1, and double bond locations are designated by the number of the carbon atom on the carboxyl side of it. These designations of double bonds are in parentheses after the rest of the symbol.

Most Fatty Acids in Humans Occur as Triacylglycerols

Fatty acids occur primarily as esters of glycerol, as shown in Figure 9.4, when they are stored for future use. Compounds with one **(monoacylglycerols)** or two **(diacylglycerols)** acids esterified are present only in relatively minor amounts and occur largely as metabolic intermediates in biosynthesis and degradation of glycerol-containing lipids. Most fatty acids in humans exist as **triacylglycerols,** in which all three hydroxyl groups on glycerol are esterified with a fatty acid. These compounds have been called "neutral fats or triglycerides." There are other types of "neutral fats" in the body, and the terms "triglyceride," "monoglyceride," and "diglyceride" are chemically incorrect and should not be used.

The distribution of different fatty acids in the three positions of the glycerol moiety of triacylglycerols in the body at any given time is influenced by many

TABLE 9.1 Fatty Acids of Importance to Humans

Numerical Symbol	*Structure*	*Trivial Name*	*Systematic Name*
16:0	$CH_3-(CH_2)_{14}-COOH$	Palmitic	Hexadecanoic
16:1(9)	$CH_3-(CH_2)_5-CH=CH-(CH_2)_7-COOH$	Palmitoleic	*cis*-9-Hexadecenoic
18:0	$CH_3-(CH_2)_{16}-COOH$	Stearic	Octadecanoic
18:1(9)	$CH_3-(CH_2)_7-CH=CH-(CH_2)_7-COOH$	Oleic	*cis*-9-Octadecenoic
18:2(9,12)	$CH_3-(CH_2)_3-(CH_2-CH=CH)_2-(CH_2)_7-COOH$	Linoleic	*cis,cis*-9,12-Octadecadienoic
18:3(9,12,15)	$CH_3-(CH_2-CH=CH)_3-(CH_2)_7-COOH$	Linolenic	*cis,cis,cis*-9,12,15-Octadecatrienoic
20:4(5,8,11,14)	$CH_3-(CH_2)_3-(CH_2-CH=CH)_4-(CH_2)_3-COOH$	Arachidonic	*cis,cis,cis,cis*-5,8,11,14-Eicosatetraenoic

factors, including diet and anatomical location of the triacylglycerol. Compounds with the same fatty acid in all three positions of glycerol are rare; the usual case is for a complex mixture.

The Hydrophobic Nature of Lipids Is Important for Their Biological Function

One significant property of fatty acids and triacylglycerols is their lack of affinity for water. Long hydrocarbon chains have negligible possibility for hydrogen bonding. Acids, whether unesterified or in a complex lipid, have a much greater tendency to associate with each other or other hydrophobic structures, such as sterols and hydrophobic side chains of amino acids, than they do with water or polar organic compounds. This hydrophobic character is essential for construction of complex biological structures such as membranes.

The **hydrophobic nature** of triacylglycerols and their highly reduced state make them efficient compounds in comparison to glycogen for storing energy. Three points deserve emphasis. First, on a weight basis pure triacylglycerols yield near two and one-half times the amount of ATP on complete oxidation than does pure glycogen. Second, triacylglycerols can be stored without associated water, whereas glycogen is very hydrophilic and binds about twice its weight of water when stored in tissues. Thus the equivalent amount of metabolically recoverable energy stored as hydrated glycogen would weigh about four times as much as if it were stored as triacylglycerols. Third, the average 70-kg person stores about 350 g of carbohydrate as liver and muscle glycogen. This represents about 1400 kcal of available energy, barely enough to sustain bodily functions for 24 hours of fasting. By contrast, a normal complement of fat stores will provide sufficient energy to allow several weeks of survival during total food deprivation.

In humans most of the fatty acids are either saturated or contain only one double bond. Although they are readily catabolized by appropriate enzymes and cofactors, they are fairly inert chemically. The highly unsaturated fatty acids in tissues are much more susceptible to oxidation.

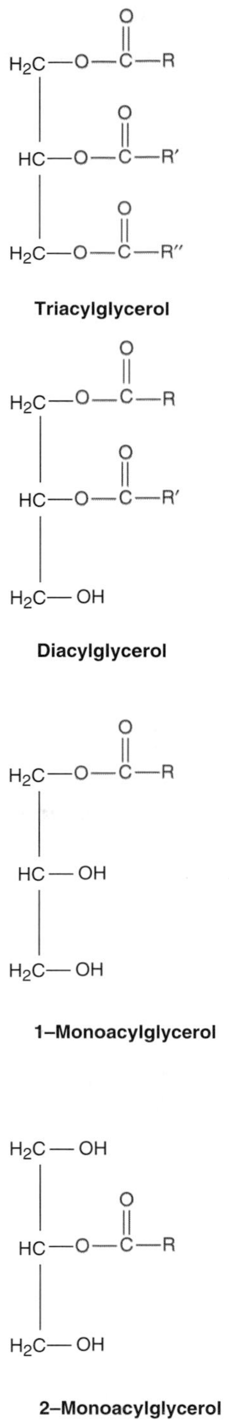

Triacylglycerol

Diacylglycerol

1–Monoacylglycerol

2–Monoacylglycerol

FIGURE 9.4
Acylglycerols.

9.3 ■ SOURCES OF FATTY ACIDS

Both diet and biosynthesis supply the fatty acids needed by the human body for energy and for construction of hydrophobic parts of biomolecules. Excess amounts of protein and carbohydrate in the diet are readily converted to fatty acids and stored as triacylglycerols.

Most Fatty Acids Are Supplied in the Diet

Various animal and vegetable lipids are ingested, hydrolyzed at least partially by digestive enzymes, and absorbed through the intestinal mucosa to be distributed through the body, first in the lymphatic system and then in the bloodstream. These processes are discussed in Chapter 25. To a large extent dietary supply governs the composition of fatty acids in body lipids. Metabolic processes in various tissues modify both dietary and *de novo* synthesized fatty acids to produce nearly all the required structures. With one exception, the actual composition of fatty acids supplied in the diet is relatively unimportant. This exception involves the need for appropriate proportions of relatively highly unsaturated fatty acids because many higher mammals, including humans, are unable to synthesize fatty acids with double bonds near the methyl end of the molecule. Certain **polyunsaturated acids** with double bonds within the last seven linkages toward the methyl end are essential for specific functions. Although all

$$CH_3-(CH_2)_3-(CH_3-CH{=}CH)_n-(CH_2)_m-COOH$$

Basic formula of the linoleic acid series

$$CH_3-(CH_2-CH{=}CH)_n-(CH_2)_m-COOH$$

Basic formula of the linolenic acid series

FIGURE 9.5
Linoleic and linolenic acid series.

the reasons for this need are not yet explained, one is that some of these acids are precursors of prostaglandins, very active oxidation products (see p. 431).

In humans a dietary precursor is essential for two series of fatty acids. These are the linoleic series and the linolenic series (Figure 9.5).

Palmitate Is Synthesized from Acetyl CoA

The second major source of fatty acids for humans is their biosynthesis from small-molecule intermediates derived from metabolic breakdown of sugars, some amino acids, and other fatty acids. In a majority of instances the saturated, straight-chain C16 acid, **palmitic acid,** is first synthesized, and all other fatty acids are made by modification of palmitic acid. Acetyl CoA is the direct source of all carbon atoms for this synthesis. Fatty acids are synthesized by sequential addition of two-carbon units to the activated carboxyl end of a growing chain. In mammalian systems the sequence of reactions is carried out by **fatty acid synthase.**

Fatty acid synthase is a fascinating enzyme complex that is still studied intensely. In bacteria it is a complex of several proteins, whereas in mammalian cells it is a single multifunctional protein. Either acetyl CoA or butyryl CoA is the priming unit for fatty acid synthesis, and the methyl end of these primers becomes the methyl end of palmitate. Addition of the rest of the two-carbon units requires activation of the methyl carbon of acetyl CoA by carboxylation to malonyl CoA. However, CO_2 added in this process is lost when condensation of malonyl CoA to the growing chain occurs, so carbon atoms in the palmitate chain originate only from acetyl CoA.

Formation of Malonyl CoA Is the Commitment Step of Fatty Acid Synthesis

The reaction that commits acetyl CoA to fatty acid synthesis is its carboxylation to **malonyl CoA** by the enzyme **acetyl-CoA carboxylase** (Figure 9.6). This reaction is similar in many ways to carboxylation of pyruvate, which starts the process of gluconeogenesis. The reaction requires ATP and HCO_3^- as the source of CO_2. As with pyruvate carboxylase, the first step is formation of activated CO_2 on the biotin moiety of acetyl-CoA carboxylase using energy from ATP. This is then transferred to acetyl CoA.

Acetyl-CoA carboxylase, a key control point in the overall synthesis of fatty acids, can be isolated in a protomeric state that is inactive. The protomers aggregate to form enzymatically active polymers upon addition of citrate *in*

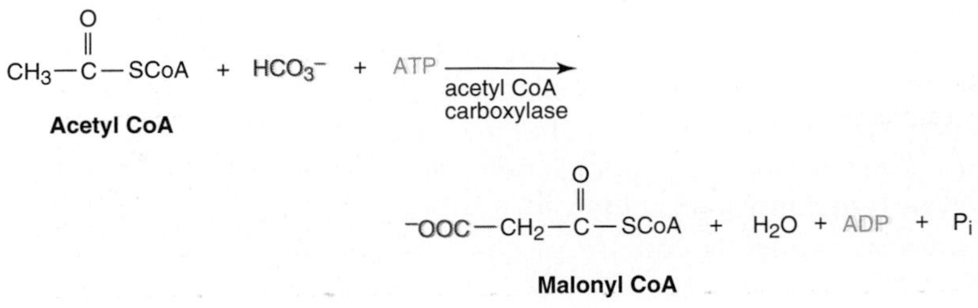

$$\underset{\text{Acetyl CoA}}{CH_3-\overset{O}{\overset{\|}{C}}-SCoA} + HCO_3^- + ATP \xrightarrow[\text{carboxylase}]{\text{acetyl CoA}} \underset{\text{Malonyl CoA}}{^-OOC-CH_2-\overset{O}{\overset{\|}{C}}-SCoA} + H_2O + ADP + P_i$$

FIGURE 9.6
Acetyl-CoA carboxylase reaction.

vitro. Pamitoyl CoA *in vitro* inhibits the active enzyme. The action of these two effectors is very logical. Increased synthesis of fatty acids to store energy is desirable when citrate is in high concentration, and decreased synthesis is necessary if high levels of product accumulate. However, the degree to which these regulatory mechanisms actually operate *in vivo* is still unclear.

Acetyl-CoA carboxylase is also controlled by a cAMP-mediated phosphorylation–dephosphorylation mechanism in which the phosphorylated enzyme is less active than the dephosphorylated one. There is evidence suggesting that phosphorylation is promoted by glucagon (via cAMP) as well as by AMP (via an AMP-activated kinase) and that the active form is fostered by insulin. These effects of hormone-mediated phosphorylation are separate from the allosteric effects of citrate and palmitoyl CoA (see Table 9.2).

TABLE 9.2 Regulation of Fatty Acid Synthesis

Enzyme		*Regulatory Agent*	*Effect*
		Palmitate Biosynthesis	
Acetyl-CoA carboxylase	Short term	Citrate	Allosteric activation
		C16–C18 acyl CoAs	Allosteric inhibition
		Insulin	Stimulation
		Glucagon	Inhibition
		cAMP-mediated phosphorylation	Inhibition
		Dephosphorylation	Stimulation
	Long term	High-carbohydrate diet	Stimulation by increased enzyme synthesis
		Fat-free diet	Stimulation by increased enzyme synthesis
		High-fat diet	Inhibition by decreased enzyme synthesis
		Fasting	Inhibition by decreased enzyme synthesis
		Glucagon	Inhibition by decreased enzyme synthesis
Fatty acid synthase		Phosphorylated sugars	Allosteric activation
		High-carbohydrate diet	Stimulation by increased enzyme synthesis
		Fat-free diet	Stimulation by increased enzyme synthesis
		High-fat diet	Inhibition by decreased enzyme synthesis
		Fasting	Inhibition by decreased enzyme synthesis
		Glucagon	Inhibition by decreased enzyme synthesis
		Biosynthesis of Fatty Acids Other than Palmitate	
Fatty acid synthase		High ratio of methylmalonyl CoA/malonyl CoA	Increased synthesis of methylated fatty acids
		Thioesterase cofactor	Termination of synthesis with short-chain product
Stearyl CoA desaturase		Various hormones	Stimulation of unsaturated fatty acid synthesis by increased enzyme synthesis
		Dietary polyunsaturated fatty acids	Decreased activity

The rate of synthesis of acetyl-CoA carboxylase is also regulated. More enzyme is produced by animals on high-carbohydrate or fat-free diets, whereas on fasting or high-fat diets the rate of enzyme synthesis is decreased.

Reaction Sequence for Synthesis of Palmitic Acid

The first step catalyzed by fatty acid synthase in bacteria is transacylation of the primer molecule, either acetyl CoA or butyryl CoA, to a 4′-phosphopantetheine moiety on a protein constituent of the enzyme complex. This protein is ***acyl carrier protein* (ACP),** and its phosphopantetheine unit is identical with that in CoA. The mammalian enzyme also contains a phosphopantetheine. Six or seven two-carbon units are then added sequentially to the enzyme complex until the palmitate molecule is completed. After each addition of a two-carbon unit a series of reductive steps takes place. The reaction sequence starting with an acetyl CoA primer and leading to butyryl-ACP is as presented in Figure 9.7.

The next round of synthesis is initiated by transfer of the newly formed fatty acid chain from 4′-phosphopantetheine moiety of ACP to a functional —SH group of ***β*-ketoacyl-ACP synthase** (analogous to Reaction 3a). This liberates the —SH group of ACP for acceptance of a second malonyl unit from

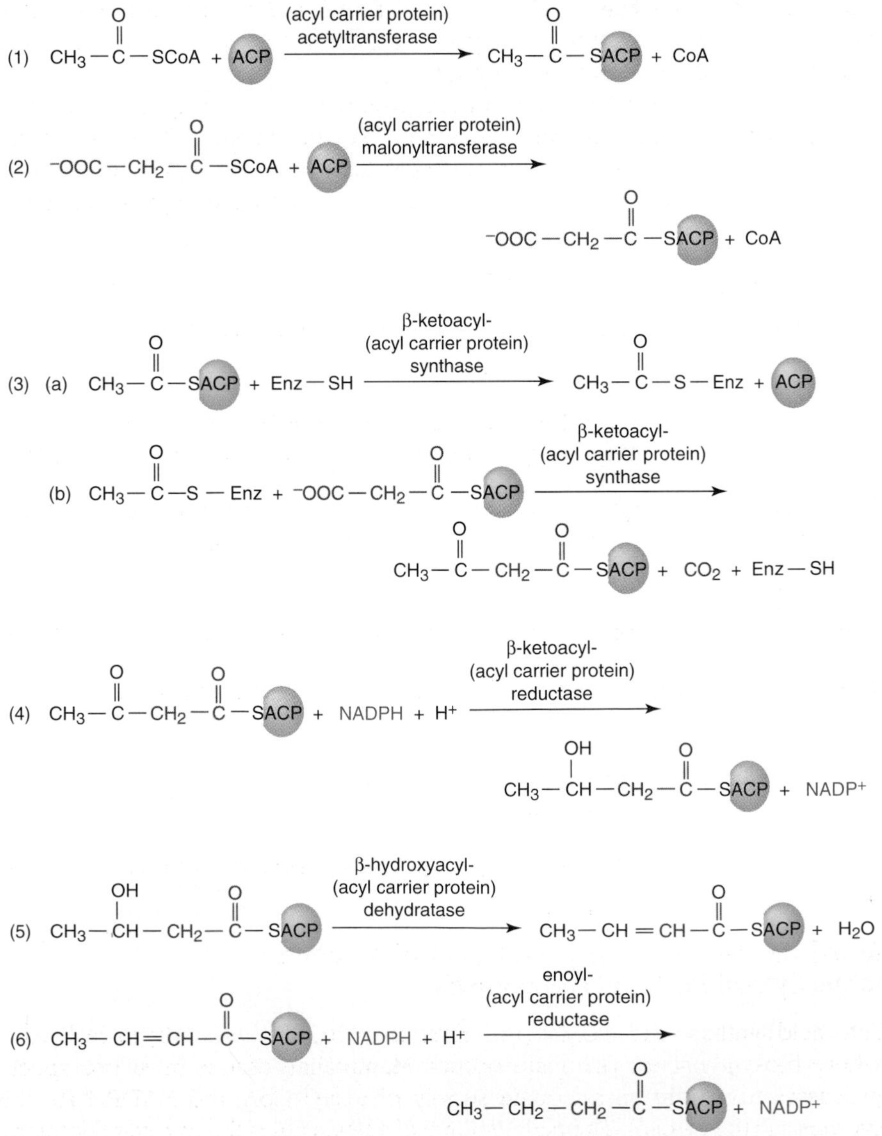

(1) $CH_3-CO-SCoA$ + ACP —(acyl carrier protein) acetyltransferase→ $CH_3-CO-SACP$ + CoA

(2) $^{-}OOC-CH_2-CO-SCoA$ + ACP —(acyl carrier protein) malonyltransferase→ $^{-}OOC-CH_2-CO-SACP$ + CoA

(3) (a) $CH_3-CO-SACP$ + Enz—SH —β-ketoacyl-(acyl carrier protein) synthase→ $CH_3-CO-S-Enz$ + ACP

(b) $CH_3-CO-S-Enz$ + $^{-}OOC-CH_2-CO-SACP$ —β-ketoacyl-(acyl carrier protein) synthase→ $CH_3-CO-CH_2-CO-SACP$ + CO_2 + Enz—SH

(4) $CH_3-CO-CH_2-CO-SACP$ + NADPH + H^+ —β-ketoacyl-(acyl carrier protein) reductase→ $CH_3-CH(OH)-CH_2-CO-SACP$ + $NADP^+$

(5) $CH_3-CH(OH)-CH_2-CO-SACP$ —β-hydroxyacyl-(acyl carrier protein) dehydratase→ $CH_3-CH=CH-CO-SACP$ + H_2O

(6) $CH_3-CH=CH-CO-SACP$ + NADPH + H^+ —enoyl-(acyl carrier protein) reductase→ $CH_3-CH_2-CH_2-CO-SACP$ + $NADP^+$

FIGURE 9.7
Reactions catalyzed by fatty acid synthase.

malonyl CoA (Reaction 2) and allows Reactions 3b to 6 to generate hexanoyl-ACP. The process is repeated five more times at which point palmitoyl-ACP is acted on by a **thioesterase** with production of free palmitic acid (Figure 9.8). Note that at this stage the sulfhydryl groups of ACP and β-ketoacyl-ACP synthase are both free so that another cycle of fatty acid synthesis can begin.

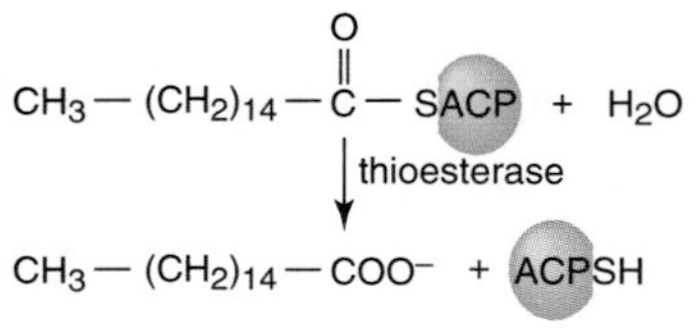

$$CH_3-(CH_2)_{14}-\overset{O}{\overset{\|}{C}}-SACP + H_2O \xrightarrow{\text{thioesterase}} CH_3-(CH_2)_{14}-COO^- + ACPSH$$

FIGURE 9.8
Release of palmitic acid from fatty acid synthase.

Mammalian Fatty Acid Synthase Is a Multifunctional Polypeptide

The reaction sequence given above is the basic pattern for fatty acid biosynthesis in living systems. The details of the reaction mechanisms are still unclear and may vary between species. The enzyme complex termed fatty acid synthase catalyzes all these reactions, but its structure and properties vary considerably. The individual enzymes in *Escherichia coli* are dissociable. By contrast, **mammalian synthase** is composed of two possibly identical subunits, each of which is a multienzyme polypeptide containing all of the necessary catalytic activities in a linear array. Even between mammalian species and tissues there are variations.

It appears that the growing fatty acid chain is continually bound to the multifunctional protein and is sequentially transferred between the 4′-phosphopantetheine group of ACP, a domain on the protein, and the sulfhydryl group of a cysteine residue on β-ketoacyl-ACP synthase during the condensation reaction (Reaction 3, Figure 9.7) (see also Figure 9.9). An intermediate acylation to a serine residue probably takes place when acyl CoA units add to enzyme-bound ACP in the transacylase reactions.

Regulation of palmitate biosynthesis probably occurs primarily by controlling the rate of synthesis and degradation of the enzyme. The agents and conditions that do this are given in Table 9.2. They are logical in terms of balancing an efficient utilization of the various biological energy substrates.

Stoichiometry of Fatty Acid Biosynthesis

If acetyl CoA is the primer for palmitate biosynthesis, the overall reaction is

$$CH_3-\overset{O}{\overset{\|}{C}}-SCoA + 7\,{}^-OOC-CH_2-\overset{O}{\overset{\|}{C}}-SCoA + 14\ NADPH + 14\ H^+ \longrightarrow CH_3-(CH_2)_{14}-COO^- + 7\ CO_2 + 14\ NADP^+ + 8\ CoASH + 6\ H_2O$$

To calculate the energy needed for the overall conversion of acetyl CoA to palmitate, we must add the ATP used in formation of malonyl CoA:

$$7\ CH_3-\overset{O}{\overset{\|}{C}}-SCoA + 7\ CO_2 + 7\ ATP \longrightarrow 7\ OOC-CH_2-\overset{O}{\overset{\|}{C}}-SCoA + 7\ ADP + 7\ P_i$$

Then the stoichiometry for conversion of acetyl CoA to palmitate is

$$8\ CH_3-\overset{O}{\overset{\|}{C}}-SCoA + 7\ ATP + 14\ NADPH + 14\ H^+ \longrightarrow CH_3-(CH_2)_{14}-\overset{O}{\overset{\|}{C}}-O + 8\ CoASH + 7\ ADP + 7\ P_i + 6\ H_2O + 14\ NADP^+$$

Acetyl CoA Must Be Transported from Mitochondria to the Cytosol for Palmitate Synthesis

Fatty acid synthase and acetyl-CoA carboxylase are found primarily in the cytosol where biosynthesis of palmitate occurs. Mammalian tissues must use special processes to ensure an adequate supply of acetyl CoA and NADPH for this synthesis in the cytosol. The major source of acetyl CoA is the pyruvate dehydro-

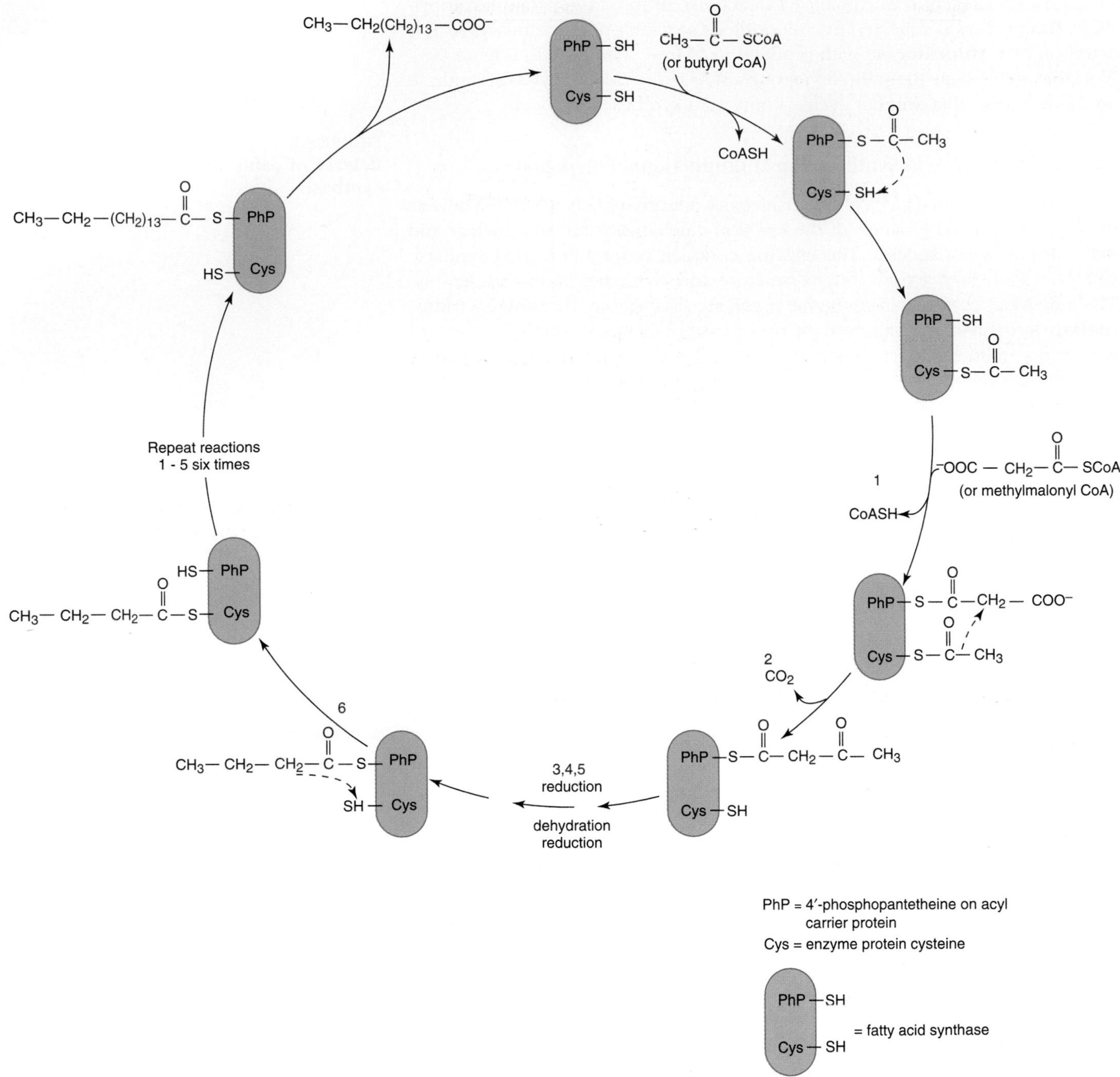

FIGURE 9.9
Proposed mechanism of elongation reactions taking place on mammalian fatty acid synthase.

genase reaction in the matrix of mitochondria. Since the mitochondrial inner membrane is not readily permeable to acetyl CoA, a process involving citrate moves the C2 unit to the cytosol for palmitate biosynthesis. This mechanism (Figure 9.10) takes advantage of the facts that citrate exchanges freely from mitochondria to cytosol (see p. 243) and that an enzyme exists in cytosol to convert citrate to acetyl CoA and oxaloacetate. When there is an excess of citrate from the TCA cycle, this intermediate will pass into the cytosol and supply acetyl CoA for fatty acid biosynthesis. The cleavage reaction, which is

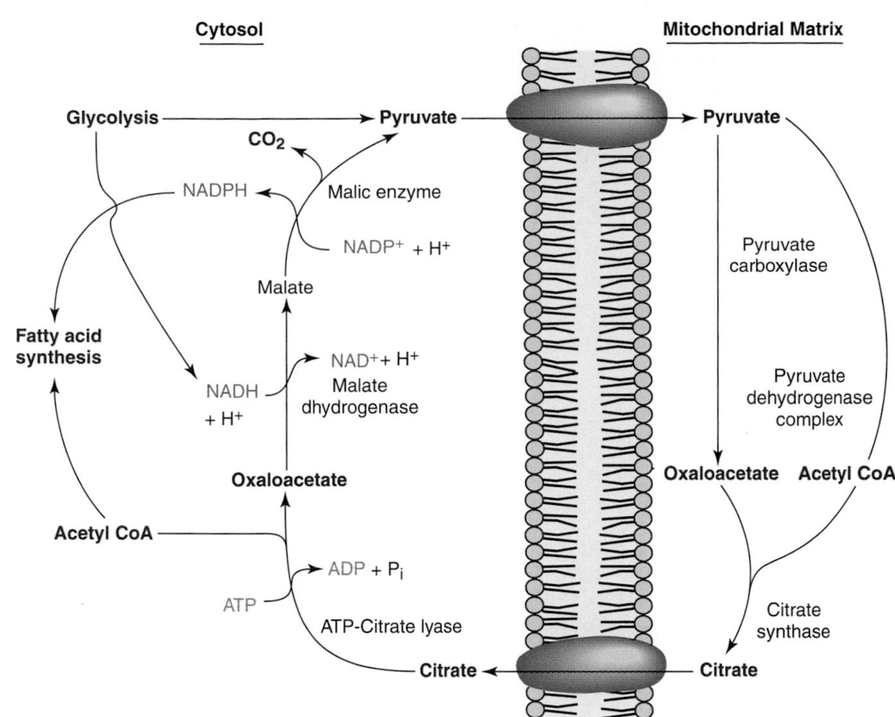

FIGURE 9.10
Mechanism for transfer of acetyl CoA from mitochondria to cytosol for fatty acid biosynthesis.

energy requiring, is catalyzed by **ATP-citrate lyase:**

$$\text{Citrate} + \text{ATP} + \text{CoA} \longrightarrow \text{acetyl CoA} + \text{ADP} + \text{P}_i + \text{oxaloacetate}$$

This mechanism has other advantages because CO_2 and NADPH for synthesis of palmitate can be produced from excess cytosolic oxaloacetate. As shown in Figure 9.10, NADH reduces oxaloacetate to malate via **malate dehydrogenase,** and malate is then decarboxylated by **NADP-linked malic enzyme** (malate : $NADP^+$oxidoreductase-decarboxylating) to produce NADPH, pyruvate, and CO_2. Thus NADPH is produced from NADH generated in glycolysis. The cycle is completed by return of pyruvate to the mitochondrion where it can be carboxylated to regenerate oxaloacetate, as described in the process of gluconeogenesis (see p. 299).

In summary, 1 NADH is converted to NADPH for each acetyl CoA transferred from mitochondria to cytosol, each transfer requiring 1 ATP. The transfer of the 8 acetyl CoA used for each molecule of palmitate supplies 8 NADPH. Since palmitate biosynthesis requires 14 NADPH mol^{-1}, the other 6 NADPH must be supplied by the cytosolic pentose phosphate pathway. This stoichiometry is, of course, hypothetical. The *in vivo* relationships are complicated because transport of citrate and other di- and tricarboxylic acids across the inner mitochondrial membrane occurs by one-for-one exchanges. The actual flow rates are probably controlled by a composite of the concentration gradients of several of these exchange systems.

Palmitate Is the Precursor of Other Fatty Acids

Humans can synthesize all of the fatty acids they need from palmitate except the essential, polyunsaturated fatty acids (see p. 365). These syntheses involve a variety of enzyme systems in a number of locations. Palmitate produced by fatty acid synthase is modified by three processes: elongation, desaturation, and hydroxylation.

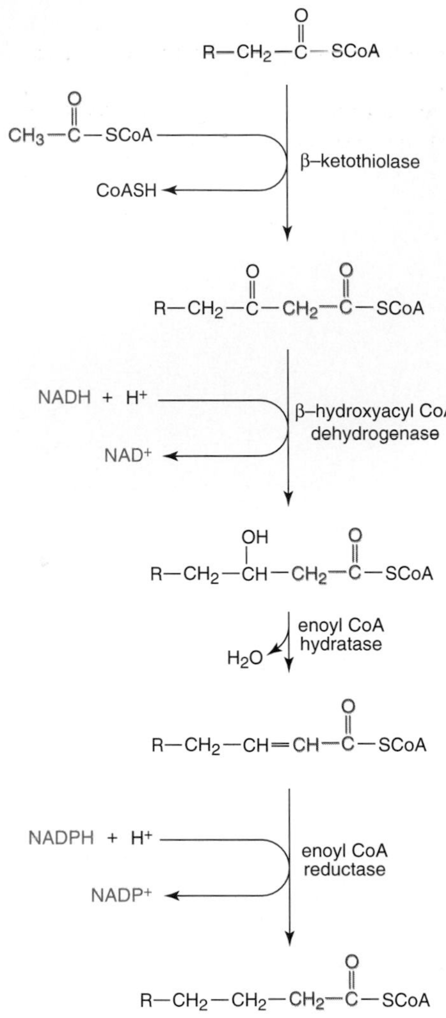

Elongation Reactions

In mammals **elongation of fatty acids** occurs in either the endoplasmic reticulum or mitochondria; the processes are slightly different in these two loci. In the endoplasmic reticulum the sequence of reactions is similar to that occurring in the cytosolic fatty acid synthase with malonyl CoA as the source of two-carbon units and NADPH providing the reducing power. The preferred substrate for elongation is palmitoyl CoA. In contrast to palmitate synthesis, intermediates in subsequent reactions are CoA esters rather than attached to a protein, suggesting that the process is carried out by separate enzymes rather than a complex like fatty acid synthase. In most tissues this elongation system in the endoplasmic reticulum converts palmitate to stearate almost exclusively. Brain, however, contains one or more additional elongation systems, which synthesize longer chain acids (up to C24) needed for brain lipids. These other systems also use malonyl CoA as substrate.

The elongation system in mitochondria differs in that acetyl CoA is the source of the added two-carbon units and both NADH and NADPH serve as reducing agents (Figure 9.11). This system operates by reversal of the pathway of fatty acid β-oxidation (see Section 9.6) with the exception that NADPH-linked enoyl-CoA reductase (last step of elongation) replaces FAD-linked acyl-CoA dehydrogenase (first step in β-oxidation). The process has little activity with acyl CoA substrates of C16 atoms or longer, suggesting that it serves primarily in elongation of shorter chain species.

$R{-}CH_2{-}C(=O){-}SCoA$

$CH_3{-}C(=O){-}SCoA$ → CoASH (β-ketothiolase)

$R{-}CH_2{-}C(=O){-}CH_2{-}C(=O){-}SCoA$

$NADH + H^+$ → NAD^+ (β-hydroxyacyl CoA dehydrogenase)

$R{-}CH_2{-}CH(OH){-}CH_2{-}C(=O){-}SCoA$

H_2O (enoyl CoA hydratase)

$R{-}CH_2{-}CH{=}CH{-}C(=O){-}SCoA$

$NADPH + H^+$ → $NADP^+$ (enoyl CoA reductase)

$R{-}CH_2{-}CH_2{-}CH_2{-}C(=O){-}SCoA$

FIGURE 9.11
Mitochondrial elongation of fatty acids.

Formation of Monoenoic Acids by Stearoyl CoA Desaturase

In higher animals **desaturation of fatty acids** occurs in the endoplasmic reticulum, and the oxidizing system used to introduce cis double bonds is significantly different from the main fatty acid oxidation process in mitochondria. The systems in endoplasmic reticulum have sometimes been termed **"mixed function oxidases"** because the enzymes simultaneously oxidize two substrates. In fatty acid desaturation one of these substrates is NADPH and the other is the fatty acid. Electrons from NADPH are transferred through a specific flavoprotein reductase and a cytochrome to "active" oxygen so that it will then oxidize the fatty acid. Although the complete mechanism has not been determined, this latter step may involve a hydroxylation. The three components of the system are the **desaturase enzyme, cytochrome b_5,** and **NADPH-cytochrome b_5 reductase.** The overall reaction is

$$R{-}CH_2{-}CH_2{-}(CH_2)_7{-}COOH + NADPH + H^+ + O_2 \longrightarrow R{-}CH{=}CH{-}(CH_2)_7{-}COOH + NADP^+ + 2\,H_2O$$

The enzyme specificity is such that the R group must contain at least six carbon atoms.

The regulatory mechanisms that govern the conversion of palmitate to unsaturated fatty acids are largely unexplored. An important consideration is the control of the proportions of unsaturated fatty acids for proper maintenance of the physical state of stored triacylglycerols and membrane phospholipids. A committed step in the formation of unsaturated fatty acids from palmitate or stearate is introduction of the first double bond between C-9 and C-10 atoms by **stearoyl CoA desaturase** to produce palmitoleic or oleic acid, respectively. The activity of this enzyme and its synthesis are controlled by both dietary and hormonal mechanisms. Increasing the amounts of polyunsaturated fatty acids in the diet of experimental animals decreases the activity of stearoyl CoA desaturase in liver, and insulin, triiodothyronine, and hydrocortisone cause its induction.

Formation and Modification of Polyunsaturated Fatty Acids

A variety of **polyunsaturated fatty acids** are synthesized by humans through a combination of elongation and desaturation reactions. Once the initial double

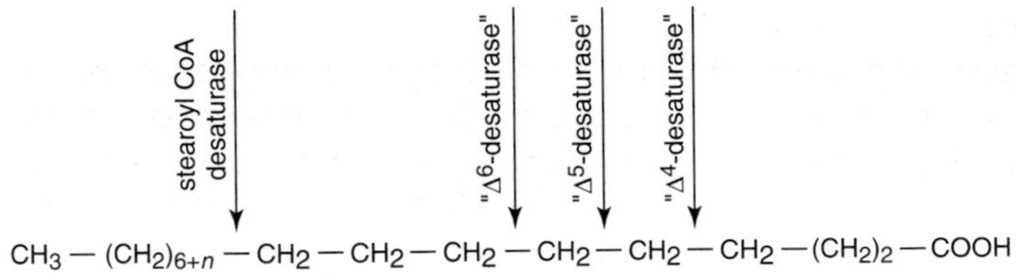

FIGURE 9.12
Positions in the fatty acid chain where desaturation can occur in the human.
There must always be at least six single bonds in the chain toward the methyl end of the molecule just beyond the bond being desaturated.

bond has been placed between carbons 9 and 10 by stearoyl CoA desaturase, additional double bonds can be introduced just beyond C-4, C-5, or C-6 atoms. Desaturation at C-8 probably occurs also in some tissues. The positions of these desaturations are shown in Figure 9.12. The relative specificities of the various enzymes are still to be determined completely, but it seems likely that elongation and desaturation can occur in either order. Conversion of linolenic acid to all *cis*-4, 7, 10, 13, 16, 19-docosahexaenoic acid in brain is a specific example of such a sequence.

$$CH_3-(CH_2-CH{=}CH)_3-CH_2-CH_2-CH_2-CH_2-CH_2-CH_2-CH_2-COOH$$
Linolenic acid

"Δ6-desaturase" ↓

$$CH_3-(CH_2-CH{=}CH)_3-CH_2-CH{=}CH-CH_2-CH_2-CH_2-CH_2-COOH$$

elongation ↓

$$CH_3-(CH_2-CH{=}CH)_3-CH_2-CH{=}CH-CH_2-CH_2-CH_2-CH_2-CH_2-CH_2-COOH$$

"Δ5-desaturase" ↓

$$CH_3-(CH_2-CH{=}CH)_3-CH_2-CH{=}CH-CH_2-CH{=}CH-CH_2-CH_2-CH_2-COOH$$

elongation ↓

$$CH_3-(CH_2-CH{=}CH)_3-CH_2-CH{=}CH-CH_2-CH{=}CH-CH_2-CH_2-CH_2-CH_2-CH_2-COOH$$

"Δ4-desaturase" ↓

$$CH_3-(CH_2-CH{=}CH)_3-CH_2-CH{=}CH-CH_2-CH{=}CH-CH_2-CH{=}CH-CH_2-CH_2-COOH$$

All-*cis*-4,7,10,13,16,19-docosahexaenoic acid

Polyunsaturated fatty acids, particularly arachidonic acid, are precursors of the highly active prostaglandins and thromboxanes. Different classes of prostaglandins are formed depending on the precursor fatty acid and the sequence of oxidations that convert the acids to active compounds. A detailed discussion of these substances and their formation is found in Chapter 10. Polyunsaturated fatty acids in living systems have a significant potential for auto-oxidation, a process that may have important physiological and/or pathological consequences. Auto-oxidation reactions cause rancidity in fats and curing of linseed oil in paints.

Formation of Hydroxy Fatty Acids in Nerve Tissue

There are apparently two different processes that produce **α-hydroxy fatty acids** in higher animals. One occurs in the mitochondria of many tissues and acts on relatively short-chain fatty acids (see Section 9.6). The other has been demonstrated only in tissues of the nervous system where it produces long-chain fatty acids with a hydroxyl group on C-2. These are needed for the formation of some myelin lipids. The specific case of α-hydroxylation of lignoceric acid to cerebronic acid has been studied. These enzymes preferentially use C22 and C24 fatty acids and show characteristics of the "mixed function oxidase" systems, requiring molecular oxygen and NADH or NADPH. This synthesis may be closely coordinated with biosynthesis of sphingolipids that contain hydroxylated fatty acids.

Fatty Acid Synthase Can Produce Fatty Acids Other than Palmitate

The schemes outlined, which synthesize and modify palmitate, account for the great bulk of fatty acid biosynthesis in the human body, particularly that involved in energy storage. There are, however, many special instances where smaller amounts of different fatty acids are needed for specific structural or functional purposes. These acids are produced by modification of the process carried out by fatty acid synthase. Two examples are production of fatty acids shorter than palmitate in mammary glands and synthesis of branched-chain fatty acids in certain secretory glands.

Milk produced by many animals contains varying amounts of fatty acids with shorter chain lengths than palmitate. The amounts produced by **mammary gland** apparently vary with species and especially with the physiological state of the animal. This is probably true of humans, although most investigations have been carried out with rats, rabbits, and various ruminants. The same fatty acid synthase that produces palmitate synthesizes shorter chain acids when the linkage of the growing chain with acyl carrier protein is split before the full C16 chain is completed. This hydrolysis is caused by soluble **thioesterases** whose activity is under hormonal control.

There are relatively few branched-chain fatty acids in higher animals. Until recently, their metabolism has been studied mostly in primitive species such as mycobacteria, where they are present in greater variety and amount. Simple branched-chain fatty acids are synthesized by tissues of higher animals for specific purposes, such as the production of waxes in sebaceous glands and avian preen glands and the elaboration of structures in echo-locating systems of porpoises.

The majority of branched-chain fatty acids in higher animals are synthesized by fatty acid synthase and are methylated derivatives of saturated, straight-chain acids. When **methylmalonyl CoA** is used as a substrate instead of malonyl CoA, a methyl side chain is inserted in the fatty acid, and the reaction is as follows:

$$CH_3\text{—}(CH_2)_n\text{—}\overset{\overset{\displaystyle O}{\|}}{C}\text{—SACP} + HOOC\text{—}\overset{\overset{\displaystyle CH_3}{|}}{CH}\text{—}\overset{\overset{\displaystyle O}{\|}}{C}\text{—SCoA} \longrightarrow$$

$$CH_3\text{—}(CH_2)_n\text{—}\overset{\overset{\displaystyle O}{\|}}{C}\text{—}\overset{\overset{\displaystyle CH_3}{|}}{CH}\text{—}\overset{\overset{\displaystyle O}{\|}}{C}\text{—SACP} + CO_2 + CoA$$

Regular reduction steps then follow. Apparently these reactions occur in many tissues normally at a rate several orders of magnitude lower than the utilization of malonyl CoA to produce palmitate. The proportion of branched-chain fatty acids synthesized is largely governed by the relative availability of the two precursors. An increase in branching can occur by decreasing the ratio of malonyl CoA to methylmalonyl CoA. A malonyl-CoA decarboxylase capable of causing this decrease occurs in many tissues. It has also been suggested that increased levels of methylmalonyl CoA in pathological situations, such as vitamin B_{12} deficiency, can lead to excessive production of branched-chain fatty acids.

Fatty Acyl CoAs May Be Reduced to Fatty Alcohols

As discussed in Chapter 10, many phospholipids contain fatty acid chains in ether linkage rather than ester linkage. The biosynthetic precursors of these ether-linked chains are **fatty alcohols** (Figure 9.13) rather than fatty acids. These alcohols are formed in higher animals by a two-step, NADPH-linked reduction of fatty acyl CoAs in the endoplasmic reticulum. In organs that produce relatively large amounts of ether-containing lipids, the concurrent production of fatty acids and fatty alcohols is probably closely coordinated.

$CH_3—(CH_2)_n—CH_2OH$

FIGURE 9.13
Fatty alcohol.

9.4 ■ STORAGE OF FATTY ACIDS AS TRIACYLGLYCEROLS

Most tissues in the body can convert fatty acids to triacylglycerols (Figure 9.14) by a common sequence of reactions, but liver and adipose tissue carry out this process to the greatest extent. Adipose tissue is a specialized connective tissue designed for synthesis, storage, and hydrolysis of triacylglycerols. This is the main system for long-term energy storage in humans. We are concerned here with white adipose tissue as opposed to brown adipose tissue, which occurs in much lesser amounts and has other specialized functions. Triacylglycerols are stored as liquid droplets in the cytoplasm, but this is not "dead storage" since they turn over with an average half-life of only a few days. Thus, in a homeostatic situation, there is continuous synthesis and breakdown of triacylglycerols in adipose tissue. Some storage also occurs in skeletal and cardiac muscle, but only for local consumption.

Triacylglycerol synthesis in liver is used primarily for production of blood lipoproteins, although the products can serve as energy sources for other liver

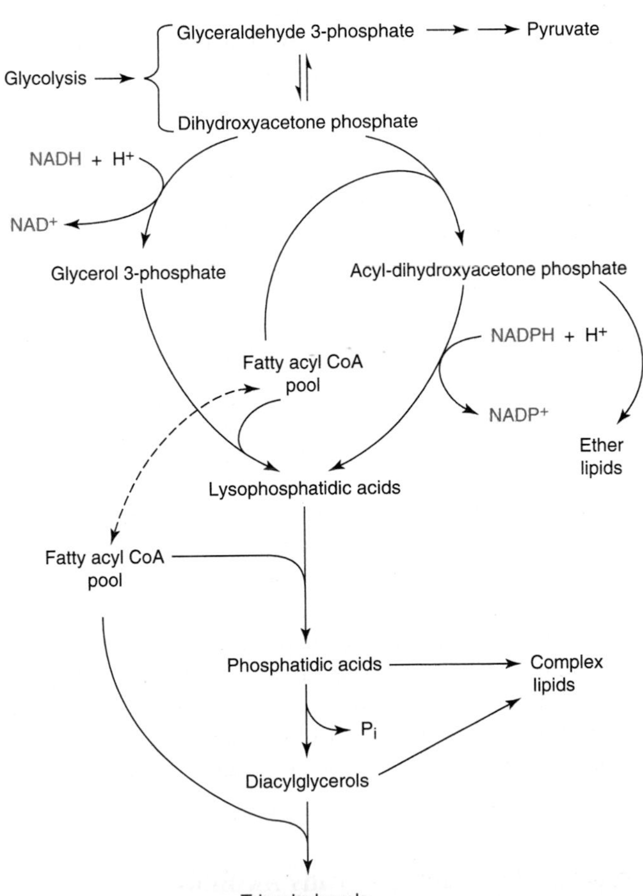

FIGURE 9.14
Alternative pathways for biosynthesis of triacylglycerols from dihydroxyacetone phosphate.

functions. Required fatty acids may come from the diet, from adipose tissue via blood transport, or from *de novo* biosynthesis. Acetyl CoA for biosynthesis is derived principally from glucose catabolism.

Triacylglycerols Are Synthesized from Fatty Acyl CoAs and Glycerol 3-Phosphate in Most Tissues

Triacylglycerols are synthesized in most tissues from activated fatty acids and a phosphorylated three-carbon product of glucose catabolism (see Figure 9.14), which can be either **glycerol 3-phosphate** or **dihydroxyacetone phosphate.** Glycerol 3-phosphate is formed either by reduction of dihydroxyacetone phosphate produced in glycolysis or by phosphorylation of glycerol. White adipose tissue contains little or no glycerol kinase, so it derives glycerol phosphate from glycolytic intermediates. Fatty acids are activated by conversion to their CoA esters in the following reaction:

$$R-\overset{O}{\overset{\|}{C}}-O^- + ATP + CoASH \xrightarrow[\text{synthetase}]{\text{acyl-CoA}} R-\overset{O}{\overset{\|}{C}}-SCoA + AMP + PP_i + H_2O$$

This two-step reaction has an acyl adenylate as intermediate and is driven by hydrolysis of pyrophosphate to P_i.

Synthesis of triacylglycerols from phosphorylated three-carbon fragments involves formation of **phosphatidic acid,** which is a key intermediate in synthesis of other lipids as well (see Chapter 10). This may be formed by two sequential acylations of glycerol 3-phosphate, as shown in Figure 9.15. Alternatively, dihydroxyacetone phosphate may be acylated directly at C-1 followed by reduction at C-2. The resultant lysophosphatidic acid can then be further esterified, as illustrated in Figure 9.16. If phosphatidic acid from either of these routes is used for synthesis of triacylglycerol, the phosphate group is next hydrolyzed by **phosphatidate phosphatase** to yield diacylglycerol, which is then acylated to triacylglycerol (Figure 9.17).

There is at least one tissue, **intestinal mucosa,** in which the synthesis of triacylglycerols does not require formation of phosphatidic acid as described above. A major product of intestinal digestion of lipids is 2-monoacylglycerols, which are absorbed as such into mucosa cells. An enzyme in these cells catalyzes acylation of these monoacylglycerols with acyl CoA to form 1,2-diacylglycerols, which then can be further acylated as shown above.

The specificity of the acylation reactions in all these steps is still quite controversial. Analysis of **fatty acid patterns** in triacylglycerols from various human tissues shows that the distribution of different acids on the three positions of glycerol is neither random nor absolutely specific. The patterns in different tissues show some characteristic tendencies. Palmitic acid tends to be concentrated in position 1 and oleic acid in positions 2 and 3 of human adipose tissue triacylglycerols. Two main factors that determine localization of a particular fatty acid to a given position on glycerol are the specificity of acyltransferase involved and relative availability of different fatty acids in the fatty acyl CoA pool. Other factors are probably involved but their relative importance has not been determined.

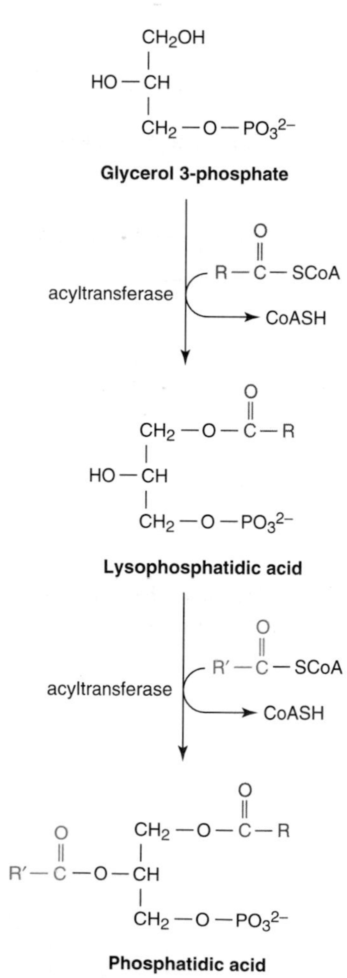

Glycerol 3-phosphate: $CH_2OH-CH(OH)-CH_2-O-PO_3^{2-}$

acyltransferase: $R-\overset{O}{\overset{\|}{C}}-SCoA \rightarrow CoASH$

Lysophosphatidic acid: $CH_2(-O-\overset{O}{\overset{\|}{C}}-R)-CH(OH)-CH_2-O-PO_3^{2-}$

acyltransferase: $R'-\overset{O}{\overset{\|}{C}}-SCoA \rightarrow CoASH$

Phosphatidic acid: $CH_2(-O-\overset{O}{\overset{\|}{C}}-R)-CH(-O-\overset{O}{\overset{\|}{C}}-R')-CH_2-O-PO_3^{2-}$

FIGURE 9.15
Synthesis of phosphatidic acid from glycerol 3-phosphate.

Mobilization of Triacylglycerols Requires Hydrolysis

The first step in recovering stored fatty acids for energy production is hydrolysis of triacylglycerols. A variety of lipases catalyze this reaction, the sequence of hydrolysis from the three positions on glycerol depending on the specificities of the particular lipases involved.

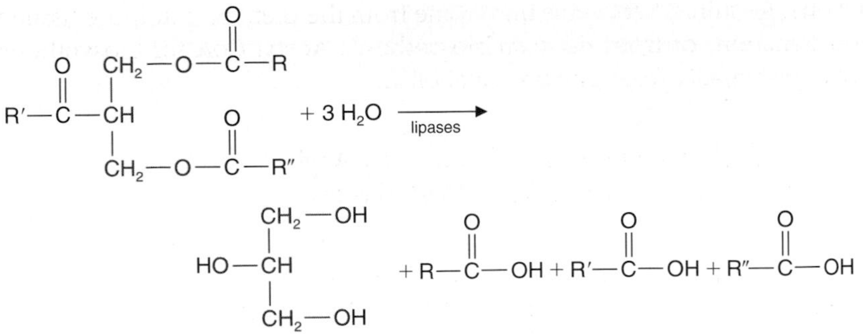

$$\text{Triacylglycerol} + 3\,H_2O \xrightarrow{\text{lipases}} \text{Glycerol } (CH_2OH-CHOH-CH_2OH) + R-COOH + R'-COOH + R''-COOH$$

Lipases in adipose tissue are, of course, key enzymes for release of the major energy stores. The lipase that removes the first fatty acid is a controlled enzyme, which is sensitive to a variety of circulating hormones. This control of triacylglycerol hydrolysis must be balanced with the process of triacylglycerol synthesis to assure adequate energy stores and avoid obesity (see Clin. Corr. 9.1 and 9.2). Fatty acids and glycerol produced by adipose tissue lipases are released to circulating blood, where fatty acids are bound by serum albumin and transported to tissues for use. Glycerol returns to liver, where it is converted to dihydroxyacetone phosphate and enters glycolytic or gluconeogenic pathways.

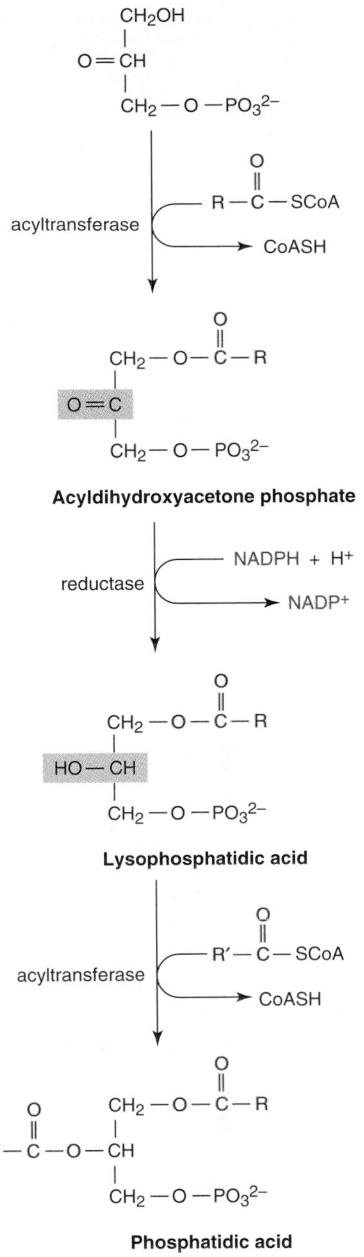

Dihydroxyacetone phosphate (CH_2OH, $O{=}CH$, $CH_2-O-PO_3^{2-}$)

acyltransferase ($R-CO-SCoA$ → CoASH)

Acyldihydroxyacetone phosphate

reductase (NADPH + H^+ → $NADP^+$)

Lysophosphatidic acid

acyltransferase ($R'-CO-SCoA$ → CoASH)

Phosphatidic acid

FIGURE 9.16
Synthesis of phosphatidic acid from dihydroxyacetone phosphate.

Phosphatidic acid

phosphatidate phosphatase

Diacylglycerol + P_i

acyltransferase ($R''-CO-SCoA$ → CoASH)

Triacylglycerol

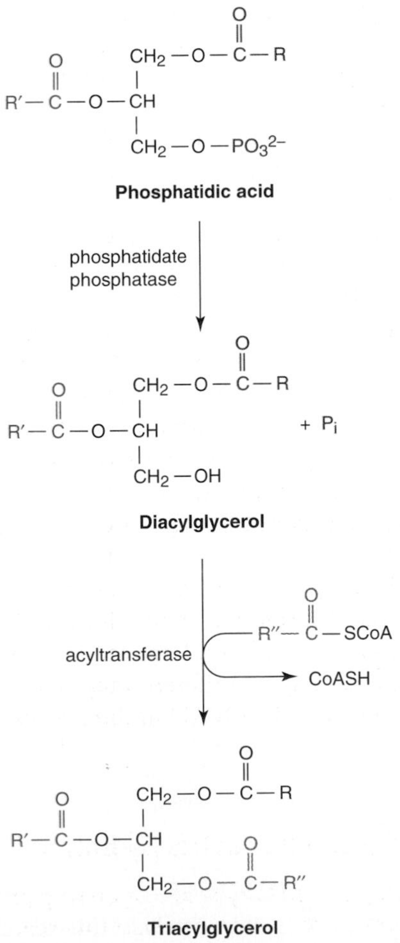

FIGURE 9.17
Synthesis of triacylglycerol from phosphatidic acid.

CLINICAL CORRELATION 9.1

Obesity

The terms obesity and overweight refer to excess in body weight relative to height. Their definitions are arbitrary and are based on actuarial estimates of ideal body weight (IBW), that is, body weight associated with the lowest morbidity and mortality. Relative weight is body weight relative to IBW: overweight is defined as relative weight up to 20% above normal and obesity is relative weight over 20% above IBW. The body mass index (BMI) is well correlated with measures of body fat and is defined as weight (kg) divided by height^2 (m^2). Overweight is defined as a BMI of 25–30 kg per m^2 and obesity as a BMI > 30 kg per m^2. Skinfold thickness also is a measure of body fat stores.

The cause of most cases of obesity is not known. Endocrine diseases such as hypothyroidism or Cushing's disease (overproduction of corticosteroids) are rare causes. Genetic factors interact with environmental factors: 80% of children of two obese parents will be obese, while only 14% of children of normal weight parents are obese. The major mechanism of weight gain is consumption of calories in excess of daily energy requirements, but the normal processes controlling food intake are not very well understood. Rarely, tumors of the hypothalamus result in pathological overeating (hyperphagia). However, a specific defect in most cases of human obesity has not been demonstrated.

The treatment of obesity revolves about dietary restriction, increased physical activity, and behavior modification. The real problem is to modify the patients' eating patterns long term, and even in those who lose weight, regain of the weight is very common. Currently, no pharmacological agents are effective in promoting long-term weight control. Surgery to limit the size of the gastric reservoir can be considered for patients over 100% above IBW. Medical complications of obesity include a two- to threefold increase in hypertension, gallstones, and diabetes, and fivefold increase in risk of endometrial carcinoma. Obese patients have decreased plasma antithrombin III levels, which predisposes them to venous thrombosis (see Clin. Corr. 8.8).

Bray, G. A. Complications of obesity. *Ann. Intern. Med.* 103:1052, 1985; and Bray, G. A. The syndromes of obesity: an endocrine approach. In: L. J. DeGroot (Ed.), *Endocrinology*, Vol. 3, 3rd ed. Philadelphia: Saunders, 1995, p. 2624.

9.5 METHODS OF INTERORGAN TRANSPORT OF FATTY ACIDS AND THEIR PRIMARY PRODUCTS

Lipid-Based Energy Is Transported in Blood in Different Forms

The energy available in fatty acids needs to be distributed throughout the body from the site of fatty acid absorption, biosynthesis, or storage to functioning tissues that consume them. This transport is closely integrated with that of other lipids, especially cholesterol, and is intimately involved in pathological processes leading to atherosclerosis. Various mechanisms are being intensively studied, but many important questions are still unanswered.

In humans, three types of substances are used as vehicles to transport lipid-based energy: (1) chylomicrons and other plasma lipoproteins in which

CLINICAL CORRELATION 9.2

Leptin and Obesity

In 1994 the *OB* gene of mice, its protein product, and their human homologues were identified. The human gene encodes a polypeptide of 166 amino acids that is expressed in adipose tissue in proportion to the severity of the obesity. The secreted protein, called leptin, contains 146 amino acids, can be measured by immunoassay, and is highly homologous to the murine protein.

Mice of the ob/ob strain that inherit a nonsense mutation in the leptin gene, leading to a truncated protein of 104 amino acids that is not secreted, are obese, diabetic, and exhibit reduced activity, metabolism, and body temperature. Injection of recombinant leptin into mice homozygous for this mutation lowered their food intake, body weight, percentage of body fat, and serum glucose and insulin concentrations, and increased their metabolic rate, body temperature, and activity level.

There is no difference in the structure of leptin between lean and obese human subjects. This suggests that the problem in obese individuals might be decreased sensitivity to leptin. Interestingly, a leptin receptor present in the hypothalamus has been shown to be defective in the db/db mouse and the fa/fa Zucker rat. In both cases the phenotype is similar to that of the ob/ob mouse. Whether an analogous situation applies in human obesity remains to be established.

Considine, R. V., Sinha, M. K., Heiman, M. L., et al. Serum immunoreactive-leptin concentrations in normal-weight and obese humans. *N. Engl. J. Med.* 334:292, 1996; and Lee, G. H., Proenca, R., Montez, J. M., et al. Abnormal splicing of the leptin receptor in diabetic mice. *Nature* 379:632, 1996.

triacylglycerols are carried in protein-coated lipid droplets, both of which contain other lipids; (2) fatty acids bound to serum albumin; and (3) so-called ketone bodies, acetoacetate and β-hydroxybutyrate. These three vehicles are used in varying proportions to carry energy in the bloodstream via three routes. One is transport of dietary fatty acids as chylomicrons throughout the body from the intestine after absorption. Another is transport of lipid-based energy processed by or synthesized in liver and distributed either to adipose tissue for storage or to other tissues for use; this includes "ketone bodies" and plasma lipoproteins other than chylomicrons. Finally, there is transport of energy released from storage in adipose tissue to the rest of the body in the form of fatty acids that are bound to serum albumin.

The proportion of energy being transported in any one of the modes outlined above varies considerably with metabolic and physiological state. At any time, the largest amount of lipid in blood is in the form of triacylglycerols in various lipoproteins. Fatty acids bound to albumin, however, are utilized and replaced very rapidly so total energy transport for a given period by this mode may be very significant.

Plasma Lipoproteins Carry Triacylglycerols and Other Lipids

Plasma lipoproteins are synthesized in both intestine and liver and are a heterogeneous group of lipid–protein complexes composed of various types of lipids and apoproteins (see p. 56 for a detailed discussion of structure). The two most important vehicles for delivery of lipid-based energy are **chylomicrons** and **very low density lipoprotein (VLDL),** because they contain relatively large amounts of triacylglycerols. Chylomicrons are formed in the intestine and function in absorption and transport of dietary triacylglycerol, cholesterol, and fat-soluble vitamins. The exact precursor–product relationships between the other types of plasma lipoproteins have yet to be completely defined, as do the roles of various protein components. Liver synthesizes VLDL and fatty acids from triacylglycerols in VLDL are taken up by adipose tissue and other tissues. In the process VLDLs are converted to **low density lipoproteins (LDLs).** The role of **high density lipoprotein (HDL)** in transport of lipid-based energy is yet to be clarified. All of these lipoproteins are integrally involved in transport of other lipids, especially cholesterol. Lipid components can interchange to some extent between different classes of lipoprotein, and some apoproteins probably have functional roles in modifying enzyme activity during exchange of lipids between plasma lipoproteins and tissues. Other apoproteins serve as specific recognition sites for cell surface receptors. Such interaction constitutes the first step in receptor-mediated endocytosis of certain lipoproteins. Studies of rare genetic abnormalities have been helpful in explaining the roles of some of these apoproteins (see Clin. Corr. 9.3).

Fatty Acids Are Bound to Serum Albumin

Serum albumin acts as a carrier for a number of substances in blood, some of the most important being fatty acids. These acids are water insoluble in themselves, but when they are released into plasma during triacylglycerol hydrolysis they are quickly bound to albumin. This protein has a number of binding sites for fatty acid, some of them having very high affinity. At any one time the number of sites on albumin actually occupied with fatty acids is far from maximal, but the turnover of these fatty acids is high, so binding by this mechanism constitutes a major route of energy transfer.

Ketone Bodies Are a Lipid-Based Energy Supply

The third mode of transport of lipid-based energy-yielding molecules is in the form of small water-soluble molecules, **acetoacetate** and ***β*-hydroxybutyrate** (Figure 9.18), produced primarily by liver during oxidation of fatty acids. The reactions involved in their formation and utilization will be discussed later.

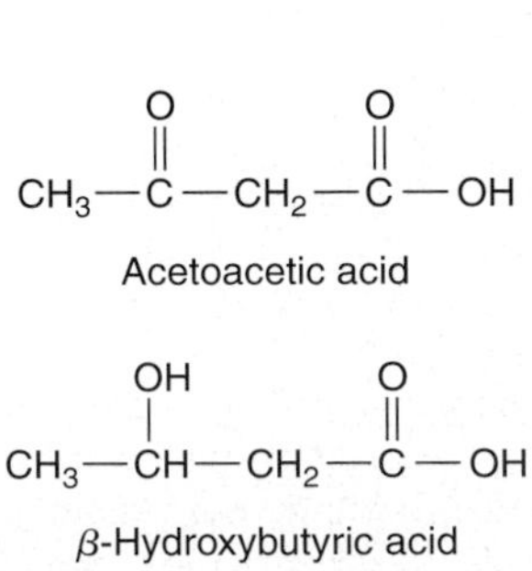

$CH_3-C(=O)-CH_2-C(=O)-OH$

Acetoacetic acid

$CH_3-CH(OH)-CH_2-C(=O)-OH$

β-Hydroxybutyric acid

FIGURE 9.18
Structures of ketone bodies.

CLINICAL CORRELATION 9.3

Genetic Abnormalities in Lipid-Energy Transport

Diseases that affect the transport of lipid-based energy frequently result in abnormally high plasma triacylglycerols, cholesterol, or both. They are classified as hyperlipidemias. Some of them are genetically transmitted, and presumably they result from the alteration or lack of one or more proteins involved in the production or processing of plasma lipids. The nature and function of all of these proteins are yet to be determined, so the elucidation of exact causes of the pathology in most of these diseases is still in the early stages. However, in several cases a specific protein abnormality has been associated with altered lipid transport in the patient's plasma.

In the extremely rare disease, analbuminemia, there is an almost complete lack of serum albumin. In a rat strain with analbuminemia, a 7 base-pair deletion in an intron of the albumin gene results in the inability to process the nuclear mRNA for albumin. Despite the many functions of this protein, the symptoms of the disease are surprisingly mild. Lack of serum albumin effectively eliminates the transport of fatty acids unless they are esterified in acylglycerols or complex lipids. However, since patients with analbuminemia do have elevated plasma triacylglycerol levels, presumably the deficiency in lipid-based energy transport caused by the absence of albumin to carry fatty acids is filled by increased use of plasma lipoproteins to carry triacylglycerols.

A more serious genetic defect is the absence of lipoprotein lipase. The major problem here is the inability to process chylomicrons after a fatty meal. Pathological fat deposits occur in the skin (eruptive xanthomas) and the patients typically suffer from pancreatitis. If patients are put on a low-fat diet they respond reasonably well.

Another rare but more severe disease, abetalipoproteinemia, is caused by defective synthesis of apoprotein B, an essential component in the formation of chylomicrons and VLDL. Under these circumstances the major pathway for transporting lipid-based energy from the diet to the body is unavailable. Chylomicrons, VLDL, and LDL are absent from the plasma and fat absorption is deficient or nonexistent. There are other serious symptoms, including neuropathy and red cell deformities, whose etiology is less clear.

Havel, R. J., and Kane, J. P. Structure and metabolism of plasma lipoproteins. In: C. R. Scriver, A. L. Beaudet, W. S. Sly, and D. Valle (Eds.), *The Metabolic and Molecular Bases of Inherited Disease,* Vol. II, 7th ed. New York: McGraw-Hill, 1995, p. 1841; and Brunzell, J. D. Familial lipoprotein lipase deficiency and other causes of the chylomicronemia syndrome. In: C. R. Scriver, A. L. Beaudet, W. S. Sly, and D. Valle (Eds.), *The Metabolic and Molecular Bases of Inherited Disease,* Vol. II, 7th ed. New York: McGraw-Hill, 1995, p. 1913.

Under certain conditions, these substances can reach excessive concentrations in blood, leading to ketosis and acidosis. Spontaneous decarboxylation of acetoacetate to **acetone** also occurs, which is detectable as the smell of acetone in the breath when acetoacetate concentrations are high. This led early investigators to call the group of soluble products **"ketone bodies."** In fact, β-hydroxybutyrate and acetoacetate are continually produced by liver and, to a lesser extent, by kidney. Skeletal and cardiac muscle utilize them to produce ATP. Nervous tissue, which normally obtains almost all of its energy from glucose, is unable to take up and use fatty acids bound to albumin for energy production. However, it can use ketone bodies when glucose supplies are insufficient.

Lipases Must Hydrolyze Blood Triacylglycerols for Their Fatty Acids to Become Available to Tissues

Fatty acids bound to albumin and ketone bodies are readily taken up by various tissues for oxidation and production of ATP. The energy in fatty acids stored or circulated as triacylglycerols, however, is not directly available, but rather triacylglycerols must be enzymatically hydrolyzed to release the fatty acids and glycerol. Two types of lipases are involved: (1) **lipoprotein lipase,** which hydrolyzes triacylglycerols in plasma lipoproteins; and (2) **"hormone-sensitive triacylglycerol lipase,"** which initiates hydrolysis of triacylglycerols in adipose tissue and release of fatty acids and glycerol into plasma.

Lipoprotein lipase is located on the surface of endothelial cells of capillaries and possibly of adjoining tissue cells. It hydrolyzes fatty acids from the 1 and/or 3 position of tri- and diacylglycerols present in VLDL or chylomicrons. One of the lipoprotein apoproteins (ApoC-II) must be present to activate the process. Fatty acids released are either bound to serum albumin or taken up by the tissue. Monoacylglycerol products may either pass into the cells or be further hydrolyzed by serum **monoacylglycerol hydrolase.**

A completely distinct type of lipase controls mobilization of fatty acids from triacylglycerols stored in adipose tissue. One of them is hormonally controlled

TABLE 9.3 Regulation of Triacylglycerol Metabolism

Enzyme	*Regulatory Agent*	*Effect*
	Triacylglycerol Mobilization	
"Hormone-sensitive" lipase	"Lipolytic hormones," e.g., epinephrine, glucagon, and ACTH	Stimulation by cAMP-mediated phosphorylation of relatively inactive enzyme
	Insulin	Inhibition
	Prostaglandins	Inhibition
Lipoprotein lipase	Apolipoprotein C-II	Activation
	Insulin	Activation
	Triacylglycerol Biosynthesis	
Phosphatidate phosphatase	Steroid hormones	Stimulation by increased enzyme synthesis

by a cAMP-mediated mechanism. There are a number of lipase activities in the tissue, but the enzyme attacking triacylglycerols initiates the process. Two other lipases then rapidly complete the hydrolysis of mono- and diacylglycerols, releasing fatty acids to plasma where they are bound to serum albumin. Triacylglycerol metabolism is tightly controlled by both hormones and required cofactors. Some of the key regulatory factors are presented in Table 9.3.

9.6 ■ UTILIZATION OF FATTY ACIDS FOR ENERGY PRODUCTION

Fatty acids that arrive at the surface of cells are taken up and used for energy production primarily in mitochondria in a process intimately integrated with energy generation from other sources. Energy-rich intermediates produced from fatty acids are the same as those obtained from sugars, that is, NADH and $FADH_2$. The final stages of the oxidation process are exactly the same as for carbohydrates, that is, the metabolism of acetyl CoA by the TCA cycle and production of ATP in the mitochondrial electron transport system.

The degree of utilization of fatty acids for energy production varies considerably from tissue to tissue and depends to a significant extent on the metabolic status of the body, whether it is fed or fasted, exercising or at rest, and so on. For instance, nervous tissue oxidizes fatty acids to a minimal degree, if at all, but cardiac and skeletal muscle depend heavily on fatty acids as a major energy source. During prolonged fasting most tissues can use fatty acids or ketone bodies for their energy requirements.

β-Oxidation of Straight-Chain Fatty Acids Is the Major Energy-Producing Process

For the most part, fatty acids are oxidized by a mechanism that is similar to, but not identical with, a reversal of the process of palmitate synthesis. That is, two-carbon fragments are removed sequentially from the carboxyl end of the acid after steps of **dehydrogenation, hydration,** and **oxidation** to form a β-keto acid, which is split by **thiolysis.** These processes take place while the acid is activated in a thioester linkage to the 4′-phosphopantetheine of CoA.

Fatty Acids Are Activated by Conversion to Fatty Acyl CoA

The first step in oxidation of a fatty acid is its activation to a fatty acyl CoA. This is the same reaction described for synthesis of triacylglycerols in Section 9.4 and occurs in the endoplasmic reticulum or the outer mitochondrial membrane.

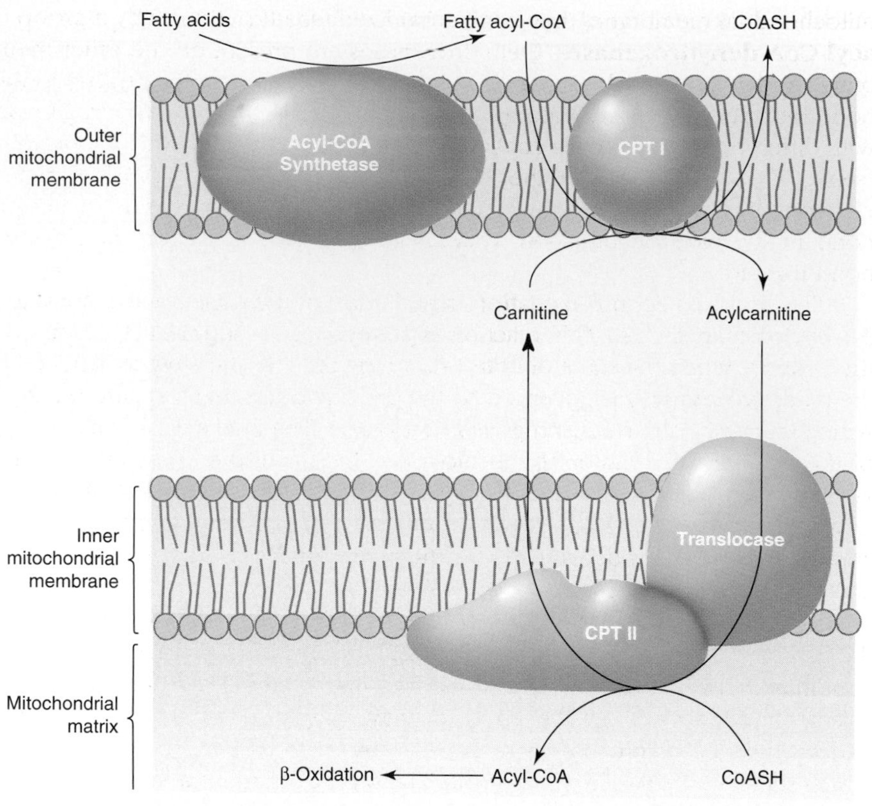

FIGURE 9.19
Mechanism for transfer of fatty acids from the cytosol through the inner mitochondrial membrane for oxidation.

Carnitine Carries Acyl Groups Across the Mitochondrial Membrane

Whereas most fatty acyl CoAs are formed outside mitochondria, the oxidizing machinery is inside the inner membrane, which is impermeable to CoA and its derivatives. The cell overcomes this problem by using **carnitine (4-trimethylamino-3-hydroxybutyrate)** as the carrier of acyl groups across the membrane. The steps involved are outlined in Figure 9.19. Enzymes on both sides of the membrane transfer fatty acyl groups between CoA and carnitine.

$$CH_3-(CH_2)_n-\overset{O}{\overset{\|}{C}}-SCoA + HO-\underset{\underset{\underset{\overset{+}{N}-(CH_3)_3}{|}}{CH_2}}{\overset{}{CH}}-CH_2-COOH \underset{\text{carnitine palmitoyl-transferase}}{\rightleftharpoons} CH_3-(CH_2)_n-\overset{O}{\overset{\|}{C}}-O-\underset{\underset{\underset{\overset{+}{N}-(CH_3)_3}{|}}{CH_2}}{\overset{}{CH}}-CH_2-COOH + CoASH$$

On the outer mitochondrial membrane the acyl group is transferred to carnitine catalyzed by **carnitine palmitoyltransferase I (CPT I).** Acyl carnitine then exchanges across the inner mitochondrial membrane with free carnitine by a carnitine–acylcarnitine antiporter translocase. Finally, the fatty acyl group is transferred back to CoA by **carnitine palmitoyltransferase II (CPT II)** located on the matrix side of the inner membrane. This process functions primarily in mitochondrial transport of fatty acyl CoAs with chain lengths of C12–C18. Genetic abnormalities in the system lead to serious pathology (see Clin. Corr. 9.4). By contrast, entry of shorter chain fatty acids is independent of carnitine because they cross the inner mitochondrial membrane directly and become activated to their CoA derivatives in the matrix compartment.

β-Oxidation Is a Sequence of Four Reactions

The four reactions of β-oxidation are presented in Figure 9.20. Once the fatty acyl groups have been transferred back to CoA at the inner surface of the inner mitochondrial membrane, they can be oxidized (see Reaction 1) by a group of **acyl-CoA dehydrogenases.** Dehydrogenases are present on the inner membrane and remove hydrogen atoms to form enoyl CoA with a trans double bond between C-2 and C-3 atoms. There are several different dehydrogenases with different specificities for chain length of the acyl CoA. All are flavoproteins (see Clin. Corr. 9.5). As in the TCA cycle, enzyme-bound $FADH_2$ transfers electrons through several other electron-transferring flavoproteins to ubiquinone in the electron transport system, yielding two ATPs for each double bond formed.

The second step in β-oxidation is hydration of the trans double bond to a **3-L-hydroxyacyl CoA.** This reaction is stereospecific, in that the L isomer is the product when the trans double bond is hydrated. The stereospecificity of the oxidative pathway is governed by the enzyme catalyzing the third reaction, which is specific for the L isomer as its substrate. The final step is the cleavage of the two-carbon fragment by a thiolase, which, like the preceding two enzymes, has relatively broad specificity with regard to chain length of the acyl group being oxidized. In the overall process then, an acetyl CoA is produced and the acyl CoA product is ready for the next round of oxidation starting with acyl-CoA dehydrogenase.

It has been impossible to show conclusively that any of the enzymes in the β-oxidation scheme are control points, although under rather rigid *in vitro* conditions some apparently have slower maximum rates of reaction than others. It is assumed that control is exerted by availability of substrates and cofactors and by the rate of processing of acetyl CoA by the TCA cycle. One way in which substrate availability is controlled is by regulation of the carnitine shuttle mechanism that transports fatty acids into mitochondria, a phenomenon of central importance in the regulation of hepatic ketone body production (see p. 387).

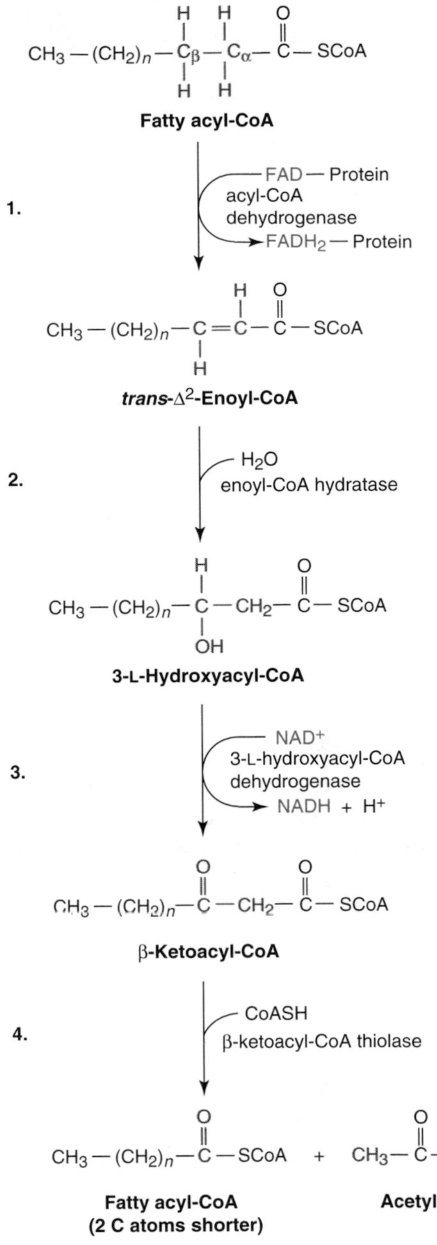

$CH_3-(CH_2)_n-C_\beta H_2-C_\alpha H_2-C(=O)-SCoA$

Fatty acyl-CoA

1. FAD — Protein; acyl-CoA dehydrogenase; → $FADH_2$ — Protein

$CH_3-(CH_2)_n-CH=CH-C(=O)-SCoA$

***trans*-Δ^2-Enoyl-CoA**

2. H_2O; enoyl-CoA hydratase

$CH_3-(CH_2)_n-CH(OH)-CH_2-C(=O)-SCoA$

3-L-Hydroxyacyl-CoA

3. NAD^+; 3-L-hydroxyacyl-CoA dehydrogenase; → $NADH + H^+$

$CH_3-(CH_2)_n-C(=O)-CH_2-C(=O)-SCoA$

β-Ketoacyl-CoA

4. CoASH; β-ketoacyl-CoA thiolase

$CH_3-(CH_2)_n-C(=O)-SCoA + CH_3-C(=O)-SCoA$

Fatty acyl-CoA (2 C atoms shorter) **Acetyl-CoA**

FIGURE 9.20
Pathway of fatty acid β-oxidation.

Energy-Yield from β-Oxidation of Fatty Acids

Each set of oxidations resulting in production of a two-carbon fragment yields, in addition to acetyl CoA, one reduced flavoprotein and one NADH. In the oxidation of palmitoyl CoA, seven such cleavages take place, and in the last cleavage two acetyl CoA molecules are formed. Thus the products of β-oxidation of palmitate are eight acetyl CoAs, seven reduced flavoproteins, and seven NADH. Each of the reduced flavoproteins can yield two ATP and each NADH can yield three when oxidized by the electron transport chain, so the reduced nucleotides yield 35 ATP per palmitoyl CoA. As described in Chapter 6, oxidation of each acetyl CoA through the TCA cycle yields 12 ATP, so the eight two-carbon fragments from a palmitate molecule produce 96 ATP. However, 2 ATP equivalents (1 ATP going to 1 AMP) were used to activate palmitate to palmitoyl CoA. Therefore each palmitic acid entering the cell from the action of lipoprotein lipase or from its combination with serum albumin can yield 129 ATP mol^{-1} by complete oxidation. The significance of the role of fatty acids in supplying the energy needs in humans is discussed on page 536.

Comparison of the β-Oxidation Scheme with Palmitate Biosynthesis

In living metabolic systems the reactions in a catabolic pathway are sometimes quite similar to those in a reversal of the corresponding anabolic sequence, but there are usually mechanisms that provide for separate control of the two schemes. This is true in the case of fatty acid biosynthesis and β-oxidation. The critical differences between the two pathways are outlined in Table 9.4. They include separation by subcellular compartmentation (β-oxidation occurs in the mitochondria and palmitate biosynthesis in the cytosol) and use of different cofactors (NADPH in biosynthesis, FAD and NAD^+ in oxidation).

CLINICAL CORRELATION 9.4

Genetic Deficiencies in Carnitine Transport or Carnitine Palmitoyltransferase

A number of diseases result from genetic abnormalities in the transport of long-chain fatty acids across the inner mitochondrial membrane. They stem from deficiencies either in the level of carnitine or in the functioning of the carnitine palmitoyltransferase (CPT) enzyme system.

The clinical symptoms of carnitine deficiency range from mild, recurrent muscle cramping to severe weakness and death. Two categories of the disorder, primary and secondary, are now recognized. Primary carnitine deficiency is caused by a defect in the high-affinity plasma membrane carnitine transporter in tissues such as muscle, kidney, heart, and fibroblasts (but apparently not in liver where a different transporter is operative). It results in extremely low levels of carnitine in affected tissues and also in plasma (because of failure to the kidneys to reabsorb carnitine). The very low carnitine level in heart and skeletal muscle seriously compromises long-chain fatty acid oxidation. Dietary carnitine therapy, by raising the plasma concentration of carnitine and forcing its entry into tissues in a nonspecific manner, is frequently beneficial. Secondary carnitine deficiency is often associated with inherited defects in the β-oxidation pathway that give rise to the accumulation of acyl CoAs and, in turn, acylcarnitines. The latter compounds can be excreted in the urine (see Clin. Corr. 9.5), thus draining the body's carnitine pool; in addition, they are thought to impair the tissue uptake of free carnitine.

CPT deficiency also presents as distinct clinical entities. The most common deficiency results from mutations in the CPT II gene that give rise to a partial loss of enzyme activity. The patient generally experiences muscle weakness during prolonged exercise when muscle relies heavily on fatty acids as an energy source. Myoglobinuria, due to breakdown of muscle tissue, is a frequent accompaniment. The disorder is usually referred to as the "muscular" form of CPT II deficiency. Mutations causing more severe (90% or greater) loss of CPT II activity can have serious consequences in early infancy. These are usually precipitated by periods of fasting and include hypoketotic hypoglycemia, hyperammonemia, cardiac malfunction, and sometimes death. Similar morbidity and mortality are associated with mutations in the gene for liver CPT I. To date only a few patients with hepatic CPT I deficiency have been reported, the small number possibly indicating that the disease is frequently lethal and has gone undiagnosed. Muscle CPT I is now known to be a different isoform from its liver counterpart, but no defects at this locus have yet been reported.

The first patient with carnitine–acylcarnitine translocase deficiency was described as recently as 1992. Clinical features included intermittent hypoglycemic coma, hyperammonemia, muscle weakness, and cardiomyopathy. The condition proved fatal at age 3 years. Three additional cases with similar symptomatology have since been reported.

The hallmark of treatment for all inherited disorders of the carnitine transport/CPT system is avoidance of starvation and a diet low in long-chain fatty acids. Supplementary dietary medium-chain triacylglycerols, the fatty acids of which are oxidized by a carnitine-independent mechanism, have proved beneficial.

Stanley, C. A., Hale, D. E., Berry, G. T., Deleeno, S., Boxer, J., and Bonnefont, J.-P. A deficiency of carnitine–acylcarnitine translocase in the inner mitochondrial membrane. *N. Engl. J. Med.* 327:19, 1992; and Roe, C R., and Coates, P. M. Mitochondrial fatty acid oxidation disorders. In: C. R. Scriver, A. L. Beaudet, W. S. Sly, and D. Valle (Eds.), *The Metabolic and Molecular Bases of Inherited Disease*, Vol. II, 7th ed. New York: McGraw-Hill, 1995, p. 1501.

Some Fatty Acids Require Modification of β-Oxidation for Metabolism

The β-oxidation scheme accounts for the bulk of energy production from fatty acids in the human. These reactions, however, must be supplemented by other mechanisms so that ingested odd-chain and unsaturated fatty acids can be oxidized. In addition, reactions catalyze α- and ω-oxidation of fatty acids. **α-Oxidation** occurs at C-2 instead of C-3, as in the β-oxidation scheme. **ω-Oxidation** occurs at the methyl end of the fatty acid molecule. Partial oxidation of fatty acids with cyclopropane ring structures probably occurs in humans, but the mechanisms are not worked out.

Propionyl CoA Is Produced by Oxidation of Odd-Chain Fatty Acids

Oxidation of fatty acids with an odd number of carbon atoms proceeds exactly as described above, but the final product is a molecule of propionyl CoA (Figure 9.21). For this compound to be further oxidized, it undergoes carboxylation to methylmalonyl CoA, molecular rearrangement, and conversion to succinyl CoA. These reactions are identical with those described on page 479 for the metabolism of **propionyl CoA** formed in the metabolic breakdown of some amino acids.

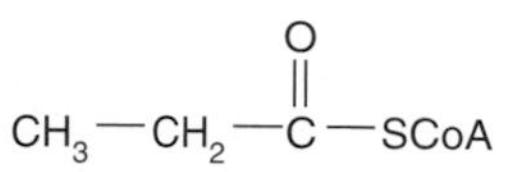

$$CH_3-CH_2-\overset{\overset{\displaystyle O}{\|}}{C}-SCoA$$

FIGURE 9.21
Propionyl CoA.

Oxidation of Unsaturated Fatty Acids Requires Additional Enzymes

Many unsaturated fatty acids in the diet are available for production of energy by humans. Structures encountered in these dietary acids may differ from those

CLINICAL CORRELATION 9.5

Genetic Deficiencies in the Acyl-CoA Dehydrogenases

The acyl-CoA dehydrogenase deficiencies represent a recently discovered group of inherited defects that impair the β-oxidation of fatty acids at different stages of the chain shortening process. The affected enzyme may be the long-chain acyl-CoA dehydrogenase (LCAD), the medium-chain acyl-CoA dehydrogenase (MCAD), or the short-chain acyl-CoA dehydrogenase (SCAD), whose substrate specificities are for acyl CoA chains of greater than C12, C6–C12, and C4–C6, respectively. The three conditions are inherited in autosomal recessive fashion and share many of the same clinical features. The best characterized is MCAD deficiency, which, though first recognized as late as 1982, is now thought to be one of the most common of all inborn errors of metabolism.

Medium-chain acyl-CoA dehydrogenase deficiency usually manifests itself within the first 2 years of life after a fasting period of 12 h or more. Typical symptoms include vomiting, lethargy, and frequently coma, accompanied by hypoketotic hypoglycemia and dicarboxylic aciduria. The absence of starvation ketosis is accounted for by the block in hepatic fatty acid oxidation, which also causes a slowdown of gluconeogenesis. This, coupled with impaired fatty acid oxidation in muscle, which promotes glucose utilization, leads to profound hypoglycemia. Accumulation of medium-chain acyl CoAs in tissues forces their metabolism through alternative pathways including ω-oxidation and transesterification to glycine or carnitine. Excessive urinary excretion of the reaction products (medium-chain dicarboxylic acids together with medium-chain esters of glycine and carnitine) provide diagnostic clues.

Most patients with this disorder do well simply by avoiding prolonged periods of starvation, which is consistent with the fact that the metabolic complications of MCAD deficiency are seen only when body tissues become heavily dependent on fatty acids as a source of energy (e.g., with carbohydrate deprivation). In retrospect, it now seems likely that many cases previously diagnosed loosely as "Reye-like syndrome" or "sudden infant death syndrome" were in fact due to MCAD deficiency.

Coates, P. M., and Tanaka, K. Molecular basis of mitochondrial fatty acid oxidation defects. *J. Lipid Res.* 33:1099, 1992.

required by the specificity of enzymes in β-oxidation pathway. Oxidation of linoleoyl CoA, outlined in Figure 9.22, illustrates two special reactions required for oxidation of unsaturated fatty acids.

One problem is that in β-oxidation of unsaturated fatty acids the sequential excision of C2 fragments can generate an acyl CoA intermediate with a double bond between C-3 and C-4 atoms instead of between C-2 and C-3 atoms as

TABLE 9.4 Comparison of Schemes for Biosynthesis and β-Oxidation of Palmitate

Parameter	*Biosynthesis*	*β-Oxidation*
Subcellular localization	Primarily cytosolic	Primarily mitochondrial
Phosphopantetheine-containing active carrier	Acyl carrier protein	Coenzyme A
Nature of small carbon fragment added or removed	C-1 and C-2 atoms of malonyl CoA after initial priming	Acetyl CoA
Nature of oxidation–reduction coenzyme	NADPH	FAD when saturated chain dehydrogenated, NAD^+ when hydroxy acid dehydrogenated
Stereochemical configuration of β-hydroxy intermediates	D-β-Hydroxy	L-β-Hydroxy
Energy equivalents yielded or utilized in interconversion of palmitate and acetyl CoA	7 ATP + 14 NADPH = 49 ATP equiv	7 $FADH_2$ + 7 NADH − 2 ATP = 33 ATP equiv

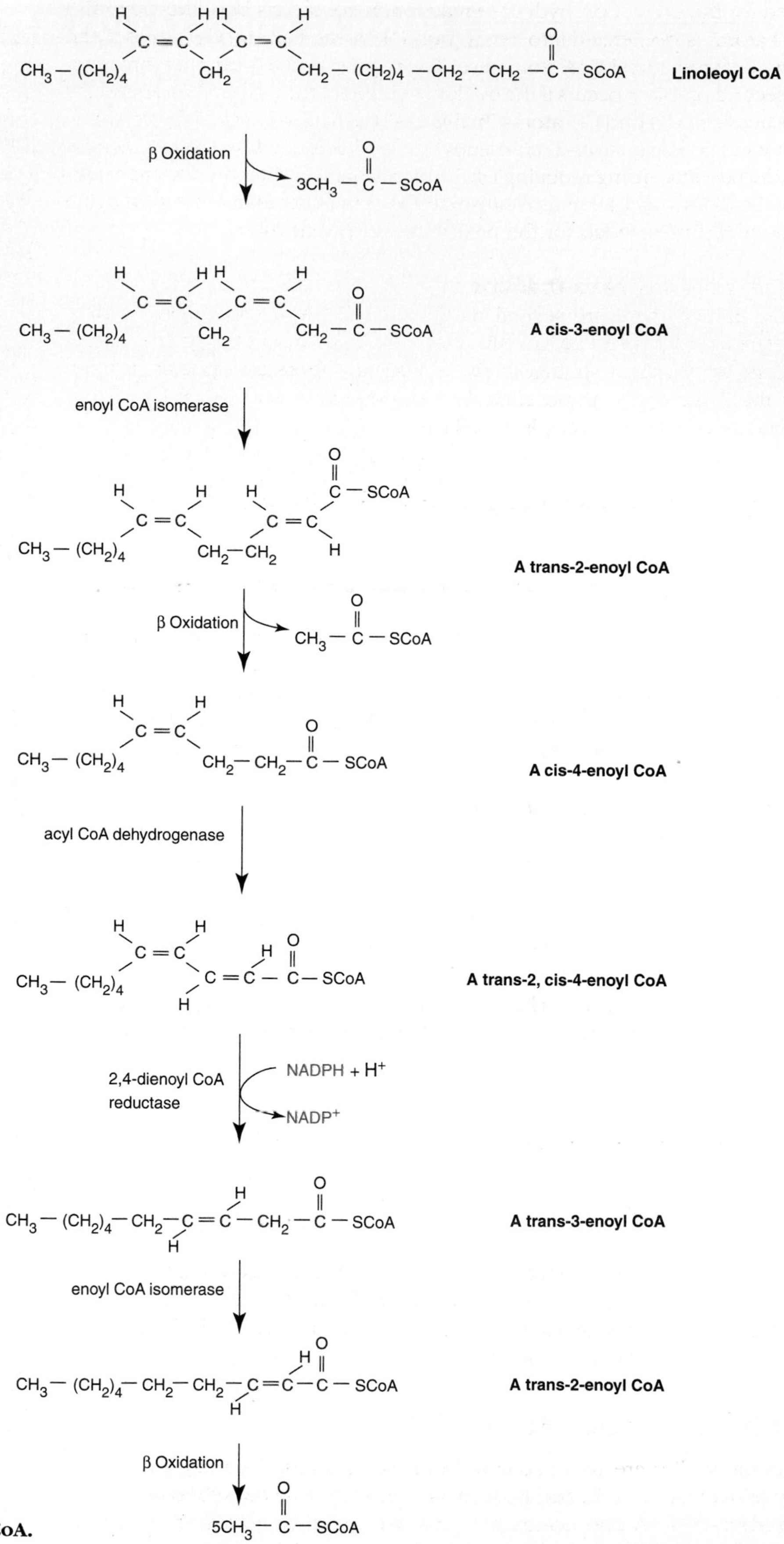

$CH_3-(CH_2)_4-CH{=}CH-CH_2-CH{=}CH-CH_2-(CH_2)_4-CH_2-CH_2-C(=O)-SCoA$ **Linoleoyl CoA**

β Oxidation → $3CH_3-C(=O)-SCoA$

$CH_3-(CH_2)_4-CH{=}CH-CH_2-CH{=}CH-CH_2-C(=O)-SCoA$ **A cis-3-enoyl CoA**

enoyl CoA isomerase

$CH_3-(CH_2)_4-CH{=}CH-CH_2-CH_2-CH{=}CH-C(=O)-SCoA$ **A trans-2-enoyl CoA**

β Oxidation → $CH_3-C(=O)-SCoA$

$CH_3-(CH_2)_4-CH{=}CH-CH_2-CH_2-C(=O)-SCoA$ **A cis-4-enoyl CoA**

acyl CoA dehydrogenase

$CH_3-(CH_2)_4-CH{=}CH-CH{=}CH-C(=O)-SCoA$ **A trans-2, cis-4-enoyl CoA**

2,4-dienoyl CoA reductase

$NADPH + H^+$ → $NADP^+$

$CH_3-(CH_2)_4-CH_2-CH{=}CH-CH_2-C(=O)-SCoA$ **A trans-3-enoyl CoA**

enoyl CoA isomerase

$CH_3-(CH_2)_4-CH_2-CH_2-CH{=}CH-C(=O)-SCoA$ **A trans-2-enoyl CoA**

β Oxidation

$5CH_3-C(=O)-SCoA$

FIGURE 9.22
Oxidation of linoleoyl CoA.

required for the enoyl CoA hydratase reaction. If so, the cis bond between C-3 and C-4 atoms is isomerized into a trans bond between C-2 and C-3 atoms by an auxiliary enzyme, enoyl CoA isomerase. The regular process can then proceed.

A second problem occurs if the cis double bond of the acyl CoA intermediate resides between C-4 and C-5 atoms. In this case the action of acyl-CoA dehydrogenase gives rise to a *trans*-2, *cis*-4-enoyl CoA. This is acted on by 2,4-dienoyl CoA reductase that, using reducing equivalents from NADPH, produces a *trans*-3-enoyl CoA. This will serve as a substrate for enoyl CoA isomerase producing *trans*-2-enoyl CoA needed for the next round of β-oxidation.

Some Fatty Acids Undergo α-Oxidation

As noted earlier, there are several mechanisms for **hydroxylation of fatty acids.** The one discussed previously is for a hydroxylation of long-chain acids needed for synthesis of sphingolipids. In addition, there are systems in other tissues that hydroxylate the α carbon of shorter chain acids in order to start their oxidation. The sequence is as follows:

$$-(CH_2)_n-CH_2-\overset{\overset{\displaystyle O}{\|}}{C}-OH \longrightarrow CH_3-(CH_2)_n-\overset{\overset{\displaystyle OH}{|}}{CH}-\overset{\overset{\displaystyle O}{\|}}{C}-OH \longrightarrow$$

$$CH_3-(CH_2)_n-\overset{\overset{\displaystyle O}{\|}}{C}-\overset{\overset{\displaystyle O}{\|}}{C}-OH \longrightarrow CH_3-(CH_2)_n-\overset{\overset{\displaystyle O}{\|}}{C}-OH + CO_2$$

These hydroxylations probably occur in the endoplasmic reticulum and mitochondria and involve the "mixed function oxidase" type of mechanism discussed previously, because they require molecular oxygen, reduced nicotinamide nucleotides and specific cytochromes. Such reactions are particularly important in oxidation of methylated fatty acids (see Clin. Corr. 9.6).

ω-Oxidation Gives Rise to a Dicarboxylic Acid

Another minor pathway for fatty acid oxidation also involves hydroxylation and occurs in the endoplasmic reticulum of many tissues. In this case hydroxylation takes place on the methyl carbon at the other end of the molecule from the carboxyl group or on the carbon next to the methyl end. It uses the "mixed function oxidase" type of reaction requiring cytochrome P450, O_2, and NADPH, as well as the necessary enzymes (see Chapter 23). Hydroxylated fatty acid can be further oxidized to a **dicarboxylic acid** via sequential action of cytosolic **alcohol** and **aldehyde dehydrogenases.** The process occurs primarily with medium-chain fatty acids. The overall reactions are

$$H_3-(CH_2)_n-\overset{\overset{\displaystyle O}{\|}}{C}-OH \longrightarrow HO-CH_2-(CH_2)_n-\overset{\overset{\displaystyle O}{\|}}{C}-OH \longrightarrow \longrightarrow$$

$$HO-\overset{\overset{\displaystyle O}{\|}}{C}-(CH_2)_n-\overset{\overset{\displaystyle O}{\|}}{C}-OH$$

The dicarboxylic acid so formed can be activated at either end of the molecule to form a CoA ester, which in turn can undergo β-oxidation to produce shorter chain dicarboxylic acids such as adipic (C6) and succinic (C4) acids. This process appears to occur primarily in peroxisomes (see p. 19).

Ketone Bodies Are Formed from Acetyl CoA

The ketone bodies are water-soluble forms of lipid-based energy and consist mainly of acetoacetic acid and its reduction product β-hydroxybutyric acid. β-Hydroxybutyryl CoA and acetoacetyl CoA are intermediates near the end of the β-oxidation sequence, and it was initially presumed that enzymatic removal

CLINICAL CORRELATION 9.6

Refsum's Disease

Although the use of the α-oxidation scheme is a relatively minor one in terms of total energy production, it is significant in the metabolism of dietary fatty acids that are methylated. A principal example of these is phytanic acid,

$$\begin{array}{l} CH_3 \\ | \\ CH-CH_3 \\ | \\ (CH_2)_3 \\ | \\ CH-CH_3 \\ | \\ (CH_2)_3 \\ | \\ CH-CH_3 \\ | \\ (CH_2)_3 \\ | \\ CH-CH_3 \\ | \\ CH_2 \\ | \\ COOH \end{array}$$

Phytanic acid

a metabolic product of phytol, which occurs as a constituent of chlorophyll. Phytanic acid is a significant constituent of ~~milk~~ lipids and animal fats, and normally it is metabolized by an initial α-hydroxylation followed by dehydrogenation and decarboxylation. β-Oxidation cannot occur initially because of the presence of the 3-methyl group, but it can proceed after the decarboxylation. The whole reaction produces three molecules of propionyl CoA, three molecules of acetyl CoA, and one molecule of isobutyryl CoA.

In a rare genetic disease called Refsum's disease, the patients lack the α-hydroxylating enzyme and accumulate large quantities of phytanic acid in their tissues and sera. This leads to serious neurological problems such as retinitis pigmentosa, peripheral neuropathy, cerebellar ataxia, and nerve deafness. The restriction of dietary dairy products and meat products from ruminants results in lowering of plasma phytanic acid and regression of neurologic symptoms.

Steinberg. D. Refsum disease. In: C. R. Scriver, A. L. Beaudet, W. S. Sly, and D. Valle (Eds.), *The Metabolic and Molecular Bases of Inherited Disease,* Vol. II, 7th ed. New York: McGraw-Hill, 1995, p. 2351.

of CoA from these compounds was the main route for production of the free acids. However, β-oxidation proceeds completely to acetyl CoA production without accumulation of any intermediates, and acetoacetate and β-hydroxybutyrate are formed subsequently from acetyl CoA by a separate mechanism.

HMG CoA Is an Intermediate in the Synthesis of Acetoacetate from Acetyl CoA

The primary site for formation of ketone bodies is liver, with lesser activity occurring in kidney. The entire process takes place within the mitochondrial matrix and begins with condensation of two acetyl CoA molecules to form acetoacetyl CoA (Figure 9.23). The enzyme involved, **β-ketothiolase,** is probably an isozyme of that which catalyzes the reverse reaction as the last step of β-oxidation. Acetoacetyl CoA then condenses with another molecule of acetyl CoA to form **β-hydroxy-β-methylglutaryl coenzyme A (HMG CoA).** Cleavage of HMG CoA then yields acetoacetic acid and acetyl CoA.

Acetoacetate Forms Both D-β-Hydroxybutyrate and Acetone

In mitochondria a fraction of the acetoacetate is reduced to D-β-hydroxybutyrate depending on the intramitochondrial [NADH]/[NAD$^+$] ratio. Note that the product of this reaction is D-β-hydroxybutyrate, whereas β-hydroxybutyryl CoA formed during β-oxidation is of the L configuration. **β-Hydroxybutyrate dehydrogenase** is tightly associated with the inner mitochondrial membrane and, because of its high activity in liver, the concentrations of substrates and products

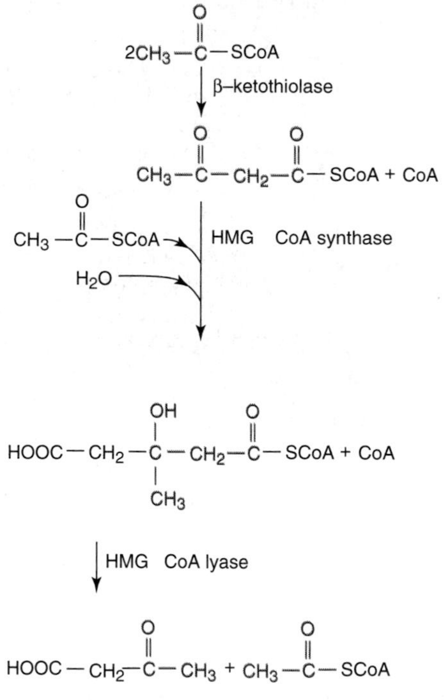

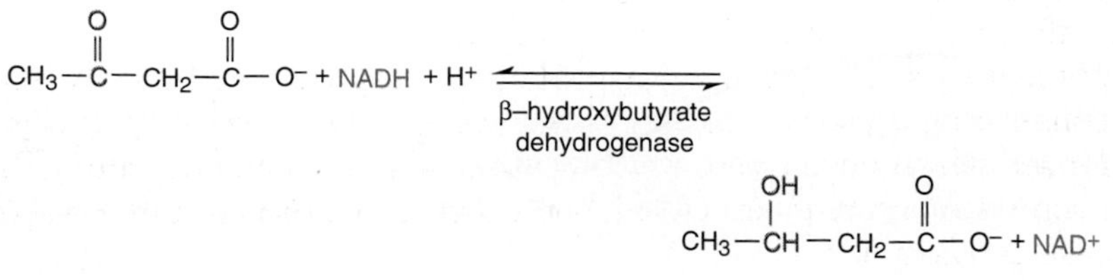

$$2CH_3{-}\overset{O}{\overset{\|}{C}}{-}SCoA$$

$\downarrow$ β–ketothiolase

$$CH_3{-}\overset{O}{\overset{\|}{C}}{-}CH_2{-}\overset{O}{\overset{\|}{C}}{-}SCoA + CoA$$

$CH_3{-}\overset{O}{\overset{\|}{C}}{-}SCoA$, H_2O $\downarrow$ HMG CoA synthase

$$HOOC{-}CH_2{-}\overset{OH}{\underset{CH_3}{C}}{-}CH_2{-}\overset{O}{\overset{\|}{C}}{-}SCoA + CoA$$

$\downarrow$ HMG CoA lyase

$$HOOC{-}CH_2{-}\overset{O}{\overset{\|}{C}}{-}CH_3 + CH_3{-}\overset{O}{\overset{\|}{C}}{-}SCoA$$

$$CH_3{-}\overset{O}{\overset{\|}{C}}{-}CH_2{-}\overset{O}{\overset{\|}{C}}{-}O^- + NADH + H^+ \rightleftharpoons CH_3{-}\overset{OH}{\overset{|}{C}H}{-}CH_2{-}\overset{O}{\overset{\|}{C}}{-}O^- + NAD^+$$

(β–hydroxybutyrate dehydrogenase)

FIGURE 9.23
Pathway of acetoacetate formation.

of the reaction are maintained close to equilibrium. Thus the ratio of β-hydroxybutyrate to acetoacetate in blood leaving liver can be taken as a reflection of the mitochondrial [NADH]/[NAD^+] ratio.

Some acetoacetate continually undergoes slow, spontaneous nonenzymatic decarboxylation to acetone:

$$CH_3{-}\overset{\displaystyle O}{\overset{\|}{C}}{-}CH_2{-}\overset{\displaystyle O}{\overset{\|}{C}}{-}O^- + H^+ \longrightarrow CH_3{-}\overset{\displaystyle O}{\overset{\|}{C}}{-}CH_3 + CO_2$$

Under normal conditions acetone formation is negligible, but when pathological accumulations of acetoacetate occur, as, for example, in severe diabetic ketoacidosis (see Clin. Corr. 9.7), the amount of acetone in blood can be sufficient to cause it to be detectable in a patient's breath.

As seen from Figure 9.24, the pathway leading from acetyl CoA to HMG CoA also operates in the cytosolic space of liver cells (indeed, this applies to essentially all tissues of the body). However, in this compartment HMG CoA lyase is absent and the HMG CoA formed is used for cholesterol biosynthesis (see Chapter 10). What distinguishes liver from nonhepatic tissues is its high complement of intramitochondrial **HMG CoA synthase,** thus providing an enzymological basis for the primacy of this organ in ketone body production.

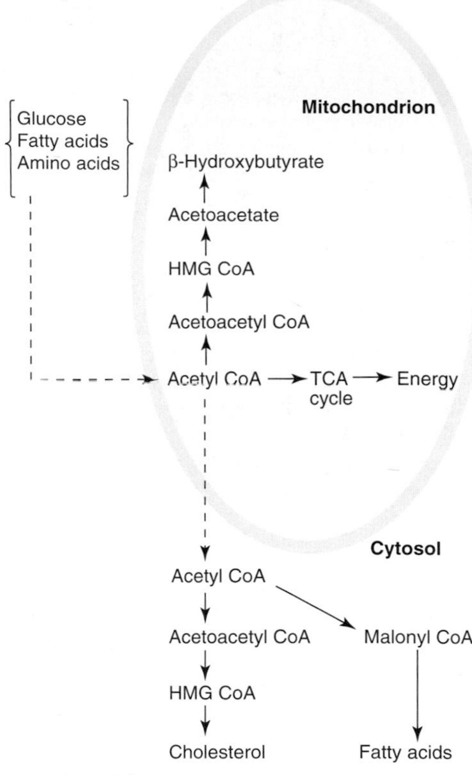

FIGURE 9.24
Interrelationships of ketone bodies with lipid, carbohydrate, and amino acid metabolism in liver.

Utilization of Ketone Bodies by Nonhepatic Tissues Requires Formation of Acetoacetyl CoA

Acetoacetate and β-hydroxybutyrate produced by liver serve as excellent fuels for a variety of nonhepatic tissues, such as cardiac and skeletal muscle, particularly when glucose is in short supply (starvation) or inefficiently used (insulin deficiency). But since under these conditions the same tissues can readily use free fatty acids (whose blood concentration rises as insulin levels fall) as a source of energy, a nagging question for many years was why liver should produce ketone bodies in the first place. The answer emerged in the late 1960s with the recognition that during prolonged starvation in humans the ketone bodies replace glucose as the major fuel of respiration for the central nervous system, which has a low capacity for fatty acid oxidation. Also noteworthy is the fact that during the neonatal period of development, acetoacetate and β-hydroxybutyrate serve as important precursors for cerebral lipid synthesis.

Use of ketone bodies requires that acetoacetate first be reactivated to its CoA derivative. This is accomplished by a mitochondrial enzyme, acetoacetate:succinyl CoA CoA transferase, present in most nonhepatic tissues but absent from liver. Succinyl CoA serves as the source of the coenzyme. The reaction is depicted in Figure 9.25. Through the action of β-ketothiolase, acetoacetyl CoA is then converted into acetyl CoA, which in turn enters the TCA cycle with production of energy. Mitochondrial β-hydroxybutyrate dehydrogenase in nonhepatic tissues reconverts β-hydroxybutyrate into acetoacetate as the concentration of the latter is decreased.

Acetoacetate + succinyl CoA

⇅ acetoacetate : succinyl CoA CoA transferase

Acetoacetyl CoA + succinate

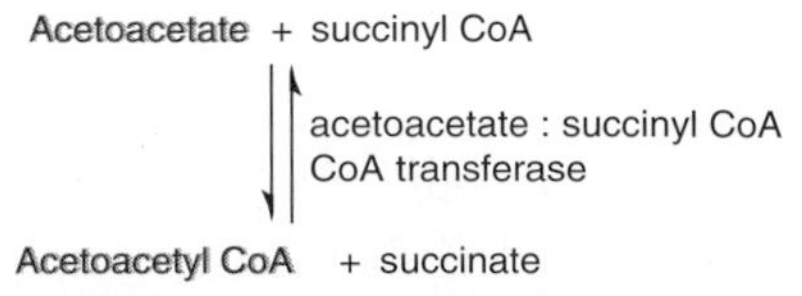

FIGURE 9.25
Initial step in utilization of acetoacetate by nonhepatic tissues.

Starvation and Certain Pathological Conditions Lead to Ketosis

Under normal feeding conditions, hepatic production of acetoacetate and β-hydroxybutyrate is minimal and the concentration of these compounds in the blood is very low (≤0.2 mM). However, with food deprivation ketone body synthesis is greatly accelerated, and the circulating level of acetoacetate plus β-hydroxybutyrate may rise to the region of 3–5 mM. This is a normal response of the body to a shortage of carbohydrate and serves a number of crucial roles. In the early stages of fasting, use of ketone bodies by heart and skeletal muscle conserves glucose for support of the central nervous system. With more prolonged starvation, increased blood concentrations of acetoacetate and β-hydroxybutyrate ensure their efficient uptake by brain, thereby further sparing glucose consumption.

CLINICAL CORRELATION 9.7

Diabetic Ketoacidosis

Diabetic ketoacidosis (DKA) is a common illness among patients with insulin-dependent diabetes mellitus. Although mortality rates have declined, they are still in the range of 6–10%. The condition is triggered by severe insulin deficiency coupled with glucagon excess and is frequently accompanied by concomitant elevation of other stress hormones, such as epinephrine, norepinephrine, cortisol, and growth hormone. The major metabolic derangements are marked hyperglycemia, excessive ketonemia, and ketonuria. Blood concentrations of acetoacetic acid plus β-hydroxybutyric acid as high as 20 mM are not uncommon. Because these are relatively strong acids (p$K \approx 3.5$), the situation results in life-threatening metabolic acidosis.

The massive accumulation of ketone bodies in the blood in DKA stems from a greatly accelerated hepatic production rate such that the capacity of nonhepatic tissues to use them is exceeded. In biochemical terms the initiating events are identical with those operative in the development of starvation ketosis; that is, increased glucagon/insulin ratio → elevation of liver cAMP → decreased malonyl CoA → deinhibition of CPT I → activation of fatty acid oxidation and ketone production (see text for details). However, in contrast to physiological ketosis, where insulin secretion from the pancreatic β cells limits free fatty acid (FFA) availability to the liver, this restraining mechanism is absent in the diabetic individual. As a result, plasma FFA concentrations can reach levels as high as 3–4 mM, which drive hepatic ketone production at maximal rates.

Correction of DKA requires rapid treatment that will be dictated by the severity of the metabolic abnormalities and the associated tissue water and electrolyte imbalance. Insulin is essential. It lowers the plasma glucagon level, antagonizes the catabolic effects of glucagon on the liver, inhibits the flow of ketogenic and gluconeogenic substrates (FFA and amino acids) from the periphery, and stimulates glucose uptake in target tissues.

Foster, J. D., and McGarry, J. D. Metabolic derangements and treatment of diabetic ketoacidosis. *N. Engl. J. Med.* 309:159, 1983; and Foster, D. W., and McGarry, J. D. Acute complications of diabetes: ketoacidosis, hyperosmolar coma, lactic acidosis. In: L. J. DeGroot (Ed.), *Endocrinology,* Vol. 2, 3rd ed. Philadelphia: Saunders, 1995, p. 1506.

In contrast to the **physiological ketosis of starvation,** certain pathological conditions, most notably **diabetic ketoacidosis** (see Clin. Corr. 9.7), are characterized by excessive accumulation of ketone bodies in the blood (up to 20 mM). Hormonal and biochemical factors operative in the overall control of hepatic ketone body production are discussed in detail in Chapter 14.

Peroxisomal Oxidation of Fatty Acids Serves Many Functions

Although the bulk of cellular fatty acid oxidation occurs in mitochondria it has recently become clear that a significant fraction also takes place in **peroxisomes** of liver, kidney, and other tissues. Peroxisomes are a class of subcellular organelles with distinctive morphological and chemical characteristics. Their initial distinguishing property was a high content of the enzyme catalase and it has been suggested that peroxisomes may function in a protective role against oxygen toxicity. Several lines of evidence suggest that they are also involved in lipid catabolism. First, the analogous structures in plants, glyoxysomes, are capable of oxidizing fatty acids. Second, a number of drugs used clinically to decrease triacylglycerol levels in patients cause a marked increase in peroxisomes. Third, liver peroxisomes, isolated by differential centrifugation, oxidize fatty acids and contain most of the enzymes needed for the β-oxidation process.

The mammalian **peroxisomal fatty acid oxidation** scheme is similar to that in plant glyoxysomes but differs from the mitochondrial β-oxidation system in three important respects. First, the initial dehydrogenation is accomplished by a cyanide-insensitive oxidase system, as shown in Figure 9.26. $\mathbf{H_2O_2}$ formed is eliminated by **catalase,** and the remaining steps are the same as in the mitochondrial system. Second, there is evidence that the peroxisomal and mitochondrial enzymes are slightly different and that the specificity in peroxisomes is for somewhat longer chain length. Third, although rat liver mitochondria will oxidize a molecule of palmitoyl CoA to eight molecules of acetyl CoA, the β-oxidation system in peroxisomes from the same organ will not proceed beyond the stage of octanoyl CoA (C8). The possibility is thus raised that one function

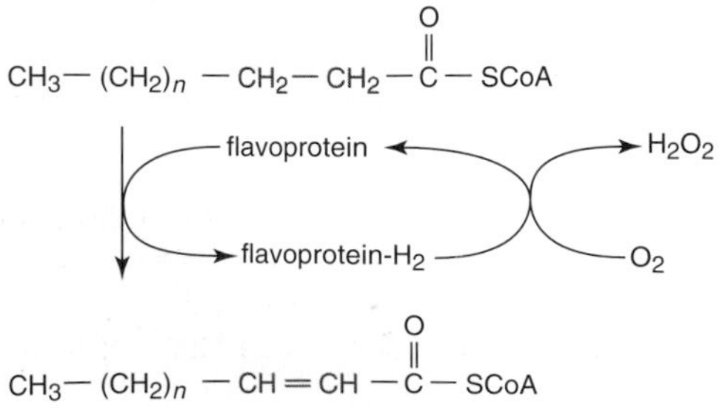

$CH_3-(CH_2)_n-CH_2-CH_2-\overset{O}{\overset{\|}{C}}-SCoA$

flavoprotein → flavoprotein-H_2; O_2 → H_2O_2

$CH_3-(CH_2)_n-CH{=}CH-\overset{O}{\overset{\|}{C}}-SCoA$

FIGURE 9.26
Initial step in peroxisomal fatty acid oxidation.

of peroxisomes is to shorten the chains of relatively long-chain fatty acids to a point at which β-oxidation can be completed in mitochondria.

Other peroxisomal reactions include chain shortening of dicarboxylic acids, as noted earlier, conversion of cholesterol into bile acids, and formation of ether lipids. Given these diverse metabolic roles it is not surprising that the congenital absence of functional peroxisomes, an inherited defect known as Zellweger syndrome, has such devastating effects (see Clin. Corr. 1.3).

BIBLIOGRAPHY

Foster, D. W., and McGarry, J. D. Acute complications of diabetes: ketogenesis, hyperosmolar coma, lactic acidosis. In: L. J. DeGroot (Ed.), *Endocrinology,* Vol. 2, 3rd ed. Philadelphia: Saunders, 1995, p. 1506.

Goldstein, J. L., Hobbs, H. H., and Brown, M. S. Familial hypercholesterolemia. In: C. R. Scriver, A. L. Beaudet, W. S. Sly, and D. Valle (Eds.), *The Metabolic and Molecular Bases of Inherited Disease,* Vol. II, 7th ed. New York: McGraw-Hill, 1995, p. 1981.

Gurr, M. I., and James, A. T. *Lipid Biochemistry, An Introduction,* 3rd ed. London: Chapman and Hall, 1980.

Kane, J. P., and Havel, R. J. Disorders of the biogenesis and secretion of lipoproteins containing the B apolipoproteins. In: C. R. Scriver, A. L. Beaudet, W. S. Sly, and D. Valle (Eds.), *The Metabolic and Molecular Bases of Inherited Disease,* Vol. II, 7th ed. New York: McGraw-Hill, 1995, p. 1853

McGarry, J. D., and Foster, D. W. Regulation of hepatic fatty acid oxidation and ketone body production. *Annu. Rev. Biochem.* 49:395, 1980.

McGarry, J. D., Woeltje, K. F., Kuwajima, M., and Foster, D. W. Regulation of ketogenesis and the renaissance of carnitine palmitoyltransferase. *Diabetes Metab. Rev.* 5:271, 1989.

Nilsson-Ehle, P., Garfinkel, A. S., and Schotz, M. C. Lipolytic enzymes and plasma lipoprotein metabolism. *Annu. Rev. Biochem.* 49:667, 1980.

Robinson, A. M., and Williamson, D. H. Physiological roles of ketone bodies as substrates and signals in mammalian tissues. *Physiol. Rev.* 60:143, 1980.

Saudubray, J.-M., Mitchell, G., Bonnefont, J.-P., Schwartz, G., et al. Approach to the patient with a fatty acid oxidation disorder. In: P. M. Coates and K. Tanaka (Eds.), *New Developments in Fatty Acid Oxidation.* New York: Wiley-Liss, 1992, p. 271.

Stanley, C. A. Plasma and mitochondrial membrane carnitine transport defects. In: P. M. Coates and K. Tanaka (Eds.), *New Developments in Fatty Acid Oxidation.* New York: Wiley-Liss, 1992, p. 289.

Wakil, S. J., Stoops, J. K., and Joshi, V. C. Fatty acid synthesis and its regulation. *Annu. Rev. Biochem.* 52:537, 1983.

QUESTIONS ■ C. N. ANGSTADT AND J. BAGGOTT

1. Fatty acids occurring in humans most commonly:
   A. are highly branched structures.
   B. have double bonds present in trans configuration.
   C. contain an even number of carbon atoms.
   D. are limited to 16 or fewer carbon atoms.
   E. if polyunsaturated, have a conjugated double-bond system.

2. Triacylglycerols:
   A. would be expected to be good emulsifying agents.
   B. yield about the same amount of ATP on complete oxidation as would an equivalent weight of glycogen.
   C. are stored as hydrated molecules.
   D. in the average individual, represent sufficient energy to sustain life for several weeks.
   E. are generally negatively charged molecules at physiological pH.

3. In humans, fatty acids:
   A. can be synthesized from excess dietary carbohydrate or protein.
   B. are not required at all in the diet.
   C. containing double bonds cannot be synthesized.
   D. must be supplied entirely by the diet.
   E. other than palmitate, must be supplied by the diet.

4. All of the following statements about acetyl-CoA carboxylase are correct EXCEPT:
   A. it undergoes protomer–polymer interconversion during its physiological regulation.
   B. it requires biotin.
   C. it is inhibited by cAMP-mediated phosphorylation.
   D. it is activated by both palmitoyl CoA and citrate.
   E. its content in a cell responds to changes in fat content in the diet.

5. In the synthesis of palmitate:
   A. the addition of malonyl CoA to fatty acid synthase elongates the growing chain by three carbon atoms.
   B. a β-keto residue on the 4′-phosphopantetheine moiety is reduced to a saturated residue by NADPH.
   C. palmitoyl CoA is released from the synthase.
   D. transfer of the growing chain from ACP to another —SH occurs after the addition of the next malonyl CoA.
   E. the first compound to add to fatty acid synthase is malonyl CoA.

6. Citrate stimulates fatty acid synthesis by all of the following EXCEPT:
   A. allosterically activating acetyl-CoA carboxylase.
   B. providing a mechanism to transport acetyl CoA from the mitochondria to the cytosol.
   C. participating in a pathway that ultimately produces CO_2 and NADPH in the cytosol.
   D. participating in the production of ATP.

7. Fatty acyl CoAs shorter than 16 carbon atoms are the preferred substrates for:
   A. fatty acid elongation in the brain.
   B. carnitine transport into the mitochondria.
   C. fatty acid elongation in mitochondria.
   D. fatty acid elongation in the endoplasmic reticulum.
   E. all of the above.

8. Fatty acid synthase:
   A. synthesizes only palmitate.
   B. yields an unsaturated fatty acid by skipping a reductive step.
   C. produces hydroxy fatty acids in nerve tissue.
   D. can stop synthesis with the release of a fatty alcohol instead of an acid.
   E. can produce a branched-chain fatty acid if methylmalonyl CoA is used as a substrate.

9. In humans, desaturation of fatty acids:
   A. occurs primarily in mitochondria.
   B. is catalyzed by an enzyme system that uses NADPH and a cytochrome.
   C. introduces double bonds primarily of trans configuration.
   D. can occur only after palmitate has been elongated to stearic acid.
   E. introduces the first double bond at the methyl end of the molecule.

10. All of the following events are usually involved in the synthesis of triacylglycerols in adipose tissue EXCEPT:
    A. addition of a fatty acyl CoA to a diacylglycerol.
    B. addition of a fatty acyl CoA to a lysophosphatide.
    C. a reaction catalyzed by glycerol kinase.
    D. hydrolysis of phosphatidic acid by a phosphatase.
    E. reduction of dihydroxyacetone phosphate.

11. Plasma lipoproteins:
    A. are the only carriers of lipid-based energy in the blood.
    B. usually have a nonpolar core containing triacylglycerols and cholesterol esters.
    C. are composed primarily of free (unesterified) fatty acids.
    D. include chylomicrons generated in the liver.
    E. include high density lipoproteins (HDL) as the major carrier of lipid-based energy.

12. Lipoprotein lipase:
    A. is an intracellular enzyme.
    B. is stimulated by cAMP-mediated phosphorylation.
    C. functions to mobilize stored triacylglycerols from adipose tissue.
    D. is stimulated by one of the apoproteins present in VLDL.
    E. readily hydrolyzes three fatty acids from a triacylglycerol.

13. A deficiency of carnitine might be expected to interfere with:
    A. β-oxidation.
    B. ketone body formation from acetyl CoA.
    C. palmitate synthesis.
    D. mobilization of stored triacylglycerols from adipose tissue.
    E. uptake of fatty acids into cells from the blood.

14. β-Oxidation of fatty acids:
    A. generates ATP only if acetyl CoA is subsequently oxidized.
    B. is controlled primarily by allosteric effectors.
    C. uses only even-chain, saturated fatty acids as substrates.
    D. uses $NADP^+$.
    E. occurs by a repeated sequence of four reactions.

15. Ketone bodies:
    A. are formed by removal of CoA from the corresponding intermediate of β-oxidation.
    B. are synthesized from cytoplasmic β-hydroxy-β-methylglutaryl coenzyme A (HMG CoA).
    C. are excellent energy substrates for liver.
    D. include both β-hydroxybutyrate and acetoacetate, the ratio reflecting the intramitochondrial [NADH]/[NAD^+] ratio in liver.
    E. form when β-oxidation is interrupted.

16. The high glucagon/insulin ratio seen in starvation:
    A. promotes mobilization of fatty acids from adipose stores.
    B. stimulates β-oxidation by inhibiting the production of malonyl CoA.
    C. leads to increased concentrations of ketone bodies in the blood.
    D. all of the above.
    E. none of the above.

17. Peroxisomal oxidation of fatty acids:
    A. is identical to β-oxidation in the mitochondria.
    B. involves a flavoprotein that produces H_2O_2.
    C. has a preference for fatty acids shorter than 12 carbons.
    D. does not use NAD^+.
    E. is effective only for dicarboxylic acids.

ANSWERS

1. C A: Some may have methyl branches but most are straight chain. B: Most naturally occurring double bonds are cis, an important factor in β-oxidation of unsaturated fatty acids. D: C18 and C20 fatty acids are very common. E: Double bonds are separated by —CH_2— (p. 363).
2. D A, C, and E: Triacylglycerols are neutral, hydrophobic molecules with no hydrophilic portion and therefore are not emulsifying agents and are stored anhydrously. B: Their more reduced state, compared to carbohydrates, makes them more energy-rich (p. 365).
3. A It is important to realize that triacylglycerol is the ultimate storage form of excess dietary intake. B–E: We can synthesize most fatty acids, including those with double bonds, except for the essential fatty acids, linoleic and linolenic acids (p. 365).
4. D A: Acetyl-CoA carboxylase shifts between its protomeric (inactive) and polymeric (active) forms under the influence of a variety of regulatory factors. C: Since cAMP increases at times when energy is needed, it is consistent that a process that uses energy would be inhibited. E: Long-term control is

related to enzyme synthesis and responds appropriately to dietary changes (Table 9.2, p. 367).

5. B A: Splitting CO_2 from malonyl CoA is the driving force for the condensation reaction so the chain grows two carbon atoms at a time. C: Palmitate is released as the free acid; the conversion to the CoA ester is by a different enzyme (p. 369). D: It is important to realize that only ACP binds the incoming malonyl CoA so it must be freed before another addition can be made. E: Acetyl CoA adds first to form the foundation for the rest of the chain (p. 368).

6. D Citrate consumes ATP when acted upon by citrate cleavage enzyme (p. 371). A: Table 9.2. B: Acetyl CoA is generated primarily in mitochondria but does not cross the membrane readily. C: Oxaloacetate generated by citrate cleavage enzyme, when converted to malate, yields CO_2 and NADPH by the malic enzyme (Figure 9.10).

7. C C and D:The role of mitochondrial fatty acid elongation seems to be to elongate short-chain fatty acids; the cytoplasmic system is most active with palmitate. A: Brain elongates 18 carbon acids to meet its needs. B: Short- and medium-chain fatty acids are capable of entering mitochondria and their activation to CoA esters occurs there (p. 372).

8. E This is much slower than reaction with malonyl CoA, but it is significant. A: In certain tissues, for example, mammary glands, shorter chain products are formed. B–D: These products are all formed by other processes. Reactions proceeding on a multienzyme complex generally do not "stop" at intermediate steps (p. 374).

9. B A: Desaturation occurs in the endoplasmic reticulum. C: Naturally occurring fatty acids are cis. D: Elongation and unsaturation can occur in any order. E: If this were true we could make linoleic acid (p. 372).

10. C This does not occur to any significant extent in adipose tissue. A, B, and D: The sequential addition of fatty acyl CoAs to glycerol 3-phosphate forms lysophosphatidic acid, then phosphatidic acid whose phosphate is removed before the addition of the third fatty acyl residue. E: This is the formation of α-glycerol phosphate in adipose tissue (p. 375).

11. B All lipoproteins (Section 9.5) have this same general structure, a nonpolar core surrounded by a more polar shell. A and C: Fatty acids bound to serum albumin and ketone bodies are other sources. D: Chylomicrons carry dietary lipid from the intestine. E: HDL function is to carry cholesterol away from tissues (p. 379).

12. D A–C: These are characteristics of hormone-sensitive lipase. E: It generally requires more than one lipase to hydrolyze all of the fatty acids (p. 381, Table 9.3).

13. A Carnitine functions in transport of fatty acyl CoA esters formed in cytosol into the mitochondria (p. 382).

14. E A and D: It is important to realize that β-oxidation, itself, generates $FADH_2$ and NADH, which can be reoxidized to generate ATP. B: Carnitine transport to provide the substrate and reoxidation of reduced cofactors control β-oxidation. C: β-Oxidation is a general process requiring only minor modifications to oxidize nearly any fatty acid in the cell (p. 385, Table 9.4).

15. D A and E: β-Oxidation proceeds to completion; ketone bodies are formed by a separate process. B and C: Ketone bodies are formed, but not used, in liver mitochondria; cytosolic HMG CoA is a precursor of cholesterol (pp. 387–389).

16. D High glucagon/insulin ratio results in cAMP-mediated phosphorylations that activate hormone-sensitive lipase and inhibit acetyl-CoA carboxylase. Both of these, as well as other events, promote ketone body formation by greatly increasing acetyl CoA production in mitochondria, thereby assuring efficient uptake and utilization by brain (pp. 377, 381, 389).

17. B A and B: This is one of the differences between the peroxisomal and mitochondrial systems. C and E: Role seems to be to oxidize longer chain fatty acids to a point where mitochondrial oxidation can work. D: Except for the flavoprotein, the reactions are the same as the mitochondrial process (p. 390).

CHAPTER

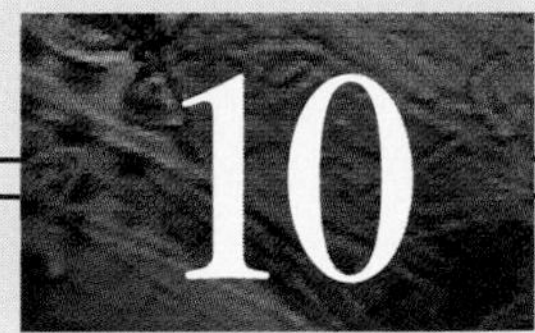

LIPID METABOLISM II: PATHWAYS OF METABOLISM OF SPECIAL LIPIDS

Robert H. Glew

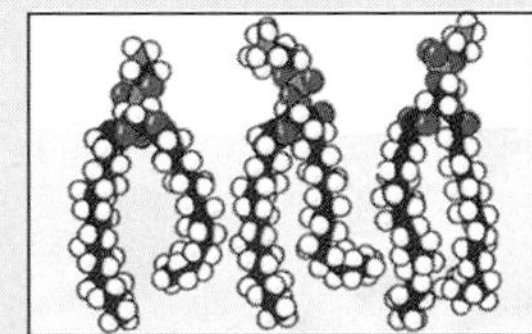

CLINICAL CORRELATIONS

10.1 ■ OVERVIEW

Lipid is a general term that describes substances that are relatively water insoluble and extractable by nonpolar solvents. Complex lipids of humans fall into one of two broad categories: nonpolar lipids, such as triacylglycerols and cholesterol esters, and polar lipids, which are amphipathic in that they contain both a hydrophobic domain and a hydrophilic region in the same molecule. This chapter discusses polar lipids including *phospholipids, sphingolipids,* and *eicosanoids*. The hydrophobic and hydrophilic regions are bridged by a glycerol moiety in glycerophospholipids and by sphingosine in sphingomyelin and glycosphingolipids. Triacylglycerol is confined largely to storage sites in adipose tissue, whereas polar lipids occur primarily in cellular membranes. Oils of soybean, oil palm, rapeseed, sunflower, cottonseed, and peanut account for 80% of worldwide plant oil production and consist mainly of palmitic, stearic, oleic, linoleic, and α-linolenic acids. Membranes generally contain 40% of their dry weight as lipid and 60% as protein.

Cell–cell recognition, phagocytosis, contact inhibition, and rejection of transplanted tissues and organs are all phenomena of medical significance that involve highly specific recognition sites on the surface of plasma membranes. Synthesis of the complex glycosphingolipids that play a role in these important biological events will be described. Glycolipids are worthy of study because ABO antigenic determinants of blood groups are primarily glycolipid in nature. In addition, various sphingolipids are the storage substances that accumulate in liver, spleen, kidney, or nervous tissue of persons suffering from certain genetic disorders called sphingolipidoses. In order to understand the basis of

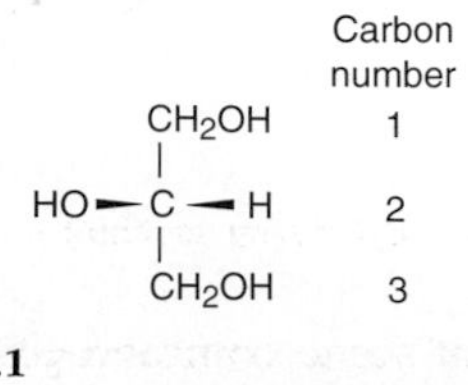

	Carbon number
CH_2OH	1
HO—C—H	2
CH_2OH	3

FIGURE 10.1
Stereospecific numbering of glycerol.

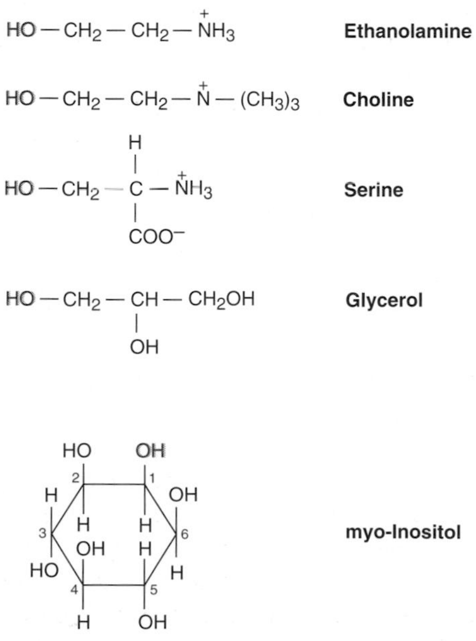

$HO-CH_2-CH_2-\overset{+}{N}H_3$ **Ethanolamine**

$HO-CH_2-CH_2-\overset{+}{N}-(CH_3)_3$ **Choline**

$HO-CH_2-CH(COO^-)-\overset{+}{N}H_3$ **Serine**

$HO-CH_2-CH(OH)-CH_2OH$ **Glycerol**

myo-Inositol

FIGURE 10.2
Structure of some common polar groups of phospholipids.

these enzyme-deficiency states, a knowledge of relevant chemical structures involved is required.

A very important lipid is *cholesterol*. This chapter describes the pathway of cholesterol biosynthesis and its regulation and shows how cholesterol functions as a precursor to bile salts and steroid hormones. Also described is the role of high-density lipoprotein (HDL) and lecithin:cholesterol acyltransferase (LCAT) in the management of plasma cholesterol.

Finally, the metabolism and function of two pharmacologically powerful classes of hormones derived from arachidonic acid, namely, prostaglandins and leukotrienes, will be discussed. See the Appendix, for a discussion of nomenclature and chemistry of lipids.

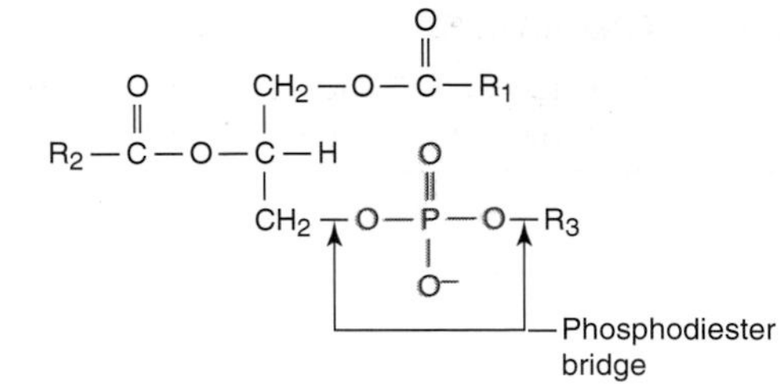

Phosphodiester bridge

FIGURE 10.3
Generalized structure of a phospholipid where R_1 and R_2 represent the aliphatic chains of fatty acids, and R_3 represents a polar group.

10.2 ■ PHOSPHOLIPIDS

Two principal classes of **acylglycerolipids** are **triacylglycerols** and **glycerophospholipids.** They are referred to as glycerolipids because the core of these compounds is provided by the C3 polyol, glycerol. Two primary alcohol groups of glycerol are not stereochemically identical and in the case of phospholipids, it is usually the same hydroxyl group that is esterified to the phosphate residue. The stereospecific numbering system is the best way to designate different hydroxyl groups. In this system, when the structure of glycerol is drawn in the Fischer projection with the C-2 hydroxyl group projecting to the left of the page, the carbon atoms are numbered as shown in Figure 10.1. When the stereospecific numbering (*sn*) system is employed, the prefix *sn*- is used before the name of the compound. Glycerophospholipids usually contain an *sn*-glycerol 3-phosphate moiety. Although each contains the glycerol moiety as a fundamental structural element, neutral triacylglycerols and charged ionic phospholipids have very different physical properties and functions.

Phospholipids Contain 1,2-Diacylglycerol and a Base Connected by a Phosphodiester Bridge

Phospholipids are polar, ionic lipids composed of 1,2-diacylglycerol and a phosphodiester bridge that links the glycerol backbone to some base, usually a nitrogenous one, such as choline, serine, or ethanolamine (Figures 10.2 and 10.3). The most abundant phospholipids in human tissues are **phosphatidylcholine** (also called lecithin), **phosphatidylethanolamine,** and **phosphatidylserine** (Figure 10.4). At physiologic pH, phosphatidylcholine and phosphatidylethanolamine have no net charge and exist as dipolar zwitterions, whereas phosphatidylserine has a net charge of −1, causing it to be an acidic phospholipid. Phosphatidylethanolamine (PE) is related to phosphatidylcholine in that trimethylation of PE produces lecithin. Most phospholipids contain more than one kind of fatty acid per molecule, so that a given class of phospholipids from any tissue actually represents a family of molecular species. Phosphatidylcholine (PC) contains mostly palmitic acid (16:0) or stearic acid (18:0) in the *sn*-1 position and primarily unsaturated C18 fatty acids oleic, linoleic, or α-linolenic in the *sn*-2 position. Phosphatidylethanolamine has the same saturated fatty acids as PC at the *sn*-1 position but contains more of the long-chain polyunsaturated fatty acids—namely, 18:2, 20:4, and 22:6—at the *sn*-2 position.

Phosphatidylinositol is an acidic phospholipid that occurs in mammalian membranes (Figure 10.5). Phosphatidylinositol is rather unusual because it often contains almost exclusively stearic acid in the *sn*-1 position and arachidonic acid (20:4) in the *sn*-2 position.

Another phospholipid comprised of a polyol polar head group is **phosphatidylglycerol** (Figure 10.5), which occurs in relatively large amounts in

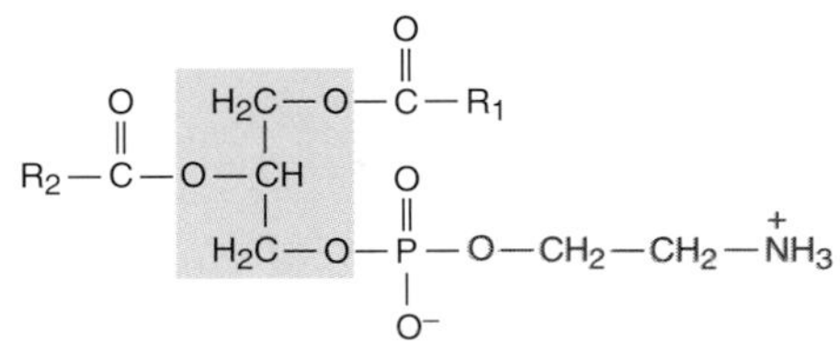

Phosphatidylethanolamine

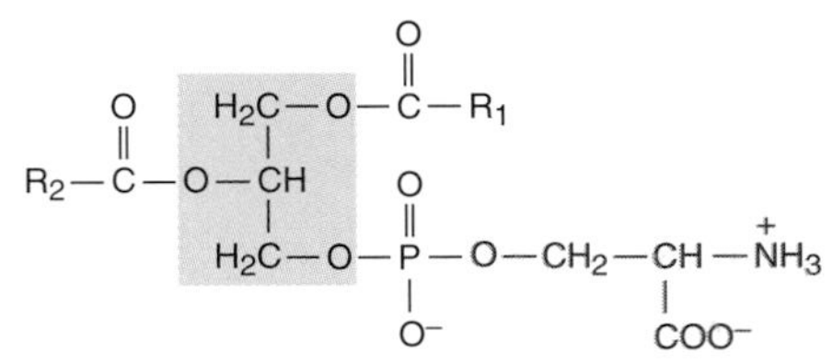

Phosphatidylserine

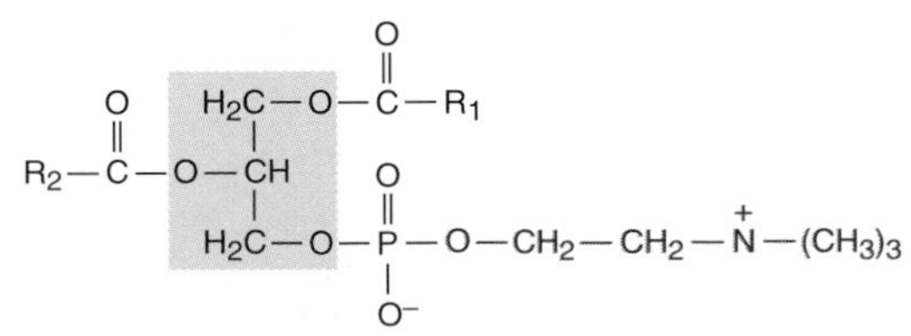

Phosphatidylcholine (lecithin)

FIGURE 10.4
Structures of some common phospholipids.

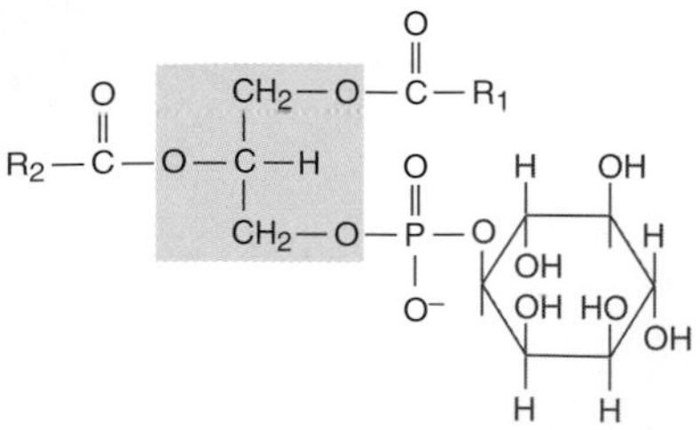

Phosphatidylinositol

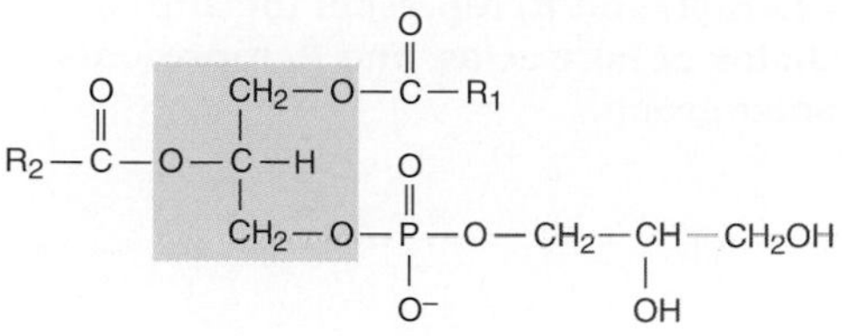

Phosphatidylglycerol

FIGURE 10.5
Structures of phosphatidylglycerol and phosphatidylinositol.

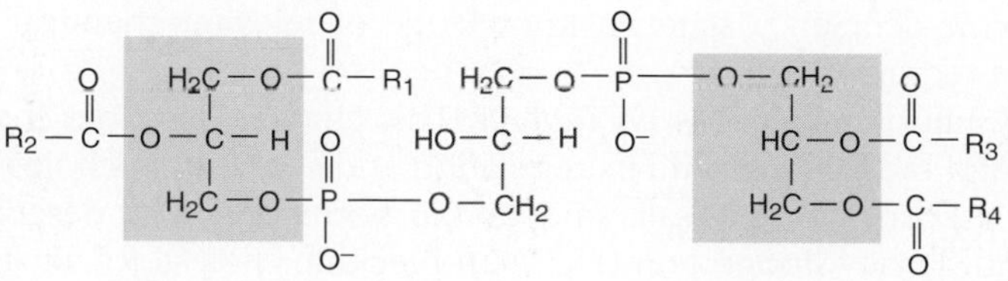

FIGURE 10.6
Structure of cardiolipin.

mitochondrial membranes and pulmonary surfactant and is a precursor of **cardiolipin.** Phosphatidylglycerol and phosphatidylinositol both carry a formal charge of −1 at neutral pH and are therefore acidic lipids. Cardiolipin, a very acidic (charge, −2) phospholipid, is composed of two molecules of phosphatidic acid linked together covalently through a molecule of glycerol (Figure 10.6). It occurs primarily in the inner membrane of mitochondria and in bacterial membranes.

Phospholipids mentioned so far contain only *O*-acyl residues attached to glycerol. *O*-(1-Alkenyl) substituents occur at C-1 of the *sn*-glycerol in phosphoglycerides in combination with an *O*-acyl residue esterified to the C-2 position; compounds in this class are known as **plasmalogens** (Figure 10.7). Relatively large amounts of ethanolamine plasmalogen (also called plasmenylethanolamine) occur in myelin with lesser amounts in heart muscle where choline plasmalogen is abundant.

An unusual phospholipid called **"platelet-activating factor"** (PAF) (Figure 10.8) is a major mediator of hypersensitivity, acute inflammatory reactions and anaphylactic shock. In hypersensitive individuals, cells of the polymorphonuclear (PMN) leukocyte family (basophils, neutrophils, and eosinophils), macrophages, and monocytes are coated with IgE molecules that are specific for a particular antigen (e.g., ragweed pollen and bee venom). Subsequent reexposure to the antigen and formation of antigen–IgE complexes on the surface of the aforementioned inflammatory cells provoke synthesis and release of PAF. Platelet-activating factor contains an *O*-alkyl moiety at the *sn*-1 position and an acetyl residue instead of a long-chain fatty acid (e.g., stearic acid) in position 2 of the glycerol moiety. PAF is not stored; it is synthesized and released when PMNs are stimulated. Platelet aggregation, cardiovascular and pulmonary changes, edema, hypotension, and PMN cell chemotaxis are affected by PAF.

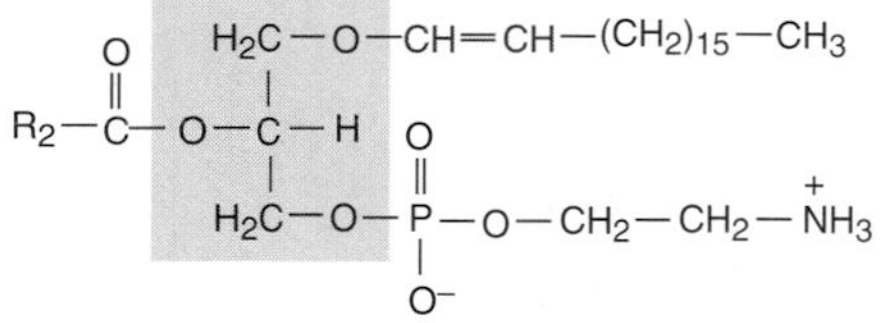

FIGURE 10.7
Structure of ethanolamine plasmalogen.

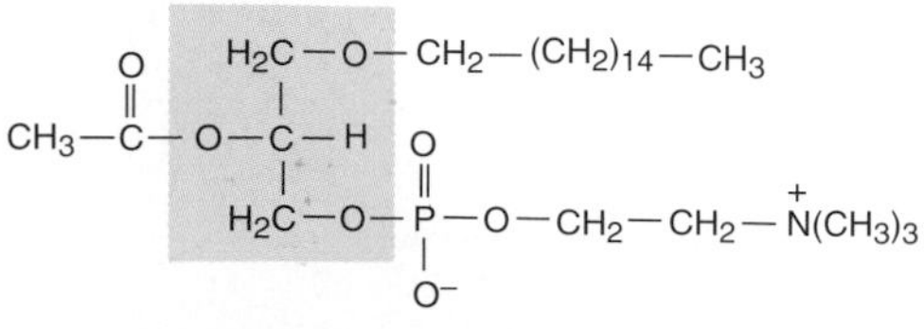

FIGURE 10.8
Structure of platelet activating factor (PAF).

Phospholipids in Membranes Serve a Variety of Roles

Although present in body fluids such as plasma and bile, phospholipids are found in highest concentration in various cellular membranes where they serve as structural and functional components. Nearly one-half the mass of the erythrocyte membrane is comprised of various phospholipids (see Chapter 5). Phospholipids also activate certain enzymes. β-Hydroxybutyrate dehydrogenase, an enzyme imbedded in the inner membrane of mitochondria (see p. 388), has an absolute requirement for phosphatidylcholine; phosphatidylserine and phosphatidylethanolamine cannot substitute.

Dipalmitoyllecithin Is Necessary for Normal Lung Function

Normal lung function depends on a constant supply of **dipalmitoyllecithin** in which the lecithin molecule contains palmitic acid (16:0) residues in both the *sn*-1 and *sn*-2 positions. More than 80% of the phospholipid in the extracellular liquid layer that lines alveoli of normal lungs is dipalmitoyllecithin. This particular phospholipid, called **surfactant,** is produced by type II epithelial cells and prevents atelectasis at the end of the expiration phase of breathing

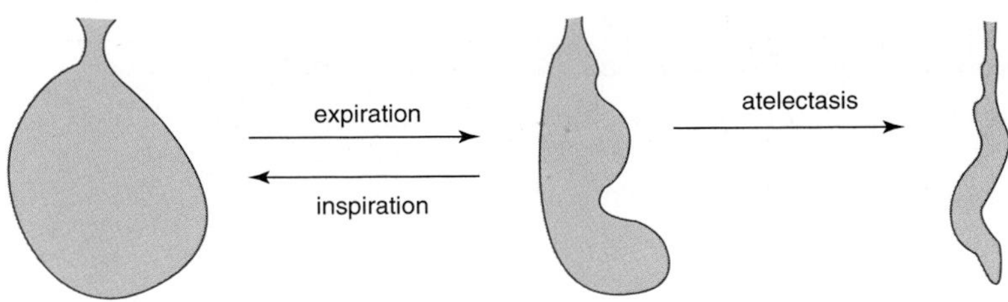

FIGURE 10.9
Role of surfactant in preventing atelectasis.

(Figure 10.9). This lipid decreases surface tension of the aqueous surface layer of the lung. Lecithin molecules that do not contain two residues of palmitic acid are not effective in lowering surface tension of the fluid layer lining alveoli. Surfactant also contains phosphatidylglycerol, phosphatidylinositol, and 18- and 36-kDa proteins (designated surfactant proteins), which contribute significantly to the surface tension lowering property of pulmonary surfactant.

During the third trimester—before the 28th week of gestation—fetal lung synthesizes primarily sphingomyelin. Normally, at this time, glycogen that has been stored in epithelial type II cells is converted to fatty acids and then to dipalmitoyllecithin. During lung maturation there is a good correlation between increase in lamellar inclusion bodies that represent the intracellular pulmonary surfactant (phosphatidylcholine) storage organelles, called lamellar bodies, and the simultaneous decrease in glycogen content of type II pneumocytes. At the 24th week of gestation the type II granular pneumocytes appear in the alveolar epithelium, and within a few days they produce their typical osmiophilic lamellar inclusion bodies. The number of type II cells increases until the 32nd week, at which time surface active agent appears in the lung and amniotic fluid. Surface tension decreases when inclusion bodies increase in the type II cells. In the few weeks before term one can perform screening tests on amniotic fluid to detect newborns that are at risk for respiratory distress syndrome (RDS) (see Clin. Corr. 10.1). These tests are useful in timing elective deliveries, in applying vigorous preventive therapy to the newborn infant, and to determine if the mother should be treated with a glucocorticoid drug to accelerate maturation of the fetal lung. Dexamethasone therapy has also been used in neonates with chronic lung disease (bronchopulmonary dysplasia); however, while such corticosteroid therapy may be effective in some cases in improving lung function, in others it causes periventricular abnormalities in the brain.

Respiratory failure due to an insufficiency in surfactant can also occur in adults whose type II cells or surfactant-producing pneumocytes have been destroyed as an adverse side effect of the use of immunosuppressive medications or chemotherapeutic drugs.

The **detergent properties** of phospholipids, especially phosphatidylcholine, play an important role in bile where they function to solubilize cholesterol. An impairment in phospholipid production and secretion into bile can result in formation of cholesterol stones and bile pigment gallstones. Phosphatidylinositol and phosphatidylcholine also serve as sources of arachidonic acid for synthesis of prostaglandins, thromboxanes, leukotrienes, and related compounds.

Inositides Play a Role in Signal Transduction

Inositol-containing phospholipids (inositides) play a central role in signal transduction systems; the most important is **phosphatidylinositol 4,5-bisphosphate** (PIP_2) (Figure 10.10). When certain ligands bind to their respective receptors on the plasma membrane of mammalian cells (see Chapter 19), PIP_2

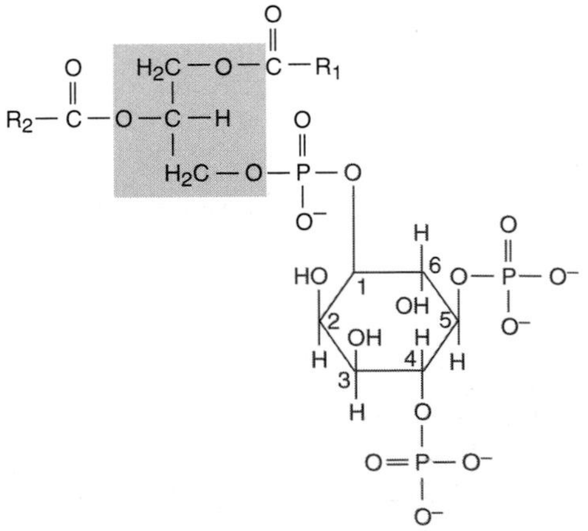

FIGURE 10.10
Structure of phosphatidylinositol 4,5-bisphosphate (PIP_2 or PtdIns $(4,5)P_2$).

CLINICAL CORRELATION 10.1

Respiratory Distress Syndrome

Respiratory distress syndrome (RDS) is a major cause of neonatal morbidity and mortality in many countries. It accounts for approximately 15–20% of all neonatal deaths in Western countries and somewhat less in developing countries. The disease affects only premature babies and its incidence varies directly with the degree of prematurity. Premature babies develop RDS because of immaturity of their lungs, resulting from a deficiency of pulmonary surfactant. The maturity of the fetal lung can be predicted antenatally by measuring the lecithin/sphingomyelin (L/S) ratio in the amniotic fluid. The mean L/S ratio in normal pregnancies increases gradually with gestation until about 31 or 32 weeks when the slope rises sharply. The ratio of 2.0 that is characteristic of the term infant at birth is achieved at the gestational age of about 34 weeks. For predicting pulmonary maturity, the critical L/S ratio is 2.0 or greater. The risk of developing RDS when the L/S ratio is 1.5–1.9 is approximately 40%, and for a ratio less than 1.5 about 75%. Although the L/S ratio in amniotic fluid is still widely used to predict the risk of RDS, the results are unreliable if the amniotic fluid specimen has been contaminated by blood or meconium obtained during a complicated pregnancy.

In recent years determinations of saturated palmitoylphosphatidylcholine (SPC), phosphatidylglycerol, and phosphatidylinositol have been found to be additional predictors of the risk of RDS. Exogenous surfactant replacement therapy using surfactant from human and animal lungs is effective in the prevention and treatment of RDS.

Merritt, T. A., Hallman, M., Bloom, B.T., et al. Prophylactic treatment of very premature infants with human surfactant. *N. Engl. J. Med.* 315:785, 1986; and Simon, N. V., Williams, G. H., Fairbrother, P. F., Elser, R. C., and Perkins, R. P. Prediction of fetal lung maturity by amniotic fluid fluorescence polarization, L/S ratio, and phosphatidylglycerol. *Obstet. Gynecol.* 57:295, 1981.

localized to the inner leaflet of the membrane becomes a substrate for a receptor-dependent phosphoinositidase C (PIC), which hydrolyzes it into two intracellular signals (Figure 10.11): **inositol 1,4,5-trisphosphate** (IP_3), which triggers release of Ca^{2+} from special vesicles of the endoplasmic reticulum, and **1,2-diacylglycerol,** which stimulates activity of protein kinase C. Regulatory functions of these products of the PIC reaction are discussed in Chapter 19. Phosphatidic acid, a product of phospholipase D action on phospholipids, has been implicated as a second messenger.

The complex pathways of inositol phosphate metabolism serve three roles: (1) removal and inactivation of the potent intracellular signal IP_3; (2) conservation of inositol; and (3) synthesis of polyphosphates such as inositol pentakis-

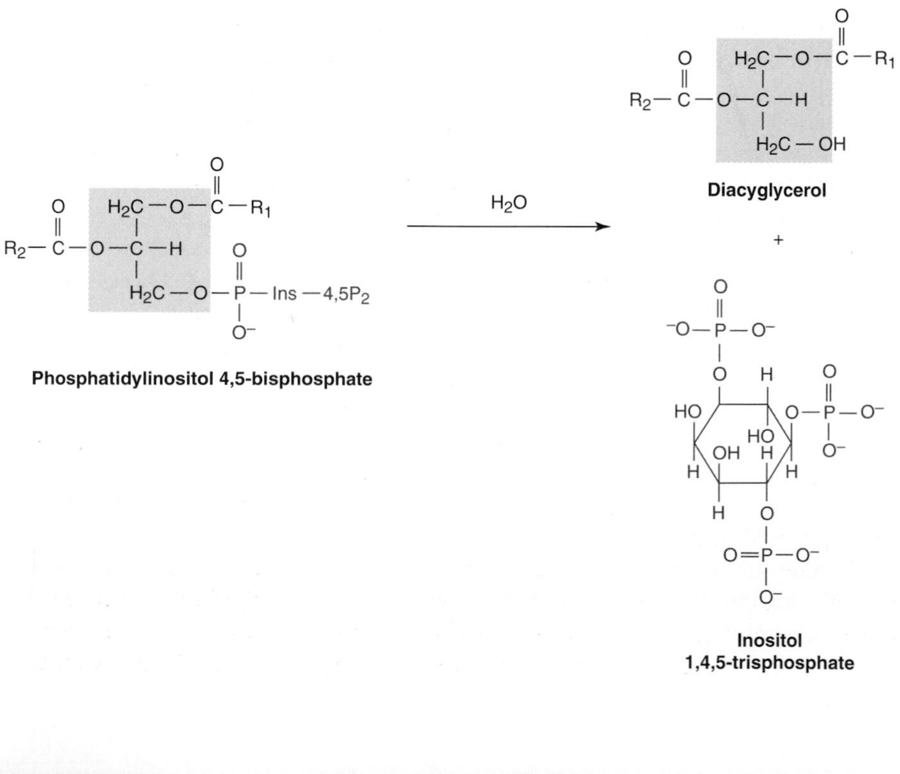

Phosphatidylinositol 4,5-bisphosphate

H_2O

Diacylglycerol

+

Inositol 1,4,5-trisphosphate

FIGURE 10.11
Generation of 1,2-diacylglycerol and inositol 1,4,5-trisphosphate by action of phospholipase C on phosphatidylinositol 4,5-bisphosphate.

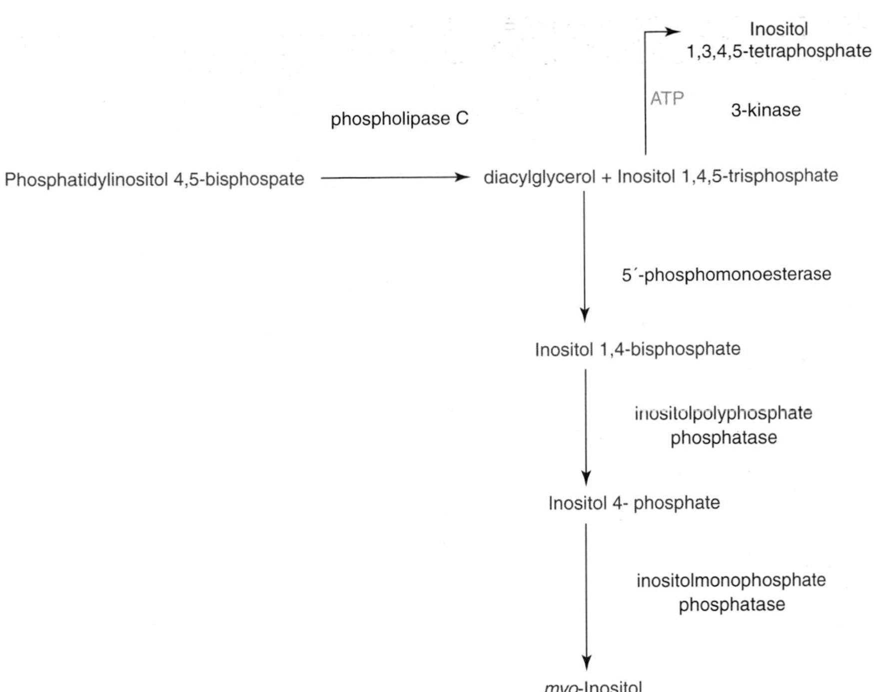

FIGURE 10.12
Pathways for the removal of intracellular inositol 1,4,5-trisphosphate.

phosphate ($InsP_5$) and inositol hexakisphosphate ($InsP_6$) whose functions have not been determined. Inositol 1,4,5-trisphosphate is metabolized by two enzymes: first a 5-phosphomonoesterase that converts IP_3 to inositol 1,4-bisphosphate and second a 3-kinase that forms inositol 1,3,4,5-tetraphosphate. A family of phosphatases in turn convert Ins(1,4)P_2 to *myo*-inositol (Figure 10.12). Inositol is eventually reincorporated into the phospholipid pool.

Phosphatidylinositol Serves to Anchor Glycoproteins to the Plasma Membrane

In addition to its role as a structural component of membranes and source of arachidonic acid for prostaglandin and leukotriene synthesis (see p. 431), phosphatidylinositol serves as an anchor to tether certain glycoproteins to the external surface of plasma membranes. In trypanosomal parasites (e.g., *Trypanosoma brucei,* which causes sleeping sickness), the external surface of the plasma membrane is coated with a protein called **variable surface glycoprotein** (VSG) linked to the membrane through a glycophospholipid anchor, specifically phosphatidylinositol (Figure 10.13). The salient structural features of the protein–lipid linkage region of the **glycosylphosphatidylinositol** (GPI) **anchor** are: (1) the diacylglyceride (DAG) moiety of phosphatidylinositol is integrated into the outer leaflet of the lipid bilayer of the plasma membrane; (2) the inositol residue is linked to DAG through a phosphodiester bond; (3) inositol is bonded to glucosamine, which contains a free, unacetylated amino group; (4) the presence of a mannose-rich glycan domain; and (5) a phosphoethanolamine residue linked to the carboxy terminus of the protein. Depending on the protein to which it is attached and the tissue or organism in which it is expressed, the GPI core may be decorated with additional carbohydrates and phosphatidylethanolamines that extend from the core mannoses; these include mannose, glucose, galactose, *N*-acetylgalactose, *N*-acetylneuraminic acid, and *N*-acetylgalactosamine. Some other proteins that are attached to the external surface of the plasma membrane include acetylcholine esterase, alkaline phosphatase, and 5′-nucleotidase.

The GPI anchor serves several functions. First, it confers on the protein to which it is attached unrestricted lateral mobility within the lipid bilayer, thereby allowing the protein to move about rapidly on the surface of the plasma membrane. Second, the presence of phospholipase C-type activity on the cell surface

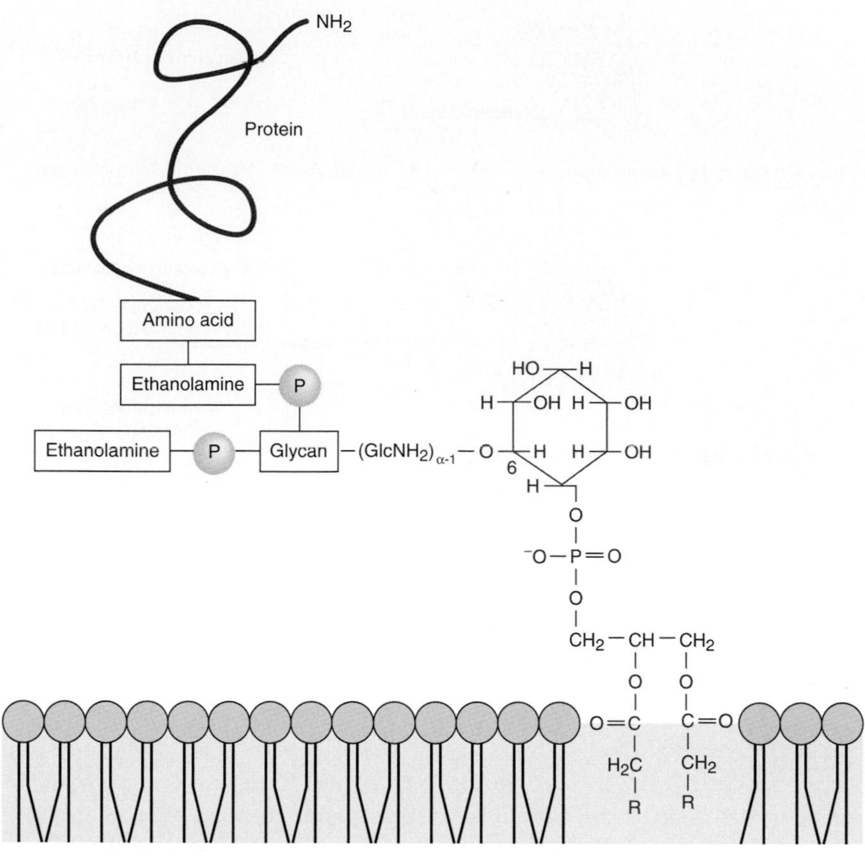

FIGURE 10.13
Structure of a typical phosphatidylinositol membrane protein anchor; $GlcNH_2$, glucosamine.

permits shedding of the phosphatidylinositol-anchored protein. As an example, this provides trypanosomes with a means for discarding surface antigens, thus changing their coat and escaping antibodies of the host's immune system. Third, the action of phospholipase C on the phosphatidylinositol anchor releases diacylglyceride, a second messenger that can activate protein kinase C (see p. 865). Biosynthesis of GPI anchors has been characterized extensively.

Other types of protein lipidation (co- or posttranslational modification of proteins by specific lipids) include *N*-myristoylation at the amino terminus of proteins, *S*-palmitoylation at internal cysteines, and *S*-prenylation by farnesyl or geranylgeranyl residues at cysteines at the carboxyl terminus of proteins.

Biosynthesis of Phospholipids

Phosphatidic Acid Is Synthesized from α-Glycerophosphate and Fatty Acyl CoA

l-α-Phosphatidic acid (commonly called phosphatidic acid) and 1,2-diacyl-*sn*-glycerol are common intermediates in the pathways of phospholipid and triacylglycerol biosynthesis (Figure 10.14) and both pathways share some of the same enzymes (see Chapter 9). Essentially all cells are capable of synthesizing phospholipids to some degree (except mature erythrocytes), whereas triacylglycerol biosynthesis occurs only in liver, adipose tissue, and intestine. In most tissues, the pathway for phosphatidic acid synthesis begins with α-glycerophosphate (*sn*-glycerol 3-phosphate). The most general source of α-glycerophosphate, particularly in adipose tissue, is from reduction of the glycolytic intermediate, dihydroxyacetone phosphate, in the reaction catalyzed by α-glycerophosphate dehydrogenase:

$$\text{Dihydroxyacetone phosphate} + \text{NADH} + \text{H}^+ \rightleftharpoons \alpha\text{-glycerol 3-phosphate} + \text{NAD}^+$$

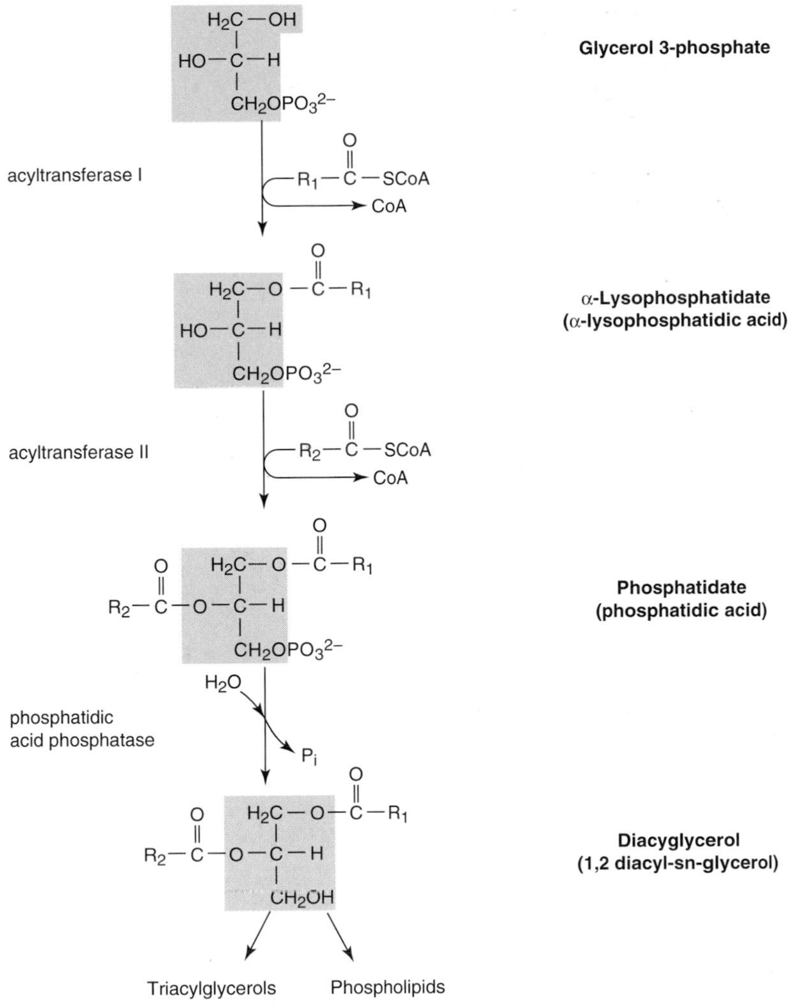

FIGURE 10.14
Phosphatidic acid biosynthesis from glycerol 3-phosphate and the role of phosphatidic acid phosphatase in synthesis of phospholipids and triacylglycerols.

A few specialized tissues, including liver and kidney, derive α-glycerophosphate by means of the glycerol kinase reaction:

$$\text{Glycerol} + \text{ATP} \overset{Mg^{2+}}{\rightleftharpoons} \alpha\text{-glycerol 3-phosphate} + \text{ADP}$$

The next two steps in phosphatidic acid biosynthesis involve stepwise transfer of long-chain fatty acyl groups from fatty acyl CoA. The first acyltransferase (I) is called **glycerol phosphate:acyltransferase** and attaches predominantly saturated fatty acids or oleic acid to the *sn*-1 to produce 1-acylglycerol phosphate or α-lysophosphatidic acid. The second enzyme (II), **1-acylglycerol phosphate:acyltransferase,** acylates the *sn*-2 position, usually with an unsaturated fatty acid (Figure 10.14). In both cases the donor of acyl groups is the CoA thioester derivative of the appropriate long-chain fatty acid.

The specificity of the two acyltransferases does not always match the fatty acid asymmetry found in the phospholipids of a particular cell. Remodeling reactions, discussed below, modify the fatty acid composition at C-1 and C-2 of the glycerol phosphate backbone.

Cytosolic phosphatidic acid phosphatase (also called phosphatidic acid phosphohydrolase) hydrolyzes phosphatidic acid (1,2-diacylglycerophosphate) that is generated on the endoplasmic reticulum, thereby yielding 1,2-diacyl-*sn*-glycerol that serves as the branch point in triacylglycerol and phospholipid synthesis (Figure 10.14). Phosphatidic acid can also be formed by a second pathway that begins with DHAP. This is usually an alternative supportive route used by some tissues to produce phosphatidic acid (see Chapter 9).

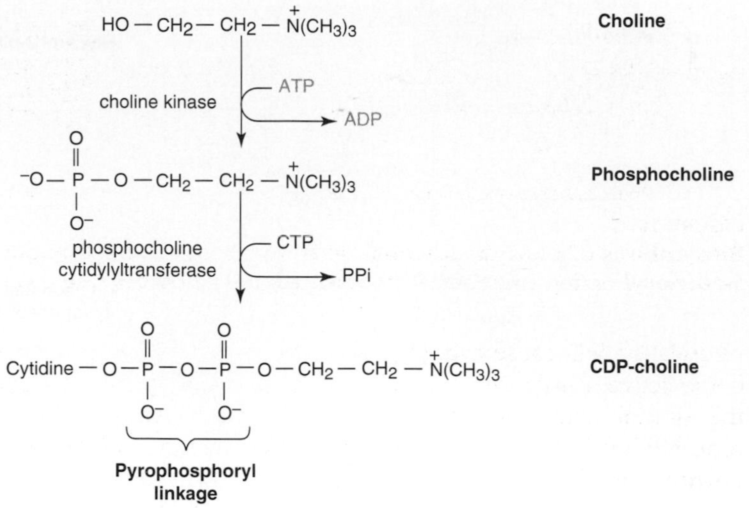

HO — CH_2 — CH_2 — $\overset{+}{N}(CH_3)_3$ Choline

choline kinase (ATP → ADP)

^-O — P(=O)(O$^-$) — O — CH_2 — CH_2 — $\overset{+}{N}(CH_3)_3$ Phosphocholine

phosphocholine cytidylyltransferase (CTP → PPi)

Cytidine — O — P(=O)(O$^-$) — O — P(=O)(O$^-$) — O — CH_2 — CH_2 — $\overset{+}{N}(CH_3)_3$ CDP-choline

Pyrophosphoryl linkage

FIGURE 10.15
Biosynthesis of CDP-choline from choline.

Specific Phospholipids Are Synthesized by Addition of a Base to Diacylglycerol

The major pathway for biosynthesis of phosphatidylcholine (lecithin) involves sequential conversion of choline to phosphocholine, CDP-choline, and phosphatidylcholine. In this pathway, the phosphocholine polar head group is activated using CTP, according to the following reactions. Free choline, a dietary requirement for most mammals, is first phosphorylated by ATP by choline kinase (Figure 10.15). Phosphocholine is converted to CDP-choline at the expense of CTP in the reaction catalyzed by **phosphocholine cytidylyltransferase.** Note inorganic pyrophosphate (PP_i) is a product of this reaction. The high-energy pyrophosphoryl bond in CDP-choline is very unstable and reactive so that the phosphocholine moiety can be transferred readily to the nucleophilic center provided by the OH group at position 3 of 1,2-diacylglycerol by choline phosphotransferase (Figure 10.16). This is the principal pathway for the synthesis of dipalmitoyllecithin in lung.

The rate-limiting step for phosphatidylcholine biosynthesis is the cytidylyltransferase reaction that forms CDP-choline (Figure 10.15). This enzyme is regulated by a novel mechanism involving exchange of enzyme between cytosol and endoplasmic reticulum. The cytosolic form of cytidylyltransferase is inactive and appears to function as a reservoir of enzyme; binding of the enzyme to the membrane results in activation. Translocation of cytidylyltransferase from the cytosol to the endoplasmic reticulum is regulated by cAMP and fatty acids. Reversible phosphorylation of the enzyme by a cAMP-dependent kinase causes it to be released from the membrane, rendering it inactive. Subsequent dephos-

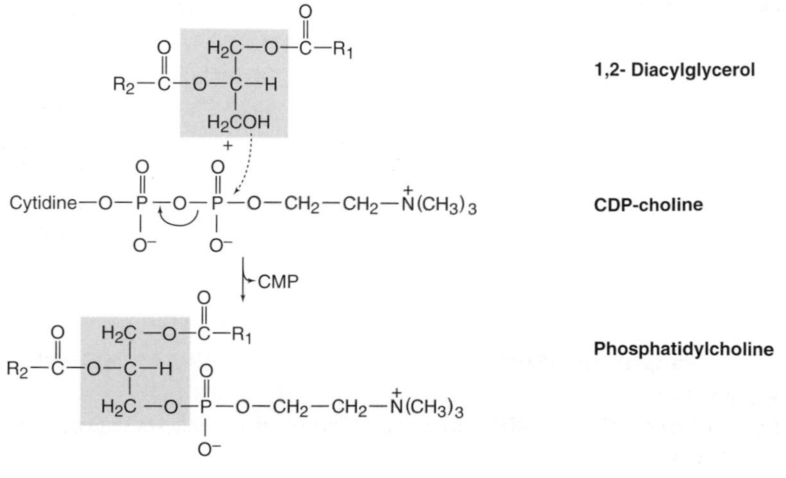

R_2—C(=O)—O—C—H with H_2C—O—C(=O)—R_1 and H_2COH 1,2- Diacylglycerol

\+

Cytidine—O—P(=O)(O$^-$)—O—P(=O)(O$^-$)—O—CH_2—CH_2—$\overset{+}{N}(CH_3)_3$ CDP-choline

→ CMP

R_2—C(=O)—O—C—H with H_2C—O—C(=O)—R_1 and H_2C—O—P(=O)(O$^-$)—O—CH_2—CH_2—$\overset{+}{N}(CH_3)_3$ Phosphatidylcholine

FIGURE 10.16
Choline phosphotransferase reaction.

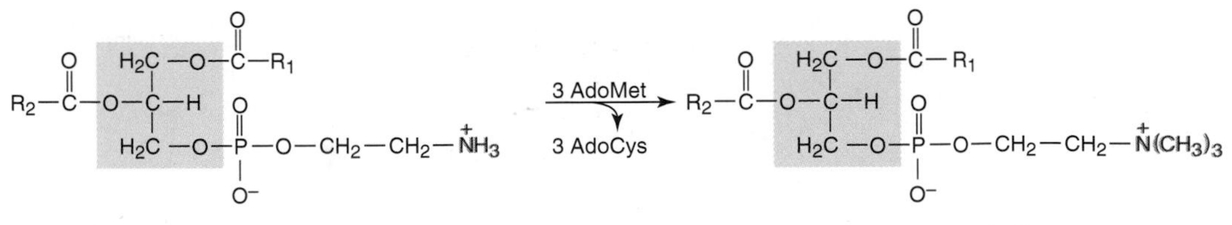

Phosphatidylethanolamine —(3 AdoMet → 3 AdoCys)→ Phosphatidylcholine

FIGURE 10.17
Biosynthesis of phosphatidylcholine from phosphatidylethanolamine and *S*-adenosylmethionine (AdoMet) and *S*-adenosylhomocysteine (AdoCys).

phorylation will cause cytidylyltransferase to rebind to the membrane and become active. Fatty acyl CoAs activate the enzyme by promoting its binding to the endoplasmic reticulum. In liver only, phosphatidylcholine is formed by repeated methylation of phosphatidylethanolamine. **Phosphatidylethanolamine *N*-methyltransferase,** an enzyme of the endoplasmic reticulum, catalyzes transfer of methyl groups one at a time from ***S*-adenosylmethionine (AdoMet)** to phosphatidylethanolamine to produce phosphatidylcholine (Figure 10.17).

The primary pathway for phosphatidylethanolamine synthesis in liver and brain involves **ethanolamine phosphotransferase** of the endoplasmic reticulum that catalyzes the reaction shown in Figure 10.18. This enzyme is particularly abundant in liver. CDP-ethanolamine is formed by **ethanolamine kinase:**

$$\text{Ethanolamine} + \text{ATP} \xrightleftharpoons{Mg^{2+}} \text{phosphoethanolamine} + \text{ADP}$$

and **phosphoethanolamine cytidylyltransferase:**

$$\text{Phosphoethanolamine} + \text{CTP} \xrightleftharpoons{Mg^{2+}} \text{CDP-ethanolamine} + PP_i$$

Liver mitochondria also generate phosphatidylethanolamine by decarboxylation of phosphatidylserine; however, this is thought to represent only a minor pathway (Figure 10.19).

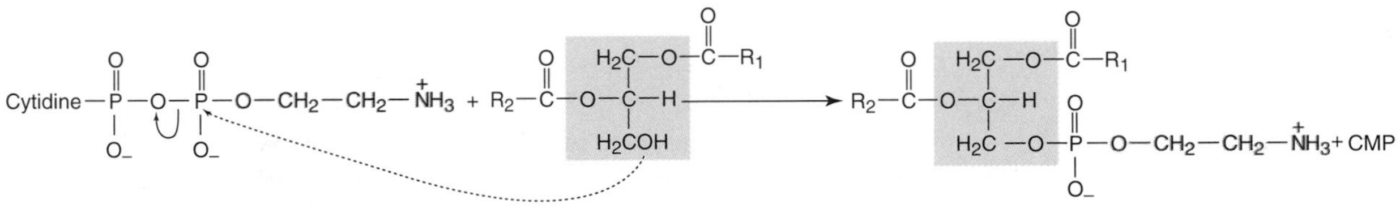

CDP-ethanolamine + 1,2- Diacylglycerol → Phosphatidylethanolamine + CMP

FIGURE 10.18
Biosynthesis of phosphatidylethanolamine from CDP-ethanolamine and diacylglycerol; the reaction is catalyzed by ethanolamine phosphotransferase.

Phosphatidylserine + H^+ → Phosphatidylethanolamine + CO_2

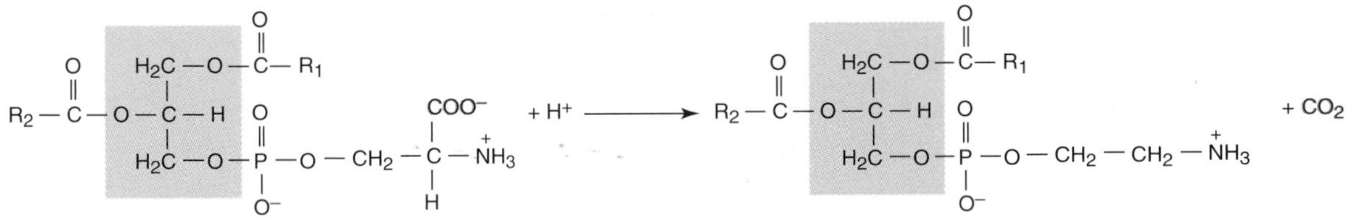

FIGURE 10.19
Formation of phosphatidylethanolamine by the decarboxylation of phosphatidylserine.

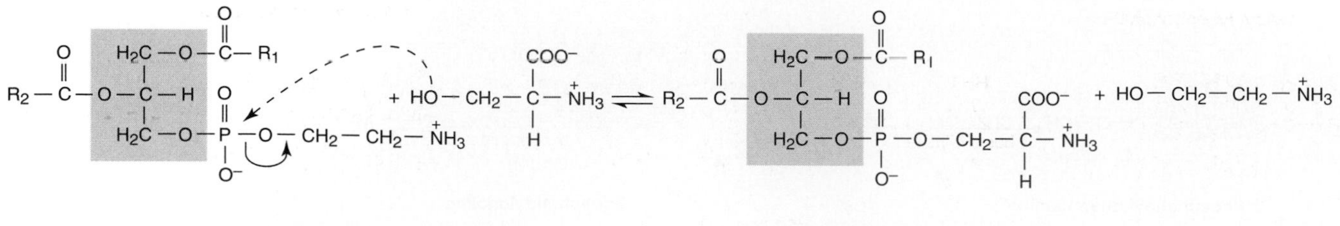

Phosphatidylethanolamine Serine Phosphatidylserine Ethanolamine

FIGURE 10.20
Biosynthesis of phosphatidylserine from serine and phosphatidylethanolamine by "base exchange."

The major source of phosphatidylserine in mammalian tissues is provided by the "base-exchange" reaction (Figure 10.20) in which the polar head group of phosphatidylethanolamine is exchanged for serine. Since there is no net change in the number or kinds of bonds, this reaction is reversible and has no requirement for ATP or any other high-energy compound. The reaction is initiated by attack on the phosphodiester bond of phosphatidylethanolamine by the hydroxyl group of serine.

Phosphatidylinositol is made via CDP-diacylglycerol and free *myo*-inositol (Figure 10.21) in a reaction catalyzed by **phosphatidylinositol synthase,** another enzyme of the endoplasmic reticulum.

The Asymmetric Distribution of Fatty Acids in Phospholipids Is Due to Remodeling Reactions

Two phospholipases, phospholipase A_1 and phospholipase A_2, occur in many tissues and play a role in the formation of specific phospholipid structures containing appropriate fatty acids in the *sn*-1 and *sn*-2 positions. Most fatty acyl CoA transferases and phospholipid synthesizing enzymes discussed above lack the specificity required to account for the asymmetric position or distribution of fatty acids found in many tissue phospholipids. The fatty acids found in the *sn*-1 and *sn*-2 positions of the various phospholipids are often not the same ones transferred to the glycerol backbone in the initial acyl transferase reactions of the phospholipid biosynthetic pathways. **Phospholipases A_1 and A_2** catalyze reactions indicated in Figure 10.22 where X represents the polar head group of a phospholipid. The products of the action of phospholipases A_1 and A_2 are called lysophosphatides.

If it becomes necessary for a cell to remove some undesired fatty acid, such as stearic acid from the *sn*-2 position of phosphatidylcholine, and replace it by a more unsaturated one like arachidonic acid, then this can be accomplished by the action of phospholipase A_2 followed by a reacylation reaction. Insertion of arachidonic acid into the 2 position of *sn*-2-lysophosphatidylcholine can

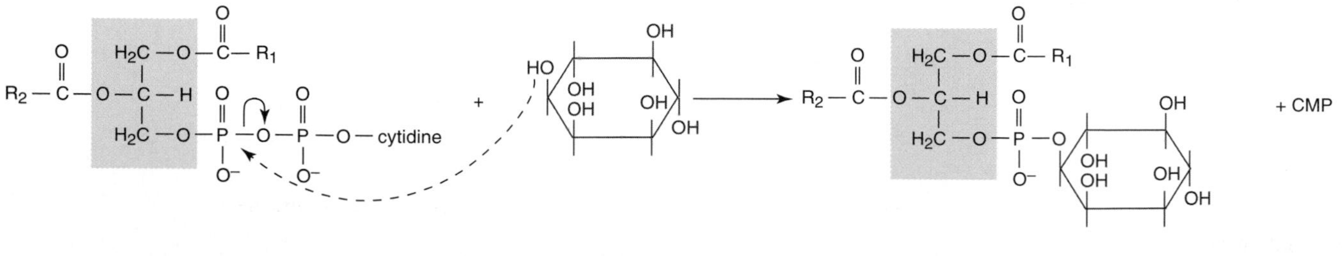

CDP-diacylglycerol Inositol Phosphatidylinositol

FIGURE 10.21
Biosynthesis of phosphatidylinositol.

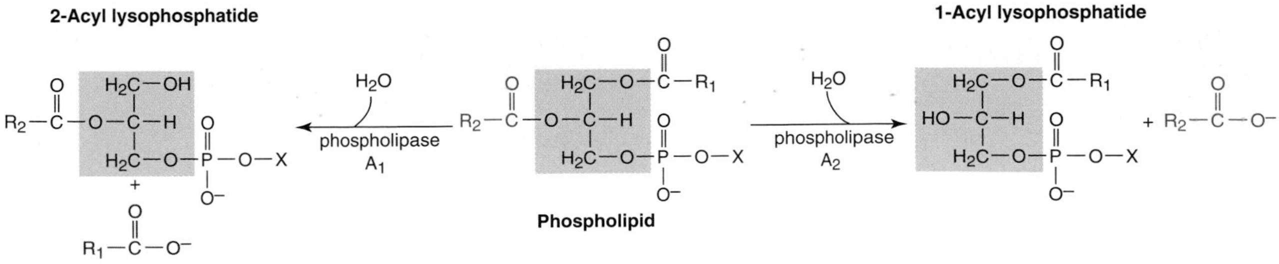

2-Acyl lysophosphatide

1-Acyl lysophosphatide

Phospholipid

phospholipase A_1

phospholipase A_2

FIGURE 10.22
Reactions catalyzed by phospholipase A_1 and phospholipase A_2.

be accomplished either by direct acylation from arachidonoyl CoA involving **arachidonic acid-specific acyl CoA transacylase** (Figure 10.23) or from some other arachidonic acid-containing phospholipid by an exchange-type reaction (Figure 10.24) catalyzed by **lysolecithin:lecithin acyltransferase** (LLAT) (Figure 10.24). Since there is no change in either number or nature of the bonds involved in products and reactants, ATP is not required. Reacylation of lysophosphatidylcholine from acyl CoA is the major route for remodeling of phosphatidylcholine.

Lysophospholipids, particularly *sn*-1-lysophosphatidylcholine, can also serve as sources of fatty acid in remodeling reactions. Those involved in synthe-

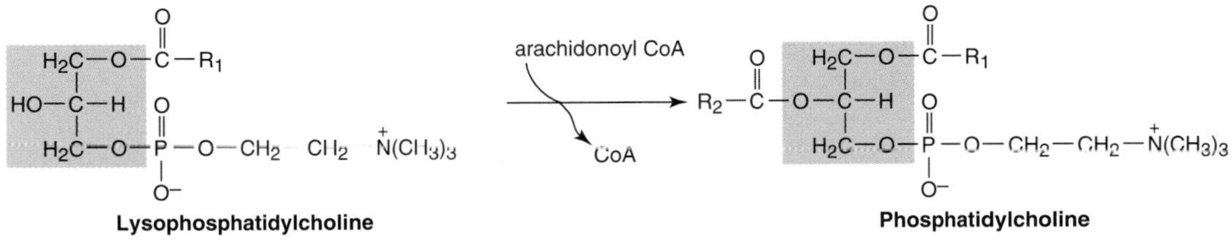

Lysophosphatidylcholine

arachidonoyl CoA

CoA

Phosphatidylcholine

FIGURE 10.23
Synthesis of phosphatidylcholine by reacylation of lysophosphatidylcholine where R_2—C(=O)—O— represents arachidonic acid.
This reaction is catalyzed by acyl CoA:1-acylglycerol-3-phosphocholine *O*-acyltransferase.

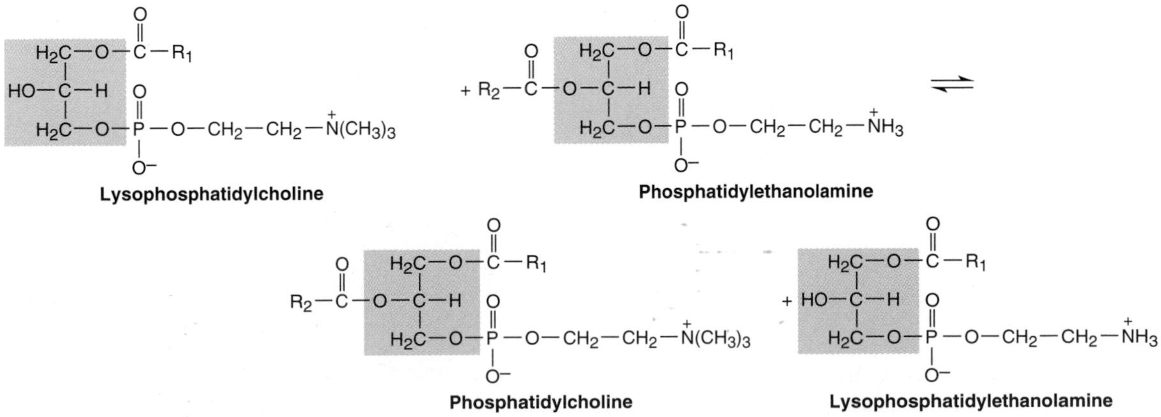

Lysophosphatidylcholine

Phosphatidylethanolamine

Phosphatidylcholine

Lysophosphatidylethanolamine

FIGURE 10.24
Formation of phosphatidylcholine by lysolecithin exchange, where R_2—C(=O)—O— represents arachidonic acid.

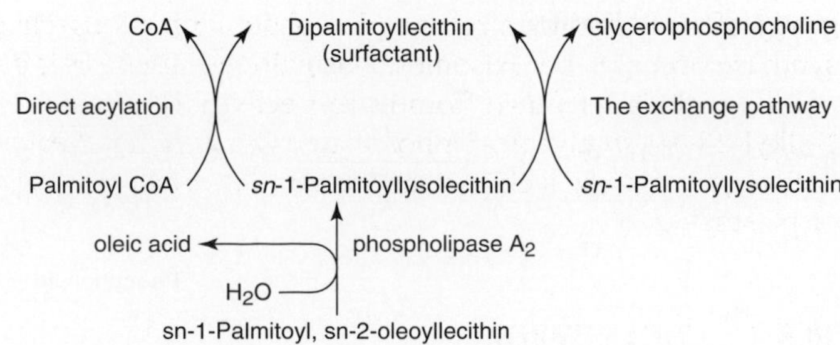

FIGURE 10.25
Two pathways for biosynthesis of dipalmitoyllecithin from *sn*-1 palmitoyl-lysolecithin.

sis of dipalmitoyllecithin (surfactant) from 1-palmitoyl-2-oleoylphosphatidylcholine are presented in Figure 10.25. Note that *sn*-1-palmitoyllysolecithin is the source of palmitic acid in the acyltransferase exchange reaction.

Plasmalogens Are Synthesized from Fatty Alcohols

Ether glycerolipids are synthesized from DHAP, long-chain fatty acids, and long-chain fatty alcohols; the reactions are summarized in Figure 10.26. Acyldihydroxyacetone phosphate is formed by **acyl CoA: dihydroxyacetone phosphate acyltransferase** (enzyme 1) acting on dihydroxyacetone phosphate and long-chain fatty acyl CoA. The ether bond is introduced by **dihydroxyacetone phosphate synthase** (Figure 10.26, enzyme 2), which exchanges the 1-*O*-acyl

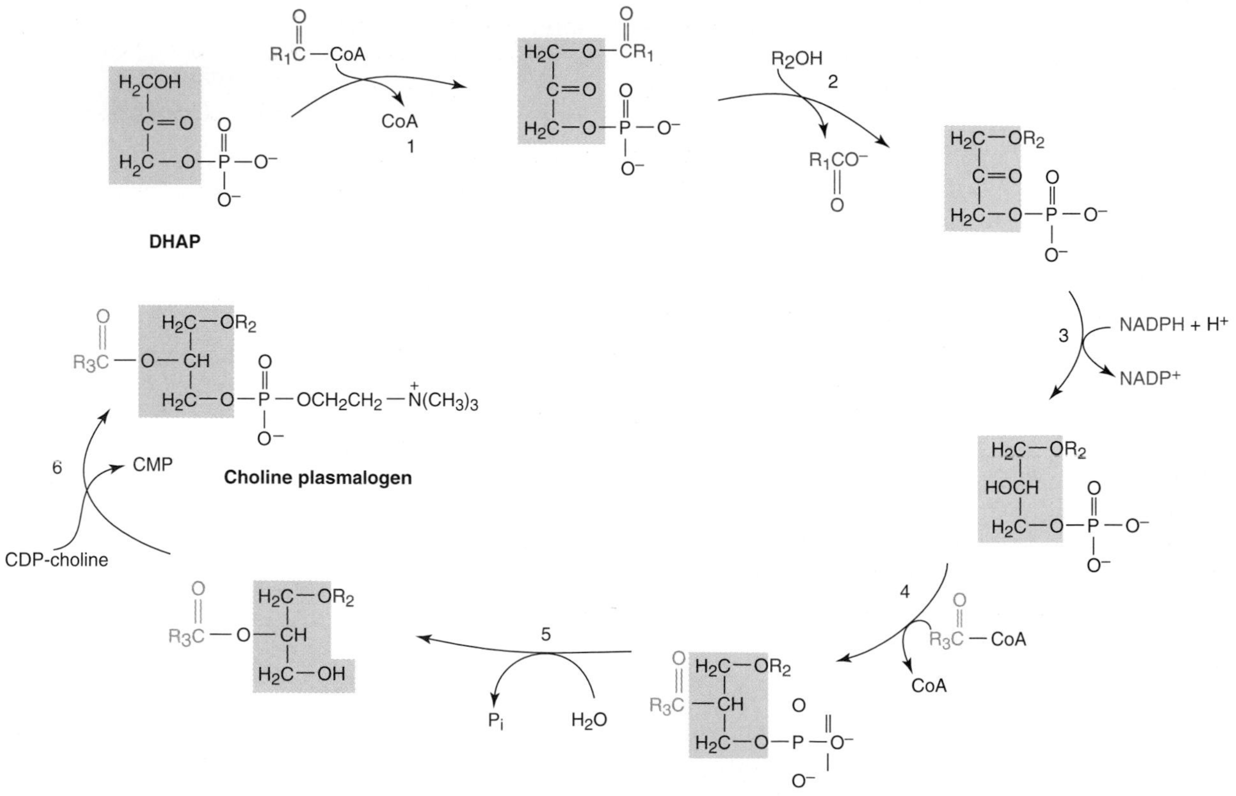

FIGURE 10.26
Pathway of choline plasmalogen biosynthesis from DHAP.
1, acyl CoA: dihydroxyacetone phosphate acyltransferase; 2, alkyldihydroxyacetone phosphate synthase; 3, NADPH: alkyldihydroxyacetone phosphate oxidoreductase; 4, acyl CoA:1-alkyl-2-lyso-*sn*-glycero-3-phosphate acyltransferase; 5, 1-alkyl-2-acyl-*sn*-glycerol-3-phosphate phosphohydrolase; 6, CDP-choline: 1-alkyl-2-acyl-*sn*-glycerol cholinephosphotransferase.

group of acyldihydroxyacetone phosphate with a long-chain fatty alcohol. The synthase occurs in peroxisomes. Plasmalogen synthesis is completed by transfer of a long-chain fatty acid from its respective CoA donor to the *sn*-2 position of 1-alkyl-2-lyso-*sn*-glycero-3-phosphate (Figure 10.26, Reaction 4). Patients with Zellweger's disease lack peroxisomes and cannot synthesize adequate amounts of plasmalogen.

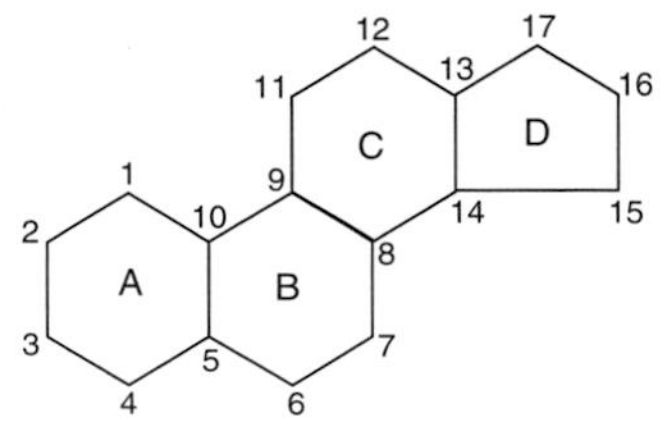

FIGURE 10.27
The cyclopentanophenanthrene ring.

10.3 ■ CHOLESTEROL

Cholesterol, an Alicyclic Compound, Is Widely Distributed in Free and Esterified Forms

Cholesterol is an alicyclic compound whose structure includes: (1) the perhydrocyclopentanophenanthrene nucleus with its four fused rings; (2) a single hydroxyl group at C-3, (3) an unsaturated center between C-5 and C-6 atoms; (4) an eight-membered branched hydrocarbon chain attached to the D ring at position 17; and (5) a methyl group (designated C-19) attached at position 10 and another methyl group (designated C-18) attached at position 13 (see Figures 10.27 and 10.28).

In terms of physical properties, cholesterol is a lipid with very low solubility in water; at 25°C, the limit of solubility is approximately 0.2 mg/100 mL. The actual concentration of cholesterol in plasma of healthy people is usually 150–200 mg/100 mL; this value is almost twice the normal concentration of blood glucose. This high solubility of cholesterol in blood is due to plasma lipoproteins (mainly LDL and VLDL) that have the ability to bind and thereby solubilize large amounts of cholesterol (see p. 56). Actually, only about 30% of the total plasma cholesterol occurs free; approximately 70% of the cholesterol in plasma lipoproteins exists in the form of **cholesterol esters** where some long-chain fatty acid, usually linoleic acid, is attached by an ester bond to the OH group on C-3 of the A ring. The long-chain fatty acid residue enhances the hydrophobicity of cholesterol (Figure 10.29). Cholesterol is a ubiquitous and essential component of mammalian cell membranes.

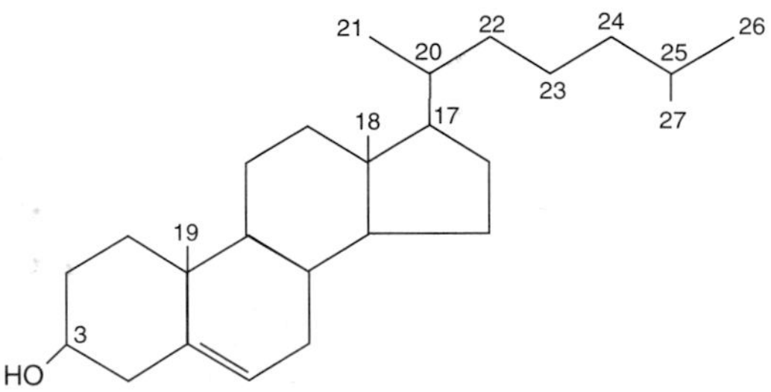

FIGURE 10.28
Structure of cholesterol (5-cholesten-3β-ol).

Cholesterol is also abundant in bile where the normal concentration is 390 mg/100 mL. Only 4% of cholesterol in bile is esterified to a long-chain fatty acid. Bile does not contain appreciable amounts of lipoproteins and solubilization of free cholesterol is achieved in part by the detergent property of phospholipids present in bile that are produced in liver (see p. 1078). A chronic disturbance in phospholipid metabolism in liver can result in deposition of cholesterol-rich gallstones. Bile salts, which are derivatives of cholesterol, also aid in keeping cholesterol in solution in bile. Cholesterol also appears to protect membranes of the gallbladder from potentially irritating or harmful effects of bile salts.

In the clinical laboratory, total cholesterol is estimated by the Liebermann–Burchard reaction. The proportions of free and esterified cholesterol can be determined by gas–liquid chromatography or reverse-phase high-pressure liquid chromatography (HPLC).

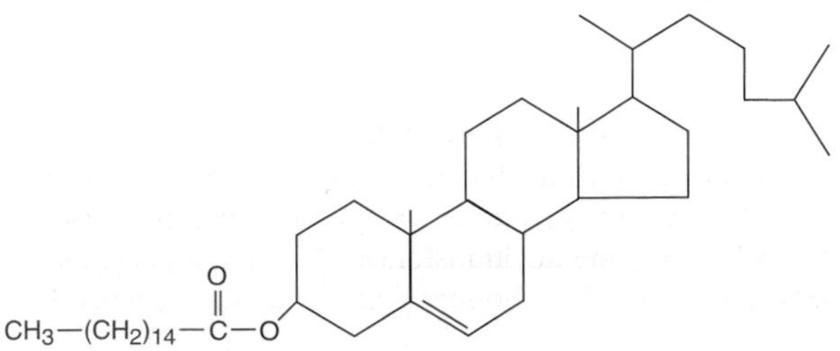

FIGURE 10.29
Structure of cholesterol (palmitoyl) ester.

Cholesterol Is a Membrane Component and Precursor of Bile Salts and Steroid Hormones

Cholesterol, derived from the diet or synthesized *de novo* in virtually all cells of humans, has a number of important roles. It is the major sterol in humans and a component of virtually all plasma and intracellular membranes. Cholesterol is especially abundant in myelinated structures of brain and central nervous system but is present in small amounts in the inner membrane of the mitochondrion (see p. 186). In contrast to the situation in plasma, most cholesterol in cellular membranes occurs in the free, unesterified form.

Cholesterol is the immediate precursor of **bile acids** synthesized in liver and that function to facilitate absorption of dietary triacylglycerols and fat-soluble vitamins (Chapter 26). It is important to realize that the ring structure of cholesterol cannot be metabolized to CO_2 and water in humans. Excretion of cholesterol is by way of the liver and gallbladder through the intestine in the form of bile acids.

Another physiological role of cholesterol is as the precursor of various **steroid hormones** (Chapter 21). Progesterone is the C_{21} keto steroid sex hormone secreted by the corpus luteum of the ovary and by placenta. The metabolically powerful corticosteroids of adrenal cortex are derived from cholesterol; these include deoxycorticosterone, corticosterone, cortisol, and cortisone. The mineralocorticoid aldosterone is derived from cholesterol in the zona glomerulosa tissue of the cortex of the adrenal gland. Cholesterol is also the precursor of female steroid hormones (estrogens, e.g., estradiol) in the ovary and of male steroids (e.g., testosterone) in the testes. Although all steroid hormones are structurally related to and biochemically derived from cholesterol, they have widely different physiological properties that relate to spermatogenesis, pregnancy, lactation and parturition, mineral balance, and energy (amino acids, carbohydrate, and fat) metabolism.

The hydrocarbon skeleton of cholesterol is also found in plant sterols, for example, **ergosterol,** a precursor of vitamin D (Figure 10.30). Ergosterol is converted in skin by ultraviolet irradiation to vitamin D_2. Vitamin D_2 is involved in calcium and phosphorus metabolism (Chapter 28).

Cholesterol Is Synthesized from Acetyl CoA

Although *de novo* biosynthesis of cholesterol occurs in virtually all cells, this capacity is greatest in liver, intestine, adrenal cortex, and reproductive tissues, including ovaries, testes, and placenta. From an inspection of its structure it is apparent that cholesterol biosynthesis will require a source of carbon atoms and considerable reducing power to generate the numerous carbon–carbon and carbon–hydrogen bonds. All carbon atoms of cholesterol are derived from acetate. Reducing power in the form of NADPH is provided mainly by glucose 6-phosphate dehydrogenase and 6-phosphogluconate dehydrogenase of the hexose monophosphate shunt (see p. 336). The pathway of cholesterol synthesis occurs in the cytosol and is driven in large part by hydrolysis of high-energy thioester bonds of acetyl CoA and phosphoanhydride bonds of ATP.

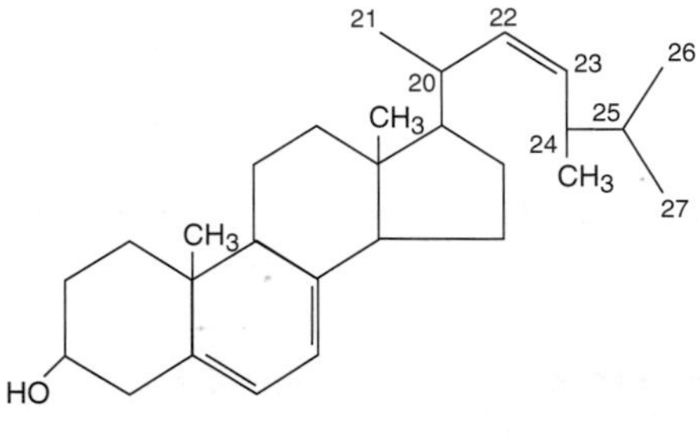

FIGURE 10.30
Structure of ergosterol.

Mevalonic Acid Is a Key Intermediate

The first compound unique to cholesterol biosynthesis is mevalonic acid derived from acetyl CoA. Acetyl CoA can be obtained from several sources: (1) the β-oxidation of fatty acids (Chapter 9); (2) the oxidation of ketogenic amino acids such as leucine and isoleucine (Chapter 11); and (3) the pyruvate dehydrogenase reaction. Free acetate can be activated to its thioester derivative at the expense of ATP by **acetokinase,** also referred to as **acetate thiokinase:**

$$\text{ATP} + \text{CH}_3\text{COO}^- + \text{CoASH} \longrightarrow \text{CH}_3\text{—}\overset{\text{O}}{\overset{\|}{\text{C}}}\text{—SCoA} + \text{AMP} + \text{PP}_i$$

The first two reactions in cholesterol biosynthesis are shared by the pathway that produces ketone bodies (see p. 387). Two molecules of acetyl CoA condense to form acetoacetyl CoA in a reaction catalyzed by acetoacetyl CoA thiolase (acetyl CoA:acetyl CoA acetyltransferase):

$$\text{CH}_3\text{—}\overset{\text{O}}{\overset{\|}{\text{C}}}\text{—SCoA} + \text{CH}_3\text{—}\overset{\text{O}}{\overset{\|}{\text{C}}}\text{—SCoA} \longrightarrow \text{CH}_3\text{—}\overset{\text{O}}{\overset{\|}{\text{C}}}\text{—CH}_2\text{—}\overset{\text{O}}{\overset{\|}{\text{C}}}\text{—SCoA} + \text{CoA}$$

Formation of the carbon–carbon bond in acetoacetyl CoA in this reaction is favored energetically by cleavage of a thioester bond and generation of free coenzyme A.

The next step introduces a third molecule of acetyl CoA into the cholesterol pathway and forms the branched-chain compound **3-hydroxy-3-methylglutaryl CoA** (HMG CoA) (Figure 10.31). This condensation reaction is catalyzed by **HMG CoA synthase** (3-hydroxy-3-methylglutaryl CoA:acetoacetyl CoA lyase). Liver parenchymal cells contain two isoenzyme forms of HMG CoA synthase; one in the cytosol is involved in cholesterol synthesis, while the other has a mitochondrial location and functions in synthesis of ketone bodies (see p. 388). In the HMG CoA synthase reaction, an aldol condensation occurs between the methyl carbon of acetyl CoA and the β-carbonyl group of acetoacetyl CoA with the simultaneous hydrolysis of the thioester bond of acetyl CoA. The thioester bond in the original acetoacetyl CoA substrate molecule remains intact. HMG CoA can also be formed from oxidative degradation of the branched-chain amino acid leucine, through the intermediates 3-methylcrotonyl CoA and 3-methylglutaconyl CoA (Chapter 11).

The step that produces the unique compound mevalonic acid from HMG CoA is catalyzed by the important microsomal enzyme **HMG CoA reductase** (mevalonate:NADP$^+$ oxidoreductase) that has an absolute requirement for NADPH as the reductant (Figure 10.32). This reductive step (1) consumes two molecules of NADPH, (2) results in hydrolysis of the thioester bond of HMG CoA, and (3) generates a primary alcohol residue in mevalonate. This reduction reaction is irreversible and produces (*R*)-(+)mevalonate, which contains six carbon atoms. HMG CoA reductase catalyzes the rate-limiting reaction in the pathway of cholesterol biosynthesis. HMG CoA reductase is an intrinsic membrane protein of the endoplasmic reticulum whose carboxyl terminus extends into the cytosol and carries the enzyme's active site. Phosphorylation regulates

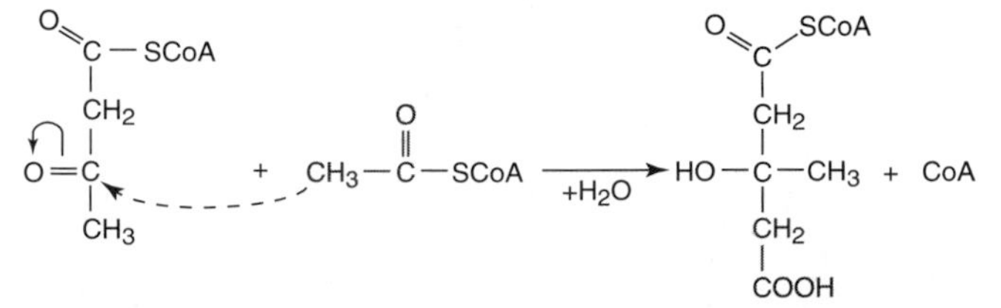

$$\underset{\text{Acetoacetyl CoA}}{\text{CH}_3\text{—CO—CH}_2\text{—CO—SCoA}} + \underset{\text{Acetyl CoA}}{\text{CH}_3\text{—}\overset{\text{O}}{\overset{\|}{\text{C}}}\text{—SCoA}} \xrightarrow{+\text{H}_2\text{O}} \underset{\text{HMG CoA}}{\text{HO—}\underset{\text{CH}_2\text{—COOH}}{\overset{\text{CH}_2\text{—CO—SCoA}}{\text{C}}}\text{—CH}_3} + \text{CoA}$$

FIGURE 10.31
HMG CoA synthase reaction.

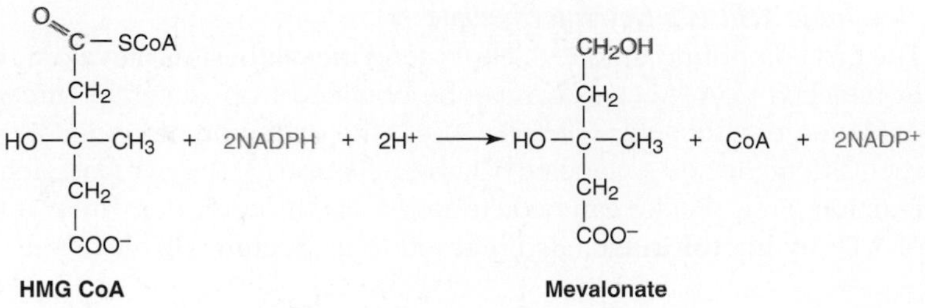

FIGURE 10.32
HMG CoA reductase reaction.

HMG CoA reductase activity of the cell by diminishing its catalytic activity (V_{max}) and enhancing the rate of its degradation by increasing its susceptibility to proteolytic attack. Increased amounts of intracellular cholesterol stimulate phosphorylation of HMG CoA reductase.

Mevalonic Acid Is a Precursor of Farnesyl Pyrophosphate

Reactions involved in conversion of mevalonate to **farnesyl pyrophosphate** are summarized in Figure 10.33. The stepwise transfer of the terminal γ-phosphate group from two molecules of ATP to mevalonate (A) to form 5-pyrophosphomevalonate (B) are catalyzed by mevalonate kinase (enzyme I) and phosphomevalonate kinase (enzyme II). The next step affects decarboxylation of 5-pyrophosphomevalonate and generates Δ^3-isopentenyl pyrophosphate (D); this reaction is catalyzed by pyrophosphomevalonate decarboxylase. In this ATP-dependent reaction in which ADP, P_i, and CO_2 are produced, it is thought that decarboxylation–dehydration proceeds by way of the triphosphate intermediate, 3-phosphomevalonate 5-pyrophosphate (C). Isopentenyl pyrophosphate is converted to its allylic isomer 3,3-dimethylallyl pyrophosphate (E) in a reversible reaction catalyzed by isopentenyl pyrophosphate isomerase. The condensation of 3,3-dimethylallyl pyrophosphate (E) and Δ^3-isopentenyl pyrophosphate (D) generates **geranyl pyrophosphate** (F).

The stepwise condensation of three C_5 isopentenyl units to form the C15 unit farnesyl pyrophosphate (G) is catalyzed by one enzyme, a cytoplasmic prenyl transferase called geranyltransferase.

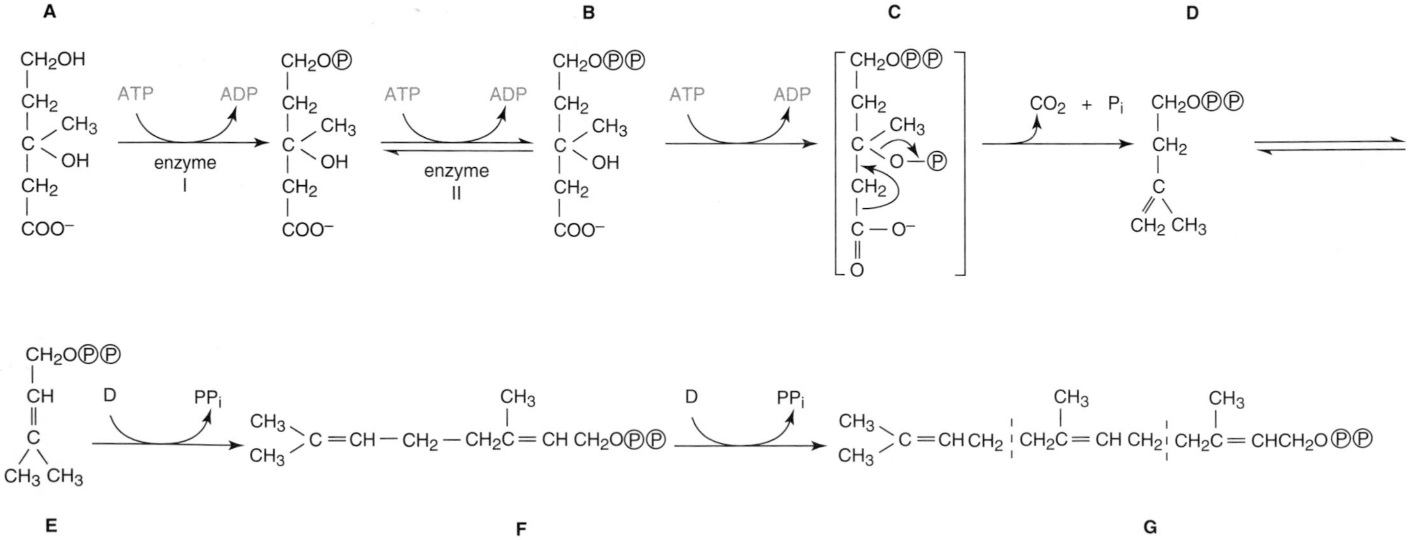

FIGURE 10.33
Formation of farnesyl pyrophosphate (F) from mevalonate (A). Dotted lines divide molecules into isoprenoid-derived units. D is 3-isopentenyl pyrophosphate.

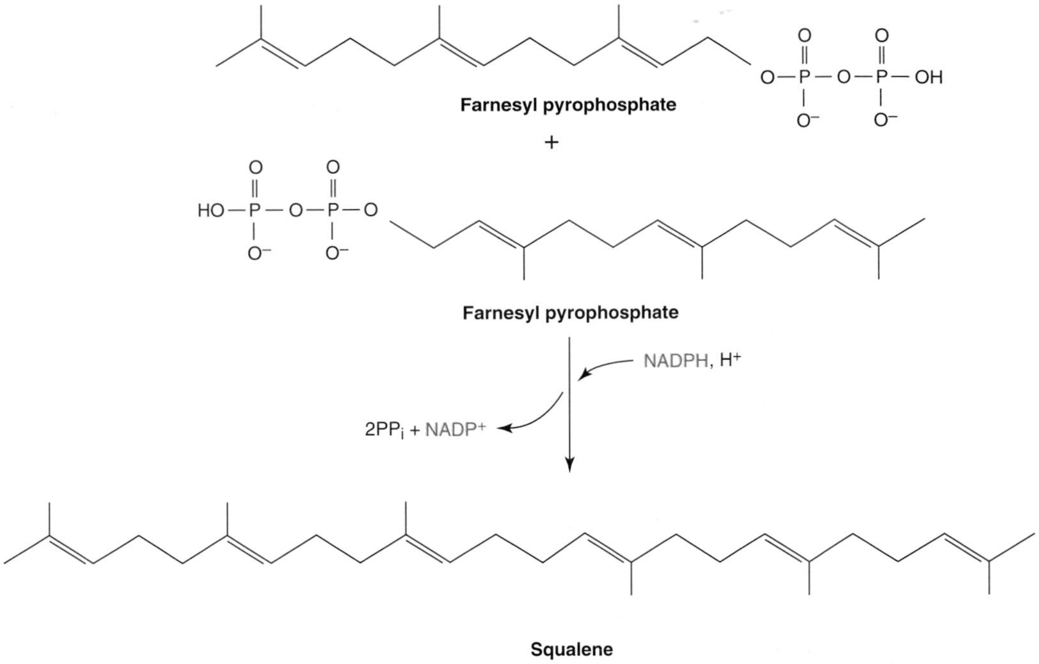

FIGURE 10.34
Formation of squalene from two molecules of farnesyl pyrophosphate.

Cholesterol Is Formed from Farnesyl Pyrophosphate via Squalene

The last steps in cholesterol biosynthesis involve "head-to-head" fusion of two molecules of farnesyl pyrophosphate to form **squalene** and finally cyclization of squalene to yield cholesterol. The reaction that produces the C_{30} squalene molecule from two C_{15} farnesyl pyrophosphate moieties (Figure 10.34) and is unlike the previous carbon–carbon bond-forming reactions in the pathway (Figure 10.33). **Squalene synthase,** present in the endoplasmic reticulum, releases two pyrophosphate groups, with loss of a hydrogen atom from one molecule of farnesyl pyrophosphate and replacement by a hydrogen from NADPH. Several different intermediates probably occur between farnesyl pyrophosphate and squalene. By rotation about carbon–carbon single bonds, the conformation of squalene indicated in Figure 10.35 can be obtained. Note the similarity of the overall shape of the compound to cholesterol and that squalene is devoid of oxygen atoms.

Cholesterol biosynthesis from squalene proceeds through the intermediate **lanosterol,** which contains the fused tetracyclic ring system and a C_8 side chain:

$$\text{Squalene} \rightarrow \text{squalene 2,3-epoxide} \rightarrow \text{lanosterol}$$

The many carbon–carbon bonds formed during cyclization of squalene are generated in a concerted fashion as indicated in Figure 10.36. The OH group

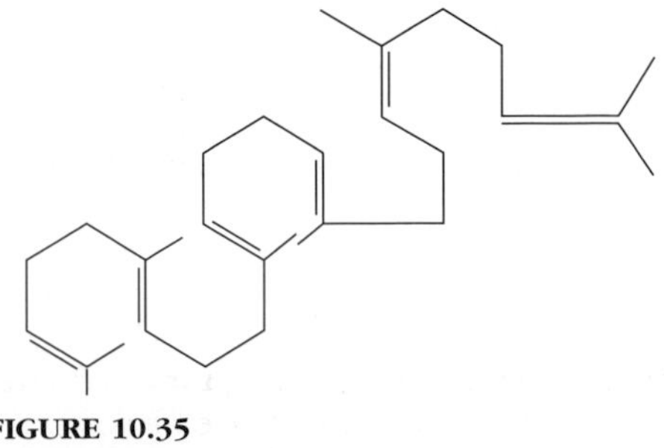

FIGURE 10.35
Structure of squalene, C_{30}.

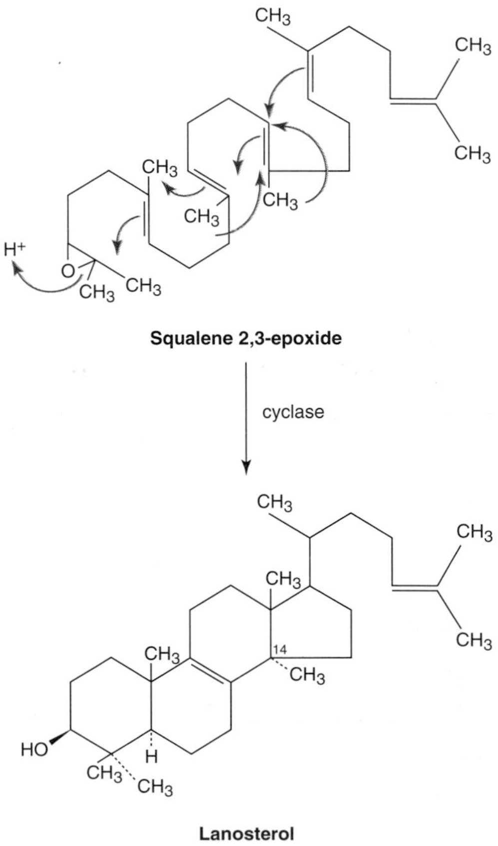

FIGURE 10.36
Conversion of squalene 2,3-epoxide to lanosterol.

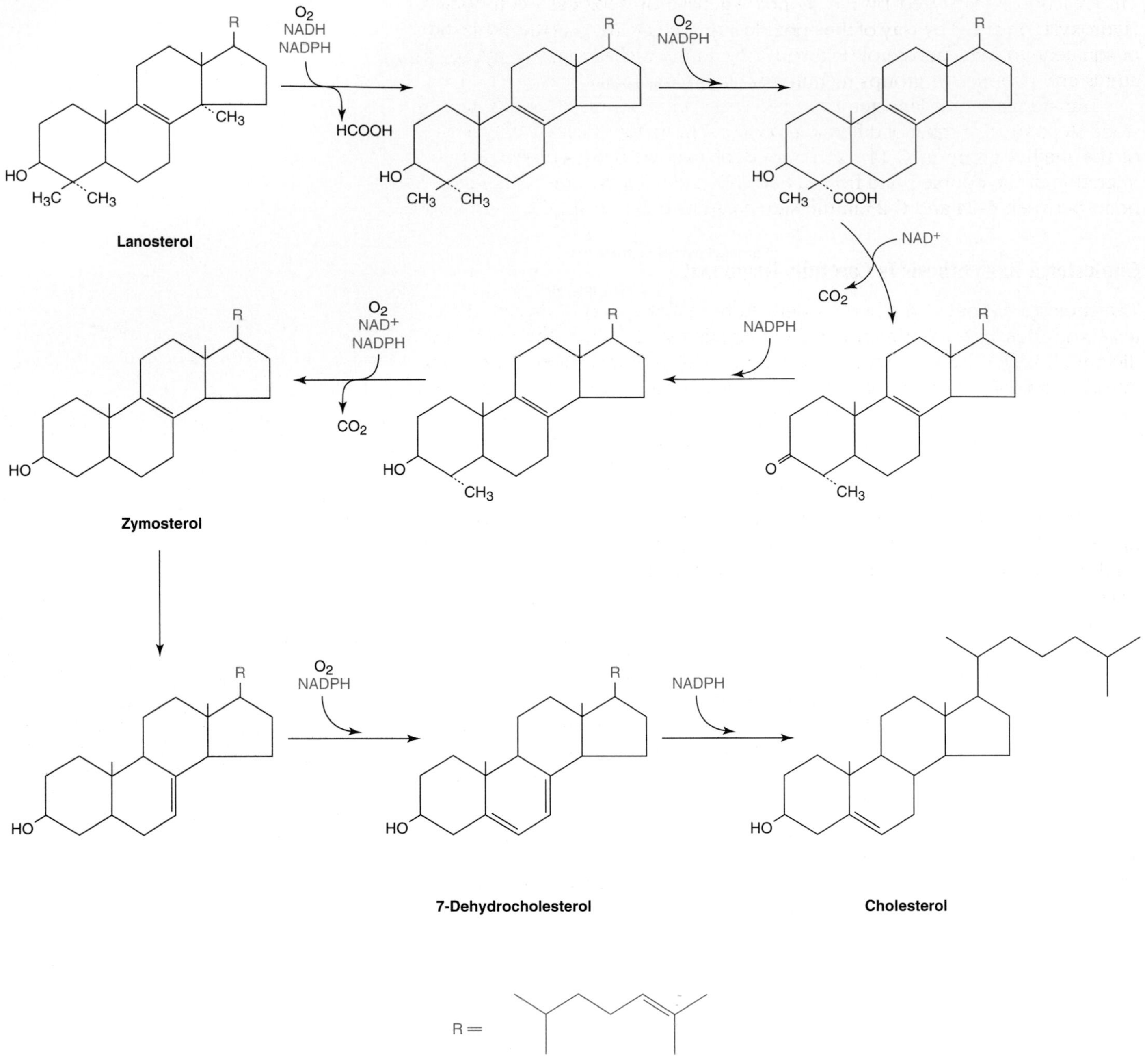

Lanosterol

Zymosterol

7-Dehydrocholesterol

Cholesterol

FIGURE 10.37
Conversion of lanosterol to cholesterol.

of lanosterol projects above the plane of the A ring; this is referred to as the β orientation. Groups that extend down below the ring in a trans relationship to the OH group are designated as α by a dotted line. During this reaction sequence an OH group is added to C-3, two methyl groups undergo shifts, and a proton is eliminated. The oxygen atom is derived from molecular oxygen. The reaction is catalyzed by an endoplasmic reticulum enzyme, **squalene oxidocyclase,** that is composed of at least two activities, squalene epoxidase or monooxygenase and a cyclase (lanosterol cyclase).

The cyclization process is initiated by epoxide formation at the expense of NADPH:

$$\text{Squalene} + O_2 + \text{NADPH} + H^+ \rightarrow \text{squalene 2,3-epoxide} + H_2O + \text{NADP}^+$$

This reaction is catalyzed by the monooxygenase or epoxidase component. Hydroxylation at C-3 by way of the epoxide intermediate triggers the cyclization of squalene to form lanosterol (Figure 10.36). In the cyclization, two hydrogen atoms and two methyl groups migrate to neighboring positions.

Transformation of lanosterol to cholesterol involves many poorly understood steps and a number of different enzymes. These steps include: (1) removal of the methyl group at C-14; (2) removal of two methyl groups at C-4; (3) migration of the double bond from C-8 to C-5; and (4) reduction of the double bond between C-24 and C-25 in the side chain (see Figure 10.37).

Cholesterol Biosynthesis Is Carefully Regulated

The cholesterol pool of the body is derived from absorption of dietary cholesterol and biosynthesis primarily in liver and intestine. When the amount of dietary cholesterol is reduced, cholesterol synthesis is increased in liver and intestine to satisfy the needs of other tissues and organs. Cholesterol synthesized *de novo* is transported from liver and intestine to peripheral tissues in the form of lipoproteins. These are the only tissues that manufacture **apolipoprotein B,** the protein component of cholesterol transport proteins LDL and VLDL. Most apolipoprotein B is secreted into the circulation as VLDL, which is converted into LDL by removal of triacylglycerol and apolipoprotein C components, probably in plasma and liver. When the quantity of dietary cholesterol increases, cholesterol synthesis in liver and intestine is almost totally suppressed. Thus the rate of *de novo* cholesterol synthesis is inversely related to the amount of dietary cholesterol taken up by the body.

The primary site for control of cholesterol biosynthesis is HMG CoA reductase, which catalyzes the step that produces mevalonic acid. This is the committed step and the rate-limiting reaction in the pathway of cholesterol biosynthesis (Figure 10.38). Cholesterol effects feedback inhibition of its own synthesis by inhibiting the activity of preexisting HMG CoA reductase and also by promoting rapid inactivation of the enzyme by mechanisms that remain to be elucidated.

In a normal healthy adult on a low-cholesterol diet, about 1300 mg of cholesterol is returned to the liver each day for disposal. This cholesterol comes from cholesterol reabsorbed from the gut by means of the enterohepatic circulation and HDL, which carries cholesterol to the liver from peripheral tissues. Liver disposes of cholesterol by: (1) excretion in bile as free cholesterol and

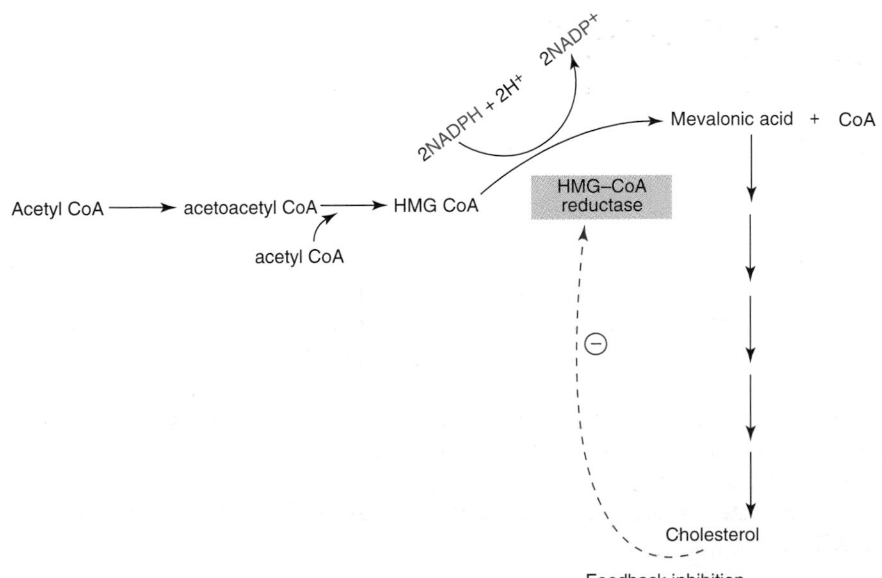

FIGURE 10.38
Summary of the pathway of cholesterol synthesis indicating feedback inhibition of HMG CoA reductase by cholesterol.

after conversion to bile salts; each day, about 250 mg of bile salts and 550 mg of cholesterol are lost from the enterohepatic circulation; (2) esterification and storage in liver as cholesterol esters; and (3) incorporation into lipoproteins (VLDL and LDL) and secretion into the circulation. On a low-cholesterol diet, liver will synthesize ~800 mg of cholesterol per day to replace bile salts and cholesterol lost from the enterohepatic circulation in the feces.

The mechanism of suppression of cholesterol biosynthesis by LDL-bound cholesterol involves specific **LDL receptors** that project from the surface of human cells. The first step of the regulatory mechanism involves the binding of the lipoprotein LDL to these LDL receptors, thereby extracting the LDL particles from the blood. The binding reaction is characterized by its saturability, high affinity, and high degree of specificity. The receptor recognizes only LDL and VLDL, the two plasma lipoproteins that contain apolipoprotein B-100. Once binding to receptor occurs at sites on the plasma membrane that contain pits coated with a protein called **clathrin,** the cholesterol-charged lipoprotein is endocytosed in the form of clathrin-coated vesicles. Intracellularly, the coated vesicle loses its clathrin and becomes an endosome (see p. 379). This process is termed **receptor-mediated endocytosis.** The next step involves the fusion of the endosome with a lysosome that contains numerous hydrolytic enzymes, including proteases and cholesterol esterase. The LDL receptor separates from LDL and returns to the cell surface. Inside the lysosome the cholesterol esters of LDL are hydrolyzed by cholesterol esterase to produce free cholesterol and a long-chain fatty acid. Free cholesterol then diffuses into the cytoplasm where, by some unknown mechanism, it inhibits the activity of HMG CoA reductase and suppresses the synthesis of HMG CoA reductase enzyme. There is evidence that cholesterol acts at the level of DNA and protein synthesis to decrease the rate of synthesis of HMG CoA reductase. At the same time, **fatty acyl CoA:cholesterol acyltransferase** (ACAT) in the endoplasmic reticulum is activated by cholesterol, promoting the formation of cholesterol esters, principally cholesterol oleate. Accumulation of intracellular cholesterol eventually inhibits the replenishment of LDL receptors on the cell surface, a phenomenon called **down regulation,** thereby blocking further uptake and accumulation of cholesterol.

The LDL receptor is a single-chain glycoprotein; numerous mutations in its gene are associated with familial hypercholesterolemia. The receptor spans the plasma membrane once with the carboxyl terminus on the cytoplasmic face and the amino terminus, which contains the LDL-binding site, extending into the extracellular space. **Apoprotein B-100** and **apoprotein E,** which is present in IDL (intermediate density lipoprotein) and some forms of HDL, are the two proteins through which particular lipoproteins bind to the LDL receptor.

The correlation between high levels of blood cholesterol, particularly LDL cholesterol, and heart attacks and strokes have led to the development of dietary and therapeutic approaches to lower blood cholesterol (see Clin. Corr. 10.2). Patients with **familial** (genetic) **hypercholesterolemia** suffer from accelerated atherosclerosis (see Clin. Corr. 10.3). In most cases, there is a lack of functional LDL receptors on the cell surface because the mutant alleles produce little or no LDL receptor protein; these patients are referred to as receptor-negative. In others the LDL receptor is synthesized and transported normally to the cell surface; an amino acid substitution or other alteration in the protein's primary structure, however, adversely affects the LDL-binding region of the receptor. As a result, there is little or no binding of LDL to the cell, cholesterol is not transferred into the cell, cholesterol synthesis is not inhibited, and the blood cholesterol level increases. Another LDL-deficient group of hypercholesterolemic patients is able to synthesize the LDL receptor but has a defect in the transport mechanism that delivers the glycoprotein to its proper location on the plasma membrane. And finally, there is another subclass of genetically determined hypercholesterolemics whose LDL receptors have a defect in the

CLINICAL CORRELATION 10.2

Treatment of Hypercholesterolemia

Many authorities recommend screening asymptomatic individuals by measuring plasma cholesterol. A level less than 200 mg% is considered desirable, and a level over 240 mg% requires lipoprotein analysis, especially determination of LDL cholesterol. Reduction of LDL cholesterol depends on dietary restriction of cholesterol to less than 300 mg day^{-1}, of calories to attain ideal body weight, and of total fat intake to less than 30% of total calories. Approximately two-thirds of the fat should be mono- or polyunsaturated. The second line of therapy is with drugs. Cholestyramine and colestipol are bile salt-binding drugs that promote excretion of bile salts in the stool. This in turn increases the rate of hepatic bile salt synthesis and of LDL uptake by the liver. Lovastatin is an inhibitor of HMG CoA reductase. Since this enzyme is limiting for cholesterol synthesis, lovastatin decreases endogenous synthesis of cholesterol and stimulates uptake and LDL via the LDL receptor. The combination of lovastatin and cholestyramine is sometimes used for severe hyperlipidemia.

Expert Panel. Evaluation and treatment of high blood cholesterol in adults. *Arch. Intern. Med.* 148:36, 1988.

cytoplasmic carboxyl terminus; they populate their cell surfaces with LDL receptors normally but are unable to internalize the LDL–LDL receptor complex due to an inability to cluster this complex in coated pits.

In specialized tissues such as the adrenal gland and ovary, the cholesterol derived from LDL serves as a precursor to the steroid hormones made by these organs, such as cortisol and estradiol, respectively. In liver, cholesterol extracted from LDL and HDL is converted into bile salts that function in intestinal fat digestion.

Plasma Cholesterol Is in a Dynamic State

Plasma cholesterol is in a dynamic state, entering the blood complexed with lipoproteins that keep the lipid in solution and leaving the blood as tissues take up cholesterol from these lipoproteins. Plasma lipoproteins contain free cholesterol and cholesterol esterified to a long-chain fatty acid. From 70% to 75% of plasma cholesterol is esterified to long-chain fatty acids. It is the free, unesterified form of cholesterol that exchanges readily between different lipoproteins and the plasma membrane of cells.

The mechanism for entry of cholesterol into liver cells from the three types of plasma lipoprotein is quite different. While the metabolism of chylomicrons and LDL has been quite well defined, that of HDL is just beginning to be understood. Chylomicrons that have had their triacylglycerol content reduced by plasma lipoprotein lipase become chylomicron remnants, which are rich in dietary cholesterol (free and esterified) and in fat-soluble vitamins. They are taken up by receptor-mediated endocytosis into liver cells, as is LDL.

High-density lipoproteins and the enzyme **lecithin:cholesterol acyltransferase** (LCAT) play important roles in the elimination of cholesterol from the body. LCAT catalyzes the freely reversible reaction (Figure 10.39), which transfers the fatty acid in the *sn*-2 position of phosphatidylcholine to the 3-hydroxyl of cholesterol. LCAT is a plasma enzyme produced mainly by liver. The actual substrate for LCAT is cholesterol contained in HDL. The LCAT–HDL system functions to protect cells, especially their plasma membrane, from the damaging effects of excessive amounts of free cholesterol. Cholesterol ester generated in the LCAT reaction diffuses into the core of the HDL particle where it is then transported from the tissues and plasma to liver, the latter being the only organ capable of metabolizing and excreting cholesterol. Thus, by this mechanism, referred to as the reverse transport of cholesterol, LCAT acting on HDL provides a vehicle for transporting cholesterol from peripheral tissues to the liver.

Cholesterol Is Excreted Primarily as Bile Acids

The bile acids are the end products of cholesterol metabolism. Primary bile acids are synthesized in hepatocytes directly from cholesterol. The most abundant bile

> **CLINICAL CORRELATION 10.3**
>
> ### Atherosclerosis
>
> Atherosclerosis is the leading cause of death in Western industrialized countries. The risk of developing it is directly related to the plasma concentration of LDL cholesterol and inversely related to that of HDL cholesterol. This explains why the former is frequently called "bad" cholesterol and the latter "good" cholesterol, though chemically there is only one cholesterol. Atherosclerosis is a disorder of the arterial wall characterized by accumulation of cholesteryl esters in cells derived from the monocyte–macrophage line, smooth muscle cell proliferation, and fibrosis. The earliest abnormality is migration of blood monocytes to the subendothelium of the artery. Once there, they differentiate into macrophages. These cells accumulate cholesterol esters derived from plasma LDL. Why these cells do not regulate cellular cholesterol stores normally is not completely understood. Some of the LDL may be taken up via pathways distinct from the classical LDL receptor pathway. For instance, receptors that mediate uptake of acetylated LDL or LDL complexed with dextran sulfate have been described and these are not regulated by cellular cholesterol content. Distortion of the subendothelium leads to platelet aggregation on the endothelial surface and release of platelet-derived mitogens such as platelet-derived growth factor (PDGF). This is thought to stimulate smooth muscle cell growth. Death of the foam cells results in the accumulation of a cellular lipid that can stimulate fibrosis. The resulting atherosclerotic plaque narrows the blood vessel and serves as the site of thrombus formation, which precipitates myocardial infarction (heart attack).
>
> Ross, R. The pathogenesis of atherosclerosis—an update. *N. Engl. J. Med.* 314:488, 1986.

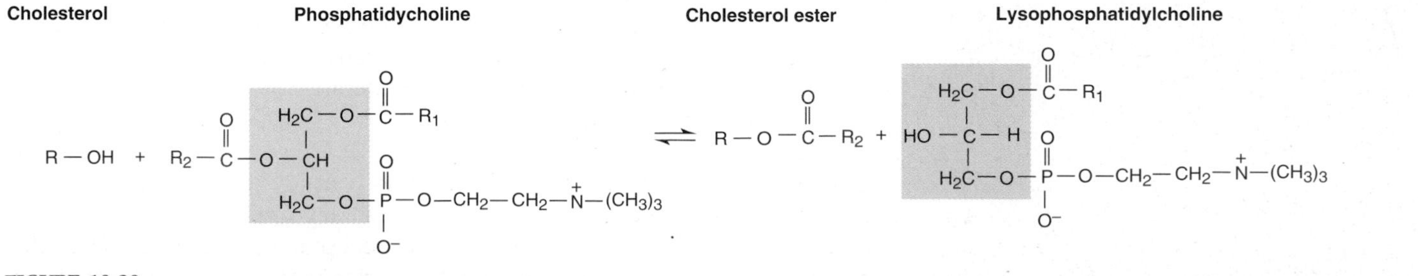

Cholesterol | Phosphatidycholine | Cholesterol ester | Lysophosphatidylcholine

$$\mathrm{R{-}OH} + \begin{array}{l} \mathrm{H_2C{-}O{-}C({=}O){-}R_1} \\ \mathrm{R_2{-}C({=}O){-}O{-}CH} \\ \mathrm{H_2C{-}O{-}P({=}O)(O^-){-}O{-}CH_2{-}CH_2{-}\overset{+}{N}{-}(CH_3)_3} \end{array} \rightleftharpoons \mathrm{R{-}O{-}C({=}O){-}R_2} + \begin{array}{l} \mathrm{H_2C{-}O{-}C({=}O){-}R_1} \\ \mathrm{HO{-}C{-}H} \\ \mathrm{H_2C{-}O{-}P({=}O)(O^-){-}O{-}CH_2{-}CH_2{-}\overset{+}{N}{-}(CH_3)_3} \end{array}$$

FIGURE 10.39
Lecithin:cholesterol acyltransferase (LCAT) reaction, where R—OH indicates cholesterol.

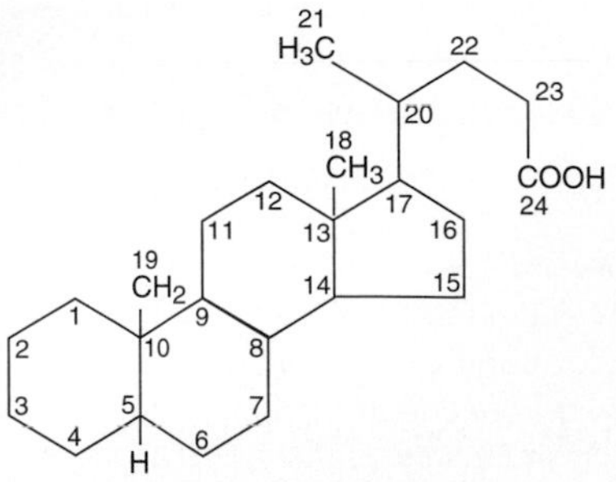

FIGURE 10.40
Structure of cholanic acid.

acids in humans are derivatives of cholanic acid (Figure 10.40), that is, **cholic acid** and **chenodeoxycholic acid** (Figure 10.41). The primary bile acids are composed of 24 carbon atoms, contain two or three OH groups, and have a side chain that ends in a carboxyl group that is ionized at pH 7.0 (hence the name bile salt). The carboxyl group of the bile acids is often conjugated via an amide bond to either glycine (NH_2-CH_2-COOH) or taurine (NH_2—CH_2—CH_2—SO_3H) to form **glycocholic** or **taurocholic acid,** respectively. The structure of glycocholic acid is shown in Figure 10.42.

When the primary bile acids undergo chemical reactions by microorganisms in the gut, they give rise to secondary bile acids that also possess 24 carbon atoms. Examples of secondary bile acids are deoxycholic acid and lithocholic acid, which are derived from cholic acid and chenodeoxycholic acid, respectively, by the removal of one OH group (Figure 10.41). Transformation of cholesterol to bile acids requires: (1) epimerization of the 3β-OH group; (2) reduction of the C-5 double bond; (3) introduction of OH groups at C-7 (chenodeoxycholic acid) or at C-7 and C-12 (cholic acid); and (4) conversion of the C-27 side chain into a C-24 carboxylic acid by elimination of a propyl equivalent.

Bile acids are secreted into bile canaliculi, specialized channels formed by adjacent hepatocytes. Bile canaliculi unite with bile ductules, which in turn come together to form bile ducts. The bile acids are carried to the gallbladder for storage and ultimately to the small intestine where they are excreted. The capacity of liver to produce bile acids is insufficient to meet the physiological demands, so the body relies on an efficient **enterohepatic circulation** that carries the bile acids from the intestine back to the liver several times each day. The primary conjugated bile acids, after removal of the glycine or taurine residue in the gut, are reabsorbed by an active transport process from the intestine, primarily in the ileum, and returned to the liver by way of the portal vein. Bile acids that are not reabsorbed are acted on by bacteria in the gut and converted into secondary bile acids; a portion of secondary bile acids, primarily deoxycholic acid and lithocholic acid, are reabsorbed passively in the colon and

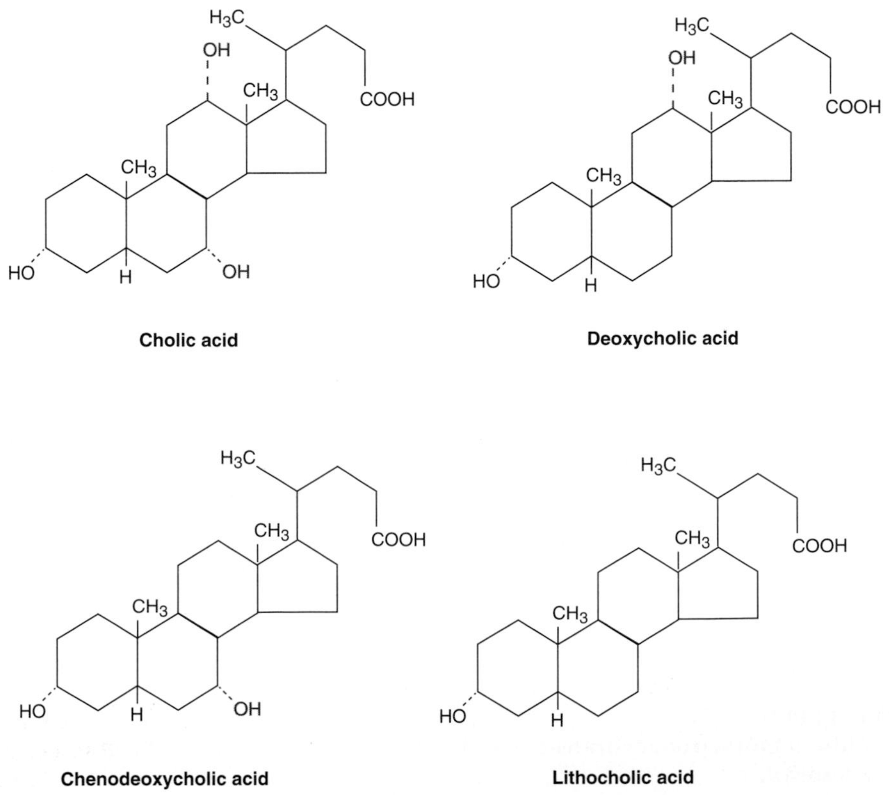

Cholic acid

Deoxycholic acid

Chenodeoxycholic acid

Lithocholic acid

FIGURE 10.41
Structures of some common bile acids.

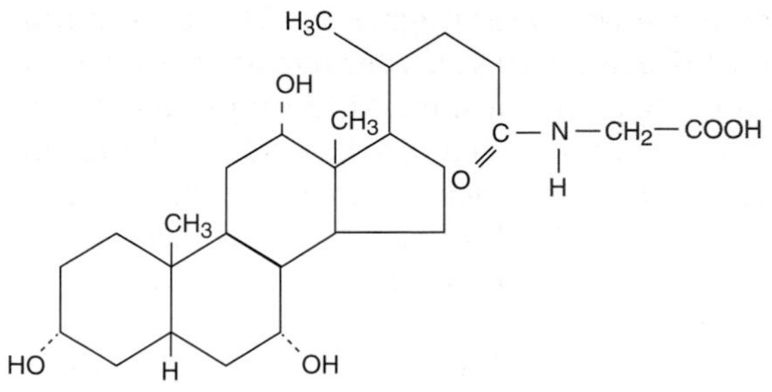

FIGURE 10.42
Structure of glycocholic acid, a conjugated bile acid.

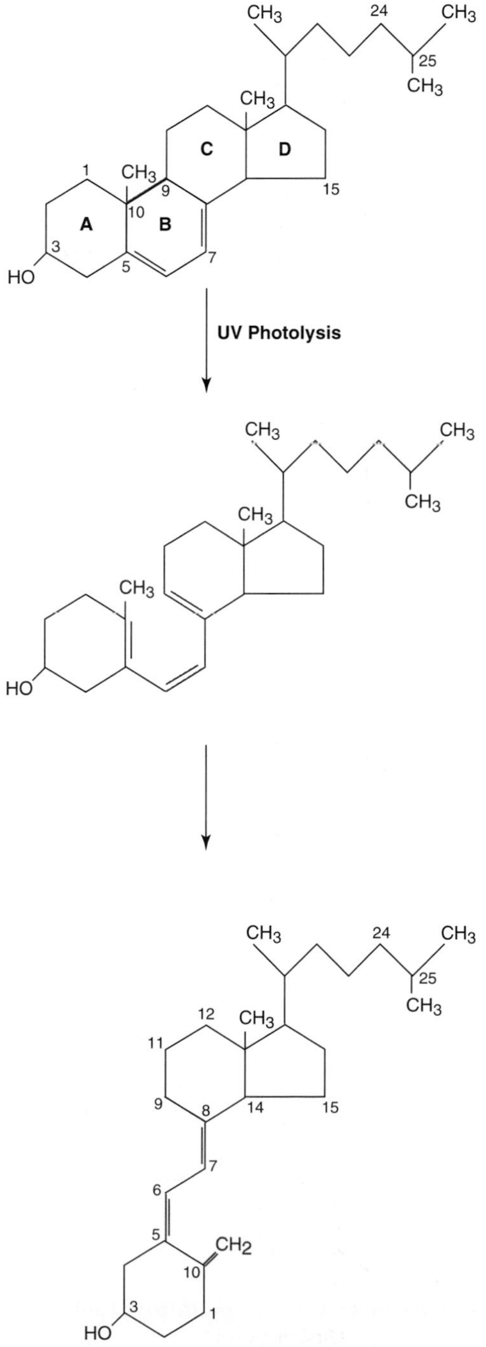

7–Dehydrocholesterol

Previtamin D_3

Vitamin D_3
(cholecalciferol)

FIGURE 10.43
Photochemical conversion of 7-dehydrocholesterol to vitamin D_3 (cholecalciferol).

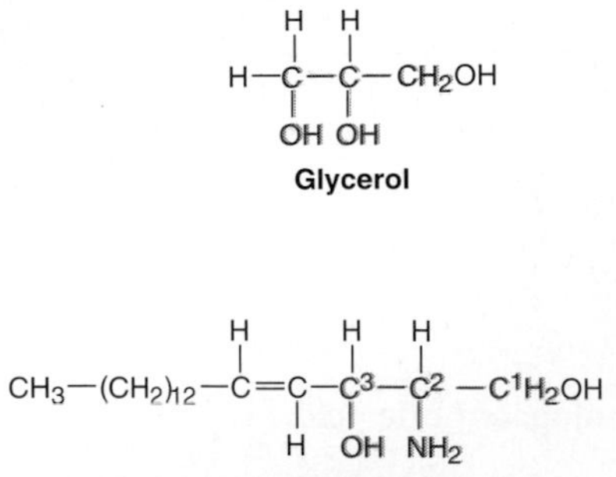

Glycerol

Sphingosine

FIGURE 10.44
Comparison of the structures of glycerol and sphingosine (*trans*-1,3,dihydroxy-2-amino-4-octadecene).

returned to the liver where they are secreted into the gallbladder. Hepatic synthesis normally produces 0.2–0.6 g of bile acids per day to replace those lost in the feces. The gallbladder pool of bile acids is 2–4 g. Because the enterohepatic circulation recycles 6–12 times each day, the total amount of bile acids absorbed per day from the intestine corresponds to 12–32 g.

Bile acids are significant in medicine for several reasons. They represent the only significant way in which cholesterol can be excreted; the carbon skeleton of cholesterol is not oxidized to CO_2 and H_2O in humans but is excreted in bile as free cholesterol and bile acids. Bile acids prevent the precipitation of cholesterol out of solution in the gallbladder. Bile acids and phospholipids function to solubilize cholesterol in bile and act as emulsifying agents to prepare dietary triacylglycerols for hydrolysis by pancreatic lipase. Bile acids may also play a direct role in activating pancreatic lipase (see Chapter 25) and they facilitate the absorption of fat-soluble vitamins, particularly vitamin D, from the intestine.

Vitamin D Is Synthesized from an Intermediate of Cholesterol Biosynthesis

Cholesterol biosynthesis provides substrate for the photochemical production of **vitamin D_3** in skin. The metabolism and function of vitamin D_3 are discussed in Chapter 27. Vitamin D_3 is a secosteroid in which the 9,10 carbon bond of the B ring of the cholesterol nucleus has undergone fission (Figure 10.43). The most important supply of vitamin D_3 is that manufactured in the skin. **7-Dehydrocholesterol** is an intermediate in the pathway of cholesterol biosynthesis and is converted in the skin to provitamin D_3 by irradiation with UV rays of the sun (285–310 nm). Provitamin D_3 is biologically inert and labile and converted thermally and slowly (~36 h) to the double-bond isomer by a nonenzymatic reaction to the biologically active vitamin, cholecalciferol (vitamin D_3). As little as 10-min exposure each day of the hands and face to sunlight will satisfy the body's need for vitamin D. Photochemical action on the plant sterol ergosterol also provides a dietary precursor to a compound designated **vitamin D_2 (calciferol)** that can satisfy the vitamin D requirement.

10.4 ■ SPHINGOLIPIDS

Biosynthesis of Sphingosine

Sphingolipids are complex lipids whose core structure is provided by the long-chain amino alcohol **sphingosine** (Figure 10.44) (4-sphingenine or *trans*-1,3-dihydroxy-2-amino-4-octadecene). Sphingosine has two asymmetric carbon atoms (C-2 and C-3); of the four possible optical isomers, naturally occurring sphingosine is of the D-erythro form. The double bond of sphingosine has the trans configuration. The primary alcohol group at C-1 is a nucleophilic center that forms covalent bonds with sugars to form glycosphingolipids and phosphocholine to form sphingomyelin. The amino group at C-2 always bears a long-

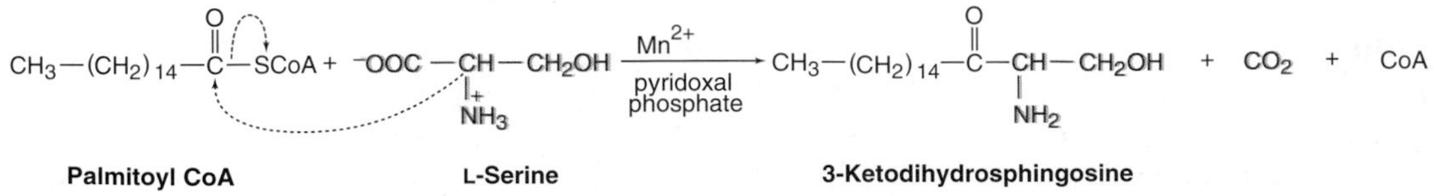

Palmitoyl CoA L-Serine 3-Ketodihydrosphingosine

FIGURE 10.45
Formation of 3-ketodihydrosphingosine from serine and palmitoyl CoA.

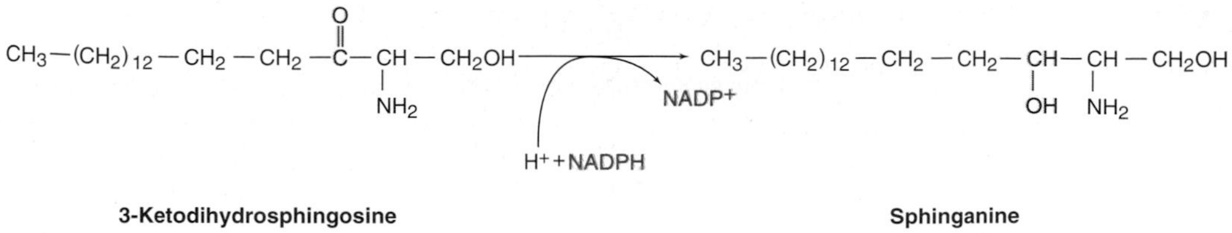

$$CH_3-(CH_2)_{12}-CH_2-CH_2-\overset{O}{\overset{\|}{C}}-\underset{NH_2}{\underset{|}{CH}}-CH_2OH \xrightarrow[H^+ + NADPH]{NADP^+} CH_3-(CH_2)_{12}-CH_2-CH_2-\underset{OH}{\underset{|}{CH}}-\underset{NH_2}{\underset{|}{CH}}-CH_2OH$$

3-Ketodihydrosphingosine — Sphinganine

FIGURE 10.46
Conversion of 3-ketodihydrosphingosine to sphinganine.

chain fatty acid (usually C_{20}–C_{26}) in amide linkage. The secondary alcohol at C-3 is always free. It is useful to appreciate the structural similarity of a part of the sphingosine molecule to the glycerol moiety of the acylglycerols (Fig. 10.44).

Sphingolipids are present in blood and nearly all body tissues. The highest concentrations are found in the white matter of the central nervous system. Various sphingolipids are components of the plasma membrane of practically all cells.

Sphingosine is synthesized by way of **sphinganine** (dihydrosphingosine) in two steps from the precursors serine and palmitoyl CoA. Serine is the source of C-1, C-2, and the amino group of sphingosine, while palmitic acid provides the remaining carbon atoms. Condensation of serine and palmitoyl CoA is catalyzed by a pyridoxal phosphate-dependent enzyme, serine palmitoyltransferase. The driving force for the reaction is provided by both cleavage of the reactive, high-energy thioester bond of palmitoyl CoA and the release of CO_2 from serine (Figure 10.45). The next step involves the reduction of the carbonyl group in 3-ketodihydrosphingosine with reducing equivalents being derived from NADPH to produce sphinganine (Figure 10.46). The insertion of the double bond into sphinganine to produce sphingosine occurs at the level of ceramide (see below).

Ceramides Are Fatty Acid Amide Derivatives of Sphingosine

Sphingosine does not occur naturally. The core structure of the natural sphingolipids is **ceramide,** a long-chain fatty acid amide derivative of sphingosine. The long-chain fatty acid is attached to the 2-amino group of sphingosine through an amide bond (Figure 10.47). Most often the acyl group is **behenic acid,** a saturated C22 fatty acid, but other long-chain acyl groups can be used. There are two long-chain hydrocarbon domains in the ceramide molecule; these hydrophobic regions are responsible for the lipid character of sphingolipids.

Ceramide is synthesized from dihydrosphingosine and a molecule of long-chain fatty acyl CoA by a microsomal enzyme with dihydroceramide as an intermediate that is then oxidized by dehydrogenation at C-4 and C-5 (Figure 10.48). Free ceramide is not a component of membrane lipids but rather is an intermediate in the biosynthesis and catabolism of glycosphingolipids and sphingomyelin. Structures of prominent sphingolipids of humans are presented in Figure 10.49 in diagrammatic form.

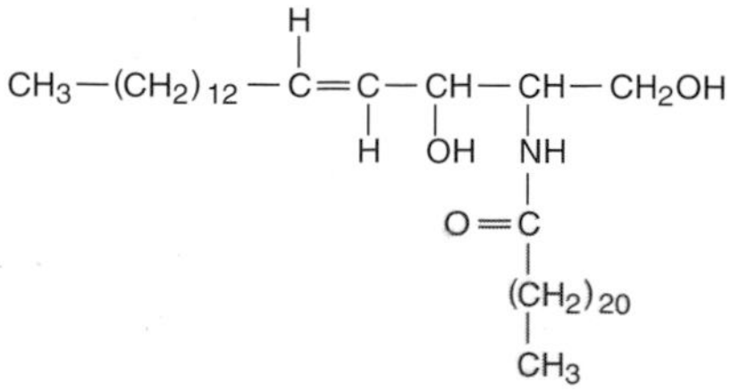

$$CH_3-(CH_2)_{12}-\overset{H}{\overset{|}{C}}=\underset{H}{\underset{|}{C}}-\underset{OH}{\underset{|}{CH}}-\underset{NH-C(=O)-(CH_2)_{20}-CH_3}{\underset{|}{CH}}-CH_2OH$$

FIGURE 10.47
Structure of a ceramide (*N*-acylsphingosine).

Sphingomyelin Is the Only Sphingolipid Containing Phosphorus

Sphingomyelin, a major structural lipid of membranes of nervous tissue, is the only sphingolipid that is a phospholipid. In sphingomyelin the primary alcohol at C-1 of sphingosine is esterified to choline through a phosphodiester bridge of the kind that occurs in the acyl glycerophospholipids and the amino group of sphingosine is attached to a long-chain fatty acid by an amide bond. Sphingomyelin is therefore a ceramide phosphocholine. It contains one negative

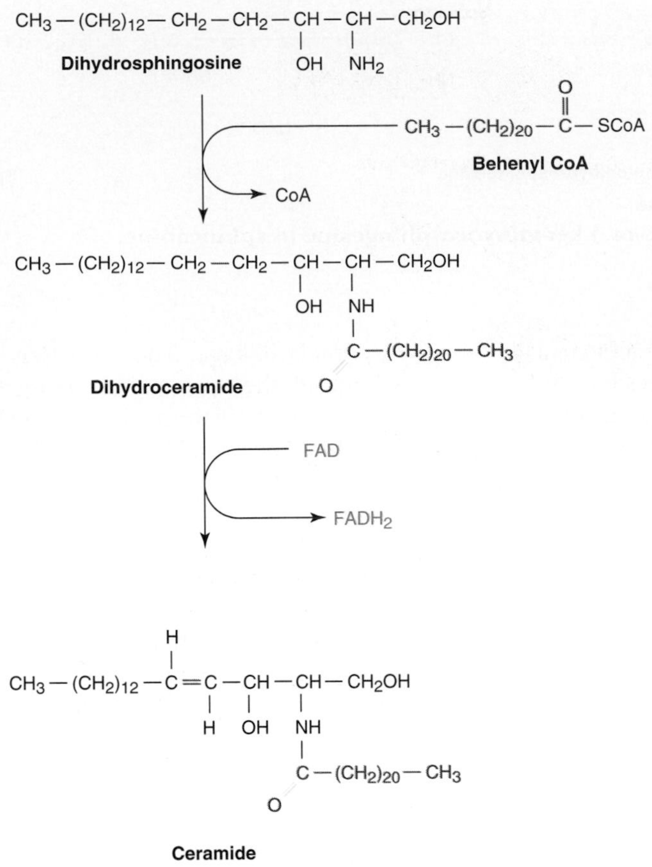

$CH_3-(CH_2)_{12}-CH_2-CH_2-CH(OH)-CH(NH_2)-CH_2OH$

Dihydrosphingosine

$CH_3-(CH_2)_{20}-C(=O)-SCoA$

Behenyl CoA

CoA

$CH_3-(CH_2)_{12}-CH_2-CH_2-CH(OH)-CH(NH-C(=O)-(CH_2)_{20}-CH_3)-CH_2OH$

Dihydroceramide

FAD

$FADH_2$

$CH_3-(CH_2)_{12}-CH=CH-CH(OH)-CH(NH-C(=O)-(CH_2)_{20}-CH_3)-CH_2OH$

Ceramide

FIGURE 10.48
Formation of ceramide from dihydrosphingosine.

and one positive charge so that it is neutral at physiological pH (Figure 10.50). The most common fatty acids in sphingomyelin are palmitic (16:0), stearic (18:0), lignoceric (24:0), and nervonic acid (24:1). The sphingomyelin of myelin contains predominantly longer chain fatty acids, mainly lignoceric and nervonic, whereas that of gray matter contains largely stearic acid. Excessive accumulations of sphingomyelin occur in Niemann–Pick disease.

Sphingomyelin Is Synthesized from a Ceramide and Phosphatidylcholine

Conversion of ceramide to sphingomyelin involves transfer of a phosphocholine moiety from phosphatidylcholine (lecithin), not from CDP–choline as was suspected for many years; this reaction is catalyzed by **sphingomyelin synthase** (Figure 10.51).

Glycosphingolipids Usually Have a Galactose or Glucose Unit

The principal glycosphingolipid classes are cerebrosides, sulfatides, globosides, and gangliosides. In the glycolipid class of compounds the polar head group is attached to sphingosine via the glycosidic linkage of a sugar molecule rather than a phosphate ester bond, as in phospholipids.

Cerebrosides Are Glycosylceramides

Cerebrosides are ceramide monohexosides; the two most common are **galactocerebroside** and **glucocerebroside.** Unless specified otherwise, the term cerebroside usually refers to galactocerebroside, also called **"galactolipid."** In Figure 10.52 note that the monosaccharide units are attached at C-1 of the sugar

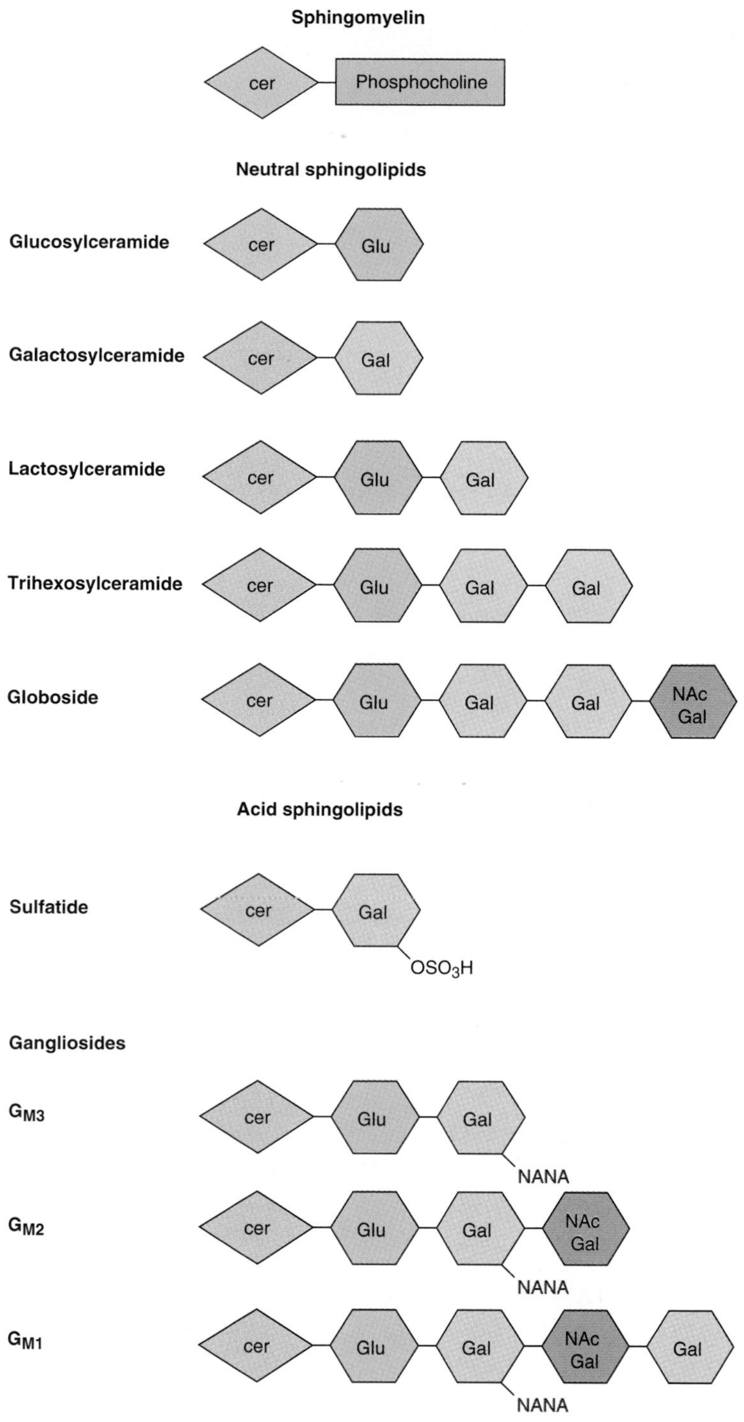

Sphingomyelin

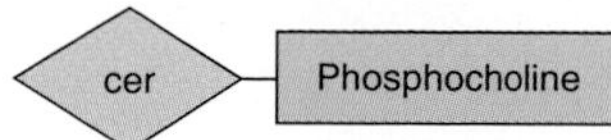

Neutral sphingolipids

Glucosylceramide

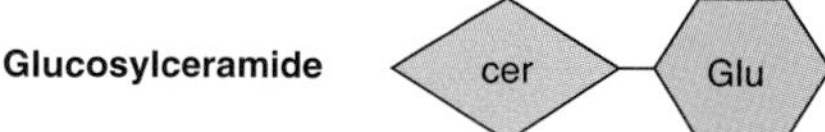

Galactosylceramide — cer — Gal

Lactosylceramide — cer — Glu — Gal

Trihexosylceramide — cer — Glu — Gal — Gal

Globoside — cer — Glu — Gal — Gal — NAc Gal

Acid sphingolipids

Sulfatide — cer — Gal — OSO_3H

Gangliosides

G_{M3} — cer — Glu — Gal (NANA)

G_{M2} — cer — Glu — Gal (NANA) — NAc Gal

G_{M1} — cer — Glu — Gal (NANA) — NAc Gal — Gal

FIGURE 10.49
Structures of some common sphingolipids in diagrammatic form.
Cer, ceramide; Glu, glucose; Gal, galactose; NAcGal, *N*-acetylgalactosamine; and NANA, *N*-acetylneuraminic acid (sialic acid).

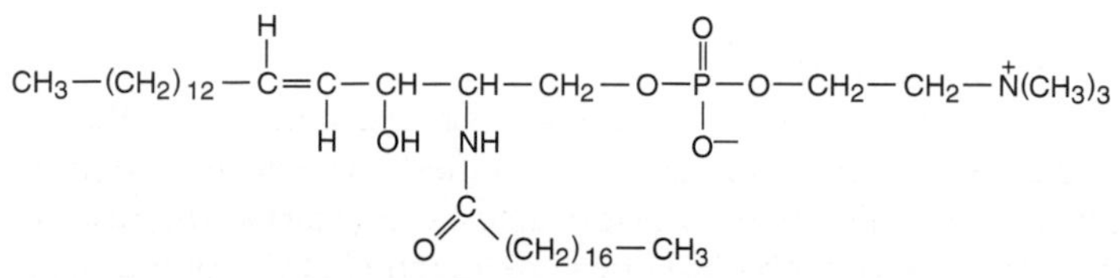

$$CH_3-(CH_2)_{12}-CH{=}CH-CH(OH)-CH(NH-C(=O)-(CH_2)_{16}-CH_3)-CH_2-O-P(=O)(O^-)-O-CH_2-CH_2-\overset{+}{N}(CH_3)_3$$

FIGURE 10.50
Structure of sphingomyelin.

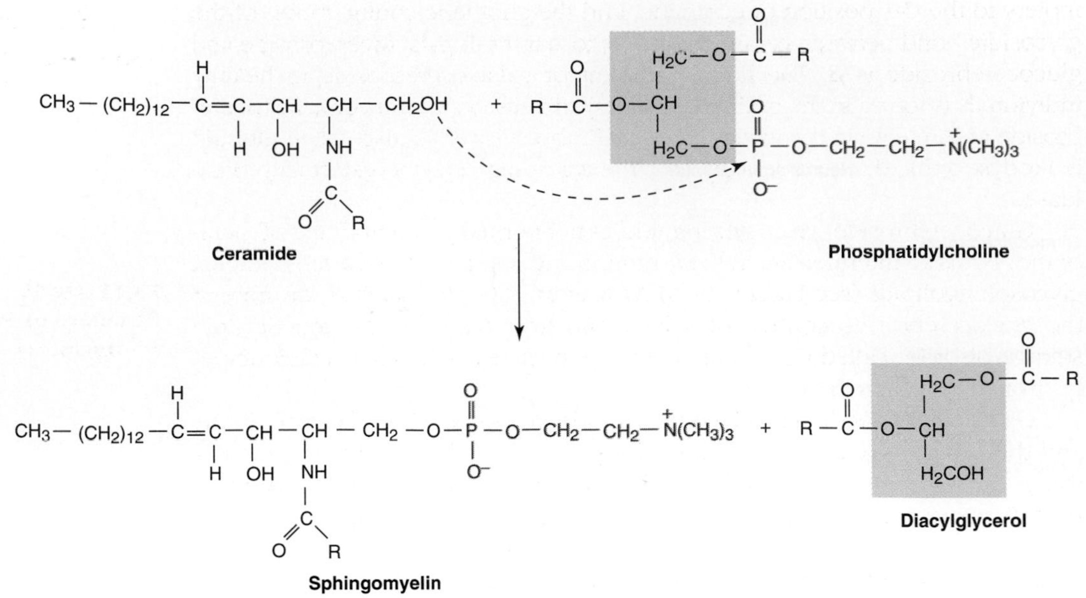

Ceramide + Phosphatidylcholine → Sphingomyelin + Diacylglycerol

FIGURE 10.51
Sphingomyelin synthesis from ceramide and phosphatidylcholine.

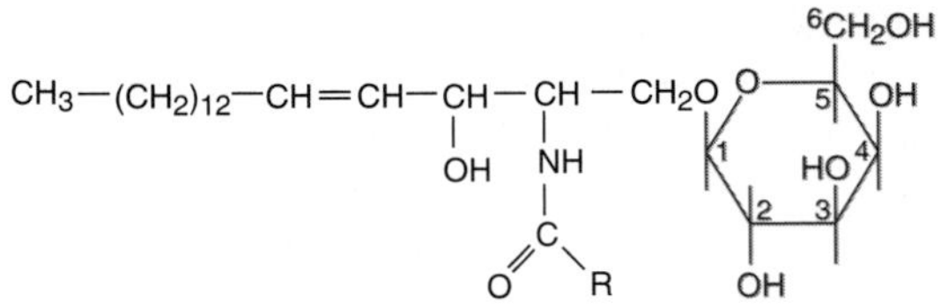

FIGURE 10.52
Structure of galactocerebroside (galactolipid).

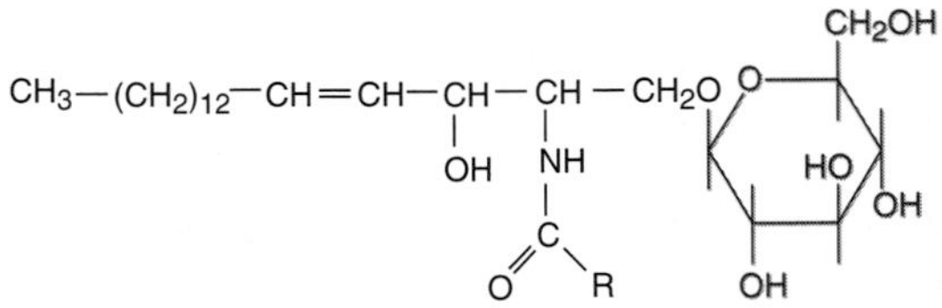

FIGURE 10.53
Structure of glucocerebroside.

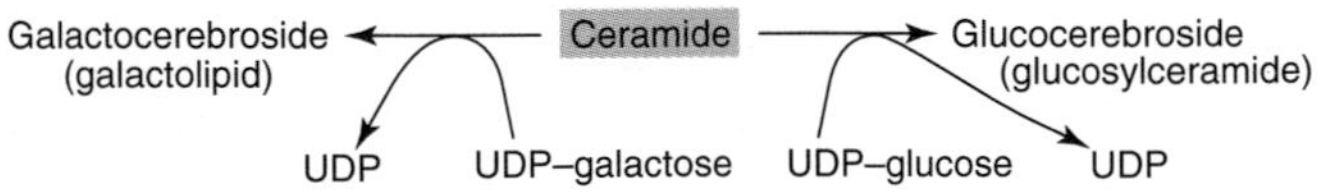

Galactocerebroside (galactolipid) ← Ceramide → Glucocerebroside (glucosylceramide)

UDP, UDP–galactose, UDP–glucose, UDP

FIGURE 10.54
Synthesis of galacto- and glucocerebrosides.

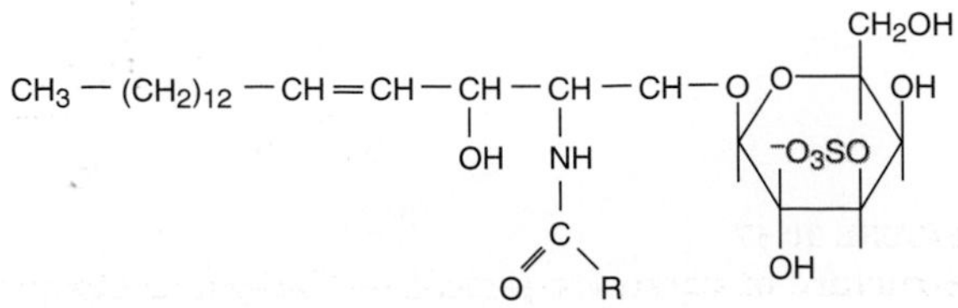

FIGURE 10.55
Structure of galactocerebroside sulfate (sulfolipid).

moiety to the C-1 position of ceramide, and the anomeric configuration of the glycosidic bond between ceramide and hexose in both galactocerebroside and glucocerebroside is β. The largest amount of galactocerebroside in healthy individuals is found in the brain. Moderately increased amounts of galactocerebroside accumulate in the white matter in Krabbe's disease, also called globoid leukodystrophy, due to a deficiency in the lysosomal enzyme galactocerebrosidase.

Glucocerebroside (glucosylceramide) is not normally a component of membranes but is an intermediate in the synthesis and degradation of more complex glycosphingolipids (see Figure 10.53). However, 100-fold increases or more in the glucocerebroside content of spleen and liver occur in the genetic lipid storage disorder called Gaucher's disease, which results from a deficiency of lysosomal glucocerebrosidase.

Galactocerebroside and glucocerebroside are synthesized from ceramide and the activated nucleotide sugars UDP-galactose and UDP-glucose, respectively. The enzymes that catalyze these reactions, **glucosyl** and **galactosyltransferases,** are associated with the endoplasmic reticulum (Figure 10.54). In some tissues, the synthesis of glucocerebroside (glucosylceramide) proceeds by glucosylation of sphingosine catalyzed by glucosyltransferase:

$$\text{Sphingosine} + \text{UDP-glucose} \rightarrow \text{glucosylsphingosine} + \text{UDP}$$

followed by fatty acylation:

$$\text{Glucosylsphingosine} + \text{stearoyl CoA} \rightarrow \text{glucocerebroside} + \text{CoASH}$$

Sulfatide Is a Sulfuric Acid Ester of Galactocerebroside

Sulfatide, or **sulfogalactocerebroside,** is a sulfuric acid ester of galactocerebroside. Galactocerebroside 3-sulfate is the major sulfolipid in brain and accounts for approximately 15% of the lipids of white matter (see Figure 10.55). Galactocerebroside sulfate is synthesized from galactocerebroside and 3′-phosphoadenosine 5′-phosphosulfate (PAPS) in a reaction catalyzed by sulfotransferase:

$$\text{Galactocerebroside} + \text{PAPS} \rightarrow \text{PAP} + \text{galactocerebroside 3-sulfate}$$

The structure of PAPS, sometimes referred to as "activated sulfate," is indicated in Figure 10.56. Large quantities of sulfatide accumulate in the central nervous system in metachromatic leukodystrophy due to a deficiency of a specific lysosomal sulfatase.

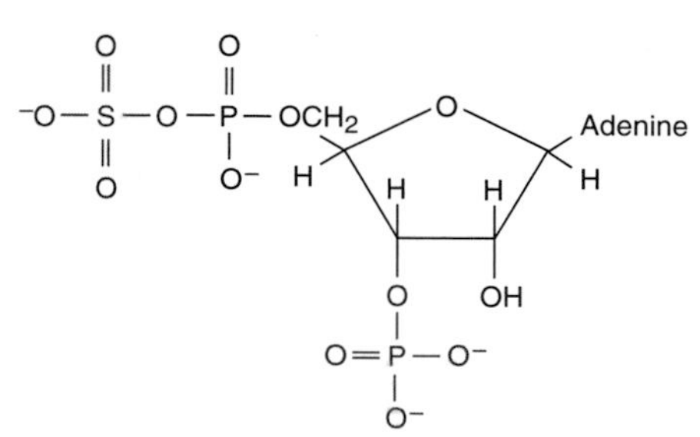

FIGURE 10.56
Structure of PAPS (3′-phosphoadenosine 5′-phosphosulfate).

Globosides Are Ceramide Oligosaccharides

Globosides are cerebrosides that contain two or more sugar residues, usually galactose, glucose, or *N*-acetylgalactosamine. The ceramide oligosaccharides are neutral compounds and contain no free amino groups. Lactosylceramide is a component of the erythrocyte membrane (Figure 10.57). Another prominent globoside is **ceramide trihexoside** or ceramide galactosyllactoside: ceramide-β-glc-(4 $\leftarrow$ 1)-β-gal(4 $\leftarrow$ 1)-α-gal. Note that the terminal galactose residue of this globoside has the α-anomeric configuration. Ceramide trihexoside accumulates in kidneys of patients with Fabry's disease who are deficient in lysosomal α-galactosidase A.

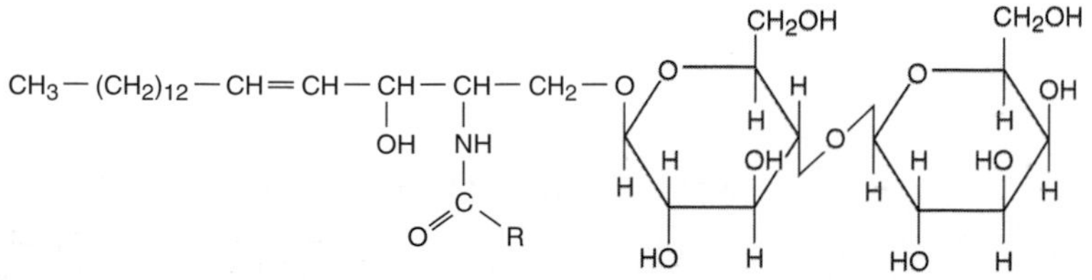

FIGURE 10.57
Structure of ceramide-β-glc(4 $\leftarrow$ 1)-β-gal (lactosylceramide).

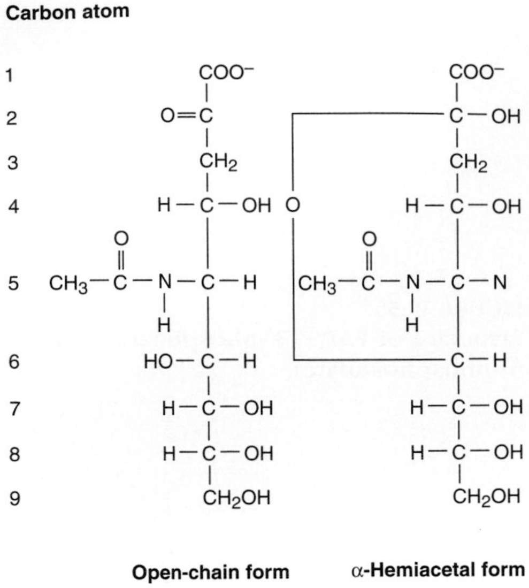

Gangliosides Contain Sialic Acid

Ganglioside are sialic acid-containing glycosphingolipids highly concentrated in the ganglion cells of the central nervous system, particularly in the nerve endings. The central nervous system is unique among human tissues because more than one-half of the sialic acid is in ceramide–lipid bound form, with the remainder of the sialic acid occurring in the oligosaccharides of glycoproteins. Lesser amounts of gangliosides are present in the surface membranes of the cells of most extraneural tissues, where they account for less than 10% of the total sialic acid.

Neuraminic acid (abbreviated Neu) is present in gangliosides, glycoproteins, and mucins. The amino group of neuraminic acid occurs most often as the *N*-acetyl derivative, and the resulting structure is called ***N*-acetylneuraminic acid** or **sialic acid,** commonly abbreviated NANA (see Figure 10.58). The OH group on C-2 occurs most often in the α-anomeric configuration and the linkage between NANA and the oligosaccharide ceramide always involves the OH group on position 2 of *N*-acetylneuraminic acid. Structures of some common gangliosides are indicated in Table 10.1. The principal gangliosides in brain are $\mathbf{G_{M1}}$, $\mathbf{G_{D1a}}$, $\mathbf{G_{D1b}}$, and $\mathbf{G_{T1b}}$. Nearly all gangliosides of the body are derived from the family of compounds originating with glucosylceramide. In the nomenclature of

Carbon atom	Open-chain form	α-Hemiacetal form
1	COO^-	COO^-
2	O=C	C—OH
3	CH_2	CH_2
4	H—C—OH	H—C—OH
5	CH_3—C(=O)—N(H)—C—H	CH_3—C(=O)—N(H)—C—N
6	HO—C—H	C—H
7	H—C—OH	H—C—OH
8	H—C—OH	H—C—OH
9	CH_2OH	CH_2OH

FIGURE 10.58
Structure of N-acetylneuraminic acid (NANA).

TABLE 10.1 Structures of Some Common Gangliosides

Code Name	*Chemical Structure*
G_{M3}	Galβ → 4Glcβ → Cer (Gal 3 ↑ αNANA)
G_{M2}	GalNAcβ → 4Galβ → 4Glcβ → Cer (Gal 3 ↑ αNANA)
G_{M1}	Galβ → 3GalNAcβ → 4Galβ → 4Glcβ → Cer (Gal 3 ↑ αNANA)
G_{D1a}	Galβ → 3GalNAcβ → 4Galβ → 4Glcβ → Cer (Gal 3 ↑ αNANA; Gal 3 ↑ αNANA)
G_{D1b}	Galβ → 3GalNAcβ → 4Galβ → 4Glcβ → Cer (Gal 3 ↑ αNANA8 ← αNANA)
G_{T1a}	Galβ → 3GalNAcβ → 4Galβ → 4Glcβ → Cer (Gal 3 ↑ αNANA8 ← αNANA; Gal 3 ↑ αNANA)
G_{T1b}	Galβ → 3GalNAcβ → 4Galβ → 4Glcβ → Cer (Gal 3 ↑ αNANA; Gal 3 ↑ αNANA8 ← αNANA)
G_{Q1b}	Galβ → 3GalNAcβ → 4Galβ → 4Glcβ → Cer (Gal 3 ↑ αNANA8 ← αNANA; Gal 3 ↑ αNANA8 ← αNANA)

the sialoglycosphingolipids, the letter G refers to the name ganglioside. The subscripts M, D, T, and Q indicate mono-, di-, tri-, and quatra (tetra)-sialic acid-containing gangliosides and subscripts 1, 2, and 3 designate the carbohydrate sequence that is attached to ceramide as indicated as follows: 1, Gal-GalNAc-Gal-Glc-ceramide; 2, GalNAc-Gal-Glc-ceramide; and 3, Gal-Glc-ceramide. Consider the nomenclature of the Tay–Sachs ganglioside; the designation G_{M2} denotes the ganglioside structure shown in Table 10.1.

A specific ganglioside on intestinal mucosal cells mediates the action of cholera toxin, a protein of mol wt 84,000, secreted by the pathogen *Vibrio cholerae*. The toxin stimulates the secretion of chloride ions into the gut lumen, resulting in the severe diarrhea characteristic of cholera. Two kinds of subunits, A and B, comprise the cholera toxin; there is one copy of the A subunit (28,000 Da) and five copies of the B subunit (~11,000 Da each). After binding to the cell surface membrane through a domain on the B subunit, the active subunit A passes into the cell. There it acts as an **ADP-ribosyltransferase** and transfers ADP-ribose of NAD^+ on to the $G_{\alpha s}$ subunit of a G-protein on the cytoplasmic side of the cell membrane (see p. 859). This leads to activation of adenylate cyclase. The cAMP generated stimulates chloride ion transport and produces diarrhea. The choleragenoid domain, as the B subunits are called, binds to the **ganglioside G_{M1}** that has the structure shown in Table 10.1.

Gangliosides are also thought to be receptors for other toxins, such as tetanus toxin, and certain viruses, such as the influenza viruses. There is also speculation that gangliosides play an informational role in cell–cell interactions by providing specific recognition determinants on the surface of cells. There are several lipid storage disorders that involve the accumulation of sialic acid-containing glycosphingolipids. The two most common gangliosidoses involve the storage of the gangliosides G_{M1} (G_{M1} gangliosidosis) and G_{M2} (Tay–Sachs disease). G_{M1} gangliosidosis is an autosomal recessive metabolic disease characterized by impaired psychomotor function, mental retardation, hepatosplenomegaly, and death within the first few years of life. The massive cerebral and visceral accumulation of G_{M1} ganglioside is due to a marked deficiency of β-galactosidase.

Sphingolipidoses Are Lysosomal Storage Diseases with Defects in the Catabolic Pathway for Sphingolipids

Sphingolipids are normally degraded within lysosomes of phagocytic cells, particularly the histiocytes or macrophages of the reticuloendothelial system located primarily in liver, spleen, and bone marrow. Degradation of the sphingolipids by visceral organs begins with the engulfment of the membranes of white cells and erythrocytes that are rich in lactosylceramide (Cer-Glc-Gal) and hematoside (Cer-Glc-Gal-NANA). In the brain, the majority of the cerebroside-type lipids are gangliosides. Particularly during the neonatal period, ganglioside turnover in the central nervous system is extensive so that glycosphingolipids are rapidly being broken down and resynthesized. The pathway of sphingolipid catabolism is summarized in Figure 10.59. Note that among the various sphingolipids that comprise this pathway, there occurs a sulfate ester (in sulfolipid or sulfogalactolipid); *N*-acetylneuraminic acid groups (in the gangliosides); an α-linked galactose residue (in ceramide trihexoside); several β-galactosides (in galactocerebroside and G_{M1}); the ganglioside G_{M2}, which terminates in a β-linked *N*-acetylgalactosamine unit; and glucocerebroside, which is composed of a single glucose residue attached to ceramide through a β linkage. The phosphodiester bond in sphingomyelin is broken to produce ceramide, which in turn is converted in sphingosine by the cleavage of an amide bond to a long-chain fatty acid. This overall pathway of sphingolipid catabolism is composed of a series of enzymes that cleave specific bonds in the compounds including α- and β-galactosidases, a β-glucosidase, a neuraminidase, hexosaminidase, a sphingomyelin-specific phosphodiesterase (sphingomyelinase), a sulfate esterase (sulfatase), and a ceramide-specific amidase (ceramidase). The important features of the sphingolipid catabolic pathway are as follows: (1) all the reactions take place within the lysosome; that is, the enzymes of the pathway are contained in lysosomes; (2) the enzymes are hydrolases; therefore one of the substrates in each reaction is water; (3) the pH optimum of each of the hydrolases is in the acid range, pH 3.5–5.5; (4) most of the enzymes are relatively stable and occur as isoenzymes; for example, **hexosaminidase** occurs in two forms: hexosaminidase A (HexA) and hexosaminidase B (HexB); (5) the hydrolases that comprise the sphingolipid pathway are glycoproteins and often occur firmly bound to the lysosomal membrane; and (6) the pathway is composed of intermediates that differ by only one sugar molecule, a sulfate group, or a fatty acid residue. The substrates are converted to products by the sequential, stepwise removal of constituents such as sugars and sulfate, by hydrolytic, irreversible reactions.

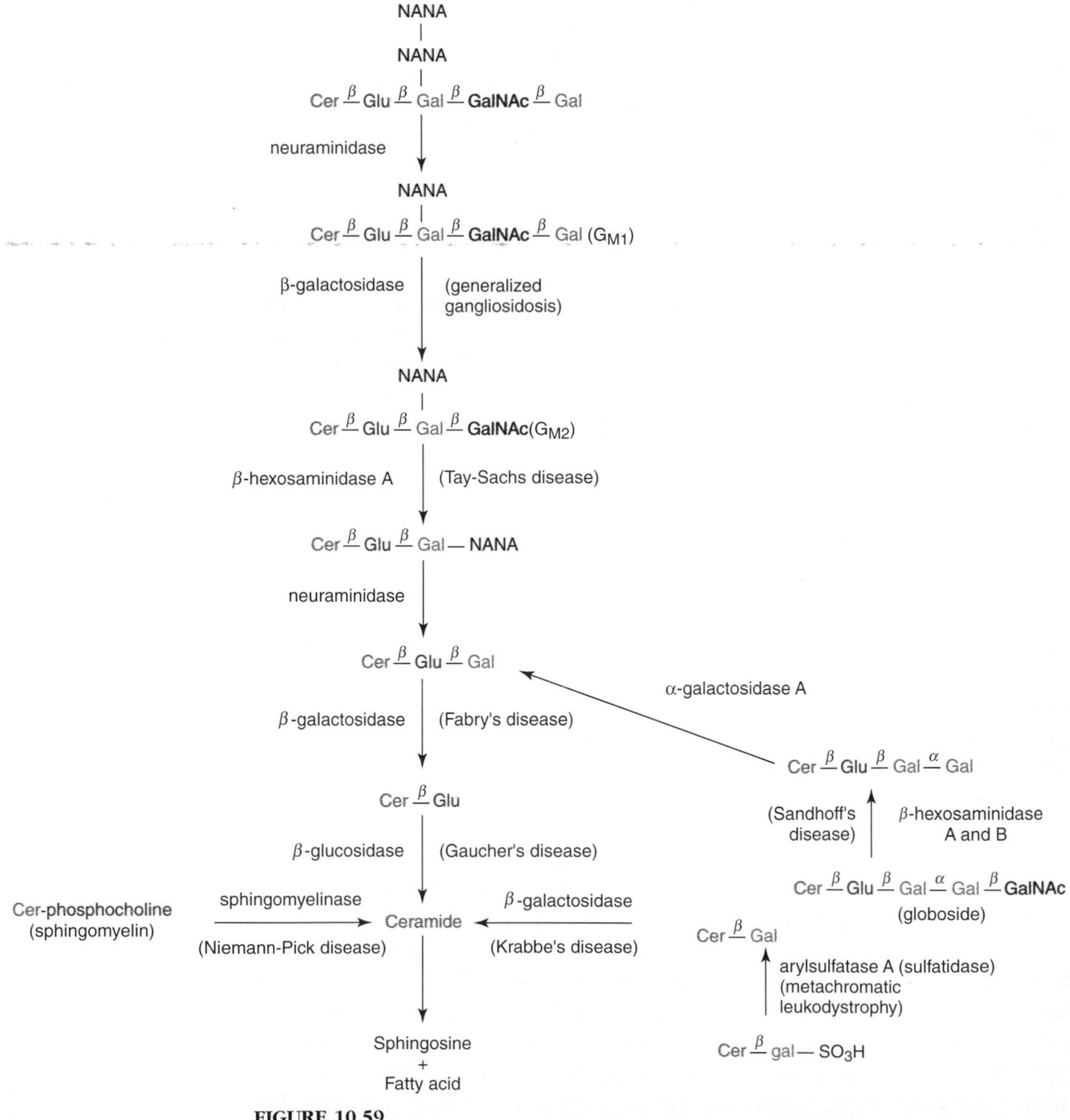

FIGURE 10.59
Summary of the pathways for catabolism of sphingolipids by lysosomal enzymes.
The genetically determined enzyme deficiency diseases are indicated in parentheses.

TABLE 10.2 Sphingolipid Storage Diseases of Humans

Disorder	*Principal Signs and Symptoms*	*Principal Storage Substance*	*Enzyme Deficiency*
1. Tay–Sachs disease	Mental retardation, blindness, cherry red spot on macula, death between second and third year	Ganglioside G_{M2}	Hexosaminidase A
2. Gaucher's disease	Liver and spleen enlargement, erosion of long bones and pelvis, mental retardation in infantile form only	Glucocerebroside	Glucocerebrosidase
3. Fabry's disease	Skin rash, kidney failure, pains in lower extremities	Ceramide trihexoside	α-Galactosidase A
4. Niemann–Pick disease	Liver and spleen enlargement, mental retardation	Sphingomyelin	Sphingomyelinase
5. Globoid leukodystrophy (Krabbe's disease)	Mental retardation, absence of myelin	Galactocerebroside	Galactocerebrosidase
6. Metachromatic leukodystrophy	Mental retardation, nerves stain yellowish brown with cresyl violet dye (metachromasia)	Sulfatide	Arylsulfatase A
7. Generalized gangliosidosis	Mental retardation, liver enlargement, skeletal involvement	Ganglioside G_{M1}	G_{M1} ganglioside: β-galactosidase
8. Sandhoff–Jatzkewitz disease	Same as 1; disease has more rapidly progressing course	G_{M2} ganglioside, globoside	Hexosaminidase A and B
9. Fucosidosis	Cerebral degeneration, muscle spasticity, thick skin	Pentahexosylfucoglycolipid	α-L-Fucosidase

In most cases, sphingolipid catabolism functions smoothly, and all of the various complex glycosphingolipids and sphingomyelin are degraded to the level of their basic building blocks, namely, sugars, sulfate, fatty acid, phosphocholine, and sphingosine. However, when the activity of one of the hydrolytic enzymes is markedly reduced due to a genetic error, then the substrate for the defective or missing enzyme accumulates and is deposited within the lysosomes of the tissue responsible for the catabolism of that sphingolipid. For most of the reactions in Figure 10.59, patients have been identified who lack the enzyme that normally catalyzes that reaction. These disorders, called **sphingolipidoses,** are summarized in Table 10.2.

We can generalize about some of the common features of **lipid storage diseases:** (1) usually only a single sphingolipid accumulates in the involved organs; (2) the ceramide portion is common to the various storage lipids; (3) the rate of biosynthesis of the accumulating lipid is normal; (4) a catabolic enzyme is missing in each of these disorders; and (5) the extent of the enzyme deficiency is the same in all tissues.

Diagnostic Enzyme Assays for Sphingolipidoses

Diagnosis of a given sphingolipidosis can be made from a biopsy of the involved organ, usually bone marrow, liver, or brain, on morphologic grounds on the basis of the highly characteristic appearance of the storage lipid within lysosomes. Assay of enzyme activity is used to confirm the diagnosis of a particular lipid storage disease. Of great practical value is the fact that, for most of the diseases, peripheral leukocytes, cultured skin fibroblasts, and chorionic villi express the relevant enzyme deficiency and can be used as a source of enzyme for diagnostic purposes. In some cases (e.g., Tay–Sachs disease) serum and even tears are a source of enzyme for the diagnosis of a lipid storage disorder. Sphingolipidoses, for the most part, are autosomal recessive, with the disease occurring only in homozygotes with a defect in both alleles. Enzyme assays can identify carriers or heterozygotes.

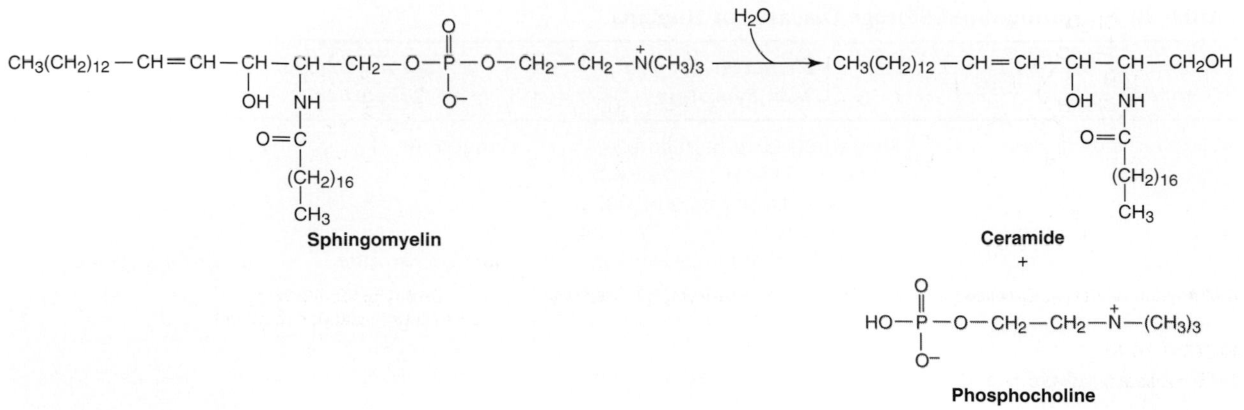

FIGURE 10.60
Sphingomyelinase reaction.

In **Niemann–Pick disease,** the deficient enzyme is **sphingomyelinase,** which normally catalyzes the reaction shown in Figure 10.60. Sphingomyelin, radiolabeled in the methyl groups of choline with carbon-14, provides a useful substrate for determining sphingomyelinase activity. Extracts of white blood cells from healthy, appropriate controls will hydrolyze the labeled substrate and produce the water-soluble product, phosphocholine. Extraction of the final incubation medium with an organic solvent such as chloroform will result in radioactivity in the upper, aqueous phase; the unused, lipid-like substrate sphingomyelin will be found in the chloroform phase. On the other hand, if the white blood cells were derived from a patient with Niemann–Pick disease, then after incubation with labeled substrate and extraction with chloroform, little or no radioactivity (i.e., phosphocholine) would be found in the aqueous phase and the diagnosis would be confirmed.

Another disease that can be diagnosed by use of an artificial substrate is **Tay–Sachs disease,** the most common form of **G_{M2} gangliosidosis.** In this fatal disorder the ganglion cells of the cerebral cortex are swollen and the lysosomes are engorged with the acidic lipid, G_{M2} ganglioside. This results in a loss of ganglion cells, proliferation of glial cells, and demyelination of peripheral nerves. The pathognomonic finding is a cherry red spot on the macula caused by swelling and necrosis of ganglion cells in the eye. In Tay–Sachs disease, the commercially available artificial substrate 4-methylumbelliferyl-β-*N*-acetyl-glucosamine is used to confirm the diagnosis. The compound is hydrolyzed by hexosaminidase A, the deficient lysosomal hydrolase, to produce the intensely fluorescent product 4-methylumbelliferone (Figure 10.61). Unfortunately, the diagnosis may be confused by the presence of hexosaminidase B in tissue extracts and body fluids. This enzyme is not deficient in the Tay–Sachs patient and will hydrolyze the test substrate, thereby confusing the interpretation of results. The problem is usually resolved by taking advantage of the relative heat lability of hexosaminidase A and heat stability of hexosaminidase B. The tissue extract or serum specimen to be tested is first heated at 55°C for 1 h and then assayed for hexosaminidase activity. The amount of heat-labile activity is a measure of hexosaminidase A, and this value is used in making the diagnosis.

Enzyme assays of serum or extracts of tissues, peripheral leukocytes, and fibroblasts have proved useful in heterozygote detection. Once carriers of a lipid storage disease have been identified, or if there has been a previously affected child in a family, the pregnancies at risk for these diseases can be monitored. All nine of the lipid storage disorders are transmitted as recessive genetic abnormalities. In all but one the allele is carried on an autosomal chromosome. Fabry's disease is linked to the X chromosome. In all of these conditions statistically one of four fetuses will be homozygous (or hemizygous in Fabry's disease), two fetuses will be carriers, and one will be completely

CLINICAL CORRELATION 10.4

Diagnosis of Gaucher's Disease in an Adult

Gaucher's disease is an inherited disease of lipid catabolism that results in deposition of glucocerebroside in macrophages of the reticuloendothelial system. Because of the large numbers of macrophages in spleen, bone marrow, and liver, hepatomegaly, splenomegaly and its sequelae (thrombocytopenia or anemia), and bone pain are the most common signs and symptoms of the disease.

Gaucher's disease results from a deficiency of glucocerebrosidase. Although this enzyme deficiency is inherited, different clinical patterns are observed. Some patients suffer severe neurologic deficits as infants, while others do not exhibit symptoms until adulthood. The diagnosis can be made by assaying leukocytes or fibroblasts for their ability to hydrolyze the β-glycosidic bond of artificial substrates (β-glucosidase activity) or of glucocerebroside (glucocerebrosidase activity). Gaucher's disease has been treated with regular infusions of purified glucocerebrosidase and the long-term efficacy of the therapy looks encouraging.

Brady, R. O., Kanfer, J. N., Bradley, R. M., and Shapiro, D. Demonstration of a deficiency of glucocerebroside-cleaving enzyme in Gaucher's disease. *J. Clin. Invest.* 45:1112, 1966.

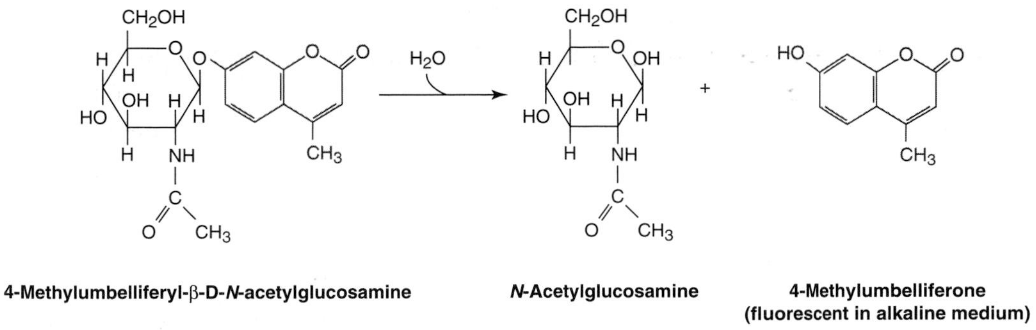

4-Methylumbelliferyl-β-D-*N*-acetylglucosamine

N-Acetylglucosamine

4-Methylumbelliferone (fluorescent in alkaline medium)

FIGURE 10.61
***β*-Hexosaminidase reaction.**

normal. The enzyme assays have been used to detect affected fetuses and carriers *in utero,* using cultured fibroblasts obtained by amniocentesis as a source of enzyme.

Except for Gaucher's disease, there is no therapy for the sphingolipidoses; the role of medicine at present is prevention through genetic counseling based on enzyme assays of the type discussed above. A discussion of the diagnosis and therapy of **Gaucher's disease** is presented in Clin. Corr. 10.4.

10.5 ■ PROSTAGLANDINS AND THROMBOXANES

Prostaglandins and Thromboxanes Are Derivatives of Twenty-Carbon, Monocarboxylic Acids

In mammalian cells two major pathways of arachidonic acid metabolism produce important mediators of cellular and bodily functions: the **cyclooxygenase** and the **lipoxygenase pathways.** The substrate for both pathways is unesteri-

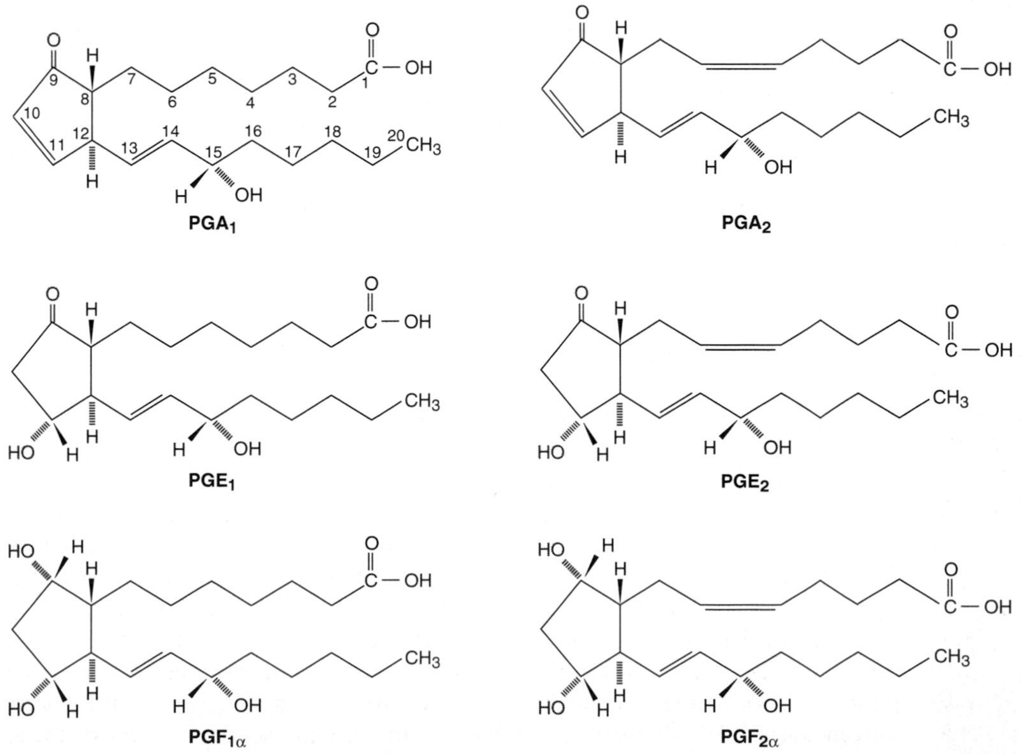

PGA$_1$

PGA$_2$

PGE$_1$

PGE$_2$

PGF$_{1\alpha}$

PGF$_{2\alpha}$

FIGURE 10.62
Structures of the major prostaglandins.

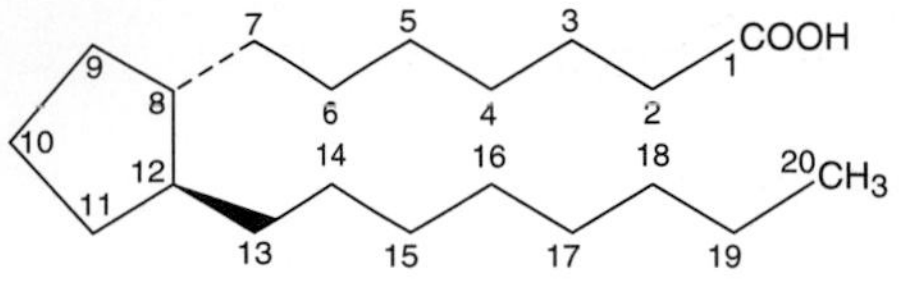

FIGURE 10.63
Structure of prostanoic acid.

fied arachidonic acid. The cyclooxygenase pathway leads to a series of compounds including prostaglandins and thromboxanes. Prostaglandins were discovered through their effects on smooth muscle, specifically their ability to promote the contraction of intestinal and uterine muscle and the lowering of blood pressure. Although the complexity of their structures and the diversity of their sometimes conflicting functions often create a sense of frustration, the potent pharmacological effects of the prostaglandins have afforded them an important place in human biology and medicine. With the exception of the red blood cell, the prostaglandins are produced and released by nearly all mammalian cells and tissues; they are not confined to specialized cells. Unlike most hormones, prostaglandins are not stored in cells but instead are synthesized and released immediately.

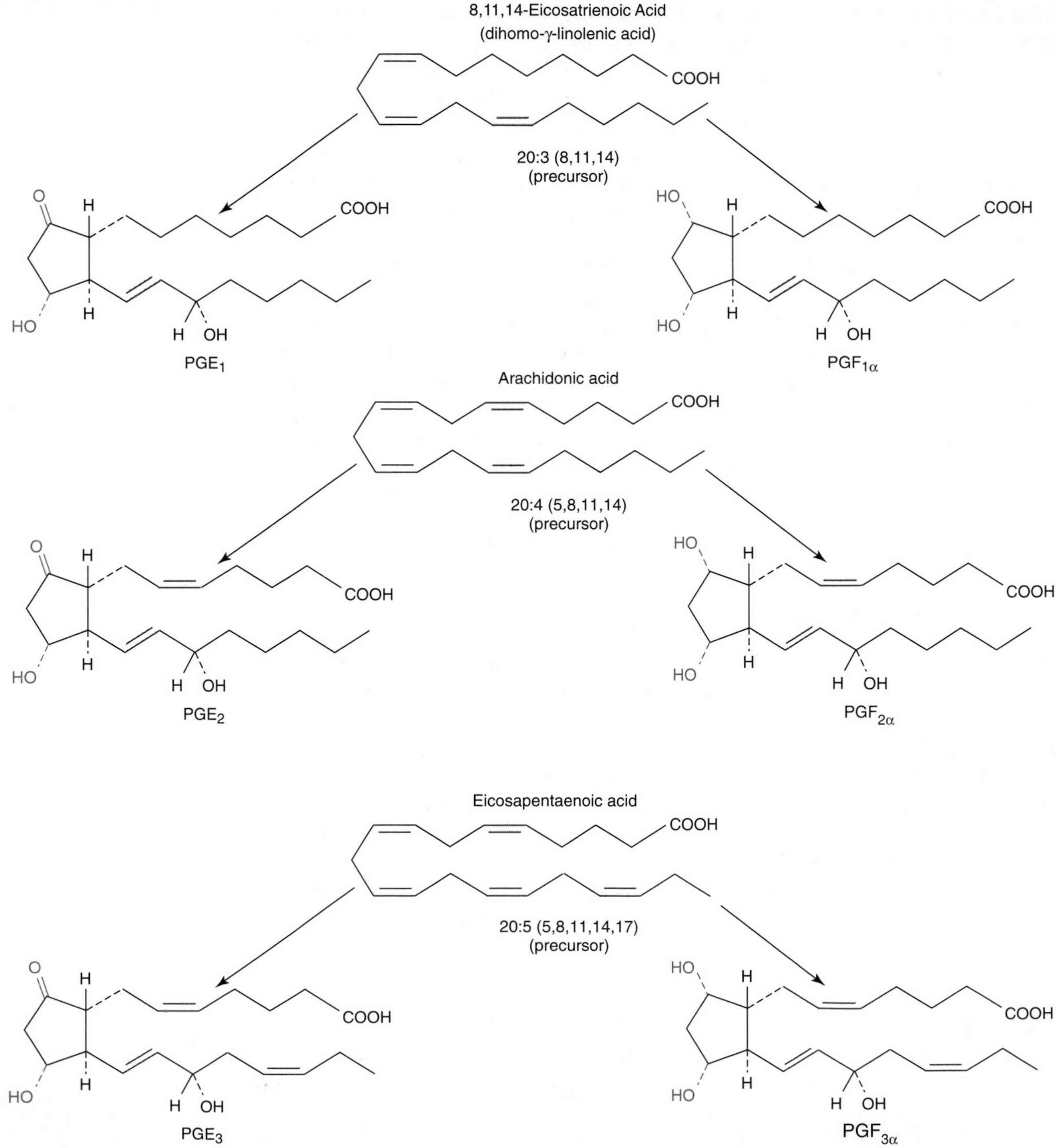

FIGURE 10.64
Synthesis of E and F prostaglandins from fatty acid precursors.

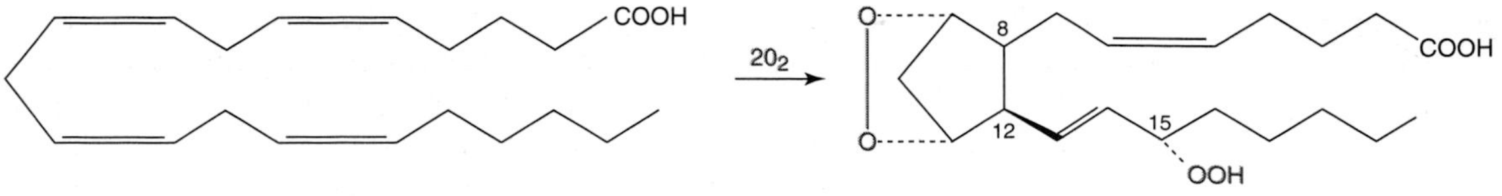

Arachidonic acid

$2O_2$

PGG_2

FIGURE 10.65
Cyclooxygenase reaction.

There are three major classes of primary **prostaglandins,** the **A, E,** and **F series.** The structures of the more common prostaglandins A, E, and F are shown in Figure 10.62 (p. 431). All are related to the hypothetical parent compound, prostanoic acid (Figure 10.63). Note that the prostaglandins contain a multiplicity of functional groups; for example, PGE_2 contains a carboxyl group, a β-hydroxyketone, a secondary alkylic alcohol, and two carbon–carbon double bonds. The three classes (A, E, and F) are distinguished on the basis of the functional groups about the cyclopentane ring (Figure 10.64): the E series contains a β-hydroxyketone, the F series are 1,3-diols, and those in the A series are α,β-unsaturated ketones. The subscript numerals 1, 2, and 3, refer to the number of double bonds in the side chains. The subscript α refers to the configuration of the C-9 OH group: an α-hydroxyl group projects "down" from the plane of the ring.

The most important dietary precursor of the prostaglandins is linoleic acid (18:2), which is an essential fatty acid. In adults linoleic acid is ingested daily in amounts of about 10 g. Only a very minor part of this total intake is converted by carbon chain elongation and desaturation in liver to arachidonic acid (eicosatetraenoic acid) and to some extent also to dihomo-γ-linolenic acid. Since the total daily excretion of prostaglandins and their metabolites is only about 1 mg, it is clear that the formation of prostaglandins is a quantitatively unimportant pathway in the overall metabolism of fatty acids. At the same time, however, the metabolism of prostaglandins is completely dependent on a regular and constant supply of linoleic acid. When the diet is deficient in linoleic acid, there is decreased production of prostaglandins. The diet also provides arachidonic acid.

Synthesis of Prostaglandins Involves a Cyclooxygenase

The immediate precursors to the prostaglandins are C_{20} polyunsaturated fatty acids containing 3, 4, and 5 carbon–carbon double bonds. Since **arachidonic acid** and most of its metabolites contain 20 carbon atoms, they are referred to as **eicosanoids.** During their transformation into various prostaglandins they are cyclized and take up oxygen. Dihomo-γ-linolenic acid (20:3(8,11,14)) is the precursor to PGE_1 and $PGF_{1\alpha}$; arachidonic acid (20:4(5,8,11,14)) is the precursor to PGE_2 and $PGF_{2\alpha}$; and eicosapentaenoic acid (20:4(5,8,11,14,17)) is the precursor to PGE_3 and $PGF_{3\alpha}$ (see Figure 10.64).

Compounds of the 2-series derived from arachidonic acid are the principal prostaglandins in humans and are of the greatest significance biologically. The

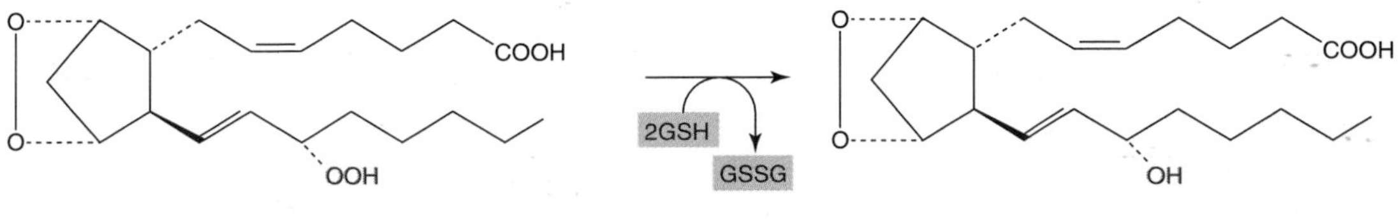

PGG_2

2GSH → GSSG

PGH_2

FIGURE 10.66
Conversion of PGG_2 to PGH_2; PG hydroperoxidase (PGH synthase) reaction.

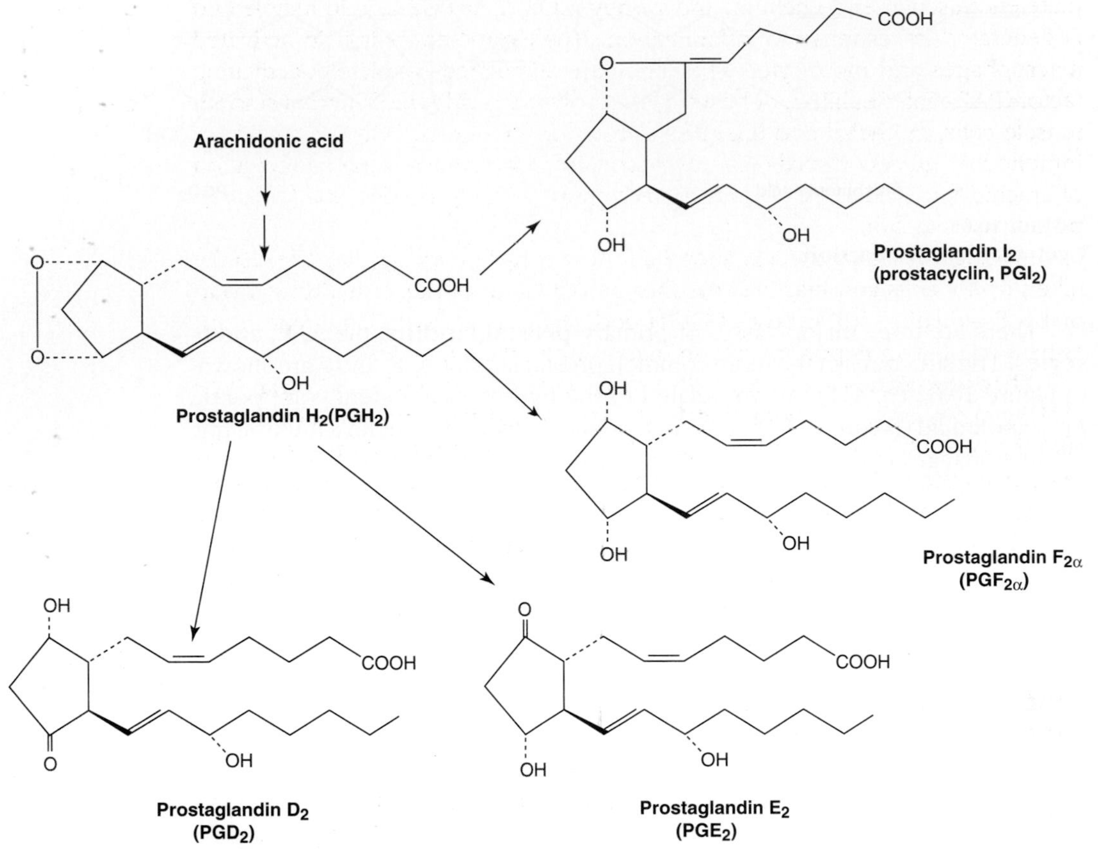

FIGURE 10.67
Major routes of prostaglandin biosynthesis.

central enzyme system in prostaglandin biosynthesis is the **prostaglandin synthase** (PGS) **complex,** which catalyzes oxidative cyclization of polyunsaturated fatty acids. Arachidonic acid is derived from membrane phospholipids by the action of the hydrolase **phospholipase A_2.** This cleavage step is the rate-limiting step in prostaglandin synthesis and some agents that stimulate prostaglandin production act by stimulating the activity of phospholipase A_2. Cholesterol esters containing arachidonic acid may also serve as a source of arachidonic acid substrate.

The **cyclooxygenase** component of the prostaglandin synthase complex catalyzes the cyclization of C-8–C-12 of arachidonic acid to form the cyclic 9,11-endoperoxide 15-hydroperoxide, PGG_2. The reaction requires two molecules of oxygen (Figure 10.65; see p. 433). PGG_2 is then converted to prostaglandin H_2 (PGH_2) by a reduced **glutathione** (GSH)-**dependent peroxidase** (PG hydroperoxidase) (Figure 10.66; see p. 433). Details of the additional steps leading to individual prostaglandins remain to be elucidated. Reactions that cyclize polyunsaturated fatty acids are found in the membranes of the endoplasmic reticulum. Major pathways of prostaglandin biosynthesis are summarized in Figure 10.67. Formation of primary prostaglandins of the D, E, and F series and of thromboxanes or prostacyclin (PGI_2) is mediated by different specific enzymes, whose presence varies depending on the cell type and tissue. This results in a degree of tissue specificity as to the type and quantity of prostaglandin produced. In kidney and spleen PGE_2 and $PGF_{2\alpha}$ are the major prostaglandins formed. In contrast, blood vessels produce mostly PGI_2 and $PGF_{2\alpha}$. In the heart PGE_2, $PGF_{2\alpha}$, and PGI_2 are formed in about equal amounts. Thromboxane A_2 (TXA_2) is the main prostaglandin endoperoxide formed in platelets.

There are two forms of cyclooxygenase (COX) or **prostaglandin synthase** (PGS). COX-1, or PGS-1, is a constitutive enzyme found in gastric mucosa, platelets, vascular endothelium, and kidney. COX-2, or PGS-2, is inducible and is generated in response to inflammation. It is expressed mainly in activated macrophages and monocytes when they are stimulated by platelet-activating factor (PAF), interleukin-1, or bacterial lipopolysaccharide (LPS), and in smooth muscle cells, epithelial and endothelial cells, and neurons. PGS-2 induction is inhibited by glucocorticoids. The two forms of PGS catalyze both oxygenation of arachidonic acid to PGG_2 and the reduction of PGG_2 to PGH_2, which is the peroxidase reaction.

Prostaglandins have a very short half-life. Soon after release they are rapidly taken up by cells and inactivated either by oxidation of the 15-hydroxy group or by β-oxidation from the C_1-COOH end of the fatty acid chain. The lungs appear to play an important role in inactivating prostaglandins.

Thromboxanes are highly active metabolites of the PGG_2- and PGH_2-type prostaglandin endoperoxides that have the cyclopentane ring replaced by a six-membered oxygen-containing (oxane) ring. The term thromboxane is derived from the fact that these compounds have a thrombus-forming potential. **Thromboxane A synthase,** present in the endoplasmic reticulum, is abundant in lung and platelets and catalyzes conversion of endoperoxide PGH_2 to TXA_2. The half-life of TXA_2 is very short in water ($t_{1/2} \sim 1$ min) as the compound is transformed rapidly into inactive thromboxane B_2 (TXB_2) by the reaction shown in Figure 10.68.

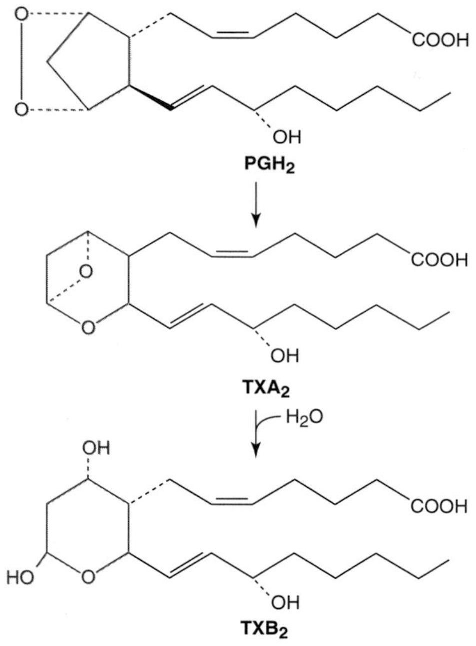

FIGURE 10.68
Synthesis of TXB_2 from PGH_2.

Prostaglandin Production Is Inhibited by Steroidal and Nonsteroidal Anti-inflammatory Agents

Two types of drugs affect prostaglandin metabolism and are therapeutically useful. The **nonsteroidal, anti-inflammatory drugs (NSAIDs),** such as aspirin (acetylsalicylic acid), indomethacin, and phenylbutazone, block prostaglandin production by inhibiting cyclooxygenase. In the case of aspirin, irreversible inhibition occurs by acetylation of the enzyme. Other NSAIDs inhibit cyclooxygenase but do so by binding noncovalently to the enzyme instead of acetylating it; they are called "non-aspirin NSAIDs." Certain NSAIDs inhibit COX-1 more than COX-2 and vice versa. These drugs are not without their undesirable side effects; aplastic anemia can result from phenylbutazone therapy. **Steroidal anti-inflammatory drugs** like hydrocortisone, prednisone, and betamethasone block prostaglandin release by inhibiting phospholipase A_2 activity so as to interfere with mobilization of arachidonic acid (see Figure 10.69). The rate-limiting step in the synthesis of prostaglandins is release of arachidonic acid from membrane phospholipid stores in response to phospholipase A_2 activation.

Factors that govern the biosynthesis of prostaglandins are poorly understood, but, in general, prostaglandin release seems to be triggered following hormonal or neural excitation or after muscular activity. For example, histamine stimulates an increase in the prostaglandin concentration in gastric perfusates. Also, prostaglandins are released during labor and after cellular injury (e.g., platelets exposed to thrombin, lungs irritated by dust).

Prostaglandins Exhibit Many Physiological Effects

Prostaglandins are natural mediators of **inflammation.** Inflammatory reactions most often involve the joints (rheumatoid arthritis), skin (psoriasis), and eyes, and inflammation of these sites is frequently treated with corticosteroids that inhibit prostaglandin synthesis. Administration of PGE_2 or PGE_1 induce the signs of inflammation that include redness and heat (due to arteriolar vasodilation) and swelling and edema resulting from increased capillary permeability. PGE_2 generated in immune tissues (e.g., macrophages, mast cells, B cells) evokes chemokinesis of T cells. PGE_2 in amounts that alone do not cause **pain,** prior to administration of the autocoids, histamine and bradykinin, enhance both the intensity and duration of pain caused by these two agents. It is thought that

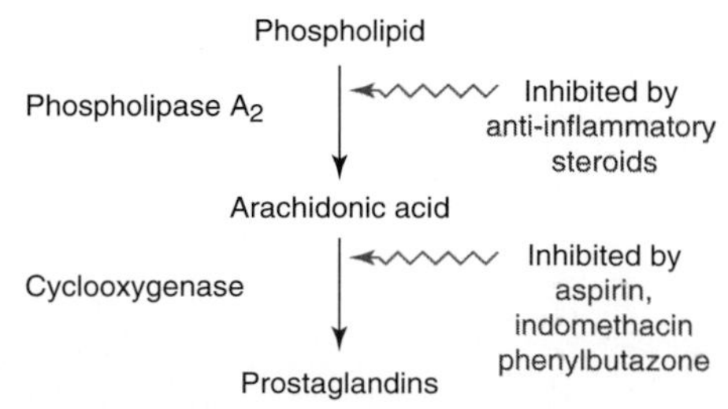

FIGURE 10.69
Site of action of inhibitors of prostaglandin synthesis.

pyrogens (**fever**-inducing agents) activate the prostaglandin biosynthetic pathway resulting in release of PGE_2 in the region of the hypothalamus where body temperature is regulated. Aspirin, which is an antipyretic drug, acts by inhibiting cyclooxygenase. The prostaglandins have been used extensively as drugs in **reproduction.** Both PGE_2 and PGF_2 have been used to induce parturition and for the termination of an unwanted pregnancy, specifically in the second trimester. There is also evidence that the PGE series of prostaglandins may play some role in infertility in males.

Synthetic prostaglandins have proved to be very effective in inhibiting **gastric acid secretion** in patients with **peptic ulcers.** The inhibitory effect of PGE compounds appears to be due to inhibition of cAMP formation in gastric mucosal cells. Prostaglandins also accelerate the healing of gastric ulcers. Prostaglandins play an important role in controlling blood vessel tone and arterial **blood pressure.** The vasodilator prostaglandins, PGE, PGA, and PGI_2, lower systemic arterial pressure, thereby increasing local blood flow and decreasing peripheral resistance. TXA_2 causes contraction of vascular smooth muscle and glomerular mesangium. There is hope that the prostaglandins may eventually prove useful in the treatment of hypertension. PGE_2 functions in the fetus to maintain the patency of the **ductus arteriosus** prior to birth. If the ductus remains open after birth, closure can be hastened by administration of the cyclooxygenase inhibitor indomethacin. In other situations it may be desirable to keep the ductus open. For example, in infants born with congenital abnormalities where the defect can be corrected surgically, infusion of prostaglandins will maintain blood flow through the ductus over this interim period.

Certain prostaglandins, especially PGI_2, inhibit **platelet aggregation,** whereas PGE_2 and TXA_2 promote this clotting process. TXA_2 is produced by platelets and accounts for the spontaneous aggregation that occurs when platelets contact some foreign surface, collagen, or thrombin. Endothelial cells lining blood vessels release PGI_2 and this may account for the lack of adherence of platelets to the healthy blood vessel wall. PGE_2 and PGD_2 dilate renal blood vessels and increase blood flow through the kidney. They also regulate sodium secretion and glomerular filtration rate.

10.6 ■ LIPOXYGENASE AND OXY-EICOSATETRAENOIC ACIDS

Cyclooxygenase directs polyunsaturated fatty acids into the prostaglandin pathway. Another equally important arachidonic acid-oxygenating enzyme, called **lipoxygenase,** is a dioxygenase. Actually, there is a family of lipoxygenases that differ in the position of the double bond on the arachidonic acid molecule at which oxygen attack initially occurs (e.g., positions 5, 11, or 15). In humans the most important leukotrienes are the 5-lipoxygenase products that are involved in the mediation of inflammatory disorders.

Monohydroperoxyeicosatetraenoic Acids Are Products of Lipoxygenase Action

The products of the lipoxygenase reaction, which arise by addition of hydroperoxy groups to arachidonic acid, are designated **monohydroperoxyeicosatetraenoic acids** (HPETEs). Figure 10.70 shows the conversion of arachidonic acid to the three major HPETEs. Thus, in contrast to the cyclooxygenase of prostaglandin endoperoxide synthase, which catalyzes the bis-dioxygenation of unsaturated fatty acids to endoperoxides, lipoxygenases catalyze the monodioxygenation of unsaturated fatty acids to allylic hydroperoxides. Hydroperoxy substitution of arachidonic acid by lipoxygenases may occur at position 5, 12, or 15. 5-HPETE is the major lipoxygenase product in basophils, polymorphonuclear (PMN) leukocytes, macrophages, mast cells, and any organ undergoing

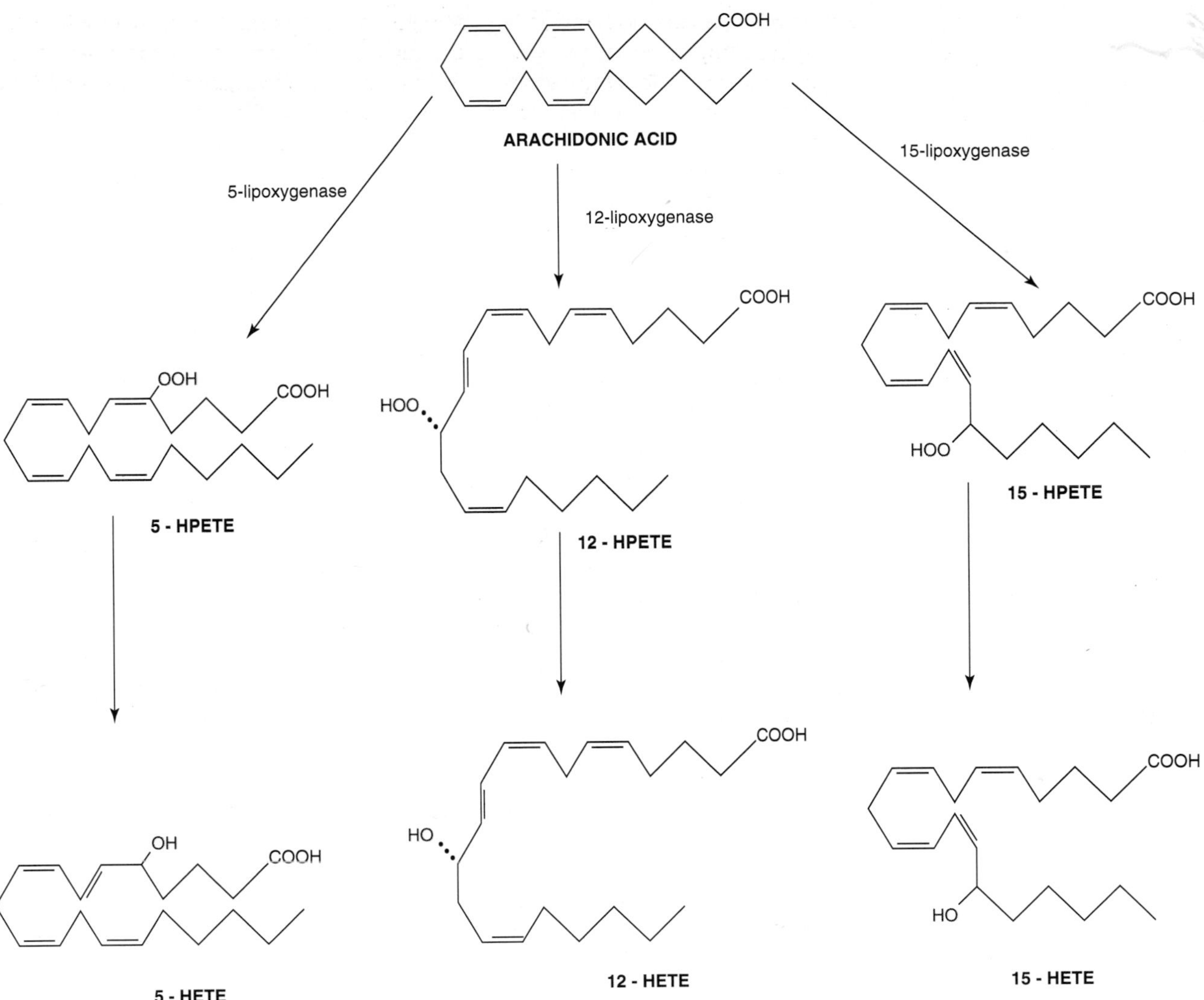

FIGURE 10.70
Lipoxygenase reaction and role of 5-hydroperoxyeicosatetraenoic acids (HPETEs) as precursors of hydroxyeicosatetraenoic acids (HETEs).

an inflammatory response; 12-HPETE predominates in platelets, pancreatic endocrine islet cells, vascular smooth muscle, and glomerular cells; 15-HPETE is the principal lipoxygenase product in reticulocytes, eosinophils, T-lymphocytes, and tracheal epithelial cells. The 5-, 12-, and 15-lipoxygenases occur mainly in the cytosol. Specific stimuli or signals determine which type of lipoxygenase product a given type of cell produces. The oxygenated carbon atom in HPETEs is asymmetric and there are two possible stereoisomers of the hydroperoxy acid, (*R*) or (*S*). All three major HPETEs are of the (*S*) configuration. 5-Lipoxygenase (5-LO) exhibits both a dioxygenase activity that converts arachidonic acid to 5-HPETE and a dehydrase activity that transforms 5-HPETE to LTA_4. 5-LO activity is restricted to a few cell types, including B lymphocytes but not T lymphocytes. It is activated by an accessory protein called 5-lipoxygenase activating protein.

Leukotrienes and Hydroxyeicosatetraenoic Acids Are Hormones Derived from HPETEs

HPETE-hydroperoxides are not hormones, but are highly reactive, unstable intermediates that are converted either to the analogous alcohol (hydroxy fatty

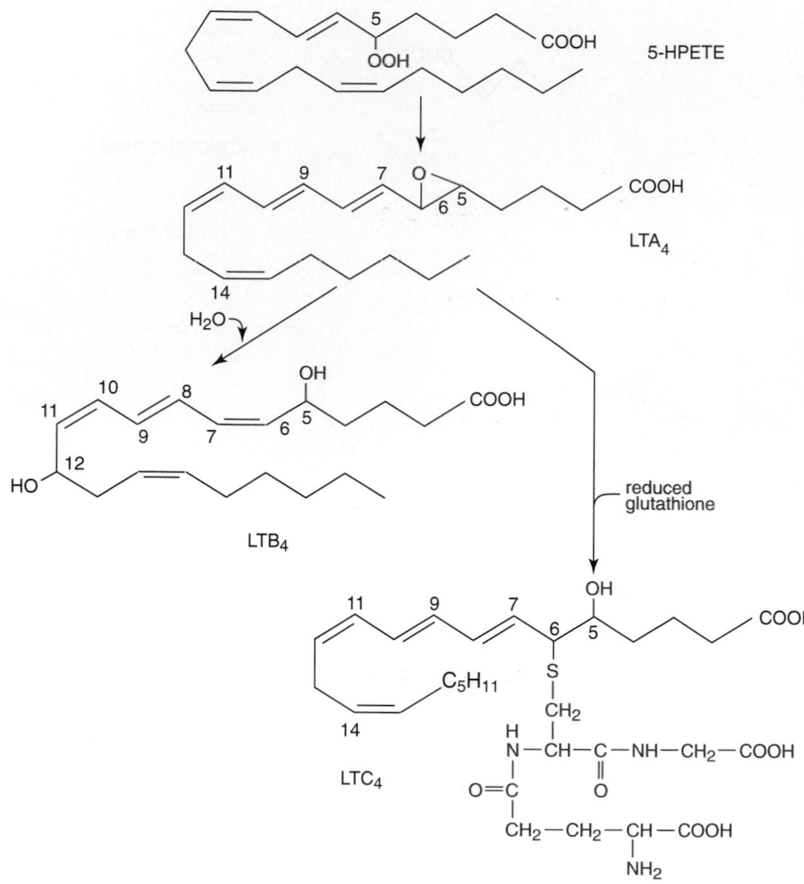

FIGURE 10.71
Conversion of 5-HPETE to LTB_4 and LTC_4 through LTA_4 as intermediate.

acid) by reduction of the peroxide moiety or to leukotrienes. Leukotrienes are lipoxygenase products containing at least three conjugated double bonds. Figure 10.71 shows how 5-HPETE rearranges to the epoxide **leukotriene A_4** (LTA_4), which is then converted to LTB_4 or LTC_4, emphasizing that 5-HPETE occurs at an important branch point in the lipoxygenase pathway.

Peroxidative reduction of 5-HPETE to the stable **5-hydroxyeicosatetraenoic acid** (5-HETE) is illustrated in Figure 10.70. Note that the double bonds in 5-HETE occur at positions 6, 8, 11, and 14, and that they are unconjugated and that the geometry of the double bonds is trans, cis, cis, and cis, respectively. Two other common forms of HETE are 12- and 15-HETE. The HPETEs are reduced either spontaneously or by the action of peroxidases to the corresponding HETEs.

Leukotrienes are derived from the unstable precursor 5-HPETE by a reaction catalyzed by **LTA_4 synthase** that generates an epoxide called LTA_4. In the leukotriene series, the subscript indicates the number of double bonds. Thus, while double-bond rearrangement may occur, the number of double bonds in the leukotriene product is the same as in the original arachidonic acid. LTA_4 occurs at a branch point (Figure 10.71) and can be converted either to 5,12-dihydroxyeicosatetraenoic acid (designated leukotriene B_4 or LTB_4) or to LTC_4 and LTD_4.

Conversion of 5-HPETE to the diol LTB_4 (Figure 10.71) is catalyzed by a cytosolic enzyme, **LTB_4 synthase** (LTA_4 hydrolase), which adds water to the double bond between C-11 and C-12. The diversion of LTA_4 to leukotrienes LTC_4, LTD_4, and LTE_4 requires the participation of reduced glutathione that opens the epoxide ring in LTA_4 to produce LTC_4 (Figure 10.71). Sequential removal of glutamic acid and glycine residues by specific dipeptidases yields

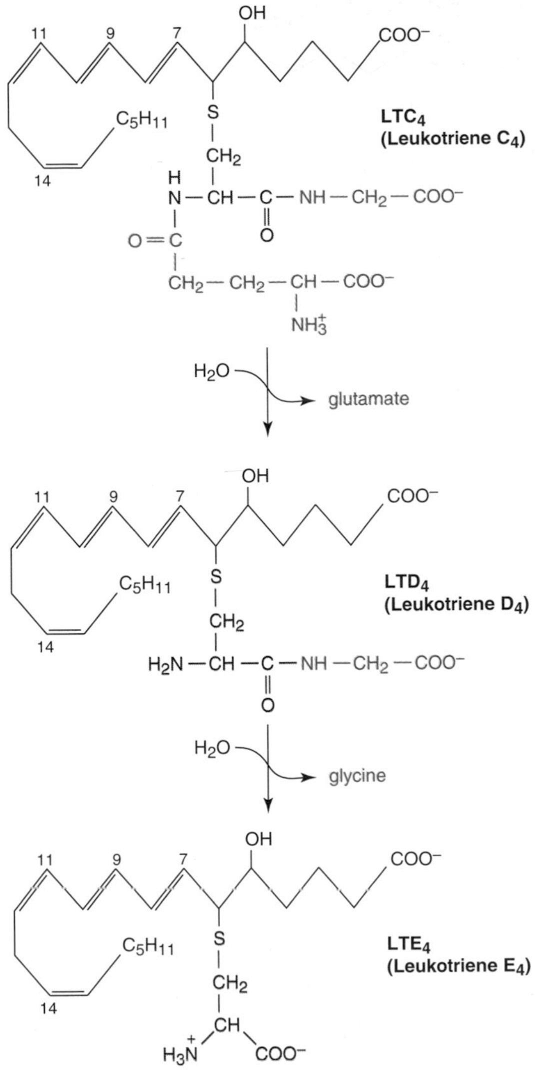

FIGURE 10.72
Conversion of LTC_4 to LTD_4 and LTE_4.

the leukotrienes LTD_4 and LTE_4 (Figure 10.72). The subscript 4 denotes the total number of double bonds.

Leukotrienes and HETEs Affect Several Physiological Processes

Leukotrienes persist for as long as 4 h in the body. Stepwise ω-oxidation of the methyl end and β-oxidation of the resulting COOH-terminated fatty acid chain are responsible for the inactivation and degradation of LTB_4 and LTE_4. These reactions occur in mitochondria and peroxisomes. The actions of the thionyl peptides LTC_4, LTD_4, and LTE_4 comprise the **slow-reacting substance of anaphylaxis** (SRS-A). They cause slowly evolving but protracted contraction of smooth muscles in the airways and gastrointestinal tract. LTC_4 is rapidly converted to LTD_4 and then slowly converted to LTE_4. These conversions are catalyzed by enzymes in plasma. LTB_4 and the sulfidopeptides LTC_4, LTD_4, and LTE_4 exert their biological actions through specific ligand–receptor interactions.

In general, HETEs (especially 5-HETE) and LTB_4 are involved mainly in regulating neutrophil and eosinophil function: they mediate chemotaxis, stimulate adenylate cyclase, and induce PMNs to degranulate and release lysosomal hydrolytic enzymes. In contrast, LTC_4 and LTD_4 are humoral agents that promote smooth muscle contraction, constriction of pulmonary airways, trachea, and intestine, and increases in capillary permeability (edema). HETEs appear to exert their effects by being incorporated into the phospholipids of target cells. It is thought that the presence of fatty acyl chains containing a polar OH group disturbs the packing of lipids and thus the structure and function of the membrane. LTB_4 has immunosuppressive activity exerted through inhibition of $CD4^+$ cells and proliferation of suppressor $CD8^+$ cells. LTB_4 also promotes neutrophil–endothelial cell adhesion.

Monohydroxyeicosatetraenoic acids that comprise the lipoxygenase pathway are potent mediators of processes involved in allergy (hypersensitivity) and inflammation, secretion (e.g., insulin), cell movement, cell growth, and calcium fluxes. The initial allergic event, namely, the binding of IgE antibody to receptors on the surface of the mast cell, causes the release of substances, including leukotrienes, that are referred to as mediators of immediate hypersensitivity. Lipoxygenase products are usually produced within minutes after the stimulus. The leukotrienes LTC_4, LTD_4, and LTE_4 are much more potent than histamine in contracting nonvascular smooth muscles of bronchi and intestine. LTD_4 increases the permeability of the microvasculature. Mono-HETEs and LTB_4 stimulate migration (chemotaxis) of eosinophils and neutrophils, making them the principal mediators of PMN–leukocyte infiltration in inflammatory reactions.

Eicosatrienoic acids (e.g., dihomo-γ-linolenic acid) and **eicosapentaenoic acid** (Figure 10.64) also serve as lipoxygenase substrates. The content of these C20 fatty acids with three and five double bonds in tissues is less than that of arachidonic acid, but special diets can increase their levels. The lipoxygenase products of these tri- and pentaeicosanoids are usually less active than LTA_4 or LTB_4. It remains to be determined if fish oil diets rich in eicosapentaenoic acid are useful in the treatment of allergic and autoimmune diseases.

Pharmaceutical research into therapeutic uses of lipoxygenase and cyclooxygenase inhibitors and inhibitors and agonists of leukotrienes in treatment of inflammatory diseases such as asthma, psoriasis, rheumatoid arthritis, and ulcerative colitis is very active.

BIBLIOGRAPHY

Phospholipid Metabolism

Downes, C. P. The cellular functions of *myo*-inositol. *Biochem. Soc. Trans.* 17:259, 1989.

Johnson, D. R., Bhatnager, R. S., Knoll, L. J., and Gordon, J. I. Genetic and biochemical studies of protein *N*-myristoylation. *Annu. Rev. Biochem.* 63:869, 1994.

Kent, C., Carman, G. M., Spence, W., and Dowhan, W. Regulation of eukaryotic phospholipid metabolism. *FASEB J.* 5:2258, 1991.

Low, M. G. Biochemistry of the glycosyl-phosphatidyl inositol membrane protein anchors. *Biochem. J.* 244:1, 1987.

McConville, M. J., and Ferguson, M. A. J. The structure, biosynthesis and function of glycosylated phosphatidylinositols in the parasitic protozoa and higher eukaryotes. *Biochem. J.* 294:305, 1993.

Nishizuka, Y. Protein kinase C and lipid signaling for sustained cellular responses. *FASEB J.* 9:484, 1995.

Raetz, C. R. H. Molecular genetics of membrane phospholipid synthesis. *Am. Rev. Genet.* 20:253, 1986.

Shears, S. B. Metabolism of the inositol phosphates produced upon receptor activation. *Biochem. J.* 260:313, 1989.

Snyder, F. Platelet-activating factor and its analogs: metabolic pathways and related intracellular processes. *Biochem. Biophys. Acta* 1254:231, 1995.

Stevens, V. L. Biosynthesis of glycosylphosphatidylinositol membrane anchors. *Biochem. J.* 310:361, 1995.

Vance, D. E., and Vance, J. E. *Biochemistry of Lipids and Membranes.* Menlo Park, CA: Benjamin/Cummings, 1985.

Cholesterol Synthesis

Brown, M. S., and Goldstein, J. L. A receptor-mediated pathway for cholesterol homeostasis. *Science* 232:68, 1986.

Edwards, P. A. Regulation of sterol biosynthesis and isoprenylation of proteins. In D. E. Vance and J. E. Vance (Eds.), *Biochemistry of Lipids, Lipoproteins and Membranes.* Amsterdam: Elsevier Science Publishers, 1991.

Goldstein, J. L., and Brown, M. S. Regulation of the mevalonate pathway. *Nature* 343:425, 1990.

Gordon, D. J., and Rifkind, B. M. High-density lipoprotein: the clinical implications of recent studies. *N. Engl. J. Med.* 321:1311, 1989.

Sphingolipids and Sphingolipidoses

Grabowski, G. A., Gatt, S., and Horowitz, M. Acid β-glucosidase: enzymology and molecular biology of Gaucher disease. *Crit. Rev. Biochem. Mol. Biol.* 25:385, 1990.

Robinson, D. Shedding light on lysosomes—applications of fluorescence techniques to cell biology and diagnosis of lysosomal disorders. *Biochem. Soc. Trans.* 16:11, 1988.

Tsuji, S., Choudary, P. V., Martin, B. M., Stubblefield, B. K., Mayor, J. A., Barranger, J. A., and Ginns, E. I. A mutation in the human glucocerebrosidase gene in neuronopathic Gaucher's disease. *N. Engl. J. Med.* 316:570, 1987.

Lung Surfactant

Caminici, S. P., and Young, S. The pulmonary surfactant system. *Hosp. Pract.* 26:87, 1991.

Konishi, M., Fujiwara, T., Naito, T., Tokeuchi, Y., Ogawa, Y., Inukai, K., Fujimura, M., Nakamura, H., and Hashimoto, T. Surfactant replacement therapy in neonatal respiratory distress syndrome. *Eur. J. Pediatr.* 147:20, 1988.

Prostaglandins, Thromboxanes, and Leukotrienes

Fitzpatrick, F. A., and Murphy, R. C. Cytochrome P-450 metabolism of arachidonic acid: formation and biological actions of "epoxygenase"-derived eicosanoids. *Pharmacol. Rev.* 40:229, 1989.

Fordhutchinson, A. W., et al. 5-Lipoxygenase. *Annu. Rev. Biochem.* 63:383, 1994.

Goetzl, E. J., An, S., and Smith, W. L. Specificity of expression and effects of eicosanoid mediators in normal physiology and human diseases. *FASEB J.* 9:1051, 1995.

Henderson, W. R. Jr. The role of leukotrienes in inflammation. *Ann. Intern. Med.* 121:684, 1994.

Mayatepek, E., and Hoffmann, G. Leukotrienes: biosynthesis, metabolism and pathophysiologic significance. *Pediatr. Res.* 37:1, 1995.

Parker, C. W. Lipid mediators produced through the lipoxygenase pathway. *Annu. Rev. Immunol.* 5:65, 1987.

Sardesai, V. M. Biochemical and nutritional aspects of eicosanoids. *J. Nutr. Biochem.* 3:562, 1992.

Yamamoto, S. Mammalian lipoxygenases: molecular and catalytic properties. *Prostaglandins Leukot. Essent. Fatty Acids* 35:219, 1989.

Bile Acids

Angelin, B., and Einarsson, K. Bile acids and lipoprotein metabolism. In: S. M. Grundy (Ed.), *Bile Acids and Atherosclerosis.* New York: Raven, 1986, p. 41.

Bjorkhem, I. Mechanism of bile acid biosynthesis in mammalian liver. In: H. Danielsson and J. Sjovall (Eds.), *New Comprehensive Biochemistry.* Amsterdam: Elsevier Science Publishers, 1985, pp. 231–278.

■ QUESTIONS ■ C. N. ANGSTADT AND J. BAGGOTT

Refer to the following structures for Questions 1–3.

1. A plasmalogen.
2. A cardiolipin.
3. An acylglycerol that would likely be liquid at room temperature.

A

```
                               O
                               ||
              O     H2C—O—C—(CH2)14CH3
              ||      |
CH3(CH2)16—C—O—CH     O
                      |     ||
                    H2C—O—C—(CH2)14CH3
```

B

```
                                                        O
                                                        ||
                                        O     H2C—O—C—(CH2)7CH=CH—(CH2)5CH3
                                        ||      |
CH3(CH2)3(CH2—CH=CH)4—(CH2)3—C—O—CH     O
                                                |     ||
                                              H2C—O—C—(CH2)14CH3
```

C

```
   O      H2C—O—CH=CH(CH2)15CH3
   ||       |
R—C—O—CH          O
            |     ||             +
          H2C—O—P—O—(CH2)2—NH3
                  |
                  O−
```

D

```
                     O
                     ||
    O      H2C—O—C—R1
    ||       |
R2—C—O—CH          O
             |     ||             +
           H2C—O—P—O—(CH2)2—N(CH3)3
                   |
                   O−
```

E

```
                     O                  O
                     ||                 ||
    O      H2C—O—C—R1   CH2—O—P—O———CH2        O
    ||       |              |       |           |        ||
R2—C—O—CH          O  HO—C—H     O−     O  HC—O—C—R3
             |     ||       |              ||  |
           H2C—O—P—O—CH2              R4C—O—CH2
                   |
                   O−
```

4. Roles of various phospholipids include all of the following EXCEPT:
   A. cell–cell recognition.
   B. a surfactant function in the lung.
   C. activation of certain membrane enzymes.
   D. signal transduction.
   E. mediator of hypersensitivity and acute inflammatory reactions.

5. Which of the following represents a correct group of enzymes involved in phosphatidylcholine synthesis in adipose tissue?
   A. choline phosphotransferase, glycerol kinase, phosphatidic acid phosphatase
   B. choline phosphotransferase, glycerol phosphate:acyltransferase, phosphatidylethanolamine *N*-methyltransferase
   C. glycerol phosphate:acyltransferase, α-glycerol-phosphate dehydrogenase, phosphatidic acid phosphatase.
   D. glycerol phosphate:acyltransferase, α-glycerol-phosphate dehydrogenase, glycerol kinase.
   E. α-glycerol-phosphate dehydrogenase, glycerol kinase, phosphatidic acid phosphatase.

6. CDP-X (where X is the appropriate alcohol) reacts with 1,2-diacylglycerol in the primary synthetic pathway for:
   A. phosphatidylcholine.
   B. phosphatidylinositol.
   C. phosphatidylserine.
   D. all of the above.
   E. none of the above.

7. Phospholipases A_1 and A_2:
   A. have no role in phospholipid synthesis.
   B. are responsible for the initial insertion of fatty acids in *sn*-1 and *sn*-2 positions during synthesis.
   C. are responsible for base exchange in the interconversion of phosphatidylethanolamine and phosphatidylserine.
   D. hydrolyze a phosphatidic acid to a diglyceride.
   E. remove a fatty acid in an *sn*-1 or *sn*-2 position so it can be replaced by another in phospholipid synthesis.

8. In the biosynthesis of cholesterol:
   A. 3-hydroxy-3-methyl glutaryl CoA (HMG CoA) is synthesized by mitochondrial HMG CoA synthase.
   B. HMG CoA reductase catalyzes the rate-limiting step.
   C. the conversion of mevalonic acid to farnesyl pyrophosphate proceeds via the condensation of three molecules of mevalonic acid.
   D. the condensation of two farnesyl pyrophosphates to form squalene is a freely reversible reaction.
   E. the conversion of squalene to lanosterol is initiated by formation of the fused ring system, followed by addition of oxygen.

9. The cholesterol present in LDL (low-density lipoprotein):
   A. binds to a cell receptor and diffuses across the cell membrane.
   B. when it enters a cell, suppresses the activity of ACAT (acyl CoA:cholesterol acyltransferase).
   C. once in the cell is converted to cholesterol esters by LCAT (lecithin:cholesterol acyltransferase).
   D. once it has accumulated in the cell, inhibits the replenishment of LDL receptors.
   E. represents primarily cholesterol that is being removed from peripheral cells.

10. Primary bile acids:
    A. are any bile acids that are found in the intestinal tract.
    B. are any bile acids reabsorbed from the intestinal tract.
    C. are synthesized in the intestinal tract by bacteria.
    D. are synthesized in hepatocytes directly from cholesterol.
    E. are converted to secondary bile acids by conjugation with glycine or taurine.

11. A ganglioside may contain all of the following EXCEPT:
    A. a ceramide structure.
    B. glucose or galactose.
    C. phosphate.
    D. one or more sialic acids.
    E. sphingosine.

12. Sphingomyelins differ from the other sphingolipids in that they are:
    A. not based on a ceramide core.
    B. acidic rather than neutral at physiological pH.
    C. the only types containing *N*-acetylneuraminic acid.
    D. the only types that are phospholipids.
    E. not amphipathic.

13. All of the following are true about the degradation of sphingolipids EXCEPT it:
    A. occurs by hydrolytic enzymes contained in lysosomes.
    B. terminates at the level of ceramides.
    C. is a sequential, stepwise removal of constituents.
    D. is inhibited in the types of diseases known as sphingolipidoses (lysosomal storage diseases).
    E. is catalyzed by enzymes that are specific for a type of linkage rather than for a particular compound.

14. Structural features that are common to all prostaglandins include:
    A. 20-carbon atoms.
    B. an oxygen-containing internal heterocyclic ring.
    C. a peroxide group at C-15.
    D. two double bonds.
    E. a ketone group.

15. The prostaglandin synthase complex:
    A. catalyzes the rate-limiting step of prostaglandin synthesis.
    B. is inhibited by anti-inflammatory steroids.
    C. contains both a cyclooxygenase and a peroxidase component.
    D. produces PGG_2 as the end product.
    E. uses as substrate the pool of free arachidonic acid in the cell.

16. Thromboxane A_2:
    A. is a long-lived prostaglandin.
    B. is an inactive metabolite of PGE_2.
    C. is the major prostaglandin produced in all cells.
    D. does not contain a ring structure.
    E. is synthesized from the intermediate PGH_2.

17. Hydroperoxy eicosatetraenoic acids (HPETEs):
    A. are derived from arachidonic acid by a peroxidase reaction.
    B. are mediators of hypersensitivity reactions.
    C. are intermediates in the formation of leukotrienes.
    D. are relatively stable compounds (persist for as long as 4 h).
    E. are the inactivated forms of leukotrienes.

ANSWERS

1. C Only one with an ether instead of an ester link at *sn*-1. D is a phosphatidylcholine (p. 397).
2. E Two phosphatidic acids connected by glycerol (p. 398).
3. B Note the two unsaturated fatty acids. A: With all saturated fatty acids, would likely be solid at room temperature.
4. A This function appears to be associated with complex glycosphingolipids (p. 427). B: Especially dipalmitoyllecithin (p. 398). C: For example, β-hydroxybutyrate dehydrogenase (p. 399). D: Especially the phosphatidylinositols (p. 400). E: Platelet activating factor (PAF) does this (p. 398).
5. C A, D, and E: Glycerol kinase is not present in adipose tissue, which must rely on the α-glycerol-phosphate dehydrogenase. This is a liver process only (p. 402).
6. A B: Phosphatidylinositol is formed from CDP-diglyceride reacting with *myo*-inositol (Figure 10.21, p. 406). C: This is formed by "base exchange" (Figure 10.20, p. 406).
7. E Phospholipases A_1 and A_2, as their names imply, hydrolyze a fatty acid from a phospholipid and so are part of phospholipid degradation. They are also important in synthesis, however, in assuring the asymmetric distribution of fatty acids that occurs in phospholipids (p. 406).
8. B A: Remember that cholesterol biosynthesis is cytosolic; mitochondrial biosynthesis of HMG CoA leads to ketone body formation. C: The rate-limiting step produces the isoprene pyrophosphates, which are the condensing units. D: Pyrophosphate is hydrolyzed, which prevents reversal. E: The process is initiated by epoxide formation (pp. 411–414).
9. D This is one of the ways to prevent overload in the cell. A: The LDL binds to the cell receptor and is endocytosed and then degraded in lysosome to release cholesterol. B: ACAT is activated to facilitate storage. C: LCAT is a plasma enzyme. E: The primary role of LDLs is to deliver cholesterol to peripheral tissues (pp. 415–417).
10. D The intestinal tract contains a mixture of primary and secondary bile acids, both of which can be reabsorbed. Secondary bile acids are formed by bacteria in the intestine by chemical reactions, such as the removal of the C-7 OH group (pp. 417 and 418).
11. C The glycosphingolipids do not contain phosphate. A and E: Ceramide, which is formed from sphingosine, is the base structure from which the glycosphingolipids are formed. D: By definition, gangliosides must contain sialic acid (p. 426).
12. D Sphingomyelins are not glycosphingolipids. They are formed from ceramides, are amphipathic, and are neutral. C is the definition of gangliosides (p. 421).
13. B Ceramides are hydrolyzed to sphingosine and the fatty acid. E: Many of the sphingolipids share the same types of bonds (e.g., a β-galactosidic bond), and one enzyme (e.g., β-galactosidase), will hydrolyze it whenever it occurs (p. 428, Figure 10.59).
14. A Prostaglandins are eicosanoids. B: This is true of thromboxanes but the prostaglandin ring contains only carbons. C: True only of the intermediate of synthesis, PGG_2. D: The number of double bonds is variable. E: True of the A and E series but not of the F series (Figures 10.64–10.68).
15. C A and B: The release of the precursor fatty acid by phospholipase A_2 is the rate-limiting step and the one inhibited by anti-inflammatory steroids. D: The peroxidase component converts the PGG_2 to PGH_2. E: Arachidonic acid is not free in the cell but is part of the membrane phospholipids (p. 433).
16. E TXA_2 is very active, has a very short half-life, contains a six-membered ring, and is the main prostaglandin in platelets but not all tissues (p. 435).
17. C A: The enzyme is a lipoxygenase. B–E: HPETEs themselves are not hormones but highly unstable intermediates that are converted to either HETEs (mediators of hypersensitivity) or leukotrienes (p. 436).

CHAPTER

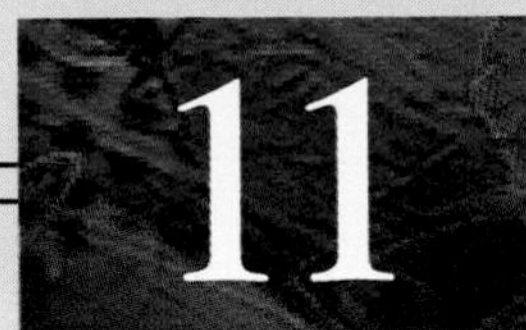

AMINO ACID METABOLISM

Marguerite W. Coomes

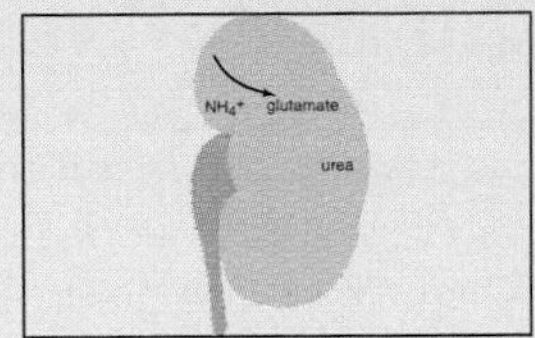

11.1 ■ OVERVIEW

Amino acids and the relationship between their structure and the structure and function of proteins were presented in Chapter 2. This chapter describes the metabolism of amino acids, emphasizing the importance of dietary protein as the major source of amino acids for humans.

Molecular nitrogen, N_2, exists in the atmosphere in great abundance. Before it can be utilized by animals it must be "fixed," that is, reduced from N_2 to NH_3 by microorganisms, plants, and electrical discharge from lightning. Ammonia is then incorporated into amino acids and proteins, and these become part of the food chain (Figure 11.1). Humans can synthesize only 11 of the 20 amino acids needed for protein synthesis. Those that cannot be synthesized *de novo* are termed **"essential"** because they must be obtained from dietary foodstuffs that contain them (Table 11.1).

This chapter includes discussion of interconversions of amino acids, removal and excretion of ammonia, and synthesis of "nonessential" amino acids

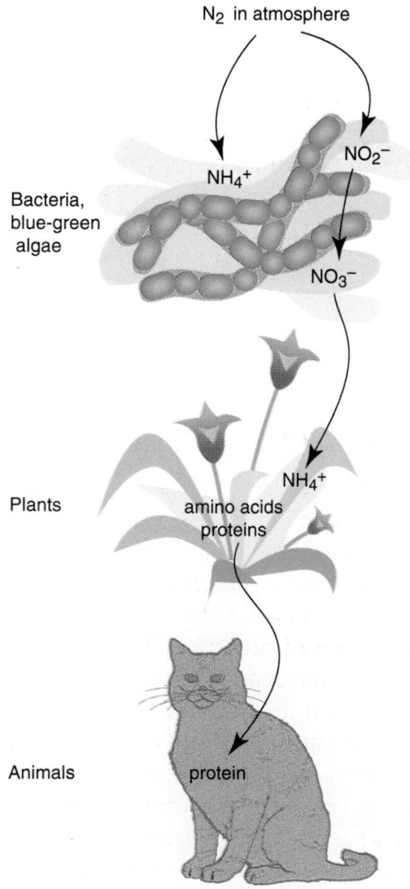

FIGURE 11.1
Outline of entry of atmospheric nitrogen into the human diet.
This occurs initially by reduction of nitrogen to ammonia by enzymes in microorganisms and plants.

TABLE 11.1 Dietary Requirements of Amino Acids

Essential	*Nonessential*
Arginine[a]	Alanine
Histidine	Aspartate
Isoleucine	Cysteine
Leucine	Glutamate
Lysine	Glycine
Methionine[b]	Proline
Phenylalanine[c]	Serine
Threonine	Tyrosine
Tryptophan	
Valine	

[a] Arginine is synthesized by mammalian tissues, but the rate is not sufficient to meet the need during growth.

[b] Methionine is required in large amounts to produce cysteine if the latter is not supplied adequately by the diet.

[c] Phenylalanine is needed in larger amounts to form tyrosine if the latter is not supplied adequately by the diet.

by the body. As part of ammonia metabolism, synthesis and degradation of glutamate, glutamine, aspartate, asparagine, alanine, and arginine are discussed. Synthesis and degradation of other nonessential amino acids are then described, as well as the degradation of the essential amino acids. Synthetic pathways of amino acid derivatives and some diseases of amino acid metabolism are also presented.

Carbons from amino acids enter intermediary metabolism at one of seven points. Glucogenic amino acids are metabolized to pyruvate, 3-phosphoglycerate, α-ketoglutarate, oxaloacetate, fumarate, or succinyl CoA. Ketogenic amino acids produce acetyl CoA or acetoacetate. Metabolism of some amino acids results in more than one of the above and they are therefore both glucogenic and ketogenic (Figure 11.2). Products of amino acid metabolism can be used to provide energy. Additional energy-generating compounds, usually NADH, are also produced during degradation of some of the amino acids.

11.2 INCORPORATION OF NITROGEN INTO AMINO ACIDS

Most Amino Acids Are Obtained from the Diet

A healthy adult eating a varied and plentiful diet is generally in **"nitrogen balance,"** a state where the amount of nitrogen ingested each day is balanced by the amount excreted, resulting in no net change in the amount of body nitrogen. In the well-fed condition, excreted nitrogen comes mostly from digestion of excess protein or from normal turnover. Protein turnover is defined as the synthesis and degradation of protein. Under some conditions the body is either in negative or positive nitrogen balance. In **negative nitrogen balance** more nitrogen is excreted than ingested. This occurs in starvation and certain diseases. During starvation carbon chains of amino acids from proteins are needed for gluconeogenesis; ammonia released from amino acids is excreted mostly as urea and is not reincorporated into protein. A diet deficient in an essential amino acid also leads to a negative nitrogen balance, since body proteins are degraded to provide the deficient essential amino acid, and the

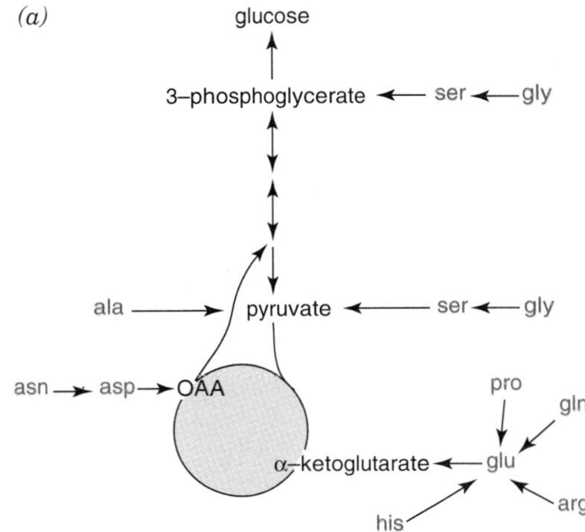

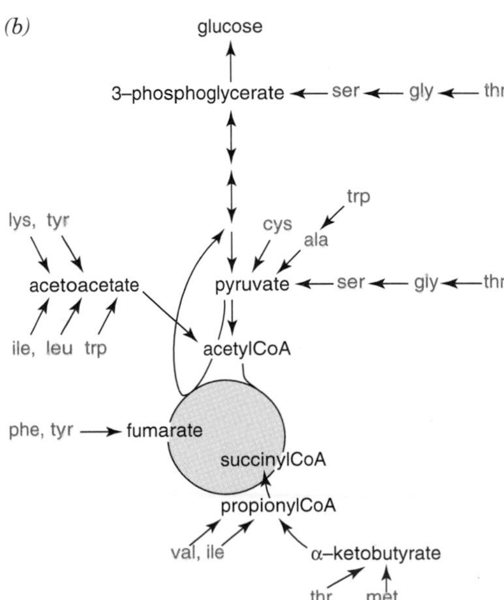

FIGURE 11.2
Metabolic fate of (*a*) nonessential amino acids; (*b*) essential amino acids plus cysteine and tyrosine.

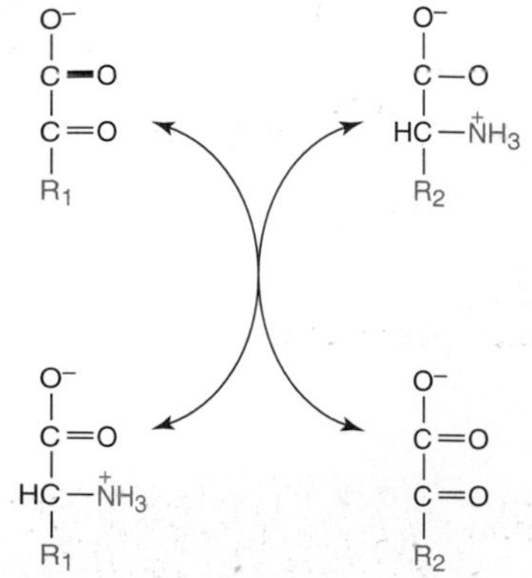

other 19 amino acids liberated are metabolized. Negative nitrogen balance may also exist in senescence. **Positive nitrogen balance** occurs in growing children, who are increasing their body weight and incorporating more amino acids into proteins than they break down. Cysteine and arginine are not essential in adults but are essential in children because they are synthesized from methionine and ornithine. These amino acids are readily available in adults but limited in children because of their greater use of all amino acids. Positive nitrogen balance also occurs in pregnancy and during refeeding after starvation.

FIGURE 11.3
Aminotransferase reaction.

Amino Groups Are Transferred from One Amino Acid to Form Another

Most amino acids used by the body to synthesize protein or as precursors for amino acid derivatives are obtained from the diet or from protein turnover. When necessary, nonessential amino acids are synthesized from α-keto acid precursors via transfer of a preexisting amino group from another amino acid by **aminotransferases,** also called **transaminases** (Figure 11.3). Transfer of amino groups also occurs during degradation of amino acids. Figure 11.4 shows how the amino group of alanine is transferred to α-ketoglutarate to form glutamate. In this reaction the pyruvate produced provides carbons for gluconeogenesis or for energy production via the TCA cycle. This reaction is necessary since ammonia cannot enter the urea cycle directly from alanine but can be donated by glutamate. The opposite reaction would occur if there were a need for alanine for protein synthesis that was not being met by dietary intake or protein turnover. Transamination involving essential amino acids is normally unidirectional since the body cannot synthesize the equivalent α-keto acid. Figure 11.5 shows transamination of valine, an essential amino acid. The resulting α-ketoisovalerate is further metabolized to succinyl CoA as discussed on page 477. Transamination is the most common reaction involving free amino acids, and only threonine and lysine do not participate in an aminotransferase reaction. An obligate amino and α-keto acid pair in all of these reactions is glutamate and α-ketoglutarate. This means that amino group transfer between alanine and aspartate would have to occur via coupled reactions, with a glutamate intermediate (Figure 11.6). The equilibrium constant for aminotransferases is close to one so that the reactions are freely reversible. When nitrogen excretion is impaired and **hyperammonemia** occurs, as in liver failure, amino acids, including the essential amino acids, can be replaced in the diet by α-keto acid analogs, with the exception of threonine and lysine as mentioned above. The α-keto acids are transaminated by aminotransferases to produce the different amino acids. Figure 11.5 shows valine formation after administration of α-ketoisovalerate as therapy for hyperammonemia.

Tissue distribution of some of the aminotransferase family is used diagnostically by measuring the release of a specific enzyme during tissue damage; for instance, the presence of glutamate oxaloacetate aminotransferase in plasma is a sign of liver damage (see p. 166).

alanine + α-ketoglutarate ⇌ pyruvate + glutamate

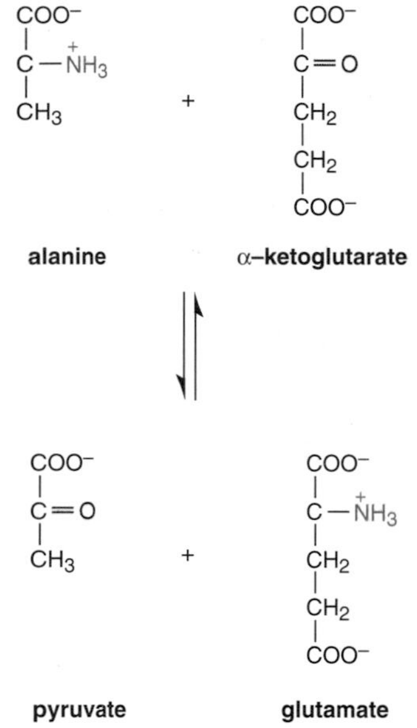

FIGURE 11.4
Glutamate–pyruvate aminotransferase reaction.

valine ⇌ α-ketoisovalerate (α-ketoglutarate → glutamate)

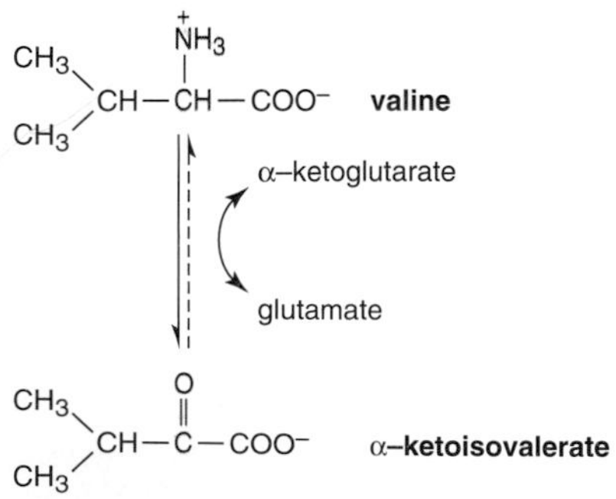

FIGURE 11.5
Transamination of valine.
Valine can be formed from α-ketoisovalerate only when this compound is administered therapeutically.

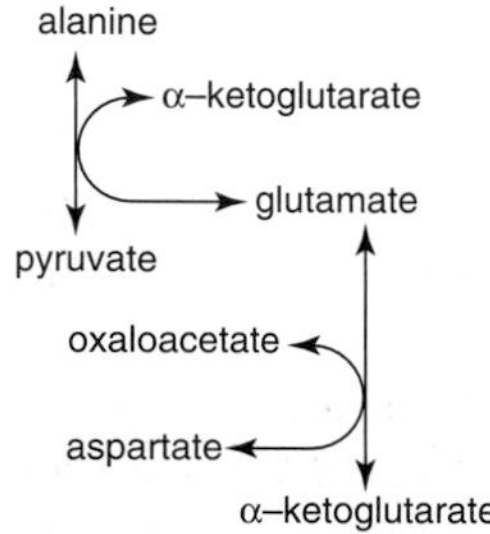

FIGURE 11.6
A coupled transamination reaction.

Pyridoxal Phosphate Is Cofactor for Aminotransferases

Transfer of amino groups occurs via enzyme-associated intermediates derived from **pyridoxal phosphate,** the functional form of vitamin B_6 (Figure 11.7). The active site of the "resting" aminotransferase contains pyridoxal phosphate covalently attached to an ε-amino group of a lysine residue that forms part of the amino acid chain of the transferase (Figure 11.8) The complex is further stabilized by ionic and hydrophobic interactions. The linkage, $-CH{=}N-$, is called a **Schiff base.** The carbon originates in the aldehyde group of pyridoxal phosphate, and the nitrogen is donated by the lysine residue. When a substrate amino acid, ready to be metabolized, approaches the active site, its amino group displaces the lysine ε-amino group and a Schiff base linkage is formed with the amino group of the amino acid substrate (Figure 11.9). At this point the pyridoxal phosphate-derived molecule is no longer covalently attached to the enzyme but is held in the active site only by ionic and hydrophobic interactions between it and the protein. The Schiff base linkage involving the amino acid substrate is in tautomeric equilibrium between an aldimine, $-CH{=}N{-}CHR_2$, and a ketimine, $-CH_2{-}N{=}CR$. Hydrolysis of the ketimine liberates an α-keto acid, leaving the amino group as part of the pyridoxamine structure. A reversal of the process is now possible; an α-keto acid reacts with the amine group, the double bond is shifted, and then hydrolysis liberates an amino acid. Pyridoxal phosphate now reforms its Schiff base with the "resting" enzyme (Figure 11.8). Most pyridoxal phosphate-requiring reactions involve transamination, but the ability of the Schiff base to transfer electrons between different atoms allows this cofactor to participate

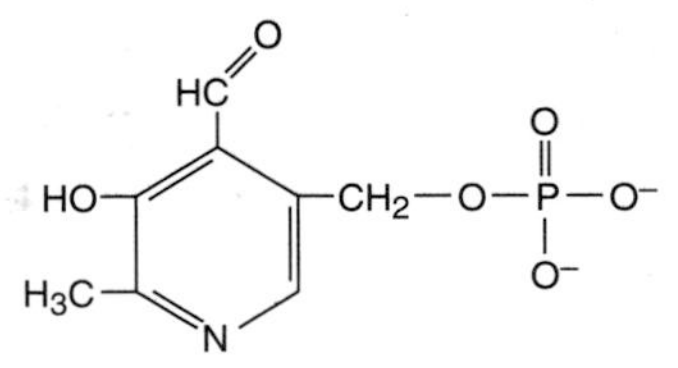

FIGURE 11.7
Pyridoxal phosphate.

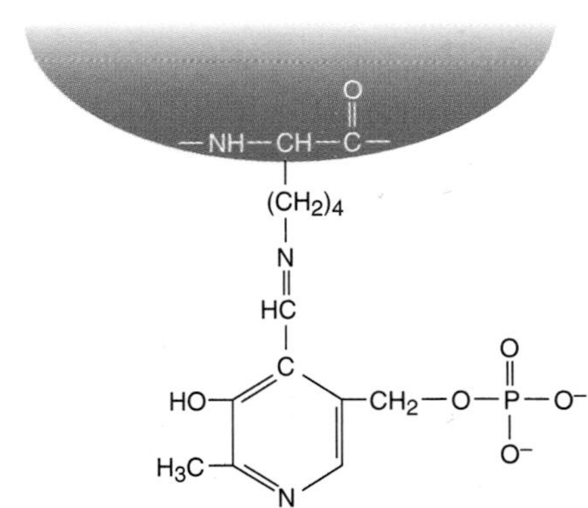

FIGURE 11.8
Pyridoxal phosphate in aldimine linkage to protein lysine residue.

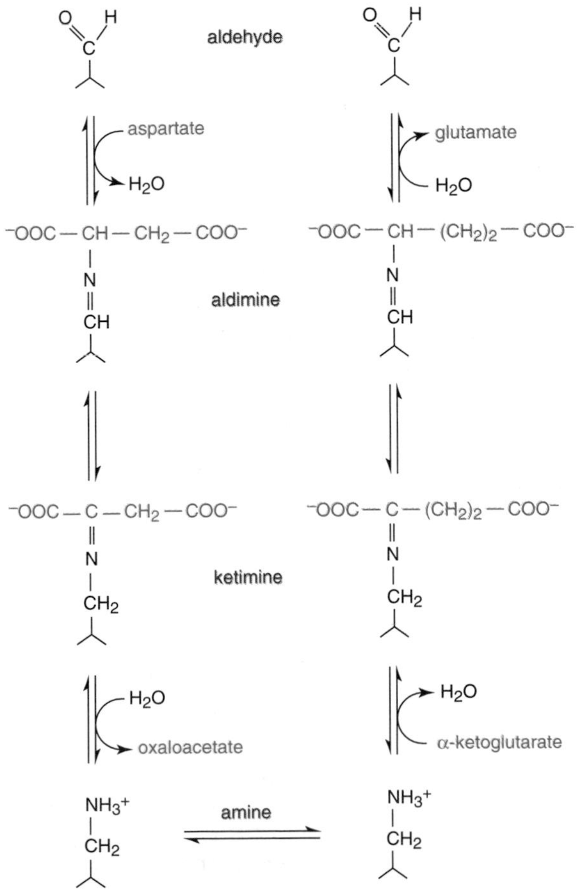

FIGURE 11.9
Different forms of pyridoxal phosphate during a transamination reaction.

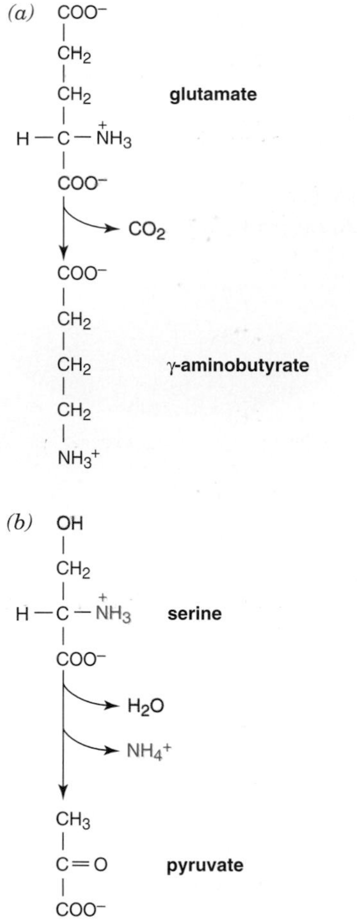

when other groups, such as carboxyls, are to be eliminated. Figure 11.10 shows the reaction of a **pyridoxal-dependent decarboxylase** and an **α-, β-elimination.**

The effective concentration of vitamin B_6 in the body may be decreased by administration of certain drugs, such as the antitubercular, isoniazid, which forms a Schiff base with pyridoxal making it unavailable for catalysis.

FIGURE 11.10
Glutamate decarboxylase and serine dehydratase are pyridoxal phosphate-dependent reactions.

Glutamate Dehydrogenase Incorporates and Produces Ammonia

In the liver ammonia is incorporated as the amino group of nitrogen by **glutamate dehydrogenase** (Figure 11.11). This enzyme also catalyzes the reverse reaction. Glutamate always serves as one of the amino acids in transaminations and is thus the "gateway" between free ammonia and amino groups of most amino acids (Figure 11.12). NADPH is used in the synthetic reaction, whereas NAD^+ is used in liberation of ammonia, a degradative reaction. The enzyme is involved in the production of ammonia from amino acids when these are needed as glucose precursors or for energy. Formation of NADH during the oxidative deamination reaction is a welcome bonus, since it can be reoxidized by the respiratory chain with formation of ATP. The reaction as shown is readily reversible in the test tube but it is likely that *in vivo* it occurs more frequently in the direction of ammonia formation. The concentration of ammonia needed for the reaction to produce glutamate is toxic and under normal conditions would rarely be attained except in the perivenous region of the liver. A major source of ammonia is **bacterial metabolism** in the intestine, the released ammonia being absorbed and transported to the liver. Glutamate dehydrogenase incorporates this ammonia, as well as that produced locally, into glutamate. The enzyme's dominant role in ammonia removal is emphasized by its location inside liver mitochondria, where the initial reactions of the urea cycle occur.

Glutamate dehydrogenase is regulated allosterically by purine nucleotides. When there is need for oxidation of amino acids for energy, the activity is increased in the direction of glutamate degradation by ADP and GDP, which are indicative of a low cellular energy level. GTP and ATP, indicative of an ample energy level, are allosteric activators in the direction of glutamate synthesis (Figure 11.13).

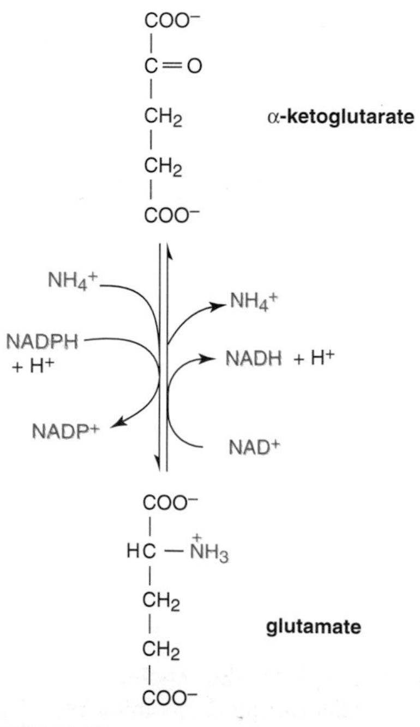

Free Ammonia Is Incorporated into and Produced from Glutamine

Free ammonia is toxic and is preferentially transported in the blood in the form of amino or amide groups. Fifty percent of circulating amino acids are **glutamine,** an ammonia transporter. The amide group of glutamine is important as a nitrogen donor for several classes of molecules, including purine bases, and the amino group of cytosine. Glutamate and ammonia are substrates for **glutamine synthetase** (Figure 11.14). ATP is needed for activation of the α-carboxyl group to make the reaction energetically favorable.

Removal of the amide group is catalyzed by **glutaminase** (Figure 11.15). There are tissue-specific isozymes. Mitochondrial glutaminase I of kidney and

FIGURE 11.11
Glutamate dehydrogenase reaction.

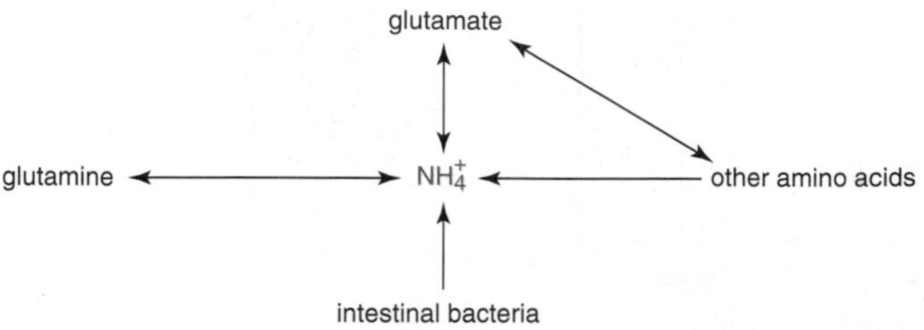

FIGURE 11.12
Role of glutamate in amino acid synthesis, degradation, and interconversion.

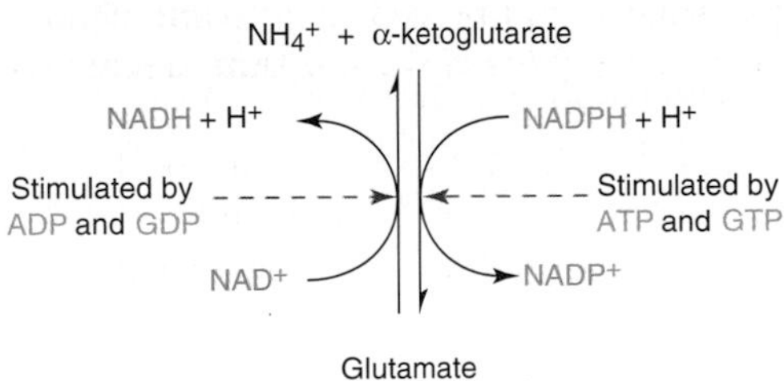

FIGURE 11.13
Allosteric regulation of glutamate dehydrogenase.

COO^-–CH_2–CH_2–HC–$\overset{+}{N}H_3$–COO^- **Glutamate**

$\downarrow$ NH_4^+, ATP → ADP + P_i

NH_2–C=O–CH_2–CH_2–HC–$\overset{+}{N}H_3$–COO^- **Glutamine**

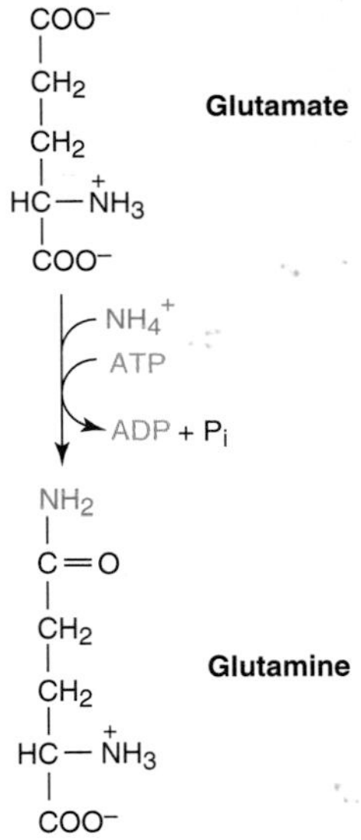

FIGURE 11.14
Reaction catalyzed by glutamine synthetase.

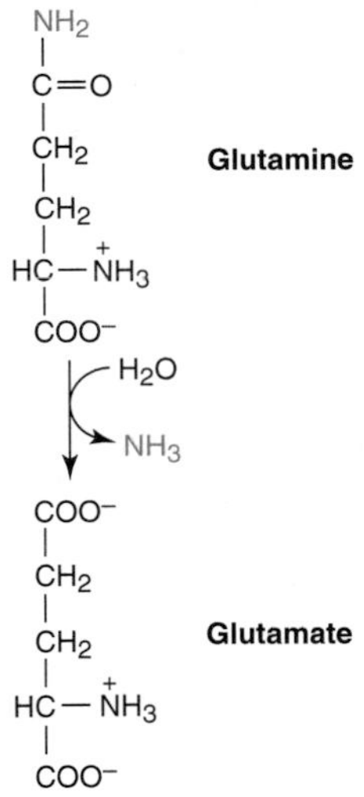

liver requires phosphate for activity. Liver contains glutamine synthetase and glutaminase but is neither a net consumer nor a net producer of glutamine. The two enzymes are confined to parenchymal cells in different segments of the liver. The **periportal region** is in contact with blood coming from skeletal muscle and contains glutaminase (and the urea cycle enzymes). The **perivenous area** represents 5% of parenchymal cells; blood from it flows to the kidney and cells in this area contain glutamine synthetase. This **"intercellular glutamine cycle"** (Figure 11.16) can be considered a mechanism for scavenging ammonia that has not been incorporated into urea. The enzymes of urea synthesis are found in the same periportal cells as glutaminase, whereas the uptake of glutamate and α-ketoglutarate for glutamine synthesis predominates in the perivenous region. The glutamine cycle makes it possible to control flux of ammonia either to urea or to glutamine and thence to excretion of ammonia by the kidney under different pH conditions (see p. 1045).

NH_2–C=O–CH_2–CH_2–HC–$\overset{+}{N}H_3$–COO^- **Glutamine**

$\downarrow$ H_2O → NH_3

COO^-–CH_2–CH_2–HC–$\overset{+}{N}H_3$–COO^- **Glutamate**

FIGURE 11.15
Reaction catalyzed by glutaminase.

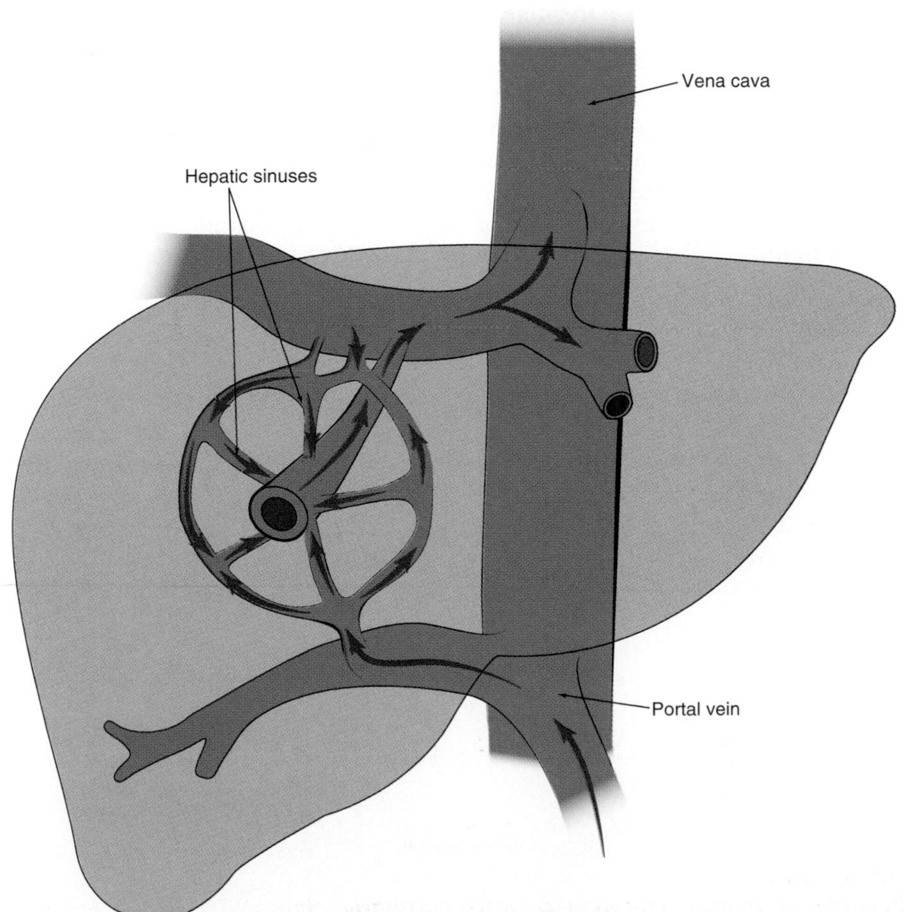

FIGURE 11.16
Intercellular glutamine cycle.
Periportal cells surround incoming blood vessels, and perivenous cells surround outgoing blood vessels.

Amide Group of Asparagine Is Derived from Glutamine

The amide group of **asparagine** comes from that of glutamine (Figure 11.17), and not from free ammonia, as in the synthesis of glutamine. ATP is needed to activate the receptor α-carboxyl group. Asparagine is readily synthesized in most cells, but some leukemic cells seem to have lost this ability. A therapeutic approach that has been tried for patients with **asparagine synthetase**-deficient tumors is treatment with exogenous **asparaginase** to hydrolyze the blood-borne asparagine on which these cells rely (Figure 11.18). Normal cells synthesize and degrade asparagine.

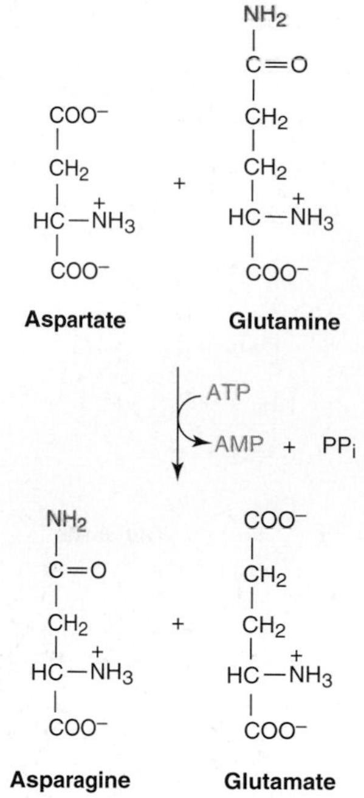

Aspartate + Glutamine → (ATP → AMP + PP_i) → Asparagine + Glutamate

FIGURE 11.17
Synthesis of asparagine.

Asparagine → (H_2O → NH_4^+) → Aspartate

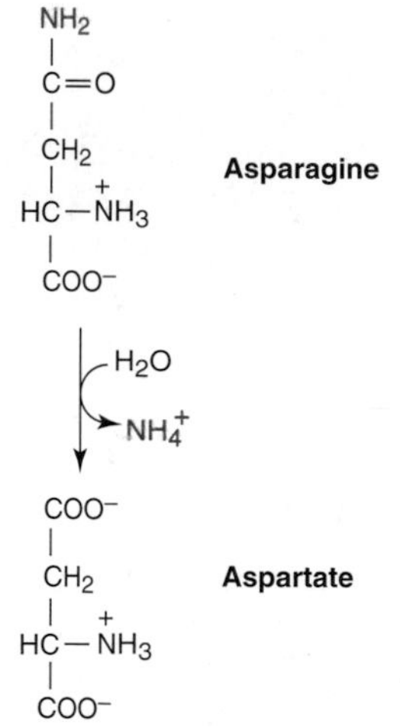

FIGURE 11.18
Reaction catalyzed by asparaginase.

Amino Acid Oxidases Remove Amino Groups

Many amino acids are substrates for **L-amino acid oxidase** (Figure 11.19). The significance of this reaction in the metabolism of amino acids is uncertain, but appears to be small. The enzyme contains flavin mononucleotide (FMN) and produces hydrogen peroxide. After the hydrogen peroxide is reduced to water, the final products are an α-keto acid, ammonia, and water, the same products as those of the glutamate dehydrogenase reaction. In the amino acid oxidase reaction, unlike the reaction catalyzed by glutamate dehydrogenase, there is no concomitant production of NADH, and therefore no production of ATP.

A **D-amino acid oxidase** also occurs in human cells. Very little of the D-amino acid isomer is found in humans and the role of D-amino acid oxidase may be in degradation of D-amino acids derived from intestinal bacteria.

11.3 ■ TRANSPORT OF NITROGEN TO LIVER AND KIDNEY

Protein Is Degraded on a Regular Basis

Whole cells die on a regular and planned basis, and their component molecules are metabolized. This **"planned cell death"** is called **apoptosis.** Individual proteins also undergo regular turnover under normal conditions. Even though the reactions involved in intracellular protein degradation have been identified, an understanding of the regulation of protein degradation is in its infancy. The half-life of a protein can be an hour or less, such as for ornithine decarboxylase, phosphokinase C, and insulin, several months for hemoglobin and histones,

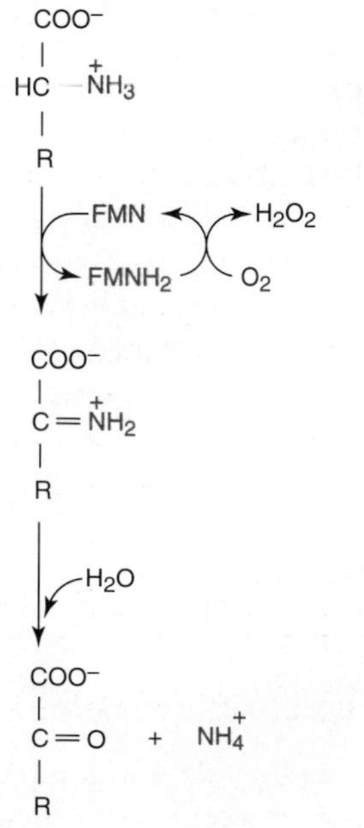

COO^-–HC–$\overset{+}{N}H_3$–R → (FMN → $FMNH_2$; O_2 → H_2O_2) → COO^-–$C{=}\overset{+}{N}H_2$–R → (H_2O) → COO^-–$C{=}O$–R + NH_4^+

FIGURE 11.19
Reaction of L-amino acid oxidase, a flavoprotein.

or the life of the organism for the crystallins of the lens. The majority, however, turn over every few days. Selection of a particular protein molecule for degradation is not well understood but may, in many cases, occur by "marking" with covalently bound molecules of an oligopeptide, termed **ubiquitin.** Ubiquitin contains 76 amino acid residues and is attached via its C-terminal glycine residue to the terminal amino group and to lysine residues in the protein to be marked for degradation. This is a nonlysosomal, ATP-dependent process and requires a complex of three enzymes known as ubiquitin protein ligase. Recently, ubiquitination and protein degradation have been found to regulate the cell cycle by influencing the availability of proteins required in the S and G_1 phases. Other protein degradation occurs in the lysosomes, or extralysosomally by calcium-dependent enzymes.

Amino Acids Are Transported from Muscle After Proteolysis

The majority of protein, and consequently of amino acids, is in skeletal muscle. Under conditions of energy need, this protein is degraded and amino groups from the amino acids are transferred to glutamine and alanine and transported to liver or kidney. Urea is produced in liver and ammonia (from glutamine) in kidney (Figure 11.20). Carbon skeletons are either used for energy or transported to the liver for gluconeogenesis. Muscle protein responds to conditions such as starvation, trauma, burns, and septicemia, by undergoing massive degradation. Of the amino acids released, most important as a source of fuel are **branched-chain amino acids** (valine, leucine, and isoleucine). The first step in their degradation is transamination, which occurs almost exclusively in muscle. Protein is, of course, degraded throughout the body, but muscle is by far the greatest source of free amino acids for metabolism.

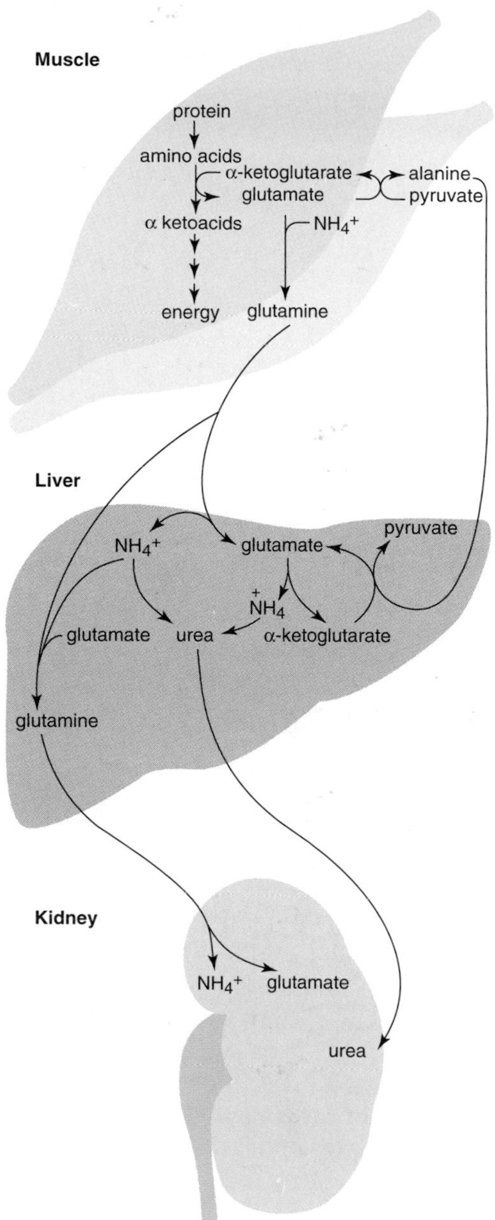

FIGURE 11.20
Major pathways of interorgan nitrogen transport following muscle proteolysis.

Ammonia Is Released in Liver and Kidney

The main destination of glutamine and alanine in the blood is the liver (see Figure 11.20). Here ammonia is released by alanine aminotransferase, glutaminase, and glutamate dehydrogenase. Glutamate dehydrogenase not only releases ammonia but also produces NADH and α-ketoglutarate, a glucogenic intermediate. Under conditions of energy need these products are very beneficial. Many tumors produce a condition called **cachexia,** characterized by wasting of muscle. This is caused not at the level of regulation of the rate of muscle protein breakdown, but rather by an increase in the rate at which liver removes amino acids from plasma, which, in turn, has a potentiating effect on muscle proteolysis. When circulating glucagon concentration is high (a signal that carbon is required by the liver for gluconeogenesis), it also potentiates amino acid metabolism by stimulating amino acid uptake by the liver.

Some glutamine and alanine is taken up by the kidney. Ammonia is released by the same enzymes that are active in liver, protonated to ammonium ion and excreted. When acidosis occurs the body shunts glutamine from liver to kidney to **conserve bicarbonate,** since formation of urea, the major mechanism for removal of NH_4^+, requires bicarbonate. To avoid use and excretion of this anion as urea during acidosis, uptake of glutamine by liver is suppressed, and more is transported to kidney for excretion as ammonium ion (see p. 1045).

11.4 UREA CYCLE

Nitrogens of Urea Come from Ammonia and Aspartate

The **urea cycle** and the tricarboxylic acid (TCA) cycle were discovered by Sir Hans Krebs and co-workers. In fact, the urea cycle was described before the

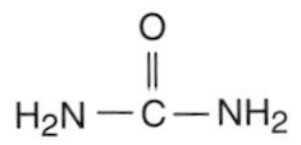

$$H_2N-C(=O)-NH_2$$

FIGURE 11.21
Urea.

$HCO_3^- + ATP + \text{enzyme}$

↓

$O=C(OH)-O-P(=O)(O^-)-O^-\cdot\text{enzyme} + ADP$

↓ NH_3, ATP → ADP + P_i

$H_2N-C(=O)-O-P(=O)(O^-)-O^- + \text{enzyme}$

Carbamoyl phosphate

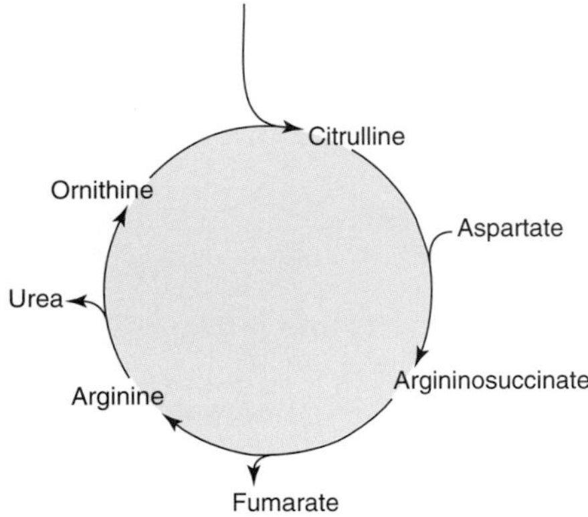

FIGURE 11.22
Synthesis of carbamoyl phosphate and entry into urea cycle.

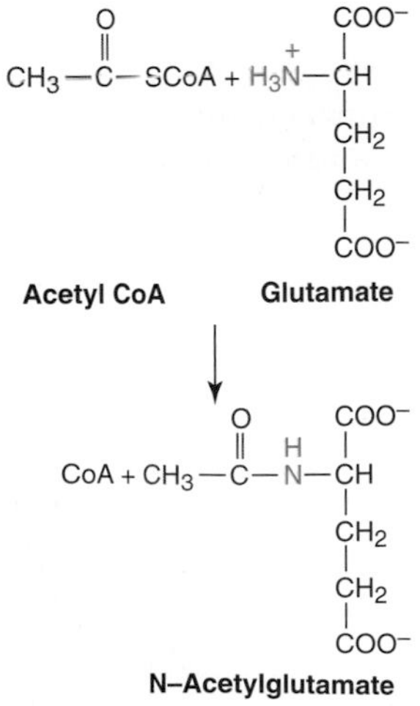

$CH_3-C(=O)-SCoA + H_3\overset{+}{N}-CH(COO^-)-CH_2-CH_2-COO^-$

Acetyl CoA Glutamate

↓

$CoA + CH_3-C(=O)-NH-CH(COO^-)-CH_2-CH_2-COO^-$

N–Acetylglutamate

FIGURE 11.23
Reaction catalyzed by *N*-acetylglutamate synthetase.

TCA cycle. In land-dwelling mammals, the urea cycle is the mechanism of choice for nitrogen excretion. The two nitrogens in each urea molecule (Figure 11.21) are derived from two sources, free ammonia and the amino group of aspartate. The cycle starts and finishes with **ornithine.** Unlike the TCA cycle, where carbons of oxaloacetate at the start are different from those at the end, the carbons in the final ornithine are the same carbons with which the molecule started.

Ammonia (first nitrogen for urea) enters the cycle after condensation with bicarbonate to form **carbamoyl phosphate** (Figure 11.22), which reacts with ornithine to form **citrulline.** Aspartate (the donor of the second urea nitrogen) and citrulline react to form **argininosuccinate,** which is then cleaved to arginine and fumarate. Arginine is hydrolyzed to urea and ornithine is regenerated. Urea is then transported to the kidney and excreted in urine. The cycle requires 4 ATPs to excrete each two nitrogen atoms. It is therefore more energy efficient to incorporate ammonia into amino acids than to excrete it. The major regulatory step is the initial synthesis of carbamoyl phosphate, and the cycle is also regulated by induction of the enzymes involved.

Synthesis of Urea Requires Five Enzymes

Carbamoyl phosphate synthetase I is technically not a part of the urea cycle, although it is essential for urea synthesis. Free ammonium ion and bicarbonate are condensed, at the expense of 2 ATPs, to form carbamoyl phosphate. One ATP activates bicarbonate, and the other donates the phosphate group of carbamoyl phosphate. Carbamoyl phosphate synthetase I occurs in the mitochondrial matrix, uses ammonia as nitrogen donor, and is absolutely dependent on ***N*-acetylglutamate** for activity (Figure 11.23). Another enzyme with similar activity, **carbamoyl phosphate synthase II,** is cytosolic, uses the amide group of glutamine, and is not affected by *N*-acetylglutamate. It participates in pyrimidine biosynthesis (see p. 505).

Formation of citrulline is catalyzed by **ornithine transcarbamoylase** (Figure 11.24) in the mitochondrial matrix. Citrulline is transported from the mitochondria, and other reactions of the urea cycle occur in the cytosol. Argininosuccinate production by **argininosuccinate synthetase** requires hydrolysis of ATP to AMP and PP_i, the equivalent of hydrolysis of two molecules of ATP. Cleavage of argininosuccinate by **argininosuccinate lyase** produces fumarate and arginine. Arginine is cleaved by **arginase** to ornithine and urea. Ornithine reenters the mitochondrion for another turn of the cycle. The inner mitochondrial membrane contains a **citrulline/ornithine exchange transporter.**

Synthesis of additional ornithine from glutamate for the cycle will be described later. Since arginine is produced from carbons and nitrogens of ornithine, ammonia, and aspartate, it is a nonessential amino acid. In growing children, however, where there is net incorporation of nitrogen into the body, *de novo* synthesis of arginine is inadequate and the amino acid becomes essential.

Carbons from aspartate, released as fumarate, may enter the mitochondrion and be metabolized to oxaloacetate by the TCA enzymes fumarase and malate dehydrogenase, transaminated, and then theoretically enter another turn of the urea cycle as aspartate. Most oxaloacetate (about two-thirds) from fumarate is metabolized via phosphoenolpyruvate to glucose (Figure 11.25). The amount of fumarate used to form ATP is approximately equal to that required for the urea cycle and gluconeogenesis, meaning that the liver itself gains no net energy in the process of amino acid metabolism.

Since humans cannot metabolize urea it is transported to the kidney for filtration and excretion. Any urea that enters the intestinal tract is cleaved by the intestinal **urease**-containing bacteria, the resulting ammonia being absorbed and used by the liver.

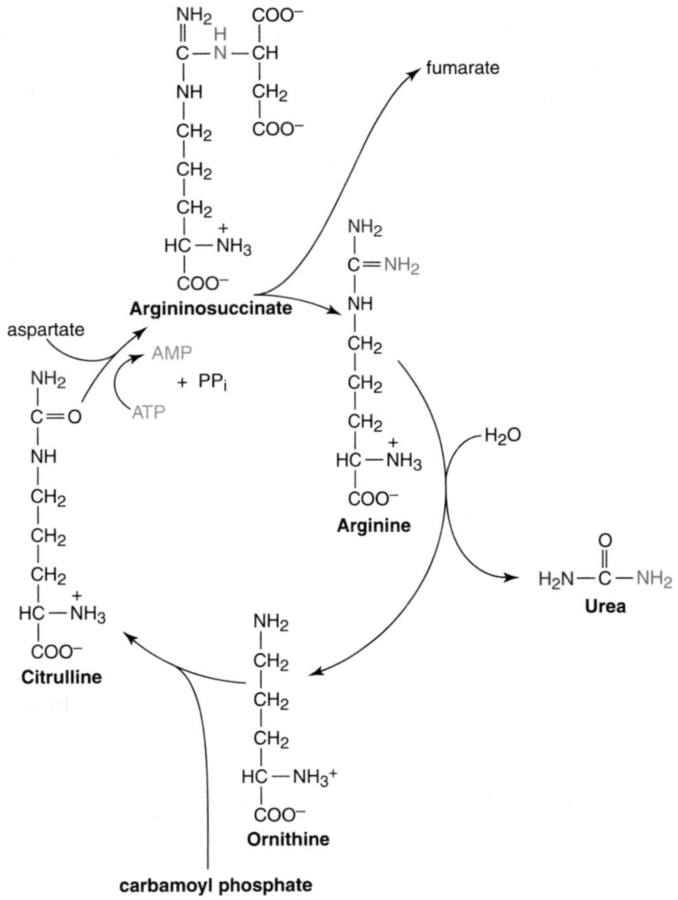

FIGURE 11.24
Urea cycle.

Urea Synthesis Is Regulated by an Allosteric Effector and Enzyme Induction

Carbamoyl phosphate synthetase has a mandatory requirement for the allosteric activator ***N*-acetylglutamate** (see Figure 11.23). This compound is synthesized from glutamate and acetyl CoA by ***N*-acetylglutamate synthetase,** which is activated by arginine. Acetyl CoA, glutamate, and arginine are needed to supply intermediates or energy for the urea cycle, and the presence of *N*-acetylglutamate indicates that they are all available. Tight regulation is desirable for a pathway that controls the plasma level of potentially toxic ammonia and that is also highly energy dependent.

Induction of urea cycle enzymes occurs (10- to 20-fold) when delivery of ammonia or amino acids to liver rises. Concentration of cycle intermediates also plays a role in its regulation through mass action. A high-protein diet (net excess amino acids) and starvation (need to metabolize excess nitrogen in order to provide carbons for energy production) result in induction of urea cycle enzymes.

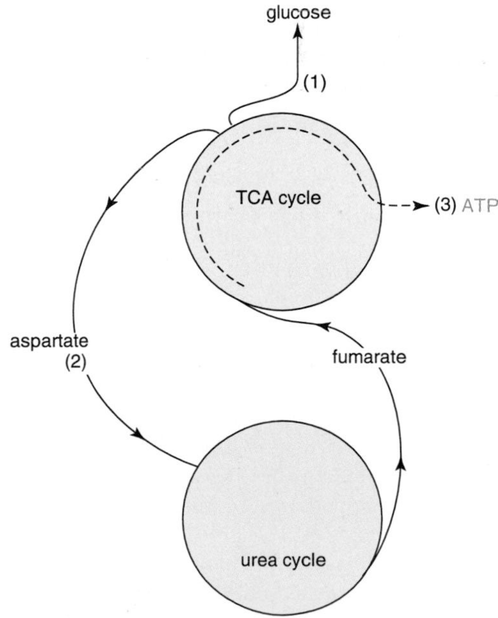

FIGURE 11.25
Fumarate from the urea cycle is a source of glucose (1), aspartate (2), or energy (3).

Metabolic Disorders of Urea Synthesis Have Serious Results

The urea cycle is the major mechanism for the elimination of ammonia, a very toxic substance. Metabolic disorders that arise from abnormal function of enzymes of urea synthesis are potentially fatal and cause coma when ammonia concentrations become high. Loss of consciousness may be a consequence of ATP depletion. The major source of ATP is oxidative phosphorylation, which

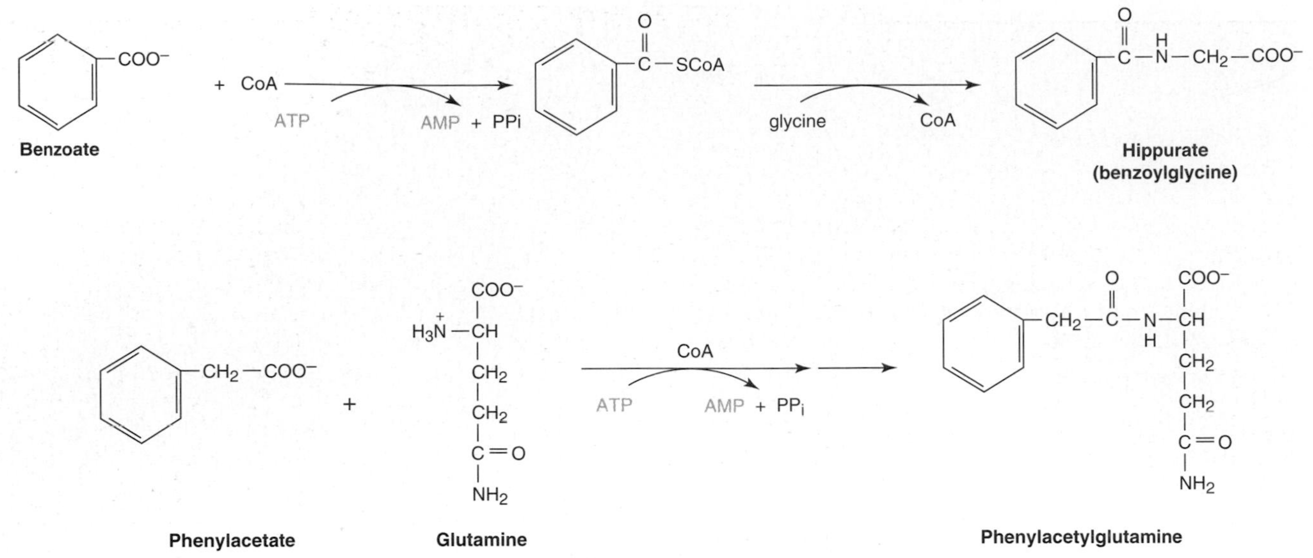

FIGURE 11.26
Detoxification reactions as alternatives to the urea cycle.

is linked to transfer of electrons from the TCA cycle down the electron transport chain. A high concentration of ammonia sequesters α-ketoglutarate to form glutamate, thus depleting the TCA cycle of important intermediates and reducing ATP production.

Patients with a deficiency in each of the urea cycle enzymes have been found. Therapy for these deficiencies has a threefold basis: (1) to limit protein intake and potential buildup of ammonia, (2) to remove excess ammonia, and (3) to replace any intermediates missing from the urea cycle. The first is accomplished by limiting ingestion of amino acids, replacing them if necessary with the equivalent α-keto acids to be transaminated *in vivo*. The bacterial source of ammonia in the intestines can be decreased by a compound that acidifies the colon, such as levulose, a poorly absorbed synthetic disaccharide that is metabolized by colonic bacteria to acidic products. This promotes the excretion of ammonia in feces as protonated ammonium ions. Antibiotics can also be administered to kill ammonia-producing bacteria. The second is achieved by compounds that bind covalently to amino acids and produce nitrogen-containing molecules that are excreted in urine. Figure 11.26 shows condensation of benzoate and glycine to form **hippurate,** and of phenylacetate and glutamine to form **phenylacetylglutamine.** Phenylacetate is extremely unpalatable and is given as the precursor sodium phenylbutyrate. Both reactions require energy for activation of the carboxyl groups by addition of CoA.

Clinical Correlations 11.1 and 11.2 give examples of therapy for specific enzyme deficiencies, which often includes administration of urea cycle intermediates.

CLINICAL CORRELATION 11.1

Carbamoyl Phosphate Synthetase and *N*-Acetylglutamate Synthetase Deficiencies

Hyperammonemia has been observed in infants with 0–50% of the normal level of carbamoyl synthetase activity in their livers. In addition to the treatments described in the text, these infants have been treated with arginine, on the hypothesis that activation of *N*-acetylglutamate synthetase by arginine would stimulate the residual carbamoyl phosphate synthetase. This enzyme deficiency generally leads to mental retardation. A case of *N*-acetylglutamate synthetase deficiency has been described and treated successfully by administering carbamoyl glutamate, an analog of *N*-acetylglutamate, that is also able to activate carbamoyl phosphate synthetase.

11.5 ■ SYNTHESIS AND DEGRADATION OF INDIVIDUAL AMINO ACIDS

Other aspects of metabolism of glutamate, glutamine, aspartate, asparagine, pyruvate, and arginine, the amino acids whose basic metabolism has already been covered, are now discussed. Synthesis of other nonessential amino acids and degradation of all the amino acids will be covered, as well as synthesis of physiologically important amino acid derivatives.

CLINICAL CORRELATION 11.2

Deficiencies of Urea Cycle Enzymes

Ornithine Transcarbamoylase Deficiency

The most common deficiency involving urea cycle enzymes is lack of ornithine transcarbamoylase. Mental retardation and death often result, but the occasional finding of normal development in treated patients suggests that the mental retardation usually associated is caused by the excess ammonia before adequate therapy. The gene for ornithine transcarbamoylase is on the X chromosome, and males generally are more seriously affected than heterozygotic females. In addition to ammonia and amino acids appearing in the blood in increased amounts, orotic acid also increases, presumably because carbamoyl phosphate that cannot be used to form citrulline diffuses into the cytosol, where it condenses with aspartate, ultimately forming orotate (Chapter 12).

Argininosuccinate Synthetase and Lyase Deficiency

The inability to condense citrulline with aspartate results in accumulation of citrulline in blood and excretion in urine (citrullinemia). Therapy for this normally benign disease requires specific supplementation with arginine for protein synthesis and for formation of creatine. Impaired ability to split argininosuccinate to form arginine resembles argininosuccinate synthetase deficiency in that the substrate, in this case argininosuccinate, is excreted in large amounts. The severity of symptoms in this disease varies greatly so that it is hard to evaluate the effect of therapy, which includes dietary supplementation with arginine.

Arginase Deficiency

Arginase deficiency is rare but causes many abnormalities in development and function of the central nervous system. Arginine accumulates and is excreted. Precursors of arginine and products of arginine metabolism may also be excreted. Unexpectedly, some urea is also excreted; this has been attributed to a second type of arginase found in the kidney. A diet including essential amino acids but excluding arginine has been used effectively.

Brusilow, S. W., Danney, M., Waber, L. J., Batshaw, M., et al. Treatment of episodic hyperammonemia in children with inborn errors of urea synthesis. *N. Engl. J. Med.* 310:1630, 1984.

Glutamate Is a Precursor of Glutathione and γ-Aminobutyrate

Glutamate is a component of **glutathione,** which is discussed at the end of this chapter (see p. 484). It is also a precursor for **γ-aminobutyric acid,** a neurotransmitter (Figure 11.27), which will be discussed in Chapter 21, and of proline and ornithine, described below.

Arginine Is Also Synthesized in Intestines

Production of arginine for protein synthesis, rather than as an intermediate in the urea cycle, occurs in kidney, which lacks arginase. The major site of synthesis of citrulline to be used as an arginine precursor is intestinal mucosa, which has all necessary enzymes to convert glutamate (via ornithine as described below) to citrulline, which is then transported to the kidney to produce arginine. Arginine is also a precursor for **nitric oxide** (Chapter 22); in brain, **agmatine,** a compound that may have antihypertensive properties, is an arginine derivative (Figure 11.28).

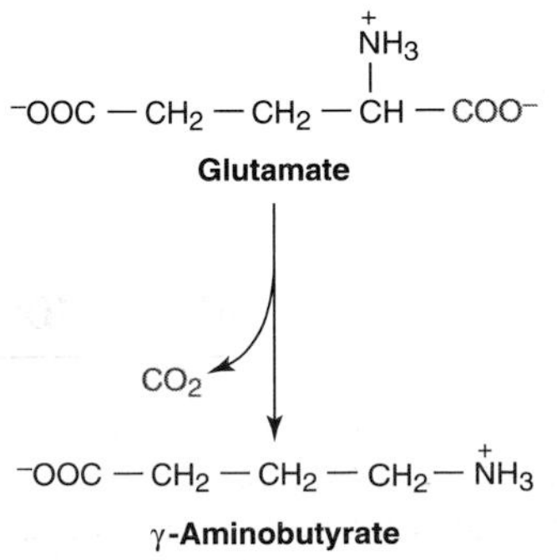

$$^{-}OOC-CH_2-CH_2-\underset{\overset{|}{\overset{+}{N}H_3}}{CH}-COO^{-}$$

Glutamate

↓ (CO_2 released)

$$^{-}OOC-CH_2-CH_2-CH_2-\overset{+}{N}H_3$$

γ-Aminobutyrate

FIGURE 11.27
Synthesis of γ-aminobutyric acid.

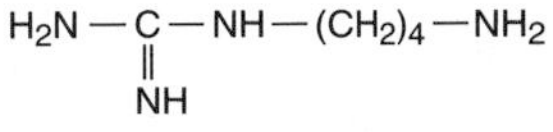

$$H_2N-\underset{\underset{NH}{\|}}{C}-NH-(CH_2)_4-NH_2$$

Agmatine

FIGURE 11.28
Agmatine.

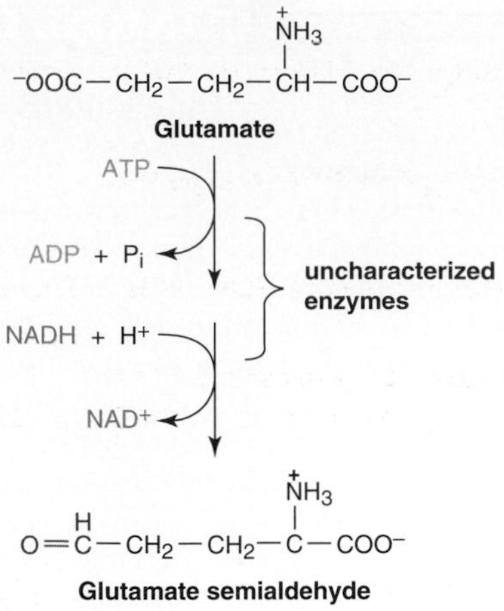

$$^{-}OOC-CH_2-CH_2-CH(\overset{+}{N}H_3)-COO^-$$

Glutamate

ATP → ADP + P_i; NADH + H^+ → NAD^+ (uncharacterized enzymes)

$$O=C(H)-CH_2-CH_2-C(\overset{+}{N}H_3)-COO^-$$

Glutamate semialdehyde

FIGURE 11.29
Synthesis of glutamic semialdehyde.

$$H_2N-CH_2-CH_2-CH_2-CH(\overset{+}{N}H_3)-COO^-$$

Ornithine

α–ketoacid / α–amino acid — aminotransferase

$$O=C(H)-CH_2-CH_2-CH(\overset{+}{N}H_3)-COO^-$$

Glutamic semialdehyde

spontaneous

Δ^1Pyrroline–5–carboxylate

NADPH + H^+ / $NADP^+$ — Pyrroline-5-carboxylate reductase

Proline

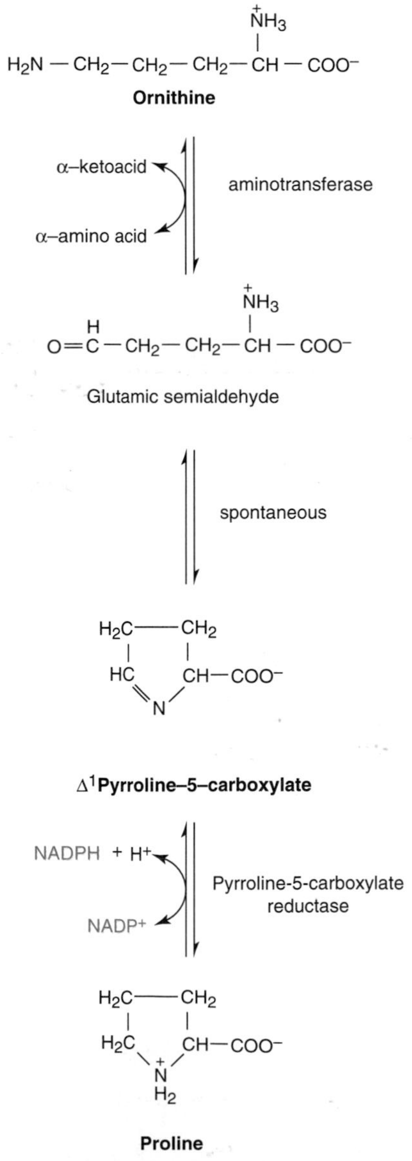

FIGURE 11.30
Synthesis of ornithine and proline from glutamic semialdehyde, a shared intermediate.

Ornithine and Proline

Ornithine, the precursor of citrulline and arginine, and **proline** are both synthesized from glutamate and degraded, by a slightly different pathway, to glutamate. Synthesis of these two nonessential amino acids starts from α-ketoglutarate with a shared reaction that uses ATP and NADH (Figure 11.29) and forms **glutamic semialdehyde.** This spontaneously will cyclize to form a Schiff base between the aldehyde and amino groups, which is then reduced by NADPH to proline. Glutamic semialdehyde can undergo transamination of the aldehyde group, preventing cyclization and producing ornithine (Figure 11.30).

Proline is converted back to the Schiff base intermediate, Δ^1-pyrroline 5-carboxylate, which is in equilibrium with glutamic semialdehyde. The transaminase reaction in the ornithine synthetic pathway is freely reversible and forms glutamic semialdehyde from ornithine (Figure 11.30). Proline residues can be hydroxylated after incorporation into a protein. This posttranslational modification forms **3-** or **4-hydroxyproline** (Figure 11.31). When these are released by protein degradation and metabolized they produce glyoxalate and pyruvate, and 4-hydroxy-2-ketoglutarate, respectively.

Ornithine is a precursor of putrescine, the foundation molecule of polyamines, highly cationic molecules that interact with DNA. Ornithine decarboxylase catalyzes this reaction (Figure 11.32). It is regulated by phosphorylation at several sites, presumably in response to specific hormones, growth factors, or cell cycle regulatory signals. It can also be induced, and this is often the first easily measurable sign that cell division is imminent, since polyamines must be synthesized before mitosis can occur. Other common **polyamines** are **spermidine** and **spermine** (see Figure 11.59), which are synthesized from putrescine by addition of propylamine, a product of methionine metabolism (see p. 472).

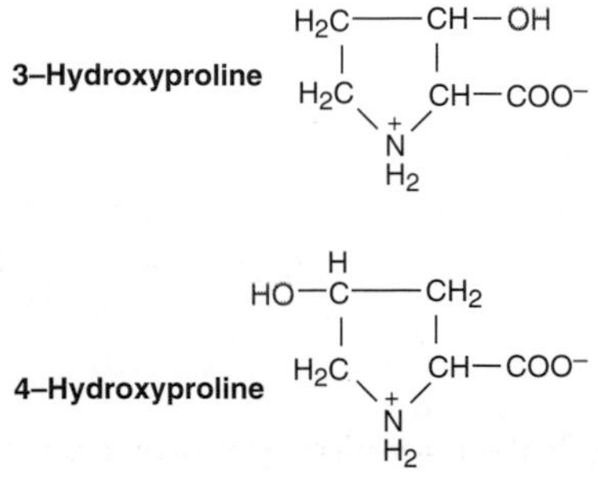

3–Hydroxyproline

4–Hydroxyproline

FIGURE 11.31
Hydroxyprolines.

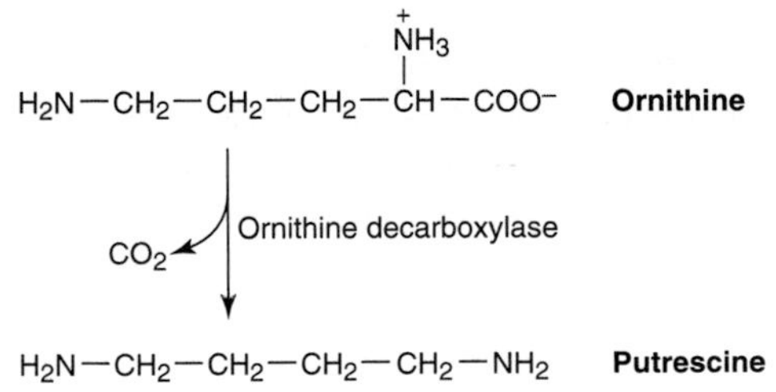

FIGURE 11.32
Decarboxylation of ornithine to putrescine.
Structures of spermidine and spermine are shown in Figure 11.59.

Serine and Glycine

Serine is synthesized *de novo* starting with 3-phosphoglycerate from the glycolytic pathway. When serine provides gluconeogenic intermediates this is also the product of its degradation, although the enzymes and intermediates in the two pathways are different. Synthesis of serine uses phosphorylated intermediates between 3-phosphoglycerate and serine (Figure 11.33*a*), loss of the phosphate being the last step. From serine to 3-phosphoglycerate the intermediates are unphosphorylated, the addition of a phosphate being the last step. The enzymes that catalyze the reactions in the two pathways are not the same (Figure 11.33*b*). Another reaction for entry of serine into intermediary metabolism is via **serine dehydratase,** which forms pyruvate with loss of the amino group as NH_4^+ (Figure 11.34). The same enzyme catalyzes a similar reaction with threonine (see p. 463).

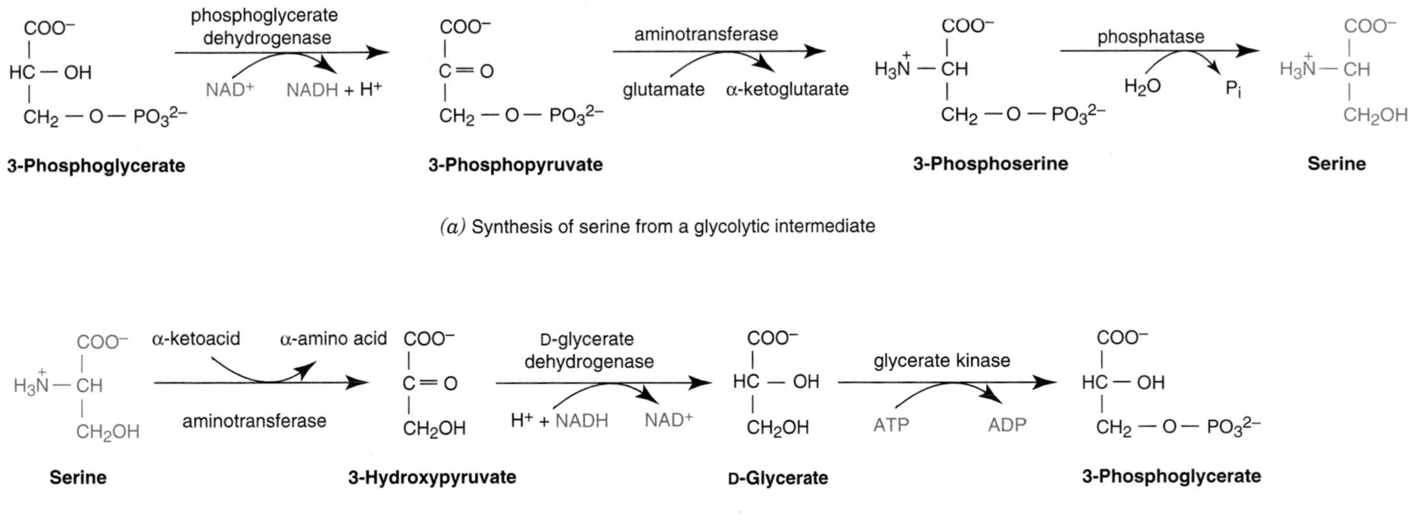

(*a*) Synthesis of serine from a glycolytic intermediate

(*b*) Reactions from serine to a gluconeogenic intermediate

FIGURE 11.33
Pathways for (*a*) synthesis of serine and (*b*) metabolism of serine for gluconeogenesis.

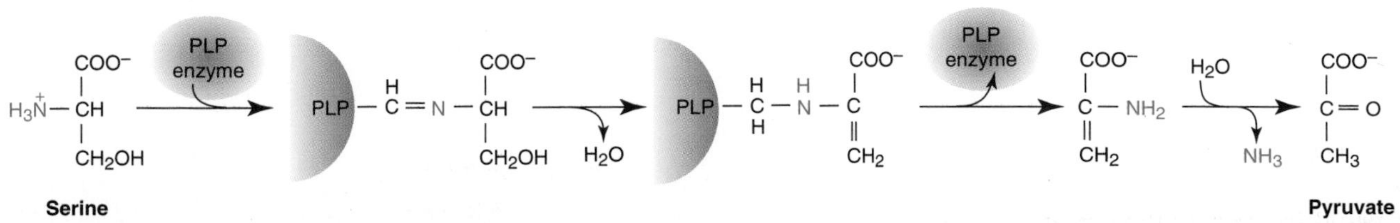

FIGURE 11.34
Reaction of serine dehydratase requires pyridoxal phosphate.

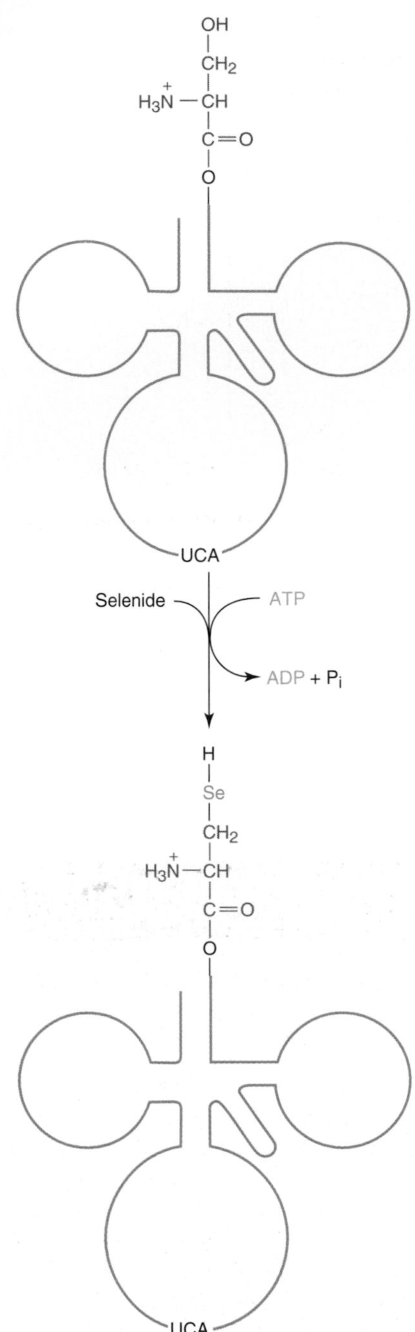

FIGURE 11.35
Formation of selenocysteinyl tRNA from seryl tRNA is via a phosphoseryl tRNA intermediate.

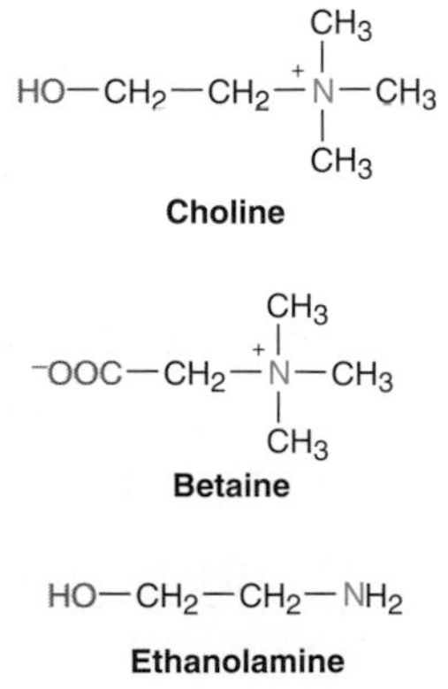

Serine is precursor of an unusual but important amino acid. Certain proteins, notably **glutathione peroxidase,** contain **selenocysteine** (Figure 11.35). In mRNA for selenoproteins the codon UGA, which generally serves as a termination codon, codes for selenocysteine. This amino acid is formed from serine after formation of the seryl–tRNA complex (serine bound to a specific $tRNA^{Ser}$ with the anticodon to UGA).

Ethanolamine, choline, and **betaine** (Figure 11.36) are derivatives of serine. Ethanolamine and choline are components of lipids, and betaine is a methyl donor in a minor pathway leading to methionine salvage (see p. 472). Serine is also a sulfhydryl group acceptor from homocysteine in cysteine synthesis (see p. 470).

In some enzymes a serine residue is modified to form a prosthetic group. In humans the only example described so far is ***S*-adenosylmethionine decarboxylase** (discussed below in relation to polyamine formation; (see p. 473). The prosthetic group formed is similar to pyruvate. *S*-Adenosylmethionine decarboxylase is synthesized in precursor form that is then cleaved autocatalytically between a glutamate and a serine residue to form two polypeptides. During cleavage other reactions convert the new N-terminal serine of one of the resulting peptides into a pyruvate (Figure 11.37). The pyruvate functions in decarboxylation by forming a Schiff base with the amino group of *S*-adenosylmethionine.

Serine is converted reversibly to **glycine** in a reaction that requires pyridoxal phosphate and **tetrahydrofolate.** $\boldsymbol{N^5,N^{10}}$**-methylenetetrahydrofolate** (N^5,N^{10}-THF) is produced (Figure 11.38). The demand for serine or glycine and the amount of N^5,N^{10}-THF available determine the direction of this reaction. Glycine is degraded to CO_2 and ammonia by a **glycine cleavage complex** (Figure 11.39; see Clin. Corr. 11.3). This reaction is reversible in the test tube, but not *in vivo,* as the K_m values for ammonia and N^5,N^{10}-THF are much higher than their respective physiological concentrations.

Glycine is the precursor of **glyoxalate,** which can be transaminated back to glycine or oxidized to **oxalate** (Figure 11.40). Excessive production of oxalate forms the insoluble calcium oxalate salt, which may lead to kidney stones. In Chapter 21 the role of glycine as a neurotransmitter is described.

Tetrahydrofolate Is a Cofactor in Many Reactions of Amino Acids

The **tetrahydrofolate** molecule is the reduced form of folic acid, one of the B vitamins, and often occurs as a polyglutamyl derivative (Figure 11.41). Tetrahydrofolate, involved in two reactions described earlier in the chapter, is a **one-carbon carrier** that facilitates interconversion of methenyl, formyl, formimino,

$HO{-}CH_2{-}CH_2{-}\overset{+}{N}(CH_3)_3$

Choline

$^{-}OOC{-}CH_2{-}\overset{+}{N}(CH_3)_3$

Betaine

$HO{-}CH_2{-}CH_2{-}NH_2$

Ethanolamine

FIGURE 11.36
Choline and related compounds.

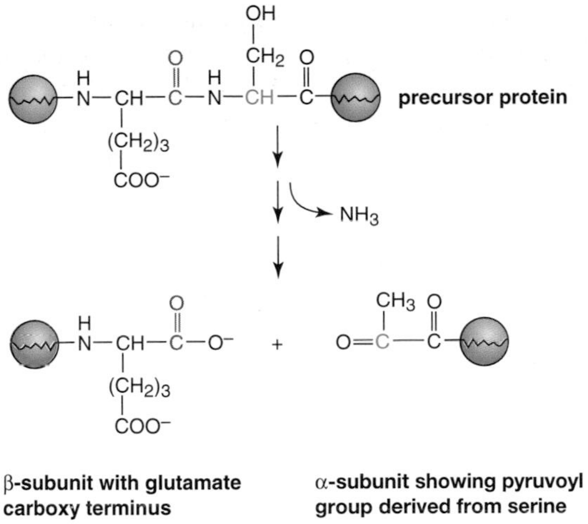

precursor protein

NH_3

β-subunit with glutamate carboxy terminus

α-subunit showing pyruvoyl group derived from serine

FIGURE 11.37
Formation of enzyme with covalently bound pyruvoyl prosthetic group.

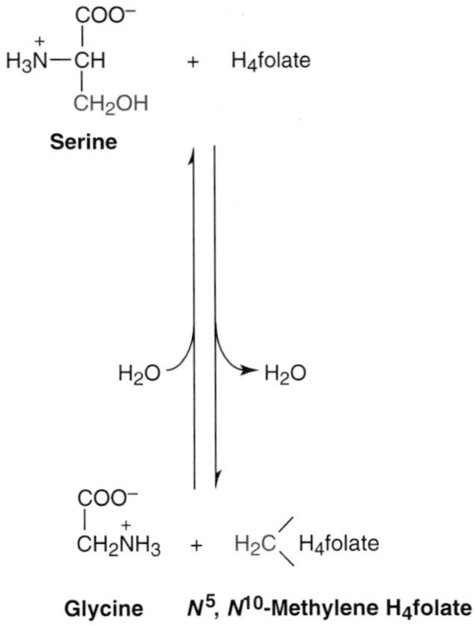

Serine + H_4folate

H_2O H_2O

Glycine + N^5, N^{10}-Methylene H_4folate

FIGURE 11.38
Serine hydroxymethyltransferase.

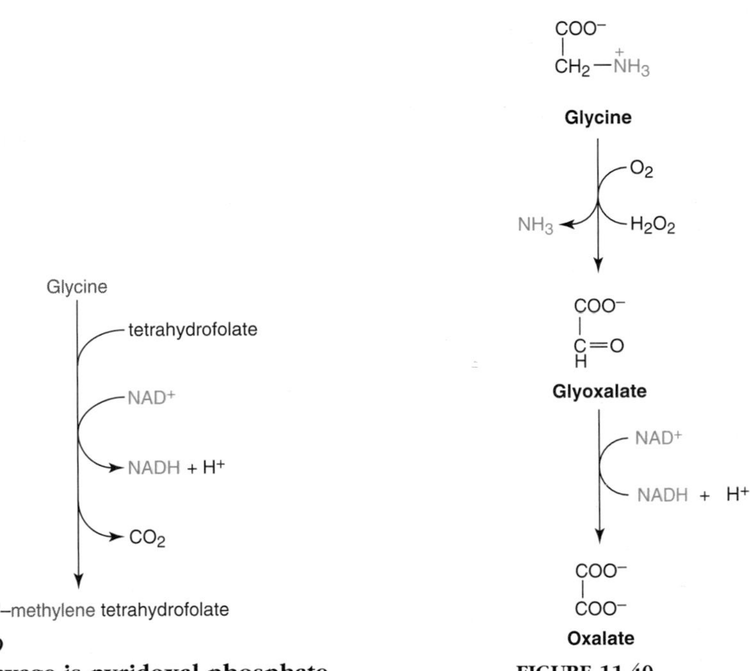

FIGURE 11.39
Glycine cleavage is pyridoxal phosphate dependent.

FIGURE 11.40
Oxidation of glycine.

2-Amino-4-hydroxy-6-methylpteridine | p-aminobenzoic acid | Glutamate

Pteroic acid

Folic acid (pteroylglutamic acid)

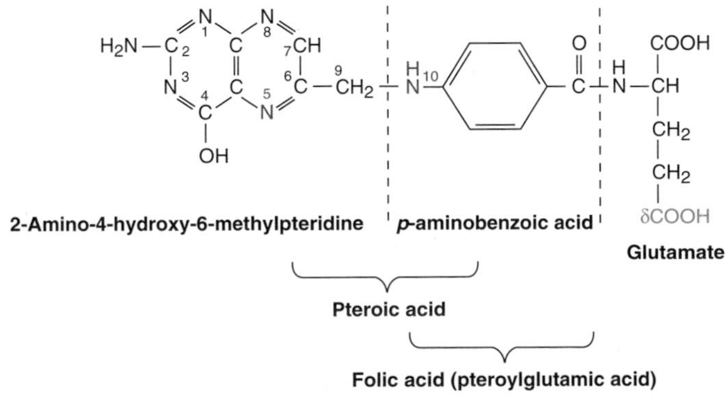

FIGURE 11.41
Components of folate.
Polyglutamate can be added to the δ-carboxyl group.

CLINICAL CORRELATION 11.3

Nonketotic Hyperglycinemia

Nonketotic hyperglycinemia is characterized by severe mental deficiency, and many patients do not survive infancy. The name of this very serious disease is meant to distinguish it from ketoacidosis in abnormalities of branched-chain amino acid metabolism in which, for unknown reasons, the glycine level in the blood is also elevated. Deficiency of glycine cleavage complex has been demonstrated in homogenates of liver from several patients, and isotopic studies *in vivo* have confirmed that this enzyme is not active in these patients. The glycine cleavage complex consists of four different protein subunits. Inherited abnormalities have been found in three of these. The severity of this disease suggests that glycine cleavage is of major importance in the catabolism of glycine. Glycine is a major inhibitory neurotransmitter, which probably explains some neurological complications of the disease. Vigorous measures to reduce the glycine levels fail to alter the course of the disease.

Nyhan, W. L. Metabolism of glycine in the normal individual and in patients with non-ketotic hyperglycinemia. *J. Inherit. Metab. Dis.* 5:105, 1982.

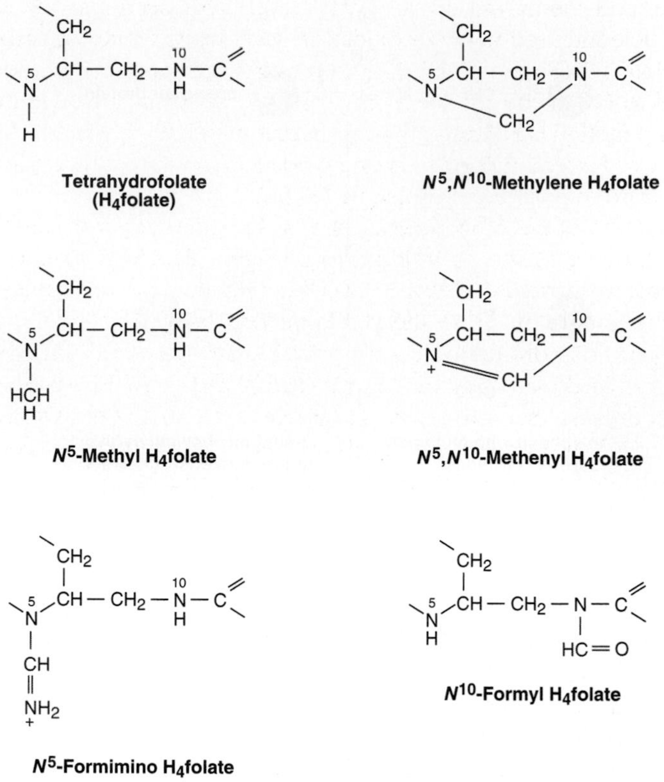

Tetrahydrofolate (H4folate)

N^5,N^{10}-Methylene H4folate

N^5-Methyl H4folate

N^5,N^{10}-Methenyl H4folate

N^5-Formimino H4folate

N^{10}-Formyl H4folate

FIGURE 11.42

Active center of THF.

N^5 is the site of attachment of methyl groups; N^{10} is the site for formyl and formimino; methylene and methenyl groups form bridges between N^5 and N^{10}.

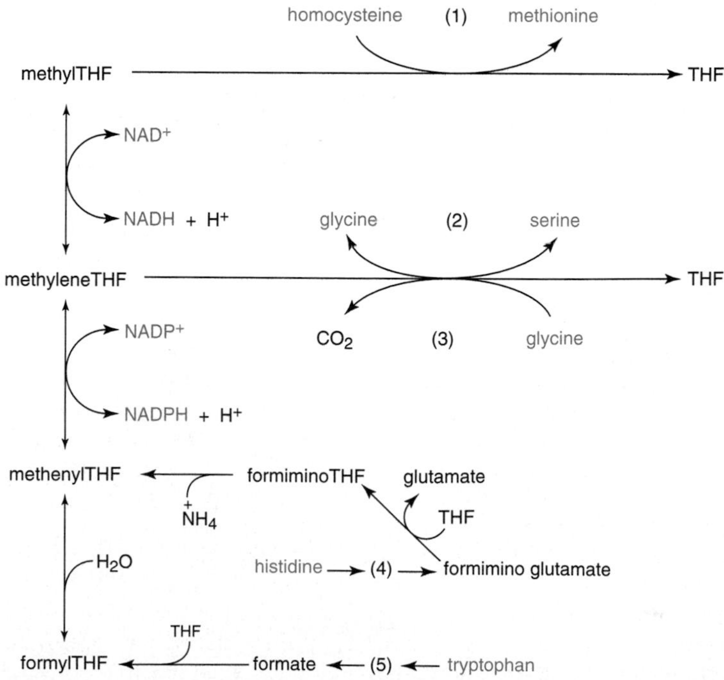

FIGURE 11.43

Interconversion of derivatized THF and roles in amino acid metabolism.

(1) Methionine salvage, (2) serine hydroxymethyltransferase, (3) glycine cleavage complex, (4) histidine degradation, and (5) tryptophan metabolism.

methylene, and methyl groups (Figure 11.42). This occurs at the expense of pyridine nucleotide reduction or oxidation and occurs while the carbon moiety is attached to THF (Figure 11.43). The most oxidized forms, formyl and methenyl, are bound to N^{10} of the pteridine ring, methylene forms a bridge between N^5 and N^{10}, and methyl is bound to N^5. The interconversions permit use of a carbon that is removed from a molecule in one oxidation state for addition in a different oxidation state to a different molecule (Fig.11.42).

In reduction of the N^5,N^{10}-methylene bridge of tetrahydrofolate to a methyl group for transfer to the pyrimidine ring (Figure 11.44), a reaction found in **thymidylate synthesis** (Chapter 12), the reducing power comes not from pyridine nucleotide but from the pteridine ring itself. The resulting oxidized form of folate, dihydrofolate, has no physiological role and must be reduced back to tetrahydrofolate. The reaction is catalyzed by NADPH-dependent dihydrofolate reductase (see Clin. Corr. 11.4). The net result of the two reactions is oxidation of NADPH and reduction of the methylene bridge to a methyl group, analogous to the one-step reactions shown in Figure 11.43.

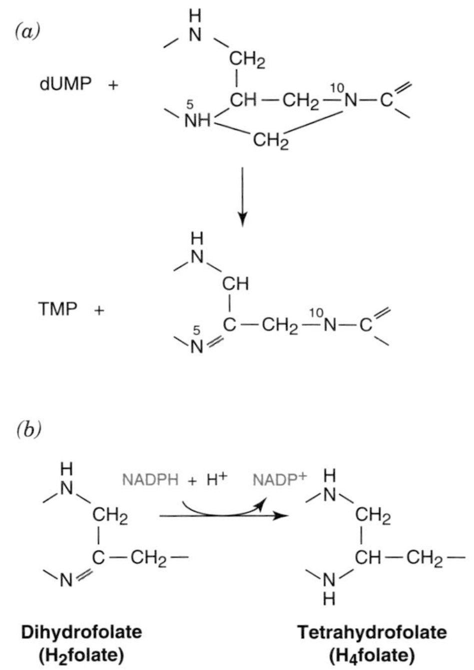

(a)

dUMP + [N^5,N^{10}-methylene-THF fragment] → TMP + [dihydrofolate fragment]

(b)

Dihydrofolate (H_2folate) —(NADPH + H^+ → $NADP^+$)→ Tetrahydrofolate (H_4folate)

FIGURE 11.44
Reduction reactions involving THF.
(a) Reduction of methylene group on THF to a methyl group and transfer to dUMP to form TMP. (b) Reduction of resulting dihydrofolate to tetrahydrofolate.

Threonine

Threonine is usually metabolized to lactate (Figure 11.45), but an intermediate in this pathway can undergo thiolysis with CoA to acetyl CoA and glycine. Thus the α-carbon atom of threonine can contribute to the one-carbon pool. In an alternative, but less common pathway, the enzyme described earlier in serine metabolism, **serine dehydratase** (see p. 459), converts threonine to α-ketobutyrate. A complex similar to pyruvate dehydrogenase metabolizes this to propionyl CoA.

Phenylalanine and Tyrosine

Tyrosine and **phenylalanine** are discussed together, since tyrosine results from hydroxylation of phenylalanine and is the first product in phenylalanine degradation. Because of this, tyrosine is not usually considered to be essential, whereas phenylalanine is. Three-quarters of ingested phenylalanine is metabo-

CLINICAL CORRELATION 11.4

Folic Acid Deficiency

The 100–200 mg of folic acid required daily by an average adult can theoretically be obtained easily from conventional Western diets. Deficiency of folic acid, however, is not uncommon. It may result from limited diets, especially when food is cooked at high temperatures for long periods, which destroys the vitamin. Intestinal diseases, notably celiac disease, are often characterized by folic acid deficiency caused by malabsorption. Inability to absorb folate is rare. Folate deficiency is usually seen only in newborns and produces symptoms of megaloblastic anemia. Of the few cases studied, some were responsive to large doses of oral folate but one required parenteral administration, suggesting a carrier-mediated process for absorption. Besides the anemia, mental and other central nervous system symptoms are seen in patients with folate deficiency, and all respond to continuous therapy although permanent damage appears to be caused by delayed or inadequate treatment. A classical experiment was carried out by a physician, apparently serving as his own experimental subject, to study the human requirements for folic acid. His diet consisted only of foods (boiled repeatedly to extract the water-soluble vitamins) to which vitamins (and minerals) were added, omitting folic acid. Symptoms attributable to folate deficiency did not appear for seven weeks, altered appearance of blood cells and formiminoglutamate excretion were seen only at 13 weeks, and serious symptoms (irritability, forgetfulness, and macrocytic anemia) appeared only after four months. Neurological symptoms were alleviated within two days after folic acid was added to the diet; the blood picture became normal more slowly. The occurrence of folic acid in essentially all natural foods makes deficiency difficult, and apparently a normal person accumulates more than adequate reserves of this vitamin. For pregnant women the situation is very different. Needs of the fetus for normal growth and development include constant, uninterrupted supplies of coenzymes (in addition to amino acids and other cell constituents). Recently, folate deficiency has been implicated in spina bifida.

Herbert, V. Experimental nutritional folate deficiency in man. *Trans. Assoc. Am. Physicians* 75:307, 1962.

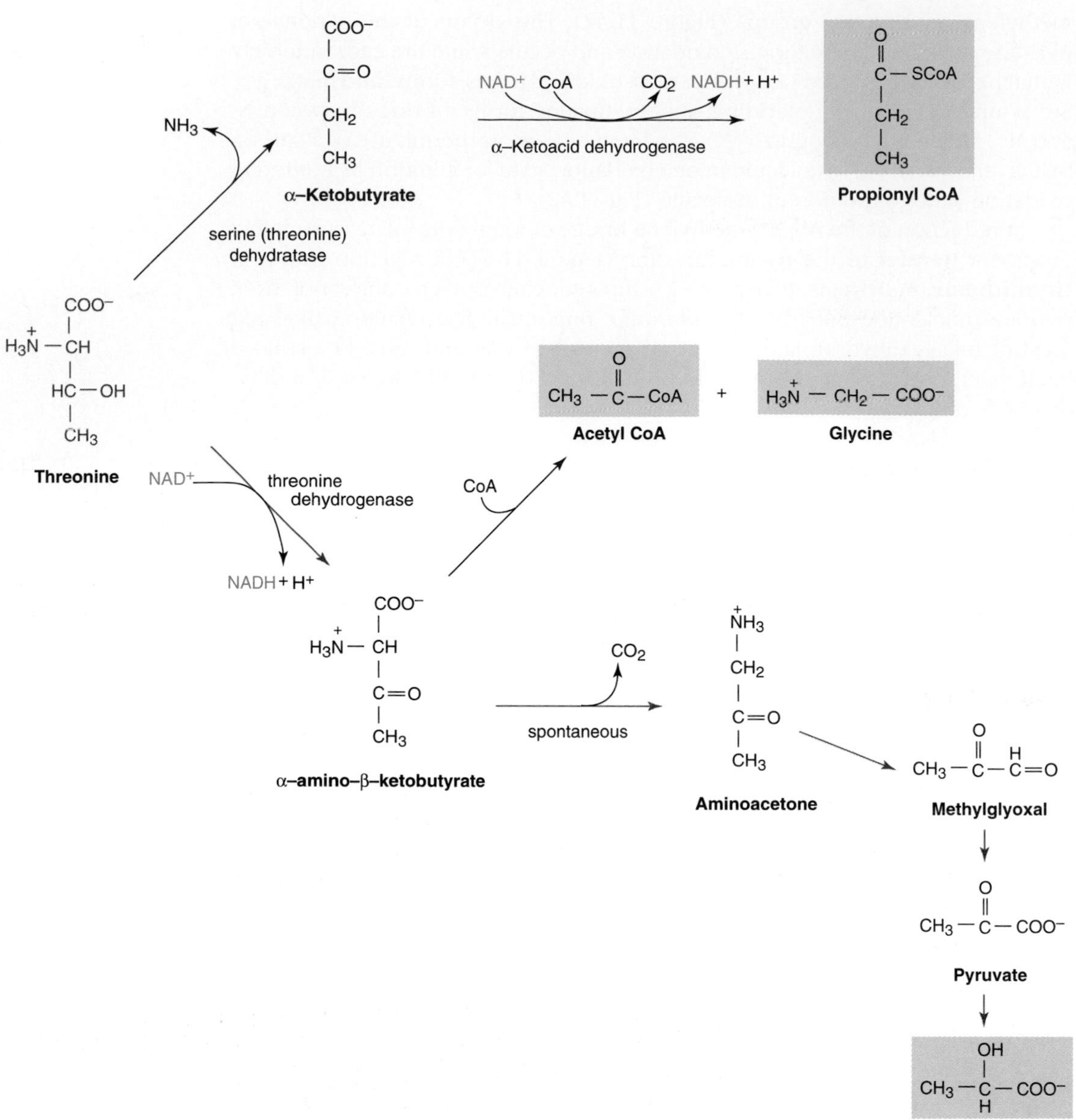

FIGURE 11.45
Outline of threonine metabolism.
Major pathway is in color.

lized to tyrosine. This is catalyzed by **phenylalanine hydroxylase** (Figures 11.46 and Clin. Corr. 11.5), which is **tetrahydrobiopterin dependent** (Figure 11.48). This reaction occurs only in the direction of tyrosine formation, and phenylalanine cannot be synthesized from tyrosine. **Biopterin,** unlike folic

Phenylalanine —(tetrahydrobiopterin, O_2 → dihydrobiopterin, H_2O; phenylalanine hydroxylase)→ Tyrosine

FIGURE 11.46
Phenylalanine hydroxylase.

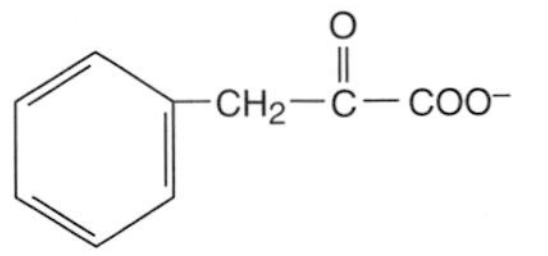

Phenylpyruvate

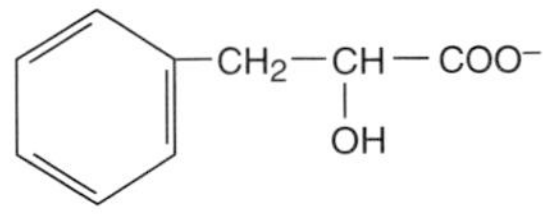

Phenyllactate

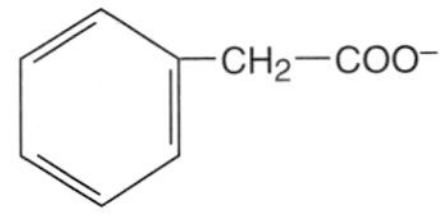

Phenylacetate

FIGURE 11.47
Minor products of phenylalanine metabolism.

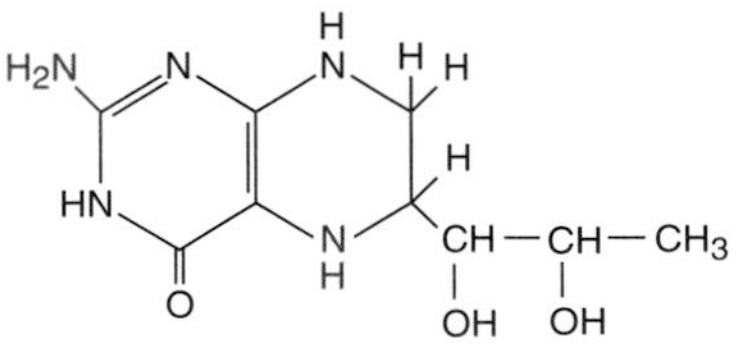

Tetrahydrobiopterin

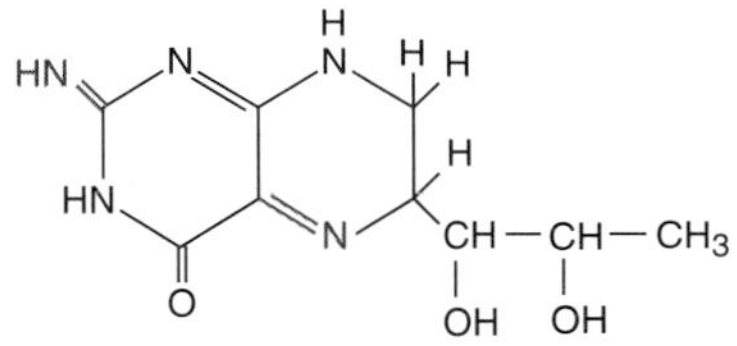

Dihydrobiopterin

FIGURE 11.48
Biopterin.
The dihydro- (quinonoid) form is produced during oxidation of aromatic amino acids and is then reduced to the tetrahydro- form by a dehydrogenase using NADH and H^+.

acid, which it resembles in containing a pteridine ring, is not a vitamin. It is synthesized from GTP. (See Clin. Corr. 11.5.)

Tyrosine Is the First Intermediate in Phenylalanine Metabolism

The first step in metabolism of tyrosine is transamination by **tyrosine aminotransferase** to *p*-hydroxyphenylpyruvate (Figure 11.49). The enzyme is inducible, its synthesis being increased by glucocorticoids and dietary tyrosine. ***p*-Hydroxyphenylpyruvate oxidase** produces **homogentisic acid.** This complex reaction involves decarboxylation, oxidation, migration of the carbon side chain, and hydroxylation. Ascorbic acid is required for at least one of these activities, but all four are catalyzed by the one enzyme. The aromatic ring is next cleaved by an iron-containing enzyme, homogentisate oxidase, to maleyla-

CLINICAL CORRELATION 11.5

Phenylketonuria

Phenylketonuria (PKU) is the most common disease caused by a deficiency of an enzyme of amino acid metabolism. The name comes from the excretion of phenylpyruvic acid, a phenylketone, in the urine. Phenyllactate is also excreted (Figure 11.47), as is an oxidation product of phenylpyruvate, phenylacetate, which gives the urine a "mousey" odor. These three metabolites are found only in trace amounts in urine in the healthy person. The symptoms of mental retardation associated with this disease can be prevented by a phenylalanine-free diet. Routine screening is required by governments in many parts of the world. Classical PKU is an autosomal recessive deficiency of phenylalanine hydroxylase. Over 170 mutations in the gene have been reported. In some cases there are severe neurological symptoms and very low IQ. These are generally attributed to toxic effects of phenylalanine, possibly because of reduced transport and metabolism of other aromatic amino acids in the brain due to competition from the high phenylalanine concentration. Another characteristic is light color of skin and eyes, due to underpigmentation because of tyrosine deficiency. Conventional treatment is to feed affected infants a synthetic diet low in phenylalanine, but including tyrosine, for about four to five years, and impose dietary protein restriction for several more years or for life. About 3% of infants with high levels of phenylalanine have normal hydroxylase but are defective in either synthesis or reduction of biopterin. Biopterin deficiency can be treated by addition to the diet. Deficiency in dihydrobiopterin reductase is more serious. Since biopterin is also necessary for the synthesis of catecholamines and serotonin, which function as neurotransmitters, central nervous system functions are more seriously affected and treatment at this time includes administration of precursors of serotonin and catecholamines.

Brewster, T. G., Moskowitz, M. A., Kaufman, S., et al. Dihydrobiopterin reductase deficiency associated with severe neurologic disease and mild hyperphenylalanemia. *Pediatrics* 63:94, 1979; Kaufman, S. Regulation of the activity of hepatic phenylalanine hydroxylase. *Adv. Enzyme Regul.* 25:37, 1986; Scriver, C. R. and Clow, L. L. Phenylketonuria: epitome of human biochemical genetics. *N. Engl. J. Med.* 303:1336,1980; Woo, S. L. C. Molecular basis and population genetics of phenylketonuria. *Biochemistry* 28:1, 1989.

cetoacetate. This will isomerize from cis to trans to give fumarylacetoacetate, in a reaction catalyzed by maleylacetoacetate isomerase, an enzyme that seems to require glutathione for activity. Fumarylacetoacetate is then cleaved to fumarate and acetoacetate. Fumarate can be further utilized in the TCA cycle for energy or for gluconeogenesis. Acetoacetate can be used, as acetyl CoA, for lipid synthesis or energy. (See Clin. Corr. 11.6.)

Dopamine, Epinephrine, and Norepinephrine Are Derivatives of Tyrosine

Most tyrosine not incorporated into proteins is metabolized to acetoacetate and fumarate. Some is used as precursor of **catecholamines.** The eventual metabolic fate of tyrosine carbons is determined by the first step in each pathway. Catecholamine synthesis (Figure 11.50) starts with **tyrosine hydroxylase,** which, like phenylalanine and tryptophan hydroxylase, is dependent on tetrahydrobiopterin. All three are affected by biopterin deficiency or a defect in dihydrobiopterin reductase (see Figure 11.48). Tyrosine hydroxylase produces dihydroxyphenylalanine, also known as DOPA, dioxophenylalanine. **DOPA decarboxylase,** with pyridoxal phosphate as cofactor, forms **dopamine,** the active neurotransmitter, from DOPA. In the substantia nigra and some other parts of the brain, this is the last enzyme in this pathway (see Clin. Corr. 11.7). The adrenal medulla converts dopamine to **norepinephrine** and **epinephrine**

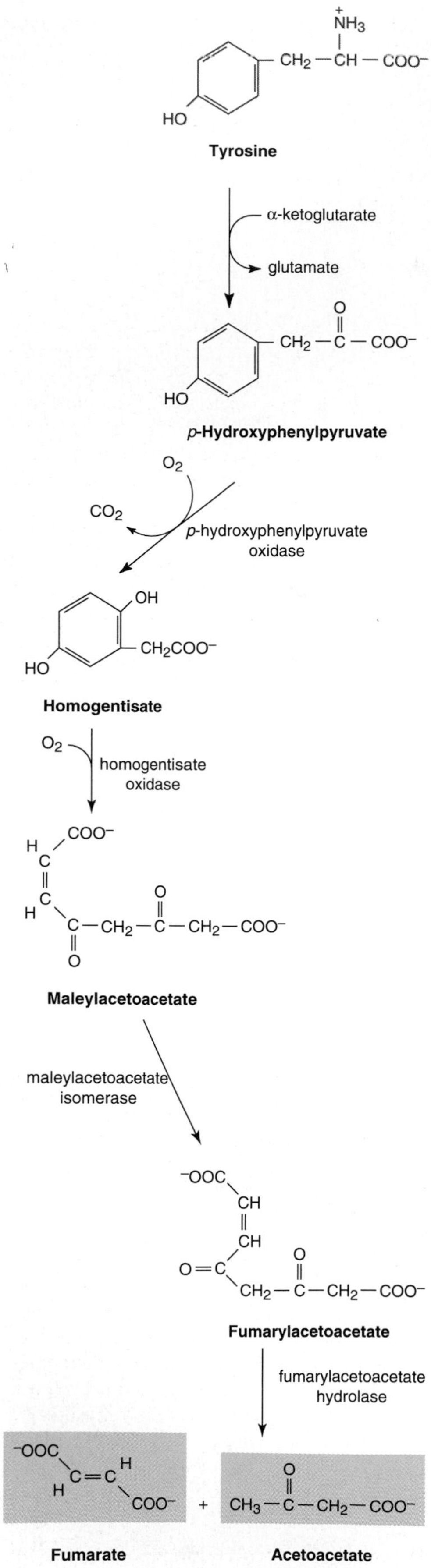

Tyrosine
α-ketoglutarate
glutamate
p-Hydroxyphenylpyruvate
O_2
CO_2
p-hydroxyphenylpyruvate oxidase
Homogentisate
O_2
homogentisate oxidase
Maleylacetoacetate
maleylacetoacetate isomerase
Fumarylacetoacetate
fumarylacetoacetate hydrolase
Fumarate
Acetoacetate

FIGURE 11.49
Degradation of tyrosine.

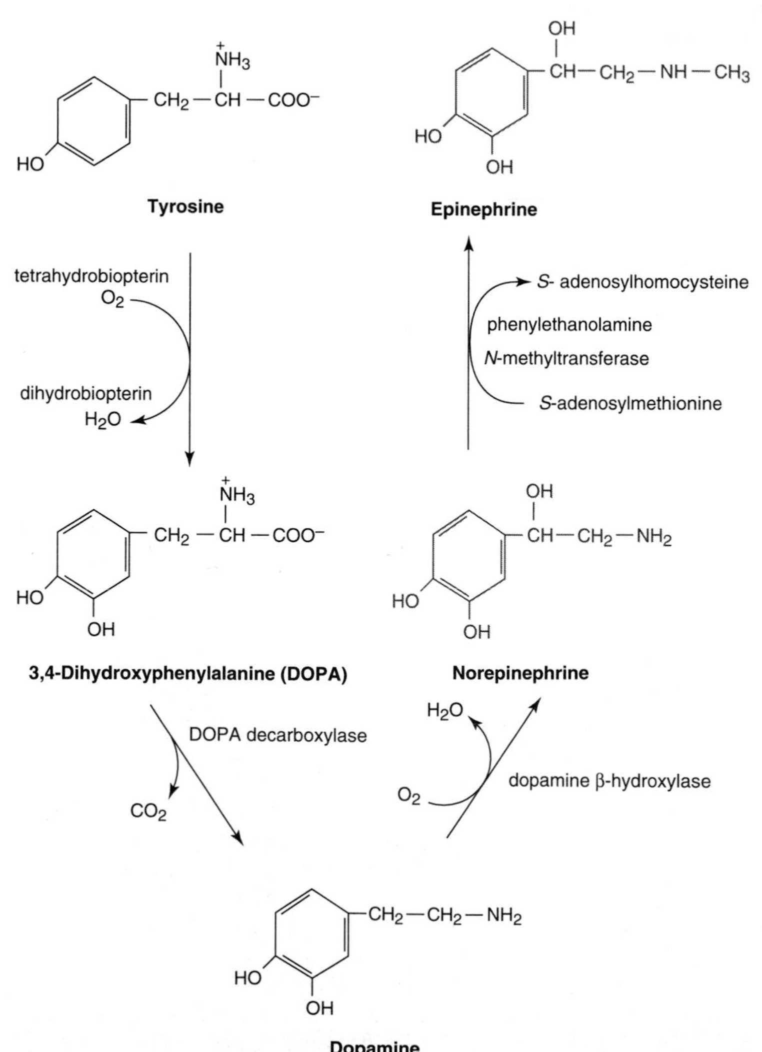

FIGURE 11.50
Synthesis of catecholamines.

CLINICAL CORRELATION 11.6

Disorders of Tyrosine Metabolism

Tyrosinemias

The absence or deficiency of tyrosine aminotransferase produces accumulation and excretion of tyrosine and metabolites. The disease, oculocutaneous or type II tyrosinemia, results in eye and skin lesions and mental retardation. Type I, hepatorenal tyrosinemia, is more serious, involving liver failure, renal tubular dysfunction, rickets, and polyneuropathy, caused by a deficiency of fumarylacetoacetate hydrolase. Accumulation of fumarylacetoacetate and maleylacetate, both of which are alkylating agents, can lead to DNA alkylation and tumorigenesis. Both diseases are autosomal recessive and rare.

Alcaptonuria

The first condition identified as an "inborn error of metabolism" was alcaptonuria. Individuals deficient in homogentisate oxidase excrete almost all ingested tyrosine as the colorless homogentisic acid in their urine. This auto-oxidizes to the corresponding quinone, which polymerizes to form an intensely dark color. Concern about the dark urine is the only consequence of this condition early in life. Homogentisate is slowly oxidized to pigments that are deposited in bones, connective tissue, and other organs, a condition called ochronosis because of the ochre color of the deposits. This is thought to be responsible for the associated arthritis, especially in males. The study of alcaptonuria by Archibald Garrod, who first indicated its autosomal recessive genetic basis, includes an unusual historical description of the iatrogenic suffering of the first patient treated for the condition, which is frequently benign.

Albinism

Skin and hair color are controlled by an unknown number of genetic loci in humans and exist in infinite variation; in mice, 147 genes have been identified in color determination. Many conditions have been described in which the skin has little or no pigment. The chemical basis is not established for any except classical albinism, which results from a lack of tyrosinase. Lack of pigment in the skin makes albinos sensitive to sunlight, increasing carcinoma of the skin in addition to burns; lack of pigment in the eyes may contribute to photophobia.

Fellman, J. H., Vanbellinghan, P. J., Jones, R. T., and Koler, R. D. Soluble and mitochondrial tyrosine aminotransferase. Relationship to human tyrosinemia. *Biochemistry* 8:615, 1969; Kvittingen, E. A. Hereditary tyrosinemia type I. An overview. *Scand. J. Clin. Lab. Invest.* 46:27, 1986

(also called **adrenaline).** The methyl group of epinephrine is derived from *S*-adenosylmethionine (see p. 469).

Brain plasma tyrosine regulates norepinephrine formation. Estrogens decrease tyrosine concentration and increase tyrosine aminotransferase activity, diverting tyrosine into the catabolic pathway. Furthermore, estrogen sulfate competes for the pyridoxal phosphate site on DOPA decarboxylase. These three effects combined may help explain mood variations during the menstrual cycle. Tyrosine is therapeutic in some cases of depression and stress. Its transport appears to be reduced in skin fibroblasts from schizophrenic patients, indicating other roles for tyrosine derivatives in mental disorders.

CLINICAL CORRELATION 11.7

Parkinson's Disease

Usually in people over the age of 60 years but occasionally earlier, tremors may develop that gradually interfere with motor function of various muscle groups. This condition is named for the physician who described "shaking palsy" in 1817. The primary cause is unknown, and there may be more than one etiological agent. The defect is caused by degeneration of cells in certain small nuclei of the brain called substantia nigra and locus caeruleus. Their cells normally produce dopamine as a neurotransmitter, the amount released being proportional to the number of surviving cells. A dramatic outbreak of parkinsonism occurred in young adult drug addicts using a derivative of pyridine (methylphenyl-tetrahydropyridine, MPTP). It (or a contaminant produced during its manufacture) appears to be directly toxic to dopamine-producing cells of substantia nigra. Symptomatic relief, often dramatic, is obtained by administering DOPA, the precursor of dopamine. Clinical problems developed when DOPA (L-DOPA, levo-DOPA) was used for treatment of many people who have Parkinson's disease. Side effects included nausea, vomiting, hypotension, cardiac arrhythmias, and various central nervous system symptoms. These were explained as effects of dopamine produced outside the central nervous system. Administration of DOPA analogs that inhibit DOPA decarboxylase but are unable to cross the blood–brain barrier has been effective in decreasing side effects and increasing effectiveness of the DOPA. The interactions of the many brain neurotransmitters are very complex, cell degeneration continues after treatment, and elucidation of the major biochemical abnormality has not yet led to complete control of the disease. Recently, attempts have been made at treatment by transplantation of fetal adrenal medullary tissue into the brain. The adrenal tissue synthesizes dopamine and improves the movement disorder.

Calne, D. B., and Langston, J. W. Aetiology of Parkinson's disease. *Lancet* 2:1457, 1983; and Cell and tissue transplantation into the adult brain. *Ann. N.Y. Acad. Sci.* 495, 1987.

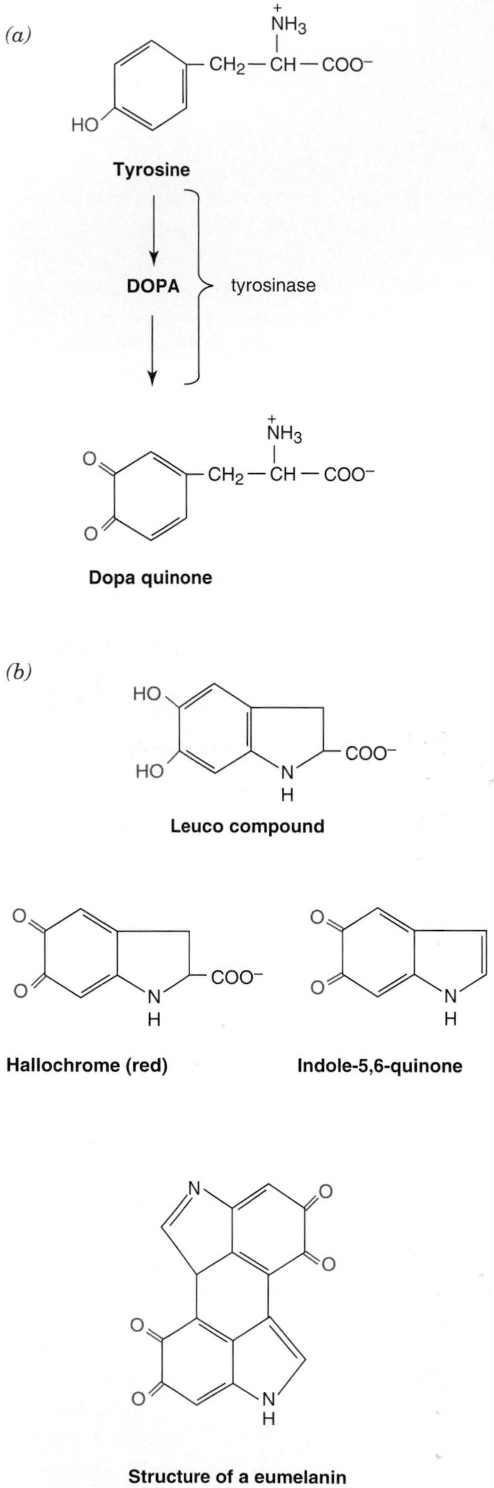

(a)

Tyrosine → DOPA → Dopa quinone (tyrosinase)

(b)

Leuco compound

Hallochrome (red)

Indole-5,6-quinone

Structure of a eumelanin

FIGURE 11.52
(*a*) Tyrosinase uses DOPA as a cofactor/intermediate; (*b*) some intermediates in melanin synthesis and an example of the family of black eumelanins.

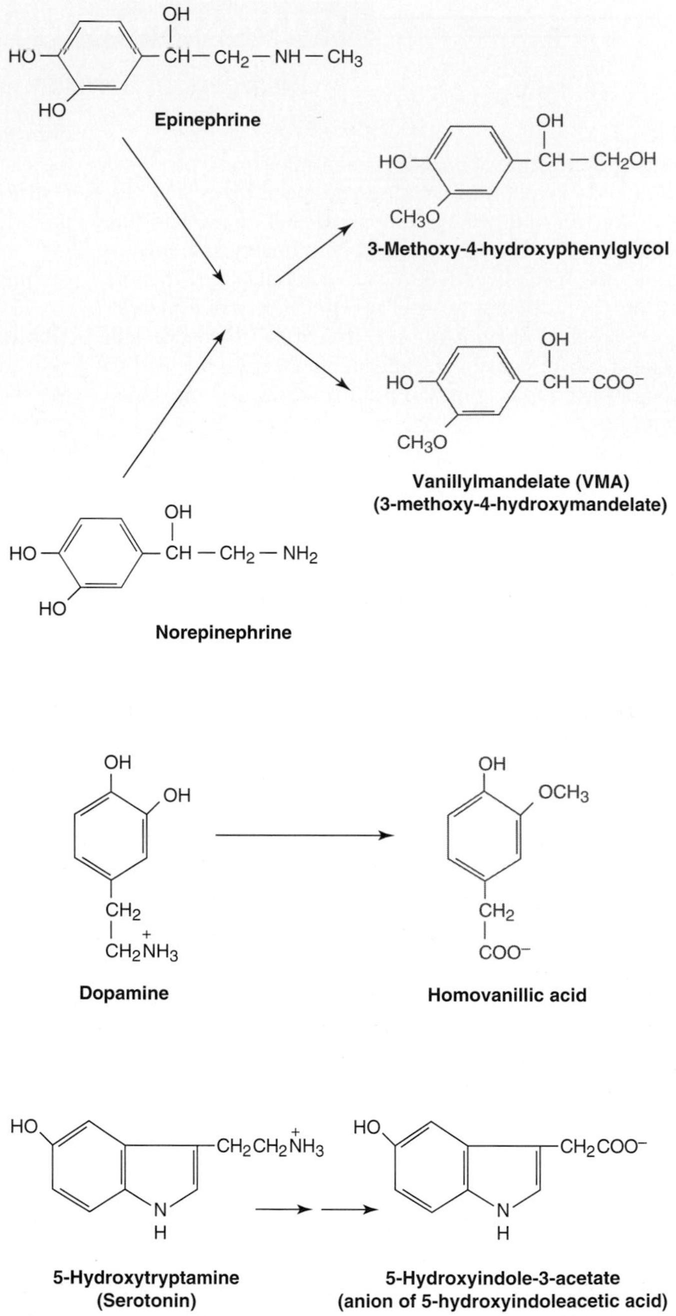

Epinephrine

3-Methoxy-4-hydroxyphenylglycol

Vanillylmandelate (VMA) (3-methoxy-4-hydroxymandelate)

Norepinephrine

Dopamine

Homovanillic acid

5-Hydroxytryptamine (Serotonin)

5-Hydroxyindole-3-acetate (anion of 5-hydroxyindoleacetic acid)

FIGURE 11.51
Major urinary excretion products of dopamine, epinephrine, norepinephrine, and serotonin.

Catecholamines are metabolized by **monoamine oxidase** and catecholamine ***O*-methyltransferase.** Major metabolites are shown in Figure 11.51. Absence of these metabolites in urine is diagnostic of a deficiency in synthesis of catecholamines. Lack of synthesis of serotonin (see p. 866) is indicated by lack of 5-hydroxyindole-3-acetic acid, shown in the same figure.

Tyrosine Is Involved in Synthesis of Melanin, Thyroid Hormone, and Quinoproteins

Conversion of tyrosine to melanin requires **tyrosinase,** a copper-containing protein (Figure 11.52*a*). The two-step reaction uses DOPA as a cofactor internal to the reaction and produces **dopaquinone.** During melanogenesis, following

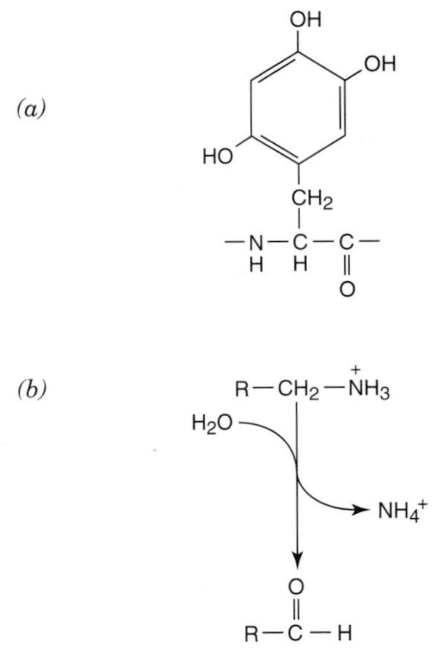

FIGURE 11.53
(*a*) Topaquinone and (*b*) amine oxidase reaction.

exposure to UVB light, tyrosinase and a protein called tyrosinase-related protein, which may function in posttranslational modification of tyrosinase, are induced. A lack of tyrosinase activity produces **albinism.**

There are various types of **melanin** (Figure 11.52*b*). All are aromatic quinones and the conjugated bond system gives rise to color. The dark pigment that is usually associated with melanin is eumelanin, from the Greek for "good melanin." Other melanins are yellow or colorless. The role of tyrosine residues of thyroglobulin in thyroid hormone synthesis is presented in the chapter on hormones (Chapter 20).

Some proteins use a modified tyrosine residue as a prosthetic group in oxidation–reduction reactions. The only example reported in humans is **topaquinone** (trihydroxyphenylalanylquinone), which is present in some plasma amine oxidases (Figure 11.53).

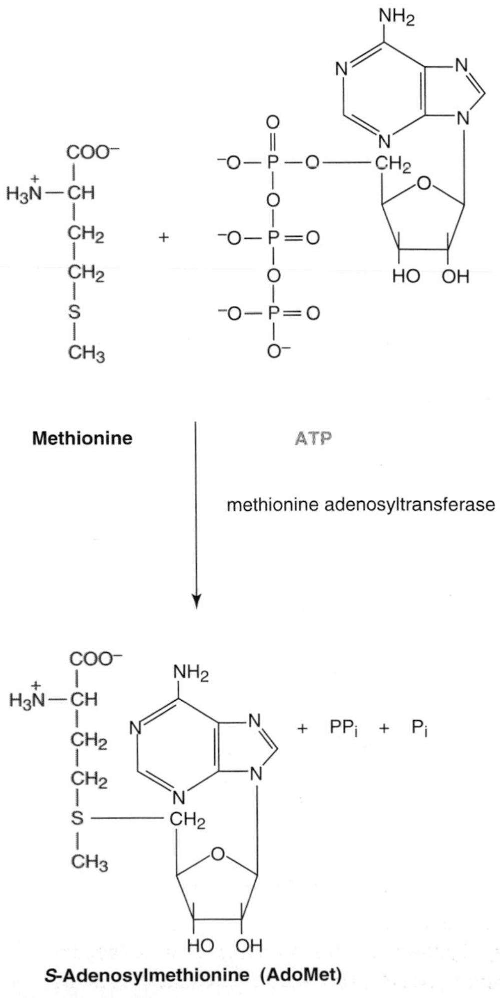

Methionine and Cysteine

De novo synthesis of **methionine** does not occur and methionine is essential. **Cysteine,** however, is synthesized by transfer of the sulfur atom derived from methionine to the hydroxyl group of serine. As long as the supply of methionine is adequate, cysteine is nonessential. The disposition of individual atoms of methionine and cysteine is a prime example of how cells regulate pathways to fit their immediate needs for energy or for other purposes. Conditions under which various pathways are given preference will be emphasized.

Methionine Is First Reacted with Adenosine Triphosphate

When excess methionine is present its carbons can be used for energy or for gluconeogenesis, and the sulfur retained as the sulfhydryl of cysteine. Figure 11.54 shows the first step, catalyzed by **methionine adenosyltransferase.** All phosphates of ATP are lost, and the product is ***S*-adenosylmethionine** (abbreviated **AdoMet,** or **SAM** in older references). The sulfonium ion is highly reactive, and the methyl is a good leaving group. AdoMet as a methyl group donor will be described below. After a methyltransferase removes the methyl group, the resulting ***S*-adenosylhomocysteine** is cleaved by **adenosylhomocysteinase** (Figure 11.55). Note that homocysteine is one carbon longer than cysteine. Although the carbons are destined for intermediary metabolism, the

FIGURE 11.54
Synthesis of AdoMet.

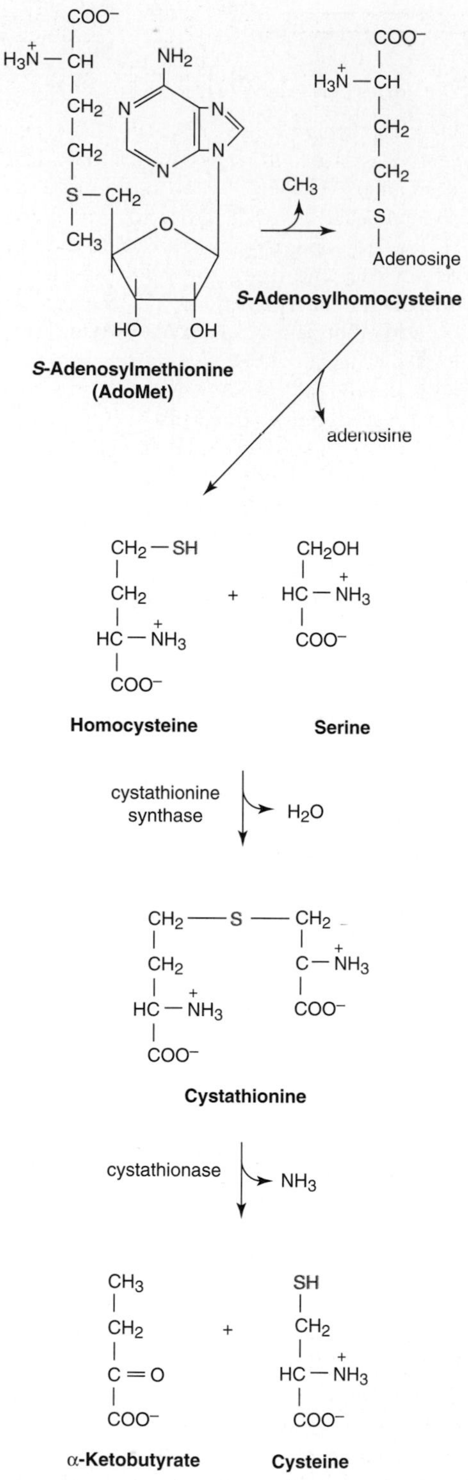

S-Adenosylmethionine (AdoMet)

S-Adenosylhomocysteine

adenosine

Homocysteine

Serine

cystathionine synthase

H_2O

Cystathionine

cystathionase

NH_3

α-Ketobutyrate

Cysteine

FIGURE 11.55
Synthesis of cysteine from *S*-adenosylmethionine.

sulfur, a more specialized atom, will be conserved through transfer to serine to form cysteine. This requires the pyridoxal phosphate-dependent **cystathionine synthase** and **cystathionase** (Figure 11.55; see Clin. Corr. 11.8). Since the bond to form cystathionine is made on one side of the sulfur, and that cleaved is on the other side, the result is a **transsulfuration** (see Clin. Corr. 11.9). Homocysteine produces α-ketobutyrate and ammonia. α-Ketobutyrate is decarboxylated by a multienzyme complex resembling pyruvate dehydrogenase to

CLINICAL CORRELATION 11.8

Hyperhomocysteinemia and Atherogenesis

Deficiency of cystathionine synthase causes homocysteine to accumulate, and remethylation leads to high levels of methionine. Many minor products of these amino acids are formed and excreted. No mechanism has been established to explain why accumulation of homocysteine should lead to some of the pathological changes. Homocysteine may react with and block lysyl aldehyde groups on collagen. The lens of the eye is frequently dislocated some time after the age of 3, and other ocular abnormalities often occur. Osteoporosis develops during childhood. Mental retardation is frequently the first indication of this deficiency. Attempts at treatment include restriction of methionine intake and feeding of betaine (or its precursor, choline). In some cases significant improvement has been obtained by feeding pyridoxine (vitamin B_6), suggesting that the deficiency may be caused by more than one type of gene mutation; one type may affect the K_m for pyridoxal phosphate and others may alter the K_m for other substrates, V_{max}, or the amount of enzyme. A theory relating hyperhomocysteinemia to atherogenesis has been proposed. Excess homocysteine can form homocysteine thiolactone, a highly reactive intermediate, which thiolates free amino groups in low density lipoproteins (LDLs) and causes them to aggregate and be endocytosed by macrophages. The lipid deposits form atheromas. Homocysteine can have other effects, including lipid oxidation and platelet aggregation, which in turn lead to fibrosis and calcification of atherosclerotic plaques. About one-quarter of patients with atherosclerosis who exhibit none of the other risk factors (such as smoking or oral contraceptive therapy) have been found to be deficient in cystathionine synthase activity.

Kaiser-Kupfer, M. I., Fujikawa, L., Kuwabara, T., et al. Removal of corneal crystals by topical cysteamine in nephrotic cystinosis. *N. Engl. J. Med.* 316:775, 1987; McCully, K. S. Chemical pathology of homocysteine I. Atherogenesis. *Ann. Clin. Lab. Sci.* 23:477, 1993.

yield propionyl CoA, which is then converted to succinyl CoA as described on page 479.

When the need is for energy, and not for cysteine, homocysteine produced in the above pathway is metabolized by **homocysteine desulfhydrase** to α-ketobutyrate, NH_3, and H_2S (Figure 11.56).

S-Adenosylmethionine Is a Methyl Group Donor

The role of tetrahydrofolate as a one-carbon group donor has been described (see p. 460). Although this cofactor could in theory serve as a source of methyl groups, the vast majority of methyltransferase reactions utilize ***S*-adenosylmethionine.** Methyl group transfer from AdoMet to a methyl acceptor is irre-

CLINICAL CORRELATION 11.9

Other Diseases of Sulfur Amino Acids

Congenital deficiency of any of the enzymes involved in transsulfuration results in accumulation of sulfur-containing amino acids. Hypermethioninemia has been attributed to deficiency of methionine adenosyltransferase, probably caused by a K_m mutant that requires higher than normal concentrations of methionine for saturation, but functions normally in methylation reactions. Lack of cystathionase does not seem to cause any clinical abnormalities other than cystathioninuria. The first reported case of this deficiency was about a mentally retarded patient and the retardation was attributed to the deficiency. Apparently the mental retardation was coincidental, the condition being benign. The amount of cysteine synthesized in these deficiencies is unknown, but treatment with a low-methionine diet for hypermethioninemia is unnecessary.

Diseases Involving Cystine

Cystinuria is a defect of membrane transport of cystine and basic amino acids (lysine, arginine, and ornithine) that results in their increased renal excretion. Extracellular sulfhydryl compounds are quickly oxidized to disulfides. Low solubility of cystine results in crystals and the formation of calculi, a serious feature of this disease. Treatment is limited to removal of stones, prevention of precipitation by drinking large amounts of water or alkalinizing the urine to solubilize cystine, or formation of soluble derivatives by conjugation with drugs. Much more serious is cystinosis in which cystine accumulates in lysosomes. The stored cystine forms crystals in many cells, with a serious loss of function of the kidneys, usually causing renal failure within ten years. The defect is believed to be in the cystine transporter of lysosomal membranes.

Seashore, M. R., Durant, J. L., and Rosenberg, L. E. Studies on the mechanisms of pyridoxine responsive homocystinuria. *Pediatr. Res.* 6:187, 1972; Mudd, S. H. The natural history of homocystinuria due to cystathione β-synthase deficiency. *Am. J. Hum. Genet.* 37:1, 1985; and Frimpter, G. W. Cystathionuria: nature of the defect. *Science* 149:1095, 1965.

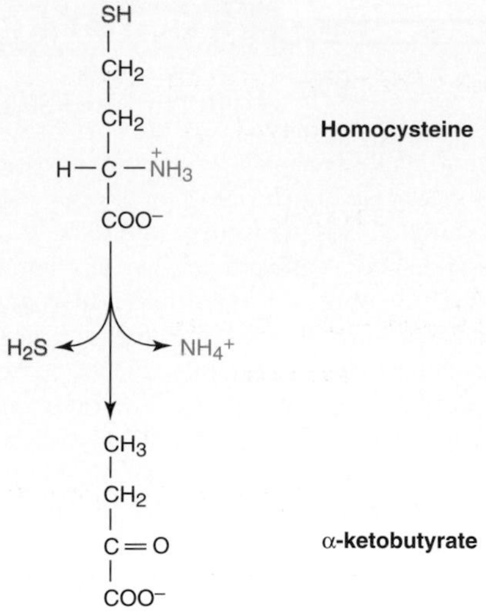

Homocysteine

H_2S NH_4^+

α-ketobutyrate

FIGURE 11.56
Homocysteine desulfhydrase.

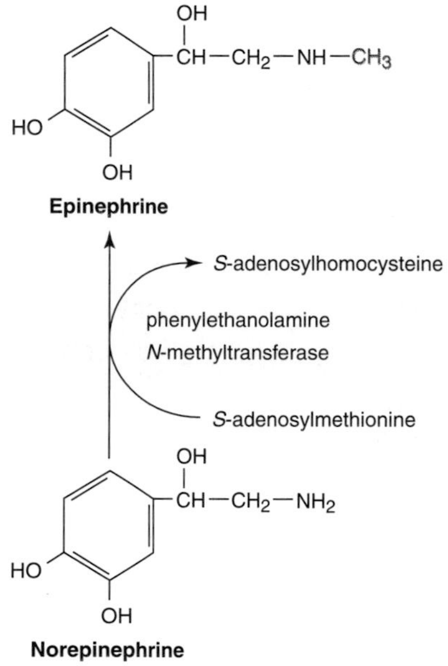

Epinephrine

S-adenosylhomocysteine

phenylethanolamine N-methyltransferase

S-adenosylmethionine

Norepinephrine

FIGURE 11.57
***S*-adenosylmethyltransferase reaction.**

versible. An example is shown in Figure 11.57. *S*-Adenosylhomocysteine left after methyl group transfer can be metabolized to cysteine, α-ketobutyrate, and ammonia. When cells need to resynthesize methionine, since the methyltransferase reaction is irreversible, another enzyme is required (Figure 11.58). **Homocysteine methyltransferase** is one of two enzymes known to require a vitamin B_{12} cofactor (the other is described on p. 479). The methyl group comes from ***N*⁵-methyltetrahydrofolate.** This is the only reaction known that uses this form of tetrahydrofolate as a methyl donor. The net result of reactions in Figures 11.57 and 11.58 is donation of a methyl group and regeneration of methionine under methionine-sparing conditions. A minor salvage pathway uses a methyl group from betaine instead of N^5-methyltetrahydrofolate.

AdoMet Is the Precursor of Spermidine and Spermine

Propylamine added to putrescine (see p. 459) to form spermidine and spermine is also derived from AdoMet, leaving methylthioadenosine. Putrescine is formed by decarboxylation of ornithine (see p. 459), and with propylamine forms spermidine. Addition of another propylamine gives spermine (Figure 11.59). The methylthioadenosine that remains can be used to resynthesize methionine. Much of the polyamine needed by the body is provided by microflora in the gut or from the diet and is carried by the enterohepatic circulation. Meat has

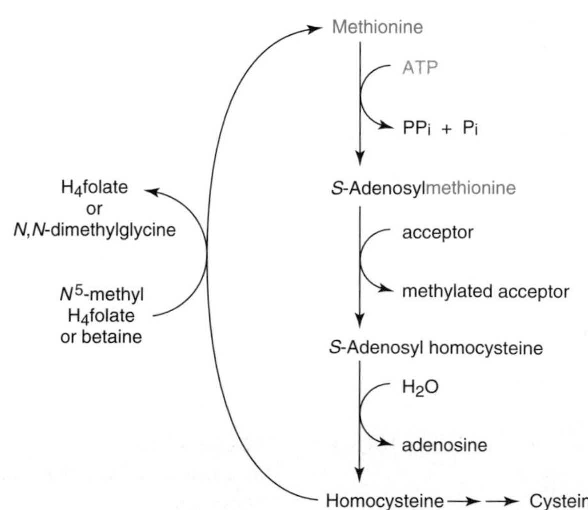

FIGURE 11.58
Resynthesis of methionine, a methylcobalamin-dependent reaction.

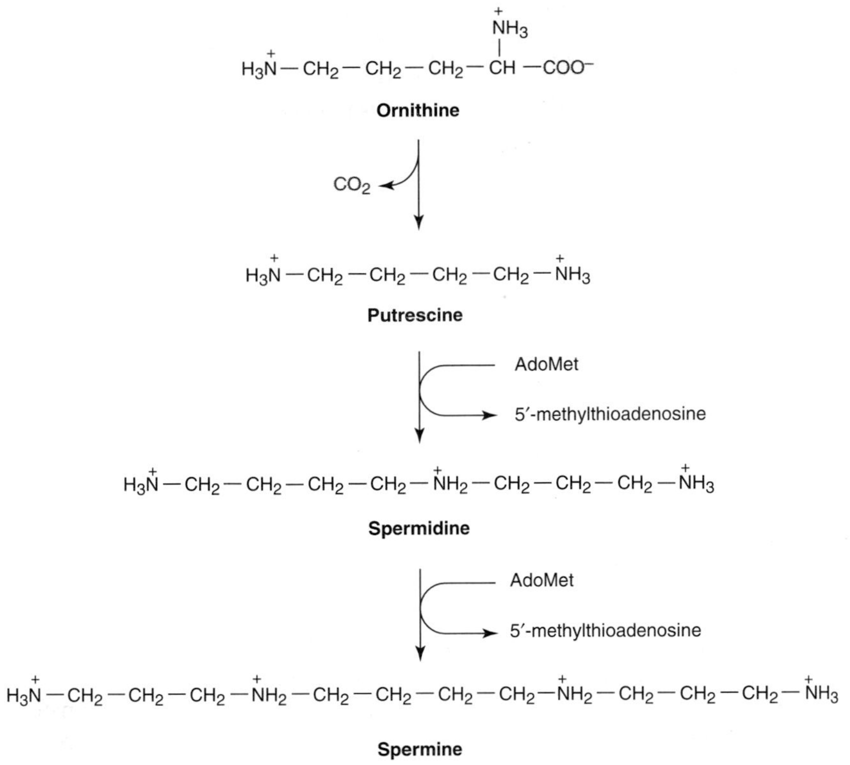

$$H_3\overset{+}{N}-CH_2-CH_2-CH_2-CH(\overset{+}{N}H_3)-COO^-$$
Ornithine

$\downarrow$ (CO_2 released)

$$H_3\overset{+}{N}-CH_2-CH_2-CH_2-CH_2-\overset{+}{N}H_3$$
Putrescine

$\downarrow$ AdoMet → 5′-methylthioadenosine

$$H_3\overset{+}{N}-CH_2-CH_2-CH_2-CH_2-\overset{+}{N}H_2-CH_2-CH_2-CH_2-\overset{+}{N}H_3$$
Spermidine

$\downarrow$ AdoMet → 5′-methylthioadenosine

$$H_3\overset{+}{N}-CH_2-CH_2-CH_2-\overset{+}{N}H_2-CH_2-CH_2-CH_2-CH_2-\overset{+}{N}H_2-CH_2-CH_2-CH_2-\overset{+}{N}H_3$$
Spermine

FIGURE 11.59
Polyamine synthesis.

a high content of putrescine, but other foods contain more spermidine and spermine.

The butylamino group of spermidine is used for posttranslational modification of a specific lysine residue in eIF-4D, an initiation factor for eukaryotic protein synthesis. The group is then hydroxylated, and the modified residue that results is called **hypusine** (Figure 11.60).

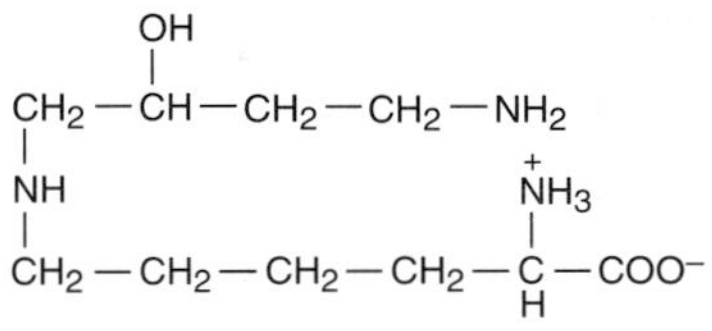

$$CH_2-CH(OH)-CH_2-CH_2-NH_2$$
$$|$$
$$NH \qquad\qquad \overset{+}{N}H_3$$
$$CH_2-CH_2-CH_2-CH_2-C(H)-COO^-$$

FIGURE 11.60
Hypusine.

Metabolism of Cysteine Produces Sulfur-Containing Compounds

Cysteine, derived from the sulfur of homocysteine and a molecule of serine, is metabolized in several ways. The pathway chosen is determined by the needs of the cell. The major metabolite is **cysteinesulfinate** (Figure 11.61). This is further metabolized to sulfite and pyruvate, or to hypotaurine and taurine.

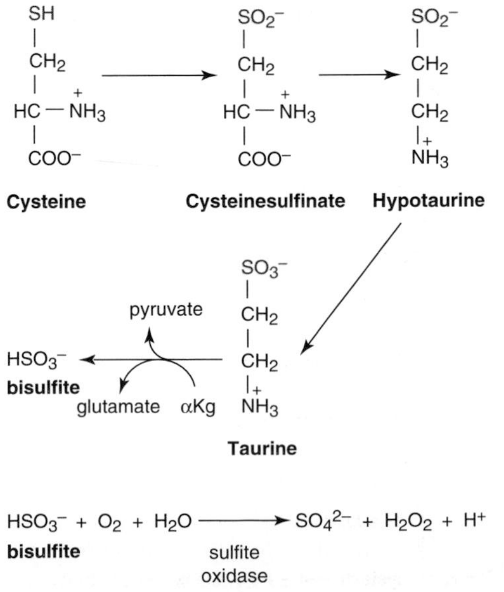

Cysteine ($SH-CH_2-HC(\overset{+}{N}H_3)-COO^-$) → **Cysteinesulfinate** ($SO_2^--CH_2-HC(\overset{+}{N}H_3)-COO^-$) → **Hypotaurine** ($SO_2^--CH_2-CH_2-\overset{+}{N}H_3$) → **Taurine** ($SO_3^--CH_2-CH_2-\overset{+}{N}H_3$)

Cysteinesulfinate → HSO_3^- **bisulfite** + pyruvate (glutamate → αKg)

$$HSO_3^- + O_2 + H_2O \xrightarrow{\text{sulfite oxidase}} SO_4^{2-} + H_2O_2 + H^+$$
bisulfite

FIGURE 11.61
Formation of taurine and sulfate from cysteine.

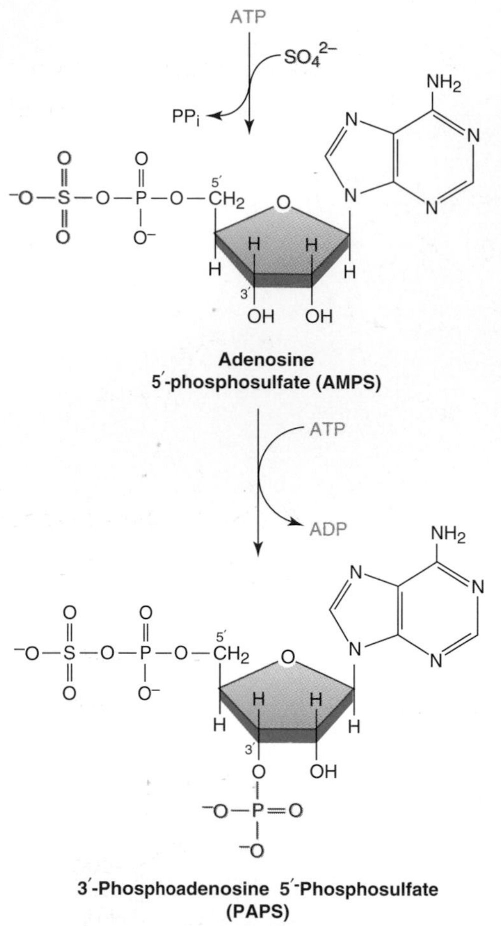

FIGURE 11.62
Synthesis of PAPS.

Taurine is an abundant intracellular free amino acid, but its exact role is unknown. It appears to play a necessary role in brain development. It forms conjugates with bile acids (see p. 418) and may enhance bile flow and increase cholesterol clearance by the liver. Taurine may also play a role in salvaging toxic intermediates, in regulating intracellular calcium, and, because of its abundance, in osmoregulation.

Sulfite produced from cysteine metabolism can be oxidized to **sulfate** (Figure 11.61), and this can be used in formation of **3′-phosphoadenosine-5′-phosphosulfate (PAPS),** the source of sulfate groups for addition to biological molecules (Figure 11.62).

Another reaction of cysteine metabolism catalyzed by cystathionase moves the sulfur from one cysteine to another cysteine (Figure 11.63) to form **thiocysteine.** Thiosulfate is formed from cysteine as shown in Figure 11.64. An enzyme called **rhodanese** can incorporate a sulfur from thiosulfate or thiocysteine into other molecules such as cyanide ion (Figure 11.65).

Tryptophan

Metabolism of **tryptophan** has many branch points. The dominant or oxidative pathway of tryptophan in the human (Figure 11.66, in color) starts with oxidation of tryptophan to *N*-formylkynurenine by a heme-containing enzyme, **tryptophan dioxygenase,** also called **tryptophan pyrrolase** or **tryptophan oxygenase,** because the pyrrole ring is cleaved in the reaction. Tryptophan dioxygenase is induced by glucocorticoids and glucagon. It is found in liver; other tissues contain a similar enzyme called indolamine dioxygenase, which is less substrate specific. Formamidase then hydrolyzes formylkynurenine to formate and kynurenine. At this point the pathway begins to branch. In the dominant pathway, reactions lead to 3-hydroxykynurenine, 3-hydroxyanthranilic acid and alanine, amino-carboxymuconic semialdehyde, and, by decarboxylation, to aminomuconic semialdehyde. This can be further metabolized in several steps to glutarate and eventually acetoacetyl CoA, or recyclized nonenzymatically to **picolinic acid,** which is excreted in the urine.

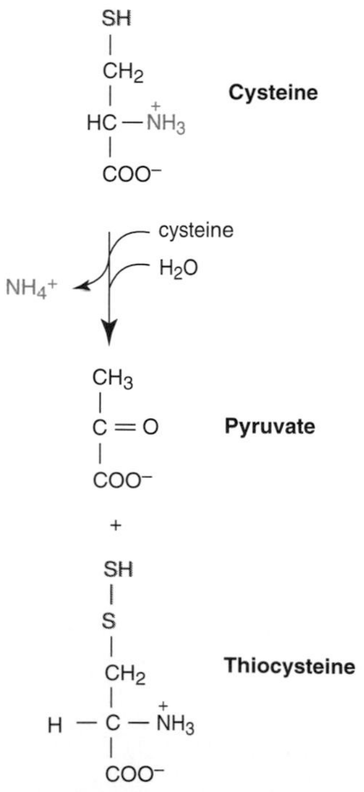

FIGURE 11.63
Synthesis of thiocysteine.

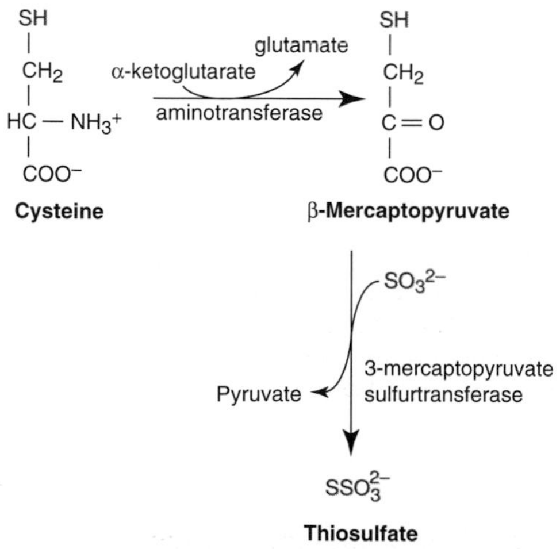

FIGURE 11.64
Formation of thiosulfate.

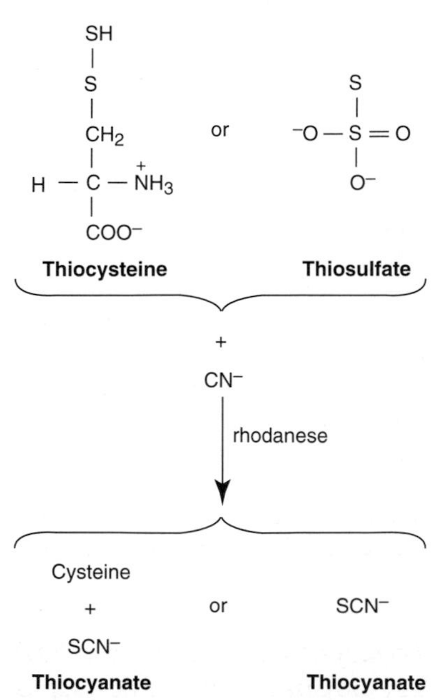

FIGURE 11.65
Detoxification of cyanide by products of cysteine metabolism.

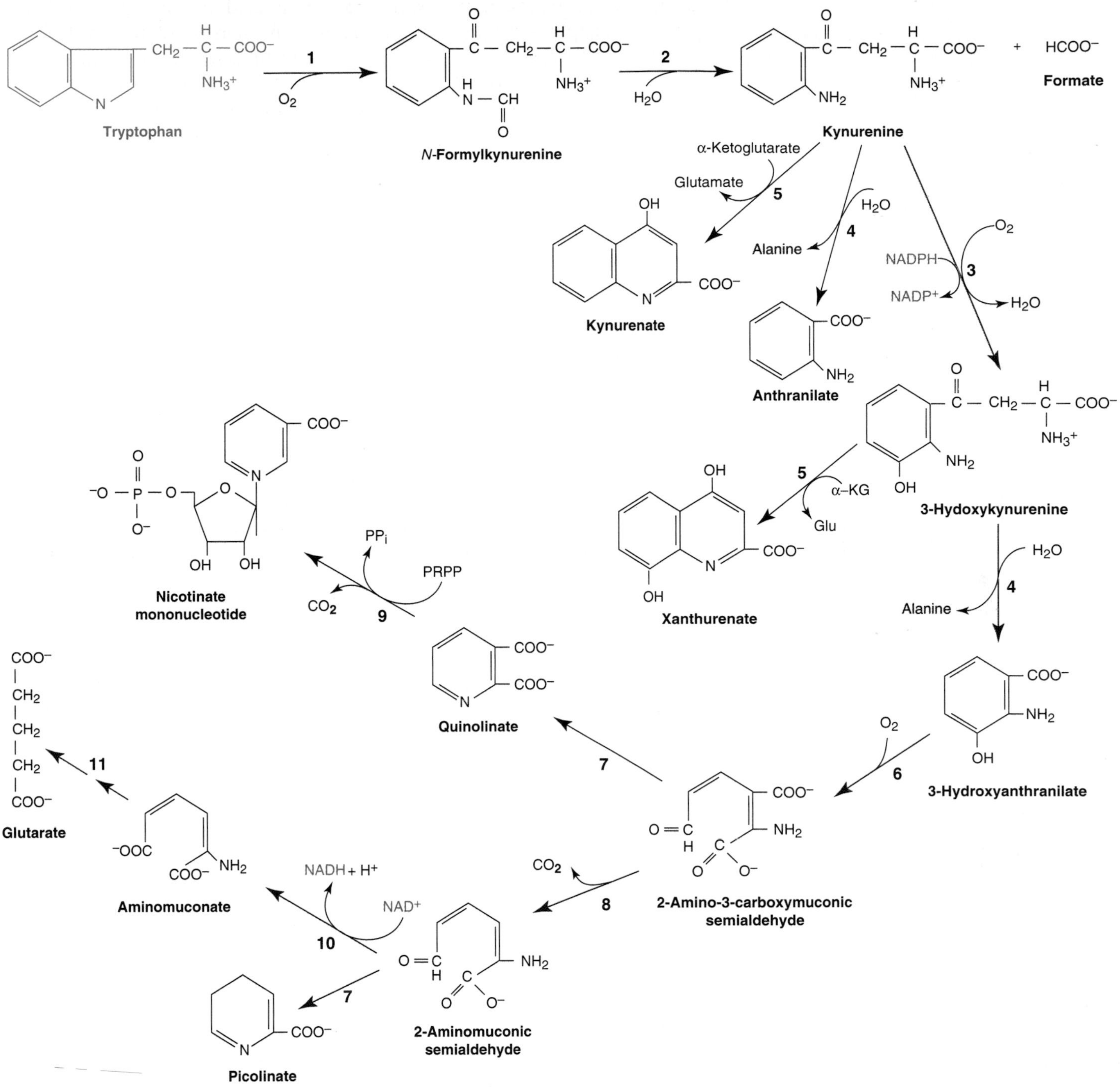

FIGURE 11.66
Metabolism of tryptophan.
Major pathway is shown in red. Enzymes indicated by number are (1) tryptophan oxygenase, (2) kynurenine formamidase, (3) kynurenine hydroxylase, (4) kynureninase, (5) aminotransferase, (6) 3-hydroxyanthranilate oxidase, (7) spontaneous nonenzymatic reaction, (8) picolinate carboxylase, (9) quinolinate phosphoribosyltransferase, (10) aldehyde dehydrogenase, and (11) complex series of reactions.

Tryptophan Is a Precursor of NAD

Tryptophan is the precursor of approximately 50% of the body's pyridine nucleotides. The rest is obtained from the diet. The branch point leading to nicotinate mononucleotide can be seen in Figure 11.66 at the stage of amino-carboxymuconic semialdehyde. The enzyme that forms 2-aminomuconic semi-

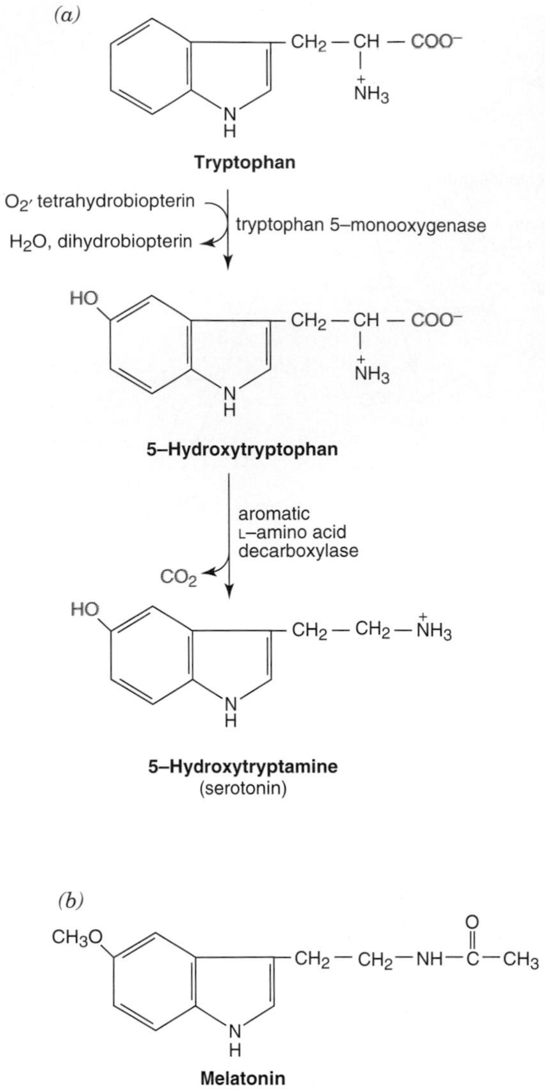

(a)

Tryptophan

O_2, tetrahydrobiopterin → H_2O, dihydrobiopterin; tryptophan 5–monooxygenase

5–Hydroxytryptophan

aromatic L–amino acid decarboxylase; CO_2

5–Hydroxytryptamine (serotonin)

(b)

Melatonin

FIGURE 11.67
(*a*) Synthesis of serotonin (5-hydroxytryptamine) and (*b*) structure of melatonin.

aldehyde, **picolinate carboxylase,** from this compound has a low K_m and is easily saturated with substrate. Since picolinate carboxylase has low activity in liver, some amino-carboxymuconic semialdehyde is cyclized in a nonenzymatic reaction to quinolinic acid. Phosphoribosylpyrophosphate provides a ribonucleotide moiety and the final step is a decarboxylation leading to nicotinate mononucleotide. Note that the nicotinic acid ring is synthesized as a part of a nucleotide. Because **kynurenine hydroxylase** is inhibited by estrogen, women are more susceptible to **pellagra,** the disease produced by niacin deficiency (from the Italian *pelle,* skin, and *agra,* rough).

Pyridoxal Phosphate Has a Prominent Role in Tryptophan Metabolism

Many enzymes in this lengthy pathway are pyridoxal phosphate dependent. **Kynureninase** is one of them and is affected by a vitamin B_6 deficiency (Figure 11.66), resulting in excess kynurenine and xanthurenate excretion and giving urine a greenish-yellow color. This is a diagnostic symptom of vitamin B_6 deficiency.

Kynurenine Gives Rise to Neurotransmitters

Another pathway that kynurenine can follow is transamination and condensation of the side chain to form a two-ring compound, kynurenic acid. This reaction is also depicted in Figure 11.66. **Kynurenic acid,** its decarboxylated metabolite **kynuramine,** and **quinolinate** have all been shown to act as tryptophan-derived neurotransmitters, possibly as antiexcitotoxics and anticonvulsives.

Serotonin and Melatonin Are Tryptophan Derivatives

Serotonin (5-hydroxytryptamine) results from hydroxylation of tryptophan by a tetrahydrobiopterin-dependent enzyme and decarboxylation by a pyridoxal phosphate-containing enzyme (Figure 11.67*a*). It is a neurotransmitter in brain and causes contraction of smooth muscle of arterioles and bronchioles. It is found widely in the body and may have other physiological roles. **Melatonin,** a sleep-inducing molecule, is ***N*-acetyl-5-methoxytryptamine** (Figure 11.67*b*). The acetyltransferase needed for its synthesis is present in pineal gland and retina. Melatonin is involved in regulation of circadian rhythm, being synthesized mostly at night. It appears to function by inhibiting synthesis and secretion of other neurotransmitters such as dopamine and GABA (see p. 866).

Tryptophan Induces Sleep

Ingestion of foods rich in tryptophan leads to sleepiness because serotonin is also sleep-inducing. Reducing availability of tryptophan in the brain can interfere with sleep. Tryptophan availability is reduced when other amino acids compete with it for transport through the blood–brain barrier. Elevated plasma concentrations of other amino acids, after a high-protein meal, diminish transport of tryptophan and induce wakefulness. The sleep-inducing effect of carbohydrates is due to decreased plasma amino acid levels, since carbohydrate stimulates release of insulin, and insulin causes removal of amino acids from plasma and uptake into muscle. This alleviates competition and increases the amount of tryptophan that can enter the brain. Strangely, extra serotonin appears to lead to sleepiness in females, but only calmness in males.

Branched-Chain Amino Acids

Metabolism of **branched-chain amino acids** (BCAAs)—**valine, isoleucine,** and **leucine**—is unusual, being initiated in muscle. NADH is formed during their metabolism, making them an excellent source of energy. BCAA aminotransferase is present at a much higher concentration in muscle than liver. Although the three amino acids produce different products, the first steps in their metabolism are similar.

Initial Reactions of BCAA Metabolism Are Shared

BCAA aminotransferase exists in three isozymes distributed differently between tissues, sometimes found in cytosol and sometimes in mitochondria (Figure 11.68). Two handle all three BCAAs, and one is specific for leucine and methionine. Starvation induces the muscle aminotransferases but does not affect these enzymes in liver. The resulting α-keto branched-chain acids are oxidatively decarboxylated by an inner mitochondrial membrane enzyme complex similar to the pyruvate dehydrogenase complex, which produces NADH and CO_2. When phosphorylated the dehydrogenase component of the complex has some activity, but this is greatly increased by dephosphorylation. All three α-keto branched-chain acids appear to be metabolized by the same enzyme. The more active form is found in liver in the fed state, and in muscle during starvation, reflecting the metabolism of dietary BCAAs by liver, and of muscle BCAAs to provide energy during fasting. The resulting CoA compounds are one carbon shorter than the original amino acids and are next acted on by an enzyme that resembles the first dehydrogenase found in fatty acid β-oxidation.

Pathways of Valine and Isoleucine Metabolism Are Similar

Valine and isoleucine continue down a common pathway, with addition of water across the double bond to form a hydroxylated intermediate (Figure 11.69). The hydroxyl group on the isoleucine derivative is oxidized by NAD^+ followed by thiolysis to give acetyl CoA and propionyl CoA. The valine derivative loses CoA and is oxidized by NAD^+ to methylmalonate semialdehyde, which is then converted to propionyl CoA.

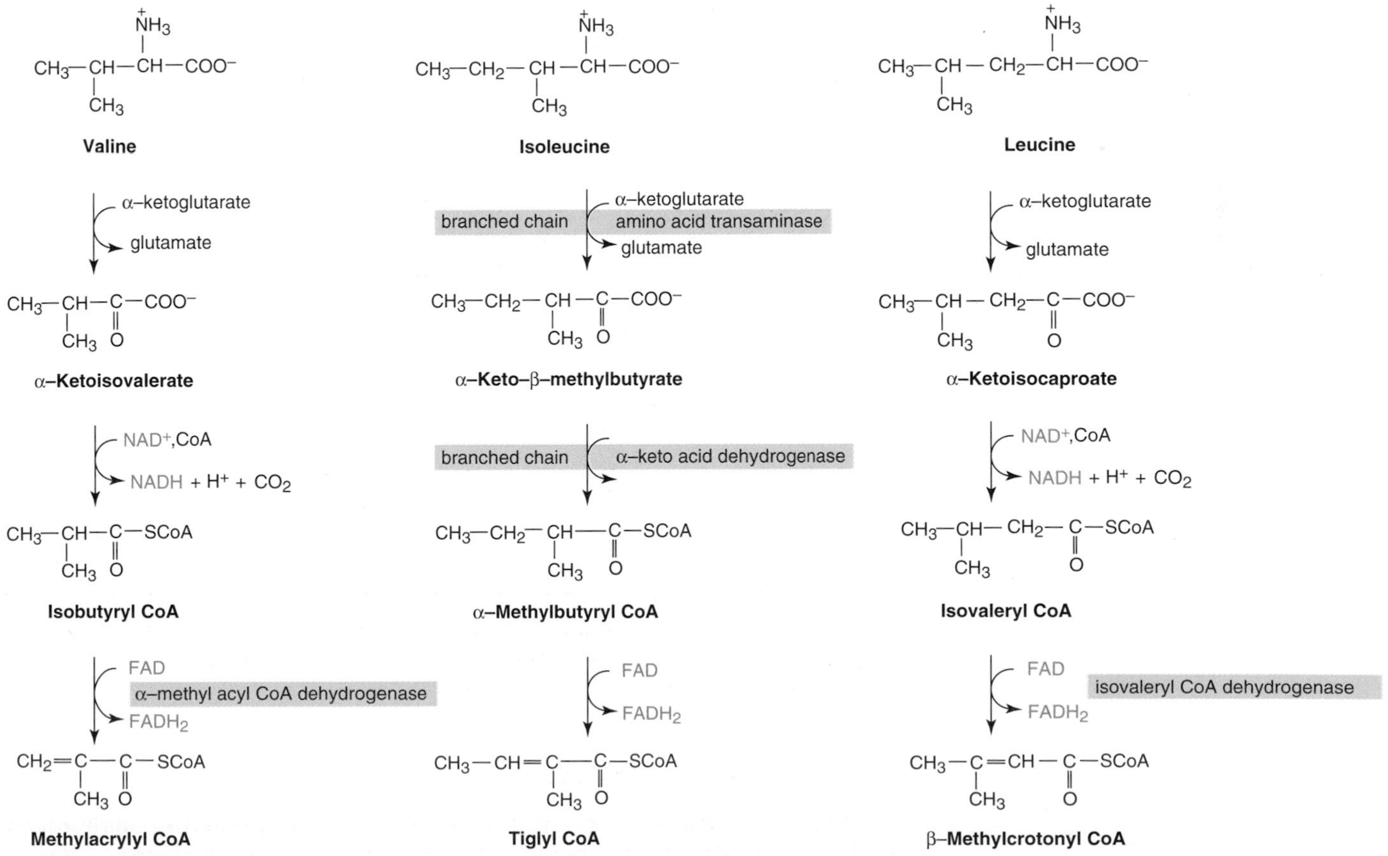

Valine | Isoleucine | Leucine

α–ketoglutarate → glutamate (branched chain amino acid transaminase)

α–Ketoisovalerate | α–Keto–β–methylbutyrate | α–Ketoisocaproate

NAD^+,CoA → NADH + H^+ + CO_2 (branched chain α–keto acid dehydrogenase)

Isobutyryl CoA | α–Methylbutyryl CoA | Isovaleryl CoA

FAD → $FADH_2$ (α–methyl acyl CoA dehydrogenase; isovaleryl CoA dehydrogenase)

Methylacrylyl CoA | Tiglyl CoA | β–Methylcrotonyl CoA

FIGURE 11.68
Common reactions in degradation of branched-chain amino acids.

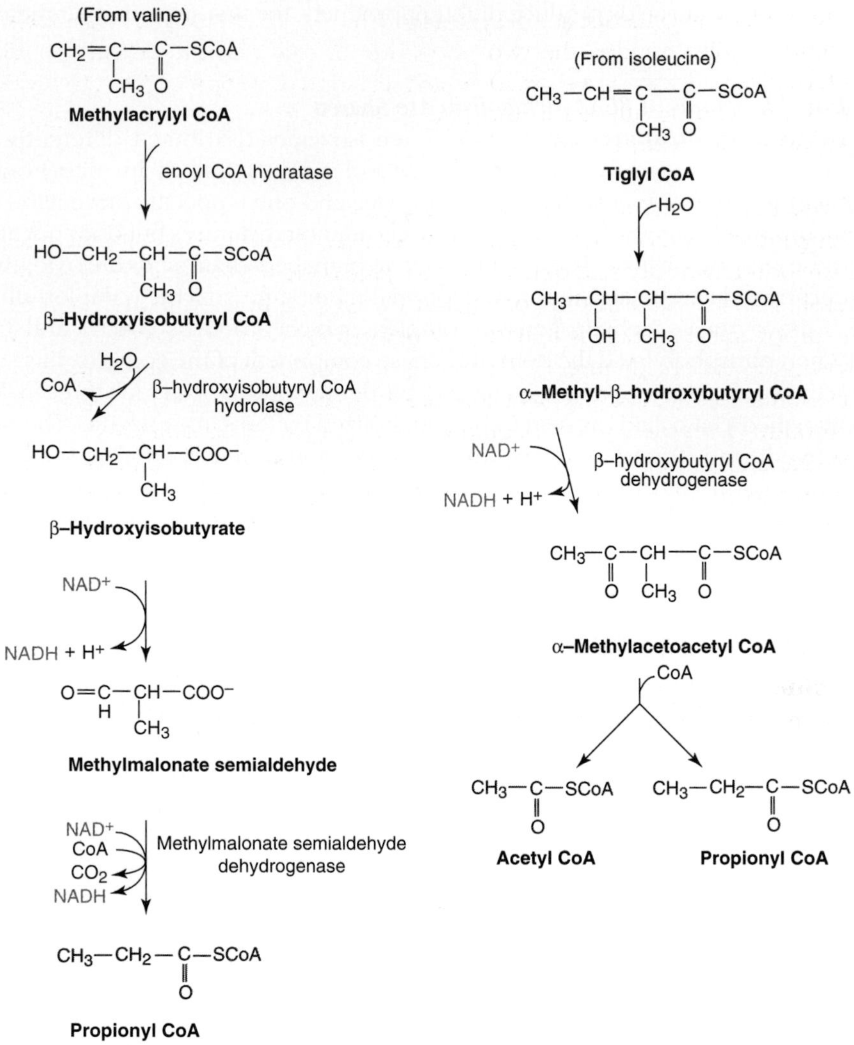

(From valine)

$CH_2{=}C(CH_3){-}C({=}O){-}SCoA$

Methylacrylyl CoA

enoyl CoA hydratase

$HO{-}CH_2{-}CH(CH_3){-}C({=}O){-}SCoA$

β-Hydroxyisobutyryl CoA

H_2O, CoA — β-hydroxyisobutyryl CoA hydrolase

$HO{-}CH_2{-}CH(CH_3){-}COO^-$

β-Hydroxyisobutyrate

NAD^+ → $NADH + H^+$

$O{=}C(H){-}CH(CH_3){-}COO^-$

Methylmalonate semialdehyde

NAD^+, CoA → CO_2, NADH — Methylmalonate semialdehyde dehydrogenase

$CH_3{-}CH_2{-}C({=}O){-}SCoA$

Propionyl CoA

(From isoleucine)

$CH_3{-}CH{=}C(CH_3){-}C({=}O){-}SCoA$

Tiglyl CoA

H_2O

$CH_3{-}CH(OH){-}CH(CH_3){-}C({=}O){-}SCoA$

α-Methyl-β-hydroxybutyryl CoA

NAD^+ → $NADH + H^+$ — β-hydroxybutyryl CoA dehydrogenase

$CH_3{-}C({=}O){-}CH(CH_3){-}C({=}O){-}SCoA$

α-Methylacetoacetyl CoA

CoA

$CH_3{-}C({=}O){-}SCoA$ **Acetyl CoA**

$CH_3{-}CH_2{-}C({=}O){-}SCoA$ **Propionyl CoA**

FIGURE 11.69
Terminal reactions in degradation of valine and isoleucine.

The Leucine Pathway Differs from Those of the Other Two Branched-Chain Amino Acids

The position of the methyl side chain in leucine prohibits the oxidation step found in the metabolism of the other BCAAs (Figure 11.70). The double bond-containing derivative is carboxylated, hydroxylated, and cleaved to acetoacetate and acetyl CoA. One intermediate is **β-hydroxy-β-methylglutaryl CoA,** an

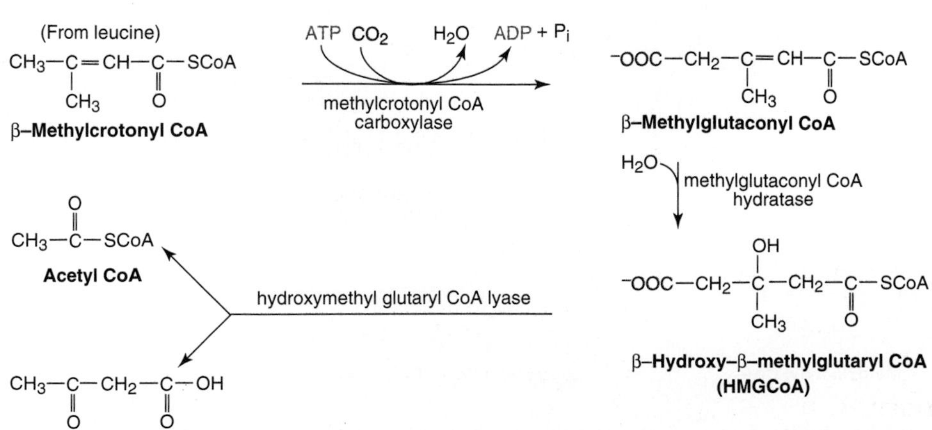

FIGURE 11.70
Terminal reactions of leucine degradation.

intermediate in cytosolic sterol synthesis (Chapter 10). Since BCAA degradation occurs in mitochondria the two pools do not mix. Leucine also has a minor alternative pathway (not shown), which results in excretion of 3-hydroxyvaleric acid, and can be utilized in the case of blockage in the leucine degradative pathway (Clin. Corr. 11.10).

Propionyl CoA Is Metabolized to Succinyl CoA

Propionyl CoA is an end product of isoleucine, valine, and methionine metabolism, odd-chain fatty acid oxidation, and degradation of the side chain of cholesterol. The first step in the conversion of the 3-carbon propionyl CoA to the 4-carbon succinyl CoA is initiated by **propionyl-CoA carboxylase,** which is biotin dependent (Figure 11.71; see 11.11). This gives D-methylmalonyl CoA, an isomerase that converts to a mixture of D- and L-methymalonyl CoA. **Methylmalonyl mutase,** which requires 5′-deoxyadenosylcobalamin (a derivative of vitamin B_{12}) converts the L-isomer to succinyl CoA. This is the second enzyme known to be dependent on vitamin B_{12} (see p. 473). The reaction is very unusual, removing a methyl side chain and inserting it as a methylene group into the backbone of the compound.

Lysine

Lysine is the other entirely ketogenic amino acid. The carbons enter intermediary metabolism as acetoacetyl CoA. Lysine has an ε- and an α-amino group.

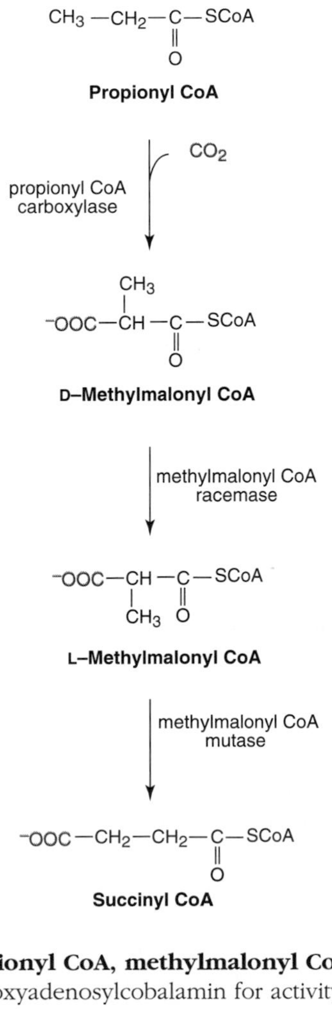

$$CH_3-CH_2-\underset{\underset{O}{\|}}{C}-SCoA$$

Propionyl CoA

propionyl CoA carboxylase (CO_2) ↓

$$^{-}OOC-\overset{\overset{CH_3}{|}}{CH}-\underset{\underset{O}{\|}}{C}-SCoA$$

D–Methylmalonyl CoA

↓ methylmalonyl CoA racemase

$$^{-}OOC-\underset{\underset{CH_3}{|}}{CH}-\underset{\underset{O}{\|}}{C}-SCoA$$

L–Methylmalonyl CoA

↓ methylmalonyl CoA mutase

$$^{-}OOC-CH_2-CH_2-\underset{\underset{O}{\|}}{C}-SCoA$$

Succinyl CoA

FIGURE 11.71
Interconversion of propionyl CoA, methylmalonyl CoA, and succinyl CoA. The mutase requires 5′-deoxyadenosylcobalamin for activity.

CLINICAL CORRELATION 11.10

Diseases of Metabolism of Branched-Chain Amino Acids

Enzyme deficiencies in catabolism of branched-chain amino acids are not common. In general, they produce acidosis in newborns or young children. Very rare instances have been reported of hypervalinemia and hyperleucine–isoleucinemia. It has been suggested that the two conditions indicate existence of specific aminotransferases for valine and for leucine and isoleucine. Alternatively, mutation could alter the specificity of a single enzyme. The most common abnormality is deficiency of branched-chain keto acid dehydrogenase complex activity. There are several variations, but all patients excrete the branched-chain α-keto acids and corresponding hydroxy acids and other side products; an unidentified product imparts characteristic odor associated with the name maple syrup urine disease. Some cases respond to high doses of thiamine. A large percentage show serious mental retardation, ketoacidosis, and short life span. Dietary treatment to reduce the branched-chain ketoacidemia is effective in some cases. Some cases have been reported of deficiency of enzymes in later reactions of branched-chain amino acids. These include a blockage of oxidation of isovaleryl CoA with accumulation of isovalerate (which gives urine a sweaty feet smell), β-methylcrotonyl CoA carboxylase deficiency (in which urine smells like that of a cat), deficiency of β-hydroxy-β-methylglutaryl CoA lyase, and deficiency of β-ketothiolase that splits α-methylacetoacetyl CoA (with no defect in acetoacetate cleavage). In the latter condition, development is normal and symptoms appear to be related only to episodes of ketoacidosis.

Zhang, B., Edenberg, H. J., Crabb, D. W., and Harris, R. A. Evidence for both a regulatory and structural mutation in a family with maple syrup urine disease. *J. Clin. Invest.* 83:1425, 1989.

CLINICAL CORRELATION 11.11

Diseases of Propionate and Methylmalonate Metabolism

Deficiencies of the three enzymes shown in Figure 11.71 contribute to ketoacidosis. Propionate is formed in the degradation of valine, isoleucine, methionine, threonine, the side chain of cholesterol, and odd-chain fatty acids. The amino acids appear to be the main precursors since decreasing or eliminating dietary protein immediately minimizes acidosis. A defect in propionyl-CoA carboxylase results in accumulation of propionate, which is diverted to alternative pathways, including incorporation into fatty acids for an acetyl group forming odd-chain fatty acids. The extent of these reactions is very limited. In one case large amounts of biotin were reported to produce beneficial effects, suggesting that more than one defect decreases propionyl-CoA carboxylase activity. Possibilities are a lack of intestinal biotinidase that liberates biotin from ingested food for absorption or a lack of biotin holocarboxylase that incorporates biotin into biotin-dependent enzymes. Children have been found with acidosis caused by high levels of methylmalonate, which is normally undetectable in blood. Enzymes analyzed from liver taken at autopsy or from cultured fibroblasts have shown that some cases were due to deficiency of methylmalonyl-CoA mutase. One group was unable to convert methylmalonyl CoA to succinyl CoA under any conditions, but another group carried out the conversion when 5′-adenosylcobalamin was added. Clearly, those with an active site defect in the enzyme cannot metabolize methylmalonate, but those with defects in handling vitamin B_{12} respond to massive doses of the vitamin. Other cases of methylmalonic aciduria suffer from a more fundamental inability to use vitamin B_{12} that leads to deficiency in methylcobalamin (coenzyme of methionine salvage) and in 5′-adenosylcobalamin deficiency (coenzyme of methylmalonyl CoA isomerization).

Mahoney, M. J., and Bick, D. Recent advances in the inherited methylmalonic acidemias. *Acta Paediatr. Scand.* 76:689, 1987.

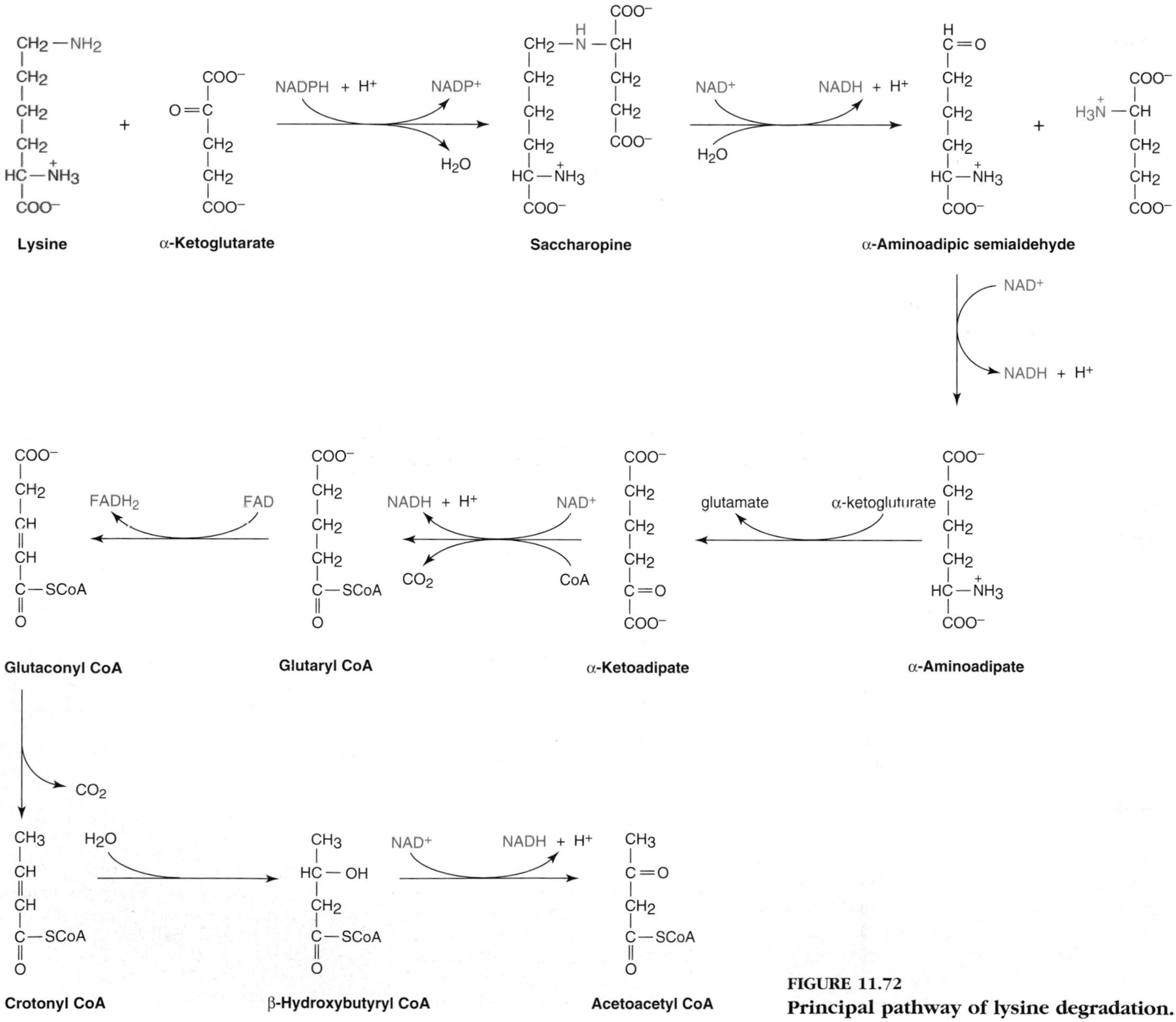

Lysine + α-Ketoglutarate → (NADPH + H^+ → $NADP^+$; H_2O) → Saccharopine → (NAD^+ → NADH + H^+; H_2O) → α-Aminoadipic semialdehyde + Glutamate

α-Aminoadipic semialdehyde → (NAD^+ → NADH + H^+) → α-Aminoadipate

α-Aminoadipate → (α-ketoglutarate → glutamate) → α-Ketoadipate → (NAD^+, CoA → NADH + H^+, CO_2) → Glutaryl CoA → (FAD → $FADH_2$) → Glutaconyl CoA

Glutaconyl CoA → (CO_2) → Crotonyl CoA → (H_2O) → β-Hydroxybutyryl CoA → (NAD^+ → NADH + H^+) → Acetoacetyl CoA

FIGURE 11.72
Principal pathway of lysine degradation.

The initial transamination of the ε-amino group requires α-ketoglutarate as acceptor and cosubstrate (Figure 11.72). Instead of the pyridoxal phosphate–Schiff base mechanism, an intermediate called **saccharopine** is formed, which is then cleaved to glutamate and a semialdehyde compound. The usual Schiff base electronic rearrangement mechanism is replaced by an oxidation and a reduction, but the products are effectively the same. The semialdehyde is then oxidized to a dicarboxylic amino acid, and a transamination of the α-amino group occurs in a pyridoxal-dependent manner. Further reactions lead to acetoacetyl CoA.

A minor pathway starts with removal of the α-amino group and goes via the cyclic compound **pipecolate** (Figure 11.73) to join the major pathway at the level of the semialdehyde intermediate. This does not replace the major pathway even in a deficiency of enzymes in the early part of the pathway (see Clin. Corr. 11.12).

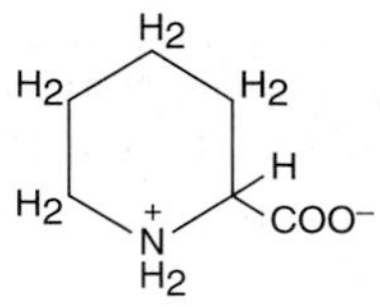

Pipecolate

FIGURE 11.73
Minor product of lysine metabolism.

Carnitine Is Derived from Lysine

Medium- and long-chain fatty acids are transported into mitochondria for β-oxidation as **carnitine** conjugates (see p. 382). Carnitine is synthesized not from free lysine but rather from lysine residues in certain proteins. The first step is trimethylation of the ε-amino group of the lysine side chain, with AdoMet as the methyl donor (Figure 11.74). Free trimethyllysine is obtained from hydrolysis of the protein and is metabolized in four steps to carnitine.

Histidine

The first reaction catalyzed by **histidase** (Clin. Corr. 11.13) removes free ammonia and leaves a compound with a double bond called urocanate (Figure 11.75). Two other reactions lead to **formiminoglutamate (FIGLU).** The formimino group is then transferred to tetrahydrofolate.

Urinary Formiminoglutamate Is Diagnostic of Folate Deficiency

The formimino group of formiminoglutamate must be transferred to tetrahydrofolate before the final product, glutamate, can be produced. When there is

CLINICAL CORRELATION 11.12

Diseases Involving Lysine and Ornithine

Lysine

Two metabolic disorders of lysine are recognized. α-Amino adipic semialdehyde synthase is deficient in a small number of patients who excrete lysine and smaller amounts of saccharopine. This has led to the discovery that the enzyme has both lysine-α-ketoglutarate reductase and saccharopine dehydrogenase activities. Single proteins with multiple enzymatic activities are also found in pyrimidine synthesis and fatty acid synthesis. It is thought that hyperlysinemia is benign. More serious is familial lysinuric protein intolerance due to failure to transport dibasic amino acids across intestinal mucosa and renal tubular epithelium. Plasma lysine, arginine, and ornithine are decreased to one-third or one-half of normal. Patients develop marked hyperammonemia after a meal containing protein. This is thought to arise from deficiency of the urea cycle intermediates ornithine and arginine in liver, limiting the capacity of the cycle. Consistent with this view, oral supplementation with citrulline prevents hyperammonemia. Other features are thin hair, muscle wasting, and osteoporosis, which may reflect protein malnutrition due to lysine and arginine deficiency.

Ornithine

Elevated ornithine levels are generally due to deficiency of ornithine δ-aminotransferase. A well-defined clinical entity, gyrate atrophy of the choroid and retina, characterized by progressive loss of vision leading to blindness by the fourth decade, is caused by deficiency of this mitochondrial enzyme. The mechanism of changes in the eye is unknown. Progression of the disease may be slowed by dietary restriction in arginine and/or pyridoxine therapy, which reduces ornithine in body fluids.

O'Donnell, J. J., Sandman, R. P., and Martin, S. R. Gyrate atrophy of the retina: inborn error of L-ornithine : 2-oxoacid aminotransferase. *Science* 200:200, 1978; Rajantil, J., Simell, O., and Perheentupa, J. Lysinuric protein intolerance. Basolateral transport defect in renal tubuli. *J. Clin. Invest.* 67:1078, 1981.

CLINICAL CORRELATION 11.13

Histidinemia

Histidinemia is due to histidase deficiency. A convenient assay for this enzyme uses skin, which produces urocanate as a constituent of sweat; urocanase and other enzymes of histidine catabolism found in liver do not occur in skin. A finding that urocanate is absent in sweat can only be interpreted as a lack of synthesis, and not as accelerated disappearance by further metabolism. Histidase deficiency can be confirmed by enzyme assay in skin biopsies. Incidence of the disorder is high, about 1 in 10,000 newborns screened. Most reported cases of histidinemia have shown normal mental development. Restriction of dietary histidine normalizes the biochemical abnormalities but is not usually required.

Scriver, C. R., and Levy, H. L. Histidinemia: reconciling retrospective and prospective findings. *J. Inherit. Metab. Dis.* 6:51, 1983.

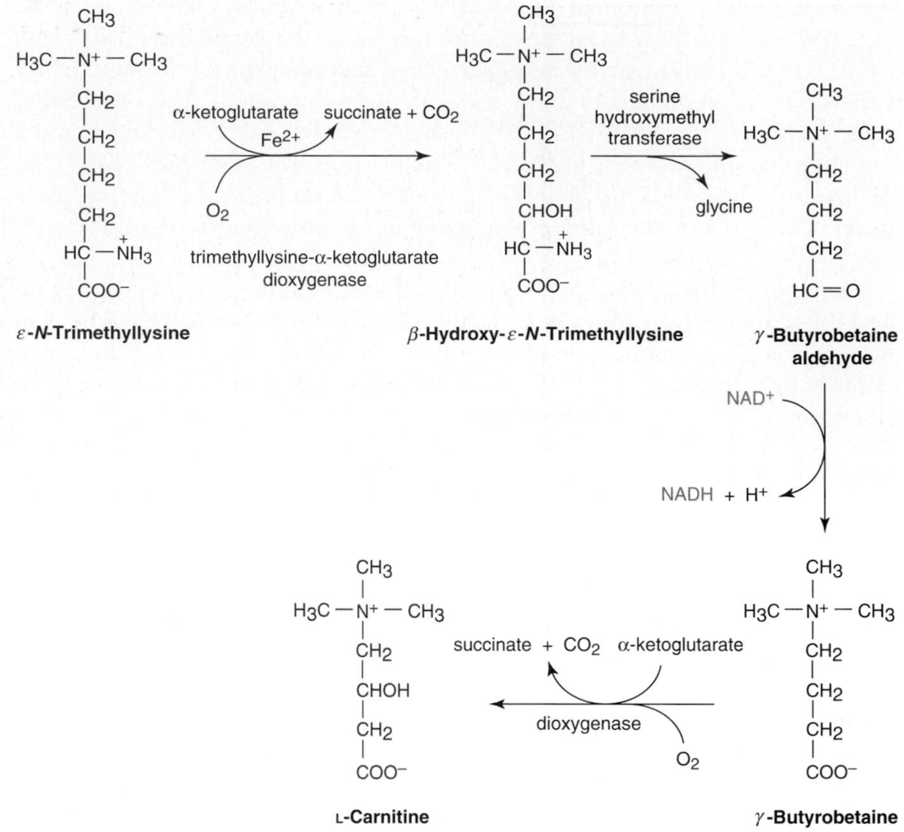

FIGURE 11.74
Biosynthesis of carnitine.

insufficient tetrahydrofolate available, this reaction decreases and FIGLU is excreted in urine. This is a diagnostic sign of folate deficiency if it happens after a test dose of histidine is ingested (see Clin. Corr. 11.14).

Histamine, Carnosine, and Anserine Are Produced from Histidine

Histamine (Figure 11.76), released from cells as part of an allergic response, is produced from histidine by **histidine decarboxylase.** Histamine has many

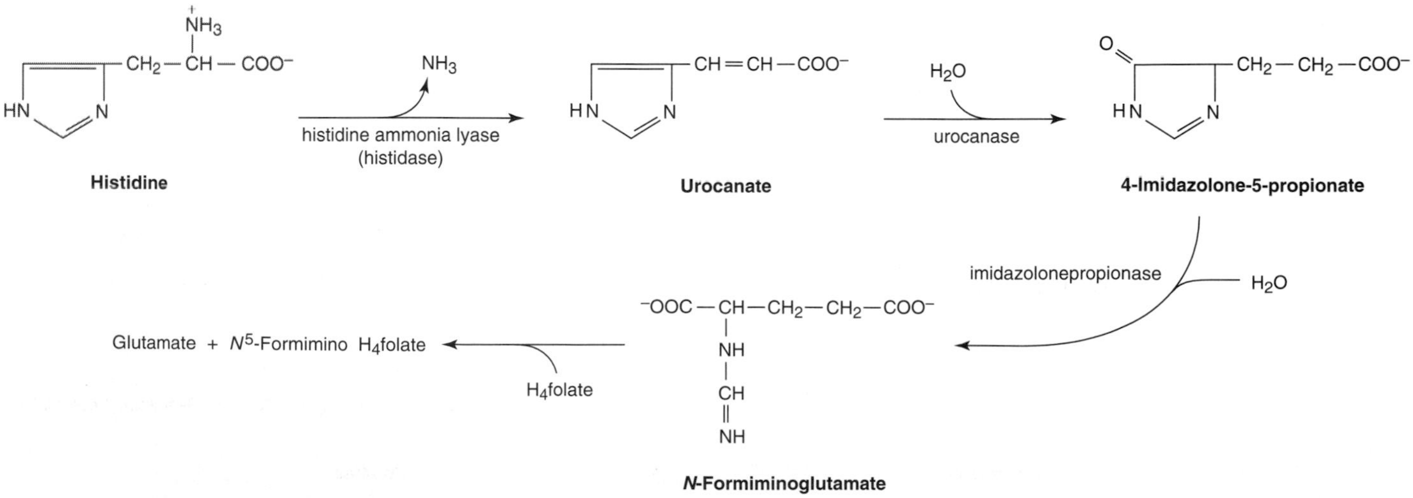

FIGURE 11.75
Degradation of histidine.

CLINICAL CORRELATION 11.14

Diseases of Folate Metabolism

A significant fraction of absorbed folic acid must be reduced to function as a coenzyme. Symptoms of folate deficiency may be due to deficiency of dihydrofolate reductase. Parenteral administration of N^5-formyltetrahydrofolate, the most stable of the reduced folates, is effective in these cases. In some cases of central nervous system abnormality attributed to deficiency of methylene folate reductase there is homocystinuria. Decreased enzyme activity lowers the N^5-methyltetrahydrofolate formed so that the source of methyl groups for the salvage of homocysteine is limiting. Large amounts of folic acid, betaine, and methionine reversed the biochemical abnormalities and, in at least one case, the neurological disorder. Patients with widely divergent presentations had shown deficiencies in transfer of the formimino group from formiminoglutamate to tetrahydrofolate. They excreted varying amounts of FIGLU; some responded to large doses of folate, but others did not. The mechanism whereby a deficiency of formiminotransferase produces pathological changes is unclear. It is not sure whether this deficiency causes a disease state. One patient showed symptoms of folate deficiency and had tetrahydrofolate methyltransferase deficiency. The associated anemia did not respond to vitamin B_{12} but showed some improvement with folate. It was suggested that the patient formed inadequate N^5-methyltetrahydrofolate to promote remethylation of homocysteine. This left the coenzyme "trapped" in the methylated form and unavailable for use in other reactions.

physiological roles, including dilation and constriction of certain blood vessels. An overreaction to histamine can lead to asthma and other allergic reactions. **Carnosine** (β-alanylhistidine) and **anserine** (β-alanylmethylhistidine) are dipeptides (Figure 11.77) found in muscle. Their function is unknown.

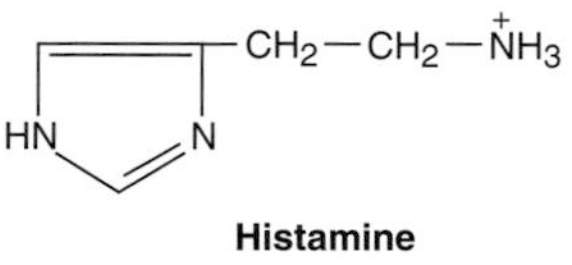

Creatine

Storage of "high-energy" phosphate, particularly in cardiac and skeletal muscle, occurs by transfer of the phosphate group from ATP to **creatine** (Figure 11.78). Creatine is synthesized by transfer of the guanidinium group of arginine to glycine, and subsequent addition of a methyl group from AdoMet. The amount of creatine in the body is related to muscle mass, and a certain percentage of this undergoes turnover each day. About 1–2% of preexisting creatine phosphate is cyclized nonenzymatically to **creatinine** (Figure 11.79) and excreted in urine, and new creatine is synthesized to replace it. The amount of creatinine excreted by an individual is therefore constant from day to day. When a 24-hour urine sample is requested, the amount of creatinine in the sample can be used to determine whether the sample truly represents a whole day's urinary output.

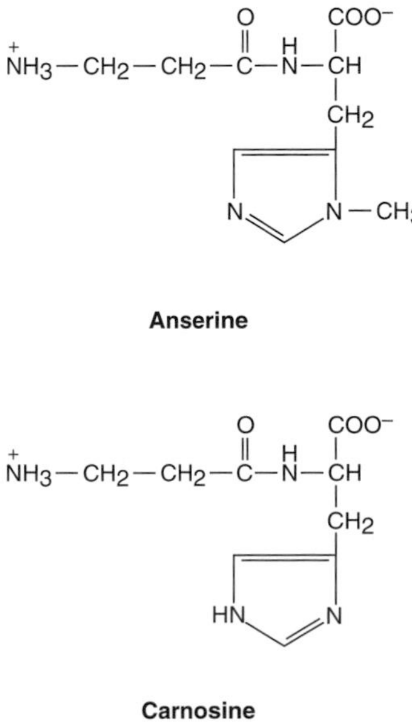

FIGURE 11.76
Histamine.

FIGURE 11.77
Anserine and carnosine.

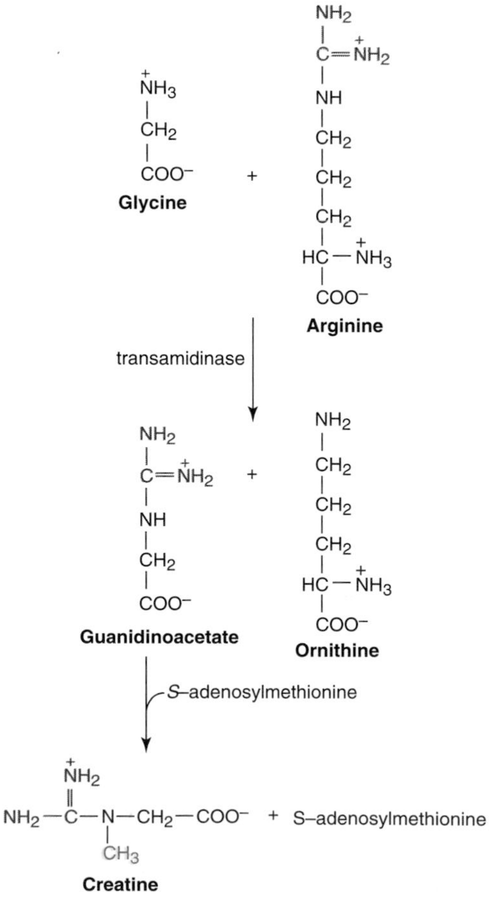

FIGURE 11.78
Synthesis of creatine.

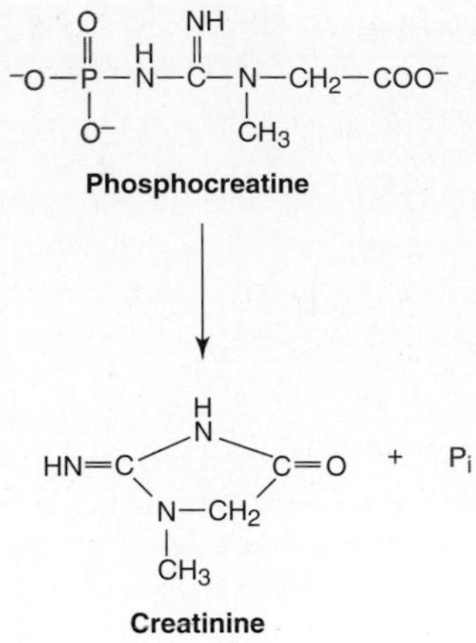

Phosphocreatine

Creatinine

FIGURE 11.79
Spontaneous reaction forming creatinine.

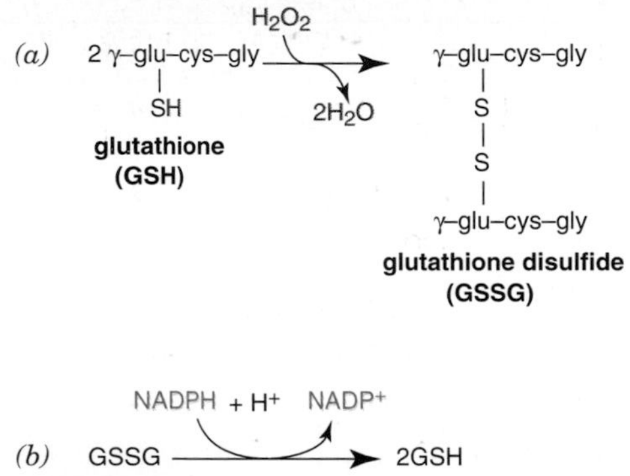

Glutathione

Glutathione, the tripeptide γ-glutamylcysteinylglycine, has several important functions. It is a reductant, conjugated to drugs to make them more water soluble, involved in transport of amino acids across cell membranes, part of some leukotriene structures (see p. 438), a cofactor for some enzymatic reactions, and an aid in the rearrangement of protein disulfide bonds.

Glutathione as reductant is very important in maintaining stability of erythrocyte membranes. Its sulfhydryl group can be used to reduce peroxides formed during oxygen transport (see p. 1026). The resulting oxidized form of GSH consists of two molecules joined by a disulfide bond. This is reduced to two molecules of GSH at the expense of NADPH (Figure 11.80). The usual steady-state ratio of GSH to GSSG in erythrocytes is 100 : 1.

Conjugation of drugs by glutathione, often after a preliminary reaction catalyzed by cytochrome P450 (Chapter 23), renders them more polar for excretion (Figure 11.81).

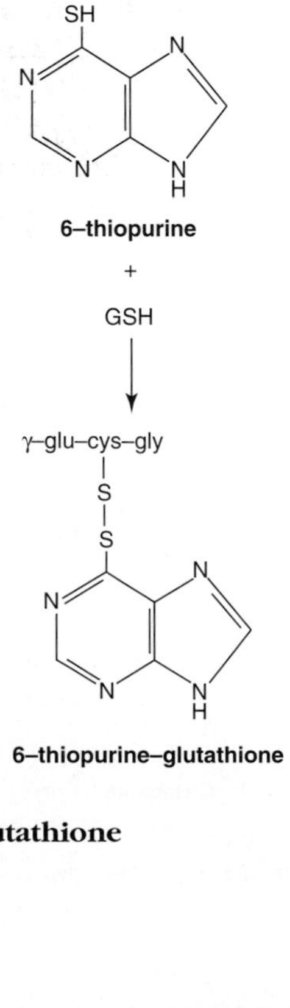

(a) 2 γ-glu-cys-gly (SH) glutathione (GSH) + H_2O_2 → $2H_2O$ + γ-glu-cys-gly–S–S–γ-glu-cys-gly glutathione disulfide (GSSG)

(b) GSSG → 2GSH (NADPH + H^+ → $NADP^+$)

FIGURE 11.80
(a) Scavenging of peroxide by glutathione peroxidase and (b) regeneration of reduced glutathione by glutathione reductase.

6–thiopurine + GSH → 6–thiopurine–glutathione

FIGURE 11.81
Conjugation of a drug by glutathione transferase.

Glutathione Is Synthesized from Three Amino Acids

Glutathione is synthesized by formation of the dipeptide γ-glutamylcysteine and the subsequent addition of glycine. Both reactions require activation of carboxyl groups by ATP (Figure 11.82). Synthesis of glutathione is largely regulated by cysteine availability.

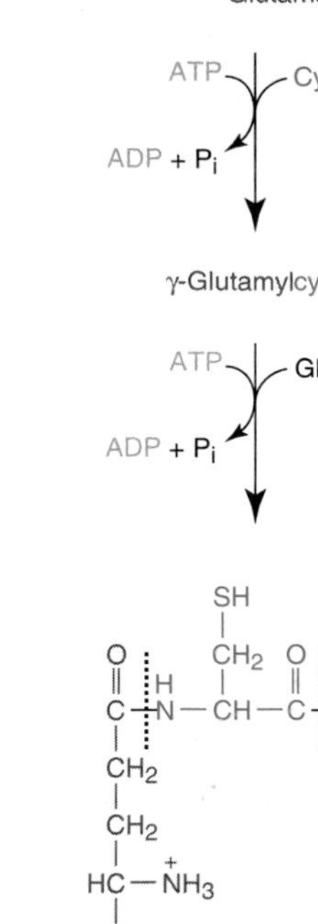

Glutathione
(γ-glutamylcysteinylglycine)

FIGURE 11.82
Synthesis of glutathione.

The γ-Glutamyl Cycle Transports Amino Acids

There are several mechanisms for transport of amino acids across cell membranes. Many are symport or antiport mechanisms (see p. 200) and are coupled to sodium transport. The **γ-glutamyl cycle** is an example of "group transfer" transport. It is more energy-requiring than other mechanisms, but is rapid and has high capacity, and functions in the kidney and some other tissues. It is particularly important in renal epithelial cells.

The enzyme **γ-glutamyl transpeptidase** is located in the cell membrane. It shuttles GSH to the cell surface to interact with an amino acid. γ-Glutamyl amino acid is transported into the cell, and the complex is hydrolyzed to liberate the amino acid (Figure 11.83). Glutamate is released as **5-oxoproline,** and cysteinylglycine is cleaved to its component amino acids. To regenerate GSH glutamate is reformed from oxoproline in an ATP-requiring reaction, and GSH is resynthesized from its three component parts. Three ATPs are used in the regeneration of glutathione, one in formation of glutamate from oxoproline and two in formation of the peptide bonds.

Glutathione Concentration Affects the Response to Toxins

When the body encounters toxic conditions such as peroxide formation, ionizing radiation, alkylating agents, or other reactive intermediates, it is beneficial to increase the level of GSH. Cysteine and methionine have been administered as GSH precursors, but they have the disadvantage of being precursors of an energy-expensive pathway to GSH. A more promising approach is administration of a soluble diester of GSH, such as γ-(α-ethyl)glutamylcysteinylethylglycinate.

Very premature infants have a very low concentration of cysteine because of low cystathionase activity in liver. This keeps the GSH concentration low and makes them more susceptible to oxidative damage, especially from hydroperoxides formed in the eye after hyperbaric oxygen treatment. Under certain circumstances, such as rendering tumor cells more sensitive to radiation or parasites more sensitive to drugs, it is desirable to lower GSH levels. This can be achieved by the glutamate analog **buthionine** sulfoximine (Figure 11.84) as a competitive inhibitor of GSH synthesis.

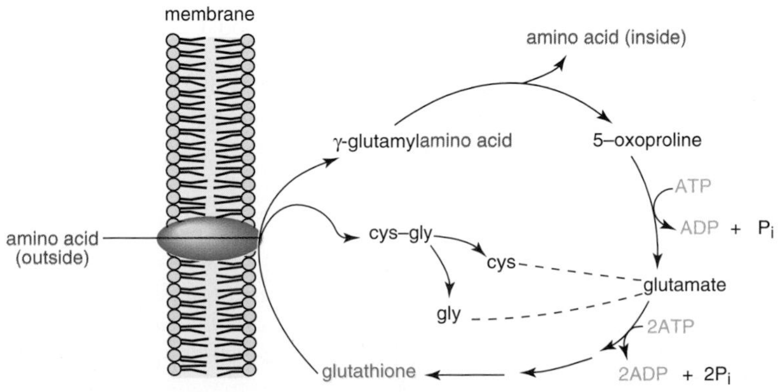

FIGURE 11.83
γ-Glutamyl cycle for transporting amino acids.

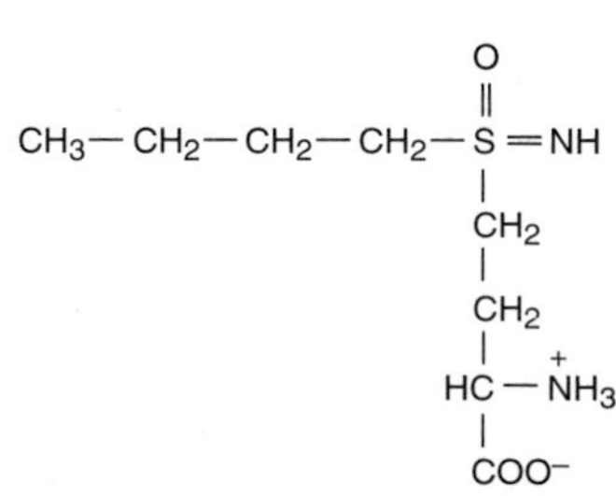

FIGURE 11.84
Buthionine sulfoximine.

BIBLIOGRAPHY

General

Meister, A. *Biochemistry of the Amino Acids,* 2nd ed. New York: Academic Press, 1965.

Wright, C. E., Tallan, H. H., Lin, Y. Y., and Gaull, G. E. Taurine: biological update. *Annu. Rev. Biochem.* 55:427, 1986.

Pyridoxal Phosphate

Dolphin, D., Poulson, R., and Avramovic, O. (Eds.). *Vitamin B_6 Pyridoxal Phosphate.* New York: Wiley, 1986.

Glutamate and Glutamine

Bode, B. L., Kaminski, D. L., Souba, W. W., and Li, A. P. Glutamine transport in human hepatocytes and transformed liver cells. *Hepatology* 21:511, 1995.

Fisher, H. F. Glutamate dehydrogenase. *Methods Enzymol.* 113:16, 1985.

Haussinger, D. Nitrogen metabolism in liver: structural and functional organization and physiological relevance. *Biochem. J.* 267:281, 1990.

Urea Cycle

Holmes, F. L. Hans Krebs and the discovery of the ornithine cycle. *Fed. Proc.* 39:216, 1980.

Jungas, R. L., Halperin, M. L., and Brosnan, J. T. Quantitative analysis of amino acid oxidation and related gluconeogenesis in humans. *Physiol. Rev.* 72:419, 1992.

Branched-Chain Amino Acids

Shander, P., Wahren, J., Paoletti, R., Bernardi, R., Rinetti, M. *Branched Chain Amino Acids.* New York: Raven Press, 1992.

Serine

Snell, K. The duality of pathways for serine biosynthesis is a fallacy. *Trends Biochem. Sci.* 11:241, 1986.

Arginine

Reyes, A. A., Karl, I. E., and Klahr, S. Editorial review: role of arginine in health and renal disease. *Am. J. Physiol.* 267:F331, 1994.

Sulfur Amino Acids

Lee, B. J., Worland, P. J., Davis, J. N., Stadtman, T. C., and Hatfield, D. L. Identification of a selenocysteyl–$tRNA^{Ser}$ in mammalian cells that recognizes the nonsense codon, UGA. *J. Biol. Chem.* 264:9724, 1989.

Stepanuk, M. H. Metabolism of sulfur-containing amino acids. *Annu. Rev. Nutr.* 6:179, 1986.

Polyamines

Perin, A., Scalabrino, G., Sessa, A., and Ferioloini, M. E. *Perspectives in Polyamine Research.* Milan: Wichtig Editore, 1988.

Tabor, C. W., and Tabor, H. Polyamines. *Annu. Rev. Biochem.* 53:749, 1984.

Folates and Pterins

Blakley, R. L., and Benkovic, S. J. *Folate and Pterins.* New York: Wiley, Vol. 1, 1984; Vol. 2, 1985.

Quinoproteins

Davidson, V. L., (Ed.). *Principles and Applications of Quinoproteins.* New York: Marcel Dekker, 1993.

Carnitine

Bieber, L. L. Carnitine. *Annu. Rev. Biochem.* 57:261, 1988.

Glutathione

Taniguchi, N., Higashi, T., Sakamoto, Y., and Meister, A. *Glutathione Centennial: Molecular Perspectives and Clinical Implications.* New York: Academic Press, 1989.

Tryptophan

Stone, T. W. *Quinolinic Acid and the Kynurenines.* Boca Raton, FL: CRC Press, 1989.

Schwarcz, R. Metabolism and function of brain kynurenines. *Biochem. Soc. Trans.* 21:77, 1993.

Disorders of Amino Acid Metabolism

Rosenberg, L. E., and Scriver, C. R. Disorders of amino acid metabolism. In: P. K. Bondy and L. E. Rosenberg (Eds.), *Metabolic Control and Disease,* 8th ed. Philadelphia: Saunders, 1980.

Scriver, C. R., Beaudet, A. L., Sly, W. S., and Valle, D. *The Metabolic and Molecular Bases of Inherited Disease,* 7th ed. New York: McGraw-Hill, 1994.

Wellner, D., and Meister, A. A survey of inborn errors of amino acid metabolism and transport. *Annu. Rev. Biochem.* 50:911, 1980.

QUESTIONS C. N. ANGSTADT AND J. BAGGOTT

1. Amino acids considered nonessential for humans are:
   A. those not incorporated into protein.
   B. not necessary in the diet if sufficient amounts of precursors are present.
   C. the same for adults as for children.
   D. the ones made in specific proteins by posttranslational modifications.
   E. generally not provided by the ordinary diet.

2. Aminotransferases:
   A. usually require α-ketoglutarate or glutamine as one of the reacting pair.
   B. catalyze reactions that result in a net use or production of amino acids.
   C. catalyze irreversible reactions.
   D. require pyridoxal phosphate as an essential cofactor for the reaction.
   E. are not able to catalyze transamination reactions with essential amino acids.

3. The production of ammonia in the reaction catalyzed by glutamate dehydrogenase:
   A. requires the participation of NADH or NADPH.
   B. proceeds through a Schiff base intermediate.
   C. may be reversed to consume ammonia if it is present in excess.
   D. is favored by high levels of ATP or GTP.
   E. would be inhibited when gluconeogenesis is active.

4. The amide nitrogen of glutamine:
   A. represents a nontoxic transport form of ammonia.
   B. is a major source of ammonia for urinary excretion.
   C. is used in the synthesis of asparagine, purines, and pyrimidines.
   D. can be recovered as ammonia by the action of glutaminase.
   E. all of the above are correct.

5. In the formation of urea from ammonia by the urea cycle, all of the following are correct EXCEPT:
   A. aspartate supplies one of the nitrogens found in urea.
   B. part of the large negative free-energy change of the process may be attributed to the hydrolysis of pyrophosphate.
   C. the rate of the cycle is independent of diet.
   D. fumarate is produced.
   E. genetic deficiency of any one of the enzymes can lead to hyperammonemia.

6. Carbamoyl phosphate synthetase I:
   A. is a flavoprotein.
   B. is controlled primarily by feedback inhibition.
   C. is unresponsive to changes in arginine.
   D. requires acetylglutamate as an allosteric effector.
   E. requires ATP as an allosteric effector.

7. All of the following are correct about ornithine EXCEPT it:
   A. may be formed from or converted to glutamic semialdehyde.
   B. can be converted to proline.
   C. plays a major role in the urea cycle.
   D. is a precursor of putrescine, a polyamine.
   E. is in equilibrium with spermidine.

8. Serine:
   A. is in equilibrium with threonine via a reaction catalyzed by a hydroxymethyltransferase.
   B. may enter intermediary metabolism either as 3-phosphoglycerate or as pyruvate.
   C. can be converted to selenoserine for incorporation into proteins.
   D. is a prosthetic group for *S*-adenosylmethionine decarboxylase.
   E. all of the above are correct.

9. In folic acid-dependent carriage of a one-carbon group:
   A. the formation of the methyl group of thymine involves a direct transfer from methyl THF.
   B. the first entry of carbons into the THF pool is via methylene THF.
   C. carbons are fixed at the oxidation level at which they enter the pool.
   D. the only acceptor for the methyl form is homocysteine.
   E. carbons are always carried on nitrogen 10 of the pteridine ring.

10. An inability to generate tetrahydrobiopterin might be expected to:
    A. inhibit the normal degradative pathway of phenylalanine.
    B. lead to albinism.
    C. directly prevent formation of melatonin.
    D. reduce the body's ability to transfer one-carbon fragments.
    E. have little or no effect on the production of catecholamines.

11. Both tyrosine aminotransferase and tryptophan oxygenase are enzymes that can be induced by adrenal glucocorticoids. This is reasonable because:
    A. tyrosine and tryptophan are precursors of physiologic amines.
    B. glucocorticoids work by inducing enzymes.
    C. tryptophan is the precursor of nicotinic acid needed for NAD^+ synthesis.
    D. tyrosine is the precursor of catecholamines in the adrenal gland.
    E. these two enzymes initiate the major catabolic pathways in the liver of tyrosine and tryptophan.

12. *S*-Adenosylmethionine:
    A. contains a positively charged sulfur (sulfonium) that facilitates the transfer of substituents to suitable acceptors.
    B. yields α-ketobutyrate in the reaction in which the methyl is transferred.
    C. donates a methyl group in a freely reversible reaction.
    D. generates H_2S by transsulfuration.
    E. provides the carbons for the formation of cysteine.

13. In humans, sulfur of cysteine may participate in all of the following EXCEPT:
    A. the conversion of cyanide to less toxic thiocyanate.
    B. the formation of thiosulfate.
    C. the formation of taurine.
    D. the donation of the sulfur for methionine formation.
    E. the formation of PAPS.

14. All of the following are true about the branched-chain amino acids EXCEPT they:
    A. are essential in the diet.
    B. differ in that one is glucogenic, one is ketogenic, and one is classified as both.
    C. are catabolized in a manner that bears a resemblance to β-oxidation of fatty acids.
    D. are oxidized by a dehydrogenase complex to branched-chain acyl CoAs one carbon shorter than the parent compound.
    E. are metabolized initially in the liver.

15. Lysine as a nutrient:
    A. may be replaced by its α-keto acid analog.
    B. produces pyruvate and acetoacetyl CoA in its catabolic pathway.
    C. is methylated by *S*-adenosylmethionine.
    D. is the only one of the common amino acids that is a precursor of carnitine.
    E. all of the above are correct.

16. Histidine:
    A. unlike most amino acids, is not converted to an α-keto acid when the amino group is removed.
    B. is a contributor to the tetrahydrofolate one-carbon pool.
    C. decarboxylation produces a physiologically active amine.
    D. forms a peptide with β-alanine.
    E. all of the above are correct.

17. Glutathione does all of the following EXCEPT:
    A. participate in the transport of amino acids across some cell membranes.
    B. scavenge peroxides and free radicals.
    C. form sulfur conjugates for detoxification of compounds.
    D. convert hemoglobin to methemoglobin.
    E. act as a cofactor for some enzymes.

ANSWERS

1. B A: All of the 20 common amino acids are incorporated into protein. B and E: Although most of our supply of nonessential amino acids comes from the diet, we can make them if necessary, given the precursors. C: Arginine is not believed to be required for adults (pp. 446–447).
2. D A: Most mammalian aminotransferases use glutamate or α-ketoglutarate. B: One amino acid is converted into another amino acid; there is neither net gain nor net loss. C: The reactions are freely reversible. E: Only lysine and threonine do not have aminotransferases (pp. 448–449).
3. C This is an important mechanism for reducing toxic ammonia concentrations. A: This would favor ammonia consumption. B: The cofactor is a pyridine nucleotide not pyridoxal phosphate. D: These are inhibitory. E: Since part of the role is to provide amino acid carbon chains for gluconeogenesis, this would be active (p. 450).
4. E It is in the form of the amide nitrogen of glutamine that much of amino acid nitrogen is made available in a nontoxic form (pp. 450–452).
5. C Rate must fluctuate to accommodate the amount of ammonia to be removed. A, B, and D: One of the nitrogen atoms is supplied as aspartate, with its carbon atoms being released as fumarate. This reaction is physiologically irreversible because of the hydrolysis of pyrophosphate. E: Since this is the main pathway for disposal of ammonia, any defect leads to hyperammonemia (pp. 454–456).
6. D B, C, and D: The primary control is by the allosteric effector, *N*-acetylglutamate. Synthesis of the effector, and therefore activity of CPSI, is increased in the presence of arginine. E: ATP is a substrate (p. 455).
7. E Spermidine is formed by adding propylamine to putrescine. A and B: Both amino acids give rise to glutamic semialdehyde and are formed from it. C: It is both a substrate and product of the cycle. D: This is a decarboxylation (p. 458).
8. B It is also synthesized from 3-phosphoglycerate. A: Threonine is an essential amino acid. C: It is converted to selenocysteine after forming a Ser-tRNA. D: It is *converted* to the prosthetic group (pyruvate) for that enzyme (p. 459).
9. D This forms methionine, which would become a general methyl donor. A: Methylene THF is reduced during the process of transfer to dUMP to form the thymine nucleotide. B: This is true for serine but not for other donors. C: An important aspect of the pool is interconvertibility of its forms. E: They can also be carried on nitrogen 5 or between nitrogens 5 and 10 (pp. 459–463).
10. A Tetrahydrobiopterin is a necessary cofactor for phenylalanine, tyrosine, and tryptophan hydroxylases. The first catalyzes the major pathway of phenylalanine catabolism. B: Albinism stems from a deficiency of tyrosinase, which, while giving the same product as tyrosine hydroxylase, is not a tetrahydrobiopterin-requiring enzyme. C: It would reduce the formation of the precursor, serotonin, but not melatonin itself. D: One-carbon fragments are transferred from either *S*-adenosylmethionine or the THF one-carbon pool. E: Catecholamine formation, catalyzed by the second enzyme, would also be deficient (pp. 464–467).
11. E Although all the statements are true, only E offers a suitable rationale. Tyrosine and tryptophan both yield a glucogenic fragment (fumarate and alanine) upon catabolism. Glucocorticoids are secreted in response to low blood glucose or stress (pp. 465 and 474).
12. A The reactive, positively charged sulfur reverts to a neutral thioether when the methyl group is transferred to an acceptor. B: The product, *S*-adenosylhomocysteine, is hydrolyzed to homocysteine. C: Transmethylations from AdoMet are irreversible. D: Transsulfuration refers to the combined action of cystathionine synthase and cystathionase transferring methionine's sulfur to serine to yield cysteine. E: Methionine provides only the sulfur; carbons are from serine (pp. 469–472).
13. D Methionine is the source of sulfur for cysteine (via homocysteine), but the reverse is not true in humans. A and B: Transamination to β-mercaptopyruvate with subsequent formation of thiosulfate and/or conversion of cystine to thiocysteine allows transfer of the sulfur to detoxify cyanide. C: Taurine is deaminated cysteine. E: SO_4^{2-}, the most oxidized form of sulfur found physiologically, is either excreted or activated as PAPS for use in detoxifying phenolic compounds or in biosynthesis (pp. 470 and 473).
14. E BCAA aminotransferase, the first enzyme, is much higher in muscle than in liver. B, C, and D: Although their catabolism is similar, the end products are different because of the differences in the branching. After transamination, the α-keto acids are oxidized by a dehydrogenase complex in a fashion similar to pyruvate dehydrogenase. The similarity to β-oxidation comes in steps like oxidation to an α,β-unsaturated CoA, hydration of the double bond, and oxidation of a hydroxyl to a carbonyl (pp. 476 and 479).
15. D A: Lysine does not participate in transamination probably in part because the α-keto acid exists as a cyclic Schiff base. B: This is one of two purely ketogenic amino acids. C and D: Free lysine is not methylated, but lysyl residues in a protein are methylated in a posttranslational modification. Intermediates of carnitine synthesis are derived from trimethyllysine liberated by proteolysis (pp. 479–481).
16. E A: Elimination of ammonia from histidine leaves a double bond (urocanate) unlike both transamination and oxidative deamination reactions. B: A portion of the ring is released as formimino THF. C and D: Histamine; carnosine (pp. 481–483).
17. D Most of the functions of glutathione listed are dependent on the sulfhydryl group (—SH). A major role of glutathione in red blood cells is reduction of methemoglobin. Glutathione reductase helps to maintain the ratio of GSH/GSSG at about 100 : 1 (p. 484).

CHAPTER

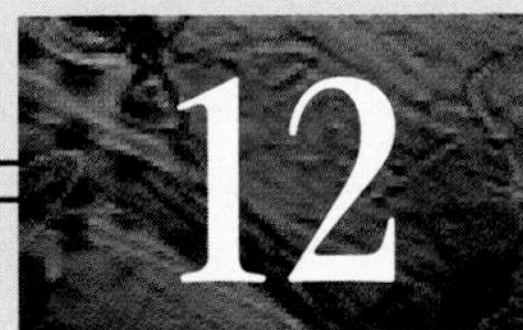

PURINE AND PYRIMIDINE NUCLEOTIDE METABOLISM

Joseph G. Cory

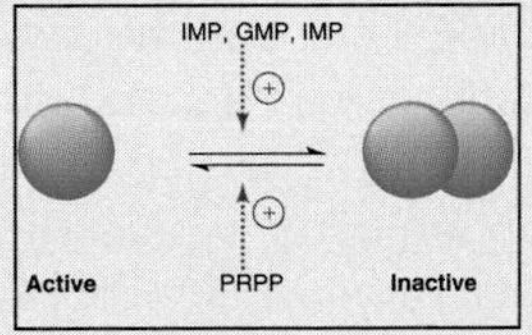

12.1 ■ OVERVIEW

The material in this chapter is limited to mammalian cells and where possible to nucleotide metabolism in humans. There are major differences between nucleotide metabolism in bacteria and mammalian cells and even some differences between humans and other mammals. Purine and pyrimidine nucleotides participate in many critical cellular functions. The metabolic roles of the nucleotides range from serving as the monomeric precursors of RNA and DNA to serving as second messengers. The sources of the purine and pyrimidine nucleotides are via *de novo* synthetic pathways and salvage of exogenous and endogenous nucleobases and nucleosides. Amino acids, CO_2, and ribose 5-phosphate (from the hexose monophosphate shunt) serve as sources for carbon, nitrogen, and oxygen atoms of purines and pyrimidine nucleotides.

The intracellular concentrations of nucleotides are finely regulated by allosterically modulated enzymes in the pathways in which nucleotide end products control key steps in the pathways. 2′-Deoxyribonucleotides required for DNA replication are generated directly from ribonucleotides and these reactions are also carefully regulated by nucleotides acting as positive and negative effectors. In addition to the regulation of nucleotide metabolism via allosteric regulation, concentrations of key enzymes in the metabolic pathway are altered during the cell cycle with many of the increases in enzyme activity occurring during late G1/early S phase just preceding DNA replication.

Defects in the metabolic pathways for *de novo* synthesis or salvage of nucleotides result in clinical diseases or syndromes. Furthermore, defects in degradation of nucleotides also lead to clinical problems. These include gout (defect in *de novo* purine nucleotide synthesis), Lesch–Nyhan syndrome (defect in purine nucleobase salvage), orotic aciduria (defect in *de novo* pyrimidine nucleotide synthesis), and immunodeficiency diseases (defects in purine nucleoside degradation). Because nucleotide synthesis is required for DNA replication and RNA synthesis in dividing cells, drugs that block *de novo* pathways of nucleotide synthesis have been used successfully as antitumor and antiviral agents.

12.2 ■ METABOLIC FUNCTIONS OF NUCLEOTIDES

Nucleotides and their derivatives play critical and diverse roles in cellular metabolism. Many different nucleotides are present in mammalian cells. Some, such as ATP, are present in the millimolar range while others, such as cyclic AMP, are orders of magnitude lower in concentration. The functions of nucleotides include the following:

1. Role in **Energy Metabolism:** As seen in earlier chapters, ATP is the principal form of chemical energy available to cells. ATP is generated in cells via either oxidative or substrate-level phosphorylation. ATP drives reactions as a phosphorylating agent and is involved in muscle contraction, active transport, and maintenance of ion gradients. ATP also serves as phosphate donor for generation of other nucleoside 5′-triphosphates.
2. **Monomeric Units of Nucleic Acids:** RNA and DNA consist of sequences of nucleotides. Nucleoside 5′-triphosphates are substrates for reactions catalyzed by RNA and DNA polymerases.
3. **Physiological Mediators:** Nucleosides and nucleotides serve as physiological mediators of key metabolic processes. Adenosine is important in control of coronary blood flow; ADP is critical in platelet aggregation and hence blood coagulation; cAMP and cGMP act as second messengers; and GTP is required for capping of mRNA, signal transduction through GTP-binding proteins, and in microtubule formation.

4. **Precursor Function:** GTP is the precursor for formation of the cofactor, tetrahydrobiopterin, required for hydroxylation reactions and nitric oxide generation.

5. **Components of Coenzymes:** The coenzymes NAD^+, $NADP^+$, FAD and their reduced forms and coenzyme A all contain as part of their structures a 5′-AMP moiety.

6. **Activated Intermediates:** Nucleotides also serve as carriers of "activated" intermediates required for a variety of reactions. UDP-glucose is a key intermediate in synthesis of glycogen and glycoproteins. GDP-mannose, GDP-fucose, UDP-galactose, and CMP-sialic acid are all key intermediates in reactions in which sugar moieties are transferred for synthesis of glycoproteins. CTP is utilized to generate CDP-choline, CDP-ethanolamine, and CDP- diacylglycerols, which are involved in phospholipid metabolism. Other activated intermediates include *S*-adenosylmethionine (SAM) and 3′-phosphoadenosine 5′-phosphosulfate (PAPS). *S*-Adenosylmethionine is a methyl donor in reactions involving methylation of sugar and base moieties of RNA and DNA and in formation of compounds such as phosphatidylcholine from phosphatidylethanolamine and carnitine from lysine. *S*-Adenosylmethionine also provides aminopropyl groups for synthesis of spermine from ornithine. PAPS is used as the sulfate donor to generate sulfated biomolecules such as proteoglycans and sulfatides.

7. **Allosteric Effectors:** Many of the regulated steps of metabolic pathways are controlled by intracellular concentrations of nucleotides. Many examples have already been discussed in previous chapters, and the roles of nucleotides in regulation of mammalian nucleotide metabolism will be discussed in this chapter.

Distributions of Nucleotides Vary with Cell Type

The principal purine and pyrimidine compounds found in cells are the 5′-nucleotide derivatives. ATP is the nucleotide found in the highest concentration in cells. The distributions of nucleotides in cells vary with cell type. In red blood cells, adenine nucleotides far exceed the concentrations of guanine, cytosine, and uridine nucleotides; in other tissues, such as liver, there is a complete spectrum of nucleotides and their derivatives, which include NAD^+ NADH, UDP-glucose, and UDP-glucuronic acid. In normally functioning cells, nucleoside 5′-triphosphates predominate, whereas in hypoxic cells the concentrations of nucleoside 5′-monophosphates and nucleoside 5′-diphosphates are greatly increased. Free nucleobases, nucleosides, nucleoside 2′- and 3′-monophosphates, and "modified" bases represent degradation products of endogenous or exogenous nucleotides or nucleic acids.

The concentrations of **ribonucleotides** in cells are in great excess over the concentrations of **2′-deoxyribonucleotides.** For example, the concentration of ATP in Ehrlich tumor cells is 3600 pmol per 10^6 cells compared to dATP concentration of 4 pmol per 10^6 cells. However, at the time of DNA replication the concentrations of dATP and other deoxyribonucleoside 5′-triphosphates are markedly increased to meet the substrate requirements for DNA synthesis.

In normal cells, the total concentrations of nucleotides are essentially constant. Thus the total concentration of AMP plus ADP plus ATP remains constant, but there can be major changes in the individual concentration such that the ratio of ATP/(ATP + ADP + AMP) is altered depending on the energy state of the cell. The same is true for NAD^+ and NADH. The total concentration of NAD^+ plus NADH is normally fixed within rather narrow concentration limits. Consequently, when it is stated that the NADH level is increased, it follows that the concentration of NAD^+ is correspondingly decreased in that cell. The basis for this "fixed" concentration of nucleotides is that *de novo* synthesis and salvage pathways for nucleotides, nucleosides, and nucleobases are very rigidly controlled under normal conditions.

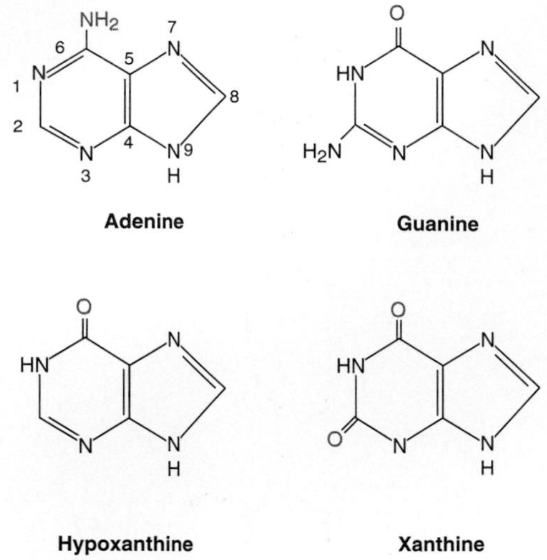

Adenine

Guanine

Hypoxanthine

Xanthine

FIGURE 12.1
Purine bases.

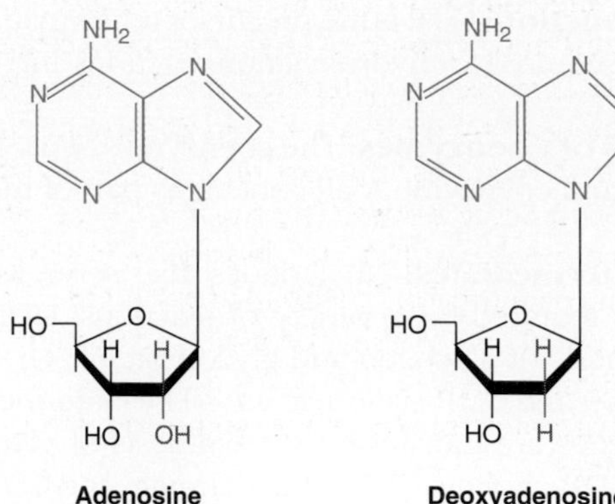

FIGURE 12.2
Adenosine and deoxyadenosine.

12.3 ■ CHEMISTRY OF NUCLEOTIDES

The major purine derivatives in cells are those of **adenine** and **guanine.** Other purine bases encountered are hypoxanthine and xanthine (Figure 12.1). Nucleoside derivatives of these molecules will contain either ribose or 2-deoxyribose linked to the purine ring through a ***β-N*-glycosidic bond** at N-9. Ribonucleosides contain ribose, while deoxyribonucleosides contain deoxyribose as the sugar moiety (Figure 12.2). Nucleotides are **phosphate esters** of purine nucleosides (Figure 12.3). 3′-Nucleotides such as adenosine 3′-monophosphate (3′-AMP) may occur in cells as a result of nucleic acid degradation. In normally functioning cells, tri- and diphosphates are found to a greater extent than monophosphates, nucleosides, or free bases.

Adenosine 5′-monophosphate (AMP)

Deoxyadenosine 5′-monophosphate (dAMP)

Adenosine 5′-diphosphate (ADP)

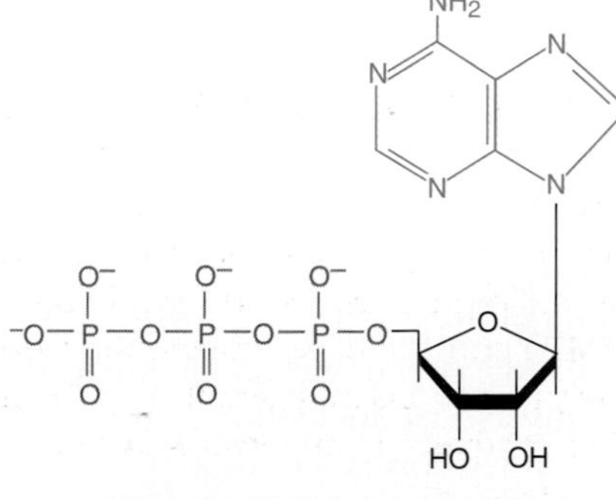

FIGURE 12.3
Adenine nucleotides.

The pyrimidine nucleotides found in highest concentrations in cells are those containing **uracil** and **cytosine.** The structures of the bases are shown in Figure 12.4. Uracil and cytosine nucleotides are the major pyrimidine components of RNA; cytosine and thymine are the major pyrimidine components of DNA. As with purine derivatives, the pyrimidine nucleosides or nucleotides contain either ribose or 2-deoxyribose. The sugar moiety is linked to the pyrimidine in a β-*N*-glycosidic bond at N-1. Nucleosides of pyrimidines are uridine, cytidine, and thymidine (Figure 12.5). **Phosphate esters** of pyrimidine nucleosides are UMP, CMP, and TMP. In cells the major pyrimidine derivatives are tri- and diphosphates (Figure 12.6).

See the Appendix for a summary of the nomenclature and chemistry of the purines and pyrimidines.

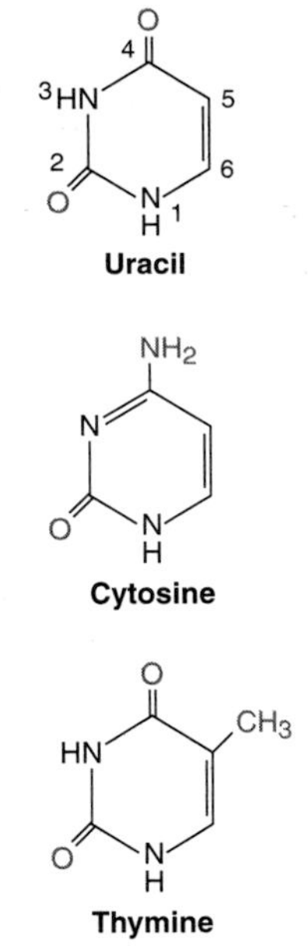

Uracil

Cytosine

Thymine

FIGURE 12.4
Pyrimidine bases.

Properties of Nucleotides

Cellular components containing either purine or pyrimidine bases can be easily detected because of their strong absorption of UV light. Purine bases, nucleosides, and nucleotides have stronger absorptions than pyrimidines and their derivatives. The wavelength of light at which maximum absorption occurs varies with the particular base component, but in most cases the UV maximum is close to 260 nm. The UV spectrum for each derivative responds differently to changes in pH. The UV absorptions provide the basis for sensitive methods in assaying these compounds. For example, deamination of adenine nucleosides or nucleotides to the corresponding hypoxanthine derivatives causes a marked shift in λ_{max} from 265 to 250 nm, which is easily determined. Because of the high molar extinction coefficients of the purine and pyrimidine bases and their high concentrations in nucleic acids, the absorbance at 260 nm can be used to quantitate the amount of nucleic acid in RNA and DNA preparations.

The *N*-glycosidic bond of nucleosides and nucleotides is stable to alkali. However, stability of this bond to acid hydrolysis differs markedly. The *N*-glycosidic bond of purine nucleosides and nucleotides is easily hydrolyzed by dilute acid at elevated temperatures (e.g., 60°C) to yield free purine base and sugar or sugar phosphate. On the other hand, the *N*-glycosidic bond of uracil, cytosine, and thymine nucleosides and nucleotides is very stable to acid treatment. Strong conditions, such as perchloric acid (60%) and 100°C, releases free pyrimidine but with complete destruction of the sugar. The *N*-glycosidic bond of dihydrouracil nucleoside and dihydrouracil nucleotide is labile in mild acid.

Because of the highly polar phosphate group, purine and pyrimidine nucleotides are much more soluble in aqueous solutions than are their nucleosides and free bases. In general, nucleosides are more soluble than free bases.

Purine and pyrimidine bases and their nucleoside and nucleotide derivatives can be easily separated by a variety of techniques. These methods include paper chromatography; thin-layer chromatography (TLC), utilizing plates with cellulose or ion-exchange resins, electrophoresis; and ion-exchange column chromatography. With high-performance liquid chromatography (HPLC) nanomole quantities of these components are easily and quickly separated and detected.

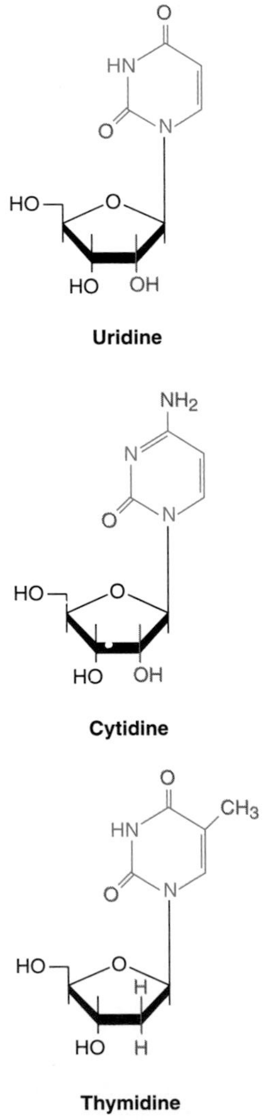

Uridine

Cytidine

Thymidine

FIGURE 12.5
Pyrimidine nucleosides.

12.4 METABOLISM OF PURINE NUCLEOTIDES

The purine ring is synthesized *de novo* in mammalian cells utilizing amino acids as carbon and nitrogen donors and also CO_2 as a carbon donor. The ***de novo* pathway** for purine nucleotide synthesis leading to **inosine 5′-monophosphate (IMP)** consists of ten metabolic steps. Hydrolysis of ATP is required to drive several reactions in this pathway. Overall, the *de novo* pathway for purine nucleotide synthesis is expensive in terms of moles of ATP utilized per mole of IMP synthesized.

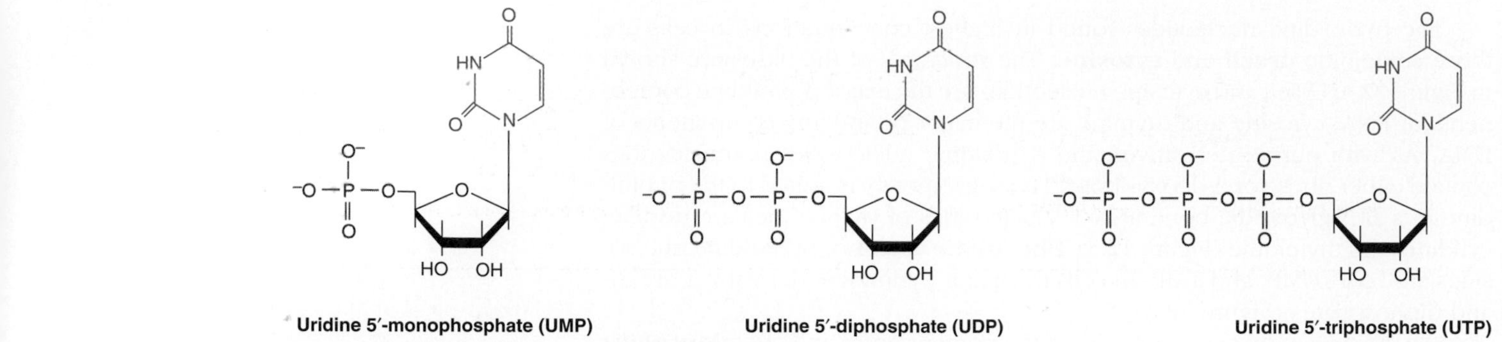

Uridine 5′-monophosphate (UMP) Uridine 5′-diphosphate (UDP) Uridine 5′-triphosphate (UTP)

FIGURE 12.6
Uracil nucleotides.

Purine Nucleotides Are Synthesized by a Stepwise Buildup of the Ring to Form IMP

All enzymes involved in synthesis of purine nucleotides are found in the cytosol of the cell. However, not all cells (e.g., red cells) are capable of *de novo* purine nucleotide synthesis. In the *de novo* pathway, a stepwise series of reactions leads to synthesis of IMP, which in turn serves as the precursor for both **adenosine 5′-monophosphate** (AMP) and **guanosine 5′-monophosphate** (GMP). Since IMP serves as the common precursor for AMP and GMP and this pathway is highly regulated by AMP and GMP, IMP is not normally found to any extent in cells.

Formation of IMP is shown in Figure 12.7. Several points should be emphasized about this pathway: phosphoribosylpyrophosphate (PRPP) is synthesized from ribose 5-phosphate generated by the hexose monophosphate pathway; the equivalent of 6 moles of ATP are utilized per mole of IMP synthesized; formation of 5-phosphoribosylamine (the first step) is the committed step. In formation of **5-phosphoribosylamine,** the N—C bond is formed that will ultimately be the *N*-glycosidic bond of the purine nucleotide; there are no known regulated steps between 5-phosphoribosylamine and IMP. **Tetrahydrofolate** serves as a "C_1" carrier (**N^{10}-formyl H_4folate,** Figure 12.8) in this pathway.

The enzyme activities catalyzing several steps in the pathway reside on separate domains of **multifunctional proteins.** The activities of 5′-phosphoribosylglycinamide synthetase, 5′-phosphoribosylglycinamide transformylase, and 5′-phosphoribosylaminoimidazole synthetase form part of a trifunctional protein. 5′-Phosphoribosylaminoimidazole carboxylase and 5′-phosphoribosyl-4-(*N*-succinocarboxamide)-5-aminoimidazole synthetase activities are on a bifunctional protein. 5′-Phosphoribosyl-4-carboxamide-5-aminoimidazole transformylase and IMP cyclohydrolase activities are present on another bifunctional protein.

To summarize, *de novo* synthesis of purine nucleotides requires amino acids as carbon and nitrogen donors, CO_2 as a carbon source, and "C_1 units" transferred via H_4folate. The contributions of these sources to the purine ring are shown in Figure 12.9. Several amino acids including serine, glycine, tryptophan, and histidine can yield "C_1 units" to H_4folate (Chapter 11) and therefore they can contribute to C-2 and C-8 of the ring. 5′-Phosphoribosyl-5-aminoimidazole carboxylase, which catalyzes the reaction in which CO_2 is used to introduce C-6 of the ring, is not a biotin-dependent carboxylase.

IMP Is the Common Precursor for AMP and GMP

IMP, the first ribonucleotide formed in the *de novo* pathway, serves as the common precursor for AMP and GMP synthesis (Figure 12.10). AMP and GMP are converted to ATP and GTP, respectively, utilizing nucleoside 5′-monophos-

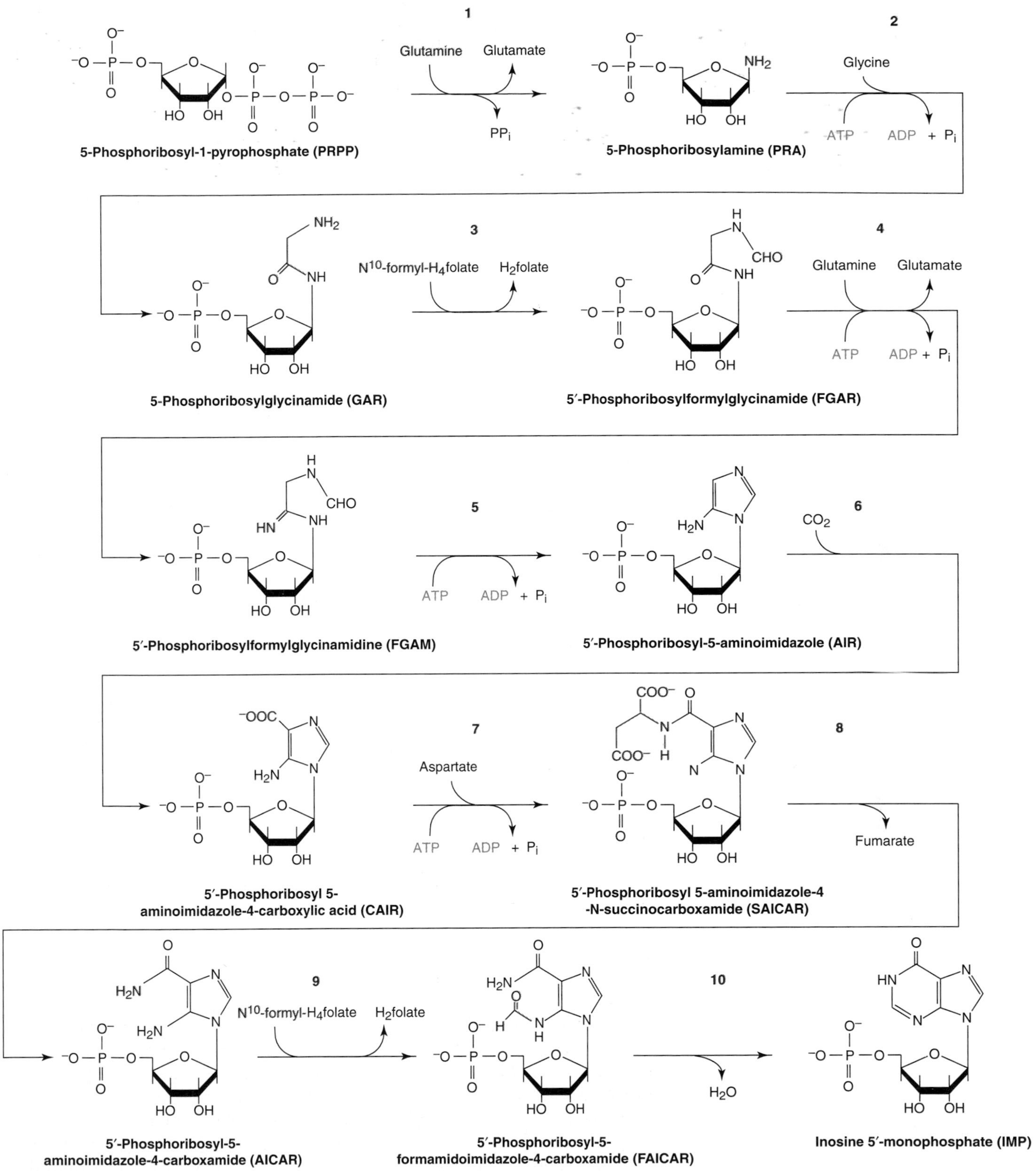

1 Glutamine → Glutamate; PP_i

5-Phosphoribosyl-1-pyrophosphate (PRPP)

2 Glycine; ATP → ADP + P_i

5-Phosphoribosylamine (PRA)

3 N^{10}-formyl-H_4folate → H_2folate

5-Phosphoribosylglycinamide (GAR)

4 Glutamine → Glutamate; ATP → ADP + P_i

5′-Phosphoribosylformylglycinamide (FGAR)

5 ATP → ADP + P_i

5′-Phosphoribosylformylglycinamidine (FGAM)

6 CO_2

5′-Phosphoribosyl-5-aminoimidazole (AIR)

7 Aspartate; ATP → ADP + P_i

5′-Phosphoribosyl 5-aminoimidazole-4-carboxylic acid (CAIR)

8 Fumarate

5′-Phosphoribosyl 5-aminoimidazole-4-N-succinocarboxamide (SAICAR)

9 N^{10}-formyl-H_4folate → H_2folate

5′-Phosphoribosyl-5-aminoimidazole-4-carboxamide (AICAR)

10 H_2O

5′-Phosphoribosyl-5-formamidoimidazole-4-carboxamide (FAICAR)

Inosine 5′-monophosphate (IMP)

FIGURE 12.7

***De novo* synthesis of purine ribonucleotides.**

The enzymes catalyzing the reactions are: ① glutamine PRPP amidotransferase; ② GAR synthetase; ③ GAR transformylase; ④ FGAM synthetase; ⑤ AIR synthetase; ⑥ AIR carboxylase; ⑦ SAICAR synthetase; ⑧ adenylosuccinate lyase; ⑨ AICAR transformylase; and ⑩ IMP cyclohydrolase.

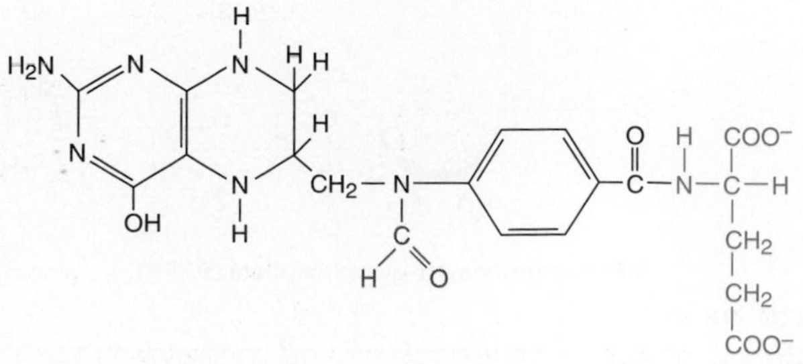

FIGURE 12.8
Structure of N^{10}-formyl H_4folate.

HCO3–
Glycine
Aspartate amino
"C1"–H4folate
"C1"–H4folate
Glutamine amide

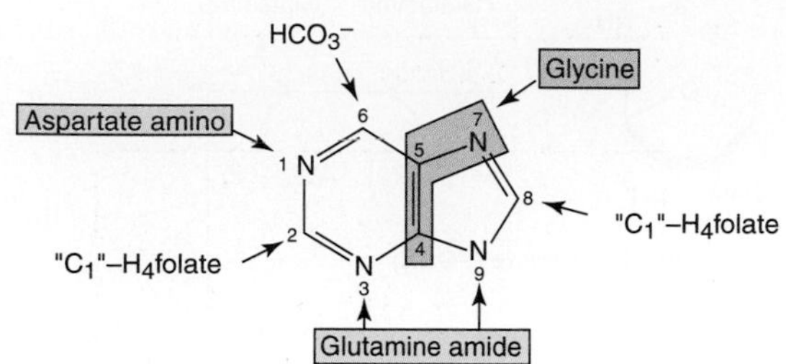

FIGURE 12.9
Sources of carbon and nitrogen atoms in the purine ring.
C-4, C-5, and N-7 are from glycine; N-3 and N-9 from glutamine; C-2 and C-8 from "C_1"-H_4folate; N-1 from aspartate; and C-6 from CO_2.

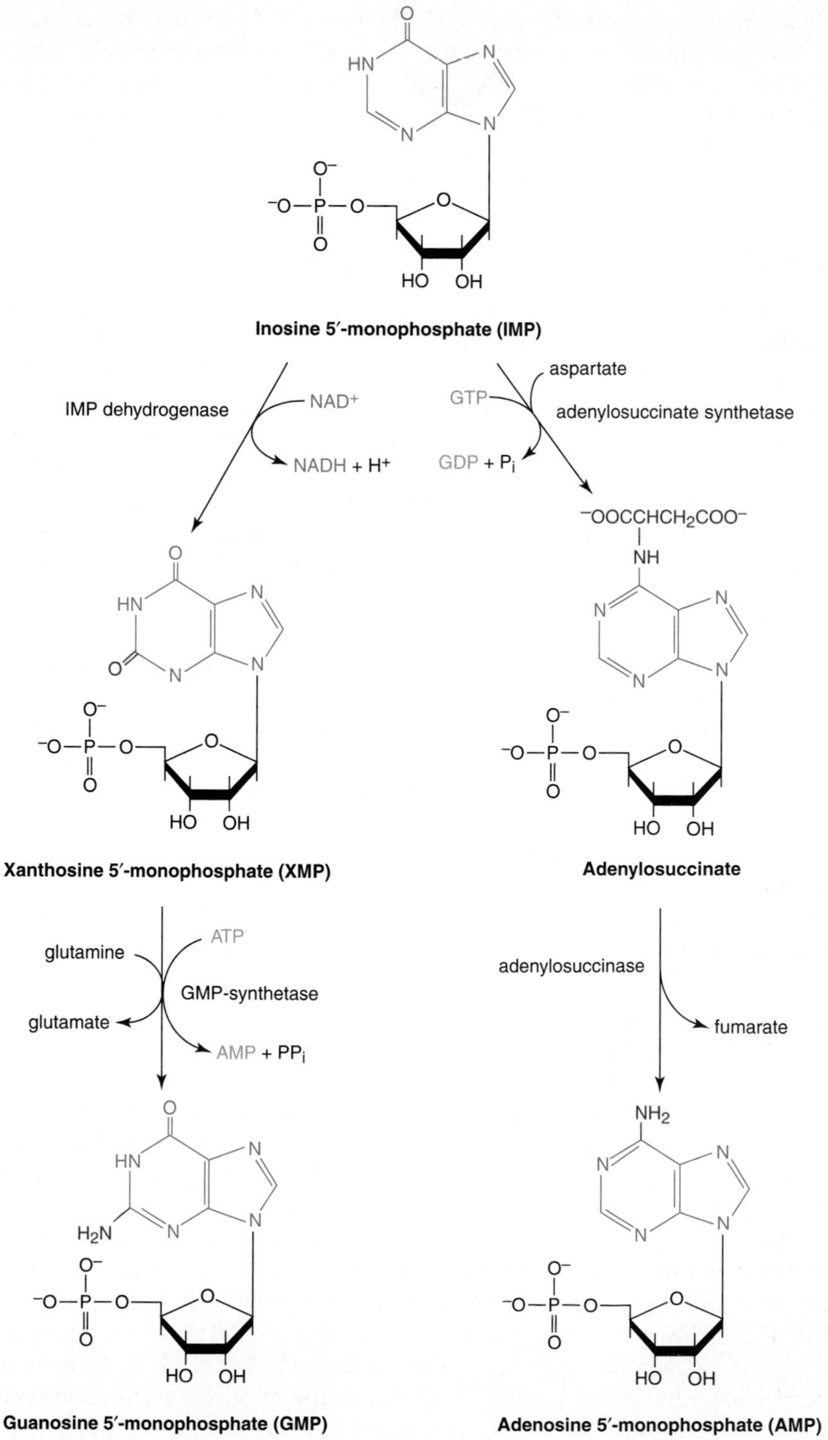

Inosine 5′-monophosphate (IMP)
IMP dehydrogenase
NAD+
NADH + H+
aspartate
GTP
adenylosuccinate synthetase
GDP + Pi
Xanthosine 5′-monophosphate (XMP)
Adenylosuccinate
glutamine
ATP
GMP-synthetase
glutamate
AMP + PPi
adenylosuccinase
fumarate
Guanosine 5′-monophosphate (GMP)
Adenosine 5′-monophosphate (AMP)

FIGURE 12.10
Formation of AMP and GMP from IMP branch point.

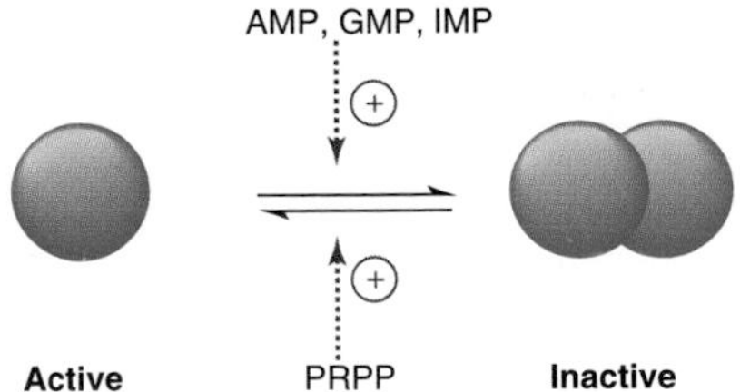

FIGURE 12.11
Effects of allosteric modulators on molecular forms of glutamine PRPP amido-transferase.

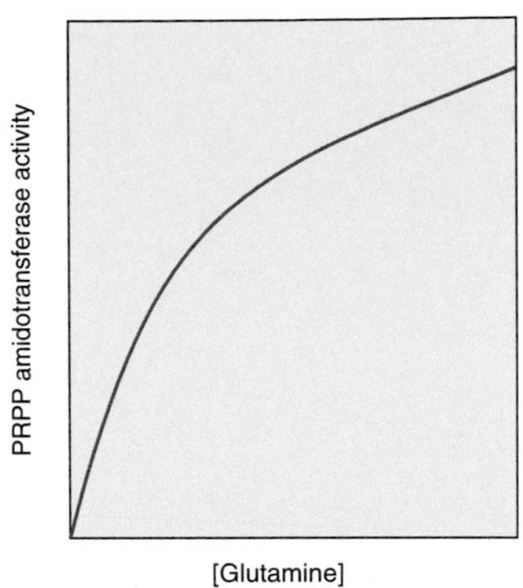

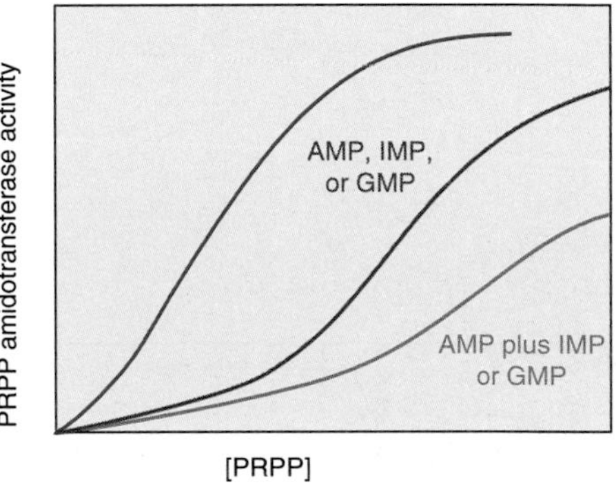

FIGURE 12.12
Glutamine PRPP amidotransferase activity as a function of glutamine or PRPP concentrations.

phate kinases and **nucleoside 5′-diphosphate kinases.** Conversion of IMP to AMP and GMP, from this branch point, does not occur randomly. Formation of GMP from IMP requires ATP as the energy source, whereas formation of AMP from IMP requires GTP as the energy source. This can be thought of as a reciprocal relationship. That is, when there is sufficient ATP in the cell, GMP will be synthesized and when there is sufficient GTP, AMP will be synthesized.

Purine Nucleotide Synthesis Is Highly Regulated

The committed step of a metabolic pathway is generally the site of metabolic regulation. In the *de novo* pathway of purine nucleotide synthesis, formation of 5-phosphoribosylamine from glutamine and **5-phosphoribosyl-1-pyrophosphate** is the committed step in IMP formation. The enzyme catalyzing this reaction, **glutamine PRPP amidotransferase,** is rate-limiting and is regulated allosterically by the end products of the pathway—IMP, GMP, and AMP. These nucleotides serve as negative effectors. On the other hand, PRPP is a positive effector. Glutamine PRPP amidotransferase is a monomer of 135 kDa that is enzymatically active. In the presence of IMP, AMP, or GMP, the enzyme forms a dimer that is much less active. The presence of PRPP favors the active monomeric form of the enzyme (Figure 12.11).

The enzyme from human tissues has distinct nucleotide-binding sites. One site specifically binds oxypurine nucleotides (IMP and GMP) while the other site specifically binds aminopurine nucleotides (AMP). When AMP and GMP or IMP are simultaneously present, the enzyme activity is synergistically inhibited. Glutamine PRPP amidotransferase displays hyperbolic kinetics with respect to glutamine as the substrate and sigmoidal kinetics with respect to PRPP (Figure 12.12). Since the intracellular concentration of glutamine is close to its K_m and the concentration varies relatively little, the glutamine concentration has little effect in regulating IMP synthesis. The intracellular concentration of PRPP, however, varies widely and can be 10 to 100 times less than the K_m for PRPP. As a result, the concentration of PRPP plays an important role in regulating synthesis of purine nucleotides.

Between the formation of 5-phosphoribosylamine and IMP, there are no known regulated steps. However, there is regulation at the branch point of IMP to AMP and IMP to GMP. From IMP to GMP, **IMP dehydrogenase** is the rate-limiting enzyme and it is regulated by GMP acting as a competitive inhibitor. **Adenylosuccinate synthetase** is the rate-limiting enzyme in conversion of IMP to AMP with AMP acting as a competitive inhibitor.

There must be other as yet unknown mechanisms that regulate the ATP/GTP ratio within relatively narrow limits. In most cells the total cellular concentration of adenine nucleotides (ATP plus ADP plus AMP) is four to six times that of guanine nucleotides (GTP plus GDP plus GMP). The overall regulation of purine nucleotide synthesis is summarized in Figure 12.13. Defects in the metabolic pathway that lead to loss of regulation of purine nucleotide synthesis result in overproduction of purine nucleotides and the end product, uric acid.

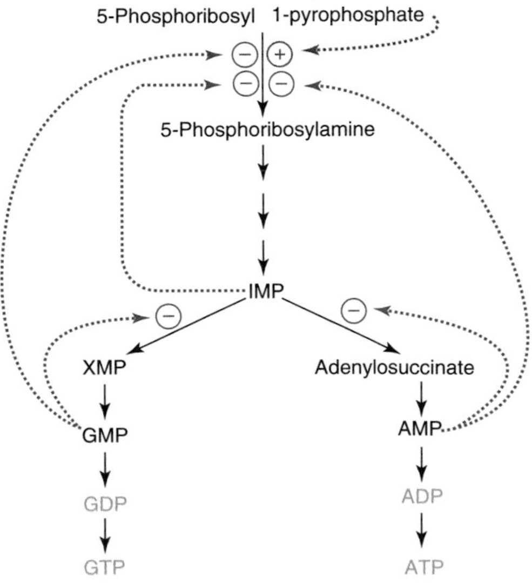

FIGURE 12.13
Regulation of purine nucleotide synthesis.
The dashed lines represent sites of active ⊕ or inhibition ⊖.

This results in a relatively common clinical condition known as gout (see Clin. Corr. 12.1).

Purine Bases and Nucleosides Can Be Salvaged to Reform Nucleotides

The efficiency of normal metabolism is shown by the presence of two distinct **"salvage pathways."** One pathway utilizes the bases, hypoxanthine, guanine, and adenine as substrates while the other pathway utilizes preformed nucleosides as the substrates. In each pathway there is specificity with respect to the base or nucleoside being "salvaged." The "salvage" of bases requires the activity of **phosphoribosyl transferases.** There are two distinct phosphoribosyl transferases. **Hypoxanthine–guanine phosphoribosyltransferase** (HGPRTase) catalyzes the reactions

$$\text{Hypoxanthine} + \text{PRPP} \rightarrow \text{IMP} + \text{PP}_i$$

and

$$\text{Guanine} + \text{PRPP} \rightarrow \text{GMP} + \text{PP}_i$$

and **adenine phosphoribosyltransferase** (APRTase) catalyzes

$$\text{Adenine} + \text{PRPP} \rightarrow \text{AMP} + \text{PP}_i$$

CLINICAL CORRELATION 12.1

Gout

Gout is characterized by elevated uric acid levels in blood and urine due to a variety of metabolic abnormalities that lead to overproduction of purine nucleotides via the *de novo* pathway. Many, if not all, of the clinical symptoms associated with elevated levels of uric acid arise because of the very poor solubility of uric acid in the aqueous environment. Sodium urate crystals deposit in joints of the extremities and in renal interstitial tissue, and these events tend to trigger the sequelae. Hyperuricemia from overproduction of uric acid via the *de novo* pathway can be distinguished from hyperuricemia that results from kidney disease or excessive cell death (e.g., increased degradation of nucleic acids from radiation therapy). Feeding of [^{15}N]glycine to a patient who is an overproducer will result in uric acid excreted in urine that is enriched in ^{15}N at the N-7 of uric acid while in a patient who is not an overproducer, there will be no enrichment of ^{15}N in uric acid from these patients.

Studies of "gouty" patients have shown that multiple and heterogeneous defects are the cause of overproduction of uric acid. In some cases, biochemical defects have not been defined. Examples of biochemical defects that result in increased purine nucleotide synthesis include the following:

1. Increased PRPP synthetase activity: Increased PRPP synthetase activity results in increased intracellular levels of PRPP. As discussed in the section on regulation of purine nucleotide synthesis, PRPP acts as a positive effector of glutamine–PRPP amidotransferase, leading to increased flux through the *de novo* pathway since activity of the rate-limiting step is markedly increased.

2. Partial HGPRTase activity: Partial decrease in HGPRTase activity has two fallouts with respect to the *de novo* pathway for purine nucleotide synthesis. First, since there is decreased salvage of hypoxanthine and guanine, PRPP is not consumed by the HGPRTase reaction and PRPP can activate glutamine–PRPP amidotransferase activity. Second, with decreased salvage of hypoxanthine and guanine, IMP and GMP are not formed via this pathway so that regulation of the PRPP amidotransferase step by IMP and GMP as negative effectors is compromised.

3. Glucose 6-phosphatase deficiency: In patients who have glucose 6-phosphatase deficiency (von Gierke's disease, type I glycogen storage disease) there is frequently hyperuricemia and gout as well. Loss of glucose 6-phosphatase activity results in more glucose 6-phosphate being shunted to the hexose monophosphate shunt. As a result of increased hexose monophosphate shunt activity, more ribose 5-phosphate is generated and the intracellular level of PRPP is increased. PRPP is a positive effector of PRPP amidotransferase.

These examples show that factors that increase the rate-limiting step in *de novo* synthesis of purine nucleotide synthesis lead to increased synthesis and degradation to uric acid.

There are different approaches to the treatment of gout that include colchicine, antihyperuricemic drugs, and allopurinol. Allopurinol and its metabolite, alloxanthine, are effective inhibitors of xanthine oxidase and will cause a decrease in uric acid levels. In "overproducers" who do not have a severe deficiency of HGPRTase activity, allopurinol treatment inhibits xanthine oxidase, thereby increasing the concentrations of hypoxanthine and xanthine. These purine bases are then salvaged to form IMP and XMP. These reactions consume PRPP and generate inhibitors of PRPP amidotransferase. The overall effect is that allopurinol treatment decreases both uric acid formation and *de novo* synthesis of purine nucleotides.

Becker, M. A., and Roessler, B. J. Hyperuricemia and gout. In: C. R. Scriver, A. L. Beaudet, W. S. Sly, and D. Valle (Eds.), *The Metabolic and Molecular Bases of Inherited Disease,* 7th ed., Vol. II, Chap. 49. New York: McGraw-Hill, 1995, pp. 1655–1677.

These two enzymes do not overlap in substrate specificity. The phosphoribosyltransferase reactions are regulated by the end products of the reactions. IMP and GMP are competitive inhibitors, with respect to PRPP, of HGPRTase while AMP is a competitive inhibitor, with respect to PRPP, of APRTase. In this way, salvage of purine bases is regulated.

The hypoxanthine and guanine for salvage arise from degradation of endogenous or exogenous purine nucleotides. On the other hand, the source of adenine utilized in the APRTase reaction appears to be mainly from synthesis of polyamines (see p. 473). For each molecule of **spermine** synthesized, two molecules of **5′-methylthioadenosine** are generated that are degraded to **5-methylthioribose-1-phosphate** and adenine via the **5′-methylthioadenosine phosphorylase**-catalyzed reaction. The adenine base is salvaged through the APRTase reaction.

Generation of AMP and GMP through these phosphoribosyltransferase reactions effectively inhibits the *de novo* pathway at the PRPP amidotransferase step. First, PRPP is consumed, decreasing the rate of formation of 5-phosphoribosylamine; and second, AMP and GMP serve as feedback inhibitors at this step.

HGPRTase activity is markedly depressed in the **Lesch–Nyhan syndrome** (see Clin. Corr. 12.2), which is characterized clinically by hyperuricemia, mental retardation, and self-mutilation.

CLINICAL CORRELATION 12.2

Lesch–Nyhan Syndrome

The Lesch–Nyhan syndrome is characterized clinically by hyperuricemia, excessive uric acid production, and neurological problems, which may include spasticity, mental retardation, and self-mutilation. This disorder is associated with a very severe or complete deficiency of HGPRTase activity. The gene for HGPRTase is on the X chromosome, hence the deficiency is virtually limited to males. In a study of the available patients, it was observed that if HGPRTase activity was less than 2% of normal, mental retardation was present, and if the activity was less than 0.2% of normal, the self-mutilation aspect was expressed. This defect also leads to excretion of hypoxanthine and xanthine.

There are more than a hundred disease-related mutations defined in the HGPRTase gene from Lesch–Nyhan patients. These have led to the loss of HGPRTase protein, loss of HGPRTase activity, "K_m mutants," HGPRTase protein with a short half-life, and so on.

The role of HGPRTase is to catalyze reactions in which hypoxanthine and guanine are converted to nucleotides. The hyperuricemia and excessive uric acid production that occur in patients with the Lesch–Nyhan syndrome are easily explained by the lack of HGPRTase activity. Hypoxanthine and guanine are not salvaged, leading to increased intracellular pools of PRPP and decreased levels of IMP or GMP. Both of these factors promote *de novo* synthesis of purine nucleotides without regard for proper regulation of this pathway.

It is not understood why a severe defect in this salvage pathway leads to neurological problems. Adenine phosphoribosyltransferase activity in these patients is normal or elevated. With this salvage enzyme, presumably the cellular needs for purine nucleotides could be met by conversion of AMP to GMP via IMP if the cell's *de novo* pathway were not functioning. The normal tissue distribution of HGPRTase activity perhaps could explain the neurological symptoms. The brain (frontal lob, basal ganglia, and cerebellum) has 10–20 times the enzyme activity found in liver, spleen, or kidney and from 4 to 8 times that found in erythrocytes. Individuals who have primary gout with excessive uric acid formation and hyperuricemia do not display neurological problems. It is argued that products of purine degradation (hypoxanthine, xanthine, and uric acid) cannot be toxic to the central nervous system (CNS). However, it is possible that these metabolites are toxic to the developing CNS or that lack of this enzyme leads to an imbalance in the concentrations of purine nucleotides at critical times during development.

If IMP dehydrogenase activity in brain were extremely low, lack of HGPRTase could lead to decreased levels of intracellular GTP due to decreased salvage of guanine. Since GTP is a precursor of tetrahydrobiopterin, a required cofactor in the biosynthesis of neurotransmitters, and is required in other functions such as signal transduction via G-proteins and protein synthesis, low levels of GTP during development could be the triggering factor in the observed neurological manifestations.

Treatment of Lesch–Nyhan patients with allopurinol will decrease the amount of uric acid formed, relieving some of the problems caused by sodium urate deposits. However, since the Lesch–Nyhan patient has a marked reduction in HGPRTase activity, hypoxanthine and guanine are not salvaged, PRPP is not consumed, and consequently *de novo* synthesis of purine nucleotides is not shut down. There is no treatment for the neurological problems. These patients usually die from kidney failure, resulting from high sodium urate deposits.

Rossiter, B. J. F., and Caskey, C. T. Hypoxanthine–guanine phosphoribosyltransferase deficiency: Lesch–Nyhan syndrome and gout. In: C. R. Scriver, A. L. Beaudet, W. S. Sly, and D. Valle (Eds.), *The Metabolic and Molecular Bases of Inherited Disease,* 7th ed., Vol II, Chap. 50. New York: McGraw Hill, 1995, pp. 1679–1706.

Overall, these salvage reactions not only conserve energy but also permit cells to form nucleotides from the bases. The erythrocyte, for example, does not have glutamine PRPP amidotransferase and hence cannot synthesize 5-phosphoribosylamine, the first unique metabolite in the pathway of purine nucleotide synthesis. As a consequence, red cells must depend on purine phosphoribosyltransferases and 5′-phosphotransferase to replenish their nucleotide pools.

Purine Nucleotides Can Be Interconverted to Maintain the Appropriate Balance of Adenine and Guanine Nucleotides

De novo synthesis of purine nucleotides is under very fine control, executed at the committed step catalyzed by **glutamine PRPP amidotransferase** and at the branch point of IMP to AMP and IMP to GMP. Additional enzymes present in mammalian cells allow for interconversions of adenine and guanine nucleotides to maintain the appropriate balance of cellular concentrations of these purine nucleotides. These interconversions occur by indirect steps. There is no direct one-step pathway for conversion of GMP to AMP or AMP to GMP. In each case, AMP or GMP is metabolized to IMP (Figure 12.14). These reactions are catalyzed by separate enzymes, each of which is under separate controls. Reductive deamination of GMP to IMP is catalyzed by **GMP reductase.** GTP activates this step while XMP is a strong competitive inhibitor of the reaction. GTP, while not required by the enzyme, increases enzyme activity by lowering the K_m with respect to GMP and by increasing V_{max}.

AMP deaminase (**5′-AMP aminohydrolase**) catalyzes deamination of AMP to IMP and is activated by K^+ and ATP and inhibited by P_i, GDP, and GTP. In the absence of K^+, the v versus [AMP] curve is sigmoidal. The presence of K^+ is not required for maximum activity; rather K^+ is a positive allosteric effector reducing the apparent K_m for AMP.

The net effect of these reactions is that cells can interconvert adenine and guanine nucleotides to meet cellular needs, while maintaining control over these reactions.

GTP Is Precursor of Tetrahydrobiopterin

GTP is the direct precursor for **tetrahydrobiopterin** synthesis (Figure 12.15). Reactions from GTP to tetrahydrobiopterin are catalyzed by **GTP cyclohydrolase I, 6-pyruvoyl-tetrahydropterin synthase,** and **sepiapterin reductase,** with GTP cyclohydrolase I being rate-limiting. Many cell types can synthesize tetrahydrobiopterin. Tetrahydrobiopterin is a required cofactor in hydroxylation reactions involving phenylalanine, tyrosine, and tryptophan (see p. 476) and is involved in the generation of nitric oxide. Inhibitors of IMP dehydrogenase cause a marked reduction in cellular levels of tetrahydrobiopterin, demonstrating the importance of GTP as the precursor of tetrahydrobiopterin and of IMP dehydrogenase as the rate-limiting enzyme in GTP formation.

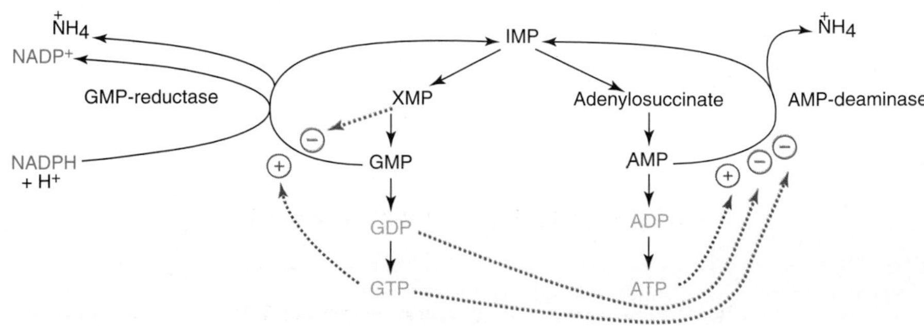

FIGURE 12.14
Interconversions of purine nucleotides.
The dashed lines represent sites of regulation; ⊕ activation or ⊖ inhibition.

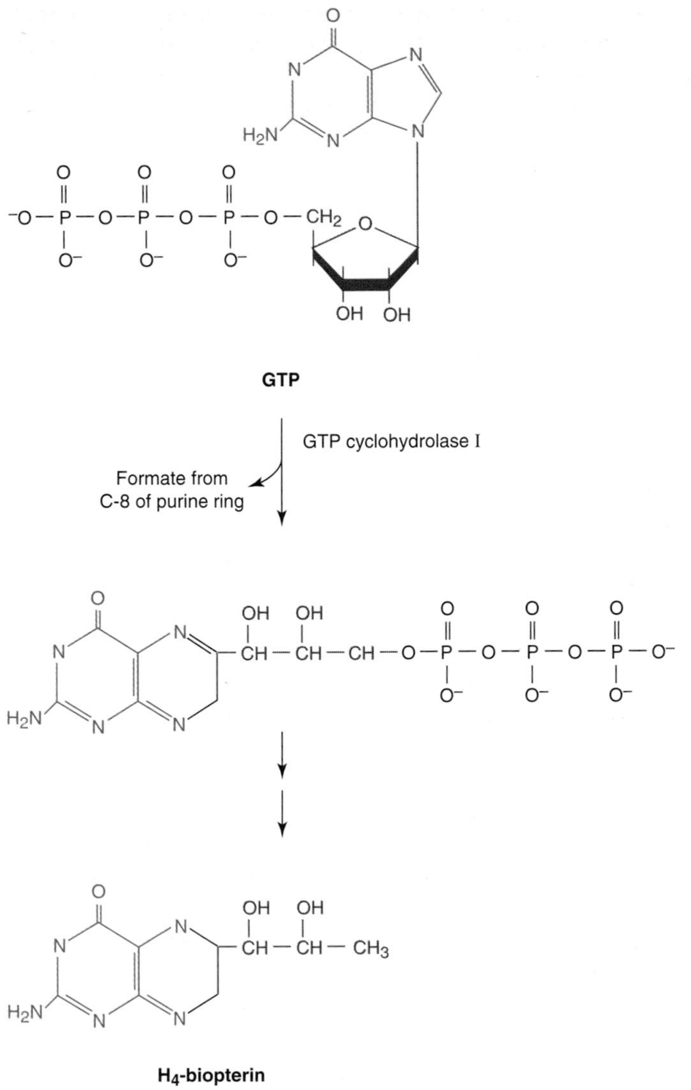

GTP

GTP cyclohydrolase I

Formate from C-8 of purine ring

H4-biopterin

FIGURE 12.15
Synthesis of tetrahydrobiopterin from GTP.

End Product of Purine Degradation in Humans Is Uric Acid

The degradation of purine nucleotides, nucleosides, and bases funnel through a common pathway leading to formation of uric acid (Figure 12.16). The enzymes involved in degradation of nucleic acids and nucleotides and nucleosides vary in specificity. **Nucleases** show specificity toward either RNA or DNA and also toward the bases and position of cleavage site at the 3′,5′-phosphodiester bonds. **Nucleotidases** range from those with relatively high specificity, such as 5′-AMP nucleotidase, to those with broad specificity, such as the acid and alkaline phosphatases, which will hydrolyze any of the 3′- or 5′-nucleotides. **AMP deaminase** is specific for AMP. **Adenosine deaminase** is less specific, since not only adenosine but also 2′-deoxyadenosine and many other 6-aminopurine nucleosides are deaminated by this enzyme.

Purine nucleoside phosphorylase catalyzes the reversible reactions

$$\text{Inosine} + P_i \rightleftharpoons \text{hypoxanthine} + \text{ribose 1-P}$$

or

$$\text{Guanosine} + P_i \rightleftharpoons \text{guanine} + \text{ribose 1-P}$$

or

$$\text{Xanthosine} + P_i \rightleftharpoons \text{xanthine} + \text{ribose 1-P}$$

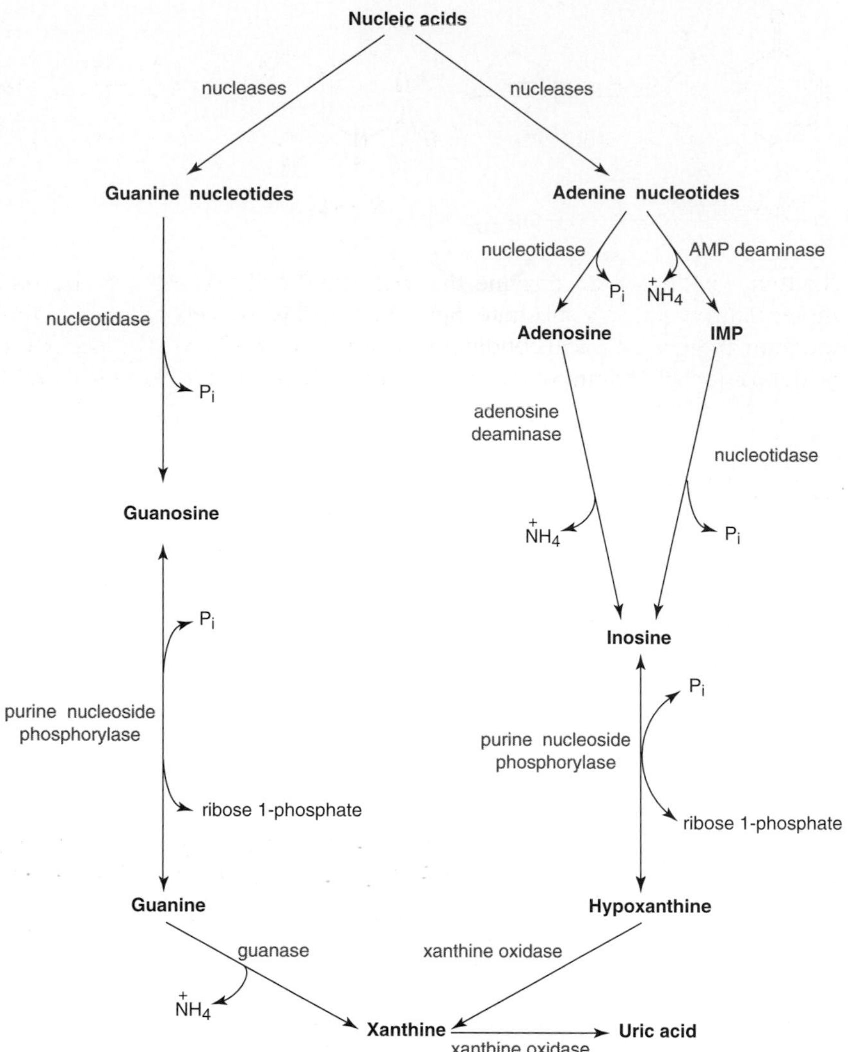

FIGURE 12.16
Degradation of purine nucleotides.

Deoxyinosine and deoxyguanosine are also excellent substrates for purine nucleoside phosphorylase. This is important for removal of deoxyguanosine to prevent uncontrolled accumulation of dGTP, which is toxic to cells at high concentrations. While the equilibrium constants for reactions catalyzed by purine nucleoside phosphorylase favor the direction of nucleoside synthesis, cellular concentrations of free purine base and ribose 1-phosphate are too low to support nucleoside synthesis under normal conditions. The main function of the enzyme is the degradative rather than synthetic pathway. Deficiencies in adenosine deaminase and purine nucleoside phosphorylase have been correlated with disease states in humans. Adenosine deaminase deficiency is associated with **severe combined immunodeficiency,** and purine nucleoside phosphorylase deficiency with a defective **T-cell immunity** but normal B-cell immunity (see Clin. Corr. 12.3).

Formation of Uric Acid

As seen in Figure 12.16, adenine nucleotides end up as hypoxanthine while guanine nucleotides are metabolized to xanthine. These purines are metabolized by **xanthine oxidase** to form **uric acid,** a unique end product of purine nucleotide degradation in humans. The reactions are as follows:

Hypoxanthine —xanthine oxidase (O_2 → H_2O_2)→ Xanthine —xanthine oxidase (O_2 → H_2O_2)→ Uric acid

Xanthine oxidase is an enzyme that contains FAD, Fe, and Mo and requires molecular oxygen as a substrate. Since uric acid is not very soluble in aqueous medium, there are clinical conditions in which elevated levels of uric acid result in deposition of sodium urate crystals primarily in joints (see Clin. Corr. 12.1).

12.5 ■ METABOLISM OF PYRIMIDINE NUCLEOTIDES

The pyrimidine ring is synthesized *de novo* in mammalian cells utilizing amino acids as carbon and nitrogen donors and CO_2 as a carbon donor. *De novo* synthesis of pyrimidine nucleotide leads to **uridine 5′-monophosphate** (UMP) in six metabolic steps. ATP hydrolysis (or equivalent) is required to drive several steps in the pathway.

CLINICAL CORRELATION 12.3

Immunodeficiency Diseases Associated with Defects in Purine Nucleoside Degradation

Two distinct immunodeficiency diseases are associated with defects in adenosine deaminase (ADA) and purine nucleoside phosphorylase (PNP), respectively. These enzymes are involved in the degradative pathways leading to formation of uric acid. Substrates for adenosine deaminase are adenosine and deoxyadenosine, while substrates for purine nucleoside phosphorylase are inosine, guanosine, deoxyinosine, and deoxyguanosine. A deficiency in ADA is associated with a severe combined immunodeficiency involving both T-cell and B-cell functions. PNP deficiency is associated with an immunodeficiency involving T-cell functions with the sparing of effects on B-cell function. In neither case is the mechanism(s) by which the lack of these enzymes leads to immune dysfunction known. However, in ADA-deficient patients, intracellular concentrations of dATP and *S*-adenosylhomocysteine are greatly increased. Several hypotheses have been put forth to explain the biochemical consequences of a lack of ADA: (1) high levels of dATP inhibit ribonucleotide reductase activity and as a consequence inhibit DNA synthesis; (2) deoxyadenosine inactivates *S*-adenosyl homocysteine hydrolase, leading to decreased *S*-adenosylmethionine required for methylation of bases in RNA and DNA; and (3) increased levels of adenosine result in increased cAMP levels. It is possible that each of these mechanisms contributes to the overall effect of immune dysfunction. There is not, however, a suitable explanation for the specificity of the effects on only T cells and B cells.

Treatment of children with ADA deficiency have included blood transfusions, bone marrow transplantation, enzyme replacement therapy with ADA–polyethylene glycol (ADA–PEG), and, most recently, gene therapy. Each of these treatments has disadvantages. Blood transfusions produce problems of "iron overload" and safety of the source. Bone marrow transplantation, while curative, requires a suitably matched donor. Enzyme replacement therapy with ADA–PEG has been the most successful to date, but the treatment requires constant monitoring of ADA levels and frequent injections of ADA–PEG, and there is considerable cost involved for the ADA–PEG. Gene therapy presents the hope for the future. While it has not been unequivocally established that gene therapy is curative, there are strong indications in early gene therapy trials that the ADA gene has been successfully transfected into stem cells of ADA-deficient children.

Cournoyer, D., and Caskey, C. T. Gene therapy of the immune system. *Annu. Rev. Immunol.* 11:297, 1993; Hershfield, M. S. PEG-ADA: an alternative to haploidentical bone marrow transplantation and an adjunct to gene therapy for adenosine deaminase deficiency. *Hum. Mutat.* 5:107, 1995; Hershfield, M. S., and Mitchell, B. S. Immunodeficiency diseases caused by adenosine deaminase deficiency and purine nucleoside phosphorylase deficiency. In: C. R. Scriver, A. L. Beaudet, W. S. Sly, and D. Valle (Eds.), *The Metabolic and Molecular Bases of Inherited Disease,* 7th ed., Vol. II, Chap. 52. New York: McGraw-Hill, 1995, pp. 1725–1768; Hoogerbrugge, P. M., von Beusechem, V. W., Kaptein, L. C., Einerhard, M. P., and Valerio, D. Gene therapy for adenosine deaminase deficiency. *Br. Med. Bull.* 51:72, 1995; Markert, M. L. Molecular basis for adenosine deaminase deficiency. *Immunodeficiency* 5:141, 1994; and Markert, M. L. Purine nucleoside phosphorylase deficiency. *Immunodeficiency Rev.* 3:45, 1991.

Pyrimidine Nucleotides Are Synthesized by a Stepwise Series of Reactions to Form UMP

In contrast to *de novo* purine nucleotide synthesis, all enzymes for *de novo* synthesis of pyrimidine nucleotides are not found in the cytosol of the cell. Reactions leading to formation of UMP are shown in Figure 12.17. The following

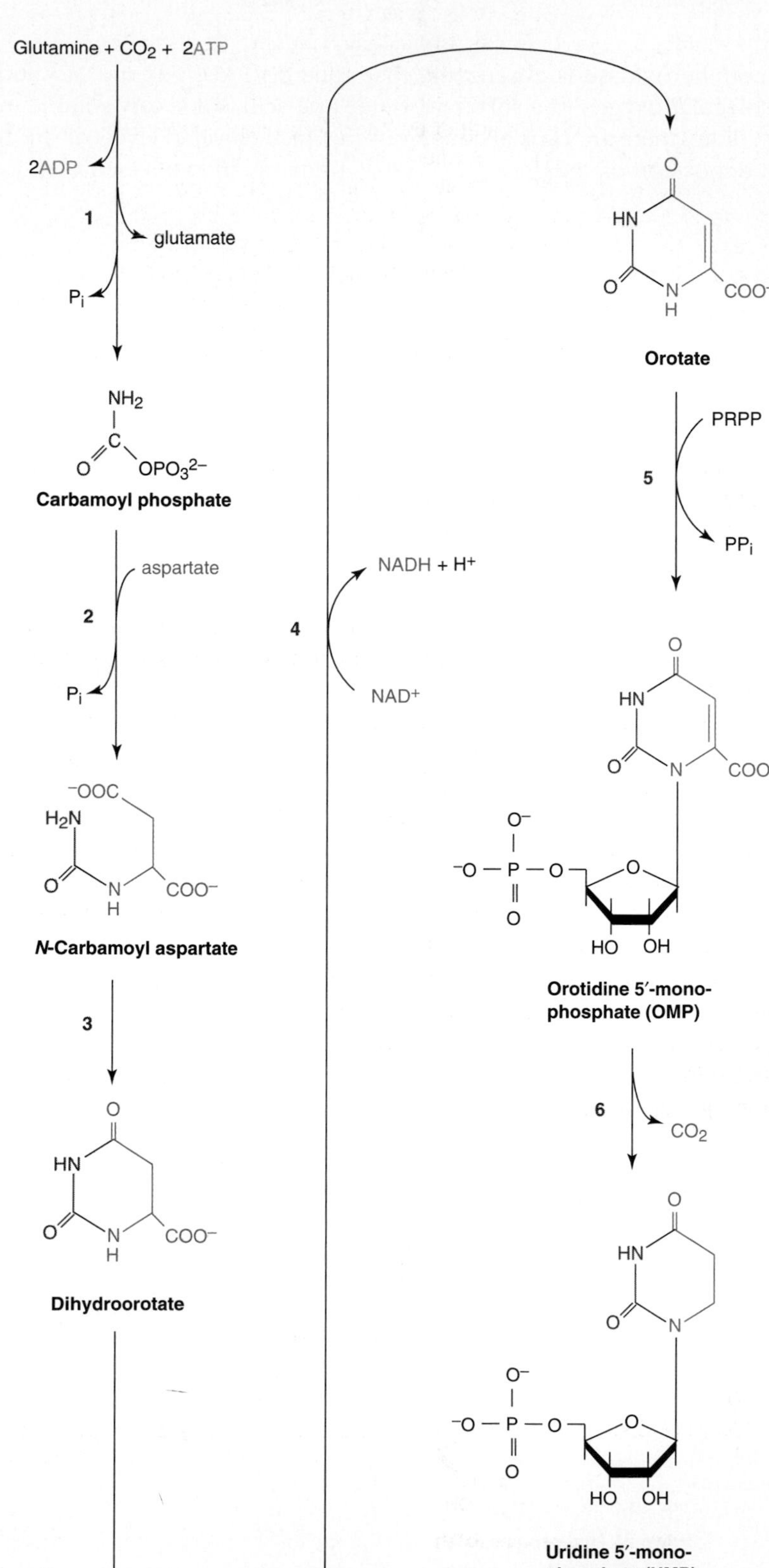

FIGURE 12.17
***De novo* synthesis of pyrimidine nucleotides.** Enzyme activities catalyzing the reactions are (1) carbamoyl phosphate synthetase II, (2) aspartate carbamoyltransferase, (3) dihydroorotase, (4) dihydroorotate dehydrogenase, (5) orotate phosphoribosyltransferase, and (6) OMP decarboxylase. The activities of (1), (2), and (3) are on a trifunctional protein (CAD); the activities of (5) and (6) are on a bifunctional protein (UMP synthase).

CLINICAL CORRELATION 12.4

Hereditary Orotic Aciduria

Hereditary orotic aciduria results from a defect in *de novo* synthesis of pyrimidine nucleotides. This genetic disease is characterized by severe anemia, growth retardation, and high levels of orotic acid excretion. The biochemical basis for this orotic aciduria is a defect in one or both of the activities (orotate phosphoribosyltransferase or orotidine decarboxylase) associated with UMP synthase, the bifunctional protein. It is a very rare disease (only 15 patients are known) but the understanding of the metabolic basis for this disease has led to successful treatment of the disorder. Patients are fed uridine, which leads not only to reversal of the hematologic problem but also to decreased formation of orotic acid. Uridine is taken up by cells and converted by uridine phosphotransferase to UMP that is converted to UDP and then to UTP. UTP formed from exogenous uridine, in turn, inhibits carbamoyl phosphate synthetase II, the major regulated step in the *de novo* pathway. As a result, orotic acid via the *de novo* pathway is markedly decreased to essentially normal levels. UTP is also a substrate for CTP synthesis. In effect, then, exogenous uridine bypasses the defective UMP synthase and supplies cells with UTP and CTP required for nucleic acid synthesis and other cellular functions. The success of treatment of hereditary orotic aciduria with uridine provides *in vivo* data regarding the importance of the carbamoyl phosphate synthase step as the site of regulation of pyrimidine nucleotide synthesis in humans.

Webster, D. R., Becroft, D. M. O., and Suttle, D. P. Hereditary orotic aciduria and other disorders of pyrimidine metabolism. In: C. R. Scriver, A. L. Beaudet, W. S. Sly, and D. Valle (Eds.), *The Metabolic and Molecular Bases of Inherited Disease,* 7th ed., Vol. II, Chap. 55. New York: McGraw-Hill, 1995, pp. 1799–1837.

important aspects of the pathway should be noted. The pyrimidine ring is formed first and then ribose 5-phosphate is added via PRPP. The enzyme catalyzing formation of carbamoyl phosphate, **carbamoyl phosphate synthetase II,** is cytosolic and is distinctly different from **carbamoyl phosphate synthetase I** found in the mitochondria as part of the urea cycle. Synthesis of *N*-carbamoylaspartate is the committed step in pyrimidine nucleotide synthesis but formation of cytosolic carbamoyl phosphate is the regulated step. Formation of **orotate** from dihydroorotate is catalyzed by a mitochondrial enzyme. Other enzymes of the pathway are found in the cytosol on multifunctional proteins. The enzyme activities of carbamoyl phosphate synthetase II, aspartate carbamoyl-transferase, and dihydroorotase are found on a trifunctional protein (CAD), and orotate phosphoribosyltransferase and OMP decarboxylase activities are found on a bifunctional protein, defined as UMP synthase. A defect in this bifunctional protein that affects either phosphoribosyltransferase activity or decarboxylase activity leads to a rare clinical condition known as hereditary orotic aciduria (see Clin. Corr. 12.4).

This series of reactions produces UMP. Other major pyrimidine nucleotides found in cells are cytidine nucleotides, which are formed from UTP; UMP is converted to UTP by **nucleotide diphosphokinase** (Figure 12.18). **CTP synthetase** catalyzes formation of CTP from UTP with glutamine being the amino group donor (Figure 12.19). CTP synthetase displays homotropic sigmoi-

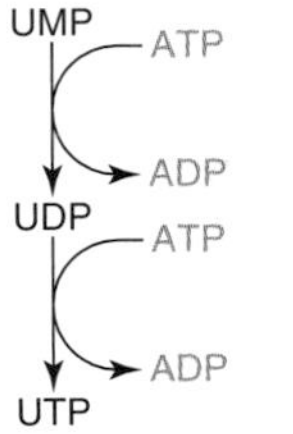

FIGURE 12.18
Formation of UTP from UMP.

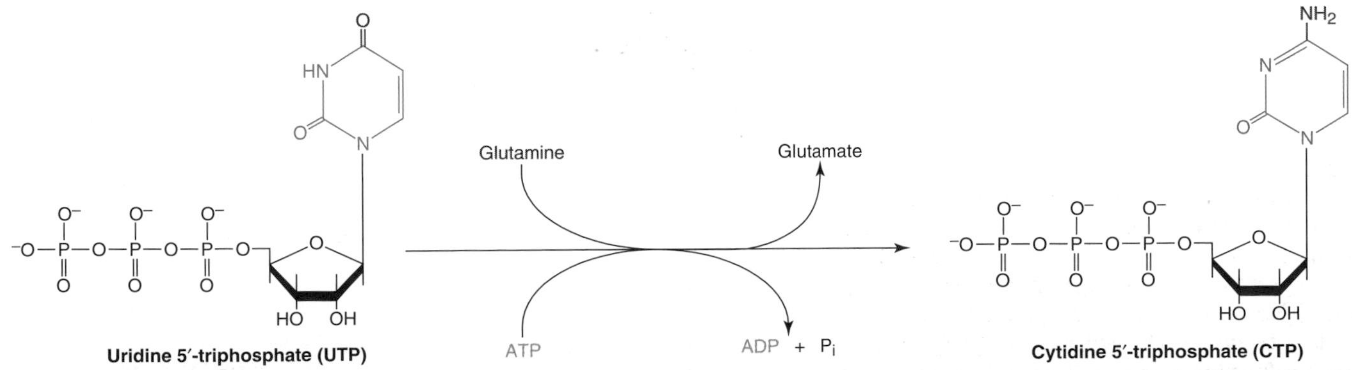

FIGURE 12.19
Formation of CTP from UTP catalyzed by CTP synthetase.

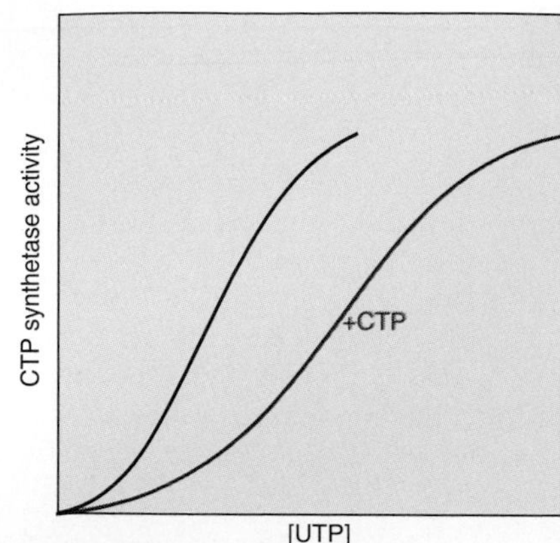

FIGURE 12.20
Regulation of CTP synthetase.

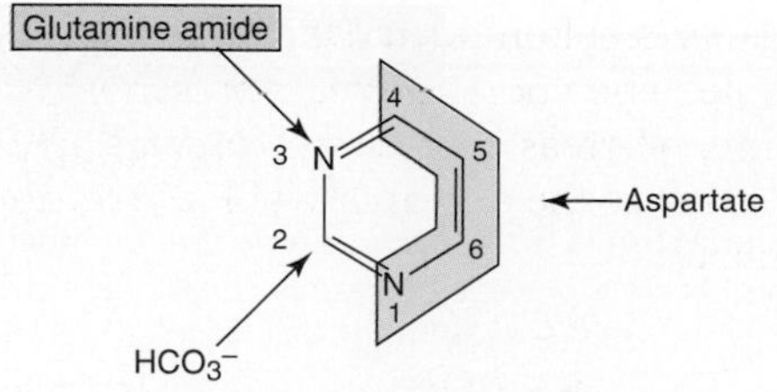

FIGURE 12.21
Sources of carbon and nitrogen atoms in pyrimidines.
C-4, C-5, and C-6, and N-1 are from aspartate; N-3 is from glutamine; and C-2 from CO_2.

dal kinetics; CTP, the product, is a negative effector of the reaction as shown in Figure 12.20.

To summarize, *de novo* synthesis of pyrimidine nucleotides requires aspartate and glutamine as carbon and nitrogen donors and CO_2 as a carbon donor (Figure 12.21). Five of the six reactions in the pathway take place in the cytosol of the cell, while the other reaction occurs in the mitochondria. The enzyme activities involved with the cytosolic reactions reside on multifunctional proteins. UTP is the direct precursor of CTP.

Pyrimidine Nucleotide Synthesis in Humans Is Regulated at the Level of Carbamoyl Phosphate Synthetase II

Regulation of pyrimidine nucleotide synthesis in mammalian cells occurs at the carbamoyl phosphate synthetase II step. As mentioned earlier, carbamoyl phosphate synthetase II is a cytosolic enzyme and distinct from carbamoyl phosphate synthetase I, which is mitochondrial, utilizes ammonia as the amino donor, and is activated by *N*-acetylglutamate. Carbamoyl phosphate synthetase II is inhibited by UTP, an end product of the pathway, and is activated by PRPP. K_i for UTP and K_a for PRPP are in the range of values that would allow intracellular levels of UTP and PRPP to have an effect on the control of pyrimidine nucleotide synthesis. Carbamoyl phosphate synthetase II is the only source of carbamoyl phosphate in extrahepatic tissues. However, in liver, under stressed conditions in which there is excess ammonia, carbamoyl phosphate synthetase I can generate carbamoyl phosphate in mitochondria, which ends up in the cytosol and serves as a substrate for pyrimidine nucleotide synthesis. This pathway serves to detoxify excess ammonia. Elevated levels of orotic acid are excreted as a result of ammonia toxicity in humans. This points to carbamoyl phosphate synthetase II as being the major regulated activity in pyrimidine nucleotide metabolism.

UMP does not inhibit carbamoyl phosphate synthetase II activity but does compete with OMP to inhibit the **OMP decarboxylase** (Figure 12.22). As discussed earlier, conversion of UTP to CTP is also regulated so that cells can maintain a balance between uridine and cytidine nucleotides.

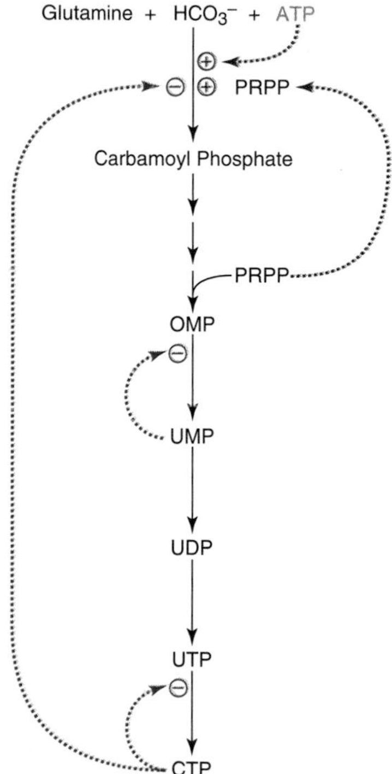

FIGURE 12.22
Regulation of pyrimidine nucleotide synthesis.
Solid arrows represent enzyme catalyzed reactions and dashed arrows represent activation ⊕ and inhibition ⊖.

Pyrimidine Bases Are Salvaged to Reform Nucleotides

Pyrimidines are "salvaged" by conversion to the nucleotide level by reactions involving **pyrimidine phosphoribosyltransferase.** The general reaction is

$$\text{Pyrimidine} + \text{PRPP} \rightarrow \text{pyrimidine nucleoside 5}'\text{-monophosphate} + \text{PP}_i$$

The enzyme from human erythrocytes can utilize orotate, uracil, and thymine as substrates but not cytosine. These salvage pathways divert the pyrimidine base from the degradative pathway to the nucleotide level for cellular utilization. As a pyrimidine base becomes available to cells, there are competing reactions that will either result in degradation and excretion or reutilization of the bases. For example, when normal liver is presented with uracil, it is rapidly degraded to β-alanine, whereas proliferating tumor cells would convert uracil to UMP. This is the result of the availability of PRPP, enzyme levels, and metabolic state of the animal.

12.6 ■ DEOXYRIBONUCLEOTIDE FORMATION

As indicated previously, the concentrations of **deoxyribonucleotides** are extremely low in nonproliferating cells. Only at the time of DNA replication (S phase) does the deoxyribonucleotide pool increase to support the required DNA synthesis.

Deoxyribonucleotides Are Formed by Reduction of Ribonucleoside Diphosphates

Nucleoside 5′-diphosphate reductase (ribonucleotide reductase) catalyzes the reaction in which 2′-deoxyribonucleotides are synthesized from the corresponding ribonucleoside 5′-diphosphate. The reaction is controlled not only by the amount of enzyme present in cells but also by a very finely regulated allosteric control mechanism. The reaction can be summarized as shown in Figure 12.23. Reduction of a particular substrate requires the presence of a specific nucleoside 5′-triphosphate as a positive effector. For example, reduction of CDP or UDP requires ATP as the positive effector, while reduction of ADP and GDP require the presence of dGTP and dTTP, respectively. A small molecular weight protein, **thioredoxin** or **glutaredoxin,** is involved in reduction at the 2′ position through oxidation of its sulfhydryl groups. To complete the catalytic cycle, NADPH is used to regenerate free sulfhydryl groups on the protein. **Thioredoxin reductase,** a flavoprotein, is required if thioredoxin is involved; glutathione and **glutathione reductase** are involved if glutaredoxin is the protein.

Mammalian ribonucleotide reductase consists of two nonidentical protein subunits (heterodimer), neither of which alone has enzymatic activity. The larger subunit has at least two different effector-binding sites. The smaller subunit contains a nonheme iron and a stable tyrosyl free radical. The two subunits make up the active site of the enzyme. The two subunits are encoded by different genes on separate chromosomes. The mRNAs for these subunits, and consequently the proteins, are differentially expressed as cells transit the cell cycle.

As mentioned earlier, the activity of ribonucleotide reductase is under allosteric control. While reduction of each substrate requires the presence of a specific positive effector, the products serve as potent negative effectors of the enzyme. DeoxyATP is a potent inhibitor of the reduction of all four substrates: CDP, UDP, GDP, and ADP; dGTP inhibits reduction of CDP, UDP, and GDP; dTTP inhibits reduction of CDP, UDP, and ADP. From this it is seen that dGTP

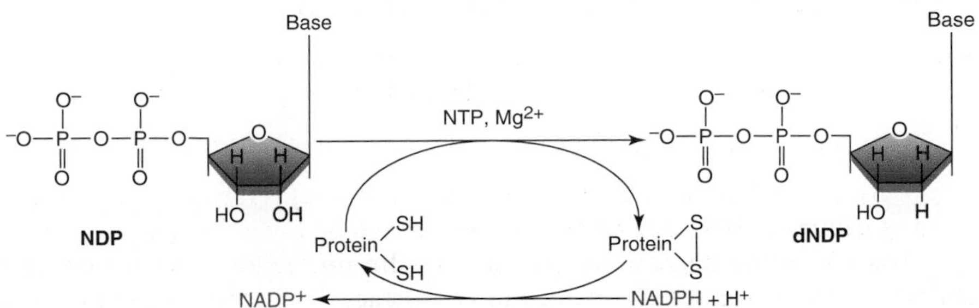

FIGURE 12.23
***De novo* synthesis of 2′-deoxyribonucleotides from ribonucleotides. This reaction is catalyzed by ribonucleotide reductase.**

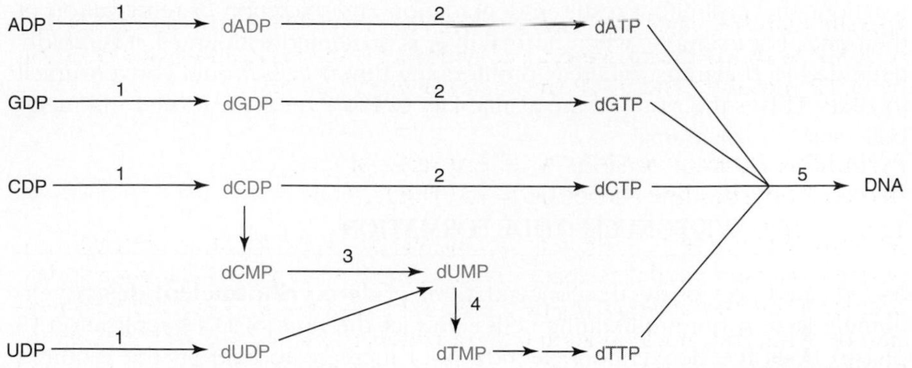

ADP →(1) dADP →(2) dATP
GDP →(1) dGDP →(2) dGTP
CDP →(1) dCDP →(2) dCTP →(5) DNA
dCDP → dCMP →(3) dUMP
UDP →(1) dUDP → dUMP →(4) dTMP → → dTTP

FIGURE 12.24
Role of ribonucleotide reductase in DNA synthesis.
The enzymes catalyzing the reactions are (1) ribonucleotide reductase, (2) nucleoside 5′-diphosphate kinase, (3) deoxycytidylate deaminase, (4) thymidylate synthase, and (5) DNA polymerase.

and dTTP can serve as either positive or negative effectors of ribonucleotide reductase. Effective inhibition of ribonucleotide reductase by dATP, dGTP, or dTTP explains the toxicity of deoxyadenosine, deoxyguanosine, and thymidine to a variety of mammalian cells.

Ribonucleotide reductase is uniquely responsible for catalyzing the rate-limiting reactions by which 2′-deoxyribonucleoside 5′-triphosphates are synthesized *de novo* for DNA replication as summarized in Figure 12.24. Effective inhibitors of ribonucleotide reductase are potent inhibitors of DNA synthesis and hence of cell replication.

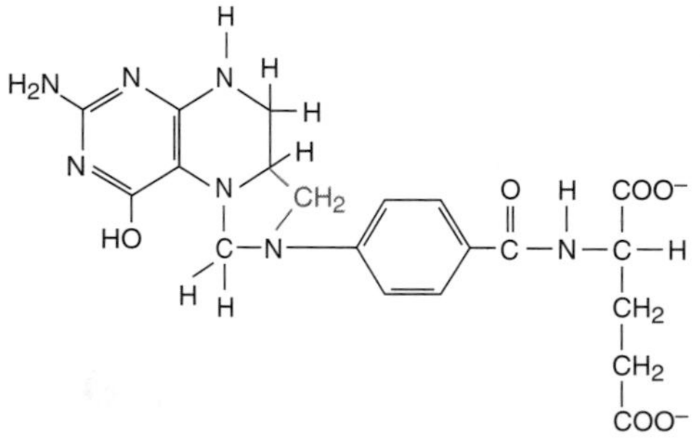

FIGURE 12.25
Structure of N^5,N^{10}-methylene H_4folate.

Deoxythymidylate Synthesis Requires N^5,N^{10}-Methylene H_4Folate

Deoxythymidylate (dTMP) is formed from 2′-deoxyuridine 5′-monophosphate (dUMP) in a reaction that is unique. **Thymidylate synthase** catalyzes the reaction in which a one-carbon unit from N^5,N^{10}-methylene H_4folate (Figure 12.25) is transferred to dUMP and simultaneously reduced to a methyl group. The reaction is presented in Figure 12.26. In this reaction, N^5,N^{10}-methylene H_4folate serves as the one-carbon donor and as a reducing agent. This is the only reaction in which H_4folate, acting as a one-carbon carrier, is oxidized to H_2folate. There are no known regulatory mechanisms for this reaction.

The substrate for this reaction can come from two different pathways as shown below:

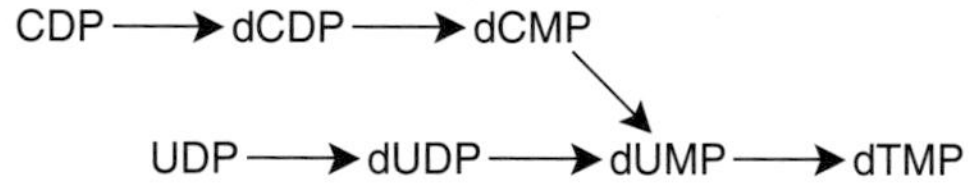

CDP → dCDP → dCMP
dCMP → dUMP
UDP → dUDP → dUMP → dTMP

In both pathways deoxyribonucleotides, dCDP or dUDP, are generated by ribonucleotide reductase. In one pathway, dUMP is generated from dUDP while in the other pathway, dCMP is deaminated to dUMP. From labeling studies it

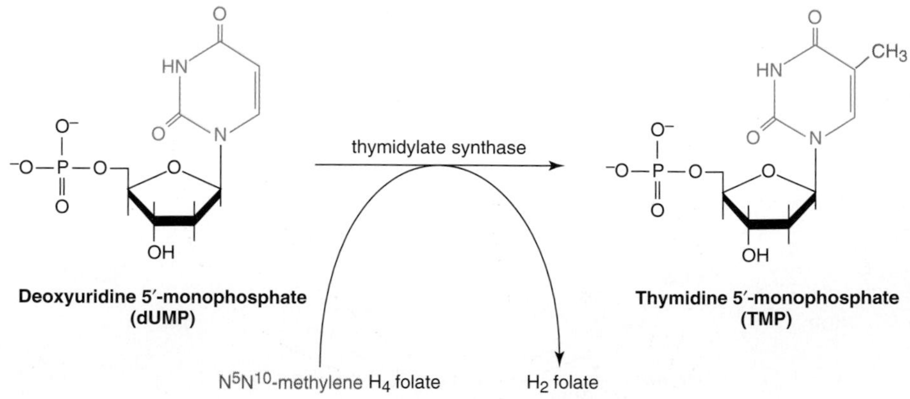

thymidylate synthase

Deoxyuridine 5′-monophosphate (dUMP)

Thymidine 5′-monophosphate (TMP)

N^5N^{10}-methylene H_4 folate → H_2 folate

FIGURE 12.26
Synthesis of deoxythymidine nucleotide.

appears that the major pathway for formation of dUMP involves deamination of dCMP by **dCMP deaminase,** an enzyme that is subject to allosteric regulation by dCTP (positive) and dTTP (negative) (Figure 12.27).

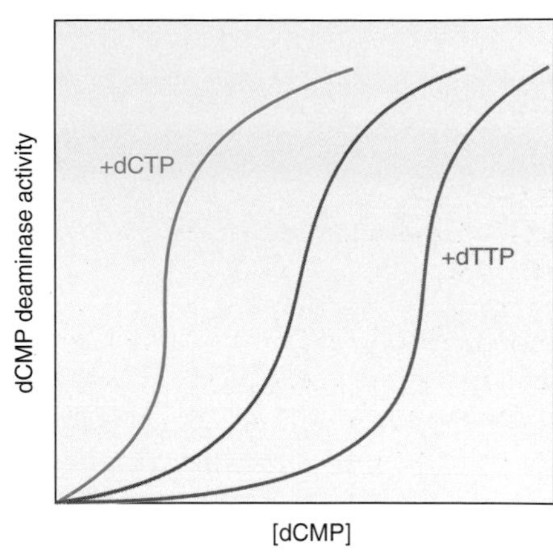

FIGURE 12.27
Regulation of dCMP deaminase.

Pyrimidine Interconversions with Emphasis on Deoxyribopyrimidine Nucleosides and Nucleotides

As shown in Section 12.4, there are metabolic pathways for interconversions of purine nucleotides and these pathways are regulated to maintain an appropriate balance of adenine and guanine nucleotides. Pathways also exist for interconversion of pyrimidine nucleotides and these pathways are of particular importance for pyrimidine deoxyribonucleosides and deoxyribonucleotide as summarized in Figure 12.28. Note that dCTP and dTTP are major positive and negative effectors of the interconversions and salvage of deoxyribonucleosides.

Pyrimidine Nucleotides Are Degraded to β-Amino Acids

Turnover of nucleic acids results in release of pyrimidine nucleotides and purine nucleotides (discussed previously). Degradation of pyrimidine nucleotides follows the pathways shown in Figure 12.29. In these degradative pathways the pyrimidine nucleotides are converted to nucleosides by nonspecific phosphatases. Cytidine and deoxycytidine are deaminated to uridine and deoxyuridine by pyrimidine **nucleoside deaminase. Uridine phosphorylase** catalyzes phosphorolysis of uridine, deoxyuridine, and thymidine resulting in formation of uracil and thymine as pyrimidine base products.

Uracil and thymine are then further degraded by analogous reactions, although the final products are different as shown in Figure 12.30. Uracil is degraded to β-alanine, NH_4^+, and CO_2. None of these products is unique to uracil degradation, and consequently the turnover of cytosine or uracil nucleotides cannot be estimated from the end products of this pathway. Thymine degradation proceeds to ***β*-aminoisobutyric acid,** NH_4^+, and CO_2. β-Aminoisobutyric acid is excreted in urine of humans and originates exclusively from degradation of thymine. Thus it is possible to estimate the turnover of DNA or thymidine nucleotides by measurement of β-aminoisobutyric acid excretion. Increased levels of β-aminoisobutyric acid are excreted in cancer patients undergoing chemotherapy or radiation therapy in which large numbers of cells are killed and DNA is degraded.

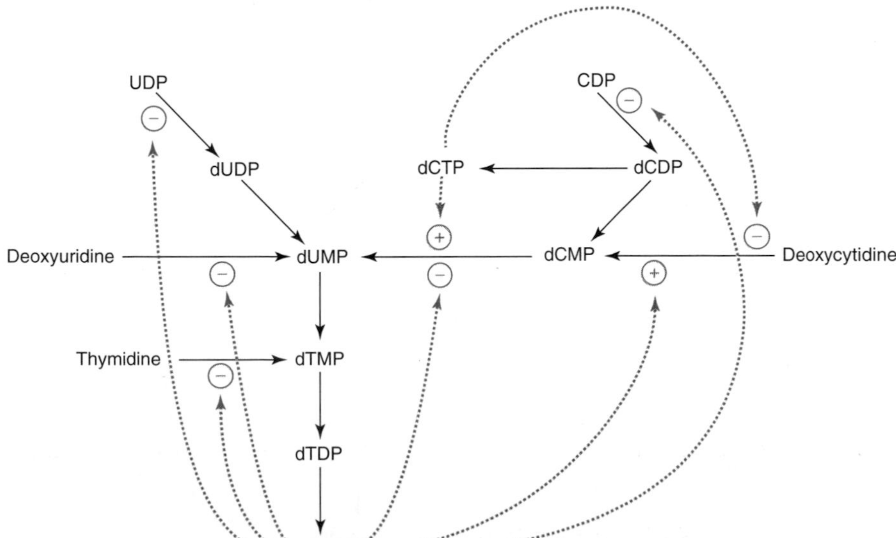

FIGURE 12.28
Interconversions of pyrimidine nucleotides with emphasis on deoxyribonucleotide metabolism.
The solid arrows indicate enzyme-catalyzed reactions; the dashed lines represent sites of activation ⊕ or inhibition ⊖.

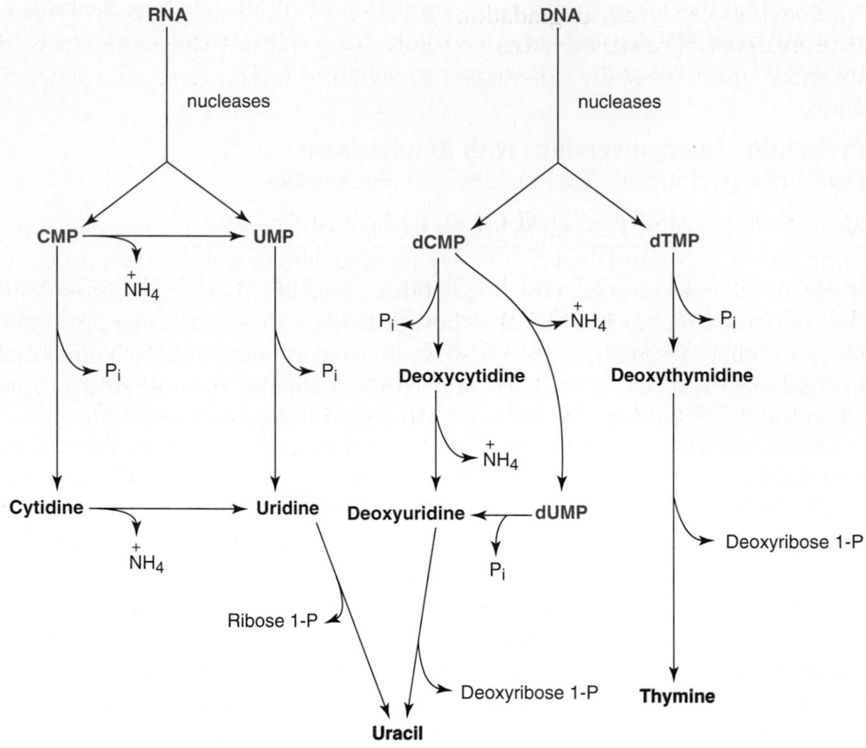

FIGURE 12.29
Pathways for degradation of pyrimidine nucleotides.

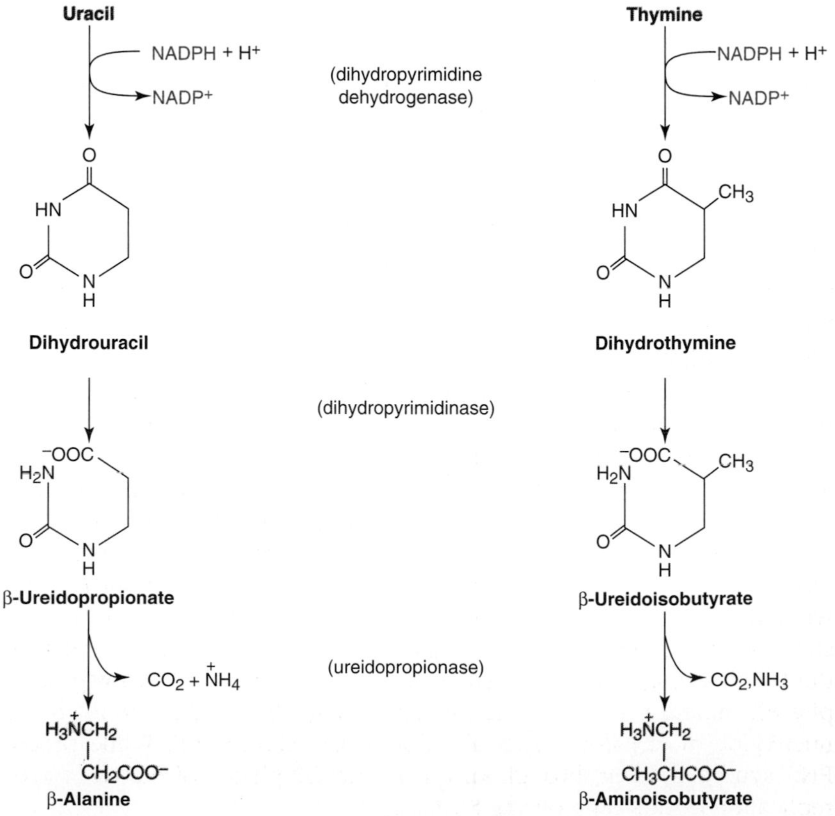

Uracil | **Thymine**

$NADPH + H^+$ → $NADP^+$ (dihydropyrimidine dehydrogenase)

Dihydrouracil | **Dihydrothymine**

(dihydropyrimidinase)

β-Ureidopropionate | **β-Ureidoisobutyrate**

(ureidopropionase)

$CO_2 + \overset{+}{N}H_4$ | CO_2, NH_3

$H_3\overset{+}{N}CH_2-CH_2COO^-$ **β-Alanine** | $H_3\overset{+}{N}CH_2-CH_3CHCOO^-$ **β-Aminoisobutyrate**

FIGURE 12.30
Degradation of uracil and thymine to end products.

Enzymes catalyzing degradation of uracil and thymine (**dihydropyrimidine dehydrogenase, dihydropyrimidinase,** and **uriedopropionase**) do not show a preference for either uracil or thymine or their degradative intermediates.

12.7 NUCLEOSIDE AND NUCLEOTIDE KINASES

As shown in Figures 12.7 and 12.17, *de novo* synthesis of both purines and pyrimidine nucleotides yields nucleoside 5′-monophosphates. Cells contain specific nucleoside kinases that utilize nucleosides from endogenous or exogenous sources to form nucleoside 5′-monophosphates. This is particularly important in a cell such as the red cell that cannot form nucleotides *de novo*.

In addition to nucleoside kinases, there are nucleotide kinases that convert a nucleoside 5′-monophosphate to nucleoside 5′-diphosphate and nucleoside 5′-diphosphates to nucleoside 5′-triphosphates. These are important reactions since most reactions in which nucleotides function require nucleoside 5′-triphosphate (primarily) or nucleoside 5′-diphosphate.

Nucleoside kinases show a high level of specificity with respect to the base and sugar moieties. There is also substrate specificity in nucleotide kinases. On the other hand, mammalian cells contain, in high concentration, nucleoside diphosphate kinase, which is relatively nonspecific for either phosphate donor or phosphate acceptor in terms of purine or pyrimidine base or the sugar. This reaction is as follows:

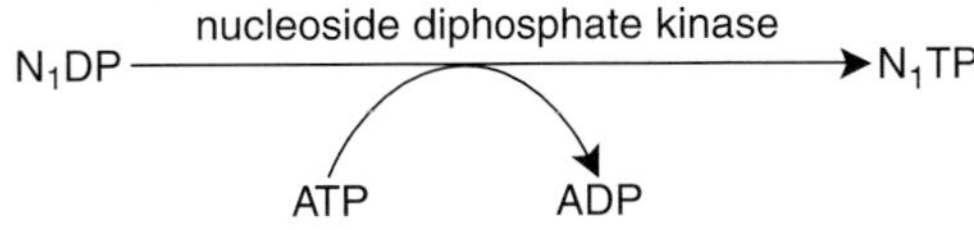

Since ATP is present in the highest concentration and most readily regenerated on a net basis via glycolysis or oxidative phosphorylation, ATP is probably the major donor for these reactions.

12.8 NUCLEOTIDE-METABOLIZING ENZYMES AS A FUNCTION OF THE CELL CYCLE AND RATE OF CELL DIVISION

For cell division to occur, essentially all of the components of cells must double. The term **cell cycle** describes the events that lead from formation of a daughter cell, as a result of mitosis, to completion of processes needed for its own division into two daughter cells. The cell cycle is represented in Figure 12.31. The phases of the cell cycle have been defined as mitosis (M), gap 1 (G1), synthesis (S) and gap 2 (G2). Some cells will enter G0, a state in which cells are viable and functional but are in a nonproliferative or quiescent phase. The total period of the cell cycle will vary with the particular cell type. In most mammalian cell types, times for the cell cycle phases of M, S, and G2 are relatively constant, while time periods for the G1 phase vary widely, causing cells to have long or short doubling times. There are many "factors" that will cause cells to leave the G0 state and reenter the cell cycle. In preparation for **DNA replication** (S phase), there are considerable increases in synthesis of enzymes involved in nucleotide metabolism, especially during late G1/early S. While protein and RNA synthesis occur throughout G1, S, and G2 phases of the cell cycle, DNA replication occurs only during S phase.

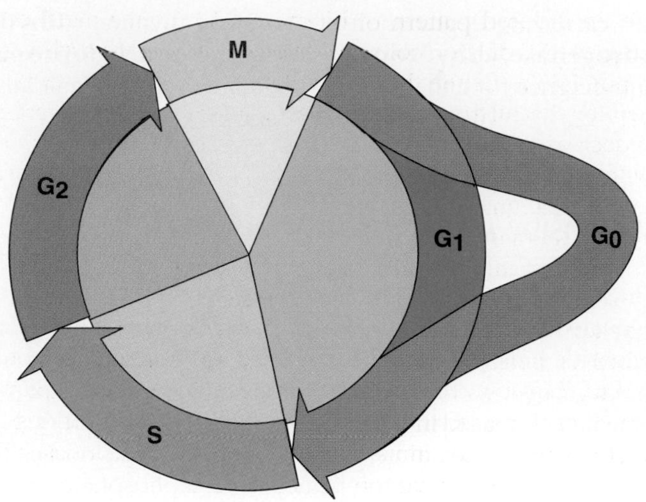

FIGURE 12.31
Diagrammatic representation of the cell cycle.
For a mammalian cell with a doubling time of 24 h, G1 would last ~12 h; S, 7 h; G2, 4 h; and M, 1 h. Cells would enter the G0 state if they became quiescent or nonproliferative.

Enzymes of Purine and Pyrimidine Nucleotide Synthesis Are Elevated During S Phase

Strict regulation of nucleotide synthesis requires that certain mechanisms must be available to the cell to meet the requirements for ribonucleotide and deoxyribonucleotide precursors at the time of increased RNA synthesis and DNA replication. To meet these needs, cells respond by increasing levels of specific enzymes involved with nucleotide formation during very specific periods of the cell cycle.

Enzymes involved in purine nucleotide synthesis and interconversions that are elevated during the S phase of the cell cycle are PRPP amidotransferase and IMP dehydrogenase. Adenylosuccinate synthetase and adenylosuccinase do not appear to increase. Enzymes involved in pyrimidine nucleotide synthesis that are elevated during the S phase of the cell cycle include aspartate carbamoyltransferase, dihydroorotase, dihydroorotate dehydrogenase, orotate phosphoribosyltransferase, and CTP synthetase. Many enzymes involved in synthesis and interconversions of deoxyribonucleotides are also elevated during the S phase of the cell cycle. Included in these enzymes are ribonucleotide reductase, thymidine kinase, dCMP deaminase, thymidylate synthase, and TMP kinase. The importance of increased levels of enzyme activities during late G1/early S phase to DNA replication is worthy of further discussion with a specific example.

As discussed previously, the deoxyribonucleotide pool is extremely small in "resting" cells (less than 1 μM). As a result of the increase in ribonucleotide reductase, deoxyribonucleotides reach levels of 10–20 μM during DNA synthesis. However, this concentration would sustain DNA synthesis for only minutes, while complete DNA replication would require hours. Consequently, levels of ribonucleotide reductase activity not only must increase but must be sustained during S phase in order to provide the necessary substrates for DNA synthesis.

If we look at a population of cells (i.e., tissue) rather than individual cells going through the cell cycle, we observe that rapidly growing tissues such as regenerating liver, embryonic tissues, intestinal mucosal cells, and erythropoietic cells are geared toward DNA replication and RNA synthesis. These tissues will show elevated levels of those key enzymes involved with purine and pyrimidine nucleotide synthesis and interconversions and complementary decreases in levels of enzymes that catalyze reactions in which these precursors are degraded. These changes reflect the proportion of cells in that tissue that are in S phase.

There is an ordered pattern of biochemical changes that occur in tumor cells. Utilizing a series of liver, colon, and kidney tumors of varying growth rates, it has been possible to define these biochemical changes (1) **transformation-linked** (meaning that all tumors regardless of growth rate show certain increased and certain decreased enzyme levels), (2) **progression-linked** (alterations that correlate with growth rate of tumors), and (3) **coincidental alterations** (not connected to the malignant state). As very limited examples, levels of ribonucleotide reductase, thymidylate synthase, and IMP dehydrogenase increase as a function of tumor growth rate. PRPP amidotransferase, UDP kinase, and uridine kinase are examples of enzymes whose activity is increased in all tumors, whether they are slow-growing or the most rapidly growing tumors.

Alterations in gene expression in tumor cells are not only quantitative changes in enzyme levels but also qualitative changes (isozyme shifts). While some enzymes are increased in both fast-growing normal tissue (e.g., embryonic and regenerating liver) and tumors, the total quantitative and qualitative patterns for normal and tumor tissue can be distinguished.

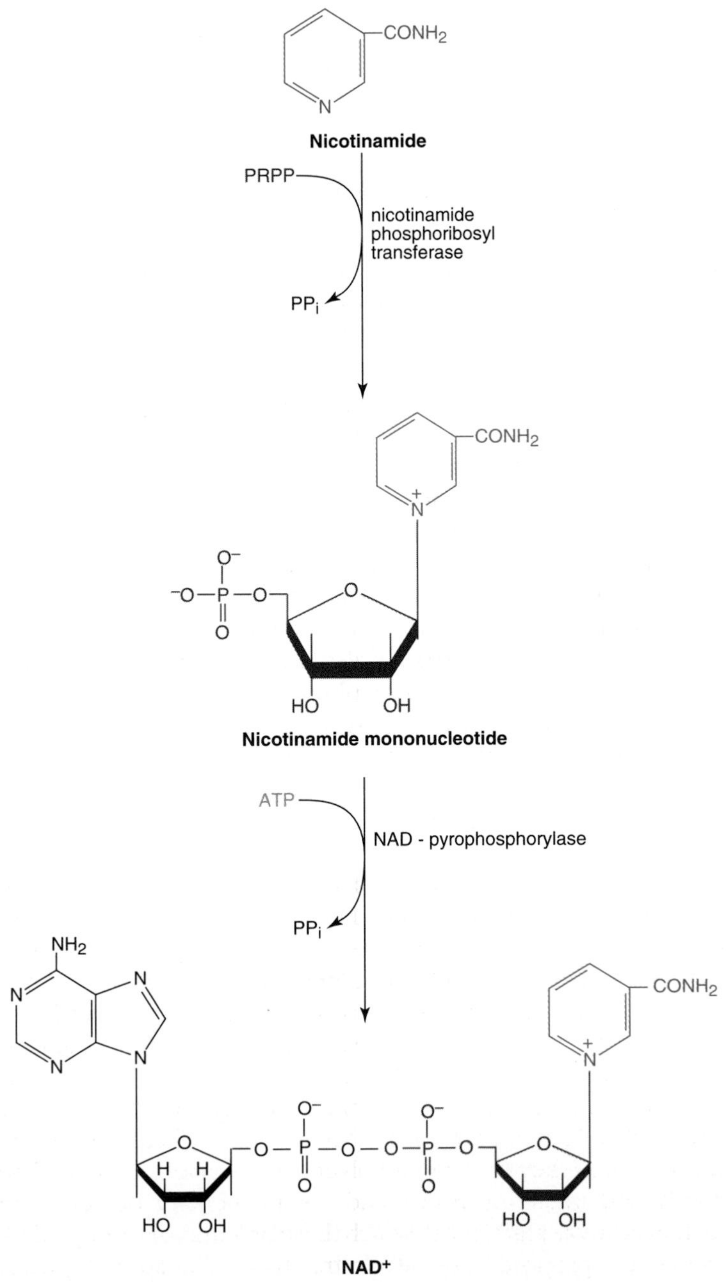

FIGURE 12.32
Pathway for NAD^+ synthesis.

12.9 ■ NUCLEOTIDE COENZYME SYNTHESIS

Nicotinamide adenine dinucleotide (NAD^+), flavin adenine nucleotide (FAD), and coenzyme A (CoA) serve as important coenzymes in intermediary metabolism. These coenzymes are synthesized by a variety of mammalian cell types. Figures 12.32 (p. 513), 12.33, and 12.34 present the biosynthetic pathways for each. NAD^+ synthesis requires niacin, FAD synthesis requires riboflavin, and CoA requires pantothenic acid. NAD can be synthesized by three different pathways starting from tryptophan (see p. 475), nicotinate, or nicotinamide. When tryptophan is in excess of the amount needed for protein synthesis and serotonin synthesis, it is used for NAD^+ synthesis. This situation is not likely in most normal diets and, consequently, niacin is required in the diet.

Each of these coenzymes has an AMP moiety as part of the molecule.

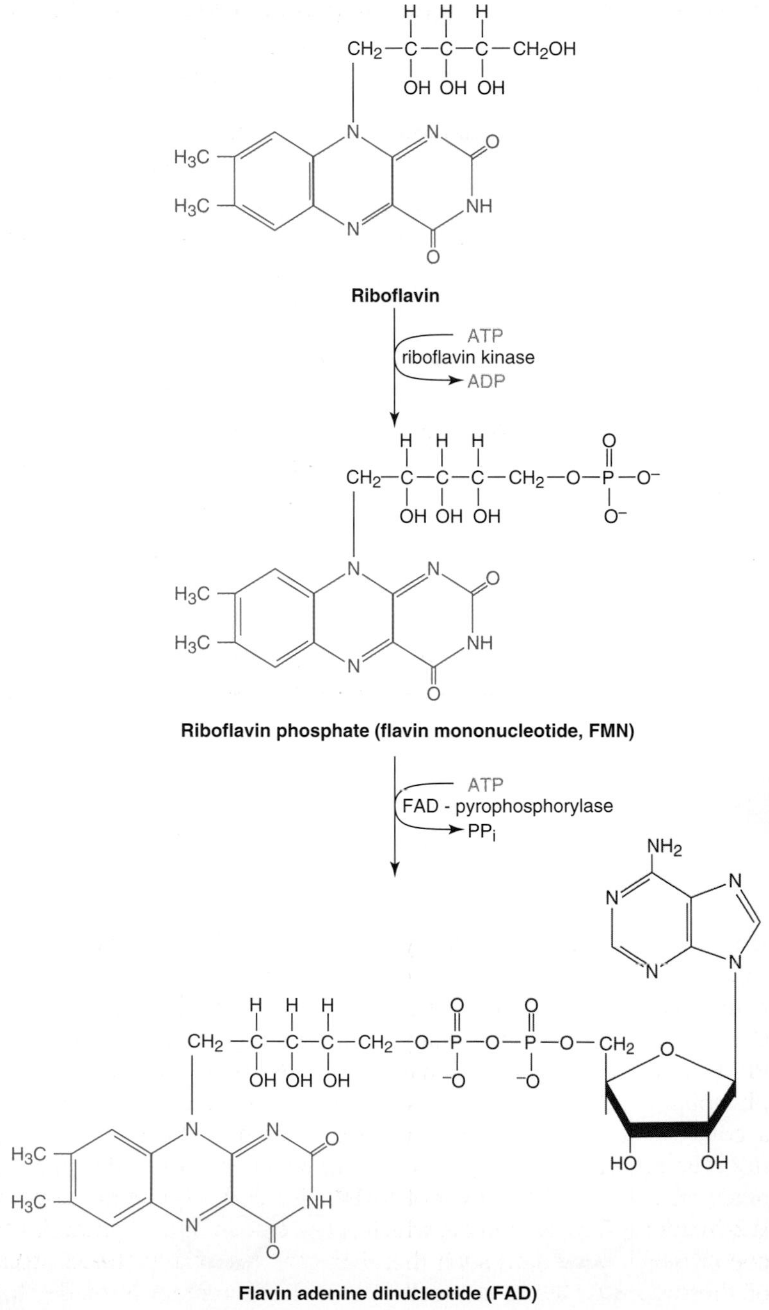

Riboflavin

ATP
riboflavin kinase
ADP

Riboflavin phosphate (flavin mononucleotide, FMN)

ATP
FAD - pyrophosphorylase
PP_i

Flavin adenine dinucleotide (FAD)

FIGURE 12.33
Synthesis of FAD.

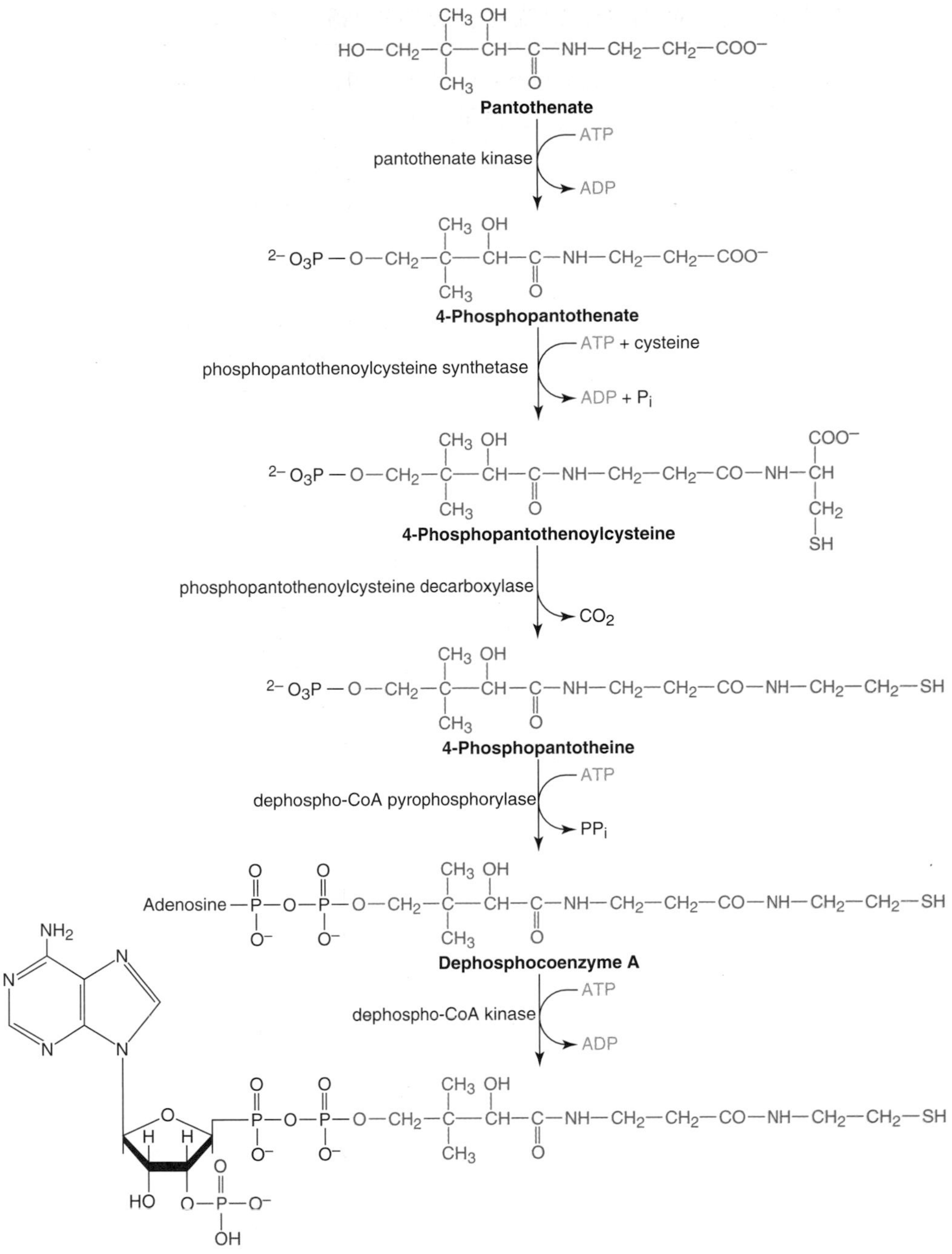

Pantothenate

pantothenate kinase (ATP → ADP)

4-Phosphopantothenate

phosphopantothenoylcysteine synthetase (ATP + cysteine → ADP + P_i)

4-Phosphopantothenoylcysteine

phosphopantothenoylcysteine decarboxylase (→ CO_2)

4-Phosphopantotheine

dephospho-CoA pyrophosphorylase (ATP → PP_i)

Dephosphocoenzyme A

dephospho-CoA kinase (ATP → ADP)

FIGURE 12.34
Synthesis of CoA.

However, the AMP is not directly involved in the functional part of the molecule since electron transfer in NAD^+ or FAD occurs via the niacin or riboflavin rings, respectively, and activation of acyl groups occurs through the —SH group of CoA. Synthesis of NAD^+ by any of the three pathways requires utilization of PRPP as the ribose 5-phosphate donor. Nicotinamide adenine dinucleotide phosphate ($NADP^+$) is synthesized from NAD^+. NAD^+ is used not only as a cofactor in oxidation–reduction reactions but also as a substrate in ADP-ribosylation reactions (e.g., DNA repair and pertussis toxin poisoning). These reactions lead to the turnover of NAD^+. The end product of NAD^+ degradation is 2-pyridone-5-carboxamide, which is excreted in urine. Synthesis of nucleotide coenzymes is regulated such that there are essentially "fixed" concentrations of these coenzymes in the cell. When the statement is made that a certain metabolic condition is favored when the concentration of NAD^+ is low, it means that the concentration of NADH is correspondingly high.

12.10 ■ SYNTHESIS AND UTILIZATION OF 5-PHOSPHORIBOSYL-1-PYROPHOSPHATE

5-Phosphoribosyl-1-pyrophosphate (PRPP) is a key molecule in *de novo* synthesis of purine and pyrimidine nucleotides, salvage of purine and pyrimidine bases, and synthesis of NAD^+. PRPP synthetase catalyzes the reaction presented in Figure 12.35. Ribose 5-phosphate used in this reaction is generated from glucose 6-phosphate metabolism via the **hexose monophosphate shunt** or from ribose 1-phosphate (generated by phosphorolysis of nucleotides) via a phosphoribomutase reaction.

The enzyme has an absolute requirement for inorganic phosphate and is strongly regulated. The v versus $[P_i]$ curve for PRPP synthetase activity is sigmoidal rather than hyperbolic, meaning that at the normal cellular concentration of P_i, the enzyme activity is depressed. The enzyme activity is further regulated by ADP, 2,3-bisphosphoglycerate, and other nucleotides. ADP serves as a competitive inhibitor of PRPP synthetase with respect to ATP; 2,3-bisphosphoglycerate is a competitive inhibitor with respect to ribose 5-phosphate; and nucleotides serve as noncompetitive inhibitors with respect to both substrates. 2,3-Bisphosphoglycerate may be important in regulating PRPP synthetase activity in red cells.

Levels of PRPP are low in "resting" or confluent cells but increase rapidly at the time of rapid cell division. Increased flux of glucose 6-phosphate through the hexose monophosphate shunt can result in increased cellular levels of PRPP and increased production of purine and pyrimidine nucleotides. PRPP is important not only because it serves as a substrate in the glutamine PRPP amidotransferase reaction and the phosphoribosyltransferase reactions, but also because it serves as a positive effector of the major regulated steps in purine and pyrimidine nucleotide synthesis, namely, PRPP amidotransferase and carbamoyl phosphate synthetase II.

Reactions and pathways in which PRPP is required are as follows:

1. *De novo* purine nucleotide synthesis

   a. PRPP + glutamine $\rightarrow$ 5-phosphoribosylamine + glutamate + PP_i

2. Salvage of purine bases

   a. PRPP + hypoxanthine (guanine) $\rightarrow$ IMP (GMP) + PP_i

   b. PRPP + adenine $\rightarrow$ AMP + PP_i

3. *De novo* pyrimidine nucleotide synthesis

   a. PRPP + orotate $\rightarrow$ OMP + PP_i

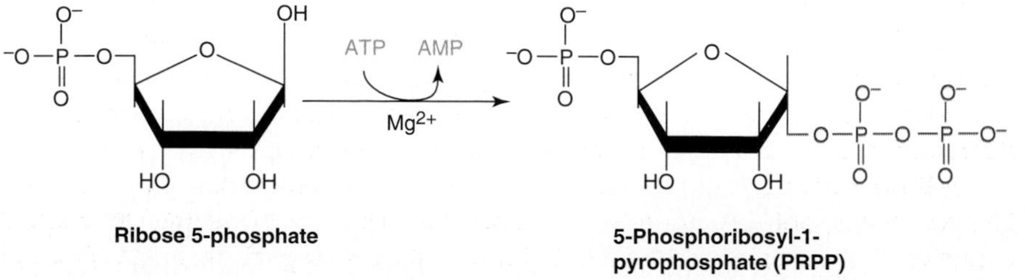

ATP AMP, Mg^{2+}

Ribose 5-phosphate → 5-Phosphoribosyl-1-pyrophosphate (PRPP)

FIGURE 12.35
Synthesis of PRPP.

4. Salvage of pyrimidine bases

a. PRPP + uracil → UMP + PP_i

5. NAD^+ synthesis

a. PRPP + nicotinate → nicotinate mononucleotide + PP_i

b. PRPP + nicotinamide → nicotinamide mononucleotide + PP_i

c. PRPP + quinolinate → nicotinate mononucleotide + PP_i

12.11 COMPOUNDS THAT INTERFERE WITH CELLULAR PURINE AND PYRIMIDINE NUCLEOTIDE METABOLISM: CHEMOTHERAPEUTIC AGENTS

De novo synthesis of purine and pyrimidine nucleotides is critical to normal cell replication, maintenance, and function. Regulation of these pathways is important since disease states arise from defects in the regulatory enzymes. Many compounds have been synthesized or isolated as natural products from plants, bacteria, or fungi that are structural analogs of the bases or nucleosides used in metabolic reactions. These compounds are relatively specific inhibitors of enzymes involved in nucleotide synthesis or interconversions and have proved to be useful in therapy of diverse clinical problems. They are generally classified as antimetabolites, antifolates, glutamine antagonists, and other compounds.

Antimetabolites Are Structural Analogs of Bases or Nucleosides

Antimetabolites, generally, are structural analogs of purine and pyrimidine bases or nucleosides that interfere with very specific metabolic sites. They include **6-mercaptopurine** and **6-thioguanine** for treatment of acute leukemia, **azathioprine** for immunosuppression in patients with organ transplants, **allopurinol** for treatment of gout and hyperuricemia, and **acyclovir** for treatment of herpesvirus infection. The detailed understanding of purine nucleotide metabolism aided in the development of these drugs. Conversely, study of the mechanism of action of these drugs has led to a better understanding of normal nucleotide metabolism in humans.

Only a few of these will be discussed to show (1) the importance of *de novo* pathways in normal cell metabolism, (2) that regulation of these pathways occurs *in vivo,* (3) the concept of the requirement for metabolic activation of the drugs, and (4) that inactivation of these compounds can greatly influence their usefulness.

6-Mercaptopurine (6-MP) (Figure 12.36) is a useful antitumor drug in humans. The cytotoxic activity of this agent is related to formation of 6-mercaptopurine ribonucleotide by the tumor cell. Utilizing PRPP and HGPRTase, 6-mercaptopurine ribonucleoside 5′-monophosphate accumulates in cells and is a negative effector of PRPP amidotransferas, the committed step in the *de novo* pathway. This nucleotide also acts as an inhibitor of the conversion of IMP to GMP at the IMP dehydrogenase step and IMP to AMP at the adenylosuccinate synthetase step. Since 6-mercaptopurine is a substrate for xanthine oxidase and is oxidized to 6-thiouric acid, allopurinol is generally administered to inhibit degradation of 6-MP and to potentiate the antitumor properties of 6-MP.

5-Fluorouracil (Fura) (Figure 12.36) is a pyrimidine analog of uracil. 5-Fluorouracil is, of itself, not the active species. It must be converted by cellular enzymes to the active metabolites 5-fluorouridine 5′-triphosphate (FUTP) and

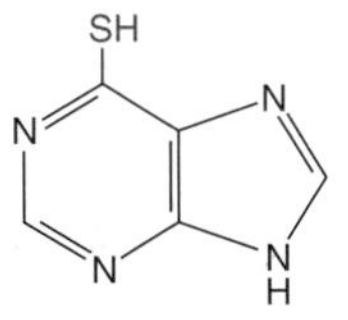

6-Mercaptopurine

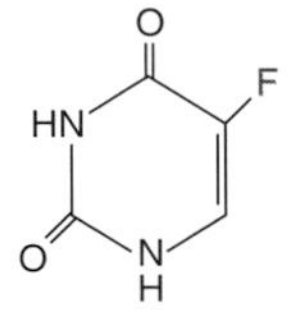

5-Fluorouracil

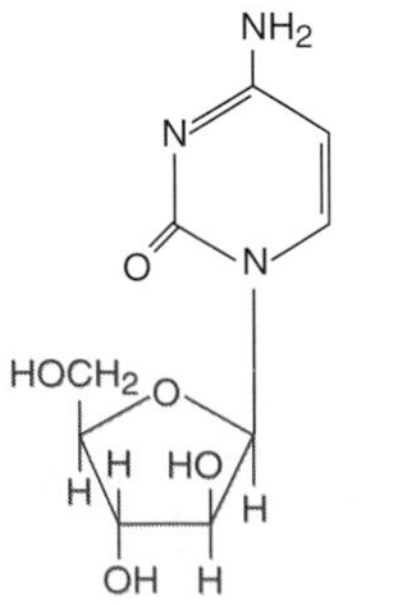

Cytosine arabinoside

FIGURE 12.36
Structures of 6-mercaptopurine, 5-fluorouracil, and cytosine arabinoside.

5-fluoro-2′-deoxyuridine 5′-monophosphate (FdUMP). FUTP is efficiently incorporated into RNA and once incorporated into RNA inhibits maturation of 45S precursor rRNA into the 28S and 18S species and alters splicing of pre-mRNA into functional mRNA. FdUMP is a potent and specific inhibitor of thymidylate synthase. In the presence of H_4folate, FdUMP, and thymidylate synthase, a ternary complex is formed that results in covalent bonding of FdUMP to thymidylate synthase. This results in inhibition of dTMP synthesis and leads, in effect, to what is called a "thymineless death" for cells.

Cytosine arabinoside (araC) (Figure 12.36) is used in treatment of several forms of human cancer. AraC must be metabolized by cellular enzymes to cytosine arabinoside 5′-triphosphate (araCTP) to exert its cytotoxic effects. AraCTP competes with dCTP in the DNA polymerase reaction and araCMP is incorporated into DNA. This results in inhibition of synthesis of the growing DNA strand. Clinically, the efficacy of araC as an antileukemic drug correlates with the concentration of araCTP that is achieved in the tumor cell, which in turn determines the level of araCMP incorporated into DNA. Formation of araCMP via deoxycytidine kinase appears to be the rate-limiting step in activation to araCTP.

Antifolates Inhibit Formation of Tetrahydrofolate

Antifolates interfere with formation of H_4folate from H_2folate or folate by inhibition of H_2folate reductase. **Methotrexate** (MTX), a close structural analog of folic acid, is used as an antitumor agent in treatment of human cancers. The comparison of the two structures is seen in Figure 12.37. Differences are at C-4 where an amino group replaces a hydroxyl group and at N-10 where a methyl group replaces a hydrogen atom. The mode of action of MTX is specific; it inhibits H_2folate reductase with a K_i in the range of 0.1 nM. The reactions inhibited are shown in Figure 12.38.

MTX at very low concentrations is cytotoxic to mammalian cells in culture. The effects can be prevented by addition of thymidine and hypoxanthine to the culture medium. Reversal of the MTX effects by thymidine and hypoxanthine indicates that MTX causes depletion of thymidine and purine nucleotides in cells. Figure 12.39 shows the relationship between H_4folate, *de novo* purine

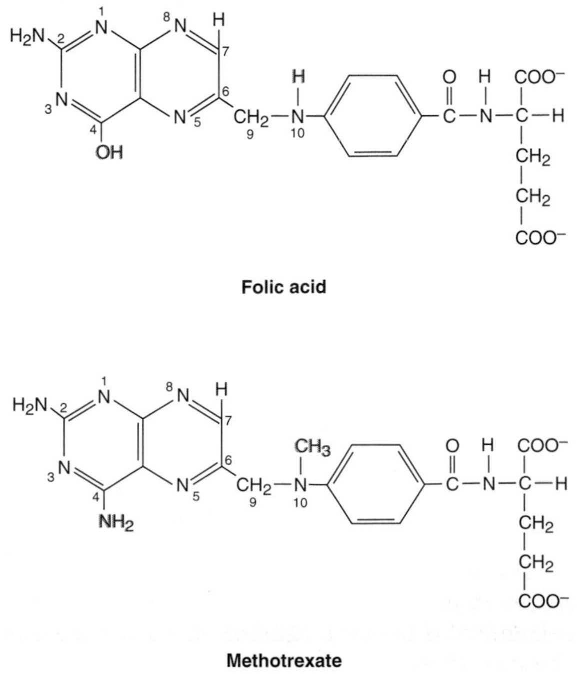

Folic acid

Methotrexate

FIGURE 12.37
Comparison of the structures of folic acid and methotrexate.

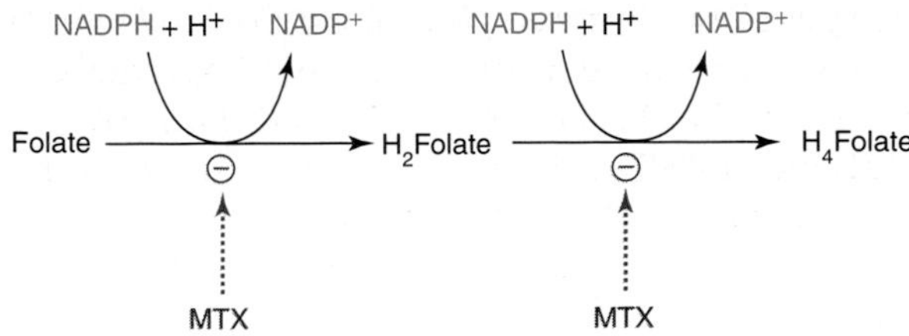

FIGURE 12.38
Sites of inhibition of methotrexate.

nucleotide synthesis, and dTMP formation. It is important to note that in the thymidylate synthase reaction, H_2folate is generated and unless it can readily be reduced back to H_4folate via dihydrofolate reductase, cells would not be capable of *de novo* synthesis of purine nucleotides or thymidylate synthesis due to depletion of H_4folate pools.

In treatment of human leukemias, normal cells can be rescued from the toxic effects of "high-dose MTX" by N^5-formyl-H_4folate **(leucovorin).** This increases the clinical efficacy of MTX treatment.

Glutamine Antagonists Inhibit Enzymes that Utilize Glutamine as Nitrogen Donors

Many reactions in mammalian cells utilize glutamine as the amino group donor. This is different from bacterial cells that primarily utilize ammonia as the amino donor in a similar reaction. These amidation reactions are critical in *de novo* synthesis of purine nucleotide (N-3 and N-9), synthesis of GMP from IMP, formation of cytosolic carbamoyl phosphate, synthesis of CTP from UTP, and synthesis of NAD^+.

Compounds that inhibit these reactions are referred to as glutamine antagonists. **Azaserine** (*O*-diazoacetyl-L-serine) and **6-diazo-5-oxo-L-norleucine** (DON) (Figure 12.40), which were first isolated from cultures of *Streptomyces,* are very effective inhibitors of enzymes that utilize glutamine as the amino donor. Since azaserine and DON inactivate the enzymes involved, addition of glutamine alone will not reverse the effects of either of these two drugs. It would necessitate that many metabolites such as guanine, cytosine, hypoxanthine (or adenine), and nicotinamide be provided to bypass the many sites blocked by these glutamine antagonists. As expected from the fact that so many key steps

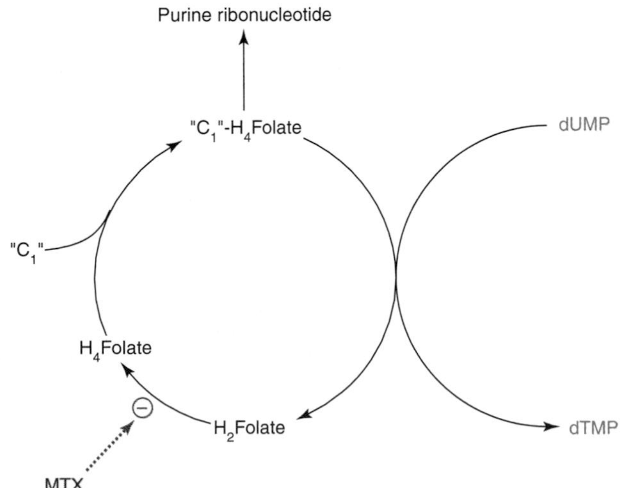

FIGURE 12.39
Relationships between H_4folate, *de novo* purine nucleotide synthesis, and dTMP synthesis.

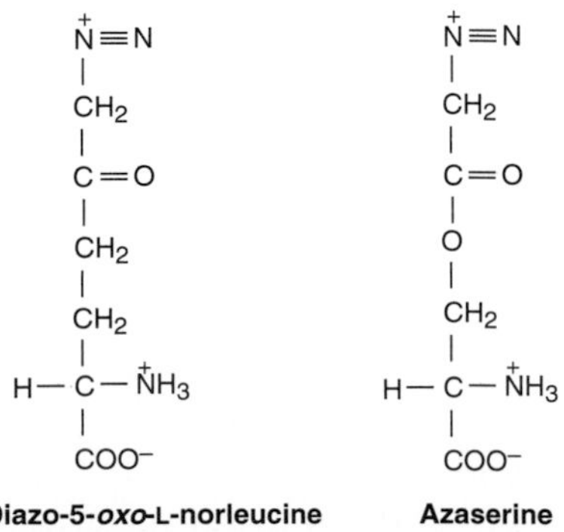

6-Diazo-5-*oxo*-L-norleucine   Azaserine

FIGURE 12.40
Structure of glutamine antagonists.

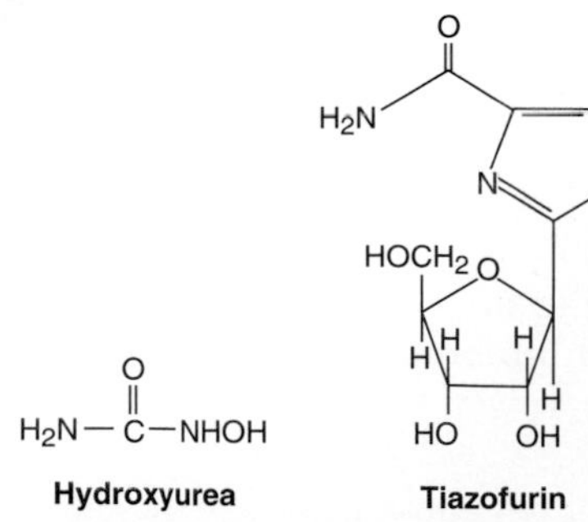

Hydroxyurea Tiazofurin

FIGURE 12.41
Structure of hydroxyurea and tiazofurin.

are inhibited by DON and azaserine, these agents are extremely toxic and not of clinical use.

Other Agents Inhibit Cell Growth by Interfering with Nucleotide Metabolism

Tumor cells treated with **hydroxyurea** (Figure 12.41) show a specific inhibition of DNA synthesis with little or no inhibition of RNA or protein synthesis. Hydroxyurea is an inhibitor of ribonucleotide reductase, blocking reduction of CDP, UDP, GDP, and ADP to the corresponding 2′-deoxyribonucleoside 5′-diphosphates. Toxicity of this drug results from depletion of 2′-deoxyribonucleoside 5′-triphosphates required for DNA replication. Although hydroxyurea is specific for inhibition of ribonucleotide reductase, its clinical use is limited because of its rapid rate of clearance and the high drug concentration required for effective inhibition.

Tiazofurin (Figure 12.41) is converted by cellular enzymes to the NAD^+ analog, **tiazofurin adenine dinucleotide** (TAD). TAD inhibits IMP dehydrogenase, the rate-limiting enzyme in GTP synthesis, with a K_i of 0.1 μM. As a result of IMP dehydrogenase inhibition, the concentration of GTP is markedly depressed.

These clinically useful drugs serve as examples in which knowledge of basic biochemical pathways and mechanisms leads to generation of effective drugs. An important point regarding many of the antimetabolites used as drugs is that they must be activated to the nucleotide level by cellular enzymes to exert their cytotoxic effects.

Purine and Pyrimidine Analogs as Antiviral Agents

Herpesvirus (HSV) and **human immunodeficiency virus** (HIV) infections (AIDS) present major clinical problems. Two antimetabolites have been identified that can be used in the control/treatment (but not cure) of HSV and HIV infections. These drugs—**acyclovir** (acycloguanosine), a purine analog, and **3′-azido-3′-deoxythymidine** (AZT), a pyrimidine analog (Figure 12.42)—require metabolism to phosphorylated compounds to yield the active drug. Acycloguanosine is activated to the monophosphate by a specific HSV–thymidine kinase, encoded by the HSV genome, which can catalyze phosphorylation of acycloguanosine. The host cellular thymidine kinase cannot utilize acyclovir as a substrate. Acycloguanosine monophosphate is then phosphorylated by the cellular enzymes to the di- and triphosphate forms. Acycloguanosine triphosphate serves as a substrate for the HSV-specific DNA polymerase and is incorporated into the growing viral DNA chain causing chain termination. The specificity of acycloguanosine and its high therapeutic index therefore reside in the fact that only HSV-infected cells can form the acycloguanosine monophosphate.

AZT is phosphorylated by cellular kinases to AZT triphosphate, which blocks HIV replication by inhibiting HIV–DNA polymerase (an RNA-dependent polymerase). The selectivity of AZT for HIV-infected versus uninfected cells occurs because DNA polymerase from HIV is at least 100-fold more sensitive to AZT triphosphate than is host cell DNA-dependent DNA polymerase.

These two antiviral agents demonstrate the diversity of responses required for selectivity. In one case, enzyme activity encoded by the viral genome is mandatory for activation of the drug (acycloguanosine); in the second example, although cellular enzymes activate the drug (AZT), the viral gene product (HIV–DNA polymerase) is the selective target.

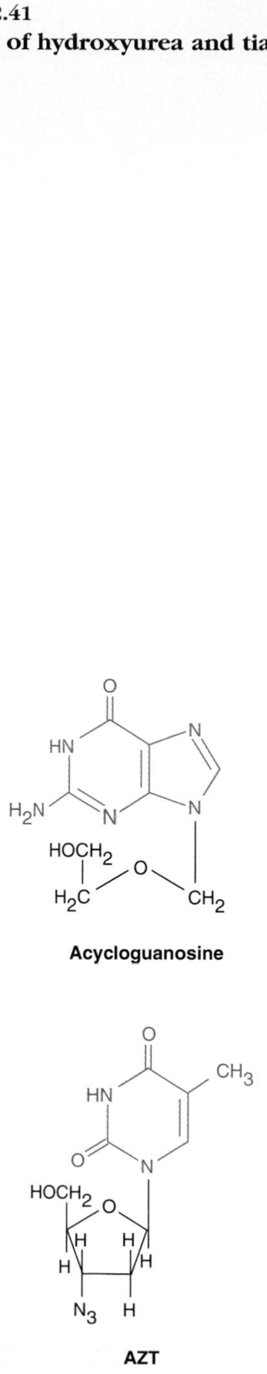

Acycloguanosine

AZT

FIGURE 12.42
Structure of the antiviral agents, acyclovir and AZT.

Biochemical Basis for Development of Drug Resistance

Failure of chemotherapy in treatment of human cancer is often related to development of tumor cell populations that are resistant to the cytotoxic effects of the particular drug. Tumors represent a very heterogenous population of cells and in many instances drug-resistant cells are present. Upon therapy, drug-sensitive cells are killed off and a resistant cell population becomes enriched. In some cases, drug treatment causes genetic alterations that result in the drug-resistant phenotype. Resistance to drugs can be categorized as "specific drug resistance" or "multidrug resistance."

Biochemical and molecular mechanisms that account for drug resistance have been determined for many drugs. For example, resistance to methotrexate can develop as a result of several different alterations. These include a defect or loss of the transporter for N^5-formyl-H_4folate and N^5-methyl-H_4folate, which results in decreased cellular uptake of MTX; amplification of the dihydrofolate reductase gene, which results in a marked increase in cellular dihydrofolate reductase, the target enzyme; alterations in the dihydrofolate reductase gene that result in a "mutant" dihydrofolate reductase that is less sensitive to inhibition by MTX; and decreased levels of folylpolyglutamate synthetase, which results in lower levels of polyglutamylated MTX, the "trapped" form of MTX. A MTX-resistant population could have any one or a combination of these alterations. The net result of any of these resistance mechanisms is to decrease the ability of MTX to inhibit dihydrofolate reductase at clinically achievable MTX concentrations. Other specific drug resistance mechanisms could be described for compounds such as cytosine arabinoside, 5-fluorouracil, and hydroxyurea.

In multiple drug resistance, the drug-resistant population is cross-resistant to a series of seemingly unrelated antitumor agents. These compounds include drugs such as the vinca alkaloids, adriamycin, actinomycin D, and etoposide. All of these drugs are natural products or derived from natural products and they are not chemically related in structure. They have different mechanisms of action as antitumor agents but appear to act on some nuclear event.

Multidrug-resistant tumor cells express high levels (compared to the drug-sensitive tumor cell phenotype) of a protein called MDR1 (P-glycoprotein) or another protein called MRP (multidrug resistance protein). These proteins are membrane bound, have a mass around 170 kDa, but are distinctly separate proteins. These proteins function as "pumps" to efflux drugs from cells. As a result of increased efflux of drugs, caused by the ATP-dependent efflux proteins, the cellular concentration of drug is decreased below its cytotoxic concentration.

Development of drug-resistant tumor cells presents major clinical problems. Study of the mechanisms of drug resistance has greatly aided in our understanding of cancer cells.

BIBLIOGRAPHY

Arner, E. S. J., and Eriksson, S. Mammalian deoxyribonucleoside kinases. *Pharmacol. Ther.* 67:155, 1995.

Cory, J. G. Role of ribonucleotide reductase in cell division. In: J. G. Cory and A. H. Cory (Eds.), *Inhibitors of Ribonucleoside Diphosphate Reductase Activity,* International Encyclopedia of Pharmacology and Therapeutics. New York: Pergamon, 1989, p. 1.

Elion, G. B. The purine path to chemotherapy. *Science* 244:41, 1989.

Scriver, C. R., Beaudet, A. L., Sly, W. S., and Valle, D. (Eds.). *The Metabolic and Molecular Bases of Inherited Disease,* 7th ed. Vol. II, Chaps. 49–55. New York: McGraw-Hill, 1995.

Weber, G. Biochemical strategy of cancer cells and the design of chemotherapy: G.H.A. Clowes Memorial Lecture. *Cancer Res.* 43:3466, 1983.

Zalkin, H., and Dixon, J. E. De novo purine nucleotide biosynthesis. *Prog. Nucleic Acid Res.* 42:259, 1992.

QUESTIONS ■ C. N. ANGSTADT AND J. BAGGOTT

1. Nucleotides serve all of the following roles EXCEPT:
   A. monomeric units of nucleic acids.
   B. physiological mediators.
   C. sources of chemical energy.
   D. structural components of membranes.
   E. structural components of coenzymes.

Refer to the following figure for Questions 2–4.

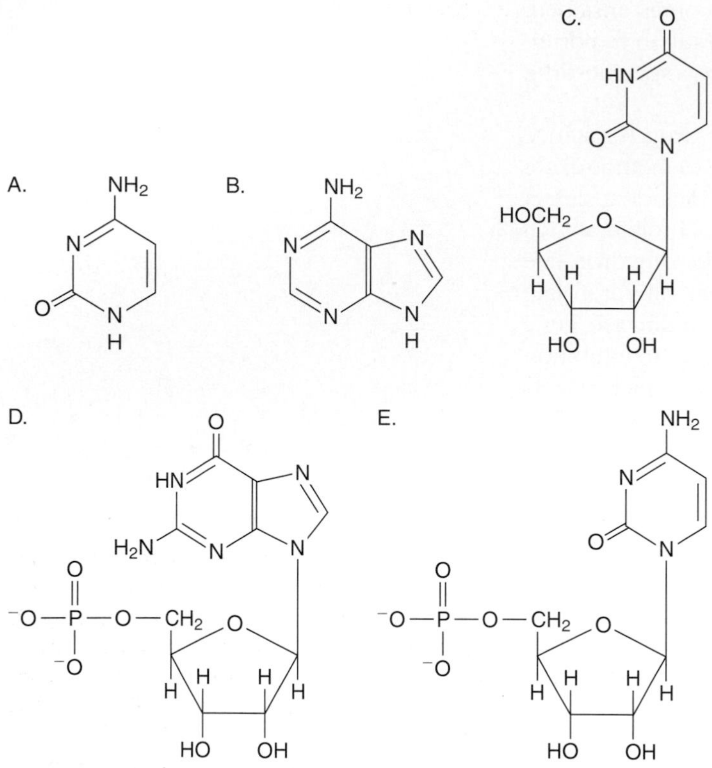

A.

B.

C.

D.

E.

2. Identify adenine.

3. Identify a pyrimidine nucleoside.

4. Identify CMP.

5. The amide nitrogen of glutamine is a source of nitrogen for the:
   A. *de novo* synthesis of purine nucleotides.
   B. *de novo* synthesis of pyrimidine nucleotides.
   C. synthesis of GMP from IMP.
   D. all of the above.
   E. none of the above.

6. The enzyme catalyzing the rate-limiting step of the *de novo* synthesis of purine nucleotides:
   A. is a multifunctional protein.
   B. uses PRPP as a substrate.
   C. requires AMP for activity.
   D. is controlled primarily by substrate availability.
   E. shows sigmoidal kinetics with respect to both of its substrates.

7. The two purine nucleotides found in RNA:
   A. are formed in a branched pathway from a common intermediate.
   B. are formed in a sequential pathway.
   C. must come from exogenous sources.
   D. are formed by oxidation of the deoxy forms.
   E. are synthesized from nonpurine precursors by totally separate pathways.

8. Which of the following is/are aspects of the overall regulation of *de novo* purine nucleotide synthesis?
   A. AMP, GMP, and IMP cause a shift of PRPP amidotransferase from a small form to a large form.
   B. PRPP levels in the cell can be severalfold less than the K_m of PRPP amidotransferase for PRPP.
   C. GMP is a competitive inhibitor of IMP dehydrogenase.
   D. All of the above are correct.
   E. None of the above is correct.

9. The type of enzyme known as a phosphoribosyltransferase is involved in all of the following EXCEPT:
   A. salvage of pyrimidine bases.
   B. the *de novo* synthesis of pyrimidine nucleotides.
   C. the *de novo* synthesis of purine nucleotides.
   D. salvage of purine bases.

10. Uric acid is:
    A. formed from xanthine in the presence of O_2.
    B. a degradation product of cytidine.
    C. deficient in the condition known as gout.
    D. a competitive inhibitor of xanthine oxidase.
    E. oxidized, in humans, before it is excreted in urine.

11. In nucleic acid degradation, all of the following are correct EXCEPT:
    A. there are nucleases that are specific for either DNA or RNA.
    B. nucleotidases convert nucleotides to nucleosides.
    C. the conversion of a nucleoside to a free base is an example of hydrolysis.
    D. because of the presence of deaminases, hypoxanthine rather than adenine is formed.
    E. a deficiency of adenosine deaminase leads to an immunodeficiency.

12. In the *de novo* synthesis of pyrimidine nucleotides:
    A. reactions take place exclusively in the cytosol.
    B. a free base is formed as an intermediate.
    C. PRPP is required in the rate-limiting step.
    D. UMP and CMP are formed from a common intermediate.
    E. UMP inhibition of OMP decarboxylase is the major control of the process.

13. Deoxyribonucleotides:
    A. cannot be synthesized so they must be supplied preformed in the diet.
    B. are synthesized *de novo* using dPRPP.
    C. are synthesized from ribonucleotides by an enzyme system involving thioredoxin.
    D. are synthesized from ribonucleotides by nucleotide kinases.
    E. can be formed only by salvaging free bases.

14. β-Aminoisobutyrate:
    A. is an intermediate in the degradation of both uracil and thymine.
    B. in the urine can be used to estimate the turnover of DNA.
    C. arises from uracil by cleavage of the pyrimidine ring.
    D. is in equilibrium with β-alanine.
    E. is the end product common to the degradation of both uracil and thymine.

15. The conversion of nucleoside 5′-monophosohates to nucleoside 5′-triphosphates:
    A. is catalyzed by nucleoside kinases.
    B. is a direct equilibrium reaction.
    C. utilizes a relatively specific nucleotide kinase and a relatively nonspecific nucleoside diphosphate kinase.
    D. generally uses GTP as a phosphate donor.
    E. occurs only during the S phase of the cell cycle.

16. If a cell were unable to synthesize PRPP, which of the following processes would likely be directly impaired?
    A. FAD synthesis
    B. NAD synthesis
    C. coenzyme A synthesis
    D. ribose 5-phosphate synthesis
    E. dTMP synthesis

17. Which of the following antitumor agents works by impairing *de novo* purine synthesis?
    A. acyclovir (acycloguanosine)
    B. 5-fluorouracil (antimetabolite)
    C. methotrexate (antifolate)
    D. hydroxyurea
    E. allopurinol

ANSWERS

1. D Both cAMP and cGMP are physiological mediators. NAD, FAD, and CoA all contain AMP as part of their structures (pp. 490–491).
2. B Adenine is the free purine. (A is a pyrimidine.)
3. C A nucleoside contains a base plus sugar but no phosphate.
4. E CMP is a pyrimidine nucleotide. (D is a purine nucleotide; pp. 492–493).
5. D Nitrogen atoms 3 and 9 of purine nucleotides (p. 495, Fig. 12.7) and N-3 of pyrimidine nucleotides (p. 504, Fig. 12.17) are supplied by glutamine in *de novo* synthesis. The 2-amino group of GMP also comes from this source.
6. B The rate-limiting step of purine nucleotide synthesis is the amido transfer between glutamine and PRPP (p. 494). A: There are several multifunctional proteins in the pathway but this is not one. C: It is inhibited by AMP. D: This is a typical allosteric enzyme. Know the things that control it. E: As expected for an allosteric enzyme, it does show sigmoidal kinetics but only with respect to PRPP. The kinetics for glutamine are hyperbolic.
7. A GMP and AMP are both formed from the first purine nucleotide, IMP, in a branched pathway (p. 494). B: The pyrimidine nucleotides UMP and CTP are formed in a sequential pathway from orotic acid (p. 505). D: Deoxy forms are formed by reduction of the ribose forms.
8. D A is the mechanism of inhibition since the large form of the enzyme is inactive (p. 497). B: PRPP amidotransferase shows sigmoidal kinetics with respect to PRPP so large shifts in concentration of PRPP have the potential for altering velocity (p. 497). C plays a major role in controlling the branched pathway of IMP to GMP or AMP (p. 497).
9. C In purine nucleotide synthesis, the purine ring is built up stepwise on ribose-5-phosphate and not transferred to it (p. 497). A, B, and D: Phosphoribosyltransferases are important salvage enzymes for both purines and pyrimidines (pp. 506–507) and are also part of the synthesis of pyrimidines since OPRT catalyzes the conversion of orotate to OMP (pp. 503–504).
10. A The xanthine oxidase reaction produces uric acid. B and E: Uric acid is an end product of purines, not pyrimidines. C: Gout is characterized by excess uric acid (p. 502, Fig. 12.16).
11. C The product is ribose 1-phosphate rather than the free sugar, a phosphorolysis. A: They can also show specificity toward the bases and positions of cleavage. B: A straight hydrolysis. D: AMP deaminase and adenosine deaminase remove the 6-NH_2 as NH_3. The IMP or inosine formed is eventually converted to hypoxanthine (p. 502, Fig. 12.16). E: This is called severe combined immunodeficiency (pp. 501–502).
12. B This is in contrast to purine *de novo* synthesis. A: One enzyme is mitochondrial. C: PRPP is required to convert orotate to OMP but this is not rate-limiting. D: OMP to UMP to CTP is a sequential process. E: This does occur but the rate-limiting step is that catalyzed by CPS II (pp. 502–506).
13. C Deoxyribonucleotides are synthesized from the ribonucleoside diphosophates by nucleoside diphosphate reductase that uses thioredoxin as the direct hydrogen-electron donor (p. 507). A, B, and E: There is a synthetic mechanism as just described but it is not a *de novo* pathway. D: Nucleotide kinases are enzymes that add phosphate to a base or nucleotide.
14. B This compound originates exclusively from thymine, which is found primarily in DNA. A and E: It is an end product of degradation but only of thymine. C and D: β-Alanine arises from cleavage of the uracil ring (p. 509).
15. C These two enzymes are important in interconverting the nucleotide forms. A: These convert nucleosides to nucleoside monophosphates. B: Two steps are required. D: ATP is present in highest concentration and is the phosphate donor. E: Occurs during the S phase but this is a general reaction for the cell (pp. 509–510).
16. D PRPP is formed from ribose 5-phosphate in an irreversible reaction. E: dTMP is formed directly from dUMP, which doesn't have to be made *de novo* (p. 507).
17. C Antifolates reduce the concentration of THF compounds that are necessary for two steps of purine synthesis. A: This is an antiviral agent that inhibits DNA synthesis. B: 5-Fluorouracil is a pyrimidine analog not a purine analog. D: Hydroxyurea inhibits the reduction of ribonucleotides to deoxyribonucleotides so it is not involved in *de novo* purine synthesis. E: Allopurinol potentiates the effect of 6-mercaptopurine but is not an inhibitor of purine synthesis (pp. 517–520).

CHAPTER

METABOLIC INTERRELATIONSHIPS

Robert A. Harris and David W. Crabb

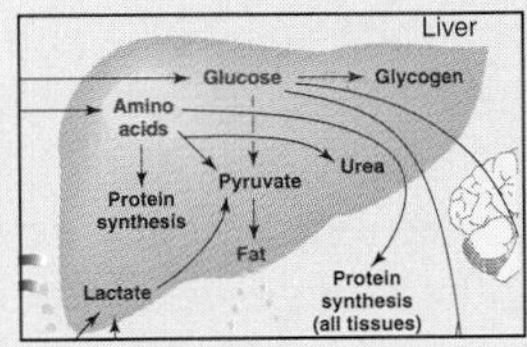

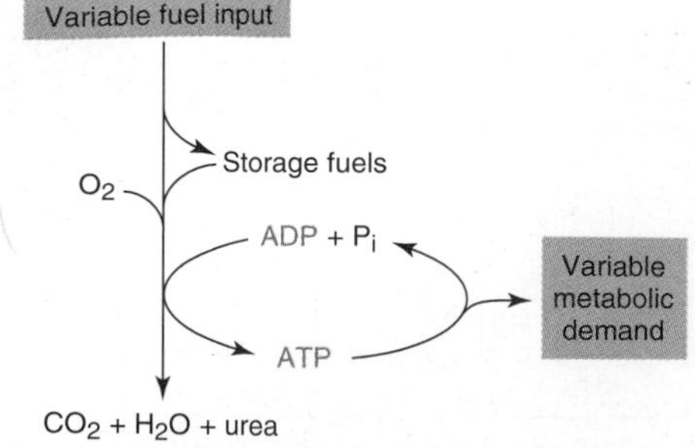

FIGURE 13.1
Humans are able to use a variable fuel input to meet a variable metabolic demand.

13.1 ■ OVERVIEW

In this chapter the interdependence of metabolic processes of the major tissues of the body will be stressed. Not all of the major metabolic pathways operate in every tissue at any given time. Given the nutritional and hormonal status of a patient, we need to be able to say qualitatively which major metabolic pathways of the body are functional and how these pathways relate to one another.

The metabolic processes with which we are concerned are glycogenesis, glycogenolysis, gluconeogenesis, glycolysis, fatty acid synthesis, lipogenesis, lipolysis, fatty acid oxidation, glutaminolysis, tricarboxylic acid cycle activity, ketogenesis, amino acid oxidation, protein synthesis, proteolysis, and urea synthesis. It is important to know (1) which tissues are most active in these various processes, (2) when these processes are most or least active, and (3) how these processes are controlled and coordinated in different metabolic states.

The best way to gain an understanding of the relationships of the pathways to one another is to become familiar with the changes in metabolism that occur during the **starve–feed cycle.** As shown in Figure 13.1, the starve–feed cycle allows a variable fuel and nitrogen consumption to meet a variable metabolic and anabolic demand. Feed refers to the intake of meals (the variable fuel input) after which we store the fuel (in the form of glycogen and fat) to be used to meet our metabolic demand while we fast. Note the participation of an **ATP cycle** within the starve–feed cycle (Figure 13.1). Adenosine triphosphate

CLINICAL CORRELATION 13.1

Obesity

Obesity is the most common nutritional problem in the United States. It can reduce life span because it is a risk factor in development of diabetes mellitus, hypertension, endometrial carcinoma, osteoarthritis, gallstones, and cardiovascular diseases. Obesity is easy to explain—an obese person has eaten more than he/she required. The accumulation of massive amounts of body fat is not otherwise possible. For unknown reasons, the neural control of caloric intake to balance energy expenditure is abnormal. Rarely, obesity is secondary to a correctable disorder, such as hypothyroidism or Cushing's syndrome. The latter is the result of increased secretion of glucocorticoids, which cause fat deposition in the face and trunk, with wasting of the limbs, and glucose intolerance. These effects are due to increased protein breakdown in muscle and conversion of the amino acids to glucose and fat. Less commonly, tumors, vascular accidents, or maldevelopment of the nervous system hunger control centers in the hypothalamus cause obesity.

Genetic models of obesity in rodents have led to breakthroughs in our understanding of the control of body mass. The obese (*ob/ob*) mouse was discovered in the 1950s, and the defective gene cloned in 1994. This *ob* gene encodes a 146 amino acid secreted protein (alternatively called OB protein or leptin, for its slimming effect) that is produced in adipocytes and detectable in blood. The *ob/ob* mice have a nonsense mutation in the gene and produce no OB protein. Injection of the OB protein into *ob/ob* mice causes increased energy expenditure and reduced eating, with marked weight loss. This effect on appetite is mimicked by intracerebroventricular injection. The OB protein also reduced appetite and weight of normal mice. Obese humans do not generally have defective *ob* genes but, like normal mice, may still respond to OB protein used as an anti-obesity drug.

In the most common type of obesity, the number of adipocytes of the body does not increase, they just get large as they become engorged with triacylglycerols. If obesity develops before puberty, however, an increase in the number of adipocytes can also occur. In the latter case, both hyperplasia (increase in cell number) and hypertrophy (increase in cell size) are contributing factors to the magnitude of the obesity. Obesity in men tends to be centered on the abdomen and mesenteric fat, while in women it is more likely to be on the hips. The male pattern, characterized by a high waist to hip circumference ratio, is more predictive of premature coronary heart disease.

The only effective treatment of obesity is reduction in the ingestion or increase in the use of calories. Practically speaking, this means dieting, since even vigorous exercise such as running only consumes 10 kcal/min of exercise. Thus an hour-long run (perhaps 5–6 miles) uses the energy present in about two candy bars. However, exercise programs can be useful to help motivate individuals to remain on their diets. Unfortunately, the body compensates for decreased energy intake with reduced formation of triiodothyronine and a corresponding decrease in the basal metabolic rate. Thus there is a biochemical basis for the universal complaint that it is far easier to gain than to lose weight. Furthermore, about 95% of people who are able to lose a significant amount of weight regain it within one year.

Bray, G. D. Effect of caloric restriction on energy expenditure in obese patients. *Lancet* 2:397, 1969; Bray, G. D. The overweight patient. *Adv. Intern. Med.* 21:267, 1976; and Baringer, M. Obese protein slims mice. *Science* 269:475, 1995.

CLINICAL CORRELATION 13.2

Protein Malnutrition

Protein malnutrition is the most important and widespread nutritional problem among young children in the world today. The clinical syndrome, called kwashiorkor, occurs mainly in children 1–3 years of age and is precipitated by weaning an infant from breast milk onto a starchy, protein-poor diet. The name originated in Ghana, meaning "the sickness of the older child when the next baby is born." It is a consequence of feeding the child a diet adequate in calories but deficient in protein. It may become clinically manifest when protein requirements are increased by infection, for example, malaria, helminth infestation, or gastroenteritis. The syndrome is characterized by poor growth, low plasma protein and amino acid levels, muscle wasting, edema, diarrhea, and increased susceptibility to infection. The presence of subcutaneous fat clearly differentiates it from simple starvation. The maintenance of fat stores is due to the high carbohydrate intake and resulting high insulin levels. In fact, the high insulin level interferes with the adaptations described for starvation. Fat is not mobilized as an energy source, ketogenesis does not take place, and there is no transfer of amino acids from the skeletal muscle to the visceral organs, that is, the liver, kidneys, heart, and immune cells. The lack of dietary amino acids results in diminished protein synthesis in all tissues. The liver becomes enlarged and infiltrated with fat, reflecting the need for hepatic protein synthesis for the formation and release of lipoproteins. In addition, protein malnutrition impairs the function of the gut, resulting in malabsorption of calories, protein, and vitamins, which accelerates the disease. The consequences of the disease depend somewhat on when in development the deficiency occurs. Children with low weight for height are called "wasted" but can make a good recovery when properly fed. Those with low height for weight are called "stunted" and never regain full height or cognitive potential.

Protein–calorie malnutrition is also a problem for the elderly when they become sick. Both the energy requirements and food intake of well elderly decline with age. On a lower calorie diet, there is the risk that insufficient intake of protein and of certain nutrients such as iron, calcium, and vitamins will be lower than needed. Deficiencies in these nutrients may accelerate loss of lean body mass and strength (leading to falls), anemia, loss of bone strength, and rarely, vitamin deficiency states.

Bistrian, B. R., Blackburn, G. L., Vitale, J., and Cochran, D. Prevalence of malnutrition in general medical patients. *JAMA* 235:1567, 1976; Chase, H. P., Kumar, V., Caldwell, R. T., and O'Brien, D. Kwashiorkor in the United States. *Pediatrics* 66:972, 1980; and Schlienger, J. L., Pradignac, A., and Grunenberger, F. Nutrition of the elderly: a challenge between facts and needs. *Horm. Res.* 43:46, 1995.

is the energy-transferring agent in the starve–feed cycle, being like money to the cell.

Humans have the capacity to consume food at a rate far greater than their basal caloric requirements, which allows them to survive from meal to meal. We thus store calories as glycogen and fat and utilize them as needed. Unfortunately, an almost unlimited capacity to consume food is matched by an almost unlimited capacity to store it as fat. **Obesity** is the consequence of excess food consumption and is the commonest form of malnutrition in affluent countries (see Clin. Corr. 13.1), whereas other forms of malnutrition are more prevalent in developing countries (see Clin. Corr. 13.2 and 13.3). The regulation of food

CLINICAL CORRELATION 13.3

Starvation

Starvation leads to the development of a syndrome known as marasmus. Marasmus is a word of Greek origin meaning "to waste." Although not restricted to any age group, it is most common in children under 1 year of age. In developing countries early weaning of infants from breast milk is a common cause of marasmus. This may result from pregnancies in rapid succession, the desire of the mother to return to work, or the use of overdiluted artificial formulas (to make the expensive formulas last longer). This practice leads to insufficient intake of calories. Likewise, diarrhea and malabsorption can develop if safe water and sterile procedures are not used.

In contrast to kwashiorkor (see Clin. Corr. 13.2), subcutaneous fat, hepatomegaly, and fatty liver are absent in marasmus because fat is mobilized as an energy source and muscle temporarily provides amino acids to the liver for the synthesis of glucose and hepatic proteins. Low insulin levels allow the liver to oxidize fatty acids and to produce ketone bodies for other tissues. Ultimately, energy and protein reserves are exhausted, and the child starves to death. The immediate cause of death is often pneumonia, which occurs because the child is too weak to cough. Adults can suffer from marasmus as a result of diseases that prevent swallowing (cancer of the throat or esophagus) or interfere with access to food (strokes or dementia).

Waterlow, J. C. Childhood malnutrition—the global problem. *Proc. Nutr. Soc.* 38:1, 1979; and Uvin, P. The state of world hunger. *Nutr. Rev.* 52:151, 1994.

consumption is complex and not well understood. Recent observations suggest that the product of the **leptin gene** (*ob* in mice) expressed in adipocytes is secreted into the blood and regulates energy expenditure and appetite through the hypothalamus (see Clin. Corr. 13.1). The tight control needed is indicated by the calculation that eating two extra pats of butter (~100 cal) per day over caloric expenditures results in a 10-lb weight gain per year. A weight gain of 10 lb may not sound excessive, but multiplied by 10 years it equals obesity!

13.2 ■ STARVE–FEED CYCLE

In the Well-Fed State the Diet Supplies the Energy Requirements

Figure 13.2 shows the fate of glucose, amino acids, and fat obtained from food. Glucose passes from the intestinal epithelial cells to the liver by way of the portal vein. Amino acids are partially metabolized in the gut before being released into portal blood. Fat, contained in **chylomicrons,** is secreted by the intestinal epithelial cells into lymphatics, which drain the intestine. The lymphatics lead to the thoracic duct, which, by way of the subclavian vein, delivers chylomicrons to the blood at a site of rapid blood flow. This rapidly distributes the chylomicrons and prevents their coalescence.

Liver is the first tissue to have the opportunity to use dietary glucose. Glucose can be converted into glycogen by glycogenesis, into pyruvate and lactate by glycolysis, or can be used in the pentose phosphate pathway for the

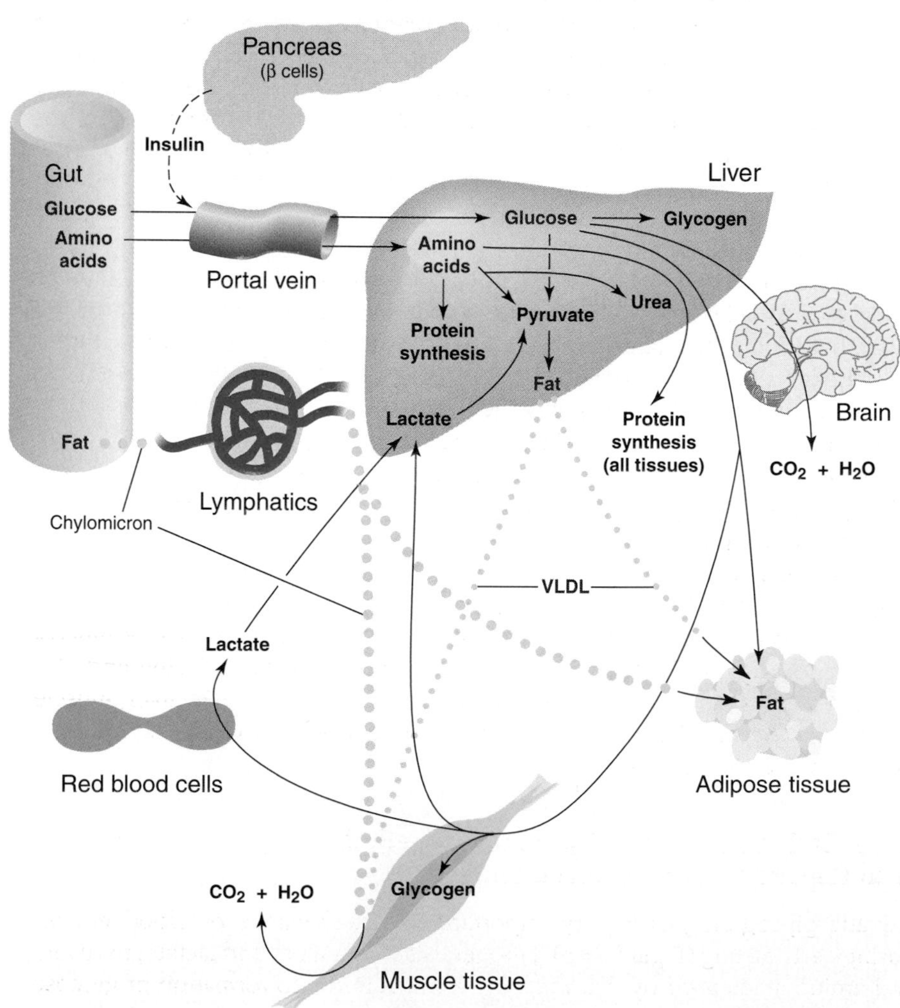

FIGURE 13.2
Disposition of glucose, amino acids, and fat by various tissues in the well-fed state.

generation of NADPH for synthetic processes. Pyruvate can be oxidized to acetyl CoA, which, in turn, can be converted into fat or oxidized to CO_2 and water by the TCA cycle. Much of the glucose coming from the intestine passes through the liver to reach other organs, including brain and testis, which are almost solely dependent on glucose for the production of ATP, red blood cells and renal medulla, which can only convert glucose to lactate and pyruvate, and the adipose tissue, which converts it into fat. Muscle also has good capacity to use glucose, converting it to glycogen or using it in the glycolytic and the TCA cycle pathways. A number of tissues produce lactate and pyruvate from circulating glucose, which are taken up by the liver and converted to fat. In the very well-fed state, the liver uses glucose and does not engage in gluconeogenesis. Thus the **Cori cycle** (the conversion of glucose to lactate in the peripheral tissues followed by conversion of lactate back to glucose in liver) is interrupted in the well-fed state.

Dietary protein is hydrolyzed in the intestine, the cells of which use some amino acids as an energy source. Most dietary amino acids are transported into the portal blood, but the intestinal cells metabolize aspartate, asparagine, glutamate, and glutamine and release alanine, lactate, citrulline, and proline into portal blood. Liver then has the opportunity to remove absorbed amino acids from the blood (Figure 13.2). The liver lets most of each amino acid pass through, unless the concentration of the amino acid is unusually high. This is especially important for the essential amino acids, needed by all tissues of the body for protein synthesis. Liver catabolizes amino acids, but the K_m values for amino acids of many of the enzymes involved are high, allowing the amino acids to be present in excess before significant catabolism can occur. In contrast, the tRNA-charging enzymes that generate **aminoacyl-tRNAs** have much lower K_m values for amino acids. This ensures that as long as all the amino acids are present, protein synthesis occurs as needed for growth and protein turnover. Excess amino acids can be oxidized completely to CO_2, urea, and water, or the intermediates generated can be used as substrates for lipogenesis. Amino acids that escape the liver are used for protein synthesis or energy in other tissues.

Glucose, lactate, pyruvate, and amino acids can support hepatic **lipogenesis** (Figure 13.2). Fat formed from these substrates is released from the liver in the form of very low density lipoproteins (VLDLs). Dietary fat is delivered to the bloodstream as **chylomicrons.** Both chylomicrons and **VLDLs** circulate in the blood until they are acted on by an extracellular enzyme attached to the endothelial cells in the lumen of the capillaries. This enzyme, **lipoprotein lipase,** is particularly abundant in the capillaries in adipose tissue. It acts on both the VLDLs and chylomicrons, liberating fatty acids by hydrolysis of the triacylglycerols. The fatty acids are then taken up by the adipocytes, reesterified with glycerol 3-phosphate to form triacylglycerols, and stored as fat droplets. Glycerol 3-phosphate is generated from glucose, using the first half of the glycolytic pathway to generate dihydroxyacetone phosphate, which is reduced to glycerol 3-phosphate by glycerol-3-phosphate dehydrogenase.

The β cells of the pancreas are very responsive to the influx of glucose and amino acids in the fed state. The β cells release insulin during and after eating, which is essential for the metabolism of these nutrients by liver, muscle, and adipose tissue. The role of insulin in the starve–feed cycle is discussed in more detail in Section 13.3.

In the Early Fasting State Hepatic Glycogenolysis Is an Important Source of Blood Glucose

Hepatic glycogenolysis is very important for maintenance of blood glucose during early fasting (Figure 13.3). Lipogenesis is curtailed, and lactate, pyruvate, and amino acids used by that pathway are diverted into formation of glucose, completing the Cori cycle. The **alanine cycle,** in which carbon and nitrogen

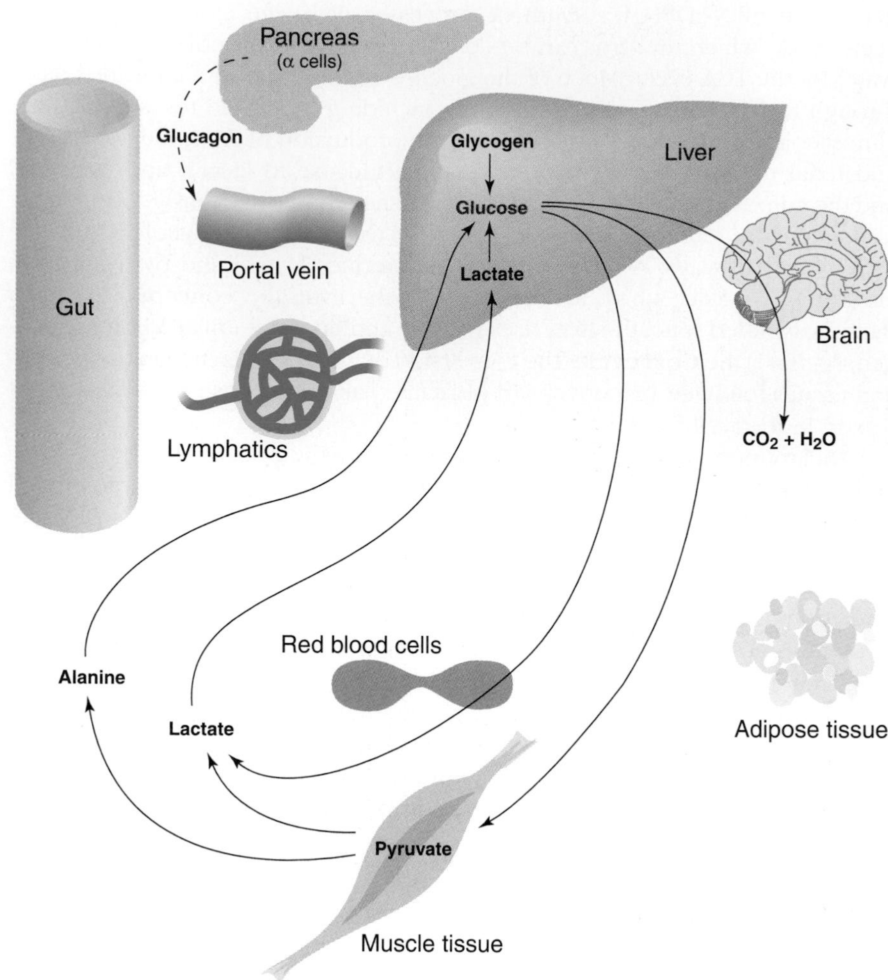

FIGURE 13.3
Metabolic interrelationships of major tissues in the early fasting state.

return to the liver in the form of alanine, also becomes important. Catabolism of amino acids for energy is greatly diminished in early fasting because less is available.

The Fasting State Requires Gluconeogenesis from Amino Acids and Glycerol

No fuel enters from the gut and little glycogen is left in the liver in the fasting state (Figure 13.4). Tissues that require glucose are dependent on hepatic **gluconeogenesis,** primarily from lactate, glycerol, and alanine. The Cori and alanine cycles play important roles but do not provide carbon for net synthesis of glucose. Glucose formed from lactate and alanine by the liver merely replaces that which was converted to lactate and alanine by peripheral tissues. In effect, these cycles transfer energy from fatty acid oxidation in the liver to peripheral tissues that cannot oxidize fat. The brain oxidizes glucose completely to CO_2 and water. Hence net glucose synthesis from some other source of carbon is mandatory in fasting. Fatty acids cannot be used for the synthesis of glucose, because acetyl CoA obtained by fatty acid catabolism cannot be converted to glucose. Glycerol, a by-product of lipolysis in adipose tissue, is an important substrate for glucose synthesis. However, protein, especially from skeletal muscle, supplies most of the carbon needed for net glucose synthesis. Proteins are hydrolyzed within muscle cells and most amino acids are partially metabolized within muscle cells. Only two amino acids—alanine and glutamine—are re-

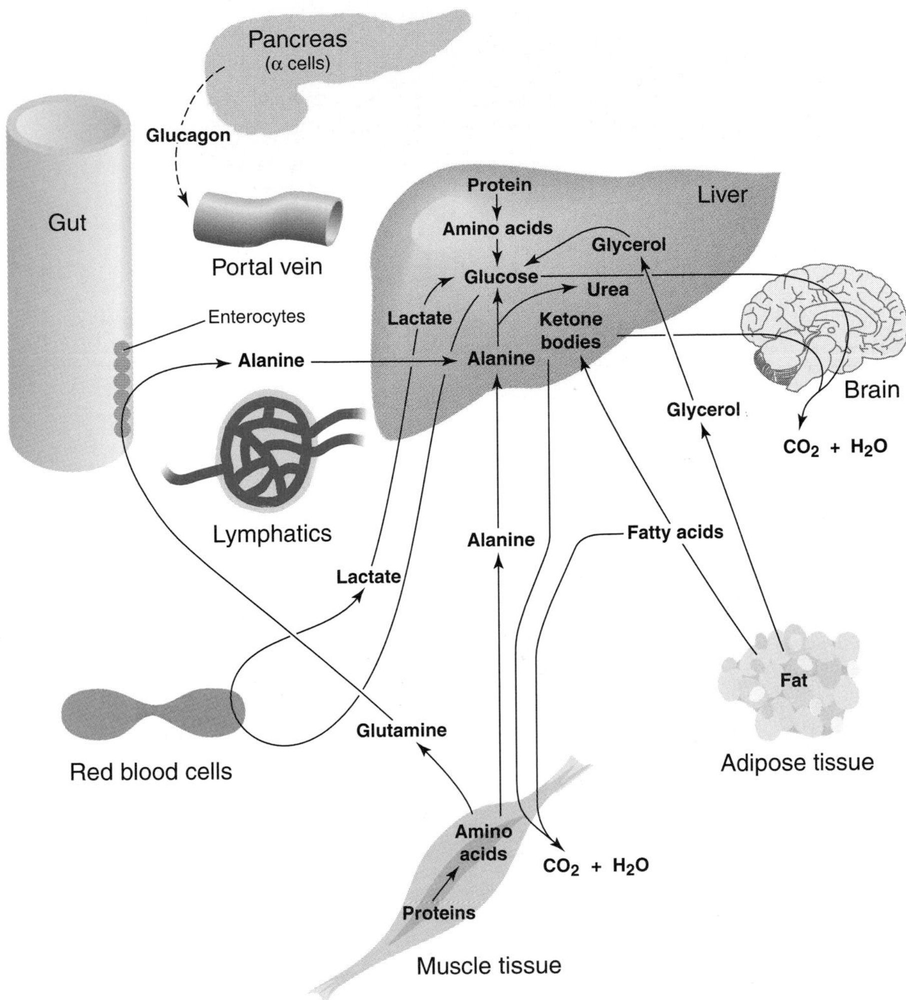

FIGURE 13.4
Metabolic interrelationships of major tissues in the fasting state.

leased in large amounts. The others are metabolized to give intermediates (pyruvate and α-ketoglutarate), which can yield alanine and glutamine. Branched-chain amino acids are a major source of nitrogen for the production of alanine and glutamine in muscle. Branched-chain α-keto acids produced from the branched-chain amino acids by transamination are partially released into the blood for uptake by the liver, which synthesizes glucose from the keto acid of valine, ketone bodies from the keto acid of leucine, and both glucose and ketone bodies from the keto acid of isoleucine.

Much of the glutamine released from muscle is converted into alanine by the intestinal epithelium. Glutamine is partially oxidized in **enterocytes** to supply energy and precursor molecules for synthesis of pyrimidines and purines, with the carbon and amino groups left over being released back into the bloodstream in part as alanine and NH_4^+. This pathway, sometimes called **glutaminolysis** because glutamine is only partially oxidized, involves formation of malate from glutamine via the TCA cycle and the conversion of malate to pyruvate by malic enzyme (Figure 13.5*a*). Pyruvate then transaminates with glutamate to give alanine, which is released from the cells.

Glutaminolysis is also used by cells of the immune system (lymphocytes and macrophages) to meet a large portion of their energy needs (Figure 13.5*b*). Aspartate rather than alanine is the major end product of glutaminolysis in **lymphocytes.** Enterocytes and lymphocytes use glutamine as their major fuel source as a way to ensure a continuous supply of the precursor molecules

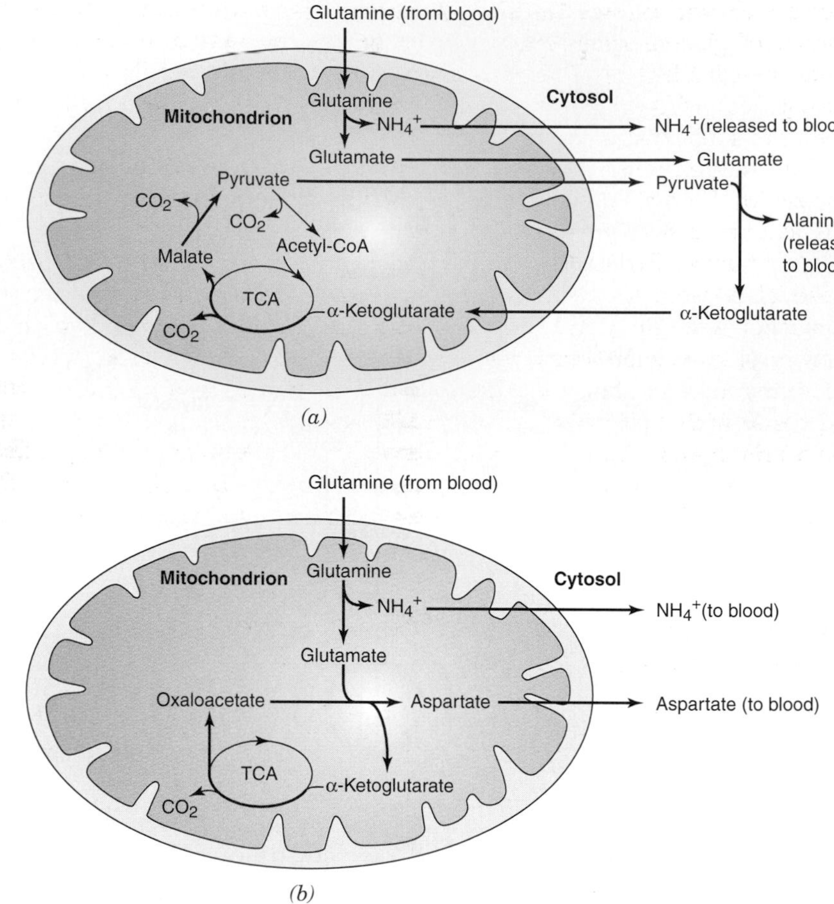

FIGURE 13.5
Glutamine catabolism by rapidly dividing cells.
(*a*) Enterocytes. (*b*) Lymphocytes.
Redrawn from Duée, P.-H., Darcy-Vrillon, B., Blachier, F., and Morel, M.-T. Fuel selection in intestinal cells. Proc. Nutr. Soc. *54:83, 1995.*

(glutamine and aspartate) required for synthesis of purines and pyrimidines, which these rapidly dividing cells need for the synthesis of RNA and DNA.

Synthesis of glucose in the liver during fasting is closely linked to synthesis of urea. Most amino acids can give up the amino nitrogen by transamination with α-ketoglutarate, forming glutamate and a new α-keto acid, which can be utilized for glucose synthesis. Glutamate provides both nitrogenous compounds required for urea synthesis: ammonia from oxidative deamination by glutamate dehydrogenase, and aspartate from transamination of oxaloacetate by aspartate aminotransferase. An additional important source of ammonia and precursors of ornithine such as citrulline is the gut mucosa (described in more detail in Section 13.4).

Adipose tissue is also very important in the fasting state. Because of low blood insulin levels during fasting, **lipolysis** is greatly activated in this tissue. This raises the blood level of fatty acids, which are used in preference to glucose by many tissues. In heart and muscle, the oxidation of fatty acids inhibits glycolysis and pyruvate oxidation. In liver, fatty acid oxidation provides most of the ATP needed for gluconeogenesis. Very little acetyl CoA generated by fatty acid oxidation in liver is oxidized completely. The acetyl CoA is converted instead into **ketone bodies** by liver mitochondria. Ketone bodies (acetoacetate and β-hydroxybutyrate) are released into the blood and are a source of energy for many tissues. Like fatty acids, ketone bodies are preferred by many tissues over glucose. Fatty acids are not oxidized by the brain because fatty acids cannot cross the blood–brain barrier. Ketone bodies can penetrate, however, and are oxidized. Once their blood concentration is high enough, ketone bodies function as an alternative fuel for the brain. They are unable, however, to completely replace the need for glucose by the brain. Ketone bodies may also suppress proteolysis and branched-chain amino acid oxidation in muscle and decrease alanine release. This both decreases muscle wasting and reduces the amount of glucose synthesized in liver. As long as ketone body levels are maintained at a high level by hepatic fatty acid oxidation, there is less need for glucose, less need for gluconeogenic amino acids, and less need for breaking down precious muscle tissue.

The interrelationships among liver, muscle, and adipose tissue in supplying glucose for the brain are shown in Figure 13.4. Liver synthesizes the glucose, muscle and gut supply the substrate (alanine), and adipose tissue supplies the ATP (via fatty acid oxidation in the liver) needed for hepatic gluconeogenesis. These relationships are disrupted in Reye's syndrome (see Clin. Corr. 13.4) and by alcohol (see Clin. Corr. 7.10). This tissue cooperation is dependent on the appropriate blood hormone levels. Glucose levels are lower in fasting, reducing the secretion of insulin but favoring release of **glucagon** from the pancreas and **epinephrine** from the adrenal medulla. In addition, fasting reduces formation of **triiodothyronine,** the active form of thyroid hormone, from **thyroxine.** This reduces the daily basal energy requirements by as much as 25%. This response is useful for survival but makes weight loss more difficult than weight gain (see Clin. Corr. 13.1).

In the Early Refed State, Fat Is Metabolized Normally, but Normal Glucose Metabolism Is Slowly Reestablished

Figure 13.6 shows what happens soon after fuel is absorbed from the gut. Fat is metabolized as described above for the well-fed state. In contrast, glucose

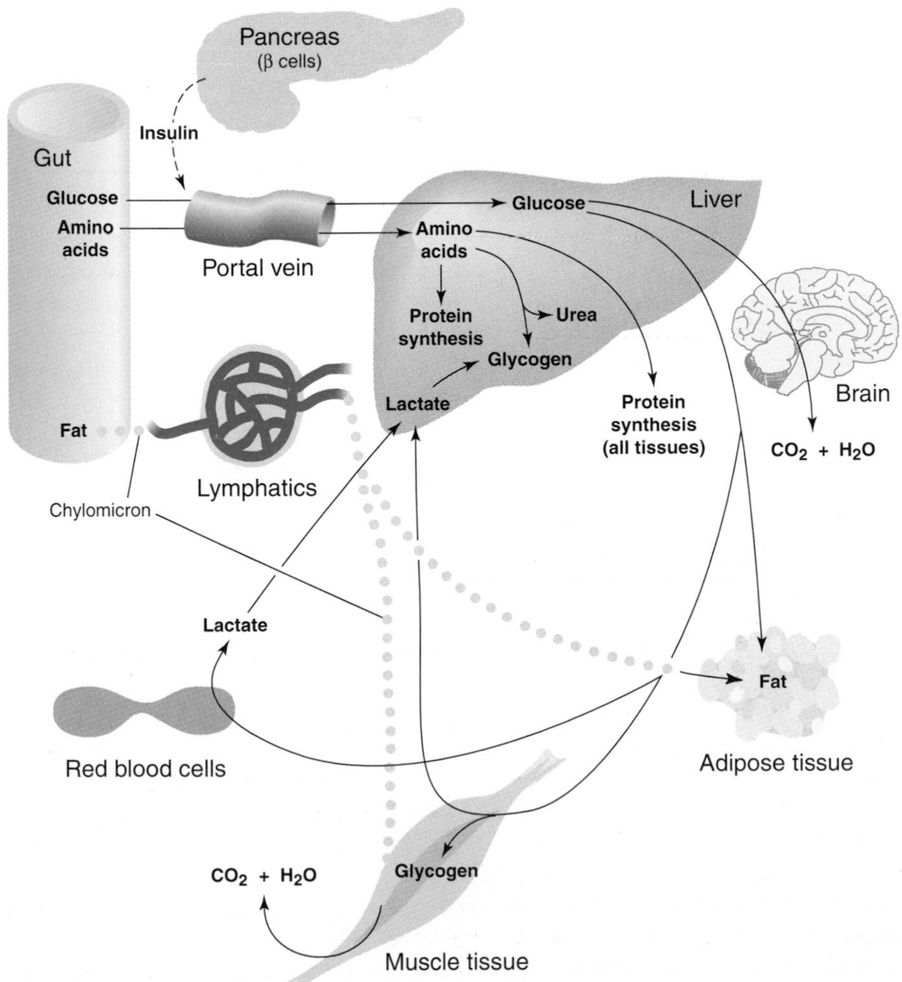

FIGURE 13.6
Metabolic interrelationships of major tissues in the early refed state.

CLINICAL CORRELATION 13.4

Reye's Syndrome

Reye's syndrome is a devastating but now rare illness of children that is characterized by evidence of brain dysfunction and edema (irritability, lethargy, and coma) and liver dysfunction (elevated plasma free fatty acids, fatty liver, hypoglycemia, hyperammonemia, and accumulation of short-chain organic acids). It appears that hepatic mitochondria are specifically damaged, which impairs fatty acid oxidation and synthesis of carbamoyl phosphate and ornithine (for ammonia detoxification) and oxaloacetate (for gluconeogenesis). On the other hand, the accumulation of organic acids has suggested that the oxidation of these compounds is defective and that the CoA esters of some of these acids may inhibit specific enzymes, such as carbamoyl phosphate synthetase I, pyruvate dehydrogenase, pyruvate carboxylase, and the adenine nucleotide transporter, all present in mitochondria. The issue has not yet been resolved. The use of aspirin by children with varicella was linked to the development of Reye's syndrome, and parents have been urged not to give aspirin to children with viral infections. The incidence of the syndrome subsequently decreased. The therapy for Reye's syndrome consists of measures to reduce brain edema and the provision of glucose intravenously. Glucose administration prevents hypoglycemia and elicits a rise in insulin levels that may (1) inhibit lipolysis in adipose cells and (2) reduce proteolysis in muscles and the release of amino acids, which (3) reduces the deamination of amino acids to ammonia.

Reye, R. D. K., Morgan, G., and Baval, J. Encephalopathy and fatty degeneration of the viscera, a disease entity in childhood. *Lancet* 2:749, 1963; and Treem, W. R. Inherited and acquired syndromes of hyperammonemia and encephalopathy in children. *Semin. Liver Dis.* 14:236, 1994.

is poorly extracted by the liver during this period of the starve–feed cycle. In fact, the liver remains in the gluconeogenic mode for a few hours after feeding. Rather than providing blood glucose, however, hepatic gluconeogenesis provides glucose 6-phosphate for glycogenesis. This means that liver glycogen is not repleted after a fast by direct synthesis from blood glucose. Rather, glucose is catabolized in peripheral tissues to lactate, which is converted in the liver to glycogen by the indirect pathway of glycogen synthesis (i.e., gluconeogenesis):

$$\begin{array}{c} \text{Glycogen} \\ \uparrow \\ \text{Glucose} \xrightarrow{\textit{direct}} \text{glucose 6-phosphate} \xleftarrow{\textit{indirect}} \text{lactate} \end{array}$$

Gluconeogenesis from specific amino acids entering from the gut also plays an important role in reestablishing normal liver glycogen levels by the indirect pathway. After the rate of gluconeogenesis declines, glycolysis becomes the predominant means of glucose disposal in the liver, and liver glycogen is sustained by the direct pathway of synthesis from blood glucose.

Other Important Interorgan Metabolic Interactions

An important pathway exists in the intestinal epithelium for the conversion of glutamine to **citrulline** (Figure 13.7). One of the enzymes (ATP-dependent glutamate reductase) necessary for this conversion is expressed only in enterocytes. Citrulline produced in the gut is metabolized by the kidney to arginine, which can be converted to creatine or released into the blood. The liver uses blood arginine to generate ornithine, which expands the capacity of the urea cycle during periods of increased protein intake. Although perhaps not immedi-

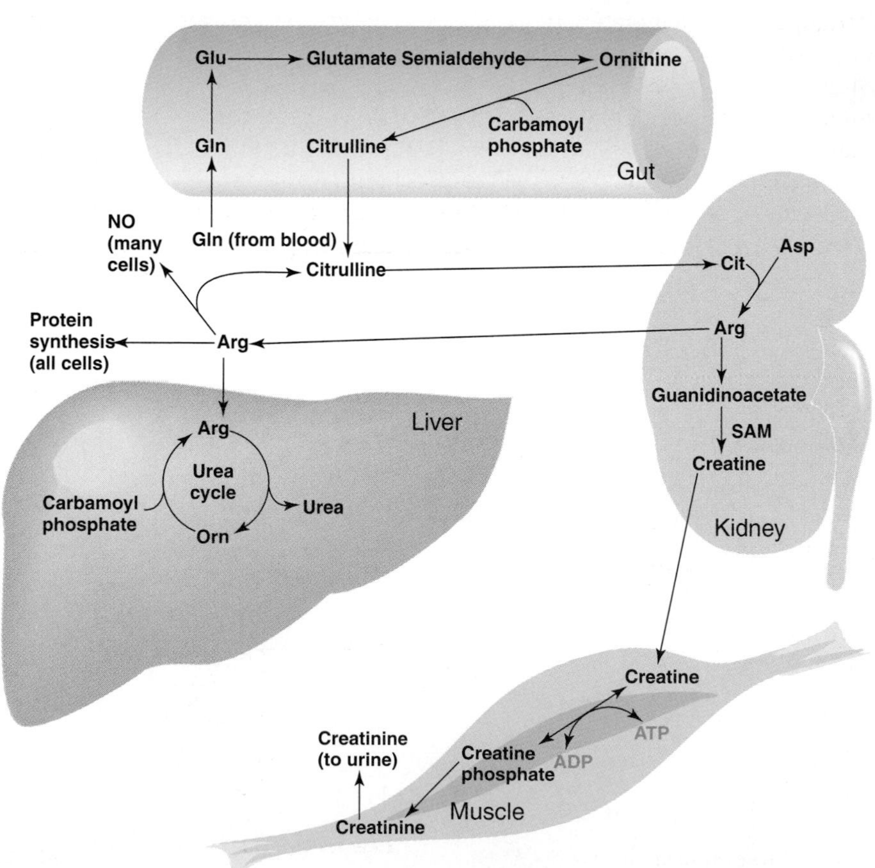

FIGURE 13.7
Gut and kidney function together in synthesis of arginine from glutamine. Abbreviations: Cit, citrulline; Arg, arginine; Asp, aspartate; Gln, glutamine; Glu, glutamate; NO, nitric oxide; Orn, ornithine; SAM, *S*-adenosylmethionine.

ately obvious, this pathway is of great importance for urea cycle activity in the liver. The liver contains an enzyme system that irreversibly converts ornithine into glutamate:

$$\text{Ornithine} \rightarrow \text{glutamate semialdehyde} \rightarrow \text{glutamate}$$

Depletion of ornithine by these reactions inhibits urea synthesis in the liver for want of ornithine, the intermediate of the urea cycle that must recycle. Replenishment of ornithine is necessary and completely dependent on a source of blood arginine. Thus urea synthesis in the liver is dependent on citrulline synthesis by the gut and arginine synthesis by the kidney. Arginine is also used by many cells for the production of **nitric oxide** (NO) (Figure 13.7), an activator of guanylate cyclase that produces cGMP, an important second messenger (see p. 995).

Citrulline participates in another interesting interorgan shuttle. The arginine generated from citrulline in the kidney can be metabolized further to **creatine** (Figure 13.7). The first enzyme in this pathway is glycine transamidinase (GTA), which generates guanidinoacetate from arginine and glycine (see p. 483). GTA is found predominantly in renal cortex, pancreas, and liver. After methylation in a reaction that requires ***S*-adenosylmethionine** (SAM), creatine is formed. This is quantitatively the most important use of **SAM** in the body. One to two grams of creatine are synthesized per day. Creatine then circulates to other tissues, especially muscle, where it serves as a high-energy reservoir when phosphorylated to creatine phosphate. Creatine phosphate undergoes nonenzymatic conversion to **creatinine.** Creatinine is released to the bloodstream and removed from the body by renal filtration. Excretion of creatinine is thus used both as a measure of muscle mass and of renal function.

Two other compounds related to amino acids participate in interorgan shuttles. **Glutathione** (GSH) is a tripeptide that is important in detoxification of endogenously generated peroxides and exogenous chemical compounds (see p. 484). Liver plays a major role in the synthesis of GSH from glutamate, cysteine, and glycine (Figure 13.8). Synthesis is limited by the availability of cysteine. Cystine present in plasma is not taken up well by liver, which utilizes dietary methionine to form cysteine via the cystathionine pathway (see p. 469). Hepatic GSH is released both to the bloodstream and to the bile. Kidney removes a substantial amount of plasma GSH. Enterocytes may be able to take up biliary-excreted GSH from the intestinal lumen. Release to plasma is the same in fed

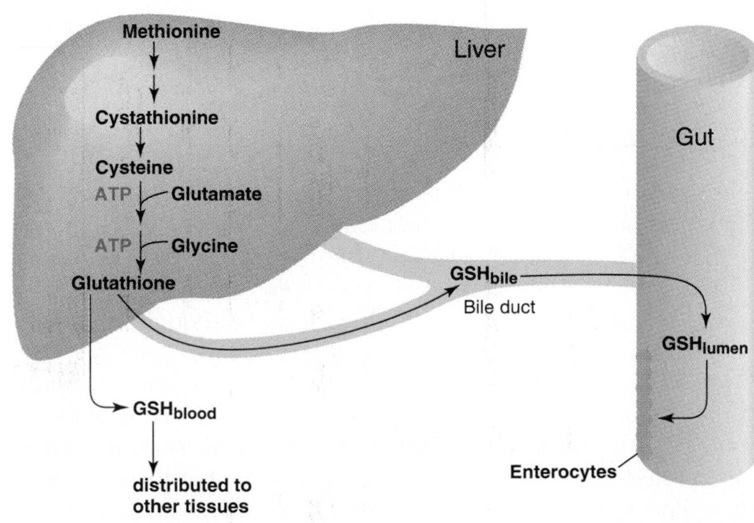

FIGURE 13.8
Liver provides glutathione for other tissues.

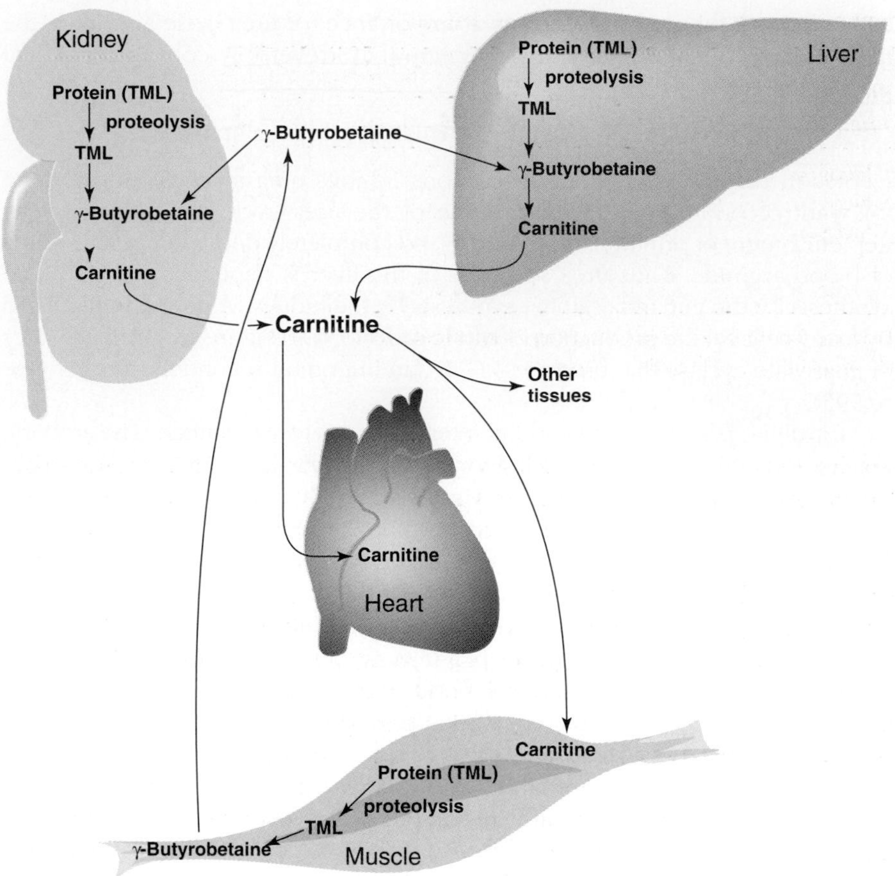

FIGURE 13.9
Kidney and liver provide carnitine for other tissues.
Abbreviations: Protein (TML), trimethyllysyl residues in protein molecules; TML, free trimethyllysine.

and fasting states, providing a stable source of this compound and its constituent amino acids, especially cysteine, for most tissues of the body.

Carnitine is derived from lysyl residues on various proteins, which are *N*-methylated utilizing SAM to form trimethyllysyl residues (Figure 13.9). Free **trimethyllysine** is released when the proteins are degraded. It is hydroxylated and then cleaved, releasing glycine and γ-butyrobetaine aldehyde. The latter is oxidized to γ-butyrobetaine and then hydroxylated to form carnitine. Both hydroxylation steps require **vitamin C** as a cofactor. Kidney and to a lesser extent liver are the only tissues that can carry out the complete pathway, and thus they supply other tissues, especially muscle and heart, with the carnitine needed for fatty acid oxidation. Skeletal muscle can form γ-butyrobetaine but must release it for its final conversion to carnitine by liver or kidney.

Energy Requirements, Reserves, and Caloric Homeostasis

The average person leading a sedentary life consumes 200–300 g of carbohydrate, 70–100 g of protein, and 60–90 g of fat daily. This meets a daily energy requirement of 1600–2400 kcal. As shown in Table 13.1, the **energy reserves** of an average-sized person are considerable. These reserves are called upon between meals and overnight to maintain blood glucose. Although the ability to mobilize glycogen rapidly is indeed very important, our glycogen reserves are minuscule with respect to our fat reserves (Table 13.1). Fat stores are only called upon during more prolonged fasting. The fat stores of obese subjects can weigh as much as 80 kg, adding another 585,000 kcal to their energy reserves. Protein is listed in Table 13.1 as an energy reserve because it can be used to provide amino acids for oxidation. On the other hand, protein is not inert like stored fat and glycogen. Proteins make up the muscles that allow us

TABLE 13.1 The Energy Reserves of Humans[a]

Stored Fuel	Tissue	Fuel Reserves (g)	Fuel Reserves (kcal)
Glycogen	Liver	70	280
Glycogen	Muscle	120	480
Glucose	Body fluids	20	80
Fat	Adipose	15,000	135,000
Protein	Muscle	6,000	24,000

[a] Data are for a normal subject weighing 70 kg. Carbohydrate supplies 4 kcal g^{-1}; fat, 9 kcal g^{-1}; protein, 4 kcal g^{-1}.

to move and breathe and the enzymes that carry out metabolism. Hence it is not as dispensable as fat and glycogen and is given up by the body more reluctantly.

The constant availability of fuels in the blood is termed **caloric homeostasis,** which, as illustrated in Table 13.2, means that regardless of whether a person is well-fed, fasting, or starving to death, the blood level of fuels that supply a comparable amount of ATP when metabolized does not fall below certain limits. Note that blood glucose concentrations are controlled within very tight limits, whereas fatty acid and ketone body concentrations in the blood can vary by one or two orders of magnitude, respectively. Glucose is carefully regulated because of the absolute need of the brain for this substrate. If the blood glucose level falls too low (<2.0 mM), coma and death will follow shortly unless the glucose concentration is restored. On the other hand, **hyperglycemia** must be avoided because glucose will be lost in the urine, resulting in dehydration and sometimes hyperglycemic, hyperosmolar coma (see Clin. Corr. 13.5). Chronic hyperglycemia results in glycation of a number of proteins, which contributes to the complications of **diabetes** (see Clin. Corr. 13.6). The changes

TABLE 13.2 Substrate and Hormone Levels in Blood of Well-Fed, Fasting, and Starving Humans[a]

Hormone or Substrate (units)	Very Well Fed	Postabsorptive 12 h	Fasted 3 days	Starved 5 weeks
Insulin (μU mL^{-1})	40	15	8	6
Glucagon (pg mL^{-1})	80	100	150	120
Insulin/glucagon ratio (μU pg^{-1})	0.50	0.15	0.05	0.05
Glucose (mM)	6.1	4.8	3.8	3.6
Fatty acids (mM)	0.14	0.6	1.2	1.4
Acetoacetate (mM)	0.04	0.05	0.4	1.3
β-Hydroxybutyrate (mM)	0.03	0.10	1.4	6.0
Lactate (mM)	2.5	0.7	0.7	0.6
Pyruvate (mM)	0.25	0.06	0.04	0.03
Alanine (mM)	0.8	0.3	0.3	0.1
ATP equivalents (mM)	313	290	380	537

Source: From Ruderman, N. B., Aoki, T. T., and Cahill, G. F. Jr. Gluconeogenesis and its disorders in man. In: R. W. Hanson and M. A. Mehlman (Eds.), *Gluconeogenesis, Its Regulation in Mammalian Species.* New York: Wiley, 1976, p. 515.

[a] Data are for normal-weight subjects except for the 5-week starvation values, which are from obese subjects undergoing therapeutic starvation. ATP equivalents were calculated on the basis of the ATP yield expected on complete oxidation of each substrate to CO_2 and H_2O: 38 molecules of ATP for each molecule of glucose; 144 for the average fatty acid (oleate); 23 for acetoacetate; 26 for β-hydroxybutyrate; 18 for lactate; 15 for pyruvate; and 13 (corrected for urea formation) for alanine.

CLINICAL CORRELATION 13.5

Hyperglycemic, Hyperosmolar Coma

Type II diabetic patients sometimes develop a condition called hyperglycemic, hyperosmolar coma. This is particularly common in the elderly and can even occur in individuals under severe metabolic stress who were not recognized as having diabetes beforehand. Hyperglycemia, perhaps worsened by failure to take insulin or hypoglycemic drugs, an infection, or a coincidental medical problem such as a heart attack, leads to urinary losses of water, glucose, and electrolytes (sodium, chloride, and potassium). This osmotic diuresis reduces the circulating blood volume, a stress that results in the release of hormones that worsen insulin resistance and hyperglycemia. In addition, elderly patients may be less able to sense thirst or to obtain fluids. Over the course of several days these patients can become extremely hyperglycemic (glucose >1000 mg dL^{-1}), dehydrated, and comatose. Ketoacidosis does not develop in these patients, possibly because free fatty acids are not always elevated or because adequate insulin concentrations exist in the portal blood to inhibit ketogenesis (although it is not high enough to inhibit gluconeogenesis). Therapy is aimed at restoring water and electrolyte balance and correcting the hyperglycemia with insulin. The mortality of this syndrome is considerably higher than that of diabetic ketoacidosis.

Arieff, A. I., and Carroll, H. J. Nonketotic hyperosmolar coma with hyperglycemia. Clinical features, pathophysiology, renal function, acid–base balance, plasma–cerebrospinal fluid equilibria, and the effects of therapy in 37 cases. *Medicine* 51:73, 1972; and Cruz-Caudillo, J. C., and Sabatini, S. Diabetic hyperosmolar syndrome. *Nephron* 69:201, 1995.

CLINICAL CORRELATION 13.6

Hyperglycemia and Protein Glycation

Glycation of enzymes is known to cause changes in their activity, solubility, and susceptibility to degradation. In the case of hemoglobin A, glycation occurs by a nonenzymatic reaction between glucose and the amino-terminal valine of the β chain. A Schiff base forms between glucose and valine, followed by a rearrangement of the molecule to give a 1-deoxyfructose molecule attached to the valine. The reaction is favored by high glucose levels and the resulting protein, called hemoglobin A_{1c}, is a good index of how high a person's average blood glucose concentration has been over the previous several weeks. The concentration of this modified protein increases in an uncontrolled diabetic and is low in patients who control their glucose level closely.

It has been proposed that glycation of proteins may contribute to the medical complications caused by diabetes, for example, coronary heart disease, retinopathy, nephropathy, cataracts, and neuropathy. Increased glycation of lens proteins may contribute to the development of diabetic cataracts. Collagen, laminin, vitronectin, and other matrix proteins can become glycated and undergo alterations in biological properties, such as self-assembly and binding of other matrix molecules. Glycated proteins and lipoproteins can also be recognized by receptors present on macrophages, which are intimately involved in the formation of atherosclerotic plaques. It is likely that these phenomena favor the accelerated atherosclerosis that occurs in diabetics. The compound aminoguanidine inhibits the formation of the glycation products and is being tested for its ability to prevent diabetic complications.

Brownlee, M. Glycation products and the pathogenesis of diabetic complications. *Diabetes Care* 15:1835, 1992; Vlassara, H. Receptor-mediated interactions with advanced glycosylation end products with cellular components within diabetic tissues. *Diabetes* 41(Suppl 2):52, 1992; and Lyons, T. J. Glycation and oxidation: a role in the pathogenesis of atherosclerosis. *Am. J. Cardiol.* 71:26B, 1993.

in insulin/glucagon ratio shown in Table 13.2 are crucial to the maintenance of caloric homeostasis. Simply stated, well-fed individuals have high insulin/glucagon ratios that favor storage of glycogen and fat, while starving individuals have low insulin/glucagon ratios that stimulate lipolysis, proteolysis, and gluconeogenesis.

Glucose Homeostasis Has Five Phases

Figure 13.10 shows the work of Cahill and his colleagues with obese patients undergoing long-term starvation for weight loss. It illustrates the effects of starvation on those processes that are used to maintain **glucose homeostasis.** For convenience, the time period involved has been divided into five phases. Phase I is the well-fed state in which glucose is provided by dietary carbohydrate. Once this supply is exhausted, hepatic glycogenolysis maintains blood glucose levels during phase II. As this supply of glucose starts to dwindle, hepatic gluconeogenesis from lactate, glycerol, and alanine becomes increasingly important until, in phase III, it is the major source of blood glucose. These changes occur within 20 or so hours of fasting, depending on how well fed the individual was prior to the fast, how much hepatic glycogen was present, and the sort of physical activity occurring during the fast. Several days of fasting move one into phase IV, where the dependence on gluconeogenesis actually decreases. As discussed above, ketone bodies have accumulated to high enough concentrations for them to enter the brain and meet some of its energy needs. Renal gluconeogenesis also becomes significant in this phase. Phase V occurs after very prolonged starvation of extremely obese individuals and is characterized by even less dependence on gluconeogenesis. The energy needs of almost every tissue are met to a large extent by either fatty acid or ketone body oxidation in this phase.

As long as ketone body concentrations are high, proteolysis will be somewhat restricted, and conservation of muscle proteins and enzymes will occur. This continues until practically all of the fat is gone as a consequence of starvation. After all of it is gone, the body has to use muscle protein. Before it is gone—you are gone (see Clin. Corr. 13.3).

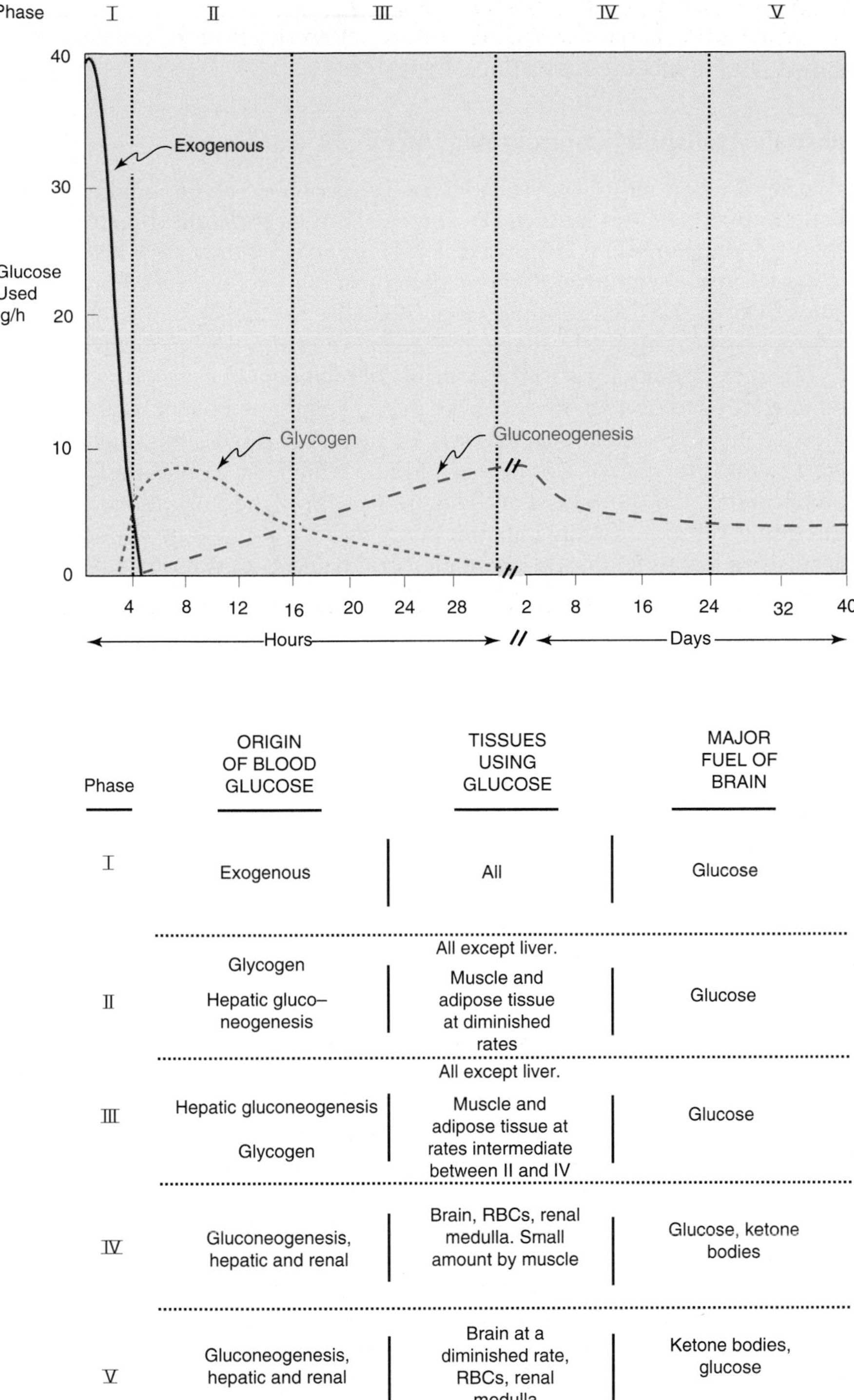

Phase	ORIGIN OF BLOOD GLUCOSE	TISSUES USING GLUCOSE	MAJOR FUEL OF BRAIN
I	Exogenous	All	Glucose
II	Glycogen Hepatic gluco–neogenesis	All except liver. Muscle and adipose tissue at diminished rates	Glucose
III	Hepatic gluconeogenesis Glycogen	All except liver. Muscle and adipose tissue at rates intermediate between II and IV	Glucose
IV	Gluconeogenesis, hepatic and renal	Brain, RBCs, renal medulla. Small amount by muscle	Glucose, ketone bodies
V	Gluconeogenesis, hepatic and renal	Brain at a diminished rate, RBCs, renal medulla	Ketone bodies, glucose

FIGURE 13.10
The five phases of glucose homeostasis in humans.
Reprinted with permission from Ruderman, N. B., Aoki, T. T., and Cahill, G. F. Jr. Gluconeogenesis and its disorders in man. In: R. W. Hanson and M. A. Mehlman (Eds.), Gluconeogenesis, Its Regulation in Mammalian Species. *New York: Wiley, 1976, p. 515.*

13.3 MECHANISMS INVOLVED IN SWITCHING THE METABOLISM OF LIVER BETWEEN THE WELL-FED STATE AND THE STARVED STATE

The liver of a well-fed person is actively engaged in processes that favor the synthesis of glycogen and fat; such a liver is glycogenic, glycolytic, and lipogenic. The liver of the fasting person is quite a different organ; it is glycogenolytic, gluconeogenic, ketogenic, and proteolytic. The strategy is to store calories when food is available, but then to mobilize these stores when the rest of the body is in need. The liver is switched between these metabolic extremes by a variety of regulatory mechanisms: substrate supply, allosteric effectors, covalent modification, and induction–repression of enzymes.

Substrate Availability Controls Many Metabolic Pathways

Because of other, more sophisticated levels of control, the importance of **substrate supply** is often ignored. However, the concentration of fatty acids in blood entering the liver is clearly a major determinant of the rate of ketogenesis. Excess fat is not synthesized unless one consumes excessive amounts of substrates that can be used for lipogenesis. Glucose synthesis by the liver is also restricted by the rate at which gluconeogenic substrates flow to the liver. Delivery of excess amino acids to the liver of the diabetic, because of accelerated and uncontrolled proteolysis, increases the rate of gluconeogenesis and exacerbates the hyperglycemia characteristic of diabetes. In addition, high glucose levels increase the rate of synthesis of sorbitol, which may contribute to diabetic complications. On the other hand, failure to supply the liver adequately with glucogenic substrate (mainly alanine) explains some types of hypoglycemia, such as that observed during pregnancy or advanced starvation.

Another pathway regulated by substrate supply is **urea synthesis.** Amino acid metabolism in the intestine provides a substantial fraction of the ammonia used by the liver for urea production. As discussed above, the intestine also releases citrulline, metabolic precursor of ornithine. A larger ornithine pool permits increased urea synthesis after a high protein meal.

We can conclude that substrate supply is a major determinant of the rate at which virtually every metabolic process of the body operates. However, variations in substrate supply are not sufficient to account for the marked changes in metabolism that must occur in the starve–feed cycle, and finer tuning of the pathways is required.

Negative and Positive Allosteric Effectors Regulate Key Enzymes

Figures 13.11 and 13.12 summarize the effects of negative and positive **allosteric effectors** important in the well-fed and starved states, respectively. As shown in Figure 13.11, glucose inactivates glycogen phosphorylase and activates glycogen synthase (indirectly; see Chapter 7, p. 326), thereby preventing degradation and promoting synthesis of glycogen; fructose 2,6-bisphosphate stimulates 6-phosphofructo-1-kinase and inhibits fructose 1,6-bisphosphatase, thereby stimulating glycolysis and inhibiting gluconeogenesis; fructose 1,6-bisphosphate activates pyruvate kinase, thereby stimulating glycolysis; pyruvate activates pyruvate dehydrogenase (indirectly by inhibition of pyruvate dehydrogenase kinase; see Chapter 6, p. 228); citrate activates acetyl-CoA carboxylase, thereby stimulating fatty acid synthesis; and malonyl CoA inhibits carnitine palmitoyltransferase I, thereby inhibiting fatty acid oxidation.

As shown in Figure 13.12, acetyl CoA stimulates gluconeogenesis in the fasted state by activating pyruvate carboxylase and inhibiting pyruvate dehydrogenase (a direct allosteric effect and also by stimulation of pyruvate dehydrogenase kinase; see Chapter 7, p. 308); long-chain acyl CoA esters inhibit acetyl-CoA carboxylase, which lowers the level of malonyl CoA and permits greater carnitine palmitoyltransferase I activity and fatty acid oxidation rates; fructose 6-phosphate acts through a regulatory protein to inhibit glucokinase; citrate, which can be increased because of fatty acid oxidation, inhibits 6-phosphofructo-1-kinase as well as 6-phosphofructo-2-kinase (not shown); and NADH produced by fatty acid oxidation inhibits TCA cycle activity.

Although not shown in Figure 13.12, **cAMP** is an important allosteric effector. Its concentration in liver is increased in the starved state. Cyclic AMP is a positive effector of cAMP-dependent protein kinase (also called **protein**

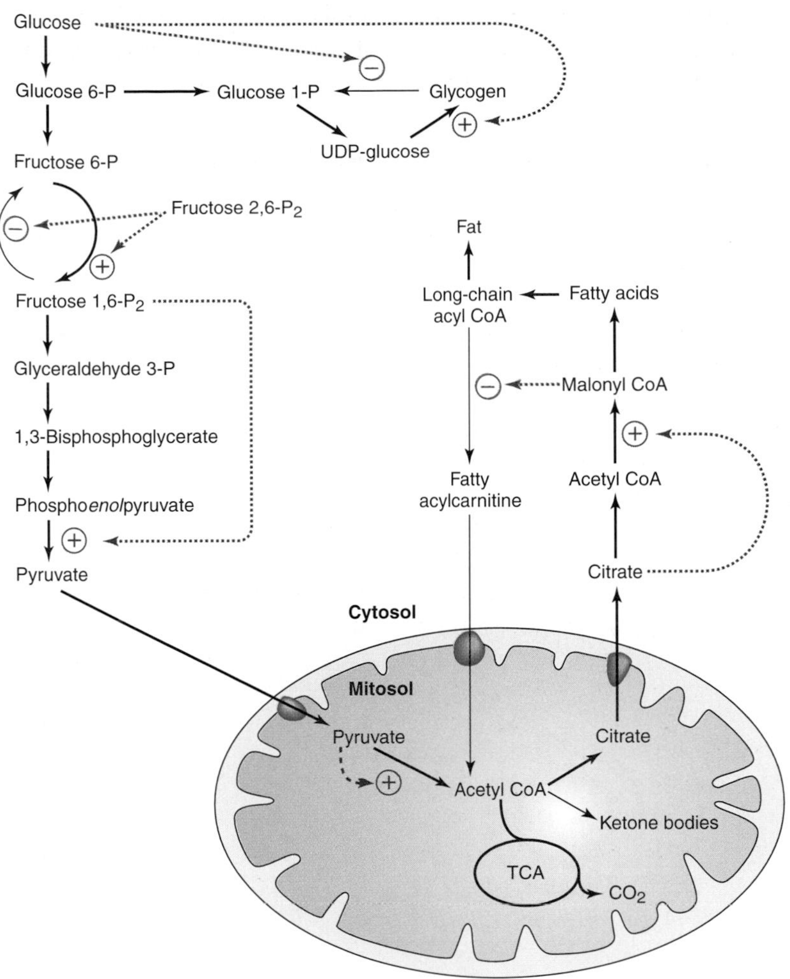

FIGURE 13.11
Control of hepatic metabolism in the well-fed state by allosteric effectors.

kinase A), which, in turn, is responsible for changing the kinetic properties of several regulatory enzymes by covalent modification, as summarized next.

Covalent Modification Regulates Key Enzymes

Figures 13.13 and 13.14 point out the interconvertible enzymes that play important roles in switching the liver between the well-fed and starved states. The regulation of enzymes by **covalent modification** has been discussed in Chapter 7. Recall that ⊡ and ⊙-P represent interconvertible forms of an enzyme in the nonphosphorylated and phosphorylated states, respectively.

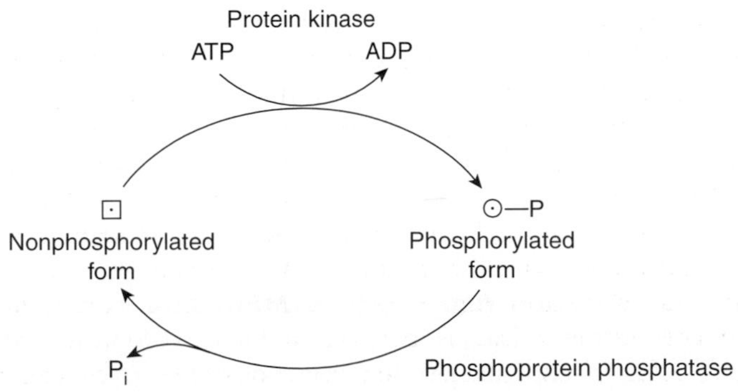

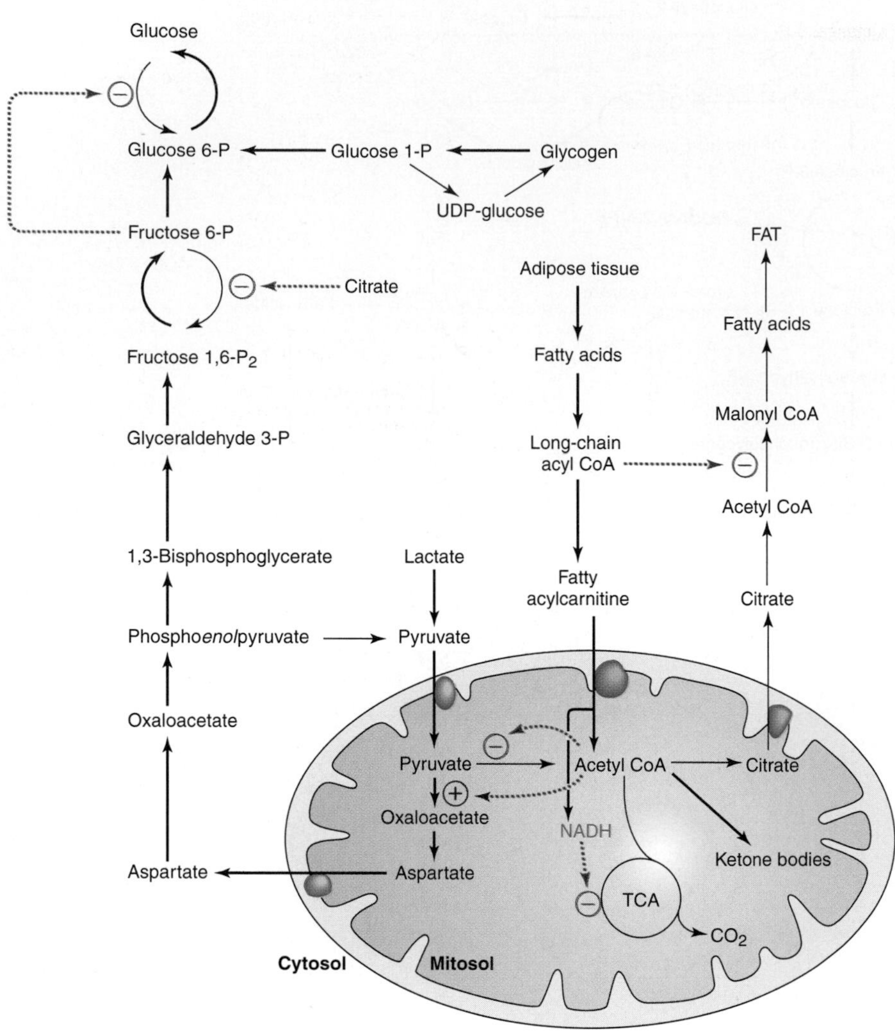

FIGURE 13.12
Control of hepatic metabolism in the fasting state by allosteric effectors.

The important points are as follows: (1) enzymes subject to covalent modification undergo phosphorylation on one or more serine residues by a protein kinase; (2) the phosphorylated enzyme can be returned to the dephosphorylated state by phosphoprotein phosphatase; (3) phosphorylation of the enzyme changes its conformation and its catalytic activity; (4) some enzymes are active only in the dephosphorylated state, others only in the phosphorylated state; (5) cAMP is the messenger that signals the phosphorylation of many, but not all, of the enzymes subject to covalent modification; (6) cAMP acts by activating protein kinase A; (7) cAMP also indirectly promotes phosphorylation of interconvertible enzymes by signaling inactivation of phosphoprotein phosphatase; (8) glucagon and β-adrenergic agonists (epinephrine) increase cAMP levels by activating adenylate cyclase; (9) insulin (see Chapter 20, p. 879) opposes the action of glucagon and epinephrine, in part by lowering cAMP and in part by mechanisms independent of cAMP; and (10) the action of insulin in general promotes dephosphorylation of interconvertible enzymes.

Hepatic enzymes subject to covalent modification are dephosphorylated in well-fed animals (Figure 13.13). Although not shown, phosphorylase kinase is also dephosphorylated in this state. Insulin/glucagon ratios are high in blood, and cAMP levels are low in liver. This results in low activity of protein kinase A and high activity of **phosphoprotein phosphatase.** Glycogen synthase, glycogen phosphorylase (via phosphorylase kinase), 6-phosphofructo-2-kinase/fructose 2,6-bisphosphatase (bifunctional enzyme), pyruvate kinase, and

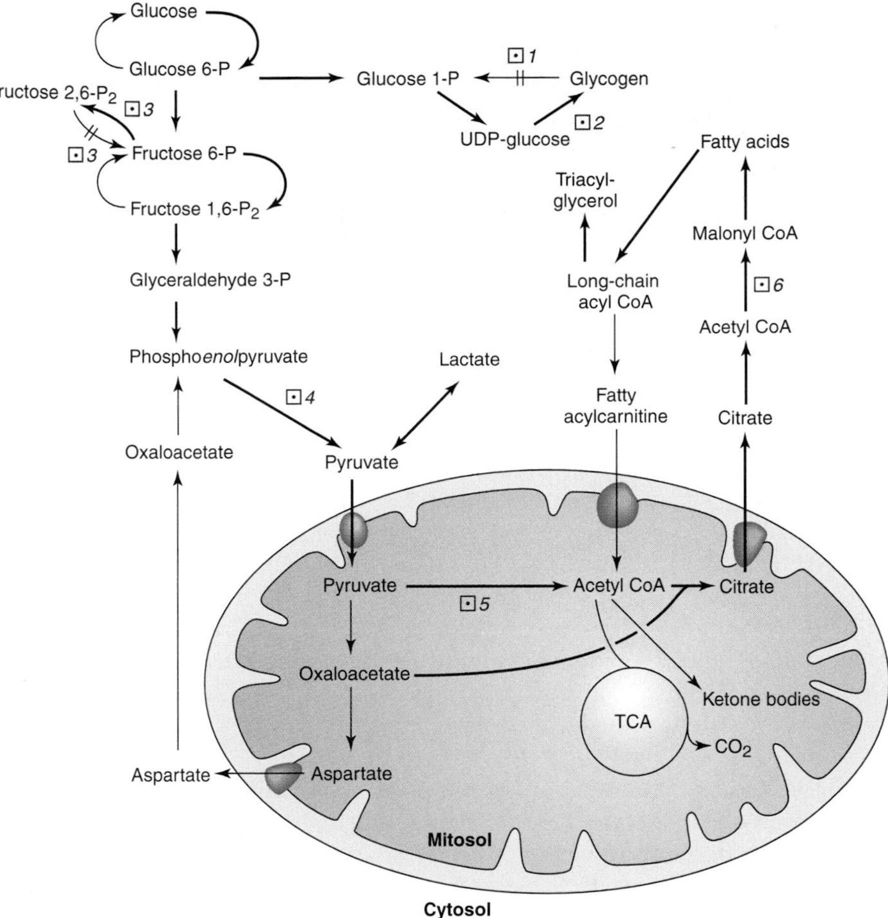

FIGURE 13.13
Activity and state of phosphorylation of enzymes subject to covalent modification in the lipogenic liver.
The dephosphorylated mode is indicated by the symbol ⊡. Interconvertible enzymes are numbered as follows: *1*, glycogen phosphorylase; *2*, glycogen synthase; *3*, 6-phosphofructo-2-kinase/fructose 2,6-bisphosphatase (bifunctional enzyme); *4*, pyruvate kinase; *5*, pyruvate dehydrogenase; and *6*, acetyl-CoA carboxylase.

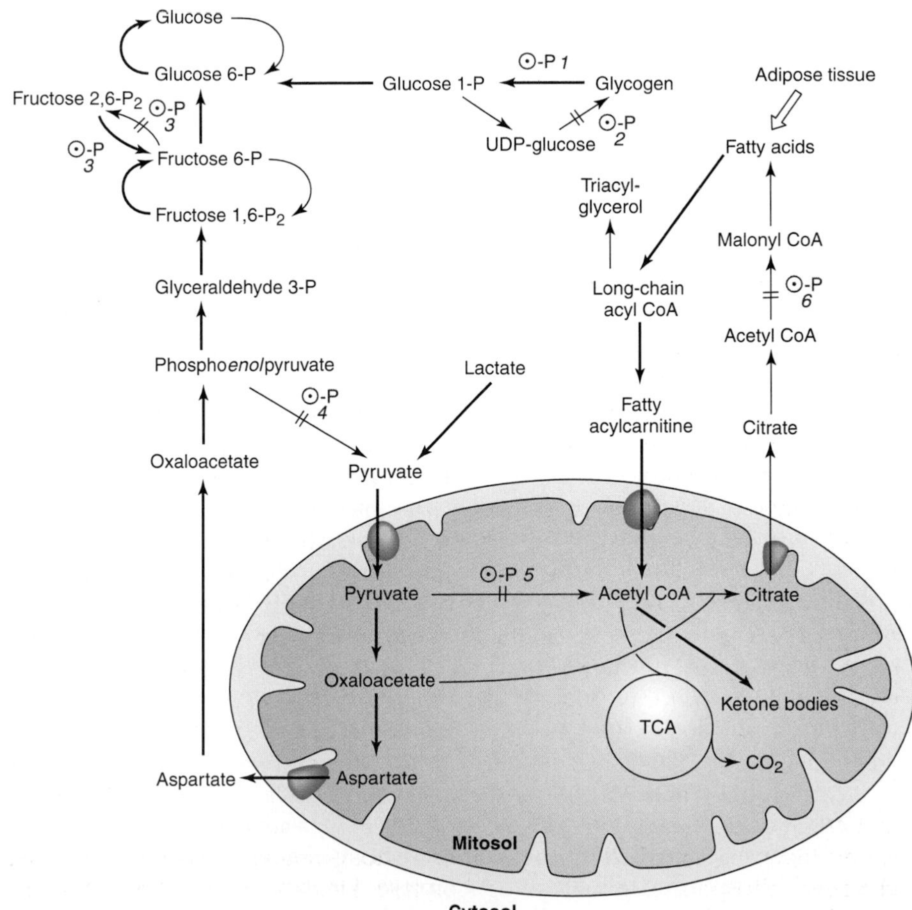

FIGURE 13.14
Activity and state of phosphorylation of enzymes subject to covalent modification in the glucogenic liver.
Phosphorylated mode is indicated by the symbol ⊙-P. Numbers refer to the same enzymes as in Figure 13.13.

acetyl-CoA carboxylase are phosphorylated by protein kinase A. However, not all interconvertible enzymes are subject to phosphorylation by protein kinase A. No link to protein kinase A for the pyruvate dehydrogenase complex has been established. Only three of the interconvertible enzymes—**glycogen phosphorylase,** phosphorylase kinase, and the **fructose 2,6-bisphosphatase** of the bifunctional enzyme—are inactive when dephosphorylated. All of the other identified interconvertible enzymes are active. Glycogenesis, glycolysis, and lipogenesis are greatly favored when these enzymes are dephosphorylated. On the other hand, the opposing pathways—glycogenolysis, gluconeogenesis, and ketogenesis—are inhibited.

As shown in Figure 13.14 (p. 543), the hepatic enzymes subject to covalent modification are in the phosphorylated mode in the liver of the fasting animal. Insulin is low but glucagon is high in the blood, resulting in an increase in hepatic cAMP levels. This activates protein kinase A and inactivates phosphoprotein phosphatase. The net effect is a greater degree of phosphorylation of interconvertible enzymes than in the well-fed state. In the starved state, three interconvertible enzymes—glycogen phosphorylase, phosphorylase kinase, and the fructose 2,6-bisphosphatase of the bifunctional enzyme—are in the active catalytic state. All the other interconvertible enzymes are inactive in the phosphorylated mode. As a result, glycogenesis, glycolysis, and lipogenesis are shut down almost completely, and glycogenolysis, gluconeogenesis, and ketogenesis predominate.

Two additional hepatic enzymes, **phenylalanine hydroxylase** and **branched-chain α-keto acid dehydrogenase,** are also controlled by phosphorylation/dephosphorylation. These enzymes catalyze rate-limiting steps in the disposal of phenylalanine and the branched-chain amino acids (leucine, isoleucine, and valine), respectively. These enzymes are not included in Figures 13.13 and 13.14 because of special features of their control by covalent modification. Phenylalanine hydroxylase, a cytosolic enzyme, is active in the phosphorylated state, and phosphorylation is stimulated by glucagon via protein kinase A. Branched-chain α-keto acid dehydrogenase, a mitochondrial enzyme, is active in the dephosphorylated state, and its activity is regulated by branched-chain α-keto acid dehydrogenase kinase and a phosphoprotein phosphatase. Phenylalanine acts as a positive allosteric effector for the phosphorylation and activation of phenylalanine hydroxylase by cAMP-dependent protein kinase. Branched-chain α-keto acids activate branched-chain α-keto acid dehydrogenase indirectly by inhibiting branched-chain α-keto acid dehydrogenase kinase. Covalent modification of these enzymes provides a very sensitive means for control of the degradation of phenylalanine and the branched-chain amino acids. The clinical experience with phenylketonuria (see Clin. Corr. 11.5) and maple syrup urine disease (see Clin. Corr. 11.10) emphasizes the importance of regulating blood and tissue levels of these amino acids. Of note, the artificial sweetener **aspartame** (NutraSweet®) is *N*-aspartylphenylalanine methyl ester. The amount in a liter of sweetened drinks may approach the amount of phenylalanine normally obtained from the daily diet. This is of no harm to normal individuals but is a threat to **phenylketonuria** patients on a low phenylalanine diet. Phenylalanine and the branched-chain amino acids cannot be synthesized in humans, making them essential amino acids that must be available continuously for protein synthesis. Thus the activities of phenylalanine hydroxylase and branched-chain α-keto acid dehydrogenase must be carefully controlled to prevent depletion of body stores. Therefore the tissue requirement for these amino acids supersedes the phase of the starve–feed cycle in establishing the phosphorylation and activity state of these interconvertible enzymes.

Adipose tissue responds almost as dramatically as liver to the starve–feed cycle because it also contains enzymes subject to covalent modification. Pyruvate kinase, pyruvate dehydrogenase, acetyl-CoA carboxylase, and hormone-sensitive lipase (not found in liver) are all in the dephosphorylated mode in the adipose tissue of the well-fed person. As in liver, the first three enzymes are active when dephosphorylated. **Hormone-sensitive lipase** is inactive when dephosphorylated. A high insulin level in the blood and a low cAMP concentration in adipose tissue are important determinants of the phosphorylation state of these enzymes, which favors lipogenesis in the well-fed state. During fasting, as a consequence of the decrease in the insulin level and an increase in epinephrine, adipocytes quickly shut down lipogenesis and activate lipolysis. This is accomplished in large part by the phosphorylation of the enzymes described above. In this manner, adipose tissue is transformed from a fat storage tissue into a source of fatty acids for oxidation in other tissues and glycerol for gluconeogenesis in the liver.

Conservation of glucose as well as three-carbon compounds that can readily be converted to glucose (lactate, alanine, and pyruvate) by the liver is crucial for survival in the starved state. Certain cells, particularly those of the central nervous system, are absolutely dependent on a continuous supply of glucose. Tissues that can use alternative fuels invariably shut down their use of glucose and three-carbon precursors. This is referred to as the glucose–fatty acid cycle in recognition that increased availability of fatty acids for oxidation spares glucose in the starved state. Inactivation of the pyruvate dehydrogenase complex by phosphorylation is an important feature of the **glucose–fatty acid cycle.** This occurs in skeletal muscle, heart, and kidney, but not in the central nervous system, when the alternative fuels (fatty acids and ketone bodies) of the starved state become abundant. Activation of pyruvate dehydrogenase kinase by products of the catabolism of the alternative fuels (acetyl CoA and NADH) is responsible for the greater degree of phosphorylation and therefore lower activity of the pyruvate dehydrogenase complex.

Covalent modification, like allosteric effectors and substrate supply, is a short-term regulatory mechanism, operating on a minute-to-minute basis. On a longer time scale, enzyme activities are controlled at the level of expression.

Changes in Levels of Key Enzymes Are a Longer Term Adaptive Mechanism

The adaptive change in enzyme levels is a mechanism of regulation involving changes in the rate of synthesis or degradation of key enzymes. Whereas allosteric effectors and covalent modification affect either the K_m or V_{max} of an enzyme, this mode of regulation involves the actual quantity of an enzyme in a tissue. Because of the influence of hormonal and nutritional factors, there are more or fewer enzyme molecules present in the tissue. For example, when a person is maintained in a well-fed or overfed condition, the liver improves its capacity to synthesize fat. This can be explained in part by increased substrate supply, appropriate changes in allosteric effectors (Figure 13.11), and the conversion of the interconvertible enzymes into the dephosphorylated form (Figure 13.13). This is not the entire story, however, because the liver also has more of those enzyme molecules that play a key role in fat synthesis (see Figure 13.15). A whole battery of enzymes is induced, including glucokinase, 6-phospho-1-fructokinase, and pyruvate kinase for faster rates of glycolysis; glucose-6-phosphate dehydrogenase, 6-phosphogluconate dehydrogenase, and malic enzyme to provide greater quantities of NADPH for reductive synthesis; and citrate cleavage enzyme, acetyl-CoA carboxylase, fatty acid synthase, and Δ^9-desaturase for more rapid rates of fatty acid synthesis. All of these enzymes are present at higher levels in the well-fed state because of an increase in the blood of the insulin/glucagon ratio and glucose. While these enzymes are induced, there is a decrease in the enzymes that favor glucose synthesis. **Phosphoenolpyruvate carboxykinase,** fructose 1,6-bisphosphatase, **glucose 6-phosphatase,** and

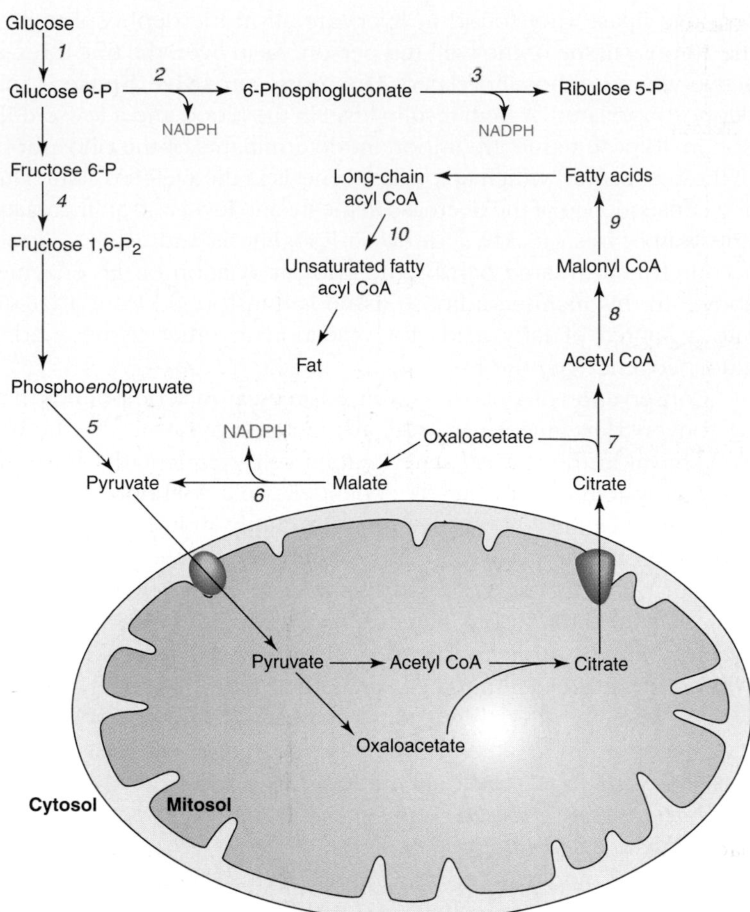

FIGURE 13.15
Enzymes induced in the liver of the well-fed individual.
Inducible enzymes are numbered as follows: *1*, glucokinase; *2*, glucose-6-phosphate dehydrogenase; *3*, 6-phosphogluconate dehydrogenase; *4*, 6-phosphofructo-1-kinase; *5*, pyruvate kinase; *6*, malic enzyme; *7*, citrate cleavage enzyme; *8*, acetyl-CoA carboxylase; *9*, fatty acid synthase; and *10*, Δ^9-desaturase.

some aminotransferases are decreased in amount; that is, their synthesis is reduced or degradation increased in response to increased circulating glucose and insulin.

In fasting, the enzyme pattern of the liver changes dramatically (Figure 13.16). The enzymes involved in lipogenesis decrease in quantity, possibly because their synthesis is decreased or degradation of these proteins is increased. At the same time a number of enzymes (glucose 6-phosphatase, fructose 1,6-bisphosphatase, phosphoenolpyruvate carboxykinase, and various aminotransferases) favoring gluconeogenesis are induced, making the liver much more effective in synthesizing glucose. In addition, the enzymes of the urea cycle and other amino acid-metabolizing enzymes such as liver **glutaminase,** tyrosine aminotransferase, serine dehydratase, proline oxidase, and histidase are induced, possibly by the presence of higher blood glucagon levels. This permits the disposal of nitrogen, as urea, from the amino acids used in gluconeogenesis.

These adaptive changes are clearly important in the starve–feed cycle, greatly affecting the capacity of the liver for its various metabolic processes. The adaptive changes also influence the effectiveness of the short-term regulatory mechanisms. For example, long-term starvation or uncontrolled diabetes decreases the level of acetyl-CoA carboxylase. Taking away long-chain acyl CoA esters that inhibit this enzyme, increasing the level of citrate that activates this enzyme, or creating conditions that activate this interconvertible enzyme by dephosphorylation will not have any effect when the enzyme is virtually absent. Another example is afforded by the **glucose intolerance** of starvation. A chronically starved person cannot effectively utilize a load of glucose because of the absence of the key enzymes needed for glucose metabolism. A glucose

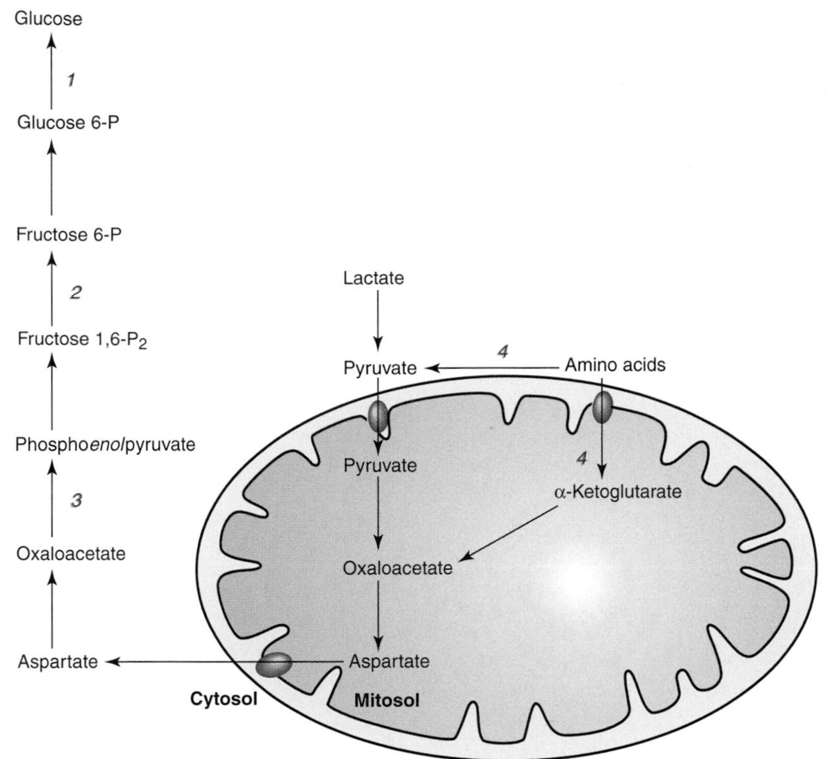

FIGURE 13.16
Enzymes induced in the liver of an individual during fasting.
Inducible enzymes are numbered as follows: *1*, glucose 6-phosphatase; *2*, fructose 1,6-bisphosphatase; *3*, phosphoenolpyruvate carboxykinase; and *4*, various aminotransferases.

load, however, will set into motion the induction of the required enzymes and the reestablishment of short-term regulatory mechanisms.

13.4 METABOLIC INTERRELATIONSHIPS OF TISSUES IN VARIOUS NUTRITIONAL AND HORMONAL STATES

Many changes that occur in various nutritional and hormonal states are variations on the starve–feed cycle and are completely predictable from what we have learned about the cycle. Some examples are given in Figure 13.17. Others are so obvious that a diagram is unnecessary; for example, in rapid growth of a child, amino acids are directed away from catabolism and into protein synthesis. However, the changes that occur in some physiologically important situations are rather subtle and poorly understood. An example of the latter is **aging,** which seems to lead to a decreased "sensitivity" of the major tissues of the body to hormones. The important consequence is a decreased ability of the tissues to respond normally during the starve–feed cycle. Whether this is a contributing factor to or a consequence of the aging process is unknown.

Staying in the Well-Fed State Results in Obesity and Insulin Resistance

Figure 13.17*a* illustrates the metabolic interrelationships prevailing in an obese person. Most of the body fat of the human is either provided by the diet or synthesized in the liver and transported to the adipose tissue for storage. Obesity is caused by a person staying in such a well-fed state that stored fat does not get used up during the fasting phase of the cycle. The body then has no option other than to accumulate fat (see Clin. Corr. 13.1).

Obesity always causes some degree of **insulin resistance.** Insulin resistance is a poorly understood phenomenon in which the tissues fail to respond to insulin. The number or affinity of insulin receptors is reduced in some patients; others have normal insulin binding, but abnormal postreceptor responses, such

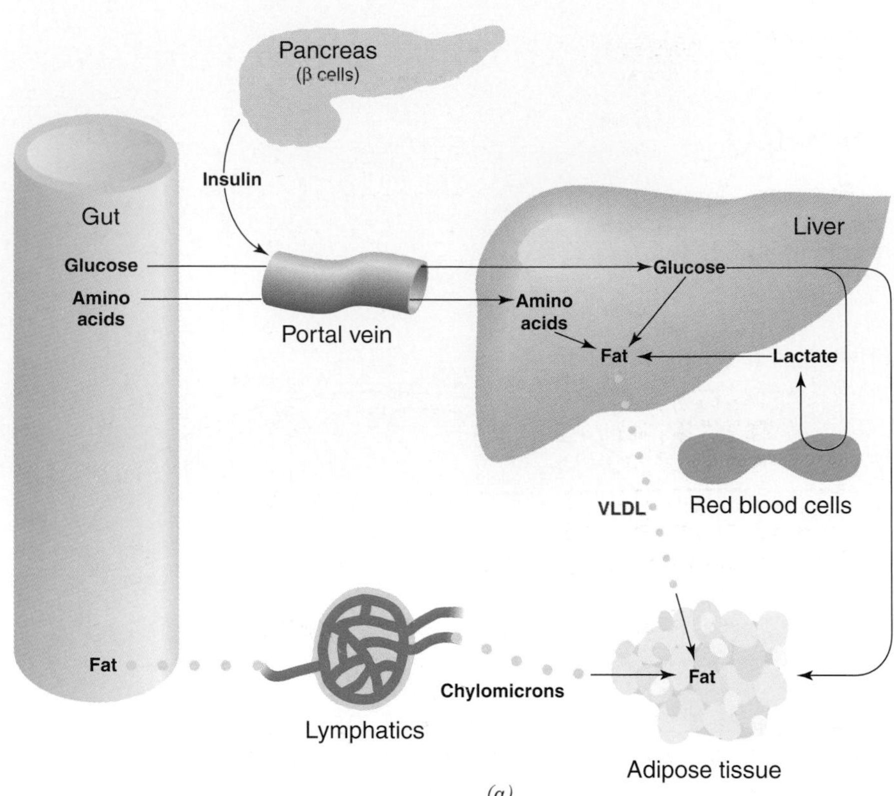

FIGURE 13.17
Metabolic interrelationships of tissues in various nutritional, hormonal, and disease states.
(*a*) Obesity.

as the activation of glucose transport. As a general rule, the greater the quantity of body fat, the greater the resistance of normally insulin-sensitive cells to the action of insulin. Current research suggests that high expression of **tumor necrosis factor-α (TNF-α)** in the fat cells of obese individuals contributes to insulin resistance. As a consequence, plasma insulin levels are greatly elevated in the blood of an obese individual. As long as the β cells of the pancreas produce enough insulin to overcome the insulin resistance, an obese individual will have relatively normal blood levels of glucose and lipoproteins. The insulin resistance of obesity can lead, however, to the development of noninsulin-dependent diabetes, as discussed next.

Noninsulin-Dependent Diabetes Mellitus

Figure 13.17b shows the metabolic interrelationships characteristic of a person with **noninsulin-dependent diabetes.** In contrast to insulin-dependent diabetes, insulin is not absent in noninsulin-dependent diabetes (see Clin. Corr. 13.7). Indeed, high levels of insulin may be observed in this form of diabetes, and the problem is primarily resistance to the action of insulin as discussed above for obese individuals. It therefore follows that the majority of patients with noninsulin-dependent diabetes mellitus are obese. Although the insulin levels of noninsulin-dependent diabetic patients may and often are high, they are not as high as those of a nondiabetic but similarly obese person. The pancreases of these diabetic patients do not produce enough insulin to overcome the insulin resistance induced by their obesity. Hence this form of diabetes is also a form of β-cell failure; exogenous insulin will reduce the hyperglycemia and very often must be administered to control blood glucose levels of noninsulin-dependent diabetic patients. Hyperglycemia results mainly because of poor uptake of glucose by peripheral tissues, especially muscle. In contrast to insulin-dependent diabetes, ketoacidosis does not develop because the adipocytes

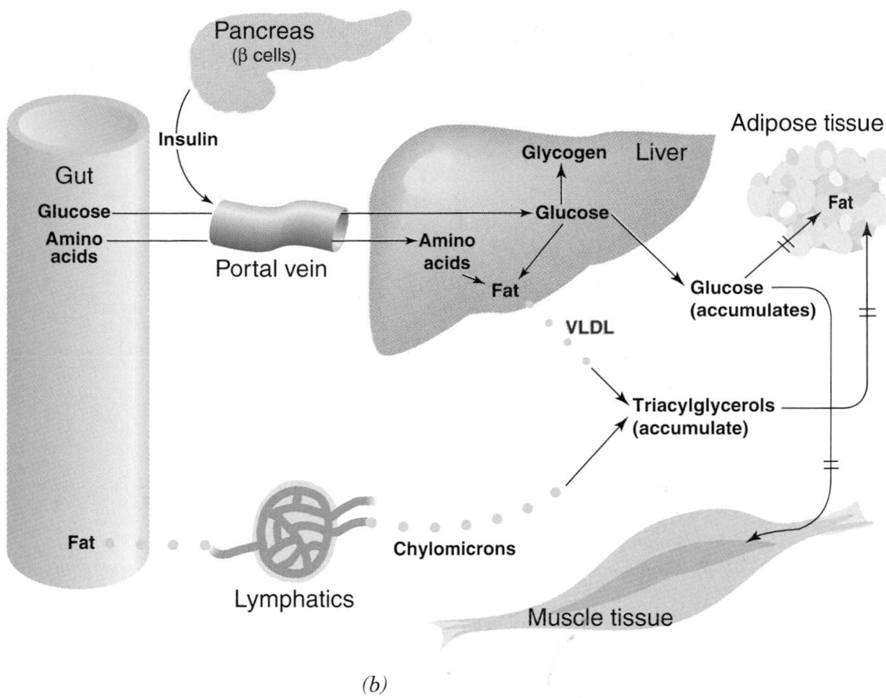

FIGURE 13.17 (continued)
(*b*) Noninsulin-dependent diabetes mellitus.

remain sensitive to the effect of insulin on lipolysis. Hypertriglyceridemia is characteristic of noninsulin-dependent diabetes but usually results from an increase in VLDLs without **hyperchylomicronemia.** This is most likely explained by rapid rates of *de novo* hepatic synthesis of fatty acids and VLDLs rather than increased delivery of fatty acids from the adipose tissue.

CLINICAL CORRELATION 13.7

Noninsulin-Dependent Diabetes Mellitus

Noninsulin-dependent diabetes mellitus (NIDDM) accounts for 80–90% of the diagnosed cases of diabetes and is also called maturity-onset diabetes to differentiate it from insulin-dependent, juvenile diabetes. It usually occurs in middle-aged obese people. Noninsulin-dependent diabetes is characterized by hyperglycemia, often with hypertriglyceridemia. The ketoacidosis characteristic of the insulin-dependent disease is not observed. Increased levels of VLDL are probably the result of increased hepatic triacylglycerol synthesis stimulated by hyperglycemia and hyperinsulinemia. Insulin is present at normal to elevated levels in this form of the disease. Obesity often precedes the development of insulin-independent diabetes and appears to be the major contributing factor. Obese patients are usually hyperinsulinemic. Very recent data implicate increased levels of expression of tumor necrosis factor-α (TNF-α) in adipocytes of obese individuals as a cause of the resistance. The greater the adipose tissue mass, the greater the production of TNF-α, which acts to impair insulin receptor function. An inverse relationship between insulin levels and the number of insulin receptors has been established. The higher the basal level of insulin, the fewer receptors present on the plasma membranes. In addition, there are defects within insulin-responsive cells at sites beyond the receptor. An example is the ability of insulin to recruit glucose transporters from intracellular sites to the plasma membrane. As a consequence, insulin levels remain high, but glucose levels are poorly controlled because of the lack of normal responsiveness to insulin. Although the insulin level is high, it is not as high as in a person who is obese but not diabetic. In other words, there is a relative deficiency in the insulin supply from the β cells. Therefore, this disease is caused not only by insulin resistance but also by impaired β-cell function resulting in relative insulin deficiency. Diet alone can often control the disease in the obese diabetic. If the patient can be motivated to lose weight, insulin receptors will increase in number, and the postreceptor abnormalities will improve, which will increase both tissue sensitivity to insulin and glucose tolerance. The noninsulin-dependent diabetic tends not to develop ketoacidosis but nevertheless develops many of the same complications as the insulin-dependent diabetic, that is, nerve, eye, kidney, and coronary artery disease.

Olefsky, J. M., and Kolterman, O. G. Mechanisms of insulin resistance in obesity and non-insulin dependent (type II) diabetes. *Am. J. Med.* 70:151, 1981; Flier, J. S. The adipocyte: storage depot or node on the energy information superhighway? *Cell* 80:15, 1995; and Ruderman, N. B., Williamson, J. R., and Brownlee, M. Glucose and diabetic vascular disease. *FASEB J.* 6:2905, 1992.

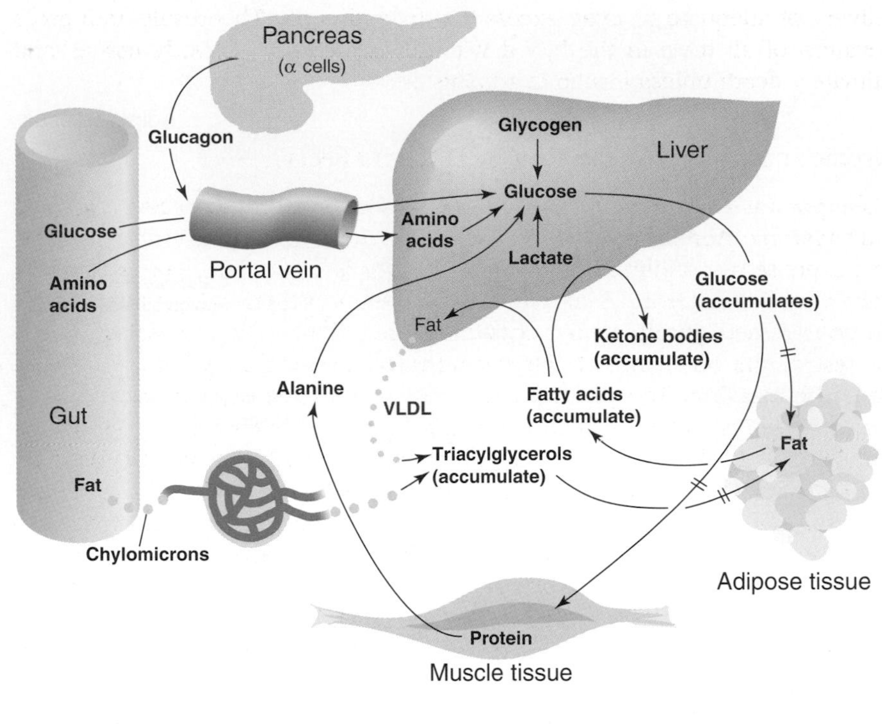

FIGURE 13.17 (continued)
(*c*) Insulin-dependent diabetes mellitus.

CLINICAL CORRELATION 13.8

Insulin-Dependent Diabetes Mellitus

Insulin-dependent diabetes mellitus (IDDM) was once called juvenile-onset diabetes because it usually appears in childhood or in the teens, but it is not limited to these patients. Insulin is absent in this disease because of defective or absent β cells in the pancreas. The β cells are destroyed by an autoimmune process. Untreated, IDDM is characterized by hyperglycemia, hyperlipoproteinemia (chylomicrons and VLDLs), and episodes of severe ketoacidosis. Far from being a disease of defects in carbohydrate metabolism alone, diabetes causes abnormalities in fat and protein metabolism in such patients as well. The hyperglycemia results in part from the inability of the insulin-dependent tissues to take up plasma glucose and in part by accelerated hepatic gluconeogenesis from amino acids derived from muscle protein. The ketoacidosis results from increased lipolysis in the adipose tissue and accelerated fatty acid oxidation in the liver. Hyperchylomicronemia is the result of low lipoprotein lipase activity in adipose tissue capillaries, an enzyme dependent on insulin for its synthesis.

Although insulin does not cure the diabetes, its use markedly alters the clinical course of the disease. The injected insulin promotes glucose uptake by tissues and inhibits gluconeogenesis, lipolysis, and proteolysis. The patient has the difficult job of trying to adjust the insulin dose to a variable dietary intake and variable physical activity, the other major determinant of glucose disposal by muscle. Tight control demands the use of several injections of insulin per day and close blood sugar monitoring by the patient. Tight control of blood sugar has now been proved to reduce the microvascular complications of diabetes (renal and retinal diseases).

National Diabetes Data Group. Classification and diagnosis of diabetes mellitus and other categories of glucose intolerance. *Diabetes* 28:1039, 1977; Atkinson, M. A., and Maclaren, N. K. The pathogenesis of insulin dependent diabetes mellitus. *N. Engl. J. Med.* 331:1428, 1994; and Clark, C. M., and Lee, D. A. Prevention and treatment of the complications of diabetes mellitus. *N. Engl. J. Med.* 332:1210, 1994.

Insulin-Dependent Diabetes Mellitus

Figure 13.17*c* shows the metabolic interrelationships that exist in **insulin-dependent diabetes mellitus** (see Clin. Corr. 13.8 and 13.9). In contrast to noninsulin-dependent diabetes, there is a complete absence of insulin production by the pancreas in this disease. Because of defective β-cell production of insulin, blood levels of insulin do not increase in response to elevated blood glucose levels. Even when dietary glucose is being delivered from the gut, the insulin/glucagon ratio cannot increase, and the liver remains gluconeogenic and ketogenic. Since it is impossible to switch to the processes of glycolysis, glycogenesis, and lipogenesis, the liver cannot properly buffer blood glucose levels. Indeed, since hepatic gluconeogenesis is continuous, the liver contributes to hyperglycemia in the well-fed state. Failure of some tissues, especially muscle, to take up glucose in the absence of insulin contributes further to the hyperglycemia. Accelerated gluconeogenesis, fueled by substrate made available by tissue protein degradation, maintains the hyperglycemia even in the starved state.

The absence of insulin in patients with insulin-dependent diabetes mellitus results in uncontrolled rates of lipolysis in adipose tissue. This increases blood levels of fatty acids and results in accelerated ketone body production by the liver. If ketone bodies are not used as rapidly as they are formed, diabetic ketoacidosis develops due to accumulation of ketone bodies and hydrogen ions. Not all the fatty acid taken up by liver can be handled by the pathway of fatty acid oxidation and ketogenesis. The excess is esterified and directed into VLDL synthesis. **Hypertriglyceridemia** results because VLDLs are synthesized and released by the liver more rapidly than these particles can be cleared from the blood by lipoprotein lipase. The quantity of this enzyme is dependent on the blood insulin level. The defect in lipoprotein lipase also results in hyperchylomicronemia, since lipoprotein lipase is required for chylomicron catabolism in adipose tissue. In summary, in diabetes every tissue continues to play the catabolic role that it was designed to play in starvation, in spite of delivery of adequate or even excess fuel from the gut. This results in a gross elevation of all fuels in the blood with severe wasting of body tissues and ultimately death unless insulin is administered.

Aerobic and Anaerobic Exercise Use Different Fuels

It is important to differentiate between two distinct types of **exercise**—aerobic and anaerobic. Aerobic exercise is exemplified by long-distance running, anaerobic exercise by sprinting or weight lifting. During anaerobic exercise there is really very little interorgan cooperation. The blood vessels within the muscles are compressed during peak contraction, thus their cells are isolated from the rest of the body. Muscle largely relies on its own stored glycogen and **phosphocreatine.** Phosphocreatine serves as a source of high-energy phosphate for ATP synthesis (Figure 13.7) until glycogenolysis and glycolysis are stimulated. Glycolysis becomes the primary source of ATP for want of oxygen. Aerobic exercise is metabolically more interesting (Figure 13.17*d*). For moderate exercise, much of the energy is derived from glycolysis of muscle glycogen. This biochemical fact is the basis for **carbohydrate loading.** Muscle glycogen content can be increased by exhaustive exercise that depletes glycogen, followed by rest and a high-carbohydrate diet. There is also stimulation of branched-chain amino acid oxidation, ammonium production, and alanine release from the exercising muscle. However, a well-fed individual does not store enough glucose and glycogen to provide the energy needed for running long distances. The **respiratory quotient,** the ratio of carbon dioxide exhaled to oxygen consumed, falls during distance running. This indicates the progressive switch from glycogen to fatty acid oxidation during a race. Lipolysis gradually increases as glucose stores are exhausted, and, as in the fasted state, muscles oxidize fatty acids in preference to glucose as the former become available.

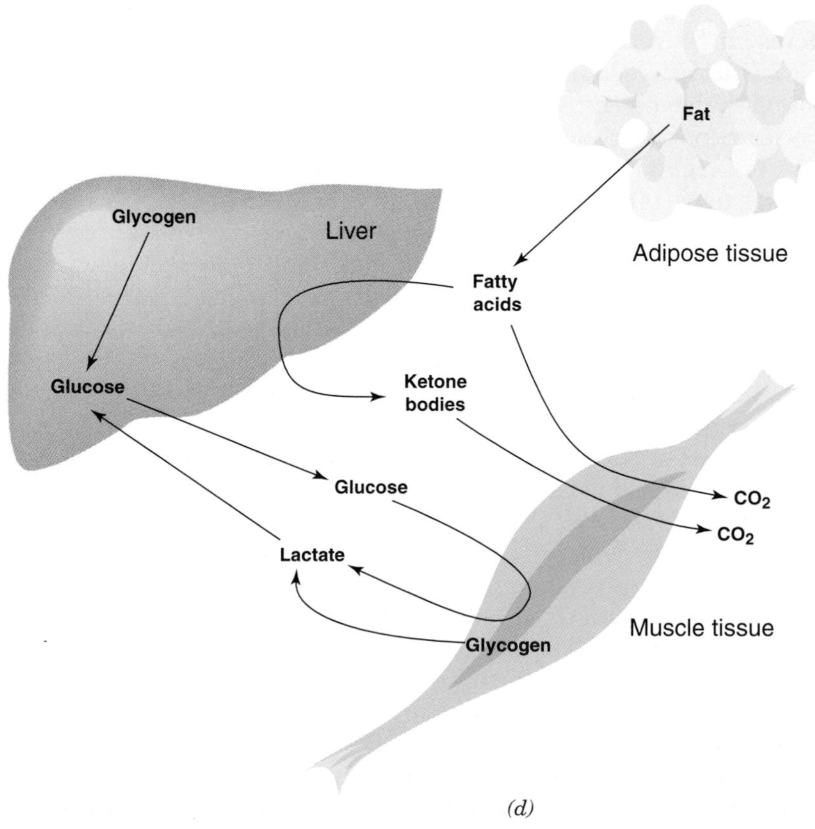

FIGURE 13.17 (continued)
(*d*) Exercise.

CLINICAL CORRELATION 13.9

Complications of Diabetes and the Polyol Pathway

Diabetes is complicated by several disorders that may share a common pathogenesis. The lens, peripheral nerve, renal papillae, Schwann cells, glomerulus, and possibly retinal capillaries contain two enzymes that constitute the polyol pathway (the term polyol refers to polyhydroxy sugars). The first is aldose reductase, an NADPH-requiring enzyme. It reduces glucose to form sorbitol. Sorbitol is further metabolized by sorbitol dehydrogenase, an NAD^+-requiring enzyme that oxidizes sorbitol to fructose. Aldose reductase has a high K_m for glucose; therefore this pathway is only quantitatively important during hyperglycemia. It is known that in diabetic animals the sorbitol content of lens, nerve, and glomerulus is elevated. Sorbitol accumulation may damage these tissues by causing them to swell. There are now inhibitors of the reductase that prevent the accumulation of sorbitol in these tissues and thus retard the onset of these complications. This is a very controversial area because differences in potency of the inhibitors, experimental designs, length of trials, and the numbers of patients enrolled have resulted in different studies reaching different conclusions. We cannot as yet confidently recommend these drugs to prevent diabetic complications.

Gabbay, K. H. Hyperglycemia, polyol metabolism, and the complications of diabetes mellitus. *Annu. Rev. Med.* 26:521, 1975; Frank, R. N. The aldose reductase controversy. *Diabetes* 43:169, 1994; and Clark, C. M., and Lee, D. A. Prevention and treatment of the complications of diabetes mellitus. *N. Engl. J. Med.* 332:1210, 1994.

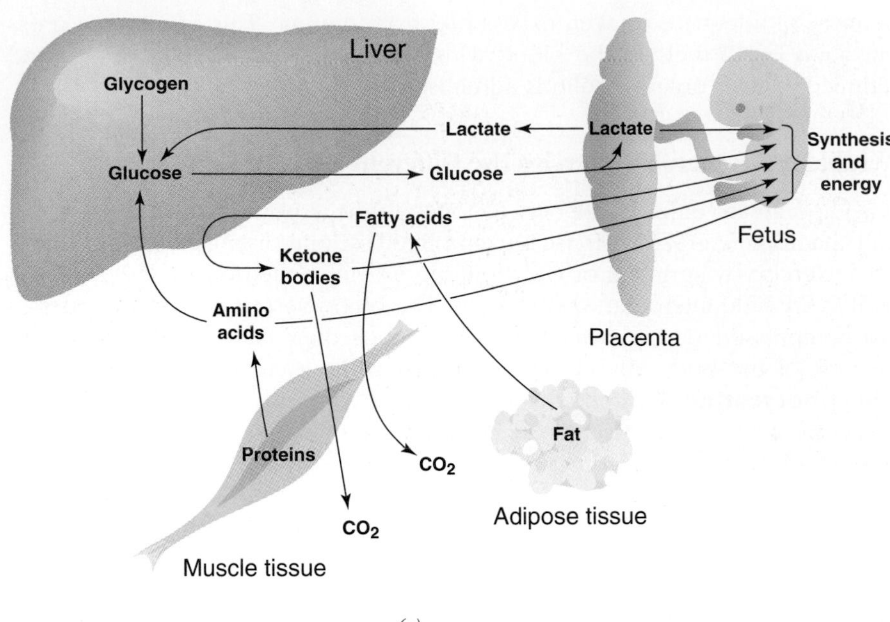

(e)

FIGURE 13.17 (continued)
(*e*) Pregnancy.

Unlike fasting, there is little increase in blood ketone body concentration. This may reflect a balance between hepatic ketone body synthesis and muscle ketone body oxidation.

Changes in Pregnancy Are Related to Fetal Requirements and Hormonal Changes

The **fetus** can be considered as another nutrient-requiring tissue (Figure 13.17*e*). It mainly uses glucose for energy but may also use amino acids, lactate, fatty acids, and ketone bodies. Lactate produced in the **placenta** by glycolysis goes in two directions. Part of it is directed to the fetus where it serves as a fuel, with the rest returning to the maternal circulation to establish a Cori cycle with the liver. Maternal LDL cholesterol is an important precursor of placental steroids (estradiol and progesterone). During **pregnancy,** the starve–feed cycle is perturbed. The placenta secretes a polypeptide hormone, **placental lactogen,** and two steroid hormones, estradiol and progesterone. Placental lactogen stimulates lipolysis in adipose tissue, and the steroid hormones induce an insulin-resistant state. Thus, in the postprandial state, pregnant women enter the starved state more rapidly than do nonpregnant women. This results from increased consumption of glucose and amino acids by the fetus. Plasma glucose, amino acids, and insulin levels fall rapidly, and glucagon and placental lactogen levels rise and stimulate lipolysis and ketogenesis. The consumption of glucose and amino acids by the fetus may be great enough to cause maternal hypoglycemia. On the other hand, in the fed state pregnant women have increased levels of insulin and glucose and demonstrate resistance to exogenous insulin. These swings of plasma hormones and fuels are even more exaggerated in pregnant diabetic women and make control of their blood glucose difficult.

Lactation Requires Synthesis of Lactose, Triacylglycerol, and Protein

In late pregnancy placental hormones induce lipoprotein lipase in the mammary gland and promote the development of milk-secreting cells and ducts. During **lactation** (see Figure 13.17*f*) the breast utilizes glucose for **lactose** and triacylglycerol synthesis, as well as its major energy source. Amino acids are taken

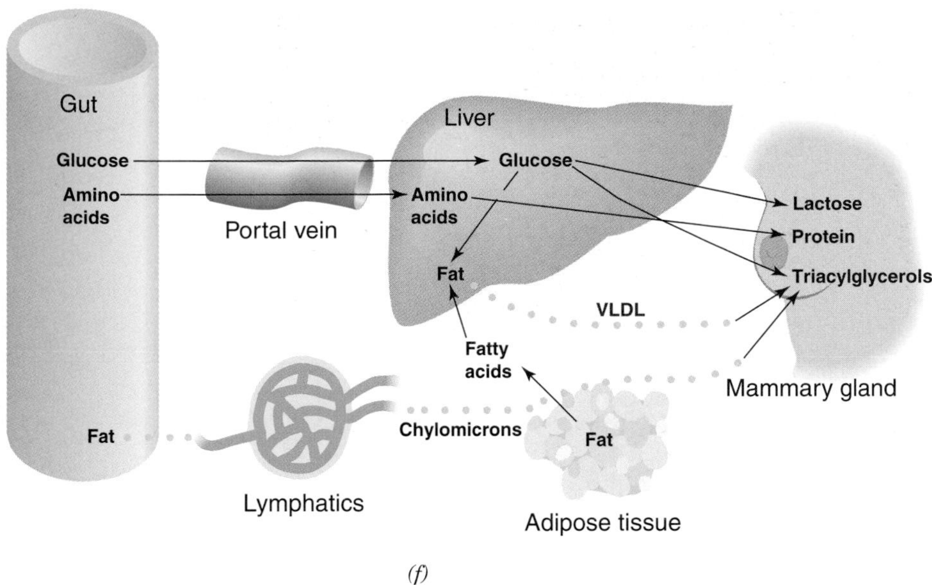

FIGURE 13.17 (continued)
(*f*) Lactation.

up for protein synthesis, and chylomicrons and VLDLs are utilized as sources of fatty acids for triacylglycerol synthesis. If these compounds are not supplied by the diet, proteolysis, gluconeogenesis, and lipolysis must supply them, resulting eventually in maternal malnutrition and poor quality milk. The lactating breast also secretes a hormone with some similarity to parathyroid hormone (see Chapter 20). This hormone probably is important for the absorption of calcium and phosphorus from the gut and bone.

Stress and Injury Lead to Metabolic Changes

Physiological stresses include **injury, surgery, renal failure, burns,** and **infections** (Figure 13.17*g*). Characteristically, blood cortisol, glucagon, **catecholamines,** and **growth hormone** levels increase. The patient is resistant to insulin. Basal metabolic rate, blood glucose, and free fatty acid levels are elevated. However, ketogenesis is not accelerated as in fasting. For incompletely understood reasons, the intracellular muscle glutamine pool is reduced, resulting in reduced protein synthesis and increased protein breakdown. It can be very difficult to reverse this protein breakdown, although now it is common to replace amino acids, glucose, and fat by infusing solutions of these nutrients intravenously. However, these solutions lack glutamine, tyrosine, and cysteine because of stability and solubility constraints. Supplementation of these amino acids, perhaps by the use of more stable dipeptides, may help to reverse the catabolic state better than can be accomplished at present.

It has been proposed that the negative nitrogen balance of injured or infected patients is mediated by monocyte and lymphocyte proteins, such as **interleukin-1,** interleukin-6, and **TNF-α** (see Clin. Corr. 13.10). These cytokines are responsible for causing fever as well as a number of other metabolic changes. Interleukin-1 activates proteolysis in skeletal muscle. **Interleukin-6** stimulates the synthesis of a number of hepatic proteins called **acute phase reactants** by the liver. Acute phase reactants include fibrinogen, complement proteins, some clotting factors, and α_2-macroglobulin, which are presumed to play a role in defense against injury and infection. TNF-α suppresses adipocyte fat synthesis, prevents uptake of circulating fat by inhibiting lipoprotein lipase, stimulates lipolysis, inhibits release of insulin, and promotes insulin resistance. These cytokines appear responsible for much of the wasting seen in chronic infections.

CLINICAL CORRELATION 13.10

Cancer Cachexia

Unexplained weight loss may be a sign of malignancy, and weight loss is common in advanced cancer. Decreased appetite and food intake contribute to but do not entirely account for the weight loss. The weight loss is largely from skeletal muscle and adipose tissue, with relative sparing of visceral protein (i.e., liver, kidney, and heart). Although tumors commonly exhibit high rates of glycolysis and release lactate, the energy requirement of the tumor probably does not explain weight loss because weight loss can occur with even small tumors. In addition, the presence of another energy-requiring growth, the fetus in a pregnant woman, does not normally lead to weight loss. Several endocrine abnormalities have been recognized in cancer patients. They tend to be insulin-resistant, have higher cortisol levels, and have a higher basal metabolic rate compared with controls matched for weight loss. Two other phenomena may contribute to the metabolic disturbances. Some tumors synthesize and secrete biologically active peptides such as ACTH, nerve growth factor, and insulin-like growth factors, which could modify the endocrine regulation of energy metabolism. It is also possible that the host response to a tumor, by analogy to chronic infection, includes release of interleukin-1 (IL-1), interleukin-6 (IL-6), and tumor necrosis factor-α(TNF-α) by cells of the immune system. TNF-α is also called cachexin because it produces wasting. TNF-α and IL-1 may act in a paracrine fashion, as plasma levels are not elevated. They do induce the synthesis of IL-6, which has been detected in cachectic patients' sera at increased levels. These cytokines stimulate fever, proteolysis, lipolysis, and the synthesis of acute phase reactants by the liver.

Beutler, B., and Cerami, A. Tumor necrosis, cachexia, shock, and inflammation: a common mediator. *Annu. Rev. Biochem.* 57:1505, 1988; and Tracey, K. J., and Cerami, A. Tumor necrosis factor: a pleiotropic cytokine and therapeutic target. *Annu. Rev. Med.* 45:491, 1994.

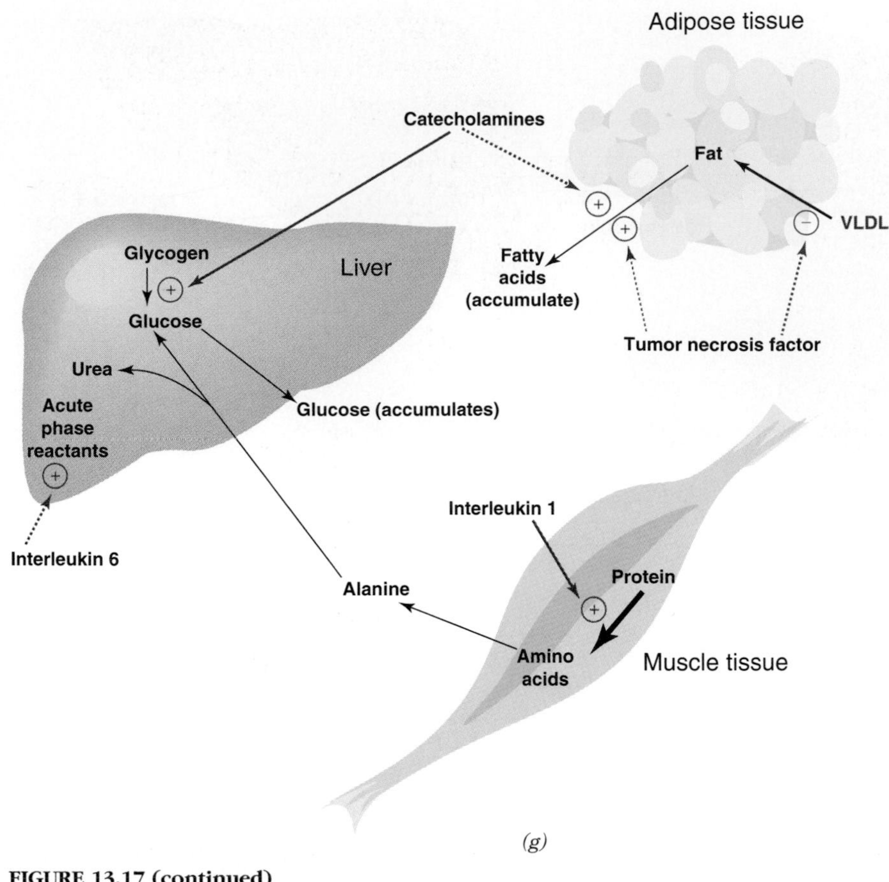

FIGURE 13.17 (continued)
(*g*) Stress.

Liver Disease Causes Major Metabolic Derangements

Since the liver is central to the body's metabolic interrelationships, advanced **liver disease** can be associated with major metabolic derangements (Figure 13.17*h*). The most important abnormalities are those in the metabolism of amino acids. The liver is the only organ capable of urea synthesis. In patients with **cirrhosis,** the liver is unable to convert ammonia into urea and glutamine rapidly enough, and the blood ammonia level rises. Part of this problem is due to abnormalities of blood flow in the cirrhotic liver, which interfere with the intercellular **glutamine cycle** (see p. 558). Ammonia arises from several enzyme reactions, such as glutaminase, glutamate dehydrogenase, and adenosine deaminase, during metabolism of amino acids by intestine and liver, and from intestinal lumen, where bacteria split urea into ammonia and carbon dioxide. Ammonia is very toxic to the central nervous system and is a major reason for the coma that sometimes occurs in patients in liver failure.

In advanced liver disease, aromatic amino acids accumulate in the blood to higher levels than branched-chain amino acids, apparently because of defective hepatic catabolism of the aromatic amino acids. This is important because aromatic amino acids and branched-chain amino acids are transported into the brain by the same carrier system. An elevated ratio of aromatic amino acids to branched-chain amino acids in liver disease results in increased brain uptake of aromatic amino acids. Increased synthesis of **neurotransmitters** such as **serotonin** in the brain as a consequence of increased availability of aromatic amino acids has been suggested to be responsible for some of the neurological abnormalities characteristic of liver disease. The liver is also a major source of insulin-like growth factor-I (IGF-I). Cirrhotics suffer muscle wasting because of deficient IGF-I synthesis in response to growth hormone. Finally, in outright

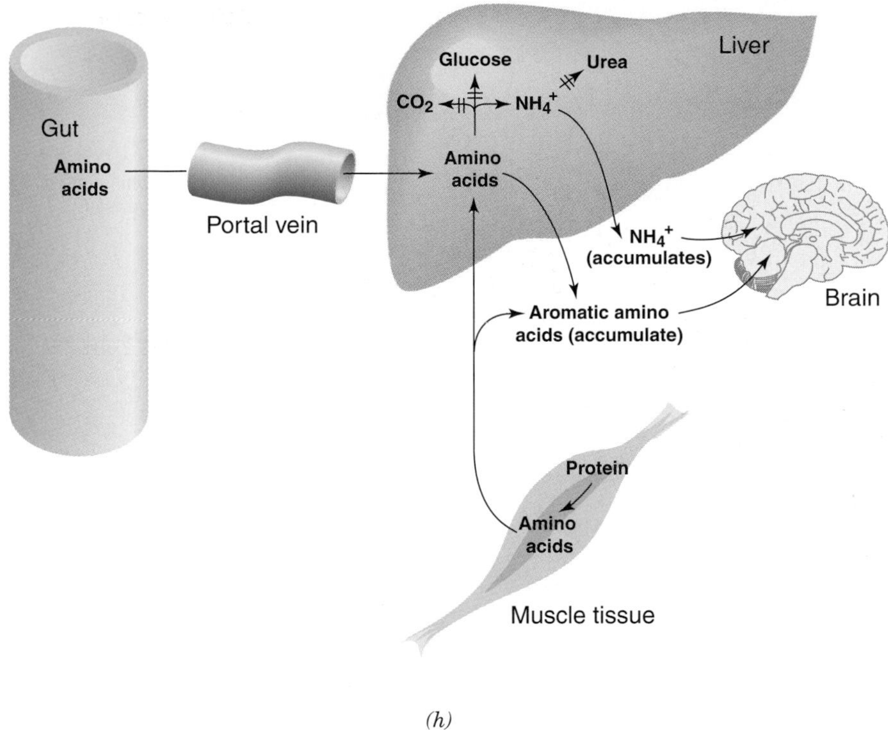

FIGURE 13.17 (continued)
(*h*) Liver disease.

liver failure, patients sometimes die of hypoglycemia because the liver is unable to maintain the blood glucose level by gluconeogenesis.

In Renal Disease Nitrogenous Wastes Accumulate

In chronic renal disease, there are many abnormalities of nitrogen metabolism. Levels of amino acids normally metabolized by kidney (glutamine, glycine, proline, and citrulline) increase. Nitrogen end products (e.g., urea, uric acid, and creatinine) also accumulate (Figure 13.17*i*). This accumulation is worsened by high dietary protein intake or accelerated proteolysis. The facts that gut bacteria can split urea into ammonia and that liver uses ammonia and α-keto acids to form nonessential amino acids have been used to control the level of nitrogenous wastes in renal patients. Patients are given a diet high in carbohydrate, and the amino acid intake is limited as much as possible to essential amino acids. Under these circumstances, the liver synthesizes nonessential amino acids from TCA cycle intermediates. This type of diet therapy may extend the time before the patient requires dialysis.

Oxidation of Ethanol in Liver Alters the NAD^+/NADH Ratio

The liver is primarily responsible for the first two steps of the **ethanol** catabolism:

$$\text{Ethanol } (CH_3CH_2OH) + NAD^+ \rightarrow \text{acetaldehyde } (CH_3CHO) + NADH + H^+$$

$$\text{Acetaldehyde } (CH_3CHO) + NAD^+ \rightarrow \text{acetate } (CH_3COO^-) + NADH + H^+$$

The first step, catalyzed by **alcohol dehydrogenases** in the cytosol, generates NADH; the second step, catalyzed by **aldehyde dehydrogenase,** also generates NADH but occurs largely in the mitochondrial matrix space. Liver disposes of NADH generated by these reactions by the only pathway it has available—the mitochondrial electron transport chain. Intake of even moderate amounts of

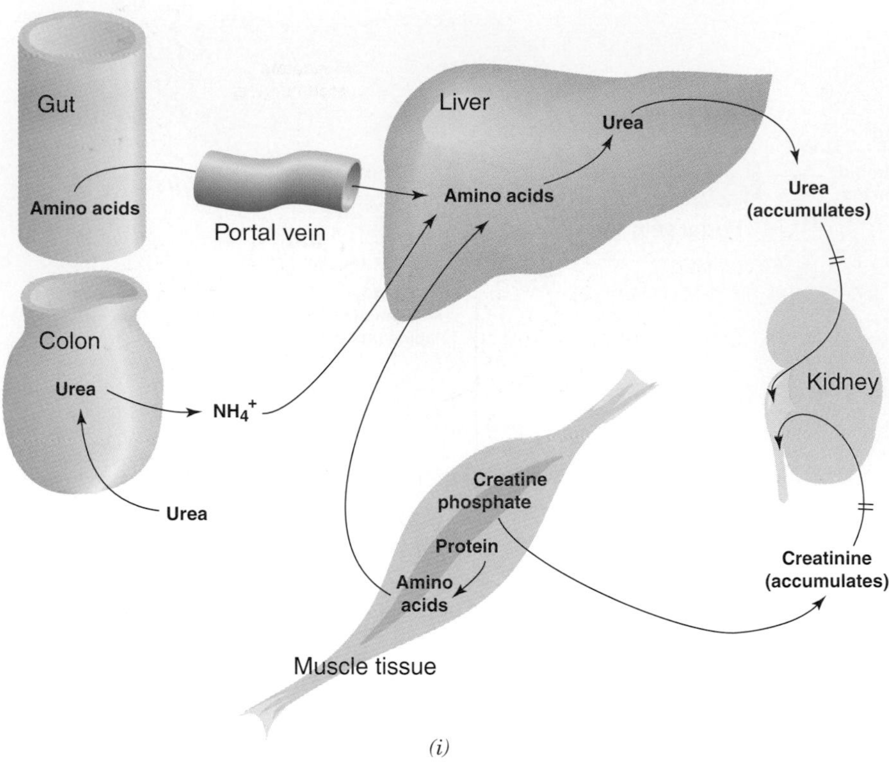

FIGURE 13.17 (continued)
(*i*) Kidney failure.

ethanol generates too much NADH. Many enzymes, for example, several involved in gluconeogenesis and fatty acid oxidation, are sensitive to product inhibition by NADH. Thus, during alcohol metabolism, these pathways are inhibited (Figure 13.17*j*), and fasting hypoglycemia and the accumulation of hepatic triacylglycerols (fatty liver) are consequences of alcohol ingestion. Lactate can accumulate as a consequence of inhibition of lactate gluconeogenesis and can result in metabolic acidosis.

Liver mitochondria have a limited capacity to oxidize acetate to CO_2, because the activation of acetate to acetyl CoA requires GTP, a product of the succinyl CoA synthetase reaction. The TCA cycle, and therefore GTP synthesis, are inhibited by high NADH levels during ethanol oxidation. Much of the acetate made from ethanol escapes the liver to the blood. Virtually every other cell with mitochondria can oxidize it to CO_2 by way of the TCA cycle.

Acetaldehyde, the intermediate in the formation of acetate from ethanol, can also escape from the liver. Acetaldehyde is a reactive compound that readily forms covalent bonds with functional groups of biologically important compounds. Formation of acetaldehyde adducts with proteins in tissues and blood of animals and humans drinking alcohol has been demonstrated. Such adducts may provide a marker for past drinking activity of an individual, just as hemoglobin A_{1c} has proved useful as an index of blood glucose control in diabetic patients.

In Acid–Base Regulation, Glutamine Plays a Pivotal Role

Regulation of acid–base balance, like that of nitrogen excretion, is shared by the liver and kidney (Figure 13.17*k*). Metabolism of proteins generates excess hydrogen ions. For example:

$$\text{Methionine or cysteine} \rightarrow SO_4^{2-} + 2\,H^+ + \text{other neutral products}$$

The kidney helps regulate blood pH by excreting hydrogen ions, which is necessary for the reabsorption of bicarbonate and the titration of phosphate

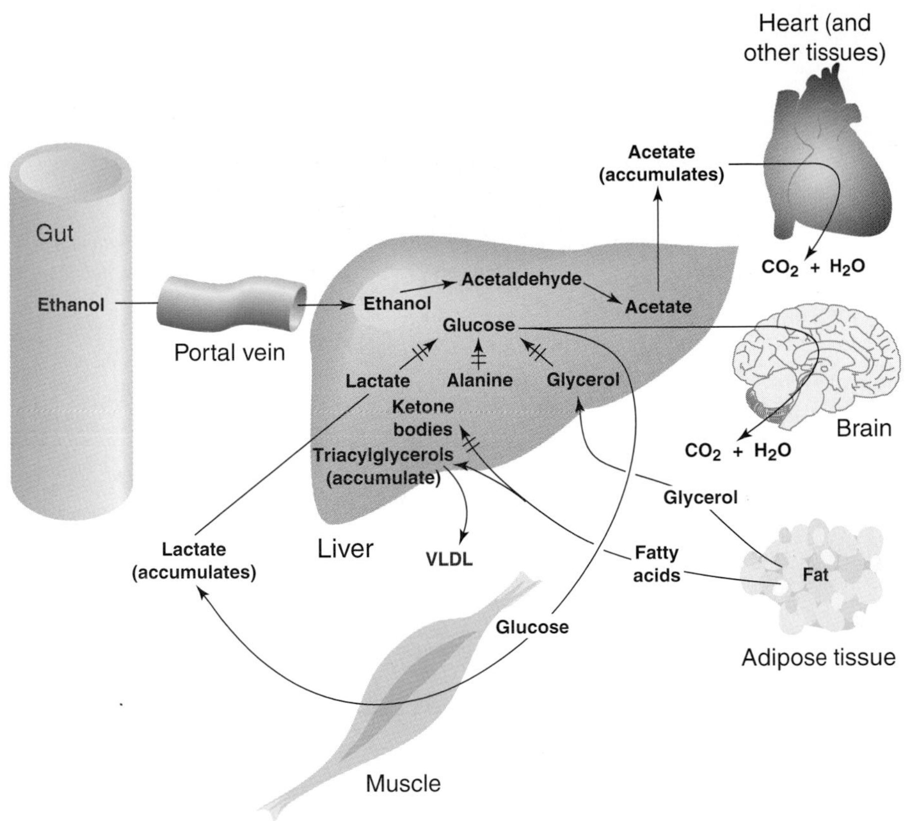

FIGURE 13.17 (continued)
(*j*) Ethanol ingestion.

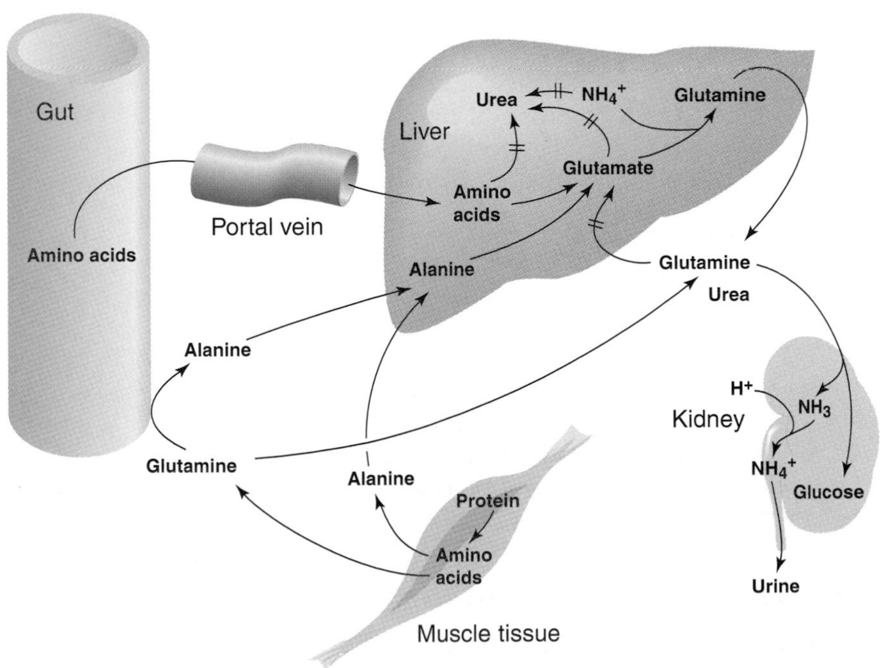

FIGURE 13.17 (continued)
(*k*) Acidosis.

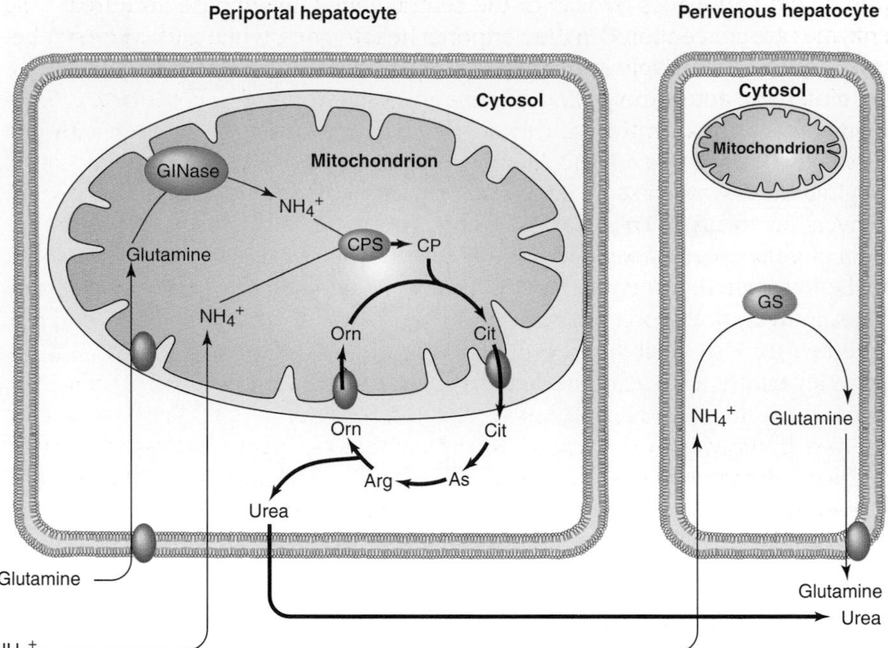

FIGURE 13.18
Intercellular glutamine cycle of the liver.
Abbreviations: GlNase, glutaminase; GS, glutamine synthetase; CPS, carbamoyl phosphate synthetase I; CP, carbamoyl phosphate; Cit, citrulline; AS, argininosuccinate; Arg, arginine; Orn, ornithine.
Redrawn from Häussinger, D. Glutamine metabolism in the liver: overview and current concepts. Metabolism *38(Suppl. 1):14, 1989.*

and ammonia in the tubular filtrate (see Chapter 25, p. 1045). Glutamine is the precursor of renal ammonia production. In chronic metabolic **acidosis,** the activities of renal glutaminase, glutamate dehydrogenase, phosphoenolpyruvate carboxykinase, and the mitochondrial glutamine transporter increase and correlate with increased urinary excretion of ammonium ions and increased renal gluconeogenesis from amino acids. Liver participates by synthesizing less urea, which makes more glutamine available for the kidney. In **alkalosis,** urea synthesis increases in the liver, and gluconeogenesis and ammonium ion excretion by the kidney decrease.

An intercellular glutamine cycle enables the liver to play a central role in the regulation of blood pH. The liver is composed of two types of hepatocytes involved in glutamine metabolism: **periportal hepatocytes** near the hepatic arteriole and portal venule and **perivenous hepatocytes** located near the central venule (Figure 13.18). Blood enters the liver by the hepatic artery and

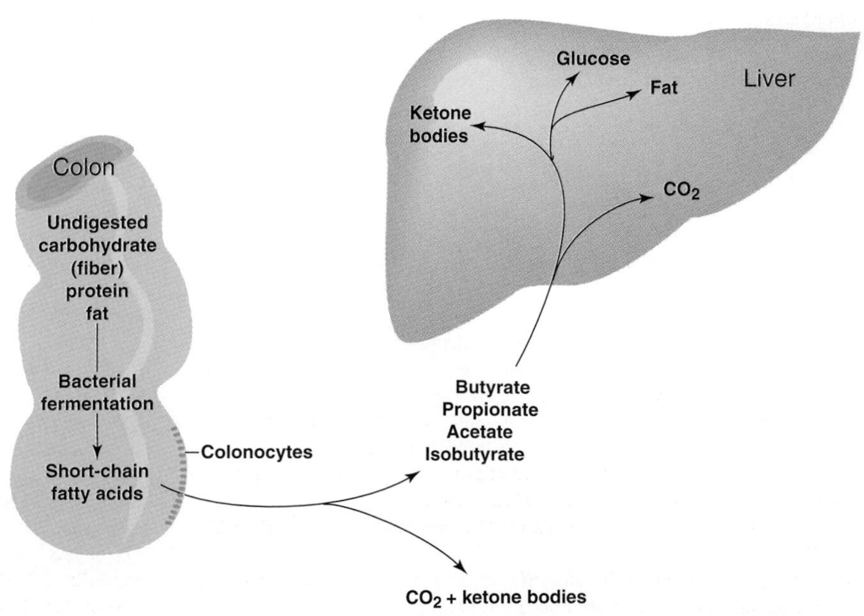

FIGURE 13.19
Bacterial fermentation generates fuel for colonocytes.

portal vein and leaves by way of the central vein. Glutaminase and urea cycle enzymes are concentrated in the periportal hepatocytes, while glutamine synthetase is found exclusively in perivenous hepatocytes (see p. 450). During alkalosis, glutamine enters the periportal cells and is hydrolyzed to contribute ammonium ion for urea synthesis. The bulk of glutamine and ammonium nitrogen entering the liver leaves the liver as urea. The perivenous cellular location of glutamine synthetase is important because some ammonium ions escape conversion to urea. This enzyme traps much of this toxic compound in the form of glutamine. Thus glutamine is released from the liver and circulates back to the liver where it reenters the glutamine cycle in the periportal hepatocytes. Thus, in liver, both donation of ammonium ion by glutamine for urea synthesis and the synthesis of glutamine are important in maintaining low blood ammonium levels. In acidosis, glutaminase of the periportal hepatocytes (unlike the renal glutaminase isozyme) is less active and much of the blood glutamine escapes hydrolysis in the liver. Likewise, carbamoyl phosphate synthetase of periportal hepatocytes is less active in acidosis, permitting perivenous cells to convert more ammonium ion to glutamine, which is then available for metabolism by the kidney to yield hydrogen ions that need to be eliminated in the urine.

The Colon Salvages Energy from the Diet

Unlike the small intestine, which uses glutamine for its major energy source, the **colon** utilizes short-chain fatty acids: **butyrate, propionate, isobutyrate,** and acetate (Figure 13.19). It obtains most of these fatty acids from the lumen of the colon, where bacteria produce them by fermentation of unabsorbed dietary components. These short-chain fatty acids would otherwise be lost in stool, so their use by cells of the colon (colonocytes) represents a way of gaining as much energy from dietary sources as possible. If produced in excess of the needs of the colon, short-chain fatty acids pass into the portal blood for use by the liver. Interestingly, colonocytes can produce ketone bodies from butyrate, presumably releasing them into the portal blood for use as fuel by extrahepatic tissues. When surgery is performed that bypasses the colon (e.g., an ileostomy), some patients develop a form of colitis called diversion **colitis.** In some cases, providing enemas containing the short-chain fatty acids has healed the colitis.

BIBLIOGRAPHY

Amiel, S. A. Organ fuel selection: brain. *Proc. Nutr. Soc.* 54:151, 1995.

Brownlee, M., Vlassara, H., and Cerami, A. Nonenzymatic glycosylation and the pathogenesis of diabetes complications. *Ann. Intern. Med.* 101:527, 1984.

Cahill, G. F. Jr. Diabetes mellitus: a brief overview. *Johns Hopkins Med. J.* 143:155, 1978.

Calder, P. C. Fuel utilization by cells of the immune system. *Proc. Nutr. Soc.* 54:65, 1995.

Cerami, A., and Koenig, R. H. Hemoglobin A_{1c} as a model for the development of the sequelae of diabetes mellitus. *Trends Biochem. Sci.* 3:73, 1978.

Cohen, P., and Cohen, P. T. W. Protein phosphatases come of age. A review. *J. Biol. Chem.* 264:21435, 1989.

Crabb, D. W., and Lumeng, L. Metabolism of alcohol and the pathophysiology of alcoholic liver disease. In: G. Gitnick (Ed.), *Principles and Practice of Gastroenterology and Hepatology. New York: Elsevier, 1988, p. 1163.*

Curthoys, N. P., and Watford, M. Regulation of glutaminase activity and glutamine metabolism. *Annu. Rev. Nutr.* 15:133, 1995.

DeLeve, L. D., and Kaplowitz, N. Glutathione metabolism and its role in hepatotoxicity. *Pharmacol. Ther.* 52:287, 1991.

Denton, R. M., and Pogson, C. I. *Metabolic Regulation.* New York: Wiley, 1976.

Duée, P.-H., Darcy-Vrillon, B., Blachier, F., and Morel, M.-T. Fuel selection in intestinal cells. *Proc. Nutr. Soc.* 54:83, 1995.

Elia, M. General integration and regulation of metabolism at the organ level. *Proc. Nutr. Soc.* 54:213, 1995.

Foster, D. W. Banting lecture 1984. From glycogen to ketones and back. *Diabetes* 33:1188, 1984.

Foster, D. W. Diabetes mellitus. In: C. R. Scriver, A. L. Beaudet, W. S. Sly, and D Vallee. (Eds), *The Metabolic Basis of Inherited Disease.* New York: McGraw-Hill, 1989.

Frayn, K. N., Humphreys, S. M., and Coppack, S. W. Fuel selection in white adipose tissue. *Proc. Nutr. Soc.* 54:177, 1995.

Fulop, M. Alcoholism, ketoacidosis, and lactic acidosis. *Diabetes Metab. Rev.* 5:365, 1989.

Geelen, M. J. H., Harris, R. A., Beynen, A. C., and McCune, S. A. Short-term hormonal control of hepatic lipogenesis. *Diabetes* 29:1006, 1980.

Goldberg, A. L., Baracos, V., Rodemann, P., Waxman, L., and Dinarello, C. Control of protein degradation in muscle by prostaglandins, calcium, and leukocytic pyrogen (interleukin 1). *Fed. Proc.* 43:1301, 1984.

Harris, R. A., Popov, K. M., and Zhao, Y. Nutritional control of the protein kinases responsible for the phosphorylation of the α-ketoacid dehydrogenase complexes. *J. Nutr.* 125:1758S, 1995.

Häussinger, D. Glutamine metabolism in the liver: overview and current concepts. *Metabolism* 38(Suppl. 1):14, 1989.

Henriksson, J. Muscle fuel selection: effect of exercise and training. *Proc. Nutr. Soc.* 54:125, 1995.

Hers, H. G., and Hue, L. Gluconeogenesis and related aspects of glycolysis. *Annu. Rev. Biochem.* 52:617, 1983.

Ingebritsen, T. S., and Cohen, P. Protein phosphatases: properties and role in cellular regulation. *Science* 221:331, 1983.

Katz, J., and McGarry, J. D. The glucose paradox. Is glucose a substrate for liver metabolism? *J. Clin. Invest.* 74:1901, 1984.

Krebs, H. A. Some aspects of the regulation of fuel supply in omnivorous animals. *Adv. Enzyme Regul.* 10:387, 1972.

Krebs, H. A., Williamson, D. H., Bates, M. W., Page, M. A., and Hawkins, R. A. The role of ketone bodies in caloric homeostasis. *Adv. Enzyme Regul.* 9:387, 1971.

Kurkland, I. J., and Pilkis, S. J. Indirect and direct routes of hepatic glycogen synthesis. *FASEB J.* 3:2277, 1989.

Larner, J. *Intermediary Metabolism and Its Regulation*. Englewood Cliffs, NJ: Prentice-Hall, 1971.

MacDonald, I. A., and Webber, J. Feeding, fasting and starvation: factors affecting fuel utilization. *Proc. Nutr. Soc.* 54:267, 1995.

McGarry, J. D., Woeltje, K. F., Kuwajima, M., and Foster, D. W. Regulation of ketogenesis and the renaissance of carnitine palmitoyltransferase. *Diabetes Metab. Rev.* 5:271, 1989.

Newsholme, E. A., and Leech, A. R. *Biochemistry for the Medical Sciences*. New York: Wiley, 1983.

Newsholme, E. A., and Start, C. *Regulation in Metabolism*. New York: Wiley, 1973.

Nosadini, R., Avogaro, A., Doria, A., Fioretto, P., Trevisan, R., and Morocutti, A. Ketone body metabolism: a physiological and clinical overview. *Diabetes Metab. Rev.* 5:299, 1989.

Pedersen, O. The impact of obesity on the pathogenesis of non-insulin-dependent diabetes mellitus: a review of current hypotheses. *Diabetes Metab. Rev.* 5:495, 1989.

Pedersen, O., and Beck-Nielsen, H. Insulin resistance and insulin-dependent diabetes mellitus. *Diabetes Care* 10:516, 1987.

Pilkis, S. J., Ed-Maghrabi, M. R., and Claus, T. H. Hormonal regulation of hepatic gluconeogenesis and glycolysis. *Annu. Rev. Biochem.* 57:755, 1988.

Randle, P. J. Metabolic fuel selection: general integration at the whole-body level. *Proc. Nutr. Soc.* 54:317, 1995.

Shulman, G. I., and Landau, B. R. Pathways of glycogen repletion. *Physiol. Rev.* 72:1019, 1992.

Sugden, M. C., Holness, M. J., and Palmer, T. N. Fuel selection and carbon flux during the starved-to-fed transition. A review article. *Biochem. J.* 263:313, 1989.

Toth, B., Bollen, M., and Stalmans, W. Acute regulation of hepatic phosphatases by glucagon, insulin, and glucose. *J. Biol. Chem.* 263:14061, 1988.

Ulwin, P. The state of world hunger. *Nutr. Rev.* 52:151, 1994.

Williamson, D. H., and Lund, P. Substrate selection and oxygen uptake by the lactating mammary gland. *Proc. Nutr. Soc.* 54:165, 1995.

QUESTIONS ■ C. N. ANGSTADT AND J. BAGGOTT

Refer to the following for Questions 1 and 2.
A. well-fed state
B. early fasting state
C. fasting state
D. early refed state

1. Hepatic glycogenolysis is a primary source of blood glucose during this period.

2. Ketone bodies supply a significant portion of the brain's fuel.

3. The fact that the K_m of aminotransferases for amino acids is much higher than that of aminoacyl-tRNA synthetases means that:
   A. at low amino acid concentrations, protein synthesis will take precedence over amino acid catabolism.
   B. the liver cannot accumulate amino acids.
   C. amino acids will undergo transamination as rapidly as they are delivered to the liver.
   D. any amino acids in excess of immediate needs for energy must be converted to protein.
   E. amino acids can be catabolized only if they are present in the diet.

4. Branched-chain amino acids:
   A. are normally completely catabolized by muscle to CO_2 and H_2O.
   B. can be catabolized by liver but not muscle.
   C. are the main dietary amino acids metabolized by intestine.
   D. are in high concentration in blood following the breakdown of muscle protein.
   E. are a major source of nitrogen for alanine and glutamine produced in muscle.

5. In the early refed state:
   A. the fatty acid concentration of blood rises.
   B. liver no longer carries out gluconeogenesis.
   C. liver replenishes its glycogen by synthesis of glucose 6-phosphate from lactate.
   D. glucose being fed is converted directly to glycogen by the liver.
   E. amino acids cannot be used.

6. All of the following statements about interorgan interactions are correct EXCEPT:
   A. ornithine for the urea cycle is synthesized from glutamate in the kidney.
   B. citrulline leads to the formation of arginine in both liver and kidney.
   C. kidney uses arginine in the synthesis of creatine for use by muscle.
   D. arginine synthesized by the kidney is the source of nitric oxide for many cells.
   E. creatinine cleared by the kidney is generated from creatine phosphate in muscle.

7. Carnitine:
   A. is formed in all cells for their own use.
   B. is synthesized from free lysine.
   C. formation requires that lysyl residues in protein be methylated by *S*-adenosylmethionine.
   D. formation is inhibited by vitamin C.
   E. is cleaved to γ-butyrobetaine.

8. The largest energy reserve (in terms of kilocalories) in humans is:
   A. blood glucose.
   B. liver glycogen.
   C. muscle glycogen.
   D. adipose tissue triacylglycerol.
   E. muscle protein.

9. All of the following represent control of a metabolic process by substrate availability EXCEPT:
   A. increased urea synthesis after a high-protein meal.
   B. rate of ketogenesis.
   C. hypoglycemia of advanced starvation.
   D. response of glycolysis to fructose 2,6-bisphosphate.
   E. sorbitol synthesis.

10. Which of the following would favor gluconeogenesis in the fasted state?
   A. fructose 1,6-bisphosphate stimulation of pyruvate kinase
   B. acetyl CoA activation of pyruvate carboxylase
   C. citrate activation of acetyl-CoA carboxylase
   D. malonyl CoA inhibition of carnitine palmitoyltransferase I
   E. fructose 2,6-bisphosphate stimulation of 6-phosphofructo-1-kinase

11. Conversion of a nonphosphorylated enzyme to a phosphorylated one:
   A. always activates the enzyme.
   B. is always catalyzed by a cAMP-dependent protein kinase.
   C. is signaled in the liver by insulin.
   D. is more likely to occur in the fasted than in the well-fed.
   E. usually occurs at threonine residues of the protein.

12. Adipose tissue responds to low insulin/glucagon ratio by:
   A. dephosphorylating the interconvertible enzymes.
   B. stimulating the deposition of fat.
   C. increasing the amount of pyruvate kinase.
   D. stimulating hormone-sensitive lipase.
   E. stimulating phenylalanine hydroxylase.

13. Changing the level of enzyme activity by changing the number of enzyme molecules:
   A. is considerably slower than allosteric or covalent modification methods.
   B. may involve enzyme induction.
   C. may override the effectiveness of allosteric control.
   D. may be caused by hormonal influences or by changing the nutritional state.
   E. all of the above are correct.

14. Muscle metabolism during exercise:
   A. is the same in both aerobic and anaerobic exercise.
   B. shifts from primarily glucose to primarily fatty acids as fuel during aerobic exercise.
   C. uses largely glycogen and phosphocreatine in the aerobic state.
   D. causes a sharp rise in blood ketone body concentration.
   E. uses only phosphocreatine in the anaerobic state.

15. In noninsulin-dependent diabetes mellitus:
   A. hypertriglyceridemia does not occur.
   B. ketoacidosis in the untreated state is always present.
   C. results because the β cells of the pancreas can no longer make insulin.
   D. may be accompanied by high levels of insulin in the blood.
   E. results in severe weight loss.

16. The elevated liver concentration of NADH produced by ingestion of ethanol:
   A. is restricted to the mitochondria.
   B. may lead to an acidosis by inhibiting gluconeogenesis from lactate.
   C. leads to "fatty liver" by stimulating fatty acid synthesis.
   D. increases the conversion of acetate to acetyl CoA.
   E. arises solely from the conversion of ethanol to acetaldehyde.

17. Glutaminase:
   A. in renal cells is unaffected by blood pH.
   B. in liver is confined to perivenous hepatocytes.
   C. activity is low in liver during alkalosis.
   D. activity is more active in both liver and kidney in acidosis.
   E. in renal cells increases in acidosis.

ANSWERS

1. B The response of glycogenolysis to fasting is rapid, and during this period there is still glycogen present. In fasting, the glycogen is depleted and in the other two states, glycogenesis would occur (p. 529).
2. C If ketone body concentration in blood is high, ketone bodies can cross the blood–brain barrier and they are a good fuel. High ketone body concentrations do not occur in the other states (p. 532).
3. A A high K_m means that a reaction will proceed slowly at low concentration, whereas a low K_m means the reaction can be rapid under the same circumstances. Protein synthesis requires only that all amino acids be present. Unless amino acids are in high enough concentration, the liver does not catabolize them (p. 529).
4. E A and B: Muscle has high levels of the aminotransferases for branched-chain amino acids, whereas liver has high levels of enzymes for the catabolism of the branched-chain α-keto acids. C: Intestine metabolizes several dietary amino acids but not these. D and E: When branched-chain amino acids are derived from muscle protein, transamination transfers the nitrogen to alanine or glutamine, which are transported to the liver and kidney (p. 531).
5. C This is the indirect pathway. A, B, and D: Fat metabolism is normal but glucose metabolism is not normal yet. E: Amino acids are also used for gluconeogenesis (p. 534).
6. A This is a pathway of intestinal epithelium (p. 534). B: This is part of the urea cycle in liver but arginine from kidney is an important source of arginine for liver. C: The reaction requires *S*-adenosylmethionine. E: Creatinine is thus a measure of both muscle mass and renal function (pp. 535–536).

7. C These trimethyllysines are released when protein is hydrolyzed. A: Only liver and kidney have the complete synthetic pathway. D: There are two hydroxylations that require this vitamin. E: This is a precursor (p. 536).
8. D The caloric content of adipose tissue fat is more than five times as great as that of muscle protein and almost 200 times as great as that of the combined carbohydrates (Table 13.1). A: Blood glucose must be maintained but is a relatively minor reserve. B and C: Glycogen is a rapidly mobilizable reserve of energy but not a large one. E: Protein can be used for energy, but that is not its primary role.
9. D Fructose 2,6-bisphosphate is an allosteric effector (activates the kinase and inhibits the phosphatase) of the enzyme controlling glycolysis. A: After a high-protein meal, the intestine produces ammonia and precursors of ornithine for urea synthesis. B: Ketogenesis is dependent on the availability of fatty acids. C: This represents lack of gluconeogenic substrates. E: This leads to complications in diabetes (p. 540).
10. B Pyruvate carboxylase is a key gluconeogenic enzyme. A and E: Stimulation of these enzymes stimulates glycolysis, opposing gluconeogenesis. C and D: Malonyl CoA inhibits transport of fatty acids into mitochondria for β-oxidation, a necessary source of energy for gluconeogenesis (p. 540).
11. D In the well-fed state, insulin/glucagon ratio is high and cAMP levels are low. A: Some enzymes are active when phosphorylated; for others the reverse is true. B: This is the most common, though not only, mechanism of phosphorylation. C: Insulin does not signal the phosphorylation of the enzymes involved. E: The most common site for phosphorylation is serine (pp. 541–544).
12. D A: Low insulin/glucagon ratio means high cAMP and, thus, high activity of cAMP-dependent protein kinase and protein phosphorylation. B and D: Phosphorylation activates hormone-sensitive lipase to mobilize fat. C: cAMP works by stimulating covalent modification of enzymes. E: This is a liver enzyme (pp. 544–545).
13. E A: Adaptive changes are examples of long-term control. B and D: Both hormonal and nutritional effects are involved in inducing certain enzymes and/or altering their rate of degradation. C: If there is little or no enzyme because of adaptive changes, allosteric control is irrelevant. This is important to keep in mind in refeeding a starved person (pp. 545–546).
14. B This is indicated by the drop in the respiratory quotient. A: Anaerobically exercised muscle uses glucose almost exclusively; aerobically exercised muscle uses fatty acids and ketone bodies. D: Ketone bodies are good aerobic substrates so the blood concentration does not increase greatly. E: Phosphocreatine is only a short-term source of ATP (p. 551).
15. D A: Hypertriglyceridemia is characteristic. B: Ketoacidosis is common only in the insulin-dependent type. C and D: The problem is insulin resistance, not failure to produce insulin. E: Most patients are obese because adipocytes remain sensitive to insulin (pp. 548 and 550).
16. B Failure to oxidize lactate to pyruvate because of the unfavorable $NAD^+/NADH$ ratio leads to lactate accumulation. A and E: The oxidation of ethanol, which also produces NADH, is cytosolic. Acetaldehyde oxidation is mitochondrial. C: "Fatty liver" is a consequence of inhibition of fatty acid oxidation by high NADH. D: Acetate activation requires GTP from the TCA cycle. Why is this cycle inhibited (pp. 555–556)?
17. E A and E: Glutamine in kidney is the primary source of ammonia for excretion of protons. B: This is the site of glutamine synthesis. C: This is when urea is formed. D: The liver activity of liver glutaminase during acidosis permits glutamine to escape liver for the kidney's use (pp. 556–559).

CHAPTER

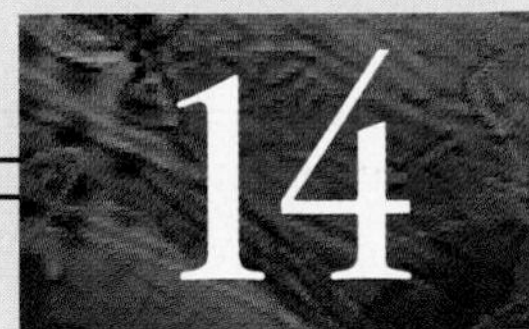

DNA I: STRUCTURE AND CONFORMATION

Stelios Aktipis

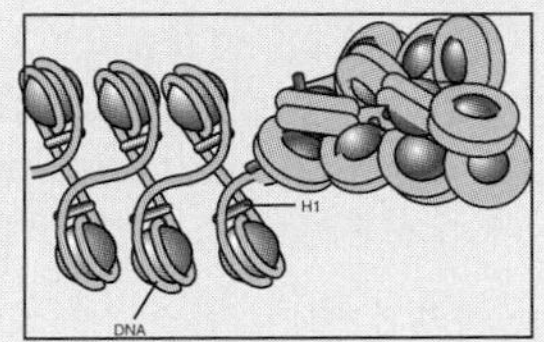

14.1 ■ OVERVIEW

One of the striking aspects of natural order is the sense of unity that exists between members of successive generations in each species. An almost totally stable bank of information must always be preserved and passed from one generation to the next if individual species are to maintain their identities relatively unchanged over millions of years. It is well established that this bank of genetic information takes the form of a macromolecule, deoxyribonucleic acid (DNA), which serves as the carrier of genetic information in both prokaryotes and eukaryotes. DNA exhibits a rare purity of function by being one of the few macromolecules known to perform, with only minor exceptions, the same basic functions across species barriers.

Properties of cells are to a large extent determined by their constituent proteins. Many proteins are indispensable structural components of cells. Other proteins, such as enzymes and certain hormones, are functional and determine many of the biochemical properties of the cell. As a result, factors that control which proteins a cell may synthesize, at what quantities, and with which sequence are the same factors that primarily determine function and destiny of every living cell.

DNA is the macromolecule that ultimately controls every aspect of cellular function, primarily through protein synthesis. DNA exercises this control as suggested by the sequence

$$\circlearrowright \text{DNA} \longrightarrow \text{RNA} \longrightarrow \text{protein}$$

Flow of biological information is clearly from one class of nucleic acid to another, from DNA to RNA, with only minor exceptions, and from there to protein. For this transfer of information to occur faithfully, each preceding macromolecule serves as a structure-specifying template for the synthesis of the subsequent member in the sequence.

In addition to regulating cellular expression, DNA plays an exclusive role in heredity. This role is suggested by a circular arrow engulfing DNA, which depicts DNA as a replicon, a molecule that can undergo self-replication. Replication permits DNA to make copies of itself as a cell divides and bestows them to daughter cells, which can thus inherit every property and characteristic of the original cell. Thus DNA ultimately determines the properties of a living cell by regulating expression of biological information, primarily by control of protein synthesis, and transfers biological information from one generation to the next; that is, it transmits genetic information.

DNA Can Transform Cells

These universally accepted principles were rejected outright not long ago. In fact, prior to the 1950s the general view was that nucleic acids are substances of somewhat limited cellular importance. The first convincing suggestion that DNA is the genetic material was made during the mid-1940s. The experiment involved transformation of a type of pneumococcus, surrounded by a polysaccharide capsule and referred to as S form because of its property of forming colonies with smooth-looking cellular perimeters, to a mutant without capsule, called R form, which forms colonies with rough-looking outlines. These two forms are genetically distinct and cannot interconvert spontaneously. **Transformation** experiments demonstrated that an extract of pure DNA from S form, when incorporated into R form of pneumococcus, conveyed to R form the specific property of synthesizing the characteristic polysaccharide capsule. Furthermore, bacteria transformed from R form to S form maintained the property of synthesizing capsule over succeeding generations. It was thus demonstrated that DNA was the **transforming agent,** as well as the material responsible for transmitting genetic information from one generation to the next. Almost three-quarters of a century elapsed from the time nucleic acids were discovered until their important biological role was generally recognized. Clinical Correlation 14.1 describes current studies in transforming mammalian cells with DNA.

CLINICAL CORRELATION 14.1

DNA Vaccines

Traditional procedures of vaccination have used purified components of an infectious organism, dead or attenuated intact cells or viruses, to provide individuals with active immunity by eliciting production of specific antibodies. Many have been successful in providing protection against diseases such as polio, smallpox, whooping cough, typhoid fever, and diphtheria.

A prototype DNA vaccine has been developed. It consists of a naked DNA that encodes the nucleoprotein of the influenza virus. This gene is the same or very similar in many strains of this virus and should afford protection against all or most of them. Naked DNA, that is, DNA freed of all its naturally associated proteins, is used. It enters cells and can be expressed without need of a complex virus system. Results of its use in mice and nonhuman primates have been very encouraging. Naked-DNA vaccines appear to stimulate cell-mediated immunity and an antibody response.

McDonnell, W. M., and Askari, F. K. DNA vaccines. *N. Engl. J. Med.* 334:42, 1996.

DNA's Information Capacity Is Enormous

A striking characteristic of DNA is its ability to encode an enormous quantity of biological information. An undifferentiated mammalian fetal cell contains only a few picograms (10^{-12} g) of DNA. Yet this minute amount of material is sufficient to direct synthesis of as many as 100,000 distinct proteins that will determine the form and biochemical behavior of a large variety of differentiated tissues in adult animals.

The compactness of information storage in DNA is unique. Even sophisticated memory elements of contemporary computers appear pitifully inadequate by comparison. How does DNA achieve such a supreme **coding effectiveness?** Answers must obviously be sought in the nature of its chemical structure. It turns out that this structure is not only consistent with the unique efficiency of DNA as a "memory bank" but also provides the basis for understanding how DNA eventually "translates" this information into proteins.

14.2 ■ STRUCTURE OF DNA

DNA is a polynucleotide produced by polymerization of deoxyribonucleotides. The structure of nucleotides and their constituent purine and pyrimidine bases are presented in Chapter 12.

The **base composition of DNA** varies considerably among species, particularly prokaryotes, which have a range of 25–75% in adenine–thymine content. This range narrows with evolution, reaching limiting values of about 45–53% in mammals.

DNA contains various **methylated bases.** These methylated derivatives are present in all prokaryotic DNA molecules examined to date but are absent in certain eukaryotes such as yeast and insects. As a rule these bases are generated by action of methylases, Dam and Dem, following synthesis of DNA. Methyl groups are transferred from *S*-adenosylmethionine. **Dam methylase** selects adenine residues on GATC sequences for methylation. **Dem methylase** acts on cytosine residues on opposite strands in the sequence

```
C C A G G
⋮ ⋮ ⋮ ⋮ ⋮
G G T C C
```

Such methylated sites are recognized by proteins involved in DNA functions such as recombination and initiation of DNA synthesis.

A base may be methylated prior to incorporation into DNA, as in transformation of cytosine to **5-hydroxycytosine. Glycosylated 5-hydroxycytosine** is found as a constituent of T-even phages of *Escherichia coli.* Other unusual base changes include the presence of uracil, a constituent of RNA, in certain *Bacillus subtilis* phages, instead of thymine. Structures of some of these bases are shown in Figure 14.1.

N^2-Dimethylguanine

N^6-Dimethyladenine

1-Methylguanine

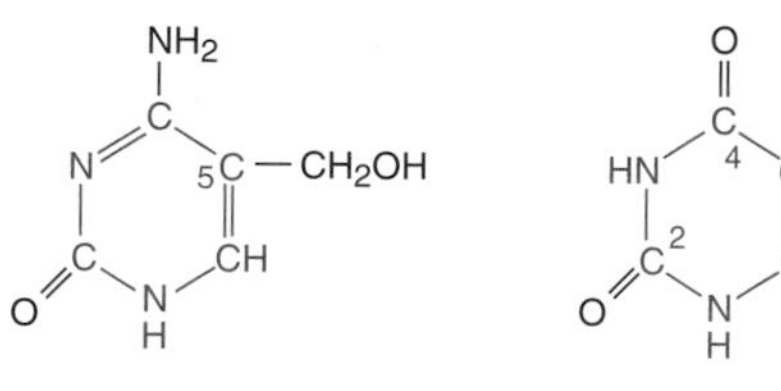

5-Hydroxymethylcytosine

Uracil (2,4-dioxypyrimidine)

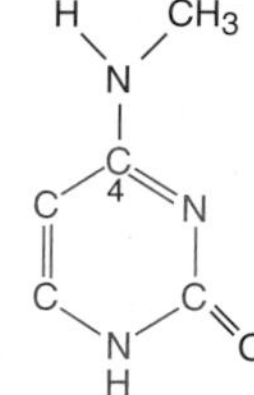

N^4-Methylcytosine

5-Methylcytosine

FIGURE 14.1
Structures of some less common bases occurring in DNA.

Nucleotides Joined by Phosphodiester Bonds Form Polynucleotides

Polynucleotides are formed by joining of nucleotides by **phosphodiester bonds.** The phosphodiester bond is the formal analog of the peptide bond in proteins. It joins by esterification of two of the three OH groups of phosphoric acid, two adjoining nucleotide residues. Deoxyribose contains two free OH groups on the C-3′ and C-5′ atoms that can participate in formation of a phosphodiester bond. Indeed, the nucleotide residues in DNA are joined by **3′,5′-phosphodiester bonds,** as shown in Figure 14.2.

Many polynucleotides are linear polymers. The last nucleotide residues at opposite ends of the polynucleotide chain serve as the two terminals of the chain. It is apparent that these terminals are not structurally equivalent, since one of the nucleotides must terminate at a 3′-OH group and the other at a 5′-OH group. These ends of the polynucleotides are referred to as 3′ and 5′ termini, and they may be viewed as corresponding to the amino and carboxyl termini in proteins. Polynucleotides also exist as cyclic structures, which contain

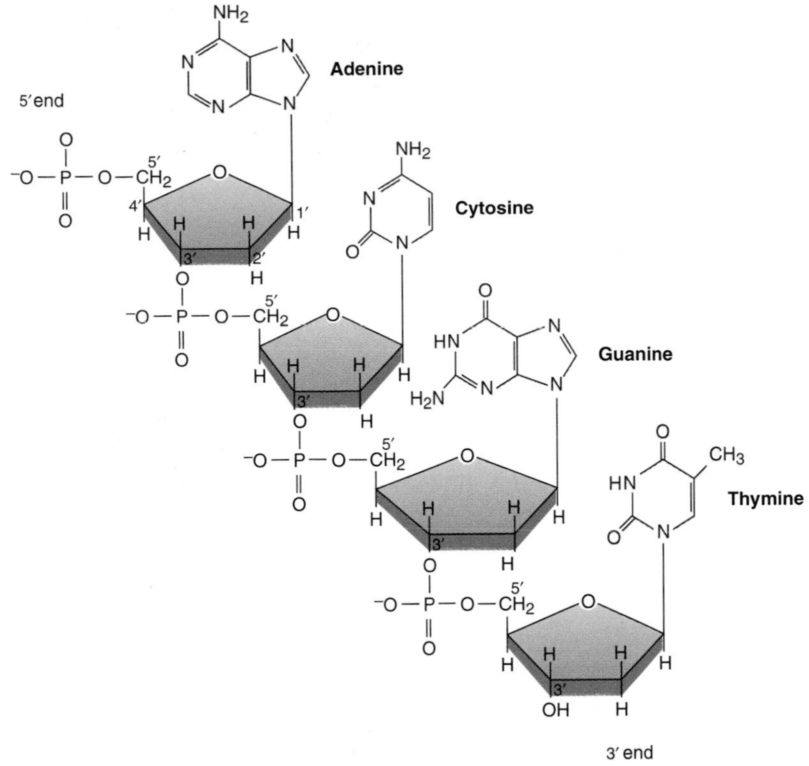

FIGURE 14.2
Structure of a DNA polynucleotide segment.
Shown is a tetranucleotide. Generally, polymers containing less than 30–40 nucleotides are referred to as oligonucleotides.

no free terminals. Esterification between the 3′-OH terminus of a polynucleotide with its own 5′-phosphate terminus can produce a cyclic polynucleotide.

Long polymers of nucleotides joined by phosphodiester bonds are called polynucleotides. **Oligonucleotides** are shorter nucleotide-containing polymers. According to formal rules of nomenclature, however, polynucleotides are named by using roots derived from the names of corresponding nucleotides, and using the ending ylyl. Polynucleotide sequences are always read in the $5' \rightarrow 3'$ direction, unless specified otherwise. For example, the polynucleotide segment in Figure 14.2, in which the 5′ terminal is on the left of each nucleotide residue, should be named from left to right as

...deoxyadenylyl, deoxycytidylyl, deoxyguanylyl, deoxythymidylyl...

However, use of complete chemical names is cumbersome and abbreviations are generally preferred. For example, the oligonucleotide shown in Figure 14.2 is usually referred to as dAdCdGdT, and a polynucleotide containing only one kind of nucleotide, for example, dA, may be written as poly(dA). Oligo- and polynucleotide structures are also written out in shorthand, as shown in Figure 14.3.

The specific sequence of bases along a polynucleotide chain determines its biological properties. Although the structure of the nucleic acid bases had been known for many years, the polymeric structure initially proposed for DNA was one of the classical errors in the history of biochemistry. Experimental data obtained from partially degraded samples of DNA, and several misconceptions, led to the erroneous conclusion that DNA consisted of repeating tetranucleotide units. Each tetranucleotide supposedly contained equimolar quantities of the four common bases. These impressions persisted to some degree until the late 1940s and early 1950s, when they were clearly shown to be in error. In the interim, however, these misconceptions were responsible for setting back acceptance of the concept that DNA of chromosomes carried genetic information. The monotonous structure of repeating tetranucleotides appeared to lack the

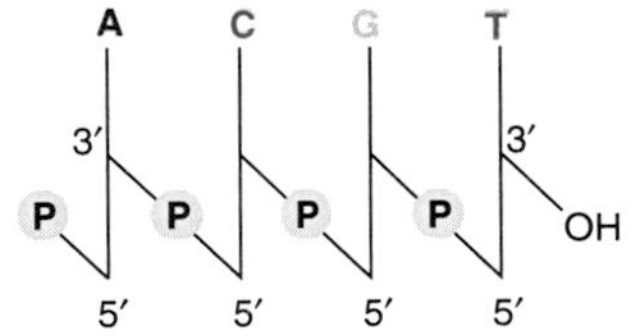

FIGURE 14.3
Shorthand form for structure of oligonucleotides.
The convention used in writing the structure of an oligo- or polynucleotide is a perpendicular bar representing the deoxyribose moiety, with the 5′-OH position of the sugar located at the bottom of the bar and the 3′-OH at a midway position. Bars joining the 3′ and 5′ positions represent the 3′,5′-phosphodiester bond, and the P on the left side of the perpendicular bar represents a 5′-phosphate ester. A 3′-phosphate ester is represented by placing the phosphate group on the right side of the bar and the base by its initial.

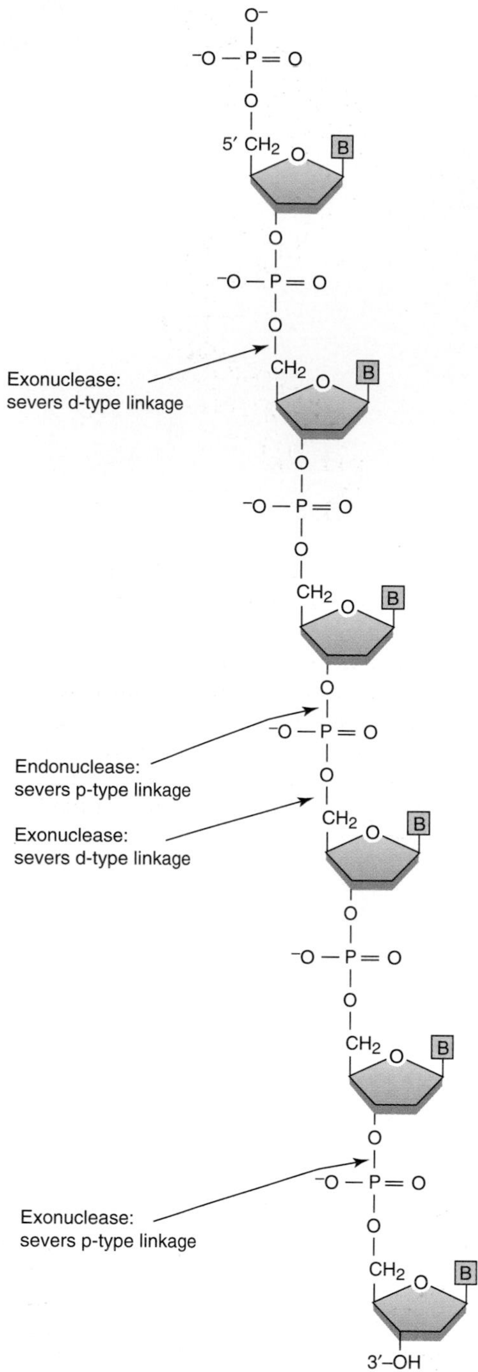

FIGURE 14.4
Specificities of nucleases.
Exonucleases remove nucleotide residues from either terminal of a polynucleotide, depending on their specificity. Endonucleases hydrolyze interior phosphodiester bonds. Both endo- and exonucleases hydrolyze either d- or p-type linkages (see text for explanation of d- and p-type linkages).

versatility to encode for the enormous number of messages necessary to convey hereditary traits. Instead proteins, which can be ordered in an almost unlimited number of amino acid sequences, were favored as the most suitable candidates for a hereditary function. Transformation experiments carried out in the mid-1940s, and the finding that DNA consists of polynucleotide and not tetranucleotide chains, were responsible for general acceptance of the hereditary role of DNA that followed.

Nucleases Hydrolyze Phosphodiester Bonds

The nature of the linkage between nucleotides to form polynucleotides was elucidated primarily by use of exonucleases, enzymes that hydrolyze these polymers in a selective manner. Exonucleases cleave the last nucleotide residue at either of the two terminals of an oligonucleotide. Oligonucleotides can thus be degraded by stepwise removal of individual nucleotides or small oligonucleotides from either the 5′ or 3′ terminus. **Nucleases** sever bonds in one of two nonequivalent positions indicated in Figure 14.4 as proximal (p) or distal (d) to the base, which occupies the 3′ end of the bond. For example, treatment of an oligodeoxyribonucleotide with snake venom diesterase, an enzyme obtained from snake venom, yields deoxyribonucleoside 5′-phosphates. In contrast, treatment with a diesterase isolated from animal spleen produces deoxyribonucleoside 3′-phosphates.

Other nucleases that cleave phosphodiester bonds located in the interior of polynucleotides are designated as endonucleases and behave similarly. For instance, DNase I cleaves only p linkages, while DNase II cleaves d linkages. Points of cleavage along an oligonucleotide chain are indicated by arrows in Figure 14.4. Some endonucleases have been particularly useful in development of methodologies for sequencing of DNA polynucleotides and have provided the basis for development of recombinant DNA techniques.

Many nucleases do not exhibit any specificity with respect to the base adjacent to the linkage that is hydrolyzed. Others, however, act very discriminately only next to specific types of bases or even specific bases. **Restriction endonucleases** act only on sequences of bases specifically recognized by each restriction enzyme. Nucleases also exhibit specificities with respect to overall structure of polynucleotides. For instance, some nucleases act on both single- or double-stranded polynucleotides, whereas others discriminate between these two structures. In addition, some nucleases exclusively designated as **phosphodiesterases** will act on either DNA or RNA, whereas other nucleases will limit their activity to only one type of polynucleotide. Nucleases listed in Table 14.1 illustrate some of the properties of these enzymes.

Periodicity Leads to Secondary Structure of DNA

Polypeptide chains of protein are often arranged in space so as to form periodic structures. For instance, in the α-helix each residue is related to the next by a translation of 1.5 Å along the helix axis and a rotation of 100°. This places 3.6 amino acid residues in each complete turn of the polypeptide helix. The property of **periodicity** is also encountered with polynucleotides, which usually occur in the form of **helices.** Such preponderance of helical conformations among macromolecules is not surprising. Formation of helices tends to accommodate effects of intramolecular forces, which in a helix can be distributed at regular intervals. The alternative, that is, a hypothetical extended linear conformation, would place successive base pairs at 0.68 nm apart and allow water molecules to be inserted between hydrophobic base pairs. Clearly such an arrangement would be thermodynamically unfavorable. The precise geometry of the polynucleotide helices varies, but the helical structure invariably results from stacking

TABLE 14.1 **Specificities of Various Types of Nucleases**

Enzyme	*Substrate*	*Specificity*[a]
EXONUCLEASES		
Snake venom phosphodiesterase	DNA or RNA single-stranded only	Cleaves all p-type linkages, starting with a free 3′-OH group and moving toward the 5′ terminal; releases nucleoside 5′-phosphates; has no base specificity
Bovine spleen phosphodiesterase	DNA or RNA single-stranded only	Cleaves all d-type linkages, starting at the free 5′-OH and proceeding to the 3′ terminal; releases nucleoside 3′-phosphates; has no base specificity
ENDONUCLEASES		
Bovine pancreas deoxyribonuclease (DNase I)	DNA single- or double-stranded	Cleaves all p-type linkages but prefers those between purine and pyrimidine bases
Calf thymus deoxyribonuclease (DNase II)	DNA single- or double-stranded	Cleaves all d-type linkages randomly

[a] See text for explanation of d- and p-type linkages.

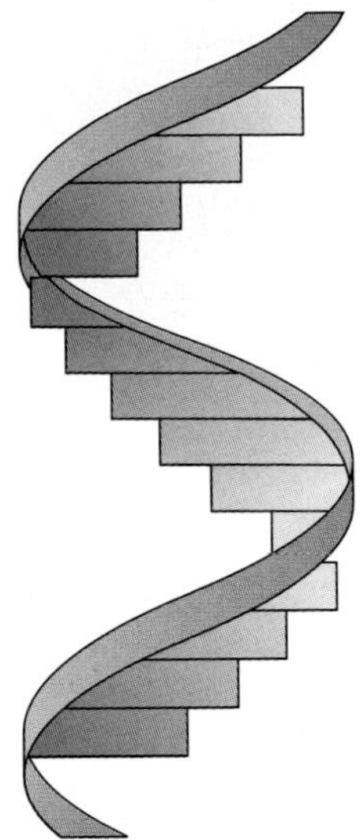

FIGURE 14.5
Conformation of a hypothetical, perfectly helical, single-stranded polynucleotide.
The helical band represents the phosphate backbone of the polynucleotide. Bases are shown in a side view as solid blocks in tight contact with their neighbors, above and below each base. Surfaces of the rings are in contact with each other and are not visible in the perspective.

of bases along the helix axis. In many instances stacking produces helices in which bases are more or less perpendicularly oriented along the helix and touch one another. This arrangement leaves no free space between two successive neighboring bases (Figure 14.5). Such stacked single-stranded helices, however, are not commonly encountered in cells. Rather, polynucleotide helices tend to associate with one another to form double helices.

Forces that Determine Polynucleotide Conformation

The hydrophobic properties of the bases are, to a large extent, responsible for forcing polynucleotides to adopt helical conformations. Molecular models of bases reveal that the edges of the rings contain polar groups (i.e., amino and OH groups) that interact with other polar groups or surrounding water molecules. The faces of the rings, however, are unable to participate in such interactions and tend to avoid any contact with water. Instead they tend to interact with one another, producing a **stacked conformation.** The stability of this arrangement is further reinforced by an interchange between electrons that circulate in π orbitals located above and below the plane of each ring.

Clearly then, single-stranded polynucleotide helices are stabilized by **hydrophobic** and **dipole-induced dipole interactions** involving the π orbitals of bases, which collectively produce base stacking. The stability of helical structures is somewhat decreased by potential repulsion among charged phosphate residues of the polynucleotide backbone. These repulsive forces introduce a certain degree of rigidity to the structure of polynucleotides. Under physiological conditions, that is, at neutral pH and relatively high concentrations of salts, the charges on the phosphate residues are partially shielded by the cations present, such as Mg^{2+}, and the structure can be viewed as a fairly flexible coil. Under more extreme conditions stacking of bases is disrupted and the helix collapses. A collapsed helix is commonly described as a **random coil.** Conversion between a stacked helix and an unstacked conformation is depicted in Figure 14.6.

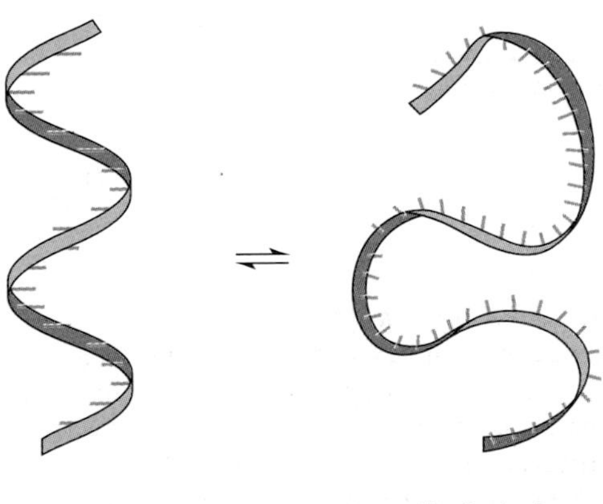

FIGURE 14.6
Stacked and unstacked conformations of a polynucleotide.
Stacking of bases decreases flexibility of a polynucleotide and tends to produce a more extended, often helical, structure.

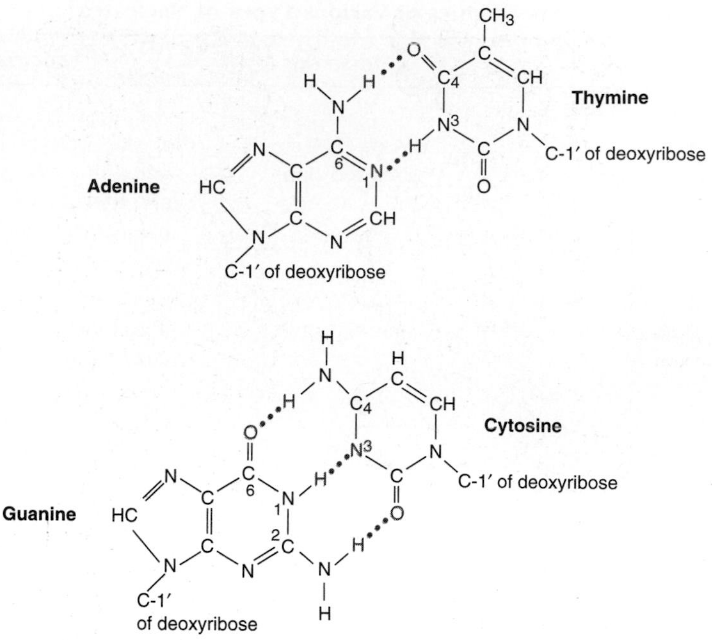

FIGURE 14.7
Formation of hydrogen bonds between complementary bases in double-stranded DNA.
Interaction between polynucleotide strands is a highly selective process. Complementarity depends not only on the geometric factors that allow the proper fitting between the complementary bases of the two strands, but also on the electronic specificity of interaction between complementary bases. Thus specificity of interaction between purines and pyrimidines has also been noted both in solution and in the crystal form, and it is expressed in terms of strong hydrogen bonding between monomers of adenine and uracil or monomers of guanine and cytosine.

DNA Double Helix

Although some forms of cellular DNA exist as **single-stranded structures,** the most widespread DNA structure is the **double helix.** The double helix can be visualized as resulting from interwinding of two right-handed helical polynucleotide strands around a common axis. The two strands achieve contact through hydrogen bonds, which are formed at the hydrophilic edges of their bases. These bonds extend between purine residues in one strand and pyrimidine residues in the other, so that the two types of resulting pairs are always adenine–thymine and guanine–cytosine. A direct consequence of these hydrogen-bonding specificities is that double-stranded DNA contains equal amounts of purines and pyrimidines. Examination of space-filling models clearly indicates structural compatibility of these bases in forming linear hydrogen bonds.

This relationship between bases in the double helix is described as **complementarity.** Bases are complementary because every base of one strand is matched by a complementary hydrogen-bonding base on the other strand. For instance, for each adenine projecting toward the common axis of the double helix, a thymine must be projected from the opposite chain so as to fill exactly the space between strands by hydrogen bonding with adenine. Neither cytosine nor guanine fits precisely in the available space across from adenine in a manner that allows formation of hydrogen bonds across strands. These **hydrogen-bonding specificities** (Figure 14.7) ensure that the entire base sequence of one strand is complementary to that of the other strand.

The double helix exists in various geometries designated as **DNA A, B, and C.** Formation of these different **conformations** depends on the base composition of DNA and on physical conditions. These forms share certain common characteristics. Specifically, the phosphate backbones are always located on the outside of the helix. Also, because diesters of phosphoric acid are fully ionized at neutral pH, the exterior of the helix is negatively charged. Bases are well packed in the interior of the helix, where their faces are protected from contact with water. In this environment the strength of hydrogen bonds that connect bases can be maximized. Interwinding of two strands produces a structure having two helical grooves that separate the winding phosphate backbone ridge.

However, the precise **geometry of the double helix** varies among the

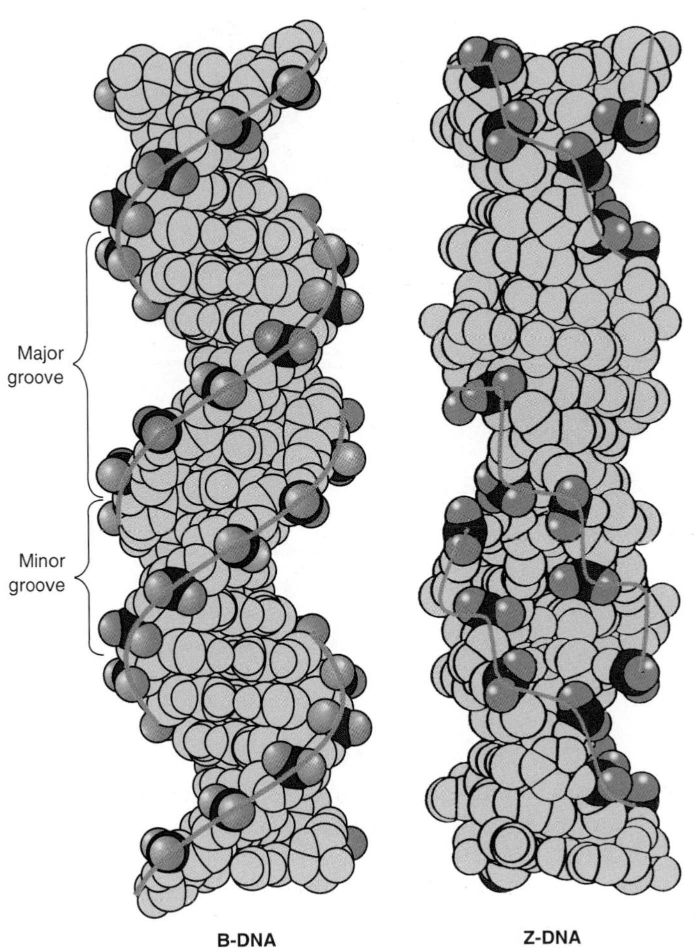

FIGURE 14.8
Space-filling molecular models of B- and Z-DNA.
The double helix is referred to as the Watson and Crick model, although this structure has been substantially refined since it was proposed. B-DNA may be the most typical form occurring in cells. Z-DNA may be present in cells as small stretches, consisting of alternating purines and pyrimidines, incorporated between long stretches of B-DNA. The zigzag nature of the Z-DNA backbone is illustrated by the heavy lines that connect phosphate residues along the chain.
Redrawn based on figure from Rich, A. J. Biomol. Struct. Dyn. *1:1, 1983.*

different forms. The original X-ray data obtained with highly oriented DNA fibers suggested occurrence of a form, later designated as B, which appears to be that commonly found in solution and *in vivo* (Figure 14.8). A characteristic of this form is that one of its grooves is wider **(major groove)** than the other **(minor groove).** Disparity in width between these two grooves results from the characteristic geometry of base pairs (bp). Glycosidic bonds between sugars and bases of each base pair are not arranged directly opposite to one another. Instead the edge of the helix, that is more than 180° from glycosidic bond to glycosidic bond, is the edge that forms part of the major groove. Clearly, the opposite edge corresponds to the minor groove. The nucleotide sequence of a polynucleotides can be discerned without dissociating the double helix by looking inside these grooves. As each of the four bases has its own orientation with respect to the rest of the helix, each base always shows the same atoms through the grooves. C-6, N-7, and C-8 of the purine rings and C-4, C-5, and C-6 of the pyrimidine rings line up in the major groove. The minor groove is paved with C-2 and N-3 of the purine and C-2 of the pyrimidine rings. Forms A and C differ from B in the pitch of the base pairs relative to the helix axis as shown in Figure 14.9, as well as in other geometric parameters of the double helix, including conformation of sugar residues, which is one of the more flexible components of the DNA molecule. Alternative forms of the double helix are the result of **conformational variations** of the sugar–phosphate groups that form the backbone of constituent polynucleotides (Figure 14.10). The conformation of the furanose ring of sugar residues exists in nonplanar (puckered) forms. This ring may be visualized in the form of an envelope with four carbon atoms at the corner of the envelope. Oxygen is positioned at the

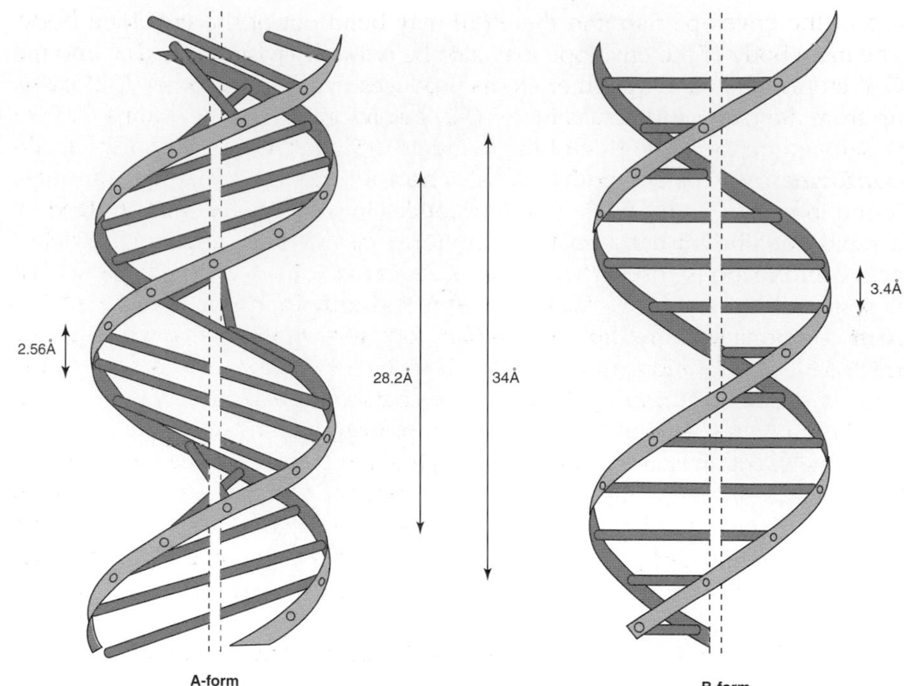

FIGURE 14.9
Various geometries of DNA double helix. Depending on conditions, the double helix can acquire various forms of distinct geometries. In the B form of DNA the centers of the bases are about 34 Å apart and produce a complete turn of a helix with a pitch of 34 Å. Such an arrangement results in a complete turn of the helix for every 10 bp. The diameter of the helix is 20 Å. Form C (not shown) is very similar to the B structure, with a pitch of 33 Å and 9 bp per turn. Form A, which is obtained from form B when the relative humidity of the fiber is reduced to 75%, differs from B in that the base pairs are not perpendicular to the helical axis but are tilted. This tilt results in a pitch of 28.2 Å and a shortening of the helix by the packing of 11 pairs per helical turn.
Redrawn based on figure from Guschelbauer, W. Nucleic Acid Structure. *Berlin: Springer-Verlag, 1976.*

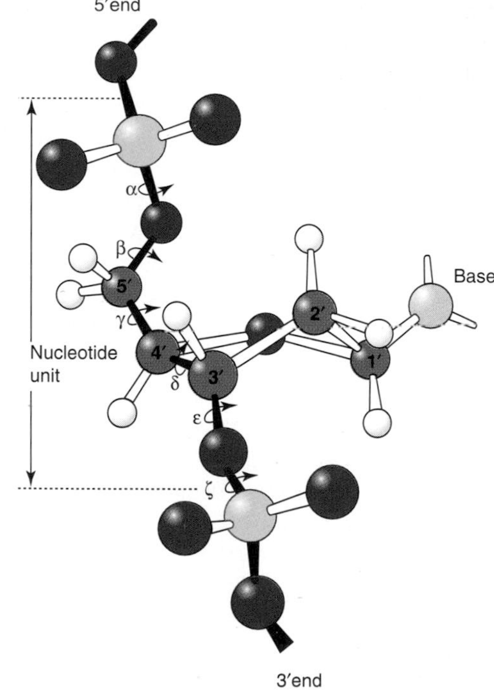

FIGURE 14.10
Structure of ribose–phosphate backbone of polynucleotides.
The polynucleotide backbone has six degrees of freedom on rotation along the bonds identified by Greek letters α to ζ. However, steric hindrance and electrostatic repulsion between the oxygen atoms of the phosphate residue restrict the number of conformational variants that can be generated by rotation along some of these bonds. Rotation is particularly limited, but still possible, around the C-5′—O bond (β bond) and the C-3′—C-4′ bond (δ bond).

top of the envelope flap and therefore may bend out of the envelope body. The main body of the envelope may also be twisted. Twisting the C-2′ and the C-3′ atoms relative to the other atoms produces two distinct forms. C-2′ twists up from the plane and results in the C-2′ **endo** form. As a rule, atoms that are positioned on the same side of the plane as C-5′ have by definition the **endo conformation.** The C-2′ **endo** and C-3′ **endo** are the most common conformers found in nucleic acids, while free nucleotides in solution are characterized by a rapid equilibrium between these conformers. Another variation in nucleic acid conformations arises from rotations about the C-1′–*N*-glycosidic bond that is responsible for variants known as **syn** and **anti** forms (see Figure 14.11). **Anti** conformations are the predominant forms in nucleic acids, while in free nucleotides in solution **syn–anti** equilibrium depends on the nature of the base. Generally, purine nucleotides are characterized by a rapid **syn–anti** equilibrium while pyrimidines usually adopt **anti** conformations.

Finally, conformational variations in DNA may result from relative orientations of the planes of the bases between strands. Differences in orientation between planes of H-bonded bases may produce double helix variants with different base **tilt, roll, twist,** or **propeller twist.** For example, DNA forms A and B differ drastically in base **tilt** and deviations of **tilt** and **roll** angles, occurring in phage tracts of adenine residues, are responsible for extensive bending of the double helix axis over certain functionally important regions of DNA. Under conditions of low salt concentration and humidity, the thin B-DNA double helix shifts to a conformation characterized by a thicker helix. In this conformation nucleotides move off center toward the major edge of each base pair, generating A-DNA, which has a narrower and deeper major groove and a wider and shallower minor groove than B-DNA. The parameters for these different DNA conformations, listed in Table 14.2, have been determined of DNA by X-ray diffraction methods. While the numbers provide very accurate information about molecular geometry and dimensions of crystalline samples, they give only average dimensions for monomeric units present in a noncrystalline macromolecule. Therefore these parameters are listed as such and the listing does not imply that the same geometry characterizes each and every individual base pair in DNA. Rather, depending on base sequence, considerable local variation in conformation of individual nucleotides may occur. Such varia-

TABLE 14.2 Structural Features of A-, B-, and Z-DNA

Features	*A-DNA*	*B-DNA*	*Z-DNA*
Helix rotation	Right-handed	Right-handed	Left-handed
Base pair per turn (crystal)	10.7	9.7	12
Base pair per turn (fiber)	11	10	—
Base pair per turn (solution)	—	10.5	—
Pitch per turn of helix	24.6 Å	33.2 Å	45.6 Å
Proportions	Short-end broad	Longer and thinner	Elongated and thin
Helix packing diameter	25.5 Å	23.7 Å	18.4 Å
Rise per base pair (crystal)	2.3 Å	3.3 Å	3.7
Rise per base pair (fiber)	2.6	3.4 Å	—
Base pair tilt	+19°	−1.2° (but varies)	−9°
Propeller twist	+18°	+16°	0°
Helix axis rotation	Major groove	Through base pairs	Minor groove
Sugar ring conformation (crystal)	C-3′ *endo*	Variable	Alternating
Sugar ring conformation (fiber)	C-3′ *endo*	C-2′ *endo*	—
Glycosyl bond conformation	anti	anti	anti at C, syn at G

tions may be important in regulation of gene expression, since they influence the extent of DNA binding with various types of regulatory proteins.

A form of DNA, which was discovered more recently, has geometric characteristics radically different from those of conventional forms. In this DNA, called **Z-DNA,** the polynucleotide phosphodiester backbone assumes a "zigzag" arrangement rather than the smooth conformation that characterizes other double-stranded forms. The Z-DNA structure is longer and much thinner than that of B-DNA and completes one turn in 12 bp rather than the 10 bp in a B-DNA turn. It forms a single groove as opposed to two grooves that characterize B-DNA. Therefore the conformation of Z-DNA may be viewed as the result of the major groove of B-DNA having "popped out" in order to form the outer convex surface of Z-DNA. This change places the stacked bases on the outer part of Z-DNA rather than in their conventional positions in the interior of the double helix. Another highly unusual property of the Z structure is that it consists of left-handed rather than right-handed helices, which characterize conventional forms. These major structural differences between B-DNA and Z-DNA (Figure 14.8) are partly the result of different conformations in nucleotide residues between the two forms. Specifically, in B- and A-DNA sugars and bases are arranged in the extended **anti** conformation. In contrast, in Z-DNA some nucleotides rotate into **syn** conformation, which places the sugar and base on the same side of the glycosidic bond (Figure 14.11). DNA sequences that consist of alternating GC nucleotides are the most prone to acquire Z conformation, which places glycosidic bonds of each G in syn, with C residues maintaining the anti conformation. The zigzag arrangement of the phosphate backbone reflects sudden turns of the backbone, as it follows the alternating arrangement of syn and anti geometries.

The **biological function of Z-DNA** is not known with certainty. Some evidence exists suggesting that Z-DNA influences gene expression and regulation. Apparently small stretches of DNA approximately 12–24 bp long with the potential of forming Z-DNA are more commonly found at the 5′ end of genes, that is, in regions that regulate transcriptional activities. These stretches consist of alternating purines and pyrimidines that favor formation of the Z conformation. Z-DNA may have a role in genetic recombination. Sites of genetic recombination in eukaryotic cells appear to be associated with DNA regions with the potential of Z-DNA formation. The Z form of DNA is stabilized by the presence of cations or polyamines and by methylation of either guanine residues in C-8 and N-7 positions or cytosine residues in C-5 position. Sequences that are not strictly alternating pu-pyr may also acquire the Z conformation as a result of methylation. For instance, the hexanucleotide ^{m5}GAT^{m5}CG, which contains two internal adjacent pairs of pu and py, forms Z-DNA. This outcome is not surprising because in Z-DNA hydrophobic methyl groups do not protrude unfavorably into the aqueous environment surrounding the double helix, as is the case with B-DNA. On this basis it might be expected that *in vivo* methylation of cytosine also induces a B $\rightarrow$ Z transition in cellular DNA. The suggestion that Z-DNA may have a role in gene regulation is supported by modification in methylation patterns that accompany the process of gene expression.

An important structural characteristic of double-stranded DNA is that its strands are **antiparallel.** Polynucleotides are asymmetric structures with an intrinsic sense of **polarity** built into them (Figure 14.12). The two strands are aligned in opposite directions; if two adjacent bases in the same strand, for example, thymine and cytosine, are connected in the 5′ $\rightarrow$ 3′ direction, their complementary bases adenine and guanine will be linked in the 3′ $\rightarrow$ 5′ direction (directions are defined by linking the 3′ and 5′ positions within the same nucleotide). This antiparallel alignment produces a stable association between strands to the exclusion of the alternate parallel arrangement.

The double-stranded structure of DNA was proposed in 1953, partly based on previously available X-ray diffraction studies suggesting that the structures

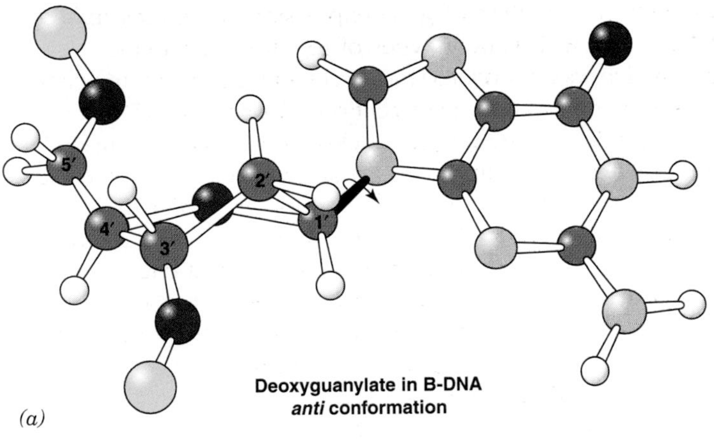

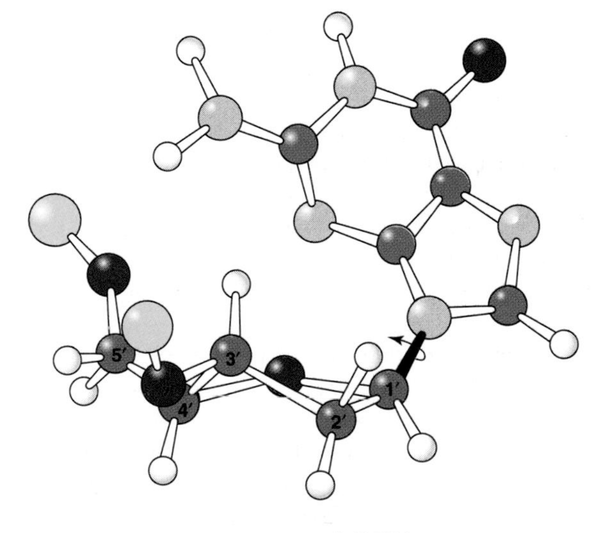

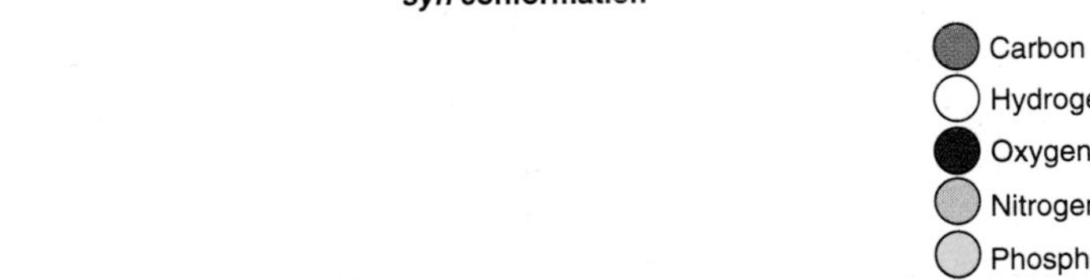

FIGURE 14.11
Conformational variants of nucleotides.
Rotation of the base plane around the C-1′—N-9 glycosyl bond gives rise to two distinct nucleotide conformations, the so-called anti and syn conformations. The anti conformation is characteristic of B-DNA. In Z-DNA the glycosyl bond rotates as shown to give the syn conformation. The B → Z DNA transformation is also accompanied by a change in the conformation of the ribose ring from the C-2′ endo to C-3′ endo conformation.

of DNA from various sources exhibited remarkable similarities. These studies also suggested that DNA had a helical structure containing two or more polynucleotides. Evidence of central importance to the proposal was the clarification of the quantitative base composition of DNA, indicating the molar equivalence between purines and pyrimidines essential for the complementarity between the two strands.

Many Factors Stabilize DNA Structure

Factors that stabilize single-stranded polynucleotides—that is, **hydrophobic interactions** and **van der Waals forces**—are also instrumental in stabilizing the double helix. Van der Waals interactions generate attractive forces among atoms that are optimally situated, that is, neither too close nor too far apart

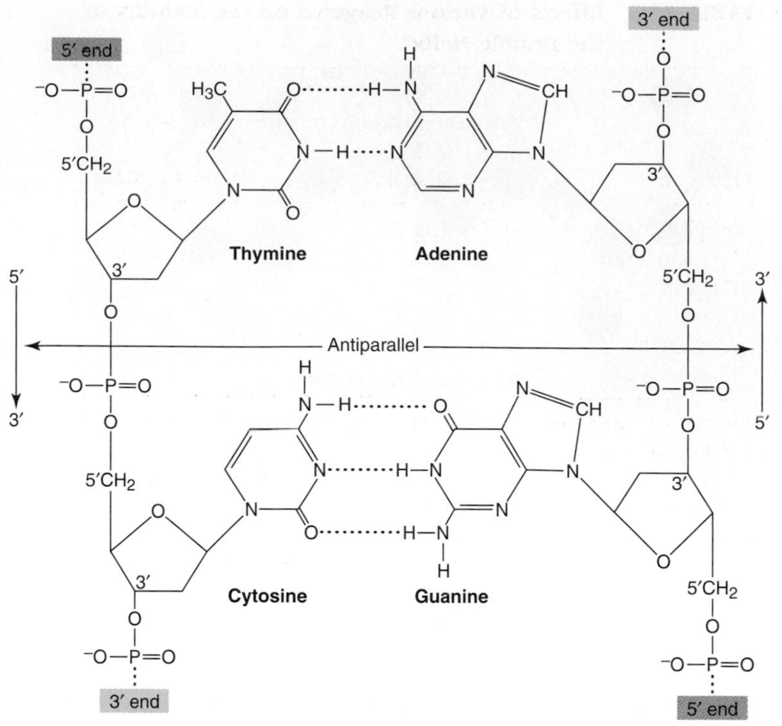

FIGURE 14.12
Antiparallel nature of DNA strands.
Note the opposite direction of the strands of a double-stranded DNA. The geometry of the helices does not prevent a parallel alignment, but such an arrangement is not found in DNA.

relative to one another, within a molecular structure. These forces are the result of **dipole–dipole interactions** and **London dispersion interactions** (transient dipole interactions) between adjacent bases. Hydrophobic interactions are also very important in stabilizing polynucleotide structures and especially the double helix. The separation between the hydrophobic core of the stacked bases and the hydrophilic exterior of the charged sugar–phosphate groups is even more striking in the double helix than with single-stranded helices. This explains the preponderance of the DNA double helix. The stacking tendency of single-stranded polynucleotides may be viewed as resulting from a tendency of the bases to avoid contact with water. The double-stranded helix is a more favorable arrangement, permitting the phosphate backbone to be highly solvated by water while the bases are essentially removed from the aqueous environment.

Collectively, hydrophobic and van der Waals forces are referred to as **stacking interactions** because they produce the stacked arrangement of the bases typical of the double helix. Stacking interactions are estimated to generate 4–15 kcal mol^{-1} for each adjacent pair of stacked bases.

Additional stabilization of both single-stranded DNA as well as the double helix results from extensive networks of **cooperative hydrogen bonding.** Typically, hydrogen bonds are relatively weak (3–7 kcal mol^{-1}) and are even weaker in DNA (2–3 kcal mol^{-1}) because of geometric constraints within the double helix. Cumulatively, however, H bonds provide substantial energies of stabilization for the double helix although the stabilization is less than what is provided by stacking interactions. However, hydrogen bonding, in contrast to stacking forces, does not confer to any significant degree preferential stabilization to the double helix relative to its constituent single-stranded polynucleotides, which can form equally effective hydrogen bonds with water molecules in an aqueous environment.

Hydrogen bonds have important biochemical consequences for the functions in which the double helix participates. In contrast to stacking forces, hydrogen bonds are highly directional and are able to provide a discriminatory function for choosing between correct and incorrect base pairs. Because of

TABLE 14.3 Effects of Various Reagents on the Stability of the Double Helix[a]

Reagent	*Adenine Solubility × 10^{-3} (in 1 M reagent)*	*Molarity Producing 50% Denaturation*
Ethylurea	22.5	0.60
Propionamide	22.5	0.62
Ethanol	17.7	1.2
Urea	17.7	1.0
Methanol	15.9	3.5
Formamide	15.4	1.9

Source: Data from Levine, L., Gordon, J., and Jencks, W. P. *Biochemistry* 2:168, 1963.

[a] The destabilizing effect of the reagents listed below on the double helix is independent of the ability of these reagents to break hydrogen bonds. Rather, the destabilizing effect is determined by the solubility of adenine. Similar results would be expected if the solubilities of the other bases were examined.

their directionality, hydrogen bonds tend to orient the bases in a way that favors stacking. Therefore the contribution of hydrogen bonds is essential for the stability of the double helix.

The relative importance of hydrogen bonding and stacking forces in stabilizing the double helix was not always appreciated. The effects of various reagents on the stability of the double helix have suggested that the destabilizing effect of a reagent is not related to the ability of the reagent to break hydrogen bonds. Rather, the stability of the double helix is determined by the solubility of the free bases in the reagent, the stability decreasing as the solubility increases. Some of these findings, summarized in Table 14.3, emphasize the importance of hydrophobic forces in maintaining the structure of double-stranded DNA.

A direct consequence of the conclusion that the relative stability of the double helix versus the single-stranded DNA depends almost exclusively on stacking forces is that differences in the stabilities of various segments of the double helix reflect variabilities in the stacking energies of different base sequences. Indeed, a large degree of variability exists among the stacking energies of various pairs of stacked bases as shown in Table 14.4. As a rule, stacking interaction involving dimers of G-C base pairs are stronger than interactions between stacked dimers of A-T base pairs.

TABLE 14.4 Base Pair Stacking Energies

Dinucleotide Base Pairs	*Stacking Energies (kcal mol^{-1} per stacked pair)*[a]
(GC) · (GC)	−14.59
(AC) · (GT)	−10.51
(TC) · (GA)	− 9.81
(CG) · (CG)	− 9.69
(GG) · (CC)	− 8.26
(AT) · (AT)	− 6.57
(TG) · (CA)	− 6.57
(AG) · (CT)	− 6.78
(AA) · (TT)	− 5.37
(TA) · (TA)	− 3.82

[a] Data from Ornstein, R. L., Reim, R., Breen, D. L., and Mc Elroy, R. D. *Biopolymers* 17:2341, 1978.

Ionic forces also have an effect on the stability and conformation of the double helix. At physiological pH, the electrostatic intrastrand repulsion between negatively charged phosphates is potentially destabilizing and it forces the double helix into a relatively rigid rod-like conformation. In addition, this repulsion tends to separate the complementary strands. In distilled water, DNA strands will separate at room temperature; near the physiological salt concentration, cations, particularly Mg^{2+} (in addition to other charged groups, e.g., the basic side chains of proteins), shield the phosphate groups and decrease repulsive forces. Therefore the flexibility of the double helix is partially restored and its stability is enhanced.

Denaturation

The double helix is disrupted during almost every important biological transformation in which DNA participates, including DNA replication, transcription, repair, and recombination. Therefore the forces that hold the two strands together are adequate for providing stability and yet weak enough to allow facile

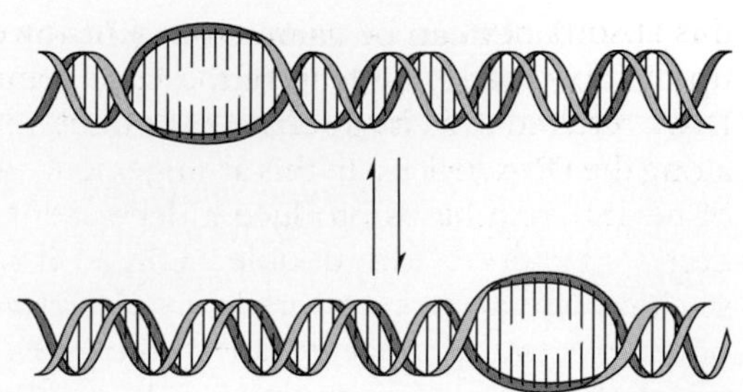

FIGURE 14.13
"Zipper" model for DNA double helix.
DNA contains short sections of open-strandedness that can "move" up and down the helix.

strand separation. In fact, the double helix is stabilized relative to the single strands by about 1 kcal per base pair. Therefore a relatively minor perturbation can produce disruption in double strandedness, provided that only a short section of the DNA is involved. As soon as the relatively few base pairs have separated, they close up again and release free energy, and then the adjacent base pairs unwind. In this manner minor disruptions of double strandedness can be propagated along the length of the double helix. Thus, at any particular moment, the large majority of the bases of the double helix remain hydrogen bonded, but all bases can pass through the single-stranded state, a few at a time. This **dynamic state** of the double helix is characterized by the movement of an "open-stranded" portion up and down the length of the helix, as indicated in Figure 14.13. The "dynamic" nature of this structure is an essential prerequisite for the biological functions of DNA as it undergoes repair or recombination.

Separation of DNA strands can be studied by increasing the temperature in solution. At relatively low temperatures a few base pairs will be disrupted, creating one or more "open-stranded bubbles." These "bubbles" form initially in sections that contain relatively higher proportions of adenine and thymine pairs because of the lower stacking energies of dimers of such pairs. As the temperature is raised, the size of the "bubbles" increases and eventually the thermal motion of the polynucleotides overcomes the forces that stabilize the double helix. This transformation is depicted in Figure 14.14. At even higher temperatures the strands separate physically and acquire a random-coil conformation (Figure 14.15). The process is most appropriately described as a **helix-to-coil transition,** but it is commonly called **denaturation.** This is accompanied by a number of physical changes, including a buoyant density increase, reduction in viscosity, change in ability to rotate polarized light, and changes in absorbancy.

Changes in absorbance are frequently used to follow the process of denaturation experimentally. DNA absorbs in the UV region due to the heterocyclic aromatic nature of its purine and pyrimidine constituents. Although each base has a unique absorption spectrum, all bases exhibit maxima at or near 260 nm. This property is responsible for the absorption of DNA at 260 nm. However,

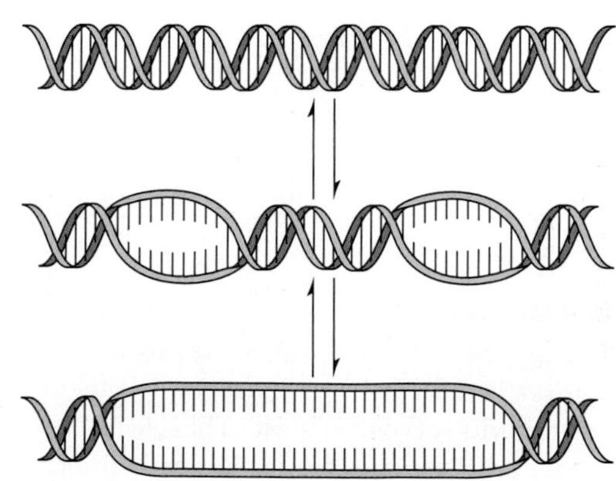

FIGURE 14.14
Structure of double-stranded DNA at increasing temperatures.
Disruptions of the double-stranded structure appear first in regions of relatively high adenine–thymine content. The size of these "bubbles" increases with increasing temperatures, leading to extensive disruptions in the structure of the double helix at elevated temperatures.

this absorbancy can be as much as 40% lower than that expected from adding up the absorbancy of each of the base components of DNA. This property of DNA, referred to as **hypochromic effect,** results from the stacking of the bases along the DNA helices. In this arrangement, interactions between the π electrons of neighboring bases produce a decrease in absorbancy. However, as the ordered structure of the double helix is disrupted at increasing temperatures, stacking interactions are gradually decreased. Therefore a totally disordered polynucleotide approaches an absorbance not very different from the sum of the absorbancies of its purine and pyrimidine constituents.

Slow heating of double-stranded DNA in solution is accompanied by a gradual change in absorbancy as the strands separate. However, since the interactions between the two strands are cooperative, the transition from double-stranded to random-coil conformation occurs over a narrow range of temperatures, as indicated in Figure 14.16. Before the rise of the **melting curve,** DNA is double stranded. In the rising section of the curve an increasing number of base pairs are interrupted as the temperature rises. Strand separation occurs at a critical temperature corresponding to the upper plateau of the curve. However, if the temperature is decreased before the complete separation of the strands, the native structure is completely restored.

The **midpoint temperature,** T_m, of this process, under standard conditions of concentration and ionic strength, is characteristic of the base content of each DNA. The higher the guanine–cytosine content, the higher the transition temperature between the double-stranded helix and the single strands. This difference in T_m values is attributed to the increased stability of guanine–cytosine pairs, as a result of the higher stacking interactions between dimers of G-C pairs relative to the dimers of A-T pairs.

Rapid cooling of a heated DNA solution normally produces denatured DNA, a structure that results from the reformation of some hydrogen bonds either between the separate strands or between different sections of the same strand. The latter must contain complementary base sequences. By and large denatured DNA is a disordered structure containing substantial amounts of **random-coil** and single-stranded regions.

DNA can also be denatured at a pH above 11.3 as the charge on several substituents on the rings of the bases is changed, preventing these groups from participating in hydrogen bonding. **Alkaline denaturation** is often used as an experimental tool in preference to heat denaturation to prevent breakage of phosphodiester bonds that can occur to some degree at high temperatures or low pH. Denaturation can also be induced at low ionic strengths, because of enhanced interstrand repulsion between negatively charged phosphates, as well as by various denaturing reagents, that is, compounds that weaken or break

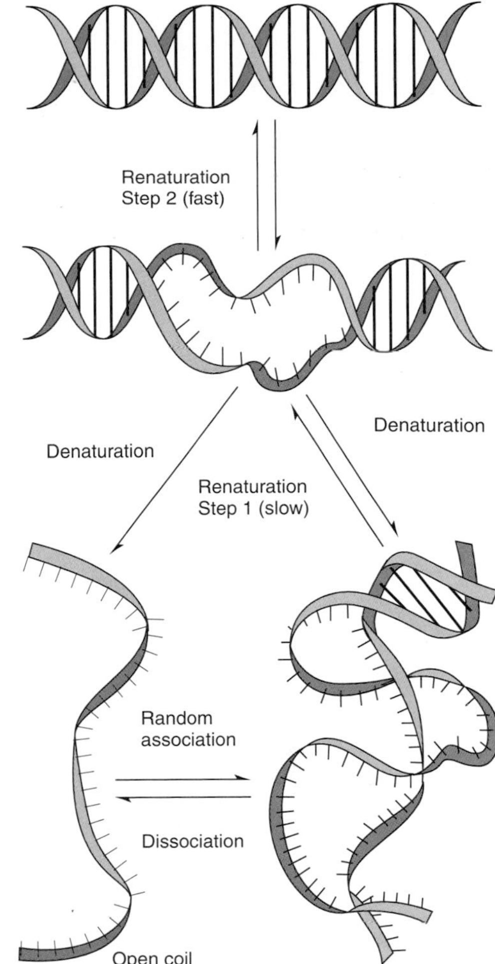

FIGURE 14.15
Denaturation of DNA.
At high temperatures the double-stranded structure of DNA is completely disrupted, with the eventual separation of the strands and the formation of single-stranded open coils. Denaturation also occurs at extreme pH ranges or at extreme ionic strengths.

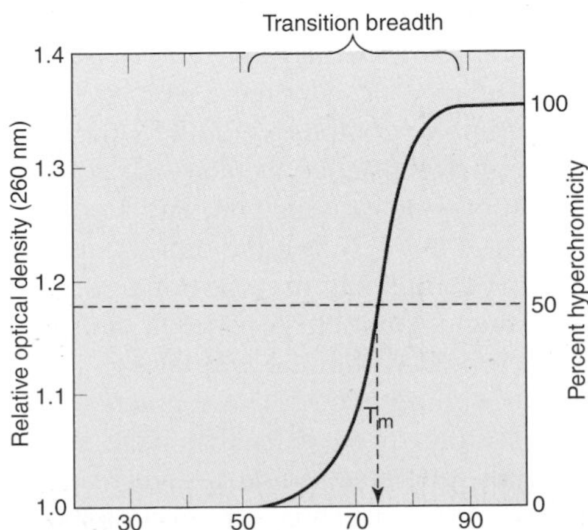

FIGURE 14.16
Temperature–optical density profile for DNA.
When DNA is heated, the optical density increases with rising temperature. A graph in which optical density versus temperature is plotted is called a "melting curve." Relative optical density is the ratio of the optical density at the temperature indicated to that at 25°C. The temperature at which one-half of the maximum optical density is reached is the midpoint temperature (T_m).
Redrawn based on figure from Freifelder, D. The DNA Molecule: Structure and Properties. *San Francisco: Freeman, 1978.*

hydrogen bonds. A complete denaturation curve similar to that shown in Figure 14.16 can be obtained at a relatively low constant temperature, for instance, room temperature, by variation of the concentration of an added denaturant.

Renaturation

Complementary DNA strands, separated by denaturation, can reform a double helix if appropriately treated. This is called **renaturation** or **reannealing.** If denaturation is not complete and only a few bases remain hydrogen bonded between the two strands, the helix-to-coil transition is rapidly reversible. **Annealing** is possible even after the complementary strands have been completely separated. Under these conditions the renaturation process depends on the meeting of complementary DNA strands in an exact manner that can lead to the reformation of the original structure, and it is a slow, concentration-dependent process. As a rule, maintaining DNA at 10–15°C below its T_m, under conditions of moderate ionic strength (0.15 M), provides the maximum opportunity for renaturation. At lower salt concentrations, the charged phosphate groups repel one another and prevent the strands from associating. As renaturation begins, some of the hydrogen bonds formed are extended between short tracts of polynucleotides that might have been distant in the original native structure. Renaturation is facilitated by the presence of short sequences, consisting of four to six base pairs, reiterated many times within every DNA strand. A large number of much longer nucleotide sequences are repeated many times within the eukaryotic genome. Such sequences provide sites for initial base pairing that produces a partially hydrogen-bonded double helix. These randomly base-paired structures are short-lived because the bases that surround the short complementary segments cannot pair and lead to the formation of a stable fully hydrogen-bonded structure. However, once the correct bases begin to pair by chance, the double helix over the entire DNA molecule is rapidly reformed. Renaturation is a two-step process. The first step determines the rate of association, involves the chance meeting of two complementary sequences on different strands, and is therefore a second-order reaction. The rate of renaturation is thus proportional to the product of the concentrations of the two homologous dissociated strands and is expressed as $dt/dc = -kc^2$, where k is the rate constant for the association. Integration of this equation gives $C/C_0 = 1/(1 + kC_0t)$, where C is the concentration of single-stranded DNA expressed as moles of nucleotide per liter at time t, and C_0 is the concentration of DNA at time zero. A plot of C/C_0 (which is proportional to DNA that is single stranded or of the DNA fraction that is reassociated) versus C_0t can be constructed (Figure 14.17), and a $C_0t_{0.5}$ **(Cot-a-half)** value, which corresponds to $C/C_0 = 0.5$ can be determined. The $C_0t_{0.5}$ value is proportional to the complexity of the genome. **Complexity** is equal to the molecular mass of the genome provided that the genome consists of unique nucleotide sequences. For example, both the complexity and molecular mass of a hypothetical genome consisting of three unique nucleotide sequences that may be represented as N_1, N_2, and N_3 is equal to the sum $N_1 + N_2 + N_3$. However, in eukaryotic genomes, which contain both unique as well as reiterated sequences, the complexity of the genome is significantly lower than the molecular mass. If, for instance, a eukaryotic genome contains 10^5 copies of sequence N_3, 10^3 copies of sequence N_2, and 1 copy of sequence N_1, the complexity will still be $N_1 + N_2 + N_3$ but the molecular mass will be equal to $10^5N_3 + 10^3N_2 + N_1$. Thus complexity may be defined as the minimum length of DNA that contains a single complete copy of all the single and **reiterated sequences** that are represented within the genome.

The C_0t curves of eukaryotic genomes with reiterated DNA segments show several kinetic components, each representing those parts that have similar reiteration frequencies (Figure 14.18). Highly reiterated sequences will reassociate the fastest; unique sequences are the slowest. Thus C_0t curves provide information on **genome complexity,** on the number of **repetitive classes,**

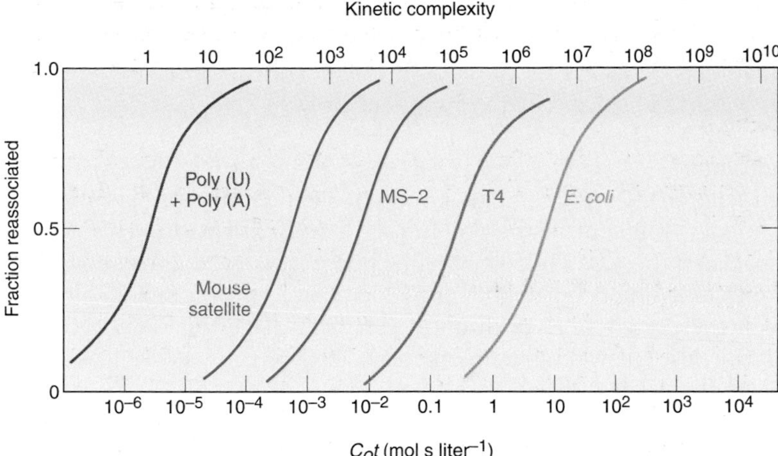

FIGURE 14.17
Reassociation kinetics for DNA isolated from various sources.
Each DNA is first fragmented to segments of approximately 400 nucleotides. The denatured segments are subsequently allowed to renature. The fraction of each polynucleotide reassociated, calculated from changes in hypochromicity, is plotted against the total concentration of nucleotides multiplied by the renaturation time (C_0t). The top scale shows the kinetic complexity of each DNA sample. Whenever a DNA contains reiterated sequences, these sequences are present in the fragments at higher concentrations than they would have been if a unique sequence had been fragmented. As a result, renaturation of fragments, obtained from DNAs containing reiterated sequences, proceeds more rapidly the higher the degree of repetition. This is exemplified by the rates of renaturation of fragments obtained from the synthetic double-stranded polynucleotide poly(A)–poly(U) and mouse satellite DNA, a DNA that contains many repeated sequences. For a homogeneous DNA, which contains a distribution of different extents of reiterated sequences, kinetic complexity can be defined as the minimum length of DNA needed to contain a whole single copy of the reiterated sequence.
Based on figure in Britten, R. J., and Kohne, D. E. Science *161:529, 1968.*

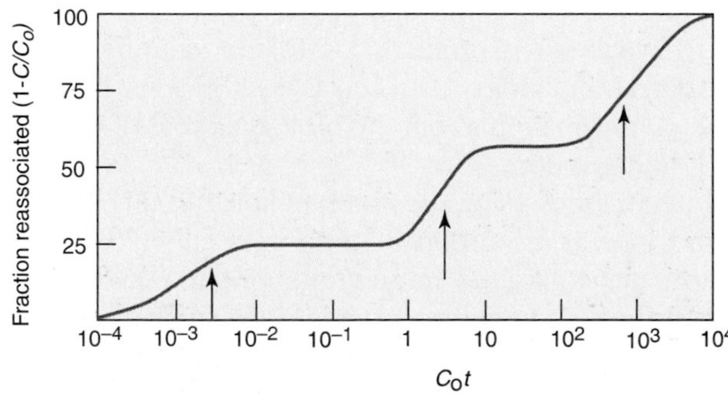

	Fast Component	Intermediate Component	Slow Component
Percent of genome	25	30	45
$C_0t_{1/2}$	0.0013	1.9	630
Complexity, bp	340	6.0×10^5	3.0×10^8
Repetition frequency	500,000	350	1

FIGURE 14.18
Reassociation kinetics of eukaryotic DNA.
This idealized $C_0t_{1/2}$ plot represents a eukaryotic DNA that consists of three distinct components with three different C_0t values. The percentage to which each one of these components is present in the DNA can be read from the ordinate (fraction-reassociated axis) of the figure. Repetition frequencies and complexities are calculated based on the principles discussed in the text. In practice, the experimental separation of different DNA components is not as pronounced and their identification not as clear-cut as shown in this hypothetical example.

and on the proportion of the total genome represented by those classes. Since most genes occur only once within a genome, separation of DNA into different repetitive classes facilitates the search for individual genes by narrowing the search within the single copy component of DNA.

Hybridization

Self-association of complementary polynucleotide strands has provided the basis for development of the technique of **hybridization.** This depends on the association between two polynucleotide chains, which may be of the same or of different origin or length, provided that a base complementarity exists between these chains. Hybridization can take place not only between DNA chains but also between complementary RNA chains as well as DNA–RNA combinations.

Appropriate techniques have been developed for measuring the maximum amount of polynucleotide that can be hybridized as well as the rates of hybridization. These techniques are important basic tools of contemporary molecular biology and are being used for the following: (1) determining whether or not a certain sequence occurs more than once in the DNA of a particular organism, (2) demonstrating a genetic or evolutionary relatedness between different organisms, (3) determining the number of genes transcribed in a particular mRNA (clearly DNA–RNA hybridizations are needed for accomplishing the last goal), and (4) determining the location of any given DNA sequence by annealing with a complementary polynucleotide, called a **probe,** that is appropriately tagged for easy detection of the hybrid.

DNA to be tested for hybridization is denatured. The resulting single strands are immobilized by binding to a suitable polymer, which is then used to pack a chromatography column. DNA formed in the presence of labeled precursors, usually tritiated thymidine, is allowed to run through the column that contains the bound, unlabeled DNA. The rate at which radioactivity is retained by the column equals the rate of annealing between complementary strands.

Determination of the maximum amount of DNA that can be hybridized can establish homologies between DNA of different species since the base sequences in each organism are unique. On this basis annealing can be used to compare the degree to which DNAs isolated from different species are related to one another. The observed homologies serve as indexes of **evolutionary relatedness** and have been particularly useful for defining phylogenies in prokaryotes. Hybridization studies between DNA and RNA have, in addition, provided very useful information about the biological role of DNA, particularly the mechanism of transcription.

Hybridization techniques using membrane filters, usually made of nitrocellulose, have found increasing application. In general, hybridization can be quantitated by either measuring the amount of hybrid in equilibrium or the rate of hybrid formation under conditions in which one nucleic acid is present in large excess. The approach used for the latter determination is analogous to the C_0t procedure and when it is used for DNA–RNA hybridization and RNA is present in excess it is referred to as the $\boldsymbol{R_0t}$ **method,** or the $\boldsymbol{D_0t}$ **method** when DNA is in excess.

A variant of filter hybridization, known as the **Southern transfer,** can be used for identifying the location of specific genes (see p. 774). Since a gene sequence represents a very small percentage of total DNA, the gene must be separated from the remaining DNA and the DNA detected by using appropriate probes. Another variation of hybridization known as ***in situ*** **hybridization** uses intact DNA molecules within metaphase chromosomes. The chromosomes are spread on slides and subjected to denaturation and then exposed to a probe labeled with a fluorescent molecule. The DNA sequence of interest is located by observation with a fluorescence microscope.

DNA Probes

Probes are short single-stranded RNA or DNA oligonucleotides that are complementary to specific sequences of interest in genomic DNA. Under proper conditions probes interact only with a segment of interest, indicating whether the segment is present in a particular sample of DNA. Probes synthesized by chemical means may appear to be limited by the degree to which the desired genomic nucleotide sequence is known, but in fact this approach has much wider applicability. As an example, if the protein product of a gene is known, the nucleotide sequence of the desired gene can be approximated by using a mixture of different synthetic oligonucleotides that represent alternate mRNA sequences that, because of degeneracy of the code, can encode for the same protein. One of these oligonucleotide sequences is therefore complementary to the desired gene. When the gene of interest is transcribed to mRNA molecules that are abundant and easily purified, mRNA can be used. Probes need to be at least 15 nucleotides long because shorter sequences may occur randomly along genomic DNA. To achieve easy detection, probes are labeled by the incorporation of ^{32}P or are identified by the use of biotin-containing nucleotides that are incorporated into the probe and serve as fluorescent labels. Probes are useful for definitive and rapid diagnosis of genetic disorders, infectious disease, and cancer as described briefly in Clin. Corr. 14.2.

Heteroduplexes

Hybridization is the basis for a technique that has permitted construction of precise physical maps of DNA genes. This technique depends on direct visualization under the electron microscope of single-stranded loops in the structures of artificially formed double-stranded DNA molecules known as **heteroduplexes** constructed by hybridization of two complementary DNA strands. One strand is selected on the basis that, as the result of a known mutation, it misses the

CLINICAL CORRELATION 14.2

Diagnostic Use of Probes in Medicine

A probe is a molecule with a strong affinity for a specific target, which can easily be detected after its interaction with the target. The specificity of DNA probes is based on interaction between complementary polynucleotide strands. Probes can be obtained by amplification of naturally occurring DNA sequences or by chemical synthesis. Use of DNA-based techniques is becoming increasingly important in laboratory diagnosis of many genetic diseases and certain types of cancers. The method is used selectively in diagnosis of bacterial infections for bacteria that are slow growing or difficult to identify by conventional culture-base methods, such as bacteria causing Lyme disease (*Borrelia burgdorferi*), certain types of syphilis (*Treponema pallidum*), or pneumonia (*Chlamydia pneumoniae*). In addition, DNA probes are indispensable for identification of bacteria that are extremely difficult or impossible to grow in culture, such as organisms responsible for Lepra (*Mycobacterium leprae*) and Whipple's disease (*Tropheryma whippellii*). DNA-based techniques also have the potential to provide faster, more versatile, and less expensive diagnostic applications for detection of more common bacterial infections. Hybridization procedures generally begin with amplification of target DNA (bacterial DNA) by cloning or more commonly by a technique known as the polymerase chain reaction (PCR). The probe hybridized with target DNA is typically detected by the Southern blot technique.

Probes are very useful for identification of mutant alleles responsible for genetic diseases, especially if the mutations are stable and few in number. Some genetic disorders are due to mutations in a single gene and in some instances appear to correlate well with a particular phenotype or symptom. Detection of mutations can be of diagnostic value. One approach used for direct identification of mutations involves hybridization with an allele-specific probe (ASP). Examples of diseases diagnosed by probes are sickle cell anemia, hemoglobin C disease, and phenylketonuria. The first two are the result of a single base change in genes coding for β-globin. By using three different probes, corresponding to the sequence of normal and two mutated hemoglobins, the presence of mutated β-globin genes can be detected. Similarly, a probe can identify a mutation in the phenylalanine 4-monooxygenase gene that is responsible for phenylketonuria. Many other genetic diseases, including cystic fibrosis, Gaucher's disease, β-thalassemia, and Tay–Sachs disease, can be diagnosed using DNA-based techniques.

Keller, G. H., and Manak, M. M. *DNA Probes*. New York: Stockton Press, 1993.

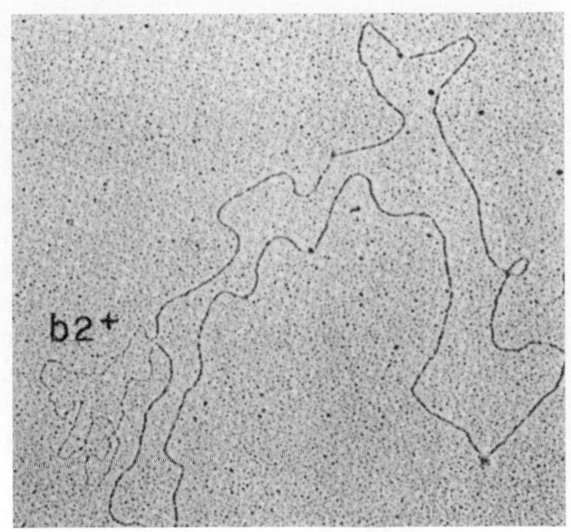

FIGURE 14.19
Heteroduplex formation in bacteriophage.
Electron micrograph of a heteroduplex DNA molecule constructed from complementary strands of bacteriophage λ and a bacteriophage λ deletion mutant (bacteriophage λb2). In λb2 a segment of DNA has been deleted, producing, at the site of deletion, a loop labeled b2+.
Reprinted with permission from Westmoreland, B. C., Szybalski, W., and Ris, H. Science 163:1343, 1969. Copyright © 1969 by the American Association for the Advancement of Science.

gene being mapped. As shown in Figure 14.19, the complementary strands of the heteroduplex pair perfectly throughout the length of the molecule except that across from the position of the missing gene in the mutant strand the complementary strand forms a visible loop. The position of the loop identifies the location of the deleted gene.

14.3 ■ TYPES OF DNA STRUCTURE

Only the essential features common to all DNAs have been presented so far. The specific structural features of DNA vary, depending on the origin and function of each DNA molecule. Molecules of DNA differ in size, conformation, and topology.

Size of DNA Is Highly Variable

The length of DNA varies from a few thousand base pairs for DNA of the small viruses, to millions for chromosomal DNA of bacteria, and to billions for the chromosomal DNA of animals. DNA size can be expressed as number of base pairs, molecular mass, the length of the strands, and even the actual mass of DNA. The units used in these expressions, however, can easily be interconverted, since a DNA of mol wt 1×10^6 contains approximately 1500 bp and is 0.5 nm long. DNA mass can be converted to molecular mass by division with the average molecular mass of a DNA nucleotide pair.

The amount of DNA per cell increases as the complexity of the cellular function increases (Table 14.5). Although mammalian cells contain some of the

TABLE 14.5 DNA Cell Content of Some Species

Type of Cell	*Organism*	*DNA per Cell (pg)*[a]
Phage	T4	2.4×10^{-4}
Bacterium	*E. coli*	4.4×10^{-3}
Fungus	*N. crassa*	1.7×10^{-2}
Avian erythrocyte	Chicken	2.5
Mammalian leukocyte	Human	3.4

Source: From Lewin, B. *Gene Expression,* Vol. 2, 2nd ed. New York: Wiley, 1980, p. 958.

[a] pg, picograms.

highest amounts of DNA per cell, some amphibian, fish, and plant cells may contain even higher amounts. In fact, lung fish cells contain more than 40 times the amount of DNA in human cells, but such extraordinary amounts of DNA reflect a **reiteration of nucleotide sequences** within the DNA macromolecule and do not represent an actual increase in the size of DNA in terms of unique sequences, that is, **DNA complexity.** The size of the DNA of higher cells is very large indeed. The DNA contained within a single human cell is packaged in the form of 46 chromatin fibers or chromosomes. In its most condensed state, that is, during metaphase, the largest of these chromosomes is about 10 μm. If the DNA packaged within this chromosome were stretched out in the conventional B-DNA form, it would be over 8 cm long, that is, 8000 times longer than it is when packed within the chromosome. This suggests that the polynucleotides are exquisitely packed in order to fit within the minute dimensions of the cell nucleus.

Because of their extraordinary length, relative to the total mass, DNA molecules are extremely sensitive to shearing forces that develop during ordinary laboratory manipulations. Even careful pipetting may shear a DNA molecule. During the process of isolation it is difficult to prevent with absolute confidence the disruption of some phosphodiester bonds by contaminating endonucleases (nicking). For these reasons the precise size of DNA of higher species could not be determined until special handling techniques were developed, both for the isolation of DNA and the measurement of its molecular mass.

Techniques for Determining DNA Size

Classical methods for determining size in proteins proved to be unsuitable for measuring the molecular mass of even relatively small DNAs. Custom-tailored methods were devised. **Equilibrium centrifugation** in a density gradient (usually a concentrated cesium chloride solution), **electron microscopy,** and **electrophoresis** in agarose gels are among the principal methods providing reliable information about the molecular masses of DNAs. Electron microscopy provides a measure of the length of DNA strands. Molecular masses can be calculated from known values of the mass per unit length. The DNA can be visualized under the electron microscope if it is first coated with protein and a metal film. Determination of molecular masses by electrophoresis depends on the molecular sieving effect of porous agarose gels. Over a limited range of molecular masses the mobility of DNA is directly proportional to the logarithm of the molecule's weight.

To determine the molecular mass of DNA by equilibrium centrifugation a small portion of a DNA solution to be analyzed is layered on top of a gradient in a centrifuge tube. Upon centrifugation, the molecules of DNA sediment to equilibrium through the gradient. Under these conditions a homogeneous high molecular mass DNA will form a Gaussian band centered at a position in the gradient that corresponds to the density of the DNA. Molecules with different densities are resolved into a series of bands that sediment independently of one another, as shown in Figure 14.20. A relationship can be demonstrated between the width of the bands at equilibrium and the molecular masses.

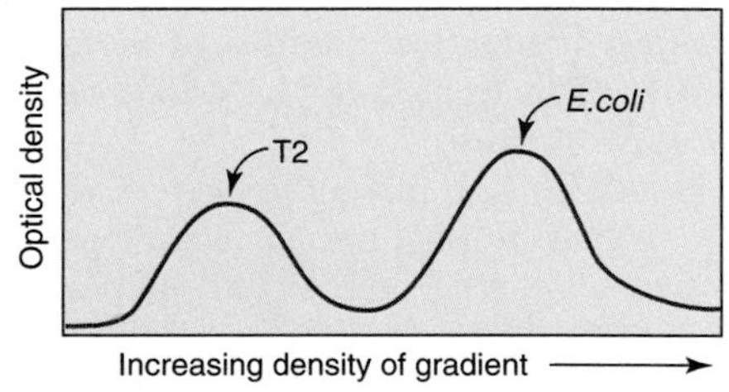

FIGURE 14.20
Equilibrium gradient centrifugation of DNA.
The DNA macromolecules travel into the increasingly dense regions of the gradient driven by centrifugal forces. The macromolecules equilibrate as soon as they reach an area of the gradient of density equal to their own. For example, bacteriophage T2 DNA and *E. coli* DNA can be resolved into two distinct bands. The width of the bands at equilibrium is related to the molecular weight of DNA.

Labeling of the terminals of DNA has been used successfully for determining molecular masses. DNA is treated with the enzyme alkaline phosphatase, which converts the 5′-phosphate nucleotide terminals of double-stranded DNA to the corresponding OH groups. These terminals are then esterified, using [γ-^{32}P]ATP with the enzyme polynucleotide kinase. The free 5′ terminus of each polynucleotide chain becomes labeled as shown in Figure 14.21. The labeled DNA is then analyzed by **zonal centrifugation** and detected from both its absorbancy at 260 nm and ^{32}P content (Figure 14.22). The molecular mass is calculated from the ratio of the amount of ^{32}P to the absorbancy, both measured at the coinciding peaks of the bands.

Gel electrophoresis (see page 773) has replaced electron microscopy and

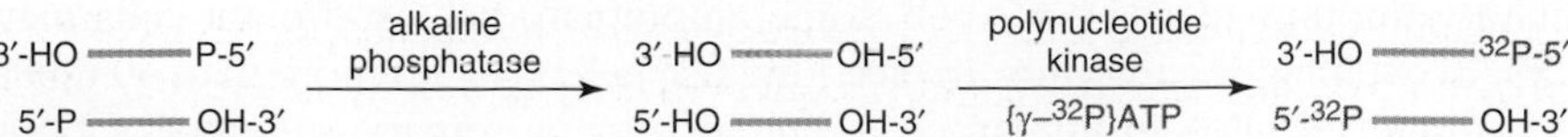

FIGURE 14.21
End-group labeling procedure.
The 5′ terminals on the opposite ends of DNA are labeled with ^{32}P by treatment with alkaline phosphatase and esterification of the resulting 5′-hydroxyl groups with ATP.

centrifugation-based methods for the routine determination of DNA molecular weights. The above methods have permitted determination of DNA molecular masses with an accuracy of at least 10%, but the usefulness of each method is limited within certain molecular mass ranges. Electrophoresis is most suitable between 7.5×10^5 and 1.5×10^7. Electron microscopy is useful for up to 2×10^8 molecular mass. The most versatile method is equilibrium centrifugation, the range of which extends between 2×10^5 and 10^9.

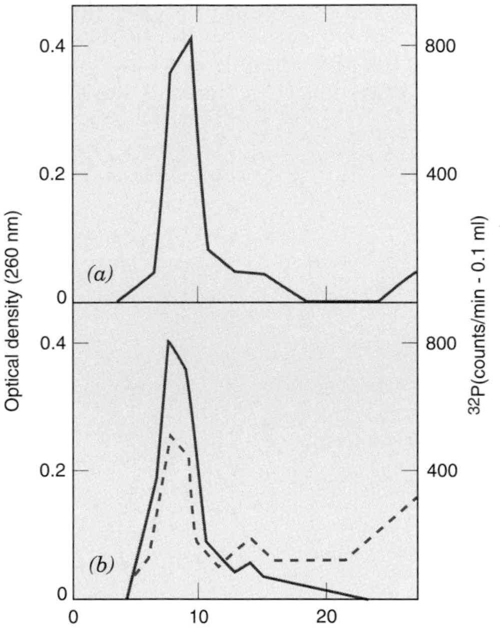

FIGURE 14.22
Zonal centrifugation profiles of denatured T7 DNA treated by the end-group labeling procedure.
Sedimentation is from right to left. (*a*) Untreated DNA. (*b*) DNA treated by the end-group labeling procedure. Zonal centrifugation is performed on a sucrose density gradient and should be distinguished from density gradient centrifugation. The latter is an equilibrium centrifugation with the macromolecules reaching equilibrium at regions within the tube at which their density equals the density of the environment. With zonal centrifugation the macromolecules move continuously until they reach the bottom of the tube or until the centrifuge is stopped. The molecular mass is calculated from the ratio of ^{32}P (dotted line) to optical density (solid line) at the peak of the curve.
Redrawn from Richardson, C. C. J. Mol. Biol. *15:49, 1966.*

DNA May Be Linear or Circular

DNAs of several small viruses are linear double-stranded helices of equal size. Some DNAs have naturally occurring interior single-stranded breaks. The breaks found in natural bacteriophage molecules result mostly from broken phosphodiester bonds, although occasionally a deoxyribonucleoside may be missing. DNA of coliphage T5 consists of one intact strand and a complementary strand, which is really four well-defined complementary fragments ordered perfectly along the intact strand. A similar regularity in the points of strand breaks is noted, for example, in *Pseudomonas aeruginosa* phage B3, but generally interior breaks seem to be randomly distributed. The double helix structure is maintained because the breaks in one strand are generally in different locations from breaks in the complementary strand.

Double-Stranded Circles

Most naturally occurring DNAs exist in circular form. In some instances **circular DNA** exists as **interlocked circles** or **catenates.** Provided that suitable precautions are taken to avoid shearing the DNA, the circular form can be isolated intact and observed by electron microscopy. The circular structure results from the circularization of a linear DNA by formation of a phosphodiester bond between the 3′ and 5′ terminals of a linear polynucleotide. Circular structures present many advantages for chromosomal DNA, protecting it from the action of exonucleases and facilitating the process of DNA replication.

The circular nature of small phage ϕX174 DNA was suspected from studies showing that no ends were available for reactions with exonucleases. Sedimentation studies also revealed that endonuclease cleavage yielded one rather than two polynucleotides. These suspicions were later confirmed by direct observation with electron microscopy.

After the circular nature of the DNA chromosome of *E. coli* was demonstrated, it became apparent that many other DNAs (e.g., those of mitochondria, chloroplasts, bacterial plasmids, and mammalian viruses) also existed as closed circles. Obviously, the strands of a circular DNA cannot be irreversibly separated by denaturation because they exist as intertwined closed circles. The absence of 3′ or 5′ termini provides an evolutionary advantage because it endows the circular DNA with complete resistance toward exonucleases, which ensures the longevity of DNA.

DNA of some bacteriophages exists in a linear double-stranded form that circularizes when it enters the host cell. The linear DNA of bacteriophage λ of *E. coli,* for instance, has single-stranded 5′ terminals consisting of 20 nucleotides each. These have complementary sequences, so that an open circle structure can be formed when the linear molecule acquires a circular shape, which allows the overlap of these complementary sequences. Subsequently, the enzyme DNA ligase, which forms phosphodiester bonds between properly aligned polynucleotides, joins the 3′- and 5′-terminal residues of each strand and forms a covalently closed circle (Figure 14.23).

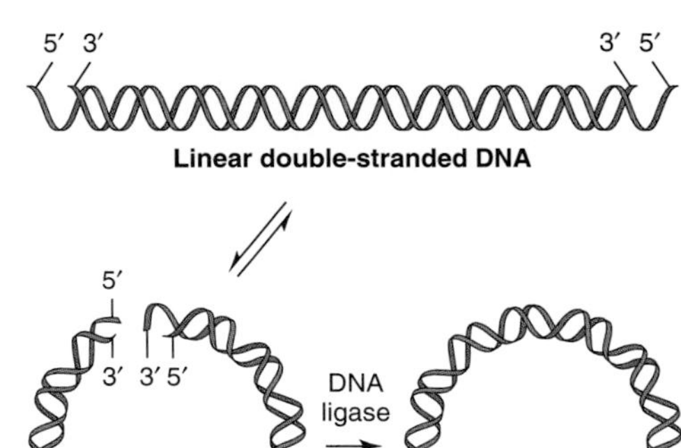

FIGURE 14.23
Circularization of λ DNA.
The DNA of bacteriophage λ exists in both linear and circular forms, which are interconvertible. The circularization of λ DNA is possible because of the complementary nature of the single-stranded 5′ terminals of the linear form.

Single-Stranded DNA

With the exception of a few small bacteriophages (e.g., ϕX174 and G4) that can acquire a single-stranded form, most circular and linear DNAs exist as double-stranded helices. The single-stranded nature of the nonreplicative form of ϕX174 DNA was suspected when it was discovered that the base composition of this DNA did not conform to the base equivalence rules; that is, A did not equal T and G did not equal C.

Circular DNA Is a Superhelix

Double-stranded circular DNA, with few exceptions, has an intriguing **topology.** The circular structure contains twists, referred to as **supercoils,** which are visualized by electron microscopy. In principle, linear DNA could be converted to a circular molecule. Circular DNA may be formed by bringing together, and joining by a phosphodiester bond, the free terminals of linear DNA. If no other manipulations are introduced, the resulting circular DNA will be **relaxed;** that is, it will have a thermodynamically favored structure of the linear double helix (B-DNA), which accommodates one complete turn of the helix for approximately 10 base pairs. However, if before sealing the circle, one DNA terminus is held steady while the other terminus is rotated in a direction that unwinds the double helix, the resulting structure will be strained. This strained structure, which is characterized by a deficit of turns, is known as **negative superhelical DNA** (Figure 14.24). Negatively supercoiled DNA is underwound in that it has fewer helical turns than what the molecule would accommodate as a linear or as a relaxed structure. The underwinding results in participation of more base pairs per helical turn, which produces a decrease in the angle of twist between adjacent base pairs. Therefore underwinding generates **torsional tension.** Torsional strain increases the standard free energy of DNA by about 10 kcal mol^{-1} per each supercoil that is introduced into the structure. The strain produced by this deficit of turns is accommodated by the disruption of hydrogen bonds

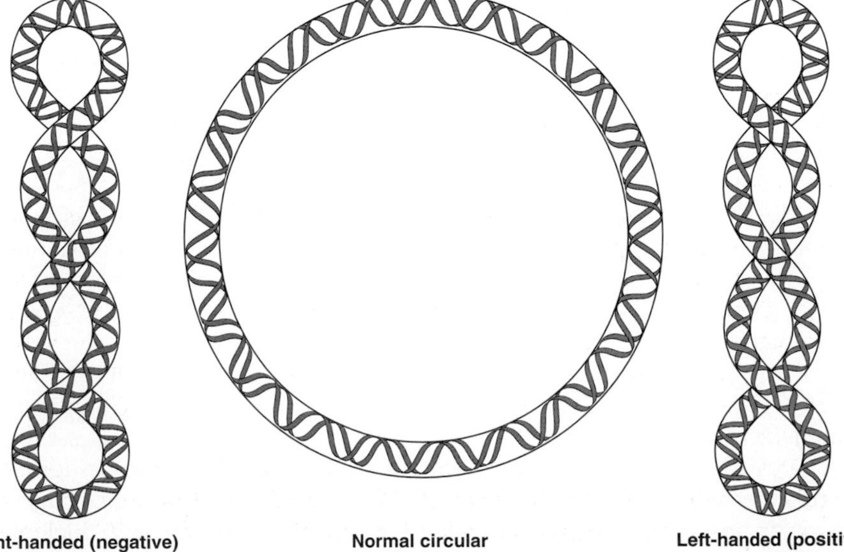

FIGURE 14.24
Relaxed and supercoiled DNA.
Relaxed DNA can be converted to either right- or left-handed superhelical DNA. Right-handed DNA (negatively supercoiled DNA) is the form normally present in cells. Left-handed DNA may also be transiently generated as DNA is subjected to enzymatically catalyzed transformations (replication, recombination, etc.) and it is also present stably in certain bacterial species. The distinctly different patterns of folding for right- and left-handed DNA are apparent in this representation of the two types of superhelices.
Redrawn from Darnell, J., Lodish, H., and Baltimore, D. Molecular Cell Biology. *New York: Freeman, 1986.*

and the opening of the double helix over a small region of the macromolecular structure. The resulting structure may be viewed as consisting of a small-stranded loop along with regions of regularly spaced double helical turns with a geometry similar to relaxed B-DNA. If, however, hydrogen bonds are not disrupted, the circular DNA will twist in a direction opposite to the one in which it was rotated initially in order to relieve the strain induced by the unwinding. Thus the rotational strain that was introduced before the circularization of DNA can be accommodated either by the disruption of H bonding or by the formation of tertiary structures with visible supercoils (Figure 14.25). These two representations of the negative superhelix should be viewed as two manifestations of the same underlying phenomenon. In general, a dynamically imposed compromise, determined by the environment and the status of circular DNA, is reached between hydrogen-bond disruption and supertwisting. In practice, this means that supercoiled DNA may consist of twisted structures with enhanced tendency to generate regions with disrupted hydrogen bonding (bubbles).

In a circular DNA that is initially relaxed, the transient strand unwinding would tend to introduce compensating supertwists. However, if DNA is superhelical to begin with, the density of the superhelix will obviously tend to fluctuate with the "breathing" of the helix. All naturally occurring DNA molecules contain a deficit of helical turns; that is, they exist as negative superhelices with a superhelical density that remains remarkably constant among different DNAs. Normally one negative twist is found for every 20 turns of the helix.

If one of the terminals of the linear polynucleotides is rotated in the direction of **overwinding** rather than **unwinding** the double helix, the resulting DNA will contain positive superhelices. While negatively superhelical DNA can accommodate unwinding stress either by unwinding (accompanied by the interruption of hydrogen bonds) or by formation of negative superhelices, the only available option for overwound DNA is to accommodate the stress by acquiring positive superhelices. Positive supercoils can be generated by specialized enzymes, the **topoisomerases,** and may be present transiently **in vivo** but are rarely present in cellular DNA.

Positive and negative supercoils can, in principle, coexist transiently within the same DNA molecule. Yet the DNA molecule, in an overall sense, may be viewed as relaxed because it may return to a relaxed state without the breaking of phosphodiester bonds. A rubber band, which in its normal unstrained form

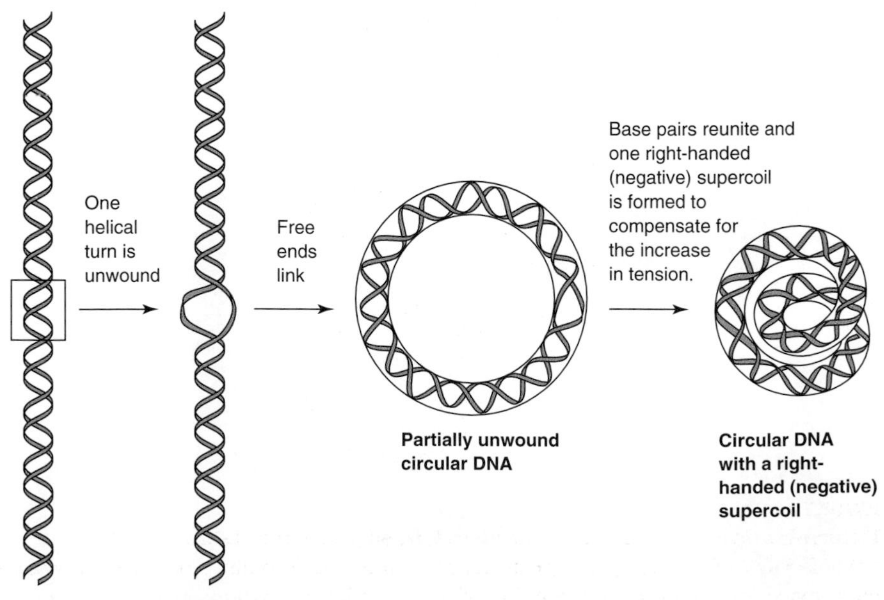

FIGURE 14.25
Right-handed (negative) DNA supercoiling.
Right-handed supercoils (negatively supercoiled DNA) are formed if relaxed DNA is partially unwound. Unwinding may lead to a disruption of hydrogen bonds or alternatively produce negative supercoils. The negative supercoils are formed to compensate for the increase in tension that is generated when disrupted base pairs are reformed. *Redrawn from Darnell, J., Lodish, H., and Baltimore, D.* Molecular Cell Biology. *New York: Freeman, W. H. 1986.*

might be visualized as a circular relaxed structure (without supercoils), can be used as such a model (Figure 14.26). Grasping this band firmly at opposite sides and twisting one side of the band generates a structure characterized by two topological domains, with twisting of opposite handedness, that are clearly visible when the two sides are pulled apart. If the opposite sides are brought back close together, each domain becomes supertwisted; that is, each domain generates a supercoil. This requires an input of energy since the supertwisted state does not represent the low-energy state of the rubber band. When the band is released from the grasping that restrains rotation, it may return to its original relaxed configuration. During these manipulations, the physical structure of the band has remained intact. A difference between the rubber band model and cellular DNA is that the latter exists almost exclusively in supercoiled form. Cellular DNA can be described on the basis of the linking number of DNA, L, an integer number defined as the number of times one strand appears to cross over the other when the DNA structure is projected onto a flat surface (Figure 14.27). Examination of Figure 14.27a further indicates that the linking number of relaxed DNA (B-DNA), L_0, can be defined as

$$L_0 = \frac{N}{10.5}$$

where N is the number of base pairs and 10.5 refers to the **average helical repeat,** that is, the number of base pairs per one complete turn of the helix.

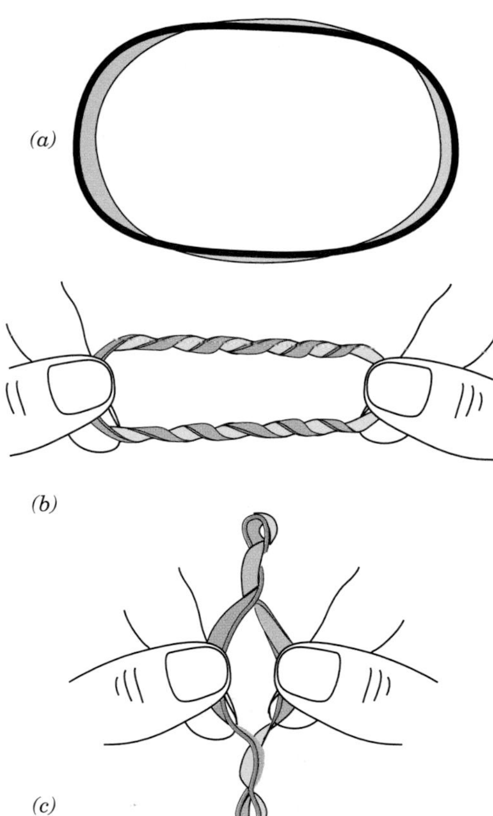

FIGURE 14.26
Superhelical model for DNA.
A rubber band represents the topological properties of double-stranded circular DNA. The relaxed form of the band, shown in (*a*), has been twisted to generate two distinct domains, separated by the pair of "thumb–forefinger anchors," as shown in (*b*). Left-handed (counterclockwise) turns have been introduced into the upper section of the band, with compensating right-handed (clockwise) turns present into the bottom section. When the "anchors" are brought into close proximity with each other as shown in (*c*), the upper section that contained the left-handed turns forms a right-handed superhelix. The bottom section produces a left-handed superhelix. Clearly, superhelicity is not the property of a DNA molecule as a whole but rather a property of specific DNA domains.
Redrawn from Sinden, R. R., and Wells, R. D. DNA structure, mutations, and human genetic disease. Curr. Opin. Biotech. *3:612, 1992.*

Geometric Description of Superhelical DNA

Conformations acquired by interlocking rings of a closed circular DNA can formally be characterized by three parameters: **linking number,** L, **number of helical turns or twist,** T, and **number of supercoils or writhing number,** W. These parameters are related by the equation $L = T + W$. The nature of T and W is self-explanatory.

Two important conclusions can be reached from consideration of these definitions and from examination of Figure 14.28. First, it is apparent that for

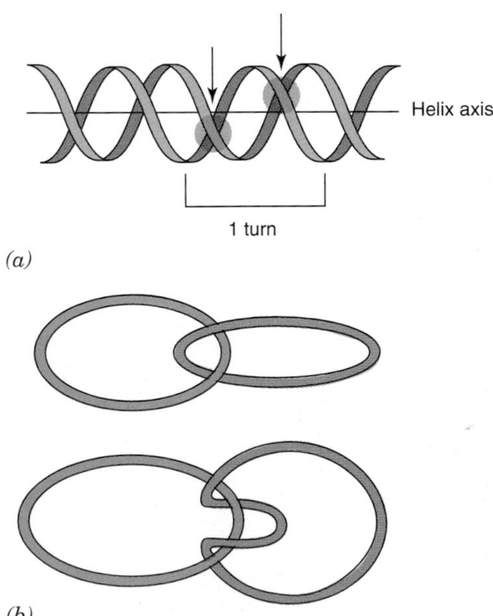

FIGURE 14.27
Determination of the linking number L in superhelical DNA.
(*a*) Side view of a schematic representation of the double helix. Note that the strands cross twice for each turn of the helix. (*b*) DNA circles interwound once and twice. Note that each pair of crossings is equivalent to one interwind.

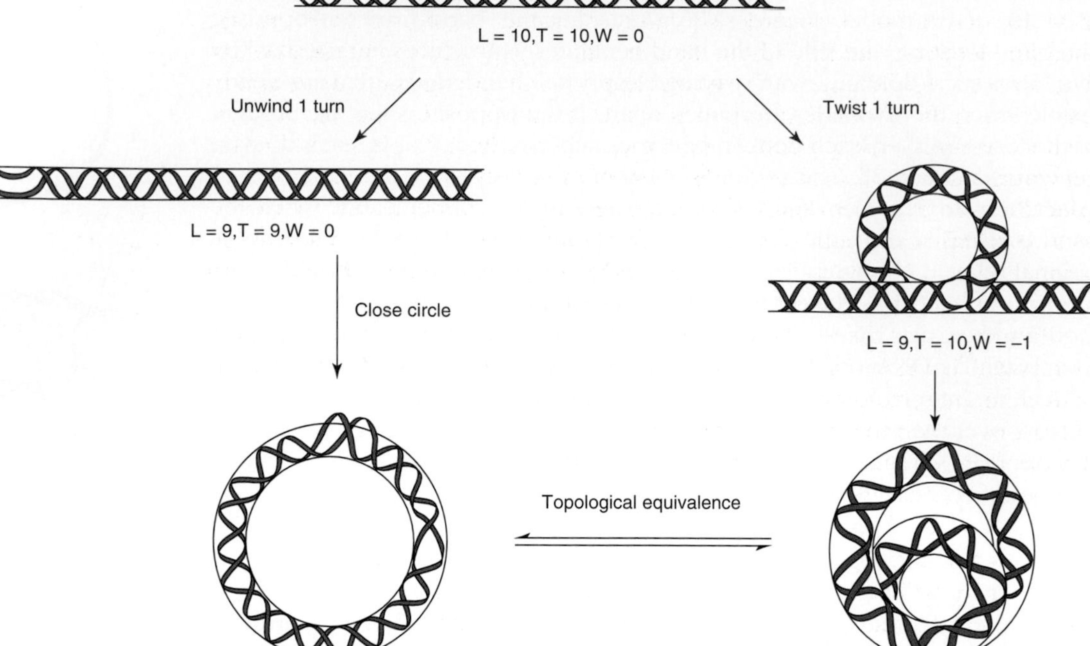

FIGURE 14.28
Various types of DNA superhelices.
An accurate representation of superhelical DNA structures can be made, using the number of helical turns or twists, *T*, and the number of supercoils or writhing number, *W*, along with a third parameter the linking number, *L*, as defined in the text. The figure shows ways of introducing one supercoil into a DNA segment of 10 duplex turns and the parameters of the resulting superhelices.
Redrawn with permission from Cantor, C. R., and Schimmel, P. R., Biophysical Chemistry, Part III. *San Francisco: Freeman, 1980. Copyright © 1980.*

every relaxed DNA the linking number *L* and the number of helical turns *T* are identical. However, as will be apparent shortly, the reverse is not true. Second, DNAs with a specific linking number can acquire various different topological conformations. Different types of supertwists (*T*) may be formed. However, all conformations with the same linking number are interconvertible without breaking any covalent bonds. Therefore linking number is a constant for any covalently closed circular DNA.

Various forms of supercoiled DNAs can be described using *L*, *T*, and *W* numbers. The mental exercise shown in Figure 14.28 illustrates how these numbers apply. It should be recalled that the turns of the typical double helix are right handed. Therefore, if a hypothetical linear DNA duplex that is 10 turns long ($L = 10$ and $T = 10$) is unwound by, say, one turn, the resulting structure will have the following characteristics: $L = 9$ and $T = 9$. A potentially equivalent structure can be formed if instead ends of the same hypothetical DNA are secured so that they cannot rotate and the molecule is looped in a counterclockwise manner. Since in this case untwisting is not permitted to occur, the number of helical turns remains unchanged; that is, $T = 10$. However, as a result of "looping" operations, linking number is now reduced by 1; that is, $L = 9$. The structure resulting from this deliberate introduction of a loop is visibly superhelical. Furthermore, application of the equation that relates values of *L*, *T*, and *W* indicates that *W* must be equal to -1; that is, the structure is a negative superhelix with one supertwist.

The two structures described above—$L = 9$, $T = 9$, $W = 0$ and $L = 9$, $T = 10$, and $W = -1$—obviously have the same linking number and are therefore interconvertible without the disruption of any phosphodiester bonds. The potential equivalence of these two types of structure becomes more apparent when ends of polynucleotides in each structure are joined into a circle without strands being allowed to rotate. Circularization produces an **interwound** circular structure (a number 8-shaped structure referred to as a **plectonemic** coil) or a doughnut-shaped superhelical arrangement referred to as a **toroidal turn,** both of which are freely interconvertible. An interwound turn, shown in Figure 14.29, can be produced by unfolding a toroidal turn along an axis that is distinct from the supercoil axis.

In summary, if the termini of a linear DNA molecule are covalently attached, a "relaxed" covalent circle results. However, if one end of the double helix is maintained in a fixed and stationary position while the other end is rotated in either direction prior to closing the circle, the resulting structure will twist in the opposite direction so as to generate a supertwisted helical structure. For each additional complete turn of the helix, DNA will acquire one more superhelical twist in the opposite direction of rotation in order to relieve intensifying strain. As a result, topologically equivalent structures, such as those shown in Figure 14.28, will be created. A real superhelical DNA exists as an equilibrium among these forms and many other intermediate arrangements in space that have the same linking number but different numbers of helical turns and supertwists. Although linking number is a constant and an integer, the number of twists can change in positive and negative increments, which are compensated by negative and positive changes in the writhing number. DNA supercoils are distributed in part as mixtures of interwound (plectonemic) and toroidal coils and as decreases in twist angle of the double helix. The interwound form is by far the more predominant structure for supercoiled DNA. In solution about 70% of the deficiency in linking numbers may be distributed as writhe change and 30% as changes in twist.

Although the closed circular form of DNA is an ideal candidate for acquiring a superhelical structure, any segment of double-stranded DNA that is in some way immobilized at both of its terminals qualifies for superhelicity. This property therefore is not the exclusive province of circular DNA. Rather, any appropriately anchored linear DNA molecule can acquire a superhelical conformation. The DNA of animal cells, for instance, normally associated with nuclear proteins, falls into this category. Animal DNA can acquire a superhelical form because its association with nuclear proteins creates numerous closed topological domains. A topological domain is defined as a DNA segment contained in a manner that restrains rotation of the double helix. In addition, circular DNAs of most bacterial phages, animal viruses, bacterial plasmids, and cell organelles, such as mitochondria and chloroplasts, contain superhelical DNAs. Existence

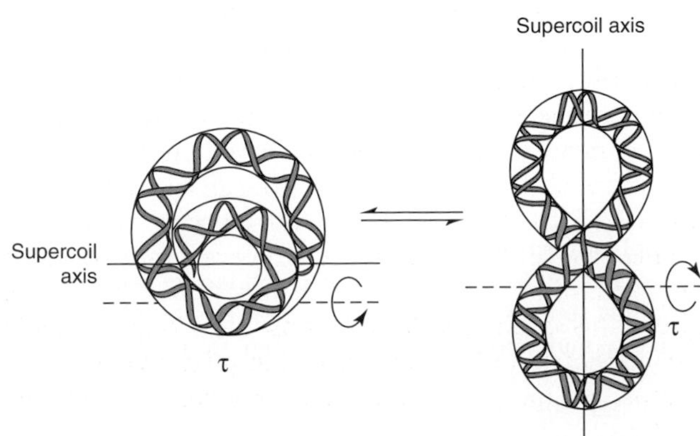

FIGURE 14.29
Equilibrium between two equivalent supercoiled forms of DNA. The forms shown are freely interconvertible by unfolding the doughnut-shaped toroidal form along an axis parallel to the supercoil axis or by folding the number 8-shaped interwound form along an axis perpendicular to the supercoil axis. The two forms have the same W, T, and L numbers.
Redrawn with permission from Cantor, C. R., and Schimmel, P. R. Biophysical Chemistry, Part III. *San Francisco: Freeman, 1980. Copyright © 1980.*

of negative superhelicity appears to be an important factor, promoting packaging of DNA within the confines of the cell because supercoils facilitate formation of compact structures. For instance, while the length of DNA in each human chromosome is of the order of centimeters, condensed mitotic chromosomes that contain this DNA are only a few nanometers long. Negative superhelicity may also be instrumental in facilitating the process of localized DNA strand separation during DNA repair, synthesis, and recombination.

Topoisomerases

Specific enzymes known as **topoisomerases** appear to regulate the formation of superhelices. These enzymes change the linking number, *L*, of DNA. Topoisomerases act by catalyzing the concerted breakage and rejoining of DNA strands, which produces a DNA that is more or less superhelical than the original DNA. Topoisomerases are classified into type I, which break only one strand, and type II, which break both strands of DNA simultaneously. **Topoisomerases I** act by making a transient single-strand break in a supercoiled DNA duplex, which changes the linking number by increments of 1 and results in relaxation of the supercoiled DNA (Figure 14.30). **Topoisomerases II** act by binding to a DNA molecule in a manner that generates two supercoiled loops, as shown in step 1 of Figure 14.31. Since one of these loops is positive and the other negative, and there is no disruption of phosphodiester bonds, the overall linking number of the DNA remains unchanged. In subsequent steps, however, the enzyme nicks both strands and passes one DNA segment through this break before resealing it. This manipulation inverts the sign of the positive supercoil, resulting in the introduction of two negative supercoils in each catalytic step and the changing of the linking number in increments of 2. This reaction occurs at the expense of ATP; that is, topoisomerases II are ATPases. Several well-studied topoisomerases are listed in Table 14.6.

Although all type II topisomerases can change the linking number of DNA, their individual properties vary considerably. A subset of type II topoisomerases (the **gyrases**—isolated from bacteria) are the only enzymes that introduce negative supercoils into relaxed DNA. Analogous eukaryotic topoisomerases have not been found. Apparently eukaryotes use alternative approaches for the

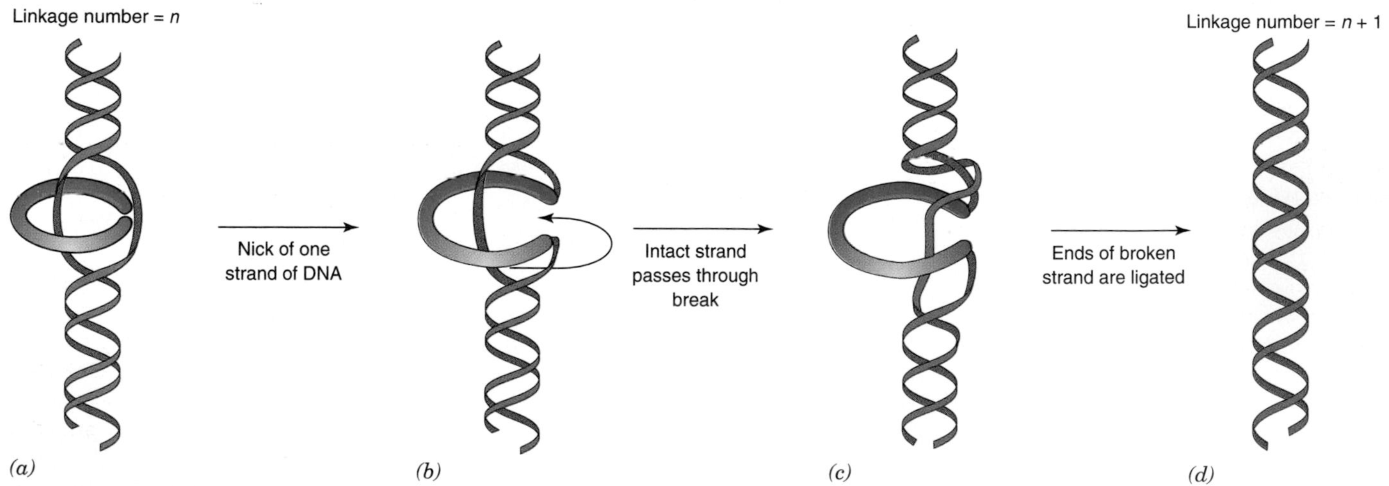

FIGURE 14.30
Mechanism of action of topoisomerases I.
Topoisomerases I can (a) relax DNA by (*a*) first binding to it and locally separating the complementary polynucleotide strands; subsequently (*b*) nick one of the strands; (*c*) bind to the newly generated termini and prevent these termini from rotating freely; and (*d*) ligate the intact strand through the gap generated by the nick, close the gap by restoring the phosphodiester bond, and give rise to a relaxed structure. *Redrawn from Dean, F., et al.* Cold Spring Harbor Symp. Quant. Biol. *47:773, 1982.*

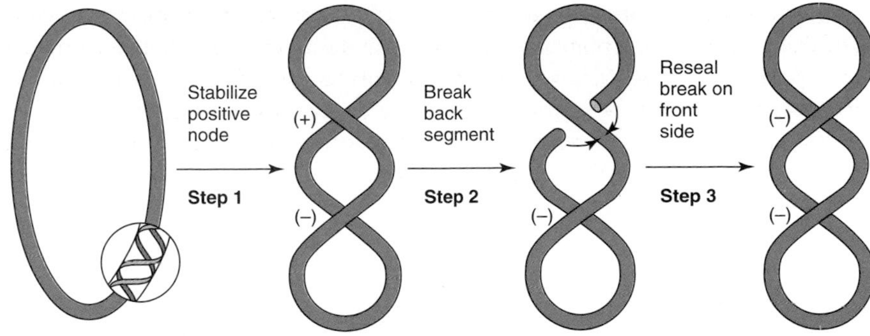

FIGURE 14.31
Mechanism of action of topoisomerases II.
Topoisomerases II (and gyrase) change the linking number of DNA by binding to a DNA molecule and passing one DNA segment through a reversible break formed at a different segment of the same DNA molecule. The mechanism of action of gyrase is illustrated above using as an example the conversion of a relaxed DNA molecule to a molecule that contains first two supercoils, one positive and one negative (step 1). Passage of a DNA segment through the positive supercoil shown on the right most part of the figure (step 3) changes the linking number, producing a molecule that contains two negative supercoils.
Redrawn with permission from Brown, P. O., and Cozzarelli, N. R. Science *206:1081, 1979. Copyright © 1979 by the American Association for the Advancement of Science.*

introduction of negative supercoils into DNA. The wrapping of DNA around chromosomal proteins followed by the action of eukaryotic topoisomerases that relax DNA may be used by eukaryotes for the generation of negative supercoiling. Bacterial type III topoisomerases are a class of topoisomerases with type I topoisomerase properties; that is, they can relax supercoils without the requirement of an energy source, such as ATP hydrolysis. These topoisomerases may specialize in the resolution of circular DNA products (catenates) that are generated just prior to the completion of DNA replication. An unusual class of topoisomerases, **reverse gyrases,** have been isolated from various species of archaebacteria. Remarkably, these gyrases introduce **positive supercoils** into DNA. Positive supercoiling may protect DNA from the denaturing conditions of high temperature and acidity under which these bacteria "exist."

TABLE 14.6 Properties of DNA Topoisomerases

Enzyme	*Type*[a]	ΔL	*Activities*
E. coli topoisomerase I (*top A*)[b]	I	Increase L $\Delta L = 1$	Relaxes negatively supercoiled DNA
Eukaryotic topoisomerase I from yeast (*top 1*)	I	Increase or decrease L $\Delta L = \pm 1$	Relaxes either positively or negatively supercoiled DNA
E. coli topoisomerase II or DNA gyrase (*gyrA, gyrB*)	II	Increase or decrease L $\Delta L = \pm 2$	Introduces negative supercoiling to DNA; relaxes either positively or negatively supercoiled DNA
E. coli topoisomerase IV (*parC, parE*)	II	Increase L $\Delta L = +2$	DNA relaxing activity; it cannot introduce negative supercoils
Eukaryotic topoisomerase II from yeast (*top 2*)	II	Increase or decrease L $\Delta L = \pm 2$	Relaxes positively or negatively supercoiled DNA
E. coli topoisomerase III (*top B*)	I	Increase L $\Delta L = +1$	Relaxes negatively supercoiled DNA; decatenation activity
Eukaryotic topoisomerase III (*top 3*)	I	Increase L $\Delta L = +1$	Specific activity on DNA with single-stranded heteroduplex

[a] Type I topoisomerases use Mg^{2+} as cofactor but do not use ATP. Type II topoisomerases require Mg^{2+} plus ATP.
[b] The name of the gene coding for the topoisomerase is shown in parentheses.

Apparently, the energy released by ATP hydrolysis is used for restoring topoisomerase II conformation, after the enzyme has catalyzed the formation of 1 mol equiv of product. The reaction is inhibited by the antibiotics **nalidixic acid** and **novobiocin.** Derivatives of nalidixic acid are used clinically in the treatment of infections caused by bacteria resistant to other more commonly used antibiotics. Various compounds that inhibit topoisomerases are also effective antitumor agents (see Clin. Corr. 14.3).

During the reaction, topoisomerases remain bound to DNA by a covalent bond between a tyrosyl residue and a phosphoryl group at the incision site (a 5′-phosphotyrosine bond). This enzyme–polynucleotide bond conserves the energy of the interrupted phosphodiester bond for the subsequent repair of the nick. The cleavage sites do not consist of unique nucleotide sequences, although certain sequences are preferentially found at cleavage sites. Gyrase, isolated from *E. coli,* is a tetrameric protein consisting of two A subunits and two B subunits. It adds negative supercoils to DNA at a rate of about 100 per minute. Topoisomerases regulate the level of supercoiling. In *E. coli* DNA such regulation requires the involvement of both gyrase and topoisomerase I activities. The balance between these two opposing enzymic activities keeps DNA at a precisely regulated cellular level of superhelicity. The ATP to ADP ratio may play a role in this process, since this ratio influences the activity of gyrase.

Other biological reactions involving DNA require participation of topoisomerases. For example, topoisomerase IV, a type II topoisomerase, may be essential for separating two circular chromosomes that become entangled by **catenation** toward the end of replication. Also, topoisomerases are involved in relaxing

CLINICAL CORRELATION 14.3

Topoisomerases in Treatment of Cancer

Topoisomerases are emerging as important targets of both antimicrobial and antineoplastic agents including camptothecin, anthracycline, and amino-acridine. These agents share a common principal mechanism of action by interfering with the enzyme-catalyzed rejoining of DNA strands, in effect inhibiting only one of the two substeps in the mechanism of action of topoisomerases. Therefore topoisomerase drugs do not act by inhibiting the overall activity of the enzyme, as is the case with most enzyme-targeting drugs. Instead, they convert topoisomerases into "DNA-breaking agents." The DNA degradation that follows leads to cell death.

Both topoisomerases I and II can be targeted with therapeutic results. Camptothesin and its derivatives modify the function of topoisomerase I. An excellent correlation has been noted between antitumor activity of various camptothecin derivatives on murine leukemia and their interference with topoisomerase activity. Camptothecins may cause potentially lethal lesions in cells in the form of drug-stabilized covalent DNA cleavage complexes. Subsequent DNA replication may be a prerequisite for cell toxicity. Increased levels of topoisomerase I found in advanced stages of colon cancer and several other human malignancies may contribute to the therapeutic efficacy of 9-amino-20(*RS*) and 10,11-methylenedioxy-20(*RS*), two camptothecin derivatives. In clinical trials these camptothecins appear to induce long-term remissions from single-agent treatment of colon cancer xenografts.

Studies with two other potent antineoplastic agents—an acridine derivative, 4′(9-acridinylamino)methanesulfon-*m*-anisidide (m-AMSA), and epipodophyllotoxin toposide—that act selectively on topoisomerases II indicate that these clinically useful drugs stabilize covalent topoisomerase II–DNA cleavage complexes by interfering with the enzyme-mediated DNA religation reaction. Indirect evidence also suggests that these drugs may stimulate formation of these complexes. Contrary to observations regarding the importance of DNA replication in the expression of the cytotoxic effect of drugs that target topoisomerase I, topoisomerase II-mediated DNA breaks can exert their cytotoxic effect in the absence of ongoing DNA synthesis. Instead, the lethal lesions induced by topoisomerase II-targeted drugs may be dependent on recombinations and mutations at sites of formation of drug-induced topoisomerase II–DNA complexes. Many anticancer agents including anthracyclines (including adriamycin and doxorubicin), synthetic intercalators, ellipticines, and podophyllotoxins exert their therapeutic effects on topoisomerases II. Hematologic neoplasms, such as lymphoid and nonlymphoid leukemias, high-grade non-Hodgkin's lymphomas, and Hodgkin's disease, are treated mostly with combinations of one or more topoisomerase II inhibitors with or without additional cytotoxic agents.

Potmesil, M., and Kohn, K. W. (Eds.). *DNA Topoisomerases in Cancer.* New York: Oxford University Press, 1991; and Ellis, A. L., Nowak, B., Plunkett, W., and Zwelling, L. A. Quantification of topoisomerase–DNA complexes in leukemia cells from patients undergoing therapy with a topoisomerase directed agent. *Cancer Chemother. Pharmacol.* 34:249, 1994.

the superhelical tension generated by the separation of DNA strands during the process of transcription.

Separation of superhelical DNA from the relaxed or linear forms can be achieved by gel electrophoresis or by equilibrium centrifugation. With the latter method separation is achieved because the density of supercoiled DNA differs from that of the relaxed forms.

Alternative DNA Conformations

Conformational variants of DNA—that is, A-, B-, and Z-DNA—are associated mainly with variation in the conformation of the nucleotide constituents of DNA. It is now recognized that DNA is not a straight, stable, monotonous, and uniform structure. Instead, DNA forms unusual structures such as **cruciforms** or **triple-stranded** arrangements and bends as it interacts with certain proteins. Such variations in DNA conformation appear to be an important recurring theme in the process of molecular recognition of DNA by proteins and enzymes. Variations in DNA structure or conformation are favored by specific motifs in the sequence of DNA referred to as **defined, ordered sequence DNA** and are abbreviated as **dos DNA.** They include such DNA elements as **inverted repeats, mirror repeats, direct repeats, homopurine–homopyrimidine sequences, phased A tracts,** and **G-rich regions.** AT-rich sequences prone to easy strand separation exist near the origins of DNA replication. The human genome is rich in homopurine–homopyrimidine sequences and alternating purine–pyrimidine tracts. DNA bending, slipped DNA, cruciform formation, triplex DNA, and **quadruplex** arrangements are among the structures reviewed in this section.

DNA Bending

DNA sequences with runs of 4 to 6 A bases phased by 10-bp spacers produce bend conformations. **DNA bending** appears to be a fundamental element in the interaction between DNA sequences and proteins that catalyze central processes, such as replication, transcription, and site-specific recombination. Bending induced by interactions of DNA with enzymes and other proteins, such as histones, does not require the exacting nucleotide sequence conditions that are needed for bending of protein-free DNA. Bending also occurs because of photochemical damage and serves as a recognition signal for the initiation of DNA repair. Contrary to the bending effect generated by phased A tracts, the presence of poly A tracts without spacers or the presence of certain arrangements of polypurine–polypyrimidine tracts may generate a DNA, known as **anisomorphic DNA,** that is less flexible than usual.

Cruciform DNA

Dos DNA is generally present within noncoding DNA regions and it consists of various symmetry elements, including **inverted repeats,** completely **symmetrical inverted repeats,** known as **palindromes** (see p. 610), **mirror repeats,** and **direct repeats** as shown in Figure 14.32. Base pairing can be disrupted and conformational variants of DNA such as **junctions, cruciforms, triplex,** and **quadruplex DNA** and **slipped mispaired** structures can be formed within the **dos** sequences.

The biological function of cruciforms has not been generally established. Inverted repeats are quite widespread within the human genome and are often found near putative control regions of genes or at origins of DNA replication. It is therefore speculated that inverted repeats may function as molecular switches for replication and transcription. In fact, in a few instances there is evidence to support the involvement of cruciforms in the control of replication and transcription. The disruption of H bonds between the complementary strands and the formation of intrastrand H bonds within the region of the inverted

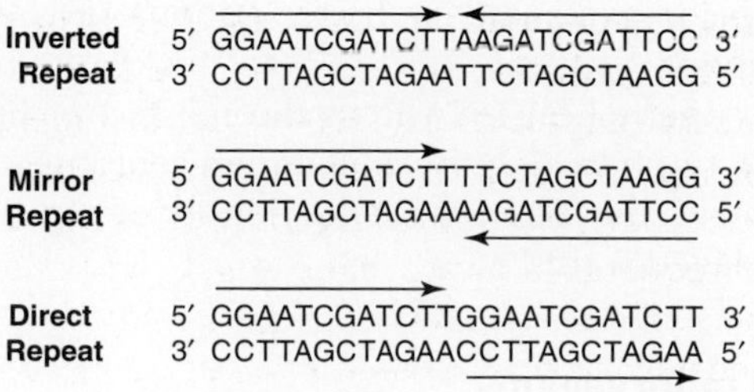

Inverted Repeat
5′ GGAATCGATCTTAAGATCGATTCC 3′
3′ CCTTAGCTAGAATTCTAGCTAAGG 5′

Mirror Repeat
5′ GGAATCGATCTTTTCTAGCTAAGG 3′
3′ CCTTAGCTAGAAAAGATCGATTCC 5′

Direct Repeat
5′ GGAATCGATCTTGGAATCGATCTT 3′
3′ CCTTAGCTAGAACCTTAGCTAGAA 5′

FIGURE 14.32
Symmetry elements of DNA sequences.
Three types of symmetry elements for double-stranded DNA sequences are shown. Arrows illustrate the special relationship of these elements in each one of these sequences. In inverted repeats, also referred to as palindromes, each single DNA strand is self-complementary within the inverted region that contains the symmetry elements. A mirror repeat is characterized by the presence of identical base pairs equidistant from a center of symmetry within the DNA segment. Direct repeats are regions of DNA in which a particular sequence is repeated. The repeats need not be adjacent to one another.

repeat produce a cruciform structure (Figure 14.33). The loops generated by cruciform formation require the unstacking of 3–4 unpaired bases at the end of the "hairpin" and therefore cruciform formation requires the expenditure of cellular energy.

Triple-Stranded DNA

Many sequences in the human genome, especially in regions involved in gene regulation, have the potential to form triple-stranded DNA structures. Such

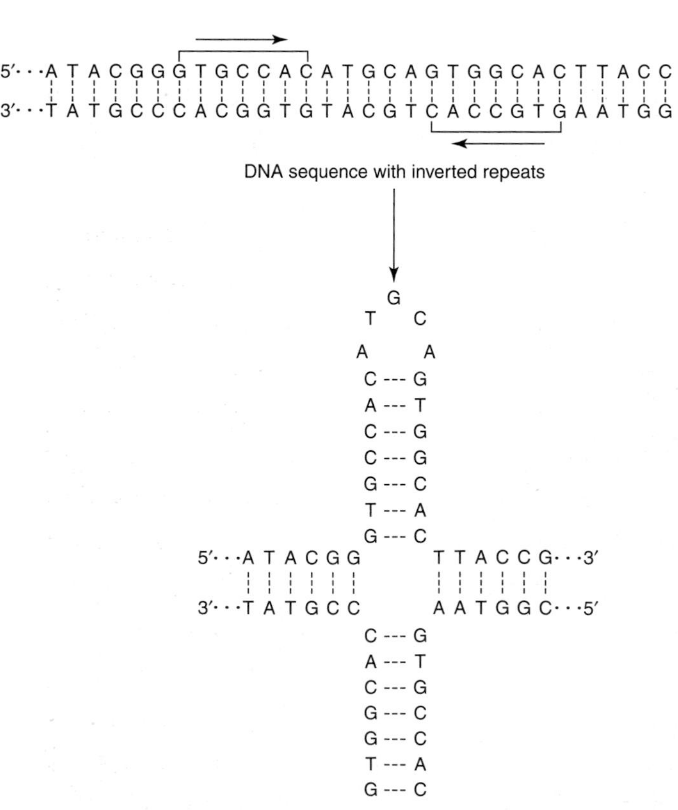

FIGURE 14.33
Formation of cruciform structures in DNA.
The existence of inverted repeats in double-stranded DNA is a necessary but not a sufficient condition for the formation of cruciform structures. In relaxed DNA, cruciforms are not likely to form because the linear DNA accommodates more hydrogen-bonded stacked base pairs than the cruciform structure, making the formation of the latter thermodynamically unfavored. Unwinding is followed by intrastrand hydrogen bond formation between the two symmetrical parts of the repeat to produce the cruciform structure. Formation of cruciform structures is not favored over DNA regions that consist of mirror repeats because such cruciforms would be constructed from parallel rather than antiparallel DNA strands. Instead, certain mirror repeats tend to form triple helices.

structures can be formed either within the same DNA structure (i.e., intramolecularly) or between DNA and a distinct or second polynucleotide (i.e., intermolecularly). In either case, **triple-stranded DNA** structures are formed, with few exceptions, in DNA regions characterized by the presence of a continuous string of purine bases, that is, **homopurine–homopyrimidine regions.** Such regions occur with frequencies much higher than expected from probability considerations alone. Polypurine tracts over 25 nucleotides long constitute as much as 0.5% of some eukaryotic genomes. Polypurine–polypyrimidine regions appear to have a multiplicity of potential biological roles, including possible effects in transcription control, in the initiation of replication, as replication terminators, as enhancers of stability at the ends of chromosomes (telomeres), and as initiators of genetic recombination.

Triple-stranded DNA is generated by the hydrogen bonding of a third strand into the major groove of B-DNA (Figure 14.34). Since base pairs are already formed in the B-DNA, the third strand forms hydrogen bonds with another surface of the double helix through so-called **Hoogsteen pairs.** The options available for the formation of a triple-stranded structure are limited to only four triplet bases—TAT, CGC, GGC, and AAT. The structure of two of these triplets is shown in Figure 14.35. Since pyrimidine does not have two H-bonding surfaces with more than one H bond, it follows that the central strand of the triplex must always be purine rich. Therefore, in practice, intermolecular triple-stranded DNA can only form within homopurine–homopyrimidine regions of DNA. Just as is the case for the Watson–Crick base pairs, formed between strands in double-stranded DNA, a polypurine–polypyrimidine region defines a unique third strand pairing sequence. Consequently, the sequence of a third strand can be designed so that it can form Hoogsteen base pairs with any specific polypurine–polypyrimidine region of DNA.

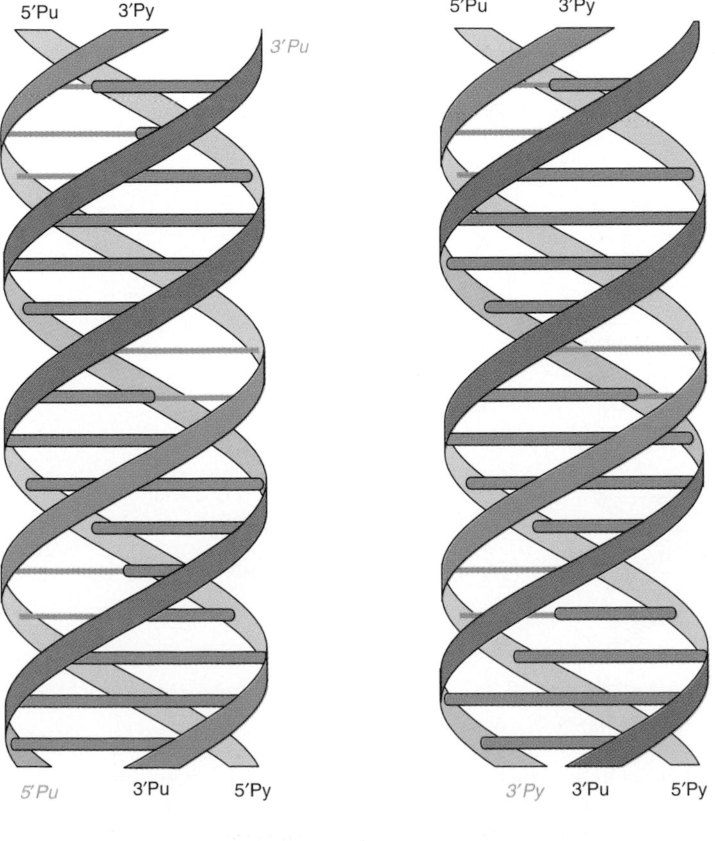

FIGURE 14.34
Structure of intermolecular triple helices.
Triple helices can form among (*a*) two polypurine strands and one polypyrimidine strand as exemplified by the polyG-polyG-polyC triplet or (*b*) among two polypyrimidine and one polypurine strand as in the case of the polyT-polyA-polyT triplet. In (*a*), held together partially by Hoogsteen base pairing, the polypurine strand is antiparallel to the polypurine strand of the original DNA duplex. In (*b*), which is characterized by reverse Hoogsteen base pairing, the polypyrimidine third strand is parallel to the polypurine strand. Brackets enclose strands held together by Watson–Crick hydrogen bonding.
Redrawn based on figure in Sinden, R. R. DNA Structure and Function. *New York: Academic Press, 1994.*

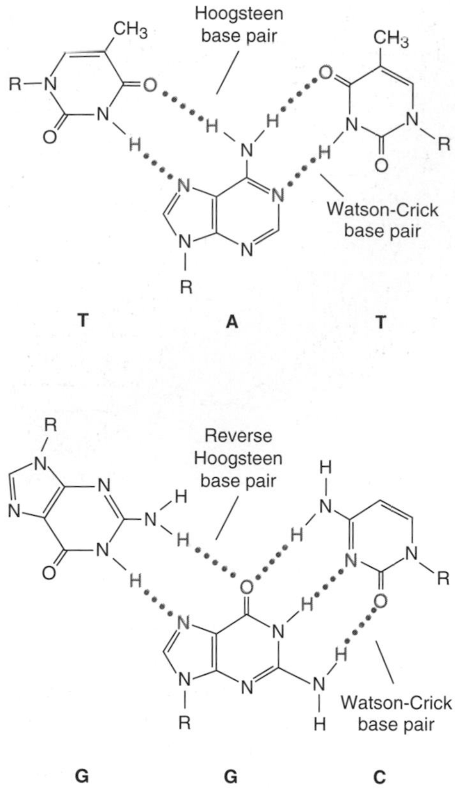

Hoogsteen base pair
Watson-Crick base pair
T A T

Reverse Hoogsteen base pair
Watson-Crick base pair
G G C

FIGURE 14.35
Base pairing in DNA triplexes.
Two examples of the type of hydrogen bonding involving the formation of triple-stranded DNA helices are shown, one for the polyG-polyG-polyC and one for the polyT-polyA-polyT triple helix. For the T-A-T triplex the purine (A) participates in a Watson–Crick base pairing to T and in an alternative type of base pairing (Hoogsteen base pairing) to a second T. In the G-G-C triplex, the purine (G) forms a Watson–Crick base pairing with C and a Hoogsteen base pairing with G. In this base pairing scheme the ribose groups of the two purines are in trans orientation, generating a so-called reverse Hoogsteen base pair. The relative orientation (polarity) of the three strands shown in Figure 14.36 depends on whether two of the participating polynucleotides form regular or reverse Hoogsteen base pairs.

Intramolecular triple helices can be formed by disruption of H bonds, over regions of DNA characterized by the presence of polypurine strands, and refolding as illustrated in Figure 14.36 to generate a triple-stranded region and a single-stranded loop. This arrangement involves disruption of base stacking interaction in the unpaired region and therefore it is not the most thermodynamically stable structure that can be formed by the double-stranded polypurine–polypyrimidine DNA segment. Yet, intramolecular triple helices are detected in cellular DNA. Apparently DNA supercoiling provides the energy to drive the unwinding of DNA that is necessary for the formation of the triple helix. Triple-strand formation produces a relaxation of negative supercoils. In addition to the general requirement that a string of purines be present, structural considerations for the formation of hydrogen bonds dictate that the polypurine–polypyrimidine region must contain **mirror repeat symmetry** for the triplex to form. A mirror repeat is a region such as AGGGGA that has the same base sequence when read, from a central point, in either direction within one of the DNA strands. There are two possible pairs of alternative structures that can form from different foldings of the polypurine–polypyrimidine region in the triple helix. One of the pairs is characterized by a pyrimidine–purine–pyrimidine arrangement in which half of the pyrimidine strand is paired as the third strand and the complementary strand remains unpaired. The other pair of possible alternative structures is characterized by the less commonly occurring purine–purine–pyrimidine arrangement.

A distinct type of intermolecular triple-stranded helix is formed by enzymatic catalysis, as an intermediate during general recombination. These intermediates are atypical triple helices in that they are not limited to polypurine–polypyrimidine regions but instead involve DNA strands of identical, or nearly identical, nucleotide sequences. These helices are unwound structures in which

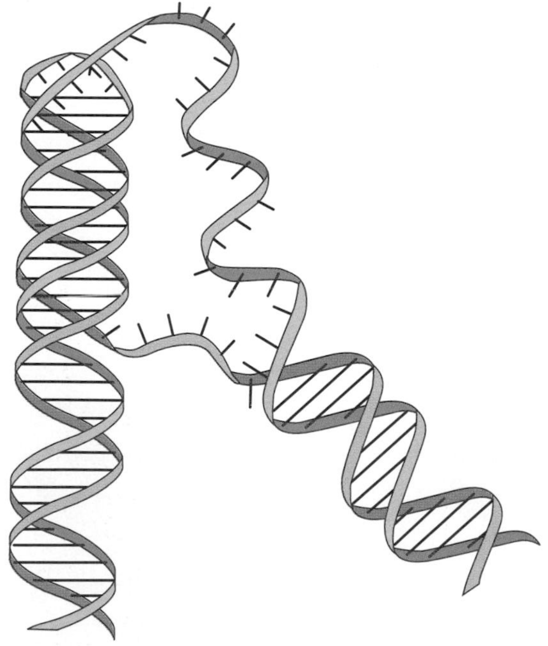

FIGURE 14.36
Intramolecular triple helices.
Polypurine–polypyrimidine regions of DNA with a mirror repeat symmetry can form an intramolecular triple helix in which the third strand lays in the major groove, whereas its complementary strand acquires a single-stranded conformation.
Redrawn based on figure in Sinden, R. R. DNA Structure and Function. *New York: Academic Press, 1994.*

the third strand binds on the major groove side of a double helix in a manner parallel to its identical strand.

Long polypurine–polypyrimidine sequences can form another variant DNA structure, the **nodule DNA,** that consists of a pair of two intermolecular triplex regions, as illustrated in Figure 14.37. Its biological significance has not been determined.

The role of DNA triplex formation in a hereditary affliction known as persistence of fetal hemoglobin is briefly reviewed in Clin. Corr. 14.4. The therapeutic potential of oligonucleotides capable of forming triplex DNA with segments of DNA having Hoogsteen base pairing potential is discussed in Clin. Corr. 14.5.

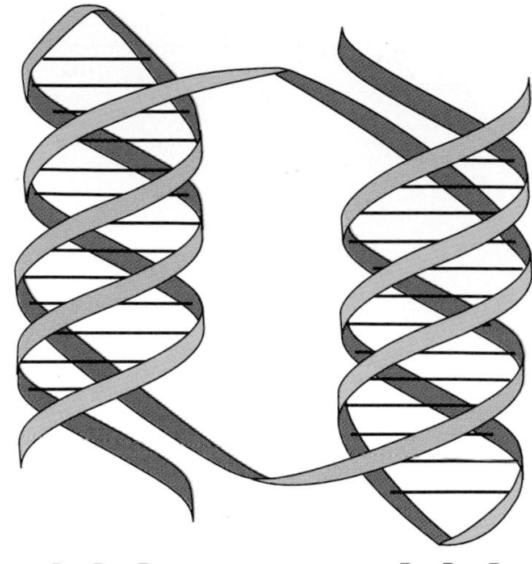

FIGURE 14.37
Nodule DNA.
Nodule DNA consisting of a combination of a Py-Pu-Py triple helix and a Pu-Pu-Py triplex can be formed within a long polypurine–polypyrimidine tract. The Py-Pu-Py structure can contribute its displaced single Pu strand to the other half of the Pu-Py region, forming the Pu-Pu-Py triplex structure.
Redrawn based on figure in Sinden, R. R. DNA Structure and Function. *New York: Academic Press, 1994.*

Four-Stranded DNA

Four-stranded DNA (quadruplex) can form as both parallel and antiparallel structures. Parallel structures may form during DNA recombination (see p. 661). A parallel four-stranded DNA may be found in an immunoglobulin heavy chain gene. The immunoglobulin genes undergo a type of recombination (specific recombination) that is responsible for the extensive diversity that characterizes antibody formation. The sequences that participate in this alternative type of DNA structure are repeated motifs high in guanine content such as GGGGAGCTGGG. A base pairing scheme for parallel four-stranded DNA, referred to as a **G-quartet DNA,** is shown in Figure 14.38. In this scheme all four DNA strands are arranged in a parallel orientation and are associated to one another through Hoogsteen base pairs. The glycosidic bonds in all nucleotides are in the **anti** configuration.

Parallel and antiparallel four-stranded DNA structures form at **telomeres.** These contain repetitive simple oligonucleotide sequences (such as G_4T_2) that are usually purine rich in one of the strands. This strand is longer and overhangs the complementary strand. The repetitive sequences make the formation of four-stranded DNA possible. One such four-stranded antiparallel structure forms when the single strand overhanging the telomere end is folded back into a hairpin structure with guanines binding to one another by Hoogsteen base pairing. Two folded double-helical regions can then interact to form four-

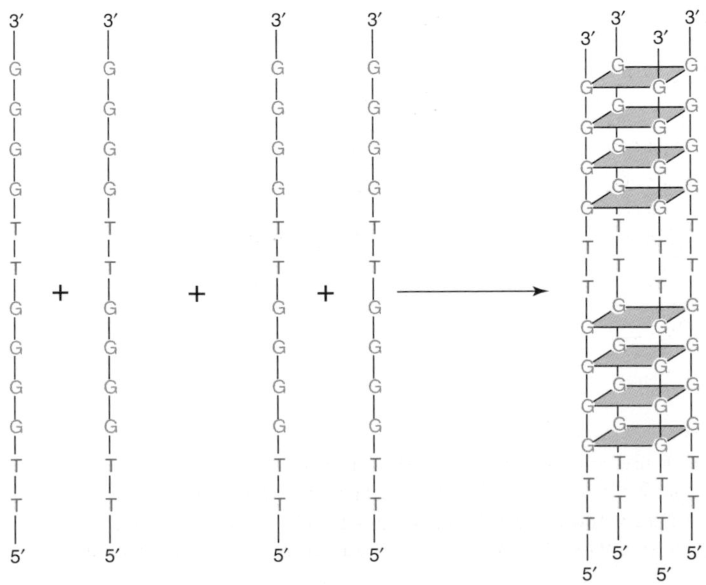

FIGURE 14.38
Parallel quadruplex DNA.
Quadruplex structures in which all four strands are parallel can form from four single-strand tracts of polyguanine. These quadruplexes, referred to as G-quartets, are associated by Hoogsteen base pairs.
Redrawn based on figure in Sinden, R. R. DNA Structure and Function. *New York: Academic Press, 1994.*

CLINICAL CORRELATION 14.4

Hereditary Persistence of Fetal Hemoglobin

Hereditary persistence of fetal hemoglobin (HPFH) is a group of conditions in which fetal hemoglobin synthesis is not turned off with development but continues into adulthood. The homozygous form of the disease is extremely uncommon, being characterized by red blood cell changes similar to those found in heterozygous β-thalassemia. HPFH, in either the homozygous or heterozygous state, is associated with mild clinical or hematologic abnormalities. Mild musculoskeletal pains may occur infrequently but HPFH patients are generally asymptomatic.

The disease is the result of failure in control of transcription from human Gγ- and Aγ-globin genes. Affected chromosomes fail to switch from γ- to β-chain synthesis. Expression of these genes appears to be affected substantially by formation of an intramolecular DNA triplex structure located about 200 bp upstream from the initiation site for transcription of genes, specifically between positions −194 and −215. 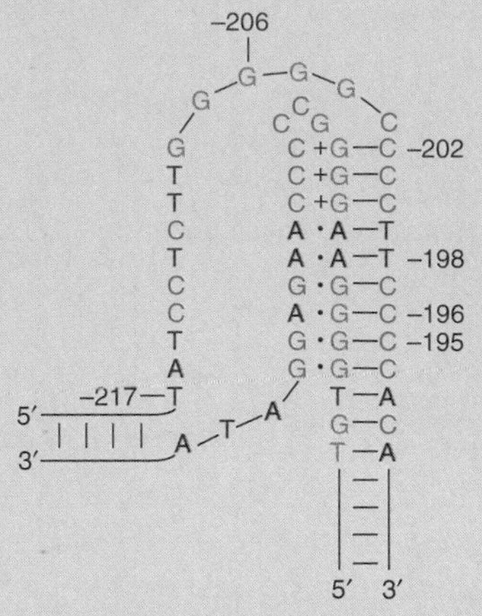
Hemoglobin genes of patients contain mutations in positions −195, −196, −198, and −202. Mutations at −202 involve changes from C to G and C to T, at −198 from T to C, at −196 from C to T, and at −195 from C to G. These mutations influence the stability of the intramolecular DNA triple helix.

In general, the presence of polypurine–polypyrimidine sequences sufficiently long to form intramolecular triple helices tends to repress transcription, while short polypurine–polypyrimidine segments that are unable to induce triple helix formation have no effect on transcription. In the case of HPFH, a remarkable correspondence is noted between base changes that destabilize formation of the triple helix and presence of the genetic disease.

Ulrich, M. J., Gray, W. J., and Ley, T. J. An intramolecular DNA triplex is disrupted by point mutations associated with hereditary persistence of fetal hemoglobin. *J. Biol. Chem.* 267:18649, 1992; and Bacolla, A., Ulrich, M. J., Larson, J. E., Ley, T. J., and Wells, R. D. An intramolecular triplex in the human gamma-globin 5′-flanking region is altered by point mutations associated with hereditary persistence of fetal hemoglobin. *J. Biol. Chem.* 270:24556, 1995.

CLINICAL CORRELATION 14.5

Therapeutic Potential of Triplex DNA Formation

Control regions of genes often contain polypurine–polypyrimidine regions. Binding of a single third strand of DNA, complementary to the polypurine strand, may under certain conditions prevent binding of regulatory proteins, such as transcription factors, and thus affect gene expression. Alternatively, triplex formation may influence regulation of gene expression by affecting the level of DNA supercoiling in the topological domain in which the triple helix forms, as shown in the figure below.

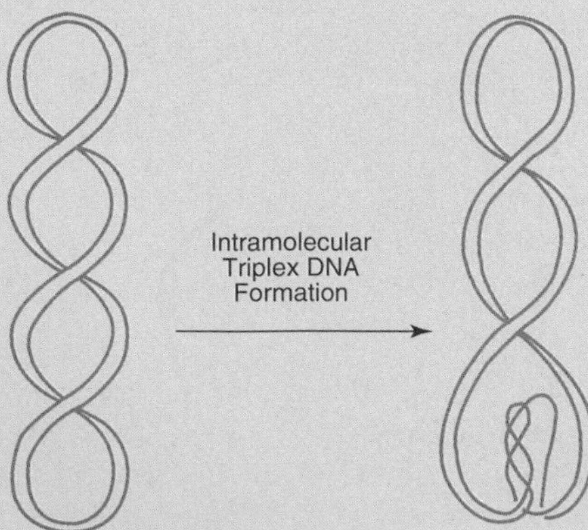

For instance, a polypurine–polypyrimidine region, which can form a triplex, is present upstream of the human *c-myc* oncogene. This region, which interacts with transcription factors, can form an intermolecular triplex with an oligonucleotide designed to provide base complementary with the polypurine–polypyrimidine region. Formation of triplex DNA results in inhibition of *c-myc* transcription *in vitro*. The above example suggests that formation of intermolecular complexes has the potential to regulate expression of specific proteins that may play important roles in health and development of disease. The great individuality inherent in the sequence of unique oligonucleotide segments provides the potential to design specific therapeutic oligonucleotides for turning certain genes off and on.

The specificity of DNA triplexes also provides another approach for the potential control of expression of certain genes. Oligonucleotide sequences that are targeted to specific regions of a eukaryotic or viral genome can be coupled with artificial nucleases or covalent modifiers of DNA. Such targeting produces endonucleolytic cutting or covalent modification of the DNA at specific sites. This approach has therapeutic potential for gene regulation and killing of virus-infected cells or other abnormal cells.

Kinniburg, A. J. A cis-acting transcription element of the *c-myc* gene can assume an H-DNA conformation. *Nucleic Acids Res.* 17:7771, 1989; and Pei, D., Corey, D. R., and Schultz, P. G. Site specific cleavage of duplex DNA by a semisynthetic nuclease via triple-helix formation. *Proc. Natl. Acad. Sci. USA* 87:9858, 1990.

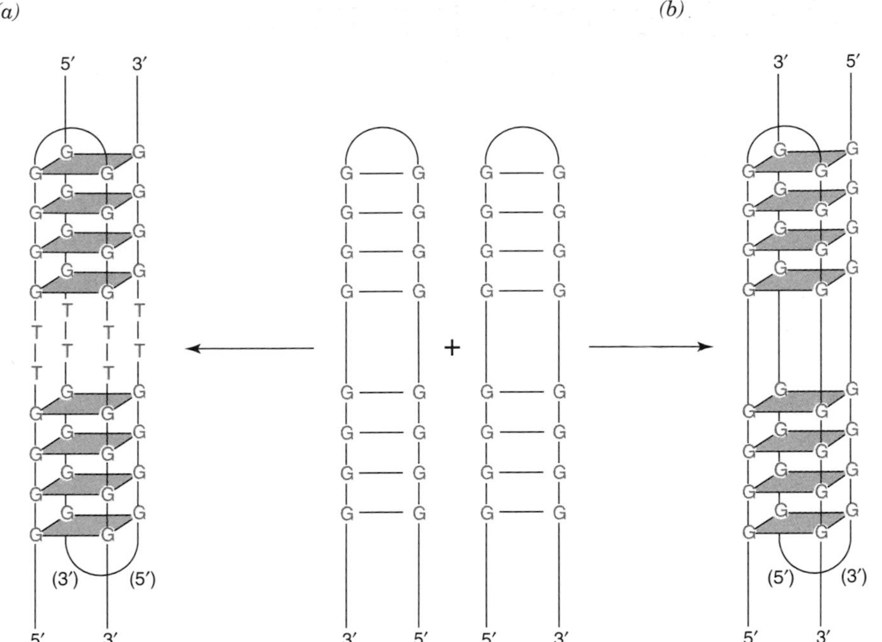

FIGURE 14.39
Antiparallel quadruplex DNA.
Several quadruplexes both of the antiparallel (*a*) and parallel (*b*) type can form at telomeres as these terminal regions are guanine-rich. *Redrawn based on figure in Sinden, R. R.* DNA Structure and Function. *New York: Academic Press, 1994.*

stranded structures held together by Hoogsteen base pairs between guanines. A number of alternative four-stranded structures can form and their existence has been confirmed by X-ray diffraction and NMR spectroscopy. An example of an antiparallel quadruplex DNA is shown in Figure 14.39.

Slipped DNA

DNA regions with direct repeat symmetry can form structures known as **slipped, mispaired DNA** (SMP-DNA). Their formation involves the unwinding of the double helix and realignment and subsequent pairing of one copy of the direct repeat with an adjacent copy on the other strand. This realignment generates a single-stranded loop (Figure 14.40). Two isomeric structures of a SMP-DNA are possible. One generates a loop consisting of the 5′ direct repeat in both strands and the other produces loops of the 3′ direct repeat. Although SMP-DNA has not yet been identified, genetic evidence suggests that this type of DNA is undoubtedly involved in spontaneous frameshift mutagenesis that is manifested as base addition or deletion occurring within runs of single bases. A mechanism that explains these mutations is shown in Figure 14.41. First, a homopolymeric sequence in one strand (template strand) unpairs from a newly synthesized complementary strand and reforms hydrogen bonds with a different set of bases, resulting in the formation of an extrahelical base on either the template strand or progeny strand. Continued replication produces a deletion when the progeny strand slips forward or a duplication when the strand slips backward. Deletions and duplications of DNA segments, longer than a single base, occur during DNA replication between direct repeats, which can form slipped-looped structures. Duplication of certain simple triplet repeats that are implicated as the basis of several human genetic diseases (see Clin. Corr. 14.6) may also occur by this mechanism.

Nucleoproteins of Eukaryotes Contain Histones and Nonhistone Proteins

DNA in eukaryotic cells is associated with various types of protein to form **chromatin.** In resting (nondividing) cells, chromatin is amorphous and dispersed within the nucleus. Just prior to cell division (mitosis), chromatin becomes organized into compact structures (fibers) called **chromosomes.** The

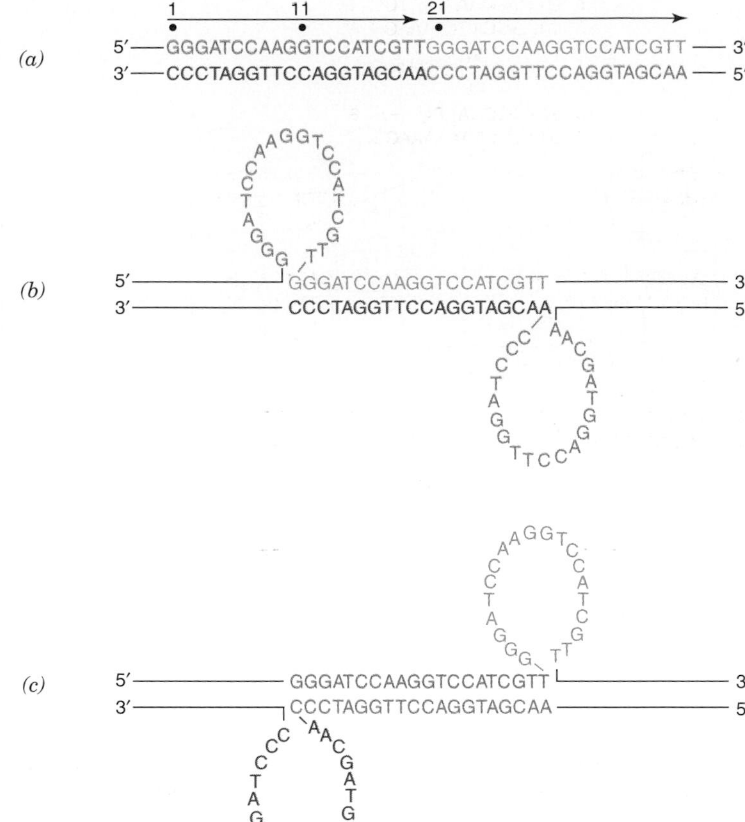

FIGURE 14.40
Slipped, mispaired DNA.
The presence of two adjacent tandem repeats (*a*) can give rise to either one of two isomers of slipped, mispaired DNA. In one of these isomers (*b*) the second copy of the direct repeat in the top strand pairs with the first copy of the repeat on the bottom strand. Pairing of the first copy of the direct repeat in the top strand with the second copy of the direct repeat in the bottom strand produces the second isomer (*c*). A pair of single-stranded loops is generated in both isomers.

CLINICAL CORRELATION 14.6

Expansion of DNA Triple Repeats and Human Disease

The presence of reiterated DNA sequences, consisting of three base pairs, has been noted in a number of human genetic diseases including fragile X syndrome, myotonic dystrophy, X-linked spinal and bulbar muscular atrophy (Kennedy syndrome), spinocerebellar ataxia, colon cancer, and more recently Huntington's disease. These diseases are associated with expansion of certain triplet nucleotide repeats that appear to be overrepresented in the human genome. For example, fragile X syndrome is characterized by expansion of a GCC triplet and spinocerebellar ataxia type I with expansion of a CAG triplet. Diseases associated with expansion of triplets are characterized by an increase in severity of the disease with successive generation, which is known as anticipation. For example, anticipation in fragile X syndrome, a leading cause of mental retardation, is associated with a major expansion of the CGG triplet. Normally, about 30 copies of this triplet are present on the 5′ side of a gene associated with the disease, the *FMR-1* gene. The site of the repeat is expanded to as many as 300 copies in males that carry fragile X gene mutations but have no symptoms of the disease. Offspring of male carriers who express the disease can have a remarkable expansion of the triplet repeat, up to thousands of copies.

The disease develops when normal expression of *FMR-1* gene is turned off. Methylation of CpG dinucleotides present in CGG triplets appears to be associated with shutting off of the *FMR-1* gene. It appears that triplet expansion is the result of slipped mispairing during DNA synthesis. Because of the massive amplification that characterizes the diseases associated with triplet expansion, repeated or multiple slippage would have to be involved to explain the high degree of expansion. What promotes repeated slippage is not known but it may be that expansion is associated with a repeated dissociation of the enzyme DNA polymerase from the DNA template. This may allow DNA breathing and repeated slippage of DNA strands that are obviously required for the observed extensive expansion of the triplets. For slippage to occur, a single-stranded break needs to be generated within the tandem repeat during replication, which can lead to addition (or deletion) of a few copies of the tandem repeat. For modest size repeats, that is, repeats of less than about 80 copies, at least one such break is expected to be generated. When a larger number of repeats are present, it is possible that two single-stranded breaks are generated during replications. The strand segment flanked by these single-stranded breaks is not anchored by a unique sequence at either end and therefore it is free to slide during synthesis, leading to triplet amplification.

Behn-Krappa, A., and Doerfler, W. Enzymatic amplification of synthetic oligodeoxyribonucleotides: implications for triplet repeat expansions in the human genome. *Hum. Mutat.* 23:19, 1994.

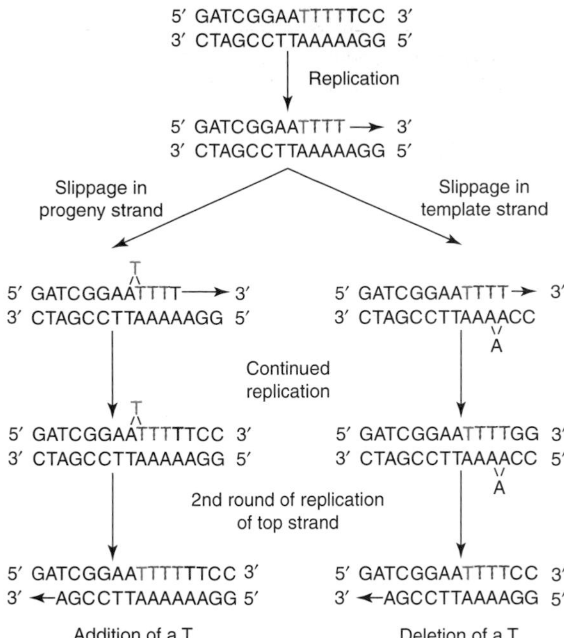

FIGURE 14.41
Frameshift mutagenesis by DNA slippage.
DNA replication within a run of a single base can produce a single base frameshift. In the example shown here, a run of five A's is replicated and, depending on whether a slippage occurs in the progeny strand or the template strand, a T may be added or deleted from the DNA.

division of genetic information into numerous independent domains, that is, chromosomes, may be necessitated by the enormous length of the genome of most eukaryotes. Each chromosome is characterized by the presence of a **centromere,** which functions as a site for attachment to proteins that link the chromosome to the mitotic spindle. Sister chromatids are connected at the centromere. **Telomeres** define the termini of linear chromosomes. A third element that characterizes chromosomes is the presence of a sequence required for the initiation of DNA replication **(origin of replication).** The number of chromosomes observed is species specific with human cells containing 46 chromosomes (chromatids) organized into 23 pairs. The average DNA length of each one of these chromosomes is 1.3×10^8 nucleotide pairs or approximately 5 cm. It is believed that each human chromosome consists of a single intact DNA molecule varying in size from 263×10^6 base pairs for chromosome 1 to less than 50×10^6 bp for chromosome 23. If the DNA of all 46 chromosomes were lined up in the B-DNA conformation, it would be more than 2 m long.

The chromosomal organization that makes it possible for DNA to fit within a cell nucleus with a diameter of approximately 5 μm requires a "condensation ratio" of more than five orders of magnitude. During metaphase the DNA molecule is very tightly wound. For example, human chromosome 16 is 2.5 μm long, whereas the DNA molecule is 3.7 cm in each of the two chromatids, giving a condensation ratio of $1.5 \times 10^4:1$. The parceling of DNA in 46 chromosomes provides for a further increase in the condensation ratio to $10^5:1$. This remarkable degree of condensation of cellular DNA is shown in Figure 14.42. The early stages of DNA packing that lead to formation of 30-nm fibers have been extensively studied. The latter stages, in which looped domains of the 30-nm fiber are organized into scaffolds and chromatid coils, are based on indirect evidence and are more speculative. At each stage of packing, shown in this model, DNA is condensed severalfold. The cumulative effect of the successive folding stages provides the large condensation ratio necessary for the **packing of DNA** within the nucleus. The first stage of organization is the formation of a **"beads-on-a-string"** structure consisting of DNA associated with a class of highly basic proteins known as **histones.** These bind tightly to DNA, forming very stable complexes. The "beads-on-a-string" arrangement is seen in chromatin treated under conditions of low ionic strength and examined

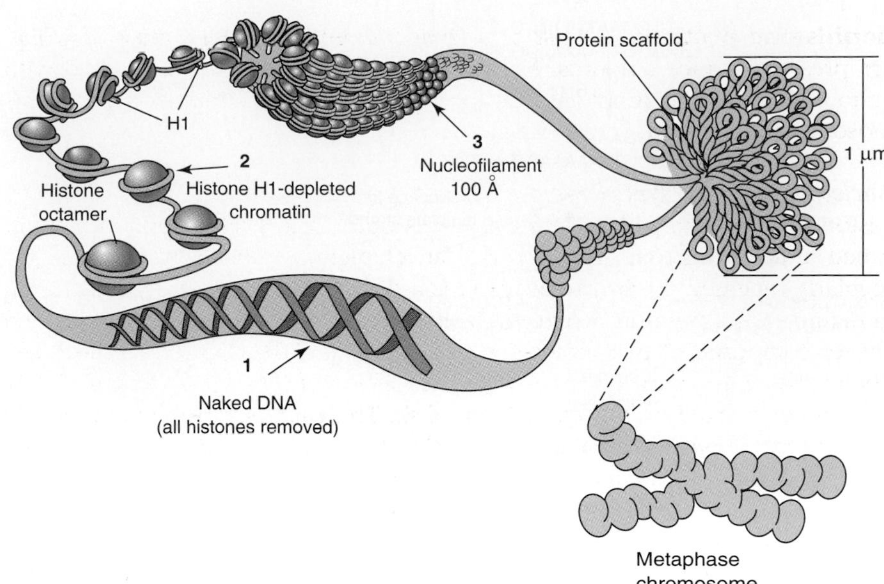

FIGURE 14.42
Organization of polynucleosomes into chromosomes.
A speculative drawing showing the condensation of polynucleosomes into the 30-nm fiber and the subsequent packaging of this fiber into a twisted, looped structure attached to a protein scaffold within the chromosome.

under the electron microscope. The "string" is free DNA and the "beads" are coiled around histones.

Histones, regardless of their source, consist of five types of polypeptides of different size and composition (Table 14.7). The most "conserved" histones are H4 and H3, which differ very little even between extremely diverse species; histones H4 from peas and cows are very similar, differing by only two amino acids, although these species diverged more than a billion years ago. The H2A and H2B histones are less highly conserved but still exhibit substantial evolutionary stability, especially within their nonbasic portions. H1 histones are quite distinct from the inner histones. They are larger, more basic, and by far the most tissue-specific and species-specific histones. Vertebrates contain an additional histone, H5, which has a function similar to H1. As a result of their unusually high content of the basic amino acids lysine and arginine, histones are highly polycationic and interact with the polyanionic phosphate backbone of DNA so as to produce uncharged nucleoproteins. All five histones are characterized by a central nonpolar domain, which forms a globular structure, and N-terminal and C-terminal regions that contain most of the basic amino acids. The basic N-terminal regions of H2A, H2B, H3, and H4 comprising 20–25% of the histone octomer are the major, but not the exclusive, sites of interaction with DNA. Nonpolar domains and C-terminal regions of histones H1, H2A, and H2B are involved in subunit and DNA and histone interactions.

A heterogeneous group of proteins with high species, and even organ, specificity is also present in chromatin. These proteins, grouped together as

TABLE 14.7 Structure of the Five Types of Histones[a]

Name	*Structure*[b]	*Residues*	*Molecular Weight*
H4	N ├────● C	102	11,300
H3	N ├────────●───┤ C	135	15,300
H2A	N ├────●───┤ C	129	14,000
H2B	N ├────●───┤ C	125	13,800
H1	N ├─────●──────────┤ C	~216	~21,000

nonhistone proteins, consist of several hundred members, most of which are present in trace amounts. Many nonhistone proteins are associated with various chromosome functions, such as replication, gene expression, and chromosome organization.

Nucleosomes and Polynucleosomes

Histones interacting with DNA form the periodic "beads-on-a-string" structure, called a **polynucleosome,** in which an elementary unit, a nucleosome, is regularly repeated. Each **nucleosome** is a disk-shaped structure about 11 nm in diameter and 6 nm in height that consists of a DNA segment and a histone cluster composed of two molecules each of H2A, H2B, H3, and H4 histones. The clusters are organized as tetramers consisting of $(H3)_2$-$(H4)_2$ with an H2A-H2B dimer stacked on each face in the disk. The DNA is wrapped around the octamer as a negative toroidal superhelix at a pitch of about 30 Å with the central $(H3)_2$-$(H4)_2$ core interacting with the central 70–80 bp of the DNA wrap. Histones are in contact with the minor groove of DNA and leave the major groove available for interaction with the proteins that regulate gene expression and other DNA functions. Two distinct structures of nucleosomes can be distinguished: the **nucleosome core** and the **chromatosome,** as presented in Figure 14.43. The chromatosome constitutes the most elementary structural unit of nucleoproteins. These two structures are obtained by the digestion of polynucleosomes with nucleases (DNases) that, depending on conditions, can re-

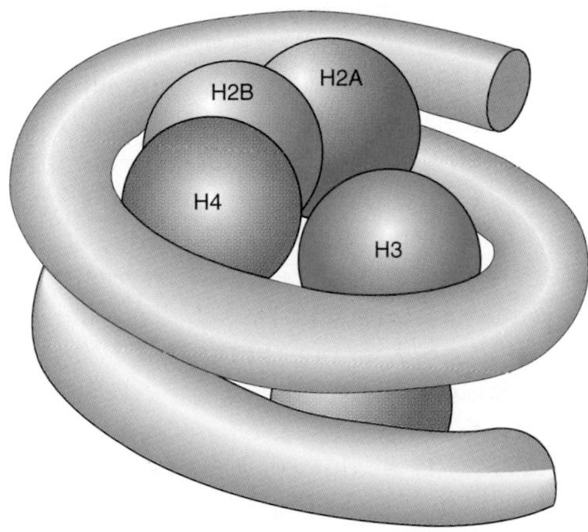

(a)

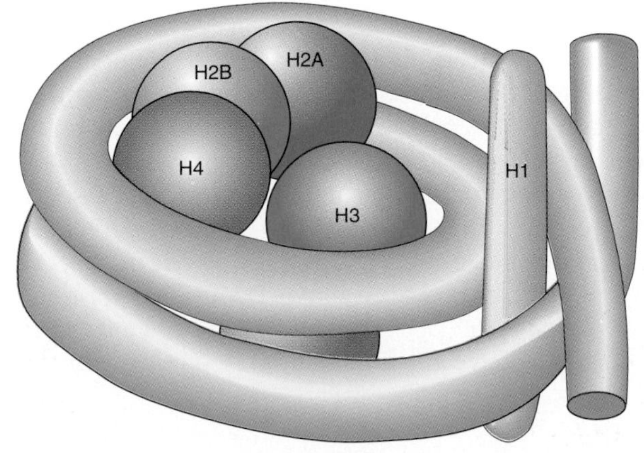

(b)

FIGURE 14.43
Postulated structures for the nucleosome and chromatosome. The nucleosome consists of approximately 146 bp of DNA corresponding to $1\frac{3}{4}$ superhelical turns wound around a histone octamer. The chromatosome (two-turn particle) consists of about 166 bp of DNA (two superhelical turns). The H1 subunit is retained by this particle and may be associated with it, as shown. Chromatosomes containing less than 166 bp do not bind the H1 subunit.

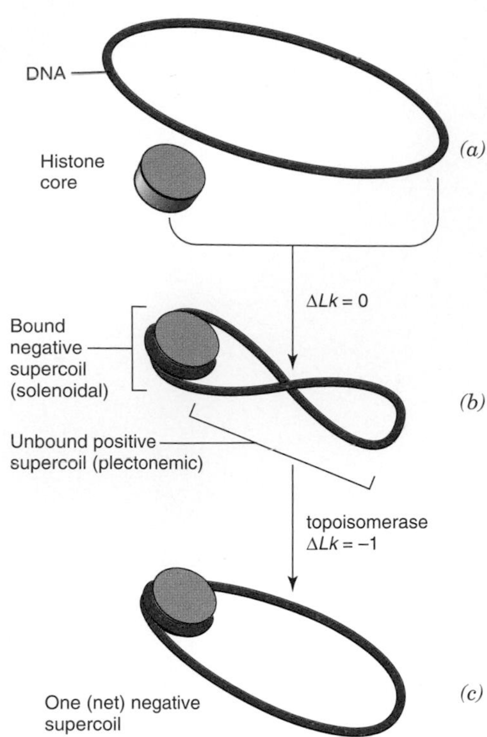

FIGURE 14.44
Generation of negative supercoiling in eukaryotic DNA.
The binding of a histone octamer to a relaxed, closed-domain DNA forces the DNA to wrap around the octamer, generating a negative supercoil. In the absence of any strand breaks, the domain remains intact and a compensating positive supercoil must be generated elsewhere within the domain. The action of a eukaryotic type I topoisomerase subsequently relaxes the positive supercoil, leaving the closed domain with one net negative supercoil.

move most or all DNA that is not tightly bound with histones. Nucleosomes obtained by nuclease digestion can be crystallized and studied by X-ray diffraction.

The structure of nucleosomes explains the puzzling finding that eukaryotic cells lack topoisomerases that can underwind DNA. It appears that negative superhelicity is, instead, introduced into eukaryotic cells as a result of DNA forming a toroidal wrapping around the histone core of nucleosomes (Figure 14.44). Such wrapping requires the removal of approximately one helical turn in DNA. Initially relaxed DNA subjected to such wrapping will generate a negative toroidal supercoil within the region bound around the histone core and a compensating positive supercoil elsewhere in the molecule, so as to maintain a constant linking number. Subsequent relaxation of the positive supercoil by eukaryotic topoisomerases leaves one net negative supercoil within the nucleosomal region.

Polynucleosomes consist of numerous nucleosomes joined by **"linker" DNA,** the size of which differs among cell types. Usually the nucleosome core is used as the elementary unit for describing the polynucleosome, in which case linker DNA size varies anywhere from about 20 to 90 bp. (Linker sequences would of course be proportionally smaller if the chromatosome were to be used as the elementary unit for the polynucleosome.) Since in addition to the linker sequence approximately 146 ± 1 bp are wrapped around the nucleosome core, the polynucleosome has a minimum nucleosome repeat frequency of about 168 ± 2 bp. Repeat frequencies for nucleosomes are found to depend on both the organism and the organ from which the cell is isolated and, as a rule, they appear to be relatively long in transcriptionally inactive cells. For example, chick erythrocytes have a repeat frequency of 212 bp. Active cells, such as yeast cells that have a frequency of 165 bp, generally have shorter linker sequences.

Periodicity of distribution of nucleosomes along the polynucleosome structure has been determined by controlled digestion with a nuclease that preferentially attacks linker DNA. The digestion pattern suggests the presence of nucleoprotein segments, which on the average contain about 200 bp of DNA or multiples of 200 that result from incomplete digestion. The relationship between size of segments and expected number of nucleosomes associated with them has been confirmed by electron microscopy. With the exception of a small amount of eukaryotic DNA, which is located in mitochondria and chloroplasts and which occurs in the form of small superhelices generally free of protein, all eukaryotic DNA is associated with histones.

Although nucleosomes are periodically positioned along the polynucleosome, their distribution is not random with respect to the base sequence of DNA. DNA does not bend uniformly but rather bends gently and then more sharply around the histone octamers. This suggests that DNA binding is sequence dependent and that **nucleosome positioning** may be influenced by the nucleotide sequence of DNA. In fact, nucleosomes tend to associate preferentially with certain DNA regions. DNA tracts that resist binding, such as long A tracts or G-C repeats, are not usually associated with nucleosomes. In contrast, certain bend DNA regions, for instance, periodically phased A tracts, associate strongly with histones. The majority of nucleosome core particles can relocate over a cluster of positions along the DNA separated by about 10 bp. The resulting mobility of these coil particles probably allows DNA polymerases and other enzymes to gain access to specific DNA sequences. The organization of DNA into nucleosomes appears to have fundamental consequences for transcription and DNA repair.

Polynucleosome Packing into Higher Structures

The wrapping of DNA around histones to form nucleosomes results in a tenfold reduction in the apparent lengths of DNA and the formation of the so-called

10-nm fiber (which is actually 11 nm wide), corresponding to the diameter of the nucleosomes. In chromosomes isolated by very gentle methods, both 10-nm fibers and thicker 30-nm fibers (in fact, 34 nm wide) can be seen in electron micrographs. The relationship between 30-nm fibers and 10-nm fibers has been further confirmed experimentally by the observation that 30-nm fibers can be dissociated into 10-nm fibers by treatment at low ionic strength. The 30-nm fibers appear to form by condensation of 10-nm fibers into a **solenoid arrangement** involving six to seven chromatosomes per solenoid turn (Figure 14.45). **Chromatosomes** are nucleosomes that contain a molecule of H1 histone. This histone is a protein consisting of three different domains that may bind DNA at the ends of the turn and at the point where DNA enters and exits the nucleosome at a ratio of one H1 per nucleosome. Adjacent H1 molecules may also bind to one another cooperatively, bringing the nucleosomes closer together in 30-nm fibers. The formation of the polynucleosome and its subsequent condensation into the 30-nm fibers provides for DNA a compaction ratio that may be as high as two orders of magnitude. The 30-nm fibers form only over selected regions of DNA that are characterized by the absence of binding with other sequence-specific (nonhistone) DNA-binding proteins. The presence of DNA-binding proteins and the effects on formation of 30-nm fibers may depend on the transcriptional status of the regions of DNA involved.

How polynucleosomes are organized into higher structures is not fully understood. Models as to the higher levels of packing of 30-nm fibers are based on indirect evidence obtained from studies of two specialized types of chromosomes—the **lampbrush chromosomes** of vertebrate oocytes and **the polytene chromosomes** of fruitfly giant secretory cells. These chromosomes are exceptional in that they maintain precisely defined higher-order structures in interphase, that is, when cells are in a resting (nondividing) state. The structural features of interphase lampbrush chromosomes have led, by extrapolation, to the proposal that chromosomes in general are organized as a series of looped, condensed domains of 30-nm fibers of variable size for different organisms. It

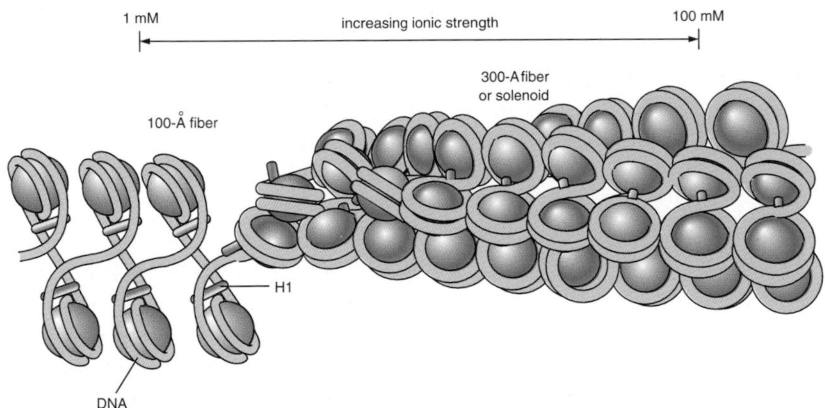

FIGURE 14.45
Nucleofilament structure.
Nucleofilament has the "string of beads" appearance, which corresponds to an extended polynucleosome chain. H1 histone is attached to the "linker" regions between nucleosomes, but in the resulting structure H1 molecules, associated to adjacent nucleosomes, are located close to one another. Furthermore, at higher salt concentrations, polynucleosomes can be transformed into the higher order structure of the 300-Å fiber. It has been proposed that at higher ionic strengths the nucleofilament forms a very compact helical structure or a helical solenoid, as illustrated in the upper part of the figure. H1 histones appear to interact strongly with one another in this structure. In fact, the organization of the 10-nm (100-Å) nucleofilament into the 30-nm (300-Å) coil or solenoid requires, and may be dependent on, the presence of H1.
Adapted from Kornberg, R. D., and Klug, A. The Nucleosome. *San Diego, CA: Academic Press, 1989.*

is estimated that these loops may contain anywhere from 5000 to 120,000 bp with an average of about 20,000. Thus the haploid human genome of 3×10^9 bp would correspond to about 60,000 loops, which is close to the estimated number of genes of 70,000 to 100,000. It appears likely that each loop contains one or a few linked genes. The domains are bound to a nuclear scaffold consisting of H1 histone and several nonhistone proteins, including two major **scaffold proteins Sc1** (a topoisomerase II) and **Sc2.** The loops are fixed at their bases and therefore they can accumulate supercoils. Specific AT-rich regions of DNA known as **SARs (scaffold attachment regions)** are preferentially associated with the scaffold. SARs also contain topoisomerase II binding sites. The presence of type II topoisomerase at the base of closed topological domains, which define the scaffold loops, suggests that supercoiling and supercoiling changes within these domains are biologically important functions. Formation of looped domains may account for as much as an additional 200-fold condensation in the length of DNA and an overall packing ratio of more than four orders of magnitude. Each loop can be coiled and then supercoiled into 0.4 μm of a 30-nm fiber. Since the thickness of a sister chromatid is about 1 μm in diameter, packing of the 20-nm fiber into a chromatid would require just one more order of folding.

The next level of chromosomal organization may therefore involve the packing of loops as suggested in Figure 14.45. The packing may be achieved by arranging the loops of the 30-nm fiber in the form of tightly stacked helical coils. It is speculated that chromatids of metaphase chromosomes consist of helically packed loops of 30-nm fibers. Packing changes, and therefore the transition between the various forms of chromatin, appear to be partially controlled by the covalent modification of core histones. Histones H3 and H4 can undergo cell-cycle-dependent reversible acetylation on the ε-amino group of lysine by two different enzymes, a **histone acetylase** and a **histone deacylase.** Acetylation appears to affect the negative superhelical tension within domains and, in certain instances, the binding of transcription factors. The hydroxyl group of the N-terminal serine residue in histone H4 is subject to phosphorylation catalyzed by a kinase. Acetylation and phosphorylation change the charge of the N-terminal region of histone H4 from +5 to −2. The overall negative charge of the core histones causes histones to bind less tightly to DNA and promotes the unraveling of 30-nm fibers and the decondensation of chromatin. Finally, phosphorylation of terminal H1 correlates with chromosome condensation into metaphase chromosome. This may result from a modulation of affinity between phosphorylated–dephosphorylated H1 with the histone octamer. The change from compact to decondensed chromatin is also promoted by the binding of proteins, known as **HMG proteins (high-mobility-group proteins),** which interact preferentially with the transcriptionally active decondensed form of chromatin, that is, the 10-nm fiber.

Control of eukaryotic transcription and replication apparently involves both histone and nonhistone protein. While dissociation of histones from chromosomal DNA may be a prerequisite for transcription, nonhistone proteins provide more finely tuned transcription controls. Whatever the details of control may be, chromosomal regions actively synthesizing RNA are least condensed, in distinction from the more compacted, inactive regions. **Active genes** must be packaged in a way that makes them accessible to regulatory proteins. At the same time permanently **repressed genes** must remain inaccessible. Packaging may also determine the accessibility of DNA to DNA-damaging agents. Finally, nonhistone proteins control gene expression during differentiation and development and may serve as sites for the binding of hormones and other regulatory molecules.

Viral DNA is almost always complexed with protein, where the function of the protein is generally one of "packaging." In essence the protein protects the DNA from mechanical damage or digestion by endonucleases.

Nucleoproteins of Prokaryotes Are Similar to Those of Eukaryotes

In prokaryotic cells DNA is generally organized as a single chromosome that is a double-stranded circular supercoil. Some bacteria contain more than one chromosome and, in some, chromosomes may have linear structures. Prokaryotes lack histones. Instead, an abundant histone-like protein, the **HU protein,** is apparently responsible for the formation of a "beaded" structure seen in prokaryotes. HU (molecular mass 18 kDa) exists as a heterodimer of two nearly identical subunits (HU-1 and HU-2). Upon binding to DNA, HU changes the shape and the supercoiling of the double helix. The binding of HU to DNA *in vitro,* compacts DNA and restrains supercoils in a concentration-dependent manner and up to an equimolar ratio. This means that the interaction of DNA with HU at an equimolar ratio prevents topoisomerases from relaxing negatively supercoiled DNA in the DNA–HU complex. It also means that HU can introduce restrained supercoils in relaxed DNA. Higher concentrations of HU do not result in the restraining of additional supercoils. From the effects of HU on DNA supercoiling and other evidence, it appears that HU bends DNA sharply into a tight circle. In addition, another abundant small histone-like protein, referred to as **H-NS,** may be involved in chromosomal organization either directly or indirectly through interaction with the HU proteins.

Bacterial chromosomes are organized into compacted structures, called **nucleoids,** by interaction of HU and H-NS proteins and participation of various cations, **polyamines** (such as spermine, spermidine, putrescine, and cadaverine), RNA, and nonhistone proteins. In the case of *E. coli* the nucleoid consists of a single supercoiled DNA molecule organized into about 40 loops, each consisting of approximately 100 kb of DNA, that merge into a scaffold rich in protein and RNA (Figure 14.46). In prokaryotic scaffolds, the loops are maintained by interactions between DNA and RNA rather than DNA–protein interactions only, as is the case with eukaryotes. The genome of *E. coli* consists of about 4.5×10^6 bp, which, if they were straightened as a linear B-DNA, would be 1.5 mm long and therefore 80 times larger than the diameter of the *E. coli* cell. As a result of a nucleoid formation, which has a diameter of only 2 μm, the *E. coli* genome can easily be fitted within the constraints of the cell. Although the nucleoid, in analogy with the chromatin of eukaryotes, is organized in the form of looped domains, the organization of domains within larger compacted structures (chromosomes) that characterize eukaryotes is absent from prokaryotes. Bacterial chromosomes are dynamic structures formed with histone-like proteins, which bind and dissociate fairly rapidly. This may reflect the need for rapid DNA synthesis, cell division, and transcription that characterize bacterial cells. In contrast, histones bind much more stably with eukaryotic DNA and may dissociate only over areas of the genome that are engaged in DNA synthesis, repair, recombination, or transcription.

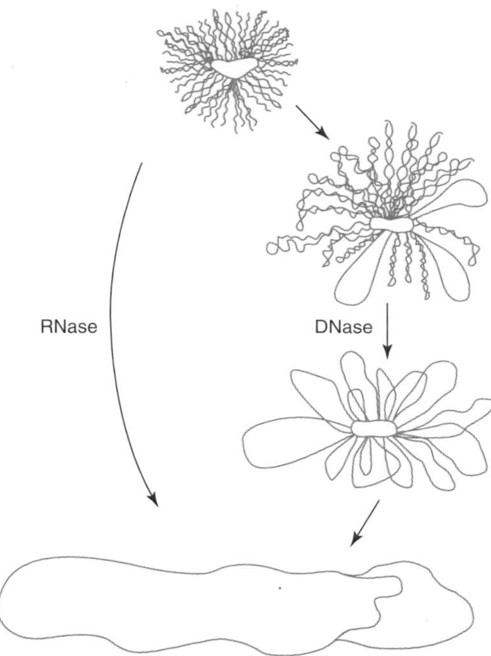

FIGURE 14.46
Schematic depiction of the folded chromosome of *E. coli.*
This chromosome contains about 50 loops of supercoiled DNA organized by a central RNA scaffold. DNase relaxes the structure progressively by opening individual loops, one at a time. RNase completely unfolds the chromosome in a single step.
Redrawn from Worcel, A., and Burgi, E. J. Mol. Biol. *71:127, 1972.*

14.4 ■ DNA STRUCTURE AND FUNCTION

Overall base composition characterizes DNA only in a very general manner. A more specific property, which characterizes any DNA in a unique way, is the nucleotide sequence. Direct determination of nucleotide sequences in DNA remained an intimidating undertaking until the discovery of the restriction endonucleases.

Restriction Endonucleases and Palindromes

Restriction endonucleases cleave DNA chains at a specific sequence, making possible the sectioning of large DNA molecules into small segments. These highly specific bacterial enzymes act by making two cuts, one in each strand

TABLE 14.8 Examples of Sites of Cleavage of DNA by Restriction Enzymes of Various Specificities[a]

Enzyme	*Microorganism*	*Specific Sequence*	*Number of Cleavage Sites for Two Commonly Used Substrates*	
			φX174	*pBR 322*
EcoRI	*E. coli*	-G↓AATT-C- -C-TTAA↓G-	25	9
HaeIII	*Haemophilus aegyptius*	-GG | CC- -CC ↓ GG-	11	22
HpaII	*Haemophilus parainfluenzae*	-C↓CG-G- -G-GC↑C-	5	26
HindIII	*Haemophilus influenzae* Rd.	-A↓AGCT-T- -T-TCGA↑A-	0	1

[a] Cleavage takes place within palindromes. The cleavage sites are indicated by arrows.

of double-stranded DNA of an invading phage, generating 3′-OH and 5′-P termini. This fragmentation exposes phage DNA to eventual degradation by bacterial exonucleases. The terminology for these endonucleases originates from the bacterial sources from which they are isolated. The first three letters of the name is an abbreviation of the species from which the enzyme is isolated. The next letter (or letters) designates the strain of the source and the Roman numeral simply refers to the order in which the enzyme was discovered from the strain. Many hundreds of restriction endonucleases have been isolated in pure form and the list of new restriction enzymes is growing daily. With few exceptions, these enzymes have been found to recognize sequences four to six nucleotides long. These sequences are completely **symmetrical inverted repeats,** known as **palindromes,** as illustrated by the examples listed in Table 14.8. The order of the bases is the same when the two strands of the palindrome are read in opposite directions. For example, in the case of the restriction enzyme EcoR1, isolated from *E. coli,* the order of the bases is GAATTC when read from the 5′ terminus of either of the strands.

Restriction endonucleases are classified into three categories. Types I and III make cuts in the vicinity of the recognition site in a unpredictable manner. Type II specifically cleaves DNA within the recognition sequence. The cuts made by type II enzymes are indicated in Table 14.8 by arrows. Examples of products generated are shown in Figure 14.47.

These enzymes recognize specific sequences that occur along large DNAs with relatively low frequencies and fragment DNA very selectively. For example, a typical bacterial DNA, which may contain about 3×10^6 bp, will be cleaved into a few hundred fragments. A small virus or plasmid may have few or

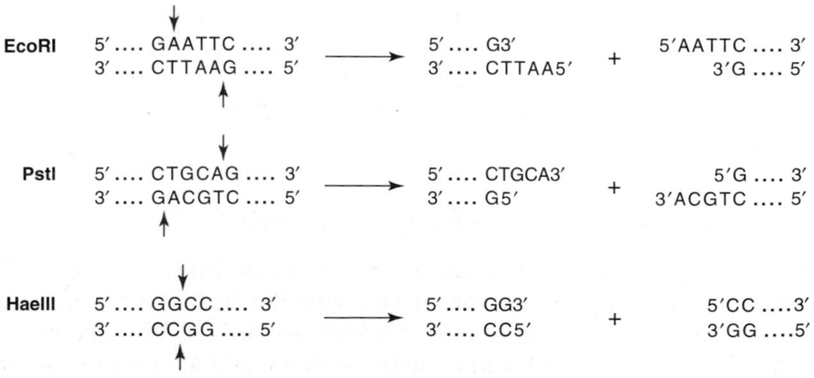

	Substrate		Product 1		Product 2
EcoRI	5′.... G↓AATTC .... 3′ 3′.... CTTAA↑G .... 5′	→	5′.... G3′ 3′.... CTTAA5′	+	5′AATTC .... 3′ 3′G .... 5′
PstI	5′.... CTGCA↓G .... 3′ 3′.... G↑ACGTC .... 5′	→	5′.... CTGCA3′ 3′.... G5′	+	5′G .... 3′ 3′ACGTC .... 5′
HaeIII	5′.... GG↓CC .... 3′ 3′.... CC↑GG .... 5′	→	5′.... GG3′ 3′.... CC5′	+	5′CC ....3′ 3′GG ....5′

FIGURE 14.47
Types of products generated by type II restriction endonucleases.
Enzymes exemplified by EcoRI and PstI nick on both sides of the center of symmetry of the palindrome, generating single-stranded stubs. Commonly used enzymes generate 5′ ends, although some produce stubs with 3′ ends as shown for PstI. Other restriction nucleases cut across the center of symmetry of the recognition sequence, producing flush or blunt ends, as exemplified by HaeIII.

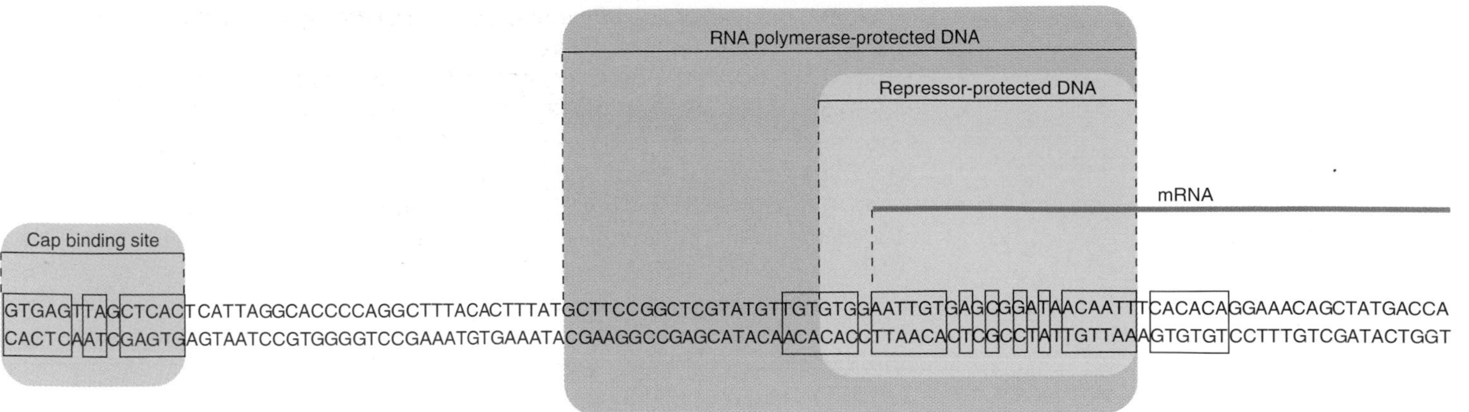

FIGURE 14.48
Nucleotide sequence of part of the DNA segment that controls synthesis of the enzyme β-galactosidase in *E. coli* (the *lac* operon).
The binding regions of the cap protein, which acts as an activator of transcription, and of the lac repressor protein, an inhibitor of transcription, are indicated. Also shown is the region of RNA polymerase interaction. Two palindromic sequences are indicated by boxes.
Redrawn from Cantor, C. R., and Schimmel, P. R. Biophysical Chemistry, Part I. *San Francisco: Freeman, 1980. Copyright © 1980.*

no cutting sites at all for a particular restriction endonuclease. The practical significance of this selectivity of restriction enzymes is that a particular enzyme generates a unique family of fragments for any given DNA molecule. This unique fragmentation pattern is called a **restriction digest.**

The availability of restriction enzymes for sectioning large DNA sequences and the development of new gel electrophoresis techniques for separating DNA segments have made the determination of sequences a simple matter. These sequencing techniques are described in Chapter 18.

Early attempts to determine DNA sequences were limited to small DNA fragments that could easily be separated from the remaining DNA. Sequences that bind selectively with various functional proteins, for example, RNA polymerase and the repressor proteins, were among the first to be determined. The binding protein protects the DNA section over which it is bound from the action of a nuclease and the protected DNA is recovered after digestion and removal of the protein. These studies indicated that many functional proteins and enzymes interact with DNA over regions of palindromic sequence (Figure 14.48).

Palindromes in DNA also serve as recognition sites for **methylases** that modify the host DNA by introducing methyl groups into two bases of the palindrome. Once methylated, these palindromes cannot be recognized by the corresponding restriction enzymes, and the DNA of the host is protected from cleavage.

Contemporary sequencing methods have made possible determination of the complete nucleotide sequences of the DNA of viruses and small bacteria and the partial sequence of many eukaryotic genomes. An ambitious current goal of DNA sequencing is the determination of the sequence of the entire human genome, which consists of almost 3×10^9 bp, and that of several other mammalian organisms.

Most Prokaryotic DNA Codes for Specific Proteins

In prokaryotes a large percentage of total chromosomal DNA codes for specific proteins. Bacterial genomes vary from about 500 kb to over 10,000 kb. More than one-half of the *E. coli* genome has been sequenced. This genome consists of about 4600 kb of DNA and contains as many as 3000 genes. The products of about one-half of *E. coli* genes have already been identified. It is possible that some of the remaining "genes" do not code for expressible functional proteins. Eighty genes code for tRNA molecules.

In an overall sense, *E. coli* DNA is densely packed with sequence information; there is little repetition of information in the genome. As much as 1% of the *E. coli* genome is composed of multiple copies of short repetitive sequences known as **repeated extragenic palindromic elements (REP elements).** REP elements are present at sites of DNA interaction with functional proteins as exemplified by the presence of such elements in the region of initiation of DNA synthesis (referred to as **OriC**). At **OriC, REP** elements with a consensus sequence of 34 nucleotides serve as sites for the binding of topoisomerase II, and REP elements with the sequence GCTGGTGG (**Chi** sites) bind the enzyme **RecBCD,** initiating DNA recombination. **Chi** sites are regularly spaced at intervals separated by about 4 kb.

Genetic information is even more densely organized in smaller organisms, such as bacteriophages, where the primary sequence of DNA reveals that structural genes—nucleotide sequences coding for protein—do not always have distinct physical locations. Rather, they frequently overlap with one another, as illustrated by the partial sequence of bacteriophage ϕX174 shown in Figure 14.49. It is believed that this type of overlap provides for the efficient and

Protein A.......................... Glu Ser Lys Asn Tyr Leu Asp Lys Ala Gly Ile Thr Thr
Origin of protein K Met Ser Arg Lys Ile Ile Leu Ile Lys Gln Glu Leu Leu Leu

Nucleotide sequence....................................... A T G A G T C G A A A A A T T A T C T T G A T A A A G C A G G A A T T A C T A C T
51 61 71 81 91

Ala Cys Leu Arg Ile Lys Ser Lys Trp Thr Ala Gly Gly Lys **Terminus of protein A**
Leu Val Tyr Glu Leu Asn Arg Ser Gly Leu Leu Ala Glu Asn Glu Lys Ile Arg Pro Ile
Origin of protein C Met Arg Lys Phe Asp Leu

G C T T G T T T A C G A A T T A A A T C G G A G T G G A C T G C T G G C G G A A A A T G A G A A A A T T C G A C C T A T
101 111 121 131 141 151

Leu Ala Gln Leu Glu Lys Leu Leu Leu Cys Asp Leu Ser Pro Ser Thr Asn Asp Ser Val
Ser Leu Arg Ser Ser Arg Ser Ser Tyr Phe Ala Thr Phe Arg His Gln Leu Thr Ile Leu

C C T T G C G C A G C T C G A G A A G C T C T T A C T T T G C G A C C T T T C G C C A T C A A C T A A C G A T T C T G T
161 171 181 191 201 211

Lys Asn **Terminus of protein K**
Ser Lys Thr.......................**Protein C continues**

C A A A A A C T ....
219

FIGURE 14.49
Partial nucleotide sequences of contiguous and overlapping genes of bacteriophage ϕX174.
The complete nucleotide sequence of ϕX174 is known. Only the sequence starting with nucleotide 51 and continuing to nucleotide 219 is shown in this figure. This sequence codes for the complete sequence of one of the proteins of ϕX174, protein K. A part of the same sequence, nucleotide 51 to nucleotide 133, codes for part of the nucleotide sequence of another protein, protein A. The sequence coding for protein K, which starts with nucleotide 133, also codes for part of a third protein, protein C. Similar overlaps are noted between other genes of ϕX174.
Adapted with permission from Smith, M. Am. Sci. *67:61, 1979.* Journal of Sigma Xi, *The Scientific Research Society.*

economic utilization of the limited DNA present in these organisms. This arrangement of genes may also be a factor in controlling the sequence in which genes are expressed.

Only a Small Percentage of Eukaryotic DNA Codes for Structural Genes

Eukaryotes have a much larger genome than prokaryotes, from about 1.5×10^7 bp for yeast to about 3.5×10^9 bp for the haploid human genome. The latter contains sufficient DNA to code for nearly 3×10^6 genes. It is estimated, however, that the human genome codes for no more than $70–100 \times 10^3$ genes. As a result, genetic information in the form of genes need not be as densely packed in eukaryotes as in bacteria. A typical mammalian DNA, with only 20 times as many genes as that of *E. coli,* contains 500 times more DNA than *E. coli*. Clearly then, structural genes—that is, genes coding for specific proteins—and sequences used to control gene expression cannot account for the entire DNA content of eukaryotic cells. In fact, only 10% of DNA present in a mammalian cell may suffice for all of its genes that are present. Some of the remaining DNA, such as DNA found in centromeres and telomeres, has well-defined function, but the majority of this uncoding DNA has been referred to as "junk" because no specific function could be assigned to it. However, there is increasing evidence that junk DNA may have a vital role in the regulation of gene expression during development.

Nucleotide sequences indicate that eukaryotic genes not only do not overlap but are instead spaced on the average 40 kb apart. However, some eukaryotic genes may be closer together in regions containing genes that are expressed in a tightly coordinated manner (gene families). As a rule eukaryotic genes are, in addition, interrupted by **intervening nucleotide sequences (IVSs),** called **introns,** as shown in Figure 14.50. The nucleotide sequences in the gene that are expressed, either in the final RNA product (mature RNA) or as a protein, are termed **exons** (see p. 703). The **intervening genomic sequences** (the **introns**), which are expressed in the initial RNA transcript and are considered part of the gene, are removed during the processing of the transcript. The remainder of the message, namely, the **exons,** is then ligated. This tailoring of the original transcript is referred to as **splicing.** The sequence and size of introns vary greatly among species, but generally these intervening segments are very large and, cumulatively, they may be five to ten times the length of the parts of the structural genes they separate. Most genes are interrupted by introns at least once, whereas others are interrupted repeatedly. Some genes, however, such as the gene for human interferon-α, contain no introns.

Introns are common in genes of vertebrates and flowering plants but occur infrequently in the genes of other species. The biological role of introns is not clear. Their presence in eukaryotes may represent a stage in the evolution of the gene, in that introns are rare in prokaryotes and much less common in lower eukaryotes, such as **yeasts.** It has been speculated that introns in eukaryo-

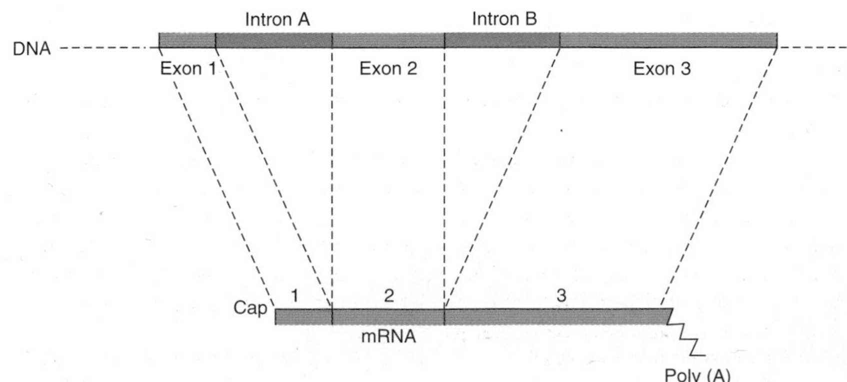

FIGURE 14.50
Schematic presentation of a eukaryotic gene. The top horizontal line represents a part of the DNA genome of a eukaryote: the bottom line represents the mRNA produced by it. In this hypothetical example the DNA consists of two introns and three exons. The intron sequences are transcribed as hnRNA (precursor mRNA) but are not present in mature mRNA.
Redrawn from Crick, F. Science *204:264, 1979. Copyright © 1979 by the American Association for the Advancement of Science.*

tic genes have arisen relatively recently in evolution as a result of migration of certain **mobile DNA elements (transposons)** from other parts of the genome and their insertion into protein-coding genes. These inserts subsequently lost, by mutation, their transposon-like character and therefore their mobility. Some repetitive DNA, such as the DNA found near centromeres and telomeres, may have well-defined structural and/or functional roles. Other repetitive DNA may simply be characterized as a leftover of evolutionary change with no identifiable function.

Repeated Sequences

As distinct from prokaryotes, where repetition of particular DNA sequences is very limited, the DNA of eukaryotes contains nucleotide sequences that are repeated anywhere from a few times, for certain coding genes, to millions of times per genome for certain simple, relatively short, sequences. Repetition of certain types of DNA sequences can be observed directly by electron microscopy, as in rRNA genes undergoing transcription. Depending on the species, **repetitive DNA** may constitute between 3% and 80% of the total DNA. In mammalian genomes, including the human, 25–35% of the DNA is repetitive.

Sequences are classified as **single copy, moderately reiterated,** and **highly reiterated.** The content of single-copy DNA varies among eukaryotes, increasing initially with genome size but reaching a plateau. Repetition classes are defined experimentally from their **rates of reassociation.** Reassociation rates also define a fourth class of DNA, **inverted repeats.**

A distinction between the terms "reiterated" and "repetitive" in describing a DNA sequence needs to be made. The term reiterated is used to describe a unique DNA sequence, usually several hundred nucleotides long, present in multiple copies in a genome. An individual DNA sequence is termed repetitive if a certain, usually short, nucleotide sequence is repeated many times over the DNA sequence.

The genome size of prokaryotic DNA can be determined by fragmenting the DNA, denaturing the fragments, and allowing them to reassociate and form double-stranded molecules. The kinetics of reassociation obey a second-order equation, indicating that essentially all the sequences in the prokaryotic genomes occur as single copies. When a mouse DNA was first studied by this method, unexpected results were obtained, which led to the realization that eukaryotic DNAs contain reiterated sequences. It was assumed that since the mammalian genome is about three orders of magnitude larger than the *E. coli* genome, the rates of reassociation of denatured mammalian DNA would be exceedingly slow. Instead, it turned out that a fraction of the mouse DNA, the highly repetitive fraction, reassociated far more rapidly than DNAs of small viruses. This is reasonable, since the probability that a fragment will encounter a complementary fragment leading to reassociation is proportional to the number of similar sequences repeated in the original DNA. The more reiterated the sequence, the more rapid the reassociation. Consequently, the reassociation kinetics of eukaryotic DNAs provided the first evidence for four classes or sequences. Inverted repeats and the highly repetitive sequences reassociate extremely rapidly. The unique sequences reassociate slowly, and the moderately reiterated at intermediate rates.

Most highly reiterated sequences have a characteristic base composition different from that of the remaining DNA. These sequences can be isolated by shearing the DNA into segments of a few hundred nucleotides each and separating the fragments by density gradient centrifugation. These fragments are termed **satellite DNA** because after centrifugation they appear as satellites of the band of bulk DNA. Other highly reiterated sequences, which cannot be isolated by centrifugation, can be identified by their property of rapid reannealing. Some of the highly reiterated sequences can also be isolated by digestion of total

DNA with restriction endonucleases that cleave at specific sites within the reiterated sequence. The exact boundaries separating the various types of reiterated DNAs do not appear to have been strictly defined.

Single-Copy DNA

About one-half of the human genome is made up of unique nucleotide sequences but, as indicated previously, only a small fraction of these sequences code for specific proteins. A part of the remaining DNA contains **pseudogenes**—that is, tracts of DNA that have significant nucleotide homology to a functional gene but contain mutations that prevent gene expression. These genes, which may be present in a frequency as high as one pseudogene for every four functional genes, significantly increase the size of eukaryotic genomes without contributing to their expressible genetic content. Additional DNA sequences are committed to serve as introns and as regions that are flanking genes.

Moderately Reiterated DNA

This class of DNA includes copies of identical or closely related sequences that are reiterated from a few to a thousand times. These sequences are relatively long, varying between a hundred to many thousand nucleotides before the same polynucleotide sequence is repeated. About 20% of mouse DNA occurs in lengths up to a few hundred base pairs that are repeated more than a thousand times. About 15% of the human genome consists of moderately reiterated DNA. Normally, single-copy and moderately reiterated sequences are present on the chromosome in an orderly pattern known as the **interspersion pattern,** which consists of alternating blocks of single-copy DNA and moderately reiterated DNA. Moderately repetitive sequences are further classified as **short interspersed repeats** that are families of related, but distinct, sequences typically 100–500 bp long and **long interspersed repeats** anywhere from about 100 bp up to several thousand base pairs long. Both short and long repeats are present at 1000 or up to 100,000 copies or more per genome. Long interspersed repeats consist of sequences several thousand nucleotides long that are present at up to 1000 copies per genome. These repeats are flanked on either side of the sequence by DNA sequences that are direct repeats (Figure 14.51). One

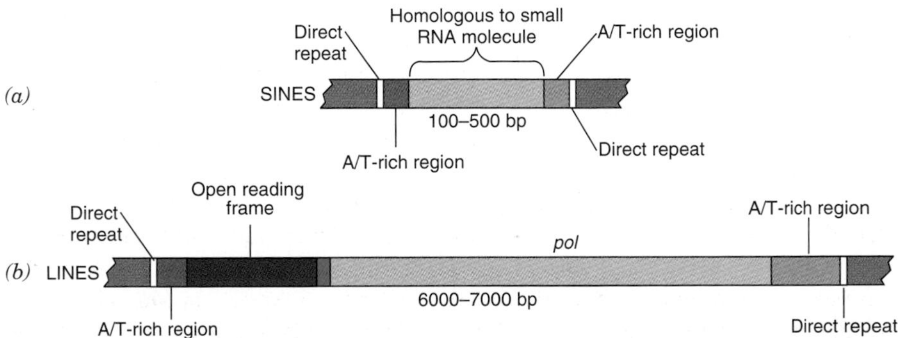

FIGURE 14.51
Short and long interspersed repeats in DNA.
Two types of interspersed repeats, short and long repeats, are found within eukaryotic DNA. (*a*) Short interspersed repeats are sequences 100–500 bp long that are homologous to small RNA molecules such as tRNA, 5SRNA or 7SLRNA (signal recognition particle). The human version of 7SLRNA is referred to as the AU sequence and accounts for approximately 10% of human DNA. (*b*) The long interspersed repeats that are present in hundreds of copies are homologous to tRNA genes and contain open reading frames with additional protein encoding sequences that resemble retroviral genes, such as the *Pol* gene. Both types of interspersed repeats contain short AT-rich sequences at the 3' terminals which are flanked by short direct repeat DNA.

example of a short interspersed repeat is the **Alu** family that constitutes a substantial portion (about 5%) of the human genome. **Alu** sequences consist of approximately 300 bp and are repeated over one-half million times. The structures of the short interspersed repeats, including the **Alu** family, are reminiscent of mobile DNA elements (transposons). The function of the **Alu** family remains to be established.

Interspersed repeats may have arisen during evolution from viruses or other transportable DNA elements that have been duplicated repeatedly and inserted into various locations within the chromosome. If this is the case, then short interspersed repeats would be nothing more than an evolutionary relic that performs no useful function for the host cell. On the assumption that this premise is correct, short interspersed repeats have been called "selfish DNA."

The interspersion pattern implicates the moderately reiterated sequences in control of transcription of structural genes since the large majority of structural genes are adjacent to reiterated sequences. A different type of moderately reiterated sequence occurs in the form of segregated tandem arrays. The two distinct types of arrangements of the moderately reiterated sequences appear to relate to different functions for these sequences. **Tandem arrays** are used for synthesis of products that must be rapidly generated in numerous copies, such as ribosomal RNA and certain proteins of specialized function. For example, in sea urchin oocyte histone, genes are amplified so that sufficient amounts of histone are available during the rapid cycles of DNA replication that follow fertilization. The genes for the five histones are arranged in tandemly repeated clusters, with each histone gene separated from its neighbor in the cluster by spacers about 400–900 nucleotides long. These spacers are AT-rich and can be separated as satellite DNA from the GC-rich DNA of the histone genes.

Single-copy and moderately repetitive sequences together normally account for more than 80% of the total nucleotide content of the eukaryotic genomes.

Highly Reiterated DNA

The remaining DNA consists of sequences constructed by the repetition, many thousand or even a million times, of a nucleotide sequence that is typically shorter than 20 nucleotides. About 10% of mouse DNA consists of 10-bp repeats that are reiterated millions of times in each cell. Because of the manner in which they are constructed, **highly reiterated DNAs** are also referred to as simple sequence DNA. Simple sequences are typically present in the DNA of most, if not all, eukaryotes. In some only one major type of simple sequence may be present. Thus in the rat the sequence 5′-GCACAC-3′ is repeated every six bases. In other eukaryotes several simple sequences are repeated up to one million times. Some considerably longer repeat units for simple sequence DNA have also been identified. For instance, in the genome of the African green monkey a 172-bp segment is highly repeated and there are few sequence repetitions within the segment. Because of its characteristic composition, simple sequence DNA can often be isolated as satellite DNA. Satellite DNA found in the centromeres of higher eukaryotes consists of thousands of tandem copies of one or a few short sequences. **Satellite sequences** have been found to be only 5–10 bp long. Simple sequence (satellite) DNA is also a constituent of telomeres where it has a well-defined role in DNA replication.

Inverted Repeat DNA

Inverted repeats are a structural motif of **dos DNA.** Short inverted repeats, consisting of up to six nucleotides, such as the palindromic sequence GAATTC, occur by chance about once for every 3000 nucleotides. Such short repeats cannot form a stable "hairpin" structure formed by longer palindromic sequences. Inverted repeat sequences that are long enough to form stable **"hair-**

CLINICAL CORRELATION 14.7

Mutations of Mitochondrial DNA: Aging and Degenerative Diseases

Somatic mutations, such as deletions of bases or oligonucleotide segments from mtDNA, are generated by oxygen damage during the life span of an individual. Somatic mutations in mtDNA are acquired at a much higher rate than in nuclear DNA. They are responsible for disorders associated with the process of oxidative phosphorylation and they may also be involved in aging and the development of degenerative diseases.

MtDNA mutations are the cause of Leber hereditary optic neuropathy (LHON). This disease, which is maternally inherited, is characterized by loss of vision in early adulthood, as a result of optic nerve degeneration. One mutation, an Arg to His substitution that leads to this disease, has been traced to a gene coding for NADH dehydrogenase (Complex I). The mutation results in mitochondria that are partially defective in electron transfer from NADH to ubiquinone and have a reduced capacity of ATP synthesis needed to support the active metabolic needs of neurons. LHON can also result from a single base change in the mitochondrial gene coding for cytochrome *b*. A mutation of the mitochondrial gene coding for a tRNA is responsible for myoclonic epilepsy and ragged-red-fiber disease (MERRF). This genetic disease, which is characterized by uncontrollable muscular jerking, is apparently caused by inadequate production of proteins that depend on mitochondrial transfer RNAs for their synthesis.

Deletions and rearrangements in mtDNA are noted with aging in both humans and mice. Five different mtDNA deletions have been noted with aged mice but these deletions are absent from young mice. The deletions involve a small portion (less than 0.01%) of total mtDNA. The deletion of a large portion of mtDNA (a 4977-bp segment), which is the most frequently noted DNA abnormality in patients with mitochondrial myopathies, is also noted, although to a much lesser degree, in tissues of healthy aging individuals.

The observations that mtDNA is easily mutated and poorly repaired have led to speculation that aging may be correlated with accumulation of somatic mutations in mtDNA. However, both environmental and genetic factors probably affect the aging process and aging is not likely to be explained solely as the result of defective mtDNA function.

Tanhauser, S. M., and Laipis, P. J. Multiple deletions are detectable in mtDNA of aging mice. *J. Biol. Chem.* 270:24769, 1995.

pins" are not likely to occur by chance, and therefore they should be classified as a separate class of eukaryotic sequences. Short repeats can easily be detected and quantitated on the basis of their extremely rapid rates of reassociation. In human DNA, about two million inverted repeats are present, with an average length of about 200 bp, although inverted sequences longer than 1000 bp have been detected. Some of these repeats may be separated by a spacer sequence that is not part of the inverted repeat. Most inverted repeat sequences are repeated 1000 or more times per cell.

Mitochondrial DNA

The **DNA of mitochondria (mtDNA)** is a small double-stranded circular structure of approximately 16,500 bp. In mammals, mtDNA makes up about 1% of total cellular DNA. Mitochondria contain multiple copies of DNA, usually distributed within several clusters. It is not known how this DNA is packaged but its structure probably resembles that of a bacterial chromosome rather than eukaryotic chromatin. The sequence of human mtDNA consists of 16,569 bp and contains 37 genes. Thirteen genes code for proteins that are subunits for factors essential for the maintenance of mitochondrial ATP synthesis. The remaining 24 genes code for mitochondria-specific RNAs, two ribosomal and 22 transfer RNAs.

The rate of mutation is one order of magnitude greater in the mitochondrial genome as compared to the nuclear genome. These high rates of mutation probably reflect a low fidelity of DNA replication, DNA repair, or both. Mitochondrial genes are maternally inherited because mitochondria from the sperm cells do not enter the fertilized egg. The effects of mtDNA mutations are discussed in Clin. Corr. 14.7.

BIBLIOGRAPHY

Bates, A. D. *DNA Topology*. Oxford, England: IRL Press, 1993.

Binden, R. R. *DNA Structure and Function*. San Diego, CA: Academic Press, 1994.

Borisova, O. F., Golova, Y. B., Gottikh, B. P., et al. Parallel double stranded helices and the tertiary structure of nucleic acids. *J. Biomol. Struct. Dyn.* 8:1187, 1991.

Bouffler, S., Silver, A., and Cox, R. The role of DNA repeats and associated secondary structures in genomic instability and neoplasia. *Bioessays* 15:409, 1993.

Bray, A. B., Lewis, J., Raff, M., Roberts, K., and Watson, J. D. *Molecular Biology of the Cell,* New York: Garland, 1994.

Calladine, C., and Drew, H. *Understanding DNA—The Molecule and How It Works*. San Diego, CA: Academic Press, 1992.

Clark, D. J., and Felsenfeld, G. Formation of nucleosomes on positively supercoiled DNA. *EMBO J.* 10:387, 1991.

Clayton, D. A. Replication and transcription of vertebrate mitochondrial DNA. *Annu.-Rev. Cell Biol.* 7:453, 1991.

Cortopassi, G., and Liu, Y. Genotypic selection of mitochondrial and oncogenic mutations in human tissue suggests mechanisms of age-related pathophysiology. *Mutat. Res.* 338:151, 1995.

Cozzarelli, N. R., Boles, T. C., and White, J. H. Primer on the topology and geometry of DNA supercoiling. In: N. R. Cozzarelli and J. C. Wang (Eds.), *DNA Topology and Its Biological Effects.* Cold Spring Harbor, NY: Cold Spring Harbor Laboratory Press, 1990.

De Vries, J. E., and de Waal Malefyt, R. *Therapeutic Applications of Oligonucleotides*. New York: Demos Vermande, 1995.

Drake, J. W. Spontaneous mutation. *Annu. Rev. Genet.* 25:125, 1991.

Drlica, K., and Riley, M. *The Bacterial Chromosome.* Washington, DC: American Society for Microbiology, 1990.

Drlica, K. Bacterial topoisomerases and the control of DNA supercoiling. *Trends Genet.* 6:433, 1990.

Drlica, K. Control of bacterial DNA supercoiling. *Mol. Microbiol.* 6:425, 1992.

Getzenberg, R. H., Pienta, K. J., Ward, W. S., and Coffey, D. S. Nuclear structure and the three-dimensional organization of DNA. *J. Cell. Biochem.* 47:289, 1991.

Han, J., Hsu, C., Zhu, Z., Longshore, J. W., and Finley, W. H. Over-representation of the disease associated (CAG) and (CGG) repeats in the human genome. *Nucleic Acids Res.* 22:1735, 1994.

Haran, T. E., Kahn, J. D., and Crothers, D. M. Sequence elements responsible for DNA curvature. *J. Mol. Biol.* 244:135, 1994.

Hardin, C. C., Henderson, E., Watson, T., and Prosser, J. K. Monovalent cation induced structural transitions in telomeric DNAs: G-DNA folding intermediates. *Biochemistry* 30:4460, 1991.

Kamenetskii, F. *Unraveling DNA*. New York: VCH, 1993.

Kim, M. G., Zhurkin, V. B., Jernigan, R. L. and Camerini-Otero, R. D. Probing the structure of a putative intermediate in homologous recombination: the third strand in the parallel DNA triplex is in contact with the major groove of the duplex. *J. Mol. Biol.* 247:874, 1995.

Leach, D. R. Long DNA palindromes, cruciform structures, genetic instability and secondary structure repair. *Bioessays* 16:893, 1994.

Lebowitz, J. Through the looking glass: the discovery of supercoiled DNA. *Trends Biochem. Sci.* 15:202, 1990.

Lee, M. S., and Garrard, W. T. Positive DNA supercoiling generates a chromatin conformation characteristic of highly active genes. *Proc. Natl. Acad. Sci. USA* 88:9675, 1991.

Lewin, B. *Genes V.* New York: Oxford University Press, 1994.

Lindsten, J., and Pettersson, U. *Etiology of Human Disease at the DNA Level.* New York: Raven Press, 1991.

Luzio, J. P., and Thompson, R. J. In: *Molecular Medical Biochemistry,* New York: Cambridge University Press, 1990.

Mitas, M., Yu, A., Dill, J., Kamp, T. J., Chambers, E. J., Haworth, I. S. Hairpin properties of single-stranded DNA containing a GC-rich triplet repeat: $(CTG)_{15}$. *Nucleic Acids Res.* 23:1050, 1995.

Neidle, S. *DNA Structure and Recognition,* 1st ed. Oxford, England: IRL Press, 1994.

Orphanides, G., and Maxwell, A. Topoisomerases. In one gate, out the other. *Curr. Biol.* 4:1006, 1994.

Owen-Hughes, T., and Workman, J. L. Experimental analysis of chromatin function in transcription control. *Crit. Rev. Eukaryot. Gene Expr.* 4:403, 1994.

Ozawa, T. Mitochondrial DNA mutations associated with aging and degenerative diseases. *Exp. Gerontol.* 30:269, 1995.

Saluz, H. P., and Wiebauer, K. *DNA and Nucleoprotein Structure in Vivo.* New York: Demos Vermande, 1995.

Soyfer, V. N., and Potaman, V. N. *Triple-Helical Nucleic Acids*. New York: Springer-Verlag, 1995.

Therman, E., and Susman, M. In: *Human Chromosomes, Structure, Behavior and Function,* 3rd ed. New York: Springer-Verlag, 1992.

Trinh, T. Q., and Sinden, R. R. Preferential DNA secondary structure mutagenesis in the lagging strand of replication in *E. coli. Nature* 352:544, 1991.

Trinh, T. Q., and Sinden, R. R. The influence of primary and secondary DNA structure in deletion and duplication between direct repeats in *Escherichia coli. Genetics* 134:409, 1993.

Turner, B. M. Histone acetylation and control of gene expression. *J. Cell. Sci.* 99:13, 1991.

Ussery, D. W., and Sinden, R. R. Environmental influences on the in vivo level of intramolecular triplex DNA in *Escherichia coli. Biochemistry* 32:6206, 1993.

Van Holde, K. E. *Chromatin*. New York: Springer-Verlag, 1989.

Vologodskii, A. V., and Cozzarelli, N. R. Conformational and thermodynamic properties of supercoiled DNA. *Annu. Rev. Biophys. Biomol. Struct.* 23:609, 1994.

Wang, C. I., and Taylor, J. S. Site-specific effect of thymine dimer formation on $dA_n \cdot dT_n$ tract bending and its biological implications. *Proc. Natl. Acad. Sci. USA* 88:9072, 1991.

Wolfe, S. L. *Molecular and Cellular Biology,* Belmont, CA: Wadsworth, 1993.

Wolffe, A. *Chromatin Structure and Function*. San Diego, CA: Academic Press, 1992.

Yu, H., Etitja, R., Bloom, L. B., and Goodman, M. F. Ionization of bromouracil and fluorouracil stimulates base mispairing frequencies with guanine. *J. Biol. Chem.* 268:15935, 1993.

QUESTIONS C. N. ANGSTADT AND J. BAGGOTT

1. A polynucleotide is a polymer in which:
   A. the two ends are structurally equivalent.
   B. the monomeric units are joined together by phosphodiester bonds.
   C. there are at least 20 different kinds of monomers that can be used.
   D. the monomeric units are not subject to hydrolysis.
   E. purine and pyrimidine bases are the repeating units.

2. The best definition of an endonuclease is an enzyme that hydrolyzes:
   A. a nucleotide from only the 3′ end of an oligonucleotide.
   B. a nucleotide from either terminal of an oligonucleotide.
   C. a phosphodiester bond located in the interior of a polynucleotide.
   D. a bond only in a specific sequence of nucleotides.
   E. a bond that is distal (d) to the base that occupies the 5′ position of the bond.

3. All of the following tend to favor a helical conformation of a single polynucleotide chain EXCEPT:
   A. hydrophobic interactions of the rings of the purine and pyrimidine bases that exclude water.
   B. interchange of electrons in the π orbitals of the purine and pyrimidine bases.
   C. charge–charge repulsion of phosphate residues of the polynucleotide backbone.
   D. hydrogen bonding between appropriate purine–pyrimidine pairs.
   E. spacing of bases in the helical conformation that excludes water.

4. In a DNA double helix:
   A. the individual strands are not helical.
   B. hydrogen bonds form between a purine and a pyrimidine base on the same strand.
   C. adenine on one strand is hydrogen-bonded to thymine on the opposite strand.
   D. phosphodiester bonds are oriented toward the interior of the helix.
   E. the outside of the helix is neutral.

5. The A helix of DNA differs from the B helix in all of the following EXCEPT:
   A. appearance of the major and minor grooves.
   B. pitch of the base pairs relative to the helix axis.
   C. thickness of the helix.
   D. tilt of the bases.
   E. polarity of the strands.

6. The Z DNA helix:
   A. has fewer base pairs per turn than the B DNA.
   B. is favored by an alternating GC sequence.
   C. tends to be found at the 3′ end of genes.
   D. is inhibited by methylation of the bases.
   E. is a permanent conformation of DNA.

Use the accompanying figure to answer Questions 7 and 8.

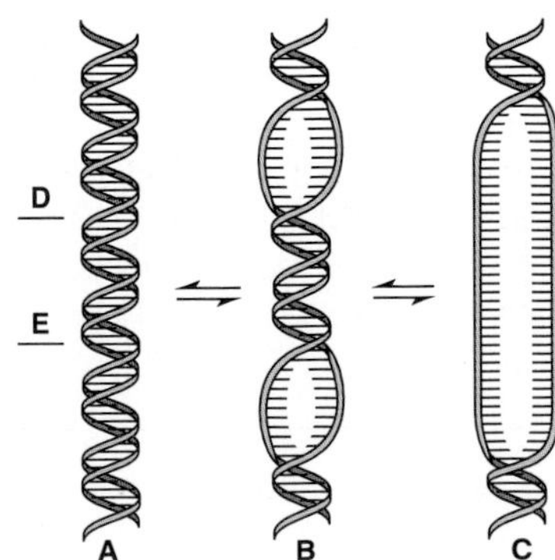

7. A, B, and C represent conformations at different temperatures. Which one represents the highest temperature?

8. Which section, D or E, has the higher content of guanine and cytosine?

Refer to the following for Questions 9–11.
A. annealing
B. electrophoresis
C. equilibrium centrifugation
D. C_0t curves

9. A technique for determining the molecular weight of large (10^5 to 10^9 Da) DNA.

10. A technique involved in locating a specific gene on DNA with a probe.

11. A technique for assessing genome complexity.

12. The superhelices that form in double-stranded circular DNA:
   A. may have fewer turns of the helix per unit length than does a linear double helix.
   B. are associated with a restricted topological domain.
   C. may exist in multiple conformations that are interconvertible without breaking covalent bonds.
   D. may be either formed or relaxed by enzymes called topoisomerases.
   E. all of the above are correct.

13. Triple-stranded DNA:
   A. generally occurs in DNA in regions that play no role in transcription.
   B. involves the formation of Hoogsteen pairs.
   C. is characterized by the presence of a string of alternating purine–pyrimidine bases.
   D. forms only intermolecularly.
   E. assumes a cruciform conformation.

Using the accompanying figure to answer Questions 14–16.

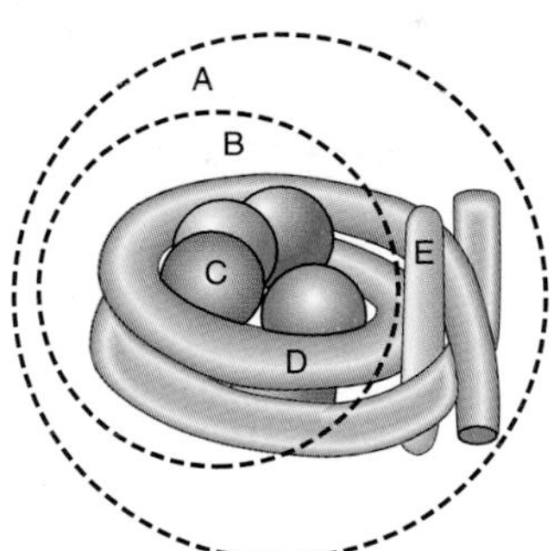

14. A chromatosome.

15. DNA.

16. H1 class of histones.

17. A palindrome is a sequence of nucleotides in DNA that:
   A. is highly reiterated.
   B. is part of the introns of eukaryotic genes.
   C. is a structural gene.
   D. has local symmetry and may serve as a recognition site for various proteins.
   E. has the information necessary to confer antibiotic resistance in bacteria.

18. An interspersion pattern in DNA consists of:
    A. highly repetitive DNA sequences.
    B. the portion of DNA composed of single copy DNA.
    C. Alu sequences.
    D. alternating blocks of single copy DNA and moderately repetitive DNA.
    E. alternating blocks of short interspersed repeats and long interspersed repeats.

ANSWERS

1. B A: The structure of a polynucleotide possesses an intrinsic sense of direction that does not depend on whether a 3′-OH or 5′-OH terminal is esterified. C and E: There are only four different monomers, and the repeating unit is the base monophosphate (p. 566).
2. C Both A and B describe exonucleases. D does refer to an endonuclease but only to a specific type, a restriction endonuclease, and is therefore not a definition of the general type. E: Both endo- and exonucleases show specificity toward the bond hydrolyzed and so this is not a definition of an endonuclease (p. 568).
3. D This is very important in holding two different polynucleotide chains together, but it is unlikely that the proper positioning would occur within a single chain. A, B, C, and E: The exclusion of water by stacking of the bases is a strong stabilizing force that is enhanced by the interaction of π orbital electrons. The repulsive forces of the phosphate groups confer a certain rigidity to the structure (pp. 568–569).
4. C This results in complementarity of the strands. A: Single strands are right-handed helices. B: Bases in a single stand interact through the hydrophobic faces of the rings. D and E: The phosphate groups are negative and on the exterior of the helix (p. 580).
5. E The two strands are always antiparallel. A: The A helix has a narrower and deeper major groove and a wider and shallower minor groove than B. B and D: Bases in the B helix are almost perpendicular to the helix axis while those in A are tilted. C: The B helix is thinner than the A (pp. 570–573).
6. B The alternating purine–pyrimidine sequence is important. A: Z DNA is longer and thinner than the B form because it has 12 bp per turn instead of 10. C: It is more likely to be found at the 5′ end, consistent with one of its proposed roles in transcriptional regulation. D: Methylation favors the Z form in which the methyl is protected from water. E: B $\rightarrow$ Z transition is influenced by such things as methylation and rotation of the G to the syn conformation (p. 574).
7. C; 8. E. The figure represents the process of denaturation with the extent of disruption increasing as temperature increases. Since a guanine–cytosine pair has three hydrogen bonds and an adenine–thymine pair only has two, higher temperatures are required to disrupt regions high in G-C (Figure 14.14).
9. C Equilibrium centrifugation is a method for determining molecular weight, but it is limited to a molecular weight of 10^9 Da or less because of the effects of shear forces on large molecules (p. 586).
10. A The probe is a labeled polynucleotide with a sequence complementary to the gene of interest. Annealing of the two permits location of the gene (pp. 580 and 582).
11. D Frequency of reassociation is dependent on amounts of highly reiterated versus unique sequences (p. 580).
12. E A describes a negative superhelix. There may also be more turns per unit length in a positive superhelix. B: Once a closed system is interrupted, a superhelix can unwind. C: All conformations with the same linking number L are interconvertible without breaking covalent bonds. D: Topoisomerase I (omega protein) from *E. coli* relaxes and gyrase (topoisomerase II) can introduce or remove superhelices (depending on the conditions) (pp. 587–592).
13. B Hoogsteen pairs, like TAT or GGC, are responsible for holding the third strand in the major groove. A: They are found frequently in regions involved in gene regulation. C: The required sequence is a homopurine string. D: They can also form intramolecularly by unfolding and refolding of the DNA. E: A cruciform is an alternate conformation of DNA but does not involve a third strand (pp. 595 and 597).
14. A; 15. D; 16. E. The chromatosome, the basic structural element of nucleoprotein, contains the nucleosome core with associated H1 histones. B: The nucleosome core is a discrete particle consisting of an octamer of specific histones with a segment of DNA wrapped around it. D: The strand depicted represents DNA; the circles, histones. E: The H1 class of histones is bound to the spacer regions between nucleosomes. C: Represents one of the histones (H2A, H2B, H3, or H4), which are part of the nucleosomes (Figure 14.43).
17. D A palindrome, by definition, reads the same forward and backward. Short palindromic segments of DNA are recognized by a variety of proteins such as restriction endonucleases and CAP-binding protein. A is not likely since it would be incompatible with specific recognition. B is possible but has not been shown. C is not correct since genes are thousands of base pairs in length, whereas palindromes are short segments. E also would not be likely because palindromes are too short (p. 610).
18. D A and B: These are two of several kinds of DNA but do not constitute patterns. C and E: Alu is a type of short interspersed repeat. Short and long interspersed repeats are the two classes of moderately repetitive DNA (p. 615).

CHAPTER

DNA II: REPAIR, SYNTHESIS, AND RECOMBINATION

Stelios Aktipis

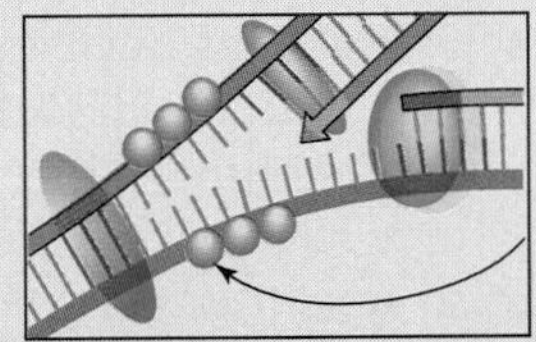

15.1 ■ OVERVIEW

Although the processes of DNA repair, DNA synthesis, and DNA recombination are presented in a somewhat independent and self-contained manner, in reality DNA repair, synthesis, and recombination are intimately connected and interdependent. Furthermore, these DNA-directed processes are also closely associated with other DNA-dependent operations and more specifically DNA transcription reviewed in Chapter 16. Some of these interconnections are indicated in this chapter. The first area to be examined is the enzymatic repair of randomly induced changes in the chemical structure of the DNA bases. A review of the processes of DNA synthesis and DNA recombination completes the chapter.

Both the repair of DNA and particularly the replication of DNA are very complex processes. Although key similarities in the mechanisms of DNA repair are discernible among different organisms, a considerable amount of diversity exists in terms of individual detail. The same is true regarding the process of DNA synthesis. This diversity defeats any attempt to present a simplified and universally applicable model of these processes. To resolve this difficulty the basic elements of the substeps of each process are first described and subsequently integrated for prokaryotes, using as an example the *Escherichia coli* replication system. Eukaryotic replication is treated separately and its similarities and differences with prokaryotic replication are highlighted.

15.2 ■ FORMATION OF THE PHOSPHODIESTER BOND *IN VIVO*

DNA-Dependent DNA Polymerases of *E. coli*

An apparent common denominator between the processes of DNA replication and repair is the enzymatically catalyzed synthesis of DNA polynucleotide segments, which can be assembled with preexisting polynucleotides, leading to repair or replication. Synthesis of these polynucleotide segments is catalyzed by a family of enzymes, **DNA-dependent DNA polymerases.** In the case of *E. coli,* DNA polymerase has been isolated in three distinct forms, polymerases I, II, and III as listed in Table 15.1. All DNA polymerases have a $3' \rightarrow 5'$ exonuclease activity in addition to the synthetic activities. Polymerase I also has a $5' \rightarrow 3'$ exonuclease activity. Generally speaking, polymerase III is involved in DNA synthesis and polymerase I is involved in both synthesis and repair. Polymerase II is also involved in DNA repair but its function is highly specialized.

TABLE 15.1 Properties of DNA Polymerases I, II, and III of *E. coli*

	Pol I	*Pol II*	*Pol III (core)*
Function			
Polymerization: $5' \rightarrow 3'$	Yes	Yes	Yes
Exonuclease: $3' \rightarrow 5'$	Yes	Yes	Yes
Exonuclease: $5' \rightarrow 3'$	Yes	No	No
Size (kDa)	103	90	(167, 130, 27.5, 10)[a]
Molecules per cell	400	—	10–20
Turnover number[b]	600	30	9000
Structural genes	*polA*	*polB*	*polC*[c]

Source: Adapted from Kornberg, A., and Baker, T. A. *DNA Replication,* 2nd ed. New York: Freeman, 1992.

[a] Sizes of the α, ε, and θ subunits.

[b] Nucleotides polymerized at 37°C/min/molecule of enzyme.

[c] Also known as dnaE, the gene for the large (α) subunit.

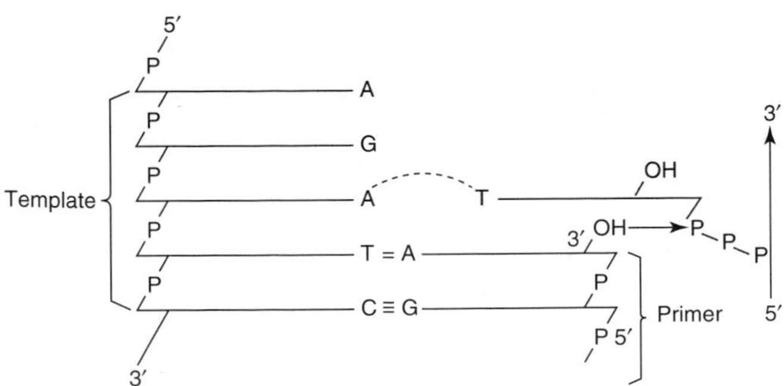

FIGURE 15.1
Synthetic activity of DNA polymerase.
DNA polymerase catalyzes polymerization of nucleotides in the $5' \rightarrow 3'$ direction. A phosphodiester bond is formed between a free 3′-hydroxyl group of the strand undergoing elongation (the primer) and an incoming deoxyribonucleoside 5′-triphosphate. Pyrophosphate is eliminated.
Redrawn based on figure in Kornberg, A. Science *163:1410, 1969. Copyright 1969 by the American Association for the Advancement of Science.*

Synthetic Activity

Figure 15.1 shows two complementary DNA strands of unequal length in which the shorter strand has a free 3′ terminus. DNA polymerase catalyzes addition of 5′-deoxynucleoside triphosphates to the 3′ terminus of the short strand, called the **primer.** The term primer applies to the terminus of a molecule, in this instance the 3′-polynucleotide end, onto which additional monomeric units can be added. The free portion of the longer complementary strand is the **template** that directs the condensation of selected 5′-deoxynucleotides onto the growing primer. The template is a single strand of nucleic acid providing the specific information necessary for the synthesis of a complementary strand. DNA polymerase requires both a primer and a template in order to function.

As seen from Table 15.2, polymerase III catalyzes the elongation of a primer with a much higher degree of efficiency than polymerase I. The enhanced catalytic efficiency of polymerase III is partially attributable to the higher **processivity** of this enzyme. After a polymerase has added a nucleotide residue on the 3′-OH terminus of the primer, it may dissociate from the primer and bind at random to another partially completed polynucleotide chain, or it may remain bound to the original template until many subsequent residues are added to it. Enzymes that tend to remain bound to their substrates through many rounds of polymerization are said to be processive. Polymerase I is less processive in that it tends to dissociate from the template after incorporating only a few nucleotides. Although processivity *per se* does not determine the catalytic rate, it is apparent that an enzyme with high catalytic activity, such as polymerase III, can achieve its optimal catalytic rate only if it is also highly processive.

DNA polymerases permit selection of 5′-deoxyribonucleoside triphosphates, one at a time, with a base complementary to that present in the corre-

TABLE 15.2 Major Subunits and Subassemblies of DNA Polymerase III

Subunit	*Mass (kDa)*	*Gene*		*Function*
α	130[a]	*dnaE*	Pol III (core)	Polymerase
ε	27.5[a]	*dnaQ* (*mutD*)		$3' \rightarrow 5'$ exonuclease
θ	10			α, ε assembly?
τ	71[a]	*dnaX*	γ Complex	Assembly of holoenzyme on DNA
γ	47.5[a]	*dnaX*		Part of the γ complex
δ	35	*holA*		(Enhances processivity; assists in replisome assembly)
δ'	33	*holB*		
χ	15	*holC*		
ψ	12	*holD*		
β	40.6[a]	*dnaN*		Sliding clamp, processivity

Source: Adapted from Kornberg, A., and Baker, T. A. *DNA Replication,* 2nd ed. New York: Freeman, 1992.
[a] Subunits γ, δ, δ', χ, and ψ form the so-called γ complex responsible for adding β subunits to DNA.

(a)

Keto Ionized

5-Bromodeoxyuracil (5-BrdU)

Ionized

2-Aminopurine

(b)

5-BrdU • Adenine

5-BrdU(ionized) • Guanine

Thymine • 2-Aminopurine

Cytosine • 2-Aminopurine (ionized)

sponding position of the template. The specificity of the polymerase reaction with respect to the template is vested in the strong association of each of the bases of the template with their normal complementary partners present in the cell as free 5′-deoxyribonucleotides. Strong binding between complementary bases is apparently achieved because the bases become confined within custom-fitted cages created by appropriate hydrophobic regions of the DNA polymerase. As a result, the reading of the template is accurate but not completely free of error. Ionized forms of the bases apparently promote **mispairing** during DNA synthesis. As an example, 5-bromodeoxyuracil pairs with guanine when present in an ionized form, as shown in Figure 15.2, instead of its normal partner, adenine. In this instance, the hydroxyl group at C-4 upon loss of a proton acquires a negative charge and changes the hydrogen-bonding properties of 5-bromouracil. Similarly, 2-aminopurine, which normally pairs with thymine in its ionized form, may mispair with cytosine. The natural bases can also undergo ionizations, giving rise to a number of alternative base pairing schemes that produce atypical base pairs leading to misincorporation of bases.

Proofreading Activity

The presence of ionized bases accounts for the incorporation into DNA of inappropriate bases at a ratio of about 1 per 10^4 to 10^5 nucleotide incorporations. Yet, the experimentally measured misincorporation of nucleotides is lower and it does not exceed an error rate of 10^{-8}. The discrepancy is accounted for by the existence of a **"proofreading"** mechanism that allows removal, by the polymerase, of erroneously introduced nucleotides. The removal is carried out by the 3′ → 5′ exonuclease activity that characterizes almost every known polymerase, suggesting that proofreading is essential for accurate DNA synthesis. Because of this activity, polymerases can temporarily reverse their synthetic activities and function as exonucleases. The proofreading activity is triggered when a mismatch between the template base sequence and a newly introduced nucleotide at the 3′-OH terminus of the primer occurs. However, some polymerases ensure that a very large percentage of mismatched bases are removed by inadvertently removing a substantial percentage of correctly introduced bases as well. Overall, proofreading fails to remove less than 1 in 10^3 improperly incorporated nucleotides.

Structure of Polymerases

Recall that **polymerase I** has three distinct enzyme activities, namely, a 5′ → 3′ synthetic activity and 3′ → 5′ and 5′ → 3′ exonuclease activities. Chemical and mutation studies of the enzyme have shown that these activities originate from three distinct active sites on the enzyme. Cleavage of polymerase I by the protease subtilisin leads to the formation of a small fragment (30-kDa mass) with 5′ → 3′ activity and a larger fragment (70-kDa mass), known as the **Klenow fragment,** having the synthetic activity (5′ → 3′ polymerization) and 3′ → 5′ exonuclease activity, which is required for **proofreading** during DNA synthesis. X-ray diffraction studies, on cocrystals of DNA and polymerase I, suggest that DNA makes a sharp bend between the 3′ → 5′ exonuclease site and the synthetic

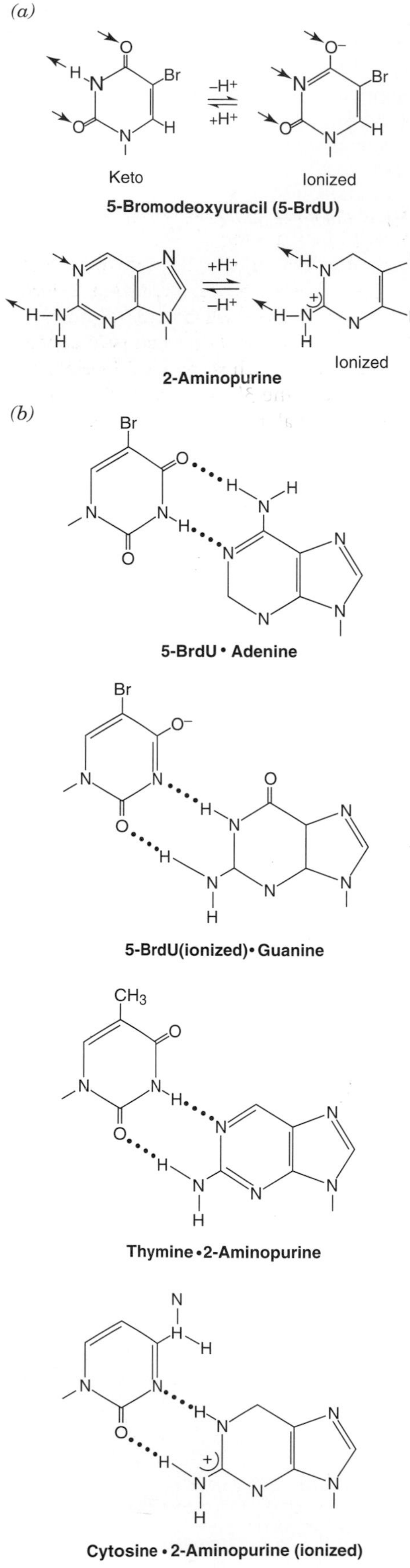

FIGURE 15.2
DNA base pairing of ionized forms of bases.
Ionization of 5′-bromodeoxyuracil (BrdU), a base analog of T, results in dissociation of a proton from the N-3 position of the pyrimidine ring whereas ionization of 2-aminopurine (2-AP), which is a base analog of A, involves dissociation of a proton from the N-1 position of the purine ring. Normal forms of these bases are in equilibrium with small amounts of the ionized forms. The ionized form of BrdU mispairs with G instead of the normal partner of T, which is A, and ionized 2-AP mispairs with C instead of the normal partner of A, which is T.

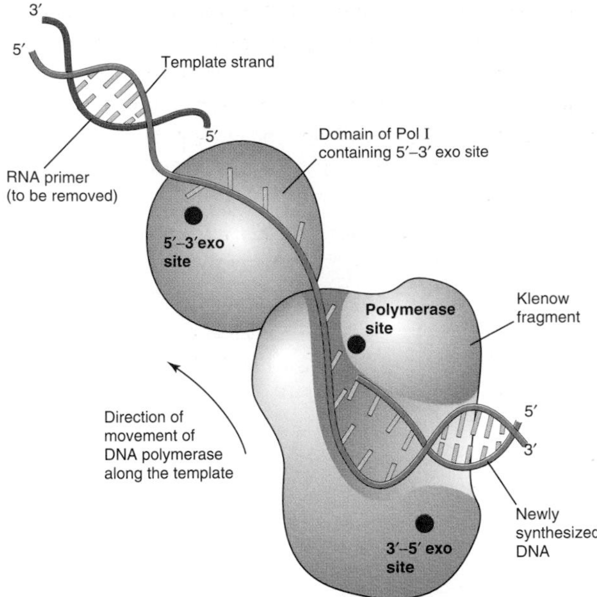

FIGURE 15.3
Model for the structure of DNA polymerase I–DNA complex. Klenow fragment of DNA polymerase I includes the 5′ → 3′ polymerization site and the 3′ → 5′ proofreading site. The remaining segment of the enzyme contains the 5′ → 3′ exonuclease site, which is used for DNA repair and the removal of RNA primers from Okazaki segments. In this drawing the 3′ growing end of a polynucleotide chain is in contact with the active site in the Klenow fragment, which is involved in elongation of the chain. The 3′ end is shifted near the 3′ → 5′ exonuclease active site, probably by sliding of the enzyme along the DNA without dissociation from the template.
Adapted from Bease, L. S., Derbyshire, V., and Steitz, T. A. Science *260:352, 1993.*

site located 3.5 nm away (Figure 15.3). When the polymerase active site detects a mismatch, the 3′ terminus of the DNA primer is guided into the 3′ → 5′ exonuclease site for removal of the mismatched base and then guided back to the polymerization site for further elongation.

Polymerase III has the same 5′ → 3′ synthetic and 3′ → 5′ exonuclease activities as polymerase I except that the processivity and polymerase activity of the former are much higher than the corresponding properties of the latter. Polymerase III is a more complex enzyme than polymerase I, consisting of at least ten different protein subunits (Table 15.2). The catalytic core of the enzyme consists of subunits α, ε, and θ and has a composite mass of about 167 kDa. Polymerization activity is vested in subunit α and 3′ → 5′ exonuclease activity in subunit ε. The function of the θ subunit is not clear but it may contribute to the interaction between α and ε or α with other subunits of the polymerase. The γ subunit participates in initiation of DNA synthesis. Subunits τ, δ, δ', χ, and ψ, appear to support the processivity properties of the enzyme. Formation of a complex of γ, δ, δ', χ, and ψ during initiation of DNA synthesis catalyzes ATP-dependent transfer of a pair of β subunits to the DNA template. These two β subunits form a clamp around the template that allows the multisubunit assembly to slide along the DNA without dissociation from the template. The subsequent binding of the catalytic core to the clamp of the β subunits generates a molecule of template-bound polymerase III holoenzyme that is a fully functional assembly (Figure 15.4). This sliding clamp is responsible for the remarkable degree of processivity exhibited by DNA polymerase III.

Eukaryotic DNA Polymerases

Less is known about **eukaryotic DNA polymerases,** relative to the *E. coli* polymerase. Five main types of polymerases have been isolated from mammalian cells (Table 15.3). With the exception of polymerase γ, which occurs in mitochondria, the remaining polymerases are involved in chromosomal DNA synthesis and repair. As with the three polymerases of *E. coli,* all five eukaryotic polymerases are characterized by 5′ → 3′ synthetic activities, but unlike the prokaryotic polymerases not all eukaryotic polymerases are vested with 3′ → 5′ exonuclease (proofreading) activities. Among eukaryotic polymerases only polymerase ε, which is primarily a repair enzyme like its counterpart in *E. coli,*

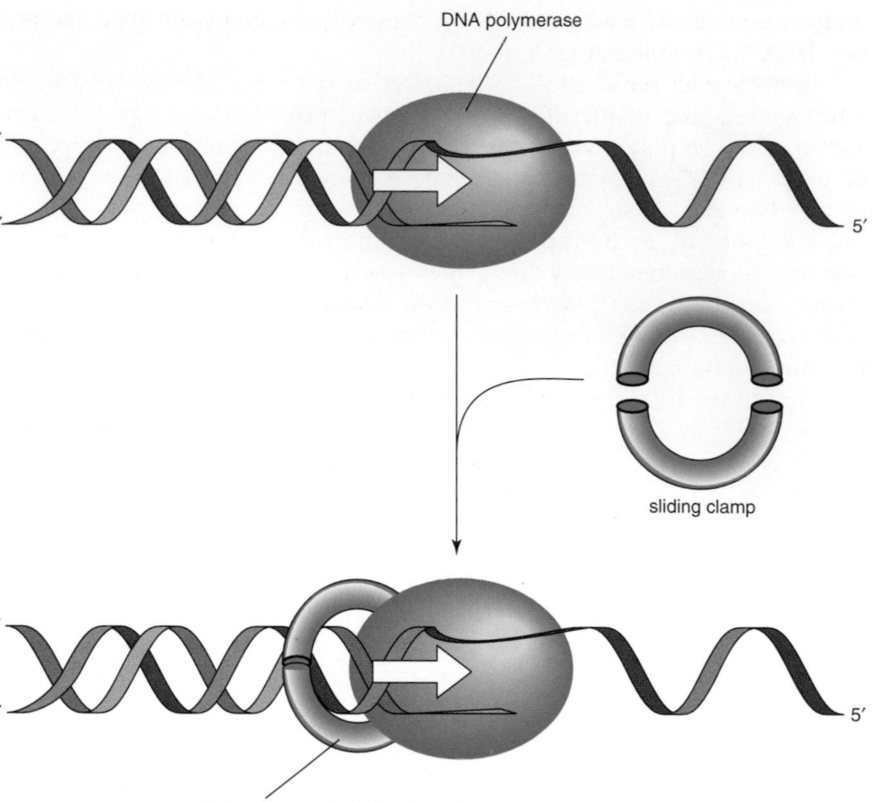

FIGURE 15.4
Model for the "clamp" that holds DNA polymerase III on the template.
The high processivity of DNA polymerase III is attributed to the formation of a sliding "clamp" that prevents the enzyme from dissociating from the template until DNA replication is completed. The sliding clamp is formed by the association of two β subunits of the polymerase that produces a donut-like structure having a hole with a diameter of about 3.5 nm. This hole easily accommodates B-DNA that has a diameter of no more than 2.5 nm. Upon completion of the synthesis, the two halves of the clamp dissociate and DNA polymerase is freed.

polymerase I, is vested with all three activities, namely, $5' \rightarrow 3'$ synthetic, $3' \rightarrow 5'$ exonuclease, and $5' \rightarrow 3'$ exonuclease activities. Polymerase β is also a repair enzyme but, since it lacks $3 \rightarrow 5'$ exonucleolytic activity necessary for proofreading, its fidelity is low. In analogy with polymerase III of *E. coli,* polymerases α and δ are the primary synthetic enzymes in eukaryotes and work in close association with each other. Of these two enzymes only polymerase α has a $3' \rightarrow 5'$ exonuclease activity that is necessary for the proofreading function. It is not clear whether polymerase δ in fact lacks $3' \rightarrow 5'$ activity or whether for some reason it is difficult to detect this activity *in vitro.* DNA polymerase δ is associated with a 37-kDa subunit, the **proliferating cell nuclear antigen (PCNA) protein,** that shows homology to the β subunit of polymerase III responsible for the high processivity of polymerase III. PCNA

TABLE 15.3 Biochemical Properties of Eukaryotic DNA Polymerases[a]

Property	α	δ	ε	β	γ
Mass (kDa)					
Native	> 250	170	256	36–38	160–300
Catalytic core	165–180	125	215	36–38	125
Other subunits	70, 50, 60	48	55	None	35, 47
Activities					
$3' \rightarrow 5'$ Exonuclease	No	Yes	Yes	No	Yes
Processivity	Low	High	High	Low	High
Fidelity	High	High	High	Low	High

Source: Adapted from Kornberg, A., and Baker, T. A. *DNA Replication,* 2nd ed. New York: Freeman, 1992.

[a] With the exception of polymerase γ, which is a mitochondrial enzyme, all other polymerases are located in the cell nucleus.

endows polymerase δ with very high processivity and is also involved in eukaryotic DNA excision repair (see p. 636).

In an overall sense DNA polymerases operate at a high level of fidelity, which is required of their function as DNA replicating and repair enzymes. *Escherichia coli* polymerases have an overall error rate in base incorporation of 10^{-7} to 10^{-8}. The experimentally observed accuracy for DNA replication in *E. coli,* however, is substantially higher, with errors made at the rate of only one for every 10^9 to 10^{10} nucleotides incorporated. The discrepancy in these numbers is accounted for by the operation of a DNA repair system that removes mismatched bases that have escaped the scrutiny of the proofreading activity of the polymerases. This repair system, known as the **mismatch repair** system, is examined on page 638.

The necessity to maintain high fidelity in replication is probably also the reason why polymerases synthesize polynucleotides only in the $5' \rightarrow 3'$ direction. If polynucleotide chains could be elongated in the $3' \rightarrow 5'$ direction, the hypothetical growing 5′ terminus, rather than the incoming nucleotide, would carry a triphosphate that is unsuitable for further elongation by the synthetic activity of the polymerase.

15.3 ■ MUTATION AND REPAIR OF DNA

Mutations Are Stable Changes in DNA Structure

One of the fundamental requirements for a structure that serves as a permanent depository of genetic information is high stability. Such stability is essential, at least in those parts that code for the genetic information. The structure of the DNA bases, however, is not totally exempt from gradual change. Normally, changes occur infrequently and they affect very few bases. Chemical and irradiation-induced reactions modify the structure of some bases, disrupt phosphodiester bonds, and sever strands. Extensive chemical changes of the bases occur spontaneously. Errors also occur during replication and DNA recombination, leading to incorporation of one or more erroneous bases. In almost every instance, however, a few cycles of DNA replication are required before a modification in the structure of a base can lead to irreversible damage. In effect, DNA polymerases must use the polynucleotide initially damaged as a template for the synthesis of a complementary strand for the initial change to become permanent. As Figure 15.5 suggests, use of the damaged strand as template extends the damage from a change of a single base to a change of a complete base pair and subsequent replication perpetuates the change. Other sources of permanent modifications of DNA include changes resulting from insertion to deletion from a DNA of short or longer nucleotide sequences during the process of DNA recombination (see p. 661). Intercalation of certain planar organic ring structures can also lead to insertion of nucleotides (see p. 631). Finally, deletions may occur as a result of chemical modification of the bases.

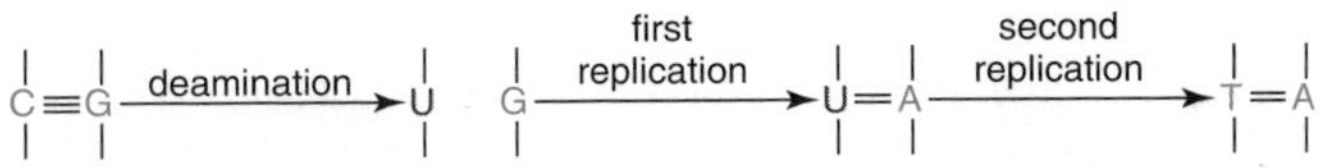

C≡G —deamination→ U G —first replication→ U=A —second replication→ T=A

FIGURE 15.5
Mutation perpetuated by replication.
Mutations introduced on a DNA strand, such as the replacement of a cytosine by a uracil resulting from deamination of cytosine, extend to both strands when the damaged strand is used as a template during replication. In the first round of replication uracil selects adenine as complementary base. In the second round of replication uracil is replaced by thymine. Similar events occur when the other bases are altered.

Irreversible alteration of a few DNA base pairs can cause drastic changes in the organism. These changes, referred to as **mutations,** may be hidden or visible, that is, **phenotypically silent** or **expressed.** Therefore a mutation is defined as a stable change in the DNA structure of a gene, which may be expressed as a phenotypic change in the organism. Mutations may be classified into two categories: **base substitutions** and **frameshift mutations.** Base substitutions include **transitions,** substitutions of one purine–pyrimidine pair by another, and **transversions,** substitutions of a purine–pyrimidine pair by a pyrimidine–purine pair. Frameshift mutations, which are the most radical, are the result of either the insertion of a new base pair or the deletion of a base pair or a block of base pairs from the DNA base sequence of the gene. These changes are illustrated in Figure 15.6.

Chemical Modification of Bases

Irradiation and certain chemical compounds are recognized as among the main mutagens. The incorporation of erroneous bases by DNA polymerase can also lead to mutations. Other mutations occur spontaneously. Bases in DNA are sensitive to the action of numerous chemicals including nitrous acid (HNO_2), hydroxylamine (NH_2OH), and various alkylating agents such as dimethyl sulfate and *N*-methyl-N^8-nitro-*N*-nitrosoguanidine. Chemical modifications of bases, brought about by these reagents, are shown in Figure 15.7.

Conversion of guanine to xanthine by nitrous acid has no effect on the hydrogen-bonding properties since xanthine, the new base, can pair with cytosine, the normal partner of guanine. However, the conversion of either adenine to hypoxanthine or the change from cytosine to uracil disrupts the normal hydrogen bonding of the double helix, because neither hypoxanthine nor uracil can form complementary pairs with the base present in the initial double helix (Figure 15.8). Subsequent replication of the DNA extends and perpetuates these base changes (Figure 15.5). Alkylating agents may affect the structure of the bases as well as disrupt phosphodiester bonds so as to lead to the fragmentation of the strands. In addition, certain alkylating agents can interact covalently with both strands, creating interstrand bridges.

DNA undergoes spontaneous changes as a result of various physical perturbations, such as thermal fluctuations or reactions with reactive forms of oxygen. Spontaneous **deamination of cytosine** in human DNA occurs at a rate of

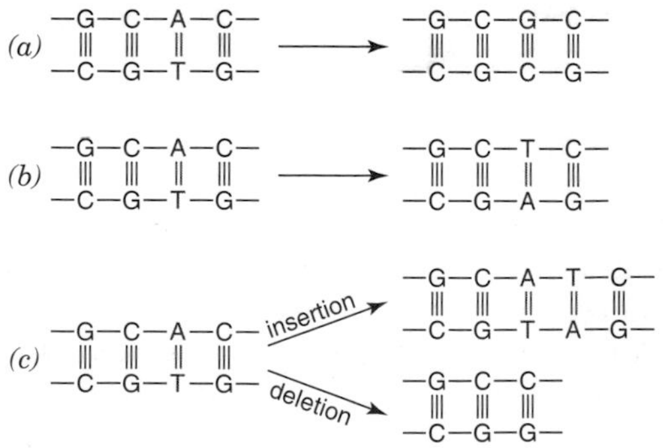

```
    —G—C—A—C—            —G—C—G—C—
(a)  |||  |||  ||  |||   ———→    |||  |||  |||  |||
    —C—G—T—G—            —C—G—C—G—

    —G—C—A—C—            —G—C—T—C—
(b)  |||  |||  ||  |||   ———→    |||  |||  ||  |||
    —C—G—T—G—            —C—G—A—G—

                                 —G—C—A—T—C—
                    insertion     |||  |||  ||  ||  |||
    —G—C—A—C—  ↗             —C—G—T—A—G—
(c)  |||  |||  ||  |||
    —C—G—T—G—  ↘              —G—C—C—
                    deletion      |||  |||  |||
                                 —C—G—G—
```

FIGURE 15.6
Mutations.
Mutations are classified as transition, transversion, and frameshift. Bases undergoing mutation are shown in color. (*a*) Transition: A purine–pyrimidine base pair is replaced by another. This mutation occurs spontaneously or can be induced chemically by such compounds as 5-bromouracil or nitrous acid. (*b*) Transversion: A purine–pyrimidine base pair is replaced by a pyrimidine–purine pair. This mutation occurs spontaneously and is common in humans. About one-half of the mutations in hemoglobin are of this type. (*c*) Frameshift: This mutation results from insertion or deletion of a base pair. Some insertions can be caused by mutagens such as acridines, proflavin, and ethidium bromide. Deletions are often caused by deaminating agents. Alteration of bases by these agents prevents pairing.

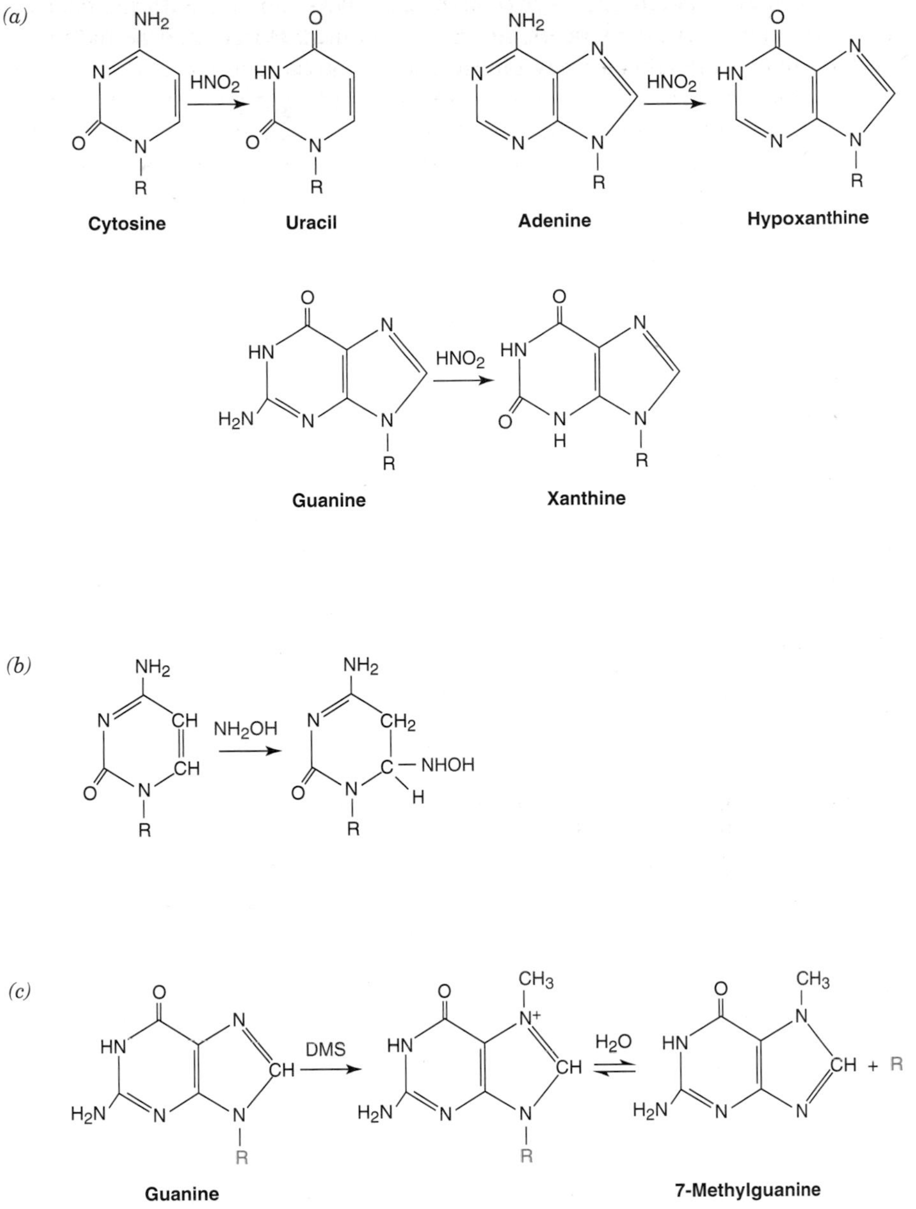

(a)

Cytosine → (HNO2) Uracil; Adenine → (HNO2) Hypoxanthine; Guanine → (HNO2) Xanthine

(b)

NH2OH

(c)

Guanine → (DMS) → ⇌ (H2O) 7-Methylguanine + R

FIGURE 15.7
Reactions of various mutagens.
(*a*) Deamination by nitrous acid (HNO_2) converts cytosine to uracil, adenine to hypoxanthine, and guanine to xanthine. (*b*) Reaction of bases with hydroxylamine (NH_2OH) as illustrated by the action of this reagent on cytosine. (*c*) Alkylations of guanine by dimethyl sulfate (DMS). Formation of a quaternary nitrogen destabilizes the deoxyriboside bond and releases deoxyribose. Among the effective agents for methylation of bases are nitrosoguanidines such as *N*-methyl-N^8-nitro-*N*-nitrosoguanidine.

about 100 base pairs per genome per day and **DNA depurination** occurs at even higher rates of 5000 bases per genome per day (Figure 15.9) as a result of thermal disruption of the *N*-glycosyl bonds of the bases. Some other changes that occur in DNA (as shown in Figure 15.10) can lead to either deletion of one or more base pairs in the daughter DNA after DNA replication or to a base pair substitution.

Radiation Damage

Ultraviolet light, including sunlight, and X-ray irradiation are also effective means of producing mutations. **Radiation energy** absorbed by the DNA induces the formation of minor amounts of the **ionized forms of the bases.** These ionized forms cannot pair with the normal partners of the base, but, instead, they engage in atypical base pairing as shown in Figure 15.11. The presence of ionized base forms at the moment of DNA replication is therefore expected to increase the frequency of mutation in the newly synthesized DNA strands. UV irradiation of DNA causes formation of dimers between adjacent pyrimidine bases. Activation of the ethylene bond of these bases frequently leads to a **photochemical**

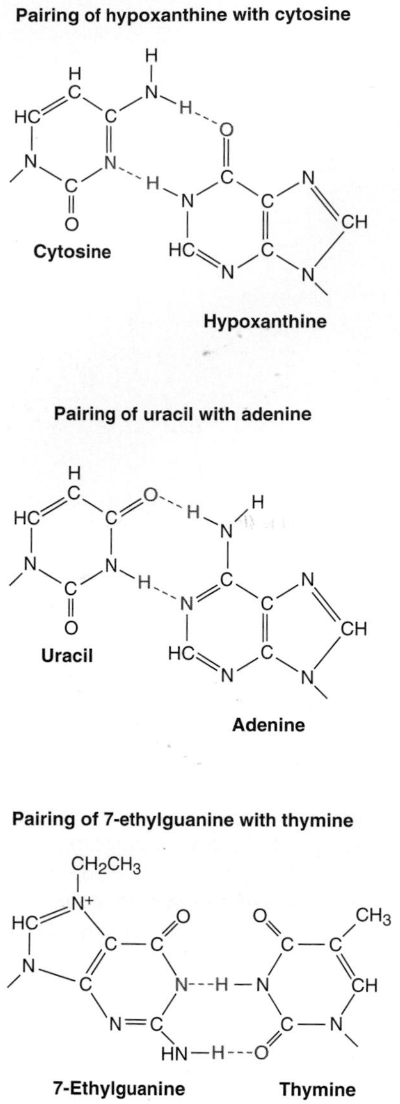

dimerization of two adjacent pyrimidines, as shown in Figure 15.12. Thymine residues are particularly susceptible to this reaction, although cytosine dimers and thymine–cytosine combinations are also produced.

High-energy radiation (X-rays or gamma rays) brings about direct modifications in the structure of the bases. Intermediates produced by electron expulsion can be rearranged, leading to the opening of the heterocyclic rings of the bases and the disruption of phosphodiester bonds. In the presence of oxygen additional reactions take place, yielding a variety of oxidation products.

DNA Polymerase Errors

With the appropriate deoxyribonucleoside triphosphates, DNA polymerases function with a high degree of fidelity. Some mutations do occur during DNA replication, but these changes are limited by the high synthetic fidelity of DNA polymerase and the "proofreading" exonuclease properties of this enzyme. The fidelity of DNA replication is further enhanced postreplicatively by an excision repair process known as the **mismatched repair system.** This system recognizes and corrects mismatches in newly replicated DNA by detecting distortions on the outside of the helix that are produced from poor fit between paired noncomplementary bases. Clearly, accurate correction of mismatched bases requires that the mismatched repair system discriminate between preexisting

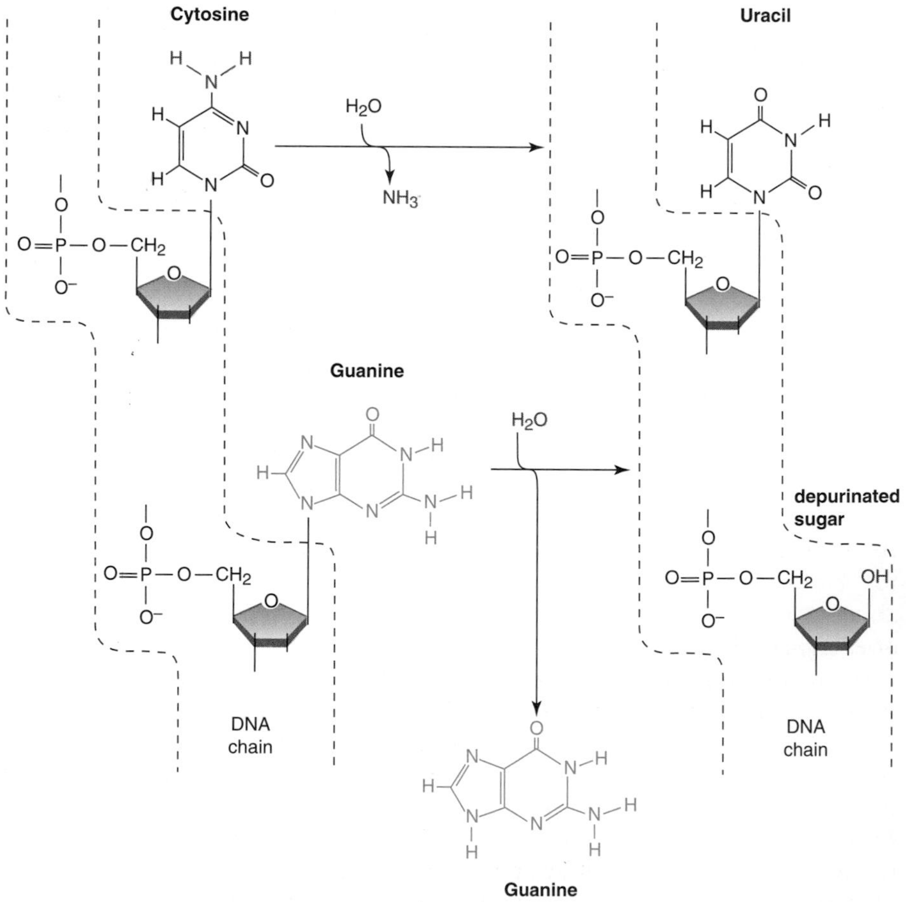

Pairing of hypoxanthine with cytosine

Cytosine

Hypoxanthine

Pairing of uracil with adenine

Uracil

Adenine

Pairing of 7-ethylguanine with thymine

7-Ethylguanine

Thymine

FIGURE 15.8
Chemical modifications that alter hydrogen-bonding properties of bases.
Hypoxanthine, obtained by deamination of adenine, has different hydrogen-bonding properties from adenine and pairs with cytosine. Similarly, uracil obtained from cytosine has a different hydrogen-bonding specificity than cytosine and pairs with adenine. Alkylation of guanine modifies hydrogen-bonding properties of the base.

Cytosine

H_2O

NH_3

Uracil

Guanine

H_2O

depurinated sugar

DNA chain

DNA chain

Guanine

FIGURE 15.9
Spontaneous deamination of pyrimidines and depurination of polynucleotides.
DNA undergoes substantial structural modifications as a result of thermal perturbations that include (1) extensive hydrolysis of the *N*-glycosyl bonds that connect purines to the deoxyribose residue and (2) deamination of cytosine residues to uracil. In absence of repair mechanisms, these changes would have disastrous consequences for cell survival because of the high frequency of their occurrence.

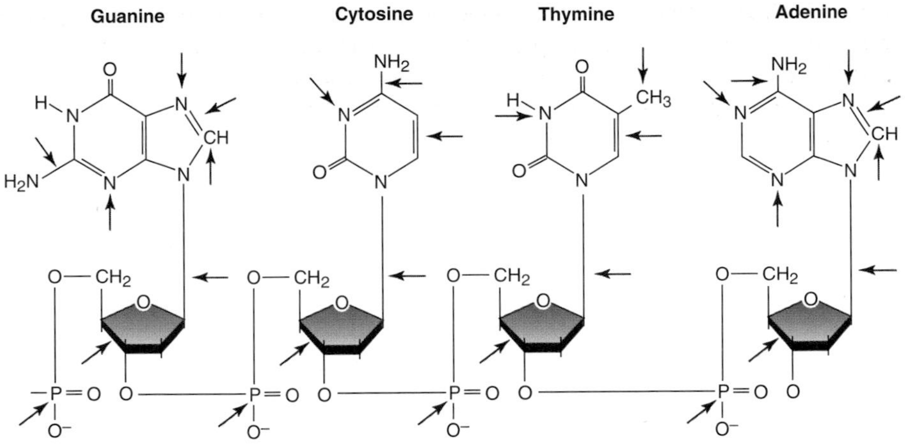

FIGURE 15.10
DNA sites subject to spontaneous chemical modifications.
Nucleotides are subject to various spontaneous chemical changes at sites indicated by arrows including (1) hydrolytic attack, (2) oxidative damage, and (3) methylation. The frequency and extent of chemical change vary from site to site.

and newly synthesized DNA strands. Such discrimination is feasible because certain adenine residues in DNA, which are part of a recurring GATC sequence, are subject to methylation that occurs posttranscriptionally, but with some delay. Mismatched proofreading is carried out by a multienzyme complex that excises mismatched nucleotides only from newly synthesized strands. The complex identifies these nucleotides by searching for unmethylated adenine residues in the GATC sequences of each strand. The mechanism of mismatched repair is described later.

DNA polymerases are unable to distinguish between the normal deoxyribonucleoside triphosphate substrates and other nucleotides with very similar structures, thus leading to their incorporation and a mutation. Classic examples of such analogs are deoxyribonucleotides of 5-bromouracil (5-BrdU) and 2-aminopurine (2-AP) that have been used experimentally for the introduction of mutations. Incorporation of 5-BrdU into DNA introduces, with a high frequency, a transition mutation in which a pu-py pair is transformed to another pu-py. Specifically, 5-BrdU paired with A is changed to a C-G pair, which amounts to a TA $\rightarrow$ GC transition. The unusual pairing properties of 5-BrdU appear to relate to the higher tendency of this base to be transformed to an ionized form, relative to T for which it is a substitute. This occurs presumably because of the higher electronegative nature of the bromine atom in comparison to the corresponding methyl group in thymine.

Stretching of the Double Helix

Organic compounds characterized by planar aromatic ring structures of appropriate size and geometry can be inserted between base pairs in double-stranded DNA. This process is referred to as **intercalation.** During intercalation neighboring base pairs in DNA are separated to allow for the insertion of the intercalating ring system, causing an elongation of the double helix by stretching. In effect the double helix is locally unwound into a ladder-like structure in which the base pairs are transiently arranged at 0.68 nm apart. This localized arrangement doubles the 0.34-nm distance characteristic of the double helix and generates sufficient space between base pairs for the insertion of the intercalator. In effect, intercalation disrupts the continuity of the base sequences in DNA and the reading of the DNA template by the DNA polymerase, producing a daughter strand with an additional base incorporated into DNA. The resulting mutation is referred to as a **frameshift.** Acridines, ethidium bromide, and other intercalators are known to be effective frameshift mutagens (Figure 15.13). Clinical Correlation 15.1 discusses mutations and the etiology of cancer.

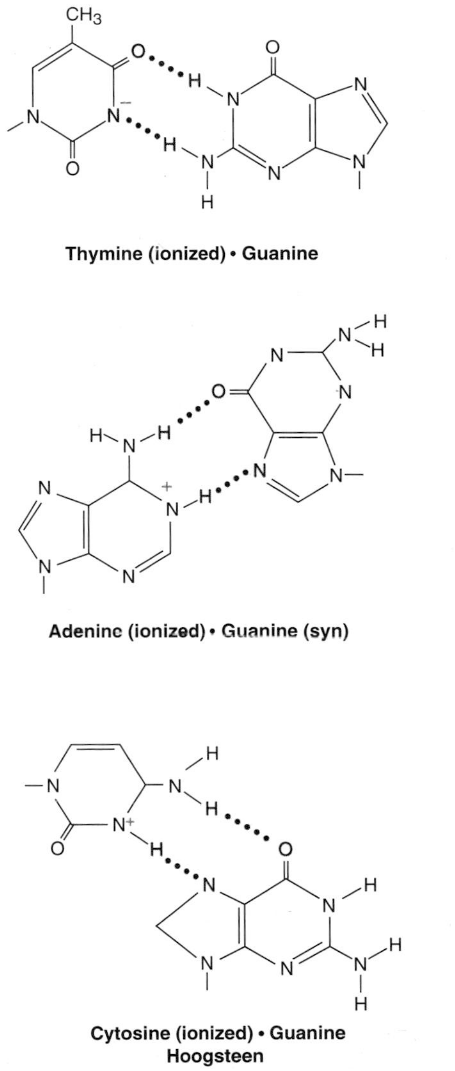

FIGURE 15.11
Base pairing between the ionized forms of the bases.
Adenine and cytosine are prone to protonation especially at lower pH. Also, an ionized form of thymine can be generated by loss of a proton. Reactions that give rise to ionized forms of bases occur readily at near-neutral pH, within certain nucleotide sequence contexts. Whereas some of the ionized complexes form with Watson–Crick hydrogen bonding, as, for instance, the T (ionized)–G pair, other ionized bases form more unusual types of H bonding. For example, the A(ionized)–G(syn) base pair involves H bonding between an A in the anti position and a G in the syn configuration.

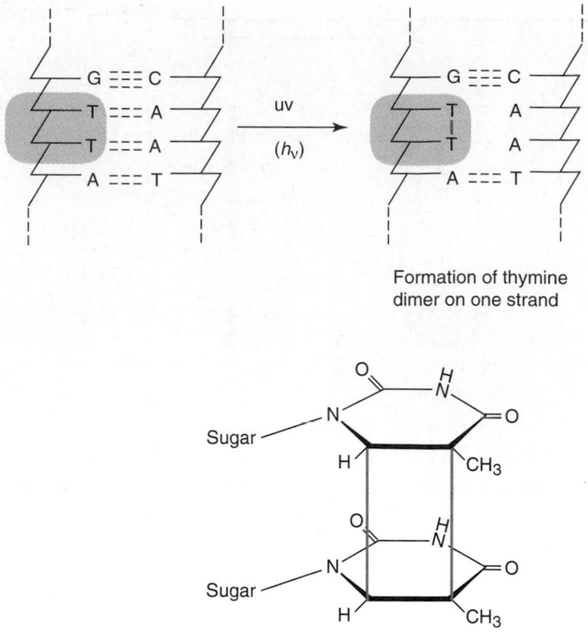

uv ($h\nu$)

Formation of thymine dimer on one strand

FIGURE 15.12
Dimerization of adjacent pyrimidines in irradiated DNA.
Thymine activated by absorption of UV light can react with a second neighboring thymine and form a thymine dimer.

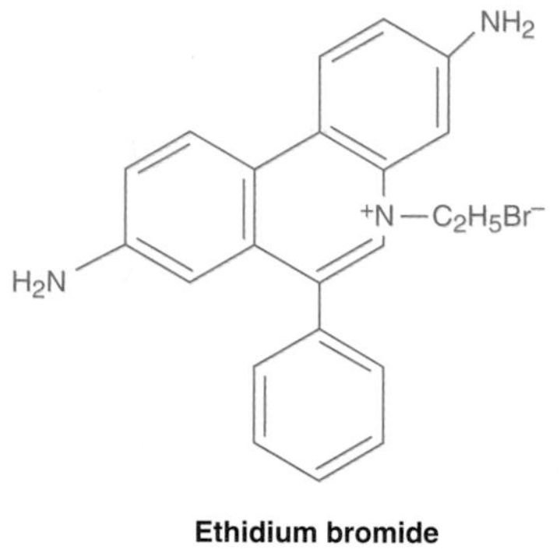

Ethidium bromide

(a)

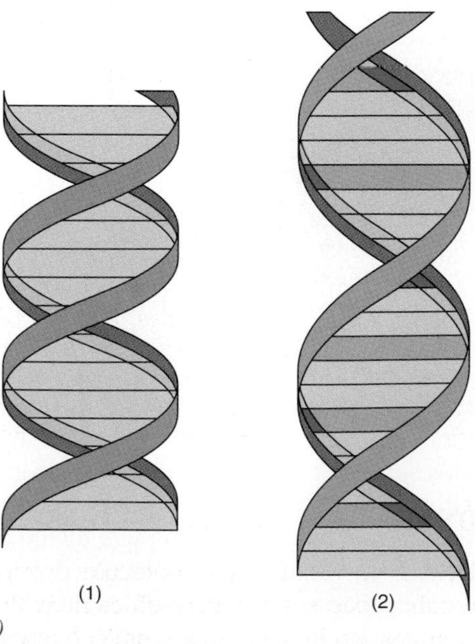

(b)

FIGURE 15.13
Intercalation between base pairs of the double helix.
(*a*) Insertion of planar ring system of intercalators between two adjacent base pairs requires stretching of the double helix (*b*). During replication this stretching apparently changes the frame used by DNA polymerase for reading the sequence of nucleotides. Consequently, newly synthesized DNA is frameshifted. (*b*-1) Original DNA helix; (*b*-2) helix with intercalative binding of ligands.
Redrawn based on figure in Lippard, S. J. Acct. Chem. Res. *11:211, 1978. Copyright © 1978 by the American Chemical Society.*

CLINICAL CORRELATION 15.1

Mutations and the Etiology of Cancer

Considerable progress in understanding the etiology of cancer has been achieved in recent years by the realization that long-term exposure to certain chemicals leads to various forms of malignancy. It is now suggested that the great majority of cancers are triggered by agents in the environment that modify underlying genetic predisposition factors.

Carcinogenic (cancer-causing) compounds are not only introduced into the environment by the increasing use of new chemicals in industrial applications but are also present in the form of natural products. For instance, the aflatoxins, produced by certain molds, and benz[*a*]anthracene, present in cigarette smoke and charcoal-broiled foods, are carcinogenic. Some carcinogens act directly, while others, such as benz[*a*]anthracene, must undergo prior hydroxylation by arylhydroxylases, present mainly in the liver, before their carcinogenic potential can be expressed.

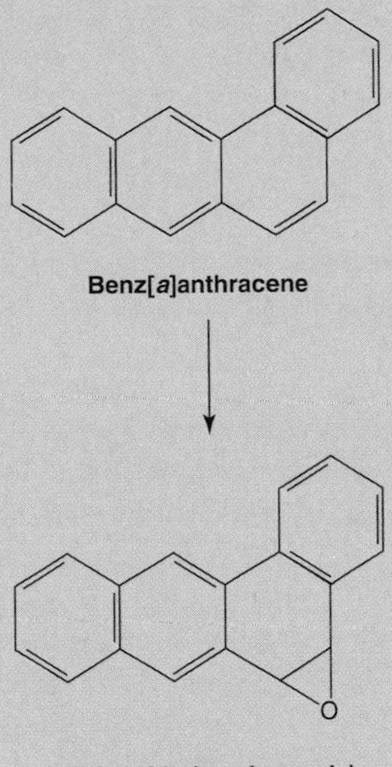

Benz[*a*]anthracene

O

5,6-Epoxide (carcinogenic)

The reactivity of many carcinogenic compounds toward guanine residues results in modification of the guanine structure, usually by alkylation at the N-7 position and by cleavage of the phosphodiester bond, events that upon replication lead to permanent mutations. Chemical mutagens are generally carcinogenic and vice versa. Vulnerability of DNA to alkylating agents and other chemicals underscores the concerns expressed by many scientists about the ever-increasing exposure of our environment to new chemicals. What is of concern is that the carcinogenic potential of new chemicals released into the environment cannot be predicted with confidence even when they appear to be chemically innocuous toward DNA.

In the past, tests for carcinogenicity, that is, the ability of a substance to cause cancer, required the use of many experimental animals treated with high doses of suspected carcinogen over a long period of time. Such tests, which are time consuming as well as expensive, are the only approach still available for testing carcinogenicity directly. A much simpler and inexpensive indirect test for carcinogenicity is also available. This test, the Ames Test, is based on the premise that carcinogenicity and mutagenicity are essentially manifestations of the same underlying phenomenon—the structural modification of DNA. The test measures the rate of mutation that bacteria undergo when exposed to chemicals suspected to be carcinogens.

A major criticism of this test is that the assumption of an equivalence between mutagenicity and carcinogenicity is not always valid. Because of economic implications of labeling a chemical with widespread use as a potential carcinogen, the scrutiny often exercised in assessing the reliability of applicable tests for labeling a chemical as a carcinogen is understandable. Certain exceptions notwithstanding, the great majority of chemicals tested have shown that a good correlation exists between the tendency of a chemical to produce bacterial mutations and animal cancer. Even the direct and very costly tests for carcinogenicity have not completely escaped criticism. The reliability of such tests has been questioned because of the relatively large doses of chemicals employed, doses that are essential for shortening the long-term chemical exposure of the animals to a practically manageable period of time. Another criticism of direct tests is that they make projections from animals, usually rodents, to humans. This criticism has some merit. During the past few years it has became apparent that rodents are less efficient than humans at repairing certain types of damage in nontranscribed regions of their DNA. Damage in nontranscribed DNA regions is more slowly repaired than damage within transcribed genes, which have first priority for repair. Although damage in nontranscribed DNA regions has few immediate consequences, it appears with time that this damage leads to cancer. The relatively large doses of chemicals used for testing are likely to exceed the capacity of rodent DNA repair systems, making the extrapolation of the results obtained from rodents to humans unreliable.

The enzymes that activate carcinogens are often members of the cytochrome P450 family (Chapter 23) that can be induced by noncarcinogenic compounds such as ethanol; hence alcohol can increase the potential risk of cancer development after exposure to carcinogens.

Ames, B., Dursto, W. E., Yamasaki, E., and Lee, F. D. Carcinogens are mutagens: a simple test system combining liver homogenates for activation and bacteria for detection. *Proc. Natl. Acad. Sci. USA* 70:2281, 1973; and Culotta, E., and Koshland, D. E. Jr. DNA repair works its way to the top. *Science* 266:1926, 1994.

DNA Is Repaired Rather than Degraded

DNA is the only macromolecule that is repaired rather than degraded. The repair processes are very efficient with fewer than 1 out of 1000 accidental changes resulting in mutations. The rest are corrected through various processes of DNA repair. Mutation rates can be estimated using two entirely different approaches, that is, from the frequency with which new mutants arise either in populations, such as fruitflies, or in specific proteins in cells growing in tissue culture. These experiments provide estimates of mutation rates of 1 base pair change per 10^9 base pairs for each cell per each generation. On this basis, for an average-sized protein, which contains about 1000 coding base pairs, a mutation may occur once in 10^6 cell generations.

DNA repair is a high-priority process for maintaining cellular function. Germ cells must be protected against high rates of mutation to preserve the species, and somatic mutation must be controlled in order to avoid uncontrolled cell growth and disease. Unchecked accumulation of damage can lead to accumulation of nonfunctional proteins or unregulated growth characteristic of malignant cells. Commonly encountered DNA lesions are listed in Table 15.4.

There are multiple DNA repair pathways and each specializes in a certain type of damage, although some repair pathways have a wider versatility than others. Generally, repair mechanisms are applicable to both prokaryotic and eukaryotic DNA repair.

Repairs may be carried out under rare circumstances as a direct reversal of the damage or, far more commonly, by the replacement of the damaged DNA section. DNA repair depends on the existence of two complementary DNA strands except for **postreplication repair of rare lesions** and **postreplication SOS repair.** Damage or imperfection on one DNA strand can be corrected since the complementary strand provides the necessary information for accurate repairs. Postreplication repair is not a true repair mechanism but rather a stop-gap measure that allows for DNA replication to occur until damage can be repaired permanently. Postreplication repair cannot use the complementary DNA strand for repairs because this strand is also altered by the replication that precedes the repair. Postreplication repair depends, instead, on another process—DNA recombination. Recombination permits the use of homologous DNA strands, namely, DNA strands with the same or almost the same sequence as the damaged strand, for carrying out the repair of the damaged DNA section. An intriguing feature of DNA repair that has been appreciated recently is its apparent intimate coupling to other central processes in which DNA participates, such as recombination, transcription, and control of the cell cycle. Enzymes involved in DNA repair participate in DNA replication, DNA recombination, and particularly DNA transcription. DNA metabolism integrates important processes that are coordinated through the use of the same molecular tools to achieve different tasks.

TABLE 15.4 DNA Lesions that Require Repair

DNA Lesion	*Cause*
Missing base	Acid and heat remove purines ($\sim 10^4$ purines per day per cell in mammals)
Altered base	Ionizing radiation; alkylating agents
Incorrect base	Spontaneous deaminations: C → U, A → hypoxanthine
Deletion–insertion	Intercalating agents (e.g., acridine dyes)
Cyclobutyl dimer	UV irradiation
Strand breaks	Ionizing radiation; chemicals (bleomycin)
Cross-linking of strands	Psoralin derivatives (light-activated); mitomycin C (antibiotic)

Source: From Kornberg, A. *DNA Replication*. San Francisco: Freeman, 1980, p. 608.

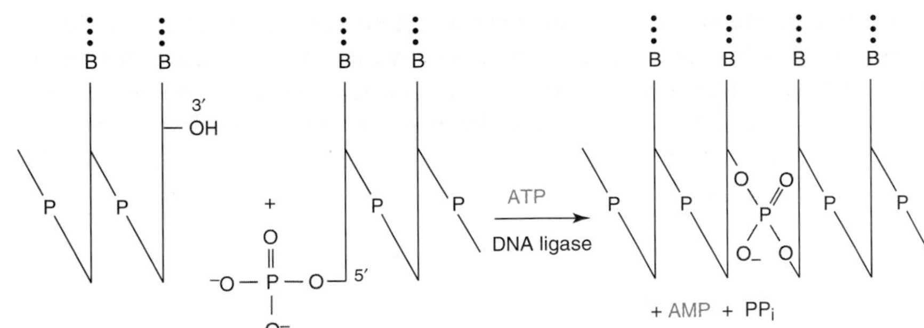

FIGURE 15.14
Action of DNA ligase.
The enzyme catalyzes the joining of polynucleotide strands that are part of a double-stranded DNA. A single phosphodiester bond is formed between 3′-OH and 5′-P ends of two strands. In *E. coli* cells, energy for formation of the bond is derived from cleavage of the pyrophosphate bond of NAD^+. In eukaryotic cells and bacteriophage-infected cells, energy is provided by hydrolysis of the α,β-pyrophosphate bond of ATP.

Excision Repair in E. coli

Excision repair is catalyzed by different enzymatic systems tailored to specific types of damage. This repair mechanism is universal, occurring in all organisms investigated. The mechanisms are characterized by four sequential steps: incision, excision, resynthesis, and ligation. Incision is the recognition step and is individualized for the specific type of damage present. It is also the rate-controlling step in the process. During excision the damaged DNA section is excised, leaving a gap in the DNA strand. In the resynthesis step the gap is filled by DNA polymerase I. This enzyme functions like DNA polymerase III in that it catalyzes the stepwise addition of nucleotide triphosphates on a 3′-OH generated by the preceding incision step. Polymerase I, however, differs from polymerase III in that it is less processive, tending to dissociate from the DNA after incorporation of 10–12 nucleotides. At this stage the gap is reduced to the size of a single phosphodiester bond. Because of the combined synthetic–nucleolytic action of polymerase I, the nick can move along the strand, undergoing repair until it is finally bridged during the ligation step by the action of DNA ligase (Figure 15.14). The ligation step appears to be very similar for all types of excision repair.

Base excision repair eliminates modified bases from DNA. The amino groups of cytosine, adenine, and guanine are susceptible to spontaneous elimination, and various chemicals lead to modifications in the structures of purines, including methylation and ring opening. In addition, ring opening may result from exposure to ionizing radiation. Bases that have been deaminated, methylated, or otherwise chemically modified are hydrolytically removed by enzymes referred to as **DNA glycosylases.** Removal of deaminated cytosine (i.e., uracil) by the enzyme **uracil DNA glycosylase** is illustrated in Figure 15.15. This enzyme removes the damaged cytosine, producing a deoxyribose residue with the base missing **[apurinic–apyrimidinic (AP) site].** AP sites are also generated without the involvement of DNA glycosylases, as in the case of spontaneous hydrolysis of purines **(depurination)** that occurs at very high rates in DNA. AP sites can also result from depyrimidination but the greater stability of the purine–glycoside bond makes this reaction almost insignificant. Once an AP site has been created, the enzyme **AP endonuclease** nicks the phosphodiester backbone at the depurinized site and excises the sugar–phosphate residue. The action of DNA polymerase I and ligase on this structure leads to the restoration of the damaged strand.

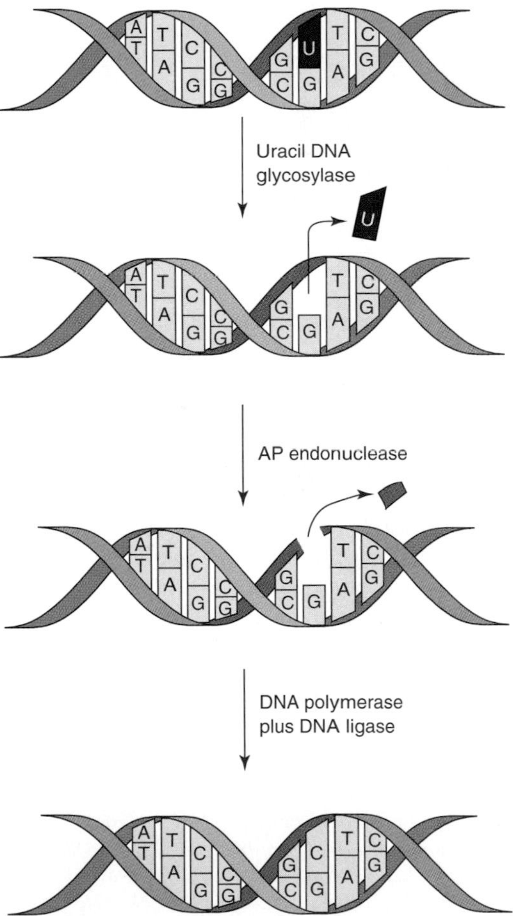

FIGURE 15.15
Uracil DNA glycosylase repair of DNA.
Uracil DNA glycosylase removes uracil, formed by accidental deamination of cytosine, by cutting the glycosidic bond, leaving DNA with a missing base. AP endonuclease subsequently cuts out the sugar–phosphate remnant. Repair is completed by DNA polymerase and ligase.

A second type of excision repair referred to as **nucleotide excision repair** is activated when DNA is damaged in a way that produces a "bulky" lesion. This occurs when DNA interacts with polycyclic aromatic hydrocarbons, such as benzo[*a*]pyrenes and dialkylbenzathracenes generated by smoking, thymine–psoralene adducts, and guanine–cisplatin adducts formed by chemotherapeutic drugs. UV light-induced dimerization of adjacent pyrimidines also causes bulky lesions. Nucleotide excision repair also corrects other lesions that do not distort the helix, such as the presence of methylated bases. Once the lesion has been located, an endonuclease activity cleaves the modified strand on both sides of

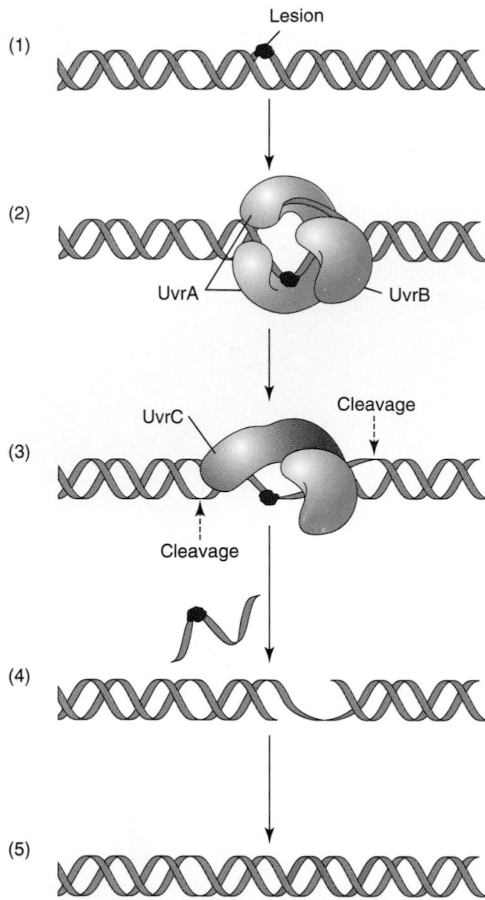

FIGURE 15.16
Nucleotide excision repair in *E. coli.*
Nucleotide excision repair in *E. coli* and in human DNA occurs in a series of analogous steps. Initial damage in *E. coli* is recognized by UvrA protein, which also serves as a "molecular matchmaker" by recruiting, at the damaged site, UvrB protein. UvrA binds to the lesion, unwinds and kinks DNA. UvrA also causes a conformational change in UvrB that promotes strong binding of UrvB at the site of the lesion. Subsequent dissociation of UvrA from UvrB–DNA complex makes the complex a target for UvrC. UvrB then makes a 3′ cut that is followed by a 5′ incision made by UvrC. Helicase II (UvrD) releases the excised oligonucleotide 12-mer and DNA polymerase displaces UvrB and fills the excision gap prior to ligation.
Redrawn based on figure in Moran, L. A., Scrimgeour, K. G., Horton, H. R., Ochs, R. S., and Rawn, J. D. Biochemistry. *Englewood Cliffs, NJ: Neil Patterson/Prentice Hall, 1994.*

the distortion and the entire lesion is removed (Figure 15.16). Repair is initiated by recognition of the distortion of the DNA by an endonuclease system consisting of the products of three *E. coli* genes *uvrA, uvrB,* and *uvrC.* A tetramer consisting of two **UvrA** and two **UvrB** proteins, which is formed on DNA during a series of preincision steps, "melts" the DNA locally at the expense of ATP and locates the bulky lesion. The complex is subsequently subjected to incision at both sides of the bulky lesion. First, UvrB makes a 3′ incision and then **UvrC** makes a 5′ incision, leading to the release of an oligonucleotide consisting of 12 or 13 residues that includes the pyrimidine dimer. This nuclease activity, which is unique to DNA repair, has been christened **excision nuclease** or **excinuclease** to clearly distinguish it from other endonucleases. For the remainder of the repair, *E. coli* makes use of the protein **UvrD** which, acting as a **helicase,** unwinds and releases the oligonucleotide that was excised by UvrB and UvrC. The repair is completed by polymerase I and ligase.

Eukaryotic Excision Repair

Excision repair in prokaryotes and eukaryotes is remarkably similar with the following distinctions. The exonuclease activity of human cells consists of a much larger number of proteins (16–17 different polypeptides) as apposed to the four proteins (UvrA, B, C, and D) that constitute the exonuclease activity of *E. coli*. Some of the protein constituents of human excinucleases are listed in Table 15.5. Proteins XPA to XPG have been identified as seven different **genetic complementation groups** (A to G) of patients with **xeroderma pigmentosum (XP),** a condition characterized by UV sensitivity and corresponding deficiencies in DNA repair. The human nucleotide repair genes are therefore referred to by an XP or ERCC (excision repair component) designation. Nucleotide excision repair of human DNA begins with the binding of XPA to a dimer between XPF and ERCC1 (Figure 15.17). XPA recognizes and binds to the damaged site along with the replication protein HSSB. An intriguing aspect of human DNA repair is involvement of an additional enzymic complex con-

TABLE 15.5 Excinuclease Activity of Human DNA

Human Gene	*Protein Function*
XPA	Damage recognition protein (binds to damaged DNA)
XPB (*ERCC3*)	DNA helicase activity; subunit of transcription factor TFIIH
XPC	Interacts with general transcription factor TFIIH
XPD (*ERCC2*)	DNA helicase activity; subunit of transcription factor TFIIH
XPF	Nuclease activity
XPG	Nuclease activity
ERCC1	Part of nuclease activity (binds to XPF and to replication protein RPA)
HSSB (*RPA*)	Binds to the XPF–ERCC1 complex and together with XPA binds to the lesion site

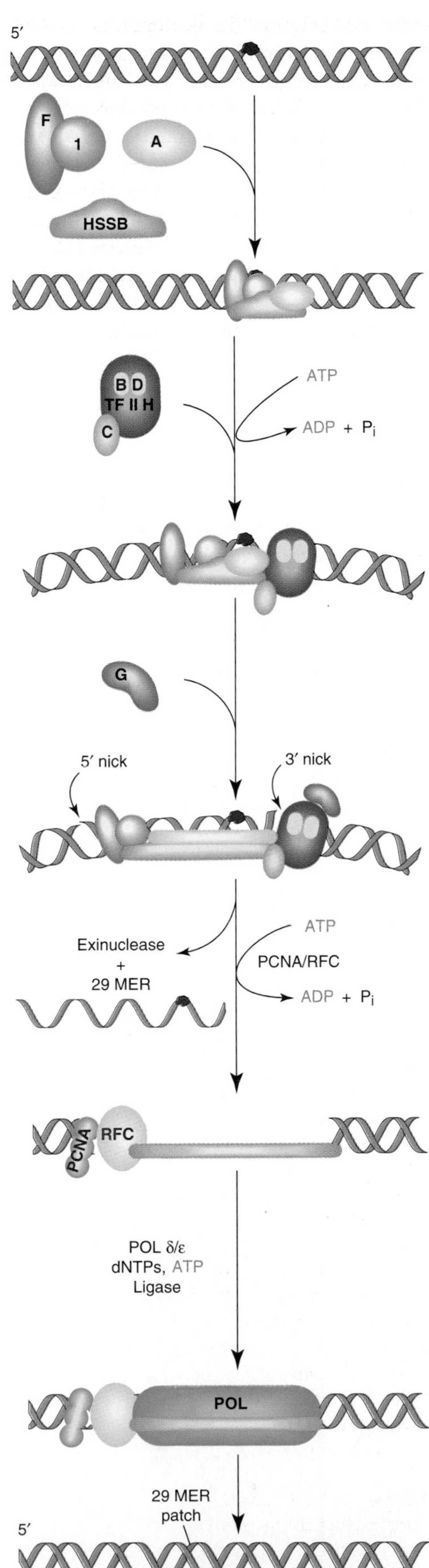

FIGURE 15.17
Nucleotide excision repair of human DNA.
In human DNA damage is recognized by the XPA factor (abbreviated in the figure as A) that recruits to the damaged site factors XPF and ERCC1 (abbreviated as F and 1, respectively) in the form of a dimer. XPF is an excinuclease that is recruited to the damaged site early on just as UvrB is recruited in the *E. coli* system. The replication protein (HSSB) binds to XPA and the lesion site. XPA also recruits to the damaged site the general transcription factor TFIIH, which, as it turns out, is also a repair protein since two of its protein subunits are repair factors XPB and XPD (abbreviated as B and D). In analogy with UvrA, TFIIH may be involved in kinking and unwinding of DNA at the damaged site and in recruiting XPC and XPG proteins, which are vested with helicase activity. Excinuclease cuts are made at the 3′ site by XPG, whereas XPF nicks at the 5′ site of the lesion, leading to the excision of a 23-mer oligonucleotide. Gap repair is carried out by polymerases δ and ε with PCNA and replication protein RFC, followed by ligation.
Redrawn based on figure in Sancar, A. Science *266:1954, 1994. Copyright © 1994 American Association for the Advancement of Science.*

sisting of eight different protein subunits and known as the **general transcription factor TFIIH.** This factor is essential for transcription initiation and for nucleotide excision repair. In fact, two of the eight subunits of TFIIH are the helicases XPB and XPD that evidently not only act in excision repair but also catalyze the opening of DNA to initiate transcription. This intimate involvement of a transcription factor suggests that DNA repair and transcription are not fully separable processes and may be coupled to each other. The TFIIH factor interacts with XPC and the entire complex is recruited to the damaged site by XPA, where it is joined by the endonuclease XPG. The two recruited endonucleases, XPF and XPG, complete the excinuclease systems with the XPG making the 3′ nick and the XPF, in the form of a complex with ERCC1, making the 5′ nick. The major XPG incision is made at the third phosphodiester bond 3′ to the lesion, whereas the XPF–ERCC1 complex incises primarily at the 25th phosphodiester bond 5′ to the lesion. The role of TFIIH is presumably to unwind the double helix at the damaged site so as to enable the endonucleases XPF and XPG to activate the excinuclease system. A protein associated with polymerase δ, PCNA **(proliferating cell nuclear antigen),** releases the excinuclease subunits and the excised oligomer, which is larger than the oligonucleotide released during *E. coli* repair (27–29 nucleotides versus 12–13 nucleotides in *E. coli*). The gap is filled by polymerases δ and ε and the DNA is ligated.

Excision repair also removes cross-links between complementary DNA strands, such as those introduced by the mustards and drugs used in cancer therapy (i.e., mitomycin D and platinum complexes). Error-free repair is not possible if the cross-link extends across directly opposing bases. Clinical Correlations 15.2 and 15.3 discuss defects in DNA repair that are associated with human disease; Clin. Corr. 15.4 examines the role of DNA repair in chemotherapy.

Mismatch Repair

Mismatch repair in both prokaryotic and eukaryotic cells deals with errors created during DNA replication. In effect, three serially operating mechanisms—base selection, exonucleolytic proofreading, and postreplicative mismatch re-

CLINICAL CORRELATION 15.2

Defects in Nucleotide Excision Repair and Hereditary Diseases

Defects in nucleotide excision repair are implicated in at least three rare hereditary disorders, xeroderma pigmentosum (XP), Cockayne's syndrome (CS), and trichothiodystrophy (TTD). XP patients exhibit sunlight-induced photodermatoses characterized by severe skin reactions that range initially from excessive freckling and skin ulcerations to the eventual development of skin cancers. Some forms are also accompanied by neurological abnormalities. The symptoms exhibited by CS and TTD patients are associated instead only with developmental abnormalities. CS syndrome is characterized by growth and mental retardation, neurological deficiencies, and photosensitivity but not an increased rate of cancer or skeletal abnormalities. TDD patients, on the other hand, have scaly skin, brittle hair, short stature, and neuroskeletal abnormalities.

Xeroderma pigmentosum is a group of closely related abnormalities in excision repair. About 80% of XP patients fall into one of seven complementation groups (different syndromes). Each group carries a mutation in a different gene and is characterized by varying levels of UV sensitivity caused by corresponding deficiencies in "excinuclease" repair activity. The remainder fall in the XPV (V for variant) group. In this variant UV irradiation produces different types of mutations compared to normal cells. During normal DNA synthesis, whenever the DNA polymerase bypasses a pyrimidine dimer in the template that has not yet been repaired, a purine (most often A) is incorporated into nascent DNA but this preference is not maintained by XPV cells. It appears that the mechanism of bypass by the DNA polymerase in XPV cells is altered possibly because of changes in one or more of the subunits of the polymerase or possibly some other protein factor that assists the polymerase to bypass the DNA lesions. The neurological abnormalities that frequently accompany XP appear to result from both abnormal gene expression and DNA deterioration caused by the accumulation of unrepaired DNA damage.

Cockayne's syndrome is associated with mutations in the *CSB/ERCC6, XPD,* and *XPB* genes. Trichothiodystrophy is caused by mutations in *XPB, XPD,* and *XPG* genes and perhaps in additional subunits of TFIIH or TFIIH-associated excision repair subunits. Obviously, different mutations in the *XPB* and *XPD* genes are responsible for each syndrome.

Tanaka, K., and Wood, R. D. Xeroderma pigmentosum and nucleotide excision repair of DNA. *TIBS* 9:83, 1994.

CLINICAL CORRELATION 15.3

DNA Ligase Activity and Bloom Syndrome

Bloom syndrome is a rare genetic disease that is characterized by chromosomal instability. Other chromosome breakage syndromes include Fanconi's anemia (FA), ataxia telangiestasia (AT), Werner's syndrome (WS), and Gardner's syndrome (GS). Deficiencies in the effective repair of DNA lesions, which can probably be attributed to defective DNA ligation, are presumably responsible for many of these syndromes. These repair deficiencies appear to increase the tendency to develop malignancies among those affected with the syndromes.

Bloom syndrome is a prototype of somatic mutation disease. The clinical features of Bloom syndrome are small body size, a sun-sensitive skin with well-defined hyper- and hypopigmented skin lesions, and increased sensitivity to bacterial infections due to immunodeficiency. Cancer, chronic lung disease, and diabetes are common complications. Cells from Bloom syndrome patients have high rates of mutation, and the excessive number of accumulated somatic mutations are responsible for many of the clinical features of this syndrome. In patients suffering from Bloom syndrome, hypermutability is responsible for the abolition of ligase I activity needed for completing DNA repair and (perhaps) DNA recombination.

German, J. *Bloom syndrome. Dermatol. Clin.* 13(1):7, 1995.

pair–participate in ensuring fidelity of replication. The mismatch repair system recognizes and eliminates mispairing from newly synthesized DNA strands, improving the fidelity of the synthesis. Base selection and proofreading act more effectively against transversion than transitions, whereas mismatch repair does the opposite. DNA replication errors are difficult to recognize because mismatches consist of erroneous but unaltered base structures. The repair system relies on other signals within the helix to identify the newly synthesized strand, which by definition harbors the replication error. Such signals are provided in *E. coli* by a methylation reaction catalyzed by **Dam methylase** that modifies GATC sequences by introducing a methyl group at the *N*-6 position of adenines. Shortly after replication these GATC sequences exist in an unmethylated state that betrays the newly synthesized nature of the DNA strand and permits strand discrimination by the mismatch repair system (Figure 15.18).

The mismatch repair system in *E. coli* includes several different protein components, which repair mismatches in the vicinity of a GATC sequence according to complementary rules dictated by the base sequence of the methylated (i.e., preexisting) parental strand. Proteins that catalyze the process of mismatch repair have been named **MutS, MutH,** and **MutL.** Repair is initiated by binding of MutS to the mismatch followed by the addition of MutL. Formation of the MutS–MutL complex activates a latent GATC endonuclease activity, vested in the MutH protein, that nicks the unmodified strand at a hemimethylated GATC site. The strand break, which can occur on either side of the mismatch, will take place as long as the mismatched base is located within the general vicinity of the GATC site, which means within a few hundred base pairs from the GATC sequence. This nick marks the strand that will be excised. When the mismatch is located on the 5′ side of the cleavage site the unmethylated strand is unwound, degraded, and replaced by new DNA synthesized in the $3' \rightarrow 5'$ direction until the mismatch is reached and excised. This reaction requires a DNA helicase II, referred to also as the **MutU** protein, a $3' \rightarrow 5'$ exonuclease (exonuclease I), DNA polymerase III, and finally DNA ligase to seal the repaired strand. If the mismatch is located on the 3′ site of the cleavage, a series of completely analogous steps takes place, except that a $5' \rightarrow 3'$ exonuclease **(RecJ)** replaces exonuclease I (an exonuclease with both $5' \rightarrow 3'$ and $3' \rightarrow 5'$ activity, exonuclease III can also substitute for RecJ in the latter repair). This unusual bidirectional excision activity of the mismatch repair system suggests that this system "keeps track" of the side on which the mispair of the GATC sequence signal is located.

Analogous mismatch repair systems have been identified in eukaryotes. Both yeast and human cells code for proteins homologous to the bacterial

CLINICAL CORRELATION 15.4

DNA Repair and Chemotherapy

Many anticancer drugs cause DNA damage. For example, cisplatin, used for treatment of several forms of cancer and particularly effective against testicular tumors, forms two intrastrand adducts with DNA. The major one, the 1,2-intrastrand d(GpG) cross-link, is repaired by excision repair. DNA adducts are believed to be the primary cytotoxic lesion and cells deficient in excision repair are very sensitive to this drug. The high mobility group (HMG)-domain proteins "shield" and specifically inhibit DNA repair of this major cisplatin–DNA adduct, thus increasing the cytotoxicity of cisplatin. The types and levels of HMG-domain proteins in a given tumor may influence the responsiveness of that cancer to cisplatin chemotherapy. This information may provide a basis for the development of new platinum anticancer drugs that may have greater therapeutic potential.

Huang, J. C., Zamble, D. B., Reardon, J. T., Lippard, S. J., and Sancar, A. HMG-domain proteins specifically inhibit the repair of the major DNA adduct of the anticancer drug cisplatin by human excision nuclease. *Proc. Natl. Acad. Sci. USA* 91:10394, 1994.

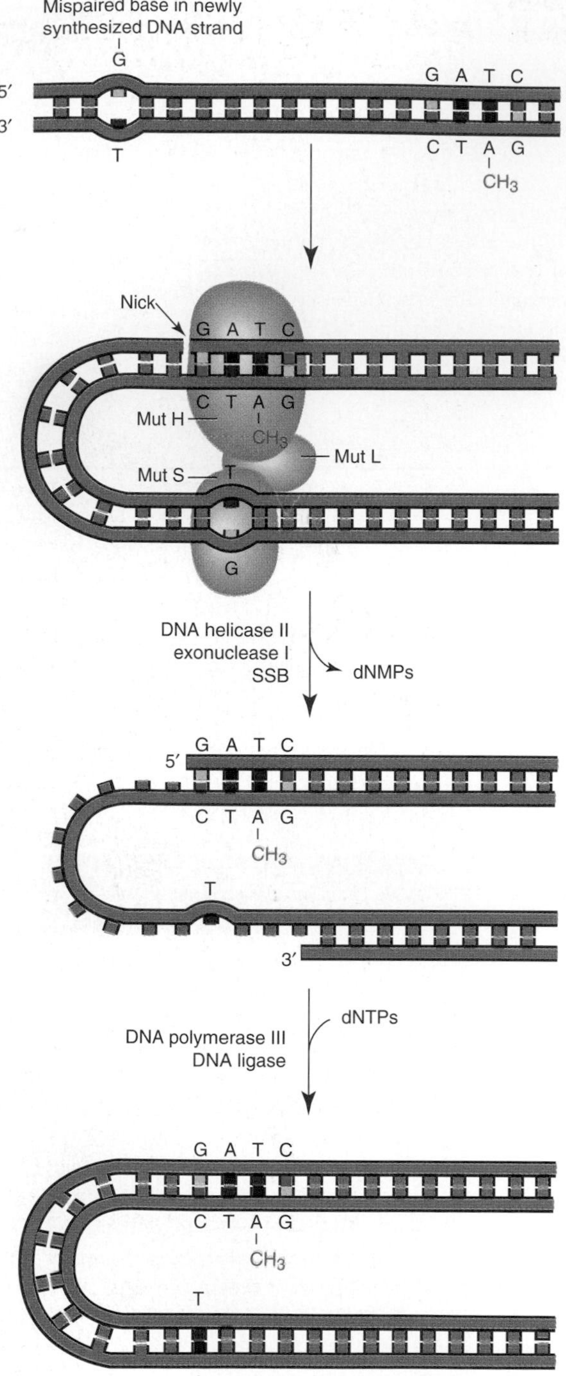

FIGURE 15.18
Mismatch DNA repair.
Methylation of adenine in palindromic 5′-GATC sequences serves to distinguish parental strands from newly synthesized strands that are methylated only after some delay. Methylation directs the mismatch repair system to repair mispaired bases. Methylated GATC sequences are recognized by MutH, which is also an endonuclease that cleaves the unmethylated strand on the 5′ site of the G in the GATC sequence, whereas the mispaired site is recognized and bound by the MutS protein. MutL, which is a molecular matchmaker, links MutH and MutS together. The segment of the unmethylated strand, which represents newly synthesized DNA between the site cleaved by MutH and a point just past the mismatched base, is then removed by the action of helicase II, exonuclease I, and SSB protein. The gap is repaired by DNA polymerase III and ligase. A similar mechanism, but based on the presence of nicks to identify newly synthesized strands, is used by eukaryotes. The eukaryotic mismatch repair system does not use MutH and depends on MutL for the degradation of newly synthesized strands that contain base mismatches.

proteins MutS and MutL but lack the MutH protein. In eukaryotic mismatch repair the role of MutL is to scan nearby DNA for the presence of nicks. Upon finding a nick, MutL degrades the nicked strand starting at the nick site and extending just past the site of the mismatched base pair. Replication errors are thereby selectively removed. Clinical Correlation 15.5 describes the role of mismatch repair in the development of certain types of cancer.

Mechanisms that Reverse Damage

Formation of dimers can be directly reversed by the action of light. Photoreversal is catalyzed by deoxyribodipyrimidine **photolyase,** which disrupts the covalent bonds that hold together the pyrimidine molecules in the dimer. Photolyases are activated by light in the range of 300–600 nm. Photolyases are present in bacteria but are not essential for DNA repair; humans lack the enzymes.

Removal of a methyl or ethyl group from the 6 position of the enol form of a guanine residue reestablishes the normal structure of guanine. A specific protein accepts alkyl groups and becomes alkylated.

Postreplication Repair

The repair processes reviewed so far deal with damage of bases on one of the two DNA strands and use of the second complementary strand as a template for repair. Such repair occurs prior to replication of DNA that turns DNA damage into permanent mutation. For example, normal DNA replication with DNA polymerase III in *E. coli* cannot proceed past most types of DNA lesions until such lesions are first repaired. These lesions cannot be excised because excision would leave breaks in both strands that replication would perpetuate. Eventually, replication resumes past the site of the lesion with the polymerase skipping over a few of the damaged bases. After synthesis the daughter strand is found to be missing a base that would normally be present across the damaged base. The lesion itself is eventually repaired by borrowing template information from a homologous DNA strand. This type of repair is illustrated in Figure 15.19.

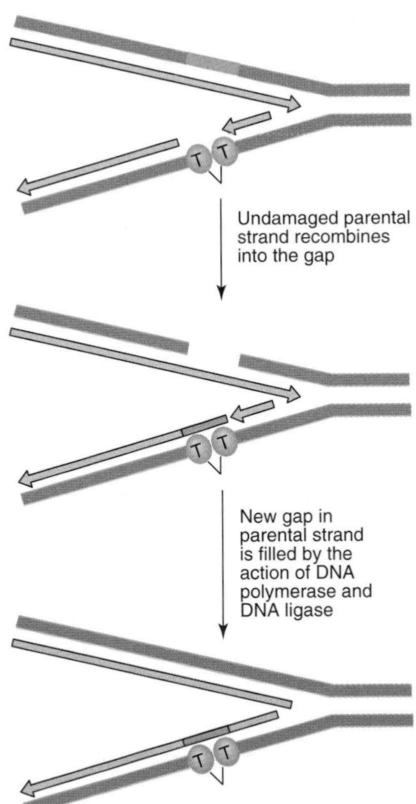

FIGURE 15.19
Postreplication repair.
Most DNA lesions in *E. coli* are repaired prior to replication. If an unrepaired lesion is encountered by the replication complex near the replication fork, replication is blocked at the site and resumes only beyond the unrepaired site. The gap, initially left behind in an unreplicated single-stranded segment of DNA, is eventually repaired by the process of recombination. Recombination allows the use of a complementary strand from another DNA as template.

CLINICAL CORRELATION 15.5

Mismatch DNA Repair and Cancer

DNA is constantly being damaged. In the absence of efficient repair, this may be the cause of as much as 90% of all human cancers. The importance of defective mismatch repair in the development of certain types of human cancer has been demonstrated recently. Tumors associated with hereditary nonpolyposis colorectal cancer (HNPCC), which causes cancer predisposition and certain sporadic cancers, have been found to be prone to mutation by as much as two orders of magnitude higher than normal human cells. These high mutation rates have been found to be consistently associated with deficiencies in mismatch repair.

That loss of mismatch repair fidelity is a central step in the development of HNPCC tumors has been concluded from the finding that the majority of these tumors are attributable to defects at any one of four different human genome loci. These are the *hMSH2* gene, which codes for a protein homolog of bacterial MutS protein, and the *hMLH1, hPMS1,* and *hPMS2* genes, which specify three similar but distinct MutL analogs. These findings demonstrate that the primary event in the development of HNPCC tumors is the loss of critical mismatch repair activity. Inefficiencies in DNA repair presumably lead to mutations that circumvent the regulatory systems controlling cell proliferation. The link between mismatch repair and the development of colon cancer provides support for the hypothesis that cancers are initiated when cells accumulate a certain mutation load. A current emphasis in studies of cancer is the search for and study of particular genes, the mutations of which appear to lead to cancer. The new findings, which demonstrate the importance of mismatch repair defects in the development of cancers, may now expand the search from simply attempting to decipher the role of certain genes in carcinogenesis to also asking why and how some cells accumulate an excessive number of mutations.

Modrich, P. Mismatch repair, genetic stability and cancer. *Science* 266:1959, 1994.

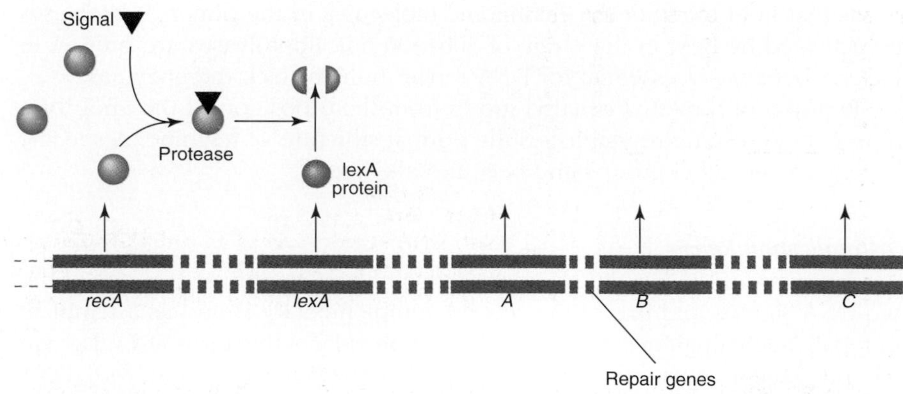

FIGURE 15.20
SOS DNA repair.
Under normal conditions the SOS repair proteins are not expressed. This is because a repressor protein, LexA, binds to promoter regions and inhibits the transcription of many genes required for DNA repair and DNA recombination. LexA also inhibits its own expression and the expression of another protein with multiple enzymatic roles, RecA. DNA damage, identified by the presence of single-stranded DNA, inactivates LexA. Inactivation of LexA is the result of proteolysis by the RecA protein, which when bound to single-stranded DNA functions as a specific protease. In the absence of LexA, genes that were previously inhibited by LexA can be expressed. After the damage of DNA is repaired, LexA begin to accumulate again, repressing the expression of SOS genes.

SOS Postreplication Repair

Many of the enzymes involved in DNA repair in *E. coli,* including the ABC excinuclease system, are inducible and regulated by proteins **LexA** and **RecA** that, together with the genes coding for the inducible proteins, form the **SOS repair** system.

Under normal conditions LexA binds tightly to the control region of genes that code for repair enzymes and several other proteins and prevents the expression. Genes in the SOS response also induce the *polB* gene encoding a polymerization subunit of DNA polymerase required for error-prone translesion replication. The SOS system is activated as a result of severe DNA damage. Activation can be described as the RecA-mediated cleavage and destruction of LexA in an autoproteolytic manner (Figure 15.20). The fragmented LexA dissociates from the DNA, allowing the efficient expression of the SOS response genes. Some of the products of the SOS response assemble at the lesion to form a specialized replication system that depends on DNA polymerase II for replicating past DNA lesions, which normally block DNA polymerase III. This **translesion replication** is made possible because of the distinct properties of polymerase II.

The signal that activates RecA is the binding of RecA onto exposed single-stranded DNA or damaged double-stranded DNA, when DNA replication is stalled because of extensive DNA damage. The SOS response to heavy DNA damage is a process that converts a lesion at a replication error-prone site and allows replication to be temporarily restored over the lesion.

15.4 ■ DNA REPLICATION

Complementary Strands Are Basic to the Mechanism of Replication

The double-stranded structure of DNA permits each strand to serve as a template for the synthesis of a new strand identical to the other strand, as suggested in Figure 15.21. The correctness of this overall scheme of replication has solidly

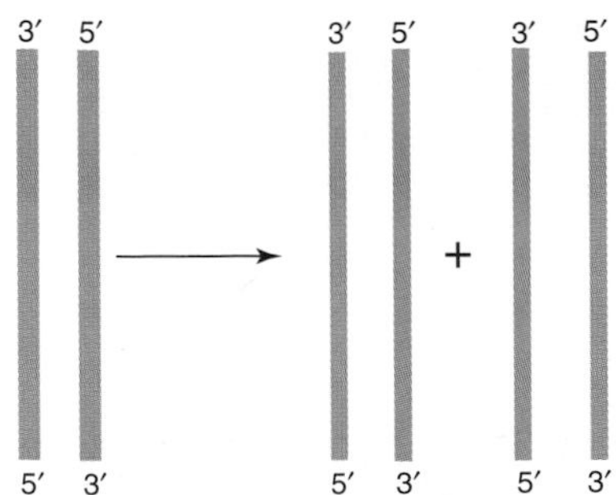

FIGURE 15.21
Each DNA strand serves as template for synthesis of a new complementary strand. Replication of DNA proceeds by a mechanism in which a new DNA strand (indicated by a red line) is synthesized that matches each of the original strands (shown by green lines).

been established. Even some bacteriophages, which contain single-stranded instead of double-stranded DNA, have been shown to convert their DNA to a double-stranded form before replication. The simplicity of the basic scheme for replication conceals a rather complex set of coordinated intricate processes. A multiplicity of enzymes and protein factors participate in these processes. The enzymes involved in replication must also deal with a variety of topological problems. DNA-dependent DNA polymerase can synthesize new strands by operating only along the $5' \rightarrow 3'$ direction, and therefore it is unable to elongate the two antiparallel strands of the helix in the same macroscopic direction. In addition, DNA polymerases are unable to start DNA synthesis in the absence of a preexisting primer and the replication cannot proceed unless the complementary strands are separated at an early stage of the synthesis. Separation requires the commitment of energy for disrupting the thermodynamically favorable double-helical arrangement and the unwinding of a highly twisted double helix at extremely rapid rates. Double-stranded DNA is normally a topologically closed domain, which, unless properly modified, will not tolerate strand unwinding to any appreciable degree. Obviously, these multiple difficulties must be dealt with before the replication of DNA can take place.

Replication Is Semiconservative

Three possibilities by which information transfer could take place during replication were initially visualized as indicated in Figure 15.22. Conservative replication could, in principle, yield a product consisting of a double helix of the original two strands and a daughter DNA consisting of completely newly synthesized chains. A second possibility, labeled dispersive, would have resulted if the nucleotides of the parental DNA were randomly scattered along the strands of the newly synthesized DNA. The synthesis of DNA eventually proved to be a **semiconservative process.** After each round of replication, the structure of parental DNA is found to preserve one of its own original strands combined with a newly synthesized complementary polynucleotide.

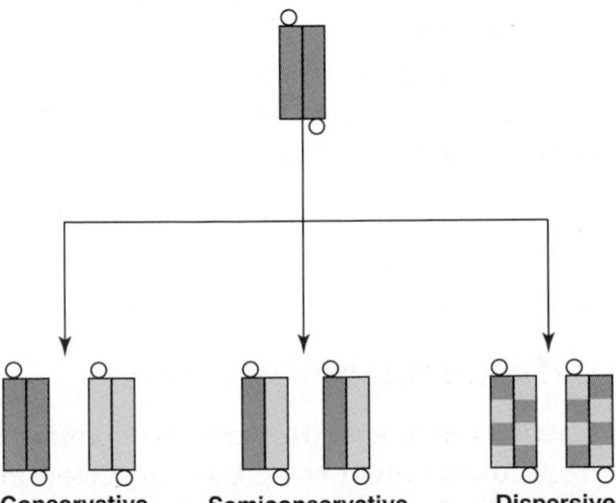

FIGURE 15.22
Three possible types of DNA replication.
Replication has been shown to occur exclusively according to the semiconservative model; that is, after each round of replication one of the parental strands is maintained intact, and it combines with one newly synthesized complementary strand. Circles represent the $5'$ terminals.

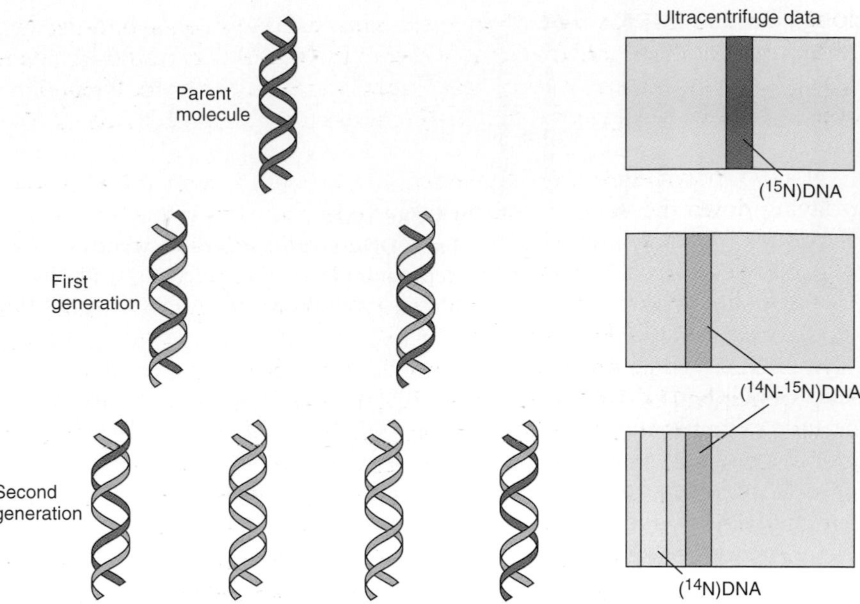

FIGURE 15.23
Semiconservative replication of DNA. Schematic representation of the experiment of Meselson and Stahl that demonstrated semiconservative replication of DNA. This model of replication requires that, if the parent molecule (dark red) contains ^{15}N, each of the molecules produced during the first generation contain ^{15}N in one strand and ^{14}N in the other. Furthermore, in the second generation two molecules must contain only ^{14}N, and two molecules must contain equal amounts of ^{14}N and ^{15}N. The results of separating DNA molecules from successive generations, shown on the right, are consistent with this model.

The semiconservative nature of replication was elegantly suggested by a classic experiment that allowed the physical separation and identification of the parental and the newly synthesized strands. *Escherichia coli* was grown in a medium containing [^{15}N]-ammonium chloride as the exclusive source of nitrogen. Several cell divisions were allowed to occur, during which the naturally occurring ^{14}N in the DNA of *E. coli* was, for all practical purposes, replaced by the heavier ^{15}N isotope. The ^{14}N-containing nutrient was then added, and cells were removed at appropriate intervals. The DNA of these cells was extracted, and the ratios of ^{14}N to ^{15}N content were determined by equilibrium density gradient centrifugation. The separation between [^{14}N]DNA and [^{15}N]DNA was achieved based on the lower density of DNA, which contained the lighter isotope. In subsequent experiments, the newly synthesized DNA was thermally denatured and the individual strands were completely separated. The results, shown in Figure 15.23, demonstrated that daughter DNA molecules consisted of two strands with different densities, corresponding to the densities of single-stranded polynucleotides containing exclusively ^{14}N or ^{15}N. Conservative and dispersive replications are clearly inconsistent with these findings.

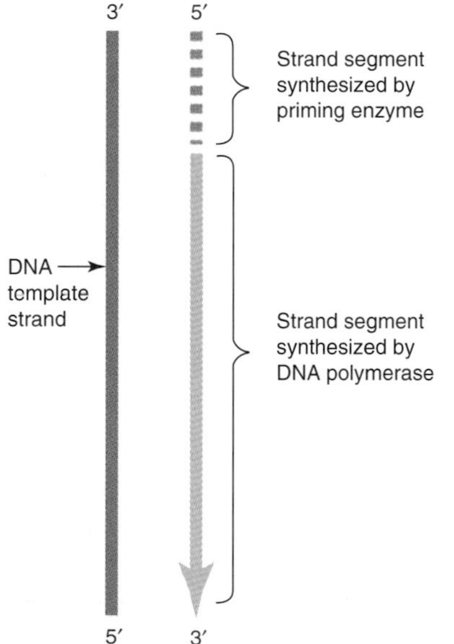

FIGURE 15.24
Synthesis of primer for DNA replication. Primer (dashed line) is synthesized by primase. A primer permits new DNA (orange line) to be synthesized by DNA polymerases. The primer is excised at the completion of DNA synthesis.

A Primer Is Required

The semiconservative nature of replication requires that each strand serve as a DNA polymerase template for the synthesis of a new complementary strand. Elongation is catalyzed by polymerase III (Table 15.1), as distinguished from polymerase I, which is primarily involved in repair. Polymerase III, which is ATP-dependent, is unable to asemble the first few nucleotides of a new strand and requires a primer. In *E. coli* primers are segments 10–60 nucleotides long. With few exceptions, the primer is an oligonucleotide synthesized by other enzymes, as indicated in Figure 15.24. **Primers** are formed by **primases,** although in a few instances **RNA polymerases** are known to synthesize a primer. In some bacterial systems and phages, the priming enzyme has activity characteristic of an RNA polymerase because the ribonucleotides condense to form the primer. In other systems the primase does not discriminate between 5′-ribonucleotides and 5′-deoxyribonucleotides. As a general rule, however, primases use ribonucleotides for incorporation into primers. Some enzymes that catalyze the synthesis of primers act exclusively as primases, while others possess additional enzymatic activities. In mammalian cells primase activity is vested in **DNA polymerase α,** an enzyme that is also involved in DNA strand elongation and in DNA repair. Once the primers have been synthesized, the DNA polymerase can move in and take over the process of synthesis. It is not clear what signal causes a switchover from primase to DNA polymerase, although it has been suggested that a specialized ribonuclease **(RNaseH)** is involved.

If DNA polymerase were the enzyme that would begin DNA synthesis by laying down the very first nucleotide complementary to the template, the efficiency of DNA synthesis would be severely reduced. Since the bases in a very short segment of a double helix have high configurational flexibility, the first nucleotide introduced into a newly synthesized DNA strand would likely be mispaired and would immediately activate the proofreading activity of DNA polymerase. The outcome would be a fruitless back-and-forth cycle of synthesis and proofreading by DNA polymerase with little net synthesis of new DNA. In contrast, primases, which have no proofreading ability, can quickly and efficiently position primers that can be elongated with DNA polymerases without appreciable backtracking. The primases ignore mismatches and produce an RNA chain long enough to allow the DNA polymerase to operate at the 3′ end of a double-stranded structure that restricts newly introduced nucleotides on the basis of strict complementary rules. The mismatches introduced by the primase are irrelevant because the characteristic RNA-like structure of primers allows for their subsequent wholesale removal and replacement by DNA of an equivalent composition.

Although primers are almost invariably short RNA or RNA-like segments (Table 15.6), RNA priming is not used universally. In the "rolling circle" replication mechanism of DNA, a 3′-OH primer is generated by endonuclease digestion of parental DNA, and with **parvoviruses** a 3′-OH primer is generated by the folding back of an existing 3′ terminus. A single deoxyribonucleotide can serve as primer in **adenovirus.** Such a nucleotide, with its 3′-OH terminus free, is attached to the end of a template strand through a virus-encoded specific protein (Figure 15.25).

TABLE 15.6 RNA Primers

Replicating System	*RNA Oligonucleotide*[a]
Bacteriophage T4	pppAC $(N)_3$
Bacteriophage T7	pppACCA
	pppACCC
Mouse polyoma virus	pppA $(N)_9$
	pppG $(N)_9$
Lymphoblastoid cells	pppA $(N)_8$
	pppG $(N)_8$

[a] N stands for any ribonucleotide. The primer lengths for the mouse polyoma virus and the animal cells are averages.

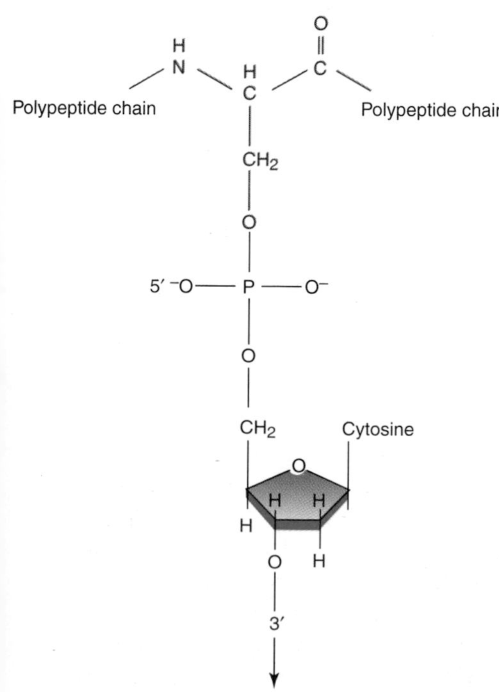

FIGURE 15.25
An unusual primer used in the replication of adenovirus DNA.
This primer is a single nucleotide attached, by its 5′-terminal phosphate, to a serine residue of a protein. Adenovirus DNA is synthesized by extension of the 3′ terminus of this nucleotide.

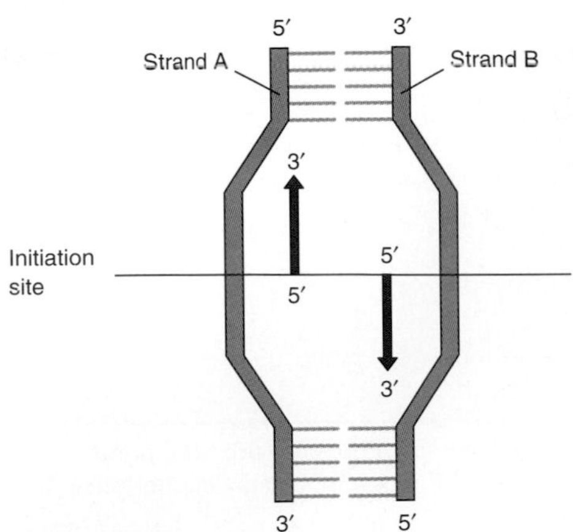

FIGURE 15.26
Both DNA strands serve as templates for DNA synthesis.
Each DNA strand must serve as a template for DNA synthesis. The new DNA can be synthesized only in the 5′ → 3′ direction. If only a single initiation origin were considered, the result of continuous synthesis would be the formation of two new nonidentical double-stranded DNA molecules (one above and one below the initiation origin). Also, the upper part of strand A and the lower part of strand B could not have been used as templates. In fact, the synthesis occurs both continuously and discontinuously.

Both Strands of DNA Serve as Templates Concurrently

In the preceding section, the events leading to the synthesis of DNA by DNA polymerase were examined and attention was directed to one of the two parental DNA strands used as template. In fact, synthetic events occur at both strands almost concurrently. This would appear to generate some problems of geometry. Specifically, if a single initiation site is considered, and the synthesis continued in the 5′ → 3′ direction until each template is completely copied, the result of the synthesis would be the creation of two new double-stranded molecules. Examination of Figure 15.26 indicates that, at least in the case of linear double-stranded DNA, neither of these two hypothetical DNA molecules would be identical to the parental DNA.

Such an outcome is not in agreement with the actual course of DNA replication. The discrepancy can be accounted for by recognizing that the microscopic synthesis of the new strands does not proceed uninterrupted. In fact, the synthesis occurs in a discontinuous fashion and in a manner that permits the assembly of the synthesized polynucleotide portions into appropriate complete DNA strands.

Synthesis Is Discontinuous

The overall process of DNA synthesis may now be considered past the immediate vicinity of initiation by examining a larger section of DNA. One of the two parts of DNA that would be generated if the macromolecule were divided at the site of chain initiation is shown in Figure 15.27. In almost every instance the synthesis is **bidirectional,** which means that the synthetic events occurring at the part of the molecule indicated by solid lines are of the same general nature as those occurring on the other site and indicated with dashed lines.

A prerequisite for the semiconservative mechanism of replication is that the two complementary strands of DNA gradually separate as the synthesis of new strands takes place. The mechanics of this separation are addressed later, but it may be apparent that as a result of separating the strands at an interior position, two topologically equivalent forks are created at the point of diversion of the two strands.

Various lines of evidence have indicated that DNA polymerase acts in a **discontinuous** manner; that is, along each DNA molecule there are numerous initiation points at which primers are formed. In eukaryotes primers may be formed at locations that are determined by nucleosome spacing. In the case of bacteriophage T7, primosomes appear to recognize TGGT and GGGT through prepriming proteins. Once a site for primer initiation has been recognized,

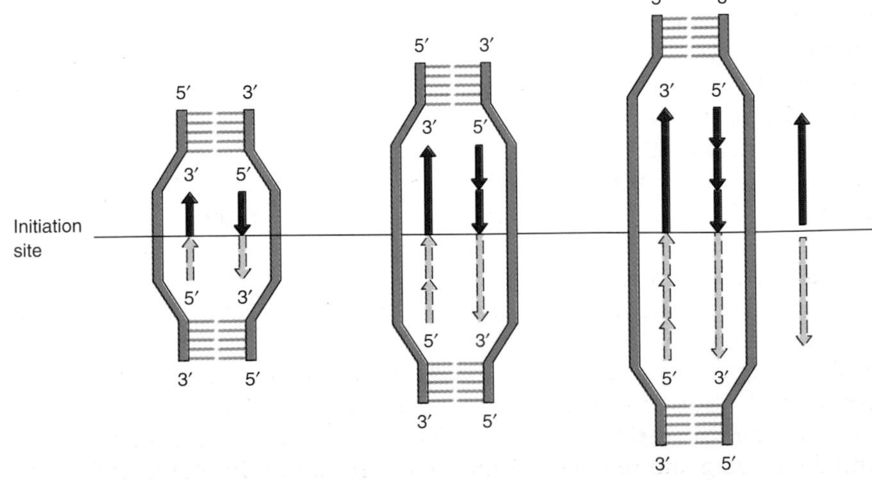

FIGURE 15.27
Discontinuous synthesis of DNA.
This figure emphasizes the synthetic events occurring at only one side of the initiation site (dark red line). The two complementary strands of DNA separate as the discontinuous synthesis of small DNA segments takes place on both strands located at different sites on the DNA. After excision of the primers, the excised parts are repaired, and the segments are joined together. Although segments are clearly synthesized in opposite directions on the two strands, overall macroscopic impression is that DNA grows in the single direction suggested by the solid red arrow on the right.

single-strand binding proteins (SSB), which interact with single-stranded polynucleotides, are displaced and the primase lays down a primer. After promoting primer initiation at one point, prepriming proteins move along the template strand in order to synthesize the adjacent primer. At each one of these locations, DNA polymerase III makes use of the assembled primers for the synthesis of DNA. When DNA polymerase reaches the end of the single-stranded template, it comes upon the next primer annealed to the template. The polymerase, as indicated by its very high processivity, can overcome this hurdle by sliding over the intervening double-stranded DNA–RNA hybrid and resuming replication at the 3′ end of this new primer.

The segments synthesized by DNA polymerase upon each primer, known as **precursor (Okazaki) fragments** or **nascent DNA,** vary in size from about 100 to 200 deoxyribonucleotides in eukaryotes to ten times as long in bacteria. Once these segments of the new DNA are synthesized on both strands of a fork (Figure 15.27), the fork opens up further, and the same process of synthesis is repeated. Shortly after synthesis, the primer portions of the Okazaki fragments are excised by the 5′ → 3′ exonuclease activity of DNA polymerase I, which also synthesizes short segments of DNA.

This discontinuous mechanism compensates for the inability of DNA polymerase to synthesize strands in the 3′ → 5′ direction. By synthesizing portions of DNA strands only in the 5′ → 3′ direction on both antiparallel strands of the parental DNA, the polymerase is able to create the illusion, when the synthesis is experimentally visualized by electron microscopy techniques, that both strands are concurrently elongated in the same macroscopic direction. In Figure 15.27 this direction is indicated by a large solid arrow. It should be noted that the first strand synthesized, often referred to as the **leading strand,** is synthesized continuously. It is the other strand, the **lagging strand,** that must be synthesized discontinuously.

Macroscopic Synthesis Is as a Rule Bidirectional

At the site of initiation of DNA synthesis two identical forks are created (Figure 15.27). Therefore two possibilities exist for the synthesis of DNA: the process may occur at only one fork and proceed in a single direction, as shown by the thick solid arrow, or alternatively it may occur at both forks and in both directions away from the starting point. The events occurring in the forks located below the starting line are simply a mirror image repetition of what occurs in the fork that is located above the line. **Bidirectional replication** is the mechanism of DNA synthesis. The only known exceptions are in a small number of phages and plasmids that replicate unidirectionally. In the case of a small linear chromosome (e.g., bacteriophage λ) each fork moves along, synthesizing new DNA, until the end of the chromosome is reached. In a circular chromosome (e.g., *E. coli*) the two forks proceed in opposite directions until they meet at a predetermined site on the other side of the chromosome, as depicted in Figure 15.28. As the two forks meet, a new copy of the parental DNA is completed and released. The average rate at which each fork moves during replication is of the order of 60,000 bases per minute at 37°C. Upon completion, new DNA is released by the action of a type II topoisomerase as illustrated in Figure 15.29.

Strands Must Unwind and Separate

Separation of the strands of the parental DNA prior to synthesis of new strands is a requirement because the bases of each template must be made accessible to the complementary deoxyribonucleotides from which the new strands are constructed. The overall process of separation consists of a number of enzymatically catalyzed, coordinated steps, including the local unwinding of the helix, and the nicking and rejoining of the strands necessary for continuation of the

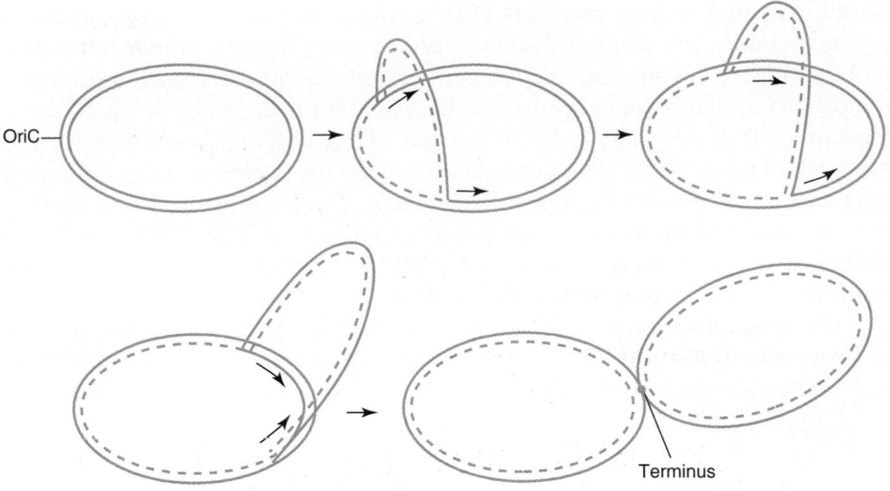

FIGURE 15.28
Bidirectional replication of a circular chromosome.
Replication starts at a fixed origin and proceeds at a constant rate in opposite directions until the two replication forks meet. Newly synthesized strands are indicated by dashed lines. After DNA synthesis is complete, two newly synthesized circular DNA molecules are separated by action of topoisomerases.

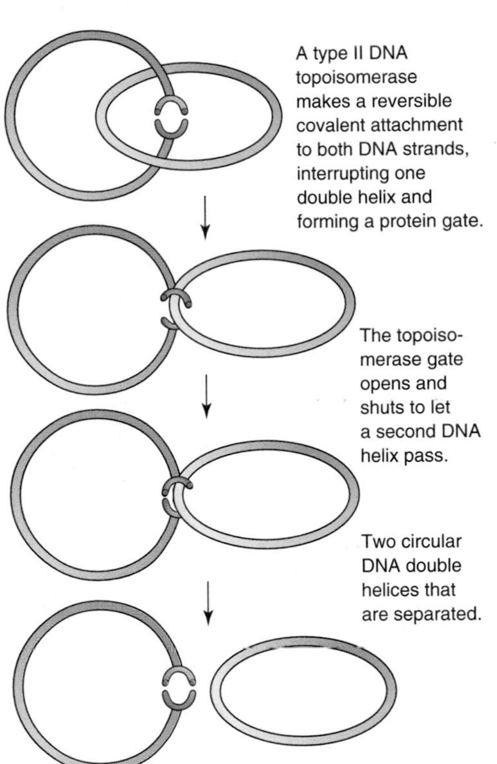

FIGURE 15.29
Function of topoisomerases II in separating interlocked DNA double helices.
Topoisomerase II attaches to both strands of DNA through reversible covalent bonds, thus forming an interrupted double helix with a topoisomerase "gate." A second DNA helix can pass through the portal using an "open-and-shut-the-gate" mechanism, leading to two separated DNA molecules. After separation of the molecules topoisomerase dissociates from DNA.

unwinding process. Once the strands are unwound, they must be kept separate so that they can operate freely as templates.

Specialized proteins accomplish rapid orderly unwinding of the strands. These proteins, **helicases,** separate DNA strands in advance of the moving replication fork and just in front of DNA polymerase. In *E. coli* they are referred to as **helicase II** and **rep protein.** Helicases move unidirectionally along DNA and separate the strands in advance of replication. They destabilize the interaction between complementary base pairs at the expense of ATP.

Once the strands have been separated, the single-stranded regions are stabilized by specific proteins, the **single-strand binding (SSB) proteins.** The DNA single strands are covered by the SSB proteins because of their high affinity for single-stranded DNA. As the helicase moves in advance of the replication fork, SSB proteins go on and off the DNA, with protein molecules that are displaced from one site reassociating with another (Figure 15.30). SSB proteins do not consume ATP and do not exhibit any enzymatic activities. Their role is only to keep the strands apart long enough for the priming process to occur.

In *E. coli* DNA, it is calculated that the parental double helix must unwind at a rate of about 6000 turns per minute. These high rates would generate insurmountable difficulties if strands were to separate over an appreciable length of DNA. The large free-energy requirements of bringing about the unwinding of large regions of DNA can, however, be reduced to manageable levels by the nicking of one or both of the DNA strands near the replicating fork. Since the fork is a moving entity, the nicking must be visualized as a reversible cut-and-rejoin process, which moves along with the fork. Nicking is indispensable for a topological reason as well. Unwinding at one of the two forks requires that the parental double helix rotate in the opposite direction to that necessary for the unwinding of the opposite fork. In the absence of a nick as the unwinding at one of the forks would progress, an increasing number of positive supercoils would have to be introduced into the double helix. Once the limit of the helix to accommodate the supercoils were reached, unwinding and replication would have to cease.

These topological restraints are overcome if DNA is maintained during replication in the **negative superhelical form.** This form could serve as a "sink" for the positive supercoils that could potentially be generated during replication. In *E. coli,* this is apparently achieved by the action of **gyrase,** a **topoisomerase** type II, which induces the formation of negative supercoils

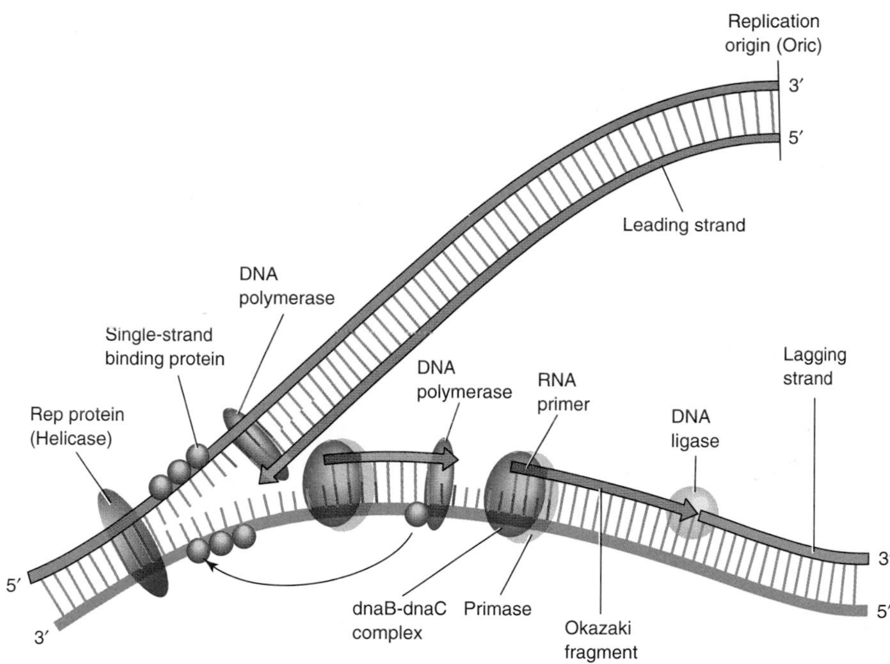

FIGURE 15.30
Model for DNA replication in *E. coli.*
The initial stages of replication are depicted. Primers are removed from newly synthesized segments of DNA at the lagging strand, and the segments are joined. Since replication is normally bidirectional, similar events take place concurrently at the other side of the initiation origin.

at the expense of ATP. **Topoisomerases type I** may also be involved. The superhelicity of DNA may be negatively regulated through a balance between topoisomerases of types I and II; that is, a diminishment of topoisomerase II activity may bring about a decrease in the amount of negative superhelicity that can be created, whereas an inhibition of topoisomerase I activity may increase it. During replication the linking number between parental strands decreases from a large value at the beginning of replication to zero at the end of a complete round of DNA synthesis.

Escherichia coli Provides Basic Model for Replication of DNA

Extensive studies in *E. coli* and its phages have permitted the proposal of a replication model that depends on the action of a large number of proteins, some of which are listed in Table 15.7. With the specific exceptions noted in the sections that follow, this model may also be viewed as a basic scheme for DNA replication in most other cells.

Initiation and Progression of DNA Synthesis

Synthesis of DNA begins at a specific site of the chromosome referred to as the **replication origin,** which in *E. coli* is referred to as **OriC** (Figure 15.30). Initiation of DNA synthesis involves participation of as many as 20–30 different proteins, many of which are needed to be present at the origin of replication in multiple copies. OriC must be recognized by specific proteins, and the origin must unwind to allow helicase, primase, and DNA polymerase III to have access to each DNA strand. OriC is a sequence of 245 base pairs that contains four sites (nucleotide 9-mers with a similar nucleotide sequence) at which **dnaA,** a tetramer consisting of four identical subunits, can initiate the stepwise assembly of all the proteins and enzymes necessary to carry out replication (Figure 15.31). In addition, the origin contains 11 methylation sites recognized by **Dam methylase** and three AT-rich direct tandem repeats consisting of 13 base pairs each. This final assembly is called a **replisome.**

Formation of a replisome begins with the binding of one dnaA molecule

TABLE 15.7 Components of the Replisome

Protein	*Function*
SSB	Single-strand binding
Protein i (dnaT), Protein n, Protein n′, Protein n″, dnaG	Primosome assembly and function
dnaG	Primase (primer synthesis)
Pol III holoenzyme	Processive chain elongation
Pol I	Gap filling and primer excision
Ligase	Ligation
Gyrase	Supercoiling
gyrA	
gyrB	
rep	Helicase
Helicase II	
dnaB	Helicase
dnaA, dnaC	Origin of replication

at each one of the 9-mers, provided that these binding sites are fully methylated. The dnaA apparently recognizes these 9-mers on the basis of their conformation, which appears to be slightly curved with the double helix somewhat elongated relative to typical B-DNA. Several more additional dnaA molecules are then added via a highly cooperative process to form a nucleosome-like structure. An additional factor, **HU protein,** participates in the formation of this complex.

The dnaA and HU protein interact with the OriC in a manner that promotes the opening of the DNA strands in the AT-rich regions adjacent to the origin. Finally, dnaA, with the aid of **dnaC,** adds **dnaB** in the complex. The dnaB, by virtue of its helicase activity, creates an initiation "bubble" consisting of a few hundred nucleotide pairs. The energy for the formation of the "bubble" is provided by ATP in a reaction catalyzed by topoisomerase II, and the 'bubble" is stabilized by SSB proteins.

Synthesis of an RNA primer begins with the formation of a prepriming complex. The prepriming assembly consists of the dnaB–dnaC complex to which four other proteins (polypeptides n, n′, n″, and i) have been added. Addition of primase, **dnaG,** converts the prepriming complex to a **primosome**

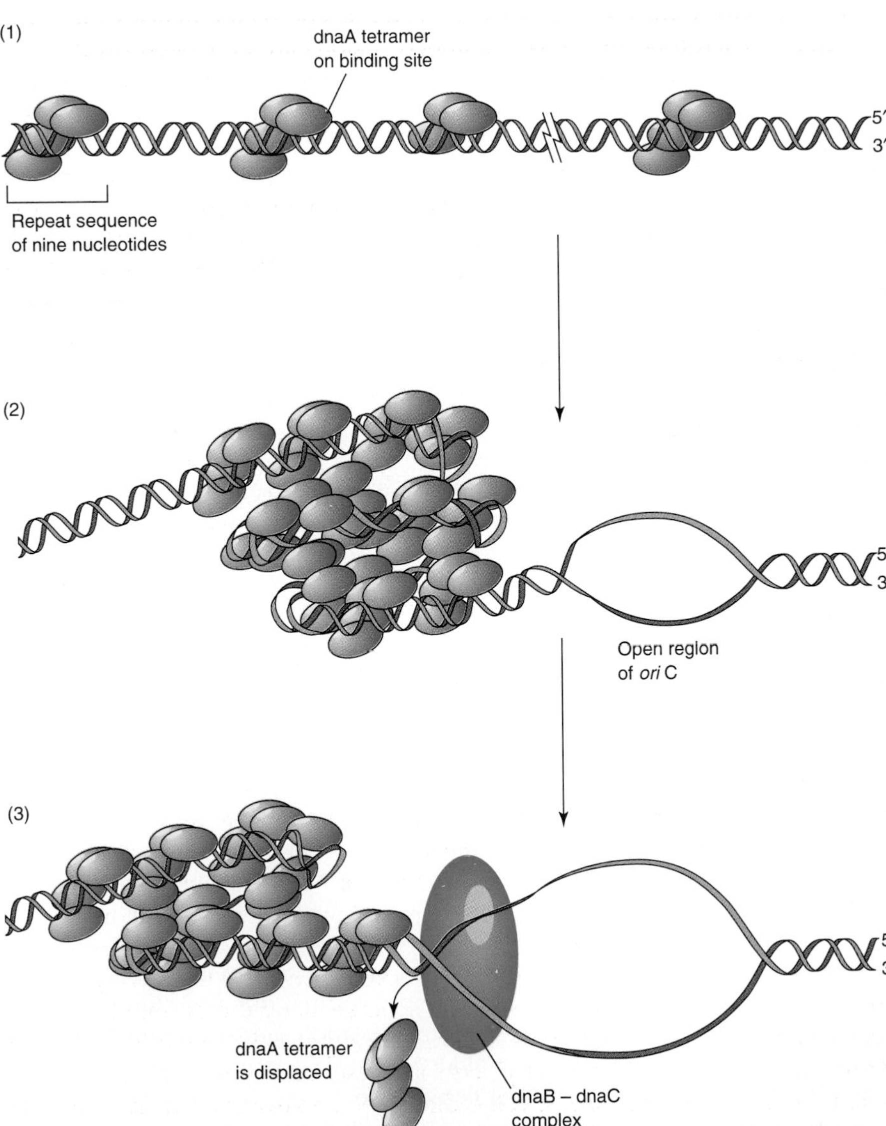

FIGURE 15.31
Model for initiation of replication in *E. coli.*
Step 1: Initiation of replication begins with binding of dnaA molecules to four sites consisting of nine-nucleotide long sequences each. These sequences are present at the origin of replication in *E. coli* (OriC). Step 2: DNA-bound dnaA molecules subsequently coalesce and are joined by additional dnaA molecules to form a nucleosome-like DNA–protein complex, which promotes nearby "melting" of the double helix. Step 3: The resulting opening of strands allows a dnaB–dnaC complex to become attached to DNA so that helicase activity of dnaB can further unwind the DNA. Unwinding is accompanied by a displacement of dnaA molecules. *Redrawn based on figure in Rawn, J. D.,* Biochemistry. *Burlington, NC: Neil Patterson Publishers, 1989.*

(Figure 15.32). The primosome interacts with a template, at each one of the two forks generated by the formation of a "bubble," and begins the synthesis of RNA primers on the two leading strands. Assembly of the replisome is completed by addition to the primosome of DNA polymerase III and **rep proteins.**

Initiation can be regulated by either restricting the availability of dnaA-binding sites at OriC or by limiting the concentration of dnaA. **Methylation** provides a switch for the availability of dnaA-binding sites. Once replication has been initiated, the dnaA near OriC binds to the plasma membrane and becomes unavailable to Dam methylase. In addition, binding of DNA in the vicinity of OriC to the cellular membrane sequesters the *dnaA* gene, which is situated near OriC (only 40 kb away). As a result, the synthesis of dnaA protein is inhibited and its cellular concentration is lowered.

Initiation of the leading DNA strand at OriC by the primosome is more complex than the subsequent initiation of synthesis of Okazaki fragments on the lagging strand initiated by primase at sites selected by the prepriming proteins. The initiation of the leading strand does not present the cell with serious topological problems, but for continuation of synthesis helicase II and rep protein are essential. These enzymes unwind and separate the strands in each of the two forks created by the initiation event. As the helicases move in advance of each fork, two single-stranded regions are generated on parental DNA. These regions are immediately covered by single-strand binding protein that keeps the fork open and allows DNA polymerase III to take over the elongation of primers. A signal for initiation of the lagging strand, uncovered on the template by the movement of helicase, leads to the binding of primase. Primase, the action of which is triggered by the prepriming proteins, synthesizes a brief complementary segment of the strand. This segment serves as a primer for covalent extension of the strand synthesized by DNA polymerase III and for formation of Okazaki fragments. DNA polymerase III complexes are endowed with similar but somewhat distinct properties, one tailored for the continuous synthesis of the leading strand and the other for the discontinuous synthesis of the lagging strand. This polymerase assembly, which appears to combine primase activity with nonidentical twin active sites for polynucleotide synthesis, allows for concurrent replication on both strands. In this scheme, looping of the lagging strand template by 180° brings it to the same orientation as the leading strand template (Figure 15.33). Thus a primer synthesized at the lagging strand is drawn past it. When a nascent (Okazaki) fragment reaches the 5′ end of the previously synthesized Okazaki fragment, the lagging strand template is released and unlooped. Removal of the primer portions at the 5′ end of the Okazaki fragments by DNA polymerase I, repair by the same enzyme, and joining of the repaired fragments by DNA ligase produces intact DNA strands.

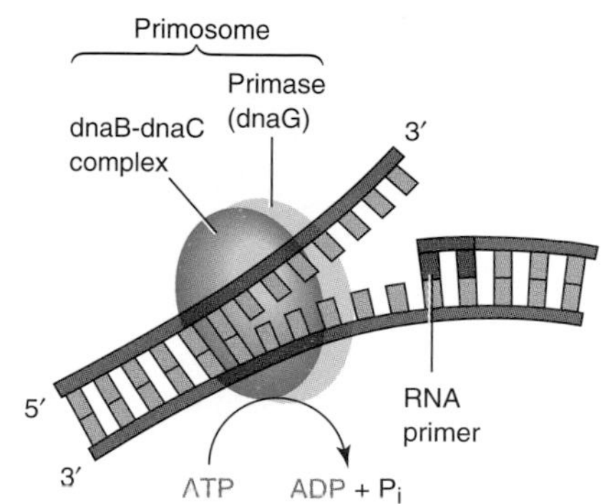

FIGURE 15.32
Primosome of *E. coli.*
The primosome is formed by binding of primase, together with a complex of dnaB and dnaC proteins, at specific sequences of DNA that serve as sites for formation of RNA primers. Additional factors, described as n proteins, are specific primosomal components that are responsible for placing the primosome at the appropriate sequences. In effect, the primosome "searches" the DNA for these sequences at the expense of ATP. Once the correct destination of the primosome is reached, RNA primer synthesis is initiated.

Termination of DNA Synthesis

Termination occurs near the center of a 270-kb region across from OriC, the **ter** or **τ locus.** This region incorporates five ter sequences, that is, loci with the core sequence GTGTGTTGT that bind the **Tus protein (terminator utilization substance)** that promotes the termination of synthesis (Figure 15.34). Tus protein is a contrahelicase in that it functions by literally interfering with the ATP-dependent and dnaB helicase-promoted unwinding of DNA rather than simply impeding the propagation of this helicase along the double helix. The organization of the ter region is shown in Figure 15.34. Each Tus site has directional properties (asymmetry) and it arrests only those replisomes that reach the Tus site from one specific direction. Replisomes arriving from the opposite direction apparently force the dissociation of the Tus protein and thus

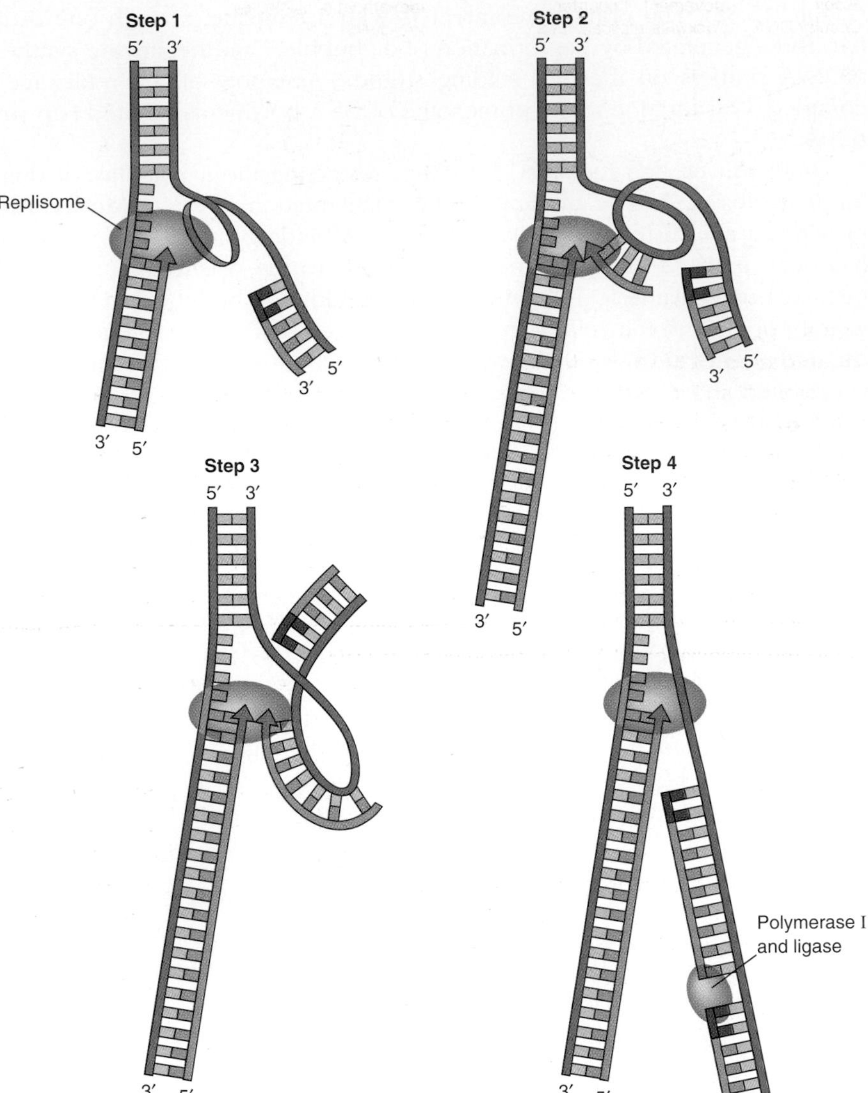

FIGURE 15.33
Model for the simultaneous synthesis of leading and lagging DNA strands by DNA polymerase.
Two molecules of DNA polymerase operating in concert, and in the same rather than the opposite direction, may be participating in the simultaneous synthesis of DNA on both strands. In this model the replisome consists of a DNA polymerase dimer associated with the primosome and helicases. The primer made by the primosome is extended by the replisome as the lagging-strand template is looped through it. The primer continues to be extended until the previously completed Okazaki fragment is reached, at which point the loop is relaxed. The stretch of unpaired lagging-strand template then loops back again to participate in the formation of the next Okazaki fragment.
Redrawn based on figure in Kornberg, A. DNA Replication. *San Francisco: Freeman, 1992.*

can proceed unimpeded past the Ter–Tus site. Because of the distribution and orientation of sites in the ter region, each replisome must first pass over all sites that are oriented the opposite way before arriving at the Tus site that is oriented in a way that causes termination. This arrangement makes it inevitable that a replisome will not dissociate from DNA until it actually collides with the replisome entering the ter region from the opposite direction. This ensures the complete replication of the chromosome and prevents overreplication. The products of replication are two **concatenated** progeny chromosomes usually interwound by as many as 30 coils. The newly synthesized DNA is untangled from the parental DNA apparently by the action of a topoisomerase II.

Rolling Circle Model for Replication

DNA synthesis directed by circular mtDNA, and in some instances by bacteria and viruses, gives rise to linear daughter DNA molecules that contain the base sequence of parental DNA repeated numerous times. These repeated linear DNAs, which are known as **concatemers,** are essential for the bacterial mating and may be involved in gene amplification. The synthesis of concatemer DNA occurs by a mechanism known as **rolling circle replication.**

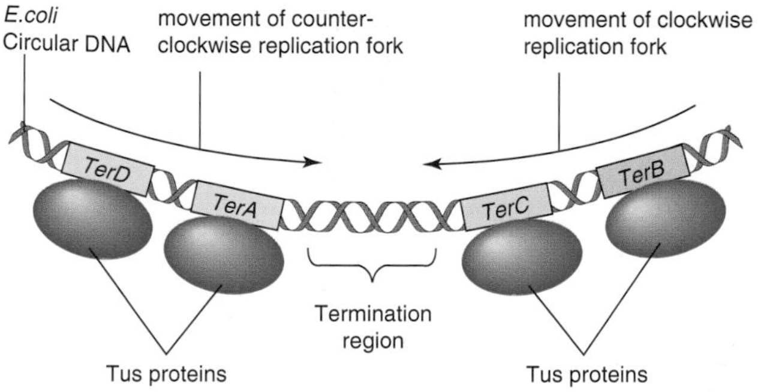

FIGURE 15.34
Termination of DNA replication in *E. coli.*
Termination region (ter) of *E. coli* incorporates five asymmetric ter sites. Each ter site can interact with Tus protein. TerB and terC are oriented in the same direction and the remaining three ter sites are oriented in the opposite direction. Because of the orientation of Tus-bound ter sites, each replisome that reaches the ter region must cross all the Tus–ter sites that are oriented the opposite way before arriving at a site that causes termination. A replisome moving in the direction shown by the arrow must first cross terE, terD, and terA before terminating replication at either the terC or terB site. This arrangement ensures that each replisome continues to synthesize DNA until it collides with a replisome entering the ter region from the opposite direction, leading to the dissociation of both replisomes from DNA.
Adapted from Hidaka, M., Kobayashi, T., and Horiuchi, T. J. Bacteriol. *173:381, 1991.*

An example is the replication of certain circular single-stranded bacteriophages such as ϕX174. When the virus enters a host bacterium the single-stranded genome is converted to a double-stranded DNA by action of primase and DNA polymerase III. The DNA strand complementary to the bacteriophage genome that is first synthesized [labeled the (−) strand] serves as the template for the genomic DNA [the (+) strand]. The atypical characteristic of this replication scheme is that the (+) strand is nicked at a specific site (by a phage-encoded endonuclease) so that it can serve as a primer for its own replication. The (+) strand is elongated from the 3′-hydroxyl end of the nick by DNA polymerase III by incrementally displacing segments of the (+) strand associated with the "helper" (−) strand (Figure 15.35).

A second characteristic is that the circular template does not dissociate from the complementary strand during the synthesis. Instead the replication of the leading strand goes on beyond the length of circle-generating linear concatemeric DNA. Appropriately sized DNA molecules are subsequently generated from concatemers by specific endonuclease cleavage.

Eukaryotic DNA Replication

The DNA synthesis in eukaryotes appears to be a process that is fundamentally similar to that occurring in prokaryotes. Formation of a replication fork, primer

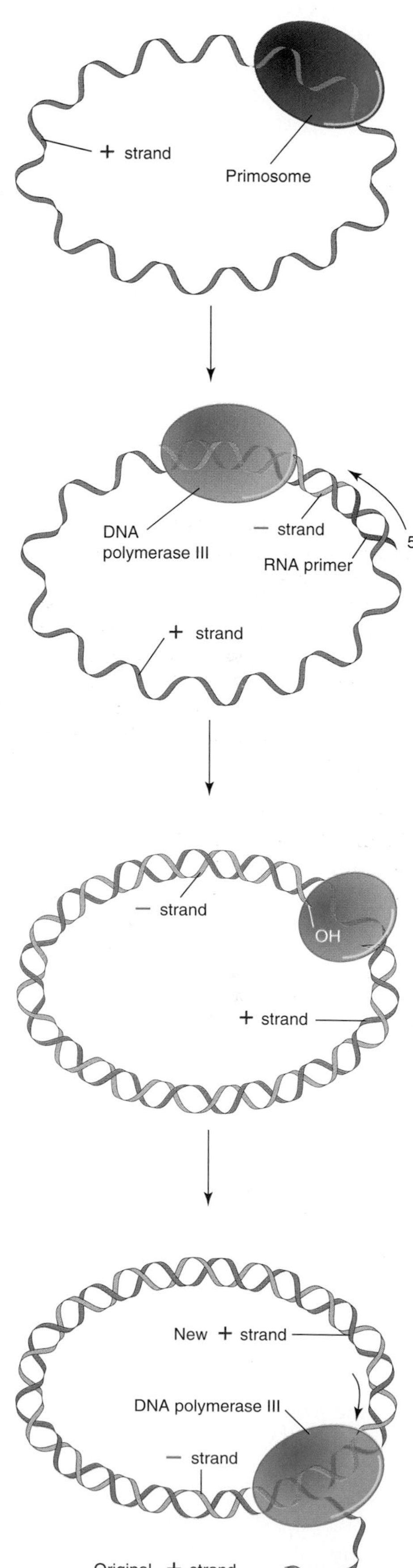

FIGURE 15.35
Replication by the rolling circle mechanism.
In ssDNA of certain bacteriophages, such as ϕX174, the (+) strand is converted into dsDNA upon injection into a host bacterium. This transformation occurs by action of primase and polymerase III upon ssDNA that synthesizes a complementary (−) strand. Replication of (+) strands begins with nicking of (+) strand so that it can serve as a primer for its own replication. The (+) strand is elongated from the 3′-hydroxyl end of the nick, as the newly synthesized strand gradually displaces from the helper-strand the original (+) strand.
Redrawn based on figure in Moran, L. A., Scrimgeour, K. G., Horton, H. R. Achs, R. S., and Rawn, S. D. Biochemistry. *Englewood Cliffs, NJ: Neil Patterson/Prentice Hall, 1994.*

synthesis, Okazaki fragments, primer removal, and gap bridging between newly synthesized DNA segments, all parallel the corresponding steps that occur in prokaryotes, but the overall process is quite a bit more complex. Replication among eukaryotes, from yeasts to humans, shares similarities.

As expected, differences are more pronounced between prokaryotes and eukaryotes. In rapidly growing prokaryotes, DNA is replicated through much of the cell cycle and cell division occurs as soon as DNA synthesis has ceased. In contrast, eukaryotic DNA synthesis (and histone synthesis) is confined to only one part of the cell cycle, specifically the synthetic (S) phase of the interphase. This phase is preceded and followed by two periods during which DNA is not synthesized (gap periods G1 and G2). Cell division occurs at a different time within the interphase, referred to as the mitotic (M) period. Beyond this characteristic limitation of eukaryotic replication to a certain period of the cell cycle, important differences in replication between prokaryotes and eukaryotes arise primarily from the larger size of eukaryotic DNA (about 10^5–10^6 kb content) as compared to prokaryotic DNA (about 5×10^3 kb for *E. coli*), the distinct packaging of eukaryotic DNA in the form of chromatin, and the slower rates of fork movement in eukaryotes. For DNA to become available to DNA polymerases, nucleosomes must disassemble, a step that slows the rates of fork movement. DNA polymerase movement does not exceed 30,000 base pairs per minute, which is considerably slower than the rates observed for *E. coli*. Based on the higher DNA content of animal cells, and the lower activities of DNA polymerases in comparison to bacteria, the replication cycle of eukaryotic cells could be expected to take as long as a month to complete. In fact, however, the replication cycle is completed within hours, because compensating factors are in operation. Eukaryotic cells contain a large number of DNA polymerase molecules (often in excess of 20,000) as compared to a few dozen in each *E. coli* cell. DNA polymerase initiates bidirectional synthesis but at several origins of replication located anywhere between 5 and 300 kilobase pairs (kb) apart within the chromosome, depending on species and cell type (Figure 15.36). DNA segments between two origins of replication are termed **replicons.** An average human chromosome contains as many as 100 replicons and replication may proceed simultaneously at as many as 200 forks. More origins can be found in developmentally active cells that carry out DNA synthesis at very rapid rates. During early embryogenesis the largest chromosome of *Drosophila melanogaster* contains as many as 6000 replicating forks, or one for every 10 kb.

Role of Eukaryotic DNA Polymerases

In prokaryotes synthesis is catalyzed by two similar but distinct subunits of DNA polymerase III. In eukaryotes, synthesis of the leading and lagging strands is carried out by different enzymes (Table 15.2). **DNA polymerase δ,** a polymerase of high processivity, catalyzes the synthesis of the leading strand. This enzyme consists of a large subunit that is vested with $5' \rightarrow 3'$ nucleotide polymerizing activity and a smaller subunit that has a $3' \rightarrow 5'$ proofreading exonuclease activity. The high processivity of DNA polymerase δ is attributed to the presence of an accessory factor, the **proliferating cell nuclear antigen (PCNA),** that is found in large amounts in the nuclei of proliferating cells. PCNA (mol wt 25,000) is a multimeric protein that can act as a "clamp" to keep the enzyme from disassociating off the leading DNA strand. The "clamp" consists of three PCNA molecules, each containing two topologically identical domains that are tightly associated to form a closed ring. This suggests that in eukaryotes PCNA is the functional equivalent of the β subunit of *E. coli* polymerase III. Another accessory protein, the **replication factor C (RFC),** also binds to polymerase δ and probably assists with association between PCNA and DNA to form the "clamp." Alternatively, RFC may be involved in setting up a link

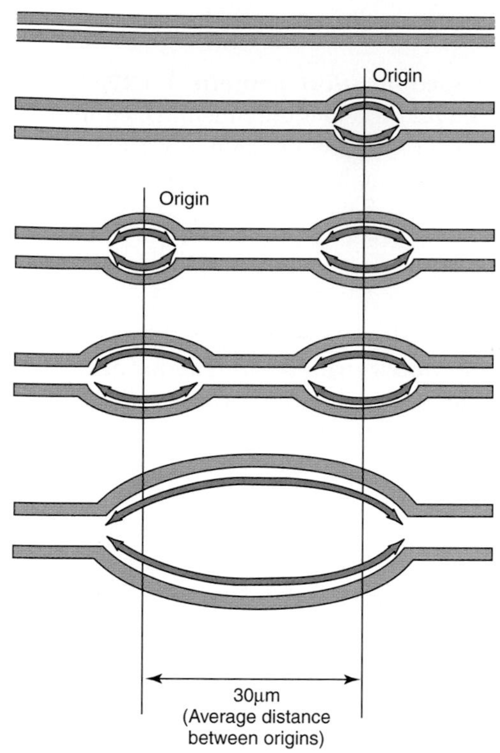

FIGURE 15.36
Replication of mammalian DNA.
Mammalian DNA replicates by using a very large number of replicating forks simultaneously. This mechanism accelerates the process of replication, which in mammalian systems is limited by rates of fork movement that are considerably slower than those characteristic of prokaryotes.
Redrawn based on figure in Huberman, J. A., and Riggs, A. D. J. Mol. Biol. *32:327, 1968.*

between polymerase δ and polymerase α. Therefore the role of RFC in DNA synthesis is analogous to the roles of the γ complex and the τ subunits of *E. coli* DNA polymerase III.

Synthesis of the lagging strand is catalyzed by **DNA polymerase α.** This polymerase has similar structure and properties in all eukaryotes. The large subunit (mol wt ~180,000) of the tetrameric DNA polymerase α is vested with the usual $5' \rightarrow 3'$ nucleotide polymerizing activity. Polymerase α, isolated from some but not most sources, also has a $3' \rightarrow 5'$ exonuclease activity. Two of the other subunits of the enzyme are **primases.** The primary proofreading function in eukaryotes appears to be carried out by polymerase δ. Polymerase δ improves the fidelity of replication by a factor of 10^2 and contributes in limiting the rates of overall error to 10^{-9} to 10^{-12}.

The relatively low processivity of DNA polymerase α is typical for an enzyme involved in synthesis of the lagging strand that is assembled from segments of DNA that are no larger than 100–200 bp. The size of these Okazaki fragments is approximately equal to the length of DNA wrapped around a nucleosome. This observation suggests that eukaryotic DNA may be releasing one nucleosome at a time for priming of the lagging chain. The primase subunit of the enzyme synthesizes Okazaki segments as a closely coordinated priming–synthesizing activity, by laying down RNA primers containing 5–15 nucleotides that are subsequently extended by the synthetic activity of polymerase α. This polymerase catalyzes the synthesis of a polynucleotide chain at a rate of 50 nucleotides per second, which is about 1/20 the rate of *E. coli* DNA polymerase III synthesis. Looping of the lagging strand allows a combined polymerase α–polymerase δ asymmetric dimer to assemble and elongate both the leading and lagging strands in the same overall direction that corresponds to the direction of the fork movement. A third large monomeric protein, **polymerase ε,** is vested with a synthetic $5' \rightarrow 3'$ polymerase activity and both a $3' \rightarrow 5'$ proofreading exonuclease activity and a $5' \rightarrow 3'$ exonuclease activity. Polymerase ε is mainly required for DNA repair and for filling the gaps between Okazaki fragments on the lagging strand.

Eukaryotic DNA synthesis requires **replication protein A (RPA),** also known as **replication factor A (RFA).** This protein is the functional equivalent of prokaryotic single strand binding (SSB) protein. While helicase activities are part of the prokaryotic chromosome, eukaryotic helicases do not appear to be associated with primase activity. Eukaryotic helicase activity appears to be associated with DNA polymerase δ.

Initiation of Eukaryotic DNA Replication

Origins of replication in eukaryotic cells have been identified in yeast (*Saccharomyces*) and are termed ARS for **autonomously replicating sequence.** ARSs are about 100–120 bp long, each of which is characterized by an AT-rich central region. The 400 or so copies of the ARS in the yeast genome have highly conserved nucleotide sequences within the central region with variations in the flanking sequences. The core sequences of ARS contain 11-bp elements known as the **ARS consensus sequence** rich in AT pairs that appear to be analogous to the AT-rich 13-mers present in the OriC of *E. coli.* The flanking elements consist of overlapping sequences that include variants of the core sequence. Protein binding to form a so-called **origin of replication complex (ORC)** promotes DNA strand unwinding over the AT-rich sequences of the ARS cores. The unwound region is stabilized by single-strand-binding protein and RPA, and is extended by helicase. Polymerases α and δ, RFC, and PCNA are thus introduced into the origin of replication and begin DNA synthesis.

Weaker binding sites identified as B1, B2, and B3 are also present near the origin. B1 and B2 serve as sites for ORC formation, while B3 is associated with a protein that promotes initiation of transcription. This observation highlights the close association between eukaryotic DNA replication and transcription. Controlled activation of variant ARS-like subgroups, consisting of ARS-like sequences with different flanking elements, may determine the order of initiation of DNA synthesis in eukaryotes. Sequences completely comparable to yeast ARS have not been identified in higher eukaryotes. In mammals it appears that initiation depends more on chromosomal context than on specific sequences. Origins of initiation may be found within a broad section of the genome that also contains a small number of "hot spots," at which initiation is favored. In spite of these differences in the origins of replication between yeast and higher eukaryotes, the rest of the replication machinery appears to be remarkably analogous. Eukaryotic genomes replicate in a definite order, and at definite times within the S phase, with some DNA regions replicating early in the S phase and other DNA regions replicating later. Genes that replicate early are found in active segments of chromosomes, and genes that replicate later are located in the inactive areas of chromosomes. This pattern of activation changes with development. Differences in the rate of replication are regulated by variations in the duration of the S phase, which can be achieved either by controlling the number of replicons activated per unit length of chromosome or by slowing down the rate of DNA unwinding and replication. Sequence elements similar to the ARS subgroups in yeast may control replicon activation in other eukaryotes through the interaction of initiating proteins with these elements. Origins that are activated simultaneously are expected to share the same DNA sequences and bind to the same control proteins.

Since eukaryotic DNA is present in packaged form as chromatin, DNA replication is sandwiched between two additional steps, namely, a carefully ordered and incomplete dissociation of the chromatin and reassociation of DNA with the histone octamers to form nucleosomes. Methylation at the 5 position of cytosine residues by a **DNA methyltransferase** appears to function by loosening up the chromatin structure and allowing DNA access of proteins and enzymes needed for DNA replication. The synthesis of new histones occurs mainly during the S phase simultaneously with DNA replication. Histone molecules appear to rarely leave the DNA to which they are bound. Instead transcription and replication forks are apparently able to move past the parental nucleosomes as they synthesize mRNA or new DNA. One possibility is that each nucleosome dissociates into two halves, thereby permitting DNA polymerase to replicate transiently uncoiled DNA. Newly synthesized DNA inherits some parental histones, which it combines with an equal amount of new histones to complete the structure of nascent nucleosomes that are formed behind the moving replication forks.

In coordinating the synthesis of DNA the eukaryotic cell copies millions of base pairs, distributed over numerous chromosomes, with remarkable accuracy and at just the right time in the cycle of cell division. Copying start at hundreds of different origins, some of which are triggered early in the S phase of the cell cycle while others are triggered late. Recent evidence indicates that the replication initiator, that is the ORC complex, does not act alone in controlling initiation. One or more additional proteins bind to the initiation origins late in mitosis and remain attached until the S phase begins. These proteins are known as **cyclin-dependent kinases** (CDKs) and operate in association with specific protein substrates **(cyclins).** Cyclins and CDKs may control the cell cycle; they push the cell to the S phase and initiation of DNA synthesis. Cyclin–CDK pair also prevents DNA synthesis from being initiated a second time, so that only one S phase occurs per cell cycle. Degradation of CDKs removes the signal that inhibits cell division and the cell cycle moves again to mitosis. This scheme suggests that DNA initiation depends upon the formation of a prereplication complex by adding to or removing from the ORC cyclins and CDKs in a cyclical manner. This scheme in which the same enzyme first activates DNA replication and then, once one round of DNA replication has begun, inhibits reformation of the prereplication complex provides an efficient arrangement for the coordination of the initiation of DNA synthesis.

DNA Replication at the End of Linear Chromosomes

Linear chromosomes cannot be fully replicated in the absence of additional steps that provide for the replication of their terminals. As a replisome falls off from the end of a linear chromosome, and the daughter DNA molecules separate, synthesis of DNA on the end of the lagging strand cannot be fully completed. A gap resulting from removal of a primer that was used to start replication is generated on the lagging strand (Figure 15.37). The exact size of this gap

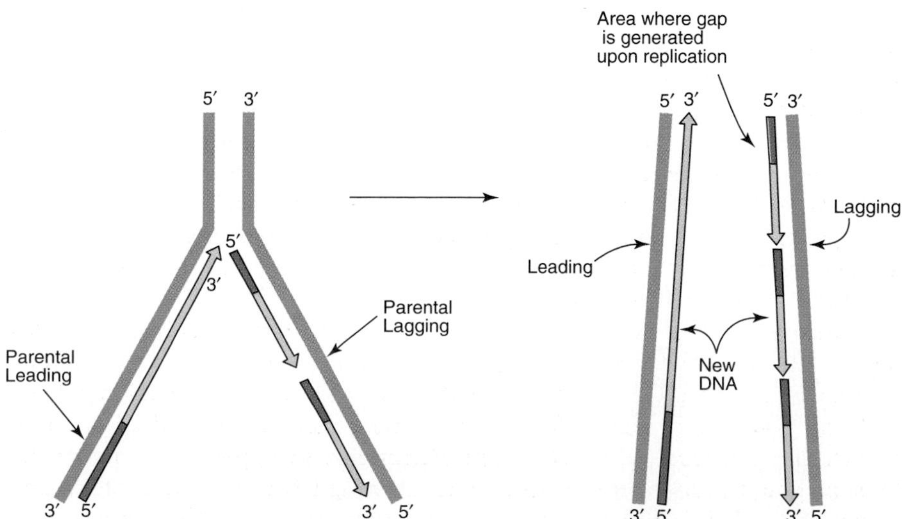

FIGURE 15.37
DNA replication at the ends of linear chromosomes.
In the absence of a special mechanism of replication operating at the ends of chromosomes, the completion of DNA synthesis of linear dsDNA would leave gaps at ends of newly synthesized strands. These gaps would result from removal of primers used to start replication. Upon each subsequent round of replication the gaps would be continuously expanded and accumulated because DNA polymerase requires a primer and therefore it cannot fill such gaps.

CLINICAL CORRELATION 15.6

Telomerase Activity in Cancer and Aging

Telomerase activity maintains appropriate length of the telomere sequences of chromosomes. Surprisingly, however, telomerase activity is absent from most somatic cells. In such cells telomere repeats gradually decrease in number with aging, as repeated cell divisions produce a substantial shortening of the telomere structure. Loss of telomerase activity in protozoans, such as *Tetrahymena,* is responsible for a gradual shortening of telomeres following each cell division, throughout the life of the cell. In human cultured fibroblast cells a linear inverse relationship exists between the length of telomeres and the age of the subject from which the cells are obtained. Eventual loss of telomeres leads to chromosomal instability and cell senescence and it may be an important factor that contributes to the process of aging. Specifically, telomere length appears to serve as a mitotic clock that limits the replication potential of mammalian cells. If it is true that the shortening of telomeres may be a contributing factor to the aging process, then the natural life span of an individual may be determined by the length of its telomere DNA. However, the possibility that telomere shortening may be the result, rather than the cause, of aging cannot be excluded. In any event, many other factors are also likely to contribute to the process of aging.

Since telomere length may serve as a mitotic clock, telomerase activity may stimulate cell division. The expression of telomerase may thus provide a selective advantage that allows tumor cells to divide indefinitely. Current understanding of telomere biology is still modest but as it improves telomerase may indeed become an important potential target for cancer chemotherapy.

Allsopp, R. C., Vaziri, H., Patterson, C. et al. Telomere length predicts replicative capacity of human fibroblasts. *Proc. Natl. Acad. Sci. USA* 89:10114, 1992; and Counter, C. M., Hirte, H. W., Bacchetti, S., and Harley, C. B. Telomerase activity in human ovarian carcinoma. *Proc. Natl. Acad. Sci. USA* 9:2900, 1994.

depends on the location of the last Okazaki fragment synthesized. As a minimum, the daughter DNA synthesized would have an 8–12 base gap generated by removal of the RNA primer for the Okazaki fragment. Without intervention this gap would be continuously regenerated and accumulated during each subsequent round of replication because it cannot be filled by DNA polymerase that requires a primer. The products of DNA replication would become shorter relative to parental DNA, leading to the gradual loss of DNA at the ends of human chromosomes. Cell senescence in humans and other mammals may be related to this chromosomal shortening as described in Clin. Corr. 15.6. In human cells that carry information to daughter cells (gamete cells) and in the linear chromosomes of bacteria and viruses, however, the integrity of DNA during replication cannot be compromised. Maintenance of intact chromosomal

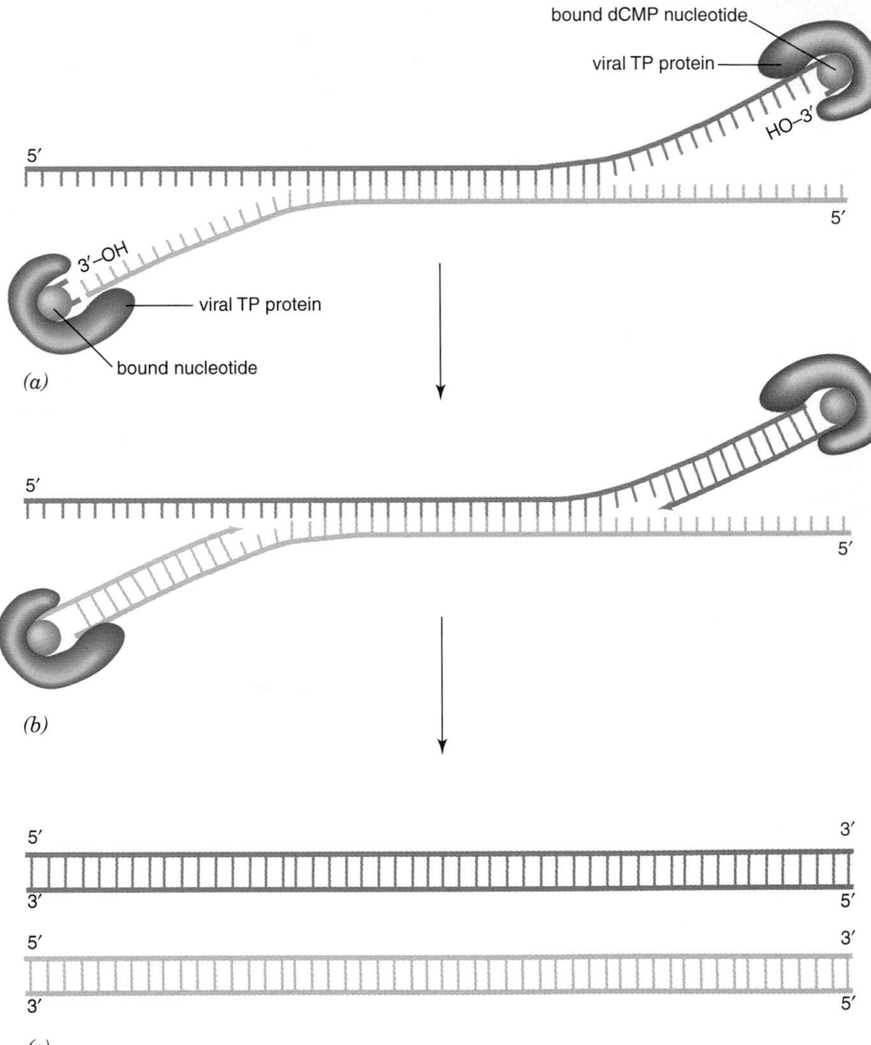

FIGURE 15.38
Replication of adenovirus DNA.
The adenovirus uses a protein as a primer, the terminal protein (TP), for synthesis of both strands of its DNA. TP, covalently associated with one dCMP, binds at the 3′ end of each template chain and the dCMP residue provides a 3′-OH for DNA polymerase-catalyzed synthesis of a complementary strand. Since both strands of the viral DNA are synthesized continuously in the 5′ → 3′ direction, DNA synthesis is complete, leaving no gaps at the ends of the chromosome.
Redrawn based on figure in Wolfe, S. L. Molecular and Cellular Biology. *Belmont, CA: Wadsworth, 1993.*

structure requires a distinct mechanism for replication at the ends of DNA molecules.

Prokaryotic Replication

Different replication strategies have evolved to deal with the problem in viruses, plasmids, and organelle DNA. One approach is the use of a primer consisting of a protein, referred to as **terminal protein, TP,** that binds covalently to the 5′ ends of viral DNA molecules via a phosphodiester bond with the hydroxyl group of a serine residue (Figure 15.38). Modified versions of TP that are distinct for different viruses also participate in replication. For instance, in the case of the mammalian adenovirus, the TP contains covalently bound dCMP. In bacteriophage ϕ29, the bound nucleotide is dAMP. These nucleotides pair with the terminal nucleotides at the 3′ end of each strand and serve as primers for replication. A special polymerase coded by each virus recognizes the TP and copies the strands unidirectionally from their 3′ to 5′ ends. With the priming limited to the ends of the parental DNA strands, both strands are replicated completely as if they both are leading strands. The TP molecule is cleaved from the primer nucleotide and it is released upon completion of the synthesis. Other viruses form circular intermediates that are copied by a rolling circle mechanism. Finally, some viruses, with identical sequences at the ends of their DNA, can hybridize their terminal sequences, forming linear repeats (linear concatenates). These concatenates are cleaved postreplicatively to generate progeny virus of the proper size (Figure 15.39).

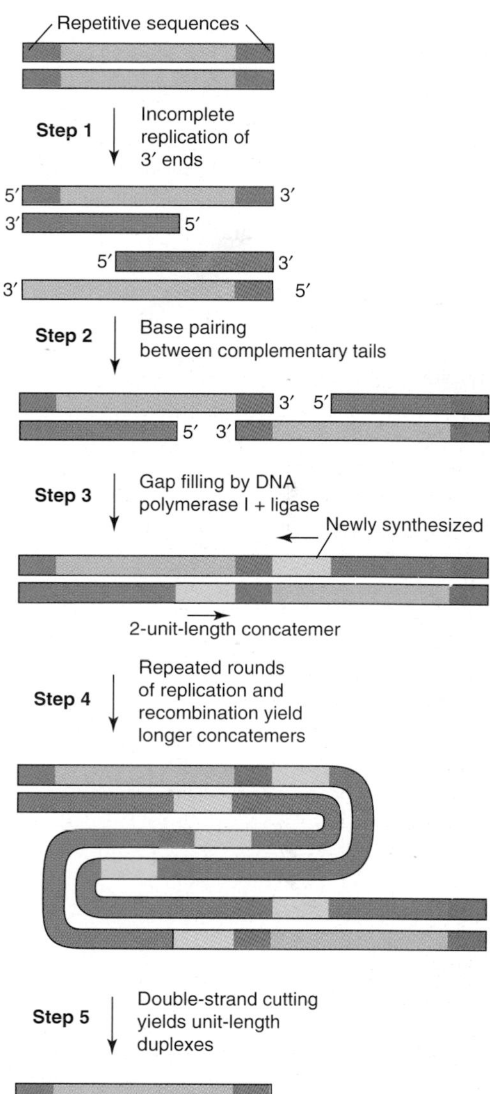

FIGURE 15.39
Replication of bacteriophage T7 DNA. Bacteriophage T7 DNA has repetitive identical sequences at its chromosomal termini so that, following replication, the daughter molecules can hybridize end to end to form dimers. During subsequent rounds of replication the process is repeated until a large linear DNA, a concatenate, is formed. A specific nuclease then cleaves the large concatenate into fully replicated genome-size DNA segments.
Redrawn based on figure in Mathews, C. K. and Van Holde, K. E. Biochemistry. *Redwood City, CA: Benjamin/Cummings, 1990.*

Eukaryotic Replication: Telomerases

Eukaryotes employ different strategies than prokaryotes and viruses for the replication of their chromosomal ends, known as **telomeres.** One approach that is used, albeit rarely, is the lengthening of chromosomal ends by the transposition of DNA segments known as **transposons.** This approach is apparently used for maintaining the chromosome ends in *Drosophila*. In most eukaryotes, however, telomere replication utilizes a specialized **reverse transcriptase enzyme** called **telomerase.** Telomerase activity depends on the presence of an RNA molecule that constitutes part of the telomerase structure and serves as an "internal" template. Maintenance of the chromosomal length depends on the action of telomerase on repetitive DNA sequences that constitute the telomeres of eukaryotic chromosomes (Figure 15.40). These telomeric tandem repeats can be several thousand nucleotides long and they consist of multiple copies of short G- and T-rich oligonucleotide sequences. Their size varies extensively from 20 bp in length for some protozoa to 150 kb in mouse telomers. For humans and other vertebrates the repetitive DNA is constructed with variants of the sequence TTAGGG. A short segment of single-stranded DNA ending in a 3′-OH group caps the end. Telomerase recognizes the G-rich single-strand at the 3′ terminus and elongates it in the 5′ → 3′ direction, by adding telomere repeats at the end of the lagging chain. The RNA of telomerase, which has a sequence of about 150 nucleotides complementary to the telomer repeats, provides a movable template that substitutes for the absence of a normal DNA template. Telomerase provides in one package all that is needed for elongation of the strand that ends in a 3′ terminus, namely, both template and enzymic activity. Extension of the telomeric sequence elongates the 3′ end of DNA by about 100 nucleotides. This is then used as template for synthesis of the complementary strand by DNA polymerase α. Telomerase is then repositioned to repeat the process as illustrated in Figure 15.40. In this manner telomerase and polymerase α serve to maintain chromosomal length during repeated rounds of DNA replication. Maintenance is affected by such factors as telomerase processivity and its frequency of action on telomers as well as the rate of degradation of telomeric DNA. Telomeres may grow, shrink, or stay fairly stable depending

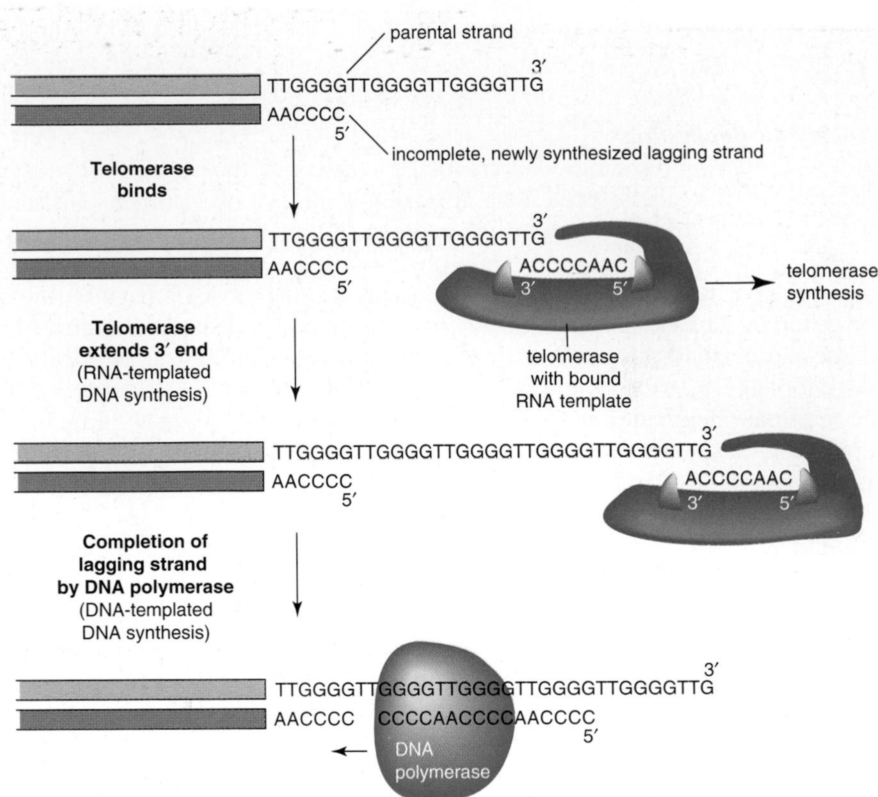

FIGURE 15.40
Telomere replication.
Telomerase contains an RNA template that codes for the extension of the ends of chromosomes and serves as a template for DNA polymerase. The DNA strand made on the lagging side of a replication fork of a linear chromosome is incomplete. For this strand to be completed, telomerase extends the 3′ end on the complementary strand at the leading side of the fork. Telomerase first binds to a TG primer at the 3′ end of this DNA strand. Binding is the result of base pairing between primer and RNA template that is part of the telomerase complex. The enzyme adds more T and G residues to the primer and repositions the RNA template so that more TG repeats can be added to the end of the primer. The extended primer is eventually recognized by DNA polymerase α, which proceeds to replicate the 5′ end of the DNA using the single-stranded 3′ end as template. Primase activity is vested in a subunit of DNA polymerase α.
Redrawn based on figure in Alberts, B., Bray, D., Lewis, J., Raff, M., Roberts, K., and Watson, J. D. Molecular Biology of the Cell. *New York: Garland, 1994.*

on genetic or nutritional changes. For example, the size of yeast telomeres can vary from about 200 to 400 bp depending on conditions.

DNA Can Be Synthesized Using an RNA Template

For many years it had been assumed without reservation that the only direction in which genetic information can flow is from DNA to RNA. This dogma had to be revised, however, when it was discovered that the genomes of certain viruses, such as the **retroviruses,** consist of RNA instead of DNA and that during viral infection this genomic RNA is copied into DNA. The DNA that is obtained can either be transcribed to produce more viruses or it may be incorporated into the DNA of the host. In the latter case the viral genome is replicated along the DNA of the host and often remains latent for many host chromosome generations.

Enzymes that use RNA templates for DNA synthesis are called **reverse transcriptases.** Reverse transcriptases are often virally encoded but they are not limited to viruses. Enzymes with reverse transcriptase activities are also found in uninfected cells and are involved in the formation of pseudogenes and in the replication of transposable elements (see p. 669). Reverse transcriptases are the most error-prone type of DNA polymerases because they lack $3' \rightarrow 5'$ exonuclease activities, thus lacking a proofreading function. Inhibitors of reverse transcriptase are used for the treatment of AIDS as described in Clin. Corr. 15.7.

DNA Replication, Repair, and Transcription Are Closely Coordinated

It has become increasingly clear that DNA replication, transcription, and repair are not separable, as most DNA lesions block both replication and transcription. Thus repair occurs with "expressed genes" as a priority, with the repair of dormant genes deferred. In addition, transcription and repair appear to cross paths at several points, with certain repair proteins participating in the activation

CLINICAL CORRELATION 15.7

Inhibitors of Reverse Transcriptase in Treatment of AIDS

AIDS is caused by a retrovirus, the human immunodeficiency virus (HIV). Treatment of AIDS is complicated by the high mutability of this virus, which reflects the low fidelity of the HIV reverse transcriptase responsible for the synthesis of the viral genome. This transcriptase is about one order of magnitude less accurate than other transcriptases and produces one or more mutations per generation, which means that any two HIV DNA molecules are almost never exactly the same in their nucleotide sequence.

The first drug that was used with some success, and continues in use, in controlling the rate of advancement of the disease is a structural analog of deoxythymidine, known as AZT.

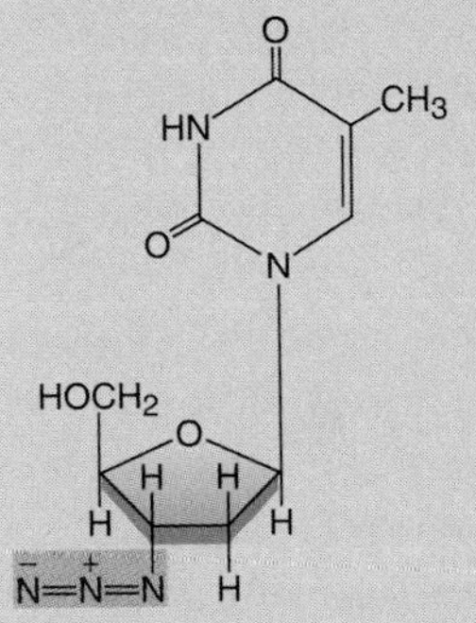

3′-Azido-2′,3′-dideoxythymidine (AZT)

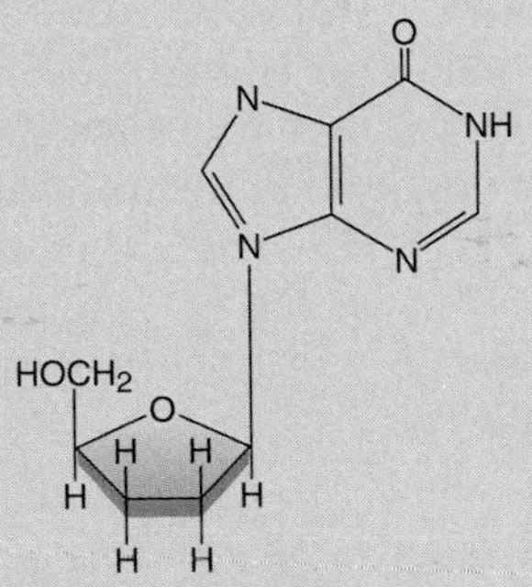

2′,3′-Dideoxyinosine (DDI)

This drug is converted to the triphosphate by cell kinases and the triphosphate is incorporated into the HIV genome in place of dTTP. AZT triphosphate competes successfully with dTTP for incorporation into the viral genome because of the higher binding affinity of AZT relative to dTTP toward the HIV reverse transcriptase. Since AZT has a lower affinity for cellular DNA polymerases than dTTP, it is not incorporated into cellular DNA. Incorporation of AZT triphosphate causes a premature termination of viral DNA synthesis because it lacks a 3′-OH site that is needed as the primer for incorporation of additional nucleotides.

Other nucleotide analogs, with similar reverse transcriptase-dependent mechanisms of actions, have been included in the treatment of AIDS. These include dideoxyinosine (ddI) dideoxycytidine (ddC), and azidothymidine (ZDV). Current approaches use ZDV or combination therapies of ZDV and ddI or ZDV and ddC. Other compounds that are not nucleotide analogs, referred to as nonnucleoside reverse transcriptase inhibitors (NNRTI), and a diverse group of other agents, such as protease inhibitors and HIV immune-based therapies, are currently under investigation for treatment of AIDS. A new class of drugs that inhibit proteases essential for HIV replication, when used in combination with reverse transcriptase inhibitors, is reported to reduce viral loads in AIDS patients to undetectable levels and in many instances reverse rather than simply arrest the symptoms of the disease.

Finkelstein, D. M., and Shoenfeld, D. A. (Eds.). *AIDS Clinical Trials*. New York: Wiley-Liss, 1995.

of initiation or elongation steps of transcription. For example, subunits of the TFIIH factor, which is essential for transcription, also participate in eukaryotic nucleotide excision repair. Repair and replication appear also to be coupled at the level of the protein factor, HSSB. This protein binds single-stranded DNA with high affinity during replication but it is also a repair protein required for the formation of the preincision complex. A protein induced as a result of DNA damage, the so-called Gadd45 protein, has regulatory effects on both DNA repair and replication. Gadd45 appears to both stimulate excision repair and inhibit DNA replication.

15.5 ■ DNA RECOMBINATION

DNA recombination refers to a number of distinct processes during which genetic material is rearranged by breaking and joining portions of the same DNA molecule or portions of different DNA molecules. Recombination also takes place between the DNAs of different organisms to generate a new "composite" DNA. Both prokaryotic and eukaryotic DNAs undergo recombination. Three well-characterized processes listed in Table 15.8 fall under this general description of genetic recombination. Other DNA rearrangements have been noted whose mechanism and function are not well-understood and are referred to as illegitimate; these will not be reviewed in this chapter. Recombination creates new combinations of genes on the chromosome, which increase the chance of survival of a population. This increase of **genetic diversity** offers no advantage for individuals within a population. Individual survival partially

TABLE 15.8 Characteristics of Different Types of Genetic Recombination

Type	*Sequence Homology*	*Heteroduplex Sequences*	*Proteins Involved*	*DNA Synthesis*
Homologous	Extensive, but the homology is DNA sequence independent	Long	RecA, RecBCD, RuvAB, RuvC, and DNA repair enzymes[a]	Some
Site-specific	Short but specific DNA sequences are required on both DNAs	Short	Recombinases	Some
Transpositional	Homology is not required; specific sequences needed on one of the DNAs	None	Transposases	Minor (only to fill gaps)

[a] Several additional protein factors including RecE (exonuclease VIII), RecF, RecG, RecJ, RecN, RecOR, RecQ, RecT, SbcCD, DNA polymerase I, DNA gyrase, DNA topoisomerase I, DNA ligase, and DNA helicases participate in catalyzing homologous recombination.

depends, instead, on the operation of DNA repair. However, certain types of DNA repair depend on DNA recombination and therefore it is possible that recombination evolved as a mechanism of repair.

Homologous genetic recombination produces an exchange between a pair of distinct DNA molecules, often two slightly variant copies of the same chromosome, or two segments of DNA generated from the same DNA molecule. The main requirement for this process to occur is that the recombining DNAs are **homologous.** This means that the two DNAs share very similar base sequences over an extended region that may contain several thousand bases. An important example of homologous recombination in eukaryotes is the exchange of sections of homologous chromosomes during the early development of gametes (egg and sperm cells). In this manner slightly different versions of the same gene (alleles) can evolve during meiosis. Gene "mixing and reassortment" by general recombination is also widespread in bacteria. Homologous recombination is quite complex and involves a multistep mechanism catalyzed by a large number of different proteins. Prominent among them is the RecA protein, which also participates in SOS DNA repair.

Conservative site-specific recombination or **site-specific recombination** requires the presence of only short homologous DNA sequences. However, site-specific recombinations occur only in specific DNA sequences present in both the participating DNA molecules. The process is catalyzed by enzymes known as **recombinases.**

Transpositional site-specific recombination, or simply **transposition,** differs from conservative site-specific recombination in that it does not require a specific DNA sequence in the "target" chromosome. Transposition is catalyzed by **transposases.** Both transposases and recombinases recognize and act on specific DNA sequences. Recombination of either type is responsible for the insertion of viruses, plasmids, and **transposable elements (transposons)** into chromosomal DNA. Transposons are DNA elements that can move from location to location within a genome, in both bacteria and eukaryotes. Viruses are related to plasmids and transposons but also differ from these genetic elements in that viruses can synthesize a protein coat that allows them more host-independent existence. Plasmids and transposons are confined to replicate only within a specific cell and the progeny of that cell.

The most common recombination is the **homologous** type. **Site-specific recombination** and **transposition** are relatively rare, but important, events in that they may control replicative function in some viruses and certain aspects of development. Homologous recombination generates new combinations of genes that can lead to genetic diversity. DNA mutation and recombination are the two principal approaches by which the cell creates variation that is required for evolution to occur. In addition, recombination events are involved in DNA repair. In those instances in which DNA damage occurs across complementary DNA sites, DNA repair can occur only through recombination. A large variety of protein structures used by the human immune system are produced by recombination as described in Clin. Corr. 15.8.

Homologous Recombination

Homologous recombination, which is accompanied by the formation of a **heteroduplex DNA** region, clearly requires breaking and rejoining of chromosomal DNA. Recombination occurs via a fairly complex multistep mechanism. A scheme that explains the outcome of recombination is shown in Figure 15.41. This scheme gives a minimal overview of recombination, in that each of the steps shown may represent more than one enzymatically catalyzed process. Numerous gene products are involved in homologous recombination.

Recombination may begin by introduction of a single-strand nick at a selected site of one of the DNA duplexes undergoing recombination. The resulting 3′-ended single-strand tail can then invade a homologous DNA duplex. Homologous DNA duplexes are chromosomes with the same linear arrangement of genes but with base sequences that may differ between the two duplexes. The variance is usually minor and may consist of no more than one different base among the millions of base pairs present in the chromosome. Single-strand invasion places the homologous DNA duplexes side by side in a process referred to as **synapsis.** Synapsis does not necessarily involve contacts between homologous sequences and further movement of the DNAs with respect to each other may be necessary until homologous sequences come into contact. This process is referred to as **homologous alignment. Strand invasion** is accompanied by **strand displacement** in the homologous DNA duplex resulting in the formation of a so-called **D-loop.** The "D-loop" strand that has been displaced by strand invasion is now nicked and it pairs with its complementary strand in the original duplex. The ends of exchanged strands are then ligated to form a stable **cross-stranded intermediate** known as **Holliday junction.** The junction can migrate in either direction by unwinding and rewinding of the two

CLINICAL CORRELATION 15.8

Immunoglobulin Genes Are Assembled by Recombination

Immunoglobulins (antibodies) are molecules that recognize and specifically bind to any substance that antibodies identify as foreign to the human body (see p. 88 for details). Because of the immense variety of infectious agents, including millions of microorganisms that are present in the environment, the human genome, which is equipped with only a limited pool of probably no more than 100,000 genes, does not have the capacity to directly produce an equivalent number of different antibodies necessary for specific recognition of all infectious agents. This inherent limitation in the gene-coding potential of the human genome is, however, overcome by recombination, which allows production, from a limited amount of gene-coding DNA, of an almost unlimited number of distinct antibodies.

Human immunoglobulins consist of two heavy and two light chains with each chain having a variable region, with a sequence that is characteristic for each immunoglobulin, and a chain with constant amino acid sequence (see p. 89). Recombination leads to diversity in the variable region of immunoglobulins. During the maturation of a bone marrow stem cell into a B lymphocyte, one V segment and one J segment are brought together by site-specific recombination. In the process the intervening DNA is deleted and a joint between the two regions is established by an RNA-splicing reaction that occurs following transcription. Since the V region consists of 300 segments and the J region of 4, at least 1200 different combinations can be generated by recombination.

Similar considerations apply to the λ light chains and the heavy chains, with the latter being assembled in as many as 5000 distinct combinations. Because individual light and individual heavy chains can subsequently be assembled in combination, at least 6×10^6 different IgG molecules can be produced. Furthermore, because some variations occur in the exact location of the V-J junction, the actual number of IgG molecules is two to three times higher than estimated above. Additional IgG diversity is produced during the process of maturation of B lymphocytes by mutational processes.

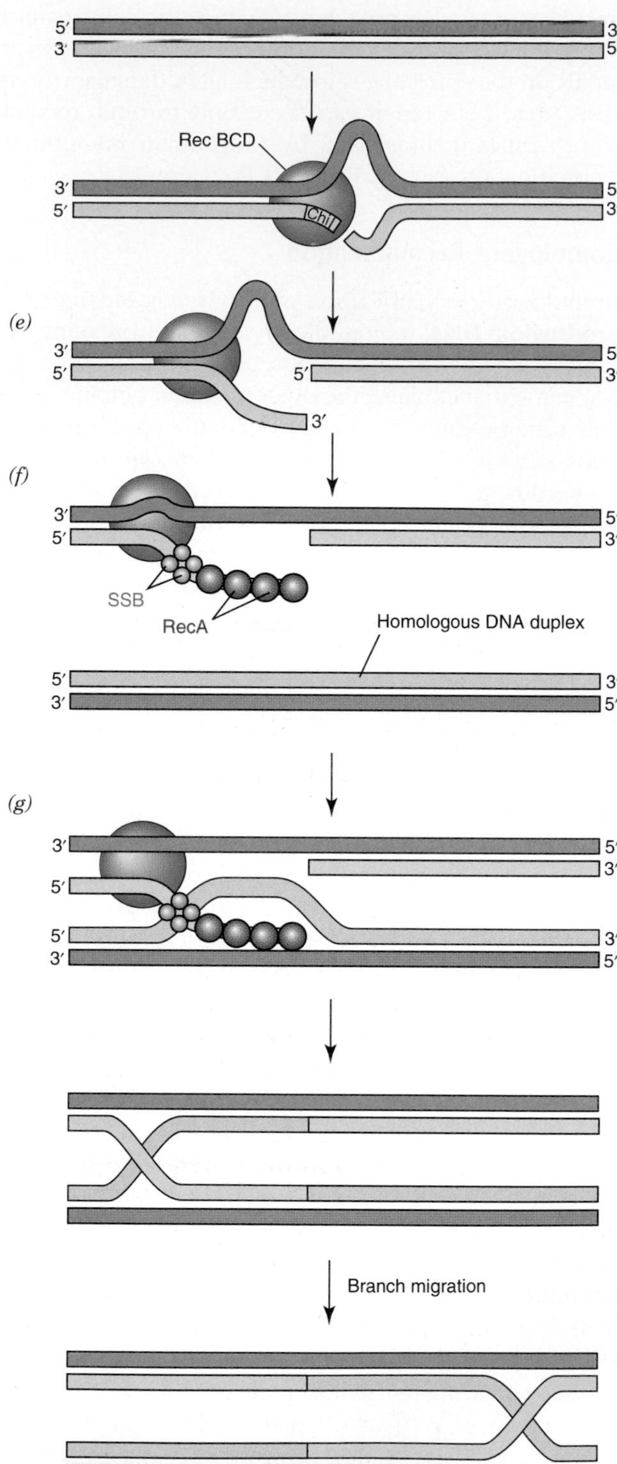

FIGURE 15.41
Overview of homologous recombination.
Transformations that can lead to formation of recombinant and nonrecombinant heteroduplexes, by participation of two homologous DNA molecules in homologous recombination are outlined. Each step indicated need not be the outcome of a single, enzymatically catalyzed or well-understood reaction. The sequence of steps shown is not necessarily universally applicable.

duplexes to produce a further exchange of single strands between interacting chromosomes. This process, known as **branch migration,** results in strand exchange and it produces **heteroduplex** regions of varying lengths. The resulting heteroduplex, shown in Figure 15.41, can also be presented in another form that is generated by merely pulling the ends of the heteroduplex together (Figure 15.42). A twist of this structure produces an isomeric heteroduplex, which is called the **Chi** form. In order to resolve the Chi form two additional single-strand nicks can be made, in either the horizontal direction or vertical

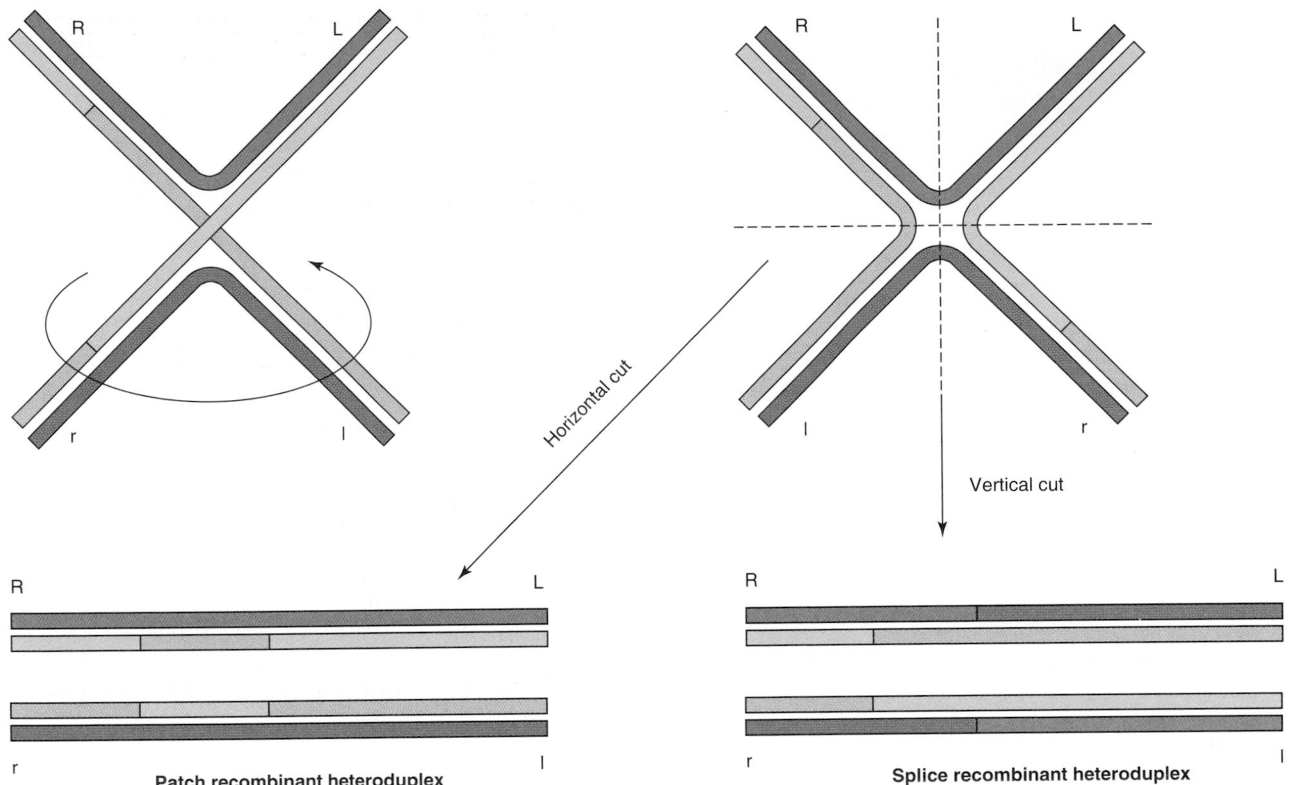

FIGURE 15.42
Patch and splice recombinant heteroduplexes.

direction, leading to two distinct products. Gaps present in these structures are repaired and ligated, leading to either one of the two products. The manner in which nicks are introduced in the horizontal and vertical directions is fundamentally different. In one case (horizontal direction) nicks are introduced again into the strands that were initially nicked, although at different sites, producing two duplexes in which one strand of each remains intact. These duplexes contain heteroduplex regions, generated by branch migration, that are misleadingly referred to as **Patch recombinant heteroduplexes.** These duplexes contain the same genes and in the same linear order as the initial duplexes. In vertical direction nicks, the complementary strands that previously were left intact are nicked again (though at different sites), producing two duplexes of true recombinant DNA, referred to as **splice recombinant heteroduplexes.** In these true recombinant heteroduplexes the linear order of DNA sequences contained in the original duplexes is clearly rearranged.

Support for this multistep recombination scheme has accumulated over the years based on genetic investigations, on electron microscopy of Holliday junctions, and by isolation of proteins and enzymes that can catalyze many of the transformations described in this recombination scheme.

Enzymes and Proteins that Catalyze Homologous Recombination

Homologous recombination in *E. coli* requires about 25 enzymes for recombination. A partial list includes **RecA** protein, **RecBCD** enzyme (which is the product of three distinct *E. coli* genes, *recB, recC,* and *recD*), **RuvAB** and **RuvC** proteins, DNA polymerase I, DNA gyrase, DNA topoisomerase I, DNA ligase, and DNA helicases (Table 15.8). Proteins homologous to RecA have also been isolated from yeast and human cells.

Homologous recombination in *E. coli* begins with RecBCD, which is a site-specific **endonuclease** and an ATP-dependent **helicase** (Figure 15.43).

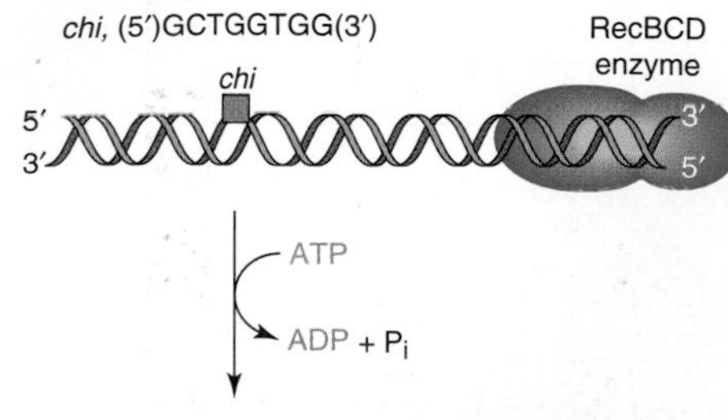

Rec BCD helicase activity of enzyme produces single-stranded bubbles.

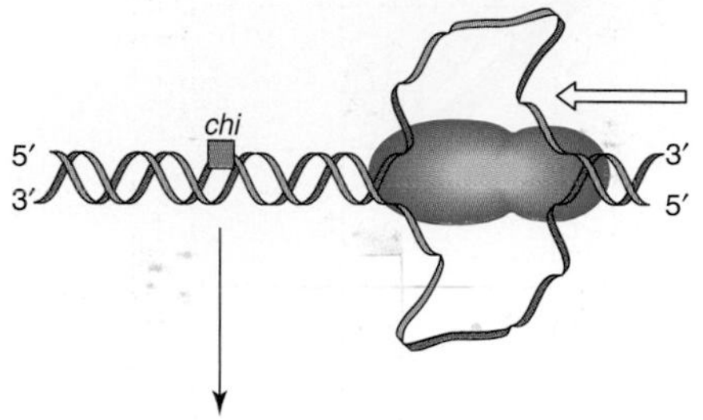

At a *chi* sequence, nuclease activity cleaves the adjacent single strand.

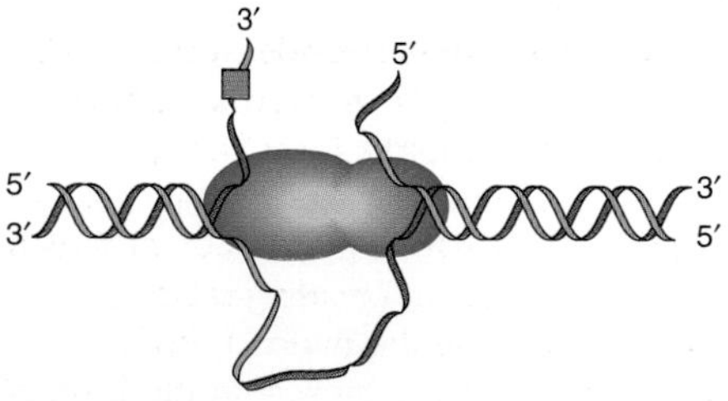

FIGURE 15.43
Activities of RecBCD protein.
RecBCD combines helicase and nuclease activities and appears to be involved in initiation of homologous genetic recombination in *E. coli*. RecBCD, using its helicase activity, enters the double helix and, using energy derived from ATP hydrolysis, travels along the helix until it encounters a Chi site, which consists of the sequence 5′-GCTGGTGG-3′. RecBCD introduces a cut, within the Chi site, that leads to displacement of a 3′-terminating single strand. This single strand initiates recombination by pairing with a homologous DNA double helix.
Redrawn based on figure in Liehninger, A. L., Nelson, D. L., and Cox, M. M. Principles of Biochemistry. *New York: Worth, 1993.*

RecBCD can initiate recombination by unwinding DNA and, on occasion, cleaving one strand. The enzyme binds to one end of linear DNA and travels along the helix at the expense of ATP, unwinding DNA as it moves and rewinding DNA behind it at a slower rate than unwinding. This produces a "bubble" consisting of two single-stranded loops that propagate on the DNA with the advance of the RecBCD. *Escherichia coli* DNA is characterized by the presence of about 1000 copies of the sequence 5′-GCTGGTGG-3′ that, on average, occurs at intervals of 4–5 kb. These Chi sites are **"hot spots" for recombination** as they increase the frequency of recombination. When the advancing RecBCD encounters a Chi site within a "bubble," it cleaves the DNA strand that incorporates the 5′-GGTGGTGG-3′ sequences 5–6 nucleotides to the 3′ side of the Chi site. The helicase activity generates a 3′ single-stranded tail of DNA that is progressively lengthened to several kilobases.

This growing single-stranded tail can then initiate the **strand invasion** process with the assistance of RecA, which catalyzes a multiplicity of reactions in DNA recombination (Figure 15.41). RecA interacts with single-stranded (ss) and double-stranded (ds) DNA and catalyzes **pairing of homologous DNA sequences, invasion of ssDNA** into the homologous double helix, formation of the **Holliday junction,** and migration of this junction (branch migration). These activities of RecA depend on the presence of a RecA site that recognizes ssDNA and promotes the cooperative binding of the protein to ssDNA. Formation of a long and relatively stiff **nucleofilament** (Figure 15.44) prevents the

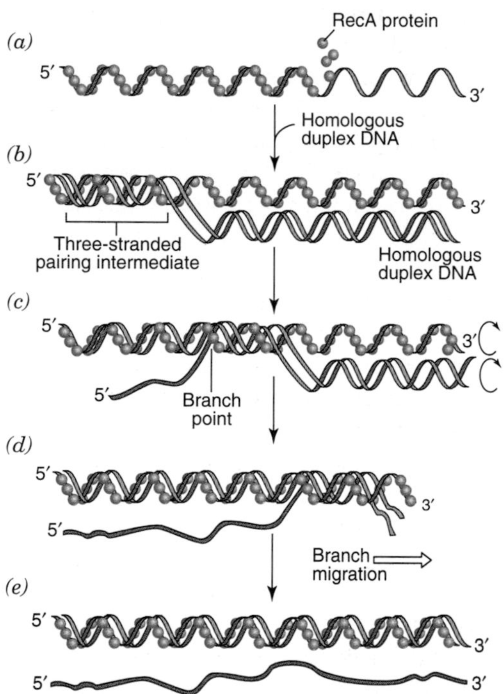

FIGURE 15.44
DNA strand exchange mediated by RecA.
Replacement of a complementary strand in a DNA duplex by a single-stranded DNA is catalyzed by RecA. RecA begins the exchange by coating both ssDNA and dsDNA by RecA (only coating of the single strand is shown). The coating modifies the conformation of both the single-stranded and double-stranded polynucleotides and catalyzes the invasion of the single-stranded intermediate. Switches in the base pairing between the strands, and the accompanying rotation of the DNA, move the three-stranded region from left to right as one strand of the DNA duplex is displaced by the identical, or nearly identical, invading ssDNA. Continuing branch migration leads to eventual separation of the displaced strand.

ssDNA tail from reassociating with the complementary strand within the DNA duplex, from which it originated, and prepares the single strand for invasion. In the resulting nucleofilament that binds one RecA molecule per 3 bases, the polynucleotide is positioned within a deep groove of the RecA protein. A second site on RecA recognizes and binds preferentially to dsDNA. In this nucleofilament each RecA monomer covers six nucleotides and each successive monomer binds to the opposite site of the DNA helix. For the sake of simplicity the dsDNA in Figure 15.44 is shown as free from RecA. The RecA–ssDNA and RecA–dsDNA nucleofilaments differ in their geometry from B-DNA, but both filaments represent partially unwound and unstacked helical structures that are extended lengthwise by 50% relative to B-DNA. DNA unwinding in the RecA–dsDNA nucleofilament (to about 18.6 bp per turn) exposes H-bond donors and acceptors in the major groove of the double helix, making them available for interaction with the ssDNA–RecA filament. Thus RecA contributes to the recognition of regions of homology between DNA strands. Once **homologous alignment** is established, a fairly stable **triple-stranded intermediate** can be formed (Figure 15.45). In this structure the third strand is in contact with the major groove of the duplex, aligned in a manner that permits RecA to flip the base pairing of the two identical strands.

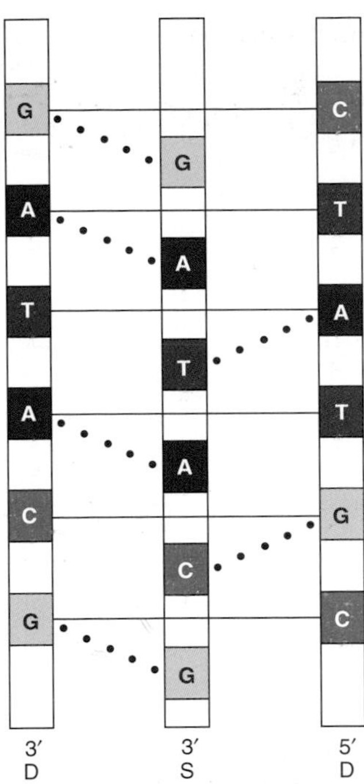

FIGURE 15.45
Model for the triple-stranded intermediate formed during DNA recombination. RecA catalyzes the formation of a triple-stranded DNA intermediate as a result of the association of a dsDNA, the strands of which are marked D, and an invading ssDNA, marked S (shown in the middle). Both dsDNA and ssDNA are present in the form of complexes with RecA. This protein catalyzes unwinding of the strands of the double helix and makes the matrix of hydrogen-bond donors and acceptors in the major groove of the double helix available for pairing with ssDNA. The ssDNA is also unwound by RecA, providing for proper alignment between dsDNA and ssDNA.

The flipping of the base pairing and the resulting invasion of the RecA–ssDNA filament involve the exchange of two identical (or nearly identical) strands between helical structures, which therefore requires an ordered rotation of two aligned strands. The polynucleotides are prepared for this exchange by "the extended" conformation generated by RecA. Strand exchange can be extended by **branch migration,** which means that progression of the exchange requires both invasion and branch migration. Branch migration may be described as a process in which an unpaired region of a single DNA strand displaces a DNA strand from a region of homologous dsDNA and moves the branching point, without appreciably increasing the total number of disrupted base pairs. Migration is achieved by RecA-catalyzed rotation of RecA-bound DNA strands involved in the exchange (Figure 15.44). The resulting "spooling" action, in which topoisomerases may be involved, moves the branch as ATP is hydrolyzed.

Branch migration also occurs at the Holliday junction that is subsequently formed. In this intermediate homologous DNA helices that were initially paired are held together by mutual exchange of two of the four strands (Figure 15.46). Stereochemistry of the intermediate is determined by the juxtaposition of the grooves and the phosphate backbones of the participating helices, and the point of exchange or actual junction can be moved back and forth along the helices. Migration of the junction can proceed in the absence of RecA. This RecA-independent migration of the junction is catalyzed by a complex of **RuvA** and **RuvB.** RuvA binds to the junction and acts as a specificity factor that targets RuvB, which is an ATPase, to the junction. The RuvAB complex promotes migration and increases the length of the heteroduplex DNA at the expense of ATP. Finally, the Holliday junction is recognized and resolved into products by the **RuvC endonuclease,** a dimer of 19-kDa subunits related to each other by a dyad axis of symmetry. The catalytic center of this **resolvase** lies at the bottom of a cleft that fits a DNA duplex. Only strands with the same polarity are cleaved and produce two types of heteroduplex molecules, one type in which only single-strand segments are exchanged **(patch recombinants)** and another type, a true recombinant, in which the ends of molecules have been exchanged **(splice recombinants).** Resolution is completed by DNA polymerase I, DNA topoisomerase I, DNA gyrase, and DNA ligase.

RecA also exhibits a highly specific protease activity that is activated by unpaired DNA strands and is directed at specific regulatory proteins. Thus RecA has unique properties for coordinating regulation of a number of cellular

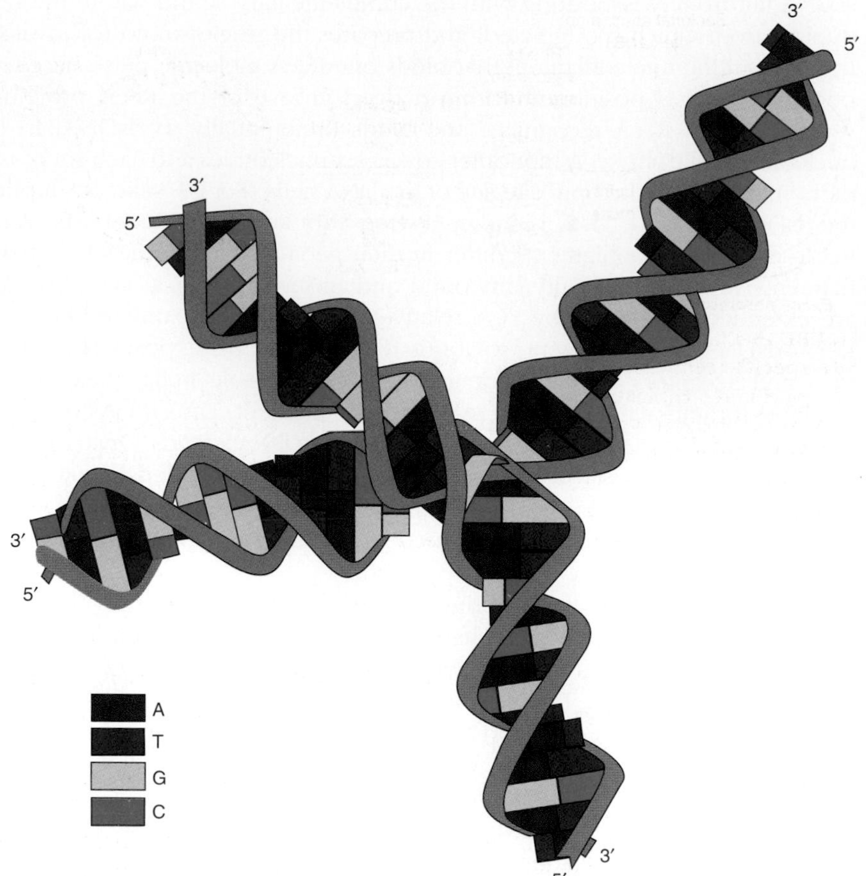

FIGURE 15.46
Structure of the Holliday junction.
The Holliday intermediate is a four-way junction that adopts a right-handed antiparallel X-shaped structure by pairwise coaxial stacking of the two double helices. The junction consists of fully stacked base pairs with the participating strands present as hydrogen-bonded DNA duplexes. *Redrawn based on figure in Moran, L. A., Scrimgeour, K. G., Horton, H. R., Ochs, R. S., and Rawn, J. D.* Biochemistry. *Englewood Cliffs, NJ: Neil Patterson/Prentice Hall, 1994.*

functions that occur when DNA damage, or the interruption of DNA replication, leads to the production of ssDNA segments. An example is the postreplication repair of DNA damaged by UV light or other mutagens.

Site-Specific Recombination

This process separates and joins dsDNA molecules at specific sites. Site-specific recombination is limited to select regions of a genome and is driven by **recombinases** that recognize short (20–200 bp) specific sequences on both recombination sites. When recombinase binds to both recombination sites on DNA molecules it can produce an insertion of DNA. A well-studied example is provided by the integration of so-called temperate phages, such as *E. coli* bacteriophage λ, into the host chromosome of the corresponding host (Figure 15.47). The circular λ chromosome becomes integrated into a specific site in the *E. coli* chromosome consisting of about 20 nucleotides, the so-called attP site. Integration requires the alignment of the λ phage in a specific orientation with the *E. coli* chromosome. The alignment is achieved by a specific recombinase known as **integrase (Int)** and the participation of a protein known as the **integration host factor (IHF)** encoded by the bacterium. Integrase brings together the attB site of the bacterium with a corresponding specific site on the phage chromosome, which consists of 230 bp and is known as the attP site. Int generates a precise wrapping of DNA to juxtapose specific nucleotide sequences for the splicing reactions that follow. Functioning as a topoisomerase, Int unwinds the attP region and forms an Int–attP nucleoprotein. A corresponding nucleoprotein is also formed between Int and attB that brings the attP and attB

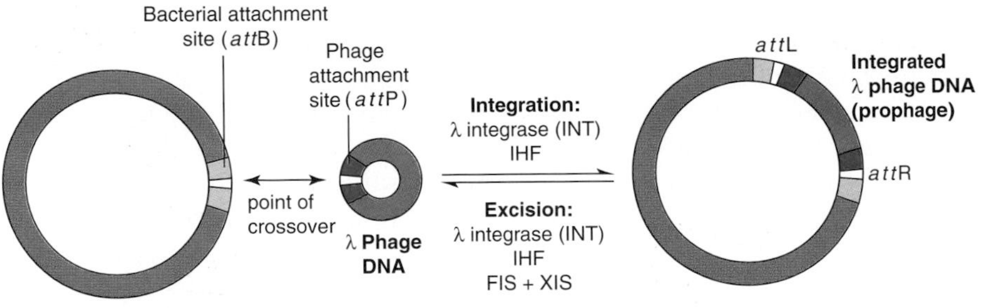

FIGURE 15.47
Site-specific recombination of λ phage.
Site-specific recombination is carried out by integrase. The phage chromosome undergoes recombination between the attP site and a corresponding site on the bacterium, attB. Integration of the phage chromosome generates two new attachment sites (attR and attL) that flank the integrated phage DNA. The reverse reaction, excision of the integrated phage chromosome, requires the participation of protein XIS produced by the bacteriophage and protein FIS encoded by the bacterium.

sites together. Integrase then generates a staggered cut, 7 base pairs apart within a core sequence of 15 bp, that is present in both the attP and attB sites and catalyzes the exchange of strands at the position of the cut to form a **Holliday intermediate.** To complete the exchange, cutting and rejoining must be repeated at a second point within each of the two recombination sites. Normally, limited branch migration is required prior to an Int-catalyzed second cleavage and strand exchange. Following ligation by Int, the original sequence of the recombination site is regenerated but the DNA on either side of the site is recombined. **Recombinases** often act in a reversible manner, restoring the sequences of original DNAs. **Integrase** also acts in a reversible manner so that the circular phage chromosome can be excised as conditions change. The forward and reverse steps of the integration reaction are separately regulated, with the reverse step being dependent on the presence of additional proteins: the XIS protein encoded by the phage and FIS encoded by the bacterium. Both reactions also require IHF.

Transposition

Transposition is a form of recombination catalyzed by recombinases called **transposases.** This type of recombination is best understood in bacteria but DNA of all cells, including eukaryotes such as *Drosophila,* maize, and yeast, contains segments that can move, generally with very low frequencies of 10^{-5}–10^{-7} per cell generation, from a **donor** site to another **target** site within a chromosome. These segments are known as **transposable elements (transposons).**

Transposition differs from homologous recombination in not requiring sequence homology between donor and target sites. Only the donor site, that is, the transposon, has specific nucleotide sequences located on both sides of the transposon that serve as binding sites for transposases. Most bacterial transposons have short repeats of about 15–25 bp at the two ends of the transposable DNA segment. In contrast, the target sites are not well defined and are not characterized by specific DNA sequences. **Heteroduplex** joints are not formed as a result of transposition.

Three classes, I, II, and III, of transposable elements are recognized. Class I transposons are called **insertion sequences (IS)** if they consist of a gene coding for transposase together, of course, with the repeats that normally flank the transposable element. IS elements vary in size between 800 and 1300 bp. When Class I transposons also contain an additional gene, such as a gene conferring antibiotic resistance to bacteria, they are called **composite transposons (Tn).** Class II transposons differ from Class I in that, in addition, they code for the gene of a second enzyme, **resolvase.** Typically, **composite transposons** and Class II transposons are several thousand base pairs long. Finally, a small group of bacteriophages, such as bacteriophage Mu, that insert their chromosome into a host chromosome are classified as Class III transposable elements.

Transposition begins by a transposase-catalyzed introduction of a staggered cut at the target DNA sequence. Cuts are also made on each side of the transposon so that it can be moved onto the target site. The relocation leaves a double-stranded break at the site from which the transposon is excised. At the target site the transposon is spliced into the staggered cut as shown in Figure 15.48. Specifically, 3–12 bp at the target site are duplicated by DNA polymerase I, to form an additional short repeat at each end of the inserted transposon, and the "tailored" transposon then is ligated within the target site. In Class II and III transposition, in addition to duplication of the short repeats, the transposon itself is replicated and one copy of it remains at the donor site while the other copy is transferred to the target site. This type of transposition, referred to as **replicative transposition,** requires the enzyme resolvase and therefore does not occur in Class I transposition. Replicative transposition can reshape the structure of a chromosome beyond the simple act of relocating a transportable element from one site to another. Because this type of transposition places two homologous sequences within the same chromosome, homologous recombination between these two sequences can produce either a deletion or an insertion, depending on whether these sequences are oriented in the same or in opposite directions, as shown in Figure 15.49.

Finally, transposition may inactivate a gene by mutation if a transposon is inserted into a coding sequence and interrupts it. Alternatively, insertion by transposition of a promoter or a transcriptional activator next to a gene may activate the gene. Clinical Correlation 15.9 reviews the role of transposition and Clin. Corr. 15.10 the role of DNA amplification in the development of drug resistance.

CLINICAL CORRELATION 15.9

Transposons and Development of Antibiotic Resistance

Genes conferring to bacteria resistance to commonly used antibiotics such as pencillin or tetracycline are usually carried on plasmids. The DNA sequences of these plasmids do not have any homology with the chromosomal DNA sequences of the host. Yet, as a result of transposition, antibiotic resistance genes can be transferred to the chromosome of bacterial hosts. The existence of genes that can move from one chromosome to another is of course of great importance in understanding the factors that produce changes in the organization of genomes. From the clinical standpoint these "transposable" genes are of critical significance for understanding how populations of antibiotic-resistant bacteria arise with use of antibiotics in the treatment of bacterial infections in humans and animals.

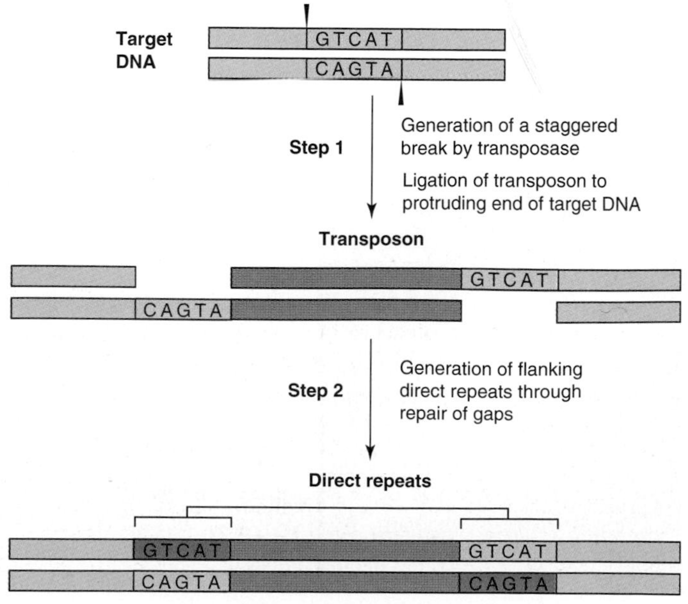

FIGURE 15.48
Direct repeats at the ends of transposons.
Transposons are inserted into gaps generated at a target sequence by introduction of a staggered cut by a transposase. Ligation of transposon to the protruding ends of target DNA leaves gaps at both sides of the transposon. Repair of these gaps is responsible for the presence of direct repeats that flank transposons.
Redrawn based on figure from Mathews, C. K. and Van Holde, K. E. Biochemistry. *Redwood City, CA: Benjamin/Cummings, 1990.*

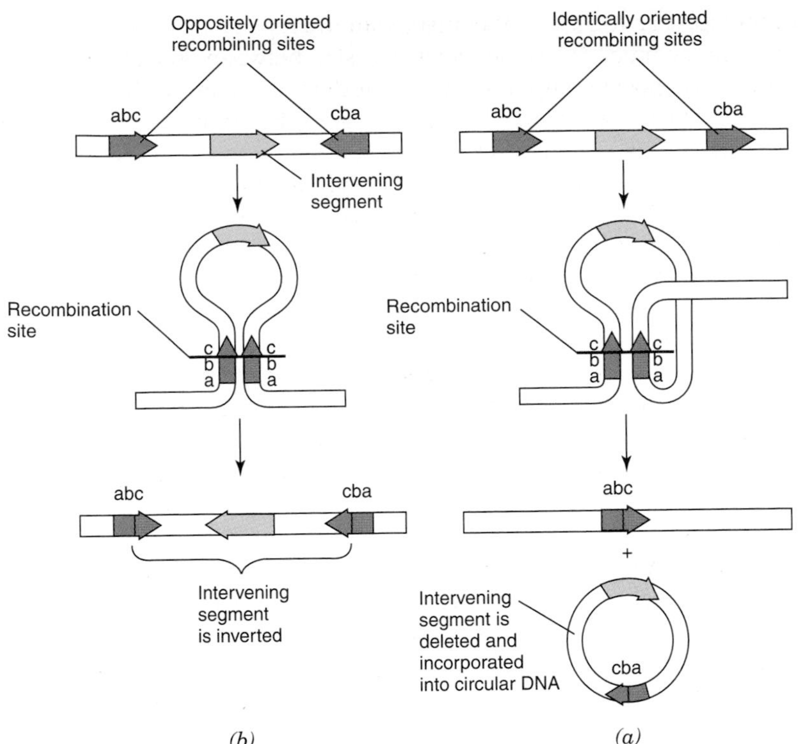

FIGURE 15.49
Genomic rearrangements promoted by transposons.
In replicative transposition a transposable element is replicated, with one copy of it remaining at the donor site and a new copy becoming inserted within a different location. This produces two homologous sequences within the same chromosome that can subsequently enter into homologous recombination. (*a*) When these homologous sequences are of the same polarity, recombination can yield a deletion of DNA by a process that is superficially analogous, but certainly not similar, to the reverse reaction occurring in site-specific recombination. (*b*) Inversion of DNA flanked by these transposons can result when transposable elements are present in the chromosome oriented in opposite direction.
Redrawn based on figure from Mathews, C. K. and Van Holde, K. E. Biochemistry. *Redwood City, CA: Benjamin/Cummings, 1990.*

15.6 ■ SEQUENCING OF NUCLEOTIDES IN DNA

Restriction Maps Give the Sequence of Segments of DNA

The sequences of many genes and adjoining DNA segments have been determined for bacteria, viruses, plants, and humans. The determination of the sequence of a large DNA molecule begins by cutting the DNA into pieces of a more manageable size with appropriate restriction endonucleases. **Restriction digests** permit the construction of a characteristic **restriction map** for each DNA. One protocol depends on the generation of partial restriction digests of end-labeled DNA. Partial digests are obtained by setting the conditions so that

CLINICAL CORRELATION 15.10

DNA Amplification and Development of Drug Resistance

An important limitation in the effectiveness of chemotoxic drugs in the treatment of cancer is the development of drug resistance. Thus cancer cells become resistant to methotrexate (see p. 520), an inhibitor of dihydrofolate reductase (DHFR). Drug resistance in cultured cells results from the specific amplification of a large DNA segment that incorporates the *DHFR* gene but the exact mechanism by which amplification occurs is not clear. It appears likely that amplification results from recombination of identically oriented homologous sequences that flank the amplified DNA. Amplification can occur by tandem duplication of DNA that contains the *DHFR* gene or alternatively the DHFR-containing segment can be excised (apparently by a recombination process), producing extrachromosomal DNA (minichromosomes). The two mechanisms of *DHFR* gene amplification are not mutually exclusive and, in fact, some resistant cells contain both types of amplified DNA.

Gene amplification is gradually reversed in the absence of methotrexate, first with the disappearance of the extrachromosomal copies. Chromosomally amplified genes, however, persist for several generations after removal of the drug. The amplification of genes is a general phenomenon not limited to methotrexate or the development of cell resistance toward other drugs. In fact, gene amplification and the accompanying resistance extend to areas well beyond clinical medicine, as, for instance, in agriculture with the development of pesticide-resistant insects.

CLINICAL CORRELATION 15.11

Nucleotide Sequence of the Human Genome

The purpose of the Human Genome Project is to provide a detailed map of the human genome and establish what DNA sequences determine human phenotypic characteristics and guide human development. A corollary to this goal is to identify genes responsible for human disease so that new approaches can be developed for diagnosis, prevention, and therapy.

The human genome is believed to consist of 70,000–100,000 different genes that determine the genetic characteristics of every cell in the human individual. The human genome consists of about three billion base-paired nucleotides that are assembled in the form of 23 pairs of chromosomes. The availability of restriction endonucleases and the development of effective physical mapping procedures for DNA, combined with the increasing rapidity of contemporary nucleotide sequencing methods, have provided strong impetus for the very ambitious undertaking of determining the nucleotide sequence of the entire human genome.

Extensive physical mapping has been completed. In addition, genetic mapping seeks to locate over 500 known genetic markers on the human chromosomes. Cumulatively over 150 million base pair sequences, representing parts of the chromosome sequences of both human DNA and that of other organisms, have been determined. Also, the sequences of certain continuous stretches of DNA, ranging from one million to several million base pairs in length, are being determined. Considering that the size of different human chromosomes varies from 263 million to less than 50 million base pairs, the determination to date of a total of about 150 million base pairs represents an important accomplishment. It is conservatively estimated that complete sequencing of the genome will take more than a decade and a half.

Because of the routine nature of determining the nucleotide sequences involved, many scientists have questioned the wisdom of diverting resources from perhaps more creative scientific endeavor, to the effort required to sequence the human genome. Others have pointed out that the project is fraught with technical uncertainties. Proponents point out the great potential benefits of determining the imprint that controls the genetic properties of the human cell at the highest possible level of resolution. Presently, as many as 4000 genetic diseases have been identified and many of them, namely, those inherited in Mendelian fashion, are caused by a single mutant gene. Searching for the imprint of human disease at the level of nucleotide sequences may permit understanding of all disease states at the genomic level. Determination of the complete sequence appears to be one of the prerequisites for understanding human disease at the molecular level. There is little doubt that the sequencing of the human genome will present us with many new challenges and opportunities in medicine.

Grant Cooper, N. (Ed.). *The Human Genome Project.* Mill Valley, CA: University Science Books, 1994.

the restriction endonuclease will not recognize all sites in every DNA molecule but will instead produce a digest that includes a collection of partial fragments. Double-stranded DNA is end-labeled by treatment with alkaline phosphatase, which removes the phosphate residue at the 5′ end, and then γ-labeled with [^{32}P]ATP and a polynucleotide kinase, which incorporates the ^{32}P into the two 5′ termini of the DNA strands. Alternately, the ^{32}P-label can be introduced at the 3′ termini by the incorporation of ^{32}P-labeled deoxyribonucleotide triphosphates using DNA polymerase. End-labeling allows for each fragment to be identified on an electrophoresis gel. The details of this procedure are presented on page 762. Thus, with a series of different site cuts, the fragments can be mapped directly relative to the labeled end. Restriction maps are used for characterization of various DNAs and for ordering of smaller DNA fragments within a particular DNA sequence. Such ordering is essential before the nucleotide sequence of large DNA molecules can be determined.

Several methods have been developed for rapid sequencing of large polydeoxyribonucleotides. They are impressively accurate. Digests obtained using different restriction enzymes produce segments with overlapping lengths of nucleotide sequences. The accuracy of sequencing methods are increased by sequencing the complementary strand. These procedures can also be used for sequencing of RNA molecules by prior conversion of the RNA sequence to a complementary DNA by use of reverse transcriptase. Sequences up to 500 bp can be determined in a single automated operation and stretches of 10,000 bp, which correspond to the average length of a gene, are now routinely determined. Clinical Correlation 15.11 discusses the application of these procedures for obtaining the sequence of the human genome.

BIBLIOGRAPHY

Adams, R. L. P. *DNA Replication*. Oxford, England: Oxford University Press; New York: IRL Press, 1991.

Alberts, B., Bray, D., Lewis, J., Raff, M., Roberts, K., and Watson, J. D. *Molecular Biology of the Cell,* 3rd ed. New York: Garland, 1994.

Bardwell, A. J., Bardwell, L., Wang, Z., Siede, W., et al. Recent insights on DNA repair: the mechanism of damaged nucleotide excision in eukaryotes and its relationship to other cellular processes. *Ann. N.Y. Acad. Sci.* 726:281, 1994.

Bell, S. P., and Stillman, B. ATP-dependent recognition of eukaryotic origins of DNA replication by a multiprotein complex. *Nature* 357:128, 1992.

Bernstein, C. *Aging, Sex and DNA Repair.* San Diego, CA: Academic Press, 1991.

Bhattacharyya, A., Murchie, A. I., von Kitzing, E., Diekmann, S., Kemper, B., and Lilley, D. M. J. A model for the interaction of DNA junctions and resolving enzymes. *J. Mol. Biol.* 221:1191, 1991.

Binden, R. R. *DNA Structure and Function.* San Diego, CA: Academic Press, 1994.

Blackburn, E. H. Telomerases. *Annu. Rev. Biochem.* 61:113, 1992.

Bootsma, D., Weeda, G., Vermeulen, W., van Vuuren, H., et al. Nucleotide excision repair syndromes: molecular basis and clinical symptoms. *Philos. Trans. R. Soc. Lond. B Biol. Sci.* 347:75, 1995.

Calladine, C., and Drew, H. *Understanding DNA—The Molecule and How It Works.* San Diego, CA: Academic Press, 1992.

Calsou, P., and Salles, B. Properties of damage-dependent DNA incision by nucleotide excision repair in human cell-free extracts. *Nucleic Acids Res.* 22:4937, 1994.

Chiu, S. K., Rao, B. J., Story, R. M., and Radding, C. M. Interactions of three strands in joints made by RecA protein. *Biochemistry* 32:13146, 1993.

Dianov, G., and Lindahl, T. Reconstitution of the DNA base excision-repair pathway. *Curr. Biol.* 4:1069, 1994.

Duckett, D. R., Murchie, A. I., Giraud-Panis, M. J., Pohler, J. R., and Lilley, D. M. Structure of the four-way DNA junction and its interaction with proteins. *Philos. Trans. R. Soc. Lond. B Biol. Sci.* 347:27, 1995.

Echols, H., and Goodman, M. F. Fidelity mechanisms in DNA replication *Annu. Rev. Biochem.* 60:477, 1991.

Fangman, W. L., and Brewer, B. J. Activation of replication origins in yeast chromosomes. *Annu. Rev. Cell Biol.* 7:375, 1991.

Friedberg, E. C., Walker, G. C., and Siede, W. *DNA Repair and Mutagenesis.* Materials Park, OH: ASM Press, 1995.

Hanawalt, P. C. Transcription-coupled repair and human disease. *Science* 266:1957, 1994.

Hiasa, H., and Marians, K. J. Tus prevents overreplication of oriC plasmid DNA. *J. Biol. Chem.* 269:26959, 1994.

Horiuchi, T., Fujimura, Y., Nishitani, H., Kobayashi, T., and Hidaka, M. The DNA replication fork blocked at the Ter site may be an entrance for the RecBCD enzyme into duplex DNA. *J. Bacteriol.* 176:4656, 1994.

Huang, J.-C., Svoboda, D. L., Reardon, J. T., and Sancar, A. Human nucleotide excision nuclease removes thymine dimers from DNA by incising the 22nd phosphodiester bond 5′ and the 6th phosphodiester bond 3′ to the photodimer. *Proc. Natl. Acad. Sci. USA* 89:3664, 1992.

Joyce, C. M., and Steitz, T. A. Function and structure relationships in DNA polymerases. *Annu. Rev. Biochem.* 63:777, 1994.

Kamenetskii, F. *Unraveling DNA.* New York: VCH Publishers, 1993.

Kim, M. G., Zhurkin, V. B., Jernigan, R. L., and Camerini-Otero, R. D. Probing the structure of a putative intermediate in homologous recombination: the third strand in the parallel DNA triplex is in contact with the major groove of the duplex. *J. Mol. Biol.* 247:874, 1995.

Kim, S. T., and Sancar, A. Photochemistry, photophysics, and mechanism of pyrimidine dimer repair by DNA photolyase. *Photochem. Photobiol.* 57:895, 1993.

Kornberg, A. *DNA Replication,* 4th ed. New York: Wiley, 1992.

Landy, A. Dynamic, structural and regulating aspects of site-specific recombination. *Annu. Rev. Biochem.* 58:913, 1989.

Lewin, B. *Genes V.* New York: Oxford University Press, 1994.

Lindsten, J., and Pettersson, U. *Etiology of Human Disease at the DNA Level.* New York: Raven Press, 1991.

Luzio, J. P., and Thompson, R. J. In: *Molecular Medical Biochemistry.* New York: Cambridge University Press, 1990.

Marians, K. J. Prokaryotic DNA replication. *Annu. Rev. Biochem.* 61:673, 1992.

Matsunaga, T., Mu, D., Park, C.-H., Reardon, J. T., and Sancar, A. Human DNA repair excision nuclease. *J. Biol. Chem.* 270:20862, 1995.

Modrich, P. Mismatch repair, genetic stability, and cancer. *Science* 266:1959, 1994.

Parsons, C. A., Stasiak, A., Bennett, R. J., and West, B. C. Structure of a multisubunit complex that promotes DNA branch migration. *Nature* 374:375, 1995.

Pederson, D. S. *Transcription Factors and DNA Replication.* Austin, TX: R. B. Landes, 1994.

Richardson, C. C., and Lehman, I. R. *Molecular Mechanisms in DNA Replication and Recombination.* New York: Wiley, 1990.

Sancar, A. Mechanisms of DNA excision repair. Science 266:1954, 1994.

Schlotterer, C., and Tautz, D. Slippage synthesis of simple sequence DNA. *Nucleic Acids Res.* 20:211, 1992.

Takahashi, M., and Nordien, B. Structure of RecA–DNA complex and mechanism of DNA strand exchange reaction in homologous recombination. *Adv. Biophys.* 30:1, 1994.

Vos, J.-M. H. *DNA Repair Mechanism: Impact on Human Disease and Cancer.* New York: Demos Vermande, 1995.

Wang, T. S. F. Eukaryotic DNA polymerases. *Annu. Rev. Biochem.* 60:513, 1991.

Wolfe, S. L. *Molecular and Cellular Biology.* Belmont, CA: Wadsworth, 1993.

Yang, S. S., Fliakas-Boltz, V., Bader, J. P., and Buckheit, R. W. Jr. Characteristics of a group of nonnucleoside reverse transcriptase inhibitors with structural diversity and potent anti-human immunodeficiency virus activity. *Leukemia* 9:575, 1995.

QUESTIONS C. N. ANGSTADT AND J. BAGGOTT

1. Which of the following statements about *E. coli* DNA polymerases is correct?
   A. All polymerases have both 3′ → 5′ and 5′ → 3′ exonuclease activity.
   B. The primary role of polymerase III is in DNA repair.
   C. Polymerases I and III require both a primer and a template.
   D. Polymerase I tends to remain bound to the template until a large number of nucleotides have been added.
   E. The specificity of the polymerase reaction is inherent in the nature of polymerases.

2. Proofreading activity to maintain the fidelity of DNA synthesis:
   A. occurs after the synthesis has been completed.
   B. is a function of the 3′ → 5′ exonuclease activity of the DNA polymerases.
   C. requires the presence of an enzyme separate from the DNA polymerases.
   D. occurs in prokaryotes but not eukaryotes.
   E. is independent of the polymerase activity in prokaryotes.

3. Which of the following would result in a frameshift mutation?
   A. formation of ionized bases by radiation.
   B. substitution of a purine–pyrimidine pair by a pyrimidine–purine pair.
   C. intercalation of ethidium bromide into the nucleotide chain.
   D. deamination of cytosine to uracil.
   E. conversion of guanine to xanthine.

4. One way of introducing a transition mutation into DNA is by:
   A. using a structural analog of a base during synthesis.
   B. the action of an acridine dye.
   C. introducing a methyl group on the adenine of a GATC sequence.
   D. blocking the proofreading action of DNA polymerase.
   E. stretching the DNA helix.

5. Which of the following is (are) step(s) in excision repair mechanisms?
   A. excision.
   B. incision.
   C. ligation.
   D. all of the above.
   E. none of the above.

6. Base excision repair:
   A. is used only for bases that have been deaminated.
   B. uses enzymes called DNA glycosylases to generate an abasic sugar site.
   C. removes about 10–15 nucleotides.
   D. requires the action of DNA polymerase III (*E. coli*).
   E. recognizes a bulky lesion.

7. All of the following are true about nucleotide excision repair EXCEPT:
   A. it is deficient in the disease xeroderma pigmentosum.
   B. it removes thymine dimers generated by UV light.
   C. it involves the activity of excision nuclease, which is an endonuclease.
   D. it requires polymerase I (*E. coli*) and ligase.
   E. it occurs in prokaryotes but not in eukaryotes.

8. Mismatch repair:
   A. recognizes and removes mismatched bases during the process of replication.
   B. occurs only if the mismatch is on a strand containing methylated bases.
   C. in *E. coli,* recognizes mismatches within a few hundred base pairs of a GATC sequence.
   D. looks for a distortion where the base structure has been altered.
   E. is characterized by all of the above being correct.

9. Both strands of DNA serve as templates concurrently in:
   A. replication.
   B. excision repair.
   C. mismatch repair.
   D. repair catalyzed by photolyase.
   E. all of the above.

10. Replication:
   A. is semiconservative.
   B. requires only proteins with DNA polymerase activity.
   C. uses $5' \rightarrow 3'$ polymerase activity to synthesize one strand and $3' \rightarrow 5'$ polymerase activity to synthesize the complementary strand.
   D. requires a primer in eukaryotes but not in prokaryotes.
   E. must begin with an incision step.

11. The discontinuous nature of DNA synthesis:
   A. requires that DNA polymerase III dissociate from the template when it reaches the end of each single-stranded region.
   B. is necessary only because synthesis is bidirectional from the initiation point.
   C. leads to the formation of Okazaki fragments.
   D. means that synthesis occurs on the second strand of DNA only after synthesis on the first strand is completed.
   E. means that both $3' \rightarrow 5'$ and $5' \rightarrow 3'$ polymerases are used.

12. All of the following are factors in the unwinding and separation of DNA strands for replication EXCEPT:
   A. the tendency of negative superhelices to partially unwind.
   B. destabilization of complementary base pairs by helicases.
   C. the action of topoisomerases.
   D. the enzymatic activity of SSB proteins.
   E. energy in the form of ATP.

13. Initiation of replication in *E. coli*:
   A. begins with dnaA binding at the OriC site if certain bases are methylated.
   B. results in the formation of several "bubbles," each consisting of a few nucleotide pairs.
   C. forms a primosome, which then uses a topoisomerase to open a replication fork.
   D. requires the action of helicase to initiate synthesis on the leading strands.
   E. begins with the formation of the replisome, followed by the formation of the primosome to begin replication.

14. In eukaryotic DNA replication:
   A. only one replisome forms because there is a single origin of replication.
   B. the leading and lagging strands are synthesized by the same enzyme.
   C. helicase dissociates from DNA as soon as the initiation bubble forms.
   D. at least one DNA polymerase has a $3' \rightarrow 5'$ exonuclease activity.
   E. the process occurs throughout the cell cycle.

15. All of the following statements about telomerase are correct EXCEPT:
   A. the RNA component acts as a template for the synthesis of a segment of DNA.
   B. it adds telomeres to the $5'$ ends of the DNA strands.
   C. it provides a mechanism for replicating the ends of linear chromosomes in most eukaryotes.
   D. telomerase recognizes a G-rich single strand of DNA.
   E. it is a reverse transcriptase.

16. Homologous recombination:
    A. occurs only between two segments from the same DNA molecule.
    B. requires that a specific DNA sequence be present.
    C. requires that one of the duplexes undergoing recombination be nicked in both strands.
    D. may result in strand exchange by branch migration.
    E. is catalyzed by transposases.

17. All of the following are true about transpositions EXCEPT:
    A. transposons move from one location to a different one within a chromosome.
    B. both the donor and target sites must be homologous.
    C. composite transposons contain an additional gene that is not present in an insertion sequence (IS).
    D. transposase introduces a staggered cut in the target DNA sequence.
    E. transposition may either activate or inactivate a gene.

ANSWERS

1. C The primer is the initial 3′ terminus of an existing strand and the template is the free portion of the complementary stand. B: Polymerase III functions in synthesis. D: Polymerase I has low processivity because it dissociates after only a few nucleotides add. E: Specificity is a function of complementary hydrogen-bonding between the base being added and the template (pp. 622–623).
2. B This activity removes a newly added base if there is a mismatch with the template. A: This is called repair. C: The polymerases are multifunctional enzymes. D: Not all eukaryotic polymerases have 3′ → 5′ exonuclease activity but some do. E: The polymerase active site seems to be the one that detects the mismatch and directs the 3′ terminus to the proofreading site (p. 624).
3. C Since the bases are read in groups of three, insertion of an additional base would shift the reading frame (p. 628). Intercalation stretches the DNA so when DNA is replicated an additional base is inserted near the intercalation site (p. 633). A: Ionized bases show atypical base pairing. B and D are both examples of base substitution type of mutations. E: This change probably wouldn't make any difference (p. 628).
4. A 5-Bromouracil and 2-aminopurine are used to deliberately introduce mutations for research. B and E: Intercalating agents stretch the helix, allowing the insertion of an extra base—a frameshift mutation. C: The mismatched repair system uses methylated adenine to distinguish between the old and newly synthesized strands. D: This could lead to a mutation but not necessarily a transition (p. 628).
5. D The other step in the process is resynthesis to fill in the gap left by the actions of A and B (p. 635).
6. B These catalyze the first step of the process. A: Methylated and other chemically modified bases can also be removed. C and E: These are characteristics of a different repair system. D: Polymerase I is the repair enzyme (p. 635).
7. E It is common to both systems. A: This is a genetic disease which requires more proteins than the prokaryotic system. B: Thymine dimers are only one cause of bulky lesions. C and D: The excision nuclease is a complex of proteins needed to unwind the DNA and remove the lesion. The polymerase and ligase fill in the gap (pp. 635–636).
8. C Methylated adenine in this sequence is a postreplicative event and signals the correct strand (i.e., unmethylated strand is newly synthesized). A: This is the function of proofreading; mismatch repair is postreplicative. B: Unmethylated sequences shortly after replication denote the newly synthesized strand. D: The bases are unaltered (p. 639).
9. A This allows for the synthesis of two identical DNA molecules. B and C: In both of these the damaged segment is removed so both strands are not available. D: This simply disrupts the inappropriate covalent bond of thymine dimers; no synthesis is involved (pp. 642 and 646).
10. A B and D: Replication requires a primer, usually synthesized by a primase. Ligases, helicases, and other proteins are required as well. C: Replication involves Okazaki fragments because synthesis occurs only in the 5′ → 3′ direction. E: Incision is the recognition step for DNA repair (p. 643).
11. C These are the segments of DNA built upon the primer. A: DNA polymerase remains bound to the template and slides over the next primer to continue synthesis. B and E: This mechanism compensates for the inability to synthesize 3′ → 5′ and would be necessary even if synthesis were unidirectional. D: Both strands are synthesized concurrently (pp. 646–647).
12. D SSB proteins stabilize the single strands after separation but have no enzymatic activity. A: This is especially true in regions of high AT pairs. B and E: This helps in the original unwinding at the expense of ATP. C: Topoisomerases nick and reseal one of the strands to prevent the introduction of an increasing number of positive supercoils (p. 648).
13. A Methylation seems to be a key in recognition of the OriC site. B: *Escherichia coli* forms only one bubble, a few hundred nucleotide pairs in size. C: The forks form and are stabilized before primase adds. D: The negative superhelicity favors initiation but helicase is necessary for the continuation of synthesis. E: The replisome is the final assembly and includes DNA polymerase III and rep proteins (pp. 649–651).
14. D Polymerase α shows this activity that provides proofreading during synthesis. δ and ε have this for proofreading. A: There are multiple initiation sites. The DNA segments between two initiation points are called replicons (p. 654). B: In prokaryotes, the DNA polymerase III does both; in eukaryotes δ synthesizes the leading strand and α the lagging strand, at least for the initiation process. C: Helicase activity is also necessary for the continuation of synthesis, that is, the opening of the forks (p. 655). E: Replication is confined to the S phase (p. 654).
15. B It is the 3′ end of each strand that cannot be conventionally replicated. A and C: Telomerase both positions itself at the 3' ends of the DNA and provides the template for extending that end (p. 660, Figure 15.40). D: This is a characteristic of the 3′-end. E: It is using an RNA template to synthesize DNA (p. 659).
16. D This is just one of the events in this complex process. A and B: It may occur between two distinct DNA molecules; the

requirement is that the two sequences be homologous but not that they be specific sequences. C: The nicks are usually on a single strand. E: These are the enzymes of transpositional site-specific recombination (p. 663).

17. B Only the donor site requires a specific nucleotide sequence; homology is not required. A: This is the definition. C: The IS contains the gene for transposon plus the flanking sequences; composite transposons have an additional gene—for example, one that confers antibiotic resistance in bacteria. D: This permits the transposon to be inserted. E: Insertion into the middle of a gene would inactivate it; insertion of a promoter next to a gene may activate it (pp. 670–671).

CHAPTER

RNA: STRUCTURE, TRANSCRIPTION, AND PROCESSING

Francis J. Schmidt

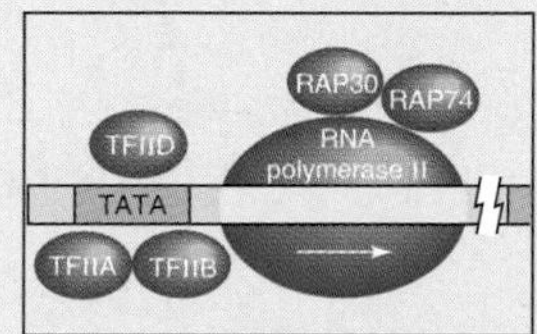

16.1 ■ OVERVIEW

The primary information store of a cell is its genetic complement, that is, its DNA. DNA information is exactly analogous to the master copies of a computer program or any database: It is the source of cellular information and therefore must be kept as error-free as possible. Chapter 14 has detailed some of the elaborate mechanisms that are employed to keep DNA information intact from one cell generation to the next. This chapter describes another type of information transfer that helps to ensure the integrity of genomic information. Just as a careful computer programmer makes working copies of a program or data set, a cell makes macromolecular copies of the information in DNA. These macromolecules, ribonucleic acids (RNAs), are linear polymers of ribonucleoside monophosphates. The sequence of DNA is copied exactly into RNA. The process by which RNA copies of selected DNA sequences are made is termed transcription. The primary role of RNA within the cell is its involvement in protein synthesis, that is, translation.

The overall process of information transfer in the cell is therefore given by the so-called **central dogma** of molecular biology:

$$\text{DNA} \xrightarrow{\text{transcription}} \text{RNA} \xrightarrow{\text{translation}} \text{protein}$$

TABLE 16.1 Characteristics of Cellular RNAs

Type of RNA	*Abbreviation*	*Function*	*Size and Sedimentation Coefficient*	*Site of Synthesis*	*Structural Features*
Messenger RNA Cytoplasmic	mRNA	Transfer of genetic information from nucleus to cytoplasm, or from gene to ribosome	Depends on size of protein 1000–10,000 nucleotides	Nucleoplasm	Blocked 5′ end; poly(A) tail on 3′ end; nontranslated sequences before and after coding regions; few base pairs and methylations
Mitochondrial	mt mRNA		9S–40S	Mitochondria	
Transfer RNA Cytoplasmic	tRNA	Transfer of amino acids to mRNA–ribosome complex and correct sequence insertion	65–110 nucleotides 4S	Nucleoplasm	Highly base paired; many modified nucleotides; common specific structure
Mitochondrial	mt tRNA		3.2S–4S	Mitochondria	
Ribosomal RNA Cytoplasmic	rRNA	Structural framework for ribosomes	28S, 5400 nucleotides 18S, 2100 nucleotides 5.8S, 158 nucleotides 5S, 120 nucleotides	Nucleolus Nucleolus Nucleolus Nucleoplasm	5.8S and 5S highly base paired; 28S and 18S have some base paired regions and some methylated nucleotides
Mitochondrial	mt rRNA		16S, 1650 nucleotides 12S, 1100 nucleotides	Mitochondria	
Heterogeneous nuclear RNA	hnRNA	Some are precursors to mRNA and other RNAs	Extremely variable 30S–100S	Nucleoplasm	mRNA precursors may have blocked 5′ ends and 3′-poly(A) tails; many have base paired loops
Small nuclear RNA	snRNA	Structural and regulatory RNAs in chromatin	100–300 nucleotides	Nucleoplasm	
Small cytoplasmic RNA [7S(L) RNA]	scRNA	Selection of proteins for export	129 nucleotides	Cytosol and rough endoplasmic reticulum	Associated with proteins as part of signal recognition particle

RNA information is occasionally **reverse transcribed** into DNA, a process important in the life cycle of infectious retroviruses such as the human immunodeficiency virus (HIV), which causes the acquired immunodeficiency syndrome (AIDS). Reverse translation of protein sequence into nucleic acid sequence information, however, does not occur in nature.

RNA molecules are classified according to the roles they play in information transfer processes (Table 16.1). In prokaryotes, transcription and translation occur close together; in fact, ribosomes can begin translating a mRNA while it is still being synthesized. In eukaryotes, these processes are spatially separated: transcription occurs in the nucleus and translation in the cytoplasmic portions of the cell. **Messenger RNAs (mRNA)** serve as templates for the synthesis of protein; they carry information from the DNA to the cellular protein synthetic machinery. Here a number of other RNA species contribute to the synthesis of the peptide bond.

The molecules that transfer specific amino acids from soluble amino acid pools to ribosomes, and ensure the alignment of these amino acids in the proper sequence prior to peptide bond formation, are **transfer RNAs (tRNA).** All tRNA molecules are approximately the same size and shape. The assembly site, or factory, for peptide synthesis involves ribosomes. These complex subcellular particles contain three or four **ribosomal RNA (rRNA)** molecules and 70–80 ribosomal proteins.

Protein synthesis requires a close interdependent relationship between mRNA, the informational template, tRNA, the amino acid adaptor molecule, and rRNA, part of the synthetic machinery. In order for protein synthesis to occur at the correct time in a cell's life, the syntheses of mRNA, tRNA, and rRNA must be coordinated with the cell's response to the intra- and extracellular environments.

All cellular RNA is synthesized on a DNA template and reflects a portion of the DNA base sequence. Therefore all RNA is associated with DNA at some time. Although DNA is the more prevalent genetic store of information, RNA can also carry genetic information. Genomic RNA is found in the RNA tumor viruses and the other small RNA viruses, such as poliovirus and reovirus.

16.2 ■ STRUCTURE OF RNA

RNA Is a Polymer of Ribonucleoside 5′-Monophosphates

Chemically, RNA is similar to DNA. Although RNA is one of the more stable components within a cell, it is not as stable as DNA. The presence of the adjacent 2′-hydroxyl group makes the RNA phosphodiester bond more susceptible to chemical and enzymatic hydrolysis than its DNA counterpart. Some RNAs, such as bacterial mRNA, are synthesized, used, and degraded within minutes, whereas others, such as rRNA, are more stable metabolically.

RNA is an unbranched linear polymer of ribonucleoside monophosphates. The purines found in RNA are *adenine* and *guanine*; the pyrimidines are *cytosine* and *uracil*. Except for uracil, which replaces thymine, these are the same bases found in DNA.

A, C, G, and U nucleotides are incorporated into RNA during transcription. Many RNAs also contain **modified nucleotides,** which are synthesized after transcription. Modified nucleotides are especially characteristic of stable RNA species (i.e., tRNA and rRNA); however, some methylated nucleotides are also present in eukaryotic mRNA. For the most part, the functions of the modified nucleotides in RNA have not been identified. Where known, the function of nucleotide modification seems to involve "fine tuning" rather than an indispensable role in the cell.

The 3′,5′-phosphodiester bonds of RNA form a chain or backbone from

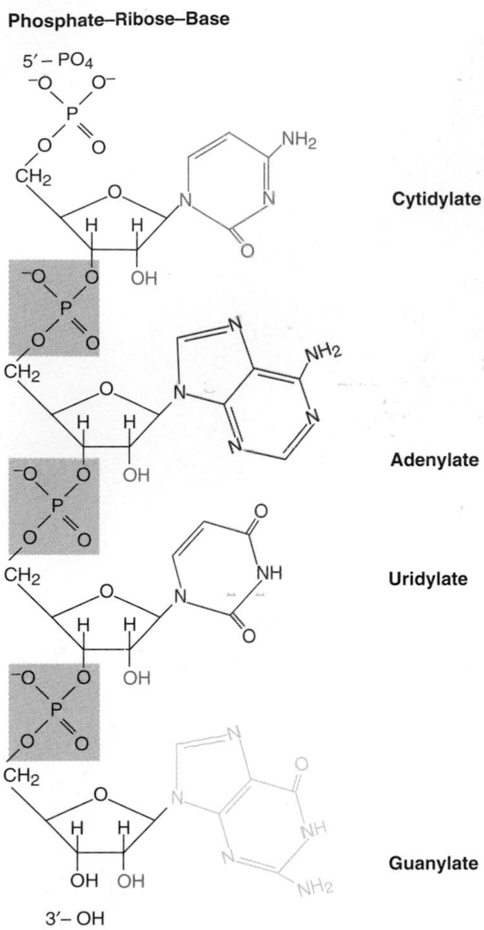

Phosphate–Ribose–Base

5′ – PO_4

Cytidylate

Adenylate

Uridylate

Guanylate

3′ – OH

FIGURE 16.1
Structure of the 3′,5′-phosphodiester bonds between ribonucleotides forming a single strand of RNA.
The phosphate joins the 3′-OH group of one ribose with the 5′-OH group of the next ribose. This linkage produces a polyribonucleotide having a sugar–phosphate "backbone." The purine and pyrimidine bases extend away from the axis of the backbone and may pair with complementary bases to form double helical base paired regions.

which the bases extend (Figure 16.1). Eukaryotic RNAs vary from approximately 65 nucleotides long to more than 200,000 nucleotides long. RNA sequences are complementary to the base sequences of specific portions of only one strand of DNA. Thus, unlike the base composition of DNA, molar ratios of A + U and G + C in RNA are not equal. All cellular RNA so far examined is linear and single stranded, but double-stranded RNA is present in some viral genomes.

Secondary Structure of RNA Involves Intramolecular Base Pairing

RNA, being single stranded rather than double stranded, does not usually form an extensive double helix. Rather, the structure in an RNA molecule arises from relatively short regions of **intramolecular base pairing.** Considerable helical structure exists in RNA even in the absence of extensive base pairing, for example, in the portions of an RNA that do not form intramolecular Watson–Crick base pairs. This helical structure is due to the strong base-stacking forces between A, G, and C residues. Base stacking is more important than simple hydrogen bonding in determining inter- and intramolecular interactions. These forces act to restrict the possible conformations of an RNA molecule (Figure 16.2). **RNA helical structures** generally are of the "A type" with 11 nucleotides per turn in a double helix.

Double helical regions in RNA are often called "hairpins." There are considerable variations in the fine structural details of **"hairpin"** structures, including the length of base paired regions and the size and number of unpaired loops (Figure 16.3). Transfer RNAs are excellent examples of base stacking and hydrogen bonding in a single-stranded molecule (Figure 16.4*a*). About 60% of the bases are paired in four double helical stems. In addition, the unpaired regions have the capability to form base pairs with free bases in the same or other looped regions, thereby contributing to the molecule's tertiary structure. The anticodon region in tRNA is an unpaired, base-stacked, loop of seven nucleotides. The partial helix caused by base stacking in this loop binds, by specific base pairing, to a complementary codon in mRNA so that translation (peptide bond formation) can occur.

RNA Molecules Have Tertiary Structures

The actual functioning structures of RNA molecules are more complex than the base-stacked and hydrogen-bonded helices mentioned above. RNAs *in vivo* are

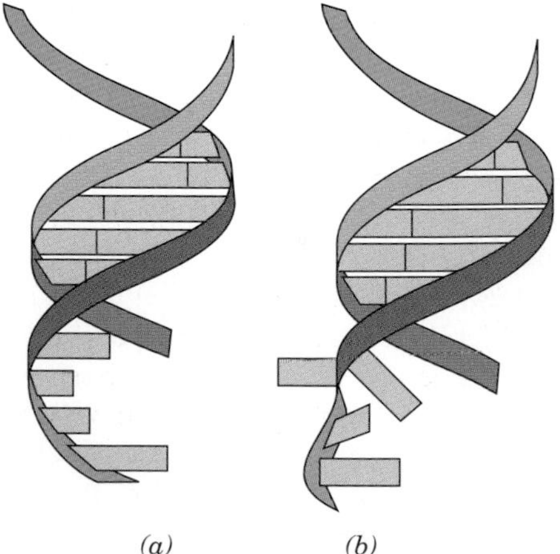

FIGURE 16.2
Helical structure of tRNA.
Models indicating a helical structure due to (a) base stacking in the CCA terminus of tRNA and (b) the lack of an ordered helix when no stacking occurs in this non-base paired region.
Redrawn from Sprinzl, M., and Cramer, F. Prog. Nucl. Res. Mol. Biol. *22:9, 1979.*

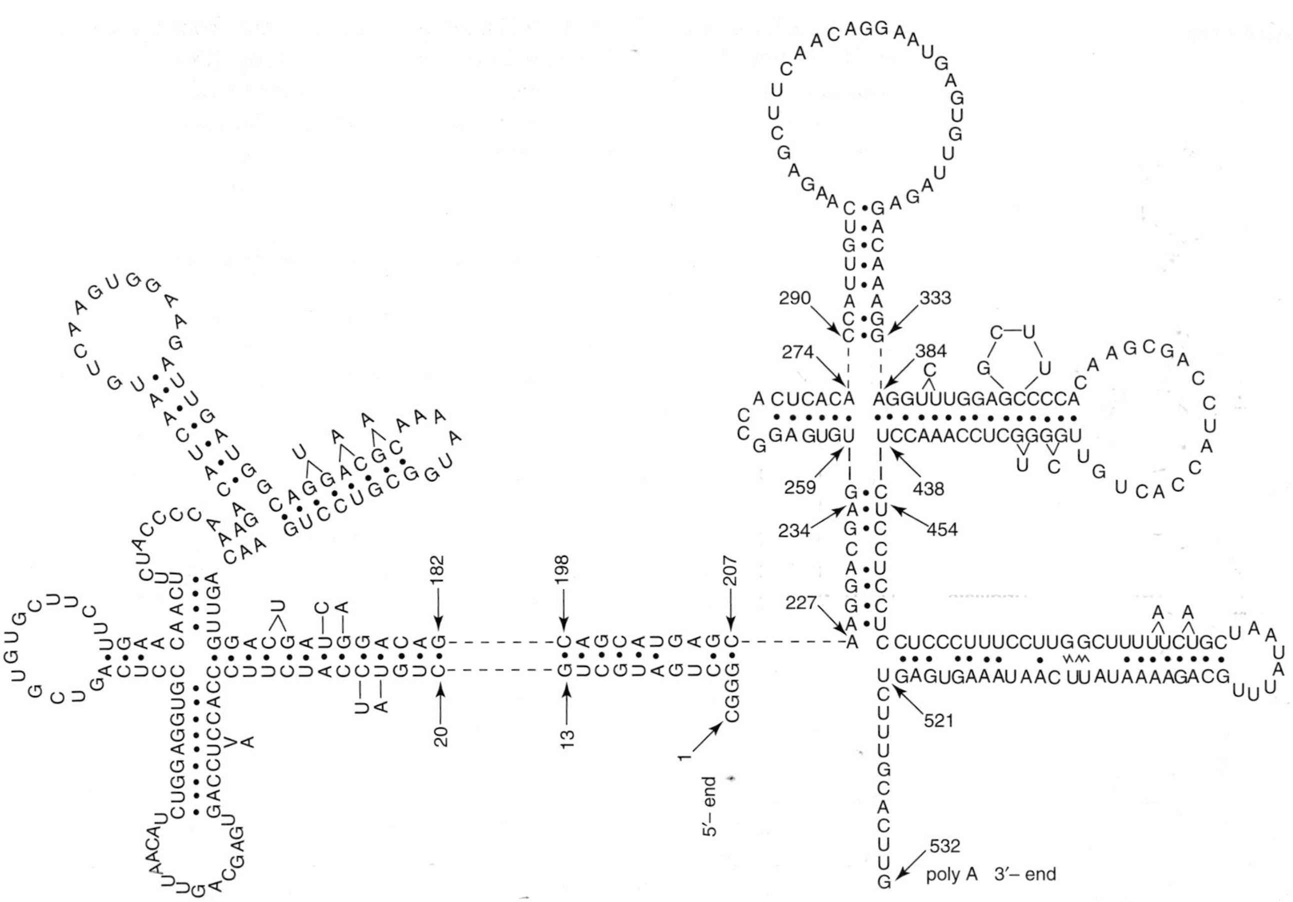

FIGURE 16.3
Proposed base pairing regions in the mRNA for mouse immunoglobulin light chain.
Base paired structures shown have free energies of at least −5 kcal. Note the variance in loop size and length of paired regions.
Redrawn from Hamlyn, P. H., Browniee, G. G., Cheng, C. C., Gait, M. J., and Milstein, C. Cell *15:1067, 1978.*

dynamic molecules that undergo changes in conformation during synthesis, processing, and functioning. Proteins associated with RNA molecules often lend stability to the RNA structure; in fact, it is perhaps more correct to think of RNA–protein complexes rather than naked RNA molecules as functioning components of the cell. In addition to the secondary, base paired structure, RNA molecules also form other hydrogen bonds to form the **tertiary structure** of the molecule. Again, the structure of tRNA provides a number of examples. In solution, tRNA is folded into a compact "L-shaped" conformation (Figure 16.4*b*). The arms and loops are folded in specific conformations held in position not only by Watson–Crick base pairing, but also by base interactions involving more than two nucleotides. Bases can donate hydrogen atoms to bond with the phosphodiester backbone. The 2′-OH of the ribose is an important donor and acceptor of hydrogens. All these interactions contribute to the folded shape of an RNA molecule.

16.3 ■ TYPES OF RNA

RNA molecules are traditionally classified as transfer, ribosomal, and messenger RNAs according to their usual function; however, we now know that RNA molecules perform or facilitate a variety of other functions in a cell.

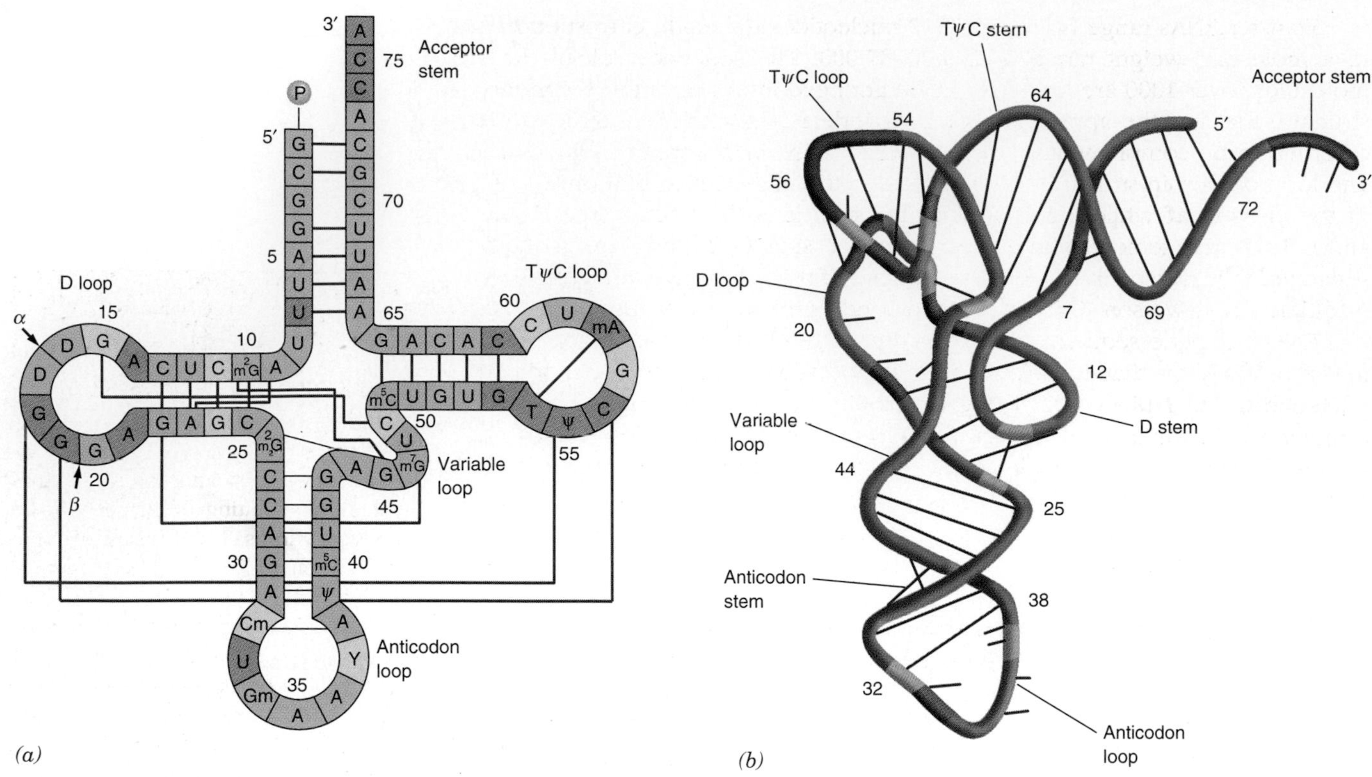

FIGURE 16.4
Coverleaf structure of tRNA
(*a*) Cloverleaf diagram of the two-dimensional structure and nucleotide sequence of yeast $tRNA^{Phe}$. Red lines connecting nucleotides indicate hydrogen-bonded residues. Insertion of nucleotides in the D loop occurs at positions α and β for different tRNAs. (*b*) Tertiary folding of the cloverleaf structure in (*a*). Hydrogen bonds are indicated by cross rungs.
Redrawn with permission from Quigley, G. J., and Rich, A. Science *194:797, 1976. Copyright © 1976 by the American Association for the Advancement of Science.*

Transfer RNA Has Two Roles: Activating Amino Acids and Recognizing Codons in mRNA

About 15% of the total cellular RNA is **tRNA.** Transfer RNA has two functions that are essential for its cellular role as an "adapter" of nucleic acid to protein information. First, tRNA molecules **activate amino acids** for protein synthesis so that formation of peptide bonds is energetically favored. The activated amino acid is transported to the polyribosome where it is transferred to the growing peptide chain (hence tRNA's name). The second function of tRNA is to recognize codons in mRNA to ensure that the correct amino acid is incorporated into the growing peptide chain. These two functions are reflected in the fact that tRNAs have two primary active sites, the 3′-OH terminal CCA, to which specific amino acids are attached enzymatically, and the **anticodon triplet,** which base pairs with mRNA codons.

Each tRNA can transfer only a single amino acid. Although there are only 20 amino acids used in protein synthesis, free-living organisms synthesize a larger set of tRNAs. For example, analysis of the recently determined genomic sequence of *Haemophilus influenzae* identified genes for 54 tRNA species. Mitochondria synthesize a much smaller number of tRNAs. Transfer RNAs that accept the same amino acid are called **isoacceptors.** A tRNA that accepts phenylalanine would be written as $tRNA^{Phe}$, whereas one accepting tyrosine would be written $tRNA^{Tyr}$.

Transfer RNAs range from 65 to 110 nucleotides in length, corresponding to a molecular weight range of 22,000–37,000. The sequences of all tRNA molecules (over 1000 are known) can be arranged into a common secondary structure that has the appearance of a cloverleaf. The cloverleaf structure is determined by complementary Watson–Crick base pairs forming three stem and loop or hairpin structures. The anticodon triplet sequence is at one "leaf" of the **cloverleaf** while the CCA acceptor stem is at the "stem" (see Figure 16.4). This arrangement where the two active sites of a tRNA are spatially separated is preserved in the tertiary structure of $tRNA^{Phe}$ shown in Figure 16.4. Additional, non-Watson–Crick, hydrogen bonds form in the L-shaped molecule.

The nucleotide sequence and structure of the $tRNA^{Phe}$ molecule depicted in Figure 16.4 show that tRNAs have several modified nucleotides. The modified nucleotides affect tRNA structure and stability but are not required for the formation or maintenance of tertiary conformation. For example, a modified base in the anticodon loop makes codon recognition more efficient but a tRNA without this modification can still be read correctly by the ribosome.

Many structural features are common to all tRNA molecules. Seven base pairs are present in the amino acid acceptor stem, which terminates with the nucleotide triplet CCA. This CCA triplet is not base paired. The dihydrouracil or "D" stem has three or four base pairs, while the anticodon and T stems have five base pairs each. Both the anticodon loop and T loop contain seven nucleotides. Differences in the number of nucleotides in different tRNAs are accounted for by the variable loop. Thus 80% of tRNAs have small variable loops of 4–5 nucleotides, while others have larger loops of 13–21 nucleotides. The positions of some nucleotides are constant in all tRNAs (see Figure 16.4*a*).

Ribosomal RNA Is Part of the Protein Synthesis Apparatus

Protein synthesis takes place on ribosomes. These complex assemblies are composed in eukaryotes of four RNA molecules, representing about two-thirds of the particle mass, and 82 proteins. The smaller subunit, the **40S particle,** contains one **18S RNA** and 33 proteins. The larger subunit, the **60S particle,** contains the **28S,** the **5.8S,** and the **5S rRNAs** and 49 proteins. The total assembly is called the **80S ribosome.** Prokaryotic ribosomes are somewhat smaller: the **30S subunit** contains a single **16S rRNA** and 21 proteins, while the larger subunit **(70S)** contains **5S** and **23S rRNAs** as well as 34 ribosomal proteins.

The rRNAs account for 80% of the total cellular RNA and are metabolically stable. This stability, required for repeated functioning of the ribosome, is enhanced by close association with the ribosomal proteins. The 28S (4718 nucleotides), 18S (1874 nucleotides), and 5.8S (160 nucleotides) rRNAs are synthesized in the nucleolar region of the nucleus. The 5S rRNA (120 nucleotides) is not transcribed in the nucleolus but rather from separate genes within the nucleoplasm (Figure 16.5). Processing of the rRNAs (see Section 16.5) includes cleavage to the functional size, internal base pairing, modification of particular nucleotides, and association with ribosomal proteins to form a stable tertiary conformation.

The larger rRNAs contain most of the altered nucleotides found in rRNA. These are primarily **methylations** on the 2′ position of the ribose, yielding 2′-*O*-methylribose. Methylation of rRNA has been directly related to bacterial antibiotic resistance in a pathogenic species (see Clin. Corr. 16.1). A small number of N^6-dimethyladenines are present in 18S rRNA. The 28S rRNA has about 45 methyl groups and the 18S rRNA has 30 methyl groups.

Biochemical studies of ribosome function indicate that rRNA molecules are more than macromolecular scaffolds for enzymatic proteins. The exact extent to which rRNA participates in protein biosynthetic reactions is the subject of current investigation. Several lines of evidence indicate that the actual formation of a peptide bond may be catalyzed by the large RNA subunit of the ribosome.

CLINICAL CORRELATION 16.1

Staphylococcal Resistance to Erythromycin

Bacteria exposed to antibiotics in a clinical or agricultural setting often develop resistance to the drugs. This resistance can arise from a mutation in the target cell's DNA, which gives rise to resistant descendants. An alternative and clinically more serious mode of resistance arises when plasmids coding for antibiotic resistance proliferate through the bacterial population. These plasmids may carry multiple resistance determinants and render several antibiotics useless at the same time.

Erythromycin inhibits protein synthesis by binding to the large ribosomal subunit. *Staphylococcus aureus* can become resistant to erythromycin and similar antibiotics as a result of a plasmid-borne RNA methylase that converts a single adenosine in 23S rRNA to N^6-dimethyladenosine. Since the same ribosomal site binds lincomycin and clindamycin, the plasmid causes cross-resistance to these antibiotics as well. Synthesis of the methylase is induced by erythromycin.

The microorganism that produces an antibiotic must also be immune to it or else it would be inhibited by its own toxic product. The producer of erythromycin, *Streptomyces erythreus,* itself possesses an rRNA methylase that acts at the same ribosomal site as the one from *S. aureus.*

Which came first? It is likely that many of the resistance genes in target organisms evolved from those of producer organisms. In several cases, DNA sequences from resistance genes of the same specificity are conserved between producer and target organisms. We may therefore look on plasmid-borne antibiotic resistance as a case of "natural genetic engineering," whereby DNA from one organism (e.g., the *Streptomyces* producer) is appropriated and expressed in another (e.g., the *Staphylococcus* target).

Cundliffe, E. How antibiotic-producing microorganisms avoid suicide. *Annu. Rev. Microbiol.* 43:207, 1989.

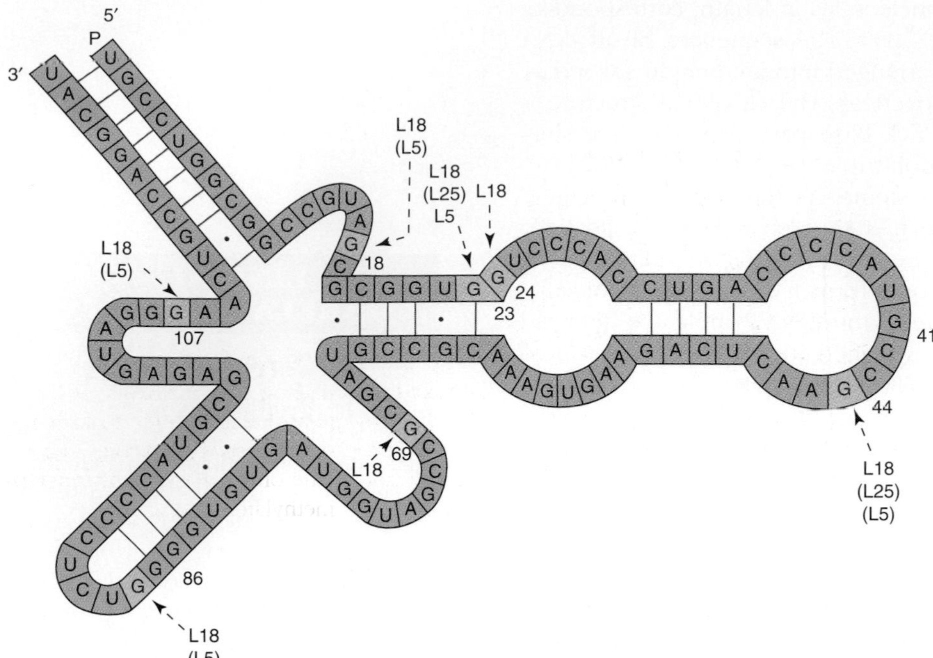

FIGURE 16.5
Secondary, base paired, structure proposed for 5S rRNA.
Arrows indicate regions protected by proteins in the large ribosomal subunit. *Combined information from Fox, G. E., and Woese, C. R.* Nature *256:505, 1975; and R. A. Garrett and P. N. Gray.*

Messenger RNAs Carry the Information for the Primary Structure of Proteins

The **mRNAs** are the direct carriers of genetic information from genomes to the ribosomes. Each eukaryotic mRNA is **monocistronic;** that is, it contains information for only one polypeptide chain. In prokaryotes, mRNA species often encode more than one protein in a **polycistronic** molecule. A cell's phenotype and functional state are related directly to its mRNA content.

In the cytoplasm mRNAs have relatively short life spans. Some mRNAs are known to be synthesized and stored in an inactive or dormant state in the cytoplasm, ready for a quick protein synthetic response. An example of this is the unfertilized egg of the African clawed toad, *Xenopus laevis*. Immediately upon fertilization the egg undergoes rapid protein synthesis in the absence of transcription, indicating the presence of preformed mRNA.

Eukaryotic mRNAs have unique structural features not found in rRNA or tRNA (see Figure 16.6). Since the information within mRNA lies in the linear sequence of the nucleotides, the integrity of this sequence is extremely im-

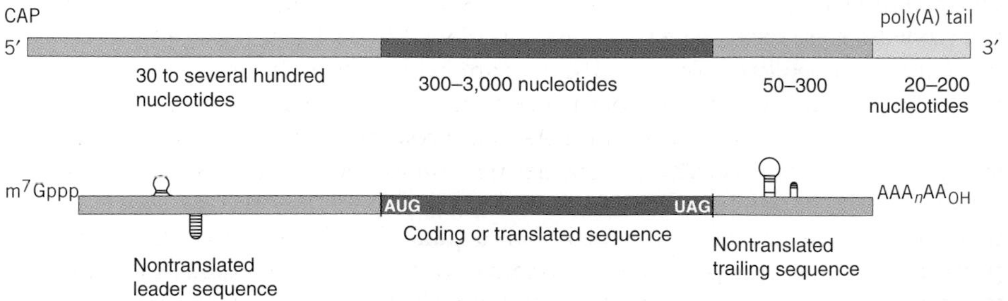

FIGURE 16.6
General structure for a eukaryotic mRNA.
There is a "blocked" 5′ terminus (cap) followed by the nontranslated leader containing a promoter sequence. The coding region usually begins with the initiator codon AUG and continues to the translation termination sequence UAG, UAA, or UGA. This is followed by the nontranslated trailer and a poly(A) tail on the 3′ end.

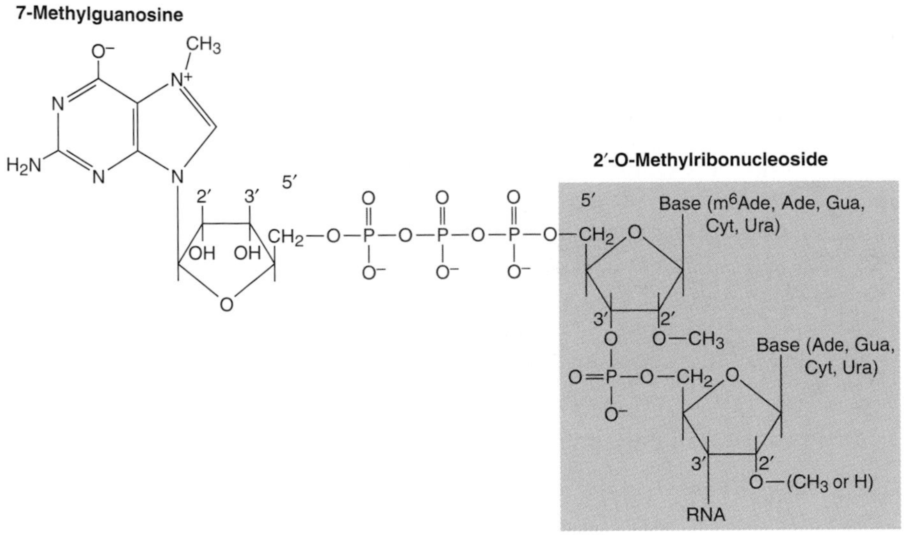

FIGURE 16.7
Diagram of the "cap" structure or blocked 5′ terminus in mRNA.
The 7-methylguanosine is inverted to form a 5′-phosphate to 5′-phosphate linkage with the first nucleotide of the mRNA. This nucleotide is often a methylated purine.

portant. Any loss or change of nucleotides could alter the protein being translated. The translation of mRNA on the ribosomes must also begin and end at specific sequences. Structurally, starting from the 5′ terminus, eukaryotic mRNA is capped with an inverted methylated base attached via **5′-phosphate–5′-phosphate bonds** rather than the usual 3′,5′-phosphodiester linkages. The **cap** is attached to the first transcribed nucleotide, usually a purine, methylated on the 2′-OH of the ribose (see Figure 16.7). The cap is followed by a nontranslated or **"leader"** sequence to the 5′ side of the coding region. Following the leader sequence are the **initiation sequence or codon,** most often AUG, and the translatable coding region of the molecule. At the end of the coding sequence is a **termination sequence** signaling termination of polypeptide formation and release from the ribosome. A second nontranslated or **"trailer"** sequence follows, terminated by a string of 20–200 adenine nucleotides, called a **poly(A) tail,** which makes up the 3′ terminus of the mRNA.

The 5′ cap has a positive effect on the initiation of message translation. In the initiation of translation of a mRNA, the cap structure is recognized by a single ribosomal protein, an initiation factor (see Chapter 17). The poly(A) sequence is correlated with the stability of the mRNA molecule; for example, **histone mRNA** molecules lack a poly(A) tail and are also present in the cell only transiently.

Mitochondria Contain Unique RNA Species

Mitochondria (mt) have their own protein-synthesizing apparatus, including ribosomes, tRNAs, and mRNAs. The mt rRNAs, 12S and 16S, are transcribed from the mitochondrial DNA (mt DNA), as are 22 specific tRNAs and 13 mRNAs, most of which encode proteins of the electron transport chain and ATP synthetase. Note that there are fewer mt tRNAs than prokaryotic or cytoplasmic tRNA species; there is only one mt tRNA species per amino acid. The mt RNAs account for 4% of the total cellular RNA. They are transcribed by a mitochondrial-specific RNA polymerase and are processed from a pair of mt RNA precursors. Each precursor is an exact copy of the entire mitochondrial genome, complementary to either the heavy (H) or light (L) strand of mt DNA. Genes for 12 tRNAs are located on the heavy mt DNA strand and 7 on the light strand. Some of the mRNAs have eukaryotic characteristics, such as 3′-poly(A) tails. A large degree of coordination exists between the nuclear and mitochondrial genomes. Most of the aminoacylating enzymes for the mt tRNAs and all of the mitochondrial ribosomal proteins are specified by nuclear genes, translated in the cytoplasm and transported into the mitochondria. The modified bases in mt tRNA species are synthesized by enzymes encoded in nuclear DNA.

RNA in Ribonucleoprotein Particles

Besides tRNA, rRNA, and mRNA, small, stable RNA species can be found in the nucleus, cytoplasm, and mitochondria. These small RNA species function as ribonucleoprotein particles (RNPs), with one or more protein subunits attached. Different RNP species have been implicated in RNA processing, splicing, transport, and control of translation, as well as in the recognition of proteins due to be exported. The actual roles of these species, where known, are described more fully in the discussion of specific metabolic events.

Some RNAs Have Catalytic Activity

RNA can be an enzyme. In several cases the RNA component of a ribonucleoprotein particle has been shown to be the catalytically active subunit of the enzyme. In other cases, *in vitro* catalytic reactions can be carried out by RNA in the absence of any protein. Enzymes whose RNA subunits carry out catalytic reactions are called **ribozymes.** There are four classes of ribozyme. Three of these RNA species carry out self-processing reactions while the fourth, **ribonuclease P (RNase P),** is a true catalyst.

In the ciliated protozoan *Tetrahymena thermophila,* an intron in the rRNA precursor is removed by a multistep reaction (Figure 16.8). A guanosine nucleoside or nucleotide reacts with the intron–exon phosphodiester linkage to displace the donor exon from the intron. This reaction, a transesterification, is promoted by the folded intron itself. The free donor exon then similarly attacks the intron–exon phosphodiester bond at the acceptor end of the intron. Introns of this type **(Group I introns)** have been found in a variety of genes in fungal mitochondria and in the bacteriophage T4. Although these introns are not true enzymes *in vivo* because they only work for one reaction cycle, they can be made to carry out catalytic reactions under specialized conditions.

Group II self-splicing introns are found in the mitochondrial RNA precursors of yeasts and other fungi. The self-splicing of these introns proceeds through a lariat intermediate similar to the lariat intermediate in the splicing of nuclear mRNA precursors (see below). Since this reaction is carried out by a ribozyme the catalytic activity of the small nucleus ribonucleoproteins (snRNPs) involved in nuclear mRNA splicing may also reside in the RNA component.

A third class of **self-cleaving RNAs** is found in the genomic RNAs of several plant viruses. These RNAs self-cleave during the generation of single genomic RNA molecules from large multimeric precursors. The three-dimensional structure of the **hammerhead ribozyme,** a member of this third class, has recently been determined (Figure 16.9). Catalysis is carried out by a bound Mg^{2+} ion positioned near the bond to be cleaved in the folded ribozyme structure. The phosphate of the cleaved bond is left at the 3′ hydroxyl position of the RNA product. A self-cleaving RNA is found in a small satellite virus, hepatitis delta virus, that is implicated in severe cases of human infectious hepatitis. All of the above self-processing RNAs can be made to act as true catalysts (i.e., exhibiting multiple turnover) *in vitro* and *in vivo.*

Ribonuclease P contains both a protein and an RNA component. It acts as a true enzyme in the cell, cleaving tRNA precursors to generate the mature 5′ end of the tRNA molecule. RNase P recognizes constant structures associated with tRNA precursors (e.g., the acceptor stem and CCA sequence) rather than using extensive base pairing to bind the substrate RNA to the ribozyme. The product of cleavage contains a 5′ phosphate in contrast to the products of hammerhead and similar RNAs. In all of these events the structure of the catalytic RNA is essential for intramolecular or enzyme catalysis.

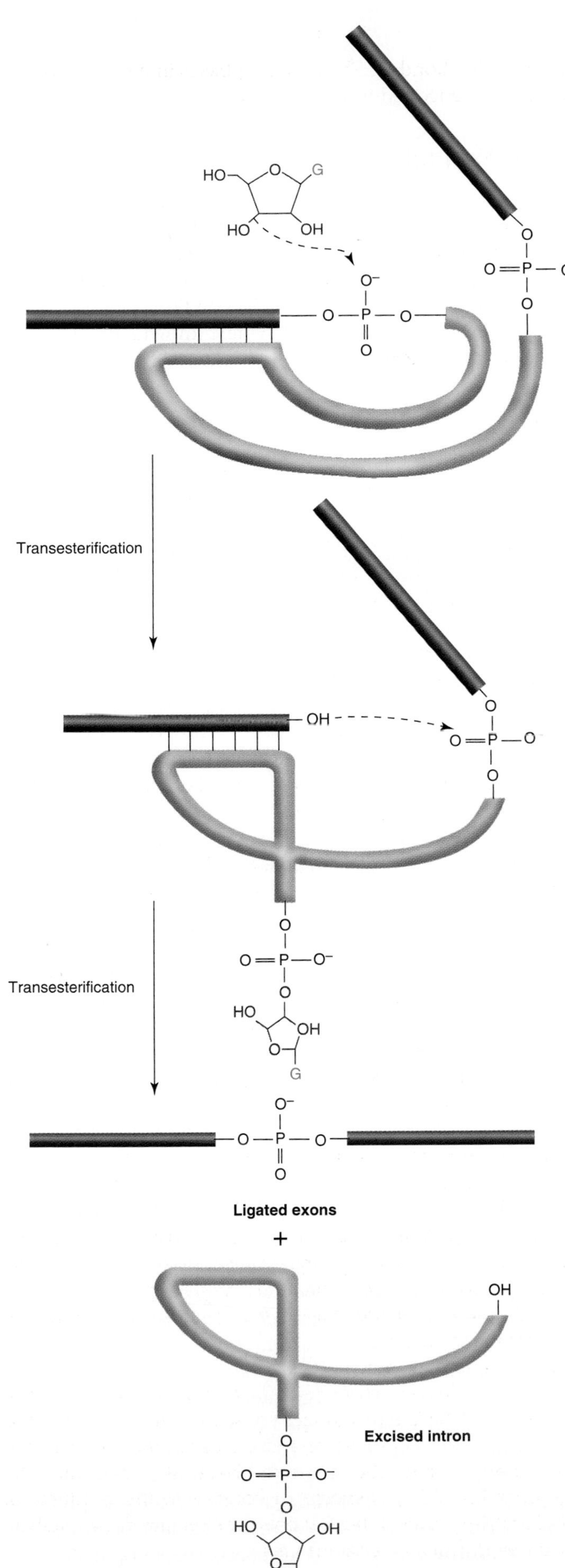

FIGURE 16.8

Mechanism of self-splicing of the rRNA precursor of *Tetrahymena.*

The two exons of the rRNA are denoted by dark blue. Catalytic functions reside in the intron, which is purple. This splicing function requires an added guanosine nucleoside or nucleotide. *Reproduced from Cech, T. R.* JAMA *260:308, 1988.*

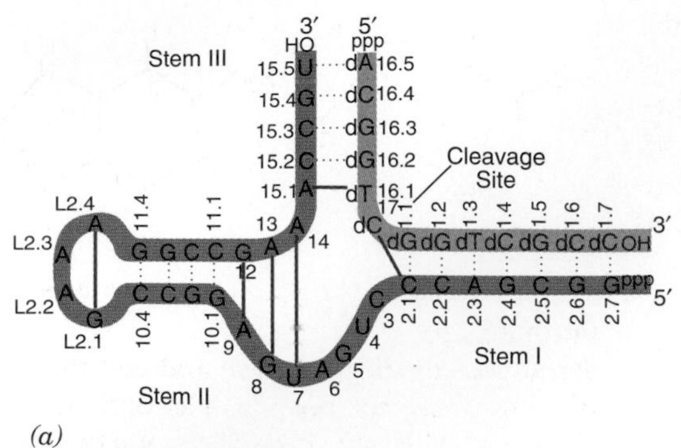

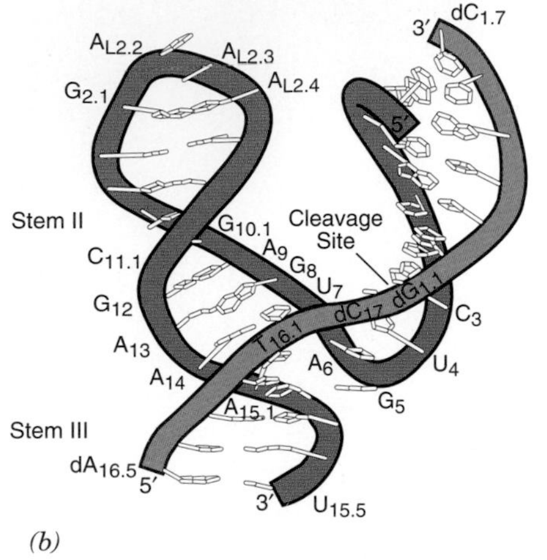

FIGURE 16.9
"Hammerhead" structure of viral RNA
(*a*) The hammerhead structure of a self-cleaving viral RNA. This artificial molecule is formed by the base pairing of two separate RNAs. The cleavage of the RNA sequence at the site indicated by the arrow in the top strand requires its base pairing with the sequence at the bottom of the molecule. The boxed nucleotides are a consensus sequence found in self-cleaving viral RNAs. (*b*) The three-dimensional folding of the hammerhead catalytic RNA. The star indicates the position of the cleaved bond while M indicates a binding site for a metal ion. Helices II and III stack to form an apparently continuous helix while non-Watson–Crick interactions position the noncomplementary bases in the hammerhead into a "uridine turn" structure identical to that found in tRNA.
Part (a) redrawn from Sampson, J. R., Sullivan, F. X., Behlen, L. S., DiRenzo, A. B., and Uhlenbeck, O. C. Cold Spring Harbor Symp. Quant. Biol. *52:267, 1987; part (b) redrawn from Pley, H. W., Flaherty, K. M., and McKay, D. B.* Nature *372:68, 1994.*

The discovery of RNA catalysis has greatly altered our concepts of biochemical evolution and the range of allowable cellular chemistry. First, we now recognize that RNA can serve as both a catalyst and a carrier of genetic information. This has raised the possibility that the earliest living organisms were based entirely on RNA and that DNA and proteins evolved later. This model is sometimes referred to as the **"RNA world."** Second, we know that many viruses, including human pathogens, use RNA genetic information; some of these RNAs have been shown to be catalytic. Thus catalytic RNA presents opportunities for the discovery of RNA-based pharmaceuticals. Third, many of the information processing events in protein synthesis and mRNA splicing require RNA components. These RNAs may also be fulfilling a catalytic function.

RNAs Can Form Binding Sites for Other Molecules

Consideration of the RNA world has led to a new type of biological chemistry based on the large number of potential sequences (4^N) that would be made if A, C, G, or U were inserted randomly in each of N positions in a nucleic acid. A set of chemically synthesized, randomized, nucleic acid molecules 25 nucleotides long would contain $4^{25} = 10^{15}$ potential members. Individual molecules within this large collection of RNAs would be expected to fold into a similarly large collection of shapes. The large number of molecular shapes implies that some member of this collection will be capable of strong, specific binding to any ligand, much as group I introns bind guanosine nucleotides specifically. Though a single molecule would be too rare to study within the original population, the RNA capable of binding can be selected and preferentially replicated *in vitro*. In one case, for example, an RNA capable of distinguishing **theophylline** from **caffeine** was selected from a complex population (see

Figure 16.10). Theophylline is used in the treatment of chronic asthma but the level must be carefully controlled to avoid side effects. The monitoring of theophylline by conventional antibody-based clinical chemistry is difficult because caffeine and theophylline differ only by a single methyl group. Therefore anti-theophylline antibodies show considerable cross-reaction with caffeine. RNA molecules have been found that bind theophylline 10,000-fold more tightly than caffeine.

Other extensions of the technology have used selection procedures to identify new, synthetic ribozymes and potential therapeutic RNAs.

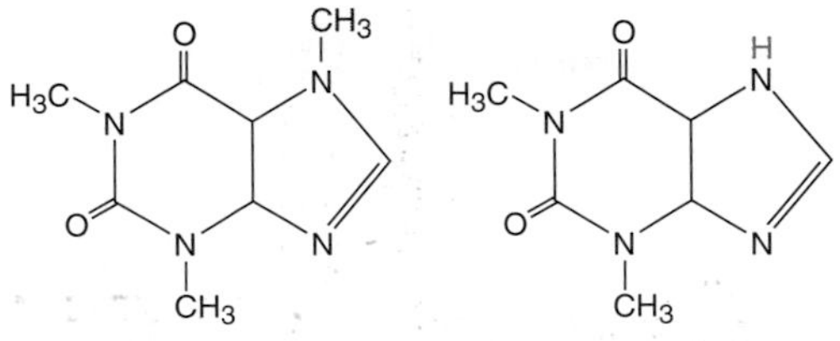

Caffeine Theophylline

FIGURE 16.10
Structures of theophylline and caffeine. Although these compounds differ only by a single methyl group, a specific synthetic RNA can bind to theophylline 10,000-fold more tightly than to caffeine.

16.4 ■ MECHANISMS OF TRANSCRIPTION

The Initial Process of RNA Synthesis Is Transcription

The process by which RNA chains are made from DNA templates is called **transcription.** All known transcription reactions take the following form:

$$\text{DNA template} + n(\text{NTP}) \rightarrow \text{pppN(pN)}_{n-1} + (n-1)\text{PP}_i + \text{DNA template}$$

Enzymes that catalyze this reaction are designated RNA polymerases; it is important to recognize that they are absolutely template dependent. In contrast to DNA polymerases, however, **RNA polymerases** do not require a primer molecule. The energetics favoring the RNA polymerase reaction are twofold: first, the 5′ α-nucleotide phosphate of the ribonucleoside triphosphate is converted from a phosphate anhydride to a phosphodiester bond with a change in free energy ($\Delta G'$) of approximately 3 kcal (12.5 kJ) mol^{-1} under standard conditions; second, the released pyrophosphate, PP_i, can be cleaved into two phosphates by pyrophosphatase so that its concentration is low and phosphodiester bond formation is more favored relative to standard conditions (see Chapter 6 for a fuller discussion of metabolic coupling).

Since a DNA template is required for RNA synthesis, eukaryotic transcription takes place in the cell nucleus or mitochondrial matrix. Within the nucleus, the *nucleolus* is the site of rRNA synthesis, whereas mRNA and tRNA are synthesized in the nucleoplasm. Prokaryotic transcription is accomplished on the cell's DNA, which is located in a relatively small region of the cell. In the case of prokaryotic plasmids, the DNA template need not be associated with the chromosome.

Structural changes occur in DNA during its transcription. In the polytene chromosomes of *Drosophila,* transcriptionally active genes are visualized in the light microscope as puffs distinct from the condensed, inactive chromatin. Furthermore, the nucleosome patterns of active genes are disrupted so that active chromatin is more accessible to, for example, DNase attack. In prokaryotes and eukaryotes, the DNA double helix is transiently opened (unwound) as the transcription complex proceeds down the DNA.

These openings and **unwindings** are a manifestation of a topological necessity. If the RNA chain were copied off DNA without this unwinding, the transcription complex and growing end of the RNA chain would have to wind around the double helix once every 10 base pairs as they travel from the beginning of the gene to its end. Such a process would wrap the newly synthesized RNA chain around the DNA double helix. Local opening and unwinding of the DNA solves this problem before it occurs by allowing transcription to proceed on a single face or side of the DNA. In addition, the opening of DNA base pairs during transcription allows Watson–Crick base pairing between template DNA and the bases in the newly synthesized RNA.

The process of transcription is divided into three parts: **initiation** refers to the recognition of an active gene starting point by RNA polymerase and the beginning of the bond formation process; **Elongation** is the actual synthesis of the RNA chain and is followed by chain **termination** and release.

$tRNA_{tyr}$	C A A C G T A A C A C T T T A C A G C G G C G C G T C A T T T G A T A T G A T G C G C C C C G C T T C C C G A T A
Str	T G T A T A T T T C T T G A C A C C T T T T C G G C A T C G C C C T A A A A T T C G G C G T C C T C A T A T T G T
Spc	T T A T T T T T T C T A C C C A T A T C C T T G A A G C G G T G T T A T A A T G C C G C G C C C T C G A T A T G G
rrn D_1	C A A A A A A A T A C T T G T G C A A A A A A T T G G G A T C C C T A T A A T G C G C C T C C G T T G A G A C G A
rrn E_1	C A A T T T T T C T A T T G C G G C C T G C G G A G A A C T C C C T A T A A T G C G C C T C C A T C G A C A C G G
rrn X_1	C A T T T T T C C G C T T G T C T T C C T G A G C C G A C T C C C T A T A A T G C G C C T C C A T C G A C A C G G
rrn $D_2E_2X_2$	G A A A T T C A G G G T T G A C T C T G A A A G A G G A A A G C G T A A T A T A C G C C A C C T C G C G A C A G T
rrn A_1	T A A A T T T C C T C T T G T C A G G C C G G A A T A A C T C C C T A T A A T G C G C C A C C A C T G A C A C G G
rrn A_2	A A A A T A A A T G C T T G A C T C T G T A G C G G G A A G G C G T A T T A T G C A C A C C C C G C G C C G C T G
SV40	G C A A T T G T T G T T G T T A A C T T G T T T A T T G C A G C T T A T A A T G G T T A C A A A T A A A G C A A
MOST COMMON	T T G A C A (17 ± 16p) T A T A A T

FIGURE 16.11
Determination of a consensus sequence for prokaryotic promoters.
A portion of the data set used for the identification of the consensus sequence for *E. coli* promoter activity. The −10 region (sometimes called the Pribnow box) is shaded in red and the −35 region nucleotides are colored. Note that none of the individual promoters has the entire consensus sequence.
Modified from Rosenberg, M., and Court, D. Ann. Rev. Genet. *13:319, 1979.*

The Template for RNA Synthesis Is DNA

Each cycle of transcription begins and ends with the recognition of specific sites in the DNA template. The DNA sequencing of a large number of transcription start regions, called **promoters,** has shown that certain **conserved sequences** occur in promoters with great regularity.

An example is shown in Figure 16.11. Similar considerations demonstrate that termination occurs at different conserved sequences. In addition, sites within a transcript may allow premature termination of transcription. These sites can act as molecular switches affecting the continuation of synthesis of an RNA molecule.

Conserved sequences near the transcription start are found for both prokaryotic and some eukaryotic promoters. In addition, eukaryotic transcription has been shown in some cases to be affected by **internal promoter** elements and other sequences called enhancers. **Enhancers** are gene-specific sequences that positively affect transcription. Enhancer sequences can stimulate transcription whether they are located at the beginning, in the middle, or at the end of a gene. An enhancer sequence must be on the same DNA strand as the transcribed gene (genetically in a cis position) but can function in either orientation. Cellular protein factors are known that specifically bind different enhancers. The most likely hypothesis is that protein factors bound to enhancers cause a structural change in the DNA template, allowing protein–protein interaction with other factors or with RNA polymerase itself. This interaction facilitates transcription.

RNA Polymerase Catalyzes the Transcription Process

RNA polymerases all synthesize RNA in the $5' \rightarrow 3'$ direction using a DNA template; in this respect, they are similar to template-dependent DNA polymerases discussed in Chapter 15. Unlike DNA polymerases, however, RNA polymerases initiate polymerization at a promoter sequence without the need of a DNA or RNA primer. Cellular RNA polymerases, both prokaryotic and eukaryotic, are large multisubunit enzymes whose mechanisms are only partially understood.

The most intensely studied prokaryotic RNA polymerase is that from *Escherichia coli,* which consists of five subunits having an aggregate molecular weight of over 500,000 (Table 16.2). Two α subunits, one β subunit, and one β' subunit constitute the **core enzyme,** which is capable of faithful transcription but not of specific (i.e., promoter-initiated) RNA synthesis. The addition of a fifth protein subunit, designated $\boldsymbol{\sigma}$**,** results in the **holoenzyme** that is capable of specific RNA synthesis *in vitro* and *in vivo*. The logical conclusion, that σ is involved in the specific recognition of promoters, has been borne out by a variety of biochemical studies and is discussed below. Specific $\boldsymbol{\sigma}$ **factors** can recognize different classes of genes. For example, a specific σ factor recognizes promoters for genes that are induced as a result of heat shock. In sporulating bacteria, specific σ factors recognize genes induced during sporulation. Some bacteriophage synthesize σ factors that allow the appropriation of the cell's RNA polymerase for transcription of the viral DNA.

The common prokaryotic RNA polymerases are inhibited by the antibiotic **rifampicin** (used in treating tuberculosis), which binds to the β subunit (see Clin. Corr. 16.2). Eukaryotic nuclear RNA polymerases are inhibited differentially by the compound $\boldsymbol{\alpha}$**-amanitin,** which is synthesized by the poisonous mushroom *Amanita phalloides*. Three nuclear RNA polymerase classes can be distinguished by these experiments. Very low concentrations of α-amanitin inhibit the synthesis of mRNA and some small nuclear RNAs (snRNAs); higher concentrations inhibit the synthesis of tRNA and other snRNAs, whereas rRNA synthesis is not inhibited at these concentrations of drug. Messenger RNA synthesis is the function of **RNA polymerase II.** Synthesis of transfer RNA, 5sRNA, and some snRNAs are carried out by **RNA polymerase III.** Ribosomal RNA genes are transcribed by **RNA polymerase I,** which is concentrated in the nucleolus. (The numbers refer to the order of elution of the enzymes from a chromatography column.) Each enzyme is highly complex structurally (Table 16.2).

In addition, a mitochondrial RNA polymerase is responsible for the synthesis of this organelle's mRNA, tRNA, and rRNA species. This enzyme, like bacterial RNA polymerase, is inhibited by rifampicin.

TABLE 16.2 Comparative Properties of Some RNA Polymerases

	Nuclear				
	I (A)	*II (B)*	*III (C)*	*Mitochondrial*	*E. coli*
High MW subunits[a]	195–197	240–214	155	65	160 (β')
	117–126	140	138		150 (β)
Low MW subunits	61–51	41–34	89		86 (σ)
	49–44	29–25	70		40 (α)
	29–25	27–20	53		10 (ω)
	19–16.5	19.5	49		
		19	41		
		16.5	32		
			29		
			19		
Variable forms	2–3 types	3–4 types	2–4 types	1	1
Specialization	Nucleolar; rRNA	mRNA Viral RNA	tRNA 5S rRNA	All mtRNA	None
Inhibition by α-amanitin	Insensitive (>1 mg mL^{-1})	Very sensitive (10^{-9}–10^{-8} M)	Sensitive (10^{-5}–10^{-4} M)	Insensitive, but sensitive to rifampicin	Rifampicin sensitive

[a] Molecular weight × 10^{-3}.

CLINICAL CORRELATION 16.2

Antibiotics and Toxins that Target RNA Polymerase

RNA polymerase is obviously an essential enzyme for life since transcription is the first step of gene expression. No RNA polymerase means no enzymes. Two natural products point out this principle; in both cases inhibition of RNA polymerase leads to death of the organism.

The "death cap" or "destroying angel" mushroom, *Amanita phalloides,* is highly poisonous and still causes several deaths each year despite widespread warnings to amateur mushroom hunters (it is reputed to taste delicious, incidentally). The most lethal toxin, α-amanitin, inhibits the largest subunit of eukaryotic RNA polymerase II, thereby inhibiting mRNA synthesis. The course of the poisoning is twofold: initial, relatively mild, gastrointestinal symptoms are followed about 48 h later by massive liver failure as essential mRNAs and their proteins are degraded but not replaced by newly synthesized molecules. The only therapy is supportive, including liver transplantation; but this latter course is clearly a desperate measure of unproven efficacy.

More benign (at least from the point of view of our own species) is the action of the antibiotic rifampicin to inhibit the RNA polymerases of a variety of bacteria, most notably in the treatment of tuberculosis. *Mycobacterium tuberculosis,* the causative agent, is insensitive to many commonly used antibiotics, but it is sensitive to rifampicin, the product of a soil streptomycetes. Since mammalian RNA polymerase is so different from the prokaryotic variety, inhibition of the latter enzyme is possible without great toxicity to the host. This consideration implies a good therapeutic index for the drug, that is, the ability to treat a disease without causing undue harm to the patient. Together with improved public health measures, antibiotic therapy with rifampicin and isoniazid (an antimetabolite) has greatly reduced the morbidity due to tuberculosis in industrialized countries. Unfortunately, the disease is still endemic in impoverished populations in the United States and in other countries. Furthermore, in increasing numbers, immunocompromised individuals, especially AIDS patients, have active tuberculosis.

Mitchel, D. H. *Amanita* mushroom poisoning. *Annu. Rev. Med.* 31:51, 1980; Gilman, A. G., Rall, T. W., Nies, A. S., and Taylor, P. (Eds.). *The Pharmacological Basis of Therapeutics,* 8th ed. New York: Pergamon Press, 1990, pp. 129–130; DeCock, K. M., Soro, B., Colibaly, I. M., Lucas, S. B. Tuberculosis and HIV infection in sub-Saharan Africa. *JAMA* 268:1581, 1992.

The Steps of Transcription in Prokaryotes Have Been Determined

Transcription is a strand-selective process; most double helical DNA is transcribed in only one direction. This is illustrated as follows:

$$
\begin{array}{ll}
\textbf{DNA:} & 5' \longrightarrow 3' \\
 & 3' \longrightarrow 5' \\
\textbf{RNA:} & \quad 5' \longrightarrow 3' \cdots
\end{array}
$$

The DNA strand that serves as the template for RNA synthesis is sometimes called the sense strand because it is complementary to the RNA transcript. Conventionally, the *sense strand* is usually the "bottom" strand of a double-stranded DNA as written. The other strand, the "top" strand, has the same direction as the transcript when read in the $5' \rightarrow 3'$ direction; this strand is sometimes (confusingly) called the *antisense strand.* When only a single DNA sequence is given in this book, the antisense strand is represented. Its sequence can be converted to the RNA transcript of a gene by simply substituting U (uracil) for T (thymine) bases. Prokaryotic transcription begins with the binding of RNA polymerase to a gene's promoter (Figures 16.11 and 16.12). RNA polymerase holoenzyme binds to one face of the DNA extending 45 bp or so upstream and 10 bp downstream from the RNA initiation site. Two short oligonucleotide sequences in this region are highly conserved. One sequence that is located about 10 bp upstream from the transcription start is the consensus sequence (sometimes called a Pribnow box):

T*A*TAAT*

The positions marked with an asterisk are the most conserved; indeed, the last T residue is always found in *E. coli* promoters.

A second consensus sequence is located upstream from the **Pribnow** or "−10" box. This "−35 sequence"

T*T*G*ACA

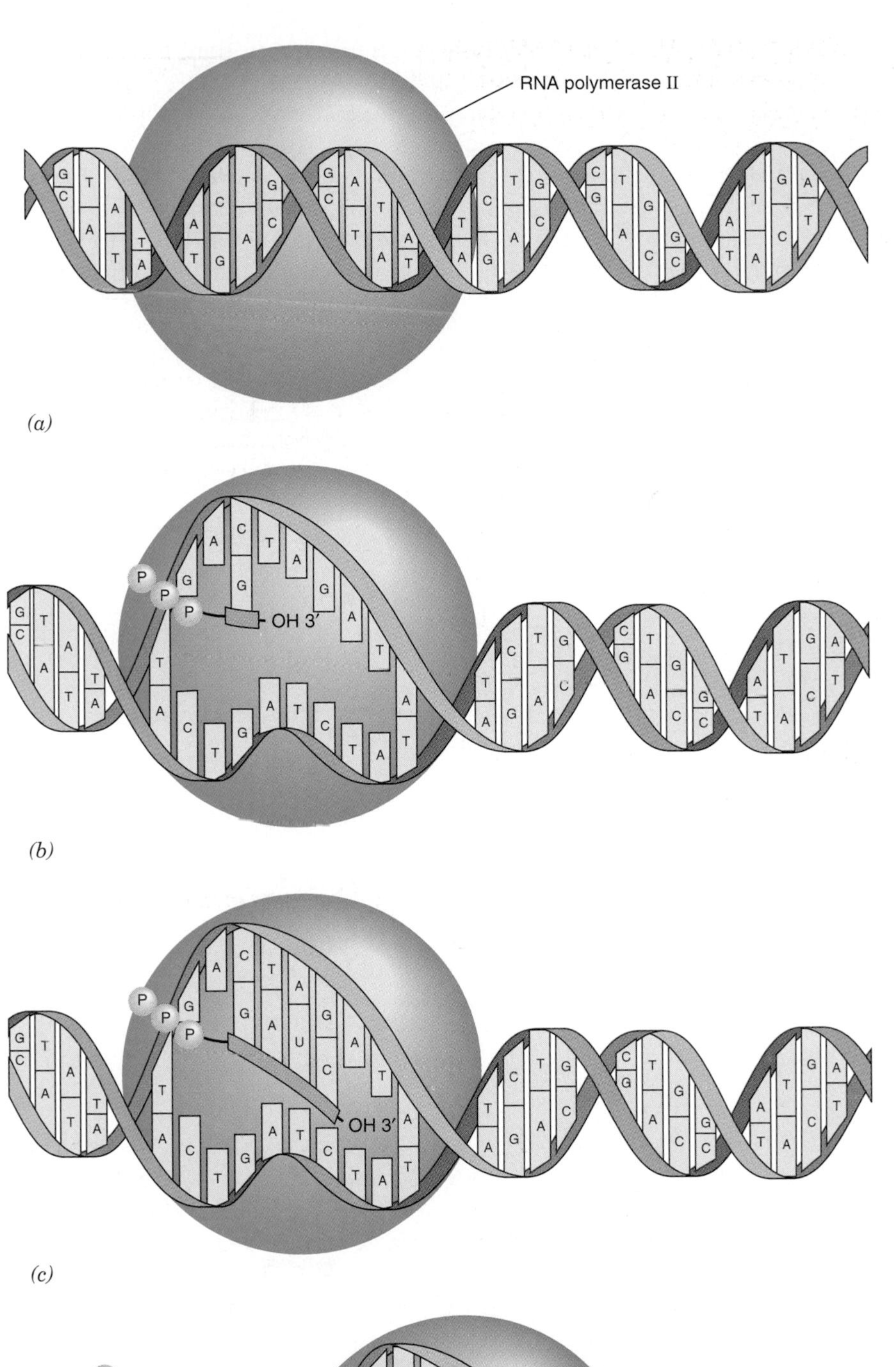

FIGURE 16.12
Early events in prokaryotic transcription. (*a*) Recognition: RNA polymerase (drawn smaller than scale) with "sigma" factor binds to a DNA promoter region in a "closed" conformation. (*b*) Initiation: The complex is converted to an "open" conformation and the first nucleoside triphosphate aligns with the DNA. (*c*) Bond formation: The first phosphodiester bond is formed and the "sigma" factor released. (*d*) Elongation: Synthesis of nascent RNA proceeds with movement of the RNA polymerase along the DNA. The double helix reforms.

is centered about 35 bp upstream from the transcription start; the nucleotides with asterisks are most conserved. The spacing between the −35 and −10 sequences is crucial with 17 bp being highly conserved. As shown in Figure 16.13, the TTGACA and TATAAT sequences are asymmetrical, that is, they do not have the same sequence if the complementary sequence is read. Thus the promoter sequence itself determines that transcription will proceed in only one direction. What difference do the consensus sequences make to a gene? Measurements of RNA polymerase binding affinity and initiation efficiency to

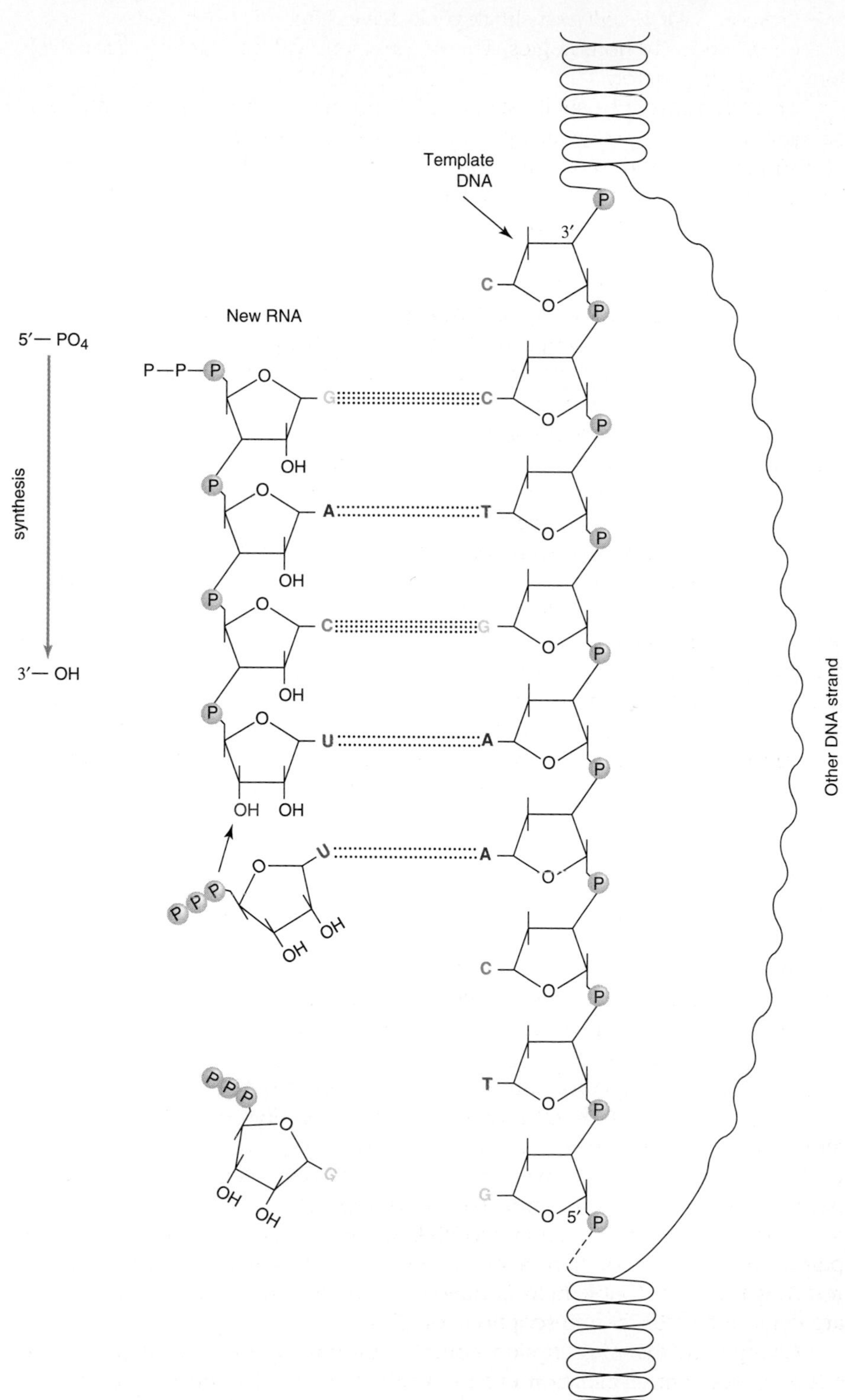

FIGURE 16.13
Biosynthesis of RNA showing asymmetry in transcription.
Nucleoside 5′-triphosphates align with complementary bases on one DNA strand, the template. RNA polymerase catalyzes the formation of the 3′,5′-phosphodiester links by attaching the 5′-phosphate of the incoming nucleotide to the 3′-OH group of the growing nascent RNA releasing P_i. The new RNA is synthesized from its 5′ end toward the 3′ end.

various promoter sequences have shown that the most active promoters fit the consensus sequences most closely. Statistical measurements of promoter homology conform closely to the measured "strength" of a promoter, that is, its kinetic ability to initiate transcription with −35 purified RNA polymerase.

Bases flanking the −35 and −10 sequences, bases near the transcription start, and bases located near the −16 position are weakly conserved. In some of these weakly conserved regions, RNA polymerase may require that a particular nucleotide not be present or that local variations in DNA helical structure be present.

Promoters for *E. coli* heat shock genes have different consensus sequences at the −35 and −10 homologies. This is consistent with their being recognized by a different σ factor.

An RNA transcript usually starts with a purine riboside triphosphate; that is, pppG··· or pppA··· , but pyrimidine starts are also known (Figures 16.11 and 16.12). The position of transcription initiation differs slightly among various promoters but usually is from five to eight base pairs downstream from the invariant T of the Pribnow box.

Initiation

Two kinetically distinct steps are required for RNA polymerase to initiate the synthesis of an RNA transcript. In the first step, RNA polymerase holoenzyme binds to the promoter DNA to form a **"closed complex."** In the second step, the holoenzyme forms a more tightly bound **"open complex,"** which is characterized by a local opening of about 10 bp of the DNA double helix. Since the consensus Pribnow box is A-T rich, it can facilitate this local unwinding. As discussed in Chapter 14, opening 10 bp of DNA is topologically equivalent to the relaxation of a single negative supercoil. As might be predicted from this observation, the activity of some promoters depends on the superhelical state of the DNA template; some promoters are more active on highly supercoiled DNA while others are more active when the superhelical density of the template is lower. The unwound DNA binds the initiating triphosphate and RNA polymerase then forms the first phosphodiester bond. The enzyme translocates to the next position (this is the rifampicin-inhibited step) and continues synthesis. At or a short time after the initial bond formation, σ factor is released and the enzyme is considered to be in an elongation mode. Other RNA polymerase molecules can now bind to the promoter so that a gene can be transcribed many times (Figure 16.14).

Elongation

RNA polymerase continues the binding–bond formation–translocation cycle at a rate of about 40 nucleotides per second. This rate is only an average, however, and there are many examples known for which RNA polymerase pauses or slows down at particular sequences, usually inverted repeats (palindrome sequence of nucleotides). As will be discussed below, these pauses can bring about transcription termination.

As RNA polymerase continues down the double helix, it continues to separate the two strands of the DNA template. As seen in Figure 16.12, this process allows the template (sense) strand of the DNA to base pair with the growing RNA chain. Thus a single mechanism of information transfer (Watson–Crick base pairing) serves several processes: DNA replication, DNA repair, and transcription of genetic information into RNA. (As will be seen in Chapter 17, base pairing is essential for translation as well.) The process of unwinding and restoring the DNA double helix is aided by DNA topoisomerases I and II, which are components of the transcription complex.

Changes in the transcription complex during the elongation phase can affect subsequent termination events. These changes depend on the binding of another cellular protein (nusA protein) to core RNA polymerase. Failure to

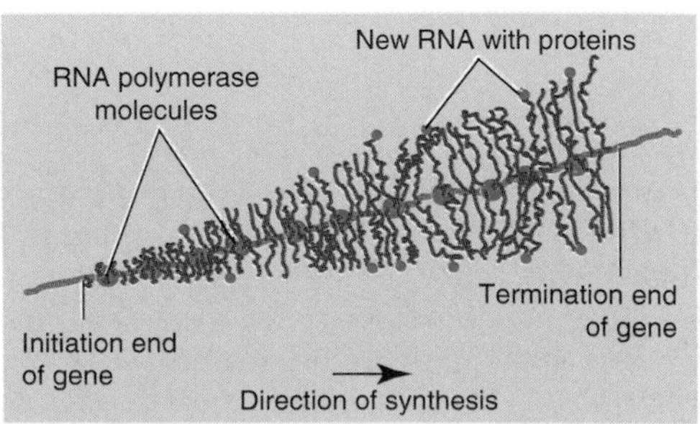

FIGURE 16.14
Simultaneous transcription of a gene by many RNA polymerases, depicting the increasing length of nascent RNA molecules.
Courtesy of Dr. O. L. Miller, University of Virginia. Reproduced with permission from Miller, O. L., and Beatty, B. R. J. Cell Physiol. *74:225, 1969.*

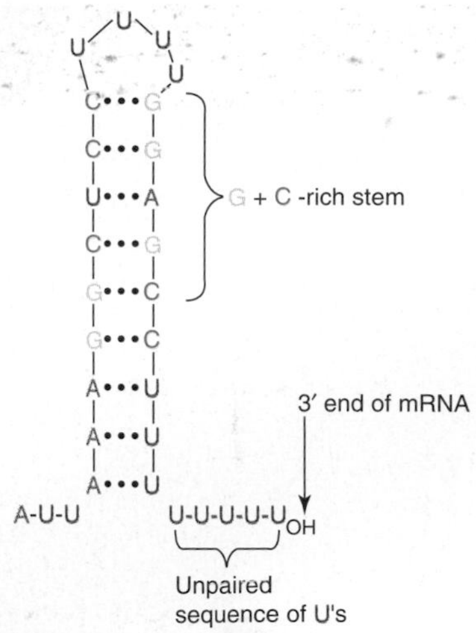

bind sometimes results in an increased frequency of termination and, consequently, a reduced level of gene expression.

Termination

The RNA polymerase complex also recognizes the ends of genes (Figure 16.15). Transcription termination can occur in either of two modes, depending on whether or not it is dependent on the protein factor rho. Terminators are thus classified as rho independent or rho dependent.

Rho-independent terminators are better characterized (Figure 16.15). A consensus-type sequence is involved here: a G-C rich palindrome (inverted repeat) precedes a sequence of 6–7 U residues in the RNA chain. As a result the RNA chain forms a stem and loop structure preceding the U residues. The secondary structure of the stem and loop is crucial for termination; base change mutations in the stem and loop that disrupt pairing also reduce termination. Furthermore, the most efficient terminators are the most G-C rich and therefore most stable. The terminator stem and loop stabilize prokaryotic mRNA against nucleolytic degradation.

Rho-dependent terminators are less well defined. Rho factor is a hexameric protein possessing an essential RNA-dependent ATPase activity. The sequences of rho-dependent termination sites feature regularly spaced C residues within a relatively unstructured length of the transcript. The nascent RNA is thought to wrap around rho factor while ATP hydrolysis leads to dissociation of the transcript from the template.

Prokaryotic ribosomes usually attach to the nascent mRNA while it is being transcribed. This coupling between transcription and translation is important in gene control by *attenuation,* which is discussed in Chapter 19.

G + C -rich stem
3′ end of mRNA
A-U-U
U-U-U-U-U$_{OH}$
Unpaired sequence of U's

FIGURE 16.15
The stem–loop structure of the RNA transcript that determines rho-independent transcriptional termination.
Note the two components of the structure: the G + C-rich stem and loop, followed by a sequence of U residues.

Transcription in Eukaryotes Involves Many Additional Molecular Events

Eukaryotic transcription is considerably more complex than the process in prokaryotes. While the information specifying a promoter is still carried in a DNA sequence, several molecular events besides RNA polymerase binding are required for transcription initiation. First, chromatin containing the promoter sequence must be spatially accessible to the transcription machinery. Second, protein **transcription factors** distinct from RNA polymerase must bind to sequences in the promoter region for a gene to be active. Third, other sequences located some distance away from the promoter affect transcription; these sequences are termed **enhancers** and they, too, bind protein factors to stimulate transcription. Finally, recall that the eukaryotic RNA polymerase consists of three distinct enzyme forms, each specific form capable of transcribing only a

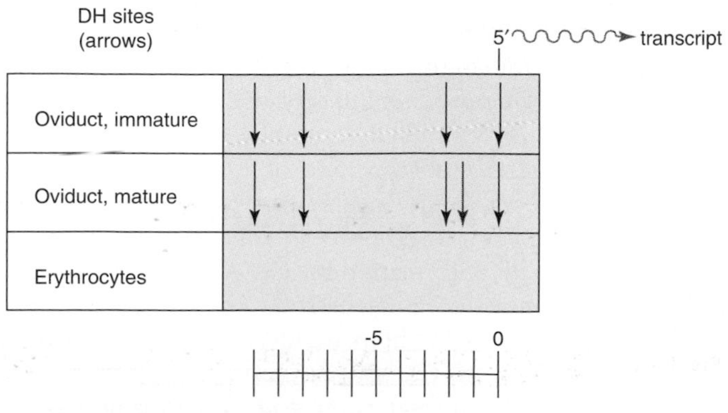

FIGURE 16.16
DNase-hypersensitive (DH) sites upstream of the promoter for the chick lysozyme gene, a typical eukaryotic transcriptional unit.
Hypersensitive sites, that is, sequences around the lysozyme gene where nucleosomes are not bound to the DNA, are indicated by arrows. Note that some hypersensitive sites are found in the lysozyme promoter whether the oviduct is synthesizing or not synthesizing lysozyme; the synthesis of lysozyme is accompanied by the opening up of a new hypersensitive site in mature oviduct. In contrast, no hypersensitive sites are present in nucleated erythrocytes that never synthesize lysozyme.
Adapted from Elgin, S. C. R. J. Biol. Chem. *263:1925, 1988.*

single class of cellular RNA. By contrast, transcription in prokaryotes requires, in the simplest case, only an appropriate sequence of DNA, RNA polymerase holoenzyme, and nucleoside triphosphate substrates.

The Nature of Active Chromatin

The structural organization of eukaryotic chromosomes was discussed in Chapter 14. Although chromatin is organized into **nucleosomes** whether or not it is capable of being transcribed, an active gene has a generally "looser" configuration than does transcriptionally inactive chromatin. This difference is most striking in the promoter sequences, parts of which are not organized into nucleosomes at all (Figure 16.16). The lack of nucleosomes is manifested experimentally by the enhanced sensitivity of promoter sequences to external reagents that cleave DNA, such as the enzyme DNase I. This enhanced accessibility of promoter sequences (termed **DNase I hypersensitivity**) ensures that transcriptional factors will be able to bind to appropriate regulatory sequences. In addition, although the transcribed parts of a gene may be organized into nucleosomes, the nucleosomes are less tightly bound than those in an inactive gene. Finally, DNA may be transcriptionally inactivated by methylation (see Clin. Corr. 16.3). The overall theme is one of partially unfolded chromatin being necessary but not sufficient for transcription.

Enhancers

Enhancer sequences increase (enhance) the expression of a gene about 100-fold, hence the name. They function only when located on the same DNA molecule (chromosome) as the promoter whose activity they affect. They can function when located in either the 5′ or 3′ direction and as much as 1000 bp away from the relevant promoter. Protein factors bind to enhancer DNA and are necessary for enhancer function.

Transcription of Ribosomal RNA Genes

Recall that rRNA genes are located in a specialized nuclear structure, the nucleolus. There are several hundred copies of each rRNA gene in a eukaryotic cell, tandemly repeated in the DNA of a specific region of one chromosome, the **nucleolar organizer.** The repeat units contain a copy of each RNA sequence (28S, 5.8S, and 18S) and are separated from each other by **nontranscribed spacer regions.** Figure 16.17 is a diagram of this arrangement. Each repeat unit is transcribed as a unit, yielding a primary transcript containing one copy each of the 28S, 5.8S, and 18S sequences, ensuring synthesis of equimolar amounts of these three RNAs. The primary transcript is then processed by ribonucleases and modifying enzymes to the three mature rRNA species (see Section 16.5). Termination of transcription occurs within the nontranscribed spacer region before RNA polymerase I reaches the promoter of the next repeat unit.

The promoter recognized by RNA polymerase I is located within the nontranscribed spacer, from about positions −40 to +10 and from −150 to −110. A transcription factor binds to the promoter and thereby directs RNA polymerase

CLINICAL CORRELATION 16.3

Fragile X Syndrome: A Chromatin Disease?

Fragile X syndrome is the single most common form of inherited mental retardation, affecting 1/1250 males and 1/2000 females. A variety of anatomical and neurological symptoms result from the inactivation of the FMR1 gene, located on the X chromosome. The genetics of the syndrome are complex due to the molecular mechanism of the Fragile X mutation.

The Fragile X condition results from the expansion of a trinucleotide repeat sequence, CGG, found at the 5′-untranslated region of the FRM1 gene. Normally, this repeat is present in 30 copies, although normal individuals can have up to 200 copies of the repeat. In individuals with Fragile X syndrome, the FMR1 gene contains many more copies, from 200 to thousands, of the CGG repeat. The complex genetics of the disease result from the potential of the CGG repeat sequence to expand from generation to generation.

The presence of an abnormally high number of CGG repeats induces extensive DNA methylation of the entire promoter region of FMR1. Methylated DNA is transcriptionally inactive, so FMR1 mRNA is not synthesized. The absence of FMR1 protein leads to the pathology of the disease.

FMR1 protein normally is located in the cytoplasm in all tissues of the early fetus and, later, especially in the fetal brain. Its sequence has some characteristics of an RNA-binding protein. One hypothesis is that the protein aids in the translation of brain-specific mRNAs during development.

Warren, S. L., and Nelson, D. L. Advances in molecular analysis of Fragile X syndrome. JAMA 271:536, 1994; and Caskey, C. T. Triple repeat mutations in human disease. *Science* 256:784, 1992.

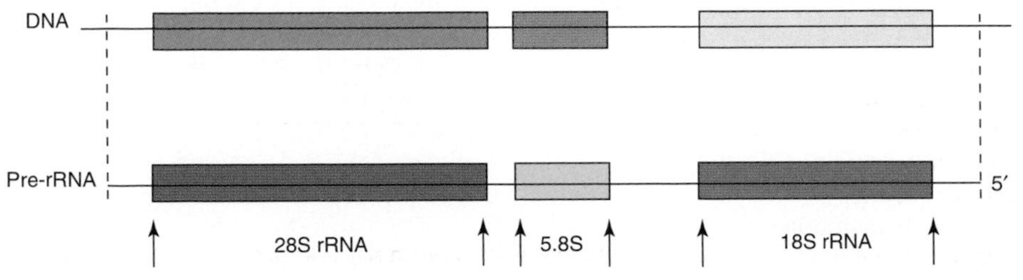

FIGURE 16.17
Structure of a rRNA transcription unit. Ribosomal RNA genes are arranged with many copies one after another. Each copy is transcribed separately and each transcript is processed into three separate RNA species. Promoter and enhancer sequences are located in the nontranscribed regions of the tandemly repeated sequences.

recognition of the promoter sequence. In addition, an enhancer element is located about 250 bp upstream from the promoter in human ribosomal DNA. The size of the nontranscribed spacer varies considerably from one organism to the next, as does the position of the enhancer element.

Transcription of rRNA can be very rapid; this reflects the fact that synthesis of ribosomes is rate-limiting for cell growth. Phosphorylation of RNA polymerase I may activate especially rapid transcription of rRNA, for example, during embryonic growth or liver regeneration.

Transcription by RNA Polymerase II

RNA polymerase II is responsible for the synthesis of mRNA in the nucleus. Three common themes have emerged from research on a large number of genes (Figure 16.18). (1) The DNA sequences controlling transcription are complex; a single gene may be controlled by as many as six or eight DNA sequence elements in addition to the promoter (RNA polymerase binding region) itself. The controlling sequence elements function in combination to give a finely tuned pattern of control. (2) The effect of the controlling sequences on transcription is mediated by the binding of protein molecules to each sequence element. These transcription factors recognize the nucleotide sequence of the appropriate controlling sequence element. (3) Bound transcription factors bind with each other and with RNA polymerase to activate transcription. The DNA binding and activation activities of the factors reside in separate domains of the proteins.

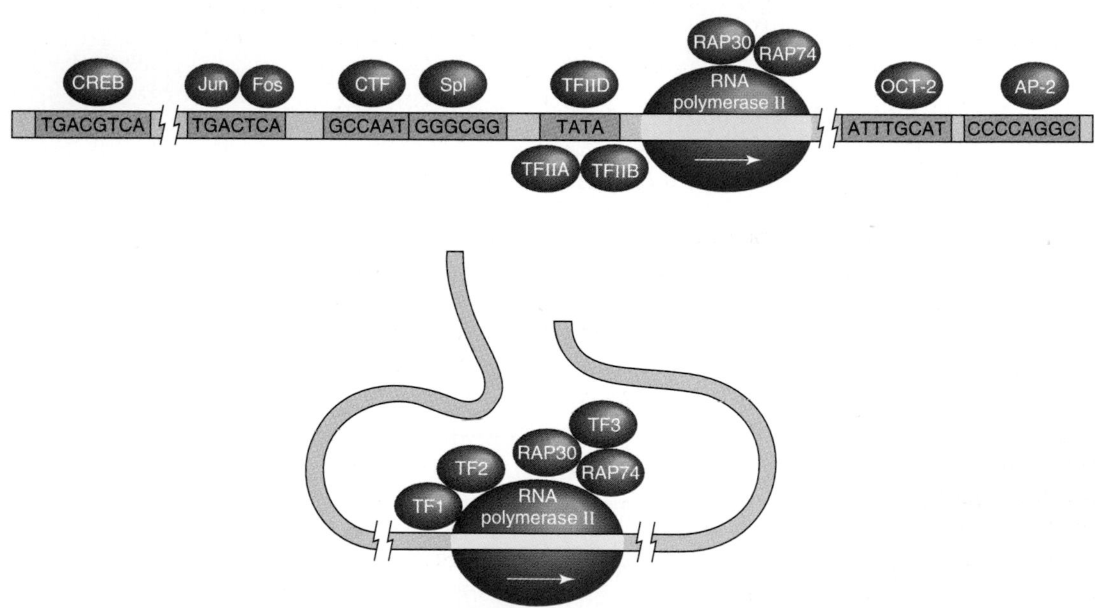

FIGURE 16.18
Interaction of transcription factors with promoters.
A large number of transcriptional factors interact with eukaryotic promoter regions. (*a*) A hypothetical array of factors that interact with specific DNA sequences near the promoter. This includes a factor, TFIID, which binds to the TATA box and the Jun and Fos proteins, which are proto-oncogenes (Clin. Corr. 16.4). The figure is not meant to imply that all of the DNA binding factors bind to the promoter simultaneously. (*b*) One way in which the DNA binding factors are hypothesized to bind to each other and to RNA polymerase. Although this model is not completely proved, it is known that proteins that bind to distant DNA sequences make protein–protein contacts with each other.
Reprinted with permission from Mitchell, P. J., and Tjian, R. Science *245:371, 1989.*

Promoters for mRNA Synthesis

In contrast to prokaryotic RNA polymerase which recognizes only a single promoter sequence, RNA polymerase II can initiate transcription by recognizing several classes of consensus sequences upstream from the mRNA start site. The first and most prominent of these, sometimes called the **TATA box,** has the sequence

A A
TATA A
T T

The TATA box is centered about 25 bp upstream from the transcription unit. Experiments in which it was deleted suggest that it is required for efficient transcription, although some promoters may lack it entirely.

A second region of homology is located further upstream, in which the **CAAT box** sequence

T
GG CAATCT
C

is found. This sequence is not as highly conserved as the TATA box, and some active promoters may not possess it. Other sequences, described in Figure 16.18, may also promote transcription. The CAAT and TATA boxes, as well as the other sequences shown in Figure 16.15, do not contact RNA polymerase II directly. Rather, they require the binding of specific transcription factors to function. The current model for the **activation of genes** in this manner is shown in Figure 16.18. Note how protein factors bind not only to their recognition sequences but also to each other and to RNA polymerase, itself a very large and complex enzyme. Despite the complexities of the detailed interactions, the three principles elaborated above account for the known mechanisms of all class II transcription factors. Mutated forms of several of these transcription factors function as nuclear oncogenes (see Clin. Corr. 16.4).

Transcription by RNA Polymerase III

The themes elaborated above for the transcription of class I and class II promoters hold for the transcription of 5S RNA and tRNA by RNA polymerase III. Transcription factors bind to DNA and direct the action of RNA polymerase. One unusual feature of RNA polymerase III action in the transcription of 5S RNA is the location of the factor-binding sequence; it can be located within the DNA sequence encoding the RNA. The DNA in the region that would normally be thought of as a promoter, that is, the sequence immediately 5′ to the transcribed region of the gene, has no specific sequence and can be substituted by other sequences without a substantial effect on transcription. Figure 16.19 diagrams this unusual sequence arrangement. In other cases, for example, tRNA transcription, the factor-binding sequence is located more conventionally at the 5′ region of the gene, that is, preceding the transcribed sequences.

16.5 ■ POSTTRANSCRIPTIONAL PROCESSING

The immediate product of transcription is a **precursor RNA molecule,** called the **primary transcript,** which is modified to a mature, functional molecule. The reactions of RNA processing can include removal of extra nucleotides, base modification, addition of nucleotides, and separation of different RNA sequences by the action of specific nucleases. Finally, in eukaryotes, RNAs must be exported from the nucleus.

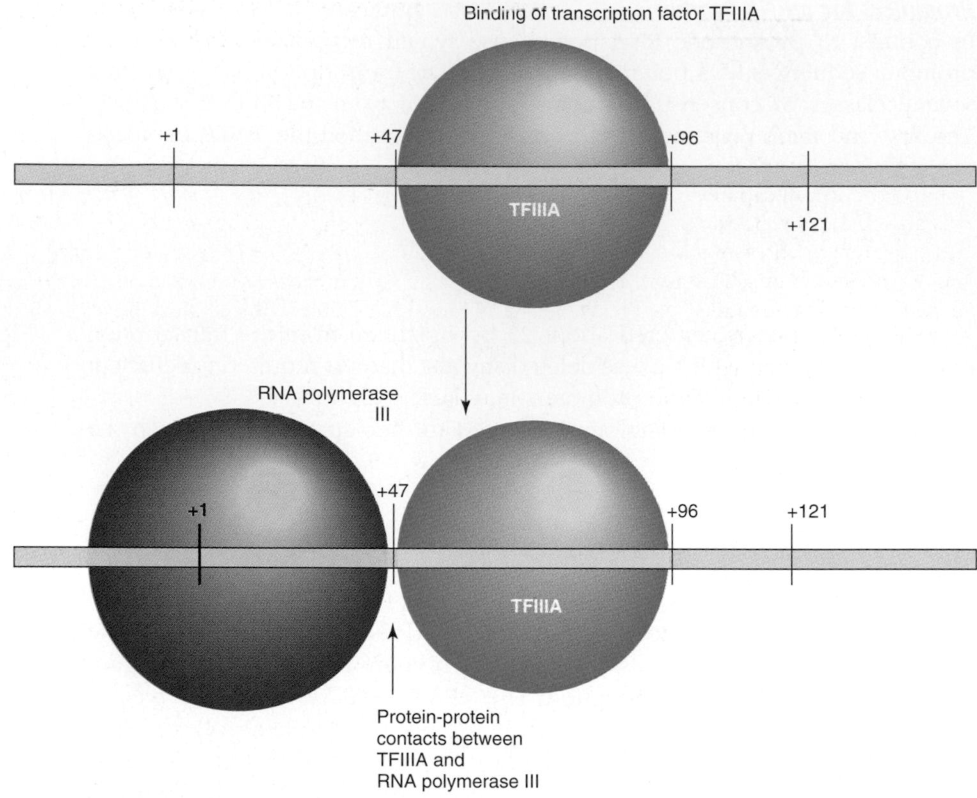

FIGURE 16.19
Transcription factor for a class III eukaryotic gene.
The transcription factor TFIIIA binds to a sequence located within the *Xenopus* gene for 5S rRNA. The RNA polymerase III then binds to the factor and initiates transcription of the 5S sequence. No specific sequence in the DNA is required other than the factor binding sequence.

Transfer RNA Precursors Are Modified by Cleavage, Additions, and Base Modification

Cleavage

The primary transcript of a tRNA gene contains extra nucleotide sequences both 5′ and 3′ to the tRNA sequence. In some cases these primary transcripts contain introns in the anticodon region of the tRNA also. Processing reactions occur in a closely defined but not necessarily rigid temporal order. First, the primary transcript is trimmed in a relatively nonspecific manner to yield a precursor molecule with shorter 5′ and 3′ extensions. Then ribonuclease P, a ribozyme (see above), removes the 5′ extension by endonucleolytic cleavage. The 3′ end is trimmed exonucleolytically, followed by synthesis of the CCA terminus. Synthesis of the modified nucleotides occurs in any order relative to the nucleolytic trimming. **Intron removal** is dictated by the secondary structure of the precursor (see Figure 16.20, p. 702) and is carried out by a soluble, two-component enzyme system; one enzyme removes the intron and the other reseals the nucleotide chain.

Additions

Each functional tRNA has the sequence CCA at its 3′ terminus. In most instances this sequence is added sequentially by the enzyme **tRNA nucleotidyltransfer-**

CLINICAL CORRELATION 16.4

Involvement of Transcriptional Factors in Carcinogenesis

The conversion of a normally well-regulated cell into a cancerous one requires a number of independent steps whose end result is a transformed cell capable of uncontrolled growth and metastasis. Insights into this process have come from recombinant DNA studies of the genes whose mutated or overexpressed products contribute to carcinogenesis. These genes are termed oncogenes. Oncogenes were first identified as products of DNA or RNA tumor viruses but normal cells have copies of these genes as well. The normal, nonmutated cellular analogs of oncogenes are termed proto-oncogenes. The products of proto-oncogenes are components of the many pathways that regulate growth and differentiation of a normal cell; mutation into an oncogenic form involves a change that makes the regulatory product less responsive to normal control.

Some proto-oncogenic products are involved in the transduction of hormonal signals or the recognition of cellular growth factors and act cytoplasmically. Other proto-oncogenes have a nuclear site of action; their gene products are often associated with the transcriptional apparatus and they are synthesized in response to growth stimuli. It is easy to visualize how the overproduction or permanent activation of such a positive transcription factor could aid the transformation of a cell to malignancy: genes normally transcribed at a low or controlled level would be overexpressed by such a deranged control mechanism.

A more subtle genetic effect predisposing to cancer is exemplified by the human tumor suppressor protein p53. This protein is the product of a dominant oncogene. A single copy of the mutant gene causes Li–Fraumeni syndrome, an inherited condition predisposing to carcinomas of the breast and adrenal cortex, sarcomas, leukemia, and brain tumors.

Somatic mutations in p53 can be identified in about half of all human cancers. Mutations represent a loss of function, affecting either the stability or DNA-binding ability of p53. Thus wild-type p53 functions as a tumor suppressor. The wild-type protein helps to control the checkpoint between the G1 and S phases of the cell cycle, activates DNA repair, and, in other circumstances, leads to programmed cell death (apoptosis). Thus the biochemical actions of p53 serve to keep cell growth regulated, maintain the information content of the genome, and, finally, eliminate damaged cells. All of these functions would counteract neoplastic transformation of a cell.

These varied roles are a function of p53's action as a transcription factor, inhibiting some genes and activating others. For example, p53 inhibits transcription of genes with TATA sequences, perhaps by binding to the complex formed between transcription factors and the TATA sequence. Alternatively, p53 is a site-specific DNA-binding protein and promotes transcription of some other genes, for example, those for DNA repair.

The three-dimensional structure of p53 has been determined. Mutations found in p53 from tumors affect the DNA-binding domain of the protein. For example, nearly 20% of all mutated residues involve mutations at two positions in p53. The crystal structure of the protein–DNA complex shows that these two amino acids, both arginines, form hydrogen bonds with DNA. Arginine 248 forms hydrogen bonds in the minor groove of the DNA helix with a thymine oxygen and with a ring nitrogen of adenine. Mutation disrupts this H-bonded network and therefore the ability of p53 to regulate transcription.

Weinberg, R. A. Oncogenes, antioncogenes, and the molecular basis of multistep carcinogenesis. *Cancer Res.* 49:3713, 1989; Cho, Y., Gorina, S., Jeffrey, P. D., and Pavletich, N. P. Crystal structure of a p53 tumor suppressor–DNA complex: understanding tumorigenic mutations. *Science* 265:346, 1994; Friend, S. p53: A glimpse at the puppet behind the shadow play. *Science* 265:334, 1994; and Harris, C. C., and Hollstein, M. Clinical implications of the p53 tumor-suppressor gene. *N. Engl. J. Med.* 329:1318, 1993.

ase. Nucleotidyltransferase uses ATP and CTP as substrates and always incorporates them into tRNA at a ratio of 2C/1A. The CCA ends are found on both cytoplasmic and mitochondrial tRNAs.

Modified Nucleosides

Transfer RNA nucleotides are the most highly modified of all nucleic acids. More than 60 different modifications to the bases and ribose, requiring well over 100 different enzymatic reactions, have been found in tRNA. Many are simple, one-step methylations, but others involve multistep synthesis. Two derivatives, **pseudouridine** and **queuosine** (7–4, 5-*cis*-dihydroxy-1-cyclopenten-3-ylamino methyl-7-deazaguanosine), actually require severing of the β-glycosidic bond of the altered nucleotide. One enzyme or set of enzymes produces a single site-specific modification in more than one species of tRNA molecule. Separate enzymes or sets of enzymes produce the same modifications at more than one location in tRNA. In other words, most modification enzymes are site or nucleotide sequence specific, not tRNA specific. Most modifications are completed before the tRNA precursors have been cleaved to mature tRNA size.

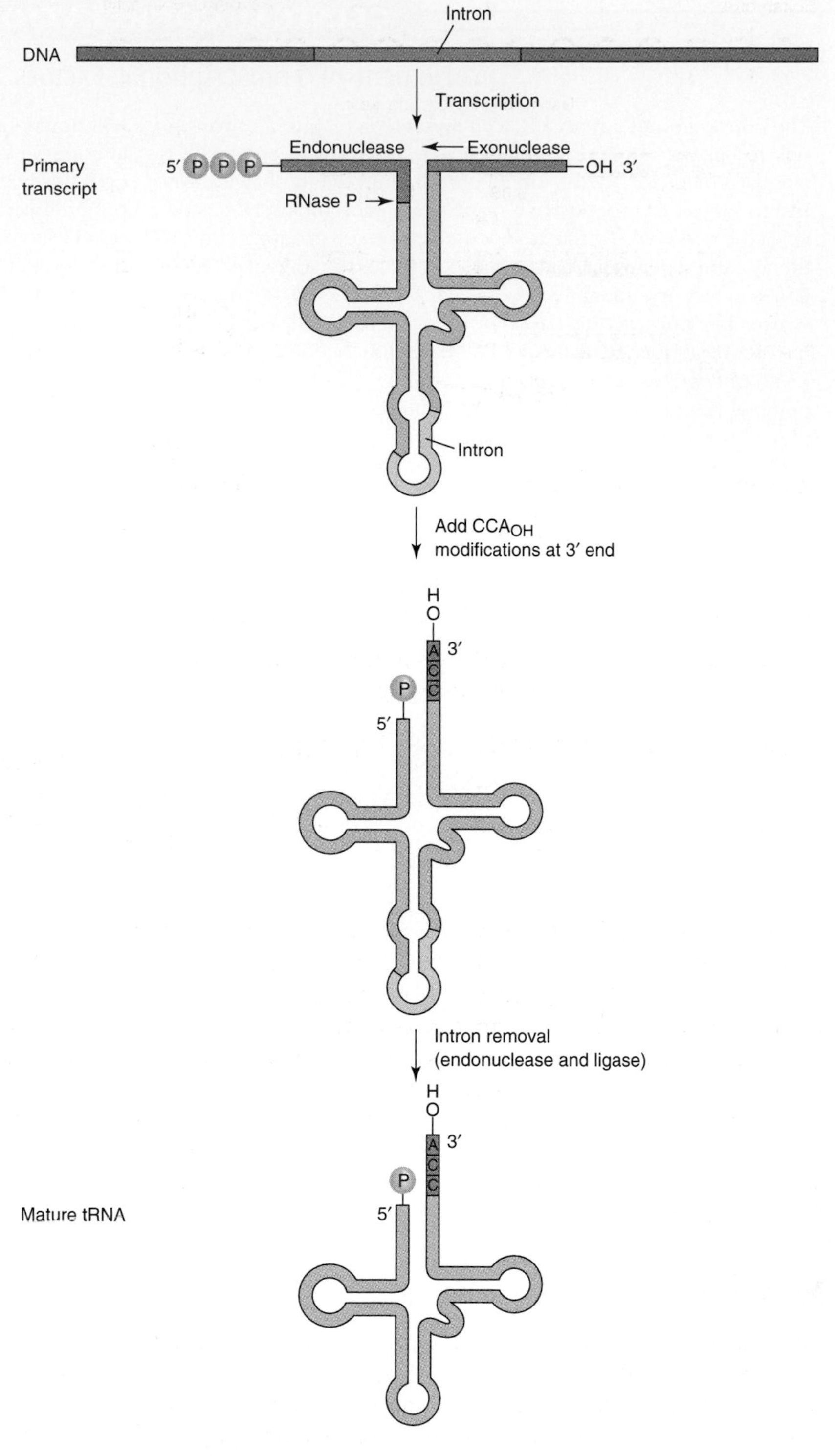

FIGURE 16.20
Scheme for processing a eukaryotic tRNA.
The primary transcript is cleaved by RNase P and a 3′-exonuclease, and the terminal CCA is synthesized by tRNA nucleotidyltransferase before the intron is removed, if necessary.

Ribosomal RNA Processing Releases the Various RNAs from a Longer Precursor

The primary product of rRNA transcription is a long RNA, termed 45S RNA, which contains the sequences of 28S, 5.8S, and 18S rRNAs. Processing of 45S RNA occurs in the nucleolus. Like the processing of mRNA precursors (see below), processing of the rRNA precursors is carried out by large multisubunit ribonucleoprotein assemblies. At least three RNA species are required for processing. These all function as **small nucleolar ribonucleoprotein complexes** (snoRNPs). Processing of the rRNAs follows a sequential order (Figure 16.21).

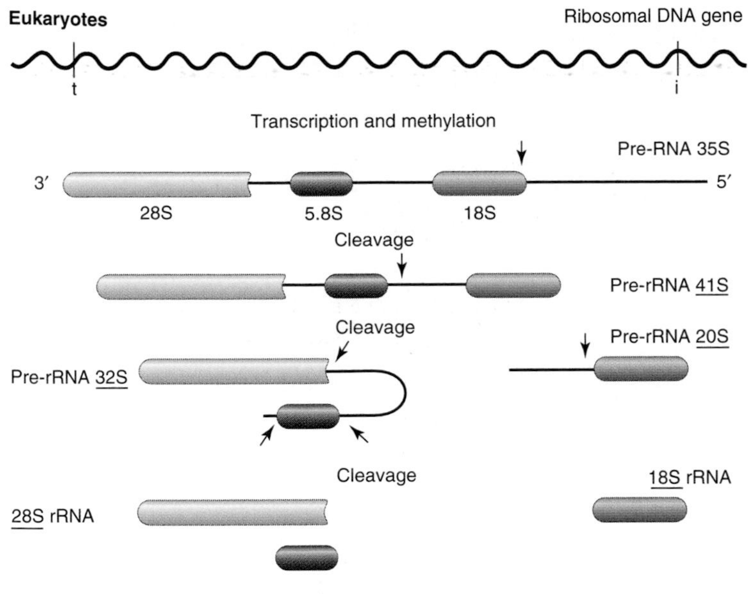

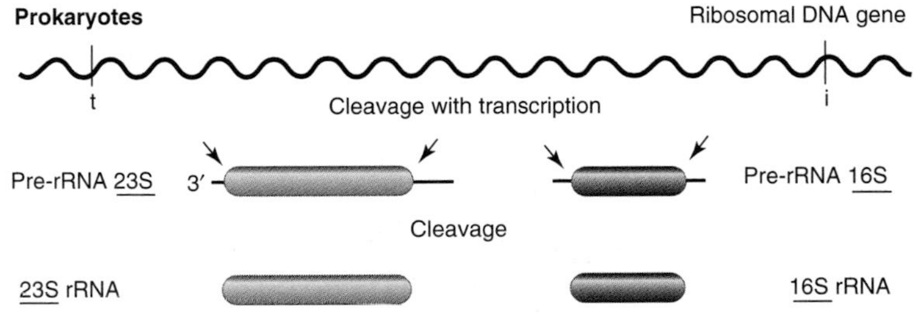

FIGURE 16.21
Schemes for transcription and processing of rRNAs.
Redrawn from Perry, R. Annu. Rev. Biochem. *45:611, 1976. Copyright © 1976 by Annual Reviews, Inc.*

Processing of pre-rRNA in prokaryotes also involves cleavage of high molecular weight precursors to smaller molecules (see Figure 16.21). Some of the bases are modified by methylation on the ring nitrogens of the bases rather than the ribose and by the formation of pseudouridine. The *E. coli* genome has seven rRNA transcriptional units dispersed throughout the DNA. Each contains one 16S, one 23S, and one 5S rRNA or tRNA sequence. Processing of the rRNA is coupled directly to transcription, so that cleavage of a large precursor primary transcript rapidly yields pre-16S, pre-23S, pre-5S, and pre-tRNAs. These precursors are slightly larger than the functional molecules and only require trimming for maturation.

Messenger RNA Processing Requires Maintenance of the Coding Sequence

Most eukaryotic mRNAs have distinctive structural features added in the nucleus by enzyme systems other than RNA polymerase. These include the 3′-terminal poly(A) tail, methylated internal nucleotides, and the cap 5′ terminus. Cytoplasmic mRNAs are shorter than their primary transcripts, which can contain additional terminal and internal sequences. Noncoding sequences present within pre-mRNA molecules, but not present in mature mRNAs, are called **intervening sequences** or **introns.** The **expressed** or **retained sequences** are called **exons.** The general pattern for mRNA processing is depicted in Figure 16.22. Incompletely processed mRNAs make up a large part of the heterogeneous nuclear RNA (hnRNA).

Processing of eukaryotic pre-mRNA involves a number of molecular reactions, all of which must be carried out with exact fidelity. This principle is most clear in the removal of introns from an mRNA transcript. An extra nucleotide in the coding sequence of mature mRNA would cause the reading frame of

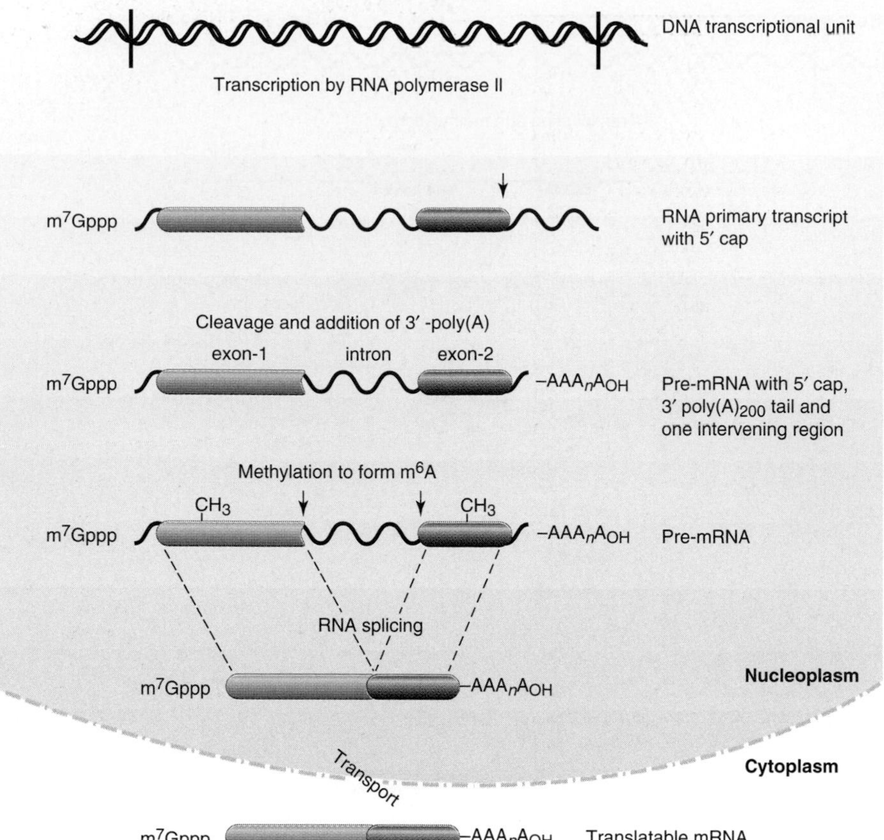

FIGURE 16.22
Scheme for processing mRNA.
The points for initiation and termination of transcription are indicated on the DNA. Arrows indicate cleavage points. The many proteins associated with the RNA and tertiary conformations are not shown.

that message to be shifted and the resulting protein will almost certainly be nonfunctional. Indeed, mutations in the β-globin gene that interfere with intron removal are a major cause of the genetic disease ***β*-thalassemia** (see Clin. Corr. 16.5). The task for the cell becomes even more daunting when seen in the light of the structure of some important human genes that consist of over 90% intron sequences. The complex reactions to remove introns are accomplished by multicomponent enzyme systems that act in the nucleus; after these reactions are completed the mRNA is exported to the cytoplasm where it interacts with ribosomes to initiate translation.

Blocking of the 5′ Terminus and Poly(A) Synthesis

Addition of the **cap structures** occurs during transcription by RNA polymerase II (Figure 16.22). As the transcription complex moves along the DNA, the capping enzyme complex modifies the 5' end of the nascent mRNA. This is the only eukaryotic pre-mRNA processing event that is known to occur cotranscriptionally, that is, while RNA polymerase is still transcribing the downstream portions of the gene.

After initiation and cap synthesis, RNA polymerase continues transcribing the gene until a **polyadenylation signal sequence** is reached (Figure 16.23). This sequence, which has the consensus AAUAAA, appears in the mature mRNA but usually does not form part of its coding region. Rather, it signals cleavage of the nascent mRNA precursor about 20 or so nucleotides downstream. The poly(A) sequence is then added by a soluble polymerase to the free 3′ end produced by this cleavage. Note that polyadenylation does not require a template. Somewhat paradoxically, RNA polymerase II continues transcription for as many as 1000 nucleotides beyond the point at which the transcript is released from chromatin. Nucleotides incorporated into RNA by this process are apparently turned over and never appear in any cytoplasmic RNA species.

CLINICAL CORRELATION 16.5

Thalassemia Due to Defects in Messenger RNA Synthesis

The thalassemias are genetic defects in the coordinated synthesis of α- and β-globin peptide chains; a deficiency of β chains is termed β-thalassemia while a deficiency of α chains is termed α-thalassemia. Patients suffering from either of these conditions present with anemia at about 6 months of age as HbF synthesis ceases and HbA synthesis would become predominant. The severity of symptoms leads to the classification of the disease into either thalassemia major, where a severe deficiency of globin synthesis occurs, or thalassemia minor, representing a less severe imbalance. Occasionally, an intermediate form is seen. Therapy for thalassemia major involves frequent transfusions, leading to a risk of complications from iron overload. Unless chelation therapy is successful, the deposition of iron in peripheral tissues, termed hemosiderosis, can lead to death before adulthood. Carriers of the disease usually have thalassemia minor, involving mild anemia. Ethnographically, the disease is common in persons of Mediterranean, Arabian, and East Asian descent. As is the case for sickle cell anemia (HbS) and glucose 6-phosphate dehydrogenase deficiency, the abnormality of the carriers' erythrocytes affords some protection from malaria. Maps of the regions where one or another of these diseases is frequent in the native population superimpose over the areas of the world where malaria is endemic.

α-Thalassemia is usually due to a genetic deletion, which can occur because the α-globin genes are duplicated; unequal crossing over between adjacent α alleles apparently has led to the loss of one or more loci. In contrast, β-thalassemia can result from a wide variety of mutations. Known events include mutations leading to frameshifts in the β-globin coding sequence, as well as mutations leading to premature termination of peptide synthesis. Many β-thalassemias result from mutations affecting the biosynthesis of β-globin mRNA. Genetic defects are known that affect the promoter of the gene, leading to inefficient transcription. Other mutations result in aberrant processing of the nascent transcript, either during splicing out of the two introns from the transcript or during polyadenylation of the mRNA precursor. Examples where the molecular defect illustrates a general principle of mRNA synthesis are discussed in the text.

Orkin, S. H. Disorders of hemoglobin synthesis: the thalassemias. In: G. Stamatoyannopoulis, A. W. Nienhuis, P. Leder, and P. W. Majerus (Eds.). *The Molecular Basis of Blood Diseases*. Philadelphia: Saunders, 1987; and Weatherall, D. J., Clegg, J. B., Higgs, D. R., and Wood, W. G. The hemoglobinopathies. In: C. R. Scriver, A. L. Beaudet, W. S. Sly, and D. Valle (Eds.). *The Metabolic and Molecular Bases of Inherited Disease*, 7th ed. New York: McGraw-Hill, 1995.

Removal of Introns from mRNA Precursors

As pre-RNA is extruded from the RNA polymerase complex, it is rapidly bound by **small nuclear ribonucleoproteins, snRNPs** (snurps), which carry out the dual steps of **RNA splicing:** (1) breakage of the intron at the 5′ donor site and (2) joining the upstream and downstream exon sequences together. All introns begin with a GU sequence and end with AG; these are termed the donor and acceptor intron–exon junctions, respectively. Not all GU or AG sequences are spliced out of RNA, however. How does the cell know which GU sequences are in introns (and therefore must be removed) and which are destined to remain in mature mRNA? This discrimination is accomplished by the formation of base pairs between **U1 RNA** and the sequence of the mRNA precursor surrounding the donor GU sequence (see Clin. Corr. 16.6). See Figure 16.24 for an illustration of this process. Another snRNP, containing **U2 RNA,** recognizes

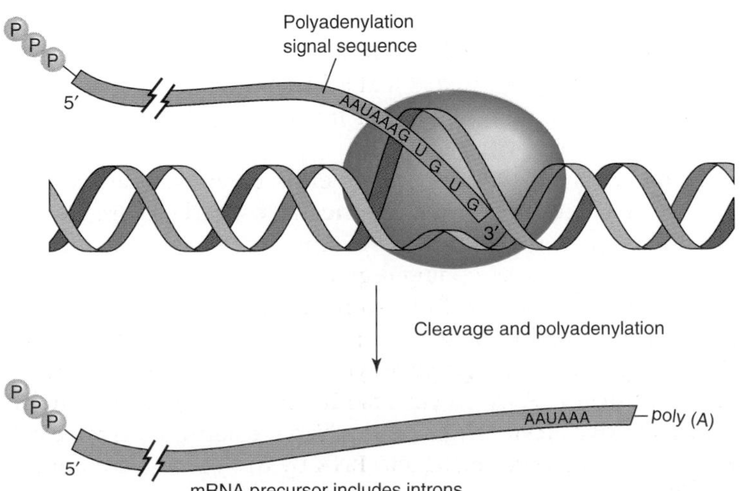

FIGURE 16.23
Cleavage and polyadenylation of eukaryotic mRNA precursors.
The 3′ termini of eukaryotic mRNA species are derived by processing. The sequence AAUAAA in the mRNA specifies the cleavage of the mRNA precursor. The free 3′-OH end of the mRNA is a primer for poly(A) synthesis.
Adapted from Proudfoot, N. J. Trends Biochem. Sci. *14:105, 1989.*

important sequences at the 3′ acceptor end of the intron. Still other snRNP species, among them U5 and U6, then bind to the RNA precursor, forming a large complex termed a **spliceosome** (by analogy with the large ribonucleoprotein assembly involved in protein synthesis, the ribosome). The spliceosome uses ATP energy to carry out the accurate removal of the intron. First, the phosphodiester bond between the exon and the donor GU sequence is broken, leaving a free 3′-OH group at the end of the first exon and a 5′ phosphate on the donor G of the intron. This pG is then used to form an unusual linkage with the 2′-OH group of an adenosine within the intron to form a branched or **lariat RNA** structure, as shown in Figure 16.25. After the lariat is formed, the second step of splicing occurs. The phosphodiester bond immediately following the AG is cleaved and the two exon sequences are ligated together. In pre-mRNAs containing a large number of introns, splicing occurs roughly in order from the 5′ to the 3′ end of the mRNA precursor. However, this is not a hard and fast rule as there is no singly preferred order for removal. The end result of processing is a fully functional coding mRNA, all introns removed, and ready to direct protein synthesis.

CLINICAL CORRELATION 16.6

Autoimmunity in Connective Tissue Disease

Humoral antibodies in sera of patients with various connective tissue diseases recognize a variety of ribonucleoprotein complexes. Patients with systemic lupus erythematosus exhibit a serum antibody activity designated Sm, and those with mixed connective tissue disease exhibit an antibody designated RNP. Each antibody recognizes a distinct site on the same RNA–protein complex, U1 RNP, that is involved in mRNA processing in mammalian cells. The U1–RNP complex contains U1 RNA, a 165-nucleotide sequence highly conserved among eukaryotes, that at its 5′ terminus includes a sequence complementary to intron–exon splice junctions. Addition of this antibody to *in vitro* splicing assays inhibits splicing, presumably by removal of the U1 RNP from the reaction. Sera from patients with other connective tissue diseases recognize different nuclear antigens, nucleolar proteins, and/or chromosomal centromeres. Sera of patients with myositis have been shown to recognize cytoplasmic antigens such as aminoacyl-tRNA synthetases. Although humoral antibodies have been reported to enter cells via Fc receptors, there is no evidence that this is part of the mechanism of autoimmune disease.

Mutations in Splicing Signals Cause Human Diseases

Messenger RNA splicing is an intricate process dependent on many molecular events. If these events are not carried out with precision, functional mRNA is not produced. This principle is illustrated in the human thalassemias, which affect the balanced synthesis of α- and β-globin chains (see Clin. Corr. 16.5). Some of the mutations leading to **β-thalassemia** interfere with the splicing of β-globin mRNA precursors. For example, we know that all intron sequences begin with the dinucleotide GU. Mutation of the G in this sequence to an A means that the splicing machinery will no longer recognize this dinucleotide as a donor site. Splicing will "pass by" the correct exon–intron junction. This could lead to two results: extra sequences that would normally be spliced out will appear in the β-globin mRNA, or, alternatively, sequences could be deleted from the mRNA product (Figure 16.26). In either event, functional β-globin will be made in reduced amounts and the anemia characteristic of the disease will result.

Alternate pre-mRNA Splicing Can Lead to Multiple Proteins Being Made from a Single DNA Coding Sequence

The existence of intron sequences is paradoxical. Introns must be removed precisely so that the mRNA can accurately encode a protein. As we have seen above, a single base mutation can drastically interfere with splicing and cause a serious disease. Furthermore, the presence of intron sequences in a gene means that its overall sequence is much larger than is required to encode its

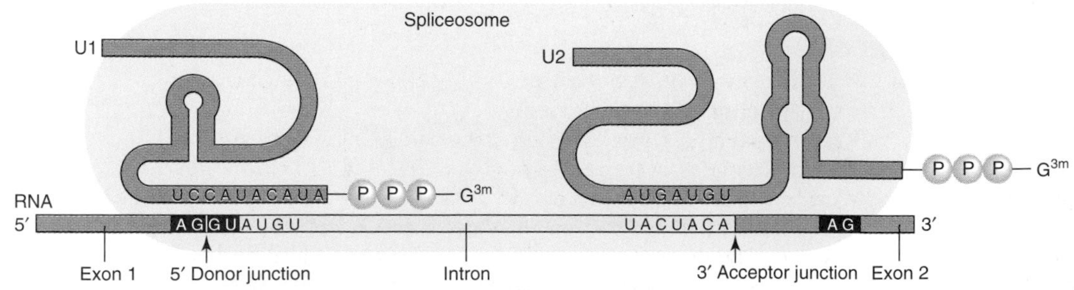

FIGURE 16.24
Mechanism of splice junction recognition.
The recognition of the 5′ splice junction involves base pairing between the intron–exon junction and the U1 RNA snRNP. This base pairing targets the intron for removal.
Adapted from Sharp, P. A. JAMA *260:3035, 1988.*

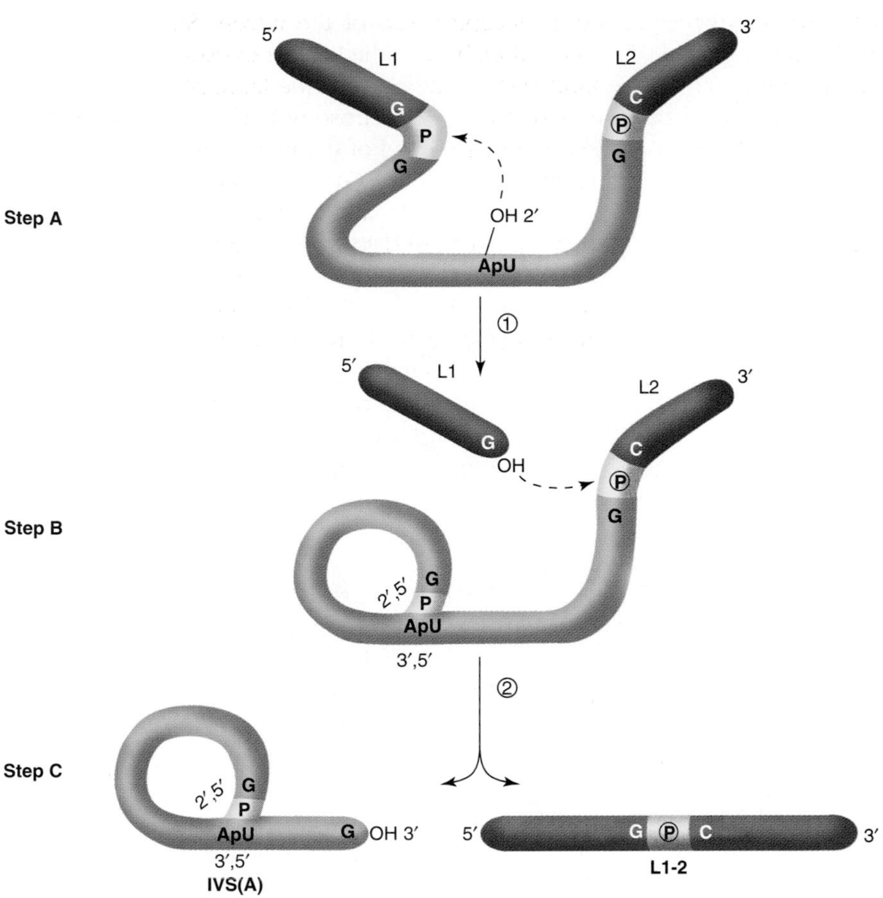

FIGURE 16.25
Proposed scheme for mRNA splicing to include the lariat structure.
A messenger RNA is depicted with two exons (in dark blue) and an intervening intron (in light blue). A 2′-OH group of the intron sequence reacts with the 5′-phosphate of the intron's 5′-terminal nucleotide producing a 2′–5′ linkage and the lariat structure. Simultaneously, the exon 1–intron phosphodiester bond is broken, leaving a 3′-OH terminus on this exon free to react with the 5′-phosphate of the exon 2, displacing the intron and creating the spliced mRNA. The released intron lariat is subsequently digested by cellular nucleases.

protein product. A large gene is a target for more mutagenic events than is a small one. Indeed, common human genetic diseases like Duchenne muscular dystrophy occur in genes that encompass millions of base pairs of DNA information. Why has nature not removed introns completely over the long time scale of eukaryotic evolution? There are no clear answers to questions of this type but some introns do have beneficial effects.

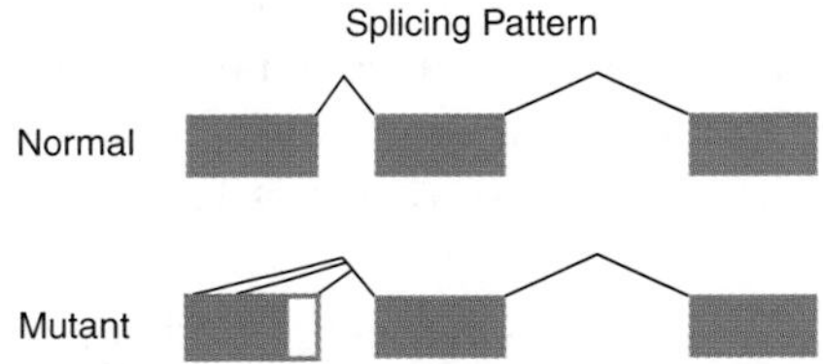

FIGURE 16.26
Nucleotide change at an intron–exon junction of the human β-globin gene, which leads to aberrant splicing and β-thalassemia.
This figure shows the splicing pattern of a mutated transcript containing a change of G-U to A-U at the first two nucleotides of the first intron. Loss of this invariant sequence means that the correct splice junction cannot be used; therefore transcript sequences that base pair with the U1 snRNA less well than the correct sequence junction are used as splice donors. The diagonal lines indicate the portions spliced together in mutant transcripts. Note that some of the mutant mRNA precursor molecules are spliced so that portions of the first intron (denoted as a white box) appear in the processed product. In other instances the donor junction lies within the first exon and portions of the first exon are deleted. In no case is wild-type globin mRNA produced.
Adapted from Orkin, S. H. In: G. Stamatoyannopoulis et al. (Eds.). The Molecular Basis of Blood Diseases. *Philadelphia: Saunders, 1987.*

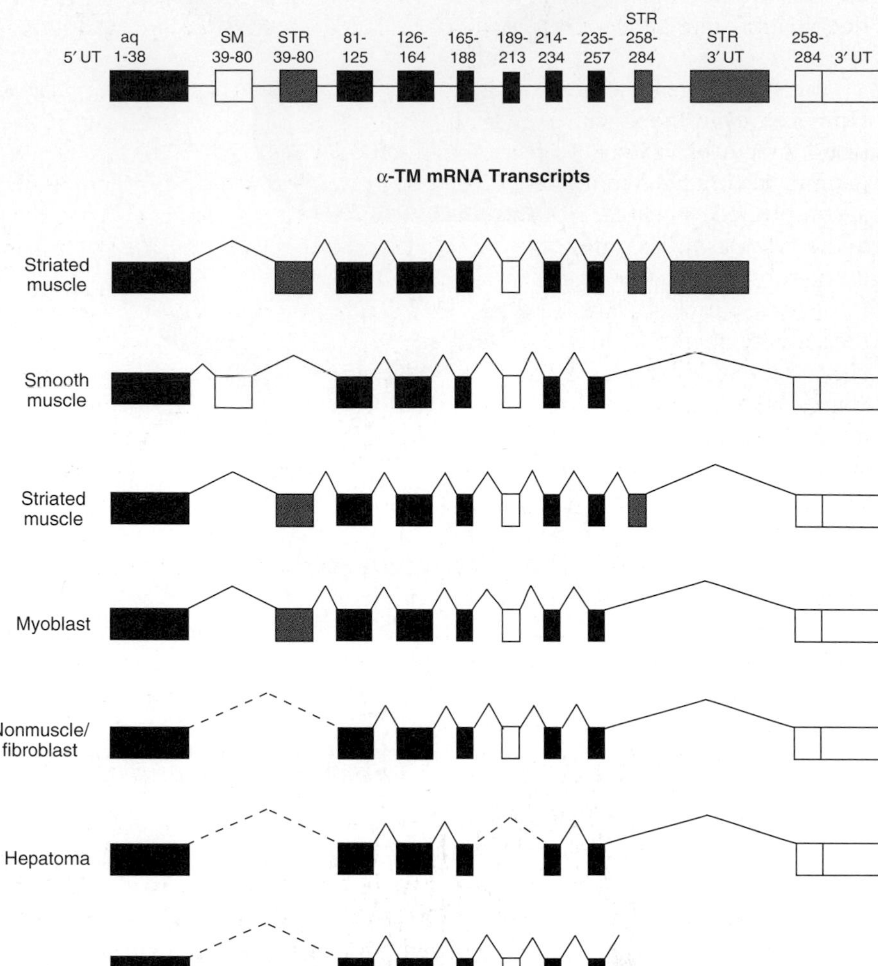

FIGURE 16.27
Alternate splicing of tropomyosin gene transcripts results in a family of tissue-specific tropomyosin proteins.
Redrawn from Breitbart, R. E., Andreadis, A., and Nadal-Ginard, B. Annu. Rev. Biochem. *56:467, 1986.*

Tropomyosin proteins are essential components of the contractile apparatus in the three types of muscle (see, p. 948) and each contractile cell type contains a specific tropomyosin type. This diversity arises from a single gene that is transcribed into a primary transcript. The transcript is then processed as diagramed in Figure 16.27. All cells containing tropomyosin make the same primary transcript but each cell type processes this transcript in a characteristic fashion. The resulting mRNA species then are translated to yield the tropomyosins characteristic of each cell type. About 40 examples are well documented of tissue-specific splicing. Thus the existence of introns supplies the organism with still another method of generating protein diversity.

16.6 NUCLEASES AND RNA TURNOVER

The different roles of RNA and DNA in genetic expression are reflected in their metabolic fates. A cell's information store (DNA) must be preserved, thus the myriad DNA repair and editing systems in the nucleus. Although individual stretches of nucleotides in DNA may turn over, the molecule as a whole is metabolically inert when not replicating. The various RNA molecules, on the other hand, are individually dispensable and can be replaced by newly synthesized species of the same specificity. It is therefore no surprise that RNA repair systems are not known. Instead, defective RNAs are removed from the cell by degradation into nucleotides, which then are repolymerized into new RNA species.

This principle is clearest for mRNA species, which are classified as unstable. However, even the so-called stable RNAs turn over; for example, the half-life of tRNA species in liver is on the order of 5 days. A fairly long half-life for a mammalian mRNA would be 30 h. Removal of RNAs from the cytoplasm is accomplished by cellular **ribonucleases.** Messenger RNAs are initially degraded in the cytoplasm. The rates vary for different mRNA species, raising the possibility of control by differential degradation.

Two examples of the role of RNA stability in gene control illustrate how the stability of mRNA influences gene expression. **Tubulin** is the major component of the microtubules found in many cell types as part of the cytoskeleton. When there is an excess of tubulin in the cell, the monomeric protein binds to and promotes the degradation of tubulin mRNA, thereby reducing tubulin synthesis. A second example is provided by **herpes simplex viruses** (HSV), the agent causing cold sores and some genital infections. An early event in the establishment of HSV infection is the ability of the virus to destabilize all the cellular mRNA molecules, thereby reducing the competition for free ribosomes. Thus the viral proteins are more efficiently translated.

Nucleases are of several types and specificities. The most useful distinction is between **exonucleases,** which degrade RNA from either the 5′ or 3′ end, and **endonucleases,** which cleave phosphodiester bonds within a molecule. The products of RNase action contain either 3′ or 5′ terminal phosphates, and both endo- and exonucleases can be further characterized by the position (5′ or 3′) at which the monophosphate created by the cleavage is located.

The structure of RNA also affects nuclease action. Most ribonucleases are less efficient on regions of highly ordered RNA structure. Thus tRNAs are preferentially cleaved in unpaired regions of the sequence. On the other hand, many RNases involved in RNA processing require a defined three-dimensional structure for enzyme activity. These enzymes are discussed more fully above in the consideration of RNA processing pathways.

BIBLIOGRAPHY

Bradshaw, R. A. (Ed.). Transcription. Special issue of *Trends Biochem. Sci.* 16, November, 1991.

Breitbart, R. E., Andreadis, A., and Nadal-Ginard, B. Alternative splicing: A ubiquitous mechanism for the generation of multiple protein isoforms from single genes. *Annu. Rev. Biochem.* 56:467, 1987.

Caskey, C.T. Triple repeat mutations in human disease. *Science* 256:784, 1992.

Cundliffe, E. How antibiotic-producing microorganisms avoid suicide. *Annu. Rev. Microbiol.* 43:207, 1989.

Das, A. Control of transcription by RNA-binding proteins. *Annu. Rev. Biochem.* 62:893, 1993.

Friend, S. p53: A glimpse at the puppet behind the shadow play. *Science* 265:334, 1994.

Gesteland, R. F., and Atkins, J. F. (Eds.). *The RNA World.* Cold Spring Harbor: Cold Spring Harbor Laboratory Press, 1993.

Gold, L., Polisky, B., Uhlenbeck, O., and Yarus, M. Diversity of oligonucleotide functions. *Annu. Rev. Biochem.* 64:763, 1995.

Koleske, A. J., and Young, R. A. The RNA polymerase II holoenzyme and its implications for gene regulation. *Trends Biochem. Sci.* 20:113, 1995.

Lai, M. M. C. The molecular biology of hepatitis delta virus. *Annu. Rev. Biochem.* 64:259, 1995.

Larson, D. E., Zahradka, P., and Sells, B. H. Control points in eucaryotic ribosome biogenesis. *Biochem. Cell. Biol.* 69:5, 1991.

Orkin, S. H. Disorders of hemoglobin synthesis: The thalassemias. In: G. Stamatoyannopoulis, A. W. Nienhuis, P. Leder, and P. W. Majerus (Eds.), *The Molecular Basis of Blood Diseases.* Philadelphia: Saunders, 1987, pp. 106–126.

Pace, N. R., and Brown, J. W. Evolutionary perspective on the structure and function of ribonuclease P, a ribozyme. *J. Bacteriol.* 177:1919, 1995.

Rosenberg, M., and Court, D. Regulatory sequences involved in the promotion and termination of RNA transcription. *Annu. Rev. Genet.* 12:319, 1979.

Soll, D., and Rajbhandary, U. L. (Eds.). *tRNA: Structure, Biosynthesis and Function.* Washington DC: American Society for Microbiology, 1994.

Weatherall, D. J., Clegg, J. B., Higgs, D. R., and Wood, W. G. The hemoglobinopathies. In: C. R. Scriver, A. L. Beaudet, W. S. Sly, and D. Valle (Eds.), *The Metabolic and Molecular Bases of Inherited Disease,* 7th ed. New York: McGraw-Hill, 1995.

Weinberg, R. A. Oncogenes, antioncogenes and the molecular basis of multistep carcinogenesis. *Cancer Res.* 49:3713, 1989.

Wise, J. A. Guides to the heart of the spliceosome. *Science* 262:1978, 1993.

QUESTIONS ■ C. N. ANGSTADT AND J. BAGGOTT

1. RNA:
   A. incorporates both modified and unmodified purine and pyrimidine bases during transcription.
   B. does not exhibit any double helical structure.
   C. structures exhibit base stacking and hydrogen-bonded base pairing.
   D. usually contains about 65–100 nucleotides.
   E. does not exhibit Watson–Crick base pairing.

Refer to the following for Questions 2–4.
   A. HnRNA
   B. mRNA
   C. rRNA
   D. snRNA
   E. tRNA

2. Has the highest percentage of modified bases of any RNA.

3. Stable RNA representing the largest percentage by weight of cellular RNA.

4. Contains both a 7-methylguanosine triphosphate cap and a polyadenylate segment.

5. Ribozymes:
   A. are any ribonucleoprotein particles.
   B. are enzymes whose catalytic function resides in RNA subunits.
   C. carry out self-processing reactions but cannot be considered true catalysts.
   D. bind to the mRNA precursor to recognize the 5′-splice site for intron removal.
   E. function only in the processing of mRNA.

6. In eukaryotic transcription:
   A. RNA polymerase does not require a template.
   B. all RNA is synthesized in the nucleolus.
   C. consensus sequences are the only known promoter elements.
   D. phosphodiester bond formation is favored, in part, because it is followed by pyrophosphate hydrolysis.
   E. RNA polymerase requires a primer.

7. An enhancer:
   A. is a consensus sequence in DNA located where RNA polymerase first binds.
   B. may be located in various places in different genes.
   C. may be located on a separate chromosome from the gene it regulates.
   D. functions by binding RNA polymerase.
   E. stimulates transcription in both prokaryotes and eukaryotes.

8. The sigma (σ) subunit of prokaryotic RNA polymerase:
   A. is part of the core enzyme.
   B. binds the antibiotic rifampicin.
   C. is inhibited by α-amanitin.
   D. must be present for transcription to occur.
   E. specifically recognizes promoter sites.

Use this schematic representation of a prokaryotic gene to answer Questions 9–11. Numbers refer to positions of base pairs relative to the beginning of transcription.

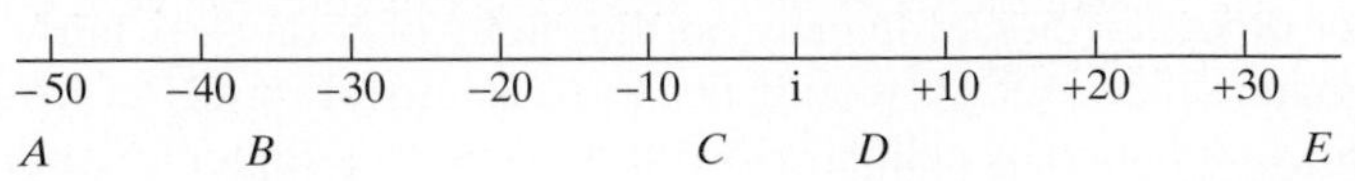

Initiation of transcription

9. Sigma (σ) factor might be released from RNA polymerase.

10. An "open complex" should form in this region.

11. Events beyond this region should be catalyzed by core enzyme.

12. Termination of a prokaryotic transcript:
    A. is a random process.
    B. requires the presence of the rho subunit of the holoenzyme.
    C. does not require rho factor if the end of the gene contains a G-C rich palindrome.
    D. is most efficient if there is an A-T rich segment at the end of the gene.
    E. requires an ATPase in addition to rho factor.

13. Eukaryotic transcription:
    A. is independent of the presence of consensus sequences upstream from the start of transcription.
    B. may involve a promoter located within the region transcribed rather than upstream.
    C. requires a separate promoter region for each of the three ribosomal RNAs transcribed.
    D. requires that the entire gene be in the nucleosome form of chromatin.
    E. is affected by enhancer sequences only if they are adjacent to the promoter.

14. All of the following are correct about a primary transcript in eukaryotes EXCEPT it:
    A. is usually longer than the functional RNA.
    B. may contain nucleotide sequences that are not present in functional RNA.
    C. will contain no modified bases.
    D. usually contains information for more than one RNA molecule.
    E. contains a TATA box.

15. The processing of transfer RNA involves all of the following EXCEPT:
    A. addition of a methylated guanosine at the 5′ end.
    B. cleavage of extra bases from both the 3′ and 5′ ends.
    C. nucleotide sequence-specific methylation of bases.
    D. addition of the sequence CCA by a nucleotidyl transferase.
    E. sometimes, removal of intron from the anticodon region.

16. Cleavage and splicing:
    A. are features of ribosomal RNA processing.
    B. always occur in the same way for a given primary transcript.
    C. remove noninformational sequences occurring anywhere within a primary transcript.
    D. are usually the first events in mRNA processing.
    E. are catalyzed by enzymes that recognize and remove specific introns.

17. In the cellular degradation of RNA:
    A. any of the nucleotides released may be recycled.
    B. regions of extensive base pairing are more susceptible to cleavage.
    C. endonucleases may cleave the molecule starting at either the 5′ or 3′ end.
    D. the products are nucleotides with a phosphate at either the 3′- or 5′-OH group.
    E. all species except rRNA are cleaved.

ANSWERS

1. C Stacking stabilizes the single-stranded helix. A: Only the four bases A, G, U, and C are incorporated during transcription. B and C: Although single stranded, RNA exhibits considerable secondary and tertiary structure. D: Only tRNA would be this small; sizes can range to more than 6000 nucleotides. E: This occurs in the intrachain helical regions (pp. 679–680).
2. E Modified bases seem to be very important in the three-dimensional structure of tRNA (p. 683).
3. C Stability of rRNA is necessary for repeated functioning of ribosomes (p. 683).
4. B These are important additions during processing that yield a functional eukaryotic mRNA (p. 685, Table 16.1).
5. B A: Ribozymes are a very specific type of particle. C: One of the four classes, RNase P, catalyzes a cleavage reaction. D: This is the function of one of the snRNPs, several of which binding to mRNA result in a spliceosome. E: Ribozymes have been implicated in the processing of ribosomal and tRNAs (p. 686).
6. D This is an important mechanism for driving reactions. A and B: Transcription is directed by the genetic code, generating rRNA precursors in the nucleolus and mRNA and tRNA precursors in nucleoplasm. C: Eukaryotic transcription may have internal promoter regions as well as enhancers. E: This is a difference from DNA polymerase (p. 689).
7. B B and C: Enhancer sequences seem to work whether they are at the beginning or end of the gene, but they must be on the same DNA strand as the transcribed gene. D: They seem to function by binding proteins which themselves bind RNA polymerase (p. 697).
8. E A, D, and E: Sigma factor is required for correct initiation and dissociates from the core enzyme after the first bonds have been formed. Core enzyme can transcribe but cannot correctly initiate transcription. B and C: Rifampicin binds to the β subunit, and α-amanitin is an inhibitor of eukaryotic polymerases (p. 691).
9. D Sigma factor is released when, or a short time after, the initial bond is formed.
10. C The high A-T content of the Pribnow box is believed to facilitate initial unwinding.
11. E Elongation, which requires only the core enzyme, is well underway in this region (p. 695, Figure 16.2).
12. C A, B, and E: There is a rho-dependent as well as a rho-independent process. Rho is a separate protein from RNA polymerase and appears to possess ATPase activity (p. 696). C and D: Rho-independent termination involves secondary structure, which is stabilized by high G-C content.
13. B RNA polymerase III uses an internal promoter. A: RNA polymerase II activity involves the TATA and CAAT boxes. C: RNA polymerase I produces one transcript, which is later processed to yield three rRNAs. D: Parts of the promoter are not in a nucleosome. E: Enhancers may be as much as 1000 bp away (pp. 696–697).
14. E The TATA box is part of the promoter, which is not transcribed. A–D: Modification of bases, cleavage, and splicing are all important events in posttranscriptional processing to form functional molecules (pp. 700–707).
15. A Capping is a feature of mRNA. B: The primary transcript is longer than the functional molecule. C: The same modifications, catalyzed by a certain (set of) enzyme(s), occurs at more than one location. D: This is a posttranscriptional modification (pp. 700–701).
16. C A: Cleavage occurs, but splicing does not. B: Alternate splicing leads to different proteins from a single gene. D: Splicing occurs after other events. E: Specificity of cleavage is related to specific sequences at the intron–exon junctions, not to the sequence of the intron itself (pp. 702–707).
17. D A: Modified bases cannot be recycled. B: Although some enzymes of maturation may require an ordered structure, degradative enzymes are less efficient on an ordered structure. C: An endonuclease cleaves an interior phosphodiester bond. E: Even rRNA turns over although it is more stable than the other species (p. 709).

CHAPTER

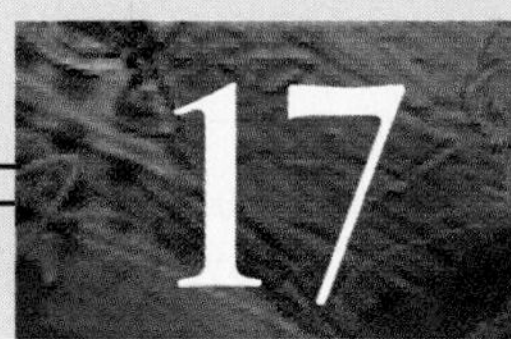

PROTEIN SYNTHESIS: TRANSLATION AND POSTTRANSLATIONAL MODIFICATIONS

Dohn Glitz

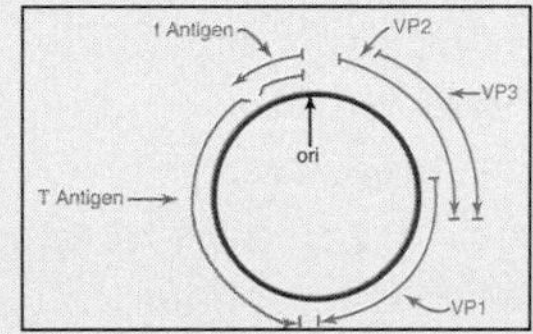

17.1 ■ OVERVIEW

Protein biosynthesis is also called **translation** since it involves the biochemical translation of information from the four-letter language and structure of nucleic acids into the 20-letter language and structure of proteins. This process has many requirements: an informational messenger RNA molecule that is exported from the nucleus, several "bilingual" transfer RNA species that read the message, ribosomes that serve as catalytic and organizational centers, a variety of protein factors, and energy. Polypeptides are formed by the sequential addition of amino acids in the specific order determined by the information carried in the nucleotide sequence of the mRNA. The protein is often then matured or processed by a variety of modifications. These may target it to a specific intracellular location or for secretion from the cell, or they may modulate its activity or function. These complex processes are carried out with considerable speed and extreme precision. Levels of translation are regulated, both globally and for specific proteins. Finally, when a protein becomes nonfunctional or is no longer needed, it is degraded and its amino acids are catabolized or recycled into new proteins.

Cells vary in their need and ability to synthesize proteins. At one extreme, terminally differentiated red blood cells have a life span of about 120 days, have no nuclei, do not divide, and do not synthesize proteins because they lack the components of the biosynthetic apparatus. Nondividing cells need to maintain levels of enzymes and other proteins and carry out limited protein synthesis. Growing and dividing cells must synthesize much larger amounts of protein. Finally, some cells synthesize proteins for export as well as for their own use. For example, liver cells synthesize large numbers of enzymes needed for their many metabolic pathways as well as proteins for export, including serum albumin, the major protein of blood plasma or serum. Liver cells are protein factories that are particularly rich in the machinery for synthesis of proteins.

17.2 ■ COMPONENTS OF THE TRANSLATIONAL APPARATUS

Messenger RNA Is the Carrier of Information Present in DNA

Genetic information is stored and transmitted in the nucleotide sequences of DNA. Selective expression of this information requires its transcription into mRNA that carries specific and precise messages from the nuclear "data bank" to the cytoplasmic sites of protein synthesis. In eukaryotes, the messengers, mRNAs, are usually synthesized as significantly larger precursor molecules that are processed prior to export from the nucleus. Eukaryotic mRNA in the cytosol has several identifying characteristics. It is almost always **monocistronic,** that is, encoding a single polypeptide. The 5′ end is capped with a specific structure consisting of **7-methylguanosine** linked through a 5′-triphosphate bridge to the 5′ end of the messenger sequence (see p. 704). A 5′-nontranslated region, which may be short or up to a few hundred nucleotides in length, separates the cap from the **translational initiation signal,** an **AUG** codon. Usually, but not always, this is the first AUG sequence encountered as the message is read 5′ → 3′. Uninterrupted sequences that specify a unique polypeptide sequence follow the initiation signal until a specific translation termination signal is reached. This is followed by a 3′-untranslated sequence, usually about 100 nucleotides in length, before the mRNA is terminated by a 100- to 200-nucleotide long polyadenylate tail.

Prokaryotic mRNA differs from eukaryotic mRNA in that the 5′ terminus is not capped but retains a terminal triphosphate from initiation of its synthesis by RNA polymerase. Also, most messengers are **polycistronic,** that is, encoding several polypeptides, and include more than one initiation AUG sequence. A ribosome-positioning sequence is located about 10 nucleotides upstream of a valid AUG initiation signal. An untranslated sequence follows the termination signal, but there is no polyadenylate tail.

Ribosomes Are Workbenches for Protein Biosynthesis

Proteins are assembled on particles called ribosomes. These have two dissimilar subunits, each of which contains RNA and many proteins. With one exception, each protein is present in a single copy per ribosome, as is each RNA species. The composition of major ribosome types is shown in Table 17.1, and characteristics of their RNAs are given in Table 16.1.

Ribosome architecture has been conserved in evolution. The similarities between ribosomes and subunits from different sources are more obvious than the differences, and functional roles for each subunit are well defined. Details of ribosome structure and its relationship to function have been learned using many techniques. Overall size and shape can be determined by electron microscopy. The location of many ribosomal proteins, some elements of the RNA, and functional sites on each subunit have been determined by electron microscopy of subunits that are complexed with antibodies against a single ribosomal component. The antibody molecule serves as a physical pointer to the site on the ribosome. Further structural information has been obtained from chemical cross-linking, which identifies near neighbors within the structure, and from neutron diffraction measurements, which quantitate the distances between pairs of proteins. Ribosomes have been crystallized and X-ray structural determination is under way. Sequence comparisons and chemical, immunological, and enzymatic probes give information about RNA conformation. Correlations of structural data with functional measurements in protein synthesis have allowed development of models, such as that in Figure 17.1, that link ribosome morphology to various functions in translation. Each subunit has an RNA core, folded into a specific three-dimensional structure, upon which proteins are positioned through protein–RNA and protein–protein interactions.

Many of these experiments were possible because prokaryotic ribosomes can **self-assemble;** that is, the native structures can be reconstituted from mixtures of purified individual proteins and RNAs. Reconstitution of subunits

TABLE 17.1 Ribosome Classification and Composition

Ribosome Source	*Monomer Size*	*Subunits*	
		Small	*Large*
Eukaryotes			
Cytosol	80S	40S: 34 proteins 18S RNA	60S: 50 proteins 28S, 5.8S, 5S RNAs
Mitochondria			
Animals	55S–60S	30S–35S: 12S RNA	40–45S: 16S RNA
		70–100 proteins	
Higher plants	77S–80S	40S: 19S RNA	60S: 25S, 5S RNAs
		70–75 proteins	
Chloroplasts	70S	30S: 20–24 proteins 16S RNA	50S: 34–38 proteins 23S, 5S, 4.5S RNAs
Prokaryotes			
Escherichia coli	70S	30S: 21 proteins 16S RNA	50S: 34 proteins 23S, 5S RNAs

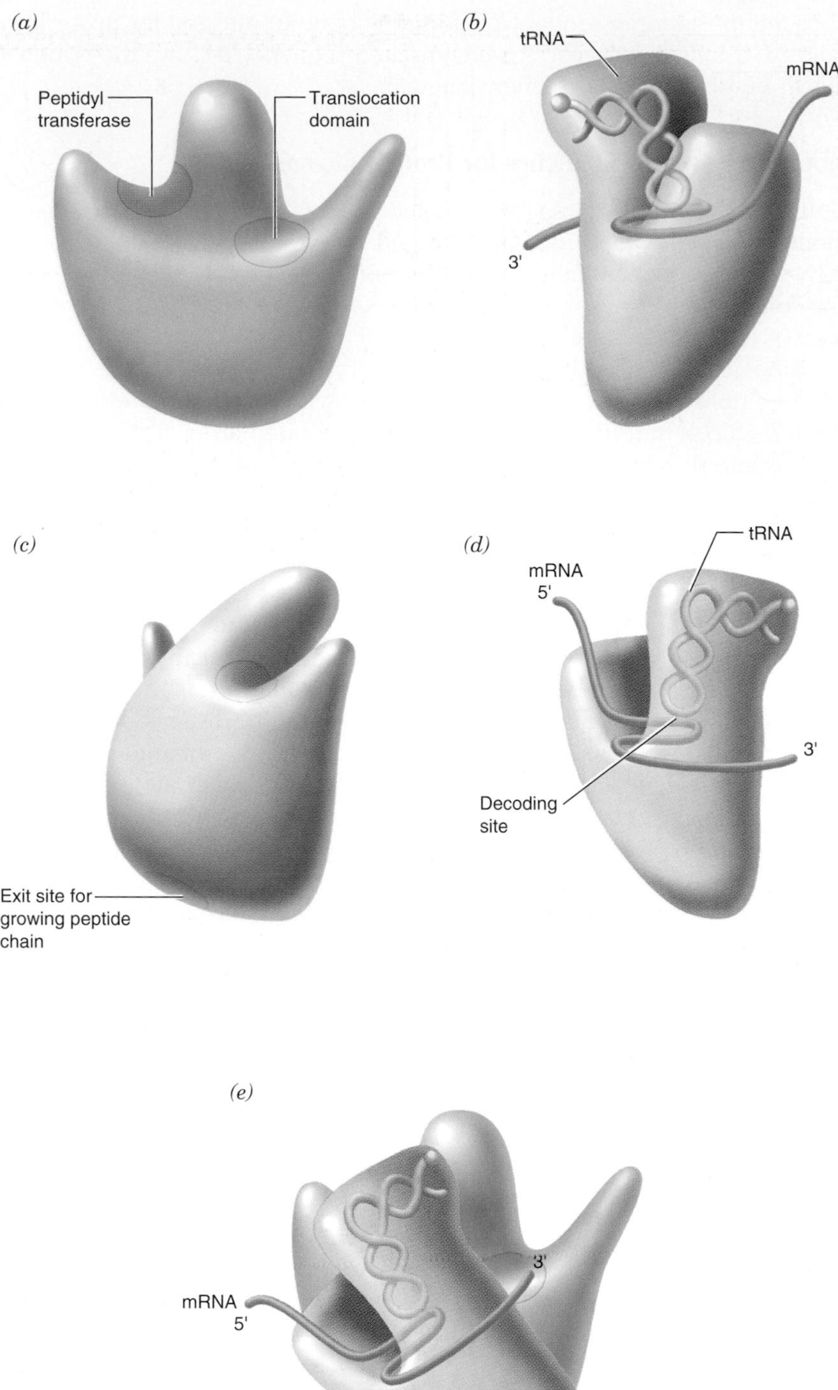

FIGURE 17.1
Ribosome structure and functional sites. Top row shows the faces of each subunit that interact in the functional ribosome. In (a) the large subunit is shown; note that sites of peptide bond formation and of binding of the elongation factors are on opposite sides of the bulbous "central protuberance." The arm-like structure is somewhat flexible or mobile and is seldom visualized in complete ribosomes. In (b) the small subunit is shown with a "platform" or ledge protruding toward the reader. mRNA and tRNA interact in a "decoding site," deep in the cleft between the platform and subunit body. The orientation of mRNA and tRNA is depicted, although their interaction in the decoding site is obscured by the platform. In (c) the large subunit has been rotated 90° and the arm projects into the page. The exit site near the base of the subunit is where newly synthesized protein emerges from the subunit. This area of the subunit is in contact with membranes in the "bound" ribosomes of rough endoplasmic reticulum. The site of peptide bond formation, the peptidyltransferase center, is distant from the exit site; the growing peptide passes through a groove or tunnel in the ribosome to reach the exit site. In (d) the small subunit has been rotated 90° such that the platform projects toward the dish-like face of the large subunit and the cleft is apparent. In (e) subunits have been brought together to show their relative orientation in the ribosome. Note that tRNA bound by the small subunit is oriented so that the aminoacyl acceptor end is near the peptidyltransferase while the translocational domain (where EF-1α and EF-2 bind) is near the decoding region and the area in which mRNA enters the complex. Drawings are based on electron microscopy of stained and unstained, frozen ribosomes. The latter technique preserves native structure and, perhaps along with X-ray crystallography, should lead to a more detailed and complete model of the ribosome.

from mixtures in which a single component is omitted or modified can show, for example, if a given protein is required for assembly of the subunit or for some specific function. An assembly map for large ribosomal subunits of *Escherichia coli* is shown in Figure 17.2. Total reconstitution of subunits from eukaryotes has not yet been achieved but the general conclusions about how ribosomes function, although determined using bacterial ribosomes, are fully applicable to eukaryotic systems.

Ribosomes are organized in two additional ways. First, several ribosomes often translate a single mRNA molecule simultaneously. Purified mRNA-linked

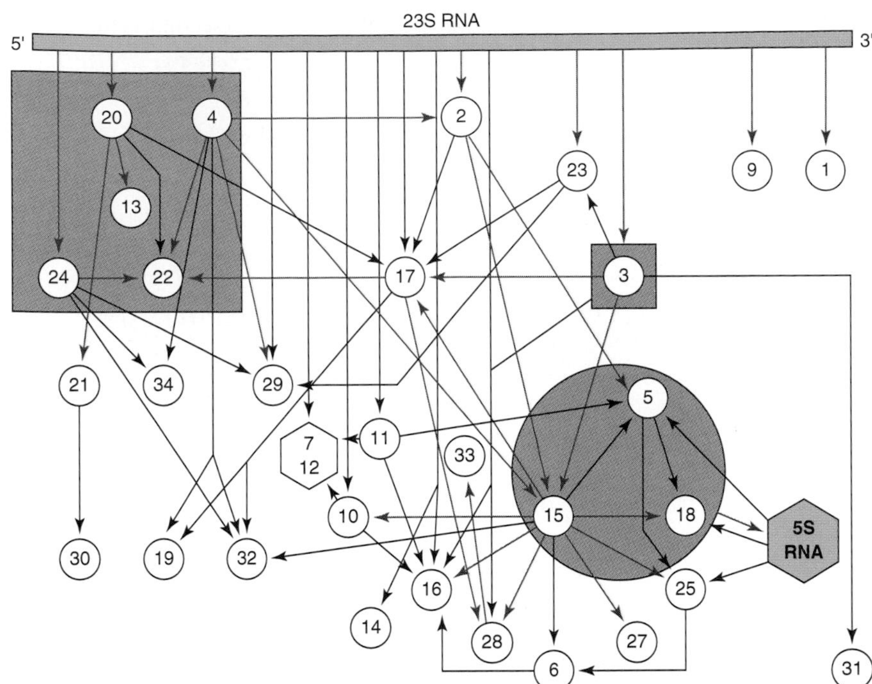

FIGURE 17.2
Assembly map of the large ribosomal subunit of *E. coli*.
The heavy bar at the top represents the 23S rRNA, and the individual ribosomal proteins are identified by numbers in circles. Arrows that connect components indicate their interaction. Red arrows from RNA to protein indicate that the protein binds directly and strongly to RNA, while black arrows indicate a weaker interaction. Similarly, red arrows between proteins show a strong binding dependence and black arrows show a lesser dependency. For example, protein L4 binds RNA strongly; it then strongly stimulates binding of proteins L2, L22, and L29. Protein L2 in turn stimulates binding of proteins L5 and L15. Proteins L5, L15, and L18 are essential for binding 5S RNA. Proteins within the boxes are required for a conformational transition that occurs during assembly. Diagram shows both orderly progression of the assembly process and interdependence of the components and their specific reactions with other components during the assembly of the subunit.
Adapted from M. Herold and K. Nierhaus, J. Biol. Chem. *262:8826, 1987. A similar assembly map for the small subunit was elucidated earlier. (M. Nomura,* Cold Spring Harbor Symp. Quant. Biol. *52:653, 1987.)*

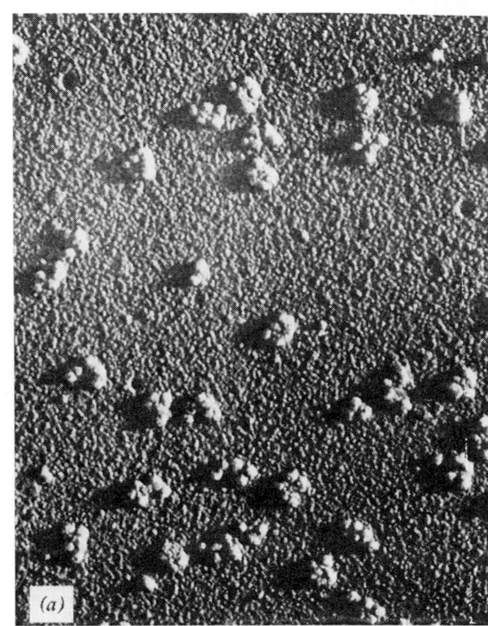

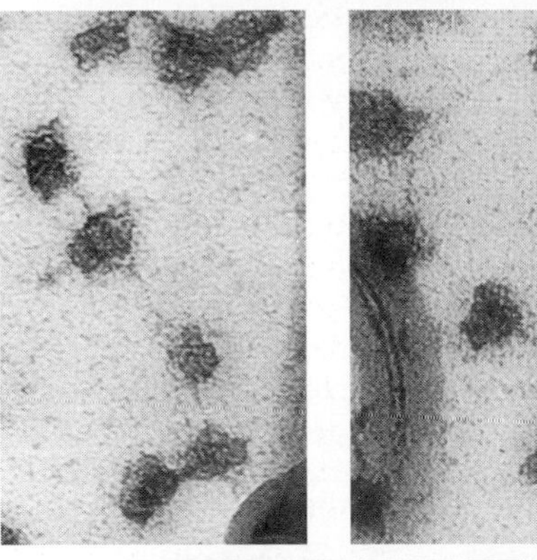

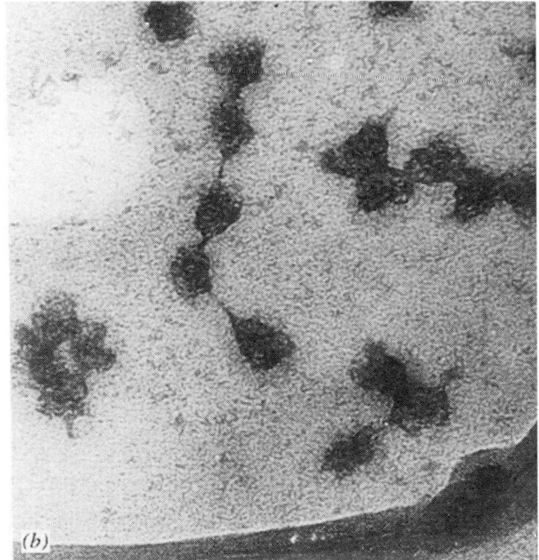

FIGURE 17.3
Electron micrographs of polysomes.
(*a*) Reticulocyte polyribosomes shadowed with platinum are seen in clusters of three to six ribosomes, a number consistent with the size of mRNA for a globin chain. (*b*) Uranyl acetate staining in addition to visualization at a higher magnification shows polysomes in which parts of the mRNA are visible.
Courtesy of Dr. Alex Rich, MIT.

polysomes can be visualized by electron microscopy (Figure 17.3). Second, in eukaryotic cells some ribosomes occur free in the cytosol, but many are bound to membranes of the rough endoplasmic reticulum. In general, **free ribosomes** synthesize proteins that remain within the cell cytosol or become targeted to the nucleus, mitochondria, or some of the other organelles. **Membrane-bound ribosomes** synthesize proteins that will be secreted from the cell or sequestered and function in other cellular membranes or vesicles. In cell homogenates, membrane fragments and the bound ribosomes constitute the **microsome** fraction; detergents that disrupt membranes release these ribosomes.

Transfer RNA Acts as a Bilingual Translator Molecule

All tRNA molecules have several common structural characteristics including the 3′-terminal CCA sequence to which amino acids are bound, a highly conserved cloverleaf secondary structure, and an L-shaped three-dimensional structure (see p. 682). But each of the many molecular species has a unique nucleotide sequence, giving it individual characteristics that allow great specificity in interactions with mRNA and with the aminoacyl-tRNA synthetase that couples one specific amino acid to it.

The Genetic Code Uses a Four-Letter Alphabet of Nucleotides

Information in the cell is stored in the form of linear sequences of nucleotides in DNA, in a manner that is analogous to the linear sequence of letters of the alphabet in the words you are now reading. The DNA language uses a simple **four-letter alphabet** that comprises the two purines, A and G (adenine and guanine), and the two pyrimidines, C and T (cytosine and thymine). In mRNA the information is encoded in a similar four-letter alphabet, but U (uracil) replaces T. The language of RNA is thus a dialect of the genetic language of DNA. Genetic information is **expressed** predominantly in the form of proteins that derive their properties from their linear sequence of amino acids and to a much lesser extent as RNA species such as tRNA and rRNA. Thus, during protein biosynthesis, the four-letter language of nucleic acids is translated into the 20-letter language of proteins. Implicit in the analogy to language is the directionality of these sequences. By convention, nucleic acid sequences are written in a $5' \rightarrow 3'$ direction, and protein sequences from the amino terminus to the carboxy terminus. These directions in mRNA and protein correspond in both their reading and biosynthetic senses.

Codons in mRNA Are Three-Letter Words

A 1:1 correspondence of nucleotides to amino acids would only permit mRNA to encode four amino acids, while a 2:1 correspondence would encode $4^2 = 16$ amino acids. Neither is sufficient since 20 amino acids occur in most proteins. The actual three-letter **genetic code** has $4^3 = 64$ permutations or words, which is also sufficient to encode start and stop signals, equivalent to punctuation. The three-base words are called **codons** and they are customarily shown in the form of Table 17.2. Only two amino acids are designated by

TABLE 17.2 The Genetic Code[a]

5′ Base	U	C	A	G	3′ Base
U	UUU Phe	UCU Ser	UAU Tyr	UGU Cys	U
	UUC Phe	UCC Ser	UAC Tyr	UGC Cys	C
	UUA Leu	UCA Ser	UAA Stop	UGA Stop	A
	UUG Leu	UCG Ser	UAG Stop	UGG Trp	G
C	CUU Leu	CCU Pro	CAU His	CGU Arg	U
	CUC Leu	CCC Pro	CAC His	CGC Arg	C
	CUA Leu	CCA Pro	CAA Gln	CGA Arg	A
	CUG Leu	CCG Pro	CAG Gln	CGG Arg	G
A	AUU Ile	ACU Thr	AAU Asn	AGU Ser	U
	AUC Ile	ACC Thr	AAC Asn	AGC Ser	C
	AUA Ile	ACA Thr	AAA Lys	AGA Arg	A
	AUG Met	ACG Thr	AAG Lys	AGG Arg	G
G	GUU Val	GCU Ala	GAU Asp	GGU Gly	U
	GUC Val	GCC Ala	GAC Asp	GGC Gly	C
	GUA Val	GCA Ala	GAA Glu	GGA Gly	A
	GUG Val	GCG Ala	GAG Glu	GGG Gly	G

[a] The genetic code comprises 64 codons, which are permutations of four bases taken in threes. Note the importance of sequence: three bases, each used once per triplet codon, give six permutations: ACG, AGC, GAC, GCA, CAG, and CGA, for threonine, serine, aspartate, alanine, glutamine, and arginine, respectively.

TABLE 17.3 Nonuniversal Codon Usage in Mammalian Mitochondria

Codon	*Usual Code*	*Mitochondrial Code*
UGA	Termination	Tryptophan
AUA	Isoleucine	Methionine
AGA	Arginine	Termination
AGG	Arginine	Termination

single codons: methionine as AUG and tryptophan as UGG. The rest are designated by two, three, four, or six codons. Multiple codons for a single amino acid represent **degeneracy** in the code. The genetic code is nearly **universal.** The same code words are used in all living organisms, prokaryotic and eukaryotic. An exception to universality occurs in mitochondria, in which a few codons have a different meaning than in the cytosol of the same organism (Table 17.3).

Punctuation

Four codons function partly or totally as punctuation, signaling the start and stop of protein synthesis. The **start signal,** AUG, also specifies methionine. An AUG at an appropriate site and within an acceptable sequence in mRNA signifies methionine as the initial, amino-terminal residue. AUG codons elsewhere in the message specify methionine residues within the protein. Three codons, UAG, UAA, and UGA, are **stop signals;** they specify no amino acid and are known as **termination codons** or, less appropriately, as **nonsense codons.**

Codon–Anticodon Interactions Permit Reading of mRNA

Translation of the codons of mRNA involves their direct interaction with complementary **anticodon sequences** in tRNA. Each tRNA species carries a unique amino acid, and each has a specific three-base anticodon sequence. Codon–anticodon base pairing is antiparallel, as shown in Figure 17.4. The anticodon is far from the amino acid-acceptor stem in both the tRNA cloverleaf and the L-shaped three-dimensional structure of all tRNA molecules. (See Chapter 16, p. 682.) Location of the anticodon and amino acid residue at opposite extremes of the molecule permits the tRNA to conceptually and physically bridge the gap between the nucleotide sequence of the ribosome-bound mRNA and the site of protein assembly on the ribosome.

Since 61 codons designate an amino acid, it might seem necessary to have 61 different tRNA species. This is **not** the case. Variances from standard base pairing are common in codon–anticodon interactions. Many amino acids can be carried by more than one tRNA species, and degenerate codons can be read by more than one tRNA (but always one carrying the correct amino acid). Much of this complexity is explained by the **"wobble" hypothesis,** which permits less stringent base pairing between the third position of a codon and the first position of its anticodon. Thus the first two positions of a codon predominate in tRNA selection and the **degenerate** (third) position is less important. A second modulator of codon–anticodon interactions is the presence of modified nucleotides at or beside the first nucleotide of the anticodon in many tRNA species. A frequent anticodon nucleotide is **inosinic acid** (I), the nucleotide of hypoxanthine, which base pairs with U, C, or A. Wobble base pairing rules are shown in Table 17.4.

If the wobble rules are followed, the 61 nonpunctuation codons could be read by as few as 31 tRNA molecules, but most cells have 50 or more tRNA

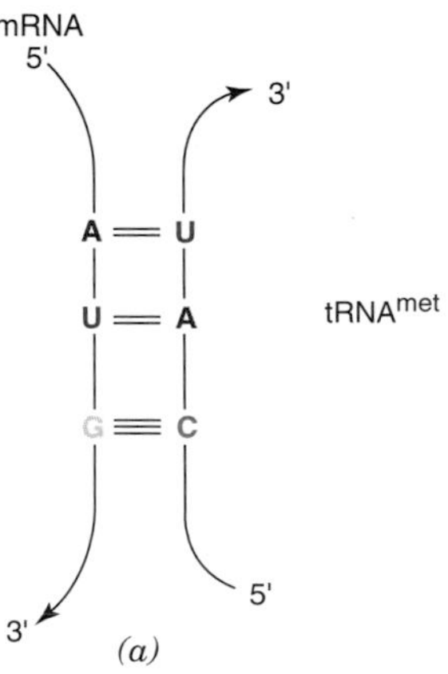

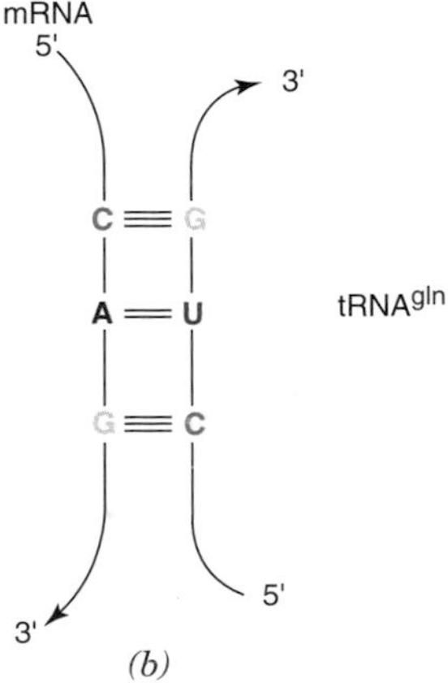

FIGURE 17.4
Codon–anticodon interactions.
Shown are interactions between (*a*) the AUG (methionine) codon and its CAU anticodon and (*b*) the CAG (glutamine) codon and a CUG anticodon. Note that these interactions involve antiparallel pairing of mRNA with tRNA.

TABLE 17.4 Wobble Base Pairing Rules

3' Codon Base	*5' Anticodon Bases Possible*
A	U or I
C	G or I
G	C or U
U	A or G or I

species. Some codons are read more efficiently by one anticodon than another. Not all codons are used equally, some being used very rarely. Examination of many mRNA sequences has allowed construction of "codon usage" tables that show that different organisms preferentially use different codons to generate similar polypeptide sequences.

"Breaking" the Genetic Code

The genetic code (Table 17.2) was determined before methods were developed to sequence natural mRNA. These code-breaking experiments provide insight into how proteins are synthesized. Important experiments used simple artificial mRNAs or chemically synthesized trinucleotide codons.

Polynucleotide phosphorylase catalyzes the template-independent and readily reversible reaction:

$$x\text{NDP} \leftrightarrows \text{polynucleotide } (\text{pN})_x + P_i$$

where NDP is any nucleoside 5′-diphosphate or a mixture of two or more. If the nucleoside diphosphate is UDP, a polymer of U designated poly(U) is formed. Under nonphysiological conditions protein synthesis can occur *in vitro* without the initiation components that are normally required. With poly(U) as mRNA, the "protein" polyphenylalanine is made. Similarly, poly(A) encodes polylysine and poly(C) polyproline. An mRNA with a random sequence of only U and C produces polypeptides that contain not only proline and phenylalanine, as predicted, but also serine (from UCU and UCC) and leucine (from CUU and CUC). Because of degeneracy in the code and the complexity of the products, experiments with random sequence mRNAs were difficult to interpret, and so synthetic messengers of defined sequence were transcribed from simple repeating DNA sequences by RNA polymerase. Thus poly(AU), transcribed from a repeating poly(dAT), produces only a repeating copolymer of Ile-Tyr-Ile-Tyr, read from successive triplets AUA UAU AUA UAU and so on. A synthetic poly(CUG) has possible codons CUG for Leu, UGC for Cys, and GCU for Ala, each repeating itself once the **reading frame** has been selected. Since selection of the initiation codon is random in these *in vitro* experiments, three different homopolypeptides are produced: polyleucine, polycysteine, and polyalanine. A perfect poly(CUCG) produces a polypeptide with the sequence (-Leu-Ala-Arg-Ser-) whatever the initiation point. These relationships are summarized in Table 17.5; they show codons to be triplets read in exact sequence, without overlap or omission. Other experiments used chemically synthesized trinucleotide codons as minimal messages. No proteins were made, but the binding of only one amino acid (conjugated to an appropriate tRNA) by the ribosome was stimulated by a given codon. It was thus possible to decipher the meaning of each possible codon and to identify termination codons. All of these conclusions were later verified by the determination of mRNA sequences.

TABLE 17.5 Polypeptide Products of Synthetic mRNAs[a]

mRNA	*Codon Sequence*	*Products*
—$(\text{AU})_n$—	— AUA UAU AUA UAU —	—$(\text{Ile-Tyr})_{n/3}$—
—$(\text{CUG})_n$—	— CUG CUG CUG CUG —	—Leu_n—
	— UGC UGC UGC UGC —	—Cys_n—
	— GCU GCU GCU GCU —	—Ala_n—
—$(\text{CUCG})_n$—	CUC GCU CGC UCG	—$(\text{Leu-Ala-Arg-Ser})_{n/3}$—

[a] The horizontal brackets accent the reading frame.

Mutations

An understanding of the genetic code and how it is read provides a basis for understanding the nature of mutations. A mutation is simply a change in a gene. **Point mutations** involve a change in a single base pair in the DNA, and thus a single base in the corresponding mRNA. Sometimes this change occurs in the third position of a degenerate codon and there is no change in the amino acid specified (e.g., UCC to UCA still codes for serine). Such **silent mutations** are only detected by gene sequence determination. They are commonly seen during comparison of genes for similar proteins, for example, hemoglobins from different species. **Missense mutations** arise from a base change that causes incorporation of a different amino acid in the encoded protein (see Clin. Corr. 17.1). Point mutations can also form or destroy a termination codon and thus change the length of a protein. Formation of a termination codon from one that encodes an amino acid (see Clin. Corr. 17.2) is often called a **nonsense mutation;** it results in premature termination and a truncated protein. Mutation of a termination codon to one for an amino acid allows the message to be "read through" until another stop codon is encountered. The result is a larger than normal protein. This phenomenon is the basis of several disorders (see Table 17.6 and Clin. Corr. 17.3).

Insertion or deletion of a single nucleotide within the coding region of a gene results in a **frameshift mutation.** The reading frame is altered at that point and subsequent codons are read in the new context until a termination codon is reached. Table 17.7 illustrates this phenomenon with the mutant hemoglobin Wayne. The significance of reading frame selection is underscored by a phenomenon in some viruses in which a single segment of DNA encodes different polypeptides that are translated using different reading frames. An example is the tumor-causing simian virus SV40 (Figure 17.5), whose small size physically limits the amount of DNA that can be packaged within it.

Aminoacylation of Transfer RNA Activates Amino Acids for Protein Synthesis

In order to be incorporated into proteins, amino acids must first be "activated" by linkage to their appropriate tRNA carriers. This is a two-step process that requires energy and is catalyzed by one of a family of aminoacyl-tRNA synthetases, each of which is specific for a single amino acid and its appropriate tRNA species. The reactions are normally written as follows:

$$\mathrm{H{-}N(H){-}CH(R){-}C({=}O){-}OH + ATP + E} \rightleftharpoons \left[\mathrm{H{-}N(H){-}CH(R){-}C({=}O) \sim AMP \cdot E}\right] + \mathrm{PP_i} \quad (1)$$

$$\left[\mathrm{H{-}N(H){-}CH(R){-}C({=}O) \sim AMP \cdot E}\right] + \mathrm{tRNA} \rightleftharpoons \mathrm{H{-}N(H){-}CH(R){-}C({=}O){-}tRNA + AMP + E} \quad (2)$$

Sum:

$$\mathrm{H{-}N(H){-}CH(R){-}C({=}O){-}OH + ATP + tRNA} \rightleftharpoons \mathrm{H{-}N(H){-}CH(R){-}C({=}O){-}tRNA + AMP + PP_i}$$

The brackets surrounding the aminoacyl-AMP–enzyme complex indicate that it is a transient, enzyme-bound intermediate. The "squiggle" (~) linkage of amino acid to AMP identifies the aminoacyl-adenylate as a high-energy intermediate, a mixed acid anhydride with carboxyl and phosphoryl components. The aminoacyl ester linkage in tRNA is lower in energy than the aminoacyl-adenylate, but still higher than that of the carboxyl group of the free amino acid. The

CLINICAL CORRELATION 17.1

Missense Mutation: Hemoglobin

Clinically, the most important missense mutation known is the change from A to U in either the GAA or GAG codon for glutamate to give a GUA or GUG codon for valine in the sixth position of the β chain for hemoglobin. An estimated 1 in 10 African-Americans are carriers of this mutation, which in its homozygous state is the basis for sickle cell disease, the most common of all hemoglobinopathies (see Clin. Corr. 2.3 for the effects of this substitution on the polymerization of deoxygenated hemoglobin). The second most common hemoglobinopathy is hemoglobin C disease, in which a change from G to A in either the GAA or GAG codon for glutamate results in an AAA or AAG codon for lysine in the sixth position of the β chain. Over 600 other hemoglobin missense mutations are now known. Methods for diagnosis of these and other genetic disorders are discussed in Clin. Corr. 16.2. A recent advance in therapy of sickle cell anemia uses hydroxyurea treatment to stimulate synthesis of γ chains and thus increase fetal hemoglobin production in affected adults. This decreases the tendency of the HbS in erythrocytes to form linear multimers that result in cell shape distortion—that is, sickling—when the oxygen tension decreases.

Charache, S. et al. Effect of hydroxyurea on the frequency of painful crises in sickle cell anemia. *N. Engl. J. Med.* 332:1317–1322, 1995.

CLINICAL CORRELATION 17.2

Disorders of Terminator Codons

In hemoglobin McKees Rocks the UAU or UAC codon normally designating tyrosine in position 145 of the β chain has mutated to the terminator codon UAA or UAG. This results in shortening of the β chain from its normal 146 residues to 144 residues. This change gives the hemoglobin molecule an unusually high oxygen affinity since the normal C-terminal sequence involved in binding 2,3-bisphosphoglycerate is modified. The response to decreased oxygen delivery is secretion of erythropoietin by the kidney and increased red blood cell production that produces a polycythemic phenotype (see Clin. Corr. 22.2).

Another illness that results from a terminator mutation is a variety of β-thalassemia. Thalassemias are a group of disorders characterized at the molecular level by an imbalance in the stoichiometry of α- and β-globin synthesis. In β^0-thalassemia no β-globin is synthesized. As a result, α-globin, unable to associate with β-globin to form hemoglobin, accumulates and precipitates in erythroid cells. The precipitation damages cell membranes, causing hemolytic anemia and stimulation of erythropoiesis. One variety of β^0-thalassemia, common in Southeast Asia, results from a terminator mutation at codon 17 of the β-globin; the normal codon AAG that designates a lysyl residue at β-17 becomes the stop codon UAG. In contrast to hemoglobin McKees Rocks, in which the terminator mutation occurs late in the β-globin message, the mutation occurs so early in the mRNA that no useful β-globin sequence can be synthesized, and β-globin is absent. This leads to anemia and aggregation of unused α-globin in the red cell precursors. In addition, β-globin mRNA levels are depressed, probably because premature termination of translation leads to instability of the mRNA.

Winslow, R. M., Swenberg, M., Gross, E., et al. Hemoglobin McKees Rocks ($\alpha_2\beta_2^{145\,\text{Tyr}\rightarrow\text{term}}$). A human nonsense mutation leading to a shortened β chain. *J. Clin. Invest.* 57:772, 1976. Chang, J. C., and Kan, Y. W. β-Thalassemia: a nonsense mutation in man. *Proc. Natl. Acad. Sci. USA* 76:2886, 1979.

CLINICAL CORRELATION 17.3

Thalassemia

There are two expressed α-globin genes on each chromosome 16. Many instances of α-thalassemia arise from the deletion of two, three, or all four copies of the α-globin gene. The clinical severity increases with the number of genes deleted. In contrast, the disorders summarized in Table 17.6 are forms of α-thalassemia that arise from abnormally long α-globin molecules, which replace normal α-globin, and are present only in small amounts. These small amounts of α-globin result from a decreased rate of synthesis or more likely from an increased rate of breakdown of the abnormally elongated α-globin. The normal stop codon, UAA, for α-globin mutates to any of four sense codons with resultant placement of four different amino acids at position 142. Normal α-globin is only 141 residues in length, but the four abnormal α-globins are 172 residues in length, presumably because a triplet of nucleotides in the normally untranslated region of the mRNA becomes a terminator codon in the abnormal position 173. Elongated globin chains can also result from frameshift mutations or insertions.

Weatherall, D. J., and Clegg, J. B. The α-chain termination mutants and their relationship to the α-thalassemias. *Philos. Trans. R. Soc. Lond.* 271:411, 1975.

reactions are written to show their reversibility. In reality, **pyrophosphatases** cleave the pyrophosphate released and the equilibrium is strongly shifted toward formation of aminoacyl-tRNA. From the viewpoint of precision in translation, the amino acid, which had only its side chain (R group) to distinguish it, becomes linked to a large, complex, and easily recognized carrier.

Specificity and Fidelity of Aminoacylation Reactions

Cells contain 20 different **aminoacyl-tRNA synthetases,** each specific for one amino acid, and at most a small family of carrier tRNAs for that amino acid. In translation, codon–anticodon interactions define the amino acid to be incorporated. If an incorrect amino acid is carried by the tRNA, it will be incorporated into the protein. Correct selection of both tRNA and amino acid by the synthetase is necessary to avoid such mistakes. Accuracy of these enzymes is central to the fidelity of protein synthesis.

Aminoacyl-tRNA synthetases share a common mechanism and many are physically associated with one another in the cell. Nevertheless, they are a diverse group of proteins that may contain one, two, or four identical subunits or pairs of dissimilar subunits. Detailed studies indicate that separate structural domains are involved in aminoacyl-adenylate formation, tRNA recognition, and, if it occurs, subunit interactions. In spite of their structural diversity, each enzyme is capable of almost error-free formation of correct aminoacyl-tRNA combinations.

TABLE 17.6 "Read Through" Mutation in Termination Codons Produce Abnormally Long α-Globin Chains

Hemoglobin	*α-Codon 142*	*Amino Acid 142*	*α-Globin Length (Residues)*
A	UAA		141
Constant Spring	CAA	Glutamine	172
Icaria	AAA	Lysine	172
Seal Rock	GAA	Glutamate	172
Koya Dora	UCA	Serine	172

Selection and incorporation of a correct amino acid require great discrimination on the part of some synthetases. While some amino acids be may easily recognized by their bulk (e.g., tryptophan) or lack of bulk (glycine), or by positive or negative charges on the side chains (e.g., lysine and glutamate), others are much more difficult to discriminate. Recognition of valine rather than threonine or isoleucine by the valyl-tRNA synthetase is difficult since the side chains differ by either an added hydroxyl or single methylene group. The amino acid-recognition and -activation sites of each enzyme have great specificity, as is characteristic of many enzymes. Nevertheless, misrecognition does occur. An additional **"proofreading"** or **"editing"** step increases discrimination. This most often occurs through hydrolysis of the aminoacyl-adenylate intermediate, with the release of amino acid and AMP. Valyl-tRNA synthetase efficiently hydrolyzes threonyl-adenylate and it hydrolyzes isoleucyl-adenylate in the presence of bound (but not aminoacylated) $tRNA^{Val}$. In other cases a misacylated tRNA is recognized and deacylated. Valyl- and phenylalanyl-tRNA synthetases deacylate tRNAs that have been mischarged with threonine and tyrosine, respectively. This proofreading is analogous to editing of misincorporated nucleotides by the $3' \rightarrow 5'$ exonuclease activity of DNA polymerases (Chapter 16). Editing is performed by many but not all aminoacyl-tRNA synthetases. The net result is an average level of misacylation of one in 10^4 to 10^5.

Each synthetase must correctly recognize one to several tRNA species that correctly serve to carry the same amino acid, while rejecting incorrect tRNA species. Given the complexity of tRNA molecules, this should be simpler than selection of a single amino acid. However, recall the conformational similarity and common sequence elements of all tRNAs (p. 682). Different synthetases recognize different elements of tRNA structure. One logical element of tRNA recognition by the synthetase is the anticodon, specific to one amino acid. For example, in the case of $tRNA^{Met}$, changing the anticodon also alters recognition by the synthetase. In other instances, this is at least partly true. Sometimes the anticodon is not a determinant of synthetase-tRNA recognition. Consider, for example, suppressor mutations that "suppress" the expression of classes of chain termination (nonsense) mutations. A point mutation in a glutamine (CAG) codon produces a termination (UAG) codon, which causes the premature termination of the encoded protein. A second **suppressor mutation** in the anticodon of a $tRNA^{Tyr}$, in which the normal GUA anticodon is changed to CUA, allows "read through" of the termination codon. The initial mutation is suppressed as a nearly normal protein is made, with the affected glutamine replaced by tyrosine. Aminoacylation of the mutant $tRNA^{tyr}$ with tyrosine shows that in this case the anticodon does not determine synthetase specificity. In *E. coli* $tRNA^{Ala}$, the primary recognition characteristic is a G_3-U_{70} base pair in the acceptor stem; even if no other changes in the $tRNA^{Ala}$ occur, any variation at this position destroys its acceptor ability with alanine-$tRNA^{Ala}$ synthetase. Incorporation of a G_3-U_{70} base pair in $tRNA^{Cys}$ makes it an alanine acceptor, and even the isolated

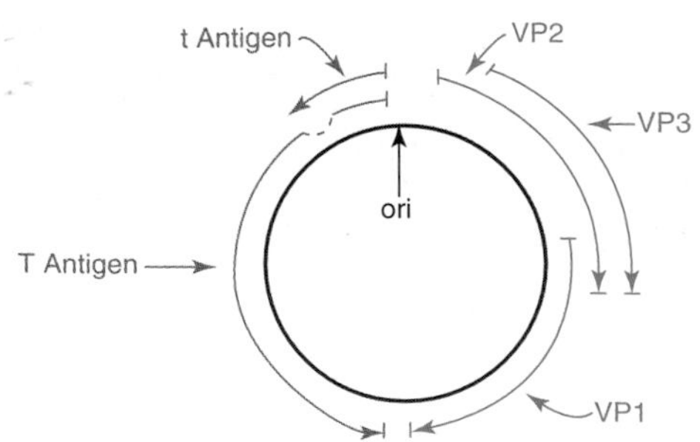

FIGURE 17.5
Map of genome of simian virus 40 (SV40).
DNA of SV40, shown in red, is a double-stranded circle of slightly more than 5000 base pairs that encodes all information needed by the virus for its survival and replication within a host cell. It is an example of extremely efficient use of the information-coding potential of a small genome. Proteins VP1, VP2, and VP3 are structural proteins of the virus; VP2 and VP3 are translated from different initiation points to the same carboxyl terminus. VP1 is translated in a different reading frame so that its amino-terminal section overlaps the VP2 and VP3 genes but its amino acid sequence in the overlapping segment is different from that of VP2 and VP3. Two additional proteins, the large T and small t tumor antigens, which promote transformation of infected cells, have identical amino-terminal sequences. The carboxyl-terminal segment of small t protein is encoded by a segment of mRNA that is spliced out of the large T message, and the carboxyl-terminal sequence of large T is encoded by DNA that follows termination of small t. This occurs through differential processing of a common mRNA precursor. The single site of origin of DNA replication (ori) is outside all coding regions of the genome.

TABLE 17.7 A Frameshift Mutation Results in Production of Abnormal Hemoglobin Wayne[a]

Position	*137*	*138*	*139*	*140*	*141*	*142*	*143*	*144*	*145*	*146*	*147*
Normal α-globin amino acid sequence	- Thr	- Ser	- Lys	- Tyr	- Arg						
Normal α-globin codon sequence	- ACP	- UC(U)	- AAA	- UAC	- CGU	- [UAA]	- GCU	- GGA	- GCC	- UCG	- GUA
Wayne α-globin codon sequence	- ACP	- UCA	- AAU	- ACC	- GUU	- AAG	- CUG	- GAG	- CCU	- CGG	- [UAG]
Wayne α-globin amino acid sequence	- Thr	- Ser	- Asn	- Thr	- Val	- Lys	- Leu	- Glu	- Pro	- Arg	

[a] The base deletion causing thre frameshift is encircled. The stop codons are boxed.

P = A, G, U, or C.

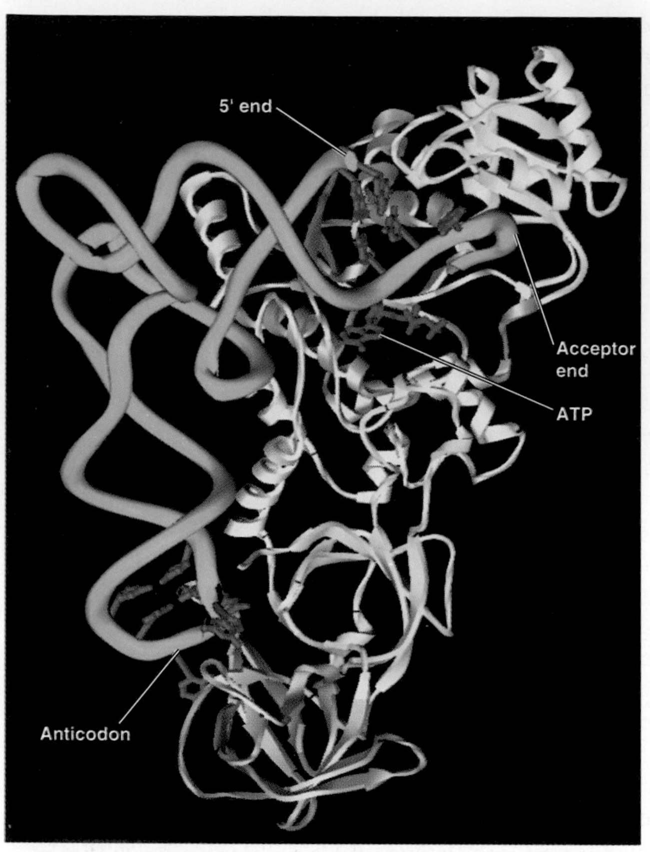

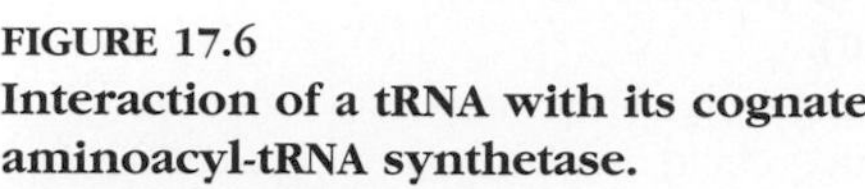

FIGURE 17.6
Interaction of a tRNA with its cognate aminoacyl-tRNA synthetase.
Figure shows sugar–phosphate backbone of *E. coli* glutaminyl tRNA in green and the peptide backbone of the glutamine $tRNA^{Gln}$ synthetase in multiple colors. Note the strong interactions of the synthetase with both the partially unwound acceptor stem and the anticodon loop of the tRNA, and placement of ATP, shown in red, within a few angstroms of the 3′ end of tRNA. Space-filling models of the enzyme and tRNA would show both molecules to be solid objects with several sites of direct contact.
Adapted from J. Perona, M. Rould, and T. Steitz, Biochemistry 32:8758, 1993.

acceptor stem of $tRNA^{Ala}$ can be aminoacylated. Other tRNA identification features include additional elements of the acceptor stem and sometimes parts of the variable loop or the D-stem/loop. Usually multiple structural elements contribute to recognition, but many are not absolute determinants. The X-ray structure of the glutaminyl synthetase–tRNA complex shown in Figure 17.6 shows binding at the concave tRNA surface, which is typical and compatible with the biochemical observations.

17.3 ■ PROTEIN BIOSYNTHESIS

Translation Is Directional and Colinear with mRNA

In the English language words are read from left to right and not from right to left. Similarly, mRNA sequences are written $5' \rightarrow 3'$ and in the translation process they are read in the same direction. Amino acid sequences are both written and biosynthesized from the amino-terminal residue to the carboxy terminus. This was first demonstrated by following the incorporation of radioactive amino acids into specific sites in hemoglobin as a function of time. Only full length, complete globin chains were isolated and analyzed. Completed chains that incorporated radioactive amino acids during the shortest exposures to the radioactive precursor were near to being finished at the time of the pulse and were found to have radioactive amino acids only in the carboxy-terminal segments. Longer pulses with radioactive amino acids resulted also in labeling of central segments of the protein, and the longest pulse time, still corresponding to less than that needed to synthesize a full-length polypeptide, showed radioactivity approaching the amino-terminal segments. Again, this amino- to carboxy-terminal directionality became obvious as details of translation were clarified.

The existence of stable polysomes and the directional nature of translation imply that each ribosome remains bound to an mRNA molecule and moves along the length of the mRNA until it is fully read. Comparison of mRNA sequences with sequences of the proteins they encode shows a perfect, colinear, gap-free correspondence of the mRNA coding sequence and that of the synthesized polypeptide. In fact, it is common to deduce the sequence of a protein solely from the nucleotide sequence of its mRNA or the DNA of the gene encoding it. However, the deduced sequence may differ from the genuine protein because of posttranslational events and modifications.

Initiation of Protein Synthesis Is a Complex Process

A good novel can be analyzed in terms of its beginning, its development or middle section, and its satisfactory ending. Protein biosynthesis will be described in a similar conceptual and mechanical framework: initiation of the process, elongation during which the great bulk of the protein is formed, and termination of synthesis and release of the finished polypeptide. We will then examine the posttranslational modifications that a protein may undergo.

Initiation requires bringing together a small (40S) ribosomal subunit, the mRNA, and a tRNA complex of the amino-terminal amino acid, all in a proper orientation. This is followed by association of the large (60S) subunit to form a completed initiation complex on an 80S ribosome. The ordered process is shown in Figure 17.7; it also requires a complex group of proteins, known as **initiation factors,** that participate only in initiation. They are not ribosomal proteins, although many of them bind transiently to ribosomes during initiation steps. There are many eukaryotic initiation factors and the specific functions of some remain unclear; prokaryotic protein synthesis provides a useful and less complex model for comparison.

As a first step, **eukaryotic initiation factor 2a (eIF-2a)** binds to GTP and one species of $tRNA^{Met}$, designated **$Met\text{-}tRNA_i^{Met}$,** to form a ternary complex. Recognition of the **initiator tRNA** by eIF-2a is in some ways analogous to the recognition of a tRNA species by its cognate aminoacyltransferase. No other aminoacyl-tRNA, including $Met\text{-}tRNA_e^{Met}$, which participates only in elongation steps of protein synthesis, normally replaces the initiation-specific $Met\text{-}tRNA_i^{Met}$ in this step. Prokaryotes also utilize a specific initiator tRNA whose methionine is modified by formylation of its amino group. Only $fMet\text{-}tRNA_i^{Met}$ is recognized by prokaryotic IF-2.

The second step in initiation requires 40S ribosomal subunits associated with a very complex protein, **eIF-3.** Mammalian eIF-3 includes eight different polypeptides and has a mass of 600–650 kDa. In electron micrographs eIF-3 is seen bound to the 40S subunit surface that will contact the larger 60S subunit, thus physically blocking association of 40S and 60S subunits. Hence eIF-3 is also called a ribosome **anti-association factor,** as is **eIF-6,** which binds to 60S subunits. A complex that includes eIF-2a · $Met\text{-}tRNA_i^{Met}$ · GTP, eIF-3 · 40S, eIF-4c, and perhaps additional protein factors now forms. This complex is able to bind mRNA and thus generate a preinitiation complex, but once again several protein factors play a role. Proteins **eIF-4a** and **eIF-4b** serve to unwind or melt secondary structure in the mRNA, and **eIF-4f** (or cap binding protein) helps place the message on the 40S subunit with the capped 5′ end correctly oriented. Hydrolysis of ATP is required in "scanning" up to 100 or more nucleotides of the mRNA in order to locate and place the initiation AUG sequence in the correct site on the 40S subunit. Usually the first AUG sequence in the mRNA is used, but sometimes the surrounding nucleotide sequence or secondary structure is not appropriate for initiation and a later AUG is selected. The final **preinitiation complex** thus includes the 40S subunit, the eIF-2a · $Met\text{-}tRNA_i^{Met}$ · GTP ternary complex, correctly oriented mRNA, and several protein factors.

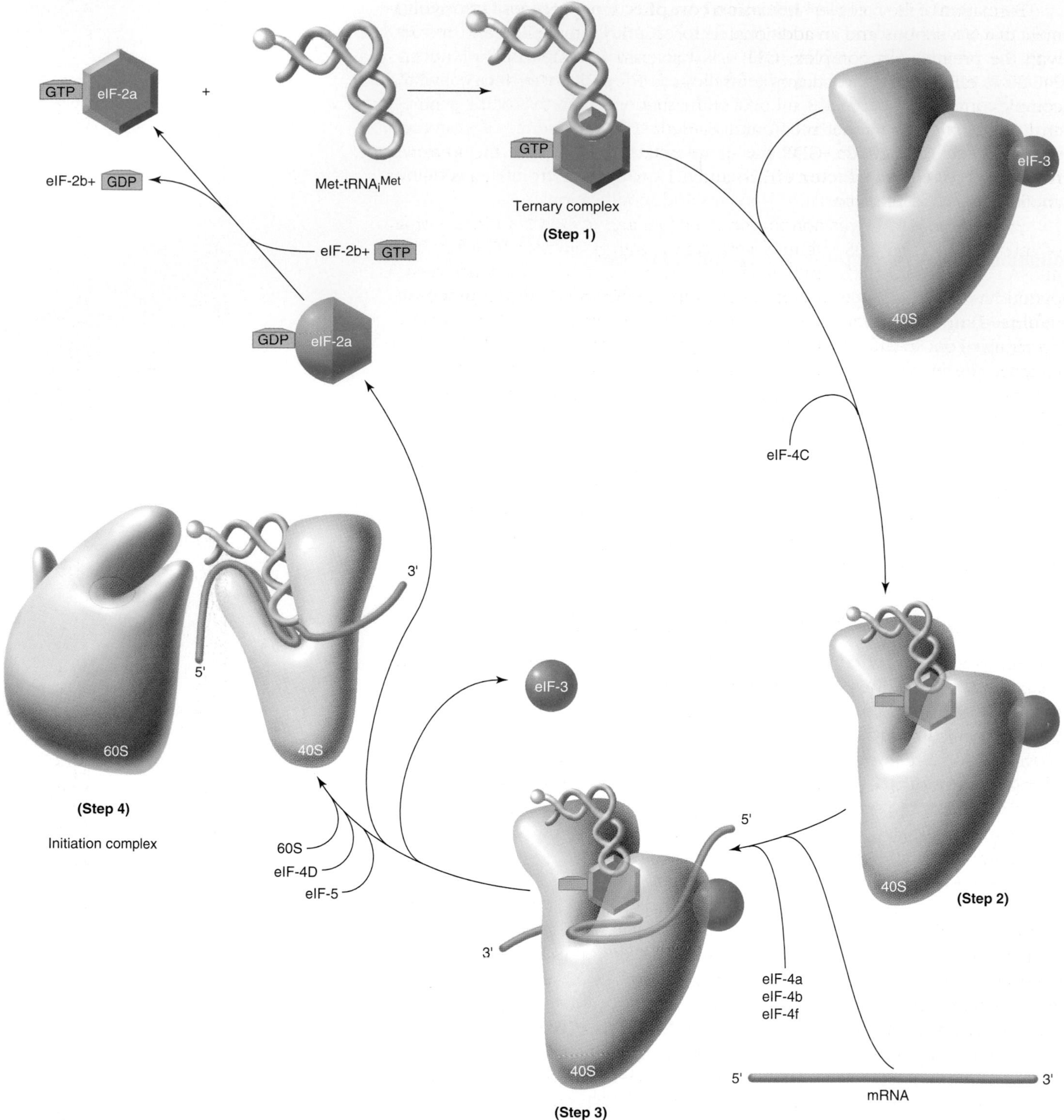

FIGURE 17.7
Initiation of translation in eukaryotes.
Details are given in the text. Ternary complex (step 1) first combines with small ribosomal subunit to place the initiator tRNA (step 2). Figure shows interaction with a naked mRNA molecule to form a preinitiation complex (step 3); additional small subunits later complex with the same mRNA as polysomes are formed. Formation of the initiation complex (is shown in step 4). The different shape of eIF-2a in complexes with GTP and GDP indicates that conformational change in the protein occurs upon hydrolysis of triphosphate.

Formation of the complete **initiation complex** now proceeds with involvement of a 60S subunit and an additional factor, **eIF-5.** Protein eIF-5 first interacts with the preinitiation complex; GTP is hydrolyzed to GDP and P_i, and eIF-2a · GDP, eIF-3, and other factors are released. The 40S · Met-$tRNA_i^{Met}$ · mRNA complex interacts with a 60S subunit and initiation factor eIF-4d to generate an 80S ribosome with the mRNA and initiator tRNA correctly positioned on the ribosome. The eIF-2a · GDP that is released interacts with the **guanine nucleotide exchange factor** eIF-2b and GTP to regenerate eIF-2a · GTP for another round of initiation.

Prokaryotes use fewer nonribosomal factors and a slightly different order of interaction. Their 30S subunits complexed with a simpler IF-3 first bind mRNA. Orientation of the mRNA relies in part on base pairing between a pyrimidine-rich sequence of eight nucleotides in 16S rRNA and a purine-rich **"Shine–Dalgarno"** sequence (named for its discoverers) about 10 nucleotides upstream of the initiator AUG codon. Complementarity between rRNA and the message-positioning sequence of an mRNA may include several mismatches but, as a first approximation, the better the complementary pairing the more efficient initiation at that AUG will be. It is interesting that eukaryotes do not utilize an mRNA–rRNA base pairing mechanism, but instead use many protein factors to position mRNA correctly. After the mRNA is bound by a 30S subunit, a ternary complex of IF-2, fMet-$tRNA_i^{Met}$, and GTP is bound. A third initiation factor, IF-1, also participates in formation of the preinitiation complex. A 50S subunit is now bound; in the process, GTP is hydrolyzed to GDP and P_i, and the initiation factors are released.

Elongation Is the Stepwise Formation of Peptide Bonds

Protein synthesis now occurs by stepwise elongation to form a polypeptide chain. At each step ribosomal **peptidyltransferase** transfers the growing peptide (or in the first step the initiating methionine residue) from its carrier tRNA to the α-amino group of the amino acid residue of the aminoacyl-tRNA specified by the next codon. Efficiency and fidelity are enhanced by nonribosomal protein **elongation factors** that utilize the energy released by GTP hydrolysis to ensure selection of the proper aminoacyl-tRNA species and to move the mRNA and associated tRNAs through the decoding region of the ribosome. Elongation is illustrated in Figure 17.8.

At a given moment, up to three different tRNA molecules may be bound at specific sites that span both ribosomal subunits. The initiating methionyl-tRNA is placed in position so that its methionyl residue may be transferred (or donated) to the free α-amino group of the incoming aminoacyl-tRNA; it thus occupies the donor site, also called the **peptidyl site** or **P site** of the ribosome. The aminoacyl-tRNA specified by the next codon of the message is bound at the acceptor site, also called the **aminoacyl site** or **A site** of the ribosome. Selection of the correct aminoacyl-tRNA is enhanced by **elongation factor 1 (EF-1);** a component of EF-1, **EF-1α,** first forms a ternary complex with aminoacyl-tRNA and GTP. The EF-1α · aminoacyl-tRNA · GTP complex binds to the ribosome and if codon–anticodon interactions are correct, the aminoacyl-tRNA is placed at the A site, GTP is hydrolyzed to GDP and P_i, and the EF-1α · GDP complex dissociates. The initiating methionyl-tRNA and the incoming aminoacyl-tRNA are now juxtaposed on the ribosome. Their anticodons are paired with successive codons of the mRNA in the **decoding region** of the small subunit, and their amino acids are beside one another at the **peptidyltransferase site** of the large subunit. Peptide bond formation now occurs. Peptidyltransferase catalyzes the attack of the α-amino group of the aminoacyl-tRNA onto the carbonyl carbon of the methionyl-tRNA. The result is transfer of the methionine to the amino group of the aminoacyl-tRNA, which then occupies a "hybrid"

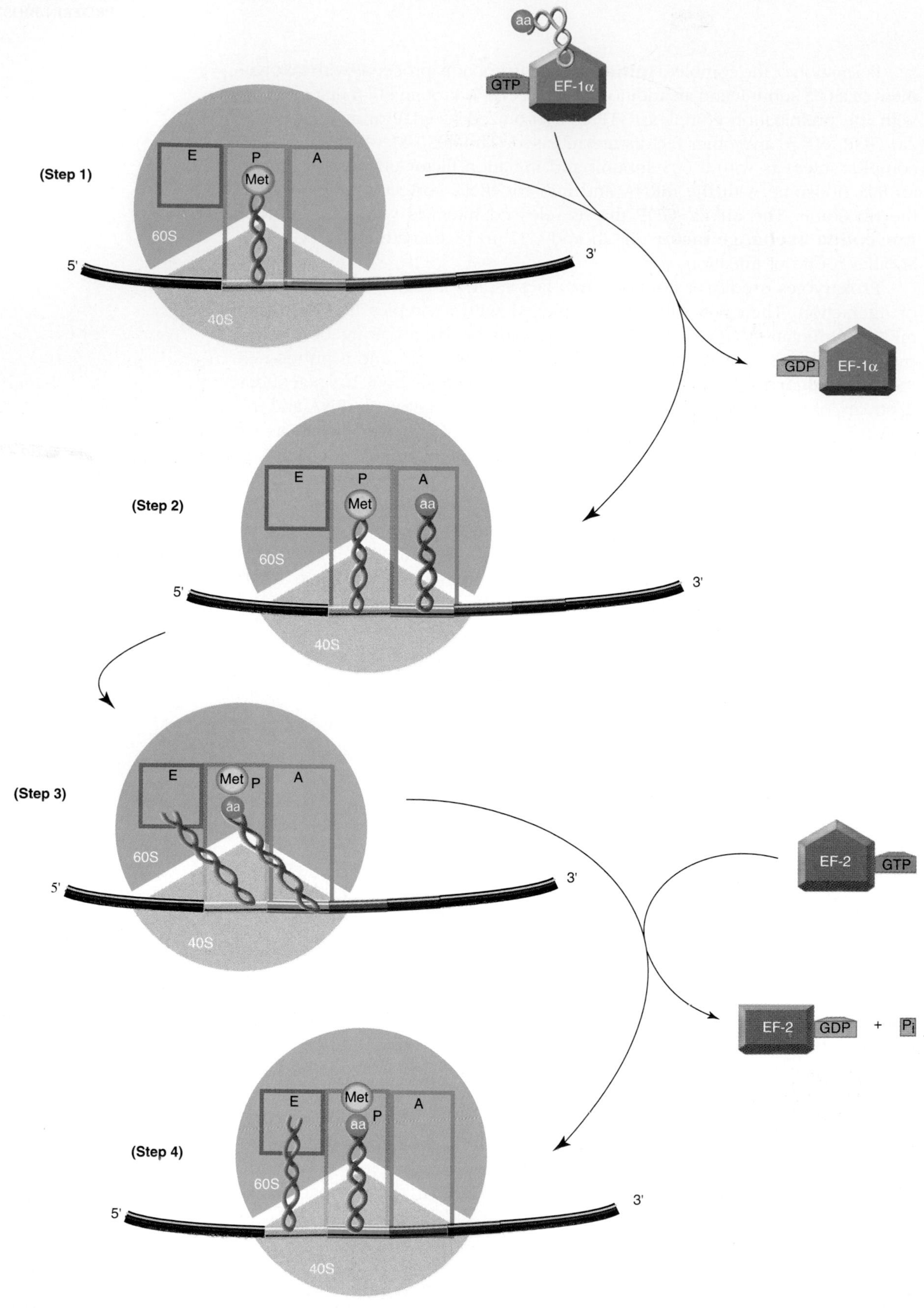

(a)

FIGURE 17.8
Elongation steps in eukaryotic protein synthesis.
(*a*) First cycle of elongation is shown. Step 1 shows completed initiation complex with methionyl $tRNA_i^{Met}$ in 80S P site. At step 2 an aminoacyl-tRNA has been placed in the ribosomal A site with participation of EF-1α. Change in shape of EF-1α shows its conformational change upon GTP hydrolysis. At step 3 the first peptide bond has been formed, new peptidyl tRNA occupies a hybrid (A/P) site on the ribosome, and the deacylated acceptor stem of the $tRNA_i^{Met}$ is displaced to the E site of the large subunit. At step

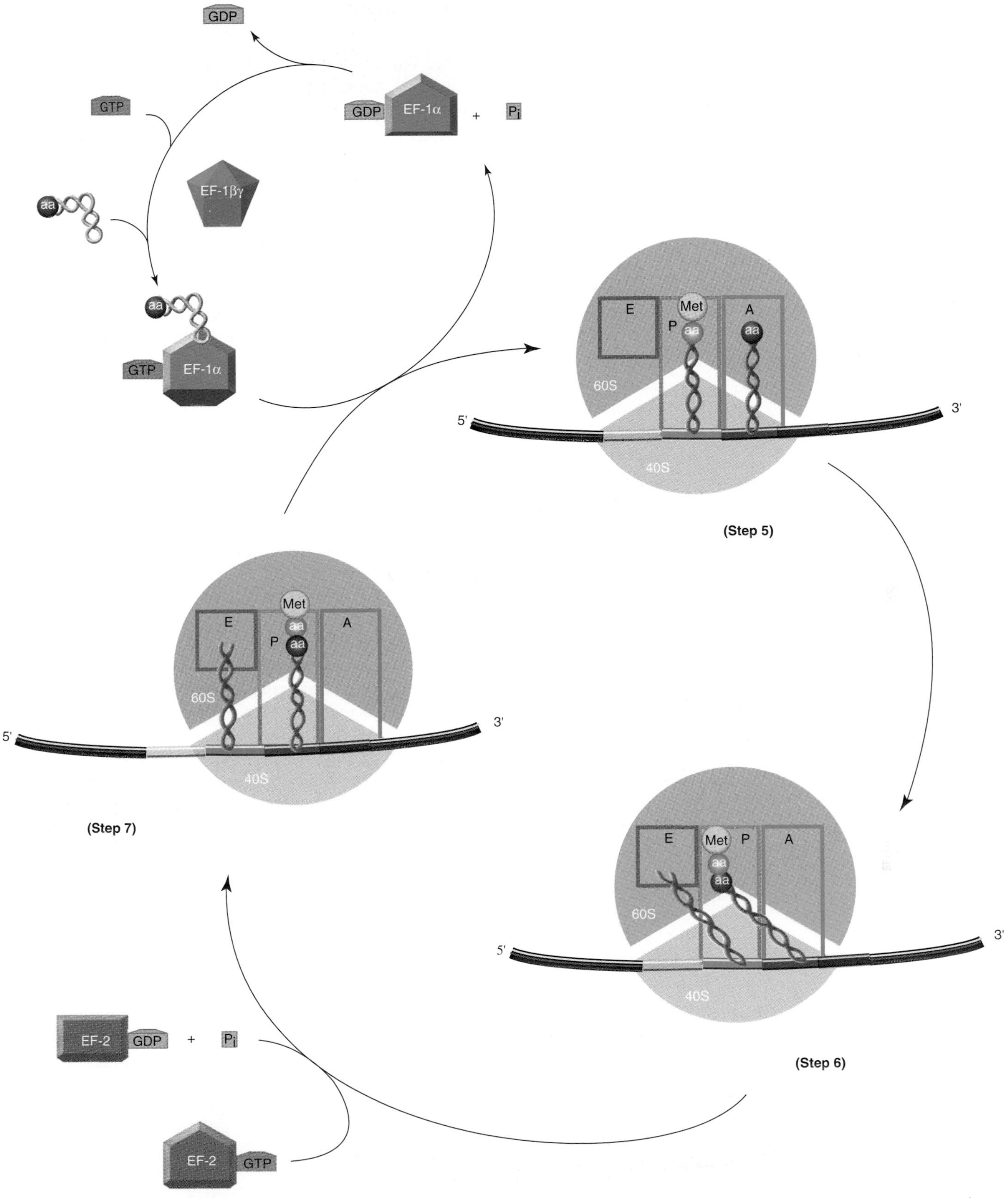

(b)

4 mRNA–peptidyl tRNA complex has been fully translocated to the P site while deacylated initiator tRNA is moved to the E site. (*b*) Further rounds of elongation are depicted. Binding of aminoacyl-tRNA probably causes concomitant release of deacylated tRNA from the E site, resulting in complex at step 5. Formation of the next peptide bond again results in the new peptidyl RNA occupying a hybrid A/P site on the ribosome (step 6), and translocation moves mRNA and new peptidyl tRNA in register into the P site (step 7). Additional amino acids are added by successive repetitions of the cycle. For further details see text.

position on the ribosome. The anticodon remains in the 40S A site, while the acceptor end and the attached peptide are in the 60S P site. The anticodon of the deacylated tRNA remains in the 40S P site, and its acceptor end is located in the 60S exit or **E site.**

The mRNA and the dipeptidyl-tRNA at the 40S A site must now be repositioned to permit another elongation cycle to begin. This is done by **elongation factor 2 (EF-2),** also called **translocase.** EF-2 moves the messenger and dipeptidyl-tRNA, in codon–anticodon register, from the 40S A site to the P site. In the process, GTP is hydrolyzed to GDP plus P_i, providing energy for the movement, and the A site is fully vacated. As the dipeptidyl-tRNA is moved to the P site, the deacylated donor (methionine) tRNA is also moved to the E site, which only exists on the 60S subunit. The ribosome can now enter a new cycle. The next aminoacyl-tRNA specified by the mRNA is delivered by EF-1α to the A site and the deacylated tRNA in the E site is probably released. Peptide transfer again occurs. Successive cycles of binding of aminoacyl-tRNA, peptide bond formation, and translocation result in the stepwise elongation of the polypeptide toward its eventual carboxyl terminus. Note that whatever the length of the growing chain, peptide bond formation always occurs through attack of the α-amino group of the incoming aminoacyl-tRNA on the peptide carboxyl-tRNA linkage; hence the geometric arrangement of the reacting molecules at the peptidyltransferase site remains constant.

Peptide bond formation does not require any additional energy source such as ATP or GTP. The energy of the methionyl (or peptidyl) ester linkage to tRNA drives the reaction toward peptide bond formation; recall that ATP is used to form each aminoacyl-tRNA and that these reactions are reversible. Isolated 60S subunits can catalyze peptidyltransferase activity, and nonribosomal factors are not involved in the reaction. Yet peptidyltransferase has never been dissociated from the large subunit or identified as a specific ribosomal protein. Reconstitution of *E. coli* peptidyltransferase activity requires only five to six different large subunit proteins and the rRNA. Omission or significant modification of the rRNA or any of these proteins causes the loss of peptidyltransferase activity, while other proteins can be deleted with little or no effect. The discovery of catalytic RNA molecules (Chapter 16) led to speculation that the primordial ribosome was an RNA particle in which peptide bond formation was catalyzed by the RNA. Experiments with very conformationally "stable" large subunit RNA from a thermophilic bacterium suggest that the rRNA may be the catalytic component of peptidyltransferase, while the proteins serve to stabilize RNA folding; however, this hypothesis remains controversial and not fully proved.

As determined with their prokaryotic equivalents, the role of GTP in the action of EF-1α and EF-2 probably relates to conformational changes in these proteins. Crystallographic studies have shown that a large rearrangement of domains with movements of several angstroms occurs upon GTP hydrolysis in **EF-Tu,** the prokaryotic equivalent of EF-1α. Both EF-1α and EF-2 bind ribosomes tightly as GTP complexes, while GDP complexes dissociate from the ribosome more easily. Viewed another way, GTP stabilizes a protein conformation that confers upon EF-1α high affinity toward aminoacyl-tRNA and the ribosome, while GDP stabilizes a conformation with lower affinity for aminoacyl-tRNA and ribosome, thus allowing tRNA delivery and factor dissociation. Restoration of the higher affinity GTP-associated conformation of EF-1α requires participation **EF-1$\beta\gamma$** (Figure 17.9). This protein displaces GDP from EF-1α, forming an EF-1α · EF-1$\beta\gamma$ complex. GTP then displaces EF-1$\beta\gamma$, forming an EF-1α · GTP complex that can successively bind an aminoacyl-tRNA and then a ribosome. Prokaryotes use a similar mechanism in which EF-Tu binds GTP and aminoacyl-tRNA and EF-Ts displaces GDP and helps recycle the carrier molecule. Prokaryotes also utilize a GTP-dependent translocase, equivalent to EF-2 but called **EF-G** or G factor.

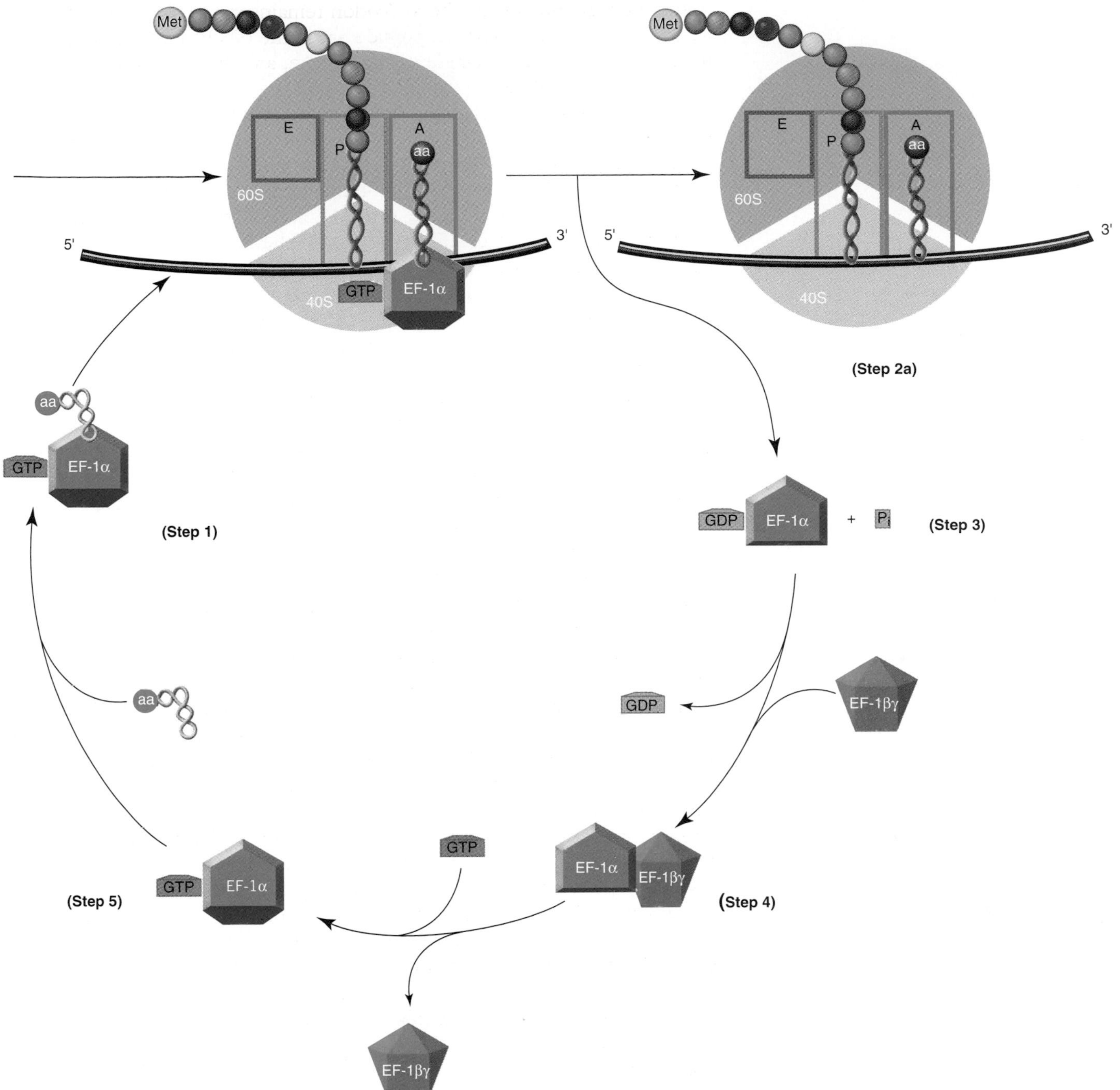

FIGURE 17.9

EF-1 in elongation cycle.

EF-1α · GTP · aminoacyl-tRNA complex (step 1) binds the ribosome (step 2) and transfers aminoacyl-tRNA to the ribosome (step 2a) with concomitant hydrolysis of GTP and a change in conformation of EF-1α (step 3) that reduces its affinity for tRNA and ribosome. The GDP is then displaced from EF-1α by EF-1$\beta\gamma$, resulting in the complex at step 4. Binding of GTP then displaces EF-1$\beta\gamma$ (step 5) and allows binding of an aminoacyl-tRNA by EF-1α in its higher affinity conformation (step 1). In prokaryotes a similar cycle exists; EF-Tu functions as the carrier of aminoacyl-tRNA and EF-Ts is guanine nucleotide exchange factor.

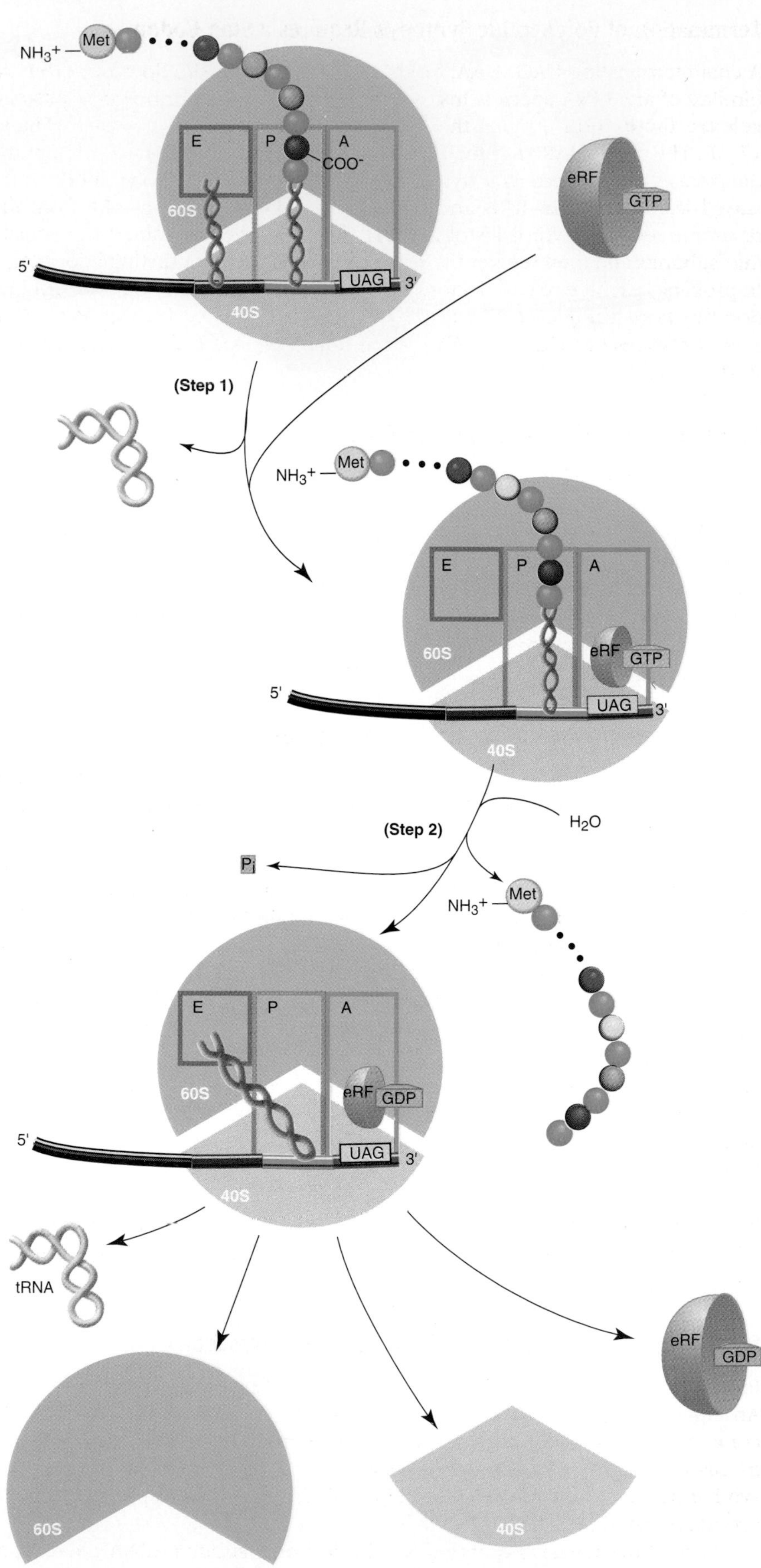

FIGURE 17.10
Model of termination of protein biosynthesis.
When a termination codon (UAG, UAA, or UGA) in mRNA occupies the ribosomal A site, binding of release factor–GTP complex occurs (step 1), probably with concomitant release of deacylated tRNA from the ribosomal E site. In step 2 peptidyltransferase now functions as a hydrolase; protein is released by hydrolysis of the ester bond linking it to tRNA, and acceptor end of deacylated tRNA is probably displaced. GTP is hydrolyzed to GDP and P_i, presumably altering the conformation of the release factor. Complex is now dissociated and components can enter additional rounds of protein synthesis.

Termination of Polypeptide Synthesis Requires a Stop Codon

A chain-terminating UAG, UAA, or UGA codon in the A site does not promote binding of any tRNA species. Instead, another complex nonribosomal protein, **release factor** (eRF), binds the ribosome as an eRF·GTP complex (Figure 17.10). The peptide–tRNA ester linkage is cleaved through the action of peptidyl transferase, acting here as a hydrolase, and the completed polypeptide is released from its carrier tRNA and the ribosome. Dissociation of eRF from the ribosome requires hydrolysis of the GTP and frees the ribosome to dissociate into subunits and then reenter the protein synthesis cycle at the initiation stage. In prokaryotes three release factors, RF-1, RF-2, and RF-3, carry out the termination function. The factor RF-1 acts in response to UAG or UAA codons, RF-2 acts in response to UGA or UAA codons, and RF-3 is a GTPase that activates RF-1 and RF-2.

Translation Has Significant Energy Cost

There is a considerable use of energy in synthesis of a polypeptide. Amino acid activation converts an ATP to AMP and pyrophosphate, which is normally hydrolyzed to P_i; the net cost is two high-energy phosphates. Two more high-energy bonds are hydrolyzed in the actions of EF-1α and EF-2, for a total of four per peptide bond formed. Posttranslational modifications may add to the energy cost, and of course energy is needed for biosynthesis of the multi-use mRNA, tRNAs, ribosomes, and protein factors, but these costs are distributed among the proteins formed during their lifetime.

Protein Synthesis in Mitochondria Differs Slightly

Many characteristics of mitochondria suggest that they are descendants of aerobic prokaryotes that invaded and set up a symbiotic relationship within a eukaryotic cell. Some of their independence and prokaryotic character are retained. Human mitochondria have a circular DNA genome of 16,569 base pairs that encodes 13 proteins, 22 tRNA species, and two mitochondrion-specific rRNA species. Their independent apparatus for protein synthesis includes RNA polymerase, aminoacyl-tRNA synthetases, tRNAs, and ribosomes. Although the course of protein biosynthesis in mitochondria is like that in the cytosol, some details are different. The synthetic components, tRNAs, aminoacyl-tRNA synthetases, and ribosomes, are unique to the mitochondrion. The number of tRNA species is small and the genetic code is slightly different (see Table 17.3). Mitochondrial ribosomes are smaller and the rRNAs are shorter than those of either the eukaryotic cytosol or of prokaryotes (see Table 17.1). An initiator Met-tRNA$_i^{Met}$ is modified by a **transformylase** that uses N^{10}-formyl H$_4$-folate to produce fMet-tRNA$_i^{Met}$. Most mitochondrial proteins are encoded in nuclear DNA and synthesized in the cytosol, but mitochondrial protein synthesis is clearly important (see Clin. Corr. 17.4). Cells must also coordinate protein synthesis within mitochondria with the cytosolic synthesis of proteins destined for import into mitochondria.

Some Antibiotics and Toxins Inhibit Protein Biosynthesis

Protein biosynthesis is central to the continuing life and reproduction of cells. An organism can gain a biological advantage by interfering in the ability of its competitors to synthesize proteins, and many antibiotics and toxins function in this way. Some are selective for prokaryotic rather than eukaryotic protein synthesis and so are extremely useful in clinical practice. Examples of antibiotic action are listed in Table 17.8.

Several mechanisms of interfering in ribosome subunit–tRNA interactions are utilized by different antibiotics. **Streptomycin** binds the small subunit of

CLINICAL CORRELATION 17.4

Mutation in Mitochondrial Ribosomal RNA Results in Antibiotic-Induced Deafness

In some regions of China a significant percentage of irreversible cases of deafness has been linked to use of normally safe and effective amounts of aminoglycoside antibiotics such as streptomycin and gentamicin. The unusual sensitivity to aminoglycosides is transmitted only through women. This maternal transmission suggests a mitochondrial locus, since sperm do not contribute mitochondria to the zygote. Aminoglycosides are normally targeted to bacterial ribosomes, so the mitochondrial ribosome is a logical place to look for a mutation site.

A single A → G point mutation at nucleotide 1555 of the gene on mitochondrial DNA for the rDNA of the large subunit has been identified in three families with this susceptibility to aminoglycosides. The mutation site is in a highly conserved region of the rRNA sequence that is known to be involved in aminoglycoside binding; some mutations in the same region confer resistance to the antibiotics, and the RNA region is part of the ribosomal A site. It is hypothesized that the mutation makes the region more "prokaryote-like," increasing its affinity for aminoglycosides and the ability of the antibiotic to interfere in protein synthesis in the mitochondrion. Proteins synthesized in the mitochondrion are needed to form the enzyme complexes of the oxidative phosphorylation system, so affected cells are starved of ATP. Aminoglycosides accumulate in the cochlea, making this a particularly sensitive target and leading to sensorineural deafness.

Fischel-Ghodsian, N., Prezant, T., Bu., X., and Öztas, S. Mitochondrial ribosomal RNA gene mutation in a patient with sporadic aminoglycoside ototoxicity. *Am. J. Otolaryngol.* 14:399, 1993. Prezant, T., Agapian, J., Bohlman. M., et al. Mitochondrial ribosomal RNA mutation associated with both antibiotic-induced and non-syndromic deafness. *Nature Genetics* 4:289, 1993.

prokaryotic ribosomes, interferes with the initiation of protein synthesis, and causes misreading of mRNA. Although streptomycin does not directly bind ribosomal protein S12 of the small subunit, mutations in this protein or in the small subunit rRNA can confer resistance to or even dependence on streptomycin. Protein S12 is involved in tRNA binding, and streptomycin alters the interactions of tRNA with the ribosomal subunit and mRNA, probably by affecting subunit conformation. Other **aminoglycoside antibiotics,** such as the **neomycins** or **gentamicins,** also cause mistranslation; they interact with the small ribosomal subunit, but at sites that differ from that for streptomycin. The aminoglycoside **kasugamycin** binds small subunits and inhibits the initiation of translation. Kasugamycin sensitivity depends on base methylation that normally occurs on two adjacent adenine moieties of small subunit rRNA. **Tetracyclines** bind directly to ribosomes and interfere in aminoacyl-tRNA binding.

Other antibiotics interfere with elongation. **Puromycin** (Figure 17.11) resembles an aminoacyl-tRNA; it binds at the ribosomal A site and acts as an acceptor in the peptidyltransferase reaction. However, since it does not interact with mRNA it cannot be translocated, and since its aminoacyl derivative is not in an ester linkage to the nucleoside it cannot serve as a peptide donor. Thus puromycin prematurely terminates translation, leading to release of peptidyl-puromycin. **Chloramphenicol** directly inhibits peptidyltransferase by binding the transferase center; no transfer occurs, and peptidyl-tRNA remains associated

TABLE 17.8 Some Inhibitors of Protein Biosynthesis

Inhibitor	*Processes Affected*	*Site of Action*
Streptomycin	Initiation, elongation	Prokaryotes: 30S subunit
Neomycins	Translation	Prokaryotes: multiple sites
Tetracyclines	Aminoacyl-tRNA binding	30S or 40S subunits
Puromycin	Peptide transfer	70S or 80S ribosomes
Erythromycin	Translocation	Prokaryotes: 50S subunit
Fusidic acid	Translocation	Prokaryotes: EF-G
Cycloheximide	Elongation	Eukaryotes: 80S ribosomes
Ricin	Multiple	Eukaryotes: 60S subunit

with the ribosome. The translocation step is also a potential target. **Erythromycin,** a macrolide antibiotic, interferes with translocation on prokaryotic ribosomes. Eukaryotic translocation is inhibited by **diphtheria toxin,** a protein toxin produced by *Corynebacterium diphtheriae*; the toxin binds at the cell membrane and a subunit enters the cytoplasm and catalyzes the ADP-ribosylation and inactivation of EF-2, as represented in the reaction:

$$\underset{\text{(active)}}{\text{EF-2}} + \text{NAD}^+ \rightleftarrows \underset{\text{(inactive)}}{\text{ADP-ribosyl EF-2}} + \text{nicotinamide} + \text{H}^+$$

ADP-ribose is attached to EF-2 at a posttranslationally modified histidine residue known as diphthamide. Posttranslational events are discussed in the next section.

A third group of toxins attack the rRNA. **Ricin** (from castor beans) and related toxins are *N*-glycosidases that cleave a single adenine from the large subunit rRNA backbone. The ribosome is inactivated by this apparently minor damage. A fungal toxin, **α-sarcin,** cleaves large subunit rRNA at a single site and similarly inactivates the ribosome. Some *E. coli* strains make extracellular toxins that affect other bacteria. One of these, **colicin E3,** is a ribonuclease that cleaves 16S RNA near the mRNA-binding sequence and decoding region; it thus inactivates the small subunit and halts protein synthesis in competitors of the colicin-producing cell.

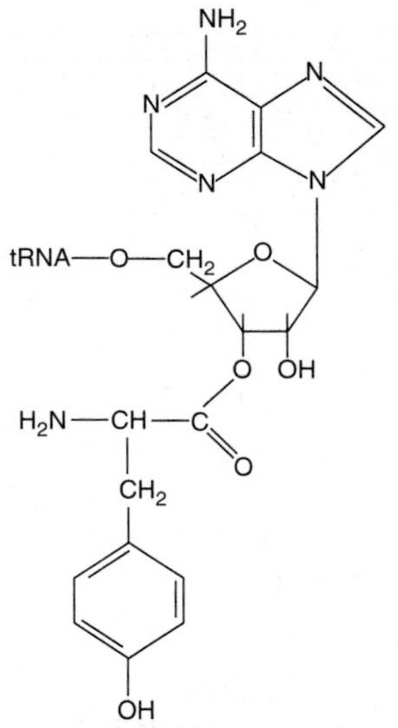

FIGURE 17.11
Puromycin (right) interferes with protein synthesis by functioning as an analog of aminoacyl-tRNA, here tyrosyl-tRNA (left) in peptidyltransferase reaction.

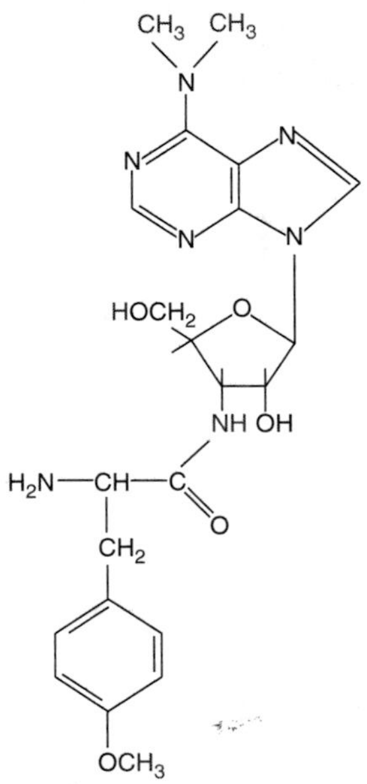

17.4 PROTEIN MATURATION: MODIFICATION, SECRETION, AND TARGETING

Some proteins emerge from the ribosome ready to function, while others undergo a variety of **posttranslational modifications.** These alterations may result in conversion to a functional form, direction to a specific subcellular compartment, secretion from the cell, or an alteration in activity or stability. Information that determines the posttranslational fate of a protein resides in its structure: that is, the amino acid sequence and conformation of the polypeptide determine whether a protein will be a substrate for a modifying enzyme and/or identify it for direction to a subcellular or extracellular location.

Proteins for Export Follow the Secretory Pathway

Proteins destined for export are synthesized on membrane-bound ribosomes of the rough endoplasmic reticulum (ER) (Figure 17.12). A ribosome has no means of classifying the polypeptide it is about to synthesize, so initiation and elongation begin on free cytosolic ribosomes. Proteins of the secretory pathway have a hydrophobic **signal peptide,** usually at or near their amino terminus. There is no unique signal peptide sequence, but its characteristics include a positively charged N terminus, a core of 8–12 hydrophobic amino acids, and a more polar C-terminal segment that eventually serves as a cleavage site for excision of the signal peptide.

The signal peptide of 15–30 amino acids emerges from the ribosome early during polypeptide synthesis. As it appears it is bound by a cytosolic **signal recognition particle (SRP)** (see Figure 17.13). The SRP is an elongated particle made up of six different proteins plus a small (7S) RNA molecule that serves as a backbone. Binding to SRP halts protein synthesis and the ribosome moves to the ER. SRP recognizes and binds to an **SRP receptor** or **"docking protein,"** localized at the cytosolic surface of the ER membrane, in a reaction that requires GTP hydrolysis and presumably involves conformational changes in the SRP and/or the receptor. The ribosome is transferred to a **"translocon,"** a ribosome receptor on the membrane that serves as a passageway through the membrane. Both SRP and docking protein are freed to direct other ribosomes to the ER,

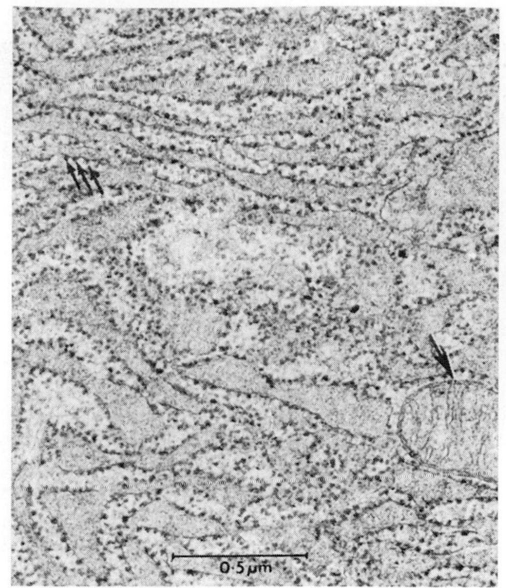

FIGURE 17.12
Rough endoplasmic reticulum of a plasma cell.
Three parallel arrows indicate three ribosomes among the many attached to the extensive membranes. Single arrow indicates a mitochondrion for comparison.
Courtesy of Dr. U. Jarlfors, University of Miami.

and the translational block caused by SRP binding is relieved. The hydrophobic signal sequence, probably complexed by a receptor protein, is inserted into the membrane, further anchoring the ribosome to the ER. Translation and extrusion into or through the membrane are now coupled. Translocon proteins form a pore or channel through which the growing polypeptide passes; even very hydrophilic or ionic segments are directed through the hydrophobic membrane into the ER lumen and folding into secondary and tertiary structures begins.

The completed export-destined protein within the ER lumen will probably be anchored to the membrane by the signal peptide. A cleavage site on the protein is hydrolyzed by **signal peptidase,** an integral membrane protein located at the luminal surface of the ER. The protein completes folding into a three-dimensional conformation, disulfide bonds can form, and components of multisubunit proteins may assemble. Other steps may include proteolytic processing and glycosylation that occur within the ER lumen and during transit of the protein through the Golgi apparatus and into secretory vesicles.

Glycosylation of Proteins Occurs in the Endoplasmic Reticulum and Golgi Apparatus

Glycosylation of proteins to form glycoproteins (see p. 60) is important for two reasons. Glycosylation alters the properties of proteins, changing their stability, solubility, and physical bulk. In addition, carbohydrates of glycoproteins act as recognition signals that are central to aspects of protein targeting and for cellular recognition of proteins and other cells. Glycosylation can involve addition of a few carbohydrate residues or the formation of large branched oligosaccharide chains. Sites and types of glycosylation are determined by the presence on a protein of appropriate amino acids and sequences, and by availability of enzymes and substrates to carry out the glycosylation reactions.

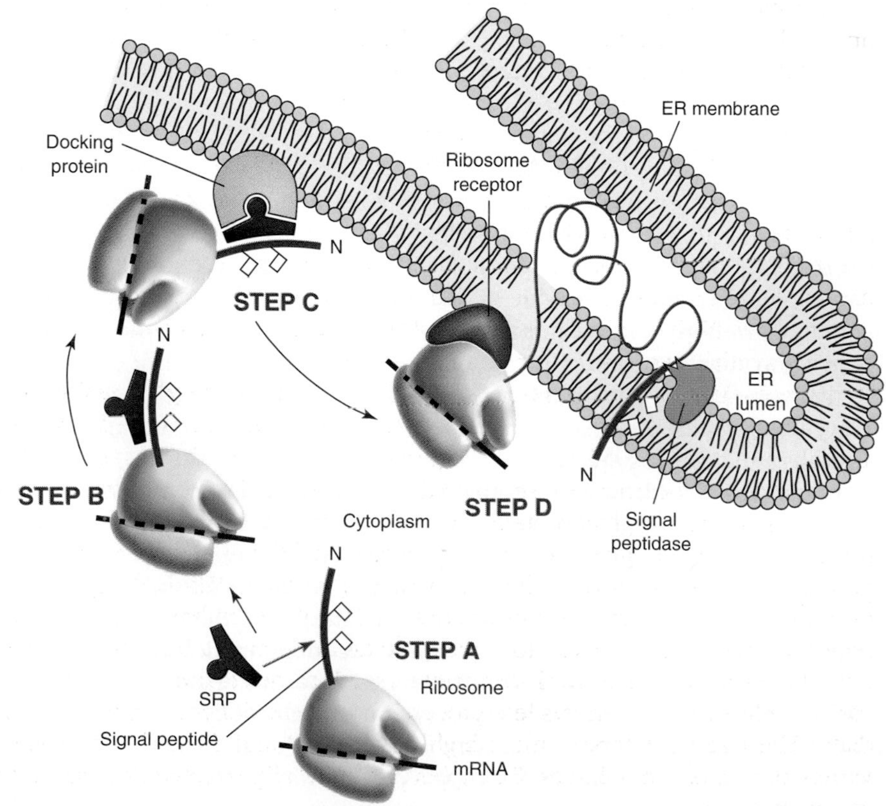

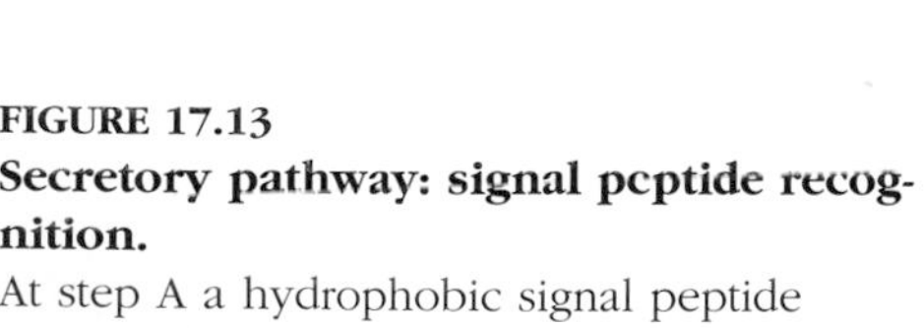

FIGURE 17.13
Secretory pathway: signal peptide recognition.
At step A a hydrophobic signal peptide emerges from the exit site of a free ribosome in the cytosol. Signal recognition particle (SRP) recognizes and binds the peptide and peptide elongation is temporarily halted (step B). The ribosome moves to the ER membrane where docking protein binds to SRP (step C). In step D the ribosome is transferred to a ribosome receptor or translocon, protein biosynthesis is resumed, and newly synthesized protein is extruded through the membrane into the ER lumen.

TABLE 17.9 Glycosyltransferases in Eukaryotic Cells

Sugar Transferred	*Abbreviation*	*Donors*	*Glycosyltransferase*
Mannose	Man	GDP-Man Dolichol-Man	Mannosyltransferase
Galactose	Gal	UDP-Gal	Galactosyltransferase
Glucose	Glc	UDP-Glc Dolichol-Glc	Glucosyltransferase
Fucose	Fuc	GDP-Fuc	Fucosyltransferase
N-Acetylgalactosamine	GalNAc	UDP-GalNac	*N*-acetylgalactosaminyltransferase
N-Acetylglucosamine	GlcNAc	UDP-GlcNAc	*N*-acetylglucosaminyltransferase
N-Acetylneuraminic acid (or sialic acid)	NANA or NeuNAc SA	CMP-NANA CMP-SA	*N*-Acetylneuraminyltransferase (sialyltransferase)

Glycosylation involves many **glycosyltransferases,** classes of which are summarized in Table 17.9. Up to 100 different enzymes each carry out a similar basic reaction in which a sugar is transferred from an activated donor substrate to an acceptor, usually another sugar residue that is part of an oligosaccharide under construction. The enzymes show three kinds of specificity: for the monosaccharide that is transferred, for structure and sequence of the acceptor molecule, and for the site and configuration of the anomeric linkage formed.

One class of glycoproteins has sugars linked through the amide nitrogen of asparagine residues in the process of ***N*-linked glycosylation.** The antibiotic **tunicamycin,** which prevents *N*-glycosylation, has been valuable in elucidating the biosynthetic pathway. Formation of *N*-linked oligosaccharides begins in the ER lumen and continues after transport of the protein to the Golgi apparatus. A specific sequence, Asn-X-Thr (or Ser) in which X may be any amino acid except proline or aspartic acid, is required for *N*-glycosylation. Not all Asn-X-Thr/Ser sequences are glycosylated because some may be unavailable due to protein conformation.

Biosynthesis of *N*-linked oligosaccharides begins with the synthesis of a lipid-linked intermediate (Figure 17.14). **Dolichol phosphate** (structure on p. 350) at the cytoplasmic surface of the ER membrane serves as glycosyl acceptor of *N*-acetylglucosamine. The GlcNAc-pyrophosphoryldolichol is an acceptor for stepwise glycosylation and formation of a branched $(Man)_5(GlcNAc)_2$-pyrophosphoryldolichol on the cytosolic side of the membrane. This intermediate is then reoriented to the luminal surface of the ER membrane, and four additional mannose and then three glucose residues are sequentially added to complete the structure. The complete oligosaccharide is then transferred from its dolichol carrier to an asparagine residue of the polypeptide as it emerges into the ER lumen. Thus *N*-glycosylation is **cotranslational,** that is, occurs as the protein is being synthesized, hence it can affect protein folding.

Processing or **modification** of the oligosaccharide by **glycosidases** involves removal of some sugar residues from the newly transferred structure. The glucose residues, which were required for transfer of the oligosaccharide from the dolichol carrier, are sequentially removed, as is one mannose. These alterations mark the glycoprotein for transport to the Golgi apparatus where further trimming by glycosidases may occur. Additional sugars may also be added by a variety of glycosyltransferases. The resulting *N*-linked oligosaccharides are diverse, but two classes are distinguishable. Each has a common core region ($GlcNAc_2Man_3$) linked to asparagine and originating from the dolichol-linked intermediate. The **high-mannose** type includes mannose residues in a variety of linkages and shows less processing from the dolichol-linked intermediate. The **complex** type is more highly processed and diverse, with a larger variety of sugars and linkages. Examples of mature oligosaccharides are shown in Figure 17.15.

The second major class of glycoproteins have sugars that are bound through either serine or threonine hydroxyl groups. Such O-linked glycosylation occurs only after the protein has reached the Golgi apparatus, hence ***O*-glycosylation** is posttranslational and occurs only on fully folded proteins. *O*-linked carbohydrates always involve *N*-acetylgalactosamine attachment to a serine or threonine residue of the protein. There is no defined amino acid sequence in which the

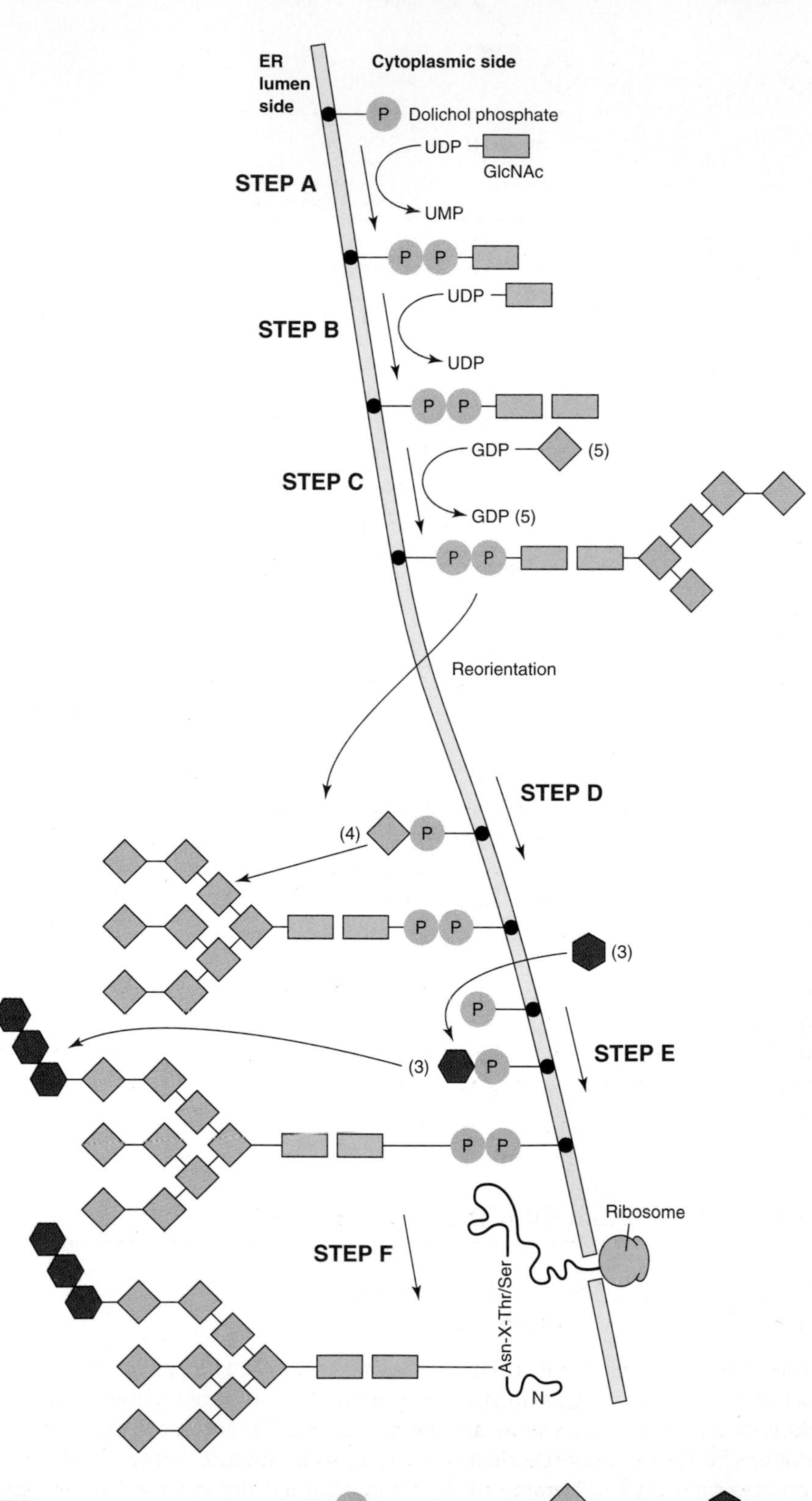

FIGURE 17.14
Biosynthesis of *N*-linked oligosaccharides at the surface of the endoplasmic reticulum.
Synthesis is initiated on the cytoplasmic face of the ER membrane by transfer of *N*-acetylglucosamine phosphate to a dolichol acceptor (step A) followed by formation of the first glycosidic bond upon transfer of a second residue of *N*-acetylglucosamine (step B). Five residues of mannose are then added sequentially (step C) from a GDP mannose carrier. At this stage lipid-linked oligosaccharide is reoriented to the luminal face of the membrane, and additional mannose (step D) and glucose (step E) residues are transferred from dolichol-linked intermediates. Dolichol sugars are generated from cytosol nucleoside diphosphate sugars. The completed oligosaccharide is finally transferred to a protein in the process of being synthesized at the membrane surface; signal peptide may have already been cleaved at this point.

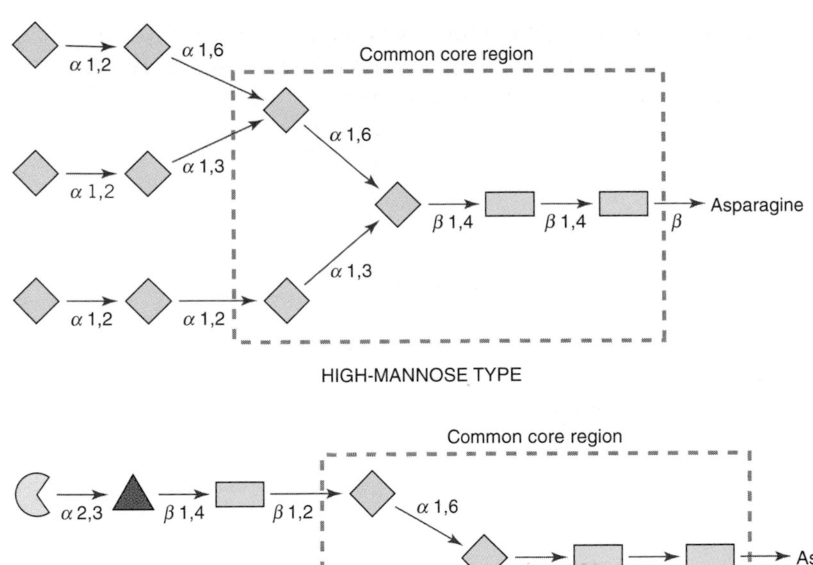

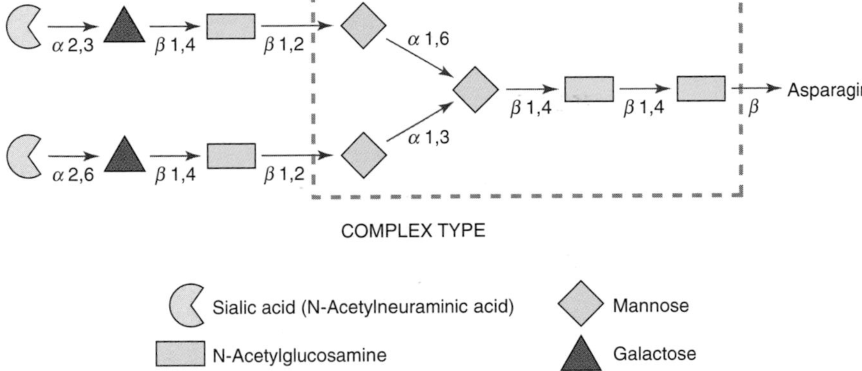

FIGURE 17.15
Structure of *N*-linked oligosaccharides. Basic structures of both types of *N*-linked oligosaccharides are shown. In each case structure is derived from that of the initial dolichol-linked oligosaccharide through action of glycosidases and glycosyltransferases. Note the variety of glycosidic linkages involved in these structures.

serine or threonine must occur, but only residues whose side chains are in an appropriate environment on the protein surface serve as acceptors for the GalNAc-transferase.

Sequential addition of sugars to the GalNAc acceptor follows, using the same glycosyltransferases that modified *N*-linked oligosaccharides in the Golgi apparatus. The structures synthesized depend on types and amounts of glycosyltransferases in a given cell. If an acceptor is a substrate for more than one transferase, the amount of each transferase controls the competition between them. Some oligosaccharides may be formed that are not acceptors for any glycosyltransferase present, hence no further growth of the chain occurs. Other structures may be excellent acceptors that continue to grow until completed by one of a number of nonacceptor termination sequences. These processes can lead to many different oligosaccharide structures on otherwise identical proteins, so heterogeneity in glycoproteins is common. Examples are shown in Figure 17.16.

17.5 ■ ORGANELLE TARGETING AND BIOGENESIS

Sorting of Proteins Targeted for Lysosomes Occurs in the Secretory Pathway

Protein transport from ER to Golgi apparatus occurs through carrier vesicles that bud from the ER. This transport requires GTP; inhibitors of oxidative phosphorylation cause proteins to accumulate in the ER and vesicles. Sorting of proteins for their ultimate destinations occurs in conjunction with their glycosylation and proteolytic trimming as they pass through the cis, medial, and trans elements of the Golgi apparatus.

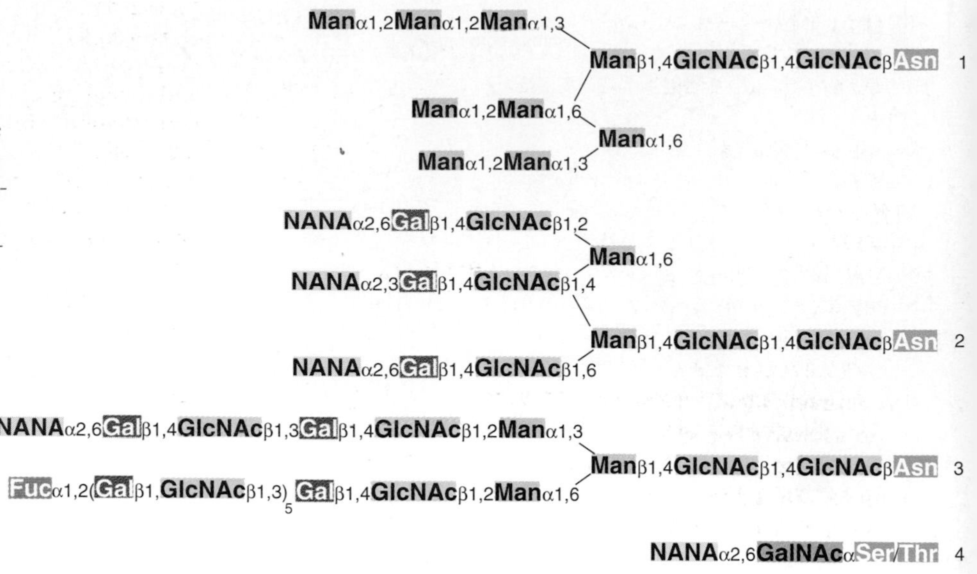

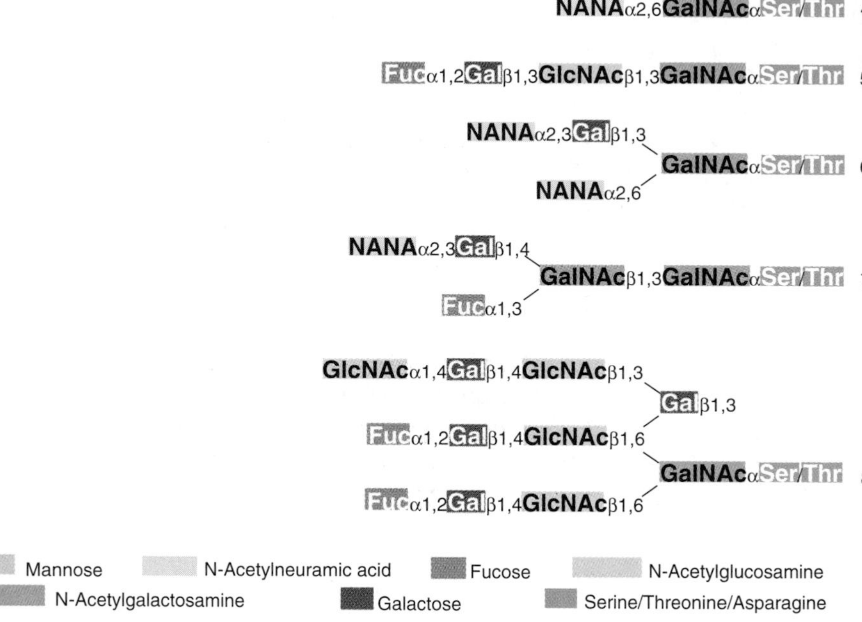

FIGURE 17.16
Examples of oligosaccharide structure. Structures 1–3 are typical *N*-linked oligosaccharides of high-mannose (1) and complex types (2, 3); note the common core structure from the protein asparagine residue through the first branch point. Structures 4–8 are common *O*-linked oligosaccharides that may be quite simple or highly complex. Note that although the core structure (GalNAc-Ser/Thr) is unlike that of *N*-linked oligosaccharides, the termini can be quite similar (e.g., structures 2 and 6, 3, and 7). Abbreviations: Man = mannose; Gal = galactose; Fuc = fucose; GlcNAc = *N*-acetylglucosamine; GalNAc = *N*-acetylgalactosamine; NANA = *N*-acetylneuraminic acid (sialic acid).
Adapted from J. Paulson, Trends Biochem. Sci. *14:272, 1989.*

CLINICAL CORRELATION 17.5

I-Cell Disease

I-cell disease (mucolipidosis II) and pseudo-Hurler polydystrophy (mucolipidosis III) are related diseases that arise from defects in lysosomal enzyme targeting because of a deficiency in the enzyme that transfers *N*-acetylglucosamine phosphate to the high mannose-type oligosaccharides of proteins destined for the lysosome. Fibroblasts from affected individuals show dense inclusion bodies (hence I-cells) and are defective in multiple lysosomal enzymes that are found secreted into the medium. Patients have abnormally high levels of lysosomal enzymes in their sera and other body fluids. The disease is characterized by severe psychomotor retardation, many skeletal abnormalities, coarse facial features, and restricted joint movement. Symptoms are usually observable at birth and progress until death, usually by age 8. Pseudo-Hurler polydystrophy is a much milder form of the disease. Onset is usually delayed until the age of 2–4 years, the disease progresses more slowly, and patients survive into adulthood. Prenatal diagnosis of both diseases is possible, but there is as yet no definitive treatment.

For a review of lysosomal enzyme trafficking, see Kornfeld, S. *J. Clin. Invest.* 77:1, 1986. For a comprehensive review of these diseases, see Kornfeld, S., and Sly, W. S., I-cEll disease and pseudo-Hurler polydystrophy. In: C. R. Scriver, A. L. Beaudet, W. S. Sly, and D. Valle (Eds.), *The Molecular and Metabolic Basis of Inherited Disease,* 7th ed. New York: McGraw-Hill, 1995, pp. 2495–2508.

The best understood sorting process is targeting of specific glycoproteins to **lysosomes.** In the cis Golgi some aspect of tertiary structure allows lysosomal proteins to be recognized by a glycosyltransferase that attaches *N*-acetylglucosamine phosphate (GlcNAc-P) to high-mannose type oligosaccharides. A glycosidase then removes the GlcNAc, forming an oligosaccharide that contains **mannose 6-phosphate** (Figure 17.17) that is recognized by a receptor protein responsible for compartmentation and vesicular transport of these proteins to lysosomes. Other oligosaccharide chains on the proteins may be further processed to form complex type structures, but the mannose 6-phosphate determines the lysosomal destination of these proteins. Patients with **I-cell disease** lack the GlcNAc-P glycosyltransferase and cannot correctly mark lysosomal enzymes for their destination. Thus the enzymes are secreted from the cell (see Clin. Corr. 17.5).

Other sorting signals are reasonably well understood. Proteins are retained in the ER lumen in response to a C-terminal KDEL (Lys-Asp-Glu-Leu) sequence, and a different sequence in an exposed C terminus signals retention in the ER membrane. Transmembrane domains have been identified that result in reten-

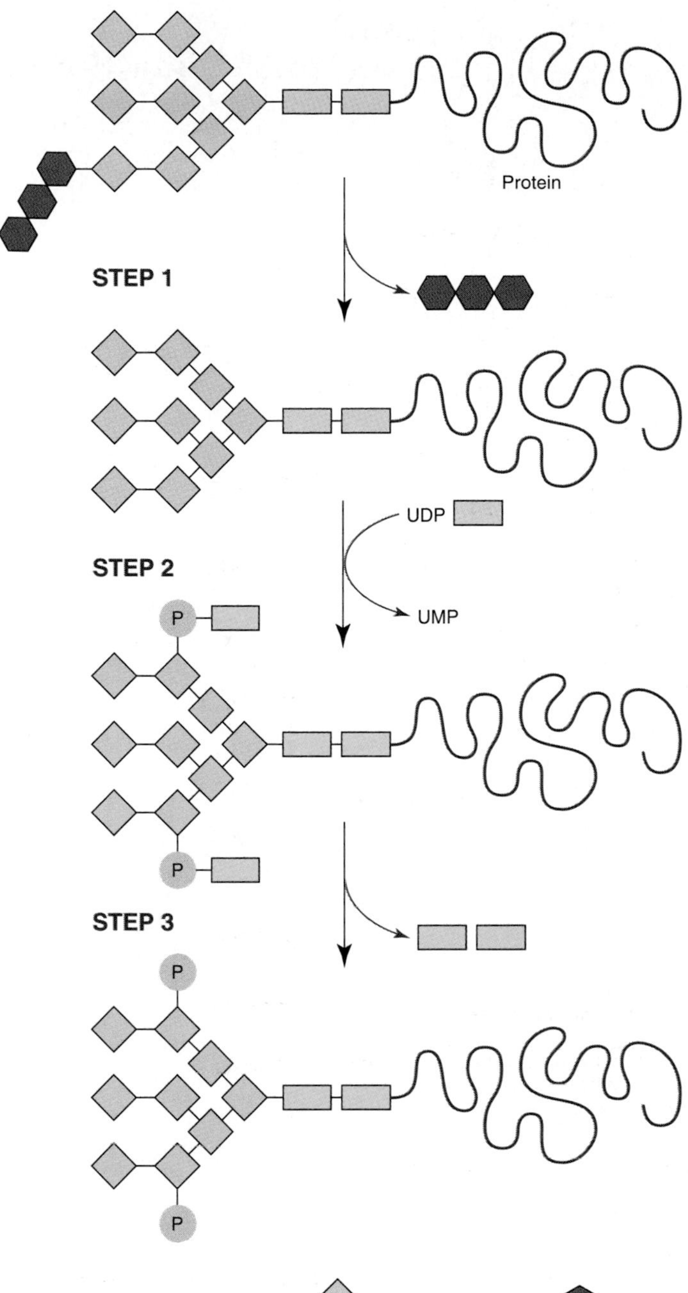

FIGURE 17.17
Targeting of enzymes to lysosomes.
Completed *N*-linked glycoprotein is released from ER membrane, and during transport to and through the Golgi apparatus the oligosaccharide is modified by glycosidases that remove glucose residues (step 1). Some mannose residues may also be removed. An element of protein structure is then recognized by a glycosyltransferase that transfers one or sometimes two *N*-acetylglucosamine phosphate residues to the oligosaccharide (step 2). A glycosidase removes *N*-acetylglucosamine, leaving one or two mannose 6-phosphate residues on the oligosaccharide (step 3). The protein is then recognized by a mannose 6-phosphate receptor and directed to lysosomes.
Adapted from R. Kornfeld and S. Kornfeld, Annu. Rev. Biochem. *54:631, 1985.*

tion in the Golgi. Polypeptide-specific glycosylation and sulfation of some glycoprotein hormones in the anterior pituitary mediate their sorting into storage granules. Polysialic acid modification of a neural cell adhesion protein appears to be both specific to the protein and regulated developmentally. Many other sorting signals must still be deciphered to explain fully how the Golgi apparatus directs proteins to its own subcompartments, various storage and secretory granules, and specific elements of the plasma membrane.

The secretory pathway directs proteins to lysosomes, the plasma membrane, or outside the cell. Proteins of the ER and Golgi apparatus are targeted through partial use of the pathway. For example, localization of proteins on either side of or spanning the ER membrane can utilize the signal recogni-

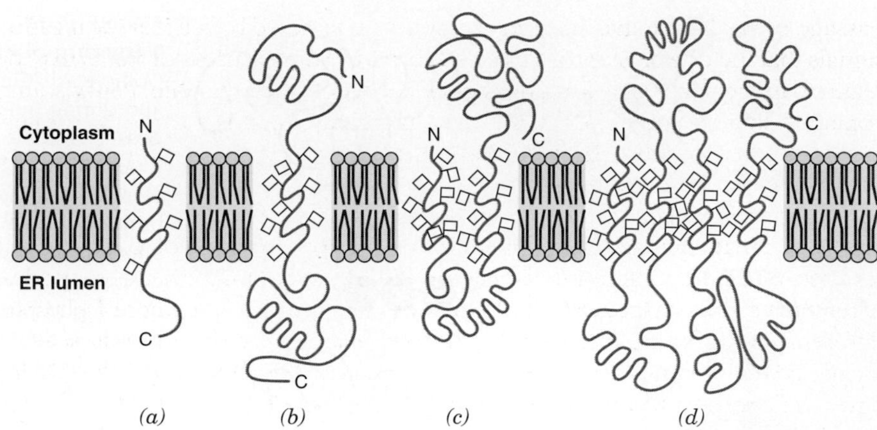

FIGURE 17.18
Topology of proteins at membranes of endoplasmic reticulum.
Proteins are shown in several orientations with respect to the membrane. In (*a*) the protein is anchored to the luminal surface of the membrane by an uncleaved signal peptide. In (*b*) the signal sequence is not near the N terminus; a domain of the protein was synthesized before emergence of signal peptide. Insertion of the internal signal sequence, followed by completion of translation, resulted in a protein with a cytoplasmic N-terminal domain, a membrane-spanning central segment, and a C-terminal domain in the ER lumen. Diagram (*c*) shows a protein with the opposite orientation: an N-terminal signal sequence, which might also have been cleaved by signal peptidase, resulted in extrusion of a segment of protein into the ER lumen. A second hydrophobic anchoring sequence remained membrane associated and prevented passage of the rest of the protein through the membrane, thus allowing formation of a C-terminal cytoplasmic domain. In (*d*), several internal signal and anchoring sequences allow various segments of the protein to be oriented on each side of the membrane.

tion particle in slightly different ways (Figure 17.18). If the signal sequence is downstream from the amino terminus of the protein, the amino end may not be inserted into the membrane and may remain on the cytoplasmic surface. Internal hydrophobic anchoring sequences within a protein can allow much of the sequence either to remain on the cytoplasmic surface or to be retained, anchored on the luminal surface of the ER membrane. Multiple anchoring sequences in a single polypeptide can cause it to span the membrane several times and thus be largely buried in it. Such hydrophobic sequences are separated by polar loops whose orientation is determined by positively charged flanking residues that predominate on the cytoplasmic side of the membrane.

Import of Proteins by Mitochondria Requires Specific Signals

Mitochondria provide a particularly complex targeting problem since specific proteins are located in the mitochondrial matrix, inner or outer membrane, or intermembrane space. Most of these proteins are synthesized in the cytosol on free ribosomes and imported into the mitochondrion, and most are synthesized as larger preproteins; N-terminal presequences mark the protein not only for the mitochondrion but also for a specific subcompartment. The **mitochondrial matrix targeting signal** is not a specific sequence, but rather a positively charged amphiphilic α-helix. With the aid of a protein chaperone, it is recognized by a **mitochondrial receptor** and the protein is translocated across both membranes and into the mitochondrial matrix in an energy-dependent reaction. Passage occurs at adhesion sites where the inner and outer membranes are close together. Proteases remove the matrix targeting signal but may leave other sequences that further sort the protein within the mitochondrion. For example, a clipped precursor of cytochrome-b_2 is moved back across the inner membrane in response to a hydrophobic signal sequence. Further proteolysis frees the protein in the intermembrane space. In contrast, cytochrome-*c* apoprotein (without heme) binds at the outer membrane and is passed into the intermembrane space. There it acquires its heme and undergoes a conformational change that prevents return to the cytosol. Outer membrane localization can utilize the matrix targeting mechanism to translocate part of the protein, but a large apolar sequence blocks full transfer and leaves a membrane-bound protein with a C-terminal domain on the surface of the mitochondrion.

Targeting to Other Organelles Requires Specific Signals

Nuclei must import many proteins involved in their own structure and for DNA replication, transcription, and ribosome biogenesis. Nuclear pores permit the passage of small proteins, but larger proteins are targeted by nuclear localization signals that include clusters of basic amino acids. Some nuclear proteins may be retained in the nucleus by forming complexes within the organelle. Peroxisomes contain a limited array of enzymes. One targeting signal is a carboxy-terminal tripeptide, Ser-Lys-Leu (SKL). An N-terminal targeting signal also exists, and others may yet be discovered.

A different targeting problem exists for proteins that reside in more than one subcellular compartment. Sometimes gene duplication and divergence have resulted in different targeting signals on closely related mature polypeptides. **Alternative transcription initiation sites** or pre-mRNA splicing can generate different messages from a single gene. An example of the latter is seen in a calcium–calmodulin-dependent protein kinase; alternatively spliced mRNAs differ with respect to an internal segment that encodes a nuclear localization signal. Without this segment, the protein remains in the cytosol. **Alternative translation initiation sites** lead to two forms of rat liver fumarase, one of which includes a mitochondrial targeting sequence while the other does not and remains in the cytosol. A suboptimal localization signal can lead to inefficient targeting and a dual location, as is seen in the partial secretion of an inhibitor of the plasminogen activator. Finally, some proteins contain more than one targeting signal, which must compete with each other.

17.6 ■ FURTHER POSTTRANSLATIONAL PROTEIN MODIFICATIONS

Several additional maturation events may modify newly synthesized polypeptides to help generate their final, functional structures. Many of these events are very common, while others are specialized to one or a few known instances.

Insulin Biosynthesis Involves Partial Proteolysis

Partial proteolysis of proteins is a common maturation step. Sequences can be removed from either end or from within the protein. Proteolysis in the ER and Golgi apparatus helps to mature the protein hormone insulin (Figure 17.19). **Preproinsulin** encoded by mRNA is inserted into the ER lumen. Signal peptidase cleaves the signal peptide to generate **proinsulin,** which folds to form the correct disulfide linkages. Proinsulin is transported to the Golgi apparatus where it is packaged into secretory granules. An internal connecting peptide **(C peptide)** is removed by proteolysis, and mature insulin is secreted. In familial hyperproinsulinemia, processing is incomplete (see Clin. Corr. 17.6).

This pathway for insulin biosynthesis has advantages over synthesis and binding of two separate polypeptides. First, it ensures production of equal amounts of A and B chains without coordination of two translational activities. Second, proinsulin folds into a three-dimensional structure in which the cysteine residues are placed for correct disulfide bond formation. Proinsulin can be reduced and denatured but refolds correctly to form proinsulin. Renaturation of reduced and denatured insulin is less efficient, and incorrect disulfide linkages are also formed. Correct formation of insulin from separately synthesized chains might have required evolution of a helper protein or molecular chaperone.

Proteolysis Leads to Zymogen Activation

Precursor protein cleavage is a common means of enzyme activation. Digestive proteases are classic examples of this phenomenon (see p. 1059). Inactive **zymogen** precursors are packaged in storage granules and activated by proteol-

CLINICAL CORRELATION 17.6

Familial Hyperproinsulinemia

Familial hyperproinsulinemia, an autosomal dominant condition, results in approximately equal amounts of insulin and an abnormally processed proinsulin being released into the circulation. Although affected individuals have high levels of proinsulin in their blood, they are apparently normal in terms of glucose metabolism, being neither diabetic nor hypoglycemic. The defect was originally thought to result from a deficiency of one of the proteases that process proinsulin. Three enzymes process proinsulin: endopeptidases that cleave the Arg31–Arg32 and Lys64–Arg65 peptide bonds, and a carboxypeptidase. In several families the defect is the substitution of Arg65 by His or Leu, which prevents cleavage between the C-peptide and the A chain of insulin, resulting in secretion of a partially processed proinsulin. In one family a point mutation (His10→Asp10) causes the hyperproinsulinemia, but how this mutation interferes with processing is not known.

Steiner, D. F., Tager, H. S., Naujo, K., Chan, S. J., and Rubenstein, A. H. Familial syndromes of hyperproinsulinemia with mild diabetes. In: C. R. Scriver, A. L. Beaudet, W. S. Sly, and D. Valle (Eds.), *The Molecular and Metabolic Basis of Inherited Disease,* 7th ed. New York: McGraw-Hill, 1995, pp. 897–904.

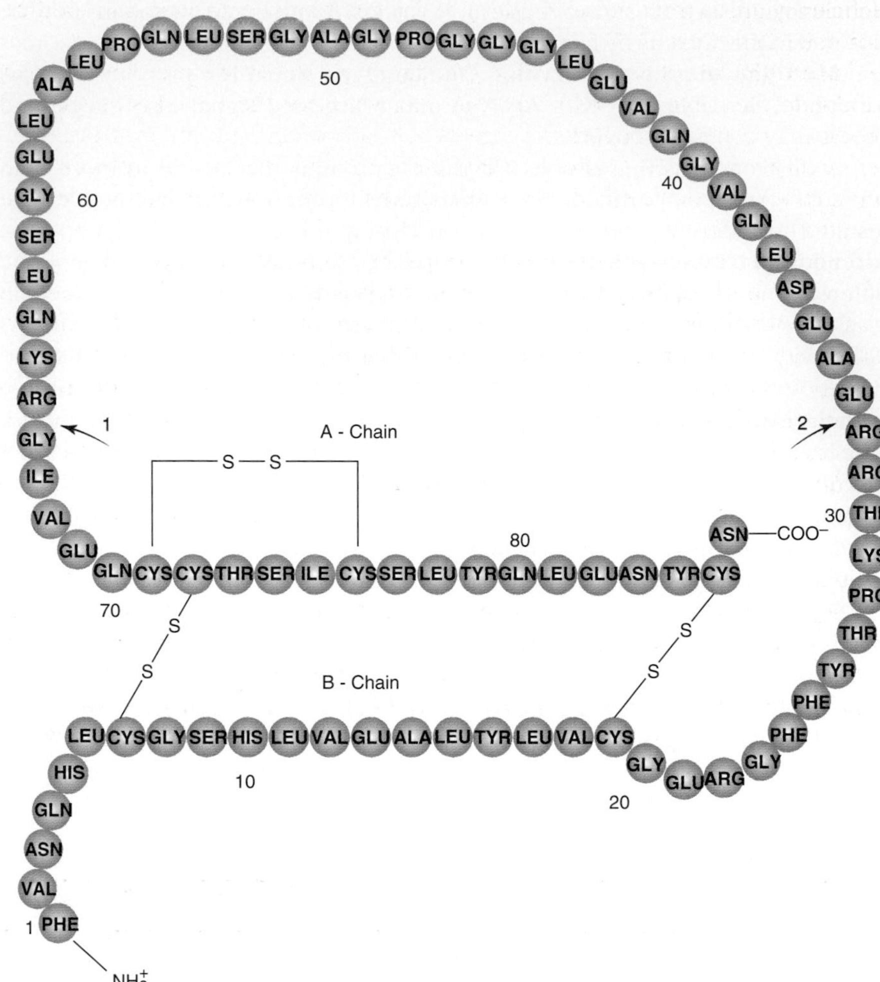

FIGURE 17.19
Maturation of human proinsulin.
After cleavage at two sites indicated by arrows, the arginine residues 31, 32, and 65 and lysine residue 64 are removed to produce insulin and C-peptide.
Redrawn from G. I. Bell, W. F. Swain, R. Pictet, B. Cordell, H. M. Goodman, and W. J. Rutter, Nature *282:525, 1979.*

ysis upon secretion. Thus trypsinogen is cleaved to give an amino-terminal peptide plus trypsin, and chymotrypsinogen is cleaved to form chymotrypsin and two peptides.

Amino Acids Can Be Modified After Incorporation into Proteins

Only 20 amino acids are encoded genetically and incorporated during translation. **Posttranslational modification** of proteins, however, leads to formation of 100 or more different amino acid derivatives in proteins. Modification may be permanent or highly reversible. The amounts of modified amino acids may be small, but they often play a major functional role in proteins. Examples are listed in Table 17.10.

Protein amino termini are frequently modified. Protein synthesis is initiated using methionine, but in the majority of proteins the amino-terminal residue is not methionine; proteolysis has occurred. The amino terminus is then sometimes modified by, for example, acetylation or myristoylation. Amino-terminal glutamine residues spontaneously cyclize; one possible result is the stabilization of the protein. Amino terminal sequences are occasionally lengthened by the addition of an amino acid (see Section 17.8, Protein Degradation and Turnover).

Posttranslational disulfide bond formation is catalyzed by a **disulfide isomerase.** The cystine-containing protein is conformationally stabilized. Disulfide formation can prevent unfolding of proteins and their passage across membranes, so it also becomes a means of localization. As seen in the case of insulin, disulfide bonds can covalently link separate polypeptides and be necessary for biological function. Cysteine modification also occurs; multiple sulfatase deficiency arises from reduced ability to carry out a posttranslational modification (see Clin. Corr 17.7).

Methylation of lysine ε-amino groups occurs in histone proteins and may modulate their interactions with DNA. A fraction of the H2A histone is also modified through isopeptide linkage of a small protein, ubiquitin, from its C-terminal glycine to a lysine ε-amino group on the histone. A role in DNA interactions is postulated. Biotin is also linked to proteins through amide linkages to lysine.

Serine and threonine hydroxyl groups are major sites of glycosylation and of reversible phosphorylation by protein kinases and protein phosphatases. A classic example of phosphorylation of a serine residue is glycogen phosphorylase, which is modified by phosphorylase kinase (see p. 322). Tyrosine kinase activity is a property of many growth factor receptors; growth factor binding stimulates cell division and the proliferation of specific cell types. Oncogenes, responsible in part for the proliferation of tumor cells, often have tyrosine kinase activity and show strong homology with normal growth factor receptors. Dozens of other examples exist; together the protein kinases and protein phosphatases control the activity of many proteins that are central to normal and abnormal cellular development.

ADP-ribosylation of EF-2 at a modified histidine residue represents a doubling of posttranslational modifications. First, a specific EF-2 histidine residue is modified to generate the diphthamide derivative (Figure 17.20) of the functional protein. This modification is probably not absolutely required since yeast mutants that cannot make diphthamide survive. ADP-ribosylation of the diphtham-

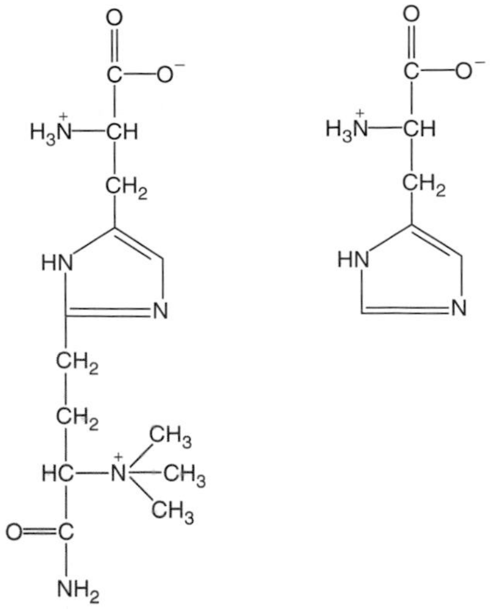

FIGURE 17.20
Diphthamide (left) is a posttranslational modification of a specific residue of histidine (right) in EF-2.

TABLE 17.10 Modified Amino Acids in Proteins[a]

Amino Acid	*Modifications Found*
Amino terminus	Formylation, acetylation, aminoacylation, myristoylation, glycosylation
Carboxyl terminus	Methylation, glycosyl-phosphatidylinositol anchor formation, ADP-ribosylation
Arginine	*N*-Methylation, ADP-ribosylation
Asparagine	*N*-Glycosylation, *N*-methylation, deamidation
Aspartic acid	Methylation, phosphorylation, hydroxylation
Cysteine	Cystine formation, selenocysteine formation, palmitoylation, linkage to heme, *S*-glycosylation, prenylation
Glutamic acid	Methylation, γ-carboxylation, ADP-ribosylation
Glutamine	Deamidation, cross-linking, pyroglutamate formation
Histidine	Methylation, phosphorylation, diphthamide formation, ADP-ribosylation
Lysine	*N*-acetylation, *N*-methylation, oxidation, hydroxylation, cross-linking, ubiquitination, allysine formation
Methionine	Sulfoxide formation
Phenylalanine	β-Hydroxylation and glycosylation
Proline	Hydroxylation, glycosylation
Serine	Phosphorylation, glycosylation, acetylation
Threonine	Phosphorylation, glycosylation, methylation
Tryptophan	β-Hydroxylation, dione formation
Tyrosine	Phosphorylation, iodination, adenylation, sulfonylation, hydroxylation

Source: Adapted from R. G. Krishna and F. Wold, Post-translational modification of proteins. In: A. Meister (Ed.), *Advances in Enzymology,* Vol. 67. New York: Wiley-Interscience, 1993, pp. 265–298.

[a] The listing is not comprehensive and some of the modifications are very rare. Note that no derivatives of alanine, glycine, isoleucine, and valine have been identified in proteins.

CLINICAL CORRELATION 17.7

Absence of Posttranslational Modification: Multiple Sulfatase Deficiency

A variety of biological molecules are sulfated; examples include glycosaminoglycans, steroids, and glycolipids. Ineffective sulfation of the glycosaminoglycans chondroitin sulfate and keratan sulfate of cartilage results in major skeletal deformities. Degradation of sulfated molecules depends on the activity of a group of related sulfatases, most of which are located in lysosomes. Multiple sulfatase deficiency is a rare lysosomal storage disorder that combines features of metachromatic leukodystrophy and mucopolysaccharidosis. Affected individuals develop slowly and from their second year of life lose the abilities to stand, sit, or speak; physical deformities and neurological deficiencies develop and death before age 10 is usual. Biochemically, multiple sulfatase deficiency is characterized by severe lack of all the sulfatases. In contrast, deficiencies in individual sulfatases are also known, and several distinct diseases are linked to single enzyme defects.

The molecular defect in multiple sulfatase deficiency arises from a deficiency in a posttranslational modification that is common to all sulfatase enzymes and is necessary for their enzymatic activity. In each case a cysteine residue of the enzyme is normally converted to 2-amino-3-oxopropionic acid; the $-CH_2SH$ side chain of cysteine becomes a $-CHO$ (aldehyde) group, which may itself react with amino or hydroxyl groups of the enzyme, a cofactor, and so on. Fibroblasts from individuals with multiple sulfatase deficiency catalyze this modification with significantly lowered efficiency, and the unmodified sulfatases are catalytically inactive.

Schmidt, B., Selmer, T., Ingendoh, A, and von Figura, K. A novel amino acid modification in sulfatases that is deficient in multiple sulfatase deficiency. *Cell* 82:271–278, 1995.

ide by diphtheria toxin then inhibits EF-2 activity. Other instances of physiological ADP-ribosylation not mediated by bacterial toxins are reversible.

Formation of γ-carboxyglutamate from glutamic acid residues occurs in several blood-clotting proteins including prothrombin and factors VII, IX, and X. The γ-carboxyglutamate residues chelate calcium ion, which is required for normal blood clotting (see p. 963). In each case the modification requires vitamin K and can be blocked by coumarin derivatives, which antagonize vitamin K. As a result, the rate of coagulation is greatly decreased.

Collagen Biosynthesis Requires Many Posttranslational Modifications

Collagen, the most abundant protein (or family of related proteins) in the human body, is a fibrous protein that provides the structural framework for tissues and organs. It undergoes a wide variety of posttranslational modifications that directly affect its structure and function, and defects in its modification result in serious diseases. Collagen is an excellent example of the importance of posttranslational modification.

Different species of collagen, designated types I, II, III, IV, and so on (see Table 2.11) are encoded on several chromosomes and expressed in different tissues. Their amino acid sequences differ, but their overall structural similarity suggests a common evolutionary origin. Each collagen polypeptide, designated an α chain, has a repeating sequence Gly-X-Y that is about 1000 residues long. Every third residue is glycine, about one-third of the X positions are occupied by proline and a similar number of Y positions are 4-hydroxyproline, a posttranslationally modified form of proline. Proline and hydroxyproline residues impart considerable rigidity to the structure, which exists as a polyproline type II helix (Figure 17.21; see also p. 52). A collagen molecule includes three α chains intertwined in a collagen triple helix in which the glycine residues occupy the center of the structure.

Procollagen Formation in the Endoplasmic Reticulum and Golgi Apparatus

Collagen α chain synthesis starts in the cytosol, where the amino-terminal signal sequences bind signal recognition particles. Precursor forms, designated, for example, prepro $\alpha 1(I)$, are extruded into the ER lumen and the signal peptides are cleaved. Hydroxylation of proline and lysine residues occurs **cotranslationally,** before assembly of a triple helix. Prolyl 4-hydroxylase requires an -X-Pro-

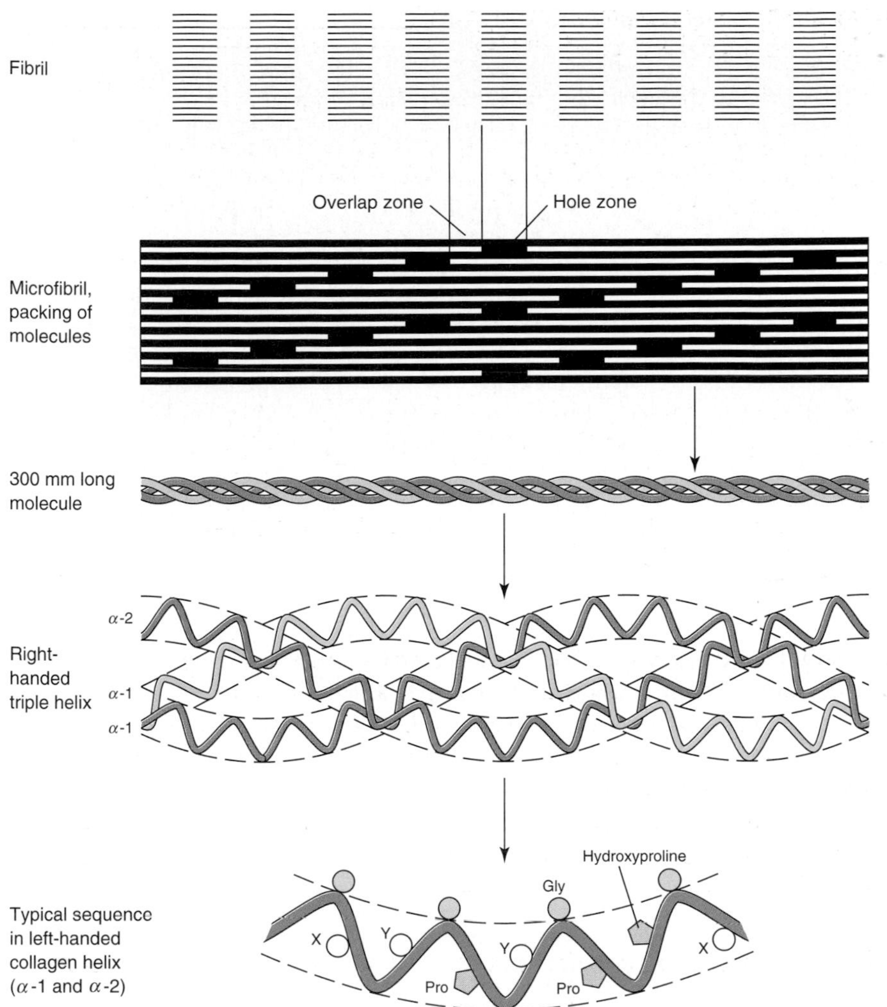

FIGURE 17.21
Collagen structure, illustrating the regularity of the primary sequence, the left-handed helix, the right-handed triple helix, the 300-nm molecule, and the organization of molecules in a typical fibril, within which collagen molecules are cross-linked.

Gly- sequence (hence 4-hydroxyproline is found only at Y positions in the -Gly-X-Y- sequence). Also present in the ER is a prolyl 3-hydroxylase, which modifies a smaller number of proline residues, and a lysyl hydroxylase, which modifies some of the Y-position lysine residues. These hydroxylases require Fe^{2+} and ascorbic acid, the extent of modification depending on the specific α-chain type. Proline hydroxylation stabilizes collagen and lysine hydroxylation provides sites for interchain cross-linking and for glycosylation by specific glycosyl transferases of the ER. Asparagine residues are also glycosylated at this point, eventually leading to high mannose-type oligosaccharides.

Triple helix assembly occurs after the polypeptide chains have been completed. Carboxy-terminal globular proprotein domains fold and disulfide bonds are formed. Interaction of these domains initiates winding of the triple helix from the carboxyl end toward the amino terminus. The completed triple helix, with globular proprotein domains at each end, moves to the Golgi apparatus where oligosaccharides are processed and matured. Sometimes tyrosine residues are modified by sulfation and some serines are phosphorylated. The completed procollagen is then released from the cell via secretory vesicles.

Collagen Maturation

Conversion of procollagen to collagen occurs extracellularly. The amino-terminal and carboxyl-terminal propeptides are cleaved by separate proteases that may also be type specific. Concurrently, the triple helices assemble into fibrils

TABLE 17.11 Selected Disorders in Collagen Biosynthesis and Structure

Disorder	*Collagen Defect*	*Clinical Manifestations*
Osteogenesis imperfecta 1	Decreased synthesis of type I	Long bone fractures prior to puberty
Osteogenesis imperfecta 2	Point mutations and exon rearrangements in triple helical regions	Perinatal lethality; malformed and soft,fragile bones
Ehlers–Danlos IV	Poor secretion, premature degradation of type III	Translucent skin, easy bruising, arterial and colon rupture
Ehlers–Danlos VI	Decreased hydroxylysine in types I and III	Hyperextensive skin, joint hypermobility
Ehlers–Danlos VII	Type I procollagen accumulation: N-terminal propeptide not cleaved	Joint hypermobility and dislocation
Cutis laxa (occipital horn syndrome)	Decreased hydroxylysine due to poor Cu distribution	Lax, soft skin; occipital horn formation in adolescents

and the collagen is stabilized by extensive cross-linking (see Figure 2.39). Lysyl oxidase converts some lysine or hydroxylysine to the reactive aldehydes, allysine, or hydroxyallysine. These residues condense with each other or with lysine or hydroxylysine residues in adjacent chains to form Schiff's base and aldol cross-links. Further and less well-characterized reactions can involve other residues including histidines and can link three α chains. Defects at many of these steps are known. Some of the best characterized are listed in Table 17.11 and described in Clin. Corr. 17.8.

17.7 ■ REGULATION OF TRANSLATION

Translation requires considerable energy, and the formation of functioning proteins has significant consequences for the cell. It is logical that the process is carefully controlled, both globally and for specific proteins. The most efficient and common mechanism of regulation is at the initiation stage.

The best understood means of overall regulation of translation involves the reversible phosphorylation of eIF-2a. Under conditions that include nutrient starvation, heat shock, and viral infection, eIF-2a is phosphorylated by a specific kinase. Phosphorylated eIF-2a · GDP binds tightly to eIF-2b, the guanine nucleotide exchange factor, which is present in limiting amounts. Since eIF-2b is unavailable for nucleotide exchange, no eIF-2a · GTP is available for initiation. Phosphorylation can be catalyzed by a **heme-regulated inhibitor kinase,** which, in the absence of heme, is activated by autophosphorylation. This kinase is present in many cells but is best studied in reticulocytes that synthesize hemoglobin. Deficiencies in energy supply or any heme precursor activate the kinase. A related **double-stranded RNA-dependent kinase** is autophosphorylated and activated in response to binding of ds-RNA that results from many viral infections. Production of this kinase is also induced by interferon. Initiation factor eIF-4e (a component of the cap binding protein eIF-4f) is activated by phosphorylation in response to, for example, growth factors and is inactivated by a protein phosphatase following, for example, viral infection. These effects may be greatest in the translation of mRNAs with long, highly structured leader sequences that need to be unwound to allow identification of a translational start site.

Regulation of translation of specific genes also occurs. A clear example is the regulation by iron of synthesis of the iron-binding protein, ferritin. In

CLINICAL CORRELATION 17.8

Defects in Collagen Synthesis

Ehlers–Danlos Syndrome, Type IV

Ehlers–Danlos syndrome is a group of at least ten disorders that are clinically, genetically, and biochemically distinguishable, but that share manifestations of structural weaknesses in connective tissue. The usual problems are fragility and hyperextensibility of skin and hypermobility of the joints. The weaknesses result from defects in collagen structure. For example, type IV Ehlers–Danlos syndrome is caused by defects in type III collagen, which is particularly important in skin, arteries, and hollow organs. Characteristics include thin, translucent skin through which veins are easily seen, marked bruising, and sometimes an appearance of aging in the hands and skin. Clinical problems arise from arterial rupture, intestinal perforation, and rupture of the uterus during pregnancy or labor. Surgical repair is difficult because of tissue fragility. The basic defects in type IV Ehlers–Danlos appear to be due to changes in the primary structure of type III chains. These arise from point mutations that result in replacement of glycine residues and thus disruption of the collagen triple helix, and from exon-skipping, which shortens the polypeptide and can result in inefficient secretion and decreased thermal stability of the collagen, and in abnormal formation of type III collagen fibrils. In some cases type III collagen is accumulated in the rough ER, overmodified, and degraded very slowly.

Superti-Furga, A., Gugler, E., Gitzelmann, R., and Steinmann, B. Ehlers–Danlos syndrome type IV: a multi-exon deletion in one of the two COL 3A1 alleles affecting structure, stability, and processing of type III procollagen. *J. Biol. Chem.* 263:6226, 1988.

Osteogenesis Imperfecta

Osteogenesis imperfecta is a group of at least four clinically, genetically, and biochemically distinguishable disorders, all characterized by multiple fractures with resultant bone deformities. Several variants result from mutations producing modified α(I) chains. In the clearest example a deletion mutation causes absence of 84 amino acids in the α1(I) chain. The shortened α1(I) chains are synthesized, because the mutation leaves the reading frame in register. The short α1(I) chains associate with normal α1(I) and α2(I) chains, thereby preventing normal collagen triple helix formation, with resultant degradation of all the chains, a phenomenon aptly named "protein suicide." Three-fourths of all the collagen molecules formed have at least one short (defective) α1(I) chain, an amplification of the effect of a heterozygous gene defect. Other forms of osteogenesis imperfecta result from point mutations that substitute another amino acid for one of the glycines. Since glycine has to fit into the interior of the collagen triple helix, these substitutions destabilize that helix.

Barsh, G. S., Roush, C. L., Bonadio, J., Byers, P. H., and Gelinas, R. E. Intron mediated recombination causes an α(I) collagen deletion in a lethal form of osteogenesis imperfecta. *Proc. Natl. Acad. Sci. USA* 82:2870, 1985.

Scurvy and Hydroxyproline Synthesis

Scurvy results from dietary deficiency of ascorbic acid. Most animals can synthesize ascorbic acid from glucose but humans have lost this enzymatic mechanism. Among other problems, ascorbic acid deficiency causes decreased hydroxyproline synthesis because prolyl hydroxylase requires ascorbic acid. The hydroxyproline provides additional hydrogen-bonding atoms that stabilize the collagen triple helix. Collagen containing insufficient hydroxyproline loses temperature stability, becoming less stable than normal collagen at body temperature. The resultant clinical manifestations are distinctive and understandable: suppression of the orderly growth process of bone in children, poor wound healing, and increased capillary fragility with resultant hemorrhage, particularly in the skin. Severe ascorbic acid deficiency leads secondarily to a decreased rate of procollagen synthesis.

Crandon, J. H., Lund, C. C., and Dill, D. B. Experimental human scurvy. *N. Engl. J. Med.* 223:353, 1940.

Deficiency of Lysyl Hydroxylase

In type VI Ehlers–Danlos syndrome lysyl hydroxylase is deficient. As a result type I and III collagens in skin are synthesized with decreased hydroxylysine content, and subsequent cross-linking of collagen fibrils is less stable. Some cross-linking between lysine and allysine occurs but these are not as stable and do not mature as readily as do hydroxylysine-containing cross-links. In addition, carbohydrates add to the hydroxylysine residues but the function of this carbohydrate is unknown. The clinical features include marked hyperextensibility of the skin and joints, poor wound healing, and musculoskeletal deformities. Some patients with this form of Ehlers–Danlos syndrome have a mutant form of lysyl hydroxylase with a higher Michaelis constant for ascorbic acid than the normal enzyme. Accordingly, they respond to high doses of ascorbic acid.

Pinnell, S. R., Krane, S. M., Kenzora, J. E., and Glimcher, M. J. A heritable disorder of connective tissue: hydroxylysine-deficient collagen disease. *N. Engl. J. Med.* 286:1013, 1972.

Ehlers–Danlos Syndrome, Type VII

In Ehlers–Danlos syndrome, type VII, skin bruises easily and is hyperextensible, but the major manifestations are dislocations of major joints, such as hips and knees. Laxity of ligaments is caused by incomplete removal of the amino-terminal propeptide of the procollagen chains. One variant of the disease results from deficiency of procollagen *N*-protease. A similar deficiency occurs in the autosomal recessive disease called dermatosparaxis of cattle, sheep, and cats, in which skin fragility is so extreme as to be lethal. In other variants the proα1(I) and proα2(I) chains lack amino acids at the cleavage site because of skipping of one exon in the genes. This prevents normal cleavage by procollagen *N*-protease.

Cole, W. G., Chan, W., Chambers, G. W., Walker, I. D., and Bateman, J. F. Deletion of 24 amino acids from the proα(I) chain of type I procollagen in a patient with the Ehlers–Danlos syndrome type VII. *J. Biol. Chem.* 261:5496, 1986.

Occipital Horn Syndrome

In type IX Ehlers-Danlos syndrome and in Menke's (kinky-hair) syndrome there is thought to be a deficiency in lysyl oxidase activity. In type IX Ehlers–Danlos syndrome there are consequent cross-linking defects manifested in lax, soft skin and in the appearance during adolescence of bony occipital horns. Copper-deficient animals have deficient cross-linking of elastin and collagen, apparently because of the requirement for cuprous ion by lysyl oxidase.

(*continued*)

In Menke's (kinky-hair) syndrome there is a defect in intracellular copper transport that results in low activity of lysyl oxidase, and in occipital horn syndrome there is also a defect in intracellular copper distribution. A woman taking high doses of the copper-chelating drug, *d*-penicillamine, gave birth to an infant with an acquired Ehlers–Danlos-like syndrome, which subsequently cleared. Side effects of *d*-penicillamine therapy include poor wound healing and hyperextensible skin.

Peltonen, L., Kuivaniemi, H., Palotie, A., et al. Alterations of copper and collagen metabolism in the Menkes syndrome and a new subtype of Ehlers–Danlos syndrome. *Biochemistry* 22:6156, 1983. For a detailed overview of collagen disorders see: Byers, P. H. Disorders of collagen biosynthesis and structure. In: C. R. Scriver, A. L. Beaudet, W. S. Sly, and D. Valle (Eds.) *The Metabolic and Molecular Basis of Inherited Disease*, Vol. III, 7th ed. New York: McGraw-Hill, 1995, pp. 4029–4077.

the absence of iron, a repressor protein binds to the **iron-responsive element** (IRE), a stem-loop structure in the 5′ leader sequence of ferritin mRNA . This mRNA is sequestered for future use. δ-Aminolevulinic acid synthase, an enzyme of heme biosynthesis, is also regulated by a 5′-IRE in its mRNA. In contrast, more ferritin receptor mRNA is needed if iron is limited; it has IREs in its 3′-nontranslated region. Binding of the repressor protein stabilizes the mRNA and prolongs its useful lifetime. Many growth-regulated mRNAs, including those for ribosomal proteins, have a polypyrimidine tract in their leader sequence. A polypyrimidine-binding protein helps regulate their translation.

17.8 ■ PROTEIN DEGRADATION AND TURNOVER

Proteins have finite lifetimes. They are subject to environmental damage such as oxidation, proteolysis, conformational denaturation, or other irreversible modifications. Equally important, cells need to change their protein complements in order to respond to different needs and situations. Specific proteins have very different lifetimes. Cells of the eye lens are not replaced and their proteins are not recycled. Hemoglobin in red blood cells lasts the life of these cells, about 120 days. Other proteins have lifetimes measured in days, hours, or even minutes. Some blood-clotting proteins survive for only a few days, so hemophiliacs are only protected for a short period by transfusions or injections of required factors. Diabetics require insulin injections regularly since the hormone is metabolized. Metabolic enzymes vary quantitatively depending on need; for example, urea cycle enzyme levels change in response to diet. Most amino acids produced by protein degradation are recycled to synthesize new proteins but some degradation products will be excreted. In either case, proteolysis first reduces the proteins in question to peptides and eventually amino acids. Several proteolytic systems accomplish this end.

Intracellular Digestion of Some Proteins Occurs in Lysosomes

Digestive proteases such as pepsin, trypsin, chymotrypsin, and elastase hydrolyze dietary protein and have no part in intracellular protein turnover within an organism (see Chapter 25). Intracellular digestion of proteins from the extracellular environment occurs within **lysosomes.** Material that is impermeable to the plasma membrane is imported by endocytosis. In **pinocytosis** large particles, molecular aggregates, or other molecules present in the extracellular fluid are ingested by engulfment. Macrophages ingest bacteria and dead cells by this mechanism. **Receptor-mediated endocytosis** uses cell surface receptors to bind specific molecules. Endocytosis occurs at pits in the cell surface that are coated internally with the multisubunit protein clathrin. Uptake is by invagination of the plasma membrane and the receptors to form intracellular coated vesicles. One fate of such vesicles is fusion with a lysosome and degradation of the contents. Some intracellular protein turnover may also occur within lysosomes, and under some conditions significant amounts of cellular material can be mobilized via lysosomes. For example, serum starvation of fibroblasts in culture or starvation of rats leads to the lysosomal degradation of a subpopulation of cellular proteins. Recognition of a specific peptide sequence is involved, indicating that the lifetime of a protein is ultimately encoded in its sequence. This concept will be more apparent in the next section on ubiquitin-dependent proteolysis.

Although lysosomal degradation of cellular proteins occurs, it is not the main route of protein turnover. Calcium-dependent proteases, also called calpains, are present in most cells. Activators and inhibitors of these enzymes are also present, and calpains are logical candidates for enzymes involved in protein turnover. However, their role in these processes is not quantitatively established. Golgi and ER proteases degrade peptide fragments that arise during maturation of proteins in the secretory pathway. They could also be involved in turnover of ER proteins. **Apoptosis,** programmed cell death, requires several proteases. It is likely that other uncharacterized mechanisms exist in both the cytosol and in the mitochondrion.

Ubiquitin Is a Marker in ATP-Dependent Proteolysis

One well-described proteolytic pathway requires ATP hydrolysis and the participation of **ubiquitin,** a highly conserved protein containing 76 amino acids. One function of ubiquitin is to mark proteins for degradation. Ubiquitin has other roles; as an example, linkage of ubiquitin to histones H2A and H2B is unrelated to turnover since the proteins are stable, but modification may affect chromatin structure or transcription.

The ubiquitin-dependent proteolytic cycle is shown in Figure 17.22. Ubiquitin is activated by enzyme E1 to form a thioester; ATP is required and a transient AMP–ubiquitin complex is involved. The ubiquitin is then passed to enzyme E2, and finally via one of a group of E3 enzymes it is coupled to a targeted protein. Linkage of ubiquitin is through isopeptide bonds between ε-amino groups of lysine residues of the protein and the carboxyl-terminal glycine residues of ubiquitin. Several ubiquitin molecules may be attached to the protein and to each other. ATP-dependent proteases then degrade the tagged protein and free the ubiquitin for further degradation cycles.

Ubiquitin-dependent proteolysis plays a major role in the regulation of cellular events. **Cyclins** are involved in control of progress through the cell cycle. The ubiquitin-dependent destruction of a cyclin allows cells to pass from the M phase into G1. Other proteins known to be degraded by ubiquitin-dependent proteolysis include transcription factors, the p53 tumor suppressor and other oncoproteins, a protein kinase, and immune system and other cell surface receptors.

Damaged or mutant proteins are rapidly degraded via the ubiquitin pathway. In **cystic fibrosis** a mutation that results in deletion of one amino acid greatly alters the stability of a protein (see Clin. Corr. 17.9), but it is not always clear how native proteins are identified for degradation. Selectivity occurs at the level of the E3 enzyme, but most specific recognition signals are obscure. One determinant is simply the identity of the amino-terminal amino acid. Otherwise identical β-galactosidase proteins with different amino-terminal residues are degraded at widely differing rates. Amino termini may be modified to alter the lifetime of the protein, and some residues serve as aminoacyl acceptors for a destabilizing residue from an aminoacyl-tRNA. Internal sequences and conformation are also likely to be important; destabilizing PEST sequences (rich in Pro, Glu, Ser, and Thr) have been identified in several short-lived proteins.

The ATP-dependent degradation of ubiquitin-marked proteins occurs in a 26S organelle called the **proteasome.** Proteasomes are dumbbell-shaped complexes of about 25 polypeptides; a proteolytically active 20S cylindrical

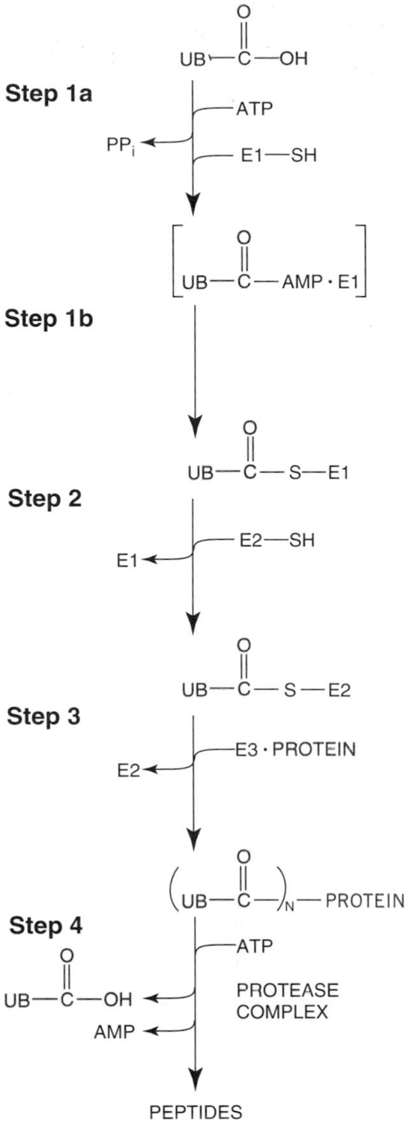

FIGURE 17.22
ATP and ubiquitin-dependent protein degradation.
Ubiquitin is first activated in a two-step reaction involving formation of a transient mixed anhydride of AMP and the carboxy terminus of ubiquitin (step 1a), followed by generation of a thioester with enzyme E1 (step 1b). Enzyme E2 can now form a thioester with ubiquitin (step 2) and serve as a donor in E3-catalyzed transfer of ubiquitin to a targeted protein (step 3). Several ubiquitin molecules are usually attached to different lysine residues of a targeted protein at this stage. Ubiquitinylated protein is now degraded by ATP-dependent proteolysis (step 4); ubiquitin is not degraded and can reenter the process at step 1.

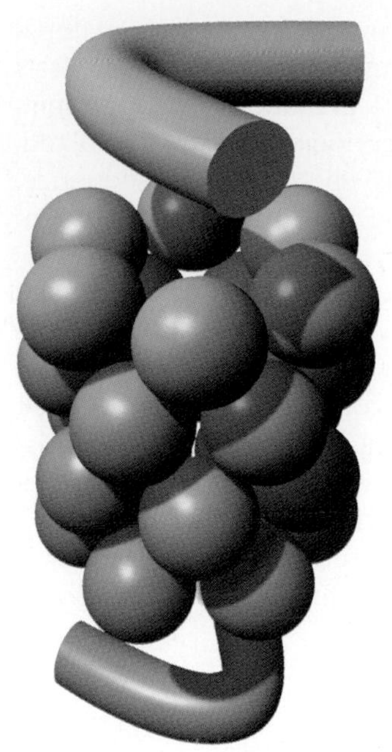

FIGURE 17.23
Model of proteasome.
A 20S central segment is made up of four stacked heptameric rings of two types. The core is hollow and includes 12–15 different polypeptides; several proteases with different specificities are localized within the rings. V-shaped segments at each end cap the cylinder and are responsible for ATP-dependent substrate recognition, unfolding, and translocation into the proteolytic core. Upper cap structure is also in contact with the central segment but it is shown displaced from it in order to illustrate the hollow core of the cylinder.
Adapted from D. Rubin and D. Finley, Curr. Biol. *5:854,* 1995; *and J.-M. Peters,* Trends Biochem. Sci. *19:377, 1994.*

core is capped at each end by V-shaped complexes that bestow ATP dependence (Figure 17.23). It is speculated that the cap structure is involved in recognizing and unfolding polypeptides and transporting them to the proteolytic core. The complex *E. coli* proteases Lon and Clp and similar enzymes in other microorganisms (and in mitochondria) also require ATP hydrolysis for their action, but ubiquitin is absent in prokaryotes and the means of identification of proteins for degradation is still obscure. It is likely that protein degradation will turn out to be as complex and important a problem as protein biosynthesis.

CLINICAL CORRELATION 17.9

Deletion of a Codon, Incorrect Posttranslational Modification, and Premature Protein Degradation: Cystic Fibrosis

Cystic fibrosis (CF) is the most common autosomal recessive disease in Caucasians, with a frequency of almost 1 per 2000. The CF gene is 230 kb in length and includes 27 exons encoding a protein of 1480 amino acids. The protein known as the cystic fibrosis transmembrane conductance regulator or CFTR is a member of a family of ATP-dependent transport proteins and it includes two membrane-spanning domains, two nucleotide-binding domains that interact with ATP, and one regulatory domain that includes several phosphorylation sites. CFTR functions as a cyclic AMP-regulated chloride channel. CF epithelia are characterized by defective electrolyte transport. The organs most strongly affected include the lungs, pancreas, and liver, and the most life-threatening effects involve thick mucous secretions that lead to chronic obstructive lung disease and persistent infections of lungs.

In about 70% of affected individuals the problem is traced to a three-nucleotide deletion that results in deletion of a single amino acid, phenylalanine 508, normally located in ATP-binding domain 1 on the cytoplasmic side of the plasma membrane. As with several other CF mutations, the Phe 508 deletion protein is not properly glycosylated or transported to the cell surface. Instead, it is only partially glycosylated, and it is degraded within the endoplasmic reticulum. It is postulated that the mutant protein does not fold properly and is marked for degradation rather than movement to the plasma membrane.

Ward, C., Omura, S., and Kopito, R. Degradation of CFTR by the ubiquitin–proteasome pathway. Cell 83:121, 1995.

BIBLIOGRAPHY

Ribosomes and Transfer RNA

Filonenko, V. V., and Deutscher, M. P. Evidence for similar structural organization of the multienzyme aminoacyl-tRNA complex *in vivo* and *in vitro*. *J. Biol. Chem.* 269:17375, 1994.

Frank, J., Zhu, J., Penczek, P., et al. A model of protein synthesis based on a new cryo-electron microscopy reconstruction of the *E. coli* ribosome. *Nature* 376:441, 1995.

Freist, W. Mechanisms of aminoacyl-tRNA synthetases: a critical consideration of recent results. *Biochemistry* 28:6787, 1989.

Gesteland, R. F., and Atkins, J. F. (Eds.). *The RNA World.* Cold Spring Harbor, NY: Cold Spring Harbor Press, 1993.

Herold, M., and Nierhaus, K. H. Incorporation of six additional proteins to complete the assembly map of the 50S subunit from *Escherichia coli* ribosomes. *J. Biol. Chem.* 262:8826, 1987.

Hou, Y.-M., Francklyn, C., and Schimmel, P. Molecular dissection of a transfer RNA and the basis for its identity. *Trends Biochem. Sci.* 14:233, 1989.

Jakubowski, H., and Goldman, E. Editing errors in selection of amino acids for protein synthesis. *Microbiol. Rev.* 56:412, 1992.

Nierhaus, K. H., Franceschi, F., Subramanian, A. R., Erdmann, V. A., and Wittmann-Liebold, B. (Eds.). *The Translational Apparatus: Structure, Function, Regulation, Evolution.* New York: Plenum Press, 1993.

Nomura, M. The role of RNA and protein in ribosome function: a review of early reconstitution studies and prospects for future studies. *Cold Spring Harbor Symp. Quant. Biol.* 52:653, 1987.

Perona, J., Rould, M., and Steitz, T. Structural basis for transfer RNA aminoacylation by *Escherichia coli* glutaminyl-tRNA synthetase. *Biochemstry* 32:8758, 1993.

Stark, H., Mueller, F., Orleva, E. V., et al. The 70S *Escherichia coli* ribosome at 23Å resolution: fitting the ribosomal RNA. *Structure* 3:815, 1995.

Verschoor, A., and Frank, J. Three-dimensional structure of the mammalian cytoplasmic ribosome. *J. Mol. Biol.* 214:737, 1990.

Protein Biosynthesis and Its Regulation

Barrell, B., Anderson, S., Bankier, A. T., et al. Different pattern of codon recognition by mammalian mitochondrial tRNAs. *Proc. Natl. Acad. Sci. USA* 77:3164, 1980.

Berchtold, H., Reshetnikova, L., Reiser, C. O., et al. Crystal structure of active elongation factor T_u reveals major domain rearrangements. *Nature* 365:126, 1993.

Gnirke, A., Geigenmuller, U., Rheinberger, H., and Nierhaus, K. The allosteric three-site model for the ribosomal elongation cycle. *J. Biol. Chem.* 264:7291, 1989.

Merrick, W. C. Mechanism and regulation of eukaryotic protein synthesis. *Microbiol. Rev.* 56:291, 1992.

Merrick, W. C. Eukaryotic protein synthesis: an *in vitro* analysis. *Biochimie* 76:822, 1994.

Rhoads, R. E. Regulation of eukaryotic protein biosynthesis by initiation factors. *J. Biol. Chem.* 268:3017, 1993.

Samuel, C. E. The eIF2a protein kinases as regulators of protein synthesis in eukaryotes from yeasts to humans. *J. Biol. Chem.* 268:7603, 1993.

Zhouravleva, G., Frolova, L., LeGoff, X., et al. Termination of translation in eukaryotes is governed by two interacting polypeptide chain release factors, eRF1 and eRF3. *EMBO J* 14:4065, 1995.

Ziff, E. B. Transcription and RNA processing by the DNA tumour viruses. Nature 287:491, 1980.

Protein Targeting and Posttranslational Modification

Dahms, N. M., Lobel, P., and Kornfeld, S. Mannose 6-phosphate receptors and lysosomal enzyme targeting. *J. Biol. Chem.* 264:12115, 1989.

Danpure, C. J. How can products of a single gene be localized to more than one subcellular compartment? *Trends Cell Biol.* 5:230, 1995.

Kornfeld, R., and Kornfeld, S. Assembly of asparagine-linked oligosaccharides. *Annu. Rev. Biochem.* 54:631, 1985.

Krishna, R. G., and Wold, F. Post-translational modification of proteins. *Adv. Enzymol.* 67:265, 1993.

Kuhn, K. The classical collagens. In: R. Mayne and R. E. Burgeson (Eds.), *Structure and Function of Collagen Types.* Orlando, FL: Academic Press, 1987, pp. 1–42.

Nothwehr, S. F., and Stevens, T. H. Sorting of membrane proteins in the yeast secretory pathway. *J. Biol. Chem.* 269:10185, 1994.

Paulson, J. C. Glycoproteins: what are the sugar chains for? *Trends Biochem. Sci.* 14:272, 1989.

Paulson, J. C., and Colley, K. J. Glycosyltransferases: structure, localization, and control of cell type-specific glycosylation. *J. Biol. Chem.* 264:17615, 1989.

Pfanner, N., Craig, E., and Meijer, M. The protein import machinery of the mitochondrial inner membrane. *Trends Biochem. Sci.* 19:368, 1994.

Pfeffer, S. R., and Rothman, J. E. Biosynthetic protein transport and sorting by the endoplasmic reticulum and Golgi. *Annu. Rev. Biochem.* 56:829, 1987.

Rachubinski, R. A., and Subramani, S. How proteins penetrate peroxisomes. *Cell* 83:525, 1995.

Rogenkamp, R. Targeting signals for protein import into peroxisomes. *Cell Biochem. Function* 10:193, 1992.

Rudd, P. M., et al. The effects of variable glycosylation on the functional activities of ribonuclease, plasminogen and tissue plasminogen activator. *Biochim. Biophys. Acta* 1248:1, 1995.

von Heijne, G. Signals for protein targeting into and across membranes. In: A. H. Maddy and J. R. Harris (Eds.), *Subcellular Biochemistry, Vol. 22: Membrane Biochemistry.* New York: Plenum Press, 1994, pp. 1–19.

Walter, P., and Johnson, A. E. Signal sequence recognition and protein targeting to the endoplasmic reticulum membrane. *Annu. Rev. Cell Biol.* 10:87, 1994.

Wolin, S. From the elephant to *E. coli*: SRP-dependent protein targeting. *Cell* 77:787, 1994.

Protein Turnover and Proteasomes

Ciechanover, A. The ubiquitin–proteasome proteolytic pathway. *Cell* 79:13, 1994.

Dice, J. F. Molecular determinants of protein half-lives in eukaryotic cells. *FASEB J.* 1:349, 1987.

Gonda, D. K., Bachmair, A., Wünning, I., et al. Universality and structure of the *N*-end rule. *J. Biol. Chem.* 264:16700, 1989.

Jentsch, S. The ubiquitin-conjugation system. *Annu. Rev. Genet.* 26:179, 1992.

Kessel, M., Maurizi, M. R., Kim, B., et al. Homology in structural organization between *E. coli* C1pAP protease and the eukaryotic 26S proteasome. *J. Mol. Biol.* 250:587, 1995.

Löwe, J., Stock, D., Jap, B., et al. Crystal structure of the 20S proteasome from the archaeon *T. acidophilum* at 3.4Å resolution. *Science* 268:533, 1995.

Rechsteiner, M. Natural substrates of the ubiquitin proteolytic pathway. *Trends Biochem. Sci.* 66:615, 1991.

Rock, K., Gramm, C., Rothstein, L., et al. Inhibitors of the proteasome block the degradation of most cell proteins and the generation of peptides presented on MHC class II molecules. *Cell* 78:761, 1994.

Rogers, S., Wells, R., and Rechsteiner, M. Amino acid sequences common to rapidly degraded proteins: the PEST hypothesis. *Science* 234:364, 1986.

Wlodawer, A. Proteasome: a complex protease with a new fold and a distinct mechanism. *Structure* 3:417, 1995.

QUESTIONS ■ J. BAGGOTT AND C. N. ANGSTADT

1. Degeneracy of the genetic code denotes the existence of:
   A. multiple codons for a single amino acid.
   B. codons consisting of only two bases.
   C. base triplets that do not code for any amino acid.
   D. different protein synthesis systems in which a given triplet codes for different amino acids.
   E. codons that include one or more of the "unusual" bases.

2. Deletion of a single base from a coding sequence of mRNA may result in a polypeptide product with any of the following EXCEPT:
   A. a sequence of amino acids that differs from the sequence found in the normal polypeptide.
   B. more amino acids.
   C. fewer amino acids.
   D. a single amino acid replaced by another amino acid.

3. During initiation of protein synthesis.
   A. methionyl-tRNA appears at the A site of the 80S initiation complex.
   B. eIF-3 and the 40S ribosomal subunit participate in forming a preinitiation complex.
   C. eIF-2 is phosphorylated by GTP.
   D. the same methionyl-tRNA is used as is used during elongation.
   E. a complex consisting of mRNA, the 60S ribosomal subunit, and certain initiation factors is formed.

4. Requirements for eukaryotic protein synthesis include all of the following EXCEPT:
   A. mRNA.
   B. ribosomes.
   C. GTP.
   D. 20 different amino acids in the form of aminoacyl-tRNAs.
   E. fMet-$tRNA_i^{Met}$.

5. During the elongation stage of eukaryotic protein synthesis:
   A. the incoming aminoacyl-tRNA binds to the P site.
   B. a new peptide bond is synthesized by peptidyl transferase site of the large ribosomal subunit in a GTP-requiring reaction.
   C. the peptide, still bound to a tRNA molecule, is translocated to a different site on the ribosome.
   D. streptomycin can cause premature release of the incomplete peptide.
   E. peptide bond formation occurs by the attack of the carboxyl group of the incoming aminoacyl-tRNA on the amino group of the growing peptide chain.

6. Diphtheria toxin:
   A. acts catalytically.
   B. releases incomplete polypeptide chains from the ribosome.
   C. inhibits translocase.
   D. prevents release factor from recognizing termination signals.
   E. attacks the RNA of the large subunit.

7. How many high-energy bonds are expended in the formation of one peptide bond?
   A. 1
   B. 2
   C. 3
   D. 4
   E. 5

8. Formation of mature insulin includes all of the following EXCEPT:
   A. removal of a signal peptide.
   B. folding into a three-dimensional structure.
   C. disulfide bond formation.
   D. removal of a peptide from an internal region.
   E. γ-carboxylation of glutamate residues.

9. 4-Hydroxylation of specific prolyl residues during collagen synthesis requires all of the following EXCEPT:
   A. Fe^{2+}.
   B. a specific amino acid sequence.
   C. ascorbic acid.
   D. succinate.
   E. individual α-chains, not yet assembled into a triple helix.

10. In the formation of an aminoacyl-tRNA:
    A. ADP and P_i are products of the reaction.
    B. aminoacyl adenylate appears in solution as a free intermediate.
    C. the aminoacyl-tRNA synthetase is believed to recognize and hydrolyze incorrect aminoacyl-tRNAs it may have produced.
    D. there is a separate aminoacyl-tRNA synthetase for every amino acid appearing in the final, functional protein.
    E. there is a separate aminoacyl-tRNA synthetase for every tRNA species.

11. During collagen synthesis, events that occur extracellularly include all of the following EXCEPT:
    A. modification of prolyl residues.
    B. amino-terminal peptide cleavage.
    C. carboxyl-terminal peptide cleavage.
    D. modification of lysyl residues.
    E. covalent cross-linking.

12. In the functions of ubiquitin all of the following are true EXCEPT:
    A. ATP is required for activation of ubiquitin.
    B. ubiquitin-dependent degradation of proteins occurs in the lysosomes.
    C. linkage of a protein to ubiquitin does not always mark it for degradation.
    D. the identity of the N-terminal amino acid is one determinant of selection for degradation.
    E. ATP is required by the protease that degrades the tagged protein.

Match each of the following numbered markers with the appropriate lettered target site.

A. export from the cell
B. lysosomes
C. mitochondria
D. nucleus
E. peroxisomes

13. Clusters of lysine and arginine amino acid residues.
14. Mannose 6-phosphate.
15. Positively charged amphiphilic α-helix.
16. Ser-Lys-Leu (SKL).

ANSWERS

1. A This is the definition of degeneracy (p. 719). B and E are not known to occur, although sometimes tRNA reads only the first two bases of a triplet (wobble), and sometimes unusual bases occur in anticodons (p. 719). C denotes the stop (nonsense) codons (p. 719). D is a deviation from universality of the code, as found in mitochondria (p. 719).
2. D Deletion of a single base causes a frameshift mutation (p. 721). The frameshift would destroy the original stop codon; another one would be generated before or after the original location. In contrast, replacement of one base by another would cause replacement of one amino acid (missense mutation), unless a stop codon is thereby generated (p. 721).
3. B A: Methionyl-$tRNA_i^{Met}$ appears at the P site. C: Phosphorylation of eIF-2 inhibits initiation. D: Methionyl-$tRNA_e^{Met}$ is used internally. E: mRNA associates first with the 40S subunit (p. 725).
4. E fMet-$tRNA_i^{Met}$ is involved in initiation of protein synthesis in prokaryote (p. 725).
5. C A: The incoming aminoacyl-tRNA binds to the A site. B: Peptide bond formation requires no energy source other than the aminoacyl-tRNA (pp. 727 and 730). D: Streptomycin inhibits formation of the prokaryotic 70S initiation complex (analogous to the eukaryotic 80S complex) and causes misreading of the genetic code when the initiation complex is already formed (p. 734). E: The electron pair of the amino group carries out a nucleophilic attack on the carbonyl carbon.
6. A This toxin catalyzes the formation of an ADP ribosyl derivative of translocase, which irreversibly inactivates the translocase (p. 735).
7. D One ATP is converted to AMP during activation of an amino acid (p. 721), and two GTP are converted to GDP during elongation (pp. 727 and 730). The ATP $\rightarrow$ AMP counts as two high-energy bonds expended.
8. E See p. 743. γ-Carboxylation is of special importance in several blood clotting proteins (p. 746).
9. D See pp. 746–747.
10. C Bonds between a tRNA and an incorrect smaller amino acid may form but are rapidly hydrolyzed (p. 723). A and B: ATP and the amino acid react to form an enzyme-bound aminoacyl adenylate; PP_i is released into the medium (p. 721). D: Some amino acids, such as hydroxyproline and hydroxylysine, arise by co- or posttranslational modification (p. 747). E: An aminoacyl-tRNA synthetase may recognize any of several tRNAs specific for a given amino acid (p. 722).
11. A See p. 747. Some modification of lysyl residues also occurs intracellularly (p. 747).
12. E A–D: True (see p. 751). C: Linkage to histones does not result in their degradation.
13. D (see p. 743).
14. B (see p. 740).
15. C (see p. 742).
16. E (see p. 743). This tripeptide must occur at the carboxyl terminal.

CHAPTER

RECOMBINANT DNA AND BIOTECHNOLOGY

Gerald Soslau

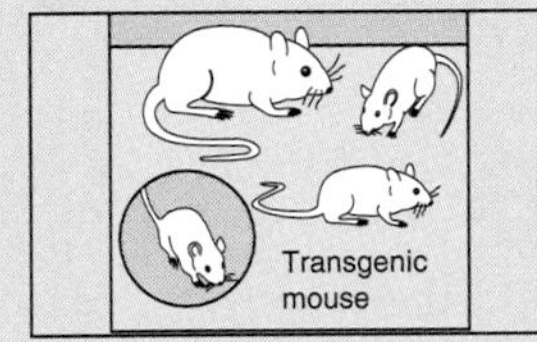

18.1 ■ OVERVIEW

By 1970, the stage was set for modern molecular biology based on studies of numerous scientists in the previous 30 years, during which ignorance of what biochemical entity orchestrated the replication of life forms with such fidelity gave way to a state where sequencing and manipulating the expression of genes would be feasible. The relentless march toward a full understanding of gene regulation under normal and pathological conditions has moved with increasing rapidity since the 1970s. Deoxyribonucleic acid, composed of only four different nucleotides covalently linked by a sugar–phosphate backbone, is deceptively complex. Complexity is conferred on the DNA molecule by the nonrandom sequence of its bases, multiple conformations that exist in equilibrium in the biological environment, and specific proteins that recognize and associate with selected regions. By the 1970s biochemical knowledge of the cellular processes and their macromolecular components had established several facts required for the surge forward. It was clear that gene expression was highly regulated. Enzymes involved in DNA replication and RNA transcription had been purified and their function in the synthetic process defined. The genetic code had been broken. Genetic maps of prokaryotic chromosomes had been established based on gene linkage studies with thousands of different mutants. Finally, RNA species could be purified, enzymatically hydrolyzed into discrete pieces, and laboriously sequenced. It was evident that further progress in the understanding of gene regulation would require techniques to selectively cut DNA into homogeneous pieces. Even small, highly purified viral DNA genomes were too complex to decipher. The thought of tackling the human genome with more than 3×10^9 base pairs was all the more onerous.

Identification, purification, and characterization of restriction endonucleases that faithfully hydrolyze DNA molecules at specific sequences permitted the development of recombinant DNA methodologies. Development of DNA sequencing opened the previously tightly locked molecular biology gates to the secrets held within the organization of diverse biological genomes. Genes could finally be sequenced, but perhaps more importantly so could the flanking regions that regulate their expression. Sequencing regulatory regions of numerous genes defined consensus sequences such as those found in promoters, enhancers, and many binding sites for regulatory proteins (see Chapter 19). Each gene contains an upstream promoter where a DNA-dependent RNA polymerase binds prior to initiation of transcription. While some DNA regulatory sites lie just upstream of the transcription initiation site, other regulatory regions are hundreds to thousands of bases removed and still others are downstream.

This chapter presents many of the sophisticated techniques, developed in the past 25 years, that allow for the dissection of complex genomes into defined fragments with the complete analysis of the nucleotide sequence and function of these DNA regions. The modification and manipulation of genes, that is, genetic engineering, facilitates the introduction and expression of genes in both prokaryotic and eukaryotic cells. Many methodological approaches in genetic engineering have been greatly simplified by employment of a method that rapidly amplifies selected regions of DNA—the polymerase chain reaction (PCR). Proteins for experimental and clinical uses are readily produced by these procedures and it is anticipated that in the not too distant future these methods will allow for the rapid increase of treatment modalities of genetic diseases with gene replacement therapy. Current and potential uses of recombinant DNA technologies are also described. The significance to our society of advancements in the understanding of genetic macromolecules and their manipulation cannot be overstated.

18.2 ■ POLYMERASE CHAIN REACTION

The rapid production of large quantities of a specific DNA sequence took a leap forward with the development of the **polymerase chain reaction (PCR).** The PCR requires two nucleotide oligomers that hybridize to the complementary DNA strands in a region of interest. The oligomers serve as primers for a DNA polymerase that extends each strand. Repeated cycling of the PCR yields large amounts of each DNA molecule of interest in a matter of hours as opposed to days and weeks associated with cloning techniques.

The PCR *amplification of a specific DNA sequence* can be accomplished with a purified DNA sample or a small region within a complex mixture of DNA. The principles of the reaction are shown in Figure 18.1. The nucleotide sequence of the DNA to be amplified must be known or it must be cloned in a vector (see p. 778) where the sequence of the flanking DNA has been established. The product of PCR is a double-stranded DNA molecule and the reaction is completed in each cycle when all of the template molecules have been copied. In order to initiate a new round of replication the sample is heated to melt the double-stranded DNA and, in the presence of excess oligonucleotide primers, cooled to permit hybridization of the single-stranded template with free oligomers. A new cycle of DNA replication will initiate in the presence of DNA polymerase and all four dNTPs. Heating to about 95°C as required for melting DNA inactivates most DNA polymerases, but a heat stable polymerase,

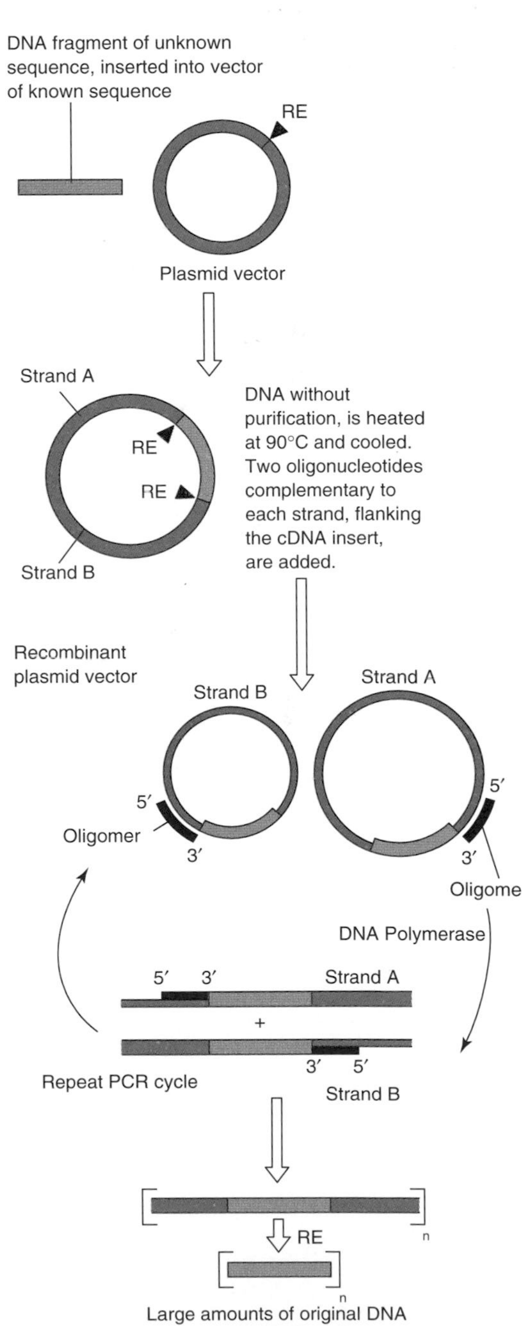

FIGURE 18.1
Polymerase chain reaction (PCR).
A DNA fragment of unknown sequence is inserted into a vector of known sequence by normal recombinant methodologies. The recombinant DNA of interest does not need to be purified from contaminating DNA species. The DNA is heated to 90°C to dissociate the double strands and cooled in the presence of excess amounts of two different complementary oligomers that hybridize to the known vector DNA sequences flanking the foreign DNA insert. Only recombinant single-stranded DNA species can serve as templates for DNA replication, yielding double-stranded DNA fragments of foreign DNA bounded by the oligomer DNA sequences. The heating–replication cycle is repeated many times to rapidly produce greatly amplified amounts of the original foreign DNA. The DNA fragment of interest can be purified from the polymerase chain reaction mixture by cleaving it with the original restriction endonuclease (RE), electrophoresing the DNA mixture through an agarose gel, and eluting the band of interest from the gel.

CLINICAL CORRELATION 18.1

Polymerase Chain Reaction and Screening for Human Immunodeficiency Virus

Use of the polymerase chain reaction (PCR) to amplify minute quantities of DNA has revolutionized the ability to detect and analyze DNA species. With PCR it is possible to synthesize sufficient DNA for analysis. Conventional methods for detection and identification of the human immunodeficiency virus (HIV), such as Southern blot–DNA hybridization and antigen analysis, are labor intensive, expensive, and have low sensitivity. An infected individual, with no sign of AIDS (acquired immunodeficiency syndrome), may test false negative for HIV by these procedures. Early detection of HIV infections in these individuals is crucial to initiate treatment and/or monitor the progression of their disease. In addition, a sensitive method is required to be certain that contributed blood from donors does not contain HIV. PCR amplification of potential HIV DNA sequences within DNA isolated from an individual's white blood cells permits the identification of viral infections prior to the presence of antibodies, the so-called seronegative state. Current methodologies are too costly to apply this testing to large-scale screening of donor blood samples. PCR can also be used to increase the sensitivity to detect and characterize DNA sequences of any other human infectious pathogen.

Kwok, S., and Sninsky, J. J. Application of PCR to the detection of human infectious diseases. In: H. A. Erlich (Ed.), *PCR Technology*. New York: Stockton Press, 1989, p. 235.

termed Taq DNA polymerase isolated from *Thermus aquaticus,* is now employed, obviating the need for fresh polymerase after each cycle. This has permitted the automation of PCR with each DNA molecule capable of being amplified one million-fold.

When the DNA to be amplified is present in very low concentrations relative to the total DNA in the sample, it is possible to amplify the DNA region of interest along with other spurious sequences. In this situation the specificity of the amplification reaction can be enhanced by **nested PCR.** After conducting the first PCR with one set of primers for 10–20 cycles, a small aliquot is removed for a second PCR. However, the second PCR is conducted with a new set of primers that are complementary to the template DNA just downstream of the first set of primers, or "nested" between the original set of primers. This process amplifies the DNA region of interest twice with a greatly enhanced specificity.

PCR has many applications including gene diagnosis, forensic investigations where only a drop of dried blood or a single hair is available, and evolutionary studies with preserved biological material. Use of PCR for screening for human immunodeficiency virus is presented in Clin. Corr. 18.1.

18.3 ■ RESTRICTION ENDONUCLEASE AND RESTRICTION MAPS

Restriction Endonucleases Permit Selective Hydrolysis of DNA to Generate Restriction Maps

Nature possesses a diverse set of tools, the **restriction endonucleases,** capable of selectively dissecting DNA molecules of all sizes and origin into smaller fragments. These enzymes confer some protection on bacteria against invading viruses, that is, bacteriophage. The bacterial DNA sequences normally recognized by the restriction endonuclease may be protected from cleavage in the host cell by methylation of bases within the enzyme recognized palindrome while the unmethylated viral DNA is recognized as foreign and is hydrolyzed. Numerous Type II restriction endonucleases, with differing sequence specificities, have been identified and purified; many are now commercially available (see p. 609 for discussion of restriction endonuclease activities).

Restriction endonuclease permits construction of a new type of genetic map, the **restriction map,** in which the site of enzyme cleavage within the DNA is identified. Purified DNA species that contain restriction endonuclease sequences are subjected to restriction endonuclease cleavage. By regulating the time of exposure of the purified DNA molecules to restriction endonuclease cleavage, a population of DNA fragments that are partially to fully hydrolyzed can be generated. Separation of these enzyme-generated fragments by agarose gel electrophoresis allows for the construction of restriction maps; an example of this procedure with circular DNA is presented in Figure 18.2. Analysis of a DNA completely hydrolyzed by a restriction endonuclease establishes how many sites the restriction endonuclease recognizes within the molecule and what size fragments are generated. The size distribution of composite fragments generated by the partial enzymatic cleavage of the DNA molecules demonstrates linkage of all potential fragments. The sequential use of different restriction endonucleases has permitted a detailed restriction map of numerous circular DNA species including bacterial plasmids, viruses, and mitochondrial DNA. The method is also equally amenable to linear DNA fragments that have been purified to homogeneity.

Restriction Maps Permit the Routine Preparation of Defined Segments of DNA

Restriction maps may yield little information as to the genes or regulatory elements within the various DNA fragments. They have been used to demonstrate sequence diversity of organelle DNA, such as mitochondrial DNA, within species (see Clin. Corr. 18.2). Restriction maps can also be used to detect deletion mutations where a defined DNA fragment from the parental strain

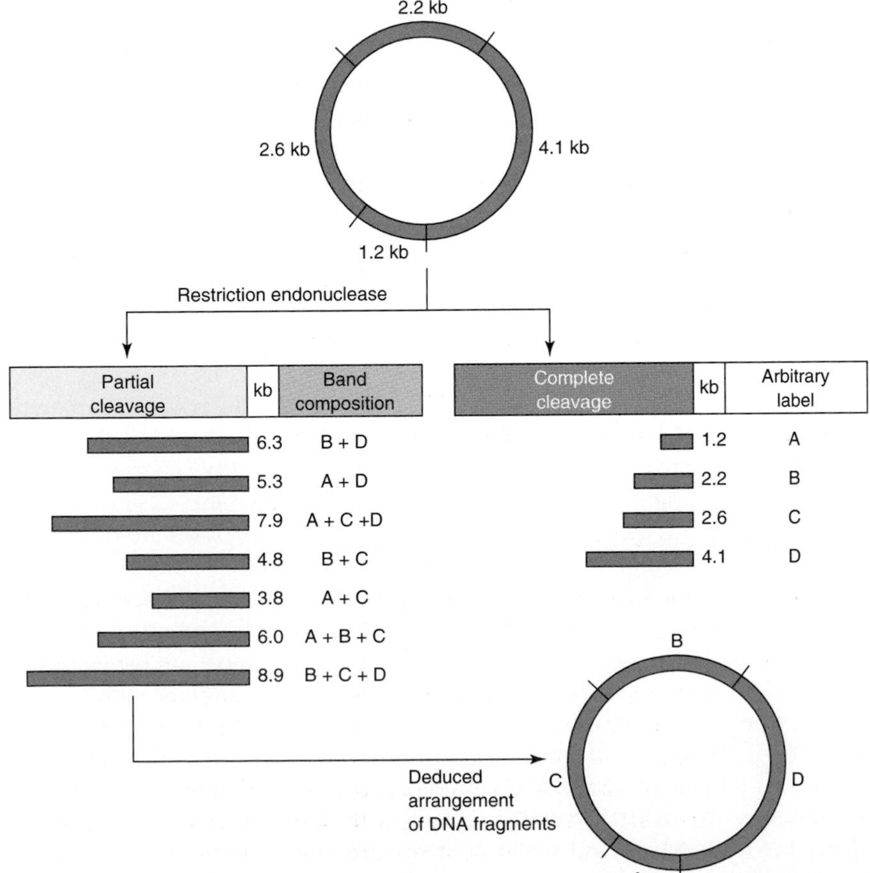

FIGURE 18.2
Restriction endonuclease mapping of DNA. Purified DNA is subjected to restriction endonuclease digestion for varying times, which generates partially to fully cleaved DNA fragments. The DNA fragments are separated by agarose gel electrophoresis and stained with ethidium bromide. The DNA bands are visualized with a UV light source and photographed. The size of the DNA fragments is determined by the relative migration through the gel as compared to co-electrophoresed DNA standards. The relative arrangement of each fragment within the DNA molecule can be deduced from the size of the incompletely hydrolyzed fragments.

CLINICAL CORRELATION 18.2

Restriction Mapping and Evolution

In the past, evolutionary studies of species have depended solely on anatomical changes observed in fossil records and on carbon dating. More recently, these studies are being supported by molecular analysis of the sequence and size of selected genes or whole DNA molecules. Evolutionary alterations of a selected DNA molecule from different species can be rapidly assessed by restriction endonuclease mapping. Generation of restriction endonuclease maps requires a pure preparation of DNA. Mammalian mitochondria contain a covalently closed circular DNA molecule of approximately 16,000 base pairs that can rapidly be purified from cells. The mitochondrial DNA (mtDNA) can be employed directly for the study of evolutionary changes in DNA without the need of cloning a specific gene.

Mitochondrial DNA has been purified from the Guinea baboon, rhesus macaque, guenon, and human and cleaved with 11 different restriction endonucleases. Restriction maps were constructed for each species. The maps were all aligned relative to the direction and nucleotide site where DNA replication is initiated. A comparison of shared and altered restriction endonuclease sites allowed for calculation of the degree of divergence in nucleotide sequence between species. It was found that the rate of base substitution (calculated from the degree of divergence versus the time of divergence) has been about tenfold greater than changes in the nuclear genome. This high rate of mutation of the readily purified mtDNA molecule makes it an excellent model to study evolutionary relationships between species.

Brown, W. M., George, M. Jr., and Wilson, A. C. Rapid evolution of animal mitochondrial DNA. *Proc. Natl. Acad. Sci. USA* 76:1967, 1979.

migrates as a smaller fragment in the mutated strain. Most importantly, the enzymatic microscissors used to generate restriction maps cut DNA into defined homogeneous fragments that can be readily purified. These maps are crucial for cloning and for sequencing genes and their flanking DNA regions.

18.4 ■ DNA SEQUENCING

To determine the complexities of regulation of gene expression and to seek the basis for genetic diseases, techniques were necessary to determine the exact sequence of bases in DNA. In the late 1970s two different sequencing techniques were developed, one by A. Maxam and W. Gilbert, the chemical cleavage approach, and the other by F. Sanger, the enzymatic approach. Both procedures may employ the labeling of a terminal nucleotide, followed by the separation and detection of generated oligonucleotides.

Chemical Cleavage Method: Maxam–Gilbert Procedure

Requirements for this procedure include (1) labeling of the terminal nucleotide, (2) selective hydrolysis of the phosphodiester bond for each nucleotide separately to produce fragments with 1, 2, 3, or more bases, (3) quantitative separation of the hydrolyzed fragments, and (4) a qualitative determination of the label added in Step 1. The following describes one approach of the **Maxam–Gilbert procedure.** The overall approach is presented in Figure 18.3.

One end of each strand of DNA can be selectively radiolabeled with ^{32}P. This is accomplished when a purified double helix DNA fragment contains restriction endonuclease sites on either side of the region to be sequenced. Hydrolysis of the DNA with two different restriction endonucleases then results in different staggered ends, each with a different base in the first position of the single-stranded region. Labeling of the 3′ end of each strand is accomplished with addition of the next nucleotide as directed by the corresponding base sequence on the complementary DNA strand. A fragment of *E. coli* DNA polymerase I, termed the **Klenow fragment,** will catalyze this reaction. The Klenow fragment, produced by partial proteolysis of the polymerase holoenzyme, lacks $5' \rightarrow 3'$ exonuclease activity but retains the $3' \rightarrow 5'$ exonuclease and polymerase activity. Each strand can therefore be selectively labeled in separate experiments. The complementary unlabeled strand will not be detectable when analyzing the sequence of the labeled strand.

The hydrolysis of the labeled DNA into different lengths is accomplished by first selectively destroying one or two bases of the four nucleotides. The procedure used exposes the phosphodiester bond connecting adjoining bases and permits selective cleavage of the DNA at the altered base. In separate chemical treatments, samples of labeled DNA are treated to alter purines and pyrimidines without disrupting the sugar–phosphate backbone; a method is not currently available to specifically alter adenine or thymine. Conditions for base modification are selected such that only one or a few bases are destroyed randomly within any one molecule. The four separate DNA samples are then reacted with piperidine, which chemically breaks the sugar–phosphate backbone at sites where a base has been destroyed, generating fragments of different sizes. Since labeling is specific at the end while the chemical alteration of the base is random and not total, some of the fragments will be end labeled. For example, wherever a cytosine residue had been randomly destroyed in the appropriate reaction tube a break will be introduced into the DNA fragment. The series of chemically generated, end-labeled DNA fragments from each of the four tubes are electrophoresed through a polyacrylamide gel. Bases destroyed near the end-labeled nucleotide will generate fragments that migrate faster through the gel, as low molecular weight species, while fragments derived

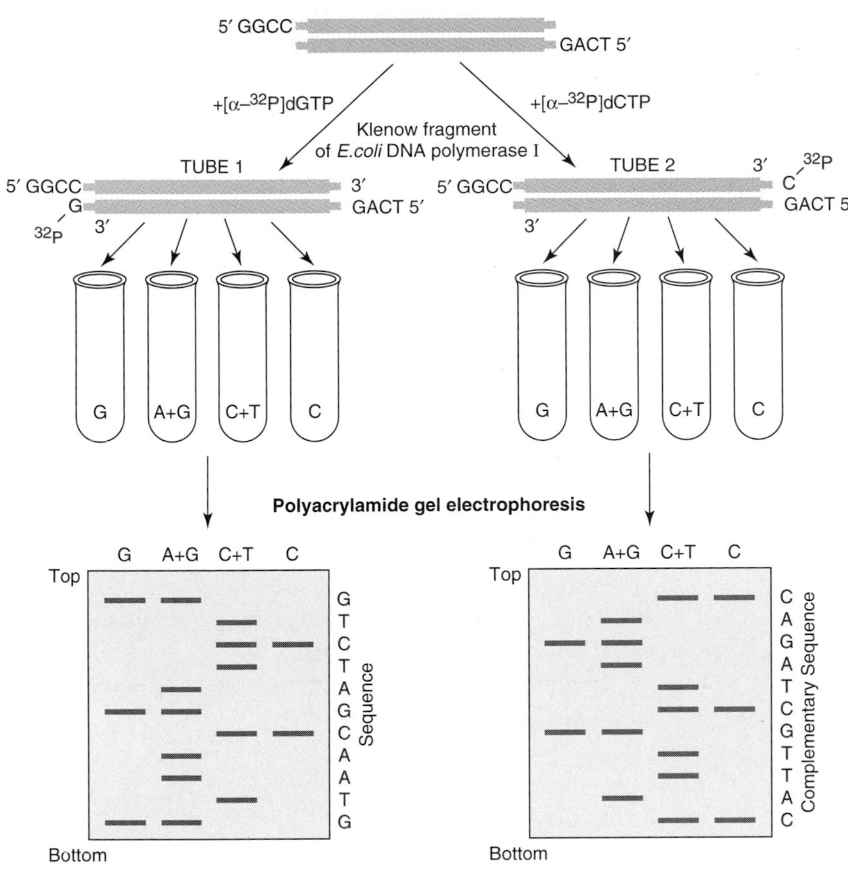

FIGURE 18.3
Maxam–Gilbert chemical method to sequence DNA.
A double-stranded DNA fragment to be sequenced is obtained by restriction endonuclease cleavage and purified. Both strands are sequenced by selectively labeling the ends of each DNA strand. One strand of DNA is end-labeled with [^{32}P]dGTP in reaction tube 1 while the other is end-labeled with [^{32}P]dCTP in reaction tube 2. The end-labeled DNA is then subdivided into four fractions where the different bases are chemically destroyed at random positions within the single-stranded DNA molecule. The less selective chemical destruction of adenine simultaneously destroys G and the destruction of thymine destroys the C bases. The single-stranded DNA is cleaved at the sites of the destroyed bases. This generates end-labeled fragments of all possible lengths corresponding to the distance from the end to the sites of base destruction. Labeled DNA fragments are separated according to size by electrophoresis. The DNA sequence can then be determined from the electrophoretic patterns detected on autoradiograms.

from bases destroyed more distant from the end will migrate through the gel more slowly as higher molecular weight molecules. The gel is then exposed to X-ray film, which detects the ^{32}P, and the radioactively labeled bands within the gel can be visualized. The sequence can be read manually or by automated methods directly from the X-ray autoradiograph beginning at the bottom (smaller fragments) and proceeding toward the top of the film (larger fragments). Sequencing the complementary strand checks the correctness of the sequence.

Interrupted Enzymatic Cleavage Method: Sanger Procedure

The **Sanger procedure** of DNA sequencing is based on the random termination of a DNA chain during enzymatic synthesis. The technique is possible because the dideoxynucleotide analog of each of the four normal nucleotides (Figure 18.4) can be incorporated into a growing DNA chain by DNA polymerase. The ribose of the **dideoxynucleotide triphosphate (ddNTP)** has the OH group at both the 2′ and 3′ positions replaced with a proton, whereas dNTP has only a single OH group replaced by a proton at the 2′ position. Thus the ddNTP incorporated into the growing chain is unable to form a phosphodiester bond with another dNTP because the 3′ position of the ribose does not contain an OH group. The growing DNA molecule can be terminated at random points, from the first nucleotide incorporated to the last, by including in the reaction system both the normal nucleotide and the ddNTP (e.g., dATP and ddATP) at concentrations such that the two nucleotides compete for incorporation.

Identification of DNA fragments requires labeling of the 5′ end of the DNA molecules or the incorporation of labeled nucleotides during synthesis. The technique, outlined in Figure 18.5, is best conducted with pure single-stranded DNA; however, denatured double-stranded DNA can be used. Today, the DNA

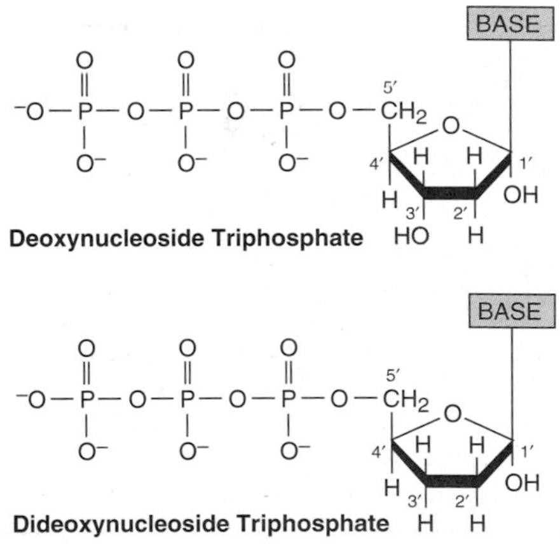

Deoxynucleoside Triphosphate

Dideoxynucleoside Triphosphate

FIGURE 18.4
Structure of deoxynucleoside triphosphate and dideoxynucleoside triphosphate.
The 3′-OH group is lacking on the ribose component of the dideoxynucleoside triphosphate (ddNTP). This molecule can be incorporated into a growing DNA molecule through a phosphodiester bond with its 5′-phosphates. Once incorporated, the ddNTP blocks further synthesis of the DNA molecule since it lacks the 3′-OH acceptor group for an incoming nucleotide.

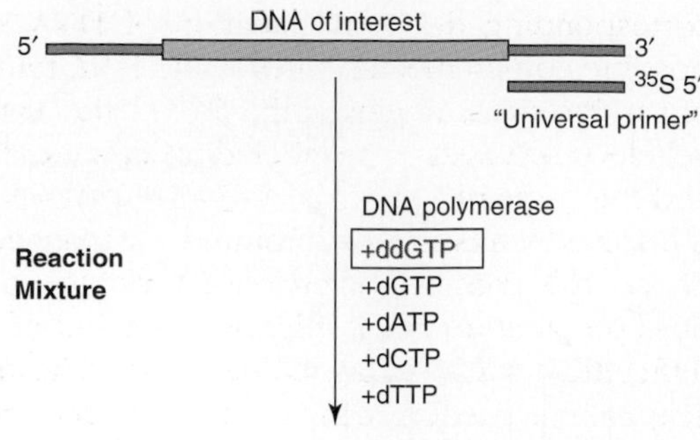

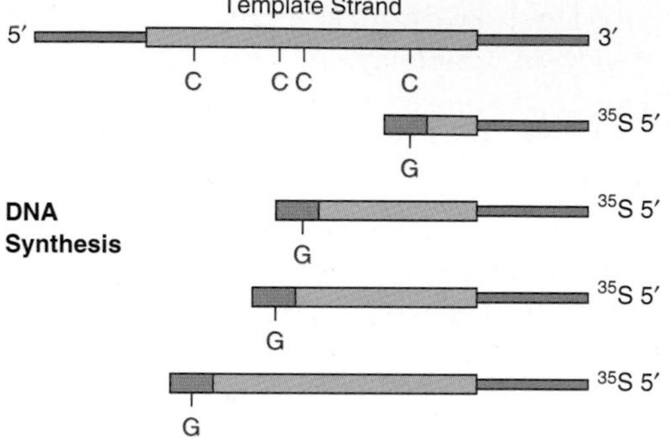

(a) Recombinant M13 bacteriophage

(b) Polyacrylamide gel electrophoresis of reaction mixture

FIGURE 18.5
Sanger dideoxynucleoside triphosphate method to sequence DNA.
The DNA region of interest is inserted into bacteriophage DNA molecule. Replicating bacteriophage produces a single-stranded recombinant DNA molecule that is readily purified. The known sequence of the bacteriophage DNA downstream of the DNA insert serves as a hybridization site for an end-labeled oligomer with a complementary sequence, a universal primer. Extension of this primer is catalyzed with a DNA polymerase in the presence of all four deoxynucleoside triphosphates plus one dideoxynucleoside triphosphate, for example, ddGTP. Synthesis stops whenever a dideoxynucleoside triphosphate is incorporated into the growing molecule. Note that the dideoxynucleotide competes for incorporation with the deoxynucleotide. This generates end-labeled DNA fragments of all possible lengths that are separated by electrophoresis. The DNA sequence can then be determined from the electrophoretic patterns.

to be sequenced is frequently isolated from a recombinant single-stranded bacteriophage (see p. 778) where a region flanking the DNA of interest contains a sequence that is complementary to a universal primer. The primer can be labeled with either ^{32}P or ^{35}S nucleotide. Primer extension is accomplished with one of several different available DNA polymerases; one with great versatility is a genetically engineered form of the bacteriophage T7 DNA polymerase. The reaction mixture, composed of the target DNA, labeled primer, and all four deoxynucleoside triphosphates, is divided into four tubes, each containing a different dideoxynucleoside triphosphate. The ddNTPs are randomly incorporated during the enzymatic synthesis of DNA and cause termination of the chain.

Since the ddNTP is present in the reaction tube at a low level, relative to the corresponding dNTP, termination of DNA synthesis occurs randomly at all possible complementary sites to the DNA template. This yields DNA molecules of varying sizes, labeled at the 5′ end, that can be separated by polyacrylamide gel electrophoresis. The labeled species are detected by X-ray autoradiography and the sequence is read.

Initially, this method required a single-stranded DNA template, production of a specific complementary oligonucleotide primer, and the need for a relatively pure preparation of the Klenow fragment of *E. coli* DNA polymerase I. These difficulties have been overcome and modifications have simplified the approach. The Sanger method can rapidly sequence as many as 400 bases while the Maxam–Gilbert method is limited to about 250 bases.

The PCR and Sanger methods can be combined for **direct sequencing** of small DNA regions of interest. The double-stranded PCR product is employed directly as template. Conditions are set such that one strand of melted DNA (template) anneals with the primer in preference to reannealing of template with its complementary strand, which would reform the original double-stranded DNA. Sequencing then follows the standard dideoxy chain termination reaction (typically with Sequenase in lieu of the Klenow polymerase) with synthesis of random-length chains occurring as extensions of the PCR primer. This method has been employed successfully for the diagnosis of genetic disorders (see Clin. Corr. 18.3).

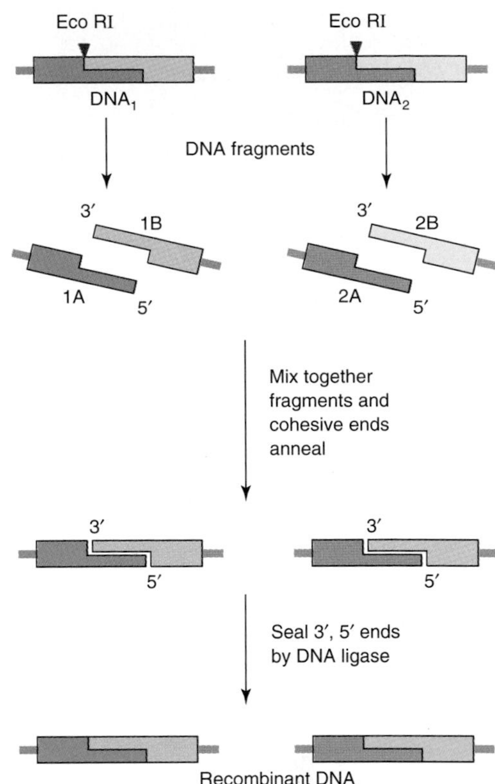

FIGURE 18.6
Formation of recombinant DNA from restriction endonuclease-generated fragments containing cohesive ends.
Many restriction endonucleases hydrolyze DNA in a staggered fashion, yielding fragments with single-stranded regions at their 5′ and 3′ ends. DNA fragments generated from different molecules with the same restriction endonuclease have complementary single-stranded ends that can be annealed and covalently linked together with a DNA ligase. All different combinations are possible in a mixture. When two DNA fragments of different origin combine it results in a recombinant DNA molecule.

18.5 ■ RECOMBINANT DNA AND CLONING

DNA from Different Sources Can Be Ligated to Form a New DNA Species: Recombinant DNA

The ability to selectively hydrolyze a population of DNA molecules with a battery of restriction endonucleases led to the development of a technique for joining two different DNA molecules termed **recombinant DNA.** This technique combined with the various techniques for replication, separation, and identification permits the production of large quantities of purified DNA fragments. The combined techniques, referred to as **recombinant DNA technologies,** allow the removal of a piece of DNA out of a larger complex molecule, such as the genome of a virus or human, and amplification of the DNA fragment. Recombinant DNAs have been prepared with DNA fragments from bacteria combined with fragments from humans, viruses with viruses, and so on. The ability to join two different pieces of DNA together at specific sites within the molecules is achieved with two enzymes, a restriction endonuclease and a **DNA ligase.** There are a number of different restriction endonucleases, varying in their nucleotide sequence specificity, that can be used (Section 18.3). Some hydrolyze the two strands of DNA in a staggered fashion, producing "*sticky or cohesive*" *ends* (Figure 18.6), while others cut both strands symmetrically, producing a *blunt end.* A specific restriction enzyme cuts DNA at exactly the same nucleotide sequence site regardless of the source of the DNA (bacteria, plant, mammal, etc.). A DNA molecule may have one, several, hundreds, thousands, or no recognition sites for a particular restriction endonuclease. The staggered cut results in a fragmented DNA molecule with ends that are single stranded. When different DNA fragments generated by the same restriction endonuclease are mixed, their single-stranded ends can hybridize, that is, anneal together. In the presence of DNA ligase the two fragments are connected covalently, producing a recombinant DNA molecule.

The DNA fragments produced from restriction endonuclease that form blunt ends can also be ligated but with much lower efficiency. The efficiency can be increased by enzymatically adding a poly(dA) tail to one species of DNA and a poly(dT) tail to the ends of the second species of DNA. The DNA fragments with complementary tails can be annealed and ligated in the same manner as fragments with restriction enzyme-generated cohesive ends.

Recombinant DNA Vectors Can Be Produced in Significant Quantities by Cloning

Synthesis of a recombinant DNA opens the way for production of significant quantities of interesting DNA fragments. By incorporating a recombinant DNA into a cellular system that allows replication of recombinant DNA, amplification of DNA of interest can be achieved. A carrier DNA, termed a **cloning vector,** is employed. Bacterial plasmids are ideally suited as recombinant DNA vectors. Many bacteria contain a single circular chromosome of approximately 4 million base pairs and minicircular DNA molecules called **plasmids.** Plasmids are usually composed of only a few thousand base pairs and are rarely associated with the large chromosomal molecule. Genes within the plasmid have various functions; one of the most useful is the ability to confer antibiotic resistance to the bacterium, an attribute useful in selecting specific colonies of the bacteria. Plasmids replicate independently of replication of the main bacterial chromosome. One type of plasmid, the **relaxed-control** plasmids, may be present in tens to hundreds of copies per bacterium, and replication is dependent solely on host enzymes that have long half-lives. Therefore replication of **"relaxed" plasmids** can occur in the presence of a protein synthesis inhibitor. Bacteria can accumulate several thousand plasmid copies per cell under these conditions. Other plasmid types are subjected to **stringent control** and their replication is dependent on the continued synthesis of plasmid-encoded proteins. These plasmids replicate at about the same rate as the large bacterial chromosome, and only a low number of copies occur per cell. The former plasmid type is routinely used for recombinant DNA studies.

The first practical recombinant DNA molecule that could be cloned involved as a vector the *E. coli* **plasmid pSC101,** which contains a single EcoRI restriction endonuclease site and a gene that encodes for a protein that confers antibiotic resistance to the bacteria. This plasmid contains an origin of replication and associated DNA regulatory sequences that are referred to as a **replicon.** This vector, however, suffers from a number of limiting factors. The single restriction endonuclease site limits the DNA fragments that can be cloned and the one antibiotic-resistance selectable marker reduces the convenience in selection; in addition, it replicates poorly.

Plasmid vectors with broad versatilities have been constructed using recombinant DNA technology. The desirable features of a plasmid vector include a relatively low molecular weight (3–5 kb) to accommodate larger fragments; several different restriction endonuclease sites useful in cloning a variety of restriction enzyme-generated fragments; multiple selectable markers to aid in selecting bacteria with recombinant DNA molecules; and a high rate of replication. The first plasmid constructed (Figure 18.7) to satisfy these requirements was **pBR322** and this plasmid has been used for the subsequent generation of newer vectors in use today. Most currently employed vectors contain an inserted sequence of DNA termed **polylinker, restriction site bank,** or **polycloning site,** which contains numerous restriction endonuclease sites unique to the plasmid.

DNA Can Be Inserted into Vector DNA in a Specific Direction: Directional Cloning

Directional cloning reduces the number of variable "recombinants" and enhances the probability of selection of the desired recombinant. Insertion of foreign DNA, with a defined polarity, into a plasmid vector in the absence of the plasmid resealing itself can be accomplished by employing two restriction

CLINICAL CORRELATION 18.3

Direct Sequencing of DNA for Diagnosis of Genetic Disorders

The X-linked recessive hemorrhagic disorder hemophilia B is caused by a coagulation factor IX deficiency. The factor IX gene has been cloned and sequenced and contains 8 exons spanning 34 kb that encode a glycoprotein secreted by the liver. Over 300 mutations of the gene have been discovered of which about 85% are single base substitutions and the rest are complete or partial gene deletions. Several methods have been employed to identify carriers of a defective gene copy and for prenatal diagnoses. Unfortunately, these methods were costly, time consuming, and all too often inaccurate. Direct sequencing of PCR amplified genomic DNA has been employed to circumvent these diagnostic shortcomings. Between 0.1 and 1 μg of genomic DNA can readily be isolated from patient blood samples and each factor IX exon can be PCR amplified with appropriate primers. The amplified DNA can then be used for direct sequencing to determine if a mutation in the gene exists that would be diagnostic of one of the forms of hemophilia B. For example, a patient with a moderate hemophilia B (London 6) had an A → G transition at position 10442 that led to a substitution of Asp 64 by Gly.

Green, P. M., Bentley, D. R., Mibashan, R. S., Nilsson, I. M., and Gianelli, F. Molecular pathology of hemophilia b. *EMBO J.* 8:1067, 1989.

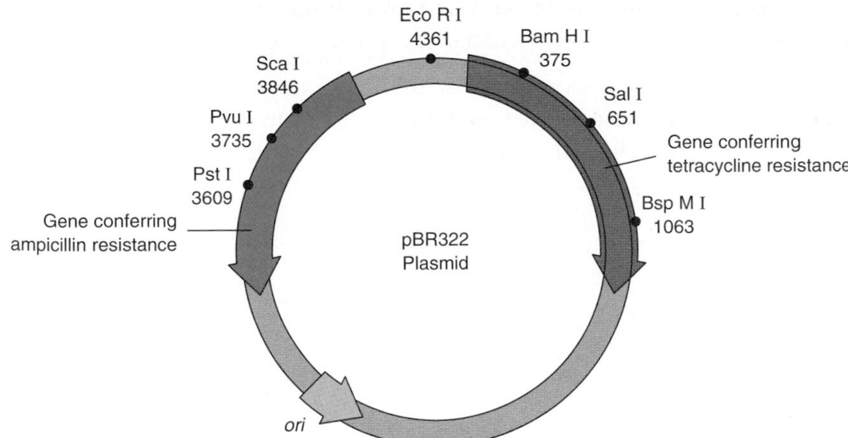

FIGURE 18.7
The pBR322 plasmid constructed in the laboratory to contain features that facilitate cloning foreign DNA fragments.
By convention, the numbering of the nucleotides begins with the first T in the unique EcoRI recognition sequence (GAATTC) and the positions on the map refer to the 5′ base of the various restriction endonuclease-recognition sequences. Only a few of the unique restriction sites within the antibiotic resistance genes and none of the numerous sites where an enzyme cuts more than once within the plasmid are shown.

endonucleases to cleave the plasmids (Figure 18.8); vectors with polylinkers are ideally suited for this purpose. The use of two enzymes yields DNA fragments and linearized plasmids with different "sticky" ends. Under these conditions the plasmid is unable to reanneal with itself. In addition, the foreign DNA can be inserted into the vector in only one orientation. This is extremely important when one clones a potentially functional gene downstream from the promoter-regulatory elements in expression vectors (see p. 778).

Bacteria Can Be Transformed with Recombinant DNA

The process of artificially introducing DNA into bacteria is referred to as **transformation.** It is accomplished by briefly exposing the cells to divalent cations that make them transiently permeable to small DNA molecules. Recombinant plasmid molecules, containing foreign DNA, can be introduced into bacteria where it would replicate normally.

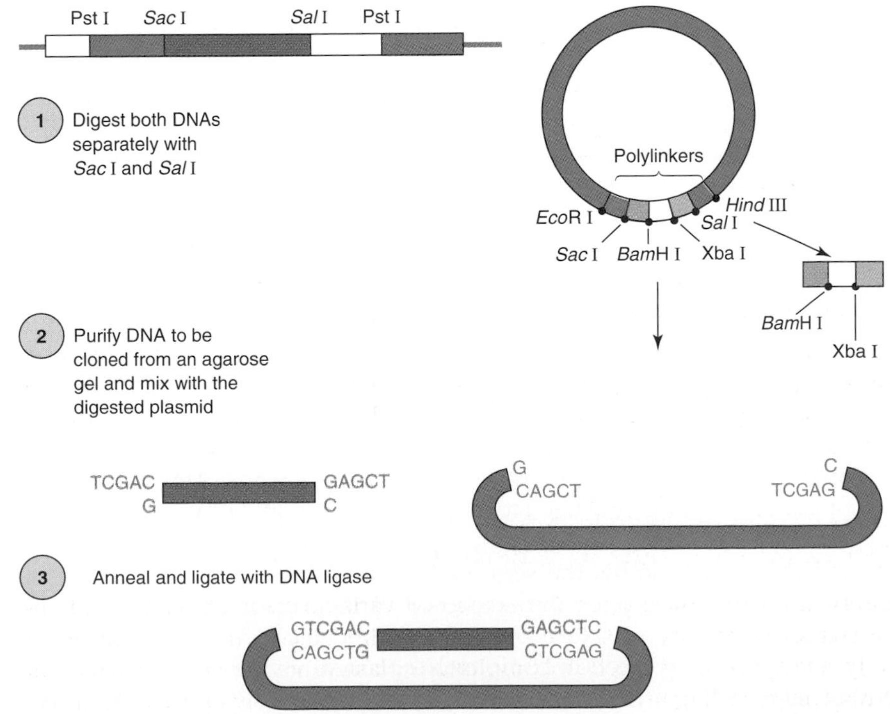

FIGURE 18.8
Directional cloning of foreign DNA into vectors with a specified orientation.
Insertion of a foreign DNA fragment into a vector with a specified orientation requires two different annealing sequences at each end of the fragment and the corresponding complementary sequence at the two ends generated in the vector. A polylinker with numerous unique restriction endonuclease sites within the vector facilitates directional cloning. Knowledge of the restriction map for the DNA of interest allows for selection of appropriate restriction endonucleases to generate specific DNA fragments that can be cloned in a vector.

It Is Necessary to Be Able to Select Transformed Bacteria

Once the plasmid has been introduced into the bacterium, both can replicate. Methods are available to select those bacteria that carry the recombinant DNA molecules. In the recombinant process some bacteria may not be transformed or may be transformed with a vector not carrying foreign DNA; in preparing the vector some may reanneal without inclusion of the DNA of interest. In some experimental conditions one can generate DNA fragments that can be readily purified for recombinant studies. Such fragments can be generated from small, highly purified DNA species, for example, some DNA viruses. More typically, however, a single restriction endonuclease will generate hundreds to hundreds of thousands of DNA fragments, depending on the size and complexity of DNA being studied. Individual fragments cannot be isolated from these samples to be individually incorporated into the plasmid. Methods have therefore been developed to select those bacteria containing the desired DNA.

Restriction endonucleases do not necessarily hydrolyze DNA into fragments containing intact genes. If the fragment contains an entire gene it may not contain the required flanking regulatory sequences, such as the promoter region. If the foreign gene is of mammalian origin, its regulatory sequences would not be recognized by the bacterial synthetic machinery. The primary gene transcript (pre-mRNA) can also contain introns that cannot be processed by the bacteria.

Recombinant DNA Molecules in a Gene Library

When a complex mixture of thousands of different genes, arranged on different chromosomes, as in the human genome, is subjected to hydrolysis with a single restriction endonuclease, thousands of DNA fragments are generated. These DNA fragments are annealed with a plasmid vector that has been cleaved to a linear molecule with the same restriction endonuclease. By adjusting the ratio of plasmid to foreign DNA the probability of joining at least one copy of each DNA fragment within a cyclized recombinant-plasmid DNA approaches one. Usually, only one out of the multiple DNA fragments is inserted into each plasmid vector. Bacteria are transformed with the recombinant molecules such that only one plasmid is taken up by a single bacterium. Each recombinant molecule can now be replicated within the bacterium and the bacterium will give rise to progeny, each carrying multiple copies of the recombinant DNA. The total population of bacteria now contain fragments of DNA that may represent the entire human genome. This is termed a **gene library.** As in any library containing thousands of volumes, a selection system must be available to retrieve the book or gene of interest.

Plasmids are commonly employed to clone DNA fragments generated from molecules of limited size and complexity, such as viruses, and to subclone large DNA fragments previously cloned in other vectors. Genomic DNA fragments are usually cloned from other vectors capable of carrying larger foreign DNA fragments than plasmids (see p. 780).

PCR May Circumvent the Need to Clone DNA

Cloning and amplification of a DNA fragment carried within a vector may be employed for subcloning, mutagenesis, and sequencing. The PCR has, in many instances, replaced the need to amplify recombinant DNA in a replicating biological system, greatly reducing the time and preparative steps required. It is not necessary to know the sequence of the DNA insert (up to 6 kb) to amplify it by the PCR, since the sequence of the vector DNA flanking the insert is known.

In some instances the PCR completely circumvents the need to clone the DNA of interest. For instance, a gene that has previously been cloned and sequenced can readily be analyzed in patient DNA for the detection of mutations

Step 1

Amplification of the DNA region of interest by the PCR

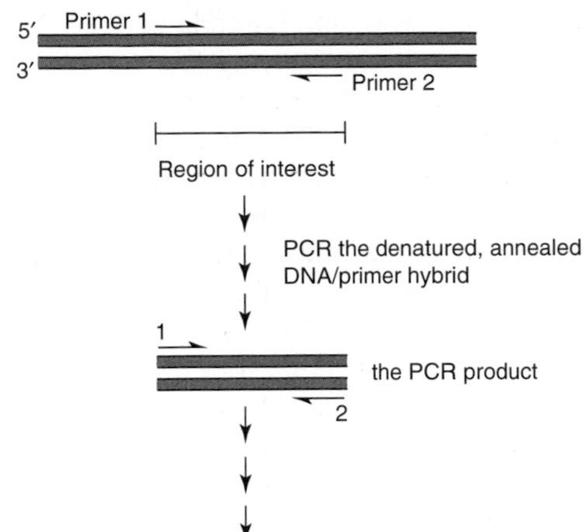

Step 2a

Employ multiple primers (1′ – 6′) simultaneously with the isolated PCR product to yield secondary PCR products of varying sizes

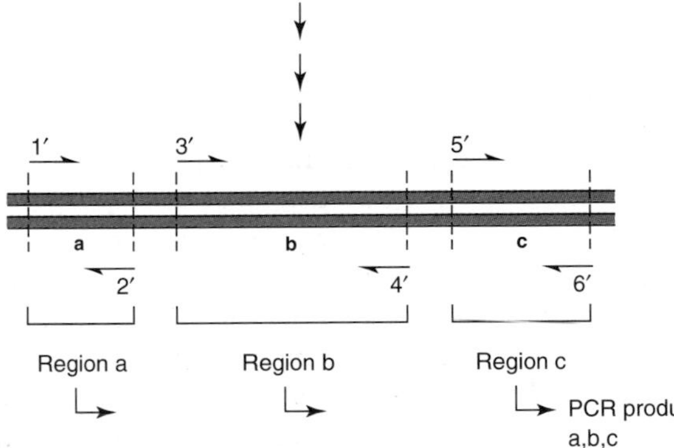

Step 2b

Repeat steps 1 and 2a with products from patient material containing a potentially deleted region b

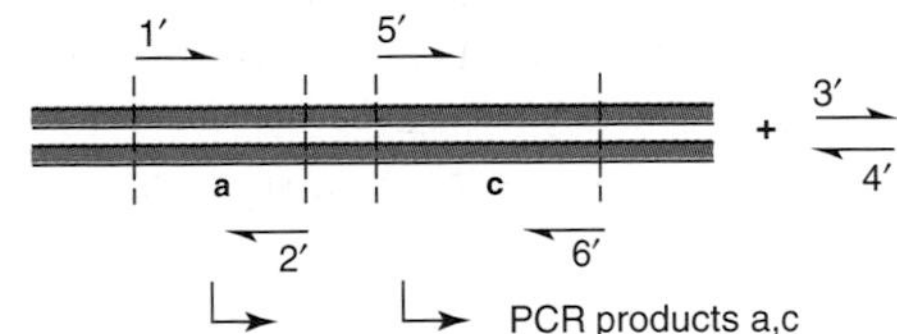

Step 3

Separate and detect the PCR products from control and patient samples by agarose gel electrophoresis and ethidium bromide staining to demonstrate the deletion of region b in the patient DNA

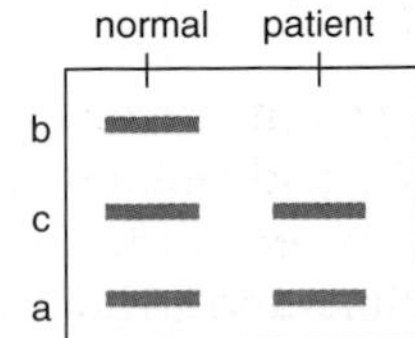

FIGURE 18.9
A multiplex PCR strategy to analyze a DNA region of interest for mutated alterations.
A region of DNA within a complex DNA molecule, derived from any source, can be amplified by the PCR with specific primers that are complementary to sequences flanking the DNA region of interest (Step 1). After multiple PCR cycles the amplified DNA (PCR product) can then be used as a template simultaneously for multiple pairs of primers (Step 2a) that are complementary throughout the DNA (here they cover three segments—a, b, and c). This procedure requires prior knowledge of the sequence of the normal DNA/gene. Step 2a is repeated for DNA derived from a patient with potential mutation(s) in the DNA region of interest (Step 2b). The amplified DNA products from the multiplex PCR step (Steps 2a and 2b) are then analyzed by agarose gel electrophoresis to ascertain if the patient sample contains a mutation (Step 3).

within this gene by a **multiplex PCR strategy.** DNA is isolated from patient blood cells and multiple pairs of oligonucleotide primers are synthesized to amplify the entire gene or selected regions within the gene (Figure 18.9). Analysis of the amplified DNA fragments by agarose gel electrophoresis would

CLINICAL CORRELATION 18.4

Multiplex PCR Analysis of HGPRTase Gene Defects in Lesch–Nyhan Syndrome

Lesch–Nyhan syndrome, as described in Clin. Corr. 12.2, results from a deficiency in hypoxanthine–guanine phosphoribosyltransferase (HGPRTase) activity. Several variant forms of HGPRTase defects have been detected. Multiplex PCR amplification of the *HGPRT* gene locus has been employed to analyze this gene in cells derived from Lesch–Nyhan patients and results account for the variability of the HGPRTase. The gene, comprised of 9 exons, can be multiplex amplified using 16 different primers in a single PCR. The products can be separated by agarose gel electrophoresis. Analysis of the *HGPRT* gene locus by multiplex amplification of DNA derived from cells of several patients detected great variations in deletions of different exons to total absence of the exons.

Rossiter, B. J. F., et al. In: M. J. McPherson, P. Quirke, and G. R. Taylor (Eds.), *PCR. A Practical Approach,* Vol. 1. Oxford, England: Oxford University Press, 1994, p. 67.

allow one to detect any potential deletion mutation as compared to the normal gene products. Direct sequencing of multiple PCR products can be employed to detect point mutations in the patient gene. Multiplex PCR has been used to detect various defects in the HGPRTase gene in Lesch–Nyhan patients (see Clin. Corr. 18.4).

18.6 ■ SELECTION OF SPECIFIC CLONED DNA IN LIBRARIES

Loss of Antibiotic Resistance Is Used to Select Transformed Bacteria

When a single transformed bacterium carrying a recombinant molecule multiplies, its progeny are all genetically the same. If the transformed bacterium carries a recombinant DNA, all progeny will carry copies of the same recombinant plasmid. The foreign DNA has been amplified and is derived from a single cloned DNA fragment. The problem is how to identify the one colony containing the desired plasmid in a field of thousands to millions of different bacterial colonies. The plasmid construct pBR322 and its descendants carry two genes that confer antibiotic resistance. Within these antibiotic-resistant genes are DNA sequences sensitive to restriction endonuclease. When a fragment of foreign DNA is inserted into a restriction site within the gene for antibiotic resistance, the gene becomes nonfunctional. Bacteria carrying this recombinant plasmid are sensitive to the antibiotic (Figure 18.10). The second antibiotic resistance gene within the plasmid, however, remains intact and the bacteria will be resistant to this antibiotic. This technique of **insertional inactivation** of plasmid gene products affords a method to select bacteria that carry recombinant plasmids.

pBR322 contains genes that confer resistance to ampicillin (amp^r) and tetracycline (tet^r). A gene library with cellular DNA fragments inserted within the tet^r gene can be selected and screened in two stages (Figure 18.10). First, the bacteria are grown in an ampicillin-containing growth medium. Bacteria that are not transformed by a plasmid (they lack a normal or recombinant plasmid) during the construction of the gene library will not grow in the presence of the antibiotic, thus eliminating this population of bacteria. This, however, does not indicate which of the remaining viable bacteria carry a recombinant plasmid vector versus a plasmid with no DNA insert. The second step is to identify bacteria carrying recombinant vectors with nonfunctional tet^r genes, which are therefore sensitive to tetracycline.

Bacteria insensitive to ampicillin are plated and grown on agar plates containing ampicillin (Figure 18.10). Replica plates can be made by touching the colonies on the original agar plate with a filter and then touching additional sterile plates with the filter. All the plates will contain portions of each original colony at identifiable positions on the plates. The replica plate can contain tetracycline, which will not support the growth of bacteria harboring recombinant plasmids with their tet^r gene disrupted. Comparison of replica plates with and without tetracycline will indicate which colonies on the original ampicillin plate contain recombinant plasmids. Thus individual colonies containing the recombinant DNA can be selected, cultured, and analyzed.

Either **DNA** or **RNA probes** (see pp. 583 and 773) can be utilized to identify the DNA of interest. Ampicillin-resistant bacterial colonies on agar can be replica plated onto a nitrocellulose filter and adhering cells from each colony can be lysed with NaOH (Figure 18.10). DNA within the lysed bacteria is also denatured by the NaOH and becomes firmly bound to the filter. A labeled DNA or RNA probe that is complementary to the DNA of interest can be hybridized to the nitrocellulose-bound DNA. The filter is exposed to X-ray autoradiography. Any colony carrying the cloned DNA of interest will appear as a developed signal on the X-ray film. These spots would then correspond to the colony on the

1 Insertional Inactivation

ampʳ pBR322 tetʳ

Restriction endonuclease

Genomic DNA

Restriction endonuclease

ampʳ

n DNA fragments

ampʳ tetʳ

ampʳ tetʳ tetʳ

Reannealed plasmid without a foreign DNA fragment

Recombinant plasmid with DNA insert inactive *tetʳ* gene

Recombinant DNA linear arrays

2 Transformation of Interest

ampʳ tetʳ

Bacteria with normal plasmid

ampʳ tetʳ

Bacteria with recombinant plasmid GENE LIBRARY

no growth

Nontransformed bacteria

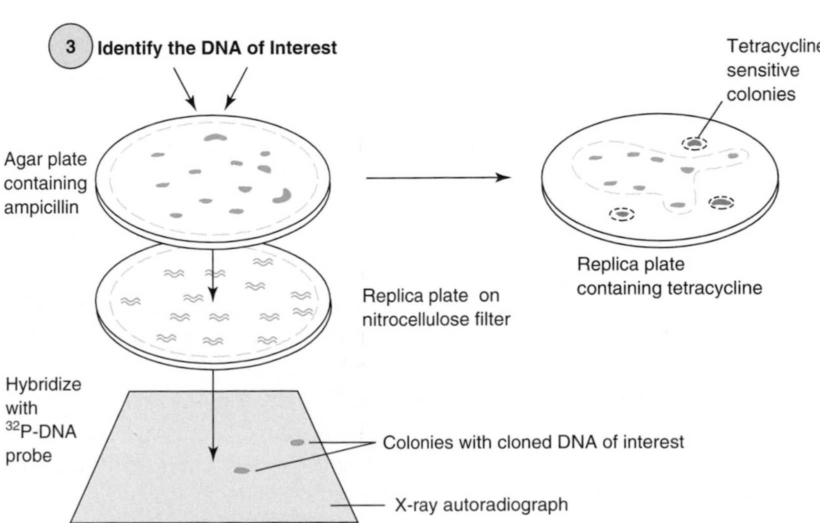

FIGURE 18.10

Insertional inactivation of recombinant plasmids and detection of transformed bacteria carrying a cloned DNA of interest. When the insertion of a foreign DNA fragment into a vector disrupts a functional gene sequence, the resulting recombinant DNA does not express the gene. The gene that codes for antibiotic resistance to tetracycline (*tetʳ*) is destroyed by DNA insertion while the ampicillin resistance gene (*ampʳ*) remains functional. Destruction of one antibiotic resistance gene and retention of a second antibiotic resistance gene allow for the detection of bacterial colonies carrying the foreign DNA of interest within the replicating recombinant vector.

original agar plate that can then be grown in a large-scale culture for further manipulation.

Cloned and amplified DNA fragments usually do not contain a complete gene and are not expressed. The DNA inserts, however, can readily be purified for sequencing or used as probes to detect genes within a mixture of genomic DNA, transcription levels of mRNA, and pathological conditions via clinical diagnostic tests.

α-Complementation for Selecting Bacteria Carrying Recombinant Plasmids

Other selection techniques can identify bacteria carrying recombinant DNA molecules. Vectors have been constructed (the pUC series) such that selected bacteria transformed with these vectors carrying foreign DNA inserts can be identified visually (Figure 18.11). The pUC plasmids contain the regulatory sequences and a portion of the 5′-end coding sequence (N-terminal 146 amino acids) for the β-galactosidase gene (*lacZ* gene) of the *lac* operon (Chapter 19, p. 802). The translated N-terminal 146 amino acid fragment of β-galactosidase is an inactive polypeptide. Mutant *E. coli* that code for the missing inactive carboxy-terminal portion of β-galactosidase can be transformed with the pUC plasmids. The translation of the host cell and plasmid portions of the β-galactosidase in response to an inducer, isopropylthio-β-D-galactoside, complement each other, yielding an active enzyme. The process is referred to as ***α*-complementation.** When these transformed bacteria are grown in the presence of a chromogenic substrate (5-bromo-4-chloro-3-indolyl-β-D-galactoside[X-gal]) for β-galactosidase they form blue colonies. If, however, a foreign DNA fragment is inserted into the base sequence for the N-terminal portion of β-galactosidase,

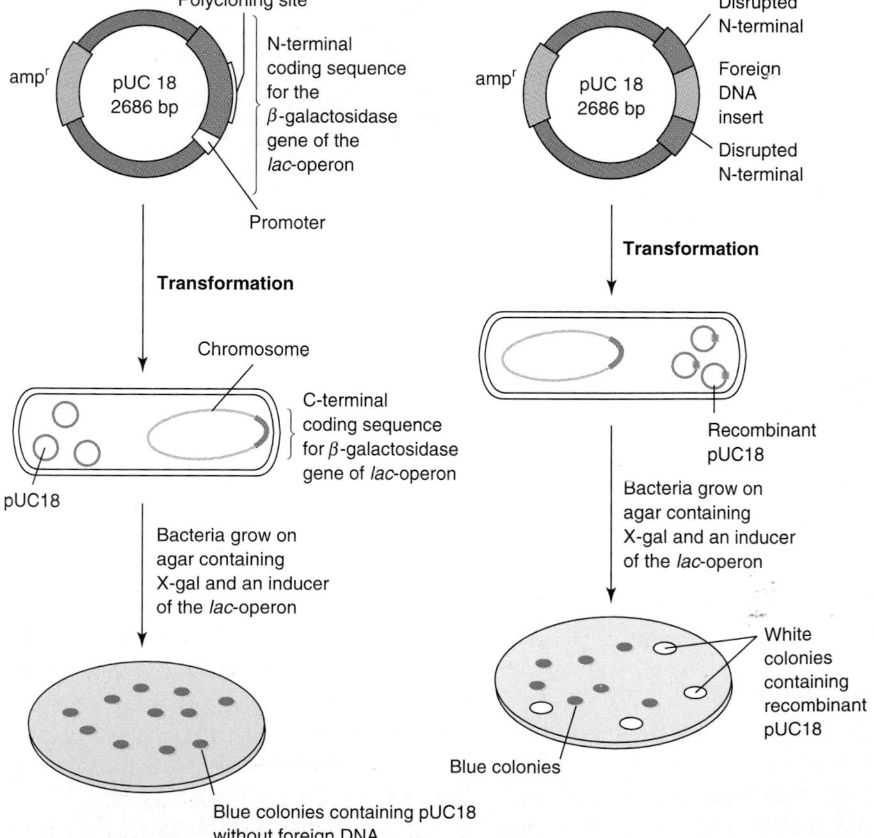

FIGURE 18.11
***α*-Complementation for detection of transformed bacteria.**
A vector has been constructed (pUC 18) that expresses the N-terminal coding sequence for the enzyme β-galactosidase of the *lac* operon. Bacterial mutants coding for the C-terminal portion of β-galactosidase are transformed with pUC 18. These transformed bacteria, grown in the presence of a special substrate for the intact enzyme (X-gal), result in blue colonies because they contain the enzyme to react with substrate. The functional N-terminal and C-terminal coding sequences for the gene complement each other to yield a functional enzyme. If, however, a foreign DNA fragment insert disrupts the pUC 18 N-terminal coding sequence for β-galactosidase, bacteria transformed with this recombinant molecule will not produce a functional enzyme. Bacterial colonies carrying these recombinant vectors can then be visually detected as white colonies.

the active enzyme cannot be formed. Bacteria transformed with these recombinant plasmids and grown on X-gal will yield white colonies and can be selected visually from nontransformed blue colonies.

18.7 TECHNIQUES FOR DETECTION AND IDENTIFICATION OF NUCLEIC ACIDS

Nucleic Acids Can Serve as Probes for Specific DNA or RNA Sequences

Selection of bacteria harboring recombinant DNAs of interest, analysis of mRNAs expressed in a cell, or identification of the presence of DNA sequences within a genome require sensitive and specific detection methods. DNA and RNA **probes** meet these requirements. These probes contain nucleotide sequences complementary to the target nucleic acid and will thus hybridize with the nucleic acid of interest. The degree of complementarity of a probe with the DNA under investigation determines the tightness of binding of the probe. The probe does not need to contain the entire complementary sequence of the DNA. The probe, RNA or DNA, can be labeled, usually with ^{32}P. Nonradioactive labels are also employed that depend on enzyme substrates coupled to nucleotides, which when incorporated into the nucleic acid can be detected by an enzyme-catalyzed reaction.

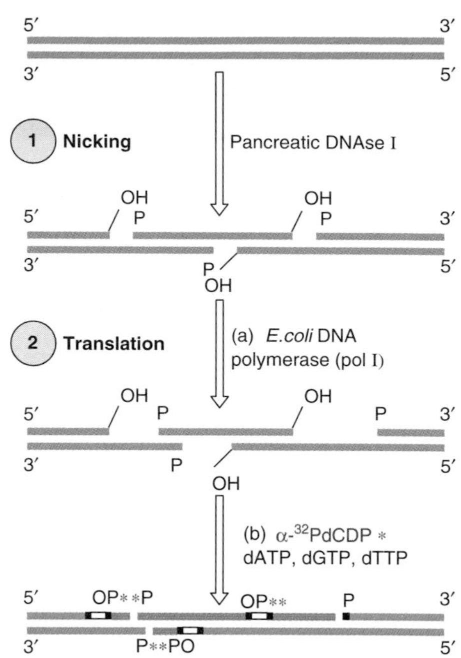

FIGURE 18.12
Nick translation to label DNA probes. Purified DNA molecules can be radioactively labeled and used to detect, by hybridization, the presence of complementary RNA or DNA in experimental samples. (1) Nicking step: introduces random single-stranded breaks in the DNA. (2) Translation step: (a) *E. coli* DNA polymerase (pol I) has 5′ → 3′ exonucleolytic activity that hydrolyzes nucleotides from the 5′ end of the nick; (b) pol I simultaneously fills in the single-stranded gap with radioactively labeled nucleotides using the 3′ end as a primer.

Labeled probes can be produced by **nick translation** of double-stranded DNA. Nick translation (Figure 18.12) involves the random enzymatic hydrolysis of a phosphodiester bond in the backbone of one strand of DNA by DNase I; the enzymatic breaks in the DNA backbone are referred to as nicks. A second enzyme, *E. coli* DNA polymerase I, with its 5′ → 3′ exonucleolytic activity and its DNA polymerase activity, creates single-strand gaps by hydrolyzing nucleotides from the 5′ side of the nick and then filling in the gaps with its polymerase activity. The polymerase reaction is usually carried out in the presence of one α-^{32}P-labeled deoxynucleotide triphosphate and three unlabeled deoxynucleotide triphosphates. The DNA employed in this method is usually purified and is derived from cloned DNA, viral DNA, or cDNA.

Another method to label DNA probes, **random primer labeling of DNA,** has distinct advantages over the nick translation method. The random primer method typically requires only 25 ng of DNA as opposed to 1–2 μg of DNA for nick translation and results in labeled probes with a specific activity ($>10^9$ cmp μg^{-1}) approximately ten times higher. This method generally produces longer labeled DNA probes. The double-stranded probe is melted and hybridized with a mixture of random hexanucleotides containing all possible sequences (ACTCGG, ACTCGA, ACTCGC, etc.). The hybridized hexanucleotides serve as primers for DNA synthesis with a DNA polymerase, such as the Klenow enzyme, in the presence of one or more radioactively labeled deoxynucleoside triphosphates.

Labeled RNA probes have advantages over DNA probes. For one, relatively large amounts of RNA can be transcribed from a template, which may be available in very limited quantities. A double-stranded DNA (dsDNA) probe must be denatured prior to hybridization with the target DNA and rehybridization with itself competes for hybridization with the DNA of interest. No similar competition occurs with the single-stranded RNA probes that hybridize with complementary DNA or RNA molecules. Synthesis of an RNA probe requires DNA as a template. To be transcribed the template DNA must be covalently linked to an upstream promoter that can be recognized by a DNA-dependent RNA polymerase. Vectors have been constructed that are well suited for this technique.

A labeled DNA or RNA probe can be hybridized to nitrocellulose-bound nucleic acids and identified by the detection of the labeled probe. The nucleic acids of interest can be transferred to nitrocellulose from bacterial colonies grown on agar or from agarose gels where the nucleic acid species have been electrophoretically separated by size.

Southern Blot Technique Is Useful for Identifying DNA Fragments

A technique to transfer DNA species, separated by agarose gel electrophoresis, to a filter for analysis was developed in the 1970s, and it is an indispensable tool. The method, developed by E. M. Southern, is referred to as the **Southern blot technique** (Figure 18.13). A DNA mixture of discrete restriction endonuclease-generated fragments from any source and complexity can be separated according to size by electrophoresis through an agarose gel. The DNA is dena-

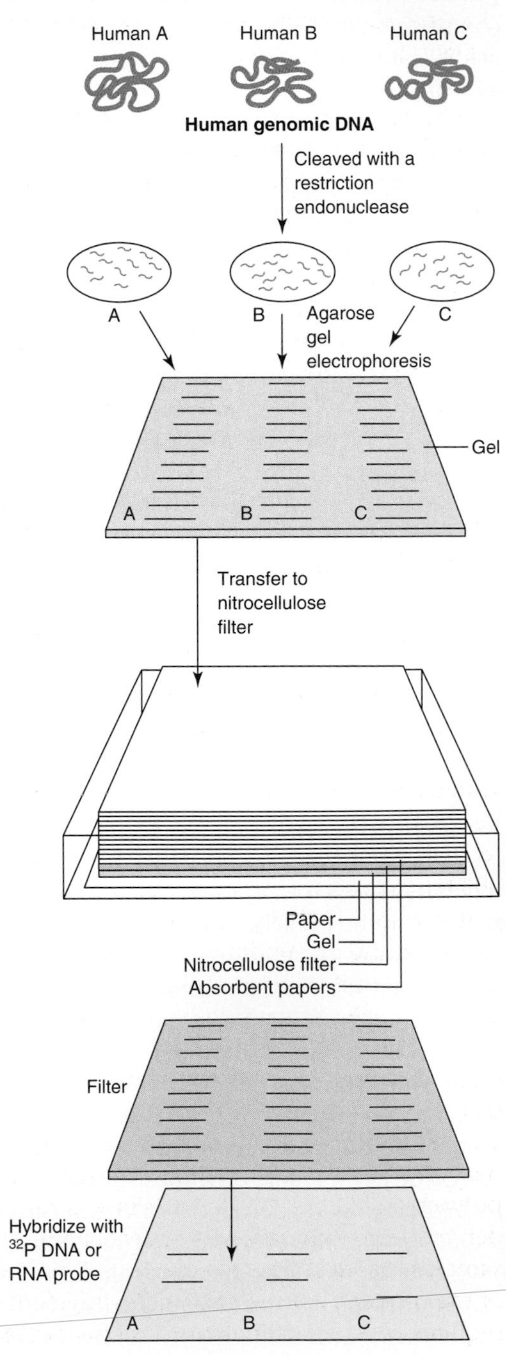

FIGURE 18.13
Southern blot to transfer DNA from agarose gels to nitrocellulose.
Transfer of DNA to nitrocellulose, as single-stranded molecules, allows for the detection of specific DNA sequences within a complex mixture of DNA. Hybridization with nick translated labeled probes can demonstrate if a DNA sequence of interest is present in the same or different regions of the genome.

tured by soaking the gel in alkali. The gel is then placed on absorbent paper and a nitrocellulose filter placed directly on top of the gel. Several layers of absorbent paper are placed on top of the nitrocellulose filter. The absorbent paper under the gel is kept wet with a concentrated salt solution that by capillary action is pulled up through the gel, the nitrocellulose, and into the absorbent paper layers above. The DNA is eluted from the gel by the upward movement of the high salt solution onto the nitrocellulose filter directly above, where it becomes bound. The position of the DNA bound to the nitrocellulose filter is exactly that which was present in the agarose gel. In its single-stranded membrane-bound form, the DNA can be analyzed with labeled probes.

The Southern blot technique is invaluable in analytical procedures for detection of the presence and determination of the number of copies of particular sequences in complex genomic DNA, confirming DNA cloning results, and demonstrating the polymorphic DNA arrangements of the human genome that correspond to pathological states. An example of the use of Southern blots is shown in Figure 18.13. Here whole human genomic DNA, isolated from three individuals, was digested with a restriction endonuclease, generating thousands of fragments. These fragments were distributed throughout the agarose gel according to size in an electric field. The DNA was transferred (blotted) to a nitrocellulose filter and hybridized with a ^{32}P-labeled DNA or RNA probe that represents a portion of a gene of interest. The probe detected two bands in all three individuals, indicating that the gene of interest is cleaved at one site within its sequence. Individuals A and B presented a normal pattern while patient C had one normal band and one lower molecular weight band. This is an example of altered DNA within different individuals of a single species, **restriction fragment length polymorphism (RFLP),** and implies a deletion in a segment of the gene that may be associated with a pathological state. The gene from this patient can be cloned, sequenced, and fully analyzed to characterize the altered nature of the DNA (see Clin. Corr. 18.5).

Other techniques that employ the principles of Southern blot are the transfer of RNA (Northern blots) and of proteins (Western blots) to nitrocellulose filters or nylon membranes.

Single-Strand Conformation Polymorphism

Southern blot analysis and detection of base changes in DNA from different individuals by RFLP analysis is dependent on alteration of a restriction endonuclease site. Often a base substitution, deletion, or insertion does not occur within a restriction endonuclease site. However, these modifications can readily be detected by **single-strand conformation polymorphism (SSCP).** This technique takes advantage of the fact that single-stranded DNA, smaller than 400 bases long, subjected to electrophoresis through a polyacrylamide gel migrates with a mobility partially dependent on its conformation. A single base alteration usually modifies the DNA conformation sufficiently to be detected as a mobility shift upon electrophoresis through a nondenaturing polyacrylamide gel. The analysis of a small region of genomic DNA or cDNA for SSCP can be accomplished by PCR amplification of the region of interest. Sense and antisense oligonucleotide primers are synthesized that flank the region of interest and this DNA is amplified by PCR in the presence of radiolabeled nucleotide(s). The resulting purified radiolabeled double-stranded PCR product is then heat denatured in 80% formamide and immediately loaded onto a nondenaturing polyacrylamide gel. The mobilities of control products are compared to samples derived from experimental/patient samples. Detection of mutations in patient samples can identify genetic lesions. This method depends on prior knowledge of the sequence of the gene/gene fragment of interest, while analysis by RFLP requires only restriction map analysis of DNA.

CLINICAL CORRELATION 18.5

Restriction Fragment Length Polymorphisms Determine the Clonal Origin of Tumors

It is generally assumed that most tumors are monoclonal in origin; that is, a rare event alters a single somatic cell genome in such a fashion that the cells grow abnormally into a tumor mass with all-daughter cells carrying the identically altered genome. Proof that a tumor is of monoclonal origin versus polyclonal in origin can help to distinguish hyperplasia (increased production and growth of normal cells) from neoplasia (growth of new or tumor cells). The detection of restriction fragment length polymorphisms (RFLPs) of Southern blotted DNA samples allows one to define the clonal origin of human tumors. If tumor cells were collectively derived from different parental cells they should contain a mixture of DNA markers characteristic of each cell of origin. However, an identical DNA marker in all tumor cells would indicate a monoclonal origin. The analysis is limited to females where one can take advantage of the fact that each cell carries only one active X chromosome of either paternal or maternal origin with the second X chromosome being inactivated. Activation occurs randomly during embryogenesis and is faithfully maintained in all-daughter cells with one-half the cells carrying an activated maternal X chromosome and the other one-half an activated paternal X chromosome.

Analysis of the clonal nature of a human tumor depends on the fact that activation of an X chromosome involves changes in the methylation of selected cytosine (C) residues within the DNA molecule. Several restriction endonucleases, such as Hha I, which cleaves DNA at GCGC sites, will not cleave DNA at their recognition sequences if a C is methylated within this site. Therefore the methylated state (activated versus inactivated) of the X chromosome can be probed with restriction endonucleases. Furthermore, the paternal X chromosome can be distinguished from the maternal X chromosome in a significant number of individuals based on differences in the electrophoretic migration of restriction endonuclease generated fragments derived from selected regions of the chromosome. These DNA fragments are identified on a Southern blot by hybridization with a DNA probe that is complementary to this region of the X chromosome. An X-linked gene that is amenable to these studies is the hypoxanthine phosphoribosyltransferase (*HPRTase*) gene. The *HPRTase* gene consistently has two BamHI restriction endonuclease sites (B_1 and B_3 in figure), but in many individuals a third site (B_2) is also present (see figure).

The presence of site B_2 in only one parental X chromosome HPRT allows for the detection of restriction enzyme-generated polymorphisms. Therefore a female cell may carry one X chromosome with the *HPRT* gene possessing two BamHI sites (results in a single detectable DNA fragment of 24 kb) or three BamHI sites (results in a single detectable DNA fragment of 12 kb). This figure depicts the expected results for the analysis of tumor cell DNA to determine its monoclonal or polyclonal origin. As expected, three human tumors examined by this method were shown to be of monoclonal origin.

Vogelstein, B., Fearon, E. R., Hamilton, S. R., and Feinberg, A. B. Use of restriction fragment length polymorphism to determine the clonal origin of tumors. *Science* 227:642, 1985.

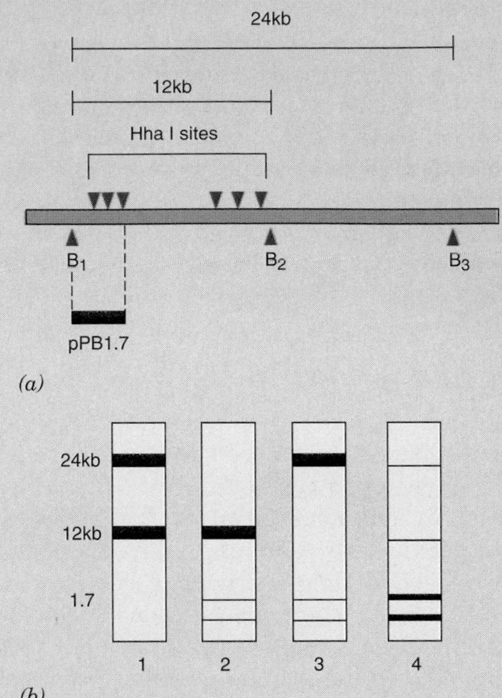

Analysis of genomic DNA to determine the clonal origin of tumors.
(*a*) The X chromosome-linked *HPRTase* gene contains two invariant BamHI restriction endonuclease sites (B_1 and B_3) while in some individuals a third site, B_2, is also present. The *HPRTase* gene also contains several HhaI sites; however, all of these sites, except H1, are usually methylated in the active X chromosome. Therefore only the H1 site would be available for cleavage by HhaI in the active X chromosome. A cloned, labeled probe, pPB1.7, is employed to determine which form of the HPRTase gene is present in a tumor and if it is present on an active X chromosome. (*b*) Restriction endonuclease patterns predicted for monoclonal versus polyclonal tumors are as follows: (1) Cleaved with BamHI alone; 24-kb fragment derived from *HPRTase* gene containing only B_1 and B_3 sites and 12-kb fragment derived from *HPRTase* gene containing extra B_2 site. Pattern is characteristic for heterozygous individual. (2) Cleaved with BamHI plus HhaI, monoclonal tumor with the 12-kb fragment derived from an active X chromosome (methylated). (3) Cleaved with BamHI plus HhaI; monoclonal tumor with the 24-kb fragment derived from an active X chromosome (methylated). (4) Cleaved with BamHI plus HhaI; polyclonal tumor. All tumors studied displayed patterns as in Lane 2 or Lane 3.

18.8 COMPLEMENTARY DNA AND COMPLEMENTARY DNA LIBRARIES

The insertion of specific functional eukaryotic genes into vectors that can be expressed in a prokaryotic cell could produce large amounts of "genetically engineered" proteins with significant medical, agricultural, and experimental potential. Hormones and enzymes are currently produced by these methods, including insulin, erythropoietin, thrombopoietin, interleukins, interferons, and tissue plasminogen activator. Unfortunately, it is impossible, except in rare instances, to clone functional genes from genomic DNA. One reason for this is that most genes within the mammalian genome yield transcripts that contain introns that must be spliced out of the primary mRNA transcript. Prokaryotic systems cannot splice out the introns to yield functional mRNA transcripts. This problem can be circumvented by synthesizing **complementary DNA (cDNA)** from functional eukaryotic mRNA.

mRNA Is Used as a Template for DNA Synthesis Using Reverse Transcriptase

Messenger RNA can be reverse transcribed to cDNA and the cDNA inserted into a vector for amplification, identification, and expression. Mammalian cells normally contain 10,000–30,000 different species of mRNA molecules at any time during the cell cycle. In some cases, however, a specific mRNA species may approach 90% of the total mRNA, such as mRNA for globin in reticulocytes. Many mRNAs are normally present at only a few (1–14) copies per cell. A **cDNA library** can be constructed from the total cellular mRNA but if only a few copies per cell of mRNA of interest are present, the cDNA may be very difficult to identify. Methods that enrich the population of mRNAs or their corresponding cDNAs permit reduction of the number of different cDNA species within a cDNA library and greatly enhance the probability of identifying the clone of interest.

Desired mRNA in a Sample Can Be Enriched by Separation Techniques

Messenger RNA can be separated by size by gel electrophoresis or centrifugation. Utilization of mRNA in a specific molecular size range will enrich several-fold an mRNA of interest. Knowledge of the molecular weight of the protein encoded by the gene of interest gives a clue to the approximate size of the mRNA transcript or its cDNA; variability in the predicted size, however, will arise from differences in the length of the untranslated regions of the mRNAs.

Enrichment of a specific mRNA molecule can also be accomplished by immunological procedures but requires the availability of antibodies against the protein encoded by the gene of interest. Antibodies added to an *in vitro* protein synthesis mixture will react with the growing polypeptide chain associated with the polysome and precipitate it. The mRNA can be purified from the immunoprecipitated polysomal fraction.

Complementary DNA Synthesis

An isolated mRNA mixture is used as a template to synthesize a complementary strand of DNA using RNA-dependent DNA polymerase, reverse transcriptase (Figure 18.14). A primer is required for the reaction; advantage is taken of the poly(A) tail at the 3′ terminus of eukaryotic mRNA. An oligo(dT) with 12–18 bases is employed as the primer that will hybridize with the poly(A) sequence. After cDNA synthesis, the hybrid is denatured or the mRNA hydrolyzed in alkali in order to obtain the single-stranded cDNA. The 3′ termini of single-stranded cDNAs form a hairpin loop that serves as a primer for the synthesis of the second strand of the cDNA. Either the Klenow fragment or a reverse transcriptase can be used for this step. The resulting double-stranded cDNA contains a single-

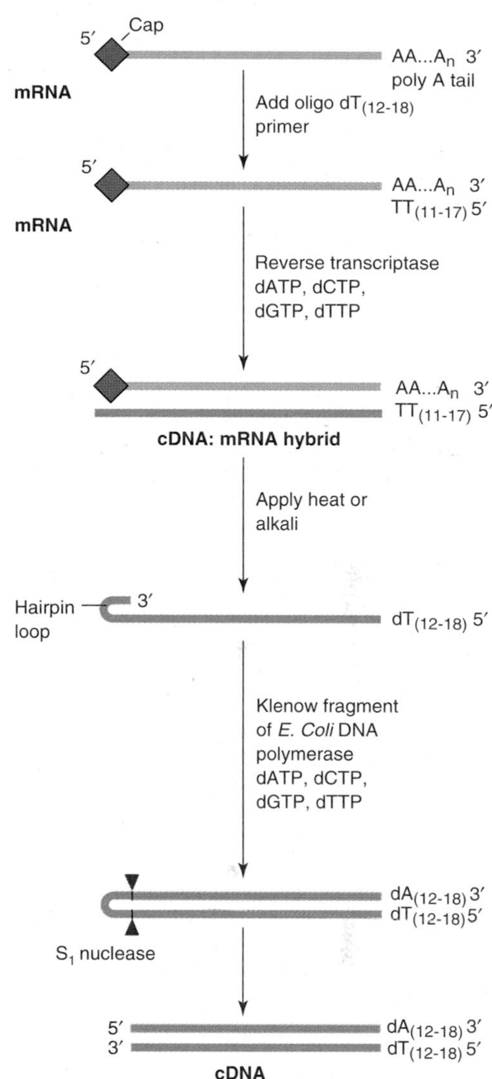

FIGURE 18.14
Synthesis of cDNA from mRNA.
The 3′ poly(A) tail of mRNA is hybridized with an oligomer of dT [oligo(dT)12–18] that serves as a primer for reverse transcriptase, which catalyzes the synthesis of the complementary DNA (cDNA) strand in the presence of all four deoxynucleotide triphosphates (dNTPs). The resulting cDNA–mRNA hybrid is separated into single-stranded cDNA by melting with heat or hydrolyzing the mRNA with alkali. The 3′ end of the cDNA molecule forms a hairpin loop that serves as a primer for the synthesis of the second DNA strand catalyzed by the Klenow fragment of *E. coli* DNA polymerase. The single-stranded unpaired DNA loop is hydrolyzed by S_1 nuclease to yield a double-stranded DNA molecule.

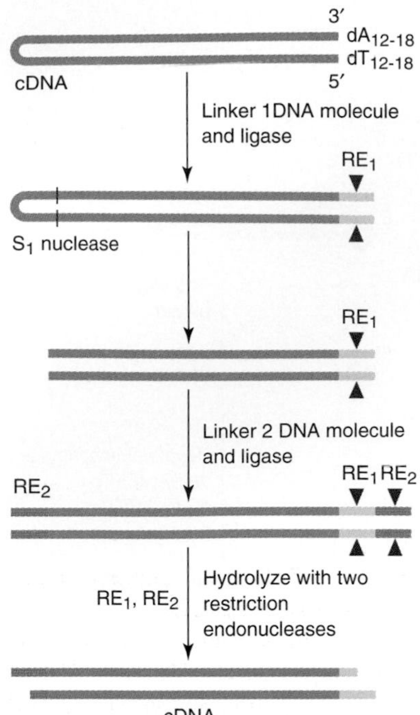

FIGURE 18.15
Modification of cDNA for cloning.
The procedure begins with double-stranded DNA containing a hairpin loop. A linker DNA containing a restriction endonuclease site (RE_1) is added to the free end of the cDNA by blunt-end ligation. The single-stranded hairpin loop is next hydrolyzed with S_1 nuclease. A second linker with a different restriction endonuclease site within (RE_2) is blunt-end ligated to the newly created free cDNA. The second linker will probably bind to both ends but will not interfere with the first restriction endonuclease site. The modified DNA is hydrolyzed with the two restriction endonucleases and can be inserted into a plasmid or bacteriophage DNA by directional cloning.

stranded loop that is selectively recognized and digested by S1 nuclease. The ends of the cDNA must be modified prior to cloning in a vector. One method involves incubating blunt-ended cDNA molecules with linker molecules and a bacteriophage T4 DNA ligase that catalyzes the ligation of blunt-ended molecules (Figure 18.15). The synthetic linker molecules contain restriction endonuclease sites that can now be hydrolyzed with the appropriate enzyme for insertion of the cDNA into a compatibly cut vector.

Bacteriophage DNA (see p. 779) is the most convenient and efficient vector to create cDNA libraries because they can readily be amplified and stored indefinitely. Two bacteriophage vectors, **λgt10** and **λgt11,** and their newer constructs have been employed to produce cDNA libraries. The cDNA libraries in λgt10 can be screened only with labeled nucleic acid probes, whereas those in λgt11, an expression vector, can also be screened with antibody for the production of the protein or antigen of interest.

Total Cellular RNA May Be Used as a Template for DNA Synthesis Using RT-PCR

Alternative methods to construct cDNA libraries employ a **reverse transcriptase–PCR (RT-PCR) technique** and obviate the need to purify mRNA. One such strategy is depicted in Figure 18.16 and begins with the reverse transcriptase production of a DNA–mRNA hybrid. The method then adds a dG homopolymer tail to the 3′ end catalyzed by terminal transferase and the subsequent hydrolysis of the mRNA. PCR primers are synthesized to hybridize with the dG, dA tails and terminate with two different restriction endonuclease sequences. The resulting PCR-amplified cDNA can then be hydrolyzed with the two different restriction endonucleases for directional cloning (see p. 765, Section 18.5) into an appropriate vector.

18.9 ■ BACTERIOPHAGE, COSMID, AND YEAST CLONING VECTORS

Detection of noncoding sequences in most eukaryotic genes and distant regulatory regions flanking the genes necessitated new cloning strategies to package larger DNA fragments than could be cloned in plasmids. Plasmids can accommodate foreign DNA inserts with a maximum length in the range of 5–10 kb (kilobases). Portions of recombinant DNA fragments larger than this are randomly deleted during replication of the plasmid within the bacterium. Thus alternate vectors have been developed.

Bacteriophage as Cloning Vectors

Bacteriophage λ (λ phage)—a virus that infects and replicates in bacteria—is an ideal vector for DNA inserts of approximately 15-kb lengths. The λ phage selectively infects bacteria and can replicate by either a lytic or nonlytic (lysogenic) pathway. The λ phage contains a self-complementary 12-base single-stranded tail (cohesive termini) at both ends of its 50-kb double-stranded DNA molecule. Upon infection of the bacteria the cohesive termini (cos sites) of a single λ phage DNA molecule self-anneal and the ends are covalently linked with the host cell DNA ligase. The circular DNA molecule serves as a template for transcription and replication. The λ phage, with restriction endonuclease-generated fragments representing a cell's whole genomic DNA inserted into it, is used to infect bacteria. Recombinant bacteriophages, released from the lysed cells, are collected and constitute a genomic library in λ phage. The phage library can be screened more rapidly than a plasmid library due to the increased size of the DNA inserts.

Numerous λ phage vectors have been constructed for different cloning strategies. For the sake of simplicity only a generic λ phage vector will be

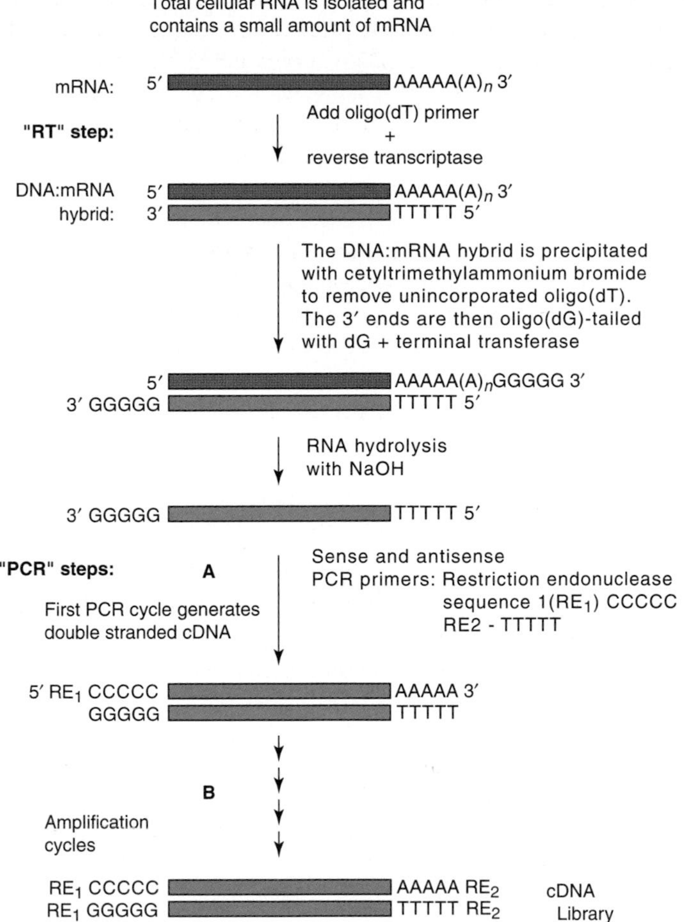

FIGURE 18.16
Generation of cDNA by reverse transcriptase–PCR (RT-PCR).
Total cellular RNA or mRNA can be used to generate cDNA by RT-PCR. The mRNA with an oligo rA tail is reverse transcribed with an oligo dT primer. An oligo dG tail is added to the 3′ ends of the RNA and DNA strands and the RNA strand is subsequently hydrolyzed with NaOH. Sense and antisense primers, modified with restriction site sequences, are then employed to amplify the cDNA by the PCR. The products can be hydrolyzed with the specific restriction endonucleases (RE_1 and RE_2) for cloning and subsequent studies.

described here. Cloning large fragments of DNA in λ phage takes advantage of the fact that a 15–25 kb segment of the phage DNA can be replaced without impairing its replication in *E. coli* (Figure 18.17). Packaging of phage DNA into the virus particle is constrained by its total length, which must be approximately 50 kb. The linear phage λ DNA can be digested with specific restriction endonucleases that generate small terminal fragments with their **cos sites** (arms), which are separated from the larger intervening fragments. Cellular genomic DNA is partially digested with the appropriate restriction enzymes to permit annealing and ligation with the phage arms. Genomic DNA is not enzymatically hydrolyzed completely in order to randomly generate fragments that can be properly packaged into phage particles. The DNA fragments that are smaller or larger than 15–25 kb can hybridize with the cos arms but are excluded from being packaged into infectious bacteriophage particles. All of the information required for phage infection and replication in bacteria is carried within the cos arms. The recombinant phage DNA is mixed with λ phage proteins *in vitro,* which assemble into infectious virions. The infectious recombinant λ phage particles are then propagated in an appropriate *E. coli* strain to yield a **λ phage library.** Many different *E. coli* strains have been genetically altered to sustain replication of specific recombinant virions.

Screening Bacteriophage Libraries

The bacteriophage library can be screened by plating the virus on a continuous layer of bacteria (a bacterial lawn) grown on agar plates (Figure 18.18). The individual phage will infect, replicate, and lyse one cell. The progeny virions will then infect and subsequently lyse bacteria immediately adjacent to the site of the first infected cell, creating a clear region or plaque in the opaque bacterial

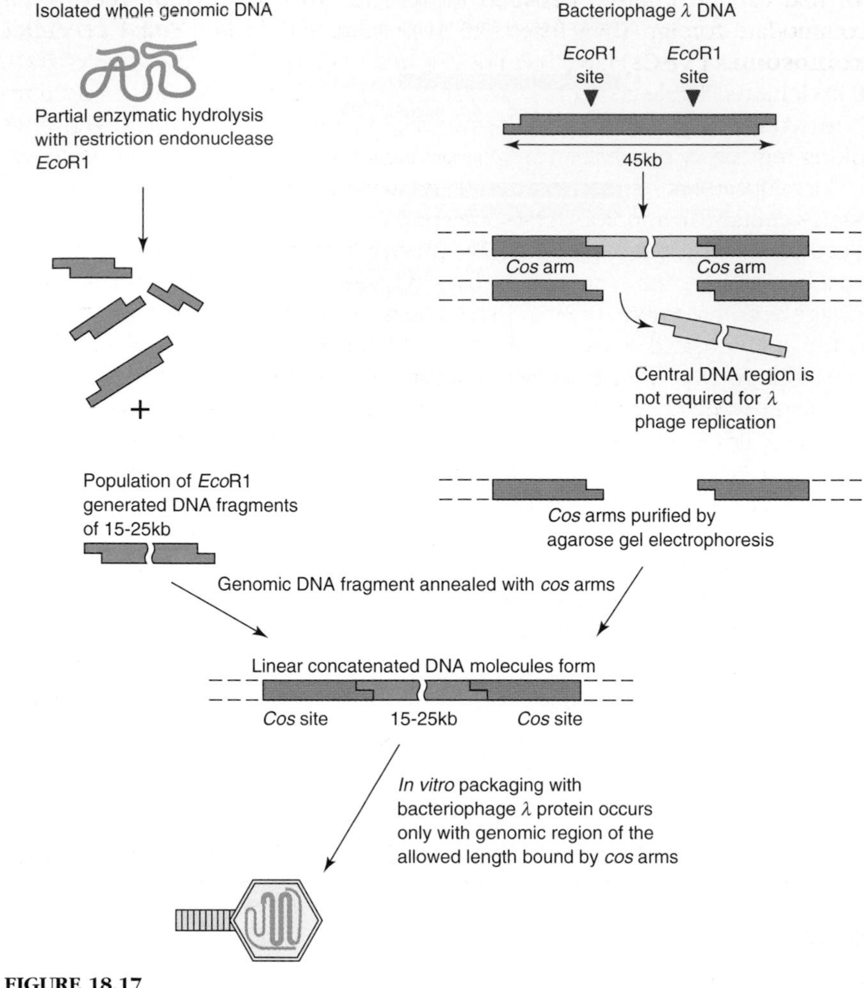

FIGURE 18.17
Cloning genomic DNA in bacteriophage λ.
Whole genomic DNA is incompletely digested with a restriction endonuclease (e.g., EcoRI). This results in DNA of random size fragments with single-stranded sticky ends. DNA fragments, cos arms, are generated with the same restriction endonuclease from bacteriophage λ DNA. The purified cos arm fragments carry sequence signals required for packaging DNA into a bacteriophage virion. The genomic fragments are mixed with the cos arms, annealed, and ligated, forming linear concatenated DNA arrays. The *in vitro* packaging with bacteriophage λ proteins occurs only with genomic DNA fragments of allowed lengths (15–25 kb) bounded by cos arms.

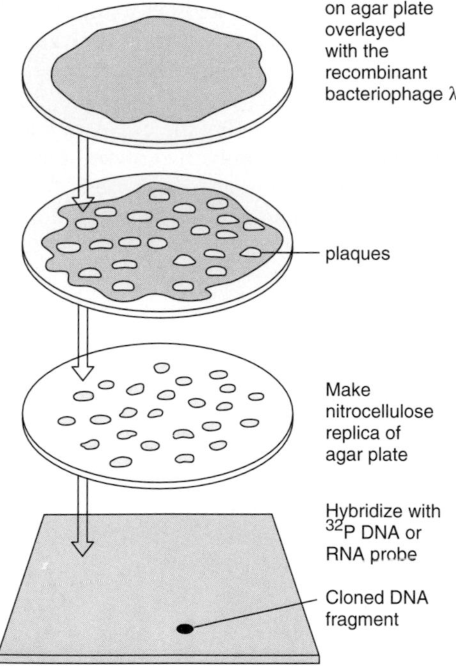

FIGURE 18.18
Screening genomic libraries in bacteriophage λ.
Competent *E. coli* are grown to confluence on an agar plate and then overlayed with the recombinant bacteriophage. Plaques develop where bacteria are infected and subsequently lysed by the phage λ. Replicas of the plate can be made by touching the plate with a nitrocellulose filter. The DNA is denatured and fixed to the nitrocellulose with NaOH. The fixed DNA is hybridized with a ^{32}P-labeled probe and exposed to X-ray film. The autoradiograph identifies the plaque(s) with recombinant DNA of interest.

field. Phage, within each plaque, can be picked up on a nitrocellulose filter (as for replica plating) and the DNA fixed to the filter with NaOH. The location of cloned DNA fragments of interest is determined by hybridizing the filter-bound DNA with a labeled DNA or RNA probe followed by autoradiography. Bacteriophages in the plaque corresponding to the labeled filter-bound hybrid are picked up and amplified in bacteria for further analysis. Complementary DNA libraries in bacteriophage are also constructed that contain the phage cos arms. If the cDNA is recombined with phage DNA that permits expression of the gene, such as λ*gt11*, then plaques can be screened immunologically with antibodies specific for the antigen of interest.

Cloning DNA Fragments into Cosmid and Yeast Artificial Chromosome Vectors

Even though λ phage are the most commonly used vectors to construct genomic DNA libraries, the lengths of many genes exceed the maximum size of the

DNA that can be inserted between the phage arms. A **cosmid vector** can accommodate foreign DNA inserts of approximately 45 kb. **Yeast artificial chromosomes (YACs)** have been developed to clone DNA fragments of 200–500 kb lengths. While cosmid and yeast artificial chromosome vectors are difficult to work with, their libraries permit the cloning of large genes with their flanking regulatory sequences, as well as families of genes or contiguous genes.

Cosmid vectors are a cross between plasmid and bacteriophage vectors. Cosmids contain an antibiotic-resistance gene for selection of recombinant DNA molecules, an origin of replication for propagation in bacteria, and a cos site for packaging of recombinant molecules in bacteriophage particles. The bacteriophage with recombinant cosmid DNA can infect *E. coli* and inject its DNA into the cell. Cosmid vectors contain only approximately 5 kb of the 50-kb bacteriophage DNA and therefore cannot direct replication and assembly of new infectious phage particles. Instead, the recombinant cosmid DNA circularizes and replicates as a large plasmid. Bacterial colonies with recombinants of interest can be selected and amplified by methods similar to those described for plasmids.

Standard cloning procedures and some novel methods are employed to construct YACs. Very large foreign DNA fragments are joined to yeast DNA sequences, one that functions as a telomere (distal extremity of chromosome arm) and another that functions as a centromere and as an origin of replication. The recombinant YAC DNA is introduced into the yeast by transformation. The YAC constructs are designed so that yeast transformed with recombinant chromosomes grow as visually distinguishable colonies. This facilitates selection and analysis of cloned DNA fragments.

18.10 ■ TECHNIQUES TO FURTHER ANALYZE LONG STRETCHES OF DNA

Subcloning Permits Definition of Large Segments of DNA

Complete analysis of functional elements in a cloned DNA fragment requires sequencing of the entire molecule. Current techniques can sequence 200–400 bases in a DNA fragment, yet cloned DNA inserts are frequently much larger. Restriction maps of the initial DNA clone are essential for cleaving the DNA into smaller pieces to be recloned, or **subcloned** for further analysis. The sequences of each of the small subcloned DNA fragments can be determined. Overlapping regions of the subcloned DNA properly align and confirm the entire sequence of the original DNA clone.

Sequencing can often be accomplished without subcloning. Antisense primers can be synthesized that are complementary to the initially sequenced 3′ ends of the cloned DNA. This process is repeated until the full length of the cloned DNA has been sequenced. This method obviates the need to prepare subclones but it requires synthesis/purchase of numerous primers. On the other hand, the subcloned DNA is always inserted back into the same region of the plasmid. Therefore one set of primers complementary to the plasmid DNA sequences flanking the inserted DNA can be used for all of the sequencing reactions with subcloned DNA.

Chromosome Walking Is a Technique to Define Gene Arrangement in Long Stretches of DNA

Knowledge of how genes and their regulatory elements are arranged in a chromosome should lead to an understanding of how sets of genes may be coordinately regulated. Currently, it is difficult to clone DNA fragments large enough to identify contiguous genes. The combination of several techniques allows for the analysis of very long stretches of DNA (50–100 kb). The method, **chromosome walking,** is possible because λ phage or cosmid libraries contain

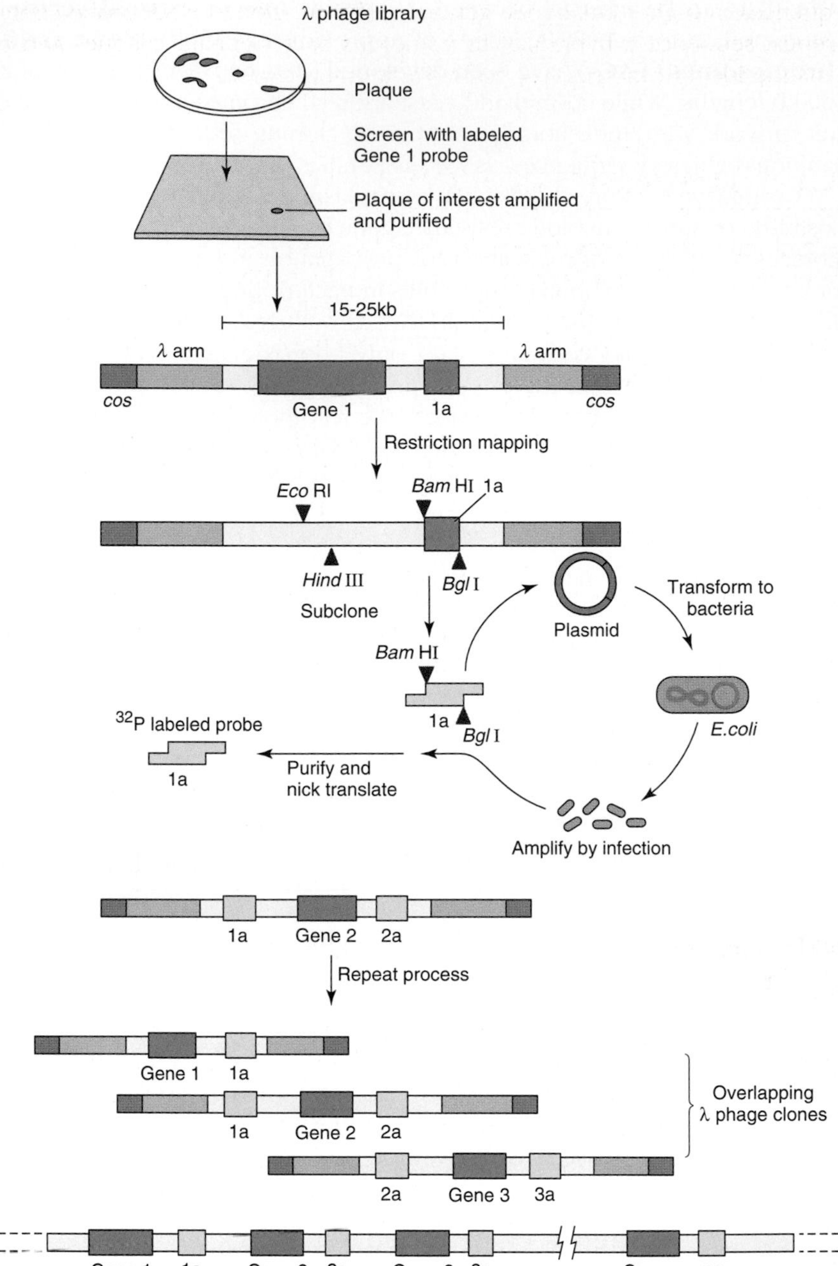

FIGURE 18.19
Chromosome walking to analyze contiguous DNA segments in a genome.
Initially, a DNA fragment is labeled by nick translation to screen a library for recombinant λ phage carrying a gene of interest. The amplified DNA is mapped with a battery of restriction endonucleases to select a new region (1a) within the original cloned DNA that can be recloned (subcloned). The subcloned DNA (1a) is used to identify other DNA fragments within the original library that would overlap the initially amplified DNA region. The process can be repeated many times to identify contiguous DNA regions upstream and downstream of the initial DNA (gene 1) of interest.

partially cleaved genomic DNA cut at specific restriction endonuclease sites. The cloned fragments will contain overlapping sequences with other cloned fragments. Overlapping regions are identified by restriction mapping, subcloning, screening λ phage or cosmid libraries, and sequencing procedures.

The overall procedure of chromosome walking is shown in Figure 18.19. Initially the λ phage library is screened for a sequence of interest with a DNA or RNA probe. The cloned DNA is restriction mapped and a small segment is subcloned in a plasmid, amplified, purified, and labeled by nick translation. This labeled probe is then used to rescreen the λ phage library for complementary sequences, which are then cloned. The newly identified overlapping cloned DNA is then treated in the same fashion as the initial DNA clone to search for other overlapping sequences. Caution must be taken that the subcloned DNA does not contain a sequence common to the large numbers of repeating DNA sequences in higher eukaryotic genomes. If a subcloned DNA probe contains a repeat sequence it hybridizes to numerous bacteriophage plaques and prevents the identification of a specific overlapping clone.

18.11 ■ EXPRESSION VECTORS AND FUSION PROTEINS

Recombinant DNA methodology described to this point has dealt primarily with screening, amplification, and purification of cloned DNA species. An important goal of recombinant DNA studies, as stated earlier, is to have a foreign gene expressed in bacteria with the product in a biologically active form. Sequencing the DNA of many bacterial genes and their flanking regions has identified the spatial arrangement of regulatory sequences required for expression of genes. A promoter and other regulatory elements upstream of the gene are required to transcribe a gene (Chapter 19, Section 19.3). mRNA transcript of a recombinant eukaryotic gene, however, is not translated in a bacterial system because it lacks the bacterial recognition sequence, the Shine–Dalgarno sequence, required to properly orient it with a functional bacterial ribosome. Vectors that facilitate the functional transcription of DNA inserts, termed **expression vectors,** have been constructed such that a foreign gene can be inserted into the vector downstream of a regulated promoter but within a bacterial gene, commonly the *lacZ* gene. The mRNA transcript of the recombinant DNA contains the *lacZ* Shine–Dalgarno sequence, codons for a portion of the 3′ end of the *lacZ* gene protein, followed by the codons of the complete foreign gene of interest. The protein product is a **fusion protein** that contains a few N-terminal amino acids of the *lacZ* gene protein and the complete amino acid sequence of the foreign gene product.

Foreign Genes Can Be Expressed in Bacteria Allowing Synthesis of Their Encoded Proteins

Many plasmid and bacteriophage vectors have been constructed to permit expression of eukaryotic genes in bacterial cells. Rapidly replicating bacteria can serve as a biological factory to produce large amounts of specific proteins, which have research, clinical, and commercial value. As an example, human protein hormones are produced by recombinant technologies, which serve as replacement or supplemental hormones in patients with aberrant or missing hormone production. Figure 18.20 depicts a generalized plasmid vector for the expression of a mammalian gene. Recall that the inserted foreign gene must be in the form of cDNA from its corresponding mRNA since the bacterial system cannot remove the introns in the pre-mRNA transcript. The DNA must be inserted in register with the codons of the 3′-terminal codons of the bacterial protein when creating a fusion protein. That is, insertion must occur after a triplet codon of the bacterial protein and at the beginning of a triplet codon of the eukaryotic gene protein to ensure proper translation. Finally, the foreign gene must be inserted in the proper orientation relative to the promoter to yield a functional transcript. This can be achieved by directional cloning.

Eukaryotic proteins synthesized within bacteria are often unstable and are degraded by intracellular proteases. Fusion protein products, however, are usually stable. The fusion protein amino acids encoded by the prokaryotic genome may be cleaved from the purified protein of interest by enzymatic or chemical procedures. An alternative cloning strategy to circumvent the intracellular instability of some proteins is to produce a foreign protein that is secreted. This requires cloning the foreign gene in a vector such that the fusion protein synthesized contains a signal peptide that can be recognized by the bacterial signal peptidase that properly processes the protein for secretion.

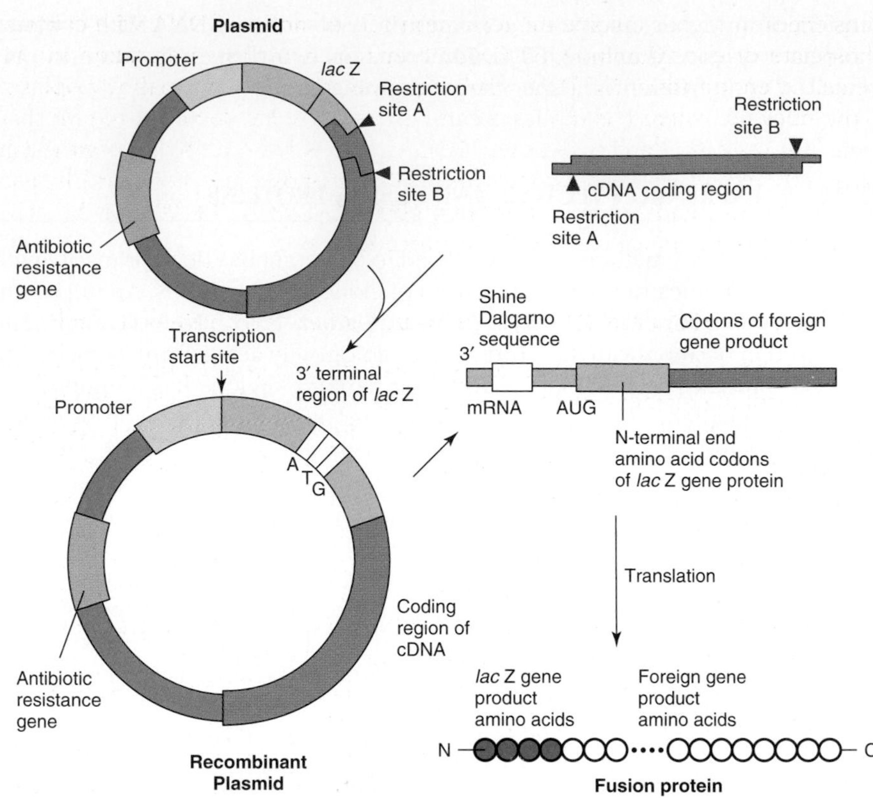

FIGURE 18.20
Construction of a bacterial expression vector.
A cDNA coding region of a protein of interest is inserted downstream of bacterial regulatory sequences (promoter, P) for the *lacZ* gene, the coding sequence for the mRNA Shine–Dalgarno sequence, the AUG codon, and a few codons for the N-terminal amino acids of the *lacZ* gene protein. The mRNA produced from this expression vector will therefore direct synthesis of a foreign protein in the bacterium with a few of its N-terminal amino acids of bacterial protein origin (a fusion protein).

18.12 ■ EXPRESSION VECTORS IN EUKARYOTIC CELLS

Mammalian genetic diseases result from missing or defective intracellular proteins. To utilize recombinant techniques to treat these diseases, vectors have to be constructed that can be incorporated into mammalian cells. In addition, these vectors have to be selective for the tissue or cells containing the aberrant protein. Numerous vectors permit the expression of foreign DNA genes in mammalian cells grown in tissue culture. These vectors have been used extensively for elucidation of the posttranslational processing and synthesis of proteins in cultured eukaryotic cells. Unfortunately, the goal to selectively express genes in specific tissues or at specific developmental stages within an animal has met with very limited success.

Several types of expression vectors have been developed that allow the replication, transcription, and translation of foreign genes in eukaryotic cells grown *in vitro*, including both RNA and DNA viral vectors that contain a foreign DNA insert. These viral vectors are able to infect and then replicate in a host cell. Experimentally constructed vectors that contain essential DNA elements, usually derived from a viral genome, permit expression of foreign gene inserts. **Shuttle vectors** contain both bacterial and eukaryotic replication signals, thus permitting replication of the vector in both bacteria and mammalian cells. A shuttle vector allows a gene to be cloned and purified in large quantities from a bacterial system and then the same recombinant vector can be expressed in a mammalian cell. Some expression vectors become integrated into the host cell genome while others remain as extrachromosomal entities (episomes) with stable expression of their recombinant gene in the daughter cells. Other expression vectors remain as episomal DNA, permitting only transient expression of their foreign gene prior to cell death.

Foreign DNA, such as viral expression vectors, may be introduced into the cultured eukaryotic cells by **transfection,** a process that is analogous to transformation of DNA into bacterial cells. The most commonly employed transfection methods involve the formation of a complex of DNA with calcium phosphate or diethylaminoethyl (DEAE)-dextran, which is then taken up by the cell by endocytosis. The DNA is subsequently transferred from the cytoplasm to the nucleus, where it is replicated and expressed. The details of the mechanism of transfection are not known. Both methods are employed to establish transiently expressed vectors while the calcium phosphate procedure is also used for permanently expressed foreign genes. Typically, 10–20% of the cells in culture can be transfected by these procedures.

DNA Elements Required for Expression of Vectors in Mammalian Cells

Expression of recombinant genes in mammalian cells requires the presence of DNA-controlling elements within the vector that are not necessary in the bacterial system. To be expressed in a eukaryotic cell the cloned gene is inserted in the vector in the proper orientation relative to control elements, including a promoter, polyadenylation signals, and an enhancer sequence. Expression may be improved by the inclusion of an intron. Some or all of these DNA elements may be present in the recombinant gene if whole genomic DNA is used for cloning. A particular cloned fragment generated by restriction endonuclease cleavage, however, may not contain the required controlling elements. A cDNA would not possess these required DNA elements. It is therefore necessary that the expression vector to be used in mammalian cells be constructed such that it contains all of the required controlling elements.

An expression vector can be constructed by insertion of required DNA-controlling elements into the vector by recombinant technologies. Enhancer and promoter elements, engineered into an expression vector, should be recognized by a broad spectrum of cells in culture for the greatest applicability of the vector. Controlling elements derived from viruses with a broad host range are used for this purpose and are usually derived from the **papovavirus, simian virus 40 (SV40), Rous sarcoma virus,** or the **human cytomegalovirus.**

The vector must replicate so as to increase the number of copies within each cell or to maintain copies in daughter cells. The vector therefore is constructed to contain DNA sequences that promote its replication in the eukaryotic cell. This DNA region is usually derived from a virus and is referred to as the origin of replication (Ori). Specific protein factors, encoded by genes engineered into the vector or previously introduced into the host genome, recognize and interact with the ori sequences to initiate DNA replication.

Transfected Eukaryotic Cells Can Be Selected by Utilizing Mutant Cells that Require Specific Nutrients

It is important to have a means of selectively growing the transfected cells since they often represent only 10–20% of the cell population. As was the case for the bacterial plasmid, a gene can be incorporated into the vector that encodes an enzyme that confers resistance to a drug or confers selective growth capability to the cells carrying the vector. Constructing vectors that express both a selectable marker and a foreign gene is difficult. **Cotransfection** circumvents this problem. Two different vectors are efficiently taken up by those cells capable of being transfected. In most cases greater than 90% of transfected cells carry both vectors, one with the selectable marker and the second carrying the gene of interest.

Two of the more commonly employed selectable markers are the thymidine kinase (*tk*) and the dihydrofolate reductase gene. The *tk* gene product, thymidine kinase, is expressed in most mammalian cells and participates in the salvage pathway for thymidine. Several mutant cell lines have been isolated that lack a functional thymidine kinase gene (tk^-) and in growth medium containing hypoxanthine, aminopterin, and thymidine these cells will not survive. Only

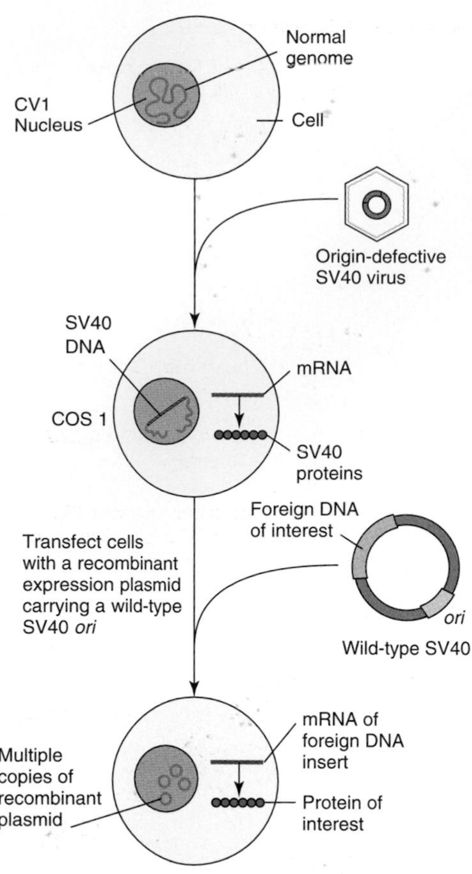

FIGURE 18.21
Expression of foreign genes in the eukaryotic COS cell.
CV1, an established tissue culture cell line of simian origin, can be infected and supports the lytic replication of the simian DNA virus, SV40. Cells are infected with an origin (ori)-defective mutant of SV40 whose DNA permanently integrates into the host CV1 cell genome. The defective viral DNA continuously codes for proteins that can associate with a normal SV40 ori to regulate replication. Due to its defective ori, the integrated viral DNA will not produce viruses. The SV40 proteins synthesized in the permanently altered CV1 cell line, COS-1, can, however, induce the replication of recombinant plasmids carrying a wild-type SV40 ori to a high copy number (as high as 105 molecules per cell). The foreign protein synthesized in the transfected cells may be detected immunologically or enzymatically.

those *tk*⁻ mutant cells cotransfected with a vector carrying a *tk* gene, usually of herpes simplex virus origin, will grow in the medium. In most instances, these cells have been cotransfected with the gene of interest.

The dihydrofolate reductase gene (*dhfr*) is required to maintain cellular concentrations of tetrahydrofolate for nucleotide biosynthesis (see Chapter 13). Cells lacking this enzyme will only survive in media containing thymidine, glycine, and purines. Mutant cells (*dhfr*⁻), which are transfected with the *dhfr* gene, can therefore be selectively grown in a medium lacking these supplements. Expressing foreign genes in mutant cells, cotransfected with selectable markers, is limited to cell types that can be isolated with the required gene defect. Normal cells, however, transfected with a vector carrying the *dhfr* gene, are also resistant to methotrexate, an inhibitor of dihydrofolate reductase, and these cells can be selected for by growth in methotrexate.

Another approach for selecting nonmutated cells involves the use of a bacterial gene coding for aminoglycoside 3′-phosphotransferase (APH) for cotransfection. Cells expressing APH are resistant to aminoglycoside antibiotics such as neomycin and kanamycin, which inhibits protein synthesis in both prokaryotes and eukaryotes. Vectors carrying an *APH* gene can therefore be used as a selectable marker in both bacterial and mammalian cells.

Foreign Genes Can Be Expressed in Eukaryotic Cells by Utilizing Virus Transformed Cells

Figure 18.21 depicts the transient expression of a transfected gene in COS cells, a commonly used system to express foreign eukaryotic genes. The COS cells are permanently cultured simian cells, transformed with an origin-defective SV40 genome. The defective viral genome has integrated into the host cell genome and constantly expresses viral proteins. Infectious viruses, which are normally lytic to infected cells, are not produced because the viral origin of replication is defective. The SV40 proteins expressed by the transformed COS cell will recognize and interact with a normal SV40 ori carried in a vector transfected into these cells. These SV40 proteins will therefore promote the repeated replication of the vector. A transfected vector containing both an SV40 ori and a gene of interest may reach a copy number in excess of 10^5 molecules/cell. Transfected COS cells die after 3–4 days, possibly due to a toxic overload of the episomal vector DNA.

18.13 ■ SITE-DIRECTED MUTAGENESIS

By mutating selected regions or single nucleotides within cloned DNA, it is possible to define the role of DNA sequences in gene regulation and amino acid sequences in protein function. **Site-directed mutagenesis** is the controlled alteration of selected regions of a DNA molecule. It may involve the insertion or deletion of selected DNA sequences or the replacement of a specific nucleotide with a different base. A variety of chemical methods mutate DNA *in vitro* and *in vivo* usually at random sites within the molecule.

Role of Flanking Regions in DNA Can Be Evaluated by Deletion and Insertion Mutations

Site-directed mutagenesis can be carried out in various regions of a DNA sequence including the gene itself or the flanking regions. Figure 18.22 depicts a simple deletion mutation strategy where the sequence of interest is selectively cleaved with restriction endonuclease, the specific sequence removed, and the altered recombinant vector recircularized with DNA ligase. The role of the deleted sequence can be determined by comparing the level of expression (translation) of the gene product, measured immunologically or enzymatically, to the unaltered recombinant expression vector. A similar technique is used to insert new sequences at the site of cleavage. Deletion of a DNA sequence within the flanking region of a cloned gene can help to define its regulatory role in gene expression. The presence or absence of a regulatory sequence may not be sufficient to evaluate its role in controlling expression. The spatial arrangement of regulatory elements to one another, to the gene, and to its promoter may be important in the regulation of gene expression (see Chapter 19).

Analysis of potential regulatory sequences is conveniently conducted by inserting the sequence of interest upstream of a reporter gene in an expression vector. A **reporter gene,** usually of prokaryotic origin, encodes for a gene product that can readily be distinguished from proteins normally present in the nontransfected cell and for which there is a convenient and rapid assay. A commonly used reporter gene is the chloramphenicol acetyltransferase (*CAT*) gene of bacteria. The gene product catalyzes the acetylation and inactivation of chloramphenicol, a protein synthesis inhibitor of prokaryotic cells. The ability of a regulatory element to enhance or suppress expression of the *CAT* gene can be determined by assaying the level of acetylation of chloramphenicol in extracts prepared from transfected cells. The regulatory element can be mutated prior to insertion into the vector carrying the reporter gene to determine its spatial and sequence requirements as a regulator of gene expression.

A difficulty encountered in analysis of regulatory elements is the lack of restriction endonuclease sites at useful positions within the cloned DNA. **Deletion mutations** can be made, in the absence of appropriately positioned restriction endonuclease sites, by linearizing cloned DNA with a restriction endonuclease downstream of the potential regulatory sequence of interest. The DNA can then be systematically truncated with an exonuclease, which hydrolyzes nucleotides from the free end of both strands of the linearized DNA. Increasing times of digestion generates smaller DNA fragments. Figure 18.23 demonstrates how larger deletion mutations (yielding smaller fragments) can be tested for functional activity. The enzymatic hydrolysis of the double strand of DNA occurs at both ends of the linearized recombinant vector, destroying the original restriction endonuclease site (RE_2). A unique restriction endonuclease site is reestablished to recircularize the truncated DNA molecule for further manipulations to evaluate the function of the deleted sequence. This is accomplished by ligating the blunt ends with a linker DNA, a synthetic oligonucleotide containing one or more restriction endonuclease sites. The ligated linkers are cut with the appropriate enzyme permitting recircularization and ligation of the DNA.

Site-Directed Mutagenesis of a Single Nucleotide

The previously discussed procedures can elucidate the functional role of small to large DNA sequences. Frequently, however, one wants to evaluate the role of a single nucleotide at selected sites within the DNA molecule. A single base change permits evaluation of the role of specific amino acids in a protein (see Clin. Corr. 18.6). This method also allows one to create or destroy a restriction endonuclease site at specific locations within a DNA sequence. The site-directed mutagenesis of a specific nucleotide is a multistep process that begins with cloning the normal type gene in a bacteriophage (Figure 18.24). The M13 series of recombinant bacteriophage vectors are commonly employed for these studies. M13 is a filamentous bacteriophage that specifically infects male *E. coli* that express sex pili encoded for by a plasmid (F factor). M13 bacteriophage contains DNA in a single-stranded or replicative form, which is replicated to double-stranded DNA within an infected cell. The double-stranded form of the

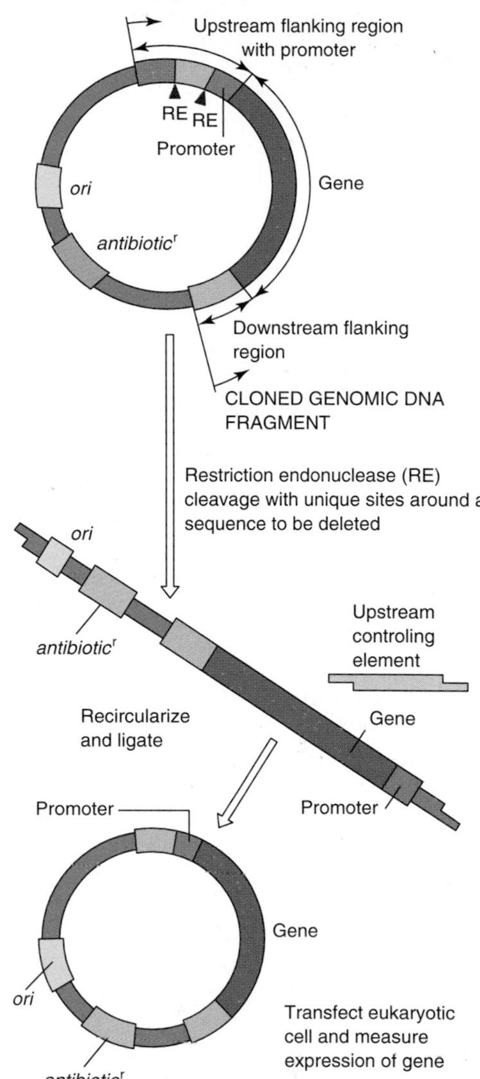

FIGURE 18.22
Use of expression vectors to study DNA regulatory sequences.
The gene of interest along with upstream and/or downstream DNA flanking regions is inserted and cloned in an expression vector and the baseline expression of the gene in an appropriate cell is determined. Defined regions of potential regulatory sequences can be removed by restriction endonuclease cleavage and the truncated recombinant DNA vector can be recircularized, ligated, and transfected into an appropriate host cell. The level of gene expression in the absence of the potential regulator is determined and compared to controls to ascertain the regulatory role of the deleted flanking DNA sequence.

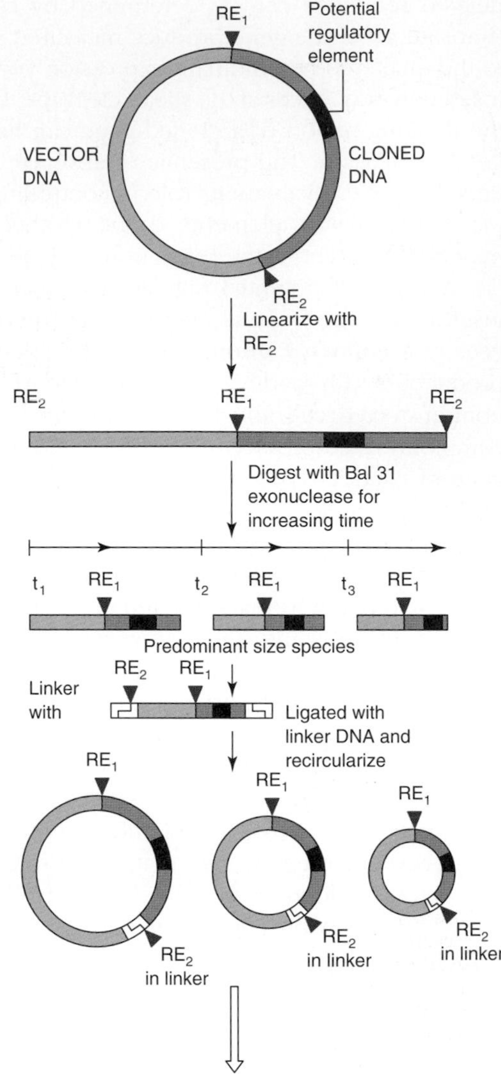

FIGURE 18.23
Enzymatic modification of potential DNA regulatory sequences.
A purified recombinant DNA molecule with a suspected gene regulatory element within flanking DNA regions is cleaved with a restriction endonuclease (RE_2). The linearized recombinant DNA is digested for varying time periods with the exonuclease, Bal31, reducing the size of the DNA flanking the potential regulatory element. The resulting recombinant DNA molecules of varying reduced sizes have small DNA oligomers (linkers) containing a restriction endonuclease sequence for RE_2 ligated to their ends. The linker-modified DNA is hydrolyzed with RE_2, creating complementary single-stranded sticky ends that permit recircularization of recombinant vectors. The potential regulatory element, bounded by various reduced-sized flanking DNA sequences, can be amplified, purified, sequenced, and inserted upstream of a competent gene in an expression vector. Modification of expression of the gene in an appropriate transfected cell can then be monitored to evaluate the role of the potential regulatory element placed at varying distances from the gene.

DNA is isolated from infected cells and used for cloning the gene to be mutated. The plaques of interest can be visually identified by α-complementation (see p. 772).

The M13 carrying the cloned gene of interest is used to infect susceptible *E. coli*. The progeny bacteriophages are released into the growth medium and contain single-stranded DNA. An oligonucleotide (18–30 nucleotides long) is synthesized that is complementary to a region of interest except for the nucleotide to be mutated. This oligomer, with one mismatched base, will hybridize to the single-stranded gene cloned in the M13 DNA and serves as a primer. Primer extension is accomplished with the bacteriophage T4 DNA polymerase and the resulting double-stranded DNA can be transformed into susceptible *E. coli,* where the mutated DNA strand serves as a template to replicate new (+) strands now carrying the mutated nucleotide.

The bacteriophage plaques, containing the mutated DNA, are screened by hybridizing with a labeled probe of the original oligonucleotide. By adjusting the wash temperature of the hybridized probe only the perfectly matched hybrid will remain complexed while the wild-type DNA–oligomer with mismatched nucleotide will dissociate. The M13 carrying the mutated gene is then replicated in bacteria, the DNA purified, and the mutated region of the gene sequenced

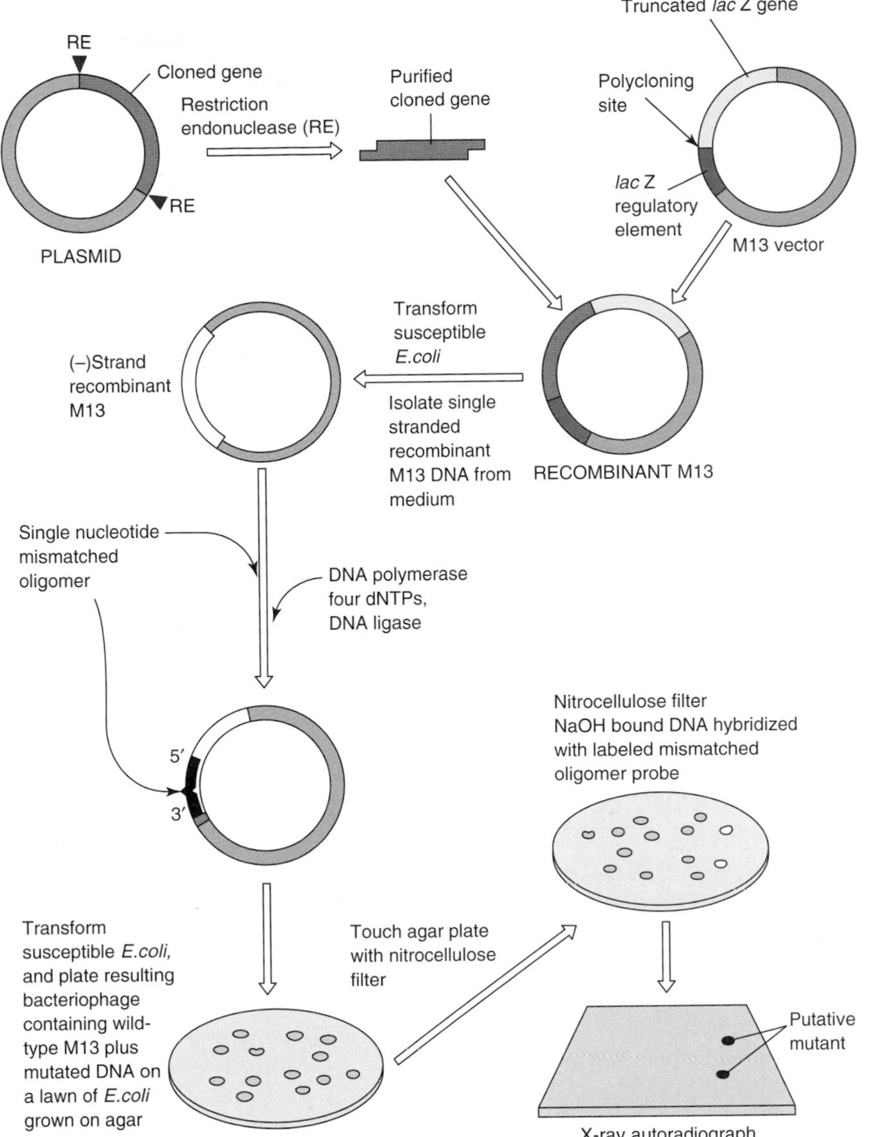

FIGURE 18.24
Site-directed mutagenesis of a single nucleotide and detection of the mutated DNA.
The figure is a simplified overview of the method. This process involves the insertion of an amplified pure DNA fragment into a modified bacteriophage vector, M13. Susceptible *E. coli,* transformed with the recombinant M13 DNA, synthesize the (+) strand DNA packaged within the viron bacteriophage proteins. The bacteriophages are isolated from the growth medium and the single-stranded recombinant M13 DNA is purified. The recombinant M13 DNA serves as a template for DNA replication in the presence of DNA polymerase, deoxynucleoside triphosphates (dNTPs), DNA ligase, and a special primer. The DNA primer (mismatched oligomer) is synthesized to be exactly complementary to a region of the DNA (gene) of interest except for the one base intended to be altered (mutated). The newly synthesized M13 DNA therefore contains a specifically mutated base, which when reintroduced into susceptible *E. coli* will be faithfully replicated. The transformed *E. coli* are grown on agar plates with replicas of the resulting colonies picked up on a nitrocellulose filter. DNA associated with each colony is denatured and fixed to the filter with NaOH and the filter-bound DNA is hybridized with a ^{32}P-labeled mismatched DNA oligomer probe. The putative mutants are then identified by exposing the filter to X-ray film.

CLINICAL CORRELATION 18.6

Site-Directed Mutagenesis of HSV I gD

The structural and functional roles of a carbohydrate moiety covalently linked to a protein can be studied by site-directed mutagenesis. The gene that codes for a glycoprotein whose asparagine residue(s) is normally glycosylated (N-linked) must first be cloned. The herpes simplex virus type I (HSV I) glycoprotein D (gD) may contain as many as three N-linked carbohydrate groups. The envelope bound HSV I gD appears to play a central role in virus absorption and penetration. Carbohydrate groups may play a role in these processes.

The cloned *HSV I gD* gene has been modified by site-directed mutagenesis to alter codons for the asparagine residue at the three potential glycosylation sites. These mutated genes, cloned within an expression vector, were transfected into eukaryotic cells (COS-1), where the gD protein was transiently expressed. The mutated HSV I gD, lacking one or all of its normal carbohydrate groups, can be analyzed with a variety of available monoclonal anti-gD antibodies to determine if immunological epitopes (specific sites on a protein recognized by an antibody) have been altered. Altered epitopes would indicate that the missing carbohydrate moiety is directly associated with the normal recognition site or played a role in the protein's native conformation. An altered protein conformation can impact on immunogenicity (e.g., for vaccines) and protein processing (movement of the protein from the endoplasmic reticulum, where it is synthesized, to the membrane, where it is normally bound). Mutations at two of the glycosylation sites altered the native conformation of the protein such that it was less reactive with selected monoclonal antibodies. Alteration at a third site had no apparent effect on protein structure, and loss of the carbohydrate chain at all three sites did not prevent normal processing of the protein.

Sodora, D. L., Cohen, G. H., and Eisenberg, R. J. Influence of asparagine-linked oligosaccharides on antigenicity, processing, and cell surface expression of herpes simplex virus type I glycoprotein D. *J. Virol.* 63:5184, 1989.

to confirm the identity of the mutation. Many modifications have been developed to improve the efficiency of site-directed mutagenesis of a single nucleotide including a method to selectively replicate the mutated strand. M13 bacteriophage, replicated in a mutant *E. coli,* incorporates some uracil residues into its DNA in place of thymine due to a metabolic defect in the synthesis of dTTP from dUTP and the lack of an enzyme that normally removes uracil residues from DNA. The purified single-stranded M13 uracil-containing DNA is hybridized with a complementary oligomer containing a mismatched base at the nucleotide to be mutated. The oligomer serves as the primer for DNA replication *in vitro* with the template (+) strand containing uracils and the new (−) strand containing thymines. When this double-stranded M13 DNA is transformed into a wild-type *E. coli,* the uracil-containing strand is destroyed and the mutated (−) strand serves as the template for the progeny bacteriophages, most of which will carry the mutation of interest.

The polymerase chain reaction can also be employed for site-directed mutagenesis. Strategies have readily been developed to incorporate a mismatched base into one of the oligonucleotides that primes the PCR. Some of these procedures employ M13 bacteriophage and follow the principles described in Figure 18.24. A variation of these PCR methods, **inverse PCR mutagenesis,** has been applied to small recombinant plasmids (4–5 kb) (Figure 18.25). The method is very rapid with 50–100% of the generated colonies containing the mutant sequence. The two primers are synthesized so that they anneal back-to-back with one primer carrying the mismatched base.

18.14 ■ APPLICATIONS OF RECOMBINANT DNA TECHNOLOGIES

The practical uses of recombinant DNA methods in biological systems are limited only by one's imagination. Recombinant DNA methods are applicable to numerous biological disciplines including agriculture, studies of evolution, forensic biology, and clinical medicine. Genetic engineering can introduce new or altered proteins into crops (e.g., corn), so that they contain amino acids essential to humans but often lacking in plant proteins. Toxins that are lethal to specific insects but harmless to humans can be introduced into crops to protect plants without the use of environmentally destructive pesticides. The DNA isolated from cells in the amniotic fluid of a pregnant woman can be analyzed for the presence or absence of genetic defects in the fetus. Minuscule quantities of DNA can be isolated from biological samples that have been preserved in ancient tar pits or frozen tundra and can be amplified and sequenced for evolutionary studies at the molecular level. The DNA from a single hair, a drop of blood, or sperm from a rape victim can be isolated, amplified, and mapped to aid in identifying felons. Current technologies in conjunction with future invented methods should permit the selective introduction of genes into cells with defective or absent genes. Developing methodologies are also likely to become available to introduce nucleic acid sequences into cells to selectively turn off the expression of detrimental genes.

Antisense Nucleic Acids Hold Promise as Research Tools and in Therapy

Recently, a new tool, **antisense nucleic acids,** has been introduced to study the intracellular expression and function of specific proteins. Natural and synthetic antisense nucleic acids that are complementary to mRNAs will hybridize within the cell, inactivate the mRNA, and block translation. The introduction of antisense nucleic acids into cells has opened new avenues to explore how proteins, whose expression has been selectively repressed in a cell, function within that cell. This method also holds great promise in control of diseased processes

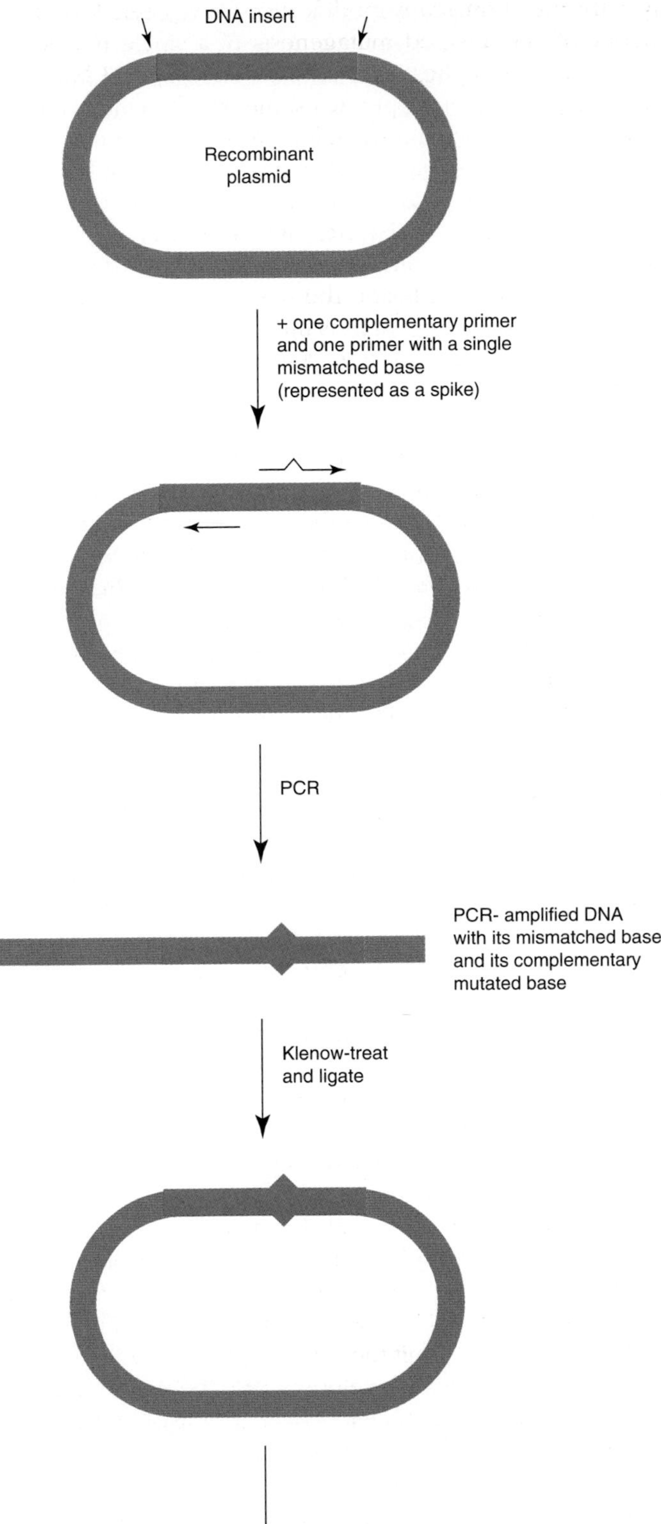

FIGURE 18.25
Inverse PCR mutagenesis.
A single base can be mutated in recombinant DNA plasmids by inverse PCR. Two primers are synthesized with their antiparallel 5′ ends complementary to adjacent bases on the two strands of DNA. One of the two primers carries a specific mismatched base that is faithfully copied during the PCR amplification steps, yielding ultimately a recombinant plasmid with a single mutated base.

such as viral infections. Antisense technology, along with site-directed mutagenesis, are part of a new approach termed **reverse genetics.** Reverse genetics (from gene to phenotype) selectively modifies a gene to evaluate its function, as opposed to classical genetics, which depends on the isolation and analysis of cells carrying random mutations that can be identified. A second use of the term reverse genetics refers to the mapping and ultimate cloning of a human gene associated with a disease where no prior knowledge of the molecular agents causing the disease exists. The use of the term "reverse genetics" in this latter case is likely to be modified.

Antisense RNA can be introduced into a cell by common cloning techniques. Figure 18.26 demonstrates one method. A gene of interest is cloned in an expression vector in the wrong orientation. That is, the sense or coding strand that is normally inserted into the expression vector downstream of a promoter is intentionally inserted in the opposite direction. This now places the complementary or antisense strand of the DNA under the control of the promoter with expression or transcription yielding antisense RNA. Transfection of cells with the antisense expression vector introduces antisense RNA that is capable of hybridizing with normal cellular mRNA. The mRNA–antisense RNA complex is not translated due to a number of reasons, such as its inability to bind to ribosomes, blockage of normal processing, and rapid enzymatic degradation.

DNA oligonucleotides have also been synthesized that are complementary to the known sequences of mRNAs of selected genes. Introduction of specific DNA oligomers to cells in culture have inhibited viral infections including infections by the human immunodeficiency virus (HIV). It is conceivable that one day bone marrow cells will be removed from AIDS patients and antisense HIV nucleic acids will be introduced into their cells in culture. These "protected" cells can then be reintroduced into the AIDS patient's bone marrow (autologous bone marrow transplantation) and replace those cells normally destroyed by

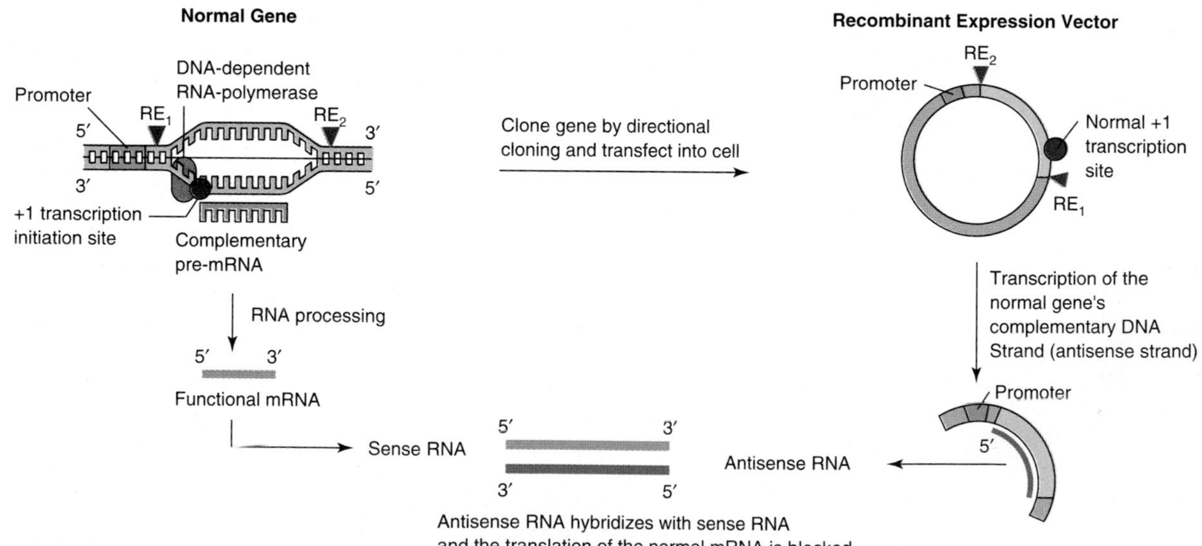

FIGURE 18.26
Production of antisense RNA.
A gene, or a portion of it, is inserted into a vector by directional cloning downstream of a promoter and in the reversed orientation to that normally found in the cell of origin. Transfection of this recombinant DNA into the parental cell carrying the normal gene results in the transcription of RNA (antisense RNA) from the cloned reversed-polarity DNA along with a normal cellular mRNA (sense RNA) transcript. The two antiparallel complementary RNAs hybridize within the cell, resulting in blocked expression (translation) of the normal mRNA transcript.

the virus. Experimental progress is also being made with antisense nucleic acids that can regulate the expression of oncogenes, genes involved in the cancer-forming process. Harnessing antisense technologies holds great promise for treatment of human diseases.

Normal Genes Can Be Introduced into Cells with a Defective Gene in Gene Therapy

It is sometimes desirable for the transfected recombinant DNA to replicate to high copy numbers independent of the cell cycle. In other situations it is preferable for only one or few copies to integrate into the host genome with its replication regulated by the cell cycle. Individuals who possess a defective gene resulting in a debilitating or fatal condition could theoretically be treated by supplying their cells with a normal gene. **Gene therapy** is in its infancy; however, the successful transfer of a normal gene to humans has been accomplished employing retroviral vectors (see Clin. Corr 18.7). The success of gene transfer depends, in part, on integration of the gene into the host genome. This is directed by the retroviral integration system. Integration, however, is normally a random event that could result in deleterious sequelae. Exciting studies are in progress that indicate that the viral integration machinery can be selectively tethered to specific target sequences within the host DNA by protein–protein interactions to obviate these potential problems.

CLINICAL CORRELATION 18.7

Normal Genes Can Be Introduced into Cells with Defective Genes in Gene Therapy

More than 4000 different genetic diseases are known, many of which are debilitating or fatal. Most are currently incurable. With the advent of new technologies in molecular biology, the clinical application of gene transfer and gene therapy is becoming a reality. Adenosine deaminase (ADA) deficiency and Gaucher's disease are but two of many genetic diseases that may readily be cured by gene therapy.

ADA is important in purine salvage, catalyzing the conversion of adenosine to inosine or deoxyadenosine to deoxyinosine. It is a protein of 363 amino acids with highest activity in thymus and other lymphoid tissues. A defect in the *ADA* gene is inherited as an autosomal recessive disorder. Over 30 mutations are associated with the disease. ADA deficiency causes a severe combined immunodeficiency disease (SCID), by an unknown mechanism. These immune-compromised children usually die in the first few years of life due to overwhelming infections. The first authorized gene therapy in humans began on September 14, 1990 with the treatment of a four-year-old girl with ADA deficiency. The patient's peripheral blood T cells were expanded in tissue culture with appropriate growth factors. The *ADA* gene was introduced within these cells by retroviral mediated gene transfer. A modified retrovirus was constructed to contain the human *ADA* gene such that it would be expressed in human cells without virus replication. (These viruses that cannot replicate are first propagated in a cell line that contains a helper virus to produce "infectious" viruses. The "infectious" viruses with foreign genetic information can now infect and transfer information to cells without helper virus functions and, therefore, cannot replicate.) Transfer of the *ADA* gene to the patient's T cells was mediated by retroviral infection. Modified T cells carrying a normal *ADA* gene were then reintroduced to the patient by autologous transfusion. Levels of ADA as low as 10% of normal are sufficient to normalize the patient.

Gaucher's disease is an autosomal recessive lysosomal storage disorder caused by a deficiency of lysosomal glucocerebrosidase (GC). Clinical problems include hepatosplenomegaly, pancytopenia, and bone deterioration. The enzyme is a lysosomal membrane glycoprotein that contains 497 amino acids. Over 36 mutations, mostly missense, that decrease catalytic activity are associated with the disease. The disorder can be treated with enzyme replacement; however, this is very expensive and the patient must be subjected to intravenous therapy throughout life. Viral constructs, similar to the ADA protocol, have been made that carry the *GC* gene and have been successfully transduced into a Gaucher patient's hematopoietic cells in culture with very high efficiencies. These studies indicate that Gaucher patients may be normalized by gene therapy in the near future. The genetically altered cells would become endogenous factories capable of continuously synthesizing *GC*, thus obviating the need for intravenous delivery of the missing enzyme.

Blaese, R. M. Progress toward gene therapy. *Clin. Immunol. Immunopathol* 61:574, 1991; Mitani, K., Wakamiya, M., and Caskey, C. T. Long-term expression of retroviral-transduced adenosine deaminase in human primitive hematopoietic progenitors. *Hum. Gene Ther.* 4:9, 1993; and Xu, L., Stahl, S. K., Dave, H. P., Schiffman, R., Correll, P. H., Kessler, S., and Karlsson, S. Correction of the enzyme deficiency in hematopoietic cells of Gaucher patients using a clinically acceptable retroviral supernatant transduction protocol. *Exp. Hematol.* 22:223, 1994.

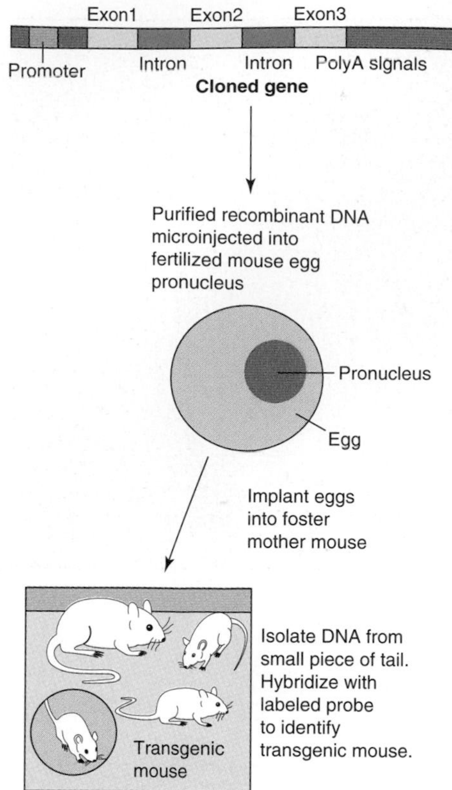

FIGURE 18.27
Production of transgenic animals. Cloned, amplified, and purified functional genes are microinjected into several fertilized mouse egg pronuclei *in vitro*. The eggs are implanted into a foster mother. DNA is isolated from a small piece of each offspring pup's tail and hybridized with a labeled probe to identify animals carrying the foreign gene (transgenic mouse). The transgenic mice can be mated to establish a new strain of mice. Cell lines can also be established from tissues of transgenic mice to study gene regulation and the structure/function of the foreign gene product.

Transgenic Animals

Recombinant DNA methods allow production of large amounts of foreign gene products in bacteria and cultured cells. These methods also facilitate evaluation of the role of a specific gene product in cell structure or function. In order to investigate the role of a selected gene product in the growth and development of a whole animal, the gene must be introduced into the fertilized egg. Foreign genes can be inserted into the genome of a fertilized egg. Animals that develop from a fertilized egg with a foreign gene insert carry that gene in every cell and are referred to as **transgenic animals.**

The most commonly employed method to create transgenic animals is outlined in Figure 18.27. The gene of interest is usually a cloned recombinant DNA molecule that includes its own promoter or is cloned in a construct with a different promoter that can be selectively regulated. Multiple copies of the foreign gene are microinjected into the pronucleus of the fertilized egg. The foreign DNA inserts randomly within the chromosomal DNA. If the insert disrupts a critical cellular gene the embryo will die. Usually, nonlethal mutagenic events result from the insertion of the foreign DNA into the chromosome.

Transgenic animals are currently being used to study several different aspects of the foreign gene, including the analysis of DNA regulatory elements, expression of proteins during differentiation, tissue specificity, and the potential role of oncogene products on growth, differentiation, and induction of tumorigenesis. Eventually, it is expected that these and related technologies will allow for methods to replace defective genes in the developing embryo (see Clin. Corr. 18.8).

Recombinant DNA in Agriculture Will Have Significant Commercial Impact

Perhaps the greatest gain to all humanity would be the practical use of recombinant technologies to improve our agricultural crops. Genes must be identified and isolated that code for properties that include higher crop yield, rapid plant growth, resistance to adverse conditions such as arid conditions or cold periods, and plant size. New genes, not common to plants, may be engineered into plants that confer resistance to insects, fungi, or bacteria. Finally, genes encoding existing structural proteins can be modified to contain essential amino acids not normally present in the plant, without modifying the protein function. The potential to produce plants with new genetic properties depends on the ability to introduce genes into plant cells that can differentiate into whole plants.

New genetic information carried in **crown gall plasmids** can be introduced into plants infected with soil bacteria known as agrobacteria. Agrobacteria naturally contain a crown gall or Ti (tumor-inducing) plasmid whose genes integrate into an infected cell's chromosome. The plasmid genes direct the host plant cell to produce new amino acid species that are required for bacterial growth. A crown gall, or tumor mass of undifferentiated plant cells, develops at the site of bacterial infection. New genes can be engineered into the Ti plasmid, and the recombinant plasmid introduced into plant cells upon infection with the agrobacteria. Transformed plant cells can then be grown in culture and under proper conditions can be induced to redifferentiate into whole plants. Every cell would contain the new genetic information and would represent a transgenic plant.

Some limitations in producing plants with improved genetic properties must be overcome before significant advances in our world food supply can be realized. Clearly, proper genes must yet be identified and isolated for desired characteristics. Also, important crops such as corn and wheat cannot be transformed by Ti plasmids; therefore other vectors must be identified. However, significant success has been achieved in recent years in designing crop plants

CLINICAL CORRELATION 18.8

Transgenic Animal Models

Transgenic animal model systems hold promise for future methodologies to correct genetic diseases early in fetal development. These animals are used to study the regulation of expression and function of specific gene products in a whole animal and have the potential for creating new breeds of commercially valuable animals. Transgenic mice have been developed from fertilized mouse eggs with rat growth hormone (*GH*) genes microinjected into their male pronuclei (see p. 835). The rat *GH* gene DNA, fused to the mouse metallothionein-I (MT-I) promoter region, was purified from the plasmid in which it had been cloned. Approximately 600 copies of the promoter–gene complex were introduced into each egg, which was then inserted into the reproductive tract of a foster mother mouse. The resulting transgenic mouse was shown to carry the rat *GH* gene within its genome by hybridizing a labeled DNA probe to mouse DNA that had been purified from a slice of the tail, restriction endonuclease digested, electrophoresed, and Southern blotted. The diet of the animals was supplemented with $ZnSO_4$ at 33 days postparturition. The $ZnSO_4$ presumably can activate the mouse MT-I promoter to initiate transcription of the rat *GH* gene. The continuous overexpression of rat GH in some transgenic animals produced mice nearly twice the size of littermates that did not carry the rat *GH* gene. A transgenic mouse transmitted the rat *GH* gene to one-half of its offspring, indicating that the gene stably integrated into the germ cell genome and that new breeds of animals can be created.

Palmiter, R. D., Brinster, R. L., Hammer, R. E., et al. Dramatic growth of mice that develop from eggs microinjected with metallothionein-growth hormone fusion genes. *Nature* 300:611, 1982.

with resistance to insects and viruses. Of equal importance is the very recent genetic engineering feat of inserting a foreign gene into pea plants that now produce a protein that inhibits the feeding of weevil larvae on the pea seeds. Peas and other legume seeds will be able to be stored without the need of protective chemical fumigants (currently Brazilian farmers lose 20–40% of their stored beans to pests).

18.15 ■ CONCLUDING REMARKS

The old cliché, so close and yet so far away, seems appropriate for our current juncture in molecular biology. The eukaryotic yeast genome, which consists of approximately 14 million base pairs of DNA distributed among 16 chromosomes, will be entirely sequenced by the mid-1990s. Equally impressive is the fact that the entire human genome will likely be sequenced in the next decade or so (see Clin. Corr. 15.11). Two human chromosomes, 16 and 19, have been fully mapped and it is anticipated they will be the first chromosomes to be fully sequenced. More than 100,000 cDNA clones are available for sequencing, which ultimately will provide landmarks of the huge human genetic map. More than 100 clinical trials in gene therapy have been initiated since the apparent success with ADA. Genetic diseases now identified and to be identified should eventually be curable by gene replacement therapy when the technical roadblocks are surmounted. If one looks at the enormous advances made in molecular biology in just the past two decades it is reasonable to believe the "when" will not be that far off.

BIBLIOGRAPHY

Askari, F. K., and McDonnell, W. M. Molecular medicine: Antisense oligonucleotide therapy. *N. Engl. J. Med.* 334:316, 1996.

Brown, W. M., George, M. Jr., and Wilson, A. C. Rapid evolution of animal mitochondrial DNA. *Proc. Natl. Acad. Sci. USA* 76:1967, 1979.

Bushman, F. Targeting retroviral integration. *Science* 267:1443, 1995.

Davis, L. G., Kuehl, W. M., and Battey, J. F. *Basic Methods in Molecular Biology*, 2nd ed. Norwalk, CT: Appleton & Lange, 1994.

Erlich, H. A. (Ed.). *PCR Technology. Principles and Applications for DNA Amplification*. New York: Stockton Press, 1989.

Feinberg, A., and Vogelstein, B. Addendum: A technique for radiolabeling DNA restriction endonuclease fragments to high specific activity. *Anal. Biochem.* 137:266, 1984.

Jaenisch, R. Transgenic animals. *Science* 240:1468, 1988.

Kreeger, K. Y. Influential consortium's cDNA clones praised as genome research time-saver. *The Scientist* 9:1, 1995.

Kunkel, T. A. Rapid and efficient site-specific mutagenesis without phenotypic selection. *Proc. Natl. Acad. Sci. USA* 82:488, 1985.

Marshall, E. Gene therapy's growing pains. *Science* 269:1050, 1995.

Maxam, A. M., and Gilbert, W. A new method of sequencing DNA. *Proc. Natl. Acad. Sci. USA* 74:560, 1977.
McPherson, M. J., Quirke, P., and Taylor, G. R. (Eds.). *PCR. A Practical Approach,* Vol. 1. Oxford, England: Oxford University Press, 1994.
Mulligan, R. C. The basic science of gene therapy. *Science* 260:926, 1993.
Palmiter, R. D., Brinster, R. L., Hammer, R. E., et al. Dramatic growth of mice that develop from eggs microinjected with metallothionein–growth hormone fusion genes. *Nature* 300:611, 1982.
Rigby, P. W. J., Dieckmann, M., Rhodes, C., and Berg, P. Labelled deoxyribonucleic acid to high specific activity in vitro by nick translation with DNA polymerase I. *J. Mol. Biol.* 113:237, 1977.
Sambrook, J., Fritsch, E. F., and Maniatis, T. *Molecular Cloning. A Laboratory Manual,* 2nd ed. New York: Cold Spring Harbor Laboratory Press, 1989.
Sanger, F., Nicklen, S., and Coulson, A. R. DNA sequencing with chain-terminating inhibitors. *Proc. Natl. Acad. Sci. USA* 74:5463, 1977.
Southern, E. M. Detection of specific sequences among DNA fragments separated by gel electrophoresis. *J. Mol. Biol.* 98:503, 1975.
Vogelstein, B., Fearon, E. R., Hamilton, S. R., and Feinberg, A. P. Use of restriction fragment length polymorphism to determine the clonal origin of human tumors. *Science* 227:642, 1985.
Watson, J. D., Tooze, J., and Kurtz, D. T. *Recombinant DNA: A Short Course.* San Francisco: Scientific American Books/Freeman, 1983.
Weintraub, H. M. Antisense RNA and DNA. *Sci. Am.* 262:40, 1990.
Williams, N. Closing in on the complete yeast genome sequence. *Science* 268:1560, 1995.
Zhang, Y., and Yunis, J. J. Improved blood RNA extraction micro-technique for RT-PCR. *Biotechniques* 18:788, 1995.

QUESTIONS ■ J. BAGGOTT AND C. N. ANGSTADT

1. Development of recombinant DNA methodologies is based on discovery of:
   A. the polymerase chain reaction (PCR).
   B. restriction endonucleases.
   C. plasmids.
   D. complementary DNA (cDNA).
   E. yeast artificial chromosomes (YACs).

2. The essential property of the DNA polymerase employed in the polymerase chain reaction (PCR) is that it:
   A. does not require a primer.
   B. is unusually active.
   C. is thermostable.
   D. replicates double-stranded DNA.
   E. can replicate both eukaryotic and prokaryotic DNA.

3. Construction of a restriction map of DNA requires all of the following EXCEPT:
   A. partial hydrolysis of DNA.
   B. complete hydrolysis of DNA.
   C. electrophoretic separation of fragments on a gel.
   D. staining of an electrophoretic gel to locate DNA.
   E. cyclic heating and cooling of the reaction mixture.

4. In the Maxam–Gilbert method of DNA sequencing:
   A. cleavage of the DNA backbone occurs randomly at only some of the sites where the base had been destroyed.
   B. all nucleotides produced during cleavage of the DNA backbone are detected by radioautography.
   C. electrophoretic separation of DNA fragments is due to differences in both size and charge.
   D. the sequence of bands in the four lanes of the autoradiogram contains the base sequence information.
   E. dideoxynucleoside triphosphates are used.

5. The Sanger and Maxam–Gilbert methods of DNA sequencing differ in that:
   A. the Maxam–Gilbert method involves labeling the 5′ end, while the Sanger method requires labeling the 3′ end of the DNA.
   B. only the Maxam–Gilbert method involves electrophoresing a mixture of fragments of different sizes.
   C. the Sanger method employs DNA cleavage, while the Maxam–Gilbert method employs interrupted DNA synthesis.
   D. only the Maxam–Gilbert method uses radioautography to detect fragments in which one of the termini is radioactively labeled.
   E. in the Maxam–Gilbert method, a complete DNA chain is cleaved, while in the Sanger method, synthesis of the chain is interrupted at different points.

6. Preparation of recombinant DNA requires:
   A. restriction endonucleases that cut in a staggered fashion.
   B. restriction endonucleases that cleave to yield blunt-ended fragments.
   C. poly (dT).
   D. DNA ligase.
   E. cDNA.

7. In the selection of colonies of bacteria that carry cloned DNA in plasmids, such as pBR322, that contain two antibiotic resistance genes:
   A. one antibiotic resistance gene is nonfunctional in the desired bacterial colonies.
   B. untransformed bacteria are antibiotic resistant.
   C. both antibiotic resistance genes are functional in the desired bacterial colonies.
   D. radiolabeled DNA or RNA probes play a role.
   E. none of the above.

8. A technique for defining gene arrangement in very long stretches of DNA (50–100 kb) is:
   A. RFLP.
   B. chromosome walking.
   C. nick translation.
   D. Southern blotting.
   E. SSCP.

9. Which of the following pairs of vectors and DNA insert sizes is correct?
   A. plasmids 5–10 kb
   B. cosmids 15 kb
   C. YACs 2000–5000 kb
   D. bacteriophage λ 45 kb
   E. none of the above

10. Expression of a eukaryotic gene in prokaryotes involves which of the following:
    A. a SD sequence in mRNA.
    B. absence of introns.
    C. regulatory elements upstream of the gene.
    D. a fusion protein.
    E. all of the above.

Refer to the following for Questions 11–15.
    A. antisense nucleic acid
    B. polymerase chain reaction
    C. site-directed mutagenesis
    D. shuttle vector
    E. transfecton

11. Contains both bacterial and eukaryotic replication signals.

12. Complementary to mRNA and will hybridize to it, thus blocking translation.

13. Can rapidly produce large quantities of a specific DNA.

14. Oligomer with one mismatched base is used as a primer.

15. A process that introduces foreign DNA into a eukaryotic genome.

ANSWERS

1. B The ability to cleave DNA predictably at specific sites is essential to recombinant DNA technology (p. 760).
2. C PCR requires cycling between low temperatures, where hybridization of template DNA and oligomer primers occurs, and high temperatures, where DNA melts (p. 759). The Taq DNA polymerase, isolated from a thermophilic organism discovered in a hot spring on federal land, is stable at high temperatures and makes the cycling possible with no addition of fresh polymerase after each cycle. The lucrative commercialization of this publicly owned natural resource, with no royalties accruing to the public (i.e., taxpayers') coffers, has evoked criticism from some observers.
3. E Cyclic heating and cooling are part of the PCR process, not of restriction mapping (p. 761). A and B: Restriction mapping involves all degrees of hydrolysis. Partial hydrolysis gives fragments of varying sizes, and complete hydrolysis gives the smallest possible fragments. C and D: Fragments are electrophoretically separated by size on agarose gel, which is stained to reveal the DNA.
4. D The relative positions of G are given by the bands in the lane corresponding to the destruction of G; of A by the bands in the AG lane that are not duplicated in the G lane; of C by the bands in the C lane; of T by the bands in the CT lane that are not duplicated in the C lane. A: Cleavage occurs at all such sites. Limited destruction of the bases is random (p. 762). B: Only the nucleotides that contain the labeled 5′ terminal are detected. Other nucleotides are produced but are not detected by the method and do not contribute information to the analysis (p. 762). C: Although charge is, of course, required to produce movement of a particle in a field, the separation of these fragments is not due to charge differences, but to size differences, with the smallest fragments migrating farthest (pp. 762–763). E: This is part of the Sanger method (p. 763).
5. D They both use radioautography to detect fragments in which one of the termini is radioactively labeled. A: The Sanger method involves a labeled 5′ end. With the Maxam–Gilbert method either end could be labeled. Here we show labeling of the 3′ end. B: Both methods do this. C: This statement reverses the methodologies. E: See pp. 762–765.
6. D DNA ligase covalently connects fragments held together by interaction of cohesive ends (p. 765). A: This is the most desirable type of restriction endonuclease to use, but it is not essential. B: Restriction nucleases that make blunt cuts can also be used if necessary. C: This is used in conjunction with poly (dA) if restriction endonucleases that make blunt cuts are employed, but it is not essential to all of recombinant DNA preparation.
7. A The foreign DNA is inserted into one antibiotic resistance gene, thus destroying it (p. 770). B: Resistance is due to the plasmids. C: See the comment for A above. D: Radiolabeling detects the DNA of interest, not the colonies that contain cloned DNA (p. 770).
8. B A: Restriction fragment length polymorphism (RFLP) is a characteristic of DNA, not a technique (p. 775). C: Nick translation is used to label DNA during chromosome walking (p. 773). D: Southern blotting is a method for analyzing DNA (p. 774). E: Single-strand conformation polymorphism (SSCP) is a method for detecting base changes in DNA that do not alter restriction endonuclease sites.
9. A B: Cosmids will accept a 45-kb insert (p. 781). C: YACs will accept a 200–500 kb insert (p. 781). D: Bacteriophage λ will accept a 15-kb insert (p. 779).
10. E A: The SD sequence is necessary for the bacterial ribosome to recognize the mRNA. B: Bacteria do not have the intracellular machinery to remove introns from mRNA. C: Appropriate regulatory elements are necessary to allow the DNA to be transcribed. D: A fusion protein may be a product of the reaction (p. 783).
11. D (see p. 784).
12. A (see p. 790).
13. B (see p. 759).
14. C (see p. 788).
15. E (see p. 784).

CHAPTER

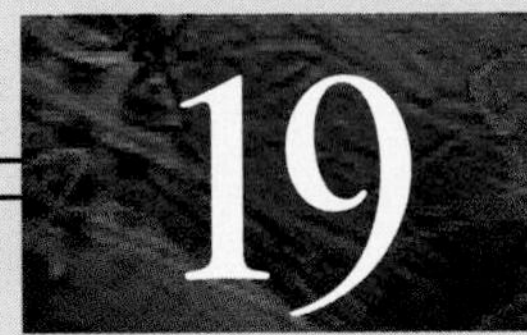

REGULATION OF GENE EXPRESSION

John E. Donelson

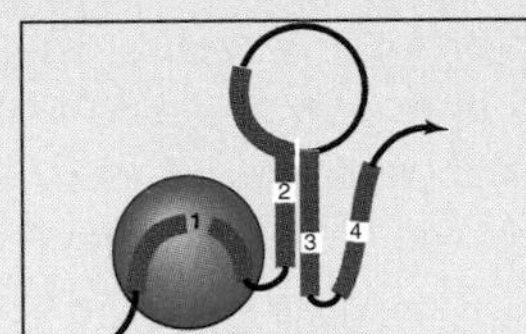

19.1 ■ OVERVIEW

To survive, a living cell must be able to respond to changes in its environment. One of many ways in which cells adjust to changes is to alter expression of specific genes, which, in turn, affects the number of corresponding protein molecules in the cell. This chapter focuses on some of the molecular mechanisms that determine when a given gene will be expressed and to what extent. The attempt to understand how expression of genes is regulated is one of the most active areas of biochemical research today.

It makes sense for a cell to vary the amount of a given gene product available under different conditions. For example, the bacterium *Escherichia coli* (*E. coli*) contains genes for about 3000 different proteins, but it does not need to synthesize all of these proteins at the same time. Therefore it regulates the number of molecules of these proteins that are made. The classic illustration of this phenomenon is the regulation of the number of **β-galactosidase** molecules in the cell. This enzyme converts the disaccharide lactose into the monosaccharides, glucose and galactose. When *E. coli* is growing in a medium containing glucose as the carbon source, β-galactosidase is not required and only about five molecules of the enzyme are present in the cell. When lactose is the sole carbon source, however, 5000 or more molecules of β-galactosidase occur in the cell. Clearly, the bacteria respond to the need to metabolize lactose by increasing the synthesis of β-galactosidase molecules. If lactose is removed from the medium, the synthesis of this enzyme stops as rapidly as it began.

The complexity of eukaryotic cells means that they have even more extensive mechanisms of gene regulation than do prokaryotic cells. The differentiated cells of higher organisms have a much more complicated physical structure and often a more specialized biological function that is determined, again, by the expression of their genes. For example, **insulin** is synthesized in β cells of the pancreas and not in kidney cells even though the nuclei of all cells of the body contain the insulin genes. Molecular regulatory mechanisms facilitate the expression of insulin in pancreas and prevent its synthesis in kidney and other cells. In addition, during development of the organism appearance or disappearance of proteins in specific cell types is tightly controlled with respect to timing and sequence of developmental events.

As expected from the differences in complexities, far more is understood about the regulation of genes in prokaryotes than in eukaryotes. However, studies on the control of gene expression in prokaryotes often provide exciting new ideas that can be tested in eukaryotic systems. Sometimes, discoveries about eukaryotic gene structure and regulation alter the interpretation of data on the control of prokaryotic genes.

Several of the best studied examples of gene regulation in bacteria will be discussed, followed by some illustrations of the organization and regulation of related genes in the human genome. Finally, the use of recombinant DNA techniques to express some human genes of clinical interest will be presented.

19.2 ■ UNIT OF TRANSCRIPTION IN BACTERIA: THE OPERON

The single *E. coli* chromosome is a circular double-stranded DNA molecule of about four million base pairs. Most of the approximately 3000 *E. coli* genes are not distributed randomly throughout this DNA; instead, the genes that code for the enzymes of a specific metabolic pathway are clustered in one region of the DNA. In addition, genes for associated structural proteins, such as the 70 or so proteins that comprise the ribosome, are frequently adjacent to one another. Members of a set of clustered genes are usually coordinately regulated; they are transcribed together to form a "polycistronic" mRNA species that contains the coding sequences for several proteins. The term **operon** describes the complete regulatory unit of a set of clustered genes. An operon includes the adjacent **structural genes** that code for the related enzymes or associated proteins, a **regulatory gene** or genes that code for regulator protein(s), and **control elements** that are sites on the DNA near the structural genes at which regulator proteins act. Figure 19.1 shows a partial genetic map of the *E. coli* chromosome that gives locations of structural genes of some of the different operons.

When transcription of the structural genes of an operon increases in response to the presence of a specific substrate in the medium, the effect is known as **induction.** The increase in transcription of the β-galactosidase gene when lactose is the sole carbon source is an example of induction. Bacteria also respond to nutritional changes by quickly turning off the synthesis of enzymes that are no longer needed. As will be described below, *E. coli* synthesizes the amino acid tryptophan as the end product of a specific biosynthetic pathway. However, if tryptophan is supplied in the medium, the bacteria do not need to make it themselves, and synthesis of enzymes for this metabolic pathway is stopped. This process is called **repression.** It permits the bacteria to avoid using their energy for making unnecessary and even harmful proteins.

Induction and repression are manifestations of the same phenomenon. In one case the bacterium changes its enzyme composition so that it can utilize a specific substrate in the medium; in the other it reduces the number of enzyme

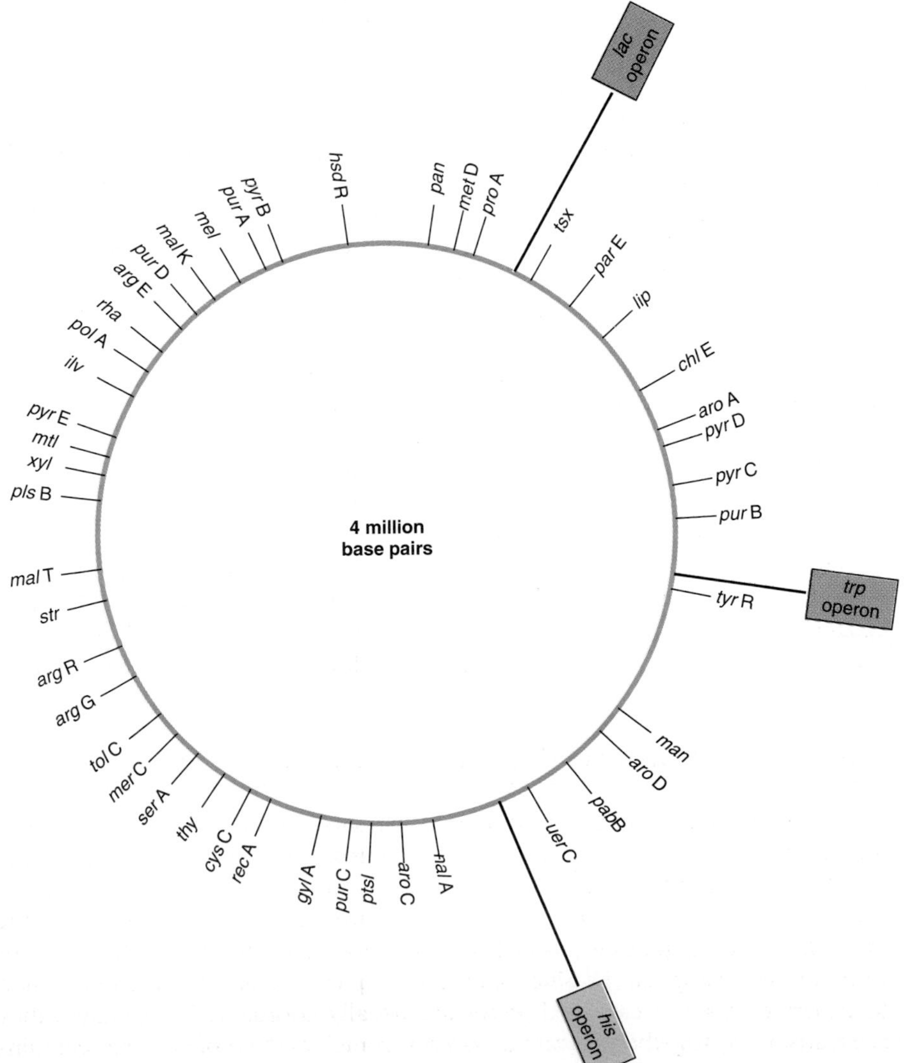

FIGURE 19.1
Partial genetic map of *E. coli*.
The locations of only a few of the genes identified and mapped in *E. coli* are shown here. Three operons discussed in this chapter are indicated.
Reproduced with permission from Stent, G. S., and Calendar, R. Molecular Genetics, An Introductory Narrative. *San Francisco: Freeman, 1978, p. 289; modified from Bachmann, B. J., Low, K. B., and Taylor, A. L.* Bacteriol. Rev. *40:116, 1976.*

molecules so that it does not overproduce a specific metabolic product. The signal for each type of regulation is the small molecule that is a substrate for the metabolic pathway or a product of the pathway, respectively. These small molecules are called **inducers** when they stimulate induction and **corepressors** when they cause repression to occur.

Section 19.3 will describe in detail the lactose operon, the best studied example of a set of inducible genes. Section 19.4 will present the tryptophan operon, an example of a repressible operon. Sections 19.5–19.7 will briefly describe some other operons as well as some gene systems in which physical movement of the genes themselves within the DNA (i.e., gene rearrangements) plays a role in their regulation.

19.3 ■ LACTOSE OPERON OF *E. COLI*

The lactose operon contains three adjacent structural genes as shown in Figure 19.2. *Lac*Z codes for the enzyme β-galactosidase, which is composed of four identical subunits of 1021 amino acids. *Lac*Y codes for a permease, which is a 275-amino acid protein that occurs in the cell membrane and participates in the transport of sugars, including lactose, across the membrane. The third gene, *lac*A, codes for β-galactoside transacetylase, a 275-amino acid enzyme that transfers an acetyl group from acetyl CoA to β-galactoside. Of these three proteins, only β-galactosidase actually participates in a known metabolic pathway. However, the permease is clearly important in the utilization of lactose since it is involved in transporting lactose into the cell. The acetylation reaction may be associated with detoxification and excretion reactions of nonmetabolized analogs of β-galactosides.

Mutations in *lac*Z or *lac*Y that destroy the function of β-galactosidase or permease prevent cells from cleaving lactose or acquiring it from the medium, respectively. Mutations in *lac*A that destroy transacetylase activity do not seem to have an identifiable effect on cell growth and division. Perhaps there are other related enzymes in the cell that serve as backups for this enzyme, or perhaps it has an unknown function that is required only under certain conditions.

A single mRNA species containing the coding sequences of all three structural genes is transcribed from a promoter that occurs just upstream from the *lac*Z gene. Induction of these three genes occurs during initiation of their

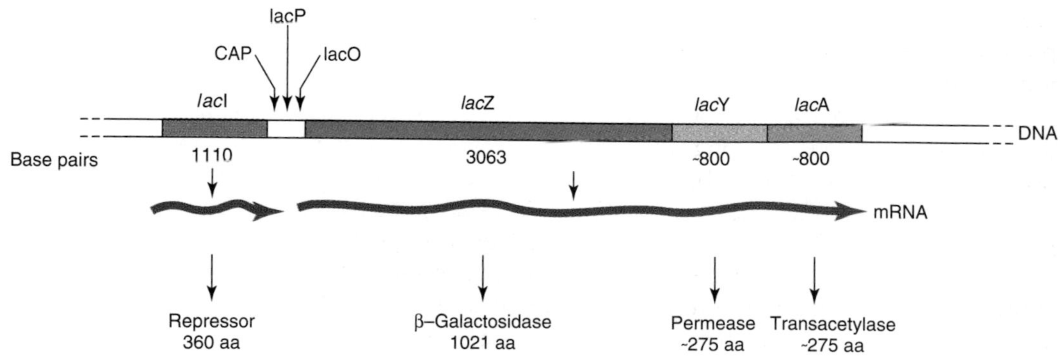

FIGURE 19.2
Lactose operon of *E. coli*.
The lactose operon is composed of the *lacI* gene, which codes for a repressor, the control elements of *CAP, lacP,* and *lacO,* and three structural genes, *lacZ, lacY,* and *lacA,* which code for β-galactosidase, a permease, and a transacetylase, respectively. The *lacI* gene is transcribed from its own promotor. Three structural genes are transcribed from the promoter, *lacP,* to form a polycistronic mRNA from which the three proteins are translated.

transcription. Without the inducer, transcription of the gene cluster occurs only at a very low level. In the presence of the inducer, transcription begins at the **promoter,** called *lac*P, and goes through all three genes to a transcription terminator located slightly beyond the end of *lac*A. Therefore the genes are **coordinately expressed**; either all three are transcribed in unison or none is transcribed.

The presence of three coding sequences on the same mRNA molecule suggests that the relative amounts of the three proteins are always the same under varying conditions of induction. An inducer that causes a high rate of transcription will result in a high level of all three proteins; an inducer that stimulates only a little transcription of the operon will result in a low level of the proteins. The inducer can be thought of as a molecular switch that influences synthesis of the single mRNA species for all three genes. The number of molecules of each protein in the cell may be different, but this does not reflect differences in transcription; it reflects differences in translation rates of the coding sequences or in degradation of the proteins themselves.

The mRNA induced by lactose is very unstable; it is degraded with a half-life of about 3 min. Therefore expression of the operon can be altered very quickly. Transcription ceases as soon as inducer is no longer present, existing mRNA molecules disappear within a few minutes, and cells stop making the proteins.

Repressor of the Lactose Operon Is a Diffusible Protein

The regulatory gene of the lactose operon, *lac*I, codes for a protein whose only function is to control the transcription initiation of the three *lac* structural genes. This regulator protein is called the *lac* **repressor.** The *lac*I gene is located just in front of the controlling elements for the *lac*ZYA gene cluster. However, it is not obligatory that a regulatory gene be physically close to the gene cluster it regulates. In some of the other operons it is not. Transcription of *lac*I is not regulated; instead, this single gene is always transcribed from its own promoter at a low rate that is relatively independent of the cell's status. Therefore affinity of the *lac*I promoter for **RNA polymerase** seems to be the only factor involved in its transcription initiation.

The lac repressor is initially synthesized as a monomer of 360 amino acids and four monomers associate to form a tetramer, the active form of the repressor. Usually there are about 10 tetramers per cell. The repressor has a strong affinity for a specific DNA sequence that lies between *lac*P and the start of *lac*Z. This sequence is called the **operator** and is designated *lac*O. The operator overlaps the promoter somewhat so that presence of repressor bound to the operator physically prevents RNA polymerase from binding to the promoter and initiating transcription.

In addition to recognizing and binding to the lac operator DNA sequence, the repressor also has a strong affinity for the inducer molecules of the *lac* operon. Each monomer has a binding site for an inducer molecule. Binding of inducer to the monomers causes an **allosteric change** in the repressor that greatly lowers its affinity for the operator sequence (Figure 19.3). In other words, when inducer molecules are bound to their sites on the repressor, a conformational change in the repressor occurs that alters the binding site for the operator. The result is that repressor no longer binds to the operator so that RNA polymerase, in turn, can begin transcription from the promoter. A repressor molecule that is already bound to the operator when the inducer becomes available can still bind to inducer so that the repressor–inducer complex immediately disassociates from the operator.

A study of the lactose operon has been greatly facilitated by the discovery that some small molecules fortuitously serve as inducers but are not metabolized by β-galactosidase. Isopropylthiogalactoside **(IPTG)** is one of several thiogalac-

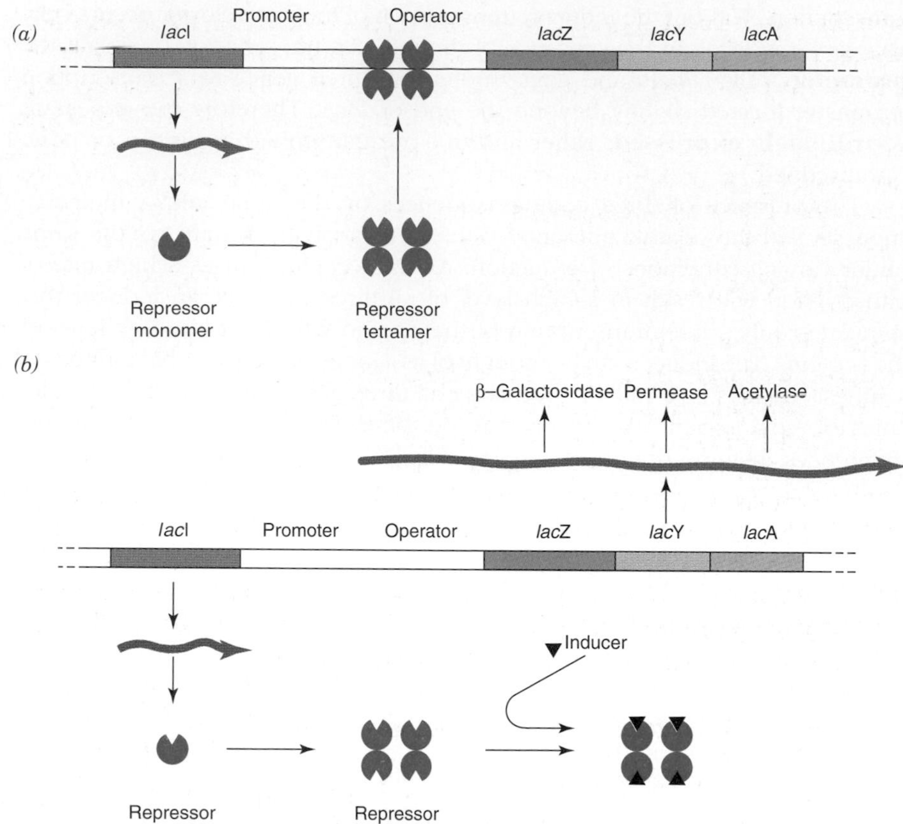

FIGURE 19.3
Control of *lac* operon.
(*a*) Repressor tetramer binds to operator and prevents transcription of structural genes. (*b*) Inducer binds to repressor tetramer, which prevents repressor from binding to operator. Transcription of three structural genes can occur from the promoter.

tosides with this property. They are called **gratuitous inducers.** They bind to inducer sites on the repressor molecule causing the conformational change but are not cleaved by the induced β-galactosidase. Therefore they affect the system without themselves being altered (metabolized) by it. If it were not possible to manipulate experimentally the system with these gratuitous inducers, it would have been much more difficult to reach our current understanding of the lactose operon in particular and bacterial gene regulation in general.

The product of the *lac*I gene, the repressor protein, acts in trans; that is, it is a diffusible product that moves through the cell to its site of action. Therefore mutations in the *lac*I gene can exert an effect on the expression of other genes located far away or even on genes located on different DNA molecules. *Lac*I mutations can be of several types. One class of mutations changes or deletes amino acids of the repressor that are located in the binding site for the inducer. These changes interfere with interaction between the inducer and the repressor but do not affect the affinity of repressor for the operator. Therefore the repressor is always bound to the operator, even in the presence of inducer, and the *lac*ZYA genes are never transcribed above a very low basal level. Another class of *lac*I mutations changes the amino acids in the operator-binding site of the repressor. Most of these mutations lessen the affinity of the repressor for the operator. This means that repressor does not bind to the operator and *lac*ZYA genes are always being transcribed. These mutations are called **repressor-constitutive mutations** because *lac* genes are permanently turned on. Interestingly, a few rare *lac*I mutants actually increase the affinity of repressor for the operator over that of wild-type repressor. In these cases inducer molecules can still bind to repressor, but they are less effective in releasing repressor from the operator.

Repressor-constitutive mutants illustrate the features of a negative control system. An active repressor, in the absence of an inducer, shuts off the expression of the *lac* structural genes. An inactive repressor results in the constitutive, unregulated, expression of these genes. It is possible, using the recombinant DNA techniques described in Chapter 18, to introduce into constitutive *lac*I mutant cells a recombinant plasmid containing the wild-type *lac*I gene (but not the rest of the *lac* operon). Therefore these cells have one wild-type and one mutant *lac*I gene and will synthesize both active and inactive repressor molecules. Under these conditions, normal wild-type regulation of the lactose operon occurs. In genetic terms, the wild-type induction is dominant over the mutant constitutivity. This property is the main feature of a negative control system.

Operator Sequence of the Lactose Operon Is Contiguous on DNA with a Promoter and Three Structural Genes

The known control elements in front of the structural genes of the lactose operon are the operator and promoter. The operator was originally identified, like the *lac*I gene, by mutations that affected the transcription of the *lac*ZYA region. Some of these mutations also result in the constitutive synthesis of lac mRNA; that is, they are **operator-constitutive mutations.** In these cases the operator DNA sequence has undergone one or more base pair changes so that the repressor no longer binds as tightly to the sequence. Thus the repressor is less effective in preventing RNA polymerase from initiating transcription.

In contrast to mutations in the *lac*I gene that affect the diffusible repressor, mutations in the operator do not affect a diffusible product. They exert their influence on the transcription of only the three *lac* genes that lie immediately downstream of the operator on the same DNA molecule. This means that if a second lac operon is introduced into a bacterium on a recombinant plasmid, the operator of one operon does not influence action on the other operon. Therefore an operon with a wild-type operator will be repressed under the usual conditions, whereas in the same bacterium a second operon that has an operator-constitutive mutation will be transcribed continuously.

Operator mutations are frequently referred to as **cis-dominant** to emphasize that these mutations affect only adjacent genes on the same DNA molecule and that they are not influenced by the presence in the cell of other copies of the unmutated sequence. Cis-dominant mutations occur in DNA sequences that are recognized by proteins rather than in DNA sequences that code for the diffusible proteins. **Trans-dominant** mutations occur in genes that specify the diffusible products. Therefore cis-dominant mutations also occur in promoter and transcription termination sequences, whereas trans-dominant mutations also occur in the genes for the subunit proteins of RNA polymerase, the ribosomes, and so on.

Figure 19.4 shows the sequence of both the *lac* operator and promoter. The operator sequence has an axis of dyad symmetry. The sequence of the upper strand on the left side of the operator is nearly identical to the lower strand on the right side; only three differences occur between these inverted

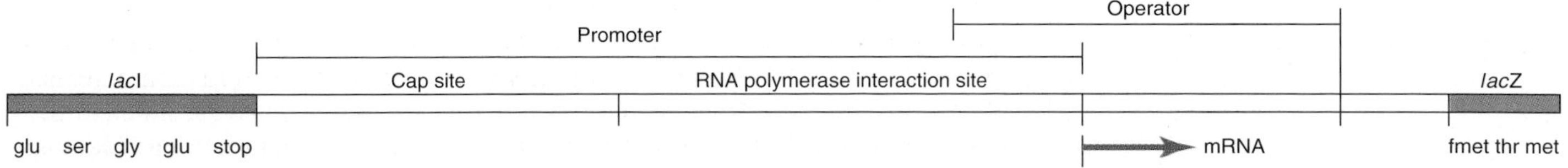

5′ GGAAAGCGGGCAGTGAGCGCAACGCAATTAATGTGAGTTAGCTCACTCATTAGGCACCCCAGGCTTTACACTTTATGCTTCCGGCTCGTATGTTGTGTGGAATTGTGAGCGGATAACAATTTCACACAGGAAACAGCTATGACCATG 3′
3′ CCTTTCGCCCGTCACTCGCGTTGCGTTAATTACACTCAATCGAGTGAGTAATCCGTGGGGTCCGAAATGTGAAATACGAAGGCCGAGCATACAACACACCTTAACACTCGCCTATTGTTAAAGTGTGTCCTTTGTCGATACTGGTAC 5′

FIGURE 19.4
Nucleotide sequence of control elements of lactose operon.
The end of the *lacI* gene (coding for the lactose repressor) and the beginning of the *lacZ* gene (coding for β-galactosidase) are also shown. Lines above and below the sequence indicate symmetrical sequences within the CAP site and operator.

DNA repeats. This symmetry in the DNA recognition sequence reflects symmetry in the tetrameric repressor. It probably facilitates the tight binding of the subunits of the repressor to the operator, although this has not been definitively demonstrated. A common feature of many protein-binding or recognition sites on double-stranded DNA, including most recognition sites for restriction enzymes, is a **dyad symmetry** in the nucleotide sequence.

The 30 bp that constitute the *lac* operator are an extremely small fraction of the total *E. coli* genome of 4×10^6 bp and occupy an even smaller fraction of the total volume of the cell. Therefore it would seem that the approximately 10 tetrameric repressors in a cell might have trouble finding the *lac* operator if they just randomly diffuse about the cell. Although this remains a puzzling consideration, there are factors that confine the repressor to a much smaller space than the entire volume of the cell. First, it probably helps that the repressor gene is very close to the *lac* operator. This means that the repressor does not have far to diffuse if its translation begins before its mRNA is fully synthesized. Second, and more importantly, the repressor possesses a low general affinity for all DNA sequences. When the inducer binds to the repressor, its affinity for the operator is reduced about a 1000-fold, but its low affinity for random DNA sequences is unaltered. Therefore all of the *lac* repressors of the cell probably spend the majority of the time in loose association with the DNA. As the binding of the inducer releases a repressor molecule from the operator, it quickly reassociates with another nearby region of the DNA. Therefore induction redistributes the repressor on the DNA rather than generates freely diffusing repressor molecules. This confines the repressor to a smaller volume within the cell.

Another question is how does lactose enter a *lac*-repressed cell in the first place if the *lac*Y gene product, the permease, is repressed yet is required for lactose transport across the cell membrane? The answer is that even in the fully repressed state, there is a very low basal level of transcription of the *lac* operon that provides five or six molecules of the permease per cell. Perhaps this is just enough to get a few molecules of lactose inside the cell and begin the process.

An even more curious observation is that, in fact, lactose is not the natural inducer of the lactose operon as we would expect. When the repressor is isolated from fully induced cells, the small molecule bound to each repressor monomer is **allolactose,** not lactose. Allolactose, like lactose, is composed of galactose and glucose, but the linkage between the two sugars is different. It turns out that a side reaction of β-galactosidase (which normally breaks down lactose to galactose and glucose) converts these two products to allolactose. Therefore it appears that a few molecules of lactose are taken up and converted by β-galactosidase to allolactose, which then binds to the repressor and induces the operon. Further confirmation that lactose itself is not the real inducer comes from experiments indicating that lactose binding to the purified repressor slightly increases the repressor's affinity for the operator. Therefore, in the induced state, a small amount of allolactose must be present in the cell to overcome this "anti-inducer" effect of the lactose substrate.

Promoter Sequence of Lactose Operon Contains Recognition Sites for RNA Polymerase and a Regulator Protein

Immediately in front of the *lac* operator sequence is the promoter sequence. This sequence contains the recognition sites for two different proteins, RNA polymerase and the **CAP-binding protein** (Figure 19.4). The site at which RNA polymerase interacts with the DNA to initiate transcription has been identified using several different genetic and biochemical approaches. Point mutations in this region frequently affect the affinity to which RNA polymerase will bind the DNA. Deletions (or insertions) that extend into this region also dramatically affect the binding of RNA polymerase to the DNA. The end points of the sequence to which RNA polymerase binds were identified by **DNase protection** experiments. Purified RNA polymerase was bound to the *lac* promoter region cloned in a bacteriophage DNA or a plasmid, and this protein–DNA complex was digested with DNase I. The DNA segment protected from degradation by DNase was recovered and its sequence determined. The ends of this protected segment varied slightly with different DNA molecules but corresponded closely to the boundaries of the RNA polymerase interaction site shown in Figure 19.4.

The sequence of the RNA polymerase interaction site is not composed of symmetrical elements similar to those described for the operator sequence. This is not surprising since RNA polymerase must associate with the DNA in an asymmetrical fashion for RNA synthesis to be initiated in only one direction from the binding site. However, that portion of the promoter sequence recognized by the CAP-binding protein does contain some symmetry. A **DNA–protein interaction** at this region enhances transcription of the lac operon as described in the next section.

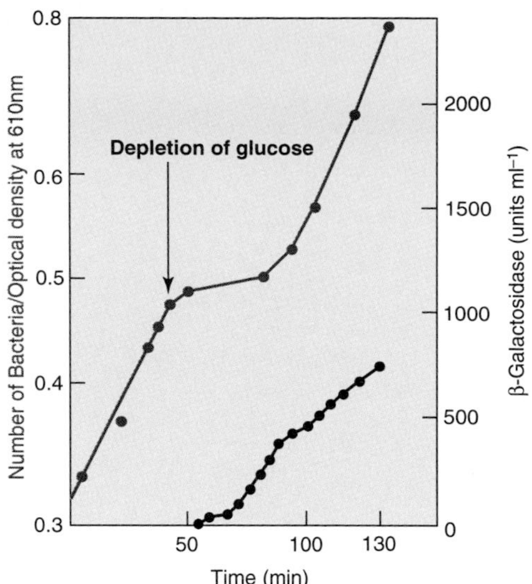

FIGURE 19.5
Lack of synthesis of β-galactosidase in *E. coli* when glucose is present.
The bacteria are growing in a medium containing initially 0.4 mg mL^{-1} of glucose and 2 mg mL^{-1} lactose. The left-hand ordinate indicates the optical density of the growing culture, an indicator of the number of bacterial cells. The right-hand ordinate indicates the units of β-galactosidase per milliliter. Note that the appearance of β-galactosidase is delayed until the glucose is depleted.
Redrawn from Epstein, W., Naono, S., and Gros, F. Biochem. Biophys. Res. Commun. *24:588, 1966.*

Catabolite Activator Protein Binds at a Site on the Lactose Promoter

Escherichia coli prefers to use glucose instead of other sugars as a carbon source. For example, if the concentrations of glucose and lactose in the medium are the same, the bacteria will selectively metabolize the glucose and not utilize the lactose. This phenomenon is illustrated in Figure 19.5, which shows that the appearance of β-galactosidase, the *lac*Z product, is delayed until all of the glucose in the medium is depleted. Only then can lactose be used as the carbon source. This delay indicates that glucose interferes with the induction of the lactose operon. This effect is called **catabolite repression** because it occurs during the catabolism of glucose and may be due to a catabolite of glucose rather than glucose itself. An identical effect is exerted on a number of other inducible operons, including the arabinose and galactose operons, which code for enzymes involved in the utilization of various substances as energy sources. It probably is a general coordinating system for turning off synthesis of unwanted enzymes whenever the preferred substrate, glucose, is present.

Catabolite repression begins in the cell when glucose lowers the concentration of intracellular **cyclic AMP** (cAMP). The exact mechanism by which this reduction in the cAMP level is accomplished is not known. Perhaps glucose influences either the rate of synthesis or degradation of cAMP. At any rate, cAMP can bind to another regulatory protein, which has not been discussed yet, called CAP (for **catabolite activator protein**) or CRP (for cAMP receptor protein). CAP is an **allosteric protein,** and when it is combined with cAMP, it is capable of binding to the CAP regulatory site that is at the promoter of the *lac* (and other) operons. The CAP–cAMP complex exerts positive control on the transcription of these operons. Its binding to the CAP site on the DNA facilitates the binding of RNA polymerase to the promoter (Figure 19.6). Alternatively, if the CAP site is not occupied, RNA polymerase has more difficulty binding to the promoter, and transcription of the operon occurs much less efficiently. Therefore, when glucose is present, the cAMP level drops, the CAP–cAMP complex does not form, and the positive influence on RNA polymerase does not occur. Conversely, if glucose is absent, the cAMP level is high, a CAP–cAMP complex binds to the CAP site, and transcription is enhanced.

19.4 TRYPTOPHAN OPERON OF *E. COLI*

Tryptophan is essential for bacterial growth; it is needed for the synthesis of all proteins that contain tryptophan. Therefore, if tryptophan is not present in sufficient amount by the medium, the cell must make it. In contrast, lactose is not absolutely required for the cell's growth; many other sugars can substitute for it, and, in fact, as we saw in the previous section, the bacterium prefers to

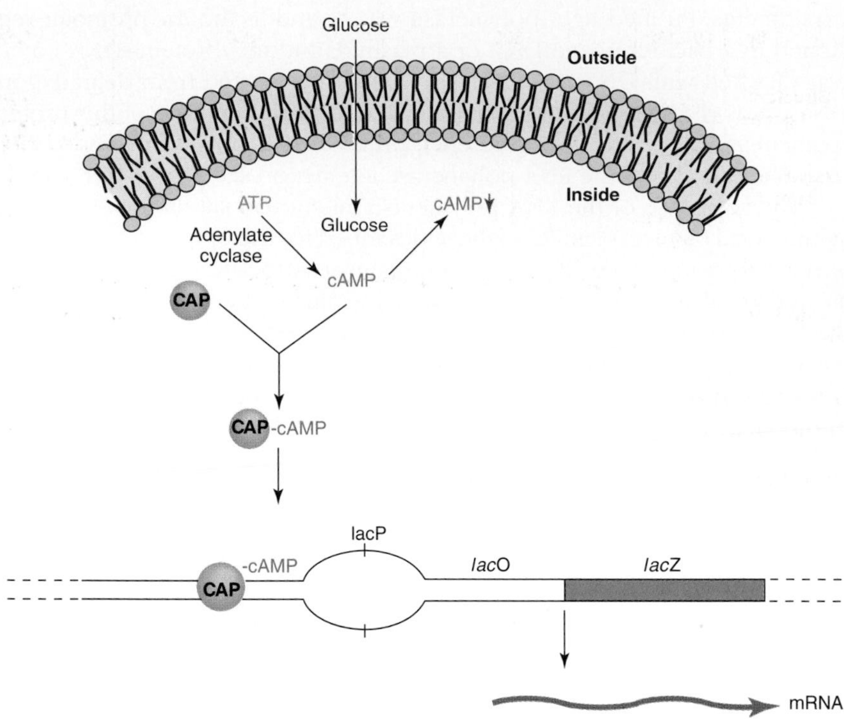

FIGURE 19.6
Control of *lacP* by cAMP.
A CAP–cAMP complex binds to the CAP site and enhances transcription at *lacP*. Catabolite repression occurs when glucose lowers the intracellular concentration of cAMP. This reduces the amount of the CAP–cAMP complex and decreases transcription from *lacP* and from the promoters of several other operons.

use some of these other sugars for the carbon source. As a result, synthesis of the tryptophan biosynthetic enzymes is regulated differently than synthesis of the proteins encoded by the lactose operon.

Tryptophan Operon Is Controlled by a Repressor Protein

In *E. coli* tryptophan is synthesized from chorismic acid in a five-step pathway that is catalyzed by three different enzymes as shown in Figure 19.7. The **tryptophan operon** contains the five structural genes that code for these three enzymes (two of which have two different subunits). Upstream from this gene cluster is a promoter where transcription begins and an operator to which binds a repressor protein encoded by the unlinked *trp*R gene. Transcription of the lactose operon is generally "turned off" unless it is induced by the small molecule inducer. The tryptophan operon, on the other hand, is always "turned on" unless it is repressed by the presence of a small molecule **corepressor** (a term used to distinguish it from the repressor protein). Hence the lac operon is inducible, whereas the *trp* operon is repressible. When the *trp* operon is being actively transcribed, it is said to be **derepressed;** that is, the trp repressor is not preventing RNA polymerase from binding. This is mechanistically the same as an induced lactose operon in which the *lac* repressor is not interfering with RNA polymerase.

The biosynthetic pathway for tryptophan synthesis is regulated by mechanisms that affect both the synthesis and activity of the enzymes that catalyze the pathway. For example, anthranilate synthetase, which catalyzes the first step of the pathway, is encoded by the *trp*E and *trp*D genes of the trp operon. The number of molecules of this enzyme that is present in the cell is determined by the transcriptional regulation of the *trp* operon. However, the catalytic activity of the existing molecules of the enzyme is regulated by **feedback inhibition.** This is a common short-term means of regulating the first committed step in a metabolic pathway. In this case, tryptophan, the end product of the pathway, can bind to an allosteric site on the anthranilate synthetase and interfere with its catalytic activity at another site. Therefore, as the concentration of tryptophan

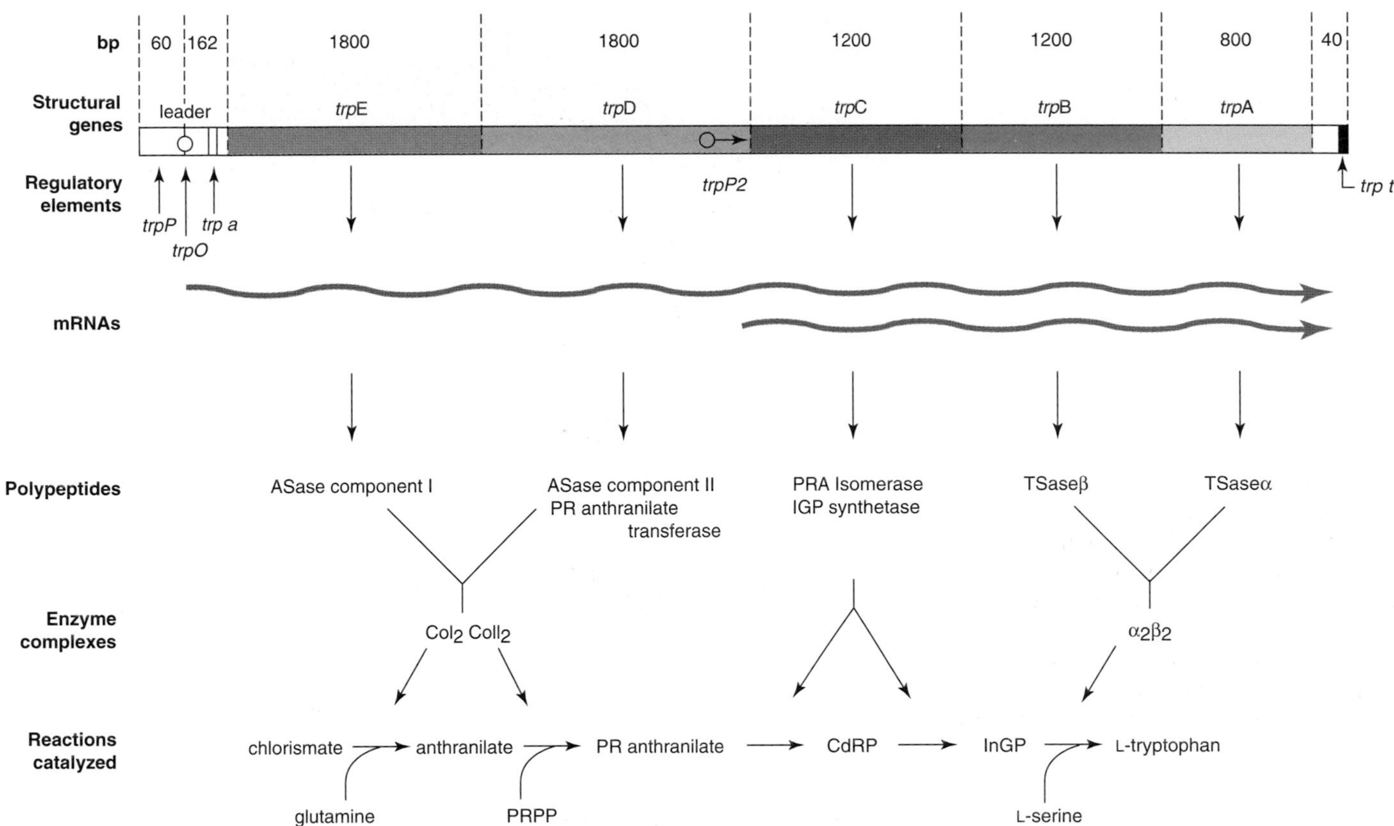

FIGURE 19.7
Genes of tryptophan operon of *E. coli*.
Regulatory elements are the primary promoter (*trpP*), operator (*trpO*), attenuator (*trp* a), secondary internal promoter (*trpP2*), and terminator (*trp t*). Direction of mRNA synthesis is indicated on the wavy lines representing mRNAs. CoI_2 and $CoII_2$ signify components I and II, respectively, of the anthranilate synthetase (ASase) complex; PR-anthranilate is *N*-5′-phosphoribosyl-anthranilate; CdRP is 1-(*o*-carboxy-phenylamino)-1-deoxyribulose-5-phosphate; InGP is indole-3-glycerol phosphate; PRPP is 5-phosphoribosyl-1-pyrophosphate; and TSase is tryptophan synthetase.
Redrawn from Platt, T. The tryptophan operon. In: J. H. Miller and W. Reznikoff (Eds.), The Operon. *Cold Spring Harbor, NY: Cold Spring Harbor Laboratory Press, 1978, p. 263.*

builds up in the cell, it begins to bind to anthranilate synthetase and immediately decreases its activity on the substrate, chorismic acid. In addition, tryptophan also acts as a **corepressor** to shut down the synthesis of new enzyme molecules from the *trp* operon. Thus feedback inhibition is a short-term control that has an immediate effect on the pathway, whereas repression takes a little longer but has the more permanent effect of reducing the number of enzyme molecules.

The *trp* repressor is a tetramer of four identical subunits of about 100 amino acids each. Under normal conditions about 20 molecules of the repressor tetramer are present in the cell. The repressor by itself does not bind to the *trp* operator. It must be complexed with tryptophan in order to bind to the operator and therefore acts *in vivo* only in the presence of tryptophan. This is exactly the opposite of the *lac* repressor, which binds to its operator only in the absence of its small molecule inducer. Interestingly, *trp* repressor also regulates transcription of *trp*R, its own gene. As *trp* repressor accumulates in cells, the repressor–tryptophan complex binds to a region upstream of this gene, turning off its transcription and maintaining the equilibrium of 20 repressors per cell. Another difference from the *lac* operon is that the *trp* operator occurs entirely within the *trp* promoter rather than adjacent to it, as shown in Figure 19.8. The operator sequence is a region of dyad symmetry, and the mechanism

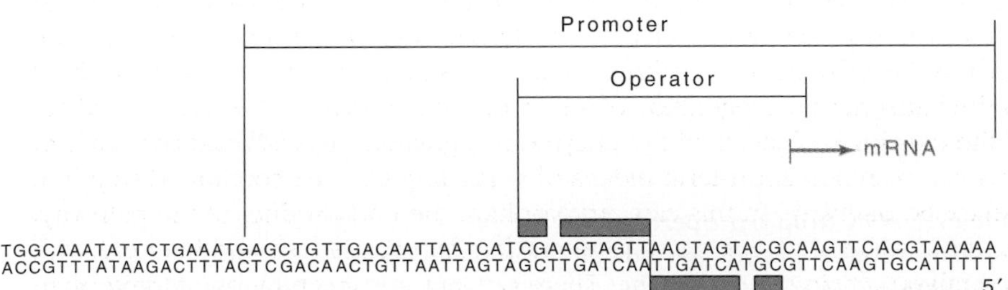

FIGURE 19.8
Nucleotide sequence of control elements of the tryptophan operon.
Lines above and below sequence indicate symmetrical sequences within operator.

of preventing transcription is the same as in the *lac* operon. Binding of the repressor–corepressor complex to the operator physically blocks the binding of RNA polymerase to the promoter.

Repression results in about a 70-fold decrease in the rate of transcription initiation at the *trp* promoter. (In contrast, the basal level of *lac* gene products is about 1000-fold lower than the induced level.) However, the *trp* operon contains additional regulatory elements that impose further control on the extent of its transcription. One of these additional control sites is a secondary promoter, designated *trp*P2, which is located within the coding sequence of the *trp*D gene (shown in Figure 19.7). This promoter is not regulated by the *trp* repressor. Transcription from it occurs constitutively at a relatively low rate and is terminated at the same location as transcription from the regulated promoter for the whole operon, *trp*P. The resulting transcription product from *trp*P2 is an mRNA that contains the coding sequences for *trp*CBA, the last three genes of the operon. Therefore two polycistronic mRNAs are derived from the *trp* operon, one containing all five structural genes and one possessing only the last three genes. Under conditions of maximum repression the basal level of mRNA coding sequence for the last three genes is about five times higher than the basal mRNA level for the first two genes.

The reason for a second internal promoter is unclear. Perhaps the best alternative comes from the observation that three of the five proteins do not contain tryptophan; only the *trp*B and *trp*C genes contain the single codon that specifies tryptophan. Therefore, under extreme tryptophan starvation, these two proteins would not be synthesized, which would prevent the pathway from being activated. However, since both of these genes lie downstream of the unregulated second promoter, their protein products will always be present at the basal level necessary to maintain the pathway.

Tryptophan Operon Has a Second Control Site: The Attenuator Site

Another important control element of the *trp* operon not present in the *lac* operon is the **attenuator** site (Figure 19.9). It lies within 162 nucleotides between the start of transcription from *trp*P and the initiator codon of the *trp*E gene. Its existence was first deduced by the identification of mutations that mapped in this region and increased transcription of all five structural genes. Within the 162 nucleotides, called the **leader sequence,** are 14 adjacent codons that begin with a methionine codon and end with an in-phase termination codon. These codons are preceded by a canonical ribosome-binding site and

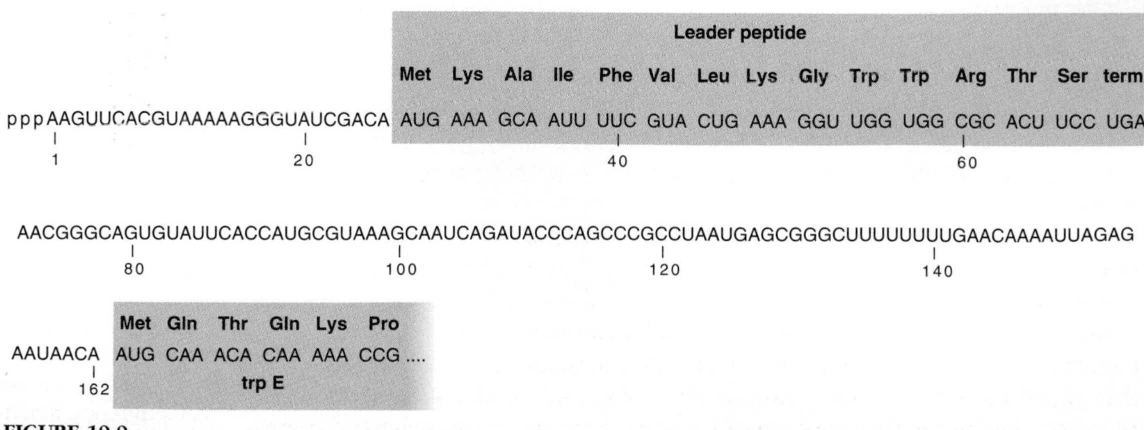

FIGURE 19.9
Nucleotide sequence of leader RNA from *trp* operon.
The 14 amino acids of the putative leader peptide are indicated over their codons.
Redrawn with permission from Oxender, D. L., Zurawski, G., and Yanofsky, C. Proc. Natl. Acad. Sci. USA *76:5524, 1979.*

could potentially specify a 14-residue leader peptide. This peptide has never been detected in bacterial cells, perhaps because it is degraded very rapidly. The ribosome-binding site does function properly when its corresponding DNA sequence is ligated upstream of a structural gene using recombinant DNA techniques.

The attenuator region provides RNA polymerase with a second chance to stop transcription if the trp enzymes are not needed by the cell. In the presence of tryptophan, it acts like a rho-independent transcription termination site to produce a short 140-nucleotide transcript. In the absence of tryptophan, it has no effect on transcription, and the entire polycistronic mRNA of the five structural genes is synthesized. Therefore, at both the operator and attenuator, tryptophan exerts the same general influence. At the operator it participates in repressing transcription, and at the attenuator it participates in stopping transcription by those RNA polymerases that have escaped repression. It has been estimated that attenuation has about a 10-fold effect on transcription of the trp structural genes. When multiplied by the 70-fold effect of derepression at the operator, about a 700-fold range exists in the level at which the *trp* operon can be transcribed.

The molecular mechanism by which transcription is terminated at the attenuator site is a marvelous example of cooperative interaction between bacterial transcription and translation to achieve desired levels of a given mRNA. The first hints that ribosomes were involved in the mechanism of attenuation came from the observation that mutations in the gene for **tRNA^{Trp} synthetase** (the enzyme that charges the tRNA with tryptophan) or the gene for an enzyme that modifies some bases in the tRNA prevent attenuation. Therefore a functional tRNA^{Trp} must participate in the process.

The leader peptide (Figure 19.9) of 14 residues contains two adjacent tryptophans in positions 10 and 11. This is unusual because tryptophan is a relatively rare amino acid in *E. coli.* It also provides a clue about the involvement of tRNA^{Trp} in attenuation. If the tryptophan in the cell is low, the amount of charged tRNA^{Trp} will also be low and the ribosomes may be unable to translate through the two *trp* codons of the leader peptide region. Therefore they will stall at this place in the leader RNA sequence.

It turns out that the RNA sequence of the attenuator region can adopt several possible secondary structures (Figure 19.10). The position of the ribosome within the leader peptide-coding sequence determines the secondary structure that will form. This secondary structure, in turn, is recognized (or sensed) by the RNA polymerase that has just transcribed through the attenuator coding region and is now located a small distance downstream. The RNA secondary structure that forms when a ribosome is not stalled at the *trp* codons is a termination signal for the RNA polymerase. Under these conditions the cell does not need to make tryptophan, and transcription stops after the synthesis of a 140-nucleotide transcript, which is quickly degraded. On the other hand, the secondary structure that results when the ribosomes are stalled at the *trp* codons is not recognized as a termination signal, and the RNA polymerase continues on into the *trpE* gene. Figure 19.11 shows these different secondary structures in detail.

The structure in Figure 19.11*a* shows the situation when a ribosome does not stall at the two tandem *trp* codons, UGG-UGG, near the beginning of region 1, but instead moves on to region 2. When the ribosome is in region 2, regions 1 and 2 cannot base pair but regions 3 and 4 can form base pairs, resulting in a hairpin loop followed by eight U residues, a structure common to sequences that signal transcription termination. Thus when the leader RNA sequence is being synthesized in the presence of sufficient tryptophan (and charged tryptophanyl-tRNA^{Trp}), it is likely that a loop between regions 3 and 4 will occur and be recognized as a signal for termination by the RNA polymerase.

A different structure occurs if the ribosome is stalled at the *trp* codons and

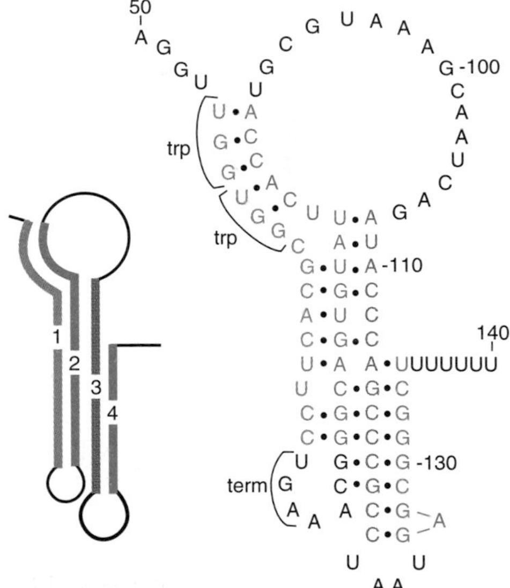

FIGURE 19.10
Schematic diagram showing the proposed secondary structures in *trp* leader RNA from *E. coli.*
Four regions can base pair to form three stem-and-loop structures. These are shown as 1–2, 2–3, and 3–4.
Reproduced with permission from Oxender, D. L., Zurawski, G., and Yanofsky, C. Proc. Natl. Acad. Sci. USA *76:5524, 1979.*

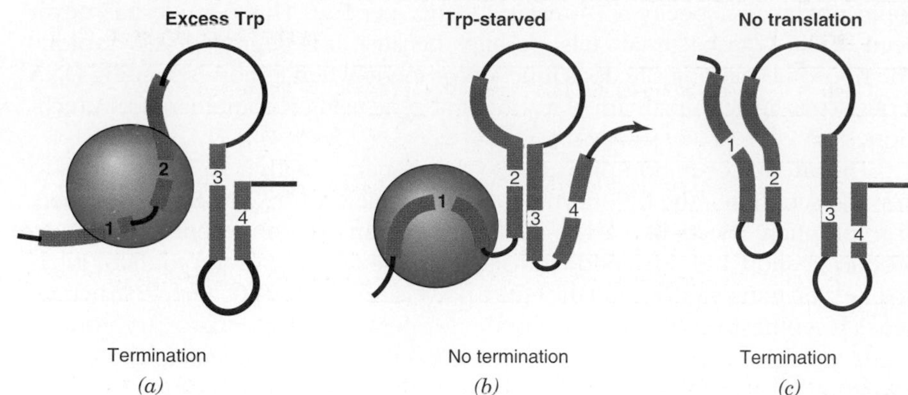

FIGURE 19.11
Schematic diagram showing the model for attenuation in the *trp* operon of *E. coli.*
(*a*) Under conditions of excess tryptophan, the ribosome (green sphere) translating the newly transcribed leader RNA will synthesize the complete leader peptide. During this synthesis the ribosome will bind to regions 1 and 2 of the RNA and prevent formation of stem and loop 1–2 or 2–3. Stem and loop 3–4 will be free to form and signal the RNA polymerase molecule (not shown) to terminate transcription. (*b*) Under conditions of tryptophan starvation, tryptophanyl-tRNA^{Trp} will be limiting, and the ribosome will stall at the adjacent *trp* codons at the beginning of region 1 in the leader peptide-coding region. Because region 1 is bound to the ribosomes, stem and loop 2–3 will form, excluding formation of stem and loop 3–4, which is required as the signal for transcription termination. Therefore RNA polymerase will continue transcription into the structural genes. (*c*) Under conditions in which the leader peptide is not translated, stem and loop 1–2 will form, preventing formation of stem and loop 2–3, and thereby permit formation of stem and loop 3–4. This will signal transcription termination.
Reproduced with permission from Oxender, D. L., Zurawski, G., and Yanofsky, C. Proc. Natl. Acad. Sci. USA *76:5524, 1979.*

region 1 is prevented from base pairing with region 2 (Figure 19.11*b*). Under these circumstances, region 2 now can base pair with region 3. This region 2 and 3 hairpin ties up the sequence complementary to region 4, so that region 4 remains single stranded. Therefore the region 3 and 4 hairpin loop that serves as the termination signal does not form, and the RNA polymerase continues on with its transcription. Thus for transcription to proceed past the attenuator, region 1 must be prevented from pairing with region 2. This is accomplished if the ribosome stalls in region 1 due to an insufficient amount of charged tryptophan-tRNA for translation of the leader peptide to continue beyond two *trp* codons. When this happens, region 1 is bound within the ribosome and cannot pair with region 2. Since regions 2 and 3 are synthesized before region 4, they, in turn, will base pair before region 4 appears in the newly transcribed RNA. Therefore region 4 remains single stranded, the termination hairpin does not form, and RNA polymerase continues transcription into the structural genes.

Since the two *trp* codons occur in region 1, if the ribosome happens to stall at an earlier codon in the leader sequence, it will have little effect on attenuation. For example, starvation for lysine, valine, or glycine would be expected to reduce the amount of the corresponding charged tRNA and stall the ribosome at that codon, but a deficiency in these amino acids has no effect on transcription of the *trp* operon. An exception is arginine whose codon occurs immediately after the *trp* codons. Starving for arginine does attenuate transcription termination somewhat, probably because of ribosome stalling at this codon, but to less of an extent than a deficiency in tryptophan.

Cis-acting mutations in the attenuator region support this alternate hairpin model. Most of these mutations result in increased transcription because they disrupt base pairing in the double-stranded portion of the termination hairpin

Operon	Leader peptide sequence	Regulatory amino acids
his	Met-Thr-Arg-Val-Gln-Phe-Lys-His-His-His-His-His-His-His-Pro-Asp	His
pheA	Met-Lys-His-Ile-Pro-Phe-Phe-Phe-Ala-Phe-Phe-Phe-Thr-Phe-Pro	Phe
thr	Met-Lys-Arg-Ile-Ser-Thr-Thr-Ile-Thr-Thr-Thr-Ile-Thr-Ile-Thr-Thr-Gly-Asn-Gly-Ala-Gly	Thr Ile
leu	Met-Ser-His-Ile-Val-Arg-Phe-Thr-Gly-Leu-Leu-Leu-Leu-Asn-Ala-Phe-Ile-Val-Arg-Gly-Arg-Pro-Val-Gly-Gly-Ile-Gln-His	Leu
ilv	Met-Thr-Ala-Leu-Leu-Arg-Val-Ile-Ser-Leu-Val-Val-Ile-Ser-Val-Val-Val-Ile-Ile-Ile-Pro-Pro-Cys-Gly-Ala-Ala-Leu-Gly-Arg-Gly-Lys-Ala	Leu, Val, Ile

FIGURE 19.12
Leader peptide sequences specified by biosynthetic operons of *E. coli.*
All contain multiple copies of amino acid(s) synthesized by enzymes coded for by operon.

and render it less stable. Some mutations, however, increase termination at the attenuator. One of these interferes with base pairing between regions 2 and 3, allowing region 3 to be available for pairing with region 4 even when region 1 is bound to a stalled ribosome. Another mutation occurs in the AUG initiator codon for the leader peptide so that the ribosome cannot begin its synthesis.

Transcription Attenuation Is a Mechanism of Control in Operons for Amino Acid Biosynthesis

Attenuation is a common phenomenon in bacterial gene expression; it occurs in at least six other operons that code for enzymes catalyzing amino acid biosynthetic pathways. Figure 19.12 shows the corresponding **leader peptide** sequences specified by each of these operons. In each case, the leader peptide contains several codons for the amino acid product of the biosynthetic pathway. The most extreme case is the 16-residue leader peptide of the histidine operon that contains seven contiguous histidines. Starvation for histidine results in a decrease in the amount of histidinyl-$tRNA^{His}$ and a dramatic increase in transcription of the *his* operon. As with the *trp* operon, this effect is diminished by mutations that interfere with the level of charged histidinyl-$tRNA^{His}$. Furthermore, the nucleotide sequence of the attenuator region suggests that ribosome stalling at the histidine codons also influences the formation of alternate hairpin loops, one of which resembles a termination hairpin followed by several U residues. In contrast to the *trp* operon, transcription of the *his* operon is regulated entirely by attenuation; it does not possess an operator that is recognized by a repressor protein. Instead, the **ribosome** acts rather like a positive regulator protein, similar to the cAMP–CAP complex discussed with the *lac* operon. If the ribosome is bound to (i.e., stalled at) the attenuator site, then transcription of the downstream structural genes is enhanced. If the ribosome is not bound, then transcription of these genes is greatly reduced.

Transcription of the other operons shown in Figure 19.12 can be attenuated by more than one amino acid. For example, the *thr* operon is attenuated by either threonine or isoleucine; the *ilv* operon is attenuated by leucine, valine, or isoleucine. This effect can be explained in each case by stalling of the ribosome at the corresponding codon, which, in turn, interferes with the formation of a termination hairpin. Although not proved, it is possible that in the cases of the longer leader peptides, stalling at more than one codon is necessary to achieve maximal transcription through the attenuation region.

19.5 OTHER BACTERIAL OPERONS

Synthesis of Ribosomal Proteins Is Regulated in a Coordinated Manner

Many other bacterial operons have been studied and found to possess the same general regulatory mechanisms as the *lac, trp,* and *his* operons, as discussed

Operon	Regulator protein	Proteins specified by the operon
Spc	S8	L14-L24-L5-S14-S8-L6-L18-S5-L15-L30
S10	L4	S10-L3-L2-L4-L23-S19-L22-S3-S17-L16-L29
str	S7	S12-S7-EF•G-EF•Tu
α	S4	S13-S11-S4-α-L17
L11	L1	L11-L1
rif	L10	L10-L7-β–β′

FIGURE 19.13
Operons containing genes for ribosomal proteins *E. coli*. Genes for the protein components of the small (S) and large (L) ribosomal subunits of *E. coli* are clustered on several operons. Some of these operons also contain genes for RNA polymerase subunits α, β, and β', and protein synthesis factors EF·G and EF·Tu. At least one of the protein products of each operon usually regulates expression of that operon (see text).

in Section 19.4. However, each operon has evolved its own distinctive quirks. For example, one interesting group of operons are those containing the structural genes for the 70 or more proteins that comprise the ribosome (Figure 19.13). Each ribosome contains one copy of each **ribosomal protein** (except for protein L7-L12, which is probably present in four copies). Therefore all 70 proteins are required in equimolar amounts, and it makes sense that their synthesis is regulated in a coordinated fashion. Characterization of this set of operons is not yet complete, but six operons, containing about one-half of the ribosomal protein genes, occur in two major gene clusters. One cluster contains four adjacent operons (*str, Spc, S10,* and *a*), and the other two operons are near each other elsewhere in the *E. coli* chromosome. There is no obvious pattern to distribution of these genes among different operons. Some operons contain genes for proteins of just one ribosomal subunit; others code for proteins of both subunits. In addition to structural genes for ribosomal proteins, these operons also contain genes for other (related) proteins. For example, *str* operon contains genes for the two soluble **translation elongation factors,** EF·Tu and EF·G, as well as genes for some proteins in the 30S ribosomal subunit. The α operon has genes for proteins of both 30S and 50S ribosomal subunits plus a gene for one of the subunits of RNA polymerase. The *rif* operon has genes for two other protein subunits of RNA polymerase and genes for ribosomal proteins.

A common theme among the six ribosomal operons is that their expression is regulated by one of their own structural gene products; that is, they are **self-regulated.** The precise mechanism of this self-regulation varies considerably with each operon and is not yet understood in detail. However, in some cases the regulation occurs at the level of translation, not transcription as discussed for the *lac* and *trp* operons. After the polycistronic mRNA is made, the "regulatory" ribosomal protein binds to this mRNA and determines which regions, if any, are translated. In general, the ribosomal protein that regulates expression of its own operon, or part of its own operon, is a protein that is associated with one of the ribosomal RNAs (rRNAs) in the intact ribosome. This ribosomal protein has a high affinity for the rRNA and a lower affinity for one or more regions of its own mRNA. Therefore a competition between the rRNA and the operon's mRNA for binding with the ribosomal protein occurs. As the ribosomal protein accumulates to a higher level than the free rRNA, it binds to its own mRNA and prevents the initiation of protein synthesis at one or more of the coding sequences on this mRNA (Figure 19.14). As more ribosomes are formed, the excess of this particular ribosomal protein is used up and translation of its coding sequence on the mRNA can begin again.

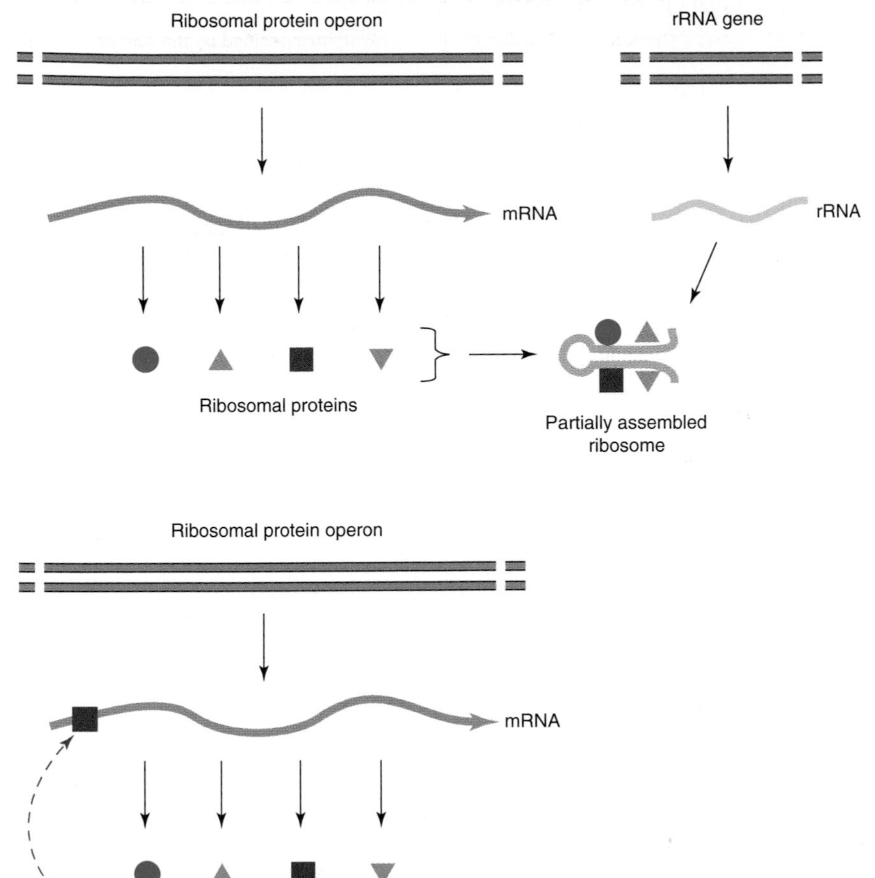

FIGURE 19.14
Self-regulation of ribosomal protein synthesis.
If free rRNA is not available for assembly of new ribosomal subunits, individual ribosomal proteins bind to polycistronic mRNA from their own operon, blocking further translation.

Stringent Response Controls Synthesis of rRNAs and tRNAs

Bacteria have several ways in which to respond molecularly to emergency situations; that is, times of **extreme general stress.** One of these situations is when the bacterium does not have a sufficient pool of amino acids to maintain protein synthesis. Under these conditions the cell invokes what is called the **stringent response,** a mechanism that reduces the synthesis of the rRNAs and tRNAs about 20-fold. This places many of the activities within the cell on hold until conditions improve. The mRNAs are less affected, but there is also about a three-fold decrease in their synthesis.

The stringent response is triggered by the presence of an uncharged tRNA in the A site of the ribosome. This occurs when the concentration of the corresponding charged tRNA is very low. The first result, of course, is that further peptide elongation by the ribosome stops. This event causes a protein called the **stringent factor,** the product of the *rel*A gene, to synthesize **guanosine tetraphosphate** (ppGpp) and **guanosine pentaphosphate** (pppGpp), from ATP and GTP or GDP as shown in Figure 19.15. Stringent factor is loosely associated with a few, but not all, ribosomes of the cell. Perhaps a conformational change in the ribosome is induced by occupation of the A site by an uncharged tRNA, which, in turn, activates the associated stringent factor. The exact functions of ppGpp and pppGpp are unknown. However, they seem to inhibit transcription initiation of the rRNA and tRNA genes. In addition they affect transcription of some operons more than others.

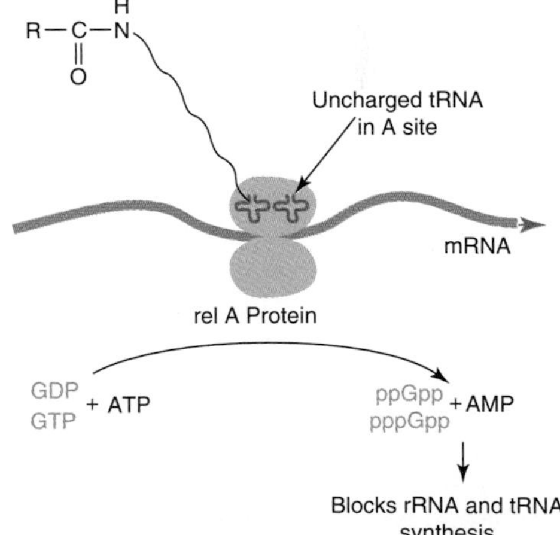

FIGURE 19.15
Stringent control of protein synthesis in *E. coli.*
During extreme amino acid starvation, an uncharged tRNA in the A site of the ribosome activates the relA protein to synthesize ppGpp and pppGpp, which, in turn, are involved in decreasing transcription of the genes coding for rRNAs and tRNAs.

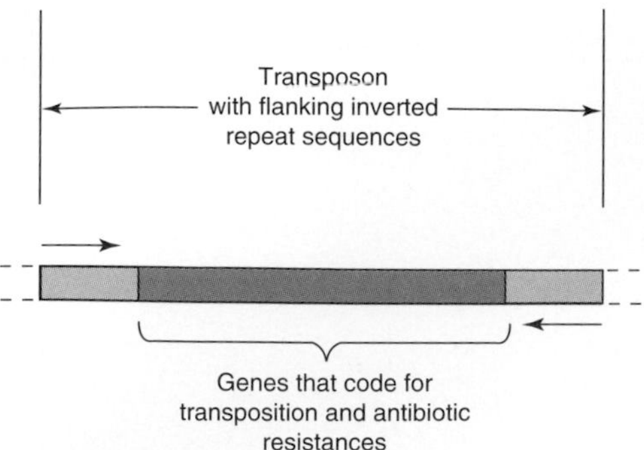

FIGURE 19.16
General structure of transposons.
Transposons are relatively rare mobile segments of DNA that contain genes coding for their own rearangement and (usually) genes that specify resistance to various antibiotics.

19.6 ■ BACTERIAL TRANSPOSONS

Transposons Are Mobile Segments of DNA

So far we have only discussed the regulation of bacterial genes whose locations are fixed in the chromosome. Their positions relative to the neighboring genes do not change. The vast majority of bacterial genes are of this type. In fact, genetic maps of *E. coli* and *Salmonella typhimurium* are quite similar, indicating the lack of much evolutionary movement of most genes within the bacterial chromosome. There is a class of bacterial genes, however, in which newly duplicated gene copies "jump" to another genomic site with a frequency of about 10^{-7} per generation, the same rate as spontaneous point mutations occur. The mobile segments of DNA containing these genes are called **transposable elements** or **transposons** (Figure 19.16). Transposons were first detected as rare insertions of foreign DNA into structural genes of bacterial operons. Usually, these insertions interfere with the expression of the structural gene into which they have inserted and all downstream genes of the operon. This is not surprising since they can potentially destroy the translation reading frame, introduce transcription termination signals, affect the mRNA stability, and so on. Many transposons and the sites into which they insert have been isolated using recombinant DNA techniques and have been extensively characterized. These studies have revealed many interesting features about the mechanisms of transposition and the nature of genes located within transposons.

Transposons vary tremendously in length. Some are a few thousand base pairs and contain only two or three genes; others are many thousands of base pairs long, containing several genes. Several small transposons can occur within a large transposon. All active transposons contain at least one gene that codes for a **transposase,** an enzyme required for the transposition event. Often they contain genes that code for resistance to antibiotics or heavy metals. Most transpositions involve generation of an addition copy of the transposon and insertion of this copy into another location. The original transposon copy is the same after the duplication as before; that is, the donor copy is unaffected by insertion of its duplicate into the recipient site. Transposons contain short inverted **terminal repeat sequences** that are essential for the insertion mechanism, and in fact these inverted repeats are often used to define the two boundaries of a transposon. The multiple target sites into which most transposons can insert seem to be fairly random in sequence; other transposons have a propensity for insertion at specific "hot spots." The duplicated transposon can be located in a different DNA molecule than its donor. Frequently, transposons are found on plasmids that pass from one bacterial strain to another and are the source of a suddenly acquired resistance to one or more antibiotics by a bacterium (Clin. Corr. 19.1).

As with bacterial operons, each transposon or set of transposons has its own distinctive characteristics. The well-characterized transposon *Tn3* will be discussed as an example of their general properties.

CLINICAL CORRELATION 19.1

Transmissible Multiple Drug Resistances

Pathogenic bacteria are becoming increasingly resistant to a large number of antibiotics, which is viewed with alarm by many physicians. Many cases have been documented in which a bacterial strain in a patient being treated with one antibiotic suddenly became resistant to that antibiotic and, simultaneously, to several other antibiotics even though the bacterial strain had never been previously exposed to these other antibiotics. This occurs when the bacteria suddenly acquire from another bacterial strain a plasmid that contains several different transposons, each containing one or more antibiotic-resistance genes. Examples include the genes encoding β-lactamase, which inactivates penicillins and cephalosporins, chloramphenicol acetyltransferase, which inactivates chloramphenicol, and phosphotransferases, which modify aminoglycosides such as neomycin and gentamycin.

Neu, H. C. The crisis in antibiotic resistance. *Science* 257: 1064, 1992.

Tn3 Transposon Contains Three Structural Genes

The **transposon Tn3** has been cloned using recombinant DNA techniques and its complete sequence determined. It contains 4957 base pairs including 38 base pairs at one end that occur as an inverted repeat at the other end (Figure 19.17). Three genes are present in *Tn3*. One gene codes for the enzyme β-lactamase, which hydrolyzes ampicillin and renders the cell resistant to this antibiotic. The other two genes, *tnp*A and *tnp*R, code for a transposase and a repressor protein, respectively. The transposase has 1021 amino acids and binds to single-stranded DNA. Little else is known about its action, but it is thought

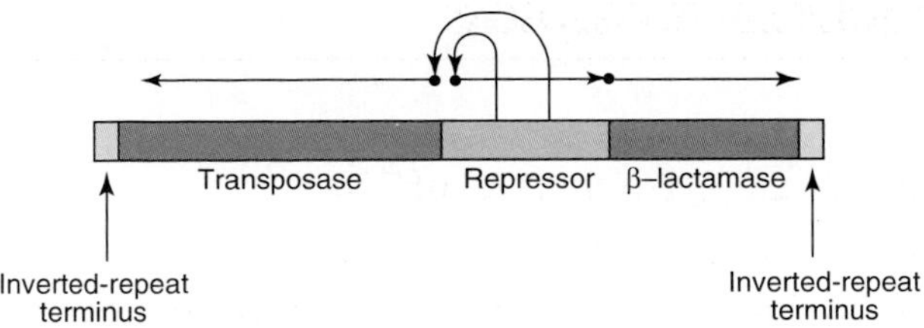

FIGURE 19.17
Functional components of the transposon *Tn3*.
Genetic analysis shows there are at least four kinds of regions: the inverted repeat termini; a gene for the enzyme β-lactamase, which confers resistance to ampicillin and related antibiotics; a gene encoding an enzyme required for transposition (transposase); and a gene for a repressor protein that controls transcription of genes for transposase and for repressor itself. The horizontal arrows indicate direction in which DNA of various regions is transcribed.
Redrawn from Cohen, S. N., and Shapiro, J. A. Sci. Am. *242:40, 1980. W. H. Freeman and Company, Copyright © 1980.*

to recognize the repetitive ends of the transposon and to participate in the cleavage of the recipient site into which the new transposon copy inserts. The *tnp*R gene product is a protein of 185 amino acids. In its role as a repressor it controls transcription of both the transposase gene and its own gene. The *tnp*A and *tnp*R genes are transcribed divergently from a 163 base pair control region located between the two genes that is recognized by the repressor. The *tnp*R product also participates in the recombination process that results in the insertion of the new transposon. Transcription of the ampicillin-resistance gene is not affected by the *tnp*R gene product.

Mutations in the transposase gene generally decrease the frequency of Tn3 transposition, demonstrating its direct role in the transposition process. Mutations that destroy the repressor function of the *tnp*R product cause an increased frequency of transposition. These mutations derepress the *tnp*A gene, resulting in more molecules of the transposase, which increases the formation of more transposons. They also derepress the *tnp*R gene but, since the repressor is inactive, this has no effect on the system.

When a transposon, containing its terminal inverted repeats, inserts into a new site, it generates short (5–10 bp) direct repeats of the sequences at the recipient site that flank the new transposon. This is due to the mechanism of recombination that occurs during the insertion process (Figure 19.18). The first step is the generation of staggered nicks at the recipient sequence. These staggered single-strand, protruding 5′ ends then join covalently to the inverted repeat ends of the transposon. The resulting intermediate resembles two replicating forks pointing toward each other and separated by the length of the transposon. The replication machinery of the cell fills in the gaps and continues the divergent elongation of the two primers through the transposon region. This ultimately results in two copies of the transposon sequence. Reciprocal recombination within the two copies regenerates the original transposon copy at its original position and completes the process of forming a new copy at the recipient site that is flanked by direct repeats of the recipient sequence.

The practical importance of transposons located on plasmids has taken on increased significance for the use of antibiotics in treatment of bacterial infections. Plasmids that have not been altered for experimental use in the laboratory usually contain genes that facilitate their transfer from one bacterium to another. As the plasmids transfer (e.g., between different infecting bacterial strains), their transposons containing **antibiotic-resistance genes** are moved into new bacterial strains. Once inside a new bacterium, the transposon can be duplicated onto the chromosome and become permanently established in that cell's lineage.

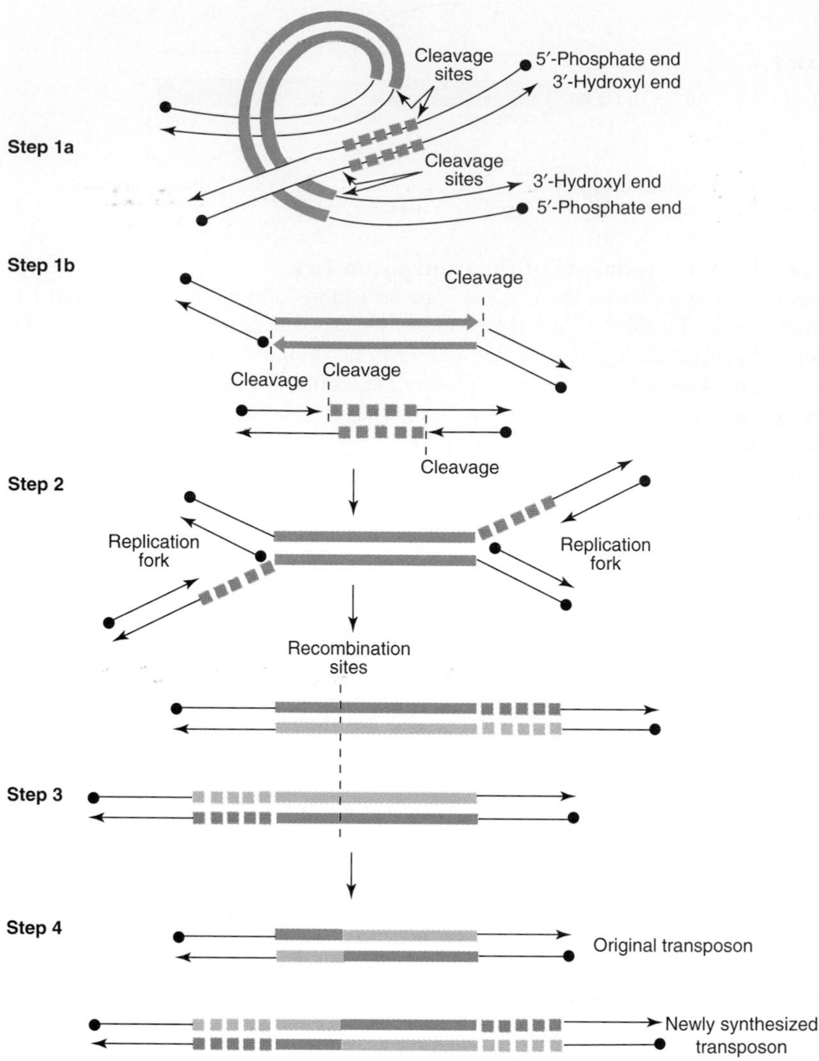

FIGURE 19.18
Proposed molecular pathway for transposition and chromosome rearrangements.
Donor DNA, including the transposon, shown in red, recipient DNA contains small light green. The pathway has four steps, beginning with staggered, single-strand cleavages (Step 1a) at each end of the transposable element and at each end of the "target" nucleotide sequence to be duplicated. The cleavages expose (Step 1b) the DNA strand ends involved in the next step: the joining of DNA strands from donor and recipient molecules in such a way that the double-stranded transposable element has a DNA replication fork at each end (Step 2). DNA synthesis (Step 3) replicates transposon (red bars) and target sequence (light green squares), accounting for the observed duplication. This step forms two new complete double-stranded molecules; each copy of the transposable element joins a segment of the donor molecule and a segment of the recipient molecules. (Copies of the element serve as linkers for the recombination of two unrelated DNA molecules.) In the final Step 4, reciprocal recombination between copies of the transposable element inserts the element at a new genetic site and regenerates the donor molecule.
Redrawn from Cohen, S. N., and Shapiro, J. A. Sci. Am. *252:40, 1980. W. H. Freeman and Company, Copyright © 1980.*

The result is that more and more pathogenic bacterial strains become resistant to an increasing number of antibiotics.

19.7 ■ INVERSION OF GENES IN *SALMONELLA*

A different mechanism of differential gene regulation has been discovered for one set of genes in *Salmonella*. Similar control mechanisms exist for the expression of other genes in other prokaryotes (e.g., a bacteriophage called μ).

Bacteria move by waving their **flagella** that are composed predominantly of subunits of a protein called flagellin. Many *Salmonella* species possess two different flagellin genes and express only one of these genes at a time. Bacteria are said to be in phase 1 if they are expressing the H1 flagellin gene and in phase 2 if they are expressing the H2 flagellin gene. A bacterial clone in one phase switches to the other phase about once every 1000 divisions. This switch is called **phase variation,** and its occurrence is controlled at the level of transcription of *H1* and *H2* genes.

Organization of the flagellin genes and their regulatory elements are shown in Figure 19.19. A 995-bp segment of DNA flanked by 14-bp repeats is adjacent to the *H2* gene and a *rhl* gene that codes for a repressor of *H1*. The *H2* and

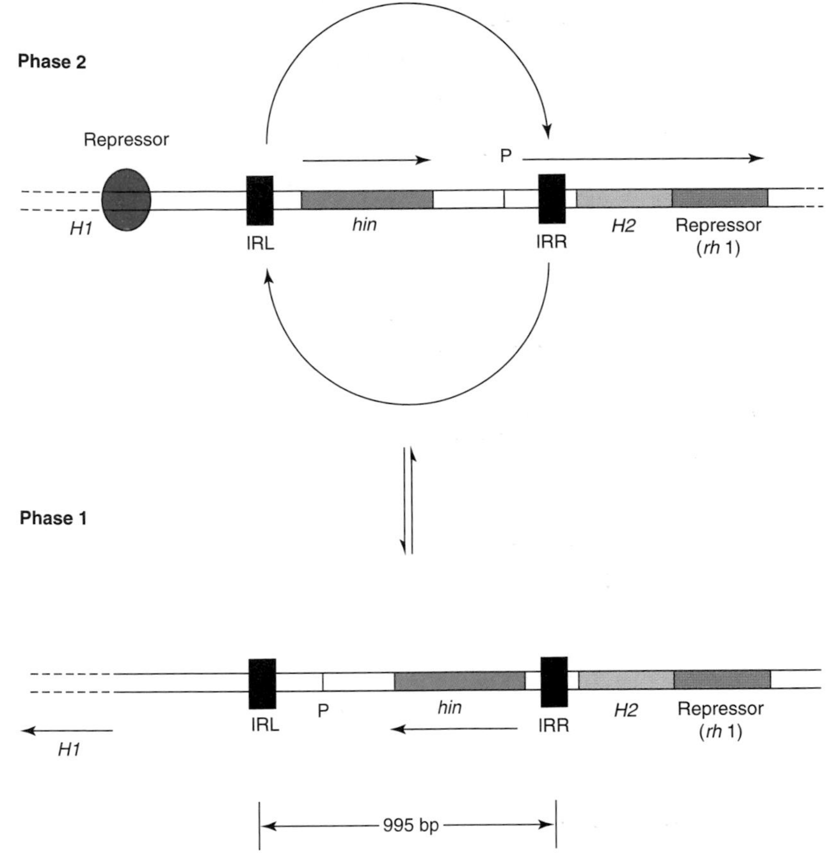

FIGURE 19.19
Organization of the flagellin genes of *Salmonella*.
Orientation of a 995-bp DNA segment flanked by 14-bp inverted repeats (IRL and IRR) controls the expression of *H1* and *H2* flagellin genes. In phase 2, transcription initiates at promoter P within the invertible segment and continues through *H2* and *rh1* genes. In phase 1, the orientation is reversed so that transcription of *H2* and *rh1* genes does not occur.

rhl genes are coordinately transcribed. Therefore, when *H2* is expressed, the repressor is also made and turns off *H1* expression. When H2 protein and the repressor are not made, the H1 gene is derepressed and *H1* synthesis occurs.

The promoter for the operon containing *H2* and *rhl* lies near one end of the 995-bp segment, just inside one copy of the 14-bp repeats. This segment can undergo inversions between the 14-bp repeats. In one orientation of the segment, the promoter is upstream of the *H2–rhl* transcription unit; in the other orientation it points toward the opposite direction so that *H2* and *rhl* are not transcribed. In addition to containing this promoter, the invertible segment of DNA possesses the *hin* gene whose product is an enzyme that catalyzes the inversion event itself. The *hin* gene seems to be transcribed constitutively at a low rate. Mutations in *hin* reduce the rate of inversion by 10,000-fold. Therefore phase variation is controlled by physical inversion of the segment of DNA that removes a promoter from its position in front of the *H2–rhl* operon. When the promoter is in the opposite direction, it presumably still initiates transcription, but the fate of that RNA is unknown. It does not initiate transcription of the *H1* that maps in this direction. That gene apparently has its own promoter controlled directly by the *rhl* repressor.

Inversion of the *hin* segment probably occurs via recombination between the 14-bp inverted repeats that is similar to recombination events involved in the transposition of a transposon. In fact, transposons do invert relative to their flanking sequences in a fashion exactly analogous to the *hin* inversion. Furthermore, the amino acid sequence of the *hin* product shows considerable similarity to that of the *tnp*R product of the *Tn3* transposon, which participates in the integration of the transposon into a new site. Thus it is possible, and even likely, that the two processes are evolutionarily related.

19.8 ■ ORGANIZATION OF GENES IN MAMMALIAN DNA

The past 20 years have seen a virtual explosion of new information about the organization, structure, and regulation of genes in eukaryotic organisms. The reason for this enormous increase in our knowledge about eukaryotic genes has been the concurrent development of recombinant DNA techniques and DNA sequencing techniques (Chapter 18). Experiments undreamed of a few years ago are now routine accomplishments.

The human haploid genome contains 3×10^9 bp of DNA, about 1000 times more DNA than the *E. coli* chromosome. All available evidence suggests that each of the 23 haploid chromosomes in the human genome has a single unique DNA molecule. Since the distance between two adjacent base pairs is 3.4×10^{-10} meters (3.4 Å), if these 23 human chromosomal DNA molecules were stretched out end-to-end, they would extend about 1 meter. Each mammalian cell contains virtually a complete copy of this genome, and all except the haploid germline cells contain two copies.

Different types of mammalian cells express widely different proteins even though each contains the same complement of genes. In addition, widely different patterns of protein synthesis occur at different developmental stages of the same type of cells. Therefore extremely intricate and complicated mechanisms of regulation for these genes must exist, and, in fact, these mechanisms are not understood for even one mammalian gene to the extent that they are understood for many bacterial operons. Despite the great advances of the past 20 years, our understanding of gene regulation in mammals, and indeed all eukaryotes, remains fragmentary at best and probably is still very naive.

Only a Small Fraction of Eukaryotic DNA Codes for Proteins

It was appreciated even before the advent of recombinant DNA methodology that eukaryotic cells, including mammalian cells, contain far more DNA than seems necessary to code for all of the required proteins. Furthermore, organisms that appear rather similar in complexity can have a several-fold difference in cellular DNA content. A housefly, for example, has about six times the cellular DNA content of a fruitfly. Some plant cells have almost ten times more DNA than human cells. Therefore DNA content does not always correlate with the complexity and diversity of functions of the organism.

It is difficult to obtain an accurate estimate of the number of different proteins, and therefore genes, in a mammalian cell or in the entire mammalian organism. However, nucleic acid hybridization procedures indicate that a maximum of 5000–10,000 different mRNA species may be present in a mammalian cell at a given time. Most of these mRNAs code for proteins that are common to many cell types. Therefore a generous estimate is that there are approximately 100,000 genes for the entire mammalian genome. If the average coding sequence is 1500 nucleotides (specifying a 500 amino acid protein), this accounts for 5% of the mammalian genome. DNA regulatory elements, repetitive genes for rRNAs, and so on may account for another 5–10%. However, as much as 85–90% of the mammalian genome may not have a direct genetic function. This remarkable conclusion is in contrast to the bacterial genome in which virtually all of the DNA is consumed by genes and their regulatory elements.

Eukaryotic Genes Usually Contain Intervening Sequences (Introns)

As discussed in Chapter 16, coding sequences **(exons)** of eukaryotic genes are frequently interrupted by intervening sequences or **introns** that do not code for a product. These introns are transcribed into a **precursor RNA** species found in the nucleus and are removed by **RNA splicing** events during the processing of the nuclear precursor RNA to the mature mRNA in the cytoplasm.

The number and length of the introns in a gene can vary tremendously. Histone genes and interferon genes lack introns; they contain a continuous coding sequence for the protein as do bacterial genes. The mammalian collagen gene, on the other hand, has more than 50 different introns that collectively consume 90% of the gene. The largest human gene discovered to date is 2400 kb, or more than half the size of the entire *E. coli* genome of 4000 kb. This gene contains 79 introns of about 30-kb average size and encodes a 427-kDa muscle protein called **dystrophin** (Figure 19.20). Despite the fact that dystrophin is a very large protein, the dystrophin gene's introns consume more than 99% of the gene's length. Mutations in this huge dystrophin gene are responsible for **Duchenne/Becker muscular dystrophy** (see Clin. Corr. 19.2). On the basis of the many mammalian genes analyzed to date, it appears that most have three or four introns and that the presence of 50 or more introns in a single gene represents an extreme case. Nevertheless, introns of genes clearly account for some of the "excess" DNA present in eukaryotic genomes.

The significance of introns and their potential biological functions, if any, are the subject of much speculation and experimentation. In a few genes, including those for the **α- and β-globin subunits** of hemoglobin (see below), introns separate the coding regions for functional domains of the protein. In many other genes, however, no obvious correlation exists between the intron positions of a gene and the three-dimensional domains of its encoded protein. In fact, the number of introns in a given gene sometimes is not the same in different mammalian species, or even within a single species. For example, the rat haploid genome has two insulin genes, one with two introns and one with a single intron. The haploid genomes of other rodents have a single insulin gene with two introns.

One widely quoted hypothesis for the possible function of introns is that they may have served to facilitate the mixing and matching of exons during the course of evolution so that occasionally new protein-encoding genes are created, which provide a selective advantage for the organism. Some circumstantial evidence exists to support this possibility. For example, **chicken collagen** has a larger number of repeating Gly-X-Y triplets and most of the exons in its genes are multiples of 9 bp (i.e., 45, 54, 99, 108, or 162 bp per exon) beginning with a glycine codon and ending with a Y codon. Thus the collagen gene may have evolved via multiple duplications of an exon–intron unit. Genes of unicellular lower eukaryotes, such as **yeast,** have either no introns or a small number of introns that tend to be short compared to introns of higher eukaryotes. Perhaps these lower eukaryotes, which reproduce much faster than do higher organisms, have to be more efficient in their DNA and RNA metabolism and

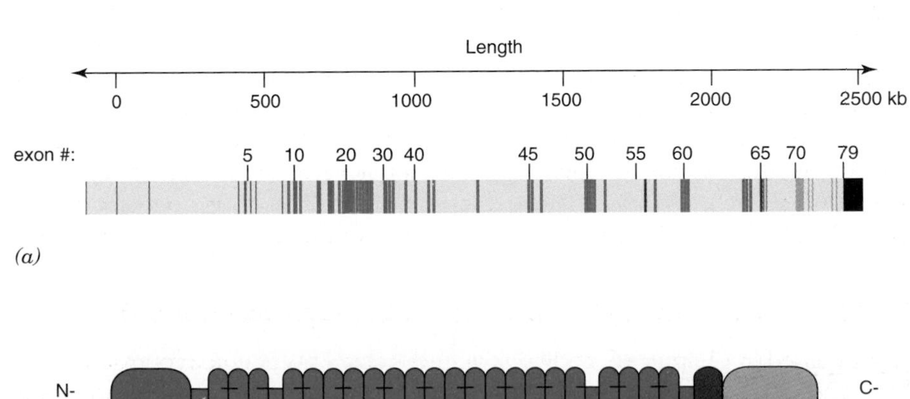

FIGURE 19.20
Human dystrophin gene and its protein. (*a*) The 79 exons (dark thin vertical lines) of human dystrophin gene span 2.4 × 10^6 bp (2400 kb), more than one-half the length of the *E. coli* genome. The average dystrophin exon is 140 bp and the average dystrophin intron (light gray background regions) is more than 30,000 bp. (*b*) Dystrophin (427 kDa) has 3685 amino acids. It contains an actin-binding domain blue, 24 tandem repeats of about 109 amino acids that likely form a rod-like domain (green), a cysteine-rich domain (purple), and a C terminus that may associate with the membrane (red).
Redrawn from Ahn, A. H., and Kunkel, L. M. Nature Genetics *3:283, 1993.*

CLINICAL CORRELATION 19.2

Duchenne/Becker Muscular Dystrophy and the Dystrophin Gene

Both Duchenne muscular dystrophy (DMD) and the milder Becker muscular dystrophy (BMD) are inherited as X-linked recessive diseases. They result in degenerative disorders of skeletal muscle and are the most common of all lethal neuromuscular genetic diseases, affecting 1 in 3500 males. They are associated with abnormally high levels of serum creatine kinase levels from birth. Although most afflicted males inherit the defect from their unaffected, heterozygous mother, 30% of the cases exhibit no previous family history and appear to be "spontaneous" new mutations in the germline of either the mother or her parents. Both forms of muscular dystrophy are caused by defects in the dystrophin gene on the X chromosome. This gene is huge and complicated. It has 79 exons and spans 2.4×10^6 bp and encodes a membrane-associated cytoskeleton protein. Its expression is regulated in a cell-specific and developmentally controlled manner from at least five different promoters. Many mutations responsible for DMD and BMD are large deletions that remove one or more of the 79 exons, but the size of the deletion does not necessarily correlate with the severity of the disorder. In DMD patients, dystrophin is undetectable or absent, whereas in BMD patients, it is reduced or altered. Genetic, biochemical, and anatomical studies suggest that dystrophin may serve diverse roles in many other tissues besides muscle. It is hoped that future studies of dystrophin may lead to an understanding of the cause and perhaps a rational treatment for muscular dystrophy.

Ahn, A. H., and Kunkel, L. M. The structural and functional diversity of dystrophin. *Nature Genetics* 3:283, 1993.

cannot tolerate large numbers of large introns. In many ways, however, introns remain as big an enigma as when first discovered.

19.9 ■ REPETITIVE DNA SEQUENCES IN EUKARYOTES

Another curiosity about mammalian DNA, and the DNA of most higher organisms, is that, in contrast to bacterial DNA, it contains repetitive sequences in addition to single copy sequences. This repetitive DNA falls into two general classes—**highly repetitive** simple sequences and **moderately repetitive** longer sequences of several hundred to several thousand base pairs.

Importance of Highly Repetitive Sequences Is Unknown

The highly repetitive sequences range from 5 to about 300 bp and occur in tandem. Their contribution to the total genomic size is extremely variable, but in most organisms they are repeated millions of times and in a few organisms they consume 50% or more of the total DNA. These highly repetitive sequences are sometimes called **satellite DNAs** because when total DNA isolated from a eukaryote is sheared slightly and centrifuged in a CsCl gradient, they can be separated as "satellites" of the bulk of the DNA on the basis of their differing buoyant densities. They are concentrated primarily at the **centromeres** and to a lesser extent at **telomeres** (i.e., ends of chromosomes). Figure 19.21 shows the three main repeat units of the highly repetitive sequences at the chromosomal centromeres of the fruitfly, *Drosophila virilis*. Repeats of these three sequences of 7 bp comprise 41% of the organism's DNA. They are obviously related evolutionarily since two of the repeats can be derived from the third by a single base pair change. Relatively little transcription occurs from the highly repetitive sequences, and their biological importance remains, for the most part, a mystery (see Clin. Corr. 19.3). Those repetitive sequences that occur near the telomeres are probably required for the replication of the ends of the linear DNA molecules. The ones at the centromeres might play a structural role since these regions attach to the **microtubules** of the **mitotic spindle** during chromosome pairing and segregation in mitosis and meiosis. Highly repetitive sequences occur in human DNA at both centromeres and telomeres but their repeat units at centromeres are longer and more variable in sequence than those of *Drosophila virilis* shown in Figure 19.21.

A Variety of Repeating Units Are Defined as Moderately Repetitive Sequences

The moderately repetitive sequences consist of a large number of different sequences repeated to such different extents that it is somewhat misleading to group them under one heading. Some are clustered in one region of the genome;

Genome (%)	Number of copies in genome	Predominant sequence
25	1×10^7	5′ -ACAAACT- 3′ 3′ -TGTTTGA- 5′
8	3.6×10^6	5′ -ATAAACT- 3′ 3′ -TATTTGA- 5′
8	3.6×10^6	5′ -ACAAATT- 3′ 3′ -TGTTTAA- 5′

FIGURE 19.21
Main repeat units of repetitive sequences of the fruitfly *Drosophila virilis*.
Approximately 41% of genomic DNA of *Drosophila virilis* is comprised of three related repeat sequences of 7 bp. The bottom two sequences differ from the top sequence at one base pair shown in box.

many are scattered throughout the DNA. Some moderate repeats are several thousand base pairs in length; other repeats come in a unit size of only a hundred base pairs. Sometimes the sequence is highly conserved from one repeat to another; in other cases, different repeat units of the same basic sequence will have undergone considerable divergence. Two examples from the human genome will be described.

In mammalian cells the 18S, 5.8S, and 28S rRNAs are transcribed as a single precursor transcript that is subsequently processed to yield the mature rRNAs. In humans the length of this precursor is 13,400 nucleotides, about one-half of which is comprised of the three mature rRNA sequences. Several **posttranscriptional cleavage** steps remove the extra sequences from the ends and the middle of the precursor RNA, releasing the mature rRNA species. DNA that contains the rRNA genes is a moderately repetitive sequence of about 43,000 bp of which 30,000 bp are nontranscribed spacer DNA. Clusters of this entire DNA unit occur on five chromosomes. In total, there are about 280 repeats of this unit, which comprise about 0.3% of the total genome (Figure 19.22). The 5S rRNA genes are repeated about 2000 times but in different clusters. The need for so many rRNA genes is because the rRNAs are structural RNAs. Each transcript from the gene yields only one copy of each rRNA molecule. On the other hand, each mRNA molecule derived from a ribosomal protein gene can be translated repeatedly to give many protein molecules.

In contrast to tandemly repetitive rRNA genes clustered at a few chromosomal sites, most moderately repetitive sequences in the mammalian genome do not code for a stable gene product and are interspersed with nonrepetitive sequences that occur only once or a few times in the genome. The average size of these interspersed repetitive sequences is about 300 bp. Almost one-half of these sequences are members of a general family of moderately repetitive sequences called the **Alu family** because they can be cleaved by the restriction enzyme *Alu*I. There are about 300,000 Alu sequences scattered throughout the human haploid genome (on the high side of being moderately repetitive). Individual members are related in sequence but are frequently not identical. Their average homology with a consensus sequence is about 87%.

Additional repeat symmetry occurs within an Alu sequence. The sequence appears to have arisen by tandem duplication of a 130-bp sequence with a 31-bp insertion in one of the two adjacent repeats. Some members of the Alu family resemble bacterial transposons in that they are flanked by short direct repeats. This does not prove that an Alu repeat can be duplicated and transposed to another site like true transposons, but it suggests that such events may occur.

The biological function of Alu sequences is unknown. One suggestion is that they serve as multiple origins for the DNA replication during S phase, but more sequences occur than seem necessary for this function. Alu sequences appear in the introns of some genes and are transcribed as part of large precursor RNAs in which the Alu sequences are removed during RNA splicing. Other Alu sequences are transcribed into small RNA molecules whose function is unknown. All mammalian genomes appear to have a counterpart to the human interspersed Alu sequence family although the size of the repeat and its distribution can vary considerably between species.

CLINICAL CORRELATION 19.3

Huntington's Disease and Trinucleotide Repeat Expansions

Huntington's disease is an autosomal dominant neurodegenerative disorder characterized by increasing behavioral disturbance, involuntary movements, cognitive impairment, and dementia. It can be inherited from either parent. Disease onset often does not occur until age 40 and death results 10–15 years later from aspiration, trauma, or pneumonia. The defective gene on chromosome 4 responsible for the disease is dominant over the normal gene, suggesting the defect causes the gene's protein to gain a deleterious function. This gene encodes a large protein called "huntingtin" that contains 3144 amino acids found in many tissues but whose function is unknown. Near the beginning of the gene is a run of CAGs that encodes a polyglutamine tract in huntingtin. The length of this polyglutamine tract is 11–34 in normal individuals and 37–121 in Huntington's disease patients. The larger the number of repeats, the sooner the onset of the disease. Furthermore, the child of a parent with an abnormally large number of repeats will often have an even larger number of repeats, resulting in a "genetic anticipation" of the disease. Neither the cause of the trinucleotide repeat expansions nor the abnormal function of huntingtin with an expanded polyglutamine is known. However, at least seven other neurological disorders are caused by trinucleotide repeat expansions in other genes, including X-linked spinal and bulbar muscular atrophy, fragile X syndrome, and myotonic dystrophy. The reason for this neuronal toxicity is currently the subject of intense research. These diseases can be diagnosed molecularly by tests based on the polymerase chain reaction.

La Spada, A. R., Paulson, H. L., and Fischbeck, K. H. Trinucleotide repeat expansion in neurological disease. *Ann. Neurol.* 36:814, 1994.

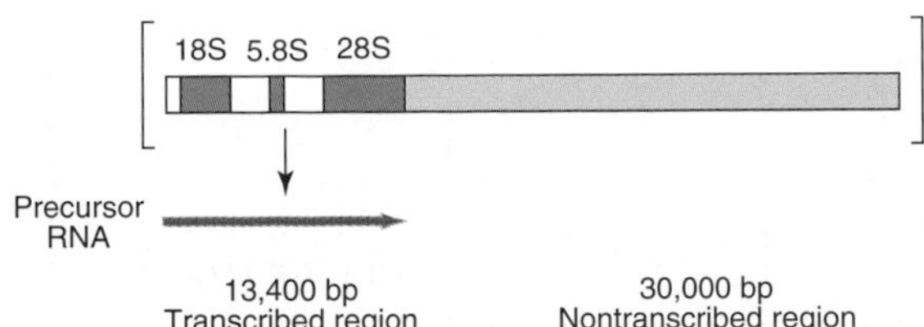

FIGURE 19.22
Repetitive sequence in human DNA for rRNA.
In human cells a single transcription unit of 13,400 nucleotides is processed to yield the 18S, 5.8S, and 28S rRNAs. About 280 copies of the corresponding rRNA genes are clustered on five chromosomes. Each repeat contains a nontranscribed spacer region of about 30,000 bp.

19.10 ■ GENES FOR GLOBIN PROTEINS

Recombinant DNA Technology Has Been Used to Clone Genes for Many Eukaryotic Proteins

Many mammalian structural genes that have been cloned by recombinant DNA techniques specify proteins that either occur in large quantity in a specific cell type, such as the **globin subunits** in the red blood cell, or after induction of a specific cell type, for example, **growth hormone** or **prolactin** in the pituitary. As a result, more is known about the regulation of these genes than of other genes whose protein products occur at lower levels in many different cell types. Increasingly, however, information is being gained about mammalian genes for "rare" proteins with low abundances in the cell. We will discuss organization, structure, and regulation of the related members of two gene families—the genes for the globin subunits and the growth hormone-like proteins.

The first step in characterizing a eukaryotic gene is usually to use recombinant DNA techniques to clone a **complementary DNA** (cDNA) copy of that gene's corresponding mRNA. In fact, this is the reason that the most extensively studied mammalian genes code for the major proteins of specific cells; a large fraction of the total mRNA isolated from these cells codes for protein of interest. **Hemoglobin** is comprised of two **α-globin** subunits (141 amino acids) and two **β-globin** subunits (146 amino acids). Almost all of the mRNA isolated from immature red cells **(reticulocytes)** codes for these two subunits of hemoglobin.

There are several experimental variations of the procedure for synthesizing double-stranded cDNA copies of isolated mRNA *in vitro*. As discussed in Chapter 18, many different plasmid and viral DNA vectors are available for cloning the (passenger) cDNA molecules. Figure 19.23 shows one protocol for constructing and cloning cDNAs prepared from mRNA of reticulocytes.

A synthetic **oligonucleotide** composed of 12–18 residues of deoxythymidine is hybridized to the 3′-polyadenylate tail of the mRNA and serves as a primer for **reverse transcriptase,** an enzyme that copies an RNA sequence into a DNA strand in the presence of the four deoxynucleoside triphosphates. The resulting RNA–DNA heteroduplex is treated with NaOH, which degrades the RNA strand and leaves the DNA strand intact. The 3′ end of the remaining DNA strand can then fold back and serve as a primer for initiating synthesis of a second DNA strand at random locations by reverse transcriptase, the same enzyme used to synthesize the first strand. The hairpin loop is then nicked by **S1 nuclease,** an enzyme that cleaves single-stranded DNA but has little activity against double-stranded DNA. The ends of the resulting double-stranded cDNAs are ligated to small synthetic "linker" oligonucleotides that contain the recognition site for the restriction enzyme *Hind*III. Digestion of the resulting DNA with *Hind*III generates DNA fragments that contain *Hind*III-specific ends. These fragments can be ligated into the *Hind*III site of a plasmid, and when the resulting circular "recombinant" DNA species are incubated with *E. coli* in the presence of cations such as calcium or rubidium, a few molecules will be taken up by the bacteria. The incorporated **recombinant DNAs** will be replicated and maintained in the progeny of the original transformed bacterial cell.

The collection of cloned cDNAs synthesized from the total mRNA in a given tissue or cell type is called a cDNA library, for example, a liver cDNA library or a reticulocyte cDNA library. Since most of the mRNAs of a reticulocyte code for either α- or β-globin, it is relatively easy to identify these globin cDNAs in a reticulocyte cDNA library using procedures discussed in Chapter 16. Once identified, the nucleotide sequences of the cDNAs can be determined to confirm that they do code for the known amino acid sequences of the α- and β-globins. In cases in which the amino acid sequence of the protein is not known, other procedures (sometimes immunological) are used to confirm the identification of the desired cDNA clone.

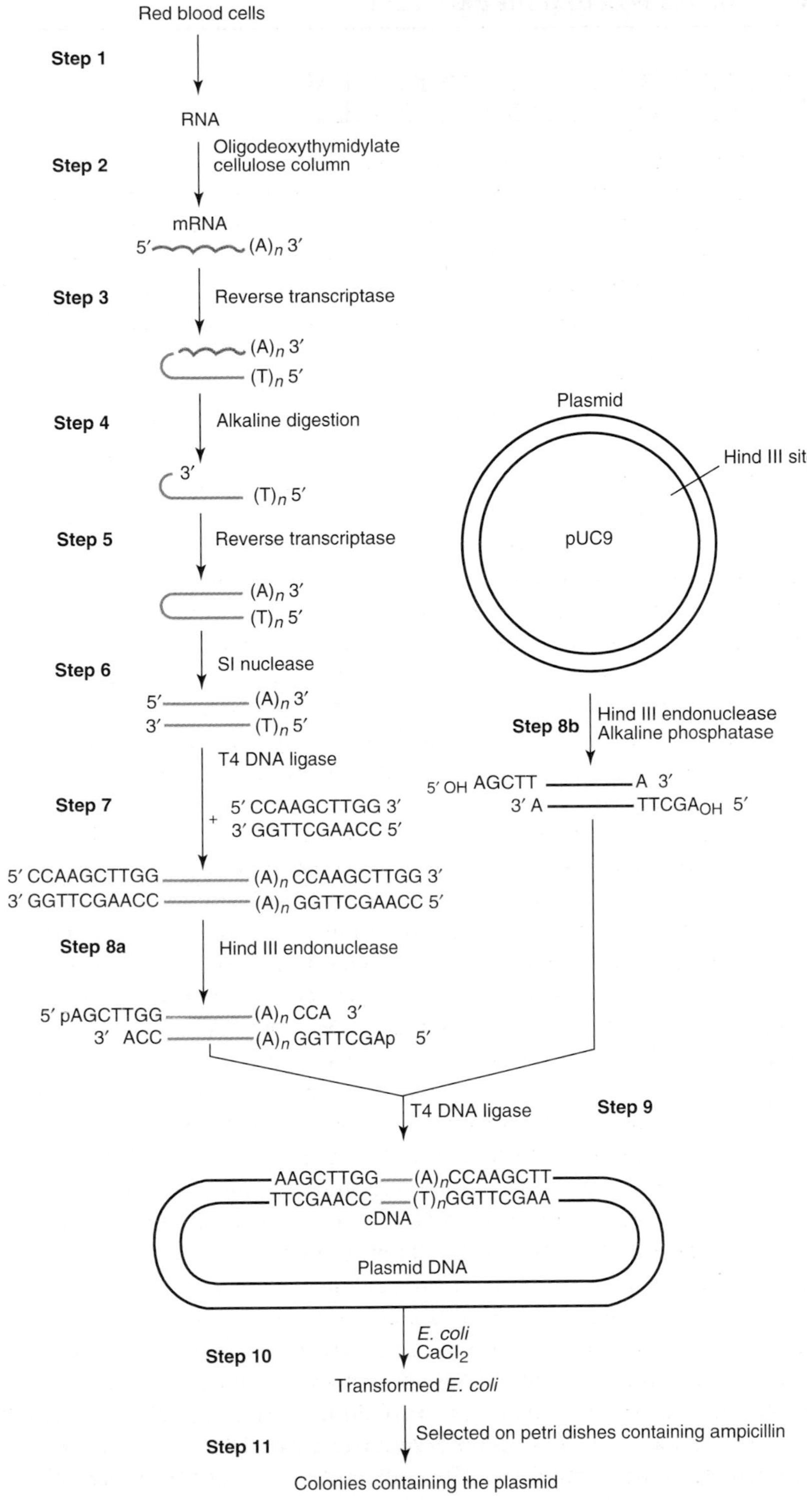

FIGURE 19.23
Cloning of globin cDNA.
Step 1: Total RNA is extracted from red blood cells. Step 2: The total RNA is passed through an oligodeoxythymidylate cellulose column, which separates polyadenylated mRNA (see Chapter 15) from rRNA and tRNA. Polyadenylated mRNA of red blood cells contains predominantly hemoglobin mRNA. Step 3: The mRNA is reverse-transcribed into first-strand cDNA using reverse transcriptase, the viral enzyme that synthesizes DNA from RNA templates (see Chapter 15). Step 4: The mRNA is hydrolyzed with alkali whereas the DNA is unaffected. Step 5: The single-stranded cDNA is converted into double-stranded DNA by reverse transcriptase. Step 6: The resulting double helix contains a single-stranded hairpin loop that is removed by S1 nuclease, an enzyme that hydrolyzes single-stranded DNA. Step 7: The cDNA is now a double helix with A-T base pairs at one end. To generate cohesive ends for the ligation of this cDNA into a plasmid, a chemically synthesized decanucleotide is attached to both ends using DNA ligase from bacteriophage T4. This decanucleotide contains the sequence recognized by *Hind*III restriction nuclease. Step 8a: Treatment with *Hind*III produces a cDNA molecule with *Hind*III cohesive ends. Step 8b: The plasmid pUC9, which contains an ampicillin-resistance gene, is cleaved with *Hind*III and exposed to bacterial alkaline phosphatase, an enzyme that removes the phosphates from the cleaved 5′-terminal ends of the plasmids at the *Hind*III site. This prevents the cleaved plasmid from recircularizing without the insertion of the cDNA. Step 9: The linear plasmid and the cDNA molecules are mixed with T4 DNA ligase, and circular, dimeric, "recombinant" DNA molecules are formed. Step 10: This ligation mixture is used to transform *E. coli*. Step 11: Individual *E. coli* cells that take up the plasmid are selected by their ability to grow on ampicillin. The globin cDNA is confirmed by determining the nucleotide sequence of the small DNA fragment released from the plasmid DNA by *Hind*III; if the observed nucleotide sequences corresponded to those expected based on the known amino acid sequence of α- and β-globin, then the cDNA is identified.

Comparison of the α- and β-globin cDNA sequences with the corresponding globin genes, which have also been cloned using recombinant DNA techniques, reveals that all members of both sets of genes contain two introns at approximately the same positions relative to the coding sequences (Figure 19.24). The α (and α-like) genes have an intron of 95 bp between codons 31 and 32 and a second intron of 125 bp between codons 99 and 100. The β (and β-like) genes have introns of 125–150 bp and 800–900 bp located between codons 30

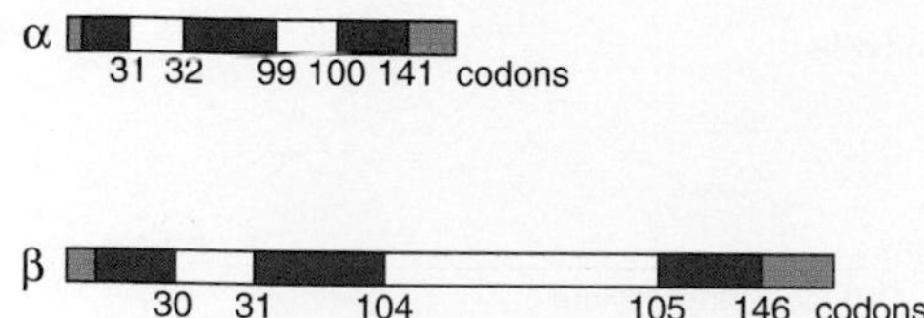

FIGURE 19.24
Structures of human globin genes.
Structures for the human α-like and β-like globin genes are drawn to approximate scale. Red rectangles and open rectangles represent exons and introns, respectively. Gray rectangles indicate the (5′) upstream and (3′) downstream nontranslated regions in the DNA. The α-like globin genes contain introns of approximately 95 and 125 bp, located between codons 31 and 32, and 99 and 100, respectively. The β-like globin genes contain introns of approximately 125–150 and 800–900 bp, located between codons 30 and 31, and 104 and 105, respectively.

and 31 and codons 104 and 105, respectively. Introns separate the coding sequences of different functional domains of a few proteins, including the globins. The coding region between the two globin introns specifies the region of the protein that interacts with the heme group. The final coding region (after the second intron) encodes the region of the protein that serves as the interface with the opposite subunit, that is, the α- globin-β-globin interaction. This separation of the coding sequences for functional domains of a protein by introns is not a general phenomenon, however. The positioning of introns in other genes seems to bear little relationship to the final three-dimensional structure of the encoded protein.

Different α-like and β-like globin subunits are synthesized at different developmental stages. These developmentally distinct subunits have slightly different amino acid sequences and oxygen affinities but are closely related. In humans there are two α-like chains—that is, ζ, which is expressed in the embryo during the first 8 weeks, and α itself, which replaces ζ in the fetus and continues through adulthood. There are four β-like chains. Epsilon (ε) and γ are expressed in the embryo, γ in the fetus, and δ plus β in the adult.

Each of the different globin chains is coded by at least one gene in the haploid genome. The α-like genes are clustered on the short arm of human **chromosome 16,** and the β-like genes are clustered on the short arm of **chromosome 11.** The gene organization within these two clusters is shown in Figure 19.25. The genes within both clusters are positioned relative to one another in the order of both their transcriptional direction and their developmental expression; that is, 5′–embryonic–fetal–adult–3′.

The α-gene cluster spans about 28 kb and includes three functional genes and two **pseudogenes.** The functional genes are the embryonic ζ gene and two α genes, $\alpha 1$ and $\alpha 2$, that code for identical α-globin proteins but have different 3′ untranslated regions. The two pseudogenes, $\psi\zeta$ and $\psi\alpha$, occur between the ζ and $\alpha 1$ genes. They have sequences very similar to the functional genes, but various mutations prevent them from coding for an active globin subunit. Pseudogenes are common in eukaryotic genomes. They do not seem to be deleterious and probably arose via a duplication of a segment of DNA followed by mutations.

The β-gene cluster encompasses about 60 kb and has five active genes and one pseudogene. Of the five functional genes, two are for the γ subunit and specify proteins that differ only at position 136, which is a glycine in the G variant and an alanine in the A variant. Only a single haploid gene exists for the ε-, δ-, and β-globin subunits. Alu repetitive sequences and other moderately repetitive sequences are scattered between some genes of the α- and β-gene clusters.

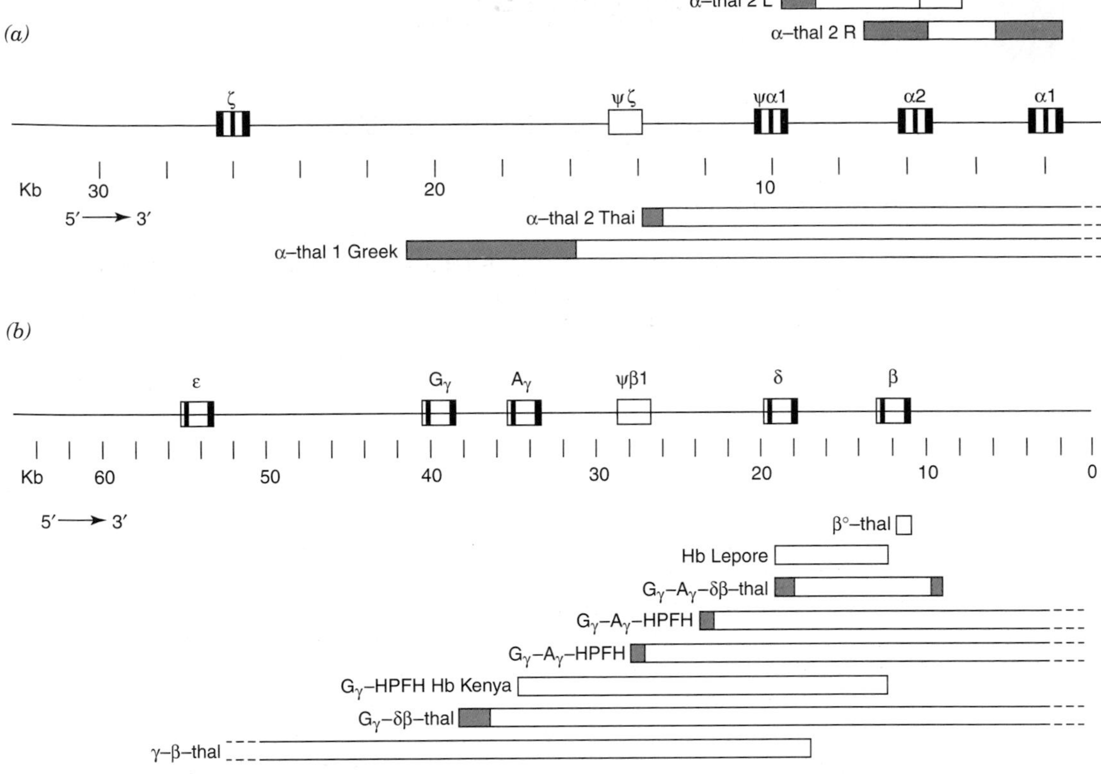

FIGURE 19.25

Gene organization for α-like and β-like genes of human hemoglobin.

(a) Linkage of human α-like globin genes on chromosome 16 and locations of some known deletions within α-like gene cluster. The positions of adult ($\alpha1$, $\alpha2$) and embryonic (ζ) α-like globin genes and two pseudogenes ($\psi\zeta$, $\psi\alpha1$) are shown. Pseudogenes have mutations that prevent the formation of functional proteins from them. For each functional gene the black and white boxes represent exons and introns, respectively. Horizontal arrow indicates the direction of transcription of each gene. The locations of DNA deletions associated with the leftward and rightward types of α-thalassemia 2 are indicated above the linkage map by the rectangles labeled α-thal 2 L and α-thal 2 R. Red areas at the ends of these rectangles indicate the deletion end points have not been mapped precisely. Locations of deletions associated with two cases of α-thalassemia 1 (α-thal 1 Thai and α-thal 1 Greek) are shown below the linkage map. The light green areas and dashed lines indicate uncertainties in the left and right endpoints, respectively, of each deletion. (b) Linkage of the human β-like globin genes on chromosome 11 and locations of deletions within the β-like gene cluster. The positions of the embryonic (ε), fetal (G_γ, A_γ), and adult (δ, β) β-like globin genes and one β-like pseudogene ($\psi\beta1$) are shown. For each functional gene the black and white boxes represent the exons and introns, respectively. The locations of various known deletions within the gene cluster are shown below the map. Open rectangles represent areas known to be deleted; Red areas and dashed lines indicate that the endpoints of the deletion have not been determined. For $\delta\beta$-thalassemia and hereditary persistence of fetal hemoglobin (HPFH), the type of fetal globin chain produced (G_γ and/or A_γ) is indicated in the name of each syndrome (e.g., in G_γ-A_γ-$\delta\beta$-thalassemia, the G_γ- and A_γ-globin chains are produced).

Redrawn from Maniatis, T., Fritsch, E. F., Lauer, J., and Lawn, R. M. Annu. Rev. Genet. *14:145, 1980. Copyright © 1980 by Annual Reviews, Inc.; and from Karlsson, S., and Nienhuis, A. W.* Annu. Rev. Biochem. *54:1071, 1985. Copyright © 1985 by Annual Reviews, Inc.*

Other mammalian species often have a different number of globin-like genes within the two clusters. For example, rabbits have only four β-like genes, goats have seven, and mice have as many as nine. Some of these additional genes are pseudogenes.

Many patients have been identified who have abnormalities in hemoglobin structure or expression. In many cases the precise molecular defect responsible for these abnormalities is known. The two that have been the most extensively studied are **sickle cell anemia** and a family of diseases collectively called **thalassemias.**

CLINICAL CORRELATION 19.4

Prenatal Diagnosis of Sickle Cell Anemia

Sickle cell anemia can be diagnosed from fetal DNA obtained by amniocentesis. This genetic disease is caused by a single base pair change that converts a glutamate to a valine in the sixth position of β-globin. In the normal β-globin gene, the sequence that specifies amino acids 5, 6, and 7 (Pro-Glu-Glu) is CCT-GAG-GAG. In a heterozygous carrier of sickle cell anemia, this sequence is CCT-GTG-GAG. An A in the middle of the sixth codon has been changed to a T. The restriction enzyme *Mst*II recognizes and cleaves the sequence CCT-GAG-G, which is present at this position in normal DNA but not the mutated DNA. Therefore digestion of fetal DNA with *Mst*II followed by the Southern blot technique (see p. 774) using β-globin cDNA as the radioactive probe reveals whether this restriction site is present in one or both allelic copies of the gene. If it is absent in both copies, the fetus will be homozygous for the sickle trait; if it is missing in only one copy, the fetus will be heterozygous for the trait. The difference in restriction enzyme patterns observed between individuals is often called a restriction fragment length polymorphism (RFLP). Polymerase chain reaction methods can be used to amplify the desired chromosomal DNA region and greatly speed up the RFLP analysis.

Other methods are necessary if the disease mutation does not cause a change in a restriction site or is not linked to an RFLP. For example, the DNA carrying the mutation can be amplified by the polymerase chain reaction, and the alleles can be detected by hybridization with allele-specific oligonucleotides (ASOs). Two ASOs differing at usually one nucleotide are made so that one ASO matches the normal allele perfectly while the other ASO matches the abnormal allele. Hybridization conditions are used in which only the ASO matching perfectly remains bound to the DNA.

Sickle Cell Anemia Is Due to a Single Base Pair Change

A **single base pair change** within the coding region for the β-globin subunit is responsible for sickle cell anemia. This occurs in the second position of the codon for position 6 of the β chain. In the mRNA the codon, GAG, which specifies glutamate in normal β chains, is converted to GUG, which specifies valine. The resultant hemoglobin, called **hemoglobin S** (HbS), has altered surface charge properties (because the negative charge of glutamate has been replaced by valine's nonpolar group), which is responsible for clinical symptoms. This mutation occurs mainly in peoples of equatorial African descent and is the classic example of a mutation that confers an adaptive advantage as well as a **genetically inheritable disease.** Individuals heterozygous for HbS are resistant to infection by the parasites that cause **malaria** but do not acquire the symptoms of sickle cell disease exhibited by individuals homozygous for HbS. The life cycle of the malaria-causing parasites includes an obligatory stage that occurs inside erythrocytes and they do not survive in erythrocytes containing HbS. Carriers of the mutation can be detected by restriction enzyme digestion of a sample of the potential carrier's DNA followed by **Southern hybridization** technique with the β-globin cDNA as described in Clin. Corr. 19.4.

Thalassemias Are Caused by Mutations in Genes for the α or β Subunits of Globin

Thalassemias are a family of related genetic diseases that occur in people who frequently originate from the Mediterranean areas and Asia. If there is a reduced synthesis or a total lack of synthesis of α-globin mRNA, the disease is classified as **α-thalassemia;** if the β-globin mRNA level is affected, it is called **β-thalassemia.** Thalassemias can be due to the deletion of one or more globin-like genes in either of the globin gene clusters or be caused by a defect in the transcription or processing of a globin gene's mRNA.

Since each chromosome 16 contains two adjacent α-globin genes, a normal diploid individual has four copies of this gene. α-Thalassemic patients may be missing one to four α-globin genes. The condition in which one α-globin gene is missing is referred to as **α-thal 1;** when two α-globin genes are gone, the condition is **α-thal 2.** In both cases the individuals can experience mild to moderate anemia but may have no additional symptoms. When three α-globin genes are missing, many more β-globin molecules are synthesized than α-globin molecules, resulting in the formation of a globin tetramer of four β-globins, which causes **HbH disease** and accompanying anemia. When all four α-globin genes are absent, the disease **hydrops fetalis** occurs, which is fatal at or before birth. Some chromosomal deletions that have been mapped in the α-globin gene cluster are shown in Figure 19.25.

β-Thalassemias also exhibit different degrees of severity and can be caused by a variety of defects or deletions. In one case the β globin gene is present but has undergone a mutation in the codon 17, which generates a termination codon. In another case the β-globin gene is transcribed in the nucleus but no β-globin mRNA occurs in the cytoplasm. Thus a defect has occurred in the processing and/or transport of the primary transcript of the gene.

Other β-thalassemias are caused by deletions within the β-globin gene cluster on chromosome 11 (Figure 19.25). In some cases these deletions remove the DNA between two adjacent genes, resulting in a new fusion gene. For example, in the normal person the linked δ-globin and β-globin genes differ in only about 7% of their positions. In **Hb Lepore** a deletion has placed the front portion of the δ-globin gene in register with the back portion of the β-globin gene. From this fusion gene a new β-like globin is produced in which the N-terminal sequence of δ-globin is joined to the C-terminal sequence of β-globin. Several variants of Hb Lepore are known, and in each case the globin product is a composite of the δ and β sequence, but the actual fusion junction is different.

Another fusion β-like globin is **Hb Kenya.** This deletion results in a gene product that contains the N-terminal sequence of the γ-globin gene and the C-terminal sequence of the β-globin gene. Still another series of deletions has been found in which both the δ- and β-globin genes are removed, causing HPFH **(hereditary persistence of fetal hemoglobin).** Frequently, there are no clinical symptoms of this condition because fetal hemoglobin ($\alpha_2\gamma_2$) continues to be synthesized after the time at which γ-globin gene expression is normally turned off (see Clin. Corr. 19.5.)

19.11 ■ GENES FOR HUMAN GROWTH HORMONE-LIKE PROTEINS

Human growth hormone (hGH, also called somatotropin) is a polypeptide of 191 amino acids. A larger precursor is synthesized in the somatotrophs of the anterior pituitary, and the mature form is secreted into the circulatory system. Growth hormone induces liver (and perhaps other) cells to produce other hormones called **somatomedins,** which are insulin-like growth factors that stimulate proliferation of mesodermal tissues such as bone, cartilage, and muscle. Infants with a deficiency in growth hormone become dwarfs, whereas those who produce too much become giants.

A closely related protein of 191 amino acids, having 85% homology with growth hormone, is human **chorionic somatomammotropin** (hCS, also called placental lactogen) synthesized in the placenta. The complete role of this hormone in normal fetal–maternal physiology is still unclear, but it participates in placental growth and contributes to mammary gland preparation for lactation during pregnancy.

The hormones hGH and hCS are examples of two very similar proteins that serve different biological functions and are synthesized in different tissues. It is to be expected that their genes also are closely related but expressed in a tissue-specific fashion. The genes for hGH and hCS are very similar and occur in the same region of chromosome 17 (Figure 19.26).

Five related genes comprise the human growth hormone gene family. They occur over a distance of about 55 kb and share a common structure of five exons and four introns, with the exon–intron boundaries always in the same locations. Alu repetitive sequences occur between some of the genes, as in the globin gene clusters. The order of the genes is 5′ *hGH-N, ψhCS-L, hCS-A, hGH-V, hCS-B* 3′. The first gene in this cluster, *hGH-N,* is expressed in the anterior

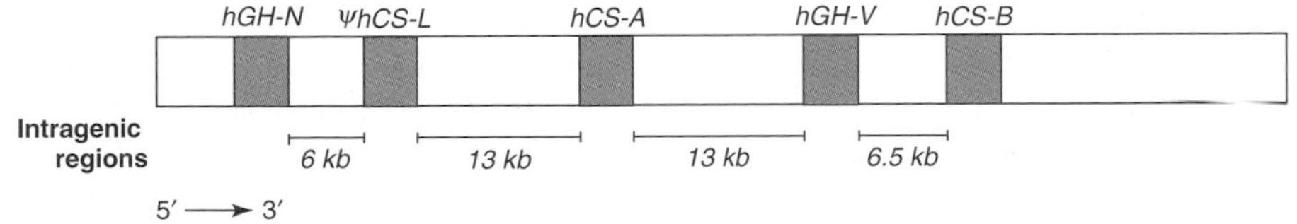

FIGURE 19.26
Organization of human growth hormone (*hGH*) gene family.
The five structural genes of this family occur as a linear array over about 55 kb on the long arm of chromosome 17. Two genes (*hGH-N* and *hGH-V*) code for growth hormone, two genes code for the closely related human chorionic somatomammotropin (*hCS-A* and *hCS-B*), and one gene appears to be a pseudogene (*ψhCS-L*). Only *hGH-N* is expressed in the pituitary; other genes are expressed in the placenta. The order of the genes in the array (red boxes) is 5′ *hGH-N, ψhCS-L, hCS-A, hGH-V, hCS-B* 3′, and all are transcribed in the same direction. Each gene has the same basic structure of five exons and four introns (not shown).
Redrawn from Chen, E. Y., Liao, Y. C., Smith, D. H., Barrera-Saldana, H. A. et al. Genomics *2:479, 1989.*

CLINICAL CORRELATION 19.5

Prenatal Diagnosis of Thalassemia

If a fetus is suspected of being thalassemic because of its genetic background, recombinant DNA techniques can be used to determine if one or more globin genes are missing from its genome. Fetal DNA can easily be obtained (in relatively small quantities) from amniotic fluid cells aspirated early during the second trimester of pregnancy. Regions of interest are amplified from the fetal DNA by polymerase chain reactions and digested with restriction enzymes that divide the globin genes among restriction fragments of several hundred to 2000 base pairs. These fragments are separated by electrophoresis through an agarose gel and hybridized with radioactive cDNA for α- and/or β-globin using the Southern blot technique (see p. 774). If one or more globin genes are missing, the corresponding restriction fragment will not be detected or its hybridization to the radioactive cDNA probe will be reduced (in the case when only one of two diploid genes is absent).

Benž, E. J. The hemoglobinopathies. In: W. N. Kelly (Ed.), *Textbook of Internal Medicine*. Philadelphia: Lippincott, 1989, pp. 1423–1432.

pituitary, whereas the others are expressed in the placenta. The *hGH* and *hCS* genes have different sequences about 100 bp beyond their polyadenylation sites. The *hGH-N* gene codes for normal growth hormone of 22 kDa. Alternative splicing of intron 3 of this gene occurs in about 10% of the primary transcripts, giving rise to a 20-kDa version of growth hormone whose significance is not known. (See Chapter 16.) The *hGH-V* gene codes for a variant growth hormone that can be expressed in transgenic animals (see Section 19.14), but whose function in the placenta is unknown. The *hCS-A* and *hCS-B* genes specify the same mature hormone but are expressed at different levels in the placenta. The ψhCS-L pseudogene has a single base substitution at an exon–intron splice site that appears to prevent normal maturation of its primary transcript into mRNA.

Expression of *hGH* and *hCS* genes is under the regulation of other hormones. **Thyroxine** and **cortisol** stimulate increased transcription of these genes. In cultured rat pituitary tumor cells these hormones act in a synergistic fashion to induce growth hormone mRNA synthesis. Pituitary cells that have only about two molecules of growth hormone mRNA per cell can be stimulated to a level of 1000 growth hormone mRNA molecules per cell, a 500-fold increase comparable in magnitude to the induction of many bacterial operons.

Only some of the details by which thyroxin and cortisol stimulate this increased transcription are known. Their regulatory effect at the molecular level is clearly more complicated than is the control of bacterial operon transcription. Two promoter sites lie just upstream of *hGH-N* and a specific transcription factor, GHF-1 (also called Pit-1), contributes to this gene's pituitary-specific expression. GHF-1 belongs to a family of **homeodomain transcription factors** found in organisms as diverse as yeast and fruitflies. The regulatory hormones are transported into the nucleus and in association either with their receptors or with a binding protein, such as GHF-1, affect transcription initiation at *hGH-N*. Alternatively, these other hormones may interact with additional factors in the cell that in turn regulate the level of transcription. The DNA regulatory site influenced by glucocorticoid hormones is known to be upstream of the site at which transcription of *hGS-N* begins. An example of the many transcription initiation protein factors that can interact with the DNA in the vicinity of eukaryotic genes is shown in Figure 16.18.

Deletions can occur within the growth hormone gene family. Deletions of *hGH-N* in both copies of chromosome 17 have been detected in some cases of severe growth hormone deficiency. These individuals are very short and do not have detectable serum growth hormone. Some such children initially respond very well to treatment with recombinant human growth hormone synthesized in the bacterium *E. coli* (see p. 834 and Figure 19.29) but they often develop antibodies against the growth hormone. Deletions also have been detected in which *hCS-A*, *hGH-V*, and *hCS-B* are lost from both chromosome 17 copies. Despite the fact that maternal sera of these individuals lack these hormones, fetal development usually proceeds normally, suggesting they either are unnecessary or can be compensated for by other hormones or factors.

19.12 ■ MITOCHONDRIAL GENES

About 0.3% of the DNA of human cells occurs in the mitochondria. Human mitochondrial DNA (mtDNA) is a double-stranded circular molecule of 16,569 bp whose sequence has been completely determined. As many as 100 molecules of mtDNA can occur in a metabolically active cell. Each mtDNA codes for 2 rRNAs, 22 tRNAs, and 13 proteins, most of which are subunits of multi-subunit complexes in the mitochondrial inner membrane that catalyze oxidative phosphorylation (Figure 19.27). For example, Complex I (NADH dehydrogenase), the first of three proton-pumping complexes involved in oxidative phosphorylation, is comprised of 26 proteins. Seven of these proteins are encoded by the

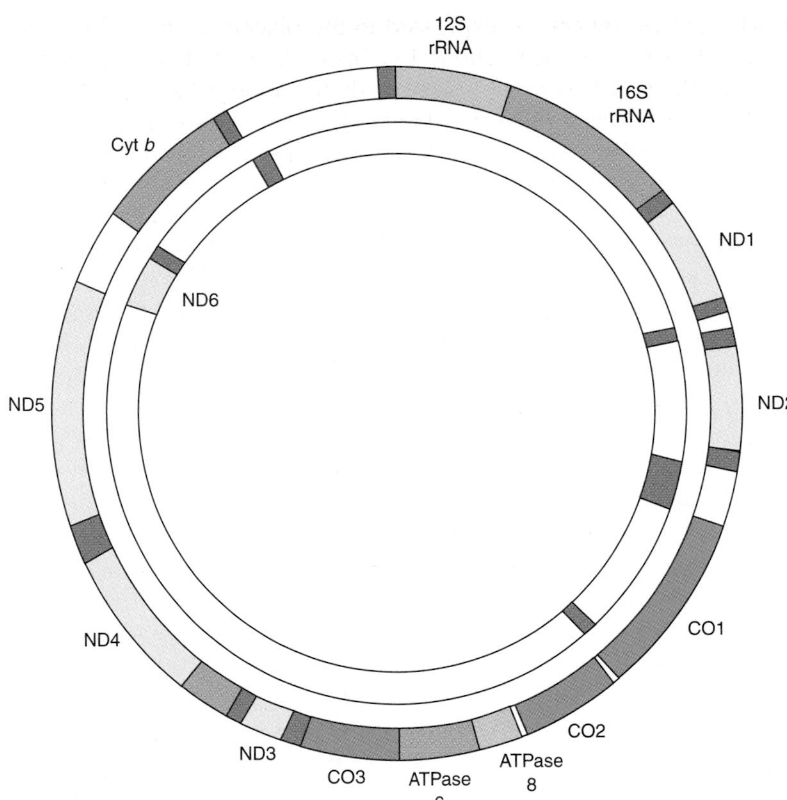

FIGURE 19.27
Human mitochondrial DNA.
The 16,569-bp human mtDNA molecule codes for two ribosomal RNAs (12 S and 16 S rRNA), some of the subunits for NADH dehydrogenase (ND), cytochrome oxidase (CO), ATP synthase (ATPase), and cytochrome *b* (cyt *b*), and 22 tRNAs (dark gray regions). Most genes occur on the outer DNA strand but genes for ND6 and a few tRNAs are on the inner strand.

mtDNA. Mitochondrial DNA also contains genes for three cytochrome oxidase subunits, two ATP synthase subunits, and cytochrome *b*. In contrast to the nucleus, where much of the chromosomal DNA seems to have no genetic function, virtually every base pair in mtDNA is essential. Regions between the protein-coding genes usually encode tRNAs and sometimes the last nucleotide of one gene will be the first nucleotide of the adjacent gene. Polyadenylation at the 3′ ends of some of the mitochondrial mRNAs adds the last two A residues of the termination codon, UAA, to create the end of the reading frame.

Even more remarkable, the genetic code of mammalian mtDNA is not identical to the genetic code of nuclear or prokaryotic DNA. UGA codes for tryptophan instead of for termination, AUA codes for methionine rather than isoleucine, and AGA and AGG serve as stop codons instead of specifying arginine. It is not clear why mitochondria have their own altered genetic system. Perhaps mtDNA is an evolutionary vestige of an early symbiotic relationship between a bacterium and the progenitor of eukaryotic cells. What is clear is that cells makes a large investment to express the 13 mitochondria-encoded proteins. To produce those proteins a large group of nucleus-encoded ribosomal proteins and associated translation factors must be imported into the mitochondrion and assembled, as well as all of the enzymes and binding proteins required for mtDNA replication and transcription. More than 100 nucleus-encoded proteins are probably necessary to maintain the mtDNA and express its gene products.

Since mitochondria are in the cytoplasm, mtDNA molecules are maternally inherited. mtDNA sequences can be used as markers for maternal lineages. In addition, mutations in mtDNA can lead to genetic diseases that are inherited only from the mother. For example, a single base pair change in mtDNA has been found to be responsible for **Leber's hereditary optic neuropathy** (see Clin. Corr. 19.6). Similar mtDNA mutations may be the cause of two other maternally inherited genetic diseases, **myoclonic epilepsy** and **infantile bilateral striatal necrosis.**

CLINICAL CORRELATION 19.6

Leber's Hereditary Optic Neuropathy (LHON)

Leber's hereditary optic neuropathy, first described in 1871, is a maternally inherited genetic disease that usually strikes young adults and results in complete or partial blindness from optic nerve degeneration. Other neurological disorders such as cardiac dysrhythmia can also be associated with the disease. The cause of this defect in many patients has been traced to a single base pair mutation in the mitochondrial DNA that changes an arginine to a histidine at amino acid 340 in NADH dehydrogenase subunit 4 of Complex I in the inner mitochondrial membrane. Although it is not clear why this mutation leads to blindness, the eyes require a high level of mitochondrial activity and perhaps become sensitive over time to a small decrease in ATP synthesis by oxidative phosphorylation.

Singh, G., Lott, M. T., and Wallace, D. C. A mitochondrial DNA mutation as a cause of Leber's Hereditary Optic Neuropathy. *N. Eng. J. Med.* 320:1300, 1989.

19.13 BACTERIAL EXPRESSION OF FOREIGN GENES

Recombinant DNA techniques are now frequently used to construct bacteria that are "factories" for making large quantities of specific human proteins useful in the diagnosis or treatment of disease. The two examples to be illustrated here are the construction of bacteria that synthesize human insulin and human growth hormone.

Many factors must be considered in designing recombinant plasmids that contain a eukaryotic gene to be expressed in bacteria. First, the cloned eukaryotic gene cannot have any introns since the bacteria do not have the RNA-splicing enzymes that correctly remove introns from the initial transcript. Thus the actual eukaryotic chromosomal gene is usually not used for these experiments; instead, the cDNA or a synthetic equivalent of the coding sequence, or a combination of both, is placed in the bacterial plasmid.

Another consideration is that different nucleotide sequences comprise the binding sites for RNA polymerase and ribosomes in bacteria and eukaryotes. Therefore, to achieve expression of the desired protein, it is necessary to insert the eukaryotic coding sequence directly behind a set of bacterial regulatory elements. This has the advantage that the foreign gene is now under the regulation of the bacterial control elements, but its disadvantage is that considerable recombinant DNA manipulation is required to make the appropriate plasmid. Still other factors to be considered are that the foreign gene product must not be degraded by bacterial proteases or require modification before it is active (e.g., specific glycosylation events that the bacteria cannot perform) and must not be toxic to the bacteria. Even when the bacteria do synthesize the desired product, it must be isolated from the 1000 or more endogenous bacterial proteins.

Recombinant Bacteria Can Synthesize Human Insulin

Insulin is produced by the β cells of the pancreatic islets of Langerhans. It is initially synthesized as **preproinsulin,** a precursor polypeptide that possesses an N-terminal signal peptide and an internal C peptide of 33 amino acids that are removed during the subsequent maturation and secretion of insulin (see p. 40). The **A peptide** (21 amino acids) and **B peptide** (30 amino acids) of mature insulin are both derived from this initial precursor and are held together by two disulfide bridges. Bacteria do not have the processing enzymes that convert the precursor form to mature insulin. Therefore the initial strategy for bacterial synthesis of human insulin involved the production of the A and B chains by separate bacteria followed by purification of the individual chains and subsequent formation of the proper disulfide linkages.

The first step was to use synthetic organic chemistry methods to prepare a series of single-stranded oligonucleotides (11–18 nucleotides) that were both complementary and overlapping with each other. When these oligonucleotides were mixed together in the presence of **DNA ligase** under proper conditions, they formed a double-stranded fragment of DNA with termini equivalent to those formed by specific restriction enzymes (Figure 19.28). The sequences of the oligonucleotides were carefully chosen so that one of the two strands contained a methionine codon followed by the coding sequence of the A chain of insulin and a termination codon. A second set of overlapping complementary oligonucleotides were prepared and ligated together to form another double-stranded DNA fragment that contained a methionine codon followed by 30 codons specifying the B chain of insulin and a termination codon.

These two double-stranded fragments were then individually cloned at a restriction site in the β-galactosidase gene of the lactose operon in a plasmid. These two recombinant plasmids were introduced into bacteria. The bacteria could now produce a fusion protein of β-galactosidase and the A chain (or B chain) whose expression was under control of the lactose operon. In the absence

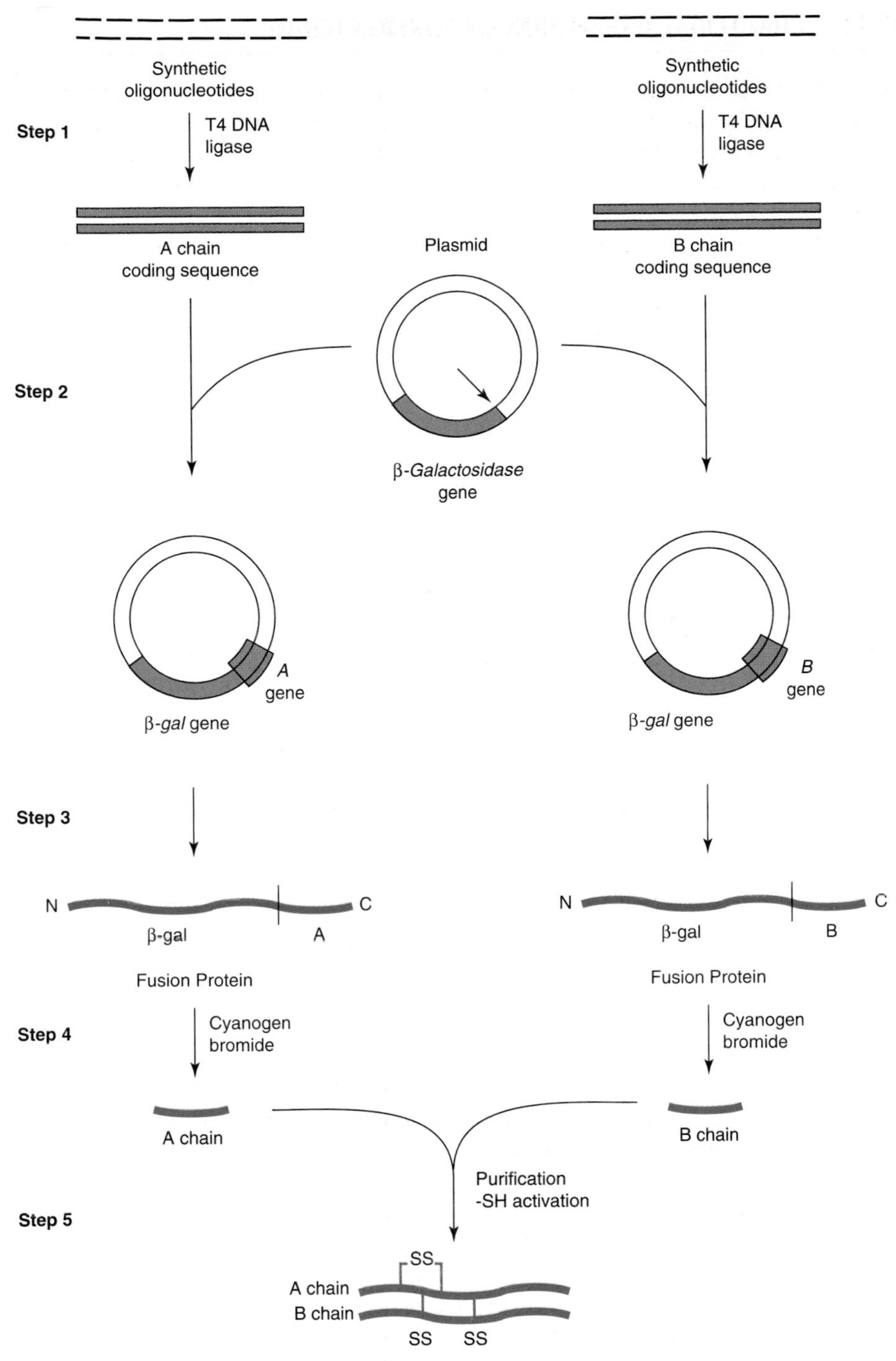

FIGURE 19.28
Bacterial expression of the A and B chains of human insulin.
Step 1: A series of overlapping, complementary oligonucleotides (11 for the A chain and 18 for the B chain) were synthesized and ligated together. One strand of the resulting small DNA fragments contained a methionine codon followed by coding sequence for A chain and B chain, respectively. Step 2: The small DNA fragments were ligated into a restriction site near the end of the β-galactosidase gene of the lactose operon in a plasmid. Step 3: Recombinant plasmids were introduced into *E. coli* and the β-galactosidase gene was induced with IPTG, an inducer of the lactose operon. A fusion protein was produced that contained most of the β-galactosidase sequence at the N terminus and the A chain (or B chain) at the C terminus. Step 4: Bacterial cell lysates containing the fusion protein were treated with cyanogen bromide, which cleaves peptide bonds following methionine residues. Step 5: A and B chains were purified away from all other cyanogen bromide peptides using biochemical and immunological separation techniques. The —SH groups on the cysteines were activated and reacted to form intra- and interchain disulfide bridges found in mature human insulin.
Redrawn from Crea, R., Krazewski, A., Hirose, T., and Itakura, K. Proc. Natl. Acad. Sci. USA *75:5765, 1980.*

of lactose in the bacterial medium, the lactose operon is repressed and only very small amounts of the fusion protein are synthesized. Using induction with IPTG and some additional genetic tricks, the bacteria can be forced to synthesize as much as 20% of their protein as the fusion protein. The A peptide (or B peptide) can be released from this fusion protein by treatment with cyanogen bromide, which cleaves on the carboxyl side of methionine residues. Since neither the A nor B peptide contains a methionine, they will be liberated intact and can subsequently be purified to homogeneity. The final steps involve chemically activating the free —SH groups on the cysteines and mixing the activated A and B chains together in a way that the proper disulfide linkages form to generate molecules of mature human insulin.

Recombinant Bacteria Can Synthesize Human Growth Hormone

The strategy for generating a recombinant DNA plasmid from which bacteria can synthesize human growth hormone is somewhat different than for insulin synthesis. First, human growth hormone is 191 amino acids long so the synthetic construction of the corresponding DNA coding sequence is more difficult (although certainly not impossible) than in the insulin case. On the other hand, growth hormone is a single polypeptide so it is not necessary to deal with the production of two chains and their subsequent dimerization to form a protein with biological activity. Because of these considerations, the coding sequence was initially cloned into a bacterial expression plasmid using part of a cloned growth hormone cDNA and several synthetic oligonucleotides (Figure 19.29). The overlapping oligonucleotides were prepared so that, when ligated together, they would form a small double-stranded DNA containing the codons for the first 24 amino acids of mature human growth hormone. One end of this DNA

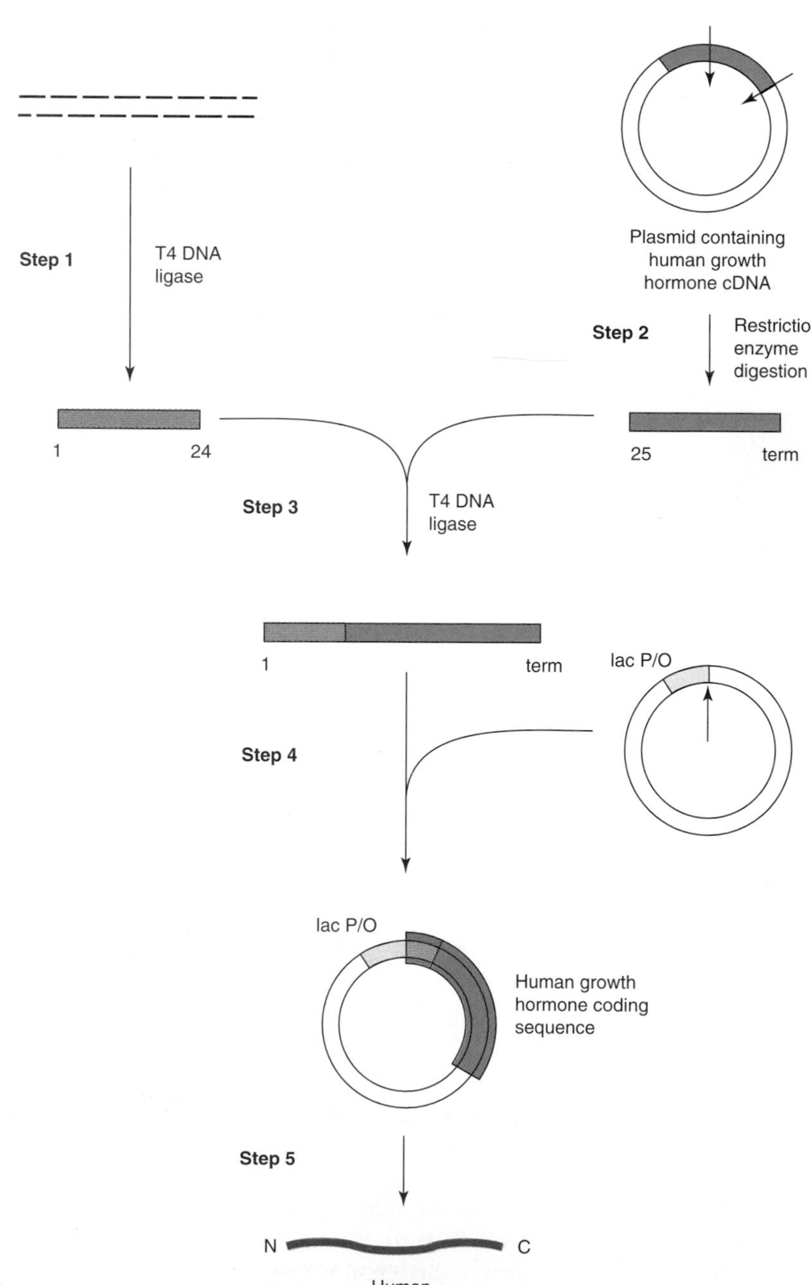

FIGURE 19.29
Expression of human growth hormone in *E. coli*.
Step 1: Several overlapping, complementary, oligonucleotides were synthesized and ligated together. One strand of the resulting small DNA fragment contains the coding sequence for the first 24 amino acids of mature human growth hormone (after removal of the N-terminal signal peptide). Step 2: A recombinant plasmid with a full length human growth hormone (hGH) cDNA, which is not expressed, is cleaved with restriction enzymes that release a fragment containing the complete growth hormone coding sequence after codon 24. Step 3: The synthetic fragment and the partial cDNA-containing fragment are ligated together to yield a new fragment containing the complete coding sequence of mature hGH. Step 4: The new fragment is ligated into a restriction site just downstream from the lactose promoter–operator region cloned in a plasmid. Step 5: The resulting recombinant DNA plasmid is introduced into bacteria in which synthesis of hGH can be induced with IPTG, an inducer of the lactose operon.

fragment was designed so that the fragment could be ligated in front of a restriction fragment of growth hormone cDNA that provided the rest of the coding sequence, including the termination codon. The other end of the synthetic fragment was chosen so that the composite coding sequence could easily be inserted into a site immediately downstream of the promoter–operator–ribosome binding site of the lactose operon cloned in a plasmid. After the introduction into bacteria, the bacteria were induced with IPTG to transcribe this foreign coding region and the greatly overproduced human growth hormone subsequently was purified away from the bacterial proteins.

19.14 INTRODUCTION OF RAT GROWTH HORMONE GENE INTO MICE

The previous section described the use of bacteria to produce large quantities of human proteins for treatment of disease. It is possible to microinject molecules of purified RNA or DNA directly into eukaryotic cells. This provides a very powerful approach for identifying conditions under which specific genes are expressed in eukaryotic cells. One of the most dramatic illustrations of this approach was the microinjection of a chromosomal DNA fragment containing the structural gene for rat growth hormone into the **pronuclei** of fertilized mouse eggs. The eggs were then reimplanted into the reproductive tracts of foster mouse mothers. Some of the mice that developed from this procedure were **transgenic;** one or more copies of the microinjected growth hormone gene integrated into a host mouse chromosome at an early stage of embryo development. These foreign genes were transmitted through the germline and became a permanent feature in the host chromosomes of the progeny (Figure 19.30).

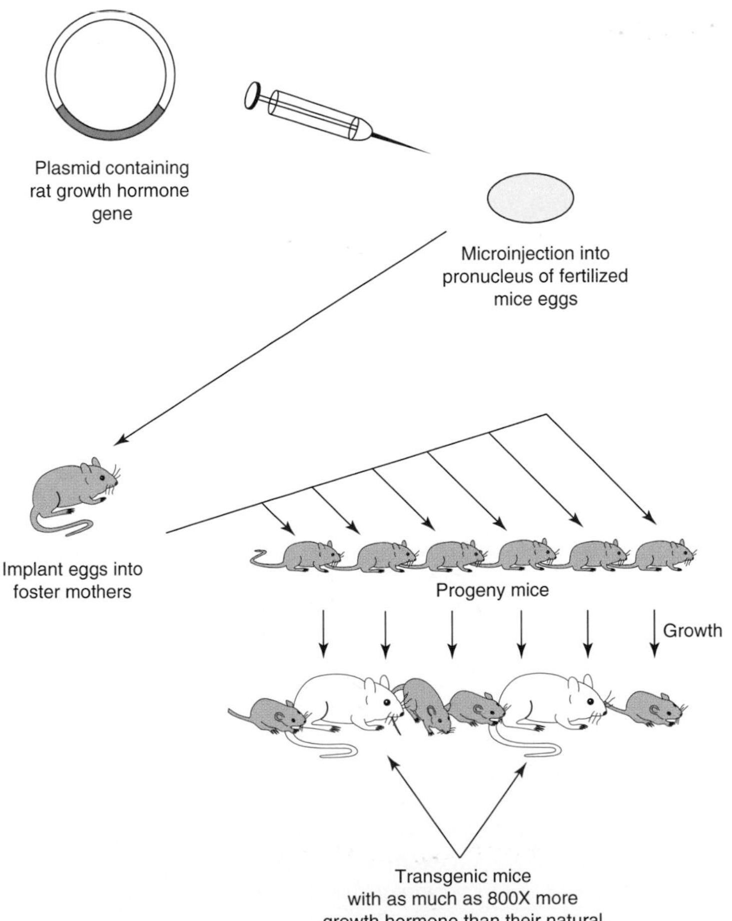

FIGURE 19.30
Schematic illustration of the introduction of rat growth hormone gene into mice.
Copies of a recombinant plasmid DNA containing rat growth hormone gene were microinjected into fertilized mouse eggs that were reimplanted into foster mothers. Some of the resulting progeny contained the foreign gene integrated into their own genome and greatly overexpressed growth hormone, growing much larger than their normal-sized littermates.
Redrawn from Palmiter, R. D., Brinster, R. L., Hammer, R. E. et al. Nature *300:611, 1982.*

Analysis of these transgenic mice revealed that in some cases several tandem copies of the rat growth hormone gene had integrated into a mouse chromosome; in other cases only one gene copy was present. In all cases at least some transcription occurred from the integrated gene(s), and in a few cases a dramatic overproduction of rat growth hormone resulted. In these latter cases, as much as 800 times more growth hormone was present in the transgenic mice than in normal mice, resulting in animals more than three times the size and weight of their unaffected littermates.

These results present many potential experimental possibilities for the future and raise a number of issues. One implied possibility is the use of similar growth hormone gene insertions to stimulate rapid growth of commercially valuable animals. This could result in a shorter production time and increased efficiency of food utilization. Another long-term possibility is the use of this approach to correct certain human genetic diseases or mimic the diseases in experimental animals so that they can be studied more carefully. One obvious human disease that is a candidate for this **"gene therapy"** approach is thalassemia. For example, an individual with two to three missing α-globin genes might benefit tremendously from receiving bone marrow transplants of his/her own cells that have been established in culture and microinjected with additional copies of the normal α-globin gene. This approach to gene therapy is being investigated. Insertion of normal genes into human somatic cells of a defective tissue or organ does not result in transmission of these genes to the progeny. This lessens the ethical considerations for experiments that do not alter germline characteristics.

BIBLIOGRAPHY

Prokaryotic Gene Expression

Cohen, S. N., and Shapiro, J. A. Transposable genetic elements. *Sci. Am.* 242:40, 1980.

Miller, J. H. The *lac* gene: its role in *lac* operon control and its use as a genetic system. In: J. H. Miller and W. S. Resnikoff (Eds.), *The Operon*. Cold Spring Harbor, NY: Cold Spring Harbor Laboratory Press, 1978, p. 31.

Platt, T. Regulation of gene expression in the tryptophan operon of *Escherichia coli*. In: J. H. Miller and W. S. Resnikoff (Eds.), *The Operon*. Cold Spring Harbor, NY: Cold Spring Harbor Laboratory Press, 1978, p. 263.

Simon, M., Zieg, J., Silverman, M., Mandel, G., and Doolittle, R. Phase variation: evolution of a controlling element. *Science* 209:1370, 1980.

Eukaryotic Gene Expression

Ahn, A. H., and Kunkel, L. M. The structural and functional diversity of dystrophin. *Nature Genetics* 3:283, 1993.

Chen, E. Y., Liao, Y.-C., Smith, D. H., Barrera-Saldaña, H. A., Gelinas, R. E., and Seeburg, P. H. The human growth hormone locus: nucleotide sequence, biology and evolution. *Genomics* 4:479, 1989.

Enver, T., and Greaves, D. R. Globin gene switching: a paradigm or what? *Curr. Opin. Biotech.* 2:787, 1991.

Johns, D. R. Mitochondrial DNA and disease. *N. Engl. J. Med.* 333:638, 1995.

Karlsson, S., and Nienhuis, A. W. Developmental regulation of human globin genes. *Annu. Rev. Biochem.* 54:1071, 1985.

Maniatis, T., Fritsch, E. F., Laurer, J., and Lawn, R. M. The molecular genetics of human hemoglobins. *Annu. Rev. Genet.* 14:145, 1980.

Mitchell, P. J., and Tjian, R. Transcription regulation in mammalian cells by sequence-specific DNA binding proteins. *Science* 245:371, 1989.

Palmiter, R. D., Brinster, R. L., Hammer, R. E., et al. Dramatic growth of mice that develop from eggs microinjected with metallothionein-growth hormone fusion genes. *Nature* 300:611, 1982.

Singh, G., Lott, M. T., and Wallace, D. C. A mitochondrial DNA mutation as a cause of Leber's hereditary optic neuropathy. *N. Engl. J. Med.* 320:1300, 1989.

Struhl, K. Chromatin structure and RNA polymerase II connection: implications for transcription. *Cell* 84:179, 1996.

The Huntington's Disease Collaborative Research Group. A novel gene containing a trinucleotide repeat that is expanded and unstable on Huntington's disease chromosomes. *Cell* 72:971, 1993.

QUESTIONS ■ J. BAGGOTT AND C. N. ANGSTADT

1. Full expression of the *lac* operon requires:
   A. lactose and cAMP.
   B. allolactose and cAMP.
   C. lactose alone.
   D. allolactose alone.
   E. absence or inactivation of the *lac* corepressor.

2. In an operon:
   A. each gene of the operon is regulated independently to achieve levels of expression required by the cell.
   B. control may be exerted via induction or via repression.
   C. operator and promoter may be trans to the genes they regulate.

D. the structural genes are either not expressed at all or are fully expressed.
E. control of gene expression consists exclusively of induction and repression.

3. The *E. coli lacZYA* region will be upregulated if:
A. there is a defect in binding of the inducer to the product of the *lacI* gene.
B. glucose and lactose are both present in the growth medium, but there is a defect in the cell's ability to bind the CAP protein.
C. glucose and lactose are both readily available in the growth medium.
D. the operator has mutated so it can no longer bind repressor.
E. the *lac* corepressor is not present.

4. All of the following describe an operon EXCEPT:
A. control mechanism for eukaryotic genes.
B. includes structural genes.
C. expected to code for polycistronic mRNA.
D. contains control sequences such as an operator.
E. can have multiple promoters.

Refer to the following for Questions 5–9:
A. repression
B. corepression
C. attenuation
D. stringent response
E. RNA splicing

5. Associated with guanosine tetraphosphate and guanosine pentaphosphate.

6. Not found in prokaryotes.

7. Involves rho-independent transcription termination.

8. Involves a leader peptide containing several occurrences of the same amino acid.

9. The only regulatory mechanism for the *his* operon.

10. Ribosomal operons:
A. all contain genes for proteins of just one ribosomal subunit.
B. all contain genes for proteins of both ribosomal subunits.
C. all contain genes for only ribosomal proteins.
D. can have their expression regulated at the level of translation.
E. are widely separated in the *E. coli* chromosome.

11. All of the following phrases describe transposons EXCEPT:
A. a means for the permanent incorporation of antibiotic resistance into the bacterial chromosome.
B. contain short inverted terminal repeat sequences.
C. code for an enzyme that synthesizes guanosine tetraphosphate and guanosine pentaphosphate, which inhibit further transposition.
D. include at least one gene that codes for a transposase.
E. contain varying numbers of genes, from two to several.

12. Introns:
A. are of approximately uniform size.
B. are skipped over during translation.
C. are found in all eukaryotic genes.
D. function to separate functional domains of proteins.
E. are smaller and shorter in unicellular lower eukaryotes than in higher, more complicated eukaryotes.

13. Repetitive DNA:
A. is common in bacterial and mammalian systems.
B. is uniformly distributed throughout the genome.
C. includes DNA that codes for rRNA.
D. consists mostly of DNA that codes for enzymes catalyzing major metabolic processes.
E. is resistant to the action of restriction endonucleases.

14. The β-gene cluster contains:
A. one haploid ζ gene.
B. one haploid β gene.
C. one haploid γ gene.
D. two haploid δ genes.
E. two haploid ε genes.

15. The number of α genes in the haploid α-gene cluster is
A. one.
B. two.
C. three.
D. four.
E. five.

16. In designing a recombinant DNA for the purpose of synthesizing an active eukaryotic polypeptide in bacteria all of the following should be true EXCEPT:
A. the eukaryotic gene may contain its usual complement of introns.
B. the foreign polypeptide should be resistant to degradation by bacterial proteases.
C. glycosylation of the polypeptide should be unnecessary.
D. the foreign polypeptide should be nontoxic to the bacteria.
E. bacterial controlling elements are necessary.

ANSWERS

1. B A: The true inducer is allolactose, not lactose (p. 806). C: Lactose is converted in the cell to allolactose. D: In addition, cAMP must bind to the CAP protein, and the cAMP–CAP complex serves as a positive control of transcription (p. 807). E: The *lac* operon does not involve corepression.
2. B Induction and repression are among the mechanisms used to control operons. A: In an operon the structural genes are under coordinate control. C: The operator and promoter are elements of the same strand of DNA as the operon they control; they are not diffusible. D: Typically, regulation of operators is somewhat leaky; some gene product is produced even in the repressed state. E: Another mechanism for regulation of an operon is attenuation (p. 810).

3. D If the operator is unable to bind repressor, the rate of transcription is greater than the basal level (p. 804). A: The product of the *lac*I gene is the repressor protein. When this protein binds an inducer, it changes its conformation, no longer binds to the operator site of DNA, and transcription occurs at an increased rate. Failure to bind an inducer prevents this sequence. B and C: In the presence of glucose catabolite repression occurs. Glucose lowers the intracellular level of cAMP. The catabolite activator protein (CAP) then cannot complex with cAMP, so there is no CAP–cAMP complex to activate transcription. The same would occur if the cell had lost its capacity to synthesize cAMP (p. 808). E: The *lac* operon does not involve corepression.
4. A Operons are prokaryotic mechanisms. B–D: An operon is the complete regulatory unit of a set of clustered genes, including the structural genes (which are transcribed together to form a polycistronic mRNA), regulatory genes, and control elements, such as the operator (p. 801). E: An operon may have more than one promoter, as does the tryptophan operon of *E. coli* (p. 810).
5. D The exact functions of these species are not yet known, but their production is very rapid after the onset of amino acid starvation (p. 815).
6. E Splicing is a eukaryotic phenomenon (p. 820).
7. C The hairpin loop that forms between regions 3 and 4 (Figure 19.11) is followed by an oligo-U region (Figure 19.10). This constellation compromises the signal for rho-independent termination of transcription. (See pp. 811–812.)
8. C Synthesis of the leader peptide depends strongly on availability of this amino acid, since it must be incorporated several times. When it is insufficiently available, the ribosome stalls, in region 1 (Figure 19.11), allowing the 2–3 hairpin to form. This in turn prevents formation of the 3–4 hairpin, which would signal termination of transcription.
9. C In this operon the stalled ribosome acts rather like a positive regulator protein, that is, the cAMP–CAP complex (p. 813).
10. D Excess ribosomal protein binds to its own mRNA, preventing initiation of further synthesis of that protein (p. 814). A, B, C, and E: The genes for one half of the ribosomal proteins are in two major clusters. There is no pattern to the distribution of genes for the proteins of the two ribosomal subunits, and they are intermixed with genes for other proteins involved in protein synthesis.
11. C These guanosine phosphates are synthesized by the product of the *relA* gene; they inhibit initiation of transcription of the rRNA and tRNA genes, shutting off protein synthesis in general. This is the stringent response (p. 815).
12. E A: Introns are of various sizes. B: They are excised during splicing, not skipped over during translation. C: Although they are common, some genes do not have them, for example, the histone and interferon genes (p. 821). D: Sometimes they occur between functional domains of proteins, but not always.
13. C This makes sense, since many copies of these structural elements are needed (p. 823). A and B: Highly repetitive and moderately repetitive DNA are found only in eukaryotes. Highly repetitive sequences tend to be clustered, as are some moderately repetitive sequences (p. 822). D: Most repetitive DNA does not code for a stable gene product (p. 822). E: The Alu family of moderately repetitive DNA is named for the restriction endonuclease that cleaves them (p. 823).
14. B This means that there are only two β genes per diploid cell. As a result, in β-thalassemia, one defective β-globin gene gives rise to a minor form of the disease, while two defective genes cause the major form. (See p. 828.)
15. B As a result, α-thalassemia is more complicated than β-thalassemia because there are four α-globin genes per diploid cell, and anywhere between zero and four of them can be defective. (See p. 828.)
16. A A and C: The bacterial system has no mechanism for posttranscriptional modification of mRNA or for posttranslational (or cotranslational) modification of protein. E: Bacterial systems need bacterial promoters, and so on (p. 832).

CHAPTER

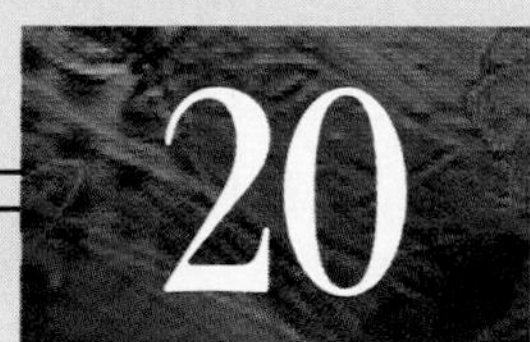

BIOCHEMISTRY OF HORMONES I: POLYPEPTIDE HORMONES

Gerald Litwack and Thomas J. Schmidt

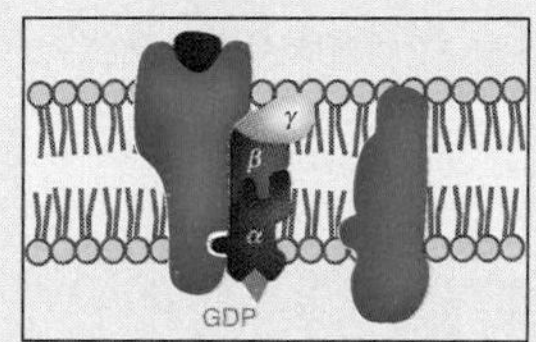

20.1 ■ OVERVIEW

Cells are regulated by many hormones, growth factors, neurotransmitters, and certain toxins through interactions of these diverse ligands with their **cognate receptors** located at the cell surface. This collection of receptors is the major mechanism through which **peptide hormones** and **amino acid-derived hormones** exert their effects at the cellular level. Another important mechanism involves permeation of the cell membrane by **steroid hormones** that subsequently interact with their intracellular cognate receptors (Chapter 21). These two sites, the plasma membrane and the intracellular milieu, represent the principal locations of the initial interaction between ligands and cellular receptors and are diagrammed in Figure 20.1. Polypeptide hormones and several amino acid-derived hormones bind to cognate receptors in the plasma membrane. One exception is thyroid hormone, which binds to a receptor that resides in the nucleus much like certain steroid hormone receptors.

The **hormonal cascade system** is applicable to many, but not all, hormones. It begins with signals in the central nervous system (CNS), followed by hormone secretion by the hypothalamus, pituitary, and end target organ. In this chapter major polypeptide hormones are summarized and the synthesis of specific hormones is described. Synthesis of the amino acid-derived hormones, epinephrine and triiodo-L-thyronine, is also outlined. Examples of hormone inactivation and degradation are presented. The remainder of this chapter focuses on receptors, **signal transduction,** and **second messenger pathways.** Receptor internalization is described and examples of cyclic hormonal cascade systems are introduced. Finally, a discussion of oncogenes and receptor function is presented.

In terms of receptor mechanisms, aspects of hormone–receptor interactions are presented with a brief mathematical analysis. Signal transduction is considered, especially in reference to GTP-binding proteins. Second messenger systems discussed include cAMP and the protein kinase A pathway, inositol triphosphate–diacylglycerol and the Ca^{2+}–protein kinase C pathway, and cGMP and

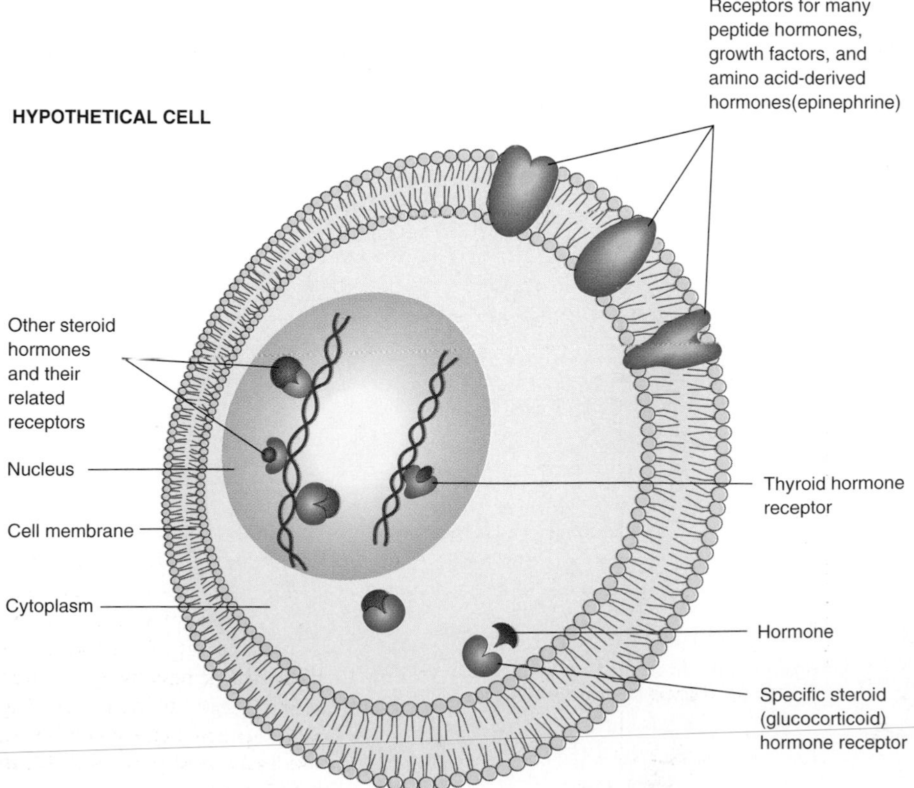

FIGURE 20.1
Diagram showing the different locations of classes of receptors expressed by a target cell.

the protein kinase G pathway. These pathways are discussed in the context of representative hormone action. Newly identified components of these signal transduction pathways are defined in terms of the kinase system(s) involved. In addition, the insulin receptor and its tyrosine kinase and second messenger pathways are considered.

20.2 HORMONES AND THE HORMONAL CASCADE SYSTEM

The definition of a hormone has been expanded over the last several decades. Hormones secreted by endocrine glands were originally considered to represent all of the physiologically relevant hormones. Today, the term **hormone** refers to any substance in an organism that carries a signal to generate some sort of alteration at the cellular level. Thus **endocrine hormones** represent a class of hormones that arise in one tissue, or "gland," and travel a considerable distance through the circulation to reach a target cell expressing cognate receptors. **Paracrine hormones** arise from a cell and travel a relatively small distance to interact with their cognate receptors on another neighboring cell. **Autocrine hormones** are produced by the same cell that functions as the target for that hormone (neighboring cells may also be targets). Thus we can classify hormones based on their radii of action. Often, endocrine hormones that travel long distances to their target cells may be more stable than autocrine hormones that exert their effects over very short distances.

Cascade System Amplifies a Specific Signal

For many hormonal systems in higher animals, the signal pathway originates with the brain and culminates with the ultimate target cell. Figure 20.2 outlines the sequence of events in this cascade. A stimulus may originate in the external environment or within the organism in this cascade. This signal may be transmitted as an electrical pulse (action potential) or as a chemical signal or both. In many cases, but not all, such signals are forwarded to the limbic system and subsequently to the hypothalamus, the pituitary, and the target gland that secretes the final hormone. This hormone then affects various target cells to a degree that is frequently proportional to the number of cognate receptors

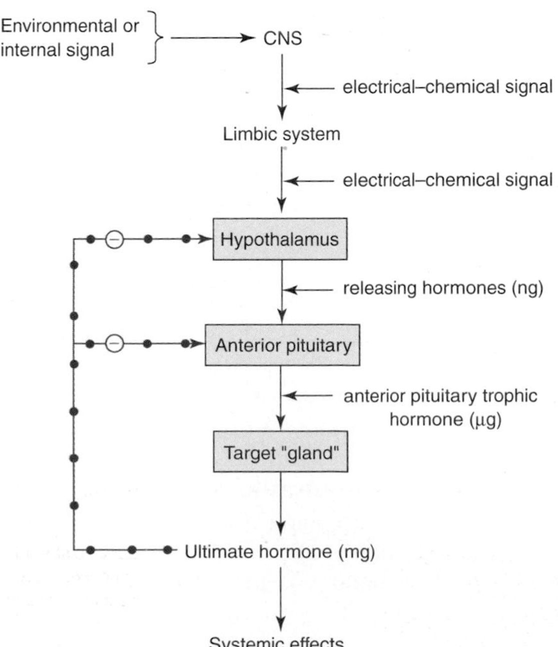

FIGURE 20.2
Hormonal cascade of signals from CNS to ultimate hormone.
The target "gland" refers to the last hormone-producing tissue in the cascade, which is stimulated by an appropriate anterior pituitary hormone. Examples would be thyroid gland, adrenal cortex, ovary, and testis. Ultimate hormone feeds back negatively on sites producing intermediate hormones in the cascade. Amounts [nanogram (ng), microgram (mg), and milligram (mg)] represent approximate quantities of hormone released.
Redrawn from Norman, A. W., and Litwack, G. Hormones. *New York: Academic Press, 1987, p. 38.*

expressed by that cell. This may be a true **cascade** in the sense that increasing amounts of hormones are generated at successive levels (hypothalamus, pituitary, and target gland) and also because the half-lives of these blood-borne hormones tend to become longer in progression from the hypothalamic hormone to the ultimate hormone. In the case of environmental stress, for example, there is a single stressor (change in temperature, noise, trauma, etc.). This stress results in a signal to the hippocampal structure in the limbic system that signals the hypothalamus to release a hypothalamic releasing hormone, corticotropin-releasing hormone (CRH), which is usually secreted in nanogram amounts and may have a $t_{1/2}$ in the bloodstream of several minutes. This hormone travels down a closed portal system to gain access to the **anterior pituitary,** where it binds to its cognate receptor in the cell membrane of corticotropic cells and initiates a set of metabolic changes resulting in the release of adrenocorticotropic hormone (ACTH) as well as β-lipotropin. This hormone, which is released in microgram amounts and has a longer $t_{1/2}$ than CRH, circulates in the bloodstream until it binds to its cognate receptors expressed in the membranes of cells located in the inner layer of the cortex of the adrenal gland (target gland). Here it affects metabolic changes leading to the synthesis and release in 24 h of the ultimate hormone, cortisol, in multimilligram amounts and this active glucocorticoid hormone has a substantial $t_{1/2}$ in blood. Cortisol is taken up by a wide variety of cells that express varying amounts of the intracellular glucocorticoid receptor. The ultimate hormone, in this case cortisol, feeds back negatively on cells of the anterior pituitary, hypothalamus, and perhaps higher levels to shut down the overall pathway in a process that is also mediated by the glucocorticoid receptor. At the **target cell** level these cortisol–receptor complexes mediate specific transcriptional responses and the individual hormonal effects summate to produce the systemic effects of the hormone. The cascade is represented in this example by a single environmental stimulus generating a series of hormones in progressively larger amounts and with increasing stabilities, and by the ultimate hormone that affects most of the cells in the body. Many other systems operate similarly, there being different specific **releasing hormones, anterior pituitary tropic hormones,** and ultimate hormones involved in the process. Clearly, the final number of target cells affected may be large or small depending on the distribution of receptors for each ultimate hormone.

A related system involves the **posterior pituitary hormones,** oxytocin and vasopressin (antidiuretic hormone), which are stored in the posterior pituitary gland but are synthesized in neuronal cell bodies located in the hypothalamus. This system is represented in Figure 20.3; elements of Figure 20.2 appear in the central vertical pathway. The posterior pituitary system branches to the right from the hypothalamus. Oxytocin and vasopressin are synthesized in separate cell bodies of hypothalamic neurons. More cell bodies dedicated to synthesis of vasopressin are located in the supraoptic nucleus and more cell bodies dedicated to synthesis of oxytocin are located in the paraventricular nucleus. Their release from the posterior pituitary gland along with **neurophysin,** a stabilizing protein, occurs separately via specific stimuli impinging on each of these types of neuronal cells.

There are highly specific signals dictating the release of polypeptide hormones along the cascade of this system. Thus there are a variety of **aminergic neurons** (secreting amine-containing substances like dopamine and serotonin) which connect to neurons involved in the synthesis and release of the **releasing hormones** of the hypothalamus. Releasing hormones are summarized in Table 20.1. These aminergic neurons fire depending on various types of internal or external signals and their activities account for **pulsatile release patterns** of certain hormones, such as the gonadotropin-releasing hormone (GnRH), and the **rhythmic cyclic release** of other hormones like cortisol.

Another prominent feature of the hormonal cascade (Figure 20.3) is the **negative feedback** system operating when sufficiently high levels of the ultimate hormone have been secreted into the circulation. Generally, there are three feedback loops—the **long feedback,** the **short feedback,** and the **ultra-**

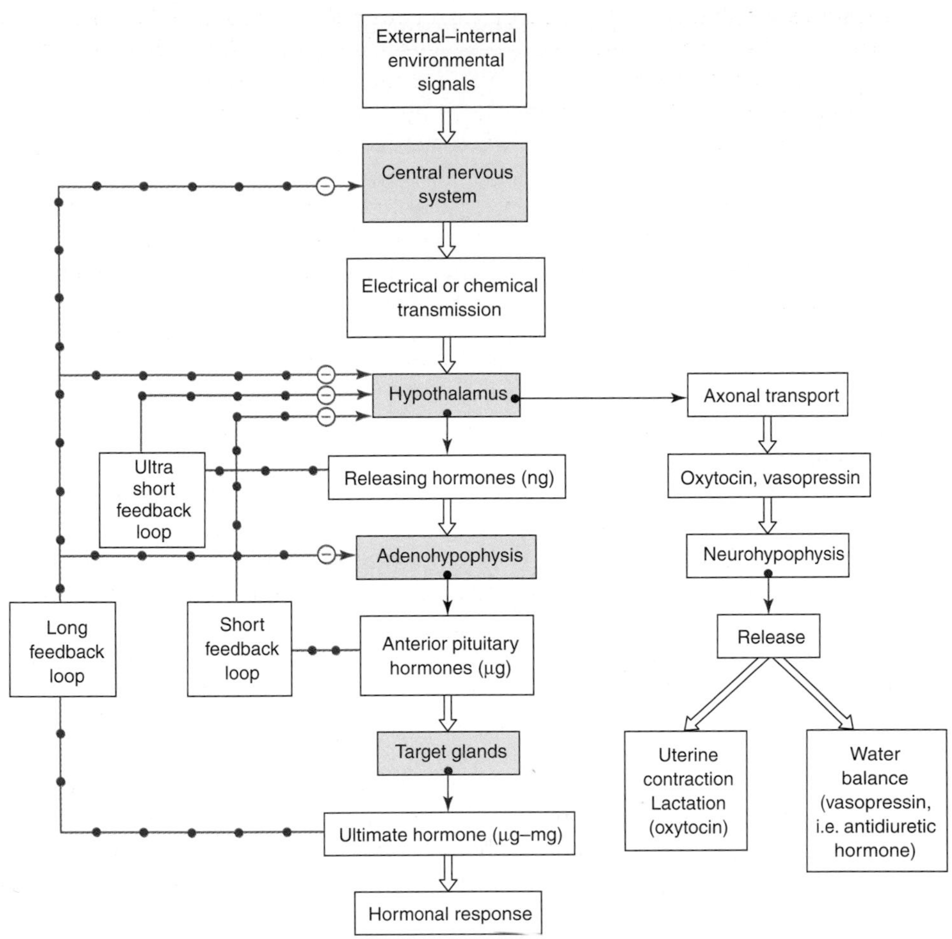

FIGURE 20.3
Many hormonal systems involve the hypothalamus.
Cascade of hormonal signals starting with an external or internal environmental signal. This is transmitted first to the CNS and may involve components of the limbic system, such as the hippocampus and amygdala. These structures innervate the hypothalamus in a specific region, which responds with secretion of a specific releasing hormone, usually in nanogram amounts. Releasing hormones are transported down a closed portal system connecting the hypothalamus and anterior pituitary, bind to cell membrane receptors and cause the secretion of specific anterior pituitary hormones, usually in microgram amounts. These access the general circulation through fenestrated local capillaries and bind to specific target gland receptors. The interactions trigger release of an ultimate hormone in microgram to milligram daily amounts, which generate the hormonal response by binding to receptors in several target tissues. In effect, this overall system is an amplifying cascade. Releasing hormones are secreted in nanogram amounts and they have short half-lives on the order of a few minutes. Anterior pituitary hormones are produced often in microgram amounts and have longer half-lives than releasing hormones. Ultimate hormones can be produced in daily milligram amounts with much longer half-lives. Thus the products of mass × half-life constitute an amplifying cascade mechanism. With respect to differences in mass of hormones produced from hypothalamus to target gland, the range is nanograms to milligrams, or as much as one million-fold. When the ultimate hormone has receptors in nearly every cell type, it is possible to affect the body chemistry of virtually every cell by a single environmental signal. Consequently, the organism is in intimate association with the external environment, a fact that we tend to underemphasize. Solid arrows indicate a secretory process. Long arrows studded with open or closed circles indicate negative feedback pathways (ultra-short, short, and long feedback loops).
Redrawn from Norman, A. W., and Litwack, G. Hormones. *New York: Academic Press, 1987, p. 102.*

TABLE 20.1 Hypothalamic Releasing Hormones[a]

Releasing Hormone	*Number of Amino Acids in Structure*	*Anterior Pituitary Hormone Released or Inhibited*
Thyrotropin-releasing hormone (TRH)	3	Thyrotropin (TSH); can also release prolactin (PRL) experimentally
Gonadotropin-releasing hormone (GnRH)	10	Luteinizing and follicle-stimulating hormones (LH and FSH) from the same cell type; leukotriene C_4 (LTC_4) can also release LH and FSH by a different mechanism
Gonadotropin release-inhibiting factor (GnRIF)	12.2 kDa molecular weight	LH and FSH release inhibited
Corticotropin-releasing hormone (CRH)	41	ACTH, β-lipotropin (β-LPH), and some β-endorphin
Arginine vasopressin (AVP)	9	Stimulates CRH action in ACTH release
Angiotensin II (AII)	8	Stimulates CRH action in ACTH release; releases ACTH weakly
Somatocrinin (GRH)	44	Growth hormone (GH) release
Somatostatin (GIH)	14	GH release inhibited
Hypothalamic gastrin-releasing peptide		Inhibits release of GH and PRL
Prolactin-releasing factor (PRF)		Releases prolactin (PRL)
Prolactin release-inhibiting factor (PIF)		Evidence that a new peptide may inhibit PRL release; dopamine also inhibits PRL release and was thought to be PIF for some time; dopamine may be a secondary PIF: oxytocin may inhibit PRL release

[a] Melanocyte-stimulating hormone (MSH) is a major product of the *pars intermedia* (Figure 20.5) in the rat and is under the control of aminergic neurons. Humans may also secrete α-MSH from *pars intermedia*-like cells although this structure is anatomically indistinct in the human.

CLINICAL CORRELATION 20.1

Testing Activity of the Anterior Pituitary

Releasing hormones and chemical analogs, particularly of the smaller peptides, are now routinely synthesized. The gonadotropin-releasing hormone, a decapeptide, is available for use in assessing the function of the anterior pituitary. This is of importance when a disease situation may involve either the hypothalamus, the anterior pituitary, or the end organ. Infertility is an example of such a situation. What needs to be assessed is which organ is at fault in the hormonal cascade. Initially, the end organ, in this case the gonads, must be considered. This can be accomplished by injecting the anterior pituitary hormone LH or FSH. If sex hormone secretion is elicited, then the ultimate gland would appear to be functioning properly. Next, the anterior pituitary would need to be analyzed. This can be done by i.v. administration of synthetic GnRH; by this route GnRH can gain access to the gonadotropic cells of the anterior pituitary and elicit secretion of LH and FSH. Routinely, LH levels are measured in the blood as a function of time after the injection. These levels are measured by radioimmunoassay (RIA) in which radioactive LH or hCG is displaced from binding to an LH-binding protein by LH in the serum sample. The extent of the competition is proportional to the amount of LH in the serum. In this way a progress of response is measured that will be within normal limits or clearly deficient. If the response is deficient, the anterior pituitary cells are not functioning normally and are the cause of the syndrome. On the other hand, normal pituitary response to GnRH would indicate that the hypothalamus was nonfunctional. Such a finding would prompt examination of the hypothalamus for conditions leading to insufficient availability/production of releasing hormones. Obviously, the knowledge of hormone structure and the ability to synthesize specific hormones permit the diagnosis of these disease states.

Marshall, J. C., and Barkan, A. L. Disorders of the hypothalamus and anterior pituitary. In: W. N. Kelley (Ed.), *Internal Medicine*. New York: Lippincott, 1989, p. 2159; and Conn, P. M. The molecular basis of gonadotropin-releasing hormone action. *Endocr. Rev.* 7:3, 1986.

short feedback loops. In the long feedback loop, the final hormone binds a cognate receptor in/on cells of the anterior pituitary, hypothalamus, and CNS to prevent further elaboration of hormones from those cells that are involved in the cascade. The short feedback loop is accounted for by the pituitary hormone that feeds back negatively on the hypothalamus operating through a cognate receptor. In ultra-short feedback loops the hypothalamic releasing factor feeds back at the level of the hypothalamus to inhibit further secretion of this releasing factor. These mechanisms provide tight controls on the operation of the cascade, responding to stimulating signals as well as negative feedback, and render this system highly responsive to the hormonal milieu. Clinical Correlation 20.1 describes approaches for testing the responsiveness of the anterior pituitary gland.

Polypeptide Hormones of the Anterior Pituitary

The polypeptide hormones of the anterior pituitary are shown in Figure 20.4 together with their controlling hormones from the hypothalamus. The major

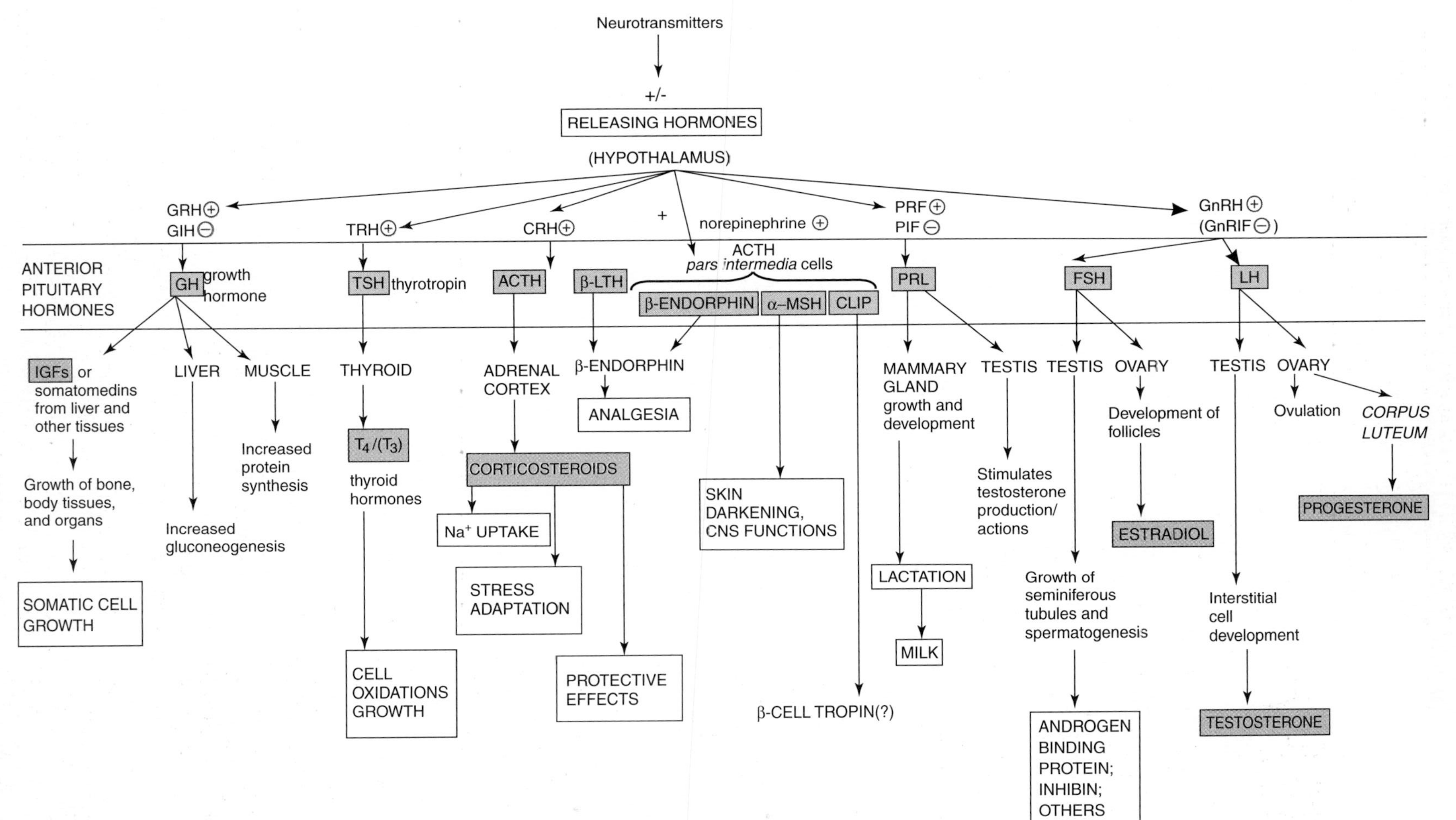

FIGURE 20.4
Overview of anterior pituitary hormones with hypothalamic releasing hormones and their actions.

CLINICAL CORRELATION 20.2

Hypopituitarism

The hypothalamus is connected to the anterior pituitary by a delicate stalk that contains the portal system through which releasing hormones, secreted from the hypothalamus, gain access to the anterior pituitary cells. In the cell membranes of these cells are specific receptors for releasing hormones. In most cases, different cells express different releasing hormone receptors. The connection between the hypothalamus and anterior pituitary can be disrupted by trauma or tumors. Trauma can occur in automobile accidents or other local damaging events that may result in severing of the stalk and preventing the releasing hormones from reaching their target anterior pituitary cells. When this happens, the anterior pituitary cells no longer have their signaling mechanism for the release of anterior pituitary hormones. In the case of tumors of the pituitary gland, all of the anterior pituitary hormones may not be shut off to the same degree or the secretion of some may disappear sooner than others. In any case, if hypopituitarism occurs this condition may result in a life-threatening situation in which the clinician must determine the extent of loss of pituitary hormones, especially ACTH. Posterior pituitary hormones—oxytocin and vasopressin—may also be lost, precipitating a problem of excessive urination (vasopressin deficiency) that must be addressed. The usual therapy involves administration of the end organ hormones, such as thyroid hormone, cortisol, sex hormones, and progestin; with female patients it is also necessary to maintain the ovarian cycle. These hormones can easily be administered in oral form. Growth hormone deficiency is not a problem in the adult but would be an important problem in a growing child. The patient must learn to anticipate needed increases of cortisol in the face of stressful situations. Fortunately, these patients are usually maintained in reasonably good condition.

Marshall, J. C., and Barkan, A. L. Disorders of the hypothalamus and anterior pituitary. In: W. N. Kelley (Ed.), *Internal Medicine.* New York: Lippincott, 1989, p. 2159; and Robinson, A. G. Disorders of the posterior pituitary. In: W. N. Kelley (Ed.), *Internal Medicine,* New York: Lippincott, 1989, p. 2172.

hormones of the anterior pituitary are growth hormone (GH), thyrotropin or thyroid-stimulating hormone (TSH), adrenocorticotropic hormone (ACTH),β-lipotropin (β-LTH), β-endorphin (from *pars intermedia*-like cells), α-MSH (from *pars intermedia*-like cells), β-MSH (from *pars intermedia*-like cells), corticotropin-like intermediary peptide (CLIP; from *pars intermedia*-like cells), prolactin (PRL), follicle-stimulating hormone (FSH), and luteinizing hormone (LH). Of these, all are single polypeptide chains, except TSH, FSH, and LH, which are dimers that share a similar or identical subunit, the α subunit. Since the intermediate lobe in humans is rudimentary, the circulating levels of free α- and β-MSH are relatively low. It is of interest, particularly in the human, that MSH receptors recognize and are activated by ACTH, since the first 13 amino acids of ACTH contain the α-MSH sequence. For this reason, ACTH may be an important contributing factor to skin pigmentation and may exceed the importance of MSH, especially in conditions where the circulating level of ACTH is high. The clinical consequences of hypopituitarism are presented in Clin. Corr. 20.2.

20.3 ■ MAJOR POLYPEPTIDE HORMONES AND THEIR ACTIONS

Since cellular communication is so specific, it is not surprising that there are a large number of hormones in the body and new hormones continue to be discovered. Limitations of space permit a summary of only a few of the well-characterized hormones. Table 20.2 presents some major polypeptide hormones and their actions. By inspection of Table 20.2 it becomes evident that many hormones cause the release of other substances, some of which may themselves be hormones. This is particularly the case for hormonal systems that are included in cascades like that presented in Figures 20.2 and 20.3. Other activities of receptor–hormone complexes located in cell membranes are to increase the flux of ions into cells, particularly calcium ions, and to activate or suppress activities of enzymes in contact with the receptor or a transducing protein with which the receptor interacts. Examples of these kinds of activities are discussed later in this chapter. In the functioning of most membrane–receptor complexes,

TABLE 20.2 Important Polypeptide Hormones in the Body and Their Actions[a]

Source	*Hormone*	*Action*
Hypothalamus	Thyrotropin-releasing hormone (TRH)	Acts on thyrotrope to release TSH
	Gonadotropin-releasing hormone (GnRH)	Acts on gonadotrope to release LH and FSH from the same cell
	Growth hormone-releasing hormone or somatocrinin (GRH)	Acts on somatotrope to release GH
	Growth hormone release inhibiting hormone or somatostatin (GIH)	Acts on somatotrope to prevent release of GH
	Corticotropin-releasing hormone (CRH)	Acts on corticotrope to release ACTH and β-lipotropin
	Vasopressin is a helper hormone to CRH in releasing ACTH; angiotensin II also stimulates CRH action in releasing ACTH	
	Prolactin-releasing factor (PRF) (not well established)	Acts on lactotrope to release PRL
	Prolactin release inhibiting factor (PIF) (not well established; may be a peptide hormone under control of dopamine or may be dopamine itself)	Acts on lactotrope to inhibit release of PRL
Anterior pituitary	Thyrotropin (TSH)	Acts on thyroid follicle cells to bring about release of T_4 (T_3)
	Luteinizing hormone (LH) (human chorionic gonadotropin, hCG, is a similar hormone from the placenta)	Acts on Leydig cells of testis to increase testosterone synthesis and release; acts on corpus luteum of ovary to increase progesterone production and release
	Follicle-stimulating hormone (FSH)	Acts on Sertoli cells of seminiferous tubule to increase proteins in sperm and other proteins; acts on ovarian follicles to stimulate maturation of ovum and production of estradiol
	Growth hormone (GH)	Acts on a variety of cells to produce IGFs (or somatomedins), cell growth, and bone sulfation
	Adrenocorticotropic hormone (ACTH)	Acts on cells in the adrenal gland to increase cortisol production and secretion
	β-Endorphin	Acts on cells and neurons to produce analgesic and other effects
	Prolactin (PRL)	Acts on mammary gland to cause differentiation of secretory cells (with other hormones) and to stimulate synthesis of components of milk
	Melanocyte-stimulating hormone (MSH)	Acts on skin cells to cause the dispersion of melanin (skin darkening)
Ultimate gland hormones	Insulin-like growth factors (IGF)	Respond to GH and produce growth effects by stimulating cell mitosis
	Thyroid hormone (T_4/T_3) (amino acid-derived hormone)	Responds to TSH and stimulates oxidation in many cells
	Opioid peptides	May derive as breakdown products of γ-lipotropin or β-endorphin or from specific gene products; can respond to CRH or dopamine and may produce analgesia and other effects
	Inhibin	Responds to FSH in ovary and in Sertoli cell; regulates secretion of FSH from anterior pituitary. Second form of inhibin (activin) may stimulate FSH secretion
	Corticotropin-like intermediary peptide (CLIP)	Derives from intermediate pituitary by degradation of ACTH; contains β-cell tropin activity, which stimulates insulin release from β cells in presence of glucose

(*continued*)

TABLE 20.2 (*Continued*)

Source	*Hormone*	*Action*
Peptide hormones responding to other signals than anterior pituitary hormones	Arginine vasopressin (AVP; antidiuretic hormone, ADH)	Responds to increase in osmoreceptor, which senses extracellular [Na^+]; increases water reabsorption from distal kidney tubule
	Oxytocin	Responds to suckling reflex and estradiol; causes milk "let down" or ejection in lactating female, involved in uterine contractions of labor; luteolytic factor produced by *corpus luteum*; decreases steroid synthesis in testis
β Cells of pancreas respond to glucose and other blood constituents to release insulin	Insulin	Increases tissue utilization of glucose
α Cells of pancrease respond to low levels of glucose and falling serum calcium	Glucagon	Decreases tissue utilization of glucose to elevate blood glucose
Derived from circulating blood protein by actions of renin and converting enzyme	Angiotensin II and III (AII and AIII)	Renin initially responds to decreased blood volume or decreased [Na^+] in the *macula densa* of the kidney. AII/AIII stimulate outer layer of adrenal cells to synthesize and release aldosterone
Released from heart atria in response to hypovolemia; regulated by other hormones	Atrial natriuretic factor (ANF) or atriopeptin	Acts on outer adrenal cells to decrease aldosterone release; has other effects also
Generates from plasma, gut, or other tissues	Bradykinin	Modulates extensive vasodilation resulting in hypotension
Hypothalamus and intestinal mucosa	Neurotensin	Effects on gut; may have neurotransmitter actions
Hypothalamus, CNS, and intestine	Substance P	Pain transmitter, increases smooth muscle contractions of the GI tract
Nerves and endocrine cells of gut; hypothermic hormone	Bombesin	Increases gastric acid secretion
	Cholecystokinin (CCK)	Stimulates gallbladder contraction and bile flow; increases secretion of pancreatic enzymes
Stomach antrum	Gastrin	Increases secretion of gastric acid and pepsin
Duodenum at pH values below 4.5	Secretin	Stimulates pancreatic acinar cells to release bicarbonate and water to elevate duodenal pH
Hypothalamus and GI tract	Vasointestinal peptide (VIP)	Acts as a neurotransmitter in peripheral autonomic nervous system; relaxes smooth muscles of circulation; increases secretion of water and electrolytes from pancreas and gut
Kidney	Erythropoietin	Acts on bone marrow for terminal differentiation and initiates hemoglobin synthesis
Ovarian corpus luteum	Relaxin	Inhibits myometrial contractions; its secretion increases during gestation
	Human placental lactogen (hPL)	Acts like PRL and GH because of large amount of hPL produced
Salivary gland	Epidermal growth factor	Stimulates proliferations of cells derived from ectoderm and mesoderm together with serum; inhibits gastric secretion
Thymus	Thymopoietin (α-thymosin)	Stimulates phagocytes; stimulates differentiation of precursors into immune competent T cells

TABLE 20.2 (*Continued*)

Source	*Hormone*	*Action*
Parafollicular C cells of thyroid gland	Calcitonin (CT)	Lowers serum calcium
Parathyroid glands	Parathyroid hormone (PTH)	Stimulates bone resorption; stimulates phosphate excretion by kidney; raises serum calcium levels
Endothelial cells of blood vessels	Endothelin	Vasoconstriction

Source: Part of this table is reproduced from Norman, A. W., and Litwack, G. *Hormones*. Orlando, FL: Academic Press, 1987.

[a] This is only a partial list of polypeptide hormones in humans. TSH, thyroid-stimulating hormone or thyrotropin; LH, luteinizing hormone; FSH, follicle-stimulating hormone; GH, growth hormone; ACTH, adenocorticotropic hormone; PRL, prolactin; T_4, thyroid hormone (also T); IGF, insulin-like growth factor. For the releasing hormones and for some hormones in other categories, the abbreviation may contain "H" at the end when the hormone has been well characterized, and "F" in place of H to refer to "Factor" when the hormone has not been well characterized. Names of hormones may contain "tropic" or "trophic" endings; tropic is mainly used here. Tropic refers to a hormone generating a change, whereas trophic refers to growth promotion. Both terms can refer to the same hormone at different stages of development. Many of these hormones have effects in addition to those listed here.

stimulation of enzymes or flux of ions is followed by a chain of events, which may be described as intracellular cascades, during which a high degree of amplification is obtained.

20.4 GENES AND FORMATION OF POLYPEPTIDE HORMONES

Genes for polypeptide hormones contain the information for the hormone and the control elements upstream of the transcriptionally active sequence. In some cases, more than one hormone is encoded in a gene. One example is **proopiomelanocortin,** a hormone precursor that encodes the following hormones: ACTH, β-lipotropin, and other hormones like γ-lipotropin, γ-MSH, α-MSH, CLIP, β-endorphin, and potentially β-MSH and enkephalins. In the case of the posterior pituitary hormones, oxytocin and vasopressin, information for these hormones are each encoded on a separate gene together with information for each respective **neurophysin,** a protein that binds to the completed hormone and stabilizes it.

Proopiomelanocortin Is a Precursor Polypeptide for Eight Hormones

Proopiomelanocortin, as schematized in Figure 20.5, can generate at least eight hormones from a single gene product. All products are not expressed simultaneously in a single cell type, but occur in separate cells based on their content of specific proteases required to cleave the propeptide, specific metabolic controls, and the presence of different positive regulators. Thus, while proopiomelanocortin is expressed in both the corticotropic cell of the anterior pituitary and the *pars intermedia* cell, the stimuli and products are different as summarized in Table 20.3. The *pars intermedia* is a discrete anatomical structure located between the anterior and posterior pituitary in the rat (Figure 20.6). In the human, however, the *pars intermedia* is not a discrete anatomical structure, although the cell type may be present in the equivalent location.

Many Polypeptide Hormones Are Encoded Together in a Single Gene

An example of another gene and gene products encoding more than one peptide are the genes for vasopressin and oxytocin and their accompanying neurophysin proteins, products that are released from the posterior pituitary upon specific stimulation. In much the same manner that ACTH and β-lipotropin

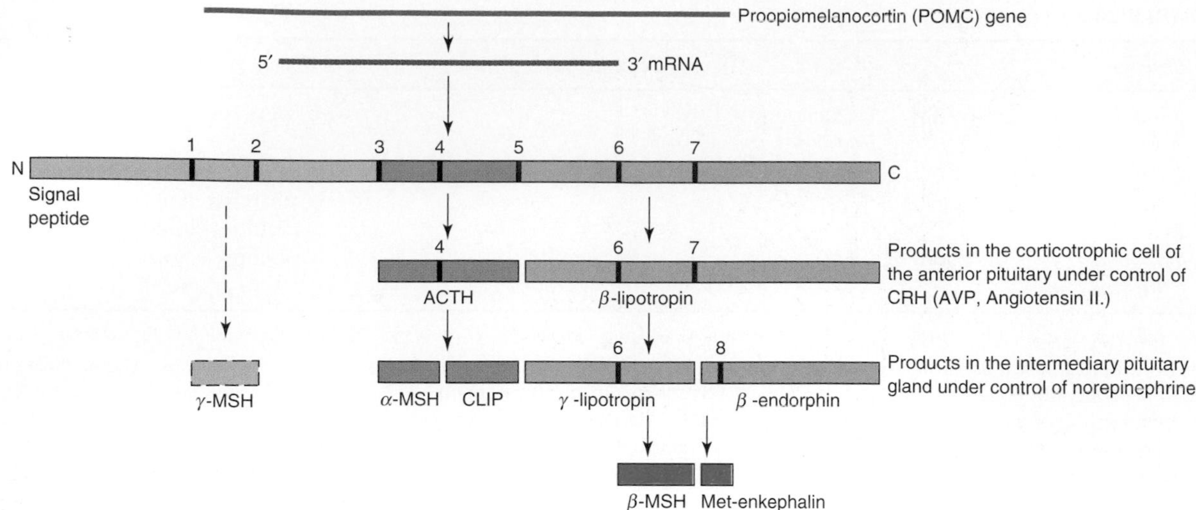

FIGURE 20.5
Proopiomelanocortin is a polypeptide product encoded by a single gene. The dark vertical bars represent proteolytic cleavage sites for specific enzymes. The cleavage sites are Arg-Lys, Lys-Arg, or Lys-Lys. Some specificity also may be conferred by neighboring amino acid residues. In the corticotropic cell of the anterior pituitary, enzymes are present that cleave at sites 3 and 5, releasing the major products, ACTH and β-lipotropin, into the general circulation. In the pars intermedia, especially in vertebrates below humans, these products are further cleaved at major sites 4, 6, and 7 to release α-MSH, CLIP, γ-lipotropin, and β-endorphin into the general circulation. Some β-lipotropin arising in the corticotroph may be further degraded to form β-endorphin. These two cell types appear to be under separate controls. The corticotropic cell of the anterior pituitary is under the positive control of the CRH and its auxiliary helpers, arginine vasopressin (AVP) and angiotensin II. AVP by itself does not release ACTH but enhances the action of CRH in this process. The products of the intermediary pituitary, α-MSH, CLIP (corticotropin-like intermediary peptide), γ-lipotropin, and β-endorphin, are under the positive control of norepinephrine, rather than CRH, for release. Obviously there must exist different proteases in these different cell types in order to generate a specific array of hormonal products. β-Endorphin also contains a pentapeptide, enkephalin, which potentially could be released at some point (hydrolysis at 8).

TABLE 20.3 Summary of Stimuli and Products of Proopiomelanocortin[a]

Cell type	Corticotroph	Pars intermedia
Stimulus	CRH (+) (Cortisol (−))	Dopamine (−) Norepinephrine (+)
Auxiliary stimulus	AVP, AII	
Major products	ACTH, β-lipotropin (β-endorphin)	α-MSH, CLIP, γ-lipotropin, β-endorphin

[a] CRH, corticotropin-releasing hormone; AVP, arginine vasopressin; AII, angiotensin II; ACTH, adrenocorticotropin; α-MSH, α melanocyte-stimulating hormone; CLIP, corticotropin-like intermediary peptide.

Note: Although there are pars intermedia cells in the human pituitary gland, they do not represent a distinct lobe.

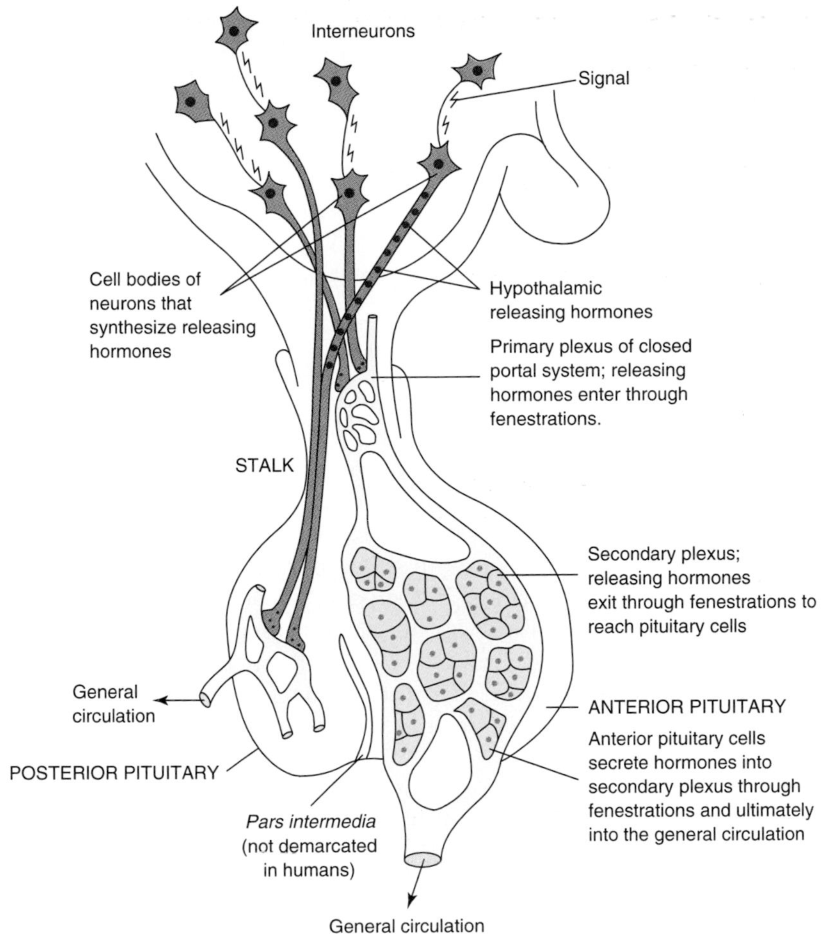

FIGURE 20.6
The hypothalamus with nuclei in various locations in which the hypothalamic releasing hormones are synthesized.
Shown is the major vascular network consisting of a primary plexus where releasing hormones enter its circulation through fenestrations and the secondary plexus in the anterior pituitary where the releasing hormones are transported out of the circulation, again through fenestrations in the vessels, to the region of the anterior pituitary target cells. Also shown are the resultant effects of the actions of the hypothalamic releasing hormones causing the secretion into the general circulation of the anterior pituitary hormones.
Adapted from Norman, A. W., and Litwack, G. Hormones. *New York: Academic Press, 1987, p. 104.*

(β-LPH) are split out of the proopiomelanocortin precursor peptide, so are the products vasopressin, neurophysin II, and a glycoprotein of as yet unknown function split out of the vasopressin precursor. A similar situation exists for oxytocin and neurophysin I (Figure 20.7).

Vasopressin and **neurophysin II** are released by the activity of baroreceptors and osmoreceptors, which sense a fall in blood pressure or a rise in extracellular sodium ion concentration, respectively. Generally, **oxytocin** and

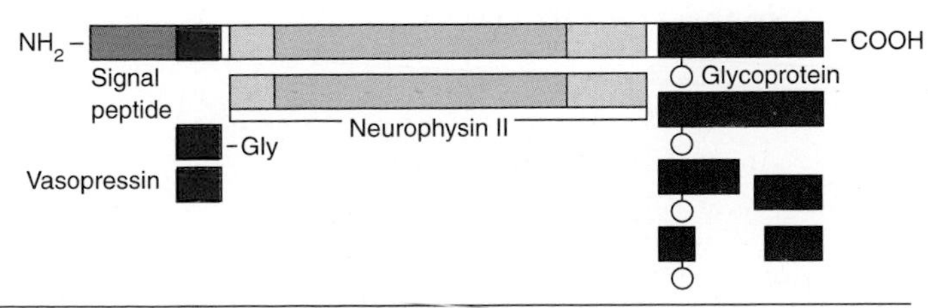

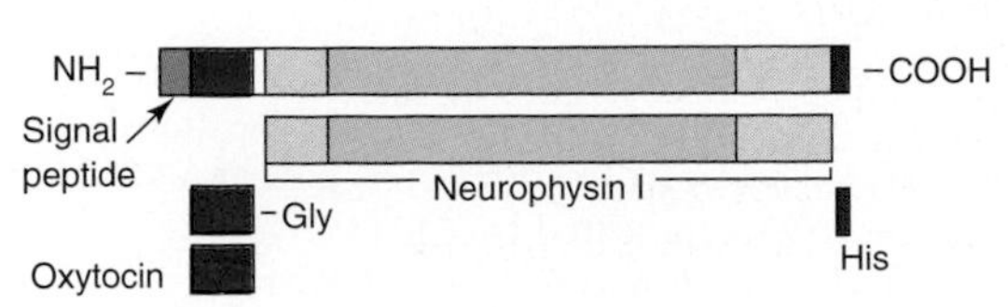

FIGURE 20.7
Prepro-vasopressin and prepro-oxytocin.
Proteolytic maturation proceeds from top to bottom for each precursor. The organization of the gene translation products is similar in either case except that a glycopeptide is included on the proprotein of vasopressin in the C-terminal region. Orange bars of the neurophysin represent conserved amino acid regions; gray bars represent variable C and N termini.
Redrawn with permission from Richter, D. VP and OT are expressed as polyproteins. Trends *Biochem. 8:278, 1983.*

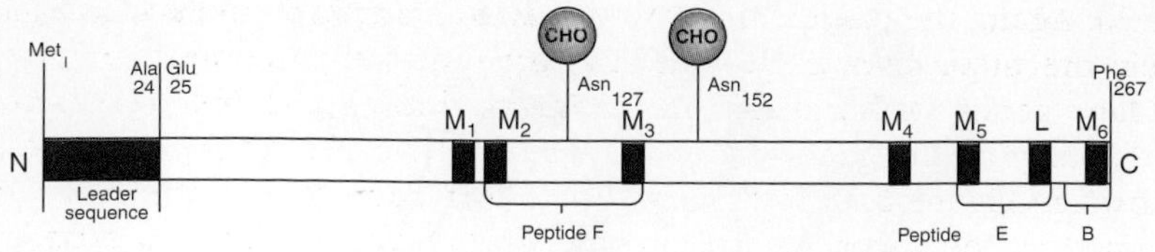

FIGURE 20.8
Model of enkephalin precursor.
The distribution of Met-enkephalin sequences (M_1–M_6) and Leu-enkephalin (L) sequences within the protein precursor of bovine adrenal medulla. CHO, potential carbohydrate attachment sites.
Redrawn from Comb, M., Seeburg, P. H., Adelman, J., Eiden, L., and Herbert, E. Nature *295:663, 1982.*

neurophysin I are released from the posterior pituitary by the suckling response in lactating females or by other stimuli mediated by a specific cholinergic mechanism. Oxytocin–neurophysin I release can be triggered by injection of estradiol. Release of vasopressin–neurophysin II can be stimulated by administration of nicotine. The two separate and specific releasing agents, estradiol and nicotine, prove that oxytocin and vasopressin, together with their respective neurophysins, are synthesized and released from different cell types. Although oxytocin is well known for its milk-releasing action in the lactating female, in the male it seems to have a separate role associated with an increase in testosterone synthesis in the testes.

Other polypeptide hormones are being discovered that are co-encoded together by a single gene. An example is the discovery of the gene encoding GnRH, a decapeptide that appears to reside to the left of a gene for the GnRH-associated peptide (GAP), which, like dopamine, may be capable of inhibiting prolactin release. Thus both hormones—GnRH and the prolactin release inhibiting factor GAP—appear to be co-secreted by the same hypothalamic cells.

Multiple Copies of a Hormone Can Be Encoded on a Single Gene

An example of multiple copies of a single hormone encoded on a single gene is the gene product for enkephalins located in the chromaffin cell of the adrenal medulla. **Enkephalins** are pentapeptides with opioid activity; methionine-enkephalin (Met-ENK) and leucine-enkephalin (Leu-ENK) have the structures:

Tyr-Gly-Gly-Phe-Met (Met-ENK)

Tyr-Gly-Gly-Phe-Leu (Leu-ENK)

A model of enkephalin precursor in adrenal medulla is presented in Figure 20.8, which encodes several Met-ENK (M) molecules and a molecule of Leu-

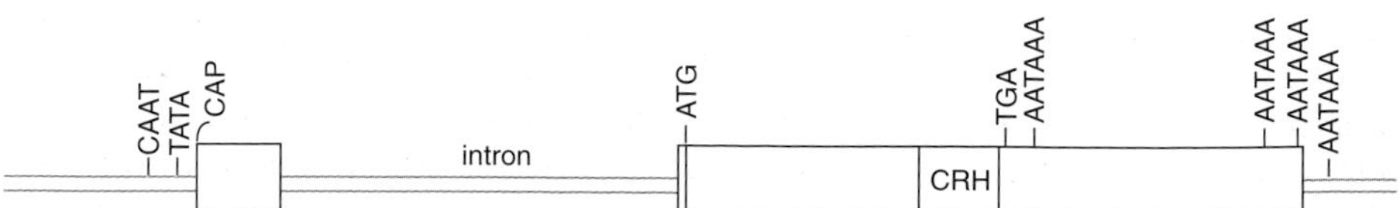

FIGURE 20.9
Nucleic acid sequence for rat *proCRH* genes.
Representation of the rat *proCRH* gene. Exons are shown as blocks and the intron by a double red line. The TATA and CAAT sequence, putative cap site, translation initiation ATG, translation terminator TGA, and poly(A) addition signals (AATAAA) are indicated. The location of the CRH peptide is indicated by CRH.
Redrawn from Thompson, R. D., Seasholz, A. F., and Herbert, E. Mol. Endocrinol. *1:363, 1987.*

ENK (L). Again, the processing sites to release enkephalin molecules from the protein precursor involve Lys–Arg, Arg–Arg, and Lys–Lys bonds.

Many genes for hormones are constructed to encode only one hormone and this may be the general situation. An example of a single hormone gene is shown in Figure 20.9. In this case the information for the hormone CRH is contained in the second exon and the information in the first exon is not expressed. Having cDNAs for use as probes that contain the information for expression of CRH allows for the localization of the hormone in tissues. Previously it was thought that the hormone should be restricted to the hypothalamus, the anterior pituitary, and the stalk, which contains the closed vascular transporting system (Figure 20.6). However, RNA extracts from different tissues probed with this DNA reveal the location of CRH mRNA in testis, brain stem, and adrenal gland in addition to pituitary and hypothalamus. The presence of the hormone in extrahypothalamic–pituitary axis tissues and its functions there are subjects of active investigation.

20.5 SYNTHESIS OF AMINO ACID-DERIVED HORMONES

Many hormones and neurotransmitters are derived from amino acids, principally from tyrosine and phenylalanine. Glutamate, aspartate, and other compounds are important neurotransmitter substances as well. Although there may be some confusion about which compounds are neurotransmitters and which are hormones, it is clear that epinephrine from the adrenal medulla is a hormone, whereas norepinephrine is a neurotransmitter. This section considers epinephrine and thyroxine or triiodothyronine. The other biogenic amines, such as dopamine, which are considered to be neurotransmitters, are discussed in Chapter 22.

Epinephrine Is Synthesized from Phenylalanine/Tyrosine

The synthesis of epinephrine occurs in the adrenal medulla. A number of steroid hormones, including aldosterone, cortisol, and dehydroepiandrosterone (sulfate), are produced in the adrenal cortex and are discussed in Chapter 21. The biochemical reactions leading to the formation of **epinephrine** from tyrosine or phenylalanine are presented in Figure 20.10. Epinephrine is a principal hormone secreted from the adrenal medulla chromaffin cell along with some norepinephrine, enkephalins, and some of the enzyme *dopamine-β-hydroxylase*. Secretion of epinephrine is signaled by the neural response to stress, which is transmitted to the adrenal medulla by way of a preganglionic acetylcholinergic neuron (Figure 20.11). Release of acetylcholine by the neuron increases the availability of intracellular calcium ion, which stimulates exocytosis and release of the material stored in the **chromaffin granules** (Figure 20.11*b*). This overall system of epinephrine synthesis, storage, and release from the adrenal medulla is regulated by neuronal controls and also by glucocorticoid hormones synthesized in and secreted from the adrenal cortex in response to stress. Since the products of the adrenal cortex are transported through the adrenal medulla on their way out to the general circulation, cortisol becomes elevated in the medulla and induces **phenylethanolamine *N*-methyltransferase (PNMT),** a key enzyme catalyzing the conversion of norepinephrine to epinephrine. Thus, in biochemical terms, the stress response at the level of the adrenal cortex ensures the production of epinephrine from the adrenal medulla (Figure 20.12). Presumably, epinephrine once secreted into the bloodstream not only affects α receptors of hepatocytes to ultimately increase blood glucose levels as indicated, but also interacts with α receptors on vascular smooth muscle cells and on pericytes to cause cellular contraction and increase blood pressure.

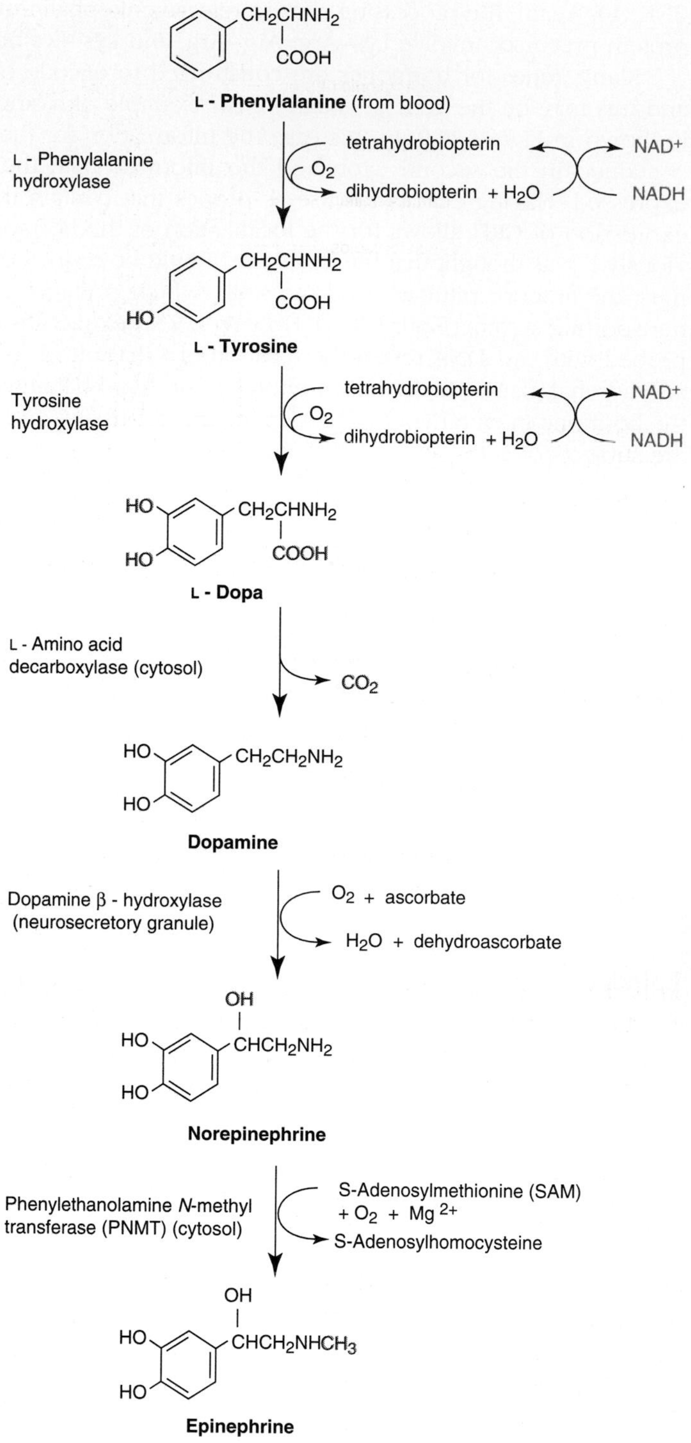

FIGURE 20.10
Biochemical steps in synthesis of epinephrine by chromaffin cell of adrenal medulla.

Synthesis of Thyroid Hormone Requires Incorporation of Iodine into a Tyrosine of Thyroglobulin

An outline of the biosynthesis and secretion of thyroid hormone, **tetraiodo-L-thyronine (T_4),** also called **thyroxine,** and its active cellular counterpart, **triiodo-L-thyronine (T_3)** (structures presented in Figure 20.13) is presented in Figure 20.14. The thyroid gland is differentiated to concentrate iodide from the blood and through the series of reactions shown in Figures 20.13 and 20.14, monoiodotyrosine (MIT), diiodotyrosine (DIT), T_4, and T_3 are produced within **thyroglobulin** (TG). Thus the iodinated amino acids and thyronines are stored in the thyroid follicle as part of thyroglobulin. Recent work indicates that there

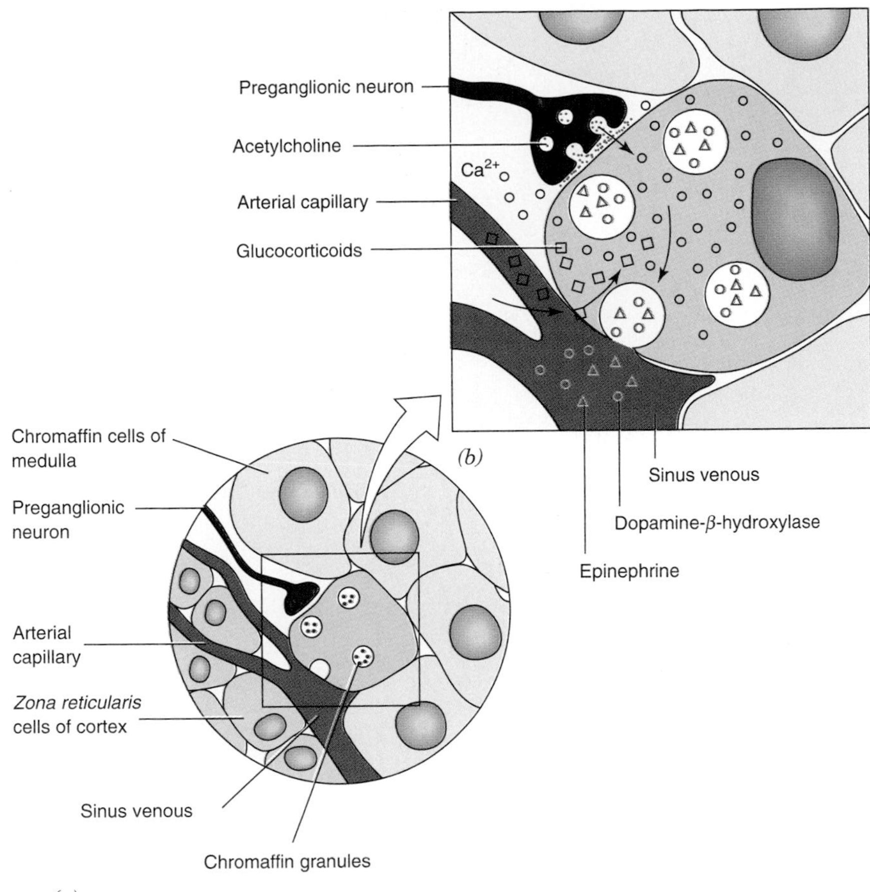

FIGURE 20.11
Relationship of adrenal medulla chromaffin cells to preganglionic neuron innervation and the structural elements involved in the synthesis of epinephrine and the discharge of catecholamines in response to acetylcholine.
(*a*) Functional relationship between cortex and medulla for control of synthesis of adrenal catecholamines. Glucocorticoids that stimulate enzymes catalyzing the conversion of norepinephrine to epinephrine reach the chromaffin cells from capillaries shown in (*b*). (*b*) Discharge of catecholamines from storage granules in chromaffin cells after nerve fiber stimulation, resulting in the release of acetylcholine. Calcium enters the cells as a result, causing the fusion of granular membranes with the plasma membrane and exocytosis of the contents.
Reprinted with permission from Krieger, D. T., and Hughes, J. C. (Eds.). Neuroendocrinology. *Sunderland, MA: Sinauer Associates, 1980.*

are hot spots (regions for very active iodination) in the thyroglobulin sequence for the incorporation of iodine. Apparently, the sequences around iodotyrosyls occur in three consensus groups: Glu/Asp-Tyr, associated with the synthesis of thyroxine or iodotyrosines; Ser/Thr-Tyr-Ser, associated with the synthesis of

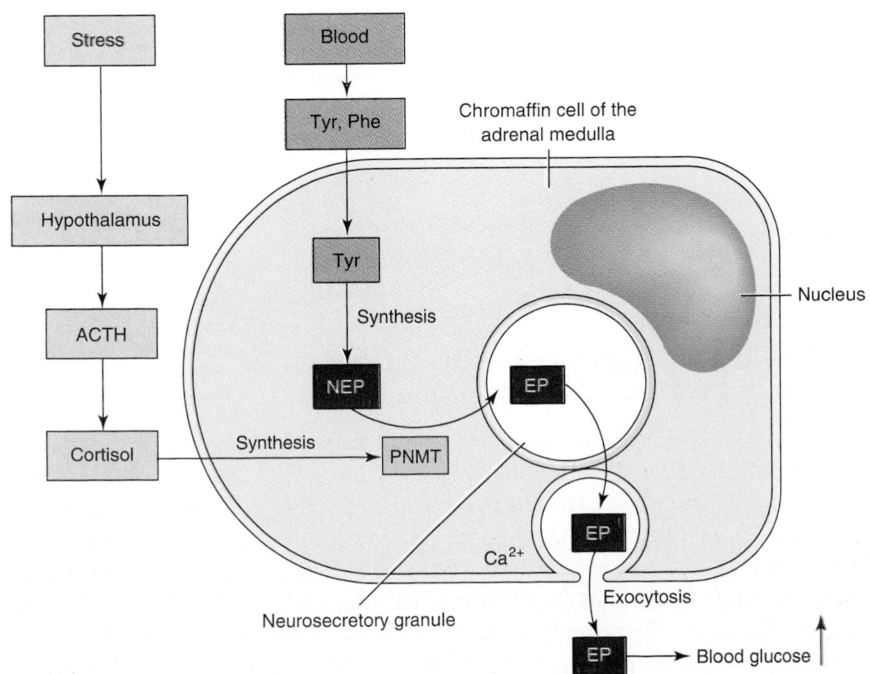

FIGURE 20.12
Biosynthesis, packaging, and release of epinephrine in the adrenal medulla chromaffin cell.
PNMT, phenylethanolamine *N*-methyltransferase; EP, epinephrine; NEP, norepinephrine. Neurosecretory granules contain epinephrine, dopamine β-hydroxylase, ATP, Met- or Leu-enkephalin, as well as larger enkephalin-containing peptides or norepinephrine in place of epinephrine. Epinephrine and norepinephrine are stored in different cells. Enkephalins could also be contained in separate cells, although that is not completely clear.
Adapted from Norman, A. W., and Litwack, G. Hormones. *New York: Academic Press, 1987, p. 464.*

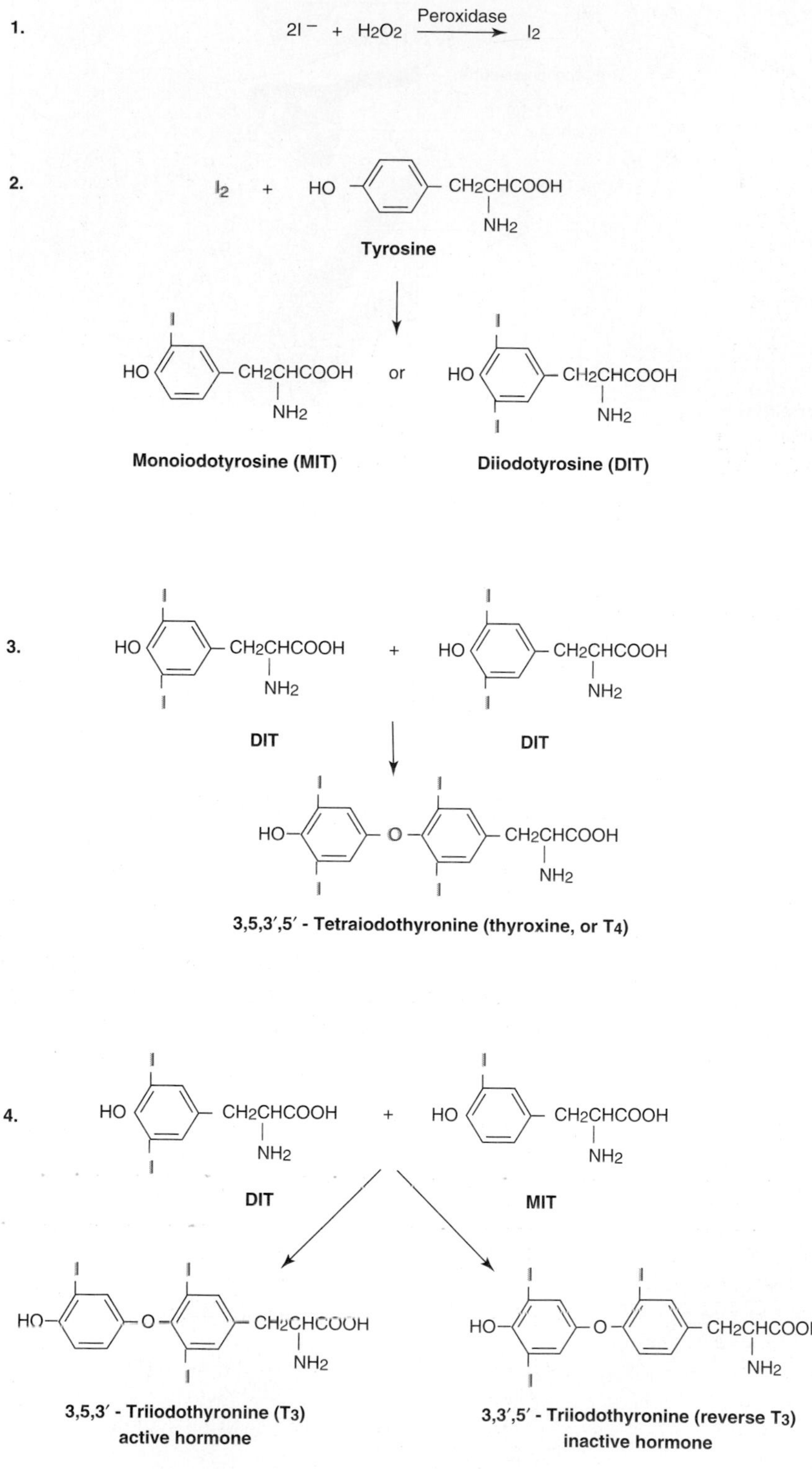

1. $2I^- + H_2O_2 \xrightarrow{\text{Peroxidase}} I_2$

2. I_2 + HO–(tyrosine ring)–$CH_2CHCOOH$ (NH_2)

Tyrosine

Monoiodotyrosine (MIT) or Diiodotyrosine (DIT)

3. DIT + DIT → 3,5,3′,5′ - Tetraiodothyronine (thyroxine, or T_4)

4. DIT + MIT → 3,5,3′ - Triiodothyronine (T_3) active hormone; 3,3′,5′ - Triiodothyronine (reverse T_3) inactive hormone

FIGURE 20.13
Synthesis and structures of thyroid hormones T_4, T_3, and reverse T_3.
Step 1, oxidation of iodide: Step 2, iodination of tyrosine residues; Step 3, coupling of DIT to DIT; Step 4, coupling of DIT to MIT (coupling may be intramolecular or intermolecular).

iodothyronine and iodotyrosine; and Glu-X-Tyr, associated with the remaining iodotyrosyls in the sequence. As depicted in Figure 20.14, secretion of T_3 and T_4 into the bloodstream requires endocytosis of the thyroglobulin stored in the follicle and subsequent proteolysis within the epithelial cell. The released DIT and MIT are then deiodinated and the released iodide ions are recycled and reutilized for hormone synthesis.

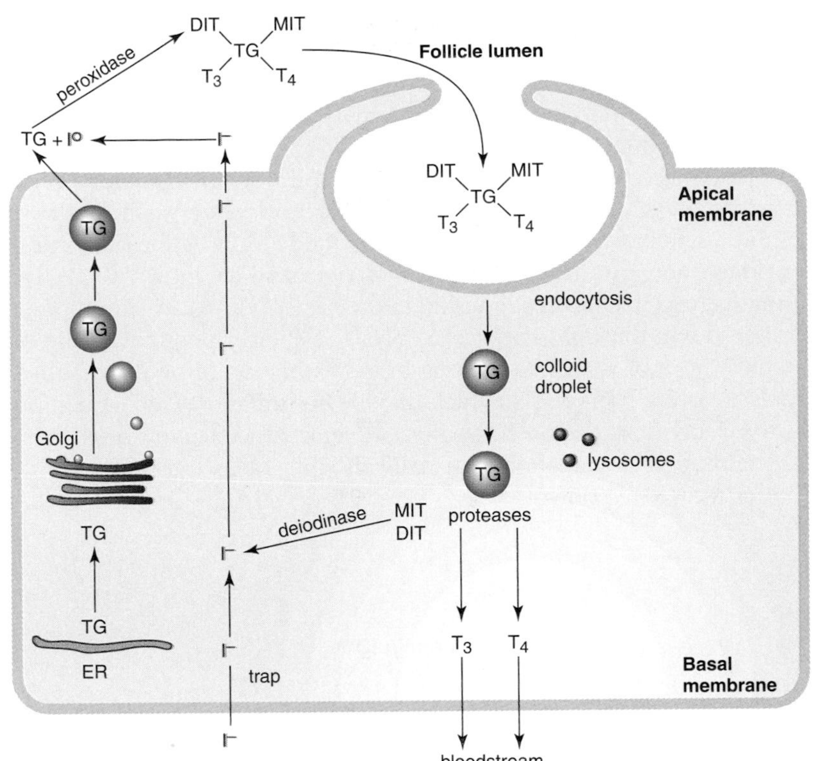

FIGURE 20.14
Cellular mechanisms for T_3 and T_4 release into the bloodstream.
Iodide trapping at basal membrane of thyroid epithelium concentrates iodide approximately 30-fold. Secretion of T_3 and T_4 into bloodstream requires endocytosis of thyroglobulin and subsequent proteolysis. DIT and MIT are deiodinated and the released iodide ions are reutilized for hormone synthesis.

20.6 INACTIVATION AND DEGRADATION OF HORMONES

Most polypeptide hormones are degraded to amino acids by hydrolysis, which presumably occurs in the **lysosome.** Partial hydrolysis by proteinases is a principal pathway for degradation. Certain hormones, however, contain modified amino acids; for example, among the hypothalamic releasing hormones, the N-terminal amino acid can be **cycloglutamic acid** (or pyroglutamic acid) (Table 20.4) and a C-terminal amino acid amide. Some of the releasing hormones

TABLE 20.4 Hypothalamic Releasing Hormones Containing an N-Terminal Pyroglutamate,[a] a C-Terminal Amino Acid Amide, or Both

Hormone	*Sequence*[b]
Thyrotropin-releasing hormone (TRH)	pGlu-H-Pro-NH_2
Gonadotropin-releasing hormone (GnRH)	pGlu-HWSYGLRP-Gly-NH_2
Corticotropin-releasing hormone (CRH)	SQEPPISLDLTFHLLREVLEMTKADQLAQQAHSNRKLLDI-Ala-NH_2
Somatocrinin (GRH)	YADAIFTNSYRKVLGQLSARKLLQDIMSRQQGESNQERG-ARAR-Leu-NH_2

[a] The pyroglutamate structure is

$$\text{pyroglutamyl ring (}H_2C\text{–}CH_2\text{, }O{=}C\text{–}NH\text{–}CH\text{)}\text{–}C(=O)\text{--->Peptide}$$

[b] Single-letter abbreviations used for amino acids: Ala, A; Arg, R; Asn, N; Asp, D; Cys, C; Glu, E, Gln, Q; Gly, G; His, H; Ile, I; Leu, L; Lys, K; Met, M; Phe, F; Pro, P; Ser, S; Thr, T; Trp, W; Tyr, Y; Val, V.

TABLE 20.5 Examples of Hormones Containing a Cystine Disulfide Bridge Structure

Hormone	*Sequence*[a]
Somatostatin (GH)	FFNKCGA[1] / W—K / S—S / TFTSC[14] (ring: A[1]…C[14] joined by S—S)
Oxytocin	YC[1] / I—E / S—S / NCPLG—NH_2
Arginine vasopressin	YC / F—Q / S—S / NCPRG—NH_2

[a] Letters refer to single-letter amino acid abbreviations (see Table 20.4)

that have either or both of these amino acid derivatives are listed in Table 20.4. Apparently, breakage of the cyclic glutamate ring or cleavage of the C-terminal amide can lead to inactivation of many of these hormones and such enzymic activities have been reported in blood. This activity probably accounts, in part, for the short half-life of many of these hormones.

Some hormones contain a ring structure joined by a cystine disulfide bond. A few examples are given in Table 20.5. Peptide hormones, such as those shown in Table 20.5, may be degraded initially by the random action of **cystine aminopeptidase** and **glutathione transhydrogenase** as shown in Figure 20.15. Alternatively, as has been suggested in the case of oxytocin, the peptide may be broken down through partial proteolysis to shorter peptides, some of which may have hormonal actions on their own. Maturation of **prohormones** in many cases involves proteolysis, which may be considered as a degradation process in the sense that the prohormone is degraded to active forms (e.g., Figure 20.5), although degradation is usually thought of as the reduction of active peptides to inactive ones.

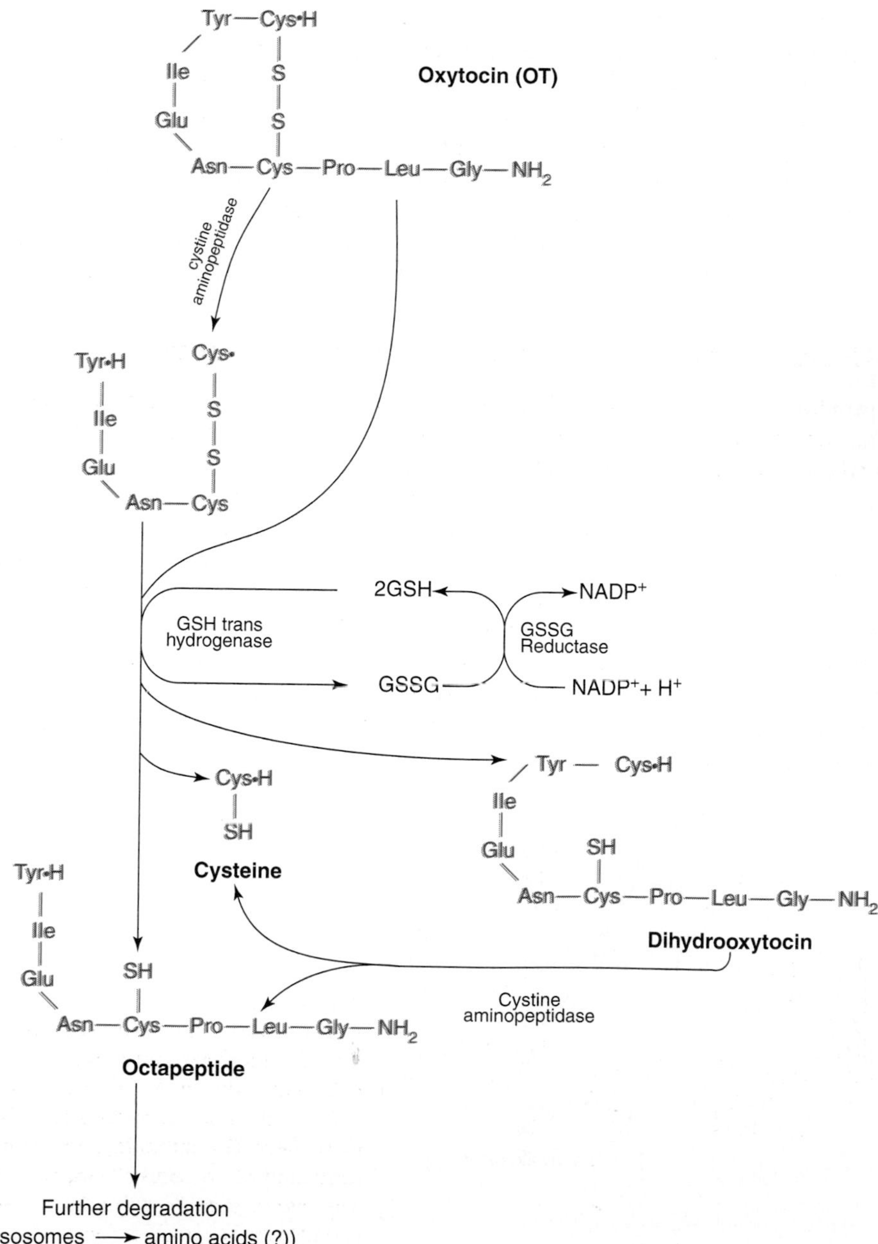

FIGURE 20.15
Degradation of posterior pituitary hormones.
Oxytocin transhydrogenase is similar to degrading enzymes for insulin; presumably, these enzymes also degrade vasopressin. *Redrawn from Norman, A. W., and Litwack, G.* Hormones. *New York: Academic Press, 1987, p. 167.*

20.7 ■ CELL REGULATION AND HORMONE SECRETION

Hormonal secretion is under specific control. In the cascade system displayed in Figures 20.2 and 20.3, hormones must emanate from one source, cause hormonal release from the next cell type in line, and so on, down the cascade system. The correct responses must follow from a specific stimulus. The precision of these signals is defined by the hormone and the receptor as well as by the activities of the CNS, which precedes the first hormonal response in many cases. Certain generalizations can be made. Polypeptide hormones generally bind to their cognate receptors located in cell membranes. The receptor recognizes structural features of the hormone to generate a high degree of specificity and affinity. The affinity constants for these interactions are in the range of 10^9–10^{11} M^{-1}, representing tight binding. This interaction usually activates or complexes with a transducing protein in the membrane, such as a **G-protein** (GTP-binding protein), or other transducer and causes an activation of some enzymatic function on the cytoplasmic side of the membrane. In some cases receptors undergo **internalization** to the cell interior; these receptors may or may not (e.g., the insulin receptor) be coupled to transducing proteins in the cell membrane. A discussion of internalization of receptors is presented in Section 20.11. The "activated" receptor complex could physically open a membrane ion channel or have other profound impacts on membrane structure and function. For example, binding of the hormone to the receptor may cause conformational changes in the receptor molecule, enabling it to associate with transducer in which further conformational changes may occur to permit interaction with an enzyme on the cytoplasmic side of the plasma membrane. This interaction may cause conformational changes in an enzyme so that its catalytic site becomes active.

G-Proteins Serve as Cellular Transducers of Hormone Signals

Most transducers of receptors in the plasma membrane are GTP-binding proteins and are referred to as **G-proteins.** G-Proteins consist of three types of **subunits—α, β, and γ.** The **α subunit** is the guanine nucleotide-binding component and is thought to interact with the receptor indirectly through the β and γ subunits and then directly with an enzyme, such as adenylate cyclase, resulting in enzyme activation. Actually there are two forms of the α subunit, designated α_s for a stimulatory subunit and α_i for an inhibitory subunit. Two types of receptors, and thus hormones, control the adenylate cyclase reaction: hormone–receptors that lead to a stimulation of the adenylate cyclase and those that lead to an inhibition of the cyclase. This is depicted in Figure 20.16 with an indication of the role of α_s and α_i and some of the hormones that interact with the stimulatory and inhibitory receptors.

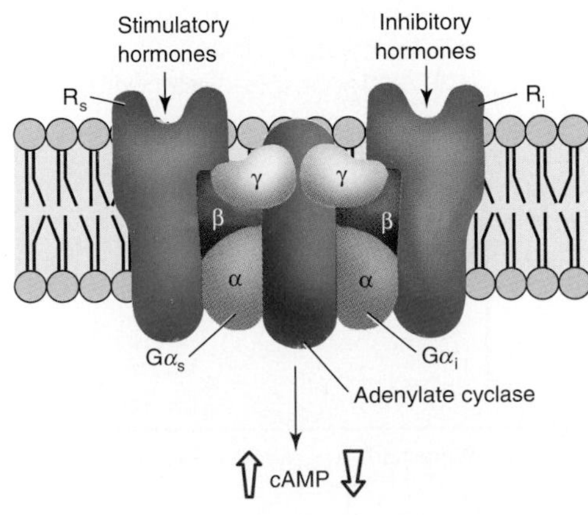

FIGURE 20.16
Components that constitute a hormone-sensitive adenylate cyclase system and the subunit composition.
Adenylate cyclase is responsible for conversion of ATP to cAMP. The occupancy of R_s by stimulatory hormones stimulates adenylate cyclase via formation of an active dissociated $G\alpha_s$ subunit. The occupancy of R_i by inhibitory hormones results in the formation of an "active" $G\alpha_i$ complex and concomitant reduction in cyclase activity. The fate of β and γ subunits in these dissociation reactions is not yet known. R_s, stimulatory hormone receptor; R_i, inhibitory hormone receptor.

The sequence of events that occurs when hormone and receptor interact is presented in Figure 20.17 and is as follows: receptor binds hormone in the membrane (Step 1); which produces a conformational change in receptor to expose a site for G-protein (β, γ subunit) attachment (Step 2); G-protein can be either stimulatory, G_s, or inhibitory, G_i, referring to the ultimate effects on the activity of adenylate cyclase; the receptor interacts with β, γ subunit of G-protein, enabling the α subunit to exchange GTP for bound GDP (Step 3); dissociation of GDP causes separation of G-protein α subunit from β, γ subunit and the α-binding site for interaction with adenylate cyclase appears on the surface of the G-protein α subunit (Step 4); α subunit binds to adenylate cyclase and activates the catalytic center, so that ATP is converted to cAMP (Step 5); GTP is hydrolyzed to GDP by the GTPase activity of the α subunit, returning it to its original conformation and allowing its interaction with β, γ subunit once again (Step 6); GDP associates with the α subunit and the system is returned to the unstimulated state awaiting another cycle of activity. It is important to note that there is also evidence suggesting that the β,γ complexes may play important roles in regulating certain effectors including adenylate cyclase.

In the case where an inhibitory G-protein is coupled to the receptor, the events are similar but inhibition of adenylate cyclase activity may arise by direct interaction of the inhibitory α subunit with adenylate cyclase or, alternatively, the inhibitory α subunit may interact directly with the stimulatory α subunit on the other side and prevent the stimulation of adenylate cyclase activity indirectly. Immunochemical evidence suggests multiple G_i subtypes and molecular cloning of complementary DNAs encoding putative α subunits has also provided evidence for multiple α_i subtypes.

Purification and biochemical characterization of G-proteins (G_s as well as G_i) have revealed somewhat unanticipated diversity in this subfamily. Polymerase chain reaction-based cloning has now brought the number of distinct genes encoding mammalian α subunits to at least 15. With regard to α subunits, further diversity is achieved by alternative splicing of the α_s (four forms) gene. There also appears to be diversity among the mammalian β and γ subunits. At least four distinct β subunit cDNAs and probably as many γ subunits have been described. What is not clear is how these complexes combine to form distinct β,γ complexes. Some data suggest that different β,γ complexes may have distinct properties with respect to α subunit and receptor interactions, but additional research will be required to fully describe these unique interactions.

Table 20.6 lists some activities transduced by G-protein subfamilies.

TABLE 20.6 Activities Transduced by G-Protein Subfamilies

α Subunit	*Expression*	*Effector*
G_s	Ubiquitous	↑ Adenylate cyclase, Ca^{2+} channel
G_{olf}	Olfactory	↑ Adenylate cyclase
G_{+1} (transducin)	Rod photoreceptors	↑ cGMP-phosphodiesterase
G_{+2} (transducin)	Cone photoreceptors	↑ cGMP-phosphodiesterase
G_{i1}	Neural > other tissues	↓ Adenylate cyclase
G_{i2}	Ubiquitous	
G_{i3}	Other tissues > neural	
G_o	Neural, endocrine	↓ Ca^{2+} channel
G_q	Ubiquitous	↑ Phospholipase C
G_{11}	Ubiquitous	
G_{14}	Liver, lung, kidney	
$G_{15/16}$	Blood cells	

Source: Adapted from Spiegel, A. M., Shenker, A., and Weinstein, L. S. *Endocr. Rev.* 13:536, 1992.

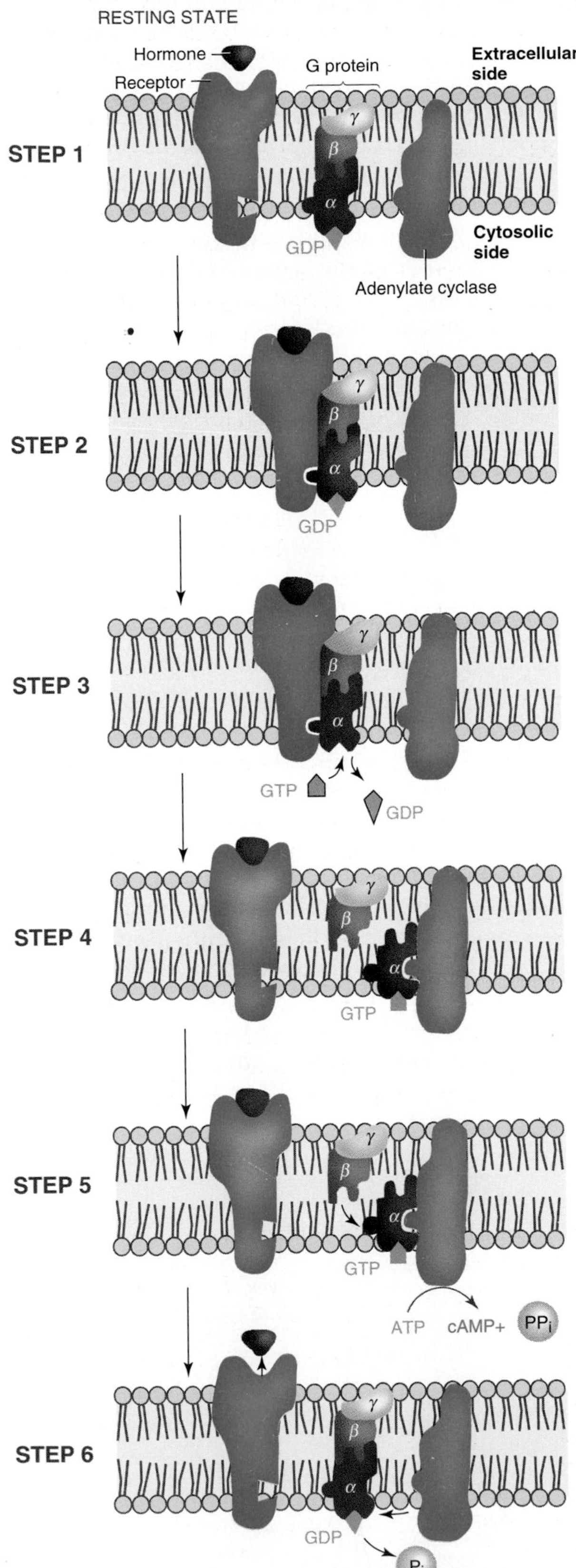

FIGURE 20.17

Activation of adenylate cyclase by binding of a hormone to its receptor.

The cell membrane is depicted, which contains on its outer surface a receptor protein for a hormone. On the inside surface of the membrane is adenylate cyclase protein and the transducer protein G. In the resting state GDP is bound to the α subunit of the G-protein. When a hormone binds to the receptor, a conformational change occurs (Step 1). The activated receptor binds to the G-protein (Step 2), which activates the latter so that it releases GDP and binds GTP (Step 3), causing the α and the complex of β and γ subunits to dissociate (Step 4). Free G_α subunit binds to the adenylate cyclase and activates it so that it catalyzes the synthesis of cAMP from ATP (Step 5); this step may involve a conformational change in G_α. In some cases the β,γ complex may play an important role in regulation of certain effectors including adenylate cyclase. When GTP is hydrolyzed to GDP, a reaction most likely catalyzed by G_α itself, G_α is no longer able to activate adenylate cyclase (Step 6), and G_α and $G_{\beta\gamma}$ reassociate. The hormone dissociates from the receptor and the system returns to its resting state.
Redrawn from Darnell, J., Lodish, H., and Baltimore, D. Molecular Cell Biology. *New York: Scientific American Books, 1986, p. 682.*

Cyclic AMP Activates Protein Kinase A Pathway

The generation of cAMP in the cell usually activates protein kinase A, referred to as the **protein kinase A pathway.** The overall pathway is presented in Figure 20.18. Four cAMP molecules are used in the reaction to complex two regulatory subunits (R) and liberating two protein kinase catalytic subunits (C). The liberated catalytic subunits are able to phosphorylate proteins to produce a cellular effect. In many cases the cellular effect leads to the release of preformed hormones. For example, ACTH binds to membrane receptors, elevates intracellular **cAMP** levels, and releases cortisol from the *zona fasciculata* cells of the adrenal gland by this general mechanism. Part of the mechanism of release of thyroid hormones from the thyroid gland involves the cAMP pathway as outlined in Figure 20.19. TSH has been shown to stimulate numerous key steps in this secretory process, including iodide uptake and endocytosis of thyroglobulin (Figure 20.14). The protein kinase A pathway is also responsible for the release of testosterone by testicular Leydig cells as presented in Figure 20.20. There are many other examples of hormonal actions mediated by cAMP and the protein kinase A pathway.

Inositol Triphosphate Formation Leads to Release of Calcium from Intracellular Stores

Uptake of calcium from the cell exterior through calcium channels may be affected directly by hormone–receptor interaction at the cell membrane. In some cases, ligand–receptor interaction is thought to open calcium channels directly in the cell membrane (Chapter 5, Section 5.5). Another system to increase intracellular Ca^{2+} concentration derives from hormone–receptor activation of **phospholipase C** activity transduced by a G-protein (Figure 20.21).

A hormone operating through this system binds to a specific cell membrane receptor, which interacts with a G-protein in a mechanism similar to that of the protein kinase A pathway and transduces the signal, resulting in stimulation of phospholipase C. This enzyme catalyzes the hydrolysis of **phosphatidylinositol-4,5-bisphosphate** (PIP_2) to form two **second messengers, diacylglycerol (DAG)** and **inositol 1,4,5-triphosphate (IP_3).**

Inositol 1,4,5-triphosphate diffuses to the cytosol and binds to an IP_3 receptor on the membrane of a particulate **calcium** store, either separate from or

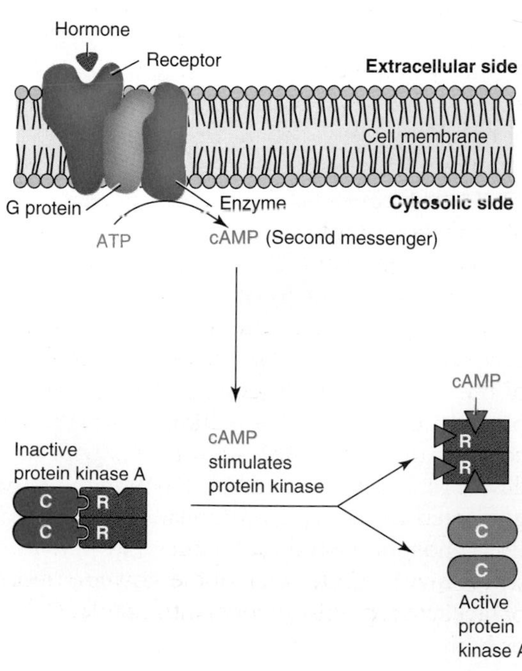

FIGURE 20.18
Activation of protein kinase A.
Hormone–receptor mediated stimulation of adenylate cyclase and subsequent activation of protein kinase A. C, catalytic subunit; R, regulatory subunit.

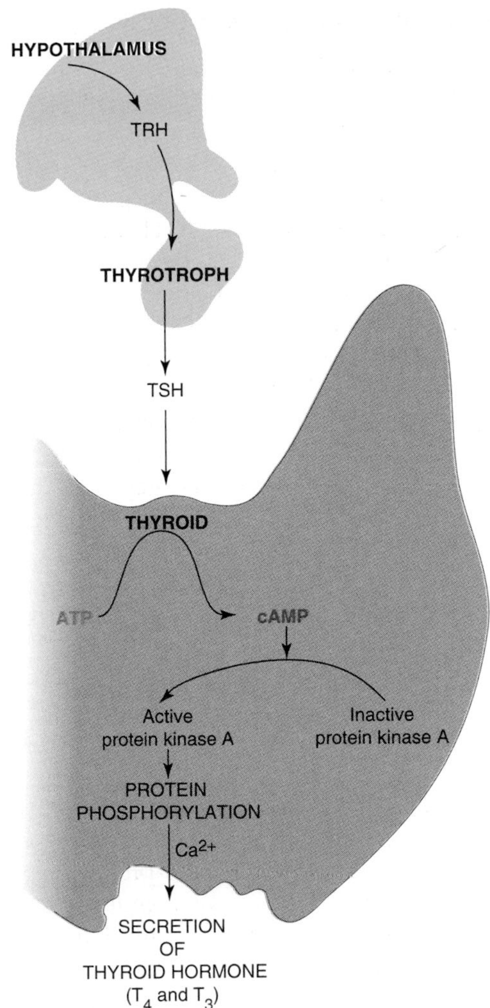

FIGURE 20.19
Overview of secretion controls of thyroid hormone.

part of the endoplasmic reticulum. IP_3 binding results in the release of calcium ions contributing to the large increase in cytosolic Ca^{2+} levels. Calcium ions may be important to the process of exocytosis by taking part in the fusion of secretory granules to the internal cell membrane, in microtubular aggregation or in the function of contractile proteins, which may be part of the structure of the exocytotic mechanism, or all of these.

The IP_3 is metabolized by stepwise removal of phosphate groups (Figure 20.21) to form inositol. This combines with phosphatidic acid (PA) to form phosphatidylinositol (PI) in the cell membrane. PI is phosphorylated twice by a kinase to form PIP_2, which is ready to undergo another round of hydrolysis and formation of second messengers (DAG and IP_3) upon hormonal stimulation. If the receptor is still occupied by hormone, several rounds of the cycle could occur before the hormone–receptor complex dissociates or some other feature of the cycle becomes limiting. It is interesting that the conversion of inositol phosphate to inositol is inhibited by **lithium ion** (Li^+) (Figure 20.21). This could be the metabolic basis for the beneficial effects of Li^+ in manic–depressive illness (see Clin. Corr. 20.3). Finally, it is important to note that not all of the generated IP_3 is dephosphorylated during hormonal stimulation. Some of the IP_3 is phosphorylated via IP_3 kinase to yield inositol 1,3,4,5-tetraphosphate (IP_4), which may mediate some of the slower or more prolonged hormonal responses or facilitate replenishment of intracellular Ca^{2+} stores from the extracellular fluid, or both.

CLINICAL CORRELATION 20.3

Lithium Treatment of Manic–Depressive Illness: The Phosphatidylinositol Cycle

Lithium has been used for years in the treatment of manic depression. Our newer knowledge suggests that lithium therapy involves the phosphatidylinositol (PI) pathway. This pathway generates the second messengers inositol 1,4,5-triphosphate (IP_3) and diacylglycerol following the hormone/neurotransmitter–membrane receptor interaction and involves the G-protein complex and activation of phospholipase C. IP_3 and its many phosphorylated derivatives are ultimately dephosphorylated in a stepwise fashion to generate free inositol. Inositol is then used for the synthesis of phosphatidylinositol monophosphate. The phosphatase that dephosphorylates IP to inositol is inhibited by Li^+. In addition, Li^+ may also interfere directly with G-protein function. The result of Li^+ inhibition is that the PI cycle is greatly slowed even in the face of continued hormonal/neurotransmitter stimulation and the cell becomes less sensitive to these stimuli. Manic–depressive illness may occur through the overactivity of certain CNS cells, perhaps as a result of abnormally high levels of hormones or neurotransmitters whose actions are to stimulate the PI cycle. The chemotherapeutic effect of the Li^+ could be to decrease the cellular responsiveness to elevated levels of agents that might promote high levels of PI cycle and precipitate manic–depressive illness.

Avissar, S., and Schreiber, G. Muscarinic receptor subclassification and G-proteins: significance for lithium action in affective disorders and for the treatment of the extrapyramidal side effects of neuroleptics. *Biol. Psychiatry* 26:113, 1989; Hallcher, L. M., and Sherman, W. R. The effects of lithium ion and other agents on the activity of myoinositol 1-phosphatase from bovine brain. *J. Biol. Chem.* 255:896, 1980; and Pollack, S. J., Atack, J. R., Knowles, M. R., McAllister, G., Ragan, C. I., Baker, R., Fletcher, S. R., Iversen, L. L., and Broughton, H. B. Mechanism of inositol monophosphatase, the putative target of lithium therapy. *Proc. Natl. Acad. Sci. USA* 91:5766, 1994.

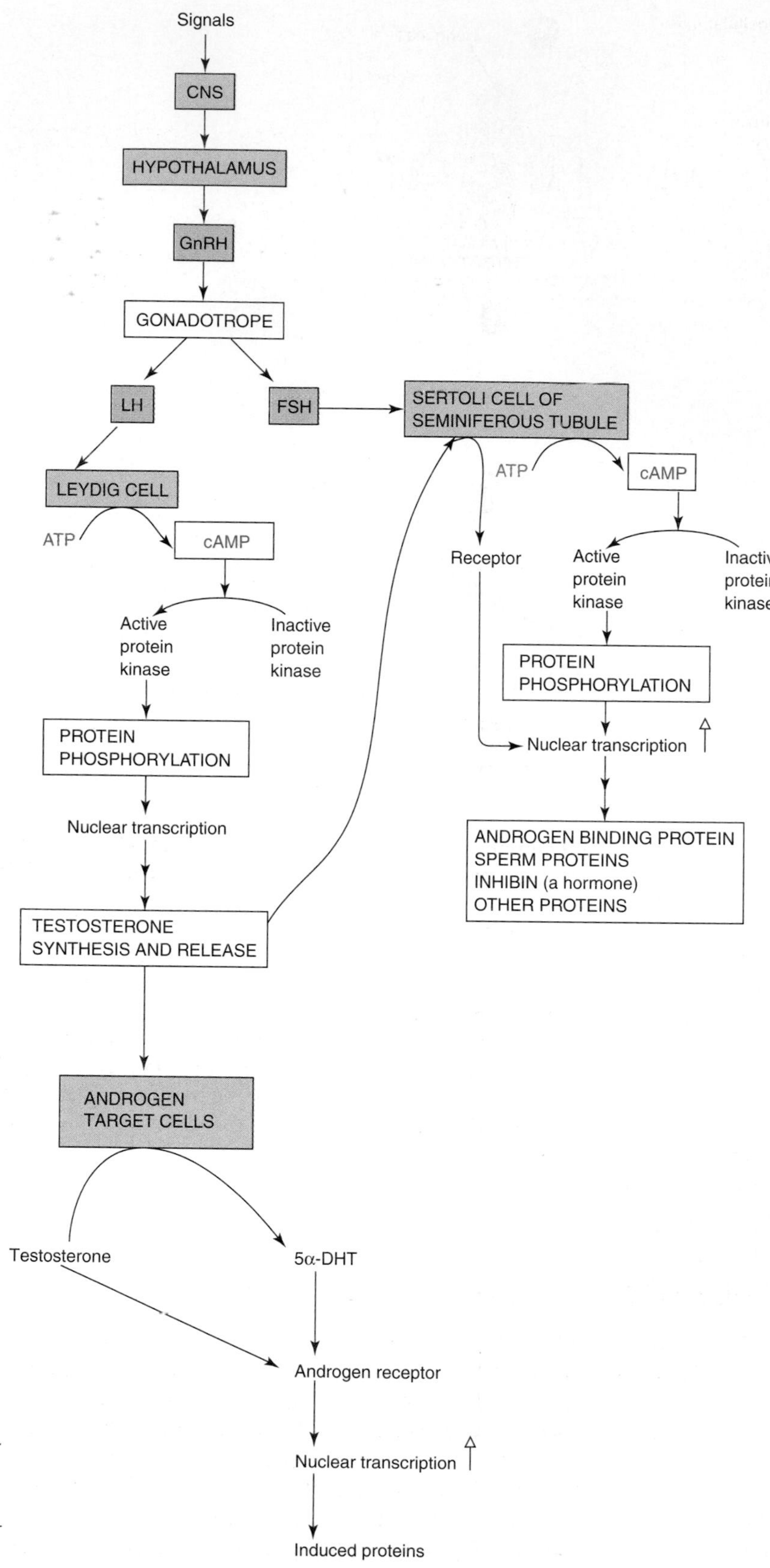

FIGURE 20.20
Overview of the secretion controls and some general actions of the gonadotropes and testosterone release in males.
In some, but not all, androgen target cells, testosterone is reduced to the more potent androgen, 5α- dihydrotestosterone (5α-DHT).

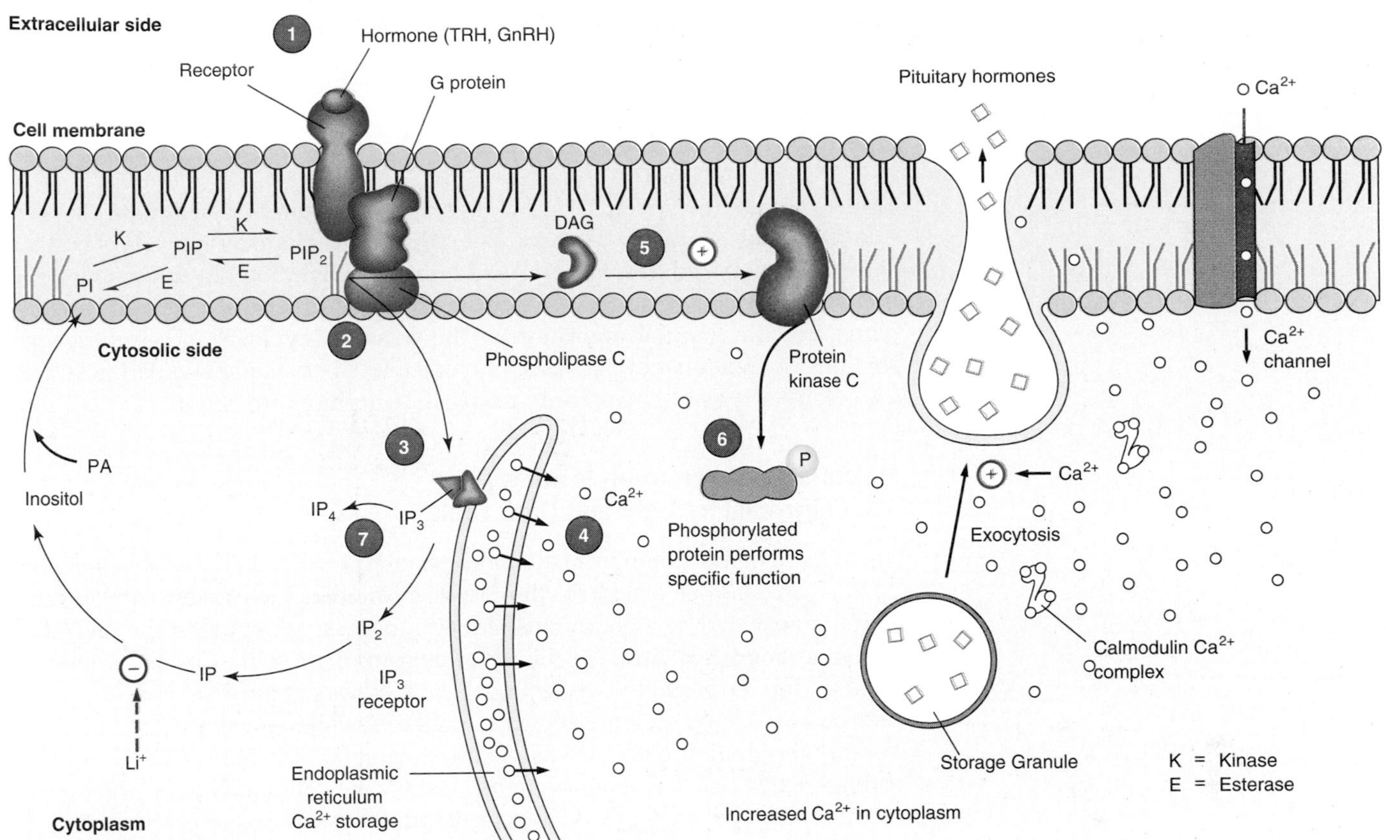

FIGURE 20.21
Overview of hormonal signaling through the phosphatidylinositol system generating the second messengers, inositol 1,4,5-trisphosphate (IP_3) and diacylglycerol (DAG).
The action of IP_3 is to increase cytosol Ca^{2+} levels by a receptor-mediated event in the cellular calcium store. Steps in pathway: (1) binding of hormone to cell membrane receptor; (2) production of IP_3 from PIP_2; (3) binding of IP_3 to receptor on calcium storage site; (4) release of free calcium to the cytosol; (5) release of DAG and subsequent binding to protein kinase C; (6) phosphorylation of protein substrates by protein kinase C activated by DAG and Ca^{2+}; and (7) phosphorylation of IP_3 to yield IP_4. DAG, diacylglycerol; PA, phosphatidic acid; IP, inositol phosphate; IP_2, inositol bisphosphate; IP_3, inositol 1,4,5-triphosphate; IP_4, inositol 1,3,4,5-tetrakisphosphate; PIP, phosphatidylinositol phosphate; PIP_2, phosphatidylinositol 4,5-bisphosphate; K, kinase; E, esterase.

Diacylglycerol Activates Protein Kinase C Pathway

At the same time that the IP_3 produced by hydrolysis of PIP_2 is increasing the concentration of Ca^{2+} in the cytosol, the other cleavage product, DAG, mediates different effects. Importantly, DAG activates a crucial serine/threonine protein kinase called **protein kinase C** because it is Ca^{2+} dependent (details of protein kinase C discussed on p. 883). The initial rise in cytosolic Ca^{2+} induced by IP_3 is believed to somehow alter kinase C so that it translocates from the cytosol to the cytoplasmic face of the plasma membrane. Once translocated, it is activated by a combination of Ca^{2+}, DAG, and the negatively charged membrane phospholipid, phosphatidylserine. Once activated, protein kinase C then phosphorylates specific proteins in the cytosol or, in some cases, in the plasma membrane. These phosphorylated proteins perform specific functions that they could not mediate in their nonphosphorylated states. For example, a phosphorylated protein could potentially migrate to the nucleus and stimulate mitosis and growth. It is also possible that a phosphorylated protein could play a role in the secretion of preformed hormones.

20.8 ■ CYCLIC HORMONAL CASCADE SYSTEMS

Hormonal cascade systems can be generated by external signals as well as by internal signals. Examples of this are the **diurnal variations** in levels of cortisol secreted from the adrenal gland probably initiated by serotonin and vasopressin, the day and night variations in the secretion of **melatonin** from the pineal gland and the internal regulation of the **ovarian cycle.** Some of these biorhythms operate on a cyclic basis, often dictated by daylight and darkness, and are referred to as **chronotropic control** of hormone secretion.

Melatonin and Serotonin Synthesis Are Controlled by Light and Dark Cycles

The release of melatonin from the pineal gland, presented in overview in Figure 20.22, is an example of a biorhythm. Here, as in other such systems, the internal signal is provided by a neurotransmitter, in this case norepinephrine produced by an adrenergic neuron. In this system, control is exerted by light entering the eyes and is transmitted to the pineal gland by way of the CNS. The adrenergic neuron innervating the pinealocyte is inhibited by light transmitted through the eyes. Norepinephrine released as a neurotransmitter in the dark stimulates cAMP formation through a β receptor in the pinealocyte cell membrane, which leads to the enhanced synthesis of ***N*-acetyltransferase.** The increased activity of this enzyme causes the conversion of **serotonin** to ***N*-acetylserotonin,** and **hydroxyindole-*O*-methyltransferase (HIOMT)** then catalyzes the conversion of *N*-acetylserotonin to **melatonin,** which is secreted in the dark hours but not during light hours. Melatonin is circulated to cells containing receptors that generate effects on reproductive and other functions. For example, melatonin has been shown to exert an antigonadotropic effect, although the physiological significance of this effect is unclear.

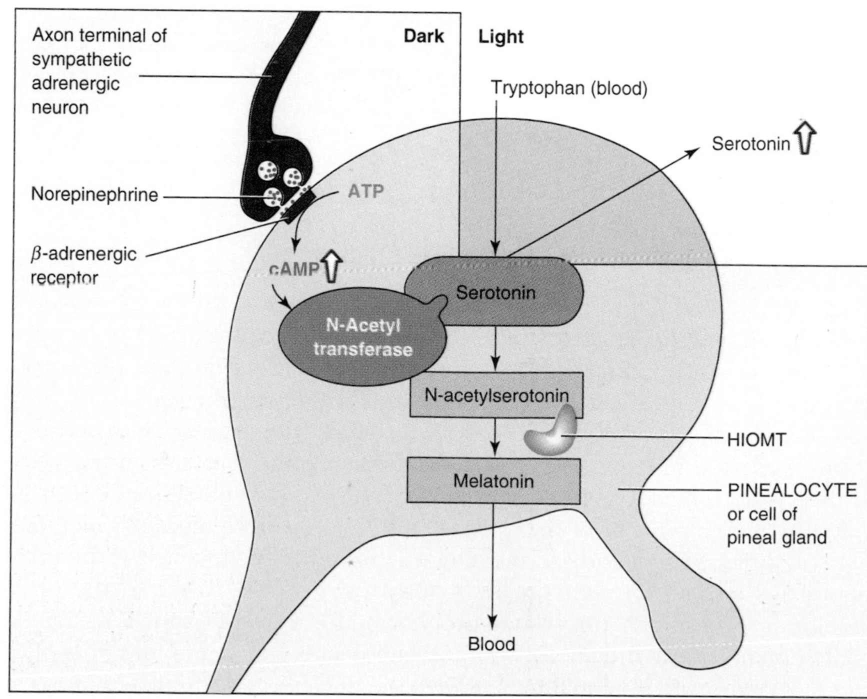

FIGURE 20.22
Biosynthesis of melatonin in pinealocytes. HIOMT, hydroxyindole-*O*-methyltransferase. *Redrawn from Norman, A. W., and Litwack, G.* Hormones. *New York: Academic Press, 1987, p. 710.*

Ovarian Cycle Is Controlled by Gonadotropin-Releasing Hormone

An example of a pulsatile release mechanism is regulation of the periodic release of GnRH. A periodic control regulates the release of this substance at definitive periods (of about 1 h in higher animals) and is controlled by aminergic neurons, which may be adrenergic (norepinephrine secreting) in nature. The initiation of this function occurs at puberty and is important in both the male and female. While the male system functions continually, the female system is periodic and known as the **ovarian cycle.** This system is presented in Figure 20.23. In the

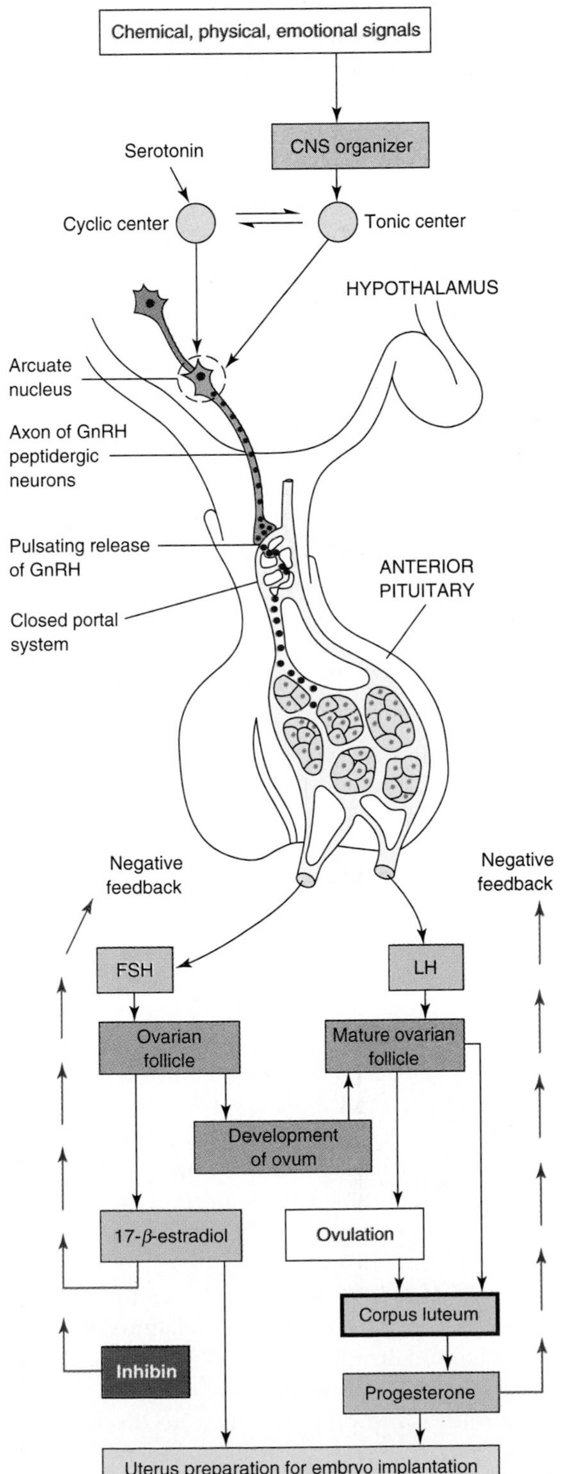

FIGURE 20.23
Ovarian cycle in terms of generation of hypothalamic hormone, pituitary gonadotropic hormones, and sex hormones.
To begin the cycle at puberty, several centers in the CNS coordinate with the hypothalamus so that hypothalamic GnRH can be released in a pulsatile fashion. This causes the release of the gonadotropic hormones, LH and FSH, which in turn affect the ovarian follicle, ovulation, and the corpus luteum. The hormone inhibin selectively inhibits FSH secretion. Products of the follicle and corpus luteum, respectively, are β-estradiol and progesterone. GnRH, gonadotropin-releasing hormone; FSH, follicle-stimulating hormone; LH, luteinizing hormone.

male, the cycling center in the CNS does not develop because its development is blocked by androgens before birth.

In the female, a complicated set of signals needs to be organized in the CNS before the initial secretion of GnRH occurs at puberty. The higher centers (CNS organizer) must harmonize with the tonic and cycling centers and these interact with each other to prime the hypothalamus. The pulsatile system, which innervates the arcuate nucleus of the hypothalamus, must also function for GnRH to be released, and this system apparently must be functional throughout life for these cycles to be maintained. Release of GnRH from the axon terminals of the cells that synthesize this hormone is followed by entry of the hormone into the primary plexus of the closed portal system connecting the hypothalamus and the anterior pituitary (Figure 20.23). The blood–brain barrier preventing peptide transport is overcome in this process by allowing GnRH to enter the vascular system through fenestrations, or openings in the blood vessels, that permit such transport. The GnRH is then carried down the **portal system** and leaves the secondary plexus through fenestrations, again, in the region of the target cells **(gonadotropes)** of the anterior pituitary. The hormone binds to its cognate membrane receptor and the signal, mediated by the phosphatidylinositol metabolic system, causes the release of both FSH and LH from the same cell. The **FSH** binds to its cognate membrane receptor on the ovarian follicle and, operating through the protein kinase A pathway via cAMP elevation, stimulates synthesis and secretion of 17β-estradiol, the female sex hormone, and maturation of the follicle and ovum. Other proteins, such as **inhibin,** are also synthesized. Inhibin is a negative feedback regulator of FSH production in the gonadotrope. When the follicle reaches full maturation and the ovum also is matured, LH binds to its cognate receptor and plays a role in ovulation together with other factors, such as prostaglandin $F_{2\alpha}$. The residual follicle remaining after ovulation becomes the functional *corpus luteum* under primary control of LH (Figure 20.23). The **LH** binds to its cognate receptor in the *corpus luteum* cell membrane and, through stimulation of the protein kinase A pathway, stimulates synthesis of progesterone, the progestational hormone. **Estradiol** and **progesterone** bind to intracellular receptors (Chapter 21) in the uterine endometrium and cause major changes resulting in the thickening of the wall and vascularization in preparation for implantation of the fertilized egg. Estradiol, which is synthesized in large amount prior to production of progesterone, induces the progesterone receptor as one of its inducible phenotypes. This induction of progesterone receptors primes the uterus for subsequent stimulation by progesterone secreted by the *corpus luteum.*

Absence of Fertilization

If fertilization of the ovum does not occur, the *corpus luteum* involutes as a consequence of diminished LH supply. Progesterone levels fall sharply in the blood with the regression of the *corpus luteum.* Estradiol levels also fall due to the cessation of its production by the *corpus luteum.* Thus the stimuli for a thickened and vascularized uterine endometrial wall are lost. *Menstruation* occurs through a process of programmed cell death of the uterine endometrial cells until the endometrium reaches its unstimulated state. Ultimately, the fall in blood steroid levels releases the negative feedback inhibition on the gonadotropes and hypothalamus and the cycle starts again with release of FSH and LH by the gonadotropes in response to GnRH.

The course of the ovarian cycle is shown in Figure 20.24 with respect to the relative blood levels of hormones released from the hypothalamus, anterior pituitary, ovarian follicle, and corpus luteum. In addition, changes in the maturation of the follicle and ovum as well as the uterine endometrium are shown. Aspects of the steroid hormones, estradiol and progesterone, are discussed in Chapter 21.

The cycle first begins at puberty when GnRH is released, corresponding

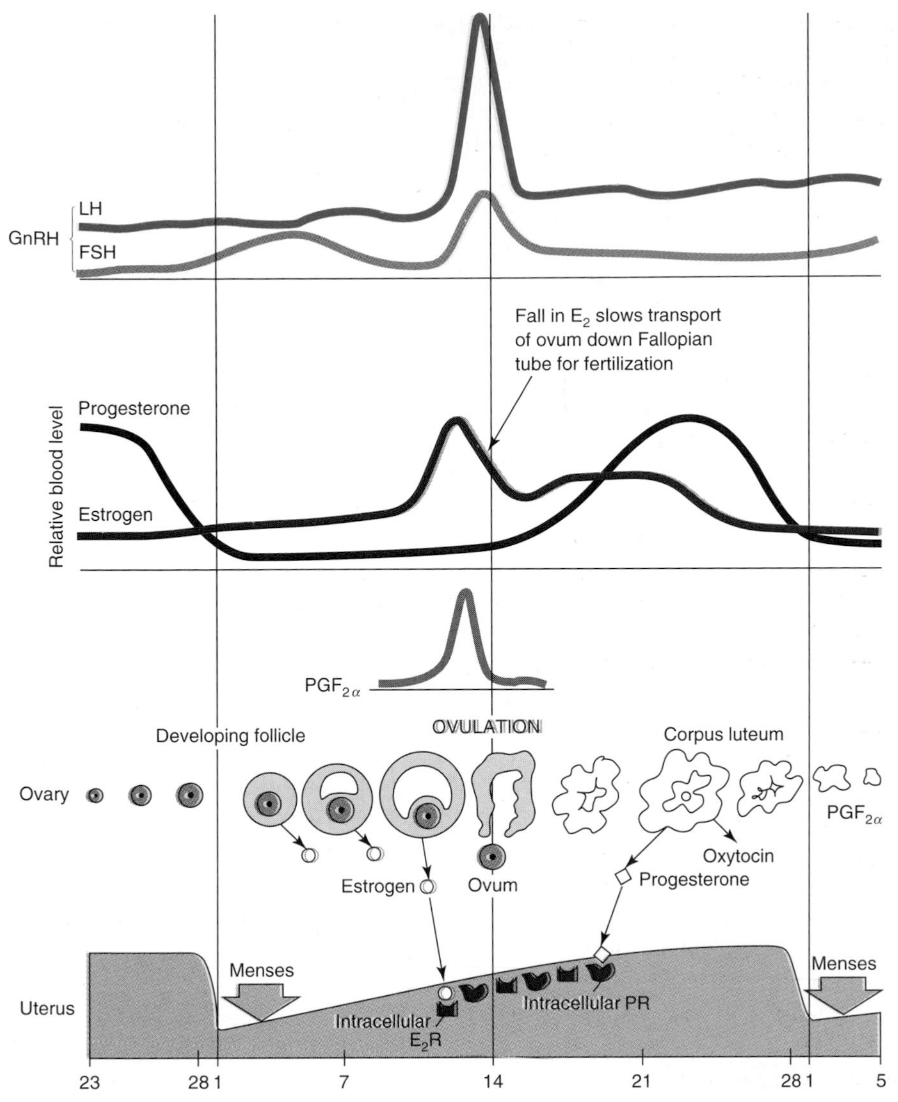

FIGURE 20.24
The ovarian cycle.
In the upper diagram, relative blood levels of GnRH, LH, FSH, progesterone, estrogen, and $PGF_{2\alpha}$ are shown. In the lower diagram, events in the ovarian follicle, corpus luteum, and uterine endometrium are diagrammed. GnRH, gonadotropin-releasing hormone; LH, luteinizing hormone; FSH, follicle-stimulating hormone; $PGF_{2\alpha}$, prostaglandin $F_{2\alpha}$; E_2, estradiol; E_2R, intracellular estrogen receptor; PR, intracellular progesterone receptor.

to day 1 in Figure 20.24. GnRH is released in a pulsatile fashion, causing the gonadotrope to release FSH and LH; there is a rise in the blood levels of these gonadotropic hormones in subsequent days. Under the stimulation of FSH the follicle begins to mature (lower section of Figure 20.24) and estradiol (E_2) is produced. In response to estradiol the uterine endometrium begins to thicken (there would have been no prior menstruation in the very first cycle). Eventually, under the continued action of FSH, the follicle matures with the maturing ovum, and extraordinarily high levels of estradiol are produced (around day 13 of the cycle). These levels of estradiol, instead of causing feedback inhibition, now generate, through **feedback stimulation,** a huge release of LH and to a lesser extent FSH from the gonadotrope. The FSH responds to a smaller extent due to the ovarian production of the hormone inhibin under the influence of FSH. Inhibin is a specific negative feedback inhibitor of FSH, but not of LH, and probably suppresses the synthesis of the β subunit of FSH. The high midcycle peak of LH is referred to as the "LH spike." Ovulation then occurs at about day 14 (midcycle) through the effects of high LH concentration together with other factors, such as $PGF_{2\alpha}$. Both LH and $PGF_{2\alpha}$ act on cell membrane receptors. After ovulation, the function of the follicle declines as reflected by the fall in blood estrogen levels. The spent follicle now differentiates into the functional corpus luteum driven by the still high levels of blood LH (Figure 20.23, top).

Under the influence of prior high levels of estradiol (estrogen) and the high levels of progesterone produced by the now functional *corpus luteum,* the uterine endometrial wall reaches its greatest development in preparation for implantation of the fertilized egg, should fertilization occur. Note that the previous availability of estradiol in combination with the estrogen receptor (E_2R) produces elevated levels of progesterone receptor (PR) within the cells of the uterine wall. The blood levels of estrogen fall with the loss of function of the follicle but some estrogen is produced by the *corpus luteum* in addition to the much greater levels of progesterone. In the absence of fertilization the *corpus luteum* continues to function for about 2 weeks, then involutes because of the loss of high levels of LH. The production of oxytocin by the *corpus luteum* itself and the production or availability of $PGF_{2\alpha}$ cause inhibition of progesterone synthesis and enhances luteolysis by a process of programmed cell death (Chapter 21). With the death of the *corpus luteum* there is a profound decline in blood levels of estradiol and progesterone so that the thickened endometrial wall can no longer be maintained and menstruation occurs, followed by the start of another cycle with a new developing follicle.

Fertilization

The situation changes if fertilization occurs as shown in Figure 20.25. The *corpus luteum,* which would have ceased function by 28 days, remains viable due to the production of **chorionic gonadotropin,** which resembles and acts like LH, from the trophoblast. Eventually, the production of **human chorionic gonadotropin** (hCG) is taken over by the placenta, which continues to produce the hormone at very high levels throughout most of the gestational period. Nevertheless, the *corpus luteum,* referred to as the "*corpus luteum* of pregnancy," eventually dies and, by about 12 weeks of pregnancy, the placenta has taken over the production of progesterone, which is secreted at high levels throughout pregnancy. Although both progesterone and estrogen are secreted in progressively greater quantities throughout pregnancy, from the seventh month onward estrogen secretion continues to increase while progesterone secretion remains constant or may even decrease slightly (Figure 20.25). The increased production of a progesterone-binding protein may also serve to lower the effective concentration of free progesterone in the myometrium. Thus the estrogen/progesterone ratio increases toward the end of pregnancy and may

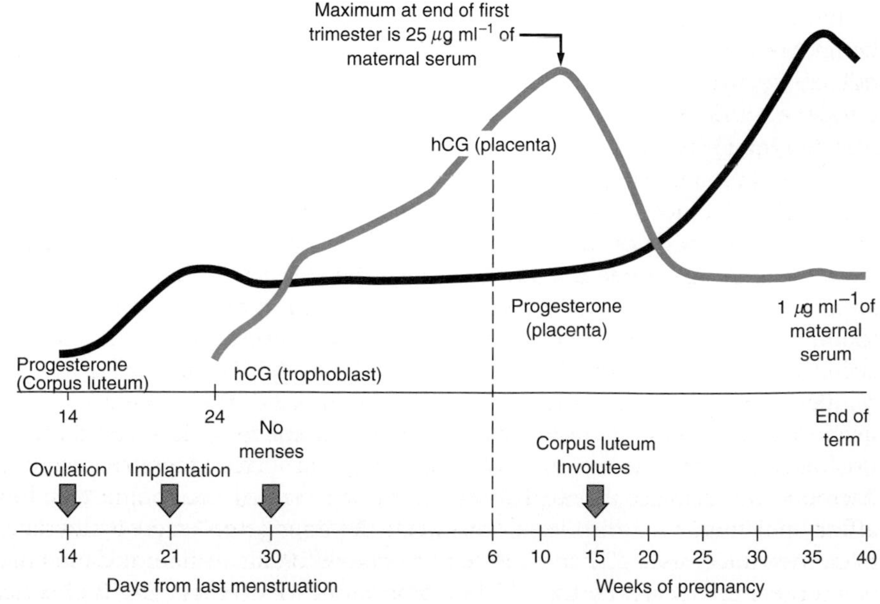

FIGURE 20.25
Effect of fertilization on ovarian cycle in terms of progesterone and secretion of human chorionic gonadotropin (hCG).

be partly responsible for the increased uterine contractions. Oxytocin secreted by the posterior pituitary also contributes to these uterine contractions. The fetal membranes also release prostaglandins ($PGF_{2\alpha}$) at the time of parturition and they also increase the intensity of uterine contractions. Finally, the fetal adrenal glands secrete cortisol, which not only stimulates fetal lung maturation by inducing surfactant but may also stimulate uterine contractions.

As mentioned before, the system in the male is similar, but less complex in that cycling is not involved, and it progresses much as outlined in Figure 20.25. This is only one example of biorhythmic and pulsatile systems.

20.9 HORMONE–RECEPTOR INTERACTIONS

Receptors are proteins and differ by their specificity for ligands and by their location in the cell (see Figure 20.1). The interaction of ligand with receptor essentially resembles a semienzymatic reaction:

$$\text{Hormone} + \text{receptor} \rightleftharpoons \text{hormone–receptor complex}$$

The **hormone–receptor complex** usually undergoes conformational changes resulting from interaction with the hormonal ligand. These changes allow for a subsequent interaction with a transducing protein (G-protein) in the membrane or for activation to a new state in which active domains become available on the surface of the receptor. The mathematical treatment of the interaction of hormone and receptor is a function of the concentrations of the reactants, hormone [H] and receptor [R], in the formation of the hormone–receptor complex [RH], and the rates of formation and reversal of the reaction:

$$[\mathrm{H}] + [\mathrm{R}] \underset{k-1}{\overset{k+1}{\rightleftharpoons}} [\mathrm{RH}]$$

The reaction can be studied under conditions, such as low temperature, that will further reduce reactions involving the hormone–receptor complex. The equilibrium can thus be expressed in terms of the association constant, K_a, which is equal to the inverse of the dissociation constant, K_d:

$$K_a = \frac{[\mathrm{RH}]}{[\mathrm{H}][\mathrm{R}]} = \frac{k_{+1}}{k_{-1}} = \frac{1}{K_d}$$

The concentrations are equilibrium concentrations that can be restated in terms of the forward and reverse velocity constants, k_{+1} being the on-rate and k_{-1} being the off-rate (**on** refers to hormone association with the receptor and **off** refers to hormone dissociation). Experimentally, equilibrium under given conditions is determined by a progress curve of binding that reaches saturation. A saturating amount of hormone is determined using variable amounts of free hormone and measuring the amount bound with some convenient assay. The half-maximal value of a plot of receptor-bound hormone (ordinate) versus total free-hormone concentration (abscissa) approximates the dissociation constant, which will have a specific hormone concentration in molarity as its value. Hormone bound to receptor is corrected for nonspecific binding of the hormone to the membrane or other nonreceptor intracellular proteins. This can be measured conveniently if the hormone is radiolabelled, by measuring receptor binding using labeled hormone ("hot" or "uncompeted") and receptor binding using labeled hormone after the addition of an excess (100–1000 times) of unlabeled hormone ("hot" + "cold" or competed). The excess of unlabeled hormone will displace the high-affinity hormone-binding sites but not the low-affinity nonspecific binding sites. Thus when the "competed" curve is subtracted from the "uncompeted" curve, as seen in Figure 20.26, an intermediate curve will represent specific binding of labeled hormone to receptor. This is of critical

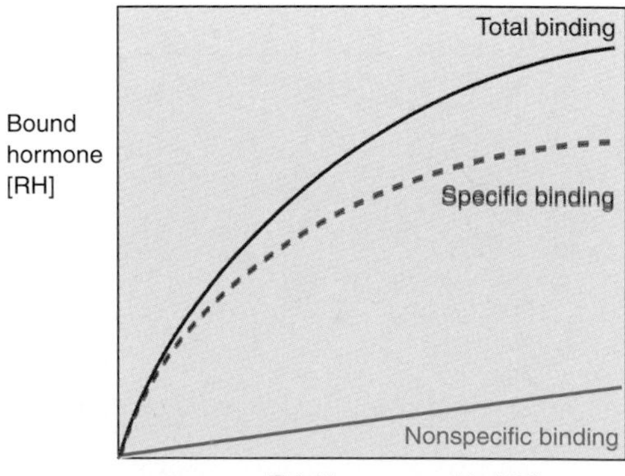

FIGURE 20.26
Typical plot showing specific hormone binding.

importance when receptor is measured in a system containing other proteins. As an approximation, 20 times the K_d value of hormone is usually enough to saturate the receptor.

Scatchard Analysis Permits Determination of the Number of Receptor-Binding Sites and Association Constant for Ligand

Most measurements of K_d are made using **Scatchard analysis,** which is a manipulation of the equilibrium equation. The equation can be developed by a number of routes but can be envisioned from mass action analysis of the equation presented above. At equilibrium the total possible number of binding sites (B_{max}) equals the unbound plus the bound sites, so that $B_{max} = R + RH$, and the unbound sites (R) will be equal to $R = B_{max} - RH$. To consider the sites left unbound in the reaction the equilibrium equation becomes

$$K_a = \frac{[RH]}{[H](B_{max} - [RH])}$$

Thus

$$\frac{\text{bound}}{\text{free}} = \frac{[RH]}{[H]} = K_a(B_{max} - ([RH]) = \frac{1}{K_d}(B_{max} - [RH])$$

The Scatchard plot of bound/free = [RH]/[H] on the ordinate versus bound on the abscissa yields a straight line, as shown in Figure 20.27. When the line is extrapolated to the abscissa, the intercept gives the value of B_{max} (the total number of specific receptor-binding sites). The slope of the negative straight line is $-K_a$ or $-1/K_d$.

These analyses are sufficient for most systems but become more complex when there are two components in the Scatchard plot. In this case the straight line usually curves as it approaches the abscissa and a second phase is observed somewhat asymptotic to the abscissa while still retaining a negative slope (Figure 20.28*a*). In order to obtain the true value of K_d for the steeper, higher-affinity sites, the low-affinity curve must be subtracted from the first set, which also corrects the extrapolated value of B_{max}. From these analyses information is obtained on K_d, the number of classes of binding sites (usually one or two), and the maximal number of high-affinity receptor sites (receptor number) in the system (see Figure 20.28*b*). These curvilinear Scatchard plots can result not only from the existence of more than one distinct binding component but also as a consequence of what is referred to as **negative cooperativity.** This term refers to the fact that in some systems the affinity of the receptor for its ligand is gradually decreased as more and more ligand binds. From application to a wide variety of systems it appears that K_d values for many hormone receptors range from 10^{-9} to 10^{-11} M, indicating very tight binding. These interactions are generally marked by a high degree of specificity so that both parameters describe interactions of a high order, indicating the uniqueness of receptors and the selectivity of signal reception.

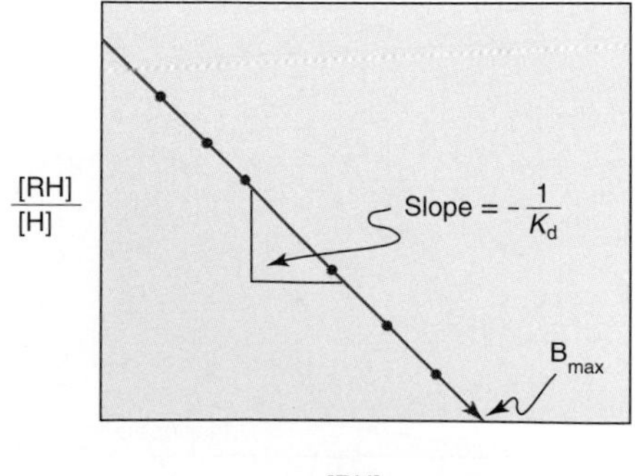

FIGURE 20.27
Typical plot of Scatchard analysis of specific binding of ligand to receptor.

Some Hormone–Receptor Interactions Involve Multiple Hormone Subunits

Interaction of hormone and receptor can be exemplified by the anterior pituitary hormones, **thyrotropin (TSH), luteinizing hormone (LH),** and **follicle-stimulating hormone (FSH).** These hormones each contain two subunits, an α and a β subunit. The α subunit for all three hormones is nearly identical and the α subunit of any of the three can substitute for the other two. Consequently, the α subunit performs some function in common to all three hormones in their interaction with receptor but is obviously not responsible for the specificity

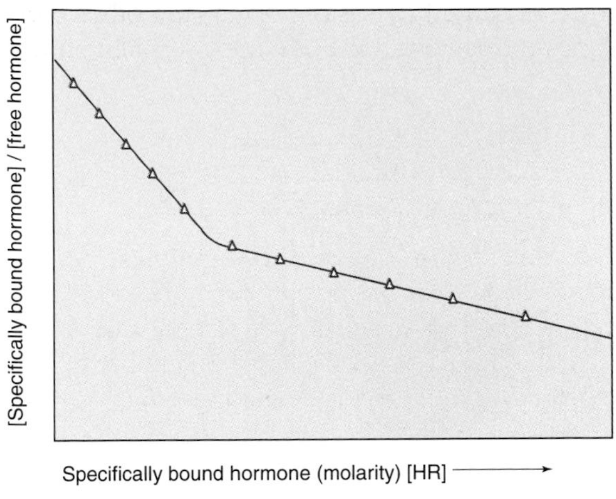

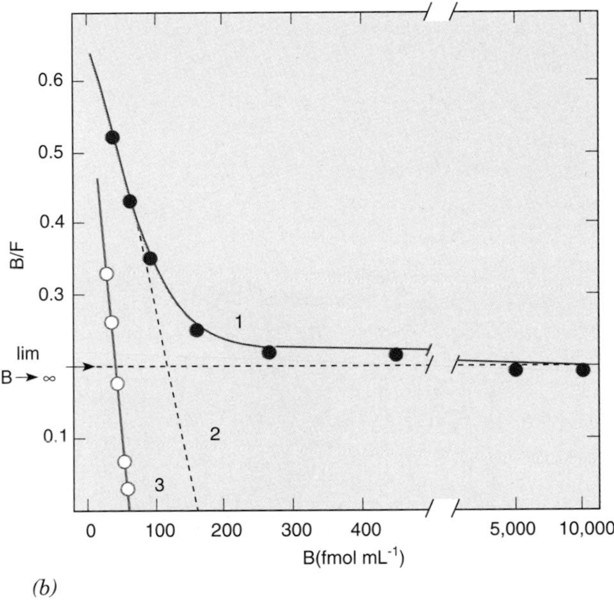

FIGURE 20.28
Scatchard analysis of curves representing two components. (*a*) Scatchard curve showing two components. (*b*) Scatchard plot with correction of high-affinity component by subtraction of nonspecific binding attributable to the low-affinity component. Curve 1: total binding. Curve 2: Linear extrapolation of high-affinity component that includes contribution from low-affinity component. Curve 3: Specific binding of high-affinity component after removal of nonspecific component.
Redrawn from Chamness, G. C., and McGuire, W. L. Steroids *26:538, 1975.*

required for each cognate receptor. The hormones cannot replace each other in binding to their specific receptor. Thus the specificity of receptor recognition is imparted by the β subunit, whose structure is unique for the three hormones.

On the basis of topological studies with monoclonal antibodies, a picture of the interaction of LH with its receptor has been suggested as shown in Figure 20.29. In this model, the receptor recognizes both subunits of the hormonal ligand, but the β subunit is specifically recognized by the receptor to lead to a response. With the TSH–receptor complex there may be more than one second messenger generated. In addition to the stimulation of adenylate cyclase and the increased intracellular level of cAMP, the phosphatidylinositol pathway (Figure 20.21) is also turned on. The preferred model is one in which there is a single receptor whose interaction with hormone activates both the adenylate cyclase and the phospholipid second messenger systems, as shown in Figure 20.30. Thus a variety of reactions could follow the hormone–receptor interaction through the subsequent stimulation of cAMP levels (protein kinase A pathway) and stimulation of phosphatidylinositol turnover (protein kinase C pathway).

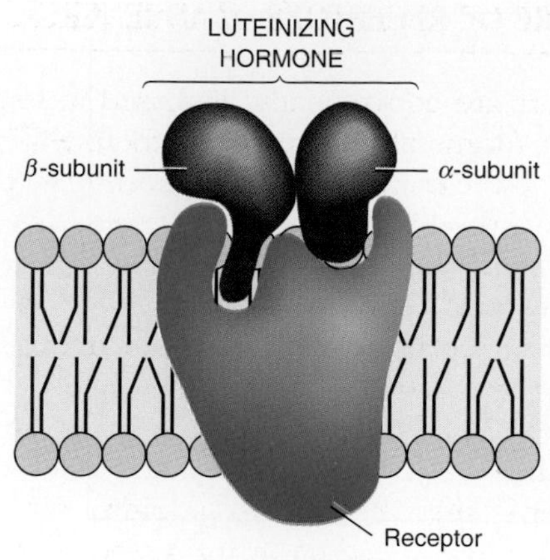

FIGURE 20.29
Interaction of the α and β subunits of LH with the LH receptor of rat Leydig cells.
The interaction was determined by topological analysis with monoclonal antibodies directed against epitopes on the α and β subunits of the hormone. Both α and β subunits participate in LH receptor binding.
Adapted from Alonoso-Whipple, C., Couet, M. L., Doss, R., Koziarz, J., Ogunro, E. A., and Crowley, W. E. Jr. Endocrinology *123:1854, 1988.*

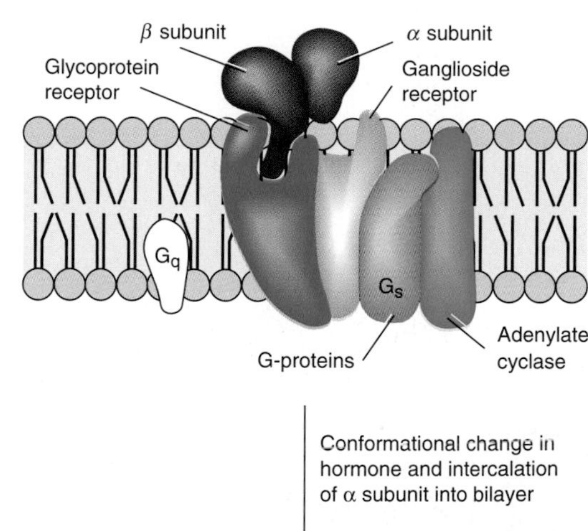

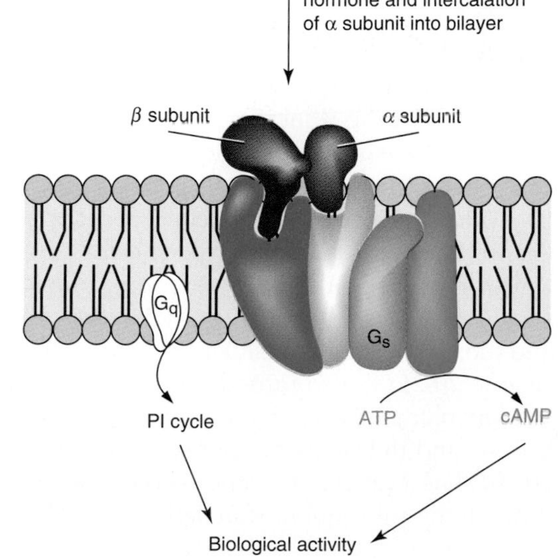

FIGURE 20.30
Model of TSH receptor, which is composed of glycoprotein and ganglioside component.
After the TSH β subunit interacts with receptor, the hormone changes its conformation and the α subunit is brought into the bilayer, where it interacts with other membrane components. The β subunit of TSH may carry primary determinants recognized by the glycoprotein receptor component. It is suggested that the TSH signal to adenylate cyclase is via the ganglioside; the glycoprotein component appears more directly linked to phospholipid signal system. PI, phosphatidylinositol; G_s, G-protein linked to activation of adenylate cyclase; G_q G-protein linked to PI cycle.
Adapted with modifications from L. D. Kohn, et al. Biochemical Actions of Hormones, *12. G. Litwack (Ed.). Academic Press, 1985, p. 466.*

20.10 STRUCTURE OF RECEPTORS: β-ADRENERGIC RECEPTOR

Structures of receptors are conveniently discussed in terms of functional domains. Consequently, for membrane receptors there will be functional **ligand-binding domains** and the **transmembrane domains,** which for many membrane receptors involve protein kinase activities. In addition, specific **immunological domains** contain primary epitopes of antigenic regions. Several membrane receptors have been cloned and studied with regard to structure and function, including the β receptors (β_1 and β_2), which recognize catecholamines, principally norepinephrine, and stimulate adenylate cyclase. The β_1 and β_2 receptors are subtypes that differ in affinities for norepinephrine and for synthetic antagonists. Thus β_1-adrenergic receptor binds norepinephrine with a higher affinity than epinephrine, whereas the order of affinities is reversed for the β_2-adrenergic receptor. The drug isoproterenol has a greater affinity for both receptors than the two hormones. In Figure 20.31 the amino acid sequence is shown (with single letter abbreviations for amino acids; see Table 20.4 for list) for the β_2-adrenergic receptor. A polypeptide stretch extending from α helix I extends to the extracellular space. There are seven membrane-spanning domains and these appear also in the β_1 receptor, where there is extensive homology with the β_2 receptor. Cytosolic peptide regions extend to form loops between I and II, III and IV, and V and VI and an extended chain from VII.

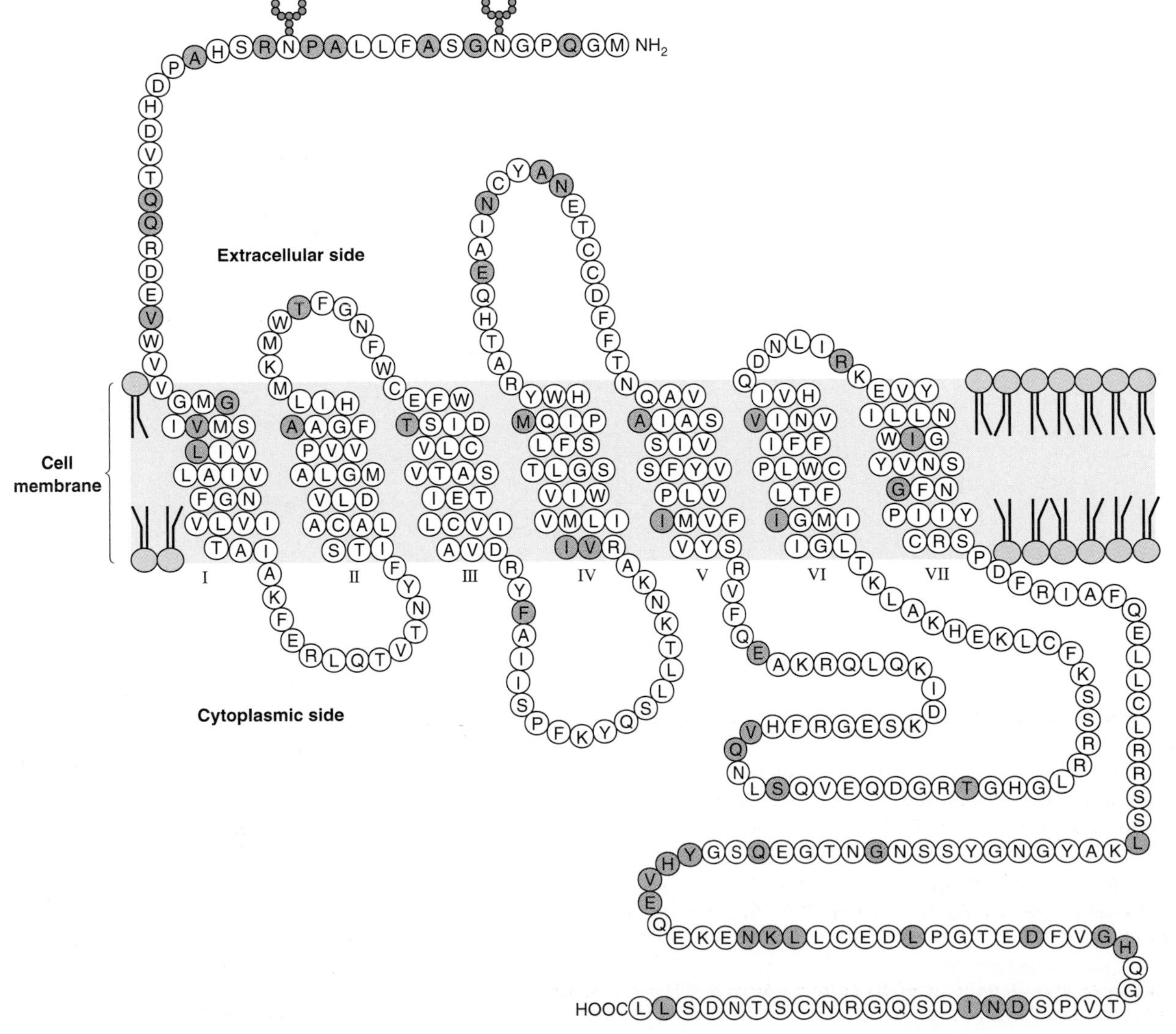

FIGURE 20.31
Proposed model for insertion of the β_2-adrenergic receptor (AR) in the cell membrane.
The model is based on hydropathicity analysis of the human β_2-AR. Standard one-letter codes for amino acid residues are used. Hydrophobic domains are represented as transmembrane helices. Pink circles with black letters indicate residues in the human sequence that differ from those in hamster. Also noted are the potential sites of N-linked glycosylation.
Redrawn from Kobilka, B. K., Dixon, R. A., Frielle, T., Dohlman, H. G., et al. Proc. Natl. Acad. Sci. USA *84:46, 1987.*

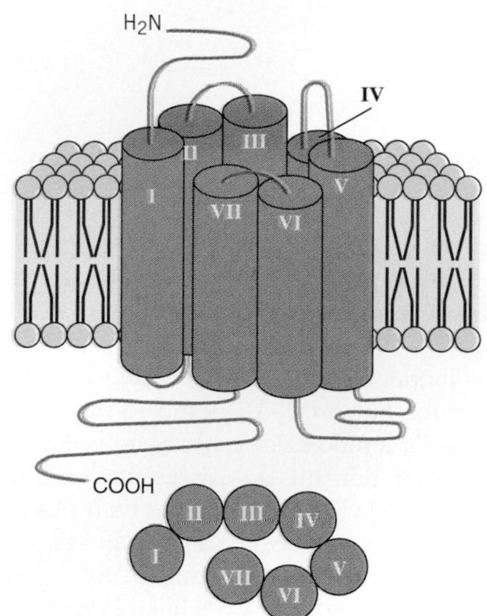

FIGURE 20.32
Proposed arrangement of β-adrenergic receptor helices in the membrane.
Lower portion of the figure is a view from above the plane of the plasma membrane. It is proposed that helices IV, VI, and VII are arranged in the membrane in such a way as to delineate a ligand-binding pocket, with helix VII centrally located.
Adapted from Frielle, T., Daniel, K. W., Caron, M. G., and Lefkowitz, R. J. Proc. Natl. Acad. Sci. USA *85:9494, 1988.*

The long extended chain from VII may contain phosphorylation sites (serine and threonine residues) of the receptor, which are important in terms of the receptor regulatory process involving receptor desensitization. Phosphorylation of these residues within the cytoplasmic tail of the receptor results in the binding of an inhibitory protein, called β arrestin, which blocks the receptor's ability to activate G_s. Cell exterior peptide loops extend from II to III, IV to V, and VI to VII, but mutational analysis suggests that the external loops do not take part in ligand binding. It appears that ligand binding may occur in a pocket arranged by the location of the membrane-spanning cylinders I–VII, which for the β_1 receptor appear to form a ligand pocket, as shown from a top view in Figure 20.32. Recently reported work suggests that transmembrane domain VI may play a role in the stimulation of adenylate cyclase activity. By substitution of a specific cysteine residue in this transmembrane domain, a mutant was generated that displays normal ligand-binding properties but a decreased ability to stimulate the cyclase.

20.11 ■ INTERNALIZATION OF RECEPTORS

Up to now we have described receptor systems that transduce signals through other membrane proteins, such as G-proteins, which move about in the fluid

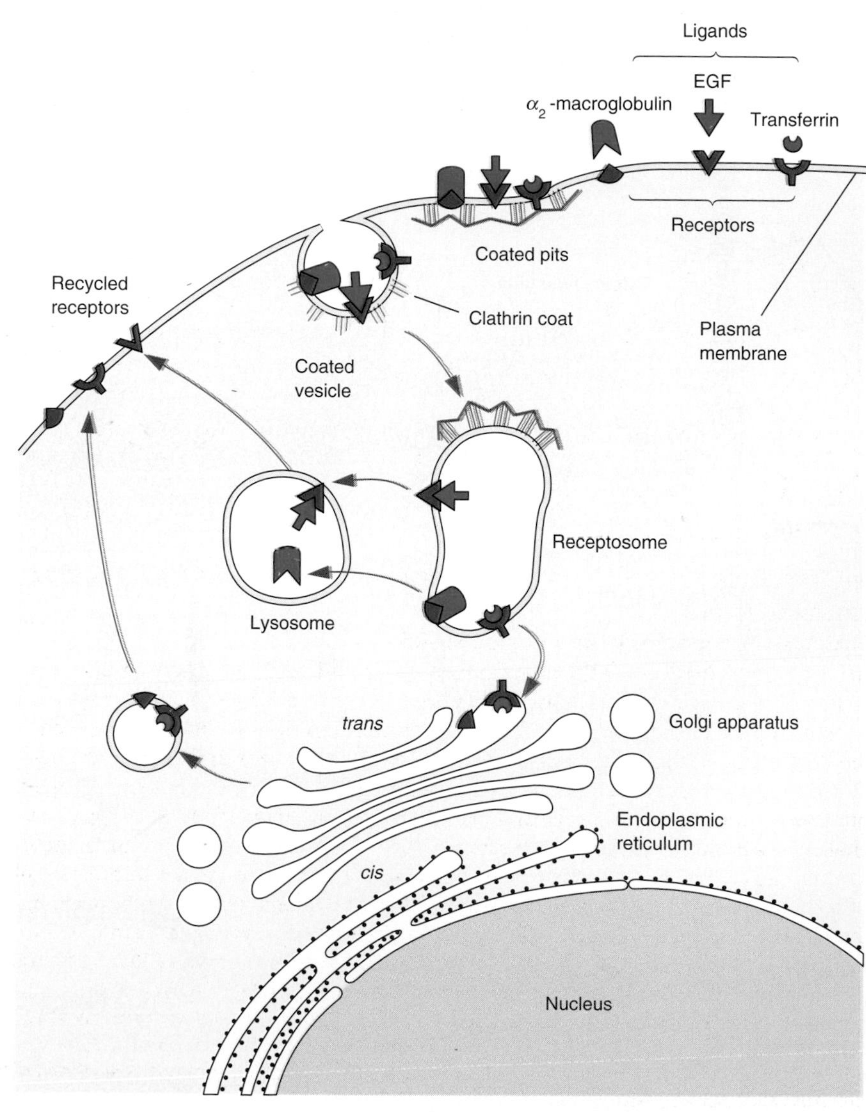

FIGURE 20.33
Diagrammatic summary of the morphological pathway of endocytosis in cells.
The morphological elements of the pathway of endocytosis are not drawn to scale. The ligands shown as examples are EGF, transferrin, and α_2-macroglobulin. EGF is an example of a receptor system in which both ligand and receptor are delivered to lysosomes; transferrin is shown as an example of a system in which both the ligand and receptor recycle to the surface; α_2-macroglobulin is shown as an example of a system in which the ligand is delivered to lysosomes but the receptor recycles efficiently back to the cell surface via the Golgi apparatus.
Adapted from Pastan, I., and Willingham, M. C. (Eds.). Endocytosis. *New York: Plenum Press, 1985, p. 3.*

cell membrane. However, many types of cell membrane hormone–receptor complexes are internalized, that is, moved from the cell membrane to the cell interior by a process called **endocytosis.** This would represent the opposite of exocytosis in which components within the cell are moved to the cell exterior. The process of endocytosis as presented in Figure 20.33 involves the polypeptide–receptor complex bound in **coated pits,** which are indentations in the plasma membrane that invaginate into the cytosol and pinch off from the membrane to form **coated vesicles.** The vesicles shed their coats, fuse with each other, and form vesicles called receptosomes. The receptors and ligands on the inside of these **receptosomes** can have different fates. Receptors can be recycled to the cell surface following fusion with the Golgi apparatus. Alternatively, the vesicles can fuse with lysosomes for degradation of both the receptor and hormone. In addition, some hormone–receptor complexes are dissociated in the lysosome and only the hormone is degraded, while the receptor is returned intact to the membrane. In some systems, the receptor may also be concentrated in coated pits in the absence of exogenous ligand and cycle in and out of the cell in a constitutive, nonligand-dependent manner.

Clathrin Forms a Lattice Structure to Direct Internalization of Hormone–Receptor Complexes from the Plasma Membrane

The major protein component of the coated vesicle is **clathrin,** a nonglycosylated protein of mol wt 180,000 whose amino acid sequence is highly conserved. The coated vesicle contains 70% clathrin, 5% polypeptides of about 35 kDa, and 25% polypeptides of 50–100 kDa. Aspects of the structure of a coated vesicle are shown in Figure 20.34. Coated vesicles have a lattice-like surface

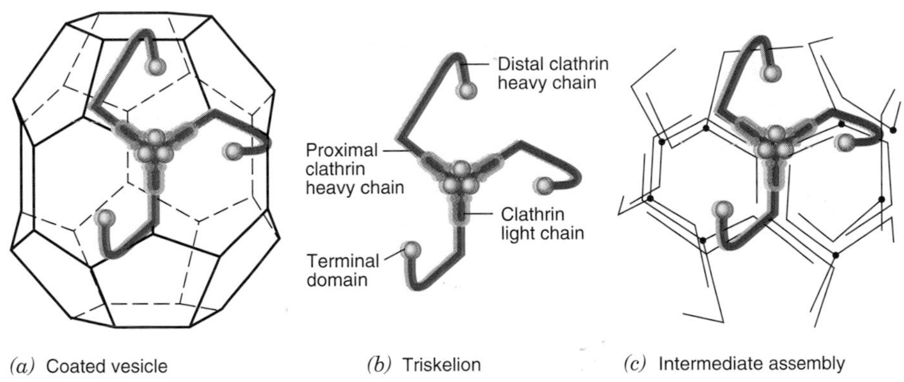

FIGURE 20.34
Structure and assembly of a coated vesicle.
(*a*) A typical coated vesicle contains a membrane vesicle about 40 nm in diameter surrounded by a fibrous network of 12 pentagons and 8 hexagons. The fibrous coat is constructed of 36 clathrin triskelions. One clathrin triskelion is centered on each of the 36 vertices of the coat. Coated vesicles having other sizes and shapes are believed to be constructed similarly: each vesicle contains 12 pentagons but a variable number of hexagons. (*b*) Detail of a clathrin triskelion. Each of three clathrin heavy chains is bent into a proximal arm and a distal arm. A clathrin light chain is attached to each heavy chain, most likely near the center. (*c*) An intermediate in the assembly of a coated vesicle, containing 10 of the final 36 triskelions, illustrates the packing of the clathrin triskelions. Each of the 54 edges of a coated vesicle is constructed of two proximal and two distal arms intertwined. The 36 triskelions contain $36 \times 3 = 108$ proximal and 108 distal arms, and the coated vesicle has precisely 54 edges.
See Crowther, R. A., and Pearse, B. M. F. J. Cell. Biol. *91:790, 1981. Redrawn from Nathke, I. S., Heuser, J., Lupas, A., Stock, J., Turck, C. W., and Brodsky, E. M.* Cell *68:899, 1992. Redrawn from Darnell, J., Lodish, H., and Baltimore, D.* Molecular Cell Biology. *New York: Scientific American Books, 1986, p. 647.*

structure comprised of hexagons and pentagons. Three clathrin molecules generate each polyhedral vertex and two clathrin molecules contribute to each edge. The smallest such structure would contain 12 pentagons with 4–8 hexagons and 84 or 108 clathrin molecules. A 200-nm diameter coated vesicle contains about 1000 clathrin molecules. Clathrin can form flexible lattice structures that can act as scaffolds for vesicular budding. Completion of the budding process results in the mature vesicle being able to enter the cycle.

The events following endocytosis are not always clear with respect to a specific membrane receptor system. This process can be a means to introduce the intact receptor or ligand to the cell interior in cases where the nucleus is thought to contain a receptor or ligand-binding site. Consider, for example, growth factors that are known to bind to a cell membrane receptor but trigger events leading to mitosis. It is possible that signal transmission occurs by the alteration of a specific cytosolic protein, perhaps by membrane growth factor receptor-associated protein kinase activity, resulting in the nuclear translocation of the covalently modified cytosolic protein. In the case of internalization, delivery of an intact ligand (or portion of the ligand) could interact with a nuclear receptor. Such mechanisms are speculative. Nevertheless, these ideas could constitute a rationale for the participation of endocytosis in signal transmission to intracellular components.

Endocytosis renders a cell less responsive to hormone. Removal of the receptor to the interior, or cycling of membrane components, alters responsiveness or metabolism (e.g., glucose receptors can be shuttled between the cell interior and the cell membrane under the control of hormones in certain cells). In another type of downregulation, a hormone–receptor complex translocated to the nucleus can repress its own receptor mRNA levels by interacting with a specific DNA sequence. More about this form of receptor downregulation is mentioned in Chapter 21.

20.12 INTRACELLULAR ACTION: PROTEIN KINASES

Many amino acid-derived hormones or polypeptides bind to cell membrane receptors (except for thyroid hormone) and transmit their signal by (1) elevation of cAMP and transmission through the **protein kinase A pathway;** (2) triggering of the hydrolysis of phosphatidylinositol 4,5-bisphosphate and stimulation of the **protein kinase C** and IP_3–Ca^{2+} pathways; or (3) stimulation of intracellular levels of cGMP and activation of the **protein kinase G pathway.** There are also other less prevalent systems for signal transfer, which, for example, affect molecules in the membrane like phosphatidylcholine. As previously discussed in the case of TSH–receptor signaling, it may be possible that two of these pathways are activated.

The cAMP system operating through protein kinase A activation has been described. Specific proteins are expected to be phosphorylated by this kinase compared to other protein kinases, such as protein kinase C. Both protein kinase A and C phosphorylate proteins on **serine** or **threonine** residues. An additional protein kinase system involves phosphorylation of **tyrosine,** which occurs in cytoplasmic domains of some membrane receptors especially growth factor receptors. This system is important for the insulin receptor, IGF receptor, and certain oncogenes discussed below. The cellular location of these protein kinases is presented in Figure 20.35.

The catalytic domain in the protein kinases is similar in amino acid sequence, suggesting that they have all evolved from a common primordial kinase. The three **tyrosine-specific kinases** shown in Figure 20.35 are transmembrane receptor proteins that, when activated by the binding of specific extracellular ligands, phosphorylate proteins (including themselves) on tyrosine residues inside the cell. Both chains of the insulin receptor are encoded by a single

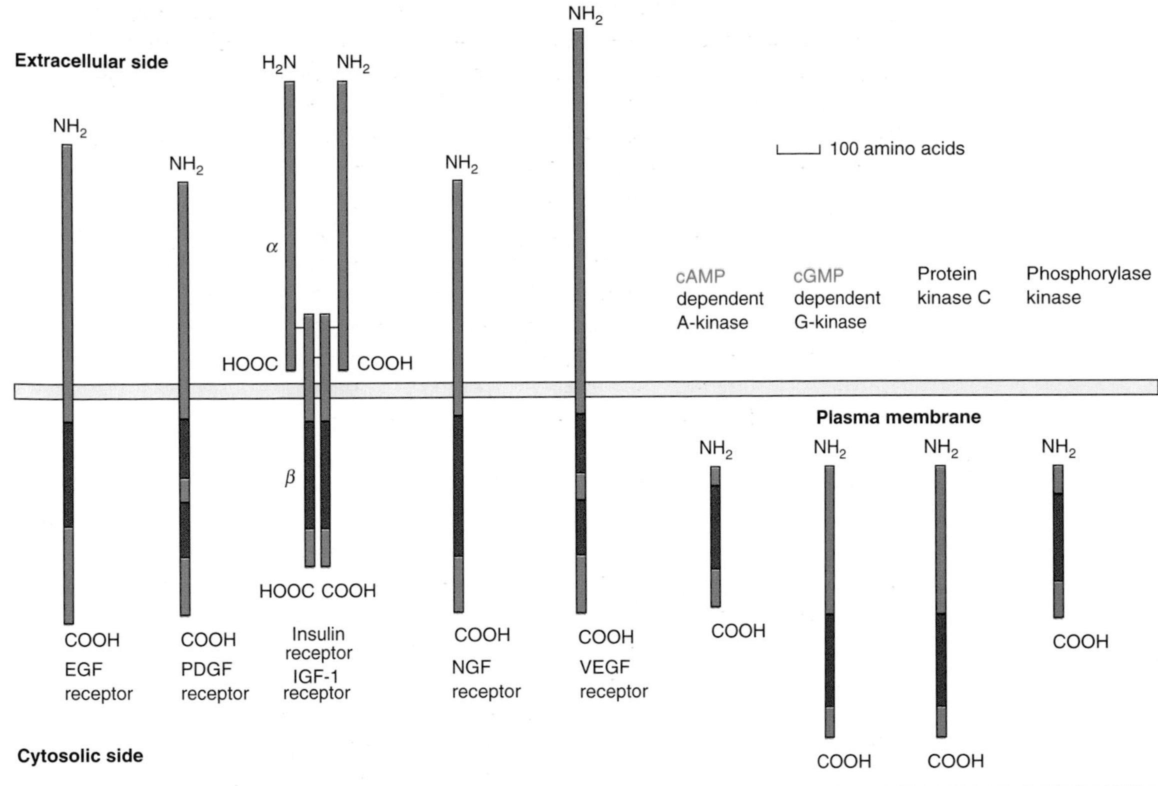

FIGURE 20.35
Protein kinases showing the size and location of their catalytic domain.
In each case the catalytic domain (red region) is about 250 amino acid residues long. The regulatory subunits normally associated with A-kinase and with phosphorylase kinase are not shown. EGF, epidermal growth factor; NGF, nerve growth factor; VEGF, vascular endothelial growth factor.
Redrawn from Alberts, B., Bray, D., Lewis, J., Raff, M., Roberts, K., and Watson, J. D. Molecular Biology of the Cell, *3rd ed. New York: Garland Publishing, 1994, p. 760.*

gene, which produces a precursor protein that is cleaved into the two disulfide-linked chains. The extracellular domain of the PDGF receptor is thought to be folded into five immunoglobulin (Ig)-like domains, suggesting that this protein belongs to the Ig superfamily.

Proteins that are regulated by phosphorylation–dephosphorylation can have multiple phosphorylation sites and may be phosphorylated by more than one class of protein kinase.

Insulin Receptor: Transduction Through Tyrosine Kinase

From Figure 20.35 it is seen that the α subunits of the **insulin receptor** are located outside the cell membrane and apparently serve as the insulin-binding site. The insulin–receptor complex undergoes an activation sequence probably involving conformational changes and phosphorylation **(autophosphorylation)** of tyrosine residues located in the cytoplasmic portion of the receptor (β subunits). This results in activation of the tyrosine kinase activity located in the β subunit, which is now able to phosphorylate cytosolic proteins that may carry the insulin signal to the interior of the cell. The net results of these phosphorylation events include a series of short-term metabolic effects, such as increased uptake of glucose, as well as longer-term effects of insulin on cellular differentiation and growth. Although, as already indicated, the insulin receptor itself is a tyrosine kinase that is activated upon hormone binding, the

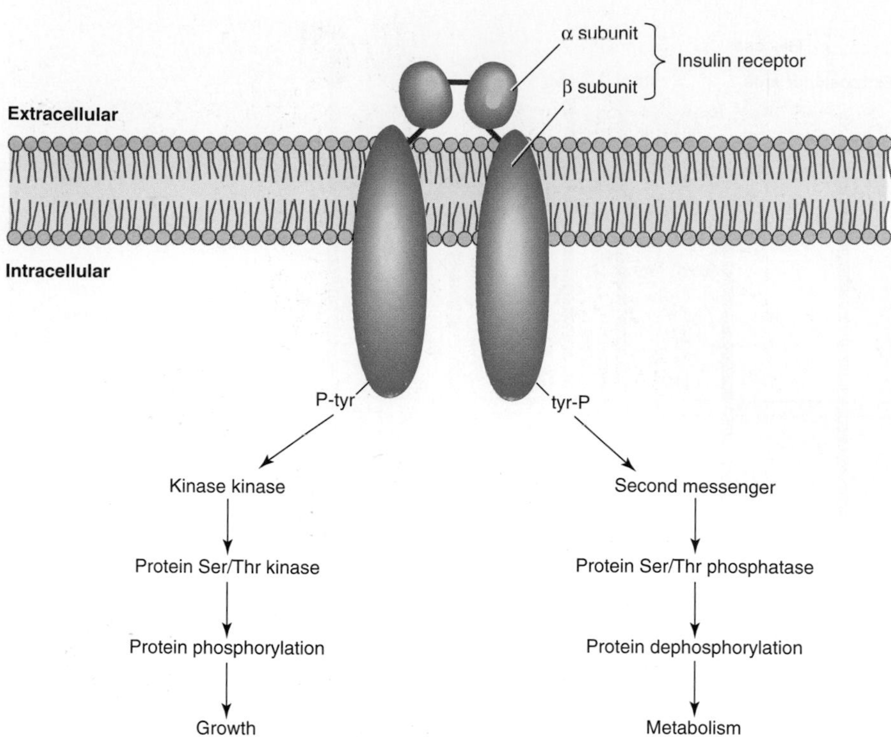

FIGURE 20.36
Hypothetical model depicting two separate biochemical pathways to explain paradoxical effects of insulin on protein phosphorylation.
Insulin simultaneously produces increases in the serine/threonine phosphorylation of some proteins and decreases in others. This paradoxical effect may result from activation of both kinases and phosphatases. Model explains (1) the generation of a soluble second messenger that directly or indirectly activates serine/threonine phosphatase and (2) the stimulation of a cascade of protein kinases, resulting in phosphorylation of cellular proteins.
Redrawn from Saltiel, A. R. The paradoxical regulation of protein phosphorylation in insulin action. FASEB J. *8:1034, 1994.*

subsequent changes in phosphorylation occur predominantly on serine and threonine residues, as indicated in Figure 20.36. As also shown, insulin can simultaneously stimulate the phosphorylation of some proteins and the dephosphorylation of other proteins. Either of these biochemical events can lead to activation or inhibition of specific enzymes involved in mediating the effects of insulin. These opposite effects (phosphorylation and dephosphorylation) mediated by insulin suggest that perhaps separate signal transduction pathways may originate from the insulin receptor to produce these pleiotropic actions. A hypothetical scheme for this bifurcation of signals in insulin's action is presented in Figure 20.37. The substrates of the insulin–receptor tyrosine kinase are an important current research effort since phosphorylated proteins could produce the long-term effects of insulin. On the other hand, there is evidence that an insulin second messenger may be developed at the cell membrane to account for the short-term metabolic effects of insulin. The substance released as a result of insulin–insulin receptor interaction may be a glycoinositol derivative that, when released from the membrane into the cytosol, could be a stimulator of phosphoprotein phosphatase. This activity would dephosphorylate a variety of enzymes, either activating or inhibiting them, and produce effects already known to be associated with the action of insulin. In addition, this second messenger, or the direct phosphorylating activity of the receptor tyrosine kinase, might explain the movement of glucose receptors (transporters) from the cell interior to the surface to account for enhanced cellular glucose utilization in cells that utilize this mechanism to control glucose uptake. These possibilities are reviewed in Figure 20.37. Activation of the enzymes indicated in this figure leads to increased metabolism of glucose while inhibition of the enzymes indicated leads to decreased breakdown of glucose or fatty acid stores.

Activity of Vasopressin: Protein Kinase A

An example of the activation of the **protein kinase A** pathway by a hormone is the activity of arginine vasopressin (AVP) on the distal kidney cell. Here the action of **vasopressin (VP),** also called the antidiuretic hormone (Table 20.5),

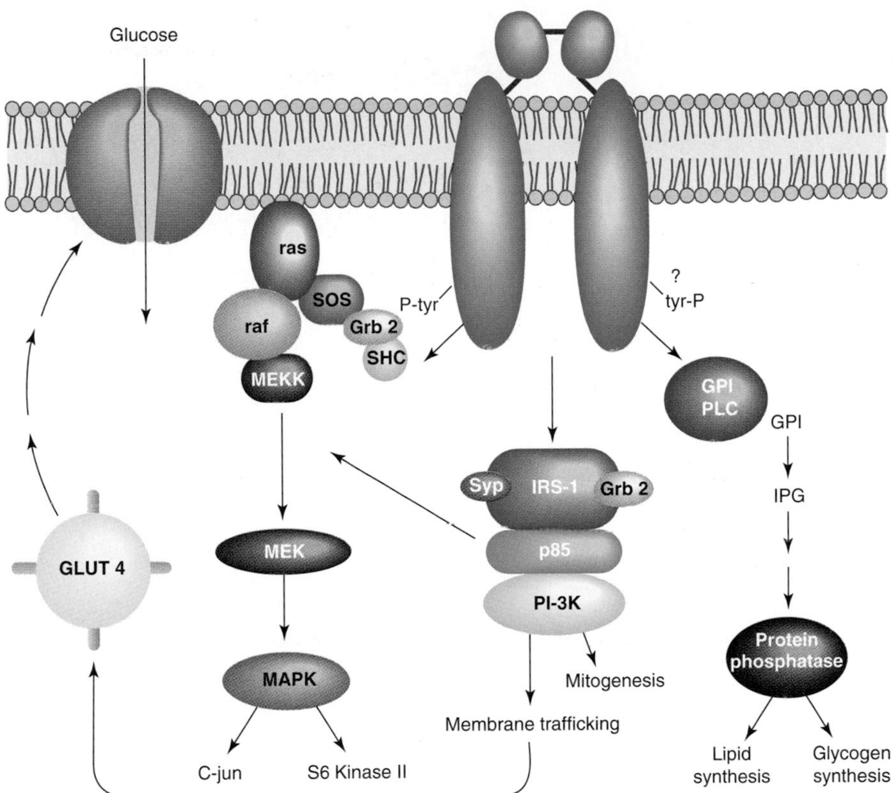

FIGURE 20.37
Hypothetical scheme for signal transduction in insulin action.
The insulin receptor undergoes tyrosine autophosphorylation and subsequent kinase activation upon hormone binding. The receptor phosphorylates intracellular substrates including IRS-1 and Shc proteins, which associate with SH2-containing proteins like p85, SYP, or Grb2 upon phosphorylation. Formation of the IRS-1–p85 complex activates PI 3-kinase; the IRS-1–SYP complex activates SYP, leading to MEK activation. Formation of the Shc–Grb2 complex mediates the stimulation of $P21^{Ras}$ GTP binding, leading to a cascade of phosphorylations. These phosphorylations probably occur sequentially and involve *raf* proto-oncogene, MEK, MAP kinase, and S6 kinase II. The receptor is probably separately coupled to activation of a specific phospholipase C that catalyzes the hydrolysis of the glycosyl-PI molecules in the plasma membrane. A product of this reaction, inositol phosphate glycan (IPG), may act as a second messenger, especially with regard to activation of serine/threonine phosphatases and the subsequent regulation of lipid and glucose metabolism. Abbreviations: IRS-1, insulin receptor substrate-1; SH, *src* homology; MAP kinase, mitogen-activated protein kinase; MEK, MAP kinase kinase; GPI, glycosylphosphatidylinositol; PLC, phospholipase; SOS, son of sevenless.
Redrawn from Saltiel, A. R. The paradoxical regulation of protein phosphorylation in insulin action. FASEB J. *8:1034, 1994.*

is to cause increased water reabsorption from the urine in the distal kidney. A mechanism for this system is shown in Figure 20.38. Neurons synthesizing AVP (vasopressinergic neurons) are signaled to release AVP from their nerve endings by interneuronal firing from a **baroreceptor** responding to a fall in blood pressure or from an **osmoreceptor** (probably an interneuron), which responds to an increase in extracellular salt concentration. The high extracellular salt concentration apparently causes shrinkage of the osmoreceptor cell and generates an electrical signal transmitted down the axon of the osmoreceptor to the cell body of the VP neuron generating an action potential. This signal is then transmitted down the long axon from the VP cell body to its nerve ending where, by depolarization, the VP–neurophysin II complex is released in to the

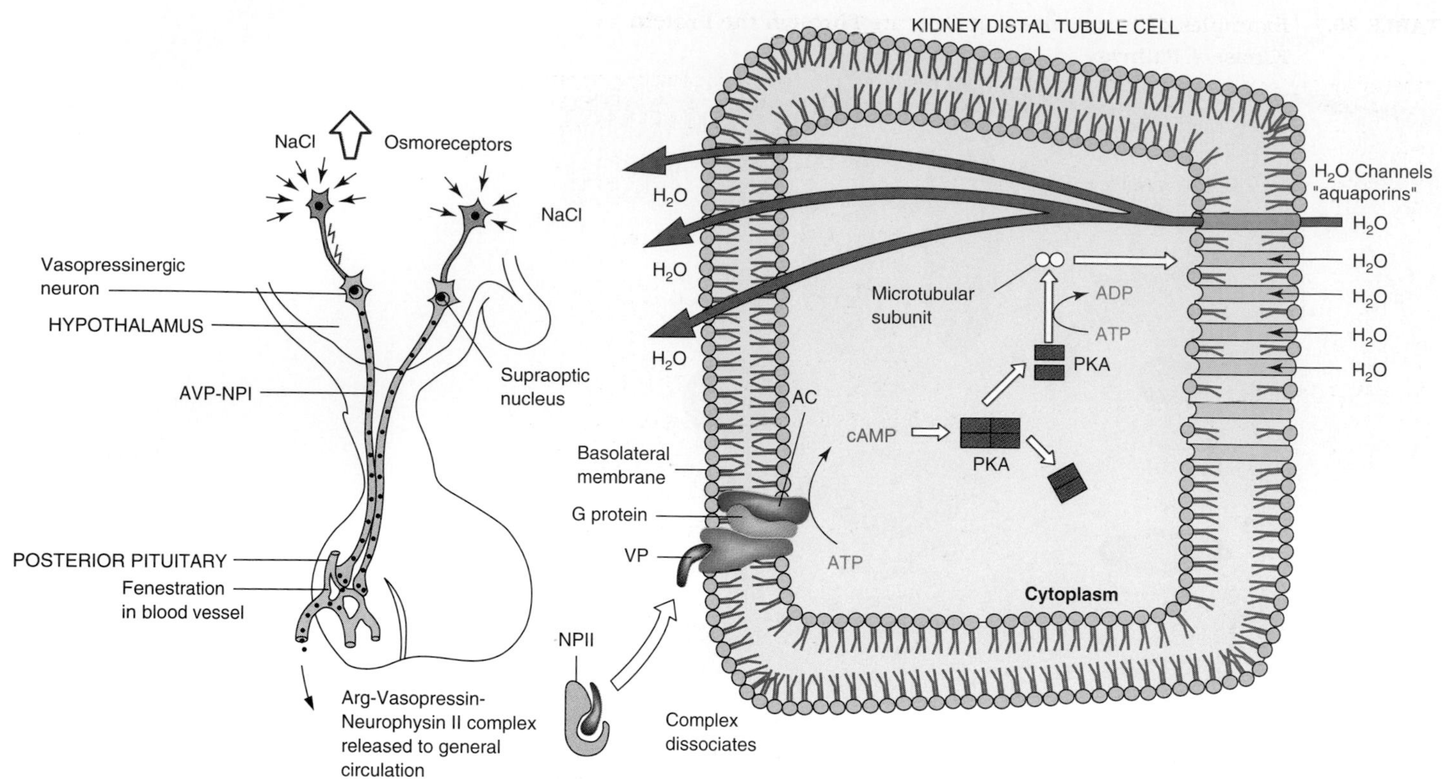

FIGURE 20.38
Secretion and action of arginine vasopressin in the distal kidney.
The release of arginine vasopressin (AVP or VP) from the posterior pituitary begins with a signal from the osmoreceptor, or baroreceptor (not shown), in the upper right-hand corner of figure. The signal can be an increase in the extracellular concentration of sodium chloride, which causes the osmoreceptor neuron to shrink and send an electrical message down its axon, which interfaces with the vasopressinergic cell body. This signal is transmitted down the long axon of the vasopressinergic neuron and depolarizes the nerve endings causing the release, by exocytosis, of the VP–neurophysin complex stored there. They enter the local circulation through fenestrations in the vessels and perfuse the general circulation. Soon after release, neurophysin dissociates from VP and VP binds to its cognate receptor in the cell membrane of the kidney distal tubule cell (other VP receptors are located on the corticotrope of the anterior pituitary and on the hepatocytes and their mechanisms in these other cells are different from the one for the kidney tubule cell). NPII, neurophysin II; VP, vasopressin; R, receptor; AC, adenylate cyclase; MF, myofibril; GP, glycogen phosphorylase; PK_i, inactive protein kinase; PK_a, active protein kinase; R-Ca, regulatory subunit–cyclic AMP complex; TJ, tight junction; PD, phosphodiesterase. Vasopressin–neurophysin complex dissociates at some point and free VP binds to its cell membrane receptor in the plasma membrane surface. Through a G-protein adenylate cyclase is stimulated on the cytoplasmic side of the cell membrane, generating increased levels of cAMP from ATP. Cyclic AMP-dependent protein kinases are stimulated and phosphorylate various proteins (perhaps including microtubular subunits) which, through aggregation, insert as water channels (aquaporins) in the luminal plasma membrane, thus increasing the reabsorption of water by free diffusion.
Redrawn in part from Dousa, T. P., and Valtin, H. Cellular actions of vasopressin in the mammalian kidney. Kidney Int. *10:45, 1975.*

extracellular space. The complex enters local capillaries through fenestrations and progresses to the general circulation. The complex dissociates and free VP is able to bind to its cognate membrane receptors in the distal kidney, anterior pituitary, hepatocyte, and perhaps other cell types. After binding to the kidney receptor, VP causes stimulation of adenylate cyclase through the stimulatory G-protein and activates protein kinase A. The protein kinase phosphorylates

TABLE 20.7 Examples of Hormones that Operate Through the Protein Kinase A Pathway

Hormone	*Location of Action*
CRH	Corticotrope of anterior pituitary
TSH (also phospholipid metabolism?)	Thyroid follicle
LH	Leydig cell of testis Mature follicle at ovulation and *corpus luteum*
FSH	Sertoli cell of seminiferous tubule Ovarian follicle
ACTH	Inner layers of cells of adrenal cortex
Opioid peptides	Some in CNS function on inhibitory pathway through G_i
AVP	Kidney distal tubular cell (the AVP hepatocyte receptor causes phospholipid turnover and calcium ion uptake; the AVP receptor in anterior pituitary causes phospholipid turnover)
PGI_2 (prostacyclin)	Blood platelet membrane
Norepinephrine/epinephrine	β-Receptor

microtubular subunits that aggregate to form specific water channels, referred to as aquaporins, which are inserted into the luminal membrane for admission of larger volumes of water than would occur by free diffusion. Water is transported across the kidney cell to the basolateral side and to the general circulation, causing a dilution of the original high salt concentration (signal) and an increase in blood pressure. These aquaporins, which are a family of integral membrane proteins that function as selective water channels, consist of six transmembrane α helical domains. Although aquaporin monomers function as water channels or pores, their stability and proper functioning may require a tetrameric assembly. Specific mutations in the amino acid sequences of the intracellular and extracellular loops of these proteins result in nonfunctional aquaporins and the development of diabetes insipidus, which is characterized by increased thirst and production of a large volume of urine.

Some hormones that operate through the protein kinase A pathway are listed in Table 20.7.

Gonadotropin-Releasing Hormone (GnRH): Protein Kinase C

Table 20.8 presents examples of polypeptide hormones that stimulate the phosphatidylinositol pathway. An example of a system operating through stimulation of the phosphatidylinositol pathway and subsequent activation of the **protein kinase C** system is **GnRH** action, shown in Figure 20.39. Probably under aminergic interneuronal controls, a signal is generated to stimulate the cell body of the GnRH-ergic neuron where GnRH is synthesized. The signal is transmitted down the long axon to the nerve ending where the hormone is stored. The hormone is released from the nerve ending by exocytosis resulting from depolarization caused by signal transmission. The GnRH enters the primary plexus of the closed portal system connecting the hypothalamus and anterior pituitary through fenestrations. Then GnRH exits the closed portal system through fenestrations in the secondary plexus and binds to cognate receptors in the cell membrane of the gonadotrope (see enlarged view in Figure 20.39). The signal from the hormone–receptor complex is transduced (through a G-protein) and phospholipase C is activated. This enzyme catalyzes the hydrolysis of PIP_2 to form DAG and IP_3. Diacylglycerol activates protein kinase C, which phosphoryl-

TABLE 20.8 **Examples of Polypeptide Hormones that Stimulate the Phosphatidylinositol Pathway**

Hormone	*Location of Action*
TRH	Thyrotrope of the anterior pituitary releasing TSH
GnRH	Gonadotrope of the anterior pituitary releasing LH and FSH
AVP	Corticotrope of the anterior pituitary; assists CRH in releasing ACTH; hepatocyte: causes increase in cellular Ca^{2+}
TSH	Thyroid follicle: releasing thyroid hormones causes increase in phosphatidylinositol cycle as well as increase in protein kinase A pathway
Angiotensin II/III	*Zona glomerulosa* cell of adrenal cortex: releases aldosterone
Epinephrine (thrombin)	Platelet: releasing ADP/serotonin; hepatocyte via α receptor: releasing intracellular Ca^{2+}

ates specific proteins, some of which may participate in the resulting secretory process to transport LH and FSH to the cell exterior. The product IP_3, which binds to a receptor on the membrane of the calcium storage particle, probably located near the cell membrane, stimulates the release of calcium ion. Elevated cytosolic Ca^{2+} causes increased stimulation of protein kinase C and participates in the exocytosis of LH and FSH from the cell.

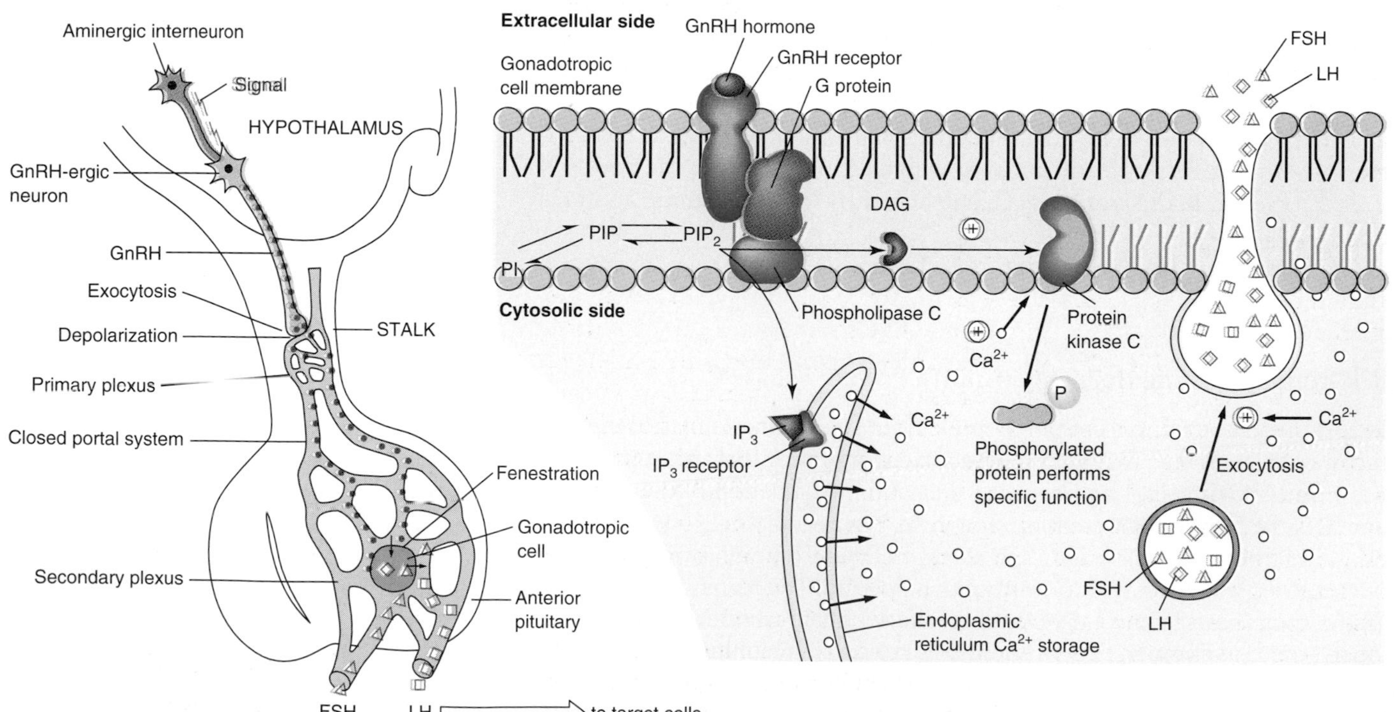

FIGURE 20.39
Overview of regulation of secretion of LH and FSH.
A general mode of action of GnRH to release the gonadotropes from the gonadotropic cell of the anterior pituitary is presented. GnRH, gonadotropin-releasing hormone; FSH, follicle-stimulating hormone; LH, luteinizing hormone; DAG, diacylglycerol.

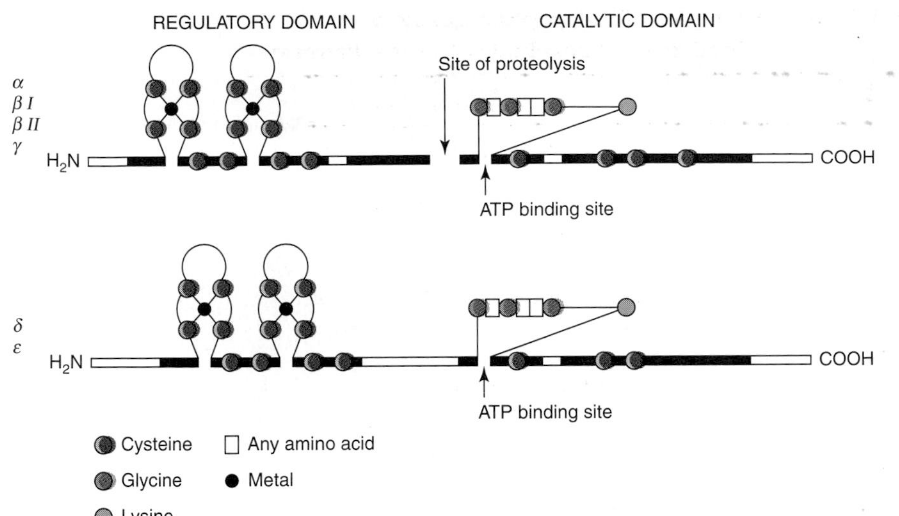

FIGURE 20.40
Common structure of protein kinase C subspecies.
Modified from U. Kikkawa, A. Kishimoto, and Y. Nishizuka, Annu. Rev. Biochem. *58:31, 1989.*

Much recent work has focused on protein kinase C. It has been shown to have a number of subspecies; such heterogeneity may indicate that there are multiple functions for this critical enzyme (Figure 20.40). The enzyme consists of two domains, a regulatory and a catalytic domain, which can be separated by proteolysis at a specific site. The free catalytic domain, formerly called **protein kinase M,** can phosphorylate proteins free of the regulatory components. The free catalytic subunit, however, may be degraded. More needs to be learned about the dynamics of this system and the translocation of the enzyme from one compartment to another. The regulatory domain contains two Zn^{2+} fingers usually considered to be hallmarks of DNA-binding proteins (see Chapter 3). This DNA-binding activity has not yet been demonstrated for protein kinase C and metal fingers may participate in other types of interactions. The ATP-binding site in the catalytic domain contains the G box, GXGXXG, which is a consensus sequence for ATP binding with a downstream lysine residue.

Activity of Atrial Natriuretic Factor (ANF): Protein Kinase G

The third system is the **protein kinase G** system, which is stimulated by the elevation of cytosolic cGMP (Figure 20.41). **Cyclic GMP** is synthesized by guanylate cyclase from GTP. Like adenylate cyclase, guanylate cyclase is linked to a specific biological signal through a membrane receptor. The guanylate cyclase extracellular domain may serve the role of the hormone receptor. This is directly coupled to the cytosolic domain through one membrane-spanning domain (Figure 20.42), which may be applicable to the **atrial natriuretic factor** (ANF; also referred to as atriopeptin) **receptor–guanylate cyclase system.** Thus the hormone-binding site, transmembrane domain, and guanylate cyclase activities are all served by a single polypeptide chain.

This hormone is a family of peptides, as shown in Figure 20.43; a sequence of human ANF is shown at the bottom. The functional domains of the ANF receptor are illustrated in Figure 20.44. Atrial natriuretic factor is released from atrial cells of the heart under control of several hormones. Data from atrial cell culture suggest that ANF secretion is stimulated by activators of protein kinase C and decreased by activators of protein kinase A. These opposing actions may be mediated by the actions of α- and β-adrenergic receptors, respectively. An overview of the secretion of ANF and its general effects is shown in Figure 20.45. ANF is released by a number of signals, such as blood volume expansion, elevated blood pressure directly induced by vasoconstrictors, high salt intake,

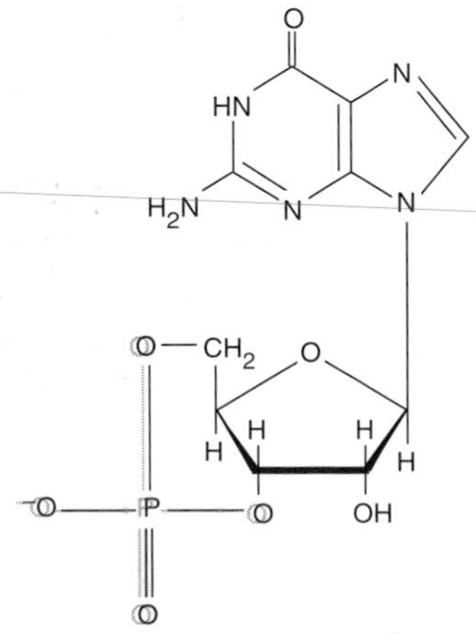

FIGURE 20.41
Structure of cGMP.

Extracellular side
Guanylate cyclase
Plasma membrane
Cytosolic side
P
Guanylate cyclase
Peptide hormone
GTP
cGMP + P_i
Hormone
Dephosphorylated guanylate cyclase

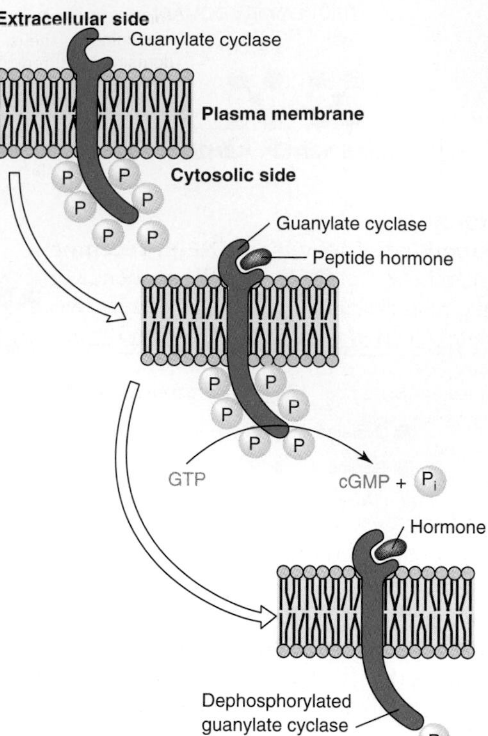

FIGURE 20.42
Model for the regulation of guanylate cyclase activity after peptide hormone binding.
The enzyme exists in a highly phosphorylated state under normal conditions. Binding of hormone markedly enhances enzyme activity, followed by a rapid dephosphorylation of guanylate cyclase and a return of activity to basal state despite continued presence of hormonal peptide.
Redrawn from Schultz, S., Chinkers, M., and Garbers, D. L. FASEB J. *3:2026, 1989.*

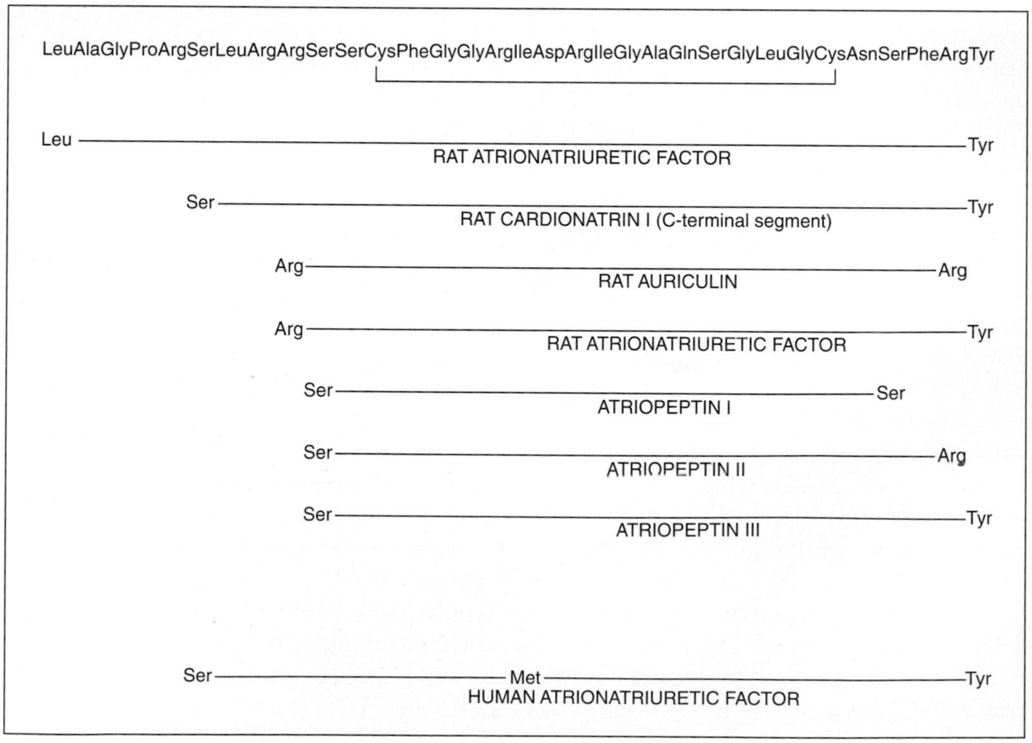

LeuAlaGlyProArgSerLeuArgArgSerSerCysPheGlyGlyArgIleAspArgIleGlyAlaGlnSerGlyLeuGlyCysAsnSerPheArgTyr
Leu
Tyr
RAT ATRIONATRIURETIC FACTOR
Ser
Tyr
RAT CARDIONATRIN I (C-terminal segment)
Arg
Arg
RAT AURICULIN
Arg
Tyr
RAT ATRIONATRIURETIC FACTOR
Ser
Ser
ATRIOPEPTIN I
Ser
Arg
ATRIOPEPTIN II
Ser
Tyr
ATRIOPEPTIN III
Ser
Met
Tyr
HUMAN ATRIONATRIURETIC FACTOR

FIGURE 20.43
Atrial natriuretic peptides.
These active peptides relax vascular smooth muscle and produce vasodilation and natriuresis as well as other effects discussed in the text.
Adapted from Carlin, M., and Genest, J. The heart and the atrial natriuretic factor. Endocr. Rev. *6:107, 1985.*

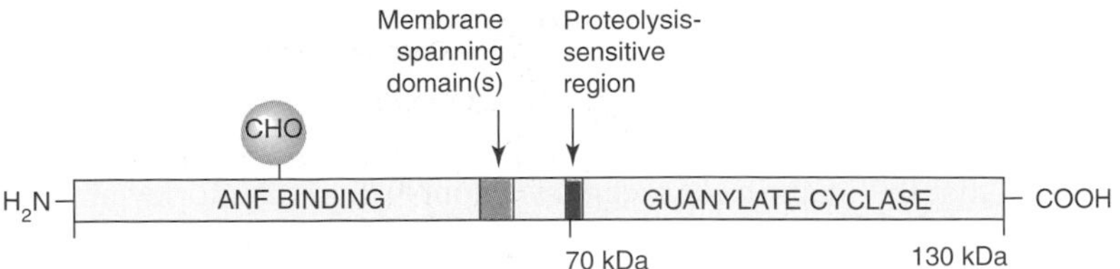

FIGURE 20.44
Functional domains of ANF-R_1 receptor.
Hypothetical model shows the sequence of an ANF-binding domain, a membrane-spanning domain(s), a proteolysis-sensitive region, a guanylate cyclase catalytic domain, glucosylation sites (CHO), and amino (H_2N) and carboxyl terminals (COOH) of receptor.
Redrawn from Liu, B., Meloche, S., McNicoll, N., Lord, C., and DeLéan, A. Biochemistry *28:5599, 1989.*

and increased heart pumping rate. ANF is secreted as a dimer that is inactive for receptor interaction and is converted in plasma to a monomer capable of interacting with receptor. The actions of ANF (Figure 20.45) are to increase the glomerular filtration rate without increasing renal blood flow, leading to increased urine volume and excretion of sodium ion. Renin secretion is also reduced and aldosterone secretion by the adrenal cortex is lowered. This action reduces aldosterone-mediated sodium reabsorption. ANF inhibits the vasoconstriction produced by angiotensin II and relaxes the constriction of the renal vessels, other vascular beds, and large arteries. ANF operates through its mem-

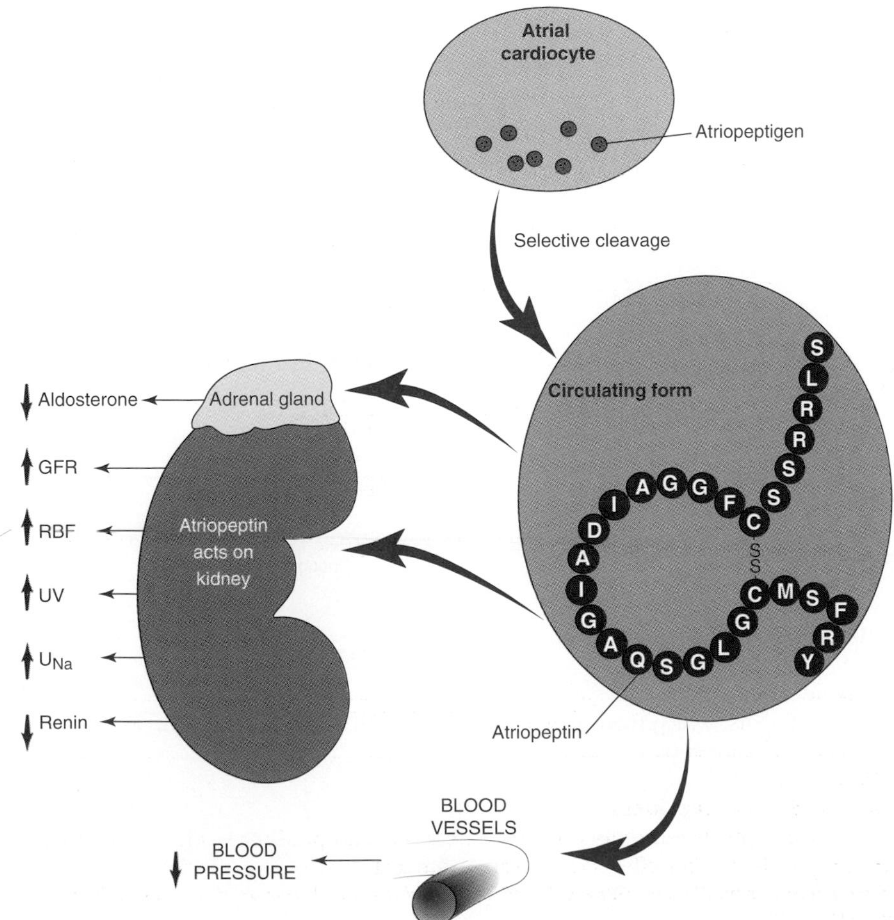

FIGURE 20.45
Schematic diagram of atrial natriuretic factor–atriopeptin hormonal system.
Prohormone is stored in granules located in perinuclear atrial cardiocytes. An elevated vascular volume results in cleavage and release of atriopeptin, which acts on the kidney (glomeruli and papilla) to increase the glomerular filtration rate (GFR), to increase renal blood flow (RBF), to increase urine volume (UV) and sodium excretion (U_{Na}), and to decrease plasma renin activity. Natriuresis and diuresis are also enhanced by the suppression of aldosterone secretion by the adrenal cortex and the release from the posterior pituitary of arginine vasopressin. Vasodilatation of blood vessels also results in a lowering of blood pressure (BP). Diminution of vascular volume provides a negative feedback signal that suppresses circulating levels of atriopeptin.
Redrawn from Needleman, P., and Greenwald, J. E. Atriopeptin: a cardiac hormone intimately involved in fluid, electrolyte, and blood pressure homeostasis. N. Engl. J. Med. *314:828, 1986.*

brane receptor, which appears to be the extracellular domain of guanylate cyclase. The cGMP produced activates protein kinase G, which further phosphorylates cellular proteins to express many of the actions of this pathway. More needs to be learned about protein kinase G. Using analogs of ANF it has been shown that the majority of receptors expressed in the kidney are biologically silent, since they fail to elicit a physiological response. This new class of receptors may serve as specific peripheral storage–clearance binding sites and as such act as a hormonal buffer system to modulate plasma levels of ANF.

20.13 ■ ONCOGENES AND RECEPTOR FUNCTIONS

Oncogenes are genes that are expressed by cancerous transformed cells. A cancer cell may express few or many oncogenes that dictate the aberrant uncontrolled behavior of the cell. There are three mechanisms by which oncogenes allow a cell to escape dependence on exogenous growth factors; these are presented in Figure 20.46. Some oncogenes are genes for parts of receptors, most often related to growth factor hormone receptors, which can function in the absence of the hormonal ligand. Thus an oncogene may represent a truncated gene where the ligand-binding domain is missing. This would result in production of the receptor protein, insertion into the cell membrane, and continuous constitutive function in the absence or presence of ligand (Figure 20.46*b,c*). In this situation the second messengers would be produced constitutively at a high rate, instead of being regulated by ligand, and the result would be uncontrolled growth of the cell. Some oncogenes may have tyrosine protein kinase activity and therefore function like tyrosine kinase normally related to certain cell membrane receptors. Other oncogenes relate to thyroid and steroid hormone receptors (see Chapter 21) while still others are DNA-binding proteins, some of which may be transactivating factors or related to such factors. Oncogene-encoded proteins that bind to DNA may be identical with or related to transactivating factors. The oncogene *Jun,* for example, is a component of activator protein 1 (AP1), a transactivating factor that regulates transcription. Table 20.9 reviews some of the oncogenes, or cancer-causing genes, together with the functions of their proto-oncogenes (normal proliferation gene).

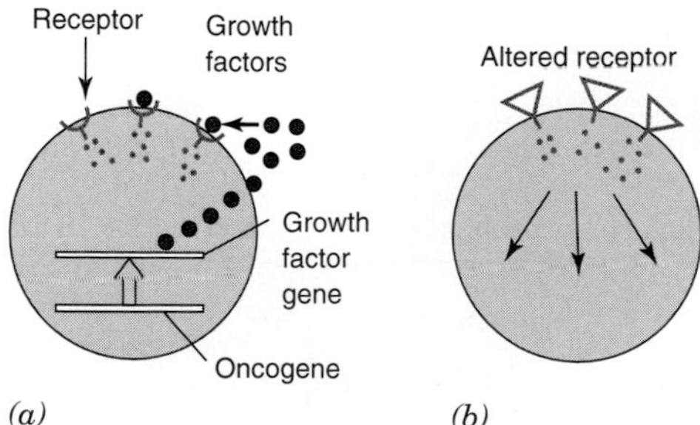

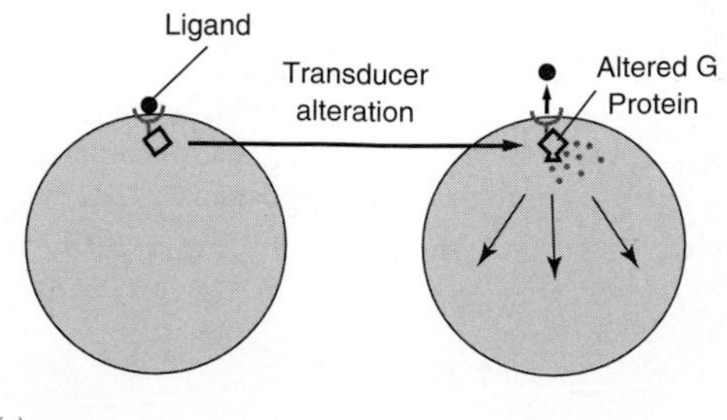

FIGURE 20.46
Mechanisms by which oncogenes can allow a cell to escape dependence on exogenous growth factors.
(*a*) By autocrine mechanism, where the cytosolic oncogene indirectly stimulates expression of growth factor gene and oversecretion of growth factors, which then overstimulates receptors on same cell; (*b*) by receptor alteration so that receptor is "permanently turned on" without a requirement for growth factor binding; and (*c*) by transducer alteration, where the intermediate between the receptor and its resultant activity, that is, the GTP-stimulatory protein, is permanently activated, uncoupling the normal requirement of ligand–receptor binding.
Redrawn from Weinberg, R. A. The action of oncogenes in the cytoplasm and nucleus. Science *230:770, 1985.*

TABLE 20.9 Known Oncogenes, Their Products and Functions[a]

Name of Oncogene	Retrovirus	Virus-Induced Tumor	Oncogenic Protein	
			Cellular Location	Proto-oncogene Function
src	Chicken sarcoma	Chicken sarcoma	Plasma membrane	Tyrosine-specific protein kinase
yes	Chicken sarcoma		Plasma membrane (?)	
fgr	Cat sarcoma		(?)	
abl	Mouse leukemia	Human leukemia	Plasma membrane	Tyrosine-specific protein kinase
fps	Chicken sarcoma		Cytoplasm (plasma membrane?)	
fes	Cat sarcoma	Sarcoma	Cytoplasm (cytoskeleton?)	Tyrosine-specific protein kinase
ros	Chicken sarcoma		(?)	
erb-B	Chicken leukemia	Erythroleukemia, fibrosarcoma	Plasma and cytoplasmic membranes	EGF receptor's cytoplasmic tyrosine-specific protein kinase domain
fms	Cat sarcoma	Sarcoma	Plasma and cytoplasmic membranes	Tyrosine-specific protein kinase; macrophage colony-stimulating factor receptor
mil	Chicken carcinoma		Cytoplasm	(?)
raf	Mouse sarcoma	Sarcoma	Cytoplasm	Protein kinase (serine/threonine) activated by Ras
mos	Mouse sarcoma	Mouse leukemia	Cytoplasm	(?)
sis	Monkey sarcoma	Monkey sarcoma	Secreted	PDGF-like growth factor, β-chain
Ha-ras	Rat sarcoma	Human carcinoma, rat carcinoma	Plasma membrane	GTP-binding protein
Ki-ras	Rat sarcoma	Human carcinoma, leukemia, and sarcoma	Plasma membrane	GTP-binding protein
N-ras	—	Human leukemia and carcinoma	Plasma membrane	
myc	Chicken leukemia	Sarcoma, myelocytoma, and carcinoma	Nucleus	DNA-binding related to cell proliferation; transcriptional control
myb	Chicken leukemia	Human leukemia	Nucleus	(?)
B-lym	—	Chicken lymphoma, human lymphoma	Nucleus (?)	(?)
ski	Chicken sarcoma		Nucleus (?)	(?)
rel	Turkey leukemia	Reticuloendotheliosis	(?)	(?)
erb-A	Chicken leukemia		(?)	Thyroid hormone receptor (c-erb-Aα1); related to steroid hormone receptors, retinoic acid receptor, and vitamin D_3 receptor
ets	Chicken leukemia		(?)	DNA binding
elk (*ets*-like)				DNA-binding protein
jun		Osteosarcoma		Products associate to form AP1 gene transcription factor
fos		Fibrosarcoma		Products associate to form AP1 gene transcription factor

Source: Adapted from Hunter, T. The proteins of oncogenes. *Sci. Am.* 251:70, 1984.

[a] The second column gives the source from which each viral oncogene was first isolated and the cancer induced by the oncogene. Some names, such as *fps* and *fes,* may be equivalent genes in birds and mammals. The third column lists human and animal tumors caused by agents other than viruses in which the *ras* oncogene or an inappropriately expressed proto-oncogene has been identified.

BIBLIOGRAPHY

Alberts, B., Bray, D., Lewis, J., Raff, R., Roberts, K., and Watson, J. D. *Molecular Biology of the Cell,* 3rd ed. New York: Garland Publishing, 1994.

Cuatrecasas, P. Hormone receptors, membrane phospholipids, and protein kinases. *The Harvey Lectures* Series 80:89, 1986.

DeGroot, L. J., (Ed.). *Endocrinology.* Philadelphia: Saunders, 1995.

Hunter, T. The proteins of oncogenes. *Sci. Am.* 251:70, 1984.

Krieger, D. T., and Hughes, J. C. (Eds.). *Neuroendocrinology.* Sunderland, MA: Sinauer Associates, 1980.

Litwack, G. (Ed.). *Biochemical Actions of Hormones,* Vols. 1–14. New York: Academic Press, 1973–1987.

Litwack, G. (Ed. in Chief) *Vitamins and Hormones,* Vol. 50. Orlando: Academic Press, 1995.

Norman, A. W., and Litwack, G. *Hormones.* Orlando: Academic Press, 1987.

Richter, D. Molecular events in expression of vasopressin and oxytocin and their cognate receptors. *Am. J. Physiol.* 255:F207, 1988.

Ryan, R. J., Charlesworth, M. C., McCormick, D. J., Milius, R. P., and Keutmann, H. T. *FASEB J.* 2:2661, 1988.

Saltiel, A. R. The paradoxical regulation of protein phosphorylation in insulin action. *FASEB J.* 8:1034, 1994.

Spiegel, A. M., Shenker, A., and Weinstein, L. S. Receptor–effector coupling by G proteins: implication for normal and abnormal signal-transduction. *Endocr. Rev.* 13:536, 1992.

Struthers, A. D. (Ed.) *Atrial Natriuretic Factor.* Boston: Blackwell Scientific Publications, 1990.

Weinberg, R. A. The action of oncogenes in the cytoplasm and nucleus. *Science* 230:770, 1985.

QUESTIONS

J. Baggott and C. N. Angstadt

1. In a cascade of hormones (e.g., hypothalamus, pituitary, and target tissue), at each successive level:
   A. the quantity of hormone released and its half-life can be expected to increase.
   B. the quantity of hormone released increases, but its half-life does not change.
   C. the quantity of hormone released and its half-life are approximately constant.
   D. the quantity of hormone released decreases, but its half-life does not change.
   E. the quantity of hormone released and its half-life can both be expected to decrease.

2. All of the following have an identical (or very similar) α subunit EXCEPT:
   A. growth hormone.
   B. thyroid-stimulating hormone.
   C. luteinizing hormone.
   D. follicle-stimulating hormone.

3. If a single gene contains information for the synthesis of more than one hormone molecule:
   A. all the hormones are produced by any tissue that expresses the gene.
   B. all of the hormone molecules are identical.
   C. cleavage sites in the gene product are typically pairs of basic amino acids.
   D. all of the peptides of the gene product have well-defined biological activity.
   E. the hormones all have similar function.

4. In the sequence of events associated with signal transduction, which one is out of place? Receptor binds hormone.
   A. Conformational change occurs in receptor.
   B. Receptor interacts with G-protein.
   C. α Subunit of G-protein hydrolyzes GTP.
   D. α Subunit of G-protein dissociates from β and γ subunits.
   E. α Subunit of G-protein binds to adenylate cyclase.

5. The direct effect of cAMP in the protein kinase A pathway is to:
   A. activate adenylate cyclase.
   B. dissociate regulatory subunits from protein kinase.
   C. phosphorylate certain cellular proteins.
   D. phosphorylate protein kinase A.
   E. release hormones from a target tissue.

6. Activation of phospholipase C initiates a sequence of events including all of the following EXCEPT:
   A. release of inositol 4,5-bisphosphate from a phospholipid.
   B. increase in intracellular Ca^{2+} concentration.
   C. release of diacylglycerol (DAG) from a phospholipid.
   D. activation of protein kinase C.
   E. phosphorylation of certain cytoplasmic proteins.

7. In the ovarian cycle:
   A. GnRH enters the vascular system via transport by a specific membrane carrier.
   B. the corpus luteum dies only if fertilization does not occur.
   C. inhibin works by inhibiting the synthesis of the α subunit of FSH.
   D. FSH activates a protein kinase A pathway.
   E. LH is taken up by the corpus luteum and binds to cytoplasmic receptors.

8. The Scatchard plot, shown in the accompanying figure, could be used to determine kinetic parameters of an enzyme. Which letter in the graph corresponds to total binding sites in a Scatchard plot or V_{max} in an enzyme kinetic plot?

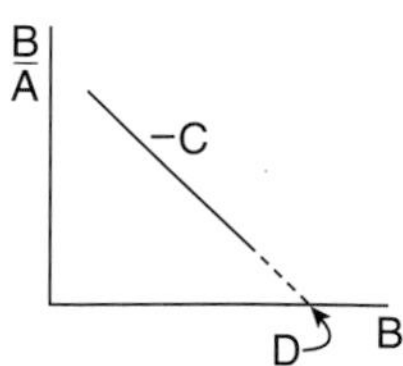

9. With the anterior pituitary hormones, TSH, LH, and FSH:
   A. the α subunits are all different.
   B. the β subunits are specifically recognized by the receptor.
   C. the β subunit alone can bind to the receptor.
   D. hormonal activity is expressed through activation of protein kinase B.
   E. intracellular receptors bind these hormones.

10. In the interaction of a hormone with its receptor, all of the following are true EXCEPT:
   A. more than one polypeptide chain of the hormone may be necessary.
   B. more than one second messenger may be generated.
   C. an array of transmembrane helices may form the binding site for the hormone.
   D. receptors have a greater affinity for hormones than for synthetic agonists or antagonists.
   E. hormones released from their receptor after endocytosis could interact with a nuclear receptor.

In the following questions, match the numbered hormone with the lettered kinase it stimulates.

   A. protein kinase A
   B. tyrosine kinase
   C. protein kinase C
   D. protein kinase G

11. Atrial natriuretic factor.

12. Gonadotropin-releasing hormone.

13. Insulin.

14. Vasopressin.

ANSWERS

1. A Each successive step typically releases a larger amount of a longer lived hormone (p. 842).
2. A All of these are anterior pituitary hormones, but only the last three, the glycoprotein hormones, have an α subunit that is similar or identical from hormone to hormone (p. 846).
3. C One or more trypsin-like proteases catalyze the reaction (Figure 20.5). A: The POMC gene product is cleaved differently in different parts of the anterior pituitary (p. 849). B: Multiple copies of a single hormone may occur (p. 852) , but not necessarily (Figure 20.5, p. 850). D: Some fragments have no known function. E: ACTH and β-endorphin, for example, hardly have similar functions (p. 847; Table 20.2).
4. C Hydrolysis of GTP returns the α subunit to its original conformation and allows it to associate with the β and γ subunits (p. 861).
5. B cAMP binding causes a conformational change in the regulatory subunits, resulting in the release of active protein kinase A (p. 862).
6. A Inositol 1,4,5-triphosphate (IP_3) is released from the phospholipid, phosphatidylinositol 4,5-bisphosphate (PIP_2) (p. 862).
7. D A: GnRH enters the vascular system through fenestrations (p. 868). B. The corpus luteum is replaced by the placenta if fertilization occurs (p. 870). C: The glycoprotein hormones share a common α subunit. Specific control of them would not involve a subunit they share. E: LH interacts with receptors on the cell membrane.
8. D A is free ligand concentration (analogous to substrate concentration), B is bound ligand concentration (analogous to v), C is the equilibrium constant (analogous to K_m), and D is the extrapolated maximum number of binding sites (analogous to V_{max}) (p. 872).
9. B A: The α subunits are identical or nearly so (p. 872). B and C: Although specificity is conferred by the β subunits, which differ among the three hormones, binding to the receptor requires both subunits (p. 873). D: It is protein kinase A, and perhaps also protein kinase C in the case of TSH (p. 873). E: These large glycoprotein hormones do not penetrate the cell membrane; they bind to receptors on the cell surface (p. 874). See Figure 20.30.
10. D β Receptors bind isoproterenol more tightly than their hormones (p. 875). A and B: These are true of the glycoprotein hormones (p. 873). C: This appears to be true for the β_1 receptor (Figure 20.31). E: This is possible, but entirely speculative; there are currently no known examples.
11. D See p. 885.
12. C See p. 883.
13. B See p. 879.
14. A See p. 880.

CHAPTER

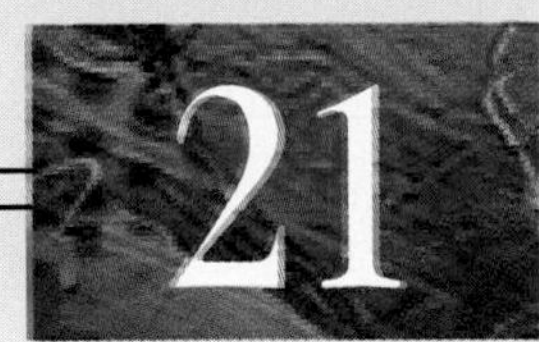

BIOCHEMISTRY OF HORMONES II: STEROID HORMONES

Gerald Litwack and Thomas J. Schmidt

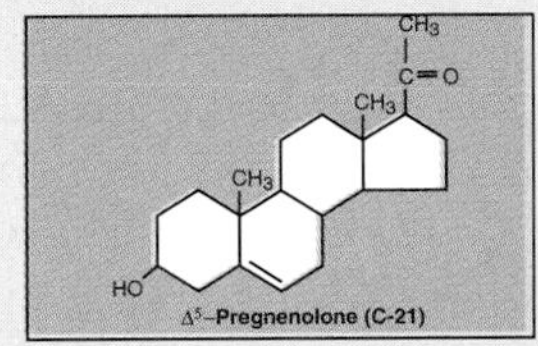

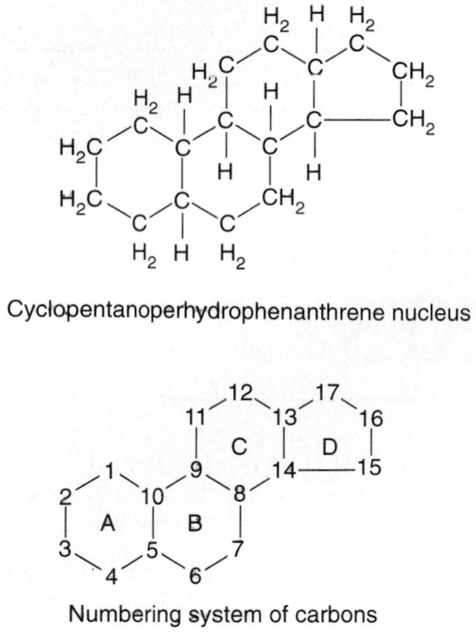

FIGURE 21.1
The steroid nucleus.

21.1 OVERVIEW

Steroid hormones in the human include cortisol as the major glucocorticoid or anti-stress hormone, aldosterone as an important regulator of Na^+ uptake, and the sex and progestational hormones. Sex hormones are 17β-estradiol in females and testosterone in males. Progesterone is the major progestational hormone. Testosterone is reduced in some target tissues to dihydrotestosterone, a higher affinity ligand for the androgen receptor. Vitamin D_3 is converted to the steroid hormone, dihydroxy vitamin D_3. Genes in the steroid receptor supergene family include retinoic acid receptors and thyroid hormone receptor, although the ligands for these additional receptors are not derivatives of cholesterol. Retinoic acid and thyroid hormone, however, have six-membered ring structures that could be considered to resemble the A ring of a steroid.

Steroidal structure will be reviewed with the synthesis and inactivation of steroid hormones. Regulation of synthesis of steroid hormones is reviewed with respect to the renin–angiotensin system for aldosterone, the gonadotropes, especially follicle-stimulating hormone for 17β-estradiol, and the vitamin D_3 mechanism. Steroid hormone transport is reviewed with respect to the transporting proteins in blood. A general model for steroid hormone action at the cellular level is presented with information on receptor activation and regulation of receptor levels. Specific examples of steroid hormone action for programmed cell death and for stress are presented. Finally, the roles of steroid hormone receptors as transcriptional transactivators and repressors are reviewed.

21.2 STRUCTURES OF STEROID HORMONES

Steroid hormones are derived in specific tissues in the body and are divided into two classes: the **sex** and **progestational hormones,** and the **adrenal hormones.** They are synthesized from cholesterol and all of these hormones pass through the required intermediate, Δ^5-pregnenolone. The structure of steroid hormones is related to the **cyclopentanoperhydrophenanthrene** nucleus. The numbering of the cyclopentanoperhydrophenanthrene ring system and the lettering of the rings is presented in Figure 21.1. The ring system of the steroid hormones is stable and not catabolized by mammalian cells. Conversion of active hormones to less active or inactive forms involves alteration of ring substituents rather than the ring structure itself. The parental precursor of the steroid is **cholesterol,** shown in Figure 21.2. The biosynthesis of cholesterol is given on p. 410.

The major steroid hormones of humans and their actions are shown in Table 21.1. Many of these hormones are similar in gross structure, although the specific receptor for each hormone is able to distinguish the cognate ligand. In the cases of cortisol and aldosterone, however, there is overlap in the ability of each specific receptor to bind both ligands. Thus the availability and concen-

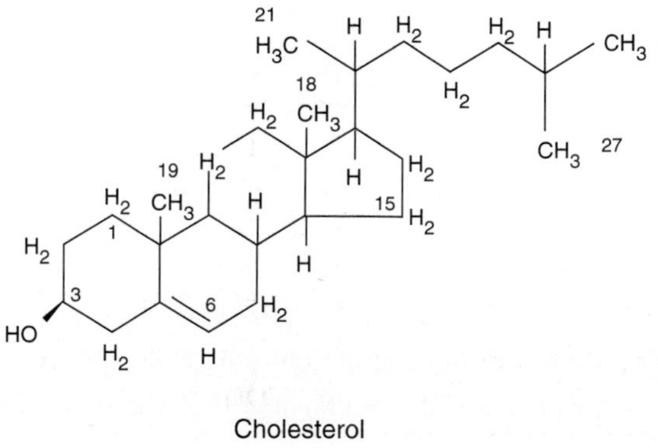

FIGURE 21.2
Structure of cholesterol.

TABLE 21.1 Major Steroid Hormones of Humans

Hormone	*Structure*	*Secretion from*	*Secretion Signal*[a]	*Functions*
Progesterone	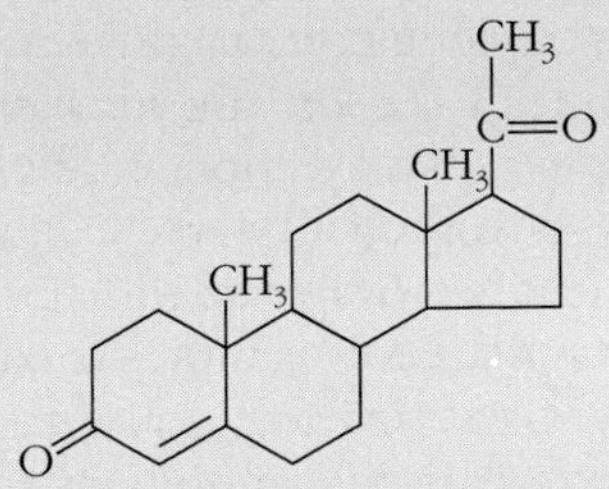	Corpus luteum	LH	Maintains (with estradiol) the uterine endometrium for implantation; differentiation factor for mammary glands
17β-Estradiol	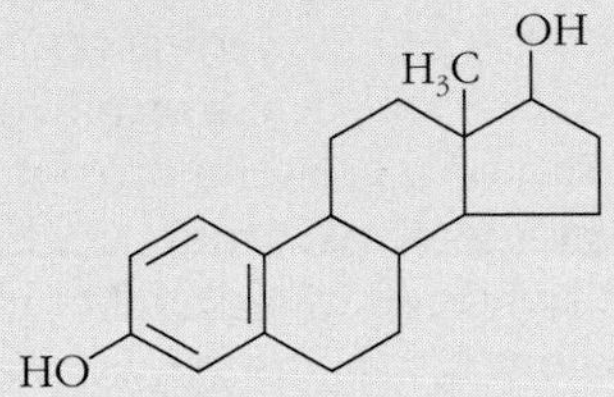	Ovarian follicle; corpus luteum; (Sertoli cell)	FSH	Female: regulates gondotropin secretion in ovarian cycle (see Chapter 20); maintains (with progesterone) uterine endometrium; differentiation of mammary gland. Male: negative feedback inhibitor of Leydig cell synthesis of testosterone
Testosterone	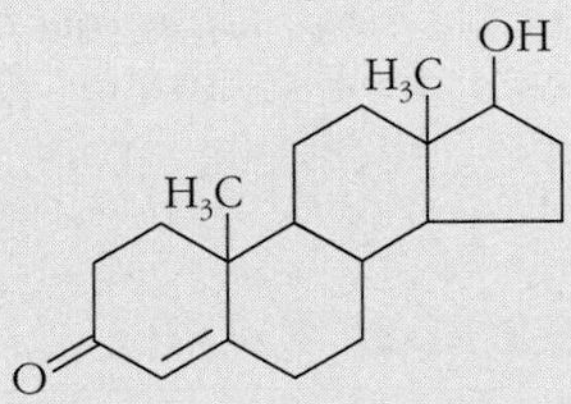	Leydig cells of testis; (adrenal gland); ovary	LH	Male: after conversion to dihydrotestosterone, production of sperm proteins in Sertoli cells; secondary sex characteristics (in some tissues testosterone is active hormone)
Dehydroepiandrosterone	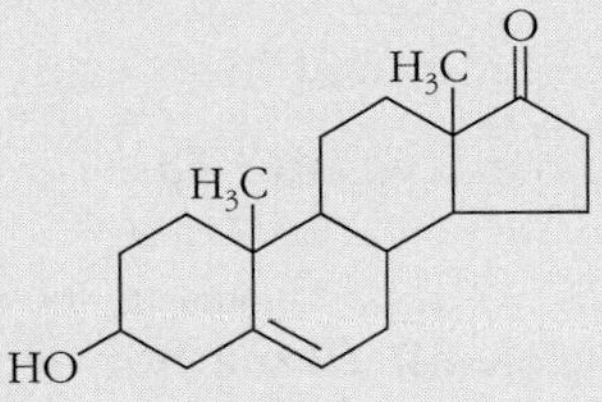	Reticularis cells	ACTH	Various protective effects; weak androgen; can be converted to estrogen; no receptor yet found; inhibitor of G6-PDH: regulates NAD^+ coenzymes
Cortisol	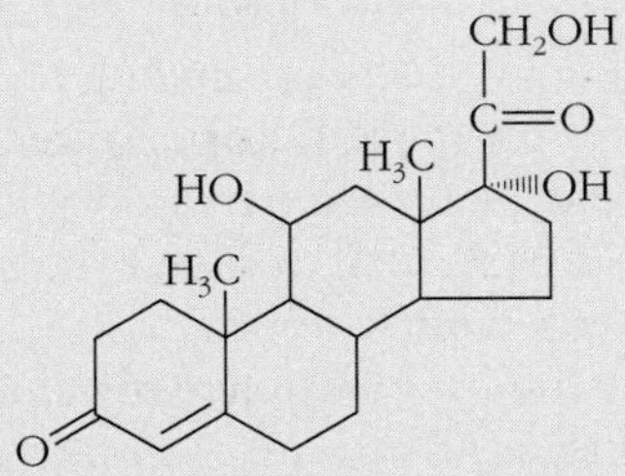	Fasciculata cells	ACTH	Stress adaptation through various cellular phenotypic expressions; slight elevation of liver glycogen; killing effect on certain T cells in high doses; elevates blood pressure; sodium uptake in luminal epithelia
Aldosterone	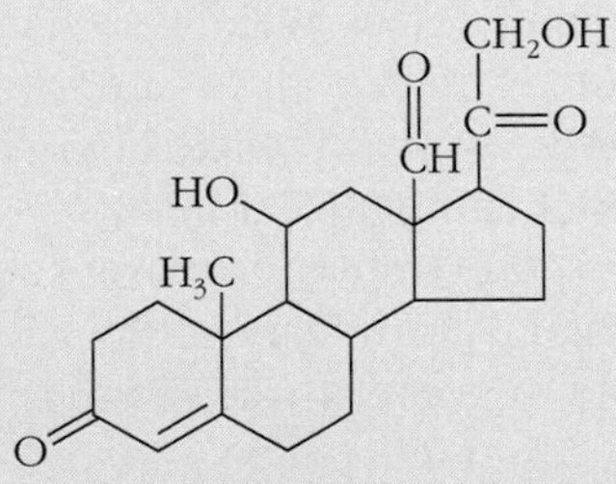	Glomerulosa cells of adrenal cortex	Angiotensin II/III	Causes sodium ion uptake via conductance channel; occurs in high levels during stress; raises blood pressure; fluid volume increased
1,25-Dihydroxyvitamin D_3	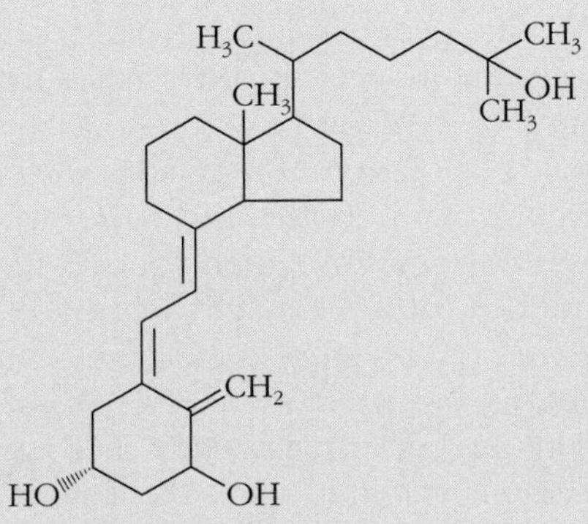	Vitamin D arises in skin cells after irradiation and then successive hydroxylations occur in liver and kidney to yield active form of hormone	PTH (stimulates kidney proximal tubule hydroxylation system)	Facilitates Ca^{2+} and phosphate absorption by intestinal epithelial cells; induces intracellular calcium-binding protein

[a] LH, luteinizing hormone; FSH, follicle-stimulating hormone; ACTH, adrenocorticotropic hormone; PTH, parathyroid hormone.

trations of each receptor and the relative amounts of each hormone in a given cell become paramount considerations. The steroid hormones listed in Table 21.1 can be described as classes based on the carbon number in their structures. Thus a C-27 steroid is 1,25$(OH)_2D_3$; C-21 steroids are **progesterone, cortisol,** and **aldosterone;** C-19 steroids are **testosterone** and **dehydroepiandrosterone;** and a C-18 steroid is **17β-estradiol.** Classes, such as sex hormones, can be distinguished easily by the carbon number, C-19 being androgens, C-18 being estrogens, and C-21 being progestational or adrenal steroids. Aside from the number of carbon atoms in a class structure, certain substituents in the ring system are characteristic. For example, glucocorticoids and mineralocorticoids (typically aldosterone) possess a C-11 OH or oxygen function. In rare exceptions, certain synthetic compounds can elicit a response without a C-11 OH group but they require a new functional group in proximity within the A-B ring system. Estrogens do not have a C-19 methyl group and the A ring is contracted by the content of three double bonds. Many receptors recognize the ligand A ring primarily, the estrogen receptor can distinguish the A ring of estradiol stretched out of the plane of the B-C-D rings compared to other steroids in which the A ring is coplanar with the B-C-D rings. These relationships are shown in Figure 21.3.

21.3 ■ BIOSYNTHESIS OF STEROID HORMONES

Steroid Hormones Are Synthesized from Cholesterol

Hormonal regulation of steroid hormone biosynthesis is generally believed to be mediated by an elevation of intracellular **cAMP** and **Ca^{2+},** although generation of **inositol triphosphate** may also be involved, as shown in Figure 21.4. The stimulatory response of cAMP is mediated via acute (occurring within seconds to minutes) and chronic (requiring hours) effects on steroid synthesis. The acute effect is to mobilize and deliver cholesterol, the precursor for all steroid hormones, to the mitochondrial inner membrane, where it is metabolized to pregnenolone by the cytochrome P450 cholesterol side chain cleavage enzyme (see Chapter 22 for discussion of P450 enzymes). In contrast, the chronic effects of cAMP are mediated via increased transcription of the genes that encode the steroidogenic enzymes and are thus responsible for maintaining optimal long-term steroid production. Data demonstrate that a protein is induced and that this newly synthesized regulatory protein actually facilitates the translocation of cholesterol from outer to inner mitochondrial membrane where the P450 enzyme is located. This 30-kDa phosphoprotein is designated as the **steroidogenic acute regulatory (StAR)** protein. In humans, StAR mRNA has been shown to be specifically expressed in testis and ovary, known sites of steroidogenesis. Patients with lipoid congenital adrenal hyperplasia (LCAH), an inherited disease in which both adrenal and gonadal steroidogenesis is significantly impaired and lipoidal deposits occur in these tissues, express truncated and nonfunctional StAR proteins. These biochemical and genetic data strongly suggest that StAR protein is the hormone-induced protein factor that mediates acute regulation of steroid hormone biosynthesis.

Pathways for conversion of cholesterol to the adrenal cortical steroid hormones are presented in Figure 21.5. Cholesterol is the major precursor and undergoes side chain cleavage to form Δ^5-pregnenolone releasing a C_6 aldehyde, isocaproaldehyde. **Δ^5-Pregnenolone** is mandatory in the synthesis of all steroid hormones. As shown in Figure 21.5, pregnenolone can be converted directly to progesterone, which requires two cytoplasmic enzymes, **3β-ol dehydrogenase** and **$\Delta^{4,5}$-isomerase.** The dehydrogenase converts the 3-OH group of pregnenolone to a 3-keto group and the isomerase moves the double bond from the B ring to the A ring to produce progesterone. In the *corpus luteum* the bulk

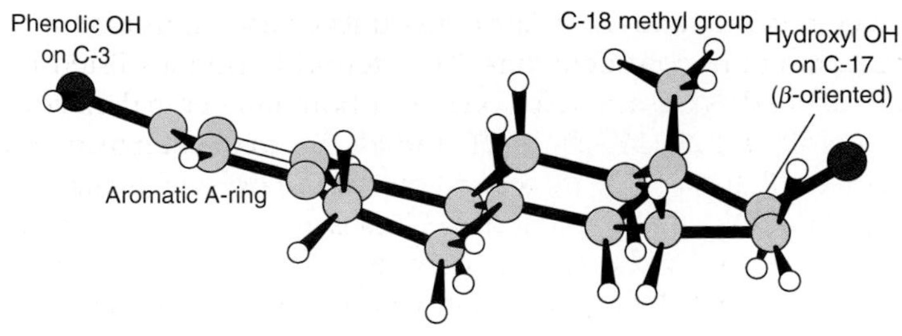

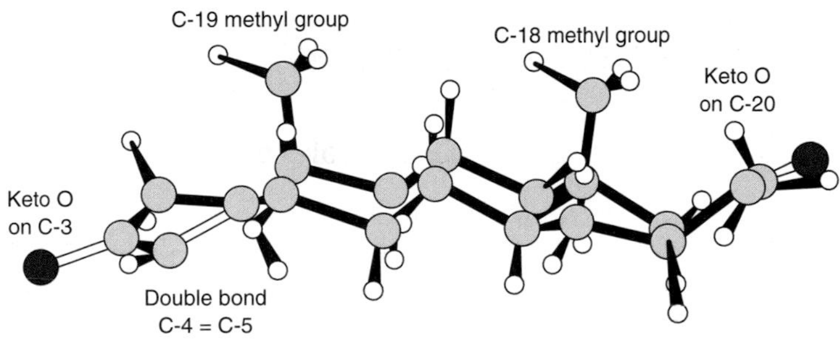

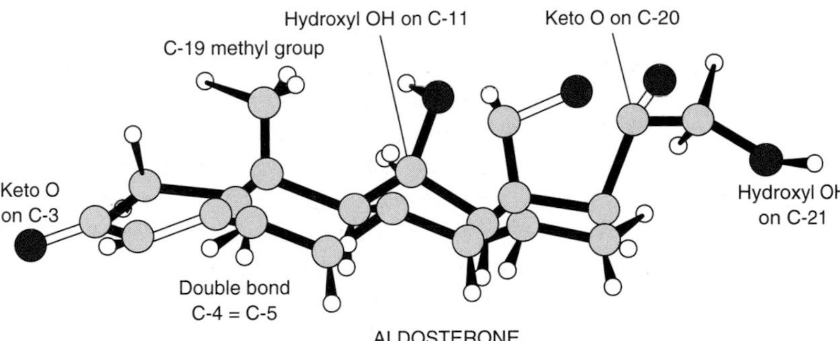

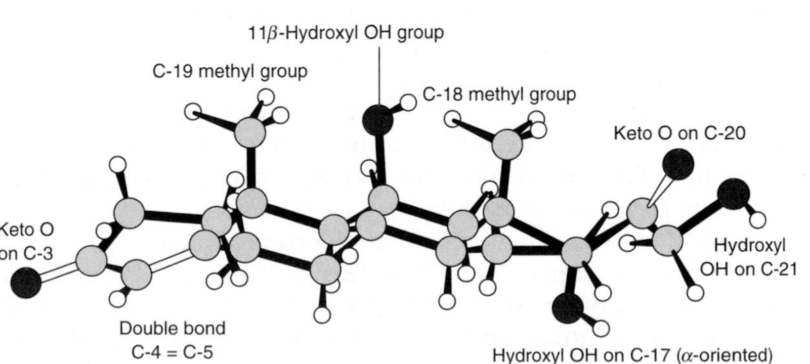

FIGURE 21.3
"Ball-and-stick" representations of the structures of some steroid hormones determined by X-ray crystallographic methods.
Details of each structure are labeled. In aldosterone the acetal grouping is

$$R\text{—}CH(OR_1)(OR_2)$$

and the hemiketal grouping is

$$(R_1)(R_2)C(OR_3)(OH)$$

where R_1, R_2, and R_3 refer to different substituents.

Reprinted with permission from Glusker, J. P. In G. Litwack (Ed.), Biochemical Actions of Hormones, *Vol. 6. New York: Academic Press, 1979, pp. 121–204.*

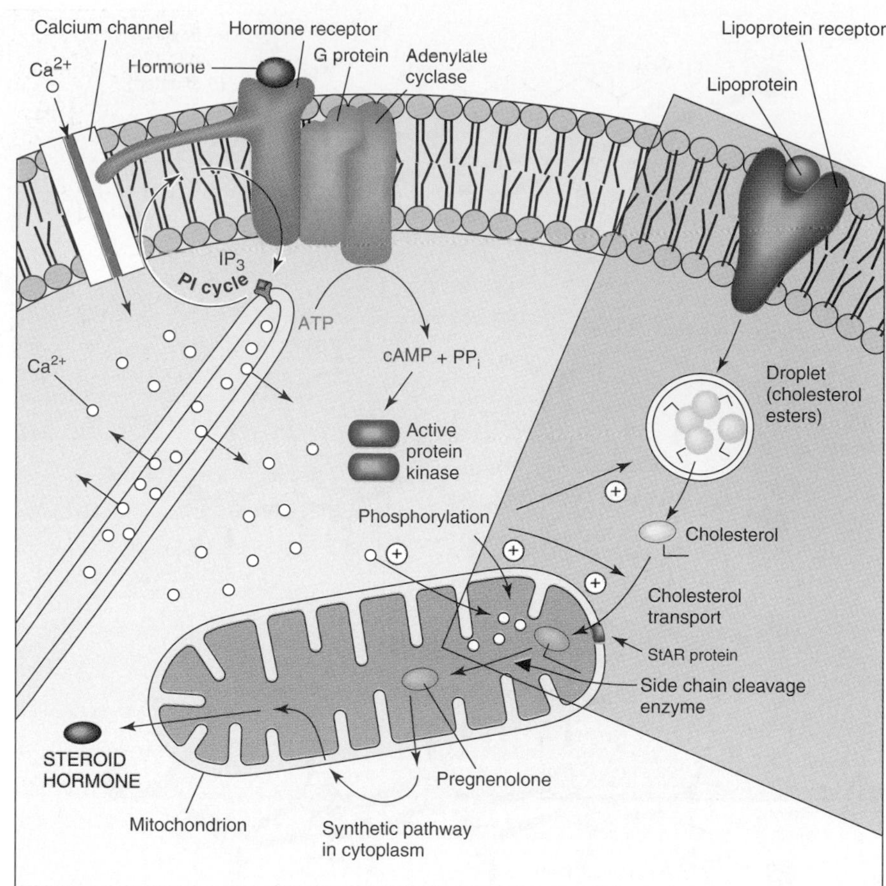

FIGURE 21.4
Overview of hormonal stimulation of steroid hormone biosynthesis.
Nature of the hormone (top of figure) depends on the cell type and receptor (ACTH for cortisol synthesis; FSH for estradiol synthesis; LH for testosterone synthesis, etc., as given in Table 20.1). It binds to cell membrane receptor and activates adenylate cyclase mediated by a stimulatory G-protein. Receptor, activated by hormone, may directly stimulate a calcium channel or indirectly stimulate it by activating the phosphatidylinositol cycle (PI cycle) as shown in Figure 20.25. If the PI cycle is concurrently stimulated, IP_3 could augment cytosol Ca^{2+} levels from the intracellular calcium store. The increase in cAMP activates protein kinase A (Figure 21.21) whose phosphorylations cause increased hydrolysis of cholesteryl esters from the droplet to free cholesterol and increase cholesterol transport into the mitochondrion. The combination of elevated Ca^{2+} levels and protein phosphorylation, as well as induction of the StAR protein, result in increased side chain cleavage and steroid biosynthesis. These combined reactions overcome the rate-limiting steps in steroid biosynthesis and more steroid is produced, which is secreted into the extracellular space and circulated to the target tissues in the bloodstream.

of steroid synthesis stops at this point. Progesterone is further converted to aldosterone or cortisol. Conversion of pregnenolone to **aldosterone,** which occurs in the adrenal *zona glomerulosa* cells, requires endoplasmic reticulum 21-hydroxylase, and mitochondrial 11β-hydroxylase and 18-hydroxylase. To form cortisol, primarily in adrenal *zona fasciculata* cells, endoplasmic reticulum **17-hydroxylase** and **21-hydroxylase** are required together with mitochondrial **11β-hydroxylase.** The endoplasmic reticulum (ER) hydroxylases are all cytochrome P450-linked enzymes (see Chapter 22). Δ^5-Pregnenolone is converted to **dehydroepiandrosterone** in the adrenal *zona reticularis* cells by the action of 17α-hydroxylase of the endoplasmic reticulum to form 17α-hydroxypregnenolone and then by the action of a carbon side chain-cleavage system to form dehydroepiandrosterone.

Cholesterol is also converted to the sex hormones by way of Δ^5-pregnenolone (Figure 21.6). **Progesterone** can be formed as described above and further converted to testosterone by the action of the endoplasmic reticulum enzymes and 17-dehydrogenase. **Testosterone,** so formed, is a major secretory product in the Leydig cells of the testis and undergoes conversion to dihydrotestosterone in some androgen target cells before binding to the androgen receptor. This conversion requires the activity of **5α-reductase** located in the ER and nuclear fractions. Pregnenolone can enter an alternative pathway to form dehydroepiandrosterone as described above. This compound can be converted to 17β-estradiol via the aromatase enzyme system and the action of 17-reductase. Also, estradiol can be formed from testosterone by the action of the aromatase system.

The hydroxylases of endoplasmic reticulum involved in steroid hormone synthesis are cytochrome P450 enzymes (Chapter 22). Molecular oxygen (O_2) is a substrate with one oxygen atom incorporated into the steroidal substrate (as an OH) and the second atom incorporated into a water molecule. Electrons

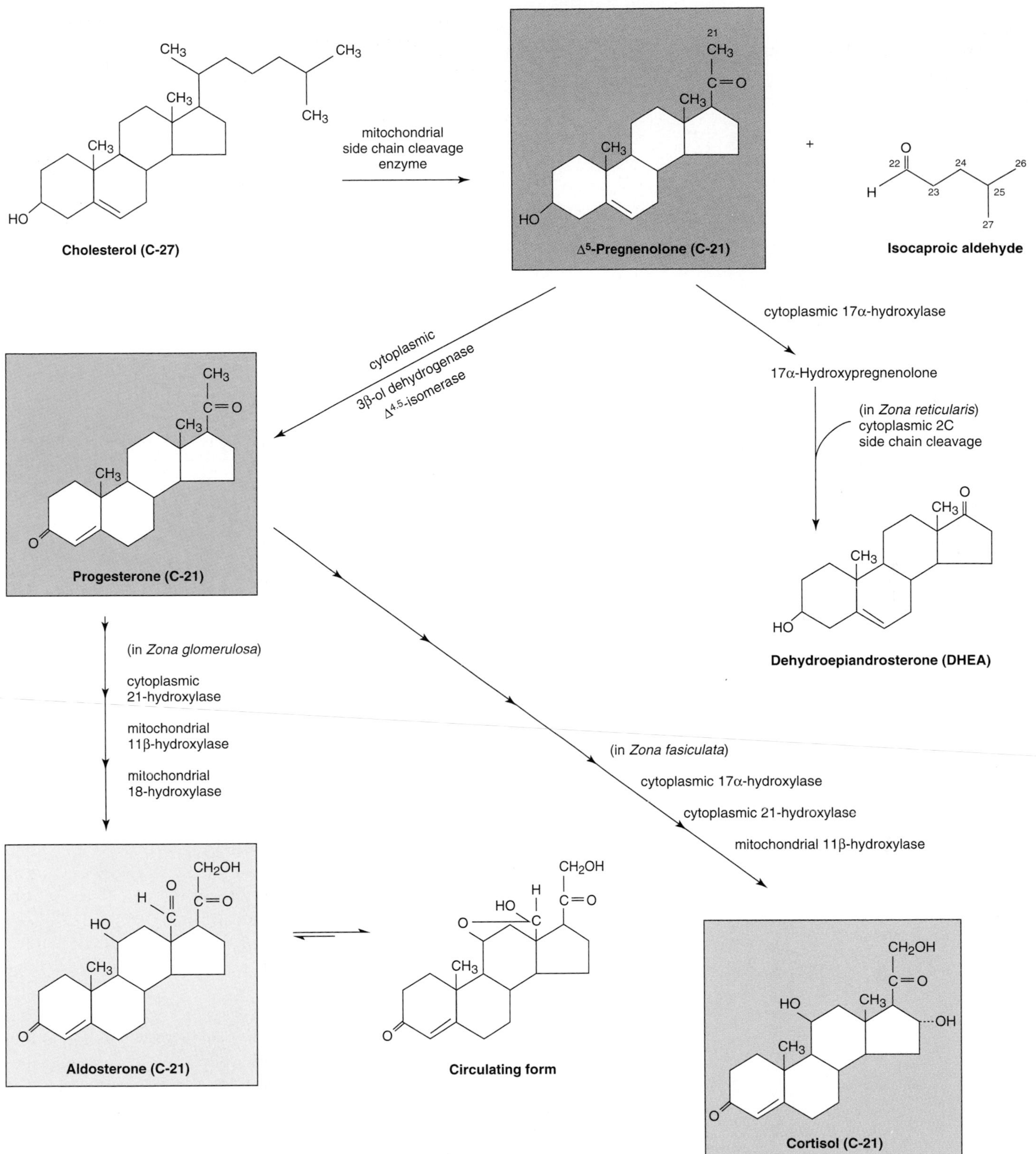

FIGURE 21.5
Conversion of cholesterol to adrenal cortical hormones.

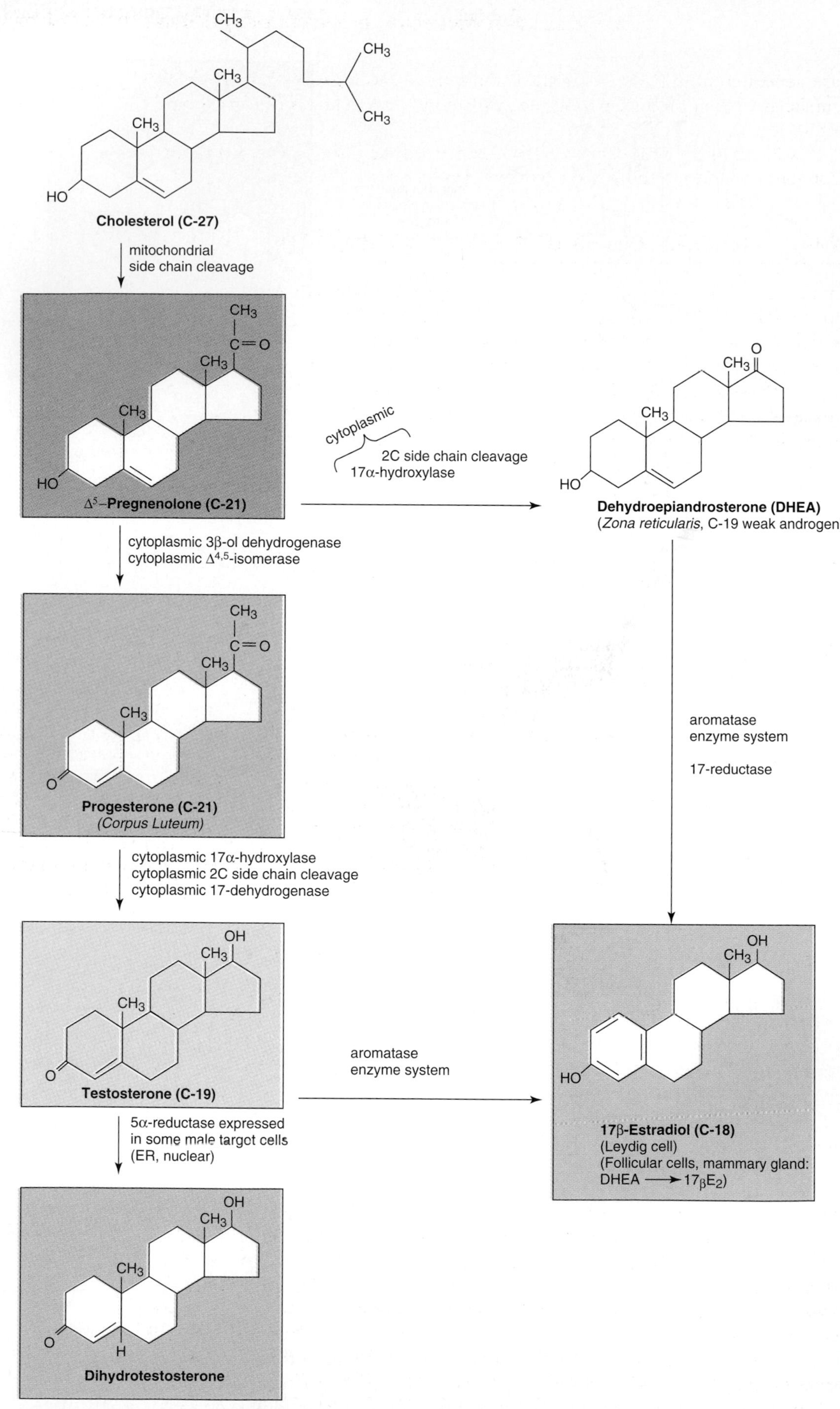

FIGURE 21.6

Conversion of cholesterol to sex hormones.

Mt, mitochondrial; cyto, cytoplasmic; and ER, endoplasmic reticulum.

are generated from NADH or NADPH through a flavoprotein to ferredoxin or similar nonheme protein. Various agents can induce the levels of cytochrome P450.

Note that there is movement of intermediates in and out of the mitochondrial compartment during the steroid synthetic process.

21.4 METABOLIC INACTIVATION OF STEROID HORMONES

A feature of the steroid ring system is its great stability. For the most part, inactivation of steroid hormones involves reduction. Testosterone is initially reduced to a more active form by the enzyme 5α-reductase to form **dihydrotestosterone,** the preferred ligand for the androgen receptor. However, further reduction similar to the other steroid hormones results in inactivation. The inactivation reactions predominate in liver and generally render the steroids more water soluble, as marked by subsequent conjugation with glucuronides or sulfates (see Chapter 22) that are excreted in the urine. Table 21.2 summarizes reactions leading to inactivation and excretory forms of the steroid hormones.

21.5 CELL–CELL COMMUNICATION AND CONTROL OF SYNTHESIS AND RELEASE OF STEROID HORMONES

Secretion of steroid hormones from cells where they are synthesized is elicited by other hormones. Many, but not all, such systems are described in Chapter 20, Figures 20.2 and 20.3. The hormones that directly stimulate the biosynthesis and secretion of the steroid hormones are summarized in Table 21.3. The signals for stimulation of biosynthesis and secretion of steroid hormones are polypeptide hormones operating through cognate cell membrane receptors. In some systems where both cAMP and the phosphatidylinositol (PI) cycle are involved, it is not clear whether one second messenger predominates. In many such systems, for example, aldosterone synthesis and secretion, probably several components (i.e., acetylcholine muscarinic receptor, atriopeptin receptor, and their second messengers) are involved in addition to the signal listed in Table 21.3.

Steroid Hormone Synthesis Is Controlled by Specific Hormones

The general mechanism for hormonal stimulation of steroid hormone synthesis is presented in Figure 21.4. Figure 21.7 (p. 903) presents the system for stimulation of cortisol biosynthesis and release. The role of Ca^{2+} in steroid synthesis and/or secretion is unclear. Rate-limiting steps in the biosynthetic process involve the availability of cholesterol from cholesteryl esters in the droplet, the transport of cholesterol to the inner mitochondrial membrane (StAR protein), and the upregulation of the otherwise rate-limiting side chain cleavage reaction.

Aldosterone

Figure 21.8 (p. 904) shows the overall reactions leading to the secretion of aldosterone in the adrenal zona glomerulosa cell. This set of regulatory controls on aldosterone synthesis and secretion is complicated. The main driving force is **angiotensin II** generated from the signaling to the **renin–angiotensin system** shown in Figure 21.9 (p. 905). Essentially, the signal is generated under conditions when blood [Na^+] and blood pressure (blood volume) are required to be increased. The N-terminal decapeptide of circulating **α_2-globulin (angiotensinogen)** is cleaved by **renin,** a protease. This decapeptide is the hormonally inactive precursor, angiotensin I. It is converted to the octapeptide hormone, angiotensin II, by the action of converting enzyme. Angiotensin II is converted to the heptapeptide, angiotensin III, by an aminopeptidase. Both angiotensins

TABLE 21.2 Excretion Pathways for Steroid Hormones

Steroid Class	*Starting Steroid*	*Inactivation Steps*	*A:B Ring Junction*	*Steroid Structure Representations of Excreted Product*	*Principal Conjugate Present*[a]
Progestins	Progesterone	1. Reduction of C-20 2. Reduction of 4-ene-3-one	(cis)	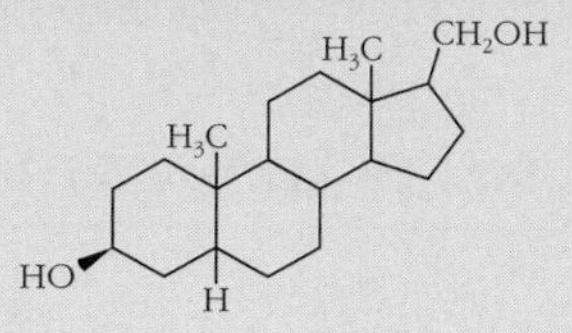 Pregnanediol (5β-pregnane-3α, 2α-diol)	G
Estrogens	Estradiol	1. Oxidation of 17β-OH 2. Hydroxylation at C-2 with subsequent methylation 3. Further hydroxylation or ketone formation at a variety of positions (e.g., C-6, C-7, C-14, C-15, C-16, C-18)		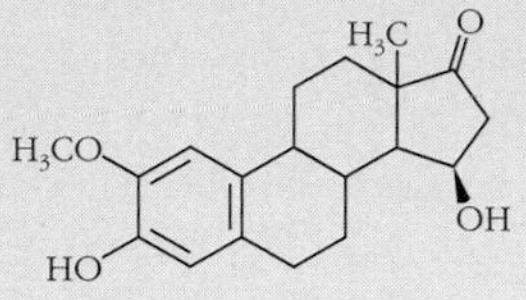 One of many possible compounds	G
Androgens	Testosterone	1. Reduction of 4-ene-3-one 2. Oxidation of C-17 hydroxyl	(cis and trans)	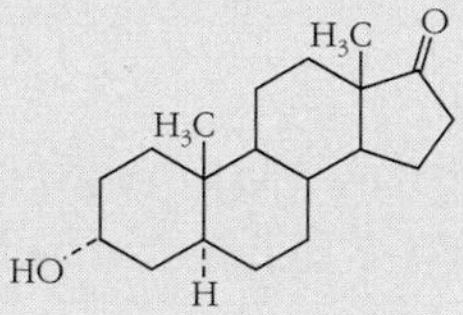 Androsterone + 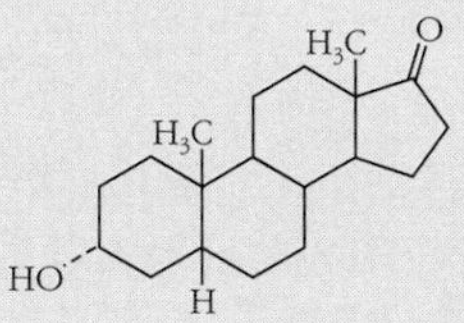 Etiocholanolone	G, S
Glucocorticoids	Cortisol	1. Reduction of 4-ene-3-one 2. Reduction of 20-oxo group 3. Side chain cleavage	(trans)	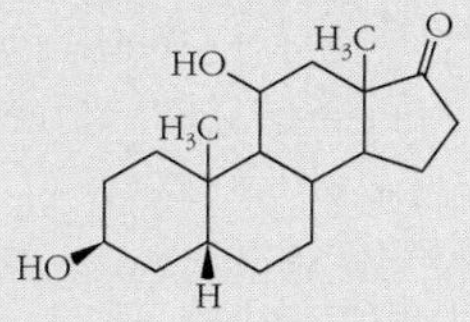 11β-OH-androsterone + 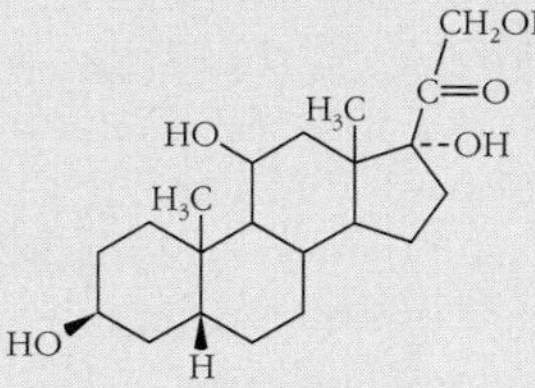 Allo tetrahydrocortisone	G
Mineralocorticoids	Aldosterone	1. Reduction of 4-ene-3-one	(trans)	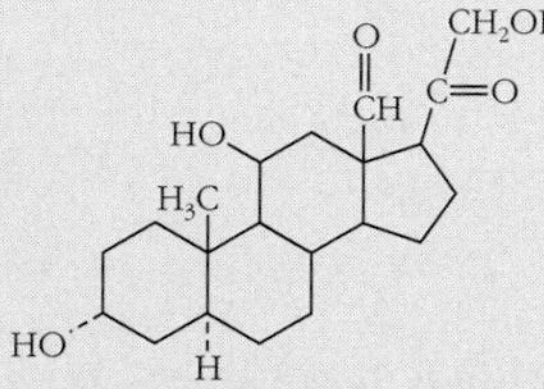 3α, 11β, 21-$(OH)_3$-20-oxo-5β-pregnane-18-al	G
Vitamin D metabolites	$1,25(OH)_2D_3$	1. Side chain cleavage between C-23 and C-24		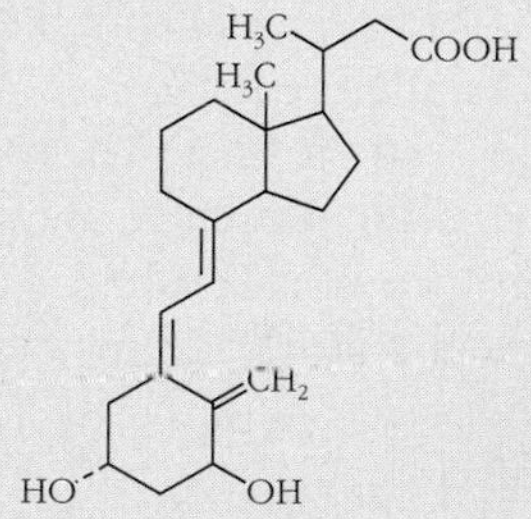 Calcitroic acid	?

Source: From Norman, A. W., and Litwack, G. *Hormones*. Orlando, FL: Academic Press, 1987.

[a] G, Glucuronide; S, sulfate.

II and III can bind to the angiotensin receptor (Figure 21.8), which activates the phosphatidylinositol cycle to generate IP_3 and DAG. IP_3 stimulates release of calcium ions from the intracellular calcium storage vesicles. In addition, the activity of the Ca^{2+} channel is stimulated by the angiotensin–receptor complex. K^+ ions are also required to stimulate the Ca^{2+} channel and these events lead to a greatly increased level of cytoplasmic Ca^{2+}. The enhanced cytoplasmic Ca^{2+}

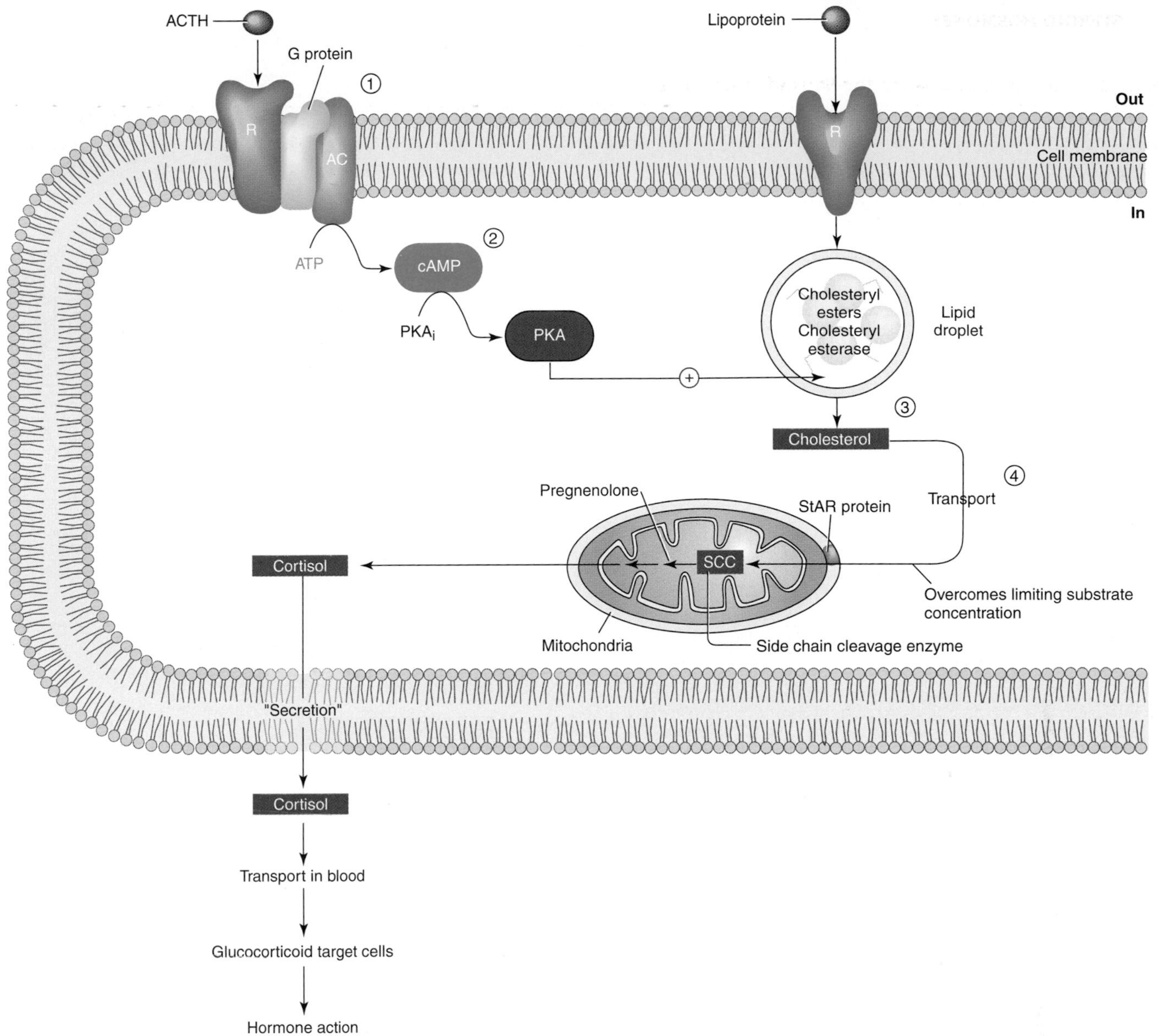

FIGURE 21.7
Action of ACTH on adrenal fasciculata cells to enhance production and secretion of cortisol.
AC, adenylate cyclase; cAMP, cyclic AMP; PKA, protein kinase A; SCC, side chain cleavage system of enzymes. StAR (steroidogenic acute regulatory) protein is a cholesterol transporter functioning between the outer and inner mitochondrial membranes.

TABLE 21.3 Hormones that Directly Stimulate Synthesis and Release of Steroid Hormones

Steroid Hormone	*Steroid-Producing Cell or Structure*	*Signal*[a]	*Second Messenger*	*Signal System*
Cortisol	Adrenal zona fasciculata	ACTH	cAMP, PI cycle, Ca^{2+}	Hypothalamic–pituitary cascade
Aldosterone	Adrenal zona glomerulosa	Angiotensin II/III	PI cycle, Ca^{2+}	Renin–angiotensin system
Testosterone	Leydig cell	LH	cAMP	Hypothalamic–pituitary cascade
17β-Estradiol	Ovarian follicle	FSH	cAMP	Hypothalamic–pituitary–ovarian cycle
Progesterone	Corpus luteum	LH	cAMP	Hypothalamic–pituitary–ovarian cycle
1,25$(OH)_2$Vitamin D_3	Kidney	PTH	cAMP	Sunlight, parathyroid glands, plasma Ca^{2+} level

[a] ACTH, adrenocorticotropic hormone; LH, luteinizing hormone; FSH, follicle-stimulating hormone; PI, phosphatidylinositol; PTH, parathyroid hormone.

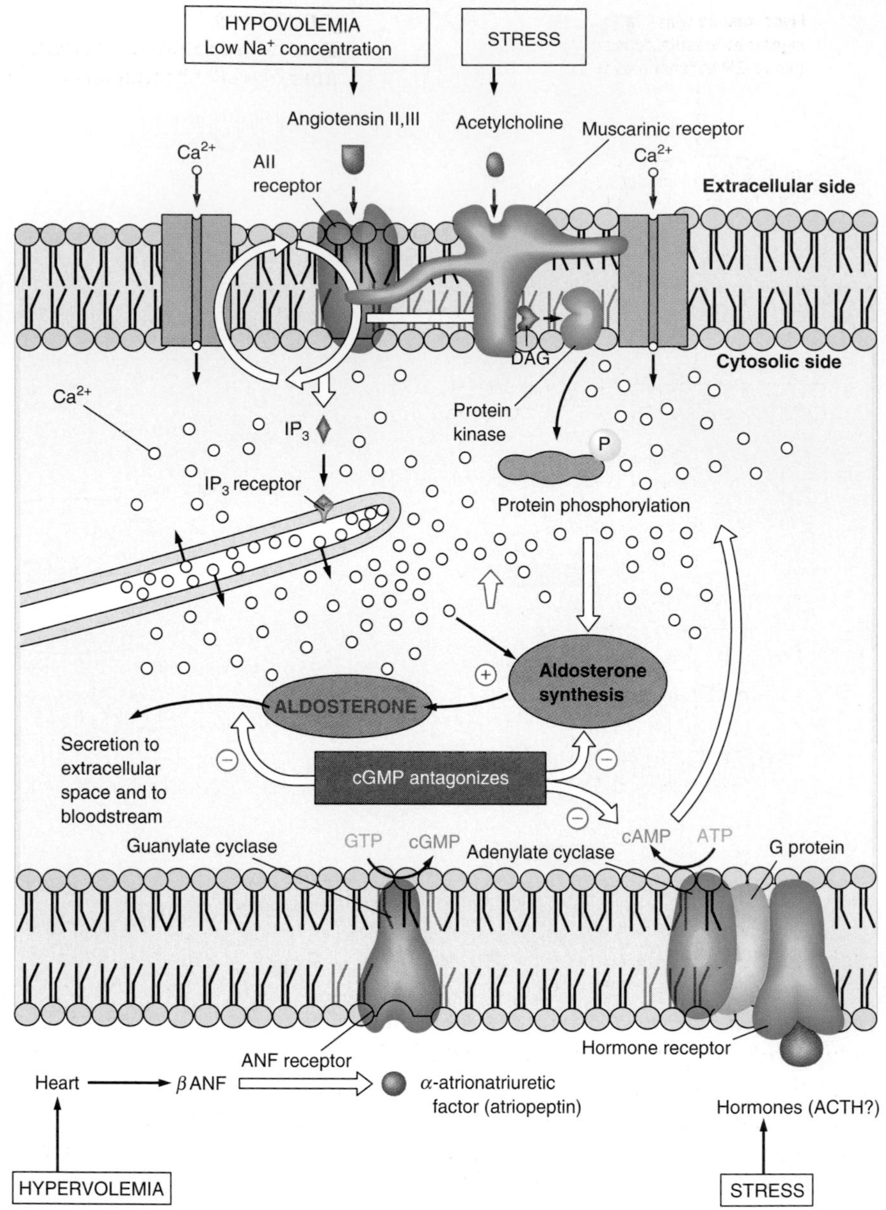

FIGURE 21.8
Reactions leading to the secretion of aldosterone in the adrenal *zona glomerulosa* cell.
cGMP, cyclic GMP; ANF, atrial natriuretic factor; see Figure 21.7 for additional abbreviations.

has a role in aldosterone secretion and together with diacylglycerol stimulates protein kinase C. **Acetylcholine** released through the neuronal stress signals has similar effects mediated by the muscarinic acetylcholine receptor to further reinforce Ca^{2+} uptake by the cell and stimulation of protein kinase C. Enhanced protein kinase C activity leads to protein phosphorylations that stimulate the rate-limiting steps of aldosterone synthesis leading to elevated levels of aldosterone, which are then secreted into the extracellular space and finally into the blood. Once in the blood aldosterone enters the distal kidney cell, binds to its receptor, which initially may be cytoplasmic, and ultimately stimulates expression of proteins that increase the transport of Na^+ from the glomerular filtrate to the blood (see p. 1043).

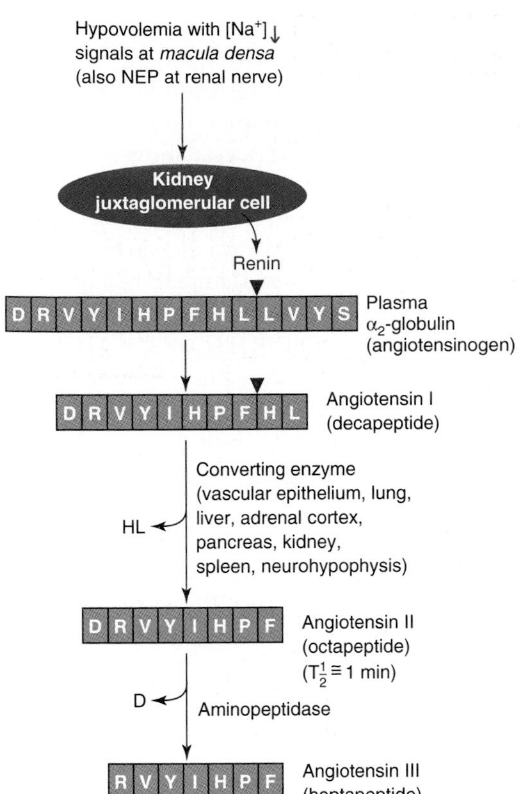

FIGURE 21.9
Renin–angiotensin system.
Amino acid abbreviations are found on p. 27. NEP, norepinephrine.

Signals opposite to those that activate the formation of angiotensin generate **atrial natriuretic factor** (ANF) or atriopeptin from the heart atria (Figure 21.8; see also Figure 20.45). ANF binds to a specific *zona glomerulosa* cell membrane receptor and activates guanylate cyclase, which is part of the same receptor polypeptide so that the cytosolic level of cGMP increases. Cyclic GMP antagonizes the synthesis and secretion of aldosterone as well as the formation of cAMP by adenylate cyclase. Involvement of ACTH in aldosterone synthesis and release may involve adenylate cyclase but may be of secondary importance.

Aldosterone should be regarded as a stress hormone since its presence in elevated levels in blood occurs as a result of stressful situations. In contrast, cortisol, also released in stress has an additional biorhythmic release (possibly under control of serotonin and vasopressin), which accounts for a substantial reabsorption of Na^+ probably through glucocorticoid stimulation of the Na^+–H^+ antiport in luminal epithelial cells in addition to the many other activities of cortisol (e.g., anti-inflammatory action, control of T-cell growth factors, synthesis of glycogen, and effects on carbohydrate metabolism).

Estradiol

Control of formation and secretion of **17β-estradiol,** the female sex hormone, is shown in Figure 21.10. During development, control centers for the steady-state and cycling levels arise in the CNS. Their functions are required to initiate the ovarian cycle at puberty. These centers must harmonize with the firing of other neurons, such as those producing a clock-like mechanism via release of catecholamines or other amines to generate the pulsatile release of gonadotropin-releasing hormone (GnRH), probably at hourly intervals. Details of these reactions are presented on page 867, Chapter 20. The FSH circulates and binds to, its cognate receptor on the cell membrane of the ovarian follicle cell and

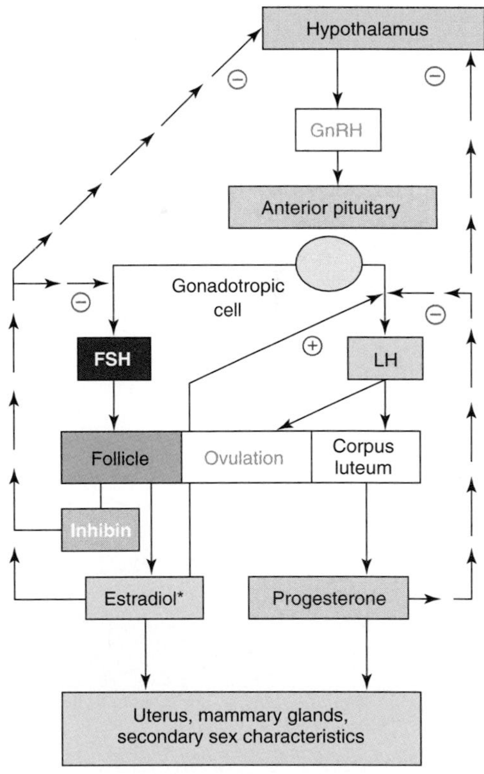

FIGURE 21.10
Formation and secretion of 17β-estradiol and progesterone.

through its second messengers, primarily cAMP and the activation of cAMP-dependent protein kinase, there is stimulation of the synthesis and secretion of the female sex hormone, 17β-estradiol. At normal stimulated levels of 17β-estradiol, there is a negative feedback on the **gonadotrope** (anterior pituitary), suppressing further secretion of FSH. Near ovarian midcycle, however, there is a superstimulated level of 17β-estradiol produced that has a positive rather than a negative feedback effect on the gonadotrope. This causes very high levels of LH to be released, referred to as the LH spike, and elevated levels of FSH. The level of FSH released is substantially lower than LH because the follicle produces **inhibin,** a polypeptide hormone that specifically inhibits FSH release without affecting LH release. The elevation of LH in the LH spike participates in the process of ovulation. After ovulation, the remnant of the follicle is differentiated into the functional *corpus luteum,* which now synthesizes progesterone (and also some estradiol), under the influence of elevated LH levels. Progesterone, however, is a feedback inhibitor of LH synthesis and release (operating through a progesterone receptor in the gonadotropic cell) and eventually the *corpus luteum* dies, owing to a fall in the level of available LH and the production of oxytocin, a luteolytic agent, by the *corpus luteum.* Prostaglandin $F_{2\alpha}$ may also be involved. With the death of the *corpus luteum,* the blood levels of progesterone and estradiol fall, causing menstruation as well as a decline in the negative feedback effects of these steroids on the anterior pituitary and hypothalamus, and the cycle begins again. Clinical Correlation 21.1 describes how oral contraceptives interrupt this sequence.

The situation is similar in males with respect to regulation of gonadotropin secretion, but LH acts principally on the Leydig cell for the stimulated production of testosterone, and FSH acts on the Sertoli cells to stimulate production of inhibin and sperm proteins. Production of testosterone is subject to the negative feedback effect of 17β-estradiol synthesized in the Sertoli cell. The 17β-estradiol so produced operates through a nuclear estrogen receptor in the Leydig cell to produce inhibition of testosterone synthesis at the transcriptional level. In all cases of steroid hormone production, the synthetic system resembles that shown in Figure 21.4.

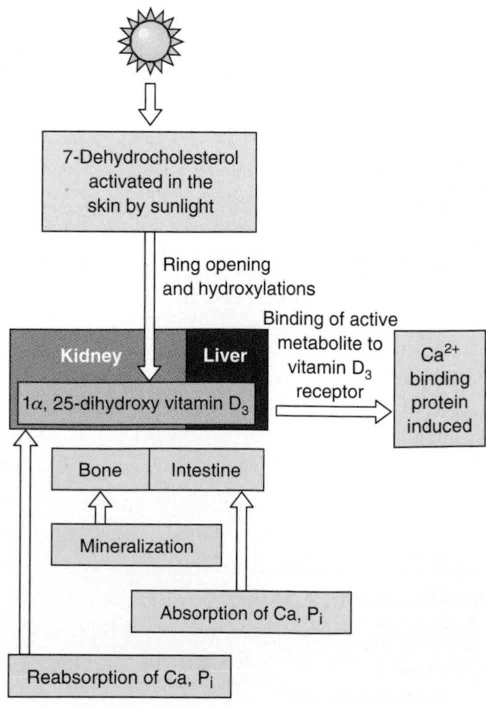

FIGURE 21.11
The vitamin D endocrine system.
P_i, inorganic phosphate.
Adapted from Norman, A. W. and Litwack, G. Hormones. *Orlando, FL: Academic Press, 1987, p. 379.*

Vitamin D_3

Activation of vitamin D to dihydroxy vitamin D_3 produces a hormone that has the general features of a steroid hormone. The active form of vitamin D stimulates intestinal absorption of dietary calcium and phosphorus, the mineralization of bone matrix, bone resorption, and reabsorption of calcium and phosphate in the renal tubule. The **vitamin D endocrine system** is diagrammed in Figure 21.11. 7-Dehydrocholesterol is activated in the skin by sunlight to form **vitamin D_3 (cholecalciferol).** This form is hydroxylated first in the liver to **25-hydroxy vitamin D_3 (25-hydroxycholecalciferol)** and subsequently in the kidney to form the **1α,25-vitamin D_3 ($1,25(OH)_2D_3$)(1α,25-dihydroxycholecalciferol).** The hormone can bind to nuclear $1,25(OH)_2D_3$ receptors in intestine, bone, and kidney and then transcriptionally activate genes encoding calcium-binding proteins whose actions may lead to the absorption and reabsorption of Ca^{2+} (as well as phosphorus). The subcellular mode of action is presented in Figure 21.12. In this scheme the active form of vitamin D_3 enters the intestinal cell from the blood side and migrates to the nucleus. Once inside it binds to the high-affinity vitamin D_3 receptor, which probably undergoes an activation event, and associates with a vitamin D_3-responsive element to activate genes responsive to the hormone. Messenger RNA is produced and translated in the cytoplasm; these RNAs encode calcium-binding proteins, Ca^{2+}-ATPase, other ATPases, membrane components, and facilitators of vesicle formation. Increased levels of calcium-binding proteins may cause increased uptake of Ca^{2+} from the intestine or may simply buffer the cytoplasm against high free Ca^{2+} levels.

With each of the steroid-producing systems discussed, feedback controls are operative whereby sufficient amounts of the circulating steroid hormone inhibit the further production and release of intermediate hormones in the pathway at the levels of the pituitary and hypothalamus, as viewed in Figure 20.3. In the case of the vitamin D systems, the controls are different since the steroid production is not stimulated by the cascade process applicable to estra-

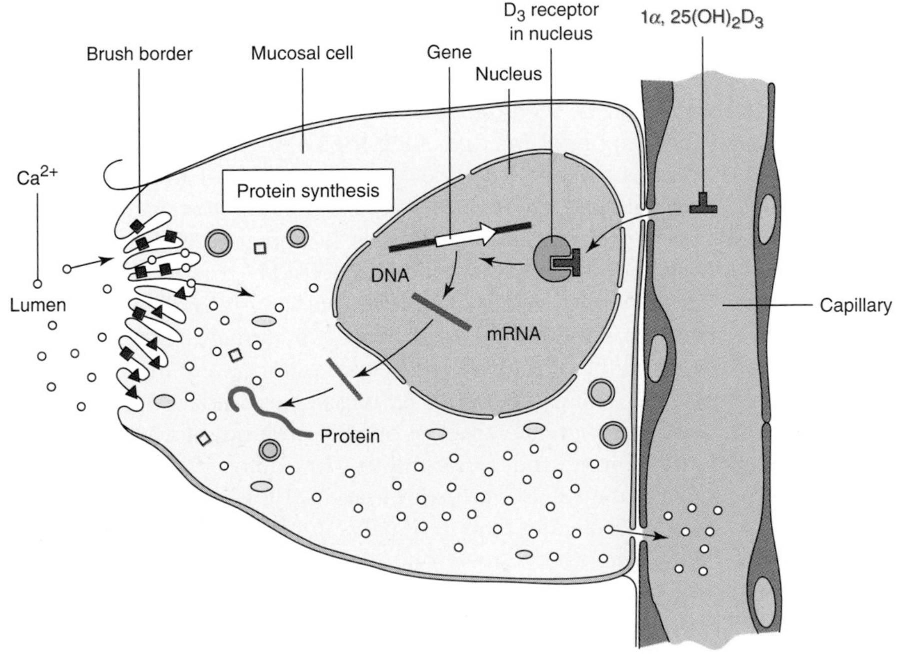

FIGURE 21.12
Schematic model to describe the action of $1,25(OH)_2D_3$ in the intestine in stimulating intestinal calcium transport.
Redrawn from Nemere, I., and Norman, A. W. Biochim. Biophys. Acta *694:307, 1982.*

CLINICAL CORRELATION 21.1

Oral Contraception

Oral contraceptives usually contain an estrogen and a progestin. Taken orally, the levels of these steroids increase in blood to a level where secretion of FSH and LH is repressed. Consequently, the gonadotropic hormone levels in blood fall and there is insufficient FSH to drive development of the ovarian follicle. As a result, the follicle does not mature and ovulation cannot occur. In addition, any *corpora lutea* cannot survive because of low LH levels. In sum, the ovarian cycle ceases. The uterine endometrium thickens and remains in this state, however, because of elevated levels of estrogen and progestin. Pills without the steroids (placebos) are usually inserted in the regimen at about the 28th day and, as a result, blood levels of steroids fall dramatically and menstruation occurs. When oral contraceptive steroids are resumed, the blood levels of estrogen and progestin increase again and the uterine endometrium thickens. This sequence creates a false "cycling" because of the occurrence of menstruation at the expected time in the cycle. The ovarian cycle and ovulation are suppressed by the oral contraceptive based on the negative feedback effects of estrogen and progestin on the secretion of the anterior pituitary gonadotropes. It is also possible to provide contraception by implanting in the skin silicone tubes containing progestins. The steroid is slowly released, providing contraception for up to 3–5 years.

Zatuchni, G. I. Female contraception. In: K. L. Becker (Ed.), *Principles and Practice of Endocrinology and Metabolism*. New York: Lippincott, 1990, p. 861; and Shoupe, D., and Mishell, D. R. Norplant: subdermal implant system for long term contraception. *Am. J. Obstet. Gynecol.* 160:1286, 1988.

diol. When the circulating levels of the active form of vitamin D (1, 25$(OH)_2D_3$) are high, hydroxylations at the 24 and 25 positions are favored and the inactive 24,25$(OH)_2$-vitamin D_3 compound is generated.

21.6 ■ TRANSPORT OF STEROID HORMONES IN BLOOD

Steroid Hormones Are Bound to Specific Proteins or Albumin in Blood

There are four major proteins in the circulation that account for much of the steroid hormones bound in the blood. They assist in maintaining a level of these hormones in the circulation and protect the hormone from metabolism and inactivation. The binding proteins of importance are corticosteroid-binding globulin protein, sex hormone-binding protein, androgen-binding protein, and albumin.

Corticosteroid-binding globulin (CBG) or **transcortin** is about 52 kDa, is 3–4 mg% in human plasma, and binds about 80% of the total 17-hydroxysteroids in the blood. In the case of cortisol, which is the principal antistress corticosteroid in humans, about 75% is bound by CBG, 22% is bound in a loose manner to albumin, and 8% is in free form. The unbound cortisol is the form that can permeate cells and bind to intracellular receptors to produce biological effects. The CBG has a high affinity for cortisol with a binding constant (K_a) of 2.4×10^7 M^{-1}. Critical structural determinants for steroid binding to CBG are the Δ^4-3-ketone and 20-ketone structures. Aldosterone binds weakly to CBG but is also bound by albumin and other plasma proteins. Normally, 60% of aldosterone is bound to albumin and 10% is bound to CBG. In human serum, albumin is 1000-fold the concentration of CBG and binds cortisol with an affinity of 10^3 M^{-1}, much lower than the affinity of CBG for cortisol. Thus cortisol will always fill CBG-binding sites first. During stress, when secretion of cortisol is very high, CBG sites will be filled but there will be sufficient albumin to accommodate excess cortisol.

Sex hormone binding globulin (SHBG) (40 kDa) binds androgens with an affinity constant of about 10^9 M^{-1}, which is much tighter than albumin binding of androgens. One to three percent of testosterone is unbound in the circulation and 10% is bound to SHBG, with the remainder bound to albumin. The level of SHBG is probably important in controlling the balance between circulating androgens and estrogens along with the actual amounts of these hormones produced in given situations. About 97–99% of bound testosterone is bound reversibly to SHBG but much less estrogen is bound to this protein in the female. As mentioned above, only the unbound steroid hormone can permeate cells and bind to intracellular receptors, thus expressing its activity. The level of SHBG before puberty is about the same in males and females, but, at puberty, when the functioning of the sex hormones becomes important, there is a small decrease in the level of circulating SHBG in females and a larger decrease in males, ensuring a relatively greater amount of the unbound, biologically active sex hormones—testosterone and 17β-estradiol. In adults, males have about one- half as much circulating SHBG as females, so that the unbound testosterone in males is about 20 times greater than in females. In addition, the total (bound plus unbound) concentration of testosterone is about 40 times greater in males. Testosterone itself lowers SHBG levels in blood, whereas 17β-estradiol raises SHBG levels in blood. These effects have important ramifications in pregnancy and in other conditions.

Androgen binding protein (ABP) is produced by Sertoli cells in response to testosterone and FSH, both of which stimulate protein synthesis in these cells. Androgen-binding protein is doubtless not of great importance in the entire blood circulation but is important because it maintains a ready supply of testosterone for the production of protein constituents of spermatozoa. Its role may be to maintain a high local concentration of testosterone in the vicinity of the developing germ cells within the tubules.

From a variety of studies it is clear that these, as well as other transport proteins, protect the circulating pool of steroid hormones. They supply free steroids that can enter cellular targets after dissociation from the bound forms as more free hormone is utilized, thus serving the needs of target cells by a mass action effect.

21.7 ■ STEROID HORMONE RECEPTORS

Steroid Hormones Bind to Specific Intracellular Protein Receptors

The general model for steroid hormone action presented in Figure 21.13 takes into account the differences among steroid receptors in terms of their location within the cell. In contrast to polypeptide hormone receptors that are generally located on/in the cell surface, steroid hormone receptors, as well as other related receptors for nonsteroids (i.e. thyroid hormone, retinoic acid, vitamin D_3), are located in the cell interior. Among the steroid receptors there appear to be some differences as to the subcellular location of the **non-DNA-binding forms** of these **receptors.** The glucocorticoid receptor and possibly the aldosterone receptor appear to reside in the cytoplasm, whereas the other receptors, for which suitable data have been collected, may be located within the nucleus, presumably in association with DNA, although not necessarily at productive acceptor sites on the DNA. Figure 21.13, Step 1, shows a bound and a free form of a steroid hormone(s). The free form may enter the cell by a process of diffusion. In the case of glucocorticoids, like cortisol, the steroid would bind

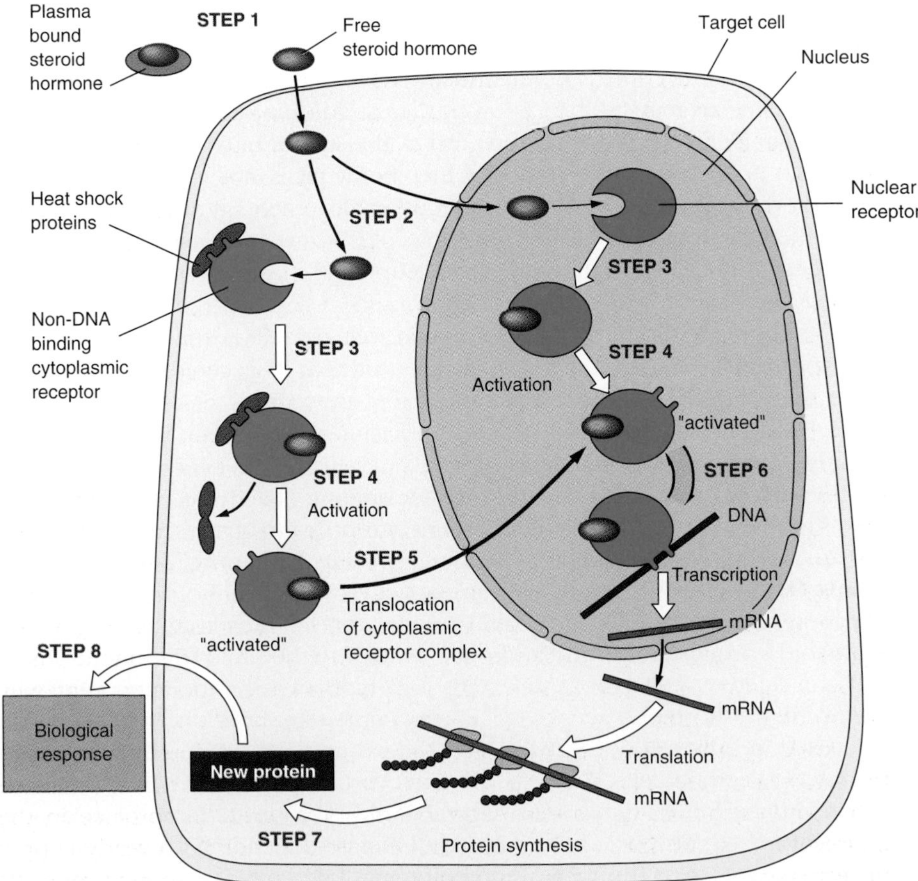

FIGURE 21.13
Model of steroid hormone action. Step 1—Dissociation of free hormone (biologically active) from circulating transport protein; Step 2—diffusion of free ligand into cytosol or nucleus; Step 3—binding of ligand to unactivated cytoplasmic or nuclear receptor; Step 4—activation of cytosolic or nuclear hormone–receptor complex to activated, DNA-binding form; Step 5—translocation of activated cytosolic hormone–receptor complex into nucleus; Step 6—binding of activated hormone–receptor complexes to specific response elements within the DNA; Step 7—synthesis of new proteins encoded by hormone-responsive genes; and Step 8—alteration in phenotype or metabolic activity of target cell mediated by specifically induced proteins.

to an unactivated receptor with an open ligand binding site (Step 3). The binding constant for this reaction is on the order of 10^9 M^{-1}, compared to about 10^7 M^{-1} for the binding to CBG (see above). The non-DNA-binding form also referred to as the unactivated or nontransformed receptor is about 300 kDa, because other proteins may be associated in the complex. Many investigators believe that a dimer of the 90-kDa protein, which is a heat shock protein that is induced when cells are stressed **(heat shock proteins),** is associated with the receptor in this form and occludes its DNA-binding domain, accounting for its non-DNA-binding activity. Associated with this dimer of hsp90 is another heat shock protein designated as hsp56, which interestingly also functions as an immunophilin and, as such, can bind to a number of potent immunosuppressive drugs. The dimer of the 90-kDa heat shock protein is depicted by the pair of red ovals attached to the cytoplasmic receptor that block the DNA-binding domain pictured as a pair of "fingers" in the subsequently activated form. Activation or transformation to the **DNA-binding form** is accomplished by release of the 90-kDa heat shock proteins (Step 4). It is not clear what actually drives the activation step(s). Clearly, the binding of the steroidal ligand is important but other factors may be involved. A low molecular weight component has been proposed to be part of the cross-linking between the nonhomologous proteins and the receptor in the DNA-binding complex. In the case of glucocorticoid receptor, only the non-DNA-binding form has a high affinity for binding steroidal ligand. Following activation and exposure of the DNA-binding domain, the receptor translocates to the nucleus (Step 5), binds to DNA, and "searches" the DNA for a high-affinity acceptor site. At this site the bound receptor complex, frequently a homodimer, acts as a transactivation factor, which together with other transactivators allows for the starting of RNA polymerase and stimulation of transcription. In some cases the binding of the receptor may lead to repression of transcription and this effect is less well understood. New mRNAs are translocated to the cytoplasm and assembled into translation complexes for the synthesis of proteins (Step 7) that alter metabolism and functioning of the target cell (Step 8).

When the unoccupied (nonliganded) steroid hormone receptor is located in the nucleus, as may be the case with the estradiol, progesterone, androgen, and vitamin D_3 receptors (see Figure 21.12), the steroid must travel through the cytoplasm and cross the perinuclear membrane. It is not clear whether this transport through the cytoplasm (aqueous environment) requires a transport protein for the hydrophobic steroid molecules. Once inside the nucleus the steroid can bind to the high-affinity, unoccupied receptor, presumably already on DNA, and cause it to be "activated" to a form bound to the acceptor site. The ligand might promote a conformation that decreases the off-rate of the receptor from its acceptor, if it is located on or near its acceptor site, or might cause the receptor to initiate searching if the unoccupied receptor associates with DNA at a locus remote from the acceptor site. Consequently, the mechanism underlying activation of nuclear receptors is less well understood as compared to activation of cytoplasmic receptors. After binding of activated receptor complexes to DNA acceptor sites, enhancement or repression of transcription occurs.

Consensus DNA sequences defining specific **hormone response elements (HREs)** for the binding of various activated steroid hormone–receptor complexes are summarized in Table 21.4. Receptors for glucocorticoids, mineralocorticoids, progesterone, and androgen all bind to the same HRE on the DNA. Thus, in a given cell type, the extent and type of receptor expressed will determine the hormone sensitivity. For example, sex hormone receptors are expressed in only a few cell types and the progesterone receptor is likewise restricted to certain cells, whereas the glucocorticoid receptor is expressed in a large number of cell types. In cases where aldosterone and cortisol receptors are coexpressed, only one form may predominate depending on the cell type. Some tissues, such as the kidney and colon, are known targets for aldosterone

TABLE 21.4 Steroid Hormone Receptor Responsive DNA Elements: Consensus Acceptor Sites

Element	*DNA Sequence*[a]
POSITIVE	
Glucocorticoid responsive element (GRE)	5′-GGTACAnnnTGTTCT-3′
Mineralocorticoid responsive element (MRE)	
Progesterone responsive element (PRE)	
Androgen responsive element (ARE)	
Estrogen responsive element (ERE)	5′-AGGTCAnnnTCACT-3′
NEGATIVE	
Glucocorticoid responsive element	5′-ATYACNnnnTGATCW-3′

Source: Data are summarized from work of Beato, M. *Cell* 56:355, 1989.

[a] n, any nucleotide; Y, a purine; W, a pyrimidine.

and express relatively high levels of mineralocorticoid receptors as well as glucocorticoid receptors. These mineralocorticoid target tissues express the enzyme **11β-hydroxysteroid dehydrogenase** (see Clin. Corr. 21.2). This enzyme converts cortisol and corticosterone, both of which can bind to the mineralocorticoid receptor with high affinity, to their 11-keto analogs, which bind poorly to the mineralocorticoid receptor. This inactivation of corticosterone and cortisol, which circulate at much higher concentrations than aldosterone, facilitates the binding of aldosterone to the mineralocorticoid receptors in these classical target tissues. In tissues that express mineralocorticoid receptors but are not considered target tissues, this enzyme may not be expressed, and in these situations the mineralocorticoid receptors may simply function as pseudoglucocorticoid receptors and mediate the effects of low circulating levels of cortisol (predominant glucocorticoid in humans). Thus the mineralocorticoid and glucocorticoid receptors may regulate the expression of an overlapping gene network in various target tissues. As also indicated in Table 21.4, the activated estrogen–receptor complex recognizes a distinct or unique response element. All of the response elements listed at the top of Table 21.4 function as positive elements, since binding of the indicated steroid receptors results in an increase in the rate of transcription of the associated gene.

Glucocorticoid hormones also repress transcription of specific genes. For example, glucocorticoids are known to repress transcription of the **proopiomelanocortin gene** (POMC) (see p. 849), which contains the ACTH sequences. Glucocorticoid-mediated repression of *POMC* gene expression thus plays a key role in the negative feedback loop regulating the rate of secretion of ACTH and ultimately cortisol. Negative glucocorticoid response elements (nGREs) mediate this repression of the *POMC* gene as well as other important genes. A general model of positive as well as negative transcriptional effects mediated by steroid receptors is shown in Figure 21.14: In (*a*) binding of a steroid receptor (R) homodimer to its response element allows it to interact synergistically with a positive transcription factor (TF) and hence induce gene transcription; in (*b*) binding of a receptor dimer to its response element displaces a positive transcription factor (TF) but has no or weak transactivation potential because no synergizing factor is nearby; and in (*c*) the DNA-AP1 (positive factor) may interact in a protein–protein fashion in such a way that the transactivating functions of both proteins are inhibited and gene transcription is repressed.

CLINICAL CORRELATION 21.2

Apparent Mineralocorticoid Excess Syndrome

Some patients (usually children) exhibit symptoms, including hypertension, hypokalemia, and suppression of the renin–angiotensin–aldosterone system, that would be expected if they were hypersecreting aldosterone. Since bioassays of plasma and urine sometimes fail to identify any excess of mineralocorticoids, these patients are said to suffer from the apparent mineralocorticoid excess (AME) syndrome. This syndrome results as a consequence of the failure of cortisol inactivation by the 11β-hydroxysteroid dehydrogenase enzyme. Inactivity of this key enzyme gives cortisol direct access to the renal mineralocorticoid receptor. Since cortisol circulates at much higher concentrations than aldosterone, this glucocorticoid saturates these mineralocorticoid receptors and functions as an agonist, causing sodium retention and suppression of the renin–angiotensin–aldosterone axis. Although this AME syndrome can result from a congenital defect in the distal nephron 11β-hydroxysteroid dehydrogenase isoform, which renders the enzyme incapable of converting cortisol to cortisone (binds poorly to mineralocorticoid receptors), it can also be acquired by ingesting excessive amounts of licorice. The major component of licorice is glycyrrhizic acid and its hydrolytic product, glycyrrhetinic acid (GE). This active ingredient (GE) acts as a potent inhibitor of 11β-hydroxysteroid dehydrogenase. By blocking activity of this inactivating enzyme, GE facilitates the binding of cortisol to renal mineralocorticoid receptors and hence induces AME syndrome.

Edwards, C. R. W. Primary mineralocorticoid excess syndromes. In: L. J. DeGroot (Ed.), *Endocrinology*. Philadelphia: Saunders, pp. 1775–1803, 1995; and Shackleton, C. H. L., and Stewart, P. M. The hypertension of apparent mineralocorticoid excess syndrome. In: E. G. Biglieri and J. C. Melby (Eds.), *Endocrine Hypertension*. New York: Raven Press, 1990, pp. 155–173.

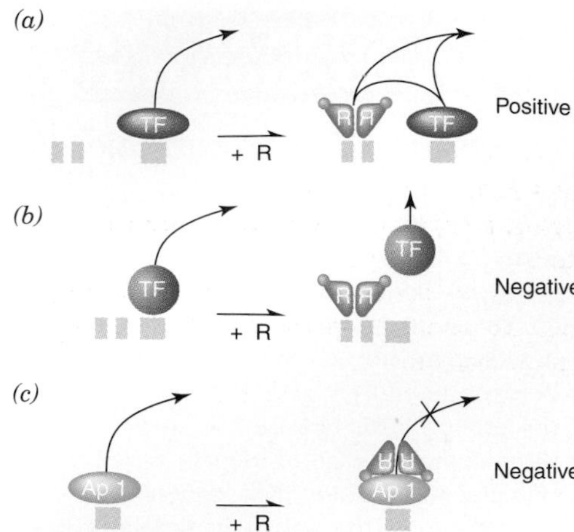

FIGURE 21.14
Positive and negative transcriptional effects of steroid receptors.
Redrawn from Renkowitz, R. Ann. N.Y. Acad. Sci. *684:1, 1993.*

Some members of this receptor supergene family can mediate gene silencing. Silencer elements, in analogy to enhancer elements, function independently of their position and orientation. The silencer for a particular gene consists of modules that independently repress gene activity. In the absence of their specific ligands, the **thyroid hormone receptor** (T_3R) and **retinoic acid receptor** (RAR) appear to bind to specific silencer elements and repress gene transcription. This silencing activity may occur via destabilization of the transcription initiation complex or via direct or indirect effects on the carboxy-terminal domain of RNA polymerase II. After binding of their respective ligands, these two receptors lose this silencing activity and are converted into transactivators of gene transcription.

As indicated in Figure 21.14, **dimerization** of receptor monomers is a prerequisite for efficient DNA binding and transcriptional activation by most steroid receptors. Strong interactions between these monomers are mediated by the ligand-binding domains of several steroid receptors. The dimerization domain of the ligand-binding domain has been proposed to form a helical structure containing a succession of hydrophobic sequences that would generate a leucine zipper-like structure or a helix–turn–zipper motif (see p. 110), which are known to be necessary for the dimerization of other transcription factors. Although the majority of receptors in this superfamily form homodimers, heterodimers have also been detected. More specifically, a distinct class of retinoic acid receptors, classified as retinoid X receptors (RXRs), regulate gene expression via heterodimerization with the other distinct form of the retinoic acid receptor (RAR), the thyroid hormone receptor, and other members of this receptor superfamily. A model for the stabilization of the transcriptional preinitiation complex by an RXR/RAR heterodimer is presented in Figure 21.15.

Thus the changes produced in different cells by the activation of steroid hormone receptors may be different in different cells that contain the relevant receptor in suitable concentration. The whole process is triggered by the entry of the steroidal ligand in amounts that supersede the dissociation constant of the receptor. The different phenotypic changes in different cell types in response to a specific hormone then summate to give the systemic or organismic response to the hormone.

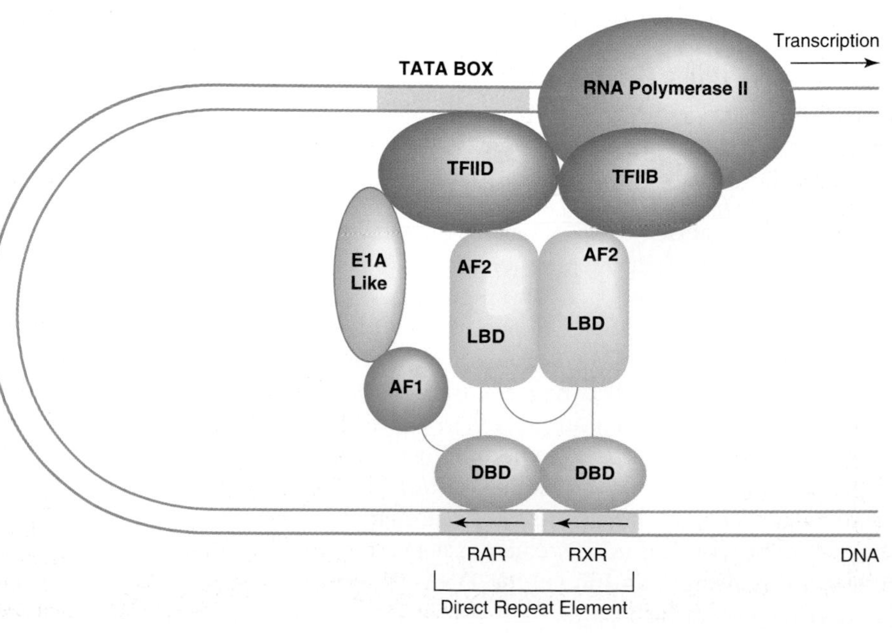

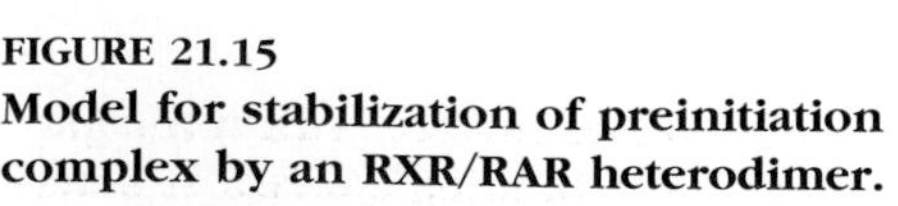
FIGURE 21.15
Model for stabilization of preinitiation complex by an RXR/RAR heterodimer.
TF, transcription factor; LBD, ligand-binding domain; DBD, DNA-binding domain; AF1, activation function located in amino-terminal region of receptor, which may provide contact with cell-specific proteins; AF2, activation function located within ligand-binding domain, which interacts directly with transcriptional machinery.

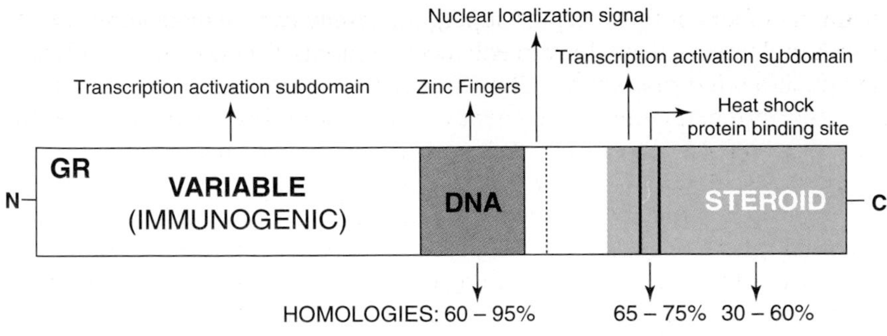

FIGURE 21.16
Model of a typical steroid hormone receptor.
The results are derived from studies on cDNA in various laboratories, especially those of R. Evans and K. Yamamoto.

Some Steroid Receptors Are Part of the *cErbA* Family of Proto-oncogenes

The glucocorticoid receptor is conveniently divided into three major **functional domains** (Figure 21.16). Starting at the C terminus, the steroid-binding domain is indicated and has 30–60% homology with the **ligand-binding domains** of other receptors in the steroid receptor family. The more alike two steroids that bind different receptors are, the greater the extent of homology to be anticipated in this domain. The steroid-binding domain contains a sequence that may be involved in the binding of molybdate and a dimer of the 90-kDa heat shock protein whose function would theoretically result in the assembly of the high molecular weight unactivated–nontransformed steroid–receptor complex. To the left of that domain is a region that modifies transcription. In the center of the molecule is the **DNA-binding domain.** Among the steroid receptors there is 60–95% homology in this domain. Two zinc fingers (see p. 108) interact with DNA. The structure of the zinc finger DNA-binding motif is shown in Figure 21.17. The N-terminal domain contains the principal **antigenic domains** and a site that modulates transcriptional activation. The amino acid sequences in this site are highly variable among the steroid receptors. These features are common to all steroid receptors. The family of steroid receptors is diagrammed in Figure 21.17. The ancestor to which these receptor genes are related is *v-erbA* or *c-erbA* (see p. 889). *v-ErbA* is an oncogene that binds to DNA but has no ligand-binding domain. In some cases the DNA-binding domains are homologous enough that more than one receptor will bind to a common responsive element (consensus sequence on DNA) as shown in Table 21.4. In addition to those genes pictured in Figure 21.18, the **aryl hydrocarbon receptor** (Ah) may also be a member of this family. The Ah receptor binds carcinogens with increasing affinity paralleling increasing carcinogenic potency and translocates the carcinogen to the cellular nucleus unless the receptor is already located in the nucleus. The N-terminal portions of the receptors usually contain major antigenic sites and may also contain a site that is active in modulating binding of the receptor to DNA.

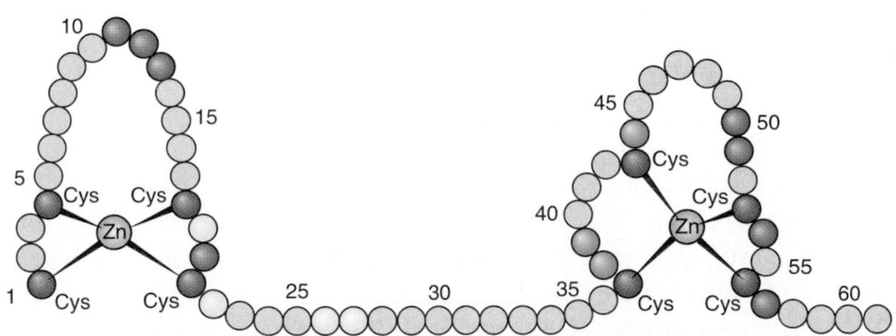

FIGURE 21.17
Structure of the zinc finger located within the glucocorticoid receptor DNA-binding domain as determined by X-ray crystallography.
Yellow circles indicate amino acid residues (located in GR monomer) that interact with base pairs. Blue circles are those making phosphate backbone contacts. Green circles are those participating in dimerization.
Redrawn from Luisi, B. F., Schwabe, J. W. R., and Freedman, L. P. In: G. Litwack (Ed.), Vitamins and Hormones, *Vol. 49. San Diego, Academic Press, 1994, pp. 1–47.*

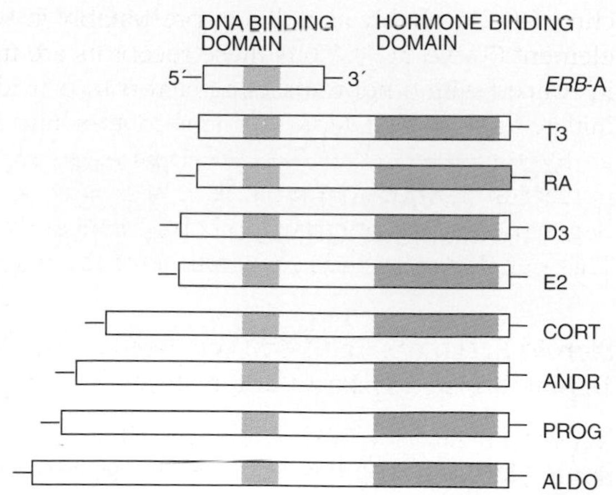

FIGURE 21.18
Steroid receptor gene superfamily.
T3, triiodothyronine; RA, retinoic acid; D3, dihydroxy vitamin D_3; E2, estradiol; CORT, cortisol; ANDR, androgen; PROG, progesterone; ALDO, aldosterone. Figure shows roughly the relative sizes of the genes for these receptors. Information derived from the laboratories of R. Evans, K. Yamamoto, P. Chambon, and others. In some cases there is high homology in DNA-binding domains and lower homology in ligand-binding domains.

Thyroid hormone and retinoic acid receptors are also members of the same superfamily of receptors although their ligands are not steroids. They do contain six-membered rings as shown in Figure 21.19. For some steroid receptors the A ring is the prominent site of recognition by the receptor, presenting the likelihood that the A ring inserts into the binding pocket of the receptor. In some cases, derivatives of the structures with a six-membered ring bind to the estradiol and glucocorticoid receptors. Thus the ring structures of thyroid hormone and retinoic acid have structural similarities not unlike many of the steroidal ligands involved in binding.

The receptors in this large gene family may act as transcriptional activators that together with other transcriptional regulators bring about gene activation.

21.8 ■ RECEPTOR ACTIVATION: UPREGULATION AND DOWNREGULATION

Little is known about activation of steroid receptors. Activation converts a non-DNA-binding form (unactivated–nontransformed) of the receptor to a form (activated–transformed) that is able to bind nonspecific DNA or specific DNA (hormone-responsive element). The likelihood that certain receptors are cytoplasmic (glucocorticoid receptor and possibly the mineralocorticoid receptor) while others seem to be nuclear (progesterone, estradiol, vitamin D_3, and androgen receptors) may have a bearing on the significance of the activation phenomena. Most information is available for cytoplasmic receptors. The current view is that the non-DNA-binding form is a heteromeric trimer consisting of one molecule of receptor and a dimer of 90-kDa heat shock protein, as shown in Figure 21.20. The DNA-binding site of the receptor is blocked by the heteromeric proteins or by some other factor or by a combination of both. Upon activation–transformation a stepwise disaggregation of this complex could occur, leading to the activated receptor having its DNA-binding site fully exposed. The reaction may be initiated by the binding of steroid to the ligand-binding site that produces a conformational change in the receptor protein.

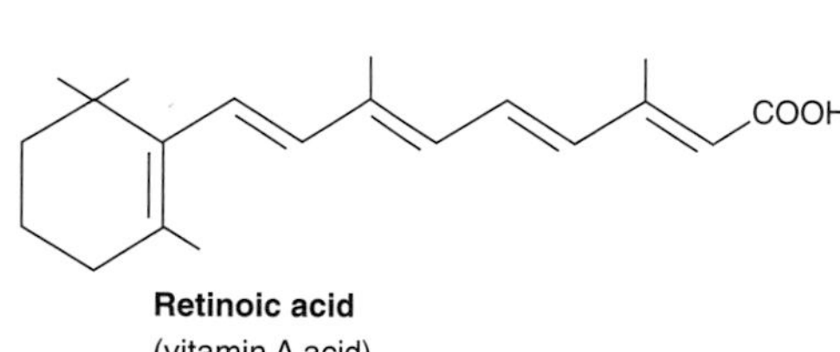

HO — O — $CH_2CHCOOH$ — NH_2 — I

3,5,3' - Triiodothyronine

FIGURE 21.19
Structures of retinoic acid (vitamin A acid) and 3,5,3′-triiodothyronine.

Although the conditions required to induce activation *in vitro* are well known, the primary signal within the cell is not. Many believe that the binding of ligand alone is not sufficient to cause the activation process. Clearly, elevated temperature is a requirement for this conformational change, since incubation of target cells with appropriate steroids at low temperatures fails to result in *in vivo* activation and subsequent translocation. Once the liberated receptor is free in the cytoplasm it crosses the perinuclear membrane, perhaps through a nucleopore, to enter the nucleus. It binds nonspecifically and specifically to chromatin, probably as a dimer, presumably in search of the specific response element (Table 21.4). Thus these receptors are transacting factors and may act in concert with other transacting factors to provide the appropriate structure to initiate transcription. Most steroid receptors have in their DNA-binding domains an SV40-like sequence (i.e., Pro-Lys-Lys-Lys-Arg-Lys-Val) known to code for nuclear translocation. Steroid receptors have variants of this sequence; some degeneracy is permitted but probably a specific lysine residue cannot be altered. This signal may provide recognition for the nucleopore.

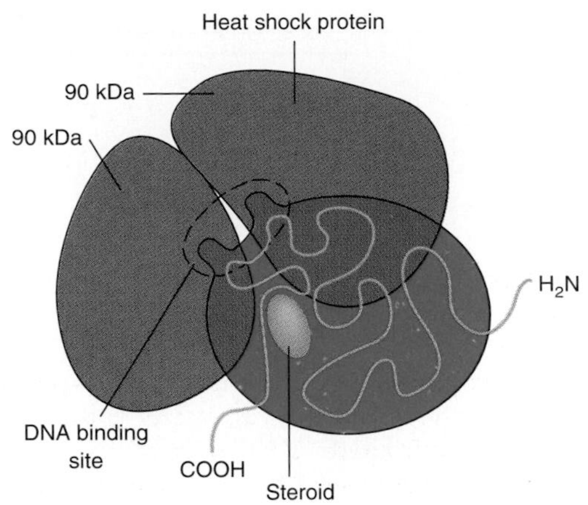

FIGURE 21.20
Hypothetical minimal model of a non-DNA-binding form of a steroid receptor. This form of the receptor cannot bind to DNA because the DNA-binding site is blocked by the 90-kDa hsp proteins or by some other constituent. Mass of this complex is approximately 300 kDa.

Steroid Receptors Can Be Upregulated or Downregulated Depending on Exposure to the Hormone

In general, many membrane or intracellular receptors are downregulated when the cell has been exposed to a certain amount of the hormonal ligand. In some cases, the downregulation is called "desensitization." **Downregulation** can take many forms. For membrane receptors the mechanism may be internalization by endocytosis of the receptors after exposure to hormone (see p. 876). Internalization reduces the number of receptors on the cell surface and renders the cell less responsive to hormone; that is, desensitizes the cell. In the case of intracellular steroid receptors, downregulation generally takes the form of reducing the level of receptor mRNA, which decreases the concentration of receptor molecules. The receptor gene may have a specific responsive element on its promoter whose action results in an inhibition of transcription of receptor mRNA or the receptor may stimulate transcription of a gene that codes for a protein that degrades the mRNA of the receptor. Sequences are now being recognized on receptor gene promoters that may bind activated steroid–receptor complexes and result in inhibition of transcription (Table 21.4). Downregulation of receptors by their own ligands plays an important physiological role because it prevents overstimulation of target cells when circulating hormone levels are elevated.

Although downregulation of steroid receptor levels by their cognate hormones appears to be the most frequently detected form of autoregulation, it is not common to all target cells. In fact, glucocorticoid-mediated upregulation has been reported in a number of responsive cells. Since all of these cells are growth inhibited by these hormones, it was initially suggested that hormone-mediated upregulation may be required for subsequent growth inhibition. However, the fact that glucocorticoid-mediated upregulation also occurs in human lymphoid cells, which express glucocorticoid receptors but are not growth inhibited by these steroids, demonstrates that this positive **autoregulation** is neither the result nor cause of hormone-mediated growth arrest.

21.9 SPECIFIC EXAMPLE OF STEROID HORMONE ACTION AT CELL LEVEL: PROGRAMMED DEATH

Programmed cell death or **apoptosis** is a suicide process by which cells die according to a program that may be beneficial for the organism. It can result from the rise or fall in the level of a specific hormone(s). Uterine endometrial cells at the beginning of menstruation are an example where programmed cell death is initiated by the fall in levels of progesterone and estradiol in the blood (see Clin. Corr. 21.3). Another case is **apoptosis** of thymus cells during development when the adrenal cortex becomes functional and begins to synthesize and secrete relatively large amounts of cortisol. A newborn has a large thymus but when cortisol is synthesized and released the thymus cortical cells begin to die until a resistant core of cells is reached and the gland achieves its adult size. Thus programmed cell death is a mechanism used in development for the maturation of certain organs as well as in cyclic systems where cells

CLINICAL CORRELATION 21.3

Programmed Cell Death in the Ovarian Cycle

During the ovarian cycle, the ovarian follicle expels the mature ovum at day 14 and the remaining cells of the follicle are differentiated into a functional *corpus luteum*. The *corpus luteum* produces some estradiol to partially replace that provided earlier by the maturing follicle. However, its principal product is progesterone. Estradiol and progesterone are the main stimulators of uterine endometrial wall thickening in preparation for implantation. One of the proteins induced by estradiol action in the endometrium is the progesterone receptor. Thus the uterine endometrial cells become exquisitely sensitive to estradiol as well as progesterone. The corpus luteum supplies the latter, but in the absence of fertilization and development of an embryo, the corpus luteum lives only for a short while and then atrophies because of lack of LH or chorionic gonadotropin, a hormone produced by the early embryo. The production of oxytocin and $PGF_{2\alpha}$ in the ovary may bring about the destruction of the corpus luteum (luteolysis). Blood levels of estradiol and progesterone fall dramatically after luteolysis and the stimulators of uterine endometrial cells disappear, causing degeneration of this thickened, vascularized layer of tissue and precipitating menstruation. These cells die by programmed cell death (apoptosis) due to the withdrawal of steroids. The hallmark of programmed cell death is internucleosomal cleavage of DNA. Thus programmed cell death appears to play specific roles in development and in tissue cycling either due to a specific hormonal stimulus or to withdrawal of hormone(s) as described here.

Erickson, G. F., and Schreiber, J. R. Morphology and physiology of the ovary. In: K. L. Becker (Ed.), *Principles and Practice of Endocrinology and Metabolism*. New York: Lippincott, 1990, p. 776; Rebar, R. W., Kenigsberg, D., and Hogden, G. D. The normal menstrual cycle and the control of ovulation. In: K. Becker (Ed.), *Principles and Practice of Endocrinology and Metabolism*. New York: Lippincott, 1990, p. 788; and Hamburger, L., Hahlin, M., Hillensjo, T., Johanson, C., and Sjogren, A. Luteotropic and luteolytic factors regulating human corpus luteum function. *Ann. N.Y. Acad. Sci.* 541:485, 1988.

proliferate and then regress until another cycle is initiated to begin the proliferation all over again, as is the case with the ovarian cycle.

Glucocorticoid-induced apoptosis in thymocytes is mediated by the intracellular glucocorticoid receptor. There are two phases to this complex process: inhibition of cell proliferation (cytostatic phase) followed by a cytolytic phase characterized by internucleosomal DNA cleavage and ultimate cell death (cytolytic phase). These two phases are not necessarily linked, since some cells are growth inhibited, but not lysed, by glucocorticoid hormones. The precise mechanism by which glucocorticoid–receptor complexes induce cell death is not fully understood. Exposure to hormone may result in a conformational change in chromatin with the unmasking of internucleosomal linker DNA regions, which are substrates for a nuclease. Treatment of thymocytes with glucocorticoids results in the activation of a constitutive, endogenous Ca^{2+}/Mg^{2+}-dependent endonuclease, while similar treatment of human leukemic T cells results in the activation of Ca^{2+}/Mg^{2+}-independent nuclease. Recent studies have demonstrated that the Ca^{2+}/Mg^{2+}-dependent nuclease that is activated by glucocorticoids in rat thymocytes is homologous with a cyclophilin. These proteins are high-affinity binding proteins for the immunosuppressive drug, cyclosporin A, and have Ca^{2+}/Mg^{2+}-dependent nuclease activity. The mechanism(s) by which glucocorticoid hormones induce lysis of thymocytes versus leukemic T cells appears to differ in several other respects. Treatment of sensitive T cells with these hormones results in upregulation of glucocorticoid receptor mRNA levels, while identical treatment of thymocytes appears to result in downregulation of mRNA levels. Also, the mRNA levels for an important growth factor, *c-myc,* are repressed in glucocorticoid-treated T cells but induced in thymocytes. Thus the cytostatic and cytolytic phases of apoptosis may be mediated by slightly different pathways in these two different cell types.

BIBLIOGRAPHY

Argentin, S., Sun, Y. L., Lihrmann, I., Schmidt, T. J., Drouin, J., and Nemer, M. Distal *cis*-acting promoter sequences mediate glucocorticoid stimulation of cardiac ANF gene transcription. *J. Biol. Chem.* 266:23315, 1991.

Baulieu, E.-E. Steroid hormone antagonists at the receptor level: a role for heat-shock protein MW 90,000 (hsp 90). *J. Cell Biochem.* 35:161, 1987.

Beato, M. Gene regulation by steroid hormones. *Cell* 56:335, 1989.

Carson-Jurica, M. A., Schrader, W. T., and O'Malley, B. W. Steroid receptor family: structure and functions. *Endocr. Rev.* 11:201, 1990.

Chrousos, G. P., Loriaux, D. L., and Lipsett, M. B. (Eds.). *Steroid Hormone Resistance.* New York: Plenum Press, 1986.

Drouin, J., Sun, Y. L. Tramblay, S., Schmidt, T. J., deLean A., and Nemer, M. Homodimer formation is rate-limiting for high affinity DNA binding by glucocorticoid receptor. *Mol. Endocrinol,* 6:1299, 1992.

Evans, R. M. The steroid and thyroid hormone receptor superfamily. *Science* 240:889, 1988.

Giguere, V., Hollenberg, S. M., Rosenfeld, M. G., and Evans, R. M. Functional domains of the human glucocorticoid receptor. *Cell* 46:645, 1986.

Green, S., Kumar, V., Theulaz, I., Wahli, W., and Chambon, P. The N-terminal DNA-binding "zinc-finger" of the estrogen and glucocorticoid receptors determines target gene specificity. *EMBO J.* 7:3037, 1988.

Gustafsson, J. A., Carlstedt-Duke, J., Poellinger, L., et al. Biochemistry, molecular biology, and physiology of the glucocorticoid receptor. *Endocr. Rev.* 8:185, 1987.

Huft, R. W., and Pauerstein, C. J. *Human Reproduction: Physiology and Pathophysiology.* New York: Wiley, 1979.

Litwack, G. (Ed.). *Biochemical Actions of Hormones,* Vols. 1–14. New York: Academic Press, 1973–1987.

Litwack, G. (Ed.). Steroids. *Vitamins and Hormones,* Vol. 49. San Diego: Academic Press, 1994.

Litwack, G. (Ed. in Chief). *Vitamins and Hormones,* Vol. 51. San Diego: Academic Press, 1995.

Mester, J., and Baulieu, E.-E. Nuclear receptor superfamily. In: L. J. DeGroot, (Ed.) *Endocrinology,* 3rd ed., Philadelphia: Saunders, 1995, pp. 93–118.

Norman, A. W., and Litwack, G. *Hormones.* Orlando, FL: Academic Press, 1987.

O'Malley, B. W., Tsai, S. Y., Bagchi, M., Weigel, N. L., Schrader, W. T., and Tsai, M.-J. Molecular mechanism of action of a steroid hormone receptor. *Recent Prog. Horm. Res.* 47:1, 1991.

Renkawitz, R. Repression mechanisms of v-*erb*A and other members of the steroid receptor superfamily. *Ann. N.Y. Acad. Sci.* 684:1, 1993.

Rusconi, S., and Yamamoto, K. R. Functional dissection of the hormone and DNA binding activities of the glucocorticoid receptor. *EMBO J.* 6:1309, 1987.

Schmidt, T. J., and Meyer, A. S. Autoregulation of corticosteroid receptors. How, when, where and why? *Receptor* 4:229, 1994.

Schwabe, J. W. R., and Rhodes, D. Beyond zinc fingers: steroid hormone receptors have a novel structural motif for DNA recognition. *Trends Biochem. Sci.* 16:291, 1991.

Wahli, W., and Martinez, E. Superfamily of steroid nuclear receptors—positive and negative regulators of gene expression. *FASEB J.* 5:2243, 1991.

QUESTIONS ■ J. BAGGOTT AND C. N. ANGSTADT

1. The C-21 steroid hormones include:
   A. aldosterone.
   B. dehydroepiandrosterone.
   C. estradiol.
   D. testosterone.
   E. vitamin D_3.

2. Side chain cleavage enzyme complex activity may be stimulated by all of the following EXCEPT:
   A. cAMP.
   B. Ca^{2+} released via stimulation of the IP_3 pathway.
   C. Ca^{2+} entering the cell through a channel.
   D. 5′-AMP.
   E. induction of the StAR protein.

3. Δ^5-Pregnenolone is a precursor of all of the following EXCEPT:
   A. aldosterone.
   B. cortisol.
   C. 17β-estradiol.
   D. progesterone.
   E. vitamin D_3.

4. Major steps in the inactivation and excretion of ALL classes of steroid hormones (except vitamin D_3) include:
   A. conjugation to glucuronic acid.
   B. conjugation to sulfuric acid.
   C. hydroxylation.
   D. oxidation.
   E. side chain cleavage.

5. All of the following may be involved in the action of steroid hormone receptors EXCEPT:
   A. binding of the hormone to an intracellular receptor.
   B. activation of a G-protein.
   C. association with a heat shock protein (hsp90) with a cytoplasmic receptor.
   D. binding to a receptor in the nucleus.
   E. translocation of a cytoplasmic hormone–receptor complex into the nucleus.

6. Retinoic acid and its derivatives:
   A. may activate genes by preventing the binding of receptor proteins to silencer elements.
   B. bind to homodimeric proteins, which in turn bind to DNA.
   C. bind to DNA via leucine zipper motifs.
   D. are vitamin derivatives and hence have no effect on regulation of gene expression.
   E. may substitute for thyroid hormones in binding to the thyroid hormone receptor.

7. Reactions in the pathway of synthesis of active vitamin D involve all of the following organs EXCEPT:
   A. skin.
   B. kidney.
   C. liver.
   D. intestine.

Refer to the following for Questions 8–11:
   A. corticosteroid binding globulin
   B. serum albumin
   C. sex hormone-binding globulin
   D. androgen-binding protein
   E. transferrin

8. Major aldosterone carrier in blood.

9. Produced by the Sertoli cells.

10. Binds about 20% of the cortisol in the plasma.

11. At puberty decreases more in males than in females.

12. Receptors for steroid hormones are found in:
   A. cell membranes.
   B. cytoplasm.
   C. ribosomes.
   D. mitochondria.
   E. Golgi apparatus.

13. Which of the following involve(s) a response element of DNA that differs from all of the other listed hormones?
A. estrogen
B. glucocorticoid
C. mineralocorticoid
D. progesterone

14. All of the following receptors may belong to the steroid receptor gene superfamily EXCEPT:
A. aryl hydrocarbon receptor.
B. erbA protein.
C. retinoic acid receptor.
D. thyroid hormone receptor.
E. α-tocopherol receptor.

Refer to the following for Questions 15 and 16:
A. programmed cell death
B. stress response
C. downregulation of steroid receptors
D. upregulation of steroid receptors
E. silencing

15. Mechanism for the maturation of certain organs.

16. Receptor mRNA is reduced.

ANSWERS

1. A B and D: These are C-19 androgens. C: Estradiol is a C-18 estrogen. E: Vitamin D_3 is a C-27 compound (pp. 899–900).
2. D See Figure 21.4, p. 898.
3. E See Figure 21.5 (p. 899) and Figure 21.6 (p. 900) for the synthesis of A–D. The synthesis of vitamin D_3 is summarized in Figure 21.11 (pp. 906–907).
4. A Oxidation (including hydroxylation) and reduction are common in steroid hormone degradation. Glucocorticoids undergo side chain cleavage. Conjugation to sulfate is important in the excretion of androgens. But conjugation to glucuronide is significant for all steroid hormones except vitamin D_3 (Table 21.2, p. 902).
5. B G-proteins are generally associated with signal transduction for receptors on the membrane surface. See Figure 21.13 for the roles of the other choices.
6. A The retinoic acid receptor (RAR) binds to specific silencer elements in the absence of the ligand, retinoic acid. When bound, transcription of the gene is repressed. In addition, there are retinoid X receptors (RXR), which also affect gene expression, via heterodimerization with RAR (p. 912, Figure 21.14*b*).
7. D Intestine is a target organ of the active hormone, but is not involved in synthesis. See Figure 21.11, p. 906. A: Light-induced cleavage of 7-dehydrocholesterol occurs in the skin. B: Hydroxylation of 25-(OH)D_3 occurs in the kidney. C: Hydroxylation of D_3 occurs in the liver.
8. B See p. 908.
9. D See p. 908.
10. B Cortisol-binding globulin carries most of the cortisol. Serum albumin, however, nonspecifically binds a large number of hydrophobic substances, including cortisol (p. 908).
11. C As a result, there is more unbound testosterone circulating in the blood of males (p. 908).
12. B B: In addition, the nucleus contains steroid hormone receptors. See Figure 21.13, p. 909. A: Membrane receptors are generally associated with nonhydrophobic hormones, such as epinephrine and peptide hormones (Figure 21.4, p. 898).
13. A The *positive* glucocorticoid response element is the same as the mineralocorticoid response element and the progesterone response element. The estrogen response element differs (Table 21.4, p. 911).
14. E Note that *c-erbA* is a protooncogene. See p. 913, Figure 21.17.
15. A Thymus cortical cells are killed by cortisol (p. 915).
16. C This contrasts with cell membrane receptors, which can be internalized to render the cell less responsive (p. 915).

CHAPTER

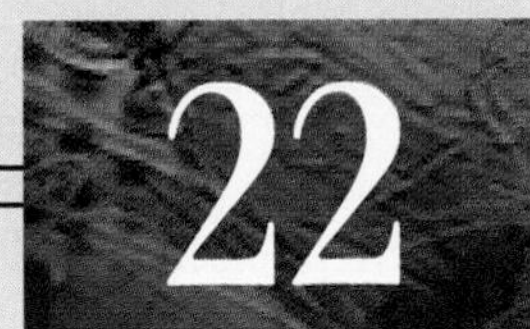

MOLECULAR CELL BIOLOGY

Thomas E. Smith

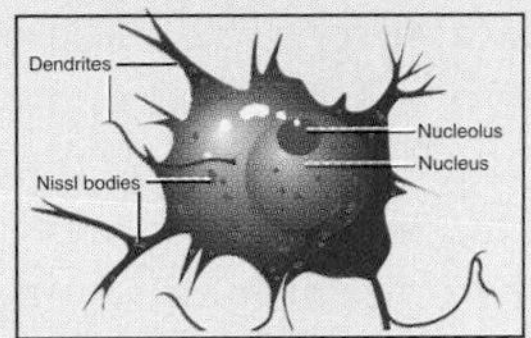

22.1 OVERVIEW

Animals sense their environment through the responses of certain organs to stimuli: touch, pain, heat, cold, intensity (light or noise), color, shape, position, pitch, quality, acid, sweet, bitter, salt, alkaline, fragrance, and so on. Externally, these generally reflect responses of the skin, eye, ear, tongue, and nose to stimuli. Some of these signals are localized to the point at which they occur; others—sound and sight—are projected in space, that is, the environment outside and distant to the animal.

Discrimination of these signals occurs at the point of reception, but acknowledgment of what they are occurs as a result of secondary stimulation of the nervous system and transmission of the signals to the brain. In many instances, a physical response is indicated, which results in muscular activity, either voluntary or involuntary. Common to these events is electrical activity associated with signal transmission along neurons and chemical activity associated with signal transmission across synaptic junctions. In all cases, stimuli received from the environment in the form of pressure (skin, feeling), light (eye, sight), noise (ear, hearing), taste (tongue), or smell (nose) are converted (transduced) into electrical impulses and to some other form of energy in order to effect the desired terminal response dictated by the brain. A biochemical component is associated with each of these events.

General biochemical mechanisms of signal transduction and amplification will be discussed as they relate to biochemical events involved in nerve transmission, vision, and muscular contraction. Finally, a specialized case of biochemical signal amplification will be discussed, namely, blood coagulation. This process is initiated on membrane surfaces as a result of the exposure of specific proteins that act as receptors and form nucleation sites for formation of multienzyme complexes. These multienzyme complexes lead to the amplification of blood coagulation through a cascade mechanism.

22.2 NERVOUS TISSUE: METABOLISM AND FUNCTION

Knowledge of the chemical composition of the **brain** began with the work of J. L. W. Thudichum in 1884 and the publication of his monogram, "A Treatise on the Chemical Composition of the Brain, Based Throughout on Original Research" (cited in West and Todd, *Textbook of Biochemistry*, MacMillan, 1957). Thudichum's research was supplemented with the work of others during those earlier years. There have been almost explosive advances during more recent years, through the use of molecular biological techniques, not only in our knowledge of the composition of the brain but also of molecular mechanisms involved in many brain/neuronal functions.

About 2.4% of an individual's body weight is nervous tissue, of which approximately 83% is the brain. The **nervous system** provides the communications network between the senses, the environment, and all parts of the body. The brain is the command center. This system is always functioning and requires a large amount of energy to keep it operational. Under normal conditions, the brain derives its **energy** from **glucose metabolism. Ketone bodies** can cross the **blood–brain barrier** and be metabolized by brain tissue. Their metabolism becomes more prominent during **starvation,** but even then they cannot replace the need for glucose. The human brain uses approximately 103 g of glucose per day. For a 1.4-kg brain, this corresponds to a rate of utilization of approximately 0.3 μmol min^{-1} g^{-1} of tissue. This rate of glucose utilization represents a capacity for **ATP production** through the **tricarboxylic acid (TCA) cycle** alone of approximately 6.8 μmol min^{-1} g^{-1} of tissue. Of course, the TCA cycle is not 100% efficient for ATP production, nor is all of the glucose metabolized through it. Most of the ATP used by the brain and other nervous tissue is generated aerobically through the TCA cycle, which functions at near maximum capacity. **Glycolysis** functions at approximately 20% capacity. Much of the energy used by the brain is to maintain ionic gradients across the plasma membranes, to effect various storage and transport processes, and for the synthesis of neurotransmitters and other cellular components.

Two features of brain composition are worth noting. It contains specialized and **complex lipids,** but they appear to function to maintain membrane integrity (see Chapter 5) rather than to have metabolic roles. There is generally a rapid **turnover rate** of **brain proteins** relative to other body proteins in spite of the fact that the cells do not divide after they have differentiated.

Cells of the nervous system responsible for collecting and transmitting messages are the **neurons.** They are very highly specialized (Figure 22.1). Each neuron consists of a cell body, **dendrites** that are short antenna-like protrusions that receive signals from other cells, and an **axon** that extends from the cell body and transmits signals to other cells. The central nervous system (CNS) is a highly integrated system where individual neurons can receive signals from a variety of different sources, including both inhibitory and excitatory stimuli.

Cells other than neurons exist in the CNS. In the brain, there are about 10 times more glial cells than there are neurons. Glial cells occupy spaces between neurons and provide some electrical insulation. Glial cells are generally not electrically active, and they are capable of division. There are basically five types of glial cells: Schwann cells, oligodendrocytes, microglia, ependymal cells, and astrocytes. Each type of glial cell has a specialized function, but only astrocytes appear to be directly associated with biochemical functions related to neuronal activity. One is metabolic (see discussion below on GABA) and the other anatomical.

Astrocytes send out processes at the external surfaces of the CNS. These processes are linked to form anatomical complexes that provide sealed barriers and isolate the CNS from the external environment. Astrocytes also send out similar processes to the circulatory system, inducing the endothelial cells of the capillaries to become sealed by forming tight junctions that prevent the passive entry into the brain of water-soluble molecules. These tight junctions form what is commonly known as the **blood–brain barrier.** Water-soluble compounds enter the brain only if there are specific membrane transport systems for them.

The normal individual has between 10^{11} and 10^{13} neurons, and communication between them is by electrical and chemical signals. Electrical signals transmit nerve impulses down the axon and chemicals transmit signals across the gap between cells. Some of the biochemical events that give the cell its electrical properties and are involved in the propagation of an impulse will be discussed.

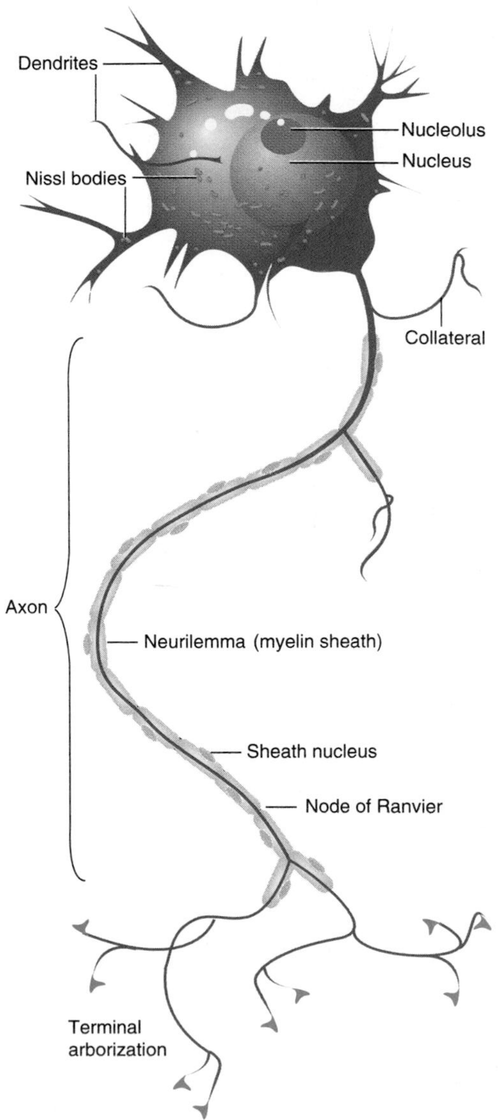

FIGURE 22.1
A motor nerve cell and investing membranes.

ATP and Transmembrane Electrical Potential in Neurons

Adenosine triphosphate generated from the metabolism of glucose is used to help maintain an **equilibrium electrical potential** across the membrane of the neuron of approximately −70 mV, with the inside being more negative than the outside. This potential is maintained by the action of the **Na^+,K^+ ion pump** (see pp. 206–207), the energy for which is derived from the hydrolysis of ATP to give ADP and inorganic phosphate. This system pumps Na^+ out of the cell by an antiport mechanism, whereas K^+ is moved into the cell. The channels through which Na^+ enters the cell are **voltage gated;** that is, the proteins of the channel undergo a charge-dependent conformation change and open when the electrical potential across the membrane decreases (specifically, becomes less negative) by a value greater than some threshold value. When the membrane becomes depolarized, Na^+, whose concentration is higher outside the cell than inside, flows into the cell and K^+, whose concentration is greater inside the cell, flows out of the cell, both going down their respective concentration gradients. The channels are open in a particular geographical

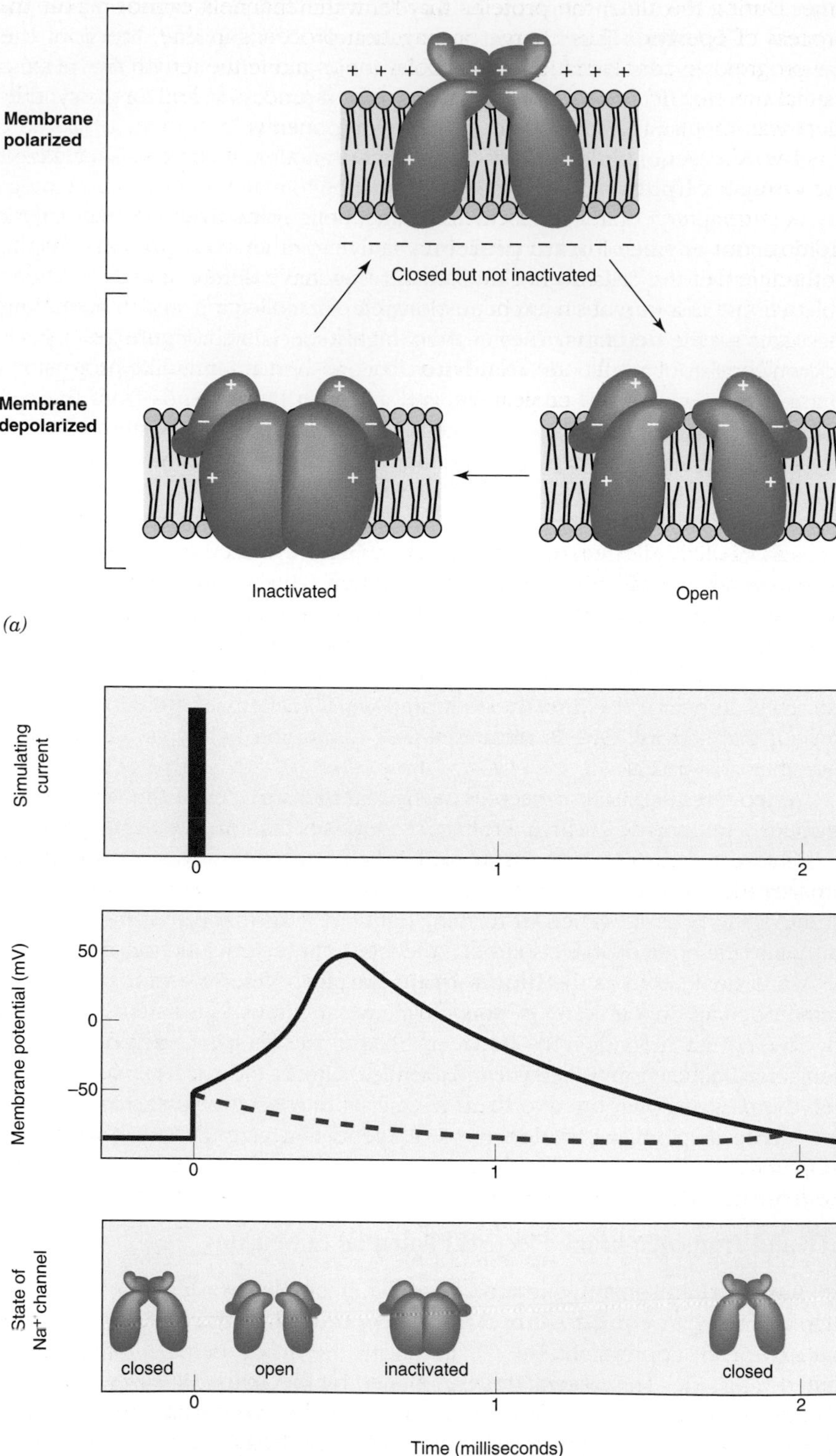

FIGURE 22.2
Schematic of Na^+ channels opening and closing during nerve impulse transmission.
Redrawn from Alberts, B., Bray, D., Lewis, J., Raff, M., Roberts, K., and Watson, J. Molecular Biology of the Cell, *2d ed. New York: Garland Publishing, 1989, p. 1071.*

region of the cell for fractions of a millisecond (Figure 22.2). The localized depolarization (voltage change) causes a conformation change in the neighboring proteins that make up the **voltage-gated ion channels.** These channels open momentarily to allow more ions in and, thus, by affecting adjacent channel proteins, allow the process to continue down the axon. There is a finite recovery time. During this time, the proteins that form the channels cannot repeat the process of opening. Thus charge propagation proceeds in one direction. It is the progressive depolarization and repolarization along the length of the axon that allow electrical impulses to be propagated undiminished in amplitude. Electrical impulse transmission is a continuous process in nervous tissue, and it is the ATP generated primarily from the metabolism of glucose that keeps the system operational.

A current area of active research in biochemistry involves the use of gene cloning and engineering techniques to isolate ion channel proteins and to determine their structures and elucidate their mechanisms of action. A considerable amount of information has been obtained in recent years on how mutations in voltage-gated ion channels may affect muscle function. Considerably less is known, however, about the relationship between structural disorders of ion channels in neurons and clinical disorders.

TABLE 22.1 Some of the Neurotransmitters Found in Nervous Tissue

EXCITATORY
Acetylcholine
Aspartate
Dopamine
Histamine
Norepinephrine
Epinephrine
ATP
Glutamate
5-Hydroxytryptamine
INHIBITORY
4-Aminobutyrate
Glycine
Taurine

Neuron–Neuron Interaction Occurs Through Synapses

There are generally two mechanisms for **neuron–neuron interaction**: through **electrical synapses** or through **chemical synapses.** Electrical synapses permit the more rapid transfer of signals from cell to cell. Chemical synapses allow for various levels of versatility in cell–cell communication. T. R. Elliot, in a paper published in 1904, was one of the first scientists to clearly express the idea that signaling between nerves could be chemical. Needless to say, considerably more information is now known about this mode of neuron–neuron communication. Chemical synapses are of two types: those that bind directly to an ion channel and cause it to open or to close, and those that bind to a receptor that releases a second messenger that reacts with the ion channel to cause it to open or to close. Primary emphasis here is on chemical synapses.

Chemical neurotransmitters fit the following criteria: they are found in the presynaptic axon terminal; enzymes necessary for their syntheses are present in the presynaptic neuron; stimulation under physiological conditions results in their release; mechanisms exist (within the synaptic junction) for rapid termination of their action; and their direct application to the postsynaptic terminal mimics the action of nervous stimulation. A sixth criterion, as a corollary of the five criteria listed above, is that drugs that modify the metabolism of the neurotransmitter should have predictable physiological effects *in vivo*, assuming that the drug is transported to the site where the neurotransmitter acts.

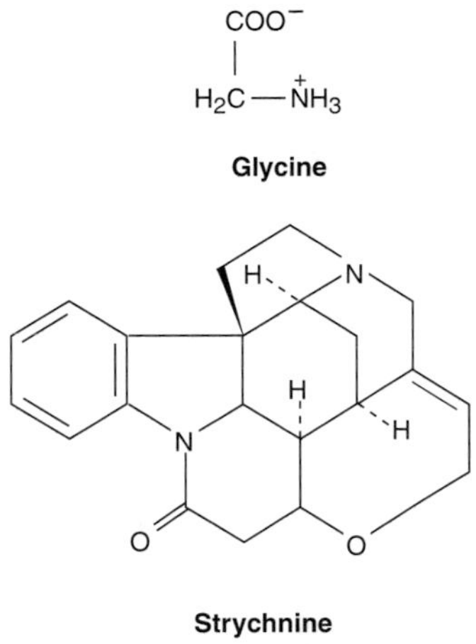

Chemical neurotransmitters may be excitatory or inhibitory. **Excitatory neurotransmitters** include acetylcholine and the catecholamines. **Inhibitory neurotransmitters** include γ-aminobutyric acid (also referred to as GABA or 4-aminobutyric acid), glycine, and taurine (Table 22.1).

The two major inhibitory neurotransmitters in the central nervous system are glycine and GABA. Glycine acts predominantly in the spinal cord and the brain stem, and γ-aminobutyric acid (GABA) acts predominantly in all other parts of the brain. **Strychnine** (Figure 22.3), a highly poisonous alkaloid obtained from *Nux vomica* and related plants of the genus *Strychnos,* binds to **glycine receptors** of the CNS. It has been used in very small amounts as a CNS stimulant. Can you propose how it works? The **GABA receptor** also reacts with a variety of pharmacologically significant agents such as benzodiazepines (Figure 22.4) and barbiturates. As with strychnine and glycine, there is little structural similarity between GABA and benzodiazepines.

The genes for the **acetylcholine receptor,** which also binds nicotinic acid, the glycine receptor, and the GABA receptor have been cloned and their amino acid sequences inferred. There is a relatively high degree of homology in their primary amino acid sequences.

A model of one-half of the GABA receptor is shown in Figure 22.5. This receptor has an $\alpha_2\beta_2$ composition. The polypeptides are synthesized with "signal

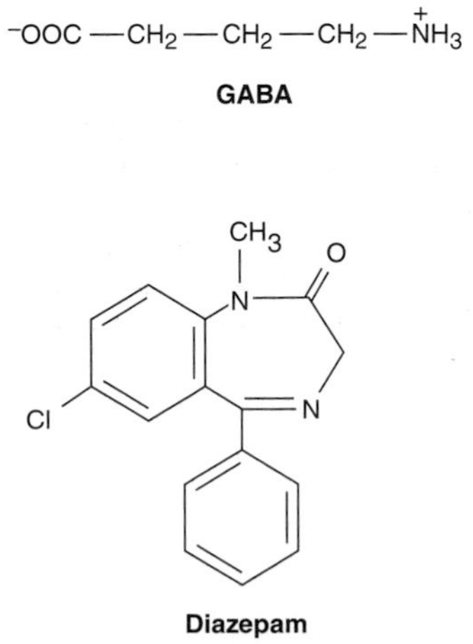

FIGURE 22.3
Structures of glycine and strychnine.

FIGURE 22.4
Structures of GABA and diazepam.

peptides" that direct their transport to the membrane. The α subunit has 456 amino acid residues and the β subunit has 474. The signal peptides are cleaved, leaving α and β subunits of 429 and 449 amino acid residues, respectively. Interestingly, the pharmaceutical agents bind to the α subunit, whereas GABA, the natural inhibitory neurotransmitter, binds to the β subunit. The protrusion of an extended length of the amino-terminal end of each polypeptide to the extracellular side of the membrane suggests that the residues to which the channel regulators bind are at the N terminal. A smaller C-terminal segment is also on the extracellular side of the membrane. The four subunits of the receptor form a channel through which small negative ions (Cl^-) can flow, depending on what is bound to the receptor end of the molecule.

All neurotransmitters are made and stored in **presynaptic neurons.** They are released after stimulation of the neuron, traverse the synapse, and bind to a specific receptor on the postsynaptic junction to elicit a response in the next cell. If the neurotransmitter is an excitatory one, it causes depolarization of the membrane as described above. If it is an inhibitory neurotransmitter, it binds to a channel-linked receptor and causes a conformation change that opens the pores and permits small negatively charged ions, specifically Cl^-, to enter. The net effect of this is to increase the chloride conductance of the postsynaptic membrane, making it more difficult for it to become depolarized—that is, effectively causing **hyperpolarization.**

Synthesis, Storage, and Release of Neurotransmitters

Nonpeptide neurotransmitters may be synthesized in almost any part of the neuron, in the cytoplasm near the nucleus, or in the axon. Most nonpeptide neurotransmitters are amino acids, derivatives of amino acids, or other intermediary metabolites. Synthesis and degradation of many of them have been discussed elsewhere, but some aspects of their metabolism relative to nerve transmission will be discussed later in this chapter.

Neurotransmitters travel rapidly across the **synaptic junction** (which is about 20 nm across), bind to receptors on the postsynaptic side, induce

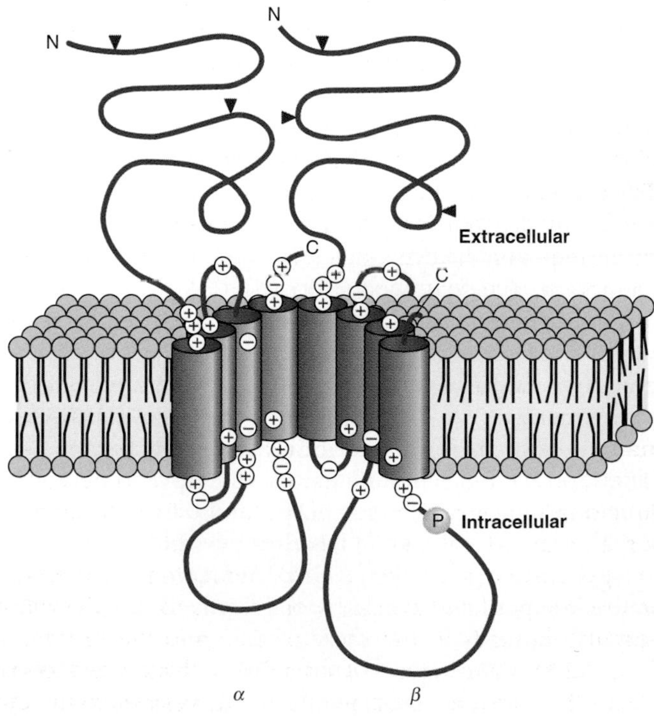

FIGURE 22.5
Schematic model of one-half of the GABA receptor embedded in the cell membrane.
The complete receptor has an $\alpha_2\beta_2$ structure and forms an ion channel. The site labeled P is a serine residue that may be phosphorylated by a cAMP-dependent protein kinase.
Redrawn from Schofield, P. R., Darlison, M. G., Fujita, N. et al. Nature *328:221, 1987.*

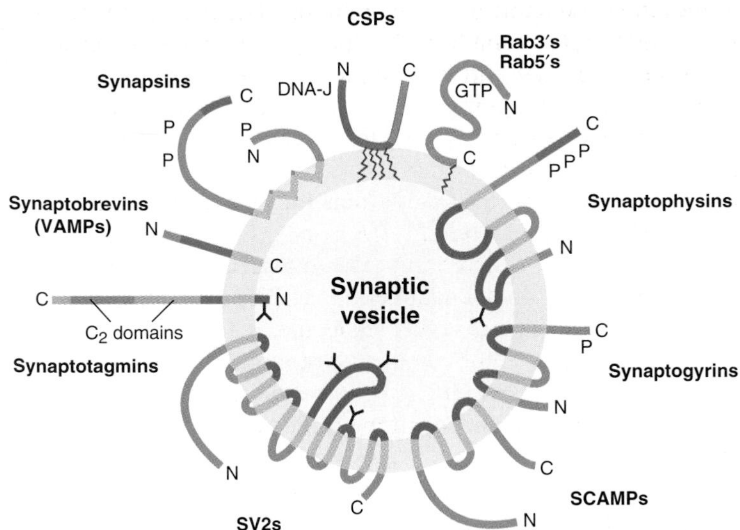

FIGURE 22.6
Schematic drawing of the relative arrangement of proteins of the synaptic vesicle (SV).
Rab proteins are attached by isoprenyl groups and cysteine string proteins by palmitoyl chains to SVs. The N and C termini of proteins are marked by N and C, respectively. Phosphorylation sites are indicated by P.
Redrawn from Sudhof, T. C. Nature *375:645, 1995.*

conformational changes in receptors and/or that membrane, and start the process of electrical impulse propagation in the postsynaptic neuron. Storage and release of neurotransmitters are intricate processes, but many details of the mechanism of these processes have begun to unfold. It has been shown by conventional techniques that some neurons contain more than one chemical type of neurotransmitter. The significance of this observation is unclear. Release of neurotransmitter is a **quantal event;** that is, a nerve impulse reaching the presynaptic terminal results in the release of transmitters from a fixed number of **synaptic vesicles.** Release of neurotransmitters involves attachment of the synaptic vesicle to the membrane and **exocytosis** of their content into the synaptic cleft.

Storage of neurotransmitters occurs in large or small vesicles in the presynaptic terminal. Small vesicles are the predominant type and exist in two pools: free and attached to cytoskeletal proteins, mainly actin. Small vesicles contain only "classical" small molecule type transmitters, whereas large vesicles may contain "classical" small molecule neurotransmitters and neuropeptides. Some may also contain enzymes for synthesis of norepinephrine from dopamine. A schematic diagram of a small synaptic vesicle is shown in Figure 22.6. The genes for many of the proteins attached to the synaptic vesicle have been cloned and significant amounts of information about their functions are known. Table 22.2 contains a list of some of those proteins. Some of their properties are briefly described. Figure 22.7 shows schematically how some of them may be arranged on the synaptic vesicle and how they may interact with the plasma membrane of the presynaptic neuron.

1. **Synapsin** exists as a family of proteins encoded by two genes. The proteins differ primarily in the C-terminal end (Figure 22.8). They constitute about 9% of the total protein of the synaptic vesicle membrane. All can be phosphorylated near their N termini by either **cAMP-dependent protein kinase** and/or **calcium–calmodulin (CaM) kinase I,** which is considered to be the physiologically important one relative to nerve transmission. Synapsins Ia and Ib can also be phosphorylated by **CaM kinase II** near their C termini, a region that is missing in synapsin IIa and IIb.

Synapsin has a major role in determining whether the synaptic vesicles are in the free pool and available for binding to the presynaptic membrane. Nerve stimulation leads to the entry of Ca^{2+} into the presynaptic vesicle (see Clin. Corr. 22.1). CaM kinase I (II also) is activated and phosphorylates synapsin. This either prevents binding of synaptic vesicles to the cytoskeletal proteins or

TABLE 22.2 List of Synaptic Vesicle Proteins

Synapsin	Ia
	Ib
	IIa
	IIb
Synaptophysin	
Synaptotagmin (p65)	
Syntaxin (p35)	
Synaptobrevin/VAMP	
Rab3 and rabphilin	
SV-2	
Vacuolar proton pump	

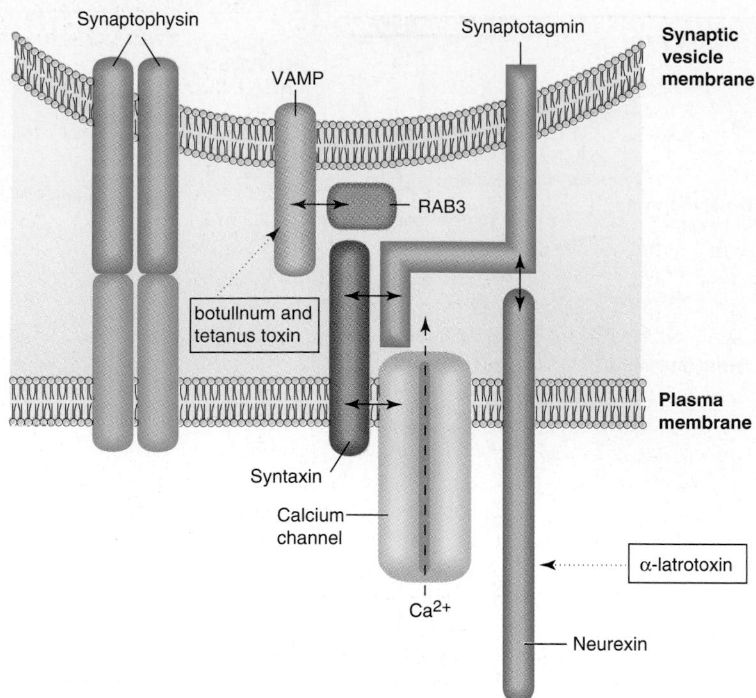

FIGURE 22.7
Schematic diagram showing how some of the synaptic vesicle proteins may interact with plasma membrane proteins to effect exocytosis.
Redrawn from Bennett, M. K., and Scheller, R. H. Proc. Natl. Acad. Sci. USA, *90:2559, 1993.*

releases them from those binding sites. The result is an increase in the free pool of synaptic vesicles. It has also been observed that **calcium–calmodulin** itself can bind synapsin and competitively block its interaction with actin. Calcium–calmodulin therefore regulates the number of free synaptic vesicles in the two pools by two mechanisms.

2. **Synaptophysin** is an integral membrane protein of synaptic vesicles that is structurally similar to gap junction proteins. It may be involved in the **formation of a channel** from the synaptic vesicle through the presynaptic membrane to permit the passage of neurotransmitters into the synaptic cleft.

3. **Synaptotagmin** is also an integral membrane protein of synaptic vesicles that interacts in a Ca^{2+}-dependent manner with specific proteins localized

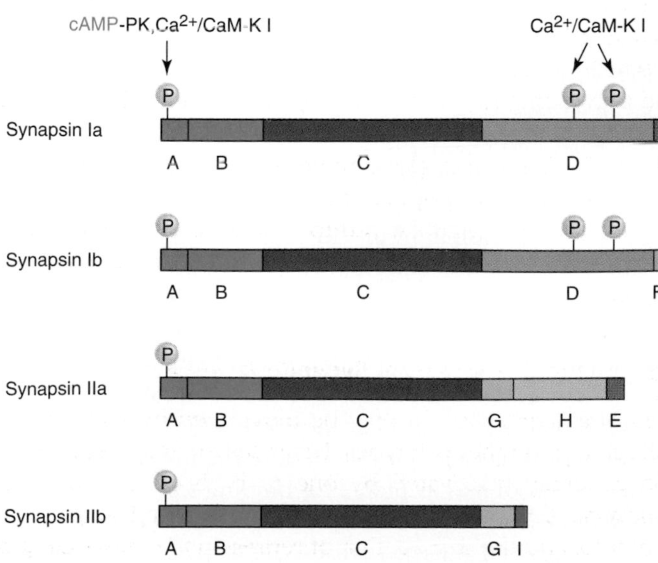

FIGURE 22.8
Structural arrangement of the synapsin family of proteins.
Redrawn from Chilcote, T. J., Siow, Y. L., Schaeffer, E., et al. J. Neurochem. *63:1568, 1994.*

CLINICAL CORRELATION 22.1

Lambert–Eaton Myasthenic Syndrome

Lambert–Eaton myasthenic syndrome (LEMS) is an autoimmune disease in which the body raises antibodies against voltage-gated calcium channels (VGCC) located on presynaptic nerve termini. Upon depolarization of presynaptic neurons, calcium channels at presynaptic nerve termini open, permitting the influx of calcium ions. This increase in calcium ion concentration initiates events of the synapsin cycle and leads to release of neurotransmitters into synaptic junctions. When autoantibodies against VGCC react with neurons at neuromuscular junctions, calcium ions cannot enter and the amount of acetylcholine released into synaptic junctions is diminished. Since action potentials to muscles may not be induced, the effect mimics that of classic myasthenia gravis.

LEMS has been observed in conjunction with other conditions such as small cell lung cancer. Some patients have shown a neurological disorder manifesting itself as subacute cerebellar degeneration (SCD). Plasma exchange (removal of antibodies) and immunosuppressive treatments have been effective for LEMS, but the latter treatment is less effective on SCD.

Diagnostic assays for LEMS depend on the detection of antibodies in patients' sera against VGCC. There are at least four subtypes of VGCC: T, L, N, and P. It has been found that the P subtype may be the one responsible for initiating neurotransmitter release at the neuromuscular junction in mammals. A peptide toxin produced by a cone snail (*Conus magnus*) binds to P-type VGCC in cerebella extracts. This small peptide has been labeled with ^{125}I, bound to VGCC in cerebella extracts, and the radiolabeled complex was precipitated by sera of patients who have been clinically and electrophysiologically defined as LEMS positive. This assay may prove useful not only in detecting LEMS but also in providing a means of finding out more about the antigenicity of the area(s) on the VGCCs to which antibodies are raised.

Goldstein, J. M., Waxman, S. G., Vollmer, T. L., et al. Subacute cerebellar degeneration and Lambert–Eaton myasthenic syndrome associated with antibodies to voltage-gated calcium channels: differential effect of immunosuppressive therapy on central and peripheral defects. *J. Neurol. Neurosurg. Psychiatry* 57:1138, 1994; and Motomura, M., Johnston, I., Lang, B., et al. An improved diagnostic assay for Lambert–Eaton myasthenic syndrome. *J. Neurol. Neurosurg. Psychiatry* 58:85, 1995.

on the presynaptic plasma membrane. It is probably involved in the process of **docking** of synaptic vesicles to the membrane.

4. **Syntaxin** is an integral membrane protein of the plasma membrane of the presynaptic neuron. Syntaxin binds synaptotagmin and mediates its interaction with Ca^{2+} channels at the site of release of the neurotransmitters. It also appears to have a role in **exocytosis.**

5. **Synaptobrevin/VAMP** (or vesicle-associated membrane protein) exists as a family of two small proteins of 18 and 17 kDa. They are anchored in the cytoplasmic side of the synaptic vesicle membrane through a single C-terminal domain and appear to be involved in **vesicle transport** and/or exocytosis. VAMPs appear to be involved in the release of synaptic vesicles from the plasma membrane of the presynaptic neuron. **Tetanus** and **botulinum toxins** bind VAMPs, causing slow and irreversible inhibition of transmitter release.

6. **Rab3** is one among a large rab family of **GTP-binding proteins**. Rab3 is specific for synaptic vesicles and is involved in the docking and **fusion process of exocytosis.** Rab3 is anchored to the membrane through a **polyprenyl side chain** near its C-terminal end. Elimination by genetic engineering of the polyprenyl side chain binding site did not alter its function *in vitro,* but it is not clear whether this is also true *in vivo.*

7. **SV-2** is a large **glycoprotein** with 12 transmembrane domains. No function has yet been assigned to it.

8. **Vacuolar proton pump** is an **ATPase** found in the vesicle membrane that is responsible for the **transport of neurotransmitters** into the synaptic vesicle.

Termination of Signals at Synaptic Junctions

Neurotransmitter action may be terminated by metabolism, reuptake, and/or diffusion into other cell types. Neurotransmitters responsible for fast responses are generally inactivated by one or both of the first two mechanisms. The following sections will outline some biochemical pathways involved in the synthesis and the degradation of representative fast-acting neurotransmitters—

specifically, acetylcholine, catecholamines, 5-hydroxytryptamine, and 4-aminobutyrate (GABA).

Acetylcholine

Reactions involving **acetylcholine** at the synapse are summarized in Figure 22.9. Acetylcholine is synthesized by the condensation of choline and acetyl CoA in a reaction catalyzed by **choline acetyltransferase** found in the cytosol of the neuron. The reaction is

$$\underset{\text{Choline}}{(CH_3)_3\overset{+}{N}CH_2CH_2OH} + CH_3CO{-}SCoA \longrightarrow \underset{\text{Acetylcholine}}{(CH_3)_3\overset{+}{N}CH_2CH_2OCOCH_3} + CoASH$$

Choline is derived mainly from the diet; however, some may come from reabsorption from the synaptic junction or from other metabolic sources (see p. 460). The major source of acetyl CoA is the decarboxylation of pyruvate by the **pyruvate dehydrogenase complex** in mitochondria. Since choline acetyltransferase is present in the cytosol, acetyl CoA must get into the cytosol for the reaction to occur. The same mechanism discussed previously (see p. 371) for getting acetyl CoA across the inner mitochondrial membrane (as citrate) operates in presynaptic neurons.

Acetylcholine is released and reacts with the **nicotinic–acetylcholine receptor** located in the postsynaptic membrane (see Clin. Corr. 22.2). The action of acetylcholine at the postsynaptic membrane is terminated by the action of the enzyme **acetylcholinesterase,** which hydrolyzes the acetylcholine to acetate and choline:

$$\text{Acetylcholine} + H_2O \rightleftharpoons \text{acetate} + \text{choline}$$

Choline is taken up by the presynaptic membrane and reutilized for synthesis of more acetylcholine. Acetate probably gets reabsorbed into the blood and is metabolized by tissues other than nervous tissue.

An X-ray crystallographic structure of acetylcholinesterase is shown in Figure 22.10. Its mechanism of action is similar to that of serine proteases (see p. 97). It too has a **catalytic triad,** but the amino acids in that triad, from N to C

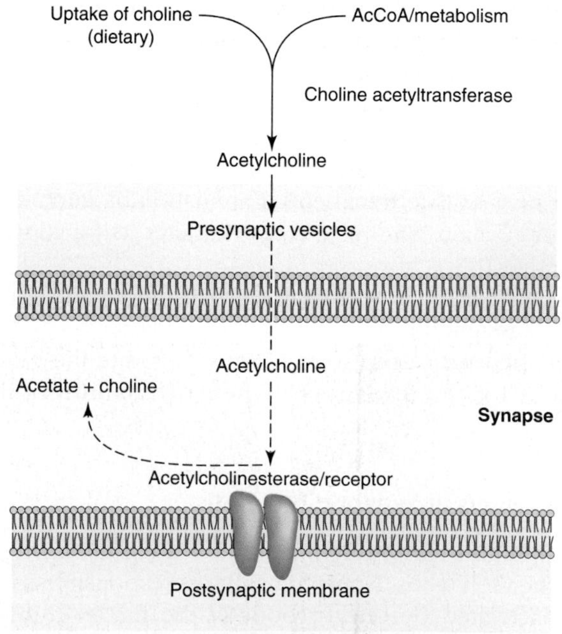

FIGURE 22.9
Summary of the reactions of acetylcholine at the synapse.
AcCoA, acetyl coenzyme A.

CLINICAL CORRELATION 22.2

Myasthenia Gravis: A Neuromuscular Disorder

Myasthenia gravis is an acquired autoimmune disease characterized by muscle weakness due to decreased neuromuscular signal transmission. The neurotransmitter involved is acetylcholine. The sera of more than 90% of patients with myasthenia gravis have antibodies to the nicotinic–acetylcholine receptor (AChR) located on the postsynaptic membrane of the neuromuscular junction. Antibodies against the AChR interact with it and inhibit its function, either its ability to bind acetylcholine or its ability to undergo conformation changes necessary to effect ion transport. Evidence in support of myasthenia gravis as an autoimmune disease affecting the AChR is the finding that the number of AChRs is reduced in patients with the disease, and experimental models of myasthenia gravis have been generated by either immunizing animals with the AChR or by injecting them with antibodies against it.

It is not known what events trigger the onset of the disease. There are a number of environmental antigens that have epitopes resembling those on the AChR. A rat monoclonal antibody of the IgM type prepared against AChRs reacts with two proteins obtained from the intestinal bacterium *Escherichia coli*. Both of the proteins are membrane proteins of 38 and 55 kDa, the smaller of which is located in the outer membrane. This does not suggest that exposure to *E. coli* proteins is likely to trigger the disease. The sera of both normal individuals and myasthenia gravis patients have antibodies against a large number of *E. coli* proteins. Some environmental antigens from other sources also react with antibodies against AChRs.

The thymus gland, which is involved in antibody production, is also implicated in this disease. Antibodies have been found in thymus glands of myasthenia gravis patients that react with AChRs and with environmental antigens. The relationship between environmental antigens, thymus antibodies against AChRs, and onset of myasthenia gravis is unclear.

Myasthenia gravis patients may receive one or a combination of several therapies. Pyridostigmine bromide, a reversible inhibitor of acetylcholine esterase (AChE) that does not cross the blood–brain barrier, has been used. The inhibition of AChE within the synapse by drugs of this type increases the half-time for acetylcholine hydrolysis. This leads to an increase in the concentration of acetylcholine, stimulation of more AChR, and increased signal transmission. Other treatments include use of immunosuppressant drugs, steroids, and surgical removal of the thymus gland to decrease the rate of production of antibodies. Future treatment may include the use of anti-idiotype antibodies to the AChR antibodies, and/or the use of small nonantigenic peptides that compete with AChR epitopes for binding to the AChR antibodies.

Stefansson, K., Dieperink, M. E., Richman, D. P., Gomez, C. M., and Marton, L. S. *N. Engl. J. Med.* 312:221, 1985; Drachman, D. B. (Ed.). Myasthenia gravis: biology and treatment. *Ann. N.Y. Acad. Sci.* 505:1, 1987; and Steinman, L., and Mantegazza, R. *FASEB J.* 4:2726, 1990.

termini, are in reverse order to those of the serine proteases, and glutamate instead of aspartate is involved.

Catecholamines

The **catecholamine neurotransmitters** are **dopamine** (3,4-dihydroxyphenylethylamine), **norepinephrine,** and **epinephrine** (Figure 22.11). Their biosynthesis has been discussed (see p. 466).

The action of catecholamine neurotransmitters is terminated by reuptake into the presynaptic neuron by specific transporter proteins. Cocaine, for example, binds to the **dopamine transporter** and blocks its reuptake. Dopamine remains within the synapse for a prolonged period of time and continues to stimulate the receptors of the postsynaptic neuron. Once inside the neuron,

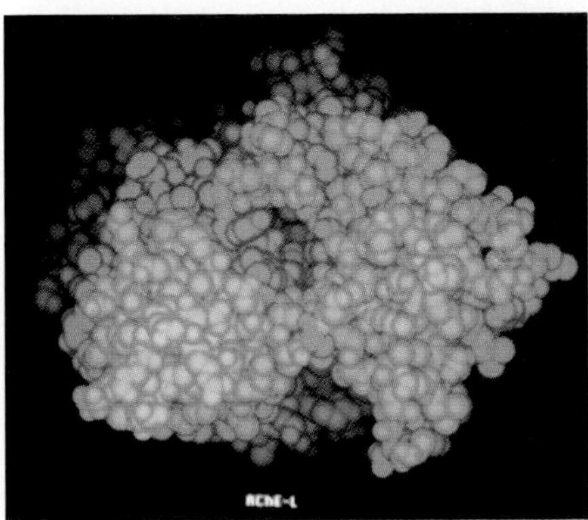

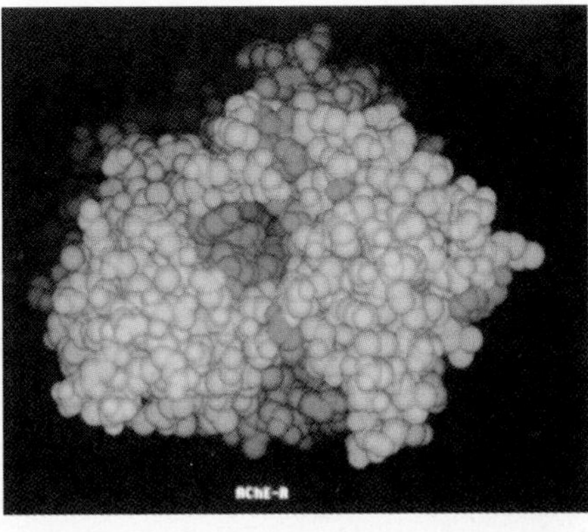

FIGURE 22.10
Space-filling stereo view of acetylcholinesterase looking down into the active site.
Aromatic residues are in green, Ser-200 is red, Glu-199 is cyan, and other residues are gray. *Reproduced with permission from Sussman, J. L., Harel, M., Frolow, F., et al.* Science *253:872, 1991. Copyright 1991 American Association for the Advancement of Science. Photograph generously supplied by Dr. J. L. Sussman.*

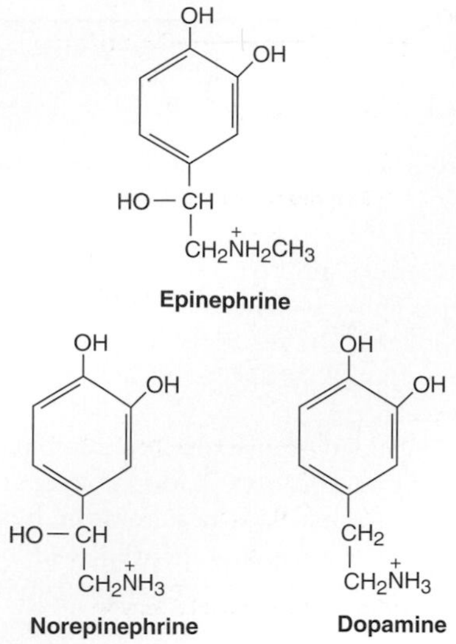

these neurotransmitters may be either repackaged into synaptic vesicles or metabolized. The two enzymes primarily involved in their metabolism are **catechol-*O*-methyltransferase** and **monoamine oxidase.** The metabolic reactions are shown in Figure 22.12. Catechol-*O*-methyltransferase catalyzes the transfer of a methyl group from *S*-adenosylmethionine to one of the phenolic OH groups. Monoamine oxidase catalyzes the oxidative deamination of these amines to aldehydes and ammonium ions. Monoamine oxidase can use them as substrates whether or not they have been altered by the methyltransferase. The end product of dopamine metabolism is homovanillic acid, and that of epinephrine and norepinephrine is 3-methoxy-4-hydroxymandelic acid.

FIGURE 22.11
Catecholamine neurotransmitters.

5-Hydroxytryptamine (Serotonin)

Serotonin, 5-hydroxytryptamine, is derived from tryptophan (see p. 476). Like dopamine, the action of serotonin is terminated by its reuptake into the presynaptic neuron by a specific transporter. Some types of depression are associated with low brain levels of serotonin. The action of some **antidepressants** such as Paxil (paroxetine hydrochloride), Prozac (fluoxetine hydrochloride), and Zoloft (sertraline hydrochloride) is linked to their ability to inhibit

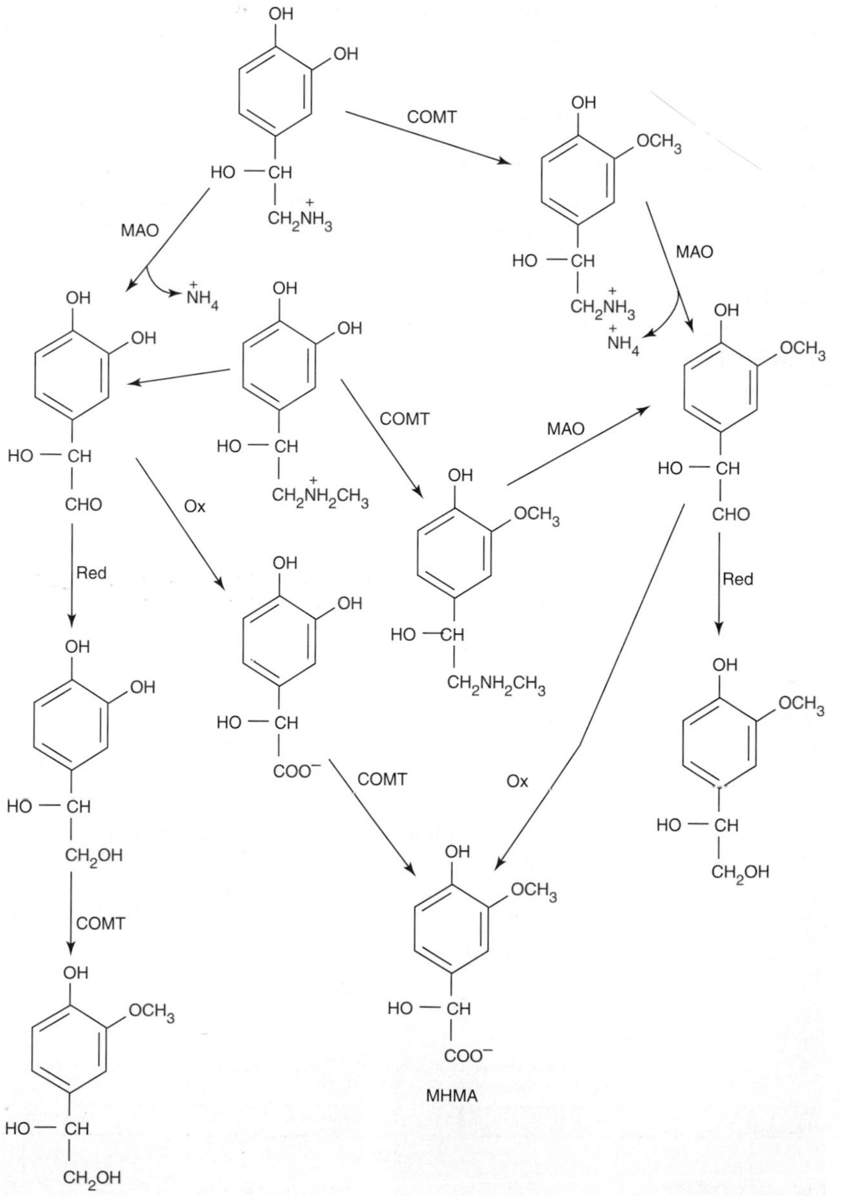

FIGURE 22.12
Pathways of catecholamine degradation.
COMT, catechol-*O*-methyltransferase (requires *S*-adenosylmethionine); MAO, monoamine oxidase; Ox, oxidation; Red, reduction. The end product of epinephrine and norepinephrine metabolism is 3-methoxy-4-hydroxymandelic acid.

serotonin reuptake. Once inside the presynaptic neuron, serotonin may be either repackaged in synaptic vesicles or metabolized. The primary route for its **degradation** is **oxidative deamination** to the corresponding acetaldehyde catalyzed by the enzyme monoamine oxidase (Figure 22.13). The aldehyde is further oxidized to 5-hydroxyindole-3-acetate by an aldehyde dehydrogenase.

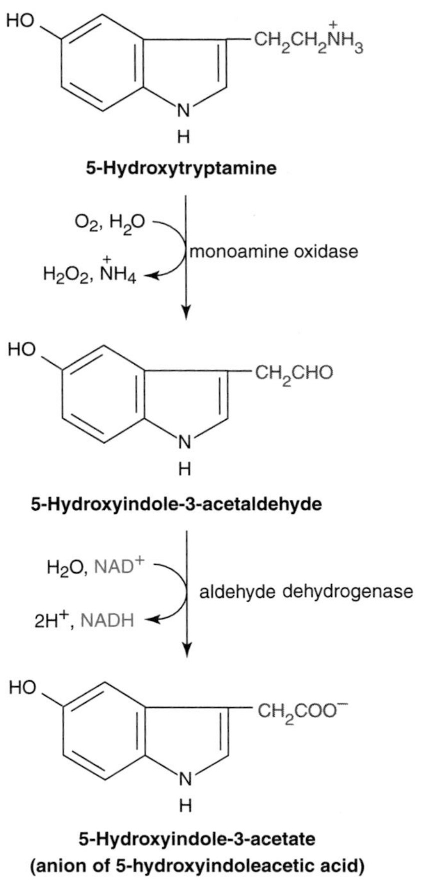

4-Aminobutyrate (γ-Aminobutyrate)

γ-Aminobutyrate (GABA), an inhibitory neurotransmitter, is synthesized and degraded through a series of reactions commonly known as the **GABA shunt.** In brain tissue, it appears that GABA and glutamate, an excitatory neurotransmitter, may share some common routes of metabolism in astrocytes (Figure 22.14). Both are taken up by astrocytes and converted to glutamine, which is then transported back into presynaptic neurons. In excitatory neurons, glutamine is converted to glutamate and repackaged in synaptic vesicles. In inhibitory neurons, glutamine is converted to glutamate and then to GABA, which is repackaged in synaptic vesicles.

It has been suggested that brain levels of GABA in some epileptic patients may be low. **Valproic acid** (2-propylpentanoic acid) apparently increases brain levels of GABA. The mechanism by which it does so is not clear. Valproic acid is metabolized primarily in the liver by glucuronidation and urinary excretion of the glucuronides, or by mitochondrial β-oxidation and microsomal oxidation.

Neuropeptides Are Derived from Precursor Proteins

Peptide neurotransmitters are generally synthesized as larger proteins and are cleaved by proteolysis to produce the neuropeptide molecules. Their synthesis requires the same biochemical machinery as does any protein synthesis and takes place in the cell body, not the axon. They travel down the axon to the presynaptic region by one of two generic mechanisms: **fast axonal transport** at a rate of about 400 millimeters per day and slow axonal transport at a rate of 1–5 millimeters per day. Since axons may vary in length from 1 millimeter to 1 meter, theoretically the total transit time could vary from 150 milliseconds to 200 days. It is highly unlikely that the latter transit time occurs under normal

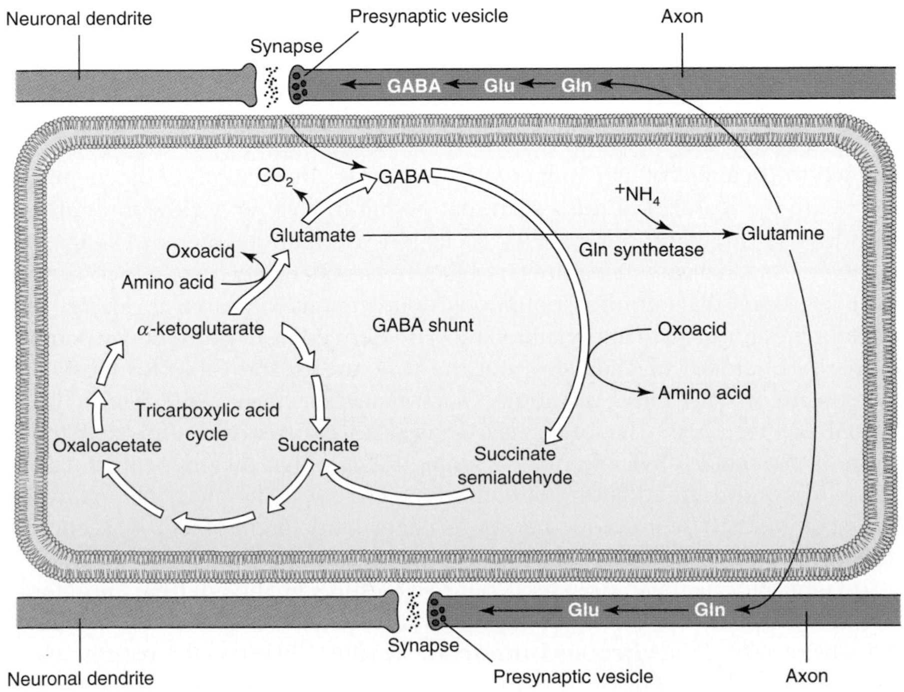

FIGURE 22.13
Degradation of 5-hydroxytryptamine (serotonin).

FIGURE 22.14
Involvement of the astrocytes in the metabolism of GABA and glutamate.

TABLE 22.3 Peptides Found in Brain Tissue[a]

Peptide	*Structure*
β-endorphin	Y G G F M T S E K S Q T P L V T L F K N A I I K N A Y K K G E
Met-enkephalin	Y G G F M
Leu-enkephalin	Y G G F L
Somatostatin	A G C K N F F W (C and C linked to) C S T F T K
Luteinizing hormone-releasing hormone	p-E H W S Y G L R P G-NH_2
Thyrotropin-releasing hormone	p-E H P-NH_2
Substance P	R P K P E E F F G L M-NH_2
Neurotensin	p-E L Y E N K P R R P Y I L
Angiotensin I	D R V Y I H P F H L
Angiotensin II	D R V Y I H P F
Vasoactive intestinal peptide	H S D A V F T D N Y T R L R K E M A V K K Y L N S I L N-NH_2

[a] Peptides with p preceding the structure indicate that the N terminal is pyroglutamate. Those with NH_2 at the end indicate that the C terminal is an amide.

physiological conditions, and the upper limit is probably hours rather than days. Recent experiments suggest that the faster transit times prevail.

Neuropeptides mediate **sensory and emotional responses** such as those associated with hunger, thirst, sex, pleasure, and pain. Included in this category are **enkephalins, endorphins,** and **substance P.** Substance P is an excitatory neurotransmitter that has a role in pain transmission, whereas endorphins have roles in eliminating the sensation of pain. Some of the peptides found in brain tissue are shown in Table 22.3. Note that Met-enkephalin is derived from the N-terminal region of β-endorphin. The N-terminal or both the N- and C-terminal amino acids of many of the neuropeptide transmitters are modified. For a further discussion of these peptides, see Chapter 20.

22.3 ■ THE EYE: METABOLISM AND VISION

The eye, our window to the outside world, allows us to view the beauties of nature, the beauties of life, and, *vide* this textbook, the beauties of biochemistry. What are the features of this organ that permit this view? A view through any window, through any camera lens, is clearest when unobstructed. The eye has evolved in such a way that a similar objective has been achieved. It is composed of live tissues that require continuous nourishment for survival. Energy and metabolites for growth and maintenance are derived from nutrients by conventional biochemical mechanisms, but the structures responsible for these processes are arranged and distributed such that they do not interfere with the visual process. Also, the brain has devised an enormously efficient filtering system that makes invisible objects within the eye that may appear to lead to visual distortion. In addition, different tissues use specific metabolic pathways to accommodate their unique needs. A schematic diagram of a cross section of the eye is shown in Figure 22.15.

Light entering the eye passes progressively through the **cornea;** the anterior chamber, which consists of the **aqueous humor;** the lens; the vitreous body, which consists of the **vitreous humor;** and finally focuses on the **retina,** which contains the visual sensing apparatus. The exterior of the cornea is bathed by

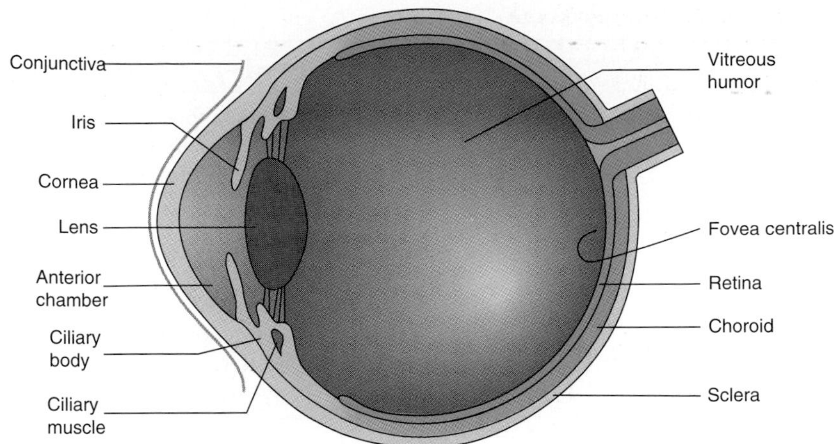

FIGURE 22.15
Schematic of a horizontal section of the left eye.

tears, while the interior is bathed by the aqueous humor, an iso-osmotic fluid containing salts, albumin, globulin, glucose, and other constituents. The aqueous humor brings nutrients to the cornea and to the lens, and it removes end products of metabolism from them. The vitreous humor is a collagenous or gelatinous mass that helps maintain the shape of the eye while allowing it to remain somewhat pliable.

The Cornea Derives ATP from Aerobic Metabolism

The eye is an extension of the nervous system, and like other tissues of the central nervous system, the major metabolic fuel is glucose. The cornea, which is not a homogeneous tissue, obtains a relatively large percentage of its ATP from aerobic metabolism. About 30% of glucose used by the cornea is metabolized by glycolysis and about 65% by the **hexose monophosphate pathway.** On a relative weight basis, the cornea has the highest activity of the hexose monophosphate pathway of any other mammalian tissue. It also has a high activity of **glutathione reductase,** an activity that requires NADPH, a product of the hexose monophosphate pathway. Corneal epithelium is permeable to atmospheric oxygen, that is necessary for various oxidative reactions. The reactions of oxygen can result in the formation of various **active oxygen species** that are harmful to the tissues, perhaps in some cases by oxidizing protein sulfhydryl groups to disulfides. Reduced glutathione (GSH) is used to reduce those disulfide bonds back to their original native states while GSH itself is converted to oxidized glutathione (GSSG). Furthermore, oxidized glutathione (GSSG) may also be formed by auto-oxidation. Glutathione reductase uses NADPH to reduce GSSG to 2GSH.

$$\text{GSSG} + \text{NADPH} + \text{H}^+ \xrightarrow{\text{GSH reductase}} \text{2GSH} + \text{NADP}^+$$

The activities of the hexose monophosphate pathway and the glutathione reductase maintain this tissue in an appropriately reduced state by effectively neutralizing the active oxygen species.

Lens Consists Mostly of Water and Protein

The **lens** is bathed on one side by the aqueous humor and supported on the other side by the vitreous humor. The lens has no blood supply, but it is metabolically active. It gets nutrients from the aqueous humor and eliminates waste into the aqueous humor. The lens is mostly water and proteins. The majority of the proteins are the **α-, β-, and γ-crystallins.** There are also albuminoids, enzymes, and membrane proteins that are synthesized in an epi-

TABLE 22.4 Eye Lens Crystallins and Their Relationships with Other Proteins

Crystallin	*Distribution*	*[Related] or Identical*
α	All vertebrates	**Small heat shock proteins** (αB) [*Schistosoma mansoni* antigen]
β	All vertebrates	[*Myxococcus xanthus* protein S]
γ	(embryonic γ not in birds)	[*Physarum polycephalum* spherulin 3a]
Taxon-specific enzyme crystallins		
δ	Most birds, reptiles	**Argininosuccinate lyase** (δ2)
ε	Crocodiles, some birds	**Lactate dehydrogenase B**
ζ	Guinea pig, camel, llama	**NADPH: quinone oxidoreductase**
η	Elephant shrew	**Aldehyde dehydrogenase I**

Source: Wistow, G. *TIBS* 18:301, 1993.

thelial layer around the edge of the lens. Some other types of proteins that are found in lens, including the lens of species other than vertebrates, are shown in Table 22.4. This shows that lens proteins may have different genetic origins and functions in other tissues. The most important physical requirement of these proteins is that they maintain a clear crystalline state. The center area of the lens, the core, consists of the lens cells that were present at birth. The lens grows from the periphery (Figure 22.16). The human lens increases in weight and thickness with age and becomes less elastic. This is accompanied by a loss of near vision (Table 22.5); a condition referred to as **presbyopia.** On average the lens may increase threefold in size and approximately $1\frac{1}{2}$-fold in thickness from birth to about age 80.

Lens proteins must be maintained in a native unaggregated state. They are sensitive to various insults such as changes in oxidation–reduction state, osmolarity, excessively increased concentrations of metabolites, and physical insults such as UV irradiation. Reactions that help maintain structural integrity of the lens are the Na^+,K^+–ATPase for osmotic balance, glutathione reductase for redox state balance, and protein synthesis for growth and maintenance. Energy for these processes comes from the metabolism of glucose. About 85% of the glucose metabolized by the lens is by glycolysis, 10% by the hexose monophosphate pathway, and 3% by the tricarboxylic acid cycle, presumably by the cells located at the periphery.

Cataract is the only known disease of the lens. Cataracts are opacities of lenses brought about by a loss of osmolarity and a change in solubility of some

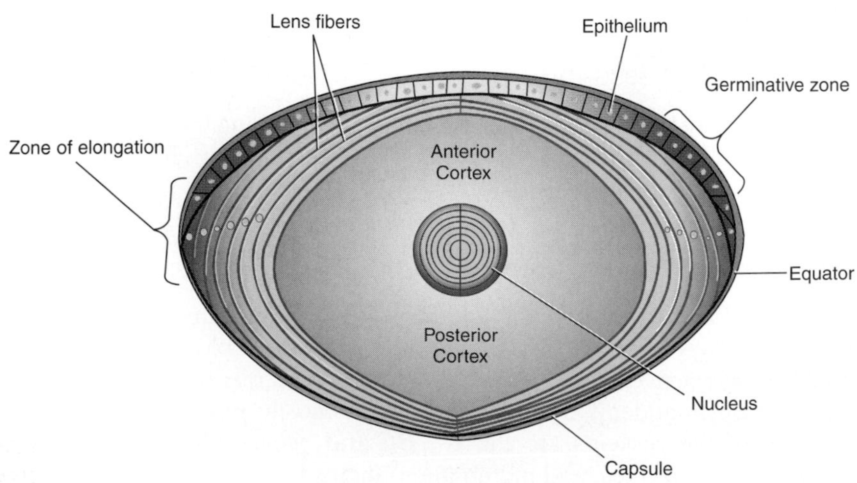

FIGURE 22.16
Schematic representation of a meridional section of a mammalian lens.

of the proteins, resulting in regions of high light scatter. Cataracts affect about 1 million people per year in the United States, and there are no known cures or preventative measures. The remedy is lens replacement, a very common operation in the United States. There are basically two types of cataracts: **senile cataracts** and **diabetic cataracts.** Both are the result of changes in the solubility and aggregation state of the lens crystallins. In senile cataracts, changes in the architectural arrangement of the lens crystallins are age-related and due to such changes as breakdown of the protein molecules starting at the C-terminal ends, deamidation, and racemization of aspartyl residues. Diabetic cataracts result from loss in osmolarity of the lens due to the activity of **aldose reductase** and **polyol (aldose) dehydrogenase** of the polyol metabolic pathway. When the glucose concentration in the lens is high, aldose reductase reduces some of it to **sorbitol** (Figure 22.17), which may be converted to **fructose** by polyol dehydrogenase. In human lens, the ratio of activities of these two enzymes favors sorbitol accumulation, especially since sorbitol is not used otherwise, and it diffuses out of the lens rather slowly. Accumulation of sorbitol in the lens increases osmolarity of the lens, affects the structural organization of the crystalline proteins within the lens, and enhances the rate of protein aggregation and denaturation. The areas where this occurs will have increased light scattering properties—which is the definition of cataracts. Normally, sorbitol formation is not a problem because the K_m of aldose reductase for glucose is about 200 mM and very little sorbitol would be formed. In diabetics, where the circulating concentration of glucose is high, activity of this enzyme can be significant.

TABLE 22.5 Changes in Focal Distance with Age

Age	*Focal Distance (in.)*
10	2.8
20	4.4
35	9.8
45	26.2
70	240.0

Source: Adapted from Koretz, J. F., and Handelman, G. H. *Sci. Am.*, 92, July 1988.

The Retina Derives ATP from Anaerobic Glycolysis

The **retina,** like the lens, depends heavily on anaerobic glycolysis for ATP production. Unlike the lens, the retina is a vascular tissue, but there are essentially no blood vessels in the area where visual acuity is greatest, the **fovea centralis** (see Clin. Corr. 22.3). Mitochondria are present in the retina, including in the rods and in the cones. There are no mitochondria in the outer segments of the rods and cones where the visual pigments are located.

NADH produced during glycolysis can be used to reduce pyruvate to lactate. The lactate dehydrogenase of the retina can use either NADH or NADPH, the

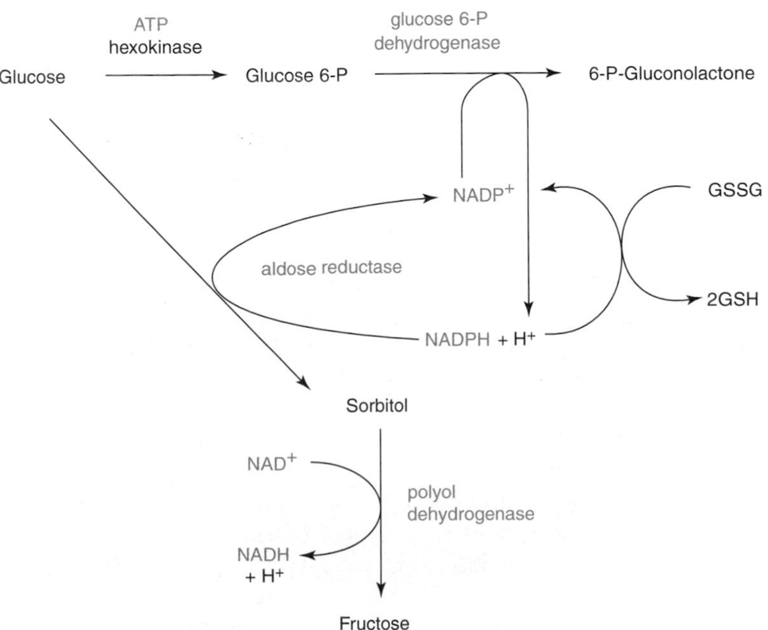

FIGURE 22.17
Metabolic interrelationships of lens metabolism.

CLINICAL CORRELATION 22.3

Macula Degeneration: Other Causes of Vision Loss

Many diseases of the eye affect vision, not all of which have clear, direct biochemical origins. The most serious eye diseases are those that result in blindness. Glaucoma is the most common and there is a direct causal relationship with diabetes, the biochemistry of which is fairly well known. Glaucoma can be treated and blindness does not have to be a result.

Macula degeneration leads to blindness and there is no cure. The macula is a circular area of the retina, the center of which is the fovea centralis, the area containing the greater concentration of cones and the one of greatest visual acuity. Macula degeneration may be among the leading causes of blindness in people over the age of 50. Macula degeneration is of two types: dry and wet. The dry form develops gradually over time, whereas the wet form develops rapidly and can lead to blindness within days. Macula degeneration occurs when blood vessels rupture under the macula, leading to a loss of the nutrient supply and a rapid loss of vision. Experimental procedures are in progress to surgically remove scar tissue that develops and to transplant tissue from the rear of the eye to restore nourishment to the photoreceptor cells.

Rupture of blood vessels that obscure macula details and result in rapid onset of blindness may be temporary in some cases. Six cases of sudden visual loss associated with sexual activity have been reported that are not associated with a sexually transmitted disease. Vision was lost in one eye apparently during, but most often reported a few days after engaging in, "highly stimulatory" sexual activity. Blindness was due to rupture of blood vessels in the macula area. When patients did see an ophthalmologist, most were reluctant to discuss what they were doing when sight loss was first observed. Four of the patients recovered with restoration of vision upon reabsorption of blood. In one case, where blood was trapped between the vitreous gel and the retinal surface directly in front of the fovea, the hemorrhage cleared only slightly during the next month, but visual acuity did not improve. The patient did not return for a follow-up examination, but there was no indication that the condition was permanent. Since most of the persons affected by this phenomenon were over the age of 39, it may be a worry more to professors than to students. It also may give a new meaning to the phrase "love is blind."

Friberg, T. R., Braunstein, R. A., and Bressler, N. M. *Arch. Ophthalmol.* 113:738, 1995.

latter being formed from the hexose monophosphate pathway. It is not clear whether lactate dehydrogenase of the retina plays any substantial role in mediating the regulation of glucose metabolism through either of these pathways by its selective use of NADH or NADPH.

Visual Transduction Involves Photochemical, Biochemical, and Electrical Events

Figure 22.18 shows an electron micrograph and schematic of the retinal membrane. Light entering the eye through the lens passes the optic nerve fibers, the ganglion neurons, the bipolar neurons, and the nuclei of the rods and cones before it reaches the outer segment of the rods and cones where the **signal transduction** process begins. The **pigmented epithelial** layer of the eye, the choroid, lies behind the retina, absorbs the excess light, and prevents reflections back into the rods and cones where it may cause distortion or blurring of the image (see Clin. Corr. 22.4).

The eye may be compared with a video camera. The camera collects images, converts them into electrical pulses, records them on magnetic tape, and allows their visualization by decoding the taped information. The eye focuses on an image by projecting that image onto the retina. A series of events begins, the first of which is photochemical, followed by biochemical events that amplify the signal, and finally electrical impulses are sent to the brain where the image is reconstructed in "the mind's eye." During this process, the initial event has been transformed from a physical event to a chemical reaction, through a series of biochemical reactions, to an electrical event, to a conscious acknowledgment of the presence of an object in the environment outside the body.

When photons of light enter the eye and are absorbed by photoreceptors in the **outer segments** of **rods** or **cones,** they cause isomerization of the visual pigment, **retinal,** from the 11-*cis* form to the all-*trans* form. This isomerization causes a conformation change in the protein moiety of the complex and affects the resting membrane potential of the cell, resulting in an electrical signal being

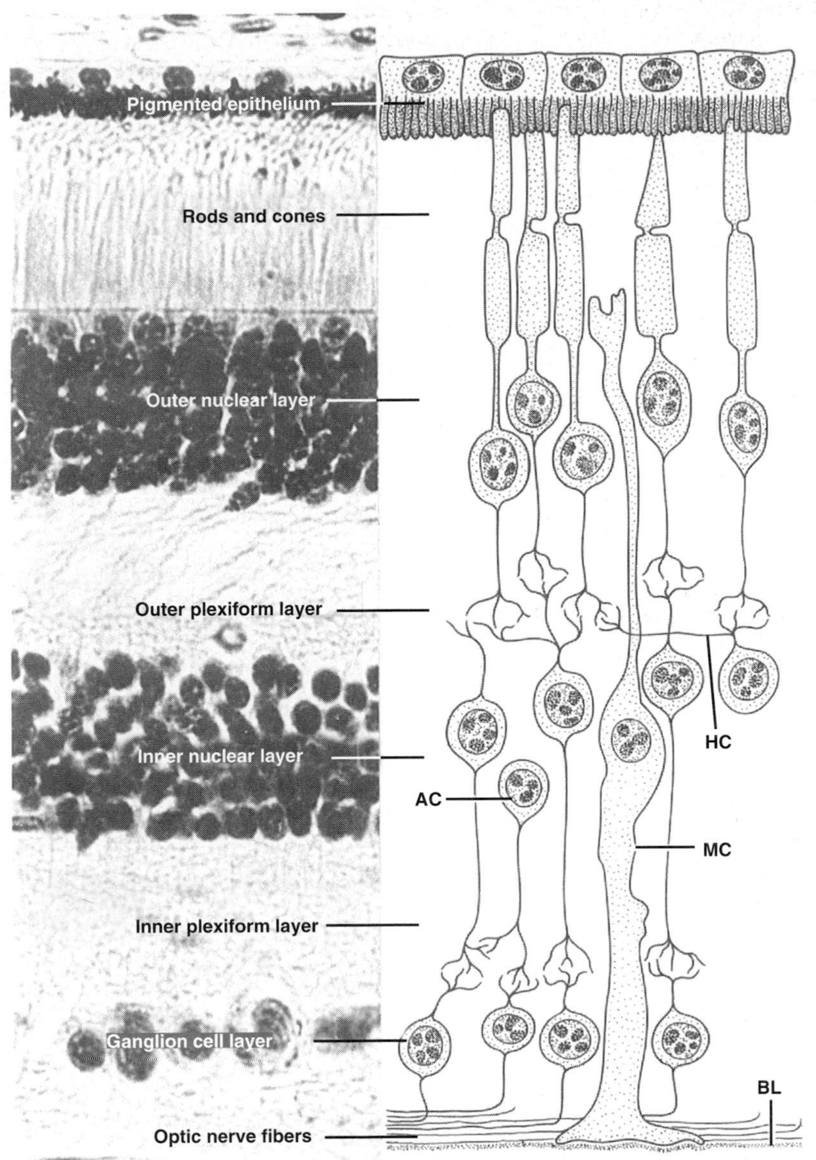

FIGURE 22.18
Electron micrograph and schematic representation of cells of the human retina. Tips of rods and cones are buried in the pigmented epithelium of the outermost layer. Rods and cones form synaptic junctions with many bipolar neurons, which in turn form synapses with cells in the ganglion layer that send axons through the optic nerve to the brain. The synapse of a rod or cone with many cells is important for the integration of information. HC, horizontal cells; AC, amacrine cell; MC, Müller cell; BL, basal lamina. *Reprinted with permission from Kessel, R. G., and Kardon, R. H.,* Tissues and Organs: A Text-Atlas of Scanning Electron Microscopy. *New York: W. H. Freeman, 1979, p. 87.*

transmitted by way of the optic nerve to the brain. These processes will be discussed later in more detail.

Photoreceptor Cells Are Rods and Cones

The **photoreceptor cells** of the eye are the **rods** and the **cones** (Figure 22.18). Each type has flattened disks that contain a photoreceptor pigment. This pigment is **rhodopsin** in the rod cells, and **red, green,** or **blue pigment** in the cone cells. Rhodopsin is a transmembrane protein to which is bound a prosthetic group, **11-*cis*-retinal.** Rhodopsin minus its prosthetic group is **opsin.** The three proteins that form the red, green, and blue pigments of cone cells are different from each other and from opsin.

Rhodopsin, an approximately 40-kDa protein, contains seven transmembrane α-helices. The 11-*cis*-retinal is attached through a protonated Schiff base to the ε-amino group of lysine-296 on the seventh helix. Lysine-296 lies about midway between the two faces of the membrane (Figure 22.19*a*). A 9-Å resolution three-dimensional (3-D) model for rhodopsin, obtained by cryomicroscopy, shows that most of the helices are perpendicular to the surface of the membrane

CLINICAL CORRELATION 22.4

Niemann–Pick Disease and Retinitis Pigmentosa

There are central nervous system disorders associated with the Niemann–Pick group of diseases that can become evident by ocular changes. Some of these are observed as abnormal macula with gray discoloration and granular pigmentation or granule opacities about the fovea.

Acute type I Niemann–Pick disease, lipidosis with sphingomyelinase deficiency and primary sphingomyelin storage, may show a cherry red spot in the retina in as many as 50% of patients. Macula halo syndrome applies to the crystalloid opacities seen in some patients with subacute type I disease. They form a halo approximately one-half the disk diameter at their outer edge and are scattered throughout the various layers of the retina. They do not interfere with vision.

In an 11-year-old girl who had type II disease, more extensive ocular involvement was observed. There was sphingomyelin storage in the keratocytes of the cornea, the lens, the retinal ganglion cells, the pigmented epithelium, the corneal tract, and the fibrous astrocytes of the optic nerve.

Retinitis pigmentosa is a secondary effect of the abnormal biochemistry associated with Niemann–Pick disease.

Spence, M. W., and Callahan, J. W. In: C. R. Schriver, A. L. Beaudet, W. Sly, and D. Volle (Eds.), *The Metabolic Basis of Inherited Disease,* New York: McGraw-Hill, 1989, pp. 1656–1676.

(Figure 22.19*b*). Some, however, are distorted from this perpendicular arrangement. It is not known whether the orientation of those distorted helices is associated with binding of 11-*cis*-retinal since this low-resolution structure will not permit tracing of the carbon backbone structure of rhodopsin. See also Clin. Corr. 22.5.

Reactions involved in the formation of 11-*cis*-retinal from **β-carotene** and rhodopsin from opsin and 11-*cis*-retinal are shown in Figure 22.20. The 11-*cis*-retinal is derived from **vitamin A** and/or β-carotene of the diet. These are

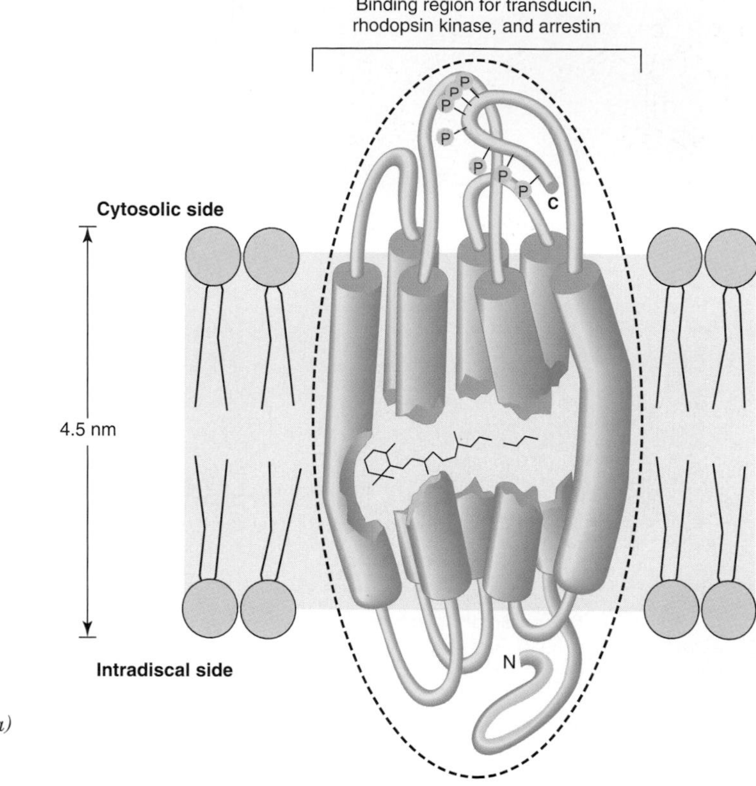

(*a*)

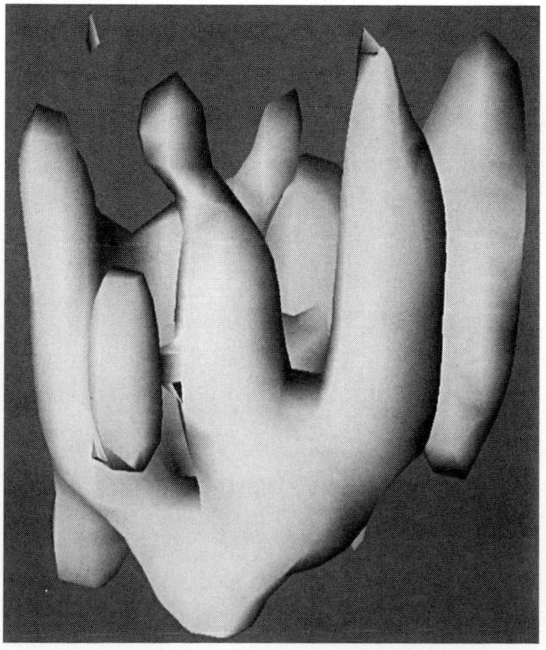

(*b*)

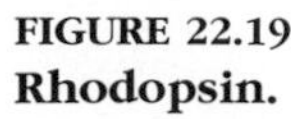

FIGURE 22.19
Rhodopsin.
(*a*) A model of the structure of vertebrate rhodopsin. (*b*) A 9-Å resolution 3-D model for rhodopsin obtained by cryomicroscopy.
(a) Redrawn from Stryer, L. Annu. Rev. Neurosci. *9:87, 1986 (based on Dratz and Hargrave, 1983). (b) Reproduced with permission from Unger, V. M. and Schertler, G. F. X.* Biophys. J. *68:1776, 1995. Photograph generously supplied by Dr. G. F. X. Schertler.*

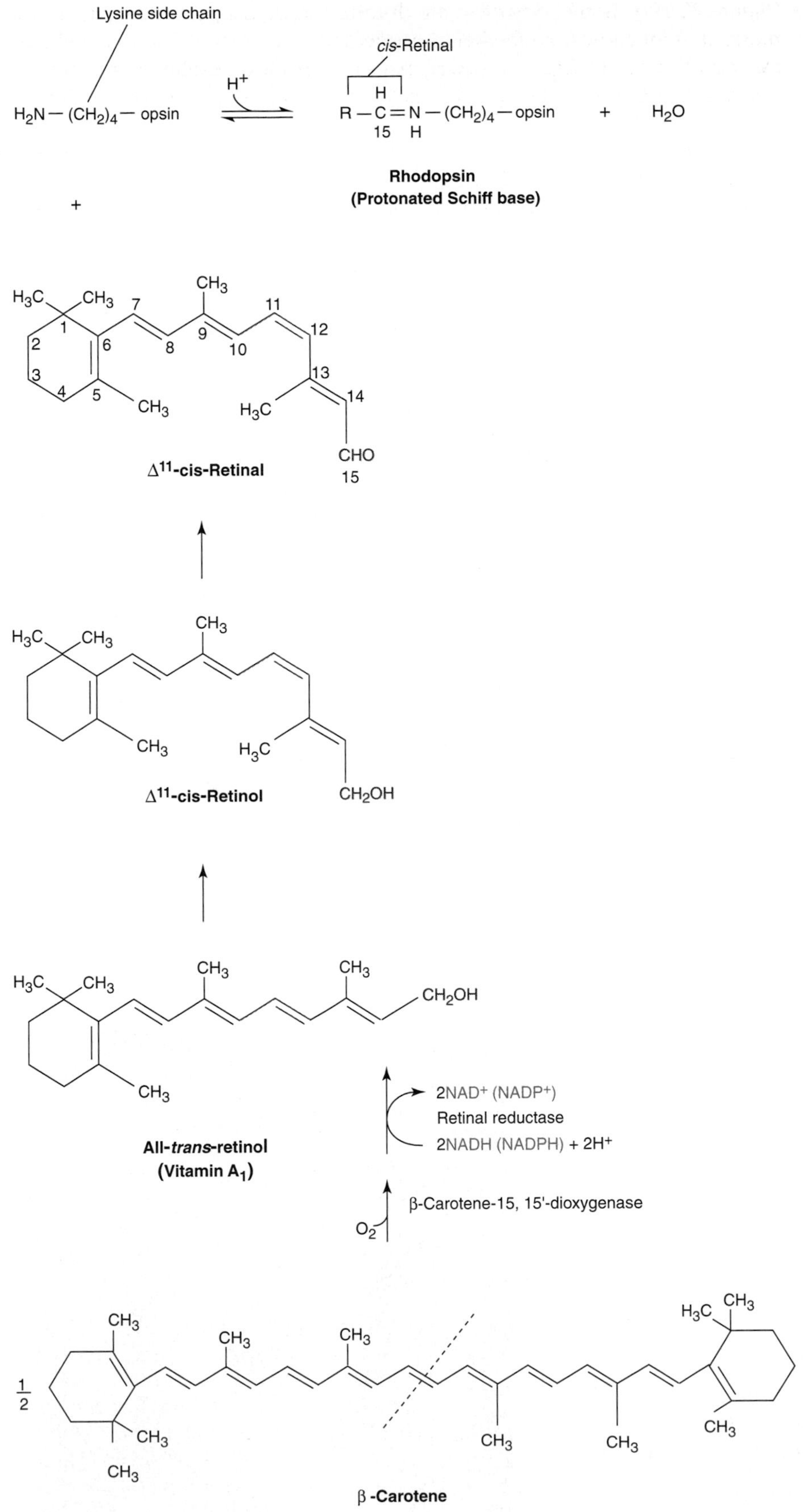

Lysine side chain

$H_2N-(CH_2)_4-$opsin + H^+ ⇌ *cis*-Retinal: $R-\overset{H}{C}=\overset{+}{N}(H)-(CH_2)_4-$opsin + H_2O (C-15)

Rhodopsin
(Protonated Schiff base)

+

Δ11-cis-Retinal

↑

Δ11-cis-Retinol

↑

All-*trans*-retinol
(Vitamin A1)

↑ 2NADH (NADPH) + 2H+ → 2NAD+ (NADP+), Retinal reductase

↑ O_2, β-Carotene-15, 15'-dioxygenase

½ **β-Carotene**

FIGURE 22.20
Formation of 11-*cis*-retinal and rhodopsin from *β*-carotene.

CLINICAL CORRELATION 22.5

Retinitis Pigmentosa Resulting from a *De Novo* Mutation in the Gene Coding for Peripherin

A group of heterogeneous diseases of variable clinical and genetic origins have been placed under the category of retinitis pigmentosa (RP). Several of these have origins in abnormal lipid metabolism. Approximately 1.5 million people throughout the world are affected by this disease. It is a slowly progressive condition associated with loss of night and peripheral vision. It can be inherited through an autosomal dominant, recessive, or X-linked mode. RP has been associated with mutations in the protein moiety of rhodopsin and in a related protein, peripherin/RDS, both of which are integral membrane proteins. Peripherin is a 344 amino acid residue protein located in the rim region of the disk membrane. Structural models of these two proteins are shown in the figure below. Filled circles and other notations in the figure mark residues or regions that have been correlated with RP or other retinal degenerations.

A case has been described where a *de novo* mutation in exon 1 of the gene coding for peripherin resulted in the onset of RP. Using molecular biological techniques, Lam et al. (1995) found the specific change in peripherin to be a C-to-T transition in the first nucleotide of codon 46. This resulted in changing an arginine to a stop codon (R46X). The pedigree of this family is shown in the figure on next page. Neither parent had the mutation and genetic typing analysis (20 different short tandem repeat polymorphisms) showed that the probability that the proband's parents are not his actual biological parents is less than 1 in 10 billion. This establishes with near certainty that the mutation is *de novo.*

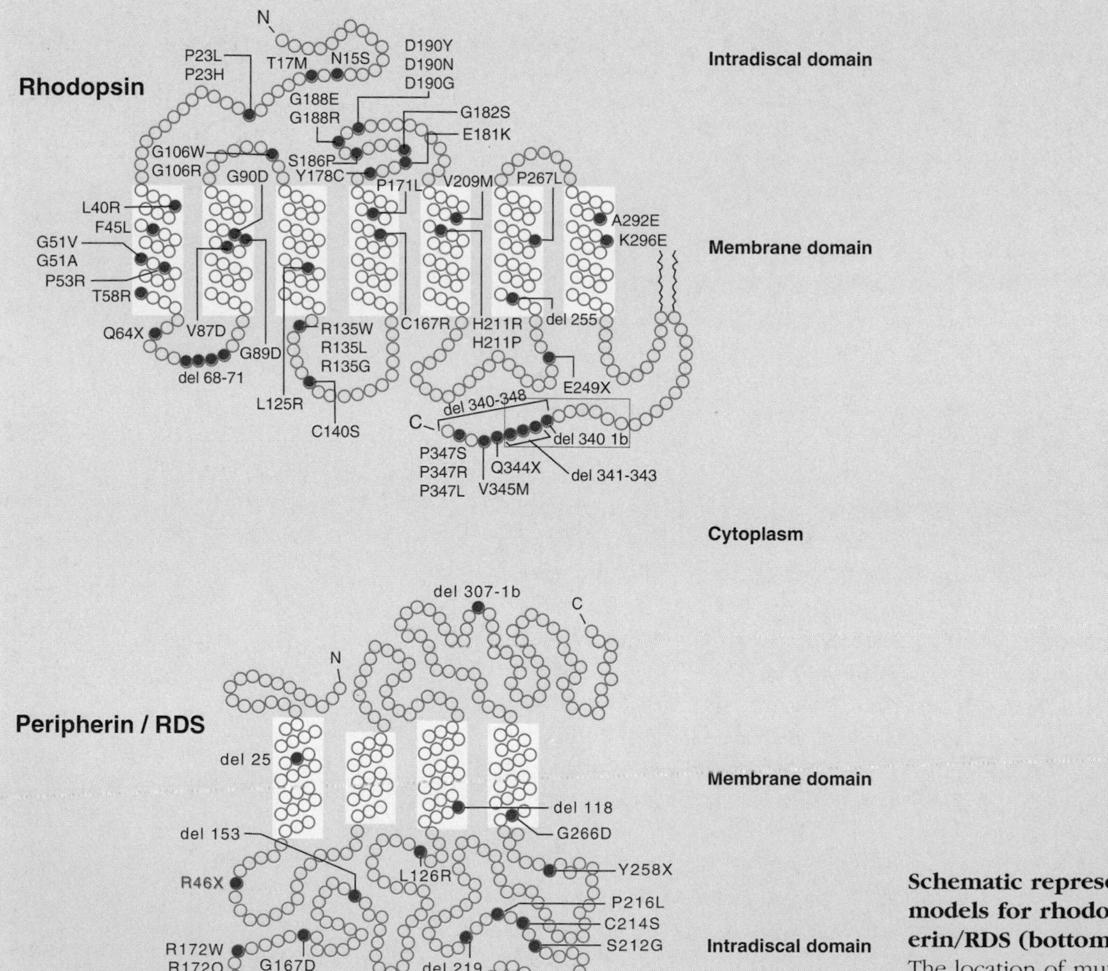

Schematic representation of structural models for rhodopsin (top) and peripherin/RDS (bottom).
The location of mutations in amino acid residues that segregate with RP or other retinal degenerations are shown as solid red circles.

Clin. Corr. 22.5 (continued)

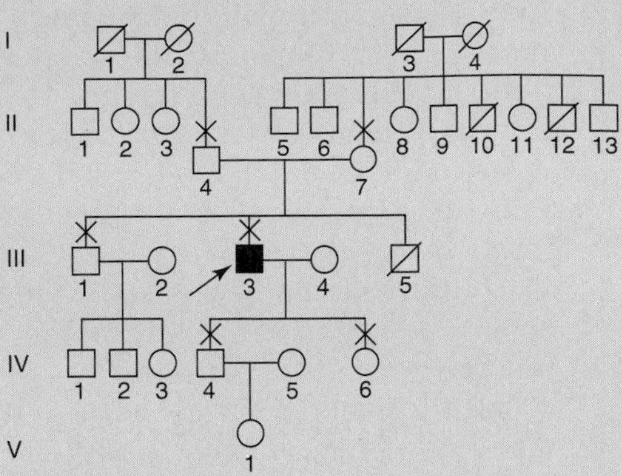

Pedigree of family.
Males are squares, females are circles. Solid square indicates the proband. A slash through a symbol indicates deceased. From Lam et al. (1995).

This R46X mutation has been observed in another unrelated patient. These observations demonstrate the importance of the use of DNA analysis to establish the genetic basis for RP, especially considering that RP symptoms have been associated with a variety of other diseases, such as those related to abnormal lipid metabolism.

Shastry, B. S. *Am. J. Med. Genet.* 52:467, 1994; and Lam, B. L., Vandenburgh, K., Sheffield, V. C., and Stone, E. M. *Am. J Ophthalmol.* 119:65, 1995.

transported to specific sites in the body while attached to specific carrier proteins. Cleavage of β-carotene yields two molecules of **all-*trans*-retinol.** There is an enzyme in the pigmented epithelial cell layer of the retina that catalyzes the isomerization of all-*trans*-retinol to **11-*cis*-retinol.** Oxidation of the 11-*cis*-retinol to 11-cis-retinal and its binding to opsin occur in the rod outer segment.

The absorption spectra of 11-*cis*-retinal and the four visual pigments are shown in Figure 22.21. There is a shift in the wavelength of maximum absorption of 11-*cis*-retinal upon binding to opsin and the protein components of the other visual pigments. Absorption bands for the pigments are coincident with their light sensitivity.

The magnitude of change in the electrical potential of photoreceptor cells following exposure to a light pulse is different in magnitude from that of neurons during depolarization. The **resting potential** of rod cell membrane is approximately **−30 mV** instead of the −70 mV observed with neurons. Excitation of rod cells causes **hyperpolarization** of the membrane, from about −30 mV to about −35 mV (Figure 22.22). It takes hundreds of milliseconds for the potential to reach its maximum state of hyperpolarization. A number of biochemical events take place during this time interval and before the potential returns to its resting state.

The initial events, absorption of photons of light and the subsequent isomerization of 11-*cis*-retinal, are rapid, requiring only picoseconds. Following this, a series of changes take place in rhodopsin, leading to various short-lived conformational states (Figure 22.23), each of which has specific absorption characteristics. Finally, rhodopsin dissociates, giving opsin and all-*trans*-retinal.

At 37°C, activated rhodopsin has decayed in slightly more than 1 millisecond through several intermediates to **metarhodopsin II.** Metarhodopsin II has a half-life of approximately 1 minute. It is the **active rhodopsin** species, R*, that is involved in the biochemical reactions of interest. Metarhodopsin II will have begun to form within hundredths of microseconds of the initial event. All of the first series of reactions shown in Figure 22.23 take place in the disk of the

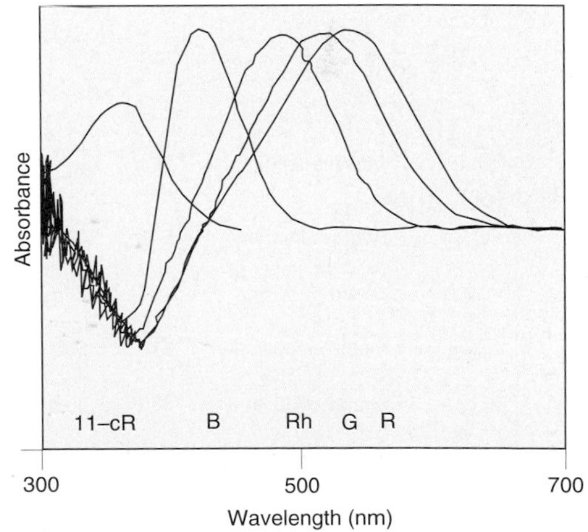

FIGURE 22.21
Absorption spectra of 11-*cis*-retinal and the four visual pigments.
Absorbance is relative and was obtained for pigments as difference spectra from reconstituted recombinant apoproteins. The spectrum for 11-*cis*-retinal (11-cR) is in the absence of protein. B, blue pigment; Rh, rhodopsin; G, green; R, red.
Adapted from Nathans, J. Cell, *78:357, 1994.*

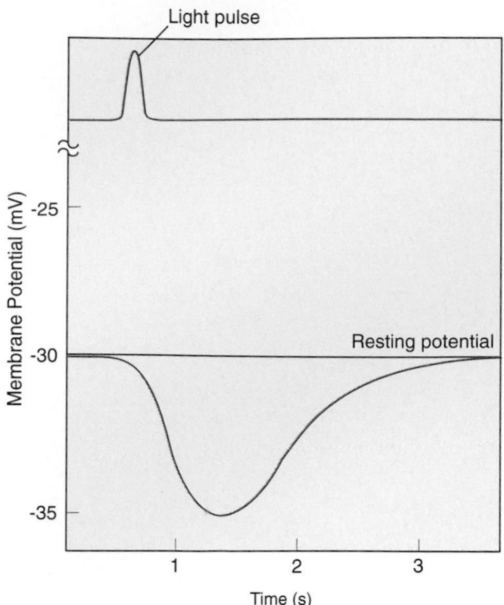

FIGURE 22.22
Changes in the potential of a rod cell membrane after a light pulse.
Redrawn from Darnell, J., Lodish, H., and Baltimore, D. Molecular Cell Biology. *New York: Scientific American Books, 1986, p. 763.*

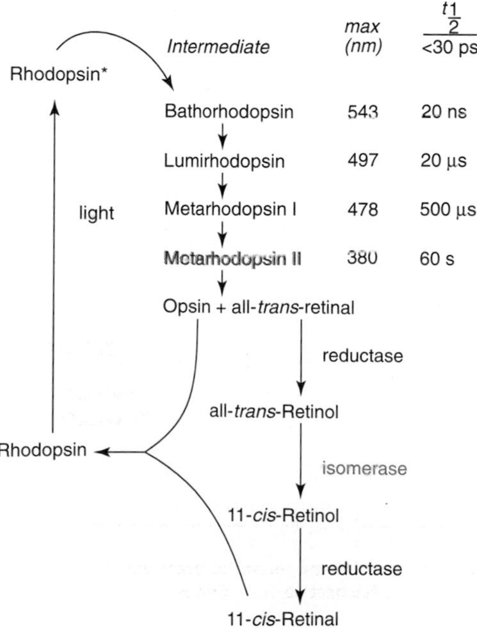

FIGURE 22.23
Light activation of rhodopsin.

rod outer segment. Upon dissociation of metarhodopsin into opsin and all-*trans*-retinal, the all-*trans*-retinal is enzymatically converted to all-*trans*-retinol by **all-*trans*-retinol dehydrogenase** that is located in the rod outer segment. All-*trans*-retinol is transported (or diffuses) into the pigmented epithelium where a specific isomerase converts it to 11-*cis*-retinol. The 11-*cis*-retinol is then transported (or diffuses) back into the rod outer segment and is reoxidized to 11-*cis*-retinal. Since the all-*trans*-retinol dehydrogenase appears to have only about 6% as much activity with 11-*cis*-retinal, it appears that another enzyme may be responsible for its oxidation. Once the aldehyde is formed, it can recombine with opsin to form rhodopsin. Rhodopsin is now in a state to begin the cycle again. The same events take place in the cones with the three proteins of the red, green, and blue pigments.

There are three interconnecting "mini" biochemical cycles involved in the conversion of light energy to nerve impulses (Figure 22.24). These cycles describe the reactions of rhodopsin, **transducin,** and **phosphodiesterase,** respectively. The net result of their operation is to cause a hyperpolarization of the plasma membrane of the rod (or cone) cells, that is, from -30 mV to approximately -35 mV. It is important to understand first what the biochemical mechanism is for maintaining the plasma membrane at -30 mV.

Rod cells of a fully dark-adapted human can detect a flash of light that emits as few as 50 photons. The rod is a specialized type of neuron in that the signal generated does not depend on an all-or-none event. The signal may be graded in intensity, reflected by the extent that the millivolt potential of the plasma membrane changes from its steady-state value of -30 mV. This **steady-state potential** is maintained at a more positive value because **Na^+ channels** of the photoreceptor cells are **ligand gated** and are maintained in a partially opened state. The ligand responsible for keeping some of the Na^+ channels open is **cyclic GMP (cGMP).** cGMP binds to them in a concentration-dependent, kinetically dynamic manner. Biochemical events that affect the concentration of cGMP within rod and cone cells also affect the number of Na^+ channels that are open and, hence, the membrane potential (Figure 22.24).

Active rhodopsin (R*, namely, metarhodopsin II) forms a complex with transducin. Transducin is a classical type of **G-protein** and functions in a manner very similar to that described on page 859 in relation to the action of some hormones. In the R*–transducin complex ($R^*–T_{\alpha,\beta,\gamma}$ complex), transducin undergoes a conformation change that facilitates an exchange of its bound **GDP** with **GTP.** When this occurs, the α subunit (T_α) of the trimeric molecule dissociates from its β, γ subunits. T_α interacts with and activates **phosphodiesterase (PDE),** which hydrolyzes cGMP to 5′-GMP, resulting in a decreased concentration of cGMP and a decrease in the number of channels held open. The membrane potential becomes more negative, that is, hyperpolarized.

The diagram of Figure 22.24 shows in cartoon form two such channels embedded in the plasma membrane, one of which has cGMP bound to it and is open. The other does not have cGMP bound to it and it is closed. By this mechanism, the concentration of Na^+ in the cell is directly linked to the concentration of cGMP and, thus, also to the membrane potential.

PDE in rod cells is a **heterotetrameric protein** consisting of one each α and β catalytic subunits and two γ regulatory subunits. T_α–GTP forms a complex with the γ subunits of PDE, resulting in their dissociation from the catalytic subunits, freeing the catalytically active α,β-dimeric PDE subunit complex. T_α has GTPase activity. Hydrolysis of bound GTP to GDP and inorganic phosphate (P_i) results in dissociation of T_α from the regulatory γ subunits of PDE, permitting them to reassociate with the catalytic subunits and to inhibit the PDE activity. The same reactions occur in cone cells, but the catalytic subunit of cone cell PDE is composed of two α catalytic subunits instead of α,β subunits as are present in rod cells.

cGMP concentration is regulated by intracellular Ca^{2+} concentration. Calcium enters rod cells in the dark through sodium channels, increasing its concentration to the 500-nM range. At these concentrations, activity of **guanylate cyclase** is low. When sodium channels are closed, Ca^{2+} entry is inhibited, but efflux mediated by the sodium/calcium–potassium exchanger is unchanged (top complex of the plasma membrane in Figure 22.24). This results in a decrease in the intracellular Ca^{2+} concentration, which in turn leads to activation of guanylate cyclase and increased production of cGMP from GTP.

Both the resynthesis of cGMP and the hydrolysis of T_α–GTP play important roles in stopping the reactions of the visual cycle. The inactivation of activated rhodopsin, R*, is also very important.

Activated rhodopsin, R*, is phosphorylated by **rhodopsin kinase** in the presence of ATP (Figure 22.24). The R*–P_i has high binding affinity for the cytosolic protein, **arrestin.** The arrestin–R*–P_i complex is no longer capable of interacting with transducin. The kinetics of arrestin binding to the activated-phosphorylated rhodopsin is sufficiently rapid *in vivo* to stop the cascade of reactions.

Rhodopsin is regenerated through another series of reactions and the cycle can be initiated again by photons of light. Figure 22.23 shows that the series of reactions leading to the regeneration of rhodopsin includes the dissociation of all-*trans*-retinal from metarhodopsin. The regeneration of 11-*cis*-retinal from all-*trans*-retinal occurs by reactions previously described and occurs before it is used again to form rhodopsin.

Major proteins involved in the visual cycle are listed in Table 22.6.

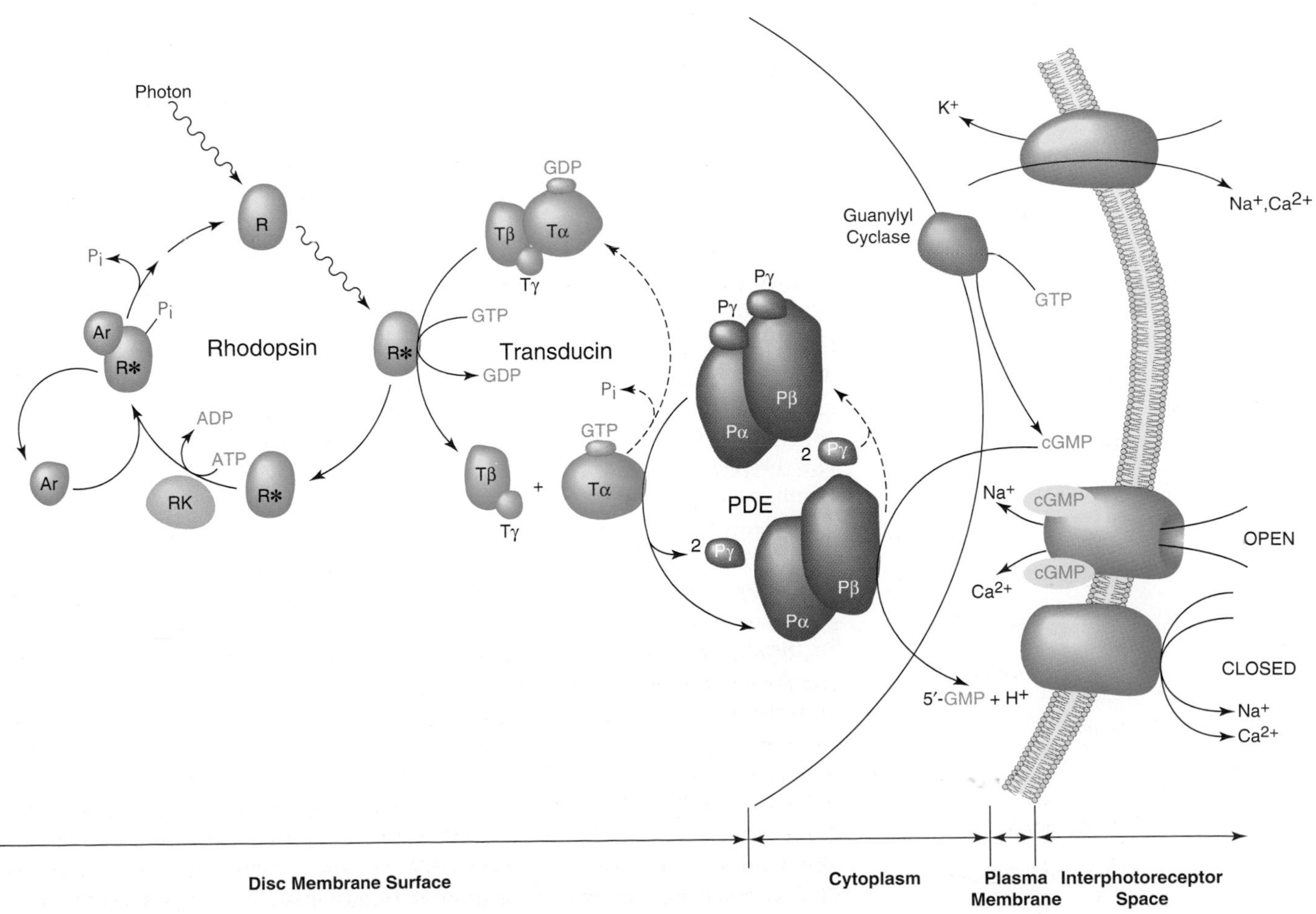

FIGURE 22.24
Cascade of biochemical reactions involved in the visual cycle.
Redrawn from Farber, D. B. Invest. Ophthalmol. Vis. Sci. *36:263, 1995.*

TABLE 22.6 Major Proteins Involved in the Phototransduction Cascade

Protein	*Relation to Membrane*	*Molecular Mass (kDa)*	*Concentration in Cytoplasm (μM)*
Rhodopsin	Intrinsic	39	—
Transducin ($\alpha + \beta + \gamma$)	Peripheral or soluble	80	500
Phosphodiesterase	Peripheral	200	150
Rhodopsin kinase	Soluble	65	5
Arrestin	Soluble	48	500
Guanylate cyclase	Attached to cytoskeleton	?	?
cGMP-activated channel	Intrinsic	66	?

Color Vision Originates in the Cones

Even though there are photographic artists, such as the late Ansel Adams, who make the world look beautiful in black and white, the intervention of colors in the spectrum of life's pictures brings another degree of beauty to the wonders of nature and the beauty of life . . . even the ability to make a distinction between tissues from histological staining. The ability of humans to distinguish colors resides within a relatively small portion of the visual system, the cones. The number of cones within the human eye are few compared with the number of rods. Some animals like dogs have even fewer cones, and other animals, like birds, have many more.

The general mechanism by which light stimulates cone cells is exactly the same as it is for rod cells. There are **three types of cone cells,** defined by the visual pigments they contain, which are either blue, green, or red. Normally, only one type of visual pigment occurs in a single cell. The blue pigment has optimum absorbance at 420 nm, the green pigment at 535 nm, and the red pigment at 565 nm (Figure 22.21). Each of these pigments has 11-*cis*-retinal as the prosthetic group, and, when activated by light, the 11-*cis*-retinal isomerizes to all-*trans*-retinal in exactly the same manner as it does in the rod cells. Colors other than those of the visual pigments are distinguished by graded stimulation of the different cones and comparative analysis by the brain. Color vision is **trichromatic.**

The characteristic of color discrimination by cone cells is an inherent property of the proteins of the visual pigments to which the 11-*cis*-retinal is attached. The 11-*cis*-retinal is attached to each of the proteins through a protonated Schiff base. The conjugated double-bond system of 11-*cis*-retinal influences the absorption spectrum of the pigment (Figure 22.21). When 11-*cis*-retinal is bound to different visual proteins, amino acid residues in the local areas around the protonated base and the conjugated π-bond system influence the energy level and give different absorption spectra with absorption maxima that are different for the different color pigments.

Genes for the color pigments have been cloned and their amino acid sequences inferred from the gene sequences. A structural comparison of the sequences of the visual pigments is shown in Figure 22.25. Open circles represent amino acids that are the same, and closed circles represent amino acids that are different. A string of closed circles at either end may represent an extension of the chain of one protein relative to the other. The red and green pigments show the greatest degree of homology, about 96% identity, whereas the degree of homology between different pairs of the others is between 40% and 45%.

Genes encoding the **visual pigments** have been mapped to specific chromosomes (see Clin. Corr. 22.6). The rhodopsin gene resides on the third chromo-

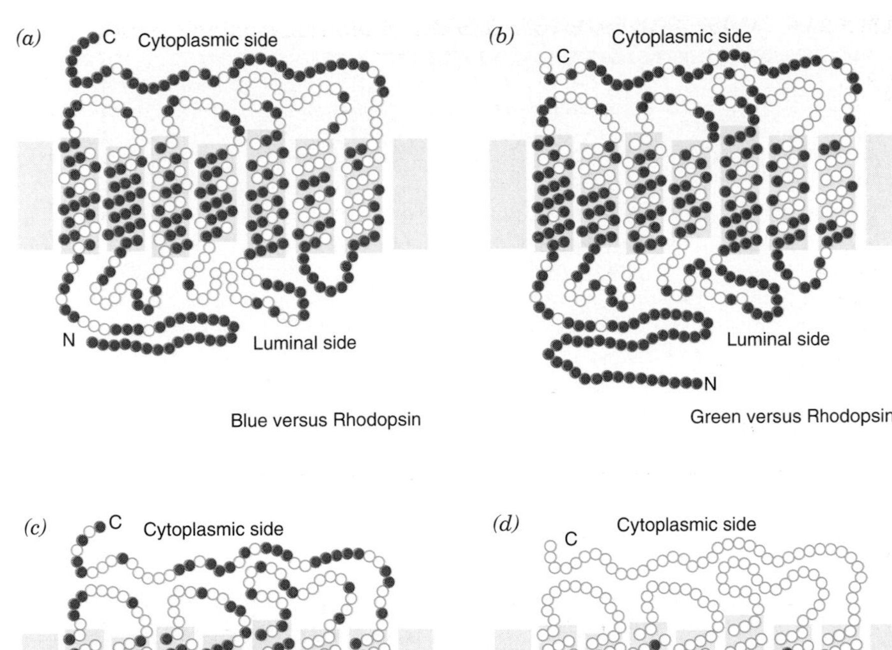

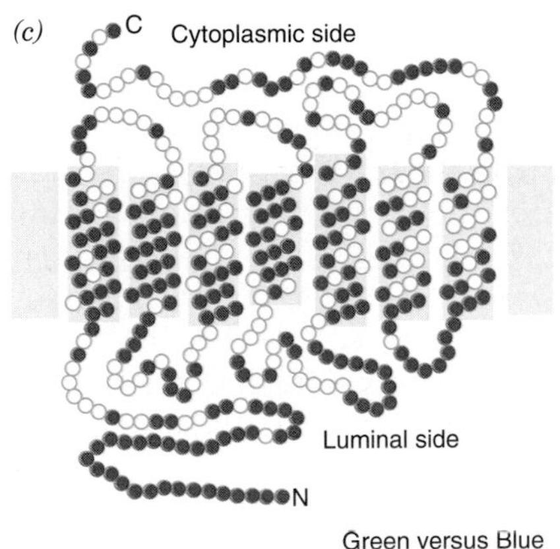

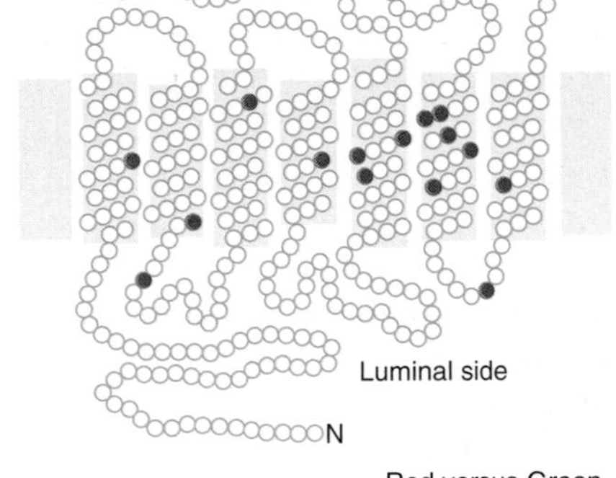

FIGURE 22.25
Comparisons of the amino acid sequences of the human visual pigments. Each red dot indicates an amino acid difference.
Adapted from Nathans, J. Annu. Rev. Neurosci. *10:163, 1987.*

some, the gene encoding the blue pigment resides on the seventh chromosome, and the two genes for the red and green pigments reside on the X chromosome. Abnormal color vision results from mutations in one or more of these genes (see Clin. Corr. 22.6). In spite of their great similarity, the red and green pigments are distinctly different proteins. Individuals have been identified with inherited variations that affect one but not both pigments simultaneously. In addition, there may be more than one gene for the green pigment, but it appears that only one is expressed.

The person who developed the atomic theory of chemistry, John Dalton (1766–1844), was color blind. He thought his color blindness was due to the vitreous humor being tinted blue, selectively absorbing longer wavelengths of light. He instructed that after his death his eyes be examined to determine whether his theory was correct. An autopsy revealed that the vitreous humor was "perfectly pellucid," normal. Using DNA analysis on his preserved eyes obtained from the British Museum, it has now been demonstrated that Dalton was missing the blue pigment. Thus, instead of having trichromatic vision, he was dichromatic with a vision type referred to as **deuteranopia.** The type of color blindness of one who is missing the green pigment is **protanopia.**

Other Physical and Chemical Differences Between Rods and Cones

The sensitivity and the response time of the rods are different from that of the cones. Absorption of a single photon by photoreceptors in rod cells generates a current of approximately 1–3 picoamperes ($1–3 \times 10^{-12}$ pA), whereas the same event in the cones generates a current of approximately 10 femtoamperes (10×10^{-15} fA), about 1/100th of the rod response. The response time of cone cells, however, is about four times faster than that of rod cells. Thus the cones

CLINICAL CORRELATION 22.6

Abnormalities in Color Perception

The chromosomal arrangement of genes for vision precludes inheritance of a single defective gene from one parent that would render recipients sightless. Genes that code for visual pigments occur on chromosomes that exist in pairs except in males where there is a single X chromosome containing the genes for red and green pigments. In females, there is a pair of X chromosomes and, therefore, color vision abnormalities in females are rare, affecting only about 0.5% of the population. By contrast, about 8% of males have abnormal color vision that affects red or green perception and, on rare occasions, both. For the sake of simplicity, the proteins coded for by the different genes will be referred to as pigments in spite of the fact that they become visual pigments only when they form complexes with 11-*cis*-retinal.

The gene that codes for the protein moiety of rhodopsin, the rod pigment, is located on the third chromosome. Genes that code for the three pigment proteins of cone cells are located on two different chromosomes. The gene for the blue pigment is on the seventh chromosome. The genes for the red and green pigments are tightly linked and are on the X chromosome, which normally contains one gene for the red pigment and from one to three genes for the green pigment. In a given set of cones, only one of these gene types is expressed, either the gene for the red pigment or one of the genes for the green pigment.

Genetic mutations may cause structural abnormalities in the proteins that influence the binding of retinal or the environment in which retinal resides. In addition, the gene for the protein of a specific pigment may not be expressed. If 11-cis-retinal does not bind or one of the proteins is not expressed, the individual will have dichromatic color vision and be color blind for the color of the missing pigment. If the mutation changes the environment around the 11-*cis*-retinal, shifting the absorption spectrum of the pigment, the individual will have abnormal trichromatic color vision; that is, the degree of stimulation of one or more of the three cone pigments will be abnormal. This will result in a different integration of the signal and hence a different interpretation of color.

Vollrath, D., Nathans, J., and Davis, R. W. *Science* 240:1669, 1988; and Nathans, J. *Cell* 78:357, 1994.

are better suited for discerning rapidly changing events and the rods are better suited for low-light visual sensitivity.

22.4 ■ MUSCLE CONTRACTION

On the basis of an extensive evaluation of electron micrographs of skeletal muscle tissue, the **sliding filament model** for muscle contraction was proposed. This simple but eloquent model has weathered the test of time. Genes for many of the proteins found in muscle tissue have been cloned, and the amino acid sequences of the proteins they encode inferred from their cDNA sequences. Three-dimensional structures of some of these proteins have also been published. Although the detailed picture of muscle contraction has not been completed, a clearer understanding of the process is emerging. In this section, some biochemical aspects of the mechanism of muscle contraction will be discussed. Primary emphasis will be on skeletal muscle rather than cardiac and smooth muscles.

Skeletal Muscle Contraction Follows an Electrical to Chemical to Mechanical Path

The signal for skeletal muscle contraction begins with an electrical impulse from a nerve. This is followed by a chemical change occurring within the unit cell of the muscle, and is followed by contraction, a mechanical process. Thus the **signal transduction** process goes from **electrical** to **chemical** to **mechanical.**

Figure 22.26 is a schematic diagram showing the structural organization of skeletal muscle. Muscle consists of bundles of fibers (diagram *c*). Each bundle is called a **fasciculus** (diagram *b*). The fibers are made up of **myofibrils** (diagram *d*), and each myofibril is a continuous series of muscle cells or units called **sarcomeres.** The muscle cell is multinucleated and is no longer capable of division. Most muscle cells survive for the life of the animal, but they can be replaced when lost or lengthened by fusion of **myoblast cells.**

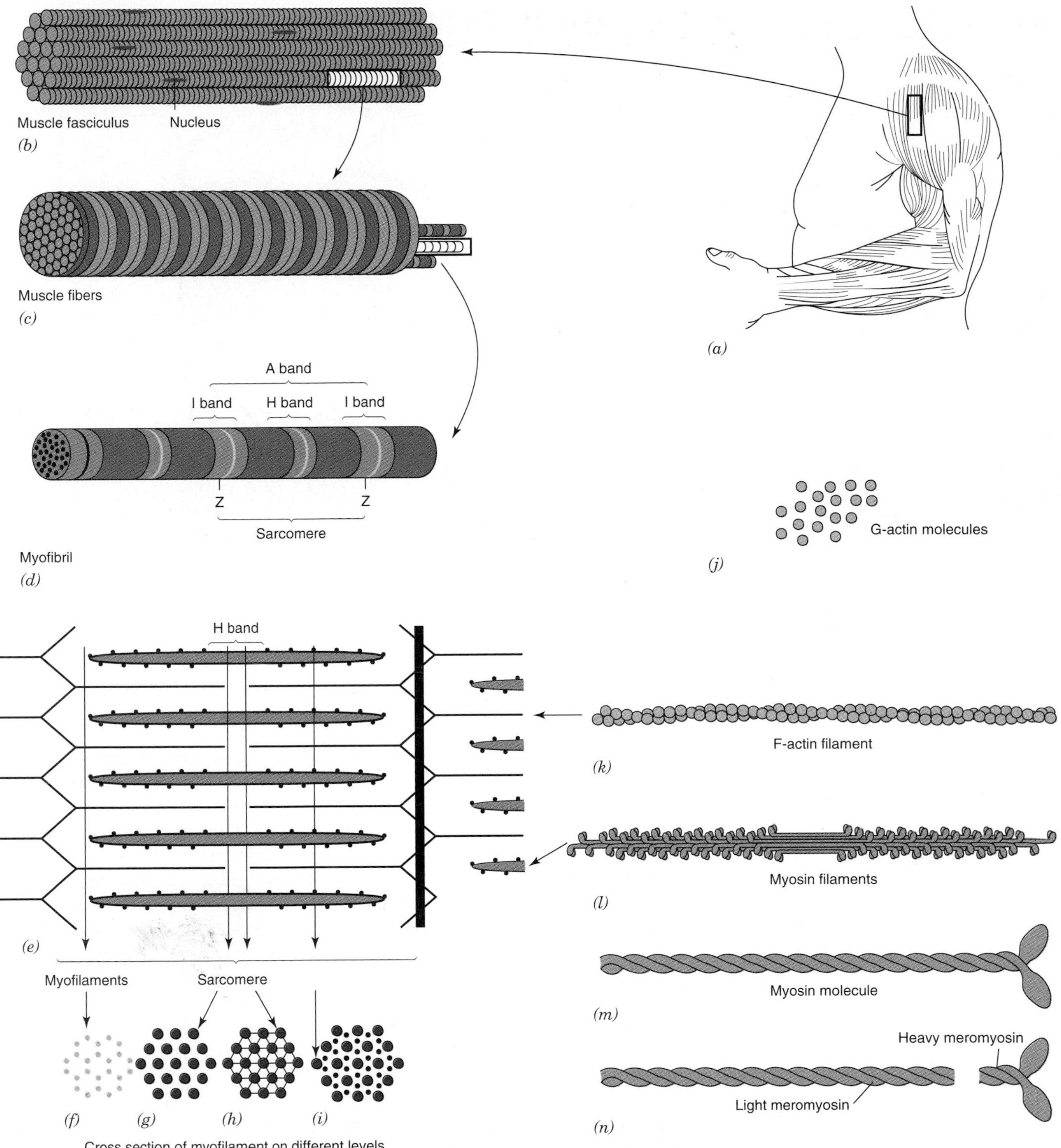

FIGURE 22.26
Structural organization of skeletal muscle.
Redrawn from Bloom, W. D., and Fawcett, D. W. Textbook of Histology, *10th ed. Philadelphia: Saunders, 1975.*

A muscle cell is shown diagrammatically in Figure 22.27. Note that the myofibrils are surrounded by a membranous structure called the **sarcoplasmic reticulum.** At discrete intervals along the fasciculi and connected to the terminal cisterna of the sarcoplasmic reticulum are **transverse tubules.** The transverse tubules are connected to the external plasma membrane that surrounds the

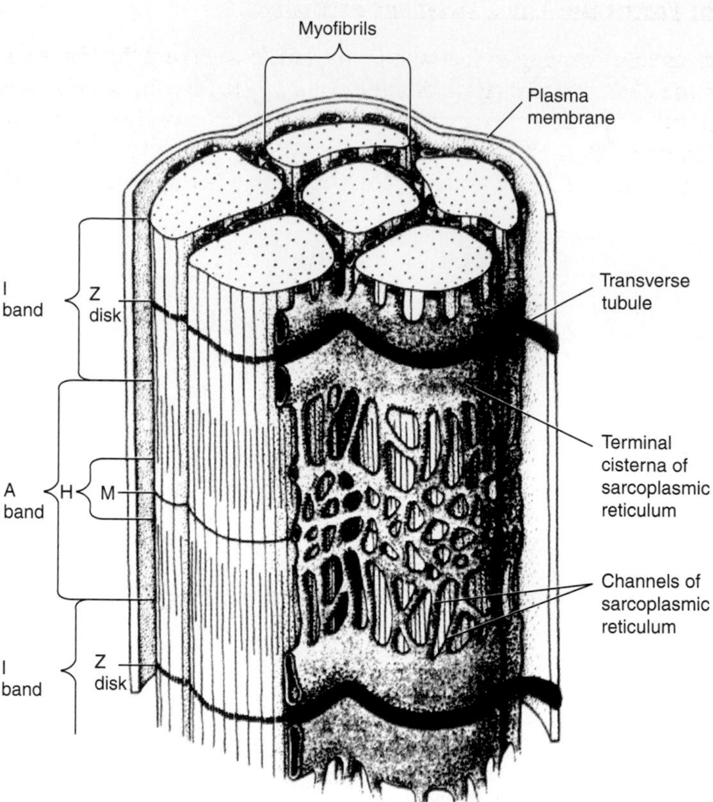

FIGURE 22.27
Schematic representation of a bundle of six myofibrils.
The lumen of the transverse tubules connects with the extracellular medium and enters the fibers at the Z disk.
Reprinted with permission from Darnell, J., Lodish, H., and Baltimore, D. Molecular Cell Biology. *New York: Scientific American Books, 1986, p. 827.*

entire structure. The nuclei and the mitochondria lie just inside the plasma membrane.

The single contractile unit, the sarcomere, extends from Z line to Z line (Figures 22.26*d* and 22.27). Bands seen in the sarcomere are due to the arrangement of specific proteins (Figure 22.26*e*). Two types of fibers are apparent: long thick ones with protrusions on both ends lie near the center of the sarcomere, and long thin ones are attached to the **Z line.** The **I band (isotropic)** extends for a short distance on both sides of the Z line. This region contains only **thin filaments** that are attached to a protein band within the Z line. The **H band** is in the center of the sarcomere. There are no thin filaments within this region. In the middle of the H band, there is a somewhat diffuse band due to the presence of other proteins that assist in cross-linking the fibers of the **heavy filaments** (Figure 22.26, pattern h). The **A band (anisotropic)** is located between the inner edges of the I bands. When the muscle contracts, the H and I bands shorten, but the distance between the Z line and the near edge of the H band remains constant. The distance between the innermost edges of the I bands on both ends of the sarcomere also remains constant. This occurs because the length of the thin filaments and the thick filaments does not change during contraction. Contraction therefore results when these filaments "slide" past each other.

The contractile elements, sarcomeres, consist of many different proteins, eight of which are listed in Table 22.7. The two most abundant proteins in the sarcomere are **myosin** and **actin.** About 60–70% of the muscle protein is myosin and about 20–25% is actin. The thick filament is mostly myosin and the thin filament is mostly actin. Three other proteins listed in Table 22.7 are associated with thin filaments, and two are associated with thick filaments.

TABLE 22.7 Molecular Weights of Skeletal Muscle Contractile Proteins

Protein	Molecular Weight
Myosin	500,000
Heavy chain	200,000
Light chain	20,000
Actin monomer (G-actin)	42,000
Tropomyosin	70,000
Troponin	76,000
Tn-C subunit	18,000
Tn-I subunit	23,000
Tn-T subunit	37,000
α-Actinin	200,000
C-protein	150,000
β-Actinin	60,000
M-protein	100,000

Myosin Forms the Thick Filament of Muscle

The schematic drawing of the myosin molecule in Figure 22.28*a* is a representation of the electron micrographs in Figure 22.28*b*. Myosin, a long molecule with two globular heads on one end, is composed of two heavy chains of about 230 kDa each. Bound to each heavy chain in the vicinity of the head group is a dissimilar pair of **light chains,** each of which is approximately 20 kDa. The

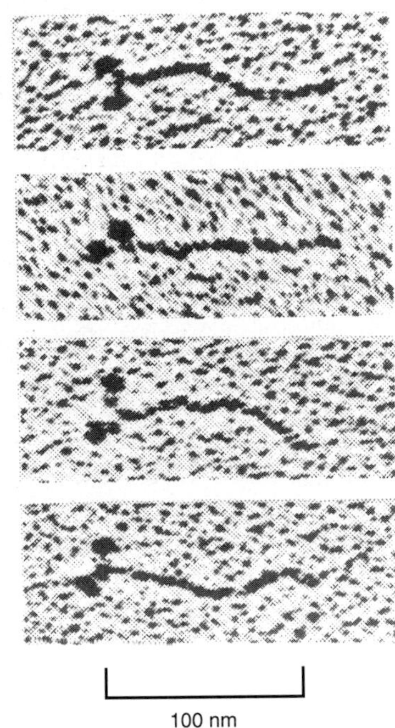

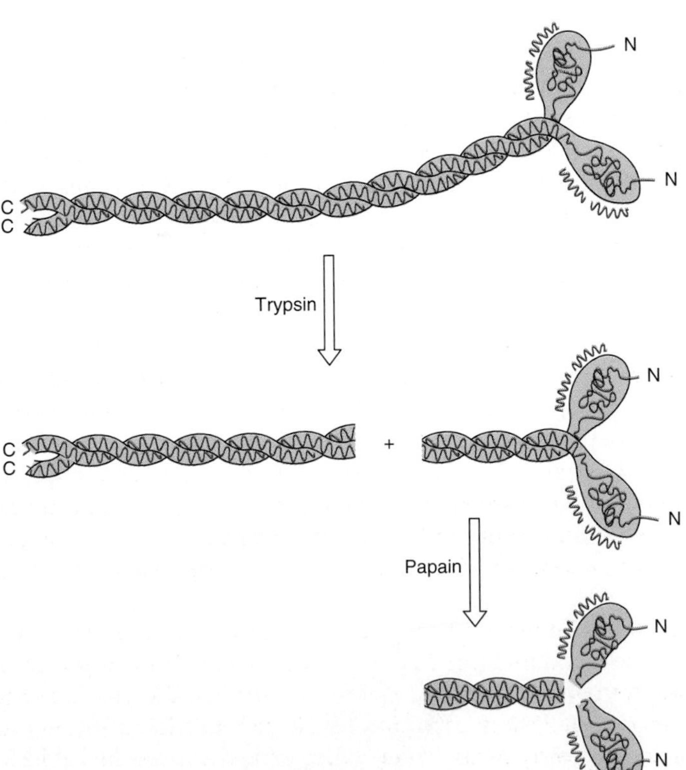

FIGURE 22.28
Myosin.
(*a*) Electron micrographs of the myosin molecule. (*b*) Schematic drawing of a myosin molecule. Diagram shows the two heavy chains and the two light chains of myosin. Also shown are the approximate positions of cleavage by trypsin and papain.
Reprinted with permission from Alberts, B., Bray, D., Lewis, J., Raff, M., Roberts, K., and Watson, J. Molecular Biology of the Cell, *2nd ed. New York: Garland Publishing, 1983.*

light chains are **"calmodulin-like"** proteins that bind calcium. One from each myosin can be removed easily without affecting *in vitro* function.

The carboxyl end of myosin is located in the tail section. The tail section of the two heavy chains are coiled around each other in an α-helical arrangement (Figure 22.28*a*). Trypsin cleaves the tail section at about one-third of its length from the head to produce **heavy meromyosin** (the head group and a short tail) and **light meromyosin** (the remainder of the tail section). Only light meromyosin has the ability to aggregate under physiological conditions, suggesting that aggregation is one of its roles in heavy chain formation. The head section can be separated from the remainder of the tail section by treatment with **papain.** The myosin head group resulting from this cleavage is referred to as **subfragment 1** or **S-1.** Action of these proteases also demonstrates that the molecule has at least two hinge points in the vicinity of the head–tail junction (Figure 22.28*a*).

cDNAs for myosin from many different species and from different types of muscle have been cloned and amino acid sequences for these myosin molecules inferred. Myosin has evolved very slowly, and there is a very high degree of homology among them, particularly within the head, or globular, region. There is somewhat less sequence homology within the tail region, but functional homology exists to an extraordinarily high degree regardless of length, which ranges from about 86 to about 150 nm for different species. The myosin head group contains nearly one-half of the total number of amino acid residues of the entire molecule in mammals, and it varies in the number of residues from only about 839 to about 850.

Myosin forms a **symmetrical tail-to-tail aggregate** around the M line of the H zone in the sarcomere. Its tail sections are aligned in a parallel manner on both sides of the M line with the head groups pointing towards the Z line. Each thick filament contains about 400 molecules of myosin. The C-protein (Table 22.7) is involved in their assembly. The M-protein is also involved, presumably to hold the tail sections together as well as to anchor them to the M line of the H zone.

The globular head section of myosin contains the **ATPase** activity that provides energy for contraction and the **actin binding site.** The S-1 fragment also contains the binding sites for the **essential light chain** and the **regulatory light chain.** A space-filling model of the three-dimensional structure of the myosin S-1 fragment is shown in Figure 22.29. The actin binding region is located at the lower right-hand corner and the cleft, visible in that region of the molecule, points toward the active site region where ATP binds. The 25-, 50-, and 20-kDa domains of the heavy chain are colored green, red, and blue, respectively. The essential light chain (ELC) and the regulatory light chain (RLC) are shown in yellow and magenta, respectively.

The active (ATP binding) site is also an open cleft about 13 Å deep and 13 Å wide. It is separated from the actin binding site by approximately 35 Å.

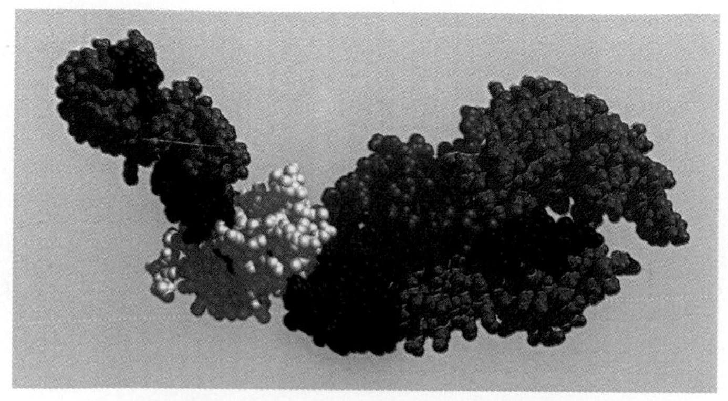

FIGURE 22.29
Space-filling model of the amino acid residues in myosin S-1 fragment.
The 25-, 50-, and 20-kDa domains of the heavy chain are green, red, and blue, respectively. The essential and regulatory light chains are yellow and magenta, respectively.
Reprinted with permission from Rayment, I., Rypniewski, W. R., Schmidt-Bäse, K., Smith, R., et al. Science *261:50, 1993. Copyright 1993 American Association for the Advancement of Science. Photograph generously supplied by Dr. I. Rayment.*

Myosin binding to actin shows stereo specificity. The ELC and RLC are associated with a single long helix that connects the head region with the tail section. There is room for flexibility, which requires only a low energy expenditure, between the ELC and the connecting single helix. The conformation of myosin that has ATP bound to it has an affinity for actin that is 1/10,000 that of the conformation of myosin that does not have ATP bound to it! Thus the process of chemical energy transduction to mechanical work depends on the primary event of protein conformation changes that occur upon binding of ATP, its hydrolysis, and product dissociation.

Actin, Tropomyosin, and Troponin Are Thin Filament Proteins

Actin is a major protein of the thin filament and makes up about 20–25% of muscle protein. It is synthesized as a 42-kDa globular protein. It has a better than 90% conserved amino acid sequence among a variety of species. This is shown in Table 22.8 for skeletal muscle, smooth muscle, and cardiac muscle actin in three different species of animals. Differences are observed at most in about seven different positions. In fact, the primary amino acid sequences of more than 30 different actin isotypes, with the longest containing 375 amino acid residues, reveal that a maximum of only 32 residues in any of them had been substituted. A significant number of them occurred at the N terminal, which may be predicted considering that all actin molecules are posttranscriptionally modified at the N terminal. The N-terminal methionine is acetylated and removed, and the next amino acid is acetylated. The process may end at this stage or it may be repeated one or two additional times. In all cases, the N-terminal amino acid will be acetylated.

As first synthesized, actin is called **G-actin** for globular actin. The structure in Figure 22.30 shows that it is not strictly globular. Actin has two distinct domains of approximately equal size that, historically, have been designated as large (left) and small (right) domains. Each of these domains consists of two subdomains. Both the N-terminal and C-terminal amino acid residues are located within subdomain 1 of the small domain. The molecule has polarity, and when it aggregates to form **F-actin,** or fibrous actin, it does so with a specific directionality. This is important for the "stick and pull" processes involved in sarcomere shortening during muscular contraction.

G-actin contains a specific binding site, located between the two major domains, for ATP and a divalent metal ion. Mg^{2+} ion is most likely the physiologically important cation, but Ca^{2+} also binds tightly and competes with Mg^{2+} for the same tight binding site. It is the **G-actin–ATP–Mg^{2+} complex** that aggregates to form the **F-actin polymer** (see Figure 22.34). Aggregation can occur from either direction, but kinetic data indicate that the preferred direction of aggregation is

TABLE 22.8 Summary of the Amino Acid Differences Between Chicken Gizzard Smooth Muscle Actin, Skeletal Muscle Actin, and Bovine Cardiac Actin

	Residue Number						
Actin Type	*1*	*2*	*3*	*17*	*89*	*298*	*357*
Skeletal muscle[a]	Asp	Glu	Asp	Val	Thr	Met	Thr
Cardiac muscle[b]		Asp	Glu			Leu	Ser
Smooth muscle[c]	Absent		Glu	Cys	Ser	Leu	Ser

Source: Adapted from Vandekerckhove, J., and Weber K. *FEBS Lett.* 102:219, 1979.

[a] From rabbit, bovine, and chicken skeletal muscle.

[b] From bovine heart.

[c] From chicken gizzard.

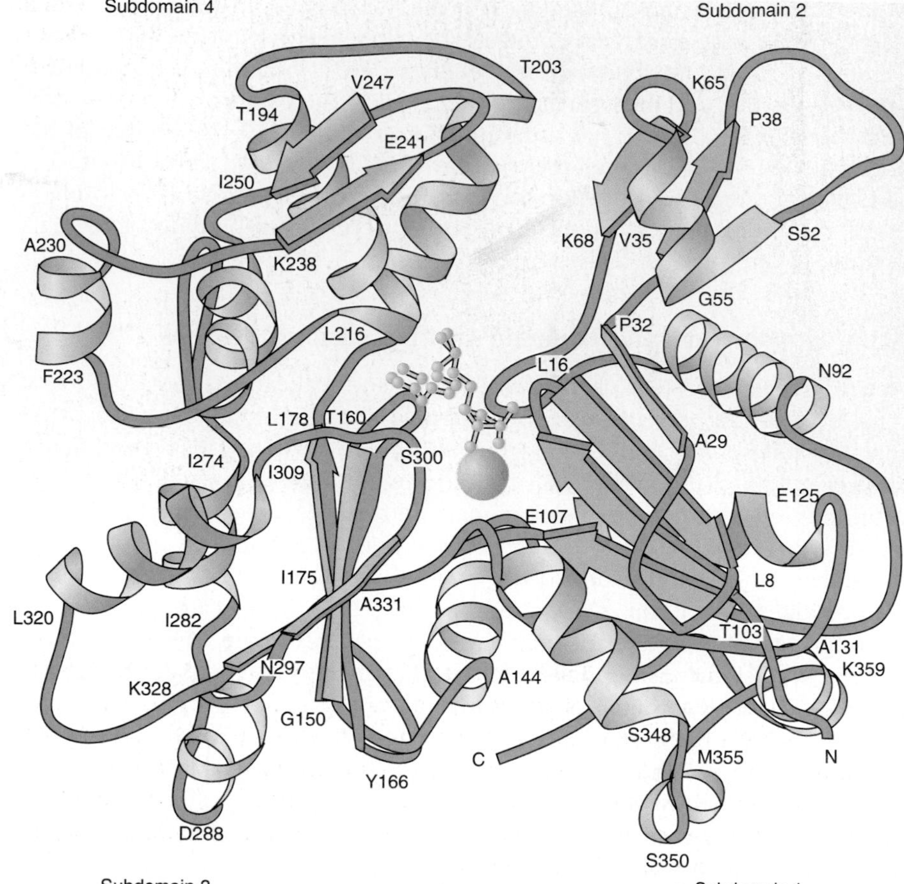

FIGURE 22.30
Secondary structural elements of G-actin crystal structure.
ADP and the metal ion are shown in the cleft between the two large domains.
Redrawn with permission from Lorenz, M., Popp, D., and Holmes, K. C. J. Mol. Biol. 234:826, 1993. By permission of the publisher, Academic Press Limited, London.

by extension from the large end of the molecule where the rate is diffusion controlled. ATP hydrolysis occurs by orders of magnitude faster in the aggregated actin than it does in the monomer. G-actin–ADP–Mg^{2+} also aggregates to form F-actin but at a slower rate. Orientation of G-actin molecules in F-actin is such that subdomains 1 and 2 are to the outside where myosin binding sites are located. F-actin may be viewed as either (1) a single-start, left-handed helix with rotation of the monomers through an approximate 166° with a rise of 27.5 Å or (2) a two-start, right-handed helix with a half pitch of 350–380 Å.

There are a number of proteins in the cytosol that bind actin. **β-Actinin** binds to F-actin and plays a major role in limiting the length of the thin filament. **α-Actinin,** a homodimeric protein with a subunit molecular weight of 90–110 kDa, binds adjacent actin monomers of F-actin at positions 86–117 and 350–375 and strengthens the fiber. It also helps to anchor the actin filament to the Z line of the sarcomere. There are two other major proteins associated with the thin filament, **tropomyosin** and **troponin.**

Tropomyosin is a rod-shaped protein consisting of two dissimilar subunits, each of about 35 kDa. It forms aggregates in a head-to-tail configuration. This polymerized protein interacts in a flexible manner with the thin filament throughout its entire length. It fits within the groove of the helical assembly of the actin monomers of F-actin. Each of the single tropomyosin molecules interacts with about seven monomers of actin. The site on actin with which tropomyosin interacts is between subdomains 1 and 3. Tropomyosin helps to stabilize the thin filament and to transmit signals for conformation change to other components of the thin filament upon Ca^{2+} binding. Bound to each individual tropomyosin molecule is one molecule of troponin.

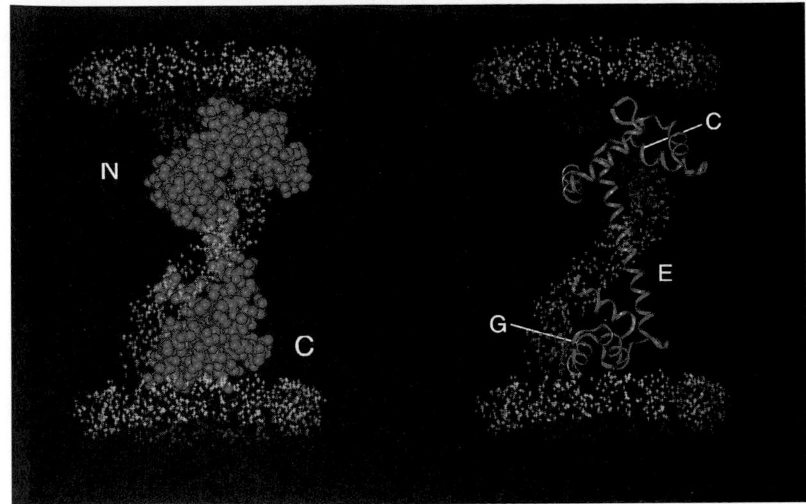

FIGURE 22.31
Best fit model for the 4 Ca^{2+} · Tn-C · Tn-I complex.
A model for the complex of 4 Ca^{2+} · troponin C · troponin I based on neutron scattering studies with deuterium labeling and contrast variation (Olah, C. A., and Trewhella, J., *Biochemistry* 33:12800, 1994). (Right) A view showing the spiral path of troponin I (green crosses) winding around the 4 Ca^{2+} · troponin C that is represented by an α-carbon backbone trace (red ribbon) with the C, E, and G helices labeled. (Left) The same view with 4 Ca^{2+} · troponin C represented as a CPK model.
Photograph generously supplied by Dr. J. Trewhella. The publisher recognizes that the U. S. Government retains a nonexclusive, royalty-free license to publish or reproduce the published form of this contribution or to allow others to do so, for U. S. Government purposes.

Troponin has three dissimilar subunits designated Tn-C, Tn-I, and Tn-T with molecular weights of about 18 kDa, 21 kDa, and 37 kDa, respectively. The Tn-T subunit binds to tropomyosin. The Tn-I subunit is involved in the inhibition of the binding of actin to myosin in the absence of Ca^{2+}. The Tn-C subunit, a calmodulin-like protein, binds Ca^{2+} and induces a conformation change that alters the conformation of Tn-I and tropomyosin, resulting in exposure of the actin–myosin binding sites.

A three-dimensional structure of Tn-C shows it to be a dumbbell-shaped molecule with much similarity to calmodulin. A structural model of the calcium saturated Tn-C–Tn-I complex is shown in Figure 22.31. The Tn-I subunit fits around the central region of Tn-C in a helical coil conformation and forms caps over it at each end. The cap regions of Tn-I are in close contact with Tn-C when Tn-C is fully saturated with calcium ions. Tn-C has four divalent metal ion binding sites. Two are in the N-terminal region, are high affinity (K_{dissoc} of about 10^{-7} M), and are presumed to be always occupied since this is about the concentration of calcium ions in resting cells. Under these conditions, Tn-I has a conformation that permits its interaction with binding sites on actin, inhibiting myosin binding and preventing contraction. Upon excitation, the calcium ion concentration increases to about 10^{-5} M, high enough to effect calcium binding to sites within the N-terminal region of Tn-C. Tn-I now binds preferentially to Tn-C in a capped structural conformation as shown in Figure 22.31. Myosin binding sites on actin are now exposed. The relatively loose interaction of tropomyosin with actin gives it the flexibility to alter its conformation as a function of calcium ion concentration and to assist in blockage of the myosin binding sites on actin. (See Clin. Corr. 22.7 for additional information about troponin.)

Figure 22.26*i* shows schematically a cross section of the sarcomere and the relative arrangement of the thin and thick filaments. There are six thin filaments surrounding each thick filament. The arrangement of myosin head groups around the thick filaments and the flexibility of those head groups make it possible for each thick filament to interact with multiple thin filaments. When **cross-bridges** are formed between the thick and thin filaments, they do so in patterns consistent with that shown in the electron micrograph of Figure 22.32. This figure shows a two-dimensional view of the myosin of the thick filament interacting with the actin of the thin filaments lying on either side of it. Similar interactions of myosin occur with the actin of the other four thin filaments that surround it.

CLINICAL CORRELATION 22.7

Troponin Subunits as Markers for Myocardial Infarction

Troponin has three subunits (Tn-T, Tn-I, and Tn-C) each of which is expressed by more than one gene. Two genes code for skeletal muscle Tn-I, one in fast- and one in slow-skeletal muscle; and one gene codes for cardiac muscle Tn-I. The genes that code for Tn-T have the same distribution pattern. They differ in that the slow-skeletal muscle gene for Tn-I is also expressed in fetal heart tissue. The gene for the cardiac form of Tn-I appears to be specific for heart tissue. Tn-C is encoded by two genes, but neither gene appears to be expressed only in cardiac tissue.

The cardiac form of Tn-I in humans is about 31 amino acids longer than the skeletal muscle form, which makes it easy to differentiate from others. Serum levels of Tn-I increase within four hours of an acute myocardial infarction and remain high for about seven days in about 68% of patients tested. Almost 25% of one group of patients tested also showed a slight increase in the cardiac-form of Tn-I after acute skeletal muscle injury. This would be a good but not a very sensitive test for myocardial infarction.

Two isoforms of cardiac Tn-T, Tn-T_1 and Tn-T_2, are present in adult human cardiac tissue. Two additional isoforms are also present in fetal heart tissue. Speculation is that the isoforms are the result of alternative splicing of mRNA. Serum levels of Tn-T_2 increase within four hours of acute myocardial infarction and remain high for up to 14 days. The appearance of Tn-T_2 in serum is 100% sensitive and 95% specific for detection of myocardial infarction. In the United States, the Food and Drug Administration has given approval for marketing of the first Tn-T assay for acute myocardial infarction. Myocardial infarcts are either undiagnosed or misdiagnosed in hospital patients admitted for other causes, or in 5 million or more people who go to doctors for episodes of chest pain. It is believed that this test will be sufficiently specific to diagnose myocardial incidents and to help direct doctors to proper treatment of these individuals.

Anderson, P. A. W., Malouf, N. N., Oakeley, A. E., Pagani, E. D., and Allen, P. D. *Circ. Res.* 69:1226, 1991; and Ottlinger, M. E., and Sacks, D. B. *Clin. Lab. News,* 33, 1994.

Muscle Contraction Requires Ca^{2+} Interaction

Contraction of skeletal muscle is initiated by transmission of **nerve impulses** across the **neuromuscular junction** mediated by release into the synaptic cleft of the neurotransmitter **acetylcholine.** The **acetylcholine receptors** are associated with the plasma membrane and are **ligand gated.** Binding of acetylcholine causes them to open and to permit Ca^{2+}/Na^{+} to enter the sarcomere. The electron micrograph and accompanying diagrams of Figure 22.33 provide a picture of the anatomical relationship between the presynaptic nerve and the sarcomere. There are transverse tubules along the membrane in the vicinity of the Z lines that are connected to the terminal cisternae of the sarcoplasmic reticulum. Nerve impulses result in a depolarization of the plasma membrane and the transverse tubules, and an influx of Ca^{2+} into the sarcomere. As indicated above, Ca^{2+} concentration increases about 100-fold, permitting it to bind to the low-affinity sites of Tn-C and to initiate the contraction process. (See Clin. Corr. 22.8.)

Energy for Muscle Contraction Is Supplied by ATP Hydrolysis

ATP is an absolute requirement for muscular contraction. ATP hydrolysis by the **myosin–ATPase** to give the myosin–ADP complex and inorganic phos-

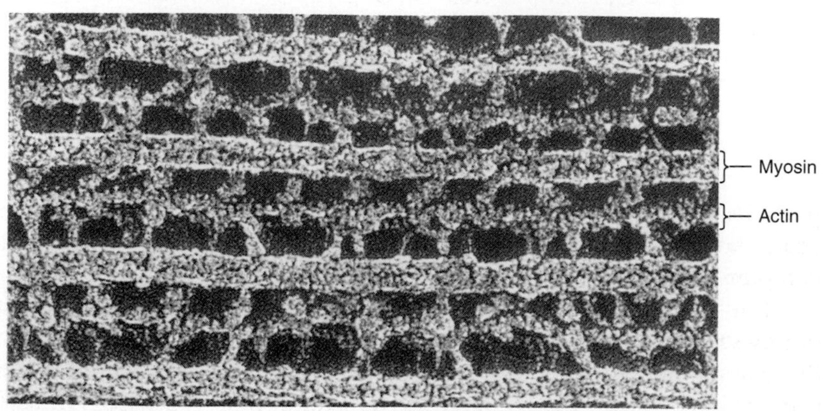

FIGURE 22.32
Electron micrograph of actin–myosin cross-bridges in a striated insect flight muscle.
Reproduced with permission from Darnell, J., Lodish, H., and Baltimore, D. Molecular Cell Biology. *New York: Scientific American Books, 1986.*

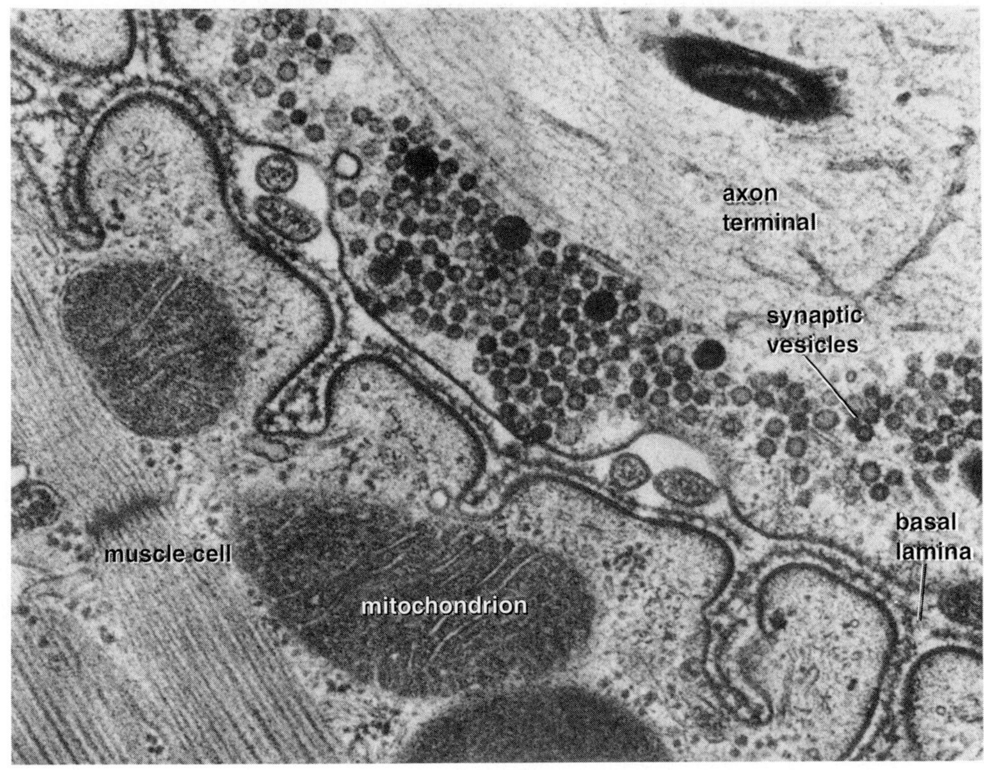

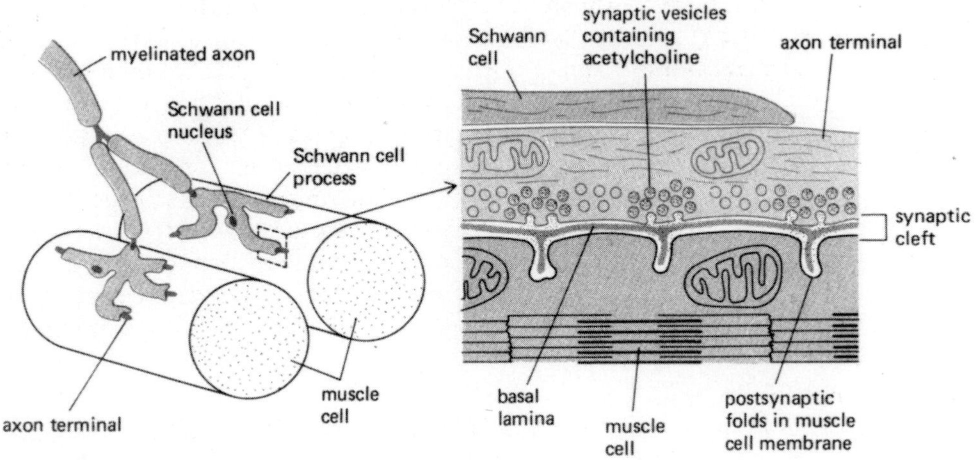

FIGURE 22.33
Neuromuscular junction.
(*a*) Electron micrograph of a neuromuscular junction. (*b*) Schematic diagram of the neuromuscular junction shown in (*a*).
Reproduced with permission from Alberts, B., Bray, D., Lewis, J., Raff, M., Roberts, K., and Watson, J. Molecular Biology of the Cell. *New York: Garland Publishing, 1983.*

phate leads to a myosin conformation that has an increased binding affinity for actin. Additional ATP is required for the dissociation of the myosin–actin complex.

The concentration of ATP in the sarcomere remains fairly constant even during strenuous muscle activity, because of increased metabolic activity and of the action of two enzymes: **creatine phosphokinase** and **adenylate kinase.** Creatine phosphokinase catalyzes the transfer of phosphate from phosphocre-

CLINICAL CORRELATION 22.8

Voltage-Gated Ion Channelopathies

Action potentials in nerve and muscle are propagated by the operation of voltage-gated ion channels. Generally, there are three recognized types of voltage-gated cation channels: Na^+, Ca^{2+}, and K^+. Each of these has been cloned, primary sequence inferred from the DNA sequence, and a model constructed of how each may be assembled in the membrane. Each is a heterogeneous protein

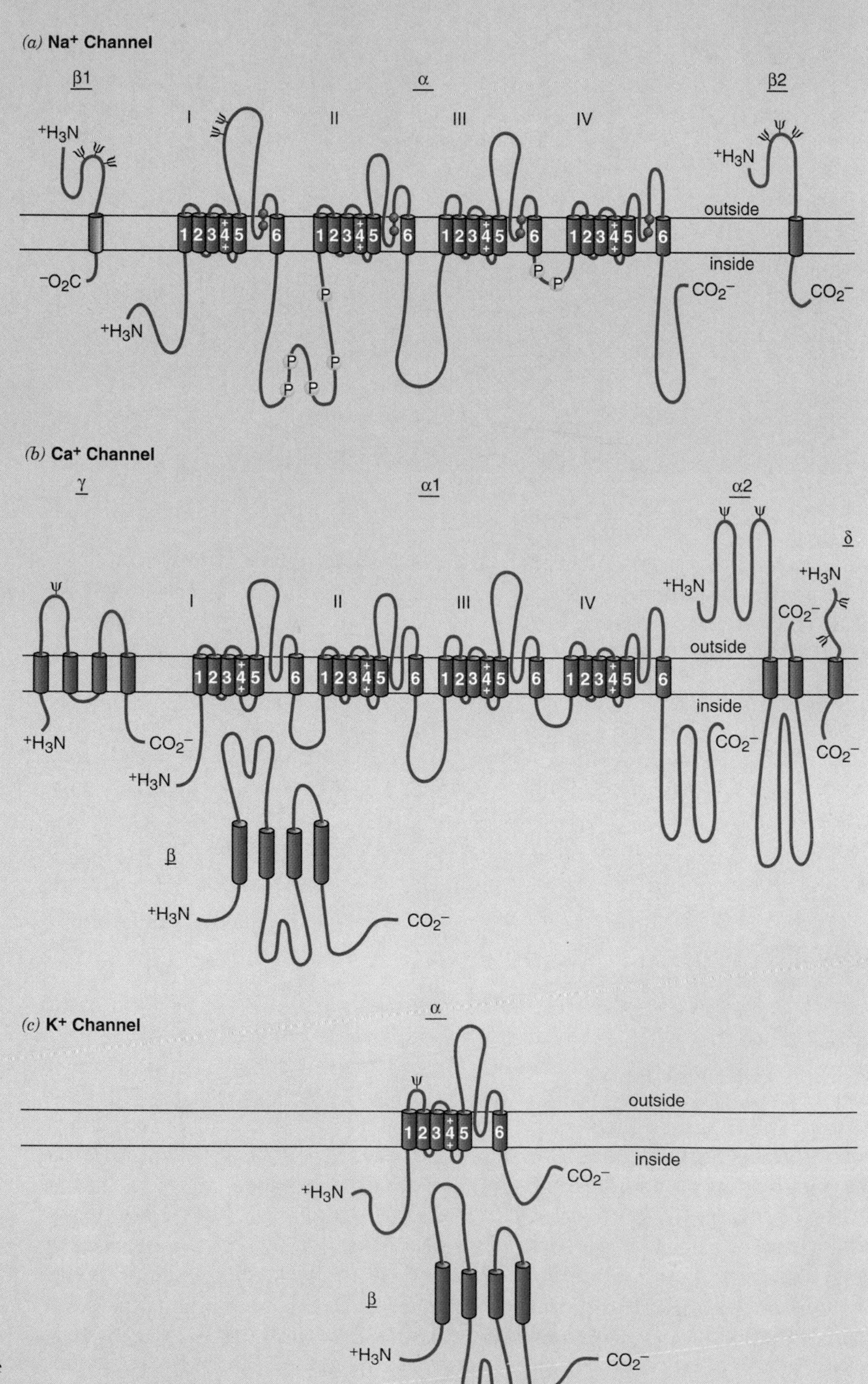

Transmembrane organization of ion channel subunits.
Glycosylation and phosphorylation sites are marked. From Catterall (1995).

consisting of various numbers of α and β subunits. A linear model of the arrangement of each of these is shown in the figure above. In actual fact, they are arranged in a more-or-less circular manner with a channel formed through the middle of the α subunits. Roles of the β subunits are still being elucidated, but they appear to help stabilize and/or regulate activity of α subunits.

Toxins are being used to study subunit function. Tetrodotoxin and saxitoxin block Na^+ channel pores of the α subunit. Scorpion toxins also bind to the α subunit and appear to affect activation and inactivation gating. Experiments of this type suggest that the α subunit is involved in both conductance and gating.

Even though the Na^+ channel was first cloned from nerve tissue, the electroplax of the eel, more is known about how mutations affect its function in muscle. Voltage-gated channels from nerve and muscle tissue show high homology in many of the transmembrane domains but are less conserved in the intracellular connecting loops. A common effect of mutations in Na^+ channels is muscle weakness or paralysis. Some inherited sodium voltage-gated ion channelopathies are listed below. Each of these is reported to result from a single amino acid change in the α subunit. The inheritance pattern generally is dominant.

Disorder	***Unique Clinical Feature***
Hyperkalemic periodic paralysis	Induced by rest after exercise, or the intake of K^+
Paramyotonia congenita	Cold-induced myotonia
Sodium channel myotonia	Constant myotonia

It has been surmised (by Hoffman, 1995; see Catterall, 1995) that if the membrane potential is slightly more positive (i.e., changes from −70 to −60 mV), the myofiber can reach the threshold more easily and the muscle becomes hyperexcitable. If the membrane potential becomes even more positive (i.e., up to −40 mV) the fiber cannot fire an action potential. This inability to generate an action potential is synonymous with paralysis. The fundamental biochemical defect in each case is a mutation in the channel protein.

Catterall, W. A. *Annu. Rev. Biochem.* 64:493, 1995; and Hoffmann, E. P. *Annu. Rev. Med.* 46:431, 1995.

atine to ADP in an energetically favored manner:

$$\text{Phosphocreatine} + \text{ADP} \rightleftharpoons \text{ATP} + \text{creatine}$$

If the metabolic process is insufficient to keep up with the energy demand, the creatine phosphokinase system serves as a "buffer" to maintain cellular levels of ATP. The second enzyme is adenylate kinase that catalyzes the reaction

$$2\ \text{ADP} \rightleftharpoons \text{ATP} + \text{AMP}$$

ATP depletion brings about rather rigid consequences to muscle cells. When the ATP supply of the muscle is exhausted and the intracellular Ca^{2+} concentration is no longer controlled, myosin will exist exclusively bound to actin, a condition called **rigor mortis.** The function of ATP binding in muscular contraction is to promote dissociation of the actin–myosin complex, not to promote its association.

Model for Skeletal Muscle Contraction

A model of the **actin–myosin complex** is shown in Figure 22.34. The myosin head undergoes conformation changes upon binding of ATP, hydrolysis of ATP, and release of products. ATP binding leads to closure of the active site cleft and opening of the cleft in the region of the actin binding site. Hydrolysis of ATP and release of inorganic phosphate result in closure of the cleft in the actin binding region. The conformation change that occurs is evident by the movement of two cysteine-containing helices. The distance between the two cysteine residues (697 and 707) changes from about 19 Å to about 2 Å. If further conformation change is prevented by cross-linking these two cysteines, ADP is trapped within its binding site. A stereo view of myosin showing the reactive cysteine pocket is shown in Figure 22.34*b*.

The sequence of events leading to muscle contraction from its resting state, following Ca^{2+} entry into the cell, probably begins with the hydrolysis of bound ATP. Myosin–ATP complex has a very low affinity for actin. Thus, even with exposed actin binding sites, any interaction between myosin and actin would be weak. The first significant interaction between myosin and actin probably

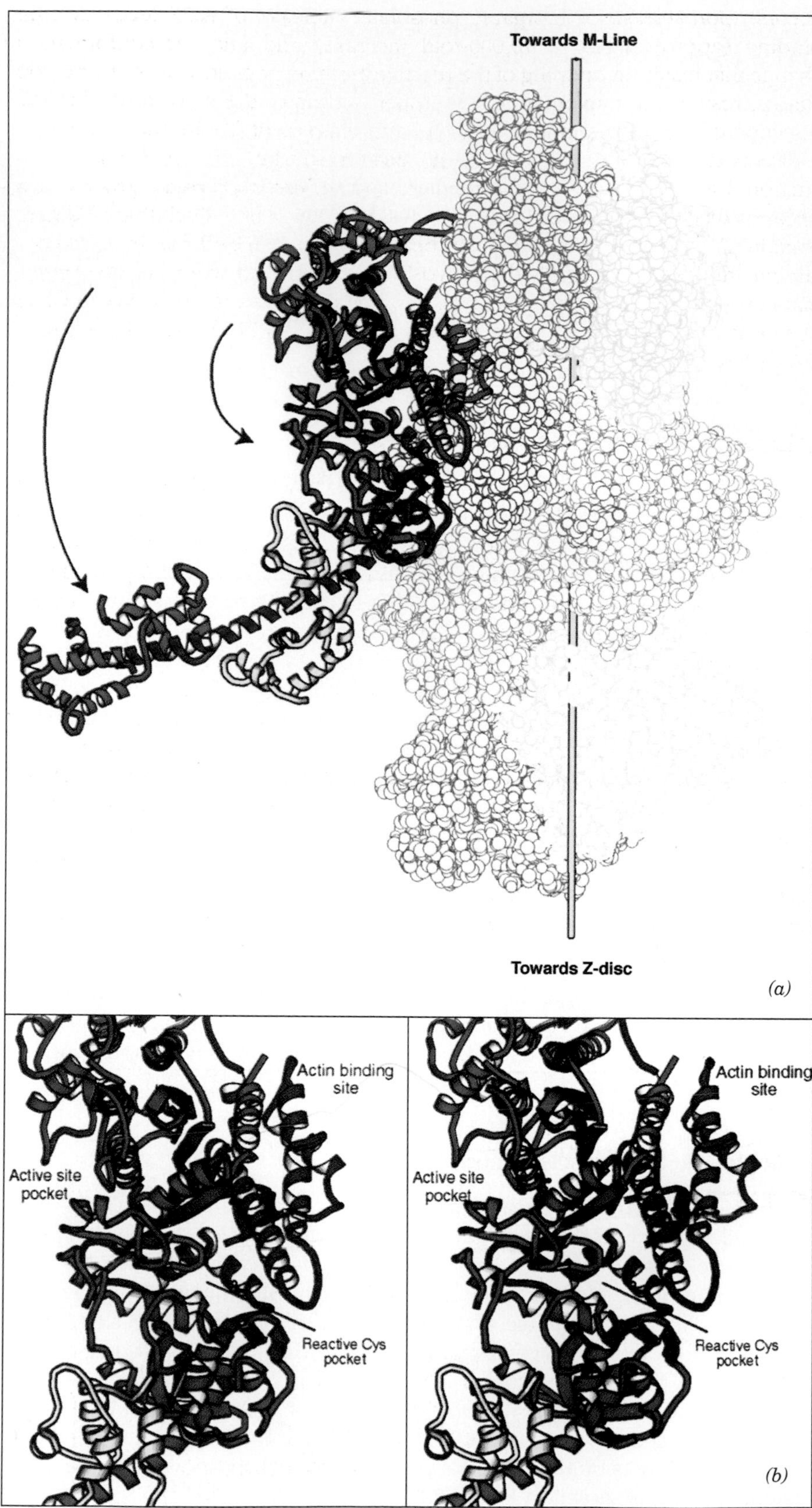

FIGURE 22.34
Model of actin–myosin interaction. (*a*) Myosin is shown as a ribbon structure and actin as space-filling. Each G-actin monomer is represented by different colors. (*b*) Stereo view of myosin showing the pocket that contains the mobile "reactive" cysteine residues.
Reproduced with permission from Rayment, I., and Holden, H. M. TIBS *19:129, 1994. Photograph generously supplied by Dr. I. Rayment.*

occurs upon release of inorganic phosphate. Release of ADP leads to tight binding (approximately a 10,000-fold increase) and another conformation change that results in opening of the reactive cysteine pocket. The conformation change results in a movement of the upper portion of the myosin head in the direction of the arrows in Figure 22.34*a* and movement of the thin filament in a direction away from the Z line, the **power stroke.** The thick filament is anchored in the center of the sarcomere and the **myosin head groups are polarized** in opposite directions on each side of the M line. Each thick filament contains hundreds of S-1 or myosin head units surrounded by six actin-containing thin filaments. Individual myosin units function in an asynchronous manner—possibly like changes in the position of hands on a rope in the game of tug-of-war. Thus when some myosin head groups bind with high affinity, others have low affinity.

Calcium Regulates Smooth Muscle Contraction

Calcium ions play an important role in **smooth muscle contraction** also, but there are some important differences in the mechanism by which it acts. A mechanism for calcium regulation of smooth muscle contraction is shown in Figure 22.35. Key elements of this mechanism are as follows. (1) A phosphorylated form of **myosin light chain** stimulates **Mg-ATPase,** which supplies energy for the contractile process. (2) Myosin light chain is phosphorylated by a **myosin light chain kinase (MLCK).** (3) MLCK is activated by a Ca^{2+}–calmodulin (CaM) complex. (4) Formation of the Ca^{2+}–CM complex is dependent on the concentration of intracellular Ca^{2+}. Release of Ca^{2+} from its intracellular stores or an increase in its flux across the plasma membrane is important for control. (5) Contraction is stopped by the action of a **myosin phosphatase** or the transport of Ca^{2+} out of the cell. It is apparent that, in smooth muscle, many more biochemical steps are involved in the regulation of contraction, steps that can be regulated in a progressive manner by hormones and other agents. These serve the function of smooth muscles well, namely, giving them the ability to develop various degrees of tension and to retain it for prolonged periods of time.

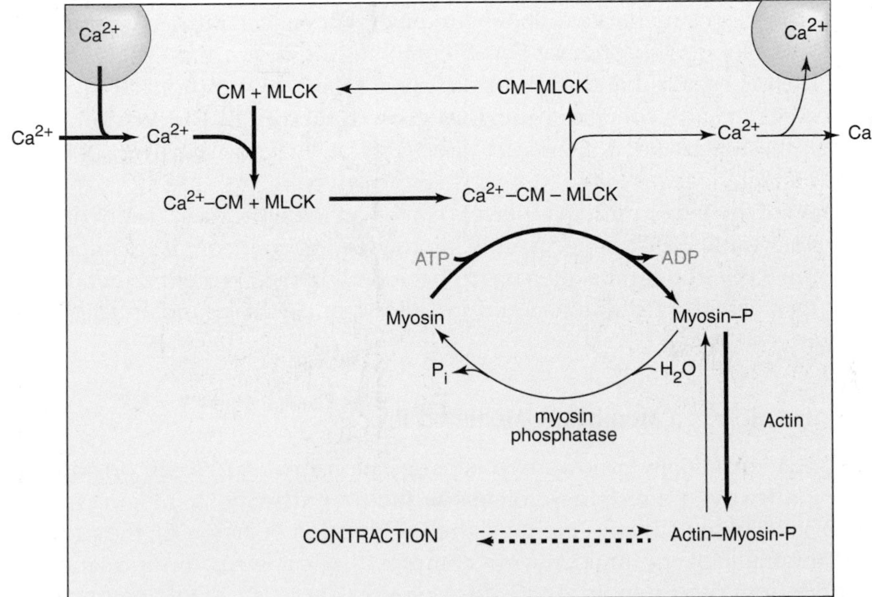

FIGURE 22.35
Schematic representation of the mechanism of regulation of smooth muscle contraction.
Heavy arrows show the pathway for tension development and light arrows show the pathway for release of tension. The Mg^{2+}-ATPase activity is highest in the actin–myosin-P complex. CaM, calmodulin; MLCK, myosin light chain kinase.
Adapted from Kramm, K. E., and Stull, J. T. Annu. Rev. Pharmacol. Toxicol. *25:593, 1985.*

22.5 ■ MECHANISM OF BLOOD COAGULATION

The circulation of blood is essential for life, and the integrity of the process must be maintained. Some aspects of the importance of blood circulation in the maintenance of pH, in the transport of oxygen and nutrients to cells, and in the transport of carbon dioxide and waste products from cells are well known. This section deals primarily with a description of the system responsible for clot formation and dissolution.

Blood circulation occurs in a very specialized type of closed system in which the volume of circulating fluid is maintained fairly constant. This system is also one in which the transfer of solutes across its boundaries is a necessary function. Like any system of pipes and tubes, leaks can occur and must be repaired. The process of **blood clotting** primarily addresses the question of stopping the leaks. Secondarily, small clots may form due to disease and other abnormalities that are independent of total rupture of vesicles. Discussion of the function of the process must therefore extend beyond the primary one of leak prevention to include **clot dissolution.**

The purpose of this section is to give a general picture of the mechanism of blood clotting from a biochemical viewpoint. To this end, this section will focus on the relationship between blood clot formation, blood clot dissolution, and the enzymes and other proteins involved—their activation, regulation, inhibition, and synthesis. Blood clotting is not a process of signal transduction in the same sense as are the other topics of this chapter. Instead, it is a dynamic process of signal amplification and modulation. Some of the primary questions to be addressed are: (1) What initiates the clotting process? (2) What substances, reactions, and mechanisms are responsible for forming the clot? (3) What factors and mechanisms are involved in inhibiting the clotting process once it is initiated? (4) How is the clot dissolved?

It is important for the body to maintain **hemostasis,** that is, no bleeding. Thus the process of blood clotting is designed to stop as rapidly as possible the loss of blood following vascular injury. When such an injury occurs, three major events take place: (1) **aggregation** of a protein, **fibrin,** into an insoluble network, or clot, to cover the ruptured area to prevent the loss of blood; (2) **clumping** of **blood platelets** at the site of injury in an effort to form a physical plug to stop the leak; and (3) **vasoconstriction** in an effort to reduce the blood flow through the area. Equally important is regulation of the process to prevent excessive clot formation.

The processes mentioned above are emergency mechanisms for stopping the loss of blood. The process is not complete, however, until the ruptured vessel itself is repaired and the clot dissolved. Many of the proteins involved in blood coagulation contain **epidermal growth factor (EGF)-like domains.** Whether these EGF-like domains act directly to facilitate the regrowth of blood vesicles is not clear.

Some of the major proteins (players) involved in this process (silent drama) are listed in Table 22.9, not necessarily in order of appearance. All are important and, as time goes on, others are sure to be added. In fact, protein Z that occurs to a larger extent in children could be added but its role and function are not clear.

Clot Formation Is a Membrane-Mediated Process

Clot formation initially follows two separate pathways: **intrinsic** or **contact factor pathway** and **extrinsic** or **tissue factor pathway** (see Figures 22.36 and 22.38). These pathways merge with the formation of factor Xa, the proteinase component of the multienzyme complex that catalyzes the formation of thrombin from prothrombin. From this point on, there is a single pathway for clot formation. Historically, the term intrinsic pathway came from the observa-

TABLE 22.9 Some of the Factors Involved in Blood Coagulation, Control, and Clot Dissolution

Factor	*Name*	*Pathway*	*Characteristic*	*Concentration*[a]
I	Fibrinogen	Both		9.1
II	Prothrombin	Both	Contains N-terminal Gla residues	1.4
III	Tissue factor	Extrinsic	Transmembrane protein	—
IV	Calcium	Both		
V	Proaccelerin	Both	Protein cofactor	0.03[b]
VII	Proconvertin	Extrinsic	Endopeptidase with Gla residues	0.010[c]
VIII	Antihemophilic	Intrinsic	Protein cofactor	0.0003[b]
IX	Christmas factor	Intrinsic	Endopeptidase with Gla residues	0.089
X	Stuart factor	Both	Endopeptidase with Gla residues	0.136
XI	Thromboplastin antecedent	Intrinsic	Endopeptidase	0.031
XII	Hageman factor	Intrinsic	Endopeptidase	0.375
XIII	Proglutamidase	Both	Transpeptidase	0.031[b]
	Protein C	(*Both*)	Endopeptidase with Gla residues	0.065
	Protein S	(*Both*)	Cofactor with Gla residues	0.30
	Prekallikrein	Intrinsic	Zymogen/activator factor-XII	0.581
	HMWK[d]	Intrinsic	Receptor protein	0.636
	Antithrombin III	Both	Thrombin inhibitor	3.0
	Plasminogen		Zymogen/clot dissolution	2.4
	Heparin Co-II	Both	Thrombin inhibitor	1.364
	α_2-Antiplasmin		Plasmin inhibitor	0.952
	Protein C inhibitor		Protein C inhibitor	0.070
	α_2-Macroglobulin		Proteinase inhibitor	2.9
	LACI[e]		Extrinsic pathway inhibitor	0.003

[a] Concentrations are approximate and shown in micromolar.
[b] These values approximate solution concentrations since some are complexed with other proteins in platelets.
[c] This factor probably circulates as both VII and VIIa.
[d] HMWK is high molecular weight kininogen.
[e] LACI is lipoprotein-associated coagulation factor.

tion that blood clotting would occur spontaneously when blood was placed in clean glass test tubes, leading to the idea that all components for the clotting process were intrinsic to the circulating blood. Glass contains **anionic surfaces** that formed the nucleation points that initiate the process. In mammals, anionic surfaces are exposed upon rupture of the **endothelial lining** of the blood vessels and are the binding sites for specific factors that initiate clotting in the intrinsic pathway. Similarly, the term extrinsic came from the observation that there was another factor extrinsic to circulating blood that facilitates blood clotting. This factor was identified as **factor III, tissue factor** (see Figure 22.39*a*). Whether intrinsic or extrinsic, the process of blood coagulation is initiated on the membrane and is continued on the membrane surface at the site of injury.

Reactions of the Intrinsic Pathway

Reactions of the intrinsic pathway are shown in Figure 22.36. Upon injury to the endothelial lining of blood vessels and exposure of external membrane surfaces, the proteinase zymogen **factor XII** binds directly to anionic surfaces and undergoes a conformation change that increases its catalytic activity 10^4- to 10^5-fold. **Prekallikrein** and **factor XI,** also zymogens, circulate in blood as separate complexes with **high molecular weight kininogen (HMWK):** either a factor XI–HMWK complex or a prekallikrein–HMWK complex. In Figure 22.37 is a schematic diagram showing the functional regions of HMWK. The binding site on HMWK for prekallikrein consists of approximately 31 amino acid residues. Factor XI binds to approximately 58 amino acid residues that include the

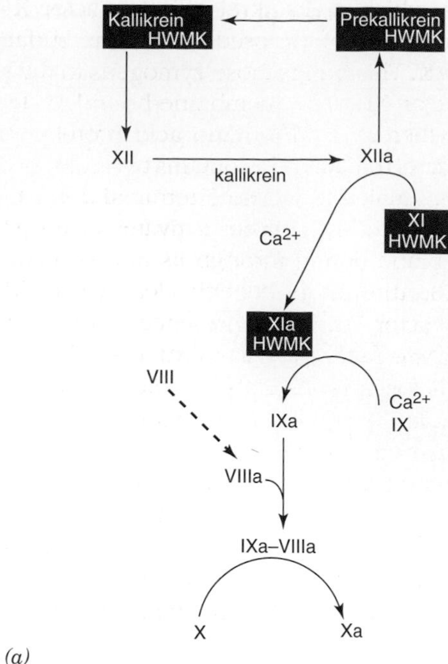

(a)

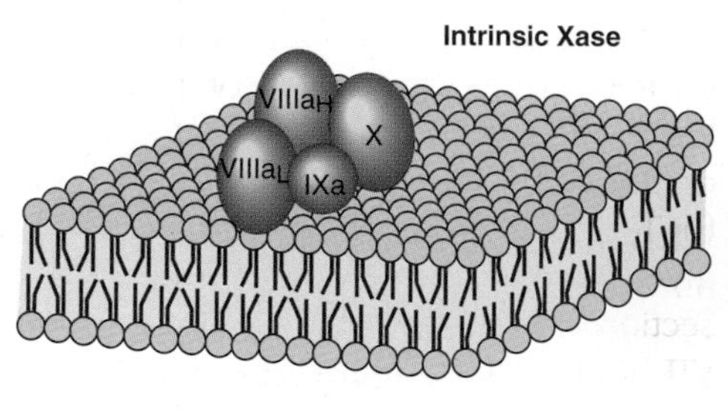

(b)

FIGURE 22.36
Intrinsic pathway of blood coagulation.
HWMK, high molecular weight kininogen. Activated factors are designated with an "a."
Adapted from Kalafatis, M., Swords, N. A., Rand, M. D., and Mann, K. G. Biochim. Biophys. Acta *1227:113, 1994.*

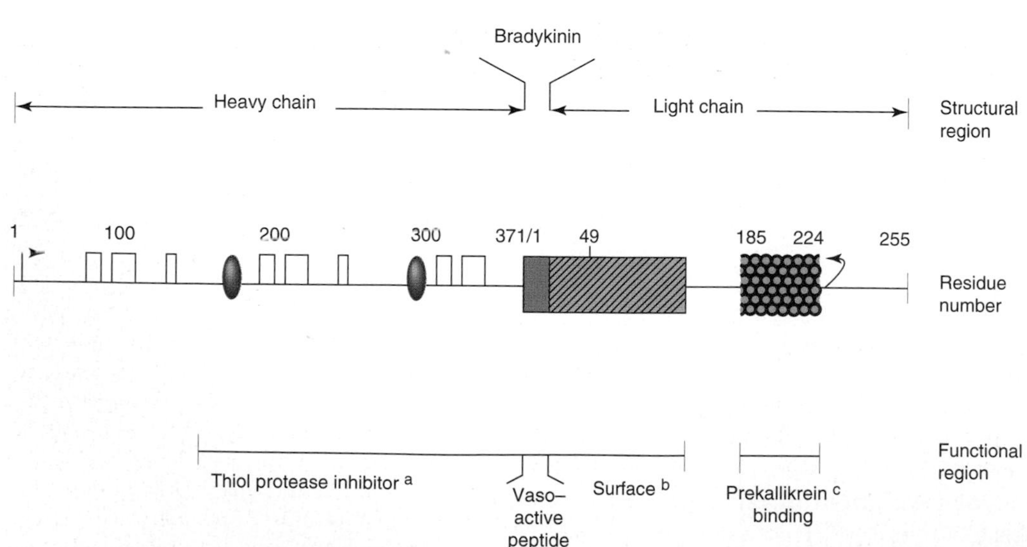

FIGURE 22.37
Schematic diagram of the functional regions of human high molecular weight kininogen (HMWK).
Bradykinin is derived from near the middle of HMWK by proteolysis. The resulting two chains are held together by disulfide bonds (horizontal arrows).
Redrawn from Tait. J. F., and Fujikawa, K. J. Biol. Chem. *261:15396, 1986.*

31 to which prekallikrein binds. Factor XI and prekallikrein are attached to anionic sites of exposed membrane surfaces through their interactions with HMWK. This brings those zymogens to the site of injury and in direct proximity to factor XII. The membrane-bound "activated" form of factor XII activates prekallikrein, a 619 amino acid protein, by cleavage at Arg^{371}–Ile^{372}, to yield **kallikrein.** Kallikrein contains two chains covalently linked by a single disulfide bond. Kallikrein, whose C-terminal domain (248 amino acid residues) contains the catalytic site, further activates factor XII to give XIIa. Factor XI, which is membrane bound through its noncovalent attachment to HMWK, is activated by XIIa through proteolytic cleavage to XIa. Factor XIa activates **factor IX** to IXa. Factor IXa in the presence of **factor VIIIa,** a protein cofactor, forms the **intrinsic factor ten'ase (intrinsic Xase)** that can now activate **factor X** to Xa. Factor Xa is the catalytic moiety of the proteinase complex responsible for the activation of prothrombin to thrombin (see Clin. Corr. 22.9). This is essentially a four-step cascade started by the "contact" activation of factor XII and the **autocatalytic** action between factor XII and kallikrein to give XIIa (step 1). Factor XIIa activates factor XI (step 2); factor XIa activates factor IX (step 3); and factor IXa, in the presence of VIIIa, activates factor X (step 4). If each enzyme molecule activated also catalyzed the formation of 100 others before it is inactivated, the **amplification factor** would be 1×10^6.

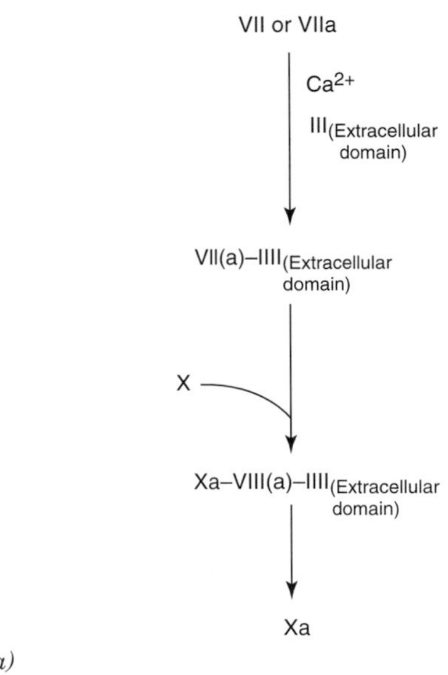

(a)

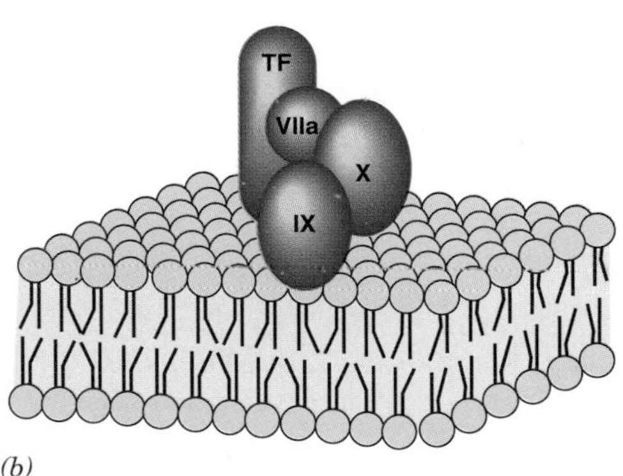

(b)

FIGURE 22.38
Extrinsic pathway of blood coagulation.

Reactions of the Extrinsic Pathway

A diagram of the extrinsic pathway is shown in Figure 22.38. The membrane receptor that initiates this process is factor III or tissue factor. Tissue factor (Figure 22.39*a*) is a transmembrane protein of 263 amino acids. Residues 243–263 are located on the cytosolic side of the membrane. Residues 220–242 are hydrophobic residues and represent the transmembrane sequence. Residues 1–219 are on the outside of the membrane, are exposed after injury, and form the receptor for formation of the initial complex of the extrinsic pathway. This domain is glycosylated and contains four cysteine residues. A stereo representation of a section of it highlighting some of the amino acid residues involved in factor VII binding is shown in Figure 22.39*b*.

Tissue factor (factor III or TF) and factor VII are unique to the **extrinsic pathway** and are essentially all of its major components. Factor VII is a **γ-carboxyglutamyl** or Gla-containing protein that binds to tissue factor only

CLINICAL CORRELATION 22.9

Intrinsic Pathway Defects: Prekallikrein Deficiency

Components of the intrinsic pathway include factor XII (Hageman factor), factor XI, prekallikrein (Fletcher factor), and high molecular weight kininogen. Clinical disorders have been associated with defects in each of these components. Inherited disorders in each appear to be autosomal recessive. Each appears to be associated with an increase in activated partial thromboplastin time (APTT). The only one of these components directly associated with a clinical bleeding disorder is factor XI deficiency.

In some cases where there is a prekallikrein (Fletcher factor) deficiency, autocorrection after prolongation of the preincubation phase of the APTT test occurs. This phenomenon is explained by the ability of factor XII to be activated by an autocatalytic mechanism. The reaction is very slow in prekallikrein deficiency since the rapid reciprocal autoactivation between factor XII and prekallikrein cannot take place. Prekallikrein deficiency may be due to a decrease in the amount of the protein synthesized, to a genetic alteration in the protein itself that interferes with its ability to be activated, or its ability to activate factor XII. A lack of knowledge of the structure of the gene for prekallikrein precludes definitive explanations of the mechanisms operational in patients with prekallikrein deficiency. Specific deficiencies of the intrinsic pathway, however, can be localized to a specific factor if the appropriate number of tests are performed. These may include a direct measurement of the amount of each of the factors present in the patient's plasma in addition to APTT test performed with and without prolonged preincubation time. Use of these direct measurements helped diagnose a prekallikrein deficiency in a 9-year-old girl who had a prolonged APTT. The functional level of prekallikrein in this patient was less than 1/50th of the minimum normal value. Immunological test (ELISA) showed an antigen level of 20–25%, suggesting that she was synthesizing a dysfunctional molecule.

Coleman, R. W., Rao, A.K ., and Rubin, R. N. *Am. J. Hematol.* 48:273, 1995.

in the presence of Ca^{2+}. The resulting TF–VII–Ca^{2+} complex is the catalytically active species. It catalyzes the formation of factor Xa from X.

The zymogen form of factor VII is initially **activated through protein–protein interaction** as a result of its binding to tissue factor. Additional factor VII is **activated by Xa** of the complex through proteolytic cleavage. Unlike other proteinases of the blood coagulation scheme, factor VIIa has a long half-life in circulating blood. Once dissociated from tissue factor, VIIa is not catalytically active, and its presence in blood would be harmless. Formation of the initial complex with TF could involve some of the already preformed factor VIIa, making it difficult to state with absolute certainty whether the zymogen form of VII in complex with tissue factor is totally responsible for the initial activation of factor X. A 3-D ribbon structural representation of factor VIIa is shown in Figure 22.40. The region for tissue factor interaction, Ca^{2+} binding, and the substrate binding pocket are highlighted.

Thrombin Converts Fibrinogen to Fibrin

The final phase in the formation of the fibrin clot (Figure 22.41) begins with action of the complex, **factor Xa–Va,** on **prothrombin.** A stereo view of factor

(a)

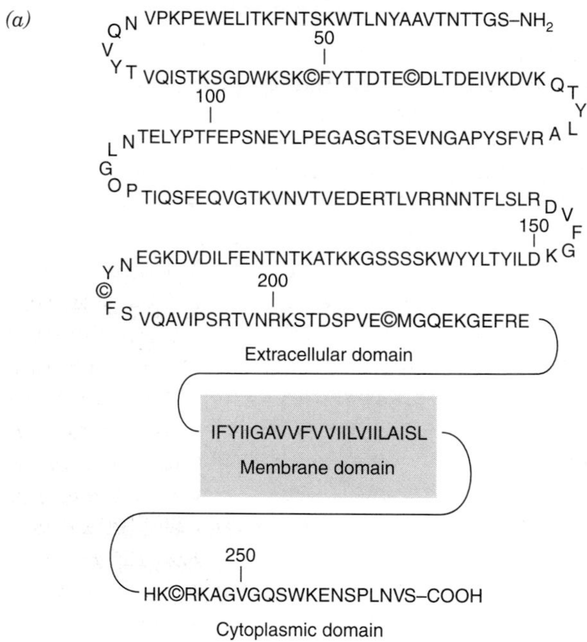

(b)

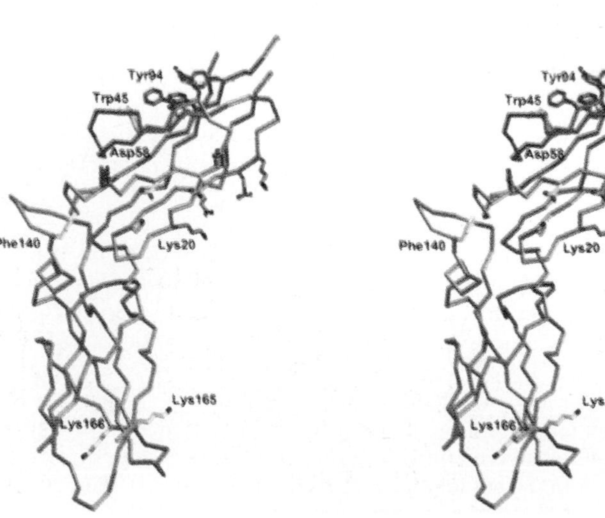

FIGURE 22.39
Tissue factor.
(*a*) Amino acid sequence of human tissue factor derived from its cDNA sequence. (*b*) A stereo representation of the carbon chain of the extracellular domain of tissue factor. Residues important for binding of factor VII are shown in yellow. Clusters of aromatic and charged residues are shown in light blue.
(a) Redrawn from Spicer, E. K., Horton, R., Bloem, L., et al. Proc. Natl. Acad. Sci. USA *84:5148, 1987. (b) Reproduced with permission from Muller, Y. A., Ultsch, M. H., Kelley, R. F., and deVos, A. M.* Biochemistry *33:10864, 1994. Copyright 1994 American Chemical Society. Photograph generously supplied by Dr. A. de Vos.*

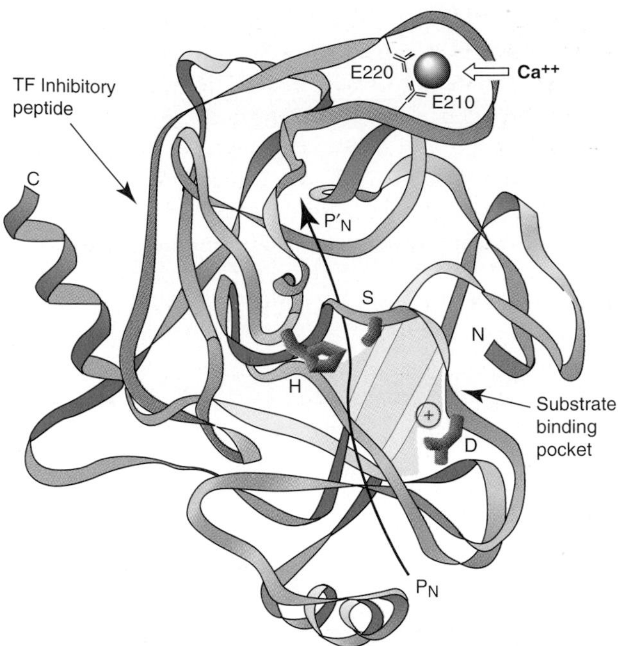

FIGURE 22.40
Ribbon structural representation of the protease domain of factor VIIa.
The dark ribbon labeled "TF inhibitory peptide" represents a section involved in binding to tissue factor. The catalytic triad is shown in the substrate binding pocket as H, S, and D for His[193], Ser[344], and Asp[338], respectively. The arrow labeled P_N–P'_N lies in the putative extended substrate binding region.
Redrawn with permission from Sabharwal, A. K., Birktoft, J. J., Gorka, J., et al. J. Biol. Chem. *270:1553, 1995.*

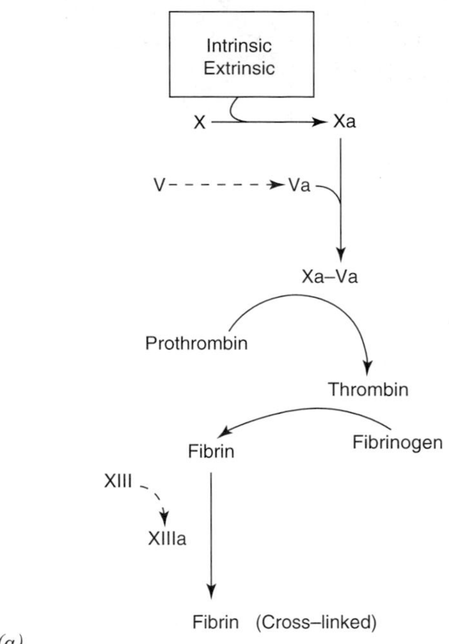

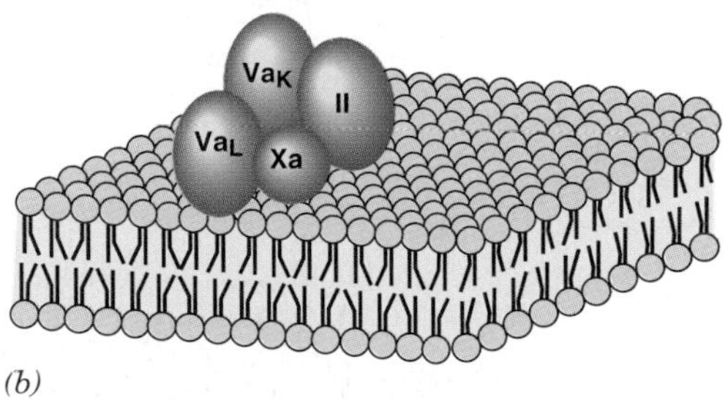

FIGURE 22.41
Clot forming pathway.
Adapted from Kalafatis, M., Swords, N. A., Rand, M. D., and Mann, K. G. Biochim. *Biophys. Acta 1227:113, 1994.*

Xa is shown in Figure 22.42. Factor Xa is formed by both the extrinsic and the intrinsic pathways by cleavage of factor X at positions 145 and 151 with elimination of a six amino acid peptide. Although the enzyme primarily responsible for activation of **factor V** is **thrombin,** factor Xa also catalyzes formation of Va. Thus the **prothrombinase complex, Xa–Va,** appears early in the process.

Thrombin, which circulates in plasma as prothrombin, catalyzes the conversion of **fibrinogen** to **fibrin.** Prothrombin, a 72-kDa protein (Figure 22.43), contains ten γ-carboxyglutamate (Gla) residues in its N-terminal region. Binding of calcium ions to these residues facilitates binding of prothrombin to membrane surfaces and to the Xa–Va complex at the site of injury. The prothrombinase complex (Xa–Va) activates prothrombin by making two proteolytic cleavages on the carboxyl side of arginine residues, first at position 320 and then at position 284. The active thrombin molecule (α-thrombin) consists of two chains, one of 6 kDa and the other of 31 kDa, that are covalently linked by a disulfide

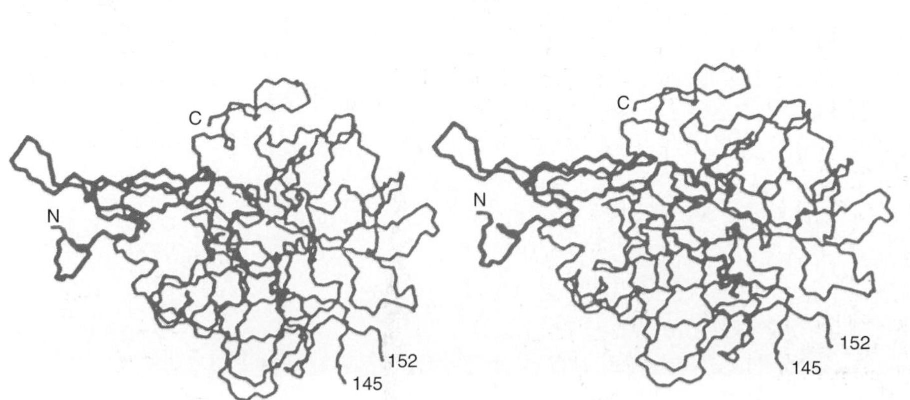

FIGURE 22.42
Stereo view of the CN-backbone structure of factor Xa.
The EGF-like domain is in bold.
Redrawn from Padmanabhan, K., Padmanabhan, K. P., Tulinsky, A., et al. J. Mol. Biol *232:947, 1993.*

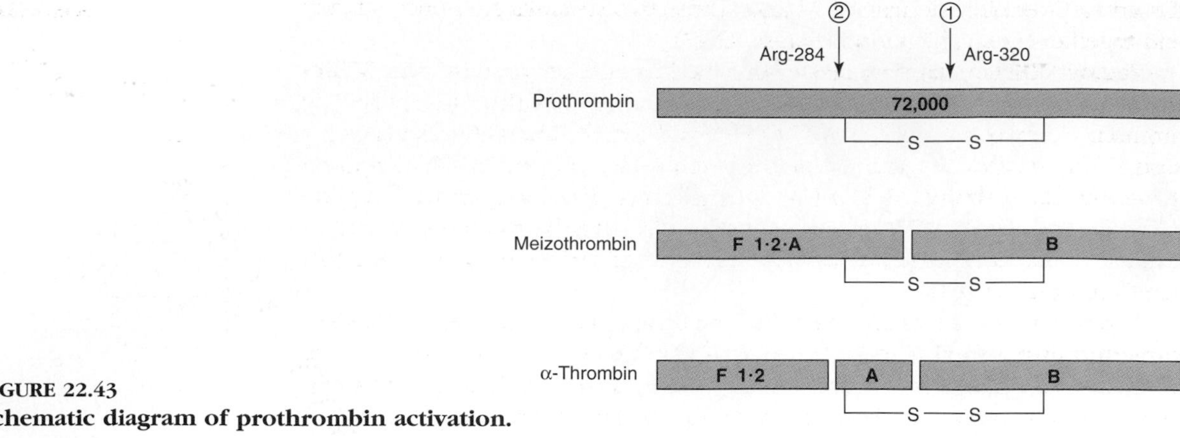

FIGURE 22.43
Schematic diagram of prothrombin activation.

bond. A stereo view of the active α-thrombin molecule is shown in Figure 22.44. Regions involved in some of its functions are highlighted. The substrate for thrombin is fibrinogen.

Fibrinogen is a large molecule of approximately 340 kDa consisting of two tripeptide units with α,β,γ structure (Figure 22.45). The subunits are "tied" together at their N-terminal regions by a group of disulfide bonds. Fibrinogen has three globular domains, one on each end and one in the middle where the chains are joined. The globular domains are separated by rod-like domains. A short segment of the free N-terminal regions projects out from the central globular domain. The N-terminal region of the $\alpha\alpha'$ and the $\beta\beta'$ subunits, through charge–charge repulsion, prevent aggregation of fibrinogen. Thrombin cleaves these N-terminal peptides and allows the resulting fibrin molecules to aggregate and to form the **"soft" clot.** The soft clot is stabilized and strengthened by the action of **factor XIIIa, transglutamidase.** This enzyme catalyzes the formation of an **isopeptide linkage** by replacing the Δ-amide group of glutamine residues of one chain with the ε-amino group of lysine residues of another chain (Figure 22.46) with the release of ammonia. This cross-linking of fibrin completes the steps involved in the formation of the hard clot.

Major Roles of Thrombin

α-Thrombin activates the protein cofactors V and VIII and it is also involved in **platelet aggregation.** Factor V is a 330,000 molecular weight protein. Activation of factor V by thrombin occurs through proteolytic cleavage at Arg^{709} and Arg^{1545}. Factor Va is a heterodimer consisting of an N-terminal domain of 105

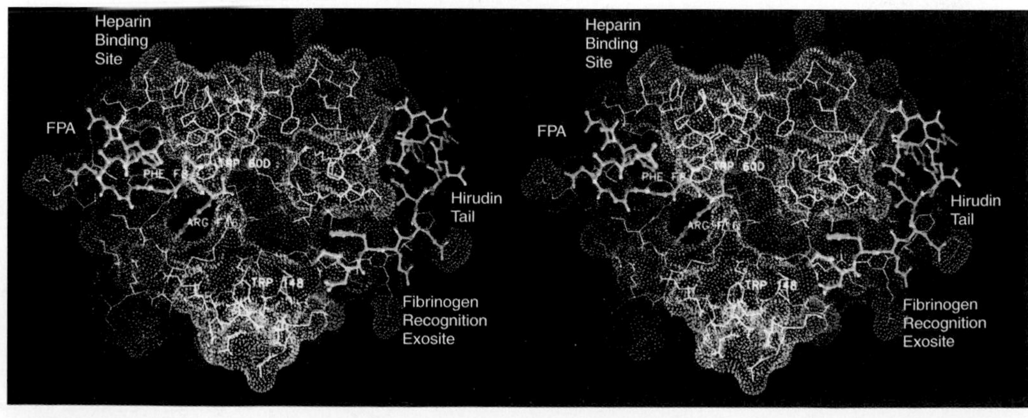

FIGURE 22.44
Stereo view of the active site cleft of human α-thrombin. Dark blue, basic amino acids; red, acid; light blue, neutral. The active site goes from left to right. *Figure courtesy of Dr. M. T. Stubbs II, Max-Planck Institut für Biochemie, Martinsreid, Germany.*

kDa and a C-terminal domain of 74 kDa. These two subunits are noncovalently held together by a calcium ion (Figure 22.47).

Factor VIII circulates in plasma attached to another protein, **von Willebrand's factor (vWF).** Factor VIII is a 285-kDa protein that is activated by thrombin cleavage at Arg^{372}, Arg^{740}, Arg^{1648}, and Arg^{1689}. The latter cleavage releases VIIIa from vWF. Factor VIIIa is a heterotrimer (Figure 23.47) composed of N-terminal peptides of 40 kDa (A_2) and 50 kDa (A_1), and a C-terminal peptide of 74 kDa (A_3). Factor VIIIa also contains a Ca^{2+} bridge between the N- and C-terminal domains. Classic hemophilia results from a deficiency in factor VIII (see Clin. Corr. 22.10).

Thrombin also activates factor XIII, transglutamidase (Figure 22.48). **Protransglutamidase** exists in both plasma and platelets. The structural form of the platelet enzyme is α_2, whereas that of the plasma form is $\alpha_2\beta_2$. Thrombin cleaves the α subunit of both the platelet and the plasma forms of transglutaminase. Cleavage of the α subunit of the plasma form of the enzyme leads to dissociation of the β subunit, which is not catalytically active. The platelet form of the enzyme is released at the site of fibrin aggregation and is activated just by cleavage of the α subunit.

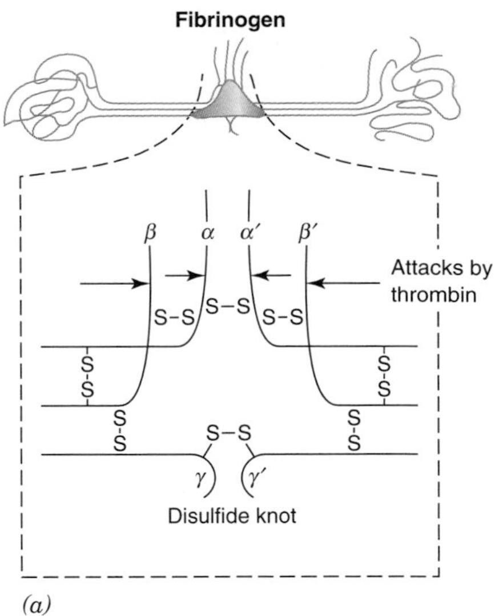

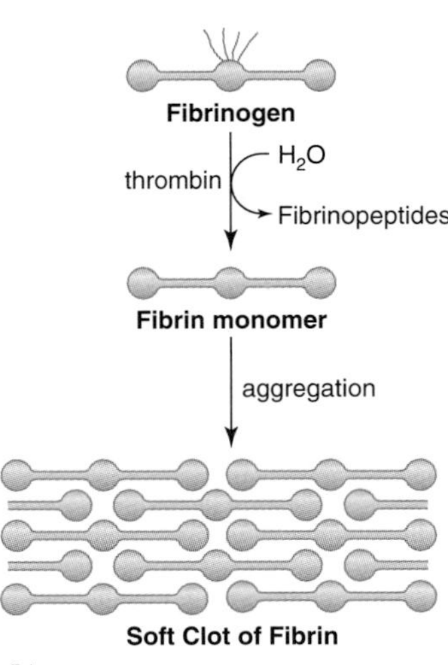

FIGURE 22.45
Diagrammatic representation of the fibrinogen molecule and its conversion to the soft clot of fibrin.

Formation of a Platelet Plug

The clumping of platelets at the site of injury is mediated by the presence of thrombin. There is a **thrombin receptor**, a member of the seven-transmembrane-domain family of receptors, on the outside of endothelial cells. This receptor is exposed upon injury and is activated by α-thrombin. **Aggregation of platelets** is facilitated by their initial binding to this activated receptor. In addition to the formation of a physical plug, platelets undergo a morphological change and release other chemicals that elicit other actions (Figure 22.49): ADP, serotonin, some types of phospholipids, and proteins that aid in coagulation and tissue repair. A glycoprotein, von Willebrand's factor (vWF) is released, concentrates in the area of the injury, and also forms a link between the exposed receptor and the platelets. von Willebrand's factor also serves as a carrier for factor VIII. Activation and release of factor VIII from vWF have been discussed.

FIGURE 22.46
Reactions catalyzed by transglutamidase.

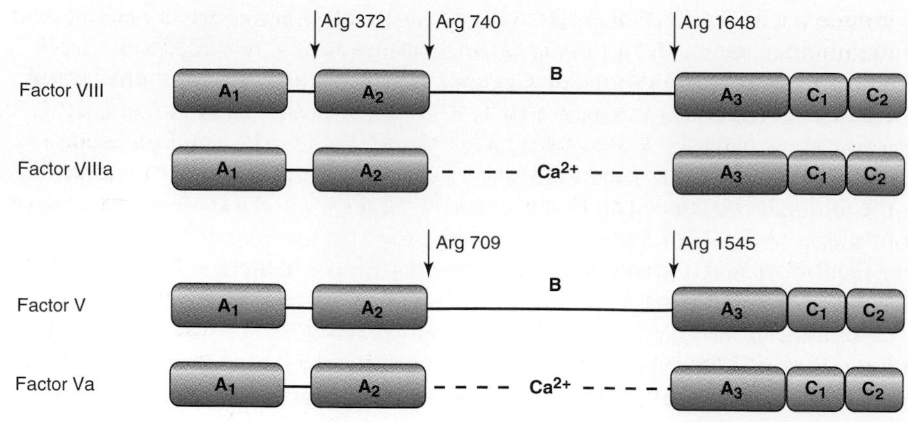

FIGURE 22.47
Organizational structure of cofactor proteins, factors VIII and V.
Positions for thrombin cleavage are shown. A's and C's represent structural domains.
Redrawn from Kalafatis, M., Swords, N. A., Rand, M. D., and Mann, K. G. Biochim. Biophys. Acta *1227:113, 1994.*

Platelet aggregation becomes autocatalytic with the release of ADP and **thromboxane A_2.** Platelet factor IV, **heparin binding protein,** prevents heparin–antithrombin III complexes from inhibiting serine proteinase coagulation factors, and it attracts cells with anti-inflammatory activity to the site of injury. About 20% of factor V exists in platelets as does one form of factor XIII, the transglutamidase.

Intact vascular endothelium does not normally initiate platelet aggregation since receptors and other elements are not exposed and activators such as ADP are rapidly degraded or are not in blood in sufficient concentration to be effective. The endothelium also secretes **prostacyclin (PGI_2),** a potent inhibitor of platelet aggregation.

Properties of Some of the Proteins Involved in Coagulation

Calcium ions have at least two important functions in blood coagulation. They form complexes with factors that contain γ-carboxyglutamyl (Gla) residues and

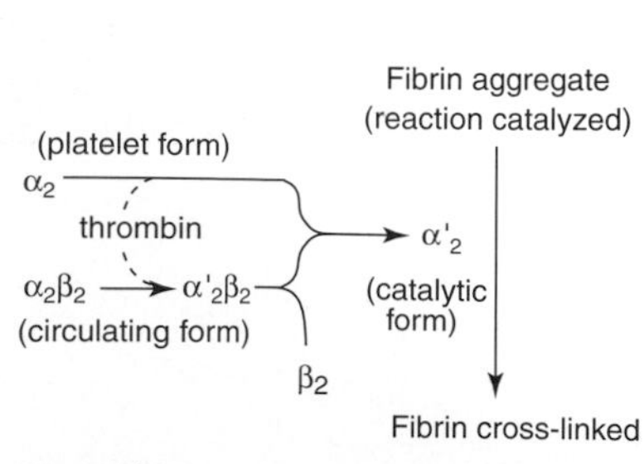

FIGURE 22.48
Activation of transglutamidase by thrombin.

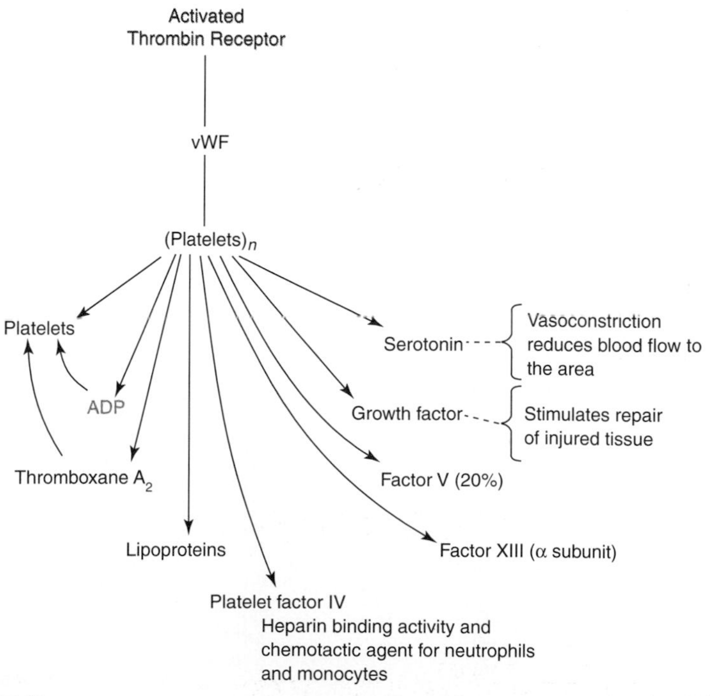

FIGURE 22.49
Action of platelets in blood coagulation.

induce conformational and electronic states that facilitate their interaction with membrane "receptors" for initiation and localization of their reactions. Calcium ions also bind at sites other than Gla residues, producing protein conformational changes that enhance catalytic activity. Evidence for this second role for calcium ions comes from the observation that activation of at least one of the enzymes leads to both the cleavage and elimination of the N-terminal region containing the Gla residues, but calcium ions are still required for its effective participation in blood coagulation.

A schematic representation of the structural arrangement of five of the **Gla-containing proteins** listed in Table 22.9 is shown in Figure 22.50. Gla-containing residues are located in the N-terminal region of the molecules followed by a structural component that resembles epidermal growth factor. The position of proteolytic cleavage by activation proteinases is generally at an amino acid residue located between cysteine residues that form a disulfide bond. Activation may or may not result in loss of a small peptide. *Prothrombin is the only one whose activation is by cleavage outside the bridging disulfide bond and results in elimination of the Gla peptide.* Factor VII is activated by cleavage of a single Arg^{152}–Ile^{153} bond. Factor IX is activated by cleavages at Arg^{145} and Arg^{180} with the release of an approximately 11-kDa peptide. Factor X consists of two chains connected by a disulfide bridge. It is activated by cleavage of its heavy chain at Arg^{194}–Ile^{195}. The Gla residues are located in the light chain. Protein C also consists of a heavy and a light chain connected by a disulfide bond. Cleavage of an Arg–Ile bond at position 169 results in its activation.

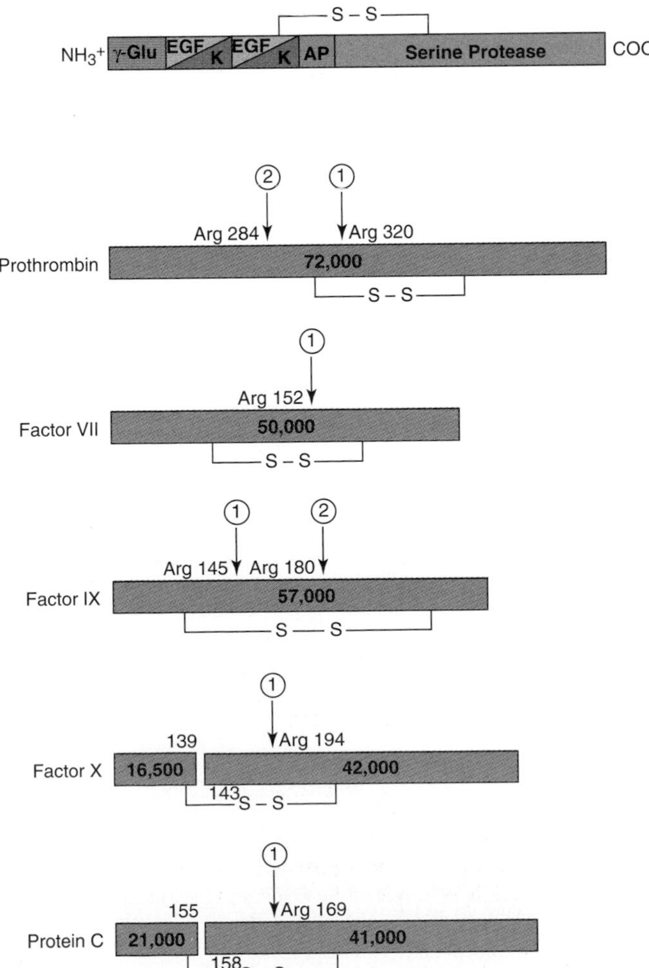

FIGURE 22.50
Gla-containing proteins.
(*a*) General structure of the γ-carboxyglutamyl-containing proteins. (*b*) Structural organization of the zymogens and their cleavage sites for activation.

CLINICAL CORRELATION 22.10

Classic Hemophilia

Hemophilia is an inherited disorder characterized by a permanent tendency for hemorrhages, spontaneous or traumatic, due to a defective blood clotting system. Classic hemophilia, hemophilia A, is an X-linked recessive disorder characterized by a deficiency of factor VIII. About 1 in 10,000 males is born with a deficiency of factor VIII. Of the approximate 25,000 hemophiliacs in the United States, more than 80% are of the A type. Hemophilia B is due to a dysfunction in factor IX.

Some hemophilia A patients may have a normal prothrombin time if the concentration of tissue factor is high. One possible explanation for this is that factor V in human plasma is much lower in concentration than factor X. Activation of an amount of factor X to Xa in excess of that required to bind all of factor Va would initiate blood clotting by the extrinsic pathway and give a normal prothrombin time. The intrinsic pathway would not function normally due to the deficiency in factor VIII. Without the two pathways operating in concert, the overall process of blood clotting would be impaired. Both factor Xa and thrombin activate factor V and are involved in a number of other reactions. If the overall process is not accelerated at its onset by intervention of the intrinsic pathway, due to kinetics of the interaction of thrombin and factor Xa with the normally low concentration of factor V, the clotting disorder is expressed. The blood levels of factor VIII in severe hemophilia A patients are less than 5% of normal. These patients have generally been treated by blood transfusion with its associated dangers: the possibility of contraction of hepatitis or HIV, and the 6% possibility of patients making autoantibodies. Treatment of hemophiliacs has been made much safer as a result of cloning and expression of the gene for factor VIII. The pure protein can be administered to patients with none of the associated dangers mentioned above.

Nemerson, Y. *Blood* 71:1, 1988.

Role of Vitamin K in Protein Carboxylase Reactions

Modification of prothrombin, **protein C, protein S,** and factors VII, IX, and X to form Gla residues occurs during **synthesis** by a **carboxylase** located on the luminal side of the rough endoplasmic reticulum. **Vitamin K** (phytonadione, the "koagulation" vitamin) is an essential **cofactor** for this carboxylase. During the reaction, the dihydroquinone or reduced form of vitamin K (Figure 22.51), vit K(H_2), is oxidized to the epoxide form, vit K(O), using molecular oxygen. A plausible mechanism involves the addition of molecular oxygen to the C-1 position of dihydro-vitamin K and its subsequent rearrangement to an alkoxide with a pK_a of ~20. This intermediate serves as a strong base and abstracts a

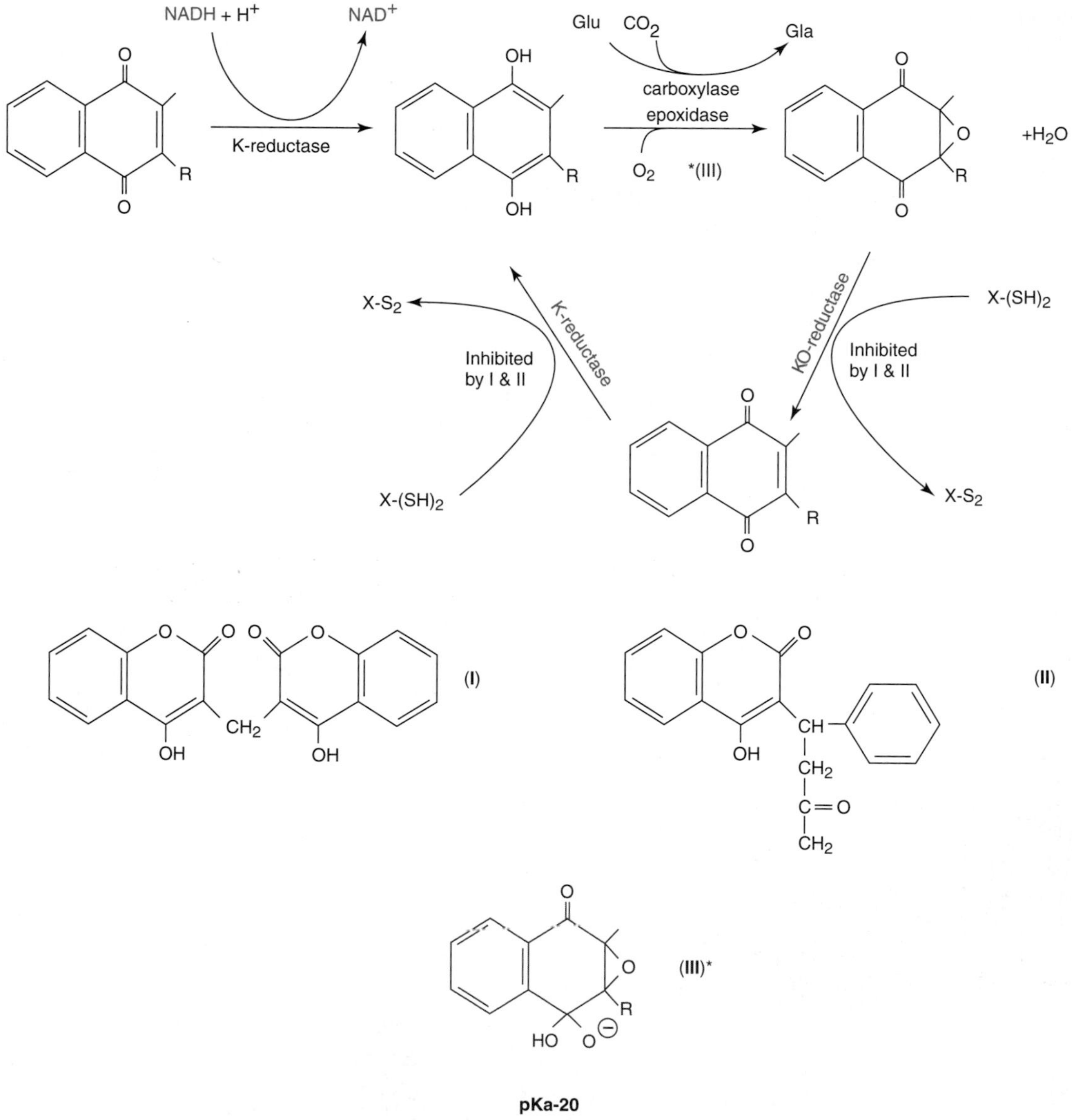

FIGURE 22.51
The vitamin K cycle as it functions in protein glutamyl carboxylation reaction.
X-$(SH)_2$ and X-S_2 represent the reduced and oxidized forms, respectively, of a thioredoxin. The NADH-dependent and the dithiol-dependent vitamin K reductases are different enzymes. The dithiol-dependent K and KO reductases are inhibited by dicumarol (I) and warfarin (II). *Possible alkoxide intermediate (III).
Redrawn and modified from Vermeer, C. Biochem. J. *266:625, 1990.*

proton from the γ-methylene carbon of glutamate, yielding a carbanion that can add to CO_2 by a nucleophilic mechanism (Figure 22.51). The **vitamin K epoxide** formed is converted back to the **dihydroquinone** by enzymes that require dithiols like **thioredoxin** as cofactors. Analogs of vitamin K inhibit dithiol-requiring vitamin K reductases and result in conversion of all available vitamin K to the epoxide form that is not functional in this reaction. The overall carboxylation reaction is

$$\mathrm{HOOC{-}CH_2{-}CH_2{-}CH(NHR_1){-}C({=}O){-}R_2} \xrightarrow[\text{Protein carboxylase}]{\text{vitamin K}(H_2) + O_2 + CO_2} \mathrm{(HOOC)_2CH{-}CH_2{-}CH(NHR_1){-}C({=}O){-}R_2} + \text{vitamin K(O)} + H_3O^+$$

The structure of two analogs, **dicumarol** and **warfarin,** that interfere with the action of vitamin K are shown in Figure 22.51. In animals treated with these compounds, prothrombin, protein C, protein S, and factors VII, IX, and X are not posttranslationally modified, are deficient in Ca^{2+} binding, and cannot participate in blood coagulation. Dicumarol and warfarin have no effect on blood coagulation in the test tube.

Control of the Synthesis of Gla-Proteins

Gla-peptides that are released from prothrombin upon activation are removed from circulation by the liver. These N-terminal Gla-containing peptides stimulate the *de novo* synthesis of Gla-requiring proteins of the blood coagulation scheme (Figure 22.52). The proteins are synthesized even in the absence of vitamin K

CLINICAL CORRELATION 22.11

Thrombosis and Defects of the Protein C Pathway

Four major proteins are involved in the action of protein C in regulating blood coagulation: protein C itself; protein S, a cofactor for protein C action; factor Va; and factor VIIIa. The latter two are substrates for catalytic action of the protein C–protein S complex. Mutations, generally inherited, in any of them can result in venous thrombosis with various degrees of severity.

De novo mutations have also been identified in patients showing type I protein C deficiency. One was the result of a missense mutation, a transition of T to C, resulting in the change of a codon for amino acid residue 270 from TCG to CCG. This gave Pro instead of Ser at that position, resulting in a conformational change that affected activity. The gene for protein C is on chromosome 2 and has 9 exons and 8 introns. In another patient, a *de novo* mutation located at the exon VI–intron f junction was detected. A 5-bp deletion (underlined below) occurred, resulting in a "read through" of sections of the intron.

Exon VI <> Intron f

Normal sequence: **CAC CCC GCA** G<>GTGAGAAGCCCCCAATAT
His Pro Ala

Mutated sequence: **CAC CCC GCA** GGA GCC CCC AAT AT
His Pro Ala Gly Ala Pro Asn

The normally translated sequence is in bold type. The degree of severity of thrombotic events depends on the extent to which the gene inherited from the other parent is normal and the extent to which it is expressed.

Resistance to the action of activated protein C as a result of single point mutations in its substrates, factor Va and factor VIIIa, can occur. This prevents or retards their inactivation through the proteolytic action of protein C. The most commonly identified cause of inherited resistance to the action of activated protein C is single point mutations in the gene for factor V.

A third cause of protein C-related thrombosis is a defect in protein S. Fewer specific details are available that permit a definition of the mechanism of the interaction between protein C and protein S, and likewise of the mutations that affect its function. It is quite clear, however, that protein S deficiency leads to thrombotic events. Venous thrombosis occurs in almost one-half of patients at some stage of their lives if they have deficiencies in functional amounts of protein S.

Gandrille, S., Jude, B., Alhenc-gelas, M., et al. *Blood* 84:2566, 1994; Zoller, B., Berntsdotter, A., Garcia de Frutos, P., et al. *Blood* 85:3518, 1995; and Reitsma, P. H., Bernardi, F., Doig, R. G., et al. *Thromb. Haemost.* 73:876, 1995.

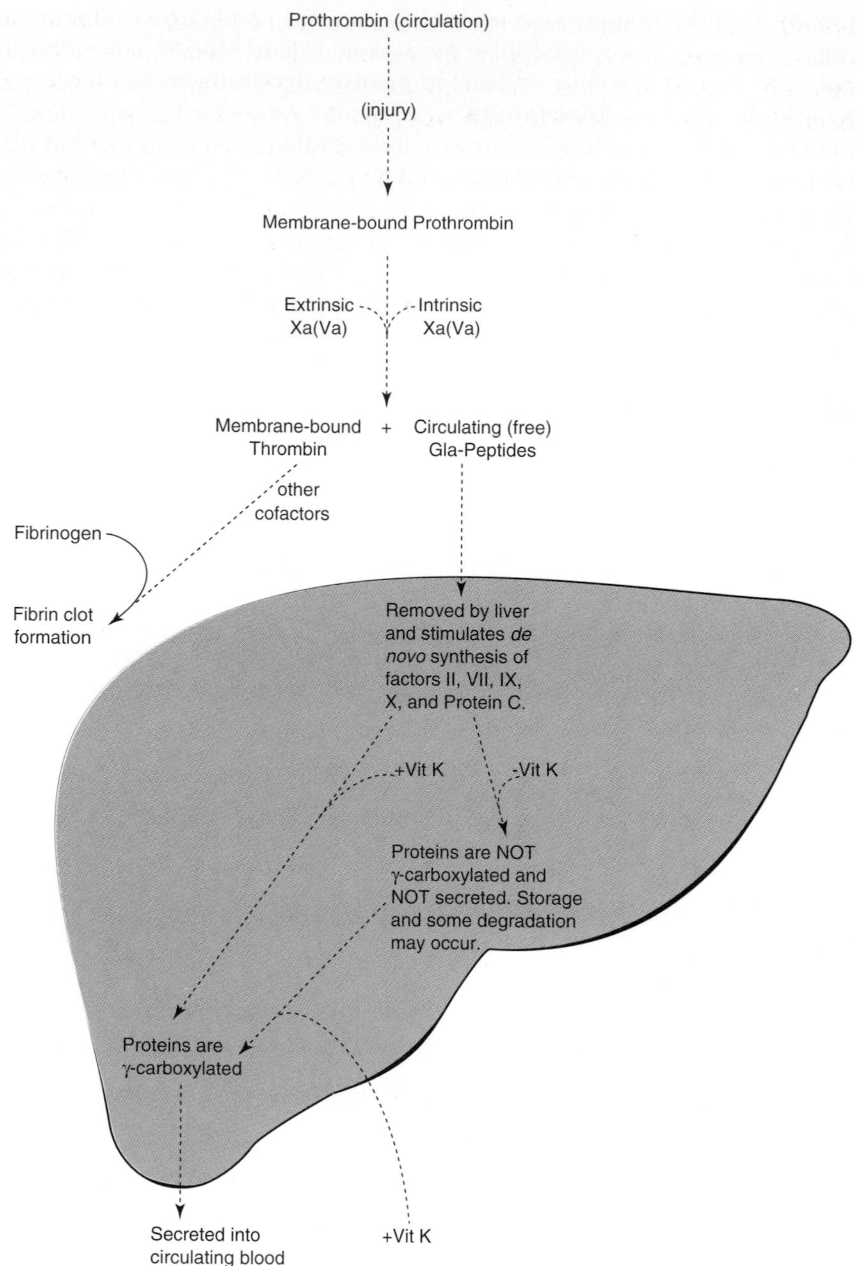

FIGURE 22.52
Role of Gla peptides in the regulation of *de novo* synthesis of coagulation factors.

or in the presence of antagonists of vitamin K. They are not secreted into the circulation, however. When vitamin K is restored, or is added in high enough concentrations to overcome the effects of antagonists, the preformed proteins are carboxylated and secreted into the circulation.

Activation of blood coagulation is a one-way process. The use of the activation peptides released from prothrombin to signal the liver to synthesize more of these proteins is an efficient mechanism for maintaining their concentrations in blood at effective levels. Monitoring of patients on long-term therapy with vitamin K antagonists is necessary to assure that posttranslational modification to produce the Gla-containing proteins is not shut down completely.

Dual Role of Thrombin in Promoting Coagulation and Clot Dissolution

The process of blood coagulation is self-controlling. One protein involved is **protein C.** Protein C, a Gla-containing protein, is activated in a membrane-bound complex of thrombin, **thrombomodulin,** and calcium. Thrombomodulin is an integral glycoprotein of the endothelial cell membrane that contains 560 amino acid residues. Thrombomodulin shows amino acid **sequence homology** with the **low-density lipoprotein receptor** but very little with tissue factor. There is, however, a great deal of similarity in functional domains between tissue factor and thrombomodulin, each of which functions as a receptor and activator for a proteinase. Thrombomodulin carries out this function for thrombin for activation of the proteinase, protein C. Binding of thrombin to thrombomodulin reduces its catalytic specificity for fibrinogen and enhances its specificity for protein C. Protein C inhibits coagulation by

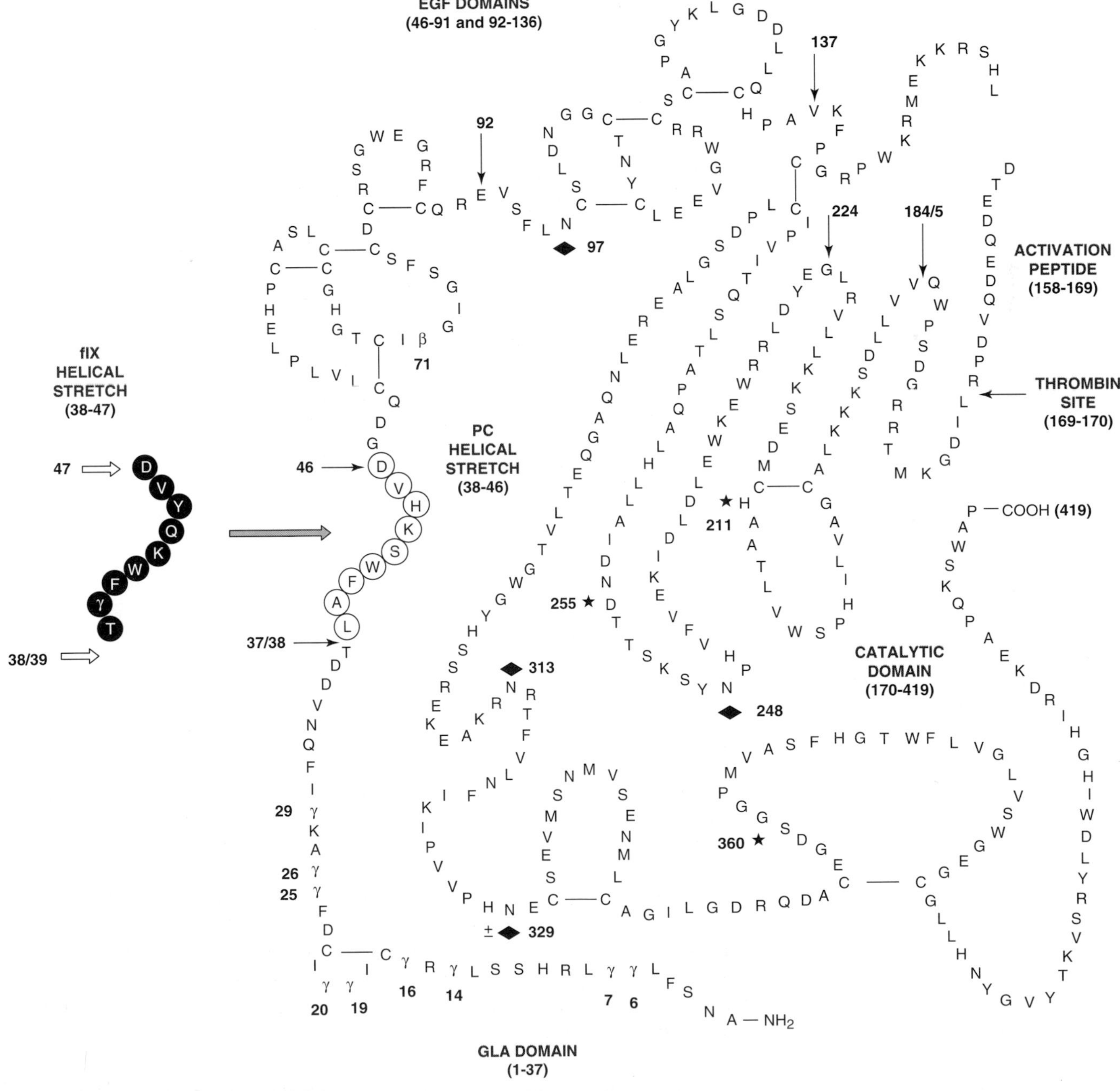

FIGURE 22.53
Primary structure of recombinant protein C.
Redrawn with permission from Christiansen, W. T., Geng, J. P., and Castillino, F. J. Biochemistry *34:8082, 1995. Copyright 1995 American Chemical Society.*

inactivating factors Va and VIIIa. Another Gla-containing protein, **protein S** (a 75-kDa protein), is a cofactor for protein C. Deficiency in protein S and/or protein C, leads to **thrombotic diseases** (see Clin. Corr. 22.11). A schematic representation of protein C showing some of its reactive regions is depicted in Figure 22.53.

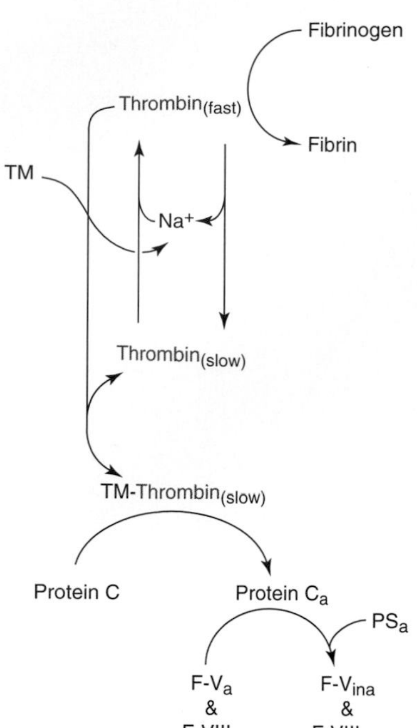

FIGURE 22.54
Allosteric reactions of thrombin and its actions on fibrinogen and protein C.

The Allosteric Role of Thrombin in Controlling Coagulation

Important reactions of thrombin relative to its dual role in the processes of promoting and stopping coagulation are summarized in Figure 22.54. Thrombin exists in two conformational forms: one is stabilized by Na^+ and has high

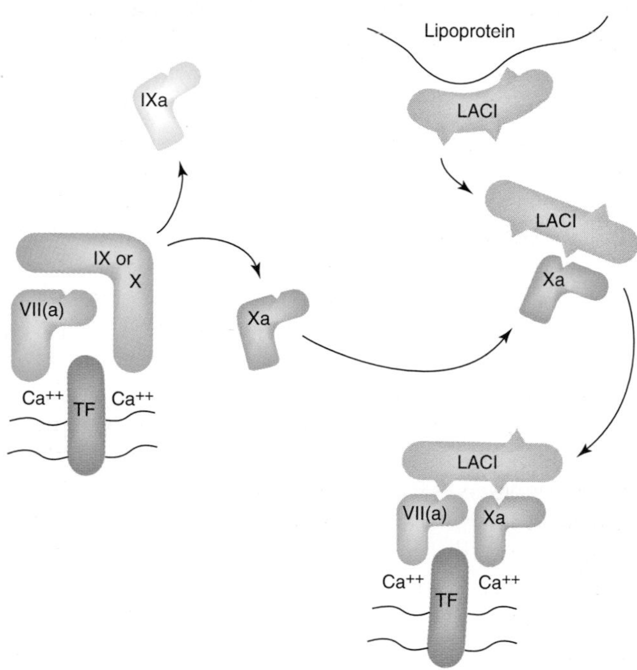

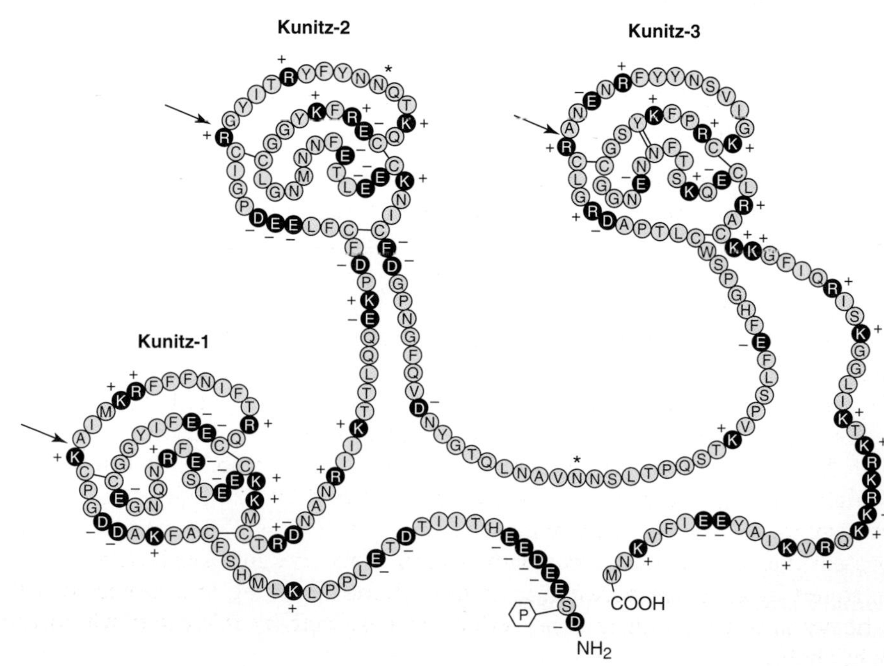

FIGURE 22.55
Proposed mechanism of inhibition of the extrinsic pathway.
LACI is lipoprotein-associated coagulation factor whose structure is shown in (*b*). Kunitz domain 1 inhibits factor VIIa and Kunitz domain 2 inhibits factor Xa. Arrows indicate the presumed location of the active-site inhibitor region for each domain.
Redrawn with permission from Broze, G. J., Girard, T. J., and Novotny, W. F. Biochemistry *29:7539, 1990. Copyright 1990 American Chemical Society.*

specificity for catalyzing the conversion of fibrinogen to fibrin; the other conformational form predominates in the absence of sodium, has low specificity for fibrinogen conversion, but high specificity for thrombomodulin binding and activity on protein C. These forms are referred to as "fast" and "slow," respectively. This dynamic **"feedback" mechanism** is important for stopping the clotting process at its point of origin. Many thrombotic diseases are associated with mutations in protein C that affect its activation by thrombin.

Inhibitors of the Plasma Serine Proteinases

Proteinase inhibitors in blood interact with enzymes of the blood coagulation system. Most of these fit into the serpin family of inhibitors. The term **serpin** was coined by Carrell and Travis and stands for **ser**ine **p**roteinase **in**hibitor. There is a tertiary structural similarity between them with a common core domain of about 350 amino acids. **Antithrombin III** is one of the major serpins and inhibits most of the serine proteinases of coagulation. Inhibition of the proteinases is a **kinetic process** that can begin almost as soon as coagulation itself begins. Initially, formation of inhibitor complexes is slow because the concentrations of the enzymes with which the inhibitors interact are low. As activation of the enzymes proceeds, inhibition increases and becomes more prominent. These reactions, and destruction of protein cofactors, eventually stop the coagulation process completely. In general, **proteinase–inhibitor complexes** do not dissociate readily and are removed intact from blood by the liver.

Inhibition of the extrinsic pathway, that is, the TF–VIIa–Ca^{2+}–Xa complex, is unique and involves specific interaction with a **lipoprotein-associated coagulation inhibitor (LACI),** formerly known as **anticonvertin.** LACI is a 32-kDa protein that contains three tandem domains (Figure 22.55, p. 974). Each domain is a functionally homologous protease inhibitor that resembles other individual protease inhibitors such as the bovine **pancreas trypsin inhibitor.** LACI inhibits the extrinsic pathway by interacting specifically with the TF–VIIa–Ca^{2+}–Xa complex. Domain 1 binds to factor Xa and domain 2 binds to factor VIIa of the complex. Binding of LACI to VIIa does not occur unless Xa is present. The uniqueness of this reaction is that LACI is a multi-enzyme inhibitor in which each of its separate domains inhibits the action of one of the enzymes of the multi-enzyme complex of the extrinsic pathway.

Fibrinolysis Requires Plasminogen and Tissue Plasminogen Activator (t-PA) to Produce Plasmin

Reactions of **fibrinolysis** are shown in Figure 22.56. Lysis of the fibrin clot occurs through action of the enzyme **plasmin,** which is formed from **plasminogen** through the action of **tissue plasminogen activator (t-PA** or **TPA).** Plasminogen has high affinity for fibrin clots and forms complexes with fibrin throughout various regions of the fibrin network. t-PA also binds to fibrin clots and activates plasminogen to plasmin by specific bond cleavage. The clot is then solubilized by the action of plasmin.

t-PA is a 72-kDa protein with several functional domains. It has a growth factor domain near its N terminus, two adjacent **Kringle domains** that interact with fibrin, and a domain with protease activity that is close to its C terminus. Kringle domains are conserved sequences that fold into large loops stabilized by disulfide bonds. These domains are important structural features for protein–protein interactions that occur with several blood coagulation factors. t-PA is activated by cleavage between an Arg–Ile bond, resulting in a molecule with a heavy and a light chain. The serine protease activity is located within the light chain.

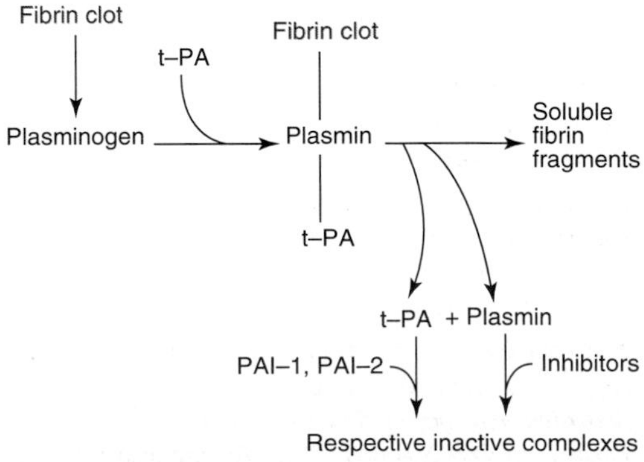

Fibrin clot
t-PA
Fibrin clot
Plasminogen
Plasmin
Soluble fibrin fragments
t-PA
t-PA + Plasmin
PAI–1, PAI–2
Inhibitors
Respective inactive complexes

FIGURE 22.56
Reactions involved in clot dissolution.

Activity of t-PA is regulated by protein inhibitors. Four immunologically distinct types of inhibitors have been identified, two of which are of greater physiological significance because they react rapidly with t-PA and are specific for it. They are **plasminogen activator-inhibitor type 1 (PAI-1)** and **plasminogen activator-inhibitor type 2 (PAI-2).** The human PAI-2 is a 415 amino acid protein.

Starting and stopping blood coagulation follow essentially the same type process, binding and proteolysis. Both are one-way processes and the only mechanism for replenishing the proteins once they are used is by resynthesis.

BIBLIOGRAPHY

General

Alberts, B., Bray, D., Lewis, J., Raff, M., Roberts, K., and Watson, J. *Molecular Biology of the Cell,* 2nd ed. New York: Garland Publishing, 1989.

Nerve

Bennett, M. K., and Scheller, R. H. The molecular machinery for secretion is conserved from yeast to neurons. *Proc. Natl. Acad. Sci. USA* 90:2559, 1993.

Fried, G. Synaptic vesicles and release of transmitters: new insights at the molecular level. *Acta Physiol. Scand.* 154:1, 1995.

Greengard, P., Valtorta, F., Czernik, A. J., and Benfenati, F. Synaptic vesicle phosphoproteins and regulation of synaptic function. *Science* 259:780, 1993.

Grenningloh, G., Rienitz, A., Schmitt, D., et al. The strychnine-binding subunit of the glycine receptor shows homology with nicotinic acetylcholine receptors. *Nature* 328:215, 1987.

Goodman, S. R., Zimmer, W. E., Clark, M. B., Zegon, I. S., Barker, J. E., and Bloom, M. L. Brain spectrin: of mice and men. *Brain Res. Bull.* 36:593, 1995.

Pleribone, V. A., Shupllakov, O., Brodin, L., Hilfiker-Rothenfluh, S., Czernik, A. J., and Greengard, P. Distinct pools of synaptic vesicles in neurotransmitter release. *Nature* 375:493, 1995.

Sudhof, T. The synaptic vesicle cycle: a cascade of protein–protein interactions. *Nature* 375:645, 1995.

Taylor, P. The cholinesterases. *J. Biol. Chem.* 266:4025, 1991.

Vision

Abrahamson, E. W., and Ostroy, S. E. (Eds.). *Molecular Processes in Vision,* Benchmark Papers in Biochemistry/3. Stroudsburg, PA: Hutchinson Ross Publishing, 1981.

Farber, D. B. From mice to men: the cyclic GMP phosphodiesterase gene in vision and disease. *Invest. Ophthalmol. Vis. Sci.* 36:263, 1995.

Nathans, J. Molecular biology of visual pigments. *Annu. Rev. Neurosci.* 10:163, 1987.

Nathans, J., Davenport, C. M., Maumenee, I. H., et al. Molecular genetics of human blue cone monochromacy. *Science* 245:831, 1989.

Palczewski, K. Is vertebrate phototransduction solved? New insights into the molecular mechanism of phototransduction. *Invest. Ophthalmol. Vis. Sci.* 35:3577, 1994.

Stryer, L. Visual excitation and recovery. *J. Biol. Chem.* 266:10711, 1991.

Zigler, J. S. Jr., and Goosey, J. Aging of protein molecules: lens crystallins as a model system. *Trends Biochem. Sci.* 7:133, 1981.

Muscle

Anderson, P. A. W., Malouf, N. N., Oakley, A. E., Pagani, E. D., and Allen, P. D. Troponin T isoform expression in humans: a comparison among normal and failing adult heart, fetal heart, and adult and fetal skeletal muscle. *Circ. Res.* 69:1226, 1991.

Carlier, M.-F. Actin: protein structure and filament dynamics. *J. Biol. Chem.* 266:1, 1991.

da Silva, A. C. R., and Reinach, F. C. Calcium binding induces conformational changes in muscle regulatory proteins. *Trends Biochem. Sci.* 16:53, 1991.

dos Remedios, C. G., and Moens, P. D. J. Actin and the actomyosin interface: a review. *Biochim. Biophys. Acta* 1228:99, 1995.

Ebashi, S. Excitation–contraction coupling and the mechanism of muscle contraction. *Annu. Rev. Physiol.* 53:1, 1991.

Gerisch, G., Noegel, A. A., and Schleicher, M. Genetic alteration of proteins in actin-based motility systems. *Annu. Rev. Psychol.* 53:607, 1991.

Hirose, K., Franzini-Armstrong, C., Goldman, Y. E., and Murray, J. M. Structural changes in muscle crossbridges accompanying force generation. *J. Cell Biol.* 127:763, 1994.

Huxley, H. E. The mechanism of muscular contraction. *Science* 164:1356, 1969.

Lorenz, M., Popp, D., and Holmes, K. C. Refinement of the F-actin model against X-ray fiber diffraction data by the use of a directed mutation algorithm. *J. Mol. Biol.* 234:826, 1993.

Blood

Antalis, T. M., Clark, M. A., Barnes, T., et al. Cloning and expressing of a cDNA coding for a human monocyte-derived plasminogen activator inhibitor. *Proc. Natl. Acad. Sci. USA* 85:985, 1988.

Colombatti, A., and Bonaldo, P. The superfamily of proteins with von Willebrand factor type A-like domains: one theme common to components of extracellular matrix, hemostasis, cellular adhesion, and defense mechanisms. *Blood* 77:2305, 1991.

Cooper, D. N. The molecular genetics of familial venous thrombosis. *Blood Rev.* 5:55, 1991.

Dowd, P., Hershline, R., Ham, S. W., and Naganathan, S. Vitamin K and energy transduction: a base strength amplification mechanism. *Science* 269:1684, 1995.

Hessing, M. The interaction between complement component C4b-binding protein and the vitamin K-dependent protein S forms a link between blood coagulation and the complement system. *Biochem. J.* 277:581, 1991.

Kalafatis, M., Sworde, N. A., Rand, M. D., and Mann, K. G. Membrane-dependent reactions in blood coagulation: role of the vitamin K-dependent enzyme complexes. *Biochim. Biophys. Acta* 1227:113, 1994.

Kuliopulus, A., Hubbard, B. R., Lam, Z., Koski, I. J., Furie, B., Furie, B. C., and Walsh, C. T. Dioxygen transfer during vitamin K-dependent carboxylase catalysis. *Biochemistry* 31:7722, 1992.

McClure, D. B., Walls, J. D., and Grinnell, B. W. Post-translational processing events in the secretion pathway of human protein C, a complex vitamin K-dependent antithrombotic factor. *J. Biol. Chem.* 267:19710, 1992.

Ny, T., Elgh, F., and Lund, B. The structure of the human tissue-type plasminogen activator gene: correlation of intron and exon structures to functional and structural domains. *Proc. Natl. Acad. Sci. USA* 81:5355, 1984.

Palston, P. A., and Gettings, P. G. W. A database of recombinant wild-type and mutant serpins. *Thromb. Haemost.* 72:166, 1994.

Reitsma, P. H., Bernardi, F., Doig, R. G., et al. Protein C deficiency: a database of mutations, 1995 update. *Thromb. Haemost.* 73:876, 1995.

Vermeer, C. γ-Carboxyglutamate-containing proteins and the vitamin K-dependent carboxylase. *Biochem. J.* 266:625, 1990.

Zeheb, R., and Gelehrter, T. D. Cloning and sequencing of cDNA for the rat plasminogen activator inhibitor-1. *Gene* 73:459, 1988.

QUESTIONS ■ C. N. ANGSTADT AND J. BAGGOTT

1. In the propagation of a nerve impulse by an electrical signal:
   A. the electrical potential across the membrane maintained by the ATP-driven Na^+,K^+ ion pump becomes more negative.
   B. local depolarization of the membrane causes protein conformational changes that allow Na^+ and K^+ to move down their concentration gradients.
   C. charge propagation is bidirectional along the axon.
   D. "voltage-gated" ion channels have a finite recovery time so the amplitude of the impulse changes as it moves along the axon.
   E. astrocytes are the antenna-like protrusions that receive signals from other cells.

2. All of the following are characteristics of nonpeptide neurotransmitters EXCEPT:
   A. they transmit the signal across the synapse between cells.
   B. they must be made in the cell body and then travel down the axon to the presynaptic terminal.
   C. electrical stimulation increasing Ca^{2+} in the presynaptic terminal fosters their release from storage vesicles.
   D. binding to receptors on the postsynaptic terminal induces a conformational change in proteins of that membrane.
   E. their actions are terminated by specific mechanisms within the synaptic junction.

Refer to the following for Questions 3–5.
   A. acetylcholine
   B. 4-aminobutyrate (GABA)
   C. catecholamines
   D. 5-hydroxytryptamine (serotonin)

3. Binding to its receptor opens a channel for Cl^-, causing hyperpolarization of the cell.

4. Termination of the signal typically involves the actions of both methyltransferase and monoamine oxidase, as well as reuptake into the presynaptic neuron.

5. Action is terminated by an esterase.

6. Which of the following is a correct statement about biochemical events occurring in the eye is (are) true?
   A. Glucose in the lens is metabolized by the TCA cycle in order to provide ATP for the Na^+, K^+–ATPase.
   B. Controlling the blood glucose level might reduce the incidence of diabetic cataracts by allowing the production of sorbitol.
   C. The high rate of the hexose monophosphate pathway in the cornea is necessary to provide NADPH as a substrate for glutathione reductase.
   D. The retina contains mitochondria so it depends on the TCA cycle for its production of ATP.
   E. Cataracts are the result of increasing blood flow in the lens leading to disaggregation of lens proteins.

7. Which of the following statements about rhodopsin is true?
   A. Rhodopsin is the primary photoreceptor of both rods and cones.
   B. The prosthetic group of rhodopsin is all-*trans*-retinol derived from cleavage of β-carotene.
   C. Conversion of rhodopsin to activated rhodopsin, R*, by a light pulse requires depolarization of the cell.
   D. Rhodopsin is located in the cytosol of the cell.
   E. Absorption of a photon of light by rhodopsin causes an isomerization of 11-*cis*-retinal to all-*trans*-retinal.

8. All of the following statements about the transduction of the light signal on rhodopsin are true EXCEPT:
   A. cGMP is involved in the transmission of the signal between the disk membrane and the plasma membrane.
   B. it involves the G-protein, transducin.
   C. cGMP concentration is increased in the presence of an activated rhodopsin–transducin–GTP complex.
   D. the signal is turned off, in part, by the GTPase activity of the α subunit of transducin.
   E. both guanylate cyclase and phosphodiesterase are regulated by calcium concentration.

9. The cones of the retina:
   A. are responsible for color vision.
   B. are much more numerous than the rods.
   C. have red, blue, and green light-sensitive pigments that differ because of small differences in the retinal prosthetic group.
   D. do not use transducin in signal transduction.
   E. are better suited for discerning rapidly changing visual events because a single photon of light generates a stronger current than it does in the rods.

10. When a muscle contracts, the:
    A. transverse tubules shorten, drawing the myofibrils and sarcoplasmic reticulum closer together.
    B. thin filaments and the thick filaments of the sarcomere shorten.
    C. light chains dissociate from the heavy chains of myosin.
    D. H bands and I bands of the sarcomere shorten because the thin filaments and thick filaments slide past each other.
    E. cross-linking of proteins in the heavy filaments increases.

11. All of the following statements about actin and myosin are true EXCEPT:
    A. the globular head section of myosin has domains for binding ATP and actin.
    B. actin is the major protein of the thick filament.
    C. the binding of ATP to the actin–myosin complex promotes dissociation of actin and myosin.
    D. F-actin, formed by aggregation of G-actin–ATP–Mg^{2+} complex, is stabilized when tropomyosin is bound to it.
    E. binding of calcium to the calmodulin-like subunit of troponin induces conformational changes that permit myosin to bind to actin.

12. ATP concentration is maintained relatively constant during muscle contraction by:
    A. increasing the metabolic activity.
    B. the action of adenylate kinase.
    C. the action of creatine phosphokinase.
    D. all of the above.
    E. none of the above.

13. The nerve impulse that initiates muscular contraction:
   A. begins with the binding of acetylcholine to receptors in the sarcoplasmic reticulum.
   B. causes both the plasma membrane and the transverse tubules to undergo hyperpolarization.
   C. causes opening of calcium channels, which leads to an increase in calcium concentration within the sarcomere.
   D. prevents Na^+ from entering the sarcomere.
   E. prevents Ca^{2+} from binding to troponin C.

14. Platelet aggregation:
   A. is initiated at the site of an injury by conversion of fibrinogen to fibrin.
   B. is inhibited in uninjured blood vessels by the secretion of prostacyclin by intact vascular endothelium.
   C. causes morphological changes and a release of the vasodilator, serotonin.
   D. is inhibited by the release of ADP and thromboxane A_2.
   E. is inhibited by von Willebrand factor (vWF).

15. In the formation of a blood clot:
   A. proteolysis of γ-carboxyglutamate residues from fibrinogen to form fibrin is required.
   B. the clot is stabilized by the cross-linking of fibrin molecules by the action of factor XIII, transglutamidase.
   C. antagonists of vitamin K inhibit the formation of γ-carboxyglutamate residues in various proteins, thus facilitating the clotting process.
   D. tissue factor, factor III, must be inactivated for the clotting process to begin.
   E. the role of calcium is primarily to bind fibrin molecules together to form the clot.

16. Factor Xa, necessary for conversion of prothrombin to thrombin, is formed by the action of the TF–VII–Ca^{2+} complex on factor X:
   A. only in the extrinsic pathway for blood clotting.
   B. only in the intrinsic pathway for blood clotting.
   C. as part of both the extrinsic and intrinsic pathways.
   D. only if the normal blood clotting cascade is inhibited.

17. Lysis of a fibrin clot:
   A. is in equilibrium with formation of the clot.
   B. begins when plasmin binds to the clot.
   C. requires the hydrolysis of plasminogen into heavy and light chains.
   D. is regulated by the action of protein inhibitors on plasminogen.
   E. requires the conversion of plasminogen to plasmin by t-PA (tissue plasminogen activator).

ANSWERS

1. B This is the mechanism for impulse propagation. A: The potential becomes less negative. C: It is unidirectional. D: "Voltage-gated" channels do have a finite recovery time so the amplitude remains constant. E: This describes dendrites. Astrocytes are glial cells that are involved in processes isolating the CNS from the external environment (pp. 921–923).
2. B This is true for neuropeptides, but many nonpeptide neurotransmitters are synthesized in the presynaptic terminal (pp. 923–924). A: This is a difference between electrical and chemical signals (p. 921). C: What is the role of synapsin I in this process (p. 925)? E: Make sure you know the three types of processes involved (p. 927).
3. B GABA is an inhibitory neurotransmitter. All the others are excitatory ones that cause depolarization of the cells (p. 931).
4. C Methylation by catecholamine-*O*-methyltransferase is an important part of the metabolism of the catecholamines. A: Acetylcholinesterase terminates the action of this (p. 928). B: GABA is converted into an intermediate of the TCA cycle (p. 931). D: Monoamine oxidase is the primary enzyme responsible for terminating serotonin's action (p. 930).
5. A The enzyme is acetylcholinesterase (p. 928).
6. C Make sure you understand the role of glutathione in protecting against harmful by-products from atmospheric oxygen (p. 933). A: Most of the ATP (85%) in the lens is generated by glycolysis (p. 934). B: Controlling glucose reduces sorbitol formation (p. 935). D: Its metabolism is similar to that of other eye tissues directly involved in the visual process. Thus its major source of energy is from glycolysis (p. 935). E: Lens has no blood supply. In diabetic cataracts there is increased aggregation of lens proteins because of increasing sorbitol (p. 935).
7. E This causes the conformational change of the protein that affects the resting membrane potential and initiates the rest of the events. A: Cones have the same prosthetic group but different proteins, so rhodopsin is in rods only (p. 937). B: This is the precursor of the prosthetic group 11-*cis*-retinal (p. 938). C: Isomerization of the prosthetic group leads to hyperpolarization (p. 939 Figure 22.20). D: Rhodopsin is a transmembrane protein (p. 937).
8. C The transducin complex activates the phosphodiesterase, thus lowering [cGMP] (p. 942). A: This is an example of a second messenger type chemical synapse. B and D: Transducin meets the criteria for a typical G-protein. E: The enzymes are regulated in opposite directions by Ca^{2+}, thus controlling [cGMP] (p. 943).
9. A Rods are responsible for low light vision. C: All three pigments have 11-*cis*-retinal; the proteins differ and are responsible for the slightly different spectra (pp. 937 and 944). D: The biochemical events are believed to be the same in rods and cones (p. 944). E: Cones are better suited for rapid events because their response rate is about four times faster than rods, even though their sensitivity to light is much less (p. 945).
10. D This occurs because of association–dissociation of actin and myosin (pp. 948 and 957). A: Depolarization in the transverse tubules may be involved in transmission of the signal but not directly in the contractile process (p. 954). B: The filaments do not change in length, but slide past each other (p. 948). C: This is not physiological. E: Cross-linking occurs in the H band of the sarcomere but does not change during the contractile process (p. 953).
11. B A: See Figure 22.28. C: Note that the role of ATP in contraction is to favor dissociation, not formation, of the actin–myosin

complex (p. 957). D and E: Tropomyosin, troponin, and actin are the three major proteins of the filament. Their actions are closely interconnected (pp. 951–953).

12. D Make sure you know the reactions catalyzed by these two enzymes (pp. 954–957).
13. C A: Acetylcholine receptors are on the plasma membrane. B: The impulse results in depolarization of both of these structures. D: Both Ca^{2+} and Na^{2+} enter the sarcomere when the channels open. E: Binding of Ca^{+2} to Tn-C initiates contraction (p. 954).
14. B The "ying–yang" nature of PGI_2 and TXA_2 help to control platelet aggregation until there is a need for it. A: Initiation is by contact with an activated receptor at the site of injury. Clot formation requires activation of various enzymes (pp. 960–961). C: Serotonin is a vasoconstrictor. Vasodilation would be contraindicated in this situation (p. 967). D: TXA_2 facilitates aggregation. E: vWF forms a link between the receptor and platelets, promoting aggregation (p. 967).
15. B The cross-linking occurs between a glutamine and a lysine (Figure 22.46). A and E: γ-Carboxyglutamate residues are on various enzymes; they bind calcium and facilitate the interaction of these proteins with membranes that form the sites for initiation of reaction (pp. 968–969). C: Vitamin K is an activator for the γ-carboxylation reaction, which is a necessary posttranslational modification of some of the enzymes involved in clot formation (p. 970). D: TF, factor III, is the primary receptor for initiation of the clotting process (p. 963).
16. A Tissue factor and factor VII are unique to the extrinsic pathway. B,C: The membrane interaction with the intrinsic pathway is with high-molecular-weight kininogen and prekallikrein (p. 961).
17. E The clot is solubilized by plasmin. A: Both formation and lysis of clots are unidirectional. B: Both plasminogen and t-PA bind to the clot. C and D: Both of these refer to t-PA (pp. 975–976).

CHAPTER

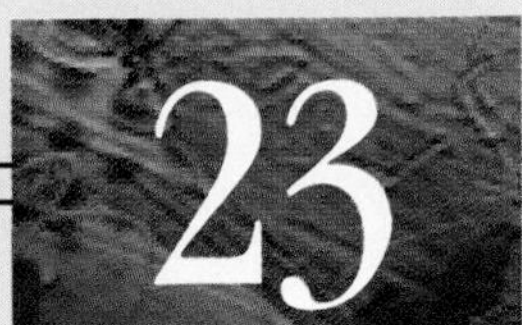

BIOTRANSFORMATIONS: THE CYTOCHROMES P450

Richard T. Okita and Bettie Sue Siler Masters

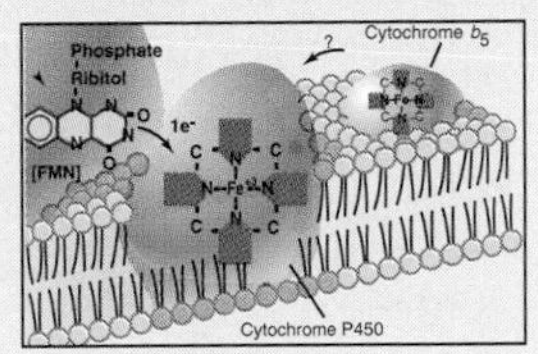

23.1 OVERVIEW

The term **cytochrome P450** refers to a family of **heme proteins** present in all mammalian cell types, except mature red blood cells and skeletal muscle cells, which catalyze oxidation of a wide variety of structurally diverse compounds. Cytochrome P450 also occurs in prokaryotes. Substrates for this enzyme system include endogenously synthesized compounds, such as steroids and fatty acids (including prostaglandins and leukotrienes), and exogenous compounds, such as drugs, food additives, or industrial by-products that enter the body through food sources, injection, inhalation from the air, or absorption through the skin. The cytochrome P450 system has far-reaching effects in medicine. It is involved in (1) inactivation or activation of therapeutic agents; (2) conversion of chemicals to highly reactive molecules, which may produce unwanted cellular damage, cell death, or mutations; (3) production of steroid hormones; and (4) metabolism of fatty acids and their derivatives. Other heme-binding, cysteine thiolate-containing proteins also exist, including thromboxane, prostacyclin, and allene oxide synthases, as well as the **nitric oxide synthases.** This chapter will address the cytochromes P450 in detail and will introduce the isoforms of nitric oxide synthase. Clinical implications of these oxygenation systems will be presented.

23.2 CYTOCHROMES P450: NOMENCLATURE AND OVERALL REACTION

Designation of a particular protein as a cytochrome P450 originated from its spectral properties before its catalytic function was known. This group of proteins has a unique absorbance spectrum that is obtained by adding a reducing agent, such as sodium dithionite, to a suspension of **endoplasmic reticulum** vesicles, frequently referred to as **microsomes,** followed by bubbling of carbon monoxide gas into the solution. Carbon monoxide is bound to the reduced heme protein and produces an absorbance spectrum with a peak at approximately 450 nm (Figure 23.1); thus the name P450 for a pigment with an absorbance at 450 nm. Specific forms of cytochrome P450 differ in their maximum absorbance wavelengths, with a range between 446 and 452 nm. The many forms of cytochrome P450 are classified, according to their sequence similarities, into various **gene subfamilies;** this system of **nomenclature** is being adopted almost universally. Individual cytochrome P450 forms are given an Arabic number to designate a specific family, followed by a capital letter to identify its subfamily, followed by another Arabic number designating the individual P450 form, for example, 1A2 or 2D6. The term **CYP,** which represents the first two letters of *cy*tochrome and the first letter in *P*450, is used as a preface to designate a gene or protein as a cytochrome P450 form. Thus cytochromes P450 1A2 and P450 2D6 are designated CYP1A2 and CYP2D6 in this nomenclature system. Members of the same family share at least 40% amino acid sequence homology and members of the same subfamily share at least 55% sequence homology. Table 23.1 lists several human cytochrome P450 forms. In certain families several subfamilies have been identified such as in CYP2 (CYP2A and CYP2B) and CYP4 (CYP4A and CYP4B), whereas in others only a single gene has been reported (CYP17, CYP19, and CYP21).

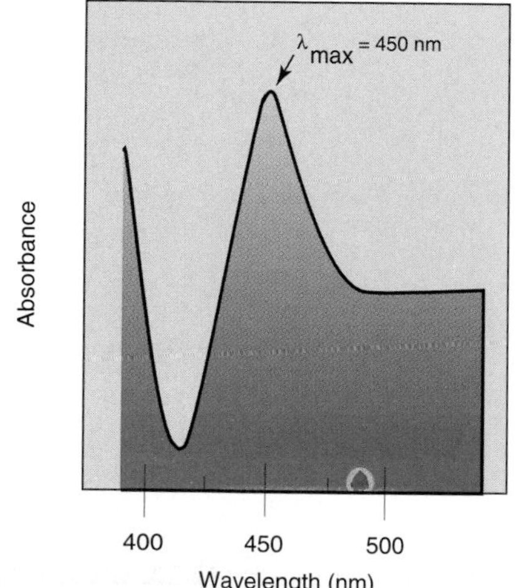

FIGURE 23.1
Absorbance spectrum of the carbon monoxide-bound cytochrome P450.
The reduced form of this heme protein binds carbon monoxide to produce a maximum absorbance at approximately 450 nm. Hence this cytochrome was designated P450.

The general reaction catalyzed by cytochrome P450 is written as follows:

$$NADPH + H^+ + O_2 + SH \rightarrow NADP^+ + H_2O + SOH$$

where the substrate (S) may be a steroid, fatty acid, drug, or other chemical that has an alkane, alkene, aromatic ring, or heterocyclic ring substituent that can serve as a site for oxygenation. The reaction is referred to as a monooxygenation and the enzyme as a **monooxygenase** because only one of the two oxygen atoms is incorporated into the substrate. In mammalian cells, cytochromes P450

TABLE 23.1 Human Cytochrome P450 Forms

CYP1	*CYP2*	*CYP3*	*CYP4*	*CYP11*	*CYP17*	*CYP19*	*CYP21*
			Cytochrome P450 Subfamilies / *Individual Forms*				
1A1	2A6	3A3	4A9	11A1			21A2
1A2	2A7	3A4	4A11	11B1			
	2B6	3A5	4B1	11B2			
	2C8	3A7	4F2				
	2C9		4F3				
	2C10						
	2C18						
	2C19						
	2D6						
	2E1						

serve as terminal electron acceptors in **electron transport systems,** which are present either in the endoplasmic reticulum or **inner mitochondrial membrane.** The cytochrome P450 proteins contain a single iron **protoporphyrin IX** prosthetic group (see p. 1009), which binds oxygen, and the resulting heme protein contains binding sites for the substrate. Heme iron of all known cytochromes P450 is bound to the four pyrrole nitrogen atoms of the porphyrin ring and two axial ligands, one of which is a sulfhydryl group from a cysteine residue located toward the carboxyl end of the molecule (Figure 23.2). Heme iron may exist in two different spin states: (1) a hexa-coordinated low-spin

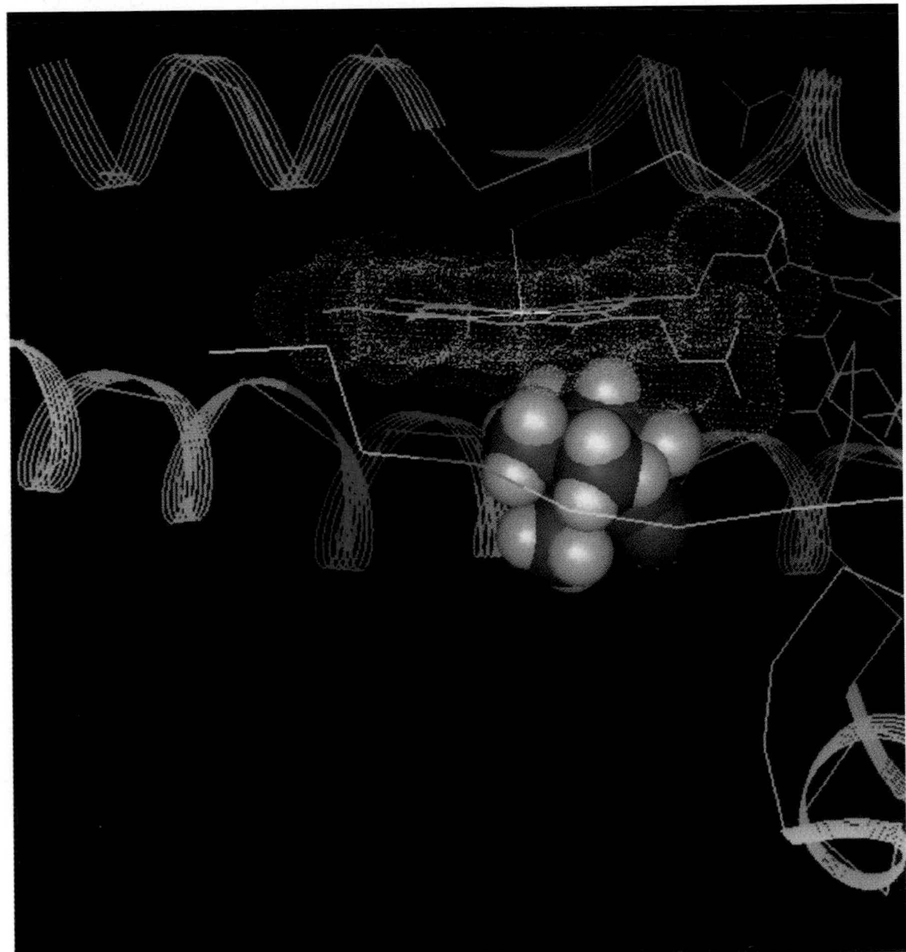

FIGURE 23.2
Binding of protoporphyrin IX prosthetic group of cytochromes P450.
The cysteine thiolate ligand (Cys 357) liganded to the heme iron is shown in the top of the figure and the space-filling model shows the camphor in the active site of the cytochrome $P450_{cam}$. Generated by Dr. John Salerno from Dr. Tom Poulos' $P450_{cam}$ structure using Biosym's Insight program run on a Silicon Graphics Indigo Extreme platform.

iron or (2) a penta-coordinated high-spin state. Low- and high-spin states are descriptions of the electronic shells within the iron atom. When a cytochrome P450 molecule binds a substrate, there is a perturbation of the structure surrounding heme iron such that a more positive reduction potential (−170 mV) results than in the absence of substrate (−270 mV). This accelerates the rate at which cytochrome P450 may be reduced by electrons donated from NADPH through the flavoprotein enzyme **NADPH–cytochrome P450 reductase** (Figure 23.3). In order for **hydroxylation** (monooxygenation) to occur, heme iron must be reduced from the ferric (Fe^{3+}) to its ferrous (Fe^{2+}) state so that oxygen may bind to the heme iron. A total of two electrons is required for the **monooxygenation reaction.** Electrons are transferred to the cytochrome P450 molecule individually, the first to allow oxygen binding and the second to cleave the oxygen molecule to generate the active oxygen species for insertion into the reaction site of the substrate.

23.3 ■ CYTOCHROMES P450: MULTIPLE FORMS

Since the mid-1950s it has been known that one atom of molecular O_2 is inserted into a substrate being metabolized. This process of monooxygenation is also performed by other specialized proteins such as flavoprotein monooxygenases (hydroxylases). None of the other proteins classified as **oxygenases,** however, displays the versatility of the members of the cytochrome P450 family. In the past decade, information on the sequence and structure of cytochromes P450 has led to a further understanding of their evolution and regulation.

Multiplicity of Genes Produces Many Forms of Cytochrome P450

Many cytochrome P450 forms have emerged due to **gene duplication** events occurring in the last 5–50 million years. The different forms of cytochrome P450 among various animal species have likely arisen from the selective pressure of environmental influences, such as dietary habits or exposure to environmental agents. It is logical that the primordial genes gave rise to those cytochromes P450 that metabolized endogenous substrates. Examination of the phylogenetic tree, generated by comparing amino acid sequences and assuming a constant evolutionary change rate, leads to the conclusion that the earliest cytochromes P450 evolved to metabolize cholesterol and fatty acids. Therefore they may have played a role in the maintenance of membrane integrity in early eukaryotes.

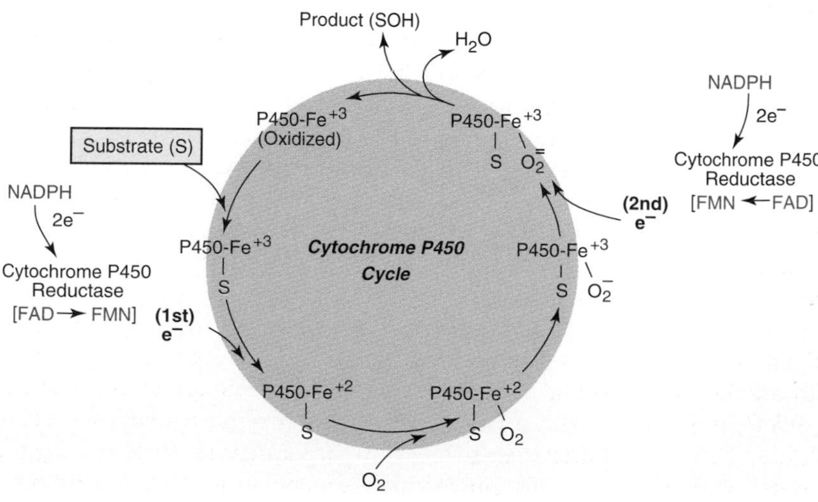

FIGURE 23.3
Sequence of reactions at cytochrome P450.
Diagram demonstrates the binding of substrate, transfer of the first and second electrons from NADPH–cytochrome P450 reductase, and binding of molecular oxygen.

Substrate Specificity

By the mid-1990s, nucleotide sequences for over 300 cytochrome P450 genes, coding for different proteins catalyzing the oxygenation of a variety of endogenous and exogenous substrates, had been characterized. There remain other members of this **gene superfamily** for which sequences have not yet been determined. One of the ways of characterizing these enzymes is the determination of **substrate specificity.** While this has been possible with many of the members of this family, the similarity of molecular weights and other molecular properties has made purification of individual cytochromes P450 from the same organ or even the same subcellular organelle very difficult, if not impossible. One way of determining the substrate specificity of a cytochrome P450 has been to express the cDNA for the particular protein via an expression vector in an appropriate cellular **expression system** in which that specific cytochrome P450 form is not expressed constitutively. This has been achieved in bacterial, insect, yeast, and mammalian cell systems and permits the unequivocal determination of substrate specificity uncomplicated by impurities of protein purification. The assumption is that knowing the nucleotide sequences of the expressed genes leaves little doubt as to the source of enzyme activity expressed in those cells.

Induction of Cytochromes P450

Induction of various cytochromes P450 by both endogenous and exogenous compounds has been known since the mid-1960s. The mechanisms of induction of cytochromes P450 have been demonstrated to be at either the **transcriptional** or **posttranscriptional** level and it is not possible to predict the mode of induction based on the inducing compound. For example, a single cytochrome P450 can be induced by different mechanisms. In one case, induction occurs at the transcriptional level and, in the other, it involves posttranscriptional events, that is, stabilization of mRNA. An example of the complexity of the induction process occurs with rat CYP2E1 as a result of treatment with small organic molecules, such as ethanol, acetone, or pyrazole, or during fasting or diabetic conditions. Administration of these small organic compounds produces larger amounts of the CYP2E1 protein without affecting the levels of mRNA. While the mechanism is not completely understood, pyrazole may stabilize this specific cytochrome P450 from proteolytic degradation. However, in diabetic rats the sixfold induction of CYP2E1 protein is accompanied by a tenfold increase in mRNA in the absence of an increase in gene transcription, suggesting stabilization of the mRNA.

The role of specific cytosolic receptor proteins has been indicated in the case of some of the known inducing agents. One of the most extensively studied is the interaction of **2,3,7,8-tetrachlorodibenzo-*p*-dioxin** (TCDD) with its cytosolic receptor, called the **aryl hydrocarbon (or Ah) receptor,** which functions in the induction of CYP1A1 and CYP1A2 forms. **Polycyclic aromatic hydrocarbons** serve as ligands which bind to the Ah receptor, producing a complex that is translocated to the nucleus and is involved in binding to the upstream regulatory regions (specific **response elements**) of cytochrome P450 genes. A second protein called the **Ah receptor nuclear translocator** or **Arnt protein** was found to interact with the ligand bound Ah receptor. The Arnt protein was essential for enabling this ligand–Ah receptor complex to recognize and bind to its specific DNA response element. Utilizing cytochrome P450 gene transfection and expression vector technology, it has been possible to express those portions of the cytochrome P450 genomic DNA representing the RNA polymerase II promoter region and the upstream DNA sequences in conjunction with another gene coding for an enzyme that is not expressed constitutively in eukaryotes. In an assay of the prokaryotic enzyme activity, for example, chloramphenicol acetyltransferase (CAT) in the expression system, it is possible to determine which specific nucleotide sequences of DNA are involved in

CLINICAL CORRELATION 23.1

Consequences of Induction of Drug-Metabolizing Enzymes

Induction of the cytochrome P450 system may result in altered efficacy of therapeutic drugs, as the accelerated rate of hydroxylation will increase the inactivation and/or enhance the excretion rate of drugs. Induction of this protein system may also produce unexpected and unwanted side effects of therapeutic agents due to increased formation of toxic metabolites that may cause cell injury if produced in large enough concentrations. The induction of different cytochrome P450 forms by a drug may stimulate the metabolism of itself or other drugs that are substrates for the cytochrome P450 system. Clinical problems may develop as a consequence of cytochrome P450 induction.

The increase in clearance of oral contraceptives by rifampicin, an antituberculosis drug and CYP3A4 inducer, has been shown to decrease the effectiveness of the contraceptive agent and increase the incidence of pregnancy in women who are prescribed both drugs. Fatalities have been reported in patients who are simultaneously treated with phenobarbital, a long-acting sedative and potent cytochrome P450 inducer, and warfarin, an anticoagulant, which is prescribed to patients with clotting disorders. Higher doses of warfarin are required in these patients to maintain the same effective concentration of the drug to delay coagulation because warfarin is a substrate for the cytochrome P450 induced by phenobarbital. Consequently, the drug is metabolized and cleared at a faster rate, which reduces its therapeutic efficacy. Clinical problems are created when phenobarbital is removed from the treatment regimen with no corresponding decrease in warfarin levels. With time, cytochrome P450 levels decrease to the noninduced state but the high concentrations of warfarin, proper under conditions of accelerated metabolism and clearance, are in excess and produce unwanted hemorrhaging.

Induction of CYP2E1 by chronic alcohol use has led to a warning for consumers of acetaminophen, a common over-the-counter analgesic agent, because this cytochrome P450 will metabolize acetaminophen to a toxic metabolite that may lead to liver cell damage. These represent classic examples of cytochrome P450–drug interactions that can lead to unwanted and unexpected clinical problems.

regulating these genes. These nucleotide sequences are referred to as **xenobiotic regulatory elements** or XREs.

Another much studied inducer of cytochrome P450 genes is **phenobarbital,** which increases the transcription rate of certain cytochrome P450 forms. A receptor that binds phenobarbital has not been described, but a specific DNA response element that is essential for phenobarbital-mediated induction has been identified in the upstream regulatory region of *CYP2B2* and *CYP3A1* genes. Although the mechanism by which phenobarbital increases transcription is unknown, the intracellular messenger, adenosine 2′,3′-cyclic monophosphate (cAMP), is a negative modifier, suppressing phenobarbital-mediated cytochrome P450 gene expression. An increase in cAMP levels in rat hepatocytes was found to prevent the phenobarbital-directed induction of CYP2B2 and CYP3A1 by activating protein kinase A activity. Some clinical consequences of induction of drug-metabolizing enzymes are presented in Clin. Corr. 23.1.

Polymorphisms

In addition to exposure to different inducing agents, individuals may differ in their rates of metabolism of a particular drug because of differences in the cytochrome P450 genes they possess. Different forms of a cytochrome P450 gene may exist in a given population, which will alter the functional activity of the complement of cytochromes P450. These **genetic polymorphisms** may be present in a small percentage of the population and cause an individual to be unable to metabolize a drug at a sufficient rate, thereby producing significantly elevated drug levels. These **"poor metabolizers"** may be at risk for a dose-dependent toxicity if the unmetabolized form of the drug is pharmacologically active. Examples of genetic polymorphisms in drug metabolism are described in Clin. Corr. 23.2.

23.4 ■ INHIBITORS OF CYTOCHROMES P450

Due to the many forms of cytochrome P450, it is of interest to examine the metabolic roles of these various enzymes in the organs in which they function. Several inhibitors have been utilized to demonstrate that cytochrome(s) P450 may be involved in a metabolic pathway, for example, the metabolism of steroids in the adrenal or specific reproductive organs. As has been discussed, the detection of cytochrome P450 in most tissues can be ascertained by the reduced-**carbon monoxide difference spectrum.** Carbon monoxide (CO) binds to the heme iron, in lieu of oxygen, with a much higher binding affinity and thereby is a potent inhibitor of its function. The identity of a cytochrome P450 in the catalysis of a putative substrate in a metabolic pathway rested on the reversal of CO inhibition by light at 450 nm, corresponding to the reduced-CO absorption maximum. This was first demonstrated for steroids as substrates for adrenal mitochondrial cytochromes P450 and later for drugs metabolized by liver microsomal cytochromes P450. However, this is a nonspecific inhibition characteristic of most cytochromes P450 and does not differentiate among the various forms.

More specific inhibitors are needed that can determine the role of a specific cytochrome P450 in a particular metabolic pathway. Although monospecific polyclonal and monoclonal antibodies have been developed to a number of cytochromes P450, it is not always possible to determine that a single form is responsible because of inhibition of a given reaction. The strong structural homology among the various forms may allow cross-reactivity among cytochromes P450. This is particularly true of members of the same gene family that exhibit immune cross-reactivity.

Recently, efforts have been directed to develop **mechanism-based inhibitors,** so-called **suicide substrates,** which bear strong resemblance to the sub-

CLINICAL CORRELATION 23.2

Genetic Polymorphisms of Drug-Metabolizing Enzymes

Genetic polymorphisms of cytochromes P450 result in the expression of cytochromes P450 that are nonfunctional or exhibit lower enzymatic activities. This may result in unwanted side effects because of the inability to eliminate the active form of the drug, causing elevated concentrations in the body. It may also result in the absence of a therapeutic effect because the active form of a drug is not formed.

The discovery of an individual who suffered exaggerated hypotensive effects when administered the antihypertensive drug, debrisoquine, led to the characterization of individuals who metabolized substrates catalyzed by the CYP2D6 form inefficiently. Approximately 5–10% of the Caucasian population, 2% of the Asian, and 1% of the Arabic populations were deficient for the catalytically active CYP2D6 form. In addition to debrisoquine, other drugs that are metabolized by CYP2D6 are sparteine, amitriptyline, dextromethorphan, and codeine. In the case of codeine, CYP2D6 catalyzes the *O*-demethylation of codeine to morphine. Approximately 10% of the dose of codeine is metabolized to morphine in individuals who have a normal CYP2D6 and this metabolism is responsible for the analgesic effects of this drug. Individuals who lack the normal gene for CYP2D6 are unable to catalyze this reaction and are unable to achieve the analgesic effects associated with codeine.

Another genetic polymorphism was demonstrated in individuals who were poor metabolizers of the drug mephenytoin. This drug is used in the treatment of epilepsy. Poor metabolizers of this drug suffer greater sedative effects at normal dosages. The 4-hydroxylation of the *S*-enantiomer of mephenytoin is carried out by CYP2C19. Approximately 14–22% of the Asian population are reported to be poor metabolizers of the *S*-isomer of mephenytoin whereas only 3–6% of the Caucasian population are affected. These genetic polymorphisms may explain some of the interindividual or interracial differences in the way individuals respond to therapeutic drugs.

Eichelbaum, M., and Gross, A. S. The genetic polymorphism of debrisoquine/sparteine metabolism—clinical aspects. In: W. Kalow (Ed.), *Pharmacogenetics of Drug Metabolism*. New York: Pergamon Press, 1992, Chap. 21, p. 625; and Meyer, U. A., Skoda, R. D., Zanger, U. M., Heim, M., and Broly, F. The genetic polymorphism of debrisoquine/sparteine metabolism—molecular mechanism. In: W. Kalow (Ed.), *Pharmocogenetics of Drug Metabolism*. New York: Pergamon Press, 1992, Chap. 20, p. 609.

strate(s) of the specific cytochrome P450, but which during catalytic turnover form an irreversible inhibition product with the enzyme prosthetic group or protein. Because of their structural resemblance to the substrate(s), these inhibitors become highly specific for that particular form of cytochrome P450. These inhibitors contain functional groups that are metabolized to intermediates that result in their covalent binding to the enzymes, thereby accounting for their irreversibility. This represents a possible tactical approach to drug design.

23.5 ■ CYTOCHROME P450 ELECTRON TRANSPORT SYSTEMS

Although cytochrome P450-catalyzed reactions require two electrons to accomplish the tasks of heme iron reduction, oxygen binding, and oxygen cleavage, a basic mechanistic problem is the direct and simultaneous transfer of electrons from NADPH to the cytochrome P450. Pyridine nucleotides are two electron donors (see p. 250), but cytochrome P450, with its single heme prosthetic group, may only accept one electron at a time. Thus a protein that serves to transfer electrons from NADPH to the cytochrome P450 molecule must have the capacity to accept two electrons but serve as a one-electron donor. This problem is solved by the presence of a NADPH-dependent flavoprotein reductase, which accepts two electrons from NADPH simultaneously but transfers the electrons individually either to an intermediate **iron–sulfur protein** (mitochondria) or directly to cytochrome P450 (endoplasmic reticulum). The active redox group of the flavin moiety is the isoalloxazine ring (see p. 251). The isoalloxazine nucleus is uniquely suited to perform this chemical task since it can exist in oxidized and one- and two-electron reduced states (Figure 23.4). The transfer of electrons from NADPH to cytochrome P450 is accomplished by two distinct electron transport systems that reside almost exclusively in either mitochondria or endoplasmic reticulum.

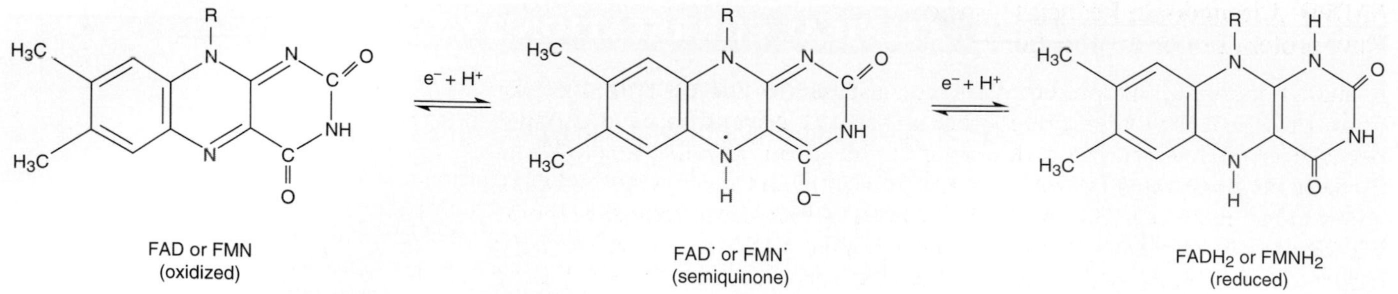

$e^- + H^+$ ⇌ $e^- + H^+$ ⇌

FAD or FMN (oxidized)

FAD˙ or FMN˙ (semiquinone)

$FADH_2$ or $FMNH_2$ (reduced)

FIGURE 23.4
Isoalloxazine ring of FMN or FAD in its oxidized, semiquinone ($1e^-$ reduced), or fully reduced ($2e^-$ reduced) states.

NADPH–Cytochrome P450 Reductase Is the Flavoprotein Donor in the Endoplasmic Reticulum

In the endoplasmic reticulum, NADPH donates electrons to a flavoprotein called NADPH–cytochrome P450 reductase. The rat enzyme has a mass of 76,962 Da and contains both flavin adenine dinucleotide (FAD) and flavin mononucleotide (FMN) as prosthetic groups. Until the recent characterization of nitric oxide synthases, it was the only mammalian flavoprotein known to contain both FAD and FMN. A significant number of residues at the amino end of the molecule are hydrophobic, and this segment of the protein is embedded in the endoplasmic reticulum (Figure 23.5). FAD serves as the entry point for electrons from NADPH, and FMN serves as the exit point, transferring electrons individually to cytochrome P450. Because the flavin molecule may exist as one- or two-electron-reduced forms and two flavin molecules are bound per reductase molecule, the enzyme may receive electrons from NADPH and store them between the two flavin molecules before transferring them individually to the cytochrome P450.

In certain reactions catalyzed by the microsomal cytochrome P450, the transfer of the second electron may not be directly from **NADPH–cytochrome P450 reductase** but may occur from **cytochrome b_5**, a small heme protein of molecular mass 15,330 Da. Cytochrome b_5 is reduced either by NADPH–cytochrome P450 reductase or another microsome-bound flavoprotein, **NADH–cytochrome b_5 reductase.** It is not known why reactions catalyzed by specific cytochromes P450 apparently require cytochrome b_5 for optimal enzymatic activity. In addition, NADH–cytochrome b_5 reductase and cytochrome b_5 constitute the electron transfer system for NADH to the iron–sulfur protein, **fatty acid desaturase,** which catalyzes the formation of double bonds in fatty acids (see p. 372).

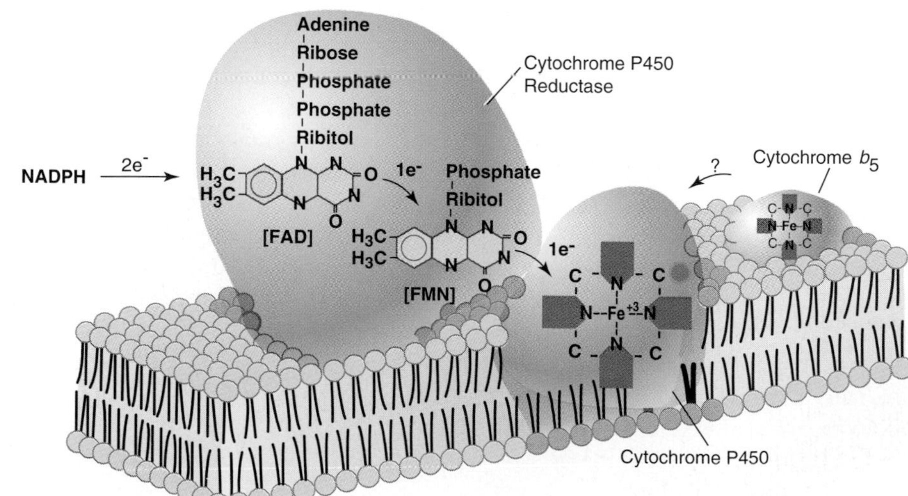

FIGURE 23.5
Components of the endoplasmic reticulum (microsomal) cytochrome P450 system.
NADPH–cytochrome P450 reductase is bound by its hydrophobic tail to the membrane, whereas cytochrome P450 is deeply embedded in the membrane. Also shown is cytochrome b_5, which may participate in selected cytochrome P450-mediated reactions.

NADPH–Adrenodoxin Reductase Is the Flavoprotein Donor in Mitochondria

In mitochondria, a flavoprotein reductase also acts as the electron acceptor from NADPH. This protein is referred to as **NADPH–adrenodoxin reductase** because its characteristics were described for the flavoprotein first isolated from the adrenal gland. This protein contains only FAD and the bovine NADPH–adrenodoxin reductase has a mass of 50,709 Da. Adrenodoxin reductase is only weakly associated with its membrane milieu, unlike NADPH–cytochrome P450 reductase of endoplasmic reticulum. Adrenodoxin reductase cannot directly transfer either the first or second electron to heme iron of cytochrome P450 (Figure 23.6). A small molecular weight protein, called **adrenodoxin** (12,500 Da), serves as an intermediate between the adrenodoxin reductase and **mitochondrial cytochrome P450.** The adrenodoxin molecule is also weakly associated with the inner mitochondrial membrane through interaction with the membrane-bound cytochrome P450. Adrenodoxin contains two iron–sulfur clusters, which serve as redox centers for this molecule and function as an electron shuttle between the adrenodoxin reductase and the mitochondrial cytochromes P450. One adrenodoxin molecule receives an electron from its mitochondrial flavoprotein reductase and interacts with a second adrenodoxin, which then transfers its electron to the cytochrome P450 (Figure 23.6). Components of the mitochondrial cytochrome P450 system are synthesized in the cytosol as larger molecular weight precursors, transported into mitochondria, and processed by proteases into smaller molecular weight, mature proteins.

23.6 PHYSIOLOGICAL FUNCTIONS OF CYTOCHROMES P450

Cytochromes P450 metabolize a variety of lipophilic compounds of endogenous or exogenous origin. These enzymes may catalyze simple hydroxylations of the carbon atom of a methyl group, insertion of a hydroxyl group into a methylene carbon of an alkane, hydroxylation of an aromatic ring to form a phenol, or addition of an oxygen atom across a double bond to form an **epoxide.** In dealkylation reactions, the oxygen is inserted into the carbon–hydrogen bond, but the resulting product is unstable and rearranges to the primary alcohol, amine, or sulfhydryl compound. Oxidation of nitrogen, sulfur, and phosphorus atoms and dehalogenation reactions are also catalyzed by cytochromes P450. Reactions catalyzed by cytochrome P450 forms are shown in Figure 23.7.

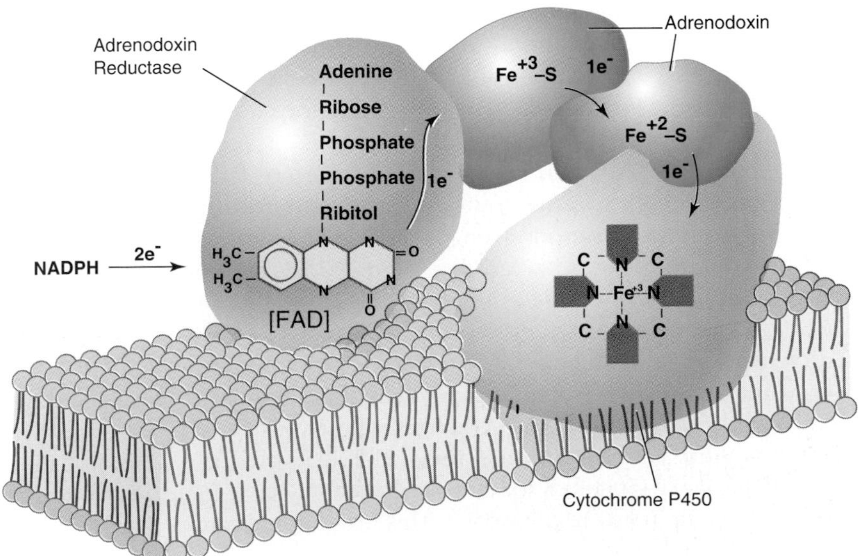

FIGURE 23.6
Components of mitochondrial cytochrome P450 system.
Cytochrome P450 is an integral protein of the inner mitochondrial membrane. NADPH–adrenodoxin reductase and adrenodoxin (ADR) are peripheral proteins and are not embedded in the membrane.

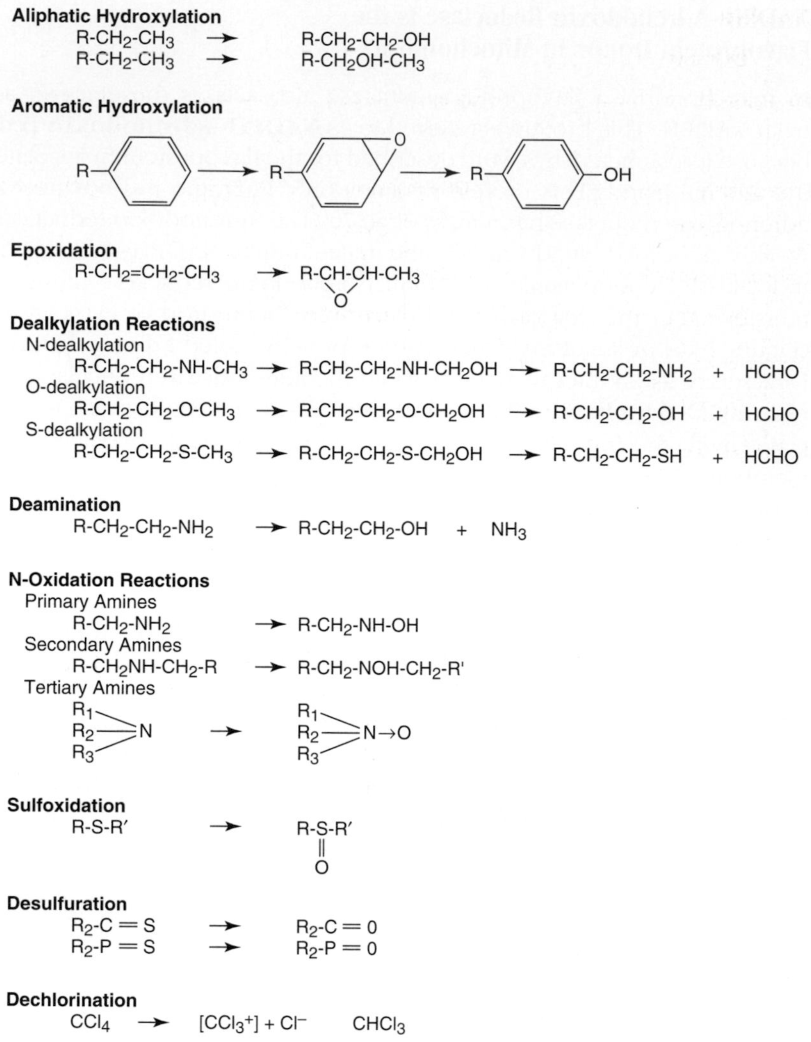

Aliphatic Hydroxylation

$R\text{-}CH_2\text{-}CH_3 \rightarrow R\text{-}CH_2\text{-}CH_2\text{-}OH$

$R\text{-}CH_2\text{-}CH_3 \rightarrow R\text{-}CH_2OH\text{-}CH_3$

Aromatic Hydroxylation

R–(benzene ring) → R–(benzene ring epoxide, O) → R–(benzene ring)–OH

Epoxidation

$R\text{-}CH_2\text{=}CH_2\text{-}CH_3 \rightarrow R\text{-}CH\text{-}CH\text{-}CH_3$ (with O bridging the two CH carbons)

Dealkylation Reactions

N-dealkylation

$R\text{-}CH_2\text{-}CH_2\text{-}NH\text{-}CH_3 \rightarrow R\text{-}CH_2\text{-}CH_2\text{-}NH\text{-}CH_2OH \rightarrow R\text{-}CH_2\text{-}CH_2\text{-}NH_2 + HCHO$

O-dealkylation

$R\text{-}CH_2\text{-}CH_2\text{-}O\text{-}CH_3 \rightarrow R\text{-}CH_2\text{-}CH_2\text{-}O\text{-}CH_2OH \rightarrow R\text{-}CH_2\text{-}CH_2\text{-}OH + HCHO$

S-dealkylation

$R\text{-}CH_2\text{-}CH_2\text{-}S\text{-}CH_3 \rightarrow R\text{-}CH_2\text{-}CH_2\text{-}S\text{-}CH_2OH \rightarrow R\text{-}CH_2\text{-}CH_2\text{-}SH + HCHO$

Deamination

$R\text{-}CH_2\text{-}CH_2\text{-}NH_2 \rightarrow R\text{-}CH_2\text{-}CH_2\text{-}OH + NH_3$

N-Oxidation Reactions

Primary Amines

$R\text{-}CH_2\text{-}NH_2 \rightarrow R\text{-}CH_2\text{-}NH\text{-}OH$

Secondary Amines

$R\text{-}CH_2NH\text{-}CH_2\text{-}R \rightarrow R\text{-}CH_2\text{-}NOH\text{-}CH_2\text{-}R'$

Tertiary Amines

$R_1R_2R_3N \rightarrow R_1R_2R_3N \rightarrow O$

Sulfoxidation

$R\text{-}S\text{-}R' \rightarrow R\text{-}S(=O)\text{-}R'$

Desulfuration

$R_2\text{-}C=S \rightarrow R_2\text{-}C=0$

$R_2\text{-}P=S \rightarrow R_2\text{-}P=0$

Dechlorination

$CCl_4 \rightarrow [CCl_3^+] + Cl^- \quad CHCl_3$

FIGURE 23.7
Reaction types catalyzed by cytochromes P450.

Cytochromes P450 Participate in Synthesis of Steroid Hormones and Oxygenation of Eicosanoids

The importance of cytochrome P450-catalyzed reactions is illustrated by the synthesis of **steroid hormones** from cholesterol in the adrenal cortex and sex organs. Mitochondrial and endoplasmic reticulum cytochrome P450 systems are required to metabolize cholesterol stepwise into **aldosterone** and **cortisol** in adrenal cortex, **testosterone** in testes, and **estradiol** in ovaries.

Cytochromes P450 are responsible for several steps in the adrenal synthesis of aldosterone, the mineralocorticoid responsible for regulating salt and water balance, and cortisol, the glucocorticoid that governs protein, carbohydrate, and lipid metabolism. In addition, adrenal cytochromes P450 catalyze the synthesis of small quantities of the androgen, **androstenedione,** a precursor of both estrogens and testosterone (see p. 900). Production of androstenedione regulates secondary sex characteristics. Figure 23.8 presents a summary of these pathways.

In adrenal mitochondria, a cytochrome P450 (CYP11A1) catalyzes the **side chain cleavage** converting cholesterol to pregnenolone, a committed step in steroid synthesis. The removal of isocaproic aldehyde results from a cytochrome P450-catalyzed reaction involving sequential hydroxylation at C-22 and C-20 to produce 22-hydroxycholesterol and then 20,22-dihydroxycholesterol (Figure 23.9). An additional P450-catalyzed step is necessary to cleave the bond between C-20 and C-22 to produce pregnenolone. This reaction sequence, which requires

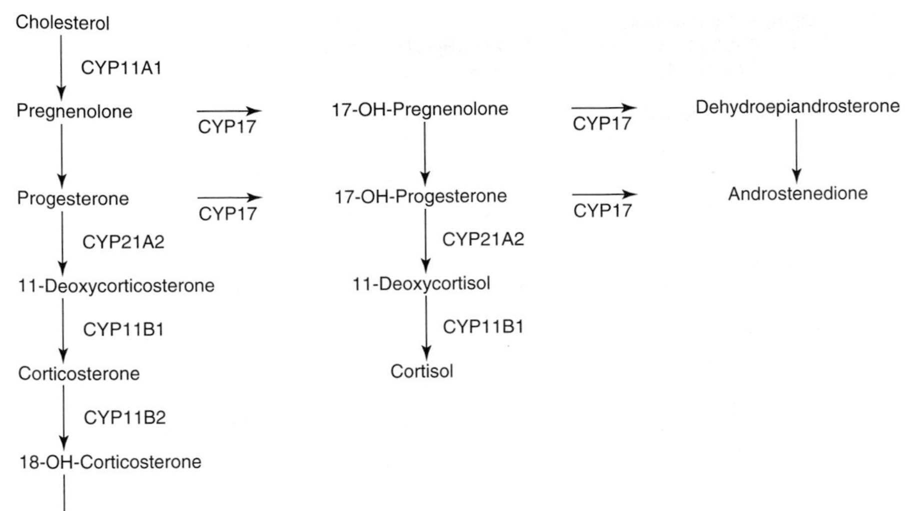

FIGURE 23.8
Steroid hormone synthesis in the adrenal gland.
The reactions catalyzed by cytochromes P450 (CYP) are indicated.

3 NADPH and 3 O_2 molecules, results in the breakage of a carbon–carbon bond and is catalyzed by a single cytochrome P450 enzyme, CYP11A1. After pregnenolone is produced in mitochondria, it is transported into the cytosol where it is oxidized by 3β-hydroxysteroid dehydrogenase/$\Delta^{4,5}$-isomerase to progesterone. Progesterone is metabolized to **11-deoxycorticosterone (DOC)** by an endoplasmic reticulum cytochrome P450 **(CYP21),** which catalyzes the 21-hydroxylation reaction. DOC is hydroxylated by an additional mitochondrial

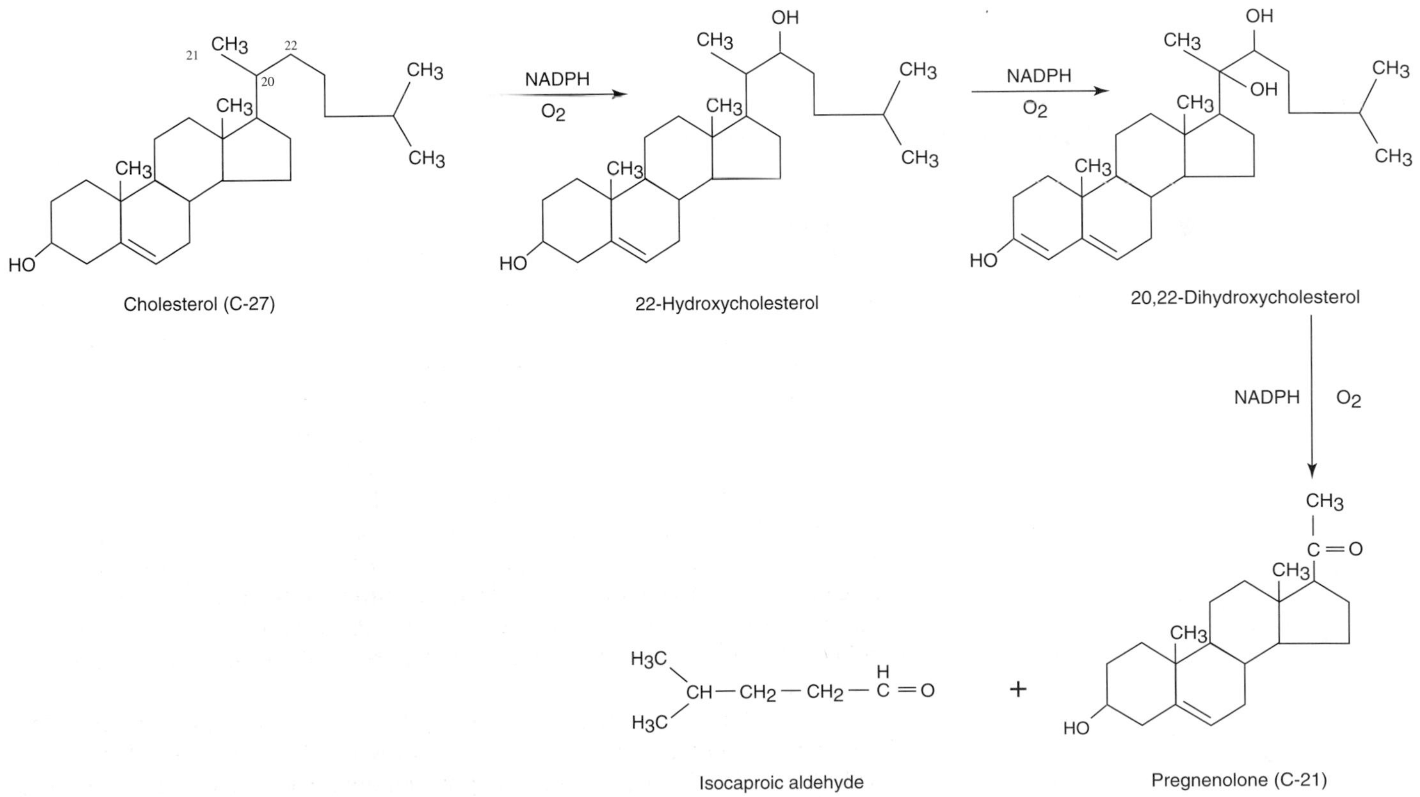

Cholesterol (C-27) → (NADPH, O_2) → 22-Hydroxycholesterol → (NADPH, O_2) → 20,22-Dihydroxycholesterol → (NADPH, O_2) → Isocaproic aldehyde + Pregnenolone (C-21)

FIGURE 23.9
Side chain cleavage reaction of cholesterol.
Three sequential reactions are catalyzed by cytochrome P450 to produce pregnenolone and isocaproic aldehyde.

cytochrome P450 **(CYP11B2),** which catalyzes both the 11β-hydroxylase and 18-hydroxylase activities to form the mineralocorticoid, aldosterone, in the zona glomerulosa (Chapter 21, p. 899).

Synthesis of cortisol proceeds from either pregnenolone or progesterone and involves a cytochrome P450 **(CYP17),** an endoplasmic reticulum cytochrome P450, which catalyzes the 17α-hydroxylation reaction. Hydroxylation of the C-21 of 17α-hydroxyprogesterone by CYP21 produces 11-deoxycortisol, which is transported into mitochondria where it is hydroxylated at carbon atom 11 by **CYP11B1** to form cortisol. These reactions occur primarily in the zona fasciculata of the adrenal cortex. The consequences of a genetic polymorphism in CYP21 is presented in Clin. Corr. 23.3.

Synthesis of steroids containing 19 carbon atoms from 17α-hydroxypregnenolone or 17α-hydroxyprogesterone is the result of the loss of the acetyl group at C-17. This reaction is catalyzed by CYP17, identified as the same cytochrome P450 that hydroxylates C-17. Thus cleavage of the bond between C-17 and C-20 with loss of the acetyl group is also catalyzed by a cytochrome P450 molecule. The factors that determine whether this cytochrome P450 performs only a single hydroxylation step to produce the 17-OH product or proceeds further to cleave the C-17–C-20 bond has not been determined. The products are **dehydroepiandrosterone** (DHEA) from 17α-hydroxypregnenolone or androstenedione from 17α-hydroxyprogesterone. DHEA in the sex organs may be metabolized by dehydrogenation of the 3-OH group to androstenedione, a potent androgenic steroid that serves as the immediate precursor of testosterone.

Another physiologically important reaction catalyzed by cytochromes P450 is synthesis of estrogens from androgens, collectively called **aromatization** because an aromatic ring is introduced into the product. This is a complex reaction not unlike the side chain cleavage of cholesterol in which multiple hydroxylation reactions are carried out by a single cytochrome P450 enzyme to form the aromatic ring and remove the methyl group at C-19. Figure 23.10 outlines the aromatization reaction of ring A. Two cytochrome P450-mediated hydroxylation reactions at the methyl carbon atom at position 19 introduce an aldehyde group. It has been proposed that the final step involves a peroxidative attack at C-19 with loss of the methyl group and elimination of the hydrogen atom to produce the aromatic ring. The reaction steps of this sequence are catalyzed by the same cytochrome P450 and the enzyme is called aromatase or $P450_{arom}$. $P450_{arom}$ is a member of the CYP19 subfamily. The complexity of steroid hormone production and the role of cytochromes P450 are illustrated in Clin. Corr. 23.4.

Other cytochromes P450 metabolize **vitamin D_3** to produce the **1,25-dihydroxy vitamin D_3,** which is the active form of this important hormone (see p. 907), leukotriene B_4 to produce 20-hydroxy-leukotriene B_4, which is the less active form of this chemotactic agent (see p. 438), and arachidonic acid to produce epoxides, hydroxy and dihydroxy derivatives of arachidonic acid, which may have important regulatory functions (see p. 433).

CLINICAL CORRELATION 23.3

Deficiency of Cytochrome P450 Steroid 21-Hydroxylase (CYP21A2)

The adrenal cortex is a major site of steroid hormone production during fetal and adult life. The adrenal gland is metabolically more active in fetal life and may produce 100–200 mg of steroids per day in comparison to the 20–30 mg produced per day in the nonstressed adult adrenal gland. A number of enzymes are required for the production of cortisol, and enzyme deficiencies have been reported at all steps of cortisol production. Diseases associated with insufficient cortisol production are referred to as congenital adrenal hyperplasias (CAHs). The enzyme deficiency that is most common in CAH is the cytochrome P450-dependent 21-hydroxylase or CYP21A2. A deficiency in a functional 21-hydroxylase enzyme prevents the metabolism of 17α-hydroxyprogesterone to 11-deoxycortisol and subsequently to cortisol. This causes an increase in ACTH secretion, the pituitary hormone that regulates adrenal cortex production of cortisol. Prolonged periods of elevated ACTH levels causes adrenal hyperplasia and an increased production of the androgenic hormones, DHEA and androstenedione. Clinical problems arise because the additional production of androgenic steroids causes virilization in females, precocious sex organ development in prepubertal males, or diseases related to salt imbalance because of decreased levels of aldosterone. Clinical consequences of severe 21-hydroxylase deficiency may be recognizable at birth, particularly in females, because the excessive buildup of androgenic steroids may cause obvious irregular development of their genitalia. In male newborns, a deficiency in 21-hydroxylase activity may be overlooked, because male genitalia will appear normal, but there will be precocious masculinization and physical development. In late onset CAH, individuals are born without obvious signs of prenatal exposure to excessive androgen levels, and clinical symptoms may vary considerably from early development of pubic hair, early fusion of epiphyseal growth plates causing premature cessation of growth, or male baldness patterns in females.

Donohoue, P. A., Parker, K., and Migeon, C. J. Congenital adrenal hyperplasia. In: C. S. Scriver, A. L. Beaudet, W. S. Sly, and D. Valle (Eds.), *The Metabolic and Molecular Bases of Inherited Disease,* 7th ed., Vol. II. New York; McGraw-Hill, 1995, Chap. 94, p. 2929.

Cytochromes P450 Oxidize Exogenous Lipophilic Substrates

Exogenous substrates are often referred to as **xenobiotics,** meaning "foreign to life." They include therapeutic drugs, chemicals used in the workplace, industrial by-products that become environmental contaminants, and food additives. Cytochromes P450 oxidize a variety of xenobiotics, particularly lipophilic compounds. The addition of a hydroxyl group makes the compound more polar and thus more soluble in the aqueous environment of the cell. Many exogenous compounds are highly lipophilic and accumulate within cells, interfering with cellular function over a period of time. Examples of xenobiotics that are oxidized by cytochromes P450 are presented in Tables 23.2 and 23.3 (p. 994). In many cases the action of the cytochromes P450 leads to a compound

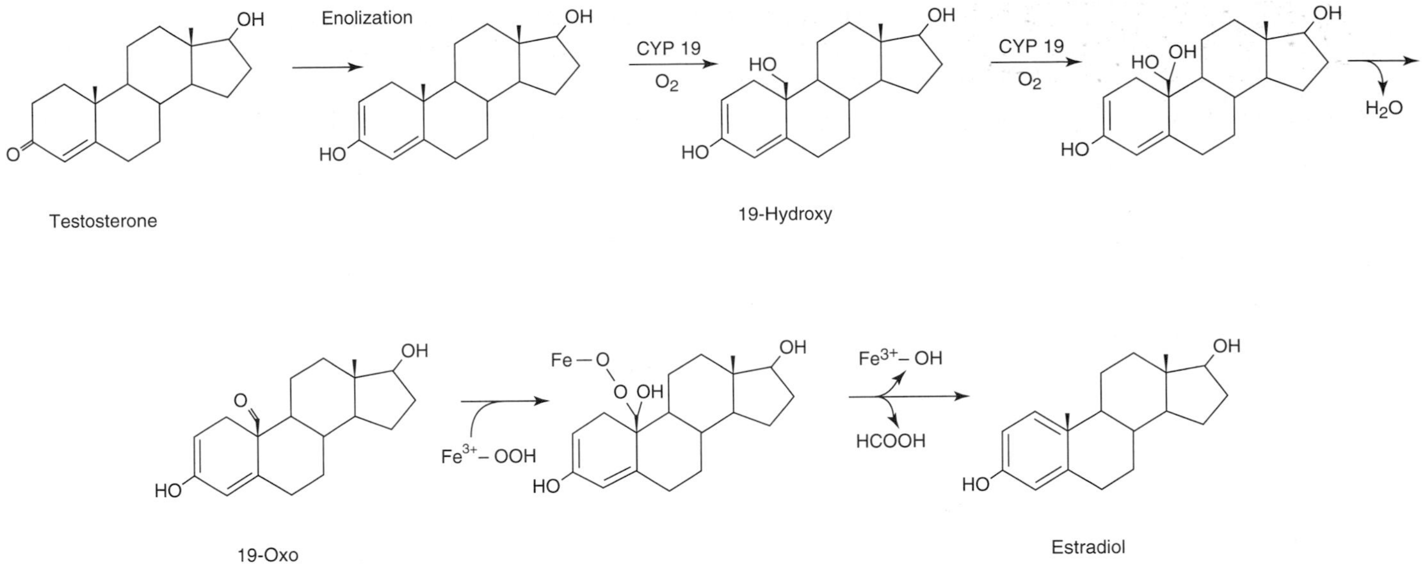

Testosterone → (Enolization) → (CYP 19, O_2) → 19-Hydroxy → (CYP 19, O_2) → (H_2O) → 19-Oxo → (Fe^{3+}–OOH) → (Fe^{3+}–OH, HCOOH) → Estradiol

FIGURE 23.10
Sequence of reactions leading to aromatization of androgens to estrogens.
Adapted from Graham-Lorence, S., Amarneh, B., White, R. E., Peterson, J. A., and Simpson E. R. Protein Sci. *4:1065, 1995.*

with reduced pharmacological activity or toxicity, which can readily be excreted in the urine or bile. Modified and unmodified xenobiotics can be altered chemically by a variety of conjugating enzyme systems forming products that are even less toxic and that can readily be eliminated from the body. A list of enzymes that metabolize xenobiotics is presented in Table 23.3; many occur primarily in the liver.

One xenobiotic that has received considerable attention is **benzo[*a*]pyrene,** a common environmental contaminant produced from the burning of

CLINICAL CORRELATION 23.4

Steroid Hormone Production During Pregnancy

Steroid hormone production increases dramatically during pregnancy and, at term, the pregnant woman produces 15–20 mg of estradiol, 50–100 mg of estriol, and approximately 250 mg of progesterone per 24-h period. The amount of estrogens synthesized during pregnancy far exceeds the amount synthesized by nonpregnant women. For example, the pregnant woman at the end of gestation produces 1000 times more estrogen than premenopausal women per day.

Production of progesterone and estrogens in pregnant women is decidedly different from that in the nonpregnant woman. The corpus luteum of the ovary is the major site for estrogen production in the first few weeks of pregnancy, but at approximately 4 weeks of gestation, the placenta begins synthesizing and secreting progesterone and estrogens. After 8 weeks of gestation, the placenta becomes the dominant source for the synthesis of progesterone. An interesting difference between the steroid hydroxylating systems in the placenta and the ovary is that the human placenta lacks the cytochrome P450 (CYP11A1) that catalyzes the 17α-hydroxylation reaction and the cleavage of the 17,20 carbon–carbon bond (see Chapter 21, p. 898, for details of synthesis of steroid hormones). Thus the placenta cannot, by itself, synthesize estrogens from cholesterol. The placenta catalyzes the side chain cleavage reaction to form pregnenolone from cholesterol and oxidizes pregnenolone to progesterone but releases this hormone into the maternal circulation. How then does the placenta produce estrogens if it cannot synthesize DHEA or androstenedione from progesterone? This is accomplished in the fetal adrenal gland, which represents a significant proportion of the total fetal weight compared to its adult state. The fetal adrenal gland catalyzes the synthesis of DHEA from cholesterol and releases it into the fetal circulation. A large proportion of the fetal DHEA is metabolized by the fetal liver to 16α-hydroxy-DHEA, and this product is aromatized in the placenta to the estrogen, estriol. This is an elegant demonstration of the cooperativity of the cytochrome P450-mediated hydroxylating systems in the fetal and maternal organ systems leading to the progressive formation of estrogens during the gestational development of the human fetus.

Cunningham, F. G., MacDonald, P. C., Gant, N. F., Leveno, K. J., and Gilstrap, L. C. The placental hormones. In: *Williams Obstetrics,* 19th ed. East Norwalk, CT: Appleton & Lange, 1993, Chap. 6, p. 139.

TABLE 23.2 Xenobiotics Metabolized by Cytochromes P450

Reaction	*Examples*
Aliphatic hydroxylation	Valproic acid, pentobarbital
Aromatic hydroxylation	Debrisoquine, acetanilide
Epoxidation	Benzene, benzo[*a*]pyrene
Dealkylation	Aminopyrine, phenacetin, 6-methyl-thiopurine
Oxidative deamination	Amphetamine
Nitrogen or sulfur oxidation	2-Acetylaminofluorene, chlorpromazine
Dehalogenation	Halothane
Alcohol oxidation	Ethanol

coal, from the combustion of plant materials in tobacco, from food barbecued on charcoal, and as an industrial by-product. Benzo[*a*]pyrene binds to the **aryl hydrocarbon receptor** and induces cytochromes P450 in the 1A subfamily, thus increasing its own metabolism. Several sites of the molecule may be hydroxylated by different forms of cytochrome P450. Benzo[*a*]pyrene is metabolized to a **carcinogen** in animals and a mutagen in bacteria, prompting considerable work in identifying the enzymes involved in this process. The product found to represent the ultimate carcinogen is **benzo[*a*]pyrene-7,8-dihydrodiol-9,10-epoxide,** the formation of which is illustrated in Figure 23.11. The initial step involves a cytochrome P450-catalyzed epoxidation at the 7,8 position, hydrolysis by **epoxide hydrolase** to the vicinal hydroxylated compound, benzo[*a*]pyrene-7,8-dihydrodiol, and then another epoxidation reaction to form benzo[*a*]pyrene-7,8-dihydrodiol-9,10-epoxide. The parent compound, benzo[*a*]pyrene, is a weak carcinogen and, like most carcinogens that have been characterized, requires metabolic activation to its more potent carcinogenic form.

In a number of cases, the cytochrome P450 system is responsible for generation of the ultimate carcinogen. Formation of toxic compounds by the cytochrome P450 system, however, does not mean that cell damage or cancer will occur, because many other factors will determine whether or not the toxic metabolite will cause cell injury. These include the involvement of detoxification enzyme systems, the status of the immune system, nutritional state, genetic predisposition, and environmental factors. One may ask why the body should possess an enzyme system that would create highly toxic compounds? As indi-

TABLE 23.3 Xenobiotic-Metabolizing Enzymes

Type of Reaction	*Enzyme*	*Representative Substrate*
Oxidation	Cytochrome P450	Toluene
	Alcohol dehydrogenase	Ethyl alcohol
	Flavin-containing monooxygenase	Dimethylaniline
Reduction	Ketone reductase	Metyrapone
Hydration	Epoxide hydrolase	Benzo[*a*]pyrene-7,8-epoxide
Hydrolysis	Esterase	Procaine
Conjugation	UDP-glucuronyltransferase	Acetaminophen
	Sulfotransferase	β-Naphthol
	N-acetyltransferase	Sulfanilamide
	Methyltransferase	Thiouracil
	Glutathionetransferase	Acetaminophen

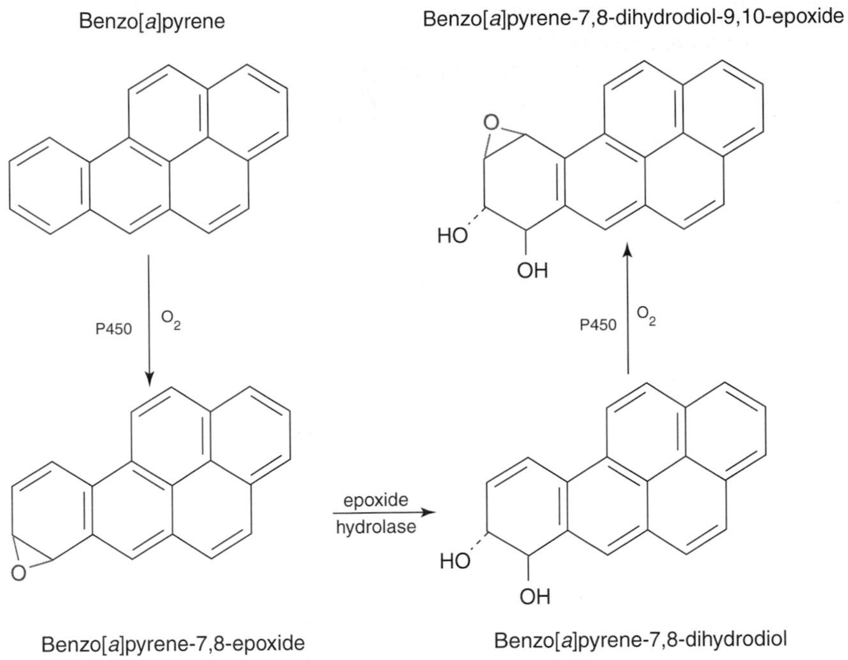

Benzo[*a*]pyrene

Benzo[*a*]pyrene-7,8-dihydrodiol-9,10-epoxide

P450 O_2

epoxide hydrolase

Benzo[*a*]pyrene-7,8-epoxide

Benzo[*a*]pyrene-7,8-dihydrodiol

FIGURE 23.11
Metabolism of benzo[*a*]pyrene by cytochrome P450 and epoxide hydrolase to form benzo[*a*]pyrene-7,8-dihydrodiol-9,10-epoxide.

cated, the purpose of the cytochrome P450 system is to add or expose functional groups making the molecule more polar and/or more susceptible to attack by additional detoxification enzyme systems. In addition, many of these compounds resemble hormones that are our natural communication signals and would interfere with cell–cell or organ–organ communication.

Thus the cytochrome P450 system plays a significant role in the health and disease of humans. Different cytochromes P450 are responsible for generation of essential steroid hormones, the regulation of blood levels of therapeutic agents, the removal of unwanted chemicals that would accumulate because of their lipophilicity, and the generation of potentially toxic metabolites that may cause acute cell injury or damage to genetic material and lead to production of tumors.

23.7 OTHER HEMOPROTEIN- AND FLAVOPROTEIN-MEDIATED OXYGENATIONS: THE NITRIC OXIDE SYNTHASES

Three Distinct Nitric Oxide Synthase Gene Products Display Diverse Physiological Functions

Release of nitric oxide from therapeutic drugs has been used as a treatment for angina pectoris since 1867, when Sir Thomas Lauder Brunton reported the use of nitroglycerin and amyl nitrate in his patients. However, it was not known until the 1980s that **nitric oxide,** or NO·, was the active agent in the dilation of blood vessels. The demonstration that this free radical diatomic gas was the primary endogenous vasodilator released by the vascular endothelium led to the search for an enzymatic source of NO·. The source of NO· is the guanidino group of the naturally occurring amino acid, L-arginine. The reaction catalyzed by the enzymes responsible for the conversion of L-arginine to L-citrulline and NO· is shown below:

$$\text{L-Arginine} + \text{NADPH} \rightarrow \text{L-citrulline} + \text{NO}\cdot + \text{NADP}^+$$

Nitric oxide synthases have been examined in whole animals, tissues, and cells for functional properties and recently three genes have been identified for

CLINICAL CORRELATION 23.5

Clinical Aspects of Nitric Oxide Production

Although the role of NO• in the tumoricidal and bactericidal functions of macrophages is essential in these cells, the overproduction of NO• (from the inducible isoform of nitric oxide synthase, iNOS or NOS-II) has been implicated in septic/cytokine-induced circulatory shock in humans through the activation of guanylate cyclase. This mechanism is responsible for profound hypotension in patients after abdominal surgery or abdominal trauma complicated by bacterial infections that produce endotoxins, as well as in patients with neoplasias treated by IL-2 chemotherapy. Hypotension in these patients is often refractory to treatment with conventional vasoconstrictor drugs. Therapeutic interventions using NOS inhibitors are being examined in gastrointestinal inflammatory diseases, such as pancreatitis and ulcerative colitis, and in arthritis. Administration of NOS inhibitors (e.g., specific to iNOS) might be a treatment of choice in such patients.

The endothelial isoform of nitric oxide synthase, eNOS or NOS-III, is thought to play a critical role in maintaining a basic vasotonus in hemodynamic regulation such that an imbalance in the production of NO• could result in hypertension, thrombosis, or atherosclerosis. Direct application of NO• gas may also be beneficial in the treatment of pulmonary hypertension. In addition, recent experiments with mice in which the gene for the neuronal isoform of nitric oxide synthase, nNOS or NOS-I, has been deleted have resulted in animals with distended stomachs due to constriction of the pyloric sphincter. This work has unexpectedly produced a model for the clinical disease, infantile hypertrophic pyloric stenosis. It has also been shown that these nNOS-deficient mice are resistant to brain damage as a result of ischemic injury usually resulting in vascular strokes. While the direct connection to human disease has not yet been made, in this instance, it presents a paradigm that can now be examined in clinical and pathological settings.

The development of potent, specific inhibitors of the isoforms of nitric oxide synthase is an active area of research being pursued collaboratively by investigators in academia and the pharmaceutical industry.

the isoforms responsible for the activities in various tissues. Accordingly, the respective enzymes have been designated as **neuronal (NOS-I), macrophage** or **induced (NOS-II),** or **endothelial (NOS-III).** Any tissue or cell may contain more than one isoform of nitric oxide synthase, thus contributing to the production of NO• under various physiological circumstances. Studies of the macrophage type of nitric oxide synthase led to the conclusion that, upon treatment of animals with cytokines or lipopolysaccharide, the increase in production of NO• was due to this isoform, since it is quantitatively the major source of NO•. Subsequently, L-arginine was shown to be the precursor of NO• in both endothelial and neuronal cells. Production of NO• is necessary for maintenance of vascular tone, platelet aggregation, neural transmission, and bacterial and/or tumor cytotoxicity (see Clin. Corr. 23.5).

As further evidence of the importance of heme enzymes, signaling events require binding to the heme prosthetic group of guanylate cyclase of NO• produced in neuronal and endothelial cells for activation of signaling events. The formation of cGMP leads to the subsequent downregulation of intracellular **Ca^{2+}** concentrations and to a cellular response appropriate to the specific cell involved. For example, the production of cGMP in vascular smooth muscle cells resulting from NO• production leads to the lowering of Ca^{2+} concentrations, resulting in vasodilatation due to smooth muscle relaxation.

Structural Aspects of Nitric Oxide Synthases

Although the written reaction does not reveal the overall stoichiometry, it is representative of a monooxygenation reaction and the mechanism is similar to that catalyzed by cytochromes P450. The oxygen atoms incorporated into both L-citrulline and NO• are derived from atmospheric oxygen. It was originally assumed that oxygenation was occurring through mediation of **tetrahydrobiopterin (BH_4),** a required cofactor for the overall reaction, analogous to the phenylalanine hydroxylase reaction (see p. 464). The discovery that **heme** (iron protoporphyrin IX) is a functional prosthetic group associated with all three isoforms of nitric oxide synthase has directed subsequent studies to include interactions between the flavoprotein and hemoprotein domains of these enzymes. These complex proteins must now be understood from the standpoint of the roles of the flavins, heme, and BH_4, under the control of Ca^{2+}/calmodulin in the case of the neuronal (NOS-I) and endothelial (NOS-II) isoforms. Figure 23.12 shows the overall structural organization of the neuronal NOS isoform. In addition to the various protein modules or domains of NOS-I which are involved in electron transfer, substrate binding, oxygen activation, and calcium binding, a four-amino acid motif (glycine–leucine–glycine–phenylalanine, GLGF) has been identified in the amino terminal region of NOS-I. Although the function of this amino acid motif in NOS-I has not been established, studies on other proteins containing this motif indicate that it may serve to target proteins to specific sites in the cell.

The flow of electrons is assumed to occur in an analogous fashion to that of cytochrome P450-mediated electron systems. The electron donor is NADPH, which donates two electrons to the enzyme-bound entry FAD, which, in turn, reduces the exit FMN. It is the latter flavin that reduces the heme iron prosthetic group to Fe^{2+} to which oxygen can now bind for the oxygenation of the substrate, L-arginine. The overall reaction is inhibited by carbon monoxide and enzyme activity is totally dependent on bound calmodulin, which requires high concentrations of Ca^{2+} for the neuronal and endothelial isoforms. **Calmodulin** is involved in the control of electron flow between the flavin prosthetic groups and between the exit flavin, FMN, and the heme prosthetic group in the oxygenase module. While the precise residues constituting the binding site of BH_4 have not been identified, its location has been narrowed to the

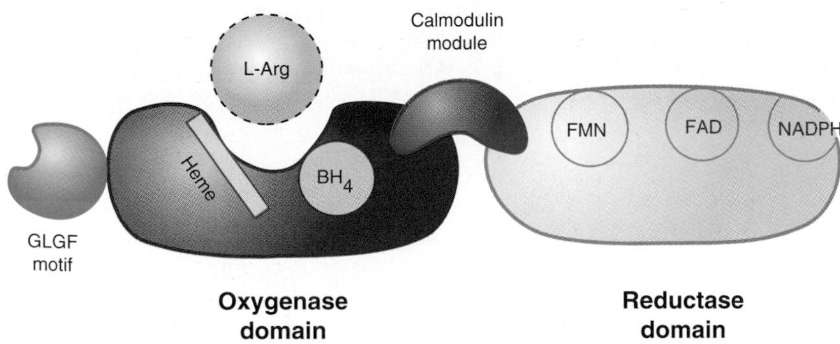

FIGURE 23.12
Modular structure of neuronal nitric oxide synthase showing approximate locations of prosthetic groups and cofactors.
Adapted from Masters, B.S.S., McMillan, K., Sheta, E. A., Nishimura, J. S. et al. FASEB J., *10:552, 1996.*

oxygenase module in the vicinity of the heme-binding site. The analogy between the systems synthesizing nitric oxide and the cytochrome P450-mediated systems is remarkable, but the differences are significant and the oxygenase module probably represents an example of convergent evolution with the cytochromes P450. The three-dimensional structures of mammalian representatives of either the cytochromes P450 or the nitric oxide synthases are yet to be determined.

BIBLIOGRAPHY

Drug Metabolism and Cytochrome P450

Eichelbaum, M., and Gross, A. S. The genetic polymorphism of debrisoquine/sparteine metabolism—clinical aspects. In: W. Kalow (Ed.), *Pharmacogenetics of Drug Metabolism*. New York: Pergamon Press, 1992, Chap. 21, p. 625.

Gibson, G. G., and Skett, P. *Introduction to Drug Metabolism,* 2nd ed. London: Blackie Academic & Professional, 1994.

Guengerich, F. J. Reactions and significance of cytochrome P-450 enzymes. *J. Biol. Chem.* 266:10019, 1991.

Meyer, U. A., Skoda, R. C., Zanger, U. M., Heim, M., and Broly, F. The genetic polymorphism of debrisoquine/sparteine metabolism—molecular mechanism. In: W. Kalow (Ed.), *Pharmacogenetics of Drug Metabolism*. New York: Pergamon Press, 1992, Chap. 20, p. 609.

Nelson, D. R., Koymans, L., Kamataki, T., Stegeman, J. J., Feyereisen, R., Waxman, D. J., Waterman, M. R., Gotoh, O., Coon, M. J., Estabrook, R. W., Gunsalus, I. C., and Nebert, D. W. The P450 superfamily: update on new sequences, gene mapping, accession numbers and nomenclature. *Pharmacogenetics* 6:1, 1996.

Parkinson, A. Biotransformation of xenobiotics In: C. D. Klassen (Ed.), *Casarett and Doull's Toxicology. The Basic Science of Poisons.* New York: McGraw-Hill, 1996, Chap. 6, p. 113.

Wilkinson, G. R., Guengerich, F. P., and Branch, R. A. Genetic polymorphism of *S*-mephenytoin hydroxylation. In: W. Kalow (Ed.), *Pharmacogenetics of Drug Metabolism*. New York: Pergamon Press, 1992, Chap. 23, p. 657.

Electron Transport and Cytochrome P450

Estabrook, R. W., Cooper, D. Y., and Rosenthal, O. The light reversible carbon monoxide inhibition of the steroid C21-hydroxylase system of the adrenal cortex. *Biochem. Zeit.* 338:741, 1963.

Peterson, J. A., and Prough, R. A. Cytochrome P-450 reductase and cytochrome b_5 in cytochrome P-450 catalysis. In: P. R. Ortiz de Montellano (Ed.), *Cytochrome P-450 Structure, Mechanism, and Biochemistry*. New York: Plenum Press, 1986, Chap. 4, p. 89.

Induction of Cytochrome P450

Denison, M. S., and Whitlock, J. P. Xenobiotic-inducible transcription of cytochrome P450 genes. *J. Biol. Chem.* 270:18175, 1995.

Sidhu, J. S., and Omiecinski, C. J. cAMP-associated inhibition of phenobarbital-inducible cytochrome P450 gene expression in primary rat hepatocyte cultures. *J. Biol. Chem.* 270:12762, 1995.

Endogenous Substrates and Cytochrome P450

Cunningham, F. G., MacDonald, P. C., Gant, N. F., Leveno, K. J., and Gilstrap, L. C. The placental hormones. In: *Williams Obstetrics,* 19th ed. East Norwalk, CT: Appleton & Lange, 1993, Chap. 6, p. 139.

Donohoue, P. A., Parker, K., and Migeon, C. J. Congenital adrenal hyperplasia. In: C. R. Scriver, A. L. Beaudet, W. S. Sly, and D. Valle (Eds.), *The Metabolic and Molecular Bases of Inherited Disease,* 7th ed., Vol. II. New York: McGraw-Hill, 1995, Chap. 94, p. 2929.

Graham-Lorence, S., Amarneh, B., White, R. E., Peterson, J. A., and Simpson, E. R. A three-dimensional model of aromatase cytochrome P450. *Protein Sci.* 4:1065, 1995.

Masters, B. S. S., Muerhoff, A. S., and Okita, R. T. Enzymology of extrahepatic cytochromes P450. In: F. P. Guengerich (Ed.), *Mammalian Cytochromes P450.* Boca Raton, FL: CRC Press, 1987, Chap. 3, p. 107.

Waterman, M. R., John, M. E., and Simpson, E. R. Regulation of synthesis and activity of cytochrome P-450 enzymes in physiological pathways. In: P. R. Ortiz de Montellano (Ed.), *Cytochrome P-450. Structure, Mechanism, and Biochemistry.* New York: Plenum Press, 1986, Chap. 10, p. 315.

Biochemistry and Physiology of Nitric Oxide Formation

Bredt, D. S., and Snyder, S. H. Nitric oxide: a physiologic messenger molecule. *Annu. Rev. Biochem.* 63:175, 1994.

Garthwaite, J., and Boulton, C. L. Nitric oxide signalling in the central nervous system. *Annu. Rev. Physiol.* 57:683, 1995.

Griffith, O. W., and Stuehr, D. J. Nitric oxide synthases—properties and catalytic mechanism. *Annu. Rev. Physiol.* 57:707, 1995.

Ignarro, L. J., Buga, G. M., Wood, K. S., Byrns, R. E., and Chaudhuri, G. Endothelium-derived relaxing factor produced and released from artery and vein is nitric oxide. *Proc. Natl. Acad. Sci. USA* 84:9265, 1987.

Khan, M. T., and Furchgott, R. F. Additional evidence that endothelium-derived relaxing factor is nitric oxide. In: M. J. Rand and C. Raper (Eds.), *Pharmacology.* Amsterdam: Elsevier, 1987, p. 341.

Marletta, M. A. Approaches toward selective inhibition of nitric oxide synthase. *J. Med. Chem.* 37:1899, 1994.

Masters, B. S. S. Nitric oxide synthases: Why so complex? *Annu. Rev. Nutr.* 14:131, 1994.

Masters, B. S. S., McMillan, K., Sheta, E. A., Nishimura, J. S., Roman, L. J., and Martasek, P. Neuronal nitric oxide synthase, a modular enzyme formed by convergent evolution: structure studies of a cysteine thiolate-liganded heme protein that hydroxylates L-arginine to produce NO as a cellular signal. *FASEB J.* 10:552, 1996.

Palmer, R. M. J., Ferrige, A. G., and Moncada, S. Nitric oxide release acccounts for the biological activity of endothelium-derived relaxing factor. *Nature* 327:524, 1987.

QUESTIONS ■ C. N. ANGSTADT AND J. BAGGOTT

1. All of the following are correct about a molecule designated as a cytochrome P450 EXCEPT:
   A. it contains a heme as a prosthetic group.
   B. it catalyzes the hydroxylation of a hydrophobic substrate.
   C. it may accept electrons from a substance such as NADPH.
   D. it undergoes a change in the heme iron upon binding a substrate.
   E. it comes from the same gene family as all other molecules designated as cytochromes P450.

2. Known roles for cytochromes P450 include all of the following EXCEPT:
   A. synthesis of steroid hormones.
   B. conversion of some chemicals to mutagens.
   C. hydroxylation of an amino acid.
   D. inactivation of some hydrophobic drugs.
   E. metabolism of fatty acid derivatives.

3. The induction of cytochromes P450:
   A. occurs only by endogenous compounds.
   B. occurs only at the transcriptional level.
   C. necessarily results from increased transcription of the appropriate mRNA.
   D. necessitates the formation of an inducer–receptor protein complex.
   E. may occur by posttranscriptional processes.

4. Flavoproteins are usually intermediates in the transfer of electrons from NADPH to cytochrome P450 because:
   A. NADPH cannot enter the membrane.
   B. flavoproteins can accept two electrons from NADPH and donate them one at a time to cytochrome P450.
   C. they have a more negative reduction potential than NADPH and so accept electrons more readily.
   D. as redox proteins, they can directly reducc cytochromes P450 while the nonprotein NADPH cannot.
   E. they contain iron–sulfur centers.

5. NADPH–cytochrome P450 reductase:
   A. uses both FAD and FMN as prosthetic groups.
   B. is found in mitochondria.
   C. requires an iron–sulfur center for activity.
   D. always passes its electrons to cytochrome b_5.
   E. can use NADH as readily as NADPH.

6. The system necessary for the formation of double bonds in fatty acids:
   A. is the cytochrome P450 electron transport system in the endoplasmic reticulum.
   B. is the cytochrome P450 electron transport system in the mitochondria.
   C. contains NADH–cytochrome b_5 reductase.
   D. uses NADPH–adrenodoxin reductase to reduce cytochrome b_5.
   E. uses both FAD and FMN as prosthetic groups.

7. NADPH–adrenodoxin reductase:
   A. is located in the endoplasmic reticulum
   B. passes its electrons to a protein with iron–sulfur centers.
   C. has a stretch of hydrophobic amino acid residues at the N-terminal end.
   D. reacts directly with cytochrome P450.
   E. reacts directly with cytochrome b_5.

8. Cytochrome P450 systems are able to oxidize:
   A. $—CH_2—$ groups.
   B. benzene rings.
   C. nitrogen atoms in an organic compound.
   D. sulfur atoms in an organic compound.
   E. all of the above.

9. In the conversion of cholesterol to steroid hormones in the adrenal gland:
   A. all of the cytochrome P450 oxidations occur in the endoplasmic reticulum.
   B. all of the cytochrome P450 oxidations occur in the mitochondria.
   C. side chain cleavage of cholesterol to pregnenolone is one of the cytochrome P450 systems that uses adrenodoxin reductase.
   D. cytochrome P450 is necessary for the formation of aldosterone and cortisol but not for the formation of the androgens and estrogens.
   E. aromatization of the first ring of the steroid does not use cytochrome P450 because it involves removal of a methyl group, not a hydroxylation.

10. Many xenobiotics (exogenous substrates) are oxidized by cytochromes P450 in order to:
    A. make them carcinogenic.
    B. increase their solubility in an aqueous environment.
    C. enhance their deposition in adipose tissue.
    D. increase their pharmacological activity.
    E. all of the above.

11. Benzo[a]pyrene, a xenobiotic produced by combustion of a variety of substances:
    A. induces the synthesis of cytochrome P450.
    B. undergoes epoxidation by a cytochrome P450.
    C. is converted to a potent carcinogen in animals by cytochrome P450.
    D. would be rendered more water-soluble after the action of cytochrome P450.
    E. all of the above.

12. Phenobarbital is a potent inducer of cytochrome P450. Warfarin, an anticoagulant, is a substrate for cytochrome P450 with the result that the drug is metabolized and cleared from the body more rapidly than normal. If phenobarbital is added to the therapeutic regimen of a patient, with no change in the dosage of warfarin, the expected consequence would be:
    A. no change in the clinical results.
    B. an increased possibility of clot formation.
    C. an increased possibility of hemorrhaging.

13. Nitric oxide:
    A. is formed spontaneously by a reduction of NO_2.
    B. is synthesized only in macrophages.
    C. is synthesized from arginine.
    D. acts as a potent vasoconstrictor.
    E. has three isoforms.

14. Nitric oxide synthase:
    A. catalyzes a dioxygenase reaction.
    B. is similar mechanistically to phenylalanine hydroxylase since it requires tetrahydrobiopterin.
    C. accepts electrons from NADH.
    D. uses a flow of electrons from NADPH to FAD to FMN to heme iron.
    E. is inhibited by Ca^{2+}.

ANSWERS

1. E Several gene families are known. The number after CYP designates the family. B: The types of substrates are hydrophobic. It is classified as a monooxygenase. C: See Figure 23.3. D: The change from hexa to penta coordinated gives the compound a more positive reduction potential (pp. 982–984).
2. C Cytochromes P450 are not the only hydroxylases and other types are active with amino acids (pp. 982, 989–995).
3. E There may be a stabilization of mRNA (as seen in diabetic rats) or decrease in the degradation of the protein, which may be a mechanism for pyrazole (p. 985). A: One of the roles of cytochromes P450 is in the metabolism of exogenous substances. B and C: Transcriptional modification is only one of the mechanisms of induction (see E). D: This has been shown with induction by some compounds, but with others, like phenobarbital, this is not so (p. 985).
4. B Heme can accept only one electron at a time while NADPH always donates two at a time. A: NADPH passes only electrons; it does not have to enter the membrane. C: If this were true, the flow of electrons would not occur in the way it does. D: Protein–protein binding is not known to play a role here. E: Iron–sulfur centers play a role in some, but not all, systems. Flavoproteins are not the only system with iron–sulfur centers (p. 987).
5. A This enzyme is one of two mammalian proteins known to do so. B: This is in the endoplasmic reticulum. C: Some reductases do so but not this one. D: Only certain reactions catalyzed by the enzyme do. E: There are NADH-dependent reductases but they are different enzymes (p. 988).
6. C This enzyme reduces desaturase. A: Desaturase does not react with cytochrome P450. B: Desaturase is in the endoplasmic reticulum. D: This is a mitochondrial system. E: This is not one of the two enzymes that use both flavins (p. 988).
7. B The iron–sulfur protein is adrenodoxin, which passes the electron to cytochrome P450. A and C: This is a mitochondrial enzyme. D and E: See B (p. 989).
8. E See Figure 23.7, p. 989.
9. C This is a mitochondrial process (Figure 23.8, p. 990). A and B: Hormone synthesis involves a series of reactions that move back and forth between mitochondria and endoplasmic reticulum (p. 991). D and E: Removal of side chains frequently begins with oxidation reactions (p. 992).
10. B The types of xenobiotics oxidized by cytochrome P450 are usually highly lipophilic but must be excreted in the aqueous urine or bile. A: This may happen but is certainly not the purpose. C: They do that prior to oxidation. D: Oxidation tends to reduce pharmacological activity (p. 992).
11. E A: It is not uncommon for xenobiotics to induce synthesis of something that will enhance their own metabolism. B and C: Epoxidation is the first step in the conversion of this compound to one that is carcinogenic—again, a common occurrence (p. 994). D: Benzo[a]pyrene, with its four fused benzene rings, is highly hydrophobic; introducing oxygens increases water solubility (p. 993).
12. B If warfarin is metabolized and cleared more rapidly by cytochrome P450, its therapeutic efficiency is decreased. Therefore, at the same dosage, it will be less effective as an anticoagulant. Think what would happen if the warfarin dosage were adjusted for a proper response, and then phenobarbital were withdrawn without adjusting the warfarin dose (see Clin. Corr. 23.1).
13. C The other product is citrulline. A and E: Three isoforms of nitric oxide synthase have been identified. B: One of the isoforms of NO synthase has been found in macrophages but neuronal and endothelial isoforms also exist. D: Nitric oxide is a vasodilator, which is the basis for the use of nitroglycerin in angina pectoris (p. 995).
14. D This is the second mammalian enzyme known to use both FAD and FMN. A: The reaction is a monooxygenation. B: BH_4 is required but the action of the enzyme is similar to a cytochrome P450-mediated system. C: The donor is NADPH. E: The system requires Ca^{2+}–calmodulin, at least the neuronal and endothelial isoforms (p. 996).

CHAPTER

24

IRON AND HEME METABOLISM

William M. Awad, Jr.

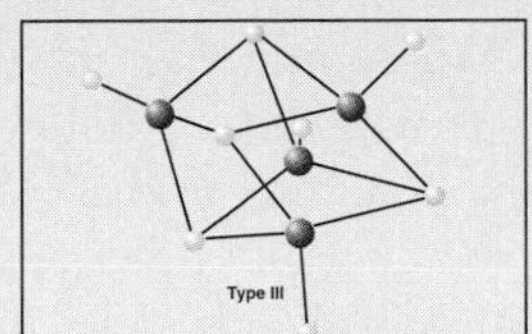

24.1 ■ IRON METABOLISM: OVERVIEW

Iron is closely involved in the metabolism of oxygen, permitting the transportation and participation of oxygen in a variety of biochemical processes. The common **oxidation states** are either **ferrous** (Fe^{2+}) or **ferric** (Fe^{3+}); higher oxidation levels occur as short-lived intermediates in certain redox processes. Iron has an affinity for electronegative atoms such as oxygen, nitrogen, and sulfur, which provide the electrons that form the bonds with iron. These can be of very high affinity when favorably oriented on macromolecules. In forming complexes, no bonding electrons are derived from iron. There is an added complexity to the structure of iron: the nonbonding electrons in the outer shell of the metal (the incompletely filled 3*d* orbitals) can exist in two states. Where bonding interactions with iron are weak, the outer nonbonding electrons will avoid pairing and distribute throughout the 3*d* orbitals. Where bonding electrons interact strongly with iron, however, there will be pairing of the outer nonbonding electrons, favoring lower-energy 3*d* orbitals. These two different distributions for each oxidation state of iron can be determined by electron spin resonance measurements. Dispersion of 3*d* electrons to all orbitals leads to the high-spin state, whereas restriction of 3*d* electrons to lower energy orbitals, because of electron pairing, leads to a low-spin state. Some iron–protein complexes reveal changes in spin state without changes in oxidation during chemical events (e.g., binding and release of oxygen by hemoglobin).

At neutral and alkaline pH ranges, the redox potential for iron in aqueous solutions favors the Fe^{3+} state; at acid pH values, the equilibrium favors the Fe^{2+} state. In the Fe^{3+} state iron slowly forms large polynuclear complexes with hydroxide ion, water, and other anions that may be present. These complexes can become so large as to exceed their solubility products, leading to their aggregation and precipitation with pathological consequences.

Iron can bind to and influence the structure and function of various macromolecules, with deleterious results to the organism. To protect against such reactions, several iron-binding proteins function specifically to store and transport iron. These proteins have both a very high affinity for the metal and, in the normal physiological state, also have incompletely filled iron-binding sites. The interaction of iron with its ligands has been well characterized in some proteins (e.g., hemoglobin and myoglobin), whereas for others (e.g., transferrin) it is presently in the process of being defined. The major area of ignorance in the biochemistry of iron lies in the *in vivo* transfer processes of iron from one macromolecule to another. Several proposed mechanisms may explain the process of iron transfer. Two are supported by excellent model studies but have varying degrees of relevance to the physiological state. The proposed processes are the following. First, the redox change of iron has been an attractive mechanism because it is supported by selective *in vitro* studies and because in some cases macromolecules have a very selective affinity for Fe^{3+}, binding Fe^{2+} poorly. Thus reduction of iron would permit ferrous ions to dissociate, and reoxidation would allow the iron to redistribute to appropriate macromolecules. Redox mechanisms have only been defined in a very few settings, some of which will be described below. An alternative hypothesis involves chelation of ferric ions by specific small molecules with high affinities for iron; this mechanism has been supported also by selective *in vitro* studies. The chelation mechanism suffers from the lack of a demonstrably specific *in vivo* chelator. Because the redox potential strongly favors ferric ion at almost all tissue sites and because Fe^{3+} binds so strongly to liganding groups, the probability is that there are cooperating mechanisms regulating the intermolecular transfer of iron.

24.2 ■ IRON-CONTAINING PROTEINS

Iron binds to proteins either by incorporation into a **protoporphyrin IX** ring (see below) or by interaction with other protein ligands. Ferrous- and ferric-protoporphyrin IX complexes are designated **heme** and **hematin,** respectively. Heme-containing proteins include those that transport (e.g., hemoglobin) and store (e.g., myoglobin) oxygen, and certain enzymes that contain heme as part of their prosthetic groups (e.g., catalase, peroxidases, tryptophan pyrrolase, prostaglandin synthase, guanylate cyclase, NO synthase, and the microsomal and mitochondrial cytochromes.). Discussions on structure–function relationships of heme proteins are presented in Chapters 6 and 25.

Nonheme proteins include transferrin, ferritin, a variety of redox enzymes that contain iron at the active site, and iron–sulfur proteins. A significant body of information has been acquired that relates to the structure–function relationships of some of these molecules.

Transferrin Transports Iron in Serum

The protein in serum involved in the transport of iron is **transferrin,** a β1-glycoprotein synthesized in the liver, consisting of a single polypeptide chain of 78,000 Da with two noncooperative iron-binding sites. The protein is a product of gene duplication derived from a putative ancestral gene coding for a protein binding only one atom of iron. Several metals bind to transferrin; the highest affinity is for Fe^{3+}; Fe^{2+} ion is not bound. The binding of each Fe^{3+} ion is absolutely dependent on the coordinate binding of an anion, which in the physiological state is carbonate as indicated below:

$$\text{Transferrin} + Fe^{3+} + Co_3{}^{2-} \rightarrow \text{transferrin} \cdot Fe^{3} \cdot CO_3{}^{2-}$$
$$\text{Transferrin} \cdot Fe^{3+} \cdot CO_3{}^{2-} \rightarrow \text{transferrin} \cdot 2\,(Fe^{3+}CO_3{}^{2-})$$

Estimates of the association constants for the binding of Fe^{3+} to transferrins from different species range from 10^{19} to $10^{31}\,M^{-1}$, indicating for practical purposes that wherever there is excess transferrin free ferric ions will not be found. In the normal physiological state, approximately one-ninth of all transferrin molecules are saturated with iron at both sites; four-ninths of transferrin molecules have iron at either site; and four-ninths of circulating transferrin are free of iron. Unsaturated transferrin protects against infections (see Clin. Corr. 24.1). The two iron-binding sites show differences in sequences and in affinities for other metals. Transferrin binds to specific cell surface receptors that mediate the internalization of the protein.

The **transferrin receptor** is a transmembrane protein consisting of two subunits of 90,000 Da each, joined by a disulfide bond. Each subunit contains one transmembrane segment and about 670 residues that are extracellular and bind a transferrin molecule, favoring the diferric form. Internalization of the receptor–transferrin complex is dependent on receptor phosphorylation by a Ca^{2+}–calmodulin–protein kinase C complex. Release of the iron atoms occurs within the acidic milieu of the lysosome after which the receptor–apotransferrin complex returns to the cell surface where the apotransferrin is released to be reutilized in the plasma.

Lactoferrin Binds Iron in Milk

Milk contains iron that is bound almost exclusively to a glycoprotein, **lactoferrin,** closely homologous to transferrin, with two sites binding the metal. The iron content of the protein varies, but it is never saturated. Studies on the function of lactoferrin have been directed toward its antimicrobial effect, protecting the newborn from gastrointestinal infections. Microorganisms require iron for

CLINICAL CORRELATION 24.1

Iron Overload and Infection

If an individual is overloaded with iron by any of several causes, the serum transferrin value can be close to saturation, making small amounts of free serum iron available. Microorganisms that are usually nonpathogenic, because they are iron dependent and cannot compete against partially saturated transferrin in the normal individual, can now become pathogenic under these circumstances. For example, *Vibrio vulnificus,* a marine halophile, is found in a small percentage of oysters and commercial shellfish. Individuals who are iron overloaded can develop a rapidly progressive infection, with death ensuing within 24 h after ingestion of the offending meal, whereas normal individuals consuming the same food are entirely free of symptoms.

Muench, K. H. Hemochromatosis and infection: alcohol and iron, oysters and sepsis. *Am. J. Med.* 87:3, 1989.

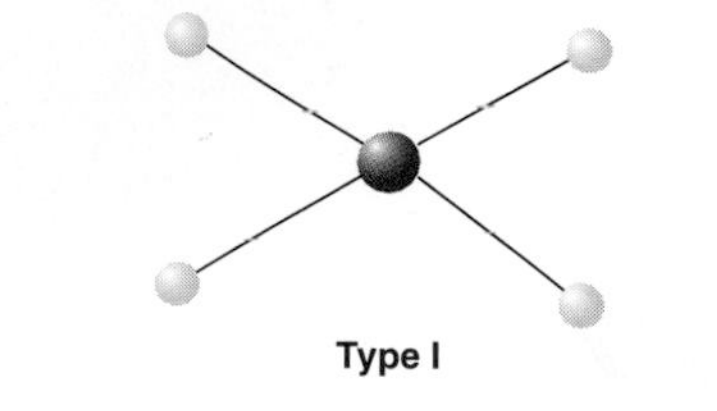

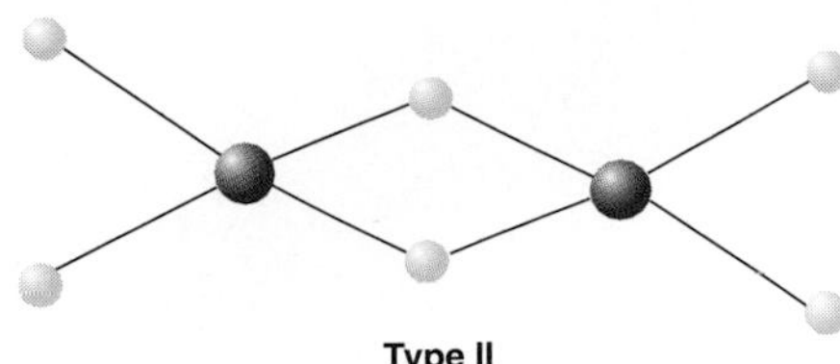

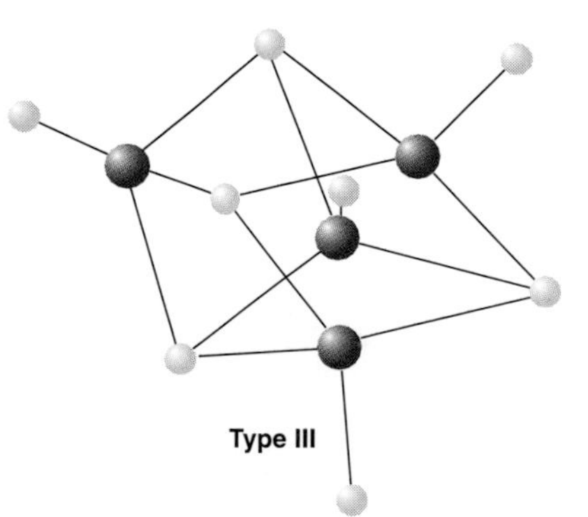

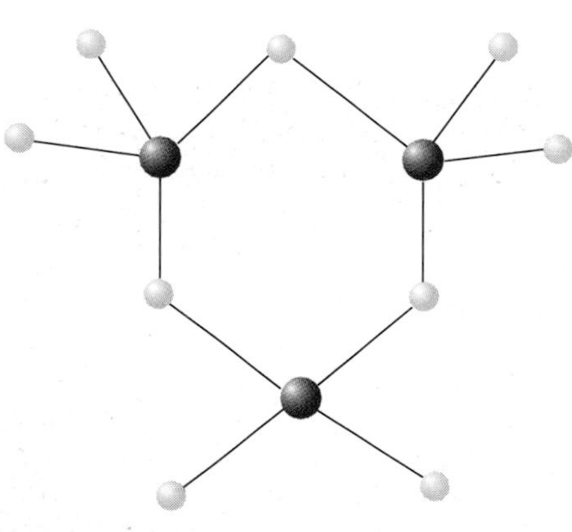

FIGURE 24.1
Structure of ferredoxins.
Dark red circles represent iron atoms; light red circles represent the inorganic sulfur atoms; and small gray circles represent the cysteinyl sulfur atoms derived from the polypeptide chain. Variation in type IV ferredoxins can occur where one of the cysteinyl residues can be substituted by a solvent oxygen atom of an OH group.

replication and function. Presence of incompletely saturated lactoferrin results in the rapid binding of any free iron, leading to the inhibition of microbial growth by preventing a sufficient amount of iron from entering these microorganisms. Other microbes, such as *Escherichia coli,* which release competitive iron chelators, are able to proliferate despite the presence of lactoferrin, since the chelators transfer the iron specifically to the microorganism. Lactoferrin is present in granulocytes being released during bacterial infections. It is also present in mucous secretions. Besides its bacteriostatic function it is believed to facilitate iron transport and storage in milk. Lactoferrin has been found in urine of premature infants fed human milk.

Ferritin Is a Protein Involved in Storage of Iron

Ferritin is the major protein involved in the storage of iron. The protein consists of an outer polypeptide shell 130 Å in diameter with a central ferric-hydroxide-phosphate core 60 Å across. The apoprotein, **apoferritin,** consists of 24 subunits of a varying mixture of H subunits (178 amino acids) and L subunits (171 amino acids) that provide various isoprotein forms. H subunits predominate in nucleated blood cells and heart, L subunits in liver and spleen. Synthesis of the subunits is regulated mainly by the concentration of free intracellular iron. The bulk of iron storage occurs in hepatocytes, reticuloendothelial cells, and skeletal muscle. The ratio of iron to polypeptide is not constant, since the protein has the ability to gain and release iron according to physiological needs. With a capacity of 4500 iron atoms, the molecule contains usually less than 3000. Channels from the surface permit the accumulation and release of iron. When iron is in excess, the storage capacity of newly synthesized apoferritin may be exceeded. This leads to iron deposition adjacent to ferritin spheres. Histologically, such amorphous iron deposition is called **hemosiderin.** The H chains of ferritin oxidize ferrous ions to the ferric state. Ferritins derived from different tissues of the same species differ in electrophoretic mobility in a fashion analogous to the differences noted with isoenzymes. In some tissues ferritin spheres form lattice-like arrays, which are identifiable by electron microscopy. Plasma ferritin (low in iron, rich in L subunits) has a half-life of 50 h and is cleared by reticuloendothelial cells and hepatocytes, and its concentration, although very low, correlates closely to the size of the body iron stores.

Other Nonheme Iron-Containing Proteins Are Involved in Enzymatic Processes

Many iron-containing proteins are involved in enzymatic processes, most of which are related to oxidation mechanisms. The structural features of the ligands binding the iron are not well known, except for a few components involved in mitochondrial electron transport. These latter proteins, termed **ferredoxins,** are characterized by iron being bonded, with one exception, only to sulfur atoms. Four major types of such proteins are known (see Figure 24.1). The smallest, type I (e.g., nebredoxin), found only in microorganisms, consists of a small polypeptide chain with a mass of about 6000 and contains one iron atom bound to four cysteine residues. Type II consists of ferredoxins found in both plants and animal tissues where two iron atoms are found, each liganding to two separate cysteine residues and sharing two sulfide anions. The most complicated of the iron–sulfur proteins are the bacterial ferredoxins, type III, which contain four atoms of iron, each of which is linked to single separate cysteine residues but also shares three sulfide anions with neighboring iron molecules to form a cube-like structure. In some anaerobic bacteria, a family of ferredoxins may contain two type III iron–sulfur groups per macromolecule. Type IV ferredoxins contain structures with three atoms of iron, each linked to two separate cysteine residues and each sharing two sulfide anions, forming a planar ring. In one example of this ferredoxin type, an exception of iron atoms being liganded only to sulfur atoms was found where the sulfur of a cysteinyl residue was substituted by a solvent oxygen atom. The redox potential afforded by these different ferredoxins varies widely and is in part dependent on the environment of the surrounding polypeptide chain that envelops these iron–sulfur groups. In nebredoxin the iron undergoes ferric–ferrous conversion during electron transport. With the plant and animal ferredoxins (type II iron–sulfur proteins) both irons are in the Fe^{3+} form in the oxidized state; upon reduction only one iron goes to Fe^{2+}. In the bacterial ferredoxin (type III iron–sulfur protein) the oxidized state can be either 2 $Fe^{3+} \cdot$ 2 Fe^{2+} or 3 $Fe^{3+} \cdot Fe^{2+}$, with corresponding reduced forms of $Fe^{3+} \cdot$ 3 Fe^{2+} or 2 $Fe^{3+} \cdot$ 2 Fe^{2+}.

24.3 INTESTINAL ABSORPTION OF IRON

The high affinity of iron for both specific and nonspecific macromolecules leads to the absence of significant formation of free iron salts, and thus this metal is not lost via usual excretory routes. Rather, excretion of iron occurs only through the normal sloughing of tissues that are not reutilized (e.g., epidermis and gastrointestinal mucosal cells). In the healthy adult male the loss is about 1 mg day^{-1}. In premenopausal women, the normal physiological events of menses and parturition substantially augment iron loss. A wide variation of such loss exists, depending on the amounts of menstrual flow and the multiplicity of births. In the extremes of the latter settings, a premenopausal woman may require an amount of iron that is four to five times that needed in an adult male for prolonged periods of time. The postmenopausal woman who is not iron-deficient has an iron requirement similar to that of the adult male. Children and patients with blood loss naturally have increased iron requirements.

Cooking of food facilitates the breakdown of ligands attached to iron, increasing the availability of the metal in the gut. The low pH of stomach contents permits the reduction of Fe^{3+} to Fe^{2+}, facilitating dissociation from ligands. The latter requires the presence of an accompanying **reductant,** which is usually achieved by adding **ascorbate** to the diet. The absence of a normally functioning stomach reduces substantially the amount of iron that is absorbed. Some iron-containing compounds bind the metal so tightly that it is not available for assimilation. Contrary to popular belief, spinach is a poor source of iron because of an earlier erroneous record of the iron content and because some of the iron is bound to phytate (inositol hexaphosphate), which is resistant to the chemical actions of the gastrointestinal tract. Specific protein cofactors derived from the stomach or pancreas have been suggested as being facilitators of iron absorption in the small intestine.

The major site of **absorption of iron** is in the small intestine, with the largest amount being absorbed in the duodenum and a gradient of lesser absorption occurring in the more distal portions of the small intestine. The metal enters the mucosal cell either as the free ion or as heme; in the latter case the metal is split off from the porphyrin ring in the mucosal cytoplasm. The large amount of bicarbonate secreted by the pancreas neutralizes the acidic material delivered by the stomach and thus favors the oxidation of Fe^{2+} to Fe^{3+}. The major barrier to the absorption of iron is not at the luminal surface of the duodenal mucosal cell. Whatever the requirements of the host are, in the face of an adequate delivery of iron to the lumen, a substantial amount of iron will enter the mucosal cell. Regulation of iron transfer occurs between the mucosal cell and the capillary bed (see Figure 24.2 and Clin. Corr. 24.2). In the normal state, certain processes define the amount of iron that will be transferred. Where there is **iron deficiency,** the amount of transfer increases; where there is **iron overload** in the host, the amount transferred is curtailed substantially. One mechanism that has been demonstrated to regulate this transfer of iron across the mucosal–capillary

CLINICAL CORRELATION 24.2

Duodenal Iron Absorption

Mucin in the duodenal lumen helps to solubilize ferric ions with presentation of the metal to an integrin, a transmembrane protein consisting of a heterodimer of 230 kDa. The cytosolic surface of the integrin interacts with a 56-kDa protein known as mobilferrin. The integrin transfers the iron from the luminal to cytoplasmic surface of the cell, where it is bound by mobilferrin. Mobilferrin acts as a cytosolic shuttle, transferring iron either to cytosolic ferritin or to the opposite pole of the duodenal cell where the iron is transported by an as yet undefined mechanism to capillaries to be picked up by transferrin.

Conrad, M. D., and Umbreit, J. N. Iron absorption—the mucin–mobilferrin–integrin pathway. A competitive pathway for metal absorption. *Am. J. Hematol.* 42:67, 1993.

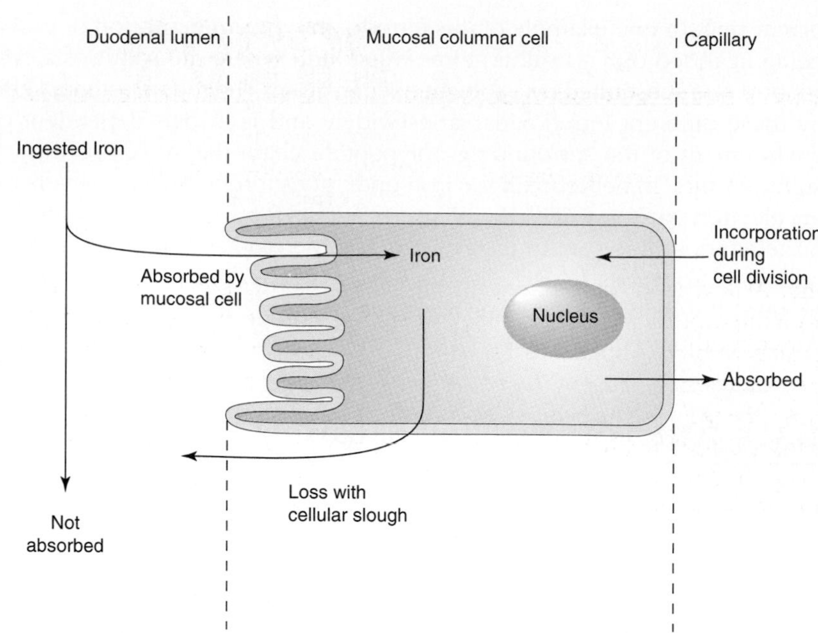

FIGURE 24.2
Intestinal mucosal regulation of iron absorption.
The flux of iron in the duodenal mucosal cell is indicated. A fraction of the iron that is potentially acceptable is transferred from the intestinal lumen into the epithelial cell. A large portion of ingested iron is not absorbed, in part because it is not presented in a readily acceptable form. Some iron is retained within the cell, bound by apoferritin to form ferritin. This iron is sloughed into the intestinal lumen with the normal turnover of the cell. A portion of the iron within the mucosal cell is absorbed and transferred to the capillary bed to be incorporated into transferrin. During cell division, which occurs at the bases of the intestinal crypts, iron is incorporated for cellular requirements. These fluxes change dramatically in iron-depleted or iron-excess states.

interface is the synthesis of apoferritin by the mucosal cell. In situations in which little iron is required by the host, a large amount of apoferritin is synthesized to trap the iron within the mucosal cell and prevent transfer to the capillary bed. As the cells turn over (within a week), their contents are extruded into the intestinal lumen without absorption occurring. In situations in which there is iron deficiency, virtually no apoferritin is synthesized so as not to compete against the transfer of iron to the deficient host. There are other as yet undefined positive mechanisms that increase the rate of iron absorption in the iron-deficient state. Iron transferred to the capillaries is trapped exclusively by transferrin.

24.4 MOLECULAR REGULATION OF IRON UTILIZATION

Cytosol contains at least two proteins that respond to changes in iron concentration. They act as effector molecules controlling the translation of mRNAs, which are important in iron metabolism. These **iron regulatory proteins (IRPs)** bind to specific **stem–loop structures** on certain mRNAs. IRP-1 is the best defined of these proteins. It contains an Fe_4S_4 cubane group when the cellular concentration of iron is high. This prosthetic group activates IRP-1 so that it possesses an **aconitase** activity. However, since neither citrate nor isocitrate is present in significant amounts in the cytosol, the activity is only a potential

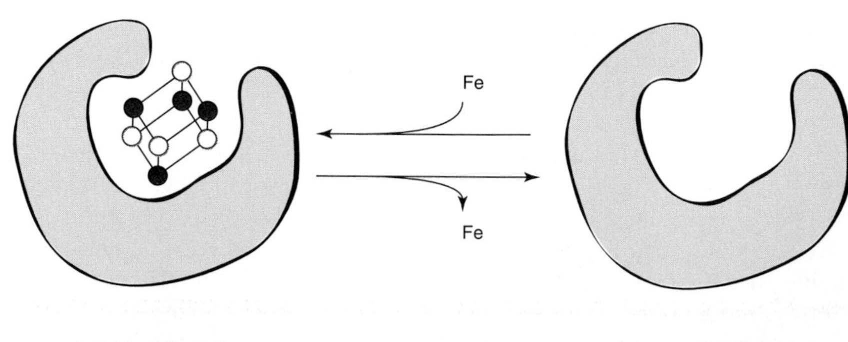

FIGURE 24.3
Iron-responsive protein-1.
Dark blue circles represent iron atoms and open circles inorganic sulfur atoms.

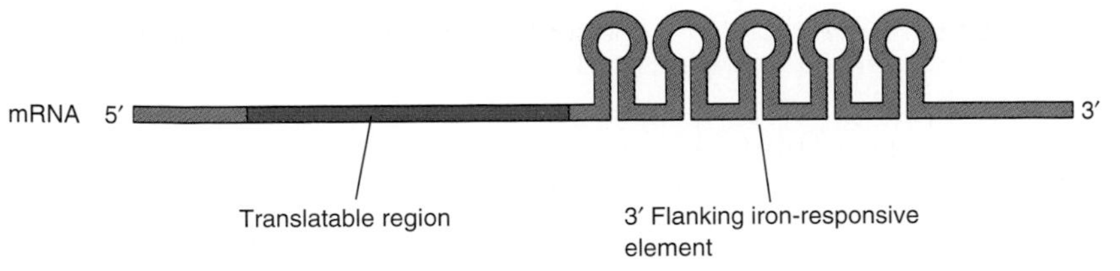

mRNA 5′ 3′

Translatable region

3′ Flanking iron-responsive element

FIGURE 24.4
Structure of transferrin receptor mRNA.

one. At low iron concentrations, the cubane structure collapses, dissociating from the protein and leaving an apoenzyme without catalytic activity. However, it can now bind to specific mRNA stem–loop structures, known as **iron-responsive elements (IREs)** (Figure 24.3). Five mRNAs are known to contain IREs: those for the light and heavy chains of ferritin, the erythrocytic form of aminolevulinic acid synthase, the mitochondrial form of aconitase, and transferrin receptor. (Mitochondrial aconitase, the physiologically active isozyme, has no IRP function.) The first four mRNAs have single IREs in the 5′ flanking region, which bind a single IRP. In contrast, the transferrin receptor has five tandem IREs that bind IRPs in the 3′ flanking region. The binding of the 5′ and 3′ flanking IREs leads to different translational effects. In the iron-deprived state, binding to the 3′ IRE of transferrin receptor (Figure 24.4) leads to stabilization of the mRNA with reduced turnover and, therefore, an increased number of receptor-specific RNA molecules, thereby leading to the increased synthesis of receptor protein. The single 5′ stem–loop of ferritin mRNA (Figure 24.5) is homologous to the 3′ stem–loops of the transferrin receptor mRNA. However, in the former case, binding of the IRP leads to a decreased rate of translation of the mRNA and, thereby, to a decreased concentration of ferritin molecules. Note that the molecular events that are controlled are different in the syntheses of transferrin receptor and apoferritin (see Clin. Corr. 24.3).

In summary, low iron concentrations lead to activation of an IRP that binds to the mRNAs for transferrin receptor and ferritin. In the former case, more receptor is synthesized, while in the latter case less apoferritin is synthesized. The net effect is utilization of iron by proliferating cells. In contrast, high iron concentrations lead to loss of binding by the IRPs to IREs, with a shift of iron from uptake by proliferating cells to storage in the liver.

IRP-1 is regulated by its change from active to inactive states in mRNA-binding properties as noted above. **IRP-2,** a second regulatory protein, also responds to varying concentrations of iron, but in this case, the protein is regulated by increased synthesis at low iron concentrations and increased degradation by a proteasome at high iron concentrations. In addition to the effects of changed iron concentration, increased production of NO (see p. 995) also acts to regulate IRPs.

CLINICAL CORRELATION 24.3

Mutant Iron-Responsive Element

Single mutations have been described of two adjacent bases in the loop segment of the iron-responsive element of ferritin light chain mRNA with an increased amount of apoferritin being synthesized but without an increase in total body iron. This mutation leads to a 28-fold lower affinity for IRP-1 in one case and perhaps an even lower affinity in the other. The reason why these patients have cataracts is unknown. The gene for MP-19, an abundant protein in the lens, which is very close to the light chain gene on chrosomome 19, might possibly be affected by the regulatory process on the mRNA. However, it is more probable that a greatly increased synthesis of ferritin in the lens leads to an increased amount of iron-catalyzed reactions with well-described oxidative lenticular damage.

Girelli, D., Corrocher, R., Bisceglia, L., et al. Molecular basis for the recently described hereditary hyperferritinemia–cataract syndrome: a mutation in the iron-responsive elements of ferritin L-subunit gene (the "Verona mutation"). *Blood* 86:4050, 1995; and Beaumont, C., Leneuve, P., Devaux, I., Scoazec, J. Y., et al. Mutation in the iron responsive element of the L ferritin mRNA in a family with dominant hyperferritinaemia and cataract. *Nature Genet.* 11:444, 1995.

24.5 ■ IRON DISTRIBUTION AND KINETICS

A normal 70-kg male has 3–4 g of iron, of which only 0.1% (3.5 mg) is in the plasma. Approximately 2.5 g are in hemoglobin. Table 24.1 lists the distribution

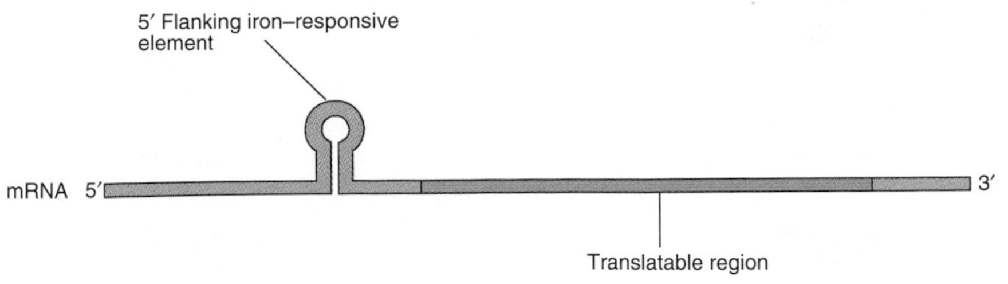

FIGURE 24.5
Structure of apoferritin H-subunit mRNA.

TABLE 24.1 Approximate Iron Distribution: 70–kg Man

	g	%
Hemoglobin	2.5	68
Myoglobin	0.15	4
Transferrin	0.003	0.1
Ferritin, tissue	1.0	27
Ferritin, serum	0.0001	0.004
Enzymes	0.02	0.6
Total	3.7	100

of iron in humans. Normally about 33% of the sites on transferrin contain iron. Iron picked up from the intestine is delivered primarily to the marrow for incorporation into the hemoglobin of red blood cells. The mobilization of iron from the mucosa and from storage sites involves in part the reduction of iron to the ferrous state and its reoxidation to the ferric form. The reduction mechanisms have not been well described. On the other hand, conversion of the Fe^{2+} back to Fe^{3+} state is regulated by serum enzymes called ferroxidases as indicated below:

$$Fe^{2+} + \text{ferroxidase} \rightarrow Fe^{3+} + \text{reduced ferroxidase}$$

Ferroxidase I is also known as **ceruloplasmin** (see Clin. Corr. 24.4). Another serum protein, **ferroxidase II**, appears to be the major serum component that oxidizes ferrous ions. In any disease process in which iron loss exceeds iron repletion, a sequence of physiological responses occurs. The initial events are without symptoms to the subject and involve depletion of iron stores without compromise of any physiological function. This depletion will be manifested by a reduction or absence of iron stores in the liver and in the bone marrow and also by a decrease in the content of the very small amount of ferritin that is normally present in plasma. Serum ferritin levels reflect slow release from storage sites during the normal cellular turnover that occurs in the liver; measurements are made by radioimmunoassays. Serum ferritin is mostly apoferritin in form, containing very little iron. During this early phase, the level and percentage saturation of serum transferrin are not distinctly abnormal. As the iron deficiency progresses, the level of hemoglobin begins to fall and morphological changes appear in the red blood cells. Concurrently, the serum iron falls with a rise in the level of total serum transferrin, the latter reflecting a physiological adaptation in an attempt to absorb more iron from the gastrointestinal tract. At this state of iron depletion a very sensitive index is the percentage saturation of serum transferrin with iron (normal range, 21–50%). At this point the patient usually comes to medical attention, and the diagnosis of iron deficiency is made. In countries in which iron deficiency is severe without available corrective medical measures, a third and severe stage of iron deficiency can occur, where a depletion of iron-containing enzymes leads to very pronounced metabolic effects (see Clin. Corr. 24.5).

Iron overload can occur in patients so that the iron content of the body can be elevated to values as high as 100 g. This may happen for a variety of reasons. Some patients have a recessive heritable disorder associated with a marked inappropriate increase in iron absorption. In such cases the serum transferrin can be almost completely saturated with iron. This state, which is known as **idiopathic hemochromatosis,** is more commonly seen in men because women with the abnormal gene are protected somewhat by menstrual and childbearing events. The accumulation of iron in the liver, pancreas, and heart can lead to cirrhosis and liver tumors, diabetes mellitus, and cardiac failure, respectively. Treatment for these patients is periodic withdrawals of large amounts of blood, where the iron is contained in the hemoglobin. Another group of patients has severe anemias, among the most common of which are the thalassemias, a group of hereditary **hemolytic anemias.** In these cases the subjects require transfusions throughout their lives, leading to the accumulation of large amounts of iron derived from the transfused blood. Clearly bleeding would be an inappropriate measure in these cases; rather, the patients are treated by the administration of iron chelators, such as desferrioxamine, which leads to the excretion of large amounts of complexed iron in the urine. Rarely, a third group of patients will acquire excess iron because they ingest large amounts of both iron and ethanol, the latter promoting iron absorption. In these cases excess stored iron can be removed by bleeding (see Clin. Corr. 24.6).

CLINICAL CORRELATION 24.4

Ceruloplasmin Deficiency

A deficiency of ceruloplasmin, a copper-containing protein, but not its absence, is associated with Wilson's disease in which there is progressive hepatic failure and degeneration of the basal ganglia, associated with a characteristic copper deposition in the cornea (Kayser–Fleischer rings). Because there was no evidence for significant impairment of mobilization of iron in Wilson's disease, it was originally thought that the ferroxidase activity of ceruloplasmin was not physiologically important. However, a recently discovered very rare genetic defect in ceruloplasmin biosynthesis, where the protein was virtually absent in serum, leads to a marked elevation of liver-iron content and serum ferritin levels. These patients develop diabetes, retinal degeneration, and central nervous system findings. The diabetes and central nervous system findings are associated with increased iron in the pancreas and brain, respectively. Thus, in contrast to earlier considerations, it appears that ceruloplasmin has a significant role in iron metabolism.

Harris, E. D. The iron–copper connection: the link to ceruloplasmin grows stronger. *Nutr. Rev.* 53:226, 1995.

CLINICAL CORRELATION 24.5

Iron-Deficiency Anemia

Microscopic examination of a blood smear in patients with iron-deficiency anemia usually reveals the characteristic findings of microcytic (small in size) and hypochromic (underpigmented) red blood cells. These changes in the red cell result from decreased rates of globin synthesis when heme is not available. A bone marrow aspiration will reveal no storage iron to be present and serum ferritin values are virtually zero. The serum transferrin value (expressed as the total iron-binding capacity) will be elevated (upper limits of normal: 410 $\mu g\ dL^{-1}$) with a serum iron saturation of less than 16%. Common causes for iron deficiency include excessive menstrual flow, multiple births, and gastrointestinal bleeding that may be occult. The common causes of gastrointestinal bleeding include medications that can cause ulcers or erosion of the gastric mucosa (especially aspirin or cortisone-like drugs), hiatal hernia, peptic ulcer disease, gastritis associated with chronic alcoholism, and gastrointestinal tumor. The management of such patients must include both a careful examination for the cause and source of bleeding and supplementation with iron. The latter is usually provided in the form of oral ferrous sulfate tablets; occasionally, intravenous iron therapy may be required. Where the iron deficiency is severe, transfusion with packed red blood cells may also be indicated.

Finch, C. A., and Huebers, H. Perspectives in iron metabolism. *N. Engl. J. Med.* 306:1520, 1982.

24.6 ■ HEME BIOSYNTHESIS

Heme is produced in virtually all mammalian tissues. Its synthesis is most pronounced in the bone marrow and liver because of the requirements for incorporation into hemoglobin and the cytochromes, respectively. As depicted in Figure 24.6, heme is largely a planar molecule. It consists of one ferrous ion and a tetrapyrrole ring, **protoporphyrin IX.** The diameter of the iron atom is a little too large to be accommodated within the plane of the porphyrin ring, and thus the metal puckers out to one side as it coordinates with the apical nitrogen atoms of the four pyrrole groups. Heme is one of the most stable compounds, reflecting its strong resonance features.

Figure 24.7 depicts the pathway for heme biosynthesis. The following are the important aspects to be noted. First, the initial and last three enzymatic steps are catalyzed by enzymes that are in the mitochondrion, whereas the intermediate steps take place in the cytoplasm. This is important in considering the regulation by heme of the first biosynthetic step; this aspect is discussed below. Second, the organic portion of heme is derived totally from eight residues each of glycine and succinyl CoA. Third, the reactions occurring on the side groups attached to the tetrapyrrole ring involve the colorless intermediates known as **porphyrinogens.** The latter compounds, though exhibiting reso-

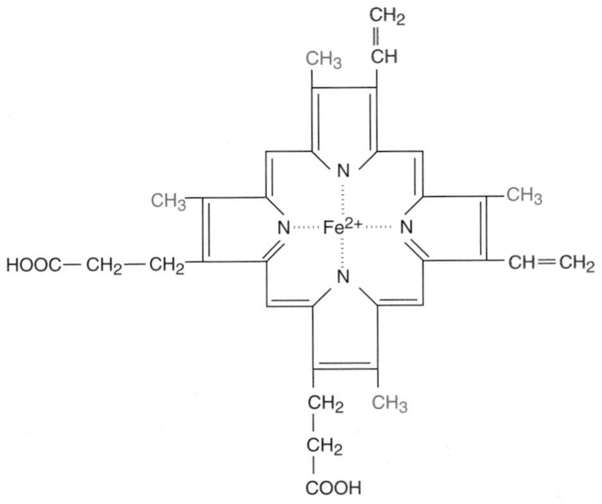

FIGURE 24.6
Structure of heme.

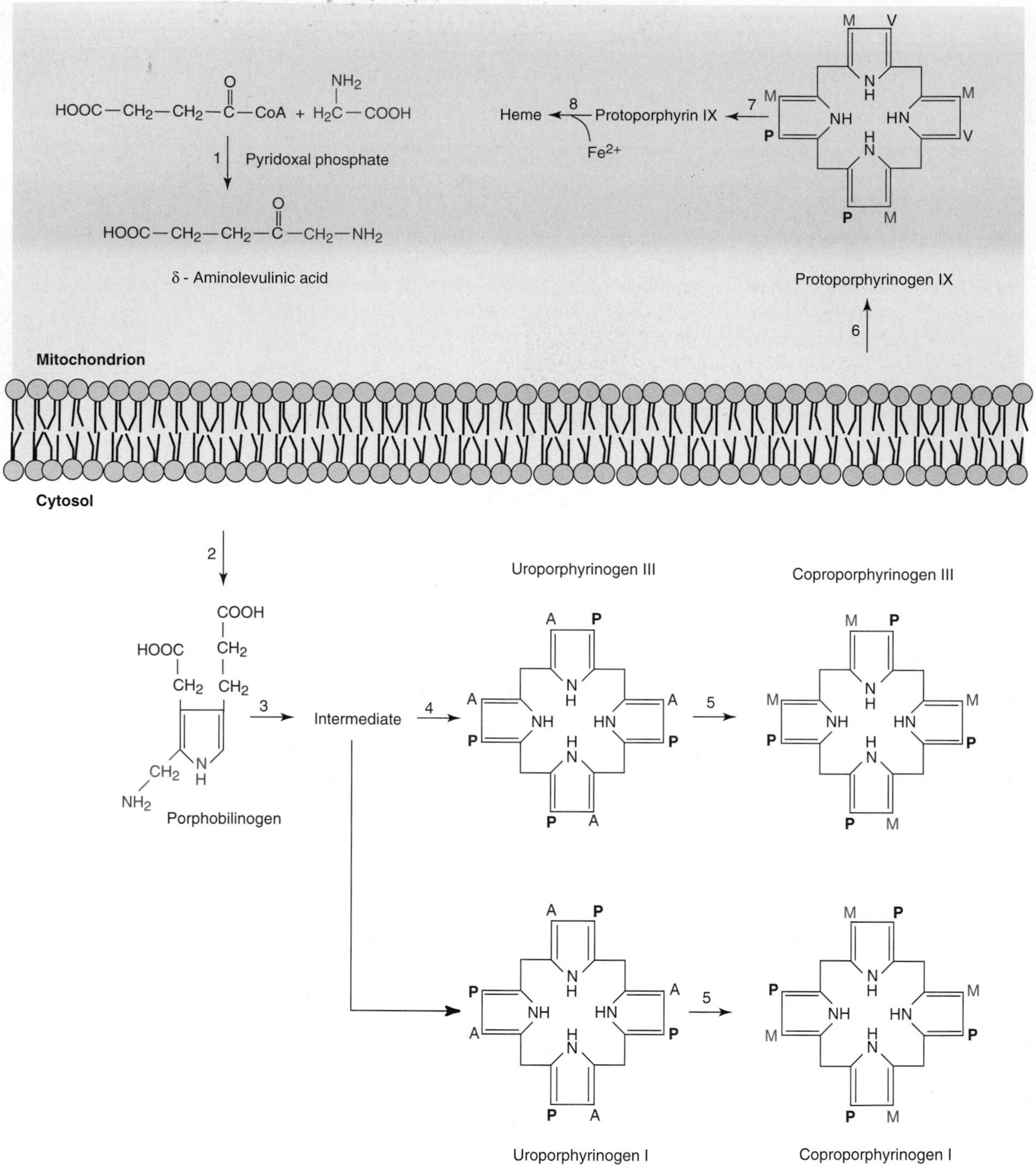

FIGURE 24.7
Pathway for heme biosynthesis.
Numbers indicate enzymes involved in each step as follows: 1, ALA synthase; 2, ALA dehydratase; 3, porphobilinogen deaminase; 4, uroporphyrinogen III cosynthase; 5, uroporphyrinogen decarboxylase; 6, coproporphyrinogen III oxidase; 7, protoporphyrinogen IX oxidase; 8, ferrochelatase. Pyrrole ligands are indicated as follows: P, propionic (β-carboxyethyl); A, acetic (carboxymethyl); M, methyl; V, = vinyl.

nance features within each pyrrole ring, do not demonstrate resonance between the pyrrole groups. As a consequence, the porphyrinogens are unstable and can readily be oxidized, especially in the presence of light, by nonenzymatic means to their stable **porphyrin** products. In the latter cases resonance between pyrrole groups is established by oxidation of the four methylene bridges. Figure 24.8 depicts the enzymatic conversion of protoporphyrinogen to protoporphyrin

CLINICAL CORRELATION 24.6

Hemochromatosis: Molecular Genetics and the Issue of Iron-Fortified Diets

The hemochromatosis gene is heterozygous in about 9% of the population. The disease is expressed primarily in the homozygous state; about 0.25% of all individuals are at risk. Normal individuals have a major histocompatibility complex class-1 gene (HLA-H) with unknown function that encodes for the α-chain, containing three immunoglobulin-like domains. The normal gene product has a structure that cannot present an antigen. Most individuals with hemochromatosis are homozygous for a Cys_{282}-Tyr mutation which prevents the normal conformation of an immunoglobulin domain.

A controversy has developed as to whether food should be fortified with iron because of the prevalence of iron-deficiency anemia, especially among premenopausal women. It was suggested that dietary iron deficiency would be reduced if at least 50 mg of iron was incorporated per pound of enriched flour. Others suggested that toxicity from excess iron absorption through iron fortification was too great. Sweden has mandated iron fortification for 45 years and about 42% of the average daily intake of iron is derived from these sources. However, 5% of males had elevation of serum iron values, with 2% having iron stores consonant with the distribution found in early stages of hemochromatosis, pointing out the danger of iron-fortified diets. In countries where iron deficiency is widespread, however, fortification may still be the most appropriate measure.

McLaren, C. E., Gorddeuk, V. R., Looker, A. C., et al. Prevalence of heterozygotes for hemochromatosis in the white population of the United States. *Blood* 86:2021, 1995; Feder, J. N., Gnirki, A., Thomas, W., et al. A novel MHC class 1-like gene is mutated in patients with hereditary haemochromatosis. *Nature Genetics* 13:399, 1996; Olsson, K. S., Heedman, P. A., and Staugard, F. Preclinical hemochromatosis in a population on a high-iron-fortified diet. *J. Am. Med. Assoc.* 239:1999, 1978; Olsson, K. S., Marsell, R., Ritter, B., Olander, B., et al. Iron deficiency and iron overload in Swedish male adolescents. *J. Intern. Med.* 237:187, 1995.

by this oxidation mechanism. This is the only known porphyrinogen oxidation that is enzyme regulated in humans; all other porphyrinogen → porphyrin conversions are nonenzymatic and catalyzed by light rather than catalyzed by specific enzymes. Fourth, once the tetrapyrrole ring is formed, the order of the R groups as one goes clockwise around the tetrapyrrole ring defines which of the four possible types of **uro-** or **coproporphyrinogens** are being synthesized. These latter compounds have two different substituents, one each for every pyrrole group. Going clockwise around the ring, the substituents can be arranged as ABABABAB (where A is one substituent and B the other), forming a type I porphyrinogen, or the arrangement can be ABABABBA, forming a type III porphyrinogen. In principle, two other arrangements can occur to form porphyrinogens II and IV, and these can be synthesized chemically; however, they do not occur naturally. In protoporphyrinogen and protoporphyrin there are three types of substituents, and the classification becomes more complicated; type IX is the only form that is synthesized naturally.

Derangements of porphyrin metabolism are known clinically as the **porphyrias.** This family of diseases is of great interest because it has revealed that the regulation of heme biosynthesis is complicated. The clinical presentations of the different porphyrias provide a fascinating exposition of biochemical regulatory abnormalities and their relationship to pathophysiological processes. Table 24.2 lists the details of the different porphyrias (see Clin. Corr. 24.7).

Enzymes in Heme Biosynthesis Occur in Both Mitochondria and Cytosol

Aminolevulinic Acid Synthase

Aminolevulinic acid (ALA) synthase controls the rate-limiting step of heme synthesis in all tissues studied. Synthesis of the enzyme is not directed by mitochondrial DNA but occurs rather in the cytosol, being directed by mRNA derived from the nucleus. The enzyme is incorporated into the matrix of the mitochondrion. Succinyl CoA is one of the substrates and is found only in the mitochondrion. This protein has been purified to homogeneity from rat liver mitochondria. The cytosolic protein is a dimer of a 71,000-Da subunit, containing a basic N-terminal signaling sequence that directs the enzyme into the mitochondrion. An ATP-dependent 70,000-Da cytostolic component, known as a chaperone protein, maintains ALA synthase in the unfolded extended state, the only form that can pass through the mitochondrial membrane. Thereafter, the N-

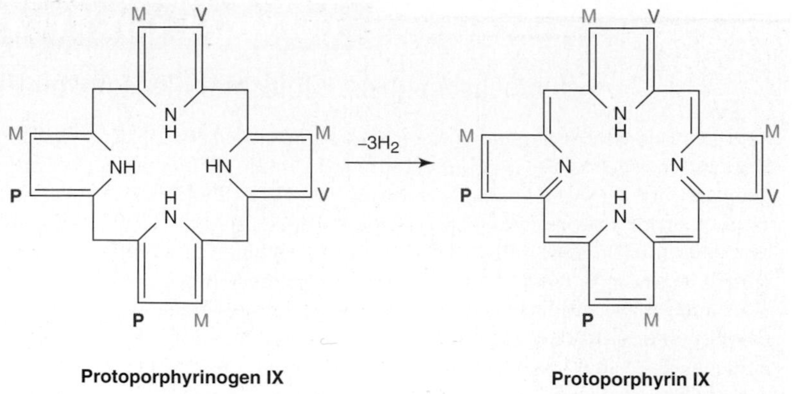

FIGURE 24.8
Action of protoporphyrinogen IX oxidase, an example of the conversion of a porphyrinogen to a porphyrin.

terminal signaling sequence is cleaved by a metal-dependent protease in the mitochondrial matrix, yielding an ALA synthase with subunits of 65,000 Da each. Within the matrix another oligomeric chaperone protein, of 14 subunits of 60,000 Da each, catalyzes the correct folding of the protein in a second ATP-dependent process (Figure 24.9, p. 1014). The ALA synthase has a short biological half-life (~60 min). Both the synthesis and activity of the enzyme are subject to regulation by a variety of substances; 50% inhibition of activity occurs in the presence of 5 mM of hemin, and virtually complete inhibition is noted at a 20-mM concentration. The enzymatic reaction involves the condensation of a **glycine** residue with a residue of **succinyl CoA.** The reaction has an absolute requirement for **pyridoxal phosphate.** Two isoenzymes exist for ALA synthase; only the erythrocytic form contains an IRE.

ALA Dehydratase

Aminolevulinic acid dehydratase (280 Da) (or porphobilinogen synthase) is a cytosol component consisting of eight subunits, of which only four interact with the substrate. This protein also interacts with the substrate to form a Schiff base, but in this case the ε-amino group of a lysine residue binds to the ketonic carbon of the substrate molecule (Figure 24.10, p. 1015). Two molecules of

TABLE 24.2 Derangements in Porphyrin Metabolism

Disease State	*Genetics*	*Tissue*	*Enzyme*	*Activity*	*Organ Pathology*
Acute intermittent porphyria	Dominant	Liver	1. ALA synthase 2. Porphobilinogen deaminase 3. Δ^4-5α-Reductase	Increase Decrease Decrease	Nervous system
Hereditary coproporphyria	Dominant	Liver	1. ALA synthase 2. Coproporphyrinogen oxidase	Increase Decrease	Nervous system; skin
Variegate porphyria	Dominant	Liver	1. ALA synthase 2. Protoporphyrinogen oxidase	Increase Decrease	Nervous system; skin
Porphyria cutanea tarda	Dominant	Liver	1. Uroporphyrinogen decarboxylase	Decrease	Skin, induced by liver disease
Hereditary protoporphyria	Dominant	Marrow	1. Ferrochelatase	Decrease	Gallstones, liver disease, skin
Erythropoietic porphyria	Recessive	Marrow	1. Uroporphyrinogen III cosynthase	Decrease	Skin and appendages; reticuloengothelial system
Lead poisoning	None	All tissues	1. ALA dehydrase 2. Ferrochelatase	Decrease Decrease	Nervous system; blood; others

CLINICAL CORRELATION 24.7

Acute Intermittent Porphyria

A 40-year-old woman appears in the emergency room in an agitated state, weeping and complaining of severe abdominal pain. She has been constipated for several days and has noted marked weakness in the arms and legs and that "things do not appear to be quite right." Physical examination reveals a slightly rapid heart rate (100/min) and moderate hypertension (blood pressure of 160/110 mmHg). There have been earlier episodes of severe abdominal pain; operations undertaken on two occasions revealed no abnormalities. The usual laboratory tests are normal. The neurological complaints are not localized to an anatomical focus. The decision is made that the present symptoms are largely psychiatric in origin and have a functional rather than an organic basis. The patient is sedated with 60 mg of phenobarbital; a consultant psychiatrist agrees by telephone to see the patient in about 4 h. The staff notices a marked deterioration; generalized weakness rapidly appears, progressing to a compromise of respiratory function. This ominous development leads to immediate incorporation of a ventilatory assistance regimen, with transfer to intensive care for physiological monitoring. Her condition deteriorates and she dies 48 h later. A urine sample of the patient is reported later to have a markedly elevated level of porphobilinogen. This patient had acute intermittent porphyria, a disease of incompletely understood derangement of heme biosynthesis. There is a dominant pattern of inheritance associated with an overproduction of the porphyrin precursors, ALA and porphobilinogen. Three enzyme abnormalities are noted in the cases that have been studied carefully. These include (1) a marked increase in ALA synthase, (2) a reduction by one-half of activity of porphobilinogen deaminase, and (3) a reduction of one-half of the activity of steroid Δ^4-5α-reductase. The change in content of the second enzyme is consonant with a dominant expression. The change in content of the third enzyme is acquired and not apparently a heritable expression of the disease. It is believed that a decrease in porphobilinogen deaminase leads to a minor decrease in content of heme in liver. The lower concentration of heme leads to a failure both to repress the synthesis and to inhibit the activity of ALA synthase. Almost never manifested before puberty, the disease is thought to appear only with the induction of Δ^4-5β-reductase at adolescence. Without a sufficient amount of Δ^4-5α-reductase, the observed increase in the 5β steroids is due to a shunting of Δ^4 steroids into the 5β-reductase pathway. The importance of abnormalities of this last metabolic pathway in the pathogenesis of porphyria is controversial. Pathophysiologically, the disease poses a great riddle: the derangement of porphyrin metabolism is confined to the liver, which anatomically appears normal, whereas the pathological findings are restricted to the nervous system. In the present case, involvement of (1) the brain led to the agitated and confused state and the respiratory collapse, (2) the autonomic system led to the hypertension, increased heart rate, constipation, and abdominal pain, and (3) the peripheral nervous system and spinal cord led to the weakness and sensory disturbances. Experimentally, no known metabolic intermediate of heme biosynthesis can cause the pathology noted in acute intermittent porphyria. There should have been a greater suspicion of the possibility of porphyria early in the patient's presentation. The analysis of porphobilinogen in the urine is a relatively simple test. The treatment would have been glucose infusion, the exclusion of any drugs that could cause elevation of ALA synthase (e.g., barbiturates), and, if her disease failed to respond satisfactorily despite these measures, the administration of intravenous hematin to inhibit the synthesis and activity of ALA synthase. Acute hepatic porphyria is of historic political interest. The disease has been diagnosed in two descendants of King George III, suggesting that the latter's deranged personality preceding and during the American Revolution could possibly be ascribed to porphyria.

Meyer, U. A., Strand, L. J., Doss, M., et al. Intermittent acute porphyria: demonstration of a genetic defect in porphobilinogen metabolism. *N. Engl. J. Med.* 286:1277, 1972; and Stein, J. A., and Tschudy, D. D. Acute intermittent porphyria: a clinical and biochemical study of 46 patients. *Medicine (Baltimore)* 49:1, 1970.

ALA condense asymmetrically to form **porphobilinogen.** The ALA dehydratase is a sulfhydryl enzyme and is very sensitive to inhibition by heavy metals. A characteristic finding of **lead poisoning** is the elevation of ALA in the absence of an elevation of porphobilinogen.

Porphobilinogen Deaminase

Synthesis of the porphyrin ring is a complicated process. A sulfhydryl group on porphobilinogen deaminase forms a thioether bond with a porphobilinogen residue through a deamination reaction. Thereafter, five additional porphobilinogen residues are deaminated successively to form a linear hexapyrrole adduct with the enzyme. The adduct is cleaved hydrolytically to form both an enzyme–dipyrromethane complex and the linear tetrapyrrole, hydroxymethylbilane. The enzyme–dipyrromethane complex is then ready for another cycle of addition of four porphobilinogen residues to generate another tetrapyrrole. Thus dipyrromethane is the covalently attached novel cofactor for the enzyme. Porphobilinogen deaminase has no ring-closing function; hydroxymethylbilane closes in an enzyme-independent step to form uroporphyrinogen I if no additional factors are present. However, the deaminase is closely associated with a second protein,

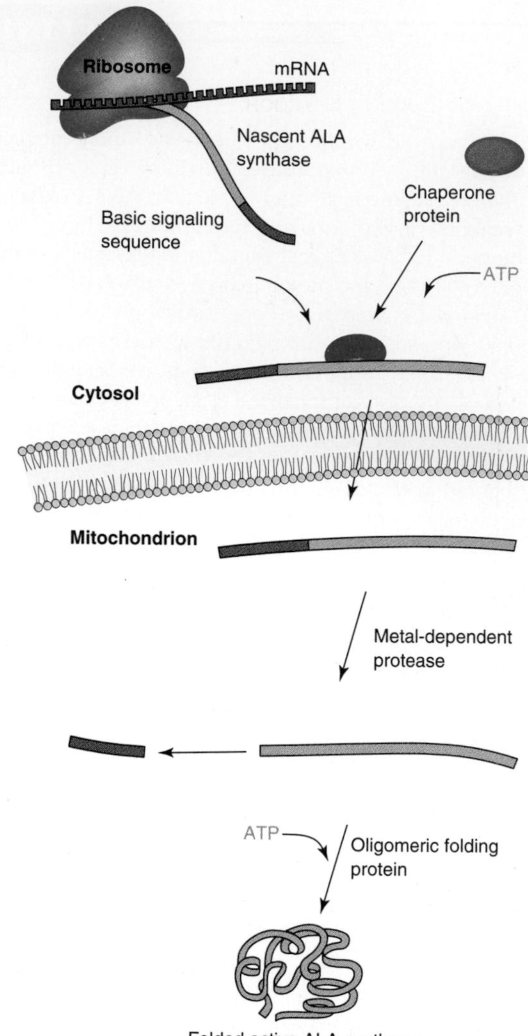

FIGURE 24.9
Synthesis of Δ-aminolevulinic acid synthase.

uroporphyrinogen III cosynthase, which directs the synthesis of the III isomer. The formation of the latter involves a spiro intermediate generated from hydroxymethylbilane; this allows inversion of one of the pyrrole groups (Figure 24.11, p. 1016). In the absence of the cosynthase, uroporphyrinogen I is synthesized slowly; in its presence, the III isomer is synthesized rapidly. A rare recessively inherited disease, **erythropoietic porphyria,** associated with marked cutaneous light sensitization, is due to an abnormality of red blood cell cosynthase. Here, large amounts of the type I isomers of uroporphyrinogen and coproporphyrinogen are synthesized in the bone marrow. Two isoenzymes exist for porphobilinogen deaminase due to alternative splicing of exon 1 or exon 2 to the rest of the mRNA.

Uroporphyrinogen Decarboxylase

This enzyme acts on the side chains of the uroporphyrinogens to form the coproporphyrinogens. The protein catalyzes the conversion of both I and III isomers of uroporphyrinogen to the respective coproporphyrinogen isomers. Uroporphyrinogen decarboxylase is inhibited by iron salts. Clinically, the most common cause of porphyrin derangement is associated with patients who have a single gene abnormality for this enzyme, leading to 50% depression of the enzyme's activity. This disease, which shows cutaneous manifestations primarily with sensitivity to light, is known as **porphyria cutanea tarda.** The condition

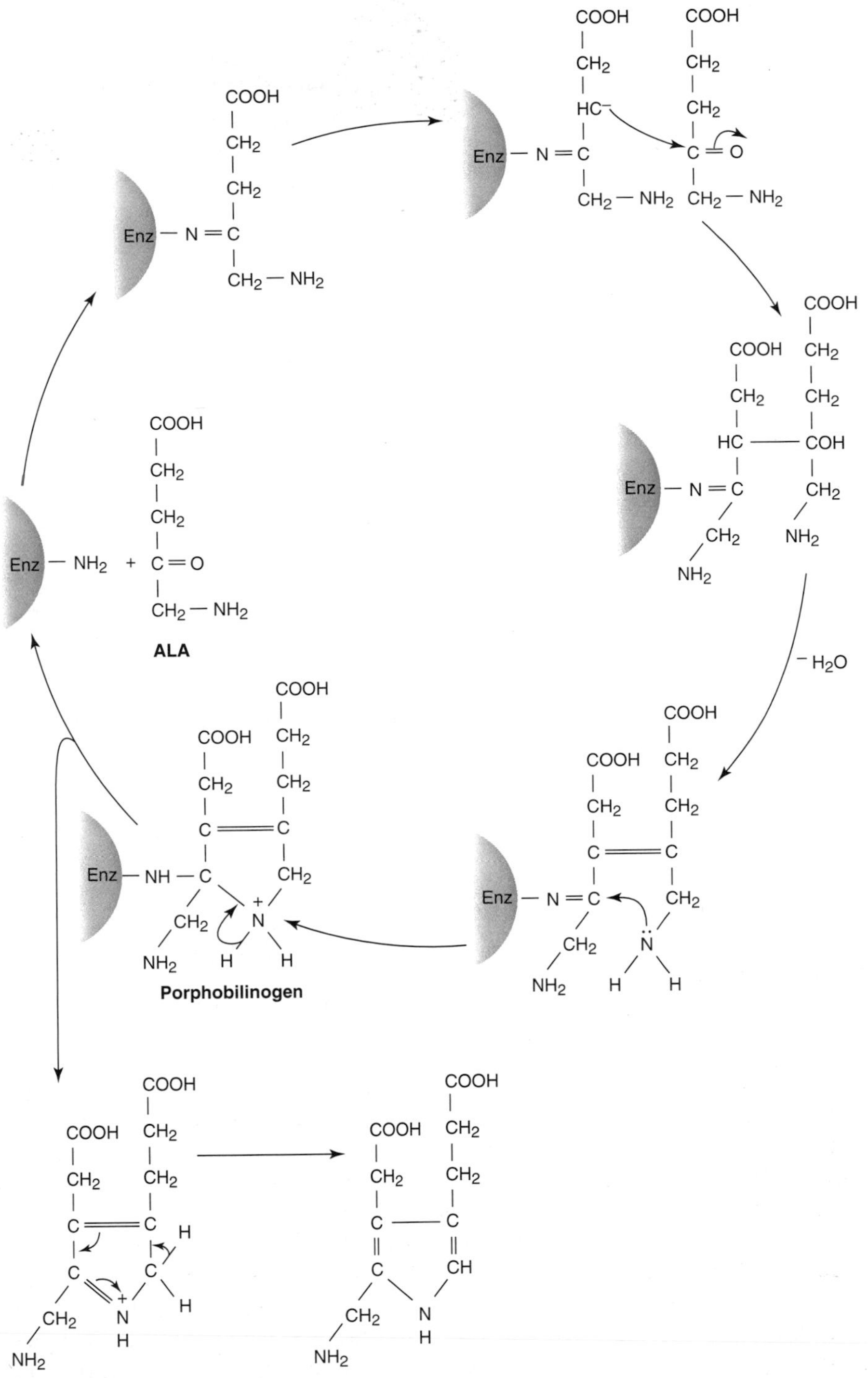

ALA

$-H_2O$

Porphobilinogen

FIGURE 24.10
Synthesis of porphobilinogen.

is not expressed unless patients either take drugs that cause an increase in porphyrin synthesis or drink large amounts of alcohol, leading to the accumulation of iron, which then acts to inhibit further the activity of uroporphyrinogen decarboxylase.

Coproporphyrinogen Oxidase

This mitochondrial enzyme is specific for the type III isomer of coproporphyrinogen, not acting on the type I isomer. Coproporphyrinogen III enters the mitochondrion and is converted to protoporphyrinogen IX. The mechanism of action is not understood. A dominant disease associated with a deficiency of this

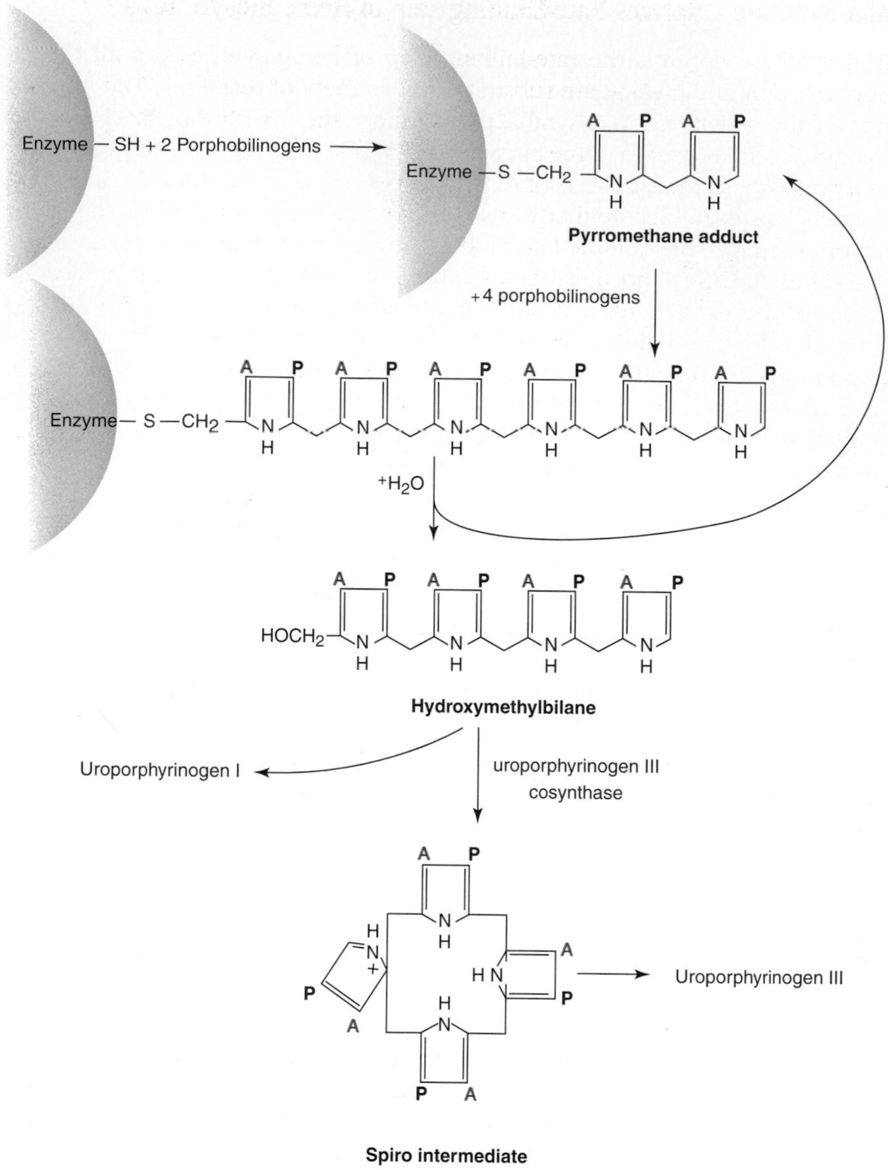

FIGURE 24.11
Synthesis of uroporphyrinogens I and III.
Enzyme in blue is uroporphyrinogen I synthase.

enzyme leads to a form of hereditary hepatic porphyria, known as **hereditary coproporphyria.**

Protoporphyrinogen Oxidase

This mitochondrial enzyme generates a product, protoporphyrin IX, which, in contrast to the other heme precursors, is very water-insoluble. Excess amounts of protoporphyrin IX that are not converted to heme are excreted by the biliary system into the intestinal tract. A dominant disease, **variegate porphyria,** is due to a deficiency of protoporphyrinogen oxidase.

Ferrochelatase

Ferrochelatase inserts ferrous iron into protoporphyrin IX in the final step of the synthesis of heme. The protein is sensitive to the effects of heavy metals (especially lead) and, of course, to iron deprivation. In these latter instances, zinc instead of iron is incorporated to form a zinc–protoporphyrin IX complex. In contrast to heme, the zinc–protoporphyrin IX complex is brilliantly fluorescent and easily detectable in small amounts. The enzyme contains an Fe_2S_2 group and has been proposed as an IRP-3 that controls translation of the erythrocytic ALA synthase mRNA.

ALA Synthase Catalyzes Rate-Limiting Step of Heme Biosynthesis

ALA synthase controls the rate-limiting step of heme synthesis in all tissues. Succinyl CoA and glycine are substrates for a variety of reactions. The modulation of the activity of ALA synthase determines the quantity of the substrates that will be shunted into heme biosynthesis. Heme (and also hematin) acts both as a repressor of the synthesis of ALA synthase and as an inhibitor of its activity. Since heme resembles neither the substrates nor the product of the enzyme's action, it is probable that the latter inhibition occurs at an allosteric site. Almost 100 different drugs and metabolites can cause induction of ALA synthase; for example, a 40-fold increase is noted in the rat after treatment with 3,5-dicarbethoxy-1,4-dihydrocollidine. The effect of pharmacological agents has led to the important clinical feature where some patients with certain kinds of porphyria have had exacerbations of their condition following the inappropriate administration of certain drugs (e.g., barbiturates). ALA dehydratase is also inhibited by heme; but this is of little physiological consequence, since the activity of ALA dehydrase is about 80-fold greater than that of ALA synthase, and thus heme-inhibitory effects are reflected first in the activity of ALA synthase.

Glucose or a proximal metabolite serves to inhibit heme biosynthesis in a mechanism that is not yet defined. This is of clinical relevance, since some patients manifest their porphyric state for the first time when placed on a very low caloric (and therefore glucose) intake. Other regulators of porphyrin metabolism include certain steroids. Steroid hormones (e.g., oral contraceptive pills) with a double bond in ring A between C-4 and C-5 atoms can be reduced by two different reductases. The product of 5α-reduction has little effect on heme biosynthesis; however, the product of 5β-reduction serves as a stimulus for the synthesis of ALA synthase.

24.7 HEME CATABOLISM

Catabolism of heme-containing proteins presents two requirements to the mammalian host: (1) development of a means of processing the hydrophobic products of porphyrin ring cleavage and (2) retention and mobilization of the contained iron so that it may be reutilized. Red blood cells have a life span of approximately 120 days. Senescent cells are recognized by their membrane changes and removed and engulfed by the reticuloendothelial system at extravascular sites. The globin chains denature, releasing heme into the cytoplasm. The globin is degraded to its constituent amino acids, which are reutilized for general metabolic needs.

Figure 24.12 depicts the events of heme catabolism. Heme is degraded primarily by a microsomal enzyme system in reticuloendothelial cells that requires molecular oxygen and NADPH. **Heme oxygenase** is substrate inducible and catalyzes the cleavage of the α-methene bridge, which joins the two pyrrole residues containing the vinyl substituents. The α-methene carbon is converted quantitatively to carbon monoxide. The only endogenous source of **carbon monoxide** in humans is the α-methene carbon. A fraction of the carbon monoxide is released via the respiratory tract. Thus the measurement of carbon monoxide in an exhaled breath provides an index to the quantity of heme that is degraded in an individual. The oxygen present in the carbon monoxide and in the newly derivatized lactam rings are generated entirely from molecular oxygen. The stoichiometry of the reaction requires 3 mol of oxygen for each ring cleavage. Heme oxygenase will only use heme as a substrate, with the iron possibly participating in the cleavage mechanism. Thus free protoporphyrin IX is not a substrate. The linear tetrapyrrole **biliverdin IX** is the product formed by the action of heme oxygenase. Biliverdin IX is reduced by **biliverdin reductase** to bilirubin IX.

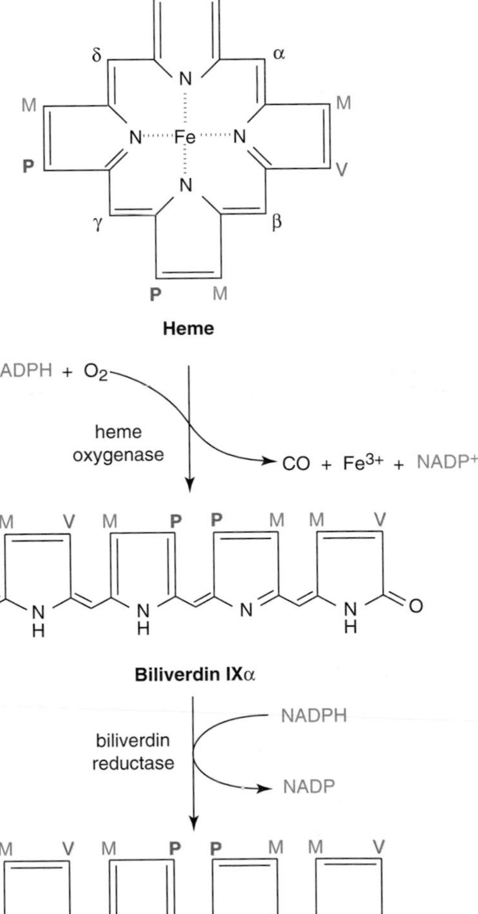

FIGURE 24.12
Formation of bilirubin from heme. Greek letters indicate the labeling of the methene carbon atoms in heme.

Bilirubin Is Conjugated to Form Bilirubin Diglucuronide in Liver

Bilirubin is derived not only from senescent red cells but also from the turnover of other heme-containing proteins, such as the cytochromes. Studies with labeled glycine as a precursor have revealed that an early-labeled bilirubin, with a peak within 1–3 h, appears a very short time after a pulsed administration of the labeled precursor. A larger amount of bilirubin appears much later at about 120 days, reflecting the turnover of heme in red blood cells. Early-labeled bilirubin can be divided into two parts: an early–early part, which reflects the turnover of heme proteins in the liver, and a late–early part, which consists of both the turnover of heme-containing hepatic proteins and the turnover of bone marrow heme, which is either poorly incorporated or easily released from red blood cells. The latter is a measurement of ineffective erythropoiesis and can be very pronounced in disease states such as pernicious anemia (see Chapter 28) and the thalassemias.

Bilirubin is poorly soluble in aqueous solutions at physiological pH values. When transported in plasma, it is bound to serum albumin with an association constant greater than 10^6 M^{-1}. Albumin contains one such high-affinity site and another with a lesser affinity. At the normal albumin concentration of 4 g dL^{-1}, about 70 mg of bilirubin per deciliter of plasma can be bound on the two sites. However, bilirubin toxicity **(kernicterus),** which is manifested by the transfer of bilirubin to membrane lipids, commonly occurs at concentrations greater than 25 mg dL^{-1}. This suggests that the weak affinity of the second site does not allow it to serve effectively in the transport of bilirubin. Bilirubin on serum albumin is rapidly cleared by the liver, where there is a free bidirectional flux of the tetrapyrrole across the sinusoidal–hepatocyte interface. Once in the hepatocyte, bilirubin is bound to several cytostolic proteins, of which only one has been well characterized. The latter component, **ligandin,** is a small basic component making up to 6% of the total cytosolic protein of rat liver. Ligandin has been purified to homogeneity from rat liver and characterized as having two subunits with molecular masses of 22 kDa and 27 kDa. Each subunit contains glutathione *S*-epoxidetransferase activity, a function important in detoxification mechanisms of aryl groups. The stoichiometry of binding is one bilirubin molecule per complete ligandin molecule. The functional role of ligandin and other hepatic bilirubin-binding proteins remains to be defined.

Once in the hepatocyte the propionyl side chains of bilirubin are conjugated to form a diglucuronide (Figure 24.13). The reaction utilizes uridine diphosphoglucuronate derived from the oxidation of uridine diphosphoglucose. The former serves as a glucuronate donor to bilirubin. In normal bile, the diglucuronide is the major form of excreted bilirubin, with only small amounts of the monoglucuronide or other glycosidic adducts present. **Bilirubin diglucuronide** is much more water-soluble than free bilirubin, and thus the transferase facilitates excretion of the bilirubin into bile. Bilirubin diglucuronide is poorly absorbed by the intestinal mucosa. The glucuronide residues are released in the terminal ileum and large intestine by bacterial hydrolases; the released free bilirubin is reduced to the colorless linear tetrapyrroles known as **urobilinogens.** Urobilinogens can be oxidized to colored products known as **urobilins,** which are excreted in the feces. A small fraction of urobilinogen can be reabsorbed by the terminal ileum and large intestine to be removed by hepatic cells and resecreted in bile. When urobilinogen is reabsorbed in large amounts in certain disease states, the kidney serves as a major excretory site.

In the normal state, plasma bilirubin concentrations are 0.3–1 mg dL^{-1}, and this is almost all in the unconjugated state. In the clinical setting, conjugated bilirubin is expressed as **direct bilirubin** because it can be coupled readily with diazonium salts to yield azo dyes; this is the direct **van den Bergh reaction.** Unconjugated bilirubin is bound noncovalently to albumin and will not react until it is released by the addition of an organic solvent such as

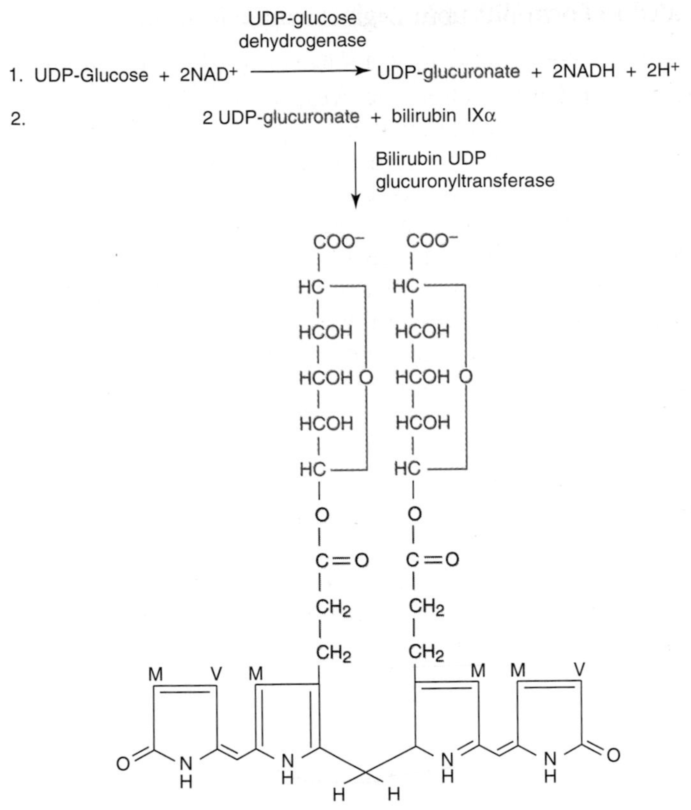

FIGURE 24.13
Biosynthesis of bilirubin diglucuronide.

ethanol. The reaction with diazonium salts yielding the azo dye after the addition of ethanol is the indirect van den Bergh reaction, and this measures the **indirect bilirubin** or the unconjugated bilirubin. Unconjugated bilirubin binds so tightly to serum albumin and lipid that it does not diffuse freely in plasma and therefore does not lead to an elevation of bilirubin in the urine. Unconjugated bilirubin has a high affinity for membrane lipids, which leads to the impairment of cell membrane function, especially in the nervous system. In contrast, conjugated bilirubin is relatively water-soluble, and elevations of this bilirubin form lead to high urinary concentrations with the characteristic deep yellow-brown color. The deposition of conjugated and unconjugated bilirubin in skin and the sclera gives the yellow to yellow-green color seen in patients with jaundice.

A third form of plasma bilirubin occurs only with hepatocellular disease in which a fraction of the bilirubin binds so tightly that it is not released from serum albumin by the usual techniques and is linked covalently to the protein. In some cases up to 90% of total bilirubin can be in this covalently bound form.

The normal liver has a very large capacity to conjugate and mobilize the bilirubin that is delivered. As a consequence, **hyperbilirubinemia** due to excess heme destruction, as in hemolytic diseases, rarely leads to bilirubin levels that exceed 5 mg dL^{-1}, except in situations in which functional derangement of the liver is present (see Clin. Corr. 24.8). Thus marked elevation of unconjugated bilirubin reflects primarily a variety of hepatic diseases, including those that are heritable and those that are acquired (see Clin. Corr. 24.9).

Elevations of conjugated bilirubin level in plasma are attributable to liver and/or biliary tract disease. In simple uncomplicated biliary tract obstruction, the major component of the elevated serum bilirubin is the diglucuronide form, which is released by the liver into the vascular compartment. Biliary tract disease may be extrahepatic or intrahepatic, the latter involving the canaliculi and biliary ductules (see Clin. Corr. 24.10).

CLINICAL CORRELATION 24.8

Neonatal Isoimmune Hemolysis

Rh-negative women pregnant with Rh-positive fetuses will develop antibodies to Rh factors. These antibodies will cross the placenta to hemolyze fetal red blood cells. Usually this is not of clinical relevance until about the third Rh-positive pregnancy, in which the mother has had antigenic challenges with earlier babies. Antenatal studies will reveal rising maternal levels of IgG antibodies against Rh-positive red blood cells, indicating that the fetus is Rh-positive. Before birth, placental transfer of fetal bilirubin occurs with excretion through the maternal liver. Because hepatic enzymes of bilirubin metabolism are poorly expressed in the newborn, infants may not be able to excrete the large amounts of bilirubin that can be generated from red cell breakdown. At birth these infants usually appear normal; however, the unconjugated bilirubin in the umbilical cord blood is elevated up to 4 mg dL^{-1}; due to the hemolysis initiated by maternal antibodies. During the next 2 days the serum bilirubin rises, reflecting continuing isoimmune hemolysis, leading to jaundice, hepatosplenomegaly, ascites, and edema. If untreated, signs of central nervous system damage can occur, with the appearance of lethargy, hypotonia, spasticity, and respiratory difficulty, constituting the syndrome of kernicterus. Treatment involves exchange transfusion with whole blood, which is serologically compatible with both the infant's blood and maternal serum. The latter requirement is necessary to prevent hemolysis of the transfused cells. Additional treatment includes external phototherapy, which facilitates the breakdown of bilirubin. The entire problem can be prevented by treating Rh-negative mothers with anti-Rh globulin. These antibodies recognize the fetal red cells, block the Rh antigens, and cause them to be destroyed without stimulating an immune response in the mothers.

Mauer, H. M., Shumway, C. N., Draper, D. A., and Hossaini, A. A. Controlled trial comparing agar, intermittent phototherapy, and continuous phototherapy for reducing neonatal hyperbilirubinemia. *J. Pediatr.* 82:73, 1973; and Bowman, J. J. Management of Rh-isoimmunization. *Obstet. Gynecol.* 52:1, 1978.

Intravascular Hemolysis Requires Scavenging of Iron

In certain diseases destruction of red blood cells occurs in the intravascular compartment rather than in the extravascular reticuloendothelial cells. In the former case the appearance of free hemoglobin and heme in the plasma potentially could lead to the excretion of these substances through the kidney with a substantial loss of iron. To prevent this occurrence, specific plasma proteins are involved in scavenging mechanisms. Transferrin binds free iron and thus permits its reutilization. Free hemoglobin, after oxygenation in the pulmonary capillaries, dissociates into α,β dimers, which are bound to a family of circulating

CLINICAL CORRELATION 24.9

Bilirubin UDP-Glucuronosyltransferase Deficiency

Bilirubin UDP-glucuronosyltransferase has two isoenzyme forms, derived from alternative mRNA splicing between variable forms of exon 1 and common exons 2, 3, 4, and 5. The latter exons define the part of the protein that binds the UDP-glucuronate, whereas the various exons 1 have defined specificities for either bilirubin or other acceptors, such as phenol. Two exons have bilirubin specificity leading to two forms of bilirubin UDP-glucuronosyltransferase forms. Two major families of diseases are seen with deficiencies of the enzyme. Crigler–Najjar syndrome is seen in infants and is associated with extraordinarily high serum unconjugated bilirubin due to an autosomal recessive inheritance of mutations on both alleles in exons 2, 3, 4, or 5. Gilbert's syndrome is also associated with a deficiency of the enzyme's activity, but only to about 25% of normal. The patients appear jaundiced but without other clinical symptoms. The major complication is an exhaustive search by the physician looking for some serious liver disease and failing to recognize the benign condition. Two different findings that may be restricted to different populations account for the condition. In Japan a dominant pattern of inheritance is noted with a mutation on only one allele. The 75% reduction of activity is ascribed to the fact that the enzyme exists as an oligomer, where mutant and normal monomers might associate to form heterooligomers. The explanation is that not only is the mutant monomer inactive, but it forces conformational effects on the normal subunit, reducing its activity substantially. In contrast, in the Western world the condition is due largely to a homozygous expansion of the bases in the promoter region with less efficient transcription of the gene.

Aono, S., Adachi, Y., Uyama, S., et al. Analysis of genes for bilirubin UDP-glucuronosyltransferase in Gilbert's syndrome. *Lancet* 345:958, 1995; and Bosma, P. J., Chowdhury, J. R., Bakker, C., et al. The genetic basis of the reduced expression of bilirubin UDP-glucuronosyltransferase 1 in Gilbert's syndrome. *N. Engl. J. Med.* 333:1171, 1995.

plasma proteins, the **haptoglobins,** having a high affinity for the oxyhemoglobin dimer. Since deoxyhemoglobin does not dissociate into dimers in physiological settings, it is not bound by haptoglobin. The stoichiometry of binding is two α,β-oxyhemoglobin dimers per haptoglobin molecule. Interesting studies have been made with rabbit antihuman-hemoglobin antibodies on the haptoglobin–hemoglobin interaction. Human haptoglobin interacts with a variety of hemoglobins from different species. The binding of human haptoglobin with human hemoglobin is not affected by the binding of rabbit antihuman-hemoglobin antibody. These studies suggest that haptoglobin binds to sites on hemoglobin that are highly conserved in evolution and therefore are not sufficiently antigenic to generate antibodies. The most likely site for the molecular interaction of hemoglobin and haptoglobin is the interface of the α and β globins of the tetramer that dissociates to yield α,β dimers. Sequence determinations have indicated that these contact regions are highly conserved in evolution.

The haptoglobins are **α_2-globulins.** Synthesized in the liver, they consist of two pairs of polypeptide chains (α being the lighter and β the heavier). The genes for the α and β chains are linked so that a single mRNA is synthesized, generating a single polypeptide chain that is cleaved to form the two different chains. The β chains are glycopeptides of 39 kDa and are invariant in structure; α chains are of several kinds. The haptoglobin peptide chains are joined by disulfide bonds between the α and β chains and between the two α chains.

Interaction of haptoglobin with hemoglobin forms a complex that is too large to be filtered through the renal glomerulus. Free hemoglobin (appearing in renal tubules and in urine) will occur during intravascular hemolysis only when the binding capacity of circulating haptoglobin has been exceeded. Haptoglobin delivers hemoglobin to the reticuloendothelial cells. The heme in free hemoglobin is relatively resistant to the action of heme oxygenase, whereas the heme residues in an α,β dimer of hemoglobin bound to haptoglobin are very susceptible.

The measurement of serum haptoglobin is used clinically as an indication of the degree of intravascular hemolysis. Patients who have significant intravascular hemolysis will have little or no levels of haptoglobin because of the removal of haptoglobin–hemoglobin complexes by the reticuloendothelial system. Haptoglobin levels can also be low in severe extravascular hemolysis, in which the large load of hemoglobin in the reticuloendothelial system leads to the transfer of free hemoglobin into plasma.

Free heme and hematin appearing in plasma are bound by a β-globulin, **hemopexin** (57 kDa). One heme residue binds per hemopexin molecule. Hemopexin transfers heme to liver, where further metabolism by heme oxygenase occurs. Normal plasma hemopexin contains very little bound heme, whereas in intravascular hemolysis, the hemopexin is almost completely saturated by heme and is cleared with a half-life of about 7 h. In the latter instance, excess heme binds to albumin, with newly synthesized hemopexin serving as a mediator for the transfer of the heme from albumin to the liver. Hemopexin also binds free protoporphyrin.

CLINICAL CORRELATION 24.10

Elevation of Serum Conjugated Bilirubin

Elevations of serum conjugated bilirubin are attributable to liver and/or biliary tract disease. In simple uncomplicated biliary tract obstruction, the major component of the elevated serum bilirubin is the diglucuronide form, which is released by the liver into the vascular compartment. Biliary tract disease may be extrahepatic or intrahepatic, the latter involving the canaliculi and biliary ductules. Dubin–Johnson syndrome is an autosomal recessive disease involving a defect in the biliary secretory mechanisms in liver. Excretion through the biliary tract of a variety of (but not all) organic anions is affected. Retention of melanin-like pigment in the liver in this disorder leads to a characteristic gray-black color of this organ. A second heritable disorder associated with elevated levels of serum conjugated bilirubin is Rotor's syndrome. In this poorly defined disease no hepatic pigmentation occurs.

Kitamura, T., Alroy, J., Gatmaitan, Z., et al. Defective biliary excretion of epinephrine metabolites in mutant (TR-) rats: relation to the pathogenesis of black liver in the Dubin–Johnson syndrome and Corriedale sheep with an analogous excretory defect. *Hepatology* 15:1154, 1992.

BIBLIOGRAPHY

Battersby, A. R. The Bakerian Lecture, 1984. Biosynthesis of the pigments of life. *Proc. R. Soc. Lond. B Biol. Sci.* 225:1, 1985.

Bothwell, T. H., Charlton, R. W., and Motulsky, A. G. Hemochromatosis. In: C. R. Scriver, A. L. Beaudet, W. S. Sly, and D. Valle (Eds.), *The Metabolic and Molecular Bases of Inherited Disease,* 7th ed., Vol. II. New York: McGraw-Hill, 1995, p. 2237.

Braig, K., Otwinowski, Z., Hegde, R., Boisvert, D. C., Joachimiak, A., Horwich, A. L., and Sigler, P. B. The crystal structure of the bacterial chaperonin GroEL at 2.8 Å. *Nature* 371:578, 1994.

Casey, J. L., Hentze, M. W., Koeller, D. H., Caughman, S., Rouault, T. A., Klausner, R. D., and Harford, J. B. Iron-responsive elements: regulatory RNA sequences that control mRNA levels and translation. *Science* 240:924, 1988.

Chowdhury, J. R., Wolkoff, A. W., Chowdhury, N. R., and Arias, I. M. Hereditary jaundice and disorders of bilirubin metabolism. In: C. R. Scriver, A. L. Beaudet, W. S. Sly, and D. Valle (Eds.), *The Metabolic and Molecular Bases of Inherited Disease,* 7th ed., Vol. II. New York: McGraw-Hill, 1995, p. 2161.

Fenton, W. A., Kashi, Y., Furtak, K., and Horwich, A. L. Residues in chaperonin GroEL required for polypeptide binding and release. *Nature* 371:614, 1994.

Ferreira, G. C. Ferrochelatase binds the iron-responsive element present in the erythroid 5-aminolevulinate synthase mRNA. *Biochem. Biophys. Res. Commun.* 214:875, 1995.

Fleet, J. C. A new role for lactoferrin: DNA binding and transcription activation. *Nutr. Rev.* 53:226, 1995.

Guo, B., Phillips, J. D., Yu, Y., and Leibold, E. A. Iron regulates the intracellular degradation of iron regulatory protein 2 by the proteasome. *J. Biol. Chem.* 270:21645, 1995.

Hartl, F. U. Molecular chaperones in cellular protein folding. *Nature* 381:571, 1996.

Huebers, H. A., and Finch, C. A. Transferrin: physiologic behavior and clinical implications. *Blood* 64:763, 1984.

Kappas, A., Sassa, S., Galbraith, R. A., and Nordmann, Y. The porphyrias. In: C. R. Scriver, A. L. Beaudet, W. S. Sly, and D. Valle (Eds.), *The Metabolic and Molecular Bases of Inherited Disease,* 7th ed., Vol. II. New York: McGraw-Hill, 1995, p. 2103.

Lustbader, J. W., Arcoleo, J. P., Birken, S., and Greer, J. Hemoglobin-binding site on haptoglobin probed by selective proteolysis. *J. Biol. Chem.* 258:1227, 1983.

Maeda, N., Yang, F., Barnett, D. R., Bowman, B. H., and Smithies, O. Duplication within the haptoglobin *Hp2* gene. *Nature* 309:131, 1984.

Mascotti, D. P., Rup, D., and Thach, R. E. Regulation of iron metabolism: translational effects mediated by iron, heme, and cytokines. *Annu. Rev. Nutr.* 15:239, 1995.

May, W. S., Sahyoun, N., Jacobs, S., Wolf, M., and Cuatracasas, P. Mechanism of phorbol-diester-induced regulation of surface transferrin receptor involves the action of activated protein kinase C and an intact cytoskeleton. *J. Biol. Chem.* 260:9419, 1985.

Melefors, O., and Hentze, M. W. Iron regulatory factor—the conductor of cellular iron regulation. *Blood Rev.* 7:251, 1993.

Osterman, J., Horwich, A. L., Neupert, W., and Hartl, F.-U. Protein folding in mitochondria requires complex formation with hsp60 and ATP hydrolysis. *Nature* 341:125, 1989.

Pantopoulos, K., Gray, N. K., and Hentze, M. W. Differential regulation of two related RNA-binding proteins, iron regulatory protein (IRP) and IRP_B. *RNA* 1:155, 1995.

Pantopoulos, K., and Hentze, M. W. Nitric oxide signalling to iron-regulatory protein: direct control of ferritin mRNA translation and transferrin receptor mRNA stability in transfected fibroblasts. *Proc. Natl. Acad. Sci. USA* 92:1267, 1995.

Weiss, J. S., Gautam, A., Lauff, J. J., et al. The clinical importance of a protein-bound fraction of serum bilirubin in patients with hyperbilirubinemia. *N. Engl. J. Med.* 309:147, 1983.

Yamashiro, D. J., Tycko, B., Fluss, S. R., and Maxfield, F. R. Segregation of transferrin to a mildly acidic (pH 6.5) para-golgi compartment in the recycling pathway. *Cell* 37:789, 1984.

QUESTIONS ■ C. N. ANGSTADT AND J. BAGGOTT

Refer to the following for Questions 1–3:

A. ferritin
B. ferredoxin
C. hemosiderin
D. lactoferrin
E. transferrin

1. A type of protein in which iron is specifically bound to sulfur.

2. Exhibits an antimicrobial effect in the intestinal tract of newborns because of its ability to bind iron.

3. Delivers iron to tissues by binding to specific cell surface receptors.

4. In the intestinal absorption of iron:
   A. the presence of a reductant like ascorbate enhances the availability of iron.
   B. regulation of uptake occurs between the lumen and mucosal cells.
   C. the amount of apoferritin synthesized in the mucosal cell is directly related to the need for iron by the host.
   D. iron bound tightly to a ligand, such as phytate, is more readily absorbed than free iron.
   E. low pH in the stomach inhibits absorption by favoring Fe^{3+}.

5. Which of the following statements about iron distribution is correct?
   A. Iron overload cannot occur because very efficient excretory mechanisms are available.
   B. Cells cannot regulate their uptake of iron with changing iron content.
   C. Transferrin decreases in iron deficiency to facilitate storage of iron.
   D. Iron homeostasis is maintained in part by iron regulatory proteins binding to iron-responsive elements in mRNA.
   E. In the early stages of iron depletion, serum ferritin levels rise rapidly as iron is released from storage forms.

6. The biosynthesis of heme requires all of the following EXCEPT:
   A. propionic acid.
   B. succinyl CoA.
   C. glycine.
   D. ferrous ion.

7. Uroporphyrin III:
   A. is an intermediate in the biosynthesis of heme.
   B. does not contain a tetrapyrrole ring.
   C. differs from coproporphyrin III in the substituents around the ring.
   D. is formed from uroporphyrinogen III by an oxidase.
   E. formation is the primary control step in heme synthesis.

8. Aminolevulinic acid synthase:
   A. requires NAD for activity.
   B. is allosterically activated by heme.
   C. synthesis is inhibited by steroids.
   D. is synthesized in mitochondria.
   E. synthesis can be induced by a variety of drugs.

9. Lead poisoning would be expected to result in an elevated level of:
   A. aminolevulinic acid.
   B. porphobilinogen.
   C. protoporphyrin I.
   D. heme.
   E. bilirubin.

10. Ferrochelatase:
   A. is an iron-chelating compound.
   B. releases iron from heme in the degradation of hemoglobin.
   C. binds iron to sulfide ions and cysteine residues.
   D. is inhibited by heavy metals.
   E. is involved in the cytoplasmic portion of heme synthesis.

11. Heme oxygenase:
   A. can oxidize the methene bridge between any two pyrrole rings of heme.
   B. requires molecular oxygen.
   C. produces bilirubin.
   D. produces carbon dioxide.
   E. can use either heme or protoporphyrin IX as substrate.

12. The substance deposited in skin and sclera in jaundice is:
   A. biliverdin.
   B. only unconjugated bilirubin.
   C. only direct bilirubin.
   D. both bilirubin and bilirubin diglucuronide.
   E. hematin.

13. Hepatic disease leads to major elevation of the blood level of:
   A. heme.
   B. biliverdin.
   C. bilirubin.
   D. bilirubin diglucuronide.
   E. direct bilirubin.

14. Biliary obstruction leads to major elevation of the blood level of:
   A. only direct bilirubin.
   B. only indirect bilirubin.
   C. both direct and indirect bilirubin.
   D. heme but not bilirubin.
   E. biliverdin but not bilirubin.

15. Acute intermittent porphyria is accompanied by an increased urinary level of:
   A. biliverdin.
   B. direct bilirubin.
   C. heme.
   D. indirect bilirubin.
   E. porphobilinogen.

16. Haptoglobin binds:
   A. a globin monomer.
   B. an oxyhemoglobin molecule.
   C. α,β-oxyhemoglobin dimers.
   D. a deoxyhemoglobin molecule.
   E. α,β-deoxyhemoglobin dimers.

17. Haptoglobin:
   A. helps prevent loss of iron following intravascular red blood cell destruction.
   B. levels in serum are elevated in severe intravascular hemolysis.
   C. inhibits the action of heme oxygenase.
   D. binds heme and hematin as well as hemoglobin.
   E. is a β-globulin.

ANSWERS

1. B Animal ferredoxins, also known as nonheme iron-containing proteins, have two irons bound to two cysteine residues and sharing two sulfide ions (p. 1004).
2. D As long as lactoferrin is not saturated, its avid binding of iron diminishes the amount available for growth of microorganisms (p. 1003).
3. E Internalization of the receptor–transferrin complex is mediated by a Ca^{2+}–calmodulin–protein kinase C complex. Internalization is followed by release of the iron and recycling of the apotransferrin to the plasma (p. 1003). Ferritin and hemosiderin (p. 1004) are storage forms of iron.
4. A A and D: Ascorbate facilitates reduction to the ferrous state and, therefore, dissociation from ligands and absorption. B: Substantial iron enters the mucosal cell regardless of need, but the amount transferred to the capillary beds is controlled. C: Iron bound to apoferritin is trapped in mucosal cells and not transferred to the host. E: Oxidation to Fe^{3+} is favored by higher pH (p. 1005).
5. D B and D: In the presence of low iron this mechanism leads to increased synthesis of transferrin receptor and decreased synthesis of apoferritin. A: The high affinity of many macromolecules for iron prevents efficient excretion. C: Transferrin increases in iron deficiency to improve absorption. E: Serum ferritin is normally small and decreases (pp. 1007–1008).
6. A B and C: The organic portion of heme comes totally from glycine and succinyl CoA; the propionic acid side chain comes from the succinate. D: The final step of heme synthesis is the insertion of the ferrous ion (p. 1010, Figure 24.7).
7. C A, B, and D: The tetrapyrrole porphyrins (except for protoporphyrin IX) are not intermediates but end products formed from the porphyrinogens nonenzymatically. E: Synthesis of aminolevulinic acid is the rate-limiting step (p. 1010, Figure 24.7).
8. E The enzyme is induced in response to need (many drug detoxifications are cytochrome P450-dependent). A: The mechanism involves a Schiff base with glycine. B: Heme both allosterically inhibits and suppresses synthesis of the enzyme. C: One reduction product of catabolic steroids stimulates synthesis. D: The gene for this enzyme is on nuclear DNA (pp. 1009–1012).
9. A A–D: Lead inhibits ALA dehydratase so it inhibits synthesis of porphobilinogen and subsequent compounds. Heme certainly would not be elevated, because lead also inhibits ferrochelatase. E: Bilirubin is a breakdown product of heme, not an intermediate in synthesis (p. 1013).
10. D This enzyme, in the mitochondria, catalyzes the last step of heme synthesis, the insertion of Fe^{2+}, and is sensitive to the effects of heavy metals (p. 1016).
11. B Oxygenases usually use O_2. A: The enzyme is specific for the methene between the two rings containing the vinyl groups (α-methene bridge). C and D: The products are biliverdin and CO; the measurement of CO in the breath is an index of heme degradation. E: Iron is necessary for activity (p. 1017).
12. D Both conjugated (direct) and unconjugated (indirect) bilirubin are deposited (p. 1019).

13. C Since the liver is responsible for conjugating bilirubin, hepatic disease leads to the elevation of unconjugated (indirect) bilirubin in blood. A and B: Catabolism of heme to bilirubin occurs in reticuloendothelial cells. D and E: These are the same and require conjugation by the liver (p. 1019).
14. A Conjugated (direct) bilirubin is excreted in the bile. B and C: As long as the liver is functioning, bilirubin (indirect) will be conjugated. D and E: These occur in the reticuloendothelial cells so bilirubin will be formed (pp. 1020–1021).
15. E The disease is characterized by increased ALA synthase and decreased porphobilinogen deaminase activities. A, B, and E: These all represent heme catabolism. D: Heme synthesis is reduced (p. 1013).
16. C Haptoglobin binds dimers, two per haptoglobin molecule, specifically the oxyhemoglobin dimers since deoxyhemoglobin does not dissociate to dimers physiologically (p. 1021).
17. A Haptoglobin is part of the scavenging mechanism to prevent urinary loss of heme and hemoglobin from intravascular degradation of red blood cells. B: Since the scavenged complex is taken up by the reticuloendothelial system, the haptoglobin levels in serum are low. C: Heme residues in the dimers bound to haptoglobin are more susceptible than free heme to oxidation by heme oxygenase. D and E: Heme and hematin are bound by a β-globulin, while haptoglobin is an α-globulin (p. 1021).

CHAPTER

GAS TRANSPORT AND pH REGULATION

James Baggott

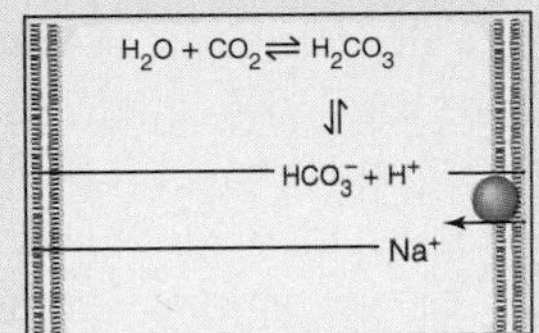

25.1 ■ INTRODUCTION TO GAS TRANSPORT

Large organisms, especially terrestrial ones, require a relatively tough, impermeable outer covering to help shield them from dust, twigs, nonisotonic fluids like rain and seawater, and other elements in the environment that might be harmful to living cells. One of the consequences of being large and having an impermeable covering is that individual cells of the organism cannot exchange gases directly with the atmosphere. Instead there must exist a specialized exchange surface, such as a lung or a gill, and a system to circulate the gases (and other materials, such as nutrients and waste products) in a manner that will meet the needs of every living cell in the body.

The existence of a system for the transport of gases from the atmosphere to cells deep within the body is not merely necessary, it has definite advantages. Oxygen is a good oxidizing agent, and at its partial pressure in the atmosphere, about 160 mmHg or 21.3 kPa, it would oxidize and inactivate many components of the cells, such as essential sulfhydryl groups of enzymes. By the time O_2 gets through the transport system of the body its partial pressure is reduced to a much less damaging 20 mmHg (2.67 kPa) or less. In contrast, CO_2 is relatively concentrated in the body and becomes diluted in transit to the atmosphere. In the tissues, where it is produced, its partial pressure is 46 mmHg (6.13 kPa) or more. In the lungs it is 40 mmHg (5.33 kPa), and in the atmosphere only 0.2 mmHg (0.03 kPa), less abundant than the rare gas, argon. Its relatively high concentration in the body permits it to be used as one component of a physiologically important buffering system, a system that is particularly useful because, upon demand, the concentration of CO_2 in the extracellular fluid can be varied over a rather wide range. This is discussed in more detail later in the chapter.

Oxygen and CO_2 are carried between the lungs and the other tissues by the blood. In the blood some of each gas is present in simple physical solution, but mostly each is involved in some sort of interaction with hemoglobin, the major protein of the red blood cell. There is a reciprocal relation between hemoglobin's affinity for O_2 and CO_2, so that the relatively high level of O_2 in the lungs aids the release of CO_2, which is to be expired, and the high CO_2 level in other tissues aids the release of O_2 for their use. Thus a description of the physiological transport of O_2 and CO_2 is the story of the interaction of these two compounds with hemoglobin.

CLINICAL CORRELATION 25.1

Diaspirin Hemoglobin

Shock is a condition of inadequate tissue perfusion due, for example, to loss of blood. Hemorrhagic shock is a major cause of death following trauma. Rapid blood transfusion can be life-saving, but cross-matching must be done before transfusing blood, and transfusion is associated with a significant risk of disease. In addition, blood (or blood of the correct type) may be in short supply under certain circumstances. Hence there is considerable interest in developing a safe, effective blood substitute.

Hemoglobin in plasma has a very short lifetime. It rapidly dissociates into $\alpha\beta$ dimers, which bind to the plasma protein, haptoglobin, and are removed from circulation. Hemoglobin can be specifically cross-linked with bis(3,5-dibromosalicyl) fumarate at the Lys 99 of the α chains; the product is called diaspirin cross-linked hemoglobin (DCLHb). DCLHb has a longer lifetime in plasma than hemoglobin, and its lifetime can be extended still further by polymerizing the DCLHb. DCLHb has performed well as a blood replacement in experimental animals, and the possibility of using it in humans is being pursued.

25.2 ■ NEED FOR A CARRIER OF OXYGEN IN BLOOD

An O_2 carrier is needed in blood because O_2 is not soluble enough in blood plasma to meet the body's needs. At 38°C, 1 L of plasma dissolves only 2.3 mL of O_2. Whole blood, because of its **hemoglobin,** has a much greater oxygen capacity (see Clin. Corr. 25.1). One liter of blood normally contains about 150 g of hemoglobin (contained within the erythrocytes), and each gram of hemoglobin can combine with 1.34 mL of O_2. Thus the hemoglobin in 1 L of blood can carry 200 mL of O_2, 87 times as much as plasma alone would carry. Without an O_2 carrier, the blood would have to circulate 87 times as fast to provide the same amount of O_2. As it is, the blood makes a complete circuit of the body in 60 s under resting conditions, and in the aorta it flows at the rate of about 18.6 m s^{-1}. An 87-fold faster flow would require a fabulous high-pressure pump, would produce tremendously turbulent flow and high shear forces in the plasma, would result in uncontrollable bleeding from wounds, and would not even allow the blood enough time in the lungs to take up O_2. The availability of a carrier not only permits us to avoid these impracticalities, but also gives us a way of controlling oxygen delivery, since the O_2 affinity of the carrier is responsive to changing physiological conditions.

Respiratory System Anatomy Affects Blood Gas Concentration

The respiratory system includes the trachea, in the neck, which bifurcates in the thorax into right and left bronchi, as shown schematically in Figure 25.1. The bronchi continue to bifurcate into smaller and smaller passages, ending with tiny bronchioles, which open into microscopic gas-filled sacs called alveoli. It is in the alveoli that gas exchange takes place with the alveolar capillary blood.

As we inhale and exhale, the alveoli do not appreciably change in size. Rather, it is the airways that change in length and diameter as the air is pumped into and out of the lungs. Gas exchange between the airways and the alveoli then proceeds simply by diffusion. These anatomical and physiological facts have two important consequences. In the first place, since the alveoli are at the ends of long tubes that constitute a large dead space, and the gases in the alveoli are not completely replaced by fresh air with each breath, the gas composition of the alveolar air differs from that of the atmosphere, as shown in Table 25.1. Oxygen concentration is lower in the alveoli because it is removed by the blood. Carbon dioxide concentration is higher because it is added. Since we do not usually breathe air that is saturated with water vapor at 38°C, water vapor is generally added in the airways. The concentration of nitrogen is lower in the alveoli, not because it is taken up by the body, but simply because it is diluted by the CO_2 and water vapor.

A second consequence of the existence of alveoli of essentially constant size is that the blood that flows through the pulmonary capillaries during expiration, as well as the blood that flows through during inspiration, can exchange gases. This would not be possible if the alveoli collapsed during expiration and contained no gases, in which case the composition of the blood gases would fluctuate widely, depending on whether the blood passed through the lungs during an inspiratory or expiratory phase of the breathing cycle.

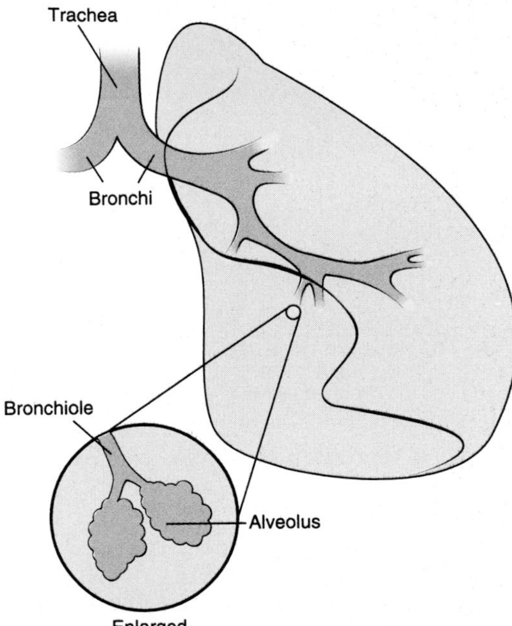

FIGURE 25.1
Diagram showing the respiratory tract.

A Physiological Oxygen Carrier Must Have Unusual Properties

We have seen that an O_2 carrier is necessary. Clearly this carrier would have to be able to bind oxygen at an O_2 tension of about 100 mmHg (13.3 kPa), the partial pressure of oxygen in the alveoli. The carrier must also be able to release O_2 to the extrapulmonary tissues. The O_2 tension in the capillary bed of an active muscle is about 20 mmHg (2.67 kPa). In resting muscle it is higher, but during extreme activity it is lower. These O_2 tensions represent the usual limits within which an oxygen carrier must work. An efficient carrier would be nearly fully saturated in the lungs but should be able to give up most of this to a working muscle.

Let us first see whether a carrier that binds O_2 in a simple equilibrium represented by

$$\text{Oxygen} + \text{carrier} \leftrightharpoons \text{oxygen} \cdot \text{carrier}$$

TABLE 25.1 Partial Pressures of Important Gases Given in Millimeters of Hg (kPa)

	In the Atmosphere		*In the Alveoli of the Lungs*	
Gas	*mmHg*	*kPa*	*mmHg*	*kPa*
O_2	159	21.2	100	13.3
N_2	601	80.1	573	76.4
CO_2	0.2	0.027	40	5.33
H_2O	0	0	47	6.27
Total	760	101	760	101

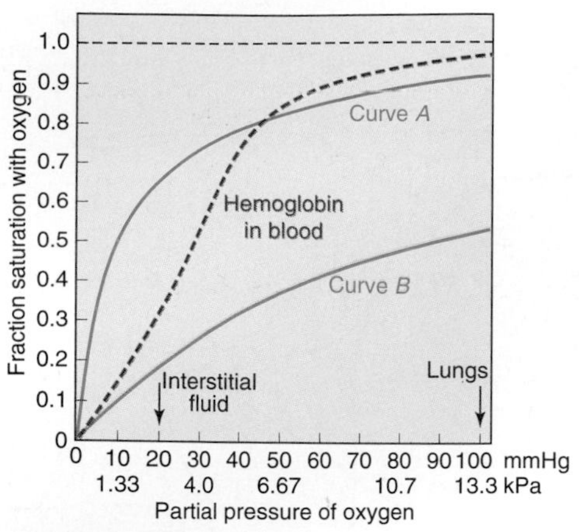

FIGURE 25.2
Oxygen saturation curves for two hypothetical oxygen carriers and for hemoglobin.
Curve *A:* Hypothetical carrier with hyperbolic saturation curve (a simple carrier), 90% saturated in the lungs and 66% saturated at the partial pressure found in interstitial fluid. Curve *B:* Hypothetical carrier with hyperbolic saturation curve (another simple carrier), 56% saturated in the lungs and 20% saturated at the partial pressure found in interstitial fluid. Dashed curve: Hemoglobin in whole blood.

would be satisfactory. For this type of carrier the dissociation constant would be given by the simple expression

$$K_d = \frac{[\text{oxygen}][\text{carrier}]}{[\text{oxygen} \cdot \text{carrier}]}$$

and the saturation curve would be a **rectangular hyperbola.** This model would be valid even for a carrier with several oxygen-binding sites per molecule, which we know is the case for hemoglobin, as long as each site were independent and not influenced by the presence or absence of O_2 at adjacent sites.

If such a carrier had a dissociation constant that permitted 90% saturation in the lungs, then, as shown in Figure 25.2, curve *A,* at a partial pressure of 20 mmHg (2.67 kPa) it would still be 66% saturated and would have delivered only 24% of its O_2 load. This would not be very efficient.

What about some other simple carrier, one that bound O_2 less tightly and therefore released most of it at low partial pressure, so that the carrier was, say, only 20% saturated at 20 mmHg (2.67 kPa)? Again, as shown in Figure 25.2, curve *B,* it would be relatively inefficient; in the lungs this carrier could fill only 56% of its maximum O_2 capacity and would deliver only 36% of what it could carry. It appears then that the mere fivefold change in O_2 tension between the lungs and the unloading site is not compatible with efficient operation of a simple carrier. Simple carriers are not sensitive enough to respond massively to a signal as small as a fivefold change.

Figure 25.2 also shows the oxygen-binding curve of hemoglobin in normal blood. The curve is **sigmoid,** not hyperbolic, and it cannot be described by a simple equilibrium expression. Hemoglobin, however, is a very good physiological O_2 carrier. It is 98% saturated in the lungs and only about 33% saturated in the working muscle. Under these conditions it delivers about 65% of the O_2 it can carry.

It can be seen in Figure 25.2 that hemoglobin is 50% saturated with O_2 at a partial pressure of 27 mmHg (3.60 kPa). The partial pressure corresponding to 50% saturation is called the $\boldsymbol{P_{50}}$. The term P_{50} is the most common way of expressing hemoglobin's O_2 affinity. By analogy with K_m for enzymes, a relatively high P_{50} corresponds to a relatively low O_2 affinity.

The Steep Part of the Curve Lies in the Physiological Range

Note that the steep part of hemoglobin's saturation curve lies in the range of O_2 tensions that prevail in the extrapulmonary tissues. This means that relatively small decreases in oxygen tension in these tissues will result in large increases in O_2 delivery, this effect becoming more pronounced as the partial pressure of O_2 diminishes within the physiological range. Furthermore, small shifts of the curve to the left or right will also strongly influence O_2 delivery. In Sections 25.3, 25.5, and 25.6 we see how physiological signals effect such shifts and result in enhanced delivery under conditions of increased O_2 demand. Small decreases of O_2 tension in the lungs, however, such as occur at moderately high altitudes, do not seriously compromise hemoglobin's ability to bind oxygen. This will be true as long as the alveolar partial pressure of O_2 remains in a range that corresponds to the relatively flat region of hemoglobin's O_2 dissociation curve (see Clin. Corr. 25.2).

Finally, we can see from Figure 25.2 that the binding of oxygen by hemoglobin is cooperative. At very low O_2 tension the hemoglobin curve tends to follow the hyperbolic curve, which represents relatively weak O_2 binding, but at higher tensions it actually rises above the hyperbolic curve that represents tight binding. Thus hemoglobin binds O_2 weakly at low oxygen tension and tightly at high tension. The binding of the first O_2 to each hemoglobin molecule enhances the binding of subsequent O_2 molecules.

CLINICAL CORRELATION 25.2

Cyanosis

Cyanosis is a condition in which a patient's skin or mucous membrane appears gray or (in severe cases) purple-magenta. It is due to an abnormally high concentration of deoxyhemoglobin below the surface, which is responsible for the observed color. The familiar blue of superficial veins is due to their deoxyhemoglobin content and is a normal manifestation of this color effect.

Cyanosis is most commonly caused by diseases of the cardiac or pulmonary systems, resulting in inadequate oxygenation of the blood. It can also be caused by certain hemoglobin abnormalities. Severely anemic individuals cannot become cyanotic; they do not have enough hemoglobin in their blood for the characteristic color of its deoxy form to be apparent.

Albert, R. K. Approach to the patient with cyanosis and/or hypoxemia. In: W. N. Kelley (Ed.), *Textbook of Internal Medicine.* Philadelphia: Lippincott, 1989, pp. 2041–2044.

Hemoglobin's ability to bind O_2 cooperatively is reflected in its **Hill coefficient,** which has a value of about 2.7. (The Hill equation is derived and interpreted on p. 119.) Since the maximum value of the Hill coefficient for a system at equilibrium is equal to the number of cooperating binding sites, a value of 2.7 means that hemoglobin, with its four oxygen-binding sites, is more cooperative than would be possible for a system with only two cooperating binding sites, but it is not as cooperative as it could be.

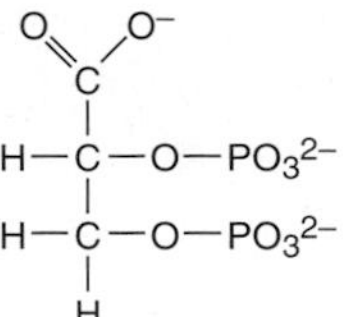

FIGURE 25.3
2,3-Bisphosphoglycerate (BPG).

25.3 HEMOGLOBIN AND ALLOSTERISM: EFFECT OF 2,3-BISPHOSPHOGLYCERATE

Hemoglobin's binding of O_2 was the original example of a **homotropic effect** (cooperativity and allosterism are discussed in Chapter 4), but hemoglobin also exhibits a **heterotropic effect** of great physiological significance. This involves its interaction with **2,3-bisphosphoglycerate** (BPG) (Figure 25.3), which is closely related to the glycolytic intermediate, 1,3-bisphosphoglycerate, from which it is biosynthesized.

It had been known for many years that hemoglobin in the red cell bound oxygen less tightly than purified hemoglobin could (Figure 25.4). It had also been known that the red cell contained high levels of BPG, nearly equimolar with hemoglobin. Finally, the appropriate experiment was done to demonstrate the relationships between these two facts. It was shown that the addition of BPG to purified hemoglobin produced a shift to the right of its oxygen-binding curve, bringing it into congruence with the curve observed for whole blood. Other organic polyphosphates, such as ATP and inositol pentaphosphate, also have this effect. Inositol pentaphosphate is the physiological effector in birds, where it replaces BPG, and ATP plays a similar role in some fish.

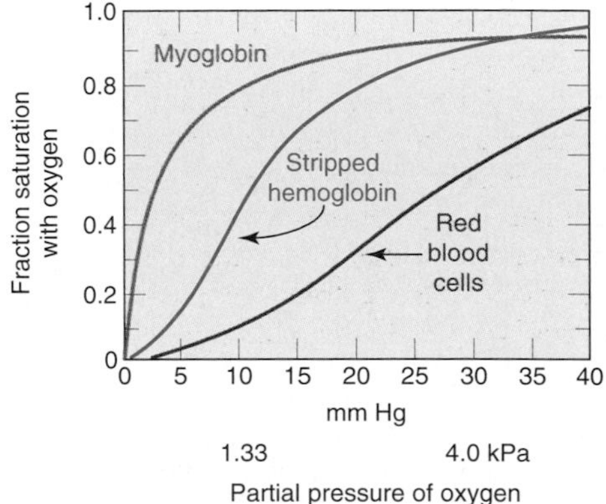

FIGURE 25.4
Oxygen dissociation curves for myoglobin, for hemoglobin that has been stripped of CO_2 and organic phosphates, and for whole red blood cells.
Data from Brenna, O., Luzzana, M., Pace, M., et al. Adv. Exp. Biol. Med. *28:19, 1972. Adapted from McGilvery, R. W.* Biochemistry: A Functional Approach, *2nd ed. Philadelphia: Saunders, 1979, p. 236.*

Monod's model of allosterism explains heterotropic interaction. Applying this model to hemoglobin, in the deoxy conformation (the **T state**) a cavity large enough to admit BPG exists between the β chains of hemoglobin. This cavity is lined with positively charged groups and firmly binds one molecule of the negatively charged BPG. In the oxy conformation (the **R state**) this cavity is smaller, and it no longer accommodates BPG as easily. The result is that the binding of BPG to oxyhemoglobin is much weaker. Since BPG binds preferentially to the T state, the presence of BPG shifts the R–T equilibrium in favor of the T state; the deoxyhemoglobin conformation is thus stabilized over the oxyhemoglobin conformation (Figure 25.5). For oxygen to overcome this and bind to hemoglobin, a higher concentration of oxygen is required. Oxygen tension in the lungs is sufficiently high under most conditions to saturate hemoglobin almost completely, even when BPG levels are high. The physiological effect of BPG can, therefore, be expected to be upon release of oxygen to the extrapulmonary tissues, where O_2 tensions are low.

The significance of a high BPG concentration is that the efficiency of O_2 delivery is increased. Concentrations of BPG in the red cell rise in conditions associated with **tissue hypoxia,** such as various anemias, cardiopulmonary insufficiency, and high altitude. These high levels of BPG enhance the formation of deoxyhemoglobin at low partial pressures of oxygen; hemoglobin then delivers more of its O_2 to the tissues. This effect can result in a substantial increase in the amount of O_2 delivered because the venous blood returning to the heart of a normal individual is (at rest) at least 60% saturated with O_2. Much of this O_2 can dissociate in the peripheral tissues if the BPG concentration rises.

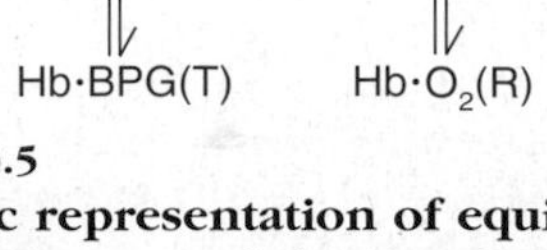

$$\begin{array}{ccc} \text{Hb(T)} & \rightleftharpoons & \text{Hb(R)} \\ + & & + \\ \text{BPG} & & O_2 \\ \updownarrow & & \updownarrow \\ \text{Hb·BPG(T)} & & \text{Hb·}O_2\text{(R)} \end{array}$$

FIGURE 25.5
Schematic representation of equilibria among BPG, O_2, and the T and R states of hemoglobin.

The BPG mechanism works very well as a compensation for tissue hypoxia as long as the partial pressure of oxygen in the lungs remains high enough that oxygen binding in the lungs is not compromised. Since, however, BPG shifts the oxygen-binding curve to the right, the mechanism will not compensate for tissue hypoxia when the partial pressure of O_2 in the lungs falls too low. Then

CLINICAL CORRELATION 25.3

Chemically Modified Hemoglobins: Methemoglobin and Sulfhemoglobin

Methemoglobin is a form of hemoglobin in which the iron is oxidized from the iron (II) state to the iron (III) state. A tendency for methemoglobin to be present in excess of its normal level of about 1% may be due to a hereditary defect of the globin chain or to exposure to oxidizing drugs or chemicals. Sulfhemoglobin is a species that forms when a sulfur atom is incorporated into the porphyrin ring of hemoglobin. Exposure to certain drugs or to soluble sulfides produces it. Sulfhemoglobin is green. Hemoglobin subunits containing these modified hemes do not bind oxygen, but they change the oxygen-binding characteristics of the normal subunits in hybrid hemoglobin molecules containing some normal subunits and one or more modified subunits. The accompanying figure shows the oxygen-binding curve of normal HbA, 15% methemoglobin and 12% sulfhemoglobin. The presence of methemoglobin shifts the curve to the left, impairing the delivery of the decreased amount of bound oxygen. In contrast, the sulfhemoglobin curve is shifted to the right, a BPG-like effect. As a result, oxygen delivery is enhanced, partially compensating for the inability of the sulfur-modified hemes to bind oxygen.

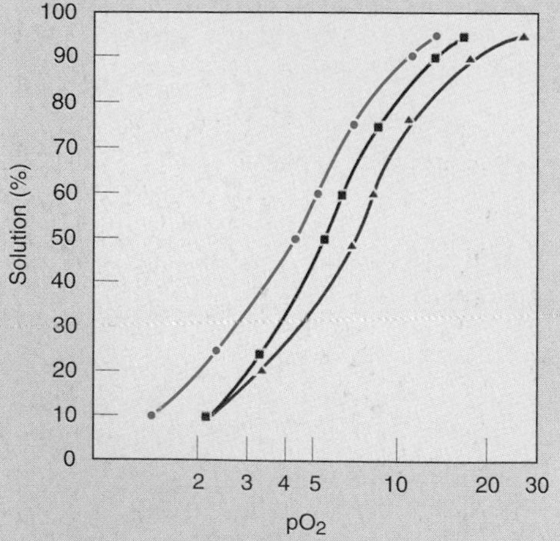

Oxygenation curves of unmodified hemoglobin A (squares) of a 15% oxidized hemolysate (circles) and of a hemolysate containing 12% sulfhemoglobin (triangles) in 0.1 M phosphate, pH 7.35, at 20°C.

Data from Park, C. M., and Nagel, R. L., N. Engl. J. Med. *310:1579, 1984.*

the increased efficiency of O_2 unloading to the tissues is counterbalanced by a decrease in the efficiency of loading in the lungs. This may be a factor in determining the maximum altitude at which people choose to establish permanent dwellings, which is about 18,000 ft (~5500 m). There is evidence that a better adaptation to extremely low ambient partial pressures of O_2 would be a shift of the curve to the left.

25.4 ■ OTHER HEMOGLOBINS

Although hemoglobin A is the major form of hemoglobin in adults and in children over seven months of age, accounting for about 90% of their total hemoglobin, it is not the only normal hemoglobin species. Normal adults also have 2–3% of **hemoglobin A_2,** which is composed of two α chains like those in hemoglobin A and two δ chains. It is represented as $\alpha_2\delta_2$. The δ chains differ in amino acid sequence from the β chains and are under independent genetic control. Hemoglobin A_2 does not appear to be important in normal individuals.

Several species of modified hemoglobin A also occur normally. These are designated A_{1a1}, A_{1a2}, A_{1b}, and A_{1c}. They are adducts of hemoglobin with various sugars, such as glucose, glucose 6-phosphate, and fructose 1,6-bisphosphate. The quantitatively most significant is **hemoglobin A_{1c},** formed by covalent binding of a glucose residue to the N terminal of the β chain at a rate that depends on the concentration of glucose. As a result, hemoglobin A_{1c} forms more rapidly in uncontrolled diabetics and can comprise up to 12% of their total hemoglobin. Hemoglobin A_{1c} or total glycosylated hemoglobin levels are a useful measure of how well diabetes has been controlled during the days and weeks before the measurement is taken; measurement of blood glucose only indicates how well diabetes is under control when the blood sample is taken. Chemical modification of hemoglobin A can also occur from interaction with drugs or environmental pollutants (see Clin. Corr. 25.3).

Fetal hemoglobin, **hemoglobin F,** is the major hemoglobin in newborn infants. It contains two γ chains in place of the β chains and is represented as $\alpha_2\gamma_2$. Shortly before birth γ-chain synthesis diminishes and β-chain synthesis is initiated, and by the age of seven months well over 90% of the infant's hemoglobin is hemoglobin A.

Hemoglobin F is adapted to the environment of the fetus, who gets oxygen from maternal blood, a source that is far poorer than the atmosphere. To compete with the maternal hemoglobin for O_2, fetal hemoglobin must bind O_2 more tightly; its oxygen-binding curve is thus shifted to the left relative to hemoglobin A. This is accomplished through a difference in the influence of BPG upon the maternal and fetal hemoglobins. In hemoglobin F two of the groups that line the BPG-binding cavity have neutral side chains instead of the positively charged ones that occur in hemoglobin A. Consequently, hemoglobin F binds BPG less tightly and thus binds oxygen more tightly than hemoglobin A does. Also, about 15–20% of the hemoglobin F is acetylated at the N terminals; this is referred to as hemoglobin F_1. Hemoglobin F_1 does not bind BPG, and its affinity for oxygen is not affected at all by BPG. The postnatal change from hemoglobin F to hemoglobin A, combined with a rise in red cell BPG that peaks three months after birth, results in a gradual shift to the right of the infant's oxygen-binding curve (Figure 25.6). The result is greater delivery of oxygen to the tissues at this age than at birth, in spite of a 30% decrease in the infant's total hemoglobin concentration.

In many inherited anomalies of hemoglobin synthesis there is formation of a structurally abnormal hemoglobin; these are called **hemoglobinopathies.** They may involve the substitution of one amino acid in one type of polypeptide chain for some other amino acid or they may involve absence of one or more amino acid residues of a polypeptide chain. In some cases the change is clinically insignificant, but in others it causes serious disease (see Clin. Corr. 25.4).

25.5 ■ PHYSICAL FACTORS THAT AFFECT OXYGEN BINDING

High Temperature Weakens Hemoglobin's Oxygen Affinity

Temperature has a significant effect on O_2 binding by hemoglobin (Figure 25.7). At below-normal temperatures the binding is tighter, resulting in a leftward shift of the curve; at higher temperatures the binding becomes weaker, and the curve is shifted to the right. The effect of elevated temperature is like that of high levels of BPG, in that both enhance unloading of oxygen. The temperature effect is physiologically useful, as it makes additional O_2 available to support the high metabolic rate found in fever or in exercising muscle with its elevated temperature. The relative insensitivity to temperature of O_2 binding at high partial pressure of oxygen minimizes compromise of O_2 uptake in the lungs under these conditions.

The tighter binding of O_2 that occurs in hypothermic conditions is not important in hypothermia induced for surgical purposes. Decreased O_2 utilization by the body and increased solubility of O_2 in plasma at lower temperatures, as well as the increased solubility of CO_2, which acidifies the blood, compensate for hemoglobin's diminished ability to release O_2.

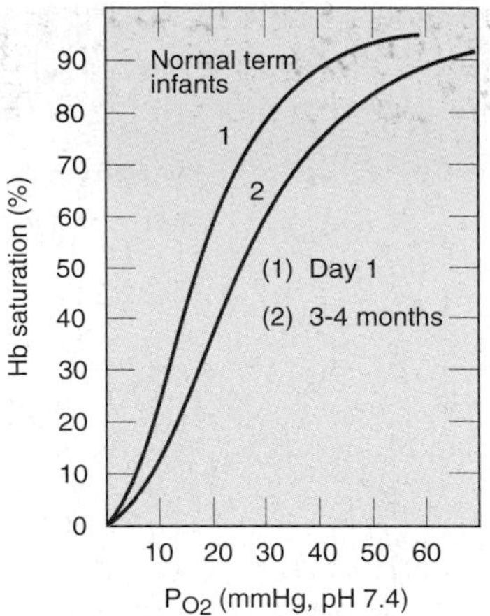

FIGURE 25.6
Oxygen dissociation curves after birth.
Adapted from Oski, F. A., and Delivoria-Papadopoulos, M. J. Pediatr. *77:941, 1970.*

Low pH Weakens Hemoglobin's Oxygen Affinity

Hydrogen ion concentration influences hemoglobin's O_2 binding. As shown in Figure 25.8, low pH shifts the curve to the right, enhancing O_2 delivery, whereas high pH shifts the curve to the left. It is customary to express O_2 binding by hemoglobin as a function of plasma pH because it is this value, not the pH within the erythrocyte, that is usually measured. Erythrocyte cell sap pH is lower than the plasma pH, but these two fluids are in equilibrium, and changes in one reflect changes in the other.

The influence of pH upon O_2 binding is physiologically significant, since a decrease in pH is often associated with increased oxygen demand. Increased metabolic rate increases production of carbon dioxide and, as in muscular exercise and hypoxic tissue, lactic acid. These acids produced by metabolism help release oxygen to support that metabolism.

The increase in acidity of hemoglobin as it binds O_2 is known as the **Bohr effect;** an equivalent statement is that the Bohr effect is the increase in basicity of hemoglobin as it releases oxygen. The effect may be expressed by the equation

$$HHb + O_2 \leftrightharpoons HbO_2 + H^+$$

This equation gives the same information as Figure 25.8—that increases in hydrogen ion concentration favor formation of free oxygen from oxyhemoglobin, and conversely, that oxygenation of hemoglobin lowers the pH of the solution.

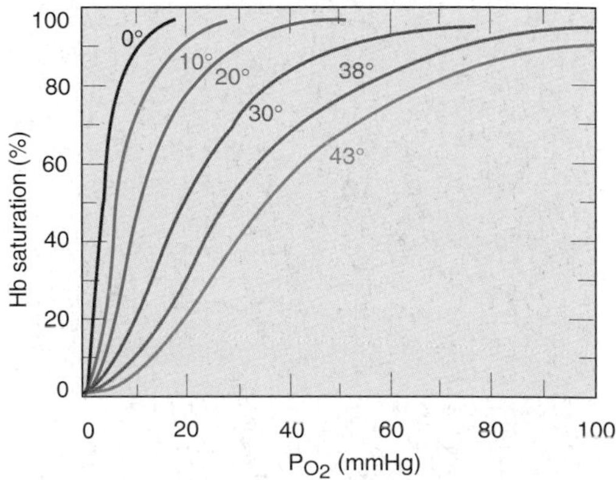

FIGURE 25.7
Oxygen dissociation curve for whole blood at various temperatures.
From Lambertson, C. J. In: P. Bard (Ed.), Medical Physiology, *11th ed. St. Louis, MO: Mosby, 1961, p. 596.*

25.6 ■ CARBON DIOXIDE TRANSPORT

The carbon dioxide we produce is excreted by the lungs, to which it is transported by the blood. Carbon dioxide transport is closely tied to hemoglobin and to the problem of maintaining a constant pH in the blood, a problem that will be discussed subsequently.

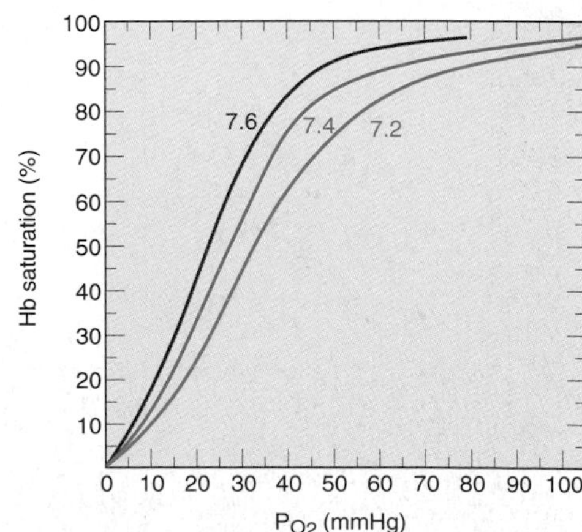

FIGURE 25.8
Oxygen dissociation curve for whole blood at various values of plasma pH.
Adapted from Lambertson, C. J. In: P. Bard (Ed.), Medical Physiology, *11th ed. St. Louis, MO: Mosby, 1961, p. 596.*

Blood CO_2 Is Present in Three Major Forms

Carbon dioxide is present in the blood in three major forms, as dissolved CO_2, as HCO_3^- (formed by ionization of H_2CO_3 produced when CO_2 reacts with H_2O), and as carbaminohemoglobin (formed when CO_2 reacts with amino groups of protein). Each of these is present both in arterial blood and in venous blood

CLINICAL CORRELATION 25.4

Hemoglobins with Abnormal Oxygen Affinity

Some abnormal hemoglobins have an altered affinity for oxygen. If oxygen affinity is increased (P_{50} decreased), oxygen delivery to the tissues will be diminished unless some sort of compensation occurs. Typically, the body responds by producing more erythrocytes (polycythemia) and more hemoglobin. Hb Rainier is an abnormal hemoglobin in which the P_{50} is 12.9 mmHg, far below the normal value of 27 mmHg.

In the accompanying figure the oxygen content in volume percent (mL of O_2 per 100 mL of blood) is plotted versus partial pressure of oxygen, both for normal blood (curve *a*) and for the blood of a patient with Hb Rainier (curve *b*). Obviously, the patient's blood carries more oxygen; this is because it contains 19.5 g of Hb per 100 mL instead of the usual 15 g per 100 mL.

Since the partial pressure of oxygen in mixed venous blood is about 40 mmHg, the volume of oxygen the blood of each individual can deliver may be obtained from the graph by subtracting the oxygen content of the blood at 40 mmHg from its oxygen content at 100 mmHg. As shown in the figure, the blood of the patient with Hb Rainier delivers nearly as much oxygen as normal blood does, although Hb Rainier delivers a significantly smaller fraction of the total amount it carries. Evidently, polycythemia is an effective compensation for this condition, at least in the resting state.

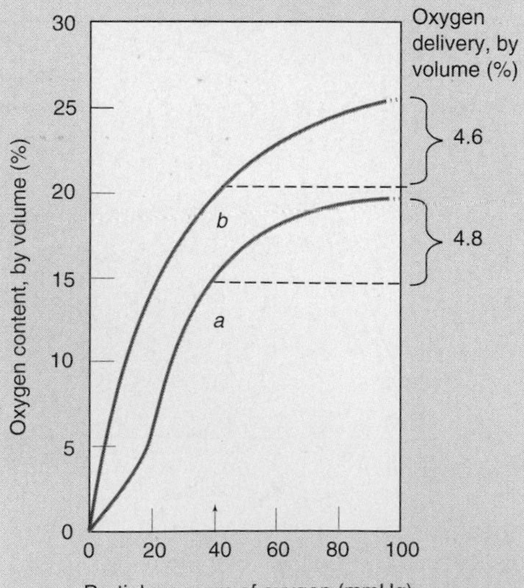

Oxygen content plotted against partial pressure of oxygen. (continued)

(see the top three lines of Table 25.2). Net transport to the lungs for excretion is represented by the concentration difference between arterial and venous blood, shown in the last column. Note that for each form of carbon dioxide the arterial–venous difference is only a small fraction of the total amount present; venous blood contains only about 10% more **total carbon dioxide** (total CO_2 is the sum of HCO_3^-, dissolved CO_2, and carbaminohemoglobin) than arterial blood.

After carbon dioxide enters the bloodstream for transport, it generates hydrogen ions. Most come from formation of bicarbonate ion, which occurs in the following manner.

Bicarbonate Formation

Carbon dioxide enters the blood and diffuses into erythrocytes, whose membranes, like most biological membranes, are freely permeable to dissolved CO_2. Within the erythrocytes most of the carbon dioxide is acted on by the intracellular enzyme, **carbonic anhydrase,** which catalyzes the reaction

$$CO_2 + H_2O \underset{\text{anhydrase}}{\overset{\text{carbonic}}{\rightleftharpoons}} H_2CO_3$$

This reaction proceeds in the absence of a catalyst, as is well known to all who drink carbonated beverages. Without the catalyst, however, it is too slow to meet the body's needs, taking over 100 s to reach equilibrium. Recall that at rest the blood makes a complete circuit of the body in 60 s. Carbonic anhydrase is a very active enzyme, having a turnover number of the order of 10^6, and inside the erythrocytes the reaction reaches equilibrium within 1 s, less than the time spent by the blood in the capillary bed. The enzyme contains zinc and accounts in part for our dietary requirement for this metal.

The ionization of carbonic acid, $H_2CO_3 \rightleftharpoons H^+ + HCO_3^-$, is a rapid, spontaneous reaction. It produces equivalent amounts of H^+ and HCO_3^-. Since, as shown in the last column of line 2 in Table 25.2, 1.69 meq of bicarbonate was added to each liter of blood by this process, 1.69 meq of H^+ must also have been generated per liter of blood. Addition of this much acid, over 10^{-3} equiv of H^+, to 1 L of water would give a final pH below 3. Since the pH of venous plasma averages 7.37, most of the H^+ generated during HCO_3^- production must be consumed by buffer action and/or other processes. This is discussed below.

Because of the compartmentalization of carbonic anhydrase, essentially all conversion of CO_2 to H_2CO_3, and ultimately to HCO_3^-, occurs inside the erythrocyte. Negligible amounts of CO_2 react nonenzymatically in the plasma. Thus virtually all of the increase in HCO_3^- in venous as compared to arterial blood is generated in erythrocytes. Most of this diffuses into the plasma, so that venous plasma HCO_3^- is higher than the arterial, but the erythrocyte was the site of its formation.

Carbaminohemoglobin Formation

It has been observed that in the presence of carbonic anhydrase inhibitors, such as acetazolamide or cyanide, blood will still take up a certain amount of carbon dioxide rapidly. This is due to the reaction of carbon dioxide with amino groups of proteins within erythrocytes to form **carbamino groups** (Figure 25.9). Hemoglobin is quantitatively the most important protein involved in this reaction. Deoxyhemoglobin forms **carbamino hemoglobin** more readily than oxyhemoglobin. Oxygenation causes release of CO_2 in carbaminohemoglobin.

Carbaminohemoglobin formation occurs only with uncharged aliphatic amino groups, not with the charged form, $R{-}NH_3^+$. The pH within erythrocytes is normally about 7.2, somewhat more acidic than the plasma. Since protein amino groups have p*K* values well to the alkaline side of 7.2, they will be mostly in the charged (undissociated acid) form. Removal of some of the uncharged form via carbamino group formation shifts the equilibrium, generating more uncharged amino groups and an equivalent amount of H^+, as shown in Figure 25.10. Carbamination, like HCO_3^- formation, generates H^+.

The N-terminal α-amino groups of proteins have p*K* values in the range of 7.6–8.4. The N terminals of hemoglobin's polypeptide chains are the principal sites of carbamination. If they are blocked chemically by reaction with cyanate, carbamino formation does not occur.

The N-terminal amino groups of the β-globin chains are part of the binding site for BPG. Since they cannot bind BPG and also form carbamino groups, a competition arises. Carbon dioxide diminishes the effect for BPG and, conversely, BPG diminishes the ability of hemoglobin to form carbaminohemoglobin. Ignorance of the latter interaction led to a major overestimation of the role of carbaminohemoglobin in carbon dioxide transport. Prior to the discovery of the BPG effect, careful measurements were made of the capacity of purified hemoglobin (no BPG present) to form carbaminohemoglobin. The results were assumed to be applicable to hemoglobin in the erythrocyte, leading to the erroneous conclusion that carbaminohemoglobin accounted for 25–30% or more of CO_2 transport. It now appears that 13–15% of CO_2 transport is via carbaminohemoglobin. Table 25.3 summarizes the contribution of each major form of blood carbon dioxide to overall CO_2 transport.

Curve *a* shows the oxygen dissociation curve of normal blood with a hemoglobin of 15 g dL^{-1}, P_{50} 27 mmHg, n 2.8, at pH 7.4, 37°C. Curve *b* shows that of blood from a patient with Hb Rainier, having a hemoglobin of 19.5 g dL^{-1}, P_{50} 12.9 mmHg, n 1.2, at the same pH and temperature. (1 mmHg ≈ 133.3 Pa.) On the right is shown the oxygen delivery. The compensatory polycythemia and hyperbolic curve of Hb Rainier result in practically normal arterial and venous oxygen tensions. Arrow indicates normal mixed venous oxygen tension.
From Bellingham, A. J. Br. Med. Bull. *32:234, 1976.*

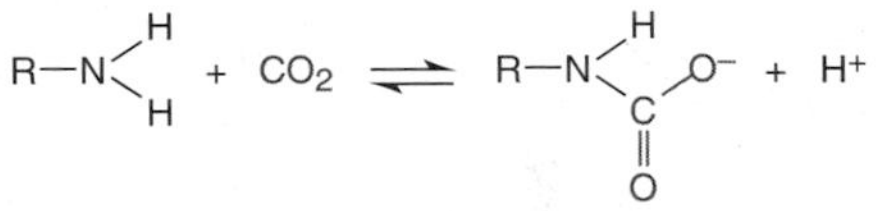

$$R{-}NH_2 + CO_2 \rightleftharpoons R{-}NH{-}COO^- + H^+$$

FIGURE 25.9
Carbamino formation from a free amino group and carbon dioxide.

$$R{-}NH_3^+ \rightleftharpoons R{-}NH_2 + H^+$$

FIGURE 25.10
Dissociation of an ammonium ion to yield a free amino group and H^+.

Two Processes Regulate [H^+] Derived from CO_2 Transport

Buffering

Hemoglobin, besides carrying O_2 and CO_2 in the covalently bound form of a carbamino group, also plays the major role in handling the H^+ produced in CO_2 transport. It does this by buffering and by the isohydric mechanism (discussed below). **Hemoglobin's buffering** power resides in its ionizable groups with p*K* values close to the intraerythrocyte pH. These include the four N-terminal amino groups and the imidazole side chains of the histidine residues. There are 38 histidines per hemoglobin tetramer; these provide most of hemoglobin's buffering ability.

In whole blood, buffering takes up about 60% of the acid generated in normal carbon dioxide transport. Although hemoglobin is by far the most important nonbicarbonate buffer in blood, the organic phosphates in the eryth-

TABLE 25.2 Properties of Blood of Humans at Rest[a]

	Arterial			*Venous*			*A–V Difference*		
	Serum	*Cells*	*Blood*	*Serum*	*Cells*	*Blood*	*Serum*	*Cells*	*Blood*
Hb carbamino groups (meq L^{-1} of blood)		1.13	1.13		1.42	1.42		+0.29	+0.29
HCO_3^- (meq L^{-1} of blood)	13.83	5.73	19.56	14.84	6.41	21.25	+1.01	+0.68	+1.69
Dissolved CO_2 (meq L^{-1} of blood)	0.71	0.48	1.19	0.82	0.56	1.38	+0.11	+0.08	+0.19
Total CO_2 (meq L^{-1} of blood)	14.54	7.34	21.88	15.66	8.39	24.05	+1.12	+1.05	+2.17
Free O_2 (mmol L^{-1} of blood)			0.10			0.04			−0.06
Bound O_2 (mmol L^{-1} of blood)			8.60			6.01			−2.59
Total O_2 (mmol L^{-1} of blood)			8.70			6.05			−2.65
P_{O_2} (mmHg)			88.0			37.2			−50.8
P_{CO_2} (mmHg)			41.0			47.5			+6.5
pH	7.40	7.19		7.37	7.17		−0.03	−0.02	
Volume (cc L^{-1} of blood)	551.7	448.3	1000	548.9	451.1	1000	−2.8	+2.8	0.0
H_2O (cc L^{-1} of blood)	517.5	322.8	840.0	514.7	325.6	840.0	−2.8	+2.8	0.0
Cl^- (meq L^{-1} of blood)	57.71	24.30	82.01	56.84	25.17	82.01	−0.88	+0.88	0.0

Source: From Baggott, J. *Trends Biochem. Sci.* 3:N207, 1978, with permission of the publisher.
[a] Hemoglobin, 9 mM; serum protein, 39.8 g L^{-1} of blood; respiratory quotient, 0.82.

TABLE 25.3 Major Forms of Carbon Dioxide Transport

Species	*Transport (%)*
HCO_3^-	78
CO_2 (dissolved)	9
Carbaminohemoglobin	13

TABLE 25.4 Processes Occurring at the N Terminals of the α Chains and β Chains of Hemoglobin

	N Terminals	
Process	*α Chains*	*β Chains*
Carbamino formation	Yes	Yes
BPG binding	No	Yes
H^+ binding in the Bohr effect	Yes	No

TABLE 25.5 Control of the Excess H^+ Generated During Normal Carbon Dioxide Transport

Buffering	
By hemoglobin	50%
By other buffers	10%
Isohydric mechanism (hemoglobin)	40%

rocytes, the plasma proteins, and so on also make a significant contribution. Buffering by these compounds accounts for about 10% of the H^+, leaving about 50% of acid control specifically attributable to buffering by hemoglobin. These buffer systems minimize the change in pH that occurs when acid or base is added but do not altogether prevent that change. A small difference in pH between arterial and venous blood is therefore observed.

Isohydric Mechanism

The remainder of the H^+ arising from carbon dioxide is taken up by hemoglobin, but not by buffering. Recall that when hemoglobin becomes oxygenated it becomes a stronger acid and releases H^+ (the Bohr effect). In the capillaries, where O_2 is released, the opposite occurs:

$$HbO_2 + H^+ \leftrightharpoons HHb + O_2$$

Simultaneously, CO_2 enters the capillaries and is hydrated:

$$CO_2 + H_2O \leftrightharpoons H^+ + HCO_3^-$$

Addition of these two equations gives

$$HbO_2 + CO_2 + H_2O \leftrightharpoons HHb + HCO_3^- + O_2$$

revealing that to some extent this system can take up H^+ arising from CO_2, and can do so without a change in H^+ concentration (i.e., with no change in pH). Hemoglobin's ability to do this, through the operation of the Bohr effect, is referred to as the **isohydric carriage of CO_2**. As already pointed out, there is a small A–V difference in plasma pH. This is because the isohydric mechanism cannot handle all the acid generated during normal CO_2 transport; if it could, no such difference would occur. Figure 25.11 is a schematic representation of

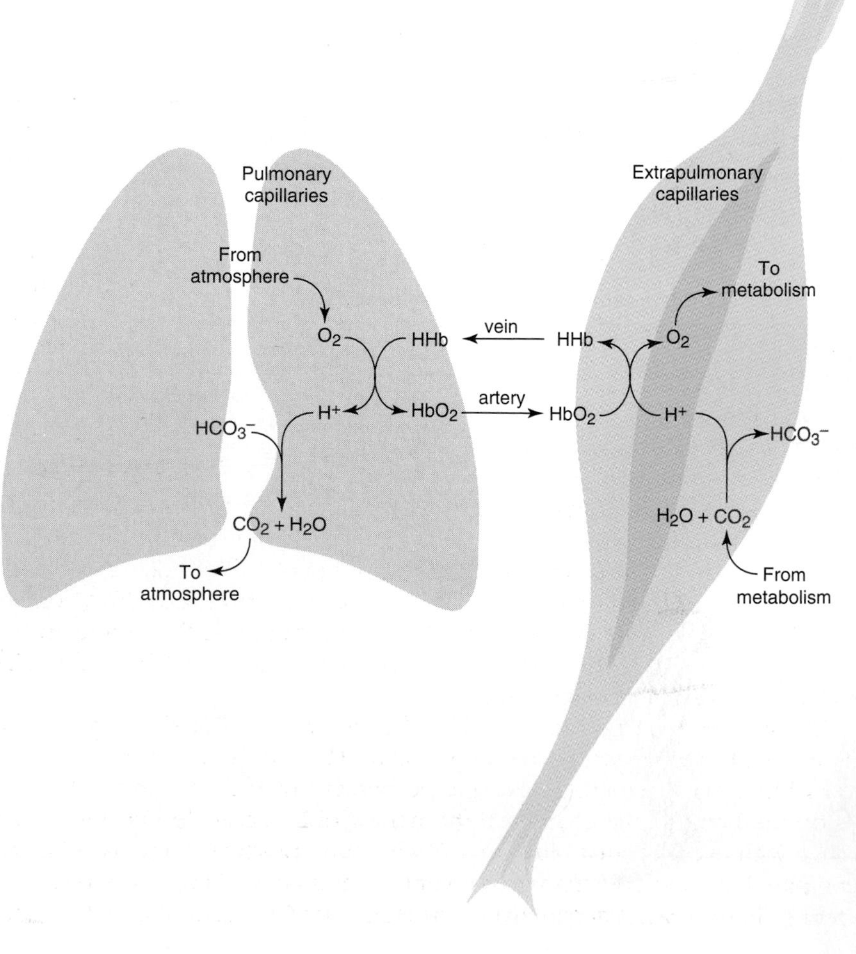

FIGURE 25.11
Schematic representation of oxygen transport and the isohydric carriage of CO_2 by hemoglobin.
In the lungs (left) O_2 from the atmosphere reacts with deoxyhemoglobin, forming oxyhemoglobin and H^+. The H^+ combines with the HCO_3^- to form H_2O and CO_2. The CO_2 is exhaled. Oxyhemoglobin is carried to extrapulmonary tissues (right), where it dissociates in response to low P_{O_2}. The O_2 is used by metabolic processes, and CO_2 is produced. CO_2 combines with H_2O to give HCO_3^- and H^+. H^+ can then react with deoxyhemoglobin to give HHb, which returns to the lungs, and the cycle repeats.

O_2 transport and the isohydric mechanism, showing what happens in the lungs and in the other tissues.

Estimates of the importance of the isohydric mechanism in handling normal respiratory acid production have changed upward and downward over the years. The older, erroneous estimates arose out of a lack of knowledge of the multiple interactions in which hemoglobin participates. The earliest experiments, titrations of purified oxyhemoglobin and purified deoxyhemoglobin, revealed that oxygenation of hemoglobin resulted in release of an average of 0.7 H^+ for every O_2 bound. This figure still appears in textbooks, and much is made of it. Authors point out that with a Bohr effect of this magnitude the isohydric mechanism alone could handle all of the acid produced by the metabolic oxidation of fat (RQ of fat is 0.7), and buffering would be unnecessary. Unfortunately, the experimental basis for this interpretation is physiologically unrealistic; the titrations were done in the total absence of carbon dioxide, which we now know binds to some of the Bohr groups, forming carbamino groups and diminishing the effect. When later experiments were carried out in the presence of physiological amounts of carbon dioxide, there was a drastic diminution of the Bohr effect, so much so that at pH 7.45 the isohydric mechanism was able to handle only the amount of acid arising from carbamino group formation. This work, however, was done prior to our appreciation of the competition between BPG and CO_2 for the same region of the hemoglobin molecule (see Table 25.4). Finally, in 1971, careful titrations of whole blood under presumably physiological conditions were carried out, yielding a value of 0.31 H^+ released per O_2 bound. This value is the basis of the present assertion that the isohydric mechanism accounts for about 40% of the H^+ generated during normal carbon dioxide transport. The quantitative contributions of various mechanisms to the handling of H^+ arising during carbon dioxide transport are summarized in Table 25.5. The major role of hemoglobin in handling this acid is obvious.

HCO_3^- Distribution Between Plasma and Erythrocytes

We have seen that essentially all of HCO_3^- formation is intracellular, catalyzed by carbonic anhydrase, and that the vast bulk of the H^+ generated by CO_2 is handled within the erythrocyte. These two observations bear upon the final distribution of HCO_3^- between plasma and the erythrocyte.

Intracellular formation of HCO_3^- increases its intracellular concentration. Since HCO_3^- and Cl^- exchange freely across the erythrocyte membrane, HCO_3^- will diffuse out of the erythrocyte, increasing the plasma HCO_3^- concentration. Electrical neutrality must be maintained across the membrane as this happens. Maintenance of neutrality can be accomplished in principle either by having a positively charged ion accompany HCO_3^- out of the cell or by having some other negatively charged ion enter the cell in exchange for the HCO_3^-. Since the distribution of the major cations, Na^+ and K^+, is under strict control, it is the latter mechanism that is seen, and the ion that is exchanged for HCO_3^- is Cl^-. Thus as HCO_3^- is formed in red cells during their passage through the capillary bed, it moves out into the plasma and Cl^- comes in to replace it. The increase in intracellular Cl^- is shown in the last line of Table 25.2. In the lungs, all events that occur in the peripheral capillary beds are reversed; HCO_3^- enters the erythrocytes to be converted to CO_2 for exhalation, and Cl^- returns to the plasma. The exchange of Cl^- and HCO_3^- between the plasma and the erythrocyte is called the **chloride shift** (Figure 25.12).

The intraerythrocytic buffering of H^+ from carbon dioxide causes these cells to swell, giving venous blood a slightly (0.6%) higher hematocrit than arterial blood. (Hematocrit is the volume percent of red cells in the blood.) This occurs because the charge on the hemoglobin molecule becomes more positive with every H^+ that binds to it. Each bound positive charge requires an accompanying negative charge to maintain neutrality. Thus as a result of buffering there is a net accumulation of HCO_3^- or Cl^- inside the erythrocyte.

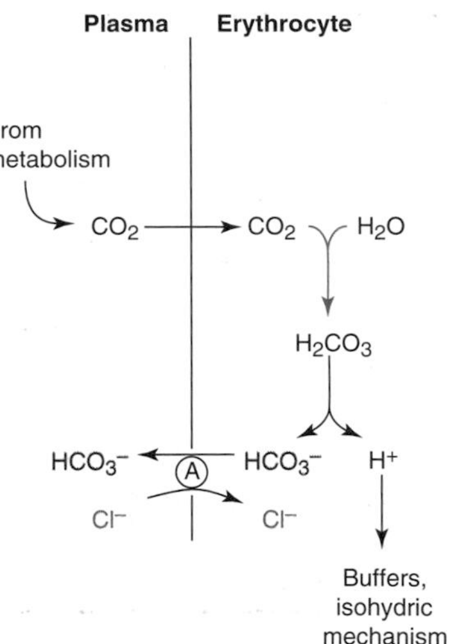

(*a*) Bicarbonate efflux from and chloride influx into erythrocytes in extrapulmonary tissues.

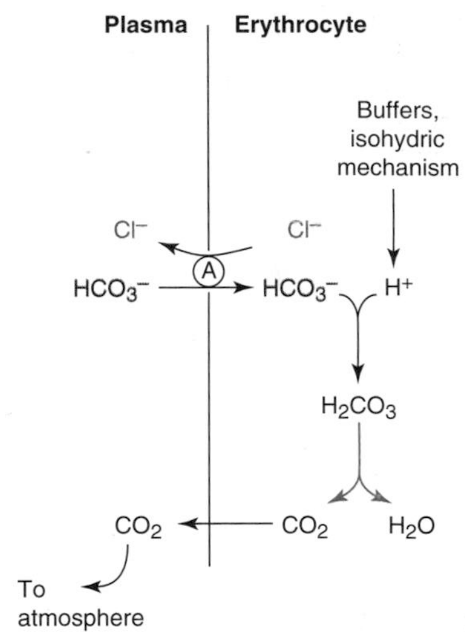

(*b*) Chloride efflux from and bicarbonate influx into erythrocytes in pulmonary tissues.

FIGURE 25.12
Schematic representation of the chloride shift.
(*a*) In the capillaries of the extrapulmonary tissues, CO_2 produced by tissue metabolism is converted to HCO_3^- in the erythrocytes. This HCO_3^- exits the erythrocytes in exchange for Cl^-. (*b*) In the capillaries of the lungs, HCO_3^- enters the erythrocytes in exchange for Cl^-. Within the erythrocytes HCO_3^- is converted to CO_2. CO_2 subsequently diffuses out of the erythrocytes and is exhaled.

$$HHb\begin{matrix}BPG\\CO_2\end{matrix} + O_2 \rightleftharpoons HbO_2 + CO_2 + BPG + H^+$$

FIGURE 25.13
Interaction of H^+, BPG, CO_2, and O_2 with hemoglobin.
This is a schematic, intended to denote the direction of the equilibrium, not the stoichiometry of the reaction.

An increase in the osmotic pressure of the intracellular fluid results from this increase in concentration of particles. As a consequence, water enters the cells, causing them to swell slightly. Typically, an arterial hematocrit might be 44.8 and a venous hematocrit 45.1, as shown in Table 25.2 by the line labeled "volume (cc L^{-1} of blood)."

25.7 ■ INTERRELATIONSHIPS AMONG HEMOGLOBIN, OXYGEN, CARBON DIOXIDE, HYDROGEN ION, AND 2,3-BISPHOSPHOGLYCERATE

By now it should be clear that multiple interrelationships of physiological significance exist among the ligands of hemoglobin. These interrelationships are summarized schematically in Figure 25.13. This equation shows that changes in the concentration of H^+, BPG, or CO_2 have similar effects on O_2 binding. The equation will help you remember the effect of changes in any one of these variables upon hemoglobin's O_2 affinity.

BPG levels in the erythrocytes are controlled by product inhibition of its synthesis and by pH. Hypoxia results in increased levels of deoxyhemoglobin on a time-averaged basis. Since deoxyhemoglobin binds BPG more tightly, in hypoxia there is less free BPG to inhibit its own synthesis, and so BPG levels will rise due to increased synthesis. The effect of pH is that high pH increases BPG synthesis and low pH decreases BPG synthesis; this reflects the influence of pH on the activity of **BPG mutase,** the enzyme that catalyzes BPG formation. Since changes in BPG levels take many hours to become complete, this means that the immediate effect of a decrease in blood pH is to enhance oxygen delivery by the Bohr effect. If the acidosis is sustained (most causes of chronic metabolic acidosis are not associated with a need for enhanced oxygen delivery), diminished BPG synthesis leads to a decrease in intracellular BPG concentration, and hemoglobin's oxygen affinity returns toward normal (Figure 25.14). This system can respond appropriately to acute conditions, such as vigorous exercise, but when faced with a prolonged abnormality of pH, it readjusts to restore normal (and presumably optimal) oxygen delivery.

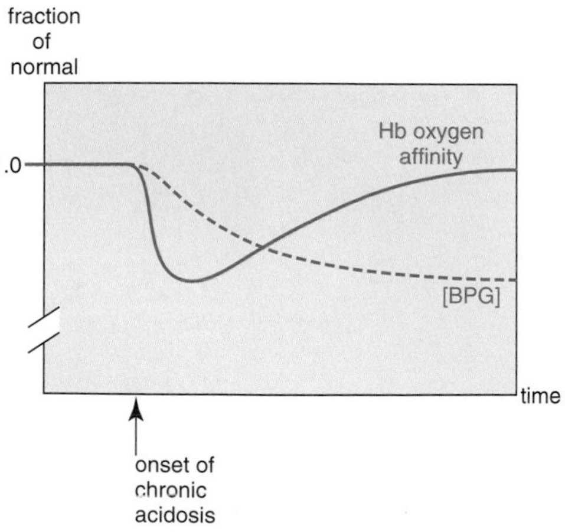

FIGURE 25.14
In chronic acidosis, BPG concentration decreases, returning hemoglobin's oxygen affinity toward normal.
This schematic diagram illustrates the rapid decrease in hemoglobin's oxygen affinity due to decreased pH. Lowering pH immediately lowers the activity of BPG mutase. In consequence, the concentration of BPG gradually diminishes as normal degradation proceeds. As BPG concentration diminishes, hemoglobin's oxygen affinity rises.

25.8 ■ INTRODUCTION TO pH REGULATION

We have noted the large amount of H^+ generated by carbon dioxide transport, and we considered the ways in which the blood pH is controlled. This is important because changes in blood pH will affect intracellular pH, which in turn may profoundly alter metabolism. Protein conformation is affected by pH, as is enzyme activity. In addition, the equilibria of important reactions that consume or generate hydrogen ions, such as any of the oxidation–reduction reactions involving pyridine nucleotides, are shifted by changes in pH.

Normal arterial plasma pH is 7.40 ± 0.05; the pH range compatible with life is about 6.8–7.8. Intracellular pH varies with cell type; that of the erythrocyte is nearly 7.2, but that of most other cells is lower, about 7.0. Values as low as 6.0 have been reported for skeletal muscle.

It is fortunate for both diagnosis and treatment of diseases that the acid–base status of intracellular fluid influences and is influenced by the acid–base status of the blood. Blood is readily available for analysis, and when alteration of body pH becomes necessary, intravenous administration of acidifying or alkalinizing agents is efficacious.

25.9 ■ BUFFER SYSTEMS OF PLASMA, INTERSTITIAL FLUID, AND CELLS

Each body water compartment is defined spatially by one or more differentially permeable membranes. Each contains characteristic kinds and concentrations

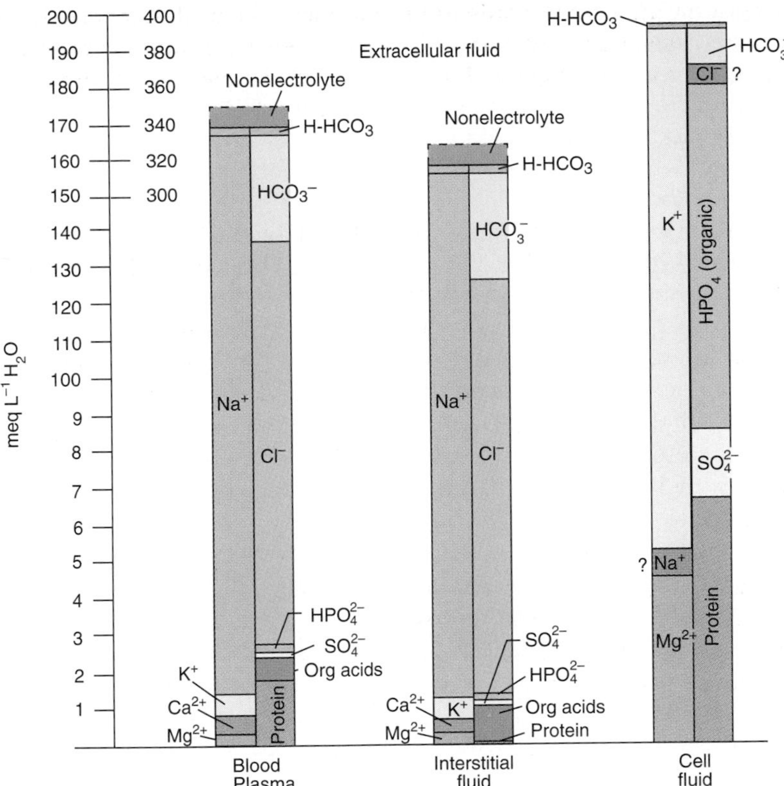

FIGURE 25.15
Chief chemical constituents of the three fluid compartments.
Height of left half of each column indicates total concentration of cations; that of right half, concentration of anions. Both are expressed in milliequivalents per liter (meq L^{-1}) of water. Note that chloride and sodium values in cell fluid are questioned. It is probable that, at least in muscle, the intracellular phase contains some sodium but no chloride.
Adapted from Gregersen, M. I. In: P. Bard (Ed.), Medical Physiology, *11th ed. St. Louis, MO: Mosby, 1961, p. 307.*

of solutes, some of which are buffers in the physiological range of pH. Although the solutes in each type of cell are different, most cells are similar enough to be considered together for purposes of acid–base balance. Thus there are, from this point of view, three major body water components: plasma, within the circulatory system; interstitial fluid, the fluid that bathes the cells; and intracellular fluid.

The compositions of these fluids are given in Figure 25.15. In plasma the major cation is Na^+; small amounts of K^+, Ca^{2+}, and Mg^{2+} are also present. The two dominant anions are HCO_3^- and Cl^-; smaller amounts of protein, phosphate, and SO_4^{2-} are also present, along with a mixture of organic anions (amino acids, etc.), each of which would be insignificant if taken separately. The sum of the anions equals, of course, the sum of the cations. It is apparent at a glance that the composition of interstitial fluid is very similar. The major difference is that interstitial fluid contains much less protein than plasma contains (capillary endothelium is not normally permeable to plasma proteins) and, correspondingly, a lower cation concentration. Plasma and interstitial fluid together comprise the extracellular fluid, and low molecular weight components equilibrate fairly rapidly between them. For example, H^+ equilibrates between the plasma and interstitial fluid within about $\frac{1}{2}$ h. The composition of intracellular fluid is strikingly different. The major cation is K^+, while organic phosphates (ATP, BPG, glycolytic intermediates, etc.) and protein are the major anions.

Because of these differences among the fluid compartments, each fluid makes a different contribution to buffering. The major buffer of extracellular fluid, for example, is the HCO_3^-/CO_2 system. Since its pK is 6.1 (Table 25.6 lists the major physiological buffers and their pK values), extracellular fluid at a pH of 7.4 is not very effective in resisting changes in pH arising from changes in P_{CO_2}. Intracellular fluid, with its high levels of protein and organic phosphates, is responsible for most of the buffering that occurs when P_{CO_2} changes. We have already seen the importance of buffering by hemoglobin and organic phosphates within erythrocytes. On the other hand, for reasons that will be explained

TABLE 25.6 Acid Dissociation Constants of Major Physiological Buffers

Buffer System	*pK*
HCO_3^-/CO_2	6.1
Phosphate	
$HPO_4^{2-}/H_2PO_4^-$	6.7–7.2
Organic phosphate esters	6.5–7.6
Protein	
Histidine side chains	5.6–7.0
N-terminal amino groups	7.6–8.4

TABLE 25.7 Buffering of Metabolic Acids

Tissue	*Buffering (%)*
Extracellular fluids	42
Red cells	6
Tissue cells	52

in Section 25.10, the bicarbonate buffer system is quite effective in controlling pH changes from causes other than changes in P_{CO_2}. Extracellular and intracellular fluids share almost equally in buffering strong organic or inorganic acids (see Table 25.7). Plasma is therefore an excellent indicator of the whole body's capacity to handle additional loads of these acids.

Since acid–base imbalance arising from metabolic production of organic acids is common and potentially life-threatening, and since plasma is such a good indicator of the whole body's capacity to handle further metabolic acid loads, plasma composition is of major clinical concern. It is hydrogen ion concentration that must be kept within acceptable limits, but measuring pH alone is like walking on thin ice while observing merely whether or not you are still on the surface. Knowledge of $[HCO_3^-]$ tells you how close the ice is to the breaking point and how deep the water is underneath.

Because of the importance of the bicarbonate buffer system and its interaction with the other buffers of blood and other tissues, we will consider blood as a buffer in some detail. We will begin with a brief consideration of a model buffer.

Every buffer consists of a weak acid, HA, and its **conjugate base,** A^-. Examples of conjugate base/weak acid pairs are acetate$^-$/acetic acid, NH_3/NH_4^+, and $HPO_4^{2-}/H_2PO_4^-$. Note that the weak acid may be neutral, positively charged, or negatively charged, and that its conjugate base must (since a H^+ has been lost) have one less positive charge (or one more negative charge) than the weak acid. The degree of ionization of a weak acid depends on the concentration of free hydrogen ions. This may be expressed in the form of the **Henderson–Hasselbalch equation** (derived on p. 9) as follows:

$$\mathrm{pH} = \mathrm{p}K + \log \frac{[\text{conjugate base}]}{[\text{acid}]}$$

This is a mathematical rearrangement of the fundamental equilibrium equation. It states that there is a direct relationship between pH and the ratio [conjugate base]/[acid]. It is important to realize that this ratio, not the absolute concentration of any particular species, is the factor that is related to pH. Use of this equation will help you to understand the operation of and to predict the effects of various alterations upon acid–base balance in the body.

Blood plasma is a mixed buffer system; in the plasma the major buffers are HCO_3^-/CO_2, $HPO_4^{2-}/H_2PO_4^-$, and protein/Hprotein. The pH is the same throughout the plasma, so each of these buffer pairs distributes independently according to its own Henderson–Hasselbalch equation, shown in Figure 25.16. Because each pair has a different pK, the [conjugate base]/[acid] ratio is also different for each. Note, though, that if the ratio is known for any given buffer pair, information about the others can be calculated (assuming the pK values are known).

$$\begin{aligned}\mathrm{pH} &= \mathrm{p}K_1 + \log \frac{[HCO_3^-]}{[CO_2]}\\ &= \mathrm{p}K_2 + \log \frac{[HPO_4^{2-}]}{[H_2PO_4^-]}\\ &= \mathrm{p}K_3 + \log \frac{[\text{protein}^-]}{[\text{Hprotein}]}\end{aligned}$$

FIGURE 25.16
Some of the Henderson–Hasselbalch equations that are obeyed simultaneously in plasma.

25.10 ■ THE CARBON DIOXIDE–BICARBONATE BUFFER SYSTEM

As we have seen, the major buffer of plasma and interstitial fluid is the **bicarbonate buffer system.** The bicarbonate system has two peculiar properties that make its operation unlike that of typical buffers. We will examine this important buffer in some detail, since a firm understanding of it is the key to a grasp of acid–base balance.

The Chemistry of the System

The Equilibrium Expression Involves an Anhydride Instead of an Acid

In the first place, the component that we consider to be the acid in this buffer system is CO_2, which is an acid anhydride, not an acid. It reacts with water to form carbonic acid, which is indeed a typical weak acid:

$$CO_2 + H_2O \leftrightharpoons H_2CO_3$$

Carbonic acid rapidly ionizes to give H^+ and HCO_3^-:

$$H_2CO_3 \leftrightharpoons H^+ + HCO_3^-$$

If these two equations are added, H_2CO_3 cancels out, and the sum is

$$CO_2 + H_2O \leftrightharpoons H^+ + HCO_3^-$$

Elimination of H_2CO_3 from formal consideration is realistic, since not only does it simplify matters, but H_2CO_3 is, in fact, quantitatively insignificant. Because the equilibrium of the reaction,

$$CO_2 + H_2O \leftrightharpoons H_2CO_3$$

lies far to the left, H_2CO_3 is present only to the extent of 1/200 of the concentration of dissolved CO_2. Since the concentration of H_2O is virtually constant, it need not be included in the equilibrium expression for the reaction, and we may write:

$$K = \frac{[H^+][HCO_3^-]}{[CO_2]}$$

The value of K is 7.95×10^{-7}.

The concentration of a gas in solution is proportional to its partial pressure. Thus we measure partial pressure of CO_2 (P_{CO_2}). P_{CO_2} multiplied by a **conversion factor,** α, gives the millimolar concentration of dissolved CO_2.

$$\alpha P_{CO_2} = \text{meq L}^{-1}$$

α has a value of 0.03 meq L^{-1} $mmHg^{-1}$ (or 0.225 meq L^{-1} kPa^{-1}) at 37°C. The equilibrium expression thus becomes

$$K = \frac{[H^+][HCO_3^-]}{0.03 \cdot P_{CO_2}}$$

and the Henderson–Hasselbalch equation for this buffer system becomes

$$pH = 6.1 + \log \frac{[HCO_3^-]}{0.03 \cdot P_{CO_2}}$$

with $[HCO_3^-]$ expressed in units of meq L^{-1} (see Clin. Corr. 25.5).

The Carbon Dioxide–Bicarbonate Buffer System Is an Open System

We said earlier that the bicarbonate buffer system, with a pK of 6.1, is not effective against carbonic acid in the pH range of 7.8–6.8 but is effective against noncarbonic acids. The usual rules of chemical equilibrium dictate that a buffer is not very useful in a pH range more than about one unit beyond its pK. Thus we need to explain how the bicarbonate system can be effective against noncarbonic acids; its failure to buffer carbonic acid is expected. The way it buffers noncarbonic acids in a pH range far from its pK is the second unusual property of this buffer system. Note that the explanation of this property in the following paragraph involves the flow of materials in a living system, and so departs from mere equilibrium considerations.

Consider first a typical buffer, consisting of a mixture of a weak acid and its conjugate base. When a strong acid is added, most of the added H^+ combines with the conjugate base. As a result, [weak acid] increases and simultaneously [conjugate base] diminishes. The ratio [conjugate base]/[weak acid] changes, and so does the pH, but much less than if there were no buffer present. Now imagine that the weak acid, as it is generated by reaction of added strong acid with conjugate base, is somehow removed so that while [conjugate base] diminishes, [weak acid] remains nearly constant. In this case the ratio of [conjugate base]/[weak acid] would change much less for a given addition of strong acid, and the pH would also change much less. This is exactly what happens with the body's bicarbonate buffer system. As strong acid is added, $[HCO_3^-]$

CLINICAL CORRELATION 25.5

The Case of the Variable Constant

In clinical laboratories plasma pH and P_{CO_2} are commonly measured with suitable electrodes, and plasma $[HCO_3^-]$ is then calculated from the Henderson–Hasselbalch equation using pK = 6.1. Although this procedure is generally satisfactory, there have been several reports of severely erroneous results in patients whose acid–base status was changing rapidly.* Clinicians who are attuned to this phenomenon urge that direct measurements of all three variables be made in acutely ill patients.

The clinical literature discusses this problem in terms of departure of the value of pK from 6.1. Studies of model systems suggest that this interpretation is incorrect; pK does change with ionic strength, temperature, and so on, and so does α, but not enough to account for the magnitude of the clinical observations.

Astute commentators have speculated that the real basis of the phenomenon is disequilibrium. The detailed nature of the putative disequilibrium has not yet been established, but it is probably related to the difference in pH across the erythrocyte membrane. Normally, the pH of the erythrocyte is about 7.2, and the plasma pH is 7.4. If the plasma pH changes rapidly in an acute illness, the pH of the erythrocyte will also change, but the rate of change within the erythrocyte is not known. If the change within the erythrocyte lags sufficiently behind the change in the plasma, the system would indeed be in gross disequilibrium, and equilibrium calculations would not apply.

*See Hood, I., and Campbell, E. J. M. *N. Engl. J. Med.* 306:864, 1982.

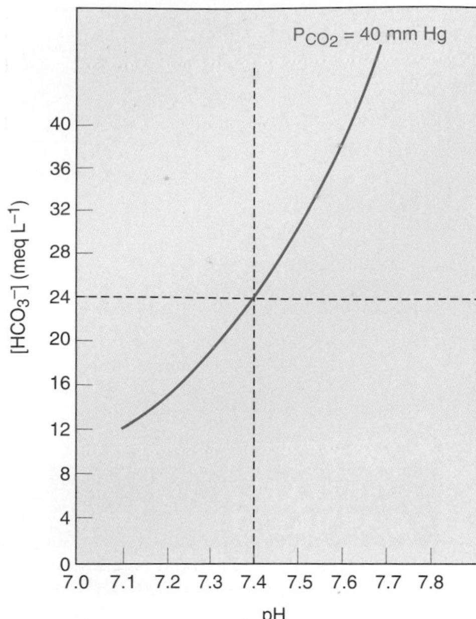

FIGURE 25.17
pH–Bicarbonate diagram including the 40-mmHg (5.33-kPa) CO_2 isobar, and showing the normal values of plasma pH and bicarbonate ion concentration.

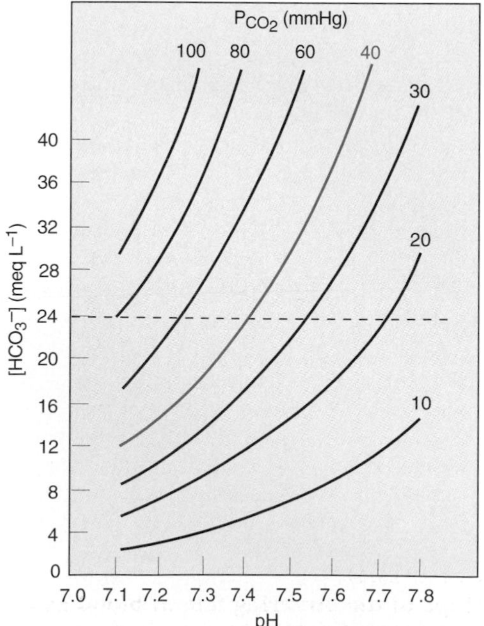

FIGURE 25.18
pH–Bicarbonate diagram showing CO_2 isobars from 10 to 100 mmHg.

diminishes and CO_2 is formed. But the excess CO_2 is exhaled, so that the ratio of [HCO_3^-]/αP_{CO_2} does not change so dramatically. In like manner, if strong base is added to the body, it will be neutralized by carbonic acid, but CO_2 will be replaced by metabolism, and, again, the ratio of [HCO_3^-]/P_{CO_2} will not change as much as would be expected. The body's bicarbonate buffer system is thus an **open system** in which P_{CO_2} is adjusted to meet the body's needs. If respiration cannot accomplish this adjustment, P_{CO_2} changes strikingly, and the bicarbonate system would be relatively ineffective, in keeping with the prediction of chemical equilibrium.

Graphical Representation: The pH–Bicarbonate Diagram

A graphical representation of the Henderson–Hasselbalch equation for the bicarbonate buffer system assists in learning and understanding how this system reflects the body's acid–base status. A common representation is the **pH–bicarbonate diagram,** shown in Figure 25.17. [HCO_3^-] up to 40 meq L^{-1} is shown on the ordinate; enough to deal with most situations. Since plasma pH does not exceed 7.8 or (except transiently) fall below 7.0 in living patients, the abscissa is limited to 7.0–7.8. The normal plasma [HCO_3^-], 24 meq L^{-1}, and the normal plasma pH, 7.4, are indicated. The third variable, CO_2, can be shown on a two-dimensional graph by assigning a fixed value to P_{CO_2} and then showing, for that value, the relationship between pH and [HCO_3^-]. Figure 25.17 shows that relationship when P_{CO_2} is normal, that is, 40 mmHg (5.33 kPa). The line is called the 40-mmHg (5.33-kPa) isobar. Whenever P_{CO_2} is 40 mmHg (5.33-kPa), pH and [HCO_3^-] must be somewhere on that line.

Similarly, we can plot isobars for various abnormal values of P_{CO_2} (Figure 25.18). The range of values given covers those found in patients. Any point on the graph gives the values of the three variables of the Henderson–Hasselbalch equation for the bicarbonate system at that point. Since only two variables are needed to locate a point, the third can be read directly from the graph.

Let us now see how the bicarbonate buffer system behaves when it is in the presence of other buffers, as it is in whole blood. First, let us acidify the system by increasing the concentration of the acid-producing component, CO_2. For every CO_2 that reacts with water to produce a H^+, one HCO_3^- forms. Most of the H^+, however, is buffered by protein and phosphate. As a result, [HCO_3^-] rises much more than [H^+]. Similarly, if acid is removed from this system by decreasing P_{CO_2}, [HCO_3^-] decreases. The [H^+] does not decrease by an equivalent amount, though, because the other buffers dissociate to resist the pH change. The results of these processes as they occur in whole blood, with its various intracellular and extracellular buffers, are shown in Figure 25.19. Let us start at the point that represents the normal values: pH of 7.4, [HCO_3^-] of 24 meq L^{-1}, and P_{CO_2} of 40 mmHg (5.33 kPa). As P_{CO_2} rises to 80 mmHg (10.7 kPa), bicarbonate goes up to 28 meq L^{-1}, an increase of 4 meq L^{-1}. This means H_2CO_3 must have increased by 4 meq L^{-1}, and that it immediately ionized to give H^+ and HCO_3^-. The pH, however, drops to 7.18; this represents an increase in [H^+] of only 26×10^{-6} meq L^{-1}. The other 3.999974 meq L^{-1} of H^+ produced by the ionization of carbonic acid were taken up by the phosphate, hemoglobin, plasma protein, and other buffer systems. If P_{CO_2} were to decrease, the opposite would occur. Thus by altering P_{CO_2} in the presence of HCO_3^- and other buffers, a line is generated with a definite nonzero slope. For the blood system, this is called the **buffering line of blood.** Note that if P_{CO_2} is the only variable that is changed, the response of the system is confined to movements along this line.

The slope of the buffering line depends on the concentration of the nonbicarbonate buffers. If they were more concentrated, they would better resist changes in pH. An increase in P_{CO_2} to 80 mmHg (10.7 kPa) would then cause a smaller drop in pH, and since the more concentrated buffers would react with more hydrogen ions (produced by the ionization of carbonic acid), [HCO_3^-] would rise higher. Thus the slope of the buffering line would be steeper.

Hemoglobin is quantitatively the second most important blood buffer, exceeded only by the bicarbonate buffer system. Since hemoglobin concentration in the blood can fluctuate widely in various disease states, it is the most important physiological determinant of the slope of the blood buffer line. Figure 25.20 shows how this slope varies with hemoglobin concentration.

Having now seen how the bicarbonate buffer system in blood responds to changes in P_{CO_2} and how this response is modified by changing the hemoglobin concentration, let us examine the response of blood to the addition of noncarbonic acids such as HCl and acetoacetic acid. We will continue to analyze the situation in terms of the pH–bicarbonate diagram. The starting point will again be the normal state: pH = 7.4, $[HCO_3^-]$ = 24 meq L^{-1}, and P_{CO_2} = 40 mmHg (5.33 kPa). As acid is added, it reacts with all the blood buffers, and the concentrations of their conjugate bases decrease. Since the bicarbonate system is the major blood buffer, the decrease in $[HCO_3^-]$ is substantial. If P_{CO_2} is held constant at 40 mmHg (5.33-kPa) as a noncarbonic acid is added, the changes in the system can be represented by a point sliding down the 40-mmHg (5.33-kPa) isobar, as shown in Figure 25.21. If alkali is added to the blood, all the undissociated acids of the various buffer systems participate in neutralizing it. Again, if this occurs at a fixed P_{CO_2} of 40 mmHg (5.33 kPa), the changes in the system are represented by a point sliding up the 40-mmHg (5.33-kPa) isobar. Note that, just as changes in P_{CO_2} were represented by points confined to the blood buffer line, changes due to the addition of acid or base at a fixed P_{CO_2} are represented by points confined to the CO_2 isobar.

The effects on blood of changing P_{CO_2} or of adding acid or alkali, as we have just described, are realistic qualitative models of what happens in certain disease states. We next see how these changes occur in the body and how the body compensates for them.

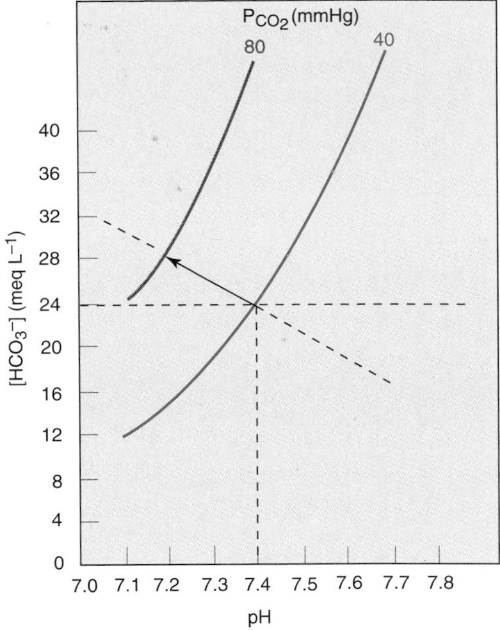

FIGURE 25.19
The buffering line of blood.
This pH–bicarbonate diagram shows the changes in pH that occur in whole blood *in vitro* when P_{CO_2} is changed. Note that the relationship between pH and $[HCO_3^-]$ is described by a straight line with a nonzero slope.

25.11 ACID–BASE BALANCE AND ITS MAINTENANCE

It should come as no surprise that mechanisms exist whereby the body normally rids itself of excess acid or alkali. The physiological implication is that if a patient is in a state of continuing **acidosis** (excess acid or deficiency of alkali in the body) or **alkalosis** (excess alkali or deficiency of acid in the body), there must be a continuing cause of the imbalance. In such a situation the body's first task is to somehow compensate so plasma pH does not exceed the limits compatible with life. Assistance from the physician is sometimes necessary. The body's second task is to eliminate the primary cause of the imbalance, that is, to cure the disease, so that a normal acid–base status can be reestablished. Again, intervention by the physician may be needed.

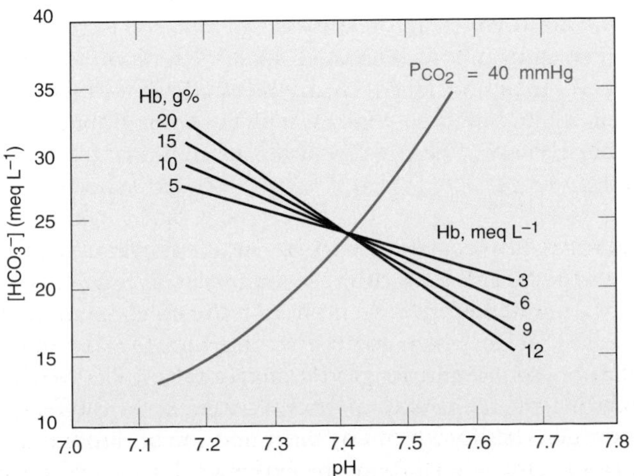

FIGURE 25.20
Slope of the buffering line of blood as it varies with hemoglobin concentration.
From Davenport, H. W. The ABC of Acid–Base Chemistry, *6th ed. revised. Chicago: University of Chicago Press, 1974, p. 55.*

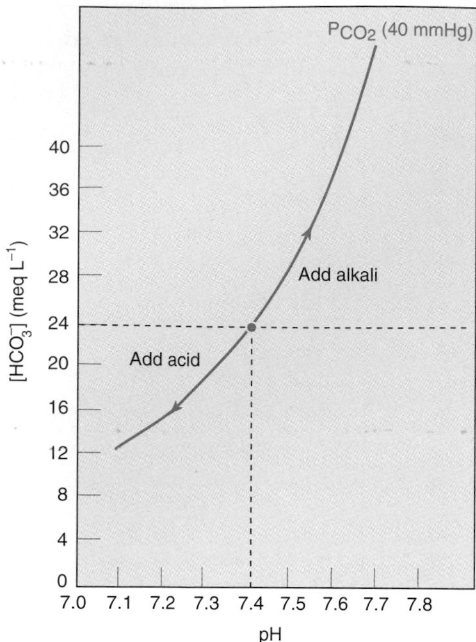

FIGURE 25.21
Effect of adding noncarbonic acid or alkali to whole blood with P_{CO_2} fixed at 40 mmHg.

All individuals, in sickness or in health, produce large amounts of acids every day. The major acid is CO_2, the amount depending on the individual's caloric expenditure, and ranging between 12,500 and nearly 50,000 meq day^{-1}. In an average young adult male, about 22,000 meq of CO_2 are produced daily. This acid is volatile and is normally excreted by the lungs. Inability of the lungs to do this adequately leads to **respiratory acidosis** or alkalosis. Respiratory acidosis is the result of hypoventilation of the alveoli, so that CO_2 accumulates in the body. Alveolar hypoventilation occurs when the depth or rate of respiration diminishes. Airway obstruction, neuromuscular disorders, and diseases of the central nervous system are common causes of acute respiratory acidosis. Chronic respiratory acidosis is seen in patients with chronic obstructive lung disease, such as emphysema. Obviously, since the common element in all these conditions is increased alveolar P_{CO_2}, inhalation of a gas mixture with a high P_{CO_2} would also cause respiratory acidosis.

Respiratory alkalosis, on the other hand, arises from decreased alveolar P_{CO_2}. Hyperventilation due to anxiety is probably the most common cause. Central nervous system injury involving the respiratory center, salicylate poisoning, fever, and artificial ventilation are other causes. At high altitude, due to the decrease in total atmospheric pressure, alveolar P_{CO_2} also falls, producing chronic respiratory alkalosis.

Nonvolatile acids are also produced by the body. The diet and physiological state of the individual determine the kinds and amounts of these acids. Oxidation of sulfur-containing amino acids produces H^+ and SO_4^{2-}, the equivalent of sulfuric acid. Hydrolysis of phosphate esters is equivalent to the formation of phosphoric acid. The contribution of these processes depends on the amount of acid precursors ingested; on an average American diet, net acid production is about 60 meq day^{-1}.

Metabolism normally produces lactic acid, acetoacetic acid, and β-hydroxybutyric acid. In some physiological or pathological states these are produced in excess, and accumulation of the excess causes acidosis. When an ammonium salt of a strong acid, such as ammonium chloride, or when arginine hydrochloride or lysine hydrochloride is administered, it is converted to urea, and the corresponding strong acid (HCl) is synthesized. Ingestion of salicylates, methyl alcohol, or ethylene glycol results in production of strong organic acids. Accumulation of any of these nonvolatile acids leads to **metabolic acidosis.**

While it is obvious that excess acid production can cause acidosis, the same net effect can arise from abnormal loss of base, as predicted from the Henderson–Hasselbalch equation for the bicarbonate buffer system. Renal tubular acidosis is a condition in which this occurs. Abnormal amounts of HCO_3^- escape from the blood into the urine, leaving the body acidotic (see Clin. Corr. 25.6). A more common cause of bicarbonate depletion is severe diarrhea. In this chapter it will be assumed that kidney function is normal.

Mammals do not synthesize alkaline compounds from neutral starting materials. **Metabolic alkalosis** therefore arises from intake of excess alkali or abnormal loss of acid. A commonly ingested alkali is sodium bicarbonate. A less obvious source of alkali is the salt of any metabolizable organic acid. Sodium lactate is often administered to combat acidosis; normal metabolism converts it to sodium bicarbonate. The net reaction is as follows:

$$Na^+ + CH_3CHOHCOO^- + 3O_2 \rightarrow Na^+ + HCO_3^- + 2CO_2 + 2H_2O$$

Most dietary fruits and vegetables have a net alkalinizing effect on the body for this reason. They contain a mixture of organic acids, which are metabolized to CO_2 and H_2O, and therefore have no long-term effect on acid–base balance, and salts of organic acids, which give rise to bicarbonate. Abnormal loss of acid, as occurs in prolonged vomiting or gastric lavage, causes alkalosis. Alkalosis may also be produced by rapid loss of body water, as in diuresis, which may temporarily increase $[HCO_3^-]$ in the plasma and extracellular fluid. Table 25.8 summarizes the causes of acid–base imbalances.

CLINICAL CORRELATION 25.6

The Role of Bone in Acid–Base Homeostasis

The average adult skeleton contains 50,000 meq of Ca^{2+} in the form of salts that are alkaline relative to the pH of plasma. In chronic acidosis this large reservoir of base is drawn upon to help control the plasma pH. Thus people with chronic kidney disease and severely impaired renal acid excretion do not experience a continuous decline in plasma pH and $[HCO_3^-]$. Rather, the pH and $[HCO_3^-]$ stabilize at some below-normal level. The resulting change in bone composition is not inconsequential, and clinical and roentgenologic evidence of rickets or osteomalacia often appear. Bone healing has been shown in these patients after prolonged administration of alkali in the form of sodium bicarbonate or citrate sufficient to restore plasma $[HCO_3^-]$.

Lemann, J. Jr. and Lennon, E. J. Kidney Int. *1:275, 1972.*

The Kidney Plays a Critical Role in Acid–Base Balance

Excess nonvolatile acid and excess bicarbonate are excreted by the kidney. As a result, urine pH varies as a function of the body's need to excrete these materials. For an individual on a typical American diet, urine pH is about 6, indicating a net acidification as compared to plasma. This is consistent with our knowledge that the typical diet results in a net production of acid. Urine pH can range from 4.4 to 8.0.

A typical daily urine volume is about 1.2 L. At the minimum urine pH of 4.4, $[H^+]$ is only 0.04 meq L^{-1}, and it would take 1250 L of urine to excrete 50 meq of acid as free hydrogen ions. Clearly, most of the acid we excrete must be in a form other than H^+. A form that can be excreted in a reasonable concentration, such as $H_2PO_4^-$ or NH_4^+, is needed.

TABLE 25.8 Causes of Acid–Base Imbalance Summarized

Acidosis
Respiratory
Alveolar hypoventilation
Metabolic
H^+ overproduction
HCO_3^- overexcretion
Alkalosis
Respiratory
Alveolar hyperventilation
Metabolic
Alkali ingestion
H^+ overexcretion

Urine Formation Occurs Primarily in the Nephron

Let us now see how the kidney accomplishes the excretion of acid or base. Figure 25.22 shows the fundamental functioning unit of the kidney, a nephron. Each human kidney contains at least a million, which first filter the blood and then modify the filtrate into urine.

Filtration occurs in the glomerulus, a tuft of capillaries enclosed by an epithelial envelope called the glomerular capsule (formerly Bowman's capsule). Water and low molecular weight solutes, such as inorganic ions, urea, sugars, and amino acids (but not normally substances with molecular weights above 70,000, such as plasma proteins), pass from these capillaries into the capsular space. This ultrafiltrate of plasma then passes through the proximal convoluted tubule, where most of the water and solutes are reabsorbed. The tubule fluid continues through the loop of the nephron (loop of Henle) and through the distal convoluted tubule, where further reabsorption of some solutes or secretion of others occurs. The tubule fluid then passes into the collecting tubule, where additional concentration can occur if necessary. The fluid may now be called urine; it contains 1% or less of the water and solutes of the original glomerular filtrate.

The kidney regulates acid–base balance by controlling bicarbonate reabsorption and by secreting acid. Both processes depend on formation of H^+ and HCO_3^- from CO_2 and H_2O within the tubule cells, shown in Figure 25.23*a*. The H^+ formed in this reaction is actively secreted into the tubule fluid in exchange for Na^+. Na^+ uptake by the tubule cell is partly passive, with Na^+ flowing down the electrochemical gradient, and partly active, via a Na^+,H^+-antiport system. At this point Na^+ has been reabsorbed in exchange for H^+, and sodium bicarbonate has been generated within the tubule cell. The sodium bicarbonate is then transported out of the cell into the interstitial fluid, which equilibrates with the plasma.

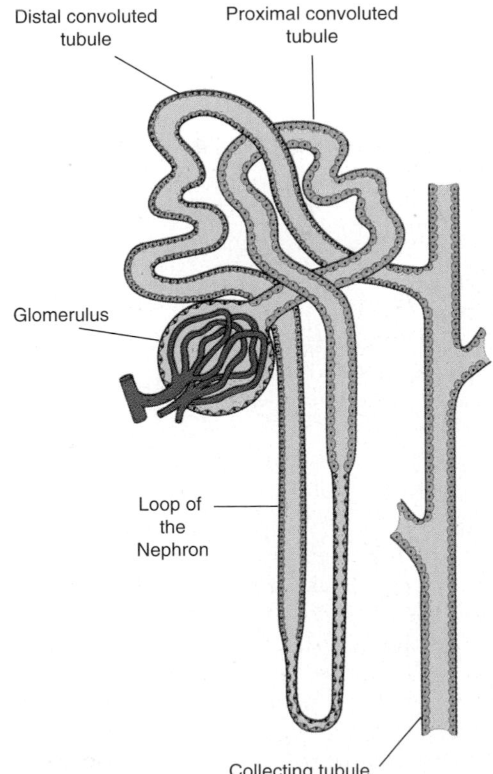

FIGURE 25.22
Essential features of a typical nephron in the human kidney.
Reprinted with permission from Smith, H. W. The Physiology of the Kidney. *London: Oxford University Press, 1937, p. 6.*

The Three Fates of Excreted H^+

The H^+ that has been secreted into the tubule fluid can now experience one of three fates. First, it can react with a HCO_3^-, as shown in Figure 25.23*b*, to form CO_2 and H_2O. The overall net effect of this process is to move sodium bicarbonate from the tubule fluid back into the interstitial fluid. The name given to this is **reabsorption of sodium bicarbonate.**

As reabsorption of sodium bicarbonate proceeds, the tubule fluid becomes depleted of HCO_3^-, and the pH drops from its initial value, which was identical to the pH of the plasma from which it was derived. As HCO_3^- becomes less available and the pH comes closer to the p*K* of the $HPO_4^{2-}/H_2PO_4^-$ buffer system, more and more of the H^+ will be taken up by this buffer. **Buffering** is the second fate of H^+, represented in Figure 25.23*c*. $H_2PO_4^-$ is not readily reabsorbed by the kidney. It passes out in the urine, and its loss represents net excretion of H^+.

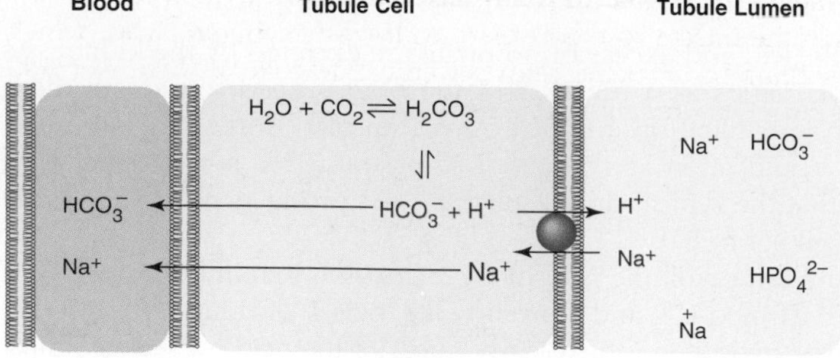

(a) Basic ion exchange mechanism

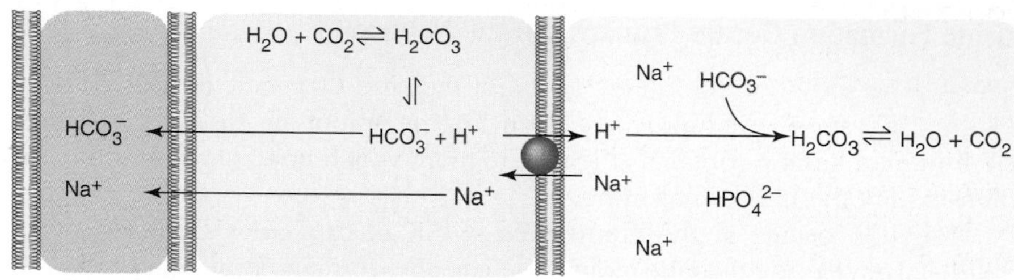

(b) Reabsorption of bicarbonate

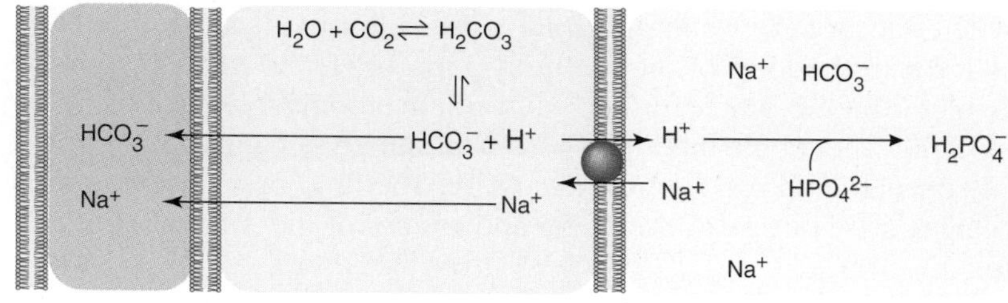

(c) Excretion of titratable acidity

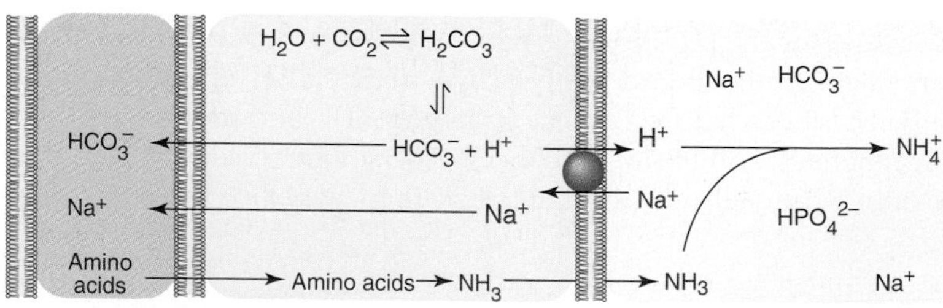

(d) Excretion of ammonia

FIGURE 25.23
Role of the exchange of tubular cell H^+ ions in tubular fluid in renal regulation of acid–base balance.
(a) Basic ion exchange mechanism. (b) Reabsorption of bicarbonate. (c) Excretion of titratable acid. (d) Excretion of ammonia.
Adapted from Pitts, R. E. N. Engl. J. Med. 284:32, 1971, with permission of the publisher.

Although phosphate is normally the most important buffer in the urine, other ions can become significant. For example, in diabetic ketoacidosis, plasma levels of acetoacetate and β-hydroxybutyrate are elevated. These pass into the glomerular filtrate and appear in the tubule fluid. Since acetoacetic acid has a $pK = 3.6$ and β-hydroxybutyric acid has a $pK = 4.7$, as the urine pH approaches its minimum of 4.4, these begin to serve as buffers.

The effect of buffering is not only to excrete acid but to regenerate the bicarbonate that was lost when the acid was first neutralized. Let us consider a situation in which the metabolic defect of a diabetic patient has produced the elements of β-hydroxybutyric acid. The protons are neutralized by sodium bicarbonate, leaving sodium β-hydroxybutyrate. In the kidney, then, β-hydroxybutyrate appears in the filtrate, it is converted to β-hydroxybutyric acid, which is excreted, and sodium bicarbonate returns to the extracellular fluid. Net acid excretion and bicarbonate regeneration occur no matter what anion in the tubule fluid acts as the H^+ acceptor.

The amount of acid excreted as the acid component of a urinary buffer is measured by titrating the urine back to the normal pH of the plasma, 7.4. The amount of base required is identical to the amount of acid excreted in this form and is called the **titratable acidity** of the urine.

The formation of titratable acidity accounts for about one-third to one-half of our normal daily acid excretion. It is thus an important mechanism for acid excretion and can put out as much as 250 meq of acid daily. There is, however, a limit to the amount of acid that can be excreted in this manner. Titratable acidity can be increased only by lowering the pH of the urine or by increasing the concentration of buffer in the urine, and neither of these processes can proceed indefinitely. The urine pH cannot go below about 4.4; evidently the Na^+/H^+ exchange mechanism is incapable of pumping H^+ out of the tubule cells against more than a 1000-fold concentration gradient. Buffer excretion is limited not only by the solubility of the buffer, but by limitations to the supply of the buffer ion and of the cations that are necessarily part of the important buffer systems. If a 600 meq day^{-1} of acid were excreted as NaH_2PO_4, the body would be totally depleted of sodium in less than one week.

The third fate that H^+ can experience in the tubule fluid is neutralization by NH_3. Tubule cells produce NH_4^+ from amino acids, particularly glutamine, as shown in Figure 25.23*d*. **Elimination of NH_4^+** in the urine contributes to net acid excretion.

NH_4^+ is normally a major urinary acid. Typically, one-half to two-thirds of our daily acid load is excreted as NH_4^+. For three reasons it becomes even more important in acidosis. In the first place, since the pK of NH_4^+ is 9.3, acid can be excreted in this form without lowering the pH of the urine, whereas formation of titratable acidity requires a decrease in urine pH. Second, enormous amounts of acid can be excreted in this form. Ammonia is readily available from amino acids, and in prolonged acidosis the NH_4^+ excretion system becomes activated. This activation, however, takes several days; it does not begin to adapt until after 2–3 days, and the process is not complete until 5–6 days after the onset of acidosis. Once complete, though, amounts of acid in excess of 500 meq can be excreted daily as NH_4^+. The third role of NH_4^+ in acidosis is that it spares the body's stores of Na^+ and K^+. Excretion of titratable acid, such as $H_2PO_4^-$, and of the anions of strong acids, such as acetoacetate, requires simultaneous excretion of a cation to maintain electrical neutrality. At the onset of acidosis this is Na^+, but as the body's Na^+ stores become depleted, K^+ excretion rises. If NH_4^+ were not available, even a moderate acidosis could quickly become fatal.

Total Acidity of the Urine

Total acid excretion, the **total acidity of the urine,** is the sum of titratable acidity and NH_4^+. Strictly speaking, we should subtract from this sum the urinary HCO_3^-, but this is seldom done in practice, since in severe metabolic acidosis, where the total acid excretion would be of greatest interest, the urine would be so acidic that $[HCO_3^-]$ would be nil.

In alkalosis the kidney's role is simply to allow HCO_3^- to escape. Metabolic alkalosis is therefore seldom long-lasting unless alkali is continuously administered or HCO_3^- elimination is somehow prevented. HCO_3^- elimination may be restricted if the kidney receives a strong signal to conserve Na^+ at a time when there is a deficiency of an easily reabsorbable anion, such as Cl^-, to be reabsorbed with it. Some diuretics cause this. The first renal response is to put out K^+ in exchange for Na^+ from the tubule fluid. When K^+ stores are depleted, H^+ is exchanged for Na^+. This results in the production of an acidic urine by an alkalotic patient. If NaCl is administered, alkalosis associated with volume and Cl^- depletion may correct itself.

25.12 ■ COMPENSATORY MECHANISMS

We have defined four primary types of acid–base imbalances and we have seen their chemical causes. Respiratory acidosis arises from an increased plasma P_{CO_2}. Respiratory alkalosis is caused by a decreased plasma P_{CO_2}. In metabolic acidosis addition of strong organic or inorganic acid (or loss of HCO_3^-) results in decreased plasma $[HCO_3^-]$. Conversely, in metabolic alkalosis loss of acid from the body or ingestion of alkali raises the plasma $[HCO_3^-]$. Recall that in an acute respiratory acid–base imbalance, as long as there is no attempt to compensate, pH will be abnormal, and $[HCO_3^-]$ will be somewhere on the buffer line. In an acute metabolic acid–base imbalance, if there is no attempt to compensate, pH will be abnormal and $[HCO_3^-]$ will be somewhere on the 40-mmHg (5.33-kPa) isobar.

Principles of Compensation

When the plasma pH deviates from the normal range, various compensatory mechanisms begin to operate. The general principle of compensation is that, since an abnormal condition has directly altered one term of the $[HCO_3^-]/[CO_2]$ ratio, plasma pH can be readjusted back toward normal by a compensatory alteration of the other term. For example, if a diabetic patient becomes acidotic due to excess production of ketone bodies, plasma $[HCO_3^-]$ will decrease. Compensation would involve decreasing plasma $[CO_2]$ so that the $[HCO_3^-]/[CO_2]$ ratio, and therefore the pH, is readjusted back toward normal. Note that compensation does not involve a return of $[HCO_3^-]$ and $[CO_2]$ toward normal. Rather, compensation is a secondary alteration in one of these that counteracts the primary alteration in the other. The result is that the plasma pH is readjusted toward normal. That this is necessarily so is evident from the Henderson–Hasselbalch equation.

$$pH = 6.1 + \log \frac{[HCO_3^-]}{0.03 \cdot P_{CO_2}}$$

If $[HCO_3^-]$ changes, the only way to restore the original $[HCO_3^-]/[CO_2]$ ratio is to change P_{CO_2} in the same direction. If the primary change is in P_{CO_2}, the original ratio can be restored only by altering $[HCO_3^-]$ in the same direction.

The Three States of Compensation Defined

Although some compensatory mechanisms begin to operate rapidly and produce their effects rapidly, others are slower and show stages of compensation. First is the acute stage, before any significant degree of compensation could possibly occur. After the acid–base imbalance has been in effect for a period of time the patient may become **compensated.** This means the compensatory mechanisms have come into play in a normal manner, as expected on the basis of experience with other individuals with an acid–base imbalance of similar type and degree. The "compensated state" does not necessarily imply that the plasma pH is within the normal range. Alternatively, the patient may show no sign of compensation and may be in the **uncompensated** state; this occurs because compensation cannot occur due to some other abnormality. Finally, there is an intermediate state where compensation is occurring but is not yet as complete as it should be. This is the **partially compensated** state. Factors that limit the compensatory processes will be discussed at the end of this section.

Specific Compensatory Processes

Respiratory Acidosis

Let us now follow the course of acute onset of each type of acid–base imbalance and of the compensatory process. Each of these will be schematically illustrated in a pH–bicarbonate diagram. Imagine an individual in normal acid–base balance who goes into acute respiratory acidosis from breathing a gas mixture containing a high level of CO_2. As P_{CO_2} rises, plasma pH drops and [HCO_3^-] rises. (If a decrease in pH and a simultaneous rise in [HCO_3^-] suddenly seems anomalous, turn back to Figure 25.19 and the text on p. 1040 and review the blood buffer line.) The point describing his/her condition follows the buffer line to point *A*, as shown in Figure 25.24. Eventually a new steady-state P_{CO_2} is established in the alveoli and in the blood, and no further change in P_{CO_2} will occur. The abnormal condition has fixed this patient on an abnormally high CO_2 isobar. If the condition is returned to normal, he/she can drop back to the 40-mmHg (5.33-kPa) isobar and all will be well, but until that time all compensatory processes are confined to the higher CO_2 isobar. Compensation, of course, consists of renal excretion of H^+. Since this is a bicarbonate-producing process, [HCO_3^-] should rise, even though it is already above normal. This could have been predicted from the pH–HCO_3^- diagram with no knowledge of the renal mechanism of compensation. Since it is assumed that the individual is fixed on the high CO_2 isobar by the abnormal condition, the only way the pH can possibly be adjusted toward normal is by sliding up the isobar to point *B* in Figure 25.24. This movement is necessarily linked to an increase in [HCO_3^-]. Thus the correct analysis of this compensation could be made either from an understanding of the nature of the compensatory mechanism or from an appreciation of the physical chemistry of the bicarbonate buffer system as expressed in the pH–HCO_3^- diagram.

Although the path we have described, up the buffer line to point *A* and then up the isobar to point *B*, is a real possibility, it is also possible that a respiratory acidosis would develop gradually, with compensation occurring simultaneously. The points describing this progress would fall on a curved line from the normal state to point *B*.

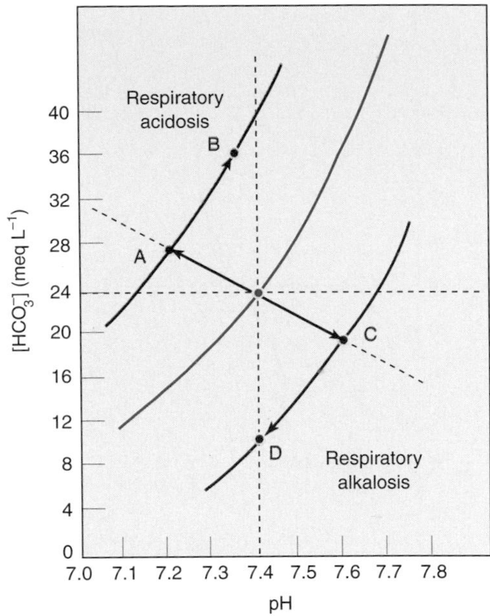

FIGURE 25.24
pH–Bicarbonate diagram showing compensation for respiratory acidosis (normal state to point *B*) and for respiratory alkalosis (normal state to point *D*).

Respiratory Alkalosis

In sudden onset respiratory alkalosis P_{CO_2} drops rapidly. The pH rises and [HCO_3^-] falls, following the buffer line to point *C* in Figure 25.24 (see Clin. Corr. 25.7 for a case of acute respiratory alkalosis). As with respiratory acidosis, unless the cause of the decreased alveolar P_{CO_2} is removed, the patient is fixed on an abnormal CO_2 isobar. Compensation consists of renal excretion of HCO_3^-; plasma [HCO_3^-] diminishes (at a fixed, subnormal P_{CO_2}), and the plasma pH

CLINICAL CORRELATION 25.7

Acute Respiratory Alkalosis

An anesthetized surgical patient with a urethral catheter in place was hyperventilated as an adjunct to the general anesthesia. Prior to hyperventilation normal values of plasma P_{CO_2} and pH were obtained. Alveolar ventilation was then increased mechanically, and a new steady state was reached, in which the plasma P_{CO_2} was 25 mmHg and the pH was 7.55. Plasma HCO_3^- was not directly measured, but interpolation from a pH–bicarbonate diagram (e.g., Figure 25.17) or calculation from the Henderson–Hasselbalch equation reveals that the plasma [HCO_3^-] decreased to 21.2 meq L^{-1}. Analysis of the urine showed negligible loss of HCO_3^- through the kidneys. It can be concluded that the decrease in [HCO_3^-] was due to titration of bicarbonate by the acid components of the body's buffer systems. The point representing the patient's new steady-state condition clearly must be on the buffering line that represents whole body buffering. (Since the buffers of the whole body are not identical in type or concentration to the blood buffers, the buffer line for the whole body will be analogous, but not identical, to the blood buffer line.)

Magarian, G. J. *Medicine (Baltimore)* 61:219, 1982.

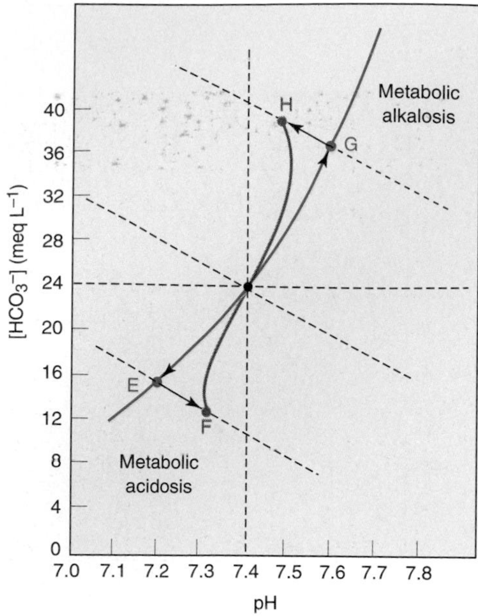

FIGURE 25.25
pH–Bicarbonate diagram showing compensation for metabolic acidosis (normal state to point *F*) and for metabolic alkalosis (normal state to point *H*).

CLINICAL CORRELATION 25.8

Chronic Respiratory Acidosis

H.W. was admitted to the hospital with marked dyspnea, cyanosis, and signs of mental confusion. As his acute problems were relieved by appropriate treatment, his symptoms disappeared except for a continuing dyspnea. Blood gas analysis performed eight days later yielded the following data: pH, 7.32; P_{CO_2}, 70 mmHg; [HCO_3^-], 34.9 meq L^{-1}. This is a typical compensation for this degree of chronic respiratory acidosis.

Another patient, C.Q., with chronic obstructive lung disease was found to have arterial plasma pH, 7.40; [HCO_3^-], 35.9 meq L^{-1}; and P_{CO_2}, 60 mmHg. A return of the plasma pH to 7.4 is not expected in the average patient with respiratory acidosis. Some patients are capable of attaining it, although it becomes less and less likely as P_{CO_2} increases. In this case, with a P_{CO_2} of 60 mmHg, a plasma pH of 7.4 lies outside the 95% probability range. Close questioning of the patient revealed that he had surreptitiously been taking a relative's thiazide diuretic, which superimposed a metabolic alkalosis upon respiratory acidosis.

Rastegar, A., and Thier, S. O. *Chest* 63:355, 1972.

decreases toward normal. This is described in Figure 25.24 by movement along the isobar from point *C* to point *D*. With a gradual onset of respiratory alkalosis, the bicarbonate buffer system would follow points along the curved line from the normal state to point *D*.

Metabolic Acidosis

In metabolic acidosis two mechanisms are usually available for dealing with the excess acid. One is that kidneys increase their H^+ excretion, but this is slow and inadequate to return [HCO_3^-] and pH to normal. The other, which begins to operate almost instantly, is respiratory compensation. Acidosis stimulates the respiratory system to hyperventilate, decreasing the P_{CO_2}. Thus, if onset of a primary metabolic acidosis is represented in Figure 25.25 by a fall in plasma [HCO_3^-] along the 40-mmHg (5.33-kPa) isobar from the normal state to point *E*, the compensatory decrease in P_{CO_2} and the concomitant rise in pH will follow the line from *E* to *F*. Note that this line is parallel to the buffer line, and that compensation for metabolic acidosis involves not only the expected decrease in P_{CO_2} but also a further small decrease in [HCO_3^-]. This is due to the same factor that causes the buffer line to have a slope: titration of nonbicarbonate buffers. The inevitability and magnitude of the further decrease in [HCO_3^-] can be seen clearly in the pH–bicarbonate diagram.

Metabolic Alkalosis

The principles governing compensation for metabolic alkalosis are like those for metabolic acidosis, but operate in the opposite direction. In metabolic alkalosis the primary defect is an increase in plasma [HCO_3^-]; it rises from the normal state to point *G* in Figure 25.25. The immediate physiological response is hypoventilation, followed by increased renal excretion of HCO_3^-. As a result of hypoventilation P_{CO_2} increases along the line from *G* to *H*, and a further small rise in [HCO_3^-] occurs.

The respiratory response to metabolic acid–base imbalance is rapid, and the bicarbonate buffer system would in most cases be expected to follow points along the curved line from the normal state to the compensated state. An acute metabolic imbalance will not generally be seen outside the experimental laboratory. Indeed, if a physician sees a patient whose plasma pH, [HCO_3^-], and P_{CO_2} are consistent with an acute metabolic imbalance, the physician concludes that the patient's compensatory mechanisms are impaired and that the patient cannot compensate. The patient would be suffering from a mixed respiratory and metabolic acidosis or a mixed respiratory and metabolic alkalosis. Obviously, if a patient had a primary acidosis of one type (respiratory or metabolic) and a primary alkalosis of the other, both caused by independent diseases, the effects of the two on plasma pH would tend to cancel. Even if the pH were within the normal range in such a circumstance, [HCO_3^-] and P_{CO_2} would be abnormal.

How complete can compensation be? Can the body totally compensate (bring the pH back to the normal range) for any imbalance? Generally, the answer is no. The compensatory organs, the lungs and kidneys, do not exist exclusively to deal with acid–base imbalance. There is a limit to how much one can hyperventilate; it is simply impossible to move air into and out of the lungs at an indefinitely high rate for an indefinitely long time. Also, one cannot suspend respiration merely to raise P_{CO_2} to some desired level. The kidney also has limits. As P_{CO_2} rises above 70 mmHg (9.33 kPa) in respiratory acidosis, renal mechanisms for reabsorbing HCO_3^- fail to keep pace, and further increases in plasma [HCO_3^-] are only about what could be expected from titration of nonbicarbonate buffers (see Clin. Corr. 25.8). In respiratory alkalosis renal excretion of excess HCO_3^- can, with time, be sufficient to return plasma pH to within the normal range. Individuals who dwell at high altitude are typically in compensated respiratory alkalosis, with their plasma pH within the normal range. For the other types of acid–base imbalance, the exact degree of compensation expected of a patient with a given clinical picture is well worked out, but a detailed discussion is beyond the scope of this chapter. Suffice it to say that if a patient is compensating, but not as well as expected, this is taken to mean that the patient cannot compensate appropriately and must therefore have a mixed acid–base disturbance.

25.13 ALTERNATIVE MEASURES OF ACID–BASE IMBALANCE

Modern clinical laboratories generally report plasma bicarbonate concentration, and the value is used by physicians just as we have used it here. Some laboratories, however, report **total plasma CO_2,** that is, the sum of bicarbonate and dissolved CO_2, and this is always slightly higher than $[HCO_3^-]$. At pH 7.4, for example, the ratio of $[HCO_3^-]$ to $[CO_2]$ is 20 : 1 (dissolved CO_2 is only 1 : 21 of the total CO_2); if $[HCO_3^-]$ is 24 meq L^{-1}, $[CO_2]$ is 1.2 meq L^{-1} and total CO_2 is 25.2 meq L^{-1}. At pH 7.1, HCO_3^- is still 10 times as concentrated as dissolved CO_2. Because the major contributor to total CO_2 is HCO_3^-, total CO_2 is often used in the same manner as bicarbonate to make clinical judgments. Strictly speaking, total CO_2 also includes that in carbamino proteins, but current clinical laboratory practice is to ignore this when making a blood gas and pH report. If it were included in a total CO_2 measurement, it would not change the interpretation of the measurement, since the CO_2 in carbamino proteins, like dissolved CO_2, represents only a small fraction of the total CO_2.

The clinical importance of bicarbonate as a gauge of the whole body's ability to buffer further loads of metabolic acid (see Clin. Corr. 25.9) has led to several ways of expressing what the $[HCO_3^-]$ would be if there were no respiratory component or respiratory compensation involved in a patient's condition. **Base excess** is one of these expressions. It is defined as the amount of acid that would have to be added to blood to titrate it to pH 7.4 at a P_{CO_2} of 40 mmHg (5.33 kPa) at 37°C. Since the titration is carried out at the normal P_{CO_2}, only the metabolic contribution to acid–base imbalance (primary metabolic imbalance and nonrespiratory compensatory processes) would be measured. If a blood sample were acidic under the conditions of the titration, alkali would have to be added instead of acid, and the base excess would be negative.

The concept and the quantitation of base excess are most easily understood from the pH–bicarbonate diagram. In our discussion of the blood buffer line we saw how increasing the P_{CO_2} in blood, where other buffers are present, would result in a rise in $[HCO_3^-]$ and a virtually identical decrease in the concentration of other buffer bases. This was because equivalent amounts of the other buffer bases were consumed as they buffered carbonic acid. Since virtually all the carbonic acid formed was buffered, for every HCO_3^- formed one conjugate base of some other system was consumed. In this situation the total base in the blood is not measurably changed; only the distribution of HCO_3^- and nonbicarbonate buffer conjugate base is changed. Thus, as long as one remains on the blood buffer line, $[HCO_3^-]$ can change but total base will not. There will be no positive or negative base excess.

If, however, renal activity, diet, or some metabolic process adds or removes HCO_3^-, then a positive or negative base excess will occur. The patient's status will no longer be described by a point on the buffer line, and the base excess will be the difference between the observed plasma $[HCO_3^-]$ and the $[HCO_3^-]$ on the buffer line at the same pH (Figure 25.26). To calculate this difference, the position of the buffer line, which can be determined from knowledge of the slope and the point representing the normal state, must be known. In the

CLINICAL CORRELATION 25.9

Salicylate Poisoning

Salicylates are the most common cause of poisoning in children. A typical pathway of salicylate intoxication is plotted in the accompanying figure. The first effect of salicylate overdose is stimulation of the respiratory center, resulting in respiratory alkalosis. Renal compensation occurs, lowering the

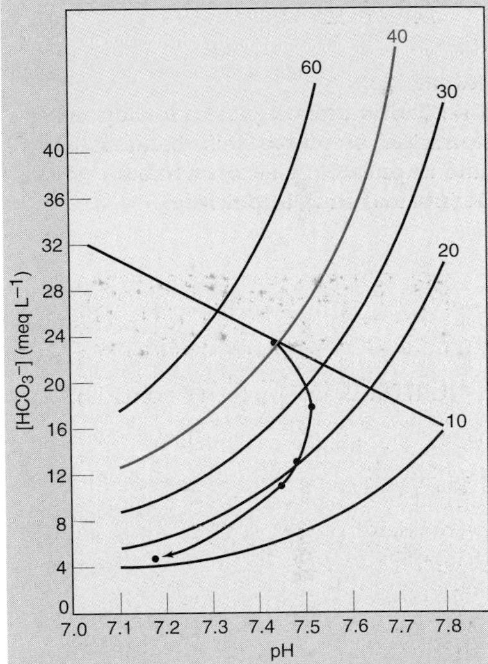

A typical pathway of salicylate intoxication.

Data replotted from Singer, R. B. Medicine *(Baltimore) 33:1, 1954.*

plasma $[HCO_3^-]$. A second, delayed effect of salicylate may then appear, metabolic acidosis. Since $[HCO_3^-]$ had been lowered by the previous compensatory process, the victim is at a particular disadvantage in dealing with the metabolic acidosis. In addition, but not shown in the graph, respiratory stimulation sometimes persists after the acidosis has run its course. Rational management of salicylate intoxication requires knowledge of the plasma pH and the plasma $[HCO_3^-]$ or its equivalent throughout the course of the condition.

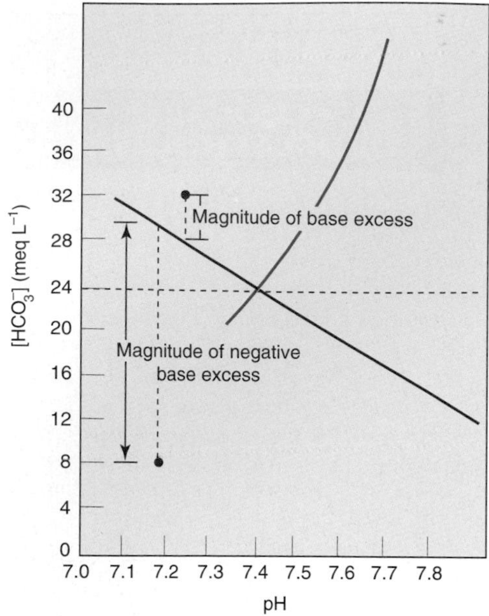

FIGURE 25.26
Calculation of base excess for a point above the blood buffer line, and calculation of negative base excess for a point below the blood buffer line.
Base excess is 32 − 28 = 4 meq L^{-1}. Negative base excess is 30 − 8 = 22 meq L^{-1}.

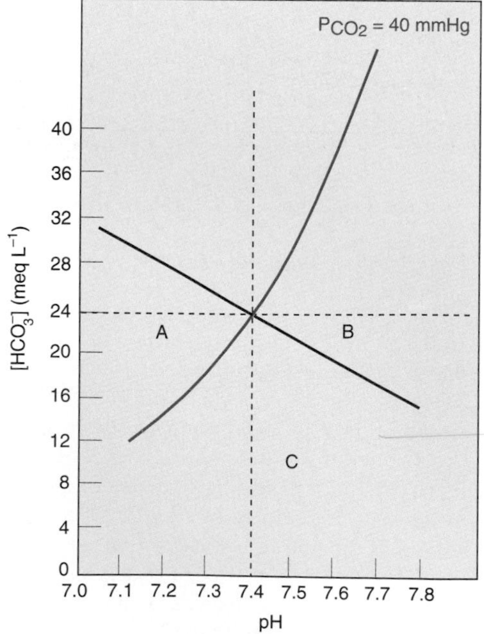

FIGURE 25.27
Examples showing the sign of the base excess at various points.
At points *A* and *C* there is a negative base excess. At point *B* the base excess is positive.

clinical laboratory it can be estimated from hemoglobin concentration and assuming that it is the major nonbicarbonate buffer.

The buffer line, then, is the dividing line between positive and negative base excess. Any point above it is in the region of positive base excess, and any point below it is in the region of negative base excess. This gives rise to situations that may seem peculiar at first. In Figure 25.27 the $[HCO_3^-]$ at point *A* is normal, but the patient has a negative base excess. A positive or negative base excess occurs as a result of compensation for a respiratory acid–base imbalance or directly from a metabolic one. Respiratory compensation for a metabolic acid–base imbalance, since it involves movement along a line parallel to the buffer line (Figure 25.25), would cause no further change in the value of the base excess. Clinical Correlation 25.10 involves consideration of base excess.

25.14 ■ THE SIGNIFICANCE OF Na^+ AND Cl^- IN ACID–BASE IMBALANCE

An important concept in diagnosing certain acid–base disorders is the **anion gap.** Most clinical laboratories routinely measure plasma Na^+, K^+, Cl^-, and HCO_3^-. A glance at the graph in Figure 25.15 confirms that in the plasma of a normal individual the sum of the concentrations of Na^+ and K^+ is greater than the sum of the concentrations of Cl^- and HCO_3^-. This difference is called A, the anion gap; it represents the other plasma anions (Figure 25.15), which are not routinely measured. It is calculated as follows:

$$A = (Na^+ + K^+) - (Cl^- + HCO_3^-)$$

The normal value of A is in the range of 12–16 meq L^{-1}. In some clinical laboratories K^+ is not measured; then the normal value is 8–12 meq L^{-1}. The gap is changed only by conditions that change the sum of the cations or the sum of the anions, or by conditions that change both sums by different amounts. Thus administration or depletion of sodium bicarbonate would not change the anion gap because $[Na^+]$ and $[HCO_3^-]$ would be affected equally. Metabolic acidosis due to HCl or NH_4Cl administration would also leave the anion gap unaffected; here $[HCO_3^-]$ would decrease, but $[Cl^-]$ would increase by an equivalent amount, and the sum of $[HCO_3^-]$ plus $[Cl^-]$ would be unchanged. In contrast, diabetic ketoacidosis or methanol poisoning involves production of organic acids, which react with HCO_3^-, decreasing its concentration. But since the $[HCO_3^-]$ is replaced by some organic anion, the sum of $[HCO_3^-]$ plus $[Cl^-]$ decreases, and the anion gap increases.

The anion gap is most commonly used to establish a differential diagnosis for metabolic acidosis. In a metabolic acidosis with an increased anion gap, H^+ must have arisen in the body with some anion other than chloride. Metabolic acidosis without an increased anion gap must be due either to accumulation of H^+ with chloride or to a decrease in the concentration of sodium bicarbonate. Thus, on the basis of the anion gap, certain diseases can be ruled out, while others would have to be considered. This information can be especially important in dealing with patients who cannot give good histories due to language barriers, unconsciousness, and so on.

Electrolytes of body fluids interact in a multitude of ways. One important way involves the capacity of K^+ and H^+ to substitute for one another under certain circumstances. This can occur in cells, where K^+ is the major cation. In acidosis intracellular $[H^+]$ rises, and it replaces some of the intracellular K^+. The displaced K^+ appears in plasma and is excreted by the kidneys. This leaves the patient with normal plasma $[K^+]$ (normokalemia), but with seriously depleted body K^+ stores (hypokalia). Subsequent excessively rapid correction of the acidosis may then reverse events. As plasma pH rises, K^+ flows back into the cells, and plasma $[K^+]$ may decline to the point where muscular weakness sets in and respiratory insufficiency may become life-threatening.

CLINICAL CORRELATION 25.10

Evaluation of Clinical Acid–Base Data

In a 1972 study of total parenteral nutrition of infants, it was found that infants who received amino acids in the form of a hydrolysate of the protein fibrin maintained normal acid–base balance. In contrast, infants receiving two different mixtures of synthetic amino acids, FreAmine and Neoaminosol, became acidotic. Both synthetic mixtures contained adequate amounts of all the essential amino acids, but neither contained aspartate or glutamate. The fibrin hydrolysate contained all of the common amino acids.

The accompanying figure shows the blood acid–base data from these infants. Note that the normal values for infants, given by the dashed lines, are not quite the same as normal values for adults. (A child is *not* a small adult.) The blood pH data show that the infants receiving synthetic mixtures were clearly acidotic. The low [HCO_3^-] of the Neoaminosol group immediately suggests a metabolic acidosis, and the P_{CO_2} and base excess data are compatible with this interpretation. The FreAmine group, however, shows nearly normal [HCO_3^-], and all of these infants have elevated P_{CO_2} values. The P_{CO_2} values indicate respiratory acidosis, but a simple respiratory acidosis should be associated with a slightly elevated [HCO_3^-]. The absence of this finding in most of the infants indicates that the acidosis must also have a metabolic component. This is confirmed by the observation that all the infants receiving FreAmine have a significant negative base excess.

The infants with mixed acid–base disturbances did, in fact, have pneumonia or respiratory distress syndrome. The metabolic acidosis, which all the infants receiving synthetic mixtures experienced, was due to synthesis of aspartic acid and glutamic acid from a neutral starting material (presumably glucose). Subsequent incorporation of these acids into body protein imposed a net acid load on the body. Addition of aspartate and/or glutamate to the synthetic mixtures was proposed as a solution of the problem.

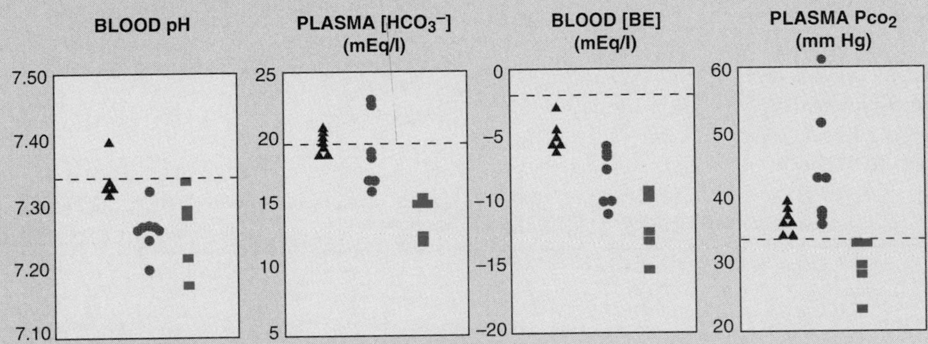

Blood acid–base data of patients receiving fibrin hydrolysate (▲) and of those receiving synthetic L-amino acid mixtures, FreAmine (●) and Neoaminosal (■).

Values are those observed at the time of the lowest blood base excess. Dashed lines represent accepted normal values for infants.
Adapted from W. C. Heird, N. Engl. J. Med. *287:943, 1972.*

In kidneys the reciprocal relationship between K^+ and H^+ results in an association between metabolic alkalosis and hypokalemia. If hypokalemia arises from long-term insufficiency of dietary potassium or long-term diuretic therapy, intracellular K^+ levels diminish, and intracellular [H^+] will increase. This leads to increased acid excretion, acidic urine, and an alkaline arterial plasma pH. We have already seen how in an alkalotic individual a hormonal signal to absorb Na^+ can lead to K^+ loss and then to an exacerbation of the metabolic alkalosis (p. 1045). The opposite also occurs, with alkalosis leading to hypokalemia. In this case increased amounts of $Na^+ + HCO_3^-$ are presented to the distal convoluted tubules, where all K^+ secretion normally takes place (all filtered K^+ is reabsorbed; K^+ loss is due to distal tubular secretion). The distal tubules take up some Na^+, but since HCO_3^- does not readily follow across that membrane, the increased Na^+ uptake is linked to increased K^+ secretion. K^+ excretion is complicated, being controlled by a variety of hormones and other

CLINICAL CORRELATION 25.11

Metabolic Alkalosis

Prolonged gastric lavage produces a metabolic alkalosis that is a good experimental model of the metabolic alkalosis that results from repeated vomiting. The following table gives plasma and urine acid–base and electrolyte data from a healthy volunteer on a low-sodium diet who, after a control period, was subjected to gastric lavage for two days. After a five day recovery period, he was placed on a low-potassium diet and given a sodium (130 meq day^{-1}) and chloride (121 meq day^{-1}) supplement. During the control period the data are within normal limits. After gastric lavage that selectively removed HCl (Na^+, K^+, and H_2O lost with the gastric juice were restored), an uncomplicated metabolic alkalosis developed. Note that the subject excreted an alkaline urine, containing a substantial amount of HCO_3^-. The Na^+ excretion increased, depleting the body's Na^+ stores. Plasma P_{CO_2} was not measured, but plotting the values of pH and [HCO_3^-] on a pH–bicarbonate diagram (e.g., Figure 25.18) allows one to interpolate a value of about 47 mmHg. Clearly, respiratory compensation was occurring. Plasma [K^+] was decreased. Plasma [Cl^-] decreased, but no more than would be expected on the basis of the changes in [Na^+], [K^+], and [HCO_3^-].

When the subject was placed on a low-potassium diet the alkalosis grew worse, and plasma [HCO_3^-] rose. Additional compensatory hypoventilation evidently prevented a further rise in plasma pH. Note, though, that the urine became acidic, in spite of the increased severity of the alkalosis. The Na^+ was conserved, not in exchange for K^+, but in exchange for H^+. After several days of Na^+ and Cl^- administration, however, the subject was able to restore the depleted Cl^-, excrete the excess HCO_3^-, and repair the acid–base imbalance with no other treatment.

	Control	*After Lavage*	*Low KCl*	*After NaCl*
Plasma				
pH	7.4	7.50	7.48	7.41
HCO_3^-	29.3	35.3	38.1	26.1
Na^+ (meq L^{-1})	138	134	141	144
K^+ (meq L^{-1})	4.2	3.2	2.9	3.2
Cl^- (meq L^{-1})	101	88	85	108
Urine				
pH				
HCO_3^- (meq/	6.12	7.48	5.70	7.19
day^{-1})	3	51	1	17
NH_4^+ (meq/day^{-1})	22	4	36	14
Titratable acidity (meq/day^{-1})	10	0	14	1
Total acidity (meq/day^{-1})	29	−49	49	−2
Na^+ (meq/day^{-1})	2	28	1	95

Source: Data from Kassirer, J. P., and Schwartz, W. B., *Am. J. Med.* 40:10, 1966.

factors. The end result, however, is that metabolic alkalosis and hypokalemia go hand in hand, so that the term "hypokalemic alkalosis" is often used synonymously with metabolic alkalosis. Clinical Correlation 25.11 discusses a case of experimental metabolic alkalosis in which this occurred.

BIBLIOGRAPHY

Gas Transport

Bunn, H. F., and Forget, B. G. *Hemoglobin: Molecular, Genetic, and Clinical Aspects.* Philadelphia: Saunders, 1986.

Bunn, H. F., Gabbay, K. H., and Gallop, P. M. The glycosylation of hemoglobin: relevance to diabetes mellitus. *Science* 200:21, 1978.

Kilmartin, J. V. Interaction of haemoglobin with protons, CO_2 and 2,3-diphosphoglycerate. *Br. Med. Bull.* 32:209, 1976.

Perutz, M. F., and Lehmann, H. Molecular pathology of human haemoglobin. *Nature* 219:902, 1968.

Steffes, M. W., and Mauer, S. M. Toward a basic understanding of diabetic complications. *N. Engl. J. Med.* 325:883, 1991.

pH Regulation

Davenport, H. W. *The ABC of Acid–Base Chemistry,* 6th ed. Chicago: University of Chicago Press, 1974.

Gabow, P. A., Kaehny, W. D., Fennessey, P. V., et al. Diagnostic importance of an increased serum anion gap. *N. Engl. J. Med.* 303:854, 1980.

Gamble, J. L. Jr., and Bettice, J. A. Acid–base relationships in the different body compartments: the basis for a simplified diagnostic approach. *Johns Hopkins Med. J.* 140:213, 1977.

Masoro, E. J., and Siegel, P. D. *Acid–Base Regulation: Its Physiology, Pathophysiology and the Interpretation of Blood–Gas Analysis,* 2nd ed. Philadelphia: Saunders, 1977.

Siggaard-Andersen, O. *The Acid–Base Status of the Blood,* 4th ed. Baltimore: Williams & Wilkins, 1974.

QUESTIONS J. BAGGOTT AND C. N. ANGSTADT

1. During a breathing cycle:
   A. the alveolar gases are completely exchanged for atmospheric gases.
   B. gas exchange between the alveoli and the capillary blood can occur at all times.
   C. gas exchange with the capillary blood occurs at the surface of all the airways.
   D. there is net uptake of nitrogen by the blood.
   E. atmospheric water vapor is taken up by the lungs.

2. From an oxygen saturation curve for normal blood we can determine that:
   A. P_{50} is in the P_{O_2} range found in extrapulmonary tissues.
   B. oxygen binding is hyperbolic.
   C. an oxygen carrier is necessary.
   D. tighter oxygen binding occurs at lower P_{O_2}.
   E. shifts of the curve to the left or right would have little effect on oxygen delivery.

Refer to the following for Questions 3–5.
   A. hemoglobin α-chains
   B. hemoglobin β-chains
   C. hemoglobin γ-chains
   D. hemoglobin δ-chains
   E. hemoglobin ε-chains

3. Found in HbA, HbA_2, and HbF.

4. Modified in HbA_{1c}.

5. Form the major binding sites for 2,3-bisphosphoglycerate (BPG).

6. At a P_{O_2} of 30 mmHg hemoglobin's percent saturation will:
   A. increase with increasing temperature.
   B. increase with decreasing pH.
   C. increase with increasing P_{CO_2}.
   D. increase with increasing 2,3-bisphosphoglycerate concentration.
   E. none of the above.

7. Significant contributors to the total carbon dioxide of whole blood include all of the following EXCEPT:
   A. bicarbonate ion.
   B. dissolved carbon dioxide (CO_2).
   C. carbaminohemoglobin.
   D. carbonic acid (H_2CO_3).

8. 2,3-Bisphosphoglycerate (BPG):
   A. is absent from the normal erythrocyte.
   B. is a homotropic effector for hemoglobin.
   C. binds more tightly to HbF than to HbA.
   D. synthesis increases when hemoglobin's T $\leftrightarrow$ R equilibrium is shifted in favor of the T state.
   E. synthesis decreases when the erythrocyte pH rises.

9. Which of the following buffer systems is far less effective in controlling changes in physiological pH due to CO_2 than changes due to metabolic acids, like acetoacetic acid?
   A. bicarbonate
   B. inorganic phosphate
   C. organic phosphate esters
   D. intracellular protein
   E. extracellular protein

10. The slope of the blood buffer line is most sensitive to pathological changes in the blood concentration of:
   A. plasma bicarbonate.
   B. plasma phosphate.
   C. hemoglobin.
   D. plasma proteins.
   E. organic phosphates of the erythrocyte.

11. As P_{CO_2} is increased in a normal individual:
   A. the plasma [CO_2] remains unchanged.
   B. plasma bicarbonate increases.
   C. the slope of the blood buffer line changes.
   D. the base excess increases.
   E. the base excess decreases.

12. All of the following produce H^+ EXCEPT:
   A. formation of bicarbonate ion from CO_2 and water.
   B. formation of carbaminohemoglobin from CO_2 and hemoglobin.
   C. binding of oxygen by hemoglobin.
   D. oxidation of sulfur-containing amino acids.
   E. metabolism of sodium lactate.

13. A substantial fraction of the urinary titratable acidity of a normal individual consists of:
   A. H_2CO_3.
   B. NH_4^+.
   C. acetoacetic acid.
   D. $H_2PO_4^-$.
   E. HCO_3^-.

14. In a patient with diabetic ketoacidosis of long duration:
   A. the major urinary acid is $H_2PO_4^-$.
   B. hemoglobin's oxygen dissociation curve would be shifted to the right.
   C. the distribution of hemoglobin species would be the same as in a normal individual.
   D. 1 mol of bicarbonate is regenerated for every mole of $H_2PO_4^-$ formed in the renal tubule.
   E. hypoventilation would be expected.

15. The following laboratory data are obtained from a patient: $P_{CO_2} = 60$ mmHg, $HCO_3^- = 27$ meq L^{-1}, pH = 7.28. These values define a point on the patient's blood buffer line. We conclude:
   A. The patient has an acute condition.
   B. The condition would lead to production of an alkaline urine.
   C. Of the blood buffers, the bicarbonate buffer system is the most important in resisting this pH change.
   D. Increasing the alveolar P_{CO_2} could restore the plasma to normal.
   E. Hyperventilation due to anxiety could cause this.

16. During compensation for a metabolic acid–base imbalance, which of the following would become increasingly abnormal?
   A. plasma pH
   B. blood P_{CO_2}
   C. base excess
   D. total hemoglobin
   E. none of the above

17. In respiratory alkalosis:
   A. the acute state is associated with an abnormally low plasma [HCO_3^-].
   B. the mechanism of compensation causes an increase in the plasma [HCO_3^-].
   C. the plasma pH never returns to the normal range in the fully compensated state.
   D. in the partially compensated state, there will be a negative base excess equal to the difference between 24 meq L^{-1} and the actual plasma [HCO_3^-].
   E. compensation involves changing P_{CO_2}.

18. Hypokalemia can be expected to:
    A. occur if the plasma pH is rapidly raised.
    B. lead to increased urine acidity.
    C. be associated with a high plasma [HCO_3^-].
    D. decrease the value of the anion gap slightly.
    E. all of the above.

ANSWERS

1. B A and C: The alveoli, where gas exchange with the blood occurs, are of constant size and exchange gases with the airways by diffusion. D and E: Water vapor and CO_2 are added to the alveolar gases by the lung tissue, diluting the nitrogen (p. 1027).
2. A P_{O_2} is typically in the neighborhood of 20 mm in active muscle and is higher in less active tissues. The normal P_{50}, 27 mm, is in this range (p. 1028). B and D: The curve is sigmoid, with tighter binding at higher P_{O_2} (p. 1028, Figure 25.2). C: If O_2 were soluble enough in plasma, no carrier would be necessary (p. 1026). E: Shifts profoundly affect delivery (p. 1028).
3. A It is the non-α-chain that differs among these (p. 1030).
4. B The β-chains are nonenzymatically glycosylated in HbA_{1c} (p. 1030).
5. B BPG binds between the N terminals of the β-chains (p. 1029).
6. E All effects are opposite to those proposed in the question. A–C: High temperature, low pH (and therefore high P_{CO_2}) favor dissociation; that is, decreased saturation (p. 1031). D: High BPG has the same effect (p. 1029).
7. D Carbonic acid is present in very small amounts; the equilibrium strongly favors CO_2 and H_2O (p. 1033, Table 25.2; see also p. 1039).
8. D A and B: BPG is a normal component of the red cell, where it serves as a heterotropic effector of HbA (p. 1029, Figure 25.4). C: It binds weakly or not at all to the HbF (p. 1030). D and E: BPG binds to the T state, relieving product inhibition of BPG synthesis; BPG synthesis is inhibited by low pH (p. 1036).
9. A The bicarbonate system is a major extracellular buffer; with a pK of 6.1 it is ineffective toward CO_2. The other buffers (phosphates and protein) are, effective (p. 1037, Table 25.6). All of these buffers, however, are effective against noncarbonic acids. The bicarbonate buffer system is included here because the response of the respiratory system to low pH, exhaling CO_2, compensates for the innate ineffectiveness of this system at a pH fairly distant from its pK (p. 1039).
10. C The slope of the blood buffer line is determined by the concentration of the nonbicarbonate buffers. Of these, hemoglobin is quantitatively the most important and is susceptible to change (i.e., anemias from any cause) (p. 1040).
11. B This is because the resulting H_2CO_3 is buffered by various nonbicarbonate buffers, producing HCO_3^- (p. 1040).
12. E Metabolism of sodium lactate produces sodium bicarbonate and is used clinically to control acidosis (p. 1042). A and B are reactions whose products include H^+ (pp. 1032–1033). C is the Bohr effect (p. 1031). D is a major source of acid in the typical American diet (p. 1042).
13. D A: The level of H_2CO_3 is very low. B: NH_4^+ is an important urinary acid, but its pK is too high to be titrated at pH 7.4, the endpoint. C: Acetoacetic acid would appear only in some kinds of severe acidosis. E: HCO_3^- is physiologically a base; its dissociable H^+ has a pK that is far above the physiological range (pp. 1043 and 1045).
14. D See pp. 1043–1045. A: After adaptation to acidosis NH_4^+ excretion rises enormously, becoming the major urinary acid (p. 1045). B: True only in acidosis of short duration; decreasing BPG in prolonged acidosis tends to restore the normal position (p. 1036). C: Large amounts of HbA_{1c} would be expected (p. 1030). E: Hyperventilation, to expel CO_2, would be expected (p. 1048).
15. A High P_{CO_2}, low pH point on the blood buffer line define an acute respiratory acidosis. Buffering by nonbicarbonate buffer systems and excretion of acid in the urine would be the physiological responses (p. 1047).
16. B P_{CO_2} would decrease during compensation for acidosis or rise during compensation for alkalosis. A: Plasma pH would be restored. C: Base excess would be unchanged. D: Hemoglobin would participate in buffering, but its total concentration would not be expected to change (pp. 1048–1050, Figures 25.25 and 25.26).
17. A A and B: See p. 1047, Figure 25.24. C: This is the only acid–base abnormality in which compensation is expected to restore the plasma pH to 7.4 (p. 1047). D: There is a negative base excess equivalent to the difference between the patient's [HCO_3^-] and the [HCO_3^-] of the point on the blood buffer line at the same pH, a point that will be less than 24 meq L^{-1} (p. 1050, Figure 25.26). E: This would either be a cure or an exacerbation, depending on the direction of the change; it would not be compensation.
18. E A, B, and C: See p. 1050. D: Decreasing K^+ would lower the anion gap by a small amount (p. 1050).

CHAPTER

26

DIGESTION AND ABSORPTION OF BASIC NUTRITIONAL CONSTITUENTS

Ulrich Hopfer

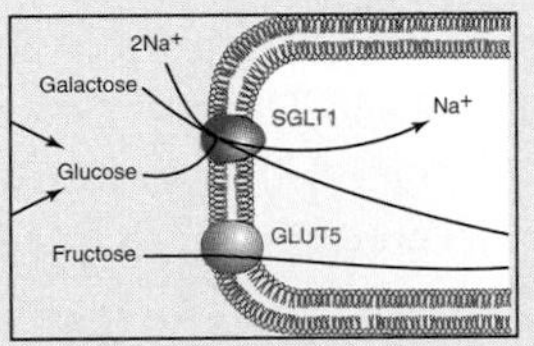

26.1 ■ OVERVIEW

Secretion of digestive fluids and digestion of food were some of the earliest biochemical events to be investigated at the beginning of the era of modern science. Major milestones were the discovery of hydrochloric acid secretion by the stomach and enzymatic hydrolysis of protein and starch by gastric juice and saliva, respectively. The discovery of gastric HCl production goes back to the American physician William Beaumont (1785–1853). In 1822 he treated a patient with a stomach wound. The patient recovered from the wound, but retained a gastric fistula (abnormal opening through the skin). Beaumont seized the opportunity to obtain and study gastric juice at different times during and after meals. Chemical analysis revealed, to the surprise of chemists and biologists, the presence of the inorganic acid HCl. This discovery established the principle of unique secretions into the gastrointestinal tract, which are elaborated by specialized glands.

Soon thereafter, the principle of enzymatic breakdown of food was recognized. In 1836 Theodor Schwann, a German anatomist and physiologist (1810–1882), noticed that gastric juice degraded albumin in the presence of dilute acid. He recognized that a new principle was involved and coined the word pepsin from the Greek *pepsis,* meaning digestion. Today the process of secretion of digestive fluids, digestion of food, and absorption of nutrients and of electrolytes can be described in considerable detail.

The basic nutrients fall into the classes of proteins, carbohydrates, and fats. Many different types of food can satisfy the nutritional needs of humans, even though they differ in the ratios of proteins to carbohydrates and to fats and in the ratio of digestible to nondigestible materials. Unprocessed plant products are especially rich in **fibrous material** that can be neither digested by human enzymes nor easily degraded by intestinal bacteria. The fibers are mostly carbohydrates, such as **cellulose** (β-1,4-glucan) or **pectins** (mixtures of methyl esters of polygalacturonic acid, polygalactose, and polyarabinose). High-fiber diets enjoy a certain popularity nowadays because of a postulated preventive effect on development of colonic cancer.

Table 26.1 describes average contributions of different food classes to the diet of North Americans. The intake of individuals may substantially deviate from the average, as food consumption depends mainly on availability and individual tastes. The ability to utilize a wide variety of food is possible because of the great adaptability and digestive reserve capacity of the gastrointestinal tract.

Knowledge of the nature of proteins and carbohydrates in the diet is important from a clinical point of view. Certain proteins and carbohydrates, although good nutrients for most humans, cannot be properly digested by some individuals and produce gastrointestinal ailments. Omission of the offending

TABLE 26.1 Contribution of Major Food Groups to Daily Nutrient Supplies in the United States

Type of Nutrient	*Total Daily Consumption (g)*	*Dairy Products, Except Butter (%)*	*Meat, Poultry, Fish (%)*	*Eggs (%)*	*Fruits, Nuts, Vegetables (%)*	*Flour, Cereal (%)*	*Sugar, Sweeteners (%)*	*Fats, Oils (%)*
Protein	100	22	42	6	12	18	0	0
Carbohydrate	381	7	0.1	0.1	19	36	37	0
Fat	155	13	35	3	4	1	0	42

material and change to another diet can eliminate these gastrointestinal problems. Examples of food constituents that can be the cause of gastrointestinal disorders are **gluten,** one of the protein fractions of wheat, and **lactose,** the disaccharide in milk.

Gastrointestinal Organs Have Multiple Functions in Digestion

The bulk of ingested nutrients consists of large **polymers** that have to be broken down to **monomers** before they can be absorbed and made available to all cells of the body. The complete process from food intake to absorption of nutrients into the blood consists of a complicated sequence of events, which at the minimum includes (Figure 26.1):

1. Mechanical homogenization of food and mixing of ingested solids with fluids secreted by the glands of the gastrointestinal tract.
2. Secretion of digestive enzymes that hydrolyze macromolecules to oligomers, dimers, or monomers.
3. Secretion of electrolytes, acid, or base to provide an appropriate environment for optimal enzymatic digestion.
4. Secretion of bile acids as detergents to solubilize lipids and facilitate their absorption.
5. Hydrolysis of nutrient oligomers and dimers by enzymes on the intestinal surface.
6. Transport of nutrient molecules and of electrolytes from the intestinal lumen across the epithelial cells into blood or lymph.

To accomplish these functions, the gastrointestinal tract contains specialized glands and surface epithelia:

Organ	Major Function in Digestion and Absorption
Salivary glands	Elaboration of fluid and digestive enzymes
Stomach	Elaboration of HCl and proteases
Pancreas	Elaboration of $NaHCO_3$ and enzymes for intraluminal digestion
Liver	Elaboration of bile acids
Gallbladder	Storage and concentration of bile
Small intestine	Terminal digestion of food, absorption of nutrients and electrolytes
Large intestine	Absorption of electrolytes

The **pancreas** and **small intestine** are essential for digestion and absorption of all basic nutrients. Fortunately, both organs have large reserve capacities. For example, maldigestion due to pancreatic failure becomes a problem only when the pancreatic secretion rate of digestive enzymes drops below one-tenth of the normal rate. The secretion of the liver **(bile)** is important for efficient lipid absorption, which depends on the presence of bile acids. In contrast, gastric digestion of food is nonessential for adequate nutrition, and loss of this function can be compensated for by the pancreas and the small intestine. Yet normal gastric digestion greatly increases the smoothness and efficiency of the total digestive process. The stomach aids in the digestion through its reservoir function, its churning ability, and initiation of protein hydrolysis, which, although small, is important for stimulation of pancreatic and gallbladder output. Peptides and amino acids liberated in the stomach stimulate the coordinated release of pancreatic juice and bile into the lumen of the small intestine, thereby ensuring efficient digestion of food.

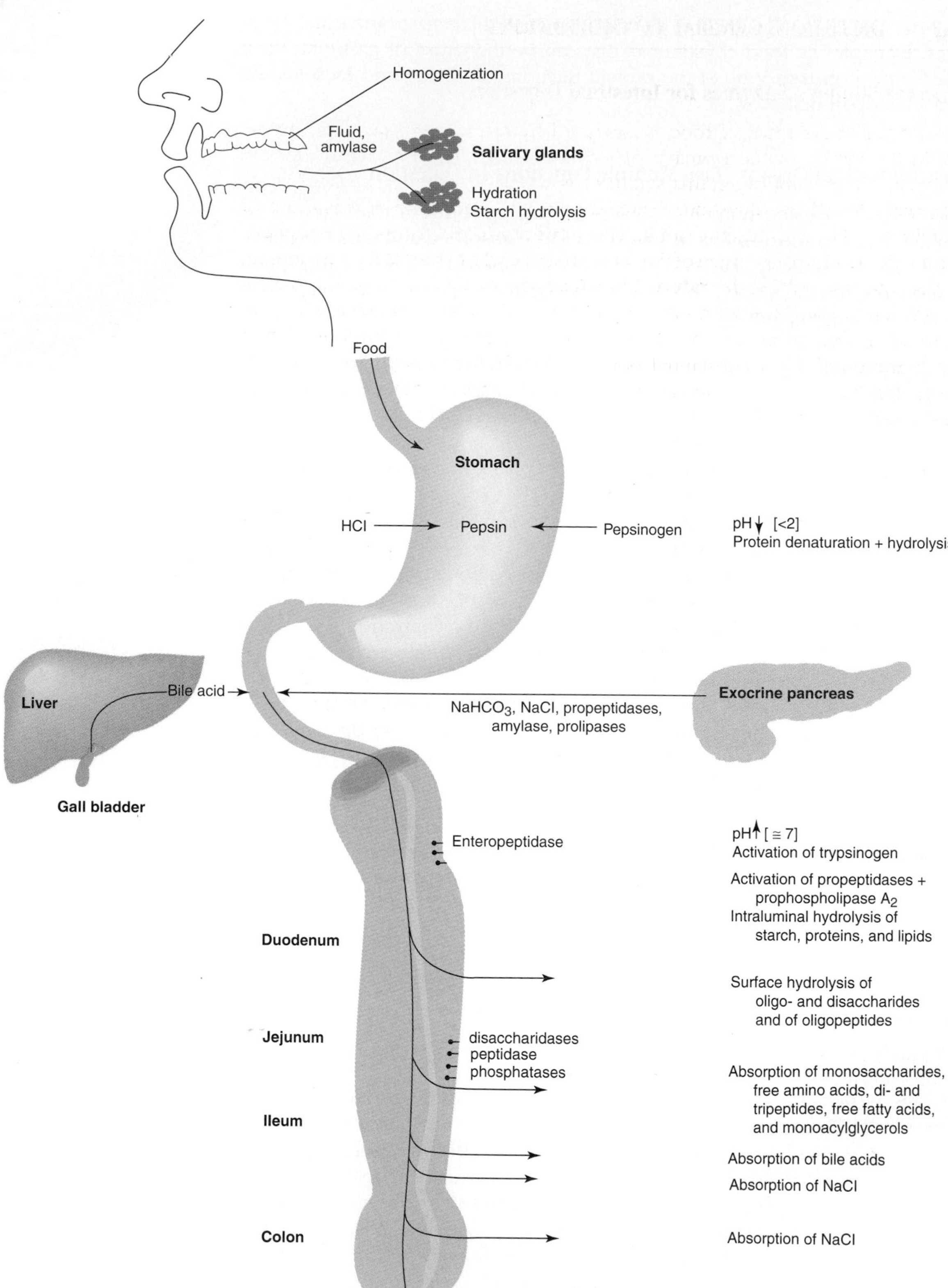

FIGURE 26.1
Gastrointestinal organs and their functions.

26.2 ■ DIGESTION: GENERAL CONSIDERATIONS

Pancreas Supplies Enzymes for Intestinal Digestion

Most of the breakdown of food is catalyzed by soluble enzymes and occurs within the lumen of the stomach or small intestine. The **pancreas,** not the stomach, is the major organ that synthesizes and secretes the large amounts of enzymes needed for digestion. Secreted enzymes amount to at least 30 g of protein per day in a healthy adult. The **pancreatic enzymes** together with bile are poured into the lumen of the second (descending) part of the duodenum, so that the bulk of the **intraluminal digestion** occurs distal to this site in the small intestine. However, pancreatic enzymes cannot completely digest all nutrients to forms that can be absorbed. Even after exhaustive contact with pancreatic enzymes, a substantial portion of carbohydrates and amino acids are present as dimers and oligomers that depend for final digestion on enzymes present on the luminal surface or within the chief epithelial cells that line the lumen of the small intestine **(enterocytes).**

The luminal plasma membrane of enterocytes is enlarged by a regular array of projections, termed microvilli, which give it the appearance of a brush and have led to the name **brush border** for the luminal pole of enterocytes. This membrane contains many **di- and oligosaccharidases, amino- and dipeptidases,** as well as **esterases** (Table 26.2). Many of these enzymes protrude up to 100 Å into the intestinal lumen, attached to the plasma membrane by an anchoring polypeptide that itself has no role in the hydrolytic activity. The substrates for these enzymes are the oligomers and dimers that result from pancreatic digestion. The surface enzymes are glycoproteins that are relatively stable against digestion by pancreatic proteases or the effects of detergents.

A third site of digestion is the cytoplasm of enterocytes. **Intracellular digestion** is of some importance for the hydrolysis of di- and tripeptides, which can be absorbed across the luminal plasma membrane.

Digestive Enzymes Are Secreted as Proenzymes

Salivary glands, gastric mucosa, and pancreas contain specialized cells that synthesize and store digestive enzymes until the enzymes are needed during

TABLE 26.2 Digestive Enzymes of the Small Intestinal Surface

Enzyme (Common Name)	*Substrate*
Maltase	Maltose
Sucrase/isomaltase	Sucrose/α-limit dextrin
Glucoamylase	Amylose
Trehalase	Trehalose
β-Glucosidase	Glucosylceramide
Lactase	Lactose
Endopeptidase 24.11	Protein (cleavage at internal hydrophobic amino acids)
Aminopeptidase A	Oligopeptide with acidic NH_2 terminus
Aminopeptidase N	Oligopeptide with neutral NH_2 terminus
Dipeptidyl aminopeptidase IV	Oligopeptide with X-Pro or X-Ala at NH_2 terminus
Leucine aminopeptidase	Peptides with neutral amino acid at NH_2 terminus
γ-Glutamyltransferase	Glutathione + amino acid
Enteropeptidase (enterokinase)	Trypsinogen
Alkaline phosphatase	Organic phosphates

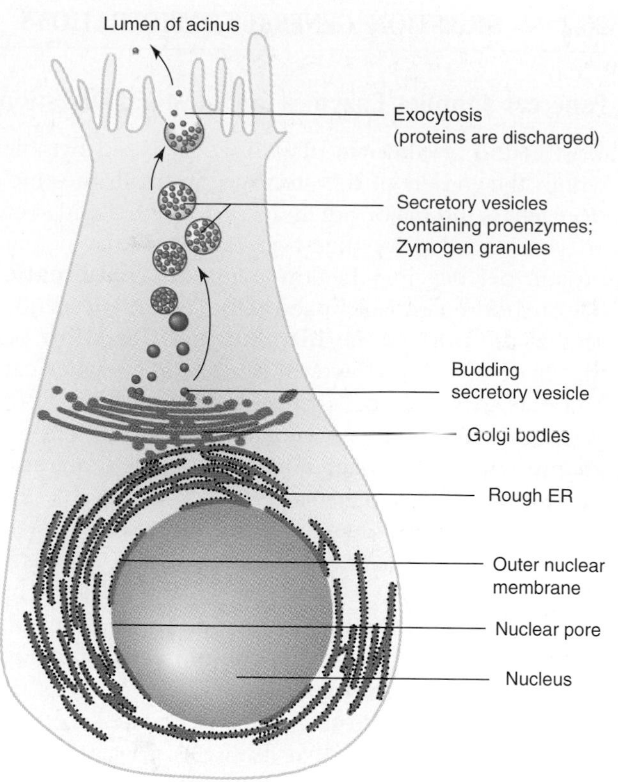

FIGURE 26.2
Exocrine secretion of digestive enzymes.
Redrawn with permission from Jamieson, J. D. Membrane and secretion. In: G. Weissmann and R. Claiborne (Eds.), Cell Membranes: Biochemistry, Cell Biology and Pathology. *New York: HP Publishing Co., 1975. Figure by B. Tagawa.*

a meal. The enzymes are then released into the lumen of the gastrointestinal tract (Figure 26.2). This secretion is termed **exocrine** because of its direction toward the lumen. Proteins destined for secretion are synthesized on the polysomes of the rough endoplasmic reticulum (see p. 739 for synthesis and glycosylation of membrane and secreted proteins) and transported via the Golgi complex to storage vesicles in the apical cytoplasm. The storage vesicles **(zymogen granules)** have a diameter of about 1 μm. Most digestive enzymes are produced and stored as inactive **proenzymes (zymogens)** (see p. 101). The zymogen granules are bounded by a typical cellular membrane. When an appropriate stimulus for secretion is received by the cell, the granules move closer to the luminal plasma membrane, where their membranes fuse with the plasma membrane and release the contents into the lumen **(exocytosis).** Activation of proenzymes occurs only after they are released from the cells.

Regulation of Secretion Occurs Through Secretagogues

The processes involved in the secretion of enzymes and electrolytes are regulated and coordinated. Elaboration of electrolytes and fluids simultaneously with that of enzymes is required to flush any discharged digestive enzymes out of the gland into the gastrointestinal lumen. The physiological regulation of secretion occurs through **secretagogues** that interact with receptors on the surface of the **exocrine cells** (Table 26.3). Neurotransmitters, hormones, pharmacological agents, and certain bacterial toxins can be secretagogues. Different exocrine cells, for example, in different glands, usually possess different sets of receptors. Binding of the secretagogues to receptors sets off a chain of signaling events that ends with fusion of zymogen granules with the plasma membrane. Two major signaling pathways have been identified (Figure 26.3): (1) activation of phosphatidylinositol-specific **phospholipase C** with liberation of **inositol 1,4,5-triphosphate** and **diacylglycerol** (see p. 862); in turn, triggering Ca^{2+} release into the cytosol and activation of protein kinase C, respec-

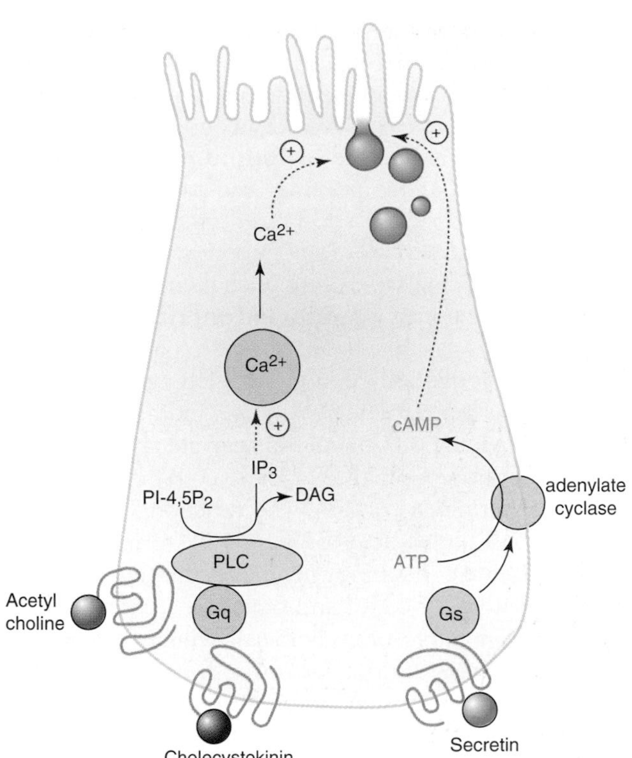

FIGURE 26.3
Cellular regulation of exocrine secretion in the pancreas.
Abbreviations: PI-4,5P$_2$, phosphatidylinositol-4,5-bisphosphate; DG, diacylglycerol; IP$_3$, inositol-1,4,5-triphosphate; PLC, phospolipase C.
Adapted from Gardner, J. D. Annu. Rev. Physiol. *41:63, 1979. Copyright © 1979 by Annual Reviews, Inc.*

tively; and (2) activation of **adenylate** or **guanylate cyclase,** resulting in elevated cAMP or cGMP levels, respectively (see p. 859). Secretion can be stimulated through either pathway.

Acetylcholine (Figure 26.4) elicits salivary, gastric, and pancreatic enzyme and electrolyte secretion. It is the major neurotransmitter for stimulating secretion, with input from the central nervous system in salivary and gastric glands, or via local reflexes in gastric glands and the pancreas. The acetylcholine receptor of exocrine cells is of the muscarinic type; that is, it can be blocked by atropine (Figure 26.5). Most people have experienced the effect of atropine because it is used by dentists to "dry up" the mouth for dental work.

Another class of secretagogues are the **biogenic amines,** consisting of **histamine** and **5-hydroxytryptamine. Histamine** (Figure 26.6) is a potent stimulator of HCl secretion. It interacts with a gastric-specific histamine receptor, also referred to as the H$_2$ receptor, on the contraluminal plasma membrane of parietal cells. Histamine is normally secreted by specialized regulatory cells in the stomach wall (**enterochromaffin-like cells,** ECC). Histamine analogs that are antagonists at the H$_2$ receptor are used medically to decrease HCl output during treatment for peptic ulcers. **5-Hydroxytryptamine (serotonin)** is pres-

$CH_3-C(=O)-O-CH_2-CH_2-N^{+}-(CH_3)_3$

FIGURE 26.4
Acetylcholine.

(a) (b)

FIGURE 26.5
(*a*) L(+)-Muscarine and (*b*) atropine.

FIGURE 26.6
Histamine.

TABLE 26.3 Physiological Secretagogues

Organ	*Secretion*	*Secretagogue*
Salivary gland	NaCl, amylase	Acetylcholine, (catecholamines?)
Stomach	HCl, pepsinogen	Acetylcholine, histamine, gastrin
Pancreas—acini	NaCl, digestive enzymes	Acetylcholine, cholecystokinin (secretin)
Pancreas—duct	$NaHCO_3$, NaCl	Secretin
Small intestine	NaCl	Acetylcholine, serotonin, vasoactive intestinal peptide (VIP), guanylin

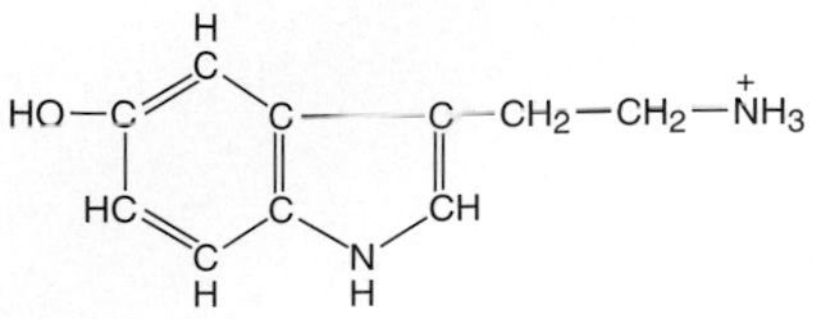

FIGURE 26.7
5-OH-Tryptamine (serotonin).

ent in relatively high amounts in the gastrointestinal tract (Figure 26.7). It stimulates secretion of NaCl by the small intestinal mucosa.

A third class of secretagogues consists of peptide-neurotransmitters and -hormones (Table 26.4). The intestinal nerve cells are rich in peptide-neurotransmitters that stimulate NaCl secretion. **Vasoactive intestinal peptide (VIP)** is a particularly potent one in this respect in the intestines and pancreas. Furthermore, the gastrointestinal tract contains many specialized epithelial cells that produce biologically active amines and peptides. The peptides are localized in granules, usually close to the contraluminal pole of these cells, and are released into the blood. Hence these cells are classified as **epithelial endocrine cells.** Of particular importance are the peptides gastrin, cholecystokinin (pancreozymin), and secretin. In contrast, a recently identified peptide—namely, **guanylin**—is released into the lumen and stimulates NaCl secretion by binding to a brush border receptor that activates guanylate cyclase and thus elevates cGMP levels.

Gastrin occurs as either a peptide of 34 amino acids (G-34) or one of 17 residues (G-17) from the COOH terminus of G-34. The functional portion of gastrin resides mainly in the last five amino acids of the COOH terminus. Thus pentagastrin, an artificial pentapeptide containing only the last five amino acids, can be used specifically to stimulate gastric HCl and pepsin secretion. Gastrin as well as cholecystokinin have an interesting chemical feature, a **sulfated tyrosine,** which considerably enhances the potency of both hormones.

Cholecystokinin and **pancreozymin** denote the same peptide. The different names allude to the different functions elicited by the peptide and had been coined before purification. The peptide stimulates gallbladder contraction (cholecystokinin) as well as secretion of pancreatic enzymes (pancreozymin). It is secreted by epithelial endocrine cells of the small intestine, particularly in the duodenum, and this secretion is stimulated by luminal amino acids and peptides, usually derived from gastric proteolysis, by fatty acids, and by an acid pH. Cholecystokinin and gastrin are thought to be related in an evolutionary sense, as both share an identical amino acid sequence at the COOH terminus.

TABLE 26.4 Structure of Human Intestinal Peptide Hormones

Vasoactive intestinal peptide (VIP)
His-Ser-Asp-Ala-Val-Phe-Thr-Asp-Asn-Tyr-Thr-Arg-Leu-Arg-Lys-Gln-Met-Ala-Val-Lys
Asn-Leu-Ile-Ser-Asn-Leu-Tyr-Lys
Secretin
His-Ser-Asp-Gly-Thr-Phe-Thr-Ser-Glu-Leu-Ser-Arg-Leu-Arg-Glu-Gly-Ala-Arg-Leu-Gln
[c]NH_2-Val-Leu-Gly-Gln-Leu-Leu-Arg
Guanylin
Pro-Gly-Thr-Cys-Glu-Ile-Cys-Ala-Tyr-Ala-Ala-Cys-Thr-Gly-Cys
Gastrin G-34-II[a] G-17-II
[b]Glp-Leu-Gly-Pro-Gln-Gly-Pro-Pro-His-Leu-Val-Ala-Asp-Pro-Ser-Lys-Lys-Gln
[c]NH_2-Phe-Asp-Met-Trp-Gly-Tyr(SO_3H)-Ala-$(Glu)_5$-Leu-Trp-Pro-Gly
Cholecystokinin
Lys-Ala-Pro-Ser-Gly-Arg-Met-Ser-Ile-Val-Lys-Asn-Leu-Gln-Asn-Leu-Asp-Pro
[c]NH_2-Phe-Asp-Met-Trp-Gly-Met-Tyr(SO_3H)-Asp-Arg-Asp-Ser-Ile-Arg-His-Ser

Source: Yanaihara, C. In: B. B. Rauner, G. M. Makhlouf, and S. G. Schultz (Eds.), *Handbook of Physiology. Section 6: Alimentary Canal. Vol. II: Neural and Endocrine Biology*. Bethesda, MD: American Physiological Society, 1989, pp. 45–62.

[a] Gastrin I is not sulfated.

[b] Glp = pyrrolidino carboxylic acid, derived from Glu through internal amide formation.

[c] NH_2 = amide of carboxy-terminal amino acid.

Secretin is a polypeptide of 27 amino acids. This peptide is secreted by yet other endocrine cells of the small intestine. Its secretion is stimulated particularly by luminal pH less than 5. The major biological activity of secretin is stimulation of secretion of pancreatic juice rich in $NaHCO_3$. Pancreatic $NaHCO_3$ is essential for neutralization of gastric HCl in the duodenum. Secretin also enhances pancreatic enzyme release, acting synergistically with cholecystokinin.

26.3 EPITHELIAL TRANSPORT

Solute Transport May Be Transcellular or Paracellular

Solute movement across an epithelial cell layer is determined by the properties of epithelial cells, particularly their plasma membranes, and by the intercellular tight junctional complexes (Figure 26.8). The **tight junctions** extend in a belt-like manner around the perimeter of each epithelial cell and connect neighboring cells. Therefore the tight junctions constitute part of the barrier between the two extracellular spaces on either side of the epithelium, that is, the lumen of the gastrointestinal tract and the intercellular (interstitial) space on the other (blood or serosal) side. The tight junction marks the boundary between the luminal and contraluminal region of the plasma membrane of epithelial cells.

Two potentially parallel pathways for **solute transport** across epithelial cell layers can be distinguished: through the cells **(transcellular)** and through the tight junctions between cells **(paracellular)** (Figure 26.8). The transcellular route in turn consists mainly of two barriers in series, formed by the luminal and contraluminal plasma membranes. Because of this combination of different barriers in parallel (cellular and paracellular pathways) and in series (luminal and contraluminal plasma membranes), biochemical and biophysical information on all three barriers as well as their mutual influence is required for understanding the overall transport properties of the epithelium.

A major function of gastrointestinal epithelial cells is **active transport** of nutrients, electrolytes, and vitamins. The cellular basis for this vectorial solute movement lies in the different properties of the luminal and contraluminal regions of the plasma membrane. The small intestinal cells provide a prominent example of the differentiation and specialization of the two types of membrane. The luminal and contraluminal plasma membranes differ in morphological appearance, enzymatic composition, chemical composition, and transport functions (Table 26.5). The luminal membrane is in contact with the nutrients in the chyme (the semifluid mass of partially digested food) and is specialized for terminal digestion of nutrients through its digestive enzymes and for nutrient absorption through transport systems that accomplish concentrative uptake. Transport systems are present for monosaccharides, amino acids, peptides, and electrolytes. In contrast, the contraluminal plasma membrane, which is in contact with the intercellular fluid, capillaries, and lymph, has properties similar to the

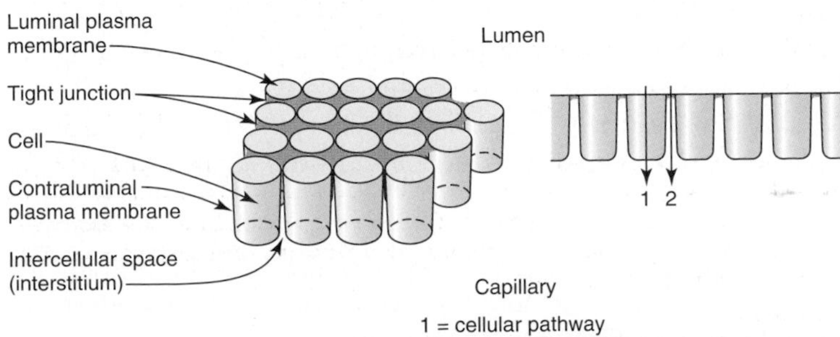

FIGURE 26.8
Pathways for transport across epithelia.

TABLE 26.5 Characteristic Differences Between Luminal and Contraluminal Plasma Membrane of Small Intestinal Epithelial Cells

Parameter	*Luminal*	*Contraluminal*
Morphological appearance	Microvilli in ordered arrangement (brush border)	Few microvilli
Enzymes	Di- and oligosaccharidases Aminopeptidase Dipeptidases γ-Glutamyltransferase Alkaline phosphatase Guanylate cyclase	Na^+,K^+–ATPase Adenylyl cyclase
Transport systems	Na^+–monosaccharide cotransport (SGLT1)	Facilitated monosaccharide transport (GLUT2)
	Facilitated fructose transport (GLUT5) Na^+–neutral amino acid cotransport Na^+–bile acid cotransport	Facilitated neutral amino acid transport

plasma membrane of most cells. It possesses receptors for hormonal or neuronal regulation of cellular functions, a Na^+,K^+–ATPase for removal of Na^+ from the cell, and transport systems for the entry of nutrients for consumption by the cell. In addition, the contraluminal plasma membrane contains the transport systems necessary for exit of the nutrients derived from the lumen so that the digested food can become available to all cells of the body. Some of the transport systems in the contraluminal plasma membrane may fulfill both the function of catalyzing exit when the intracellular nutrient concentration is high after a meal and that of mediating their entry when the blood levels are higher than those within the cell.

NaCl Absorption Has Both Active and Passive Components

Transport of Na^+ plays a crucial role not only for epithelial NaCl absorption or secretion, but also in the energization of nutrient uptake. The **Na^+,K^+–ATPase** provides the dominant mechanism for transduction of chemical energy in the form of ATP into osmotic energy of a concentration (chemical) or a combined concentration and electrical (electrochemical) ion gradient across the plasma membrane. In epithelial cells this enzyme is located exclusively in the contraluminal plasma membrane (Figure 26.9). The stoichiometry of the Na^+,K^+–ATPase reaction is 1 mol of ATP coupled to the outward pumping of 3 mol of Na^+ and the simultaneous inward pumping of 2 mol of K^+. The Na^+,K^+–ATPase maintains the high K^+ and low Na^+ concentrations in the cytosol and is directly or indirectly responsible for an electrical potential of about -60 mV of the cytoplasm relative to the extracellular solution. The direct contribution comes from the charge movement when $3Na^+$ ions are replaced by $2K^+$; the indirect contribution is by way of the K^+ gradient, which becomes the dominant force for establishing the potential by the movement of K^+ through K^+ channels.

Transepithelial NaCl movements are produced by the combined actions of the Na^+,K^+–ATPase and additional "passive" transport systems in the plasma membrane, which allow the entry of Na^+ or Cl^- into the cell. NaCl absorption results from Na^+ entry into the cell across the luminal plasma membrane and its extrusion by the Na^+,K^+–ATPase across the contraluminal membrane. Epithelial cells of the lower portion of the large intestine possess a luminal **Na^+ channel (epithelial Na^+ channel** or **ENaC)** that allows the uncoupled entry of Na^+ down its electrochemical gradient (Figure 26.10). This Na^+ flux is **electrogenic;** that is, it is associated with an electrical current, and it can be inhibited by

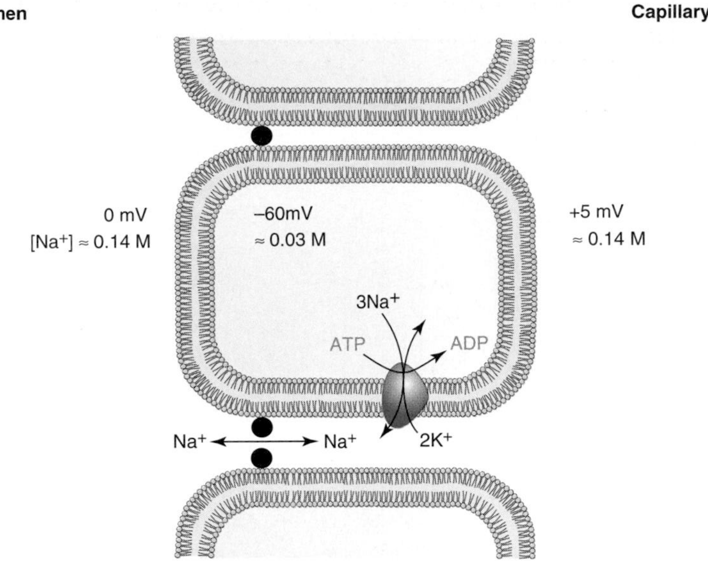

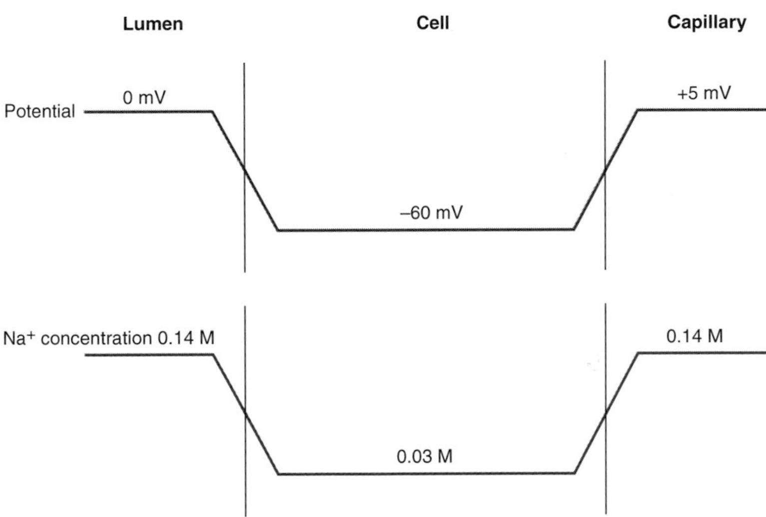

FIGURE 26.9
Na^+ concentrations and electrical potentials in enterocytes.

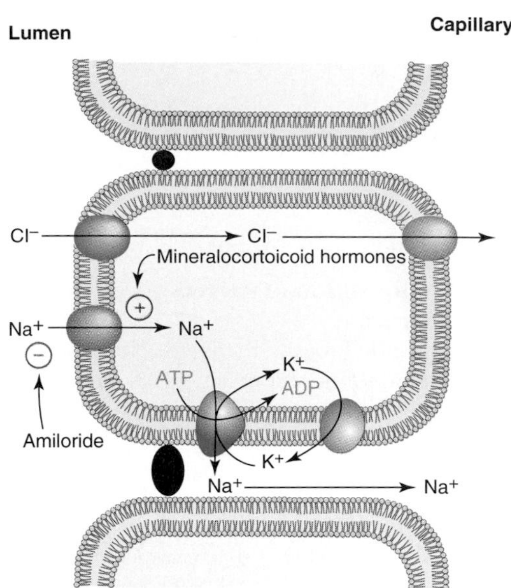

FIGURE 26.10
Model for electrogenic NaCl absorption in the lower intestine.

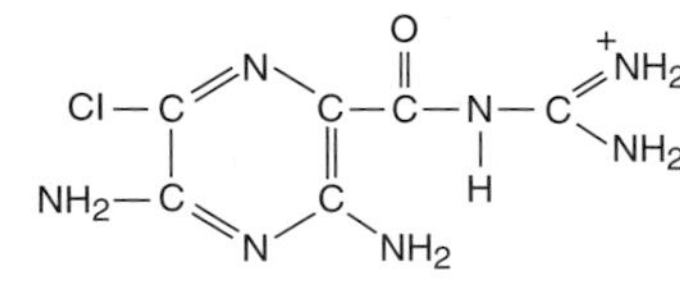

FIGURE 26.11
Amiloride.

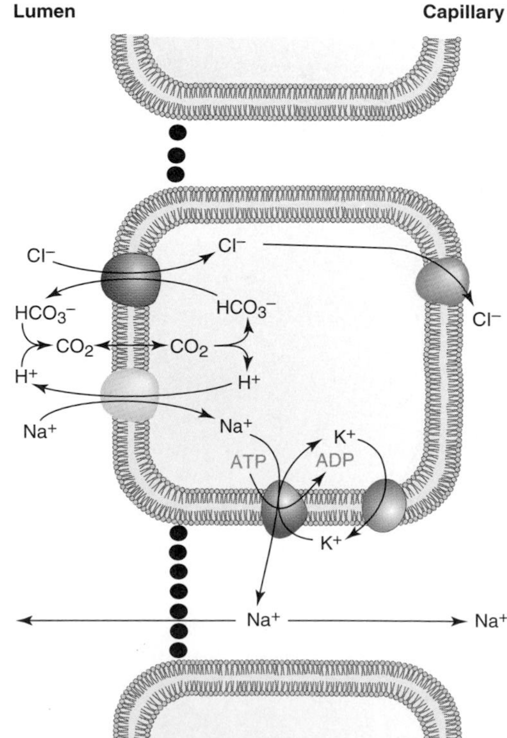

FIGURE 26.12
Model for electrically neutral NaCl absorption in the small intestine.

the diuretic drug amiloride at micromolar concentrations (Figure 26.11). The presence of this transport system, and hence NaCl absorption, is regulated by mineralocorticoid hormones of the adrenal cortex.

Epithelial cells of the small intestine possess a transport system in the brush border membrane, which catalyzes an electrically neutral **Na^+/H^+ exchange (Na/H exchanger or NHE)** (Figure 26.12). The exchange is not affected by low concentrations of amiloride and not regulated by mineralocorticoids. The Na^+ absorption secondarily drives Cl^- absorption through a specific **Cl^-/HCO_3^- exchanger (anion exchanger or AE)** in the luminal plasma membrane, as illustrated in Figure 26.12. The necessity for two types of NaCl absorption may arise from the different functions of upper and lower intestine, which require different regulation. The upper intestine reabsorbs the bulk of NaCl from the diet and from secretions of the exocrine glands after each meal, while the lower intestine participates in the fine regulation of NaCl retention, depending on the overall electrolyte balance of the body.

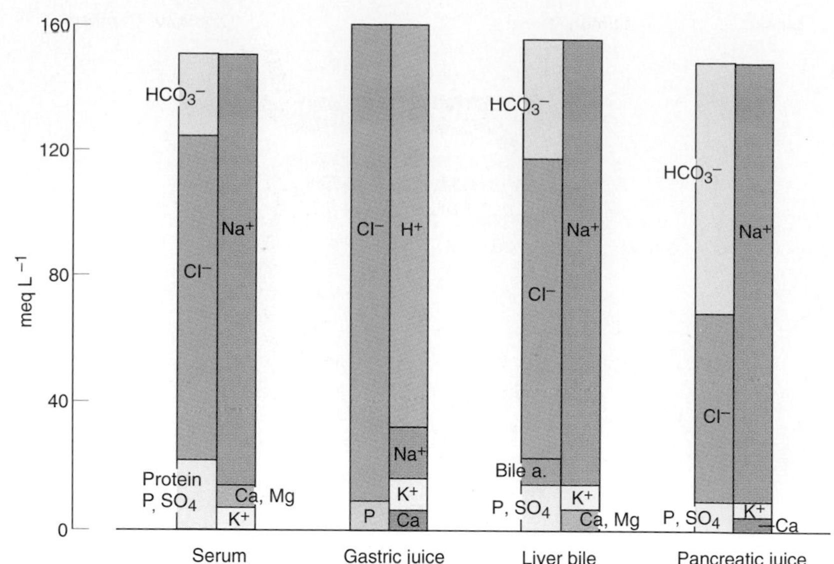

FIGURE 26.13
Ionic composition of secretions of the gastrointestinal tract.
Serum included for comparisons. Note the high H^+ concentration in gastric juice (pH = 1) and the high HCO_3^- concentration in pancreatic juice. P, organic and inorganic phosphate; SO_4, inorganic and organic sulfate; Ca, calcium; Mg, magnesium; bile a., bile acids.
Adapted from Biological Handbooks. Blood and Other Body Fluids. *Federation of American Societies for Experimental Biology, 1961.*

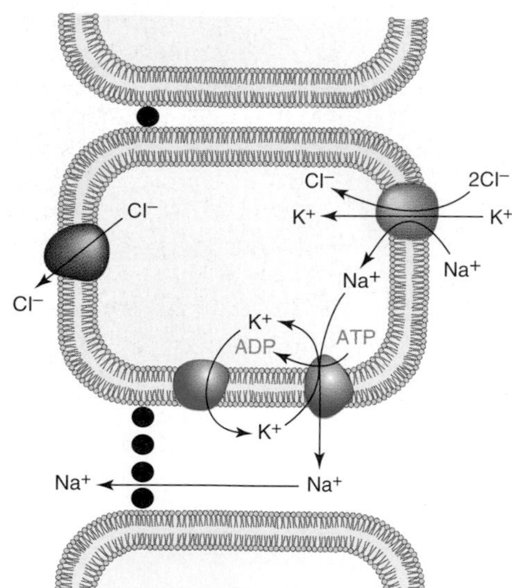

FIGURE 26.14
Model for epithelial NaCl secretion.

NaCl Secretion Depends on Contraluminal Na^+,K^+–ATPase

The epithelial cells of most regions of the gastrointestinal tract have the potential for electrolyte and fluid secretions. The major secreted ions are Na^+ and Cl^-. Water follows passively because of the osmotic forces exerted by any secreted solute. Thus NaCl secretion secondarily results in fluid secretion. The fluid may be either hypertonic or isotonic, depending on the contact time of the secreted fluid with the epithelium and the tissue permeability to water. The longer the contact and the greater the water permeability, the closer the secreted fluid gets to osmotic equilibrium, that is, isotonicity. Ionic compositions of gastrointestinal secretions are presented in Figure 26.13.

The cellular mechanisms for NaCl secretion involve the Na^+,K^+–ATPase located in the contraluminal plasma membrane of epithelial cells (Figure 26.14). The enzyme is implicated because cardiac glycosides, inhibitors of this enzyme, abolish salt secretion. However, the involvement of Na^+,K^+–ATPase does not provide a straightforward explanation for a NaCl movement from the capillary side to the lumen because the enzyme extrudes Na^+ from the cell toward the capillary side. Thus the active step of Na^+ transport across one of the plasma membranes has a direction opposite to that of overall transepithelial NaCl movements. The apparent paradox is resolved by an electrical coupling of Cl^- secretion across the luminal plasma membrane and Na^+ movements via the paracellular route, illustrated in Figure 26.14. The Cl^- secretion depends on coupled uptake of 2 Cl^- ions with Na^+ and K^+ via a specific cotransporter in the contraluminal plasma membrane and specific luminal **Cl^- channels.** The **$Na^+,K^+,2\ Cl^-$-cotransporter,** which can be identified by specific inhibitors such as the common diuretic **furosemide** (Figure 26.15), utilizes the energy of the Na^+ gradient to accumulate Cl^- within the cytoplasmic compartment above its electrochemical equilibrium concentration. Subsequent opening of luminal Cl^- channels allows efflux of Cl^- together with a negative charge (see Clin. Corr. 26.1 and 26.2).

In the pancreas a fluid rich in Na^+ and Cl^- is secreted by acinar cells. This fluid provides the vehicle for the movement of digestive enzymes from the acini, where they are released, to the lumen of the duodenum. The fluid is modified in the ducts by the additional secretion of $NaHCO_3$ (Figure 26.16). The HCO_3^- concentration in the final pancreatic juice can reach concentrations of up to 120 mM.

The permeability of the tight junction to H_2O, Na^+, or other ions modifies

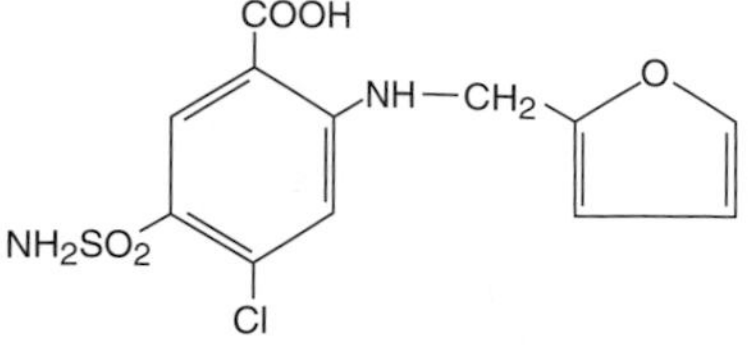

FIGURE 26.15
Furosemide.

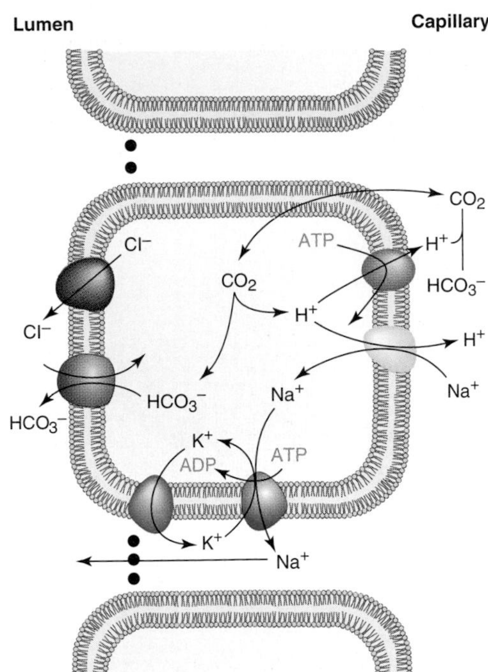

FIGURE 26.16
Model for epithelial $NaHCO_3$ secretion.
Note that two different mechanisms for H^+ secretion exist in the contraluminal plasma membrane: (1) Na^+/H^+ exchange and (2) H^+–ATPase.

active transepithelial solute movements. For example, a high permeability is necessary to allow Na^+ to equilibrate between extracellular solutions of the intercellular and luminal compartments during NaCl or $NaHCO_3$ secretion. Different regions of the gastrointestinal tract differ not only with respect to the transport systems that determine the passive entry (see above for amiloride-sensitive Na^+ channel and Na^+/H^+ exchange), but also with respect to the permeability characteristics of the tight junction. The distal portion (colon) is much tighter so as to prevent leakage of Na^+ from blood to lumen, in accordance with its function of scavenging of NaCl from the lumen.

Concentration Gradients or Electrical Potentials Drive Transport of Nutrients

Many solutes are absorbed across the intestinal epithelium against a concentration gradient. Energy for this "active" transport is directly derived from the Na^+ concentration gradient or the electrical potential across the luminal plasma membrane, rather than from the chemical energy of a covalent bond change, such as ATP hydrolysis. Glucose transport provides an example of uphill solute transport that is driven directly by the electrochemical Na^+ gradient and only indirectly by ATP (Figure 26.17).

Glucose is absorbed from the intestinal lumen into the blood against a concentration gradient. This vectorial transport is the combined result of several separate membrane events (Figure 26.18): (1) ATP-dependent Na^+ transport out of the cell at the contraluminal pole that establishes an electrochemical Na^+ gradient across the plasma membrane; (2) K^+ channels that convert a K^+ gradient into a membrane potential; (3) asymmetric insertion of two different transport systems for glucose into the luminal and contraluminal plasma membranes; and (4) coupling of Na^+ and glucose transport across the luminal membrane.

The luminal plasma membrane contains a transport system that facilitates a tightly coupled movement of Na^+ and D-glucose or structurally similar sugars

CLINICAL CORRELATION 26.1

Cystic Fibrosis

Cystic fibrosis is an autosomal recessive inherited disease due to a mutation in the cystic fibrosis transmembrane regulatory (CFTR) protein. This protein contains 1480 amino acids organized into two membrane-spanning portions, which contain six transmembrane regions each, two ATP-binding domains, and a regulatory domain that undergoes phosphorylation by cAMP-dependent protein kinase. Some 400 mutations have been discovered since the gene was cloned in 1989.

The normal form of this protein is a Cl^- channel that is found in the luminal plasma membrane of epithelial cells in many tissues. The channel is normally closed but opens when phosphorylated by protein kinase A, thus providing regulated Cl^- and fluid secretion. The most common and severe mutation lacks one amino acid (ΔF508 CFTR), which prevents the protein from properly maturing and reaching the plasma membrane. People who inherit this mutant CFTR from both parents lack Cl^- and fluid secretion in tissues that depend on CFTR for this function. Failure to secrete fluid, in turn, can lead to gross organ impairment due to partial or total blockage of passageways, for example, the ducts in the pancreas, the lumen of the intestine, or airways. (See Clin. Corr. 26.2 for activation of the CFTR Cl^- channel.)

CLINICAL CORRELATION 26.2

Bacterial Toxigenic Diarrheas and Electrolyte Replacement Therapy

Voluminous, life-threatening intestinal electrolyte and fluid secretion (diarrhea) occurs in patients with cholera, an intestinal infection by *Vibrio cholerae*. Certain strains of *E. coli* also cause (traveler's!) diarrhea that can be serious in infants. The secretory state is a result of enterotoxins produced by the bacteria. The mechanisms of action of some of these enterotoxins are well understood at the biochemical level. Cholera toxin activates adenylyl cyclase by causing ADP-ribosylation of the $G_{\alpha s}$-protein, which stimulates the cyclase (see p. 859). Elevated cAMP levels in turn activate protein kinase A, which opens the luminal CFTR Cl^- channel and inhibits the Na^+/H^+ exchanger by protein phosphorylation. The net result is gross NaCl secretion. *Escherichia coli* produces a heat-stable toxin that binds to the receptor for the physiological peptide "guanylin," namely, the brush border guanylyl cyclase. When the receptor is occupied on the luminal side by either guanylin or the heat-stable *E. coli* toxin, the guanylyl cyclase domain of the protein on the cytosolic side is activated and cGMP levels rise. Elevated cGMP levels have the same effect on Cl^- secretion as elevated cAMP levels, except that a cGMP-activated protein kinase is involved in protein phosphorylation.

Modern, oral treatment of cholera takes advantage of the presence of Na^+–glucose cotransport in the intestine, which is not regulated by cAMP and remains fully active in this disease. In this case, the presence of glucose allows uptake of Na^+ to replenish body NaCl. Composition of solution for oral treatment of cholera patients is glucose 110 mM, Na^+ 99 mM, Cl^- 74 mM, HCO_3^- 29 mM, and K^+ 4 mM. The major advantages of this form of therapy are its low cost and ease of administration when compared with intravenous fluid therapy.

Carpenter, C. C. J. In: M. Field, J. S. Fordtran, and S. G. Schultz (Eds.), *Secretory Diarrhea*. Bethesda, MD: American Physiological Society, 1980, pp. 67–83.

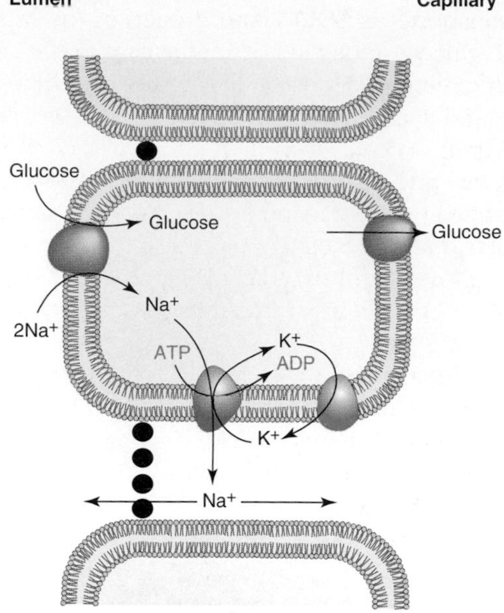

Glucose concentration profile normal to epithelial plane

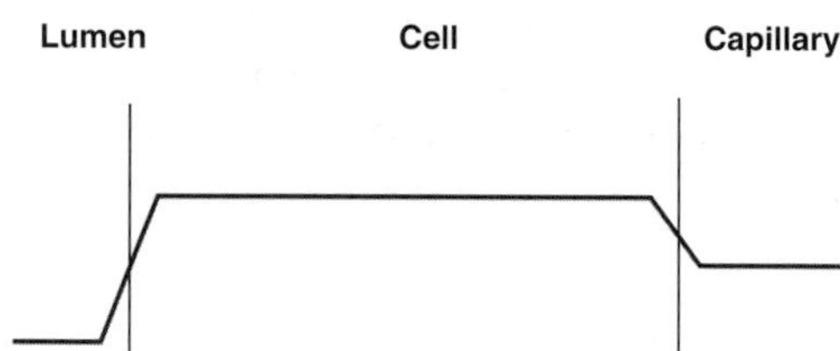

FIGURE 26.17
Model for epithelial glucose absorption.

2X	$3Na^+_{cell} + 2K^+_{interstitium} + ATP_{cell} \xrightarrow{Na^+,\,K^+\text{–ATPase}} 3Na^+_{interstitium} + 2K^+_{cell} + ADP_{cell} + P_{cell}$
4X	$K^+_{cell} \xrightleftharpoons{K^+\ \text{channel}} K^+_{interstitium}$
3X	$2Na^+_{lumen} + Glc_{lumen} \xrightleftharpoons{SGLT1} 2Na^+_{cell} + Glc_{cell}$
3X	$Glc_{cell} \xrightleftharpoons{GLUT2} Glc_{interstitium}$
6X	$Na^+_{interstitium} \rightleftharpoons Na^+_{lumen}$
Sum	$3Glc_{lumen} + 2ATP_{cell} \longrightarrow 3Glc_{interstitium} + 2ADP_{cell} + 2P_{cell}$

FIGURE 26.18
Transepithelial glucose transport as translocation reactions across the plasma membranes and the tight junction.
SGLT1 (sodium glucose transporter 1) and GLUT2 (glucose transporter 2) are specific intestinal gene products mediating Na^+–glucose cotransport and facilitated glucose transport, respectively. Numbers in the left column indicate the minimal turnover of individual reactions to balance the overall reaction.

(Sodium GLucose Transporter or **SGLT).** The most common intestinal sodium–glucose cotransporter is **SGLT1** and it couples the movement of 2 Na^+ ions with that of 1 glucose molecule. It mediates glucose and Na^+ transport equally well in both directions. However, because of the higher Na^+ concentration in the lumen and the negative potential within the cell, the observed direction is from lumen to cell, even if the cellular glucose concentration is higher than the luminal one. In other words, downhill Na^+ movement normally supports concentrative glucose transport. Concentration ratios of up to 20-fold between intracellular and extracellular glucose have been observed *in vitro* under conditions of blocked efflux of cellular glucose. In some situations Na^+ uptake via this route is actually more important than glucose uptake (see Clin. Corr. 26.2).

The contraluminal plasma membrane contains a member of the **GLUcose Transporter** (or **GLUT**) family, which facilitates glucose exit and entry. The intestine contains the **GLUT2** transporter, which accepts many monosaccharides, including glucose. The direction of net flux is determined by the sugar concentration gradient. The two glucose transport systems SGLT1 and GLUT2 in the luminal and contraluminal plasma membranes, respectively, share glucose as substrate, but otherwise differ considerably in terms of amino acid sequence, secondary protein structure, Na^+ as cosubstrate, specificity for other sugars, sensitivity to inhibitors, or biological regulation. Since both SGLT and GLUT are not inherently directional, "active" transepithelial glucose transport can be maintained under steady-state conditions only if the Na^+,K^+–ATPase continues to move Na^+ out of the cell. Thus the active glucose transport is indirectly dependent on a supply of ATP and an active Na^+,K^+–ATPase.

The advantage of an electrochemical Na^+ gradient serving as intermediate is that the Na^+,K^+–ATPase can energize the transport of many different nutrients. The only requirement is presence of a transport system catalyzing cotransport of the nutrient with Na^+.

Gastric Parietal Cells Secrete HCl

The parietal (oxyntic) cells of gastric glands are capable of secreting HCl into the gastric lumen. Luminal H^+ concentrations of up to 0.14 M (pH 0.8) have been observed (see Figure 26.13). As the plasma pH = 7.4, the parietal cell transports protons against a concentration gradient of $10^{6.6}$. The free energy required for **HCl secretion** under these conditions is minimally 9.1 kcal mol^{-1} of HCl (= 38 J mol^{-1} of HCl), as calculated from

$$\Delta G' = RT\,2.3 \log 10^{6.6} \qquad RT = 0.6 \text{ kcal mol}^{-1} \text{ at } 37°\text{C}$$

A K^+-activated ATPase **(K^+,H^+–ATPase)** is intimately involved in the mechanism of active HCl secretion. This enzyme is unique to the parietal cell and is found only in the luminal region of the plasma membrane. It couples the hydrolysis of ATP to an electrically neutral obligatory exchange of K^+ for H^+, secreting H^+ and taking K^+ into the cell. The stoichiometry appears to be 1 mol of transported H^+ and K^+ for each mole of ATP.

$$\text{ATP}_{\text{cell}} + \text{H}^+_{\text{cell}} + \text{K}^+_{\text{lumen}} \rightleftharpoons \text{ADP}_{\text{cell}} + \text{P}_{\text{i,cell}} + \text{H}^+_{\text{lumen}} + \text{K}^+_{\text{cell}}$$

As the K^+,H^+–ATPase generates a very acidic solution, protein reagents that are activated by acid can become specific inhibitors of this enzyme. Figure 26.19 shows an example of such a reagent used to treat peptic ulcers. In the steady state, HCl can be elaborated by K^+, H^+–ATPase only if the luminal membrane is permeable to K^+ and Cl^- and the contraluminal plasma membrane catalyzes an exchange of Cl^- for HCO_3^- (Figure 26.20). The exchange of Cl^- for HCO_3^- is essential to resupply the cell with Cl^- and to prevent accumulation of base within the cell. Thus, under steady-state conditions, secretion of HCl into the gastric lumen is coupled to movement of HCO_3^- into the plasma.

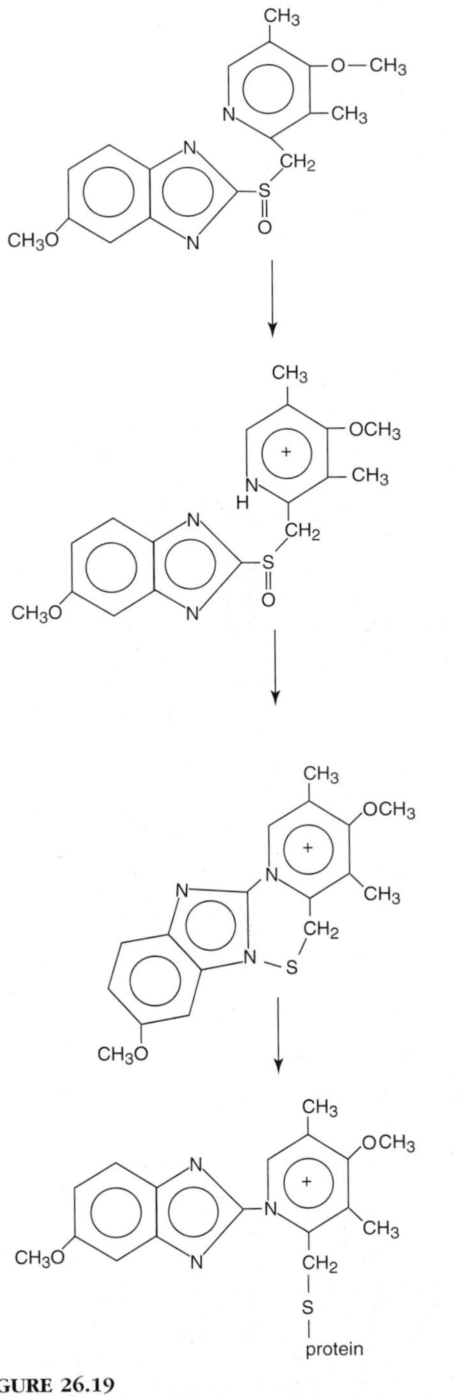

FIGURE 26.19
Omeprazole, an inhibitor of K^+,H^+–ATPase.
This drug accumulates in an acidic compartment ($pK_a \sim 4$) and is converted to a reactive sulfenamide, which reacts with cysteine SH groups.
From Sachs, G. The gastric H,K–ATPase. In. L. R. Johnson (Ed.), Physiology of the Gastrointestinal Tract. *New York: Raven Press, 1994, p. 1133.*

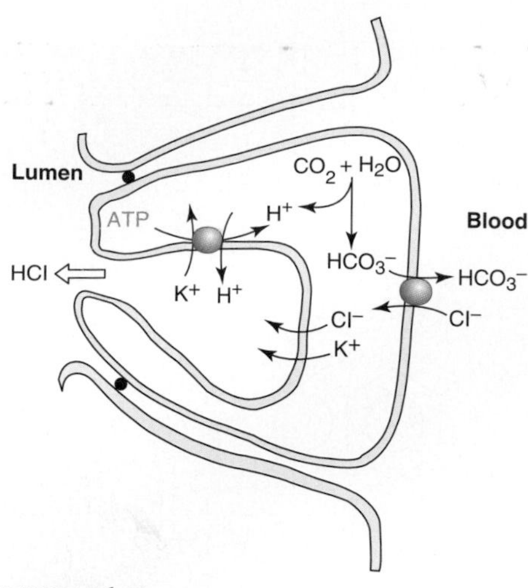

FIGURE 26.20
Model for secretion of hydrochloric acid.

26.4 ■ DIGESTION AND ABSORPTION OF PROTEINS

Mixture of Peptidases Assures Efficient Protein Digestion

The total daily protein load to be digested consists of about 70–100 g of dietary proteins and 35–200 g of endogenous proteins from digestive enzymes and sloughed-off cells. Digestion and absorption of proteins are very efficient processes in healthy humans, since only about 1–2 g of nitrogen are lost through feces each day, which is equivalent to 6–12 g of protein.

Except for a short period after birth, oligo- and polypeptides (proteins) are not absorbed intact in appreciable quantities by the intestine. Proteins are broken down by hydrolases with specificity for the peptide bond, that is, by peptidases. This class of enzymes is divided into **endopeptidases** (proteases), which attack internal bonds and liberate large peptide fragments, and **exopeptidases,** which cleave off one amino acid at a time from either the COOH **(carboxypeptidases)** or the NH_2 terminus **(aminopeptidases).** Endopeptidases are important for an initial breakdown of long polypeptides into smaller products, which can then be attacked more efficiently by exopeptidases. The final products are free amino acids and di- and tripeptides, which are absorbed by epithelial cells (Figure 26.21).

The process of protein digestion can be divided into a gastric, a pancreatic, and an intestinal phase, depending on the source of peptidases.

Pepsins Catalyze Gastric Digestion of Protein

Gastric juice is characterized by the presence of HCl and therefore a low pH less than 2 as well as the presence of proteases of the pepsin family. The acid serves to kill off microorganisms and also to **denature proteins.** Denaturation makes proteins more susceptible to hydrolysis by proteases. **Pepsins** are unique in that they are acid stable; in fact, they are active at acid but not at neutral pH. The catalytic mechanism that is effective for peptide hydrolysis at the acid pH depends on two carboxylic groups at the active site of the enzymes. Pepsin A, the major gastric protease, prefers peptide bonds formed by the amino group of aromatic acids (Phe, Tyr) (Table 26.6).

Active pepsin is generated from the proenzyme **pepsinogen** by the removal of 44 amino acids from the NH_2 terminus (pig enzyme). Cleavage between residues 44 and 45 of pepsinogen occurs as either an intramolecular reaction **(autoactivation)** below pH 5 or by active pepsin (autocatalysis). The liberated peptide from the NH_2 terminus remains bound to pepsin and acts as "pepsin

FIGURE 26.21
Digestion and absorption of proteins.

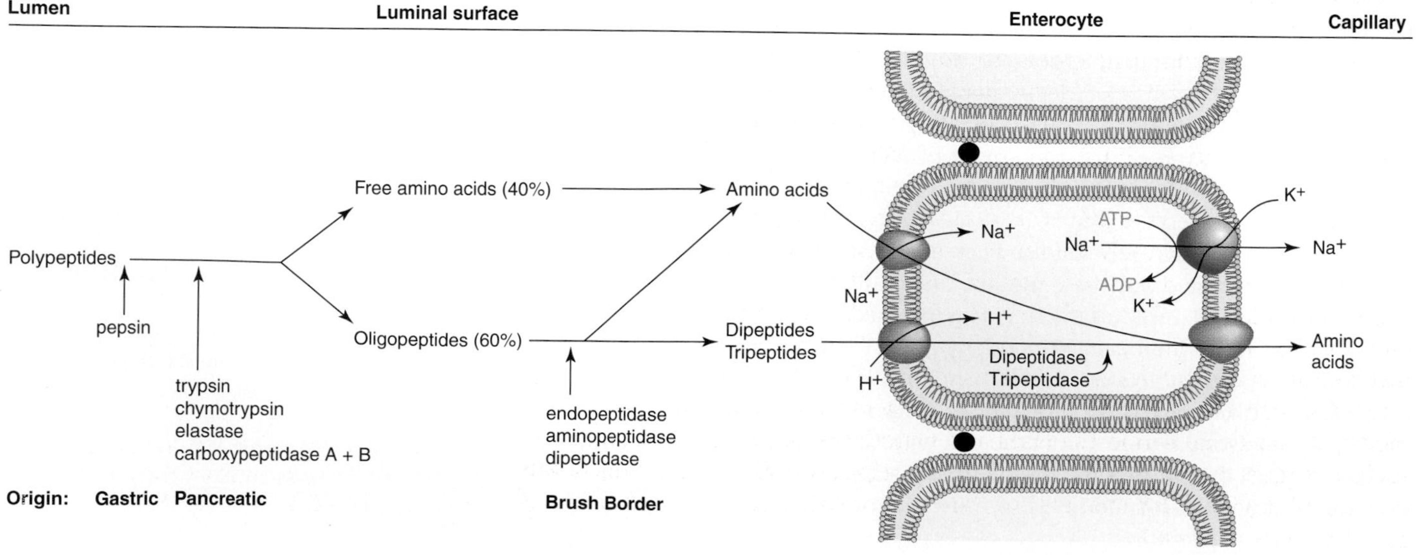

TABLE 26.6 Gastric and Pancreatic Peptidases

Enzyme	*Proenzyme*	*Activator*	*Cleavage Point*	*R*
CARBOXYL PROTEASES				
Pepsin A	Pepsinogen A	Autoactivation, pepsin	—CO—↓NHCH(R)CO—↓NHCH(R′)CO—	Tyr, Phe, Leu
SERINE PROTEASES				
Trypsin	Trypsinogen	Enteropeptidase, trypsin	—CO—NHCH(R)CO—↓NHCH(R′)CO—	Arg, Lys
Chymotrypsin	Chymotrypsinogen	Trypsin	—CO—NHCH(R)CO—↓NHCH(R′)CO—	Tyr, Trp, Phe, Met, Leu
Elastase	Proelastase	Trypsin	—CO—NHCH(R)CO—↓NHCH(R′)CO—	Ala, Gly, Ser
ZINC PEPTIDASES				
Carboxypeptidase A	Procarboxypeptidase A	Trypsin	—CO—↓NHCH(R)COO$^-$	Val, Leu, Ile, Ala
Carboxypeptidase B	Procarboxypeptidase B	Trypsin	—CO—↓NHCH(R)COO$^-$	Arg, Lys

inhibitor" above pH 2. This inhibition is released either by a drop of the pH below 2 or further degradation of the peptide by pepsin. Thus, once favorable conditions are reached, pepsinogen is converted to pepsin by autoactivation and subsequent autocatalysis at an exponential rate.

The major products of pepsin action are large peptide fragments and some free amino acids. The importance of gastric protein digestion does not lie so much in its contribution to the breakdown of ingested macromolecules, but rather in the generation of peptides and amino acids that act as stimulants for **cholecystokinin** release in the duodenum. The gastric peptides therefore are instrumental in the initiation of the pancreatic phase of protein digestion.

Pancreatic Zymogens Are Activated in Small Intestine

Pancreatic juice is rich in proenzymes of **endopeptidases** and **carboxypeptidases** (Figure 26.22), which are activated after they reach the lumen of the small intestine. **Enteropeptidase** (old name: enterokinase), a protease produced by duodenal epithelial cells, activates pancreatic **trypsinogen** to **trypsin** by scission of a hexapeptide from the NH_2 terminus. Trypsin in turn autocatalytically activates more trypsinogen to trypsin and also acts on the other proenzymes, thus liberating the endopeptidases chymotrypsin and elastase and the **carboxypeptidases A and B.** Since trypsin plays a pivotal role among pancreatic enzymes in the activation process, pancreatic juice normally contains a small-molecular-weight peptide that acts as a **trypsin inhibitor** and neutralizes any trypsin formed prematurely within the pancreatic cells or pancreatic ducts.

Trypsin, chymotrypsin, and elastase have different substrate specificity, as shown in Table 26.6. They are active only at neutral pH and depend on pancreatic $NaHCO_3$ for neutralization of gastric HCl. Their mechanism of catalysis involves an **essential serine residue** (see p. 97) and is thus similar to serine esterases, such as acetyl choline esterase. Reagents that interact with serine and modify it, inactivate serine esterases and peptidases. A prominent example of such a reagent is the highly toxic diisopropylphosphofluoridate, which was developed originally for chemical warfare (neurotoxic because of inhibition of acetyl choline esterase).

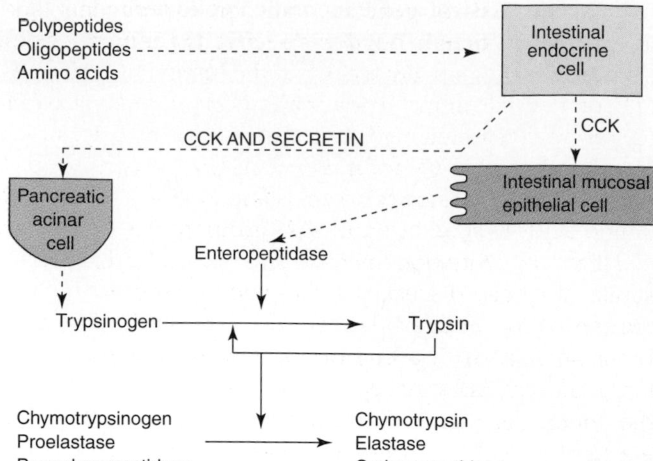

FIGURE 26.22
Secretion and activation of pancreatic enzymes.
Abbreviation: CCK, cholecystokinin.
Reproduced with permission from Freeman, H. J., and Kim, Y. S. Annu. Rev. Med. *29:102, 1978. Copyright © 1978 by Annual Reviews, Inc.*

Polypeptides generated from ingested proteins are degraded within the small intestinal lumen by **carboxypeptidases A** and **B.** The **pancreatic carboxypeptidases** are $\mathbf{Zn^{2+}}$ metalloenzymes and possess a different type of catalytic mechanism than the carboxyl or serine peptidases. The combined action of pancreatic peptidases results in the formation of free amino acids and small peptides of 2–8 residues. Peptides account for about 60% of the amino nitrogen at this point.

Intestinal Peptidases Digest Small Peptides

Since pancreatic juice does not contain appreciable aminopeptidase activity, final digestion of di- and oligopeptides depends on small intestinal enzymes. The luminal surface of epithelial cells is particularly rich in endopeptidase and aminopeptidase activity, but also contains dipeptidases (Table 26.2). The end products of the cell surface digestion are free amino acids and di- and tripeptides, which are absorbed via specific **amino acid** or **peptide transport systems.** Transported di- and tripeptides are generally hydrolyzed within the cytoplasmic compartment before they leave the cell. The cytoplasmic dipeptidases explain why practically only free amino acids are found in the portal blood after a meal. The virtual absence of peptides had previously been taken as evidence that luminal protein digestion had to proceed all the way to free amino acids before absorption could occur. However, it is now established that a large portion of dietary amino nitrogen is absorbed in the form of small peptides with subsequent intracellular hydrolysis. However, di- and tripeptides containing proline and hydroxyproline or unusual amino acids, such as β-alanine as carnosine (β-alanylhistidine) or anserine (β-alanyl 1-methylhistidine), are absorbed without intracellular hydrolysis because they are not good substrates for the intestinal cytoplasmic dipeptidases. β-Alanine is present in chicken meat.

Free Amino Acids and Dipeptides Are Absorbed by Carrier-Mediated Transport

The small intestine has a high capacity to absorb free amino acids and small peptides. Most L-amino acids can be transported across the epithelium against a concentration gradient, although the need for concentrative transport *in vivo* is not obvious, since luminal concentrations are usually higher than the plasma levels of 0.1–0.2 mM. Amino acid and peptide transport in the small intestine has all the characteristics of carrier-mediated transport, such as discrimination between D- and L-amino acids and energy and temperature dependence. In addition, genetic defects are known to occur in humans (see Clin. Corr. 26.3).

On the basis of genetics, transport experiments, and expression cloning, at least seven **brush border specific transport systems** for the uptake of L-amino acids or small peptides in the luminal membrane can be distinguished: (1) for neutral amino acids with short or polar side chains (Ser, Thr, Ala); (2) for neutral amino acids with aromatic or hydrophobic side chains (Phe, Tyr, Met, Val, Leu, Ile); (3) for imino acids (Pro, Hyp); (4) for β-amino acids (β-Ala, taurine); (5) for basic amino acids and cystine (Lys, Arg, Cys-Cys); (6) for acidic amino acids (Asp, Glu); and (7) for dipeptides (Pept1) (Gly-sarcosine).

The concentration mechanisms for neutral L-amino acids appear to be similar to those discussed for D-glucose (see Figure 26.17). **Na^+-dependent transport systems** have been identified in the luminal (brush border) membrane and **Na^+-independent transporters** in the contraluminal plasma membrane of small intestinal epithelial cells. Similarly, as for active glucose transport, the energy for concentrative amino acid transport is derived directly from the electrochemical Na^+ gradient and only indirectly from ATP. Amino acids are not chemically modified during membrane transport, although they may be metabolized within the cytoplasmic compartment. The brush border transport for the other amino acids is energized in more complicated ways. For example, the **acidic amino acid transporter** mediates cotransport of the amino acid with 2 Na^+ ions and counter transport with 1 K^+ ion.

Neutral dipeptides are cotransported across the brush border membrane with a proton and thus are energized through the proton electrochemical gradient across this membrane. However, because of the Na^+/H^+ exchange, both gradients tend to be similar and interdependent. The dipeptide transporter also accepts β-lactam antibiotics (aminopenicillins) and is important for absorption of orally administered antibiotics of this class.

Fetus and Neonate Can Absorb Intact Proteins

The fetal and neonatal small intestines can absorb intact proteins. The uptake occurs by endocytosis, that is, the internalization of small vesicles of plasma membrane, which contain ingested macromolecules. The process is also termed **pinocytosis** because of the small size of vesicles. The small intestinal pinocytosis of protein is thought to be important for the transfer of maternal antibodies (γ-globulins) to the offspring, particularly in rodents. The pinocytotic uptake of proteins is not important for nutrition, and its magnitude usually declines after birth. Persistence of low levels of this process beyond the neonatal period may, however, be responsible for absorption of sufficient quantities of macromolecules to induce antibody formation.

CLINICAL CORRELATION 26.3

Neutral Amino Aciduria (Hartnup Disease)

Transport functions, like enzymatic functions, are subject to modification by mutations. An example of a genetic lesion in epithelial amino acid transport is Hartnup disease, named after the family in which the disease entity resulting from the defect was first recognized. The disease is characterized by the inability of renal and intestinal epithelial cells to absorb neutral amino acids from the lumen. In the kidney, in which plasma amino acids reach the lumen of the proximal tubule through the ultrafiltrate, the inability to reabsorb amino acids manifests itself as excretion of amino acids in the urine (amino aciduria). The intestinal defect results in malabsorption of free amino acids from the diet. Therefore the clinical symptoms of patients with this disease are mainly those due to essential amino acid and nicotinamide deficiencies. The pellagra-like features (see p. 1121) are explained by a deficiency of tryptophan, which serves as precursor for nicotinamide. Investigations of patients with Hartnup disease revealed the existence of intestinal transport systems for di- or tripeptides, which are different from the ones for free amino acids. The genetic lesion does not affect transport of peptides, which remains as a pathway for absorption of protein digestion products.

Silk, D. B. A. Disorders of nitrogen absorption. In: J. T. Harries (Ed.), *Clinics in Gastroenterology: Familial Inherited Abnormalities,* Vol. 11: London: Saunders, 1982, pp. 47–73.

26.5 DIGESTION AND ABSORPTION OF CARBOHYDRATES

Di- and Polysaccharides Require Hydrolysis

Dietary carbohydrates provide a major portion of the daily caloric requirement. They consist of mono-, di-, and polysaccharides (Table 26.7). **Monosaccharides** need not be hydrolyzed for absorption. Disaccharides require the small intestinal surface enzymes for hydrolysis into monosaccharides, while polysaccharides depend on **pancreatic amylase** for degradation (Figure 26.23).

Starch, a major nutrient, is a plant polysaccharide with a molecular mass of more than 100 kDa. It consists of a mixture of linear chains of glucose molecules linked by α-1,4-glucosidic bonds **(amylose)** and of branched chains with branch points made up by α-1,6 linkages **(amylopectin).** The ratio of 1,4- to 1,6-glucosidic bonds is about 20 : 1. **Glycogen** is an animal polysaccharide similar in structure to amylopectin. The two compounds differ in terms of the number of branch points, which occur more frequently in glycogen.

TABLE 26.7 Dietary Carbohydrates

Carbohydrate	*Typical Source*		*Structure*
Amylopectin	Potatoes, rice, corn, bread	α-Glc(1 → 4)$_n$Glc with α-Glc(1 → 6) branches	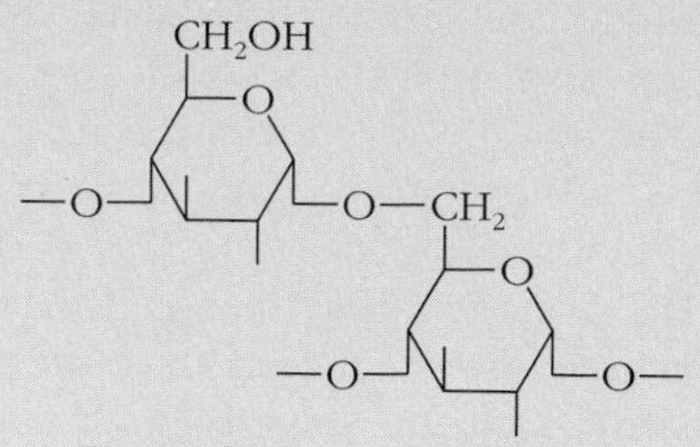
Amylose	Potatoes, rice, corn, bread	α-Glc(1 → 4)$_n$Glc	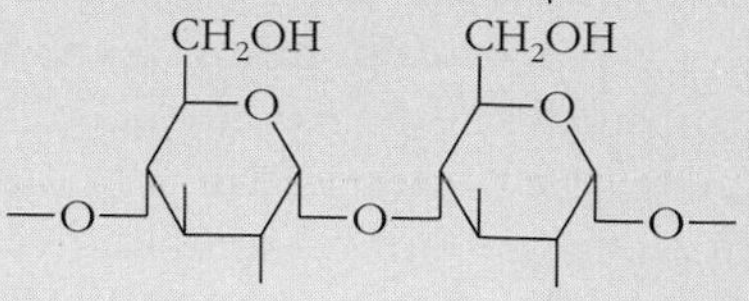
Sucrose	Table sugar, desserts	α-Glc(1 → 2)β-Fru	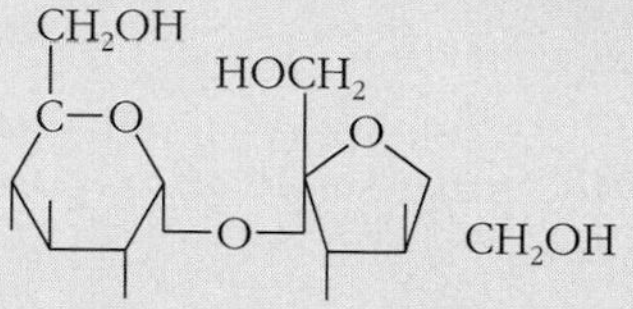
Trehalose	Young mushrooms	α-Glc(1 → 1)α-Glc	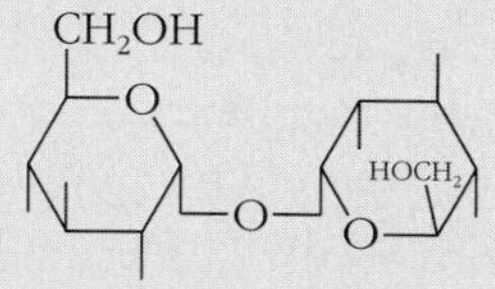
Lactose	Milk, milk products	β-Gal(1 → 4)Glc	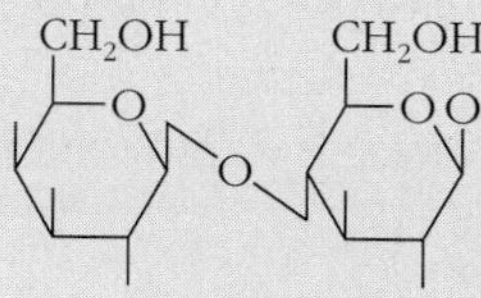
Fructose	Fruit, honey	Fru	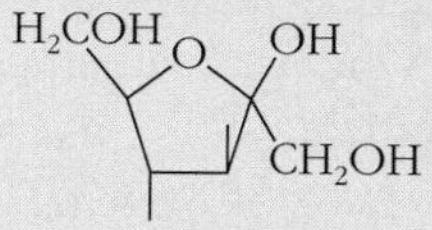
Glucose	Fruit, honey, grape	Glc	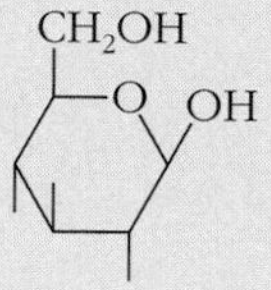
Raffinose	Leguminous seeds	α-Gal(1 → 6)α-Glc (1 → 2)β-Fru	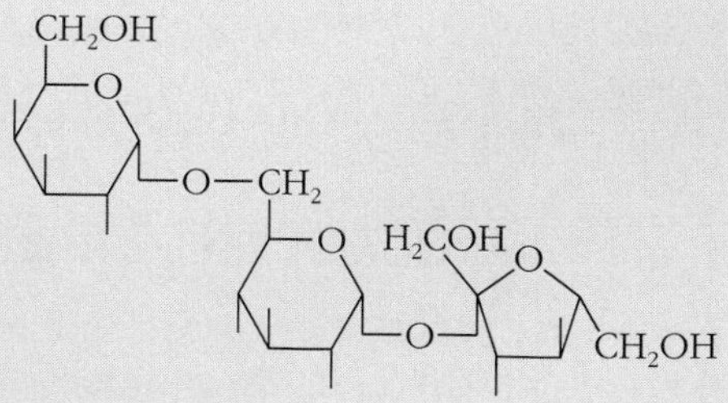

Hydrated starch and glycogen are attacked by the endosaccharidase **α-amylase** present in saliva and pancreatic juice (Figure 26.24). Hydration of the polysaccharides occurs during heating and is essential for efficient digestion. Amylase is specific for internal α-1,4-glucosidic bonds; α-1,6 bonds are not attacked, nor are α-1,4 bonds of glucose units that serve as branch points. The pancreatic isoenzyme is secreted in large excess relative to starch intake and

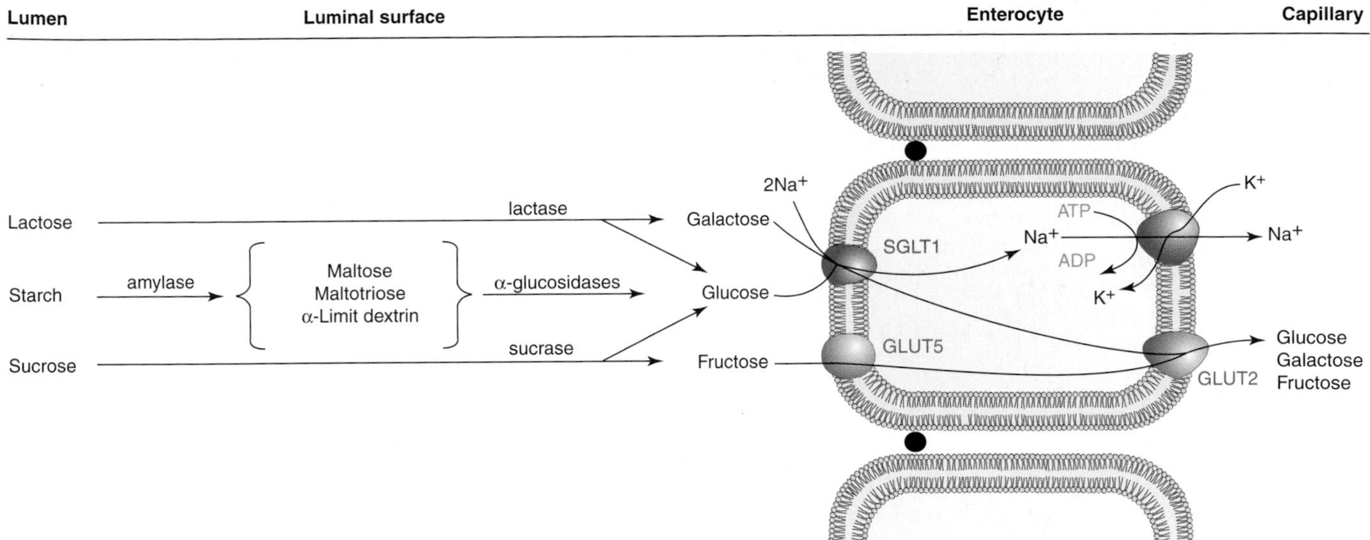

FIGURE 26.23
Digestion and absorption of carbohydrates.

is more important than the salivary enzyme from a digestive point of view. The products of the digestion by α-amylase are mainly the **disaccharide maltose,** the **trisaccharide maltotriose,** and so-called **α-limit dextrins** containing on average eight glucose units with one or more α-1,6-glucosidic bonds.

Final hydrolysis of di- and oligosaccharides to monosaccharides is carried out by surface enzymes of the small intestinal epithelial cells (Table 26.8). Most of the surface oligosaccharidases are exoenzymes that cleave off one monosaccharide at a time from the nonreducing end. The capacity of the **α-glucosidases** is normally much greater than that needed for completion of the digestion of starch. Similarly, there is usually excess capacity for sucrose (table sugar) hydrolysis relative to dietary intake. In contrast, **β-galactosidase (lactase)** can be rate-limiting in humans for hydrolysis and utilization of lactose, the major milk carbohydrate (see Clin. Corr. 26.4).

Di-, oligo-, and polysaccharides that are not hydrolyzed by α-amylase and/or intestinal surface enzymes cannot be absorbed; therefore they reach the lower tract of the intestine, which from the lower ileum on contains bacteria. Bacteria can utilize many of the remaining carbohydrates because they possess many more types of saccharidases than humans. Monosaccharides that are released as a result of **bacterial enzymes** are predominantly metabolized anaerobically by the bacteria themselves, resulting in degradation products such as short-chain fatty acids, lactate, hydrogen gas (H_2), methane (CH_4), and carbon

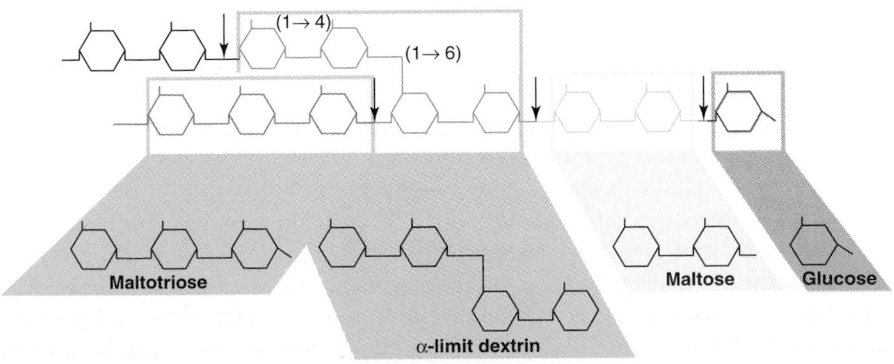

FIGURE 26.24
Digestion of amylopectin by salivary and pancreatic α-amylase.

CLINICAL CORRELATION 26.4

Disaccharidase Deficiency

Intestinal disaccharidase deficiencies are encountered relatively frequently in humans. Deficiency can be present in one enzyme or several enzymes for a variety of reasons (genetic defect, physiological decline with age, or the result of "injuries" to the mucosa). Of the disaccharidases, lactase is the most common enzyme with an absolute or relative deficiency, which is experienced as milk intolerance. The consequences of an inability to hydrolyze lactose in the upper small intestine are inability to absorb lactose and bacterial fermentation of ingested lactose in the lower small intestine. Bacterial fermentation results in the production of gas (distension of gut and flatulence) and osmotically active solutes that draw water into the intestinal lumen (diarrhea). The lactose in yogurt has already been partially hydrolyzed during the fermentation process of making yogurt. Thus individuals with lactase deficiency can often tolerate yogurt better than unfermented dairy products. The enzyme lactase is commercially available to pretreat milk so that the lactose is hydrolyzed.

Buller, H. A., and Grant, R. G. Lactose intolerance. *Annu. Rev. Med.* 41:141, 1990.

TABLE 26.8 Saccharidases of the Surface Membrane of the Small Intestine

Enzyme	*Specificity*	*Natural Substrate*	*Product*
exo-1,4-α-Glucosidase (glucoamylase)	α-(1 → 4)Glucose	Amylose	Glucose
Oligo-1,6-glucosidase (isomaltase)	α-(1 → 6)Glucose	Isomaltose, α-dextrin	Glucose
α-Glucosidase (maltase)	α-(1 → 4)Glucose	Maltose, maltotriose	Glucose
Sucrose-α-Glucosidase (sucrase)	α-Glucose	Sucrose	Glucose, fructose
α,α-Trehalase	α-(1 → 1)Glucose	Trehalose	Glucose
β-Glucosidase	β-Glucose	Glucosylceramide	Glucose, ceramide
β-Galactosidase (lactase)	β-Galactose	Lactose	Glucose, galactose

dioxide (CO_2). These compounds can cause fluid secretion, increased intestinal motility, and cramps, either because of increased intraluminal osmotic pressure, and distension of the gut, or a direct irritant effect of the bacterial degradation products on the intestinal mucosa.

The well-known problem of flatulence after ingestion of leguminous seeds (beans, peas, and soya) is caused by oligosaccharides, which cannot be hydrolyzed by human intestinal enzymes. The leguminous seeds contain modified sucrose to which one or more galactose moieties are linked. The glycosidic bonds of galactose are in the α configuration, which can only be split by bacterial enzymes. The simplest sugar of this family is **raffinose** (see Table 26.7).

Trehalose, a disaccharide that occurs in young mushrooms, requires a special disaccharidase, **trehalase.**

Monosaccharides Are Absorbed by Carrier-Mediated Transport

The major monosaccharides that result from digestion of di- and polysaccharide are D-glucose, D-galactose, and D-fructose. Absorption of these and other minor monosaccharides are carrier-mediated processes that exhibit such features as substrate specificity, stereospecificity, saturation kinetics, and inhibition by specific inhibitors.

At least two types of monosaccharide transporters catalyze monosaccharide uptake from the lumen into the cell: (1) a **Na^+-monosaccharide cotransporter,** existing probably as a tetramer of 75-kDa peptides, has high specificity for D-glucose and D-galactose and catalyzes "active" sugar absorption (SGLT); and (2) a **Na^+-independent, facilitated-diffusion** type of monosaccharide transport system with specificity for D-fructose (GLUT5). In addition, a **Na^+-independent monosaccharide transporter** (GLUT2), consisting of 57-kDa peptide(s), which accepts all three monosaccharides, is present in the contraluminal plasma membrane. GLUT2 is also located in the liver and kidney, and other members of the GLUT family of glucose transporters are found in all cells. All GLUT transporters mediate uncoupled D-glucose flux down its concentration gradient. GLUT2 of gut, liver, and kidney moves D-glucose out of the cell into the blood under physiological conditions, while in other tissues GLUT1 (in erythrocytes and brain) or the insulin-sensitive GLUT4 (in fat and muscle tissue) are mainly involved in D-glucose uptake. Properties of intestinal SGLT1 and of GLUT2 are compared in Table 26.9, and their role in transepithelial glucose absorption is illustrated in Figure 26.18.

TABLE 26.9 Characteristics of Glucose Transport Systems in the Plasma Membranes of Enterocytes

Characteristic	*Luminal*	*Contraluminal*
Designation	SGLT1	GLUT2
Subunit molecular weight (kDa)	75	57
Effect of Na^+	Cotransport with Na^+	None
Good substrates	D-Glc, D-Gal, α-methyl-D-Glc	D-Glc, D-Gal, D-Man, 2-deoxy-D-Glc
Inhibitor	Phlorizin (Figure 26.25)	Cytochalasin B (Figure 26.26)

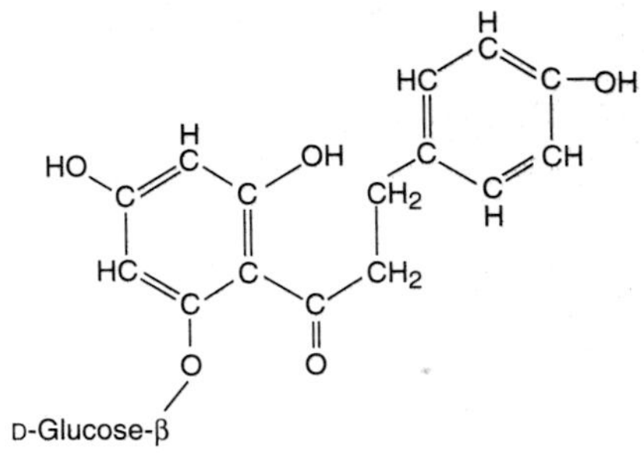

FIGURE 26.25
Phlorizin (phloretin-2′-β-glucoside).

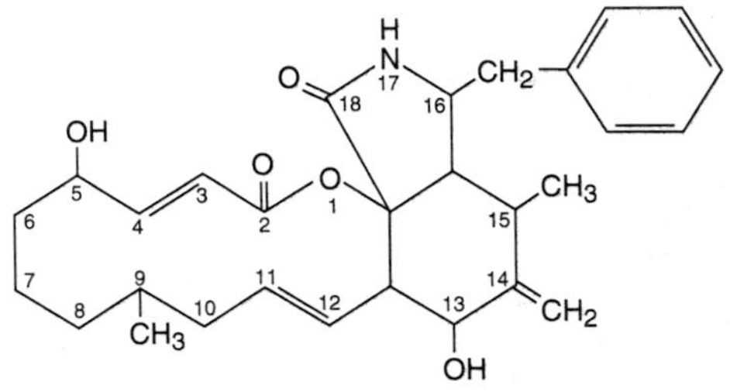

FIGURE 26.26
Cytochalasin B.

26.6 DIGESTION AND ABSORPTION OF LIPIDS

Lipid Digestion Requires Overcoming the Limited Water Solubility of Lipids

An adult man ingests about 60–150 g of lipid per day. **Triacylglycerols** constitute more than 90% of the dietary fat. The rest is made up of phospholipids, cholesterol, cholesterol esters, and free fatty acids. In addition, 1–2 g of cholesterol and 7–22 g of phosphatidylcholine (lecithin) are secreted into the small intestine lumen as constituents of bile.

Lipids are defined by their good solubility in organic solvents and their sparing or lack of solubility in aqueous solutions. The poor water solubility presents problems for digestion because the substrates are not easily accessible to the digestive enzymes in the aqueous phase. In addition, even if ingested lipids are hydrolyzed into simple constituents, the products tend to aggregate to larger complexes that make poor contact with the cell surface and therefore are not easily absorbed. These problems are overcome by (1) increases in the interfacial area between the aqueous and lipid phase and (2) "solubilization" of lipids with **detergents.** Thus changes in the physical state of lipids are intimately connected to chemical changes during digestion and absorption.

At least five different phases can be distinguished (Figure 26.27): (1) hydrolysis of triacylglycerols to free fatty acids and monoacylglycerols; (2) solubilization by detergents (bile acids) and transport from the intestinal lumen toward the cell surface; (3) uptake of free fatty acids and monoacylglycerols into the cell and resynthesis to triacylglycerols; (4) packaging of newly synthesized triacylglycerols into special lipid-rich globules, called chylomicrons; and (5) exocytosis of chylomicrons from cells and release into lymph.

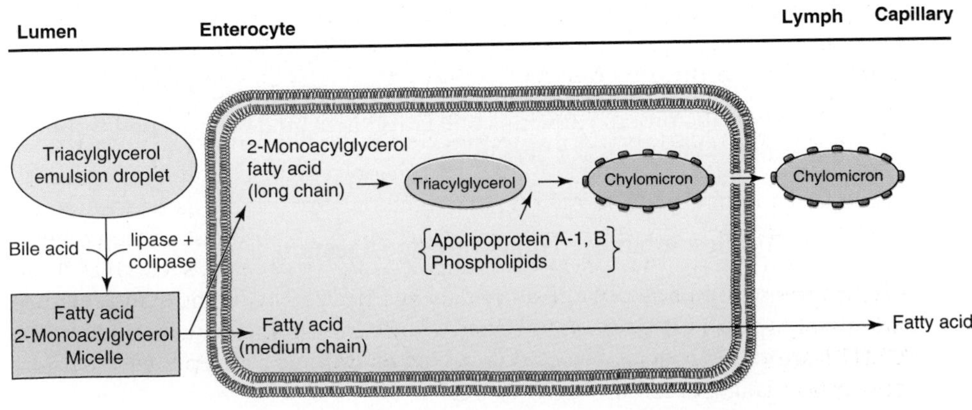

FIGURE 26.27
Digestion and absorption of lipids.

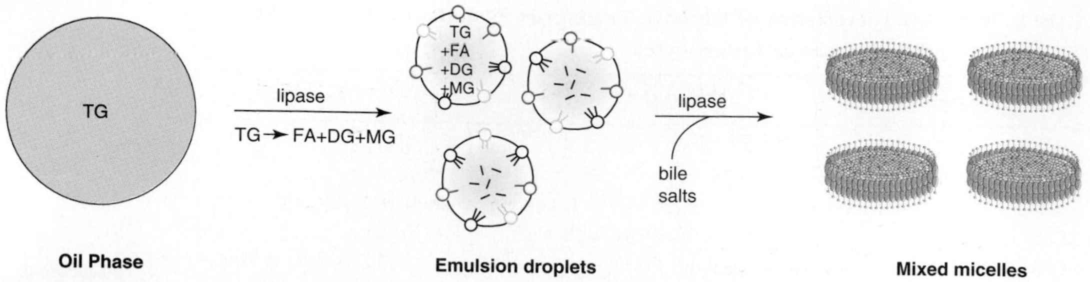

FIGURE 26.28
Changes in physical state during triacylglycerol digestion.
Abbreviations: TG, triacylglycerol; DG, diacylglycerol; MG, monoacylglycerol; FA, fatty acid.

Lipids Are Digested by Gastric and Pancreatic Lipases

Digestion of lipids is initiated in the stomach by an **acid-stable lipase,** most of which is thought to originate from glands at the back of the tongue. However, the rate of hydrolysis is slow because the ingested triacylglycerols form a separate lipid phase with a limited water–lipid interface. The lipase adsorbs to that interface and converts triacylglycerols into fatty acids and diacylglycerols (Figure 26.28). The importance of the initial hydrolysis is that some of the water-immiscible triacylglycerols are converted to products that possess both polar and nonpolar groups. Such surfactive products spontaneously adsorb to water–lipid interfaces and confer a hydrophilic surface to lipid droplets thereby providing a stable interface with the aqueous environment. At constant volume of the lipid phase, any increase in interfacial area produces dispersion of the lipid phase into smaller droplets (emulsification) and provides more sites for adsorption of more lipase molecules.

The major enzyme for triacylglycerol hydrolysis is the **pancreatic lipase** (Figure 26.29). This enzyme is specific for esters in the α-position of glycerol and prefers long-chain fatty acids with more than ten carbon atoms. Hydrolysis by the pancreatic enzyme also occurs at the water–lipid interface of emulsion droplets. The products are **free fatty acids** and **β-monoacylglycerols.** The purified form of the enzyme is strongly inhibited by the bile acids that normally are present in the small intestine during lipid digestion. The problem of inhibition is overcome by **colipase,** a small protein (12 kDa) that binds to both the water–lipid interface and to lipase, thereby anchoring and activating the enzyme. It is secreted by the pancreas as procolipase and depends on tryptic removal of a NH_2-terminal decapeptide for full activity.

Pancreatic juice also contains another less **specific lipid esterase,** which acts on cholesterol esters, monoglycerides, or other lipid esters, such as esters of vitamin A with carboxylic acids. In contrast to triacylglycerol lipase, this lipid esterase requires bile acids for activity.

Phospholipids are hydrolyzed by specific phospholipases. Pancreatic secretions are especially rich in the proenzyme for **phospholipase A_2** (Figure 26.30). As other pancreatic proenzymes, this one is also activated by trypsin. Phospholipase A_2 requires bile acids for activity.

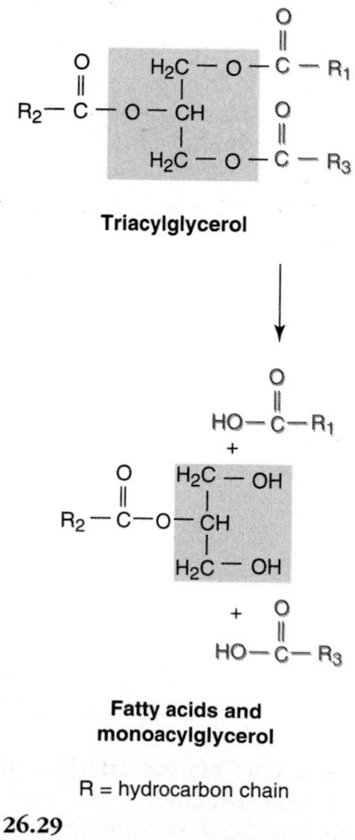

FIGURE 26.29
Mechanism of action of lipase.

Bile Acid Micelles Solubilize Lipids During Digestion

Bile acids are biological detergents that are synthesized by the liver and secreted as conjugates of **glycine** or **taurine** with the bile into the duodenum. At physiological pH values, they are present as anions, which have detergent

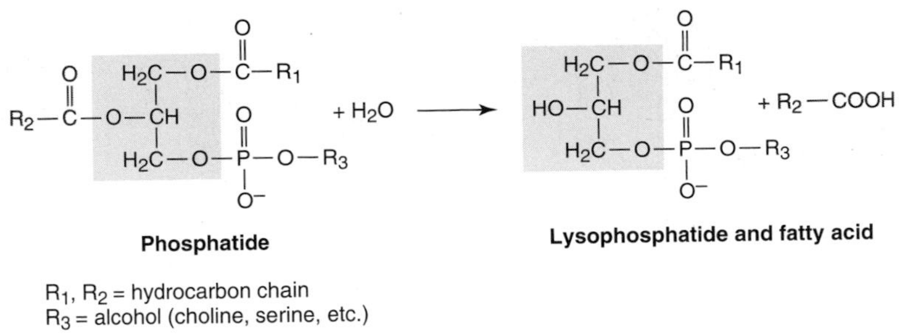

Phosphatide + H_2O → Lysophosphatide + $R_2{-}COOH$

Phosphatide

Lysophosphatide and fatty acid

R_1, R_2 = hydrocarbon chain
R_3 = alcohol (choline, serine, etc.)

FIGURE 26.30
Mechanism of action of phospholipase A_2.

properties. Therefore the terms **bile acids** and **bile salts** are often used interchangeably (Figure 26.31). Bile acids at pH values above the p*K* (Table 26.10) reversibly form aggregates at concentrations above 2–5 mM. These aggregates are called **micelles,** and the minimal concentration necessary for micelle formation is the **critical micellar concentration** (Figure 26.32). The bile acids in micelles are in equilibrium with those free in solution. Thus micelles, in contrast to emulsified lipids, are equilibrium structures with well-defined sizes that are much smaller than emulsion droplets. Micelle sizes typically range between 40 and 600 μm depending on bile acid concentration and the ratio of bile acids to lipids.

The arrangements of bile acids in micelles is such that the hydrophobic portions are removed from contact with water, while hydrophilic groups remain exposed to the water. The hydrophobic region of bile acids is formed by one surface of the fused ring system, while the carboxylate or sulfonate ion and the hydroxyl groups on the other side of the ring system are hydrophilic. Since the major driving forces for micelle formation are the removal of apolar, hydrophobic groups from and the interaction of polar groups with water molecules, the distribution of polar and apolar regions places some constraints on the stereochemical arrangements of bile acid molecules within a micelle. Four bile acid molecules are sufficient to form a very simple micelle as shown in Figure 26.33. Bile salt micelles can solubilize other lipids, such as phospholipids and fatty acids. These **mixed micelles** have disk-like shapes, whereby the phospholipids and fatty acids form a bilayer and the bile acids occupy the edge positions, rendering the edge of the disk hydrophilic (Figure 26.34). Within the mixed phospholipid–bile acid micelles, other water-insoluble lipids, such as cholesterol, can be accommodated and thereby "solubilized" (for potential problems see Clin. Corr. 26.5).

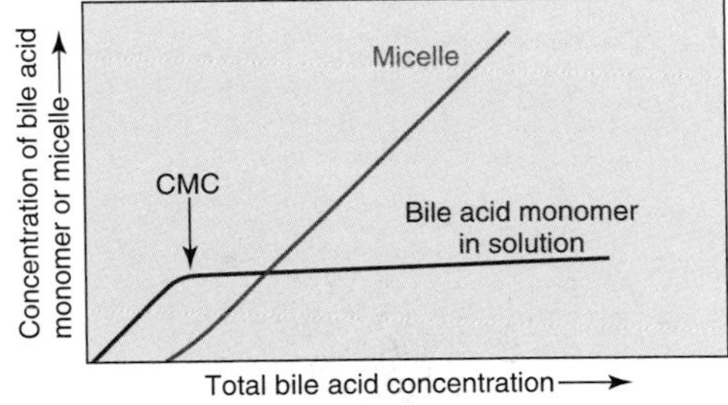

FIGURE 26.32
Solubility properties of bile acids in aqueous solutions.
Abbreviation: CMC, critical micellar concentration.

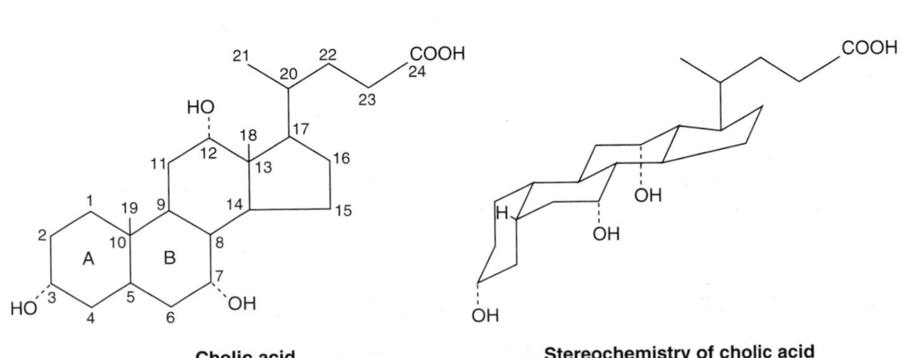

FIGURE 26.31
Cholic acid, a bile acid.

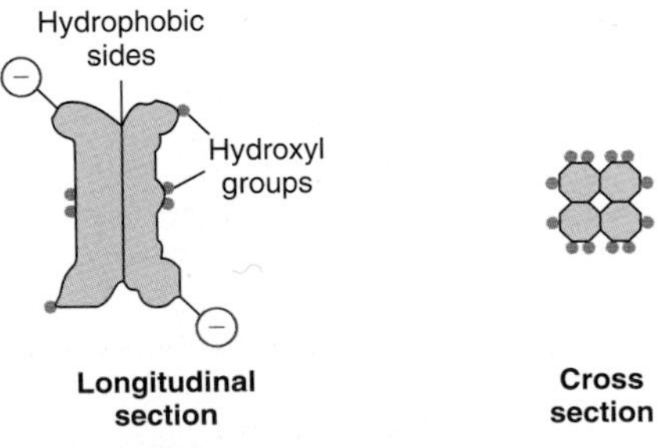

FIGURE 26.33
Diagrammatic representation of a Na^+ cholate micelle.
Adapted from Small, D. M. Biochim. Biophys. Acta *176:178, 1969.*

TABLE 26.10 Effect of Conjugation on the Acidity of Cholic, Deoxycholic, and Chenodeoxycholic Acids

Bile Acid	*Ionized Group*	pK_a
Unconjugated bile acids	$—COO^-$ of cholestanoic acid	≃5
Glycoconjugates	$—COO^-$ of glycine	≃3.7
Tauroconjugates	$—SO_3^-$ of taurine	≃1.5

Primary: Cholic (COOH; OH, HO, OH); Chenic (COOH; HO, OH)

Secondary: Deoxycholic (COOH; OH, HO)

→ $NH_3^+CH_2COO^-$ + glycine → $R—C(=O)—N(H)—CH_2COO^-$: Cholylglycine, Chenylglycine, Deoxycholylglycine

→ $NH_3^+(CH_2)_2SO_2O^-$ + taurine → $R—C(=O)—N(H)—(CH_2)_2SO_2O^-$: Cholyltaurine, Chenyltaurine, Deoxycholyltaurine

Source: Reproduced with permission from Hofmann, A. F. *Handbook of Physiology* 5:2508, 1968.

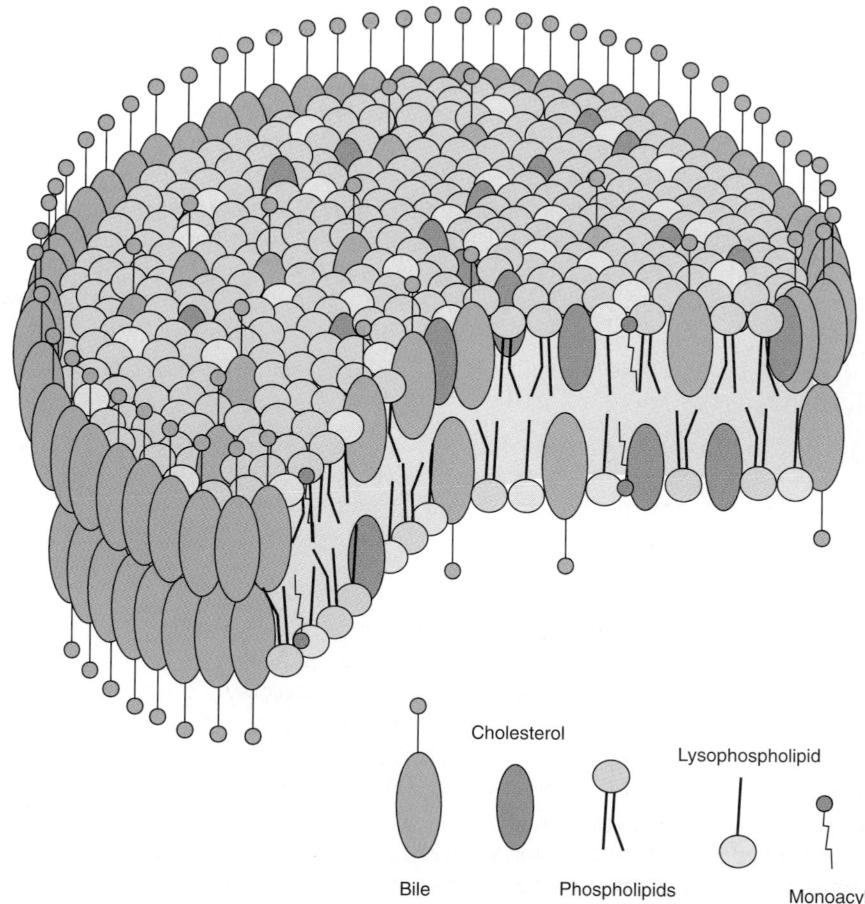

FIGURE 26.34
Proposed structure of the intestinal mixed micelle.
The bilayer disk has a band of bile salt at its periphery and other, more hydrophobic components (fatty acids, monoacylglycerol, phospholipids, and cholesterol) protected within its interior.
Redrawn based on figure from Carey, M. C. In: A. M. Arias, H. Popper, D. Schachter, et al. (Eds.), The Liver: Biology and Pathology, *New York: Raven Press, 1982.*

CLINICAL CORRELATION 26.5

Cholesterol Stones

Liver secretes phospholipids and cholesterol together with bile acids into the bile. Because of the limited solubility of cholesterol, its secretion in bile can result in cholesterol stone formation in the gallbladder. Stone formation is a relatively frequent complication; up to 20% of North Americans will develop stones during their lifetime.

Cholesterol is practically insoluble in aqueous solutions. However, it can be incorporated into mixed phospholipid–bile acid micelles up to a mole ratio of 1 : 1 for cholesterol/phospholipids and thereby "solubilized" (see accompanying figure). The liver can produce supersaturated bile with a higher ratio than 1 : 1 of cholesterol/phospholipid. This excess cholesterol has a tendency to come out of solution and to crystallize. Such bile with excess cholesterol is considered lithogenic, that is, stoneforming. Crystal formation usually occurs in the gallbladder, rather than the hepatic bile ducts, because contact times between bile and any crystallization nuclei are greater in the gallbladder. In addition, the gallbladder concentrates bile by absorption of electrolytes and water. The bile salts chenodeoxycholate and ursodeoxycholate are now available for oral use to dissolve gallstones. Ingestion of these bile salts reduces cholesterol excretion into the bile and allows cholesterol in stones to be solubilized.

The tendency to secrete bile supersaturated with respect to cholesterol is inherited and found more frequently in females than in males, often associated with obesity. Supersaturation also appears to be a function of the size and nature of the bile acid pool as well as the secretion rate.

Schoenfield, L. J., and Lachin, J. M. Chenodiol (chenodeoxycholic acid) for dissolution of gallstones: The National Cooperative Gallstone Study. A controlled trial of safety and efficacy. *Ann. Intern. Med.* 95:257, 1981; and Carey, M. C., and Small, D. M. The physical chemistry of cholesterol solubility in bile. *J. Clin. Invest.* 61:998, 1978.

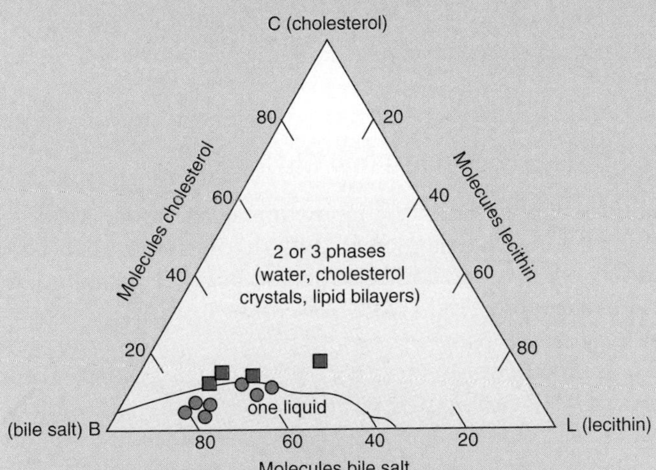

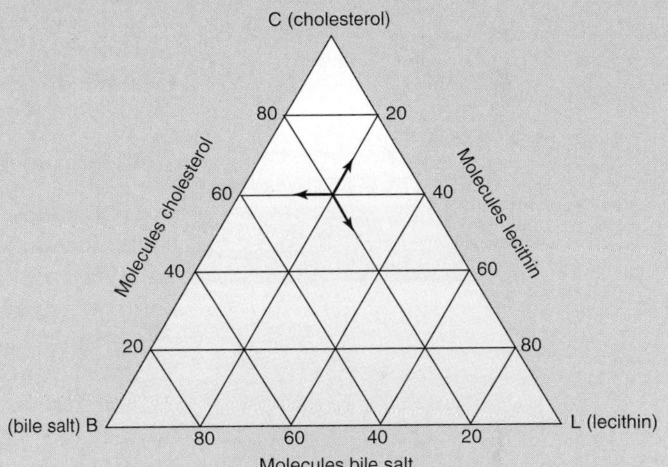

Diagram of the physical states of mixtures of 90% water and 10% lipid.
The 10% lipid is made up of bile acids, lecithin, and cholesterol, and the triangle represents all possible ratios of the three lipid constituents. Each point within the triangle corresponds to a particular composition of the three components, which can be read off the graph as indicated; each point on one of the sides corresponds to a particular composition of just two components. The left triangle contains the composition of gallbladder bile samples from patients without stones (red ○) and with cholesterol stones (blue ■). Lithogenic bile has a composition that falls outside the "one liquid" area in the lower left corner.
Redrawn from Hofmann, A. F., and Small, D. M. Annu. Rev. Med. *18:362, 1967. Copyright © 1967 by Annual Reviews, Inc.*

During triacylglycerol digestion, free fatty acids and monoacylglycerols are released at the surface of fat emulsion droplets. In contrast to triacylglycerols, which are water-insoluble, free fatty acids and monoacylglycerols are slightly water-soluble, and molecules at the surface equilibrate with those in solution. The latter in turn become incorporated into bile acid micelles. Thus the products of triacylglycerol hydrolysis are continuously transferred from emulsion droplets to the micelles (see Figure 26.27).

Micelles provide the major vehicle for moving lipids from the intestinal lumen to the cell surface where absorption occurs. Because the fluid layer next to the cell surface is poorly mixed, the major transport mechanism for solute flux across this "unstirred" fluid layer is diffusion down the concentration gradient. With this type of transport mechanism, the delivery rate of nutrients at the cell surface is proportional to their concentration difference between luminal bulk phase and cell surface. Obviously, the unstirred fluid layer presents problems for sparingly soluble or insoluble nutrients, in that reasonable delivery rates cannot be achieved. Bile acid micelles overcome this problem for lipids by increasing their effective concentration in the unstirred layer. The increase in transport rate is nearly proportional to the increase in effective concentration and can be 1000-fold over that of individually solubilized fatty acids, in accordance with the different solubility of fatty acids as micelles or as individual molecules. This relationship between flux and effective concentration holds because the diffusion constant, another parameter that determines the flux, is only slightly smaller for the mixed micelles as compared to lipid molecules free in solution. Thus efficient lipid absorption depends on the presence of sufficient bile acids to "solubilize" the ingested and hydrolyzed lipids in micelles. In the absence of bile acids, the absorption of triacylglycerols does not completely stop, although the efficiency is drastically reduced. The residual absorption depends on the slight water solubility of the free fatty acids and monoacylglycerols. Unabsorbed lipids reach the lower intestine where a small part can be metabolized by bacteria. The bulk of unabsorbed lipids, however, is excreted with the stool (this is called **steatorrhea**).

Micelles also transport cholesterol and the lipid-soluble vitamins A, D, E, and K through the unstirred fluid layers. Bile acid secretion is absolutely essential for their absorption.

Most Absorbed Lipids Are Incorporated into Chylomicrons

Uptake of lipids by the epithelial cells occurs by diffusion through the plasma membrane. Absorption is virtually complete for fatty acids and monoacylglycerols, which are slightly water-soluble. It is less efficient for water-insoluble lipids. For example, only 30–40% of the dietary cholesterol is absorbed.

Within the intestinal cells, the fate of absorbed fatty acids depends on chain length. **Fatty acids** of **medium chain length** (6–10 carbon atoms) pass through the cell into the portal blood without modification. Long-chain fatty acids (>12 carbon atoms) become bound to a cytosolic, specifically **intestinal fatty acid-binding protein** (I-FABP) and are transported to the endoplasmic reticulum, where they are resynthesized into triacylglycerols. Glycerol for this process is derived from the absorbed 2-monoacylglycerols and, to a minor degree, from glucose. The resynthesized triacylglycerols form lipid globules to which surface-active phospholipids and special proteins, termed **apolipoproteins,** adsorb. The lipid globules migrate within membrane-bounded vesicles through the Golgi to the basolateral plasma membrane. They are finally released into the intercellular space by fusion of the vesicles with the basolateral plasma membrane. Because the lipid globules can be several micrometers in diameter and because they leave the intestine via lymph vessels, they are called **chylomicrons** (chyle = milky lymph that is present in the intestinal lymph vessels, lacteals, and the thoracic duct after a lipid meal; chyle is derived from the Greek *chylos,* which means juice). The intestinal apolipoproteins are distinctly different from those of the liver and are designated A-1 and B. **Apolipoprotein B** is essential for chylomicron release from enterocytes (see Clin. Corr. 26.6).

While dietary medium-chain fatty acids reach the liver directly with the portal blood, the long-chain fatty acids bypass the liver by being released in the form of chylomicrons into the lymphatics. The intestinal lymph vessels drain into the large body veins via the thoracic duct. Blood from the large veins first reaches the lungs and then the capillaries of the peripheral tissues, including adipose tissue and muscle, before it comes into contact with the liver. Fat and

CLINICAL CORRELATION 26.6

A-β-Lipoproteinemia

A-β-lipoproteinemia is an autosomal recessive disorder characterized by the absence of all lipoproteins containing apo-β-lipoprotein, that is, chylomicrons, very low density lipoproteins (VLDLs), and low density lipoproteins (LDLs). Serum cholesterol is extremely low. This defect is associated with severe malabsorption of triacylglycerol and lipid-soluble vitamins (especially tocopherol and vitamin E) and accumulation of apo B in enterocytes and hepatocytes. The defect does not appear to involve the gene for apo B, but rather one of several proteins involved in processing of apo B in liver and intestinal mucosa, or in assembly and secretion of triacylglycerol-rich lipoproteins, that is, chylomicrons and VLDLs from these tissues, respectively.

Kane, J. P. Apolipoprotein B: structural and metabolic heterogeneity. *Annu. Rev. Physiol.* 45:673, 1983; and Kane, J. P., and Havel, R. J. In: C. R. Scriver, A. L. Beaudet, W. S. Sly, and D. Valle (Eds.), *The Metabolic and Molecular Bases of Inherited Disease,* Vol. 1, 7th ed. New York: McGraw-Hill, 1995, p. 1853.

muscle cells in particular take up large amounts of dietary lipids for storage or metabolism. The bypass of the liver may have evolved to protect this organ from a lipid overload after a meal.

The differential handling of medium- and long-chain fatty acids by intestinal cells can be specifically exploited to provide the liver with high-caloric nutrients in the form of fatty acids. Short- and medium-chain fatty acids are not very palatable; however, triacylglycerols synthesized from these fatty acids are quite palatable and can be used as part of the diet.

26.7 BILE ACID METABOLISM

All bile acids are synthesized within the liver from cholesterol but can be modified by bacterial enzymes in the intestinal lumen. **Primary bile acids** synthesized by the liver are **cholic** and **chenodeoxycholic** (or chenic) acid. The **secondary bile acids** are derived from the primary bile acids by bacterial dehydroxylation in position 7 of the ring structure, resulting in **deoxycholate** and **lithocholate,** respectively (Figure 26.35).

Primary and secondary bile acids are reabsorbed by the intestine into the portal blood, taken up by the liver, and then resecreted into bile. Within the liver, primary as well as secondary bile acids are linked to either glycine or

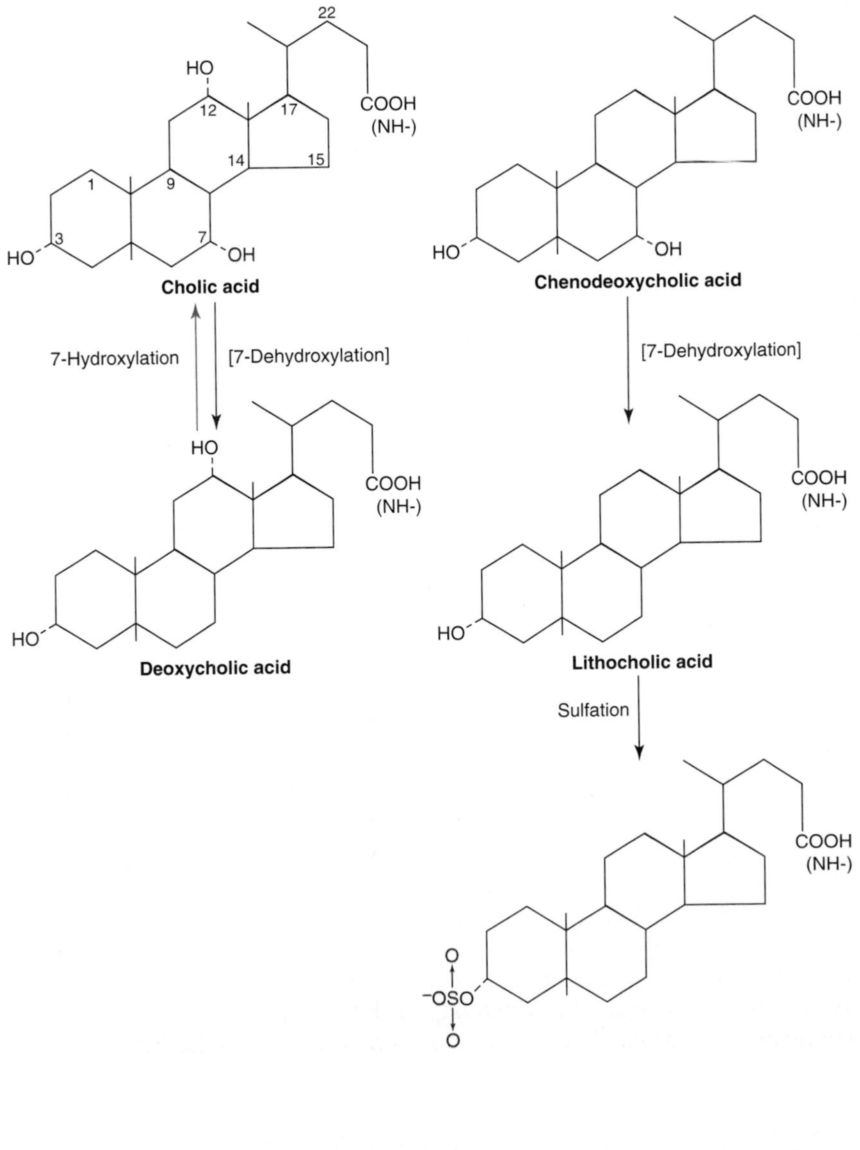

Cholic acid

Chenodeoxycholic acid

7-Hydroxylation

[7-Dehydroxylation]

[7-Dehydroxylation]

Deoxycholic acid

Lithocholic acid

Sulfation

FIGURE 26.35
Bile acid metabolism in the rat.
Green and black arrows indicate reactions catalyzed by liver enzymes; red arrows indicate those of bacterial enzymes within the intestinal lumen. (NH—), glycine or taurine conjugate of the bile acids.

taurine via an isopeptide bond. These derivatives are called **glyco-** and **tauro-conjugates,** respectively, and constitute the forms that are secreted into bile. With the conjugation, the carboxyl group of the unconjugated acid is replaced by an even more polar group. The p*K* values of the carboxyl group of glycine and of the sulfonyl group of taurine are lower than that of unconjugated bile acids, so that conjugated bile acids remain ionized over a wider pH range (see Table 26.10). The conjugation is partially reversed within the intestinal lumen by hydrolysis of the isopeptide bond.

The total amount of conjugated and unconjugated bile acids secreted per day by the liver is 16–70 g for an adult. As the total body pool is only 3–4 g, bile acids have to recirculate 5–14 times each day between the intestinal lumen and the liver. Reabsorption of bile acids is important to conserve the pool. Most of the uptake is probably by passive diffusion along the entire small intestine. In addition, the lower ileum contains a specialized **Na^+-bile acid cotransport system** for concentrative reuptake. Thus during a meal, bile acids from the gallbladder and liver are released into the lumen of the upper small intestine, pass with the chyme down the small intestinal lumen, are reabsorbed by the epithelium of the lower small intestine into the portal blood, and are then extracted from the portal blood by the liver parenchymal cells. The process of secretion and reuptake is referred to as the **enterohepatic circulation** (Figure 26.36). Reabsorption of bile acids by the intestine is quite efficient as only about 0.5 g of bile acids escapes reuptake each day and is secreted with the feces. Serum levels of bile acids normally vary with the rate of reabsorption and therefore are highest during a meal.

Cholate, deoxycholate, chenodeoxycholate, and their conjugates continuously participate in the enterohepatic circulation. In contrast, most of the **lithocholic acid** that is produced by bacterial enzymes is sulfated during the next passage through the liver. The sulfate ester of lithocholic acid is not a substrate for the bile acid transport system in the ileum and therefore is excreted in the feces.

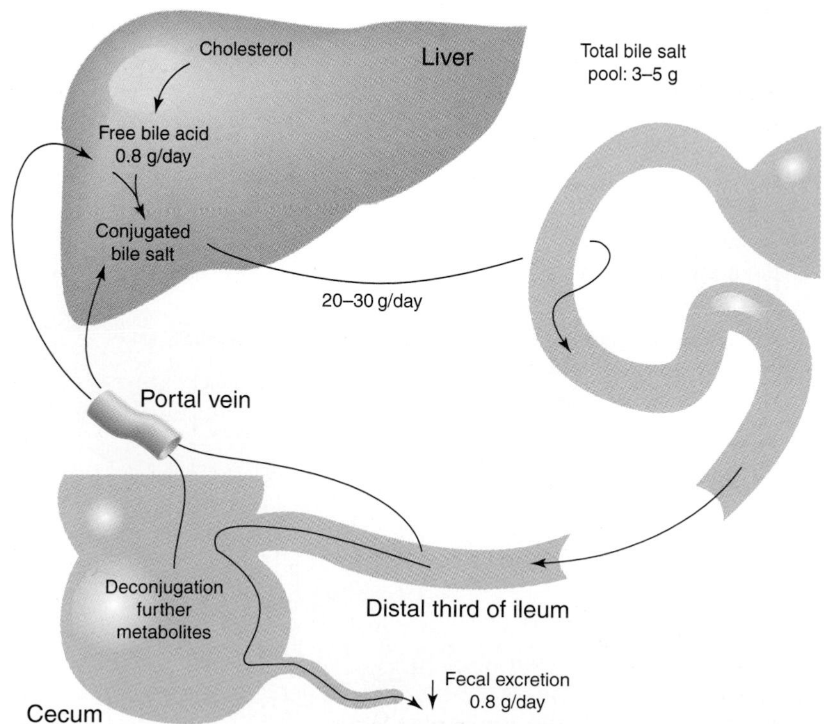

FIGURE 26.36
Enterohepatic circulation of bile acids.
Redrawn from Clark, M. L., and Harries, J. T. In: I. McColl and G. E. Sladen (Eds.), Intestinal Absorption in Man. *New York: Academic Press, 1975, p. 195.*

BIBLIOGRAPHY

Cristofaro, E., Mottu, F., and Wuhrmann, J. J. Involvement of the raffinose family of oligosaccharides in flatulence. In: H. L. Sipple and K. W. McNutt (Eds.), *Sugars in Nutrition*. New York: Academic Press, 1974, p. 314.

Field, M., and Semrad, C. E. Toxigenic diarrheas, congenital diarrheas, and cystic fibrosis. *Annu. Rev. Physiol.* 55:631–655, 1993.

Hediger, M. A., and Rhoads, D. B. Molecular physiology of sodium-glucose cotransporters. *Physiol. Rev.* 74:993–1026, 1994.

Johnson, L. R. (ed.-in-chief). *Physiology of the Gastrointestinal Tract*, Vols. 1 and 2, 2nd and 3rd eds. New York: Raven Press, 1987, 1994.

Mathews, D. M. *Protein Absorption*. New York: Wiley-Liss, 1991.

Pandol, S., and Raybauld, H. E. Integrated response to a meal. The Undergraduate Teaching Project in Gastroenterology and Liver Disease. Unit #29. American Gastroenterological Assoc. Timonium, MD: Milner-Fenwick, Inc., 1995.

Porter, R., and Collins, G. M. *Brush Border Membranes*. Volume 95, Ciba Foundation Symposium. London: Pitman, 1983.

Schultz, S. G. (section ed.). *Handbook of Physiology. Section 6: The Gastrointestinal System. Vol. IV. Intestinal Absorption and Secretion* (M. Field and R. A. Frizzell, Eds.). Bethesda, MD: American Physiological Society, 1991

Sleisenger, M. H. Malabsorption and nutritional support. *Clin. Gastroenterol.* 12:323, 1983.

Thomson, A. B. R., Schoeller, C., Keelan, M., Smith, L., and Clandinin, M. T. Lipid absorption: passing through the unstirred layers near the brush border membrane, and beyond. *Can. J. Physiol. Pharmacol.* 71:531–555, 1993.

QUESTIONS J. BAGGOTT AND C. N. ANGSTADT

Refer to the following for Questions 1–5:
A. liver
B. pancreas
C. spleen
D. stomach
E. none of the above

1. Has no role in digestion.

2. Synthesizes an essential emulsifier of lipids.

3. Participates in a nonessential manner in protein digestion.

4. Transports HCO_3^- from the cytoplasm across the contraluminal plasma membrane.

5. Site of chymotrypsinogen synthesis.

6. Active forms of enzymes that digest food may normally be found in all of the following EXCEPT:
   A. in soluble form in the lumen of the stomach.
   B. in the saliva.
   C. attached to the luminal surface of the plasma membrane of intestinal epithelial cells.
   D. dissolved in the cytoplasm of intestinal epithelial cells.
   E. in zymogen granules of pancreatic exocrine cells.

7. Histamine is a physiologically important secretagogue of:
   A. amylase by the salivary glands.
   B. HCl by the stomach.
   C. gastrin by the stomach.
   D. hydrolytic enzymes by the pancreas.
   E. $NaHCO_3$ by the pancreas.

8. The contraluminal membranes of small intestinal epithelial cells contain:
   A. aminopeptidases.
   B. Na^+,K^+–ATPase.
   C. disaccharidases.
   D. GLUT5.
   E. Na^+–monosaccharide transport (SGLT1).

9. Oral administration of large amounts of tyrosine could be expected to interfere with the intestinal absorption of:
   A. leucine.
   B. lysine.
   C. glycine.
   D. aspartate.
   E. none of the above.

10. Which of the following has two carboxyl groups essential for peptidase activity?
   A. carboxypeptidase
   B. chymotrypsin
   C. elastase
   D. pepsin
   E. trypsin

11. Starch digestion is more efficient after heating the starch with water because heating:
   A. hydrates the starch granules, making them more susceptible to pancreatic amylase.
   B. converts α-1,4 links to β-1,4 links, which are more susceptible to attack by mammalian amylases.
   C. partly hydrolyzes α-1,6 links.
   D. converts the linear amylose to branched amylopectin, which resembles glycogen.
   E. inactivates amylase inhibitors, which are common in the tissues of starchy plants.

12. In the cytoplasm of intestinal cells:
   A. all di- and tripeptides are hydrolyzed.
   B. aminopeptidases are especially active.
   C. during the neonatal period ingested proteins may be found.
   D. most disaccharides are hydrolyzed.
   E. raffinose and related sugars are degraded to yield hydrogen, methane, and carbon dioxide.

13. In the digestion and absorption of triacylglycerols:
   A. a pancreatic lipase initiates the process.
   B. an important colipase is activated by tryptic hydrolysis.
   C. hydrolysis occurs in the interior of the lipid droplets.
   D. most of the triacylglycerol hydrolysis is carried out by a lipase of gastric origin.
   E. efficiency is greatly increased if bile acids are absent.

14. Micelles:
    A. are the same as emulsion droplets.
    B. form from bile acids at all bile acid concentrations.
    C. although they are formed during lipid digestion, do not significantly enhance utilization of dietary lipid.
    D. always consist of only a single lipid species.
    E. are essential for the absorption of vitamins A and K.

15. In the metabolism of bile acids:
    A. the liver synthesizes the primary bile acids, cholic, and deoxycholic acids.
    B. secondary bile acids are produced by conjugation of primary bile acids to glycine or taurine.
    C. physiologically active bile acids are formed from primary bile acids by intestinal bacteria.
    D. daily bile acid secretion by the liver is approximately equal to daily bile acid synthesis.
    E. conjugation reduces the polarity of bile acids, enhancing their ability to interact with lipids.

ANSWERS

1. C The spleen has no role in the digestion of food, though it does participate in other degradation processes.
2. A Bile acids are synthesized in the liver and are stored in the gallbladder (p. 1057).
3. D Loss of the stomach function can be compensated for by the intestinal processes (p. 1057).
4. D This occurs in the parietal (oxyntic) cells during HCl secretion (p. 1069).
5. B
6. E Zymogen granules contain inactive proenzymes or zymogens, which are not activated until after release from the cell (p. 1060).
7. B Stimulation of H_2 receptors of the stomach causes HCl secretion (p. 1061).
8. B. Only the contraluminal surface contains the Na^+,K^+–ATPase. All other activities are associated with the luminal surface (Table 26.5, p. 1064).
9. A Tyrosine shares a transport system with Val, Leu, Met, Phe, and Ile (p. 1073).
10. D The carboxylic acid groups are involved in the mechanism that depends on an acid pH (p. 1070).
11. A α-Amylase attacks hydrated starch more readily than unhydrated; heating hydrates the starch granules (p. 1074).
12. C They are taken up by pinocytosis (p. 1073).
13. B This colipase is required to overcome bile acid inhibition of pancreatic lipase, the major enzyme of lipid digestion. The colipase is secreted by the pancreas as a procolipase and must be activated by tryptic cleavage (p. 1078). A: Lipid digestion is initiated in the stomach by acid-stable lipase (p. 1078).
14. E The lipid-soluble vitamins must be dissolved in mixed micelles as a prerequisite for absorption (p. 1082). A: Micelles are of molecular dimensions and are highly ordered structures; emulsion droplets are much larger and are random (p. 1078, Figure 26.28; p. 1080, Figure 26.34). B: Micelle formation occurs only above the critical micellar concentration (CMC); below that concentration the components are in simple solution (p. 1079, Figure 26.32). C: See item 13. D: Micelles may consist of only one component, or they may be mixed (p. 1079.)
15. C The primary bile acids (cholic and chenodeoxycholic acids) are synthesized in the liver. In the intestine they may be dehydroxylated by bacteria to form the secondary bile acids—deoxycholate and lithocholate. Only a small fraction of the bile acid escapes reuptake; this must be replaced by synthesis. Both are reabsorbed and recirculated (enterohepatic circulation). Both are conjugated to glycine or taurine, increasing their polarity (p. 1078).

CHAPTER

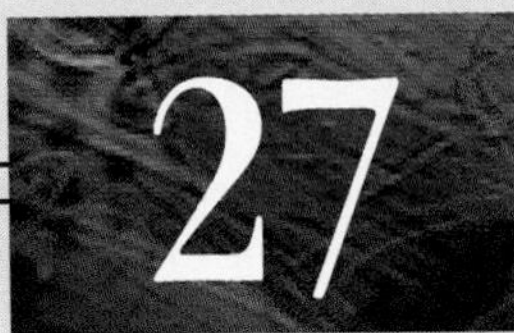

PRINCIPLES OF NUTRITION I: MACRONUTRIENTS

Stephen G. Chaney

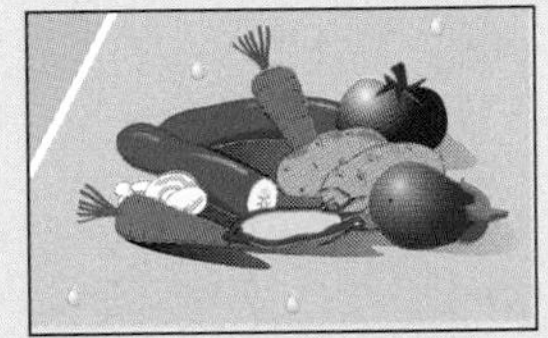

27.1 ■ OVERVIEW

Nutrition is best defined as the utilization of foods by living organisms. Since the process of food utilization is biochemical, the major thrust of the next two chapters is a discussion of basic nutritional concepts in biochemical terms. Simply understanding basic nutritional concepts is no longer sufficient. Nutrition attracts more than its share of controversy in our society, and a thorough understanding of nutrition almost demands an understanding of the issues behind these controversies. These chapters also explore the biochemical basis for some of the most important nutritional controversies.

Study of human nutrition can be divided into three areas: undernutrition, overnutrition, and ideal nutrition. **Undernutrition** is not a primary concern in this country because nutritional deficiency diseases are now quite rare. **Overnutrition** is a particularly serious problem in developed countries. Current estimates suggest that between 15% and 30% of the U.S. population is obese, and obesity is known to have a number of serious health consequences. Finally, there is increasing interest today in the concept of ideal or **optimal nutrition.** This is a concept that has meaning only in an affluent society. Only when food supply becomes abundant enough so that deficiency diseases are a rarity does it become possible to consider long-range effects of nutrients on health. This is probably the most exciting area of nutrition today.

27.2 ■ ENERGY METABOLISM

Energy Content of Food Is Measured in Kilocalories

You should be well acquainted with the energy requirements of the body. Much of the food we eat is converted to ATP and other high-energy compounds, which are utilized to drive biosynthetic pathways, generate nerve impulses, and power muscle contraction. We generally describe the energy content of foods in terms of **calories.** Technically speaking, we are actually referring to **kilocalories** of heat energy released by combustion of that food in the body. Some nutritionists prefer the term kilojoule (a measure of mechanical energy), but since the American public is likely to be counting calories rather than joules in the foreseeable future, we will restrict ourselves to that term. Caloric values of protein, fat, carbohydrate, and alcohol are roughly 4, 9, 4, and 7 kcal g^{-1}, respectively. Given these data and the composition of the food, it is simple to calculate the caloric content (input) of the foods we eat. Calculating caloric content of foods does not appear to be a major problem in this country. Millions of Americans are able to do it with ease. The problem lies in balancing caloric input with caloric output. Where do these calories go?

Energy Expenditure Is Influenced by Four Factors

There are four principal factors that affect individual energy expenditure: surface area (which is related to height and weight), age, sex, and activity level. (1) The effects of surface area are thought to be simply related to the rate of heat loss by the body—the greater the surface area, the greater the rate of heat loss. While it may seem surprising, a lean individual actually has a greater surface area, and thus a greater energy requirement, than an obese individual of the same weight. (2) Age may reflect two factors: growth and lean muscle mass. In infants and children more energy expenditure is required for rapid growth, and this is reflected in a higher **basal metabolic rate** (rate of energy utilization in resting state). In adults (even lean adults), muscle tissue is gradually replaced with fat and water during the aging process, resulting in a 2% decrease in basal metabolic rate (BMR) per decade of adult life. (3) As for sex, women tend to have a lower BMR than men due to a smaller percentage of lean muscle mass and the effects of female hormones on metabolism. (4) The effect of activity levels on energy requirements is obvious. However, most of us overemphasize the immediate, as opposed to the long-term, effects of exercise. For example, one would need to jog for over an hour to burn up the calories found in one piece of apple pie.

Yet, the effect of a regular **exercise** program on energy expenditure can be quite beneficial. Regular exercise increases lean muscle mass, which has a higher basal metabolic rate than adipose tissue, allowing one to burn up calories more rapidly 24 hours a day. A regular exercise program should be designed to increase lean muscle mass and should be repeated 3–5 days a week but need not be aerobic exercise to have an effect on basal metabolic rate. For an elderly or infirm individual, even daily walking may, with time, help to increase basal metabolic rate slightly.

Hormone levels are important also, since thyroxine, sex hormones, growth hormone, and, to a lesser extent, epinephrine and cortisol increase BMR. The effects of epinephrine and cortisol probably explain in part why severe stress and major trauma significantly increase energy requirements. Finally, energy intake itself has an inverse relationship to expenditure in that during periods of **starvation** or semistarvation BMR can decrease up to 50%. This is of great survival value in cases of genuine starvation, but not much help to the person who wishes to lose weight on a calorie-restricted diet.

27.3 PROTEIN METABOLISM

Dietary Protein Serves Many Roles Including Energy Production

Protein carries a certain mystique as a "body-building" food. While it is true that protein is an essential structural component of all cells, protein is equally important for maintaining the output of essential secretions such as digestive enzymes and peptide or protein hormones. Protein is also needed to synthesize plasma proteins, which are essential for maintaining osmotic balance, transporting substances through the blood, and maintaining immunity. However, the average adult in this country consumes far more protein than needed to carry out these essential functions. Excess protein is treated as a source of energy, with the glucogenic amino acids being converted to glucose and the ketogenic amino acids converted to fatty acids and keto acids. Both kinds of **amino acids** will eventually be converted to triacylglycerol in adipose tissue if fat and carbohydrate supplies are already adequate to meet energy requirements. Thus for most of us the only body-building obtained from high-protein diets is in adipose tissue.

It has always been popular to say that the body has no storage depot for protein, and thus adequate dietary protein must be supplied with every meal. However, in actuality, this is not quite accurate. While there is no separate class of "storage" protein, there is a certain percentage of body protein that undergoes a constant process of breakdown and resynthesis. In the fasting state the breakdown of this store of body protein is enhanced, and the resulting amino acids are utilized for glucose production, synthesis of nonprotein nitrogenous compounds, and synthesis of the essential secretory and plasma proteins described above (see also Chapter 14). Even in the fed state, some of these amino acids are utilized for energy production and as biosynthetic precursors. Thus the turnover of body protein is a normal process—and an essential feature of what is called nitrogen balance.

Nitrogen Balance Relates Intake of Nitrogen to Its Excretion

Nitrogen balance (Figure 27.1) is a comparison between intake of nitrogen (chiefly in the form of protein) and excretion of nitrogen (chiefly in the form of undigested protein in the feces and urea and ammonia in urine). A normal adult is in nitrogen equilibrium, with losses just balanced by intake. Negative nitrogen balance results from inadequate dietary intake of protein, since amino acids utilized for energy and biosynthetic reactions are not replaced. It also occurs in injury when there is net destruction of tissue and in major trauma or illness when the body's adaptive response causes increased catabolism of body protein stores. Positive nitrogen balance is observed whenever there is a net increase in the body protein stores, such as in growing children, pregnant women, or convalescing adults.

Essential Amino Acids Must Be Present in the Diet

In addition to the amount of protein in the diet, several other factors must be considered. One is the complement of essential amino acids present in the diet. **Essential amino acids** are those amino acids that cannot be synthesized by the body (Chapter 11). If just one of these essential amino acids is missing from the diet, the body cannot synthesize new protein to replace the protein lost due to normal turnover, and a negative nitrogen balance results (Figure 27.1).

(a) Positive nitrogen balance (growth, pregnancy, lactation and recovery from metabolic stress).

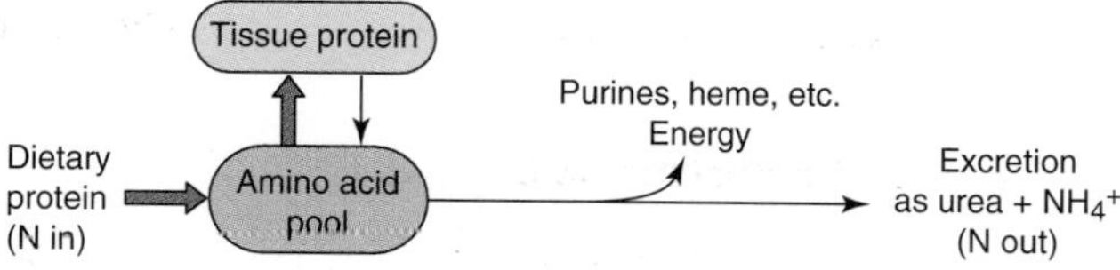

(b) Negative nitrogen balance (metabolic stress).

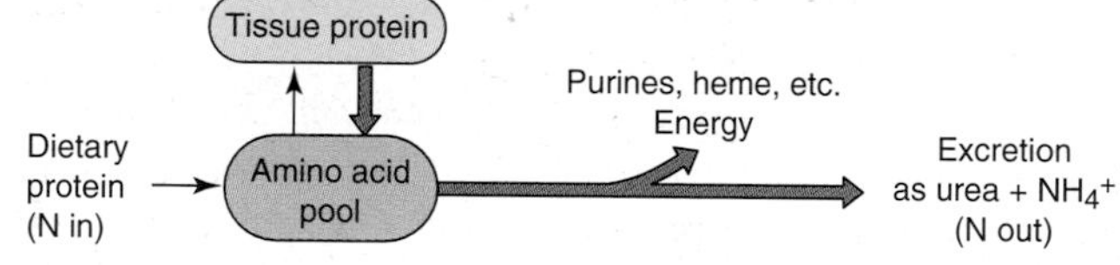

(c) Negative nitrogen balance (inadequate dietary protein).

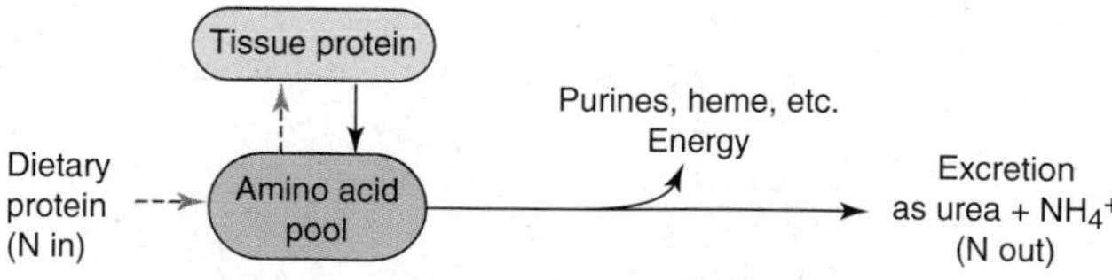

(d) Negative nitrogen balance (lack of an essential amino acid).

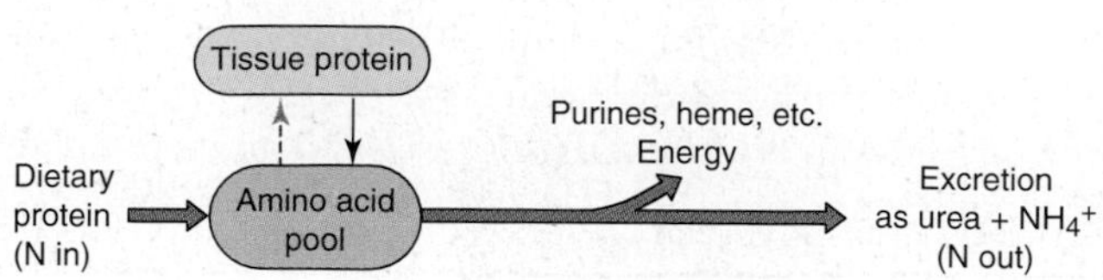

FIGURE 27.1
Factors affecting nitrogen balance.
Schematic representations of the metabolic interrelationship involved in determining nitrogen balance. Each figure represents the nitrogen balance resulting from a particular set of metabolic conditions. The dominant pathways in each situation are indicated by heavy red arrows.

Obviously then, the complement of essential amino acids in any dietary protein will determine how well it can be used by the body.

Generally, most animal proteins contain all essential amino acids in about the quantities needed by the human body. Vegetable proteins, on the other hand, often lack one or more essential amino acids and may, in some cases, be more difficult to digest. Even so, **vegetarian diets** can provide adequate protein provided enough extra protein is consumed to provide sufficient quantities of the essential amino acids and/or two or more different proteins are consumed together, which complement each other in amino acid content. For example, if corn (which is deficient in lysine) is combined with legumes (deficient in methionine but rich in lysine), the efficiency of utilization for the combination of the two vegetable proteins approaches that of animal protein. The adequacy of vegetarian diets with respect to protein and calories is discussed more fully in Clin. Corr. 27.1, and the need for high-quality protein in low-protein diets in renal disease is discussed in Clin. Corr. 27.2.

Protein Sparing Is Related to Dietary Content of Carbohydrate and Fat

Another factor that must be considered in determining protein requirements is dietary intake of fat and carbohydrate. If these components are present in insufficient quantities, some dietary protein must be used for energy generation and is unavailable for building and replacing tissue. Thus as energy (calorie) content of the diet from carbohydrate and fat increases, the need for protein decreases. This is referred to as **protein sparing.** Carbohydrate is somewhat more efficient at protein sparing than fat—presumably because carbohydrate can be used as an energy source by almost all tissues, whereas fat cannot.

Normal Adult Protein Requirements Depend on Diet

Assuming adequate calorie intake and 75% efficiency of utilization, which is typical of mixed protein in the average American diet, the **recommended**

CLINICAL CORRELATION 27.1

Vegetarian Diets and Protein–Energy Requirements

One of the most important problems of a purely vegetarian diet (as opposed to a lacto-ovo vegetarian diet) is the difficulty in obtaining sufficient calories and protein. Potential caloric deficit results from the fact that the caloric densities of fruits and vegetables are much less than the meats they replace (30–50 cal per 100 g versus 150–300 cal per 100 g). The protein problem is generally threefold: (1) most plant products contain much less protein (1–2 g of protein per 100 g versus 15–20 g per 100 g); (2) most plant protein is of low biological value; and (3) some plant proteins are incompletely digested. Actually, well-designed vegetarian diets usually provide enough calories and protein for the average adult. In fact, the reduced caloric intake may well be of benefit because strict vegetarians do tend to be lighter than their nonvegetarian counterparts.

However, whereas an adult male may require about 0.8 g of protein and 40 cal kg^{-1} of body weight, a young child may require 2–3 times that amount. Similarly, a pregnant woman needs an additional 10 g of protein and 300 cal day^{-1} and a lactating woman an extra 15 g of protein and 500 cal. Thus both young children and pregnant and lactating women run a risk of protein–energy malnutrition. Children of vegetarian mothers generally have a lower birth weight than children of mothers consuming a mixed diet. Similarly, vegetarian children generally have a slower rate of growth through the first 5 years, but generally catch up by age 10.

It is possible to provide sufficient calories and protein even for these high-risk groups provided the diet is adequately planned. Three principles should be followed to design a calorie–protein-sufficient vegetarian diet for young children: (1) whenever possible, include eggs and milk in the diet; they are both excellent sources of calories and high-quality protein; (2) include liberal amounts of those vegetable foods with high-caloric density in the diet, including nuts, grains, dried beans, and dried fruits; and (3) include liberal amounts of high-protein vegetable foods that have complementary amino acid patterns. It used to be thought that these complementary proteins must be present in the same meal. Recent animal studies, however, suggest that a meal low in (but not devoid of) an essential amino acid may be supplemented by adding the limiting amino acid at a subsequent meal.

First International Congress on Vegetarian Nutrition. *Proc. Am. J. Clin. Nutr.* 48(Suppl. 1):707, 1988; and Saunders, T. A. B. Vegetarian diets and children. *Pediatr. Nutr.*, 42:955, 1995.

CLINICAL CORRELATION 27.2

Low-Protein Diets and Renal Disease

Chronic renal failure is characterized by the buildup of the end products of protein catabolism, mainly urea. Some degree of dietary protein restriction is usually necessary because these toxic end products are responsible for many of the symptoms associated with renal failure. The amount of protein restriction is dependent on the severity of the disease. It is easy to maintain patients in nitrogen balance for prolonged periods on diets containing as little as 40 g of protein/day if the diet is calorically sufficient. Diets containing less than 40 g/day pose problems. Protein turnover continues and a balance must be found between enough protein to avoid negative nitrogen balance and little enough to avoid buildup of waste products.

The strategy employed in such diets is twofold: (1) provide a minimum of protein, primarily protein of high BV, and (2) provide the rest of the daily calories as carbohydrates and fats. The goal is to provide just enough essential amino acids to maintain positive nitrogen balance. In turn, the body should be able to synthesize the nonessential amino acids from other nitrogen-containing metabolites. Enough carbohydrate and fat are provided so that essentially all dietary protein can be spared from energy metabolism. With this type of diet, it is possible to maintain a patient on 20 g of protein per day for considerable periods. Because of the difficulty in maintaining nitrogen equilibrium at such low-protein intakes, the patient's protein status should be monitored. This can be done by measuring parameters such as serum albumin and transferrin.

Moreover, such diets are extremely monotonous and difficult to follow. A typical 20-g protein diet is shown below:

1. One egg plus $\frac{3}{4}$ cup milk or 1 additional egg or 1 oz of meat.
2. One-half pound of deglutenized (low-protein) wheat bread; all other breads and cereals must be avoided—this includes almost all baked goods.
3. A limited amount of low-protein, low-potassium fruits and vegetables.
4. Sugars and fats to make up the rest of the needed calories; however, cakes, pies, and cookies need to be avoided.

The palatability of these diets can be improved considerably by starting with a vegan diet and supplementing it with a mixture of essential amino acids and ketoacid analogs of the essential amino acids. Recent studies indicate that this technique will help preserve renal function and allow a somewhat greater variety of foods.

Goodship, T. H. J., and Mitch, W. E. Nutritional approaches to preserving renal function. *Adv. Intern. Med.* 33:377, 1988; Dwyer, J. Vegetarian diets for treating nephrotic syndrome. *Nutr. Rev.* 51:44, 1993; and Barsotti, G., Morrell, E., Cupisti, A., Bertoncini, P., and Giovannetti, S. A special supplemented "vegan" diet for nephrotic patients. *Am. J. Nephrol.* 11:380, 1991.

protein intake is 0.8 g/kg^{-1} (body weight) day^{-1}. This amounts to about 58 g protein day^{-1} for a 72-kg (160-lb) man and about 44 g day^{-1} for a 55-kg (120-lb) woman. These recommendations would need to be increased on a vegetarian diet if overall efficiency of utilization were less than 75%.

Protein Requirement Increases During Growth and Recovery from Illness

Because dietary protein is essential for synthesis of new body tissue, as well as for maintenance and repair, the need for protein increases markedly during periods of rapid growth. Such growth occurs during pregnancy, infancy, childhood, and adolescence.

Once growth requirements have been considered, age does not seem to have much effect on protein requirements. If anything, the protein requirement may decrease slightly with age. However, older people need and generally consume less calories, so high-quality protein should provide a larger percentage of their total calories. Furthermore, some older people may have special protein requirements due to malabsorption problems.

Illness, major trauma, and surgery all cause a major **catabolic response.** Energy needs are very large, and the body responds by increasing production of glucagon, glucocorticoids, epinephrine, and certain cytokines. In these situations breakdown of body protein is greatly accelerated and a negative nitrogen balance results unless protein intake is increased (Figure 27.1). Although this increased protein requirement is of little significance in short-term illness, it can be vitally important in the recovery of hospitalized patients as discussed in the next section (see also Clin. Corr. 27.3).

CLINICAL CORRELATION 27.3

Providing Adequate Protein and Calories for the Hospitalized Patient

The normal metabolic response to infection, trauma, and surgery is a complex and carefully balanced catabolic state. As discussed in the text, epinephrine, glucagon, cortisol, and cytokines are released, greatly accelerating the rates of lipolysis, proteolysis, and gluconeogenesis. The net result is an increased supply of fatty acids, amino acids, and glucose to meet the increased energy demands of such major stress. The high serum glucose results in elevation of circulating insulin levels, which is more than counterbalanced by increased levels of epinephrine and other hormones. Skeletal muscle, for example, uses very little of the serum glucose but continues to rely on free fatty acids and its own catabolized protein as a primary source of energy. It also continues to export amino acids, primarily alanine, for use elsewhere in the body, resulting in a very rapid depletion of body protein stores.

A highly catabolic hospitalized patient may require 35–45 kcal kg^{-1} day^{-1} and 2–3 g of protein kg^{-1} day^{-1}. A patient with severe burns may require even more. A physician has a number of options available to provide this postoperative patient with sufficient calories and protein to ensure optimal recovery. When the patient is simply unable to ingest enough food, it may be adequate to supplement the diet with high-calorie–high-protein preparations, which are usually mixtures of homogenized cornstarch, egg, milk protein, and flavorings. When the patient is unable to ingest solid food or unable to digest complex mixtures of foods adequately, elemental diets are usually administered via a nasogastric tube. Elemental diets consist of small peptides or purified amino acids, glucose and dextrins, some fat, vitamins, and electrolytes. These diets are sometimes sufficient to meet most of the short-term caloric and protein needs of a moderately catabolic patient.

When a patient is severely catabolic or unable to digest and absorb foods normally, parenteral (intravenous) nutrition is necessary. The least invasive method is to use a peripheral, slow-flow vein in a manner similar to any other i.v. infusion. The main limitation of this method is hypertonicity. However, a solution of 5% glucose and 4.25% purified amino acids can be used safely. This solution will usually provide enough protein to maintain positive nitrogen balance but will rarely provide enough calories for long-term maintenance of a catabolic patient.

The most aggressive nutritional therapy is total parenteral nutrition. Usually an indwelling catheter is inserted into a large fast-flow vessel such as the superior vena cava, so that the very hypertonic infusion fluid can rapidly be diluted. This allows solutions of up to 60% glucose and 4.25% amino acids to be used, providing sufficient protein and most of the calories for long-term maintenance. Intravenous lipid infusion is often added to boost calories and provide essential fatty acids. All of these methods can prevent or minimize the negative nitrogen balance associated with surgery and trauma. The actual choice of method depends on the patient's condition. As a general rule it is preferable to use the least invasive technique.

Streat, S. J., and Hill, G. L. Nutritional support in the management of critically ill patients in surgical intensive care. *World J. Surg.* 11:194, 1987; and The Veterans Affairs Total Parenteral Nutrition Cooperative Study Group. Perioperative total parenteral nutrition in surgical patients. *N. Engl. J. Med.* 325:25, 1991.

27.4 ■ PROTEIN–ENERGY MALNUTRITION

The most common form of malnutrition in the world is **protein–energy malnutrition (PEM).** In developing countries inadequate intake of protein and energy is all too common, and it is usually the infants and young children who suffer most. While the symptoms of protein–energy insufficiency vary widely from case to case, it is common to classify most cases as either marasmus or kwashiorkor. **Marasmus** is usually defined as inadequate intake of both protein and energy. **Kwashiorkor** is defined as inadequate intake of protein with adequate energy intake. Often the diets associated with marasmus and kwashiorkor may be similar, with the kwashiorkor being precipitated by conditions of increased protein demand such as infection. The marasmic infant will have a thin, wasted appearance and will be small for his/her age. If PEM continues long enough the child will be permanently stunted in both physical and mental development. In kwashiorkor the child will often have a deceptively plump appearance due to edema. Other telltale symptoms associated with kwashiorkor are dry, brittle hair, diarrhea, dermatitis of various forms, and retarded growth. Perhaps the most devastating result of both marasmus and kwashiorkor is reduced ability of the afflicted individuals to fight off infection. They have a reduced number of T lymphocytes (and thus diminished cell-mediated immune response) as well as defects in the generation of phagocytic cells and production of immunoglobulins, interferon, and other components of the immune system. Many of these individuals die from secondary infections, rather than from the starvation itself.

The most common form of PEM seen in the United States occurs in the hospital setting. A typical course of events is as follows: The patient has not been eating well for several weeks or months prior to entering the hospital due to chronic or debilitating illness. He/she enters the hospital with major trauma, severe infection, or for major surgery, all of which cause a large negative nitrogen balance. This is often compounded by difficulties in feeding the patient or by the necessity of fasting in preparation for surgery or diagnostic tests. The net result is PEM as measured by low levels of serum albumin and other serum proteins or by decreased cellular immunity tests. Recent studies have shown that hospitalized patients with demonstrable PEM have delayed wound healing, decreased resistance to infection, increased mortality, and increased length of hospitalization. Most major hospitals have programs to monitor the nutritional status of their patients and to intervene where necessary to maintain a positive nitrogen and energy balance (see Clin. Corr. 27.3).

27.5 ■ EXCESS PROTEIN–ENERGY INTAKE

Much has been said in recent years about the large amount of protein that the average American consumes. Certainly most consume far more than needed to maintain positive nitrogen balance. An average American currently consumes 99 g of protein, 68% from animal sources. However, most studies show that a healthy adult can consume that amount of protein with no apparent harm. Concern has been raised about possible effects of high-protein intake on calcium requirements. Some studies suggest that high-protein intake increases urinary loss of calcium and may accelerate bone demineralization associated with aging. However, this issue is far from settled.

Obesity Has Dietary and Genetic Components

Perhaps the more serious nutritional problem is excessive energy consumption. In fact, **obesity** is the most frequent nutritional disorder in the United States. It would, however, be unfair to label obesity as simply a problem of excess consumption. Overeating plays an important role in many individuals, as does inadequate exercise, but there is also a strong genetic component as well. While the biochemical mechanisms for this genetic predisposition are unclear, investigators have recently identified an obesity gene in mice that appears to regulate obesity through effects on both appetite and deposition of fat. A similar gene exists in humans, but its metabolic function is still not known (see p. 378). Detailed characterization of this and other genes that predispose to obesity in animals may yield valuable clues to the causes and treatment of obesity in humans.

Metabolic Consequences of Obesity Have Significant Health Implications

A discussion of the treatment of obesity is clearly beyond the scope of this chapter, but it is worthwhile to consider some of the metabolic consequences of obesity. One striking clinical feature of overweight individuals is a marked elevation of serum free fatty acids, cholesterol, and triacylglycerols irrespective of the dietary intake of fat. Why is this? Obesity is obviously associated with an increased number and/or size of adipose cells. These cells contain fewer **insulin receptors** and thus respond more poorly to insulin, resulting in increased activity of the **hormone-sensitive lipase.** The increased lipase activity along with the increased mass of adipose tissue is probably sufficient to explain the increase in circulating **free fatty acids.** These excess fatty acids are carried to the liver and metabolized to acetyl CoA, a precursor for triacylglycerol and cholesterol synthesis. Excess triacylglycerol and cholesterol are released as **very low density lipoprotein particles,** leading to higher circulating levels of both triacylglycerol and cholesterol (see Chapters 9 and 10).

A second striking finding in obese individuals is higher fasting blood sugar levels and decreased glucose tolerance. Fully 80% of **adult-onset diabetics** are overweight. Again the culprit appears to be the decrease in insulin receptors, since many adult-onset diabetics have higher than normal insulin levels. This hyperinsulinemia appears to stimulate the sympathetic nervous system, leading to sodium and water retention and vasoconstriction, which tend to increase blood pressure. Because of these metabolic changes, obesity is a primary risk factor in coronary heart disease, hypertension, and diabetes. This is nutritionally significant because all of these metabolic changes are reversible. Quite often reduction to ideal weight is the single most important aim of nutritional therapy. Furthermore, when the individual is at ideal body weight, the composition of the diet becomes a less important consideration in maintaining normal serum lipid and glucose levels.

Any discussion of weight reduction regimens should include a mention of one other metabolic consequence of obesity. As discussed above, obesity can lead to increased retention of both sodium and water. As the fat stores are metabolized, they produce water (which is denser than the fat), and the water may largely be retained. In fact, some individuals may actually observe short-term weight gain on certain diets, even though the diet is working perfectly well in terms of breaking down their adipose tissue. This metabolic fact of life can be psychologically devastating to dieters, who expect quick results for all their sacrifice.

27.6 ■ CARBOHYDRATES

The chief metabolic role of carbohydrates in the diet is for energy production. Any carbohydrate in excess of that needed for energy is converted to glycogen and triacylglycerol for long-term storage. The body can adapt to a wide range of carbohydrate levels in the diet. Diets high in carbohydrate result in higher steady-state levels of glucokinase and some of the enzymes involved in the hexose monophosphate shunt and triacylglycerol synthesis. Diets low in carbohydrate result in higher steady-state levels of some of the enzymes involved in gluconeogenesis, fatty acid oxidation, and amino acid catabolism. **Glycogen stores** are also affected by the carbohydrate content of the diet (see Clin. Corr. 27.4).

The most common nutritional problems involving carbohydrates are seen in those individuals with various **carbohydrate intolerances.** The most common form of carbohydrate intolerance is **diabetes mellitus,** caused either by lack of insulin production or lack of insulin receptors. This causes an intolerance to glucose and sugars that can readily be converted to glucose. Dietary treatment of diabetes is discussed in Clinical Correlation 27.5. **Lactase insufficiency** is also a common disorder of carbohydrate metabolism affecting over 30 million people in the United States alone. It is most prevalent among blacks, Asians, and Hispanics. Without the enzyme lactase, the lactose is not significantly hydrolyzed or absorbed. It remains in the intestine where it acts osmotically to draw water into the gut and serves as a substrate for conversion to lactic acid, CO_2, and H_2S by intestinal bacteria. The end result is bloating, flatulence, and diarrhea—all of which can be avoided simply by eliminating milk and milk products from the diet (see p. 1075).

CLINICAL CORRELATION 27.4

Carbohydrate Loading and Athletic Endurance

The practice of carbohydrate loading dates back to observations made in the early 1960s that endurance during vigorous exercise was limited primarily by muscle glycogen stores. Of course, the glycogen stores are not the sole energy source for muscle. Free fatty acids are present in the blood during vigorous exercise and are utilized by muscle along with the glycogen stores. Once the glycogen stores have been exhausted, however, muscle cannot rely entirely on free fatty acids without tiring rapidly. This is probably related to the fact that muscle becomes partially anaerobic during vigorous exercise. While glycogen stores are utilized equally well aerobically or anaerobically, fatty acids can only be utilized aerobically. Under those conditions, fatty acids cannot provide ATP rapidly enough to serve as the sole energy source.

Thus the practice of carbohydrate loading to increase glycogen stores was devised for track and other endurance athletes. Originally, it was thought that it would be necessary to trick the body into increasing glycogen stores. The original carbohydrate loading regimen consisted of a 3–4-day period of heavy exercise while on a low-carbohydrate diet, followed by 1–2 days of light exercise while on a high-carbohydrate diet. The initial low-carbohydrate–high-energy demand period caused a depletion of muscle glycogen stores. Apparently, the subsequent change to a high-carbohydrate diet resulted in a slight rebound effect, with the production of higher than normal levels of insulin and growth hormone. Under these conditions glycogen storage was favored and glycogen stores reached almost twice the normal amounts. This practice did increase endurance significantly. In one study, test subjects on a high-fat and high-protein diet had less than 1.6 g of glycogen per 100 g of muscle and could perform a standardized workload for only 60 min. When the same subjects then consumed a high-carbohydrate diet for 3 days, their glycogen stores increased to 4 g per 100 g of muscle and the same workload could be performed for up to 4 h.

While the technique clearly worked, the athletes often felt lethargic and irritable during the low-carbohydrate phase of the regimen, and the high-fat diet ran counter to current health recommendations. Fortunately, recent studies show that regular consumption of a high complex-carbohydrate–low-fat diet during training increases glycogen stores without the need for tricking the body with sudden dietary changes. Current recommendations are for endurance athletes to consume a high-carbohydrate diet (with emphasis on complex carbohydrates) during training. Then carbohydrate intake is increased further (to 70% of calories) and exercise tapered off during the 2–3 days just prior to an athletic event. This procedure increases muscle glycogen stores to levels comparable to the original carbohydrate loading regimen.

Conlee, R. K. Muscle glycogen and exercise endurance: a twenty-year perspective. *Exerc. Sport Sci. Rev.* 15:1, 1987; Ivey, J. L., Katz, A. L., Cutler, C. L., Sherman, W. M., and Cayle, E. F. Muscle glycogen synthesis after exercise: effect of time of carbohydrate ingestion. *J. Appl. Physiol.* 64:1480, 1988; and Probart, C. K., Bird, P. J., and Parker, K. A. Diet and athletic performance. *Med. Clin. North Am.* 77:757, 1993.

CLINICAL CORRELATION 27.5

High-Carbohydrate Versus High-Fat Diets for Diabetics

For years the American Diabetes Association has recommended diets that were low in fat and high in complex carbohydrates and fiber for diabetics. The logic of such a recommendation seemed to be inescapable. Diabetics are prone to hyperlipidemia with attendant risk of heart disease, and low-fat diets appeared likely to reduce risk of hyperlipidemia and heart disease. In addition, numerous clinical studies had suggested that the high-fiber content of these diets resulted in improved control of blood sugar. This recommendation has proved to be controversial. An understanding of the controversies involved illustrates the difficulties in making dietary recommendations for population groups rather than individuals. In the first place, it is very difficult to make any major changes in dietary composition without changing other components of the diet. In fact, most of the clinical trials of the high-carbohydrate–high-fiber diets have resulted in significant weight reduction, either by design or because of the lower caloric density of the diet. Since weight reduction improves diabetic control, it is not entirely clear whether the improvements seen in the treated group were due to the change in diet composition *per se* or because of the weight loss. Second, there is significant individual variation in how diabetics respond to these diets. Many diabetic patients appear to show poorer control (as evidenced by higher blood glucose levels, elevated VLDL and/or LDL levels, and reduced HDL levels) on the high-carbohydrate–high-fiber diets than they do on diets high in monounsaturated fatty acids. However, diets high in monounsaturated fatty acids tend to have higher caloric density and are inappropriate for overweight individuals with type 2 (non-insulin dependent) diabetes. Thus a single diet may not be equally appropriate for all diabetics. Even the "glycemic index" concept (Table 27.2) may also turn out to be difficult to apply to the diabetic population as a whole, because of individual variation. Thus in 1994 the American Diabetes Association abandoned the concept of a single diabetic diet. Instead, their recommendations focus on achievement of glucose, lipid, and blood pressure goals, with weight reduction and dietary recommendations based on individual preferences and what works best to achieve metabolic control in that individual.

Anderson, J. W., Gustafson, N. J., Bryant, C. A., and Tietyen-Clark, J. Dietary fiber and diabetes: a comprehensive review and practical application. *J. Am. Diet Assoc.* 87:1189, 1987; Jenkins, D. J. A., Wolener, T. M. S., Jenkins, A. L., and Taylor, R. H. Dietary fiber, carbohydrate metabolism and diabetes. *Mol. Aspects Med.* 9:97, 1987; Garg, A., Grundy, S. M., and Unger, R. H. Comparison of the effects of high and low carbohydrate diets on plasma lipoproteins and insulin sensitivity in patients with mild NIDDM. *Diabetes* 41;1278, 1992; and American Diabetes Association. Nutritional recommendations and principles for people with diabetes. *Diabetes Care* 17:519, 1994.

27.7 ■ FATS

Triacylglycerols, or fats, are directly utilized by many tissues of the body as an energy source and, as phospholipids, are an important part of membrane structure. Excess fat in the diet can only be stored as triacylglycerol. As with carbohydrate, the body adapts to a wide range of fat intakes. However, problems develop at the extremes (either high or low) of fat consumption. At the low end, **essential fatty acid (EFA)** deficiencies may become a problem. The fatty acids linoleic, linolenic, and arachidonic acid cannot be made by the body and thus are essential components of the diet. These EFAs are needed for maintaining the function and integrity of membrane structure, for fat metabolism and transport, and for synthesis of **prostaglandins.** The most characteristic symptom of essential fatty acid deficiency is a scaly dermatitis. EFA deficiency is very rare in the United States, occurring primarily in low-birth-weight infants fed artificial formulas lacking EFA and in hospitalized patients maintained on total parenteral nutrition for long periods of time. At the high end of the scale, there is concern that excess dietary fat causes elevation of serum lipids and thus an increased risk of heart disease. Recent studies also suggest that high-fat intakes are associated with increased risk of colon, breast, and prostate cancer, but it is not yet certain whether the cancer risk is associated with fat intake *per se* or with the excess calories associated with a high-fat diet. To the extent that fat intake is associated with cancer risk, animal studies suggest that polyunsaturated fatty acids of the ω-6 series may be more tumorigenic than other unsaturated fatty acids. The reason for this is not known, but it has been suggested that prostaglandins derived from the ω-6 fatty acids may stimulate tumor progression.

27.8 ■ FIBER

Dietary fiber is defined as those components of food that cannot be broken down by human digestive enzymes. It is incorrect, however, to assume that fiber is indigestible since some fibers are, in fact, at least partially broken down by intestinal bacteria. Knowledge of the role of fiber in human metabolism has expanded significantly in the past decade. Our current understanding of the metabolic roles of dietary fiber is based on three important observations: (1) there are several different types of dietary fiber, (2) they each have different chemical and physical properties, and (3) they each have different effects on human metabolism, which can be understood, in part, from their unique properties.

The major types of fiber and their properties are summarized in Table 27.1. **Cellulose** and most **hemicelluloses** increase stool bulk and decrease transit time. These are the types of fiber that should most properly be associated with the effects of fiber on regularity. They decrease intracolonic pressure and appear to play a beneficial role with respect to diverticular diseases. By diluting out potential carcinogens and speeding their transit through the colon, they may also play a role in reducing the risk of colon cancer. **Lignins** have a slightly different role. In addition to their bulk-enhancing properties, they adsorb organic substances such as cholesterol and appear to have a cholesterol-lowering effect. **Mucilaginous fibers,** such as pectin and gums, tend to form viscous gels in the stomach and intestine and slow the rate of gastric emptying, thus slowing the rate of absorption of many nutrients. The most important clinical role of these fibers is to slow the rate at which carbohydrates are digested and absorbed. Thus both the rise in blood sugar and the subsequent rise in insulin levels are significantly decreased if these fibers are ingested along with carbohydrate-containing foods. **Water-soluble fibers** (pectins, gums, some hemicelluloses, and storage polysaccharides) also help to lower serum cholesterol levels in most people. Whether this is due to their effect on insulin levels (insulin

TABLE 27.1 Major Types of Fiber and Their Properties

Type of Fiber	*Major Source in Diet*	*Chemical Properties*	*Physiological Effects*
Cellulose	Unrefined cereals Bran Whole wheat	Nondigestible Water insoluble Absorbs water	Increases stool bulk Decreases intestinal transit time Decreases intracolonic pressure
Hemicellulose	Unrefined cereals Some fruits and vegetables Whole wheat	Partially digestible Usually water insoluble Absorbs water	Increases stool bulk Decreases intestinal transit time Decreases intracolonic pressure
Lignin	Woody parts of vegetables	Nondigestible Water insoluble Absorbs organic substances	Increases stool bulk Bind cholesterol Bind carcinogens
Pectin	Fruits	Digestible Water soluble Mucilaginous	Decreases rate of gastric emptying Decreases rate of sugar uptake Decreases serum cholesterol
Gums	Dried beans Oats	Digestible Water soluble Mucilaginous	Decreases rate of gastric emptying Decreases rate of sugar uptake Decreases serum cholesterol

stimulates cholesterol synthesis and export) or to other metabolic effects (perhaps caused by end products of partial bacterial digestion) is unknown. Vegetables, wheat, and most grain fibers are the best sources of the water-insoluble cellulose, hemicellulose, and lignin. Fruits, oats, and legumes are the best source of the water-soluble fibers. Obviously, a balanced diet should include food sources of both soluble and insoluble fiber.

27.9 ■ COMPOSITION OF MACRONUTRIENTS IN THE DIET

From the foregoing discussion it is apparent that there are relatively few instances of macronutrient deficiencies in the American diet. Thus much of the interest in recent years has focused on whether there is an ideal diet composition consistent with good health. It would be easy to pass off such discussions as purely academic, yet our understanding of these issues could well be vital. Heart disease, stroke, and cancer kill many Americans each year, and if some experts are even partially correct, many of these deaths could be preventable with prudent diet.

Composition of the Diet Affects Serum Cholesterol

With respect to heart disease, the current discussion centers around two key issues: (1) Can serum cholesterol and triacylglycerol levels be controlled by diet? (2) Does lowering serum cholesterol and triacylglycerol levels protect against heart disease? The controversies centered around dietary control of cholesterol levels illustrate perfectly the trap one falls into by trying to look too closely at each individual component of the diet instead of the diet as a whole. For example, there are at least four dietary components that can be identified as having an effect on serum cholesterol: cholesterol itself, **polyunsaturated fatty acids (PUFAs), saturated fatty acids (SFAs),** and fiber. It would seem that the more cholesterol one eats, the higher the serum cholesterol should be. However, cholesterol synthesis is tightly regulated via a feedback control at the hydroxymethylglutaryl-CoA reductase step, so decreases in dietary cholesterol have relatively little effect on serum cholesterol levels (see p. 415). One can obtain a more significant reduction in cholesterol and triacylglycerol levels by increasing the ratio of PUFA/SFA in the diet. Finally, some plant fibers, especially the water-soluble fibers, appear to decrease cholesterol levels significantly.

While the effects of various lipids in the diet can be dramatic, the biochemistry of their action is still uncertain. Saturated fats inhibit receptor-mediated uptake of LDL, but the mechanism is complex. Palmitic acid (saturated, C16) raises cholesterol levels while stearic acid (saturated, C18) is neutral. Polyunsaturated fatty acids lower both LDL and HDL cholesterol levels, while oleic acid (monounsaturated, C18) appears to lower LDL without affecting HDL levels. Furthermore, the ω-3 and ω-6 polyunsaturated fatty acids have slightly different effects on lipid profiles (see Clin. Corr. 27.6). However, these mechanistic complexities do not significantly affect dietary recommendations. Most foods high in saturated fats contain both palmitic and stearic acid and are atherogenic. The data showing oleic acid lowers LDL levels mean that olive oil, and possibly peanut oil, may be considered as beneficial as polyunsaturated oils.

There is very little disagreement with respect to these data. The question is, what can be done with the information? Much of the disagreement arises from the tendency to look at each dietary factor in isolation. For example, it is debatable whether it is worthwhile placing a patient on a highly restrictive 300-mg cholesterol diet (1 egg = 213 mg of cholesterol) if his serum cholesterol is lowered by only 5–10%. Likewise, changing the **PUFA/SFA ratio** from 0.3 (the current value) to 1.0 would either require a radical change in the diet by elimination of foods containing saturated fat (largely meats and fats) or an addition of large amounts of rather unpalatable polyunsaturated fats to the diet. For many Americans this would be unrealistic. Fiber is another good example. One could expect, at the most, a 5% decrease in serum cholesterol by adding any reasonable amount of fiber to the diet. (Very few people would eat the

CLINICAL CORRELATION 27.6

Polyunsaturated Fatty Acids and Risk Factors for Heart Disease

Recent studies confirming that reduction of elevated serum cholesterol levels can reduce risk of heart disease have rekindled interest in the effects of diet on serum cholesterol levels and other risk factors for heart disease. We have known for years that one of the most important dietary factors regulating serum cholesterol levels is the ratio of polyunsaturated fats (PUFAs) to saturated fats (SFAs) in the diet. One of the most interesting recent developments is the discovery that different types of polyunsaturated fatty acids have different effects on lipid metabolism and on other risk factors for heart disease. As discussed in Chapter 9, there are two families of polyunsaturated essential fatty acids—the ω-6, or linoleic family, and the ω-3, or linolenic family. Recent clinical studies have shown that the ω-6 PUFAs (chief dietary source is linoleic acid from plants and vegetable oils) primarily decrease serum cholesterol levels, with only modest effects on triacylglycerol levels. The ω-3 PUFAs (chief dietary source is eicosapentaenoic acid from certain ocean fish and fish oils) cause modest decreases in serum cholesterol levels and significantly lower triacylglycerol levels. The biochemical mechanism behind these different effects on serum lipid levels is unknown.

The ω-3 PUFAs have yet another unique physiological effect that may decrease the risk of heart disease—they decrease platelet aggregation. The mechanism of this effect is a little clearer. Arachidonic acid (ω-6 family) is known to be a precursor of thromboxane A_2 (TXA_2), which is a potent proaggregating agent, and prostaglandin I_2 (PGI_2), which is a weak antiaggregating agent (see p. 436). The ω-3 PUFAs are thought to act by one of two mechanisms: (1) Eicosapentaenoic acid (ω-3 family) may be converted to thromboxane A_3 (TXA_3), which is only weakly proaggregating, and prostaglandin I_3 (PGI_3), which is strongly antiaggregating. Thus the balance between proaggregation and antiaggregation would be shifted toward a more antiaggregating condition as the ω-3 PUFAs displace ω-6 PUFAs as a source of precursors to the thromboxanes and prostaglandins. (2) The ω-3 PUFAs may also act by simply inhibiting the conversion of arachidonic acid to TXA_2.

The unique potential of eicosapentaenoic acid and other ω-3 PUFAs in reducing the risk of heart disease is being tested in numerous clinical trials. Although the results may affect dietary recommendations in the future, it is well to keep in mind that no long-term clinical studies of the ω-3 PUFAs have been carried out. No major health organization has recommended that we replace ω-6 with ω-3 PUFAs in the American diet.

Holub, B. J. Dietary fish oils containing eicosapentaenoic acid and the prevention of atherosclerosis and thrombosis. *Can. Med. Assoc. J.* 139:377, 1988; Simopoulos, A. P. Omega-3 fatty acids in health and disease and in growth and development. *Am. J. Clin. Nutr.* 54:438, 1991; and Gapinski, J. P., Van Ruiswyk, J. V., Heudebert, G. R., and Schectman, G. S. Preventing restenosis with fish-oils following coronary angioplasty. A meta-analysis. *Arch. Intern. Med.* 153:1595, 1993.

ten apples per day needed to lower serum cholesterol by 15%.) Are we to conclude then that any dietary means of controlling cholesterol levels is useless? Only if each element of the diet is examined in isolation. For example, recent studies have shown that vegetarians, who have lower cholesterol intakes plus higher PUFA/SFA ratios and higher fiber intakes, may average 25–30% lower cholesterol levels than their nonvegetarian counterparts. Perhaps, more to the point, diet modifications of the type acceptable to the average American have been shown to cause a 10–15% decrease in cholesterol levels in long-term studies. A 7-year clinical trial sponsored by the National Institutes of Health has proved conclusively that lowering serum cholesterol levels reduces the risk of heart disease in men. It is important to keep in mind that serum cholesterol is just one of many risk factors.

Effects of Refined Carbohydrate in the Diet Are Not Straightforward

Much of the nutritional dispute in the area of carbohydrates centers around the amount of *refined carbohydrate* in the diet. In the past, simple sugars (primarily sucrose) have been blamed for almost every ill from tooth decay to heart disease and diabetes. In the case of tooth decay, these assertions were clearly correct. In the case of heart disease, however, the linkage is more obscure (see Clin. Corr. 27.7). The situation with respect to diabetes is probably even less direct. Whereas restriction of simple sugars is often desirable in patients who already have diabetes, recent studies show less than expected correlation between the type of carbohydrate ingested and the subsequent rise in serum glucose levels (Table 27.2). Ice cream, for example, causes a much smaller increase in serum glucose levels than either potatoes or whole wheat bread. It turns out that other components of food—such as protein, fat, and the soluble fibers—are much more important than the type of carbohydrate present in determining how rapidly glucose will enter the bloodstream.

CLINICAL CORRELATION 27.7

Metabolic Adaptation: The Relationship Between Carbohydrate Intake and Serum Triacylglycerols

In evaluating the nutrition literature, it is important to be aware that most clinical trials are of rather short duration (2–6 weeks), while some metabolic adaptations may take considerably longer. Thus even apparently well-designed clinical studies may lead to erroneous conclusions that will be repeated in the popular literature for years to come. For example, several studies carried out in the 1960s and 1970s tried to assess the effects of carbohydrate intake on serum triacylglycerol levels. Typically, young college-age males were given a diet in which up to 50% of their fat calories were replaced with sucrose or other simple sugars for a period of 2–3 weeks. In most cases serum triacylglycerol levels increased markedly (up to 50%). This led to the tentative conclusion that high intake of simple sugars, particularly sucrose, might increase the risk of heart disease, a notion that was popularized by nutritional best sellers such as "Sugar Blues" and "Sweet and Dangerous." Unfortunately, while the original conclusions were promoted in the lay press, the experiments themselves were questioned. Subsequent studies showed that if these trials were continued for longer periods of time (3–6 months), the triacylglycerol levels usually normalized. The nature of this slow metabolic adaptation is unknown.

It should be noted that while the interpretation of the original clinical trials may have been faulty, the ensuing dietary recommendations may not have been entirely incorrect. Many of the snack and convenience foods in the American diet that are high in sugar are also high in fat and in caloric density. Thus removing some of these foods from the diet can aid in weight control, and being overweight is known to contribute to hypertriacylglycerolemia. Also, some individuals exhibit carbohydrate-induced hypertriacylglycerolemia. Triacylglycerol levels in these individuals respond dramatically to diets that substitute foods containing complex carbohydrates and fiber for these foods containing primarily simple sugars as a carbohydrate source.

MacDonald, I. Effects of dietary carbohydrates on serum lipids. *Prog. Biochem. Pharmacol.* 8:216, 1973; and Vrana, A., and Fabry, P. Metabolic effects of high sucrose or fructose intake. *World Rev. Nutr. Diet* 42:56, 1983.

TABLE 27.2 Glycemic Index[a] of Some Selected Foods

Grain and cereal products		Root vegetables	
Bread (white)	69 ± 5	Beets	64 ± 16
Bread (whole wheat)	72 ± 6	Carrots	92 ± 20
Rice (white)	72 ± 9	Potato (white)	70 ± 8
Sponge cake	46 ± 6	Potato (sweet)	48 ± 6
Breakfast cereals		Dried legumes	
All bran	51 ± 5	Beans (kidney)	29 ± 8
Cornflakes	80 ± 6	Beans (soy)	15 ± 5
Oatmeal	49 ± 8	Peas (blackeye)	33 ± 4
Shredded wheat	67 ± 10		
Vegetables		Fruits	
Sweet corn	59 ± 11	Apple (Golden Delicious)	39 ± 3
Frozen peas	51 ± 6	Banana	62 ± 9
		Oranges	40 ± 3
Dairy products		Sugars	
Ice cream	36 ± 8	Fructose	20 ± 5
Milk (whole)	34 ± 6	Glucose	100
Yogurt	36 ± 4	Honey	87 ± 8
		Sucrose	59 ± 10

Source: Data from Jenkins, D. A., et al. Glycemic index of foods: a physiological basis for carbohydrate exchange. *Am. J. Clin. Nutr.* 34:362, 1981.

[a] Glycemic index is defined as the area under the blood glucose response curve for each food expressed as a percentage of the area after taking the same amount of carbohydrate as glucose (mean: 5–10 individuals).

Mixed Vegetable and Animal Proteins Meet Nutritional Protein Requirements

Concern has been voiced recently about the type of protein in the American diet. Epidemiologic data and animal studies suggest that consumption of animal protein is associated with increased incidence of heart disease and various forms of cancer. One could assume that it is probably not the animal protein itself that is involved, but the associated fat and cholesterol. What sort of protein should we consume? Although the present diet may not be optimal, a strictly vegetarian diet may not be acceptable to many Americans. Perhaps a middle road is best. Clearly, there are no known health dangers associated with a mixed diet that is lower in animal protein than the current American standard.

An Increase in Fiber from Varied Sources Is Desirable

Because of our current knowledge about effects of fiber on human metabolism, most suggestions for a prudent diet recommend an increase in dietary fiber. The main question is: "How much is enough?" The current fiber content of the American diet is about 14–15 g per day. Most experts feel that an increase to at least 25–30 g would be safe and beneficial. Since we know that different fibers have different metabolic roles, this increase in fiber intake should come from a wide variety of fiber sources—including fresh fruits, vegetables, and legumes as well as the more popular cereal sources of fiber (which are primarily cellulose and hemicellulose).

Current Recommendations Are for a "Prudent Diet"

Several private and governmental groups have made specific recommendations with respect to the ideal dietary composition for the American public in recent years. This movement was spearheaded by the Senate Select Committee on Human Nutrition, which first published its *Dietary Goals for the United States* in 1977. The Senate Select Committee recommended that the American public reduce consumption of total calories, total fat, saturated fat, cholesterol, simple sugars, and salt to "ideal" goals more compatible with good health (Figure 27.2). In recent years the USDA, the American Heart Association, the American Diabetes Association, the National Research Council, and the Surgeon General all have published similar recommendations, and the USDA has used these recommendations to design revised recommendations for a balanced diet (Figure 27.3). These recommendations have become popularly known as the **prudent diet.** How valid is the scientific basis of the recommendations for a prudent diet? Is there evidence that a prudent diet will improve the health of the general public? These remain controversial questions.

An important argument against such recommendations is that we presently do not have enough information to set concrete goals. We might be creating some problems while solving others. For example, the goals of reducing total fat and saturated fat in the diet are best met by replacing animal protein with vegetable protein. This might reduce the amount of available iron and vitamin B_{12} in the diet. It is also quite clear that the same set of guidelines do not apply for every individual. For example, exercise is known to raise serum HDL cholesterol and obesity is known to elevate cholesterol and triacylglycerols and reduce glucose tolerance. Thus the very active individual who maintains ideal body weight can likely tolerate higher fat and sugar intakes than an obese individual.

On the "pro" side, however, it clearly can be argued that all of the dietary recommendations are in the right direction for reducing nutritional risk factors in the general population. Besides, similar diets have been consumed by our ancestors and by people in other countries with no apparent harm. Whatever

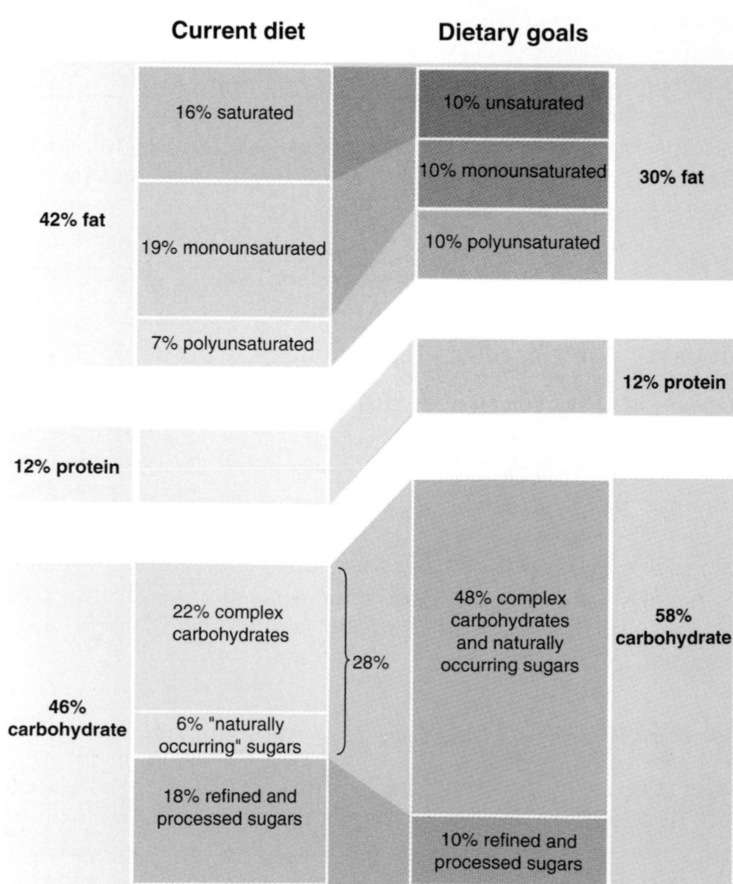

FIGURE 27.2
United States dietary goals.
Graphical comparison of the composition of the current U.S. diet and the dietary goals for the U.S. population suggested by the Senate Select Committee on Human Nutrition.
From Dietary Goals for the United States, *2nd ed. Washington, DC: U.S. Government Printing Office, 1977.*

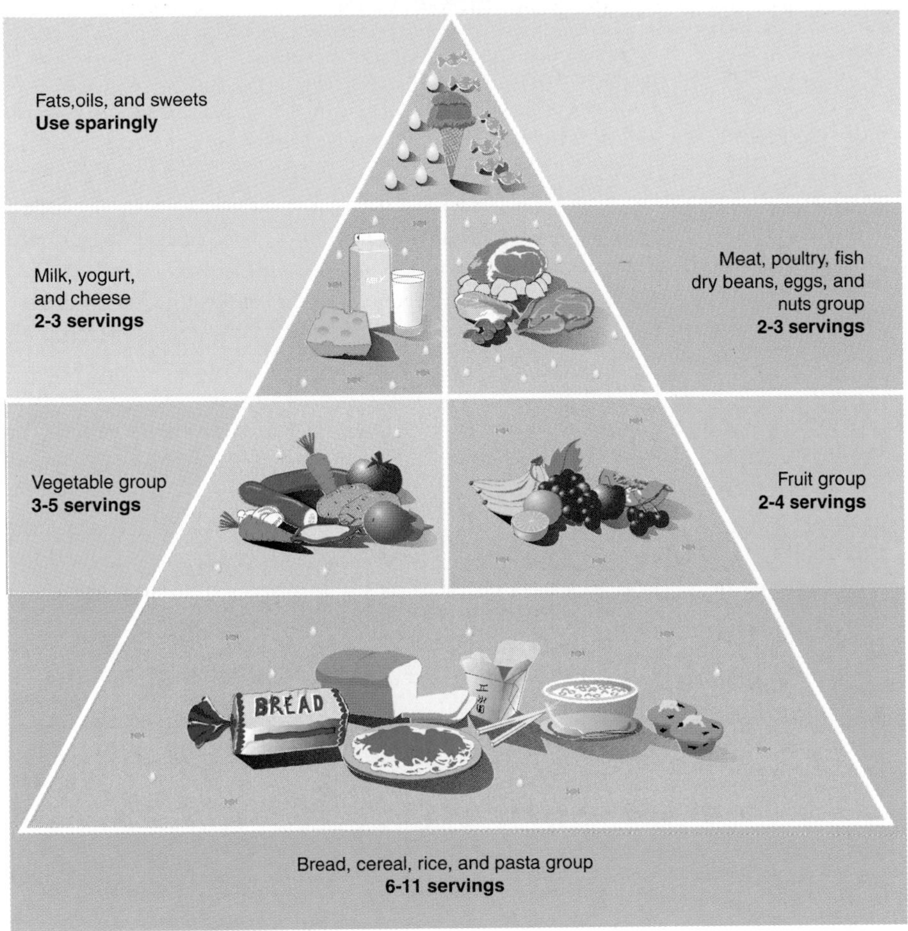

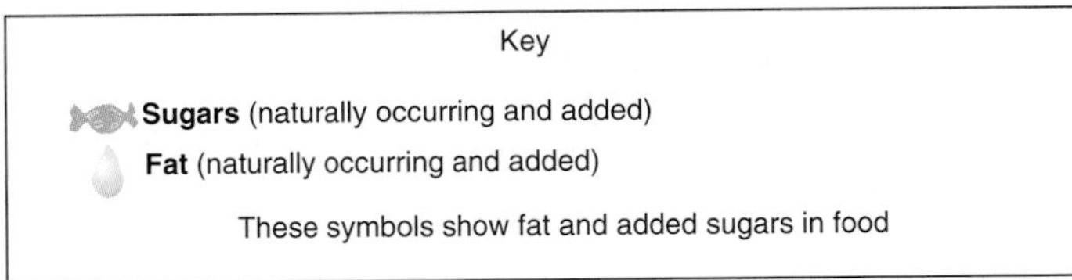

FIGURE 27.3
USDA food pyramid.
Graphical representation of USDA recommendations for a balanced diet.
HG Bulletin #252. Washington, DC: U.S. Government Printing Office, 1992.

the outcome of this debate, it will undoubtedly shape much of our ideas concerning the role of nutrition in medicine.

BIBLIOGRAPHY

Protein Energy Malnutrition in Hospitalized Patients

The Veterans Affairs Total Parenteral Nutrition Cooperative Study Group. Perioperative total parenteral nutrition in surgical patients. *N. Engl. J. Med.* 325:525, 1991.

Metabolic Consequences of Obesity

Hershcopf, R. J., and Bradlow, H. L. Obesity, diet, endogenous estrogens, and the risk of hormone-sensitive cancer. *Am. J. Clin. Nutr.* 45:283, 1987.

Maxwell, M. H., and Waks, A. U. Obesity and hypertension. *Bibl. Cardiol.* 41:29, 1987.

Pi-Sunyer, F. X. Health implications of obesity. *Am. J. Clin. Nutr.* 53:15955, 1991.

Simopoulos, A. P. Obesity and carcinogenesis: historical perspective. *Am. J. Clin. Nutr.* 45:271, 1987.

Metabolic Predisposition to Obesity

Bjorntorp, P. Fat cell distribution and metabolism. *Ann. N.Y. Acad. Sci.* 499:66, 1987.

Bray, G. A. Obesity—a disease of nutrient or energy balance? *Nutr. Rev.* 45:33, 1987.

Campfield, L. A., Smith, F. J., Guisez, Y., Devos, R., and Burn, P. Recombinant mouse OB protein: evidence for a peripheral signal linking adiposity and central neural networks. *Science* 269:546, 1995.

Dulloo, A. G., and Miller, D. S. Obesity: a disorder of the sympathetic nervous system. *World Rev. Nutr. Diet.* 50:1, 1987.

Halaas, J. L., Gajiwala, K. S., Maffei, M., Cohen, S. L., Chait, B. T., Rabinowitz, D., Lallone, R. L., Burley, S. K., and Friedman, J. M. Weight-reducing effects of the plasma protein encoded by the obese gene. *Science* 269:543, 1995.

Complex Carbohydrates and Fiber

Anderson, J. W. Fiber and health: an overview. *Am. J. Gastroenterol.* 81:892, 1986.

Eastwood, M. Dietary fiber and the risk of cancer. *Nutr. Rev.* 45:193, 1987.

Miller, J. C. B. Importance of glycemic index in diabetes. *Am. J. Clin. Nutr.* 59(Suppl.):747S, 1994.

Shankar, S., and Lanza, E. Dietary fiber and cancer prevention. *Hematol. Oncol. Clin. North Am.* 5:25, 1991.

Wolever, T. M. S., Jenkins, D. J. A., Jenkins, A. L., and Josse, R. G. The glycemic index: methodology and clinical implications. *Am. J. Clin. Nutr.* 54:846, 1991.

Macronutrient Composition and Health

Gardener, C. D., and Kraemer, H. C. Monounsaturated versus polyunsaturated dietary fat and serum lipids. *Arterioscler. Thromb. Vasc. Biol.* 15:1917,1995.

Gorlin, R. The biological actions and potential clinical significance of dietary ω-3 fatty acids. *Arch. Intern. Med.* 148:2043, 1988.

Grundy, S. M. Monounsaturated fatty acids, plasma cholesterol, and coronary heart disease. *Am. J. Clin. Nutr.* 45:1168, 1987.

Grundy, S. M., et al. Rationale of the diet—heart statement of the American Heart Association, news from the American Heart Association. *Circulation* 65:839A, 1982.

Kisselbah, A., and Schetman, G. Polyunsaturated and saturated fat, cholesterol, and fatty acid supplementation. *Diabetes Care* 11:129, 1988.

Kritchevsky, D., and Klurfeld, D. M. Caloric effects in experimental mammary tumorigenesis. *Am. J. Clin. Nutr.* 45:236, 1987.

Rasmussen, O. W., Thomsen, C., Hansen, K. W., Vesterland, M., Winther, E., and Hermansen, K. Effects on blood pressure, glucose, and lipid levels of a high monounsaturated fat diet compared with a high-carbohydrate diet in NIDDM subjects. *Diabetes Care* 16:156S, 1993.

Simopoulus, A. P. Omega-3 Fatty Acids in Health and Disease and in Growth and Development. *Am. J. Clin. Nutr.* 54:438, 1991.

Welsh, C. W. Enhancement of mammary tumorigenesis by dietary fat: review of potential mechanisms. *Am. J. Clin. Nutr.* 45:191, 1987.

Dietary Recommendations

American Heart Association. *Recommendations for Treatment of Hyperlipidemia in Adults.* Dallas: American Heart Association, 1984.

Food and Nutrition Board of the National Academy of Sciences. *Towards Healthful Diets.* Washington, DC: U.S. Government Printing Office, 1980.

National Research Council. *Diet, Nutrition and Cancer.* Washington, DC: National Academy Press, 1982.

Senate Select Committee on Human Nutrition. *Dietary Goals for the United States,* 2nd ed., Stock No. 052-070-04376-8. Washington, DC: U.S. Government Printing Office, 1977.

Truswell, A. S. Evolution of dietary recommendations, goals, and guidelines. *Am. J. Clin. Nutr.* 45:1060, 1987.

U.S. Department of Agriculture. *Nutrition and Your Health, Dietary Guidelines for Americans,* Stock No. 017-001-00416-2. Washington, DC: U.S. Government Printing Office, 1980.

U.S. Department of Agriculture. *The Food Guide Pyramid,* Stock No. HSG-252. Hyattsville, MD: Human Nutrition Information Service, 1992.

U.S. Department of Health and Human Services. *The Surgeon General's Report on Nutrition and Health,* Stock No. 017-001-00465-1. Washington, DC: U.S. Government Printing Office, 1988.

QUESTIONS ■ C. N. ANGSTADT AND J. BAGGOTT

1. Of two people with approximately the same weight, the one with the higher basal energy requirement would most likely be:
   A. taller.
   B. female if the other were male.
   C. older.
   D. under less stress.
   E. all of the above.

2. Basal metabolic rate:
   A. is not influenced by energy intake.
   B. increases in response to starvation.
   C. may decrease up to 50% during periods of starvation.
   D. increases in direct proportion to energy expenditure.
   E. is not responsive to changes in hormone levels.

3. The primary effect of the consumption of excess protein beyond the body's immediate needs will be:
   A. excretion of the excess as protein in the urine.
   B. an increase in the "storage pool" of protein.
   C. an increased synthesis of muscle protein.
   D. an enhancement in the amount of circulating plasma proteins.
   E. an increase in the amount of adipose tissue.

4. Which of the following individuals would most likely be in nitrogen equilibrium?
   A. a normal, adult male
   B. a normal, pregnant female
   C. a growing child
   D. an adult male recovering from surgery
   E. a normal female on a very low protein diet

5. Vegetarian diets:
   A. cannot meet the body's requirements for all of the essential amino acids.
   B. contain only protein that is very readily digestible.
   C. are adequate as long as two different vegetables are consumed in the same meal.
   D. would require less total protein than meat proteins to meet the requirement for all of the essential amino acids.
   E. require that proteins consumed have essential amino acid contents that complement each other.

6. In which of the following circumstances would a protein intake of 0.8 g of protein kg^{-1} (body weight) day^{-1} probably be adequate?
   A. vegetarian diet
   B. infancy
   C. severe burn
   D. about 85–90% of total calories supplied by carbohydrate and fat
   E. pregnancy

7. Kwashiorkor is:
   A. the most common form of protein–calorie malnutrition in the United States.
   B. characterized by a thin, wasted appearance.
   C. an inadequate intake of food of any kind.

D. an adequate intake of total calories but a specific deficiency of protein.
E. an adequate intake of total protein but a deficiency of the essential amino acids.

8. An excessive intake of calories:
   A. usually does not have adverse metabolic consequences.
   B. leads to metabolic changes that are usually irreversible.
   C. frequently leads to elevated serum levels of free fatty acids, cholesterol, and triglycerides.
   D. is frequently associated with an increased number of insulin receptors.
   E. is the only component of obesity.

9. A diet very low in carbohydrate:
   A. would cause weight loss because there would be no way to replenish citric acid cycle intermediates.
   B. would result in no significant metabolic changes.
   C. could lead to a chronic ketosis.
   D. would lead to water retention.
   E. would be the diet of choice for a diabetic.

10. Lactase insufficiency:
    A. is a more serious disease than diabetes mellitus.
    B. has no clinical symptoms.
    C. causes an intolerance to glucose.
    D. causes an intolerance to milk and milk products.
    E. affects utilization of milk by the liver.

11. Dietary fat:
    A. is usually present, although there is no specific need for it.
    B. if present in excess, can be stored as either glycogen or adipose tissue triacylglycerol.
    C. should include linoleic and linolenic acids.
    D. should increase on an endurance training program in order to increase the body's energy stores.
    E. if present in excess, does not usually lead to health problems.

12. Which of the following statements about dietary fiber is/are correct?
    A. Water-soluble fiber helps to lower serum cholesterol in most people.
    B. Mucilaginous fiber slows the rate of digestion and absorption of carbohydrates.
    C. Insoluble fiber increases stool bulk and decreases transit time.
    D. All of the above are correct.
    E. None of the above is correct.

13. Which one of the following dietary regimens would be *most* effective in lowering serum cholesterol?
    A. restrict dietary cholesterol
    B. increase the ratio of polyunsaturated to saturated fatty acids
    C. increase fiber content
    D. restrict cholesterol and increase fiber
    E. restrict cholesterol, increase PUFA/SFA, increase fiber

14. Most nutrition experts currently agree that an excessive consumption of sugar causes:
    A. tooth decay.
    B. diabetes.
    C. heart disease.
    D. permanently elevated triacylglycerol levels.
    E. all of the above.

Refer to the following for Questions 15 and 16:
   A. 10% of total calories
   B. 12% of total calories
   C. 30% of total calories
   D. 48% of total calories
   E. 58% of total calories

15. The dietary goal recommended by the Senate Select Committee on Human Nutrition for Polyunsaturated fatty acids.

16. The dietary goal recommended by the Senate Select Committee on Human Nutrition for complex carbohydrates and naturally occurring sugars.

17. A complete replacement of animal protein in the diet by vegetable protein:
    A. would be expected to have no effect at all on the overall diet.
    B. would reduce the total amount of food consumed for the same number of calories.
    C. might reduce the total amount of iron and vitamin B_{12} available.
    D. would be satisfactory regardless of the nature of the vegetable protein used.
    E. could not satisfy protein requirements.

ANSWERS

1. A A taller person with the same weight would have a greater surface area. B: Males have higher energy requirements than females. C: Energy requirements decrease with age. D: Stress, probably because of the effects of epinephrine and cortisol, increase energy requirements (pp. 1088–1089).
2. C This is part of the survival mechanism in starvation. A and B: BMR decreases when energy intake decreases. D: BMR as defined (p. 1088) is independent of energy expenditure. Only when the exercise is repeated on a daily basis so that lean muscle mass is increased does BMR also increase. E: Many hormones increase BMR (p. 1089).
3. E Excess protein is treated like any other excess energy source and stored (minus the nitrogen) eventually as adipose tissue fat (p. 1089). A: Protein is not found in normal urine except in very small amounts. The excess nitrogen is excreted as NH_4^+ and urea, whereas the excess carbon skeletons of the amino acids are used as energy sources. B–D: There is no discrete storage form of protein, and although some muscle and structural protein is expendable, there is no evidence that increased intake leads to generalized increased protein synthesis.

4. A B, C, and D: Although normal, pregnancy is also a period of growth, requiring positive balance, as does a period of convalescence. E: Inadequate protein intake leads to negative balance (p. 1100).
5. E A–E: It is possible to have adequate protein intake on a vegetarian diet provided enough is consumed (protein content is generally low and may be more difficult to digest) and there is a mixture of proteins that supplies all of the essential amino acids since individual proteins are frequently deficient in one or more foods (Clin. Corr. 27.1, p. 1091).
6. D This level of calories from carbohydrate and fat is more than adequate for protein sparing. A: Essential amino acids are low in vegetable protein. B, C, and E: Periods of rapid growth require extra protein, as does major trauma (p. 1092).
7. D A: The most common protein–calorie malnutrition occurs in severely ill, hospitalized patients who would be more likely to have generalized malnutrition. B and C: These are the characteristics of marasmus. E: This would lead to negative nitrogen balance but does not have a specific name (p. 1093).
8. C Probably because an increased number and/or size of adipose cells will contain fewer insulin receptors. A: Excess caloric intake will lead to obesity if continued long enough. B: Fortunately, most of the changes accompanying obesity can be reversed if weight is lost. D: Many of the adverse effects of obesity are associated with an increased number of adipocytes that are deficient in insulin receptors. E: Inadequate exercise and genetic components also play roles in obesity (pp. 1094–1095).
9. C A: This is a popular myth but untrue because many amino acids are glucogenic. B and C: The liver adapts by increasing gluconeogenesis, fatty acid oxidation, and ketone body production. D: Low carbohydrate leads to a depletion of glycogen with its stored water, accounting for rapid initial weight loss on this kind of diet (p. 1095, Clin. Corr. 27.4). E: Diabetic diets need to be individualized. There is currently no generalized recommendation for the carbohydrate content of a diabetic diet (p. 1095 and Clinical Correlation 27.5).
10. D B, D, and E: Lactase insufficiency is an inability to digest the sugar in milk products, causing intestinal symptoms, but is easily treated by eliminating milk products from the diet. A and C: Diabetes, caused by inadequate insulin or insulin receptors, inhibits appropriate utilization of glucose (p. 1095).
11. C A and C: Linoleic and linolenic acids are essential fatty acids and so must be present in the diet. B and D: Excess carbohydrate can be stored as fat but the reverse is not true. D: Carbohydrate loading has been shown to increase endurance. E: High-fat diets are associated with many health risks (p. 1096, Clin. Corr. 27.5).
12. D These each illustrate the different properties and roles of the common kinds of fiber (p. 1097).
13. E Any of the measures alone would decrease serum cholesterol slightly, but to achieve a reduction of more than 15% requires all three (pp. 1098–1100).
14. A This is the only direct linkage shown. B and C: There may be an association with these conditions but not a direct cause–effect relationship. D: Transient elevations may occur on an isocaloric switch from a high-starch to a high-simple-sugar diet but not a permanent elevation (p. 1100).
15. A See Figure 27.2, p. 1102.
16. D See Figure 27.2, p. 1102.
17. C A and C: This would reduce the amount of fat, especially saturated fat, but could also reduce the amount of necessary nutrients that come primarily from animal sources. B: The protein content of vegetables is quite low, so much larger amounts of vegetables would have to be consumed. D and E: It is possible to satisfy requirements for all of the essential amino acids completely if vegetables with complementary amino acid patterns, in proper amounts, are consumed (p. 1101, Clin. Corr. 27.1).

CHAPTER

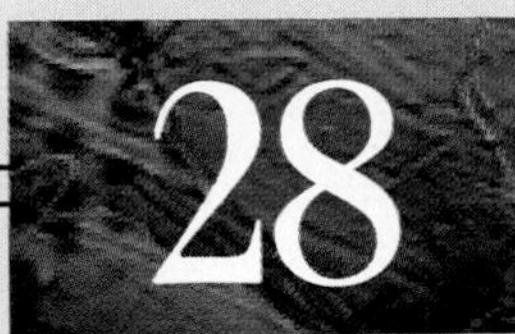

PRINCIPLES OF NUTRITION II: MICRONUTRIENTS

Stephen G. Chaney

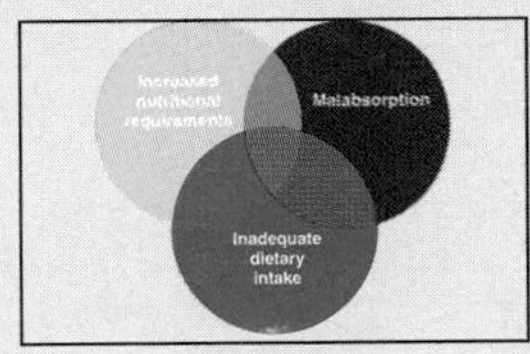

28.1 ■ OVERVIEW

Micronutrients play a vital role in human metabolism, being involved in almost every known biochemical reaction and pathway. However, the biochemistry of these nutrients is of little interest unless we also know if dietary deficiencies are likely. The American diet is undoubtedly the best it has ever been. Our current food supply provides us with an abundant variety of foods all year long and deficiency diseases have become medical curiosities. However, our diet is far from optimal. The old adage that we get everything we need from a balanced diet is true only if we eat a balanced diet. Unfortunately, most Americans do not consume a balanced diet. Foods of high caloric density and low nutrient density (often referred to as empty calories or junk food) are an abundant and popular part of the American diet, and our nutritional status suffers because of these food choices. Obviously then, neither alarm nor complacency is justified. We need to know how to evaluate the adequacy of our diet.

28.2 ■ ASSESSMENT OF MALNUTRITION

There are three increasingly stringent criteria for measuring **malnutrition.**

1. **Dietary intake studies,** which are usually based on a 24-hour recall, are the least stringent. The 24-hour recalls almost always tend to overestimate the number of people with deficient diets. Also, poor dietary intake alone is usually not a problem in this country unless the situation is compounded by increased need.

2. **Biochemical assays,** either direct or indirect, are a more useful indicator of the nutritional status of an individual. At their best, they indicate **subclinical nutritional deficiencies** that can be treated before actual deficiency diseases develop. However, all biochemical assays are not equally valid—an unfortunate fact that is not sufficiently recognized. Changes in biochemical parameters due to stress need to be interpreted with caution. The distribution of many nutrients in the body changes dramatically in a stress situation such as illness, injury, and pregnancy. A drop in level of a nutrient in one tissue compartment (usually blood) need not signal a deficiency or an increased requirement. It could simply reflect a normal metabolic adjustment to stress.

3. The most stringent criterion is the appearance of **clinical symptoms.** However, it is desirable to intervene long before symptoms became apparent.

The question remains: When should dietary surveys or biochemical assays be interpreted to indicate the necessity of nutritional intervention? The following general guidelines are useful. Dietary surveys are seldom a valid indication of general malnutrition unless the average intake for a population group falls significantly below the standard (usually two-thirds of the Recommended Dietary Allowance) for one or more nutrients. However, by looking at the percentage of people within a population group who have suboptimal intake, it is possible to identify high-risk population groups that should be monitored more closely. Biochemical assays can definitely identify subclinical cases of malnutrition where nutritional intervention is desirable provided (a) the assay has been shown to be reliable, (b) the deficiency can be verified by a second assay, and (c) there is no unusual stress situation that may alter micronutrient distribution. In assessing nutritional status, it is important for the clinician to be aware of those population groups at risk, the most reliable biochemical assays for monitoring nutritional status, and the symptoms of deficiencies if they should occur.

biochemical changes take place, resulting in the generation of a nerve impulse, conversion of the retinal to the all-trans form, and its dissociation from the visual protein (see p. 943). Regeneration of more visual pigments requires isomerization back to the Δ^{11}-*cis* form (Figure 28.3).

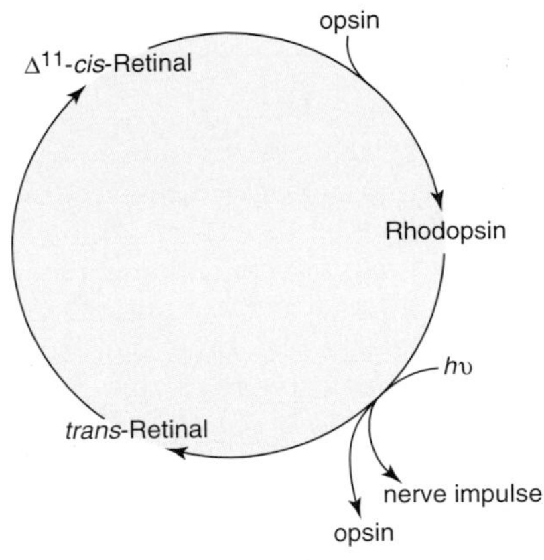

FIGURE 28.3
Role of vitamin A in vision.

Based on what is known about the biochemical mechanisms of vitamin A action, its biological effects are easier to understand. For example, vitamin A is required for the maintenance of healthy epithelial tissue. Retinol and/or retinoic acid are required to prevent the synthesis of high molecular weight forms of **keratin** and retinyl phosphate is required for the synthesis of glycoproteins (an important component of the mucus secreted by many epithelial tissues). The lack of mucus secretion leads to a drying of these cells, and the excess keratin synthesis leaves a horny keratinized surface in place of the normal moist and pliable epithelium. Vitamin A deficiency can lead to **anemia** caused by impaired mobilization of iron from the liver because retinol and/or retinoic acid are required for the synthesis of the iron transport protein transferrin.

Finally, vitamin A-deficient animals are more susceptible to both infections and cancer. Decreased resistance to infections is thought to be due to keratinization of mucosal cells lining the respiratory, gastrointestinal, and genitourinary tracts. Under these conditions fissures readily develop in the mucosal membranes, allowing microorganisms to enter. Vitamin A deficiency may impair the immune system as well. The protective effect of vitamin A against many forms of cancer probably results from the antioxidant potential of β-carotene and the effects of retinol and retinoic acid in regulating cell growth.

Since vitamin A is stored in the liver, deficiencies of this vitamin can develop only over prolonged periods of inadequate uptake. Mild **vitamin A deficiencies** are characterized by **follicular hyperkeratosis** (rough keratinized skin resembling "goosebumps"), anemia (biochemically equivalent to iron deficiency anemia, but in the presence of adequate iron intake), and increased susceptibility to infection and cancer. **Night blindness** is also an early symptom of vitamin A deficiency. Severe vitamin A deficiency leads to a progressive keratinization of the cornea of the eye known as xerophthalmia in its most advanced stages. In the final stages, infection usually sets in, with resulting hemorrhaging of the eye and permanent loss of vision.

For most people (unless they happen to eat liver) the dark green and yellow vegetables are the most important dietary source of vitamin A. Unfortunately, these are the foods most often missing from the American diet. Nationwide, dietary surveys indicate that between 40% and 60% of the population consumes less than two-thirds of the RDA for vitamin A. Clinical symptoms of vitamin A deficiency are rare in the general population, but vitamin A deficiency is a fairly common consequence of severe liver damage or diseases that cause fat malabsorption (see Clin. Corr. 28.1).

Vitamin A accumulates in the liver and over prolonged periods large amounts of this vitamin can be toxic. Doses of 25,000–50,000 RE per day over months or years will prove to be toxic for many children and adults. The usual symptoms include bone pain, scaly dermatitis, enlargement of liver and spleen, nausea, and diarrhea. It is, of course, virtually impossible to ingest toxic amounts of vitamin A from normal foods unless one eats polar bear liver (6000 RE/g) regularly. Most instances of **vitamin A toxicity** are due to the use of massive doses of vitamin A supplements. Fortunately, this practice is relatively rare because of increased public awareness of vitamin A toxicity.

Vitamin D Synthesis in the Body Requires Sunlight

Technically, vitamin D should be considered a hormone rather than a vitamin. **Cholecalciferol (D_3)** is produced in skin by UV irradiation of 7-dehydrocholesterol (Figure 28.4). Thus, as long as the body is exposed to adequate sunlight,

CLINICAL CORRELATION 28.1

Nutritional Considerations for Cystic Fibrosis

Patients with malabsorption diseases often develop malnutrition. As an example, let us examine the nutritional consequences of one disease with malabsorption components. Cystic fibrosis (CF) involves a generalized dysfunction of the exocrine glands that leads to formation of a viscid mucus, which progressively plugs the ducts. Obstruction of the bronchi and bronchioles leads to pulmonary infections, which are usually the direct cause of death. In many cases, however, the exocrine glands of the pancreas are also affected, leading to a deficiency of pancreatic enzymes and sometimes a partial obstruction of the common bile duct.

The deficiency (or partial deficiency) of pancreatic lipase and bile salts leads to severe malabsorption of fat and fat-soluble vitamins. Calcium tends to form insoluble salts with the long-chain fatty acids, which accumulate in the intestine. While these are the most severe problems, some starches and proteins are also trapped in the fatty bolus of partially digested foods. This physical entrapment, along with the deficiencies of pancreatic amylase and pancreatic proteases, can lead to severe protein–calorie malnutrition as well. Excessive mucus secretion on the luminal surfaces of the intestine may also interfere with the absorption of several nutrients, including iron.

Fortunately, microsphere preparations of pancreatic enzymes are now available that can greatly alleviate many of these malabsorption problems. With these preparations, protein and carbohydrate absorption rates are returned to near normal. Fat absorption is improved greatly but not normalized, since deficiencies of bile salts and excess mucus secretion persist. Because dietary fat is a major source of calories, these patients have difficulty obtaining sufficient calories from a normal diet. This is complicated by increased protein and energy needs resulting from the chronic infections often seen in these patients. Thus many experts recommend energy intakes ranging from 120–150% of the RDA.

Since inadequate energy intake results in poor growth and increased susceptibility to infection, inadequate caloric intake is of great concern for cystic fibrosis patients. Thus the current recommendations are for high-energy–high-protein diets without any restriction of dietary fat (50% carbohydrate, 15% protein, and 35% fat). If caloric intake from the normal diet is inadequate, dietary supplements or enteral feedings may be used. The dietary supplements most often contain easily digested carbohydrates and milk protein mixtures. Medium-chain triglycerides are sometimes used as a partial fat replacement since they can be absorbed directly through the intestinal mucosa in the absence of bile salts and pancreatic lipase.

Since some fat malabsorption is present, deficiencies of the fat-soluble vitamins often occur. Children aged 2–8 years need a standard adult multiple-vitamin preparation containing 400 IU of vitamin D and 5000 IU of vitamin A per day. Older children, adolescents, and adults need a standard multivitamin at a dose of 1–2 per day. If serum vitamin A levels become low, water-miscible vitamin A preparations should be used. For vitamin E the recommendations are: ages 0–6 mo, 25 IU day^{-1}; 6–12 mo, 50 IU day^{-1}; 1–4 years, 100 IU day^{-1}; 4–10 years, 100–200 IU day^{-1}; and >10 years, 200–400 IU day^{-1}; in water-soluble form. Vitamin K deficiency has not been adequately studied, but the current recommendations are: ages 0–12 mo, 2.5 mg $week^{-1}$ or 2.5 mg twice a week if on antibiotics; ages >1 year, 5.0 mg twice weekly when on antibiotics or if cholestatic liver disease is present. Iron deficiency is fairly common in cystic fibrosis patients but iron supplementation is not usually recommended because of concern that higher iron levels in the blood might encourage systemic bacterial infections. Calcium levels in the blood are usually normal. However, since calcium absorption is probably suboptimal, it is important to make certain that the diet provides at least RDA levels of calcium.

Littlewood, J. M., and MacDonald, A. Rationale of modern dietary recommendations in cystic fibrosis. *J. R. Soc. Med.* 80(Suppl. 15):16, 1987; and Ramsey, B. W, Farrell, P. M., and Pencharz, P. Nutritional assessment and management in cystic fibrosis; a consensus report. *Am J. Clin. Nutr.* 55:108, 1992.

there is little or no dietary requirement for vitamin D. The best dietary sources of vitamin D_3 are saltwater fish (especially salmon, sardines, and herring), liver, and egg yolk. Milk, butter, and other foods are routinely fortified with **ergocalciferol (D_2)** prepared by irradiating ergosterol from yeast. Vitamin D potency is measured in terms of milligrams of cholecalciferol (1 mg cholecalciferol or ergocalciferol = 40 IU).

Both cholecalciferol and ergocalciferol are metabolized identically. They are carried to the liver where the 25-hydroxy derivative is formed. **25-Hydroxycholecalciferol** [25-(OH)D] is the major circulating derivative of vitamin D, and it is in turn converted into the biologically active **1-α,25-dihydroxycholecalciferol** (also called calcitriol) in the proximal convoluted tubules of kidney (see Clin. Corr. 28.2).

The compound 1,25-$(OH)_2D$ acts in concert with **parathyroid hormone (PTH),** which is also produced in response to low serum calcium. Parathyroid hormone plays a major role in regulating the activation of vitamin D. High PTH levels stimulate the production of 1,25-$(OH)_2D$, while low PTH levels induce formation of an inactive 24,25-$(OH)_2D$. Once formed, the 1,25-$(OH)_2D$ acts

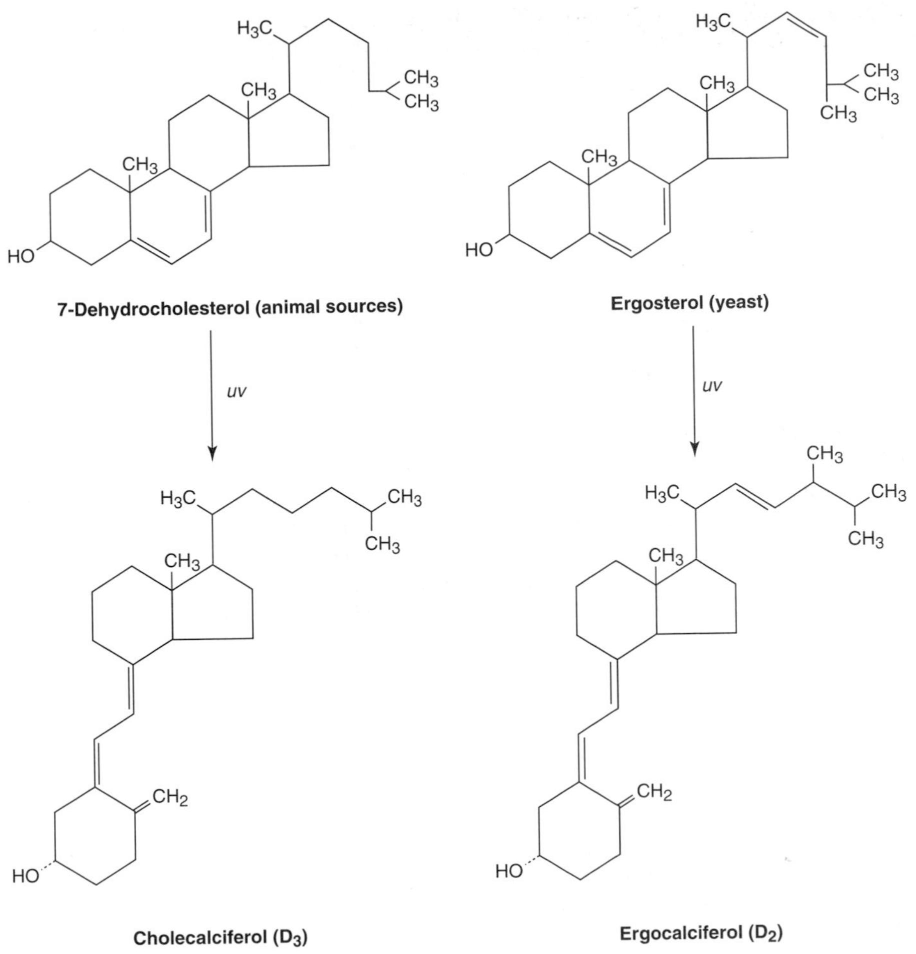

7-Dehydrocholesterol (animal sources)

Ergosterol (yeast)

uv

Cholecalciferol (D_3)

Ergocalciferol (D_2)

FIGURE 28.4
Structures of vitamin D and related compounds.

CLINICAL CORRELATION 28.2

Renal Osteodystrophy

In chronic renal failure, a complicated chain of events leads to a condition known as renal osteodystrophy. The renal failure results in an inability to produce 1,25-$(OH)_2D$, and thus bone calcium becomes the only important source of serum calcium. In the later stages of renal failure, the situation is complicated further by increased renal retention of phosphate and resulting hyperphosphatemia. The serum phosphate levels are often high enough to cause metastatic calcification (i.e., calcification of soft tissue), which tends to lower serum calcium levels further (the solubility product of calcium phosphate in the serum is very low and a high serum level of one component necessarily causes a decreased concentration of the other). The hyperphosphatemia and hypocalcemia stimulate parathyroid hormone secretion, and the resulting hyperparathyroidism further accelerates the rate of bone loss. One ends up with both bone loss and metastatic calcification. In this case, simple administration of high doses of vitamin D or its active metabolites would not be sufficient since the combination of hyperphosphatemia and hypercalcemia would only lead to more extensive metastatic calcification. The readjustment of serum calcium levels by high calcium diets and/or vitamin D supplementation must be accompanied by phosphate reduction therapies. The most common technique is to use phosphate-binding antacids that make phosphate unavailable for absorption. Orally administered 1,25-$(OH)_2D$ is effective at stimulating calcium absorption in the mucosa but does not enter the peripheral circulation in significant amounts. Thus patients with severe hyperparathyroidism may need to be treated with intravenous 1,25-$(OH)_2D$.

Johnson, W. J. Use of vitamin D analogs in renal osteodystrophy. *Semin. Nephrol.* 6:31, 1986; McCarthy, J. T., and Kumar, R. Behavior of the vitamin D endocrine system in the development of renal osteodystrophy. *Semin. Nephrol.* 6:21, 1986; and Delmez, J. M., and Siatopolsky, E. Hyperphosphatemia: its consequences and treatment in patients with chronic renal disease. *Am. J. Kidney Dis.* 19:303, 1992.

alone as a typical steroid hormone in intestinal mucosal cells, where it induces synthesis of a protein, calbinden, required for calcium transport. In the bone 1,25-$(OH)_2$D and PTH act synergistically to promote bone resorption (demineralization) by stimulating osteoblast formation and activity. Finally, PTH and 1,25-$(OH)_2$D inhibit calcium excretion in the kidney by stimulating calcium reabsorption in the distal renal tubules. The overall response of calcium metabolism to several different physiological situations is summarized in Figure 28.5. The response to low serum calcium levels is characterized by elevation of PTH and 1,25-$(OH)_2$D, which act to enhance calcium absorption and bone resorption and to inhibit calcium excretion (Figure 28.5*a*). High serum calcium levels block production of PTH. The low PTH levels allow 25-(OH)D to be metabolized to 24,25-$(OH)_2$D instead of 1,25-$(OH)_2$D. In the absence of PTH and 1,25-$(OH)_2$D bone resorption is inhibited and calcium excretion is enhanced. High levels of serum calcium and phosphate increase the rate of bone mineralization (Figure 28.5*b*). Thus bone is a very important reservoir of the calcium and phosphate needed to maintain homeostasis of serum levels. When vitamin D and dietary calcium are adequate, no net loss of bone calcium occurs. However, when dietary calcium is low, PTH and 1,25-$(OH)_2$D will cause net demineralization of bone to maintain normal serum calcium levels. Vitamin D deficiency also causes net demineralization of bone due to elevation of PTH (Figure 28.5*c*).

The most common symptoms of **vitamin D deficiency** are **rickets** in young children and **osteomalacia** in adults. Rickets is characterized by continued formation of osteoid matrix and cartilage, which are improperly mineralized, resulting in soft, pliable bones. In the adult demineralization of preexisting bone takes place, causing the bone to become softer and more susceptible to fracture. This osteomalacia is easily distinguishable from the more common osteoporosis, by the fact that the osteoid matrix remains intact in the former, but not in the latter. Vitamin D may be involved in more than regulation of calcium homeostasis. Receptors for 1,25-$(OH)_2$D have been found in many tissues including parathyroid gland, islet cells of pancreas, keratinocytes of skin, and myeloid stem cells in bone marrow. The role of vitamin D in these tissues is the subject of active investigation.

Because of fortification of dairy products with vitamin D, dietary deficiencies are very rare. The cases of dietary vitamin D deficiency that do occur are most often seen in low-income groups, the elderly (who often also have minimal exposure to sunlight), strict vegetarians (especially if their diet is also low in calcium and high in fiber), and chronic alcoholics. Most cases of vitamin D deficiency, however, are a result of diseases causing **fat malabsorption** or severe liver and kidney disease (see Clin. Corr. 28.1 and 28.2). Certain drugs also interfere with vitamin D metabolism. For example, corticosteroids stimulate the conversion of vitamin D to inactive metabolites and have been shown to cause bone demineralization when used for long periods of time.

Vitamin D can also be toxic in doses 10–100 times the RDA. The mechanism of **vitamin D toxicity** is summarized in Figure 28.5*d*. Enhanced calcium absorption and bone resorption cause hypercalcemia, which can lead to metastatic calcification. The enhanced bone resorption also causes bone demineralization similar to that seen in vitamin D deficiency. Finally, the high serum calcium leads directly to hypercalciuria, which predisposes the patient to formation of renal stones.

Vitamin E Is a Mixture of Tocopherols

For many years **vitamin E** was described as the "vitamin in search of a disease." While vitamin E deficiency diseases are still virtually unknown, its metabolic role in the body has become better understood in recent years. Vitamin E occurs in the diet as a mixture of several closely related compounds, called tocopherols.

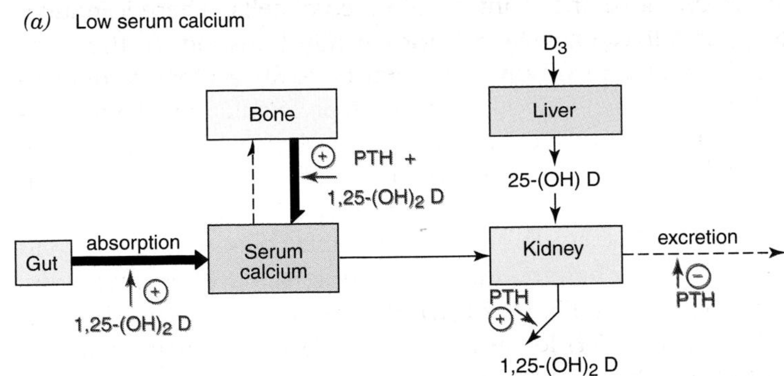

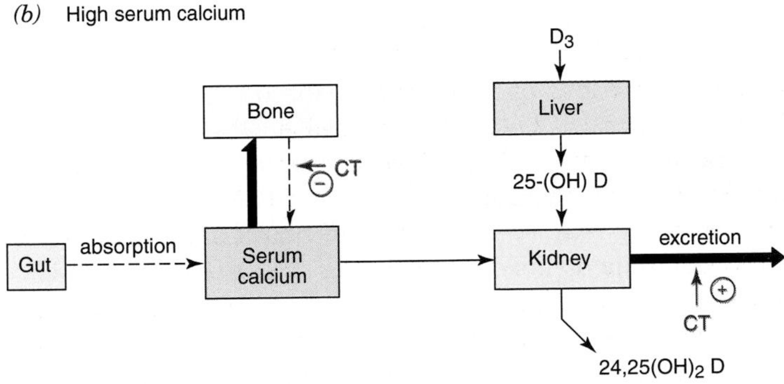

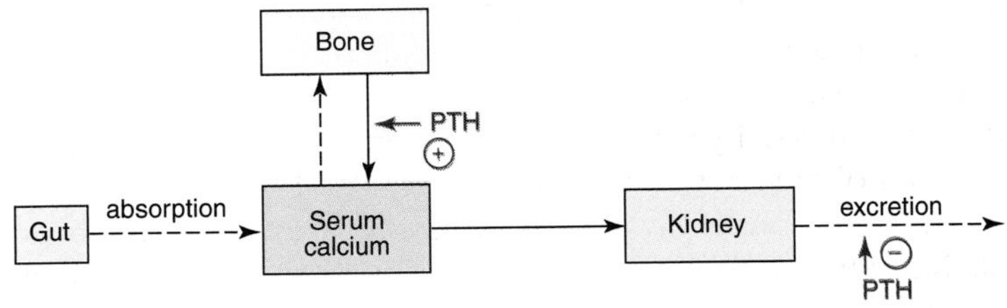

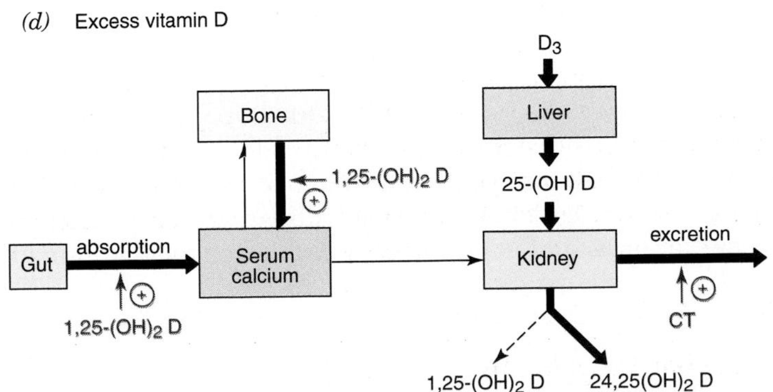

FIGURE 28.5
Vitamin D and calcium homeostasis.
Dominant pathways of calcium metabolism under each set of metabolic conditions are shown with heavy arrows. The effect of various hormones on these pathways is shown by red arrows for stimulation or blue arrows for repression. PTH, parathyroid hormone; D, cholecalciferol; 25-(OH)D, 25-hydroxycholecalciferol; and 1,25-$(OH)_2$D, 1-α,25-dihydroxycholecalciferol.

α-Tocopherol is the most potent and is used as the measure of vitamin E potency (1 α-tocopherol equiv = 1 mg α-tocopherol).

First and foremost, vitamin E is an important naturally occurring **antioxidant.** Due to its lipophilic character it accumulates in circulating lipoproteins, cellular membranes, and fat deposits, where it reacts very rapidly with molecular oxygen and free radicals. It acts as a scavenger for these compounds, protecting unsaturated fatty acids (especially those in the membranes) from peroxidation reactions. Vitamin E appears to play a role in cellular respiration, either by stabilizing coenzyme Q or by helping transfer electrons to coenzyme Q. It also appears to enhance heme synthesis by increasing the levels of δ-aminolevulinic acid (ALA) synthetase and ALA dehydratase. Most of these vitamin E effects are thought to be an indirect effect of its antioxidant potential, rather than its actual participation as a coenzyme in any biochemical reactions. For example, an important role of vitamin E in humans is to prevent oxidation of **LDL,** since it appears to be the oxidized form of LDL that is atherogenic. Finally, neurological symptoms have been reported following prolonged vitamin E deficiency associated with malabsorption diseases.

Studies on the recommended levels of vitamin E in the diet have been hampered by the difficulty of producing severe vitamin E deficiency in humans. In general, it has been assumed that the vitamin E levels in the American diet are sufficient, since no major vitamin E deficiency diseases have been found. However, vitamin E requirements increase as intake of polyunsaturated fatty acids (PUFAs) increases. While the recent emphasis on high PUFA diets to reduce serum cholesterol may be of benefit in controlling heart disease, the propensity of PUFA to form free radicals on exposure to oxygen may lead to an increased cancer risk. Thus it appears only prudent to increase vitamin E intake in high PUFA diets.

Premature infants fed on formulas low in vitamin E sometimes develop a form of hemolytic anemia that can be corrected by vitamin E supplementation. Adults suffering from fat malabsorption show a decreased red blood cell survival time. Hence vitamin E supplementation may be necessary with premature infants and in cases of fat malabsorption. In addition, recent studies have suggested that supplementation with at least 100 mg day^{-1} of vitamin E may decrease the risk of heart disease. This is well above the current RDA and is far greater than can be obtained from even a very well balanced diet. These findings have rekindled the debate as to whether dietary recommendations should consider optimal levels of nutrients rather than the levels needed to prevent deficiency diseases. As a fat-soluble vitamin, E has the potential for toxicity. However, it does appear to be the least toxic of the fat-soluble vitamins. No instances of toxicity have been reported at doses of 1600 mg day^{-1} or less.

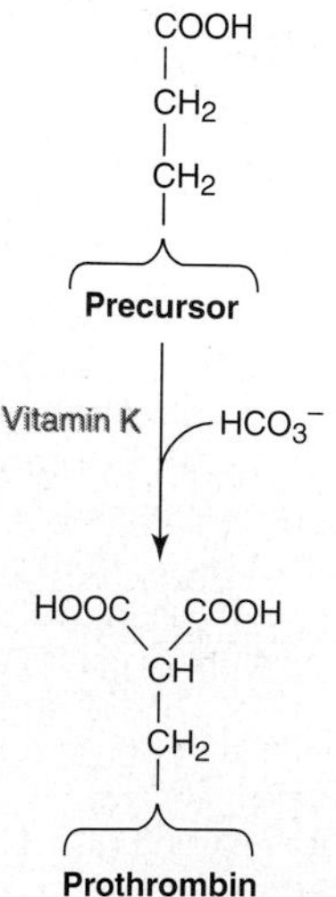

FIGURE 28.6
Function of vitamin K.

Vitamin K Is a Quinone Derivative

Vitamin K is found naturally as $\mathbf{K_1}$ (phytylmenaquinone) in green vegetables and $\mathbf{K_2}$ (multiprenylmenaquinone), which is synthesized by intestinal bacteria. The body converts synthetically prepared menaquinone (menadione) and a number of water-soluble analogs to a biologically active form of vitamin K. Dietary requirements are measured in terms of micrograms of vitamin K_1 with the RDA for adults being in the range of 60–80 μg day^{-1}.

Vitamin K_1 is required for the conversion of several **clotting factors** and **prothrombin** to the active state. The mechanism of this action has been most clearly delineated for prothrombin (see p. 970). Prothrombin is synthesized as an inactive precursor called preprothrombin. Conversion to the active form requires a vitamin K-dependent **carboxylation** of specific glutamic acid residues to **γ-carboxyglutamic acid** (Figure 28.6). The γ-carboxyglutamic acid residues are good chelators and allow prothrombin to bind calcium. The prothrombin–Ca^{2+} complex in turn binds to the phospholipid membrane, where proteolytic conversion to thrombin can occur *in vivo*. The mechanism of the carboxylation reaction has not been fully clarified but appears to involve the intermediate formation of a 2,3-epoxide derivative of vitamin K. **Dicumarol,** a naturally occurring anticoagulant, inhibits the reductase, which converts the epoxide back to the active vitamin.

Recently, vitamin K has been shown to be essential for the synthesis of γ-carboxyglutamic acid residues in the protein **osteocalcin,** which accounts for 15–20% of the noncollagen protein in the bone of most vertebrates. As with prothrombin, the γ-carboxyglutamic acid residues are responsible for most of the calcium-binding properties of osteocalcin. Because osteocalcin synthesis is controlled by vitamin D and osteocalcin is thought to play an important role in bone remodeling, vitamin K may be important for bone formation.

The only readily detectable symptom of **vitamin K deficiency** in humans is increased coagulation time, but some studies have suggested that vitamin K deficiency may be a factor in **osteoporosis** as well. Since vitamin K is synthesized by bacteria in the intestine, deficiencies have long been assumed to be rare. However, recent studies have suggested that intestinally synthesized vitamin K may not be efficiently absorbed and marginal vitamin K deficiencies may be more common than originally thought. The most common deficiency occurs in newborn infants (see Clin. Corr. 28.3), especially those whose mothers have been on anticonvulsant therapy (see Clin. Corr. 28.4). Vitamin K deficiency also occurs in patients with **obstructive jaundice** and other diseases leading to severe **fat malabsorption** (see Clin. Corr. 28.1) and patients on long-term **antibiotic therapy** (which may destroy vitamin K-synthesizing organisms in the intestine). Finally, vitamin K deficiency is sometimes seen in the elderly,

CLINICAL CORRELATION 28.3

Nutritional Considerations in the Newborn

Newborn infants are at special nutritional risk. In the first place, this is a period of very rapid growth, and needs for many nutrients are high. Some micronutrients (such as vitamins E and K) do not cross the placental membrane well and tissue stores are low in the newborn infant. The gastrointestinal tract may not be fully developed, leading to malabsorption problems (particularly with respect to the fat-soluble vitamins). The gastrointestinal tract is also sterile at birth and the intestinal flora that normally provide significant amounts of certain vitamins (especially vitamin K) take several days to become established. If the infant is born prematurely, the nutritional risk is slightly greater, since the gastrointestinal tract will be less well developed and the tissue stores will be less.

The most serious nutritional complications of newborns appear to be hemorrhagic disease. Newborn infants, especially premature infants, have low tissue stores of vitamin K and lack the intestinal flora necessary to synthesize the vitamin. Breast milk is also a relatively poor source of vitamin K. Approximately 1 out of 400 live births shows some signs of hemorrhagic disease. One milligram of the vitamin at birth is usually sufficient to prevent hemorrhagic disease.

Iron is another potential problem. Most newborn infants are born with sufficient reserves of iron to last 3–4 months (although premature infants are born with smaller reserves). Since iron is present in low amounts in both cow's milk and breast milk, iron supplementation is usually begun at a relatively early age by the introduction of iron-fortified cereal. Vitamin D levels are also somewhat low in breast milk and supplementation with vitamin D is usually recommended. However, some recent studies have suggested that iron in breast milk is present in a form that is particularly well utilized by the infant and that earlier studies probably underestimated the amount of vitamin D available in breast milk. Other vitamins and minerals appear to be present in adequate amounts in breast milk as long as the mother is getting a good diet. Recent studies have suggested that in situations in which infants must be maintained on assisted ventilation with high oxygen concentrations, supplemental vitamin E may reduce the risk of bronchopulmonary dysplasia and retrolental fibroplasia, two possible side effects of oxygen therapy. Studies have also suggested that anemia of prematurity may respond to supplemental folate and vitamin B_{12}.

In summary, most infants are provided with supplemental vitamin K at birth to prevent hemorrhagic disease. Breast-fed infants are usually provided with supplemental vitamin D, with iron being introduced along with solid foods. Bottle-fed infants are provided with supplemental iron. If infants must be maintained on oxygen, supplemental vitamin E may be beneficial.

Barness, L. A. Pediatrics. In: H. Schneider, C. E. Anderson, and D. B. Coursin (Eds.), *Nutritional Support of Medical Practice,* 2nd ed. New York: Harper & Row, 1983, pp. 541–561; Huysman, M. W., and Sauer, P. J. The vitamin K controversy. *Curr. Opin. Pediatr.* 6:129, 1994; Worthington-White, D. A., Behnke, M., and Gross, S. Premature infants require additional folate and vitamin B_{12} to reduce the severity of anemia of prematurity. *Am. J. Clin. Nutr.* 60:930, 1994; and Mueller, D. P. R. Vitamin E therapy in retinopathy of prematurity. *Eye* 6:221, 1992.

CLINICAL CORRELATION 28.4

Anticonvulsant Drugs and Vitamin Requirements

Anticonvulsant drugs such as phenobarbital or diphenylhydantoin (DPH) present an excellent example of the type of drug–nutrient interactions that are of concern to the physician. Metabolic bone disease appears to be the most significant side effect of prolonged anticonvulsant therapy. Whereas children and adults on these drugs seldom develop rickets or severe osteomalacia, as many as 65% of those on long-term therapy will have abnormally low serum calcium and phosphorus and abnormally high serum alkaline phosphatase. Some bone loss is usually observed in these cases. While the cause of the hypocalcemia and bone loss is thought to be an effect of the anticonvulsant drugs on vitamin D metabolism, not all of the studies have shown decreased levels of 25-(OH)D and 1,25-$(OH)_2$D in patients on these drugs. However, supplemental vitamin D in the range of 2000–10,000 units per day appears to correct both the hypocalcemia and osteopenia. Anticonvulsants also tend to increase needs for vitamin K, leading to an increased incidence of hemorrhagic disease in infants born to mothers on anticonvulsants. In addition, anticonvulsants appear to increase the need for folic acid and B_6. Low serum folate levels are seen in 75% of patients on anticonvulsants and megaloblastic anemia may occur in as many as 50% without supplementation. By biochemical parameters, 30–60% of the children on anticonvulsants exhibit some form of B_6 deficiency. Clinical symptoms of B_6 deficiency are rarely seen, however. From 1 to 5 mg of folic acid and 10 mg of vitamin B_6 appear to be sufficient for most patients on anticonvulsants. Since folates may speed up the metabolism of some anticonvulsants, it is important that excess folic acid not be given.

Moslet, U., and Hansen, E. S. A review of vitamin K, epilepsy and pregnancy. *Acta Neurol. Scand.* 85:39, 1992: Rivery, M. D., and Schottelius, D. D. Phenytoin–folic acid: a review. *Drug Intelligence Clin. Pharm.* 18:292, 1984; and Tjellesen, L. Metabolism and action of vitamin D in epileptic patients on anticonvulsant treatment and healthy adults. *Dan. Med. Bull.* 41:139, 1994.

who are prone to poor liver function (reducing preprothrombin synthesis) and fat malabsorption. Clearly, vitamin K deficiency should be suspected in patients demonstrating easy bruising and prolonged clotting time.

28.5 ■ WATER-SOLUBLE VITAMINS

Water-soluble vitamins differ from fat-soluble vitamins in several important aspects. Most are readily excreted once their concentration surpasses the renal threshold. Thus toxicities are rare. Deficiencies of these vitamins occur relatively quickly on an inadequate diet. Their metabolic stores are labile and depletion can often occur in a matter of weeks or months. Since the water-soluble vitamins are coenzymes for many common biochemical reactions, it is often possible to assay vitamin status by measuring one or more enzyme activities in isolated red blood cells. These assays are especially useful if one measures both the endogenous enzyme activity and the stimulated activity following addition of the active coenzyme derived from that vitamin.

Most of the water-soluble vitamins are converted to coenzymes, which are utilized either in the pathways for energy generation or hematopoiesis. Deficiencies of the energy-releasing vitamins produce a number of overlapping symptoms. In many cases the vitamins participate in so many biochemical reactions that it is impossible to pinpoint the exact biochemical cause of any given symptom. However, it is possible to generalize that because of the central role these vitamins play in energy metabolism, deficiencies show up first in rapidly growing tissues. Typical symptoms include **dermatitis, glossitis** (swelling and reddening of the tongue), **cheilitis** at the corners of the lips, and **diarrhea.** In many cases nervous tissue is also involved due to its high energy demand or specific effects of the vitamin. Some of the common neurological symptoms include **peripheral neuropathy** (tingling of nerves at the extremities), depression, mental confusion, lack of motor coordination, and **malaise.** In some cases demyelination and degeneration of nervous tissues also occur. These deficiency symptoms are so common and overlapping that they can be considered as properties of the energy-releasing vitamins as a class, rather than being specific for any one.

28.6 ■ ENERGY-RELEASING WATER-SOLUBLE VITAMINS

Thiamine (Vitamin B_1) Forms the Coenzyme Thiamine Pyrophosphate (TPP)

Thiamine

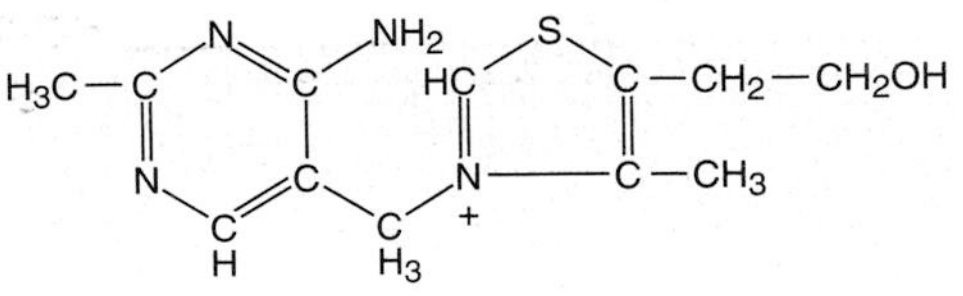

FIGURE 28.7
Structure of thiamine.

Thiamine (Figure 28.7) is rapidly converted to the coenzyme **thiamine pyrophosphate (TPP),** which is required for the key reactions catalyzed by pyruvate dehydrogenase complex and α-ketoglutarate dehydrogenase complex (Figure 28.8). Cellular energy generation is severely compromised in thiamine deficiency. TPP is also required for the transketolase reactions of the pentose phosphate pathway. While the pentose phosphate pathway is not quantitatively important in terms of energy generation, it is the sole source of ribose for the synthesis of nucleic acid precursors and the major source of NADPH for fatty acid biosynthesis and other biosynthetic pathways. Red blood cell transketolase is also the enzyme most commonly used for measuring thiamine status in the body. TPP appears to function in transmission of nerve impulses. TPP (or a related metabolite, thiamine triphosphate) is localized in peripheral nerve membranes. It appears to be required for acetylcholine synthesis and may also be required for ion translocation reactions in stimulated neural tissue.

Although the biochemical reactions involving TPP are fairly well characterized, it is not clear how these biochemical lesions result in the symptoms of **thiamine deficiency.** The pyruvate dehydrogenase and transketolase reactions are the most sensitive to thiamine levels. Thiamine deficiency appears to selectively inhibit carbohydrate metabolism, causing an accumulation of pyruvate. Cells may be directly affected by lack of available energy and NAPDH or

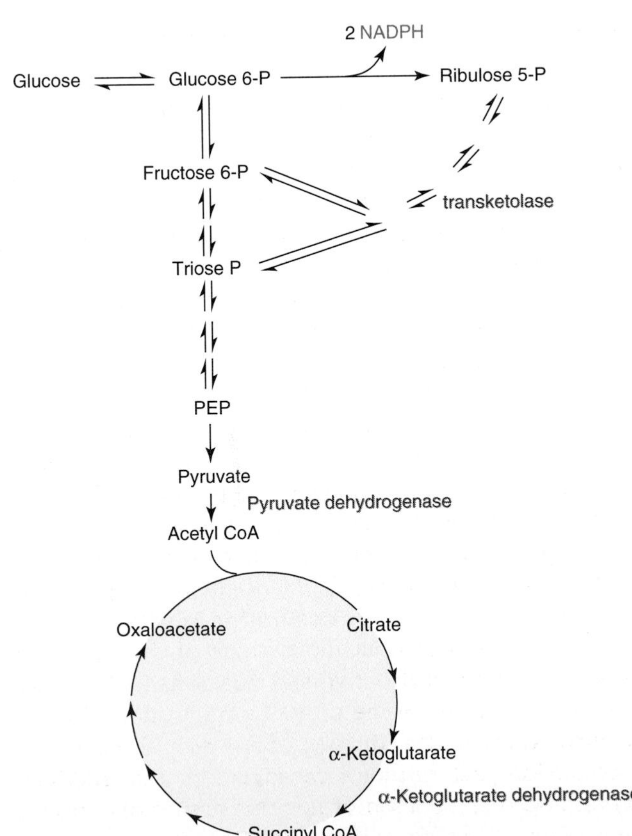

FIGURE 28.8
Summary of important reactions involving thiamine pyrophosphate.
The reactions involving thiamine pyrophosphate are indicated in red.

may be poisoned by the accumulated pyruvate. Other symptoms of thiamine deficiency involve the neural tissue and probably result from the direct role of TTP in nerve transmission.

Loss of appetite, constipation, and nausea are among the earliest symptoms of **thiamine deficiency.** Mental depression, peripheral neuropathy, irritability, and fatigue are other early symptoms and probably directly relate to the role of thiamine in maintaining healthy nervous tissue. These symptoms of thiamine deficiency are most often seen in the elderly and low-income groups on restricted diets. Symptoms of moderately severe thiamine deficiency include **mental confusion, ataxia** (unsteady gait while walking and general inability to achieve fine control of motor functions), and **ophthalmoplegia** (loss of eye coordination). This set of symptoms is usually referred to as **Wernicke–Korsakoff syndrome** and is most commonly seen in chronic **alcoholics** (see Clin. Corr. 28.5). Severe thiamine deficiency is known as **beriberi.** Dry beriberi is characterized primarily by advanced neuromuscular symptoms, including atrophy and weakness of the muscles. When these symptoms are coupled with edema, the disease is referred to as wet beriberi. Both forms of beriberi can be associated with an unusual type of heart failure characterized by high cardiac output. Beriberi is found primarily in populations relying exclusively on polished rice for food, although cardiac failure is sometimes seen in alcoholics as well.

The thiamine requirement is proportional to caloric content of the diet and is in the range of 1.0–1.5 mg per day for the normal adult. This requirement should be raised somewhat if carbohydrate intake is excessive or if the metabolic rate is elevated (due to fever, trauma, pregnancy, or lactation). Coffee and tea

CLINICAL CORRELATION 28.5

Nutritional Considerations in the Alcoholic

Chronic alcoholics run considerable risk of nutritional deficiencies. The most common problems are neurologic symptoms associated with thiamine or pyridoxine deficiencies and hematological problems associated with folate or pyridoxine deficiencies. The deficiencies seen with alcoholics are not necessarily due to poor diet alone, although it is often a strong contributing factor. Alcohol causes pathological alterations of the gastrointestinal tract that often directly interfere with absorption of certain nutrients. The liver is the most important site of activation and storage of many vitamins. The severe liver damage associated with chronic alcoholism appears to interfere directly with storage and activation of certain nutrients.

Up to 40% of hospitalized alcoholics are estimated to have megaloblastic erythropoiesis due to folate deficiency. Alcohol appears to interfere directly with folate absorption and alcoholic cirrhosis impairs storage of this nutrient. Another 30% of hospitalized alcoholics have sideroblastic anemia or identifiable sideroblasts in erythroid marrow cells characteristic of pyridoxine deficiency. Some alcoholics also develop a peripheral neuropathy that responds to pyridoxine supplementation. This problem appears to result from impaired activation and increased degradation of pyridoxine. In particular, acetaldehyde (an end product of alcohol metabolism) displaces pyridoxal phosphate from its carrier protein in the plasma. The free pyridoxal phosphate is then rapidly degraded to inactive compounds and excreted.

The most dramatic nutritionally related neurological disorder is Wernicke–Korsakoff syndrome. The symptoms include mental disturbances, ataxia (unsteady gait and lack of fine motor coordination), and uncoordinated eye movements. Congestive heart failure similar to that seen with beriberi is also seen in a small number of these patients. While this syndrome may only account for 1–3% of alcohol-related neurologic disorders, the response to supplemental thiamine is so dramatic that it is usually worth consideration. The thiamine deficiency appears to arise primarily from impaired absorption, although alcoholic cirrhosis may also affect the storage of thiamine in the liver.

While those are the most common nutritional deficiencies associated with alcoholism, deficiencies of almost any of the water-soluble vitamins can occur and cases of alcoholic scurvy and pellagra are occasionally reported. Chronic ethanol consumption causes an interesting redistribution of vitamin A stores in the body. Vitamin A stores in the liver are rapidly depleted while levels of vitamin A in the serum and other tissues may be normal or slightly elevated. Apparently, ethanol causes both increased mobilization of vitamin A from the liver and increased catabolism of liver vitamin A to inactive metabolites by the hepatic P450 system. Alcoholic patients have decreased bone density and an increased incidence of osteoporosis. This probably relates to a defect in the 25-hydroxylation step in the liver as well as an increased rate of metabolism of vitamin D to inactive products by an activated cytochrome P450 system. Dietary calcium intake is also often poor. In fact, alcoholics generally have decreased serum levels of zinc, calcium, and magnesium due to poor dietary intake and increased urinary losses. Iron-deficiency anemia is very rare unless there is gastrointestinal bleeding or chronic infection. In fact, excess iron is a more common problem with alcoholics. Many alcoholic beverages contain relatively high iron levels, and alcohol appears to enhance iron absorption.

Hayumpa, A. M. Mechanisms of vitamin deficiencies in alcoholism. *Alcohol. Clin. Exp. Res.* 10:573, 1986; and Lieber, C. S. Alcohol, liver and nutrition. *J. Am. Coll Nutr.* 10:602, 1991.

contain substances that destroy thiamine, but this is not a problem for individuals consuming normal amounts of these beverages. Routine enrichment of cereals has assured that most Americans have an adequate intake of thiamine on a normal mixed diet.

Riboflavin Is Part of FAD and FMN

Riboflavin is the precursor of the coenzymes flavin adenine dinucleotide (FAD) and flavin mononucleotide (FMN), both of which are involved in a wide variety of redox reactions. The flavin coenzymes are essential for energy production and cellular respiration. The most characteristic symptoms of **riboflavin deficiency** are angular cheilitis, glossitis, and scaly dermatitis (especially around the nasolabial folds and scrotal areas). The best flavin-requiring enzyme for assaying riboflavin status appears to be erythrocyte glutathione reductase. The recommended riboflavin intake is 1.2–1.7 mg day^{-1} for the normal adult. Foods rich in riboflavin include milk, meat, eggs, and cereal products. Riboflavin deficiencies are quite rare in this country. When riboflavin deficiency does occur, it is usually seen in chronic **alcoholics.** Hypothyroidism has recently been shown to slow the conversion of riboflavin to FMN and FAD. It is not known whether this affects riboflavin requirements, however.

Niacin Is Part of NAD and NADP

Niacin is not a vitamin in the strictest sense of the word, since some niacin can be synthesized from tryptophan. However, conversion of tryptophan to niacin is relatively inefficient (60 mg of tryptophan is required for the production of 1 mg of niacin) and occurs only after all of the body requirements for tryptophan (protein synthesis and energy production) have been met. Since synthesis of niacin requires thiamine, pyridoxine, and riboflavin, it is also very inefficient on a marginal diet. Thus most people require dietary sources of both tryptophan and niacin. Niacin (nicotinic acid) and niacinamide (nicotinamide) are both converted to the ubiquitous oxidation–reduction coenzymes NAD^+ and $NADP^+$ in the body.

Borderline **niacin deficiencies** are first seen as a glossitis (redness) of the tongue, somewhat similar to riboflavin deficiency. Pronounced deficiencies lead to **pellagra,** which is characterized by the three Ds: dermatitis, diarrhea, and dementia. The dermatitis is characteristic in that it is usually seen only in skin areas exposed to sunlight and is symmetric. The neurologic symptoms are associated with actual degeneration of nervous tissue. Because of food fortification, pellagra is a medical curiosity in the developed world. Today it is primarily seen in **alcoholics,** patients with severe **malabsorption** problems, and **elderly** on very restricted diets. Pregnancy, lactation, and chronic illness lead to increased needs for niacin, but a varied diet will usually provide sufficient amounts.

Since tryptophan can be converted to niacin, and niacin can exist in a free or bound form, the calculation of available niacin for any given food is not a simple matter. For this reason, niacin requirements are expressed in terms of niacin equivalents (1 niacin equiv = 1 mg free niacin). The current recommendation of the Food and Nutrition Board for a normal adult is 13–19 niacin equivalents (NE) per day. The richest food sources of niacin are meats, peanuts and other legumes, and enriched cereals.

Pyridoxine (Vitamin B_6) Forms the Coenzyme Pyridoxal Phosphate

Pyridoxine, pyridoxamine, and **pyridoxal** are all naturally occurring forms of vitamin B_6 (Figure 28.9). All three forms are efficiently converted by the body to **pyridoxal phosphate,** which is required for the synthesis, catabolism, and interconversion of amino acids. The role of pyridoxal phosphate in amino

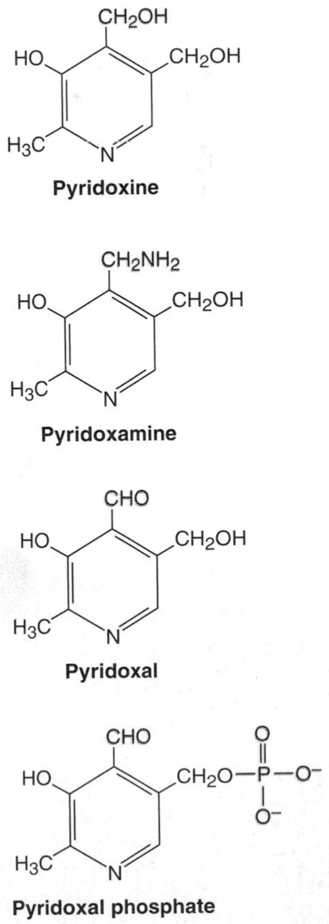

CH_2OH, HO, CH_2OH, H_3C, N

Pyridoxine

CH_2NH_2, HO, CH_2OH, H_3C, N

Pyridoxamine

CHO, HO, CH_2OH, H_3C, N

Pyridoxal

CHO, HO, $CH_2O-P(=O)(O^-)-O^-$, H_3C, N

Pyridoxal phosphate

FIGURE 28.9
Structures of vitamin B_6.

acid metabolism has been discussed previously (see p. 449). While pyridoxal phosphate-dependent reactions are legion, there are a few instances in which the biochemical lesion seems to be directly associated with the symptoms of **B_6 deficiency** (Figure 28.10). Pyridoxal phosphate is essential for energy production from amino acids and can be considered an energy-releasing vitamin. Thus some of the symptoms of severe B_6 deficiency are similar to those of the other energy-releasing vitamins. Pyridoxal phosphate is also required for the synthesis of the neurotransmitters **serotonin** and **norepinephrine** and for synthesis of the sphingolipids necessary for myelin formation. These effects are thought to explain the irritability, nervousness, and depression seen with mild deficiencies and the peripheral neuropathy and convulsions observed with severe deficiencies. Pyridoxal phosphate is required for the synthesis of Δ-aminolevulinic acid, a precursor of heme. B_6 deficiencies occasionally cause **sideroblastic anemia,** which is characteristically a microcytic anemia seen in the presence of high serum iron. Pyridoxal phosphate is also an essential component of glycogen phosphorylase; it is covalently linked to a lysine residue and stabilizes the enzyme. This role of B_6 may explain the decreased glucose tolerance associated with deficiency, although B_6 appears to have some direct effects on the glucocorticoid receptor as well. Vitamin B_6 is also required for the conversion of homocysteine to cysteine, and **hyperhomocysteinemia** appears to be a risk factor for cardiovascular disease. Finally, pyridoxal phosphate is one of the cofactors required for the conversion of tryptophan to NAD. While this may not be directly related to the symptomatology of B_6 deficiency, a tryptophan load test is a sensitive indicator of vitamin B_6 status (see Clin. Corr. 28.6, p. 1124).

The requirement for B_6 in the diet is roughly proportional to the protein content of the diet. Assuming that the average American consumes close to 100 g of protein per day, the RDA for vitamin B_6 has been set at 1.4–2.0 mg day^{-1} for a normal adult. This requirement is increased during pregnancy and lactation and may increase somewhat with age as well. Vitamin B_6 is fairly widespread in foods, but meat, vegetables, whole-grain cereals, and egg yolks are among the richest sources.

Evaluation of B_6 nutritional status has become a controversial topic in recent years. Some of this controversy is discussed in Clin. Corr. 28.6. It has usually been assumed that the average American diet is adequate in B_6 and it is not routinely added to flour and other fortified foods. However, recent nutritional surveys have cast doubt on this assumption. A significant fraction of the survey population was found to consume less than two-thirds of the RDA for B_6.

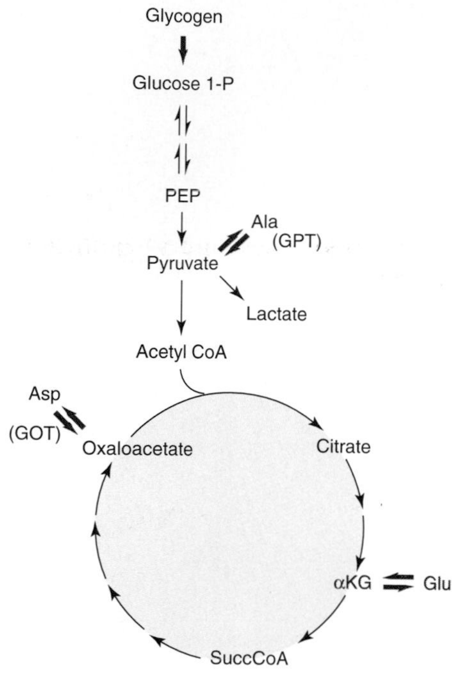

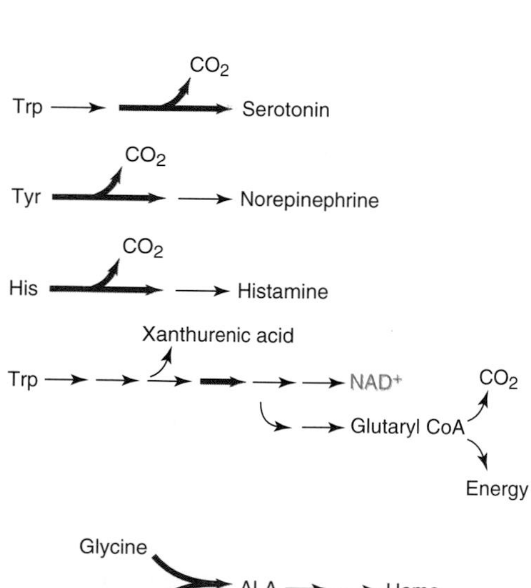

FIGURE 28.10
Important metabolic roles of pyridoxal phosphate.
Reactions requiring pyridoxal phosphate are indicated with red arrows. ALA, δ-aminolevulinic acid; αKG, α-ketoglutarate; GPT, glutamate pyruvate aminotransferase; and GOT, glutamate oxaloacetate aminotransferase.

Pantothenic Acid and Biotin Are Also Energy-Releasing Vitamins

Pantothenic acid is a component of coenzyme A (CoA) and the phosphopantetheine moiety of fatty acid synthase and thus is required for the metabolism of all fat, protein, and carbohydrate via the citric acid cycle. More than 70 enzymes have been described to date that utilize CoA or its derivatives. In view of the importance of these reactions, one would expect pantothenic acid deficiencies to be a serious concern in humans. This does not appear to be the case for two reasons: (1) pantothenic acid is very widespread in natural foods, probably reflecting its widespread metabolic role, and (2) most symptoms of pantothenic acid deficiency are vague and mimic those of other B vitamin deficiencies.

Biotin is the prosthetic group for a number of carboxylation reactions, the most notable being pyruvate carboxylase (needed for synthesis of oxaloacetate for gluconeogenesis and replenishment of the citric acid cycle), acetyl-CoA carboxylase (fatty acid biosynthesis), and propionyl-CoA carboxylase (methione, leucine, and valine metabolism). Biotin is found in peanuts, chocolate, and eggs and is synthesized by intestinal bacteria.

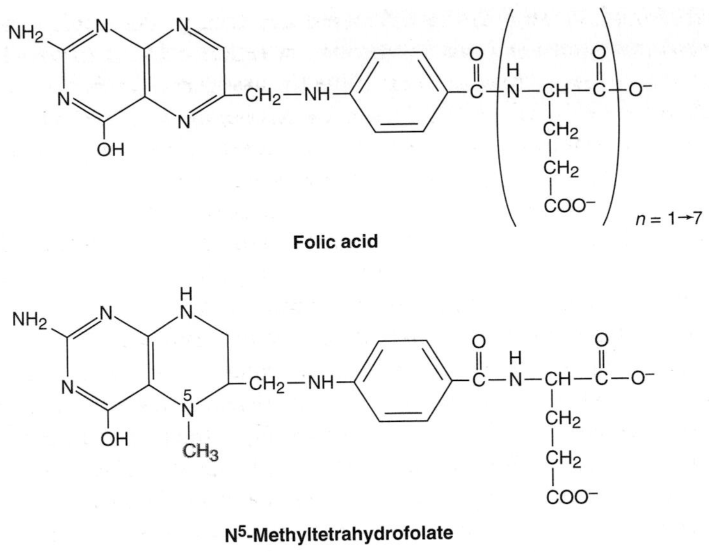

Folic acid

N^5-Methyltetrahydrofolate

FIGURE 28.11
Structure of folic acid and N^5-methyltetrahydrofolate.

28.7 HEMATOPOIETIC WATER-SOLUBLE VITAMINS

Folic Acid (Folacin) Functions as Tetrahydrofolate in One-Carbon Metabolism

The simplest form of **folic acid** is pteroylmonoglutamic acid. However, folic acid usually occurs as polyglutamate derivatives with from 2 to 7 glutamic acid residues (Figure 28.11). These compounds are taken up by intestinal mucosal cells and the extra glutamate residues are removed by **conjugase,** a lysosomal enzyme. The free folic acid is then reduced to **tetrahydrofolate** by the enzyme dihydrofolate reductase and circulated in the plasma primarily as the free N^5-methyl derivative of tetrahydrofolate (Figure 28.11). Inside cells, tetrahydrofolates are found primarily as polyglutamate derivatives, and these appear to be the biologically most potent forms. Folic acid is also stored as a polyglutamate derivative of tetrahydrofolate in the liver.

Various one-carbon tetrahydrofolate derivatives are used in biosynthetic reactions (Figure 28.12). They are required, for example, in the synthesis of choline, serine, glycine, purines, and dTMP. Since adequate amounts of choline and the amino acids can usually be obtained from the diet, the participation of folates in purine and dTMP synthesis appears to be metabolically the most

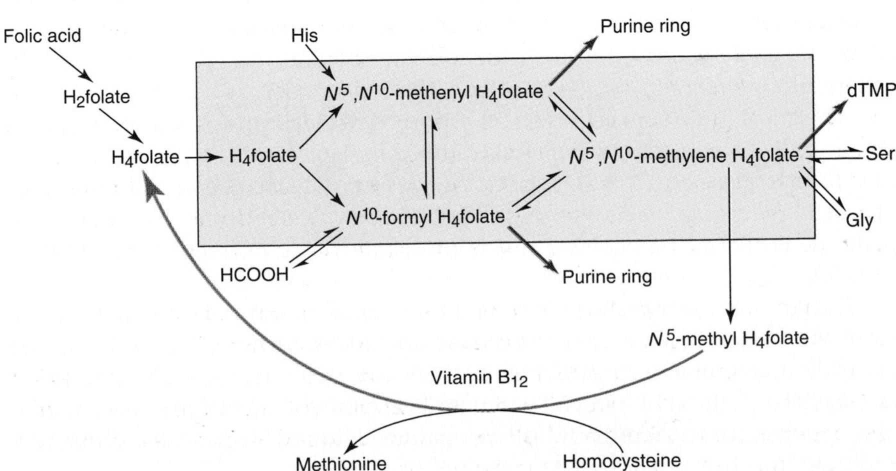

FIGURE 28.12
Metabolic roles of folic acid and vitamin B_{12} in one-carbon metabolism.
The metabolic interconversions of folic acid and its derivatives are indicated with black arrows. Pathways relying exclusively on folate are shown with red arrows. The important B_{12}-dependent reaction converting N^5-methyl H_4folate back to H_4folate is shown with a blue arrow. The box encloses the "pool" of C_1 derivatives of H_4folate.

CLINICAL CORRELATION 28.6

Vitamin B_6 Requirements for Users of Oral Contraceptives

The controversy over B_6 requirements for users of oral contraceptives best illustrates the potential problems associated with biochemical assays. For years, one of the most common assays for vitamin B_6 status had been the tryptophan load assay. This assay is based on the observation that when tissue pyridoxal phosphate levels are low, the normal catabolism of tryptophan is impaired and most of the tryptophan is catabolized by a minor pathway leading to synthesis of xanthurenic acid. Under many conditions, the amount of xanthurenic acid recovered in a 24-h urine sample following ingestion of a fixed amount of tryptophan is a valid indicator of vitamin B_6 status. When the tryptophan load test was used to assess the vitamin B_6 status of oral contraceptive users, however, alarming reports started appearing in the literature. Not only did oral contraceptive use increase the excretion of xanthurenic acid considerably but the amount of pyridoxine needed to return xanthurenic acid excretion to normal was 10 times the RDA and almost 20 times the level required to maintain normal B_6 status in control groups. As might be expected, this observation received much popular attention in spite of the fact that most classical symptoms of vitamin B_6 deficiency were not observed in oral contraceptive users.

More recent studies using other measures of vitamin B_6 have painted a slightly different picture. For example, erythrocyte glutamate pyruvate aminotransferase and erythrocyte glutamate oxaloacetate aminotransferase are both pyridoxal phosphate-containing enzymes. One can also assess vitamin B_6 status by measuring the endogenous activity of these enzymes and the degree of stimulation by added pyridoxal phosphate. These types of assays show a much smaller difference between nonusers and users of oral contraceptives. The minimum level of pyridoxine needed to maintain normal vitamin B_6 status as measured by these assays was only 2.0 mg day^{-1}, which is slightly greater than the RDA and about twice that needed by nonusers.

Why the large discrepancy? For one thing, it must be kept in mind that enzyme activity can be affected by hormones as well as vitamin cofactors. Kynureninase is the key pyridoxal phosphate-containing enzyme of the tryptophan catabolic pathway. The activity of kynureninase is regulated both by pyridoxal phosphate availability and by estrogen metabolites. Even with normal vitamin B_6 status most of the enzyme exists in the inactive apoenzyme form. However, this does not affect tryptophan metabolism because tryptophan oxygenase, the first enzyme of the pathway, is rate limiting. Thus the small amount of active holoenzyme is more than sufficient to handle the metabolites produced by the first part of the pathway. However, kynureninase is inhibited by estrogen metabolites. Thus with oral contraceptive use its activity is reduced to a level where it becomes rate limiting and excess tryptophan metabolites are shunted to xanthurenic acid. Higher than normal levels of vitamin B_6 overcome this problem by converting more apoenzyme to holoenzyme, thus increasing the total amount of enzyme. Since the estrogen was having a specific effect on the enzyme used to measure vitamin B_6 status in this assay, it did not necessarily mean that pyridoxine requirements were altered for other metabolic processes in the body.

Does this mean that vitamin B_6 status is of no concern to users of oral contraceptives? Oral contraceptives do appear to increase vitamin B_6 requirements slightly. Several dietary surveys have shown that a significant percentage of women in the 18–24-year age group consume diets containing less than 1.3 mg of pyridoxine per day. If these women are also using oral contraceptives, they are at some increased risk for developing a borderline deficiency. Thus, while the tryptophan load test was clearly misleading in a quantitative sense, it did alert the medical community to a previously unsuspected nutritional risk.

Bender, D. A. Oestrogens and vitamin B_6—actions and interactions. *World Rev. Nutr. Diet.* 51:140, 1987; and Kirksey, A., Keaton, K., Abernathy, R. P., and Grager, J. L. Vitamin B_6 nutritional status of a group of female adolescents. *Am. J. Clin. Nutr.* 31:946, 1978.

significant of those reactions. In addition, tetrahydrofolate and vitamin B_{12} are required, along with vitamin B_6, for the conversion of homocysteine to methionine. As mentioned earlier, this may also be significant because **hyperhomocysteinemia** appears to be a risk factor for cardiovascular disease. Methionine, of course, is also converted to *S*-adenosylmethionine, which is used in many methylation reactions.

The most pronounced effect of **folate deficiency** is inhibition of DNA synthesis due to decreased availability of purines and dTMP. This leads to arrest of cells in S phase and a characteristic "megaloblastic" change in size and shape of nuclei of rapidly dividing cells. The block in DNA synthesis slows down maturation of red blood cells, causing production of abnormally large "macrocytic" red blood cells with fragile membranes. Thus a **macrocytic anemia** associated with megaloblastic changes in the bone marrow is characteristic of folate deficiency. In addition, **hyperhomocysteinemia** is fairly common in the elderly population and appears to be due to inadequate intake and/or decreased utilization of folate, vitamin B_6, and vitamin B_{12}. Elevated homocysteine levels usually respond to supplementation with RDA levels of those vitamins.

There are many causes of **folate deficiency,** including inadequate intake, impaired absorption, increased demand, and impaired metabolism. Some dietary surveys have suggested that inadequate intake may be more common than previously supposed. However, as with most other vitamins, inadequate intake is probably not sufficient to trigger symptoms of folate deficiency in the absence of increased requirements or decreased utilization. Perhaps the most common example of increased need occurs during **pregnancy and lactation.** As the blood volume and the number of rapidly dividing cells in the body increase, the need for folic acid increases. By the third trimester the folic acid requirement has almost doubled. In the United States almost 20–25% of otherwise normal pregnancies are associated with low serum folate levels, but actual megaloblastic anemia is rare and is usually seen only after multiple pregnancies. However, recent studies have shown that inadequate folate levels during the early stages of pregnancy increase the risk for **neural tube defects,** a type of birth defect. Normal diets seldom supply the 400 μg of folate needed during pregnancy, so most physicians routinely recommend supplementation for women during the child-bearing years. Folate deficiency is common in **alcoholics** (see Clin. Corr. 28.5). Folate deficiencies are also seen in a number of malabsorption diseases and are occasionally seen in the elderly, due to a combination of poor dietary habits and poor absorption.

There are a number of drugs that also directly interfere with folate metabolism. **Anticonvulsants** and **oral contraceptives** may interfere with folate absorption and anticonvulsants appear to increase catabolism of folates (see Clin. Corr. 28.4). Oral contraceptives and estrogens also appear to interfere with folate metabolism in their target tissue. Long-term use of any of these drugs can lead to folate deficiencies unless adequate supplementation is provided. For example, 20% of patients using oral contraceptives develop megaloblastic changes in the cervicovaginal epithelium, and 20–30% show low serum folate levels.

Vitamin B_{12} (Cobalamine) Contains Cobalt in a Tetrapyrrole Ring

Pernicious anemia, a megaloblastic anemia associated with neurological deterioration, was invariably fatal until 1926 when liver extracts were shown to be curative. Subsequent work showed the need for both an **extrinsic factor** present in liver and an **intrinsic factor** produced by the body: **vitamin B_{12}** was the extrinsic factor. Chemically, vitamin B_{12} consists of **cobalt** in a coordination state of six—coordinated in four positions by a tetrapyrrole (or corrin) ring, in one position by a benzimidazole nitrogen, and in the sixth position by one of several different ligands (Figure 28.13). The crystalline forms of B_{12} used in supplementation are usually hydroxycobalamine or cyanocobalamine. In foods B_{12} usually occurs bound to protein in the methyl or 5′-deoxyadenosyl forms. To be utilized the B_{12} must first be removed from the protein by acid hydrolysis in the stomach or trypsin digestion in the intestine. It then must combine with **intrinsic factor,** a protein secreted by the stomach, which carries it to the ileum for absorption.

In humans there are two major symptoms of B_{12} deficiency (hematopoietic and neurological), and only two biochemical reactions in which B_{12} is known to participate (Figure 28.14). Thus it is very tempting to speculate on exact cause and effect mechanisms. The methyl derivative of B_{12} is required for conversion of homocysteine to methionine and the 5-deoxyadenosyl derivative is required for the methylmalonyl-CoA mutase reaction (methylmalonyl CoA → succinyl CoA), which is a key step in the catabolism of some branched-chain amino acids. The neurologic disorders seen in B_{12} deficiency are due to progressive demyelination of nervous tissue. It has been proposed that the

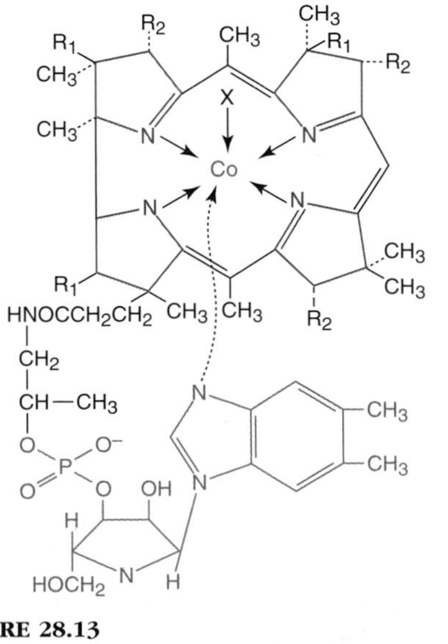

FIGURE 28.13
Structure of vitamin B_{12} (cobalamine).

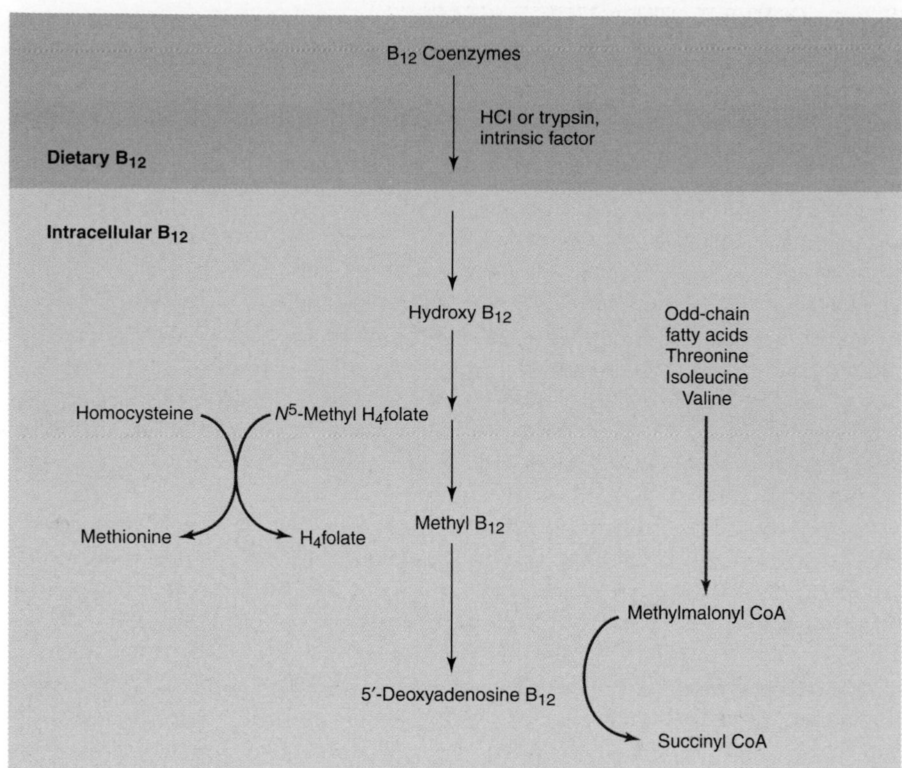

FIGURE 28.14
Metabolism of vitamin B_{12}.
Metabolic interconversions of B_{12} are indicated with light arrows, and B_{12}-requiring reactions are indicated with red arrows. Other related pathways are indicated with a blue arrow.

methylmalonyl CoA that accumulates interferes with myelin sheath formation in two ways.

1. Methylmalonyl CoA is a competitive inhibitor of malonyl CoA in fatty acid biosynthesis. Since the myelin sheath is continually turning over, any severe inhibition of fatty acid biosynthesis will lead to its eventual degeneration.
2. In the residual fatty acid synthesis, methylmalonyl CoA can substitute for malonyl CoA in the reaction sequence, leading to branched-chain fatty acids, which might disrupt normal membrane structure. There is some evidence supporting both mechanisms.

Megaloblastic anemia associated with B_{12} deficiency is thought to reflect the effect of B_{12} on folate metabolism. The B_{12}-dependent homocysteine to methionine conversion (homocysteine + N^5-methyl THF $\rightarrow$ methionine + THF) appears to be the only major pathway by which N^5-methyltetrahydrofolate can return to the tetrahydrofolate pool (Figure 28.14). Thus in B_{12} deficiency there is a buildup of N^5-methyltetrahydrofolate and a deficiency of the tetrahydrofolate derivatives needed for purine and dTMP biosynthesis. Essentially all of the folate becomes "trapped" as the N^5-methyl derivative. Vitamin B_{12} also may be required for uptake of folate by cells and for its conversion to the biologically more active polyglutamate forms. High levels of supplemental folate can overcome the megaloblastic anemia associated with B_{12} deficiencies but not the neurological problems. Hence caution must be taken in using folate to treat megaloblastic anemia.

Vitamin B_{12} is widespread in foods of animal origin, especially meats. Liver stores up to a 6-year supply of vitamin B_{12}. Thus **deficiencies** of B_{12} are extremely rare. They are occasionally seen in older people due to insufficient production of intrinsic factor and/or HCl in the stomach. B_{12} deficiency can also be seen in patients with severe malabsorption diseases and in long-term **vegetarians.**

28.8 ■ OTHER WATER-SOLUBLE VITAMINS

Ascorbic Acid Functions in Reduction and Hydroxylation Reactions

Vitamin C or ascorbic acid is a six-carbon compound closely related to glucose. Its main biological role is as a reducing agent in several important hydroxylation reactions in the body. Ascorbic acid is required for the hydroxylation of lysine and proline in protocollagen. Without this hydroxylation protocollagen cannot properly cross-link into normal collagen fibrils. Thus vitamin C is obviously important for maintenance of normal connective tissue and for wound healing, since the connective tissue is laid down first. Vitamin C is also necessary for bone formation, since bone tissue has an organic matrix containing collagen as well as the inorganic, calcified portion. Finally, collagen appears to be a component of the ground substance surrounding capillary walls, so vitamin C deficiency is associated with **capillary fragility.**

Since vitamin C is concentrated in the adrenal gland, especially in periods of stress, it may be required for hydroxylation reactions in synthesis of some corticosteroids. Ascorbic acid has other important properties as a reducing agent, which appear to be nonenzymatic. For example, it aids in **absorption of iron** by reducing it to the ferrous state in the stomach. It spares vitamin A, vitamin E, and some B vitamins by protecting them from oxidation. Also, it enhances the utilization of folic acid, either by aiding the conversion of folate to tetrahydrofolate or the formation of polyglutamate derivatives of tetrahydrofolate. Finally, vitamin C appears to be a biologically important antioxidant. The National Research Council has recently concluded that adequate amounts (RDA levels) of antioxidants such as β-carotene and vitamin C in the diet reduce the risk of **cancer.** The data for other naturally occurring antioxidants such as vitamin E and selenium are not yet conclusive.

Most of the symptoms of **vitamin C deficiency** can be directly related to its metabolic roles. Symptoms of mild vitamin C deficiency include easy bruising and formation of petechiae (small, pinpoint hemorrhages in skin) due to increased capillary fragility and decreased immunocompetence. **Scurvy** is associated with decreased wound healing, osteoporosis, hemorrhaging, and anemia. Osteoporosis results from the inability to maintain the collagenous organic matrix of the bone, followed by demineralization. Anemia results from extensive hemorrhaging coupled with defects in iron absorption and folate metabolism.

Since vitamin C is readily absorbed, deficiencies almost invariably result from poor diet and/or increased need. There is uncertainty over the need for vitamin C in periods of stress. In severe stress or trauma there is a rapid drop in serum vitamin C levels. In these situations most of the body's supply of vitamin C is mobilized to the adrenals and/or the area of the wound. Does this represent an increased demand for vitamin C, or merely a normal redistribution to those areas where it is needed most? Do the lowered serum levels of vitamin C impair its functions in other tissues in the body? The current consensus seems to be that the lowered serum vitamin C levels indicate an increased demand, but there is little agreement as to how much.

Smoking causes lower serum levels of vitamin C. In fact, the 1989 RDAs recommend that smokers consume 100 mg of vitamin C per day instead of the 60 mg day^{-1} needed by nonsmoking adults. **Aspirin** appears to block uptake of vitamin C by white blood cells. **Oral contraceptives** and **corticosteroids** also lower serum levels of vitamin C. While there is no universal agreement as to the seriousness of these effects, the possibility of marginal vitamin C deficiencies should be considered with any patient using these drugs over a long period of time, especially if dietary intake is less than optimal.

The most controversial question surrounding vitamin C is its use in megadoses to prevent and cure the **common cold.** Ever since this use of vitamin C was first popularized by Linus Pauling in 1970, the issue has generated considerable controversy. However, some double-blind studies have suggested that while vitamin C supplementation does not appear to be useful in preventing the common cold, it may moderate its symptoms. The mechanism by which vitamin C ameliorates the symptoms of the common cold is not known. It has been suggested that vitamin C is required for normal leukocyte function or for synthesis and release of histamine during stress situations.

While **megadoses of vitamin C** are probably no more harmful than the widely used over-the-counter cold medications, some potential side effects of high vitamin C intake should be considered. For example, oxalate is a major metabolite of ascorbic acid. Thus high ascorbate intakes could theoretically lead to the formation of oxalate kidney stones in predisposed individuals. However, most studies have shown that excess vitamin C is primarily excreted as ascorbate rather than oxalate. Pregnant mothers taking megadoses of vitamin C may give birth to infants with abnormally high vitamin C requirements. Earlier suggestions that megadoses of vitamin C interfered with B_{12} metabolism have proved to be incorrect.

28.9 ■ MACROMINERALS

Calcium Has Many Physiological Roles

Calcium is the most abundant mineral in the body. Most is in bone, but the small amount of calcium outside of bone functions in a number of essential processes. It is required for many enzymes, mediates some hormonal responses, and is essential for **blood coagulation.** It is also essential for muscle contractility and normal neuromuscular irritability. In fact, only a relatively narrow range of serum calcium levels is compatible with life. Since maintenance of constant serum calcium levels is so vital, an elaborate homeostatic control system has evolved (see pp. 862 and 1112). Low serum calcium stimulates formation of 1,25-dihydroxycholecalciferol, which enhances calcium absorption. If dietary calcium intake is insufficient to maintain serum calcium, 1,25-dihydroxycholecalciferol and parathyroid hormone stimulate bone resorption. Long-term dietary calcium insufficiency, therefore, almost always results in net loss of calcium from the bones.

Dietary **calcium requirements,** however, vary considerably from individual to individual due to the existence of other factors that affect availability of calcium. For example, vitamin D is required for optimal utilization of calcium. Excess dietary protein may upset calcium balance by causing more rapid excretion of calcium. Exercise increases the efficiency of calcium utilization for bone formation. Calcium balance studies carried out on Peruvian Indians, who have extensive exposure to sunlight, get extensive exercise, and subsist on low-protein vegetarian diets, indicate a need for only 300–400 mg calcium day^{-1}. However, calcium balance studies carried out in this country consistently show higher requirements and the RDA has been set at 800–1200 mg day^{-1}.

The chief symptoms of **calcium deficiency** are similar to those of vitamin D deficiency, but other symptoms such as muscle cramps are possible with marginal deficiencies. A significant portion of low-income children and adult females in this country do not have adequate calcium intake. This is of particular concern because these are the population groups with particularly high needs for calcium. For this reason, the U.S. Congress has established the WIC (Women and Infant Children) program to assure adequate protein, calcium, and iron for indigent families with pregnant/lactating mothers or young infants.

Dietary surveys show that 34–47% of the over-60 population consumes less than one-half the RDA for calcium. This is the group most at risk of developing **osteoporosis,** characterized by loss of bone organic matrix as well as progressive demineralization. Causes of osteoporosis are multifactorial and largely unknown, but it appears likely that part of the problem has to do with calcium metabolism (see Clin. Corr. 28.7). Recent studies have also suggested that inadequate intake of calcium may result in elevated blood pressure. Although this hypothesis has not been conclusively demonstrated, it is of great concern because most low-sodium diets (which are recommended for patients with high blood pressure) severely limit dairy products, the main source of calcium for Americans.

Magnesium Is Another Important Macromineral

Magnesium is required for many enzyme activities and for neuromuscular transmission. Deficiency is most often observed in conditions of alcoholism, use of certain diuretics, and metabolic acidosis. The main symptoms of magnesium deficiency are weakness, tremors, and cardiac arrhythmia. There is some evidence that supplemental magnesium may help prevent the formation of calcium oxalate stones in the kidney.

CLINICAL CORRELATION 28.7

Diet and Osteoporosis

The controversies raging over the relationships between calcium intake and osteoporosis illustrate the difficulties we face in making simple dietary recommendations for complex biological problems. Based on the TV ads and wide variety of calcium-fortified foods on the market, it would be easy to assume that all an older woman needs to prevent osteoporosis is a diet rich in calcium. However, that may be like closing the barn door after the horse has left. There is strong consensus that the years from age 10 to 35, when the bone density is reaching its maximum, are the most important for reducing the risk of osteoporosis. The maximum bone density obtained during these years is clearly dependent on both calcium intake and exercise and dense bones are less likely to become seriously depleted of calcium following menopause. Unfortunately, most American women are consuming far too little calcium during these years. The RDA for calcium is 1200 mg day^{-1} (4 glasses of milk per day) for women from age 11 to 24 and 800 mg day^{-1} (2 glasses of milk per day) for women over 24. The median calcium intake for women in this age range is only about 500 mg day^{-1}. Thus it is clear that increased calcium intake should be encouraged in this group.

But what about postmenopausal women? After all, many of the advertisements seem to be targeted at this group. Do they really need more calcium? The 1994 NIH consensus panel on osteoporosis recommended that postmenopausal women consume up to 1500 mg of calcium per day, but this recommendation has been vigorously disputed by other experts in the field. Let's examine the evidence. Calcium balance studies have shown that many postmenopausal women need 1200–1500 mg of calcium per day to maintain a positive calcium balance (more calcium coming in than is lost in the urine), but that does not necessarily mean that the additional calcium will be stored in their bones. In fact, some recent studies have failed to find a correlation between calcium intake and loss of bone density in postmenopausal women while others have reported a protective effect. All of those studies have been complicated by the discovery that calcium intake may have different effects on different types of bones. Calcium intakes in the range of 1000–1500 mg day^{-1} appear to slow the decrease in density of cortical bone, such as that found in the hip, hand, and some parts of the forearm. Similar doses, however, appear to have little or no effect on loss of density from the trabecular bone found in the spine, wrist, and other parts of the forearm. At least some of the confusion in the earlier studies appears to have resulted from differences in the site used for measurement of bone density. Thus the effect of high calcium intakes alone on slowing bone loss in postmenopausal women remains controversial at present. It is clear that elderly women should be getting at least the RDA for calcium in their diet. With the recent concern about the fat content of dairy products, calcium intakes in this group appear to be decreasing rather than increasing. Furthermore, even with estrogen replacement therapy, calcium intake should not be ignored. Recent studies have shown that with calcium intakes in the range of 1000–1500 mg day^{-1}, the effective dose of estrogen can be reduced significantly.

While the advertisements and much of the popular literature focus on calcium intake, we also need to remember that bones are not made of calcium alone. If the diet is deficient in other nutrients, the utilization of calcium for bone formation will be impaired. Vitamin C is needed to form the bone matrix and the macrominerals magnesium and phosphorus are an important part of bone structure. Recent research has also shown that vitamin K and a variety of trace minerals, including copper, zinc, manganese, and boron, are important for bone formation. Thus calcium supplements may not be optimally utilized if the overall diet is inadequate. Vitamin D is important for absorption and utilization of calcium. It deserves special mention since it may be a particular problem for the elderly (see Clin. Corr. 28.9). Finally, an adequate exercise program is just as important as estrogen replacement therapy and an adequate diet for preventing the loss of bone density.

Schaafsma, G., Van Berensteyn, E. C. H., Raymakers, J. A., and Dursma, S. A. Nutritional aspects of osteoporosis. *World Rev. Nutr. Diet.* 49:121, 1987; Heaney, R. P. Calcium in the prevention and treatment of osteoporosis. *J. Intern. Med.* 231:169, 1992; and National Institutes of Health. Optimal calcium intake. *NIH Consens. Statement,* 12 (Nov. 4), 1994.

28.10 ■ TRACE MINERALS

Iron Is Efficiently Reutilized

Iron metabolism is unique in that it operates largely as a closed system, with iron stores being efficiently reutilized by the body. Iron losses are minimal (<1 mg day^{-1}), but iron absorption is also minimal under the best of conditions. Iron usually occurs in foods in the ferric form bound to protein or organic acids. Before absorption can occur, the iron must be split from these carriers (a process that is facilitated by the acid secretions of the stomach) and reduced to the ferrous form (a process that is enhanced by ascorbic acid). Only 10% of the iron in an average mixed diet is usually absorbed, but the efficiency of absorption can be increased to 30% by severe iron deficiency. Iron absorption and metabolism have been discussed in Chapter 24 and are summarized in Figure 28.15.

Iron plays a number of important roles in the body. As a component of hemoglobin and myoglobin, it is required for O_2 and CO_2 transport. As a component of cytochromes and nonheme iron proteins, it is required for oxidative phosphorylation. As a component of the essential lysosomal enzyme myeloperoxidase, it is required for proper phagocytosis and killing of bacteria by neutrophils. The best-known symptom of iron deficiency is a **microcytic hypochromic** anemia. Iron deficiency is also associated with **decreased immunocompetence.**

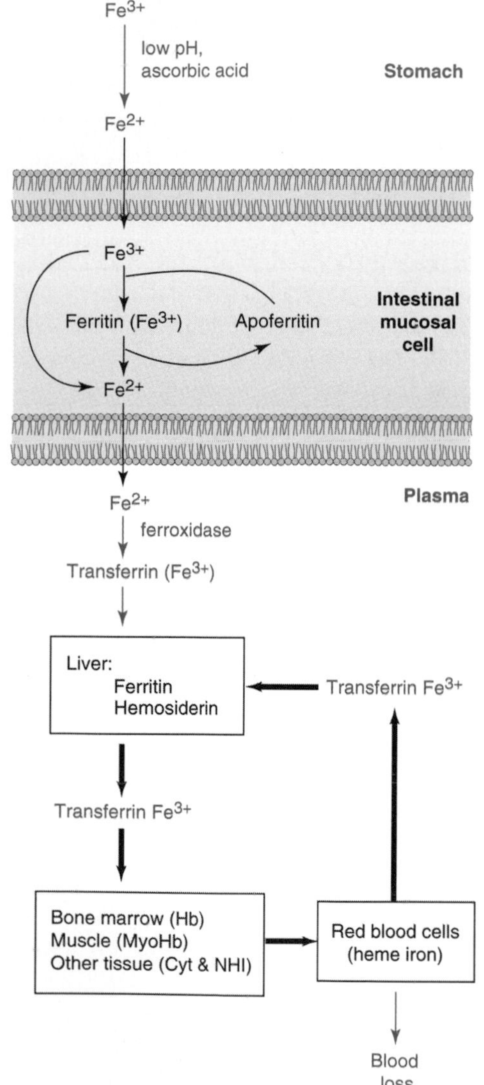

FIGURE 28.15
Overview of iron metabolism.
This figure reviews some of the features of iron metabolism discussed previously in Chapter 24. The red arrows indicate that most of the body's iron is efficiently reutilized by the pathway shown. Hb, hemoglobin; MyoHb, myoglobin; Cyt, cytochromes; and NHI, nonheme iron.

Assuming a 10–15% efficiency of absorption, the Food and Nutrition Board has set a recommended dietary allowance of 10 mg day^{-1} for normal adult males and 15 mg day^{-1} for menstruating females. For pregnant females this allowance is raised to 30 mg day^{-1}. While 10 mg of iron can easily be obtained from a normal diet, 15 mg is marginal at best and 30 mg can almost never be obtained. The best dietary sources are meats, dried legumes, dried fruits, and enriched cereal products.

Iron-deficiency anemia is considered the most prevalent nutritional disorder in the United States. Young children and pregnant females need enough iron for a continuing increase in blood volume. Menstruating females lose iron through blood loss and lactating females through production of lactoferrin. Thus iron deficiency anemia is primarily a problem for these population groups. This is reflected in dietary surveys, which indicate that 95% or more of children and menstruating females are not obtaining adequate iron in their diet. It is also reflected in biochemical measurements of a 10–25% incidence of iron deficiency anemia in this same group. Iron-deficiency anemia is also occasionally a problem with the elderly due to poor dietary intake and increased frequency of achlorhydria.

Because of the widespread nature of iron-deficiency anemia, government programs of nutritional intervention such as the WIC program have emphasized iron-rich foods. There has also been discussion of more extensive iron fortification of foods. There is concern among some nutritionists that iron deficiency has been overemphasized. Some recent studies suggest that **excess iron** intake may increase the risk of cardiovascular disease. Thus iron supplementation and the consumption of iron-fortified foods may be inappropriate for adult men and postmenopausal women. Excess iron can also lead to a rare condition called **hemochromatosis** in which iron deposits are found in abnormally high levels in many tissues. This can lead to liver, pancreatic, and cardiac dysfunction as well as pigmentation of the skin. This condition is usually only seen in hemolytic anemias and liver disease.

Iodine Is Incorporated into Thyroid Hormones

Dietary **iodine** is efficiently absorbed and transported to the **thyroid** gland, where it is stored and used for synthesis of the thyroid hormones triiodothyronine and thyroxine. These hormones function in regulating the **basal metabolic rate** of adults and the growth and development of children. Saltwater fish are the best natural food sources of iodine and in earlier years population groups living in inland areas suffered from the endemic deficiency disease **goiter.** The most characteristic symptom of goiter is the enlargement of the thyroid gland to the point where a large nodule is visible on the neck. Since iodine has been routinely added to table salt, goiter has become relatively rare. However, in some inland areas, mild forms of goiter may still be seen in up to 5% of the population.

Zinc Is a Cofactor for Many Enzymes

Zinc absorption appears to be proportional to **metallothionein** levels in intestinal mucosa cells. The exact function of metallothionein in zinc transport is uncertain, but it may serve as a buffer for zinc ions as the metal transverses the intestinal cells. Over 300 zinc metalloenzymes have been described to date, including a number of regulatory proteins and both RNA and DNA polymerases. **Zinc deficiencies** in children are usually marked by poor growth and impairment of sexual development. In both children and adults zinc deficiencies result in poor wound healing. Zinc is also present in **gustin,** a salivary polypeptide that appears to be necessary for normal development of taste buds. Thus zinc deficiencies also lead to decreased taste acuity.

The few dietary surveys that have been carried out in this country have indicated that zinc intake may be marginal for many individuals. However, few symptoms of zinc deficiency other than decreased taste acuity can be demonstrated in those individuals. Severe zinc deficiency is seen primarily in **alcoholics** (especially if they have cirrhosis), patients with **chronic renal disease** or severe malabsorption diseases, and occasionally in people after long-term parenteral nutrition (TPN). The most characteristic early symptom of zinc-deficient patients on TPN is dermatitis. Zinc is occasionally used therapeutically to promote wound healing and may be of some use in treating gastric ulcers.

Copper Is Also a Cofactor for Important Enzymes

Copper absorption may also be dependent on the protein **metallothionein,** since excess intake of either copper or zinc interferes with the absorption of the other. Copper is present in a number of important metalloenzymes, including cytochrome *c* oxidase, dopamine β-hydroxylase, superoxide dismutase, lysyl oxidase, and Δ^9-desaturase. Δ^9-Desaturase is responsible for converting stearic acid (a C_{18} saturated fatty acid) to oleic acid (a C_{18} monounsaturated fatty acid). This may be responsible for the fact that dietary stearic acid does not have the cholesterol-raising property of the other saturated fatty acids. Lysyl oxidase is necessary for the conversion of certain lysine residues in collagen and elastin to allysine, which is needed for cross-linking. Some of the symptoms of **copper deficiency** include **hypercholesterolemia,** demineralization of bones, leukopenia, anemia, fragility of large arteries, and demyelination of neural tissue. Anemia appears to be due to a defect in iron metabolism. The copper-containing enzyme ferroxidase is necessary for conversion of iron from the Fe^{2+} state (in which form it is absorbed) to the Fe^{3+} state (in which form it can bind to the plasma protein transferrin). The bone demineralization and blood vessel fragility can be traced directly to defects in collagen and elastin formation. The hypercholesterolemia may be related to increases in the ratio of saturated to monounsaturated fatty acids of the C_{18} series due to reduced activity of the C_{18}, Δ^9-desaturase.

Copper balance studies carried out with human volunteers seem to indicate a minimum requirement of 1.0–2.6 mg day^{-1}. The RDA has been set at 1.5–3 mg day^{-1}. Most dietary surveys find the average American diet provides only 1 mg at <2000 cal day^{-1}. This remains a puzzling problem. Few symptoms of copper deficiency have been identified in the general public. It is not known whether there exist widespread marginal copper deficiencies, or whether the copper balance studies are inaccurate. Recognizable symptoms of copper deficiency are usually seen only as a result of excess zinc intake and in **Menkes' syndrome,** a relatively rare X-linked hereditary disease associated with a defect in copper transport. **Wilson's disease,** an autosomal recessive disease, is associated with abnormal accumulation of copper in various tissues and can be treated with the naturally occurring copper chelating agent penicillamine.

Chromium Is a Component of Glucose Tolerance Factor

Chromium probably functions primarily as a component of **glucose tolerance factor (GTF),** a naturally occurring coordination complex between chromium, nicotinic acid, and the amino acids glycine, glutamate, cysteine, or glutathione. GTF potentiates the effects of insulin, presumably by facilitating its binding to cell receptor sites. The chief symptom of **chromium deficiency** is impaired glucose tolerance, a result of the decreased insulin effectiveness. The frequency of chromium deficiency is unknown. The RDA for chromium has been set at 50–200 μg for a normal adult. The best current estimate is that the average consumption of chromium is around 30 μg day^{-1} in the United States. Unfortunately, the range of intakes is very wide (5–100 μg) even for individuals otherwise consuming balanced diets. Those most likely to have marginal or low intakes of chromium are individuals on low-caloric intakes or consuming large amounts of processed foods. Some concern has been voiced that many Americans may be marginally deficient in chromium.

Selenium Is a Scavenger of Peroxides

Selenium functions primarily in the metalloenzyme glutathione peroxidase, which destroys peroxides in the cytosol. Since the effect of vitamin E on peroxide formation is limited primarily to the membrane, both selenium and vitamin E appear to be necessary for efficient scavenging of peroxides. Selenium is one of the few nutrients not removed by the milling of flour and is usually thought to be present in adequate amounts in the diet. The selenium levels are very low in the soil in certain parts of the country, however, and foods raised in these regions will be low in selenium. Fortunately, this effect is minimized by the current food distribution system, which assures that the foods marketed in any one area are derived from a number of different geographical regions.

Manganese, Molybdenum, Fluoride, and Boron Are Other Trace Elements

Manganese is a component of pyruvate carboxylase and probably other metalloenzymes as well. **Molybdenum** is a component of xanthine oxidase. **Fluoride** is known to strengthen bones and teeth and is usually added to drinking water. **Boron** may also play an important role in bone formation.

28.11 ■ THE AMERICAN DIET: FACT AND FALLACY

Much has been said about the supposed deterioration of the American diet. How serious a problem is this? Clearly Americans are eating much more processed food than their ancestors. These foods differ from simpler foods in that they have a higher caloric density and a lower nutrient density than the foods they replace. However, these foods are almost uniformly enriched with iron, thiamine, riboflavin, and niacin. In many cases they are even fortified (usually as much for sales promotion as for nutritional reasons) with as many as 11–15 vitamins and minerals. Unfortunately, it is simply not practical to replace all of the nutrients lost, especially the trace minerals. Imitation foods present a special problem in that they are usually incomplete in more subtle ways. For example, imitation cheese and imitation milkshakes that are widely sold in this country usually contain the protein and calcium one would expect of the food they replace, but often do not contain the riboflavin, which one would also obtain from these items. Fast food restaurants have also been much maligned in recent years. Some of the criticism has been undeserved, but fast food meals do tend to be high in calories and fat and low in certain vitamins and trace minerals. For example, the standard fast food meal provides over 50% of the calories the average adult needs for the entire day, while providing <5% of the vitamin A and <30% of biotin, folic acid, and pantothenic acid. Unfortunately, much of the controversy in recent years has centered around whether these trends are "good" or "bad." This simply obscures the issue at hand. Clearly it is possible to obtain a balanced diet which includes processed, imitation, and fast foods if one compensates by selecting foods for the other meals that are low in caloric density and rich in nutrients. Without such compensation the "balanced diet" becomes a myth.

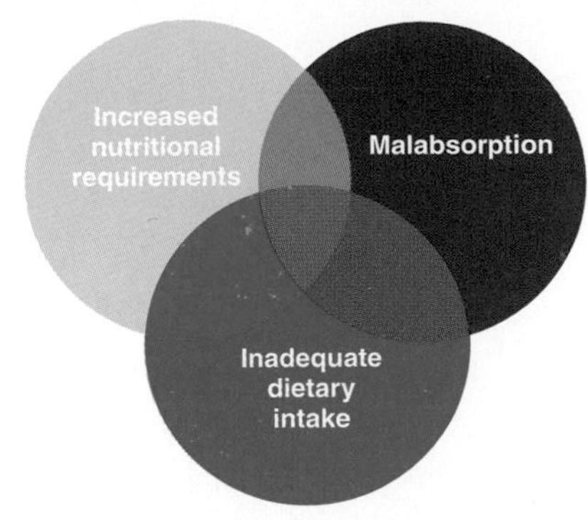

FIGURE 28.16
Factors affecting individual nutritional status.
Schematic representation of three important risk factors in determining nutritional status. A person on the periphery would have very low risk of any nutritional deficiency, whereas people in the green, orange, purple, or center areas would be much more likely to experience some symptoms of nutritional deficiencies.

28.12 ASSESSMENT OF NUTRITIONAL STATUS IN CLINICAL PRACTICE

Having surveyed the major micronutrients and their biochemical roles, it might seem that the process of evaluating the **nutritional status** of an individual patient would be an overwhelming task. It is perhaps best to recognize that there are three factors that can add to nutritional deficiencies: poor diet, malabsorption, and increased nutrient need. Only when two or three components overlap in the same person (Figure 28.16) do the risks of symptomatic deficiencies become significant. For example, infants and young children have increased needs for iron, calcium, and protein. Dietary surveys show that many of them consume diets inadequate in iron and some consume diets that are low in calcium. Protein is seldom a problem unless the children are being raised as strict vegetarians (see Clin. Corr. 28.8). Thus the chief nutritional concerns for most children are iron and calcium. **Teenagers** tend to consume diets low in calcium, magnesium, vitamin A, vitamin B_6, and vitamin C. Of all these nutrients, their needs are particularly high for calcium and magnesium during the teenage years, so these are the nutrients of greatest concern. **Young women** are likely to consume diets low in iron, calcium, magnesium, vitamin B_6, folic acid, and zinc—and all these nutrients are needed in greater amounts during pregnancy and lactation. **Adult women** often consume diets low in calcium, yet they may have a particularly high need for calcium to prevent rapid bone loss. Finally, the elderly have unique nutritional needs (see Clin. Corr. 28.9) and tend to have poor nutrient intake due to restricted income, loss of appetite, and loss of the ability to prepare a wide variety of foods. They are also more prone to suffer from malabsorption problems and to use multiple prescription drugs that increase nutrient needs (Table 28.1).

Illness and metabolic stress often cause increased demand or decreased utilization of certain nutrients. For example, diseases leading to fat malabsorption cause a particular problem with absorption of calcium and the fat-soluble vitamins. Other malabsorption diseases can result in deficiencies of many nutrients depending on the particular malabsorption disease. Liver and kidney disease can prevent activation of vitamin D and storage or utilization of many other nutrients including vitamin A, vitamin B_{12}, and folic acid. Severe illness or trauma increases the need for calories, protein, and possibly some micronutrients such as vitamin C and certain B vitamins. Long-term use of many drugs in the treatment of chronic disease states can affect the need for certain micronutrients. Some of these are summarized in Table 28.1.

Who then is at a nutritional risk? Obviously, the answer depends on many

TABLE 28.1 Drug–Nutrient Interactions

Drug	*Potential Nutrient Deficiencies*
Alcohol	Thiamine Folic acid Vitamin B_6
Anticonvulsants	Vitamin D Folic acid Vitamin K
Cholestyramine	Fat-soluble vitamins Iron
Corticosteroids	Vitamin D and calcium Zinc Potassium
Diuretics	Potassium Zinc
Isoniazid	Vitamin B_6
Oral contraceptives and estrogens	Vitamin B_6 Folic acid and B_{12}

CLINICAL CORRELATION 28.8

Nutritional Considerations for Vegetarians

A vegetarian diet poses certain problems in terms of micronutrient intake that need to be recognized in designing a well-balanced diet. Vitamin B_{12} is of special concern, since it is found only in foods of animal origin. Vitamin B_{12} should be obtained from fortified foods (such as some brands of soybean milk) or in tablet form. However, surprisingly few vegetarians ever develop pernicious anemia, perhaps because an adult who has previously eaten meat will have a 6–10-year store of B_{12} in their liver.

Iron is another problem. The best vegetable sources of iron are dried beans, dried fruits, whole grain or enriched cereals, and green leafy vegetables. Vegetarian diets can provide adequate amounts of iron provided that these foods are regularly selected and consumed with vitamin C-rich foods to promote iron absorption. However, iron supplementation is usually recommended for children and menstruating women.

When milk and dairy products are absent from the diet, certain other problems must be considered as well. Normally, dietary vitamin D is obtained primarily from fortified milk. While some butters and margarines are fortified with vitamin D, they are seldom consumed in sufficient quantities to supply significant amounts of vitamin D. Although adults can usually obtain sufficient vitamin D from exposure to sunlight, dietary sources are often necessary during periods of growth and for adults with little exposure to sunlight. Vegetarians may need to obtain their vitamin D from fortified foods such as cereals, certain soybean milks, or in tablet form. Riboflavin is found in a number of vegetable sources such as green leafy vegetables, enriched breads, and wheat germ. However, since none of these sources supply more than 10% of the RDA in normal serving sizes, fortified cereals or vitamin supplements may become an important source of this nutrient. The important sources of calcium for vegetarians include soybeans, soybean milk, almonds, and green leafy vegetables. Those green leafy vegetables without oxalic acid (mustard, turnip, and dandelion greens, collards, kale, romaine lettuce, and loose leaf lettuce) are particularly good sources of calcium. None of these sources, however, is equivalent to cow's milk in calcium content, so calcium supplements are usually recommended during periods of rapid growth.

Specker, B. L. Nutritional concerns of lactating women consuming vegetarian diets. *Am. J. Clin. Nutr.* 59:1182S, 1994; Sanders, T. A. B. and Reddy, S. Vegetarian diets and children. *Am. J. Clin. Nutr.* 59:1176S, 1994; Weaver, C. M., and Plawecki, K. L. Dietary calcium: adequancy of a vegetarian diet. *Am. J. Clin. Nutr.* 59:1238S, 1994; Craig, W. J. Iron status of vegetarians. *Am. J. Clin. Nutr.* 59:1233S, 1994; Gibson, R. S. Content and bioavailability of trace elements in the vegetarian diet. *Am J. Clin. Nutr.* 59:1223S, 1994.

CLINICAL CORRELATION 28.9

Nutritional Needs of Elderly Persons

If current trends continue, one out of five Americans will be over the age of 65 by the year 2030. With this projected aging of the American population, there has been increased interest in defining the nutritional needs of the elderly. Recent research shows altered needs of elderly persons for several essential nutrients. For example, the absorption and utilization of vitamin B_6 has been shown to decrease with age. Dietary surveys have consistently shown that B_6 is a problem nutrient for many Americans and the elderly appear to be no exception. Many older Americans get less than 50% of the RDA for B_6 from their diet. Vitamin B_{12} deficiency is also more prevalent in the elderly. Many older adults develop a condition called atrophic gastritis, which results in decreased acid production in the stomach. That along with a tendency toward decreased production of intrinsic factor leads to poor absorption of B_{12}. Recent research has suggested that elevated blood levels of the amino acid homocysteine may be a risk factor for atherosclerosis. Homocysteine is normally metabolized to methionine and cysteine in reactions requiring folic acid, B_{12} and B_6. Vitamin D can be a problem as well. Many elderly do not spend much time in the sunlight and to make matters worse the conversion of both 7-dehydrocholesterol to vitamin D in the skin and 25-(OH)D to 1,25-$(OH)_2$D in the kidney decreases with age. These factors often combine to produce significant deficiencies of 1,25-$(OH)_2$D in the elderly, which can in turn lead to negative calcium balance. These changes do not appear to be the primary cause of osteoporosis but they certainly may contribute to it.

There is some evidence for increased need for chromium and zinc as well. Chromium is not particularly abundant in the American diet and many elderly appear to have difficulty converting dietary chromium to the biologically active glucose tolerance factor. The clinical relevance of these observations is not clear but chromium deficiency could contribute to adult-onset diabetes. Similarly, dietary surveys show that most elderly consume between one-half and two-thirds the RDA for zinc. Conditions such as atrophic gastritis can also interfere with zinc absorption. Symptoms of zinc deficiency include loss of taste acuity, dermatitis, and a weakened immune system. All of these symptoms are common in the elderly population and it has been suggested that zinc deficiency might contribute.

Not all of the news is bad, however. Vitamin A absorption actually increases as we age and the ability of the liver to clear vitamin A from the blood decreases, so it remains in the circulation for a longer time. In fact, not only does the need for vitamin A decrease as we age, but the elderly also need to be particularly careful to avoid vitamin A toxicity. While this does not restrict their choice of foods or multivitamin supplements, they should generally avoid separate vitamin A supplements.

Munro, H. N., Suter, P. M., and Rusell, R. M. Nutritional requirements of the elderly. *Annu. Rev. Nutr.* 7:23, 1987; Russell, R. M., and Suter, P. M. Vitamin requirements of elderly people: an update. *Am. J. Clin. Nutr.* 58:4, 1993; Ubbink, J. B., Vermoak, W. J., van der Merne, A., and Becker, P. J. Vitamin B_{12}, Vitamin B_6 and folate nutritional status in men with hyperhomocysteinemia. *Am. J. Clin. Nutr.* 57:47, 1993; Joosten, E., van der Berg. A., Riezler, R., Neurath, H. J., Linderbaum, J. Stabler, S. P., and Allen, R. H. Metabolic evidence that deficiencies of vitamin B_{12}, folate and vitamin B_6 occur commonly in elderly people. *Am. J. Clin. Nutr.* 58:468, 1993.

factors. Nutritional counseling is an important part of treatment for infants, young children, and pregnant/lactating females. A brief analysis of a dietary history and further nutritional counseling are important when dealing with high-risk patients.

BIBLIOGRAPHY

Recommended Dietary Allowances

Food and Nutrition Board of the National Academy of Sciences. *Recommended Daily Allowances,* 10th Edition. Washington, DC: National Academy of Sciences, 1989.

Vitamin A

Goodman, D. S. Vitamin A and retinoids in health and disease. *N. Engl. J. Med.* 310:1023–1031, 1984.

Wolf, G. Mutiple functions of vitamin A. *Physiol. Rev.* 64:873–935, 1984.

van Poppel, G., and Goldbohm, R. A. Epidemiologic evidence for β-carotene and cancer prevention. *Am. J. Clin. Nutr.* 62:1393S, 1995.

Vitamin D

Darwish, H., and DeLuca, H. F. Vitamin D—regulated gene expression. *Crit. Rev. Eukaryot. Gene Expr.,* 3:89, 1993.

DeLuca, H. F. The vitamin D story. A collaborative effort of basic science and clinical medicine. *FASEB J.* 2:224–236, 1988.

Vitamin E

Bieri, J. G., Coresh, L., and Hubbard, V. S. Medical uses of vitamin E. *N. Engl. J. Med.* 308:1063–1072, 1983.

Das, S. Vitamin E in the genesis and prevention of cancer. A review. *Acta Oncol.* 33:615, 1994.

Meydani, S. N., Wu, D., Santos, M. S., and Hayek, M. C. Antioxidants and immune response in aged persons: overview of present evidence. *Am. J. Clin. Nutr.* 62:1462S, 1995.

Nyyssonen, K., Porkkala, E., Salonen, R., Korpela, H., and Salonen, J. T. Increase in oxidation resistance of atherogenic serum lipoproteins following antioxidant supplementation: a randomized double-blind placebo-controlled clinical trial. *Eur. J. Clin. Nutr.* 48:633–642, 1994.

Stampfer, M. J., and Rimm, E. B. Epidemiologic evidence for vitamin E in prevention of cardiovascular disease. *Am. J. Clin. Nutr.* 62:1365S, 1995.

Vitamin K

Binkley, N. C., and Suttie, J. W. Vitamin K nutrition and osteoporosis. *J. Nutr.* 125:1812, 1995.

Lipsky, J. J. Nutritional sources of vitamin K. *Mayo Clin. Proc.* 69:462, 1994

Vitamin B_6

Merril, A. H. Jr., and Henderson, J. M. Diseases associated with defects in vitamin B_6 metabolism or utilization. *Annu. Rev. Nutr.* 7:137–156, 1987.

Tully, D. B., Allgood, V. E., and Cidlowski, J. A. Modulation of steroid receptor-mediated gene expression by vitamin B_6. *FASEB J.* 8:343, 1994.

Folate

Blakely, R. L., and Whitehead, V. M. (Eds.). *Folate and Pterins,* Vol 3. New York: Wiley, 1986.

Landgren, F., Israelsson, B., Lindgren, A., Hultsberg, B., Anderson, A., and Brettstrom, L. Plasma homocysteine in acute myocardial infarction: homocysteine-lowering effects of folic acid. *J. Intern. Med.* 237:381, 1995.

Milunsky, A., Jick, H., Jick, S. S., Bruell, C. L., MacLaugin, D. S., Rothman, K. J., and Willet, W. Multivitamin/folic acid supplementation in early pregnancy reduces the prevalence of neural tube defects. *JAMA* 262:2847, 1989

Vitamin C

Hemila, H. Does vitamin C alleviate the symptoms of the common cold? A review of current evidence. *Scand. J. Infect Dis.* 26:1, 1994.

Third International Conference on Vitamin C. *Ann. N.Y. Acad. Sci.* 498:1–534, 1987.

Simon, J. A. Vitamin C and cardiovascular disease: a review. *J. Am. Coll. Nutr.* 11:107, 1992.

Calcium

Hatton, D. C., and McCarron, D. A. Dietary calcium and blood pressure in experimental models of hypertension. *Hypertension* 23:513, 1994.

National Institutes of Health. Optimal calcium intake. *NIH Consens. Statement,* 12(4), 1994.

Iron

Dollman, P. R. Biochemical basis for the manifestations of iron deficiency. *Annu. Rev. Nutr.* 6:13, 1986.

Chromium

Mertz, W. Chromium in human nutrition: a review. *J. Nutr.* 123:626, 1993

Other Trace Minerals

Symposium on metal metabolism and disease. *Clin. Physiol. Biochem.* 4:1–111, 1986.

Dietary Surveys

Block, G. Dietary guidelines and the results of food consumption surveys. *Am. J. Clin. Nutr.* 53:3565, 1991.

Kritchevsy, D. Dietary guidelines. The rationale for intervention. *Cancer* 72:1011, 1993.

Pao, E. M., and Mickle, S. J. Problem nutrients in the United States. *Food Technol.* 35:58–67, 1981.

QUESTIONS ■ J. BAGGOTT AND C. N. ANGSTADT

1. Recommended dietary allowances (RDAs):
   A. are standards for all individuals.
   B. meet special dietary needs arising from chronic diseases.
   C. include all nutritional needs.
   D. define optimal levels of nutrients.
   E. are useful only as general guides in evaluating the adequacy of diets.
2. The effects of vitamin A may include all of the following EXCEPT:
   A. prevention of anemia.
   B. serving as an antioxidant.
   C. cell differentiation.
   D. the visual cycle.
   E. induction of certain cancers.

3. All of the following organs are associated with vitamin D metabolism or effects of vitamin D on calcium metabolism EXCEPT:
   A. bone.
   B. erythrocytes.
   C. gut.
   D. kidney.
   E. liver.

Refer to the following for Questions 4–8:
   A. vitamin A
   B. vitamin K
   C. niacin
   D. vitamin D
   E. vitamin B_{12} (cobalamine)

4. Requirement may totally be supplied by intestinal bacteria.

5. Precursor is synthesized by green plants.

6. Tryptophan is a precursor.

7. Deficiency may be seen in long-term adherence to a strict vegetarian diet.

8. Is required for normal regulation of calcium metabolism.

9. Ascorbic acid may be associated with all of the following EXCEPT:
   A. iron absorption.
   B. bone formation.
   C. acute renal disease when taken in high doses.
   D. wound healing
   E. participation in hydroxylation reactions.

10. In assessing the adequacy of a person's diet:
   A. age of the individual usually has little relevance.
   B. trauma decreases activity, and hence decreases need for calories and possibly some micronutrients.
   C. a 24-h dietary intake history provides an adequate basis for making a judgment.
   D. currently administered medications must be considered.
   E. intestine is the only organ whose health has substantial bearing on nutritional status.

Refer to the following for Questions 11–15:
   A. calcium
   B. iron
   C. iodine
   D. copper
   E. selenium

11. Absorption is inhibited by excess dietary zinc.

12. Excess dietary protein causes rapid excretion.

13. Risk of nutritional deficiency is high in young children.

14. Unsupplemented diets of populations living in inland areas may be deficient.

15. Essential component of glutathione peroxidase.

ANSWERS

1. E A: RDAs are designed for most individuals; exceptions occur. B: Diseases often change dietary requirements. C: Some nutritional needs may be unknown; the requirements for all known nutrients are not even clear. D: Optimal levels of nutrients are hard to define; it depends on the criterion for optimal. (See pp. 1108–1109.)
2. E Vitamin A deficiency is linked to increased susceptibility to certain cancers. A: Retinyl phosphate serves as a glycosyl donor in the synthesis of certain glycoproteins (p. 1110), including transferrin (p. 1111). B: β-Carotene functions as an antioxidant. See p. 1110. C: Retinol and retinoic acid may function like steroid hormones (p. 1110). D: Retinol cycles between the Δ^{11}-cis and all-trans forms in the visual cycle (p. 1111).
3. B A: Calcium mobilization from bone is increased by 1,25-$(OH)_2D$. C: 1,25-$(OH)_2D$ regulates calcium absorption by the gut. D: Kidney converts inactive 25-(OH)D to the active 1,25-$(OH)_2D$ or to the inactive 24,25-$(OH)_2D$. E: Liver converts D to 25-(OH)D. See Figure 28.5 and p. 1114.
4. B See p. 1117.
5. A β-Carotene, from green plants, is converted to vitamin A (p. 1110).
6. C See p. 1121.
7. E This vitamin is from animal sources (p. 1126).
8. D 1,25-Dihydroxyvitamin D is required for calcium absorption and, along with parathyroid hormone, regulates bone resorption and calcium excretion.
9. C There has been speculation, not borne out by studies designed to shed light on the issue, that high levels of ascorbic acid could lead to oxalate kidney stones. A: Ascorbic acid aids in iron absorption by reducing iron. B: Ascorbic acid is essential for collagen synthesis, which is critical in bone formation. D and E: Ascorbic acid is required for the hydroxylation of lysine and proline residues in protocollagen and, therefore is required for wound healing. (See pp. 1127–1128.)
10. D Corticosteroids stimulate vitamin D inactivation. (p. 1114). A: Dramatic differences may occur at different ages. B: Trauma increases caloric requirements and probably requirements for specific micronutrients. C: You cannot be sure that any 24-h diet history is either accurate or representative of the individual's typical diet. E: While the intestine must function well enough to absorb nutrients, further metabolic changes are typically required. The metabolism of vitamin D by the liver and kidney (p. 1115) and the conversion of β-carotene to vitamin A exemplify these interorgan interrelations.
11. D See p. 1131.
12. A See p. 1128.
13. B Rapid growth in children causes high demands for iron (p. 1130).
14. C The problem is rare in the United States due to the common use of iodized salt (p. 1131).
15. E See p. 1132.

APPENDIX

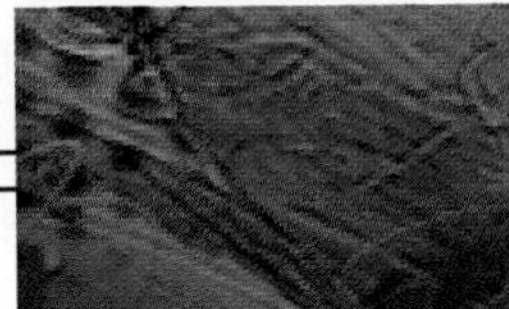

REVIEW OF ORGANIC CHEMISTRY

Carol N. Angstadt

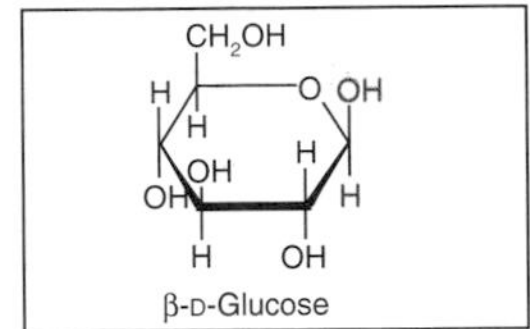

β-D-Glucose

FUNCTIONAL GROUPS

Alcohols

The general formula of **alcohols** is R—OH, where R equals an alkyl or aryl group. They are classified as *primary, secondary,* or *tertiary,* according to whether the hydroxyl (OH)-bearing carbon is bonded to no carbon or one, two, or three other carbon atoms:

$$-\mathrm{C}-\mathrm{CH_2}-\mathrm{OH} \qquad -\mathrm{C}-\mathrm{CH}(-\mathrm{C}-)-\mathrm{OH} \qquad -\mathrm{C}-\mathrm{C}(-\mathrm{C}-)_2-\mathrm{OH}$$

Primary Secondary Tertiary

Aldehydes and Ketones

Aldehydes and **ketones** contain a carbonyl group:

$$-\mathrm{C}(=\mathrm{O})-$$

Aldehydes are

$$\mathrm{R}-\mathrm{C}(=\mathrm{O})-\mathrm{H}$$

and a *ketone* has two alkyl groups at the carbonyl group

$$\mathrm{R}-\mathrm{C}(=\mathrm{O})-\mathrm{R'}$$

Acids and Acid Anhydrides

Carboxylic acids contain the functional group

$$-\mathrm{C}(=\mathrm{O})-\mathrm{OH}$$

(—COOH). Dicarboxylic and tricarboxylic acids contain two or three carboxyl groups. A carboxylic acid ionizes in water to a negatively charged carboxylate ion:

$$\underset{\text{Carboxylic acid}}{\mathrm{R}-\mathrm{C}(=\mathrm{O})-\mathrm{OH}} \rightarrow \underset{\text{Carboxylate ion}}{\mathrm{R}-\mathrm{C}(=\mathrm{O})-\mathrm{O}^- + \mathrm{H}^+}$$

Names of carboxylic acids usually end in -ic and the carboxylate ion in -ate. **Acid anhydrides** are formed when two molecules of acid react with loss of a molecule of water. An acid anhydride may form between two organic acids, two inorganic acids, or an organic and an inorganic acid:

$$\underset{\text{Organic anhydride}}{\mathrm{R}-\mathrm{C}(=\mathrm{O})-\mathrm{O}-\mathrm{C}(=\mathrm{O})-\mathrm{R}} \qquad \underset{\text{Inorganic anhydride}}{\mathrm{HO}-\mathrm{P}(=\mathrm{O})(\mathrm{OH})-\mathrm{O}-\mathrm{P}(=\mathrm{O})(\mathrm{OH})-\mathrm{OH}}$$

$$\underset{\text{Organic–inorganic anhydride}}{\mathrm{R}-\mathrm{C}(=\mathrm{O})-\mathrm{O}-\mathrm{P}(=\mathrm{O})(\mathrm{OH})-\mathrm{OH}}$$

Esters

Esters form in the reaction between a carboxylic acid and an alcohol:

$$R{-}COOH + R'{-}OH \rightarrow R{-}\overset{\overset{\displaystyle O}{\|}}{C}{-}OR'$$

Esters may form between an inorganic acid and an organic alcohol, for example, glucose 6-phosphate.

Hemiacetals, Acetals, and Lactones

A reaction between an aldehyde and an alcohol gives a **hemiacetal,** which may react with another molecule of alcohol to form an **acetal:**

$$R{-}CHO \xrightarrow{R'-OH} R{-}\underset{H}{\overset{OH}{C}}{-}OR' \xrightarrow{R''-OH} R{-}\underset{H}{\overset{OR''}{C}}{-}OR'$$

Hemiacetal Acetal

Lactones are cyclic esters formed when an acid and an alcohol group on the same molecule react and usually require that a five- or six-membered ring be formed.

Unsaturated Compounds

Unsaturated compounds are those containing one or more carbon–carbon multiple bonds, for example, a double bond: $-C{=}C-$

Amines and Amides

Amines, $R{-}NH_2$, are organic derivatives of NH_3 and are classified as *primary, secondary,* or *tertiary,* depending on the number of alkyl groups (R) bonded to the nitrogen. When a fourth substituent is bonded to the nitrogen, the species is positively charged and called a *quaternary ammonium ion:*

$$R{-}NH_2 \qquad R{-}\underset{H}{N}{-}R' \qquad R{-}\underset{R''}{N}{-}R' \qquad R{-}\underset{R''}{\overset{H(\text{or } R''')}{N^+}}{-}R'$$

Primary amine, Secondary amine, Tertiary amine, Quaternary ammonium ion

Amides contain the functional group

$$-\overset{\overset{\displaystyle O}{\|}}{C}{-}\overset{H}{N}{-}X$$

where X can be H (simple) or R (*N* substituted). The carbonyl group is from an acid, and the *N* is from an amine. If both functional groups are from amino acids, the amide bond is referred to as a **peptide bond.**

TYPES OF REACTIONS

Nucleophilic Substitutions at an Acyl Carbon

If the acyl carbon is on a carboxylic group, the leaving group is water. Nucleophilic substitution on carboxylic acids usually

$$\overset{R}{\underset{L}{>}}C{=}\ddot{O}{:} + {:}X{-}H \rightleftharpoons R{-}\underset{L}{\overset{XH^+}{C}}{-}\ddot{O}{:} \rightleftharpoons R{-}\underset{LH^+}{\overset{X}{C}}{-}\ddot{O}{:}^- \longrightarrow \overset{X}{\underset{R}{>}}C{=}O + LH$$

New compound, Leaving group

requires a catalyst or conversion to a more reactive intermediate; biologically this occurs via enzyme catalysis. X—H may be an alcohol (R—OH), ammonia, amine ($R{-}NH_2$), or another acyl compound. Types of nucleophilic substitutions include *esterification, peptide bond* formation, and *acid anhydride* formation.

Hydrolysis and Phosphorolysis Reactions

Hydrolysis is the cleavage of a bond by water:

$$R{-}\overset{\overset{\displaystyle O}{\|}}{C}{-}OR' + H_2O \longrightarrow R{-}\overset{\overset{\displaystyle O}{\|}}{C}{-}OH + R'{-}OH$$

Hydrolysis is often catalyzed by either acid or base. *Phosphorolysis* is the cleavage of a bond by inorganic phosphate:

$$\text{glucose–glucose} + HO{-}\underset{O^-}{\overset{\overset{\displaystyle O}{\|}}{P}}{-}O^- \longrightarrow \text{glucose 1-phosphate} + \text{glucose}$$

Oxidation–Reduction Reactions

Oxidation is the loss of electrons; **reduction** is the gain of electrons. Examples of oxidation are as follows:

1. Fe^{2+} + acceptor → Fe^{3+} + acceptor · e^-
2. S(ubstrate) + O_2 + DH_2 → S—OH + H_2O + D
3. S—H_2 + acceptor → S + acceptor · H_2

Some of the group changes that occur on oxidation–reduction are:

1. $-CH_2OH \rightleftharpoons -\overset{H}{C}{=}O$
2. $>C{-}OH \rightleftharpoons >C{=}O$

3. $-\overset{H}{\underset{|}{C}}=O \rightleftharpoons -\overset{O}{\overset{\|}{C}}-OH$

4. $-CH_2NH_2 \rightleftharpoons -\overset{H}{\overset{|}{C}}=O + NH_3$

5. $-CH_2-CH_2- \rightleftharpoons -CH=CH-$

STEREOCHEMISTRY

Stereoisomers are compounds with the same molecular formulas and order of attachment of constituent atoms but with different arrangements of these atoms in space.

Enantiomers are stereoisomers in which one isomer is the mirror image of the other and requires the presence of a chiral atom. A chiral carbon (also called an asymmetric carbon) is one that is attached to four different groups:

B above C; D and A on either side of C; E below C — and its mirror image: B above C; A and D on either side of C; E below C.

Enantiomers will be distinguished from each other by the designations *R* and *S* or D and L. The maximum number of stereoisomers possible is 2^n, where *n* is the number of chiral carbon atoms. A molecule with more than one chiral center will be an achiral molecule if it has a point or plane of symmetry.

Diastereomers are stereoisomers that are not mirror images of each other and need not contain chiral atoms. **Epimers** are diastereomers that contain more than one chiral carbon and differ in configuration about *only one* asymmetric carbon.

Anomers are a special form of carbohydrate epimers in which the difference is specifically about the anomeric carbon (see p. 1140). Diastereomers can also occur with molecules in which there is restricted rotation about carbon–carbon bonds. Double bonds exhibit **cis–trans isomerism.** The double bond is in the cis configuration if the two end groups are on the same side and is trans if the two ends of the longest chain are on opposite sides. Fused ring systems, such as those found in steroids (see p. 1145), also exhibit cis–trans isomerism.

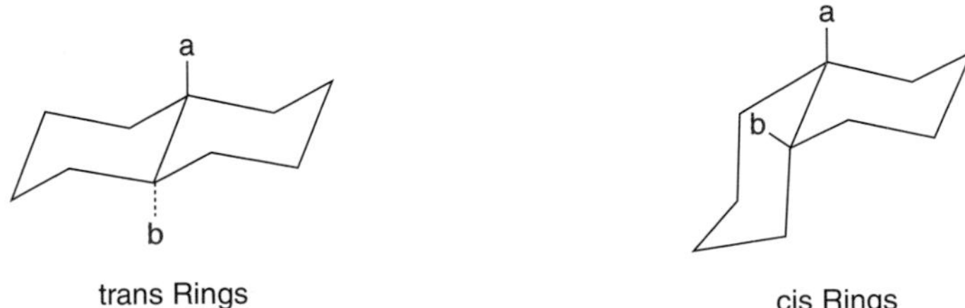

trans Rings   cis Rings

TYPES OF FORCES INVOLVED IN MACROMOLECULAR STRUCTURES

A **hydrogen bond** is a dipole–dipole attraction between a hydrogen atom attached to an electronegative atom and a nonbonding electron pair on another electronegative atom: Hydrogen bonds of importance in macromolecular structures occur between two nitrogen atoms, two oxygen atoms, or an oxygen and a nitrogen atom.

$$:\ddot{X}-H.......:\ddot{X}-H$$
$$\delta^-\ \delta^+ \qquad\qquad \delta^-\ \delta^+$$

A **hydrophobic interaction** is the association of nonpolar groups in a polar medium. *Van der Waals* forces consist of dipole and induced-dipole interactions between two nonpolar groups. A nonpolar residue dissolved in water induces a highly ordered, thermodynamically unfavorable, solvation shell. Interaction of nonpolar residues with each other, with the exclusion of water, increases the entropy of the system and is thermodynamically favorable.

Ionic (electrostatic) interactions between charged groups can be attractive if the charges are of opposite signs or repulsive if they are of the same sign. The strength of an electrostatic interaction in the interior of a protein molecule may be high. Most charged groups on the surface of a protein molecule interact with water rather than with each other.

A **disulfide bond** (S—S) is a covalent bond formed by the oxidation of two sulfhydryl (SH) groups.

CARBOHYDRATES

Carbohydrates are polyhydroxy aldehydes or ketones or their derivatives. **Monosaccharides** (simple sugars) are those carbohydrates that cannot be hydrolyzed into simpler compounds. The generic name of a monosaccharide includes the type of function, a Greek prefix indicating the number of carbon atoms, and the ending -ose; for example, *aldohexose* is a six-carbon aldehyde and *ketopentose* is a five-carbon ketone. Monosaccharides may react with each other to form larger molecules. With fewer than eight monosaccharides, either a Greek prefix indicating the number or the general term *oligosaccharide* may be used. **Polysaccharide** refers to a polymer with more than eight monosaccharides. Oligo- and polysaccharides may be either homologous or mixed.

Most *monosaccharides* are asymmetric, an important consideration since enzymes usually work on only one isomeric form. The simplest carbohydrates are glyceraldehyde and dihydroxyacetone, whose structures, shown as Fischer projections, are as follows:

H—C=O	H—C=O	CH_2OH
H—C—OH	HO—C—H	C=O
CH_2OH	CH_2OH	CH_2OH
D-Glyceraldehyde	L-Glyceraldehyde	Dihydroxyacetone

D-Glyceraldehyde may also be written as follows:

$$\begin{array}{c} H \\ C=O \\ | \\ H-C-OH \\ | \\ CH_2OH \end{array}$$

In the Cahn–Ingold–Prelog system, the designations are (*R*) (rectus; right) and (*S*) (sinister, left).

The configuration of monosaccharides is determined by the stereochemistry at the asymmetric carbon furthest from the carbonyl carbon (number 1 for an aldehyde; lowest possible number for a ketone). Based on the *position* of the OH on the highest number asymmetric carbon, a monosaccharide is D if the OH projects to the *right* and L if it projects to the *left*. The D and L monosaccharides with the same name are *enantiomers*, and the substituents on all asymmetric carbon atoms are reversed as in

D-Glucose	L-Glucose
H—C=O	H—C=O
H—C—OH	HO—C—H
HO—C—H	H—C—OH
H—C—OH	HO—C—H
H—C—OH	HO—C—H
CH_2OH	CH_2OH

Epimers (e.g., glucose and mannose) are stereoisomers that differ in the configuration about *only one* asymmetric carbon. The relationship of OH groups to *each other* determines the specific monosaccharide. Three aldohexoses and three pentoses of importance are

D-Glucose	D-Mannose	D-Galactose
H—C=O	H—C=O	H—C=O
H—C—OH	HO—C—H	H—C—OH
HO—C—H	HO—C—H	HO—C—H
H—C—OH	H—C—OH	HO—C—H
H—C—OH	H—C—OH	H—C—OH
CH_2OH	CH_2OH	CH_2OH

D-Ribose	D-Ribulose	D-Xylulose
H—C=O	CH_2OH	CH_2OH
H—C—OH	C=O	C=O
H—C—OH	H—C—OH	HO—C—H
H—C—OH	H—C—OH	H—C—OH
CH_2OH	CH_2OH	CH_2OH

Fructose, a ketohexose, differs from glucose only on carbon atoms 1 and 2:

1 CH_2OH
2 C=O
HO—3 C—H
H—4 C—OH
H—5 C—OH
6 CH_2OH

Five- and six-carbon monosaccharides form **cyclic hemiacetals** or *hemiketals* in solution. A new asymmetric carbon is generated so two isomeric forms are possible:

Both five-membered (furanose) and six-membered (pyranose) ring structures are possible, although pyranose rings are more common. A furanose ring is written as follows:

β-D-Fructose

The isomer is designated α if the OH group and the CH_2OH group on the two carbon atoms linked by the oxygen are trans to each other and β if they are cis. The hemiacetal or hemiketal forms may also be written as modified *Fischer projection formulas*: α if OH on the acetal or ketal carbon projects to the same side as the ring and β if on the opposite side:

β-D-Glucose	α-D-Glucose
HO—C—H	H—C—OH
H—C—OH	H—C—OH
HO—C—H	HO—C—H
H—C—OH	H—C—OH
H—C (ring O)	H—C (ring O)
CH_2OH	CH_2OH

Haworth formulas are used most commonly:

α-D-Glucose β-D-Glucose

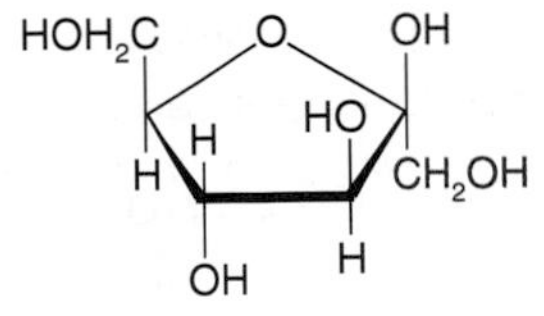

β-D-Fructose

The ring is perpendicular to the plane of the paper with the oxygen written to the back (upper) right, C-1 to the right, and substituents above or below the plane of the ring. The OH at the acetal or ketal carbon is below in the α isomer and above in the β. Anything written to the right in the Fischer projection is written down in the Haworth formula.

The α and β forms of the same monosaccharide are special forms of epimers called *anomers*, differing only in the configuration about the anomeric (acetal or ketal) carbon. Monosaccharides exist in solution primarily as a mixture of the hemiacetals (or hemiketals) but react chemically as aldehydes or ketones. *Mutarotation* is the equilibration of α and β forms through the free aldehyde or ketone. Substitution of the H of the anomeric OH prevents mutarotation and fixes the configuration in either the α or β form.

Monosaccharide Derivatives

A **deoxymonosaccharide** is one in which an OH has been replaced by H. In biological systems, this occurs at C-2 unless otherwise indicated. An **amino monosaccharide** is one in which an OH has been replaced by NH_2, again at C-2 unless otherwise specified. The amino group of an amino sugar may be *acetylated*:

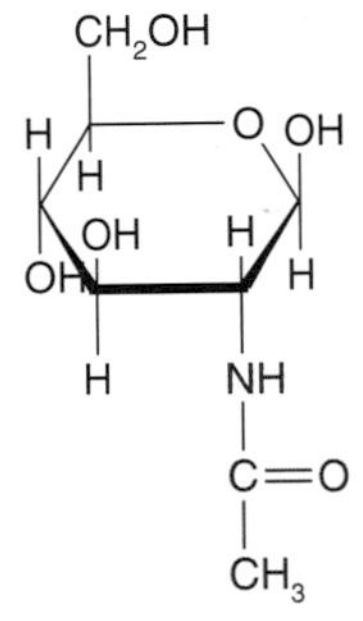

β-*N*-Acetylglucosamine

An aldehyde is reduced to a primary and a ketone to a secondary **monosaccharide alcohol (alditol).** Alcohols are named with the base name of the sugar plus the ending *-itol* or with a trivial name (glucitol = sorbitol). Monosaccharides that differ around only two of the first three carbon atoms yield the same alditol. D-Glyceraldehyde and dihydroxyacetone give glycerol:

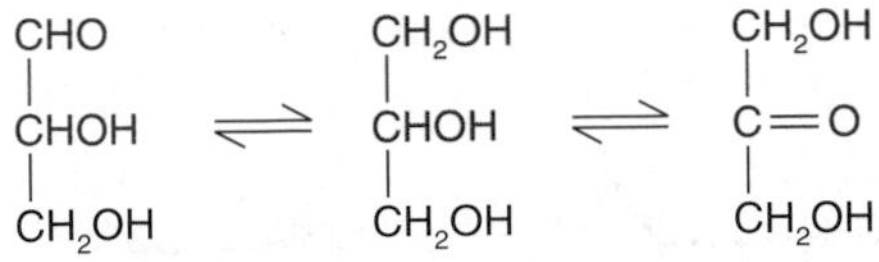

$$\begin{array}{c}CHO\\ |\\ CHOH\\ |\\ CH_2OH\end{array} \rightleftharpoons \begin{array}{c}CH_2OH\\ |\\ CHOH\\ |\\ CH_2OH\end{array} \rightleftharpoons \begin{array}{c}CH_2OH\\ |\\ C{=}O\\ |\\ CH_2OH\end{array}$$

D-Glucose and D-fructose give D-sorbitol; D-fructose and D-mannose give D-mannitol. Oxidation of the terminal CH_2OH, but not of the CHO, yields a-**uronic acid,** a *monosaccharide acid:*

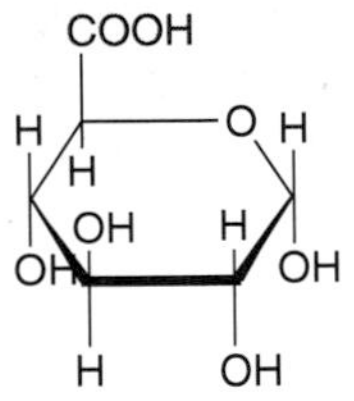

D-Glucuronic acid

Oxidation of the CHO, but not the CH_2OH, gives an **-onic acid:**

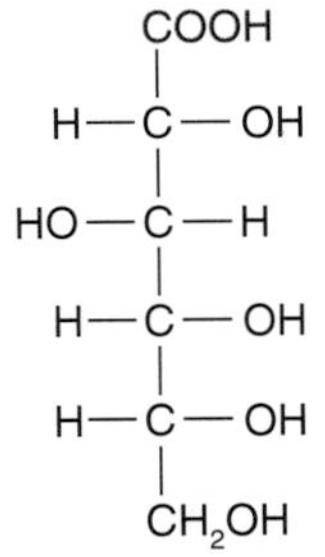

D-Gluconic acid

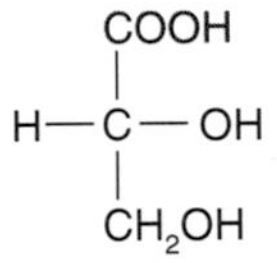

D-Glyceric acid

Oxidation of both the CHO and CH_2OH gives an **-aric acid**:

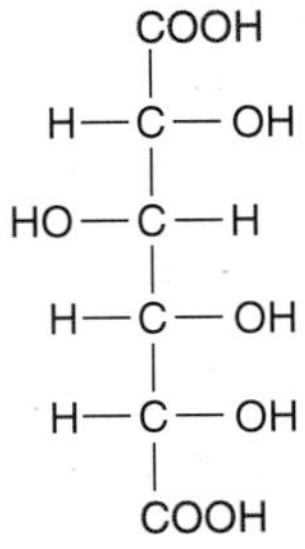

D-Glucaric acid

Ketones do not form acids. Both -onic and -uronic acids can react with an OH in the same molecule to form a **lactone** (see p. 1138):

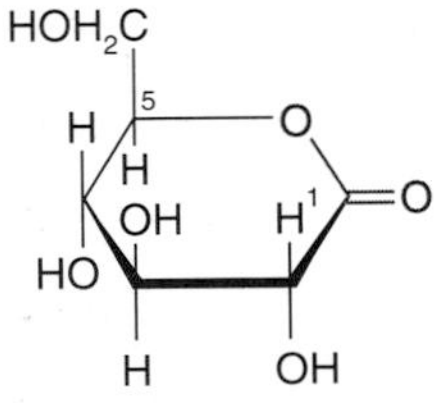

D-Glucono-5-lactone

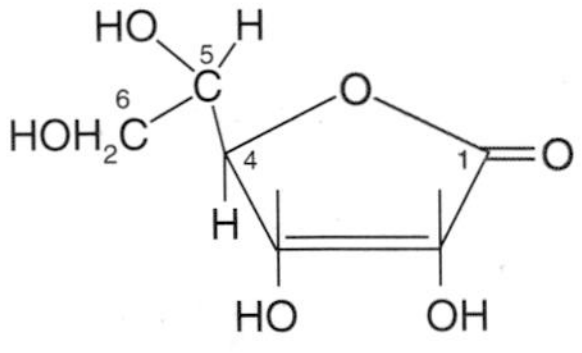

L-Ascorbic acid (derivative of L-gulose)

Reactions of Monosaccharides

The most common *esters* of monosaccharides are phosphate esters at carbon atoms 1 and/or 6:

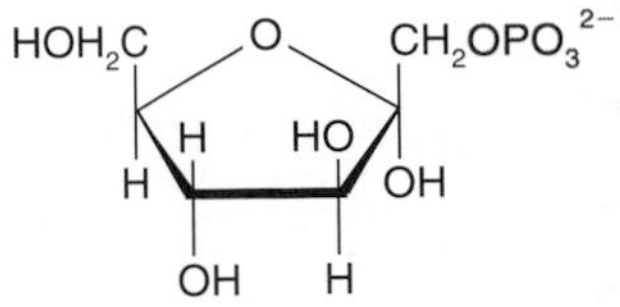

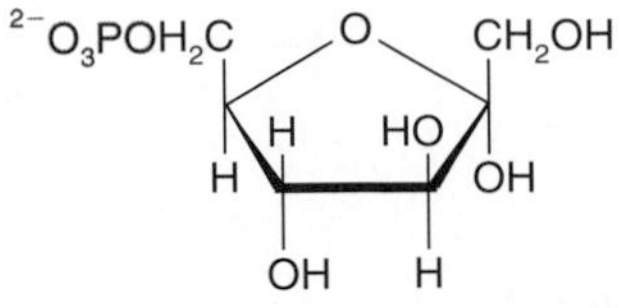

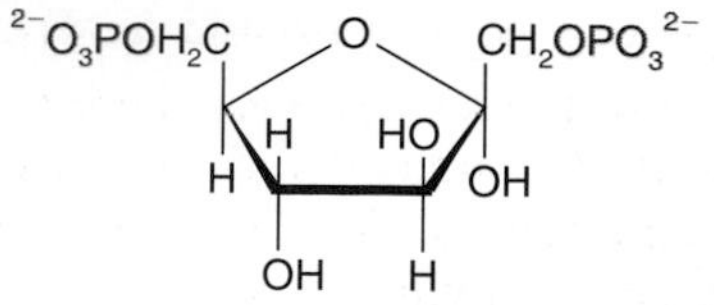

To be a **reducing sugar,** mutarotation must be possible. In alkali, enediols form that may migrate to 2,3 and 3,4 positions:

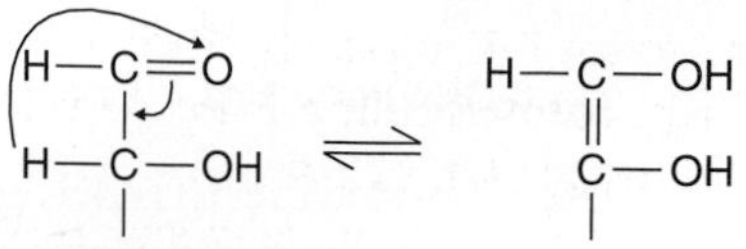

$$\mathrm{H{-}C{=}O,\ H{-}C{-}OH \rightleftharpoons H{-}C{-}OH,\ C{-}OH\ (C{=}C)}$$

Enediols may be oxidized by O_2, Cu^{2+}, Ag^+, and Hg^{2+}. Reducing ability is more important in the laboratory than physiologically. A hemiacetal or hemiketal may react with the OH of another monosaccharide to form a disaccharide (*acetal*: *glycoside*) (see below):

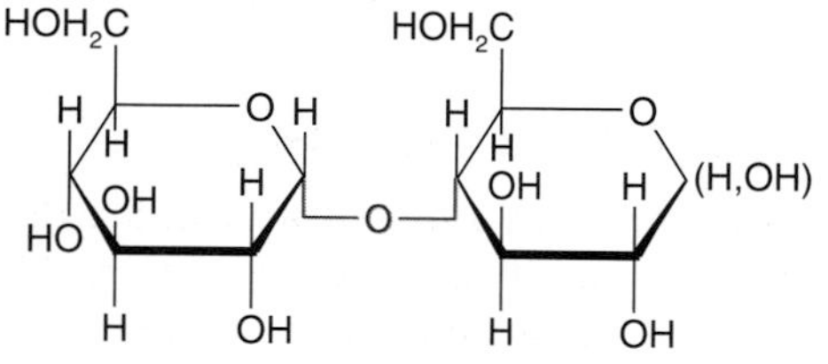

(May be either α or β)

α-1,4-Glycosidic linkage

One monosaccharide still has a free anomeric carbon and can react further. Reaction of the anomeric OH may be with any OH on the other monosaccharide, including the anomeric one. The anomeric OH that has reacted is fixed as either *α* or *β* and cannot mutarotate or reduce. If the glycosidic bond is not between two anomeric carbon atoms, one of the units will still be free to mutarotate and reduce.

Oligo- and Polysaccharides

Disaccharides have two monosaccharides, either the same or different, in glycosidic linkage. If the glycosidic linkage is between the two anomeric carbon atoms, the disaccharide is nonreducing:

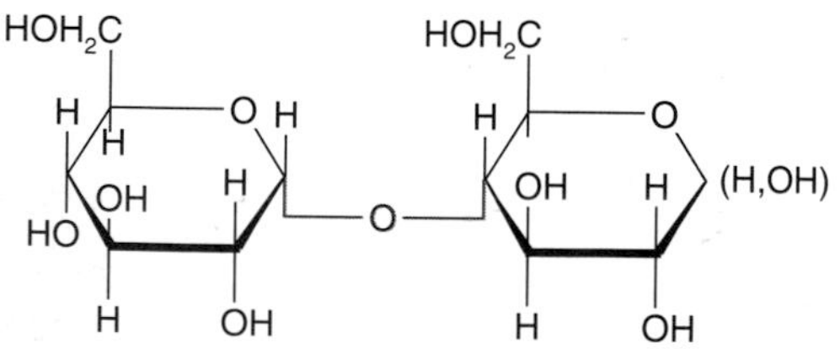

Maltose

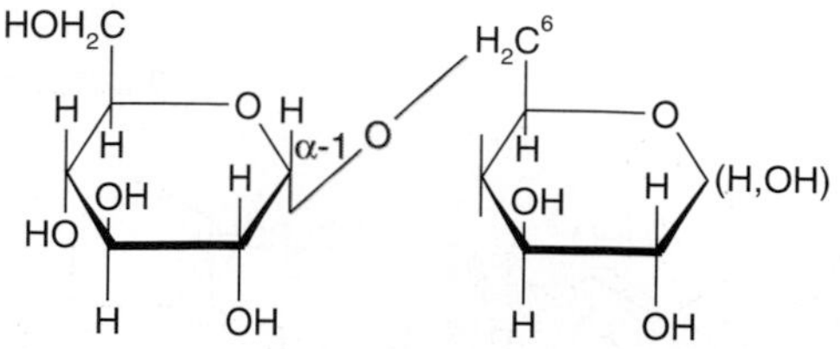

Isomaltose

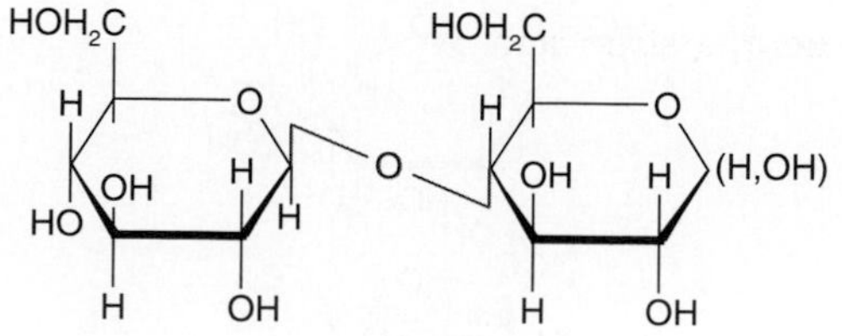

Cellobiose

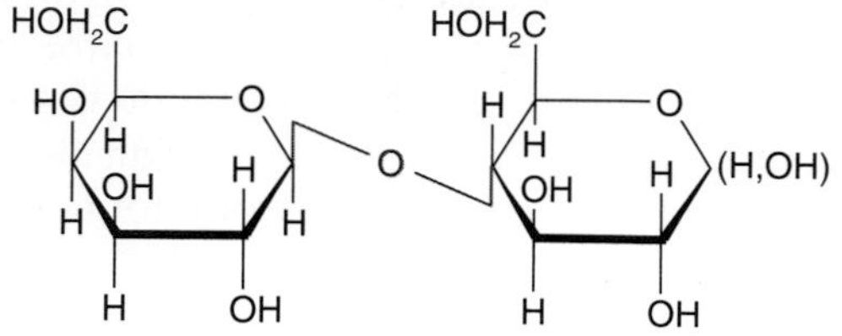

Lactose

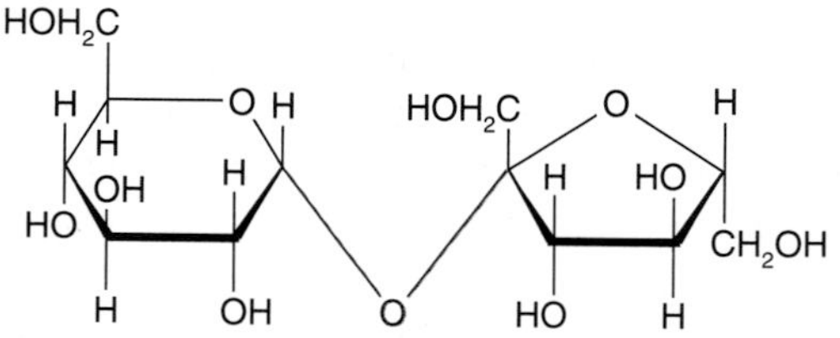

Sucrose

Maltose = 4-*O*-(*α*-D-glucopyranosyl)D-glucopyranose; reducing

Isomaltose = 6-*O*-(*α*-D-glucopyranosyl)D-glucopyranose; reducing

Cellobiose = 4-*O*-(*β*-D-glucopyranosyl)D-glucopyranose; reducing

Lactose = 4-*O*-(*β*-D-galactopyranosyl)D-glucopyranose; reducing

Sucrose = *α*-D-glucopyranosyl-*β*-D-fructofuranoside; nonreducing

As many as thousands of monosaccharides, either the same or different, may be joined by glycosidic bonds to form *polysaccharides.* The anomeric carbon of one unit is usually joined to C-4 or C-6 of the next unit. The ends of a polysaccharide are not identical (reducing end = free anomeric carbon; nonreducing = anomeric carbon linked to next unit; branched polysaccharide = more than one nonreducing end). The most common carbohydrates are homopolymers of glucose; for example, starch, glycogen, and cellulose. Plant starch is a mixture of **amylose,** a linear polymer of maltose units, and **amylopectin,** branches of repeating maltose units (glucose–glucose in *α*-1,4 linkages) joined via isomaltose linkages. **Glycogen,** the storage form of carbohydrate in animals, is similar to amylopectin, but the branches are shorter and occur more frequently. **Cellulose,** in plant cell walls, is a linear polymer of repeating cellobioses (glucose–glucose in *β*-1,4 linkages).

Mucopolysaccharides contain amino sugars, free and acetylated, uronic acids, sulfate esters, and sialic acids in addition to the simple monosaccharides. ***N*-Acetylneur-**

aminic acid, a sialic acid, is

LIPIDS

Lipids are a diverse group of chemicals related primarily because they are insoluble in water, soluble in nonpolar solvents, and found in animal and plant tissues.

Saponifiable lipids yield salts of fatty acids upon alkaline hydrolysis. *Acylglycerols* = glycerol + fatty acid(s); *phosphoacylglycerols* = glycerol + fatty acids + HPO_4^{2-} + alcohol; *sphingolipids* = sphingosine + fatty acid + polar group (phosphorylalcohol or carbohydrate); *waxes* = long-chain alcohol + fatty acid. *Nonsaponifiable lipids* (*terpenes, steroids, prostaglandins,* and related compounds) are not usually subject to hydrolysis. *Amphipathic* lipids have both a polar "head" group and a nonpolar "tail." Amphipathic molecules can stabilize emulsions and are responsible for the lipid bilayer structure of membranes.

Fatty acids are monocarboxylic acids with a short (<6 carbon atoms), medium (8–14 carbon atoms), or long (>14 carbon atoms) aliphatic chain. Biologically important ones are usually linear molecules with an even number of carbon atoms (16–20). Fatty acids are numbered using either arabic numbers (COOH is 1) or the Greek alphabet (COOH is not given a symbol; adjacent carbon atoms are α, β, γ, etc.). **Saturated fatty acids** have the general formula $CH_3(CH_2)_nCOOH$. (*Palmitic acid* = C_{16}; *stearic acid* = C_{18}.) They tend to be extended chains and solid at room temperature unless the chain is short. Both trivial and systematic (prefix indicating number of carbon atoms + *anoic acid*) names are used. $CH_3(CH_2)_{14}COOH$ = palmitic acid or hexadecanoic acid.

Unsaturated fatty acids have one or more double bonds. Most naturally occurring fatty acids have cis double bonds and are usually liquid at room temperature. Fatty acids with trans double bonds tend to have higher melting points. A double bond is indicated by Δ^n, where n is the number of the first carbon of the bond. *Palmitoleic* = Δ^9-hexadecenoic acid; *oleic* = Δ^9-octadecenoic acid; *linoleic* = $\Delta^{9,12}$-octadecadienoic acid; *linolenic* = $\Delta^{9,12,15}$-octadecatrienoic acid; *arachidonic* = $\Delta^{5,8,11,14}$-eicosatetraenoic acid. Since fatty acids are elongated *in vivo* from the carboxyl end, biochemists use alternate terminology to assign these fatty acids to families: omega (ω) minus x (or $n - x$), where x is the number of carbon atoms from the methyl end where a double bond is first encountered. *Palmitoleic* and *oleic* are $\omega - 9$ acids, *linoleic* and *arachidonic* are $\omega - 6$ acids, and *linolenic* is an $\omega - 3$ acid. Addition of carbon atoms does not change the family to which an unsaturated fatty acid belongs.

Since the p*K* values of fatty acids are about 4–5, in physiological solutions, they exist primarily in the ionized form, called salts or "soaps." Long-chain fatty acids are insoluble in water, but soaps form micelles. Fatty acids form esters with alcohols and thioesters with CoA.

The following are biochemically significant reactions of unsaturated fatty acids:

1. *Reduction*

$$-CH{=}CH- + XH_2 \rightarrow -CH_2CH_2- + X$$

2. *Addition of water*

$$-CH{=}CH- + H_2O \rightarrow -CH(OH){-}CH_2-$$

3. *Oxidation*

$$R{-}CH{=}CH{-}R' \rightarrow R{-}CHO + R'{-}CHO$$

Prostaglandins, thromboxanes, and *leukotrienes* are derivatives of C_{20}, polyunsaturated fatty acids, especially arachidonic acid. Prostaglandins have the general structure:

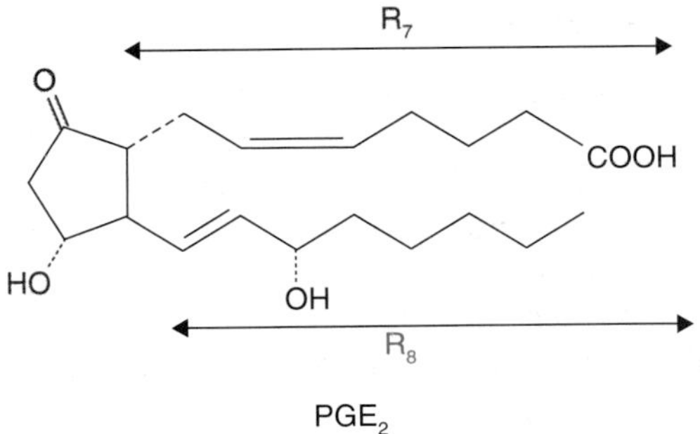

PGE2

The series differ from each other in the substituents on the ring and whether C-15 contains an OH or O · OH group. The subscript indicates the number of double bonds in the side chains. Substituents indicated by —(β) are above the plane of the ring; · · · (α) below:

PGA PGB PGE PGF

PGG(X=OH); PGH(X=OOH)

Thromboxanes have an oxygen incorporated to form a six-membered ring:

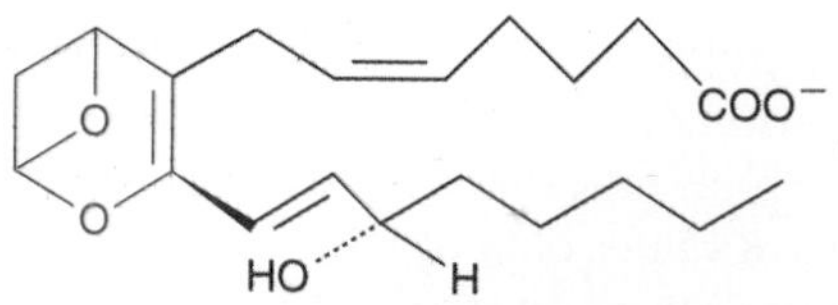

TXA$_2$

Leukotrienes are substituted derivatives of arachidonic acid in which no internal ring has formed; R is variable:

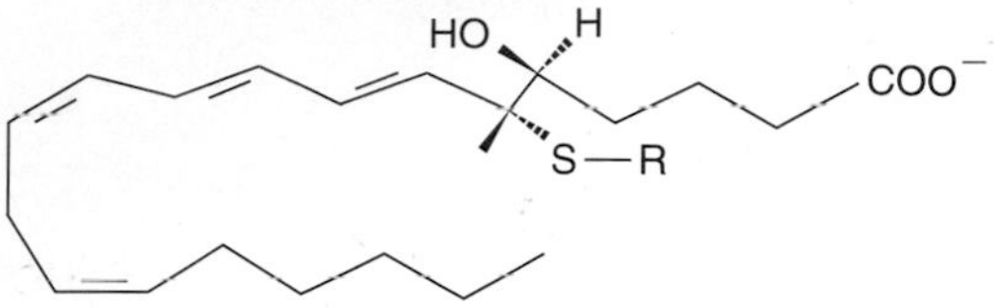

Leukotriene C, D, or E

Acylglycerols are compounds in which one or more of the three OH groups of glycerol are esterified. In **triacylglycerols** (triglycerides) all three OH groups are esterified to fatty acids. At least two of the three R groups are usually different. If R_1 is not equal to R_3, the molecule is asymmetric and of the L configuration:

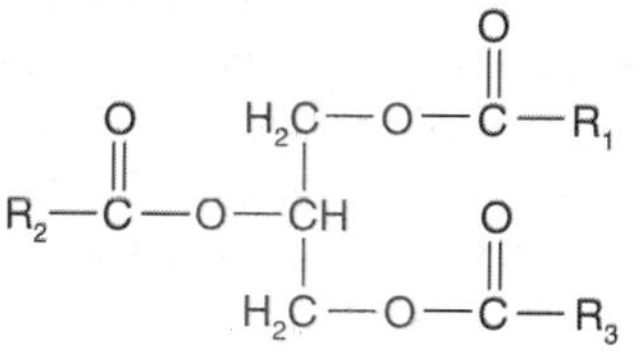

$$\begin{array}{l} H_2C-O-C(=O)-R_1 \\ R_2-C(=O)-O-CH \\ H_2C-O-C(=O)-R_3 \end{array}$$

The properties of the triacylglycerols are determined by those of the fatty acids they contain, with *oils* being liquid at room temperature (preponderance of short-chain and/or cis-unsaturated fatty acids) and *fats* being solid (preponderance of long-chain, saturated, and/or trans-unsaturated).

Triacylglycerols are hydrophobic and do not form stable micelles. They may be hydrolyzed to glycerol and three fatty acids by strong alkali or enzymes (lipases). *Mono-* [usually with the fatty acid in the β(2) position] and *diacylglycerols* also exist in small amounts as metabolic intermediates. Mono- and diacylglycerols are slightly more polar than triacylglycerols. *Phosphoacylglycerols* are derivatives of L-α-glycerolphosphate (L-glycerol 3-phosphate):

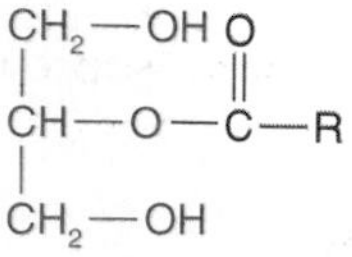

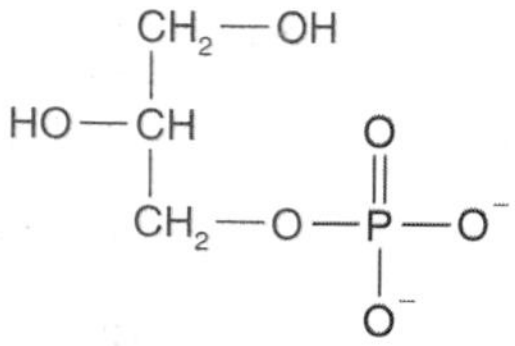

$$\begin{array}{l} CH_2-OH \\ CH-O-C(=O)-R \\ CH_2-OH \end{array} \qquad \begin{array}{l} CH_2-OH \\ HO-CH \\ CH_2-O-P(=O)(O^-)-O^- \end{array}$$

The parent compound, **phosphatidic acid** (two OH groups of L-α-glycerolphosphate esterified to fatty acids), has its phosphate esterified to an alcohol (XOH) to form several series of phosphoacylglycerols. These are amphipathic molecules, but the net charge at pH 7.4 depends on the nature of X—OH.

X—OH	Phosphoacylglycerol
$HO-CH_2-CH_2-\overset{+}{N}-(CH_3)_3$	Phosphatidylcholines (lecithins)
$HO-CH_2-CH_2-\overset{+}{N}H_3$	Phosphatidylethanolamines (cephalins)
$HO-CH_2-CH(\overset{+}{N}H_3)-COO^-$	Phosphatidylserines
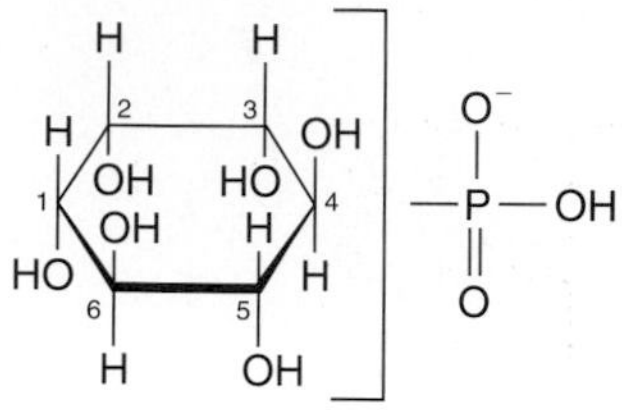 Inositol (positions 1–6) $-P(=O)(O^-)-OH$	Phosphatidylinositols phosphate on 4, or 4 and 5

In **plasmalogens,** the OH on C-1 is in *ether*, rather than ester, linkage to an alkyl group. If *one* fatty acid (usually β) has been hydrolyzed from a phosphoacylglycerol, the compound is a *lyso*-compound; for example, lysophosphatidylcholine (lysolecithin):

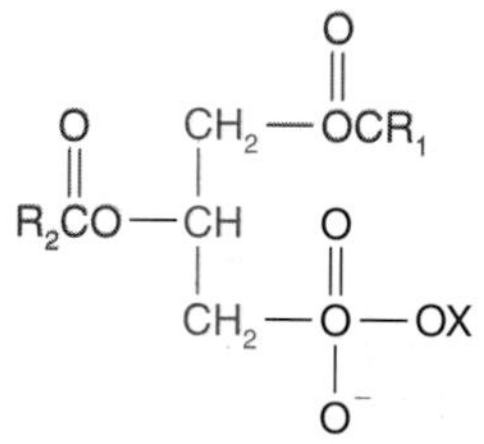

$$\begin{array}{l} CH_2-OC(=O)R_1 \\ R_2C(=O)O-CH \\ CH_2-O-P(=O)(O^-)-OX \end{array} \qquad \begin{array}{l} CH_2-OC(=O)R_1 \\ HO-CH \\ CH_2-O-P(=O)(O^-)-OX \end{array}$$

A phosphoacylglycerol 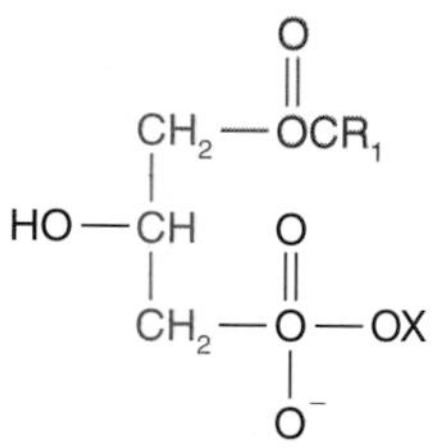   A lyso-compound

Sphingolipids are complex lipids based on the C-18, unsaturated alcohol, sphingosine. In *ceramides*, a long-chain fatty acid is in amide linkage to sphingosine:

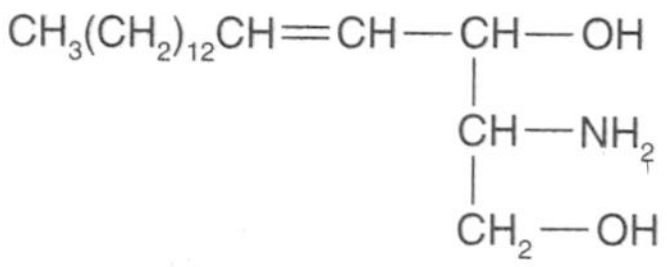

$$\begin{array}{l} CH_3(CH_2)_{12}CH=CH-CH-OH \\ \quad CH-NH_2 \\ \quad CH_2-OH \end{array}$$

Sphingosine

$$\begin{array}{l} CH_3(CH_2)_{12}CH=CH-CH-OH \\ \quad CH-NH-C(=O)-R \\ \quad CH_2-OH \end{array}$$

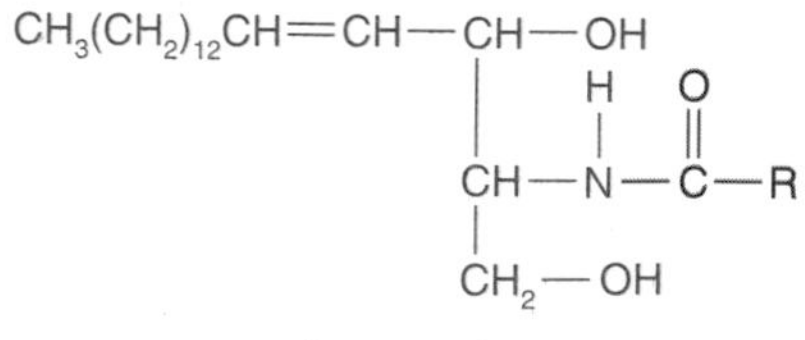

A ceramide

Sphingomyelins, the most common sphingolipids, are a family of compounds in which the primary OH group of a ceramide is esterified to phosphorylcholine (phosphorylethanolamine):

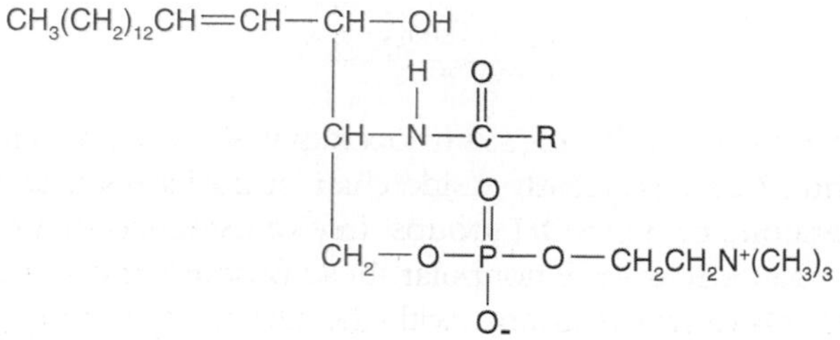

$$\begin{array}{l} CH_3(CH_2)_{12}CH=CH-CH-OH \\ \quad CH-NH-C(=O)-R \\ \quad CH_2-O-P(=O)(O^-)-O-CH_2CH_2N^+(CH_3)_3 \end{array}$$

They are amphipathic molecules, existing as zwitterions at pH 7.4 and the only sphingolipids that contain phosphorus. *Glycosphingolipids* do not contain phosphorus but contain carbohydrate in glycosidic linkage to the primary alcohol of a ceramide. They are amphipathic and either neutral or acidic if the carbohydrate moiety contains an acidic group. **Cerebrosides** have a single glucose or galactose linked to a ceramide. *Sulfatides* are galactosylceramides esterified with sulfate at C-3 of the galactose:

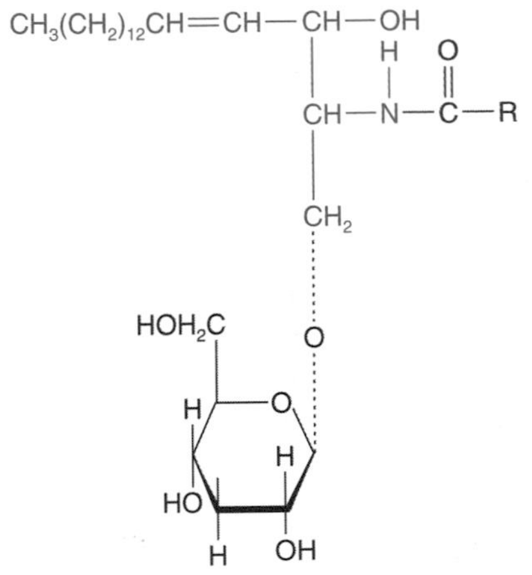

Glucosylceramide (glucocerebroside)

Globosides (*ceramide oligosaccharides*) are ceramides with two or more neutral monosaccharides, whereas **gangliosides** are an oligosaccharide containing one or more sialic acids.

Steroids are derivatives of cyclopentanoperhydrophenanthrene. The steroid nucleus is a rather rigid, essentially planar structure with substituents above or in the plane of the rings designated β (solid line) and those below called α (dotted line):

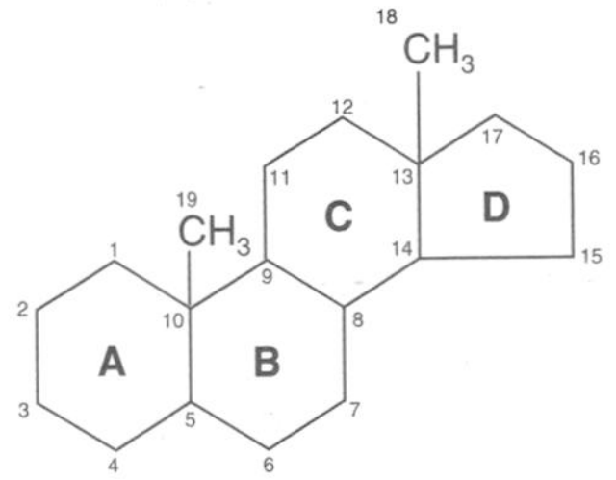

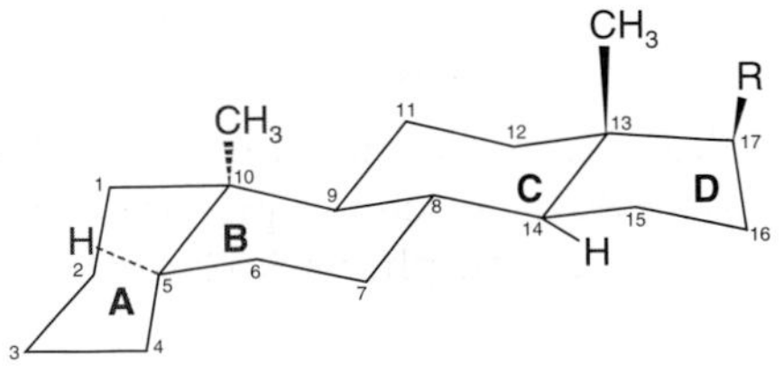

A and B rings—cis;
the others—trans

Most steroids in humans have methyl groups at positions 10 and 13 and frequently a side chain at position 17. *Sterols* contain one or more OH groups, free or esterified to a fatty acid. Most steroids are nonpolar. In a liposome or cell membrane, **cholesterol** orients with the OH toward any polar groups; cholesterol esters do not. **Bile acids** (e.g., cholic acid) have a polar side chain and so are amphipathic:

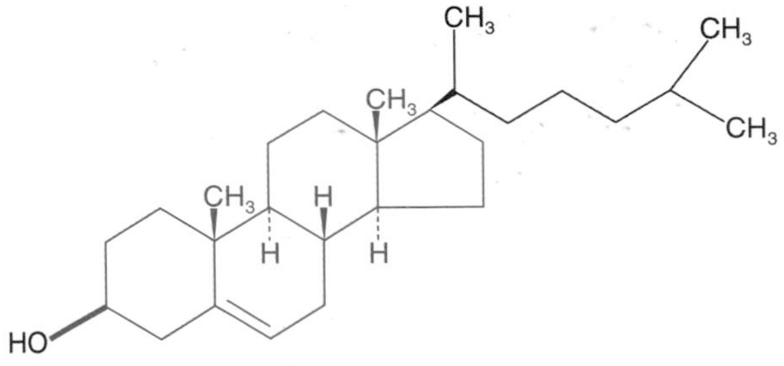

Cholesterol

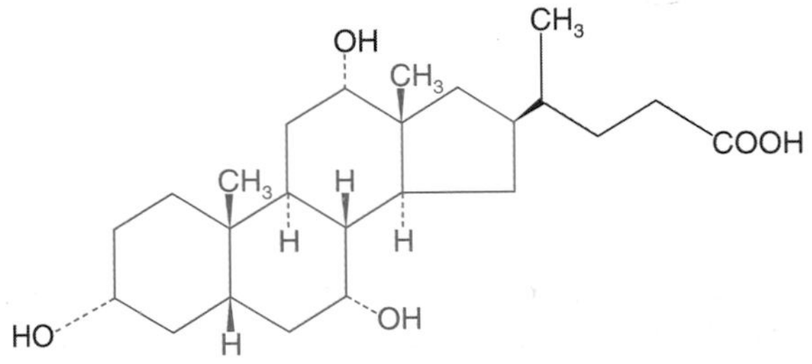

Cholic acid

Steroid hormones are oxygenated steroids of 18–21 carbon atoms. *Estrogens* have 18 carbon atoms, an aromatic ring A, and no methyl at C-10. *Androgens* have 19 carbon atoms and no side chain at C-17. *Glucocorticoids* and *mineralocorticoids* have 21 carbon atoms, including a C_2, of oxygenated side chain at C-17. *Vitamin D_3* (*cholecalciferol*) is not a sterol but is derived from 7-dehydrocholesterol in humans:

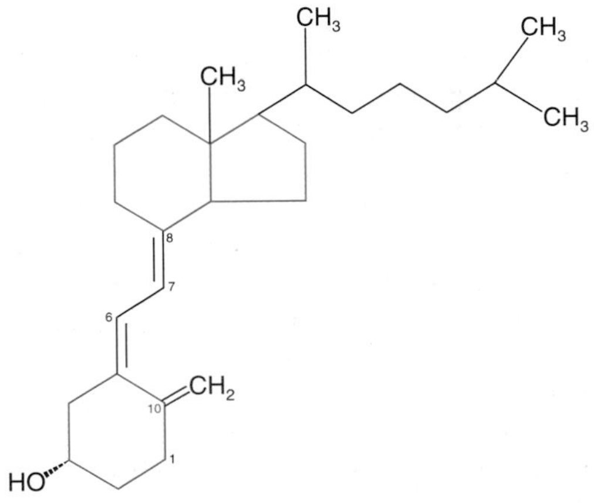

Cholecalciferol

Terpenes are polymers of two or more isoprene units. **Isoprene** is

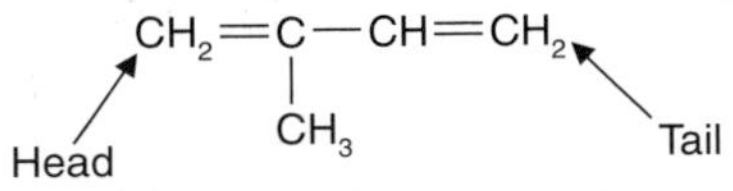

$$CH_2{=}C(CH_3){-}CH{=}CH_2$$

Head Tail

Terpenes may be linear or cyclic, with the isoprenes usually linked head to tail and most double bonds trans (but may be cis as in vitamin A). *Squalene*, the precursor of cholesterol, is a linear terpene of six isoprene units. Fat-soluble *vitamins* (A, D, E, and K) contain isoprene units:

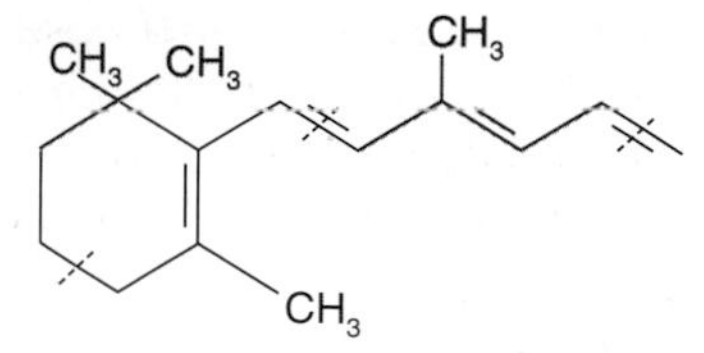

Vitamin A

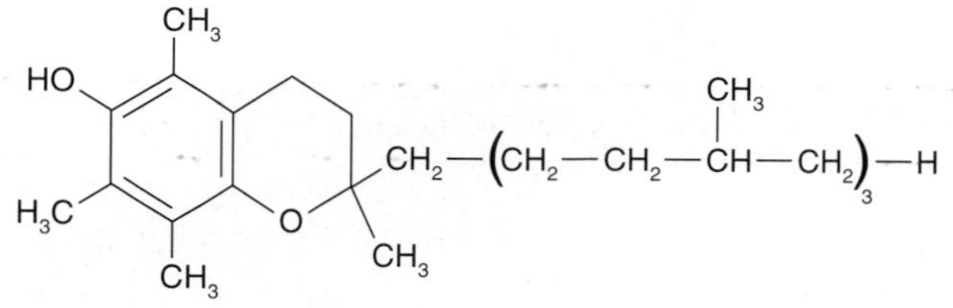

Vitamin E (α-tocopherol)

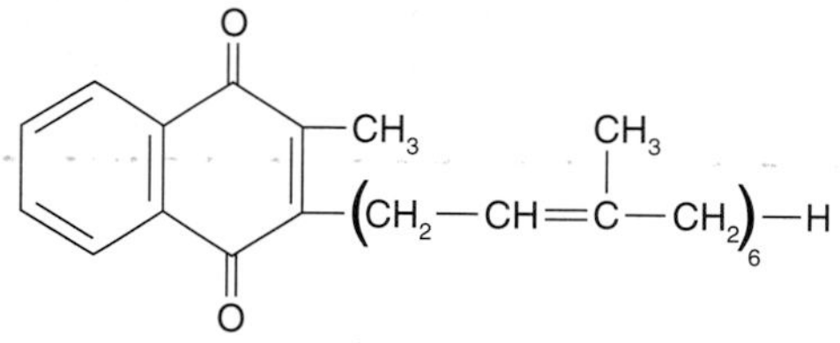

Vitamin K_2

AMINO ACIDS

Amino acids contain both an *amino* (NH_2) and a *carboxylic acid* (COOH) group. Biologically important amino acids are usually α-amino acids with the formula

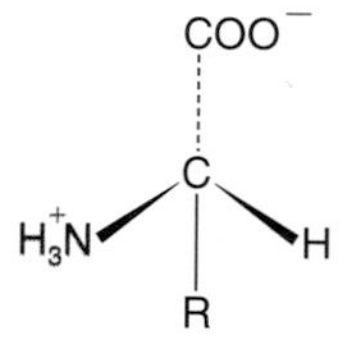

L-α-Amino acid

The amino group, with an unshared pair of electrons, is basic, with a pK_a of about 9.5, and exists primarily as $—NH_3^+$ at pH values near neutrality. The carboxylic acid group ($pK \approx 2.3$) exists primarily as a carboxylate ion. If R is anything but H, the molecule is asymmetric with most naturally occurring ones of the L configuration (same relative configuration as L-glyceraldehyde: see p. 1139).

The *polarity* of amino acids is influenced by their side chains (R groups) (see p. XX for complete structures). *Nonpolar* amino acids include those with large, aliphatic, aromatic, or undissociated sulfur groups (aliphatic = Ala, Ile, Leu, Val; aromatic = Phe, Trp; sulfur = Cys, Met). *Intermediate* polarity amino acids include Gly, Pro, Ser, Thr, and Tyr (undissociated).

Amino acids with ionizable side chains are *polar.* The pK values of the side groups of arginine, lysine, glutamate, and aspartate are such that these are nearly always charged at physiological pH, whereas the side groups of histidine (pK = 6.0) and cysteine (pK = 8.3) exist as both charged and uncharged species at pH 7.4 (acidic = Glu, Asp, Cys; basic = Lys, Arg, His). Although undissociated cysteine is nonpolar, cysteine in dissociated form is polar.

All amino acids are at least *dibasic acids* because of the presence of both the α-amino and α-carboxyl groups, the ionic state being a function of pH. The presence of another ionizable group will give a tribasic acid as shown for cysteine.

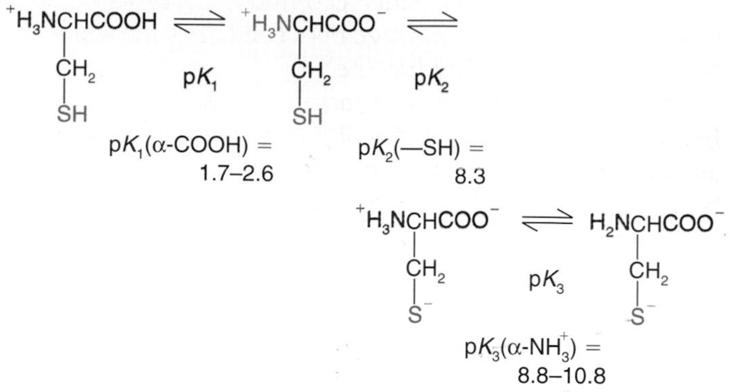

pK_1(α-COOH) = 1.7–2.6

pK_2(—SH) = 8.3

pK_3(α-NH_3^+) = 8.8–10.8

The **zwitterionic form** is the form in which the *net* charge is zero. The *isoelectric point* is the average of the two pK values involved in the formation of the zwitterionic form. In the above example this would be the average of $pK_1 + pK_2$.

PURINES AND PYRIMIDINES

Purines and **pyrimidines,** often called *bases,* are nitrogen-containing heterocyclic compounds with the structures

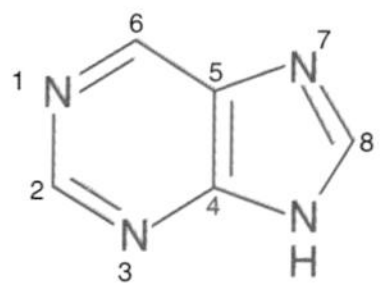

Purine

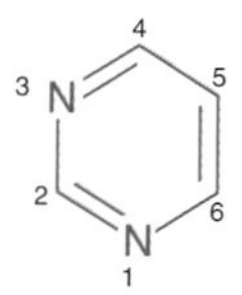

Pyrimidine

Major bases found in nucleic acids and as cellular nucleotides are the following:

Purines	*Pyrimidines*
Adenine: 6-amino	Cytosine: 2-oxy, 4-amino
Guanine: 2-amino, 6-oxy	Uracil: 2,4-dioxy
	Thymine: 2,4-dioxy, 5-methyl
Other important bases found primarily as intermediates of synthesis and/or degradation are	
Hypoxanthine: 6-oxy	Orotic acid: 2,4-dioxy, 6-carboxy
Xanthine: 2,6-dioxy	

Oxygenated purines and pyrimidines exist as *tautomeric* structures with the keto form predominating and involved in hydrogen bonding between bases in nucleic acids:

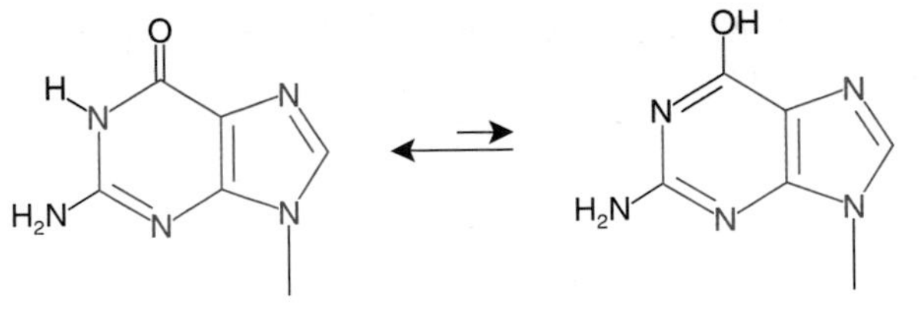

Keto ⟷ Enol

Nucleosides have either β-D-ribose or β-D-2-deoxyribose in an *N*-glycosidic linkage between C-1 of the sugar and N-9 (purine) or N-1 (pyrimidine).

Nucleotides have one or more phosphate groups esterified to the sugar. Phosphates, if more than one are present, are usually attached to each other via phosphoanhydride bonds. Monophosphates may be designated as either the base monophosphate or as an *-ylic acid* (AMP: adenylic acid):

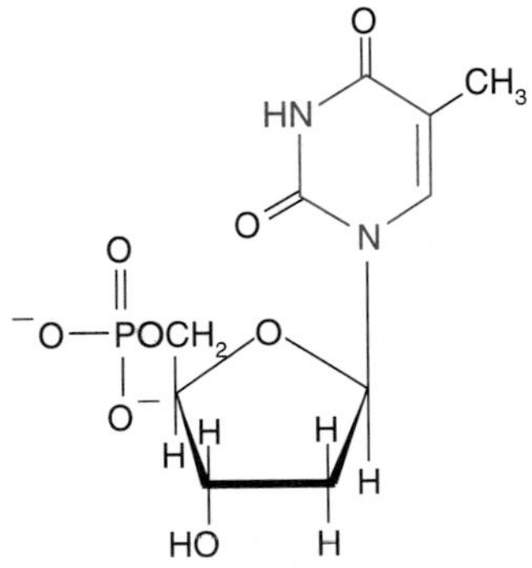

By conventional rules of *nomenclature*, the atoms of the base are numbered 1–9 in purines or 1–6 in pyrimidines and the carbon atoms of the sugar 1′–5′. A nucleoside with an unmodified name indicates that the sugar is ribose and the phosphate(s) is/are attached at C-5′ of the sugar. Deoxy forms are indicated by the prefix d (dAMP = deoxyadenylic acid). If the phosphate is esterified at any position other than 5′, it must be so designated [3′-AMP; 3′-5′-AMP (cyclic AMP = cAMP)]. The nucleosides and nucleotides (ribose form) are named as follows:

Base	*Nucleoside*	*Nucleotide*
Adenine	Adenosine	AMP, ADP, ATP
Guanine	Guanosine	GMP, GDP, GTP
Hypoxanthine	Inosine	IMP
Xanthine	Xanthosine	XMP
Cytosine	Cytidine	CMP, CDP, CTP
Uracil	Uridine	UMP, UDP, UTP
Thymine	dThymidine	dTMP, dTTP
Orotic acid	Orotidine	OMP

Minor (modified) bases and nucleosides also exist in nucleic acids. *Methylated* bases have a methyl group on an amino group (*N*-methyl guanine), a ring atom (1-methyl adenine), or on an OH group of the sugar (2′-*O*-methyl adenosine). *Dihydrouracil* has the 5–6 double bond saturated. In *pseudouridine*, the ribose is attached to C-5 rather than to N-1.

In **polynucleotides** (*nucleic acids*), the mononucleotides are joined by phosphodiester bonds between the 3′-OH of one sugar (ribose or deoxyribose) and the 5′-OH of the next (see p. 567 for the structure).

INDEX

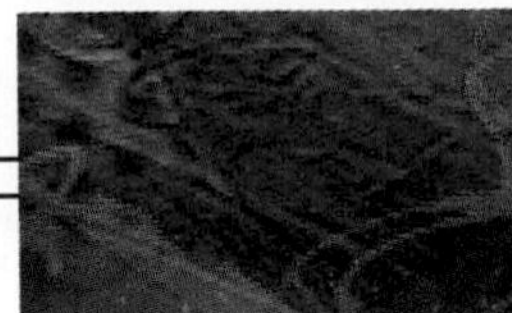

HOW TO USE THIS INDEX: The letter "*f*" after a page number designates a figure; "*t*" designates tabular material; "cc" designates a Clinical Correlation. **Boldface** page numbers show where terms are explained. "*See*" cross-references direct the reader to the synonymous term. "*See also*" cross-references direct the reader to (1) related topics or (2) the synonym under which a more detailed topic breakdown may be found.